Defensive Coping*
Ineffective Denial*
Ineffective Family Coping: Disabling
Ineffective Family Coping: Compromised
Family Coping: Potential for Growth
Noncompliance (Specify)
Decisional Conflict (Specify)*
Health Seeking Behaviors (Specify)*

PATTERN 6 MOVING

Impaired Physical Mobility
Activity Intolerance
Fatigue*
Potential Activity Intolerance
Sleep Pattern Disturbance
Diversional Activity Deficit
Impaired Home Maintenance Management
Altered Health Maintenance
Feeding Self Care Deficit†
Impaired Swallowing
Ineffective Breastfeeding*
Bathing/Hygiene Self Care Deficit†
Dressing/Grooming Self Care Deficit†
Toileting Self Care Deficit†
Altered Growth and Development

PATTERN 7 PERCEIVING

Body Image Disturbance†
Self Esteem Disturbance†**
Chronic Low Self Esteem*
Situational Low Self Esteem*
Personal Identity Disturbance†
Sensory/Perceptual Alterations (Specify) (Visual, auditory, kinesthetic, gustatory, tactile, olfactory)
Unilateral Neglect
Hopelessness
Powerlessness

PATTERN 8 KNOWING

Knowledge Deficit (Specify)
Altered Thought Processes

PATTERN 9 FEELING

Pain†
Chronic Pain
Dysfunctional Grieving
Anticipatory Grieving
Potential for Violence: Self-directed or directed at others
Post-Trauma Response
Rape-Trauma Syndrome
Rape-Trauma Syndrome: Compound Reaction
Rape-Trauma Syndrome: Silent Reaction
Anxiety
Fear

*New diagnostic categories approved 1988
**Revised diagnostic categories approved 1988
†Categories with modified label terminology

Fundamentals of Nursing

Concepts and Procedures

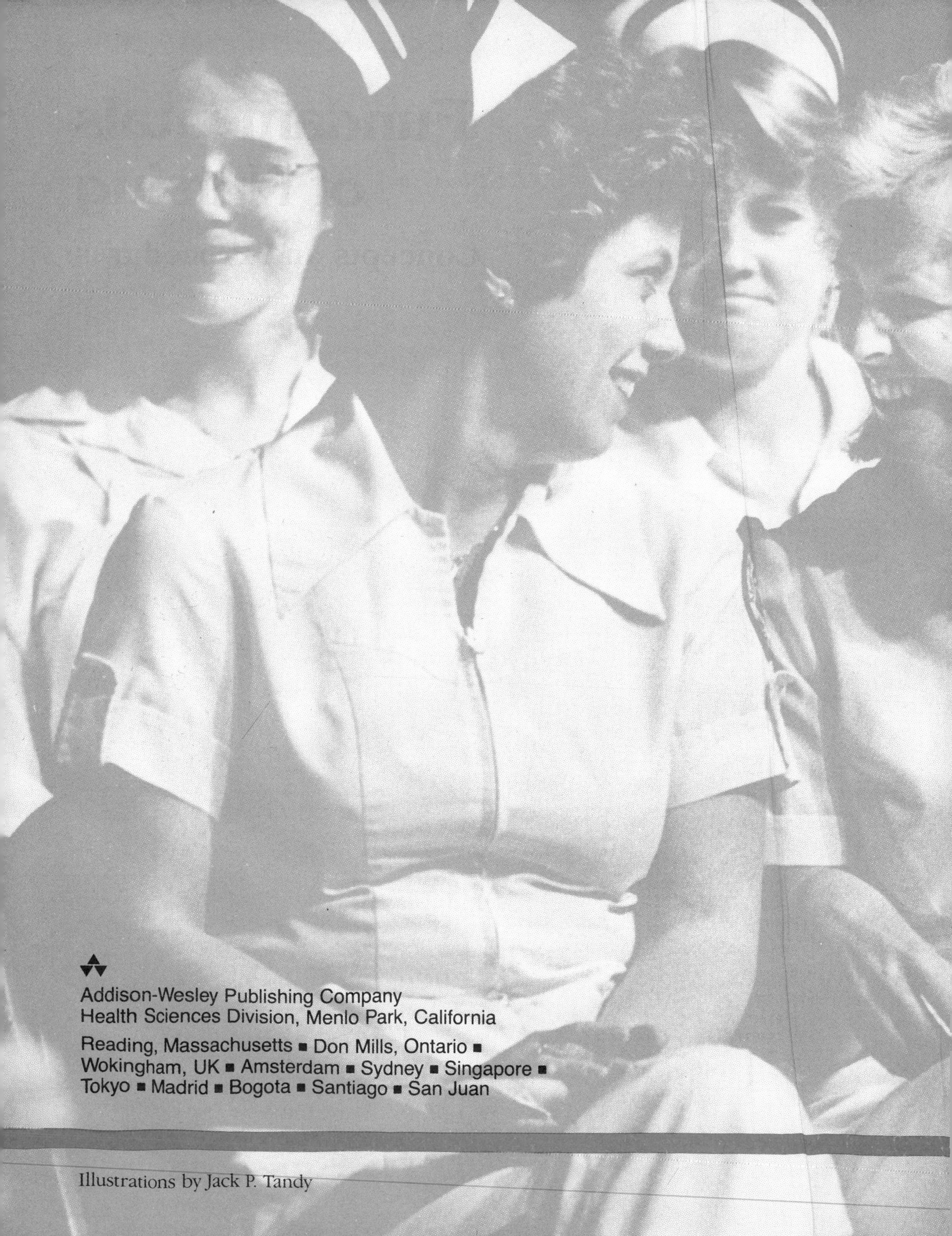

Addison-Wesley Publishing Company
Health Sciences Division, Menlo Park, California

Reading, Massachusetts ■ Don Mills, Ontario ■
Wokingham, UK ■ Amsterdam ■ Sydney ■ Singapore ■
Tokyo ■ Madrid ■ Bogota ■ Santiago ■ San Juan

Illustrations by Jack P. Tandy

Fundamentals of Nursing

Concepts and Procedures

Third Edition

Barbara Kozier
BA, BSN, RN, MN

Glenora Erb
BSN, RN

To Our Parents

Executive editor: *Debra S. Hunter*
Assistant editor: *S. Jamie Spencer*
Production supervisor: *Judith Johnstone*
Production assistant: *Brian Jones*
Cover and interior designer: *Michael A. Rogondino*
Illustrator: *Jack P. Tandy*
Photographers: *Karen Stafford Rantzman, William Thompson, Jeffry Collins, Suzanne Arms, Marianne Gontarz, Frank Keillor, Mark Tuschman, George Fry, Hank Lebo, Margorie McClory, Paul Fusco, Bill Murphy, Christopher Scott, David Barnett, Chuck Savadelis*
Copyeditors: *Antonio Padial, Elliot Simon*
Proofreaders: *Helene Harrington, Elliot Simon Associates*
Indexer: *Steven Sorensen*

The photograph on the title page is by Frank Keillor.

Epigram credits:

Curtin, L: Packaging the professional for success. *Nursing Management* (April) 1985: 16:4:9.

Diers, D: Between science and humanity: Nursing reclaims its role. *Yale Alumni Magazine* (March) 1982; 45 (5):8–12.

Fagin, C and Diers, D: Nursing as metaphor. *NE J Med* (July 14) 1983:309:116–117.

Henderson, V: The nature of nursing. *Amer J Nursing:* (August) 84:8:1112.

Kelly, L S: Coalition: Power for the powerless. *Nursing Outlook* July-August 1985: 33:4:169.

Leone, L P: Quoted in Safier G: *Contemporary American Leaders in Nursing: A History.* New York: McGraw-Hill, 1977.

Levine, ME: On creativity in nursing. *Image* 1973:5:3:16.

Masson, V: On power and vision in nursing. *Nurs Outlook* December 1979: 27:782–784.

McBride, A B: Personal communication. 1986.

Styles, M M: On Nursing: Toward a new endowment. St. Louis: Mosby. 1982.

Schorr, T: Keynote speech, Illinois Nurses' Association Annual Convention, November 7, 1985.

Library of Congress Cataloging-in-Publication Data

Kozier, Barbara.
Fundamentals of nursing.

Includes bibliographies and index.
1. Nursing. I. Erb, Glenora Lea, 1937- II. Title. [DNLM:
1. Nursing Care. WY 100K88fa] RT41.K72
1987 610.73 86-26528
ISBN 0-201-11774-6

FGHIJKL-RN-89

0-201-11774-6

The authors and publishers have exerted every effort to ensure that drug selections and dosages set forth in this text are in accord with current recommendations and practice at the time of publication. However, in view of ongoing research, changes in government regulations, and the constant flow of information relating to drug therapy and drug reactions, the reader is urged to check the package insert for each drug for any change in indications of dosage and for added warnings and precautions. This is particularly important where the recommended agent is a new and/or infrequently employed drug.

Addison-Wesley Publishing Company
Health Sciences Division
2725 Sand Hill Road
Menlo Park, California 94025

Contributors

Phyllis Carroll, RN, MS
Chairperson
Medical-Surgical Nursing
School of Nursing
Saint Joseph Medical Center
Joliet, Illinois
Care Plans

Janice Denehy, RN, PhD
Assistant Professor
School of Nursing
University of Iowa
Iowa City, Iowa
Chapter 20, The Family

Thomas Eoyang, BA, MA
San Francisco, California
Chapter 50, Loss and Grieving

Barbara Germino, RN, PHd
Associate Professor
School of Nursing
University of North Carolina
Chapel Hill, North Carolina
Chapter 4, Home Health Care

Margaret J. Herman, RN, MN
St. John's Hospital
Santa Monica, California
Research Boxes

Diana Mason, RN, MSN
Lecturer and Director of Faculty Practice Unit
Lienhard School of Nursing
Pace University
New York, New York
Chapter 6, Power and Politics

Mary Kelly Memmer, RN, BS, MNEd
Professor
School of Nursing
California State University at Chico
Chico, California
Chapter 37, Mobility and Immobility
Chapter 38, Body Alignment
Chapter 39, Body Mechanics and Ambulation

Rita Olivieri, RN, BS, MS
Assistant Professor
School of Nursing
Boston College
Chestnut Hill, Massachusetts
Chapter 31, Computers in Nursing and Health

Ross A. Stewart, RPN, RN, MHSC
Director, Department of Psychiatric Nursing
Douglas College, New Westminster, British Columbia
Independent Practitioner, Psychiatric Nursing
Vancouver, British Columbia
Chapter 19, Sexuality
Chapter 50, Loss and Grieving

Susan Talbott, RN, MA, MBA
Principal
Nurse Management Institute
Baltimore, Maryland
Chapter 6, Politics and Power

Holly Skodol Wilson, RN, PhD
Professor
Department of Mental Health, Community and Administrative Nursing
University of California, San Francisco
San Francisco, California
Chapter 5, Research in Nursing

Reviewers

Elizabeth Abernathy
Hillsborough Community College

Marilyn Bayne
University of Maryland

Nancy Bradley/Ruth Ludwick/Carol Sedlak
Kent State University

Jean Buckley
Middlesex Community College

Barbara Butera
Ohio State University

Verna Carson
University of Maryland

Patricia Chin
California State University at Los Angeles

Diane Cline
Victor Valley College

Ivory Coleman
Community College of Philadelphia

Shirley Cooley
Ohio State University

Emily Cornett
University of Texas at Austin

Judy Davy
California State University, Humboldt

Susan DeRosa
University of Rochester

Katherine Detherage
University of Rochester

Carol Dicks
Indiana University

Karen Lee Fontaine
Purdue University, Calumet

Michele Fox
San Jose State University

Barbara Gruendenmann
Mountain States Surgery Center

Connie Hill
Owens Technical College

Shirley Howard
University of Nevada, Reno

Donna Ignatavicius
University of Maryland

Andrew Irish
Gay Nurses Alliance

Rebecca James
University of North Carolina at Greensboro

Sandy Joseph
Santa Monica College

Christine Kasper
University of Wisconsin at Madison

Teresa Kellerman
Southeastern Massachusetts University

Betty Lesser
Massasoit Community College

Brenda Lyon
Indiana University

Cathy Malek
Boston College

Nancy Manley
Ohlone College

Mary Memmer
California State University at Chico

Janice Olson
Veterans Administration Hospital, Des Moines

A. Elfin Moses
University of Tennessee

Susan Poorman
University of Pittsburgh

Susan Roe
University of Manitoba

Kendra Ross
Saint Joseph Medical Center

Anna Sabol
Bergen Community College

Sharon Shipton
Youngstown State University

Lina Sims
Saint Joseph Medical Center

Judith Snyder
Mills Hospital

Barbara Soule
Saint Peter Hospital

Dana Stahl
El Centro College

Marcia Stevens
University of San Francisco

Helen Vandenberg
Bergen Community College

Christine Westphal
Mercy College

Susan Wilkins
Anne Arundel Community College

Ann Windsor
University of Wisconsin at Madison

Marian Yoder
San Jose State University

Preface

No matter where care is delivered, no matter what the pathophysiologic process, no matter how many lines, medications, or pieces of equipment are involved, nursing's unique role is to care for the person.

Sarah Sanford

Caring for the person has never held greater challenges than during today's high-tech health care revolution. Nursing's unique role demands a blend of skill, sensitivity, and commitment based on broad knowledge and the application of that knowledge in practice. This text provides a foundation on which students can build their professional repertoire of skills and values. It integrates essential knowledge from the physical and behavioral sciences with clinical nursing procedures, presented within the context of nursing theory, concepts, history, trends, and issues.

Contemporary in Approach and Content

Though unchanged in approach and purpose from the two preceding editions, this third edition has been redesigned in a two-color format and incorporates both major and minor revisions throughout. These revisions reflect the movement of health care from hospital to home and community, changes in consumer attitudes and values, new research and technology, and nursing's increasing responsibility, accountability and autonomy. They also represent the many valuable comments and suggestions from reviewers and instructors using the text.

New features include:

- Six new chapters on: health promotion; home health care; the family; research; computers in nursing; and politics and power
- Increased coverage of basic nursing theories and concepts
- Expanded discussion of wellness, health maintenance, and the nurse's role in health promotion through the life span
- Individual chapters devoted to each step of the nursing process and more in-depth application of the nursing process throughout
- Nursing diagnoses approved in the 1986 NANDA conference
- Comprehensive coverage of health assessment
- Every procedure presented in nursing process format
- Notes on nursing research and legal/ethical issues throughout the text
- Nursing care plans
- Glossary, plus key terms in boldface type where explained in the text
- Thorough revision and updating of every chapter
- New tables, charts, photographs, and drawings

Reorganized into Eleven Units

This third edition has been reorganized into eleven units plus appendixes, glossary, and index. The steps of the nursing process are emphasized as a major organizational element throughout.

Unit I, Nursing and Health, introduces the student to the nursing profession and its role within the health care system. In addition to the totally new chapter on home health care, much new material has been added on professionalism, conceptual models, and the economics of health care.

Unit II, Concepts for Professional Nursing Practice, highlights the realities of contemporary nursing practice. Two new chapters discuss research in nursing and the politics of nursing. More attention is focused on values (both personal and client values) and resolving ethical dilemmas.

Unit III, Nursing Process, systematically develops the five-step nursing process. Through all the chapters, the discussion follows one client, building a nursing care plan. The thorough explanation of this key problem-solving process lays the groundwork for application of the process throughout the remainder of the text.

Unit IV, Concepts About Humans, discusses the holistic person; homeostasis, stress and adaptation; ethnicity and culture; and sexuality. Revised throughout, this unit includes a wealth of new information.

Unit V, Health Promotion Through the Life Span, features two new chapters: health promotion, and the family; and demonstrates the nurse's role in providing health education and enhancing behavioral change. Developmental concepts introduced here are amplified in subsequent chapters that apply nursing assessment and intervention to clients of all ages, with a sensitivity to the nurse's responsibility in fostering healthful behaviors.

Unit VI, Communication Processes, helps students develop the various types of communication skills essential to their daily practice. New material in this unit and throughout the book assists students in developing nonjudgmental attitudes toward clients regardless of values, ethnicity, culture, religion, occupation, or sexual orientation. Also new to this unit is information on working with self-help groups, teaching strategies for clients and support persons, nursing care rounds, and conferences. A new chapter describes the computer as a communication and information management tool.

Unit VII, Health Protection, teaches students principles and techniques to prevent the transfer of microorganisms, and reduce environmental hazards. The latest CDC guidelines and health protection measures are reflected in this material.

Unit VIII, Health Assessment, clearly describes and illustrates this important aspect of nursing care, from assessment of vital signs to more complex physical health assessment procedures. More than 100 photographs and drawings offer explicit detail; complete rationale is included throughout.

Unit IX, Physiologic Concepts, comprises 11 chapters discussing these concepts and their implementation through use of the nursing process. New material includes 1986 CPR guidelines, urinary diversions and ostomies, bowel diversions and ostomies, and tracheostomy care.

Unit X, Psychosocial Concepts, addresses caring for the person. It includes thoroughly revised chapters on self-concept, and loss and grieving.

Unit XI, Special Nursing Interventions, discusses medications, wound care, perioperative care, and special procedures. All chapters have been carefully revised to reflect the most recent CDC guidelines. Nursing practice is emphasized in these chapters.

Appendices include rights of special groups; root words, prefixes, and suffixes; Canada's Food Guide; recommended daily dietary allowances; recommended nutrient intakes; and equivalents.

Revised In-Text Learning Aids

Many tables, boxes, and other summary devices are used to highlight essential data. Key features and in-text learning aids are highlighted through use of a second color. Each chapter opens with behavioral objectives using the early parts of Bloom's taxonomy. The behavioral objectives are stated as broad learning outcomes followed by specific objectives that clarify them. Students may find it helpful to add the words "by being able to" at the end of each general objective. A list of key terms appear in bold face where they are defined in the text and where they appear in the index. Many also appear in the glossary.

- Notes on current research studies and legal/ethical issues highlight their relevance to nursing practice. Nursing care plans spell out rationales for every nursing intervention.
- Chapter highlights summarize key points at the conclusion of each chapter, followed by annotated readings and selected references. Chapters are designed so that they may be used independently and thus in any order. A glossary at the end of the book helps the students learn nursing and medical terminology and facilitates using the chapters in any sequence.

Outstanding Art Program

Hundreds of photographs and drawings contribute to thorough student understanding. Color has been added to many of the drawings to enhance their teaching value by showing action or highlighting a focal point.

Though the art program has been highly praised in previous editions, this revision is especially enriched by the inclusion of a number of photographs from *The Addison-Wesley Photo-Atlas of Nursing Procedures* by Pamela L. Swearingen. The clarity and clinical excellence of these photographs is unsurpassed.

All-New Teaching/Learning Package

To assist instructors in gaining maximum usefulness from this new edition, a comprehensive new supplements package has been developed. This package now includes:

1. PROCEDURES SUPPLEMENT, containing many additional procedures, which may have been described or mentioned in the text, but were not found there in

tabular format. This unique supplement is part of our commitment to allow instructors and students maximum flexibility and utility of print resources. Each procedure is presented in a step-by-step format that systematically reinforces the nursing process. Illustrations further define the techniques.

2. INSTRUCTORS' MANUAL, which covers key concepts and rationales. Teaching objectives are tied to discussion questions, review exercises and student activities. Special troubleshooting and helpful hint sections offer suggestions for teaching content, which many instructors have told us can be problematic. The manual includes transparency masters, audiovisual resources, and guidelines for finding primary resource materials.

3. Student LEARNING GUIDE by Lina K. Sims and Kendra A. Ross, the first care-planning study guide in fundamentals of nursing. It contains learning objectives, chapter overviews, and study questions based on case studies for each chapter. Exercises challenge students to synthesize, apply, and extend text knowledge as they complete care plans from information provided in the case studies.

4. TESTBANK provides 1000 new items covering a broad range of levels. All questions are presented in NCLEX format. A computerized version is available for IBM-PC or Apple II users on Addison-Wesley's new and powerful TestGen II software

5. TRANSPARENCY KIT includes 40 two-color transparencies, featuring some illustrations not found in the main text.

As nursing continues to redefine itself in response to the dynamic world it serves, one thing will endure: caring for the person. Only within the context of caring does the science of nursing become meaningful; thus we have tried to make that caring central to this text.

Just as nursing is shaped by forces from within and from without, this book's development will continue to be shaped by comments from instructors and students who use it and by our own experience as educators and practitioners. The wide acceptance of the preceding editions has been most gratifying, and we welcome suggestions for ways in which this book might more effectively and enjoyably communicate the essense of nursing: caring for the person.

Barbara Kozier
Glenora Erb

Acknowledgments

We would like to extend our warmest appreciation and thanks to:

- The friends and colleagues who offered us so much support and assistance during the preparation of this manuscript.
- The nursing students and teachers who used previous editions of *Fundamentals* and who sent us many helpful suggestions for this edition. In particular we wish to thank Barbara Butera, Katherine Detherage, and Sue DeRosa for their diary review of the second edition.
- The contributors who generously provided this new edition with chapters in their areas of nursing expertise: Janice Denehy, Thomas Eoyang, Barbara Germino, Diana Mason, Susan Talbott, Mary Memmer, Rita Olivieri, Ross Stewart, and Holly Wilson. We are grateful to these people for their willingness to share their knowledge and enthusiasm in this book.
- Ilka Abbott, formerly librarian at the Registered Nurses' Association of British Columbia, for her willing assistance in acquiring reference material for the manuscript.
- Valerie Nicholson, who provided many valuable suggestions in the areas of moral development and self-concept.
- Allankah Goldy, typist *extraordinaire* and friend, who typed the entire manuscript, making it presentable for publication. Her understanding of the manuscript greatly assisted the authors with this revision.
- Illustrator Jack Tandy, of St. Louis, Missouri, who again provided the line drawings. His illustrations not only help nursing students to learn more easily, but also contribute immeasureably to the appearance of the book.
- Designer Michael Rogondino, for his talent in bringing contemporary design concepts to the cover and interior of the new edition.
- Photographers William Thompson, Karen Stafford Rantzman, Jeffry Collins, Suzanne Arms, Marianne Gontarz, and others, for their sensitive and explicit photographs.
- The nurses of the University of British Columbia Health Sciences Centre Hospital, Vancouver, British Columbia, and in particular Miss Rose Murakami, Vice President, Nursing, for all their assistance to the authors.
- The nursing staffs and clients who generously gave of their time for the photographs of this text: The Medical Center of the University of California at San Francisco, the Stanford University Hospitals, Highland General Hospital, Oakland, and the Washington Healthguard Urgent Care Clinic, Fremont, California.
- Pamela Swearingen, who generously gave her permission for the use of numerous photographs from *The Addison-Wesley Photo-Atlas of Nursing Procedures.*
- The University of California at San Francisco School of Nursing, Stanford University Hospitals, and El Camino Hospitals, who provided sample forms.
- Andrew C. Irish, Gay Nurses Alliance and A. Elfin Moses, University of Tennessee for their helpful suggestions regarding sexuality content throughout the book.
- Phyllis Carroll, who has written innovative and meaningful nursing care plans for many of the chapters.
- Margaret J. Herman, who contributed many of the research notes throughout the text.
- Edith P. Lewis, former editor of *Nursing Outlook,* for her contribution of the Significant Events in Nursing History on the inside front and back covers.
- All the nurses who reviewed portions of the manuscript for this edition. Their time, thought, and constructive comments are greatly appreciated.

We are grateful to the entire staff of the Health Sciences Division, Addison-Wesley Publishing Company, who extended themselves to bring this book to its final form. In particular we wish to thank:

- Nick Keefe, general manager, Debra Hunter, executive editor, and Glenda Epting, production manager, for their continuing support.

- Senior editor Nancy Evans, who contributed so many good ideas to this revision.
- Jamie Spencer, whose commitment and enthusiasm were unflagging throughout the editorial process.
- Brian Jones, for invaluable help in organizing and managing the art program.
- Antonio Padial, who as copyeditor gave us consistently good advice on style and syntax.
- Elliot Simon, his associates, and Helene Harrington, for their careful attention to reading the proofs.
- Steven Sorensen, who brought a high level of professionalism to the indexing.
- Judith Johnstone, whose flair for design and ability to coordinate a million details during production—always with a sense of humor—were of great assistance to the authors.

Barbara Kozier
Glenora Erb

Contents in Brief

Contents in Detail

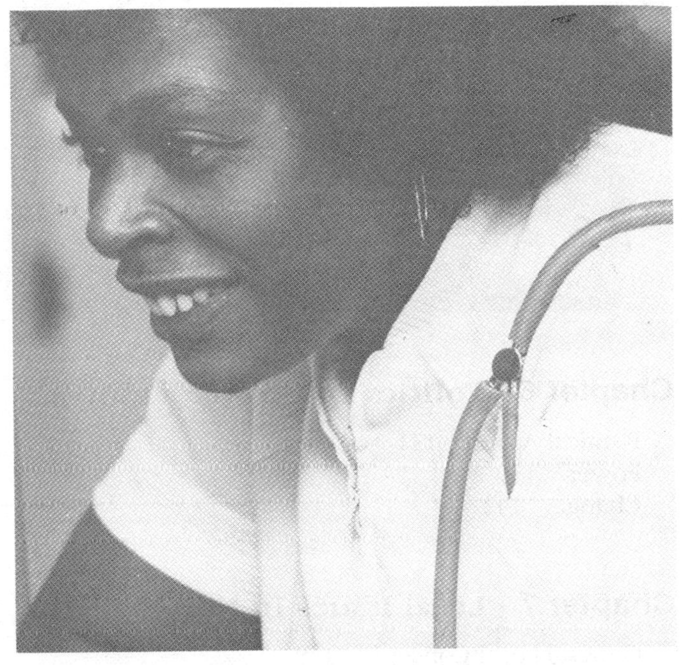

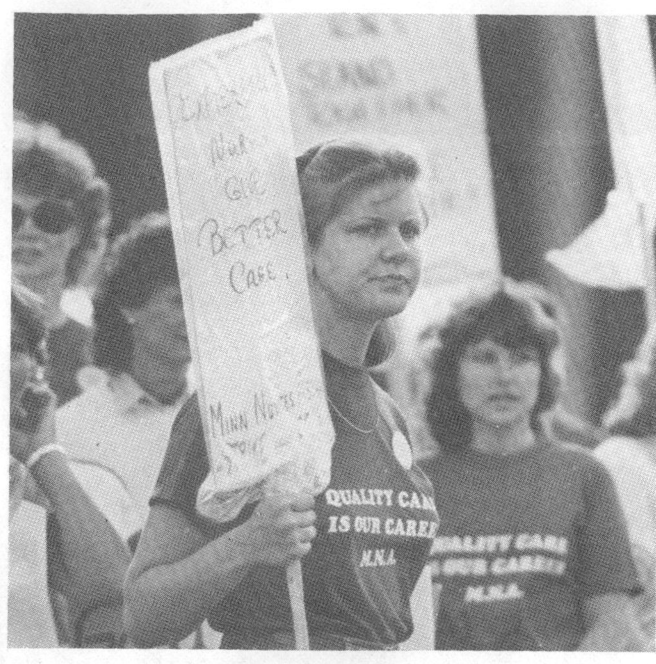
BETTER
CARE
M.N.A.

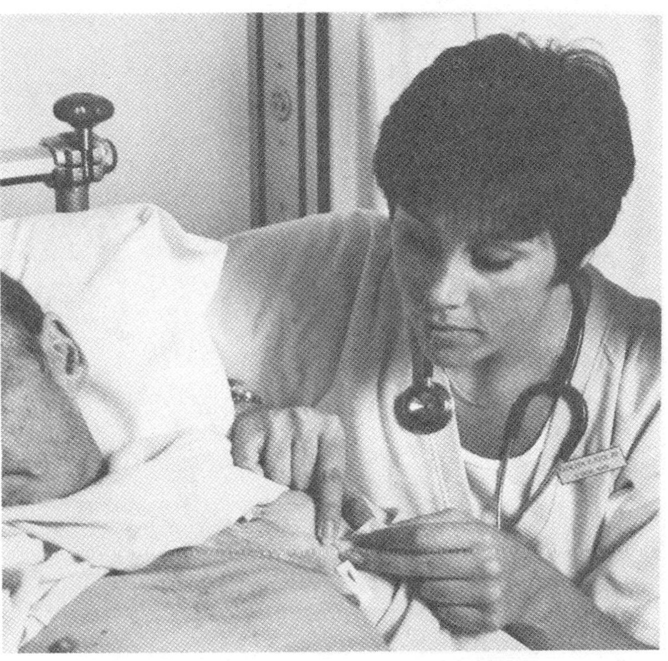

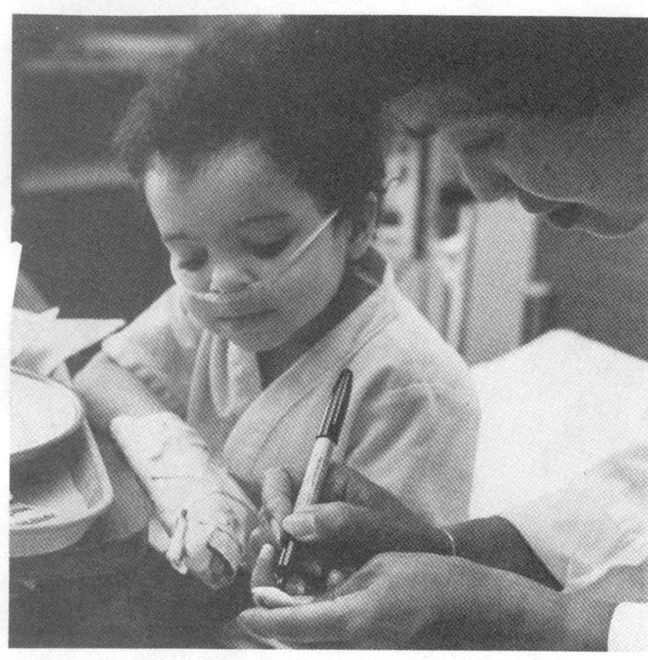

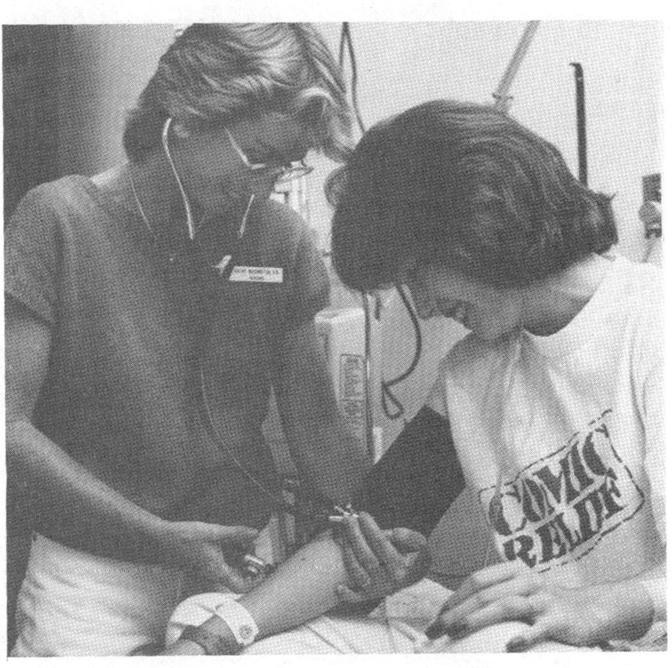

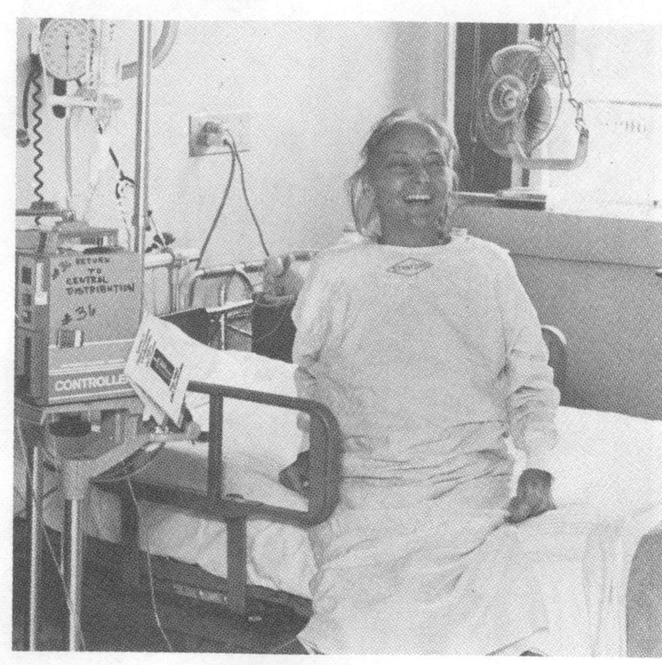

Unit 9 *Physiologic Concepts* 901

Chapter 36 Personal Hygiene 903

Chapter 37 Mobility and Immobility 964

Chapter 38 Body Alignment 1026

Chapter 39 Body Mechanics and Ambulation 1052

Chapter 40 Rest and Sleep 1098

Chapter 41 Pain 1115

Chapter 42 Nutrition 1138

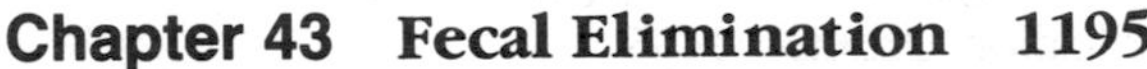

Chapter 43 Fecal Elimination 1195

Chapter 44 Urinary Elimination 1232

Chapter 45 Oxygenation 1283

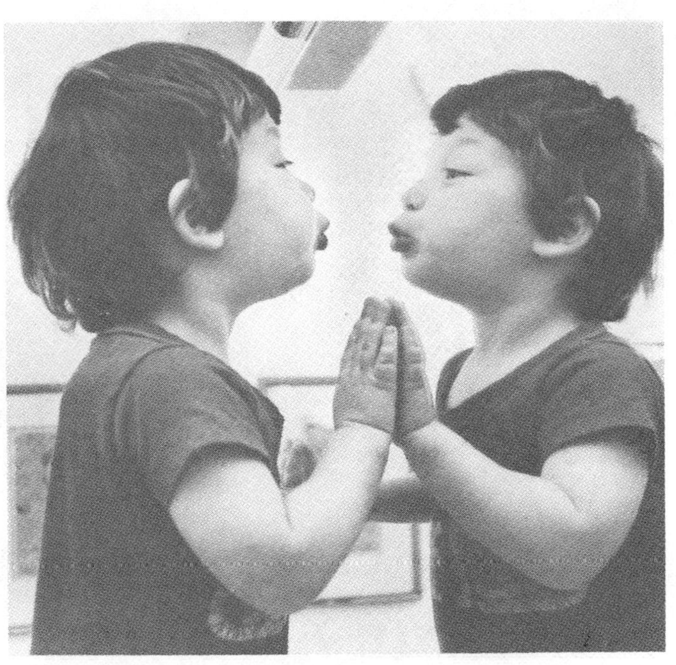

Chapter 46 Fluids and Electrolytes 1345

Unit 10 *Psychosocial Concepts 1401*

Chapter 47 Stimulation 1403

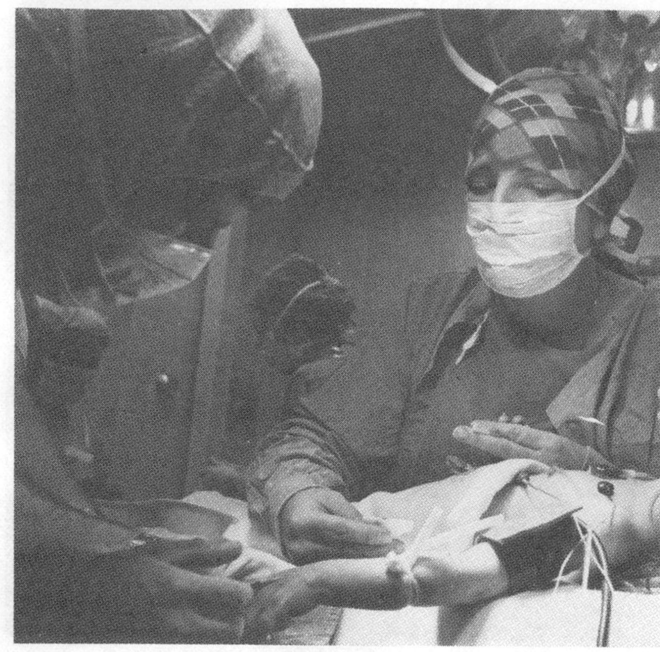

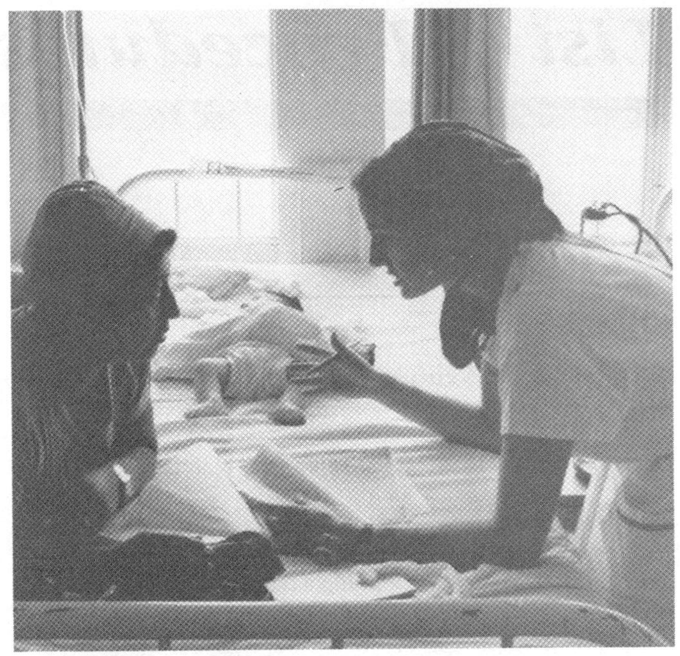

List of Procedures

More than 60 additional procedures may be found in the Procedures Supplement to this text.

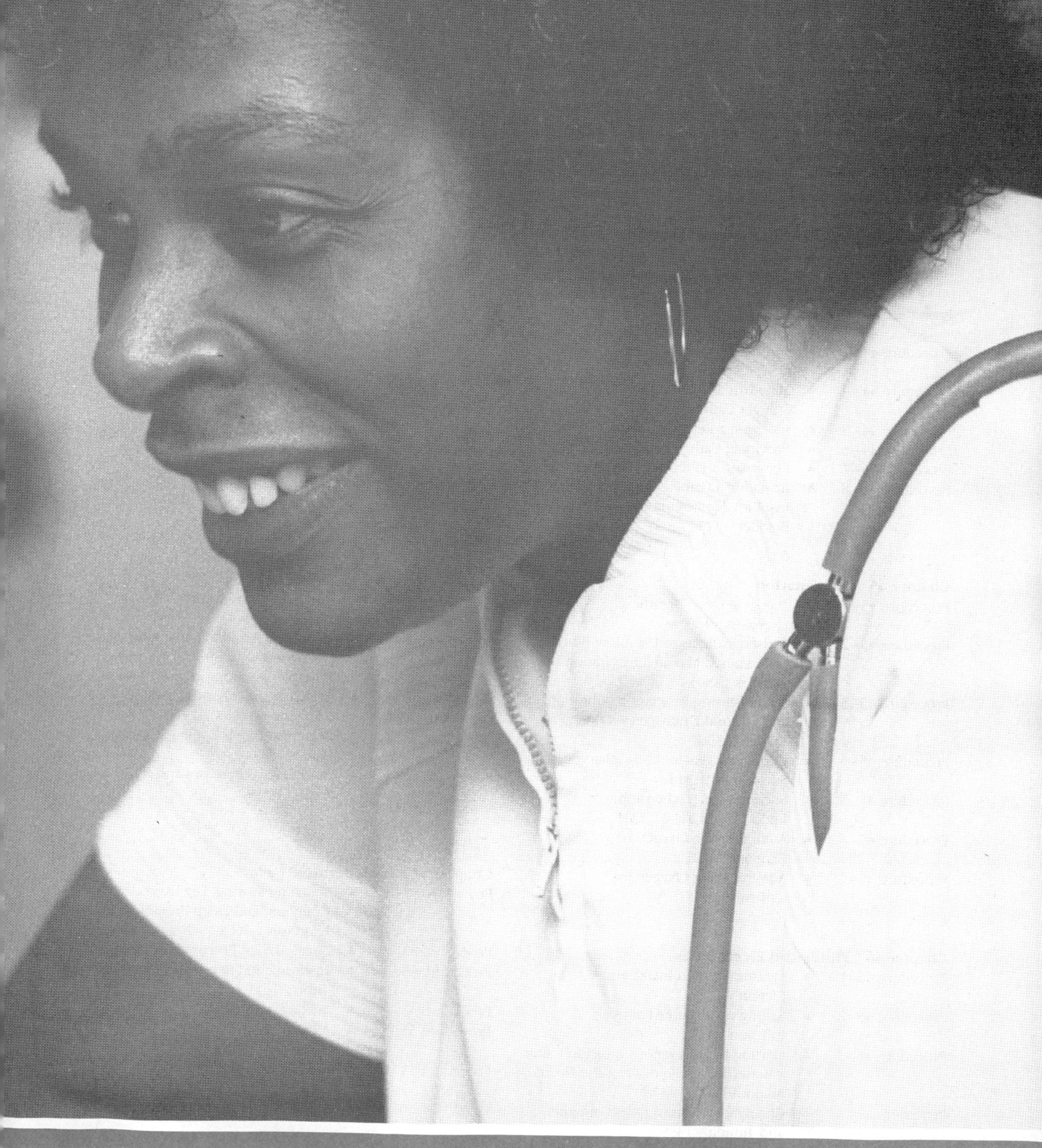

We think of ourselves as Florence Nightingale—tough, canny, powerful, autonomous, and heroic. (Claire Fagin and Donna Diers)

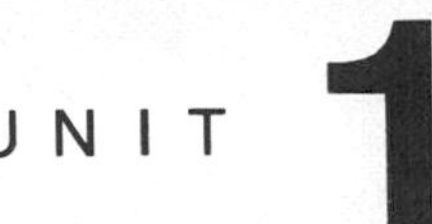

UNIT 1

Nursing and Health

WILLIAM THOMPSON

Contents

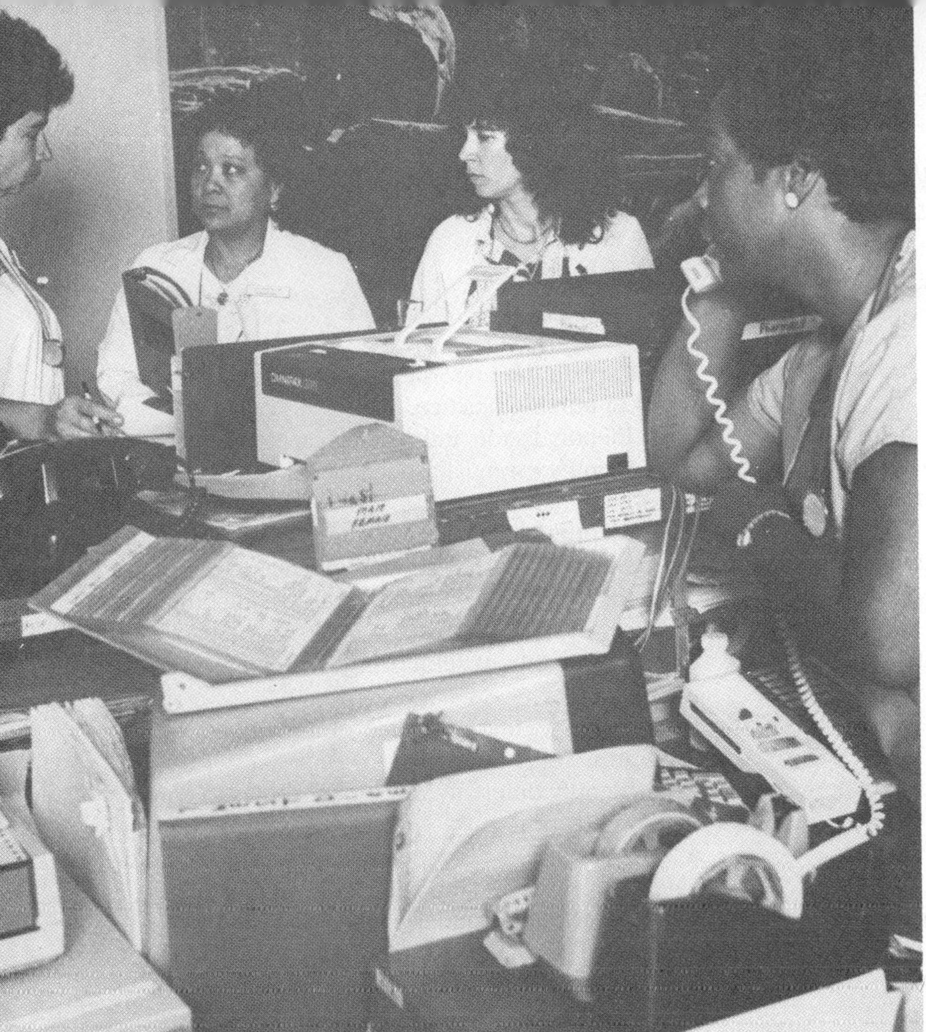

KAREN STAFFORD RANTZMAN

CHAPTER 1

Nursing and Nurses

Contents

1 *Nursing and Nurses*

Objectives

1. Understand essential facts about the nursing profession.
   1.1 Identify essential aspects of nursing included in nursing definitions cited in this chapter.
   1.2 Compare the terms *profession, occupation,* and *vocation.*
   1.3 Identify the functions that Styles cites as necessary for the preservation and development of a profession.
   1.4 Name Hall's four stages in the evolution of an occupation into a profession.
   1.5 Identify the six elements of a profession as described by Moore and Rosenblum.
   1.6 Identify the behavioral characteristics of a professional as described by Miller.
   1.7 Describe factors indicating professional growth.
2. Understand essential facts about conceptual frameworks and theories of nursing.
   2.1 Explain the purpose of conceptual frameworks and theories of nursing.
   2.2 Identify essential concepts that influence nursing.
   2.3 Differentiate a theory from a conceptual framework.
   2.4 Identify three essential elements of a theory.
   2.5 Identify three essential components of a conceptual model of nursing.
   2.6 Describe seven major units of a conceptual model of nursing.
   2.7 Explain advantages of several different conceptual models and one universally accepted model.
   2.8 Describe the relationship of the nursing process to conceptual models of nursing.
   2.9 Describe the relationship of nursing theory to nursing research.
3. Understand essential facts about nursing practice.
   3.1 Identify four foci of nursing practice.
   3.2 Identify differences in the nurse's role in various practice settings.
   3.3 Explain the significance of nurse practice acts.
   3.4 Explain the importance of established standards of nursing practice.
   3.5 Identify factors influencing career mobility.
   3.6 Identify essential aspects of expanded nursing roles.
   3.7 Identify contributions of selected nurses and factors that influenced nursing practice in the past.
   3.8 Identify factors currently influencing nursing practice.
   3.9 Describe how influencing factors affect nursing.
4. Understand significant aspects of nursing education programs.
   4.1 Identify different educational routes to enter nursing practice.
   4.2 Identify some competencies expected of graduates of various nursing education programs.
   4.3 Describe the ladder concept in nursing education.
   4.4 Compare the purposes of continuing education programs to those of in-service education programs.
   4.5 Discuss attributes of and approaches to self-directed learning.
   4.6 Discuss current professional and economic issues in nursing education.
5. Appreciate the role and functions of nursing organizations.
   5.1 Identify the functions of the National Student Nurses' Association.
   5.2 Compare the functions of national and international nurses' associations.
   5.3 Describe the unique contribution of special interest organizations.
6. Appreciate past, present, and future factors influencing nursing practice.
   6.1 Identify the significance of selected historic aspects of nursing.
   6.2 Explain the significance of factors currently influencing nursing practice.
   6.3 Explain the significance of selected trends in nursing practice.

Terms

altruism
client
concept
conceptual framework
consumer
credentialing
demography
expanded role
framework
governance
metaparadigm of nursing
model
morbidity
mortality
nurse theorist
occupation

patient
primary nursing
profession
professional
propositions
role
socialization
team nursing
theory
trend
vocation

An Emerging Definition

Nursing today is far different from nursing as it was practiced 50 years ago. It takes a vivid imagination to envision how the nursing profession will change in the next 50 years. Ours is an ever-changing world. To comprehend present-day nursing and at the same time prepare for nursing in tomorrow's world, one must understand not only past events but also contemporary nursing practice and the sociologic factors affecting it.

Florence Nightingale defined nursing over 100 years ago as "the act of utilizing the environment of the patient to assist him in his recovery" (Nightingale 1860). Nightingale considered a clean, well-ventilated, and quiet environment essential for recovery. Often considered the first nurse theorist, Nightingale raised the status of nursing to an occupation. Nurses were no longer untrained housekeepers but people trained in the care of the sick. Virginia Henderson was one of the first modern nurses to define nursing. In 1960, she wrote, "The unique function of the nurse is to assist the individual, sick or well, in the performance of those activities contributing to health or its recovery (or to peaceful death) that he would perform unaided if he had the necessary strength, will, or knowledge, and to do this in such a way as to help him gain independence as rapidly as possible" (Henderson 1966, p. 3).

The American Nurses' Association describes nursing practice as "direct service, goal oriented, and adaptable to the needs of the individual, the family, and community during health and illness" (ANA 1973, p. 2). In 1980, the ANA published this definition of nursing: "Nursing is the diagnosis and treatment of human responses to actual or potential health problems" (ANA 1980, p. 9). The Canadian Nurses' Association (CNA) published this definition in 1984:

> "Nursing" or "the practice of nursing" means the identification and treatment of human responses to actual or potential health problems and includes the practice of and supervision of functions and services that, directly or indirectly, in collaboration with a client or providers of health care other than nurses, have as their objectives the promotion of health, prevention of illness, alleviation of suffering, restoration of health and optimum development of health potential and includes all aspects of the nursing process (CNA Connection 1984, p. 8).

A number of nurse theorists have their own views of nursing. A **nurse theorist** is a person who seeks to define the basis and principles of nursing practice systematically. See Table 1–1 for definitions of nursing by selected nurse theorists.

Certain themes are common to a number of the definitions of nursing:

1. Nursing is caring for and caring about people.
2. Nursing is adapted to individual needs. Each person has unique characteristics and attributes that nurses must consider when planning care.
3. Nurses take a holistic view of the person when they plan care; that is, they view the client as a total person who is more than the sum of his or her parts and who responds as such.
4. Teaching people is an important nursing function.
5. Nursing involves individuals, families, and the community; these entities are interrelated.
6. Nursing is involved in health and in illness.
7. Nursing implementation can involve direct contact between the nurse and the client and/or support persons.
8. Nursing is involved in health promotion, health maintenance, health restoration, and the care of the dying.
9. Nursing as a science involves critical thinking.

An Evolving Profession

The history of nursing is one of constant evolution. The nursing profession owes much to the influence of Florence Nightingale (1820–1910), a woman with a vision. In an era when nursing was regarded with vehement contempt, Nightingale crusaded to change the world's view of the nurse. No longer is nursing held in disrepute as it was in the 19th century. Nightingale's belief in education, her development of theories of nursing practice and

Table 1–1 Definitions and Descriptions of Nursing

Nursing Theorist and Theory	Definition/Description
Faye Abdellah (1960): Twenty-one nursing problems	Service to individuals and families; therefore, to society. An art and science that mold the attitudes, intellectual competencies, and technical skills of the individual nurse into the desire and ability to help people, sick or well, cope with their health needs. May be carried out under general or specific medical direction.
Virginia Henderson (1960): Fourteen basic needs	The unique function of the nurse: to assist clients, sick or well, in the performance of those activities contributing to health, its recovery, or peaceful death that clients would perform unaided if they had the necessary strength, will, or knowledge. Also, to do so in such a way as to help clients gain independence as rapidly as possible.
Dorothy E. Johnson (1980): Behavioral system theory	An external regulatory force that acts to preserve the organization and integration of the client's behavior at an optimal level under those conditions in which the behavior constitutes a threat to physical or social health, or in which illness is found.
Imogene King (1971, 1981): Goal attainment theory	A helping profession that assists individuals and groups in society to attain, maintain, and restore health. If this is not possible, nurses help individuals die with dignity. Nursing is perceiving, thinking, relating, judging, and acting vis-a-vis the behavior of individuals who come to a nursing situation. A nursing situation is the immediate environment, spatial and temporal reality, in which nurse and client establish a relationship to cope with health states and adjust to changes in activities of daily living if the situation demands adjustment. It is an interpersonal process of action, reaction, interaction, and transaction whereby nurse and client share information about their perceptions in the nursing situation.
Madeleine Leininger (1984): Transcultural care theory	A learned humanistic art and science that focuses on personalized (individual and group) care behaviors, functions, and processes directed toward promoting and maintaining health behaviors or recovery from illness. Behaviors have physical, psychocultural, and social significance or meaning for those being assisted generally by a professional nurse or one with similar role competencies.
Myra Levine (1973): Four conservation principles	A human interaction; a discipline rooted in the organic dependency of the individual on relationships with other human beings. A subculture reflecting ideas and values unique to nurses, even though the values mirror the social template that created them.
Bette Neuman (1982): Systems theory	A unique profession in that it is concerned with all of the variables affecting an individual's response to stressors, which are intra-, inter-, and extrapersonal in nature. The concern of nursing is to prevent stress invasion, or, following stress invasion, to protect the client's basic structure and obtain or maintain a maximum level of wellness. The nurse helps the client, through primary, secondary, and tertiary prevention modes, to adjust to environmental stressors and maintain client system stability.
Dorothea Orem (1985): Self-care theory	A helping or assisting service to persons who are wholly or partly dependent—infants, children, and adults—when they, their parents, guardians, or other adults responsible for their care are no longer able to give or supervise their care. A creative effort of one human being to help another human being. Nursing is deliberate action, a function of the practical intelligence of nurses, and action to bring about humanely desirable conditions in persons and their environments. It is distinguished from other human services and other forms of care by its focus on human beings.
Hildegard Peplau (1952): Psychodynamic nursing	A significant, therapeutic, interpersonal process. It functions cooperatively with other human processes that make health possible for individuals in communities. An educative instrument, a maturing force that aims to promote forward movement of the personality in the direction of creative, constructive, productive, personal, and community living.
Martha Rogers (1970): Unitary human beings, an energy field	A humanistic science dedicated to compassionate concern with maintaining and promoting health, preventing illness, and caring for and rehabilitating the sick and disabled. Nursing seeks to promote symphonic interaction between the environment and the person, to strengthen the coherence and integrity of the human beings, and to direct and redirect patterns of interaction between the person and the environment for the realization of maximum health potential.
Sister Callista Roy (1976, 1984): Adaptation theory	A theoretical system of knowledge that prescribes a process of analysis and action related to the care of the ill or potentially ill person. As a science, nursing is a developing system of knowledge about persons used to observe, classify, and relate the processes by which persons positively affect their health status. As a practice discipline, nursing's scientific body of knowledge is used to provide an essential service to people, that is, to promote ability to affect health positively.

hygiene techniques, and her campaign to emphasize prevention in health care are important facets of nursing today.

In the early 20th century, however, people lost view of some of Nightingale's ideals temporarily. Medicine, in its zeal to control disease, frequently emphasized cure rather than prevention. Nurses were trained rather than educated, frequently working long hours performing hospital chores rather than spending time and energy with clients. Nurses all too often were allowed only to follow orders, not to make independent decisions about client care. Nightingale's intentions for the nursing profession were ignored but fortunately not forgotten. Her vision was shared by nursing pioneers in the years that followed, and this vision is the motivating force behind the campaign today for similar aims. Our changing society, advances in medicine, current goals for human rights, and Nightingale's vision continue to spur change in the nursing profession.

Today one of the issues before nursing is the degree of professionalism it has attained. The traditional nursing role was one of humanistic caring, nurturing, comforting, and supporting. To these must be added specific characteristics of true professionalism, including education, a code of ethics, mastery of a craft, an informed membership involved in the organized profession, and accountability for actions (Flaherty 1979, p. 61).

Criteria of a Profession

There are a number of ways to differentiate a profession from an occupation. A **profession** is a calling that requires special knowledge, skill, and preparation. Medicine and law have consistently been recognized as learned professions. The terms *vocation* and *occupation* are often used synonymously. A **vocation** is the work that a person regularly performs or the work that especially suits him or her. An **occupation** is an activity in which one engages, e.g., a business or a vocation. Thus, an occupation does not necessarily hold a special interest for the person and may be temporary, whereas a vocation often denotes employment in an area of interest on a regular basis. In this chapter, the more commonly used term *occupation* will be used to denote nonprofessions.

A profession is generally distinguished from other kinds of occupations by (a) its requirement of prolonged, specialized training to acquire a body of knowledge pertinent to the role to be performed and (b) an orientation of the individual toward service, either to a community or to an organization. The standards of training and practice for the profession are determined by the members of the profession, rather than by outsiders. The training of the professional involves a complete socialization process, more far-reaching in its social and attitudinal aspects and its technical features than is usually required in other kinds of occupations. A profession also enforces a self-discipline that is often more stringent than any legal controls to which it is subject. Thus, it tends to be relatively free from control by nonmembers. Members of a profession strongly identify with it, and they seldom change to another occupation. A **professional**, then, is a person who practices a learned profession.

Ordinarily, the professional makes little or no distinction between his or her professional role and the rest of his or her life. In contrast, the nonprofessional worker "puts in time" on the job, and his or her life "begins" at the end of the workday. In actuality, most people's view of work falls somewhere between these two extremes. Professionalism in nursing can be viewed in two ways: relative to the profession as a whole and relative to the behavior of the individuals.

Professionalism Relative to the Nursing Profession

In 1915, Abraham Flexner stated that professions are organized primarily for the achievement of social ends and secondarily for the assertion of rights and the protection of special interests (Flexner 1915, p. 901). Styles (1983) writes that nursing organizations must perform the following functions for the preservation and development of the profession:

1. Professional definition and regulation through the setting and enforcing of standards of education and practice for the generalist and the specialist. Regulation is largely achieved in the United States and Canada through the licensure of individual nurses, certification, and accreditation. See the section on credentialing of nurses in Chapter 7. Regulation is also achieved through the adoption of codes of ethics and norms of conduct (Styles 1983, p. 570).
2. Development of the knowledge base for practice in its broadest and narrowest components. Major contributions to the development of nursing knowledge have been made by various theorists. The primary purpose of nursing theories is to generate nursing knowledge. The challenge for nurses in the future is to generate questions and formulate hypotheses from these published theories and then test the hypotheses through nursing research. Since only research can determine the usefulness of a theory, research makes a major contribution to the development of nursing knowledge. Another significant contribution to nursing knowledge is the work of the North American Nursing Diagnosis Association (NANDA) (see Chapter 12). This group is generating and expanding a taxonomy of nursing diagnoses. Research is required to determine the validity and reliability of these diagnoses.
3. Transmission of values, norms, knowledge, and skill to neophytes and members of the profession for appli-

cation in practice. This function is largely performed through the education of nurses and the socialization processes. **Socialization** is the development in the individual of those qualities (skills, beliefs, habits, requirements) necessary to belong to and function in a group.

4. Communication and advocacy of the values and contributions of the field to several publics and constituencies. This function requires that nursing organizations speak for nurses from a position of broad agreement. It is essential for nurses to participate actively in the formulation of health legislation and policy. See "Politics, Power, and Change" in Chapter 6.
5. Attendance to the social and general welfare of their members. This function is carried out by the professional nursing organizations of the country. Professional associations give their members social and moral support to perform their roles as professionals and to cope with their professional problems. Association journals, for example, disseminate updated knowledge, new ideas, and professional concerns. By participating in the collective bargaining process, nurses can improve their economic and working conditions.

Hall (1968) proposes that occupations evolve into professions through these four stages:

1. Acquiring a body of knowledge in an institution of higher learning
2. Creation of a full-time occupation
3. Formation of a professional organization
4. Formulation of a code of ethics (Miller 1985, p. 24)

In 1970, Moore and Rosenblum identified six elements of a profession. A profession should:

1. Have a systematic theory
2. Exert authority
3. Command prestige
4. Have a code of ethics
5. Have a professional culture
6. Be the major source of income of those who practice it (Moore and Rosenblum 1970)

More recently, Freidson (1977) argued that the most critical element of a profession is its power to control the terms, conditions, and content of its work.

Miller states that the critical attributes of professionalism in nursing are:

1. Gaining a body of knowledge in a university setting and a science orientation at the graduate level in nursing
2. Attaining competencies derived from the theoretical base wherein the "diagnosis and the treatment of human responses to actual or potential health problems" (ANA 1980) can be accomplished
3. Delineating and specifying the skills and competencies that are the boundaries of expertise (Miller 1985, p. 25)

Professionalism Relative to Individual Nurses

Miller states that the degree to which a person behaves as a professional is reflected in the following behaviors:

1. Assesses, plans, implements, and evaluates theory, research, and practice in nursing. These behaviors are reflected in the entire nursing process. See also Chapters 10 through 15.
2. Accepts, promotes, and maintains the interdependence of theory, research, and practice. These three elements make nursing a profession and not a task-centered activity (Miller 1985, p. 26).
3. Communicates and disseminates theoretical knowledge, practical knowledge, and research findings to the nursing community. Professionalism must be demonstrated by supporting, counseling, and assisting other nurses (Miller 1985, p. 26).
4. Upholds the service orientation of nursing in the eyes of the public. This orientation differentiates nursing from an occupation pursued primarily for profit. Many consider altruism the hallmark of a profession. (**Altruism** is selfless concern for others.) Nursing has a tradition of service to others. This service, however, must be guided by certain rules, policies, or code of ethics (Miller 1985, p. 26). The nursing code of ethics is formulated by national nursing associations. In addition, society is protected by licensure and accreditation of nurses. These self-regulatory provisions give nurses the autonomy to function in the public's best interests rather than in the best interests of an institution or other profession.
5. Preserves and promotes the professional organization as the major referent. Operation under the umbrella of professional organization differentiates a profession from an occupation (Miller 1985, p. 26). In nursing, the American Nurses' Association in the United States and the Canadian Nurses' Association in Canada perform the self-regulatory functions.

Growth of Professionalism

The growth of professionalism in nursing can be viewed in relation to specialized education, knowledge base, ethics, and autonomy.

Specialized Education

Historically, nurses were educated in hospitals; however, increasingly nurses are obtaining baccalaureates in colleges and universities (see the discussion of the education of nurses later in this chapter). In addition, more nurses are obtaining master's degrees and doctorates in nursing.

People are the theoretical focus and concern of nursing, and the education of nurses should reflect this fact. Many nursing educators believe that the undergraduate nursing curriculum should include 2 years of liberal arts education. The ANA's position paper on education for nurses (1965, p. 107) states: "Education for those who work in nursing should take place within the general education system." In 1978, the ANA passed a resolution that by 1985 a baccalaureate degree be a condition of entry to professional practice (ANA 1979). In 1983, the National League for Nursing (NLN) voted at its convention to retain the baccalaureate degree as academic preparation for the professional nurse (Lewis 1983, p. 246).

In the United States today, there are five levels of entry into registered nursing: hospital diploma, associate degree, baccalaureate degree, master's degree, and doctoral degree (DeYoung 1985, p. 101).

The first preparation of registered nurses led to a diploma in nurse education. Nursing education programs offering a baccalaureate date back to 1909; their greatest growth has been since the 1950s. Associate degree programs began in 1952 and now graduate the largest number of RNs (DeYoung 1985).

A fourth approach designed specifically for the non-nurse college graduate is the master's degree in nursing, which provides basic nursing education. In May 1982, there were six such programs in the country (Slavinsky and Diers 1982, p. 293). Programs at Yale and Case Western Reserve University date back to 1923; there was a resurgence of interest in 1960 when Pace University at New York Medical College admitted its first class under Frances Reiter. Between 1923 and 1970, Yale and Case Western Reserve Universities continually altered their programs; for example, Case Western Reserve University first offered a basic master's degree in nursing, then a bachelor's degree, and now a nurse doctorate (DeYoung 1985, p. 101).

The newest approach, the nurse doctorate, was offered first at Case Western Reserve, Frances Payne Bolton School of Nursing, Cleveland, Ohio, and is now offered by several other universities. See also the section on education of nurses, later in this chapter.

Body of Knowledge

As a profession, nursing is establishing a well-defined body of knowledge and expertise. A number of nursing conceptual frameworks (discussed later in this chapter) contribute to the knowledge base of nursing and give direction to nursing research and nursing education.

Increasing research in nursing is contributing to this body of knowledge. In the 1940s, nursing research was at a very early stage of development. In the 1950s, increased federal funding and professional support helped to establish centers for nursing research. In 1952, *Nursing Research*, the first journal to report findings of nursing studies, was founded. Since that time, more nurses with doctorates are carrying out nursing research. The 1980 NLN survey of 263 accredited baccalaureate programs showed that 62% of programs offered a research course (Spruck 1980, p. 258).

Early research focused on the needs and resources of nursing and nursing education. In the 1960s, studies were often related to the nature and veracity of the knowledge base underlying nursing practice (Gortner 1980, p. 205). During the 1970s, research was largely practice-related, and nursing's involvement in research continues to grow. See Chapter 5 for additional information on nursing research.

Ethics

Nurses have traditionally placed a high value on the worth and dignity of others. The nursing profession requires integrity of its members; that is, a member is expected to do what is considered right regardless of the personal cost. Nurses must respect the professional judgment of others and must develop nursing standards and establish mechanisms for identifying and dealing with unethical behavior.

Ethical codes change as the needs and values of society change. Nursing has developed its own codes of ethics and in most instances has set up means to monitor the professional behavior of its members. See Chapter 8 for additional information on ethics.

Autonomy

A profession is autonomous if it regulates itself and sets standards for its members. Providing autonomy is one of the purposes of a professional association. In the United States, the ANA is responsible for defining the scope of nursing practice. If nursing is to have professional status, it must function autonomously in the formation of policy and in the control of its activity. To be autonomous, a professional group must be granted legal authority to define the scope of its practice, describe its particular functions and roles, and determine its goals and responsibilities in delivery of its services (Leddy and Pepper 1985, p. 189). The amount of autonomy a professional group possesses depends on its effectiveness at governance. **Governance** is the establishment and maintenance of social, political, and economic arrangements by which practitioners control their practice, their self-discipline, their working conditions, and their professional affairs (Leddy and Pepper 1985, pp. 189–90). Nurses, therefore, must work within their professional organizations.

To practitioners of nursing, autonomy means independence at work, responsibility, and accountability for one's actions. Autonomy is more easily achieved and maintained from a position of authority. Therefore many nurses seek administrative positions rather then expanded clinical competence as a means to assure their autonomy in the workplace.

Conceptual Frameworks and Theories of Nursing

A conceptual framework or model is a way of looking at (conceptualizing) a discipline (e.g., nursing and what it is) in clear, explicit terms that can be communicated to others. Although most nurses have a clear idea of what nursing is, its uniqueness needs to be clearly stated to other health professionals and the public. Professionalism and a desire for collegial status with other health professionals have made the need for conceptual frameworks of nursing explicit. If nurses are to be considered health professionals, they must communicate exactly what makes their place in the interdisciplinary team unique and important.

Before one discusses conceptual frameworks, the terms *concept, model, framework, conceptual model* or *framework,* and *theory* must be clarified. A **concept** is an abstract idea or mental image of phenomena or reality. Many concepts apply to nursing: concepts about human beings, health, helping relationships, and communication. The concepts that influence nursing most significantly and determine its practice include: the *person* receiving nursing care, the *environment* in which the person exists, *health* at the time of interaction with the nurse, and *nursing actions.* Together these concepts form the **metaparadigm of nursing**. The metaparadigm is the most global perspective of any discipline, its encapsulating unit or framework. It singles out the phenomena with which the discipline deals in a unique manner. Most disciplines have a single metaparadigm, but several conceptual models provide different views of the metaparadigm concepts. A **model** is a pattern of something to be made, an abstract outline or architectural sketch of a genuine article, or an approximation or simplification of reality. A toy model, such as a toy car, illustrates the definition simply. The model is not actually a car, but its parts represent the features of a real car. A model can also show the features of a discipline. Nursing models include only those concepts that the model builder considers relevant and that aid understanding by others. A **framework** is a basic structure supporting anything. A conceptual framework or model is a basic structure or outline of abstract ideas or images that represent reality. Conceptual frameworks, however, are not made up only of concepts. They are also made up of **propositions**, statements that express the relationships between concepts. A **conceptual framework**, therefore, is a set of concepts and statements that integrate the concepts into a meaningful configuration (Fawcett 1984, p. 2). For example, the four concepts of the metaparadigm of nursing are connected or related as follows:

"Nursing studies the wholeness or health of humans, recognizing that humans are in continuous interaction with their environments" (Donaldson and Crowley 1978, p. 119). Each nurse theorist's conceptual framework proposes a different view of the metaparadigm concepts. See Table 1–2 later in this chapter.

A conceptual model gives clear and explicit direction to the three areas of nursing: practice, education, and research. (Some nurses add a fourth field of nursing, administration; however, many consider administration a component of each of the three areas.) All conceptual models are frames of reference (conceptual and theoretical), but not all frames of reference are models in that some are not specific enough to give clear direction to practice, education, and research.

A **theory**, like a conceptual model, is made up of concepts and propositions; however, a theory accounts for phenomena with much greater specificity. The primary purpose of a theory, as opposed to a conceptual framework, is to generate knowledge in a field. A conceptual framework, by contrast, provides a guide for nursing practice, education, and research. Numerous definitions of theory exist in the literature. Most definitions include three elements:

1. A set of well-defined constructs or concepts. For example, the constructs in Imogene King's theory of goal attainment include perception, communication, interaction, transaction, self, role, growth and development, stress, time, and space.
2. A set of propositions that specify the relationships among the constructs. For example, here are a few examples of the eight propositions King developed to describe the relationship among the concepts in her theory of goal attainment (Austin and Champion 1983):
   a. If perceptual accuracy is present in nurse-client interactions, transactions (goal attainment) will occur.
   b. If role expectations and role performance as perceived by the nurse and client are congruent, transactions will occur.
   c. If transactions are made in nurse-client interactions, growth and development will be enhanced.
3. Hypotheses that test the relationships between the constructs and propositions. Because theory is abstract,

it cannot be applied to practice. Instead, hypotheses derived from the theory are tested. For example, here are some testable hypotheses derived from King's goal-attainment theory (King 1981):

a. Perceptual accuracy in nurse-client interactions increases mutual goal setting.
b. Communication increases mutual goal setting between nurses and clients and leads to satisfaction.
c. Goal attainment decreases stress and anxiety in nursing situations.

Some Conceptual Frameworks of Nursing

Because no consensus has been reached about the nature and structure of nursing, theories continue to be developed. Each theory bears the name of the person or group who developed it and reflects the beliefs of the developer. Some well-known theories are Virginia Henderson's (1966) complementary-supplementary model; Dorothy E. Johnson's (1980) behavioral systems model; Imogene King's (1981) open systems theory; Madeleine Leininger's (1984) transcultural care theory; Myra Levine's (1973) conservation theory; Betty Neuman's (1982) system model; Dorothea E. Orem's (1980) self-care model; Martha Roger's (1970, 1980) life process theory; and Sister Callista Roy's (1976) adaptation model. The Canadian Nurses' Association Testing Service (CNATS) also developed a model (CNA 1980). See "Components of Nursing Models" next, and Table 1–2 on page 12 or additional information. Leininger's transcultural care theory is discussed in Chapter 14.

Components of Nursing Models

Conceptual models have three components: assumptions, a value system, and major units.

Assumptions

Assumptions are statements of facts (premises) or suppositions that people accept as the underlying theoretical foundation for conceptualizations about nursing. Assumptions are derived from scientific theory or practice or both, and either have been or can be verified. Some nursing models draw assumptions from adaptation theories; others from general systems theories. Most models also draw assumptions from practice.

Assumptions differ greatly from model to model, since they are drawn from different premises. For example, assumptions about human beings (the client) vary considerably: Henderson views the client as a being with 14 fundamental needs; Roy, as a being with four modes of adaptation; Johnson, as a being with eight behavioral subsystems; and Orem, as an agent with six universal self-care requisites.

Values System

The beliefs underlying a profession are its value system. Generally, these beliefs are similar from model to model. Some of them are:

1. Nurses have a unique function even though they share certain functions with other health professionals.
2. Nursing is a service directed toward meeting the needs of well or ill persons or groups (families and communities) rather than directed toward specific aspects of disease or illness.
3. Nursing uses a systematic process (see Chapter 10) to operationalize its conceptual model.
4. Nursing involves a series of interpersonal relationships. The nurse-client relationship (helping relationship) is of major importance. See Chapter 27.

Margretta Styles believes that the nursing profession must have a common ideology, just as nations have their pledges of allegiance, societies their oaths, and religions their creeds. Styles proposes the following (1982, p. 61):

Declaration of belief about the nature and purpose of nursing*

I. I believe in nursing as an *occupational force for social good,* a force that, in the *totality of its concern* for all human health states and for mankind's responses to health and environment, provides a distinct, unique, and vital perspective, value orientation, and service.

II. I believe in nursing as a *professional discipline,* requiring a sound education and research base grounded in its own science and in the variety of academic and professional disciplines with which it relates.

III. I believe in nursing as a *clinical practice,* employing particular physiological, psychosocial, physical, and technological means for human amelioration, sustenance, and comfort.

IV. I believe in nursing as a *humanistic field,* in which the fullness, self-respect, self-determination, and humanity of the nurse engage the fullness, self-respect, self-determination, and humanity of the client.

V. I believe that nursing's *maximum contribution* for social betterment is dependent on:
   A. The well-developed *expertise* of the nurse;
   B. The *understanding, appreciation,* and *acknowledgment* of that expertise by the public;

---

*From Styles, Margretta M.: *On nursing: Toward a new endowment* (St. Louis: C. V. Mosby Co., 1982). Used by permission.

Table 1–2 Summary of Major Units from Selected Conceptual Models for Nursing

Major Units of Model	Conceptual model for nursing*: CNATS (CNA 1980): developmental-adaptation model	Henderson (1966): complementary-supplementary model	Johnson (Riehl and Roy 1980): behavioral system model	King (1971, 1981): open systems goal-oriented model
Goal of nursing	To help human beings achieve and sustain their optimal level of functioning	Independence in the satisfaction of human beings' 14 fundamental needs	Behavioral system equilibrium and dynamic stability	Attainment or maintenance of health to allow clients to function in their roles
Client (see also Table 16–1 on page 311)	A unique biopsychosocial being who functions as an integrated whole and whose modes of adaptation (patterns of responses to environmental and organismic stimuli) are both inborn and acquired	A whole, complete, and independent being who has fourteen fundamental needs: to breathe, eat and drink, eliminate, move and maintain posture, sleep and rest, dress and undress, maintain body temperature, keep clean, avoid danger, communicate, worship, work, play, and learn	A behavioral system composed of eight subsystems: affiliative, achievement, dependence, aggressive, eliminative, ingestive, restorative, and sexual	Three interacting systems: individuals (personal systems), groups (interpersonal systems), and society (social systems)
Role of the nurse	To care for clients at critical periods of life in such a way that they may develop and use those modes of adaptation (motor, physiologic, social, affective, cognitive) that enable them to achieve the optimal level of functioning	A complementary-supplementary role to maintain or restore independence in the satisfaction of clients' 14 fundamental needs.	A regulator and controller of behavioral system stability and equilibrium	An interaction process
Source of client difficulty	Actual or anticipated changes in stimulation, occurring at critical periods, which have the capacity to disrupt the optimal level of functioning	Lack of strength, will, or knowledge	Functional or structural stress	Stressors in the internal and external environment
Intervention focus	Modes of adaptation that require reinforcement (appropriate modes) or alteration (inappropriate modes) to sustain or restore the optimal level of functioning	The deficit that is the source of client difficulty	1. The mechanisms of control and regulation 2. The functional imperatives	Perception of client difficulty and goal setting
Modes of intervention	Manipulation of stimuli through the introduction of new ones, removal of existing ones, or modification of existing ones	Actions to replace, complete, substitute, add, reinforce, or increase strength, will, or knowledge	Actions to facilitate, inhibit, defend, or restrain the client in the face of functional or structural stress	Interaction process in which both client and nurse perceive and communicate, thus creating action; actions result in reactions, and, if there is no disturbance, goals may be set, means to achieve them explored and agreed upon, and transactions made
Consequences of nursing activity	Sustained optimal level of functioning	1. Increased independence in satisfaction of the client's 14 fundamental needs, or 2. Peaceful death	Efficient and effective client behavior	Goal attainment

*The models are listed in alphabetical order.

Conceptual model for nursing				
Levine (1973): conservation model	**Neuman (1982): system model**	**Orem (1980): self-care model**	**Rogers (1970): life-process model**	**Roy (1976): adaptation model**
Promotion of wholeness	Attainment and maintenance of client system stability	Achievement of optimal client self-care so that clients can achieve and maintain an optimal health state	Achievement of maximum health potential	Adaptation in each of the four adaptive modes in situations of health and illness
Holistic being: an open system of systems that in its wholeness expresses the organization of all its parts. The person retains his or her integrity through adaptive capability	A basic structure or central core of survival factors surrounded by concentric rings that are bounded by a line of resistance, a normal line of defense, and a flexible line of defense	A unity who can be viewed as functioning biologically, symbolically, and socially and who initiates and performs self-care activities on his or her own behalf in maintaining life, health and well-being; self-care activities deal with: air, water, food, elimination, activity and rest, solitude and social interaction, hazards to life and well-being, and being normal	A unified whole possessing integrity and manifesting characteristics that are more than and different from the sum of its parts	A biopsychosocial being who is in constant interaction with the environment and who has four modes of adaptation, based on: physiologic needs, self-concept, role function, and interdependence
Therapeutic, i.e., to influence adaptation favorably or move client toward renewed social well-being; or supportive, i.e., to maintain the status quo	To identify stressors and assist the individual to respond to stressors	To provide assistance to influence clients' development in achieving an optimal level of self-care	To help clients develop patterns of living that accommodate environmental changes rather than conflict with them	To promote clients' adaptive behaviors by manipulating the focal, contextual, and residual stimuli
Altered relationship with the internal and external environment	Intrapersonal, interpersonal, and extrapersonal stressors in the internal and external environments	Any interference with self care, by a person, object, condition, event, circumstance, or any combination of interferences	Unharmonious person-environment interactions that are determined by social values	Coping activity that is inadequate to maintain integrity in the face of a need deficit or excess
Enhancing patterns of adaptive response	Strengthening normal and flexible lines of defense	Inability to maintain self-care (a deficit in the self-care agency)	Coordinating environmental field and human field rhythmicities	The focal, contextual, and residual stimuli
Four conservation principles: actions to conserve energy, structural integrity, personal integrity, and social integrity	Primary intervention, i.e., strengthening the person's flexible line of defense; secondary prevention, i.e., strengthening internal lines of resistance; and tertiary prevention, i.e., maintaining the person's existing energy resources	Five general ways of assisting: acting for or doing for, guiding, supporting, providing a developmental environment, and teaching	Actions to promote harmonious interaction between the client and environment, to strengthen the integrity of the human field, and to direct and redirect patterning of the human and environmental fields	Manipulation of the stimuli by increasing, decreasing, and/or maintaining them
Adaptive responses that retain wholeness	Reconstitution, i.e., movement from a variance of wellness to the desired level of wellness and client system stability	Achievement of the client's optimal level of self-care	Maximum health potential and unity	Adaptive responses to stimuli by the client

C. The organizational, legal, economic, and political *arrangements* that enable the full and proper expression of nursing values and expertise;

D. The ability of the profession to maintain *unity* within diversity.

VI. I believe in *myself* and in my nursing *colleagues:*

A. In our *responsibility* to develop and dedicate our minds, bodies, and souls to the profession that we esteem and the people whom we serve;

B. In our *right* to be fulfilled, to be recognized, and to be rewarded as highly valued members of society.

Major Units

Seven major units of nursing models are constructed from the assumptions and values:

1. Goal of nursing
2. Client (patient)
3. Role of the nurse
4. Source of difficulty of the client
5. Intervention focus
6. Modes of intervention
7. Consequences of nursing activity

A summary of these units in the major conceptual models is given in Table 1–2.

Goal of nursing The goal is the end or aim of nursing, what nursing is trying to achieve. This goal has to agree with the goals common to all health professionals—to improve health, to maintain health, to prevent health problems, to restore health, etc. However, each health discipline has a goal distinct enough to justify the presence of that discipline on the health team. Specific nursing goals vary from model to model, depending on its assumptions about people. Goals need to be broad enough (a) to indicate what end the nursing profession is working toward, (b) to indicate what to teach future practitioners, and (c) to apply to nursing practice in all practice settings (community, hospital, home, health center, etc.). Before the 20th century, Florence Nightingale believed the goal of nursing was to make the patient as comfortable as possible and to put the patient in the best possible condition for nature to act and for the physician's treatment to take effect. For current goals of nursing, see Table 1–2.

Client The client unit refers not only to the intended recipient(s) of nursing service but also to conceptions about that person or group. Most models indicate that the client is a biopsychosocial being, but they differ in exactly how the client is conceptualized as such. Henderson views the client as a whole, complete, independent being who has 14 fundamental needs, while Johnson views the client as a behavioral system composed of eight subsystems. See Table 1–2 for further information.

Role of the nurse The role of the nurse must be wanted, needed, and accepted by society just as the physician's curative role or the lawyer's defending role is wanted and accepted. Many nurses consider their role to be one of "caring"; however, caring is a vague concept that is difficult to operationalize. In Orem's self-care model, the role of the nurse is to provide assistance to influence the client's development in achieving an optimal level of self-care; in Roy's adaptation model, the nurse's role is to promote the client's adaptive behaviors by manipulating stimuli. See Table 1–2 for additional information.

Source of difficulty The source of difficulty resides with the client, not the nurse. In other words, it is the probable origin or cause of any client problems amenable to nursing intervention. Clients in health care agencies have health problems that may be subcategorized as medical, psychologic, dietary, nursing, etc. The physician deals with medical problems, the psychologist or psychiatrist with psychologic problems, the dietitian with dietary problems, and the nurse with nursing problems. The source of difficulty is an explicit statement of the nursing problem. For example, in Henderson's model, the origin of the client's problem is lack of strength, will, or knowledge; in Johnson's model, it is functional or structural stress.

Intervention focus Another unit of each model is the target or focus of nursing intervention. The universally accepted intervention focus for the physician is the client's pathology. In Orem's self-care model, the intervention focus for nurses is a deficit in the client's ability to maintain self-care; in Roy's adaptation model, it is the stimuli the client is having difficulty adapting to. See Table 1–2 for additional information.

Modes of intervention The modes of intervention unit clarifies the means at the nurse's disposal when intervening. It is closely allied to the intervention focus and spells out specific ways in which the nurse helps the client. For example, in Roy's adaptation model the intervention focus is stimuli and the mode of intervention is manipulation of the stimuli. In contrast, Florence Nightingale believed the mode of intervention was manipulation of the environment. This was done by providing warmth, fresh air, light, food, and sanitation. See Table 1–2 for other intervention modes.

Consequences The last unit states the expected consequences of nursing actions. It reflects the nursing goal and the concept of the client. See Table 1–2 for the consequences of specific models.

One Model versus Several Models

Many nurses believe that there are advantages to having a single, universal model for nursing because:

1. It would further the development of nursing as a profession.
2. It would give all nurses a common framework, enhancing communication and research.
3. It would promote understanding about the nurse's role in nontraditional nursing settings, such as independent nurse practitioner practice, self-help clinics, and health maintenance organizations (HMOs), since many people believe nurses provide care for only sick persons.

In contrast, advocates of several different conceptual models point out that:

1. Most disciplines have several conceptual models, which allow members to explore phenomena in different ways and from different viewpoints.
2. Several models increase an understanding of the nature of nursing and its scope.
3. Several models foster development of the full scope and potential of the discipline.

It is possible that in the 21st century many more models for nursing will be developed or that existing ones will be refined in accordance with societal needs and with their tested usefulness. This competition is needed to determine the superiority of one or more models.

Relationship to the Nursing Process

The conceptual model for nursing is an abstraction that is operationalized or made a reality by the use of the nursing process. See Chapters 10–15 for detailed information. This systematic process, not unique to nursing and similar to the scientific or problem-solving process, consists of five steps:

1. *Assessing.* The specific data collected about a client's health needs relate directly to the second unit of the conceptual model for nursing, the client. For example, if the client is seen as having 14 fundamental needs, data are collected about these 14 needs.
2. *Diagnosing.* In this step, the client's actual or potential health problems are outlined or written as a nursing diagnostic statement in accordance with the nursing model used.
3. *Planning.* The planning of nursing interventions also relates directly to the conceptual nursing model. Interventions are planned in accordance with the modes of nursing intervention outlined in the conceptual model (see Table 1–2).
4. *Implementing.* Implementing the planned interventions draws on scientific knowledge that is not part of the nursing model. The nursing model instructs the nurse what to do and directly influences what nursing interventions are planned, but it does not tell the nurse how to do it.
5. *Evaluating.* Evaluating is a continuous nursing function. How is the client adjusting and reacting? What does the client see as needs? How does the client see these needs changing? Has the client achieved the desired consequences? The answers to these questions help the nurse evaluate the effectiveness of the total nursing process and the nursing model.

Relationship of Nursing Theory to Research

Because the primary purpose of nursing theory is to generate scientific knowledge, nursing theory and nursing research are closely related. Scientific knowledge is derived from testing hypotheses generated by theories for nursing. Research determines the utility of those hypotheses, and research findings may be developed into theories for nursing. In the research process, comparisons are made between the observed outcomes of research and the relationship predicted by the hypotheses.

Several approaches can be used to test or develop theory:

1. *Inductive.* Research is first conducted, and the findings are used to develop a theory. In this inductive method, a theory is developed from multiple data. The following premise and conclusion illustrate the inductive method: If X (e.g., low self-esteem) is true of persons A1, A2, . . ., A100, and if the persons are all members of the same class (e.g., rape victims) then X is true of all members of that class.
2. *Deductive.* A theory is devised, hypotheses generated, and then research is conducted. For example, in deductive research a premise (hypothesis) is first proposed, e.g., All rape victims have low self-esteem. Mary, Joan, Ellen, and Judy are rape victims, and their level of self-esteem is tested. Because it is low, it is concluded that the hypothesis is valid.
3. *Combined.* Both inductive and deductive methods are used.

Nursing Practice

Nurses practice in an ever-increasing variety of ways and settings. The actual focus of practice is determined largely by the setting, the needs of the clients, the nurse practice acts of the area, and the standards of the professional organization.

The Recipient of Nursing Care

The recipients of nursing care are sometimes called *consumers,* sometimes *patients,* and sometimes *clients.* Some distinctions among these terms follow.

A **consumer** is an individual, a group of people, or a community that uses a service or commodity. A family that uses electricity in their home is a consumer of electricity. People who use health care products or services are consumers of health care.

A **patient** is a person who is waiting for or undergoing medical treatment and care. The word *patient* comes from a Latin word meaning to suffer or to bear. Traditionally, the person receiving health care has been called a patient. Usually, people become patients when they seek assistance because of illness or surgery. Some nurses believe that the word *patient* implies passive acceptance of the decisions and care of health professionals. For this reason, professionals are increasingly referring to recipients of health care as clients.

A **client** is a person who engages the advice or services of another who is qualified to provide this service. The term *client* presents the receiver of health care less as a passive recipient and more as a collaborator in the care, i.e., as a person who is also responsible for his or her health. Thus the health status of a client is the responsibility of the individual in collaboration with health professionals. In this book, *client* is the preferred term, although *consumer* and *patient* are used in some instances.

Focus of Nursing Practice

Nursing involves an interrelationship of many people concerned with a client's responses to potential or actual health problems. Today, there is an emphasis on the whole person; people are seen not merely as physical beings but as biopsychosocial beings. Nursing practice involves a complex of knowledge and skills applied to the whole client. Nurses are also involved with support persons and the community as a whole. For this reason, nurses must be aware of how the support persons and community affect the client's well-being and consider the well-being of these support persons and the community.

Nursing practice involves four areas related to health (health is discussed in Chapter 2):

1. Health promotion. Health promotion means helping people develop resources to maintain or enhance their well-being. The goal of health promotion is to move people toward their own optimum level of health and well-being or wellness (Black and McDowell 1984, p. 19). An example of a nursing action that promotes health is explaining the benefits of an exercise program to a client. Health promotion activities largely take place in community care centers, schools, and, increasingly, industry. Health promotion is discussed in more detail in Chapter 19.

2. Health maintenance. Health maintenance nursing activities are those actions that help clients to maintain their health status. An elderly person in a long-term care facility can be taught and encouraged to exercise to maintain muscle strength and mobility. Health maintenance activities take place in homes, community clinics, long-term care facilities, and, to some degree, acute care hospitals.

3. Health restoration. Health restoration means helping people to improve health following health problems or illness. Examples of activities that help restore health are teaching a client to protect an incision and to change a surgical dressing or assisting a handicapped individual to attain the highest level of physical strength of which he or she is capable. Most nurses who work in hospitals function in this area.

4. Care of the dying. This area of nursing practice involves comforting and caring for people of all ages while they are dying. Nurses carrying out these activities work in homes, hospitals, and extended care facilities. Some agencies, called hospices, are specifically designed for this purpose.

Settings for Nursing Practice

In the past, the acute care hospital was the only practice setting open to most nurses. Today, however, there are employment opportunities not only in acute and long-term chronic or rehabilitation hospitals but also in clients' homes, community agencies, ambulatory clinics or health maintenance organizations (HMOs), and nursing practice centers, for example. Table 1–3 shows areas of registered practice in the United States.

Nurses have different degrees of nursing autonomy and nursing responsibility in the various settings. Today, nurses have a variety of career choices and can pursue any number of interests. They may specialize, for example, in intensive care nursing or respiratory nursing. In addition to providing direct care, they teach clients and support persons, serve as nursing advocates and change agents, and help determine health policies affecting consumers in the community and in hospitals.

Table 1–3 Areas of Registered Nurse Employment

Practice Setting	United States 1984 (percent*)	Canada 1984 (percent*)
Hospitals	65.7	73.0
Nursing homes/homes for the aged	8.0	6.5
Community health	6.6†	9.2
Physicians' and dentists' offices, family practice units	5.7	2.6
Nursing education	3.7	
Educational institutions (Canada)		2.7
Schools	3.5	
Occupational health	2.3	
Other, e.g., self-employed, insurance claims reviewers	4.1	3.1
Not stated	—	2.9

*Rounded to the first decimal
†These figures do not reflect the shift to home health care.

Sources: American Nurses' Association, *Facts about nursing 84–85* (Kansas City, Mo.: American Nurses' Association, 1985), p. 3 and Statistics Canada, *Revised registered nurses data series,* Health Manpower Statistics Section (Ottawa: Health Statistics, 1984), Table 6.

Hospitals

Hospitals are health institutions that vary in size and in the services they provide. General hospitals treat patients with different health problems and of different socioeconomic backgrounds. They range in size from the small hospital in a rural setting to the large metropolitan hospital of perhaps 2000 beds. A specialized hospital may be of any size, but it restricts its services to special areas of medical practice, such as obstetrics, pediatrics, or psychiatry.

In acute hospital settings, nurses interact with a variety of health personnel. They have many nursing responsibilities that are often critical to life. Because the average hospital stay of clients has become shorter, nursing care for acutely ill people has intensified. In addition, the greater complexity of medical technology has led to a dramatic increase in the need for nursing specialists in such areas as intensive care, nephrology, and neonatal nursing. As a result, nursing practice in acute care hospitals has become more complex, specialized, and intensive. Nursing in an acute care hospital usually involves many dependent and health restoration activities. (Dependent nursing activities are those that require a physician's order.)

The increasing number of elderly in the population and the increasing incidence of chronic disease in both the United States and Canada (see Chapter 2) has given rise to many long-term care facilities. These facilities are variously named, e.g., nursing homes, extended care facilities, and chronic care homes. Some are associated with hospitals, and some are independent. In these settings, nursing tends to focus on health maintenance, health promotion, and care of the dying rather than on health restoration. Another type of health agency is the rehabilitation institution. Nursing activities in such agencies tend to center on teaching clients and their support persons how to maximize a client's function. Their role is largely health promotion and maintenance and illness prevention rather than health restoration.

Home Health Care Agencies

Home health agencies provide care to clients in their homes. Home health care was traditionally for the aging or chronically ill client. However, the ANA's Division on Community Health Nursing Practice and Commission on Nursing Services defines home health care as "those health care services provided to individuals and families in their places of residence for the purpose of preventing illness; promoting, maintaining, or restoring health; or minimizing the effects of illness and disability" (ANA 1978, p. 1).

Nursing services provided to clients in their homes vary, depending on the needs of the client and the support persons. The recent boom in home health care services is due largely to three factors: more hospital outpatient facilities, earlier hospital discharges, and increase in the population age 65 or older. Arbeiter believes that the home care nurse requires the following characteristics: self-reliance, flexibility, adaptability, confidence, versatility, empathy, system-savvy, cooperation, and teaching skill (Arbeiter 1984, pp. 38–42). For additional information on home health care nursing, see Chapter 4.

Community Agencies

Community agencies employ nurses for a wide range of nursing activities. A community can be a particular geographic area or a group of people brought together because of common interests or a social system, e.g., an educational, religious, or political system. For example, a community might be a town or the teachers, students, and families associated with a school.

Community health agencies include community health clinics, public health agencies, industrial clinics, schools, and specialized agencies such as Planned Parenthood and the Cancer Society. In these settings, nurses tend to function more independently than in hospitals. Their contact with physicians is episodic. In rural areas, contact with a physician may occur only when the nurse judges that a physician's advice or intervention is required.

Community health centers usually provide comprehensive health programs encompassing health promotion, health maintenance, and health restoration as well as preventive nursing programs and coordination with other health agencies. Community health centers provide assistance to ambulatory clients and to clients in the home.

In some centers, physicians are present most of the time; in others, nurses provide most of the services.

Schools, colleges, and universities commonly provide health services. Nursing in such settings usually focuses on health promotion, disease prevention, and health restoration. An example of health promotion is teaching students about balanced nutrition; examples of disease prevention are teaching about alcohol and drug abuse and providing immunizations. Nursing activities for health restoration may include providing care for minor injuries or teaching students how to manage a cold or influenza.

Many companies offer occupational health nursing care to their employees. Nurses may be expected to develop programs that increase work safety and decrease the risk of occupational diseases, such as lung disease caused by inhaling fine dust. The occupational nurse is often responsible for developing health promotion programs, e.g., exercise programs and disease prevention programs.

Physicians' Offices

In physicians' offices, nurses have a minimum amount of independent function. The physician is generally there when the clients are present, and many of the nurse's activities are done in response to the physician's request. The nurse's function is related mainly to the physician's therapy and to such activities as teaching clients how to prepare for a special examination.

Other Career Settings

More and more career possibilities are available for today's nurse. Besides nursing education or administration, there are career opportunities in nursing research and in various clinical specialties. As physicians and other health professionals develop group practices (e.g., family practice clinics), nurses are joining other health personnel (e.g., social workers and technologists) as a vital part of groups devoted to a broad range of services and holistic health. In more states, nurses are being employed as independent nurse practitioners (described on page 22) in: (a) hospital practice settings, such as inpatient and emergency areas; (b) ambulatory care settings, such as private practice, hospital outpatient clinics, and community-based clinics; (c) institutions, such as schools for the mentally and physically handicapped, public schools, and college health programs; and (d) community settings, such as health departments and social service agencies. The vast majority (90%) of independent nurse practitioners are employed in settings b–d (ANA 1985, p. 25).

Models for Delivery of Nursing Care

Common configurations for the delivery of nursing care include the case method, the functional method, team nursing, and primary nursing.

Case Method

The case method, also referred to as total care, is one of the earliest models developed. This method is client-centered. One nurse is assigned to and is responsible for the comprehensive care of a group of clients during an 8- or 12-hour shift. For each client, the nurse assesses needs, makes nursing plans, formulates diagnoses, implements care, and evaluates the effectiveness of care. In this method, a client has consistent contact with one nurse during a shift but may have different nurses on other shifts. The case method, considered the precursor of primary nursing, continues to be used in a variety of practice settings, e.g., private duty nursing and intensive care. With the shortage of nursing personnel during World War II, the case method could no longer be the chief mode of care for clients. To meet staff shortages, managers hired personnel with less educational preparation than the professional nurse and developed on-the-job training programs for auxiliary helpers. The total care method became unfeasible in such situations.

Functional Method

This system of assignment, which evolved from concepts of scientific management used in the field of business administration, focuses on the jobs to be completed. In this task-oriented approach, personnel with less preparation than the professional nurse fulfill less complex care requirements. It is based on a production and efficiency model that gives authority and responsibility to the person assigning the work, e.g., the head nurse. Clearly defined job descriptions, procedures, policies, and lines of communication are required. The functional approach to nursing is economical and efficient and permits centralized direction and control. Its disadvantages are fragmentation of care (the client receives care from several different categories of nursing personnel) and the possibility that nonquantifiable aspects of care, such as meeting the client's emotional needs, may be overlooked.

Team Nursing

In the early 1950s, Eleanor Lambertson (1953) and her colleagues proposed a system of team nursing to overcome the fragmentation of care resulting from the task-oriented functional approach and to meet increasing demands for professional nurses created by advances in technologic aspects of care. **Team nursing** is the delivery of individualized nursing care to clients by a nursing team led by a professional nurse. A nursing team consists of registered nurses, licensed practical nurses, and often nurses' aides. This team is responsible for providing coordinated nursing care to a group of clients during an 8- or 12-hour shift. Compared to the functional system, team nursing emphasizes humanistic values and responds to the needs of both clients and employees. Individualized client care on a personal level rather than task-oriented care on an impersonal level is emphasized. Employees are stimulated to learn and develop new skills by the professional nurse leader, who instructs them, supervises them, and provides assignments that offer the potential for growth.

Basic to team nursing are the team conference, nursing care plan, and leadership skills. The conference, led by the professional nurse team leader, includes all personnel assigned to the team. Discussing the needs of clients, establishing goals, individualizing the plan of care, instructing personnel, and following up are all under the direction of the team leader. In essence, the team leader has a management role that requires a high degree of competence in coordination and leadership.

Although the team nursing approach has worked effectively in many health care agencies, these weaknesses have been observed in some settings:

1. Frequently nurses are ill-prepared to fulfill the leadership role required of a team leader.
2. The client may still perceive care as fragmented if the team leader does not establish a satisfactory relationship with the client.
3. Teams may not have the appropriate health care personnel, and team members may not have the expertise to meet the needs of a particular client population. Ideally, several professional nurses should be team members. Often, there is only one professional nurse, who must assume the role of team leader. To manage effectively, the leader reverts to using a functional mode of delivering care.

Primary Nursing

Primary nursing was introduced at the Loeb Center for Nursing and Rehabilitation, the Bronx, New York, under the leadership of Lydia Hall (1963). **Primary nursing** is a system in which one nurse is responsible for total care of a number of clients 24 hours a day, 7 days a week. It is a method of providing comprehensive, individualized, and consistent care.

Primary nursing uses the nurse's nursing knowledge and management skills. The primary nurse assesses and evaluates each client's needs, develops a plan of care with the client, and evaluates the effectiveness of care. While associates provide some care, the primary nurse coordinates it and communicates information about the client's health to other nurses and other health professionals. Primary nursing encompasses all aspects of the professional role, including teaching, advocacy, decision making, and continuity of care. The primary nurse is the first-line manager of the client's care with all its inherent accountabilities and responsibilities.

Nurse Practice Acts

Nurse practice acts or nursing licensure laws regulate the practice of nursing in the United States and Canada. Each state in the United States has its own nurse practice act, as does each province in Canada. Although nurse practice acts differ in various jurisdictions, they all have a common purpose: to protect the public. Nurse practice acts usually define what constitutes nursing practice, describe a "registered nurse" and a "practical nurse," and establish minimum educational and competency standards that individuals seeking authority to practice must meet. Nurse practice acts are a formalized contract between society and the profession. They serve a public purpose and also meet the needs of the profession. The public is granted a mechanism to ensure minimum standards for entry into the profession and to distinguish the unqualified. The profession achieves partial implementation of its goal of maintaining standards in practice through appropriate entry credentialing (Snyder and Labar 1984, p. 2).

In 1981, the ANA published a new manual entitled *The Nursing Practice Act: Suggested State Legislation*. This publication defines professional nursing service as follows: "Nursing practice includes but is not limited to administration, teaching, counseling, supervision, delegation, and evaluation of practice and execution of the medical regimen, including the administration of medications and treatments prescribed by any person authorized by state law to prescribe" (ANA 1981b, p. 6). During the past 10 years, many states have revised their nurse practice acts to permit expanded nursing roles.

Standards of Nursing Practice

Establishing and implementing standards of practice are major functions of a professional organization. Nursing practice standards provide exact criteria against which clients, nurses, and employers can evaluate care for effectiveness and excellence.

In the ANA publication *Standards of Nursing Practice,* the association comments on this responsibility of the nursing profession to society:

> Nursing's concern for the quality of its services constitutes the heart of its responsibility to the public. The more expertise required to perform the service, the greater society's dependence upon those who carry it out. Nursing must control its practice in order to guarantee the quality of its service to the public. Behind that guarantee are the standards of the profession, which are directed toward assurance that service of a good quality will be provided. This is essential both for the protection of the public and for the profession itself. A profession which does not maintain the confidence of the public will soon cease to be a social force (ANA 1973, p. 1).

The profession's responsibilities inherent in establishing and implementing standards of practice include (Phaneuf and Lang 1985, p. 2):

1. To establish, maintain, and improve standards
2. To hold members accountable for using standards
3. To educate the public to appreciate the standards
4. To protect the public from individuals who have not attained the standards or willfully do not follow them
5. To protect individual members of the profession from each other

Basic to the development of standards of nursing practice are:

1. The needs of clients and support persons to be assured that they are receiving a safe and good standard of care.
2. The need of clients and health administrators to know that the standard of care is efficiently provided at an acceptable level. The consumer, the health administrator, and the government have become increasingly concerned about the costs of health care.
3. The need of nursing personnel to have precise standards against which to measure the nursing they provide, thus protecting themselves and clients.

Nursing standards clearly reflect the specific functions and activities that nurses provide, as opposed to the functions of other health workers. The ANA's Standards of Nursing Practice are set forth in Table 1–4, and those of the CNA are summarized in Table 1–5. These standards apply to the practice of all registered nurses.

When standards of professional practice are implemented, they serve as yardsticks for the measurements used in licensure, certification, accreditation, quality assurance, peer review, and public policy (Phaneuf and Lang 1985, p. 7). Licensure, certification, and accreditation are discussed in Chapter 7. Quality assurance and peer review are discussed in Chapter 15.

Career Mobility

The public image of the nurse is that of a hospital staff nurse who has been educated in a hospital school. Many laypeople are unaware of the variety of roles and educational backgrounds of nurses. Two kinds of mobility are

Table 1–4 American Nurses' Association Standards of Nursing Practice

Standard	Rationale
1. The collection of data about the health status of the client/patient is systematic and continuous. The data are accessible, communicated, and recorded.	Comprehensive care requires complete and ongoing collection of data about the client/patient to determine the nursing care and needs of the client/patient. All health status data about the client/patient must be available for all members of the health care team.
2. Nursing diagnoses are derived from health status data.	The health status of the client/patient is the basis for determining the nursing care needs. The data are analyzed and compared to norms when possible.
3. The plan of nursing care includes goals derived from the nursing diagnoses.	The determination of the results to be achieved is an essential part of planning care.
4. The plan of nursing care includes priorities and the prescribed nursing approaches or measures to achieve the goals derived from the nursing diagnoses.	Nursing actions are planned to promote, maintain, and restore the client/patient's well-being.
5. Nursing actions provide for client/patient participation in health promotion, maintenance, and restoration.	The client'/patient and family are continually involved in nursing care.
6. The nursing actions assist the client/patient to maximize his health capabilities.	Nursing actions are designed to promote, maintain, and restore health.
7. The client/patient's progress or lack of progress toward goal achievement is determined by the client/patient and the nurse.	The quality of nursing care depends upon comprehensive and intelligent determination of nursing's impact upon the health status of the client/patient. The client/patient is an essential part of this determination.
8. The client/patient's progress or lack of progress toward goal achievement directs reassessment, reordering of priorities, new goal setting, and revision of the plan of nursing care.	The nursing process remains the same, but the input of new information may dictate new or revised approaches.

From American Nurses' Association, *Standards of nursing practice* (Kansas City, Mo.: American Nurses' Association, 1973). Reprinted with permission.

Table 1–5 Canadian Nurses' Association Standards for Nursing Practice

Criterion Variable	Nursing Standards
Standards Related to a Conceptual Model for Nursing	
The goal of nursing	Nursing practice requires the nurse, in any setting at any time, to have: 1. A clear conception of the distinct goal of nursing
The client	2. A clear conception of the client toward whom nursing is directed
The role of the nurse	3. A clear conception of her role as a health professional in response to health needs of society
The origin of difficulty	4. A clear conception of the source of the client's actual or potential difficulty
The focus and modes of intervention	5. A clear conception of the focus and modes of nursing intervention
The expected results of nursing activities	6. A clear conception of the expected results of nursing activities related to the goal of nursing as expressed in the conceptual model for nursing
Standards Related to the Nursing Process	
Collection of data	Nursing practice requires the nurse to: 1. Collect data in accord with her conception of the client, and with her interdependent and dependent functions
Analysis of data	2. Analyze data collected in accord with her conception of the client's source of difficulty and consistent with her interdependent and dependent functions
Planning of the intervention	3. Plan her nursing action based upon the identified actual and potential client problems and in accord with her conception of the focus and modes of intervention as well as nursing actions which arise from her interdependent and dependent functions
Implementation of the intervention	4. Perform nursing actions which implement the plan
Evaluation	5. Evaluate all steps of the nursing process in accord with her conceptual model for nursing and consistent with her interdependent and dependent functions.
Standards Related to the Helping Relationship	
Entry	Nursing practice requires the nurse to: 1. Initiate the helping relationship with the client
Maintenance	2. Assume responsibility for maintaining the helping relationship
Termination	3. Assume responsibility for terminating the helping relationship
Standards Related to Professional Responsibilities	
Legal responsibility	Nursing practice requires the nurse to: 1. Conform to statutes, policies, procedures and directives relevant to the practice setting
Ethical responsibility	2. Conform to the code of ethics of her profession
Administrative responsibility	3. Comply with administrative practices and procedures in a given setting

Source: Canadian Nurses' Association, Development of a definition of nursing practice and standards for nursing practice, *Canadian Nurse,* May 1980, 76:11–15. Used by permission.

open to the nurse: vertical and horizontal. Vertical mobility means advancing upward within a hierarchy, for example, from staff nurse to head nurse. Horizontal mobility refers to ability to change practice setting, such as from a nursing home to a community health agency.

Recognizing that nurses require encouragement, motivation, and recognition, some settings provide clinical ladder models for career development. Traditionally, a nurse's clinical competence was rewarded by moving the nurse away from client care into administrative roles. Clinical ladders provide nurses with recognition of their clinical competence, at the same time permitting them to continue clinical nursing practice.

Clinical ladders have at least four basic parts (Huey 1982, p. 1520):

1. *The structure.* This includes the number of levels in the ladder and its place in the agency organization. The number of clinical levels among organizations ranges from two to five levels in each of three or four pathways: clinical practice, administration, research, and education (ANA Cabinet on Nursing Service 1984, p. 16). Various labels are used to describe the levels. Examples are: clinical nurse I, II, III, IV and CNS (clinical nurse specialist); staff nurse I, II, III and nurse clinician; professional associate nurse (entry) and primary nurse III, II, and I (top clinical level). See Huey (1982) in "Suggested Readings" for further information about various levels and shapes of ladders. The relationship of the clinical ladder structure to the administrative structure most often places the person

at each clinical level under the direction of a nurse manager (head nurse, administrative nurse) in the administrative structure. Rarely is a level I or entry level clinical nurse responsible to a level II clinical nurse or are clinical levels I and II responsible to level III. Each level reports directly to or takes direction from the nurse manager.

Career ladders can include options for vertical mobility, lateral mobility, realignment (downward mobility), and job enrichment. "Some career development specialists recommend ladders that provide for relocation out of the organization and for researching, interviewing, and testing ideas and opportunities within or outside the organization to determine interest about another field" (ANA Cabinet on Nursing Service 1984, p. 17). Some clinical career tracks have two or more vertical tracks or pathways. For example, the Crawford W. Long Memorial Hospital of Emory University in Atlanta, Georgia, has a dual track ladder with five levels of clinical advancement. The first two are clinical; at the third level the nurse decides whether to advance in management through levels III, IV, and V or in clinical practice through levels III, IV, and V (Gassert et al. 1982, p. 1527). Lateral mobility broadens the nurse's existing knowledge and skills. For example, a geriatric clinical nurse specialist may be promoted laterally to a community geriatric outreach program. Downward mobility is another option. For example, a nurse may choose to return to a more satisfying previous position or change to a different area of practice.

2. *The criteria used to define clinical competencies at each level.* Traditionally levels have been based on education and longevity. Today some clinical ladders are based only on clinical behaviors (Anderson and Denyes 1975, p. 18; Knox 1980, p. 30). Other ladder programs have eliminated any reference to experience requirements, and still others are based on educational criteria in conjunction with behavioral objectives and experience (Colavecchio et al. 1974, pp. 55–57).

   Ladders based on clinical behaviors tend to define the clinical levels in terms of (ANA Cabinet on Nursing Services 1984, p. 13):
   a. Nursing process skills or activities—assessment, planning, implementation, and evaluation
   b. Other activities, such as participation in committees and special projects
   c. Professional development, e.g., continuing education.
   d. Teaching skills (client, family, and others)
   e. Communication responsibilities
   f. Evaluation skills (self and staff)
   g. Leadership and coordination ability
   h. Roles, i.e., clinical practice, administration, research, and education
   i. Research responsibilities

3. *Promotional procedures.* Promotional procedures vary considerably. Usually the interested nurse is required to request a promotion for a vacant position. Decisions to promote may be made by a head nurse, promotion committees that consist of nurses at various clinical and administrative levels, or peer review committees. Decisions are usually based on evaluations completed by the applicant, a peer, and the applicant's unit manager or leader.

4. *Incentive for advancement.* Incentives for advancement are the titles themselves, increased salaries, or both. In addition, some agencies also provide on-the-job training, paid tuition to local schools of nursing, and tutoring to facilitate career mobility (Miller 1975, p. 27).

Expanded Nursing Roles

A **role** is a pattern of behavior expected of individuals in specific social situations. An **expanded role** is one that a nurse assumes by virtue of education and experience. The nurse who assumes an expanded role has increased responsibilities and, usually, greater autonomy.

The acceptance of the nursing process as the framework for providing nursing to clients makes it possible to delineate the functions and roles of all nurses in the five phases of the process, i.e., assessing, diagnosing, planning, implementing, and evaluating. See Chapters 10 through 15 for implementing activities, such as communicating; caring; teaching; counseling; managing, which includes acting as a change agent and patient advocate; and carrying out technical skills. In addition to carrying out basic nursing functions described in Chapters 10 through 15, nurses are occupying expanding roles in both hospitals and communities.

Nurse Practitioner

The role of the nurse practitioner is an extension of the nurse's basic caregiving role. Usually, nurse practitioners have advanced educational preparation; often they have master's degrees in nursing, are graduates of a nurse practitioner program, or have advanced clinical nursing experience beyond the basic level. Nurse practitioners exercise judgment more independently than is permitted in most settings.

Nurse practitioners are employed in hospitals and in communities. They may be generalists, e.g., family nurse practitioners, or specialists, e.g., pediatric nurse practitioners. Nurse practitioners in a community may be employed in health maintenance organizations, health centers, schools, and physicians' offices. They are usually skilled at making nursing assessments, performing physical examinations, counseling, teaching, and treating (in concert with the physician) minor, self-limiting illnesses or stable, long-term illness.

The number of nurse practitioners in the United States has increased in recent years. In 1977, 401 nurse practitioner/midwives were employed in the United States (ANA 1981a, p. 39); by 1980, 16,758 were practicing (ANA 1985, p. 25).

Clinical Nursing Specialist

The clinical nursing specialist has advanced knowledge and skills in a particular area of nursing. An educational prerequisite is usually a master's degree in nursing. These nurses practice in hospitals or communities. In the hospital, such nurses give direct client care, advise other nurses, and coordinate nursing given by others. The clinical nurse specialist is a role model and is expected to keep abreast of new developments in the field.

In ambulatory care settings, e.g., a community clinic, the clinical nurse specialist functions much as a nurse practitioner, but only in her or his area of specialization. In 1980, 19,070 clinical nurse specialists practiced in the United States. Of that number, about 13,500 were employed in hospitals and 2033 in community health settings. The remainder were employed in schools of nursing and nursing homes (ANA 1985, p. 25).

Nurse Clinician

The term *nurse clinician* was first used by Frances Reiter in 1966. Such nurses provide bedside or direct care in a specialty area. They may or may not have advanced educational preparation. Today, most nurse clinicians are employed in hospitals; 43.7% have nursing diplomas, 26.7% have baccalaureate degrees, 12.9% have master's degrees, and 2.3% have doctorates (ANA 1985, p. 27).

Nurse Anesthetist

Nurse anesthetists are registered nurses with advanced preparation in an accredited program of anesthesiology. They are licensed to administer anesthetic agents under the supervision of an anesthesiologist (a physician with specialized knowledge of anesthetic agents). Nurse anesthetists often administer anesthetic agents to clients about to undergo minor surgical procedures or examinations in hospitals and community clinics.

Factors Influencing Nursing Practice

To understand nursing as it is practiced today and as it will be practiced tomorrow requires not only a historic perspective of nursing's evolution but also an understanding of some of the social forces presently influencing this profession. These forces usually affect the entire health care system, and nursing, as a major component of that system, cannot avoid the effects.

Historic Development

Nursing as an activity that provides help to the ill, to children, and to babies has existed since the earliest times. Before the early Christian period (1–500 A.D.), caring for the sick was a function women performed in their homes. Later, monastic orders provided nursing functions as part of their activities. The first nursing order, the Augustinian Sisters, was established in the Middle Ages. This was probably the first organized group to provide purely nursing services to people.

Prior to the Protestant Reformation in the 16th century, hospital facilities were organized chiefly by the Roman Catholic Church. With the Reformation, beginning in 1517, came a decline in people's interest in and support of the church and religion. This change introduced an era known in nursing history as the "dark period." Hospitals were unsanitary places, dark and foreboding. Nursing was provided by women who were frequently described as drunk, heartless, and immoral. They were expected to carry out the housework of the hospital, wash the laundry, and do all the cleaning for very little reward. No training was required of nurses, and it was not unusual for a nurse to work from 12 to 40 consecutive hours. This period of decline lasted until the middle of the 19th century.

The era of reform in nursing is marked by the work of the British nurse, Florence Nightingale, during the Crimean War (1854–56). Nightingale's efforts made nursing a respectable vocation once again. However, Nightingale's reform activities did not stop at respectability. Besides crusading for cleanliness and comfort in hospitals, Nightingale also worked toward educating the populace regarding health measures in an effort to stave off the widespread diseases resulting from poor conditions in the cities. Nightingale believed in prevention and in nursing the whole person, calling upon her fellow nurses to make sure that patients always had fresh air, good water, proper medication, quiet, mobility, and knowledge of how to care for themselves in the future. Many of Nightingale's ideas are now standards of client care. Education of nurses was a major goal of this reformer. Among her many other accomplishments was the establishment of the Nightingale School of Nurses at St. Thomas' Hospital, London, in 1860. This school is credited with providing the first planned educational program for nurses. She also assisted in establishing the first organized home nursing services.

In North America, establishment of nursing and health services was slow prior to the American Revolution (1775–83). One notable organization was the Nurse Society of Philadelphia, which gave women minimal instruction in obstetrics to enable them to provide maternity nursing services in home settings.

The late 1800s was a time of rapid reform of nursing services in the United States and Canada. Schools of nursing with planned educational programs were started. A number of their graduates became the early leaders in the profession.

Isabel Hampton Robb had been a young schoolteacher in Canada. She decided to change her profession and entered the Bellevue Hospital Training School in New York. After graduation, she nursed in Rome for two years, and then she became superintendent of the Illinois Training School at 26 years of age. Three years later she went to Baltimore to organize a new school in connection with Johns Hopkins Hospital. Among her many accomplishments was a nursing textbook, which became the standard text for nursing schools in America.

Mary Adelaide Nutting, also from Canada, was in the first class at Johns Hopkins. After graduation, she established a course of training for students prior to ward experience at Johns Hopkins. Later, she reduced the nursing students' hours from 12 to 8 and lengthened the nurses' training to three years.

Mary Agnes Snively graduated from Bellevue and returned to Canada to take charge of the nurses' training at Toronto General Hospital. She is credited largely with the direction of Canadian nursing education and was the first president of the Canadian Nurses' Association.

Two American graduates of the New York Hospital, Lillian D. Wald and Mary Brewster, were the first to offer trained nursing services to the poor in the New York slums. Their home among the poor on the upper floor of a tenement is now famous as a center of public health nursing (the Henry Street Settlement). Soon after, school nursing was established as an adjunct to visiting nursing. Again Wald was involved, along with Lina L. Rogers.

Linda Richards, who graduated in 1873 from the New England Hospital for Women and Children Training School for Nurses in Boston, is cited by many historians as America's first trained nurse (Jamieson et al. 1966, p. 224). She is credited with nursing reform in 12 major hospitals, some of which were specialized mental hospitals. She initiated training schools for students in mental health nursing. Her programs included a period of training in general hospitals. She also founded the first training school for nurses in Japan.

Some, however, dispute that Richards was the first trained nurse. Evidence in a series of reports of Women's Hospital of Philadelphia suggests that Harriet Newton Phillips was the first trained nurse to receive a certificate from that hospital in 1864 (Large 1976, p. 50). Phillips is also considered the first trained nurse in America to do community nursing, to do missionary service, and to take postgraduate training.

America's first trained black nurse was Mary Mahoney. She trained at the same hospital as Linda Richards and graduated in 1879 (Notter and Spalding 1976, p. 15).

During the late 1800s, the need for concerted actions by nurses was felt (in England first). In 1894, the Matrons' Council of Great Britain and Ireland was organized, followed by the American Society of Superintendents of Training Schools for Nurses of the United States and Canada. Alumnae associations joined to form the Nurses' Associated Alumnae of the United States and Canada in 1897. In 1908, the National Association of Colored Graduate Nurses was founded by a group of nurses who felt such an association could further not only the nursing cause but their own special interests. From these organizations current national groups were founded. The Society of Superintendents divided nationally and ultimately became the Canadian National Association of Trained Nurses in 1908 (now the Canadian Nurses' Association) and the National League of Nursing Education in 1912. The Nurses' Associated Alumnae became the American Nurses' Association in 1911. See the section on nursing organizations later in this chapter.

After World War I, the Frontier Nursing Service (FNS) was established by a notable pioneer nurse, Mary Breckinridge. In 1918, she worked with the American Committee for Devastated France, distributing food, clothing, and supplies to rural villages in France and taking care of sick children. In 1921, Breckinridge returned to the United States with plans to provide health care to the people of rural America. She initially prepared herself by taking courses at Teachers College in New York (where she met Mary Adelaide Nutting and gained her approval) and midwifery training in London, and by developing prominent social contacts for fundraising. In 1925, Breckinridge and two other nurses began the FNS in Leslie County, Kentucky. Within this organization, Breckinridge began one of the first midwifery training schools in the United States.

The general trend from the beginning of formal organization of nursing of the late 1800s to the end of World War I was rapid expansion in the establishment of hospitals, with nursing schools dependent upon them for support. Hospitals in turn depended on the schools to carry the chief nursing load. During the war, greater numbers of young women were accepted for entrance and less consideration was given to selection requirements. Most schools by this time had adopted 3-year programs, but the 8-hour day originally proposed with those programs was less quickly adopted.

By 1920, the hospital system of educating nurses was increasingly criticized. In addition, the effectiveness of the nurse as a teacher of nurses was being questioned. Thus, a special postbasic course was offered at Teachers College, Columbia University, New York, to prepare nurses as teachers. Preparations for a postbasic public health nursing program were also made, in response to an influenza epidemic and the development of broader aims by the medical profession, which now included teaching the principles of healthful living to individuals, families, and community groups.

During the early 1920s, the Rockefeller Survey (Committee for the Study of Nursing Education) recommended that nursing schools be independent of hospitals and on a college level. As a result, two university schools of nursing were set up, one at Yale University, New Haven, Connecticut, the other at Western Reserve University, Cleveland, Ohio. The purpose of these experimental schools was to prove the feasibility of planning both classroom instruction and ward practice in accordance with the educational needs of the students. Emphasis was placed on the social welfare and health aspects of nursing. Both schools demonstrated the value of university standards in the nursing field.

Another far-reaching result of the Rockefeller Survey was a proposal by the National League of Nursing Education to undertake a comprehensive study of nursing education (1926–34) that would lead to the grading of nursing schools. It was believed that grading would establish standards for education in these schools. This was the beginning of the accreditation function that the National League for Nursing now carries out. See the section on nursing organizations later in this chapter.

During this period, the concept of the clinical nurse specialist arose. In 1933, the need for "experts in the nursing art and specialists in the clinical branches they represent" was recognized (Stewart 1933, p. 363). This concept, currently seen by many as a new role in nursing, was discussed by nursing leaders in the 1930s and 1940s. In the early 1940s, it was thought that more emphasis needed to be placed on the clinical specialties in the advanced professional curricula of colleges and universities. Most advanced nursing curricula were preparing specialists in nursing school administration, teaching, and supervision, in public health, and in hospital administration and were not emphasizing clinical specialties. These specialties gained prominence in the postwar society. Nurses returning from overseas were required to work in clinical areas not familiar to them. One such area was psychiatric nursing, which helped individuals to readjust to civilian life. By 1946, many nursing programs in the United States were providing more clinical content. Today the clinical nurse specialist is a graduate of a master's or doctoral program in nursing with a major in a clinical specialty. This nurse is responsible for increasing her or his own clinical knowledge and competence and for enhancing the quality of nursing care and the quality of the organizational climate for learning and research (McPhail 1971, p. 16–18).

From its early days to the present, nursing has undergone change in every area. Rapid strides have been made in nursing education programs and in a wide variety of hospital and community nursing services. Throughout these changes, nursing has continued to provide a stable helping service to people.

Current Influences

It is difficult to escape the influences of society, science, and technology. Nursing, as a profession deeply involved with people, certainly cannot escape. Many factors influence the individual nurse, nursing practice, and, of course, clients. To function effectively amid media bombardment, rapid systems of communication, and advances in research, the nurse must develop in response to outside influences. The current major influences can be grouped into nine broad areas: (a) consumer demands, (b) family structure, (c) economics, (d) science and technology, (e) legislation, (f) demography, (g) the women's movement, (h) collective bargaining, and (i) the nursing profession.

Consumer Demands

Consumers of nursing services (the public) have become an increasingly effective force in changing nursing practice. On the whole, people have become better educated and have more knowledge about health and illness than in the past. This is in no small measure because of television and the news media. Consumers also have become more aware of the needs of others for care. The ethical and moral issues raised by poverty and neglect have caused people to be more vocal about the needs of minority groups and the poor.

The public's concepts of health and nursing have also changed. People now believe that health is a right of all people, not just a privilege of the rich. People are bombarded by the media with the message that individuals must assume responsibility for their own health by obtaining a physical examination regularly, checking for the seven danger signals of cancer, and maintaining their mental well-being by balancing work and recreation. Interest in health and nursing services is therefore greater than ever. Furthermore, many people now want more than freedom from disease—they want energy, vitality, and a feeling of wellness.

Increasingly, the consumer has become an active participant in making decisions about health and nursing care. Planning committees concerned with providing nursing services to a community usually have active consumer membership. More and more state and provincial nursing associations have consumer representatives on their governing boards.

Family Structure

The need for and provision of nursing services are being influenced by new family structures. An increasing number of people are living in structures other than the extended family and the nuclear family, and the family breadwinner is no longer necessarily the husband. An extended family consists of parents, children, grandparents, and sometimes aunts and uncles; a nuclear family consists only of parents and their children.

Today, many single men and women rear children, and in many two-parent families both parents work. It is also common for young parents to live at great distances from their parents. These families need support services such as day-care centers. Many families do not have grandparents or other relatives readily available to help in times of illness or to offer advice about childbearing and child health. The advice these parents get about their children usually comes from physicians and nurses as well as others.

Similarly, grandparents, who now may live alone and far from other members of the family, require homemaker and visiting nurse services when they are ill, to replace the care formerly provided by younger members of the family.

Adolescent mothers also need nursing services. These young mothers have the normal needs of teenagers as well as those of new mothers. In 1960, 13.9% of all births were to teenage mothers; this proportion has increased steadily, reaching epidemic proportions in 1986. Some of these young mothers, many of them unmarried, choose to keep their children rather than give them up for adoption. This creates an especially vulnerable type of single parent family. Even if married, adolescent mothers face many problems.

Economics

Another factor that has increased the demand and need for nursing is the greater financial support provided through health insurance programs in the United States and Canada. Medicare, Medicaid, and other government programs as well as other public and private financing agencies have increased the demand for broad health services. Thus, health services such as emergency room care, mental health counseling, and preventive physical examinations are increasingly being used by people who could not afford them in the past. Federal governments recognized this need and markedly increased their budgets for health care in the 1970s and early 1980s. This increase in expenditure is accompanied by an increase in the number of people who provide health services. In nursing alone, the number of employed registered nurses in the United States grew from 750,000 in 1971 to 1,404,200 in 1983, an increase of 53.4% (ANA 1985, p. 18). In Canada, the number of practicing nurses also increased during this period. In an effort to control costs, hospitals have instituted such measures as hiring temporary part-time nurses. These nurses are employed only as needed and the hospital saves such expenses as fringe benefits

However, costs of health care increased enormously during this period as well. In the United States, a recent annual cost (1983) was calculated to be $362 billion, or about a billion dollars a day (Curtin and Zurlage 1984, p. 9). As a result, the Medicare payment system to hospitals was revised in 1982. Diagnostic related categories (DRGs) are discussed in Chapter 3. The results of this legislation are that a greater proportion of clients in hospitals are more acutely ill than before and that clients once considered sufficiently ill to be hospitalized are now treated at home. This fact presents a challenge to nurses in hospital practice and in home health practice. It is expected that the health care industry will shift its emphasis from the inpatient hospital to preadmission testing, posthospitalization rehabilitation, home health care, health maintenance, and physical fitness (Powell 1984, p. 33). Nurses need to identify how their knowledge and skills can fit into these settings. Rogers (1985, p. 10) suggests that before long a large majority of nurses will not work in hospitals. This change in the area of employment has implications for nursing education, nursing research, and nursing practice as well as for each nurse. Indicators of this trend are:

1. The numbers of clients in the home requiring nursing
2. Cost containment measures in agencies providing health care
3. The separate itemizing of nursing care costs in some hospital's bills

Science and Technology

Discoveries in science and technology affect nursing practice. For example, the vaccine for poliomyelitis made obsolete the nursing skills required in the 1950s for these acutely ill clients. Advances in science also have an indirect effect on nursing. For example, as physicians acquire new knowledge and skills in cardiac surgery, nurses must acquire complementary knowledge and skills.

In some settings, technologic advances have required that nurses become highly specialized. Nurses frequently have to use sophisticated equipment for client monitoring or treatment. As technologies change, nursing education changes, and nurses require increasing education to provide effective, safe nursing practice.

New facts are being discovered in every field associated directly or indirectly with nursing. The social sciences offer a better understanding of human behavior and are building a knowledge of how the mind and the body are interrelated. Advances in technology are exemplified by the many machines now used to help clients maintain life. There seems to be no end to the discoveries and the knowledge explosion of the 20th century.

With this knowledge explosion has come the charge that medical services—and some health professionals—have become dehumanized. Yet an increasing understanding of the psychologic, emotional, and spiritual aspects of care has developed to balance the technologic advances. As science and technology create methods of treating disease, it is the responsibility of all health professionals, nurses in particular, to remember that clients are human beings requiring warmth, care, and acknowledgment of self-worth. Often equipment is frightening to clients and their support persons. Medical vocabulary appears mysterious and is frequently misunderstood. The nurse dealing daily with clients is in an ideal situation to humanize technology as much as is possible. Explanations by nurses and their communications of support and recognition of the clients' needs to understand and to be supported help to humanize highly technical care. This is the "high touch aspect of a "high tech" environment.

Scientific developments have led to other changes in the nursing profession by indirectly affecting human health. For example, some industries have proven hazardous to employees because of the dangerous equipment used or because of harmful chemical residues. Trauma (injury) and disease are frequently the direct result of advanced technology; the classic example is automobile accidents, which are among the top five causes of death in North America. In addition, our advanced society frequently produces high levels of stress and diminished mental health. These problems created by technologic change present new challenges to nurses.

Legislation

Legislation about nursing practice and in relation to health matters affects both the public and nursing. Legislation related to nursing is discussed in Chapter 7. However, changes in legislation affecting health also affect nursing. For example, the laws governing abortions have been relaxed in some states and in Canada. This change reduced maternal morbidity from self-induced abortions.

United States legislation regarding the Medicare payment system according to DRGs has had an enormous influence on nursing practice in hospitals and communities. Many clients leave hospitals sooner than they did in the past. As a result, more clients in hospitals are seriously ill, and more clients at home require more complex nursing care than in the past. While this trend had created a shortage of critical care nurses, it has opened new oportunities in home health.

Demography

Demography is the study of population statistics. It includes the distribution of the population by age and place of residence, **mortality** (death), and **morbidity** (incidence of disease) statistics. From demographic data, needs of the population for nursing services can be assessed. For example:

1. The total populations in both the United States and Canada have increased since 1900. The proportion of elderly people has also increased in both populations, creating an increased need for nursing services for this group. For further information on population, see Chapter 2, page 68.
2. Another study indicates a shift of population from rural (country) to urban (city) settings. This shift signals increased needs for nursing related to problems caused by pollution and by the effects on the environment of concentrations of people. Thus, most nursing services are now provided in urban settings.
3. Mortality and morbidity studies reveal the presence of "risk factors." Many of these "risk factors" e.g., smoking, are major causes of death and disease that can be prevented through changes in life-style. This area of health promotion is open to nurses (U.S. National Center for Health Statistics 1985, pp. 17–19). The nurse's role in assessing risk factors and helping clients to make healthy life-style changes is discussed in Chapter 20.

The Women's Movement

The women's movement has brought public attention to all human rights. Persons are seeking equality in all areas, particularly educational, political, economic, and social equality. Because the majority of nurses are women, this movement has altered the perspectives of nurses about economic and educational needs. As a result, nurses are increasingly asserting themselves as professional people who have a right to equality with men in health professions. They are demanding more autonomy in client care.

The increasing number of women physicians might also affect nursing practice. Women physicians may be less autocratic and more collegial in their professional relationships. As a result, nurses may find support in their quest for autonomy.

Collective Bargaining

More nurses are using collective bargaining to deal with their concerns. The ANA has participated in collective bargaining for years on behalf of nurses. Today, some nurses are joining other labor organizations that represent them at the bargaining table. In both the United States and Canada, nurses have gone on strike over certain demands and concerns. Often these concerns go beyond economic reward to issues about safe care for clients. Increasingly, nurses are becoming aware of the strength of organized, large numbers. DeCrosta (1985, p. 20) believes that nurses will increasingly look to unions as they attempt to resist staff cuts and perceived dilution in the quality of nursing practice as a result of cost containment.

The Nursing Profession

Professional nursing associations have provided leadership that affects many areas of nursing. The ANA has indicated support for a baccalaureate degree as minimum preparation for professional nursing practice. They recommend that this requirement be implemented in stages, starting in 1986 and reaching completion by 1995 (ANA 1985).

Accreditation of nursing education programs by the NLN and by licensing boards in each state has also influenced nursing. Many programs have steadily improved to meet the standards for accreditation over the years. As a result, nurse graduates are better prepared to meet the demands of society. See page 38 for further information about the NLN.

In 1979, the ANA published findings of a committee on credentialing, which recommended the establishment of a center for credentialing in nursing (ANA 1979, p. 682). **Credentialing** is the process of determining and maintaining competence in nursing. For more information, see Chapter 7. The credentialing of expanded nursing roles, such as that of the nurse practitioner, is carried out by the ANA, and certain nursing specialty organizations such as the American Association of Critical-Care Nurses.

In addition, a group of professional nurses has been organized formally for the purpose of taking political action in the nursing and health care arenas. Nurses for Political Action (NPA) was formed in 1971 and became an arm of the ANA in 1974, when its name changed to Nurses Coalition for Action in Politics (N-CAP). In 1986 the name was changed to ANA-PAC. Since then, nurses have lobbied actively for legislation affecting health care. See Chapter 6. Nurses now see the need to participate in decision making in the workplace and in government. A number of nursing leaders hold positions of authority in government. "An ongoing relationship with the White House will give nurses the status and power other groups already enjoy" (People 1983, p. 1205).

In 1980, the ANA adopted a social policy statement that addressed the nature and scope of nursing practice, the concerns of nursing, and specialization in nursing practice. The outcome of this statement was a definition of nursing (see the definition of nursing earlier in the chapter) and a description of two types of practitioners: a generalist and a specialist. The generalist provides the majority of the nursing care, while the specialist, who holds a master's degree or doctorate, focuses on specifics (ANA 1980).

The drive for increased autonomy comes from the nursing profession itself. During the past 20 years, the increased autonomy of nurses has been evidenced by their function in specialty care units, such as intensive care units, and in their expanded roles, such as that of the nurse practitioner. Many states have rewritten their nurse practice acts to reflect such changes in nursing practice.

In 1968, the CNA published its first statement about a clinical nurse specialist as a nurse with master's preparation in a clinical specialty. This statement was repeated in position papers published in 1970 and 1978. In 1970, the CNA did not support the category of physician-assistant in Canadian health care. In 1978, the CNA stated that specialization in nursing was necessary so that nurses could assume responsibilities in primary care, in continuing care, and in the preventive and specialized aspects of nursing. In 1985, the CNA formed a new committee on certification and published policies regarding specialization and certification in Canada (Levesque 1985, pp. 26–28).

Research Note

Important factors influencing nursing practice also reside within the individual nurse. Such personality variables as maturity, assertiveness, and sex-typed attitudes have been shown to affect job satisfaction and overall commitment to nursing. In a 1985 study of 101 nursing students and new graduates, Kinney found that nurses who best accommodate to the role complexity encountered in many work settings showed a high degree of assertiveness, both "feminine" and "masculine" personality characteristics, and a broad repertoire of coping behaviors. (Kinney 1985)

Education for Nurses

The nurse's function today is so complex that a nursing student requires knowledge in the biologic, physical, and social sciences. It is not possible for nurses to acquire a safe level of skill through empirical (experience and observation) means alone. They require specific knowledge and skills that can be gained only through an organized nursing curriculum.

The traditional focus of nursing education has been on teaching the skills required in hospitals. However, considerable evidence shows that the need for community and home services is increasing and that some negative aspects of hospitalization, such as separation from family, exist. As a result, nursing curricula now focus more broadly on health as well as illness needs, and community as well as hospital needs, in addition to appropriate knowledge from the biologic, social, and physical sciences.

State laws in the United States and provincial laws in Canada recognize two types of nurses: the licensed practical (vocational) nurse (LPN or LVN) and the registered nurse (RN).

Licensed Practical Nursing Education

Approved practical or vocational nursing programs are provided by community colleges, vocational schools, hospitals, and a variety of health agencies. These programs usually last 1 year and provide both classroom and clinical experiences. At the end of the program, the graduate takes examinations to obtain a license as a practical or vocational nurse. In some states and provinces, applicants for licensure are assessed on the basis of their nursing experience rather than their formal education in an approved school. Licensed practical nurses work in structured care settings, such as hospitals and nursing homes. Their skills are basically those required for bedside nursing under the guidance of a registered nurse, who has the knowledge and skills to make more sophisticated nursing judgments. In some areas of the United States, LPN programs are being phased out or changed to the associate degree level.

Registered Nursing Education

Basic education for registered nurses is provided in three types of programs: diploma, associate degree, and baccalaureate programs in the United States; and 2-year diploma, 3-year (or more) diploma, and baccalaureate programs in Canada.

Diploma

Nursing education originated in hospital-based programs. First developed by Florence Nightingale (circa 1860), these programs were operated by hospitals as "training" schools for nurses. Today's diploma nursing programs have changed markedly from the original Nightingale model, becoming hospital-based educational programs that provide a rich clinical experience for nursing students. These programs may last 2 or more years, and are often associated with colleges or universities. A significant number of nurses practicing today are graduates of diploma programs. Though the number of diploma nursing programs has declined since the ANA resolution in 1965 (see Figure 1-1, page 32), these programs are still providing one avenue for students desiring an education in nursing. In addition to the changes inherent in the 1965 resolution, hospitals found that the costs of operating educational programs were increasing, making them less viable financially. Canada has moved rapidly from hospital-based programs to those based in educational institutions. Of the 172 diploma nursing programs in 1964, all but one (admitting 21 students) were hospital-based, whereas in 1973, 78.5% of nursing students were in college- or university-based programs.

In 1978, the NLN approved a statement describing the roles and competencies of graduates of diploma nursing programs. See Table 1–6.

Associate Degree

Associate degree programs in nursing were suggested in 1951 by Mildred L. Montag (1980) as a solution to the acute shortage of nurses that grew out of World War II. The programs were to be college-based with a heavy emphasis on science but reduced clinical experience; further clinical experience was to be provided by the employing hospitals. Montag proposed that the "nurse technician" graduates of these programs would carry out nursing responsibilities under the supervision of a professional nurse and that these graduates would not have administrative responsibilities.

Associate degree programs are offered in the United States in junior and senior colleges and universities. Upon graduation, the graduate receives an associate degree (AD) in nursing. In Canada, associate degrees are not offered, but similar programs confer a diploma upon graduation.

The number of graduates from associate degree programs in the United States has steadily increased; in 1982–83, 54% of students graduated from these programs (ANA 1985, p. 126). In Canada, the first diploma nursing program was established within the general education system at the Ryerson Institute of Technology in Toronto in 1964. By 1973, 9001 students were in similar nursing programs across Canada (LaSor and Elliott 1977, p. 161).

Though AD programs did help relieve the nursing shortage, the reality of hospital practice did not match Montag's original intent; AD and BSN graduates were often used interchangeably. This created a discrepancy between what competencies nursing service expected of new graduates and their actual competencies. In an effort to resolve this discrepancy, differentiated competency statements (Table 1-7) were developed during two projects sponsored by the Midwest Alliance in Nursing and funded by the W. K. Kellogg Foundation (Primm 1986, pp. 135–37). The overall goal of the projects was to prepare differentiated statements of the scope of practice for ADN and BSN graduates by nursing service managers/staff developers and ADN and BSN educators. Because ADN and BSN prepared nurses currently function under the same practice acts, "these differentiated statements provide a basis for discussion of collaborative ADN and BSN nursing practice" (Primm 1986, p. 136).

Baccalaureate Degree

Although baccalaureate nursing education programs were established in universities in both the United States and Canada in the early 1900s, it was not until the 1960s that

Table 1–6 Role and Competencies of Graduates of Diploma Programs in Nursing

The graduate of the diploma program in nursing is eligible to seek licensure as a registered nurse and to function as a beginning practitioner in acute, intermediate, long-term, and ambulatory health care facilities. In order to fulfill such roles, the graduate should demonstrate the following competencies.*

Assessment
- Establishes a data base through a nursing history including a psychosocial and physical assessment.
- Utilizes knowledge of the etiology, pathophysiology, usual course, and prognosis for the prevalent illnesses and health problems.
- Establishes priorities when providing nursing care for one or more patients.
- Recognizes the significance of nonverbal communication.

Planning
- Formulates a written plan of nursing care based on the assessment of patient needs.
- Includes in the nursing care plan the effects of the family or significant others, life experiences, and social-cultural background.
- Involves the patient, family, and significant others in the development of the nursing plan of care.
- Incorporates the learning needs of the patient and family into an individualized plan of care.
- Applies principles of organization and management in utilizing the knowledge and skills of other nursing personnel.

Implementation
- Meets the health needs of individuals and families.
- Utilizes concepts, scientific facts, and principles when providing nursing care.
- Performs technical nursing procedures.
- Initiates appropriate intervention when environmental and safety hazards exist.
- Initiates preventive, habilitative, and rehabilitative nursing measures according to the needs demonstrated by patients and families.
- Performs independent nursing measures and/or seeks assistance from other members of the health team in response to the changing needs of patients.
- Collaborates with physicians and members of other disciplines to provide health care.
- Documents nursing interventions and patient responses.
- Utilizes effective verbal and written communication.
- Communicates pertinent information related to the patient through established channels.
- Assists the physician in implementing the medical plan of care.
- Applies knowledge of individual and group behavior in establishing interpersonal relationships.
- Teaches individuals and groups to achieve and maintain an optimum level of wellness.
- Utilizes the services of community agencies for continuity of patient care.
- Protects the rights of patients and families.

Evaluation
- Evaluates the effectiveness of nursing care and takes appropriate action.
- Initiates and cooperates in efforts to improve nursing practice.

Professionalism
- Recognizes the legal limits of nursing practice.
- Demonstrates ethical behavior in the performance of nursing.
- Practices nursing in a nondiscriminatory and nonjudgmental manner.
- Respects the rights of others to have their own value systems.
- Accepts responsibility and accountability for professional practice.
- Demonstrates flexibility in functioning in a changing society.
- Adjusts with minimal difficulty to the role of employee.

This revised statement by the Council of Diploma Programs in Nursing, National League for Nursing, was approved at the Council's April 1978 meeting.

*Competency, as used in this document, is the ability to apply in practice situations the essential principles and techniques of nursing and to apply those concepts, skills, and attitudes required of all nurses to fulfill their role, regardless of specific position or responsibility.

Source: National League for Nursing, *Roles and Competencies of Graduates of Diploma Programs in Nursing* (New York: The League, 1978). Used with permission.

the number of students enrolled in these programs increased markedly. The 1965 ANA position paper provided considerable impetus to move nursing education out of hospitals and into the general education system. It was followed by a study conducted by the National Commission for the Study of Nursing and Nursing Education. The commission's first report in 1970 reinforced the ANA recommendation. Since 1965, a number of diploma nursing schools have closed, while the number of baccalaureate programs has increased. By 1977–78, 31.1% of all nursing graduates were from baccalaureate programs, in contrast to 19.9% in 1968–69 (ANA 1981, p. 133). A similar but less striking movement look place in Canada: In 1976, 9.5% of all nursing graduates were from baccalaureate programs, compared to 3.8% in 1968. See Figures 1–1 and 1–2 for changes in the numbers of graduates from registered nursing programs.

Most baccalaureate programs also admit registered nurses who have diplomas or associate degrees. Some programs have special curricula to meet the needs of these students, often in 2-year programs. Some universities also offer nursing students the opportunity to pursue a self-paced or independent study program. Many accept transfer credits from other accredited colleges and universities and offer students the opportunity to take challenge examinations when they believe they have the knowledge or skills taught in a course.

Another impetus toward baccalaureate education for all nurses was a resolution of the ANA, passed in 1978, stating that the minimum educational preparation for entry

Table 1–7 Differentiated Competency Statements

ADN	BSN
General Statement	
The ADN cares for focal clients who are identified as individuals and members of a family. The level of responsibility of the ADN is for a specified work period and is consistent with the identified goals of care. The ADN is prepared to function in structured health care settings. The structured settings are geographical and/or situational environments where the policies, procedures, and protocols for provision of health care are established and there is recourse to assistance and support from the full scope of nursing expertise.	The BSN cares for focal clients who are identified as individuals, families, aggregates, and community groups. The level of responsibility of the BSN is from admission to post-discharge. The BSN is prepared to function in structured and unstructured health care settings. The unstructured setting is a geographical and/or situational environment which may not have established policies, procedures, and protocols and has the potential for variations requiring independent nursing decisions.
Provision of Direct Care Competencies	
The ADN provides direct care for the focal client with common, well-defined nursing diagnoses by:	The BSN provides direct care for the focal client with complex interactions of nursing diagnoses by:
A. Collecting health pattern data from available resources using established assessment format to identify basic health care needs.	A. Expanding the collection of data to identify complex care needs.
B. Organizing and analyzing health pattern data in order to select nursing diagnoses from an established list.	B. Organizing and analyzing complex health pattern data to develop nursing diagnoses.
C. Establishing goals with the focal client for a specified work period that are consistent with the overall comprehensive nursing plan of care.	C. Establishing goals with the focal client to develop a comprehensive nursing plan of care from admission to post-discharge.
D. Developing and implementing an individualized nursing plan of care using established nursing diagnoses and protocols to promote, maintain, and restore health.	D. Developing and implementing a comprehensive nursing plan of care based on nursing diagnoses for health promotion.
E. Participating in the medical plan of care to promote an integrated health care plan.	E. Interpreting the medical plan of care into nursing activities to formulate approaches to nursing care.
F. Evaluating focal client responses to nursing interventions and altering the plan of care as necessary to meet client goals.	F. Evaluating the nursing care delivery system and promoting goal-directed change to meet individualized client needs.
Communication Competencies	
The ADN uses basic communication skills with the focal client by:	The BSN uses complex communication skills with the focal client by:
A. Developing and maintaining goal-directed interactions to encourage expressing of needs and support coping behaviors.	A. Developing and maintaining goal-directed interactions to promote effective coping behaviors and facilitate change in behavior.
B. Modifying and implementing a standard teaching plan in order to restore, maintain, and promote health.	B. Designing and implementing a comprehensive teaching plan for health promotion.
The ADN coordinates focal client care with other health team members by:	The BSN collaborates with other health team members by:
A. Documenting and communicating data for clients with common, well-defined nursing diagnoses to provide continuity of care.	A. Documenting and communicating comprehensive data for clients with complex interactions to provide continuity of care.
B. Using established channels of communication to implement an effective health care plan.	B. Using established channels of communication to modify health care delivery.
C. Using interpreted nursing research findings for developing nursing care.	C. Incorporating research findings into practice and by consulting with nurse researchers regarding identified nursing problems in order to enhance nursing practice.
Management Competencies	
The ADN organizes those aspects of care for focal clients for whom s/he is accountable by:	The BSN manages nursing care of focal clients by:
A. Prioritizing, planning, and organizing the delivery of standard nursing care in order to use time and resources effectively and efficiently.	A. Prioritizing, planning, and organizing the delivery of comprehensive nursing care in order to use time and resources effectively and efficiently.

(continued)

Table 1–7 *(continued)*

B. Delegating aspects of care to peers, LPNs, and ancillary nursing personnel, consistent with their levels of education and expertise, in order to meet client needs.	B. Delegating aspects of care to other nursing personnel, consistent with their levels of education and expertise, in order to meet client needs and to maximize staff performance.
C. Maintaining accountability for own care and care delegated to others to assure adherence to ethical and legal standards.	C. Maintaining accountability for own care and care delegated to others to assure adherence to ethical and legal standards.
D. Recognizing the need for referral and conferring with appropriate nursing personnel for assistance to promote continuity of care.	D. Initiating referral to appropriate departments and agencies to provide service and promote continuity of care.
E. Working with other health care personnel within the organizational structure to manage client care.	E. Assuming a leadership role in health care management to improve client care.

Source: P. L. Primm, Entry into practice: Competency statements for BSNs and ADNs, *Nursing Outlook,* May/June 1986, 34:135–37. Used by permission.

into professional nursing practice by 1985 be a baccalaureate degree (BSN). The 1978 delegates also endorsed a resolution that diploma and associate degree graduates who are licensed to practice before 1985 not be affected. In 1984, the ANA House of Delegates adopted a different time frame for this change. The goal now is to implement the requirement of a BSN for entry into professional nursing practice in 5% of states by 1986, 15% by 1988, 50% by 1992, and 100% by 1995 (Hood 1985, p. 592).

In 1982, the Board of Directors of the CNA endorsed the recommendations of the Committee on Entry to Practice that the baccalaureate degree be the minimum entry level for professional nursing practice by the year 2000 (Dugas 1985, p. 17). Although most nurses recognize the move toward a baccalaureate degree as a requirement for entry into professional nursing practice, the issue of titling and licensure has yet to be resolved by individual state or provincial legislation.

In 1985, the ANA House of Delegates proposed that two and only two categories of nursing be established: the baccalaureate as the minimum educational requirement for licensure to practice professional nursing and to retain the title *registered nurse,* and the associate degree as the educational requirement to practice technical nursing. This proposal, referred to as the "1985 proposal," is yet to be enacted. See "Issues in Nursing Education," later in this chapter. BSN competency statements on entry into practice compared to ADN competencies are shown in Table 1–7. For additional BSN competencies, see Stull (1986) in "Suggested Readings."

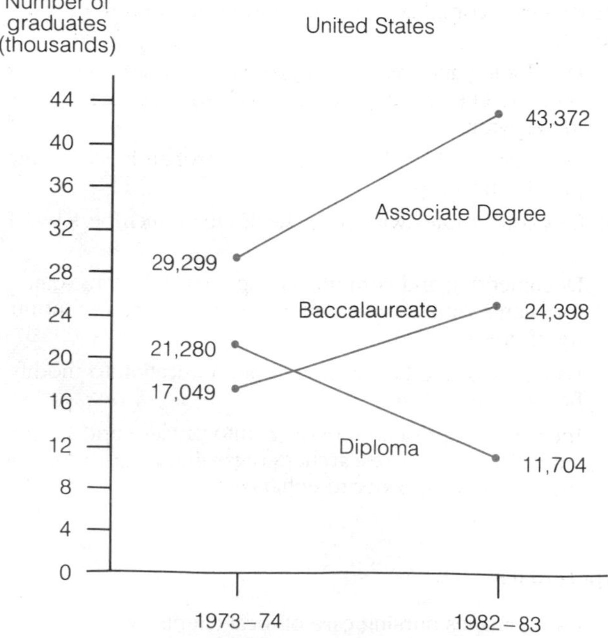

Figure 1–1 Number of graduates from registered nursing programs in the United States from 1973–74 to 1982–83

Source: American Nurses' Association, *Facts about nursing 84–85* (Kansas City, Mo.: American Nurses' Association, 1985), p. 126.

Graduate Programs

Education at the graduate level requires independent critical thinking; therefore, nurses who enter graduate study must have sufficient intellectual capacity and scholastic achievement to profit from it. Most graduate programs are conducted by departments within the graduate school of a university, and the applicant must first meet requirements established by the graduate school. Although all graduate schools have somewhat different requirements, common requirements for admission to graduate programs in nursing are (DeYoung 1985, p. 120):

1. The applicant must be a graduate registered nurse.
2. The applicant must hold a baccalaureate degree in nursing from an approved college or university and have had an acceptable upper division major in nursing at the baccalaureate level.
3. The applicant must give evidence of scholastic ability (usually a minimum grade point average of 2.7 to 3.0 on a 4.0 scale).

4. The applicant must demonstrate satisfactory achievement on a qualifying examination.

Master's Programs

Master's programs generally take from 1½ to 2 years to complete. Degrees granted are the Master of Arts in Nursing (MA), Master in Nursing (MN), or Master of Science in Nursing (MSN). In 1978, the NLN described the characteristics of these programs, which provide the student with an opportunity to:

1. Acquire advanced knowledge from the sciences and the humanities to support advanced nursing practice and role development
2. Expand knowledge of nursing theory as a basis for advanced nursing practice
3. Develop expertise in a specialized area of clinical nursing practice
4. Acquire the knowledge and skills related to a specific functional role in nursing
5. Acquire initial competence in conducting research
6. Plan and/or initiate change in the health care system, and in the practice and delivery of health care
7. Further develop and implement leadership strategies for the betterment of health care
8. Actively engage in collaborative relationships with others for the purpose of improving health care
9. Acquire a foundation for doctoral study (NLN 1978a)

Master's degree programs focus on medical-surgical nursing, maternal-child nursing, psychiatric-mental health nursing, community health nursing, and subspecialty areas such as cardiovascular nursing, gerontologic nursing, inservice, and rehabilitation. The functional focus of these programs is primarily on advanced clinical practice, but many also include teaching, supervision, and administration/management in either nursing service or education. Many programs prepare the nurse for expanded roles, such as the clinical nurse specialist and nurse practitioner.

The numbers of students receiving master's degrees in nursing has increased. In 1983, 5085 students were granted master's degrees in the United States, compared with 4217 in 1978 (ANA 1981, p. 169; ANA 1985, p. 155). In Canada, 112 students were granted master's degrees in 1983, compared with 53 students in 1974 (Statistics Canada and CNA 1985, p. 80).

Doctoral (PhD, DNS, DNSc, ND) Programs

Doctoral programs, which began in the 1960s in the United States, further prepare the nurse for advanced clinical

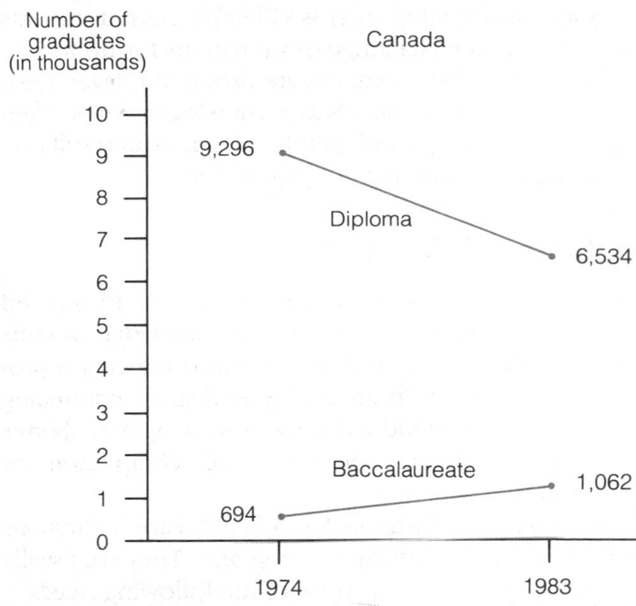

Figure 1–2 Number of graduates from registered nursing programs in Canada from 1974 to 1983 (Diploma refers to collegiate and hospital programs.)

Source: Statistics Canada and Canadian Nurses' Association, *Nursing in Canada* (Ottawa: Canadian Nurses' Association, January, 1985), p. 67.

practice, administration, education, and research. Before 1960, nurses acquired doctoral degrees in such related fields as psychology, sociology, physiology, and education.

Content and approach vary among doctoral programs. One may focus on usual clinical areas, such as medical-surgical nursing, while others emphasize such nontraditional areas as transcultural nursing. Some programs emphasize theory development, but all emphasize research (DeYoung 1985, p. 119). Although master's programs require nurses to specialize in a certain area, doctoral programs narrow the area of specialization even further. A nurse with a doctorate becomes an expert in a given area through research.

In 1984, 31 universities offered doctoral programs in nursing in the United States (DeYoung, 1985). Increasing numbers of students are receiving doctorates; 139 were granted doctorate degrees in 1983, compared with 53 in 1978 (ANA 1981, p. 169; ANA 1985, p. 155). Of all nurses in Canada, only 124 had earned doctorates by 1982 (Stinson et al. 1984, p. ii).

Ladder Programs in Nursing

The ladder concept fosters progression of an individual from one educational level to another. The nurse who wishes to progress "up the ladder" can often obtain credit for experience and/or courses at an earlier level. Although associate degree programs were originally designed to be terminal programs, some universities now give academic credit toward a baccalaureate degree for these years.

Some universities, such as Villanova, permit students to transfer or take challenge examinations for up to 50% of all credits in the baccalaureate program (Nayer 1981, p. 2057). Others admit nurses as prenursing students. Often emphasis is placed on independent learning and self-pacing for the baccalaureate nursing student.

Continuing Education

The term *continuing education* refers to formalized experiences designed to enlarge the knowledge or skills of practitioners. Compared to advanced education programs, which result in an academic degree, continuing education courses tend to be more specific and shorter and may result in certificates of completion or specialization.

A variety of educational and health care institutions conduct continuing education programs. They are usually designed to meet one or more of the following needs:

1. To keep nurses abreast of new techniques and knowledge
2. To help nurses attain expertise in a specialized area of practice, such as intensive care nursing
3. To provide nurses with information essential to nursing practice, for example, knowledge about the legal aspects of nursing

Some state laws now require a nurse to obtain a certain number of continuing education credits in order to renew her or his license. In these states, required continuing education (CE) contact hours vary from 15 to 30 hours every 2-year relicensure period. All, some, or none of these hours may be acquired through home study. Some home study courses are offered through professional journals. A few regions also require a certain number of hours of practice, either independently or in lieu of study hours, before license renewal. Examples are the state of Nebraska and the province of Alberta.

Continuing education is the responsibility of each practicing nurse. Constant updating and growth are essential to keep abreast of scientific and technologic change and changes within the nursing profession.

In-Service Education

An in-service education program is administered by an employer; it is designed to upgrade the knowledge or skills of employees. For example, an employer might offer an in-service program to inform nurses about a new piece of equipment, about specific isolation practices, or about a different method of providing nursing, such as primary nursing or implementing a nurse theorist's conceptual framework for nursing.

Self-Directed Learning

The truly professional nurse is a self-directed learner. Even though formal continuing education offerings are a condition for licensure in several American states, nurses can acquire valuable learning by assuming responsibility for their own continuing education. Because each nurse has specific personal and unique learning needs, she or he can plan a course of action to meet individual goals rather than relying on formal continuing education units or incidental and haphazard clinical experiences.

To plan a self-directed learning program:

1. Determine the weekly or monthly time you can make available to pursue educational activities.
2. Establish overall career goals—a list of learning content or skills—and a flexible time frame for achieving each. Because goals change from time to time, it is important to reassess desired skills and knowledge periodically. Also consider personal development goals as well as professional ones.
3. Assess available learning resources and determine which ones are most appropriate to achieve goals and needs. Many resources are available to the nurse:
   a. Public libraries provide films, audiotapes, and records in addition to books and articles. Some even offer educational programs.
   b. Hospital and school of nursing libraries, which are valuable sources of current journals, are often accessible even to nurses not employed in that agency.
   c. University libraries sometimes provide collect call and mailing services that give nurses information on requested topics.
   d. State or provincial nursing association libraries are a source of nursing reference literature. Through nationwide interlibrary loan programs, they also can acquire books and journal articles from universities, hospitals, and health care or allied agencies.
   e. Local community and outreach extension resources are available at many vocational and technical schools, community colleges, and tax-supported universities.
   f. Many universities offer television and teleconferencing courses. Teleconferencing is the linking, through regular telephone lines, of two or more centers in a network that is fully interactive in real time. It permits live exchange of dialogue between people in two or more centers. These courses are especially valuable for nurses practicing in remote areas.
   g. Public school systems offer adults diversified educational opportunities for personal growth and development. These programs are usually publicized through local newspapers or fliers.

h. Many nursing education institutions and professional associations provide self-study correspondence, programmed instruction, learning modules, and educational television programs.
i. Health organizations generally provide educational pamphlets, audiotapes, films, and other learning materials.
j. General community facilities, such as the YWCA and YMCA, provide many health promotion bulletins and programs.
k. Specialty nurse organizations and associations provide specific information. Through them, the nurse can locate special interest groups in a particular area of nursing.

4. Put your name on mailing lists to receive information about available educational opportunities.
5. Familiarize yourself with indexes to nursing literature. Nursing and allied health journals are often more current than books. Important indexes include:
   a. The *Cumulative Index to Nursing and Allied Health Literature* (CINAHL) indexes periodical articles, lists of book reviews, audiovisual materials, and pamphlets.
   b. The *International Nursing Index* (INI) indexes periodical articles but also lists doctoral dissertations and publications of organizations and agencies interested in nursing. Foreign language nurse journals are included.
   c. The *Nursing Studies Index* (NSI) has annotated entries about studies and research in nursing.
   d. The Medical Literature Analysis and Retrieval System (MEDLARS) provides a computer search of journal articles.
6. Become a member of health organization or professional association committees. Participation is a beneficial learning experience.
7. Periodically, at least once per year, determine your progress in achieving goals and reassess your goals.

Issues in Nursing Education

Technical and Professional Nurse

The 1985 ANA proposal discussed at right delineated two levels of nurses: technical and professional. The technical nurse is to be prepared in an associate degree program, and the professional nurse is to be prepared in a baccalaureate degree program. This proposal, if implemented by the state nursing associations, has many implications, one of which is a grandfather clause that protects those nurses already licensed to practice. Because, at present, both technical and professional nurses according to the above description are licensed as registered nurses, there is substantial agreement about grandfathering those already licensed. Even with a grandfather clause in place, many nurses are fearful that they will not be protected from discrimination when they compete with recent graduates for jobs.

Titling and Licensure

The designations *registered nurse* (RN) and *licensed practical* or *vocational nurse* (LPN, LVN) have been used since licensure laws were first enacted. In 1985, however, the ANA House of Delegates endorsed a proposal that the professional nurse with a baccalaureate degree be licensed under the legal title *registered nurse* (RN) and that the technical nurse with an associate degree be licensed under the legal title *associate nurse* (AN).

Though there is consensus at the national organizational level (Hood 1985, p. 592), controversy remains on these issues:

1. Education for nursing practice should take place in institutions of higher education that grant degrees in several disciplines.
2. Two and only two categories of nursing should be established representing professional and technical nursing practice.
3. The minimum education preparation for those newly entering professional nursing practice should be the bachelor's degree in nursing.
4. The minimum educational preparation for those newly entering technical nursing practice should be the associate degree in nursing.
5. Professional and technical nursing practice must be clearly differentiated.
6. Those engaged in professional and technical nursing practice should be titled and licensed differently.
7. *Registered nurse* (RN) should continue to be the title of those licensed to practice professional nursing in the future.

If the proposal that there be only two levels of licensure—RN and the new AN—is accepted, each state with licensure rights will need to implement changes. Such changes have major implications for diploma nurses and LPNs. In addition, this proposal will require two new standardized examinations to test the two levels of competencies.

Economic Constraints

Stevens (1985, p. 124) states that "what is best for nursing may not coincide with what is best for society at large," and that "one can no longer assume that the *best* for society—at any price—is a feasible goal." Recognizing that no discipline has ever achieved professional status outside of the traditional academic institutions, Stevens (1985, pp. 125–26) points out that (a) 4-year baccalaureate programs are more costly than 2-year programs, (b) BSN graduates require higher salaries, and (c) the financial resources of the health care industry are shrinking. For this reason, the nursing profession must substantiate to the public not only that the BSN nurse can deliver a better quality of care than an associate degree nurse but also that the BSN nurse can carry the same work load as a non-BSN graduate. The 2-year associate degree program, however, can potentially effect cost savings that can offset the high cost of training and hiring the BSN nurse. How the two roles can be redesigned to best complement each other is a question that needs to be answered.

Types of Educational Preparation Required

In the future, more nurses will be needed in home and community settings as a result of the prospective payment system in hospitals. What education will best prepare nurses to meet these needs? Because of nurses' greater autonomy in these areas, some nurse educators think that at least a baccalaureate degree is necessary. Others believe that ADN nurses can implement plans of care that are developed by a BSN primary nurse.

Financial Support

There is increasing pressure not to use Medicare dollars to support the education of health professionals in the future. This movement has serious implications for diploma schools, because the hospitals in which they are based are largely funded by Medicare.

The emphasis that hospitals are placing on reducing costs will affect the clinical base that is fundamental to the education of all health professionals. Some fear that nurses will have insufficient clinical experience in acute health care facilities. Nursing curricula will have to be scrutinized for extraneous content to ensure appropriate clinical experiences.

Curriculum Changes

Before the implementation of the Medicare prospective payment system, many nurses had little knowledge of health care and nursing care economics. Perlich (1986, p. 6) advocates that nursing school curricula be changed as follows to reflect such realities as cost containment and accountability of productivity:

1. Incorporation of communication/coordination strategies, such as the use of computers and appropriate use of statistics in health care.
2. Inclusion of planning strategies, such as discharge planning and client teaching; emphasis on disease prevention and health promotion; and the use of alternative systems of care delivery.
3. Accountability strategies, such as improved documentation and client assessment skills, and increased professional and fiscal accountability.

Post-RN Baccalaureate and Master's Programs

The thrust to make the baccalaureate degree the minimum entry level for professional nursing practice has significantly increased the need for post-RN baccalaureate programs. A survey by the University of Ottawa School of Nursing in Canada indicated that 36.4% of the respondents wished to enroll in a post-RN baccalaureate program (Dugas 1985, p. 17). The survey also indicated that many nurses already holding a baccalaureate degree were interested in a master's program of study. Ninety-three percent of the respondents wanted credit courses from the university rather than noncredit ones.

Providing programs to meet these needs and demands is a challenge for universities, especially since the profile of students indicates that most are married women in their 30s and 40s who have dependent children and hold either full-time or part-time jobs (Dugas 1985, p. 18). Students indicated a marked preference for evening classes and part-time day classes during the academic year; classroom instruction rather than correspondence, TV, or teleconference courses; and course content in the functional areas of administration, public health, and teaching followed by advanced clinical courses. Universities need flexibility to plan and provide such programs for these adult learners. Some universities now offer courses in off-campus sites for post-RN baccalaureate students and use distance delivery techniques such as teleconferencing and shipments of basic reference materials to remote areas (Kerr 1985, p. 30).

Specialization and Credentialing

Basic nursing education programs are designed to develop nurses as generalists, not specialists in any specific field of nursing. Traditionally, educators and employers have perpetuated the idea that nurses should be generalists who can rotate among services and shifts with minimal preparation. Cultural beliefs and attitudes about women have supported this idea (Baumgart 1985, p. 11). Yet over the past 10 years the market demand for nurses with specialized knowledge and skills has grown significantly.

A specialty is a defined area of clinical practice that has a narrow in-depth focus necessary for the safe delivery of a full range of services required in that area of nursing (CNA 1982, p. 23). Specialty nurses share occupational interests and desire certification that recognizes their sphere of knowledge, skills, and research. Specialty groups may include clinical specialties such as occupational health nursing, emergency and operating room nursing, enterostomal therapy nursing, intravenous therapy nursing, infection control nursing, nephrology nursing, neurology nursing, nurse midwifery, critical care nursing, oncology nursing, and palliative care nursing.

Specialty groups have proliferated in the United States, and the ANA manages most of the certification of these groups. Many U.S. groups have well-established publications, widely accepted certification mechanisms, and abundant funds for promoting research. In Canada, not all specialty groups are affiliated with or linked to a provincial or the national association. There is a bewildering array of educational programs to prepare specialists. Aims, length, and content of the programs differ. Once prepared, the specialists are employed in a wide number of capacities and have a variety of job titles. There is a need for the national association, educators, and employers to establish priorities for specialty development, program standards, credentialing mechanisms, and appropriate economic rewards for the performance of specialty services. Certification is only one form of credentialing; licensure and registration are two other forms commonly used. A more recent form is evolving with the emergence of organizations titled *academy* or *college* (Levesque 1985, p. 27).

Nursing Organizations

One way nurses can demonstrate professional commitment is active involvement in a nursing organization. There are two types of organizations: professional and nonprofessional. "A professional organization is an organization of practitioners who judge one another as professionally competent and who have banded together to perform social functions which they cannot perform in their separate capacities as individuals" (Merton 1958, p. 50). Two examples of professional organizations are the American Nurses' Association (ANA), the professional organization for RN's in the United States, and the Canadian Nurses' Association (CNA) in Canada. The National League for Nursing (NLN) is an example of a nonprofessional nursing organization; many levels of nurses and nonnurses can join. Nursing organizations are established at local, national, and international levels.

National Student Nurses' Association

The National Student Nurses' Association (NSNA) is the official preprofessional organization for nursing students. It was formed in 1953 and incorporated in 1959. Originally, the NSNA functioned under the aegis of the ANA and NLN; however, in 1968 it became an autonomous body, although it communicates with the NLN and the ANA. In 1979, the bylaws of the NSNA were revised to provide for consultants from the ANA and the NLN.

To qualify for membership in the NSNA, a student must be enrolled in a state-approved nursing education program. The NSNA offers students experience so that they will find it easier to make the transition to the ANA. The official magazine of the NSNA is the newsletter *Imprint*.

The purpose of the NSNA is to (a) assume responsibility for contribution to nursing education in order to provide for the highest quality of health care; (b) to provide programs representative of fundamental and current professional interests and concerns; and (c) to aid in the development of the whole person, her or his professional role, and her or his responsibility for the health care of people in all walks of life (NSNA 1985, p. 5).

In Canada, nursing students have a similar organization, the Canadian University Student Nurses' Association. Its members attend provincial, national, and international meetings. The provincial student nurses' associations also have programs related to the needs of nursing students and concerns within the health field in general.

Nursing International Honor Society

Sigma Theta Tau (STT) is the international honor society in nursing. It was founded in 1922 and has its headquarters in Indianapolis, Indiana. The Greek letters stand for the Greek words *storga, tharos,* and *tima* meaning love, courage, and honor. STT is a member of the association of college honor societies. The society's purpose is professional rather than social. STT membership is attained through academic achievement. Nurses in baccalaureate programs in nursing and nurses in master's, doctoral, and postdoctoral programs are eligible to join.

The official journal of STT, *Image: Journal of Nursing Scholarship,* is published quarterly. The journal publishes scholarly articles of interest to nurses.

American Nurses' Association

The ANA is the national professional organization for nursing in the United States. It was founded in 1896 as the Nurses Associated Alumnae of the United States and Canada. In 1911, the name was changed to the American Nurses' Association. It was a charter member of the International Council of Nurses along with Great Britain and

Germany in 1899. The membership is open only to registered nurses. The purposes of the ANA are to foster high standards of nursing practice and to promote the educational and professional advancement of nurses so that all people may have better nursing care. The ANA is composed of the nurses' associations from the 50 states, Guam, the Virgin Islands, Puerto Rico, and the District of Columbia. These state associations are in turn divided into regional and local chapters.

The ANA promotes programs on behalf of nurses and nursing. In 1976, the ANA revised its code of ethics. In 1978, the delegates to the ANA convention reaffirmed their support for comprehensive national health insurance and for a baccalaureate degree in nursing as the minimum preparation for professional nurses. In 1982, the organization became a federation of state nurses' associations. Individual nurses can no longer belong to the ANA, but each state nurses' association holds seats in the ANA House of Delegates. The official journal of the ANA is the *American Journal of Nursing,* and the *American Nurse* is the official means of communication with members. The functions of the ANA are shown in Table 1–8.

In 1970, the formation of the American Academy of Nursing was approved by the House of Delegates of the ANA. The purpose of the academy was to recognize those nurses who made a significant contribution to nursing practice. Members of the academy are known as fellows. In 1973, the first group of 36 nurses were admitted as fellows of the American Academy of Nursing.

Table 1–8 Functions of the American Nurses' Association

Establish standards of nursing practice, nursing education, and nursing services.
Establish a code of ethical conduct for nurses.
Ensure a system of credentialing in nursing.
Initiate and influence legislation, governmental programs, national health policy, and international health policy.
Support systematic study, evaluation, and research in nursing.
Serve as the central agency for the collection, analysis, and dissemination of information relevant to nursing.
Promote and protect the economic and general welfare of nurses.
Provide leadership in national and international nursing.
Provide for the professional development of nurses.
Conduct an affirmative action program.
Ensure a collective bargaining program for nurses.
Provide services to constituent state nurses' associations.
Maintain communication with members through official publications.
Assume an active role as consumer advocate.
Represent and speak for the nursing profession with allied health groups, national and international organizations, governmental bodies, and the public.

Source: American Nurses' Association. Bylaws, as revised July 1, 1982. Kansas City, Mo.: American Nurses' Association, 1982. Used by permission.

Canadian Nurses' Association

The Canadian Nurses' Association (CNA) is the national nursing association of Canada. Its membership is through the provincial chapters. Nurses do not join the CNA independently but obtain membership by paying a fee to the provincial chapters. In 1985, 175,000 nurses belonged to provincial chapters, i.e., to the CNA. In November 1985, the Ordre des infirmières et infirmiers du Quebec (the Quebec Nurses' Association) withdrew from the CNA. Because of the departure of the Quebec Nurses' Association, the CNA plans to reduce spending severely. At the time of writing, the CNA is considering a restructuring of the association.

The CNA has developed national standards and a code of ethics, and it offers support to all provincial associations. Through the National Testing Services, the CNA prepares licensure examinations. These examinations are available to all provinces and territories and provide a national standard for licensure of registered nurses. Through the Canadian Nurses' Foundation, research grants, fellowships, and scholarships are offered to Canadian nurses. The official journal of the CNA, *Canadian Nurse,* is published monthly and sent to each nurse member.

National League for Nursing

The National League for Nursing, formed in 1952, is an organization of both individuals and agencies. Its objective is to foster the development and improvement of all nursing services and nursing education. People who are not nurses but have an interest in nursing services, for example, hospital administrators, can be members of the league. This feature of the NLN—involving nonnurse members, consumers, and nurses from all levels of practice—is unique.

The NLN is "dedicated to meeting the health needs of the people by improving nursing education and nursing service (NLN 1975). The NLN has traditionally offered a wide range of services including institutes, workshops, seminars, consultation, accreditation of nursing education programs, testing services, and educational aid. The official journal of the NLN up to 1979 was *Nursing Outlook;* as of 1980, the official magazine became *Nursing and Health Care.*

International Council of Nurses

Illness and trauma do not respect the boundaries of countries. Although different areas of the world have different health problems, it is often in the mutual interest of countries to cooperate in health and nursing matters. Because of the ease of world travel, problems in India, for example, can quickly become problems in North America. People traveling abroad sometimes return home only to be stricken by an illness rarely seen in their own country. As the world grows closer through technologic advances and as people travel more, nurses must become increasingly concerned and involved with health matters of people all over the world. In 1973, the International Council of Nurses (ICN) stated in its Code for Nurses: "The need for nursing is universal. Inherent in nursing is respect for life, dignity and rights of man. It is unrestricted by considerations of nationality, race, creed, color, age, sex, politics or social status."

The ICN was established in 1899. Nurses from both the United States and Canada were among the founding members. The council is a federation of national nurses' associations such as the ANA and CNA. In 1985, 97 national associations from different countries were affiliated with the ICN.

The purpose of the ICN is to provide a medium through which national nursing associations can work together and share common interests. Membership in the national association automatically makes a nurse a member of the ICN. The functions of the ICN are:

1. To promote the organization of national nurses' associations and advise them in their continued development.
2. To assist national nurses' associations to play their part in developing and improving (a) health service for the public, (b) the practice of nursing, and (c) the social and economic welfare of nurses.
3. To provide means of communication among nurses throughout the world for mutual understanding and cooperation.
4. To establish and maintain liaison and cooperation with other international organizations and to serve as representatives and spokespeople of nurses at the international level.
5. To receive and manage funds and trusts that contribute to the advancement of nursing or for the benefit of nurses.
6. To do any other things incidental or conclusive to the attainment of the objective of the ICN (ICN 1973).

Special Interest Organizations

A number of nursing organizations in the United States and Canada are involved with special interests of the nurses.

Red Cross

The American Red Cross and the Canadian Red Cross are two of about 120 Red Cross, Red Crescent, Sun Societies, and Red Lion organizations around the world. The original Red Cross organization was founded by Henri Dunant in 1859. He organized a group of volunteers who worked to help the injured on the battlefield of Solferino in Italy. His work was nonpartisan, and both sides were helped by his group.

Nurses in the American Red Cross pioneered public health nursing in the United States. By 1930, however, most states had their own public health nursing services. At that time, the Red Cross extended its functions in the United States and Canada by establishing home nursing courses, organizing volunteers to assist in hospitals and nursing homes, and organizing disaster nursing and a blood program. Nursing students can volunteer their services with the Red Cross in many of these activities.

Alumni Associations

The major purpose of alumni associations is to foster the high ideals of the nursing program from which the nurses graduated. Alumni associations offer an opportunity for nurses to socialize, participate in educational programs, and raise funds for nursing students.

Other Nursing Organizations

During the past 15 years, a number of specialty organizations have formed to meet the needs of groups of nurses. A few of these organizations are the Association of Operating Room Nurses, the National Association of Pediatric Nurse Associates/Practitioners, the American Association of Nurse Anesthetists, the Canadian Orthopaedic Nurses' Association, and American Association of Nephrology Nursing.

World Health Organization (WHO)

WHO is one of the special agencies of the United Nations. It is an intergovernmental agency, formed in 1948, whose primary aim is to bring all people in the world to the highest possible level of health. As of 1985, 164 countries were members of WHO (Europa Year Book 1985, p. 87). Its major activities are to provide assistance to countries by improving health standards, education, and training; fighting disease; combating water pollution; etc.

Nurses make an essential contribution to the activities of WHO. American and Canadian nurses are frequently asked to go to countries that require assistance in nursing education and public health. About 300 nurses presently work for WHO in countries other than their own.

Trends in Nursing

A **trend** is a general direction or a prevailing tendency or inclination. Several trends are apparent in the nursing profession today. Some trends in nursing are subtle and emerge slowly, while others are obvious and seem to surface quickly. Not all trends complement one another; some may seem divergent, if not in conflict. Over time, some aspects of nursing will become prevailing trends, while others may be modified by social forces or disappear altogether. A number of trends are apparent today: the broadening focus of nursing practice, the increasingly scientific basis of nursing practice, the increasing use of technology, the drive for more education, more collaboration between nurses and other members of the health team, the push for greater autonomy in nursing practice, the increasing prevalence of home health care nursing and self-care, an increasing awareness of the need for "high touch" skills, a greater participation by nurses in the making of health policy, and intensified collective bargaining.

Broadening Focus

The focus of nursing has broadened from the care of the ill person to the care of people in illness and health, and from care of only the client to care of the family or support persons and, in some instances, the community. In the past, the nurse's main function was to care for people who were ill. Nursing care was oriented toward disease and illness. Today, there is increasing recognition of people's need for health care as distinct from illness care and of the nurse's independent functions in this area.

Nursing is also broadening to include assistance to the family and the community. Family assistance sometimes takes the form of helping a family care for an ill member, but not always. For example, the family may need assistance in providing economical but nutritious meals to growing teenagers.

Modern nursing care also has a holistic philosophy. Today's nurse deals with clients as emotional and social as well as physical beings. Care is not directed toward a particular health problem but toward the response of the total person, the health of the whole person. The broadened focus of care requires an integration of skills and concepts.

Another aspect of the broader nursing focus is the movement of nursing practice into the community. At one time, nurses worked only in institutions; increasingly, nursing services are provided in the community, often in homes and in clinics. These nursing activities not only assist those who are ill but also help those who are healthy to maintain or enhance their health. This is a major area of growth in nursing services. Rogers (1985) foresees that "nursing practice is going to take place in homes, schools, work places, playgrounds, centers for all ages, nursing homes, hospitals, clinics, moon villages, space towns. . . ."

Indicators of the broadening focus are:

1. Recognition that changes in life-style can prevent major causes of illness and death
2. Increasing numbers of health care agencies providing nursing in a community

Scientific Basis

In the past, nursing was largely either intuitive or relied on experience or observation, rather than on research. Through trial and error, the nurse sensed which measures would assist the client, and many nurses became highly skilled in providing care through experience. The past 20 years have brought an increased emphasis on nursing research and on the use of scientific data at the bedside. Indicators of this trend are:

1. The NLN requires a basic nursing research course at the baccalaureate level.
2. The number of nurses enrolled in master's programs increased from 13,105 in 1978 to 18,112 in 1983 (ANA 1985, p. 154).
3. The number of doctoral programs in nursing increased from 20 in 1978 to 31 in 1984 (DeYoung, 1985).

Technology

Technology or mechanization is being applied in the health field extensively. Certain areas of a hospital, e.g., intensive care units and coronary care units, are more technology intensive than others. Nurses find themselves in the midst of this rapidly changing, increasingly technologic environment in hospitals and in clients' homes. Many feel they need more education to obtain the knowledge and skills necessary to use the new technology. A good example is the computer, which was relatively new 10 years ago. Today, computers are used on most campuses and in many hospitals and health agencies to keep client records, record and analyze vital signs, regulate medications, diagnose and treat, and analyze laboratory data. Nurses will need to be flexible and ready to learn how to operate increasingly complex equipment.

Indicators of increasing technology are:

1. The proliferation of technologic equipment in hospitals and homes
2. The increasing costs of home and self-care equipment
3. The use of computers in many areas of health care

Education

In 1965, the ANA position paper on nursing education recommended that a baccalaureate degree be the minimum educational requirement for entry into professional nursing and that the education of nurses take place within the general educational system (ANA 1965, p. 107). The trend was slow to develop because opposition was great in many areas. However, in the late 1970s and early 1980s, a number of nursing groups endorsed this educational policy. The trend is evidenced by the following:

1. In 1960, 84% of nurses graduated from diploma programs, 3% from associate degree programs, and 13% from baccalaureate programs. In 1983, 14.9% graduated from diploma programs, 54.0% from associate degree programs, and 31.1% from baccalaureate programs (ANA 1985, p. 126).
2. In 1983, the NLN endorsed the requirement of a baccalaureate degree as minimum preparation for professional practice (Lewis 1983, p. 241).
3. In 1985, the ANA endorsed a schedule for implementing the resolution of 1985 by 1995 (AJN 1985, p. 194).
4. In 1982, the board of directors of the CNA endorsed the requirement of a baccalaureate degree as minimum preparation for professional practice by the year 2000 (Dugas 1985, p. 17).

Collaboration is "true partnership in which the power on both sides is valued by both, with recognition and acceptance of separate and combined spheres of activity and responsibility, mutual safeguarding of the legitimate interests of each party, and a commonality of goals that is recognized by both parties" (ANA 1980, p. 7). In the past, nurses have had difficulty collaborating with other health professionals and even with other nurses. Within the nursing profession, nursing educators and nursing service administrators have often had different opinions as to how to best prepare nursing students. Indicators of increasing collaboration within nursing and between nursing and other health professionals are:

1. The 1983 decision by the NLN to support the ANA's position that the baccalaureate degree be the minimum preparation for entry into professional nursing
2. Interorganizational support and communication among more than 50 different nursing groups on various issues (Breu 1984, p. 26a)
3. Recommendations of the Institute of Medicine study regarding nursing and nursing education (Institute of Medicine 1983)
4. Pharmacy practice acts protecting nursing in some Canadian provinces

Autonomy

During the past 15 years, nurses have achieved greater autonomy in practice. An early indicator was the expanded roles of nurses in specialty units of hospitals, such as intensive care units. Indicators of greater autonomy are:

1. Many states and provinces have rewritten their nurse practice acts to permit expanded roles.
2. There is increasing recognition by health care leaders in North America that more autonomy in nursing practice may be an answer to containment of health care costs.
3. A number of studies indicate that nurse practitioners can provide care as well as and sometimes better than physicians and that such care is more cost effective (Leddy and Pepper 1985, p. 298).

Home Health Care Nursing and Self-Care

There was a major increase in home health care nursing in the United States in 1983. Indicators are:

1. There were 2742 home health care agencies in 1978 and 4245 in 1983 (Arbeiter 1984, p. 42).
2. The home health and self-care market reached 6.4 billion dollars in 1983 and will reach 18.3 billion by 1990 (Mitchell 1984, p. 381).
3. Health care technology has invaded the home, whereas in the past it was restricted to hospitals. For example, clients are using ventilators and dialysis machines at home.

"High Touch"

The increasing use of technology in hospitals and homes has created an increasing need to humanize care. Nursing has traditionally been a caring and humanizing profession. Today more than ever, there is an expressed need for this "high touch" (DeCrosta 1985, p. 19). Indicators of this trend are:

1. The increasing number of professional articles about balancing caring and technical skills
2. Many studies regarding caring as an aspect of nursing
3. Increasing recognition in nursing of the needs of clients in technologic environments

Health Policy Making

Nurses are becoming increasingly involved in political action at state or provincial and federal levels. As more nurses recognize how much power they wield collectively and how they can use this power in the best interests of nurses and consumers of health care, political activity increases. Many nurses are recognizing that they must influence decision and policy making that is in the best interests of health consumers. In their practice roles, nurses are becoming more involved in decisions about their clients' care. Nursing administrators are making budgets and policies that affect nursing practice, and more nurses are influencing health policies at the state provincial and federal levels. Indicators of this trend are:

1. The number of nurses now employed in government agencies
2. The formation of a political arm, ANA-PAC, formerly N-CAP
3. The number of candidates supported by nurses and subsequently elected. In the 1984 election, 83% of candidates endorsed by N-CAP were elected on the national level (Breu 1984, p. 27a)

Collective Bargaining

Collective bargaining by nurses increased during the 1970s and 1980s. Because most nurses are women, many of the issues of the women's movement, e.g., pay, autonomy, and a voice in working conditions, are nursing issues as well. Nurses today are also confronted with cost containment, which may be perceived to affect the quality of nursing practice and employee benefits. See Chapter 7 for additional information about collective bargaining.

An indicator of this trend is the increased incidence of strikes among nurses since 1968 in the United States (Crawford et al. 1985, p. 156).

Chapter Highlights

- Florence Nightingale may be thought of as nursing's first nurse theorist, since she emphasized such independent nursing functions as preventive health care, humanistic care, comfort, and support of the client.
- There are many definitions and descriptions of nursing, but the essence of nursing is caring for and caring about people as holistic beings in matters related to health promotion, health maintenance, health restoration, and dying.
- A desired goal of nursing is professionalism, which necessitates a unique body of knowledge delineation of specific skills and competencies, autonomous regulation, enforcement of standards of education and practice, attention to the social and general welfare of nurses, formulation of a code of ethics, and an attitude of altruistic service to the public.
- Conceptual models and theories of nursing are essential in clarifying exactly how the nurse's role differs from the roles of other health professionals.
- Conceptual models of nursing have three components: assumptions about such concepts as *person, environment, health,* and *nursing;* value systems, or the beliefs that underlie the profession; and seven major model units, including the goal of nursing, the role of the nurse, and the expected consequences of nursing activity.
- Much research must be conducted before the usefulness of a conceptual model for nursing can be realized.
- Nurses use the nursing process to put a conceptual model of nursing into practice.
- Although the majority of nurses today are employed in hospital settings, more nurses are working in other areas, such as home health care and community clinics.
- Nurse practice acts vary among states and provinces, and nurses must be aware of the act governing their practice.
- Standards of nursing practice provide criteria against which the effectiveness of nursing care can be evaluated.
- The career mobility of nurses increases with their education.
- Clinical ladder systems reward nurses for their clinical competence.
- Nurses are fulfilling expanded nursing roles, for instance, those of the nurse practitioner, the clinical nursing specialist, the nurse clinician, and the nurse anesthetist, which allow greater independence and autonomy.
- Today's consumers of health care and nursing services are more aware of health issues and are taking greater responsibility for their own health; they desire a feeling of wellness and vitality rather than absence of disease.
- Needs for nursing are influenced largely by consumer demands, family structure, economic factors, advances in technology, health-related legislation, demographics, and recognition of the contribution nurses can make as individuals and as a group.
- Educational programs for nurses must reflect the health care demands and needs of a changing society, accommodate changes in the health care delivery system, and adhere to professional standards, yet be responsible to concerns about rising costs of health care.

- More nurses with baccalaureate, master's, and doctoral degrees are needed to give the profession credibility and to meet expanded nurse roles.
- Flexibility in nursing curricula and innovation in implementing curricula are needed to upgrade the educational achievement of nursing graduates from programs below the baccalaureate degree level.
- Continuous, planned, self-directed learning is not only the mark of a true professional but also helps the nurse meet her or his unique learning needs for career advancement.
- Both professional and nonprofessional nursing organizations and associations fulfill essential functions for the nursing profession and for individual nurses.
- Participation in the activities of nursing associations enhances the growth of involved individuals and helps nurses collectively influence policies affecting nursing practice.

Suggested Readings

Greiner, P. A. December 1981. What has become of the traditional nurse? *Nursing Outlook* 29:720–21.
Greiner briefly describes the changes that have taken place since the "traditional nurse" ceased to be a reality. The author explains how the contemporary nurse's function differs from the image many people have of the nurse's role.

Huey, F. L. October 1982. Looking at ladders. *American Journal of Nursing* 82:1520–26.
Huey discusses various clinical ladders in hospitals around the United States. A profile of career ladder programs, presented in tabular form, includes the name of the ladder program, number of clinical levels, salary differential between entry and top clinical level, educational or clinical requirements for top clinical level, ways clinical competencies are defined, and promotional procedures. A colored illustration indicates various shapes of ladders and reporting pathways.

McBride, A. B. September/October 1985. Orchestrating a career. *Nursing Outlook* 33:244–47.
A career in nursing—as in any other field—advances through several stages. Understanding this process can smooth the way.

McGann, M. R. March/April 1975. The clinical specialist: From hospital, to clinic, to community. *Journal of Nursing Administration* 5:33–37.
McGann describes her beliefs about the clinical specialist role. She emphasizes direct client care and follow-up of hospitalized clients discharged to clinics and their homes. Two reactions to some of her ideas are included.

Storch, J. L. January 1986. In defense of nursing theory. *The Canadian Nurse* 82:16–20.
Storch suggests that nursing theory may be the key to meeting the changing needs of health consumers. She discusses how theory can make a significant difference in the quality of client care.

Stull, M. K. May/June 1986. Entry skills for BSNs. *Nursing Outlook* 34:138, 153.
Stull, project director of the Midwest Alliance in Nursing's 3-year project, "Continuing Education for Consensus on Entry Skills," outlines the competency requirements for new baccalaureate graduates. Consensus about the skills is being reached through the collaborative efforts of 29 teams that represent nursing service and nursing education in 13 Midwestern states. Stull outlines skills related to teaching and collaboration, planning and evaluation, interpersonal relations/communication, leadership, and critical care.

Sultz, H. A.; Henry, O. M.; Bullough, B.; Buck, G. M.; and Kinyor, L. J. September/October 1983. Nurse practitioners: A decade of change. Part 3. *Nursing Outlook* 31:266–69.
Nurse practitioner students are increasingly choosing master's over certificate programs in the major specialties.

Watson, J. August 1981. Professional identity crisis: Is nursing finally growing up? *American Journal of Nursing* 81:1488–90.
The author examines some of the personal and professional problems facing nurses and the internal and external forces affecting the profession. She also analyzes six existential criteria as they apply to mature professional status.

Selected References

Abdellah, F. G., et al. 1960. *Patient-centered approaches to nursing.* New York: Macmillan Co.

Aiken, L. H. American Academy of Nursing (ed.). 1982. *Nursing in the 1980s: Crises, opportunities, challenges.* Philadelphia: J. B. Lippincott Co.

American Journal of Nursing. February 1985. ANA gears up new drive for entry-level change: Despite opposition, some SNAs see success soon. *American Journal of Nursing* 85:194, 200–201.

American Nurses' Association. December 1965. American Nurses' Association first position on education for nursing. *American Journal of Nursing* 65:106–11.

———. 1973. *Standards of nursing practice.* Kansas City, Mo.: American Nurses' Association.

———. 1978. *Health care at home: An essential component of a national health policy.* Kansas City, Mo.: American Nurses' Association.

———. April 1979. Credentialing in nursing: A new approach. Report of the Committee for the Study of Credentials in Nursing. *American Journal of Nursing* 79:674–83.

———. 1980. *Nursing: A social policy statement.* Kansas City, Mo.: American Nurses' Association.

———.1981a. *Facts about nursing 80–81.* New York: American Journal of Nursing Co.

———. 1981b. *The nursing practice act: Suggested state legislation.* Kansas City, Mo.: American Nurses' Association.

———. November/December 1982. Bylaws. *American Nurse* 14:15.

———. 1985. *Facts about nursing 84–85.* Kansas City, Mo.: American Nurses' Association.

American Nurses' Association Cabinet on Nursing Services. 1984. *Career ladders: An approach to professional productivity.* Kansas City, Mo.: American Nurses' Association.

Anderson, M. I., and Denyes, M. J. February 1975. A ladder for clinical advancement in nursing practice. *Journal of Nursing Administration* 5:16–22.

Anderson, N. D. June 1981. Ethel Fenwick's legacy to nursing and women. *Image* 13:32–33.

Arbeiter, J. S. November 1984. The big shift to home health nursing. *RN* 47:38–45.

Austin, J. K., and Champion, V. L. 1983. King's theory for nursing: Explication and evaluation. In Chinn, P. L., editor. *Advances in nursing theory development.* Rockville, Md.: Aspen Systems.

Barritt, E. R. 1973. Florence Nightingale's values and modern nursing education. *Nursing Forum* 12(1):6–47.

Baumgart, A. J. June 1985. The time is ripe. *The Canadian Nurse* 81:11.

Becktell, P. June 1981. Of women and walls. *Image* 13:34–36.

Benner, P. 1984. *From novice to expert: Excellence and power in clinical nursing practice.* Menlo Park, Calif.: Addison-Wesley Publishing Co.

Black, A., and McDowell, I. April 1984. Healthstyles: Moving beyond disease prevention. *The Canadian Nurse* 80:18–20.

Breu, C. May 1984. President's message. The end of the beginning (American Association of Critical-Care Nurses). *Heart and Lung* 13:24a–38a.

Brill, C., and Hill, L. May 1985. Giving the help that goes on giving. *Nursing 85* 15:44–47.

Canadian Nurses' Association. 1980. *A definition of nursing practice: Standards for nursing practice.* Ottawa: Canadian Nurses' Association.

———. 1982. *Credentialing in Nursing: Policy Statement and Background Paper.* Ottawa: Canadian Nurses' Association.

Chamings, P. A., and Teevan, J. February 1979. Comparison of expected competencies of baccalaureate- and associate-degree graduates in nursing. *Image* 11:16–21.

Chaska, N. L. 1978. *The nursing profession: Views through the mist.* New York: McGraw-Hill.

Check, J. F., and Wurzbach, M. E. January/February 1984. How elders view nursing. *Geriatric Nursing* 5:37–39.

Chinn, P. L., and Jacobs, M. K. 1983. *Theory and nursing: A systematic approach.* St. Louis: C. V. Mosby Co.

CNA Connection. April 1984. Canada health act. CNA appears before commons committee. *The Canadian Nurse* 80:8–9.

Cohen, H. A. 1981. *The nurse's quest for a professional identity.* Menlo Park, Calif.: Addison-Wesley Publishing Co.

Colavecchio, R.; Tescher, B.; and Scalzi, C. September/October 1974. A clinical ladder for nursing practice. *Journal of Nursing Administration* 5:54–58.

Cooper, S. S. May/June 1974. Steps in self-development. *Journal of Nursing Administration* 4:53–56.

Crawford, M.; Fisher, M.; and Kilbane, N. Collective bargaining in nursing. In DeYoung, L. 1985. *Dynamics of nursing.* 5th ed. St. Louis: C. V. Mosby Co.

Curtin, L., and Zurlage, C. 1984. *DRGs: The reorganization of health.* Chicago: S-N Publications.

DeCrosta, T. May/June 1985. Megatrends in nursing: Ten new directions that are changing your profession. *Nursing Life* 5:17–21.

DeYoung, L. 1985. *Dynamics of nursing.* 5th ed. St. Louis: C. V. Mosby Co.

Donaldson, S. K., and Crowley, D. M. February 1978. The discipline of nursing. *Nursing Outlook* 26:113–20.

Dugas, B. W. May 1985. Baccalaureate for entry to practice: A challenge that universities must meet. *The Canadian Nurse* 81:17–19.

Europa Year Book. 1985. Vol. 1. International Organizations. London: Europa Publications.

Fagin, C. M. 1982a. The national shortage of nurses: A nursing perspective. In Aiken, L. H., editor. *Nursing in the 1980s: Crises, opportunities, challenges.* Philadelphia: J. B. Lippincott Co.

———. January 1982b. Nursing as an alternative to high-cost care. *American Journal of Nursing* 82:56–60.

Fasano, M. A. April 1976. From LVN to RN in one year. *Nursing Outlook* 24:251–53.

Fawcett, J. 1980. On research and the professionalism of nursing. *Nursing Forum* 19(3):310–18.

———. 1984. *Analysis and evaluation of conceptual models of nursing.* Philadelphia: F. A. Davis Co.

Flaherty, M. J. 1979. The characteristics and scope of professional nursing. *Journal for Nursing Leadership and Management* 1:61, 63, 69.

Flexner, A. 1915. Is social work a profession? *School Society* 1(26):901.

Freidson, E. 1977. The future of professionalization. In Stacey, M., editor. pp. 14–38. *Health and the division of labor.* New York: Prodist.

Gassert, C.; Holt, C.; and Pope, K. October 1982. Building a ladder. *American Journal of Nursing* 82:1527–30.

George, J. B., editor. 1985. *Nursing theories: The base for professional nursing practice.* 2d ed. Englewood Cliffs, N.J.: Prentice-Hall.

Gortner, S. R. July/August 1980. Nursing research: Out of the past and into the future. *Nursing Research* 29:204–7.

Hale, S. L., and Boyd, B. T. September 1981. Accommodating RN students in baccalaureate nursing programs. *Nursing Outlook* 29:535–40.

Hall, L. November 1963. A center for nursing. *Nursing Outlook* 11:805–6.

Hall, R. H. 1968. Professionalization and bureaucratization. *American Sociological Review* 63:92–104.

Hart, G.; Crawford, T.; and Hicks, B. May 1985. RN to BN: Building on education and experience. *The Canadian Nurse* 81:22–23.

Henderson, V. 1966. *The nature of nursing: A definition and its implications for practice, research, and education.* New York: Macmillan Co.

———. October 1969. Excellence in nursing. *American Journal of Nursing* 69:2133–37.

———. 1972. *ICN basic principles of nursing care.* Geneva: International Council of Nurses.

Hood, G. May 1985. At issue: Titling and licensure. *American Journal of Nursing* 85:592, 594.

Huey, F. L. October 1982. Looking at ladders. *American Journal of Nursing* 82:1520–26.

Institute of Medicine. 1983. *Nursing and nursing education: Public policies and private actions.* Washington, D.C.: National Academy Press.

International Council of Nurses 1973. *Constitution and regulations.* Geneva: International Council of Nurses.

Jamieson, E. M.; Sewall, M. F.; and Suhrie, E. B. 1966. *Trends in nursing history.* 6th ed. Philadelphia: W. B. Saunders Co.

Johnson, D. E. 1980. The behavioral system model for nursing. In Riehl, J. P., and Roy, C. Conceptual models for nursing practice. 2d ed. New York: Appleton-Century-Crofts.

Kerr, J. May 1985. Taking the campus to the student. *The Canadian Nurse* 81:30–31.

King, I. M. 1971. *Toward a theory for nursing: General concepts of human behavior.* New York: John Wiley and Sons.

———. 1981. *A theory for nursing: Systems, concepts, process.* New York: John Wiley and Sons.

Kinney, C. D. May/June 1985. A reexamination of nursing role conceptions. *Nursing Research* 34(3): 170–76.

Kluge, E. H. February 1982. Nursing: Vocation or profession? *Canadian Nurse* 78:34–36.

Knox, S. L. July 1980. A clinical advancement program. *Journal of Nursing Administration* 10:29–33.

Lambertson, E. 1953. *Nursing team organization and functioning.* New York: Teachers College Press.

Lane, B. June 1985. Specialization in nursing: Some Canadian issues. *The Canadian Nurse* 81:24–25.

Large, J. T. October 1976. Harriet Newton Phillips, the first trained nurse in America. *Image* 8:49–51.

Larson, M. S. 1977. *The rise of professionalism.* Los Angeles: California Press.

LaSor, B., and Elliott, M. R. 1977. *Issues in Canadian nursing.* Scarborough, Ontario: Prentice-Hall of Canada.

Leddy, S., and Pepper, J. M. 1985. *Conceptual bases of professional nursing.* Philadelphia: J. B. Lippincott Co.

Leininger, M. 1984. *Care: The essence of nursing and health.* Thorofare, N.J.: Charles B. Slack.

Lenburg, C. B. July 1976. The external degree in nursing: The promise fulfilled. *Nursing Outlook* 24:422–29.

Levesque, V. D. June 1985. Specialization and certification: A review of CNA's activities. *The Canadian Nurse* 81:26–28.

Levine, E. November 1977. What do we know about nurse practitioners? *American Journal of Nursing* 77:1799–1803.

Levine, M. 1973. *Introduction to clinical nursing.* 2d ed. Philadelphia: F. A. Davis Co.

Lewis, E. P. September/October 1983. News outlook: The issue that won't go away. A report on the 1983 NLN convention. *Nursing Outlook* 31:246–47.

———. September/October 1985. Taking care of business: The ANA House of Delegates. *Nursing Outlook* 33:239–43.

Maraldo, P. Fall 1984. Terms of endurance: The future of nursing education. *Educational Record* 12–16.

Marram, G.; Barrett, M. W.; and Bevis, E. O. .1979. *Primary nursing: A model for individualized care.* 2d ed. St. Louis: C. V. Mosby Co.

Marriner, A. 1986. *Nursing theorists and their work.* St. Louis: C. V. Mosby Co.

McKibbin, R. 1983. Economic and employment issues in nursing education. Kansas City, Mo.: American Nurses' Association.

McPhail, J. October 1971. Reasonable expectations for the nurse clinician. *Journal of Nursing Administration* 1:16–18.

Merton, R. K. January 1958. The function of the professional organization. *American Journal of Nursing* 58:50–54.

Michelmore, E. August 1977. Distinguishing between AD and BS education. *Nursing Outlook* 25:506–10.

Miller, B. K. April 1985. Just what is a profession? *Nursing Success To-day* 2:21–27.

Miller, R. June 1975. Career ladder program: A problem-solving device. *Journal of Nursing Administration* 5:27–29.

Millis, J. S. July 1977. Primary care: Definition of, and access to. *Nursing Outlook* 25:443–45.

Mitchell, K. November/December 1984. The next economy: Where will nurses fit? *Heart and Lung* 13:381.

Montag, M. L. April 1980. Looking back: Associate degree education in perspective. *Nursing Outlook* 28:248–50.

Moore, W. E., and Rosenblum, G. W. 1970. *The professions: Roles and rules.* New York: The Russel Sage Foundation.

National Commission on Nursing: Summary report and recommendations. July 1983. American Hospital Association. Chicago: The Hospital Research and Educational Trust, and American Hospital Supply Corporation.

National League for Nursing. March/April 1975. 1974 Annual Report. *NLN News* 23:3.

———. 1978a. *Characteristics of graduate education in nursing leading to the master's degree.* New York: The League.

———. 1978b. *Competencies of the associate degree nurse on entry into practice.* New York: The League.

———. 1978c. *Roles and competencies of graduates of diploma programs in nursing.* New York: The League.

———. 1979. *Characteristics of baccalaureate education in nursing.* New York: The League.

National Student Nurses' Association. 1972. *Bylaws.* New York: National Student Nurses' Association.

———. 1985. *Getting the pieces to fit 85/86: A handbook for state associations and school chapters.* New York: National Student Nurses' Association.

Nayer, D. D. November 1981. BSN doors are opening for RN students. *American Journal of Nursing* 81:2056–57, 2062–64.

Neuman, B. 1982. *The Neuman systems model: Application to nursing education and practice.* New York:: Appleton-Century-Crofts.

Nightingale, F. 1860. *Notes on nursing: What it is, and what it is not.* London: Harrison. Reprinted in Bishop, F. L. A., and Goldie, S. 1962. *A bio-bibliography of Florence Nightingale.* London: Dawsons of Pall Mall.

Notter, L. E., and Spalding, E. K. 1976. *Professional nursing: Foundations, perspectives, and relationships.* 9th ed. New York: J. B. Lippincott Co.

Orem, D. E. 1985. *Nursing: Concepts of practice.* 3d ed. New York: McGraw-Hill.

Palmer, I. S. June 1981. Florence Nightingale and international origins of modern nursing. *Image* 8:28—31.

People. August 1983. *American Journal of Nursing* 83:1205.

Peplau, H. E. 1952. *Interpersonal relations in nursing.* New York: G. P. Putnam's Sons.

Perlich, L. J. M. January 1986. Catalyzing educational change. *Journal of Nursing Administration* 16:6.

Phaneuf, M. C., and Lang, M. 1985. *Issues in professional nursing practice 7: Standards of nursing practice.* Kansas City, Mo.: American Nurses' Association.

Pletsch, P. K. December 1981. Mary Breckinridge: A pioneer who made her mark. *American Journal of Nursing* 81:2188–90.

Poulin, M. A. 1985. *Issues in professional nursing practice 5. Configurations of nursing practice.* Kansas City, Mo.: American Nurses' Association.

Powell, D. J. January/February 1984. Nurses—"High touch" entrepreneurs. *Nursing Economics* 2:33–36.

Primm, P. L. May/June 1986. Entry into practice: Competency statements for BSNs and ADNs. *Nursing Outlook* 34:135–37.

Reiter, F. February 1966. The nurse-clinician. *American Journal of Nursing* 66:274–80.

Riehl, J. P., and Roy, C. 1980. *Conceptual models for nursing practice.* 2d ed. New York: Appleton-Century-Crofts.

Rogers, M. E. 1970. *An introduction to the theoretical basis of nursing.* Philadelphia: F. A. Davis Co.

———. 1980. Nursing: A science of unitary man. In Riehl, J. P., and Roy, C. *Conceptual models for nursing practice.* 2d ed. New York: Appleton-Century-Crofts.

———. 1985. High touch in a high-tech future. Paper presented at the National League for Nursing convention, San Antonio, Texas.

Roth, A. 1977. *National sample survey of registered nurses: A report on the nurse population and factors affecting their supply.* Springfield, Va.: National Technical Information Service.

Rothberg, J. S. The growth of political action in nursing. *Nursing Outlook* 33:133–35.

Roy, C. 1976. *Introduction to nursing: An adaptation model.* Englewood Cliffs, N.J.: Prentice-Hall.

———. 1984. *Introduction to nursing: An adaptation model.* 2d ed. Englewood Cliffs, N.J.: Prentice-Hall.

Sabina, D. J. May 1985. What are the needs of the mature RN students? *The Canadian Nurse* 81:32–33.

Segal, E. T. June 1985. Is nursing a profession? Yes no. *Nursing 85* 15:40–43.

Sheahan, D., Sr. January 1978. Scanning the seventies. *Nursing Outlook* 26:33–37.

Sims, E. February 1977. Preparation for independent practice. *Nursing Outlook* 25:114–18.

Slavinsky, A. T., and Diers, D. May 1982. Nursing education for college graduates. *Nursing Outlook* 30:292–97.

Smoyak, S. A. November 1976. Specialization in nursing: From then to now. *Nursing Outlook* 24:676–81.

Smyk, H. May 1985. The development of a post-basic certificate program—for credits! *The Canadian Nurse* 81:34–35.

Snyder, M. E., and LaBar, C. 1984. *Issues in professional nursing practice 1. Nursing: Legal authority to practice.* Kansas City, Mo.: American Nurses' Association.

Sptizer, W. O. April 19, 1984. The nurse practitioner revisited. Slow death of a good idea. *New England Journal of Medicine* 310:1049–51.

Spruck, M. July/August 1980. Teaching research at the undergraduate level. *Nursing Research* 29:257–59.

Statistics Canada. 1980. *Nursing in Canada: Canadian nursing statistics.* Ottawa: Statistics Canada.

Statistics Canada and the Canadian Nurses' Association. 1985. *Nursing in Canada.* Ottawa: Canadian Nurses' Association.

Stevens, B. J. 1979. *Nursing theory: Analysis, application, evaluation.* Boston: Little, Brown and Co.

———. May/June 1985. Does the 1985 nursing education proposal make economic sense? *Nursing Outlook* 33:124–27.

Stewart, I. April 1933. Postgraduate education—new and old. *American Journal of Nursing* 33:363.

Stinson, S. M.; Larsen, J.; and MacPhail, J. 1984. *Canadian nursing doctoral statistics: 1982 update.* Ottawa: Canadian Nurses' Association.

Storch, J. L. January 1986. In defense of nursing theory. *The Canadian Nurse* 82:16–20.

Stuart, G. W. February 1981. How professionalized is nursing? *Image* 13:18–23.

Styles, M. M. January 1978. Dialogue across the decades. *Nursing Outlook* 26:28–32.

———. 1982. *On nursing: Toward a new endowment.* St. Louis: C. V. Mosby Co.

———. November 1983. The anatomy of a profession. *Heart and Lung* 12:570–75.

Styran, P. May 1985. Winds of change: A university responds to the needs of nurses in the community. *The Canadian Nurse* 81:20–21.

U.S. Department of Health and Human Services. Public Health Service. 1985. *Charting the nation's health trends since 1960.* Hyattsville, Md.: DHHS Pub. no. (PHS) 85-1251.

U.S. National Center for Health Statistics. Public Health Service. 1985. *Vital statistics of the United States, 1982.* Vol. 11, Sec. 6. Life tables. DHHS Pub. no. (PHS) 85-1104. Washington, D.C.: U.S. Government Printing Office.

Warhola, G. August 1980. *Planning home health care services: A resource book.* Pub. no. (HRA) 80-14017. Washington, D.C.: Public Health Service. Department of Health and Human Services.

Whitman, M. January 1982. Toward a new psychology for nurses. *Nursing Outlook* 30:48–52.

Williams, C. A. April 1977. Community health nursing: What is it? *Nursing Outlook* 25:250–54.

Wright, L. M.; Watson, W. L.; and Duhamed, F. May 1985. The family nursing unit: Clinical preparation at the master's level. *The Canadian Nurse* 81:26–29.

Zimmer, M. J. 1972. Rationale for a ladder for clinical advancement. *Journal of Nursing Administration* 5:18–24.

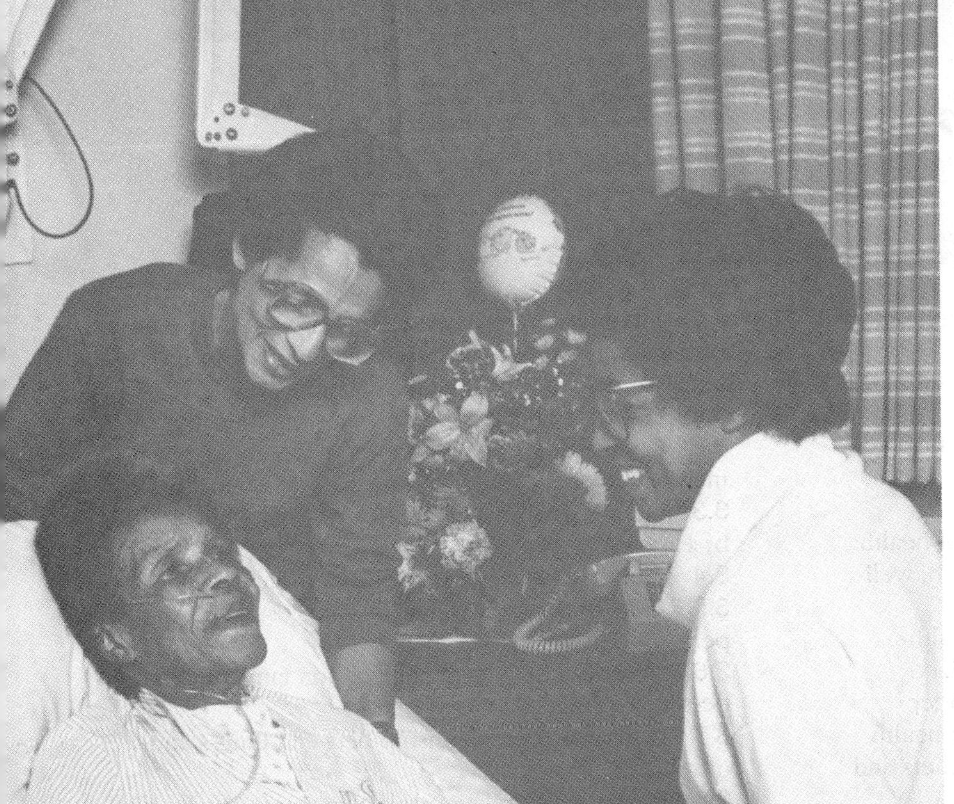

CHAPTER 2

Health and Illness

Contents

2 *Health and Illness*

Objectives

1. Understand essential facts about health, wellness, disease, and illness.
   1.1 Compare definitions of health outlined in this chapter.
   1.2 Identify characteristics basic to a positive concept of health.
   1.3 Describe selected models of health.
   1.4 Identify various theorists' concepts of health.
   1.5 Differentiate between wellness, health, well-being, illness, and disease.
   1.6 Compare varying concepts of the health-illness/normal-health continuum as theorized by Dunn, Twaddle, Jahoda, Jones, and Pender.
   1.7 Describe essential aspects of holistic health.
2. Understand essential facts about health beliefs and behaviors.
   2.1 Differentiate between health status, health belief, and health behavior.
   2.2 Identify factors that influence a person's concept of health.
   2.3 Identify variables affecting a person's state of health.
   2.4 Describe the significance of a health belief model.
   2.5 Describe how individual perceptions affect a person's health behavior.
   2.6 Describe how demographic, intrapersonal, and situational variables affect a person's health behavior.
   2.7 Identify barriers to healthy behavior.
3. Understand essential facts about illness, sick role behavior, and effects of hospitalization.
   3.1 Describe Suchman's five stages of illness.
   3.2 Compare Igun's 11 stages of illness to Suchman's 5 stages.
   3.3 Describe aspects of the sick role as delineated by Parsons.
   3.4 Identify effects of hospitalization on clients.
   3.5 Identify common behavior changes in sick persons.
   3.6 Describe the effects of illness on family members' roles and functions.
   3.7 Describe the relationship between illness and disease.
   3.8 Describe the relationship between health and illness.
4. Appreciate significant factors influencing a person's compliance with health regimens.
   4.1 Describe factors affecting compliance.
   4.2 Identify nursing interventions related to compliance.
5. Understand current health patterns and trends.
   5.1 Identify four major risk factors responsible for illness and mortality.
   5.2 Explain the health field concept.
   5.3 Relate current patterns and trends in health to people's nursing needs.

Terms

autonomy
biofeedback
client contract
compliance
complier
continuum
coping mechanism
disease
health
health behavior
health belief
health status
holistic health
illness
illness behavior
locus of control
model (paradigm)
morbidity
mortality
noncomplier
privacy
sick role behavior
well-being
wellness

Emerging Concepts

Health

Health is a changing, evolving concept that is basic to nursing. For centuries, the concept of disease was the yardstick by which health was measured. Until the late 19th century, the major concern of health professionals was the "how" of disease. Recently, there has been an increasing emphasis on health.

There is no consensus about any definition of health. There is knowledge of how to attain a certain level of health, but health itself cannot be measured.

In 1947, the World Health Organization (WHO) proposed a broad definition of **health**: "Health is a state of complete physical, mental, and social well-being, and not merely the absence of disease or infirmity" (WHO 1947, p. 1). At the time, some considered this definition impractical; some view it as a possible goal for all people, while others consider complete well-being unobtainable. However, the WHO definition of health includes three characteristics basic to a positive concept of health:

1. It reflects concern for the individual as a total person rather than as merely the sum of various parts.
2. It views health in the context of both internal and external environments.
3. It equates health with productive and creative living (Pender 1982, p. 26).

In 1953, the [United States] President's Commission on Health Needs of the Nation stated: "Health is not a condition; it is an adjustment. It is not a state but a process. The process adapts the individual not only to our physical, but also our social environment" (President's Commission 1953, p. 4).

Because health is such a complex concept, various researchers have developed models or paradigms to explain health and in some instances its relationship to illness. (A **model** or **paradigm** is an abstract outline or a theoretical depiction of a complex phenomenon.)

Clinical Model

The narrowest interpretation of health occurs in the clinical model (Smith 1981, p. 47). People are viewed as physiologic systems with related functions, and health is identified by the absence of signs and symptoms of disease or injury. In this model, the opposite of health is disease. Dunn describes health according to this model as "a relatively passive state of freedom from illness . . . a condition of relative homeostasis" (Dunn 1959b, p. 447).

In this model, the extreme of health is the absence of any signs of symptoms of disease; conversely, the conspicuous presence of such signs and symptoms is an indicator of extreme illness. Many medical practitioners use the clinical model. The focus of many medical practices is the relief of signs and symptoms of disease and the elimination of malfunctioning and pain. When the signs and symptoms of disease are no longer present in a person, the medical practitioner often considers that the individual's health is restored.

Ecologic Model

The ecologic model of health is based on the relationship of humans to their environment (see Figure 2–1). This model has three elements:

1. The host: a person or group who may or may not be at risk of acquiring an illness or disease

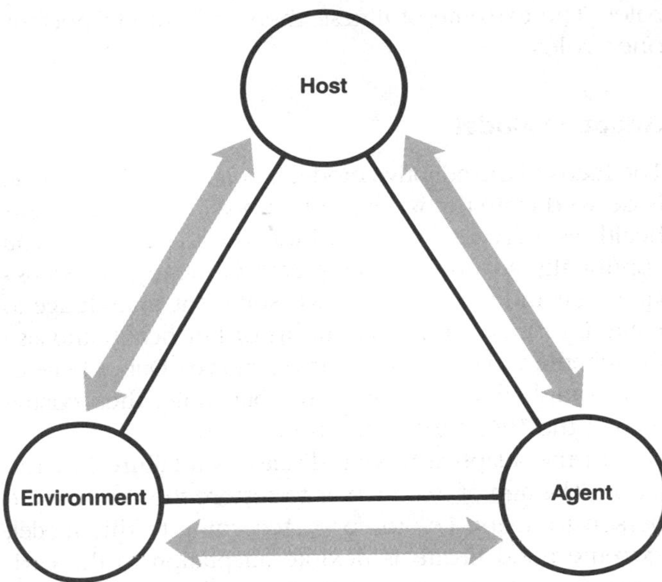

Figure 2–1 Ecologic health model showing dynamic interaction between host, agent, and environment

2. The agent: any factor in the environment that by its presence or absence can lead to illness or disease
3. The environment, including the extrinsic or intrinsic environment, which may or may not predispose the person to the development of disease (Payne 1983, p. 394)

The three elements of this model interact dynamically, and health is an ever-changing state.

Role Performance Model

The role performance model adds social and psychologic standards to the concept of health (Leddy and Pepper 1985, p. 155). Health is defined in terms of the individual's ability to fulfill his or her societal roles, i.e., to perform work. According to this model, people who can fulfill their roles are healthy even if they appear clinically ill. For example, a man who works all day at his job as expected is healthy even though an x-ray film of his lung indicates a tumor. Parsons (1972) views health in this light. Health has also been defined as "the state of optimum capacity of an individual for the effective performance of his roles and tasks" (Parsons 1972, p. 107). An emphasis in this definition is the capacity of the individual rather than a commitment to roles and tasks.

In this model, it is assumed that sickness is the inability to perform one's work. A problem with this model is the assumption that a person's most important role is his or her work role. People usually fulfill several roles, e.g., mother, daughter, friend, and certain individuals may consider nonwork roles paramount in their lives. In this model, "perfect" health is maximum performance of work roles. The extreme of illness, then, is failure to perform one's roles.

Adaptive Model

The focus of the adaptive model is adaptation. This model is derived from the writings of Dubos (1978), who views health as a creative process. Individuals are actively and continually adapting to their environments. In Dubos's view, the individual must have sufficient knowledge to make informed choices about his or her health and also the income and resources to act on choices. Dubos believes that complete well-being is unobtainable, thus contradicting the 1947 WHO definition.

In the adaptive model, disease is a failure in adaptation. The aim of treatment is to restore the ability of the person to adapt, i.e., to cope. According to this model, extreme good health is flexible adaptation to the environment and interaction with the environment to maximum advantage (Smith 1981, p. 45). The focus of this model is stability, although there is also an element of growth and change.

Wu's model of health is partly adaptive. According to Wu, health is a feeling of well-being, a capacity to perform to the best of one's ability, and the flexibility to adapt and adjust to varying situations created by the subsystems of humans or the suprasystems in which people exist (Wu 1973, p. 112). Wu also proposed that wellness (health) and illness are separate entities, each with separate behaviors. Also, both wellness and illness can exist at the same time in a person.

Murray and Zentner define health as "a state of well-being in which the person is able to use purposeful, adaptive responses and processes, physically, mentally, emotionally, spiritually, and socially, in response to internal and external stimuli (stressors) in order to maintain relative stability and comfort and to strive for personal objectives and cultural goals" (Murray and Zentner 1985, pp. 4–5).

Eudaimonistic Model

The eudaimonistic model incorporates the most comprehensive view of health (Smith 1981, p. 44). Health is seen as a condition of actualization or realization of a person's potential. Actualization is the apex of the fully developed personality. (Maslow presents this concept of health. See Chapter 16.) In this model, the highest aspiration of people is fulfillment and complete development, i.e., actualization. Illness, in this model, is a condition that prevents self-actualization.

Nursing-Based Definitions of Health

A number of nurses have provided nursing-based definitions of health. See Table 2–1 for definitions of health by selected nurse theorists.

Pender includes stabilizing and actualizing tendencies in the definition of health: "Health is the actualization of inherent and acquired human potential through satisfying relationships with others, goal-directed behavior, and competent personal care while adjustments are made as needed to maintain stability and structural integrity" (Pender 1982, p. 37). Payne proposes the following definition: "Health is the effective functioning of self-care resources which ensure the operation and adequacy of self-care actions." In Payne's view, "self-care resources" include knowledge, skills, and attitudes. "Self-care actions" are goal-directed behaviors required to regain, maintain, or promote physical, psychosocial, and spiritual functioning (Payne 1983, p. 395).

Personal Definitions of Health

Health is a highly individual perception. Meanings and descriptions of health vary considerably. An individual's personal definition of health may not agree with that of health professionals. The following factors influence an individual's definition of health:

1. *Developmental status.* The idea of health is frequently related to a person's level of development. The ability

Developing a Personal Definition of Health

The following questions can help nurses develop a personal definition of health.

- Is a person more than a biophysiologic system?
- Is health more than the absence of disease symptoms?
- Is health solely the result of the interaction between host, agent, and environment?
- Is health the ability of an individual to perform work?
- Is health the ability of an individual to adapt to the environment?
- Is health a condition of a person's actualization?
- Is health a state or a process?
- Is health effective functioning of self-care activities?
- Is health static or changing?
- Are health and wellness the same?
- Are disease and illness different?
- Are there levels of health?
- Are health and illness separate entities or points along a continuum?
- Is health socially determined?
- How do you rate your health and why?

Table 2–1 Nurse Theorists' Views of Health

Nurse Theorist and Theory	Definition/Description
Dorothy E. Johnson* Behavioral system theory	Health is an elusive, dynamic state influenced by biologic, psychologic, and social factors. Health is reflected by the organization, interaction, interdependence, and integration of the subsystems of the behavioral system. Humans attempt to achieve a balance in this system; this balance leads to functional behavior. A lack of balance in the structural or functional requirements of the subsystems leads to poor health.
Imogene King† Goal attainment theory	Health is viewed as a dynamic state in the life cycle: illness is an interference in the life cycle. Health implies continuous adaptation to stress "in the internal and external environment through optimum use of one's resources to achieve maximum potential for daily living."
Myra Levine‡ Four conservation principles	Health is socially determined. It is predetermined by social groups and is not just an absence of pathologic conditions.
Betty Neuman§ Systems model	Wellness is the condition in which all parts and subparts of an individual are in harmony with the whole system. Wholeness is based on interrelationships of variables, which determine the resistance of an individual to any stressor. Illness indicates lack of harmony among the parts and subparts of the system of the individual. Health is viewed as a point along a continuum from wellness to illness; health is dynamic, i.e., constantly subject to change. Optimal wellness or stability indicates that all a person's needs are being met. A reduced state of wellness is the result of unmet systemic needs. The individual is in a dynamic state of wellness-illness, in varying degrees, at any given time.
Florence Nightingale‖	Health means being well and using one's powers to the fullest extent. Disease is a reparative process nature institutes because of some want of attention.
Dorothea Orem¶ Self-care theory	Health is a *state* of a person that is characterized by soundness or wholeness of developed human structures and of bodily and mental functioning. *Well-being* is used in the sense of individuals' perceived condition of existence. Well-being is a state characterized by experiences of contentment, pleasure, and kinds of happiness; by spiritual experiences; by movement toward fulfillment of one's self-ideal; and by continuing personalization. Well-being is associated with health, with success in personal endeavors, and with sufficiency of resources.
Hildegard Peplau** Psychodynamic nursing	Health is "a word symbol that implies forward movement of personality and other ongoing human processes in the direction of creative, constructive, productive, personal, and community living."
Martha Rogers†† Unitary human beings, an energy field	Health is an expression of a life process. Health and illness are considered to "denote behaviors that are of high value and low value."
Sister Callista Roy‡‡ Adaptation model	Health is a state and a process of being and becoming integrated and whole.

Sources:
*D. E. Johnson, The behavioral system model for nursing. In J. P. Riehl and C. Roy, *Conceptual models for nursing practice,* 2d ed. (New York: Appleton-Century-Crofts, 1980), p. 208.
*C. Loveland-Cherry and S. Wilkerson, Dorothy Johnson's behavioral systems model. In J. Fitzpatrick and A. Whall, editors, *Conceptual models of nursing: Analysis and application* (Bowie, Md.: Robert J. Brady, 1983), pp. 119, 126.
†I. M. King, *A theory for nursing: Systems, concepts, process* (New York: John Wiley and Sons, 1981), p. 5.
‡ N. K. Leonard, Myra Estra Levine. In J. B. George, editor, *Nursing theories: The base for professional nursing practice,* 2d ed. (Englewood Cliffs, N.J.: Prentice-Hall, 1985).
§B. Neuman, *An explanation of the Betty Neuman nursing model,* paper presented at Nursing Theory in Action Conference, Edmonton, Alberta, August 23, 1985.
‖F. Nightingale, *Notes on nursing: What it is and what it is not* (New York: Dover, reprinted 1969), pp. 7, 334–35.
¶D. E. Orem, *Nursing: Concepts of practice,* 3d ed. (New York: McGraw, 1985), p. 179.
**H. E. Peplau, *Interpersonal relations in nursing* (New York: G. P. Putnam's Sons, 1952), p. 12.
††J. Fawcett, *Analysis and evaluation of conceptual models of nursing* (Philadelphia: F. A. Davis Co., 1984).
‡‡C. Roy, *An introduction to nursing. An adaptation model.* 2d ed. (Englewood Cliffs, N.J.: Prentice-Hall, 1984), pp. 22, 24.

to conceptualize a state of health and the ability to respond to changes in health are related directly to age. An infant can be aware of pain but unable to verbalize it or take measures to relieve it. The nurse's knowledge of an individual's developmental status can facilitate assessment of the appropriateness of the person's behavior and help anticipate future behaviors.

2. *Social and cultural influences.* Culture and social interactions also influence a person's notion of health. Each culture has ideas about health, and often these are transmitted from parents to children. For example, in some traditional Chinese families health is defined as a flow of energy (yin and yang). Yin is dark, cold, wet, negative, and female; yang is light, warm, dry,

positive, and male. An imbalance of yin and yang results in disease.

3. *Previous experiences.* Experiences with health and illness also affect people's perceptions of health. Some people may consider a pain or dysfunction normal because they have experienced it once or often before. In addition, knowledge gained from these experiences helps determine people's definitions of health.

4. *Expectations of self.* Some people expect to be functioning at a high level physically and psychosocially all the time when they are healthy. They perceive any change in that level of functioning, therefore, as illness. Others expect variations in their level of functioning, and their definitions of health accommodate those variations.

Another factor related to self is how the individual perceives himself or herself generally. These perceptions relate to such aspects of self as esteem, body image, needs, roles, and abilities. When there is any threat or perceived threat to these views of self, the individual usually feels some anxiety. Often the individual needs to reassess his or her health and to redefine health. For example, a 60-year-old man who can no longer play tennis as he was accustomed to do may need to examine and redefine his concept of health in view of his age and abilities.

Nurses need to understand that people have their own individual definitions of both health and illness. An individual's definition of health influences that person's understanding of health and illness as well as his or her behavior related to health and illness. By understanding clients' perceptions of health and illness, nurses can provide more meaningful assistance to help clients regain or attain a state of health.

Wellness

Wellness has received increasing attention in recent years. Some people believe *wellness* and *health* are synonymous, while others believe they differ. Wellness is similar to actualization as defined in the eudaimonistic model of health. In 1959, Dunn differentiated good health from wellness: "Good health can exist as a relatively passive state of freedom from illness in which the individual is at peace with his environment—a condition of relative homeostasis. Wellness is an integrated method of functioning which is oriented toward maximizing the potential of which the individual is capable, within the environment where he is functioning" (Dunn 1959b, p. 4).

Wellness can also be defined as an active process through which the individual becomes aware of and makes choices that lead to a more successful existence (Hettler 1982, p. 207). These choices are influenced by the individual's self-concept, culture, and environment. Hettler proposes a continuum whose extremes are total wellness and premature death. See Figure 2–2.

Well-being is a subjective perception of balance, harmony, and vitality (Leddy and Pepper 1985, p. 156). According to Leddy and Pepper, it occurs in levels. At the highest levels, a person feels satisfaction and a sense of contributing. At the lowest levels, the person sees himself or herself as ill.

Dunn describes a health grid in which a health axis and an environmental axis intersect. The resulting quadrants represent degrees of health and wellness. See Figure 2–3. This grid is intended to demonstrate the interaction of the environment with the continuum from well-being to illness.

Health, then, can be viewed as an ever-changing process, whereas well-being is a status that can be described and measured (Leddy and Pepper 1985, p. 156).

Disease

Disease is a medical term, which can be described as an alteration in body functions resulting in a reduction of capacities or a shortening of the normal life span (Twaddle 1977, p. 97). Intervention by physicians has the goal of eliminating or ameliorating disease processes. Primi-

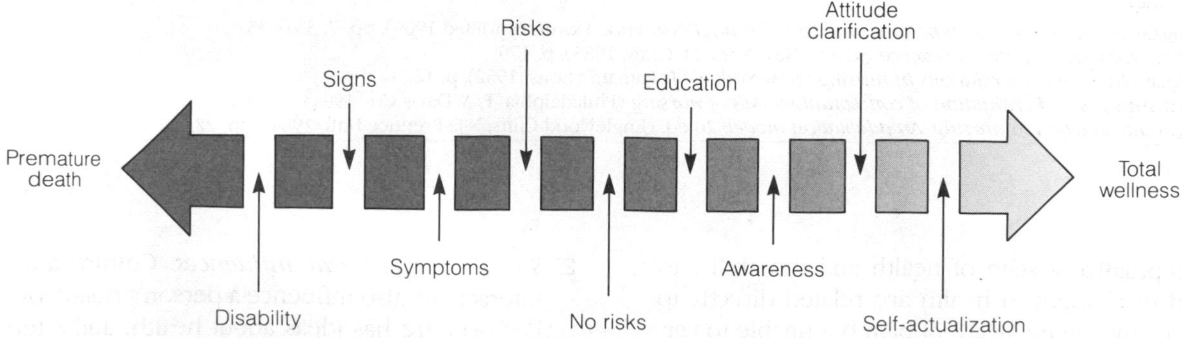

Figure 2–2 Hettler's continuum of total wellness to premature death

Source: B. Hettler, Wellness and promotion and risk reduction on a university campus. University of Wisconsin-Stevens Point.

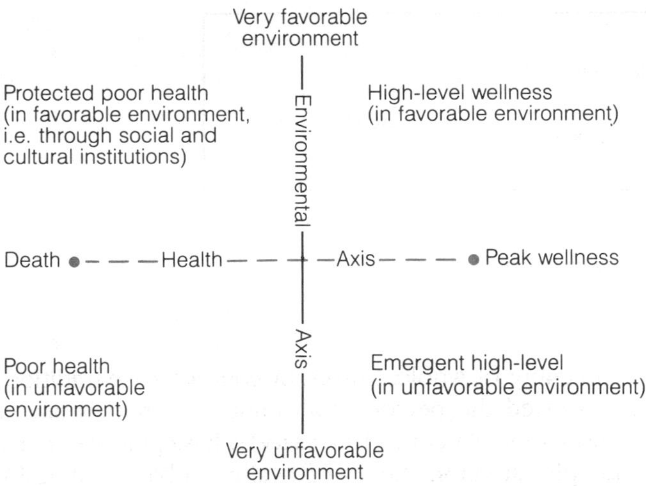

Figure 2–3 Dunn's health grid: its axes and quadrants

Source: H. L. Dunn, High-level wellness for man and society, *American Journal of Public Health,* 1959, 49:788. Reprinted with permission.

Table 2–2 Selected Definitions of Illness

- Illness is a disturbance in one or more spheres of an individual's capacity to meet minimum physical, physiologic, psychologic, and social requirements for appropriate functioning in a given sex category and at a given stage of growth and development (Hadley 1974, p. 24).
- Illness is the failure of the person's adaptive powers to maintain physical and emotional balance and to use the usual health-promoting resources in the face of internal or external stressors. It is an experience that exists when there is disturbance or failure in the biopsychosocial development or adaptation of the person, with observable or felt changes, discomforts, or impaired ability to carry out minimal physical, psychologic, or social behavioral expectations appropriate to customary roles and status (Murray and Zentner 1985, p. 5).
- Illness is the human experience of disease (Kneisl and Ames 1986, p. 18).

tive people thought disease was caused by "forces" or spirits. Later, this belief was replaced by the single-causation theory. Increasingly, a number of factors are considered to interact in causing disease and determining the individual's response to treatment.

Illness

Illness is a highly personal state in which the person feels unhealthy or ill. A person who feels pain or nausea tends to modify behavior in some way and consider himself or herself ill. Illness may or may not be related to disease. An individual could have a disease, for example, a growth in the stomach, and not feel ill. Parsons defines illness as "a state of disturbance in the normal functioning of the total human individual, including both the state of the organism as a biological system, and of his person and social adjustments" (Parsons 1972, p. 107). Leddy and Pepper suggest that society, by accepting and thus legitimizing an individual's illness, determines when a person is considered sick (Leddy and Pepper 1985, p. 154). See Table 2–2 for additional definitions of illness.

Bauman (1965, p. 206) found that people use three distinct criteria to determine whether they are ill:

1. The presence of symptoms, such as elevated temperature or pain
2. Their perceptions of how they feel; for example, good, bad, sick
3. Their ability to carry out daily activities, such as a job or schoolwork

Relationship of Health, Illness, and Disease

Health and Illness

Health and illness can be considered either as points along one continuum, as related but separate entities, or as separate entities. (A **continuum** is a grid or graduated scale.) Dunn describes a continuum of well-being (health) in which peak wellness is at one end and death is at the other. See Figure 2–3. Twaddle proposes a continuum that accommodates a range of normal health. He believes this normal range reflects the fact that no one ever attains perfect health and not everyone becomes sick. In his model, "normal" and "ill" behaviors overlap (Twaddle 1977, p. 103). See Figure 2–4. Jahoda conceptualizes health and illness along separate but coexisting continua (see Figure 2–5). The double continuum reflects the fact that people exhibit health and illness in varying degrees at the same time (Jahoda 1958, p. 75). This approach allows one to view a person's strengths (health) and illnesses at the same time.

In 1978, Jones published a framework of health and illness using the concepts of stress adaptation, Maslow's hierarchy of needs, and illness-wellness. The sides of the triangle (see Figure 2–6) represent basic needs, adaptability, and illness-wellness. Figure 2–7 shows the interaction of these three concepts in an average person. The side representing basic needs is a range from high (many unmet) needs to low (few unmet) needs. The side representing adaptability is a range from low to high adapt-

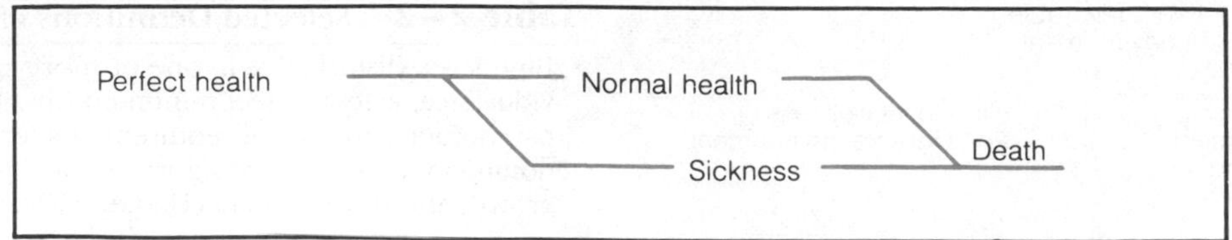

Figure 2–4 Twaddle's health continuum

Source: Twaddle, A.: *Social Science and Medicine*, 1974, 8(1), 29–38. Reprinted with permission.

ability. High adaptability intersects with high-level wellness. To determine a person's position on the illness-wellness continuum:

1. Establish a point appropriate for the individual on the basic needs continuum and draw a line from that point to the opposite apex.
2. Establish a point appropriate for the individual on the adaptability side and draw a line from that point to the opposite apex.
3. From the point where the two lines intersect draw a vertical line to the illness-wellness continuum. This point indicates the individual's position on the illness-wellness continuum (see Figure 2–8).

Jones states that few people remain at a fixed point on either of the two continua; thus, a person's position on the illness-wellness continuum is always changing (Jones 1978, p. 1902).

Pender states that health and illness are qualitatively different (separate entities) but related concepts. Illness is represented as discrete life events that are barriers to health. However, poor health can exist without illness (Pender 1982, pp. 38–39).

Illness and Disease

Traditionally, medical practitioners have dealt with disease at a subsystem level. Subsystems are those aspects of the body subsumed in the larger system of the whole body. See systems theory in Chapter 10. A subsystem may be a cell, an organ, or an organ system. Only recently have medical practitioners started looking at the person as an entity, or whole. Nurses, by contrast, have traditionally viewed the person as an entity, i.e., nurses take a holistic view of people. Nurses today base practice on the multiple-causation theory of health problems (illness). For example, unemployment, pollution, life-style, and stressful events may all contribute to illness. These can be considered suprasystem problems, i.e., problems stemming from systems in which the individual is a subsystem. See Figure 2–9. Therefore, the concept of illness must include all aspects of the total person as well as the biologic and genetic factors that contribute to disease. Illness, then, is influenced by a person's family, social network, environment, and culture (Kneisl and Ames 1986, p. 18).

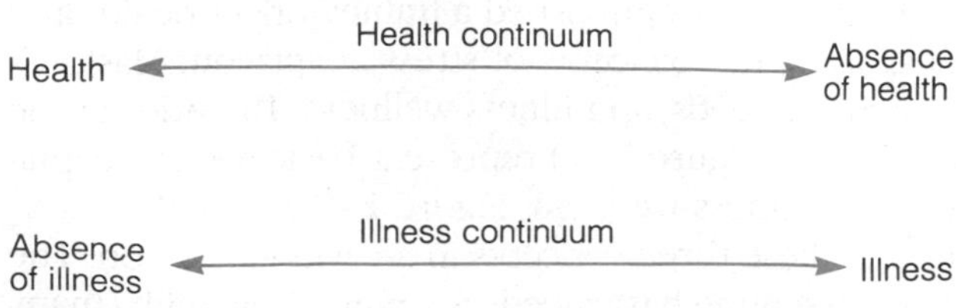

Figure 2–5 Jahoda's coexisting health and illness continua

Nontraditional Views of Health and Illness

There are a number of nontraditional views of health and illness. Some of these are influenced by culture, for example the "hot-cold" system of some Hispanic Americans. In this system, health is viewed as a balance of hot and cold qualities within a person. For example, citrus fruits

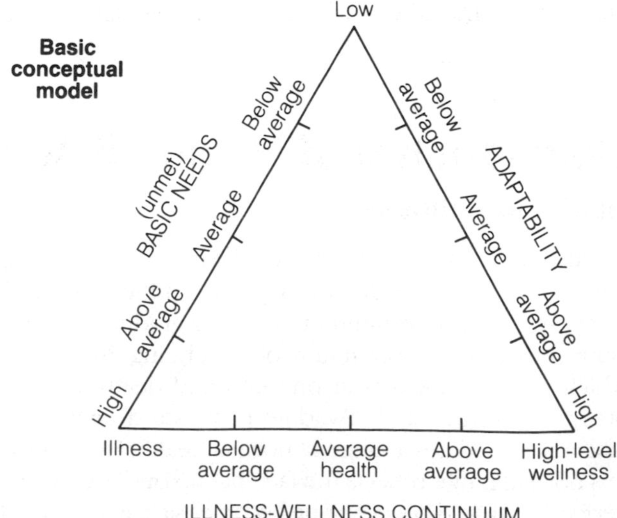

Figure 2–6 Jones's illness-wellness continuum: basic conceptual model

Source: P. S. Jones, An adaptation model for nursing practice, *American Journal of Nursing*, November 1978, 78:1901. Used by permission.

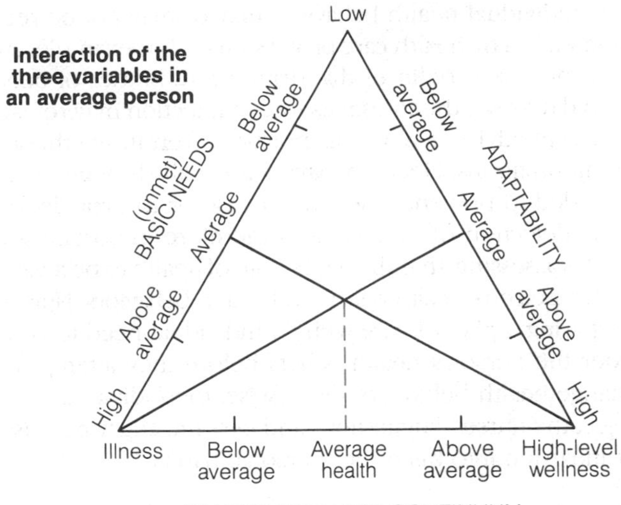

Figure 2–7 Jones's illness-wellness continuum: interaction of the three variables in an average person

Source: P. S. Jones, An adaptation model for nursing practice, *American Journal of Nursing*, November 1978, 78:1901. Used by permission.

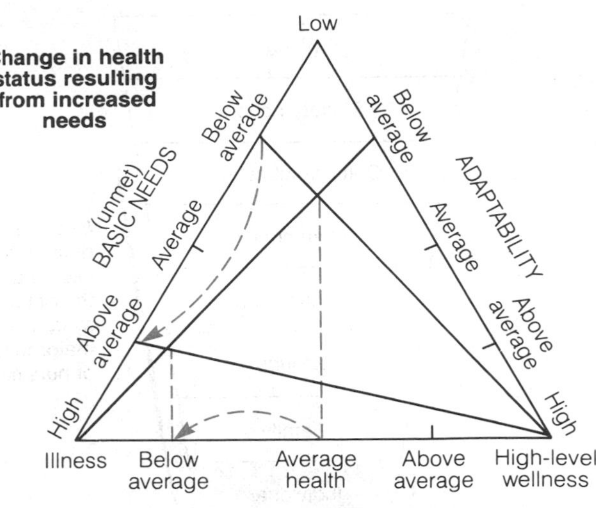

Figure 2–8 Jones's illness-wellness continuum: change in health status resulting from increased needs

Source: P. S. Jones, An adaptation model for nursing practice, *American Journal of Nursing*, November 1978, 78:1901. Used by permission.

and some fowl are cold foods, and meats and bread are hot foods. In this context, hot and cold do not denote temperature or spiciness but innate qualities of the food. For example, a fever is caused by an excess of hot foods. Another example of a nontraditional, culturally related health belief is the belief that health and illness are closely related to the amount and quality of blood in the body. For example, among some Southern whites and blacks, "high blood," caused by too much blood in the body, causes headaches and dizziness (Mitchell and Loustau 1981, pp. 41–42). For additional information about nontraditional views of health and illness, see Chapter 18.

Holistic Health

The **holistic health** model is based on the belief that the whole is more than the sum of its parts. When using a holistic health model, nurses consider an event's effect on the whole person. Illness is viewed as an opportunity for growth; health is a dynamic state of being that, for each individual, moves back and forth along a continuum. The extremes of the continuum in holistic health are highest health potential and death; good health, normal health, mild illness, illness or poor health, and critical illness are points along the continuum. See Figure 2–10.

In the holistic health model, wellness is ever-changing growth toward fulfilling an individual's potential, considering that individual's needs, abilities, and disabilities (McCann/Flynn and Heffron 1984, p. 33). A critical assumption in the holistic health model is that the perception of health is an individual decision, encouraging self-responsibility and self-control. Health can exist in the presence of illness. For example, a man who is partially paralyzed may perceive himself as being near or at the point of highest health potential along the highest health potential–death continuum if he feels he is functioning to his highest potential relative to his paralysis.

Health Beliefs and Behaviors

The **health status** (state) of an individual is the health of that person at a given time. In its general meaning, the term may refer to anxiety, depression, or acute illness and thus describes the individual as a whole: *health status* also can describe such specifics as pulse rate and body temperature. The **health beliefs** of an individual are those concepts about health that an individual believes true. Such beliefs may or may not be founded on fact. **Health**

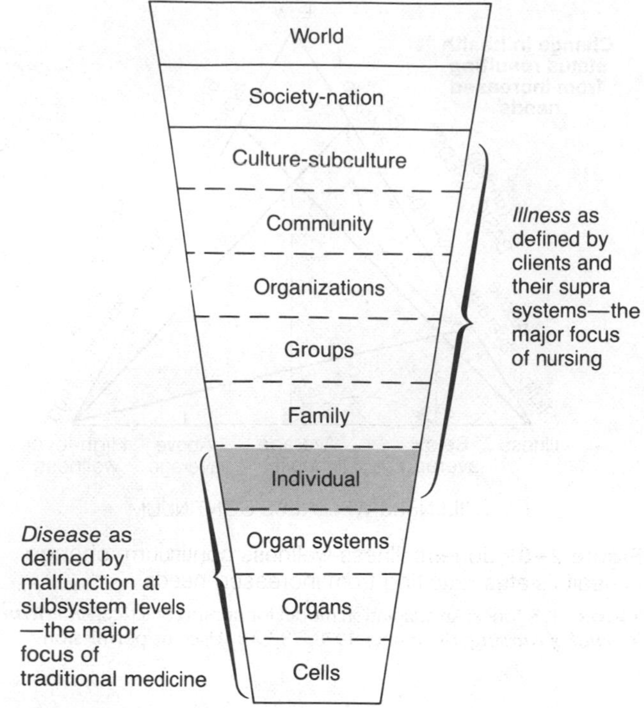

Figure 2–9 A systems hierarchy differentiating illness from disease and nursing from traditional medicine.

Source: Adapted from S. A. Ames et al., "A systems approach to curricula in primary health care nursing." In *Approaches to teaching primary health care* by Knopke/Diekelmann (eds.) St. Louis, Mosby © 1981.

behaviors are the actions a person takes to understand his or her health state, maintain an optimal state of health, prevent illness and injury, and reach his or her maximum physical and mental potential. Behaviors such as eating wisely, exercising, paying attention to signs of illness, following treatment advice, and avoiding known health hazards such as smoking are all examples. The ability to relax, emotional maturity, productivity, and self-expression also affect one's health (McCann/Flynn and Heffron 1984, p. 34).

Individual health behaviors may or may not be recommended by health care professionals. For example, an individual who believes that drinking 12 bottles of beer each day keeps the intestines free of infection may refuse to accept advice against this practice, even in life-threatening situations. Health behavior is usually thought of as intended to prevent illness or disease or to provide for early detection of disease. It is therefore important for nurses assessing an individual's state of health to be aware of that person's health beliefs and health behaviors. Nurses preparing a plan of care with an individual need to consider the person's health beliefs before they attempt to change health behaviors. Otherwise, the individual may reject the nurses' suggestions and become angry because of intrusion into his or her personal habits.

Variables Affecting Health

Multiple variables influence a person's health status. Some of these are internal factors, such as the person's genetic makeup, and others are external, such as the person's culture and physical environment (Grasser and Craft 1984, pp. 210–11; Leddy and Pepper 1985, pp. 160–65; Murray and Zentner 1985, pp. 12–19).

Genetic Makeup

Genetic makeup influences biologic characteristics, innate temperament, activity level, and intellectual potential. It has been related to susceptibility to specific diseases, such as diabetes and breast cancer.

Race

Disease distribution is associated with race. For example, blacks have a higher incidence of sickle-cell anemia and hypertension than the general population, and native American Indians have a higher rate of diabetes.

Sex

Certain acquired and genetic diseases are more common in one sex than in the other. Disorders more common

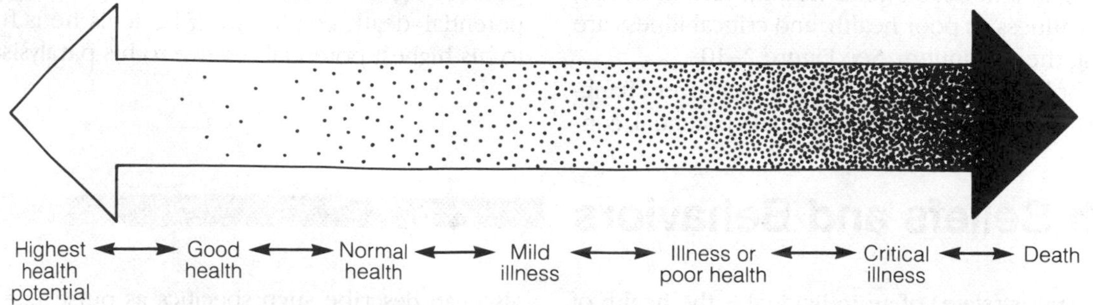

Figure 2–10 A health-illness continuum representing the holistic health model

Source: Adapted from J. B. McCann/Flynn, and P. B. Heffron, *Nursing: From concept to practice* (Bowie, Md.: Robert J. Brady Co., 1984), p. 34. Reprinted with permission of Robert J. Brady Co., Bowie, Maryland.

among females are osteoporosis; autoimmune disease, such as rheumatoid arthritis and systemic lupus erythematosus; anorexia nervosa and bulimia; diabetes mellitus; gallbladder disease; asthma; obesity; and thyroid disease. Those more common among males are stomach ulcers, abdominal hernias, respiratory diseases, arteriosclerotic heart disease, hemorrhoids, and tuberculosis. Obviously, diseases that affect reproductive organs, such as testicular or uterine tumors, are sex dependent.

Age and Developmental Level

Distribution of diseases varies with age. For example, arteriosclerotic heart disease is common in middle-aged males but occurs infrequently in younger persons; such communicable diseases as whooping cough and measles are common in children but are rare in older persons, who have acquired immunity to them. Developmental level is also a significant factor. Capabilities to respond to disease are less during the first few years of life and near the end of life. Infants lack physiologic and psychologic maturity. Declining physical and sensory-perceptual abilities in older persons limit their ability to respond to environmental hazards and stressors.

Mind-Body Relationship

Mind-body relationships—i.e., how emotional responses to stress affect body function and what emotional reactions occur in response to body conditions—also influence health. Emotional distress may increase susceptibility to organic disease or precipitate it. Emotional distress may influence the immune system through central nervous system and endocrine alterations. Alterations in the immune system are related to the incidence of infections, cancer, and autoimmune diseases. Increasing attention is being given to the mind's ability to direct the body's functioning. Relaxation, meditation, and biofeedback techniques are gaining wider recognition by individuals and health care professionals. (**Biofeedback** is the conscious control of physiologic responses under the control of the autonomic nervous system, such as heart rate and blood pressure.)

Life-Style

A person's life-style includes his or her patterns of eating; exercise; use of tobacco, drugs, and alcohol; and methods of coping with stress. Overeating, getting insufficient exercise, and being overweight are closely related to the incidence of heart disease, arteriosclerosis, diabetes, and hypertension. Excessive sugar intake increases the risk of dental caries. Abuse of drugs and alcohol is physically and mentally debilitating. Excessive use of tobacco is clearly implicated in lung cancer, emphysema, and cardiovascular diseases. See Chapter 19 for additional information.

Physical Environment

Housing and sanitation facilities affect health. Air, food, and water pollutants are often directly or indirectly related to various types of cancer. Extreme fluctuations in environmental temperature cause temporary disruptions in a person's internal environment, and the person in such an environment must expend more energy to restore physiologic stability. Persons with minimal physical coping responses are more susceptible to the effects of hypothermia and hyperthermia.

Seasonal variations also affect health and the incidence of certain illnesses. For example, drownings and insect bites occur more frequently in the summer, whereas allergic reactions occur more frequently when pollen and related allergens are present.

Standards of Living

Occupation, income, and education, which are major determinants of social class, are related to health, morbidity, and mortality. Hygiene, food habits, and the propensity to seek health care advice and follow health regimens vary among high- and low-income groups. For example, preventing illness is often not as crucial to the poor as generating and maintaining an income; they cannot afford regular medical examinations, housing, or nutritious foods that promote health. More affluent people may fulfill stressful social or occupational roles that predispose them to stress-related diseases. Such roles may also encourage overeating or social use of drugs or alcohol. Some occupational roles predispose people to certain illnesses. For instance, some industrial workers may be exposed to carcinogenic agents.

Culture

How a person perceives, experiences, and copes with health and illness is partly determined by his or her cultural beliefs. Some people may perceive home remedies or tribal health customs as superior and more dependable than the health care practices of North American society, whether or not one is more beneficial than the other. Cultural rules, values, and beliefs give people a sense of being stable and able to predict outcomes. The challenging of old beliefs and values by second-generation ethnic groups may give rise to conflict, instability, and insecurity, in turn contributing to illness.

Family

In addition to transmitting genetic predispositions, the family passes on patterns of daily living and life-styles to offspring. Physical or emotional abuse may cause long-term health problems. Emotional health depends on a social environment that is free of excessive tension and that does not isolate the person from others—a climate of open communication, sharing, and love that fosters the fulfillment of the person's optimum potential.

Self-Concept

Whether a person feels positively or negatively about self affects how that person perceives and handles situations. A person with a negative self-concept may behave according to the expectations of others rather than as he or she desires. Such attitudes can affect health practices and the times when treatment is sought. A sense of extreme hopelessness, despair, or fear may cause disease and even death. An example is the anorexic woman who deprives herself of needed nutrients because she believes she is too fat even though she is well below an acceptable weight level.

Support Network

Having a confidant, friend, or support people and job satisfaction helps people avoid illness (Grasser and Craft 1984, p. 210). Support people also help the person confirm that illness exists. Persons with inadequate support networks sometimes allow themselves to become increasingly ill before confirming the illness and seeking therapy. Support people also provide the stimulus for an ill person to become well again.

Geographic Area of Residence

Geography determines climate, and climate affects health. For instance, malaria and malaria-connected conditions, e.g., sickle-cell hemoglobin, occur more frequently in tropical than temperate climates (Overfield 1985, p. 84). Multiple sclerosis is more prevalent in northern and central Europe, southern Canada, and the northern United States, for example, than in Asia, Africa, Mexico, and Alaska (Overfield 1985, p. 127).

Factors Influencing Health Behavior

Some factors affecting health status also affect health behavior; cultural and family influences are two examples. However, people can usually control their health behaviors and can choose healthy or unhealthy activities. In contrast, people have little or no choice over their genetic makeup, age, sex, physical environments, culture, or area of residence. This section outlines the factors that affect a person's health beliefs and behavior.

In the 1950s, Rosenstock proposed a health belief model intended to predict which individuals would or would not use such preventive measures as screening for early detection of cancer. Becker modified the health belief model to include these components: individual perceptions, modifying factors, and variables likely to affect initiating action.

The health belief model is based on motivational theory. Rosenstock assumed that good health is an objective common to all people. Becker added "positive health motivation" as a consideration. Pender (1975) modified the health belief model by adding two further considerations: the importance of health as perceived by the individual and perceived control. See Figure 2–11. Pender believes that preventive well-being (health) behavior occurs in two stages: decision making and action.

Individual Perceptions

Individual perceptions include:

1. The importance of health to the person. Behavior that indicates health is perceived as something of value and includes providing special foods and vitamins to keep children well, having regular dental checkups, and participating in screening tests for cervical cancer, breast cancer, and cardiovascular disorders.
2. Perceived control. People who perceive that they have control over their own health are more likely to use preventive services than people who feel powerless. People who are internally controlled view themselves as less vulnerable to ill health (Pender 1982, p. 57). Control over health can relate to such behaviors as not smoking, maintaining an appropriate weight, using seat belts, or obtaining immunizations for influenza.
3. Perceived threat of a specific disease. For example, a man who perceives that many people around him have influenza is more likely to modify his behavior than a man who perceives that most of the people with influenza live in another city.
4. Perceived susceptibility. A family history of a certain disorder, such as diabetes or heart disease, may make the individual feel he or she is at high risk.
5. Perceived seriousness. The question here is: In the perception of the individual, does the illness cause death or have serious consequences?
6. Perceived benefits of preventive action. For example, many individuals correctly perceive that not smoking may have beneficial outcomes.
7. Perceived value of early detection. This perception can motivate the person to have screening tests and regular physical or dental examinations.

Modifying Factors

Factors that modify a person's perceptions include:

1. Demographic variables such as age, sex, and race. An infant, for example, does not perceive the importance

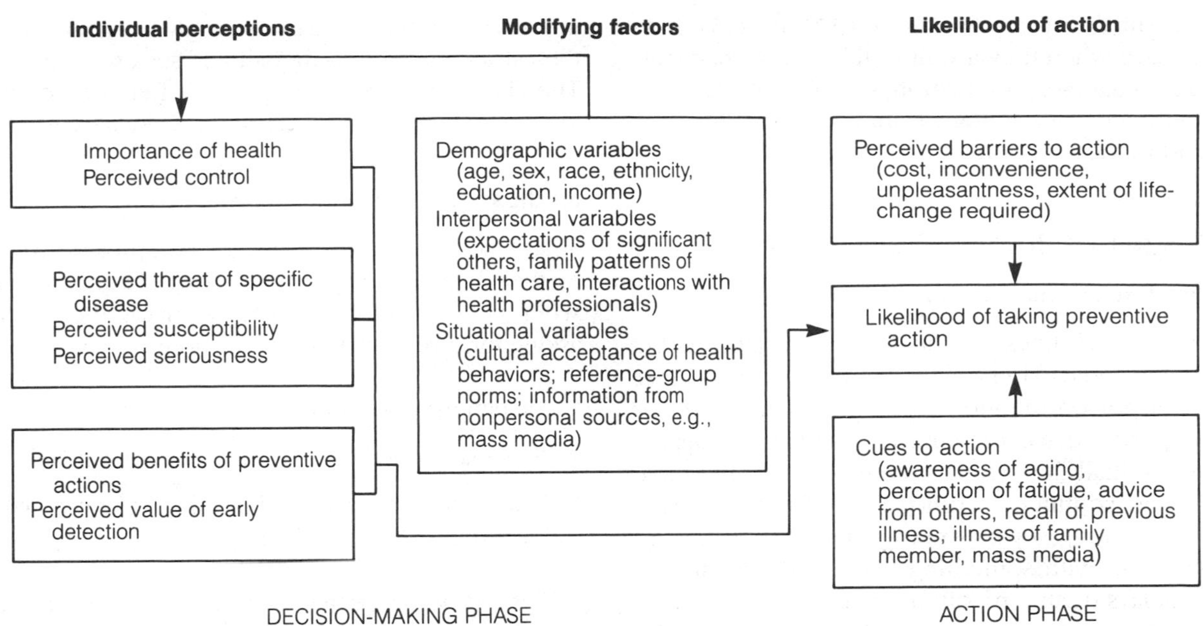

Figure 2–11 Pender's modifications to the health belief model

Source: N. J. Pender, *Health promotion in nursing practice* (Norwalk, Conn.: Appleton-Century-Crofts, 1982). Reproduced with permission.

of a healthy diet; an adolescent may perceive peer approval as more important than family approval and participate as a consequence in hazardous activities or adopt unhealthy eating and sleeping patterns.

2. Interpersonal variables. These include concern of significant others, family patterns of health care (e.g., the members of a family may have dental examinations every 6 months), and interactions with health professionals who are likely to provide information and encourage preventive behavior.

3. Situational variables. These include the cultural acceptance of specific health-related behaviors. For example, in some cultures it is considered inappropriate to seek medical advice unless one is seriously ill. Societal norms also influence behavior. For example, a group may convey disapproval when a person drives an automobile after drinking alcohol. Another situational factor that modifies behavior is information from nonpersonal sources, such as newspapers or television broadcasts, which can affect health behavior positively or negatively.

Likelihood of Action

Perceived barriers to action can include cost, inconvenience, unpleasantness, and life-style changes. By contrast, certain cues may trigger action. Such cues may be external or internal, e.g., a birthday may make a person realize that he or she is now at greater risk of developing a particular disease. If the cues are too strong, anxiety can inhibit action rather than encourage it (Pender 1975, p. 388).

Nurses play a major role during the decision-making and action phases. During decision making, nurses help clients monitor health, supply anticipatory guidance, and impart knowledge about health. During the action phase, nurses can reduce barriers to action, e.g., by minimizing inconvenience or discomfort. They can also support preventive actions. For additional information about nursing activities that promote health, see Chapter 20.

Stages of Illness

Various scientists have described the stages of illness. Suchman (1972, p. 145) describes 5 stages, and Igun (1979) describes 11 stages. By knowing these stages and the illness behaviors that accompany them, nurses can better understand their clients' behavior and determine ways to assist them.

Illness behavior is "any activity undertaken by a person who feels ill, to define the state of his health and to discover a suitable remedy" (Igun 1979, p. 445). How people behave when they are ill is affected by many variables, such as age, sex, occupation, socioeconomic status, religion, ethnicity, psychologic stability, personality, education, and modes of coping.

Five Stages of Illness (Suchman)

Symptom Experience Stage

The first stage of illness is the transition stage during which people come to believe something is wrong. Either a significant person mentions that they look unwell, or people experience some symptoms, which can appear insidiously. Initially, individuals often go through a phase of denial and continue to function as if they felt well. During this period, they may not want to bother the family or physician with something that seems trivial. This behavior delays treatment, often unwisely.

The symptom experience stage has three aspects: the physical experience of symptoms, such as pain or high temperature; the cognitive aspect, i.e., interpretation of the symptoms in terms that have some meaning to the person; and the emotional response of fear or anxiety.

During this stage, unwell persons usually consult others close to them about their symptoms or feelings. People validate with their spouses or support persons, for example, that the symptoms are real, and obtain support to seek a professional person's advice. At this stage, sick persons sometimes try home remedies, such as laxatives or cough medicines.

Assumption of the Sick Role

The second stage signals acceptance of the illness. At this time, individuals decide that their symptoms or concerns are sufficiently severe to suggest that they are sick. They seek confirmation of the illness from family and friends and then assume the sick role, discussed later in this chapter. Some people seek professional help quickly; others continue self-treatment, often following the suggestions of family and friends.

In this stage, sick people are usually afraid, but they now accept that they are ill even though they may not be able to accept the possible reasons. In conferring with people close to them, sick persons seek not only advice but also support for the decision to give up some activities and, for example, stay home from work.

At the end of this stage, sick persons experience one of two outcomes. They may find that the symptoms have changed and that they feel better. Still, they seek confirmation of improvement from the family; if family members support the perceptions of such persons, they are no longer considered or consider themselves sick. Then the recovered persons resume normal obligations, such as returning to work or attending a school concert. If, however, the symptoms persist or increase and if lack of improvement is validated by the family or significant others, then sick people know they should seek some treatment. The choice of a treatment plan is often affected by the known available alternatives and previous experience.

Medical Care Contact Stage

Sick persons seek the advice of a health professional either on their own initiative or at the urging of significant others. When people go for professional advice, they are really asking for three types of information:

1. Validation of real illness
2. Explanation of the symptoms in understandable terms
3. Reassurance that they will be all right or prediction of what the outcome will be

If the health professional does not validate illness, persons have two recourses: to return to normal activities or to seek other advice. If the symptoms disappear, people often perceive that they really are not ill. If symptoms continue, people usually return to the health professional or go to a second person for care. People who are repeatedly told that they are not ill may seek out quasi-practitioners as a last resort to alleviate the perceived symptoms. Some people will go from health professional to health professional until they find someone who provides a diagnosis that fits their own perceptions.

Most people also want an understandable explanation of their symptoms. When symptoms are not explained, people may assume the health professional does not believe them or perhaps that they are imagining the symptoms. Overly technical explanations, however, often confuse and frighten people.

People often experience anxiety about seeking help with health problems. Even minor symptoms can be construed as serious. Therefore, the client needs reassurance that he or she will be cured. Even when this reassurance cannot be given, most people want to know the likely outcome.

Dependent Patient Role Stage

When a health professional has validated that the person is ill, the individual becomes a patient, dependent on the professional for help. During this stage, sick persons may or may not be reluctant to accept a professional's recommendations. They may vacillate about what is best for them and alternately accept and reject the professional's suggestions. People vary greatly in the degree of ease with which they can give up their independence, particularly in relation to life and death. Role obligations—such as those of wage earner, father, mother, student, baseball team member, or choir member—complicate the decision to give up independence. It is also common for the client and the health professional to hold different notions of the nature of the illness, unless complete and open communication exists. During this stage, a nurse can often provide information that may allay some fears and/or provide data that support the person. Misconceptions can result from limited information, which clients interpret in the light of their experiences. For example, a client may be told by a physician that there is a small encapsulated growth in the right groin and that surgical removal is advised. If the individual's mother died after being told she had a growth in her breast, the person may assume that he or she also will die.

Most people accept their dependence on the physician, although they retain varying degrees of control over their own lives. For example, some people request precise information about their diseases, their treatment, and the cost of treatment, and they delay the decision to accept treatment until they have all this information. Others prefer that the physician proceed with treatment and do not request additional information.

During this period, sick persons often become more passive and accepting. They require a predictable environment in which people are genuinely concerned about them. In addition to being concerned about themselves, some sick people regress to an earlier behavioral stage in their development. As a result, they may have fewer **coping mechanisms** (physical and emotional adaptive or defensive abilities). Frequently reactions are related to previous experiences and to misconceptions about what will happen.

Children are accustomed to being dependent for some of their needs, although dependence varies with age and home situation. Since 1-year-old children are accustomed to being bathed and fed, this assistance is not a major adjustment when they are ill. Adults, however, are usually unaccustomed to this assistance, and they may find it difficult to relinquish independence and accept such help even when it is necessary. People have varying dependence needs. For some, illness may meet dependence needs that have never been met and thus provide satisfaction. Other people have minimal dependence needs and do everything possible to return to independent functioning. A few may even try to maintain independence to the detriment of their recovery.

Nurses need to assess the dependence needs of their clients and relate these to needs normally appropriate for their developmental stages. See Chapters 23 through 26. Client behaviors that support independent functioning need to be encouraged once the person is ready. Thus, nurses can assist clients to develop new ways of coping and decrease unhealthy dependence on others.

Recovery or Rehabilitation Stage

During the fifth stage, the client learns to give up the sick role and return to former roles and functions. For people with acute illnesses, the time as an ill person is generally short, and recovery is usually rapid. Thus they find it relatively easy to return to their former life-styles. People who have long-term illnesses and who must make adjustments in life-style find recovery more difficult. Recovery is particularly difficult for people who have to relearn skills such as walking or talking.

During this stage, readiness for social functioning often lags behind physical functioning. People may be physically able to go out to dinner but find that functioning socially is still too stressful.

Nurses can assist clients to function with increasing independence by planning with them those functions they can accomplish by themselves and those with which they need assistance. It is also important that nurses convey an attitude of hope and support. Each person, even an infant, needs hope and support to return to health.

Eleven Stages of Illness (Igun)

Igun's sequential stages vary in duration, and some may occur simultaneously.

1. *Symptoms experience.* Much like Suchman's first stage, this stage has four steps:
   a. Experiencing the actual symptoms, e.g., pain
   b. Becoming aware that there may be a problem
   c. Giving a label and meaning to the symptoms
   d. Responding with fear or anxiety

   Several factors affect how a person judges the seriousness of the symptoms: the degree to which they interfere with normal activity, the meaning of illness to the client, the client's tolerance of the symptoms, the familiarity and seriousness of the symptoms, the client's assumptions about the cause and prognosis, the speed with which the symptoms change, and other stressors in the person's life (Twaddle 1977, pp. 125–27).

2. *Self-treatment.* Often people try to treat themselves, particularly if they perceive the symptoms as not serious. Even a person who fears the symptoms are serious may deny their seriousness and hope that they will go away with certain self-treatment.

3. *Communication to significant others.* People often confide their symptoms to support persons, significant others, or health professionals. Pratt found that the poor are less likely to use personal health services than people of higher socioeconomic groups (Pratt 1971). Recent studies also indicate that two-thirds to three-quarters of all people with existing disorders remain untreated (Zola 1979, p. 85).

4. *Assessment of symptoms.* This assessment may be made by the individual, support persons, or a health care professional.

5. *Assumption of the sick role.* At this point, the person has accepted the illness, has been declared sick, and has accepted the sick role.

6. *Expression of concern.* During this stage, support persons and friends offer sympathy and express concern. Some people may recommend practitioners to their sick friend.
7. *Assessment of probable efficacy of treatment or appropriateness of treatment sources.* People who are ill may assess the variety of treatments available. A number of variables may affect this assessment, including previous experience and availability of information.
8. *Selection of a treatment plan.* A treatment plan may be selected with or without the advice of a health professional. Such factors as cost, time, knowledge, and effects are often involved in this selection. In many instances, the person accepts the recommendations of the health professional.
9. *Implementation of treatment.*
10. *Evaluation of the effects of the treatment.* The possible outcomes of treatment include full recovery, eventual recovery with a change in treatment, recovery with some disability, and no recovery. Sometimes people have unrealistic expectations, and health care professionals may need to help keep the expectations of clients similar to those of the caregiver. It is important for the health professional to remember that people have a right to reject or terminate treatment.
11. *Recovery and rehabilitation.* The return to usual social roles can be gradual or abrupt, depending on the person, the illness, and the interaction of the two.

Sick Role Behavior

Sick role behavior is "the activity undertaken by those who consider themselves ill, for the purpose of getting well (Igun 1979, p. 455). Parsons (1964, pp. 436–37) describes four aspects of the sick role:

1. Clients are not held responsible for their condition.
2. Clients are excused from certain social roles and tasks.
3. Clients are obliged to try to get well as quickly as possible.
4. Clients or their families are obliged to seek competent help.

In North America, people have traditionally not been held responsible for incurring an illness. Illness, though undesirable, is seen as beyond a person's control. Some subcultures view illness as punishment from God, and therefore consider the infirm responsible for their illnesses, because of their sins. This folk belief persists to some degree in American society. Often a client says, "What have I done to deserve this?" This remark reflects a sense that illness is a punishment. Today, people are being held increasingly responsible for some illnesses, for example, the cardiac patient who smokes or the overweight person who develops diabetes. Life-styles are being related to illness and disease (U.S. DHHS 1985, p. 17).

Nurses can help clients in the sick roles by providing factual information and not judging the client. It is important not to reinforce behaviors that exacerbate or may have helped bring about an illness and to encourage behaviors that promote health.

The sick person is also excused from some normal duties. This is true whether the person has a cold or requires surgery. Social pressures on the sick and people's expectations of the sick usually depend on the prognosis and the severity of the illness. People who are severely ill and whose prognosis is poor or uncertain are permitted more dependence than people who are less seriously ill. People who are not seriously ill and whose prognosis is good are more likely to be encouraged to fulfill personal and social responsibilities. The person with a cold may still be expected to give a scheduled speech or to take an examination. People who are chronically ill may be permanently exempted from some duties or activities by society; for example, the father confined to bed is not expected to attend his daughter's field hockey games. In this situation, arrangements are usually made in the family for another person to fulfill the father's role while he is unable to do so.

Some people may express feelings of guilt because they are unable to fulfill their normal responsibilities. Nurses can express support to clients who cannot fulfill their perceived roles and help them substitute other appropriate activities, when desirable. For example, a young father who cannot play ball with his son may be able to help his son build a model airplane, thereby fulfilling the father's role in another way.

A third aspect of the sick role is the obligation of the person to get well as quickly as possible. The sick role is a dependent one, at least in some respects. The person who fears dependence may be threatened by assuming a sick role and having to seek help. This individual might ignore advice despite the most serious consequences. Some people, however, find dependence gratifying. Some clients find dependence so satisfying that they perpetuate the sick role and do not try to get well or continue to complain of symptoms even after they are physically well. Some people in the dependent stage also find it satisfying to control others through excessive demands. With exceptions, people usually try to get well as quickly as possible.

Nurses can help clients assume a dependence appropriate to their developmental status and health. Part of the nurse's function is to reinforce both dependence and increasing independence at the appropriate times. For example, a man who is acutely ill may have to be shaved by the nurse; however, once he is stronger the nurse can assist him by providing shaving supplies and later complimenting him on his appearance.

The fourth aspect of the sick role is seeking competent help. This presupposes that competent help is available to the client. It should also be recognized that the client's notion of competent help may be different from the general population's. For example, a man with a whiplash injury may become dissatisfied with his physician's treatment because of his slow recovery and may go to a healer who uses hypnotism. Or a domineering, talkative woman may reject advice to see a therapist and decide instead to join a cult of young people, considering the members of the cult competent help.

Occasionally nurses need to encourage people to obtain competent help from health professionals. Nurses who are aware of the health facilities available in a community can assist people to obtain care. People may require considerable support before seeking assistance because, for example, they fear the health problem might be serious or they believe competent help might not be available. A nurse's function in these instances is to provide accurate information about available health facilities while recognizing clients' beliefs and their right to hold those views. For additional information on impaired role behavior, see Chapter 48.

Effects of Illness on Family Members

A person's illness affects the family or significant others. The kind of effect and its extent depend chiefly on three factors: which member of the family is ill, how serious and long the illness is, and what cultural and social customs that family holds.

The changes that can occur in the family include:

1. Role changes
2. Task reassignments
3. Increased stress due to anxiety about the outcome of the illness for the client and conflict about unaccustomed responsibilities
4. Financial problems
5. Loneliness as a result of separation and pending loss
6. Change in social customs

Each member of the family is affected differently, depending, for example, on whether a grandmother, the father of a nuclear family, or a teenager is ill. Each of these people plays a different role in the family, and each supports the family in different ways. Parents of young children, for example, have greater family responsibilities than parents of grown children.

The degree of change that family members experience is often related to their dependence on the sick person. For example, when a child is ill, there are few changes other than added responsibilities directly related to the child's illness. When the mother is ill, however, many changes are often necessary because other family members must assume her functions.

Sick Elderly Persons

When an elderly person is ill, a son or daughter often assumes the role of parent to the elderly person. Sons or daughters may find it necessary to provide housing, meals, and assistance with daily needs over a prolonged time. In other words, the parent-child roles are frequently reversed. This role reversal may be only temporary and may end when the illness ends, or it may become permanent. Since elderly people generally have few responsibilities, task reassignment is usually restricted to direct care for the sick person. The whole family, particularly the spouse of the sick person, experience stress and concern about the outcome of the illness. Younger persons in the family often deal with serious illness in an elderly person by stating, "He has led a good life" or "She had so much pain the past years." In this way, the young prepare themselves for that person's death. This same reasoning is rarely applied to a child or younger adult who is ill.

When an elderly person is ill, adult sons and daughters may face conflicting responsibilities. A daughter who lives some distance away needs to maintain her job and look after her own family, but at the same time her parents need her in another city. How often should she visit? How should she fulfill her responsibilities? These questions pose problems for a family living far apart.

The financial problems of the sick elderly can be a major problem for a family as well as a community. Because illness in this age group tends to be chronic, the costs of illness tend to be considerable.

Usually, the sick person's spouse feels a pending loss or separation most keenly. After a marriage of 50 or 60 years, elderly people find it difficult to envisage what life will be like without a husband or wife. Older people generally recognize that they are at the end of their lives, but separation and loneliness are prominent concerns. Grandchildren also experience anxiety about the outcome of a grandparent's illness, particularly if they have had long and pleasant ties. Primary ties are generally in the nuclear family (parents and children), however, and often the elderly person lives apart or in another city. When an elderly person is ill or hospitalized, the family life-style is minimally disrupted. The greatest change in life-style is that the family must now allot time for hospital visits to the elderly relative.

Sick Parents

When the sick person is a parent, the degree to which the family experiences change is related to the kinds of responsibilities the individual has and the number and age of dependents in the person's care. For example, when a father is ill for a long time, his roles are usually taken over by other members of the family, frequently the mother. Such tasks as doing chores in the house or attending a child's basketball games, for example, are either reassigned or not performed at all. Anxiety of family members about the outcome of a parent's illness is usually high, especially if the parent is the wage earner. The implications to the family of prolonged illness or death are great in almost all areas of living because of the needs of the dependents.

Prolonged illness of the mother can have equally serious consequences and be particularly disruptive if an outsider is employed to perform tasks formerly carried out by the mother. Children, especially young ones, in this situation suffer a loss in affection and feel insecure when their mother is away or too ill to function as usual. Often the children do not understand why their mother is in the hospital, and they may feel lonely and unwanted. Sometimes the mother's functions are taken over by grandparents or by aunts and uncles as well as by the father. When a young mother has a serious illness of unknown outcome, the father and family face worrisome problems of how to manage over a long period of time. Most arrangements have financial implications and involve role changes for the father and children. In this situation, the father must become both father and mother and give up many of his normal social activities. The children may also need to assume more housekeeping functions.

Sick Children

Because a child is dependent on parents for so many daily needs, both sick children and their families need to make fewer role adjustments than sick adults and their families. Task reassignments are also generally minimal. Sometimes a younger sibling takes over a paper route for a sick brother or sister, and other members of the family share the sick child's chores.

All members of the family experience anxiety if the outcome of the illness is in doubt. A permanent disability has implications for schooling, earning a living, and future needs. Financial responsibility for chronic illness or a disability often can be a serious problem for young parents. Other children may feel neglected if an unusual amount of attention is given to the ill child. Husband and wife may also expend most of their energies visiting the hospital and have little time for each other. If extended, this situation can place great stress on a marriage.

When a child is admitted to the hospital, parents and siblings may experience some sense of loss; however, children usually continue with their daily activities, and there is minimal disruption in the home.

Effects of Hospitalization

Normal patterns of behavior generally change with illness; with hospitalization, the change can be even greater. Hospitalization usually disrupts a person's privacy, autonomy, life-style, roles, and economics.

Privacy

When a client enters a hospital or nursing facility, the loss of privacy is instantly obvious. **Privacy** has been described as a comfortable feeling reflecting a deserved degree of social retreat. Its dimensions and duration are controlled by the individual seeking the privacy. It is a personal, internal state that cannot be imposed from without (Schuster 1976, p. 245).

People need varying degrees of privacy and establish boundaries for privacy; when these boundaries are crossed, they feel invaded. Hospital personnel sometimes show little concern for clients' privacy. Clients are asked to provide information that often they consider private; they may share a room with strangers; and their health is frequently discussed with many health professionals.

The boundaries of privacy are highly individual. The adult who lives alone may be used to privacy while eating, sleeping, and reading. A child from a large family may be accustomed to sharing these activities with others. It is important for nurses to ascertain what privacy means to the individual and try to support accustomed practices whenever possible.

Autonomy

Autonomy is the state of being independent and self-directed without outside control. People vary in their sense of autonomy; some are accustomed to functioning independently in most of their life activities, while others are more accustomed to direction from others. An example of the former is a writer who lives alone and works independently. By contrast, a wife in a patriarchal home may be accustomed to having decisions made by her husband and receiving direction from him.

Hospitalized people frequently give up much of their autonomy. Decisions about meals, hygienic practices, and sleeping are frequently made for them. This loss of individuality is often difficult to accept, and the client may feel dehumanized into "just a piece of machinery."

Nurses have been trying to humanize care in recent years by learning about the client as a person and by individualizing nursing care plans.

Life-Style

Hospitalization marks a change in life-style. Many hospitals determine when people wake up and when they sleep. The woman who normally rises at 8:00 A.M. and the man who usually works until 11:00 P.M. must change their habits. Food in a hospital is usually mass produced, and individual differences in taste are not always accommodated. Occasionally hospitals have relatively large populations from a particular culture and make special food arrangements, for example, a Chinese menu for traditional Chinese patients or Kosher foods for traditional Jewish patients. However, individual preferences are often not met.

Nurses can help clients adapt to life in a hospital by:

1. Making arrangements wherever possible to accommodate the client's life-style, such as providing a bath in the evening rather than in the morning
2. Providing explanations about hospital routines
3. Encouraging other health professionals to become aware of the person's life-style and to support healthy aspects of that life-style
4. Reinforcing desirable changes in practices with a view to making them a permanent part of the client's life-style

Roles

People's life roles frequently change when they are hospitalized. A man or woman may no longer be the wage earner; parents may be unable to fulfill normal parental responsibilities.

Economics

Hospitalization often places a genuine financial burden on clients and their families. Even though many people have health insurance, it may not reimburse all costs; in addition, many lose wages while they are hospitalized.

Nurses can be aware of these costs and provide care that is as economical as is safely possible; for instance, they can use only the minimum supplies necessary for safe care. Nurses also can support activities that promote health and that return clients to their normal activities as soon as possible.

Health Care Compliance

Compliance is the extent to which a person's behavior coincides with health practitioners' advice (Yoos 1981, p. 27). Shillinger states that "*compliance, adherence,* and *therapeutic alliance* are terms that, when used in a health care context, refer to the process whereby a patient assumes the various tasks that comprise a therapeutic regimen" (Shillinger 1983, p. 58). In Shillinger's view, *compliant* has overtones of coercion; *adherent* connotes conformance to some standard set by another. When the person forms an alliance, the implication is that the individual has negotiated the steps to be taken to care for himself or herself.

Clients' compliance with health care advice is of concern to all health professionals. Studies by Davis (1968) indicate that at least one-third of clients fail to follow a physician's recommendations. Yoos reports that 86% of studies of compliance report noncompliance in more than 30% of clients (Yoos 1981, p. 27). Compliance can be complete, partial, or nonexistent.

A **complier** is a person who follows a therapeutic regimen, a **noncomplier** is a person who does not. The concept of compliance is not as simple as it first appears because people have the legal right to refuse treatment, e.g., not to take prescribed medications or to rest as suggested. In addition, one's viewpoint of humans affects how one approaches compliance. Increasingly, nurses are approaching compliance with the belief that "man is capable of self-determination of goals and that in order to do this he must have a body of knowledge upon which to base his choices" (Yoos 1981, p. 29).

Whether a person complies to a therapeutic regimen depends on many variables, among them age, education, costs, the complexity of the regimen and its convenience, the individual's value of health, and the inconvenience of the illness. Trekas writes that a person's sense of control or lack of control over his or her life can influence compliance. A person who is health oriented is likely to adopt habits to promote good health and accept a regimen that will restore good health. People who see illness as a sign of weakness may deny the illness or the presence of disease. Such denial can account for noncompliance (Trekas 1984, p. 58).

In 1974, Becker published a sick role model to explain how people react to illness and to predict whether they will comply with health care advice (Becker 1974). See Figure 2–12. Becker's model indicates that compliance is related to clients' motivation to become well, the value they place on reducing the threat of illness, and their belief that compliance will reduce that threat. Modifying and enabling factors of people's behavior include age, structural factors (e.g., cost, duration, attitudes of health care personnel, and interaction with health care personnel), and enabling factors (e.g., previous health care and source of advice). One can use these, Becker believes, to anticipate compliance with health care regimens (Becker 1974).

Locus of Control

Locus of control is a concept from social learning theory. It is also relevant when determining who is most likely to take action regarding health, i.e., whether clients believe that their health status is under their own or others' control. People who believe that they have a major influence on their own health status, i.e., who believe health is largely self-determined, are called *internals*. By contrast, people who believe their health is largely controlled by outside forces, e.g., chance, are referred to as *externals*.

Locus of control is a measurable concept that can be used to predict which people are most likely to change their behavior. There are a number of scales, including the Health Locus of Control (HLC) scale developed by Wallston, Wallston, Kaplan, and Maides in 1976. This scale is intended to provide sensitive predictions of a person's

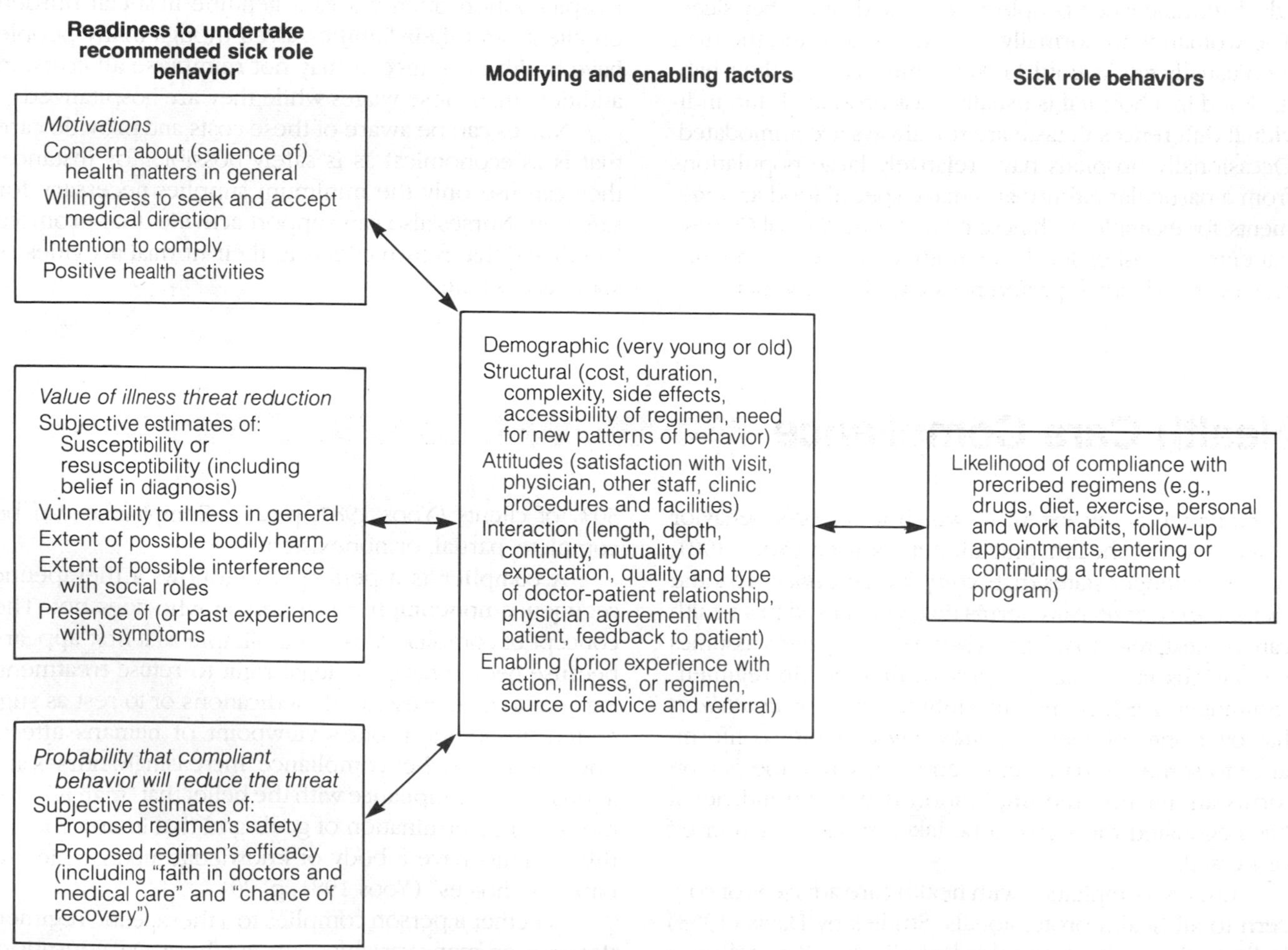

Figure 2–12 Sick role model

Source: Modified from M. H. Becker, The health belief model and sick role behavior. In M. H. Becker, editor, *The health belief model and personal health behavior* (Thorofare, N.J.: Charles B. Slack, 1974). Reprinted with permission.

locus orientation and health behaviors. It is thought that internally controlled people tend to be more assertive and are more likely to change their behavior patterns. Edelman and Mandle (1986, p. 53) suggest that externally controlled people may need assistance to become more internally controlled if behavior changes are to be successful.

The results of a study by Lewis suggest that greater personal control over one's life is associated with higher levels of self-esteem, greater purpose in life, and decreased self-report of anxiety (Lewis 1982, p. 113). Nurses can use this information about a client's locus of control to plan internal reinforcement training if necessary in order to improve client compliance. However, according to Shillinger (1983, p. 63):

> Greater emphasis should be placed on assisting the client to make his own informed decisions, helping to identify and find solutions to problems that may interfere with compliance, and giving support and guidance as needed. In essence, this means building a partnership, an alliance, with the client rather than having compliance as the major goal.

For further information on locus of control, see Chapter 20, page 433, and Chapter 29, page 611.

Enhancing Compliance

Researchers have investigated why some people comply with therapeutic regimens and others do not and how to help clients comply with therapeutic regimens. The first step is identifying noncompliance. The nurse can ask the client if he or she is following the regimen. If the client is not complying, the nurse needs to find out why. Some reasons for noncompliance have been discussed earlier. To enhance compliance, nurses can:

1. Demonstrate caring. The nurse can do so by showing sincere concern about the client's problems and decisions and at the same time accepting the client's right to a course of action. For example, a nurse might tell a client who is not taking his heart medication, "I can appreciate how you feel about this, but I am very concerned about your heart."
2. Encourage healthy behaviors through positive reinforcement. If the man who is not taking his heart medication is walking every day, the nurse might say, "You are really doing well with your walking."
3. Establish why the client is not following the regimen and where indicated provide information, correct misconceptions, attempt to decrease expense, or suggest counseling if psychologic problems are interfering with compliance.
4. Use aids to reinforce teaching. For instance, the nurse can leave pamphlets for the client to read later or make a "pill calendar," a paper with the date and number of pills to be taken.
5. Establish a relationship of freedom, mutual understanding, and mutual responsibility with the client and support persons. By providing knowledge, skills, and information, the nurse gives clients control over their health and establishes a cooperative relationship, which results in greater compliance (MacElveen-Hoehn 1983, p. 535).

Client contracts enhance compliance. A **client contract** is a written agreement between a client and a nurse regarding a behavior change. It is intended to improve client compliance through positive reinforcement: Behavior that has positive consequences is likely to be repeated (Steckel 1982, p. 493). For example, a client who feels tired most of the time but exercises very little might begin exercising by walking a mile each day. The client and the nurse agree and sign a contract regarding the walking, and the client keeps a record of the walking and sees the nurse regularly about the exercise. The client also chooses a reward, e.g., a book, another appointment time with the nurse, or a free pass to a concert.

Here is a sample client contract:

> I, Amy Martin, will walk one mile each day, keep a record of my walking, and bring the record to the clinic in return for two passes to a concert.
>
> Amy Martin (client)
> Heather Hughes (nurse)
> April 28, 19—

Health and Illness: Patterns and Trends

The health of North Americans is steadily improving. Probable reasons for this improvement are:

1. Earlier preventive efforts based on new knowledge obtained through research.
2. Improvements in sanitation, housing, nutrition, and immunization essential to disease prevention.
3. Individual measures to promote health and prevent disease. For example, increasing attention is being paid to exercise, nutrition, environmental health, and occupational health.

Four of the major risk factors responsible for illness and premature deaths cited by the surgeon general (U.S. DHEW 1979, pp. 7–8) are:

1. *Cigarette smoking.* This is clearly identified as a cause of most cases of lung cancer and a major factor increasing the risk of heart attacks.
2. *Alcohol and drug abuse.* Consumption of alcohol and drugs, even among youths, has grown substantially since the 1960s and accounts for significant illness, disability, and death.
3. *Injuries.* The highest death rate from accidents occurs among the elderly, but it is also substantial among those aged 15 to 24. Injuries from accidents may be caused by motor vehicles, firearms, falls, burns, poisons, recreational activities, and adverse drug reactions.
4. *Occupational risks.* Certain occupational hazards, such as exposure to asbestos, rubber, and plastic, are now being identified as potential cancer risks.

All of these risks present challenges to health care workers, especially nurses, in terms of prevention. Measures to enhance health include elimination of cigarette smoking; moderation of alcohol consumption; safety measures, such as using seat belts, to prevent accidents and injuries; and periodic screening for such health problems as cancer.

Health Field Concept

In 1974 Lalonde, Canadian minister of national health and welfare, introduced the health field concept, which views all causes of death and disease as having four contributing elements: (a) human biologic factors, such as genetic makeup and age; (b) behavioral factors or unhealthy life-styles; (c) environmental hazards; and (d) inadequacies in the health care system (Canadian Department of National Health and Welfare 1974, pp. 31–34). Using these four elements as a framework, a group of United States experts devised a method to assess the relative contributions of each of these elements to the ten leading causes of death in 1976. The results indicated that approximately 50% of deaths were due to unhealthy behavior or life-style; 20% to human biologic factors; 20% to environmental factors; and 10% to inadequacies in health care (U.S. DHEW 1979, p. 9). These results have implications for nursing; the most important is that a substantial number of deaths could be avoided by efforts directed at health promotion.

Trends

Evidence of current health status and changes in the last few decades are measured in various ways. Measurements are made of longevity (life expectancy); the way people feel about their health; mortality rates and causes; morbidity rates and causes; the type of health behaviors people practice; and the amount and kind of health services used. Health services are discussed in Chapter 3. The following facts and statistics are derived from *Charting the Nation's Health: Trends Since 1960* (National Center for Health Statistics 1985b) unless otherwise indicated.

Longevity

In 1960, life expectancy at birth was about 70 years. By 1983, it reached nearly 75 years. Differences, however, exist between white and black people and between males and females. In 1982, life expectancy for white males was 71.5 years; for white females, 78.8 years; for black males, 64.9 years; and for black females, 73.5 years (National Center for Health Statistics 1985a, p. 2).

Feelings about Health

The way people feel about their health is one index of health status. Over the past several years, people of all ages have generally held the same perception of their health status. When asked, "Would you say your health is excellent, good, fair, or poor compared to other persons your age?" 87.3% of the population responded *good* or *excellent* in 1981; in 1973, 87.1% said the same. Moreover, in 1981, about 70% of elderly people living in the community perceived their health as good or excellent in relation to the health of their peers.

Mortality

The infant **mortality** (death) rate has reduced by over 50% since 1960. In 1982, the rate fell to 11.5 per 1000 live births from 26.0 per 1000 in 1960. This decline is attributed largely to advances in medical science related to newborn treatment, improved socioeconomic conditions, and increased availability of maternal and infant care services. Infant mortality rates, however, are still relatively high for certain groups; rates are higher for black babies and babies with unmarried mothers, teenage mothers, and mothers over 35 years of age.

The major causes of death in infants during the first 6 days of life are immaturity (low birth weights) and birth-associated events, such as lack of oxygen. Among infants 1 year and younger, the four most important causes of death are congenital malformations, sudden infant deaths, influenza and pneumonia, and accidents.

From 1960 to 1982, children 1 to 14 years of age had the lowest death rate of any age group. In 1983, only about 35 deaths occurred per 100,000 population. Accidents cause most deaths among children (U.S. DHHS 1985, p. 4).

According to the U.S. Department of Health and Human Services (1985), the death rate increases again in people aged 15 to 24, with motor vehicle accidents, homicides, and suicides as major causes of death. In 1982, homicide was the leading cause of death among young black males age 15 to 24 years, although the rates have declined from 108.2 per 100,000 population in 1971 to 72.0 per 100,000 in 1982. The suicide rate is higher among white males than among black males, black females, or white females. Although, overall, white male suicide rates have stabilized since 1977, the rate has increased among teenagers aged 15 to 19, from 15.1 per 100,000 in 1977 to 15.5 per 100,000 in 1982 (U.S. DHHS 1985, pp. 4–7). In Canada, motor vehicle accidents (3153 deaths), suicide (2885 deaths), and homicide (385 deaths) accounted for 6423 deaths in 1983 (Minister of Supply and Services 1985, p. 12).

In people older than 24 years, accidents, heart disease, and malignant neoplasms are the major causes of death, although the deaths due to stroke and heart disease declined between 1960 and 1982. Only death rates from cancer increased 11% (U.S. DHHS 1985, p. 10). The major causes of death in the general population are shown in Table 2–3.

Table 2–3 **Major Causes of Death in the United States in 1984**

Disease	Deaths per 100,000 Residents
Diseases of the heart	183.3
Malignant neoplasms	133.1
Accidents (including motor vehicle accidents)	35.6
Cerebrovascular diseases	33.9
Chronic obstructive pulmonary disease	18.0
Pneumonia and influenza	12.2
Suicide	11.6
Diabetes mellitus	9.9
Chronic liver disease	9.8
Homicide	8.2

Source: U.S. Department of Health and Human Services, *Health United States 1985* (Hyattsville, Md.: Public Health Service, DHHS Pub. no. (PHS) 86-1232, December 1985), p. 46.

Morbidity

Morbidity means illness; the morbidity rate is the ratio of sick to well people in a population. Morbidity statistics are more difficult to obtain than mortality statistics. Two ways to measure the illness of children is to determine (a) absenteeism from school and (b) changes in average heights and weights, since growth is characteristic of healthy, well-fed children. The number of school days lost because of acute illnesses was about the same in the early 1980s as it was in the early 1960s. Influenza outbreaks account for one-third of all absences from school. Little change occurred in the heights and weights of boys and girls 6 to 17 years of age from 1960 onward. A growing concern about the physical and mental health of children today is the growing divorce rate. In 1982, 1,108,000 children were involved in divorce, compared with 463,000 children in 1960 (U.S. DHHS 1985, pp. 5–6).

The health of adults can be measured by considering the days of work lost, bed-disability days, and restricted-activity days. The rates of absenteeism from work declined for both men and women since the mid 1970s, but women had higher absenteeism rates than men. The rate of restricted-activity days increased since the late 1960s, and there has been a slight increase in bed-disability days. Because this increase correlates with increased physician utilization, the increase may reflect earlier detection of illness and better health management. Many people may be limiting their activities at the onset of illness to prevent more serious health consequences (U.S. DHHS 1985, p. 7).

In midlife, illness, disability, and impairment pose more problems. Overweight and obesity are linked to adverse effects on longevity and health. In 1976 to 1980, approximately 25% of American adults between 25 to 74 years of age were overweight. More black women were overweight than white women or men of either race. About 60% of black women aged 45 to 74 were overweight in 1976 to 1980 (U.S. DHHS 1985, p. 9).

Of the three leading causes of death in late midlife—heart disease, cancer, and stroke—the rate of death from strokes declined 60% and the rate of death from heart disease 36% from 1960 to 1982. However, rates of death from cancer increased about 11%. Respiratory cancer was a major factor in the increased cancer death rates. Of interest is the fact that the rises in deaths from respiratory cancer are greater for females. Between 1979 and 1982, the rise in the rate of death for women 54 to 64 years of age was about 20%; for men, it was 3% (U.S. DHHS 1985, p. 10).

Despite some chronic disability or impairment, most elderly people in America live in the community and maintain households with varying degrees of help. Although the elderly population living in nursing homes increased by 88% from the early 1960s through the late 1970s, the major portion of this increase was accounted for by people 85 years of age and over (U.S. DHHS 1985, p. 11).

Health Behaviors

The number of cigarette smokers in America has declined since 1964 when the Surgeon General's first *Report on Smoking and Health* was released. The sharp rise in smoking among teenage females that occurred in the 1970s has been curbed. However, the ratio of male to female smokers was about equal in 1983, whereas in 1965 male smokers outnumbered female smokers by 150%. In addition, among people who smoke, the percent who smoke 25 or more cigarettes per day has been increasing (U.S. DHHS 1985, p. 17).

Dietary practices, especially those related to the consumption of saturated fats, have had notable effects on the health of people. Over the past 20 years, the mean serum cholesterol level of adults aged 20 to 74 years has declined for every age group for both men and women. High serum cholesterol levels are associated with heart attacks and strokes. Another indicator of positive health behavior relates to hypertension control. The proportion of people with hypertension who kept their blood pressure below the level of 160/95 mm Hg nearly doubled from 1960–1962 to 1976–1980. This is thought to be due in part to adherence to prescribed medication regimens (U.S. DHHS 1985, p. 18).

Implications for Nursing

The health indicators above have the following implications for nursing:

1. Increased prenatal maternal and infant care services to reduce factors contributing to low birth weight, such as inadequate nutrition, smoking, and alcohol consumption. Services are especially required for black mothers, teenage mothers, mothers over 35 years of age, and the babies of these mothers.
2. Early identification of problems that deprive the fetus of oxygen during labor and delivery, or prompt management of such problems when they do occur.
3. Instruction in accident prevention to parents of children aged 1 to 14 years.
4. Continued child care instruction about nutrition and other factors to maintain the present trends in height and weight averages.
5. Early detection of developmental disorders in infants and children.
6. Maintenance of immunization programs to prevent infectious diseases.
7. Promotion of measures to ensure optimal childhood development.
8. Increased emphasis on supportive emotional care for children of divorced parents.
9. Instruction to young adults about motor vehicle safety and coping strategies to reduce suicide and homicide rates. Particular emphasis needs to be directed to teenagers 15 to 19 years of age since the suicide rate in that group is increasing.
10. Improved screening programs to assist in the early identification of disease.
11. Improvement in life-styles to help individuals avoid major risk factors responsible for disease.
12. Improvement in the health of adolescents and young adults; their physical, psychologic, and social attitudes; and their health habits to prevent later susceptibility to chronic diseases.
13. Education to help youths acquire skills and information to prevent pregnancy, alcohol and drug abuse, and sexually transmitted disease.
14. Investigation of the higher rate of absenteeism from work among women than men.
15. Increased instruction and supportive guidance for overweight and obese adults aged 25 to 74, especially black women over the age of 45 years.
16. Concerted efforts to reduce respiratory cancer rates by assisting people to stop smoking, especially women between 54 and 64 years of age and teenagers.
17. Increased assistance to help the elderly population with self-care and home management in their homes.
18. Guidance to help all people acquire early treatment for illness and comply with therapy.

Chapter Highlights

- The perspective from which health is viewed has changed; instead of absence of disease, health has come to mean fulfilling one's maximum potential for physical, psychosocial, and spiritual functioning.
- Holistic health practitioners relate the impact of an event to the whole person and encourage the person to take responsibility for and control over his or her health.
- Because notions of health are highly individual, the nurse must determine each client's perception of health in order to provide meaningful assistance.
- Each person's concept of health is molded by social and cultural influences, previous experiences, and expectations of self.
- The health status of a person is affected by many internal and external variables over which the person has varying degrees of control.
- Whether or not people choose to implement health behaviors depends on such factors as a perceived threat of a particular disease, perceived familial susceptibility, perceived seriousness of an illness, and perceived benefits of preventive actions.
- Whether or not people take action to improve their health often depends on the cost, inconvenience, and unpleasantness involved and on the degree of life-style change necessary.
- People realize they are ill when certain symptoms

indicate that something is wrong; they accept that they are ill when significant others or a health care professional verifies the illness.

- Increasingly, persons are being held responsible for some illnesses but are excused from certain roles and tasks during the illness; they are obliged, however, to get well as quickly as possible and to seek competent help.
- Nurses need to be aware that the illness of one member of a family affects all other members.
- Nurses need to be aware of a hospitalized client's life-style, roles, economic situation, and need for privacy and autonomy, and provide care accordingly.
- Clients may demonstrate certain behavioral changes during illness.
- People have the right and ability to make judgments about complying with health regimens after obtaining complete information.
- Health trends indicate that nurses need to assume a major role in helping people make life-style changes that will prevent accidents, suicide, obesity, heart disease, cancer, and premature death.

Suggested Readings

Birchfield, M. E. 1985. *Stages of illness: Guidelines for nursing care.* Bowie, Md.: Brady Communications Co.
Birchfield presents an in-depth study of the stages of illness: chronic, nonacute, acute, and postacute. Each stage is presented together with significant life changes, significant laboratory data, relevant nursing diagnoses, and nursing interventions.

Carey, R. L. 1984. Compliance and related nursing actions. *Nursing Forum* 21:157–61.
Carey describes how the Health Belief Model (HBM) predicts the likelihood of client compliance. The following variables figure in the prediction: high perceived severity of the relevant disease, high perceived susceptibility to the relevant disease, low perceived barriers to taking recommended action, and high perceived benefits as a result of taking the recommended action. Carey includes strategies for improving compliance and discusses the ethical issues involved. A table summarizes factors influencing compliance, possible reasons for noncompliance, and appropriate nursing strategies.

Grosser, L. R. May 1982. Health belief model aids understanding of patient behavior. *AORN Journal* 35:1056, 1058–59.
Grosser explains how a health belief model explains health behavior. The five components of the health belief model—perceived susceptibility, severity, benefits, barriers, and cues to action—are explained. Grosser states that after exploring the components of the model with a client, nurses are better able to give quality nursing care.

Payne, L. April 1983. Health: A basic concept in nursing theory. *Journal of Advanced Nursing* 8:393–95.
Payne perceives health as an evolving concept. Included is a description of some of the models (paradigms) of health, the concept of "high-level wellness," and the holistic health movement. Payne also discusses relationship of health to nursing theory.

Shaver, J. F. July/August 1985. A biopsychosocial view of human health. *Nursing Outlook* 33:186–91.
Shaver presents a brief history of the views of health. Also included is a discussion of the integrated biobehavioral fields of study and the effect of some environmental factors on biologic function. Shaver claims that a biopsychosocial perspective makes diagnostic assessment more comprehensive and differential diagnoses of human responses more specific.

Smith, J. A. April 1981. The idea of health: A philosophical inquiry. *Advances in Nursing Science* 3:43–50.
Smith describes four health models: eudaimonistic, adaptive, role-performance, and clinical. These models were chosen because of their significance to the restoration and preservation of health. Smith discusses the general structure, interrelationships, and implications of the four models.

Selected References

American Nurses' Association. November/December 1982. Bylaws as revised July 1, 1982. *American Nurse* 14:15–18.

Andreoli, K. G. November/December 1981. Self-concept and health beliefs in compliant and noncompliant hypertensive patients. *Nursing Research* 30:323–28.

Arakelian, M. 1980. An assessment and nursing application of the concept of locus of control. *Advances in Nursing Science* 3:25–42.

Baranowski, T. November/December 1981. Toward the definition of concepts of health and disease, wellness and illness. *Health Values* 5:246–56.

Bauman, B. 1965. Diversities in conceptions of health and physical fitness. In Skipper, J. K., Jr., and Leonard, R. C., editors. *Social interaction and patient care.* Philadelphia: J. B. Lippincott Co.

Becker, M. H., editor. 1974. *The health belief model and personal health behavior.* Thorofare, N.J.: Charles B. Slack.

Becker, M. H., and Maiman, L. 1975. Sociobehavioral determinants of compliance with health and medical care recommendations. *Medical Care* 13:10–24.

Brown, N. Spring 1983. The relationship among health beliefs, health values, and health promotion activity. *Western Journal of Nursing Research* 5:155–63.

Canadian Department of National Health and Welfare. 1974. *A new perspective on the health of Canadians: A working document.* Ottawa: Department of National Health and Welfare.

———. 1976. *Health field indicators, Canada and provinces.* Ottawa: Department of National Health and Welfare.

———. 1980. *Report of the task force to the conference of deputy ministers.* Ottawa: Minister of Supply and Services.

Chaska, N. L. 1983. Program for mild chronic obstructive pulmonary disease and compliance. In Chaska, N. L., editor. *The nursing profession: A time to speak.* New York: McGraw-Hill.

Coburn, D.; D'Arcy, C.; New, P.; and Torrance, G. editors. 1981. *Health and Canadian society: Sociological perspectives.* Don Mills, Ontario: Fitzhenry and Whiteside.

Davis, M. S. 1968. Variations in patients' compliance with doctors' advice: An empirical analysis of patterns of communication. *American Journal of Public Health* 58:274–88.

Dixon, J. K., and Dixon, J. P. April 1984. An evolutionary-based model of health and viability. *Advances in Nursing Science* 6:1–18.

Dubos, R. 1965. *Man adapting.* New Haven, Conn.: Yale University Press.

———. 1978. Health and creative adaptation. *Human Nature* 74(1):entire issue.

Dunn, H. L. June 1959a. High-level wellness in man and society. *American Journal of Public Health* 49:786.

———. November 1959b. What high-level wellness means. *Canadian Journal of Public Health* 50:447.

———. 1961. *High-level wellness.* Arlington, Va.: R. W. Beatty Co.

Fink, D. L. 1976. Tailoring the consensual regimen. In Sackett, D. L., and Haynes, R. B., editors. *Compliance with therapeutic regimens.* Baltimore: Johns Hopkins Press.

Grasser, C., and Craft, B. J. G. June 1984. The patient's approach to wellness. *Nursing Clinics of North America* 19:207–18.

Grosser, L. R. May 1982. Health belief model aids understanding of patient behavior. *AORN Journal* 35:1056, 1058–59.

Hadley, B. J. 1974. Current concepts of wellness and illness: Their relevance for nursing. *Image* 6:21–27.

The health of Canadians: Report of the Canada health survey. July/August 1981. 72:230–32.

Hettler, B. 1982. Wellness promotion and risk reduction on a university campus. In Faber, M. M., and Reinhardt, A. M., editors. *Promoting health through risk reduction.* New York: Macmillan Co.

Igun, U. A. 1979. Stages in health-seeking: A descriptive model. *Social Science and Medicine* 13A:445–56.

Jahoda, M. 1958. *Current concepts of positive mental health.* New York: Basic Books.

Jones, P. S. November 1978. An adaptation model for nursing practice. *American Journal of Nursing* 78:1900–6.

Kneisl, C. R., and Ames, S. W. 1986. *Adult health nursing: A biopsychosocial approach.* Menlo Park, Calif.: Addison-Wesley Publishing Co.

Laken, D. D. January 1983. Protecting patients against themselves. *Nursing 83* 13:26–27.

Leddy, S., and Pepper, J. M. 1985. *Conceptual bases of professional nursing.* Philadelphia: J. B. Lippincott Co.

Lewis, F. M. March/April 1982. Experienced personal control and quality of life in late-stage cancer patients. *Nursing Research* 31:113–18.

MacElveen-Hoehn, P. 1983. The cooperation model for care in health and illness, pp. 515–39. In Chaska, N. L., editor. *The nursing profession: A time to speak.* New York: McGraw-Hill.

McCann/Flynn, J. B., and Heffron, P. B. 1984. *Nursing: From concept to practice.* Bowie, Md.: Robert J. Brady Co.

Minister of Supply and Services. 1985. *Mortality, Vol. 3, 1983.* Cat. 84-206, ISSIV 0225-7394. Ottawa: Minister of Supply and Services.

Mitchell, P. H., and Loustau, A. 1981. *Concepts basic to nursing.* 3d ed. New York: McGraw-Hill.

Moll, J. A. January 1982. High-level wellness and the nurse. *Topics in Clinical Nursing* 3:61–67.

Murray, R. B., and Zentner, J. P. 1985. *Nursing concepts for health promotion.* 3d ed. Englewood Cliffs, N.J.: Prentice-Hall.

National Center for Health Statistics, Public Health Service. July 1985a. *Vital Statistics of the United States, 1982, Vol. 11, Section 6, Life Tables.* DHHS Pub. no. (PHS) 85-1104. Washington, D.C.: U.S. Government Printing Office.

———. August 1985b. *Charting the nation's health: Trends since 1960.* DHHS Pub. no. (PHS) 85-1251. Washington, D.C.: U.S. Government Printing Office.

Overfield, T. 1985. *Biologic variation in health and illness: Race, age, and sex differences.* Menlo Park, Calif.: Addison-Wesley Publishing Co.

Parsons, T. 1951. *The social system.* New York: Free Press.

———. 1972. Definitions of health and illness in the light of American values and social structure. In Jaco, E. G., editor. *Patients, physicians and illness.* 2d ed. New York: Free Press.

Payne, L. September 1983. Health: A basic concept in nursing theory. *Journal of Advanced Nursing* 8:393–95.

Pender, N. J. June 1975. A conceptual model for preventive health behavior. *Nursing Outlook* 23:385–90.

———. 1982. *Health promotion in nursing practice.* East Norwalk, Conn.: Appleton-Century-Crofts.

Pratt, L. 1971. The relationship of socioeconomic status to health. *American Journal of Public Health* 61:281–91.

President's Commission on Health Needs of the Nation. 1953. *Building America's health.* Vol. 2. Washington, D.C.: U.S. Government Printing Office.

Rodgers, J. A. October 1981. Health is not a right. *Nursing Outlook* 29:590–91.

Rosenstock, I. M. 1974. Historical origins of the health belief model. In Becker, M. H., editor. *The health belief model and personal health behavior.* Thorofare, N.J.: Charles B. Slack.

Schraff, S. H., editor. 1984. *Hospice: The nursing perspective.* Pub. No. 20-1967. New York: National League for Nursing.

Shaver, J. F. July/August 1985. A biopsychosocial view of human health. *Nursing Outlook* 33:186–91.

Shillinger, F. L. Spring 1983. Locus of control: Implications for clinical nursing practice. *Image: The Journal of Nursing Scholarship* 25:58–63.

Smith, J. A. April 1981. The idea of health: A philosophical inquiry. *Advanced Nursing Science* 3:43–50.

Splane, V. H. Fall 1984. Fashioning the future. *Nursing Papers* 16:12–24.

Statistics Canada. 1980. Causes of death. In *Perspectives Canada III.* Ottawa: Minister of Supply and Services.

———. 1980. *Perspectives Canada III.* Ottawa: Minister of Supply and Services.

Steckel, S. B. September 1982. Predicting, measuring, implementing and following up on patient compliance. *Nursing Clinics of North America* 17:491–98.

Suchman, E. A. 1972. Stages of illness and medical care. In Jaco, E. G., editor. *Patients, physicians and illness.* 2d ed. New York: Free Press.

Tatro, S., and Gleit, C. J. March 1983. A wellness model for nursing: Promoting high-level wellness in any setting through independent nursing functions. *Nursing Leadership* 6:5–9.

Trekas, J. September 1984. It takes two to achieve compliance. *Nursing 84* 14:58–59.

Twaddle, A. C. 1977. *A sociology of health.* St. Louis: C. V. Mosby Co.

U.S. Bureau of the Census. 1980. *Statistical abstract of the United States.* 101st ed. Washington, D.C.: U.S. Government Printing Office.

U.S. Department of Health and Human Services. December 1985. *Health United States 1985.* Pub. no. (PHS) 86-1232. Hyattsville, Md.: Public Health Service.

U.S. Department of Health, Education, and Welfare. 1979. *Healthy people: The Surgeon General's report on health promotion and disease prevention.* Pub. no. 79-55071. Washington, D.C.: U.S. Government Printing Office.

Wallston, B. S.; Wallston, K. A.; Kaplan, G. D.; and Maides, S. A. 1976. Development and validation of the health locus of control scale. *Journal of Consulting and Clinical Psychology* 44:580–85.

World Health Organization. 1947. *Constitution of the World Health Organization: Chronicle of the World Health Organization 1.* Geneva: World Health Organization.

Wu, R. 1973. *Behavior and illness.* Englewood Cliffs, N.J.: Prentice-Hall.

Yoos, L. September/October 1981. Compliance: Philosophical and ethical considerations. *Nurse Practitioner* 6:27, 29–30, 34.

Zola, I. K. Culture and symptoms: An analysis of patients presenting complaints. In Spector, R. E. 1979. *Cultural diversity in health and illness.* New York: Appleton-Century-Crofts.

CHAPTER 3

Health Care Delivery Systems

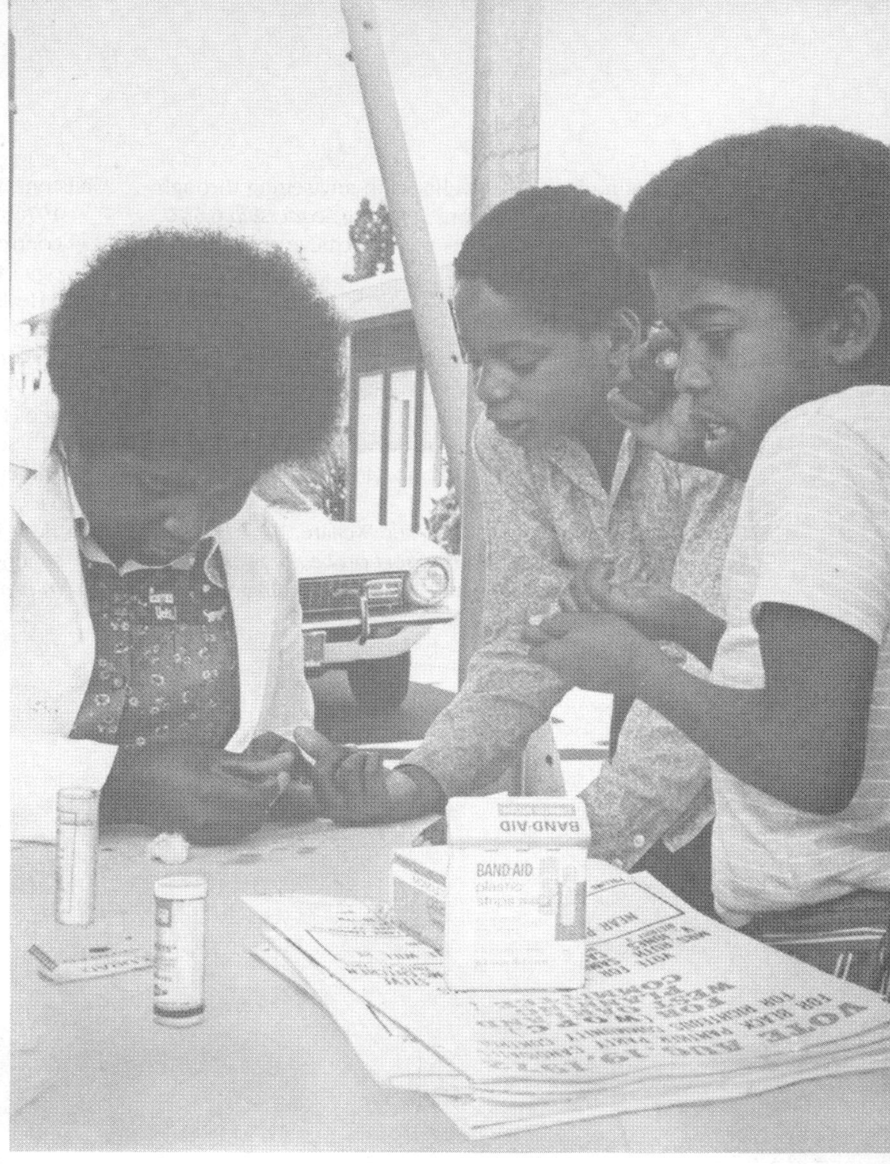

HANK LEBO/JEROBOAM, INC.

Contents

Objectives

1. Understand essential facts about the health care team and health care agencies.
   1.1 Identify the roles of various health care personnel.
   1.2 Compare official and voluntary health care agencies.
   1.3 Differentiate between the purposes of primary care, secondary care, and tertiary care.
   1.4 Identify agencies according to whether they are primary, secondary, or tertiary.
   1.5 Describe the function of various primary care centers.
   1.6 Differentiate between health maintenance organizations, preferred provider organizations, and individual practice associations.
   1.7 Describe the functions of various secondary care agencies.
   1.8 Describe the functions of various tertiary care agencies.
2. Understand essential factors about the financing of health care services.
   2.1 Differentiate between Medicare, Medicaid, and Supplemental Security Income benefits in the United States.
   2.2 Describe the National Hospital Insurance program and the National Medical Care Insurance program in Canada.
   2.3 Identify aspects of some voluntary insurance plans.
   2.4 Identify three sources of health care financing other than insurance programs.
3. Appreciate factors influencing and changing health care delivery systems and future challenges in health care delivery.
   3.1 Describe ways in which consumers are influencing changes in health care delivery.
   3.2 Describe ways in which technology affects health care delivery.
   3.3 Relate demographic influences to health care delivery.
   3.4 Describe the effects of specific social changes on health care delivery.
   3.5 Explain the effects of poverty and unemployment on health care delivery.
   3.6 Describe effects of the prospective payment system on health care delivery services.
   3.7 Explain how political decisions affect health care delivery.
   3.8 Describe the World Health Organization strategies for health care in the future.
   3.9 Discuss specific health care priorities and the requirements for promoting health and improving health care delivery services in the future.
   3.10 Identify ways to make health care more humanistic.
   3.11 Describe the implications for nursing of changes in health care delivery systems.

Terms

ambulatory care centers
clinical pharmacist
community health centers
crisis center
day-care centers
diagnostic related group (DRG)
dietitian
extended role
government (official) agency
health care
health care team
health maintenance organization (HMO)
home health care programs
hospice
individual practice association (IPA)
inhalation therapist (respiratory technologist)
long-term care facilities
Medicare
Medicaid
neighborhood health centers
nutritionist
occupational therapist
palliative measures
paramedical
pharmacist
pharmacy assistant
physician
physiatrist
physiotherapist (physical therapist)
preferred provider organization (PPO)
primary care
prospective payment system (PPS)
rehabilitation
secondary care
self-care
self-help group
Supplemental Security Income
tertiary care
voluntary health service agencies

Health Care Team

Health care is the totality of services offered by all health disciplines. The **health care team** consists of health personnel from different disciplines who coordinate their skills to assist a client and/or support persons. The choice of personnel for a particular team depends on the needs of the client. In the present system of health care in North

America, health teams commonly include physicians, nurses, dietitians, physiotherapists, social workers, occupational therapists, paramedical technologists, pharmacists, and inhalation therapists.

Physician

A **physician** is a person who is licensed to practice medicine in a particular jurisdiction. The physician has successfully completed a course of medical studies. In a hospital setting, the physician is responsible for medical diagnosis and for determining the therapy required by a person who has a disease or injury. In a community setting, the physician may be involved in diagnosis and therapy or play a consulting role. An example of the latter is the physician who specializes in public health and who serves as a consultant to the school nurse.

The traditional role of the physician is the treatment of disease and trauma (injury). However, many physicians, especially family practice physicians are now including health promotion and disease prevention in their practice.

Some physicians extend their roles by employing a physician's assistant. This person derives the authority to act from the physician. An **extended role** is one that is expanded unilaterally.

Nurse

The role of the nurse is discussed in Chapters 1 and 14. The role of the nurse varies with the needs of the situation. The advent of expanded nursing roles has established new dimensions for nursing practice. In the past, nursing was thought to comprise three types of skills: psychomotor, affective, and cognitive. Psychomotor skills are the traditional skills of nurses. The use of the hands, whether to manipulate equipment or reposition a client, for example, is a psychomotor skill. Technology has increased the psychomotor skills nurses need. Affective skills include the ability to incorporate cultural, attitudinal, and emotional elements into nursing. The nurse uses affective skills to individualize care. Caring and communicating activities (see Chapter 14) require affective skills. Cognitive skills include the ability to think, recall knowledge, apply knowledge, and evaluate. Cognitive skills are required in all aspects of the nursing process.

Today, the role of the nurse is seen more broadly. The acceptance of the nursing process as a framework for nursing practice and the recognition of other nursing roles, e.g., manager and counselor, have expanded the view of nursing practice.

A number of nursing personnel often participate actively on a health team. Sometimes nurses find it necessary to provide some services normally given by other members of the team, especially in settings where all the health services required by a client are not available 24 hours a day. For example, a nurse might assist a client who has had a cerebrovascular accident (stroke) by giving remedial exercises to restore function of the left arm. In urban hospitals, physiotherapists generally teach such exercises; however, nurses frequently teach these exercises in rural settings, where a physiotherapist's services often are not available.

Dietitian or Nutritionist

When dietary and nutritional services are required, the dietitian or nutritionist may be a member of a health team. A **dietitian** is a person who has special knowledge about the diets required to maintain health and to treat disease. A **nutritionist** is a person who has special knowledge about nutrition and food. Dietitians in hospitals design special diets—for example, for a child who has diabetes mellitus—and they supervise the preparation of the meals according to the diet. The nutritionist in a community setting recommends healthy diets and gives broad advisory services about the purchase and preparation of foods.

Hospital dietitians are generally concerned with therapeutic diets. The community nutritionist often functions at the preventive level. Such dietitians promote health and prevent disease, for example, by advising families about balanced diets for growing children and pregnant women.

Physiotherapist (Physical Therapist)

The physiotherapist assists clients with musculoskeletal problems. **Physiotherapists** treat the body by using heat, water, exercise, massage, and electric current. They provide physical therapy in response to a physician's order. The physiotherapist's functions are:

1. Assessing mobility and strength
2. Providing therapeutic measures, for example, exercises and heat applications to improve mobility and strength
3. Teaching clients new skills, for example, how to walk with an artificial leg
4. Teaching clients measures to prevent illness, for example, teaching deep breathing to a client before surgery as a preventive measure against postoperative pneumonia

Most physiotherapists provide their services in hospitals; however, independent practitioners establish offices in communities and serve clients either at the office or in the home.

Pharmacist

A **pharmacist** is a person who prepares and dispenses pharmaceuticals in hospital and community settings. The role of the pharmacist in monitoring and evaluating the actions and effects of medications on clients is becoming increasingly prominent. Pharmacists are also actively involved in preparing individual dosages for clients in hospitals that employ the unit dose system. In some settings, pharmacists prepare medications for intravenous therapy. A **clinical pharmacist** is a specialist who guides physicians in prescribing medications. A **pharmacy assistant** is also recognized in some states. This member of the health team administers medications to clients.

Inhalation Therapist

An **inhalation therapist** or respiratory technologist is skilled in therapeutic measures used in the care of clients with respiratory problems. These therapists are knowledgeable about oxygen therapy devices, intermittent positive pressure breathing respirators, artificial mechanical ventilators, and accessory devices used in inhalation therapy. Frequently they are involved in diagnostic procedures such as pulmonary function tests. Programs in inhalation therapy are offered in postsecondary educational institutions. Students complete such programs in 2 or 3 years.

Social Worker

A social worker counsels clients and support persons about social problems, such as finances, marital difficulties, and adoption of children. It is not unusual for health problems to produce problems in living. For example, an elderly woman who lives alone and has a stroke resulting in impaired walking may find it impossible to continue to live in her third-floor apartment. Finding a more suitable living arrangement can be the responsibility of the social worker if there is no support network in place.

Occupational Therapist

An occupational therapist assists clients with some impairment of function to gain the skills to perform activities of daily living. For example, a man with severe arthritis in his arms and hands might be taught how to adjust his kitchen utensils so that he can continue to cook. The therapist also teaches skills that are therapeutic and at the same time provide some satisfaction. For example, weaving is a recreational activity but also exercises the arthritic man's arms and hands. Occupational therapists coordinate their activities closely with those of other members of the health team.

Paramedical Technologist

Laboratory technologists, radiologic technologists, and nuclear medicine technologists are just three kinds of paramedical technologists in an expanding field of medical technology. **Paramedical** means having some connection with medicine. Laboratory technologists examine specimens such as urine, feces, blood, and discharges from wounds to provide the physician with exact information that facilitates the medical diagnosis and the prescription of a therapeutic regimen. The radiologic technologist assists with a wide variety of x-ray film procedures, from simple chest radiography to more complex fluoroscopy and radiography of the patient's stomach using a contrast medium. The nuclear medicine technologist, a more recent member of the technology group, uses radioactive substances to provide diagnostic information, for example, about a patient's liver, and can administer therapeutic doses of radioactive materials as part of a therapeutic regimen. These technologists have highly specialized skills and knowledge important to client care.

Health Care Agencies

Official and Voluntary Agencies

Government (official) agencies are established at the local, state (provincial), and federal levels. Local health departments (county, bicounty, or tricounty) traditionally have responsibility for (a) developing programs that are responsive to the health needs of the people, (b) providing the necessary staff and facilities to carry out these programs, and (c) continually evaluating the effectiveness of the programs and monitoring changing needs. State health organizations (approximately 60 different organizations) are responsible for assisting the local health departments. In some remote areas, state departments also provide direct services to people.

The Public Health Service (PHS) of the United States Department of Health and Human Services is an official agency at the federal level. Its functions include:

1. Research and training in the health field
2. Assistance to communities in planning and developing health facilities
3. Assistance to states and local communities through financing and provision of trained personnel

Also at the national level in the United States are research institutions such as the National Institutes of Health (NIH). The National Institute on Drug Abuse, the National Institute on Alcohol Abuse and Alcoholism, and the National Institute of Mental Health work with federal, regional, and state agencies. The Centers for Disease Control (CDC) in Atlanta, Georgia, administer a broad program related to surveillance of diseases. By means of laboratory and epidemiologic investigations, data are made available to appropriate authorities. The CDC also publishes recommendation about the prevention and control of infections, and administers a national health program.

Health agencies at the state, county, or city level vary according to the need of the area. Their funds, generally from taxes, are administered by elected or appointed officials.

The federal government also administers a number of Veterans Administration (VA) hospitals in the United States. VA hospitals are often near major medical centers. Nursing services in VA hospitals are similar to nursing services in other hospitals.

The Canadian Department of Health and Welfare (CDHW) administers such federal programs as native health in the North and health care in the Territories. However, provincial governments generally have responsibility for administering health services to the people in each province.

Voluntary health service agencies are supported by the people in a community. Examples are the National Heart Associations and Visiting Nurse Services (Associations). These nonprofit organizations rely on donations and, in some cases, on government grants for support. They are usually formed by volunteers in response to a specific recognized need, such as day care for the mentally retarded. Often they supplement official agencies' functions. Some voluntary agencies are oriented to the care of special groups in the community; others, to special programs, such as pollution control.

Once a voluntary agency has pointed out a need in a community, an official agency may take over some of the voluntary agency's functions. For example, the American Cancer Society originally funded treatment for cancer, but its treatment functions were taken over by official government agencies, such as hospitals, and the society retained its nontreatment functions, such as fund raising.

Health and Illness Services

Traditionally, the health care delivery system in North America provides two general types of services: illness care services (restorative) and health care services (preventive). Illness care services help the ill or injured. Health care services promote better health and help prevent disease and accidents. Although most facilities within the system—for example, hospitals, clinics, and physicians' offices—provide both types of services, illness care services predominate. In recent years, however, there has been increased awareness of the need to promote health and to prevent disease. Considerable emphasis has been placed on the role of the nurse in prevention. Often the community nurse's major function is to promote wellness and prevent illness, for example, through parent and child counseling.

In the past, health care facilities have been influenced largely by the needs of the people providing the service. For example, hospitals have developed in relation to medical and technologic advances and generally reflect the needs of physicians. Also, the public viewed health care facilities as sources of help primarily for the ill or injured. As a result, preventive health care facilities have been slow to develop. This delay can be attributed in great part to three factors:

1. Physicians are largely oriented to illness in their practice.
2. Consumers have been more aware of treatment of illness than of prevention and health promotion.
3. The nurse's role as the chief provider of preventive health care and health promotion has been slow to evolve, and frequently the treatment of illness takes precedence over preventive health care activities.

Agencies Providing Health Care

Health care agencies can be viewed as giving primary, secondary, and tertiary care.

Primary Care

Primary care agencies are the point of entry into the health care system—the point at which initial health care is given. This area of the health care delivery system presents many problems. Primary care is frequently inadequate in rural and economically depressed areas due to lack of physicians. Emergency departments of hospitals are often crowded and overtaxed, in many instances with nonemergency health problems.

Aydelotte writes, "The major purposes of primary care centers will be to provide: (1) entry into the system, (2) emergency care; (3) health maintenance; (4) long-term and chronic care; (5) treatment of temporary malfunctioning that does not require hospitalization" (Aydelotte 1983, p. 812). It is in this area that increased services are expected to reduce health care costs and improve health.

Primary care includes health maintenance, health promotion, and disease prevention activities. Settings for primary care are various health centers in the community, homes, schools, physicians' offices, and industry and business.

Neighborhood health centers **Neighborhood health centers** were opened by the Office of Economic Opportunity in the United States to provide health care to deprived groups, e.g., those living in ghetto areas. These centers often employ a variety of health care professionals, including social workers, nurse practitioners, and physicians. They usually offer a broad range of services, including help for both health and social problems.

Day-care centers **Day-care centers** either are attached to hospitals or operate independently to provide health services during daytime hours. Often these agencies provide a specific service. For example, the community mental health center helps clients who have emotional problems. Day-care centers often provide assistance to clients who need health care but do not require hospitalization. Such a center offers a day program, e.g., a program for elderly clients that includes physical exercise, meals, and recreational activities. Such a center serves two purposes: It provides activity and stimulation to elderly clients and frees the clients' support persons, who may work or require time for themselves.

Other types of day-care centers provide physical rehabilitation and educational programs for children with special needs, e.g., children who have cerebral palsy or arthritis.

Ambulatory care centers **Ambulatory care centers** may or may not be attached to a hospital. They usually have diagnostic and treatment facilities for people in the community. Ambulatory care centers may provide radiologic, laboratory, medical, and nursing services. Some ambulatory care centers provide services to people who require minor surgical procedures that can be performed outside the hospital. After surgery, the client returns home the same day. These centers have two advantages: They permit the client to live at home while obtaining needed health care, and they free costly hospital beds for seriously ill clients. Nurses in ambulatory care centers frequently function as nurse practitioners or clinical nurse specialists, e.g., in gastroenterology or urology.

The term *ambulatory care center* has replaced the term *clinic* in many places. The term *clinic* can refer to a department in a hospital or a group practice of physicians. Traditionally, a hospital clinic was called an outpatient clinic, serving only outpatients, not patients admitted to the hospital (inpatients). The role of the nurse in a clinic may be similar to that of a nurse practitioner or a nurse in a physician's office.

Community health centers **Community health centers** have developed slowly in Canada. They are similar in concept to neighborhood health centers, but they are not intended for a particular population group. They provide comprehensive health services and are usually staffed by a physician, nurses, social workers, and other health team members.

Home health care **Home health care programs** operate out of hospital- and community-based agencies. This is an area of enormous growth in recent years in the United States. Home health care programs provide a variety of nursing and other health services to clients and their support persons. For additional information, see Chapter 4.

Schools Schools have traditionally offered both medical and nursing services to their students. The nursing services generally focus on health services such as screening for hearing and sight problems, psychologic testing, immunizations, and counseling about health problems. Health education by school nurses involves both planned and informal teaching. Teaching is oriented to students' life-style and stresses health promotion and accident prevention.

Physicians' offices The physician's office is a traditional setting for illness care in North America. The majority of physicians either have their own offices or work with several other physicians in a group practice. People usually go to a physician because they consider themselves ill, because a relative thinks the client is ill, or because the client needs medical advice.

From 1974 to 1981, office visits to general and family practice physicians decreased from 42% to 33% of all visits. Visits to medical specialists, however, increased from 25% of all visits in 1974 to 31.3% in 1981. Visits to solo practice physicians between 1974 and 1978 accounted for about 60% of all visits; however, the percentage fell to 55% in 1981. Americans make over one billion visits to physicians per year (U.S. DHHS 1985b, pp. 14–15).

Nurses employed in physicians' offices have a variety of roles. Some nurses carry out the traditional functions of registering the client, preparing the client for an examination or treatment, and providing information. Other nurses function as nurse practitioners and have the responsibility of providing primary care to clients in stable health.

Industry and business Employee health has long been recognized as important to productivity. Today, an increasing number of companies are recognizing the value of healthy employees and encouraging healthy life-styles. Some companies provide exercise facilities, while others provide healthy snacks, such as fruit, instead of coffee. More businesses are prohibiting smoking in the work setting.

Community health nurses in the occupational setting have a variety of roles. Worker safety has been a traditional concern of occupational nurses. Today, nursing functions include health education, screening for such health problems as hypertension and obesity, counseling, and initial care after accidents.

Health maintenance organizations (HMO) A **health maintenance organization** is a group health care agency that provides basic and supplemental health maintenance and treatment services to voluntary enrollees. The enrollees prepay a fixed periodic fee that is set without regard to the amount or kind of services received. The basic idea of the HMO arose in the 1930s, when prepaid health care experiments were sponsored by unions, cooperatives, corporations, municipalities, and other organized groups. HMOs did not become popular, however, until the early 1970s with the passage, in 1973, of the Health Maintenance Organization Act. The act was a response to a proposal made in 1970 by a group near Minneapolis, Paul M. Ellwood and his associates, calling for a national "health maintenance strategy" based on competing private comprehensive health care organizations, which they called health maintenance organizations. After the concept was accepted by government, the term *HMO* was broadened to "alternative health care financing and delivery systems" or "alternative delivery systems." In 1984, 11 million people were served by HMO (Curtin and Zurlage 1984, p. 34).

To be federally qualified, an HMO company must meet certain requirements: It must offer physicians' services, hospital and outpatient services, emergency services, short-term mental health services, treatment and referral for drug and alcohol problems, laboratory and radiologic services, preventive dental services for children under 12, and preventive health services. By encouraging preventive health care and by offering ambulatory services, HMOs have reduced the cost of health insurance to the consumer.

A client of an HMO signs a contract to pay a specified amount to the HMO for unlimited care. The plan stresses wellness; the better the health of the person, the less the client needs HMO services and the greater their profit. Nurses are important employees of HMOs and function much as hospital nurses do.

Although not in every community, HMOs have been established across the United States. The largest HMO, the Kaiser-Permanente Medical Care Program, serves clients in California, Oregon, Hawaii, Ohio, and Colorado. A person with private health insurance can obtain services in most hospitals, but the clients of an HMO must use its facilities.

Preferred provider organizations (PPOs)

The **preferred provider organization** has emerged as another alternative health delivery system. It consists of a group of physicians or a hospital that provides companies with health services at a discounted rate. Hospitals, physicians, and insurance companies are the major sponsors of PPOs. PPOs were first established in 1980. As of 1985, there were 334 PPOs in the United States. Physicians can belong to one or several PPOs, and the client can choose among the physicians belonging to that PPO.

Individual practice association (IPA)

Individual practice associations are somewhat like HMOs and PPOs. The IPA provides practice in offices, just as the providers belonging to a PPO do. The difference is that clients pay a fixed prospective payment to the IPA, and the IPA pays the provider. In some instances, the health care provider bills the IPA for services; in others, the provider receives a fixed fee for services given. At the end of the fiscal year, any surplus money is divided among the providers; any loss is assumed by the IPA.

Crisis centers

Crisis centers provide emergency services. The clients are often people experiencing life crises. These centers may operate out of a hospital or in the community and usually provide 24-hour telephone service. Some also provide direct counseling to people at the center or in their homes. The primary purpose of a crisis center is to help people cope with an immediate crisis and then provide guidance and support for long-term therapy.

Nurses working in crisis centers need well-developed communication and counseling skills. The nurse must immediately identify the person's problem, offer assistance to help the person cope, and perhaps later provide guidance about resources for long-term support.

Special groups

Most communities have a number of organized support groups to assist people with special problems. Some groups help people with drug or alcohol problems. These groups, e.g., Alcoholics Anonymous, are often composed of people who have the same problem. Some organized groups employ special counselors, while others rely on the membership for this purpose.

Alcoholics Anonymous (AA) is an international organization to help alcoholics stop drinking. Members of the organization consider themselves alcoholics even if they have not had alcohol for many years. Chapters of AA meet to provide support to members. They share their experiences and have faith in a higher being. AA has 12 steps to living a life of sobriety. "Admitting you are powerless over alcohol and that life is unmanageable" is the first step. The theme of AA is "living one day at a time."

AA has developed two other groups: Al-Anon and Alateen. Al-Anon is composed of the family members of alcoholics, and their purpose is to assist other families. Alateen is a group of teenagers who have alcoholics in their families. Nurses can refer clients to AA; however, the client must want to stop drinking.

Secondary Care

Secondary care focuses on preventing complications of disease conditions. It has traditionally been the province of hospitals; however, other agencies now provide this level of service. Secondary care centers of the future will include: (a) the treatment of temporary dysfunctions that require hospitalization but not highly skilled services and high-risk interventions, (b) the evaluation of long-term illness that requires hospitalization to determine any needed change in treatment; and (c) the provision of counseling and therapy that cannot be provided in a primary care center (Aydelotte 1983, p. 813). Agencies that provide secondary care include hospitals, home health agencies, and ambulatory care centers. Home health care agencies are discussed in the section on primary care, although they are increasingly providing acute care to clients.

Ambulatory care centers Ambulatory care centers are designed to handle minor emergencies. They are an alternative to the hospital emergency department and are often preferred because no appointment is required, they are often closer to home, and they cost less. An average charge is about $50, less than half the cost of a hospital emergency visit (Kneisl and Ames 1986, p. 10).

Hospitals Hospitals traditionally have provided restorative care to the ill and injured. They vary in size from the 12-bed rural hospital to the 1500-bed metropolitan hospital with a 50-bed day surgery center. Hospitals can be classified according to their ownership or control as governmental (public) and nongovernmental (private). Governmental hospitals are either federal, state, city, or county hospitals in the United States and federal or provincial hospitals in Canada. In both countries, governments have traditionally provided hospital facilities for veterans, merchant mariners, and individuals with long-term illness.

Hospitals also are classified by the services they provide. General hospitals admit clients requiring a variety of services, including medical, surgical, obstetric, pediatric, and psychiatric services. Other hospitals offer only specialty services, such as psychiatric or pediatric care.

Although hospitals are chiefly viewed as institutions that provide care, they have other functions, such as providing resources for health-related research and teaching. Hospital personnel may conduct research and educational programs, or they may provide resources for such personnel as university teachers to carry out research and teaching responsibilities.

Hospitals can be further described as acute or chronic. An acute hospital provides assistance to clients who are acutely ill or whose illness and need for hospitalization are relatively short-term, for example, 2 days to perhaps 1 month. From 1968 to 1983, the average short stay in nonfederal United States hospitals decreased from 8.5 days to 6.9 days (U.S. DHHS 1985a, p. 15). Long-term hospitals provide health services for longer periods, sometimes for years or the remainder of the client's life.

The traditional organization of a hospital is departmental. Medical, nursing, dietary, laboratory, maintenance, pharmacy, and purchasing departments carry out their functions, which may be directly or indirectly related to client care. One of the limitations of this organizational pattern is the isolation of each department and subsequent discrepancies in personnel utilization and efficiency.

A more recent organizational structure for hospitals is the arrangement of the departments into systems and programs, each of which has a common characteristic. The systems provide a commonality among diverse functions; for example, the business system includes the functions of the business office, the accounting office, and the payroll office. Some or all of these might be separate departments in more traditional hospitals. The programs are the means of coordinating the resources of the various systems into care, teaching, and research functions.

Hospitals in the United States are undergoing massive change. In the past, hospitals were virtually the sole providers of secondary care; however, ambulatory care centers and HMOs have forced hospitals to reorganize and adopt different practices. In 1986, many acute care hospital beds remained empty, and some hospitals ran at less than 60% capacity. Some hospitals have merged or sold out to large multihospital-for-profit corporations, e.g., Humana, Inc., and Hospital Corporation of America. Other hospitals are providing innovative services, such as fitness classes, day care for elderly people, and nutrition classes. Some hospitals have even established alternative birth centers (ABCs) to attract new families.

In the United States today, all but the most seriously ill are treated outside of a hospital. Because so many of these are elderly, some general hospitals are becoming acute care hospitals solely for the elderly. Because of the increasing acuity of illness among clients, general hospitals are becoming intensive care centers.

Tertiary Care

Tertiary care is also called rehabilitation or long-term care. Tertiary care centers of the future will have two major purposes: (a) the treatment of esoteric illnesses that occur infrequently, and (b) the provision of personnel, new programs, new knowledge, and demonstrations of delivery for the total health care delivery system. Very highly skilled personnel and sophisticated equipment will be required in a tertiary center (Aydelotte 1983, p. 813).

Tertiary care today is largely provided through home health care, long-term care facilities, rehabilitation centers, and hospices. Home health care is discussed fully in Chapter 4.

Long-term care facilities There are a wide variety of long-term care facilities. Traditionally, they were all called nursing homes; however, the increase in the elderly and chronically ill population has given rise to a variety of facilities to assist these clients. Long-term care facilities include extended care, intermediate care, personal care, and nursing homes. Generally, they provide long-term care, in contrast to the acute care provided in hospitals.

Because long-term illness occurs most often in the elderly, many long-term care facilities have programs that are oriented to the needs of this age group. Nursing homes are intended for people who require not only personal services (such as assistance in bathing and dressing, and meal preparation) but also some regular nursing care and occasional medical attention. However, the type of care provided varies considerably. Some admit and retain only residents who can dress themselves and are ambulatory. Other long-term care facilities provide bed care for clients who are more incapacitated. Nursing homes can, in effect, become the clients' home, and consequently the people who live there are frequently referred to as residents rather than patients or clients.

Rehabilitation centers The concept of rehabilitation has gained considerable acceptance during the past 40 years. Before that time, it was generally associated with vocational help and social guidance for people who had physical injuries, often as a result of accidents at work. Today, the concept is applied to all illness (physical and mental), to injury, and to chemical addiction. Rehabilitation affects every age group and segment of society. **Rehabilitation** is a process of restoring people to useful function in physical, mental, social, economic, and vocational areas of their lives. Rehabilitation, then, is a process of restoring people to their previous level of health—that is, to their previous capabilities—or to the level that is possible for them. Rehabilitation, as distinct from maintenance, is an active concept and can be considered largely an educational function. Clients must participate actively in the process if it is to be effective.

The rehabilitation process involves the client and a team of health personnel who have various specialized skills. A physician, often a specialist in rehabilitation medicine, usually heads the team; this physician is referred to as a **physiatrist**. A nurse, a social worker, an occupational therapist, a physical therapist, and sometimes a psychiatrist and a speech therapist form part of the rehabilitation team. These people, together with the client and often the family and support persons, plan a program to help the client achieve maximum use of his or her capabilities.

Rehabilitation programs usually take place in independent centers in the community or in special units in hospitals. However, rehabilitation ideally starts the moment a client enters the health care system. Thus, nurses are involved in rehabilitation whether they are employed on pediatric, psychiatric, or surgical units of hospitals or in the community. A rehabilitation process usually has four broad objectives:

1. To return affected abilities to the highest possible level of function
2. To prevent further disability
3. To protect the client's present abilities
4. To assist the client to use his or her abilities

Rehabilitation centers often combine the services of physical therapists, occupational therapists, social workers, and nursing personnel. Specialists such as speech and recreational therapists and vocational counselors may also be on the staff of a center.

Hospice services A **hospice**, traditionally, was a place where travelers could rest. Recently, the term has come to mean a health care facility for the dying. The hospice movement subsumes a variety of services given to the terminally ill, their families, and support persons. The movement sprang initially from dissatisfaction with the preoccupation of health personnel with technologic care and insufficient emphasis on caring and psychologic support. In the 1970s, the movement gained momentum. It derived impetus from new attitudes toward death and from the work of such people as Elisabeth Kübler-Ross, whose books challenged prevailing attitudes, and Cicely Saunders, founder of St. Christopher's Hospice in London. Saunders believed that the physical and social environments of dying people are as important as medical interventions on their behalf.

In recent years, hospices have provided a variety of services to terminally ill clients and their families; indeed, hospices have inspired a social movement. Basic to the movement is a humanistic belief in the individuality of people and their needs. Hospice programs are institution and community based. A 1982 survey by the Joint Commission on Accreditation of Hospitals (JCAH) found that of 1145 hospice services surveyed, 40% were situated in a hospital or institution and 60% were community based (Pryga and Bachofer 1983). Some supply services in the home, either directly or through community resources. Reimbursement for these services is variable, often voluntary.

Amenta writes that four core services—nursing, medical, medical social, and counseling services—are essential in hospice care (Amenta 1984, p. 69). The hospice movement provides a model for holistic care of the dying: the care provided is continuous, i.e., care is not given only episodically at times of need, but continuously to meet the ongoing needs of clients and families.

Currently there are five forms of hospice services (Wald et al. 1980, p. 174):

1. Home care services
2. Hospice teams in hospitals
3. Palliative care units in hospitals
4. Hospices with hospital affiliations
5. Autonomous hospices

Hospices are a haven for the dying because they emphasize the needs of the individual and help clients and their families plan for death. The central concept of the hospice movement, as distinct from the acute care model, is not saving life but improving or maintaining the quality of life until death. Important in this care are **palliative measures**, measures whose aim is relief rather than cure. Comfort and relief from pain are frequently the most important needs of the dying. Hospice care addresses the needs of the mind and the spirit as well: It is truly holistic.

Financing Health Care Services

In the United States, medical costs increased 12.5% between 1981 and 1982 (Griffith 1983, p. 262). Funding for personal health care can come from a variety of sources: Governments (social insurance), the client, and health insurance are the major sources. Table 3–1 shows the costs of personal health care and the sources of funds in 1981, 1982, and 1983.

Social Insurance

Federal funding is largely through the social insurance programs Medicare and Medicaid in the United States, and the National Hospital Insurance program and the National Medical Care Insurance programs in Canada. A nationally funded program to cover the health costs of all United States citizens has been discussed for the past 15 years.

United States

In the United States, the 1965 **Medicare** amendments (Title 18) to the Social Security Act provided a national and state health insurance program for the aged. By the mid 1970s, virtually everyone over 65 years was protected by hospital insurance under Part A, which also includes posthospital extended care and home health benefits. Medicaid was established the same year under Title 19 of the Social Security Act. **Medicaid** is a federal public assistance program paid out of general taxes to people who require financial assistance, i.e., low-income groups.

In 1972, Congress directed the Department of Health, Education, and Welfare to create professional standards review organizations (PSROs) to monitor the appropriateness of hospital use under the Medicare and Medicaid programs. In 1974, the National Health Planning and Resources Development Act established health systems agencies (HSAs) throughout the United States for comprehensive health planning. In 1978, the Rural Health Clinics Act provided for the development of health care in medically underserved rural areas. This act opened the door for nurse practitioners to provide primary care.

In addition, disabled or blind persons may be eligible for special payments called **Supplemental Security Income** (SSI) benefits. These benefits are also available to people not eligible for Social Security, and payments are not restricted to health care costs. Clients often use this money to purchase medicines or to cover costs of extended health care.

To control costs of Medicare and Medicaid, the federal government passed legislation in 1983 governing a prospective pricing plan as part of a Social Security amendment. The amount of the reimbursement to hospitals is based on diagnostic related groups (DRGs). For additional information, see the discussion of DRGs on page 87.

Canada

The Canadian National Hospital Insurance program was started in 1958, and the National Medical Care Insurance program (Medicare) began in 1968. Through these programs, every Canadian can obtain health insurance. Not all hospital and medical services are insured by provincial hospital insurance or Medicare plans; there are slight differences between provinces. Also, not all physicians participate in their provincial or territorial plans, in which case the individual pays the physician directly (Crichton et al. 1984, p. 5). These insurance plans are paid for by federal and provincial governments and by individuals able to pay. In 1984, the Canada Health Act was passed by Parliament. This act mainly governs how the federal government reimburses provincial governments for health services they provide. This act replaced two acts: the Hospital Insurance and Diagnostic Services Act and the Medical Care Act. The new act penalizes provinces that permit extra billing of clients by physicians by a levy of a dollar-for-dollar assessment. The act also creates incentives for home care, community health clinics, and health pro-

Table 3–1 Personal Health Care Expenditures and Sources of Funds 1981–1983 (in billions)

		Source of Funds				
Year	Total*	Client	Federal	State and Local	Health Insurance	Other
1983	313.3	85.2	93.0	31.5	100.0	3.7
1982	284.7	90.8	84.0	29.4	77.2	3.4
1981	253.4	70.8	74.3	26.5	78.8	3.0

*Individual items may not add to totals because of rounding.

Source: American Nurses' Association, *Facts about nursing 84–85* (Kansas City, Mo.: American Nurses Association). p. 290. Original source: U.S. Department of Health and Human Services, Health Care Financing Administration, Office of Research and Demonstrations. *Health care financing review*, Winter 1984, 6(2):8. Used by permission.

motion: "Canadians can achieve further improvements in their well-being through combining individual life-styles that emphasize fitness, prevention and health promotion with collective action against the social, environmental and occupational causes of disease" (RNABC News 1984, p. 19).

Voluntary Insurance

Health care costs are also covered by private insurance plans. The costs of these insurance plans, such as Blue Shield and Blue Cross, are borne by the individual or shared by the employer and the employee. One type of voluntary health insurance is the prepaid group plan offered by HMOs. In these plans, participants pay for the services of physicians and/or nurses who participate in the plan and the facilities arranged for in the plan. An example is the Kaiser Permanente Medical Care Program in California and other states. Prepaid group plans provide for services required by the participants 24 hours a day. By advance payment, the individual takes out insurance against any health requirements in the future. These plans place heavy emphasis on promotion of health and prevention of disease and injury among participants. In 1982, Blue Cross and Blue Shield owned, operated, or were affiliated with 55 HMOs serving 1.8 million subscribers (Blue Cross and Blue Shield 1982, p. 1). In Canada, Blue Cross covers ambulance services as well as semiprivate and private accommodation in hospitals.

Client Payment

Some people do pay for their own health care costs independently. In 1983, clients paid $85.2 billion for health care. See Table 3–1 on page 83. Because costs to the client are increasing rapidly, this practice is becoming less common.

Workmen's Compensation

Workers who are injured on the job may collect workmen's compensation payments during their recovery. In some instances, all health care costs are paid by workmen's compensation. Employer companies contribute to a workmen's compensation fund to make money available when accidents occur.

Charitable Resources

Charitable resources for medical payments are supported by donations from individuals or groups and by bequests. Charitable donations are still made by some philanthropic organizations to assist the poor and to support innovations. On the whole, however, charitable donations as a means of paying for health care are declining in importance.

Current Influences and Changes in the Health Care Delivery System

Consumer Influences

Rights and Values

North Americans generally believe that all persons have a right to health care regardless of race, culture, or economic status. In addition, most believe that all persons are entitled to health care that prevents disease, treats disease, and restores ill persons to their previous state of health. In 1966, the World Health Organization stated that health care is a universal human right. This belief has led to the United States Medicare and Medicaid programs, which strive to provide health care to those who cannot afford it. In Canada, the National Hospital Insurance program and the National Medical Care Insurance program (Medicare) provide benefits for all Canadian citizens. See the section on social insurance, earlier in this chapter.

Comprehensive, holistic, and humanistic health care is being emphasized today. People want to have their health care needs met at one time at one agency—comprehensive care—rather than to seek help for an abdominal pain at one place, for a tooth problem at another place, and for an emotional problem at yet another. Holistic health practitioners emphasize the effects of one problem on the person as biopsychosocial whole. Consumers, therefore, expect health care that reflects this view of the total person and his or her roles and functions. The humanistic values desired include recognition of inherent worth, individual uniqueness, wholeness, freedom of action, equality of status, and shared decision making between the client and health care practitioner.

Mutual Support and Self-Help Groups

In North America today, there are more than 500 mutual support or **self-help groups** that focus on nearly every major health problem or life crisis people experience. Such groups arose largely because people felt their needs were not being met by the existing health care system. Alcoholics Anonymous, which formed in 1935, served as the model for many of these groups. The National Self-

Help Clearinghouse provides information on current support groups and guidelines about how to start a self-help group. Groups vary in effectiveness, but most provide education to encourage self-care as well as social and emotional support. Before referring clients to specific groups, the nurse needs to assess the group's effectiveness and availability to the client.

The consumer self-help movement has generated an abundance of newsletters, hotlines, health and medical self-help books, conferences, and workshops related to health promotion and management of chronic disease. This phenomenon indicates in part that consumers want more information and assistance to gain self-control of their primary health needs.

Self-Reliance and Self-Care

Self-reliance and independence are desired goals of people, and the elderly, chronically ill, and disabled are no exception. Increasingly, people are seeking information about **self-care** so that they can remain as independent as possible and be as useful to the community as their capacities permit. Because many consumers desire and are assuming increasing responsibility for their health, more health maintenance services and home services are now offered.

Self-care is not new. Although the role of the individual in health care is receiving increased attention, people have always independently treated minor injuries; medicated for colds, headaches, or muscle and joint pain; brushed and flossed their teeth; and carried out certain therapies, such as insulin injections for diabetes mellitus.

Health Promotion

In the past few decades, many North Americans have come to expect more of the health care system than disease prevention or cure. Consumers today are more aware and knowledgeable about the effects of life-style on health. As a result, they desire more information and services related to health promotion and illness prevention. Although the diagnosis and treatment of illness is still a necessity, the focus of health care has changed. Traditionally, health care was viewed as synonymous with professional and medical care. Now health care professionals are increasingly viewed as a supplementary resource for individuals carrying out their own health maintenance and health promotion activities. As a result, a wide range of health promotion programs have arisen. Some are provided through the traditional health care agencies, but many are developing in community facilities along with physical fitness centers. The media, too, reflect this change. It is not rare for characters in movies, for instance, to exhibit positive health behaviors, such as exercising and not smoking. In Canada, alcohol and tobacco advertisements have been restricted.

Technologic Influences

The impact of technology on health care is enormous. For example, radioisotope scanners, computed axial tomography (CAT) scanners, and ultrasound machines (see Chapter 54) are available in addition to the standard x-ray equipment; various life support and monitoring systems have been devised for the cardiac surgery client, crash victim, or premature baby; transplant surgery is now possible to replace the heart, veins, lungs, kidneys, pancreas, liver, cornea, bone marrow, and pituitary gland; and artificial implants can be inserted to replace the lens of the eye, repair damaged joints, and regulate the beating of the heart.

Immense benefits have been derived from advances since World War II. Tuberculosis and measles are no longer major causes of death; permanent disability from poliomyelitis has been eradicated; advances in anesthesiology and asepsis have allowed treatment of the acutely ill; microsurgery has made it possible to rejoin severed limbs; and people now can expect to live longer than their grandparents. The computer, too, has affected every facet of life, not just the health care system.

Advanced technology requires specialized knowledge and skills of health care practitioners. Often new medical units are created to deal with advanced technology. This sophisticated equipment and support services are costly. In addition, technology often creates complex legal and ethical questions related to prolongation of life.

Social Influences

Social influences such as the women's movement, changes in family characteristics, increasing population, environmental changes, and cultural diversity all affect the health care delivery system.

Women's Movement

The women's movement has been instrumental in changing health care practices. Examples are the provision of childbirth services in more relaxed hospital settings or the home, the provision of overnight facilities for parents in children's hospitals, and the attention being paid to premenstrual tension syndrome and unnecessary surgery performed on women, e.g., unnecessary radical mastectomies and hysterectomies. The literature on the health concerns of women and research into women's unique health experiences are growing. More nursing research is needed in every aspect of women's health. In the words of Griffith-Kenney (1986, p. xiii):

> Our understanding of the normal physiologic and psychologic changes that occur in various phases of the female life cycle is still limited. Research studies are just beginning to identify the normal physiologic patterns of men-

struation and menopause, which heretofore had been treated as pathologic. Women's reactions to stress, situational crises such as rape and battering, and occupational and environmental hazards are currently being explored. The special problems of the aging woman, including isolation and lack of mobility, are finally receiving attention, as are the stresses associated with discrimination, sex-role stereotyping, and the new expectations of the feminist era.

Family Characteristics

The characteristics of the North American family have changed considerably in the last few decades. There is a marked increase in single-parent families because of divorce and increased acceptance of children born out of wedlock. Most single-parent families are headed by women. The number of families headed by single females has doubled since 1960 and account for almost 15% of all United States families (U.S. Bureau of the Census 1980). A concern about households headed by females is that many such households have a low standard of living. The incomes of the majority of female heads of households are under the poverty level (Griffith-Kenney 1986, p. 51). Serious illness or hospitalization can create major financial and home management difficulties for single-parent families. For additional information about the family, see Chapter 21.

Increasing Population

Statistics reflect an increase in the total population and indicate the need for increased health services. In both the United States and Canada, there has been tremendous population growth, particularly since 1945. See Figure 3–1.

The impact of the growing elderly population on the health care system is a major social issue. About 30 cents of each health care dollar in the United States are allocated to this group, which now exceeds 28 million and comprises almost 12% of the population (U.S. Department of Commerce 1984). By the year 2030, it is estimated that the elderly will number 50 million, comprising 17% of the population (U.S. DHEW 1979, p. 71). In Canada, a similar increase in the number of older people is anticipated: from 1.9 million in 1976 (Statistics Canada 1980, p. 10) to 3.2 million by the year 2000. By the year 2031, 21% of the population will be over age 65 (Statistics Canada 1981). Since only 5% of older people are institutionalized because of health problems, substantial home management and nursing support services are required to assist those in their homes and communities. The frail aged population over age 85 is the second fastest growing population in North America, exceeded only by the "baby boom" generation now between 30 and 45. Numbering more than 2.6 million, this group is expected to increase to 5 million by the year 2000 (U.S. Bureau of the Census 1984). More research into the health and economic conditions of this population is needed.

Because people over 65 are becoming an increasingly large part of the population, their health needs deserve special concern. Long-term illnesses are most prevalent in this group, and these illnesses frequently make special housing, treatment services, and financial support necessary. The elderly need to feel they are still part of a community even though they are approaching the end of their lives. Feelings of being useful, wanted, and productive citizens are essential to their health. Special programs are being designed in communities so that the talents and skills of this group will be used and not lost to society. These programs—e.g., partial employment—are designed especially for the elderly person.

Environmental Change

Air and water pollution from industrial waste is a notable change in this century. Many cities publish a daily air quality index so that persons with respiratory disease will know whether the outside air is safe to breathe. Tragic industrial and nuclear leaks are also of concern.

Many work environments also pose health hazards for employees. Coal miners and textile workers are prone to lung disease. Construction workers are prone to asbestosis. Increasingly, the public is demanding smokeless air in work settings. Many corporations and cities have already banned smoking in certain work areas.

Cultural Diversity

The "high-tech" health care system of North America reflects largely Western, white values and does not adequately accommodate the values of the many different cultural groups living in this country. Language barriers and inequities in income and education hinder access of minority ethnic groups to health care. The more sophisticated and impersonal health services become, the less accessible they are to ethnic groups, who are often inwardly oriented, have a strong family tradition, and prefer personalized care from someone who understands them and their families. Many such people look on the modern health care system with distrust.

Economic Influences

The health care delivery system is very much affected by a country's total economic status. Inflation and the economic recession of the early 1980s has brought increasing concern about escalating health care costs. The United States spends $1 billion a day on health care, and costs are still rising. Medical care costs have increased more than 400% since 1965. Some reasons for this sizable increase are advanced techniques and technology, inflation, increased utilization of health services, and the system of payment for hospitals and physicians.

Prospective Payment System (PPS)

Efforts to curtail health care costs in the United States were made in 1983, when Congress passed legislation putting the **prospective payment system** into effect. This legislation limits the amount paid to hospitals that are reimbursed by Medicare. Reimbursement is made according to a classification system known as **diagnostic related groups** (DRGs). The system now has 467 categories (originally 383) that establish pretreatment diagnosis billing categories. Under this new system, the hospital is paid a predetermined amount for clients with a specific diagnosis. For example, a hospital that admits a client with a diagnosis of uncomplicated asthma is reimbursed a specified amount, such as $1300, regardless of the cost of services, the length of stay, or the acuity or complexity of the client's illness. In the past, Medicare reimbursed hospitals according to the reasonable cost of services provided to its clients. The hospital billed retrospectively, after the services were rendered. In contrast, prospective payment or billing is formulated before the client is even admitted to the hospital; thus, the record of admission, rather than the record of treatment, now governs payment. DRG rates are set in advance of the prospective year, during which they apply and are considered fixed except for major, uncontrollable occurrences. The prospective rates are paid by clients and/or third parties.

This legislation has had a tremendous impact on health care delivery in the United States, since the providers of care, rather than Medicare or other third-party payers, run the risk of monetary losses. If a hospital's cost per case exceeds the defined limit, it incurs a loss; if the cost is less than the defined limit, it receives a surplus. Thus, PPS offers financial incentives for withholding unnecessary tests or procedures and avoiding prolonged hospital stays.

Notable effects of the DRG system to date are earlier discharge of clients, a decline in admissions, and a reduction of services provided and staff, especially nurse's aides and LPN/LVN staff. With the decline in admissions, most clients now admitted are seriously ill and have multiple health problems. Many hospitals are now employing only registered nurses (RNs), believing that RNs can provide the broadest range of nursing care. The earlier discharge of clients has given rise to home care agencies that provide needed home nursing care.

Some disadvantages of the DRG system are (Bentley and Butler 1980):

1. DRGs fail to include all diagnoses and procedures.
2. Assignment to a DRG depends on the documentation of the attending physician and the conventions of the individual coder.
3. DRGs reflect the state of medical practice and technology at the time of their development and do not account for advances in diagnostic procedures or therapies.
4. DRGs provide neither a standard of what should be done nor a measure of the quality of care, since they are based solely on data about length of stay.
5. Since surgical procedures are often associated with high reimbursement rates, there is the possibility that the number of unnecessary surgical procedures will increase.

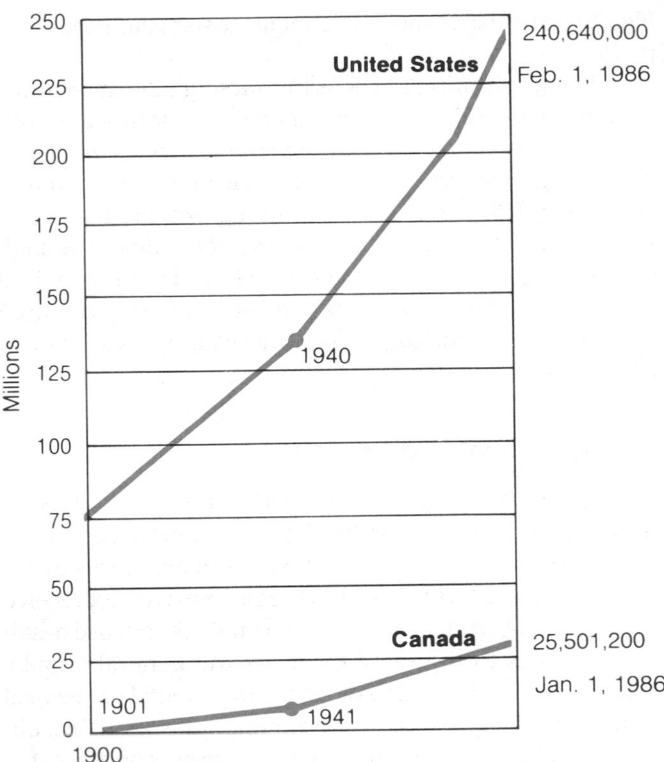

Figure 3–1 Increases in population in the United States, 1900–1986, and Canada, 1901–1986.

Source: From U.S. Department of Commerce, Bureau of the Census, *Current population reports,* Series P25, no. 983 (Washington, D.C.: U.S. Government Printing Office, February 1, 1986); U.S. Department of Commerce, Bureau of the Census, *Population profile of the United States: 1980,* Series P, no. 363 (Washington, D.C.: U.S. Government Printing Office, June 1981), p. 9; Statistics Canada, *Postcensal estimates of population* (Ottawa: Minister of Supplies and Services, January 1, 1986), table #1 91-001; and Statistics Canada, *Census of Canada* (Ottawa: Minister of Supplies and Services, 1981), p. 6.

To protect clients from DRG abuses, Medicare introduced state peer review organizations (PROs). Made up of physicians and other health care professionals, PROs are intended to monitor the hospitals and ensure high-quality care under DRGs. PROs have developed screening guidelines that govern whether admissions or procedures should occur and are used to review records, render payment decisions, and handle difficulties. Some people question the conflict of interest in the dual obligation of

PROs: to ensure quality and contain costs (Hamilton 1986, p. 43).

The implication of DRGs for nursing education, practice, and research are many, since the system was developed without explicit attention to nursing costs or the use of nursing resources. The Health Care Financing Administration (HCFA) has and is funding research to study alternative systems for classifying severity of illness through nursing diagnosis (Caterinicchio 1984, p. 130) and to shed light on the relationship between DRGs, nursing resource utilization, and nursing costs (American Nurses' Association 1985).

Unemployment and Poverty

Unemployment and poverty, whether the result of recessions, new microchip technology, or inadequate education and technical skills, affect which health services are offered and used. Because the unemployed do not receive employment-based health insurance, they do not use health care services to the same extent as the general population. Such people tend to defer needed dental or medical care. Even though some government aid is available, eligibility for government insurance programs and benefits varies considerably from state to state. Canada's economic problems are similar to those of the United States; however, the overall effects are not always as apparent because Canada has a smaller population. The National Health Care program in Canada ensures medical care and hospitalization for the poor and unemployed.

The detrimental effects of unemployment and poverty on health have not been properly determined. Some studies reveal a higher incidence of depression, asthma, headache, and backache among the unemployed and higher suicide and homicide rates. When widespread unemployment persists for 2 to 3 years, deaths from heart disease increase (O'Neill 1983, p. 139). When the breadwinner loses a job, the family is forced to change its life-style. Coping methods used to overcome stress may not always be advantageous. For example, mothers may go hungry to see that their children are well fed. Older people may skimp on food to the point of suffering vitamin deficiencies. Poverty not only results in more illness among pregnant mothers, children, and unemployed breadwinners but also exacerbates the effects of alcoholism, such as wife and child abuse (O'Neill 1983). Those who offer health care services to the poor need to consider these factors.

Political Influences

Health care is affected by political decisions. For example, political decisions affect health insurance programs, health care funding, allocation of resources (people, money, and equipment), and laws governing the duties of health care workers and the rights of clients, e.g., of women to have abortions. The attitude of people in government health ministries largely determines whether the focus of health care delivery is primary care, secondary care, or tertiary care.

Challenges for the Future

The World Health Organization Regional Office for Europe issued a warning that there could be a health care crisis by the year 2000 unless radical steps are taken by the public, the professions, industry, and governments (O'Neill 1983, p. ix). The same holds true for North America. To avoid a health care crisis, WHO recommends a new strategy of health care based on three inseparable themes:

1. Health as a way of life
2. Prevention of ill health
3. Community care for all

This strategy emphasizes the value of the individual in a caring family and community and also the responsibility of the whole nation, as well as of each citizen, for health.

Health As a Way of Life

People can become more conscious of their health by appraising their life-styles. Increased efforts by nurses, all health professionals, and government can be instrumental in helping people gain a greater awareness of health as a way of life. Greater emphasis must be given to the ill effects of smoking, excessive consumption of alcohol and narcotics, overuse of prescribed medications, failure to take regular exercise, unbalanced diets, and sexual promiscuity rather than treatment of the consequences of these activities. See Unit V, "Health Promotion throughout the Life Span," for further information.

The Prevention of Ill Health

Measures to prevent disease or reduce risks must also be emphasized. Examples are immunizing children; making childbearing more safe and natural for the mother and infant; reducing the incidence of road accidents, particularly among adolescents; and preventing accidents in the home, especially among children and older people. Prevention of ill health requires the united efforts of all citizens and health care providers. Challenges for the future are (O'Neill 1983, pp. 99–110):

1. To reduce perinatal risks and improve maternal and child health. Further development is needed in:
   a. Services for prenatal care as well as education and family planning based on genetic, biologic, and health services research
   b. Improved pregnancy tests and encouragement of women to seek prenatal care as soon as possible
   c. Services to ensure the early detection and follow-up of defects, especially for high-risk families
   d. Identification of toxic materials and other environmental causes of birth defects

2. To reduce the incidence of preventable, communicable disease. Challenges are:
   a. Expanded immunization programs, especially for people in rural areas, and encouragement for all people to seek immunization actively rather than to wait passively until they are told what to do
   b. Research on new preventive methods, including development of new vaccines and identification of new viruses

3. To reduce accidents and their consequences. Challenges are:
   a. Increased education and information about safety at work and in the home
   b. Further research into human and other factors responsible for accidents
   c. Increased vehicle safety, including compulsory use of seat belts and other restraining devices for infants and children
   d. Stricter safety regulations governing the manufacture of consumer goods, such as motorcycles and children's toys
   e. Increased provision for cyclists on the road

4. To promote balanced nutrition and safe food. Challenges are:
   a. Development of policies to ensure that low-income groups get enough food
   b. Increased cooperation among government officials who control the food industry in terms of pricing, sales, production, taxing, and inspection of public eating places

5. To reduce environmental risks. Challenges are:
   a. Increased identification and control of chemical, physical, and biologic environmental hazards, including noise and radiation
   b. Health education of the public to increase general awareness of environmental risk factors

6. To provide safe water and sanitation. Challenges are:
   a. Establishment of minimum standards of housing and hygiene
   b. Attention to housing, water, and sanitation problems in poorly equipped urban areas and rural communities

Community Care for All

Giving all people access to health care at whatever level they need it is a major goal for the future. Health professionals, working in teams, need to take an active role in promoting good health. Emphasis has traditionally been placed on cure and remedial treatment, often in a hospital, and on the family physician as the one who responds to community health needs and is responsible for meeting them. Governments have defined their role as curative rather than preventive: making sick people better rather than promoting health. Health insurance schemes, too, focus on sickness; they pay for illness treatment rather than preventive services.

Achieving the goal of equal access to appropriate health care for all people in the future requires the efforts of all people and a focus on the following (O'Neill 1983, pp. 117–18):

1. Establishment of community-based health systems in which primary health care is the major function. Such systems would need to be backed up by hospital services and other specialty services. Currently, health and welfare services are fragmented. Health and welfare centers of the future need to be planned together and cover all aspects of health. Such centers should be places that the local people can approach whatever their health requirement: health promotion, prevention, first aid, primary diagnosis, or help with problems specific to children, the elderly, working adults, or the unemployed.

2. Redistribution of health and specialty services to overcome regional inequities. Currently health care services and professionals are concentrated in urban areas. In rural and low-income areas, such as declining inner city areas, there is a notable lack of services. Some reasons for lack of services in these areas are insufficient local financial resources to support health care services, seasonal population fluctuations, a lack of social and cultural activities that attract health care workers, and a decline in the number of general and family practice physicians because of the greater number of specialists.

3. Emphasis on self-reliance and participation by the individual and community members in health matters. This will require a changed emphasis by health workers on home and community care rather than institutional care. More research will be needed about the cost-effectiveness of home and community services, self-care, and self-help approaches.

4. Increased emphasis on provision of services to specific target groups, such as children and adolescents, the elderly, the disabled, the dying, single mothers, the mentally ill, and working mothers. A whole array of services that now exist need expansion. Examples are

health education for children, home help and child care for working women, home help for the elderly and disabled, reintegration of the mentally ill into the community, and hospice care for the dying.

5. Increased involvement of existing health organizations and groups. Many existing health and social groups, e.g., AA, groups for the elderly, and paraplegic associations, can use their specialized talents to bring about change.
6. Expanded education of health professionals—medical practitioners, nurses, nurse-midwives—in community and health care as well as traditional hospital and acute care. Graduating physicians and nurses will need to think and practice in terms of health rather than disease, apply techniques of prevention and health promotion in addition to those of cure and rehabilitation, focus practice on the family and community and not the individual sick person, and work as members of a health team that invites the active participation of the consumer. In the health teams of the future, health care professionals will no longer simply assist the physician in treating passive clients. Clients are now beginning to play a critical, active role rather than their traditional, uncritical role of passively accepting everything the health professional says and does. With a new focus on teamwork and working relationships, the separate education of nurses, physicians, social workers, etc., may need to be examined. In the future, health professionals from different disciplines may receive some of their education together.
7. Expansion of traditional roles and change in the current hierarchical health profession. As O'Neill (1983, p. 72) says: "Health professionals have before them a dramatic new role in addition to the exercise of their clinical skills: that of health leaders, educators, guides, and generators of simpler and more socially acceptable technologies. To fulfill this role they will require a combination of sagacity, scientific and technical knowledge, social understanding, managerial acumen and, above all, political persuasiveness."
8. New focus by government on health rather than cure and on the roles that transportation, housing, and industry ministries can play in bringing about a healthy society.

Humanizing Health Care

Although the goal of any health care delivery system—to protect the healthy and care for the sick—is intrinsically human, the system is perceived as increasingly dehumanizing. Highly specialized techniques and new knowledge emerging during the past 30 years of research mean that an increasing number of health personnel provide specialized services. They may be highly specialized technicians or technologists who have relatively narrow but exacting jobs, such as respiratory technologists, biomedical electronic technologists, and nuclear medicine technologists. Increased specialization is evident also among physicians. All this specialization means fragmentation of care and sometimes less than desirable total care. To clients, it may mean receiving care from 5 to 30 people during their hospital experience. This seemingly endless stream of personnel is often confusing and frightening. The client feels like a cog in the wheel and asks, "Who really cares about me?" and "Who is really responsible?" This proliferation of health personnel can impede the smooth flow of information and undermine plans to help the client. Again, the client wonders, "Will someone forget to order my medication?" "Will someone help me get my meals when I return home from the hospital?" The concept of total and humanistic care is more difficult to implement when so many people are involved.

Dehumanization

Both humanization and dehumanization of care have various meanings in literature. Precise definitions are lacking; usually inferences are made about them. Dehumanization is associated with vulnerability, powerlessness, and loss of identity in large, faceless institutions. The blame usually falls on society in general, technologic change, the rat race, or bureaucratic red tape. Howard and Strauss (1975, p. 60) outline these meanings of dehumanizaiton:

1. Clients as things. People are reduced to objects with standardized needs and wants; they are quantified into elements or parts; they are done to, not doers; they cannot initiate action and must be directed; they lack feeling and are insensitive.
2. Clients as machines. This idea is encouraged by technology; the caregiver may be absent while the client interacts, for example, with a computer or electric monitor. The client thus becomes an extension of a machine, and the machine may become a substitute for people, who may spend more time adjusting parts of the machine than caring for the client.
3. Clients as guinea pigs. Dehumanization by experimentation has recently been mentioned in connection with heart transplants and in arguments about length of life versus quality of life for seriously debilitated children and adults.
4. Clients as problems. Some health personnel tend to become problem oriented or disease oriented rather than person oriented. This perception is common among clients who receive fragmented and specialized care.
5. Clients as lesser people. Dehumanization by degradation leads to depersonalization. It can occur among

groups of clients, such as those confined to mental institutions. The perception of people as somehow lesser beings is culturally determined; certain ethnic groups, the aged, and women may all be viewed in this light. Some professionals or semiprofessionals may also be perceived as lesser beings by clients or even other professionals because of an ascribed characteristic, such as sex, lack of specialized education, or practice in a less prestigious area.

6. Clients as isolates. People become isolates when overworked personnel have neither the time or the desire to speak to them. The client becomes physically or psychologically abandoned. This is often the perception of long-term clients, such as the elderly or mentally ill, or clients after long waits in outpatient clinics or private offices.
7. Clients as recipients of substandard care. Dehumanization is sometimes associated with a lower quality of care than could be provided given available knowledge and technology. An example is a nursing home whose personnel are indifferent or negligent.
8. Clients without options. Feelings of powerlessness and lack of control are sometimes the hallmark of dehumanization. The client is crushed by hierarchies of power and rendered helpless.
9. Clients "interacting" with icebergs. A common connotation of depersonalization is coldness and absence of feeling. Providers of care are encouraged to maintain emotional distance to ensure objective decision making and thus, like icebergs, keep much of themselves a mystery.
10. Clients in static, sterile environments. A depersonalized environment is seen as dehumanizing by clients. Fortunately many medical settings now approximate the warm, colorful world that is regarded as natural and humanistic.

Conditions for Humanized Care

Howard and Strauss (1975, p. 73) outline values and conditions for humanized health care as follows:

1. Ideologic dimensions. Ideologic dimensions are those based on definitions of appropriate behavior in health care environments. Three ideologic dimensions of people are inherent worth, irreplaceability, and holistic selves.
   a. Inherent worth means that human beings are of value to themselves if not to others. Health systems recognize the inherent worth of persons by trying to prolong life, reduce pain, and restore social functioning. Clients themselves emphasize that they should be treated with dignity and respect even if discriminated against in the larger society. Thus, the concept of inherent worth approximates notions of equality. The concept of inherent worth needs to apply to professional/client interactions and must be reflected in institutional policy. Are all clients treated equally? Are workers at the bottom of the professional hierarchy viewed as being inherently worthy?
   b. Irreplaceability means that each person is unique and is not stereotyped or treated in routine, uniform ways, even though all humans have some commonalities. Humanized care demands an orientation toward clients as individuals.
   c. When seen as holistic selves, clients and caregivers lead complex human lives. At any given moment, the sum of a person's past and present experience influences the person's feelings, attitudes, and actions.
2. Structural dimensions. Structural dimensions are associated more with the structure of provider-client interactions than with ideologies about them. Three structural conditions are freedom of action, status equality, and shared decision making and responsibility.
   a. Freedom of action is relative because many factors restrict the freedom of clients and practitioners. Human relations are themselves restricting because of obligations to recognize the worth and dignity of others. Clients are restricted by such factors as illness, ignorance, and financial constraints. Practitioners are restricted by institutional commitments, colleague pressures, scarce resources for therapy, and cost considerations. Humans do not have infinite freedom of action. However, most people have considerable control and choice over their destinies and need to be given the freedom to consider all options available to them.
   b. Status equality means that the people involved in an interaction are equal on some level. If either person sees himself or herself as superior or inferior to the other, the interaction cannot be fully humanizing. Various techniques—e.g., using language and terminology familiar to both, permitting informal salutations, adopting usual dress, talking with the client at eye level—can be used to equalize status.
   c. Shared decision making and responsibility reflect the ideology that all clients, regardless of education, have a right to participate as much as possible in decisions about their care. Implicit in shared responsibility are three assumptions: The client has behavioral options with respect to his or her care; the quality and duration of his or her life is at stake; and the client deserves significant control over choices of possible regimens and life-styles. Shared decision making makes the client and provider partners and therefore, in a way, equals. To share in decision making, the client must be informed

about prognoses, alternative therapies, and the rationales behind them.

The client's level of education will influence his or her desire and capacity to accept shared responsibility for care. In addition, some clients may be too sick, anxious, or irrational to analyze facts and help to make appropriate decisions.

3. Affective or emotional dimensions. The affective dimensions of humanism include empathy and positive affect.
   a. Empathy is the ability to identify and sympathize with others. Clients expect health care professionals to show sympathy and concern. Otherwise, clients feel depersonalized and dehumanized. For example, in the words of one client, "He should know how much my leg hurts and what it means to me." The dilemma of the practitioner is that too much empathy can be emotionally draining. In some instances, it may also be impossible to put oneself in the client's shoes. For example, an able-bodied nurse who cares for paraplegics knows that these clients are well aware she or he has two legs and cannot possibly identify with them as well as another paraplegic. Thus, a balance between too little and too much empathy is necessary. The means of achieving this balance needs research.
   b. Positive affect is the conveying of genuine feelings of warmth to the client. Feelings toward others may be positive, negative, or neutral. Positive feelings appear to be necessary for continued human-to-human contact, although clients may continue to consult an abusive practitioner if the talents of the practitioner are crucial, and a practitioner may continue to serve an abusive client because of professional ethics. Such interactions, however, are not humanistic.

Implications for Nursing

The changes and future trends in the health care system have many implications for nursing practice. Aydelotte (1983, pp. 814–15) described the following:

1. Greater need for nurses to function in primary care
2. Increased demands for nurses to improve their assessment and evaluation skills
3. Increased skills in communication, e.g., a second language or computer skills
4. Increased knowledge and acceptance of cultural diversity
5. Increased acceptance of change
6. Increased use of technology in teaching clients
7. Increased need for leadership skills for functioning in corporate structures

In addition nurses will need to:

1. Clarify the nurse's unique role in health care delivery. Much of the current work by nurse theorists and nurse researchers has this objective.
2. Expand the nurse's role in primary care in hospitals, homes, and industry and convince the public and government that such services would coordinate care, decrease fragmentation, and be cost efficient.
3. Design nursing strategies to meet the health promotion and health maintenance needs of people, especially the elderly, low-income persons, rural residents, the chronically ill, the unemployed, pregnant women, working women, children, and adolescents.
4. Research the costs of nursing care in relation to DRG categories and conduct research concerning quality assurance to ensure that cost containment measures do not affect the quality of nursing care provided.

Nurses in the past have prided themselves on giving high-quality care; however, ***high-quality care*** is difficult to define, and the cost of such care is impossible to quantify. In a study by Deines (1985), four levels of care were determined and then related to nursing activities. The four levels were optimum, good, fair, and safe. In this study, the frequency of mouth care, for example, varied according to the level of care, e.g., mouth care qid (optimum level); tid (good level); bid (fair level); and gd (safe level) (Deines 1985, p. 48).

Chapter Highlights

- Health care services are provided by a variety of health care personnel in a variety of settings.
- Government health care agencies, established at the local, state (provincial), and federal levels, are supported by revenues obtained through taxes.
- Voluntary nonprofit health service agencies are established to meet a specific health care need and rely on donations and government grants.
- Agencies providing health care can be viewed as giving primary, secondary, and tertiary care.
- Primary care agencies focus on health maintenance, health promotion, and disease prevention.
- Several alternative health care delivery systems, such as health maintenance organizations, preferred provider organizations, and individual practice associ-

ations, have arisen in the past decade to encourage preventive health care and to reduce the cost of health care to the consumer.

- Secondary care agencies, such as hospitals and ambulatory care clinics, focus on the treatment of illness and the prevention of complications of disease conditions.
- Tertiary care agencies provide long-term care and rehabilitation services and focus on restoring the client to optimum functioning after physical or mental illness.
- A variety of hospice services meet the special needs of the terminally ill in settings other than acute care agencies; caring and psychologic support are emphasized.
- Health care services are currently financed through social insurance, such as Medicaid and Medicare in the United States and the National Medical and Hospital Insurance programs in Canada; direct client payments; voluntary insurance plans, such as Blue Cross and Blue Shield; and charitable donations.
- The prospective payment system (PPS) was introduced in the United States to curtail the escalating costs of health care.
- Because of fewer hospital admissions, earlier discharges, and staff reductions—the results of PPS—the need for home health care has increased.
- Consumer attitudes—their view of health care as a right and their demand for comprehensive, holistic, and humanistic health care—are noticeably influencing health care delivery.
- Consumers are demanding greater emphasis on health promotion and illness prevention rather than on treatment of disease.
- The idea that health is the responsibility of each individual in society is gaining greater acceptance.
- Social changes, such as the women's movement, the rise in single-parent families and in women working outside the home, cultural diversity, and the growing elderly population are influencing the type and quantity of health care services needed.
- The unemployed and poverty-stricken have unique health care needs that require increasing attention.
- Future challenges in health care delivery are to promote health as a way of life, to prevent ill health, and to provide community care for all.
- In the future, nurses will need to be prepared to practice in primary care settings and to develop the skills to work in these settings.

Suggested Readings

Curtin, L. L. March 1980. Is there a right to health care? *American Journal of Nursing* 80:462–65.
In this thought-provoking article, Curtin discusses "human rights" as related to health care and presents these in relation to "human wants." Curtin suggests that reasonable health guidelines should be developed and that the intrusion of government in the health of people should be limited.

Griffith, H. September/October 1983. Competition in health care. *Nursing Outlook* 31:262–65.
Griffith views the effect of competition in the health care delivery system in terms of consumer involvement, free entry for qualified providers, and political prognosis of the procompetition proposals. Griffith considers the implications for nurses in legal, political, and economic areas as well as in the nurses' role in preventive and geriatric care and consumer education.

Kibrick, A. K. March 1981. Accountability, review boards, and the lay participant. *Nursing and Health Care* 2:124–29.
Kibrick describes four areas of consumer involvement in health care and recommends courses of action for consumers who wish to become members of review boards.

Maples, L. September/October 1985. Patient-family responses to the DRG system. *Geriatric Nursing* 6:271–72.
Some clients and families are experiencing the negative effects of DRGs. Although there is some consumer support for reduced hospital stays, clients need more individualization than the present system allows.

Shaffer, F. A. January 1984. A nursing perspective of the DRG world. Part 1. *Nursing and Health Care* 5:48–51.
Shaffer reviews the legislative events leading to the change in hospital reimbursement under Medicare from a per diem rate to a DRG rate. Shaffer discusses government monitoring of system abuses and implications of DRGs for nursing, nursing education, and nursing research.

Shaheen, P. P. June 1981. Nationalizing health care: A humanitarian approach. *Nursing Outlook* 29:358–63.
Shaheen briefly describes health delivery systems in Canada, the Soviet Union, China, the Arab states, and the United States. National health proposals are reviewed, and future trends are discussed. The article concludes with suggestions for reform of health care in the United States.

Selected References

Amenta, M. O. September/October 1984. Hospice U.S.A. 1984: Steady and holding. *Oncology Nursing Forum* 11:68–74.

American Demographics, P.O. Box 68, Ithaca, N.Y. 14851.

American Nurses' Association. Center for Research. June 1985. *DRGs and nursing care.* Kansas City, Mo.: American Nurses' Association.

Archer, S. E. June 1981. National health service: Rationale and implementation. *Nursing Outlook* 29:364–68.

Aydelotte, M. K. 1983. The future health care delivery system in the United States. In Chaska, N. L. *The nursing profession: A time to speak.* New York: McGraw-Hill.

Bentley, J. D., and Butler, P. 1980. Case mix reimbursements: Measures, applications, experiments. *Hospital Financial Management* 3:14.

Blue Cross and Blue Shield. December 1982. *The Blue Cross and Blue Shield consumer exchange.*

Bush, J. March 1985. DRGs challenge nursing curricula. *Journal of Nursing Education* 24:89.

Canadian Department of National Health and Welfare. 1974. *A new perspective on the health of Canadians: A working document* (Lalonde Report). Ottawa: Department of National Health and Welfare.

———. 1976. *Health field indicators, Canada and provinces.* Ottawa: Department of National Health and Welfare.

———. 1980. *Report of the task force to the conference of deputy ministers.* Ottawa: Minister of Supply and Services.

Caterinicchio, R. P., editor. 1984. *DRGs: What they are and how to survive them—A sourcebook for professional nursing.* Thorofare, N.J.: Charles B. Slack.

Colt, A. M.; Anderson, N.; Scott, H. D.; and Zimmerman, H. October 1977. Home health care is good economics. *Nursing Outlook* 25:632–36.

Crichton, A.; Lawrence, J.; and Lee, S. 1984. *Doctors and patients negotiate the system of care: Readings. The Canadian Health Care System.* Vol. 1. Ottawa: Canadian Hospital Association.

Curtin, L. L., and Zurlage, C. 1984. *DRGs: The reorganization of health.* Chicago: S-N Publications.

Deines, E. October 1985. Coping with PPS and DRGs: The levels of care approach. *Nursing Management* 16:43–44, 46–48, 52.

Diers, D. June 1985. Nursing intensity and DRGs. Unpublished paper presented at the National League for Nursing Convention.

Enthoven, A. C. 1980. *Health plan: The only practical solution to the soaring cost of medical care.* Reading, Mass.: Addison-Wesley Publishing Co.

Goldsmith, S. B. 1981. *Health care management. A contemporary perspective.* Rockville, Md.: Aspen Systems Corporation.

Griffith, H. September/October 1983. Competition in health care. *Nursing Outlook* 31:262–65.

———. May 1985. Who will become the preferred provider? *American Journal of Nursing* 85:538–42.

Griffith-Kenney, J. 1986. *Contemporary women's health: A nursing advocacy approach.* Menlo Park, Calif.: Addison-Wesley Publishing Co.

Hamilton, J. January/February 1986. Consumer alert: DRGs—Are hospitals saving money at your expense? *American Health* 41–45.

Howard, J., and Strauss, A., editors. 1975. *Humanizing health care.* New York: John Wiley and Sons.

Kneisl, C. R., and Ames, S. W. 1986. *Adult health nursing: A biopsychosocial approach.* Menlo Park, Calif.: Addison-Wesley Publishing Co.

Kron, T. 1961. *Nursing team leadership.* Philadelphia: W. B. Saunders Co.

Luft, H. S. 1981. *Health maintenance organizations: Dimensions of performance.* New York: John Wiley and Sons.

Micheletti, J. A., and Shlala, T. J. October 1985. PROs and PPS: Nursing's role in utilization management. *Nursing Management* 16:37–42.

O'Neill, P. 1983. *Health crisis 2000.* London: William Heinemann.

Porter-O'Grady, T. October 1985. Strategic planning: Nursing practice in the PPS. *Nursing Management* 16:53–56.

Pryga, E., and Bachofer, H. June 24, 1983. *Hospice care under Medicare.* Working paper. Chicago: Office of Public Policy Analysis, American Hospital Association. Cited in Amenta, M. O. September/October 1984. Hospice U.S.A. 1984: Steady and holding. *Oncology Nursing Forum* 11:68–74.

RNABC News. May/June 1984. *Key amendments part of new health act.* Vancouver: Registered Nurses' Association of British Columbia.

Rodgers, J. A. October 1981. Health is not a right. *Nursing Outlook* 29:590–91.

Rutkowski, B. L. March/April 1985. DRGs: Now all eyes are on you. *Nursing Life* 5:26–29.

Shaffer, F. A., editor. 1984. *DRGs: Changes and challenges.* New York: National League for Nursing.

Shamansky, S. L., and Clausen, C. L. February 1980. Levels of prevention: Examination of a concept. *Nursing Outlook* 28:104–8.

Smith, C. E. January 1985. DRGs: Making them work for you. *Nursing 85* 15:34–41.

Statistics Canada. 1980. *Perspectives Canada III.* Ottawa: Minister of Supply and Services.

———. 1981. *Canada year book 1980–81.* Ottawa: Statistics Canada.

U.S. Bureau of the Census. 1980. *Statistical abstract of the United States.* 101st ed. Washington, D.C.: U.S. Government Printing Office.

U.S. Department of Commerce. July 1, 1984. *Statistics on elderly population.* Washington, D.C.: Bureau of the Census.

U.S. Department of Health and Human Services. 1982. *Health United States.* Pub. no. (PHS) 83-1232. Washington, D.C.: U.S. Government Printing Office.

———. August 1985a. *Charting the nation's health trends since 1960.* Pub. no. (PHS) 85-1251. Hyattsville, Md.: Public Health Service.

———. December 1985b. *Health United States.* Pub. no. (PHS) 86-1232. Hyattsville, Md.: Public Health Service.

U.S. Department of Health, Education, and Welfare. 1979. *Healthy people: The surgeon general's report on health promotion and disease prevention.* Pub. no. 79-55071. Washington, D.C.: U.S. Government Printing Office.

Wald, F. S.; Foster, Z.; and Wald, H. J. March 1980. The hospice movement as a health care reform. *Nursing Outlook* 28:173–78.

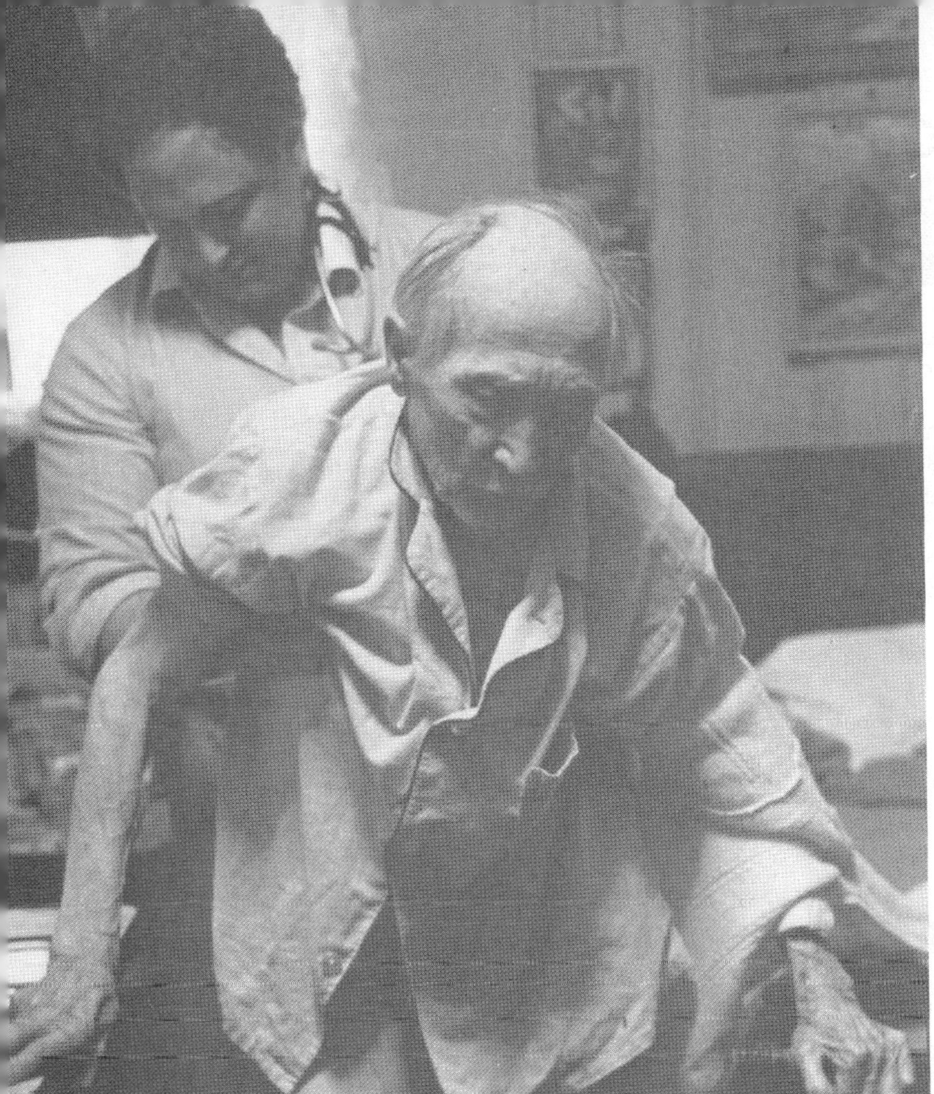

CHAPTER 4

Home Health Care

Barbara B. Germino

Contents

4 *Home Health Care*

Objectives

1. Understand essential facts about home health care.
   1.1 Define and describe the nature of home health care.
   1.2 Identify a variety of providers of home care.
   1.3 Describe three levels of home care services.
   1.4 Discuss sources of funding for home health care services.
   1.5 Compare the cost effectiveness of home health care, hospital care, and skilled nursing home care.
   1.6 Describe the recent history of home care, including legislative and policy changes and changes in providers, services provided, and client populations.
   1.7 Describe home environments that make home health care feasible.
   1.8 Define discharge planning and understand its importance in home health care.
2. Describe the use of the nursing process in home health care.
   2.1 Delineate eleven areas of client/family assessment for home health care.
   2.2 Identify issues in assessment of community needs for home health care.
   2.3 List general goals for different levels of home health care.
   2.4 Identify client/family/community variables that may affect goals for home health care.
   2.5 Discuss the processes of planning, implementing, and evaluating home health care.
   2.6 Discuss implementing home health care services to fit client and family needs.

Terms

basic services
direct services
discharge planners
discharge planning
home care
indirect services
intensive services
intermediate services
minimal services
rehabilitative services

Nature of Home Care

Home care is one aspect of comprehensive health care; it is comprised of health services provided to individuals and families in their homes. Its purposes include promoting, maintaining, and restoring health, specifically maximizing independent functioning and minimizing the disabling effects of illness, including terminal illness. Services appropriate to the needs of clients and their families are planned, coordinated, and delivered by providers organized for the delivery of home health care through the use of contractual arrangements, employed staff, or a combination of the two (Warhola 1980).

The subject of this chapter is the nature of home care. Included is a brief overview of its recent history and the impact of the national movement toward cost containment in health care. Further considerations are funding for home care; assessing needs for home care, including individual, family, and community needs; implementing home care, including hospital discharge planning; planning for acute, short-term needs, for the long-term needs of the chronically ill, and for the special needs of those dying at home; and fitting family needs and goals with services available. The role of the nurse as coordinator as well as provider of home care services is summarized.

Home care services are appropriate when an individual or family doesn't need full-time care, observation, or the special facilities of an institution such as a hospital or nursing home, yet does need care that family members or others cannot provide without assistance or teaching. Home care may or may not be associated with a hospitalization. It may precede or follow institutional care in a hospital or long-term care facility, or it may be provided along with ambulatory care (Lundberg 1984). Self-care and care given by health professionals and allied health personnel in the home account for the majority of health care provided in this country today. The time a person spends in a hospital receiving care for acute conditions is generally a very small percentage of his or her life. The need for home care services is increasing as the population of the United States ages and the incidence of chronic illness increases correspondingly (Lundberg 1984). Demand for home care services has increased for several reasons:

1. The costs of health care have inflated markedly, reflecting
   a. price increases in equipment, energy, and labor
   b. changes in supply and demand
   c. increased utilization of highly technical and specialized services
   d. little out-of-pocket expense to the consumer of health care (Davis 1983)
2. Efforts by the federal government and the health care industry to contain health care costs have resulted in shorter hospital stays and greater awareness and acceptance of home care services by providers and consumers.
3. Broader third-party coverage for care at home has become available.

The nature of home care services has broadened to include both acute, short-term care as well as long-term monitoring of problems associated with chronic illness. Comprehensive home care includes both direct and indirect services. **Direct services** involve direct contact between a caregiver and a client for the purposes of administering treatment or nursing care measures, assessment, teaching, counseling, or planning care. Direct services provided may be complex technical procedures, such as intravenous chemotherapy for cancer and respiratory therapy. Such services are becoming more widely available at home. Symptom management, teaching for self-care, monitoring adaptation to long-term illness, family counseling, physical and occupational therapy, and nutritional counseling are direct services provided by a variety of home care agencies. Such basic nursing care measures as bathing, skin care, assistance with ambulation, toileting, feeding, dressing changes, catheter care, and administration of medications have long been and continue to be direct service components of home care. Home care nursing also includes such direct services as providing ongoing assessment, anticipating and planning for problems or crises before they occur, helping clients think through problems and their options for dealing with them, managing symptoms, teaching, counseling, and assisting individuals and families to meet their health care goals.

Indirect services in home care include those measures taken to provide or facilitate direct services in nursing practice (McCorkle and Germino 1984). Consulting with other professionals and allied health personnel about client problems and needs, coordinating care within the home care agency, coordinating community resources and referrals outside the agency, supervising allied health workers providing services, and evaluating the effectiveness of care provided are all examples of indirect services currently provided by home care nurses. In addition, nurses involved in home care may be liaisons with acute care facilities and serve as facilitators and contact persons for clients and families who need access to special health care resources.

Providers of Home Care Services

Home health care services are available through a diversity of agencies and organizations. Such providers may be grouped into several general categories: government agencies (e.g., public health departments), hospital-based home care agencies, privately owned nonprofit agencies, voluntary (also nonprofit) agencies, and proprietary (for profit) agencies. Most of these agencies provide a variety of services, although their funding and financial operations differ greatly. Detailed discussion of each type of agency is beyond the scope of this chapter. However, the extent and variety of services, cost of services to the consumer, and other sources of reimbursement vary greatly. All of these agencies may coexist in a given community, serving different sectors of the population with some overlapping services.

Levels of Service

Sources for funding of home care service depend on the level of service. There are three levels: (a) intensive, (b) intermediate or rehabilitative, and (c) basic or minimal. Clients requiring **intensive services** need medical and professional nursing care as an alternative to hospitalization or skilled nursing home care. Clients are considered clinically unstable, needing a variety of therapeutic and ancillary services. Clients requiring **intermediate** or **rehabilitative services** need professional nursing supervision, direct care, physical or speech therapy, regular and periodic medical supervision, or some combination of the above. Clients are usually stable, but conditions are subject to change. Clients requiring **basic** or **minimal services** need supportive services, maintenance care, or personal care as an alternative to long-term institutionalization. Clients in this category are medically stable and have conditions unlikely to change for a period of time.

Reimbursement and Cost-Effectiveness

Medicare and most major medical insurance carriers reimburse for the intensive level of care when ordered by a physician and given by a Medicare-certified home health care agency. The intermediate level of care is also generally reimbursable when it is clearly justified by review of the client's record. It is more difficult, however, to obtain reimbursement for basic or maintenance care in the home, except on a private pay basis or from Medicaid (Lundberg 1984).

Studies documenting the cost-effectiveness of home health care services are beginning to be published, but the conditions under which home health care is most economical and the populations for whom these services are most effective are not yet clear. However, home health care in general appears to be an effective method for combating rising health care costs. The National Association for Home Care (NAHC) seeks to develop standards of care and guidelines for the administration of home care services. It also seeks to obtain and/or change health care legislation to improve services for home care clients (Weinstein 1984). The NAHC compiled these 1982 Medicare data:

Average hospital cost per day	$350
Average cost of skilled nursing home or convalescent home per day	57
Average cost of home health care visit	39

In addition, 21 home health visits cost an average of only $819 annually, as compared to 10.5 days of hospital care at an average annual Medicare cost of $3675 or 30 days in a skilled nursing facility at an average annual Medicare cost of $1710.

Although Medicare and Medicaid are major funding sources for skilled home health care, there are other ways to fund such care. States receive grants for low-income clients through Title 20. Many county and city programs support home health care for indigent or low-income clients. Some agencies receive community contributions in addition to public program reimbursements. Hospital-based home care programs participate in Medicare and Medicaid and also are supported by taxes, fees for service, and community contributions. Private agencies owned by their investors receive their major support from fees for service but also receive a return on equity payment. A number of insurance companies offer coverage for home health care. Insurance and payments by consumers for their care comprised more than half of the total home care reimbursements from 1979 through 1981 (Home Care 1984).

Funding for home care continues to change. Although more insurance companies are offering options for home care coverage, the nature of care that can be reimbursed is continually being reviewed and changed. As hospital stays become shorter and as hospital care becomes more technical, complex care is becoming more available in the home setting. A survey by the Blue Cross and Blue Shield Association showed that the number of insurance plans offering home health benefits rose from 46% of all plans in 1974 to 90% in 1983 (Home Care 1984). As private insurance rates have escalated in the last 10 to 12 years, more individuals and employees have chosen health maintenance organizations (HMOs) or preferred provider organizations (PPOs) because of their lower premiums. HMOs and PPOs specify which hospitals and physicians can provide care to their members (Yasko and Fleck 1984). Many of these organizations are beginning to offer home care provisions.

The federal government is currently reviewing Medicare payments for home care. Recent testimony in a congressional hearing by the National Association for Home Care (NAHC) reported the results of an NAHC survey of more than 2600 Medicare-certified home health agencies taken between October and December of 1985 and covering the 2 years prior. NAHC pointed out that the Department of Health and Human Services (DHHS) has, from the perspective of the home health agencies, imposed restrictive new guidelines on reimbursement for home health care. While home health agencies are rendering services to more and sicker clients, NAHC survey respondents claim that the DHHS has made it more difficult for them to do so and has decreased and slowed reimbursement to the point that some agencies are having cash flow problems (Capricious Regs 1986).

Recent History of Home Care

Nursing care has been given at home since nursing in any form first existed, and home nursing care was at times the primary mode of care delivery for all but the poorest people in Western society. Among the first significant published literature in nursing are the writings of Florence Nightingale, who discussed home care in detail. She portrayed the skilled nurse as an astute observer of both the client and the home environment—a person who could facilitate recovery from illness and maintenance of health by implementing positive changes in both the client and the home. Home care in North America has historically been part of urban public health nursing, visiting nurse services, and rural home nursing services, such as the Frontier nursing service.

Legislative and Policy Changes

Although the tradition is a long-standing one, the recent history of home care is characterized both by continuity and rapid change. Current and projected changes in funding and in types of agencies providing home care are discussed earlier in the chapter. Other changes are the result of legislation and policies enacted in the 1980s. Changes in the payment methods for hospitalized Medicare patients resulted from the Tax Equity and Fiscal Responsibility Act of 1982 (Public Law 97-248), known as TEFRA. Medicare now pays for services to hospitalized clients on an average "cost-per-case." This change was followed by adoption of a Medicare prospective payment system based on diagnosis-related groups (DRGs), a classification of clients according to how greatly they use hospital resources (Hartley and McKibbin 1983). The DRG system of classifying clients takes into account not only the client's disease but also his or her age, complicating conditions, and hospital procedures, such as surgery. Although the changes in approaches to health care financing were designed to be cost-control measures, they have far-reaching implications for the delivery of care in a variety of settings (McCorkle and Germino 1984). The new approaches reflect a change in thinking about payment for hospital services and evaluation of the variety of clients they serve (Davis 1983). The DRG idea has already been applied to the outpatient setting. Outpatient DRGs, known as APGs (ambulatory patient-related groups), were developed at Yale University in 1980 to serve as an indicator of efficiency in use of outpatient care resources (Knapp 1983).

Changes in health care financing, both philosophic and methodologic, pose a challenge to those providing home care. The careful documentation of care will be more important than ever, to sort out the costs of delivering various kinds of care and to provide data for evaluating the use of home care resources (McCorkle and Germino 1984). It has been predicted that the new prospective payment system for Medicare will spur the growth of HMOs because they have already demonstrated that they can provide quality care at affordable prices. For instance, HMOs, relying strongly on nurses, use home health care services effectively to reduce the number of hospital days of care (Davis 1983). Research is necessary to document not only the impact of home care on the health and well-being of the clients and families served but also the cost-effectiveness of that care. The research done to date indicates that although there are sometimes no significant short-term differences in cost-effectiveness, high-quality home care may enhance client and family satisfaction and offer consumers a cost-effective choice (Weissert et al. 1980).

In the current national movement toward cost containment and new models for funding of health care, nursing care services given at home will eventually be, along with other services, targeted for increased government regulation. Nurses need to be actively involved in documenting the cost-effectiveness of nursing home care services and in establishing regulations to expand those services and make them reimbursable.

Changes in Population Served, Services, and Providers

In addition to the legislative and policy changes that have affected and will continue to affect home care, there have been changes in the nature of the population being served, the services being offered, and the people providing those services. Many home care agencies, particularly those in large cities, traditionally serve the elderly ill, especially those with multiple diagnoses and those needing a range of support services, such as homemaking, home attendance, meal preparation, as well as skilled nursing care (Morris and Fonseca 1984). Services offered traditionally include coordination of support services, monitoring symptoms and side-effects of medication, client and family teaching for self-care, and basic nursing care, including catheter care and dressing changes. Another target group for home care services is the chronically ill, e.g., those with arthritis, diabetes, hypertension, heart disease, and other potentially disabling problems. Home care services for this group include, among others, monitoring symptoms, monitoring effects of treatment and medications, and teaching patients and families how to deal with illness and its effects. With the recent increase in the availability of highly technologic home care services, home care agencies are seeing a greater number of patients with remittent or progressive cancer, chronic obstructive pulmonary disease, cardiac disease, acute illnesses, and other problems requiring a variety of intravenous treatments, tube feedings, or ostomy care.

Patients with mental illnesses, such as depression and schizophrenia, may be referred for home care follow-up after hospital discharge, and home care nurses can monitor response to the home setting, administer and monitor medications, teach clients and families about medications, and offer client and family counseling as an adjunct to outpatient therapy (Weinstein 1984). With the advent of specialized programs targeting more complex ill clients, nurses carry out many procedures in the home that were once done only in the hospital. The emphasis on monitoring and maintenance, as well as primary prevention, has been expanded to include objectives such as reducing the frequency and number of hospitalizations for ill persons, reducing the incidence of infections like pneumonia, preventing and/or recognizing serious complications and taking necessary actions, arranging for 24-hour care as needed, providing more extensive teaching and demonstrations of care, managing symptoms such as pain on an ongoing basis, and administering treatments such as cancer chemotherapy and total parenteral nutrition (Weinstein 1984).

There is greater diversity in providers of home care services as well. At one time public health departments, visiting nurse associations, and private community nursing agencies (all employing nurses with general nursing backgrounds) bridged the gap between home and hospital. Now, a variety of health care professionals are more intensively involved, as are some of the manufacturers and distributors of medical products and supplies. Representatives of these companies offer coordination and support in adapting their equipment to home settings and in helping families and nurses work out reimbursement arrangements. In addition, some companies have established their own home care agencies or divisions, employing nurses and support personnel nationwide (Weinstein 1984). Many home care agencies, both private and public, employ or consult a variety of specialized providers: liaisons with hospitals and hospital teams, nurse clinical specialists, specialty nursing teams, and nurses with acute care hospital experience. New liaisons with schools and agencies offering continuing education programs are also being sought (Weinstein 1984).

Discharge Planning

Although home care is not always associated with hospitalization or a stay in a long-term care facility, home care services are often implemented as a result of such an admission. Because stays in acute care hospitals are becoming shorter due to cost-containment efforts, people are sometimes discharged still needing care. Such care is increasingly being delivered in the home. **Discharge planning**, the process of anticipating and planning for needs after discharge from a hospital or other facility, is becoming a crucial part of comprehensive health care. Effective discharge planning begins with the admission of the person and continues with ongoing assessment of both client and family needs, until discharge. It involves a comprehensive assessment not only of physical care needs but also of the availability of family and friend caregivers, the home environment as described by the client and family, client and family resources, and community resources.

Assessment of the client's and family's understanding of the health problem and subsequent needs, family values, and family health habits is also important. Some large hospitals have **discharge planners**, nurses whose primary responsibility is to assess anticipated needs after discharge. In most settings, however, staff, head nurses, and clinicians, with the help of social workers, are doing discharge planning. To facilitate the assessment needed for effective discharge planning, hospital staff may establish liaisons with community-based nurses who can visit the home before the client's discharge, thereby having the opportunity both to anticipate needs and plan with the family in advance of discharge. Effective two-way communication is obviously essential if information and planning are to be coordinated. After a thorough assessment, and preferably when the discharge date is known and the family's agreement is obtained, appropriate referrals can be made for needed home care services, including both professional and support services. The nurses can be effective in helping the family think through their typical day and week and process the changes they can anticipate when the ill person is at home. Thinking through "what-if" situations—What if the person should fall? What if there is an emergency? What if the caregiver needs to go to the store or do other essential errands?—helps families to confront what is happening to them at their own pace and in their own style and to plan for anticipated problems, thereby experiencing a sense of control and confidence (McCorkle and Germino 1984).

If at all possible, referrals and other actions are initiated before the day of discharge so that preparations for the client's return home are complete when he or she arrives. In this way, the client's and family's anxiety about the return is kept to a minimum. Referrals of a hospitalized client for home care are often initiated and implemented by the nurses caring for that client, but signed physician's orders for care are required if care is to be reimbursed by third-party payment. The physician may order treatments; medications; physical, occupational or speech therapy; and skilled nursing care. See Figure 4–1.

If a client is not hospitalized but is in need of home care services, referrals or requests for those home care services may come from the client or family, a public health or community nurse, a nurse in private practice, a physician, other health care workers, or social services personnel. Again, however, a physician's orders and signature are required for third-party reimbursement.

Assessing

Client and Family

Clients and families who need home care services often identify needs for particular kinds of help but may not be able to identify all the areas in which home care services could be helpful, either because they are not aware of problems or potential problems or because they do not understand the kinds of services available through home care agencies. The initial and ongoing assessment of clients and families, including their environments, is vital to the effectiveness of home care services. Nurses assessing a client with a potential need for home care are likely to use some or all of the following criteria (Mayers 1975):

1. *Ability to function independently.* This criterion includes the success with which the client and family have managed other health problems by themselves or with the guidance but not the direct intervention of others.
2. *Physical condition.* This assessment includes information obtained from a written referral or the client's hospital record and direct assessment of general appearance, signs and symptoms, level of growth and development, and physical functioning, especially in such activities of daily living as eating, sleeping, toileting, walking, and dressing.
3. *Feelings, behavior, and communication.* The client's mood, expression of feelings, behavior and conversation, and body language and other nonverbal cues are examined in light of the illness, the environment, and the resources available for support.
4. *Interpersonal competence.* The client's ability to make his or her needs and wishes known to others appropriately and to relate to family, friends, and caregivers are important areas for assessing how the client and family are coping with the health problem(s).
5. *Ability to meet role expectations.* Whether a client can carry out the responsibilities of job, family roles, and relationships with others and how the client feels about limitations are important aspects of assessing potential home care needs and problems.
6. *Client and family goals.* To help the client and family to achieve goals or modify them appropriately, the nurse needs information about client's and family's understanding of illness and its implications, the values held by the client and family, and their plans for the future.
7. *Cognitive functioning.* The nurse needs to assess the client's and family's ability to think through problems, level of education and intellectual ability, and decision-making skills.
8. *Economic and environmental resources.* Needs for supportive and counseling services may emerge from assessment of the adequacy of the family's economic resources, the safety and comfort of their home environment, and pending problems such as the possibility of financial burdens due to health care costs.
9. *Understanding of health problems and client/family health practices.* The nurse assesses the client's and family's basic health habits, such as nutrition, bathing, rest, and sleep; prevention practices, such as immunization; knowledge and use of health care resources in the community; and understanding of current health problems and their implications.
10. *Coping with health problems.* The nurse assesses how the client and family have adjusted to health problems and the changes they impose, e.g., by sharing tasks, taking over for the ill person, using resources to deal with problems, and seeking care as needed. The family's emotional and behavioral response to health problems is also of importance. Do some family members feel overburdened or highly stressed, fearful about the future or for each other? Are some family members' needs not being met because of the focus on the health problem(s) or on one family member?
11. *Resources for the family.* What kinds of human and other resources are available to the family? To what extent are they aware of and using these resources? How adequate are these resources in helping the family deal with the health problem(s)? What resources are unavailable? How could unmet needs be met with new resources?

Individuals and Groups at Risk

While home care services are primarily focused on individuals and families, knowledge of risk factors gained from epidemiologic research can help home health care providers identify those clients who need or potentially need particular types of intervention. Epidemiology—the study of disease, disability, and risk factor patterns in populations—provides valuable data with which to assess the home care needs of the community. Epidemiologic studies provide information on the incidence, prevalence, and the severity of disease and other conditions that cause illness and death in the population at large as well as among specific age, sex, racial, regional, or other subgroups of that population (Archer and Fleshman 1985). These data can help nurses plan for services and justify the availability and reimbursement of those services. For instance, as the percentage of the elderly in the population of the United States grows and the incidence of chronic illness rises correspondingly, the elderly's need for home care services is becoming a large portion of the total need. The increase, in many areas of the country, in the incidence of adolescent pregnancy has created a need for mother-infant and family-oriented home care services that take into account the adolescent mother's developmental level and special needs as well as the increased risk of prematurity and birth defects in the infants born to very young mothers. Epidemiologic studies show that certain groups of the population are more at risk for particular illnesses; smokers' increased risk of lung cancer is one of the most striking examples. Until some of these trends

PATIENT'S REFERRAL

4 S447652001 Inpt
NAME LAST Phillips FIRST Margaret MIDDLE P.
DATE OF BIRTH 4/18/32 SEX/COUNTY F/Lazin

Date Sent: 8/1/86 TO: agency Home Health of Lazin County

Address, (Street, Town, State, Zip Code, County -- Directions if necessary)
14 Perce Lane
Valleyville, North Carolina
(Two blocks west of town hall)
Telephone: 373 4499

I hereby authorize release of the medical information pertaining to this illness to the above named agency and to the physician accepting me as a patient.

Margaret P. Phillips
Signature of Patient (or authorized person) Date 8/1/86

Admission Date	Discharge Date	Floor or Clinic	Appointment
7/26/86	8/1/86	4 South	Date 8/10/86 Clinic Surgery

Physician to whom patient is referred for continuing care: Dr. Herbert Johnston
Address: 34 Main Street, Valleyville, North Carolina

Person responsible for patient	Relationship	Address	Telephone
Peter Phillips	husband	14 Perce Lane, Valleyville, NC	373 4499

PHYSICIAN'S ORDERS AND PLAN OF TREATMENT (including diagnosis, present condition, medications, activity, diet, plans for medical follow up, etc.)

Diagnosis: Postop modified R radical mastectomy for intraductal carcinoma breast
Present Condition: Excellent for 5 days postop.
Medications: Tylox 1 q 3-4h prn for incisional pain
Activity: Ad lib ambulation with arm exercises as taught and practiced with physical therapist; increasing distance walked each day to build strength
Diet: No restrictions; encourage adequate fluid consumption in hot weather
Incision Care: Careful cleaning with Betadine soap 1x/day and cover only open area where drain removed until it heals. Inspect incision for signs of infection.
Psychological Support: See attached

I hereby certify that this patient who is under my care:
☐ Requires care in an extended care facility
☒ Is essentially homebound and requires the specified home health services

Physician's Signature
Date 8/1/86

Known To: P.T. ☒ O.T. ☐ S.W. ☐ Dietitian ☐ Other ☐ Specify____ Additional Information Attached X

PATIENT'S NEEDS AND CARE PLAN - NOTES BY NURSE AND OTHER HEALTH WORKERS (including observations, instructions given patient/family, attitudes of patient/family regarding illness; treatment taught, etc.)

Observations: This 54 year old woman is recovering well physically from her mastectomy for breast cancer. She is walking increasing distances each day. Her incision shows no swelling, redness, induration or other signs of infection. A 5 cm. section where drain was removed is still not closed but is not draining and appears to be healing. She has some edema in her R arm but according to daily measurements it is slowly decreasing.

Client , husband, and daughter have been taught wound care, arm exercises, and given instructions for increasing activity. Restrictions currently include only bathing and extremely fatiguing activity. When wound closes, client may shower as she wishes.

Client found lump on SBE; has been encouraged to continue this practice. Diagnosis and surgery happened rapidly and unexpectedly and she appears to be experiencing some weepiness, depression, and fearfulness as the reality of the diagnosis sinks in. She needs the opportunity to continue to discuss and process her experiences, as well as to ask questions as they occur. Her physician has initiated a Reach to Recovery referral but she may need several visits from a nurse during the next two weeks. Her husband and daughter have been able to be very supportive but this has upset them too and a non-family member would be helpful as a sounding board.
(Continued on attached page)

Sara P. Jones, R.N., Head Nurse
Signature & Title

Figure 4–1 Patient's Referral Form. **Source:** From North Carolina Memorial Hospital, Chapel Hill, NC. Reprinted with permission.

Name: Phillips, Margaret P.
Unit No.: 4 S447652001

PATIENT'S REFERRAL - Continuation Sheet

Date: 8/1/86

Physician's Orders (Continued)

Psychological Support: Have ordered Reach to Recovery referral. Please follow through since this is needed as soon as possible. She is to be observed for signs of increasing depression such as loss of appetite,
1 flattened affect, inactivity, crying spells, and loss of interest in her appearance. I am concerned about this woman's psychological state.

Plans for medical follow-up: I will see in the Surgery clinic on 8/10/86 to evaluate progress. The family has my telephone number and has been encouraged to call if they are concerned about her condition. Plan followup chemotherapy as soon as possible considering both physical and psychological status.

Client's Needs and Care Plan (continued)

Please assess the following on first visit:

1. Incision, particularly open area for signs of infection
2. Status of edema in R arm. Measurement lines are still evident.
3. Physical stamina including amount of daily activity and level of fatigue. (This woman was jogging 3 miles four days a week before surgery).
4. Amount of pain or discomfort from incision or in R shoulder and arm. (Complains of joint stiffness with inactivity although she has not been diagnosed with arthritis.)

*5. Psychological/emotional status. Please assess the extent to which she has been able to process the diagnosis, the surgery, and the possible implications. She has been told she had a small tumor but two positive nodes and will have adjuvant chemotherapy. Her mood, fears, and relationships with those close to her need to be assessed. Please note her response to the Reach to Recovery volunteer's visit.

Sara P. Jones, R.N. Head Nurse
Signature & Title

can be reversed, home care services designed to meet special subpopulation needs will continue to be an essential part of comprehensive health care.

Community Needs

To determine the community need for home care services, the nurse can follow the steps recommended by the U.S. Department of Health and Human Services (Warhola 1980). These steps include consideration of the size of the elderly population (65 to 74 years of age) and the numbers of elderly over age 75 in the community. Projections are that about 9% of those 65 to 74 years of age and about 25% of those over 75 are likely to need home care services. The size of the population under age 65 is also considered in the assessment of community needs for home care, as is the number of individuals recently discharged from acute care hospitals. In addition, estimations are made of the numbers of people in the community who are being placed in skilled or intermediate care facilities but who could possibly have avoided such admissions or delayed them through home care services. Other factors that affect estimates of community need for home care services include potential needs of children, the mentally ill, the terminally ill, and other high-risk groups.

In addition to assessing specific community population characteristics, the nurse needs to assess the nature of the community itself—its structure, culture, and functioning—to best plan home care services that will be acceptable and effective in a given community. For example, the community's physical size, population density, location and resources, and topography are important. Predominant community values and styles of dealing with problems and implementing change in the community affect both the services to be offered and the structure of agencies or programs offering those services (Klein 1975).

Nursing Diagnosis

After organizing, prioritizing, and analyzing the assessment data, the nurse should next establish the nursing diagnoses for the client and/or support persons. Examples of nursing diagnoses that might be applicable are shown to the right.

Examples of Nursing Diagnoses for Home Health Care

- Ineffective individual coping related to loss of leg
- Ineffective family coping related to lack of support system
- Knowledge deficit related to medications
- Impaired home maintenance management related to impaired cognitive functioning
- Self-care deficit related to inability to bathe self secondary to visual deficit
- Self-care deficit related to inability to dress self secondary to impaired use of hands

Goals

In planning home care, both short- and long-term goals need to be established. Goals for home care vary somewhat with the type of agency and its philosophy and purposes. Most agencies, whether public or private, are committed to meeting the home care needs of the population they serve and to offering effective services at reasonable costs. General goals for home care fall in four major categories: keeping clients and families healthy and functioning as independently as possible; restoring optimal health and independent functioning after illness; assisting clients and families to deal with chronic health problems in ways that maintain optimal individual and family functioning; and assisting clients and families to deal with a terminal illness in ways that promote living to the fullest until death and, for the survivors, after the loss of a significant person. In addition, a goal for all home care is to provide continuity of care by planning for change and by coordinating services as needs and health care settings change. The idea of continuity is based on the belief that optimal care for clients and families requires ongoing

Table 4–1 General Objectives for Home Care Based on Desired Outcomes

Outcomes	Maintenance of Health and Independent Function	Recovery from Acute Illness	Adaptation to Chronic Illness
Objectives	Early diagnosis of illness	Limiting frequency and length of hospitalizations	Limiting hospitalizations
	Promoting and supporting good health habits	Preventing or limiting complications	Limiting complications and functional losses
	Encouraging regular checkups and screening	Providing supportive services for client and family	Increasing client/family understanding of the illness
	Facilitating effective development and use of support systems	Limiting both physical and psychosocial consequences of the acute illness	Assisting client and family to deal with the treatment regimen and changes imposed by the illness

contact with at least one professional caregiver who knows the client and family and who supports their right to participate in decisions affecting their health, treatment of health problems, and the circumstances of their lives.

The level of the client's health and the nature and characteristics of the client's illness determine which goals are appropriate (see Table 4–1). Maintaining health and independent functioning involves such strategies as screening and early diagnosis of illnesses; promoting and supporting good health habits, including life-style changes to improve health; encouraging regular health checkups; and helping clients to use support systems (family, friends, and professionals) effectively. When an acute or short-term illness alters individual and family health and functioning, the objectives for home care include limiting the frequency and number of hospitalizations, preventing or limiting complications, facilitating recovery, providing supportive services that allow the family to recover, and limiting the physical and psychosocial consequences of illness. Objectives for the care of clients and families dealing with chronic illnesses also include limiting hospitalizations and complications, but, in addition, involve helping individuals and families adapt over time to the changes the particular illness imposes. To facilitate such adaptation, the nurse provides teaching to help the client and family understand the illness and its signs and symptoms, and manage the required treatment regimen in a way that is effective, realistic, and tolerable to the entire family. The family with a diabetic child needs to learn about diabetes, the signs and symptoms of hypoglycemia, the administration of insulin, and appropriate diet and exercise. In addition, family members need to learn how to maintain as normal a life-style as possible, to facilitate the child's growth and development and support positive family relationships.

Discussion of family functioning, family goals, and plans for the future in light of the projected pattern and prognosis of the chronic illness is an objective in which nurses, social workers, counselors, and physicians may all be involved. Objectives for the client and family facing a chronic or terminal illness must, of necessity, be flexible and responsive to changing needs. The family may need direct physical care, teaching, respite care, referral for financial support, counseling about effects of illness on the entire family, identification of support resources, and help in making alterations in the home environment. One illness might create all these needs in one client and family over time.

Clients and families dealing with terminal illness may need help not only with providing physical care but also with handling the emotional impact of caring for a dying family member and anticipating his or her death. Research on terminal care indicates that family members not only needed help in providing physical care for the person dying at home but also expressed need for emotional support and family counseling (Rose 1976). Evaluation of the effectiveness of home care for clients and families facing terminal illness indicated that support and education for the family were as important as the physical care and comfort measures provided for the dying person (Kassakian et al. 1979).

Environment

Dealing with illness is as much an issue for the family as it is for the ill person. When one member of the family is affected by illness, all members are affected in some way; the whole family must readjust to support the ill person and continue to function effectively, both as a family and in relation to the larger society (McCorkle and Germino 1984). The nurse who assesses the ill individual's needs must also consider the needs of the family.

The client and family both live and function in several contexts. The client's family provides one context. The extent to which they are able and willing to be helpful and supportive is a part of determining whether the environment can support home care. If even one family member is willing and has the energy, time, and resources either to provide care, work with the nurse to arrange for care, and/or allow caregivers into the home and cooperate in care, the family environment can probably support the delivery of home care services. Individuals who live alone but who have family or friends who are willing to check on the ill person, provide emergency assistance, or be available to home caregivers for help or information also live in an environment that can support some kinds of home care services.

The physical environment of the client and family also may or may not support home care. For much basic nursing care, a source of clean water, clean linens and clothes, and a relatively clean and safe environment are essentials. Certainly, adequate heat in cold climates can be a significant factor in preventing complications, aiding recovery, and providing comfort. Many environments that offer less than optimum cleanliness, safety, and comfort can, with some resources and assistance, be adapted to support some home care services. In those environments that cannot be altered to support home care services, the client and family may have to consider such options as moving the ill person to another environment, for example, a friend's or relative's home, a hospital, or a convalescent or long-term care facility. This decision may be difficult and painful; the family may feel guilt at being unable to provide an environment in which home care is possible. It is extremely important that the nurse and other professionals be not only astute assessors of environments for home care but also sensitive and supportive problem solvers who work with clients and families to think through options for care that are both supportive to the ill person and acceptable to the family.

In some cultures, the importance of keeping the ill individual at home outweighs the lack of what many health care professionals might consider essentials for comfort and effective care. Cultural, religious, and family values are important considerations for nurses providing home care to families. A support system of caring family and friends, willing to work with professionals to adapt a less-than-ideal environment, can do much to make the environment conducive to home care. Such a situation provides the opportunity for families and friends to have real impact on the well-being of the ill person, to see visible results of their efforts and support. In addition, the information gained from working with health care providers may have positive long-term implications for the client and family in future health problems.

The third context or environment that must support home care is the community environment. Does the community have the resources to meet the client's and family's needs? Many smaller communities do not have the scope, variety, or specialization of services that may be required in today's home care. Sometimes, services and/or consultation can be contracted with neighboring or mobile health care programs, enabling people in such communities to have home care. For example, in some communities within 50 to 100 miles of a cancer treatment center or a hospital treating cancer patients, mobile vans staffed with nurses and sometimes physicians travel to rural areas and individuals' homes to provide intravenous cancer chemotherapy.

An environment that is supportive of home care, then, has both the human and physical resources needed by a given client and family. A large, loving family is not a prerequisite; neither is a particular kind or size of home. But home care is impossible without at least one friend or family member willing to assist, basic safety and comfort, and needed community resources.

Short-Term Goals

A recent change in the demand for home care services is the increased need for acute, short-term care for clients with time-limited illnesses or health problems. Often such clients are discharged after a short stay in an acute care hospital. Services such as surgical wound care, assistance with progressive ambulation, and prevention and early recognition of such complications as infection, thrombophlebitis, and pneumonia are examples of appropriate short-term nursing care of a postsurgical client. Short-term services might also be appropriate for an elderly person with an acute illness, such as severe influenza, pneumonia, or acute arthritis. Often, careful monitoring, adjustment of medications, rest, exercise, and respiratory therapy or similar supportive care given at home can prevent hospitalization in such a situation. Support services, e.g., homemaker services for shopping, cleaning, and meal preparation, allow the ill person to rest and recuperate without worrying about maintenance of the household or the basic needs of the family. Acute, short-term care services are often reimbursable by third-party payers although an associated hospitalization is unfortunately still sometimes required, ostensibly as evidence of the acuteness of the illness. This practice is beginning to change as insurance companies examine the cost-effectiveness of short-term home care services in preventing expensive hospital admissions and long-term problems.

Long-Term Goals

Planning for long-term care can be more complex, especially if the client requires daily, direct physical care over a long period. Insurance companies and state and federal programs of reimbursement for home care all have some limits, either on dollar amounts per unit of time, number of days of service, or number of visits. Clients and families with long-term problems are likely to have to use more than one source of reimbursement over time. The home care needs of clients and families with chronic illnesses are likely to change over time, as the demands of the illness change. During many chronic illnesses, there are periods when the client requires more care or a change in level of care. The pattern of the illness—whether one of ups and downs, relative stability, remissions and exacerbations, or progressive deterioration—is a major factor affecting home care needs. Other factors that make flexible care planning in chronic illness a necessity are the ability and willingness of the caregivers to stay involved, the health of family and friends, the family's economic resources, other family and work responsibilities, and caregivers' fatigue and the need for respite from providing care.

Long-term care planning also involves the anticipation of the eventual effects of illness, including loss of ability to work, to carry out household tasks, or even to perform such daily activities as dressing and feeding oneself. Many of these changes, if not predictable, can be anticipated, and nurses need to help clients and families deal with the changes, look at options for other care, and plan ways to make adaptation easier.

The family caring for a dying member at home has special home care needs. Due to the American public's fairly recent concern for the care of terminally ill clients and their families, more communities have hospice programs available to help clients and families meet their goal of helping the dying person stay at home. In 1984, the number of hospice organizations in the United States was estimated to be approximately 800 (Godkin et al. 1983–84). These programs offer different services. Some are freestanding institutions with inpatient services, and some are community based, home care programs with a range of professional and volunteer services. Some hospital-based hospice teams (e.g., doctors, nurses, social workers, chaplains) offer patient support in any bed in the institution and function without a special hospice unit, whereas some hospitals have special hospice units with special staff and with or without a coordinated home care program (Godkin et al. 1983–1984). The hospice philosophy promotes holistic care of dying clients and their families, including psychologic, spiritual, social, and physical care as well as support for the family in their bereavement after the death. Considerations involved in assessing whether a home death is advisable include what moral support is available to the family, what professional help is available, whether special equipment, if needed, is available, whether the family can learn the necessary skills for care, and what knowledge the family needs to determine when death is imminent and to deal with the body after death (Hine 1979–80). Effective home care for the terminally ill includes support and education for the family as well as comfort care for the client (Kassakian et al. 1979). In addition, someone, usually a family member, must be available and willing to assume responsibility for care.

Hospice services are often reimbursable through medicare and Medicaid, as well as through some private insurance plans and health maintenance organizations. The majority of hospice organizations are nonprofit, and many adopt sliding scale fee schedules based on the family's ability to pay or on available reimbursement. Many hospices are supported at least in part by community contributions through such organizations as United Way, through fundraising projects, and through private donations. In this way, they can absorb the cost of services to families that do not have the resources to pay for care.

Implementing

Fitting Needs to Services

Client- and family-centered home care services are based on the belief that the consumers of such services have the right to participate in the choices and decisions involved. It is essential to know the goals and values of the client and family to find the best possible fit of needs and services. The nurse committed to working with families at home needs to clarify her or his own philosophy of care and continually evaluate care strategies in light of that philosophy and of the goals and values of the client and family. For instance, if a client with cancer makes an informed choice to discontinue home chemotherapy treatment in a situation where the prognosis is poor, the nurse who supports the client's right to make an informed choice needs to deal with her or his own feelings of loss effectively in order to support that choice and to assist the client and family to live their lives to the fullest for the time that is left. If the agency providing the care supports client-family participation in decision making about care, that agency can respect an informed choice, even one to discontinue treatment, and shift the plan of care to fit the goals and wishes of the client and family, in this case, to live as comfortably and fully as possible for the time remaining.

The issue of personal control in care is not a simple one. Not all clients and families want to control care and participate in decision making about care. Some find it more comfortable to put themselves in the hands of experts and have choices made for them. Again, to fit the needs of the client and family to home care services, one must recognize the variability of those needs and the necessity for ongoing two-way communication between the agency care providers and the client and family.

Coordinating Services

The complexity of client and family needs for home care and the increasing number and variety of services available make coordination of care for a given client and family imperative. Coordination is essential to achieve continuity of care; it is also a practical necessity for the family with multiple needs, whose home is invaded weekly by many caregivers providing services. As professionals with a commitment to dealing with human responses to illness, nurses are highly qualified to provide such coordination of care. Client and families need continuing contact with a professional who can discuss their needs and wishes sympathetically and who has the knowledge and skills to find resources for the care she or he cannot provide. The nurse who makes a continuing commitment to a client and family can keep track of those entering the home to provide services and seek feedback from the client and family about how they are dealing with multiple caregivers. The nurse can suggest that all care providers who come make entries in a notebook; the client and family, too, can document in the notebook visits made and care received, as well as their thoughts and observations. Such a record can serve as a primary source of data both for the family and the nurse in ongoing evaluation of what care was provided, how effectively it was provided, and how well the family deals with the invasion of their home by many different people.

Evaluating

Evaluation of the extent to which the short- and long-term goals have been met is concurrent, recurrent, and terminal. As the client's and the family's needs, priorities, and goals change, caregivers must help adjust both the plan for care and the strategies for achieving client and family goals. Effective ongoing communication among nurse, client, and family is the key to responsive home health care services.

Chapter Highlights

- Home health care is services provided to individuals and families in their homes.
- The aims of home health care are promoting, maintaining, and restoring health.
- Home health care is appropriate when a client does not need the special facilities of a hospital or nursing home but does need care that household members or friends cannot provide alone.
- Home health services can be direct or indirect and provided on three levels: intensive, intermediate, or minimal.
- Government agencies, hospital-based agencies, private nonprofit agencies, voluntary nonprofit agencies, and proprietary (for profit) agencies supply home health care.
- Although proved cost-effective, home care, especially minimal care, is not always reimbursable.
- Traditionally provided to the elderly ill needing nursing, homemaking, and home attendance services, home care is now being provided to nontraditional clients, such as to chronically or acutely ill people requiring technologic services and to the mentally ill.
- Home care is sometimes planned before a client is discharged from a hospital or long-term facility; some large hospitals employ discharge planners for this purpose.
- The steps of the nursing process—assessing, diagnosing, planning, implementing, and evaluating—are carried out by those providing home care.
- Nurses assess the needs of clients and families by applying eleven criteria, such as ability to function independently, physical condition, feelings, goals, and the like.
- Nurses use demographic and epidemiologic data to assess the home care needs of groups at risk and communities.
- Nurses and clients plan short-term and long-term goals of home care; the client's level of health and the characteristics of the client's illness determine which goals are appropriate.
- Not all environments are suitable for home care; a support system of caring family and friends and dedicated professionals is more essential than an ideal physical environment.
- An essential part of implementing is fitting services to the goals, values, and needs of clients.

Suggested Readings

DeCrosta, T. March/April 1984. Home health care: It's red hot and right now. *Nursing Life*: 5:54–60.

This article surveys the growth in home health care and the opportunities for nurses inherent in this trend. Several case examples are included.

Griffith, E. March 1984. Home care today. *American Journal of Nursing*. 84:340–42.

AJN editors interview Elsie Griffith, chief executive officer,

Visiting Nurse Service of New York, and chairman, National Association for Home Care. Griffith reviews the positive and negative aspects of changes taking place in home care and the implications for nursing.

Harris, M.D. April 1981. Evaluating home care? Compare viewpoints. *Nursing and Health Care* 2:207–13.

The author reports a study conducted by one Visiting Nurse Association that compared nurses' and patients' post-discharge evaluation of the quality of care given.

Weinstein, S.M. March 1984. Specialty teams in home care. *American Journal of Nursing* 84:342–45.

This article describes how the Dallas VNA developed clinical specialty programs designed to educate patients and families in self-care. These programs included pulmonary disorders, psychiatry, enterostomal therapy, IV therapy, diabetes, and cardiology.

Selected References

Archer, S. E., and Fleshman, R. P., editors. 1985. *Community health services.* Monterey, Calif.: Wadsworth Health Sciences.

Capricious regs shred Medicare's safety net. July/August 1986. *Geriatric Nursing*: 170–71.

Davis, C. K. 1983. The federal role in changing health care financing. *Nursing Economics* 1:10–17.

Godkin, M. A.; Krant, M. J.; and Doster, N. J. 1983–84. *International Journal of Psychiatry in Medicine* 13(2):153–65.

Hartley, S. S., and McKibbin, R. C. 1983. *Hospital payment systems and nursing: Relationships and implications.* Publication D-72D. Kansas City, Mo.: American Nurses' Association.

Hine, V. H. 1979–80. Dying at home. Can families cope? *Omega* 10(2):175–87.

Home Care. 1985. *Hospitals* 59:64–66.

Kassakian, M.; Bailey, L.; Rinker, M.; Stewart, C.; and Yates, J. 1979. The cost and quality of dying: A comparison of home and hospital. *Nurse Practitioner* 2:18–23.

Klein, D. C. 1975. Assessing community characteristics. In Spradley, B. W., editor. *Contemporary community nursing.* Boston: Little, Brown and Co.

Knapp, R. E. 1983. The development of outpatient DRGs. *Journal of Ambulatory Care Management* 6(2):1–11.

Lundberg, C. J. 1984. Home health care: A logical extension of hospital services. *Topics in Health Care Financing* 11:22–33.

Mayers, M. 1975. A search for assessment criteria. In Spradley, B. W., editor. *Contemporary community nursing.* Boston: Little, Brown and Co.

McCorkle, R., and Germino, B. 1984. What nurses need to know about home care. *Oncology Nursing Forum* 11(6):63–69.

Morris, E. M., and Fonseca, J. D. 1984. Home care today: An interview. *American Journal of Nursing* 84(3):340–42.

Rose, M. 1976. Problems families face in home care. *American Journal of Nursing* 76:416–18.

Warhola, C. 1980. *Planning for home health services: A resource book.* Pub. no. (HRA) 80-14017. Washington, D.C.: Public Health Service, Department of Health and Human Services.

Weinstein, S. M. 1984. Specialty teams in home care. *American Journal of Nursing* 84(3):342–45.

Weissert, W. G.; Wan, T. T. H.; Livieratos, B. B.; and Pellegrine, J. 1980. Cost-effectiveness of homemaker services for the chronically ill. *Inquiry* 17:230–43.

Yasko, J. M., and Fleck, A. 1984. Prospective payment (DRGs): What will be the impact on cancer care? *Oncology Nursing Forum* 11(3):63–72.

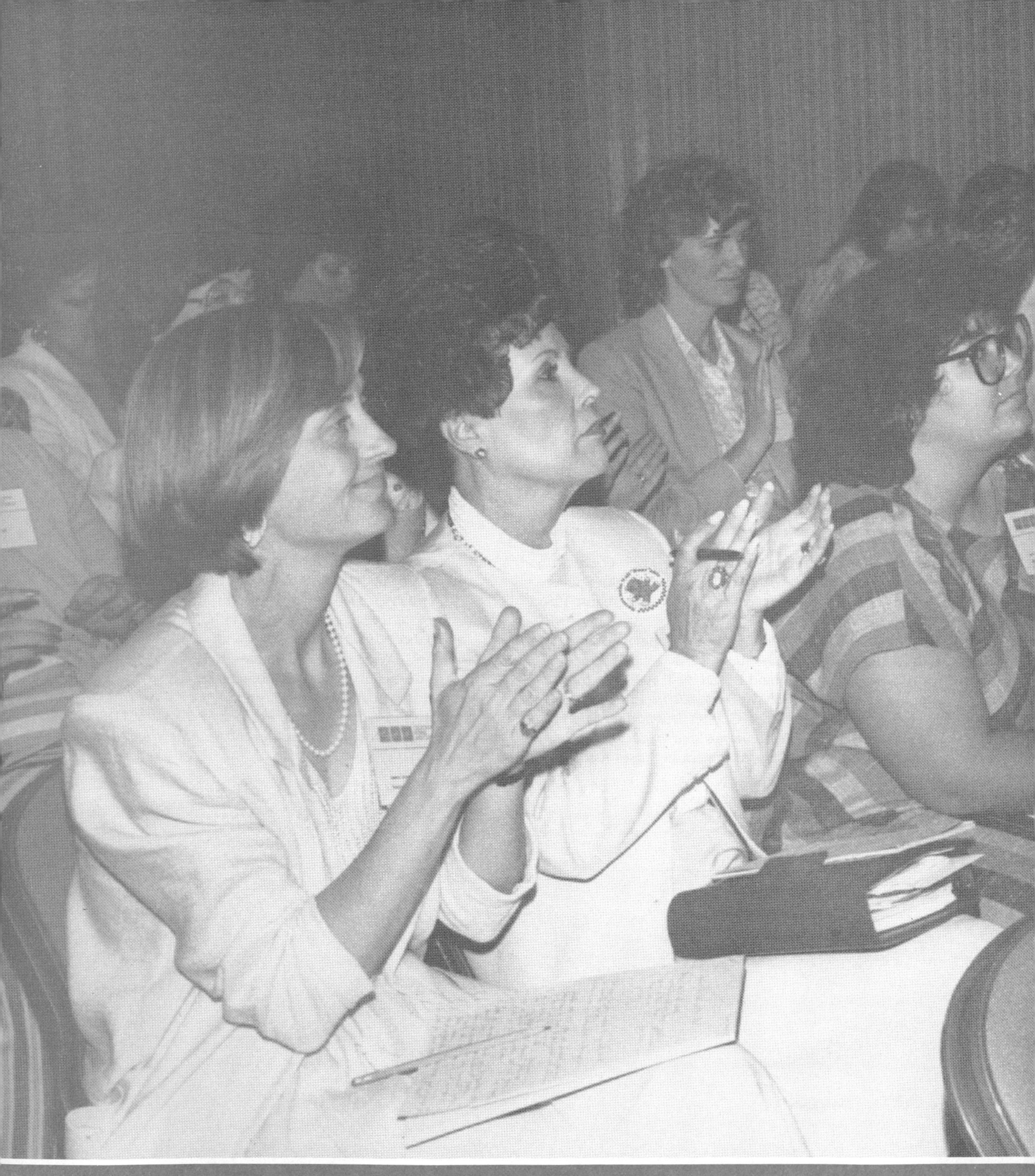

Whatever the internal issues that separate us, the most important goal is to continue to strengthen the profession. (Lucie S. Kelly)

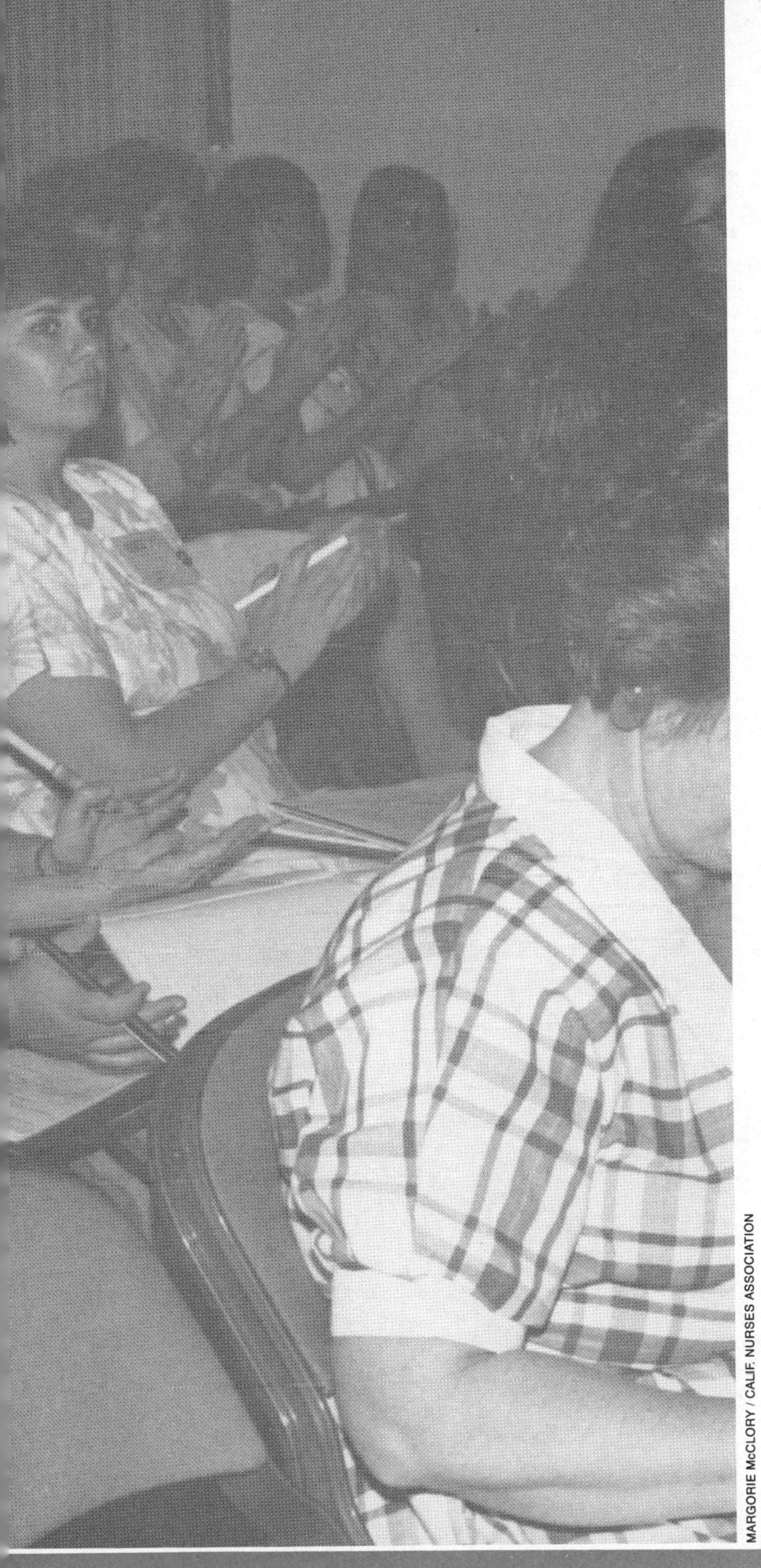

MARGORIE McCLORY / CALIF. NURSES ASSOCIATION

UNIT 2

Concepts for Professional Nursing Practice

Contents

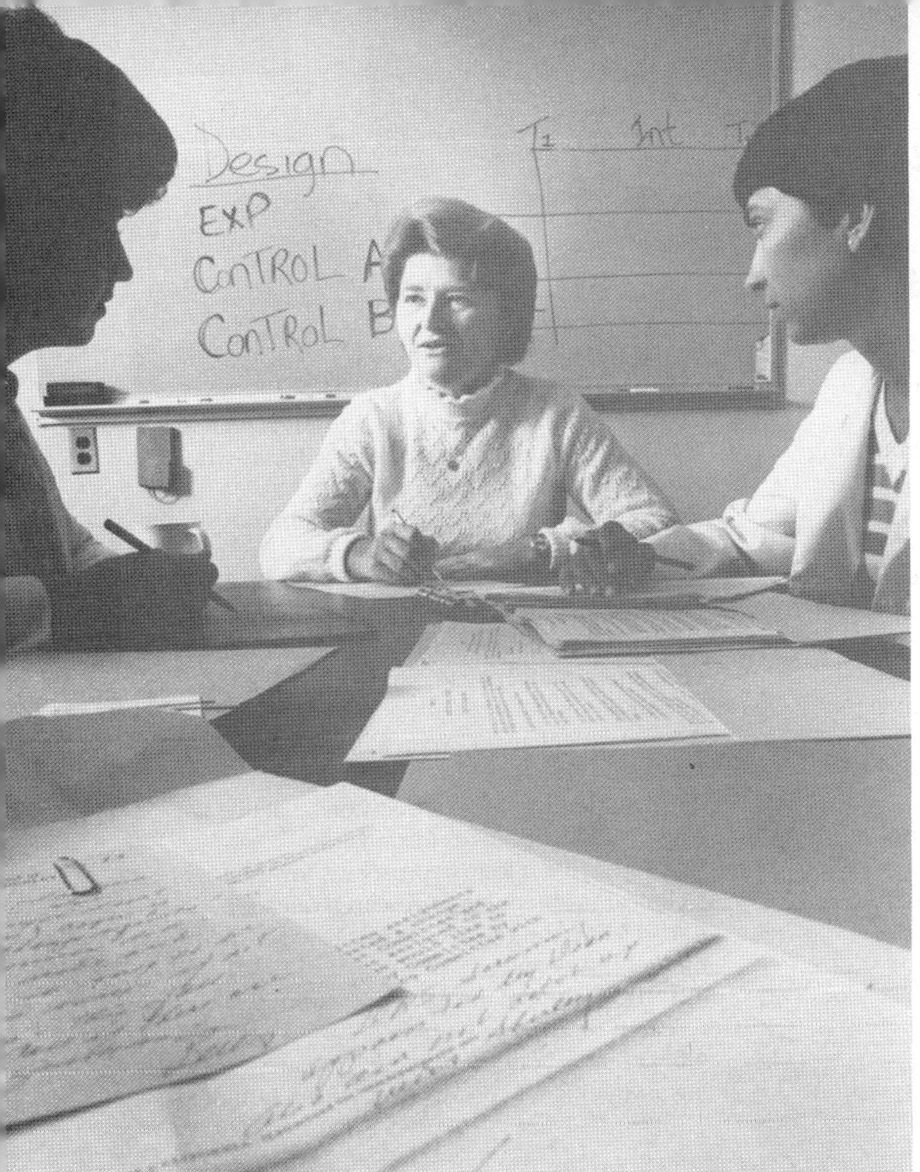

PAUL FUSCO

CHAPTER 5

Research in Nursing

Holly S. Wilson

Contents

5 *Research in Nursing*

Objectives

1. Appreciate the value of research in decision making for nursing practice and in building nursing knowledge.
   1.1 Describe the unique characteristics of nursing research.
   1.2 Differentiate nursing research from research in nursing.
   1.3 Specify the priorities for nursing research in the 1980s as identified by the ANA in 1981.
   1.4 Describe some examples of nursing studies that could influence nursing practice.
   1.5 List sources of access to published nursing research.
2. Identify the characteristics, aims, and steps of the scientific approach.
   2.1 Compare the scientific way of knowing with four other common ways of knowing.
   2.2 Identify the two major characteristics of scientific inquiry.
   2.3 List the steps of the research process.
   2.4 Discuss the primary emphasis of each step in the research process.
   2.5 Specify two major aims of science.
3. Evaluate a research study's provisions for protection of the rights of human subjects and maintenance of ethical principles.
   3.1 Define the principles of ethical research.
   3.2 Give examples of research subjects who are particularly vulnerable to risk.
   3.3 Discuss four basic rights of human research subjects.
4. Demonstrate the investigative role of all nurses in comprehending the meaning of commonly used research terminology, clinical problem identification, and intelligent use of nursing research findings.
   4.1 Differentiate between a clinical nursing problem and a researchable clinical problem.
   4.2 Name two types of questions that are not researchable without reformulation.
   4.3 Describe a four-step process for transforming a clinical problem into a research question.
   4.4 Define the research terms listed at the beginning of this chapter.
   4.5 Describe the format of a conventional research report.
   4.6 Identify some beginning strategies for becoming an intelligent consumer of research findings.

Terms

anonymity
concept
conceptual framework
confidentiality
confounding variable
construct
construct validity
data
deductive theory
dependent variable (DV)
empirical data
extraneous variable
full disclosure
grounded theory
hypotheses
independent variable (IV)
inductive theory
null hypothesis
nursing research
population
privacy
random sample
reliability
researchable problem
research ethics
research in nursing
research-practice gap
research process
rights of human subjects
risk of harm
sample
scientific inquiry
self-determination
theory
uncontrolled variable
validity
vulnerable subjects

What Is Nursing Research?

Most students recognize medicine's highly visible role in research. The public knows the role of medical research in discovering viruses, such as that responsible for acquired immune deficiency syndrome (AIDS); in facilitating surgical transplant of body organs; and in identifying habits, such as cigarette smoking, that endanger health. Until recently, however, the important impact of nursing research was not generally recognized by the public. In fact, the history of nursing research encompasses only about three decades, since its beginnings are usually traced to the early 1950s. Certain historians may point out that although nursing research had a rebirth in the 1950s and 1960s,

Florence Nightingale changed health care with her carefully researched case studies and detailed statistical accounts in the Crimea (Chenitz 1985).

Nursing research is more than just scientific investigations conducted by a person educated and credentialed as a nurse. It refers instead to research directed toward building a body of nursing knowledge about "human responses to actual or potential health problems" (ANA 1980, p. 9) and to the effects of nursing action on such human responses. The human responses of people may be (a) reactions of individuals, groups, or families to actual health problems, for example, the burden a family experiences when they must care for an elderly relative with senile dementia; and (b) concerns of individuals and groups about potential health problems, such as accident prevention or stress management in an industrial setting. The purpose of nursing research is to improve health care.

Nursing research also reflects the traditional nursing perspective. In this perspective, the client is seen as a whole person, with physiologic, psychologic, social, cultural, and economic components.

> For example, when a person has a head injury, the nurse needs to understand the body's processes for dealing with the increased pressure within the head and the changes this brings about in the patient's condition. At the same time, the nurse focuses on care that can maintain the person's cognitive, that is, thinking and feeling, processes. A nurse also would examine the person's life patterns that could lead to other head injuries (Roy 1985).

In addition to reflecting concern for the whole person, a nursing perspective implies 24-hour-a-day responsibility. Thus, this perspective encompasses all of the factors in a client's environment, such as fatigue, noise, sensory deprivation, nutrition, and positioning, that might influence coping patterns. Diers (1979) enumerates three distinguishing properties of nursing research:

1. The final focus of nursing research must be on a difference that matters for improving patient care.
2. Nursing research has the potential for contributing to theory development and the body of scientific nursing knowledge.
3. A research problem is a nursing research problem when nurses have access to and control over phenomena being studied.

Nursing Research or Research in Nursing

Some authors make a distinction between nursing research (that is, research that focuses on human responses, clinical problems, and processes of care encountered in the practice of nursing) and **research in nursing** (the broader study of the nursing profession including historic, ethical, and political studies). However, the American Nurses' Association (ANA) Commission on Nursing Research (1981b) identifies the following as priorities for nursing research in the 1980s:

1. Research on promoting health and prevention of illness
2. Research on decreasing the negative impact of health problems on coping abilities, productivity, and satisfaction
3. Research on the development of strategies that provide effective nursing care to high-risk vulnerable groups (Advancing knowledge in these priority areas could occur through both clinical investigation and policy analysis.)
4. Research on the development of cost-efficient delivery systems of nursing care

Some Illustrations of Nursing Studies

The examples in Table 5–1 give an idea of the diverse subjects, topics, and settings of actual nursing studies. The sample of contemporary nursing studies in this table only begins to show the diversity of fascinating and ultimately valuable research projects being conducted in the field of nursing. The reader can review the "Research Notes" in the other chapters in this book or glance quickly at the table of contents in any of the major journals expressly devoted to nursing research for a fuller notion of its scope.

Research Note

The findings of a 1985 study by Maxine S. Loomis clearly document the 10-year-long trend in nursing dissertation work toward clinical research and a declining emphasis on social issues. For this analysis, Loomis obtained dissertation abstracts from 25 nursing doctoral programs admitting students in the fall of 1982. She identifies distinct patterns within programs, and, happily, gives abundant evidence of active mentor relationships between faculty and students.

Loomis suggests that certain deficits still exist in the body of nursing research as a whole. Subcategories of cultural/environmental stressors, sociocultural human response systems, and the various aspects of clinical decision making all warrant more attention by researchers, in her view. Study findings also indicate that nursing research has been increasingly successful in integrating the biologic, social, and cultural domains of nursing knowledge. (Loomis 1985)

Finding Nursing Studies

Despite the fact that findings from nursing studies are being incorporated into textbooks such as this one and that clinical journals such as *The American Journal of Nursing, Heart and Lung,* and *Gerontological Nursing* are increasingly publishing the results of studies about nursing practice, only four United States nursing journals have an editorial policy that stresses science and research. These are:

Advances in Nursing Science
Journal of Research in Nursing and Health
Nursing Research
Western Journal of Nursing Research

The *Cumulative Index to Nursing and Allied Health Literature,* the *International Nursing Index,* and the *Cumulative Medical Index* are excellent resources for locating research published on a topic or problem of interest. Computerized literature searches, such as Medline and MEDLARS, are available through most school libraries. They, too, are helpful in finding relevant study reports. Since 1983, research on a variety of topics has been collected in yet another valuable source, *The Annual Review of Nursing Research.* Each volume is an excellent compilation of primary sources and references.

Why Is Nursing Research Fundamental?

In the information revolution transforming the present and shaping the future, reading and understanding nursing research is as fundamental to professional practice as knowledge of asepsis, application of the nursing process, and communication skills are. The ability to access, evaluate, and interpret findings from nursing studies is a source of power in clinical decision making and a strategy for achieving excellence in the delivery of care.

Physicians are often viewed as "men of science" who direct patient care, possess sophisticated technical skills, and provide preoperative teaching, illness management, counseling, and the like. In the popular view, the nurse retreats to the background where she (and usually, the nurse is characterized as *she*) pushes wheelchairs, answers the phone, or carries bedpans and meal trays. Research in nursing is not only a tool for discovering solutions to clinical practice problems but also a political tool. "Research provides knowledge necessary to improve practice and achieve professional status. Through research, nursing can improve the care of persons in need of health service and affect policy that directs the way health services are provided. Political wisdom is an integral part of the research act" (Chenitz 1985, p. 314).

Ways of Knowing

Do most elderly clients know the names of medications they are taking? What nursing interventions are effective in alleviating backache associated with pregnancy? Is there a circadian rhythm of intracranial pressure that can help a nurse identify the client's time of greatest vulnerability after a head injury? Should clients on oral oxygen have their temperatures taken with an oral thermometer? Does warming infant formulas increase the likelihood of gastrointestinal infection? How can the nurse teach breast self-examination most effectively to Middle Eastern immigrant women? Nurses rely on a diverse array of ways of knowing when confronted with such day-to-day clinical questions. Some may:

Retreat to established tradition and authority as reflected in a procedure book or established protocol

Use trial and error combined with their own common sense or past experience

Consult an expert

Attempt to arrive at a logically reasoned decision

The Scientific Way of Knowing

The way of knowing that is the focus of this chapter is **scientific inquiry** as evidenced in nursing research. The scientific approach is a process of learning about truth by systematically collecting and comparing observable, verifiable data through the senses to describe, explain, and/or predict events and phenomena. The scientific approach as reflected in nursing research has two characteristics that other usual ways of knowing in nursing do not: (a) It has a built-in system of checks to ensure objectivity and the potential for self-correction and (b) it relies on sensory evidence or empirical data that are collected in a systematic, carefully prescribed manner (Wilson 1985; Wilson and Hutchinson 1986).

A system of checks and balances to minimize bias is applied to knowledge generated through the research process. Nurse scientists who find that one particular hypothesis is supported also check whether alternative hypotheses are supported as well, perhaps more strongly. For instance, if data from normal volunteers indicate that receiving oral or nasal oxygen does not alter oral temperature readings significantly, a nurse researcher determines if this finding is also true of other populations, such as febrile patients. The research methods and conclusions drawn from a study's findings must always be open to the criticism of others. Following the steps in the research process is one way of determining whether a study complies with accepted conventions for conducting credible research studies.

Steps in the Research Process

The truly important discoveries made in the health care field have not been made by scientists who think in dogmatic, mechanical fashion, who focus on knowledge of irrefutable facts without interpretation, or who forget that research is most often a process that moves back and forth between ideas, hunches, existing knowledge, and carefully made observations. Yet, for the sake of clarity, the **research process** is generally conceptualized as a series of steps or phases. Although these phases are dynamic, flexible, and expandable, they can be formalized as follows:

Step 1. Stating a Research Question or Problem

An investigator's initial task is narrowing a broad area of interest to a circumscribed problem that specifies exactly what she or he intends to study. Most investigators try to define a research problem as precisely as possible. A problem is often stated in the form of a question. Here are some examples from published nursing research studies:

> How many different treatments for pressure sores are advocated by nurses, and what rationales are given for their use?
>
> How do different postoperative activity schedules affect the recovery of physical fitness among athletes?
>
> What is the relationship between types of care given to clients with indwelling urethral catheters and the incidence of urinary tract infection?
>
> What is the optimal time needed to obtain an accurate oral temperature with a glass thermometer?
>
> What is the effect of low-frequency auditory and kinesthetic stimulation on the neurologic functioning of the premature infant?

If a study problem is too broad or vague, proceeding to subsequent stages of the process becomes confusing. A research question, according to Brink and Wood (1983, p. 2), "is an explicit query about a problem or issue that can be challenged, examined, analyzed, and will yield useful new information."

Step 2. Defining the Purpose of a Study

The second step is sometimes called defining the rationale of the study. It is the researcher's statement of why the question is important and what use the answer will serve. It lets the reader or funding agency know what to expect from the study. An excellent example of the statement of a study's purpose is the report of Kathryn Barnard's (1973) classic research on the effects of environmental stimulation on the sleep of premature infants:

> Previous work with full-term neonates and older infants supports the general notion that particular kinds of stimulation assist in the regulation of sleep and arousal status. Given this evidence and the increasing evidence that quiet

Table 5–1 Examples of Nursing Studies

Baker et al. (1983) reported on the use of therapeutic touch by nurses to increase the range of motion of joints and to decrease pain in persons with arthritis.
Baker et al. (1984) studied the effect of types of thermometer and length of time inserted on oral temperature measurements of afebrile subjects.
Baum (1984) studied the physiologic determinants of a clinically successful method of enrotracheal suction.
Britten (1985) studied head nurses' perceptions of their role in a decentralized nursing department for her master's thesis at the University of Florida.
Choi-Lao (1981) measured the concentrations of halothane anesthetic vapors in the operating environments of two hospitals in Canada by analyzing air samples using a gas chromatographic technique.
Dufault (1983) used observation, interviews, and case studies to conduct a descriptive, longitudinal field study that indentifed themes and patterns of hope in elderly cancer patients.
Fehring (1983) compared the effects of a particular relaxation technique with the effects of the same technique augmented with biofeedback on the symptoms of psychologic stress among healthy college students. Findings indicate that biofeedback-augmented relaxation was more effective in lowering psychologic stress symptoms.
Hutchinson (1984) reported on the strategies used by neonatal intensive care nurses to contend with the meaninglessness and horror that is often part of their everyday work and that is a critical cause of "burnout."
Itano et al. (1983) conducted a study in which they correlated factors such as locus of control, self-esteem, anxiety, clent's understanding of the illness, client's perception of the severity of the symptoms, and client's perception of the nurse's care and concern plus several demographic factors to compliance to therapy among clients with cancer.
Martinson and Anderson (1983) studied the effects of applying different degrees of heat to the abdomens of unrestrained, unanesthetized dogs on skin surface, subcutaneous, intraperitoneal, intestinal, and colonic temperatures. Their findings indicate that a wide range of thermal applications to the abdominal skin of dogs changed skin surface and subcutaneous temperature but did not alter deep abdominal temperature.
Norbeck and Sheiner (1982) used a social support scale to identify sources of social support related to single-parent functioning.
Wilson (1982) used a method of qualitative analysis called "Discovering Grounded Theory" to explain how the presence of people can work effectively to control the behavior of unmedicated schizophrenics in an alternative healing community.

> sleep in the immature infant can improve neurological development . . . the purpose of the current investigation was to study the effect of regular, controlled stimulation on the neurological functioning in the infant born prematurely (p. 15).

Step 3. Reviewing Related Literature

If researchers want their study to build on, confirm, or even transcend the existing knowledge in a discipline and thereby qualify as a real contribution to science, they must know what has already been done. A review of the literature provides the researcher with a framework of background ideas. A theoretical framework is an essay in which the investigator relates the existing concepts, theories, research methods, and findings to his or her study question and purpose (Brink and Wood 1983). At the least, constructing such a framework provides relevant concepts for the research; at best, it gives the researcher a full awareness of facts, issues, prior findings, theories, and instruments that might be related to the study question.

Step 4. Formulating Hypotheses and Defining Variables

Hypotheses are statements of the relationship between two or more concepts, or variables. Some studies are intended to develop hypotheses (exploratory, descriptive, and grounded theory designs), and others are intended to test hypotheses using statistical procedures. Stating hypotheses requires not only sufficient knowledge about a topic to predict the outcome of the study but also definitions that specify the variables under investigation in measurable terms. Finally, the investigator must articulate the relationships among the variables. Hypotheses can be explicitly stated, as Sitzman and her colleagues (1983, p. 219) did in their study of biofeedback training:

> *Hypothesis* (H_1): Emphysema and chronic bronchitic patients who receive a biofeedback training program to decrease their respiratory rate will have a significantly decreased respiratory rate at the end of the training program and 1-month follow-up.
>
> *Hypothesis* (H_2): Emphysema and chronic bronchitic patients who decreased their respiratory rate by the end of the biofeedback training program will have significantly increased their tidal volume at the end of the training program and at 1-month follow-up.

Hypotheses (H) may be stated as null hypotheses (H_0), which essentially test the premise that there are no significant differences in the outcome or **dependent variable** other than those that can be attributed to chance. To formulate hypotheses, the investigator must specify the concepts being studied; thus, it is important at this point to determine how to define these variables for the purpose of measuring them. For example, social support might be defined as a score on a written self-report scale, or inventory. This step is called operationally defining the variables. If one does a convincing job, the study is said to have **construct** (or concept) **validity**.

Step 5. Selecting the Research Design

A research design is a well-formulated, systematic, and controlled plan for finding answers to study questions. The design is a road map or blueprint for organizing a study. Everything from methods of data collection through methods of data analysis should be spelled out in the research design.

Step 6. Selecting the Population, Sample, and Setting

After narrowing a general area of interest to a specific study question, reviewing the literature, and deciding on a research design, the researcher must choose a study population, select a sample, and decide on a setting where the sample can be located. The **population** is the group to be studied. To whom do the findings apply? Some recent studies, for instance, have focused on these populations: divorced fathers, older persons, hospitalized children, disadvantaged minorities, depressed women, nursing mothers, clients with cancer, people with AIDS, clients who have had surgery, and nursing students. The **sample** is that segment of a population from whom data will be collected. Findings from the sample are generalized to the population.

Step 7. Conducting a Pilot Study

A pilot study helps the researcher discover the strengths and weaknesses of the intended design, sample size, and data-collection instrument of the larger project. Pilot studies strengthen nursing studies by weeding out problems in advance; many funding agencies do not approve study proposals unless a pilot study has been conducted.

Step 8. Collecting the Data

The scientific method is characterized by a reliance on **empirical data**: information collected from the observable world. These data are used to make statements about what is true. Any study that goes beyond armchair speculation eventually requires the researcher to collect data. Data sources may be people, documents, or laboratory materials. Data-collection instruments include interviews, questionnaires, physiologic tests, and psychologic tests. The basic point, however, is that by moving either from observation to idea (called **inductive theory**) or from idea to observation (called **deductive theory**), the scientific method relies on empirical data to discover or test knowledge. The researcher uses the senses and measurement tools to collect data relevant to the variables being studied. The time and energy required for this step vary according to the research design. Field studies, historic research, surveys, and most experiments are time-consuming and demanding.

Step 9. Analyzing the Data

The next step in the research process is reorganizing the collected data to relate them to the study question, research objectives, or stated hypotheses. The most important part of this step is to have a procedural plan in mind, have the requisite skills for analysis (such as knowledge of statistics), and realize that analysis provides the answers to the original research questions.

Step 10. Communicating Conclusions and Implications

The researcher's challenge at the final stage is to explain the results of the investigation and link them to the existing body of knowledge in the discipline. Whether results are published or reported verbally, the study's contribution cannot be judged unless the conclusions are communicated to colleagues and critics. Communicating the conclusions, interpreting the meaning and implications of the findings, recognizing the study's limitations, and suggesting directions for future study culminate the research process. In these activities, investigators can synthesize their imaginative, insightful, and engaged style with their rigorous, systematic, and analytic one (Wilson 1985; Wilson and Hutchinson 1986).

The steps of the research process provide the tools with which scientists achieve their major aims or goals. These basic aims are: (a) to develop **theories**, or explanations of the world and (b) to find solutions to practical problems.

The Commission on Nursing Research of the American Nurses' Association (ANA 1981b) issued definitions, directions, and examples for nursing research in the 1980s. These are presented in Table 5–2.

The Investigative Roles of All Nurses

The majority of career scientists in nursing are prepared at the doctoral and postdoctoral level, although an increasing number of clinicians with master's degrees are beginning to participate in research activity as part of their nursing role. However, "if nursing is to emerge in society as a socially significant, credible, scientific, and learned profession with a commitment to high-quality patient care, then research (for all nurses) is a necessity" (Starzomski 1983). It may be unrealistic to expect each nurse to conduct a study in the clinical setting. Many constraints in clinical settings must be reckoned with before research can become a legitimate and comfortable activity. However, if nursing is to develop as a research-based practice, it is not unreasonable to expect the nurse in the clinical area to:

- Have some awareness of the process and language of research
- Be sensitive to issues related to protecting the rights of human subjects
- Participate in the identification of significant researchable problems
- Be a discriminating consumer of research findings

The nursing student must learn these investigative functions early in her or his career to establish the connection that "knowing how we know is fundamental to doing what we do" (Wilson 1985, p. viii). Bridging the **research-practice gap**, that is, bringing research into the clinical practice arena, is a key strategy in uniting the scholarly, scientific, and caring aspects of nursing in the future. Table 5–3 summarizes this position in the ANA's "Guidelines for the Investigative Function of Nurses" (1981a), which specify the generally expected research competencies of nurses with associate, bachelor's, master's, and doctoral degrees.

The Research-Practice Gap

It is apparent that nurse leaders want to make nursing practice a more frequent focus of nursing research and increase the application of valid research findings in clinical work. Yet progress toward achieving these goals is often slowed by several barriers.

Lack of Cumulative Order in the Literature

A scientist from another discipline, according to Gortner, would probably characterize most nursing research as

Table 5–2 ANA Guidelines for Nursing Research

Directions for Research	Examples
Priority should be given to nursing research that generates knowledge to guide practice in:	Examples of research consistent with these priorities include the following:
1. Promoting health, well-being, and competency for personal care among all age groups	1. Identification of determinants (personal and environmental, including social support networks) of wellness and health functioning in individuals and families, e.g., avoiding abusive behavior such as alcoholism and drug use, successfully adapting to chronic illness, and coping with the last days of life
2. Preventing health problems throughout the lifespan that have the potential to reduce productivity and satisfaction	2. Identification of phenomena that negatively influence the course of recovery and that may be alleviated by nursing practice, for example, anorexia, diarrhea, sleep deprivation, deficiencies in nutrients, electrolyte imbalances, and infections
3. Decreasing the negative impact of health problems on coping abilities, productivity, and life satisfaction of individuals and families	3. Development and testing of care strategies to do the following: • Facilitate individuals' ability to adopt and maintain health-enhancing behaviors (e.g., exercise and alterations in diet) • Enhance clients' ability to manage acute and chronic illness so as to minimize or eliminate the necessity for institutionalization and to maximize well-being • Reduce stressful responses associated with the medical management of patients (e.g., surgical procedures, intrusive examination procedures, or extensive use of monitoring devices)
4. Ensuring that the care needs of particularly vulnerable groups are met through appropriate strategies	4. Enhance the care of clients culturally different from the majority (e.g., black Americans, Mexican Americans, native Americans) and clients with special problems (e.g., teenagers, prisoners, mentally ill), and the underserved (the elderly, poor, and the rural)
5. Designing and developing health care systems that are cost-effective in meeting the nursing needs of the population	5. Design and assess, in terms of effectiveness and cost, the models for delivering nursing care strategies found to be effective in clinical studies.
6. Promoting health, well-being, and competency for personal health in all age groups	6. Provide more effective care to high-risk populations (e.g., maternal and child care service to vulnerable mothers and infants, family planning services to young teenagers, services designed to enhance self-care in the chronically ill and the very old)

Source: American Nurses' Association, Commission on Nursing Research, *Priorities for the 1980s* (Kansas City, Mo.: American Nurses' Association, 1981). Reprinted with permission.

"discrete, nonaggregated studies of isolated empirical phenomena for which the explanatory theory is not yet well known or defined" (Gortner 1980). It would be much easier for nurse generalists and clinicians with no specialized research training to apply research findings to their practice if nursing research were organized into well-defined programs that would yield cumulative discoveries. In selected instances, this pattern has been more successfully attained than in others. Walike and Walike (1977) conducted a series of studies on the undesirable effects of lactose intolerance in patients receiving tube feedings. As a result of their work, lactose has been eliminated from the formulas, and tube-fed patients with lactose intolerance need no longer experience the nausea, abdominal cramps, and distention caused by their inability to digest milk sugar. Similarly, Barnard (1983) carried out studies for over more than a decade that enabled her to specify special treatment and environmental conditions that simulate prenatal womb life and can positively affect the sleep behavior, weight gain, and development of premature infants. Because of research done by Martinson (1977) with families of leukemic children in Minnesota, hundreds of children can now remain at home with their families during the terminal phase of their illness. Other nurse scientists are striving to develop organized programs of collaborative research on clinically relevant questions such as those above.

Insufficient Preparation by Nurses

Building a cumulative, organized, scientific knowledge base to replace traditions, habits, and trial and error as the basis for practice decisions is not enough. Nurses must be motivated and competent to read, understand, evaluate, and interpret this body of work. Reports of research findings are not always easy to locate through the professional media or in the most widely read journals. Once reports are located, nurses may find their traditional scientific format and esoteric language difficult or intimidating. To read and interpret them, nurses need to become astute and proactive consumers of research findings.

Service Organization Structure

A third obstacle to bridging the research-practice gap is the fact that, until recently, the structure of most service settings rarely encouraged clinical nurses to make changes

Table 5–3 Investigative Functions of a Nurse at Various Educational Levels

Associate Degree in Nursing	Master's Degree in Nursing	Doctoral Degree in Nursing or a Related Discipline
1. Demonstrates awareness of the value or relevance of research in nursing 2. Assists in identifying problem areas in nursing practice 3. Assists in collecting data within an established, structured format **Baccalaureate in Nursing** 1. Reads, interprets, and evaluates research for applicability to nursing practice 2. Identifies nursing problems that need to be investigated and participates in the implementation of scientific studies 3. Uses nursing practice as a means of gathering data to refine and extend practice 4. Applies established findings of nursing and other health-related research to nursing practice 5. Shares research findings with colleagues	1. Analyzes and reformulates nursing practice problems so that scientific knowledge and scientific methods can be used to find solutions 2. Enhances the quality and clinical relevance of nursing research by providing expertise in clinical problems and by providing knowledge about the way in which these clinical services are delivered 3. Facilitates investigations of problems in clinical settings through such activities as contributing to a climate supportive of investigative activities, collaborating with others in investigations, and enhancing nursing's access to clients and data 4. Conducts investigations for the purpose of monitoring the quality of the practice of nursing in a clinical setting 5. Assists others to apply scientific knowledge in nursing practice	1. Provides leadership for the integration of scientific knowledge with other sources of knowledge for the advancement of practice 2. Conducts investigations to evaluate the contribution of nursing activities to the well-being of clients 3. Develops methods to monitor the quality of the practice of nursing in a clinical setting and to evaluate contributions of nursing activities to the well-being of clients **Graduate of a Research-Oriented Doctoral Program** 1. Develops theoretical explanations of phenomena relevant to nursing by empirical research and analytic processes 2. Uses analytic and empirical methods to discover ways to modify or extend existing scientific knowledge so that it is relevant to nursing 3. Develops methods for scientific inquiry of phenomena relevant to nursing

Source: American Nurses' Association, Commission on Nursing Research, *Guidelines for the investigative function of nurses* (Kansas City, Mo.: American Nurses' Association, 1981). Reprinted with permission.

in interventions based on systematic appraisals or participation in nursing research. Here are some successful strategies for introducing a research orientation into an institution whose focus is the delivery of patient care:

> Legitimize the research activities of clinical nurses by granting release time for research and recognizing nursing research through the institution's formal reward system.
>
> Form a research reference group for clinical nurses. Such a group would bring together nurses who value research, raise research consciousness among nurses, and allow members to exchange formal and informal knowledge about research.
>
> Help clinical nurse investigators explore the researcher role. In particular, give nurses access to patients for research purposes and help nurses discover differences in the rhythm of research work and clinical work. Clinical nurses are accustomed to a large volume of work that must be accomplished in a short time. Learning how much scholarly and research work to expect from oneself in a specific time represents a major shift for most clinical nurses, who must spend more time in the sedentary activities of prolonged reading and thinking (Davis 1981).

Nurses must overcome these obstacles if they are to incorporate nursing research into the practice arena and make research a fundamental area of nursing skill and expertise. The following sections address the nurse generalist's investigative roles in more detail.

Protecting the Rights of Human Subjects

Because nursing research usually focuses on humans, a major nursing responsibility is to be aware of and advocate clients' rights. All clients must be informed about the consequences of consenting to serve as research subjects. The client needs to be able to assess whether an appropriate balance exists between the risks of participating in a study and the potential benefits, either to the client or to the development of knowledge.

Research ethics not only protect the **rights of human subjects** but also encompass a broader list of characteristics. Most of these characteristics are reflected in the ANA's "Human Rights Guidelines for Nursing in Clinical and Other Research." These guidelines are based on historic documents, such as the Nuremberg Code, the Declaration of Helsinki, and United States federal regulations, all of which set standards governing the conduct of research involving human subjects. The ANA Guidelines are presented in Table 5–4.

The Nurse's Role in Protecting Subjects' Rights

All nurses who practice in settings where research is being conducted with human subjects or who participate in such research as data collectors or collaborators play an important role in safeguarding the following rights:

Right Not to Be Harmed

The Department of Health and Human Services defines **risk of harm** to a research subject as exposure to the possibility of injury going beyond everyday situations. The risk can be physical, emotional, legal, financial, or social. For instance, withholding standard care from a client in labor so as to study the course of natural childbirth clearly poses a potential physical danger. Risks can be less overt and involve psychologic factors, such as exposure to stress or anxiety, or social factors, such as loss of confidentiality, loss of privacy, and the like.

Right to Full Disclosure

Even though it may be possible to collect data about a client as part of everyday care without the client's particular knowledge or consent, to do so is considered unethical. **Full disclosure** is a basic right. It means that deception, either by withholding information about a client's participation in a study, or by giving the client false or misleading information about what participating in the study will involve, will not occur. Full disclosure involves informing study subjects about the following aspects of any study:

Table 5–4 ANA Guidelines for Nursing Research

The guidelines in this table attempt to specify several important entities: (1) the type of activities that are involved, (2) the rights that are to be protected, (3) the persons to be safeguarded, and (4) the mechanisms necessary to ensure that protection is adequate.

Guideline 1: Employment in Settings Where Research Is Conducted

Conditions of employment in settings in which clinical or other research is in progress need to be spelled out in detail for all potential workers. . . . Anyone employed in work that carries the potential of risk to others needs to be advised as to the types of risks involved, the ways of recognizing when risk is present, and the proper actions to take to counteract harmful effects and unnecessary danger.

Guideline 2: Nurses' Responsibilities for Vigilant Protection of Human Subjects' Rights

In all instances the prospective subject must be given all relevant information prior to participation in activities that go beyond established and accepted procedures necessary to meet his personal needs. . . . Nurses must be increasingly vigilant in their concern for subjects and patients who by reason of their situation and/or illness are not able to protect themselves effectively from externally imposed threat or injury. They must be sensitive to the tendency toward exploitation of "captive" populations such as students, patients, and inmates in institutions and prisons. All proposals to be used need to be discussed with the prospective subject and with any worker who is expected to participate as a subject or data collector or both. Special mechanisms must be developed to safeguard the confidentiality of information and protect human dignity.

Guideline 3: Scope of Application

The persons to whom these human rights guidelines apply include all individuals involved in research activities and include the following groups: patients, donors of organs and tissue, informants, normal volunteers including students, and vulnerable populations that are "captive" audiences, such as the mentally disordered, mentally retarded, and prisoners.

Guideline 4: Nurses' Responsibility to Support the Accrual of Knowledge

Just as nurses have an obligation to protect the human rights of patients, so do they also have an obligation to support the accrual of knowledge that broadens the scientific underpinnings of nursing practice and the delivery of nursing services.

Guideline 5: Informed Consent

To safeguard the basic rights of self-determination, nurses must obtain consent from the prospective subject or his legal representative to participate in research or unusual clinical activities. The subject needs to receive:

- A description of any benefit to the subject or the development of new knowledge that might be expected
- An offer to discuss or answer any questions about the study
- A clear statement to the subject that he is free to discontinue participation at any time he wishes to do so
- Full freedom from direct or indirect coercion and deception

Guideline 6: Representation on Human Subjects Committee

There is increasing public support for systematic accountability to ensure that individual rights are not denied to human subjects who participate in research studies. In most instances, the protective mechanism takes place through a committee judged competent to review studies and other investigative activities that involve human subjects. The profession of nursing has an obligation to publicly support the inclusion of nurses as regular members of institutional review committees of this kind.

Source: Adapted and summarized with permission from the American Nurses' Association, ***Human rights guidelines for nurses in clinical and other research*** (ANA Publication No. D-46 5M 7/75, 1975). Also found in ANA, ***Guidelines in nursing research*** (Kansas City, Mo.: ANA, 1975).

The nature, duration, and purposes of the study

The methods, procedures, and processes by which data will be collected, expressed in lay language rather than technical terms (for example, teaspoons of blood to be drawn, rather than milliliters)

The use to which the findings will be put and any benefits that could be derived

Any and all inconveniences, potential harms, or discomforts that might be expected including commitment of unreimbursed time

Any possible results or side-effects that might follow, including being sent more questionnaires

The client's alternatives to participating in the study

The right to refuse to participate or to withdraw at any point

The identities of the investigators and how to contact them

Right of Self-Determination

Many clients in dependent positions, such as people in nursing homes, feel pressured to participate in studies. They feel that they must please those doctors and nurses who are responsible for their treatment and care. The right of **self-determination** means that subjects should feel free from constraints, coercion, or any undue influence to participate in a study. Masked inducements, for instance, suggesting that they might become famous by making an important contribution to science or get special attention by taking part in the study, must be strictly avoided. Nurses must be assertive in advocating this essential right as well.

Right of Privacy and Confidentiality

Privacy enables a client to participate without worrying about later embarrassment. The **anonymity** of a study is ensured if even the investigator cannot link a specific subject to the information reported. **Confidentiality** means that any information a subject relates will not be made public or available to others. Investigators must inform research subjects about the measures that provide for these rights. Such measures may include using pseudonyms, code numbers, or reporting only aggregate or group data in published research.

Nurses who participate in scientific investigations that involve human subjects are in a key position to serve as advocates for research subjects. All of the study topics in Table 5–5 could put human subjects at risk.

Table 5–5 Research Studies with Ethical Issues at Stake

1. A nurse who had worked for 6 years on a unit for nonviable clients was concerned about the tendency for nurses to avoid certain clients. She decided to conduct a study of how nurses care for nonviable clients.
2. In a study of unprofessional behavior, several nurse informants revealed some very personal and damaging information about themselves, but this was only a pilot study and they had not signed a consent form.
3. In a study of care of mentally retarded children, the researcher found that there were some glaring deficiencies in the care of these children. For example, children were often left in uncomfortable positions for hours at a time, were rarely offered fluids, and received diaper changes infrequently.

Vulnerable Subjects

Certain subjects, including children, fetuses, the mentally disabled, the elderly, captives, the dying, and the sedated or unconscious, are considered particularly **vulnerable subjects.** The guiding principle in these cases is that the less a subject is able to give informed consent, the greater the nurse's responsibility to protect the client's rights.

The Principles of Ethical Research

The desire for scientific knowledge must be compatible with the need to preserve the dignity and rights of individuals and social groups. The following principles of ethical research (Wilson 1985) are worth remembering:

1. (S) Scientific objectivity. Objectivity ensures that the research is conducted without bias, misconduct, or fraud.
2. (C) Cooperation with duly authorized review groups, agencies, and institutional review boards (IRB). These committees are charged with reviewing provisions for protecting the rights of human subjects and interpreting law and ethics.
3. (I) Integrity in representing the research study. Integrity means that the researchers do not deceive subjects about the risks, discomforts, or potential benefits of participating as a research subject.
4. (E) Equitability in acknowledging the contributions of others. The researcher should acknowledge coauthors, research associates, and clinical nurses who provided access to clients and participated in data collection.
5. (N) Nobility in the application or processes and procedures to protect the rights of human subjects. Subjects' rights should never be compromised to facilitate the research.
6. (T) Truthfulness about a study's purpose, methods, and findings. "Undercover research" is no longer considered ethical.
7. (I) Impeccability in the use of privileges associated with the researcher's role. Researchers often have access to privileged, private information. This infor-

mation must be kept confidential and anonymous. All nurse researchers must be as discrete about patients as nurse clinicians are.

8. (F) Forthrightness about a study's funding sources and sponsorship. Any published research must disclose all sources of financial support and any special sponsorship.

9. (I) Illumination of knowledge through contributions to publications and presentations of research findings. Nurse clinicians need to be assured that efforts by nurse researchers will be available to them.

10. (C) Courage to clarify publicly any distortions or misinterpretations of research findings.

As the list acronym (SCIENTIFIC) suggests, following these principles of ethical research makes the scientific ethical (Wilson 1985). See Figure 5–1.

Finding Researchable Problems in Clinical Practice

Protecting the rights of human research subjects and advocating ethical research are crucial investigative roles for all nurses. Another important role is to identify, in the course of giving nursing care, problems and questions that call for research-based explanations. Identifying problem areas in nursing practice is an investigative skill that all nurses need to master if the interplay between research and practice urged by the ANA is to be achieved (ANA 1981b).

Sources of Research Problems

For the nurse with observation skills and an inquiring mind, each bed bath, back rub or dressing change is not only a way to meet the client's needs for hygiene and comfort but also an opportunity to recognize discrepancies between what is (existing nursing practice or patient status) and what is desirable. Every discrepancy is a potential source of research problems. Valid sources of researchable topics include one's own clinical experience, patterns or trends in someone else's observations or research, and one's own intellectual and scientific interests. Consider these examples:

> A staff nurse in a medical setting reads about the hypnotic effects of a dietary amino acid, L-tryptophan, on clients who have recently experienced a myocardial infarction. The nurse wonders if the effects of the amino acid could be approximated by serving certain amounts of dairy products and some meats to these clients (McEnany 1985).
>
> A surgical nurse battles postoperative infections and is perplexed by the various methods used in different hospitals to change subclavian line dressings. She wishes she knew which method was most effective (McEnany 1985).
>
> An outpatient clinic nurse who does physical assessments on elderly clients wonders if a program of daily hydration would improve their orientation and decrease their confusion.

Nonresearchable Problems

The examples might give the impression that a constant parade of researchable problems passes before each nurse during daily clinical work. But not all questions that are clinically relevant, important, or even interesting are necessarily researchable ones. A **researchable problem** is one that can be investigated using the steps of the *research process* (Wilson 1985). Two types of questions that are generally *not* researchable (unless they are reformulated) are "should" questions and "yes/no" questions:

> Should a baby be bathed before or after feeding?
>
> Should nurses wear white uniforms on pediatric units?
>
> Should patients be ambulated within 24 hours after surgery?

Nonresearchable questions may shed light on the facts bearing on a specific problem, but they do not address a relationship that might shed light on a broader theoretical problem applicable in other circumstances. As such, nonresearchable questions remain relevant to the problem-solving process in a specific nursing care situation, but they are not nursing research problems. "Should the nurse take a blood pressure immediately after a patient has exercised?" must be reformulated into "Among healthy adult males, what differences exist between blood pressure readings taken immediately after exercise and after periods of rest?" Likewise, the "yes/no" question "Is normal breathing silent?" can be restated as a researchable question: "What is the relationship between abnormal breathing sounds, such as wheezing, stridor, and rales, and airway constriction or fluid in the lungs?" These restatements transform clinical nursing questions into questions for clinical research. Questions of value, opinion, or policy and accumulations of specific facts and information can be very valuable to clinical problem solving. However, only questions that produce generalizable information for guiding practice under other conditions can turn a nursing care problem into a nursing research problem.

Changing a Clinical Nursing Problem to a Researchable One

Research questions usually begin with *who, what, when, where,* or *why.* Some researchers have sorted questions into different levels, suggesting that some questions are most appropriate when the existing knowledge is at a certain level. For example, if very little is known about a certain topic, it makes sense to ask a *what, who,* or *where* question to acquire descriptive information:

> What are the unmet mental health needs of the frail elderly?
>
> Where would people prefer to die?
>
> Who should assume responsibility for preoperative teaching?

When more is known about a topic, it is appropriate to ask *how* or *why* questions:

> How do nurses decide when to initiate protective asepsis?
>
> Why do clients fail to comply with drug therapy?

Research problems come from a variety of sources. In one's own clinical practice they may come from gripes, wishes, observed patterns of needs, conventions or traditions in nursing care, and the like. Changing a clinical nursing problem into a researchable one can involve four straightforward steps.

1. State the wish, gripe, etc.
2. Identify the constraints that contribute to the discrepancy between what is going on and what should occur.
3. From the brain-stormed list generated in step 2, select the most likely explanation for the discrepancy.
4. Rephrase the problem in conceptual terms so that solutions are not applicable to one case alone, but rather can be generalized to clients with similar characteristics and in similar circumstances.

A researchable problem is stated clearly and unambiguously as either a question or a statement, for example:

> What are indicators of reduced respiratory efficiency related to aging?
>
> The problem in this research is to determine the maximum extent to which exercise can strengthen weakened muscles of clients of age 50 or younger.

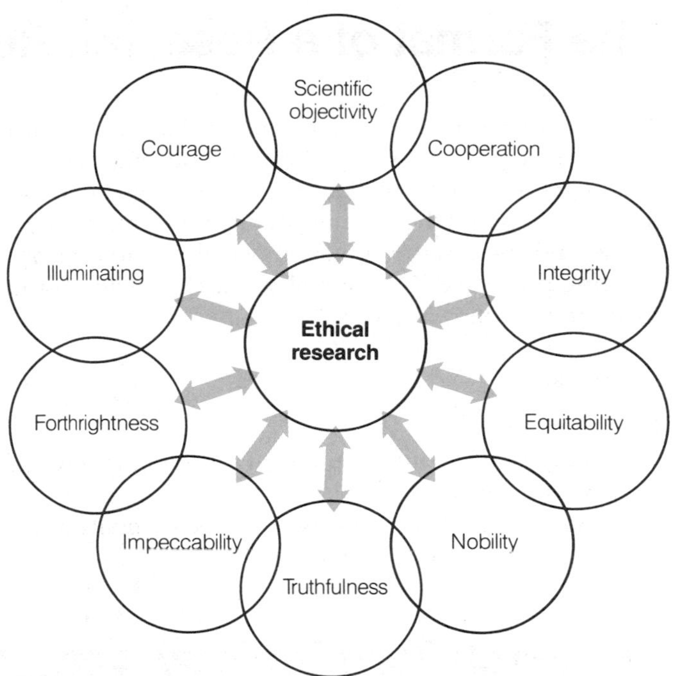

Figure 5–1 Making the scientific ethical

Probably the most important point to keep in mind when developing the skills to recognize researchable nursing problems is that much of the tradition of nursing practice is based on just that—tradition—rather than on carefully controlled research. Cardiac precautions, temperature-taking techniques, and oxygenation practices, for example, are all open to investigation through nursing research.

In the near future, nursing research will focus on the interaction of psychologic and psychosocial mechanisms in human experiences of coping with health and illness, the evaluation of nursing interventions, the application of research findings in practice, and underserved and high-risk groups, such as the elderly and minority groups. The nurse of tomorrow will be directly involved in the conduct and application of research.

Becoming an Intelligent Research Consumer

Clinical nursing research is the answer to the dilemmas that routinely face the practicing nurse, even when the questions begin with "how do I," "what if," and "what is the best way?" Before clinical nurses can evaluate the worth of a research report, however, they have to understand it. This goal is an ongoing one throughout one's nursing education, but beginning steps include: (a) understanding the format of a research journal article, (b) translating the vocabulary of scientific research, and (c) evaluating the credibility of a scientific presentation of findings.

The Format of a Research Report

Almost all reports of research findings have a standardized format. The nursing student who becomes familiar with it gets the most out of time spent reading the report; it is easier to grasp the meaning of unfamiliar terminology if one understands the context in which the information is being presented. The typical research article is organized in the following way:

1. Abstract
2. Introduction
   a. Review of related literature (including theoretical framework)
   b. Statement of the purpose or specific goals of the study (including hypotheses)
3. Methodology
   a. Procedure for selecting the study sample
   b. Study design
   c. Data collection tools or strategies
   d. Data analysis procedures
4. Results or findings
5. Discussion and implications
6. References

Once the nurse has a general idea of how a research report is organized, she or he must read it with understanding. This involves developing the skill to "come to terms with research terminology" (Wilson 1985, p. 98).

Research Terminology

Concepts, Constructs, Conceptual Frameworks, and Theory

Nurses work with **concepts** all the time. *Infection, bonding, self-care level, elimination, loss, comfort, stress, burnout, decentralization, infection,* and *deinstitutionalization* are all terms for categories of phenomena that share certain characteristics. Some phenomena, such as temperature elevation, can be measured directly with instruments. Others, because they are more abstract, call for proxy measures. For example, anxiety may be measured by a score on an anxiety scale alone or by the combination of an anxiety scale score and some physiologic measures, such as respiration and pulse rate. Certain abstract concepts are often called **constructs.** Examples of constructs from various theories are *social class* from sociology, *locus of control* from psychology, and *leadership style* from management theory. Science is concerned with identifying, refining, and explaining relationships among concepts by comparing them to empirical observations. For this reason, deciding whether a study uses appropriate, valid, and believable measures for concepts and constructs is an important step in judging the credibility of a nursing research study. **Conceptual** or theoretical **frameworks** (sometimes simply called **theories**) are systems that interrelate concepts and constructs. Most nursing students are familiar with the theories of relativity, gravity, and evolution as well as psychoanalytic theory and learning theory.

Independent and Dependent Variables

The term *variable* refers to anything that varies. The **dependent variables** (DV) in a study may also be called the output, outcome, or criterion variables. Change or the lack of it presumably depends on causes or conditions that the investigator can manipulate. In most cases, the dependent variable (sense of well-being, absence of infection, accuracy of temperature measurement, etc.) is what the researcher is trying to study. The **independent variables** (IV) are *existing* conditions or causes or those variables that the researcher manipulates to affect the dependent variable. It is possible to have multiple independent and dependent variables. Most research is designed to illumine the relationships among them. The ability to recognize the dependent and independent variables in a study is an important step in grasping a study's potential meaning and significance.

Uncontrolled Variables

Determining the dependent and independent variables in a research study is usually straightforward. Interpreting the study's findings, however, is more complicated. The researcher must take into consideration all the other relevant variables, other than the identified IV, that might effect the DV. Sometimes these other variables relate to how standardized and unbiased the data collection procedures are, and sometimes they relate to characteristics of the subjects in the sample or how they were chosen. Sometimes, unwanted variables may be introduced through the passage of time or through unforeseen events in the course of conducting the study. A well-designed study specifies the precise steps the researcher must take to be as certain as possible that the results or findings are not a result of **uncontrolled (extraneous** or **confounding)** variables. If such variables cannot be controlled through sampling procedures or analysis procedures, the researcher should report their possible influence on the findings and list them as a limitation of the study. When one reads the results of a study, it is important to ask what else could have accounted for the study findings or have influenced them in one way or another. A good practice when one is in doubt about the credibility of a research study's findings is to refer to a research critique (see for example, Wilson 1985, Chapters 6 and 7).

Data

Data is a plural noun meaning information, in this case the information that a nurse researcher collects from the subjects of a research study. Data may be physiologic measurements, such as blood pressure readings, pulse readings, ratings of pressure sores, etc.; psychologic measures, such as scores on intelligence, personality, or other mental measurement scales; or sociologic measures, such as social class reflected by such factors as educational preparation, occupation, income, and the like. Data are obtained from subjects through instruments (or tools). Many instruments are used in nursing studies, including interviews, questionnaires, intelligence tests, rating scales, and such biologic measures as body temperature or serum albumin.

Validity and Reliability

Among the most important concerns of the reader evaluating the worth of instruments used to measure variables in a nursing study are their **validity** and **reliability**. A valid instrument measures what it is supposed to measure. A reliable measure produces consistent results or data on repeated use because the researcher has established a carefully standardized procedure for administering it. If blood pressure readings are taken several times on the same subject under unchanging conditions, and the results are consistent, the measure (the procedure for taking the reading) is reliable.

Populations and Samples

The population for a study (N) is the total possible membership of the group being studied. Because it is not always possible or feasible to study everybody in a population, a microcosm of the population, called a sample (n) of participants or respondents, is usually used. When reading a study, the research consumer must attempt to determine if the findings were obtained from a sample that is representative of the study population. A **random sample** is one in which all members of a population have an equal chance of being included in the study sample.

Tables and Graphs

It is beyond the scope of this text to teach the reader how to evaluate whether qualitative or statistical analysis procedures in a nursing study were appropriate. However, a researcher consumer must learn to read and comprehend findings that customarily are presented in tables and graphs. The following guidelines should prove helpful:

Try to spot trends.

Decide if the researcher has picked the correct measure of central tendency. It can be the mean (the total divided by the number of cases); the median (the midpoint between the upper and lower halves); or the mode (the case that is most common). The consumer must determine which is the best way to describe the central tendency for any particular study question.

Pay attention to the range of numbers in charts and graphs. The range can reveal how typical the dominant response was.

Look for exceptions. Sometimes these are missing data or "outlyers": instances, observations, or scores that don't fall into the typical pattern.

Compare findings presented in the text of a research article against data presented in tables, charts, and their captions, keeping alert for any inconsistencies.

Look up unfamiliar statistical procedures in a good basic statistics book (for example, Triola 1983).

The word *criticism,* in everyday language, has negative connotations. When the nurse is analyzing, reviewing, carefully dissecting, evaluating, and even judging the merits of a research report, criticism becomes a professional responsibility. In fact, the word as Aristotle used it meant a standard for "judging well." A thoughtful research critique requires more than just following the steps of a process that begins with the question, "Is the problem clearly stated?" The beginning student must learn the standards against which to judge research reports. What are the qualities of good problem statements? How does one judge the credibility of evidence, the adequacy of explanations, the reliability and validity of a study's instruments and design? It is the professional responsibility of nursing students to acquire the investigative skills that will be required of all nurses in the future.

Chapter Highlights

- In the information revolution transforming the present and shaping the future, reading and understanding nursing research are as fundamental to professional practice as knowledge of asepsis, application of the nursing process, and communication skills are.
- The ability to access, evaluate, and interpret findings from nursing studies is a source of power in clinical

decision making and a strategy for achieving excellence in the delivery of care.

- The scientific approach is a process of learning about truth by systematically collecting and comparing observable, verifiable data through the senses to describe, explain, and/or predict events and phenomena.
- The scientific approach as reflected in nursing research has two characteristics that the major ways of knowing in nursing do not: (a) It has a built-in system of checks to ensure objectivity and the potential for self-correction and (b) it relies on sensory evidence or empirical data that are collected in a systematic, carefully prescribed manner.
- The research process is generally conceptualized as a series of steps or phases, which, however, are dynamic, flexible, and expandable.
- The steps of the research process provide the tools with which scientists achieve their major aims or goals. These basic aims are to develop explanations of the world called theories and to find solutions to practical problems.
- The *Cumulative Index to Nursing and Allied Health Literature,* the *International Nursing Index,* and the *Cumulative Medical Index* are excellent resources for locating research that has been published on a topic or problem of interest.
- If nursing is to emerge as a socially significant, credible, scientific, and learned profession with a commitment to high-quality client care, then research (for all nurses) is a necessity.
- If nursing is to develop as a research-based practice, the clinical nurse must know the process and language of research, be sensitive to protecting the rights of human subjects, participate in the identification of significant researchable problems, and be a discriminating consumer of research findings.
- Bridging the research-practice gap, that is, bringing research into the clinical practice arena, is a key strategy in uniting the scholarly, scientific, and caring aspects of nursing in the future.
- All nurses who practice in settings where research is being conducted with human subjects or who participate in such research as data collectors or collaborators play an important role in safeguarding the rights of human subjects.
- Certain subjects, including children, fetuses, the mentally disabled, the elderly, captives, the dying, and the sedated or unconscious, are considered particularly vulnerable.
- Identifying problem areas in nursing practice is an investigative skill that all nurses need to master if the interplay between research and practice urged by the ANA is to be achieved.
- A researchable problem is one that can be investigated using the steps of the research process.
- Valid sources of researchable topics include one's own clinical experience, patterns or trends in someone else's observations or research, and one's own intellectual and scientific interests.
- Criticism is a professional responsibility of readers of nursing research.

Suggested Readings

Benner, P. 1984. *From novice to expert: Excellence and power in clinical nursing practice.* Menlo Park, Calif.: Addison-Wesley Publishing Co.

This book reports descriptive research based on levels of competency identified by practicing nurses themselves through interviews and questionnaires. It is an excellent example of nursing research conducted to discover what nurse clinicians learn from their own clinical practice.

Huck, S. W., et al. 1974. *Reading statistics and research.* New York: Harper and Row.

This book is based on the premise that although a student may not conduct research, the student should be capable of understanding and evaluating the research conducted by others. This book provides the knowledge necessary to read statistically oriented research reports with confidence.

Kaplan, A. 1964. *The conduct of inquiry.* San Francisco: Chandler.

This classic behavioral science book offers a critical assessment of inquiry in the behavioral sciences from the perspective of philosophy of science.

McCall, G. J., and Simmons, J. L. 1969. *Issues in participant observation: A text and reader.* Menlo Park, Calif.: Addison-Wesley Publishing Co.

This classic volume brings together a collection of well-known articles on the problems and issues associated with conducting field research from a sociologic perspective.

Werley, H. H., and Fitzpatrick, J. J. 1983. *Annual review of nursing research.* Vol. 1. New York: Springer Publishing Co.

Since the publication of volume 1 in 1983, the *Annual Review of Nursing Research* has offered a yearly integrative review of research on selected topics. These reviews are designed to help readers identify what has been done, what has been done well, what the gaps are, and what the suggested directions for research are. Each review includes parts devoted to research on nursing practice and nursing care delivery. The first volume reviewed research that pertained to five areas of human development along the life span, from infants to the elderly and the dying.

Wilson, H. S. 1982. *Deinstitutionalized residential care for the mentally disordered: The Soteria House approach.* New York: Grune and Stratton.

This monograph presents a full report of a field study conducted in the community setting of Soteria House, a nontraditional residential alternative for diagnosed schizophrenics. A psychiatric nurse researcher used a social science methodology called the "Discovery of Grounded Theory" to explain the problems, processes, and consequences of a clinical research question concerning control.

———. 1985. *Research in nursing.* Menlo Park, Calif.: Addison-Wesley Publishing Co.
This comprehensive, up-to-date textbook stresses research as an important professional activity for all nurses. In a clear style, the author covers all key topics on the subject of research in nursing.

Wilson, H. S., and Hutchinson, S. A. 1986. *Applying research in nursing.* Menlo Park, Calif.: Addison-Wesley Publishing Co.
This resource book gives practical tools for understanding and using nursing research in everyday practice. It offers thoughtfully selected information, examples, guided activities, and resources to help the reader become an informed consumer of research and a participant in clinical nursing studies.

Selected References

American Nurses' Association. 1975. *Human rights guidelines for nurses in clinical and other research.* Kansas City, Mo.: American Nurses' Association.

———. 1980. p. 9. *Nursing: A social policy statement.* Kansas City, Mo.: American Nurses' Association.

———. Commission of Nursing Research. 1981a. *ANA guidelines for investigative functions of nurses.* Kansas City, Mo.: American Nurses' Association.

———. Commission on Nursing Research. 1981b. *Priorities for the 1980s.* Kansas City, Mo.: American Nurses' Association.

Baker, N.; Carter, M. A.; and Harrison, O. A. 1983. An experimental trial of therapeutic touch in the treatment of arthritis. *Western Journal of Nursing Research* 5(3):56.

———. April 1984. The effect of type of thermometer and length of time inserted on oral temperature measurements of afebrile subjects. *Nursing Research* 33:109–11.

Barnard, K. E. 1973. The effect of stimulation on the sleep behavior of the premature infant. *Community Nursing Research* 6:12–33.

Baun, M., et al. 1984. Physiological effects of human/companion animal bonding. *Nursing Research* 33:126–29.

Brink, P. J., and Wood, M. J. 1983. *Basic steps in planning nursing research.* Belmont, Calif.: Wadsworth, 1983.

Britten, S. May 1985. Head nurses' perceptions of their role in a decentralized nursing department. Unpublished master's thesis, University of Florida.

Chenitz, C. 1985. The politics of nursing research. In Mason, D. J. and Talbott, S. W. p. 314. *Political action handbook for nurses.* Menlo Park, Calif.: Addison-Wesley Publishing Co.

Choi-Lao, A. T. H. 1981. Trace anesthetic vapors in hospital operating room environments. *Nursing Research* 30(3):156–60.

Davis, M. March 1981. Promoting nursing research in the clinical setting. *The Journal of Nursing Administration* 122–27.

Diers, D. 1979. *Research in nursing practice.* Philadelphia: J. B. Lippincott Co.

Dufault, K. 1983. Process of hope in elderly cancer patients. *Western Journal of Nursing Research* 5(3):72.

Fehring, R. J. 1983. Effects of biofeedback relaxation on the psychological stress symptoms of college students. *Nursing Research* 32(6):362–66.

Gortner, S. July/August 1980. Out of the past and into the future. *Nursing Research* 29:204–7.

Hutchinson, S. 1984. Creating meaning out of horror. *Nursing Outlook* 32:86–90.

Itano, J., et al. 1983. Compliance of cancer patients to therapy. *Western Journal of Nursing Research* 5(3):15–25.

Loomis, M. E. March/April 1985. An analysis of dissertation abstracts and titles: 1976–1982. *Nursing Research* 34(2):113–19.

Martinson, I. M. 1977. When the patient is dying: Home care for the child. *American Journal of Nursing* 77:1815–17.

Martinson, I. M., and Anderson, S. E. 1983. Effects of thermal applications on the abdominal temperature of dogs. *Research in Nursing and Health* 6(2):89–93.

McEnany, G. 1985. *Instructor's guide to research in nursing.* Menlo Park, Calif.: Addison-Wesley Publishing Co.

Norbeck, J. S., and Sheiner, M. 1982. Sources of social support related to single-parent functioning. *Research in Nursing and Health* 5:3–12.

Roy, C. 1985. "Nursing research makes a difference." *Nurses' Educational Funds Newsletter* 4(1):2–3.

Sitzman, J., et al. July/August 1983. Biofeedback training for reduced respiratory rate in chronic obstructive pulmonary disease: A preliminary study. *Nursing Research* 32(6):218–23.

Starzomski, R. October 1983. The place of research in nursing. *The Canadian Nurse* 34–35.

Triola, M. F. 1983. *Elementary statistics.* 2d ed. Menlo Park, Calif.: Benjamin/Cummings.

Walike, B. C., and Walike, J. W. 1977. A clinical study of tube-fed patients. *Journal of American Medical Association* 238:948–51.

Wilson, H. S. 1982. *Deinstitutionalized residential care for the mentally disordered: The Soteria House approach.* New York: Grune and Stratton.

———. 1985. *Research in nursing.* Menlo Park, Calif.: Addison-Wesley Publishing Co.

Wilson, H. S., and Hutchinson, S. A. 1986. *Applying research in nursing.* Menlo Park, Calif.: Addison-Wesley Publishing Co.

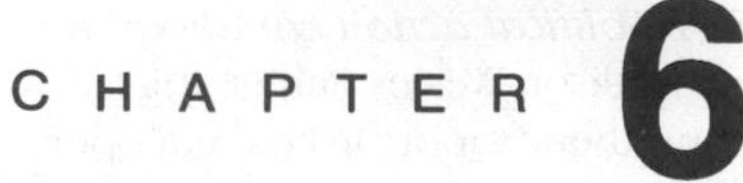

CHAPTER **6**

Politics and Power

Susan W. Talbott
Diana J. Mason

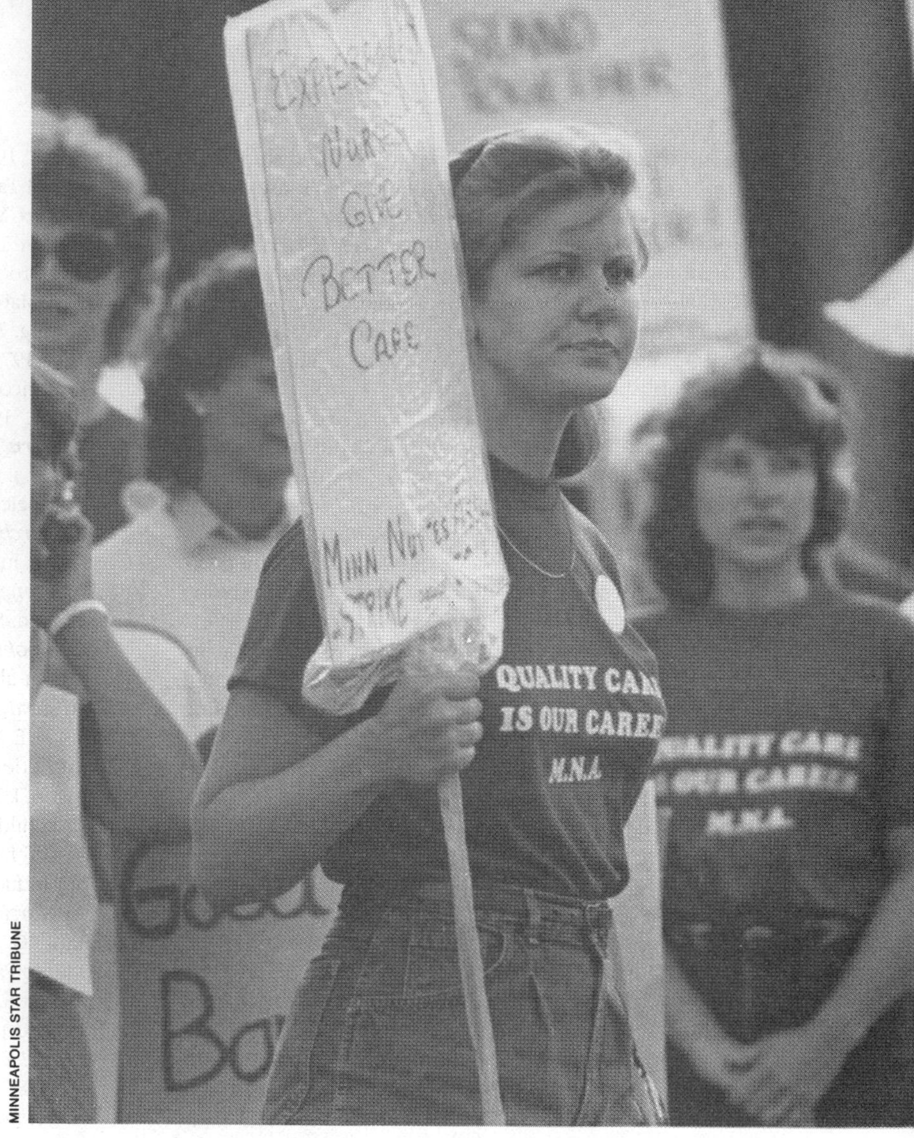

MINNEAPOLIS STAR TRIBUNE

Contents

Objectives

1. Understand how to develop and use effective political action skills.
   1.1 Define politics.
   1.2 Identify reasons why nurses are uncomfortable with politics.
   1.3 Discuss the four spheres of influence with which the nurse must be concerned.
   1.4 Identify an example of political action in each sphere of influence.
   1.5 Describe the guiding principles of political action.
2. Understand the role of power in professional nursing.
   2.1 Define power.
   2.2 Discuss the importance of power in nursing.
   2.3 Discuss sources of power.
   2.4 Discuss the importance of power images.
   2.5 Identify strategies for developing the individual and collective power of nurses.
3. Understand the change process.
   3.1 Define change.
   3.2 Discuss change theories.
   3.3 Identify the steps in the change process.
   3.4 Identify examples of change in the four spheres of influence.

Terms

change
coercive power
connection power
expert power
information power
legitimate power
political action
politics
power
referent power
reward power

The realities of the health care scene—increasingly scarce resources, governmental regulation, an aging population, the emergence of health care as big business, technological advancements, competition among providers for the health care dollar, and the developing political awareness of other health care professionals—demand that nurses become knowledgeable about and capable of influencing the development of health care policy and the delivery of patient care. Unless nurses develop their individual and collective political skills and use them to promote the profession and to become advocates for patients, patient care and the nursing profession will be jeopardized.

This chapter defines politics and discusses why nurses have been uncomfortable with political action. The four spheres of nursing influence—workplace, government, organizations, and community—are described, followed by an outline of activities for involvement in political action in each of these spheres. Two key concepts, power and change, are also discussed and illustrated.

Political Action

Politics Defined

What is politics? For many people the word *politics* evokes images of "crooked deals" hatched by men in "smoke-filled rooms," Watergate, bribes, and powerbrokers. More positive examples of **political action** are legislative initiatives to meet consumer needs and campaigns to elect nurse legislators. Although Webster's *New World Dictionary of the American Language* includes the words *crafty* and *unscrupulous* in the definition of political, a more positive definition is "having practical wisdom." Others describe politics as a means to an end, a process by which one can influence the decisions of others, thus exerting control over events (Stevens 1980).

Politics can also be defined as "influencing the allocation of scarce resources" (Talbott and Vance 1981, p. 592). Defined in this way, the word denotes more than action in the governmental arena; it is also applicable to every sphere of life where resources are limited and more than one person or group competes for them (Ehrat 1983).

The allocation of scarce resources involves everyone in some way. Consider the following examples:

- A student applying for a college loan or competing with other students for his or her fair share of a teacher's time and attention

The term *client* has been used here when referring to the person receiving care, even though it is inconsistent with my professional philosophy. In the setting in which I practice, recipients of care are considered *patients*. (Susan W. Talbott)

- A patient advocate competing for hospital education funds in order to do more preoperative teaching
- A citizen lobbying against the school board's proposal to divide one RN's time between two large schools
- A member of a professional association seeking association action on a practice issue, such as care of patients with acquired immune deficiency syndrome (AIDS).

Nurses' Discomfort with Politics

Despite nurses' experience with the political realities affecting the allocation of scarce resources, many nurses still harbor negative images of anything associated with the word *politics*. For example, it is not unusual to hear a colleague say, "I like her; she does not play politics." Although this remark is meant as a compliment, apolitical nurses in today's world hinder not only themselves and their colleagues but also the profession. For example, the nursing school dean, the head nurse, and the nurse researcher must all be politically skilled if they are to influence who gets how much of such scarce resources as funds for nursing education or nursing salaries, space for classrooms or offices, or release time to conduct research. Also, the staff nurse is in a particularly good position to influence the politics of patient care positively (Mason 1985).

Why are nurses reluctant to engage in politics? Why do many view political activity as outside the realm of the professional nurse's role and responsibility? There are a number of reasons why nurses, and many women, have avoided becoming involved in political action.

Minimal Role in Politics of Health Care

Until recently little has been written about nurses' roles in the politics of health care. Scant recognition has been given to the political nature of the social activism of many of the profession's early leaders. In addition, minimal attention has been paid to how nurses have worked together to effect legislative change in issues related to nursing and health care. Although the political knowledge and skills of successful nurses are not usually lauded in nursing journals or texts, change is occurring. For example, this text is the first of its kind to include a chapter on politics; however, others may follow suit.

Majority of Women Among Nurses

Another reason for nurses' reluctance to become involved with politics relates to the fact that a majority (97%) of nurses are women. Prior to the contemporary wave of activism in women's rights, politics was considered an aggressive, men-only endeavor. Fortunately this norm is changing, as evidenced by the nomination of Geraldine Ferraro as a candidate for Vice-President. In addition, an increasing number of nurses now serve in state legislatures across the country—a total of 40 as of January 1986.

Even though more women and nurses are becoming involved in governmental politics, many nurses have difficulty viewing the larger world of politics as an appropriate arena in which to participate. "Playing politics" in the workplace, for example, is often seen as the responsibility of those involved in collective bargaining. Although effective collective bargaining requires politically astute negotiators and staff representatives (Foley 1985), the politics of the workplace encompasses more than this singular collective political strategy. For example, the majority of nurses who must contend with a shortage of necessities such as linens, thermometers, drugs, time, or nursing staff do not view the allocation of scarce resources as an aspect of political action with which they should be involved (Mason 1985). Too often, nurses react to such predicaments with complaints but no action, and the predominantly male-dominated power structure of the health care institution supports such inaction because nurses often compete for the same resources with administrators, who are usually men. A politically astute and assertive nurse would likely review her or his knowledge of change theory (Natapoff and Loetterle 1985) and find like-minded colleagues (including nurses, physicians, social workers, physical therapists, etc.) who want to participate in solving a problem. Political skills can empower nurses to effect change in the workplace and elsewhere.

Women are socialized differently than men; for this reason, few women exert much influence on the male-dominated world of business and the professions. Research by Hennig and Jardin (1977) on the behavior of men, who generally participate in team sports while growing up, and women, who generally do not have such childhood experiences, reveals that success in business and the professional world is contingent on the ability to be a "team player." Men are trained to view the "big picture," the mission of the company or the team—e.g., to win, to get the big contract, to beat the opponent. They work together to achieve the agreed-upon goal. Their support of the leader or coach is unconditional. Even if men are not personal friends outside of work or off the playing field, they recognize that the goal is the priority. Another important element of team play is competition: Men relish the opportunity to compete in business, to do the most heart transplants, to win the big civil rights case; many women, by contrast, shy away from frank and open competition.

Are nurses good team players? Unfortunately, most nurses and their colleagues, including physicians and hospital administrators, would say nurses have a lot to learn about being effective team players. This does not mean that women and nurses must adopt the male style of power-seeking and aggressive competition. In fact, research (Miller 1982) suggests that while men strive to attain power singularly, women appear to favor "power sharing." This approach, coupled with improved skills as team players, could enable nurses to affect profoundly the design and delivery of health care as well as the future of the nursing profession.

Small Appreciation for Activist History

The fact that relatively few nurses know and appreciate their rich heritage also contributes to their discomfort with politics. Nurses who have been leaders and social activists, such as Lavinia Dock, Lillian Wald, Harriet Tubman, and Margaret Sanger, were all skilled politicians. Each had a particular style of working for change, but all knew the importance of political know-how and collective action. Indeed, they were able to make significant contributions to the profession and society because of their political skills. Maybe they had read the wise words of the founder of modern nursing, Florence Nightingale:

> When I entered into service here, I determined that, happened what would, I *never* would intrigue among the Committee. Now I perceive that I do all my business by intrigue. I propose in private to A, B, or C the resolution I think A, B, or C most capable of carrying in Committee, and then leave it to them, and I always win (Huxley 1975, p. 53).

If more nurses studied change theory along with the biographies of the influential nurses of the past, society might see more "intrigue" by nurses in behalf of health care consumers and the nursing profession.

Little Formal Political Education

Associated with the lack of appreciation of nursing history is the sparse education of nursing students, at the undergraduate and graduate level, on how to be politically astute. Fortunately, some nursing schools are adding courses that cover political action and health policy development to their curriculum (Solomon and Roe 1985). However, there is a critical need for students to have the opportunity to work with faculty and other preceptors who are skilled in the art of influencing governmental, organizational, workplace, and community politics. The need for political education of practicing nurses and current students is underscored by a study of 1086 nurse administrators by Archer and Goehner (1981):

> Respondents attribute nurses' lack of political involvement mainly to inadequate preparation, failure to realize the importance of participation, socialization of nurses into passive roles, ignorance of issues, and failure to realize our potential clout. All of these factors are related to the inability of both formal and continuing education to provide opportunities for nurses to learn the importance of political participation and how to be prepared for political effectiveness (p. 52).

Thus, a conscious effort needs to be made to educate nurses and nursing students about effective political action. Clearly, for such education to be effective, nurses must examine who they are as women and men and the values that they have been socialized to hold in relation to team play, power, and competition (Vance et al. 1985). This effort can be facilitated by learning more about how nursing leaders historically have used their political skills to bring about change, not only in the profession and health care but also in the values and actions of society as a whole.

Political Action: Four Spheres of Influence

Government

Most people think of political action in relationship to local, state, or federal government. By voting, responsible citizens convey their opinions to elected and appointed officials on matters of concern. Many women first learn about political action through the educational efforts of the League of Women Voters. Other organizations—including the American Nurses' Association (ANA), Canadian Nurses' Association (CNA), National League for Nursing (NLN), and the National Student Nurses' Association (NSNA)—publish articles on legislative matters and encourage nurses to take action in behalf of health care consumers and the nursing profession. Nursing lobbyists at the state and national level work to influence the development of health policy and legislation, but their success depends on the active support of nurses who back up these paid lobbyists by doing personal lobbying among their own elected officials.

The laws and regulations of local, state, and federal governments greatly influence nursing practice and health care. For example, federal laws and regulations establish funding of health care for the elderly, poor, and disabled (Medicare and Medicaid), authorize health care services for special groups (including American Indians, migrant workers, and veterans), set policies and formulas for reimbursement of health care services (as with prospective payment), and appropriate funding for special health care and social services (such as community health centers, the food stamp program, and the school lunch program). The federal government still plays a significant role in providing funding for nursing education and research (Osgood and Elliott 1985), but elimination of such funds has been advocated by the Reagan administration.

State laws play a similar role in determining which health care services are provided to the public and funded. An increasing number of states are passing legislation to mandate that insurance companies reimburse some categories of nurses for their services. For example, in 1983 Maine passed legislation requiring hospitals to itemize nursing services on the patient's bill. State public health codes and regulations influence the standards of public health and health care. In addition, the states are responsible for defining and regulating nursing practice. Archaic nurse practice acts in some states inhibit nurses from providing a broad range of services and can effectively limit nurses' ability to compete with other health care professionals in the provision of primary care services (Long and Mason 1985).

While the role of the local government has received less attention from nurses, its impact on health care is significant. Local public health departments provide much-needed services to a community's citizens, including school health care. Local public hospitals are frequently the only source of health care for the uninsured, a group that represents a substantial proportion of the United States population (Dallek 1985). As the societal trend toward decentralization of government continues, the local community will play an even greater role in determining and enacting its own health policies (Jordan 1985; Mason 1986).

Clearly, nurses need to learn more about political action in the governmental sphere so that, individually and collectively, they can influence the government's large role in the formulation of health policy and its enactment (Diers 1985). Just as governmental politics has been deemed appropriate for women as well as men, nurses' activities in this arena have likewise increased; however, more needs to be done, including developing an awareness of the interplay of this sphere of influence with other spheres.

Workplace

In what other spheres must nurses be involved? Earlier, the workplace was mentioned as a setting in which nurses apply political skills. In light of the facts that over 66% of nurses work in hospitals and that too few nurses derive professional satisfaction from working in these bureaucratic institutions, it seems logical that nurses would work together to change the nature of their workplace. Evidence that hospitals can be rewarding places for delivering quality care to patients is documented in the American Academy of Nursing's (1983) study of hospitals with a fine record of attracting and retaining professional nurses.

The politics of patient care impinges on the practice of every nurse. For example, as the prospective payment system becomes the norm, hospital stays will be cut more drastically in an effort to reduce health care costs (Shaffer 1984). The need for nurses to be "faster and smarter" in delivering patient care and patient education will increase. Nurses are already feeling the pressure to prepare patients for discharge days earlier than before. How can nurses ensure that the quality of nursing care is maintained under the new system? One way is for nurses to collaborate with each other and other providers to eliminate nonnursing tasks, such as answering the telephone, emptying the garbage, and transporting nonacute patients. Developing a demonstration project that compares cost and quality of care issues under different hospital unit structures can provide the necessary data and generate support from other providers and administrators for changing the role of staff nurses. This sort of "proactive" planning can empower nurses to take charge of nursing practice in ways that benefit patients and health professionals while conserving scarce resources such as money, time, and supplies.

Organizations

A third sphere of influence is the professional organization. Powerful and influential professional associations, such as the ANA and CNA and their affiliated state/province and district associations, provide a collective voice for promoting nursing and quality health care. As such, they exert influence on the individual nurse as well as in the spheres of government, the workplace, the community, and the profession. Associations monitor and influence laws and regulations affecting nursing and health care. Their role in workplace matters ranges from studying practice issues to acting as the collective bargaining agent for nurses. Additionally, the professional nursing organization is often a visible presence in the community because it presents the nursing perspective on health care issues. Indeed, the professional association works to advance nursing and nursing practice (Maraldo and Kinder 1985). How well it does this job depends largely on member participation.

There are currently over 60 national nursing associations. It is likely that a nurse will belong to at least one professional nursing organization for some time during her or his career. However, some nurses never join any nursing association; others join but fail to participate actively in the association's affairs, even though participation in the affairs of a professional association enables nurses to influence the association to work in their behalf (Talbott 1985; Skaggs 1985). Nurses can learn about the politics of the professional association from senior nursing colleagues at the local level, and students can benefit from participation in NSNA.

Community

The community in which the nurse lives and works is the fourth sphere of influence and can include the local neighborhood, the corporate world, the nation, and the international community. The community encompasses the three spheres referred to above: workplace, professional organizations, and government. Many nurses, including Lillian Wald, founder of the Henry Street Settlement and modern public health nursing, view the community as more than a practice setting. Nurses who live in the community where they work can understand and influence the complex interplay among individuals and groups that compete for scarce resources.

Many communities depend on nurses to help with a wide variety of health and social policy decisions, such as environmental pollution and the feminization of poverty (Archer 1985). For example, a nurse who serves as an elected member of her or his community school board can influence decisions that affect the health and health care of students, such as the hiring of nurses for the school system. Nurses' opinions on matters of the public health are frequently sought, and the enterprising nurse looks for opportunities to promote a positive image of nursing while serving the community (Frost 1985). She or he also identifies ways in which fellow citizens can support both consumer health and nursing agendas.

The four spheres of influence described above give each nurse ample room to develop and use political skills. All the spheres are interrelated. Efforts to effect change in one often bring about changes in the others. Learning to exert influence in each sphere takes time and is best done in concert with colleagues or a mentor.

Opportunities for Political Action

A discussion of when and where to engage in political action must be prefaced by a statement of three key assumptions:

1. *Individuals who are deeply concerned about a particular issue or cause are most likely to identify ways to take action.* Each student nurse has limited resources in time, money, and access to such support as a copying machine or telephone. Before becoming politically involved, an individual must make choices, including the conscious decision to set aside the necessary resources. For example, a student who wants her or his school to offer evening or weekend clinical practice hours may decide to seek election to the student council to work for this change from within.
2. *Political action in any sphere is best done by a group.* Individual activism is laudable, but group action is much more effective. It provides the change agents with the collegiality and support necessary to sustain a vision for change and fosters creative thinking and planning (Vance 1985).
3. *Successful political action requires the thoughtful application of change theory.* The politically astute nurse will do homework before embarking on a project by reviewing the principles of change theory. Achieving goals for change requires thoughtful planning. Effective political activists plan strategy, much as nurses use the nursing process to evaluate patients' need for care.

There are a variety of avenues to political action. The person who identifies an issue needing attention may be the one to chart the course of action. For example, a nurse who wants to see hospital policy changed to permit parents to stay overnight with their acutely ill children might begin to address the issue by discussing it with the head nurse or at a staff meeting. Consultation with peers or one's boss/instructor is a good way to initiate action. The nurse, however, may enlist the help of a more effective spokesperson for the issue.

Often, people get involved because they see others around them doing something about a problem or an opportunity of mutual interest. For example, a staff nurse agrees with her colleagues that the new nursing director seems to be a forward-thinking manager who might support their idea of organizing a staff nurse forum to address practice issues of concern to all. Together, the group of staff nurses submits a request for a meeting with the director and, once it is arranged, prepares an agenda for the meeting that includes planning and developing a welcoming reception for the new director.

Sometimes it is more difficult to get action on an issue. For example, a nurse may know "something must be done" but not know quite where to begin. The following list of avenues to action, together with some brief examples, may help the reader identify ways to become politically active.

Professional Organizations

Turning to one's professional organization for information and assistance is a logical first step, especially when the issue is related to nursing practice. For example, pediatric nurses at a large teaching hospital wanted the administration to change a policy that required nurses to hold children while x-ray films of the children were taken. When their request was denied, the nurses sought assistance from the collective bargaining representative of their state nurses' association and from Nurses' Environmental Health Watch, a national nursing organization formed to prevent and eliminate environmental health hazards. In another instance, a group of head nurses decided to organize a support group to share information on the implementation of diagnostic related categories (DRGs) with colleagues at all local hospitals. This group sought the endorsement of the district nurses' association and was granted status as a special interest group of the association.

Sometimes nursing organizations join a coalition (an alliance of several groups) formed for the purpose of collaborating on a particular problem or issue. For instance, at the national level the ANA has joined forces with other groups to take legal action in support of equal pay for work of comparable worth. Individual nurses, equally committed to achieving pay equity for women, can work through their professional associations or with other groups such as the National Organization for Women (NOW).

Workplace Organizations

Committees In most hospitals, nursing homes, and public health agencies, there exists a system of committees to deal with specific issues. For example, a nursing department has an equipment evaluation committee that selects and evaluates patient care products used by the nursing staff. A pharmacy committee in the same hospital has representatives from nursing, medicine, and the pharmacy. In addition to formal, standing committees, ad hoc committees or task forces can be appointed to deal with particular issues or problems. For example, on a nursing unit a task force might examine the best way to initiate a management development program or institute primary nursing.

Nurses who have an idea or problem they want to see addressed are advised to look for existing committees that might already be dealing with the concern or are likely to do so. For example, nurses at one Veterans' Administration hospital, concerned about staff safety in the parking lot, approached the leaders of the Staff Nurse Forum with their concern. The forum is a group of staff nurses who identify problems and the need for change. They then develop a plan for instituting the change (McKay and Lumley 1985). The forum successfully solved the parking problem, illustrating the point that employing the legitimate influence of a formal organization, such as the forum, can be very effective.

Another means to generate action is through an interdisciplinary committee (Devereux and Dirschel 1985). Nurses who find ways to work collaboratively with fellow health professionals can often successfully address problems that might otherwise be unsolvable. The collective power of nurses and physicians, working together on a patient care issue, can be very persuasive. For example, nurses and physicians on one unit were distressed about the delays in getting STAT medication orders delivered to the floor. There was no interdisciplinary pharmacy committee, and repeated calls to the pharmacy did not solve the problem. Subsequently, the problem was referred to the hospital's committee of nurses and physicians, and their proposed solution was adopted by the pharmacy. Additionally, the committee of nurses and physicians decided to ask the pharmacy director to work with them in establishing a pharmacy committee to evaluate existing policy and recommend needed changes. Student nurses might ask to attend a nursing or interdisciplinary committee meeting in a clinical site to observe such a group in action and analyze its process and effectiveness.

Nursing department newsletter Another way to generate interest in an issue is by writing an article for the hospital or nursing department newsletter. Nurses who are present at nursing grand rounds also have the opportunity to inform their colleagues of an issue of mutual concern and enlist their aid in dealing with it. What can one do if there are no newsletters or grand rounds? Form a task force of concerned nurses and, using a model for change, plan a strategy to establish ways of helping nurses communicate with one another through a newsletter, grand rounds, or possibly a support group.

Analysis of workplace structure and processes Nurses who successfully practice the politics of change in the workplace must analyze the structure and processes of this sphere to identify the available avenues for action (Talbott 1985a). Just as nurses can influence the outcome of patient care, so can they effectively alter the nature of the workplace.

The Government

Nurses are often more familiar with the avenues for action used to influence the governmental sphere. Those who want to learn more about how the government works can review excellent materials provided by the League of Women Voters or consult contemporary nursing texts on the subject (Mason and Talbott 1985; Archer and Goehner 1982; Kalisch and Kalisch 1982; Bagwell and Clements 1985). Student nurses should look for opportunities to accompany faculty on visits to legislators or to participate in a "Lobby Day," which local district nurses' associations sometimes sponsor.

Numerous ways to influence governments personally are open to nurses. Of course, the most basic step is registering to vote. Voter registration drives are sponsored by a variety of organizations, including NSNA, which has developed a kit for student nurses to hold such drives. For a copy, write to the National Student Nurses' Association, 555 West 57th Street, New York, NY 10019.

Political action committees (PACs) The collective efforts of nurses influence the federal government through the ANA's political action committee—the American Nurses' Association Political Action Committee (ANA-PAC, formerly N-CAP) (Curtis 1985). Nurses contribute funds to ANA-PAC, which supports deserving candidates for election to Congress. In 1984, N-CAP contributed $302,000 to Congressional campaigns, and 88% of those candidates endorsed by N-CAP were elected. The ANA and ANA-PAC also count on nurses at the grass roots level to work for these candidates and to serve as Congressional District Coordinators or CDCs (Ford-Roegner 1985). CDCs are responsible for organizing nurses in their Congressional district for lobbying and campaigning. This effort has been enormously successful and has provided a mechanism for nurses to influence governmental politics collectively on the federal level.

Nurses have organized PACs in most states, and information about a state PAC can be obtained from the state nurses' association. Additionally, groups of local nurses are emerging to work for candidates in city and county races. In one city, for instance, nurses worked for a woman candidate who was said to have little chance of winning. This woman won her election by fewer than 200 votes and attributed her win to the efforts of her nurse supporters.

Political parties and clubs In addition to supporting nursing PACs, nurses can become involved with political parties and local political clubs as a means to influence health policy as well as nursing practice (Hughes 1985; McCarthy 1985). Such involvement enables the nurse to exercise some control over affairs in the community and to develop a nonnursing support base for nursing and health care issues.

Work with elected officials Nurses who get to know their elected representatives, especially at the local level, often have the opportunity to work with them on health and nursing issues. Individuals who serve in elected positions review and vote on hundreds of bills each year. Nobody can be an expert on such a broad range of issues, from road building and toxic waste disposal to day care. This reality poses an opportunity for nurses. By offering to set up a health advisory committee for the legislator, the nurse can ensure that the legislator is aware of both pertinent facts and the nursing point of view. In one instance, a city councilwoman asked a nurse constituent to help her gather information about a bill related to teaching breast-feeding to new mothers in city hospitals. Although the constituent did not have the information her councilwoman needed, she consulted her network of nurse colleagues and found an expert to help the councilwoman shape a bill that best served client needs and nursing practice.

Political appointments An increasingly important avenue for nurses interested in influencing health policy and practice is the political appointment (Talbott 1985b). While such appointments generally go to experienced nurses, student nurses and new practitioners alike can help pave the way for experienced nurses to receive appointments by helping in election campaigns and/or using their political connections in behalf of nursing.

The Community

Political involvement in the community often arises out of one's own interest in living and working in a community that is supportive of the health and well-being of its citizens. For instance, a nurse may become involved with an ad hoc committee to stop unlawful dumping of hazardous wastes in the neighborhood. As a member of such a group, the nurse wears two hats: She or he is both a concerned citizen and an expert on health issues. At the same time, the nurse's position in the group enables the nurse to extend networks and expand a support base for nursing. Thus, when the administrator of the community's hospital fires the dynamic, competent, and creative director of nursing who refuses to permit a restructuring of the hospital that would place nursing under the control of medicine, the nurse can call upon these networks and support bases to protest the administrator's actions and demand reinstatement of the nursing director.

As the self-help movement expands, nurses are realizing how influential consumer groups can be. In many instances, such groups are founded by nurses who realize that consumers, often their own patients, have a need for a self-help group. Sometimes nurses who have been patients themselves start postmastectomy support groups or similar groups. Nurses contribute their leadership skills to many organizations, including the National Alliance for the Mentally Ill. The personally devastating experience of having a child with chronic schizophrenia can be a powerful motivating force toward working in behalf of others through a group such as NAMI. The political power of groups with particular health concerns—including the Gray Panthers, the American Association of Retired Persons, and the Juvenile Diabetes Association—can generate extraordinary political influence on elected and appointed officials. Such groups offer nurses a variety of avenues to learn about grass roots political activism. These groups can also be a community support base for nursing.

A variety of other opportunities for community involvement exist for nurses. Since many nurses are also parents, they can work on health issues through their school board. Those who ultimately run for government office have frequently begun their careers by running for the school board. Other nurses volunteer for community action groups, such as a community planning board or a fund raising committee for the city's art museum. Or, a nurse may get involved in the tenant's organization in her or his apartment building. Regardless of the issue, the same opportunity to organize and plan for change exists in the community as it does in the workplace, government, or professional association.

Guiding Principles for Political Action

The following list of "commandments" is designed to help newcomers to political activism consider some ideas to enhance their effectiveness.

Look at the Big Picture

Step back and take a look at the larger environment in which you live, work, and study. In the governmental sphere especially, nurses are too often described as concerned only with nursing issues rather than with a broad variety of consumer and health care issues. Nurses will not enjoy credibility as health experts unless they become more sensitive to the concerns of others and employ their expertise in all spheres. In the workplace, nurses often focus their attention on their own unit, neglecting to view their position and unit in relationship to the larger organization. Astute nurses are aware of the environmental factors that impinge on their work setting. For example, the advent of the prospective payment system has had a major effect on nursing practice and raised many issues regarding the quality of patient care. Nurses who make an effort to "take off the blinders" will see and understand the complex forces that affect their practice, the status of the nursing profession, and the nature of health care delivery. Such nurses have a better chance of influencing the allocation of scarce resources and planning for improved systems of patient care despite the seemingly hostile environment created by the realities of cost containment, DRGs, the malpractice crisis, etc.

Do Your Homework

Homework is not something that ends with graduation. Nurses must take stock of their goals and clarify their personal and professional positions on issues. Taking stock requires setting time aside for reflection. Nurses who use the nursing process as a basis for planning patient care can use the same problem-solving approach in their own behalf. For example, developing a strategy to convince the head nurse to support the development of a formal continuing education program for staff nurses requires research and planning and will be most successful if it is based on change theory.

Another aspect of doing one's homework relates to learning about the struggles and successes of our forerunners. Studying the lives and work of nurse leaders, including Lillian Wald, Margaret Sanger, and Lavinia Dock, reminds us of the power and influence these women exerted on the health systems and policies of their day and offers us models to emulate.

Nothing Ventured, Nothing Gained

Nurses have always been risk takers. Margaret Sanger risked being jailed for promoting birth control. Lavinia Dock and her colleagues chained themselves to the White House fence to call attention to their belief that women should have the vote. Clara Maas lost her life while participating in research on malaria.

A young Maryland woman—nurse, wife, and mother of two small children—was paralyzed in an automobile accident. Following months in hospitals, she decided to devote her energies to helping other neurologically impaired patients. With a colleague, she formed a self-help group. She also lobbies for the enactment of seat belt laws and speaks to school children on safety. Not many people with two good arms and legs are as productive! If you have a dream, an idea, a vision of what might be—make it a reality.

Get a Toe in the Door

Incremental changes or actions may have a better chance of success than a major project. Resistance to change is more easily overcome if change is tested by a pilot project. For example, a nursing director is more apt to agree to the introduction of primary nursing on one unit rather than an overall change in the nursing system.

A task force is another useful approach to initiating change. For example, head nurses in one hospital were concerned about an increase in *Staphylococcus* infections in their surgical division. They asked the nursing director to initiate the appointment of a multidisciplinary task force to evaluate the problem and make recommendations for controlling the spread of infection.

Quid Pro Quo

"Something for something." "Scratch my back, and I'll scratch yours." "Everything and everybody has a price." Many nurses are offended by the implications of these aphorisms, believing that they represent a cynical view of human and organizational relationships. Others, however, concede that they represent a realistic view of life. Consider how you relate to your friends and colleagues: Don't you often find yourself making tradeoffs?

When assessing your position within your school of nursing, the clinical area, or among your peers, review your friendships, connections, and pragmatic relationships. Frequently men say, "He owes me one," implying the person has received a favor and will reciprocate. Women and nurses, however, rarely use those words. In fact, they seem uncomfortable with the idea of being "in debt" or owing a favor despite the fact that they participate in give-and-take (quid-pro-quo) situations every day. It is important to develop an ease in professional and personal relationships so that one feels connected and supported rather than isolated and resentful.

Walk a Mile in Another's Moccasins

Nurses learn to evaluate patients, to assess "where they are coming from." But how often do they make similar inquiries of peers, supervisors, or friends? The politically astute nurse who wants to get ahead identifies the goals the head nurse has for the unit and finds ways to support those efforts and get help in meeting personal development goals. Identifying another's agenda can help one plan a win-win situation, one in which the staff nurse or student meets her or his own needs as well as those of the teacher or head nurse.

Strike While the Iron Is Hot

Any plan for change must include a time table that identifies the best time for a particular action. Few people would approach the head nurse to discuss the work schedule while a patient is in cardiac arrest, but a surprising number of people give little thought to what might be an opportune time to discuss such a topic. Sometimes an eagerness to take action precludes some important questions: "Is this the best time to do this? Will it be received better now or later?"

Read Between the Lines

Some people reveal a lot by the information they choose not to share. Here is one example: A high school student tells the school nurse about her family. She describes all her siblings, relatives, her mother, aunts, and neighbors. She never mentions her father, however. Although the girl is pregnant, she denies having a boy friend. After a number of meetings, the nurse's hunch is validated: The girl is a victim of sexual abuse by her father, and he has impregnated her. Just as nurses listen with a "third ear" to their clients, politically astute nurses attend to colleagues, their bosses, and the work environment for cues that help them achieve some measure of control and influence.

Half a Loaf Is Better than None

It is human nature to want it all, but the reality is that the world is far from perfect. People need to learn to share the wealth and settle, often, for less than they would like. One way to adjust to this reality is to develop an ability to identify alternative solutions or outcomes. Rather than setting one's heart on a particular goal, it is prudent to outline acceptable alternatives. For example, the head nurse has been expecting a new staff nurse assigned to her busy unit. Because of a budget crunch, all hiring has been suspended. The head nurse needs to find an alternative way to provide good patient care without the new staff nurse. She and her staff hold a brainstorming session and devise a plan to enlist the families of some patients in providing personal care and help with feeding.

Rome Was Not Built in a Day

When a student nurse or a seasoned professional gets a terrific idea, that person wants it implemented at once. Because most nurses work in bureaucratic organizations, they need to accept the fact that change does not occur rapidly. Even in a small, flexible organization, change is often slow because the nature of the change process demands that one proceed only after careful deliberation. Although it is sometimes true that he who hesitates is lost, a nurse who identifies a problem needing a solution or envisions a plan for change is well advised to remember Rome.

While political skills are gained only through practice, nurses who ponder and act on the principles that underlie political action gain the ability to view their efforts in perspective. Because nothing succeeds like success, the novice is encouraged to tackle problems and seek opportunities for change that are short term and likely to be successful.

Power

Effective political action requires an understanding of power: what it is, how to get it, and how to use it.

Power Defined

Power is another term that makes many nurses and women uncomfortable. Certainly, the negative connotations of the word *politics* extend also to the word *power.* Yet *power* is also by definition a neutral concept. Consider how two nurse leaders defined the term:

> For practical purposes, we can view power as the *capacity* to modify the conduct of others in a desired manner, while avoiding having one's own conduct modified in undesired ways by others (Stevens 1980, p. 208).

> Power is the ability to do or act. It is the possession of control or command over others. Power is access. It is the ability to deliver goods and services on your terms. Power is achievement of the desired result (Ferguson 1985, p. 89).

Clearly, power involves being in control of one's own resources and those of others. How and to what ends one uses that control determines whether power is seen as positive or negative.

Nurses' discomfort with power is also attributable to the fact that nurses are chiefly women (Vance et al. 1985). As with politics, men, not women, are socialized to seek and achieve power. A woman who even acknowledges that she wants power, let alone actively seeks it, is often deemed "unfeminine," and her conduct "inappropriate." In recent years, women have challenged the restrictive stereotypes that have limited their influence. Some feminist writers and researchers suggest that women may relate to power in different ways than most men, leading

Miller (1982, p. 3) to define **power** simply as "the capacity to produce change." Miller also suggests that women appear to be developing patterns of "power-sharing" and empowering of others that have not been characteristic of men in general.

Nurses and Power

These emerging patterns of power have enormous implications for nursing. First, as society becomes more accepting of women who seek and use power, nurses will become more comfortable with the idea of acquiring and exerting power. Second, as nurses gain and use power, different patterns of power acquisition and usage will be seen in the workplace. For example, nurses may become the driving force behind the transformation of communication patterns, change, and decision making in the workplace. Third, this transformation could foster a reconceptualization of the client as a crucial part of power relationships in health care arenas. Indeed, the power of client choice in selecting health care providers is evident today. Consider the options of a healthy pregnant woman: private physician, HMO or another prepaid group, or nurse-midwife in a freestanding birth center.

This evolving transformation of power relationships offers nurses a fine opportunity to redefine and develop their power further. Although most nurses would admit to having relatively little power within health care institutions, the majority have and use a great deal of power in relation to their clients, particularly in such institutions as hospitals and nursing homes. Many of the public's negative images of nurses undoubtedly stem from the inappropriate use of power by some nurses. For example, consider the common complaint that nurses withhold or delay pain medication because clients know (and let the nurse know that they know) when they can receive medication again. In this situation, the nurse controls the clients' level of comfort, and thus, often their sense of self-control. It is also true, however, that nurses can empower clients. For example, nursing's emphasis on client teaching suggests that the profession believes its role is one of helping clients to control their own health.

Clearly, power issues are intimately related to client care. As nurses develop greater power in the workplace, they will be in a better position to shape the power relationships there, including relationships with nurse colleagues, fellow health care professionals, and their clients.

Sources of Power

How can nurses develop their power? A number of articles describe in detail a variety of sources of power (French and Raven 1959; Hersey et al. 1979; Stevens 1980). Understanding these sources of power is prerequisite to formulating a plan for developing one's own power.

- **Legitimate** (or positional) **power** is derived from one's formal position or title in an organization. It is associated with the authority that the position gives its holder to make and enforce decisions. The title "Vice President for Nursing" implies that the holder has power by virtue of the position, regardless of who holds that position or how effective she or he is.
- **Reward power** is derived from the perception of one's ability to bestow rewards or favors on others.
- **Coercive power**, by contrast, arises from the perception of one's ability to threaten, harm, or punish others.
- **Information power** is associated with persons who are perceived to control key information.

Reward, coercive, and information power all relate to the degree an individual can control the distribution of resources.

- **Referent** (charismatic, or personal) **power** is power derived from an individual's own vision and sense of self, and her or his ability to communicate these so that others regard the person with admiration and are motivated to follow.
- **Connection power** is derived from the perception that one has important contacts or relationships with others. These connections can be an aspect of both formal and informal networks.
- **Expert** (or knowledge) **power** is power derived from one's expertise, talents, and skills. To the extent that nurses are experts at caring, one can include in this category Benner's (1984) vision of power in caring; i.e., the positive power the nurse brings to the nurse-client relationship. This power enables the nurse to transform the client's life through advocacy and other means of caring.

These sources of power involve one's own person, one's profession, and the organization in which one works. They are important in that they suggest ways for nurses to gain power.

Power Images

It should be apparent from the preceding descriptions of power sources that the *perception* of power, or power images, can be as important to one's ability to acquire power as the fact that the individual really does have a capacity to reward or punish, expertise, connections, or control over resources.

A key problem nurses face is the perception that they are powerless. Nurses, other health care providers, and the public have an image of nurses as a group comprised of individuals who lack power. For instance, while the experienced nurse ought to feel and convey a degree of expert power, the public and even other health care providers seldom recognize this expertise until they, in the role of client, receive expert nursing care. Indeed, too few nurses acknowledge their expertise and develop that source of power.

While nurses must take stock of their own power images, they must also accurately assess the power they ascribe to others. For example, physicians have exerted enormous power and influence for decades; however, in recent years, their power has been waning (Starr 1982). Overestimating the power of others can limit one's own sense of power and control.

Developing Nurses' Power

The following strategies are suggested to help nurses develop power individually and collectively:

Appraise Actual and Potential Sources of Power

What power do others think you have? What power do you actually have? Which power sources should you develop more fully?

Identify Ways to Enhance Positional Power

The title "Staff Nurse" rarely suggests positional power, yet a simple name change may bring more power and status to the position. For example, the trend toward decentralization in nursing departments is usually accompanied by changes in titles of both staff nurses and nurse managers. The title "Primary Nurse" suggests greater authority for decision making in client care than the title "Staff Nurse" does. Similarly, the corporate title "Vice-President for Nursing" connotes a broader and more influential scope of power than the title "Director of Nursing." Although nurses are becoming familiar with the greater power associated with decentralized positions, it is incumbent on the nursing department to convey this enhanced status to the other hospital departments, clients, and the public.

Recognize and Develop Nurses' Expert Power

Nurses must identify the areas of expertise they want to develop and formulate a plan to keep their knowledge base current while they become leaders in those fields. Participating in and using related research, regular reading in the field, attending continuing education programs, and collaborating with nurses and other health professionals are just a few ways to develop one's expertise.

To develop one's expertise fully as a source of power, however, one must convey this expertise to others. Some institutions have been developing career ladders to reward the nurse who stays at the bedside. "Nurse Clinician I," "Nurse Clinician II," and "Advanced Nurse Clinician" are titles that denote varying levels of nursing expertise. Similarly, the ANA's program of certification is a means for recognizing the nurse's expertise. As with positional power, nurses must communicate the meaning of these titles and credentials to the public.

One way to do so is to develop a list of "nurse experts" who can be called on to speak or write about their areas of expertise. For example, one local nursing association uses such a list when it wants to take advantage of opportunities for nurses to present testimony, be interviewed by the media, speak at a public forum on a health care topic, write an editorial for the local newspaper, etc. Such activities demand that nurses develop their speaking and writing skills.

Nurses can also convey their expertise within the institution by participating in committees, writing for the hospital newsletter, and publicizing their professional activities in that newsletter. They should also communicate their expertise to the client and family; e.g., upon the client's admission, the primary nurse might give them a business card showing her or his clinical title, area of expertise, and the telephone number of the unit. In this way, the client and family know the name of the nurse and can call for assistance.

Recognize and Expand Connection Power

Because nurses coordinate clients' care, they have more connection power than they probably realize. It is important for nurses to assess what formal and informal networks can be further developed and then to formulate a plan to build them. Most nurses' connections within an institution are mainly with individuals on the lower rungs of the institution's hierarchy. Hospital committees, social events, and dining rooms provide opportunities for developing networks up and down the entire hierarchy.

Connections outside of the workplace—in government, professional organizations, and the community—can enhance the nurse's power in all spheres of influence. Appraising one's connections in these spheres and developing a systematic plan for devising networks outside the workplace can enhance both the individual's connection power and the power image of the profession.

Reward Others and Evaluate Coercive Power

Identify ways to reward others and evaluate the extent to which others believe one has coercive power. While this source of power may be a means to an end, it must be used with caution if one is to maintain positive power images. However, creative thinking about the rewards one can bestow on others can help nurses develop such positive images. For example, writing a memo to the director of nursing about the exemplary performance of a colleague or developing a reputation as one who is willing to switch working days with colleagues to accommodate their special needs may be perceived as both rewards or favors.

Communicate Your Vision

Define and communicate a personal vision for nursing and quality health care. This requires that nurses define what their philosophy of nursing is and how it can contribute to the consumer's health. Formal and informal collegial discussions of the nursing perspective in health care and the profession's potential can help nurses describe their vision, formulate goals, and motivate and challenge others to do likewise.

It is essential for nurses to understand the fact that power is an end in itself and that the decision to exert power and produce change is based on an understanding of their goals. Clearly, nurses must develop their power if they are to stimulate positive change in the health care system.

Change

The effective and influential nurse understands and applies change theory in all four spheres: workplace, government, organization, and community. The capacity to plan and implement change is a professional responsibility as well as a largely unrealized power source that is vital to the practice of nursing. Indeed, the goal of political action, in any sphere, is to effect change.

Change Defined

What is change? Some synonyms of the verb are alter, transform, modify, convert, vary. All these terms suggest that a fundamental difference or substitution is the outcome of change. Brooten et al. (1978) define **change** as "the process which leads to alteration in individual or institutional patterns of behavior." Further, they define planned change as a "deliberative and collaborative process including a change agent and a client system," this system being "an individual, group of people, an agency, an organization, or a social institution." For additional information on change see Chapter 20, page 438.

Steps in the Change Process

The following steps are a model of planned change. The model outlines the actions one must take to plan and control change and make it serve a specific purpose (Spradley 1980).

- Identify symptoms that indicate something needs changing.
- Diagnose the problem by reviewing the symptoms and gathering additional data.
- Explore alternative solutions in terms of their risks, benefits, driving and restraining forces, advantages, disadvantages, and probable outcomes. (An effective technique often used by change agents is brainstorming.)
- Select one course of action from among the identified alternatives.
- Plan the steps in the change process:

  1. Write measurable objectives.
  2. Determine a time table.
  3. Plan a budget.
  4. Recruit individuals to carry out each aspect of the plan.
  5. Ensure ability of change agent to work with client system.
  6. Evaluate resources (driving forces) and resistance (restraining forces) and plan strategies to manage both.
  7. Design a plan to evaluate the outcomes of the change effort.
  8. Identify measures to refreeze or establish the change within the client system.

- Implement the change. (Pilot testing a new idea affords one the opportunity to evaluate it on a small scale and to "sell" it to the larger client system.)
- Evaluate the outcome(s) on the basis of the measurable objectives and make appropriate adjustments.
- Refreeze the client system so that the changes are seen as standard operating procedures and the system is once again stable.

Examples of Change

It is exciting to learn about how effective nurses can be when they determine the need for change and, using change theory, plan and effect change. The following examples outline changes initiated by nurses who have identified a need to "do something" in each of four spheres.

The Workplace*

At each of three shift meetings Mrs. Hawkins, Head Nurse, listened to nurses complain about problems with getting clients' laboratory work done and reported to the unit in a timely manner. She conferred with the attending and resident physicians on her unit and with her peers on other units within the medical division. It appeared that similar complaints were widespread. At the next head nurse meeting, Mrs. Hawkins described the problem. The group appointed a task force, with Mrs. Hawkins as Chair, and asked them to present a plan to solve the problem at their next meeting. After gathering more data, the task force invited representatives from the attending and resident staff and the laboratory director to meet with them to review the data, consider alternative solutions, and select a plan to solve the problem. By the next head nurse meeting, a preliminary plan to alter the system of laboratory reporting had been devised, and all concerned were working cooperatively to implement the plan. This example illustrates most of the steps in a system of planned change outlined above.

In another "workplace," a school of nursing, students studied the changes in the health care delivery system. They recognized a trend—many clients are now being cared for in out-of-hospital settings—and believed that their clinical placements should reflect these changes. They defined their goal, lined up faculty support, and presented a plan for expanding clinical placements to the student-faculty curriculum committee. Here, too, an idea for change was translated into action using many of the initial steps in the change model.

Organizations: The Professional Association

Nurses on the Education Committee of a district nurses' association recognized the need to make a public policy statement concerning the care of clients with AIDS. Since the Board of Directors had recently expressed interest in promulgating such policy statements, the committee sensed the timing was right and that the board would welcome their draft despite the controversial subject matter. Members of the committee researched and drafted a statement. The full committee offered a critique and selected an articulate spokesperson to seek the president's "blessing" before asking to have the statement presented to the board. Once the president had approved the statement, it was placed on the agenda for the next board meeting. After making minor additions, the board approved it for distribution to the lay and nursing press and asked the Education Committee to suggest a nurse to present the statement at a local hearing of the City Council Health Committee.

*Further examples of change that have been planned and carried out by nurses are particularly well described in case studies and vignettes in Mussallem (1983) and Mason and Talbott (1985).

The Government

While the pressure to contain health care costs escalated through the first half of the 1980s, the TRI-COUNCIL—a coalition based in Washington, D.C. and representing the shared interests of the ANA, the NLN, and the American Association of Colleges of Nursing (AACN)—mounted a campaign to convince Congress of the cost-effectiveness of a center for nursing research within the National Institutes of Health (NIH). Despite incredible odds, including opposition from the American Medical Association, the American Association of Medical Colleges, and the NIH Administration, plus a Presidential veto, the proposal was passed by Congress in the fall of 1985. The success of this effort demonstrates the effectiveness of carefully planned change including the collaboration of nursing organizations. It also illustrates the clout organized nurses can wield on any level and in any sphere.

The Community

Each nurse plays several roles besides that of registered nurse. Each resides in a community, and many are parents. Some serve on school boards, belong to the League of Women Voters, or participate in religious or club activities. There are numerous opportunities for nurses to contribute to the health and welfare of the communities in which they live. For example, Jane Chin, a psychiatric nurse-teacher at a university, knew that a policy of her state department of mental hygiene had led to the discharge of chronically mentally ill patients from state hospitals. These patients were not equipped to care for themselves in the community. She realized that she alone was powerless to effect changes in the state and local government necessary to provide the housing and health care needed by these victims of deinstitutionalization. Jane sought to position herself as a change agent by seeking an appointment to the Governor's Commission on Mental Health. She conferred with the Commissioner of Mental Health in her city, and he offered to submit her name to the governor's appointments secretary. Jane then asked others to write to the governor in support of her appointment: her state senator and assemblywoman, the president of the State Nurses' Association, and the president of the state chapter of the National Alliance for the Mentally Ill (NAMI).

Jane was a logical candidate for appointment to a key commission. She had a reputation as an expert psychiatric nurse clinician, was seen as sensitive to the needs of the mentally ill, and had lobbied in behalf of NAMI. Jane was known as a team player, an effective organizer, and a woman with political clout. She was seen as a person who had a good chance to exert positive influence as a member of the state Mental Health Commission and subsequently on the state's policies on the care of the mentally ill.

All nurses are affected by change; nobody can avoid it. Politically knowledgeable nurses make rational plans to deal with both opportunities to initiate and guide needed change as well as to respond to change that affects them in the workplace, government, organizations, and the community.

Chapter Highlights

- Politics is the process of influencing the allocation of scarce resources in the spheres of government, workplace, organizations, and community.
- Political action in one sphere often affects other spheres.
- In the four spheres, nurses both use and develop power, influence, and skills as change agents.
- Political action is like nursing—an art and science that people master individually and collectively.
- The perception of nurses as powerless is changing. Nurses are increasingly refusing to allow others to determine for them how scarce resources will be allocated.
- Student nurses can begin to develop their political skills as they deal with clinical, education, and peer issues.
- Students can also participate in their school chapter of NSNA.
- Nurses who value the nursing perspective on health issues recognize that a powerful voice for nurses is a powerful voice for health care consumers, the profession, and the nation.

Suggested Readings

Boyle, K. May/June 1984. Power in nursing: A collaborative approach. *Nursing Outlook* 32:164–67.
Boyle argues that collective power surpasses individual power. Mutual support, in her opinion, can enhance power. Nurses can empower clients and empower each other, and they can think of the solutions to nursing problems in terms of power.

Mason, D. J., and Talbott, S. W., editors. 1985. *The political action handbook for nurses: Changing the workplace, government, organizations, and community.* Menlo Park, Calif.: Addison-Wesley Publishing Co.
Eighty-five contributors from all areas of nursing discuss the nature of, and their experiences with, political action in the government, workplace, professional organizations, and community from a perspective that defines politics as influencing the allocation of scarce resources.

Rothberg, J. May/June 1985. The growth of political action in nursing. *Nursing Outlook* 33:133–35.
Rothberg describes how N-CAP evolved from a meeting of ten nurses in 1971, to the Nurses for Political Action (NPA), to the Nurses Coalition for Action in Politics (now called ANA-PAC).

Smith, F. B. November 1985. Patient power. *American Journal of Nursing* 85:1260–62.
Smith uses the term *patient power* to describe a person's ability to influence or control his or her care during illness. Clues that indicate a feeling of powerlessness include such verbal statements as "There is nothing I can do but stay here" as well as anxiety, anger, depression, and distortions of reality. Smith also describes how nurses can help clients regain a sense of power.

Selected References

American Academy of Nursing. 1983. *Magnet hospitals: Attraction and retention of professional nurses.* Kansas City, Mo.: American Nurses' Association.

Archer, S. E. 1985. Politics and the community. In Mason, D. J., and Talbott, S. W., editors. *The political action handbook for nurses.* Menlo Park, Calif.: Addison-Wesley Publishing Co.

Archer, S. E., and Goehner, P. A. November/December 1981. Acquiring political clout: Guidelines for nurse administrators. *Journal of Nursing Administration,* 11:49–55.

———. 1982. *Nurses: A political force.* Belmont, Calif.: Wadsworth Health Sciences.

Archer-Duste, H. M. 1985. When the workplace is academia: The student perspective. In Mason, D. J., and Talbott, S. W., editors. *The political action handbook for nurses.* Menlo Park, Calif.: Addison-Wesley Publishing Co.

Bagwell, M., and Clements, S. 1985. *A political handbook for health professionals.* Boston: Little, Brown and Co.

Benner, P. 1984. From novice to expert: Excellence and power. In *Clinical nursing practice.* Menlo Park, Calif.: Addison-Wesley Publishing Co.

Bennis, W. G.; Benne, K. D.; Chin, R.; and Corey, K. E. 1976. *The planning of change.* New York: Holt, Rinehart and Winston.

Brooten, D. A.; Hayman, L.; and Naylor, M. 1978. *Leadership for change: A guide for the frustrated nurse.* Philadelphia: J. B. Lippincott Co.

Curtis, B. T. 1985. Political action committees: An overview. In Mason, D. J., and Talbott, S. W., editors. *The political action handbook for nurses.* Menlo Park, Calif.: Addison-Wesley Publishing Co.

Dallek, G. May/June 1985. Six myths of American medical care: What the poor really get. *Health/PAC Bulletin* 16(3):9–15.

Devereux, P. M., and Dirschel, K. M. 1985. Interdisciplinary politics. In Mason, D. J., and Talbott, S. W., editors. *The political action handbook for nurses.* Menlo Park, Calif.: Addison-Wesley Publishing Co.

Diers, D. 1985. Policy and politics. In Mason, D. J., and Talbott, S. W., editors. *The political action handbook for nurses.* Menlo Park, Calif.: Addison-Wesley Publishing Co.

Ehrat, K. September 1983. A model for politically astute planning and decision making. *Journal of Nursing Administration* 13:29–34.

Ferguson, V. D. 1985. Power in nursing. In Mason, D. J., and Talbott, S. W., editors. *The political action handbook for nurses.* Menlo Park, Calif.: Addison-Wesley Publishing Co.

Foley, M. 1985. The politics of collective bargaining. In Mason, D. J., and Talbott, S. W., editors. *The political action handbook for nurses.* Menlo Park, Calif.: Addison-Wesley Publishing Co.

Ford-Roegner, P. 1985. Voter participation and campaigning. In Mason, D. J., and Talbott, S. W., editors. *The political action handbook for nurses.* Menlo Park, Calif.: Addison-Wesley Publishing Co.

French, J. R. P., and Raven, B. 1959. The bases of social power. In Cartwright, D., editor. *Studies in social power.* Ann Arbor: University of Michigan.

Frost, A. D. 1985. Working together: Local community action. In Mason, D. J., and Talbott, S. W., editors. *The political action handbook for nurses.* Menlo Park, Calif.: Addison-Wesley Publishing Co.

Hennig, M., and Jardim, A. J. 1977. *The managerial woman.* New York: Anchor Press/Doubleday.

Hersey, P., Blanchard, K., and Nayemeyer, W. 1979. Situational leadership: Perception and impact of power. *Group Organizational Studies,* 4:418–28.

Hughes, C. C. 1985. Political parties. In Mason, D. J., and Talbott, S. W., editors. *The political action handbook for nurses.* Menlo Park, Calif.: Addison-Wesley Publishing Co.

Huxley, E. 1975. *Florence Nightingale.* New York: G. P. Putnam's Sons.

Jordan, C. 1985. Local government. In Mason, D. J., and Talbott, S. W., editors. *The political action handbook for nurses.* Menlo Park, Calif.: Addison-Wesley Publishing Co.

Kalisch, B. J., and Kalisch, P. A. 1982. *Politics of nursing.* Philadelphia: J. B. Lippincott Co.

Levenstein, A. 1979. Effective change requires a change agent. *Journal of Nursing Administration* 9(2):12–15.

Lewin, K. 1951. *Field theory in social science.* New York: Harper and Row.

Lippitt, R.; Watson, J.; and Westley, B. 1958. *The dynamics of planned change.* Harcourt, Brace.

Long, M. N., and Mason, D. J. 1985. State government. In Mason, D. J., and Talbott, S. W., editors. *The political action handbook for nurses.* Menlo Park, Calif.: Addison-Wesley Publishing Co.

Maraldo, P., and Kinder, J. 1985. Politics and the professional organization. In Mason, D. J., and Talbott, S. W., editors. *The political action handbook for nurses.* Menlo Park, Calif.: Addison-Wesley Publishing Co.

Mason, D. J. 1985. The politics of patient care. In Mason, D. J., and Talbott, S. W., editors. *The political action handbook for nurses.* Menlo Park, Calif.: Addison-Wesley Publishing Co.

———. 1986. From bedside to White House: The local perspective. In NLN, editors. *Perspectives in nursing—1985–1987.* New York: National League for Nursing.

Mason, D. J., and Talbott, S. W., editors. 1985. *The political action handbook for nurses: Changing the workplace, government, organizations, and community.* Menlo Park, Calif.: Addison-Wesley Publishing Co.

McCarthy, A. M. 1985. Political clubs. In Mason, D. J., and Talbott, S. W., editors. *The political action handbook for nurses.* Menlo Park, Calif.: Addison-Wesley Publishing Co.

McKay, N. L., and Lumley, W. A. 1985. Nonunionized collective action: The staff nurse forum. In Mason, D. J., and Talbott, S. W., editors. *The political action handbook for nurses.* Menlo Park, Calif.: Addison-Wesley Publishing Co.

Miller, J. B. 1982. Colloquium: Women and Power. Stone Center for Developmental Services and Studies. Wellesley, Mass.: Wellesley College.

Mussallem, H. K. 1985. *Succeeding Together: Group Action by Nurses.* Geneva: International Council of Nurses.

Natapoff, J., and Loetterle, B., editors. Making a difference: The courage to change. In Mason, D. J., and Talbott, S. W., editors. *The political action handbook for nurses.* Menlo Park, Calif.: Addison-Wesley Publishing Co.

New, J. R., and Couillard, N. A. 1981. Guidelines for introducing change. *Journal of Nursing Administration* 11(3):17–21.

Osgood, G. A., and Elliott, J. E. 1985. Federal government. In Mason, D. J., and Talbott, S. W., editors. *The political action handbook for nurses.* Menlo Park, Calif.: Addison-Wesley Publishing Co.

Shaffer, F., editor. *DRGs: Changes and Challenges.* New York: National League for Nursing, 1984.

Skaggs, B. J. 1985. You and your professional association: Structure and function. In Mason, D. J., and Talbott, S. W., editors. *The political action handbook for nurses.* Menlo Park, Calif.: Addison-Wesley Publishing Co.

Solomon, S., and Roe, S., editors. 1985. *Integrating health policy into the curriculum.* New York: National League for Nursing.

Spradley, B. W. 1980. Making change creatively. *Journal of Nursing Administration* 10(5):32–37.

Starr, P. 1982. *The social transformation of American medicine.* New York: Basic Books.

Stevens, B. J. November 1980. Power and politics for the nurse executive. *Nursing and Health Care* 1(4):208–10.

Stevens, K. R. 1983. *Power and influence: A source book for nurses.* New York: John Wiley and Sons.

Talbott, S. W. 1985a. Political analysis: Structure and processes. In Mason, D. J., and Talbott, S. W., editors. *The political action handbook for nurses.* Menlo Park, Calif.: Addison-Wesley Publishing Co.

———. 1985b. Political appointments: Getting appointed. In Mason, D. J., and Talbott, S. W., editors. *The political action handbook for nurses.* Menlo Park, Calif.: Addison-Wesley Publishing Co.

———. 1985c. Influencing your association. In Mason, D. J., and Talbott, S. W., editors. *The political action handbook for nurses.* Menlo Park, Calif.: Addison-Wesley Publishing Co.

Talbott, S. W., and Vance, C. 1981. Involving nursing in a feminist group—NOW. *Nursing Outlook* 29:592–95.

Vance, C. 1985. Political influence: Building interpersonal skills. In Mason, D. J., and Talbott, S. W., editors. *The political action handbook for nurses.* Menlo Park, Calif.: Addison-Wesley Publishing Co.

Vance, C.; Talbott, S. W.; McBride, A. B.; and Mason, D. J. November/December 1985. An uneasy alliance: Nursing and the women's movement. *Nursing Outlook* 33(6):281–85.

CHAPTER 7

Legal Issues in Nursing

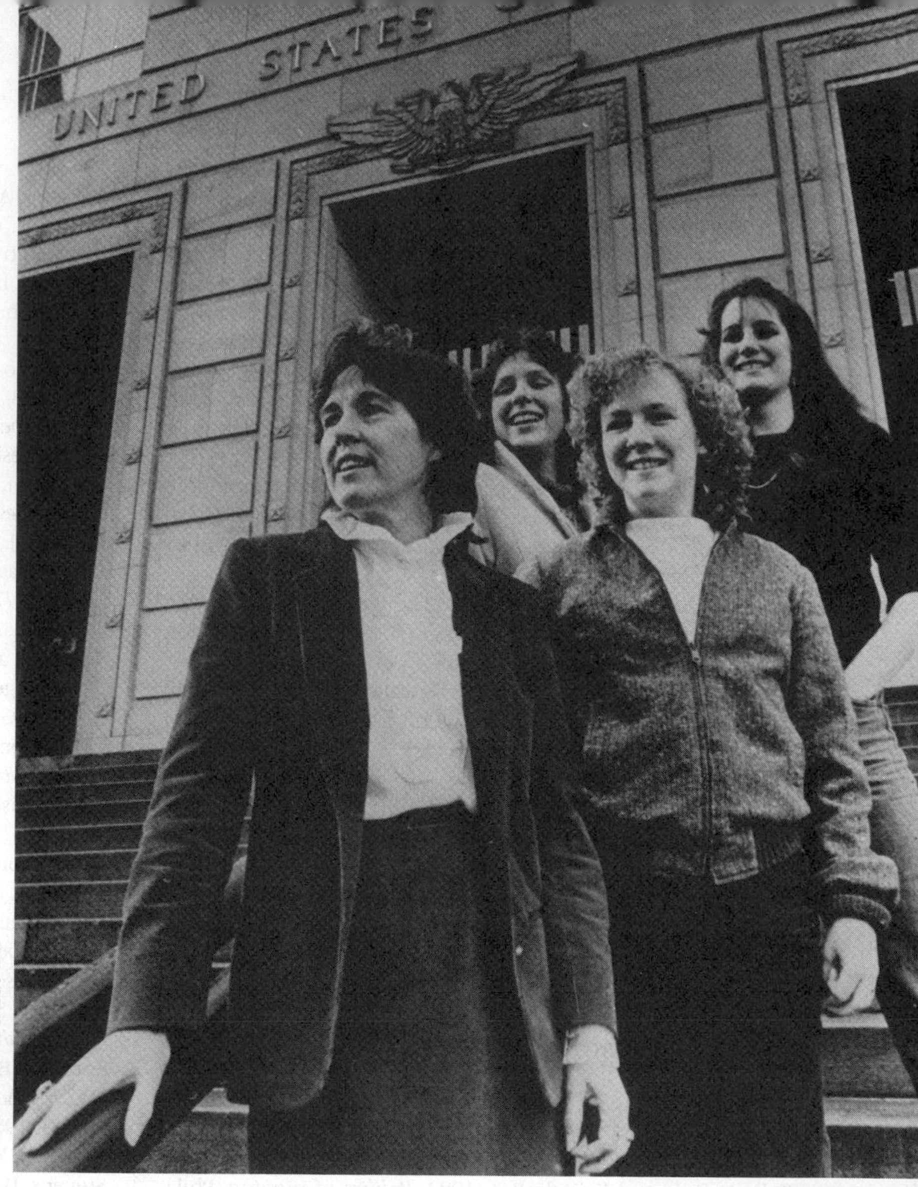

BILL MURPHY / THE OREGONIAN

Contents

Objectives

1. Understand general legal concepts as they apply to nursing.
   1.1 Define specific terms used in law.
   1.2 List four basic functions of law in society.
   1.3 List the functions of law in nursing.
   1.4 Describe three primary sources of law.
   1.5 Describe two types of law.
   1.6 Describe four basic legal principles.
   1.7 Identify two kinds of legal actions.
   1.8 Identify five steps in the judicial process.
   1.9 Identify essential aspects of the nurse's role as an expert witness.
   1.10 Identify essential aspects of privileged communications.
2. Know essential facts about the legal dimensions of nursing practice.
   2.1 Explain how nurse practice acts legally protect the nurse practitioner.
   2.2 Identify the purpose of credentialing.
   2.3 List three criteria a professional or occupation must meet to obtain the right to license its members.
   2.4 Differentiate mandatory licensure from permissive licensure.
   2.5 Differentiate certification from accreditation.
   2.6 Describe ways that standards of care, agency policies, and job descriptions affect the scope of nursing practice.
3. Understand essential aspects of contractual arrangements in nursing.
   3.1 Identify essential types and elements of contracts.
   3.2 Describe three legal roles of the nurse.
   3.3 Identify rights and obligations associated with the nurse's legal roles.
   3.4 Describe some pros and cons of collective bargaining in the nursing profession.
   3.5 Describe the process of collective bargaining.
   3.6 Describe the grievance procedure.
   3.7 Identify examples of four types of grievances.
4. Understand specific areas of potential liability in nursing.
   4.1 Differentiate crimes from torts and give examples of each in nursing.
   4.2 Differentiate intentional from unintentional torts.
   4.3 Explain the concept of fraud.
   4.4 Explain the concept of invasion of privacy.
   4.5 Compare libel to slander.
   4.6 Differentiate assault and battery from technical assault and battery.
   4.7 Compare false imprisonment to justifiable restraint.
   4.8 Differentiate malpractice from negligence.
   4.9 Give examples of types of malpractice actions.
   4.10 Describe essential steps required to report crimes, torts, and unsafe practices of others.
5. Understand essential aspects of selected legal facets of nursing practice.
   5.1 Describe essential elements of informed consent and its purpose.
   5.2 Describe the nurse's responsibilities in obtaining informed consent from competent adults, minors, mentally ill clients, and unconscious persons.
   5.3 List information that needs to be included in an incident report.
   5.4 Describe actions the nurse should take when a client is injured.
   5.5 Explain the responsibilities of the nurse in witnessing a will.
   5.6 Explain some pros and cons of living wills.
   5.7 Describe the legal implications of euthanasia.
   5.8 Describe the implications of no-code and slow-code orders for nurses.
   5.9 Compare abortion laws in the United States and Canada.
   5.10 Describe five legal issues surrounding death.
6. Appreciate various legal protections for nurses and ways nurses can protect themselves.
   6.1 Explain the intent of Good Samaritan acts.
   6.2 Describe essential aspects of professional liability insurance.
   6.3 Identify the professional nurse's legal responsibilities in relation to the nursing process and areas of potential liability.
   6.4 Identify ways the student nurse can minimize chances for liability.

Terms

accreditation
answer (legal)
assault
autopsy (postmortem examination)
battery
burden of proof
certification
civil action
collective bargaining
common law
complaint
conscience clauses
contract
contract law
contractual obligations
contractual relationships
coroner
credentialing
crime

criminal action
criminal law
decision (legal)
decisional law
defamation
defendant
discovery (legal)
due process
equal protection
euthanasia
expert witness
false imprisonment
felony
fraud
Good Samaritan acts
grievance
homicide
incident report
informed consent
inquest
law
liability
liable
libel
license
living will
lockout
malpractice
mandatory licensure
manslaughter
medical examiner
misdemeanor
negligence
no-code orders
permissive licensure
plaintiff
private (civil) law
privileged communication
probate proceedings
professional collectivism
proximate cause
public law
registration
respondant superior
slander
slow-code orders
standards of care
statute of limitations
statutory law
strike
technical assault and battery
tort
trial
verdict
will

General Legal Concepts

Nursing practice is governed by many legal concepts. It is important for nurses to know the basics of legal concepts since nurses are accountable for their professional judgments and actions. Accountability is an essential concept of professional nursing practice and the law. Knowledge of laws that regulate and affect nursing practice is needed for two reasons:

1. To ensure that the nurse's decisions and actions are consistent with current legal principles
2. To protect the nurse from liability

Nearly every society has rules and regulations that are developed and promulgated by the society itself. These rules and regulations are the laws of the country, and they provide one aspect of social control for people. **Law** can be defined as "a system of principles and processes by which people, who live in a society, attempt to control human conduct in an effort to minimize the use of force as a means of resolving conflicting interests" (Rhodes and Miller 1984, p. 1). Laws can be seen as having four basic functions in a society:

1. To define relationships among the members of a society and to state which activities are permissible and which are not permissible
2. To describe what force may be applied to maintain rules and by whom it is to be applied
3. To provide solutions to problems
4. To redefine relationships between persons and groups when conditions of life change

Functions of the Law in Nursing

The law serves a number of functions in nursing:

1. It provides a framework for establishing what nursing actions in the care of clients are legal.
2. It differentiates the nurse's responsibilities from those of other health professionals.
3. It helps to establish the boundaries of independent nursing action.
4. It assists in maintaining a standard of nursing practice by making nurses accountable under the law.

Sources of Law

The legal systems in both the United States and Canada have their origins in the English common law system. Three primary sources of law are constitutions, statutes, and decisions of courts (common law).

Constitutions

The Constitution of the United States and the Constitution of Canada are the supreme laws of each country. They establish the general organization of the federal governments, grant certain powers to them, and place limits on what federal and state or provincial governments may do. Constitutions create legal rights and responsibilities and are the foundation for a system of justice. The rights created, however, do not relate directly to the nurse-client relationship.

Constitutions have due process and equal protection clauses. The due process clause applies to state or provincial and local agencies, including public hospitals, and to actions that deprive a person of life, liberty, or property. **Due process** has two primary elements:

1. The rules being applied must be reasonable and not vague.
2. Fair procedures must be followed when enforcing the rules.

Equal protection means that like persons must be dealt with in like fashion.

Legislation (Statutes)

Laws enacted by the Congress of the United States or the Parliament of Canada or other state or provincial or local legislative bodies are called **statutory laws.** When there is a conflict between federal and state or provincial laws, federal law supersedes. Likewise, state or provincial laws supersede local laws.

The regulation of nursing is a function of state or provincial law. State or provincial legislatures pass statutes that define and regulate nursing, i.e., nurse practice acts. These acts, however, must be consistent with constitutional and federal provisions. Nurses practice acts, Good Samaritan laws, and adult or child abuse laws are examples of statutes that affect nurses.

Legislatures delegate responsibility and power to implement various laws to many administrative agencies who have the time and the expertise to address complex issues. For example, on the federal level, the U.S. Food and Drug Administration, the U.S. Department of Health and Human Services, the National Labor Relations Board (NLRB), and the Internal Revenue Service (or Revenue Canada) have been delegated quasilegislative power to adopt regulations and quasijudicial power to decide how the statutes and regulations apply to individual cases (Rhodes and Miller 1984, p. 6). The legislature retains ultimate responsibility and authority by specifying the regulations that the administrative body can make. On the state or provincial level, administrative agencies oversee the practice of the professions and regulate various aspects of commerce and public welfare. Examples pertinent to nurses are the state boards of nursing and provincial nursing associations, which implement and enforce nurse practice acts.

In the United States, there is a board of nursing in each of the 50 states and in Washington, D.C., Puerto Rico, Guam, and the Virgin Islands. These boards often have board representation and usually include nurses. Some state boards function as separate entities; others, for example, a department of health or a department of licenses, are part of a department within the state government structure. The responsibilities of state boards of nursing include examination of candidates for the profession, licensure of qualified candidates, discipline of nurses who violate the law or ethical nursing principles, and establishment of standards for, and accreditation of, basic nursing education programs.

In Canada, with the exception of Ontario and Quebec, the professional nursing associations are authorized to administer nurse practice acts. In Ontario, the responsibility rests with the College of Nurses, a separate entity. In the province of Quebec, the provincial government, in its Health Disciplines Act of 1975, established an Order of Nurses. The provincial nursing associations, the Ontario College of Nurses, and the Quebec Order of Nurses undertake the same types of tasks as those carried out by the state boards of nursing in the United States.

Common Law

The body of principles that evolves from court decisions is referred to as **common law**, or decisional laws. Although courts are called upon to interpret and apply constitutional or statutory law, they also are asked to resolve disputes between two parties. In such disputes, statutory and constitutional laws cannot support the case. Common law is continually being adapted and expanded. In deciding specific controversies, courts generally adhere to the doctrine of *stare decisis*—"to stand by things decided"—usually referred to as "following precedent." In other words, in a current case, the court applies the same rules and principles as applied in similar cases decided previously and arrives at the same ruling. Courts may depart from precedent when slight differences are noted between cases or when it is thought that a particular common-law rule no longer applies to the needs of society. Decisions made by lower courts, for example local courts, must follow the decisions of higher courts, such as state or federal courts.

Types of Law

Laws govern the relationship of private individuals with government and with each other.

Public Law

Public law refers to the body of law that deals with relationships between individuals and the government and governmental agencies. An important segment of public law is **criminal law**, which deals with actions against the safety and welfare of the public. Examples are homicide, manslaughter, and theft. Crimes are classified as felonies or misdemeanors in the United States or as indictable offenses or summary conviction offenses in Canada. See Crimes and Torts later in this chapter. Public law also includes numerous regulations designed to enhance societal objectives. Private individuals and organizations are required to follow specified courses of action in their activities. Noncompliance with these regulations can lead to criminal penalties.

Private Law

Private law, or civil law, is the body of law that deals with relationships between private individuals. It is categorized as contract law and tort law. **Contract law** involves the enforcement of agreements among private individuals or the payment of compensation for failure to fulfill the agreements. **Tort law** defines and enforces duties and rights among private individuals that are not based on contractual agreements. A **tort** is a legal wrong committed against the person or property of another. The word tort comes from the Latin word *tortus* meaning twisted. Loosely translated, it means "wrong" or "bad." Some examples of tort laws applicable to nurses are negligence and malpractice, invasion of privacy, and assault and battery. See Figure 7–1 and also Table 7–1 for selected categories of law affecting nurses.

Principles of Law

The system of law rests on four simple principles that are often cloaked in complex terminology (Fenner 1980, p. 84). These are:

1. *Law is based on a concern for justice and fairness.* The law seeks to protect the rights of one party from the transgressions of another. It sets guidelines for conduct and mechanisms to enforce those guidelines. The goal is to make known the rules of conduct that protect the rights of the parties involved and to ensure a just and fair outcome.
2. *Law is characterized by change.* Social and technologic changes occur rapidly and often without predictions of problems to follow. In response to these changes, the legal system also must change. Often the legal system reacts rather than acts. For example, after technologic devices such as respirators were developed to prolong life, it became necessary for the law to change its guidelines about indications of death—from cessation of heart function to absence of electric currents from the brain for at least 24 hours.
3. *Actions are judged on the basis of a universal standard of what a similarly educated, reasonable, and prudent person would have done under similar circumstances.* It is recognized by law that not all nurses, for example, have the same capabilities, experience, or education. Therefore, they are not all expected to function at the same level. All nurses, however, are expected to function the same way that another nurse with similar education and experience would function. This rule of reasonable and prudent conduct is the basis for evaluating a person's actions, e.g., for judging whether or not actions were negligent (see the discussion of negligence and malpractice on page 161).
4. *Each individual has rights and responsibilities.* Rights are privileges or fundamental powers that individuals possess unless they are revoked by law or given up voluntarily; responsibilities are the obligations associated with these rights. Failure to meet one's responsibilities can endanger one's rights. For example, a registered nurse has the right to practice nursing within the constraints of the law (nurse practice acts). If she or he fails to observe these constraints (e.g., prescribes medications or conducts a surgical procedure), the

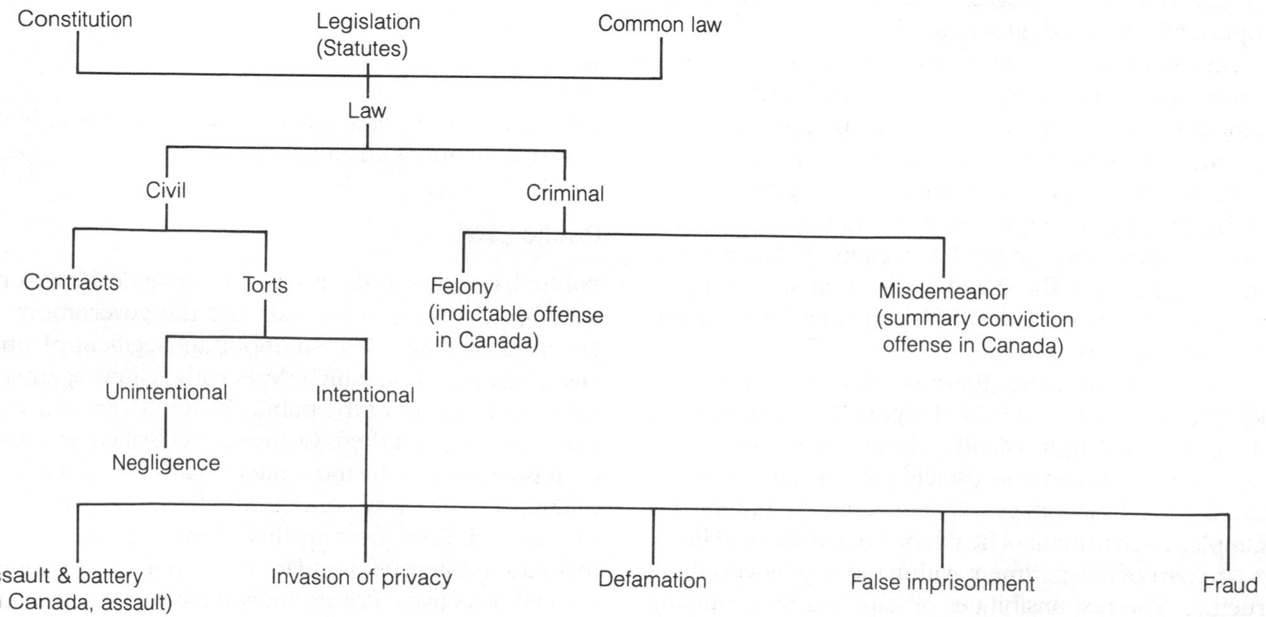

Figure 7–1 Categories of law pertinent to nurses

behavior is considered irresponsible, and the right to practice can be revoked.

Kinds of Legal Actions

There are two kinds of legal actions: civil or private actions and criminal actions. **Civil actions** deal with the relationships between individuals in society; for example, a man may file a suit against a person who he believes cheated him. Civil actions that are of concern to nurses include the torts listed in Table 7–1 and contracts. Other civil actions that might be of concern to nurses include those relating to wills and the estates of deceased persons. These cases are known as **probate proceedings. Criminal actions** deal with disputes between an individual and the society as a whole; for example, if a woman shoots a man, society brings her to trial.

The Judicial Process

The judicial process primarily functions to settle disputes peacefully and in accordance with the law. A lawsuit has strict procedural rules. There are generally five steps:

1. A document called a **complaint** is filed by a person referred to as the **plaintiff,** who claims that his or her legal rights have been infringed by one or more persons, referred to as **defendants.**
2. A written response, called an **answer,** is made by the defendants.
3. Both parties engage in pretrial activities, referred to as **discovery,** in an effort to gain all the facts of the situation.
4. In the **trial** of the case, all the relevant facts are presented to a jury or a judge.
5. The judge renders a **decision,** or the jury renders a **verdict.** If the outcome is not acceptable to one of the parties, an appeal can be made for another trial.

During a trial, a plaintiff must offer evidence of the defendant's wrongdoing. This duty of proving an assertion is called the **burden of proof.** An additional aspect of this burden of proof is that the plaintiff must have a greater amount of convincing evidence than the defendant if the plaintiff is to prevail.

Nurses as Expert Witnesses

When called into court as a witness, the nurse has a duty to assist justice as far as possible. An **expert witness** is one who, by education or experience, possesses knowledge and skill needed to understand the matter about which the person is to testify (Rhodes and Miller 1983, p. 18). Such a witness is usually called to help a judge or jury understand evidence pertaining to the extent of damage and the standard of care.

Table 7–1 Selected Categories of Laws Affecting Nurses

Category	Examples
Constitutional	Due process
	Equal protection
Statutory (legislative)	Nurse practice acts
	Good Samaritan acts
	Child and adult abuse laws
	Living wills
Criminal (public)	Homicide, manslaughter
	Theft
	Arson
	Active euthanasia
	Rape
	Illegal possession of controlled drugs
Contracts (private/civil)	Nurse and client
	Nurse and employer
	Nurse and insurance
	Client and agency
Torts (private/civil)	Negligence
	Libel and slander
	Invasion of privacy
	Assault and battery
	False imprisonment

Source: American Nurses' Association. *Standards of Nursing Practice.* Kansas City, Mo.: The Association, 1973. Used by permission.

First the nurse will be sworn in, that is, will be asked to swear to tell the truth, the whole truth, and nothing but the truth, and asked to give her or his name. Then the nurse will be asked to give information about her or his education and experience. This is intended to prove the nurse's credibility.

The witness should listen carefully to each question and answer truthfully. Information should not be volunteered; facts should be presented simply. The nurse need not be afraid to say "I don't know" if this is true; an expert witness is not expected to know everything. In addition to giving facts, an expert witness can give an opinion based on knowledge and experience.

An expert witness can expect to be cross-examined by the lawyer from the opposing side. It is important that the nurse agree to testify only if she or he is in agreement with the side who asked for the testimony.

An expert witness can be paid a reasonable professional rate for preparation time and time spent in court.

Privileged Communications

A **privileged communication** is information given to a professional person, such as a physician, who is forbidden by law from disclosing the information in a court without the consent of the person who provided it. Historically, under common law, a physician who learned, for example, that a client had a history of mental illness could be made to reveal this fact in a court. As a result, clients withheld some information from their physicians when it was not always in their best interests to do so. Many states solved this problem by enacting legislation that overrode the common law and provided that, under certain circumstances, a physician cannot be compelled to reveal confidential information. Some of these acts were later amended to include the clergy and spouses. Three states, New York, Arkansas, and New Mexico, have extended these statutes to include professional registered nurses (Creighton 1981, p. 216).

Legislation regarding privileged communications is highly complicated. A nurse would be unwise to encourage disclosures or advise a client about the subject. The privileged communication law is for the benefit of the client; a nurse who is given confidential information should be prepared to answer questions fully and honestly if required to testify in a court of law. If the law of privileged communications is to be applied, the attorney for the client will object to the question, and the judge will resolve the problem.

The matter of privileged communications is referred to in the ANA's *Code for Nurses* (1976). It advises the nurse to seek legal counsel in regard to a privileged communication and to become familiar with the rights and privileges of the client and the nurse.

In Canada, confidentiality of information is incorporated as an ethic in the legislation on nursing practice. Failure to maintain confidentiality can result in disciplinary action against the nurse. The client-physician relationship and the nurse-client relationship are not protected under the law, except in Quebec, where physicians can refuse to reveal information given by clients.

Legal Dimensions of Nursing

Nurse Practice Acts

Each state in the United States and each province of Canada has nurse practice acts, which protect the nurse's professional capacity and legally control nursing practice through licensing. Nurse practice acts legally define and describe the scope of nursing practice, which the law seeks to regulate, thereby protecting the public as well. Because of the number of acts there are many definitions and descriptions of nursing. In 1981, the ANA described nursing practice, including what is included but limited in nursing practice and what nursing practice is not. See Chapter 1, page 5, for a description of nursing by the ANA.

In 1985, the ANA recommended that the baccalaureate degree be a basic requirement for licensure to practice professional nursing and to retain the title RN. In addition, the ANA recommended that the title associate nurse (AN) be used for graduates of associate degree programs (Lewis 1985, p. 241). State nurse practice acts will need to be altered if these proposals are enacted at the state level.

Many states have an additional acts clause that pertains to acts that may be performed only by certain nurses with education beyond the minimum required for licensure under the act. For example, many of the clauses address the practice of nurse midwives or nurse anesthetists. Some address the nurse practitioner role. These clauses conflict with the ANA policy, which prohibits legal regulation of advanced or specialty nursing practice. The ANA believes it is the function of the professional association, not the law, to establish the scope and desirable qualifications required for each specialized area of practice (Snyder and Labar 1984, p. 7).

Credentialing

Credentialing is the process of determining and maintaining competence in nursing practice. The credentialing process is one way in which the nursing profession maintains standards of practice and is accountable for the educational preparation of members. Credentialing includes licensure, registration, certification, and accreditation.

In 1979, a committee of the American Nurses' Association (ANA) established to study credentialing in nursing recommended that a credentialing center be established with the purpose of monitoring the quality of nursing education and practice (ANA 1979, p. 680). The ANA enumerated the principles of credentialing; these principles reflect the belief that credentialing exists primarily to protect and benefit the public. See Table 7–2.

Licensure and Registration

Licenses are legal permits granted by a government agency to individuals to engage in the practice of a profession and to use a particular title. A particular jurisdiction or area is covered by the license. For a profession or occupation to obtain the right to license its members, it generally must meet three criteria:

1. There is a need to protect the public's safety or welfare.
2. The occupation is clearly delineated as a separate, distinct area of work.
3. There is an organization suitable in ability to assume the obligations of the licensing process.

In the United States, nurses are issued a license by the state board of nursing, which is empowered by government to grant licenses. Licenses are issued to registered nurses who have (a) successfully completed a course of studies in a school of nursing accredited by the state board, (b) passed the national qualifying examinations with a score that is acceptable to the board, and (c) paid the required fee. A state board may also grant a license to a nurse who holds an active practicing license in another state, through a process of endorsement, without the candidate having to rewrite examinations. The candidate, however, must have attained a passing score on the national examinations that is equal to, or above, that considered acceptable in the state in which she or he wishes to practice. Passing scores vary among states.

In Canada, nurses are not licensed except in the province of Quebec. They are, however, registered by their provincial nursing association and by the College of Nurses of Ontario. Nurses in the United States are also registered but must in addition be granted a license to practice. **Registration** is the listing of an individual's name and other information on the official roster of a governmental or nongovernmental agency. Nurses who are registered are permitted to use the title "Registered Nurse." To be registered, the nurse must have completed a basic course of nursing studies in a program approved by the registering body and have passed the national qualifying examinations with an acceptable grade. Canada offers a national comprehensive registered nurse examination, offered in both French and English. Ontario, Quebec, and New Brunswick offer the examination in both languages, while other provinces offer it only in English. Like state boards of nursing, provincial registering bodies vary in the score they consider an acceptable passing grade. Nurses from other provinces in Canada and from other countries may be granted registration by endorsement provided they meet the requirements of the registering body. Both licensure and registration must be renewed on an annual basis (in some states every 2 years) to be valid.

Table 7–2 Principles of Credentialing

1. In addition to benefiting and protecting the public, credentialing also benefits those who are credentialed.
2. The legitimate interests of the involved occupation or institution and of the general public should be reflected in each credentialing mechanism.
3. Accountability should be an essential component of any credentialing process.
4. A system of checks and balances within the credentialing system should assure equitable treatment for all parties involved.
5. Periodic assessments with the potential for sanction are essential components of an effective credentialing mechanism.
6. Objective standards and criteria and persons competent in their use are essential to the credentialing process.
7. Representation in credentialing systems of the community of interests directly affected by credentialing mechanisms should assure consideration of the legitimate concerns of each group.
8. Professional identity and responsibility should evolve from the credentialing process.
9. An effective system of role delineation is fundamental to any credentialing mechanism for individuals.
10. An effective system of program identification is fundamental to any credentialing mechanism for institutions.
11. Coordination of credentialing mechanisms should lead to efficiency and cost effectiveness and avoid duplication.
12. Geographic, including interstate, mobility should be improved by the credentialing of the individual.
13. Widely accepted definitions and terminology are basic to an effective credentialing system.
14. Communications and understanding between health care providers and society should be facilitated through the credentialing process.

Source: Report of the Committee for the Study of Credentialing in Nursing, American Nurses' Association.

Types of licensure/registration There are two types of licensure/registration: mandatory and permissive. Under **mandatory licensure/registration**, anyone who practices nursing must be licensed or, in Canada, registered. The only exceptions are: (a) practice in an emergency, (b) practice by nursing students as part of their education, and (c) practice by nurses employed by the federal government (nurses who practice in Veterans Administration hospitals and in public health must be currently licensed in some jurisdiction but not necessarily where the facility is located). Under **permissive licensure/registration**, the title RN is reserved for licensed or, in Canada, registered practitioners, but the practice of nursing is not prohibited to others who are not licensed or registered.

Registration is permissive in most provinces of Canada. In the United States, nursing licensure is mandatory in most states. There is a strong movement underway in Canada to make registration mandatory in all provinces.

The states and provinces also license practical nurses in much the same way as professional nurses. The major difference between the two kinds of nurses is that, through education, the registered professional nurse has more refined skills and greater knowledge and can make more complex judgments in relation to assessment and interpretation of data and therefore in the determination and provision of required nursing care.

Nursing practice acts and state board of nursing or provincial boards in Canada can affect an individual's licensure or registration. Whereas nurse practice acts are law, nursing board regulations and rulings have considerable force even though they are not enacted as law. Nursing boards often provide advisory rulings in response to a request from a nurse or an agency. These advisory opinions can be used in judicial proceedings. Nurses would be wise to know what their nurse practice acts contain and how nursing board rulings and regulations can be used.

License or registration revocation The nurses' association in each state and province has a committee, such as a board of examiners, with the power to revoke licenses (or registration in Canada) for just cause. Licenses/registration can be revoked because of incompetent nursing practice; professional misconduct; conviction of a crime, such as drug addiction or illegal sale of drugs; obtaining a license through deception, falsifying school records, or hiding a criminal history; and, in some areas, aiding in a criminal abortion. In each situation all the facts are generally reviewed by the committee at a hearing. In most places, the nurse is entitled to be represented by legal counsel at the hearing. If the nurse's license is revoked as a result of the hearing, an appeal can be made to a court, or, in some states, an agency is designated to review the decision before any court action is initiated.

Certification

Certification is the practice of determining minimum standards of nursing competence in specialty areas, such as maternal-child health, pediatrics, gerontology, mental health, and school nursing. An individual who is certified has met predetermined standards specified by the profession. Certification programs are conducted by the American Nurses' Association and by other specialty nursing organizations. The American Association of Nurse Anesthetists, for example, certifies nurse anesthetists. A certification program is not established in Canada. The Canadian Nurses' Association is currently considering the establishment of a certification program for nurses in specialized fields of nursing.

Accreditation/Approval of Basic Nursing Education Programs

Accreditation is a process by which a voluntary, nongovernmental agency or organization appraises and grants accredited status to institutions and/or programs or services that meet predetermined structure, process, and outcome criteria (ANA 1979).

Minimum standards for basic nursing education programs are established in each state of the United States and in each province in Canada. All programs preparing candidates for licensure or registration are appraised by the state boards of nursing or a designated body in the United States and by the provincial nursing associations (or the College of Nurses in Ontario or the Order of Nurses in Quebec) in Canada. State accreditation or provincial approval is granted to schools of nursing meeting the minimum criteria.

The National League for Nursing (NLN) also accredits schools of nursing in the United States. NLN accreditation is concerned with optimum, rather than minimum, standards. In other words, accreditation by the NLN certifies that an educational program has not only met minimum standards, but is considered "good" by national standards. NLN accreditation is voluntary.

Standards of Practice

Another way the nursing profession attempts to ensure that its practitioners are competent and safe to practice is through the establishment of standards of practice. The standards of practice of the ANA and the CNA are shown in Tables 1–4 and 1–5 on pages 20 and 21. These standards are often used to evaluate the quality of care provided by nurses. In addition to this basic set of standards, which are applicable in any practice setting, the ANA has developed standards of nursing practice for specific areas such as maternal-child, medical-surgical, geriatric, psychiatric, and community health nursing.

Many individual health agencies also have been attempting to determine standards of practice that nurses employed in the agency consider important. These efforts have resulted in the development of standard nursing care plans for clients with particular health problems, e.g., for those who had cerebrovascular accidents (stroke), heart attacks, or specific types of surgery. Standard care plans provide guidelines for the nurse to implement and to evaluate nursing care.

Agency Policies, Procedures, and Job Descriptions

Agency policies, procedures, and job descriptions delineate the scope of a nurse's practice more precisely than nurse practice acts. For example, in some agencies a nurse may be expected to shorten and remove a client's Penrose drain after surgery; in other agencies, this practice is not allowed. Practicing nurses must familiarize themselves with the job descriptions, policies, and procedures spelled out by each employing agency.

Other Laws Affecting Scope of Nursing Practice

Snyder and LaBar (1984, p. 17) point out the following state or district laws passed in 1983:

1. Laws permitting nurses to prescribe and dispense drugs were passed in at least three legislatures.
2. In New Jersey a new provision allows nurses under

certain conditions to pronounce a client's death and sign death certificates.

3. In the District of Columbia, a recently passed law allows nurse midwives, nurse practitioners, and nurse anesthetists to qualify for hospital privileges.
4. In Colorado, a new law adds registered nurses to the list of those who may determine that a person may be admitted for 72-hour mental health evaluation.

All of these laws have an impact on nurses' scope of practice. Other states may pass similar laws.

Contractual Arrangements in Nursing

A contract is the basis of the relationship between a nurse and an employer—for example, a nurse and a hospital or a nurse and a physician. It is also the basis of the relationship that a nurse has with a client. This latter is true whether the nurse is employed directly by the client and family or by an agency.

A **contract** is an agreement between two or more competent persons, upon sufficient consideration (remuneration), to do or not to do some lawful act. A contract may be written or oral; however, a written contract cannot be changed legally by an oral agreement. If two people wish to change some aspect of a written contract, the change must be written into the contract, because one party cannot hold the other to an oral agreement that differs from the written one.

A contract is considered to be *expressed* when the two parties discuss and agree orally or in writing to its terms, e.g., that a nurse will work at a hospital for a stated length of time and under stated conditions. An *implied* contract is one in which there has been no discussion between the parties, but the law considers that a contract exists. In the contractual relationship between nurse and client, clients have the right to expect that nurses caring for them have the competence to meet their needs. This implies that the nurse has a responsibility to remain competent. The nurse has the associated right to expect the client to provide accurate information as required.

Contract law requires that four elements be met to make a contract valid (Fenner 1980, p. 94):

1. The act contracted for must be legal. The nurse's employment must be legal, and the duties to be performed and services provided must be within the law. For example, the nurse cannot be required to provide services that are not permitted in the nurse practice act.
2. The parties to the contract must be of legal age (majority) and competent (free of mental impairment) to enter a binding agreement.
3. There must be mutual agreement about the service to be contracted for. A contract becomes invalid, for example, if the nurse does not accept an offer of hire, or if the nurse expecting to be placed in an obstetric unit is placed in a coronary intensive care unit.
4. There must be compensation (or promise of it) for the service to be provided.

These four elements are also required for contracts made by clients (with nurses, other health professionals, or health care institutions) to be valid. For example, the activity contracted for between a client and a hospital is health care, which is legal. Clients who are minors are not usually admitted for care without consent from their parents or legal guardians. The parties agree to the terms of the contract when the client gives informed consent for care and the hospital offers care. The client promises to reimburse the hospital for its services through insurance coverage or other means.

Legal Roles of Nurses

Nurses have three separate, interdependent legal roles, each with rights and associated responsibilities: (a) provider of service, (b) employee or contractor for service, and (c) private citizen (Fenner 1980, p. 86). See Table 7–3. Nurses move in and out of these roles when carrying out professional and personal responsibilities. An understanding of these roles and their rights and responsibilities promotes legally responsible conduct and practice by nurses.

Provider of Service

In the role of provider of service, the nurse is expected to provide safe and competent care so that harm (physical, psychologic, or material) to the recipient of the service is prevented. Implicit in this role are several legal concepts: (a) liability, (b) standard of care, and (c) contractual obligations.

Liability is the quality or state of being **liable**, i.e., legally responsible to account for one's obligations and actions and to make financial restitution for wrongful acts. A primary nurse or team leader, for example, has an obligation to practice and direct the practice of others under

Table 7–3 Nurses' Legal Roles, Rights, and Responsibilities

Role	Responsibilities	Rights
Provider of service	To provide safe and competent care commensurate with the nurse's preparation, experience, and circumstances	Right to adequate and qualified assistance as necessary
	To inform clients of the consequences of various alternatives and outcomes of care	Right to reasonable and prudent conduct from clients, e.g., provision of accurate information as required
	To provide adequate supervision and evaluation of subordinates for whom the nurse is responsible	
	To remain competent	
Employee or contractor for service	To fulfill the obligations of contracted service with the employer	Right to adequate working conditions, e.g., safe equipment and facilities
		Right to compensation for services rendered
	To respect the rights and responsibilities of other health care participants	Right to reasonable and prudent conduct by other health care givers
Citizen	To protect the rights of the recipients of care	Right to respect by others of the nurse's own rights and responsibilities

supervision so that harm or injury to the client is prevented and standards of care are maintained. Even when a nurse is directed by a physician, the responsibility for nursing activity is the nurse's. When a nurse is requested to carry out an activity that the nurse believes will be injurious to the client, the nurse's responsibility is to refuse to carry out the order and to report this to the responsible nurse.

The **standards of care** by which a nurse acts or fails to act are legally defined in accordance with (a) the constraints of nurse practice acts and (b) what would be done in similar circumstances by a reasonable and prudent professional with similar preparation and experience. A nurse, for example, would be acting illegally in diagnosing or treating a client for a tumor, since these functions are within the scope of the physician's practice, and nurses are constrained from engaging in them. Associated with standards of care is the nurse's right to adequate and qualified assistance as required. The nurses' standards of care are regulated further by the standards of care established by professional nursing associations and by job descriptions and other policies and procedures of the employing agency.

Contractual obligations refer to the nurse's duty of care, that is, duty to render care, established by the presence of an expressed or implied contract discussed earlier. A nurse in some circumstances cannot be held liable for care given if a valid contractual relationship with the client does not exist.

Employee or Contractor for Service

Another legal role of the nurse is that of employee or contractor for service. This role describes the nurse's rights and responsibilities as a staff nurse, private nurse, supervisor, consultant, independent practitioner, and member of a peer group of nurses. Implicit in this role are the legal concepts of contract law and contractual relationships.

A nurse who is employed by a hospital works as an agent of the hospital, and the nurse's contract with clients is an implied one. However, a nurse who is employed directly by a client, for example, a private nurse, may have a written contract with that client in which the nurse agrees to provide professional services for a certain fee. If the client is dying, the nurse can be protected by a written contract that allows collection of the fee from the client's estate.

A nurse might be prevented from carrying out the terms of the contract because of illness or death. However, personal inconvenience and personal problems, such as the nurse's car failure, are not legitimate reasons for failing to fulfill a contract. A nurse cannot be held to a contract if the terms of the contract were misrepresented. For example, a private nurse agrees to look after a client who has just had an operation; however if the client is also an alcoholic experiencing delirium tremens, and this information was withheld from the nurse at the time the contract was made, the nurse would not be held legally to the contract. In this instance, the nurse might still be ethically committed to care for the client even though the terms of the contract were misrepresented.

Contractual relationships vary among practice settings. For example, a private duty nurse who is not employed by a hospital functions within an independent contractor relationship with the client and is held individually liable for acts of malpractice. An independent nurse practitioner is a contractor for service, whose contractual relationship with the client is again an independent one. The nurse employed by a hospital functions within an employer-employee relationship, in which the nurse represents and acts for the hospital and therefore must function within the policies of the employing agency. This type of legal relationship creates the ancient legal doctrine known as **respondeat superior** ("let the master answer"). In other words, the master (employer) assumes responsibility for the conduct of the servant (employee) and can be held responsible for malpractice by the employee. By virtue of the employee role, therefore, the nurse's conduct is the hospital's responsibility.

This doctrine does not imply that the nurse cannot be held liable as an individual. Nor does it imply that the doctrine will prevail if the employee's actions are extraordinarily inappropriate, i.e., beyond those expected or foreseen by the employer. For example, if the nurse hits a client in the face, the employer could disclaim responsibility, since this behavior is beyond the bounds of expected behavior. Criminal acts, such as assisting with criminal abortions or taking tranquilizers from a client's supply for personal use would also be considered extraordinarily inappropriate behavior. Nurses can be held liable for failure to act as well. For example, if a nurse sees another nurse hitting a client and fails to do anything to protect the client, the observer is also considered negligent.

The nurse in the role of employee or contractor for service has obligations to the employer, the client, and other personnel. The nursing care provided must be within the limitations and terms specified. The nurse has an obligation to contract to meet only those responsibilities for which she or he is competent. As an employee, the nurse is expected to uphold the good name of the employer and therefore should not criticize the employer unjustifiably. The employer, in turn, is obligated to provide adequate working conditions, e.g., a safe, functional employment setting.

The nurse is expected to respect the rights and responsibilities of other health care participants. For example, although the nurse has responsibility to explain nursing activities to a client, she or he does not have the right to comment on medical practice in a way that disturbs the client or causes problems for the physician. At the same time, the nurse has the right to expect reasonable and prudent conduct from other health care participants.

Citizen

The rights and responsibilities of the nurse in the role of citizen are the same as those of any individual under the legal system. Rights of citizenship protect clients from harm and ensure consideration for their personal property rights, rights to privacy, confidentiality, and other rights discussed later in this chapter and in Chapter 9. These same rights apply to nurses. For example, nurses have the right to physical safety and need not perform functions that are considered an unreasonable risk.

Collective Bargaining

Collective bargaining is a formalized decision-making process between management and labor representatives concerning salaries, work environment, and conditions of employment (Crawford et al. 1985, p. 155). Through a written agreement, both employer and employees legally commit themselves to observe the terms and conditions of employment. Collective bargaining is a controversial issue among nurses. Some nurses argue against collective bargaining on the grounds that it is contrary to the nature of professionalism, it is not necessary, it fosters discord, and it undermines the nurse administrator's role (McClelland 1983, p. 36). Others argue that it is necessary to obtain control of nursing practice and economic security.

Two arguments support nurses' involvement in collective bargaining (Flanagan 1983, p. 17):

1. It provides the means by which nurses may achieve basic elements of professional status. Elements of a profession include promoting the welfare and well-being of its practitioners, safeguarding practitioners' interests, and accepting responsibility for the public's safety and well-being. Through the process of bargaining, nursing professionals can secure adequate compensation for services, improve employment conditions, and foster a higher quality of care.
2. There is direct correlation between working conditions and the quality of care (Flanagan 1983, p. 17). Selected working conditions that hinder delivery of nursing services are shown below. Many nurses believe that nurses can enforce standards of practice by working through the collective bargaining process.

Selected Working Conditions That Hinder the Delivery of Nursing Services

Improper use of nurses and other staff

Improper ratio of qualified nurses and unlicensed staff to clients

Lack of involvement of nurses in decision making about delivery of nursing services

Inadequate orientation, in-service, and staff development programs

Inadequate supplies and equipment

Restrictive or rigid policies and procedures

Unsafe and hazardous conditions

Assignment of nonnursing duties

Limited opportunities for nurses to work together as a group to initiate needed changes (Flanagan 1983)

Historic Review

In 1947, the United States Labor Management Relations Act (Taft-Hartley Act) was passed. In this act, collective bargaining is defined as "the performance of the mutual obligation of the employers and representative of employees to meet at reasonable times and confer in good faith with respect to wages, hours and other terms and conditions of employment—or the negotiation of any agreement or any question arising thereunder . . ." (Labor-Management Relations Act 1947). Under the Taft-Hartley Act, nonprofit hospitals were exempt from the requirement to bargain with their employees but not prevented from bargaining.

In 1974, the exemptions which had applied to nonprofit hospitals were removed by Public Law 93-360—the 1974 Health Care Amendments (U.S. Department of Labor 1979, p. 4).

The need to improve the economic and social welfare of nurses was well recognized in the 1930s. At that time, the welfare of nurses was an acute problem, largely as a result of the depression. Many nurses were unable to obtain any employment, and some nurses worked solely in exchange for room and board. Some nurses turned to unions to improve their lot. In the United States today, it is the role of state nursing associations (SNAs) to organize local units for the purpose of collective bargaining. A number of SNAs have active collective bargaining programs. Some SNAs, however, do not engage in any collective bargaining activities. The ANA supports the need for collective bargaining and assists the SNAs by giving technical and financial assistance. The national association sees collective action as a professional responsibility and refers to this ideology as **professional collectivism.** This position is based on a concern for clients as well as the working conditions of nurses.

In Canada, collective bargaining is handled by registered nurse unions, which are separate from the provincial nursing associations. This separation occurred as a result of a 1973 Supreme Court decision in Saskatchewan that a management-dominated profession could not make decisions for its members. Members of these unions include all registered nurses employed below the supervisory level. Nurse instructors are not members. Educational institutions in which instructors are employed handle collective bargaining independently.

Collective Bargaining Process

The collective bargaining process involves the recognition of a certified bargaining agent for the employees. This agent can be a union, a trade association, or a professional organization. The agent represents the employees in negotiating a contract with management.

The fundamental terms of employment about which management and labor bargain are (Barbash 1980, pp. 553–54): (a) the price of labor (e.g., wages, wage structures, methods of wage determination); (b) rules that define how labor is to be utilized, including hours, work practices, and job classifications; (c) individual job rights (e.g., seniority and discharge for cause); (d) union and management rights in bargaining relationships; and (e) methods of enforcement, interpretation, and administration of the agreement, including the resolution of grievances.

When collective bargaining breaks down because an agreement cannot be reached, the employees usually call a strike. A **strike** is an organized work stoppage by a group of employees to express a grievance, enforce a demand for changes in conditions of employment, or solve a dispute with management (Crawford et al. 1985, p. 162).

Because nursing practice is a service to people (often ill people), striking presents a moral dilemma to many nurses. Actions taken by nurses can affect the safety of people. Each nurse must make an individual decision when faced with a strike as to whether or not to cross a picket line. Nursing students may also be faced with decisions about crossing picket lines in event of a strike or in issues involving collective bargaining.

Grievance Procedures

Collective bargaining is more than the negotiation of salary terms and hours of work; it is a continuous process in which day-to-day working problems and relationships can be handled in an orderly and democratic manner. Day-to-day difficulties or grievances are handled through the grievance procedure: a formal plan established in the

Table 7–4 Categories and Examples of Grievances

Category	Examples
Contract violations	Shift or weekend work is assigned inequitably.
	A nurse is dismissed without cause.
Violations of federal and state law	A female nurse is paid less than a male nurse for the same work.
	Appropriate payment is not given for overtime work.
	Minority group nurses are not promoted.
Management responsibilities	Appropriate locker room facilities are not provided.
	Safe client care is jeopardized by inadequate staffing.
Violation of agency rules	Performance evaluations are conducted only at termination of employment, but the contract requires annual evaluations.
	A vacation period is assigned without the nurse's agreement, as required in personnel policies.

Source: American Nurses' Association, *The grievance procedure* (Kansas City, Mo.: ANA, 1985), pp. 2–4. Used by permission.

contract that outlines the channels for handling and settling of grievances through progressively higher levels of administration. A **grievance** is any dispute, difference, controversy, or disagreement arising out of the terms and conditions of employment. Grievances fall into four main categories outlined in Table 7–4.

Not all employee complaints are legitimate grievances. Complaints that fall into the categories in Table 7–4 can be considered legitimate grievances. Complaints arising from an interpersonal relationship between individual nurses do not warrant use of the grievance procedure. Other complaints may be borderline grievances, which require interpretation of unclear parts of the contract. Employed nurses need to familiarize themselves with the grievance procedures outlined in the agency's contract. Usually one or more individuals are designated to handle grievances for members in each local unit.

Areas of Potential Liability in Nursing

Crimes and Torts

Crimes

A **crime** is an act committed in violation of public (criminal) law and punishable by a fine and/or imprisonment. A crime does not have to be intended in order to be a crime. For example, a nurse may accidentally give a client an additional and lethal dose of a narcotic to relieve discomfort.

Crimes are classified as either felonies (or in Canada, indictable offenses) or misdemeanors (or in Canada, summary conviction offenses). A **felony** is a crime of a serious nature, such as murder, punishable by a term in prison. First-degree murder and second-degree murder are felonies. The former involves the intent to murder, while the latter is murder without previous intent. In some areas, second degree murder is called **manslaughter**. A nurse who accidentally gives an additional and lethal dose of a narcotic can be accused of manslaughter. Other examples of felonies are arson, armed robbery, and, in Canada, criminal abortion and attempted suicide. Crimes are punished through criminal action by the state or province against an individual. A **misdemeanor** is of a less serious nature and is usually punishable by a fine or short-term jail sentence or both. Examples of misdemeanors are soliciting for prostitution, indecent exposure (e.g., nudity on a public beach), and disturbing the peace by, for example, shouting, yelling, or swearing. A nurse who takes a bottle of wine from a client's locker would be charged with a misdemeanor.

Torts

A **tort** is a civil wrong committed against a person or a person's property. Torts may be classified as intentional and unintentional. Intentional torts include fraud, invasion of privacy, defamation (libel and slander), assault and battery, and false imprisonment. Unintentional torts are referred to as negligence. Examples of unintentional torts are: (a) the nurse improperly administers an injection to a client, causing permanent nerve damage, and (b) the nurse burns a client unable to discern skin temperature with a hot water bottle. Torts are usually litigated in court by civil action between individuals. In other words, the person or persons claimed to be responsible for the tort are sued for damages.

Tort liability almost always is based on fault, i.e., something was done incorrectly (an unreasonable act of commission) or something that should have been done was omitted (act of omission). See Table 7–5 for a summary of the differences between intentional and unintentional torts. Some torts, such as fraud or assault and battery, may be regarded as cause for criminal action instead of civil action. Whether they are considered cause for criminal or civil action depends on whether the injured person files a criminal charge or files for suit. For example, in a case of assault the injured person may charge the defendant with a criminal offense that is punishable by a fine and/or prison term. A written statement is then made by a prosecutor against the defendant. However, the injured person may choose to sue for damages, i.e., to get money for the cost of inconvenience, hospitalization, and treatment of the injuries. A lawsuit is a civil action.

Intentional Torts

Fraud

Fraud is the false presentation of some fact or facts with the intention that it will be acted upon by another person. For example, it is fraud for a person to present false records of education to gain admission to a nursing school; it is also fraud for a nurse applying to a hospital for employment to omit two employers for deceptive reasons when she or he is asked to list the previous five employers.

Invasion of Privacy

The right to privacy is the right of individuals to withhold themselves and their lives from public scrutiny. Invasion of privacy is a direct wrong of a personal nature. It injures the feelings of the person and does not take into account the effect of revealed information on the standing of the person in the community. The right to privacy can also be described as the right to be left alone. Liability can result if the nurse passes along confidential client infor-

Table 7–5 Comparison of Intentional and Unintentional Torts

Intentional	Unintentional (Negligence)
1. They involve the commission of a prohibited act.	1. They can result from either an act of commission or an act of omission.
2. The act in question is willful and deliberate (intentional).	2. The wrong results from failure to use due care.
3. They involve certain specific types of conduct listed as "wrong."	3. They are not spelled out in an all-inclusive list.

mation to others or intrudes into the client's private domain. In this context, there is a delicate balance between the need of a number of people to contribute to the diagnosis and treatment of a client and the client's right to privacy. In most situations, necessary discussion about a client's medical condition is considered appropriate, but unnecessary discussions and gossip are considered an invasion of privacy. Necessary discussion involves only those engaged in the client's care.

Most jurisdictions of the country have a variety of statutes that impose a duty to report certain confidential client information. Four major categories are:

1. Vital statistics: e.g., births and deaths
2. Infections and communicable diseases, e.g., diphtheria, syphilis, and typhoid fever
3. Child or elder abuse
4. Violent incidents, e.g., gunshot wounds and knife wounds

In addition some states, e.g., California, require that a health care provider report when a client is a danger to another person (Annas et al. 1981, pp. 176–78).

Client rights to privacy include:

1. The right to refuse to see any visitors
2. The right to refuse to see anyone not officially connected with the agency or not directly involved in his or her care and treatment, even if she or he is officially connected to the hospital
3. The right to wear religious or other medals
4. The right to wear personal clothing when it does not interfere with treatment
5. The right to have a member of the same sex present during a physical examination
6. The right to refuse to participate in clinical demonstrations for medical and nursing personnel

In teaching hospitals, it is important for health personnel to obtain the client's consent prior to any demonstration or teaching conference, to respect the right of privacy. See also the section on rights to privacy in Chapter 9.

Libel and Slander

Both libel and slander are wrongful actions that come under the heading of defamation. **Defamation** is communication that is false, or made with a careless disregard for the truth, and results in injury to the reputation of a person. **Libel** is defamation by means of print, writing, or pictures. **Slander** is defamation by the spoken word, stating unprivileged (not legally protected) or false words by which a reputation is damaged. A nurse has a qualified privilege to make statements that could be considered invasions of a client's privacy, both orally and in writing, but only as a part of nursing practice and only to a physician or another health team member caring directly for the client.

Truth is always a good defense to a charge of defamation. Care needs to be taken, however, to speak or write only the facts or the truth. A nurse, for example, may believe that a particular client had been admitted to a hospital for acquired immune deficiency syndrome (AIDS) a year earlier; in fact, it was another client. This information would be grounds for a charge of slander if the nurse shared it with nurses from another unit.

For nurses to be protected against claims of invasion of privacy, comments about clients need to be kept to a minimum and made only to health professionals involved in their care.

Assault and Battery

In the United States, the terms *assault* and *battery* are often heard together, but each has its own meaning. **Assault** can be described as an attempt or threat to touch another person unjustifiably. Assault precedes battery; it is the act that causes the person to believe a battery is about to occur. For example, the person who threatens someone by making a menacing gesture with a club or a closed fist is guilty of assault. In nursing, a client may perceive that a nurse is *about to* administer an injection without his or her consent. **Battery** is the willful or negligent touching of a person (or the person's clothes or even something the person is carrying), which may or may not cause harm. In order to be actionable at law, however, the touching must be wrong in some way, e.g., done without permission, embarrassing, or causing injury. For example, the nurse who administers a hypodermic injection to a client or ambulates a client without his or her consent could be held liable for battery. Liability applies even though the physician ordered the medication or the activity and even if the client benefits. The law recognizes a compensable injury even when the client benefits from the touching since the basis of protection from battery is the client's right to self-determination.

In Canada, the term *battery* is not used. Instead assault is classified into three categories: (a) assault with intention to injure, for example, threatening someone by making a menacing gesture with a knife, (b) assault causing bodily injury, and (c) sexual assault.

Every person has the legal right to refuse physical contact with another. While receiving health care, a client has the right to refuse such physical contact as an injection or an operation; personnel who proceed with contact despite such a refusal can be sued for battery (or, in Canada, for assault causing bodily injury).

Technical assault and battery differ from criminal assault and battery in that the latter are usually carried out with intent to injure. If a person is touched and has not given implied or actual consent (for example, when the wrong limb is operated upon), a lawsuit based on technical assault and battery can result. Consent to treat a client is therefore required.

If clients have a right to refuse medical or surgical treatments, they also have a right to refuse nursing interventions. (Curtin 1982, p. 8)

False Imprisonment

False imprisonment is unjustifiable detention that deprives a person of personal liberty for any length of time. For example, a nurse who locks a client in a room unjustifiably is guilty of false imprisonment. False imprisonment accompanied by forceful restraint or threat of restraint is assault and battery (Creighton 1981, p. 207).

Although nurses may suggest to a client under certain circumstances that he or she remain in the room or in bed, the client must not be detained against his or her will. The client has a right to insist upon leaving even though it may be detrimental to health. Detention is legal only when imposed to protect the public or perhaps to protect the individual from unintended harm, for example, when a client is high on drugs and unable to control his or her behavior. In these instances the client cannot leave when he or she wishes.

Unintentional Torts

Negligence and Malpractice

Negligence is "the omission to do something that a reasonable person, guided by those ordinary considerations which ordinarily regulate human affairs, would do, or doing something which a reasonable and prudent person would not do" (Creighton 1981, p. 154). **Malpractice** is that part of the law of negligence applied to the professional person: It is, in effect, any professional misconduct or unreasonable lack of professional skill. A nurse could be guilty of malpractice if she or he injured a client while performing a procedure differently from the way other nurses would have done it. Negligence applies to any person who, for example, drove a car too quickly in snowy weather and injured a pedestrian. Malpractice and negligence are often used interchangeably; however, malpractice is reserved for professional misconduct. It is the failure of a professional person to act within the acceptable standards of his or her profession.

Proof of a nurse's negligence includes proof of all of the following: (a) the nurse's duty to the client, (b) the nurse's failure to carry out that duty, (c) an injury incurred by the client, and (d) a causal relationship between the breach of duty by the nurse and the client's injury—a relationship referred to as **proximate cause.** In cases of proven negligence, monetary damages are awarded to the plaintiff to compensate for the inconvenience and suffering experienced and, where possible, to help the person return to the state of well-being enjoyed prior to the injury.

Nurses are responsible for their own actions even though they may be employees of a health agency. The descriptions of negligence and malpractice do not mention good intentions; it is not pertinent that the nurse did not intend to be negligent. If a nurse administers an incorrect medication, even in good faith, the fact that the nurse failed to read the label correctly indicates malpractice.

Another significant aspect of negligence and malpractice is that both omissions and commissions are included. That is, a person can be guilty of malpractice by forgetting to give a medication as well as by giving the wrong medication.

Types of Malpractice Situations

Medication errors The most common nursing errors occur in the administration of medications. With the large number of medications on the market today and the variety of methods of administration, these errors may be on the increase. Nurses are in error in not reading the label on the medication, misreading or incorrectly calculating the dosage, not identifying the client correctly, preparing the wrong concentration, or administering a medication by the wrong route (e.g., intravenously instead of orally). Some medication errors are very serious and can even cost the client's life. If, for example, a nurse gives dicumarol to a client recently returned from surgery, the patient could hemorrhage as a result. Nurses always need to check medications very carefully. Even after the nurse has done so, if a client states he or she "did not have a green pill before," the nurse is wise to check the medication order and the medication again before administering it.

Sponge counts Sponges or other small items can be left inside a client during an operation because the nurse either failed to count them before the surgeon closed the incision or counted them incorrectly. In either case, the nurse responsible for counting the sponges can be held liable for malpractice.

Burns A relatively frequent malpractice action attributed to nurses is burning a patient. Burns may be caused by hot water bottles, heating pads, and solutions that are too hot for application. Elderly, comatose, or diabetic people are particularly vulnerable to burns, due to decreased sensitivity. Hot objects can burn these people before they notice it. A nurse may also be held negligent for leaving a client without taking precautions (giving warnings or providing protections), for example, when using a steam vaporizer.

Falls Accidental falls by clients, sometimes with resultant injury, occur commonly. Side rails are used on cribs, beds, and stretchers for babies and small children, and for adults when necessary, to prevent falls. If a nurse leaves the rails down or leaves a baby unattended on a bath table, that nurse is guilty of malpractice if the client falls and is injured. Most hospitals and nursing homes have policies regarding the use of safety devices such as side rails and restraints. A nurse needs to be familiar with these policies and to take indicated precautions to prevent this type of accident.

Failure to observe and take appropriate action In some instances, nurses are guilty of malpractice by virtue of ignoring a client's complaints. If the nurse does not report a client's complaint of acute abdominal pain, the nurse is negligent, and an ensuing appendix rupture and death may be held the result of the nurse's malpractice. By failing to take the blood pressure and pulse and check the dressing of a postoperative client who has just had a kidney removed, a nurse omits important assessments. If the client hemorrhages and dies, the nurse may be held responsible for the death as a result of this malpractice.

Mistaken identity Identifying clients correctly is a problem, particularly in busy hospital units. It is not unknown for a nurse to prepare the wrong client for an operation, so that a healthy gallbladder is removed from the wrong person. These mistakes can be costly to a client and make the nurse liable for malpractice.

Loss of or damage to clients' property Items of property such as jewelry, money, and dentures are a constant concern to hospital personnel. Today, agencies are taking less responsibility for property and are generally requesting clients to sign a form on admission relieving the hospital and its employees of any responsibility for property. There are, however, situations in which the client cannot sign a waiver, and the nursing staff must follow prescribed policies about care of the client's property. On hospital units, dentures are often a major problem; they can be lost in bedding or left on a meal tray. Nurses are expected to take reasonable precautions to safeguard a client's property, and they can be held liable for its loss or damage if they do not exercise reasonable care.

Reporting Crimes, Torts, and Unsafe Practices

Nurses who believe in client health and safety may need at one time or another to report other health professionals for practices that endanger the health and safety of clients. For instance, alcohol and drug use, theft from a client or agency, and unsafe nursing practice should be reported. Reporting a colleague is not easy. The person reporting may feel disloyal to a colleague, incur the disapproval of others, or endanger her or his chances for promotion. Price and Murphy (1983) state that although nurses cannot avoid all risks, there are ways to minimize risks. They outline seven steps to do so (Price and Murphy 1983, pp. 52–53):

1. Write a clear description of the situation you believe you should report. The description should include (a) precisely what the dangerous practice entails, (b) to whom it is dangerous, and (c) how reporting the practice would be protective. For example, if a nurse observes Mrs. Kettle, another nurse, drinking alcohol while at work, the written description should state specifically that the nurse observed Mrs. Kettle taking drinks from a bottle of vodka while at work. Because alcohol impairs mental capacities and abilities to make appropriate decisions and judgments, the nurse believes this practice could endanger the clients in Mrs. Kettle's care. If the care of clients assigned to Mrs. Kettle is questionable, the nurse documents the actions or omissions specifically, e.g., an emaciated client who is prone to bedsores and who is to be turned q2h was turned only once during an 8-hour shift. As a result of the report, Mrs. Kettle could be suspended until she receives treatment. Alternatively, she could receive a warning from the nursing administrator, lose her job, or perhaps lose her nursing license. The loss of her job and license would protect the clients and the hospital; suspension and treatment protects Mrs. Kettle as well.
2. Make sure that your statements are accurate. For instance, are you sure Mrs. Kettle was drinking alcohol? Could it have been another beverage? Be sure to document your findings with dates, times, and places.
3. Make sure you are credible. Part of credibility is assessing oneself and one's motives. The nurse should ask: "Am I considered level-headed, honest, and reliable?" "Do I have other motives?" "Am I trying to get even

for Mrs. Kettle's criticism of me in the past?" Determine exactly what codes or regulations have been broken, consulting the nursing code of ethics if a nurse is involved or the medical ethical code if a physician is involved.

4. Obtain support from at least one trustworthy person before filing the report. This person must be stable but willing to take a risk: an open-minded person who appreciates the situation but can remain objective. In Mrs. Kettle's case, perhaps another nurse who has worked with her would support you.
5. Report the matter starting at the lowest possible level in the agency hierarchy. For example, report Mrs. Kettle to the nurse to whom she is directly responsible. If there is no response from that person, go up the ladder, i.e., to the nursing supervisor or manager, then to the department head, and so on. Always report to the people inside the system before going outside, e.g., to the professional association. In this way you are protecting both the agency and the clients. Going through channels minimizes damage to personal and institutional reputations.
6. Assume responsibility for reporting the individual by being open about it. An anonymous letter is more likely to make your motives suspect; also, some people do not take an anonymous complaint seriously.
7. See the problem through once you have reported it. For instance, follow through by asking "When can we expect a result?" "I'll check back with you next Friday." "I hope you understand that I think this is serious and I plan to follow this through."

Price and Murphy advocate using the first three steps "to determine whether you have a case for blowing the whistle. If you do, use the next four steps to proceed" (Price and Murphy 1983, p. 54).

Selected Legal Facets of Nursing Practice

Informed Consent

Informed consent is an agreement by a client to accept a course of treatment or a procedure after complete information, including the risks of treatment and facts relating to it, has been provided by the physician. Informed consent, then, is an exchange between a client and a physician. Usually the client signs a form provided by the agency. The form is a record of the informed consent, not the informed consent itself.

Obtaining informed consent is the responsibility of a physician. Although this responsibility is delegated to nurses in some agencies, the practice is highly questionable. The nurse's responsibility is often to witness the giving of informed consent. This involves:

1. Witnessing the exchange between the client and the physician
2. Witnessing the client's signature
3. Establishing that the client really did understand, i.e., was really informed

If a nurse witnesses only the client's signature and not the exchange between the client and the physician, the nurse should write "witnessing signature only" on the form (Northrop 1984, p. 223). If the nurse finds that the client really does not understand the physician's explanation, then it is important that the physician be notified.

Northrop (1984, p. 223) describes three major elements of informed consent:

1. The consent must be given voluntarily.
2. The consent must be given by an individual with the capacity and competence to understand.
3. The client must be given enough information to be the ultimate decision maker.

To give informed consent voluntarily, the client must not feel coerced. Sometimes fear of disapproval by a health professional can be the motivation for giving consent; such consent is not voluntarily given.

The practice of seeking informed consent is based on the belief that a client has a right to self-determination. This right is supported by both law and ethics and is grounded in three principles:

1. Humans have a unique dignity and worth.
2. Humans are never to be used merely as a means, but always as an end.
3. Humans are endowed with an inalienable right to life, liberty, and pursuit of happiness (Davis 1985, p. 40).

If a client is given sufficient information, he or she can make decisions regarding health. To do so, the client must be competent and an adult. A competent adult is a person over 18 years of age who is conscious and oriented. A person under 18 years who is considered "an emancipated minor," i.e., self-supporting or married, can also give consent. A client who is confused, disoriented, or sedated is not considered competent.

There are three groups of people who cannot provide consent. The first is minors. In most areas, consent must be given by a parent or guardian before minors can obtain treatment. The same is true of an adult who has the mental capacity of a child. In some states, however, minors are allowed to give consent for such procedures as blood donations, treatment for drug dependency and sexually transmitted disease, and procedures for obstetrical care. The second group is persons who are unconscious or injured in such a way that they are unable to give consent. In these situations, consent is usually obtained from the closest adult relative. In an emergency, if consent cannot be obtained from the client or a relative, then the law generally agrees that consent is assumed. The third group is mentally ill persons. States and province mental health acts or similar statutes generally provide definitions of mental illness and specify the rights of the mentally ill under the law as well as the rights of the staff caring for such clients.

To give informed consent, the client must receive sufficient information to make a decision; otherwise, the client's right to decide has been usurped. Information needs to include benefits, risks, and alternative procedures. It is also important that the client understand. Technical words and language barriers can inhibit understanding. If a client cannot read, the consent form must be read to him or her before it is signed. If the client does not speak English, an interpreter must be acquired.

Recordkeeping

The client's medical record is a legal document and can be produced in court as evidence. Often the record is used to remind a witness of events surrounding a lawsuit, since it usually takes several months or years for the suit to go to trial. The effectiveness of a witness's testimony can depend on the accuracy of such records. Nurses, therefore, need to keep accurate and complete records of nursing care provided to clients. Failure to keep proper records can constitute negligence and be the basis for tort liability. Insufficient or inaccurate assessments and documentation can hinder proper diagnosis and treatment and result in injury to the client. Types of records and essential facts about recording are discussed in Chapter 30. See also the section on legal safeguards for nurses, later in this chapter.

Controlled Substances

United States and Canadian laws regulate the distribution and use of controlled substances such as narcotics, depressants, stimulants, and hallucinogens. Misuse of controlled substances leads to criminal penalties. Controlled substances are kept in securely locked drawers or cupboards, and only authorized personnel have access to them. See Chapter 51 for the legal aspects of drug administration.

The Incident Report

An **incident report** is an agency record of an accident or incident. Most agencies have their own incident reports. Their purposes are (a) to make all the facts about an accident available to agency personnel, (b) to contribute to statistical data about accidents or incidents, and (c) to help health personnel plan in order to prevent future accidents. All accidents are usually reported on incident forms. Some agencies also report other incidents, e.g., the occurrence of client infection or the loss of personal affects. See below the list of information to be included in an incident report. The report should be completed as soon as possible, always within 24 hours of the incident.

Information to Include in an Incident Report

1. **Identify the client by name, initials, and hospital or identification number.**
2. **Give the date, time, and place of the incident.**
3. **Describe the facts of the incident. Avoid any conclusions or blame. Describe the incident as you saw it even if your impressions differ from those of others.**
4. **Identify all witnesses to the incident.**
5. **Identify any equipment by number and any medication by name and number.**
6. **Document any circumstance surrounding the incident, e.g., another client (Mrs. Losas) was experiencing cardiac arrest.**

Incident reports are often reviewed by an agency committee, which decides whether to investigate the incident further. The nurse may be required upon further investigation to answer such questions as: Why do you believe the accident occurred? How could it have been prevented? Should any equipment be adjusted? The nurse who believes she or he may be dismissed or that suit may be brought should obtain legal advice. Even if the agency clears the nurse of responsibility, the client or the client's family may file suit. The plaintiff, however, bears the burden of proof that the accident occurred because reasonable care was not taken. Even if the accepted standard of care was not given, the plaintiff must prove that the accident was the direct result of unacceptable standards of care and that the accident caused physical, emotional, or financial injury.

When an accident occurs and a client is injured, nurses must take steps to protect the client, themselves, and their employer. Most agencies have policies regarding acci-

Research Note

A study of all incident reports in five special-care homes of various resident capacities in Saskatchewan revealed that (a) the incidents per client day increased inversely with the size of the facility, (b) all facilities reported fewer incidents on the 2300 to 0700 hour shift, (c) in two facilities the evening shift had more incidents than the day shift, (d) in one facility there were more incidents during the day shift than the evening shift, and (e) falls accounted for the largest percentage of incidents. (Wasiuta 1982)

dents. It is important to follow these policies and not to assume one is guilty of malpractice. Although this may be the case, accidents do happen even when every precaution has been taken to prevent them.

Cournoyer (1985) describes seven nursing actions that a nurse should take after an accident:

1. Assess the client and protect him or her from further injury. Call for assistance if the client needs stabilizing or assistance before he or she is moved.
2. Notify all appropriate staff members. Most agencies indicate in written policies who is to be notified in case of an accident. These usually are the client's physician, the agency manager or administrator, and the responsible nurse. In some instances, other health personnel are notified; for example, the pharmacist is sometimes notified if the client has taken the incorrect medication.
3. Notify the family. Sometimes the physician, the agency manager, or the nurse notifies the family. Nurses should not assign blame but should explain the incident truthfully. A good policy is to explain that the matter is under investigation rather than blaming or assuming responsibility.
4. Identify everyone—including visitors, clients, and health personnel—who may have witnessed the accident. Also ask the client what happened.
5. Evaluate the circumstances surrounding the accident. Include staffing and emergencies that were taking place. It is important to remember that the legal standard of nursing practice is what a reasonably prudent nurse does in similar circumstances.
6. Identify equipment or medications involved in the accident. Attach a tag to the equipment or medication and store it safely according to agency policy. These items may be used in evidence.
7. Document all findings on the client's chart, the incident report, and personal notes. Include in the documentation assessments of the client, all medical and nursing interventions, and verbal orders. Make sure the documentation includes facts, not impressions or conclusions. Certain nursing actions that were not documented earlier can be documented now, e.g., recording a warning to the client not to walk without assistance or recording a support person's statement to remain at the bedside. Do not hide any facts. It is much easier for a lawyer to deal with the situation if all the facts are known (Cournoyer 1985, pp. 20–21).

Wills

A **will** is a declaration by a person about how the person's property is to be disposed of after his or her death. In order for a will to be valid, the following conditions must be met:

1. The person making the will must be of sound mind, that is, able to understand and retain mentally the general nature and extent of his or her property, the relationship of the beneficiaries and of relatives to whom none of the estate will be left, and the disposition he or she is making of the property. A person, therefore, who is seriously ill and unable to carry out business functions may be able to make a will.
2. The person must not be unduly influenced by anyone else.

Sometimes a client may be persuaded by someone who is close at that particular time to make that person a beneficiary. Clients sometimes are persuaded to leave their estates to persons looking after them rather than to their relatives. Frequently, the relatives will contest the will in this situation and take the matter to court, claiming undue influence.

Nurses may be requested from time to time to witness a will. In most states and provinces, a will must be signed in the presence of two witnesses. In some situations, a mark can suffice if the person making the will cannot write a signature.

In most settings, it is required that both witnesses be present at the same time when the person is signing the will. A person who is a witness to a will should not be a beneficiary, because in most jurisdictions this affects the right to take part of the estate. If a nurse is a witness to a will, the nurse should note on the client's chart that a will was made and the nurse's perception of the physical and mental condition of the client. This record will provide the nurse with accurate information if the nurse is called as a witness later. The record may also be helpful if the will is contested. If a nurse does not wish to act as a witness, for example, if in the nurse's opinion undue influence has been brought on the client, then it is the nurse's right to refuse to act in this capacity.

Euthanasia and the Right to Die (Living Wills)

Euthanasia is the act of painlessly putting to death persons suffering from incurable or distressing disease. It is commonly referred to as mercy killing. Regardless of compassion and good intentions or moral convictions, euthanasia is legally wrong and can lead to criminal charges of homicide or to a civil lawsuit for withholding treatment or providing an unacceptable standard of care. Since advanced technology has enabled the medical profession to sustain life almost indefinitely, people are increasingly considering the meaning of quality of life. For some people, the withholding of artificial life-support measures or even the withdrawal of life support is desired and acceptable practice for clients who are terminally ill or who are incurably disabled and believed unable to live their lives without some happiness and meaning.

Euthanasia is described as active, passive, or voluntary. Active euthanasia involves the administration of a lethal drug to relieve suffering. Passive euthanasia is the withdrawal of extraordinary life-prolonging techniques. Voluntary euthanasia refers to situations in which the dying individual desires some control over the time and manner of death. All forms of euthanasia are illegal except in states where right-to-die statutes and living wills exist. Right-to-die statutes legally recognize aspects of voluntary euthanasia.

Living wills (an individual's signed request to be allowed to die when life can be supported only mechanically or by heroic measures) and right-to-die statutes have received increasing attention in recent years. Most nurses agree that people have a right not to participate in medical treatment or to refuse treatment once it has started. When a person is being maintained on life-sustaining machines, however, a conflict may arise between a physician's ability to prolong life physiologically and the individual's right to die with dignity. Living wills grew out of this conflict. California was the first state to enact legislation, the California Natural Death Act of 1976, that gives legal recognition to a person's desire to control his or her right to die. As of June 1985, 23 states have enacted legislation that frees professional people from liability for honoring a person's wishes that life not be unduly prolonged (Rudy 1985, p. 51).

Some oppose these laws, for varying reasons, including: there is no need for such laws, the laws exclude family from the decision, and the law hastens death (an objection by right-to-life groups). For a sample living will, see Figure 7–2.

Since California passed the first natural death act (NDA) legally recognizing living wills, 14 other states and the District of Columbia have enacted similar legislation (Facts to know . . . 1984). Where NDAs do not exist, there is legal authority to appoint a proxy to act after a person becomes incompetent. This authority is granted through durable power of attorney (DPA) laws. *Durable* means that the proxy's authority to act continues after the client is incapacitated. Some states have both NDAs and DPAs.

Nurses need to familiarize themselves with statutes that authorize living wills in the state where they are employed. Where statutes do exist, procedures are spelled out that must be adhered to. They may include the need to obtain a court order, a medical opinion, the agreement of an ethics or medical committee, family confirmation, or some combination of these. The statutes usually grant civil and criminal immunity to those who carry out living-will requests. Living wills do *not* generally allow the withdrawal of heroic or life-support measures once they are started; they are generally considered to permit only the *withholding* of life-support measures.

In Canada, living-will or right-to-die statutes do not exist. The right to live doctrine in Canada makes it the duty of physicians and nurses to provide all necessary assistance.

No-Code and Slow-Code Orders

Physicians may order "no code" or "slow code" for clients who are in a stage of terminal, irreversible illness or expected death. **No code** means no effort is to be made to resuscitate the client. No-code orders may also be written as *"no heroics"* or DNR (do not resuscitate or do not make resuscitative efforts). **Slow code** means "half-hearted" resuscitation measures are to be initiated and implemented. The legality of no-code and slow-code orders is not yet well established; some court cases have dealt with such situations but no definitive policy exists at this time.

Experts say slow-code orders are not legally acceptable (A Nursing Life Poll Report on Ethics 1983, p. 55). If a client dies because the nurse is slow to call the code team, he or she could be charged with negligence.

The American Heart Association (AHA) *Standards and Guidelines for Cardiopulmonary Resuscitation (CPR) and Emergency Cardiac Care (ECC)* state the following medicolegal considerations and recommendations about DNR orders for physicians (American Heart Association 1986, p. 2880):

1. It is generally accepted that resuscitation is a form of medical therapy that, like most others, is indicated in some situations but not others. One of the situations in which CPR is usually not indicated is the case of the terminally ill client for whom no further therapy for the underlying disease process remains available and for whom death appears imminent. The following definitions are suggested for clarity: *Irreversible* refers to a situation in which no known therapeutic measures are effective in reversing the course of the illness; *irreparable* means the course of the illness has progressed beyond the capacity of existing knowledge and tech-

nique to stem it. *Imminent death* means that in the ordinary course of events death will probably occur within a period of 2 weeks.

2. When the decision not to resuscitate is made by the client or the client's family and physician, the physician must write a note on the client's chart and the physician's order sheet for the benefit of nursing and other personnel who may be called on to initiate or participate in resuscitation. The note should summarize the client's condition and the basis for the DNR decision.

3. DNR orders do not and should not be interpreted to imply any other change in the level of medical or nursing care. The client's family must understand and agree with the decision, although the family's opinion cannot be controlling if the client is competent. Physicians and the entire medical team should be in general agreement with the decision. Agreement may be facilitated by a confirmatory written opinion from appropriate qualified consultants.

4. If the physician desires specific types of intervention along with the DNR order, he or she should write them specifically, e.g., in the case of a child with severe pulmonary disease, "resuscitate short of intubation," if the prospect of life on a ventilator has been appropriately discussed and refused by the family.

Although these standards, like those of any professional organization, are not legally binding, they are persuasive to a judge and jury. They indicate that CPR is intended to prevent *unexpected* death.

The implications of the AHA no-code standards for nurses include:

1. Ensure that the DNR order is written on the client's order sheet and progress notes. Verbal orders can be easily misunderstood and disclaimed.

2. If the physician refuses to write such an order, follow agency policies and procedures. Some agencies have established formal protocols for nurses to follow. Because such procedures are usually carefully reviewed by legal counsel, they can minimize the risk of legal liability substantially.

3. If the agency does not have a well-established procedure, seek a legal opinion through the agency attorney or state or provincial nursing association.

4. If none of the above steps provide the nurse with sufficient guidelines, the nurse must make a personal decision based on moral values and sense of humanity. Even when there are appropriate guidelines, the guidelines may conflict with the nurse's personal ethics. Thus, DNR orders may create an ethical dilemma as well as a legal dilemma for the nurse.

■ TO MY FAMILY, MY PHYSICIAN, MY LAWYER, MY CLERGYMAN
■ TO ANY MEDICAL FACILITY IN WHOSE CARE I HAPPEN TO BE
■ TO ANY INDIVIDUAL WHO MAY BECOME RESPONSIBLE FOR MY HEALTH, WELFARE OR AFFAIRS

Death is as much a reality as birth, growth, maturity and old age—it is the one certainty of life. If the time comes when I, ____________, can no longer take part in decisions for my own future, let this statement stand as an expression of my wishes, while I am still of sound mind.

If the situation should arise in which there is no reasonable expectation of my recovery from physical or mental disability, I request that I be allowed to die and not be kept alive by artificial means or "heroic measures." I do not fear death itself as much as the indignities of deterioration, dependence and hopeless pain. I, therefore, ask that medication be mercifully administered to me to alleviate suffering even though this may hasten the moment of death.

This request is made after careful consideration. I hope you who care for me will feel morally bound to follow its mandate. I recognize that this appears to place a heavy responsibility upon you, but it is with the intention of relieving you of such responsibility and of placing it upon myself in accordance with my strong convictions that this statement is made.

Signed ____________

Date ____________

Witness ____________

Witness ____________

Copies of this request have been given to:

____

____

____

____

Figure 7–2 A sample living will

Source: For more information and a complete document contact: Concern for Dying, 250 W. 57th Street, New York, NY 10107.

Induced Abortions

Abortion laws provide specific guidelines for nurses about what is legally permissible. In 1973, when the Roe versus Wade and Doe versus Bolton cases were decided, the Supreme Court of the United States held that the constitutional rights of privacy give a woman the right to control her own body to the extent that she can abort her fetus in the early stages of pregnancy. The state, however, has a legitimate interest in controlling abortion during later stages of pregnancy. The results of the Supreme Court rulings are:

1. It is not legally permissible for the state to restrict or regulate abortions during the first trimester (first 3 months) of pregnancy except to require that the abortion be performed by a licensed physician.

2. During the second trimester of pregnancy (4 to 6 months) the mother's privacy rights must yield to *rea-*

sonable restrictions designed to protect the health and safety of the mother. Restrictions include that the facility in which the abortion is performed be licensed.

3. During the third trimester of pregnancy, the state has the right to prohibit abortion. The rationale for this ruling is that by this stage of pregnancy the state's interest in protecting the viable but unborn child outweighs the woman's right to privacy.

Since these rulings, many states have enacted statutes. In addition, the Court no longer requires that the parents of a pregnant minor consent to abortion, nor that the father of the woman's child (whether he is her husband or not) consent. Many statutes also include **conscience clauses**, upheld by the Supreme Court, designed to protect nurses and hospitals. These clauses give hospitals the right to deny admission to abortion clients and give health care personnel, including nurses, the right to refuse to participate in abortions. When these rights are exercised, the statutes also protect the agency and employee from discrimination or retaliation.

In Canada, abortion is a criminal offense that can result in up to 2 years in prison *unless* the abortion is approved by a medical abortion committee in an approved hospital.

Death and Related Issues

Legal issues surrounding death include the death certificate, labeling of the deceased, autopsy, inquest, and organ donation.

Death Certificate

By law, a death certificate must be made out when a person dies. It is usually signed by the attending physician and filed with a local health or other government office. The family is usually given a copy to use for legal matters, such as insurance claims.

Labeling the Deceased

Nurses have a duty to handle the deceased with dignity and label the corpse appropriately. Mishandling can cause emotional distress to survivors. Mislabeling can create legally libelous situations if the body is inappropriately identified and prepared incorrectly for burial or a funeral. Usually the deceased's wrist identification tag is left on, and another tag is tied to the client's ankles, in case one of the tags becomes detached. Tags tied to the ankles are preferred, since any tissue damage they cause will be concealed by bed linen or clothing. A third tag is attached to the shroud. All identification tags should include the client's name, hospital number, and physician's name.

Autopsy

An **autopsy** or **postmortem examination** is an examination of the body after death. It is performed only in certain cases. The law describes under what circumstances an autopsy must be performed, e.g., when death is sudden or when it occurs within 48 hours of admission to a hospital. The organs and tissues of the body are examined for several reasons:

1. To establish the exact cause of death
2. To learn more about a disease
3. To assist in the accumulation of statistical data

It is the responsibility of the physician or, in some instances, of a designated person in the hospital to obtain consent for autopsy. Consent must be given by the decedent (before death) or by the next of kin. Laws in many states and provinces prioritize the family members who can provide consent as follows: surviving spouse, adult children, parents, siblings. After autopsy, hospitals cannot retain any tissues or organs without the permission of the person who consented to the autopsy.

Organ Donation

Under the Uniform Anatomical Gift Act in the United States or the Human Tissue Act in Canada, any person 18 years or older and of sound mind may make a gift of all or any part of his or her body to the following persons for the following purposes (Annas et al. 1981, p. 227):

1. To any hospital, surgeon, or physician, for medical or dental education, research, advancement of medical or dental science, therapy, or transplantation.
2. To any accredited medical or dental school, college, or university for education, research, advancement of medical or dental science, or therapy.
3. To any bank or storage facility, for medical or dental education, research, advancement of medical or dental science, therapy, or transplantation.
4. To any specific individual for therapy or transplantation.

The donation can be made by a provision in a will or by signing a cardlike form in the presence of two witnesses. This card is usually carried at all times by the person who signed it. In most states and provinces, the gift can be revoked either by destroying the card or by an oral revocation in the presence of two witnesses. Nurses may serve as witnesses for persons consenting to donate organs.

Inquest

An **inquest** is a legal inquiry into the cause or manner of a death. When a death is the result of an accident, for example, an inquest will be held into the circumstances of the accident to determine any blame. The inquest is conducted under the jurisdiction of a coroner or medical examiner. A **coroner** is a public official, not necessarily a physician, appointed or elected to inquire into the causes of death, when appropriate. A **medical examiner** is a physician who usually has advanced education in pathology or forensic medicine. Agency policy dictates who is responsible for reporting deaths to the coroner or medical examiner.

Legal Protections for Nurses

Good Samaritan Acts

Good Samaritan acts are laws designed to protect physicians and other health care providers, including nurses, who provide assistance at the scene of an emergency. The health care providers in this legislation are protected against claims of malpractice unless it can be shown that there was a gross departure from the normal standard of care or willful wrongdoing on their part. Gross negligence usually involves further injury or harm to the person. For example, an injured child left on the side of the road may be struck by an automobile when the nurse leaves to obtain help.

In the United States, most state statutes do not require citizens to render aid to people in distress. Such assistance is considered more of an ethical than a legal duty. A few states, however, have enacted legislation that requires people trained in health care to stop and aid the injured. To encourage citizens to be good Samaritans, most states have now enacted legislation releasing the good Samaritan from legal liability for injuries caused under such circumstances, even if the injuries resulted from negligence of the person offering emergency aid.

In Canada, some provinces specify in traffic acts that it is the responsibility of people to give aid at the scene of an accident. Alberta is the only province that exempts physicians and nurses from liability unless gross negligence is proved. However, lawsuits against good Samaritans are rarely successful.

It is generally believed that a person who renders help in an emergency, at the level of helping that would be provided by any reasonably prudent person under similar circumstances, cannot be held liable. The same reasoning applies to nurses, who may be the people best prepared to help at the scene of an accident. If the level of care a nurse provides is of the caliber that would have been provided by any other nurse, then the nurse will not be held liable.

Professional Liability Insurance

Because of the increase in the number of malpractice lawsuits against professional people in the health field, nurses are advised in many areas to carry their own liability insurance to protect themselves.

Coverage

Most hospitals have liability insurance that adequately covers all employees, including all nurses. However, some smaller facilities, such as "walk-in" clinics, may not. Thus the nurse should always check with her employer at the time of hiring to see what kind of coverage is provided by the facility. A physician or a hospital can be sued because of the negligent conduct of a nurse, and the nurse can also be sued and held liable for negligence or malpractice. Because hospitals have been known to countersue the nurse when she or he has been found guilty of malpractice and the hospital was required to pay, nurses are advised to provide their own insurance coverage and not rely on hospital-provided insurance.

Liability insurance generally covers all costs of defending a nurse, including the costs of retaining an attorney. The insurance also covers all costs incurred by the nurse up to the face value of the policy, including a settlement made out of court. In return, the insurance company has the right to make the decisions about the claim and the settlement.

Instructor and Student Protection

Instructors of nursing and nursing students are also vulnerable to lawsuits. In hospital nursing education programs, instructors and students are often specifically covered for liability by the hospital. An instructor, however, can still be sued by a hospital in cases of negligence and malpractice.

Students and teachers of nursing employed by community colleges and universities are less likely to be covered by the insurance carried by hospitals and health agencies. It is advisable for these people to check with their employers about the coverage that applies to them. Increasingly, instructors are carrying their own malpractice insurance in both the United States and Canada. In the United States, insurance can be obtained through the American Nurses' Association or private insurance companies; in Canada, it can usually be obtained through provincial nurses' associations. Nursing students in the United States can also obtain insurance through the National Student Nurses' Association. In some states, hospitals do not allow nursing students to provide nursing care without liability insurance.

Legal Responsibilities Associated with the Nursing Process

Each step of the nursing process is associated with areas of potential liability, but the planning and evaluation phases seldom lead to liability. Failure to perform proper assessment and failure to carry out proper intervention are the focus of court decisions. Rhodes and Miller (1984; pp. 142–60) point out the following errors and responsibilities.

Assessing

The professional nurse has a responsibility to assess the health status and needs of the client and to communicate that assessment appropriately. Assessment errors can arise from:

1. Failure to take appropriate steps to gather information, e.g., asking questions, taking vital signs, and making observations. For example, if a client is admitted by ambulance to the emergency department, the nurse must obtain necessary information, e.g., the client bled profusely and has a severely depressed blood pressure, from the ambulance personnel. The nurse must also make his or her own pertinent observations of the client, take the client's vital signs, and where indicated, initiate attempts to relieve the problem. Appropriateness and frequency of observations depend on the client's needs. In a court of law, appropriateness and frequency would be determined by reference to institutional policy, physician's orders, or the standard of what a person with the same competence would do in the circumstances.

2. Failure to recognize the significance of the information gathered, within the limits of ordinary and prudent nursing knowledge. The nurse's responsibilities associated with recognizing the significance of gathered information are to communicate necessary information to the physician promptly and to initiate appropriate intervention, if necessary. In the example above, the nurse should recognize the consequences of profuse bleeding and initiate interventions to stop it. The nurse should also communicate his or her assessments, e.g., profuse bleeding, severely depressed blood pressure, and a rapid, thready pulse, to the physician immediately.

3. Failure to communicate steps taken or information gathered. Observations and knowledge gained during assessment of the client must be properly documented, and timely verbal notification must also be given when necessary. Documenting assessment data about the client is essential. Entries should be made promptly and be complete, accurate, and specific. For detailed information about recording and reporting, see Chapter 30. The nurse's responsibilities in regard to verbal communications can include:

   a. Information obtained during the initial contact with a client. For example, the nurse should communicate to the physician that a man admitted with multiple injuries stated he was receiving cortisone therapy. Failure to inform the physician of this fact could result in inappropriate medical orders with serious consequences for the client.

   b. Information derived from monitoring a client. The nurse is expected to discern abnormalities in the client's condition, decide whether assistance from a physician or others is required, and, if so, promptly inform them. For example, the nurse who notices that a client with a cast applied for a wrist fracture has fingers that are swollen, cold, blue, and lacking in sensation should report this information immediately to the physician. Failure to do so or delays in reporting can result in serious damage to the client's hand and wrist. Failure to report is not excused by the nurse's belief that the physician is not likely to respond. The physician must be notified; if he or she does not respond, the nurse must then notify the nursing supervisor or follow other necessary agency procedures so that essential care can be provided to the client.

   c. Information that should be shared with others who are working with the client at the same time or with those who are assuming responsibility for care of the client. For example, the nurse who is monitoring a client's vital signs during a special procedure conducted by the physician is obliged to inform the physician of significant changes. When a client is transferred to another unit or facility where others will be providing care, the nurse must provide appropriate and complete information.

Planning

Using the information gathered about the client, the nurse must plan what care is appropriate for the client and also how to implement the physician's orders. Few court proceedings focus on this step; rather, they focus on an intervention (or lack thereof) formulated during the planning stage.

Intervening

During the intervention phase of the nursing process, the nurse has a responsibility to interpret and carry out the physician's orders promptly and to implement nursing interventions appropriately.

Carrying Out Physician's Orders

Nurses are expected to know basic information about procedures and medications ordered by the physician. It is the nurse's responsibility to seek clarification of ambiguous or seemingly erroneous orders from the prescribing physician. Clarification from any other source is unacceptable and regarded as a departure from competent nursing practice. If the order is neither ambiguous nor apparently erroneous, the nurse is responsible for carrying it out. For example, if the physician orders oxygen to be administered at 4 liters per minute, the nurse must administer oxygen at that rate, and not at 2 or 6 liters per minute. If the orders state that the client is not to have solid food after a bowel resection, the nurse must ensure that no solid food is given to the client. Nurses who carry out orders that are neither ambiguous nor considered dangerous for the client receive significant protection from liability (Rhodes and Miller 1984, p. 152). Nurses also have a responsibility to check for changes in orders from previous shifts of duty.

Becker (1983, pp. 21–23) outlines four orders that nurses must question to protect themselves legally:

1. Question any order a client questions. For example, if a client who has been receiving an intramuscular injection tells the nurse that the doctor changed the order from an injectable to an oral medication, the nurse should recheck the order before giving the medication.

2. Question any order if the client's condition has changed. The nurse is considered responsible for notifying the physician of any significant changes in the client's condition, whether the physician requests notification or not. For example, if a client who is receiving an intravenous infusion suddenly develops a rapid pulse, chest pain, and a cough, the nurse must notify the physician immediately and question continuance of the order. If a client who is receiving morphine for pain develops severely depressed respirations, the nurse must withhold the medication and notify the physician.

3. Question and record verbal orders to avoid miscommunications. In addition to recording the time, the date, the physician's name, and the orders, the nurse documents the circumstances that occasioned the call to the physician, reads the orders back to the physician, and documents that the physician confirmed the orders as the nurse read them back.

4. Question standing orders, especially if the nurse is inexperienced. Standing orders give the nurse added responsibility to exercise appropriate judgment when implementing them. The nurse is delegated the authority to, for example, adjust the amount of a medication or other substances and make decisions about when a medication is needed. Nurses need to take the same precautions when implementing these orders as when implementing any other orders. In addition, the nurse who does not feel confident about exercising discretionary judgment should request specific guidelines from the physician or assistance from a more experienced nurse or supervisor. In some states, standing orders are not allowed except in intensive care or coronary care units.

Implementing Delegated and Independent Nursing Interventions

Nurses implementing care need to take the following precautions (Rhodes and Miller 1984, pp. 153–60) and Grane 1983, pp. 17–20):

1. Know their job description. This enables nurses to function within the scope of the description and know what is and what is not expected. Job descriptions vary from agency to agency. For example, in one agency nurses may be expected to perform venipunctures and remove Penrose drains and sutures. In another agency, the physician may be responsible for these functions.

2. Follow the policies and procedures of the agency in which they are working.

3. Always identify clients, particularly before initiating major interventions, e.g., surgical or other invasive procedures, or when administering blood transfusions.

4. Make sure the correct medications are given in the correct dose, by the right route, at the scheduled time, and to the right client. See Chapter 51 for more detailed information about the administration of medications.

5. Perform procedures appropriately. Negligent incidents during procedures generally relate to equipment failure, improper technique, and improper performance of the procedure. For instance, the nurse must know how to safeguard the client in the event that a respirator or other equipment fails. An example of improper technique is administering an intramuscular injection too near the sciatic nerve, causing pain and damage to the nerve. Nurses are advised to read procedure manuals and to ask for guidance when in doubt.

6. Promptly and accurately document all assessments and care given. Records must show that the nurse provided and supervised the client's care daily.

7. Report all incidents involving clients. Prompt reports enable those responsible to attend to the client's well-

being, to analyze why the incident occurred, and to prevent recurrences.

8. Build and maintain good rapport with clients. Keeping clients informed about diagnostic and treatment plans, giving feedback on their progress, and showing concern for the outcome of their care prevent a sense of powerlessness and a build-up of hostility in the client.
9. Maintain clinical competence in their area of practice. For students, this demands study and practice before caring for clients. For graduate nurses, it means continued study, including maintaining and updating clinical knowledge and skills. All nurses should take steps to improve their nursing care, especially if a formal performance appraisal indicates deficiencies.
10. Know their own strengths and weaknesses. A nurse who recognizes that he or she has difficulty calculating medication dosages should always ask someone to check the calculations before proceeding.
11. Nurses who delegate nursing responsibilities must make sure the person to whom they are delegating understands what to do and that the knowledge and skill required are within her or his area of competence. A nurse can be held liable if a client is harmed by actions of the person to whom the care was delegated.
12. Be alert when implementing nursing interventions and give each task their full attention and skill.

Ways nurses can protect themselves legally are summarized to the right.

Legal Precautions for Nurses

- Function within the scope of their education and job description.
- Follow the procedures and policies of the employing agency.
- Take appropriate steps to obtain complete nursing histories.
- Observe and monitor the client adequately.
- Communicate and record significant changes in the client's condition to the physician.
- Carry out physicians' orders promptly and correctly, provided the orders are not ambiguous or considered dangerous for the client.
- Check any orders that a client questions.
- Identify clients before initiating major interventions.
- Give medications as ordered to the right client.
- Perform procedures appropriately.
- Protect clients from falls and preventable injuries.
- Document all nursing assessments and interventions accurately and promptly.
- Ask for assistance and supervision in situations for which they feel inadequately prepared.
- Delegate tasks to persons with the knowledge and skill to carry them out.
- Build and maintain good rapport with their clients.

Evaluating

Although the evaluation phase of the nursing process is important, it seldom leads to liability. Since the evaluation phase involves assessment and appropriate adjustments in interventions as a result of those assessments, the nurse could be liable for failures in these areas. For example, a nurse can be held liable for failing to report increased drainage, pain, and a foul odor in a client's incision following antibiotic therapy and failing to implement appropriate measures.

Legal Responsibilities of Students

Student nurses are responsible for their own actions and liable for their own acts of negligence committed during the course of clinical experiences. When they perform duties that are within the scope of professional nursing, such as administering an injection, they are legally held to the same standard of skill and competence as a registered professional nurse (Rhodes and Miller 1984, p. 163). Lower standards are *not* applied to the actions of student nurses.

In cases arising from negligent acts by student nurses, the student nurse was traditionally treated as an employee of the hospital, which was held liable under the doctrine of *respondeat superior.* Today, associate degree and baccalaureate nursing students are not considered employees of the agencies in which they receive clinical experience, since these nursing programs contract with agencies to provide clinical experiences for students. In future cases of negligence involving such students, the hospital or agency (e.g., public health agency) and the educational institution will be held potentially liable for negligent actions by students (Rhodes and Miller 1984, p. 164).

Students in clinical situations must be assigned activity within their capabilities and be given reasonable guidance and supervision. Nursing instructors are responsible for assigning students to the care of clients and for providing reasonable supervision. Failure to provide reasonable supervision and/or the assignment of a client to a student who is not prepared and competent can be a basis for liability.

To fulfill responsibilities to clients and to minimize chances for liability, student nurses need to (Rhodes and Miller 1984, p. 164):

1. Make sure they are prepared to carry out the necessary care for assigned clients.
2. Ask for additional help or supervision in situations for which they feel inadequately prepared.
3. Comply with the policies of the agency in which they obtain their clinical experience.
4. Comply with the policies and definitions of responsibility supplied by the nursing school.

Students who work as part-time or temporary nursing assistants or aides must also remember that legally they can perform only those tasks that appear in the job description of a nurse's aide or assistant. Even though a student may have received instruction and thus acquired competence in administering injections or suctioning a tracheostomy tube, she or he cannot perform these tasks while employed as an aide or assistant.

Chapter Highlights

- Accountability is an essential concept of professional nursing practice under the law.
- Nurses need to understand laws that regulate and affect nursing practice to ensure that the nurses' actions are consistent with current legal principles and to protect the nurse from liability.
- Nurse practice acts legally define and describe the scope of nursing practice that the law seeks to regulate.
- Competence in nursing practice is determined and maintained by various credentialing methods, such as licensure, registration, certification, and accreditation, which protect the public's welfare and safety.
- Standards of care published by national and state or provincial nursing association and agency policies, procedures, and job descriptions further delineate the scope of a nurse's practice.
- The nurse has specific legal obligations and responsibilities to clients and employers and as a citizen.
- Nurses have three separate interdependent legal roles.
- As a provider of service, the nurse is expected to provide safe and competent care to the client and to protect the client from harm.
- As an employee, the nurse has rights and responsibilities within the confines of job descriptions and contractual relationships.
- As a citizen, the nurse has the same fundamental legal rights as any person in the society.
- Collective bargaining is one way nurses can improve their working conditions and economic welfare.
- Nurses can be held liable for the death of clients; for intentional torts, such as fraud, invasion of privacy, defamation, assault and battery, and false imprisonment; and for unintentional torts or negligence.
- Negligence or malpractice of nurses is established when (a) the nurse (defendant) owed a duty to the client, (b) the nurse failed to carry out that duty, (c) the client (plaintiff) was injured, and (d) the client's injury was caused by the nurse's failure to carry out her or his duty.
- One standard used to determine a nurse's liability for negligence is what would have been done in similar circumstances by a reasonable and prudent professional with similar preparation and experience.
- Nurses may on occasion be called into court as expert witnesses to confirm whether the defendant did or did not do what a reasonable prudent nurse would do under the same circumstances.
- The nurse is responsible for ensuring that the physician obtains informed consents from clients (or from the closest relative in emergencies or from parents or guardians when the client is a minor) before treatment regimens and procedures begin.
- Informed consent implies that (a) the consent was given voluntarily; (b) the client was of age and had the capacity and competence to understand; (c) consent was given after an explanation of the benefits, risks, and other facts relating to the procedure; and (d) the client understood the explanations.
- The client's medical record is a legal document and can be produced in court as evidence; nurses, therefore, must keep accurate and complete records of nursing care provided to clients.
- When a client is accidentally injured or involved in an unusual situation that may involve liability, the nurse's first responsibility is to take steps to protect the client and then to notify staff and family.

- An incident report needs to include assessment data, witnesses to the situation, descriptive facts of the incident, and surrounding circumstances.
- The nurse who witnesses a client's will must ensure that the client is of sound mind and not unduly influenced by others; the nurse must also document the client's physical and mental status on the nursing records.
- Living wills are receiving increasing attention; because statutes that authorize living wills vary, nurses need to familiarize themselves with their specifications.
- The legality of no-code and slow-code orders is not well established; nurses are advised to follow the American Heart Association standards for no-code orders.
- Induced abortion laws are clearly established in the United States; in Canada, abortion must be approved by a medical abortion committee in an approved hospital.
- Nurses must be knowledgable about their responsibilities in regard to legal issues surrounding death: death certificate, labeling of the deceased, autopsy, organ donation, and inquest.
- Good Samaritan acts protect health professionals from claims of malpractice when they provide assistance at the scene of an emergency provided there is not willful wrongdoing or gross departure from normal standards of care.
- Practicing nurses who are not covered by liability insurance in their employing agency can obtain liability insurance through professional nursing associations.
- Registered nursing students are accountable for all their actions; they are legally held to the same standard of skill and competence as registered professional nurses.
- Student nurses need to make sure they are prepared to provide the necessary care for assigned clients and ask for help or supervision in situations for which they feel inadequately prepared.
- Professional nurses can protect themselves from liability claims by conscientiously implementing the steps of the nursing process, since failure to perform proper client assessment and failure to carry out proper interventions are the focus of court decisions.
- Nurses can further protect themselves by (a) functioning within the confines of nurse practice acts, job descriptions, and agency policies and procedures; (b) documenting all nursing assessments and interventions completely and accurately; (c) maintaining clinical competence within their area of practice; and (d) implementing the physician's orders correctly provided the orders are clear and safe for the client.

Suggested Readings

Baer, O. J. May/June 1985. Protecting your patient's privacy. *Nursing Life* 5:50–53.
Baer discusses clients' rights to privacy under the law. Such problems as responding to a family's questions, responding to media inquiries, and discussing clients with others are addressed. The author reviews reporting guidelines and discusses how court decisions affect clients' right to privacy. Baer recommends that nurses secure professional liability insurance and then make sure it is never needed.

Fine, E. R. J. November/December 1982. What to do when the doctor's wrong. *Nursing Life* 2:22–24.
Fine provides several case examples and explains the nurse's duty to recognize and report. Included is a discussion of how the nurse can determine whether care is inadequate and what a prudent nurse should know. Fine provides guidelines for professional behavior and emphasizes that the nurse shares responsibility for the client with the doctor.

Huttman, B. R. January 1982. Dilemmas in practice. No code? Slow code? Show code? *American Journal of Nursing* 82:133, 135–36.
Huttman discusses the dilemma for the nurse when the physician refuses to write a no-code order or discontinue treatment when the family wishes it. Educating the public about their options is recommended.

Klimon, E. L. March/April 1985. Do you swear to tell the truth? *Nursing Economics* 3:98–102.
Klimon describes what may happen when a health professional must testify at a malpractice suit. Klimon tells nurses how to prepare for a deposition; gives advice on appearance, demeanor, and enunciation; and prepares the reader for the personal and professional information that one may need to provide. Points addressed include identifying exhibits, understanding the question, and keeping answers brief. It is exceedingly important to tell the truth and not to qualify favorable facts.

Kravitz, M. November 1985. Informed consent: Must ethical responsibility conflict with professional conduct? *Nursing Management* 16:34A–B, 34D–H.
Kravitz describes the traditional attitudes toward consent and the changes that have taken place. Topics addressed include consent in research and the need for professionals to resolve the ethical and professional issues associated with consent.

Linn, A. January/February 1982. When your patient wants to die, should you help? *Nursing Life* 2:30–33.
Although living will, the right to die, and freedom of choice seem to be reasonable as abstract ideas, how acceptable do they seem when you have to apply them to a real client? This author discusses supporting the client when you dis-

agree, supporting the client when the physician disagrees, supporting the client when the family disagrees, and supporting the client when his wishes are not clear.

Rabinow, J. September/October 1982. Delegating safely within the law. *Nursing Life* 2:48–49.
In regard to the legal risks of delegating, Rabinow discusses what tasks are appropriate to delegate, which people are appropriate to perform delegated tasks, how to choose the right person, and what responsibilities the delegator has after tasks are delegated. Rabinow lists some duties that, although not within the scope of practice of LPNs, are legally assignable to LPNs in some states and provinces.

Sklar, C. April 1984. You and the law: An act of negligence contributes to dismissal. *Canadian Nurse* 80:45.
Sklar describes a situation in which a client falls off a chair. At a hearing, witnesses give differing views. After considering the quality of care and the record of the employee, the board ruled in favor of the hospital.

Wiley, L. September 1981. Liability for death: Nine nurses' legal ordeals. *Nursing 81* 11:34–43.
Wiley presents nine nurses' highly publicized experiences in regard to liability for client deaths. The experiences provide some lessons that may help other nurses avoid such liability.

Selected References

American Heart Association. June 6, 1986. Standards and guidelines for cardiopulmonary resuscitation and emergency cardiac care. *Journal of the American Medical Association.* 255:2841–3044.

American Nurses' Association. 1961. *Legal definition of nursing.* Kansas City, Mo.: American Nurses' Association.

———. July 1973. ANA issues statement on diploma graduates. *American Journal of Nursing* 73:1135.

———. 1975. *Human rights guidelines for nurses in clinical and other research.* Publication no. D-46 5M 7/75. Kansas City, Mo.: American Nurses' Association.

———. 1976. *The code for nurses.* Kansas City, Mo.: American Nurses' Association.

———. April 1979. Credentialing in nursing. A new approach. Report of the Committee for the study of Credentialing in Nursing. *American Journal of Nursing* 79:674–83.

———. 1985. *The grievance procedure.* Kansas City, Mo.: American Nurses' Association.

American Nurses' Association Cabinet on Economic and General Welfare. 1985. *The nature and scope of ANA's economic and general welfare program.* Kansas City, Mo.: American Nurses' Association.

Annas, G. J.; Glantz, L. H.; and Katz, B. F. 1981. *The right of doctors, nurses and allied health professionals.* New York: Avon Books.

Baer, O. J. May/June 1985. Protecting your patient's privacy. *Nursing Life* 5:50–53.

Barbash, J. 1980. Collective bargaining: Contemporary American experience—A commentary. In *Collective bargaining: Contemporary American experience.* G. H. Sommers, editor. Madison, Wis.: Industrial Relations Research Association.

Becker, M. January/February 1983. Five orders you must question to protect yourself legally. *Nursing Life* 3:21–23.

Cournoyer, C. P. March/April 1985. Protecting yourself legally after a patient's injured. *Nursing Life* 5:18–22.

Crawford, M.; Fisher, M.; and Kilbane, N. 1985. Collective bargaining in nursing. In DeYoung, L. *Dynamics of nursing.* 5th ed. St. Louis: C. V. Mosby Co.

———. February 1983. Law for the nurse manager. Incident reports subject to discovery? *Nursing Management* 14:55, 57.

Creighton, H. 1981. *Law every nurse should know.* 4th ed. Philadelphia: W. B. Saunders Co.

———. November 1985. Law for the nurse manager. Relatives sue for putting patient on life support. *Nursing Management* 16:56, 60.

Curtin, L. L. October 1982. Informed consent: Rights, responsibilities, and roles. *Nursing Management* 13:7–8.

Cushing, M. August 1985. Incident reports: For your eyes only? *American Journal of Nursing* 85:873–74.

———. February 1986. How courts look at nurse practice acts. *American Journal of Nursing* 86:131.

Davis, A. January/February 1985. Informed consent: How much information is enough? *Nursing Outlook* 33:40–42.

Doe v. Bolton, 410 U.S. 179 (1973); Roe v. Wade, 410 U.S. 113 (1973).

Erickson, E. H. March/April 1973. Collective bargaining: An inappropriate technique for professionals. *Journal of Nursing Administration* 3:54–58.

Facts to know about living wills. January/February 1984. *Nursing Life* 4:26–27.

Fenner, K. 1980. *Ethics and the law in nursing.* New York: D. Van Nostrand Co.

Flanagen, L. 1983. *Collective bargaining and the nursing profession.* Kansas City, Mo.: American Nurses' Association.

Grand, N. K. March/April 1973. Nursing ideologies and collective bargaining. *Journal of Nursing Administration* 3:29–32.

Grane, N. B. January/February 1983. How to reduce your risk of a lawsuit. *Nursing Life* 3:17–20.

Instructor/student nurse/head nurse triangle: Legalities. June 1982. *Regan Report on Nursing Law* 23:2.

Labor-Management Relations Act. 1947. Section 8(d).

Lewis, E. P. September/October 1985. Taking care of business: The ANA house of delegates. *Nursing Outlook* 33:239–43.

Mackert, M. E., and Hemelt, M. D. September/October 1985. Avoiding legal risks in the E.D. *Nursing Life* 5:26–29.

Markowitz, L. A. May/June 1982. How your state board works for you. *Nursing Life* 2:25–26, 32.

McClelland, J. Q. November 1983. Professionalism and collective bargaining: A new reality for nurses and management. *Journal of Nursing Administration* 13:36–38.

Murchison, I.; Nichols, T. S.; and Janson, R. 1982. *Legal accountability in the nursing process.* 2d ed. St. Louis: C. V. Mosby Co.

Northrop, C. 1984. Legal aspects of nursing. In McCann Flynn, J. B., and Heffron, P. B. *Nursing: From concept to practice.* Bowie, Md.: Robert J. Brady Co.

———. January 1985. The ins and outs of informed consent. *Nursing 85* 15:21.

Numerof, R. E., and Abrams, M. N. Spring 1984. Collective bargaining among nurses: Current issues and future prospects. *Health Care Management Review* 9:61–67.

Nursing education and students' rights: Legalities . . . when charged with academic dishonesty. August 1983. *Regan Report on Nursing Law* 24:4.

A *Nursing Life* poll report on ethics. March/April 1983. Do you make your patient live . . . or let him die? *Nursing Life* 3:54–55.

Oberst, M. November/December 1985. Another look at informed consent. *Nursing Outlook* 33:294–95.

O'Sullivan, A. L. May 1980. Privileged communication. *American Journal of Nursing* 80:947–50.

Ozimek, D. February 1982. Rights and responsibilities of students and faculty. *Imprint* 29:50–51.

Pettengill, M. M. September/October 1985. Multilateral collective bargaining and the health care industry: Implications for nursing. *Journal of Professional Nursing* 1:275–82.

Price, D. M., and Murphy, P. January/February 1983. How—and when—to blow the whistle on unsafe practices. *Nursing Life* 3:50–54.

Rhodes, A. M., and Miller, R. D. 1984. *Nursing and the Law.* 4th ed. Rockville, Md.: Aspen Systems Corporation.

Rudy, E. B. June 1985. The living will: Are you informed? *Focus on Critical Care* 12:51–57.

Sklar, C. June 1980. Was the patient informed? *Canadian Nurse* 76:18, 20, 22.

Smith, G. R. July/August 1985. Unionization for nurses: An issue for the 1980s. *Journal of Professional Nursing* 1:192–201.

Snyder, M. E., and LaBar, C. 1984. *Issues in professional nursing practice 1. Nursing: Legal authority for practice.* Kansas City, Mo.: American Nurses' Association.

U.S. Department of Labor. 1979. *Impact of the 1974 health care amendments to the NLRA on collective bargaining in the health care industry.* Washington, D.C.: U.S. Government Printing Office.

Veninga, K., and Veninga, R. April 1982. The PATCO problem and nursing: A comparative analysis. *Nursing Outlook* 30:265–67.

Wasiuta, V. September 1982. Reporting incidents: How many is too many? *Dimensions in Health Service* 59:16–18.

Wiley, L. September 1981. Liability for death: Nine nurses' legal ordeals. *Nursing 81* 11:34–43.

Williams, R. M. March/April 1984. Collective bargaining and political lobbying: Tools to accomplish professional nursing goals. *Michigan Nurse* 57:1.

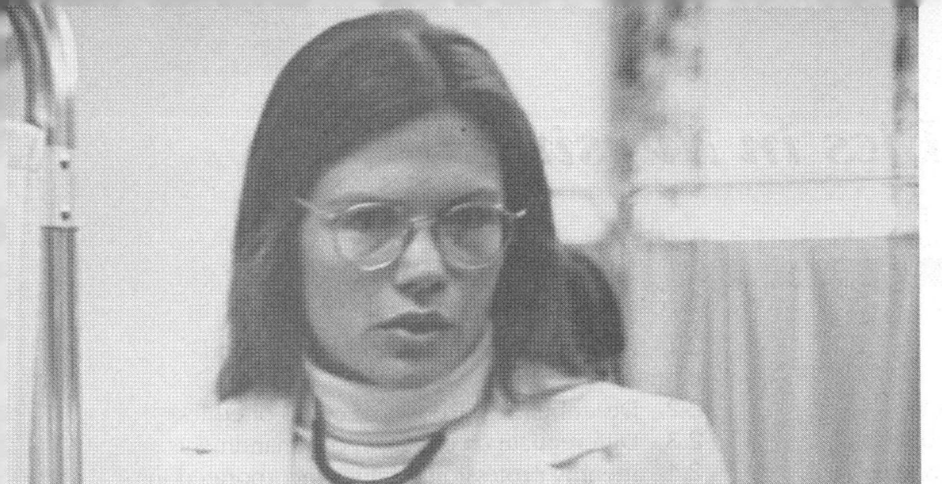

MARIANNE GONTARZ

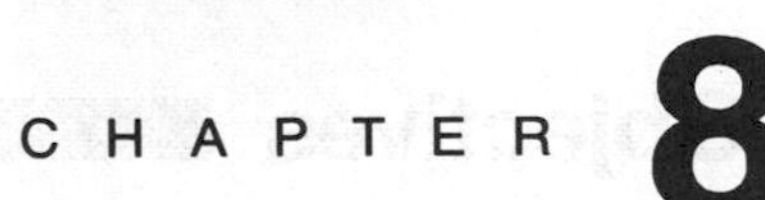

CHAPTER **8**

Values and Ethics in Nursing

Contents

8 *Values and Ethics in Nursing*

Objectives

1. Understand essential facts about values.
   1.1 Define listed terms.
   1.2 Differentiate a belief from an attitude.
   1.3 Describe the criteria to be met for beliefs, attitudes, activities, or feelings to become values.
   1.4 Differentiate morality from moral behavior.
   1.5 Identify seven criteria that must be met before beliefs and attitudes become values.
   1.6 Identify six ways in which values, beliefs, and attitudes are learned.
   1.7 Identify selected personal and professional values.
   1.8 Describe Rath's process of developing values.
   1.9 Identify five advantages of values clarification.
   1.10 Identify personal values related to specific issues such as sexuality, unwanted pregnancy, sex-role stereotypes, right to die, abortion, health, and health care.
   1.11 Describe reasons for identifying clients' values.
   1.12 Describe ways in which the nurse can help clients clarify their values.
   1.13 Differentiate a value conflict from an ethical or moral dilemma.
   1.14 State three criteria of a moral dilemma.
2. Appreciate the significance of professional ethics.
   2.1 Differentiate ethics from bioethics and morals.
   2.2 Describe the purposes of codes of ethics.
   2.3 Differentiate creeds from commandments.
   2.4 Identify professional values incorporated in nursing codes of ethics.
   2.5 Differentiate three theoretical approaches to bioethics.
3. Understand essential facts about bioethical issues in nursing.
   3.1 Explain some ways in which personal values can conflict with professional responsibilities.
   3.2 Give some examples of ethical issues between nurses and their peers.
   3.3 Give some examples of ethical issues between nurses and clients.
   3.4 Give some examples of ethical issues between nurses and other health professionals.
   3.5 Give some examples of ethical issues between nurses and agencies.
4. Understand three approaches used to resolve ethical dilemmas.
   4.1 Compare three approaches used to resolve ethical dilemmas.
   4.2 Describe a six-step approach outlined in this chapter.

Terms

attitude
autonomy
belief
beneficence
bioethics
code of ethics
commandment
creed
deontology
dilemma
ethics
extrinsic value
intrinsic value
intuitionism
justice
modeling
moral behavior
morality
moralizing
nonmaleficence
purposive behavior
socialization
teleology
value
value conflict
values clarification
value set
value system

Values, Beliefs, Attitudes, and Ethics Defined

Nurses are becoming increasingly aware of the values, beliefs, and attitudes of clients and their support persons and of the ethics involved in nursing practice. Values, beliefs, and attitudes differ from one another but are often interconnected.

A **value** can be defined as something of worth, a belief held dear by a person. A value is an affective disposition toward a person, object, or idea (Steele and Harmon 1983, p. 1). According to Simon et al. (1978), "values are a set of personal beliefs and attitudes about the truth, beauty, worth of any thought, object, or behavior. They are action oriented and give direction and meaning to one's life." Values develop from associations with people, the environment and self; they are derived from life experiences (Steele and Harmon 1983, p. 1). Values form a basis for behavior; a person's real values are shown by consistent patterns of behavior. Once one is aware of one's values, the values become an internal control for behavior.

Values common to many people are peace, truth, and

freedom, for example. Values exist in some relationship to one another within a person. A **value system** is the organization of a person's values along a continuum of relative importance. Values underlie people's purposive behavior. **Purposive behavior** refers to actions that are performed "on purpose" with the intention of reaching some goal or bringing about a certain result (Muldary 1983, p. 200). Purposive behavior, then, is based on a person's decisions or choices, and these decisions or choices are based on underlying values.

There are two types of values: intrinsic and extrinsic. An **intrinsic value** relates to the maintenance of life, e.g., food and water have intrinsic value. An **extrinsic value** originates outside the individual and is not necessary for the maintenance of life, e.g., health, holism, and humanism (Steele and Harmon 1983, p. 2).

Values can be either positive or negative. A positive value is a view about what is desirable or how something *should be*. For example, some nurses value a holistic approach to nursing; that is an approach that is desirable. Negative values, by contrast, are views of what is undesirable or how something *should not be*. For example, talking unkindly about clients is considered by many nurses to be undesirable. Therefore, being unkind is a negative value.

A **belief** (opinion) is something accepted as true by a judgment of probability rather than actuality. It is a special type of attitude whose cognitive (intellectual) component is based more on faith than on fact. People hold beliefs that may be true or that can, with reliable evidence, be proved true. Family traditions and folklore are beliefs passed from one generation to another.

Beliefs may or may not involve values. For example, a client may believe that all nurses are honest. The client has accepted that a relationship exists between "nurse" and "honesty"; nurse being the object and honesty the value. The client considers this relationship self-evident. A belief of this type is sometimes called a value judgment.

An **attitude** is a feeling tone directed toward a person, object, or idea. Attitudes have behavioral, cognitive, and affective components. The behavioral component of an attitude is exemplified by the tendency of the person to take action. It reflects the inclination of the individual to act as a result of his or her attitude. For example, a nurse who dislikes a peer's behavior toward a client is inclined to think, "If she speaks that way to Mr. B again I am going to. . . ." This is the inclination to act; a part of one's attitude toward the peer. The cognitive component of an attitude includes the beliefs and factual information associated with the attitude, e.g., nursing is a high-stress occupation. The affective component may be the central component of an attitude. It is the feelings that are associated with the belief, knowledge, and the target of the attitude. Feelings vary greatly among people; for example, one client may feel very strongly about the sound from a television in the next room, whereas another client dismisses it as unimportant. The affective component of one's attitudes is usually rooted in a person's values (Muldary 1983, p. 210).

Attitudes are made up of many beliefs (Steele and Harmon 1983, p. 3). For example, a child may learn such attitudes as cooperation and kindness from parents and in turn exhibit these in behavior. According to values clarification theory, a belief or attitude can become a value only if the belief satisfies seven criteria. See the section on values later in this chapter.

Ethics are the rules or principles that govern right conduct. The word *ethics* is derived from the Greek *ethos*, meaning custom or character. An ethic is "what ought to be." The term *bioethics* is being used increasingly in the health field. **Bioethics** are the ethics concerning life. Nurses are confronted with bioethical problems in the health care system, e.g., abortion and maintaining life with complex machinery.

Morality is a word often used interchangeably with ethics. "Morality concerns behavior which involves judgments, actions, and attitudes based on rationally conceived and effectively established norms" (Steele and Harmon 1983, p. 49). In other words, **morality** denotes what is right and wrong in conduct, character, or attitude and what individuals must do to live together in society. The way a person perceives the requirements for living together and responds to them is **moral behavior**. People learn morals during their **socialization**, the process by which individuals learn the knowledge, skills, and dispositions of their social group or society. Lawrence Kohlberg sees six stages in the moral development of individuals. See Chapter 22 for Kohlberg's theory and other theories of moral development as proposed by Kegan and Gilligan. Also see Table 8–1 for a summary of moral development.

Values

Each person, e.g., nurse, client, and physician, has a personal set of values. A **value set** is the group of values a person holds. Individuals incorporate personal values into their lives as a result of observing the behavior and attitudes of parents and teachers and interacting with their

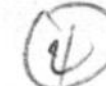
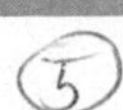
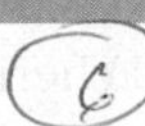

cultural, religious, and social environments. Personal values also reflect experiences, and a person's intelligence.

Professional values are a reflection and expansion of personal values (Fromer 1981, p. 15). These values are acquired as a nurse is socialized into the nursing profession.

Table 8–1 Summary of Moral Development

Developmental Stage	Moral Development	Examples of Values Developed
Infant (0 to 1 years)	The infant is generally considered not to have values but perceives emotions and the behavior of others. A mother's or caregiver's behavior toward the infant can reflect her or his values.	Parents who communicate love to their infants and convey pleasure in the infant's pleasure teach the infant the values of love and caring.
Toddler (1 to 3 years)	The toddler learns values largely through copying others; i.e., through modeling. Toddlers don't understand the meaning behind a value.	By showing appreciation and saying thank you when others give gifts and when the toddler starts to give the parent toys, objects, or food, parents teach toddlers that "giving" makes others feel good and, in turn, makes one feel good about oneself.
Preschooler (4 to 5 years)	The preschooler learns the right and wrong of singular acts but does not possess a concept of right and wrong.	By pointing out to her son that taking a toy away from a sister or friend is wrong and makes the other person feel as badly as he would if the same happened to him, a mother teachers the child to consider other person's feelings and to treat everyone as you want to be treated.
School-aged child (6 to 12 years)	People with diverse values have contact with school-aged children. Parents who provide alternatives in situations help the school-aged child solve problems, make decisions, and learn the value of self-determination.	Parents who help and encourage a child with a school project teach the child the value of industry and completing projects once started.
Adolescent (12 to 18 years)	Adolescents encounter a multitude of new values. Adolescents learn to identify some of their own significant values. Parents continue to be a major source of values.	Parents who recognize that the adolescent and other people have the right to his or her own tastes and preferences convey to the adolescent the value of respect for others.
Early adulthood	Most young adults can identify many of their own values. Although these may be tested through experience, the young adult establishes these as part of self. Some values may differ from those of his or her parents.	By moving away from home and through widening experiences, a young adult develops values associated with health, e.g., becomes a vegetarian and exercises daily.
Middle adulthood	Middle-aged adults who are secure and satisfied with their values will experience pleasure and a sense of serenity with each day. People who are dissatisfied and insecure may discard held values.	A man who values youth and helping others spends much of his time with scouts.
Late adulthood	The older adult may see his or her values challenged in a changing society. Older adults often learn to appreciate differing values of others but at the same time keep their own values.	A woman accepts that her grandson is living with his girlfriend, although for her, marriage is very important before people of the opposite sex live together.

Acquisition of Values

Raths et al. (1978) identified seven criteria that must be met for beliefs, attitudes, activities, or feelings to become values:

1. Having been freely chosen without outside pressure
2. Having been chosen from among alternatives
3. Having been chosen after reflection
4. Having been prized and cherished
5. Having been affirmed to others
6. Having been incorporated into actual behavior
7. Having been repeated in one's life (Thompson 1985, p. 77)

A value must meet the above criteria, i.e., it is a belief put into practice (Thompson and Thompson 1985, p. 78). Values are also hierarchical, i.e., each person has an individual hierarchy of values, ranging from the most important value to the least important value. For information about health values, see Chapter 20.

Values Transmission

Each person has a relatively small number of values. The origin of these values can be traced to culture, society, institutions, and personality. In addition, these few values guide virtually all aspects of behavior (Rokeach and Regan 1981, p. 576). Values are learned and are greatly influenced by a person's sociocultural environment. For example, Puerto Ricans often value treatment by a folk healer over treatment by a physician. For additional information about cultural and ethnic values relative to health and illness, see Chapter 18.

Values are learned throughout life; however, many values are learned in early childhood. Acquiring values is usually a gradual process of which the individual is unaware. People do not always realize they have a specific set of values or that they base the decisions they make on values. Values are transmitted in a variety of ways. Four approaches are modeling, laissez-faire, moralizing, and responsible choice (Simon et al. 1978, pp. 15–18).

Modeling

Modeling is a process by which a person engages in ideal behavior to serve as an example to be imitated by other persons (Johnson 1972, p. 189). There are two steps in modeling: (a) one person must engage in the ideal behavior, and (b) the second person must imitate the first person's behavior.

Parents are important models. Young children often want to be like their parents and will copy their parents' behavior. Through modeling, they behave in a manner that they perceive represents ideal values. However, modeling also can transmit socially unacceptable values. For example, a man who repeatedly hits his wife during an argument is modeling a socially unacceptable way to resolve a disagreement.

Laissez-faire

In this approach, people are left alone "to do their own thing." For example, a child is left free to have new experiences and to form his or her own values without parental guidance. The problem with this approach is that children can become confused when the adults around them do not support any behavior. For young people or people being socialized into roles, e.g., the nursing role, a laissez-faire approach to learning values can result in conflict and frustration.

Moralizing

Moralizing is a direct method of inculcating values in another person. In some religions, moralizing is the basis of indoctrination into the religion: people are told what is "right" and what is "wrong." People who learn their values through moralizing can have difficulty making responsible choices later in life because they have no experience doing so. Moralizing is a rigid approach to transmitting values: Alternatives are not provided, and the individual has no choice if he or she wishes to do or believe what is "right."

Responsible Choice

Values are also transmitted through responsible choice. The individual does not have free choice but is given limited choices. An example is the teenager who is allowed to use the family car only if it is returned by ten o'clock. The teenager has two choices that control behavior: to not use the car or to use it and return it on time. It is questionable, however, whether the teenager in this situation learns any values on which to base future behavior.

Values are also taught, usually by parents and by teachers in school and in religious organizations. For example, a parent will explain to a toddler that he or she should ask for a cookie before taking one, or a father will explain to a son how to be considerate on his first date. People also learn values through experience. For example, a young boy who drinks alcohol and then has an accident with the family car can learn from that experience to value safety and concern for others as well as himself when he drives. For additional information about teaching strategies, see Chapter 29.

Personal and Professional Values

The nurse enters the profession of nursing with values that guide personal actions. Through the process of socialization into the profession, the nurse chooses additional values. Personal and professional values are closely related and often can be the same. Hall (1973, pp. 23–32) identifies two primary values that are related to and must be in harmony with each other:

1. Self-value, or the idea that one is of worth to others
2. The idea that others are of equal worth

These primary values are not only vital as personal values in North American society but also vital as professional values, since nursing is based on relationships with clients, colleagues, and others.

Nurses' personal values influence client-nurse interactions and the practice of nursing. Steele and Harmon (1983, p. 7) believe that nurses can enact their professional roles with minimal discomfort when their personal and professional values are reasonably congruent. Thompson and Thompson (1985, p. 81) agree that nurses who are comfortable with their professional roles probably experience greater satisfaction and possibly provide better care for clients but question the latter point. A nurse who is comfortable with her or his role may not necessarily practice in an ethical manner. For example, the nurse who is comfortable in her or his role may decide not to "make waves" or may fail to take a stand against a decision that goes against her or his sense of ethics.

Personal Values

Most people derive some values from the society or subgroup of society in which they live. Values developed by society ensure its continued functioning and enable people to live harmoniously together. Examples of societal values common to Western civilization are shown below. A person may internalize some or all of these values and perceive them as personal values. In addition to internalizing societal values, people have values that are important to them as individuals. Purtilo (1978, p. 71) points out that most people find fulfillment only if they can integrate both societal and personal values into a satisfactory life-style. People need societal values to feel like an accepted part of the society and humankind, and they need personal values to individualize themselves.

Professional Values

Because nursing is a profession based on caring, professional values relate to both competence and compassion. Selected professional values are shown on page 183. Nurses develop these values during socialization into the profession and from professional codes of ethics, discussed later in this chapter.

Selected Societal and Personal Values

Societal Values	*Personal Values*
■ Human life	■ Family unity
■ Individual rights	■ Self-worth
■ Individual autonomy	■ Worth of others
■ Liberty	■ Independence
■ Democracy	■ Religion
■ Equal opportunity	■ Honesty
■ Power	■ Fairness
■ Health	■ Love
■ Wealth	■ Sense of humor
■ Youth	■ Safety
■ Vigor	■ Peace
■ Intelligence	■ Financial security
■ Imagination	■ Material things
■ Education	■ Money
■ Technology	■ Property of self
■ Conformity	■ Property of others
■ Friendship	■ Leisure time
■ Courage	■ Work
■ Compassion	■ Travel
■ Family	■ Plants
	■ Animals
	■ Physical activity
	■ Intellectual activity
	■ Artistic activity
	■ Neatness

Values Clarification

Values clarification is a process by which individuals find their own answers (values) to situations. It is not the transmission of "correct" values or rules, but a process of identifying and developing individual values. The principle of values clarification is that no one set of values is right for everyone.

The process of values clarification was formulated by Louis Raths in 1966, who built on the thinking of John Dewey. Raths was chiefly concerned with the process of valuing, not the content of the values. Valuing is composed of seven processes, which can be placed in three groups (Simon et al. 1978, p. 19):

Prizing one's beliefs and behaviors

1. Prizing and cherishing
2. Publicly affirming beliefs and behaviors when appropriate

Choosing one's beliefs and behaviors

3. Choosing from alternatives
4. Choosing after consideration of consequences
5. Choosing freely

Acting on one's beliefs

6. Acting
7. Acting with a pattern, consistency, and repetition

A belief, attitude, or feeling becomes a value when all seven steps have been satisfied. The individual applies each of the seven steps to an emerging or already formed belief, behavior pattern, or attitude.

By using these seven steps in values clarification, nurses can clarify their own values and enhance their personal growth. These steps also can be applied to client situations; the nurse can help clients identify conflict areas, examine and choose from alternatives, set goals, and act (Coletta 1978, p. 2057).

Prizing and Cherishing

Prizing or cherishing is a continuous process in which the individual asks, "Do I cherish or prize my position or belief?" Unprized beliefs may still influence behavior, but they cannot be considered values.

Publicly Affirming when Appropriate

Public affirmation or appropriate sharing is an indication of the quality of a value. Individuals who feel strongly about an issue may publicly stand up and share the value with others. For example, a nurse who values the autonomy of clients may refuse to obtain a signed consent form from a client without first explaining the procedure to the client. Thus the nurse is affirming his or her value of autonomy to others.

Choosing from Alternatives

For a belief to be a value, it must be chosen from among other alternatives. Individuals must consider the other options before they commit themselves to one choice.

Choosing after Consideration of Consequences

The individual must be able to consider the consequences of a choice, i.e., the significance of the decision. The person may reject or confirm the choice because of or in spite of the consequences. For example, a nurse may refuse to give a client a medication that the nurse believes may harm the client. This nurse considers the consequences of her or his behavior in terms of the client and of self. The nurse is concerned for the client's welfare, but the refusal could result in disciplinary action. After considering all the alternatives, the nurse may confirm the choice of not giving the medication or select another course of action, e.g., discussing the medication with a physician before making a decision. If an individual's behavior is not the consequence of considering the results of action, it cannot be considered to reflect a value.

Choosing Freely

A value must be chosen freely. Some beliefs are not freely chosen by the individual but are accepted from parents or others without much thought and without choice. These beliefs are not values. Behavior determined by fear or coercion, for example, does not reflect values.

Acting

A value involves action. Therefore a value must be incorporated into behavior. If it is not, it is not a value but a belief or an attitude.

Acting with a Pattern, Consistency, and Repetition

Behavior must be consistent over a period of time to reflect a value. The behavior is repeated in many aspects of life. For example, a nurse who values health will eat a healthful diet and get enough sleep.

It is important for nurses (a) to examine their own values and clarify them, (b) to recognize the differences in the values of clients and to accept them, and (c) to recognize the differences in the values of peers, other health care professionals, and health care organizations. Nurses need to recognize how such differences can affect them. Often values represent an ideal; when that ideal is not achievable, some adaptation or compromise has to be made. Awareness of one's own values is a first step. The next step is to learn how to make the best possible compromise of values that circumstances allow. See "Resolving Ethical Dilemmas," later in this chapter.

Selected Professional Values

- Nondiscrimination in providing care
- Honesty
- Respect for persons
- Right to privacy
- Informed consent
- Self-determination/autonomy of clients
- Safeguarding the client's welfare
- Accountability for actions
- Competence
- Participation in research
- Health promotion
- Health maintenance
- Health restoration
- Alleviation of suffering

Advantages of Values Clarification

Clarification of values has the following advantages (Steele and Harmon 1983, pp. vii, 13; Thompson and Thompson 1985, p. 78):

1. It is a process of discovery that brings to conscious awareness the values that guide one's actions.
2. It fosters the making of choices. It is not synonymous with ethical decision-making, however.
3. It leads to human growth because it fosters awareness, empathy, and insight.
4. It serves as a guide for assessing client values and provides direction for nursing interventions.
5. It gives insight into the source of a particular value. This awareness allows the individual to retain or change the value.

Approaches

A group or individual approach can be used to clarify values. The group approach often allows greater opportunities to clarify one's values, since not all members of a

Values Clarification Strategy: Values Voting

This exercise adapted from Uustal (1978, p. 2060) and Bernal (1985, p. 174) demonstrates that there are many facets to every issue. How do you determine your position? What factors influence your thoughts and feelings? How will your choice be reflected in your behavior? Talk with some colleagues. Do they feel similarly or differently?

Where do you stand on the following issues? Indicate your responses in the following manner:

SA strongly agree
A agree
U undecided
D disagree
SD strongly disagree

Do you believe:

1. _____ Clients have the right to participate in all decisions related to their health care.
2. _____ Clients have a right to refuse extraordinary treatment that is life-sustaining.
3. _____ Refusing life-sustaining treatments is a form of suicide.
4. _____ Clients have a right *not* to be interfered with in a rational act of suicide.
5. _____ Health professionals have a responsibility to assist a client in an act of rational suicide that does not cause injury to others.
6. _____ Comfort measures should always be provided.
7. _____ Health professionals should always do their best to sustain a person's life.

group hold the same values. By becoming aware of others' values and alternative viewpoints, the individual opens the door to self-learning. Individually, however, a person can examine personal values and analyze what values are most prized. Several values clarification strategies or exercises have been developed. For example, Simon et al. (1978) provide 79 specific practical strategies or exercises; Uustal (1978) provides 10. An example of a strategy called values voting is illustrated above.

Identifying Personal Values

Nurses need to know in particular what values they hold about life, health, illness, and death. To explore personal values, the nurse can begin by answering questions such as (Thompson and Thompson 1985, pp. 77–80): "What ten things do I like to do?" "What ten things do I like about myself?" "What ten things do I dislike about myself?" An awareness of things the nurse dislikes can lead to thoughts about what she or he may like to change. After initial exercises, the nurse may then list ten values that guide her or his daily interactions or activities. By comparing lists with a trusted friend or in a group that fosters trust and mutual respect, the nurse can see similarities and differences with others. Resulting discussion often reveals reasons for the items listed. Another strategy for gaining awareness of personal values is to consider individual attitudes to such issues as abortion, unwanted pregnancy, euthanasia, sex-role stereotypes, and sexuality.

Examples of some questions and issues adopted from Corey et al. (1984, pp. 57–94) follow. When considering these issues, ask yourself: "Can I accept this or live with this?" "Why does this bother me?" "What would I do or want done in this situation?"

1. *Sexuality.* What are your attitudes toward?
   a. Teenage sex
   b. Casual sex
   c. Sex as an expression of love and commitment
   d. Premarital sex
   e. Extramarital sex for males
   f. Extramarital sex for females
   g. Group sex
   h. Masturbation
   i. Homosexuality
2. *Unwanted pregnancy.* In your opinion, what should a female with an unwanted pregnancy do?
   a. Maintain the pregnancy to term
   b. Have an abortion
   c. Marry the father
   d. Put the infant up for adoption if not married
   e. Make own decision regardless of circumstances
3. *Sex-role stereotypes.* Do you agree or disagree with the following statements?
   a. A woman's place is in the home in the role of wife and mother; a man's role is to be the breadwinner.
   b. Husbands and wives should share domestic and child-rearing tasks.
   c. A wife who desires it should be allowed to combine home and a career or school.
   d. A couple should decide which spouse is to be the primary breadwinner and which is to be the primary homemaker.
   e. A woman should do the cooking, not a man.
   f. A husband should make all the financial decisions for the family.
4. *Right to die and the choice of suicide.* See the Values Voting Strategy on this page.
5. *Differences in life experiences and philosophies.* Indicate with whom you could effectively communicate:
   a. Someone from a strict religious background
   b. Someone of a different race
   c. Someone from a different ethnic group
   d. A physically handicapped person
   e. An elderly person

f. A child
g. An obese person
h. An alcoholic
i. Someone who has a different sexual orientation
j. A criminal

6. *Abortion.* Indicate whether you agree or disagree with the following statements.
   a. A woman should have the right to choose abortion.
   b. Abortion at any point during gestation is murder.
   c. Abortion is wrong.
   d. Abortion should be performed if the woman's health is endangered.
   e. A mentally handicapped woman should be encouraged to have an abortion.
   f. Abortion should not be performed after 20 weeks' gestation, when a living infant can be borne.
   g. Abortion should be encouraged when parents have genetically transmissible diseases.

7. *Health.* Various definitions of health were proposed in Chapter 2. The nurse who defines and values health as physiologic, emotional, social, cultural, and spiritual well-being does not give the same nursing care as the nurse who defines health as the absence of illness. Remember that values are what the nurse actually puts into practice. Consider whether you agree or disagree with the following:
   a. To be most effective in nursing practice, the nurse must be a role model of health.
   b. An obese nurse can effectively instruct an obese client about nutrition and exercise.
   c. A nurse who smokes can effectively help a client to stop smoking.
   d. The nurse who has been pregnant and delivered an infant is most effective in helping a client through this experience.

8. *Health care.* Aroskar (1982, p. 24) lists four mind-sets about health care that can influence ethical nursing practice. These views are shown in Table 8–2. See also the section on conditions for humanized care in Chapter 3, page 90.

Table 8–2 Mind-Sets About Health Care and Effects on the Nurse

Health Care Mind-Set	Effects on the Nurse
The medical cure of disease	The nurse is considered primarily accountable to the physician. Medical values dominate.
A commodity to be sold to others	The nurse's major accountability is to the institution. Concerns for the client may conflict with this view.
The client's right to relief from pain and other debilitating conditions	The nurse's obligation is to the clients and their needs as defined by the clients themselves. By supporting the client's autonomy, the nurse abdicates responsibility; needs as defined by the client supersede the nurse's knowledge and experience.
The promotion, maintenance, and restoration of health within a cooperative community	All participants' values are considered in decision making. Both clients and providers have rights and responsibilities.

Source: M. A. Aroskar, Are nurses' mind-sets compatible with ethical nursing practice? *Topics in Clinical Nursing,* April 1982, 4:24. Reprinted with permission of Aspen Publishers, Inc. Copyright © 1982.

Identifying Client Values

People's values change from time to time as their situation in life changes. State of health greatly influences a person's values. For example, a client with failing eyesight will probably place a high value on the ability to see; a client with failing neuromuscular ability will value the ability to stand or walk; and a client with chronic pain will value comfort. Normally, people take such things for granted. Nurses, therefore, need to identify the major values, beliefs, and behaviors of clients as they influence and relate to a particular health problem.

Reasons for identifying a client's value system include:

1. To help a client discover a new and meaningful value system following injury or illness. During prolonged illness or serious injury, the client often needs help defining values, clarifying goals, seeking solutions, and making decisions. For example, a woman with multiple sclerosis needs to learn new living patterns and find meaning in life as her physical condition deteriorates. The woman might undertake creative endeavors, such as painting or writing, to replace physical activities. Spiritual values may be strengthened to enhance meaning in life.

2. To provide information about the client's responses to injury or illness. For example, an adolescent boy who is told he has infectious mononucleosis and will have to rest for 4 weeks may respond with anger, hostility, or depression if he is scheduled to play in a soccer game the next week.

3. To help the client explore alternative goals and intervention strategies when valued goals cannot be realized. The nurse caring for the boy with mononucleosis might express sympathy at his having missed such an important event and help him explore alternative goals, such as building model airplanes, stamp collecting, or photography.

4. To plan nursing interventions that support the client's cultural and health care beliefs. Assessment of a client's cultural beliefs is discussed in detail in Chapter 18.

There are several ways of learning a client's values (Purtilo 1978, p. 75):

1. Converse with the client about his or her job, family, pets, hobbies, past achievements, goals, or material possessions. Conversation can reveal much information, since most clients are eager to talk about what they value.
2. Listen to the client's family and friends. Friends or family members often provide clues through casual remarks, such as "I'll tell you something; he used to be a great concert pianist." The nurse thus learns that the client used to value music and may still do so.
3. Review the client's health records. Information about the client's family background, religion, occupation, age, birthday, and medical history can lead to conversations that will reveal personal values.

Values clarification can be a useful tool to help clients whose unclear or conflicting values are detrimental to their health. Behaviors that may indicate the need for values clarification include:

1. Ignoring a health professional's advice. One example is the client with heart disease who values hard work and a successful career, ignoring a physician's advice to stop smoking and to exercise more. Another is the obese client who does not follow the diet plan provided by the dietitian.
2. Inconsistent communication or behavior. For example, a pregnant female says that pregnant mothers should do all they can to ensure a healthy baby but persists in smoking and shortening her rest periods by watching late night movies.
3. Numerous admissions to a health care agency for the same problem. An example is the middle-aged woman who repeatedly seeks help for back pain because she will not consistently follow an exercise program.
4. Confusion or uncertainty about which course of action to follow. An example is the middle-aged woman who has had to acquire part-time employment to meet financial obligations because her husband has lost his job. She is finding her widowed, ailing mother increasingly difficult to maintain at home. She has considered sending her to a nursing home but really does not want to do so, even though she knows she is not managing her mother's care well. What is she to do?

To help clients clarify their values, the nurse needs to help the clients think about what is and what is not important to them. It is helpful to ask the following questions, each associated with one of the seven steps in values clarification:

1. *List alternatives.* Make sure that the client is aware of all alternative actions and has thought about the consequences of each. Ask: "Are you considering other courses of action?"
2. *Examine possible consequences of choices.* Ask: "What do you think you will gain by doing that?" "What benefits do you foresee from doing that?"
3. *Choose freely.* To determine whether the client chose freely, ask: "Did you have any say in that decision?" "Did you have a choice?"
4. *Feel good about the choice.* To determine how the client feels about a decision or action, ask: "How do you feel about that decision (or action)?" Because some clients may not feel satisfied with their decision and feel badly about a bad choice, a more sensitive question may be: "Some people feel good after a decision is made; others feel bad. How do you feel?
5. *Affirm the choice.* Ask: "What will you say to others (family, friends) about this?"
6. *Act on the choice.* To determine whether the client is prepared to act on the decision, ask: "Will it be difficult to tell your wife about this?"
7. *Act with a pattern.* Help the client determine whether he or she consistently behaves in a pattern. Ask: "How many times have you done that before?" or "Would you act that way again?"

When implementing these seven steps, the nurse assists the client to think each question through, never imposing her or his own values. The nurse never offers an opinion, e.g., "It would be better to do it this way," or offer a judgment, e.g., "That's not the right thing to do." The nurse offers an opinion only when the client asks the nurse for it and then only with care.

Value Conflicts

A **value conflict** occurs when two or more values are incongruent. For example, a nurse may value life yet be expected to collaborate with a physician in disconnecting a client from a life support system. Incongruent values may not present a problem until some action must be taken, as in the example above. There is now a value conflict that may confuse the nurse and make it difficult to make a decision.

An ethical or moral **dilemma** is a choice between equally undesirable alternatives (Curtin and Flaherty 1982, p. 39). Thompson defines a dilemma as "a situation involving a choice between equally satisfactory or unsatisfactory alternatives or a difficult problem that seems to have no satisfactory solution (Thompson and Thompson 1985, p. 94). In a moral dilemma there is no right or

Steps in Values Clarification

1. List alternatives
2. Examine possible consequences of choices
3. Choose freely
4. Feel good about the choice
5. Affirm the choice
6. Act on the choice
7. Act with a pattern

wrong. For example, a nurse is alone at night on a hospital unit and two clients experience cardiac arrest at almost the same time. What does the nurse do? It may be possible to save one client, but not both. Moral dilemmas arise rarely during nursing.

Moral dilemmas are encountered in everyday life. For example, Mrs. Christian is looking after her elderly mother at home. The mother, who has lived with Mrs. Christian and her husband for 5 years, is confined to bed and needs a great deal of assistance. Mrs. Christian has told his wife to put her mother in a nursing home or he will leave her. Mrs. Christian has promised her mother she will never put her in a home and believes her mother will die as a result. Mrs. Christian wants neither to lose her husband nor break her promise and, as she believes, be responsible for her mother's death. Mrs. Christian is in a moral dilemma. Placing her mother in a nursing home or losing her husband are equally undesirable alternatives.

According to Thompson and Thompson (1985, p. 94), for a situation to be a moral dilemma, it must fulfill three criteria:

1. *Awareness of different options.* The individual must be aware of the different options that are open. The awareness may be cognitive, or it may be a feeling that something is wrong.
2. *Moral nature of the dilemma.* Is the dilemma the nurse faces a moral issue? Not all situations that appear confusing to nurses are moral dilemmas, e.g., a conflict between two nurses about how to proceed with specific client care may not be a moral dilemma but simply differing interpretation of facts or even differing assessments. For example, one nurse may believe that a client's respirations indicate the need for oxygen, while another nurse may believe that the administration of morphine sulphate, as ordered by the physician, will suppress the Hering-Breuer reflex and ease respirations. Both nurses may in fact be right.
3. *Two or more options with true choice.* For a situation to be a moral dilemma, one must have a choice between two or more actions.

For example, a physician tells a patient that when he performed the surgery he did all he could. The nurse present at the conversation knows that a resident physician performed the surgery because the client's physician could not be reached. The nurse's choices are: to tell the client his physician did not perform the surgery, say nothing, report the discussion to the charge nurse, or discuss the conversation with the physician. The nurse in this example has free choice.

Ethics

Since ethics govern right conduct, they deal with what is good and bad and with moral duty and obligation. Ethics are not unlike the law in that each deals with rules of conduct that reflect underlying principles of right and wrong and codes of morality. Ethics are designed to protect the rights of human beings. In nursing, ethics provide professional standards for nursing activities; these standards protect both the nurse and the client.

Although *ethics* and *morals* are often used interchangeably, Jameton differentiates the two. Ethics refers to publicly stated and formal sets of rules or values, while morals are values or principles to which one is personally committed (Jameton 1984, p. 5).

Nursing Codes of Ethics

A **code of ethics** provides a means by which professional standards of practice are established, maintained, and improved. It is essential to a profession. Codes of ethics are formal guidelines for professional action. They are shared by the persons within the profession and should be generally compatible with a professional member's personal values.

A code of ethics gives the members of the profession a frame of reference for judgments in complex nursing situations. No two situations are identical, and nurses are frequently in situations that require judgment about which course of action to take. A code of ethics serves as a guide in many of these situations. It identifies the values and beliefs behind ethical standards (Thompson and Thompson 1985, p. 12).

Codes of ethics are frequently a mixture of creeds and commandments. Benjamin and Curtis (1981) describe a **creed** as an affirmation of professional regard for high ideals of conduct and as a commitment of members of a profession to honor them. An example of a creed is the

Table 8–3 International Council of Nurses Code for Nurses

The fundamental responsibility of the nurse is fourfold: to promote health, to prevent illness, to restore health, and to alleviate suffering.

The need for nursing is universal. Inherent in nursing is respect for life, dignity, and rights of man. It is unrestricted by considerations of nationality, race, creed, color, age, sex, politics or social status.

Nurses render health services to the individual, the family and the community and coordinate their services with those of related groups.

Nurses and People

The nurse's primary responsibility is to those people who require nursing care.

The nurse, in providing care, promotes an environment in which the values, customs and spiritual beliefs of the individual are respected.

The nurse holds in confidence personal information and uses judgment in sharing this information.

Nurses and Practice

The nurse carries personal responsibility for nursing practice and for maintaining competence by continual learning. The nurse maintains the highest standards of nursing care possible within the reality of a specific situation.

The nurse uses judgment in relation to individual competence when accepting and delegating responsibilities.

The nurse when acting in a professional capacity should at all times maintain standards of personal conduct which reflect credit upon the profession.

Nurses and Society

The nurse shares with other citizens the responsibility for initiating and supporting action to meet the health and social needs of the public.

Nurses and Co-workers

The nurse sustains a cooperative relationship with co-workers in nursing and other fields. The nurse takes appropriate action to safeguard the individual when his care is endangered by a co-worker or any other person.

Nurses and the Profession

The nurse plays the major role in determining and implementing desirable standards of nursing practice and nursing education.

The nurse is active in developing a core of professional knowledge.

The nurse, acting through the professional organization, participates in establishing and maintaining equitable social and economic working conditions in nursing.

Source: From International Council of Nurses, *ICN Code for nurses: Ethical concepts applied to nursing* (Geneva, Switzerland: Imprimeries Populaires, 1973). Reprinted with permission of the ICN.

opening statement of the 1973 *Code for Nurses* of the International Council of Nurses (ICN): "The fundamental responsibility of the nurse is fourfold: to promote health, to prevent illness, to restore health and to alleviate suffering." See Table 8–3. As **commandments**, codes of professional ethics provide prescriptions designed to regulate conduct in more specific situations (Benjamin and Curtis 1981, p. 6). An example of a commandment is this statement in the ICN *Code for Nurses:* "The Nurse holds in confidence personal information and uses judgment in sharing this information." See Table 8–3.

International, national, state, and provincial nursing associations have established codes of ethics. If a nurse violates the code, the association may expel the nurse from membership. Increasingly, professional nursing associations are taking an active part in improving and enforcing standards.

Purposes of ethical nursing codes are:

1. Providing a basis for regulating the relationship between the nurse, the client, coworkers, society, and the profession.
2. Providing a standard basis for excluding the unscrupulous nursing practitioner and for defending a practitioner who is unjustly accused.
3. Serving as a basis for professional curricula and for orienting the new graduate to professional nursing practice.
4. Assisting the public in understanding professional nursing conduct.

In 1953, the International Council of Nurses (ICN) developed and adopted their first code of ethics. This code was revised in 1965 and again in 1973. See Table 8–3. The code should be considered together with the relevant data in each situation; thus it provides assistance in setting priorities and in taking action. For the nurse practitioner, the code specifically provides assistance in making judgments and in developing attitudes appropriate to nursing.

The American Nurses' Association (ANA) first adopted a code of ethics in 1950, which was revised in 1968 and 1976. See Table 8–4. This code is designed to provide guidance for nurses by stating principles of ethical concern. Nurses have a responsibility to be familiar with the code that governs their nursing practice. In addition, nursing practice is also defined by the particular setting. In a rural, isolated setting, a nurse may be expected to assume responsibilities not normally assumed by urban nurses. For example, the nurse may assess the progress of labor and deliver the infant if the labor is normal. Only if there is a problem is the client flown to a center for a physician's care.

In 1980, the Canadian Nurses' Association adopted a code of ethics. It was revised in 1985. See Table 8–5.

Theoretical Approaches to Bioethics

Bioethics is the ethics concerned with life, including all life in the environment. Bioethics has come to refer more precisely to the ethics concerned with health care. When referring to ethics in nursing, therefore, one is actually

Table 8–4 American Nurses' Association Code for Nurses

1. The nurse provides services with respect for human dignity and the uniqueness of the client unrestricted by considerations of social or economic status, personal attributes, or the nature of health problems.
2. The nurse safeguards the client's right to privacy by judiciously protecting information of a confidential nature.
3. The nurse acts to safeguard the client and the public when health care and safety are affected by the incompetent, unethical, or illegal practice of any person.
4. The nurse assumes responsibility and accountability for individual nursing judgments and actions.
5. The nurse maintains competence in nursing.
6. The nurse exercises informed judgment and uses individual competence and qualifications as criteria in seeking consultation, accepting responsibilities, and delegating nursing activities to others.
7. The nurse participates in activities that contribute to the ongoing development of the profession's body of knowledge.
8. The nurse participates in the profession's efforts to implement and improve standards of nursing.
9. The nurse participates in the profession's efforts to establish and maintain conditions of employment conducive to high quality nursing care.
10. The nurse participates in the profession's effort to protect the public from misinformation and misrepresentation and to maintain the integrity of nursing.
11. The nurse collaborates with members of the health professions and other citizens in promoting community and national efforts to meet the health needs of the public.

Source: From American Nurses' Association, *Code for nurses* (Kansas City, Mo.: American Nurses' Association, 1985). Reprinted with permission.

referring to bioethics, although the two terms are often used interchangeably (Thompson and Thompson 1985, p. 219).

There are three primary ways to approach bioethical issues: teleology, deontology, and intuitionism. **Teleology** is a doctrine that explains phenomena by results; a person who takes a teleologic approach to ethics is concerned with the consequences of ethical decisions. This approach is often summarized in the notion "the end justifies the means." The terms *teleology* and *utilitarianism* are sometimes used interchangeably; however, utilitarianism is also considered a type of teleology, summarized in the ideas "the end justifies the means" and "the greatest good for the greatest number." Many people in medical research support this approach to the ethics of medical problems. For example, a male surgeon who has had no experience with a particular type of surgery goes ahead and operates anyway. Although the surgeon recognizes that the surgery may not be successful largely because of his lack of experience, the knowledge he believes he will gain justifies his actions.

Deontology is the theory or study of moral obligation. A simplification of the deontologic approach is that the morality of an ethical decision is completely separate from its consequences. For instance, a nurse might believe it is necessary to tell the truth no matter who is hurt.

The difference in these approaches is shown by applying them to an ethical issue, abortion. A person who takes a teleologic approach to the ethical issue of abortion might consider that saving the mother's life (the end) justifies the abortion (the means). One taking a deontologic approach to abortion might consider any termination of life as morally bad and therefore would not harm the fetus regardless of the consequences. The approach does not determine the decision, e.g., a person taking a teleologic approach might consider that saving the life of the fetus justifies the death of the mother. The approach, however, guides the steps in the making of ethical decisions.

The third approach to ethical issues is **intuitionism**, summarized as the notion that people inherently know what is right or wrong; it is not a matter of rational thought or of learning. For example, a nurse inherently knows it is wrong to strike a client—this does not need to be taught.

Bioethical Issues in Nursing

Bioethical issues involving nurses surface in nursing practice and in the relationships nurses have with others. Ethical issues arise in almost all areas of nursing practice: community nursing, pediatric nursing, and nurse practitioner are just three. A discussion of ethical issues that nurses may need to resolve in each area of nursing practice is beyond the scope of this book. However, many ethical issues can be viewed in the context of general nursing practice and the people with whom the nurse has contact during practice.

Personal Values and Professional Practice

With the changing scope of nursing practice and medical technology, there is an increasing incidence of a nurse's personal values conflicting with practice. On the one hand, employers have needs and expectations for service from nurses; on the other hand, nurses have the right to be guided by their own personal values. An example of an area of conflict in the contemporary nursing scene is assisting with therapeutic abortions. Nurses have the right to refuse to participate in abortions or any procedure that goes against their personal values, and nurses' employment should not be jeopardized as a result. It is essential, however, that clients' welfare not suffer as a consequence.

Other areas of controversy are euthanasia, prolonging the life of nonresponsive clients by machines, and withholding blood transfusions because of an individual's

Table 8–5 Canadian Nurses' Association Code of Ethics for Nursing*

Clients

I. A nurse is obliged to treat clients with respect for their individual needs and values.

II. Based upon respect for clients and regard for their right to control their own care, nursing care should reflect respect for the right of choice held by clients

III. The nurse is obliged to hold confidential all information regarding a client learned in the health care setting.

IV. The nurse has an obligation to be guided by consideration for the dignity of clients.

V. The nurse is obligated to provide competent care to clients.

VI. The nurse is obliged to represent the ethics of nursing before colleagues and others.

VII. The nurse is obligated to advocate the client's interest.

VIII. In all professional settings, including education, research and administration, the nurse retains a commitment to the welfare of clients. The nurse bears an obligation to act in such a fashion as will maintain trust in nurses and nursing.

Health Team

IX. Client care should represent a cooperative effort, drawing upon the expertise of nursing and other health professions. Acknowledging personal or professional limitations, the nurse recognizes the perspective and expertise of colleagues from other disciplines.

X. The nurse, as a member of the health care team, is obliged to take steps to ensure that the client receives competent and ethical care.

The Social Context of Nursing

XI. Conditions of employment should contribute to client care and to the professional satisfaction of nurses. Nurses are obliged to work towards securing and maintaining conditions of employment that satisfy these connected goals.

Responsibilities of the Profession

XII. Professional nurses' organizations recognize a responsibility to clarify, secure and sustain ethical nursing conduct. The fulfillment of these tasks requires that professional organizations remain responsive to the rights, needs and legitimate interests of clients and nurses.

*This represents only one element of the code—*values. Standards,* which provide more specific directions for conduct than values, and *limitations,* which describe exceptional circumstances in which a value or standard cannot receive its usual application, are provided with each value in the publication cited above.

Source: Canadian Nurses' Association. February 1985. *Code of Ethics for Nursing.* Ottawa, Ontario. Reprinted with permission.

religious convictions. The future may hold many more conflicts of personal values with professional duty.

For example, a nurse whose personal value system does not support abortion has begun to develop a trusting relationship with a 13-year-old girl admitted to the hospital for a legal abortion. The girl is ambivalent about the abortion; because of her ambivalent feelings and her fear of the procedure, she wants to have the nurse's support. The nurse, as a professional, needs to support the client; however, as a person, the nurse is against abortion and finds it difficult to give the girl complete support. Question: Should the nurse play a strictly professional role and support the abortion, or should the nurse reveal personal feelings about abortion?

A second example is a nurse who is asked to teach birth control and who opposes birth control because of personal values. Question: What are the alternatives? Should the nurse teach the client, thereby compromising personal values? Should the nurse refuse to provide the requested information? Perhaps the nurse should tell the client that she or he doesn't agree with contraception, and then answer the client's questions. Is there a fourth alternative?

There are no easy answers in such situations. Nurses can often avoid these conflicts by clarifying during initial employment interviews, areas in which personal values may conflict with professional responsibility. The nurse can request to be assigned to nursing responsibilities that will not produce conflict. Nursing students should also make their personal values clear to teachers so as to avoid ethical issues. Students who have not anticipated a problem but find themselves facing an ethical conflict involving personal values should write down the alternative actions open to them and then discuss the alternatives with an instructor.

Nurse and Peers

A nurse who faces a problem with peers may or may not know what course of action to take.

The first example is a nurse who sees another nurse steal medications from the nursing unit drug cupboard. The nurse who is discovered cries and explains that she needs the sleeping pills to sleep during the day while her three children are home from school. She uses them only on days before she is to go on night shift. She is the sole support of her children and needs the job. Question: Does the nurse report the theft or ignore the matter?

A second situation involves a nurse newly employed at a hospital who requests Christmas leave because his father is dying and he wants to spend Christmas with him. Under the special circumstances, the nurse is granted the time. Another nurse finds out that the first nurse's father is not dying and that the nurse plans to spend Christmas vacation skiing with a friend. Question: Does the nurse report the skiing vacation to the responsible nurse or forget the information?

A third example is a white nurse who is afraid to correct a black nurse's error for fear the black nurse will report the white nurse to the Human Rights Commission. Question: Does the white nurse correct the black nurse and risk labor problems and possible firing?

A fourth situation involves a nurse who is employed on a community mental health team. Another nurse discovers that the first nurse spends most of the time at home looking after an ill mother and fabricates reports about visiting clients in their homes. Question: Does the nurse present this information to the members of the community team, discuss the situation with the first nurse, or consider another alternative?

In each of these situations, the nurse's own values or fears lead to ethical conflicts.

Nurse and Client

In some situations, nurses have ethical problems that involve a client, a family, or both. In one instance, a client requests an abortion. Her husband agrees, but he tells the nurse that he will always be tormented with the thought that he agreed to destroy a human being he helped to create. The wife tells the nurse that her husband was not the father of the unborn baby. Question: Should the nurse tell the father, the physician, or the charge nurse any of this information?

In a second example, an 18-year-old client who believes he is dying tells the nurse that he wants to die with a clear conscience and confesses that at age 15 he held his brother's head under water until he drowned. He says that his parents believe his brother drowned accidentally. Question: Should the nurse tell anyone—the physician, the nursing supervisor, or the parents—this information?

A third example involving clients and their families is a nurse caring for a woman injured in an automobile accident. The husband, also in the accident, is admitted to another hospital unit and dies. The client constantly questions the nurse about her husband. The physician directs the nurse not to tell the client but to fabricate answers; the physician gives no reason. Question: Should the nurse fabricate answers for the client, report the matter to the charge nurse, or tell the client the truth?

In the last situation, three people—the nurse, client, and physician—are involved. The situation is therefore more complex than a nurse-client problem. In this instance, the nurse's notion of ethical practice conflicts with the physician's, and the nurse's ability to provide supportive care to the client is hampered by the inability to tell the truth.

Nurse and Other Health Professionals

Ethical conflicts can arise between nurses and physicians. For example, a surgeon, the chief of staff of surgery, visits a hospital nursing unit one evening to discuss a client's surgery the next day. The nurse smells alcohol on the surgeon's breath and the surgeon's speech is slurred and his gait is unsteady. Question: Does the nurse report this or ignore it?

Another example is a physician attending elderly clients in a long-term agency. The protocol of the agency is: "Each client must be visited by his or her physician at least every 30 days and the visit documented on the client's record." A nurse at the agency observes that one physician visits the clients only every 3 months but falsely records monthly visits on the clients' records. What does the nurse do: Report the matter to the charge nurse or the agency manager? Discuss the matter with the physician?

Another example involves a nurse, client, and physician. An 87-year-old woman in a nursing home tells her nurse that she believes she is getting poor medical care and wants to change her physician. She asks the nurse what she can do. The nurse suggests that the client talk with her physician about this matter. The physician arrives while the nurse is present, and the client relates her desire to change physicians. The physician tells her, "You are just spoiled; you can't change doctors at this time." The physician then walks away. The nurse knows the client has a right to change her physician. What should the nurse do?

Nurse and Agency Practice

Health care agencies exist for a variety of reasons (see Chapter 2), and their policies often reflect the values of the members of a governing board. As an employee of an agency, a nurse may have values that conflict with institutional goals and practices. Sometimes, because of budget restrictions, there may be inadequate equipment or inadequate staff, which can create ethical dilemmas for nurses. Such nurses may work to change agency policy, or they may find it necessary to organize formally and bargain with the employer for safer working conditions. See the section on collective bargaining in Chapter 7.

Three examples of conflict between a nurse's values and agency policy follow. In one situation, the nurse is asked by a dying client not to call a clergyman, but the hospital policy is that the clergy must be called for all dying clients. Question: Should the nurse call a clergyman or discuss this with the client and the family?

In a second example, hospital policy is that all sedatives are counted at the end of each shift. The nurse has already been reprimanded for staying overtime to make the count. Question: Should the nurse not count the sedatives but just subtract those administered to clients? Should the nurse make the count and neglect a client who requires a change of dressing? Are there other alternatives?

A third example is an upset teenager who wants information about how to obtain an abortion. The agency's policy is not to discuss abortions. Question: Should the nurse give the information to the client or follow the agency's policy? Are there other alternatives?

Conflicting Responsibilities

Nurses are repeatedly faced with conflicting responsibilities. On the one hand, the nurse is frequently an employee responsible to a health agency. On the other hand, the nurse is a professional person responsible to the professional ethics of an association and the standards of nursing practice of the profession. In addition, the nurse is responsible to and for clients and is taught to respond to their needs in a therapeutic manner.

For example, a nurse is asked by a physician not to keep a record of all the supplies used for a particular client because the client will have difficulty paying the bill; however, the nurse is accountable for all supplies used. Question: Should the nurse report the matter to the hospital or follow the physician's request?

In a second situation, a nurse on the evening shift is asked by a charge nurse to administer an intramuscular antibiotic to the charge nurse, using a client's medication. Question: What should the nurse do? To whom is the nurse responsible?

Table 8–6 A Bioethical Decision Model

Step One	Review the situation to determine health problems, decision needed, ethical components, and key individuals
Step Two	Gather additional information to clarify situation
Step Three	Identify the ethical issues in the situation
Step Four	Define personal and professional moral positions
Step Five	Identify moral positions of key individuals involved
Step Six	Identify value conflicts, if any
Step Seven	Determine who should make the decision
Step Eight	Identify range of actions with anticipated outcomes
Step Nine	Decide on a course of action and carry it out
Step Ten	Evaluate/review results of decision/action

Source: J. B. Thompson, and H. O. Thompson, *Ethics in nursing.* New York: Macmillan, 1981. Used by permission.

Resolving Ethical Dilemmas

To make ethical judgments, one must rely on rational thought, not emotions. Such judgments require conscious, cognitive skills necessary to perceive the client's needs and provide client care (Sigman 1986, p. 21). Every day, nurses make decisions that affect their clients, and these decisions are frequently based on ethics (Sigman 1986, p. 22).

A number of ethical theories and ethical decision-making models can guide nurses in making ethical decisions. Purtilo and Cassel suggest a four-step process: gather relevant data, identify the dilemma, decide what to do, and complete the action (Purtilo and Cassel 1981, pp. 27–29).

Thompson and Thompson (1981) propose a ten-step bioethical decision model to help nurses examine ethical issues and make a decision. See Table 8–6.

Before a nurse can resolve ethical dilemmas, she or he should decide which ethical system is best suited to her or his views. Two prevalent theories that guide decision making are utilitarianism and deontology (Fromer 1986, p. 82). These were mentioned briefly earlier in this chapter.

Utilitarianism is summarized as "the greatest good for the greatest number." In this approach, moral decisions are based solely on the consequences of an action, not on the inherent rightness of an action. One drawback of this approach is that minority views can be ignored. For example, if three nurses agree on a course of action and the client disagrees, by the utilitarian view the client can be ignored because he or she is not in "the greatest number."

In the deontologic approach to ethical problems, certain characteristics make an act right or wrong, regardless of its consequences. These characteristics are values such as truth, justice, and love. One type of deontologic theory is pleuralistic; i.e., several principles can apply in a conflict. Principles such as autonomy and justice can be assigned different priorities, depending on the person solving the dilemma. For example, one nurse may consider the autonomy of the client more important than justice, whereas another nurse may believe just the opposite. For this reason, each would approach a problem with different priorities for resolution.

According to Fromer, the four most important principles in a deontological approach are autonomy, nonmaleficence, beneficence, and justice. **Autonomy** is personal liberty of action; it implies independence, self-reliance, freedom of choice, and the ability to make decisions (Fromer 1986, pp. 82–83). To be autonomous, a client must be able to act independently, be self-reliant, have freedom to choose a course of action, and be able to make decisions. For a client to be truly autonomous, nurses and all health professionals must respect the autonomy of the client.

Nonmaleficence means the duty to do no harm. This principle is the basis of most codes of nursing ethics. Although this would seem to be a simple principle to follow in nursing practice, in reality it is complex. Harm can mean deliberate harm, risk of harm, and harm that occurs during beneficial actions (Fromer 1986, p. 83). In nursing, intentional harm is always unacceptable. However, the risk of harm is not so clear. A client may be at risk of harm during a nursing intervention that is intended to be helpful. For example, a client may react adversely to a medication. Sometimes, the degree to which a risk is morally permissible can be a conflict.

Beneficence means "doing good." Nurses are obligated to "do good," that is to implement actions that benefit clients and their support persons. However, in an increasingly technologic health care system, "doing good" can also pose a risk of doing harm. For example, a nurse may advise a client about an exercise program to improve general health but should not do so if the client is at risk of a heart attack.

Justice, the fourth principle, is often referred to as fairness. Nurses frequently face decisions in which a sense of justice should prevail. For example, a nurse is alone on a hospital unit, and one client arrives to be admitted at the same time another client requires a medication for pain. Instead of running from one client to the other, the nurse should weigh the facts in the situation and then act based on the principle of justice.

In resolving ethical problems, nurses need to be aware of (a) the ethical theory with which she or he is most comfortable and (b) her or his own hierarchy of principles or values in that theory.

Although codes of ethics offer general guidelines for decision making, more specific guidelines are necessary in many cases to resolve the everyday ethical dilemmas encountered by nurses in practice settings. Suggested guidelines for the nurse to resolve these dilemmas are:

1. Establish a sound database.
2. Identify the conflicts presented by the situation.
3. Outline alternative actions to the proposed course of action.
4. Outline the outcomes or consequences of the alternative actions.
5. Determine ownership of the problem and the appropriate decision maker.
6. Define the nurse's obligations.

Establishing the database To establish a sound database, the nurse needs to gather as much information as possible about the situation. Aroskar (1980, p. 660) suggests that nurses get answers to the following questions:

1. What persons are involved and what is their involvement in the situation?
2. What is the proposed action?
3. What is the intent of the proposed action?
4. What are the possible consequences of the proposed action?

For example, Mrs. Green, a 67-year-old woman, is hospitalized with multiple fractures and lacerations caused by an automobile accident. Her husband, also in the accident, is admitted to the same hospital and dies. Mrs. Green, who was the driver of the automobile, constantly questions the primary nurse about her husband. The surgeon, however, has told the nurse not to tell the client about the death of her husband. The nurse is not provided with any reason for such a direction and expresses concern to the charge nurse, who says the surgeon's orders must be followed.

In this example, the database includes:

Persons involved: Client (concerned about husband's welfare), husband (deceased), surgeon, head nurse, and primary nurse.

Proposed action: Withhold information about the husband's death.

Intention of proposed action: Unknown; possibly to protect Mrs. Green from psychologic trauma, overwhelming guilt feelings, and consequent deterioration of her physical condition.

Consequences of proposed action: If information is withheld, the client may become increasingly anxious and angry and may refuse to cooperate with necessary care, delaying recovery.

Identifying conflicts A conflict is a clash between opposing elements or ideas. The conflicts for the primary nurse in the example are:

1. Need to be honest with Mrs. Green without being disloyal to the surgeon and the charge nurse
2. Need to be loyal to the surgeon and head nurse without being dishonest to Mrs. Green
3. Conflict about the effects on Mrs. Green's health if she is informed or if she is not informed.

Outlining courses of action and outcomes Alternative courses of action to the proposed action for Mrs. Green and their outcomes might include:

1. Follow the surgeon's and charge nurse's advice and do as the surgeon suggests. The outcomes for the nurse would be (a) approval from the charge nurse and surgeon, (b) risk of being seen as nonassertive, (c) violation of own value to be truthful to Mrs. Green, (d) possible benefit to Mrs. Green's health, and (e) possible detriment to her health.
2. Discuss the situation further with the charge nurse and surgeon, pointing out Mrs. Green's rights to autonomy and information. The outcomes might be: (a) the surgeon may acknowledge the client's right to be informed and may then inform the client, (b) the surgeon may state that the client's rights have no legal basis and may adhere to the action originally proposed, based on a judgment about the effects of information on Mrs. Green.

Determining ownership In some ethical dilemmas, the nurse does not make decisions about her or his own actions but assists the client to make a decision. For example, if a client states he does not want to have an operation, the question of ownership arises. In this example, it is obvious that the client owns the problem and that it is his right to choose this course of action. Associated with ownership, however, is knowledge about the probability and the risk of consequences attending various courses of actions. Therefore, the nurse does not abandon the client with this decision. The nurse has the professional knowledge and expertise to ensure that the client makes an informed decision. Thus the client needs information from the professional's frame of reference about the consequences of decisions.

A series of questions that evolve from decision-making theories can help nurses determine who owns a certain problem (Davis and Aroskar 1983, p. 218):

1. Who should be involved in making the decision and why?
2. For whom is the decision being made?
3. What criteria (social, economic, psychologic, physiologic, or legal) should be used in deciding who makes the decision?
4. What degree of consent is needed by the subject (client and other)?
5. What, if any, moral principles (rights, values) are enhanced or negated by the proposed action?

In the example of Mrs. Green, the surgeon obviously believes the decision is his or hers to make for Mrs. Green, and the charge nurse agrees. However, the criteria used to decide who the decision maker should be are not clear. If the criteria were spelled out, perhaps the conflict about the effects on Mrs. Green's health of knowing or not knowing about her husband's death could be resolved. Is it psychologically advantageous for Mrs. Green to know or not to know? Is it physically advantageous? What will the social and economic effects be?

Value systems also influence the decision about problem ownership. The value of Mrs. Green's right to information about her husband will be enhanced if she is told, negated if not. Her right to autonomy will also be affected.

This example shows that there are no clearly defined right or wrong answers to ethical dilemmas. If there were, they would not be ethical dilemmas. To resolve the ethical dilemma about Mrs. Green, it may be necessary for the involved health professionals to confer and clearly establish approaches that will be in Mrs. Green's best interests. Once an approach is agreed on, the nurses and physician can devise consistent continuing methods of support for Mrs. Green. That approach may dictate actions by the nurse that conflict with her or his own value system. However, the action chosen for Mrs. Green's best interest takes precedence.

Research Note

At times nurses confront fundamental moral dilemmas arising from their work. How do nurses respond to ethical dilemmas? McElmurry, Swider, and Yarling examined this and related questions in their study of decisions reported by 775 senior baccalaureate nursing students from 16 midwestern colleges and universities, when they were presented with an ethical dilemma in nursing practice. Loyalties to clients, institutions, and physicians were addressed and analyzed. Most of the first decisions out of the chain of decisions to follow were institution-centered. The study revealed, however, that an overall sense of confusion prevails; nurses must explore the meaning of their choices, thereby preparing to practice maturely and autonomously. (Swider et al. 1985)

Defining the nurse's obligations When nurses are determining an ethical course of action, Moser and Cox (1980, p. 43) advise them to list their nursing obligations, to assess the conflicts that will arise if all obligations are met, and to determine the alternatives from which the nurse can choose. Examples of obligations are:

1. To maximize the client's well-being
2. To balance the client's need for autonomy and family members' responsibilities for the client's well-being
3. To support each family member and enhance the family support system
4. To carry out hospital policies
5. To protect other clients' well-being
6. To protect the nurse's own standards of care

Chapter Highlights

- Values give direction and meaning to life and guide a person's behavior.
- Every person has his or her own personal set of values influenced by societal standards, parents, teachers, culture, religion, and other life experiences.
- Values are freely chosen, prized and cherished, affirmed to others, and consistently incorporated into behavior.
- The nurse enters nursing practice with a personal set of values and through socialization acquires additional professional values that influence and guide her or his actions.

- Nursing is a profession based on caring; its professional values relate to both competence and compassion.
- Clarification of personal values is important for nurses to identify values that guide one's actions and to facilitate the making of choices.
- Values often represent an ideal that is not always achieveable; compromises are thus necessary in the practice situation.
- Value conflicts do not present problems for the nurse until some action must be taken.
- Moral dilemmas are situations in which there is no right or wrong choice; the individual must choose between two equally undesirable alternatives.
- Professional standards for nursing activities are founded in ethics and designed to protect the rights of clients and nurses.
- Ethical issues in nursing may arise because of conflicts between personal values and professional responsibilities or between people involved in client care.
- To resolve an ethical dilemma, a nurse must establish a sound database, identify value conflicts, outline courses of action and outcomes, determine who owns the problem, and define the nurse's obligations.

Suggested Readings

Huttman, B. R. January 1982. Dilemmas in practice. No code? Slow code? Show code? *American Journal of Nursing* 82:133, 135–36.

Huttman discusses the dilemma for the nurse when the physician refuses to write a no-code order to discontinue treatment when the family wishes it. Educating the public about their options is recommended.

Linn, A. January/February 1982. When your patient wants to die, should you help? *Nursing Life* 2:30–33.

Although the living will, the right to die, and freedom of choice seem to be reasonable as abstract ideas, how acceptable do they seem when one must apply them to a real client? Linn discusses supporting the client when the nurse disagrees, when the physician disagrees, when the family disagrees, and when the client's wishes are not clear.

McCaffery, M.; Desmarais, C.; Storlie, F.; and Ackerman, T. F. November/December 1981. A question of ethics: Sedating the dying. *Nursing Life* 1:41–43.

A hospice nurse, a lawyer, a critical-care nurse, and a medical ethicist give advice on how to sedate the dying safely.

Moser, D., and Cox, J. M., editors. May 1980. Perspectives: Resolving an ethical dilemma. *Nursing 80* 10:39–43.

This article presents an ethical problem encountered at St. Jude's Children's Research Center. The discussion to resolve the problem is presented with consultation by Terrence Ackerman, Department of Human Values and Ethics, University of Tennessee, and Dorothy Moser, a fellow in the Program on Human Values and Ethics at the University of Tennessee.

Muyskens, J. L. July/August 1984. No easy choice resolving everyday ethical dilemmas. *Nursing Life* 4:29–32.

Should a nurse ever force clients to accept treatment, lie to them about their condition, or reveal their confidences? Muyskens advises nurses to assess their priorities when the answer is neither black nor white.

Sheehan, J. July 1985. Ethical considerations in nursing practice. *Journal of Advanced Nursing* 10:331–36.

Some ethical implications for nursing practice are considered in relation to three issues: competence, honesty, and obedience. Sheehan discusses factors that contribute to conformity, obedience, and authoritarianism and suggests respect for other people as a guiding principle for ethically acceptable conduct.

Smurl, J. F. May/June 1983. Do ethical decisions leave you wondering: "Did I do the right thing?" *Nursing Life* 3:48–55.

This test offering deals with ethical decision making for everyday nursing problems. Topics included are defining ethical duty, making judgments, setting priorities, deciding on outcomes, respecting others' rights, giving or refusing care, telling the whole truth or not, and calling a code or not.

Selected References

American Nurses' Association. 1976. *Code for nurses with interpretive statements.* Kansas City, Mo.: American Nurses' Association.

Aroskar, M. A. April 1980. Anatomy of an ethical dilemma. *American Journal of Nursing* 80:658–63.

———. April 1982. Are nurses' mind-sets compatible with ethical nursing practice? *Topics in Clinical Nursing* 4:24–26.

Bankowski, Z., and Bryant, J. H. 1985. *Health policy, ethics and human values, and international dialogue.* Proceedings of the 28th CIOMS round table conference, Athens, Greece, 29 October–2 November 1984. Geneva: Council for International Organizations of Medical Sciences.

Beauchamp, T. L., and Childless, J. F. 1983. *Principles of biomedical ethics.* 2d ed. New York: Oxford University Press.

Benjamin, M., and Curtis, J. 1981. *Ethics in nursing.* New York: Oxford University Press.

Bernal, E. W. April 1985. Values clarification: A critique. *Journal of Nursing Education* 24:174–75.

Callahan, D., and Bok, S., editor. 1980. *Ethics teaching in higher education.* New York: Plenum Press.

Callahan, D., and Engelhart, H. T. 1981. *The roots of ethics: Science, religion, and values.* New York: Plenum Press.

Chinn, P. L., editor. 1986. Ethical issues in nursing. Rockville, Md.: Aspen Systems Corporation.

Coletta, S. S. December 1978. Values clarification in nursing: Why? *American Journal of Nursing* 78:2057.

Cory, G.; Corey, M. S.; and Callahan, P. 1984. *Issues and ethics in the helping professions.* 2d ed. Monterey, Calif.: Brooks/Cole Publishing Co.

Cowart, M. E. May 1982. Moral development of health care professionals begins with sensitizing: Thirty-three sample encounters. *Journal of Nursing Education* 21:4–7.

Curtin, L., and Flaherty, M. J. 1982. *Nursing ethics: Theories and pragmatics.* Bowie, Md.: Brady Communications Co.

Davis, A. J. and Aroskar, M. A. 1978. *Ethical dilemmas and nursing practice. New York: Appleton-Century-Crofts.*

Fenner, K. M. 1980. *Ethics and law in nursing professional perspectives.* New York: D. Van Nostrand Co.

Fromer, M. J. 1981. *Ethical issues in health care.* St. Louis: C. V. Mosby Co.

———. 1986. Solving ethical dilemmas in nursing practice. In Chinn, P. L., editor. *Ethical issues in nursing.* Rockville, Md.: Aspen Systems Corporation.

Hall, B. P. 1973. *Value clarification as a learning process.* New York: Paulist Press.

Hardy, L. September 1–7, 1982. Dialogue: Values in nursing. Part 2. *Nursing Times* 78:1483–84.

International Council of Nurses. 1973. *ICN code for nurses: Ethical concepts applied to nursing.* Geneva: Imprimeries Populaires.

Jameton, A. 1984. *Nursing practice: The ethical issues.* Englewood Cliffs, N.J.: Prentice-Hall.

Johnson, D. W. 1972. *Reaching out: Interpersonal effectiveness and self-actualization.* Englewood Cliffs, N.J.: Prentice-Hall.

Moser, D., and Cox, J. M., editors. May 1980. Perspectives: Resolving an ethical dilemma. *Nursing 80* 10:39–43.

Muldary, T. W. 1983. *Interpersonal relations for health professionals: A social skills approach.* New York: Macmillan Publishing Co.

McFarlane, J. September 29–October 5, 1982. Nursing values and nursing action. *Nursing Times* 78:109–112.

Moser, D., and Cox, J. M., editors. May 1980. Perspectives: Resolving an ethical dilemma *Nursing 80* 10:39–43.

Murphy, C. P. 1985. *Ethical dilemmas in nursing practice.* Pub. no. NP-68D. Kansas City, Mo.: American Nurses' Association.

Murphy, C. P., and Hunter, H. 1983. *Ethical problems in the nurse-patient relationship.* Boston: Allyn and Bacon.

Purtilo, R. 1978. *Health professional/patient interaction.* 2d ed. Philadelphia: W. B. Saunders Co.

Purtilo, R. B., and Cassel, C. K. 1981. *Ethical dimensions in the health professions.* Philadelphia: W. B. Saunders Co.

Raths, L. E.; Harmin, M.; and Simon, S. B. 1978. *Values and teaching.* 2d ed. Columbus, Ohio: Charles E. Merrill Books.

Sheehan, J. July 1985. Ethical considerations in nursing practice: Competence, honesty, and obedience. *Journal of Advanced Nursing* 10:331–36.

Sigman, P. 1986. Ethical choice in nursing. In Chinn, P. L. (editor). *Ethical issues in nursing.* Rockville, Maryland: Aspen Systems Corporation.

Simon, S. B.; Howe, L. W.; and Kirschenbaum, H. 1978. *Values clarification: A handbook of practical strategies for teachers and students.* Rev. ed. New York: Hart Publishing Co.

Smith, S. J., and David, A. J. August 1980. Ethical dilemmas: Conflicts among rights, duties, and obligations. *American Journal of Nursing* 80:1462–66.

Steele, S. M., and Harmon, V. M. 1983. *Values clarification in nursing.* 2d ed. Norwalk, Conn.: Appleton-Century-Crofts.

Swider, S. M.; McElmurry, B. J.; and Yarling, R. R. March/April 1985. Ethical decision making in a bureaucratic context by senior nursing students. *Nursing Research* 34(2): 108–12.

Thompson, J. B., and Thompson, H. O. 1981. *Ethics in nursing.* New York: Macmillan Co.

———. 1985. *Bioethical decision making for nurses.* Norwalk, Conn.: Appleton-Century-Crofts.

Thompson, H. O., Thompson, J. B. November 1984. Learning to practice ethically synonymous with being a professional *AORN Journal* 40:778, 780, 782.

Uustal, D. B. December 1978. Values clarification: Application to practice. *American Journal of Nursing* 78:2058–63.

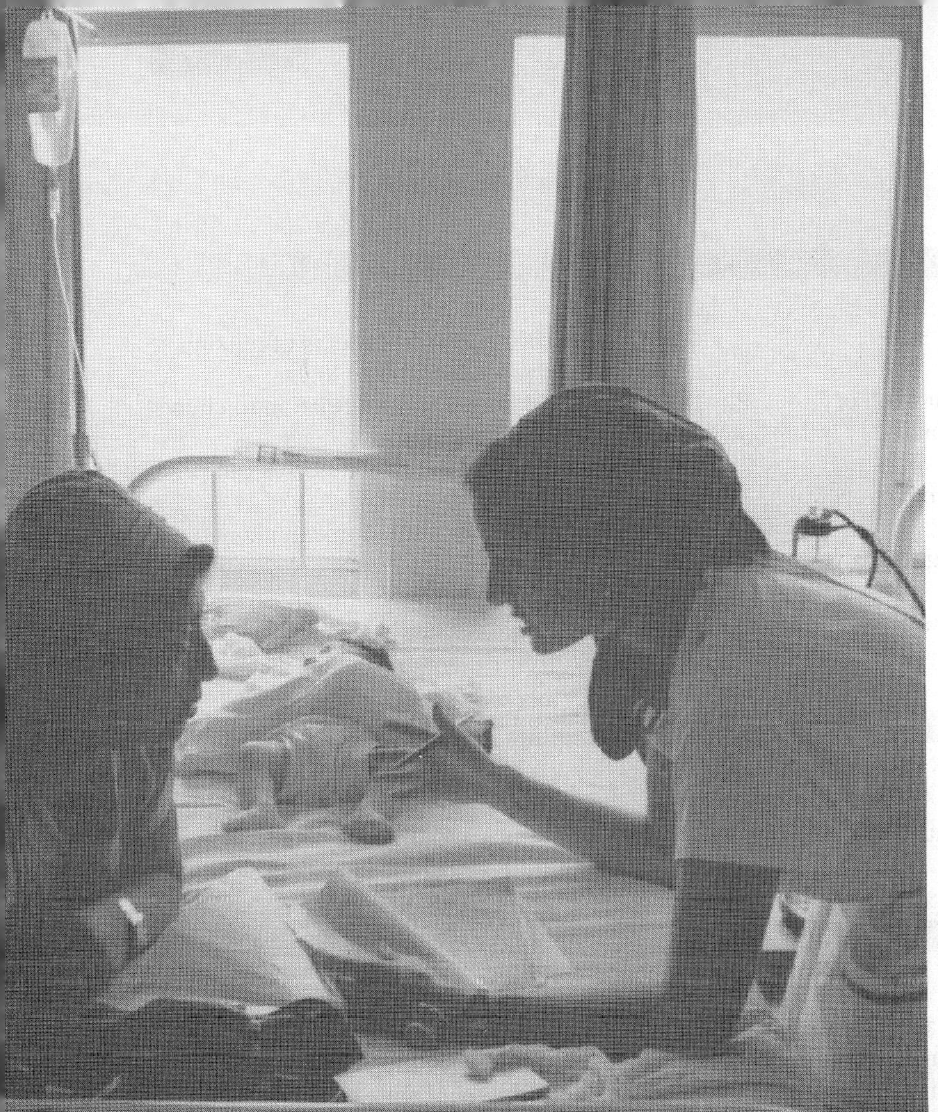

WILLIAM THOMPSON

CHAPTER **9**

Rights

Contents

9 *Rights*

Objectives

1. Know essential facts about rights.
   1.1 Define selected terms.
   1.2 Outline the essentials of the Patient's Bill of Rights established by the American Hospital Association.
   1.3 List special groups for whom statements of rights are available.
   1.4 Identify Annas and Healey's four rights that are assertable in a health care facility.
   1.5 Identify Fagin's seven rights of nurses.
   1.6 Identify five rights of students of nursing according to the Student Bill of Rights.
2. Understand the nurse's role in relation to clients' rights.
   2.1 Identify six ways by which nurses can protect clients' rights.
   2.2 Explain the role of the nurse in client advocacy.
   2.3 Explain the emergence of rights in health care.

Terms

advocate
client advocate
human rights
legislative rights
option rights
right
welfare rights

Rights Explained

Fagin (1975, p. 84) defines as a right "just claim to anything to which one is entitled, such as power or privilege." A right may be properly demanded on the basis of justice, morality, or legality. Rights are also described as "legitimate expectations of persons in a given society at a given time (Davis and Aroskar 1983, p. 70). Rights can be viewed from legal and personal perspectives. In the legal view, rights provide people with a certain power to control situations; e.g., a person has a legal right to enter a restaurant and purchase a meal. In this legal view, rights have certain attendant obligations. The individual with the right to eat in a restaurant is obliged to behave in an appropriate manner and to pay for the meal.

A right may or may not have a legal basis. For example, the American Hospital Association's "A Patient's Bill of Rights" (see Table 9–1 later in this chapter) states: "the patient has a right to considerate and respectful care"; however, lack of consideration during care is not likely to be illegal, although it might be unethical, depending on the situation. By contrast, the right of clients to have their records remain confidential is a legal right in many jurisdictions.

Having a right is not the same as exercising it. For instance, having the right to enter a theater is not the same as entering the theater.

Sometimes the rights of an individual conflict with the rights of the society. For example, a convicted felon who is sent to prison gives up the right to freedom for the protection of society.

The personal concept of rights has much to do with one's values, with the way one conducts one's life, with the decisions one makes, and with one's concept of right and wrong and of good and evil (Fromer 1981, p. 2). A number of factors influence the development of a personal concept of rights, among them social relationships, parents, culture, and information. Human rights refer to prerogatives of all humans, in particular the right to be respected as a human being. "If human beings have any natural rights at all, they have the right to be recognized and respected as human beings" (Curtin and Flaherty 1982, p. 7). These *human rights,* or the right to be treated as a human, represent a basic respect for humanity, for people as human beings. A nurse who inflicts unnecessary pain or treats a person as a piece of unfeeling machinery fails to recognize the humanity of another person. To be treated as a human is a right of all people.

The Role of Rights

1. Rights can be used as an expression of power in conflicts between people and groups. For example, a physician might tell a nurse, "I have the right to order any medication I want for my client." In this example, the physician is expressing his or her power to order medications.
2. Rights can be used to justify actions. For example, a nurse who is criticized for spending too much time

with a client may say, "I have a right to give the best nursing I can." Whether the nurse actually has this right in the situation depends on a number of variables; by claiming the right, however, the nurse is justifying the time taken with a particular client.

3. Rights can be used to settle disputes. One person can often settle a dispute by claiming a right that is also recognized by the other person. For example, a nurse suggests to a client that he should not walk downstairs. The client becomes angry, disagrees with the nurse, and says, "I have a right to walk downstairs if I wish." In this instance, the nurse should accept the client's actions if they cannot come to some agreement because to restrain the client would mean denying the client his or her freedom.

Types of Rights

There are three main types of rights: option rights, welfare rights, and legislative rights. **Option rights** are rights of freedom and choice; they express the right of people to live as they choose within prescribed boundaries (Fromer 1981, p. 2). For example, a female nurse working in a hospital can wear any uniform she wishes (her right) provided it is white, clean, and covers her body suitably (boundaries). The boundaries in this instance are probably hospital policy and a norm established by many nurses.

Welfare rights are the legal entitlement to some good, e.g., specific safety standards in a building or a number of years of education (Fromer 1981, p. 3). An example is the right of clients to health care or the right of citizens to safe water.

Legislative rights are established by law; they are based on the concept of justice. For example, a woman has the legal right not to be raped by her husband. Bandman and Bandman state that legislative rights have four roles in society: rule making, rule changing, moral constraints against unjust rules, and adjudication or dispute settling (Bandman and Bandman 1986, p. 142).

Meaning of Rights

Bandman and Bandman describe five conditions that help to define rights.

1. Freedom to exercise the right as one chooses. The individual is neither blamed nor punished for exercising or not exercising the right. For example, a client has a right to a medication prescribed by a physician, but he or she has a right to refuse or accept the medication.
2. Others have duties to facilitate an individual's exercising of the right. For example, a client has a right to his or her medication, and nurses have corresponding duties to ensure and protect the client's rights.
3. A right is in accordance with principles of justice, i.e., equality, impartiality, and fairness. For example, all clients have an equal right to medications.
4. A right is enforceable. For example, in some hospitals ethics committees have a mandate to ensure that human rights are enforced for all clients.
5. If a right is violated, set aside, or overridden, the person is given compensation. For example, if a client's name is left off a surgery schedule by mistake, the client may be compensated by being placed at the head of the list for surgery when the mistake is discovered (Bandman and Bandman 1985, pp. 57–58).

Clients' Rights

The movement for clients' rights in health care arose in the late 1960s. At that time, the broad goals of the movement were to improve the quality of health care and to make the health care system more responsive to clients' needs. Today, clients are also seeking more self-determination and control over their own bodies when they are ill. Informed consent, confidentiality, and the right of the client to refuse treatment are all aspects of this self-determination. The need for clients' rights is largely the result of two circumstances: the vulnerability of the client because of illness and the complexity of the relationships in the health care setting.

When people are ill, they are frequently unable to assert their rights as they would if they were healthy. Asserting rights requires energy and an underlying awareness of one's rights in the situation. People who are weak or preoccupied about their illness, for example, may not be able to assert their rights. In addition, individuals are not always aware of their rights because the health care environment is unfamiliar to them. The need for confidentiality of information about a client's health may not occur to a client; he or she may just not have thought about it.

The complexity and variety of health care relationships also increase the need for clients' rights. In this day of specialization, a client is often helped by a variety of health professionals. The client becomes one person among many health professionals. Thus, the client's needs or priorities, for example, can become lost in the communications among health professionals.

In traditional patterns of health care, clients experience losses, e.g., loss of the sense of independence and control. In the traditional relationship between the client and the health care provider, the care provider is seen as superordinate, an authority, and even a person to be venerated. This traditional pattern encourages client dependence: while the client seeks health or the return to health, the health care providers grant that client only limited rights. (Healey 1983, pp. 115–16.)

A new pattern of health care relationships is emerging as a result of several forces in society, including a more knowledgable consumer and recognition of the role of life-style in disease. Today, the goals of health include the return of autonomy and independence to the client and the acceptance of good health as a responsibility of the care provider, the client, and society. These goals cannot be met unless clients accept active responsibility for their health and health care and unless clients and care providers have mutual respect.

The clients' rights movement promotes this new health care relationship, and nurses today are combating the undermining of clients' rights by identifying and protecting clients' rights and helping clients assert their rights (Healey 1983, p. 116).

Annas and Healey (1974, p. 26) list four rights that are assertable in a health care facility:

1. The right to the whole truth
2. The right to privacy and personal dignity
3. The right to retain self-determination by participating in decisions regarding one's health.
4. The right of complete access to medical records, both during and after the hospital stay.

A Patient's Bill of Rights

In 1972, the American Hospital Association published "A Patient's Bill of Rights" in an effort to promote the rights of hospitalized clients. See Table 9–1. Frequently clients do not know their rights, although many hospitals today give clients upon admission a statement of their rights while in hospital.

These statements regarding the rights of clients appear to have been influenced by several factors:

1. Increased awareness on the part of the consumer about the right to health care and to greater participation in planning that care.
2. The increasing number of malpractice suits that are receiving publicity and thus coming into the public's awareness. As a result of these, the consumer is increasingly concerned about rights, often in a protective sense.
3. Legislation that has been created in other previously protected relationships, such as the employee-employer relationship, and human rights and equal rights legislation in general.
4. Consumer concern about the increasing amount of research being conducted in the health field and the increasing use of clients for educational purposes in a number of disciplines. Although clients and their families are generally willing to participate in research and educational programs, they frequently ask, "Do I have to?" In addition, some clients wonder whether the quality of their care will suffer if they do not agree to participate.

Nursing Implications

The nursing implications of the Patient's Bill of Rights are:

1. *The patient has a right to considerate and respectful care.* The client has a right to an explanation about what will happen, why, and when. The client also has the right to participate in planning his or her care. Considerate and respectful care also includes respect for the dignity of each person. Nurses can convey respect by listening carefully to clients and their support persons and reporting their concerns to the appropriate people.
2. *The patient has the right to obtain from his physician complete current information concerning his diagnosis, treatment, and prognosis, in terms the patient can be reasonably expected to understand.* The responsibility for divulging this information belongs to the physician. If a client asks a nurse for this information, the nurse should relay the questions to the physician and document the client's questions and the nurse's actions on the client's record.

   There is increased emphasis today upon "truth telling" or the disclosure of information to the client (Purtilo and Cassel 1981, p. 75). Many people believe that even when ill, clients still have a right to the whole truth, i.e., complete information about their health care. Nurses should explain independent nursing actions truthfully and completely. Because these activities are solely in the nurse's domain, the nurse has sole responsibility for explaining them. See Chapter 14 for information about independent nursing actions. However, dependent nursing functions, i.e., those nursing activities ordered by the physician, should be explained only after the nurse completely understands the physician's and client's positions. Usually, a physician has no objection to a client understanding the ordered treatments; however, occasionally a physician does not wish a client to be fully informed, e.g., about a medication for a malignancy before the client has been informed of the diagnosis.

Table 9–1 A Patient's Bill of Rights

1. The patient has the right to considerate and respectful care.
2. The patient has the right to obtain from his physician complete current information concerning his diagnosis, treatment, and prognosis, in terms the patient can be reasonably expected to understand. When it is not medically advisable to give such information to the patient, the information should be made available to an appropriate person in his behalf. He has the right to know by name the physician responsible for coordinating his care.
3. The patient has the right to receive from his physician information necessary to give informed consent prior to the start of any procedure and/or treatment. Except in emergencies, such information for informed consent should include but not necessarily be limited to the specific procedure and/or treatment, the medically significant risks involved, and the probable duration of incapacitation. Where medically significant alternatives for care or treatment exist, or when the patient requests information concerning medical alternatives, the patient has the right to such information. The patient also has the right to know the name of the person responsible for the procedures and/or treatment.
4. The patient has the right to refuse treatment to the extent permitted by law and to be informed of the medical consequences of his action.
5. The patient has the right to every consideration of his privacy concerning his own medical care program. Case discussion, consultation, examination, and treatment are confidential and should be conducted discreetly. Those not directly involved in this care must have the permission of the patient to be present.
6. The patient has the right to expect that all communications and records pertaining to his care should be treated as confidential.
7. The patient has the right to expect that within its capacity a hospital must make reasonable response to the request of a patient for services. The hospital must provide evaluation, service, and/or referral as indicated by the urgency of the case. When medically permissible, a patient may be transferred to another facility only after he has received complete information and explanation concerning the needs for and alternatives to such a transfer. The institution to which the patient is transferred must first have accepted the patient for transfer.
8. The patient has the right to obtain information as to any relationship of his hospital to other health care and educational institutions insofar as his care is concerned. The patient has the right to obtain information as to the existence of any professional relationships among individuals, by name, who are treating him.
9. The patient has the right to be advised if the hospital proposes to engage in or perform human experimentation affecting his care or treatment. The patient has the right to refuse to participate in such research projects.
10. The patient has the right to expect reasonable continuity of care. He has the right to know in advance what appointment times and physicians are available and where. The patient has the right to expect that the hospital will provide a mechanism whereby he is informed by his physician or a delegate of the physician of the patient's continuing health.
11. The patient has the right to examine and receive an explanation of his bill regardless of source of payment.
12. The patient has the right to know what hospital rules and regulations apply to his conduct as a patient.

Source: From American Hospital Association. 1973. A patient's bill of rights. *Nursing Outlook*, February 1973, 21:82, and January 1976, 24:29. Reprinted with the permission of the American Hospital Association.

Although the client has a right to be fully informed, not all jurisdictions accept the Patient's Bill of Rights as law. Therefore nurses should inform the physician about the client's questions, discuss the matter thoroughly, and document the client's questions.

3. *The patient has the right to receive from his physician information necessary to give informed consent prior to the start of any procedures and/or treatment.* The client has the right to give or withhold informed consent. Obtaining informed consent is the physician's responsibility. The nurse's role in obtaining informed consent is discussed in Chapter 7, page 163.

Before a nurse commences any nursing interventions, clients must give consent to that care. Informed consent has five aspects:

a. Explanation of the proposed treatment
b. Explanation of inherent risks and benefits
c. Alternatives to the proposed treatment
d. Adequate time for client questions
e. Option to withdraw at any time

An important nursing strategy is to "coordinate the medical, technical, and nursing activities on behalf of the patient's well-being into a meaningful process that the patient and family can utilize in the shared decision process" (Bandman and Bandman 1985, p. 74). It has been found that in most instances treatments are refused because of conflicting information (President's Commission 1982, p. 80). Therefore, when nurses and other health professionals collaborate and encourage the client's participation, the client feels more secure and more comfortable about making decisions regarding care.

A client can also withdraw consent after signing a consent form. Annas suggests that in such a case it is wise "to execute another form—this time a form of nonconsent to treatment, noting on it the date and time of day" (Annas 1975, p. 74). Because obtaining the consent is the responsibility of the physician, it is suggested that the physician obtain the nonconsent. If a nurse is about to give an injection, for example, and the client says, "I have changed my mind—I don't

Research Note

Each individual's right to self-determination, to decide what will or will not be done to his or her person, is the basis for the requirement of informed consent. Nurses are frequently called upon to give crucial information to clients, either as clinicians or researchers, and must be acutely aware of the ingredients in successful communication of benefits and risks. Silva studied the comprehension of information needed to give an informed consent to participate in a research study in a group of spouses of surgical clients. While the study showed that most spouses had been given adequate information, many did not understand that information. The study supports the idea that comprehension will be adequate if individuals are well, if they read the information carefully, if the information is short and simple, and if recall is requested shortly after presentation of the material. (Silva 1985)

want that drug," the nurse should not give the injection, report the situation to the charge nurse and/or physician, and record the client's words and the nurse's actions on the client's record.

4. *The patient has the right to refuse treatment to the extent permitted by law and to be informed of the medical consequences of his action.* Clients have the right to self-determination. Just as they have the right to informed consent, they also have the right to refuse a treatment. An adult client who is conscious and medically competent has the right to refuse any medical or surgical procedure (Annas 1975, p. 79). When the client refuses treatment, no person has to impose the treatment. The client still has the right to the best possible care within the limitations he or she imposes. In regard to a parent's refusal to allow treatment of a child, Annas states: "It is only in extreme cases involving the potential of death or permanent disability to the child that courts are likely to overrule a parent's refusal of treatment for a child" (Annas 1975, p. 87).

5. *The patient has the right to every consideration of his privacy concerning his own medical care program.* People vary in what they consider an invasion of privacy and a threat to dignity. Therefore only the client can decide whether to permit any invasion of privacy. Although a client who signs a consent form for an examination or treatment may be giving up certain aspects of privacy in the course of the examination or treatment, the invasion of the client's privacy must be kept to the minimum. For example, a client who consents to a physical examination is expected to disrobe; however, the nurse can provide some degree of privacy by supplying an appropriate gown, drapes, and a room or enclosed area. Also, by consenting to the examination, the client does not also agree to the presence of people other than those directly involved in the examination.

   The right to privacy is closely linked to the individual's personal dignity. Individuals "on exhibit" can feel demeaned and embarrassed. The experience of being viewed by a group of health professionals, e.g., nursing students, can live in a person's memory for many years as a distasteful incident. Nurses must ensure that the client fully understands and consents to the presence of health personnel not directly involved in treatment.

   The concept of privacy can be viewed as (a) an antisocial anachronism, (b) a necessary defense against the stress in society, and (c) a vital condition for personal growth (Rawnsley 1986, pp. 106–7). In the first view, privacy is considered to be dysfunctional to the group. In the second, privacy is seen as palliative and restorative, providing the individual an opportunity to build stronger defenses against the stress (Rawnsley 1986, p. 107). In the third view, privacy is seen as an opportunity to progress toward self-actualization (see Maslow's hierarchy of needs on page 314, Chapter 16).

   The right to privacy is the second item in the ANA Code (ANA 1976, p. 2). In addition, clients have a right to be examined and seen by only the people directly concerned with their care. Physicians normally have responsibility for obtaining consent if, for example, a medical student needs to examine the client. Clients have a right to privacy even after death. Privacy also means not intruding into the client's pri-

Research Note

Roosa interviewed 60 residents of a nursing home to determine how they defined privacy, what benefits it provided, and what activities required privacy. Roosa used four states of privacy in the survey:

1. Solitude: physical seclusion from others
2. Intimacy: close familiarity with people
3. Anonymity: freedom from identification when in a crowd
4. Reserve: a psychologic barrier created between oneself and others (Westin 1967, pp. 31–32)

All 60 residents selected solitude in their definition of privacy. About one-half (28) of the residents identified emotional release as a benefit and some (11) mentioned self-evaluation, e.g., reflecting on the past, concentrating, or "remaining the person I am." Nine residents stated strengthening personal autonomy as a benefit. Residents wanted privacy to read, write, conduct personal business, watch TV, and listen to music. (Roosa 1982)

vate life and disclosing confidential information. Nurses can be held legally liable for taking any action without consent that would offend a reasonable person's sensibilities (Good Intentions Gone Awry 1986, p. 55). Ways of intruding into a client's private life include eavesdropping on a conversation, searching a client's clothes or handbag, taking photographs of an unconscious client, or asking questions that have no relation to the client's health. See Chapter 7, page 159, for additional information regarding the invasion of privacy.

Another aspect of privacy of concern to nurses and other health professionals is the effect of computers on the confidentiality of records. Although computers have facilitated health care in a number of ways, any person who knows an access code can view confidential client information. Therefore, nurses and all health professionals must guard the confidentiality of client records and not give computer codes to unauthorized people.

6. *The patient has the right to expect that all communications and records pertaining to his care should be treated as confidential.* Privacy is closely related to confidentiality. Only clients have the power to let people not directly involved in their care view their medical records. Only the client has the right to provide information to support persons or others. Confidentiality is also included in the ANA ethical code. See Chapter 8.

   Confidentiality means that information disclosed to a person, e.g., a nurse, will not be disclosed to anyone not directly involved in the client's care. Disclosure of such information is a breach of confidentiality and could lead to legal action against the nurse or the health agency.

7. *The patient has the right to expect that within its capacity a hospital must make a reasonable response to the request of a patient for services.*

8. *The patient has a right to obtain information as to any relationship of his hospital to other health care and educational institutions insofar as his care is concerned.* Rights 8 and 9 are largely related to hospital administration. However, nurses are becoming increasingly involved in such matters as budget as they relate to client care. A client who believes his or her care is inadequate should communicate this fact to the appropriate person in the hospital. Every health agency should have a procedure for handling client grievances. One trend in health care is client advocacy, a function assumed by nurses in some settings. See the section on client advocacy on page 205.

9. *The patient has the right to be advised if the hospital proposes to engage in or perform human experimentation affecting his care or treatment.* Clients also have a right to consent or refuse to participate in any research or experimentation. Both the ANA and the CNA have published guidelines for nurses who participate in research. See Chapter 5.

10. *The patient has the right to expect reasonable continuity of care.* Clients have a right to know what health care they will need after they are discharged from a hospital. It is often the nurse's responsibility to teach follow-up care and to make appropriate referrals to other health agencies. Discharge planning is discussed in Chapter 4.

11. *The patient has the right to examine and receive an explanation of his bill regardless of the source of payment.* Nurses often record billable items such as dressings, medications, and the like. In some settings, it may be the nurse's responsibility to explain a bill to a client, although this task is often carried out by someone in the hospital's business office.

12. *The patient has the right to know what hospital rules and regulations apply to his conduct as a patient.* Some agencies provide pamphlets that list rules, such as those governing visiting hours, and explain services, such as cafeteria and telephone service. Often nurses clarify information and answer a client's questions about hospital rules. Nurses also explain rules associated with special procedures, such as those that apply when oxygen is in use or when a client has an infection.

Another right not mentioned specifically in the AHA Patient's Bill of Rights is the right of access to medical records. Although in some jurisdictions clients have the right of access to their health records, agency practices vary widely in this regard. Some hospitals, e.g., military hospitals, permit clients to keep records at the bedside. At the other extreme, some agencies release records to clients only if they have a subpoena. A number of state legislatures have passed laws requiring health agencies to establish reasonable policies by which clients are permitted access to their records. Laws about access to records have changed in recent years, and it is generally recognized that only clients can grant others access to their records or permit the release or transfer of their records.

Rights of Special Groups

Recently special groups have had lists of rights made public. Some of these groups are the handicapped, the dying, the retarded, and the elderly. These lists of rights reflect increased awareness of consumers' rights in general and their specific rights as members of certain groups.

In the Declaration on the Rights of Disabled Persons adopted by the General Assembly of the United Nations in December 1975, 13 points are made. See Appendix A1. This declaration defines *disability* as "deficiency, either congenital or not, in . . . physical or mental capabilities." The rights stated in this declaration do not have the force of law; however, many do have a basis in the laws of some countries. For example, statement 2 refers to the application of these rights to all people without discrimination on the basis of race, color, sex, language, religion, or other matters. This statement is similar to human rights legislation in many countries today.

The Dying Person's Bill of Rights was created at a 1975 workshop on "The Terminally Ill Patient and the Helping Person," held in Lansing, Michigan, and sponsored by the Southwestern Michigan Inservice Education Council. See Chapter 50. Amelia J. Barbus, associate professor of nursing at Wayne State University, Detroit, conducted the workshop.

The rights of the elderly were formulated as a result of a White House conference in 1961. See Appendix A2. The Declaration on the Rights of the Mentally Retarded was adopted by the United Nations in 1971. See Appendix A3. The Declaration of the Rights of the Child was adopted by the United Nations in 1979. See Appendix A4. The Pregnant Patient's Bill of Rights, published by the International Childbirth Education Association, was written by Doris B. Haire. See Appendix A5.

Nurses' Rights

The idea of nurses' rights has received considerable attention. Initially this attention was focused on the right of the nurse to refuse to carry out a specific service, such as assisting with an abortion or giving a medication that the nurse considered dangerous for the client. Now nurses' rights are being described in positive terms. Fagin (1975, pp. 82–85) lists seven rights of nurses:

1. The right to find dignity in self-expression and self-enhancement through the use of their special abilities and educational backgrounds.
2. The right to recognition for their contribution through the provision of a proper environment for practice, and through appropriate remuneration.
3. The right to a work environment that minimizes physical and emotional stress and health risks.
4. The right to control what is professional practice within the limits of the law.
5. The right to set standards of excellence in nursing.
6. The right to participate in policy making affecting nursing.
7. The right to social and political action on behalf of nursing and health care.

When a nurse's rights (ethical or legal) are violated, the nurse has an obligation to discuss the matter with the appropriate person at the employing agency. If a conflict cannot be resolved, the nurse can report her or his concerns to a professional body, such as the American Nurses' Association. Most state and provincial associations have mechanisms to deal with legal and ethical issues.

Nurses have rights as citizens and as health professionals. As a citizen, a nurse has all the rights provided under federal and state or provincial law. Upon becoming a nurse, a person does not give up any rights as a citizen. The traditional focus of the profession has been on the nurse's responsibilities and service to others, rather than on the nurse's rights and autonomy. The assertion of nurses' rights should be viewed as a means of improving nursing practice. For example, in a suitable environment, nurses can provide a professional standard of nursing care to clients, whereas in an unsuitable environment, e.g., one lacking staff or equipment, the nurse's right to provide quality care is denied.

Fenner (1980, p. 90) lists four rights of nurses:

1. *To expect own rights to be respected.* This area includes human rights—such as respect for the individual, freedom of choice, and equality—and professional rights—such as the right to set standards of excellence in nurse practice acts and to participate in policy affecting nursing and professional autonomy (Fagin 1975, pp. 82–85).
2. *To safe and functional equipment and services.* Implicit in this right is sufficient equipment and sufficient staffing to permit a high standard of professional practice. Also included in this area is the right to work in an environment that minimizes physical and emotional stress. Physical stressors, such as potentially infectious microorganisms, must be identified, and suitable precautions must be taken to protect the health of nurses and other health practitioners.
3. *To compensation for services.* The issue of compensation for services is discussed under contractual agreements in Chapter 7.
4. *To competent assistance.* This right includes not only assistance with the implementation of nursing practice but also support people such as pharmacists, dietitians, and inhalation therapists.

Davis and Aroskar (1983, p. 86) write that the assertion of nurses' rights should not be seen as an end to itself but as a means of improving nursing practice. Therefore, the recognition and implementation of nurses' rights can also result in improved care for clients and their support persons.

Nursing Students' Rights

In 1970, the Student Bill of Rights was first presented to the ANA House of Delegates. The bill indicates the minimum standards of academic and personal freedom and the rights of students in all educational communities. The National Student Nurses' Association (NSNA) also believes that students have the right to qualified instructors, the right to evaluate the performance of their teachers, the right to a curriculum that is relevant to the work situation, and the right to a voice and a vote in determining the content of nursing curricula. In addition, the NSNA supports the right of nursing students to participate in community health projects as a way to meet curriculum objectives and obtain course credits (NSNA 1985, p. 19).

In 1974, the United States Congress passed the Family Educational Rights and Privacy Act (Buckley Amendment). Its two major provisions are that the records of a student be available to that student and that the records be private.

The records available to the student are educational records, not health records or the private files of teachers. Permission to see the student's file is limited to those involved in the educational process, for example, a nursing instructor who is teaching the student, or the registrar.

In addition, letters of recommendation can be kept from the student only if the student signs a waiver giving up the right to see the letter. Students do not have the right to see confidential materials obtained from parents, such as financial statements.

When someone wishes to write a student reference, students have the right to give or withhold permission to examine the information in their files. When the teacher, for example, needs access to the central file to provide reference information about graduates, the student has the right to withhold consent. However, that teacher does not need the student's permission to write a reference without examining the central file.

According to the Buckley Amendment, students have the right to challenge factual information, and a conciliation or hearing can subsequently take place.

Students also have other general rights directly involved in their nursing education. They have the right to expect that the curriculum described in the school brochure or calendar will be followed. They have a right to competent instruction. Because students are accountable to clients for care, they must receive sufficient assistance and instruction to give safe care.

Client Advocacy

An **advocate** pleads the cause of another or argues or pleads for a cause or proposal. Advocacy involves concern for and defined actions in behalf of another person or organization to bring about a change. A **client advocate** is an advocate of clients' rights. Some nurses believe client advocacy is an essential nursing function. Others believe that a client advocate need not be a nurse. All, however, recognize the need of many clients for an advocate to protect their rights and to help them speak up for themselves.

An advocate can represent a client by presenting his or her point of view, and by interpreting and explaining his or her rights. The role of the advocate is to inform clients of their rights and options and of the consequences of these options (Kohnke 1981, p. 125). An advocate has two basic functions: to allow clients to make their own informed decisions and to support clients in their decisions. For example, Mr. Rae makes a decision not to have further chemotherapy for his malignancy after being fully informed about the treatment, the options, and the possible consequences. The client advocate informs Mr. Rae of his rights to make this decision and supports him in his decision. The client advocate does not need to approve a client's decision but must respect the client's right to make the decision.

The Patient Rights Advocate System

The goals of a program of patient advocacy are:

1. To protect patients, particularly those at a disadvantage within the hospital context (the young, the illiterate, the uncommunicative, those without relatives, those unable to speak English) by making available a series of processes and procedures.
2. To make available to those who seek it the opportunity to participate actively with one's doctor as a partner in one's personal health care program.
3. To restore to proper perspective medical technologies and pharmaceutical advances, and to confront the exaggerated expectations of the modern American medical consumer.
4. To reflect in the patient-doctor relationship the reality of the health-sickness continuum and to reassert the humanness of death as inevitable and as natural as birth.

(Annas and Healy 1974)

The role of the advocate involves influencing others. Nurses implement the advocacy role in two supportive ways: acting on behalf of the client, and giving the client full or at least mutual responsibility in decision making (Leddy and Pepper 1985, pp. 284–85). An example of acting on behalf of a client is asking a physician to talk to the client about the reasons for the immobility of the client's right arm because the client says he always forgets to ask the physician. An example of mutual responsibility for decision making is nurse and client collaboration in planning an exercise schedule. Activities that the nurse carries out in a client advocate role must be documented in the client's record.

Some people believe that the client advocate should be accountable to the client and be his or her representative. The client advocate should be able to: call in qualified consultants, participate actively in hospital committees monitoring the quality of client care, present complaints directly to the hospital director and hospital executive committee, delay discharges, and participate at the client's request and direction in discussions of the client's case (Annas 1975, pp. 209, 211).

Chapter Highlights

- A right is a legitimate expectation of a person in a given society at a given time.
- A personal concept of rights influences people's values and the conduct of their lives.
- Clients' rights are largely the result of the clients' health problems and the complex health care relationships involved in the clients' care.
- Nurses have responsibilities in regard to clients' rights.
- Client advocacy involves concern for and defined actions on behalf of another person or organization to bring about changes.
- Nurses have rights in the health care system.
- Nursing students have rights relative to their nursing education.

Suggested Readings

Baer, O. J. May/June 1985. Protecting your patients' privacy. *Nursing Life* 5:50–53.
Baer provides guidelines for helping nurses protect clients' privacy. Included are suggestions as to what to do when a client's family questions the nurse, how to respond to media inquiries, how to obey reporting laws, and what to say when called to testify about a client.

Cote, A. A. January 1981. The patient's representative: Whose side is she on? *Nursing 81* 11:26–30.
Cote discusses how the nurse and the client's representative can work together to protect the client's rights. Topics include the patient's bill of rights, informed consent, the client's right to know and not to know, the right to decline treatment, the right to privacy, and the right to information in clinical records.

Cushing, M. April 1984. Informed consent: An MD responsibility? *American Journal of Nursing* 84:437, 439–40.
Cushing explains that inherent in the concept of informed consent is the duty to give enough information so that the client can weigh the risks and benefits of a procedure. In disclosure, the physician must tell the client the diagnosis, the nature of the problem, the benefits and risks of proposed treatment, the alternatives, and the prognosis if treatment is withheld. Cushing points out that oral consent is equally as binding as written consent. Disclosure is the physician's responsibility, and nurses should not be delegated to provide medical information to clients. Cushing points out that a nurse's signature on a consent form identifies the nurse as a witness to the signature.

Ozimek, D. February 1982. Rights and responsibilities of students and faculty. *Imprint* 29:50–51, 63–64, 68–69, 72–76, 78–79.
Ozimek writes about rights in general and rights and responsibilities. Human rights are moral rights or rights derived from law. Students have rights as citizens of a community, state, and country and as members of a student body. The responsibilities of students entail liability, accountability, and answerability. Ozimek gives seven guidelines for making decisions about faculty and students' rights.

Trandel-Korenchuk, D., and Trandel-Korenchuk, K. April 1983. Nursing advocacy of patients' rights: Myth or reality. Part 2. *Nurse Practitioner* 8:37, 40–42.
The authors discuss communication in the physician-nurse relationship. Evident in communication patterns are authoritarianism (physician), acceptance of dependence (nurse), and communication control (physician). The authors relate problems in nurse-to-nurse relationships to the problems in women's relationships. It is proposed that nurses will be better able to meet medicine and hospital bureaucracy on equal ground if nursing attains unity and influence.

Selected References

American Hospital Association. January 1976. A patient's bill of rights. *Nursing Outlook* 24:29 (also February 1973, *Nursing Outlook* 21:82).

Annas, G. J. September 1973. The patient has rights: How can we protect them? *Hastings Center Report* 3:9.

———. 1975. *The rights of hospital patients: The basic ACLU guide to a hospital patient's rights.* New York: Avon Books.

Annas, G. J.; Glantz, L. H.; and Katz, B. F. 1981. *The rights of doctors, nurses and allied health professionals.* New York: Avon Books.

Annas, G. J., and Healey, J. May/June 1974. The patient rights advocate. *Journal of Nursing Administration* 4:25–31.

Bandman, E. L. 1983. Who will advocate for the nurse advocate?

In Murphy, C. P., and Hunter, H. *Ethical problems in the nurse-patient relationship.* Boston: Allyn and Bacon.

Bandman, E. L., and Bandman, B. May 1977. There is nothing automatic about rights. *American Journal of Nursing* 77:867–72.

———. January 1978. Do nurses have rights? *American Journal of Nursing* 78:84–86.

Curtin, L. L. October 1982. Informed consent: Rights, responsibilities, and roles. *Nursing Management* 13:7–8.

Curtin, L. L., and Flaherty, M. J. 1982. *Nursing ethics: Theories and pragmatics.* Bowie, Md.: Robert J. Brady Co.

Davis, A. April 1984. Patient's right to decide is new value in health care. Part 5. *American Nurse* 16:5–6, 24.

Davis, A. J., and Aroskar, M. A. 1983. *Ethical dilemmas and nursing practice.* 2d ed. Norwalk, Conn.: Appleton-Century-Crofts.

Eth, S., and Eth, C. August 1981. Can a research subject be too eager to consent? *Hastings Center Report* 11:20.

Fagin, C. M. January 1975. Nurses' rights. *American Journal of Nursing* 75:82–85.

Fromer, M. J. 1981. *Ethical issues in health care.* St. Louis: C. V. Mosby Co.

———. 1986. Solving ethical dilemmas in nursing practice. In Chinn, P. L., editor. *Ethical issues in nursing.* Rockville, Md.: Aspen Systems Corporation.

Golding, M. 1978. The concept of rights: A historical sketch. In Bandman, E., and Bandman, B., editors. *Bioethics and human rights.* Boston: Little, Brown.

Good intentions gone awry. March/April 1986. *Nursing Life* 6:55–56.

Healey, J. M. 1983. Patients' rights and nursing. In Murphy, C. P., and Hunter, H. *Ethical problems in the nurse-patient relationship.* Boston: Allyn and Bacon.

Kohnke, M. F. March 1978. The nurse's responsibility to the consumer. *American Journal of Nursing* 78:440–42.

———. 1981. Discussion of consultant/advocate for the medically hospitalized patient. *Nursing Forum* 20(2):123–36.

Leddy, S., and Pepper, J. M. 1985. *Conceptual bases of professional nursing.* Philadelphia: J. B. Lippincott Co.

Murphy, C. P., and Hunter, H. 1983. *Ethical problems in the nurse-patient relationship.* Boston: Allyn and Bacon.

National League for Nursing. 1977. *Nursing's role in patient's rights.* New York: National League for Nursing.

National Student Nurses' Association. 1985. *Getting the pieces to fit 85/86: School chapters.* New York: National Student Nurses' Association.

Ozimek, D. February 1982. Rights and responsibilities of students and faculty. *Imprint* 29:50–51, 63–64, 68–69, 72–76, 78–79.

Pollok, C. S., et al. April 1976. Students' rights. *American Journal of Nursing* 76:600–603.

———. April 1977. Faculties have rights, too. *American Journal of Nursing* 77:636–38.

President's Commission for the Study of Ethical Problems in Medicine and Biomedical and Behavioral Research: Making Health Care Decisions. 1982. Washington, D.C.: U.S. Government Printing Office.

Rawnsley, M. M. 1986. The concept of privacy. In Chinn, P. L., editor. *Ethical issues in nursing.* Rockville, Md.: Aspen Systems Corporation.

Regan, W. A. January 1984. Advocacy or unprofessional conduct? *RN* 47:23–24.

Roosa, W. M. July/August 1982. Territory and privacy. Resident views—Findings of a survey. *Geriatric Nursing* 3:241–43.

Rozovsky, L. E. 1980. *The Canadian patient's book of rights.* Toronto: Doubleday Canada.

Shephard, D. A. December 1976. The 1975 declaration of Helsinki and consent. *Canadian Medical Journal* 115:1191–92.

Silva, M. C. 1985. Comprehension of information for informed consent by spouses of surgical patients. *Research in Nursing and Health* 8:117–24.

Special poll. May/June 1985. What nurses think of computers. Part 2. *Nursing Life* 5:28–30.

Trandel-Korenchuk, D., and Trandel-Korenchuk, K. April 1983. Nursing advocacy of patients' rights: Myth or reality? Part 2. *Nurse Practitioner* 8:37, 40–42.

Zusman, J. November/December 1982. Want some good advice? Think twice about being a patient advocate. *Nursing Life* 6:46–50.

Westin, A. F. 1967. *Privacy and freedom.* New York: Atheneum.

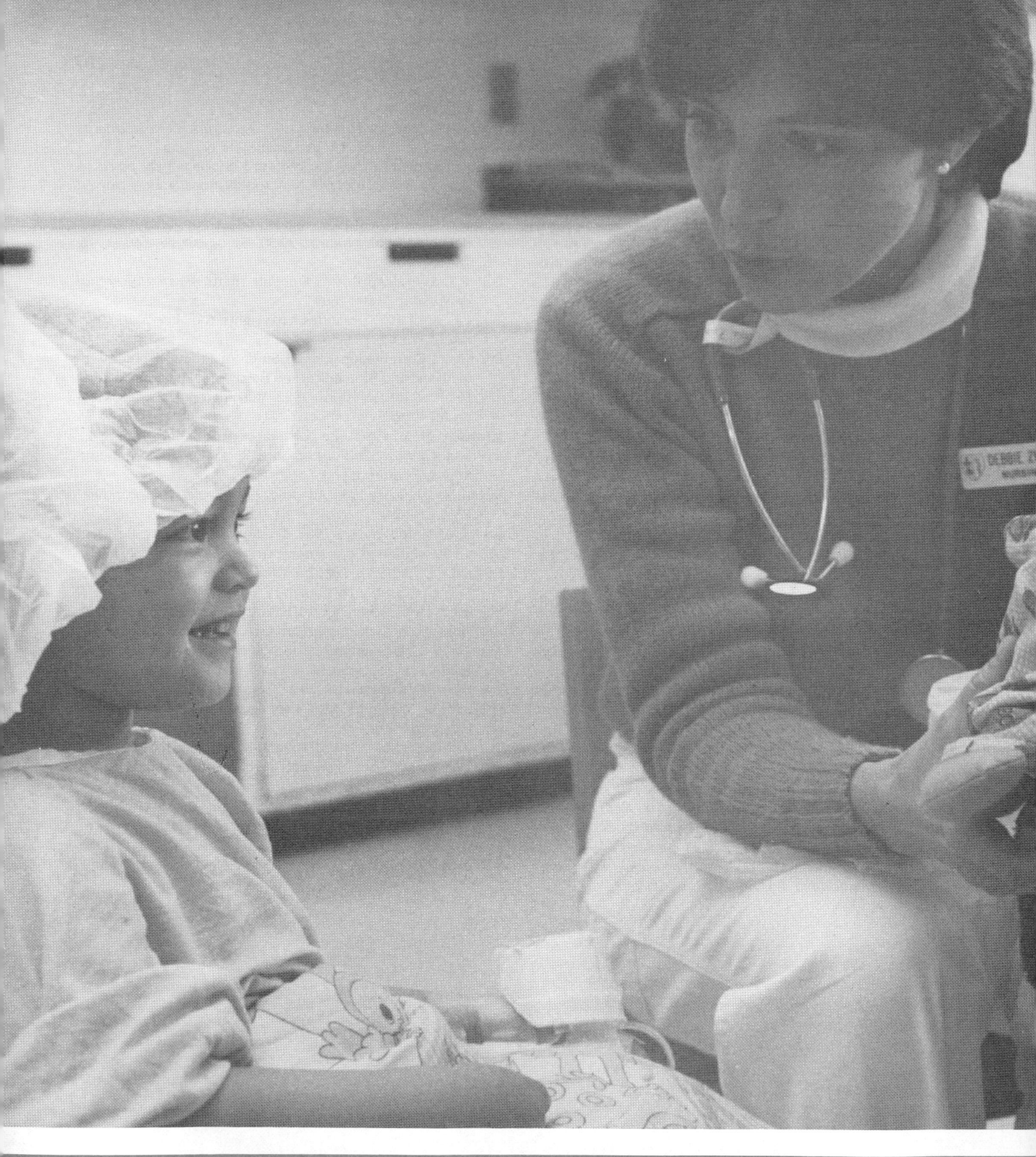

Because nursing emphasizes helping people do for themselves what they would do if they knew what to do, it seems like common sense. What we forget is that sense is not common. (Angela Barron McBride)

UNIT **3**

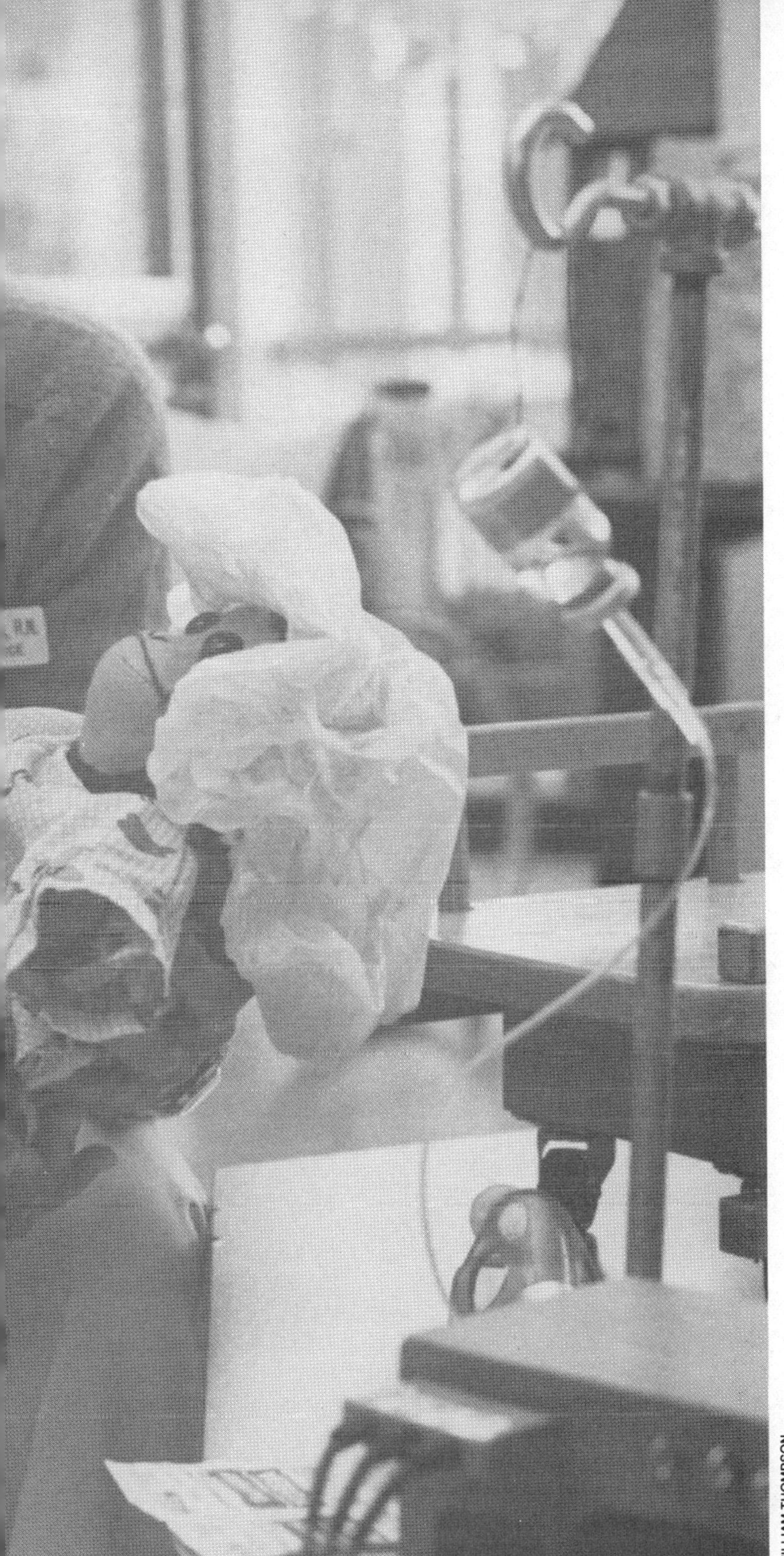
WILLIAM THOMPSON

The Nursing Process

Contents

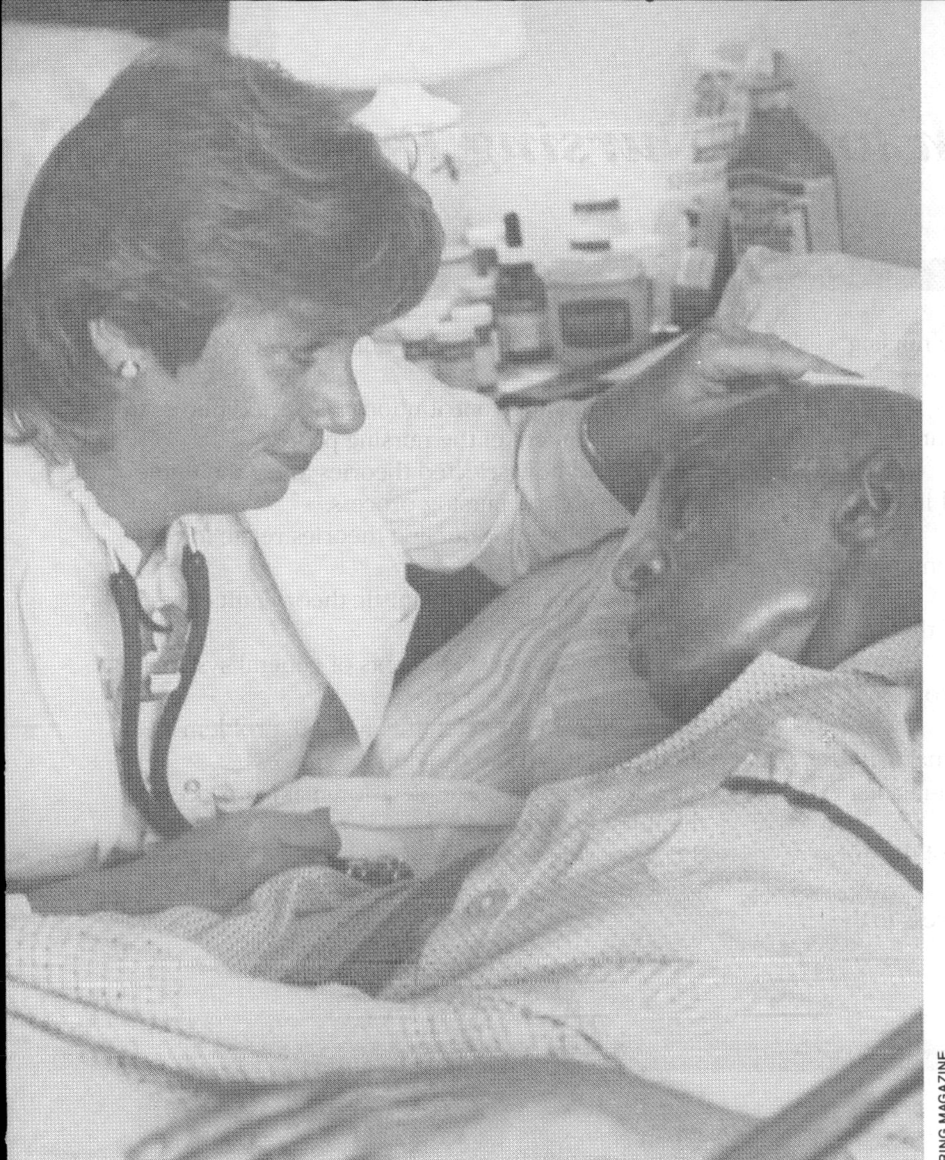

CARING MAGAZINE

CHAPTER 10

Introduction to the Nursing Process

Contents

10 *Introduction to the Nursing Process*

Objectives

1. Understand essential facts related to the nursing process.
   1.1 Define listed terms.
   1.2 Compare the four- and five-step nursing processes.
   1.3 Identify nursing activities involved in each component of the nursing process.
   1.4 Identify skills required for each component of the nursing process.
   1.5 Identify essential characteristics of the nursing process.
   1.6 Describe various approaches to problem solving.
   1.7 Describe the process of decision making.
   1.8 Differentiate between the decision-making process and problem-solving process.
2. Appreciate the history and importance of the nursing process.
   2.1 List advantages of the nursing process to the patient.
   2.2 List advantages of the nursing process to the nurse.
   2.3 Identify the contribution of selected nurses to the development of the nursing process.
3. Understand how selected theories affect the implementation of the nursing process.
   3.1 Describe how nursing theories relate to the nursing process.
   3.2 Describe how humanistic theory influences the nursing process.
   3.3 Relate essential elements of general systems theory to the nursing process.
   3.4 Compare the scientific method, problem-solving method, and the nursing process.
   3.5 Relate steps of the decision-making process to the nursing process.
   3.6 Describe how the nursing process is a framework for accountability.

Terms

accountability
analyzing
assessing
boundary (of a system)
closed system
deductive reasoning
dependent nursing intervention
dynamic equilibrium
evaluating
feedback
holism
homeodynamics
homeostasis
humanism
hypothesis
implementing
independent nursing intervention
inductive reasoning
input
interdependent nursing action
nursing diagnosis
nursing process
open system
outcome (evaluative) criteria
output
perception
planning
process
scientific method
subsystem
suprasystem
system
theory
throughput

Historical Perspective on the Nursing Process

Before the nursing process was developed, nurses tended to provide care that was based on medical orders written by physicians and focused on specific disease conditions rather than on the person being cared for. Nursing practice that was provided independently of the physician was often guided by intuition rather than a scientific method.

The term **nursing process** and the framework it implies are relatively new. In 1955, Hall originated the term *nursing process.* Since then, various nurses have described the process of nursing in different ways. Wiedenbach (1963) described three steps in nursing: observation, ministration of help, and validation. Later, Knowles (1967, pp. 248–72) suggested "five Ds" necessary for the practice of nursing: discover, delve, decide, do, and discriminate. During the first two stages, the nurse collects data about the client. During the third stage (decide), the nurse determines a plan of action; and during the fourth stage (do), the nurse implements the plan. In the fifth stage (discriminate), the nurse assesses the patient's reaction to the nursing actions.

In 1967, the Western Interstate Commission on Higher Education identified a nursing process with five steps:

perception, communication, interpretation, intervention, and evaluation. WICHE defined the nursing process as "the interrelationship between a patient and a nurse in a given setting; it incorporates the behaviors of patient and nurse and the resulting interaction" (WICHE 1967). Also in 1967, the nursing faculty of the Catholic University of America proposed four components of the nursing process: assessment, planning, intervention, and evaluation (Yura and Walsh 1983). In 1973, Gebbie and Lavin (1975) at St. Louis University School of Nursing helped to form the first national conference on the classification of nursing diagnoses. Subsequently, conferences have been held every two years. In 1982, the conference group accepted the name North American Nursing Diagnosis Association (NANDA), thus recognizing the participation and contributions of Canadian nurses. This group has currently established and accepted over 70 diagnostic categories.

In 1973, the American Nurses' Association (ANA) published Standards of Nursing Practice that followed the steps of the nursing process. See Table 1–4 on p. 20. Subsequently, a number of states revised their nurse practice acts to reflect these aspects of nursing.

In 1980, ANA declared that "nursing is the diagnosis and treatment of human responses to actual or potential health problems" (ANA 1980). Clearly, the ANA saw diagnosis as a nursing function even though it was not unusual for people to believe diagnosis was the prerogative of the physician. In 1982, the National Council of State Boards of Nursing defined and described the five-step nursing process in terms of nursing behaviors: assessing, analyzing, planning, implementing, and evaluating (National Council of State Boards of Nursing 1982). In this context, analyzing is used to describe an activity required to develop a nursing diagnosis. **Analyzing** is breaking down a whole into component parts, e.g., identifying the parts of a physician's order or the various systems (component parts) of the human body (whole). Table 10–1 lists some of the nurses who contributed to the development of the nursing process.

Table 10–1 History of the Nursing Process

Nurse	Selected Contributions
Nightingale, F.	1. Nursing separated from medicine. 2. The nurse's function defined as adjusting an inadequate environment so that it helps the client to get well (Bishop 1962, p. 18).
Henderson, V.	1. Offered definition of nursing. 2. Identified fourteen components of basic nursing as independent functions. 3. Stated that the nursing process was the same as the steps of the scientific method (Henderson 1965, pp. 3–10; Henderson 1980, p. 907).
Peplau, H.	1. Nursing is a significant therapeutic interpersonal relationship. 2. Identified four phases in an interpersonal relationship: orientation, identification, exploitation, and resolution. The phases are sequential and focus on interpersonal therapeutic interaction (George 1985, pp. 60–65).
Kreuter, F. R.	Described steps in a nursing process as coordinating, planning, and evaluating nursing care and directing the family and the nursing auxiliary as they give nursing care. These were considered to promote the quality of professional practice (Kreuter 1957, p. 302).
Hall, L.	1. Defined three components of nursing: care, core, and cure, which interact. Care was bodily care; core was the client's feelings and motivations; cure indicated the manner in which the nurse assisted the client and family. 2. Defined nursing process as having three steps: observations, ministration of help, and validation. 3. Originated the term *nursing process* (George 1985, p. 116). 4. Stated that the client, family, and nurse analyzed and solved problems. The patient/client was the leader of his or her care.
Johnson, D.	1. Viewed the human as a behavioral system. 2. Saw the nursing process as assessing situations, arriving at decisions, implementing a course of action designed to resolve nursing problems, and evaluating (Johnson 1959, p. 200). 3. Saw intervention as having four modes: restrict, defend, inhibit, and facilitate.
Orlando, P.	1. Saw the nursing process as interactive. 2. Stated that the process included three phases: client's behavior, reaction of the nurse, and nursing actions (George 1985, pp. 162–68).

(continued)

Table 10–1 *(continued)*

Nurse	Selected Contributions
Heidgerken, L.	Described steps of professional nursing care as: evaluating behavior and situations; recognizing physical symptoms; diagnosing, planning, and meeting nursing needs; and coordinating the client's regimen through all states of care (Heidgerken 1965, p. 95).
Wiedenbach, E.	1. Described nursing as a goal-directed activity. 2. Identified three concepts in her theory: central purpose, prescription, and realities. The central purpose was the nurse's professional commitment; the prescription was the nature of the action that would fulfill the nurse's central purpose; the realities were all factors (physical, physiologic, psychologic, emotional, and spiritual) involved in the situation where the nursing action occurred (Wiedenbach 1970, p. 1057–62).
McCain, R. A.	1. Was the first to use the term *assessment* in an article published in 1965. 2. Used the functional abilities of the client as the framework for assessment. 3. Collected and recorded objective and subjective data in assessment (McCain 1965, pp. 82–84).
Yura, H. and Walsh, M.	1. Described four components of the nursing process: assessment, planning, intervention, and evaluation (Yura and Walsh 1983, p. 133).
Knowles, L.	1. Described the nurse's activity as: discover, delve, decide, do, and discriminate. 2. Stated that nurses collected data about the client's health during the first two stages.
Orem, D.	1. Described nursing as a deliberate action. 2. Stated that there were three steps in nursing care: (a) initial and continuing determination of why a person requires nursing care, (b) designing nursing actions for the client that will contribute to the client's achievement of health goals and planning for the delivery of nursing care, and (c) the initiating, conducting and control of assisting actions (Orem 1985, p. 224).
Bloch, D.	Suggested a five-step nursing process that was similar to the four-step model: collection of data, definition of problem, planning of intervention, implementation of the intervention, evaluation of the intervention (Bloch 1974, p. 693).
Roy, Sr. C.	1. Used six-step nursing process: assessment of client behaviors, assessment of influencing factors, problem identification, goal setting, intervention, selection of approaches, and evaluation. 2. Advocated the use of the term *nursing diagnosis* (Roy 1976, pp. 23–38).

Components of the Nursing Process

A **process** is a series of planned actions or operations directed toward a particular result. The **nursing process** is a systematic, rational method of planning and providing nursing care. Its goal is to identify a client's actual or potential health care needs, to establish plans to meet the identified needs, and to deliver specific nursing interventions to meet those needs. The nursing process is cyclical; that is, the components of the nursing process follow a logical sequence, but more than one component may be involved at any one time. See Figure 10–1.

To carry out the nursing process, at least two people must participate: the client and the nurse. The client may be an individual, a family, or even a community. The client participates as actively as possible in all phases of the nursing process. The nurse, by contrast, requires interpersonal, technical, and intellectual skills to use the nursing process. Interpersonal skills include communicating; listening; conveying interest, compassion, knowledge, and information; developing trust and obtaining data in a manner that enhances the individuality of the client, promotes the integrity of the family, and contributes to the viability of the community. Technical skills

Research Note

It is hypothesized that client compliance with the therapeutic objectives in a nursing care plan is increased with client participation in the nursing process. The data for the study were culled from a review of the literature. The study confirmed the relationship of participation of the client in the nursing process to increased compliance with therapeutic objectives as evidenced by physical activities of the client. The hypothesis that participation of the client *increases* compliance with therapeutic objectives was unconfirmed. (Conway-Rutkowski 1982)

are manifested in the use of equipment and the performance of procedures. Intellectual skills required by a nurse include problem solving, critical thinking, and making nursing judgments. Decision making is involved in every component of the nursing process (Yura and Walsh 1983).

The nursing process consists of a series of four or five components or steps. The four-step process is assessing, planning, implementing, and evaluating. In this system, analyzing (nursing diagnosis) is included in the assessing phase. The five-step nursing process is assessing, analyzing, planning, implementing, and evaluating. See Table 10–2. Some authorities believe the five-component nursing process gives greater prominence to analyzing than the four-component process.

Both the four- and five-step nursing processes provide an organizational structure for achieving the goals of the process. In both nursing processes, interaction between the client and the nurse is essential, as illustrated in Figure 10–1.

Authorities use different terms to describe these steps. In spite of these differences, the activities of the nurse using the process are similar. To avoid misunderstanding, nurses should be familiar with alternate terms that describe steps in the process. For example, *nursing diagnosis* may be called *analysis,* and *implementation (implementing)* may be called *intervention* or *intervening.*

An overview of the five-step nursing process used in this book follows. See also Tables 10–3 and 10–4. Each of the five components of the nursing process is discussed in depth in subsequent chapters of this unit. The terms used follow the form described by the National Council of State Boards of Nursing (1982): assessing, analyzing, planning, implementing, and evaluating.

1. **Assessing** is collecting, verifying, and organizing data about a client's health status. Data about the physical, emotional, developmental, social, intellectual, and spiritual aspects of the client are obtained from a variety of sources and are the basis for actions and decisions taken in subsequent phases. Skills of observation, communication, and interviewing are essential to perform this phase of the nursing process.

2. **Diagnosing** is a process which results in a diagnostic statement or nursing diagnosis. **Nursing diagnosis** is a statement of a client's potential or actual alteration of health status. Implicit in the diagnosis is a statement of the client's response that nurses are licensed and able to treat. In this phase, the nurse sorts and clusters the data and asks, "What are the actual and potential health problems for which the client needs nursing assistance?" and "What factors contributed to this problem?" Responses to those questions establish the nursing diagnoses. An **actual health problem** is a problem that currently exists. A **potential health problem** is the presence of risk factors that predispose persons and families to a health problem.

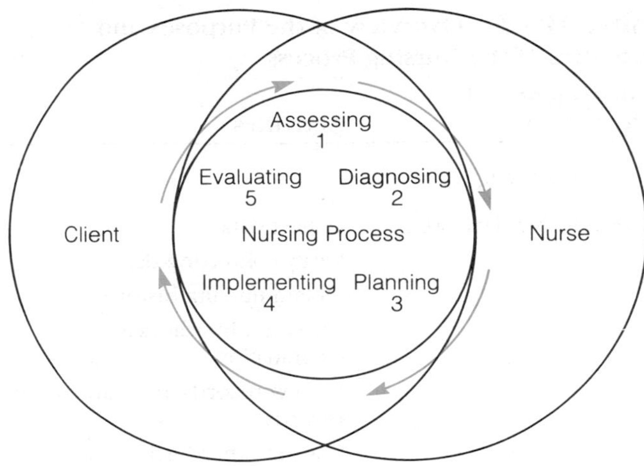

Figure 10–1 The interrelationship of the client, the nurse, and the nursing process

3. **Planning** involves a series of steps in which the nurse sets priorities, writes goals or expected outcomes, and establishes a written guide for nursing interventions designed to solve or minimize the identified problems of the client and to coordinate the care provided by all health team members. In collaboration with the client, the nurse develops specific interventions for each nursing diagnosis.

4. **Implementing** is putting the nursing care plan into action. During the implementation phase, the nurse

Table 10–2 Nursing Activities Associated with the Four- and Five-Step Nursing Process

Four-Phase Format	Nursing Behaviors	Five-Phase Format
1. Assessing	Collect data	1. Assessing
	Analyze and interpret data	2. Analyzing (nursing diagnosis)
2. Planning	Set priorities	3. Planning
	Set client goals or expected outcomes	
	Plan nursing interventions	
3. Implementing	Provide planned nursing interventions	4. Implementing
4. Evaluating	Evaluate achievement of goals or outcomes	5. Evaluating
	Reassess the nursing care plan	

Table 10–3 Overview of the Purposes and Activities of the Nursing Process

Component and Purpose(s)	Activities
Assessing	
To establish a database	Collect data Verify conflicting data Obtain nursing history Perform physical health examination Review records, e.g., laboratory records Consult other health team members Consult support persons Review literature
Analyzing (nursing diagnosis)	
To identify the client's health care needs and to prepare diagnostic statements	Validate data Sort and group data Interpret data Label groups of data with a diagnostic statement
Planning	
To identify the client's goals and appropriate nursing interventions	Set priorities Write evaluation goals and outcome criteria Select nursing strategies Consult other health personnel Write nursing care plan Delegate nursing actions
Implementing	
To carry out planned nursing interventions to help the client attain goals	Reassess client Update database Review and revise care plan Perform planned nursing interventions
Evaluating	
To determine the extent to which goals of nursing care have been achieved	Collect data about the client's response Compare the client's response to evaluation (outcome) criteria Analyze the reasons for the outcomes Modify the care plan

continues to collect data and validates the nursing care plan. Continued data collection is essential not only to keep track of changes in the client's condition but also to obtain evidence for the evaluation of goal achievement in the next phase. To validate the care plan, the nurse determines (a) whether planned nursing actions are realistic and help the client achieve the desired outcome or goal, (b) whether the client's priorities are being considered, and (c) whether the plan is individualized to meet the particular needs of the client.

5. **Evaluating** is assessing the client's response to nursing interventions and then comparing the response to predetermined standards. These standards are often referred to as **outcome criteria** or **evaluative criteria.** The nurse determines the extent to which the goals or predetermined outcomes of care have been achieved, partially achieved, or not met. If goals have not been met, reassessment of the care plan is needed. Reassessment may involve changes in any or all of the previous phases of the nursing process.

The nursing process is an adaptation of problem-solving techniques and systems theory. It can be viewed as parallel to but separate from the medical process. Table 10–5 lists the two processes for comparison. (The focus of the medical process is examining, diagnosing, planning, treating or curing disease processes, and evaluating the effectiveness of the treatment. The focus of the nursing process is gathering data, analyzing (diagnosing), planning, intervening, and evaluating the degree to which the client's goals have been met.)

Both processes begin with data gathering and analysis and base an action (intervention or treatment) on a problem statement (nursing diagnosis or medical diagnosis). Both processes include an evaluative component. Where the focus of the medical process is on the disease process, however, the nursing process is directed toward a client's *response* to illness.

The nurse can be highly creative when using the nursing process. The nurse is not bound by standard responses but may apply problem-solving skills, creativity, critical thinking, and her or his own knowledge and skills to assist clients. The nursing process can be applied in a variety of situations. It can be used with individuals of all ages, groups, and communities.

The five steps of the nursing process are not discrete entities but overlapping, continuing subprocesses. For example, assessing, the first step of the nursing process, may also be carried out during intervening and evaluating. Each step must be continually updated as the situation changes. Just as a client's health is never static but constantly changing, the nursing process, because it is responsive to the client's health, is also dynamic.

Each step or phase of the nursing process affects the others; they are closely interrelated. For example, if an inadequate database is used during assessment, the nurs-

Table 10–4 Selected Knowledge and Abilities Needed for the Nursing Process

Component	Knowledge	Abilities
Assessing	Biopsychosocial and spiritual systems of humans	Observe systematically
	Developmental needs of humans	Communicate verbally and nonverbally
	Health	Listen attentively
	Illness	Establish a helping relationship
	Pathophysiology	Develop trust
	Family system	Conduct a health interview
	Culture and values of self and client	Perform a nursing physical health assessment
Analyzing (nursing diagnosis)	Common health problems that nurses can identify and treat	Understand and evaluate cues
	Etiologic factors of health problems	Differentiate between cues* and inferences†
	Signs or characteristics of common health problems	Think critically
	Risk factors associated with potential health problems	Identify patterns and relationships
	Normal measurement standards	Organize and group data
	Individual coping mechanisms	Make inferences
		Reason inductively and deductively
		Make decisions or judgments
Planning	Client's strengths and weaknesses	Problem solve
	Values and beliefs of the client	Make decisions
	Scope of nursing practice	Write client goals that relate to the nursing diagnosis
	Resources available to implement nursing strategies	Write measurable outcome criteria that relate to the goals
	Roles of other health care personnel	Select and create nursing strategies that are safe and appropriate to meet client goals
		Write nursing orders
		Elicit the cooperation and participation of the client and other health care personnel
Implementing	Physical hazards and safety	Observe systematically
	Asepsis	Communicate effectively
	Procedures	Maintain a helping relationship
	Use of equipment	Perform psychomotor techniques
	Organization	Teach self-care
	Management	Convey caring
	Learning	Act as a client advocate
	Change theory	Counsel clients
	Advocacy	Delegate
	Client rights	Supervise and evaluate the work of others
	Client's developmental level	Implement medical orders
Evaluating	Client goals and outcome criteria	Obtain relevant data to compare with outcome criteria
	Client responses to nursing intervention	Draw conclusions about goal attainment
		Relate nursing actions to outcome criteria
		Reassess the nursing care plan

*Cue: A fact that one acquires through the use of the five senses.
†Inference: The nurse's judgment or interpretation of a cue.

ing diagnoses will be incomplete; this incompleteness will be reflected in the planning, implementation, and evaluation phases. Incomplete assessment necessarily means equivocal evaluation because the nurse will have incomplete criteria against which to evaluate changes in the client and the effectiveness of interventions.

Table 10–5 Comparison of the Nursing Process and the Medical Process

Nursing Process	Medical Process	Nursing Process	Medical Process
1. Assessing Collection of data from: a. Nursing history b. Health examination c. Review of records d. Consultation with other team members e. Review of literature	1. Assessing Collection of data from: a. Medical history b. Physical examination c. Diagnostic tests d. Review of literature	4. Implementing a. Preimplementation strategies b. Implementation c. Postimplementation strategies: update database, review and revise care plan	4. Therapy a. Physician's orders b. Medical therapy c. Referrals
2. Analyzing (nursing diagnosis) a. Analysis and synthesis of data b. Identification of the health problems c. Formulation of nursing diagnosis	2. Medical diagnosis* a. Organization of data b. Analysis and interpretation of the data c. Formulation of a diagnosis	5. Evaluating a. Collection of data about the client's response b. Comparison of the data to the established objectives and goals c. Determination of the effectiveness of the nursing plan d. Analysis of variables affecting the outcomes e. Modification of the care plan	5. Evaluating a. Establishment of the effectiveness of the medical therapy in terms of the goals b. Analysis of variables c. Revision of the plan of therapy as necessary
3. Planning a. Establishment of priorities b. Establishment of goals c. Development of objectives d. Written nursing care plan e. Delegation of nursing activities	3. Medical planning a. Establishment of priorities b. Establishment of goals for therapy c. Written plan of therapy		

*Medical diagnosis has four or five phases:
1. Suspected diagnosis following the patient's initial complaint
2. Tentative diagnosis following the medical history
3. Provisional diagnosis following the physical examination
4. Definitive diagnosis following diagnostic tests
5. Anatomical diagnosis following a postmortem

Characteristics of the Nursing Process

The following are characteristics of the nursing process:

1. The system is open, flexible, and dynamic.
2. It individualizes the approach to each client's particular needs.
3. It is planned.
4. It is goal directed.
5. It is flexible to meet the needs of client, family, or community.
6. It permits maximum flexibility and creativity for the nurse and client in devising ways to solve the stated health problem.
7. It is cyclical. Since all steps are interrelated, there is no absolute beginning or end.
8. It emphasizes feedback, which leads either to reassessment of the problem or to revision of the care plan.
9. It emphasizes validation. The stated problem must be validated by data. To validate is to confirm.

Importance of the Nursing Process

The nursing process is important to both the client and the nurse. The following advantages have been described (Atkinson and Murray 1983).

Advantages for the client

1. Quality client care. The nursing care is planned to meet the unique needs of the individual, family, or com-

munity. Continuous evaluation and reassessment of the client's changing needs ensure an appropriate level of care.

2. Continuity of care. The written care plan is accessible to all persons involved in the client's care and prevents each client from having to repeat information and preferences to each caregiver.
3. Participation by the clients in their health care. The process can help clients to develop skills related to their health care and to become more committed to the goals of care.

Advantages for the nurse

1. Consistent and systematic nursing education. The National League for Nursing (NLN), which administers a voluntary accreditation of nursing education programs, requires graduates to be competent in the use of the nursing process (NLN 1978). In addition, licensure examinations for nurses in the United States are organized around nursing process activities.
2. Job satisfaction. Well-written care plans give nurses confidence that nursing interventions are based on correct identification of the client's problems, thus preventing uncoordinated, trial-and-error nursing. Plans also can instill a sense of pride when the goals of care are accomplished.
3. Professional growth. By evaluating the effectiveness of the nursing interventions, the nurse learns which interventions are effective and which ones can be adapted to meet the needs of other clients. This process enhances the skill and expertise of the nurse. In addition, the shared knowledge and experience gained in collaborating with colleagues when formulating a care plan enhance the nurse's knowledge.
4. Avoidance of legal action (Philpott 1985, p. 79). When every step of the nursing process is used in delivering nursing care, the nurse is carrying out her or his legal obligations to the client. Failure to conduct a complete nursing assessment or failure to document data appropriately can have adverse legal consequences.
5. The nursing process holds the nurse accountable and responsible for assessing, analyzing, planning, implementing and evaluating client care.

Theories That Guide Implementation of the Nursing Process

A **theory** is a scientifically acceptable general principle that governs practice or is proposed to explain observed facts. Various theories guide how the nursing process is implemented. Some of these are nursing theory, humanistic theory, general systems theory, problem-solving and decision-making theory, perception theory, communication theory, and human needs theory. Communication theory is discussed in Chapter 27, and human needs theory in Chapter 16.

Nursing Theory

As noted in Chapter 1, the conceptual framework selected for nursing is an abstraction that is operationalized or made a reality by use of the nursing process. For example, if the client is viewed as having 14 fundamental needs, data are collected about these 14 needs. If a self-care model is used, data are collected about the client's abilities to perform self-care, and the nurse's intervention is focused on the individual's self-care deficits. Nursing theory instructs the nurse *what* to do and directly influences which interventions are planned; however, it does not tell the nurse *how* to intervene. For example, a planned intervention may be to teach a client and his wife how to give insulin. What to do is evident, but how to do it is not. To implement this plan effectively, the nurse needs further knowledge about communication, helping relationships, learning, teaching strategies, techniques for giving injections, and so on. This knowledge is drawn from sources other than the nursing model.

Humanistic Theory

Humanism is concern for human attributes, for those characteristics that are considered human. Some of these attributes are universal, that is, they occur in all cultures. Examples of humanistic behaviors are empathy, compassion, sympathy toward other people, and respect for life.

Humanism has received increased attention in nursing in response to the technologic advances that have affected nursing practice. Humanism in nursing refers to an attitude and an approach to the client and support persons recognizing them as human beings with human needs, rather than as "the appendectomy in Room 192" or "the catheterization in bed 6A." See also Humanizing Health Care in Chapter 3, p. 90.

North American societies are multiethnic (i.e., they comprise diverse ethnic groups). They are person-centered in their humanism and embody human rights concepts. This means that individuals are seen as autonomous and have certain rights and freedoms; in fact, each person has the right to be treated as an individual. By contrast, in certain societies, the tribe or the family, not the person, is the primary unit endowed with values and rights. Other characteristics of American humanism—though not necessarily unique to it—are belief in helping the poor and the suffering and respect for the ways and values of others, even if these differ from one's own.

The nurse who takes a humanistic approach to the nursing process takes into account all that is known about a client—thoughts, feelings, values, experiences, likes, desires, behavior, and body (La Monica 1985, p. 2). This humanistic approach is the traditional "caring" aspect of nursing and as important as a systems approach and problem solving to intelligent, systematic, and logical nursing care.

General Systems Theory

General systems theory or systems theory explains the breaking of whole things into parts and the working together of those parts in systems. The theory explains the relationship between wholes and parts, a description of concepts about them, and predictions about how the parts will behave and react. This theory is relevant in the nursing process as it is applied to the individual, family, and community.

The basic concepts of systems theory were proposed in the 1950s. One of its major proponents, Ludwig von Bertalanffy (1969) introduced systems theory as a universal theory that could be applied to many fields of study. Examples of disciplines that now use systems theory and its applications are psychology, biology, education, and computer science. Systems theory is being used increasingly by nurses as a way of understanding not only biologic systems but also systems in families, communities, and nursing and health care. General systems theory provides a way of examining interrelationships and deriving principles.

A **system** is a set of interacting identifiable parts or components. The **boundary** of a system is a real or imaginary line that differentiates one system from another system or a system from its environment, such as the skin around the body, the body being the system in this example. Boundaries function as a place of exchange between what goes into and what comes out of the system and therefore provide a sense of order to the overall system.

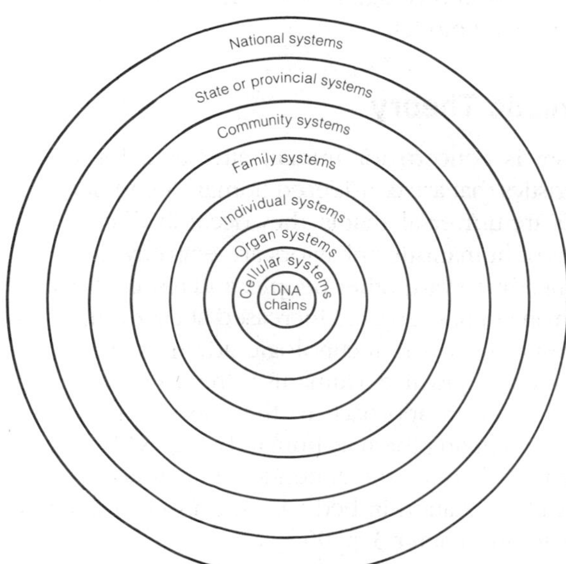

Figure 10–2 A common system hierarchy

Characteristics of Systems

1. A system is more than a sum of its parts. The system develops a character of its own with collective goals for all its parts.

2. All components of a system are interrelated. All components work together. If health care is the system, then nursing and medicine are components. The work of all health professions must be viewed as a unit, just as the body (a system) is seen as a whole and not a collection of disparate organs.

3. A system responds as a whole (holistically) to changes in one of its parts. When one aspect of a system changes, the entire system is affected. When nursing—a component of the health care delivery system—is changed, then the entire health care delivery system is affected. Similarly, a tumor of the liver affects the whole individual, that is, he or she may be nauseated, tired, anxious, etc.

4. Systems are hierarchical and composed of interrelated subsystems. Each subsystem belongs to a higher system until the highest-level **suprasystem** is reached, or at the other end, a lowest-level **subsystem.** See Figure 10–2 for a hierarchy of the human system. The designation of systems as suprasystems or subsystems is relative to the focus of study. For example, when nursing is the focus of study (the system), the health care delivery system of the country could be considered the suprasystem and individual nursing practice the subsystem. An individual is a subsystem of a larger system, the family.

5. Because systems are interrelated, the boundaries between systems are set as of a given time and may be set differently at another time. The boundaries are set according to the purposes of the people working in the system at a particular time. At one time, a health care delivery system could include nursing, medicine, social work, and clients and their families. At another time, for instance, during a research study, the same

system might include only medicine and nursing. During surgery, a physician and a nurse may view the kidney as a system even though in a larger context the kidney is a subsystem of the urinary system.

6. All systems are goal directed. A system that is not goal directed disintegrates. Although individual parts of the system may have distinct goals that are not directly consonant with the group goal, such subgoals should not conflict with the system goal.

Closed and Open Systems

There are two general types of systems: closed and open. A **closed system** does not exchange energy, matter, or information with its environment; it receives no input from the environment and gives no output to the environment. Therefore, a closed system is in a static or steady state; its components always remain in the system, and it never changes. An example of a closed system is a chemical reaction that takes place in a test tube under specified conditions. In reality, no closed systems exist. In an **open system**, energy, matter, and information move into and out of the system through the system boundary, which is often described as semipermeable because it is selective and filters what goes into and comes out of the system. All living systems—such as plants, animals, people, families, and communities—are open systems since their survival depends on a continuous exchange of energy. They are therefore in a constant state of change.

An open system depends on the quality and quantity of its input, output, and feedback for its functioning. **Input** consists of information, material, or energy that enters the system. After the input is absorbed by the system, it is processed in a way useful to the system. This process of transformation is called **throughput**. For example, in the digestive system, food is input; it is digested (throughput) so that it can be used by the body.

Output from a system is energy, matter, or information given out by the system as a result of its processes. Output from the digestive system is feces and caloric energy.

Feedback is a process that enables a system to regulate itself. Feedback gives the system the ability to control its input and output. For example, if a thirsty person drinks a glass of juice, feedback should indicate that the thirst was satisfied or unsatisfied. Feedback, which can be thought of in the context of outcome, is used to increase or decrease the system's equilibrium. Through feedback, output from the system returns to the system as input, thus forming a feedback loop. See Figure 10–3.

Numerous examples of this feedback mechanism are found within individual, family, and community systems. In the individual, for example, the autonomic nervous system relies on a feedback system to balance the effects of the sympathetic and parasympathetic centers, which regulate, among other processes, heart and respiratory rates. In the family system, parents provide feedback to children to regulate behavior. In the community, laws, rules, and regulations regulate the behavior of citizens.

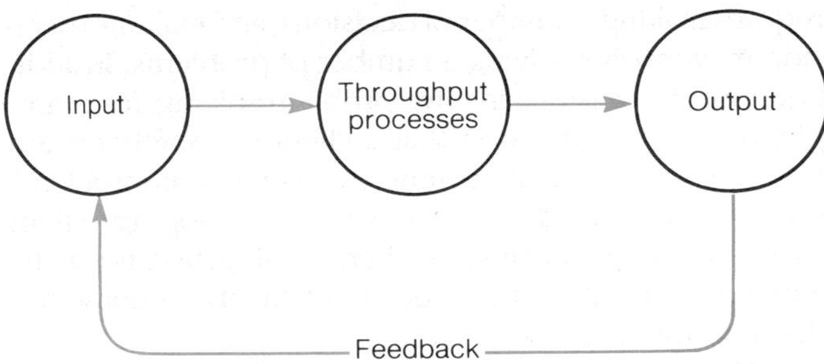

Figure 10–3 An open system with a feedback mechanism

Two types of feedback are positive and negative. Positive feedback signals change within the system, while negative feedback signals equilibrium or steadiness in the system. In this context, these two terms signify the opposite of their ordinary meanings. An example of positive feedback is pain and pallor in a postoperative client following a position change. This feedback enables the nurse to reevaluate the appropriateness of the position, perhaps change the position, and report the feedback so that the physician can relate it to the surgery and the client's diagnosis.

Open systems vary in their degree of openness. In the social sciences, families, groups, or societies are often referred to as closed systems. What is meant is that the system is *relatively* closed to outside exchange. The term *closed system* in this context is not in accordance with the definition used in general systems theory.

To survive, open systems must maintain a special balance often referred to as **dynamic equilibrium, homeostasis**, or **homeodynamics**. In the human, there are many examples of this balance. Examples are maintenance of body temperature, appropriate blood sugar levels, and pH of body fluids.

The nursing process has some of the characteristics of an open system: it is open, flexible, and dynamic; it is planned and goal directed; it interacts with the environment; and it emphasizes feedback. The nursing process can be viewed as a system with input, throughput, output, and feedback. Input (data) from the client and nurse is then transformed by the processes of analyzing, planning, implementing, all of which are throughput. The output (client's response) is then evaluated.

Problem-Solving and Decision-Making Theory

Problem solving and decision making are used in applying the nursing process. Although these two terms are often used interchangeably, they are separate processes that are related in some situations. Solving a problem may require making a number of decisions, and making a decision may involve solving a number of problems. In addition, not all decisions involve problem solving; for example, making the decision that a client can safely remain in a chair for another 15 minutes. Also, not all problems involve deliberate decision making, e.g., stopping a client from pulling out a urinary catheter. This action is usually automatic or habitual and does not involve a conscious decision by the nurse.

However, in many nursing situations decision making is an aspect of problem solving.

Problem-Solving Process

There are various approaches to problem solving. Four of the most commonly used are trial and error, intuition, experimentation, and the scientific method.

Trial-and-error problem solving One way to solve problems is to try a number of approaches until a solution is found. However, the reason one solution works is not known when alternatives in care are not considered systematically. Trial-and-error methods in nursing care can be dangerous because the client might suffer harm if an approach is inappropriate.

Intuitive problem solving Experienced nurses develop a sense of what nursing measures might help in certain situations. This sense is in part intuitive. A nurse who bases decisions on intuition alone rather than data, however, does a disservice to the client, even though in the past nurses sometimes solved problems successfully by intuition. Intuitive problem solving is not based on knowledge from research, and, as a result, it cannot be defended using any nursing care standard.

Experimentation Experimentation is more controlled than trial and error. It is based on knowledge and research, and it is therefore more ethical than trial-and-error or intuitive problem solving. Examples of experimentation are pilot projects or limited trials in an effort to solve a problem. For example, a nurse caring for a client with intractable pain may try one specific nursing intervention for 3 days to reduce the pain. If the pain is not reduced, the nurse may then implement a second plan for another 3 days.

Scientific method The **scientific method** is a logical, systematic approach to solving problems. The classic scientific method is most useful in a laboratory where the scientist is working in a controlled situation. The classic scientific method has the following steps:

1. Identifying the general problem, including defining the problem and developing hunches about it
2. Collecting all relevant data from appropriate sources
3. Formulating a **hypothesis**: an assumption made to test the logic of a proposition
4. Preparing a plan of action to test the hypothesis
5. Testing the hypothesis
6. Interpreting the test results and then evaluating the hypothesis
7. Concluding the study or revising the plan of action in the light of new data

Although the scientific method has certain applications in nursing, there are differences between the scientist's laboratory setting and the nurse's practice setting. Three of these differences are:

1. The nurse's time frame is often shorter than the scientist's. The scientist may take months or even years to carry out a study, whereas a nurse must give immediate help to a client in pain.
2. The nurse's environment makes complete scientific control impossible, while the scientist strives to establish scientific controls in experiments. For example, a visiting nurse striving to help control a client's diabetes through diet and insulin injections can outline a regimen and teach the client to administer insulin but has no control over whether the client will follow instructions later. The nurse often faces unpredictable events. For example, a client may refuse certain nursing interventions. The scientist, too, may encounter unpredictable events but strives to limit them through scientific control.
3. The nurse deals with multiple, complex problems, especially since most clients have more than one problem when they are ill. The scientist isolates and studies a single aspect of a problem.

The scientific method, therefore, must be adapted for nursing practice. The nurse requires a problem-solving system that is scientific, systematic, yet flexible enough to deal with the complex situations in the health care system.

Modified scientific method (problem-solving process) Health professionals require a modified approach of the scientific method for solving problems. This modified scientific problem-solving method is used in the nursing process but can also be used for problems relating to personnel, equipment, or other situations. Like the scientific process, it has seven steps. See Table 10–6 for a comparison of the problem-solving process, the nursing process, and the scientific method.

Table 10–6 Comparison of Steps in the Problem-Solving Process, the Nursing Process, and the Scientific Method

Problem-Solving Process	Nursing Process	Scientific Method
1. Encounter the problem	1. Assessing	1. Recognize and define the problem
2. Collect data		2. Collect data from observation and experimentation
3. Analyze information and identify exact nature of the problem	2. Analyzing (nursing diagnosis)	3. Formulate hypothesis
4. Determine a plan of action	3. Planning	4. Select plan to test the hypothesis
5. Carry out the plan	4. Implementing	5. Test the hypothesis
6. Evaluate the plan and its outcomes	5. Evaluating	6. Interpret test results (evaluate whether the hypothesis is correct)
7. Terminate or modify the plan		7. Conclude or modify hypothesis

Decision-Making Process

Decision making is a process of choosing a particular and best action to meet a desired goal. Three conditions must prevail: freedom, rationality, and voluntarity (Schaefer 1974, p. 1852). Freedom means that the individual makes the decision without pressure from others and has the authority to make the decision. Rationality, in the context of decision making, means that the best or optimal decision is made and that it is consistent with the decision maker's values and preferences. Rationality involves both deliberation and judgment. Voluntarity is making a choice voluntarily.

Decision making involves two types of reasoning: inductive and deductive. In **inductive reasoning**, generalizations are formed from a set of facts or observations. When viewed together, certain bits of information suggest a particular interpretation. For example, the nurse who observes that a client has dry skin, poor turgor, sunken eyes, and dark amber urine may make the generalization that the client is dehydrated. **Deductive reasoning**, by contrast, is reasoning from the general to the specific. The nurse starts with a conceptual framework—for example, Maslow's hierarchy of needs or a self-care action framework—and makes descriptive interpretations of the client's condition in relation to that framework. For example, the nurse who uses the needs framework might categorize data and define the client's problems in terms of elimination, nutrition, or protection needs.

Several authors have described the decision-making process. For the purposes of this text, a three-phase decision-making process is chosen: deliberation, judgment, and discrimination (choice).

Deliberation During this initial phase, the nurse considers all the available data. The data are categorized and any gaps, inconsistencies, or conflicts are identified. At this time, solutions are considered, including all alternative actions and their consequences. This step involves comparing alternative actions. For example, if the problem is that a client is not eating, the nurse and the client consider all the available data about the client's eating problem. Alternative actions for the nurse and client are then considered. Some courses of action are:

1. Client and nurse discuss the problem.
2. Nurse asks support persons to visit at meal time.
3. Nurse feeds the client.
4. Nurse tells the client "You will get stronger sooner if you eat."

After establishing the various courses of action, the consequences of each action are established. For each of the above actions the consequences might be:

1. After a discussion, the nurse might learn more and be able to help the client *or* a discussion might not affect the eating problem.
2. Support people might successfully encourage the client to eat *or* they might have no effect.
3. The client might eat *or* the client might refuse.
4. The client might accept this logic and eat *or* the client might ignore the consequences and continue to refuse.

Judgment During the judgment phase of the decision-making process, each course of action is analyzed in terms of (a) effectiveness related to the goal of the action and (b) efficiency of the action. Included in the analysis are the risk factors involved. If, for example, a client refuses to eat and the nurse asks the support persons to come at meal time, what is the risk that the client will eat only when they are present and they cannot come at each meal time? There is, then, a risk in taking this action. The efficiency of an action must also be analyzed. Is it possible for the nurse to feed the client and fulfill responsibilities to other people?

Table 10–7 A Comparison of the Steps of the Nursing Process and Decision Making

Nursing Process Steps	Decision-Making Phases
1. Assessing	Deliberation
2. Diagnosing	Judgment, discrimination
3. Planning	Discrimination
4. Implementing	Deliberation, judgment, discrimination
5. Evaluating	Deliberation, judgment, discrimination

Discrimination (choice) The third phase in the decision-making process is choosing one alternative action and the consequences. Insufficient deliberation and judgment can lead to poor choices, and inadequate consideration of the consequences can also lead to poor choices. However, thorough deliberation and judgment can lead to an effective choice of action.

Decision making, like the nursing process, is cyclical. Assessing, the gathering of data about a client, is similar to the deliberation phase of the decision-making process (see Table 10–7). The analyzing stage of the nursing process is parallel to the judgment phase of decision making. Planning, in the nursing process, is like the discrimination (choice) phase. Intervention involves continuous collection of data, analyses of the data, and nursing judgments regarding the effectiveness of the intervention. Any change in data may change the plan and the intervention. All three phases of decision making apply to this stage of the nursing process. During evaluation, the nurse continues to gather data, reassess the effectiveness of the intervention, and make decisions about it. In effect, the nurse also evaluates the effectiveness of the decision-making process itself.

Computer-assisted decision making (CADM) is a decision-making support system. There are three broad categories of decision-making support systems: support systems, expert systems, and artificial intelligence systems. Because decisions made in clinical settings are frequently complex, CADM systems to assist nurses are currently receiving much attention.

Perception Theory

Perception is a major means by which people gain information about themselves, their needs, and the environment. **Perception** is the process of selecting, organizing, and interpreting sensory stimuli into a meaningful and coherent picture of the world. When looking around, a person sees a whole range of different objects, forms, and colors. People also see depth; all objects appear three-dimensional. Why does the world look the way it does to a person? A superficial answer is that things look the way they do because that is the way they are; they mirror reality.

Perception, however, is more complex than a response to sensory stimuli. It is also the interpretation of the sensation in the light of previous learning. Perception is a person's conscious awareness of reality and is based on an individual's knowledge and past experiences.

The way people look at things, feel about them, value them, and think about them is highly individualistic. Each person has a unique perceptual field that includes not only the objective physical universe of which the person is aware but also public opinion, justice, values, love, hate, compassion, and other variables. To the individual, his or her own perceptual field allows an undistorted view of reality, while the perceptual field of another person contains error and illusion.

People tend to see what they want to see. What people anticipate as a result of past experience can become so firmly embedded into their thinking that people can be "blinded" to reality. Differences in people's perceptual fields are evident when, for example, witnesses to an accident give different reports of the same event. Often, there are as many different reports as witnesses. Observers are prone to make inferences from fragments of information, and the inferences are influenced by what the observer expects to perceive.

Three main factors influence people's perceptual fields: (a) the persons' needs, (b) their values or beliefs, and (c) their self-concept. For example, hungry shoppers perceive themselves as needing more food than those who are not hungry; people who value another's property perceive the taking of an apple from a neighbor's tree as theft, while others perceive it as all right as long as they are not seen. A person who has a low self-concept, i.e., thinks of himself as weak, will selectively ignore stimuli that refute it. The process of perception is an *inductive* learning process and consists of (Janzen 1980, p. 38):

1. Selectively attending to stimuli. Selective attention is learned. It is not possible for all stimuli to be perceived, so people learn to select certain stimuli and screen out others. They attend to those stimuli deemed valuable and meaningful by their culture and to those that meet their needs.
2. Organizing the stimuli into such categories as elements, concepts, models, or theories. Once this generalization occurs, only a few cues are needed to bring to mind whole sets of data. Thus, larger amounts of data can be processed with increasing speed and accuracy.
3. Developing relationships, for instance, among such categories as age, employment, sex, education, health, and salary. When such relationships are made, the result is perception of a "whole" phenomenon, such as a client as a biopsychosocial being.

This perceptual process is necessary for therapeutic interaction between a nurse and client. The development of perceptual skills requires inductive thinking from specifics to general rather than the deductive thinking traditionally taught in nursing.

An understanding of perceptual theory is essential for the nurse who wishes to communicate with clients and acquire and interpret data about them. Analysis of data is an inductive process. To share information accurately with a client, the nurse must perceive what the client intends to be perceived.

To enhance the ability to collect data and the accuracy of inferences made about the client, the nurse must continually strive to increase her or his observational or perceptual field. This can be achieved by:

1. Using all senses—sight, smell, hearing, touch, and taste—when collecting data.
2. Avoiding focusing attention on only particular events or aspects of a stimulus.
3. Not expecting certain types of stimulation or responses to occur.
4. Asking for feedback about the client's perceptions, sharing and comparing perceptions, and reaching a common understanding. When eliciting feedback, the nurse can say, "I don't understand" or nonverbally indicate a question with a raised eyebrow or other gesture.
5. Increasing her or his knowledge about human behavior.
6. Being aware of her or his own values, beliefs, and biases, which may affect how the nurse interprets what she or he sees and hears. Nurses need to overcome the tendency to attend only to a person's positive attributes (that is, those that are similar to the nurse's own values) or to attend overly to negative attributes (that is, those in conflict with the nurse's values).

An understanding of perception is basic to using the nursing process. Through perception, the nurse gathers data about a client, and the client gathers data about a nurse. For example, a client might say "I feel much better today." The nurse might perceive that the client is saying he is feeling stronger and happier when in fact he really means that his pain is less. As another example, a client might say, "I have always taken good care of my health." A nurse who perceives this statement in light of her or his own health values and beliefs may never learn that the client believes drinking a bottle of whiskey each day is a good health practice. A third example is this advice given to a client by a nurse: "You should go to bed early for several weeks until you are well." The client may perceive "early" to mean midnight because she was accustomed to a 2:00 A.M. bedtime. These examples show that perceived stimuli, e.g., words, when interpreted in view of an individual's values and beliefs can affect data collection and the entire nursing process.

A Framework for Accountability

Accountability is the condition of being answerable and responsible to someone for specific behaviors that are part of the nurse's professional role. The nursing process provides a framework for accountability and responsibility in nursing and maximizes accountability and responsibility for standards of care (Law 1983, p. 34). Nurses are accountable to the client (public), to their professional statutory nursing body, to colleagues, to the employing agency, and to themselves. The nursing process provides a framework for accountability in all areas. The professional nurse is accountable for activities in all five phases of the nursing process.

Assessing

The nurse is accountable for collecting information, encouraging client participation, and for judging the validity of the collected data. When assessing, the nurse is accountable for gaps in data or conflicting data, inaccurate data, and biased data.

Diagnosing

During the second phase, nurses are accountable for the judgments made about the client's health problems, i.e., the diagnostic statements. Is the health problem recognized by the client or only by the nurse? Did the nurse consider the client's values, beliefs, and cultural practices when determining the health problems? When making judgments, nurses are accountable for considering a broad spectrum of client sociocultural backgrounds.

Planning

Accountability at the planning stage involves determining priorities, establishing client goals, predicting outcomes, and planning nursing activities. These are all incorporated into a written nursing care plan available to all involved nurses. In this phase, nurses are also accountable for ensuring that the *client's* priorities are considered as well as the nurse's.

Implementing

Nurses are accountable for all their actions in delivering nursing care. These actions may be performed directly or in collaboration with others, or they may be delegated to another. Even though a nurse delegates an activity to another person, the nurse is still accountable for the delegated action as well as for the act of delegating. The nurse should be able to give reasoned answers as to why the activity was delegated, why the person was chosen to perform the activity, and how the delegated action was carried out. Nursing actions must be charted after being carried out, thereby providing a written record.

Evaluating

By establishing the degree to which the objectives have been attained, the nurse is accountable for the success or failure of the nursing actions. The nurse must be able to explain why a client goal was not met and what phase or phases of the nursing process require changing and why.

The nursing process provides the framework for nurses to help clients with their health needs and to produce a record of the actions and their effectiveness. The nursing process makes nurses responsible primarily to the client. An implicit part of applying the nursing process is having the knowledge and skills to make the required decisions and to implement the required nursing actions. Therefore, nurses are also accountable to themselves for having the knowledge and skills to use the nursing process in a specific situation.

Chapter Highlights

- The nursing process is a systematic, rational method of planning and providing nursing care.
- The goal of the nursing process is to identify a client's actual or potential health care needs, to establish plans to meet the identified needs, and to deliver specific nursing interventions to meet those needs.
- The nursing process has evolved over the past 20 to 30 years.
- The basic components of the nursing process are assessing, analyzing, planning, implementing, and evaluating.
- Specific nursing activities are associated with each component of the nursing process.
- The nursing process can be applied to individuals, families, and communities.
- Assessing is collecting, verifying, and organizing data about a client's status.
- Analyzing (nursing diagnosis) is the process of developing a statement of a client's potential or actual health problem that nurses are licensed and able to treat.
- Planning involves setting priorities, writing goals, and establishing a written guide for nursing intervention designed to solve or minimize identified problems.
- Implementing is putting the nursing care plan into action.
- Evaluating is assessing the client's response to nursing interventions and comparing the response to predetermined criteria.
- The nursing process is a system that is open, flexible, and dynamic.
- The nursing process is cyclical since all steps are interrelated.
- The nursing process individualizes care for each client's particular needs.
- The nursing process involves active participation by the client.
- The nursing process is similar to the problem-solving process and the scientific method.
- When using the nursing process, the nurse is guided by humanistic, problem-solving, decision-making, perception, communication, needs, and systems theory.
- The nursing process provides a framework for nurses' accountability and responsibility.

Suggested Readings

Leddy, S., and Pepper, J. M. 1985. The nursing process. Chapter 12 in *Conceptual bases of professional nursing,* pp. 211–26. New York: J. B. Lippincott Co.

The authors present a relationship of process to philosophy of nursing. The standards of nursing practice (ANA 1973) are then related to the nursing process. Each standard is described separately.

Masson, V. March/April 1985. Nurses and doctors as healers. *Nursing Outlook* 33:70–73.

Masson addresses the question "What is nursing?" and then contrasts nursing and medical functions. The use of logic and intuition in both areas is explained. The desire of nurses for interdependent functioning rather than autonomy in function is expressed. Masson also relates the nursing-medical relationship to the traditional female-male relationship.

Yura, H., and Walsh, M. 1984. The nursing process. In McCann Flynn, J., and Heffron, P. B. *Nursing from concept to practice,* pp. 141–75. Bowie, Md.: Robert J. Brady Co.

In this chapter, a theoretical-conceptual framework and a

theoretical base for nursing practice are presented. Following a definition of nursing and the components of nursing, the authors discuss the nursing process. Each phase of the nursing process is discussed. A needs approach is used to provide the structure and direction for the nursing activities.

Selected References

American Nurses' Association. 1973. *Standards of nursing practice.* Kansas City, Mo.: American Nurses' Association.

———. 1980. *Nursing: A social policy statement.* Publication no. NP-63. Kansas City, Mo.: American Nurses' Association.

Atkinson, L. D., and Murray, M. E. 1983. *Understanding the nursing process.* 2d ed. New York: Macmillan Co.

Bishop, W. J., and Goldie, S. 1962. *A bio-bibliography of Florence Nightingale.* London: Dawsons of Pall Mall. Citing Nightingale, F. 1860. *Notes on nursing: What it is and what it is not.* London: Harrison.

Bloch, D. November 1974. Some crucial terms in nursing: What do they really mean? *Nursing Outlook* 22:689–94.

Bowler, T. D. 1981. *General systems thinking: Its scope and applicability.* New York: Holland.

Conway-Rutkowski, B. September 1982. Patient participation in nursing process. *Nursing Clinics of North America.* 17:451–54.

deChesnay, M. Winter 1983. Problem solving in nursing. *Image: The Journal of Nursing Scholarship* 25:8–11.

George, J. B., editor. 1985. *Nursing theories: The base for professional nursing.* 2d ed. Englewood Cliffs, N.J.: Prentice-Hall.

Gordon, M. 1982. *Nursing diagnosis process and application.* New York: McGraw-Hill.

Griffith, J. W., and Christensen, P. J., editors. 1982. *Nursing process: Application of theories, frameworks, and models.* St. Louis: C. V. Mosby Co.

Hall, L. June 1955. Quality of nursing care. *Public health news.* Newark, N.J.: State Department of Health.

Heidgerken, L. E. 1965. *Teaching and learning in schools of nursing: Principles and methods.* 3d ed. Philadelphia: J. B. Lippincott.

Henderson, V. January/February 1965. The nature of nursing. *International Nursing Review* 12:23–30.

———. May 22, 1980. Nursing: Yesterday and tomorrow. *Nursing Times* 76:905–7.

Hurley, M. E., editor. 1986. *Classification of nursing diagnoses: Proceedings of the sixth conference.* St. Louis: C. V. Mosby Co.

Janzen, S. 1980. Taxonomy for development of perceptual skills. *Journal of Nursing Education* 19:33.

Johnson, D. E. April 1959. A philosophy of nursing. *Nursing Outlook* 7:198–200.

Kim, M. J., McFarland, G. K., and McLane, A. M., editors. 1984. *Pocket guide to nursing diagnoses.* St. Louis: C. V. Mosby Co.

Knowles, L. 1967. *Decision-making in nursing: A necessity for doing:* ANA Clinical Sessions, 1966. New York: Appleton-Century-Crofts.

Kreuter, F. R. May 1957. What is good nursing care? *Nursing Outlook* 5:302–304.

La Monica, E. L. 1985. *The humanistic nursing process.* Monterey, Calif.: Wadsworth Health Sciences.

Law, G. M. October 5–11, 1983. Accountability in nursing: Providing a framework . . . the nursing process and accountability are inextricably linked. Part 2. *Nursing Times* 79:34–36.

McCain, R. F. April 1965. Nursing by assessment—Not intuition. *American Journal of Nursing* 65:82–84.

McCann-Flynn, J. B., and Heffron, P. B. 1984. *Nursing: From concept to practice.* Bowie, Md.: Robert J. Brady Co.

National Council of State Boards of Nursing. 1982. *Test plan for the National Council licensure examination for registered nurses.* Chicago: National Council of State Boards of Nursing.

National League for Nursing. 1978. *Competencies of the associate degree nurse on entry into practice.* Publication no. 23-1731C. New York: National League for Nursing.

Nursing Theories Conference Group. 1980. *Nursing theories: The base for professional nursing practice.* Englewood Cliffs, N.J.: Prentice-Hall.

Orem, D. 1980. *Nursing: Concepts of practice.* 2d ed. New York: McGraw-Hill.

Orlando, I. 1961. *The dynamic nurse-patient relationship.* New York: G. P. Putnam's Sons.

Peplau, H. E. 1952. *Interpersonal relations in nursing.* New York: G. P. Putnam's Sons.

Philpott, M. 1985. *Legal liability and the nursing process.* Toronto: W. B. Saunders Co., Canada.

Riehl, J. P., and Roy, C. 1974. *Conceptual models for nursing practice.* New York: Appleton-Century-Crofts.

Roy, C. 1976. *Introduction to nursing: An adaptation model.* Englewood Cliffs, N. J.: Prentice-Hall.

Schaefer, J. October 1974. The interrelatedness of decision making and the nursing process. *American Journal of Nursing* 74:1852–55.

Smith, C. W. 1951. *Florence Nightingale, 1820–1910.* London: Constable and Co.

Sundeen, S. J., Stuart, G. W., Rankin, E. D., and Cohen, S. A. 1985. *Nurse-client interaction: Implementing the nursing process.* 3d ed. St. Louis: C. V. Mosby Co.

Torres, G. 1985. Florence Nightingale. In George, J. B., editor. *Nursing theories: The base for professional nursing practice.* 2d ed. Englewood Cliffs, N.J.: Prentice-Hall.

von Bertalanffy, L. 1969. *General system theory.* New York: George Braziller.

Western Interstate Commission on Higher Education. 1967. *Defining clinical content.* Graduate Nursing Programs, Medical and Surgical Nursing. Boulder, Colo.: Western Interstate Commission on Higher Education.

Wiedenbach, E. May 1970. Nurses' wisdom in nursing theory. *American Journal of Nursing* 70:1057–62.

Yura, H., and Walsh, M. B. 1983. *The nursing process: Assessing, planning, implementing, evaluating.* 4th ed. Norwalk, Conn.: Appleton-Century-Crofts.

CHAPTER **11**

Assessing

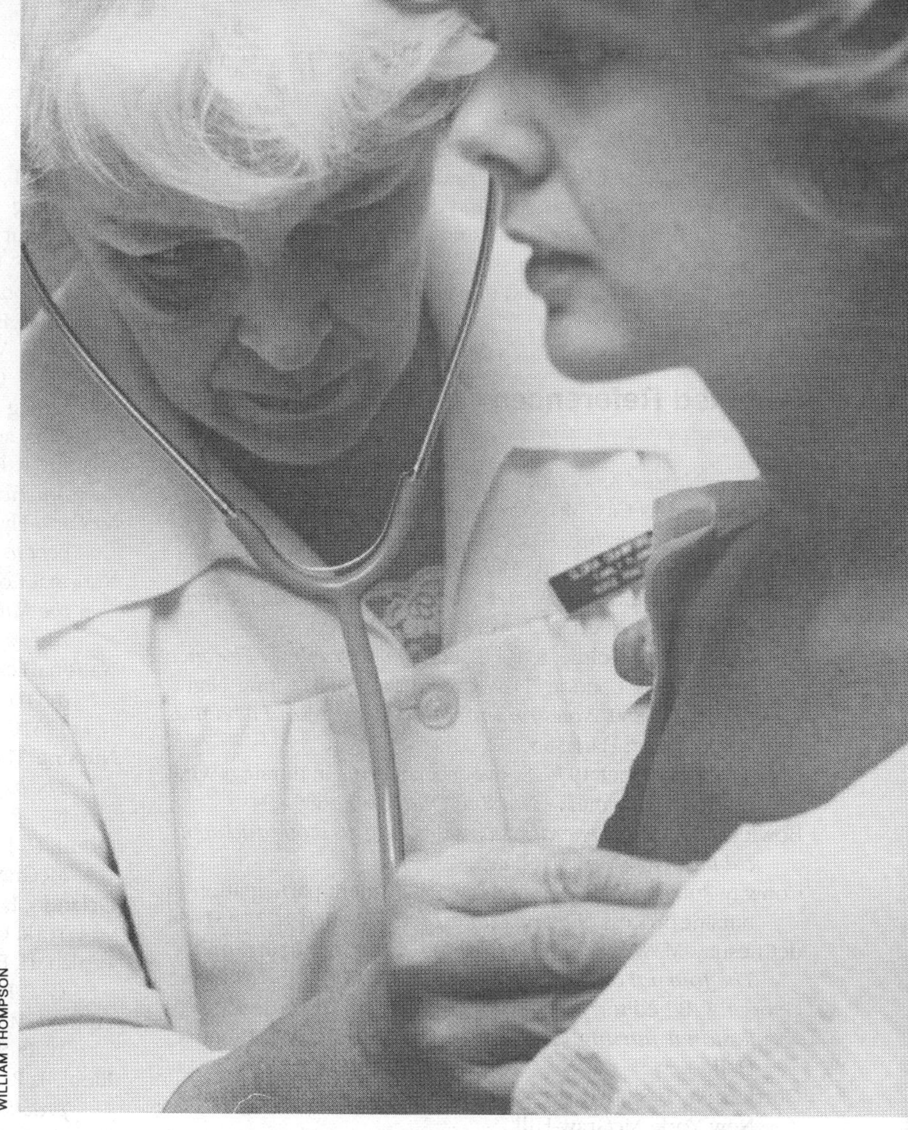

Contents

Objectives

1. Understand essential terms and facts about the assessment phase of the nursing process.
   1.1 Define listed terms.
   1.2 Identify the purpose of assessing.
   1.3 Give examples of objective and subjective data and variable and constant data.
   1.4 Identify primary and secondary sources of data.
   1.5 Name essential skills required for data collection.
   1.6 Identify five methods of data collection.
   1.7 Identify purposes of each method of data collection.
2. Understand essential aspects of the formal interview.
   2.1 Compare directive and indirective approaches to interviewing.
   2.2 Compare closed and open-ended questions.
   2.3 Give examples of closed and open-ended questions.
   2.4 List advantages and disadvantages of closed and open-ended questions.
   2.5 Identify situations in which closed or open-ended questions are appropriate.
   2.6 Describe important aspects of the interview setting.
   2.7 Differentiate the three stages of an interview.
   2.8 Describe the purposes of each interview stage.
   2.9 Identify communication guidelines for the body of the interview.
   2.10 Identify various ways to close an interview.
   2.11 Describe the process of consulting
3. Understand essential aspects of the nursing assessment (history).
   3.1 Identify purposes of the nursing assessment.
   3.2 Identify common health areas the nurse assesses.
   3.3 Compare the nursing assessment (history) and the medical history.
   3.4 Contrast various frameworks used for nursing assessment.
4. Appreciate the significance of the assessment phase of the nursing process.
   4.1 Describe the importance of assessing to nursing diagnosis.
   4.2 Describe the importance of reassessing during other phases of the nursing process.

Terms

anthropometric measurement
assessing
auscultation
cephalocaudal
closed question
constant data
consultation
coping behavior
data
database (baseline data)
data collection
direct interview
dullness (in percussion)
duration (of sound)
flatness (in percussion)
hyperresonance (in percussion)
indirect interview
intensity (of sound)
inspection
interview
leading question
neutral question
nursing assessment (nursing history)
objective data (signs, overt data)
observe
open-ended question
palpation
percussion
pitch (of sound)
pleximeter
plexor
primary questions
quality (of sound)
referring
resonance (in percussion)
secondary questions
subjective data (symptoms, covert data)
tympany (in percussion)
variable data

Purpose of Assessing

Assessing is the first phase of the nursing process, involving data collection and verification. Assessing is necessary before a nursing diagnosis can be made. In effect, assessing is also carried out during other phases of the nursing process, i.e., intervening and evaluating; some nurses refer to this as reassessing. All phases of the nursing process

Assessing is clearly an independent nursing function. In the absence of a physician's order, the frequency and comprehensiveness of assessing is within the nurse's discretion. (Philpott 1985, p. 81)

depend on the collection of data. The purpose of assessing is to establish a database about a client's health, including potential and actual health problems. Nursing is primarily accountable for the diagnosis and management of a client's health care in areas of daily living and health. Nurses also make assessments in the biomedical realm and consider the implications of that data on daily living and the achievement of developmental tasks (Carnevali 1983, p. 110–11).

The term **data** includes all relevant information about a client other than information about a disease process. It consists of information, facts, and findings, including an individual's strengths and needs. A **database** (or **baseline data**) is all the information about a client; it includes the physician's history and physical examination, the nursing assessment, physical health examination, and material contributed by other health personnel. **Data collection** is the process of gathering information about a client's health status. Data collection must be both systematic and continuous. Systematic data collection can largely prevent the omission of significant data, and continuous data collection maintains the currency of the data, reflecting a client's changing health.

Assessing involves active participation by the client and the nurse. The client may be one or more individuals, a family, or even a community. Both the nurse and the client enter the relationship with specific knowledge and previous experiences that influence their perceptions and interpretations. It is important for nurses to be aware that their interpretations may not be fact; for example, a nurse seeing a client holding his arm to his chest might believe that the client is experiencing chest pain when in fact he has a painful hand. Or a nurse might interpret a client's wish not to talk as depression when the client is in fact very tired. Another example of mistaking interpretation for fact is the assumption that a client who says "my husband died 3 weeks ago" is sad about the death when in fact his death is a great relief. Nurses need to be aware of their own biases, values, and beliefs if they are to collect data accurately.

Types of Data

Data can be objective or subjective. **Objective data** are detectable by an observer or can be tested by using an accepted standard. They can be seen, heard, felt, or smelled. For example, a discoloration of the skin, a blood pressure reading, or the act of crying are objective data. **Subjective data**, however, are apparent only to the person affected and can be described or verified only by that person. Itching, pain, and feeling worried are examples of subjective data. Objective data are sometimes called *signs* or *overt data,* and subjective data are sometimes called *symptoms* or *covert data.*

Data can also be described as **variable** or **constant.** Blood pressure, for example, varies from day to day or even by the hour and needs updating. Constant data are unchanging, for example, a date of birth. Data need to be relevant and descriptive. Data are always factual, not interpretive. It is a common error to offer opinions, generalizations, and interpretations as data. For example, a nurse may describe a client as "uncooperative" rather than record the specific behavior—perhaps a refusal to take a deep breath and to cough after surgery. A specific description of the behavior is more useful than an interpretation because the causes of specific behavior can be explored. Perhaps the client refuses to cough because she is afraid of rupturing a suture line, or perhaps she experiences severe pain upon coughing. "I do not want to cough, it hurts too much" is a noninterpretive reporting of the problem. Another common error is incomplete information, i.e., leaving out information about pain because the client does not mention it.

Clients can generalize or be nonspecific. They may describe the reason for their hospitalization as a "spell" or as "chest pain." It is important for the nurse to elicit specifics from the client. For example, the chest pain needs to be documented by how the client described it, where it was felt, how it was relieved, when it occurred, and whether it was a new experience. Data should also be concise. The nurse should briefly summarize the information collected using correct medical terms.

Sources of Data

Sources of data are *primary* or *secondary.* See Table 11–1. The client is the primary source of data. Secondary or indirect sources are significant others, other health personnel, records and reports, and relevant literature.

Client

The chief source of data is usually the client unless the client is too ill, young, or confused to communicate clearly. The client can usually provide subjective data that no one

Table 11–1 Sources of Data

Primary Source	Secondary Source
Client	Significant others Health personnel Health records Reports of diagnostic tests

Adapted from R. F. McCain, Nursing by assessment—not intuition, *American Journal of Nursing,* April 1965, 65:82. Copyright 1965 American Journal of Nursing Company.

else can offer. However, a stoic client may understate symptoms, while another person may exaggerate.

Significant Others

Significant others or support persons know the client well and often can provide data. They may supplement information or verify information provided by the client. They might convey information about the stresses the client was coping with before the illness, family attitudes to illness and health, and the client's home environment.

Significant others are an important source of data, particularly when the client is very young, unconscious, or confused. In some cases—when the client is an abused child, for example—the person giving information may wish to remain anonymous.

Health Personnel

Health personnel are often sources of information about a client's health. Nurses, social workers, physicians, and physiotherapists, for example, may have information from either previous or current contact with the client. A physician who knows the client's home setting may provide valuable data about the family and environmental stressors.

Medical Records

Medical records are often a source of a client's present and past health and illness patterns. These records can provide nurses with information about a client's coping behaviors, health practices, and previous illnesses. A **coping behavior** is behavior learned by a person in response to stress; it may be an adaptive mechanism or a task-oriented behavior. For additional information about coping see Chapter 17. The appropriateness of the information in medical records to the present situation must always be considered. For example, if the most recent medical record is 10 years old, it is likely that the client's health practices and coping behaviors have changed. Stressors in an individual's life often change, e.g., an alcoholic husband leaves home, a sick infant is now healthy.

Other Records and Reports

Other records and reports can also provide pertinent health information. Laboratory data can confirm or conflict with a nurse's findings during the nursing assessment (history) and a physical health examination. When laboratory data conflict, the nurse must collect more data to verify findings. For example, if laboratory data indicate an elevated blood sugar yet the client states he has never taken pills or injections or had a special diet, the nurse should clarify the symptoms and treatment of elevated blood sugar for the client.

Any laboratory data about a client must be compared to established norms for that particular test and for the client's age, sex, etc. Laboratory tests vary among agencies, and norms can therefore be different.

Laboratory tests are frequently ordered as part of the physician's initial examination to aid in a medical diagnosis. Laboratory tests are also used to monitor medical treatment, e.g., determination of blood glucose level to monitor the administration of oral hypoglycemic medications. In some cases, nurses can use the same laboratory test to monitor the effectiveness of nursing measures, such as teaching about diet and taking medications.

In most settings, laboratory tests are ordered by physicians and independent nurse practitioners, although this practice varies greatly. In some agencies, nurses are expected to order and/or carry out specific tests, e.g., urinalysis and routine blood tests.

Other records and reports—for example, a social agency's report on a client's living conditions or a home health care agency's report on a client's coping at home—can be helpful to the nurse.

Literature

The review of nursing and related literature, such as professional journals and reference texts, can provide additional information for the database. A literature review includes but is not limited to the following information:

1. Standards or norms against which to compare findings, e.g., height and weight tables, normal developmental tasks for an age group
2. Cultural and social health practices
3. Spiritual beliefs
4. Additional required assessment data
5. Nursing interventions and evaluation criteria relative to a client's health problems
6. Information about medical diagnoses, treatment, and prognoses

Methods of Data Collection

The major methods of collecting data are observing, interviewing, consulting, and examining. While these nursing activities are often carried out during the implementing and evaluating phases of the nursing process, they are the main nursing activities during the assessing phase. During assessment, observation occurs whenever the nurse is in contact with the client and/or support persons. The primary interviewing process during the assessment phase is the nursing assessment (nursing history). Examining during the assessment phase is the major method used in the physical health examination.

Observing

To **observe** is to gather data by using the five senses. Although nurses observe mainly through sight, all of the senses are engaged during careful observations. Observation has two aspects: (a) noticing the stimuli and (b) selecting, organizing, and interpreting the data, i.e., perceiving them. A nurse who observes that a client's face is flushed must relate that observation to, for example, body temperature, activity, environmental temperature, and blood pressure. Because observation involves selecting, organizing, and interpreting data, there is a possibility of error. For example, a nurse might not notice certain signs simply because they are unexpected in a certain client or situation or because they do not conform to preconceptions about a client's illness. Another source of error is faulty organization and misinterpretation of data. A nurse may interpret a patient's expression of sadness as fear of scheduled surgery, when in reality the client is saddened by a television program.

Observation is a conscious, deliberate skill that is developed only through effort and with an organized approach. Nurses often need to focus on specific stimuli in a clinical situation; otherwise they are overwhelmed by a multitude of stimuli. Observing, therefore, involves discriminating among stimuli, that is, separating stimuli in a meaningful manner. For example, nurses caring for newborns learn to ignore the usual sounds of machines in the nursery but respond quickly to an infant's cry or movement.

Nursing observations must be organized so that nothing significant is missed. Most nurses develop an individual sequence for observing events, for example:

1. Clinical signs of client distress; e.g., pallor or flushing, labored breathing, and behavior indicating pain or emotional distress
2. The status of the client, i.e., pulse, blood pressure, respirations, etc.
3. The functioning of associated equipment; e.g., intravenous equipment and oxygen
4. Threats to the client's safety, real or anticipated; e.g., a lowered side rail
5. The immediate environment, including people in it
6. The larger environment; i.e., the community

Interviewing

An **interview** is a planned communication or a conversation with a purpose. Some possible purposes are to gather data, to give information, to identify problems of mutual concern, to evaluate change, to teach, to provide support, and to provide counseling or therapy. Although nurses should not lose sight of these purposes during an interview, they are sometimes obliged to alter plans momentarily. If, for example, a client expresses worry about surgery, the nurse pauses to explore the client's worry and to provide support. Simply to note the worry without dealing with it can leave the impression that the nurse does not care about the client's concerns or dismisses them as unimportant. This impression could lessen the client's willingness to accept assistance from the nurse at a later date.

Interviewing can be viewed as a process that is applied in most phases of the nursing process. One example of the interview is the nursing history, which is the primary tool for data collection during the assessment phase of the nursing process.

Approaches to Interviewing

There are two approaches to interviewing: directive and nondirective.

The direct interview is highly structured and elicits specific information. The interviewer establishes the purpose of the interview and controls the interview, at least at the outset, by asking closed questions that call for specific responses. Directive interviews are frequently used to gather and to give information.

During a nondirective interview, the nurse allows the client to control the purpose, subject matter, and pacing. The nurse clarifies and encourages communication by using open-ended questions (see the next section). Nondirective interviewing is used for problem solving, counseling, and performance appraisal (Stewart and Cash 1985, p. 17).

Kinds of Interview Questions

Although there are many ways to categorize questions, in this book they are classified as open or closed, primary or secondary, and neutral or leading. The type a nurse chooses depends on the needs of the client at the time. For example, the nurse asks direct questions in an emergency because information must be obtained quickly. The nurse can ask secondary questions to elicit more information after a client answers a primary question. The direct question used in the emergency can also be primary or secondary, neutral or leading.

Closed and open-ended questions **Closed questions** are restrictive and generally require only short answers giving specific information. The highly stressed person and the person who has difficulty communicating will find closed questions easier to answer than open questions. The amount of information gained is generally limited. Examples of closed questions are: "What medication did you take?" "Are you having pain now?" "How long have you lived in the United States?" "How long has it been since you had your last physical examination?" "How old are you?" Closed questions are considered moderately closed when the person is asked to volunteer a specific piece of information. The questions listed above are examples. Highly closed questions ask the person to select an appropriate answer from among those provided in the question. An example is:

What educational level have you achieved?
——— Some high school
——— High school graduate
——— College graduate

An **open-ended question** or suggestion is broad, specifies only the topic to be discussed, and invites answers longer than one or two words. It often elicits expressions of feeling and descriptive or comparative responses. Such questions give the client the freedom to divulge only information he or she is ready to disclose. The response may also convey attitudes and beliefs the client holds. The chief disadvantages of the open-ended question is that the client may spend time conveying irrelevant information.

Examples of open-ended questions and suggestions are: "How have you been feeling lately?" "Tell me how you feel about that." "How do you feel about coming to the hospital?" Open-ended questions can be highly open, such as "Tell me about yourself," or have some restrictions, such as "Tell me about your hobbies." The nurse often finds it more effective to use a combination of directive and indirective approaches throughout an interview. See Table 11–2 for examples of directive and indirective interviewing interactions and Table 11–3 for advantages and disadvantages of closed and open-ended questions.

The interview situation often determines the type of interview approach used. For example, the nurse uses a directive approach to assess a client's health status after surgery: "Are you having any pain? What is it like? Show me where it is." The directive approach is also used in emergencies, when the nurse must assess the client's health status quickly, or learn what events preceded the emergency. For example, when a client is found lying on the floor of a hospital room, the nurse might interview others present: "When did he fall? Did he say anything? What had he been doing?" The indirective approach is used when there is no emergency and to determine the client's feelings and needs. For example, a nurse might ask: "How are you feeling today? Is there anything I can do for you? How do you feel about this I.V.?"

Table 11–2 Examples of Direct and Indirect Questions

Direct		Indirect	
Nurse:	Where is your pain?	Nurse:	Tell me about your pain.
Client:	It's in the calf of my right leg.	Client:	It's in the calf of my right leg. It starts after I've walked about a block or up a flight of stairs.
Nurse:	How long have you had this pain?	Nurse:	Uh hmm.
Client:	It started about 2 weeks ago.	Client:	It started about 2 weeks ago. I was hoping it would go away, but it's getting worse. I don't know what to do. My wife's an invalid and she relies on me to do the shopping and everything. I hope it's not serious.
Nurse:	When does the pain occur?		
Client:	After I've walked up a flight of stairs or about one block.		

Primary and secondary questions **Primary questions** introduce topics or new areas in an interview. Examples are: "What is your occupation?" "Tell me about your health this past year." **Secondary questions**, also called probing questions, are asked to obtain more information. A secondary question may be open—e.g., "What do you think happened?"—or closed—e.g., "Did you cry about that?" Secondary questions are frequently asked when the client's response to a primary question is vague, irrelevant, superficial, incomplete, or inaccurate. They are also asked when the client gives no response to a primary question (Stewart and Cash 1985, p. 86).

When a nurse asks a client about pain and the client replies, "Oh it is just a little pain," the nurse should ask a secondary question to obtain more exact information: "Tell me more about it," "Go on," or "What do you mean by a little pain?"

Table 11–3 Selected Advantages and Disadvantages of Open-Ended and Closed Questions

Open Questions		Closed Questions	
Advantages	**Disadvantages**	**Advantages**	**Disadvantages**
1. They let the interviewee do the talking. 2. The interviewer is able to listen and observe. 3. They are easy to answer and nonthreatening. 4. They reveal what the interviewee thinks is important. 5. They may reveal the interviewee's lack of information, misunderstanding of words, frame of reference, prejudices, or stereotypes. 6. They can provide information the interviewer may not ask for. 7. They can reveal the interviewee's degree of feeling about an issue. 8. They can convey interest and trust because of the freedom they provide.	1. They take more time. 2. Only brief answers may be given. 3. Valuable information may be withheld. 4. They often elicit more information than necessary. 5. Responses are difficult to document and require skill in recording. 6. The interviewer requires skill in controlling an open-ended interview. 7. Responses require psychologic insight and sensitivity from the interviewer.	1. Questions and answers can be controlled more effectively. 2. They require less effort from the interviewee. 3. They may be less threatening since they do not require explanations or justifications. 4. They take less time. 5. Information can be asked for before the information is volunteered. 6. Responses are easily documented. 7. They are easy to use and can be handled by unskilled interviewers.	1. They may provide too little information and require follow-up questions. 2. They may not reveal how the interviewee feels. 3. They do not allow the interviewee to volunteer possibly valuable information. 4. They may inhibit communication and convey lack of interest by the interviewee. 5. The interviewer may dominate the interview with questions.

Table constructed, with permission, from material on pp. 80–85 of Stewart, Charles J., and William B. Cash, Jr., *Interviewing: Principles and practices,* 4th ed.

Neutral or leading questions A client can answer a **neutral question** without direction or pressure from the nurse. Examples are: "How do you feel about that?" "Why do you think you had the operation?" "What happened then?" A **leading question** directs the client's answer. Examples are: "Wouldn't you rather have had the operation then?" "You don't think this illness is fair?" "You will take your medicine, won't you?"

Planning the Interview and Setting

It is important to plan an interview before beginning it. The nurse reviews what information is already available such as a postoperative record, information about the current illness, or literature about the client's health problem. The nurse also reviews the data collection form to make sure that the data to be collected are really needed and will serve some purpose related to the client's care. If a form is not available, most nurses prepare an interview guide to remember areas of information and determine what questions to ask. The guide includes a list of topics and subtopics rather than a series of questions.

Each interview and its setting is influenced by time, place, and seating arrangement. In all instances, the client should be made to feel comfortable and unhurried.

Time Interviews with hospitalized clients need to be scheduled for a time when the client is physically comfortable and free of pain and when interruptions by friends, family, and other health professionals are absent or minimal. Interviews with clients in their homes should be scheduled at a time selected by the client. Most people communicate best at different times during the day or week. For example, some may prefer an early morning interview, while others prefer late morning, early afternoon, or evening interviews. Monday mornings or Friday afternoons are often considered unsuitable times since motivation can be low at these times (Stewart and Cash 1985, p. 47).

Place The place of the interview must have adequate privacy to promote communication. A well-lighted, well-ventilated, moderate-sized room that is relatively free of noise, movements, and interruptions encourages communication. Constant interruptions, such as telephone calls, the noise of traffic outside a window, or people moving about in or near the location can disrupt thought patterns, concentration, and moods and may convey the impression that the nurse is too busy or uninterested. In addition, a place where others cannot overhear or, if possible, see the client is desirable. Most people are inhibited when answering personal questions in the hearing of others and expressing strong feelings in the sight of others.

Seating arrangement Seating arrangement can help or hinder the interview. A seating arrangement with the nurse behind a desk and the client seated across creates a formal setting that suggests a business meeting between a superior and a subordinate. In contrast, a seating arrangement in which the parties sit on two chairs placed at right angles to a desk or table or a few feet apart with no table between creates a less formal atmosphere, and the nurse and client tend to feel on equal terms. In groups, a horseshoe or circular chair arrangement can avoid a superior or head-of-the-table position.

When interviewing a client in bed, the nurse can sit at a 45° angle to the bed. This position is less formal than sitting behind a table in the room or standing at the foot the bed and provides room for the client to get up. During an initial admission interview, a client may feel less confronted if there is an overbed table between the client and the nurse (Davis 1984, p. 66). Sitting on a client's bed hems the client in and makes staring difficult to avoid.

Distance The distance between the interviewer and interviewee is also important. Most people feel uncomfortable when talking to someone who is too close or too far away. Most people feel comfortable 1 to 1.2 m (3 to 4 ft) apart during an interview. A distance of 1.5 to 1.8 m (5 to 6 ft) encourages a client to talk longer (Davis 1984, p. 66). For additional information, see the discussion of personal space in Chapter 28.

Height also affects communication. A nurse who stands looking down at a client can make the client feel hemmed in. Status is associated with greater space and the freedom to move about (Davis 1984, p. 68). Therefore, the nurse who stands during an interview is perceived by the client as having greater status.

Stages of an Interview

An interview has three major stages: the opening or introduction, the body or development, and the closing.

The opening The opening can be the most important part of the interview since what is said and done at that time sets the tone for the remainder of the interview. An inadequate opening can be misleading and create problems during and following the interview. The opening is a two-step process: establishing rapport and orienting the interviewee (Stewart and Cash 1985, p. 60). Either step can come first depending on the situation, the relationship between the two parties, or the interviewer's choice. The rapport and orientation stages may occur at the same time since they are often indistinguishable.

Establishing rapport is a process of creating good will and trust. It can begin with a greeting—"Good morning, John"—or a self-introduction—"Good morning. I'm Becky James, a nursing student"—accompanied by nonverbal gestures such as a smile, a handshake, and a friendly manner. Next the rapport stage is developed by asking questions about the person and proceeding with some small talk about the weather, sports, families, and the like. The nurse must be careful to not overdo this stage since too much superficial talk can arouse anxiety about what is to follow and may appear insincere.

The orientation step consists of explaining the purpose and nature of the interview, e.g. what information is needed, how long it will take, and what is expected of the client. For instance, the nurse might state that the client has the right not to provide data or might tell the client how the information will be used.

The following is an example of an interview introduction:

> Nurse: Hello, Ms. Goodwin, I'm Ms. Fellows. I'm a nursing student, and I'll be assisting with your care here.
>
> Client: Hi. Are you a student from the college?
>
> Nurse: Yes, I'm in my final year. May I sit down with you here for about 10 minutes to talk about how I can help you while you're here?
>
> Client: All right. What do you want to know?
>
> Nurse: Well, to plan your care after your operation, I'd like to get some information about your normal daily activities and what you expect here in the hospital. I'd like to make notes while we talk to get the important points and have them available to the other staff who will also look after you.
>
> Client: OK. I guess that's all right with me.
>
> Nurse: If there is anything you don't want to talk about, please feel free to say so, and if there is anything you would rather I didn't write down, just tell me. Shall we start now?
>
> Client: Sure, now is as good a time as any.

The body In the body of the interview, the client communicates what he or she thinks, feels, knows, and perceives in response to questions from the nurse. Transition from the opening stage to this stage can often be facilitated by the use of an open-ended question that is related

A client has a right to withhold any information from the nurse that the client considers to be in his or her private domain. The nurse does not have the right to intrude into a client's protected private domain.
(Morreim et al. 1982, p. 38)

to the stated purpose, is easy to answer, and does not embarrass or place stress on the person. Examples are: "Tell me what you think about being hospitalized?" "What do you think about staying in bed these days?" "Tell me how your children are managing."

Effective development of the interview demands that the nurse use communication techniques that make both parties feel comfortable and serve the purpose of the interview. Since communication techniques are discussed in detail in Chapter 28, only brief guidelines are provided here (Benjamin 1981, pp. 20–55).

1. Listen attentively, using all your senses, and speak slowly and clearly.
2. Use language the client understands and clarify points that are not understood, for instance, by asking the person to describe what a word means to him or her.
3. Plan questions to follow a logical sequence.
4. Ask only one question at a time. Double questions limit the client to one choice and may confuse both the nurse and the client. Examples are: "Do you want coffee or tea?" "Would you like to talk now or later?" These questions force the client to choose from what the nurse is pleased to offer.
5. Allow the client the opportunity to look at things the way they appear to him or her and not the way they appear to the nurse or someone else.
6. Allow the client complete self-expression even if it disagrees with your own values and morals. Do not impose your own values on the person.
7. Avoid leading the client in a direction you choose. Follow the client rather than asking him or her to follow you.
8. Use and accept silence to help the client search for more thoughts and feelings or to organize them. Silence may be necessary to absorb the depth of a heart-warming, shocking, frightening, or tragic experience.
9. Avoid interjecting your own thoughts during periods of silence.
10. Avoid using personal examples or saying, "If I were you, I should. . . ."
11. Avoid saying "I know just how you feel." This sentence conveys, "I don't know how you feel, and I'm not willing to spend the time to find out."
12. Nonverbally convey respect, concern, interest, and acceptance. Use eye contact and be calm, unhurried, and sympathetic.
13. Offer information when it is requested.
14. Use leading questions sparingly to focus on vague comments. **Leading questions** suggest the answer expected or desired, and the client often merely supplies the expected answer. Examples are: "You haven't had any emotional problems?" "You haven't ever had a venereal disease, have you?" "You classify yourself as healthy, don't you?" "You were drunk last night, weren't you?" Leading questions create difficulties if the client, from a desire to please the nurse, gives inaccurate responses.

The closing The interview is usually terminated by the nurse, although in some cases the client terminates it. Nurses normally terminate interviews when they have obtained the information they need. Clients terminate interviews when they decide not to give any more information or are unable to offer more information for some other reason—fatigue, for example. The closing is important in maintaining the rapport and trust established during the interview and in facilitating future interactions. The following ways are commonly used to close an interview (Stewart and Cash 1985, p. 72):

1. Signal that the interview is coming to an end by offering to answer questions: "Do you have any questions?" "I would be glad to answer any questions you have." Be sure to allow time for the person to answer, or the offer will be regarded as insincere.
2. Declare completion of the purpose or task by saying "Well, that's about all I need to know for now" or "Well, those are all the questions I have for now." Preceding a remark with the word *well* generally signals that the end of the interaction is near.
3. Use a clearinghouse question such as: "Is there anything else?" "I think that takes care of everything I need. Is there anything else you would like to bring up?"
4. State appreciation or satisfaction about what was accomplished: "I really enjoyed meeting you, and I think we accomplished a great deal." "Those are all the questions I have. Thank you for your time and help." "Thanks for your help. The questions you have answered will be helpful in planning your nursing care."

5. Express concern for the person's welfare and future: "Take care of yourself. I'll see you on Thursday." "I hope all goes well for you. If you run into additional problems be sure to get in touch with me."

6. Plan for the next meeting, if there is to be one. Include the day, time, place, topic, and purpose: "Let's get together again here on the fifteenth at 9:00 A.M. to see how you are managing then."

7. Reveal what will happen next. For example: "Ms. Goodwin, I will be responsible for giving you care three mornings per week while you are here. I will be in to see you each Monday, Tuesday, and Wednesday between eight o'clock and noon. At those times, we can adjust your care if we need to. When I am not here, Ms. Brown will look after you." Or: "Ms. Goodwin, it's time for you to rest. I'll come back another time to finish our talk. We need information from you and your ideas to help plan your care."

8. Make a sincere personal inquiry that does not relate to the content of the interview but brings the interview to a relaxed end. For example: "How is your son doing at college?" "What are your plans for your vacation?"

9. Signal that the time is up if a time limit was agreed upon or explain why the interview must close at that time: "Well, I see our time is up; did it ever go quickly today." Or: "I'm sorry, but we're going to have to end our discussion; I have another appointment in 10 minutes."

10. Provide a summary to verify accuracy and agreement. This is particularly helpful for clients who are anxious or who have difficulty staying with the topic. "Well, it seems to me that you are especially worried about your hospitalization and chest pain because your father died of a heart attack 5 years ago, your wife has multiple sclerosis and depends on you for support and care, and you don't want to ask for too much help from your children. Is that correct? . . . We'll do the best we can to help you with these concerns. I'll discuss this with you again tomorrow, and we'll decide what plans need to be made to help you."

Nursing Assessment

The data collected during an interview between the nurse and client constitutes a nursing assessment, formerly called a nursing health history. The nurse obtains information about the client, the client's health, responses to illness, sociocultural factors, health beliefs and practices, coping patterns, and day-to-day activities. A nursing assessment differs from a medical history in that it focuses on the meaning of illness and hospitalization to the client and the family as a basis for planning (McPhetridge 1968, p. 68).

According to Perry, the objectives of a nursing assessment are to identify the client's patterns of health and illness, the presence of risk factors for physical and behavioral health problems, any deviations from normal, and the client's available resources for adaptation (Perry 1982, p. 43).

There are many frameworks for a nursing assessment. Theories, models, frameworks, and principles are all used as approaches for the data collection. Some nursing models provide an assessment tool to help the nurse gather data. One such tool is Newman's tool, an assessment/intervention tool that has seven categories: intake summary, stressors as perceived by the client, stressors as perceived by the caregiver, intrapersonal factors, interpersonal factors, extrapersonal factors, and formulation of the problem (Cross 1985, pp. 271–72).

Abdellah (1961) and Henderson (1960) developed earlier frameworks used or adapted in many settings. More recently, Gordon (1982) established a framework of 11 functional health patterns.

Gordon's Typology of 11 Functional Health Patterns

1. *Health-perception-health-management pattern.* Describes client's perceived pattern of health and well-being and how health is managed

2. *Nutritional-metabolic pattern.* Describes pattern of food and fluid consumption relative to metabolic need and pattern indicators of local nutrient supply

3. *Elimination pattern.* Describes patterns of excretory function (bowel, bladder, and skin)

4. *Activity-exercise pattern.* Describes pattern of exercise, activity, leisure, and recreation

5. *Cognitive-perceptual pattern.* Describes sensory-perceptual and cognitive pattern

6. *Sleep-rest pattern.* Describes patterns of sleep, rest, and relaxation

7. *Self-perception–self-concept pattern.* Describes self-concept pattern and perceptions of self (e.g., body comfort, body image, feeling state)

8. *Role-relationship pattern.* Describes pattern of role-engagements and relationships

9. *Sexuality-reproductive pattern.* Describes client's patterns of satisfaction and dissatisfaction with sexuality; describes reproductive patterns

10. *Coping-stress-tolerance pattern.* Describes general coping pattern and effectiveness of the pattern in terms of stress tolerance

11. *Value-belief pattern.* Describes patterns of values, beliefs (including spiritual), or goals that guide choices or decisions (Gordon 1982, p. 81)

Gordon's framework, "A Typology of 11 Functional Health Patterns," organizes the data the nurse collects and is adaptable to all conceptual models. Three advantages of Gordon's framework are that it presents a short list of readily learned categories, organizes data in a way already familiar to most nurses, and steers the nurse toward nursing diagnoses, not medical diagnoses. Gordon uses the word *pattern* to signify a sequence of behavior. The nurse collects data about dysfunctional as well as functional behavior. Thus, using Gordon's framework to analyze data, nurses are able to discern emerging patterns.

Roy (1984) outlines the data to be collected according to the Roy Adaptation model and classifies observable behavior into four categories: physiologic, self-concept, role function, and interdependence. Orem (1985) delineates eight universal self-care requisites of humans. See Table 11–4.

Carnevali (1983, p. 93) states that "a nurse needs data in two major areas—the activities and demands of daily living associated with the presenting situation or longer-term health issues and the status of internal and external resources of the patient/family, both current and potential." The common core in a nursing database suggested by Carnevali (1983, pp. 94–112) is:

1. Activities in daily living (ADL)
2. Demands of daily living (DDL)
3. Internal resources (IR)
4. External resources (ER)
5. Needed resources
6. Usable resources
7. Health and life-style goals

Other frameworks and models from other disciplines are helpful for data collection. Some are Maslow's hierarchy of needs (see Chapter 16), Piaget's assessment of cognitive development (see Chapter 22), Selyes's stress theory (see Chapter 17). These frameworks are narrower than the model required in nursing; therefore, the nurse usually needs to combine these with other approaches to obtain a complete assessment.

Assessment records The format for a health assessment may be structured according to a specific model or theory or it may reflect a variety of concepts. It may reflect the individual as a biopsychosociospiritual being; that is a person with biophysical, psychologic, sociologic, and spiritual aspects. The form of the nursing assessment in this instance is eclectic in that it includes what is most appropriate for the situation in the realm of biophysical, psychologic, sociologic, and spiritual health. See Figure 11–1.

Table 11–4 Areas of Data Collection Delineated by Dorothea Orem and Sister Callista Roy

Orem (1985)	Roy (1984)
Universal self-care requisites	Adaptive modes
1. The maintenance of a sufficient intake of air	1. Physiological needs a. Exercise and rest b. Nutrition c. Elimination d. Fluid and electrolytes e. Oxygen and circulation f. Regulation: temperature g. Regulation: the senses h. Regulation: endocrine system
2. The maintenance of a sufficient intake of water	2. Self-concept a. Physical self b. Moral-ethical self c. Self-consistency d. Self-ideal and expectancy e. Self-esteem
3. The maintenance of a sufficient intake of food	3. Role function
4. The provision of care associated with elimination processes and excrements	4. Interdependence
5. The maintenance of a balance between activity and rest	
6. The maintenance of a balance between solitude and social interaction	
7. The prevention of hazards to human life, human functioning, and human well-being	
8. The promotion of human functioning and development within social groups in accord with human potential, known human limitations, and human desire to be normal. (Normalcy is used in the sense of that which is essentially human and that which is in accord with the genetic and constitutional characteristics and the talents of individuals.)	

All information that the nurse obtains as a result of the nurse-client relationship is considered confidential. It can be shared only with health personnel directly involved in the client's care. The client must give consent before a nurse can share the information with others even for educational purposes. (Fenner 1980, pp. 44–48)

Another type of nursing assessment record is unstructured and widely applicable, i.e., to hospitalized clients, ambulatory clients, and clients remaining at home. Nurses need to have the knowledge and skills to carry out a complete assessment without the structure. The nurse is expected to develop a format that is both appropriate for the client and useful for the nurse.

Consulting

A **consultation** is a deliberation by two or more people. Consulting differs from referring. In consulting, the responsibility for the client's care remains with the nurse who seeks the consultation. *Referring* is the transfer of a client's care to another person, e.g., a nurse practitioner may refer a client to a physician, and a hospital nurse may refer a client to a home health care agency or nurse. Nurses consult a variety of health personnel, including other nurses, throughout the nursing process. Increasingly, nurse consultants operate in many settings. These nurses have specialized knowledge and skills. For example, orthopedic nurses are consulted by nurses who require their assistance with special problems. Some nurse consultants are employed by agencies; others are in independent practice. Nurses do not consult only other nurses; they frequently consult physicians, social workers, and other health personnel. Some agencies have a protocol to be followed when consulting a health professional not presently involved in a client's care. For example, if a nurse wants to discuss a client's depression with an agency psychiatrist, she or he may need to send an agency form to the psychiatrist requesting a consultation. However, many consultations are arranged less formally. For example, a nurse may discuss a client's problem with the physician when he or she comes to see the client.

The client is not always an active participant in the consulting process. In many instances, a nurse consults on behalf of the client, e.g., when a client's desire to be discharged from the hospital is discussed with a physician. In other instances, the client is an active participant, e.g., the client, physiotherapist, and the nurse discuss the best way for the client to move from a bed to a chair.

Reasons for Consulting

Nurses generally consult for the following reasons: to verify findings, to implement change, and to obtain additional knowledge. Nurses frequently ask other nurses to verify assessment data, e.g., an extremely low blood pressure or an exceptionally fast pulse rate, when their findings are unexpected or when they are uncertain about them. Sometimes nurses discuss a client's nursing care plan with another nurse, often to make sure the best possible plan has been arranged or to implement a change in the plan. A second person's ideas can generate new approaches to the client's care. Consultation to obtain knowledge is desirable. No nurse can know everything about nursing, and another nurse may have knowledge and experience about a particular problem. A truly professional nurse does not hesitate to admit uncertainty or acknowledge that a problem is beyond the nurse's experience or knowledge. For example, a female client requires a urinary catheterization; however, the muscles of her legs are fully contracted and she is unable to abduct her legs normally. The nurse who is planning to carry out the catheterization consults with another nurse about how to position the client for the catheterization. In this example, since the client is unable to explain the position to the nurse, a consultation facilitates care and prevents undue stress for the client.

Consulting Process

The consulting process has seven steps:

Identify the problem Before consulting another person, the nurse must have the problem clearly in mind, including circumstances surrounding the problem. For example, a nursing student is unsure how to place the dressings on a draining wound to catch all the drainage because she or he did not see the previous dressing before the physician removed it. The problem is clearly described, i.e., how to place the dressing, and the circumstances include the site of the source of the drainage, the amount of drainage, and the present absence of a correct dressing.

Collect pertinent data about the client When planning to consult a health professional who is unfamiliar with the client, collect all the data relevant to the problem, e.g., the client says, "I am afraid I am bleeding all the time," and the client is thin and at risk of developing pressure sores.

Obtain the client's permission When consulting a health professional not normally involved in the client's care, it is important to obtain the client's permission before discussing the problem or providing any information. The client has a right to refuse another person's information about his health and to refuse changes in care.

Select the consultant The nurse who has identified a problem regarding nursing care should consult a recognized health professional who has the skills or knowledge required, a nurse with special knowledge and skills. For

Dear Patient:

Your nurses will be planning your hospital care to meet your individual needs. We would appreciate your help in answering the following questions. This information will help us learn about your general health and your condition. As nurses, we are concerned about your response to the diagnosis and treatment of your actual and/or potential problems.

This information is confidential. You do not have to answer any questions, or complete the form unless you want to. Thank you.

Instructions for completing the form.

1. If you have been hospitalized at UCSF within the past month, you do not need to fill out the entire form, only update the sections that have changed.
2. Complete the white sections on both sides of this page. The grey sections will be completed by your nurse.
3. A relative or friend may ask you the questions and/or write your answers for you.
4. If the question requires a yes/no answer, please circle the correct answer.
5. When you answer the questions which ask about changes or difficulties, please answer in relation to the last year.
6. After you complete the form, or if you choose not to complete it, please return it to the person who gave it to you.
7. After you are in your room your nurse will review your answers and will develop a plan of care with you.

HEALTH PERCEPTION / HEALTH MANAGEMENT

What language do you find it easiest to read & write? ✓ English; Other ______

If you have any problem completing this form, please return it to the person who gave it to you.

Who should we call in case of emergency? Joe Smith ... phone; days 345-5495 nights ______

What has caused this hospitalization? no energy and shortness of breath

What do you expect to happen during this hospitalization? get well, maybe get a new heart valve

Have you ever been in the hospital before? no yes ✓ 1984 - left hip replacement

How is your general health? good ✓ fair poor Do you have any chronic medical problems? (no) yes

What are the most important things you do to keep healthy? eat a good diet

Do you feel these things make a difference? no (yes)

Do you smoke? (no) yes... ______ packs/day ______ ...use alcohol? (no) yes ______ drinks/day no drinking

...use drugs which are not prescribed for you? (no) yes...type ______

NUTRITIONAL-METABOLIC

Do you follow a special diet? (no) yes . . . describe no sugar - I have diabetes

In the past year did you lose weight? no (yes) . . . amount? 5 lbs gain weight? (no) yes . . . amount? ______

Any changes in your appetite or thirst? (no) yes . . . describe ______

Any difficulties with food, eating, or swallowing? (no) yes . . . describe ______

ELIMINATION

Any changes or difficulties with your bowel habits? (no) yes . . . describe ______

Do you often have diarrhea or constipation? (no) yes . . . describe ______

Do you use laxatives or other aids for regularity? (no) yes . . . describe ______

Have you experienced any changes or difficulties with urinary elimination? no (yes) . . . describe go too often

ACTIVITY / EXERCISE

What is your occupation cattle rancher and farmer

Do you have enough energy for the day-to-day activities you want to do, i.e. work, recreation, fixing meals, dressing.
yes (no) . . . describe can't do my daily chores anymore

Do you feel you get enough exercise? yes no What exercise do you usually do? ______
How often? ______

For each of the following activities, please check whether you consider yourself independent, needing assistance, or unable to do. If you are not independent, please explain.

	Indep	Need Assist	Unable	
Bath/shower	✓			
Dressing yourself	✓			
Eating	✓			
Using the bathroom	✓			
Moving to/from bed or chair	✓			move slow since my operation
Have you fallen recently? no yes				

EQUIPMENT NEEDED IN

	Hospital	Home
Crutches		
Walker		
Wheelchair		
Highrise toilet seat		
Other		

Figure 11–1 Nursing Admission Assessment

Courtesy of Department of Nursing, The Medical Center at the University of California, San Francisco.

REST/SLEEP

Do you have any difficulty sleeping? (no) yes . . . describe I do not sleep much, never have

Is there anything you do or use to help you sleep? no yes . . . describe

COGNITIVE-PERCEPTUAL

Any difficulty hearing? no (yes) . . . describe a little hard of hearing

Do you use an aid? (no) yes . . . type? Do you have any difficulty seeing? no yes

When were your eyes last checked? don't know Do you wear (glasses)/contacts? no (yes) . . . type

Have you experienced any changes in your memory lately? (no) yes . . . describe

Do you sometimes have difficulty learning new things? (no) yes . . . describe

What is the easiest way for you to learn them? have people tell me – don't read much

Do you regularly experience pain or discomfort? (no) yes . . . describe/manage

ROLES-RELATIONSHIPS

With whom do you live? wife and 6 of my 13 children

Whom do you define as your family or support system? X same as above; others . . . children are ages 16-35

How does your family or significant other(s) feel about your illness/condition? scared

Are you experiencing any family difficulties as a result of your illness/condition? (no) yes . . . describe

Do others depend on you for things? no (yes) . . . how are they managing? ✓ no problems; ___ experiencing some difficulty . . . describe

Does anyone come into your home to help you (e.g. visiting nurse, housekeeper, etc.)? (no) yes . . . who and how often?

Other questions you'd like answered or specific things you'd like to learn while you're in the hospital? (no) yes . . . (if yes) list

Name of person who filled out form (if different than patient):

Relationship to patient *Date*

The following personal questions are optional. Please fill in those which you feel will assist your nurse in planning your care.

SELF-PERCEPTION/ SELF CONCEPT

Has this illness/condition caused changes in your body or the things you can do? no (yes) . . . describe too weak to do day to day work on the farm

Has it effected you emotionally? (no) yes . . . describe

Has it caused changes in the way you feel about yourself or your body? (no) yes . . . describe

Have any of these changes been a problem for you? (no) yes . . . describe

SEXUALITY-Reproduction

Some people have concern that their surgery/condition may affect their sexual relationship(s). Is this a concern for you? (no) yes...describe

(Women only) Is there a chance you might be pregnant? no yes

COPING-STRESS

Who is most helpful in talking things over? my son Tom Is s/he available to you now? no (yes)

Other than your illness/condition, have there been any big changes in your life in the last year or so? no (yes) . . . describe can't do my work

When you have problems or stress in your life, how do you generally handle them/it? no problems

Most of the time does this help? yes no . . . describe too busy to worry about things

Being in the hospital is stressful for many people. Is there anything we can do to make it easier for you? let my family visit

VALUE-BELIEF

Do you consider religion/spirituality important in your life? (yes) somewhat no

Would you like to see a hospital chaplin? no (yes)

NURSING ADMISSION ASSESSMENT

602-02 9/85

Admitted to: 525 W from: home Time: 1500 Ht: 171 Wt: 95.3 kg

T: 36.5 P: 80 R R: 16 B/P: L: 124/80 R: ___ Oriented to: ✓ phone; ✓ TV; ✓ bed; ✓ visiting hours; ✓ call light; ✓ meal times/menu; ✓ care of valuables; ✓ smoking; ✓ dentures; ✓

Completed by: Mary Jones Date/Time: 7/23/85 1400 hrs

Allergies: none

MEDICATION HISTORY

NAME	DOSE	FREQUENCY	LAST TAKEN	PURPOSE/PROBLEM TAKING
Tolinase	250 mg	qd	7/22	diabetes
Lasix	20 mg	qd	7/22	for bad heart valve
Slow K	20 mEq	qd	7/22	to replace K^+
NTG 1/150	i	prn	2 months ago	angina

GENERAL APPEARANCE: (size; posture; mobility; expression; mental status; orientation) Large, slightly obese elderly 81 year old male. Alert and oriented × 3. Moves well but stiff in joints. Pleasant but not talkative.

HEENT: (trach; eyes; cranial facial abnormalities) Wears corrective glasses for reading.

NEUROLOGICAL: (gait/balance; LOC: speech disorders) Slight limp. Independent.

MUSCULO-SKELETAL: (atrophy; swelling/edema; ROM; prosthetic devices) Ⓛ hip replacement 18 months ago s̄ complications. No pedal edema.

SCREENING EXAM

CARDIOVASCULAR: (pulses: 4+=bounding, 3+=v.strong, 2+=normal, 1+=weak/thready, 0=unable to palpate; rhythm/regularity of heart; color)

Pulse	R	L	Equal	Pulse	R	L	Equal	Rythm: (Regular)/Irregular
Temp.	2+	2+		Fem.	3+	4+		loud murmur in aortic area
Carotid	2+	2+		Pop.	2+	0	Ⓛ limb cooler than Ⓡ	
Brachial	2+	2+		D.P.	2+	0		
Radial	2+	2+		Post tib.	2+	0		

PULMONARY: (breath sounds; cough or sputum; chest symmetry; respiratory effort) Ō cough. Equal expansion. Rales in bases bilaterally which do clear with coughing.

GASTRO-INTESTINAL/GU/GYN: (size; tenderness; distention; ascites; bowel sounds; ostomy; tubes) Abdomen soft, non tender. Last BM 7/22 a.m.

GU/GYN: (date of last period, urgency, frequency, burning, vag. discharge) ↑ frequency c̄ Lasix noted by patient.

INTEGUMENTARY: (Norton Scale; on figure in box note location of any items with the appropriate letter and check in box by the letter) Pink, intact, good turgor.

S

== Numbness	B Bruise
ooo Pins and needles	D Decubitus
xxx Burning	L Laceration
+++ Aching	R Rash
/// Stabbing	S Scar

PRESSURE SORE RISK ASSESSMENT SCORING SCALE: Total score: ________ (circle #'s then total)

If ≦14, initiate a diagnosis.

Phy. Cond.	Ment. Cond.	Activity	Mobility	Incontin.
(4) (good)	(4) (alert)	(4) (ambulatory)	4 (full)	(4) (not)
3 (fair)	3 (apathetic/withdrawn)	3 (wk/help)	(3) (sl. limited)	3 (occassionally)
2 (poor)	2 (confused)	2 (chair/bound)	2 (v. limited)	2 (usual/urine)
1 (very bad)	1 (stuporous/unresponsive)	1 (bedfast)	1 (immobile)	1 (urine & stool/doubly)

Signatures Mary Jones RN Date 7/23/85

________________ ________

UNIT SPECIFIC INFORMATION

Pt. admitted for cardiac catheterization and probable aortic valve replacement. Pt has hx (6 mos.) of angina. Over past year patient has noted marked decrease in energy and episodes of SOB on exertion.

UCSF
University of California San Francisco
Hospitals and Clinics
San Francisco, CA 94143

Signature Mary Jones RN Date 7/23/85

________________ ________

example, if a client, Mrs. Kinney, has a malignancy and is experiencing acute pain in spite of analgesics, a logical consultant would be the oncology nurse specialist. This nurse is likely to have knowledge and experience to teach the nurse how to help Mrs. Kinney. As another example, a nurse might consult an enterostomal therapist about the best way to care for a client's stoma and incision.

Communicate the problem and pertinent information This information often varies with each client and each problem. However, it is important to convey information about the client's strengths as well as his or her problems. Convey the information clearly and objectively so that the consultant does not become biased yet obtains a clear picture of the situation. Make sure the data you provide are factual and not interpretive. For example, "Mrs. Marsh cries each time she moves" describes her behavior factually, but "Mrs. Marsh is seeking attention" or "Mrs. Marsh is acting like a child" interprets the crying judgmentally and conveys bias.

Discuss the recommendations with the consultant The consultant may provide recommendations at the time you describe the problem, or a later meeting may be necessary. For example, an oncology nursing consultant may give immediate recommendations regarding activity, positioning, timing of medication, or the consultant might prefer to obtain further data before making recommendations.

Include the recommendations in the client's nursing care plan Once recorded, the recommendations become part of the client's record and are available to all health professionals involved in the client's care. After implementing the recommendations, the nurse needs to evaluate their effectiveness and to record these. If they are not effective, it may be necessary to see the consultant again and make further adjustments in the client's nursing plan.

Examining

Increasingly, nurses are carrying out physical health examinations of clients during the nursing assessment phase of the nursing process to verify data obtained in the nursing assessment. The examination includes the assessment of all body parts and the taking of vital signs, height, weight, and anthropometric measurements. An **anthropometric measurement** is a measurement of the size and composition of the body. These techniques are discussed in detail in Chapters 34, 35 and 42. Instead of giving a complete examination, the nurse may focus on a specific problem area noted from the nursing assessment, such as the inability to urinate. Alternately, the nurse may perform a screening examination that includes essential functioning of various body parts or systems. An example of a screening examination is the nursing admission assessment form shown in Figure 11–1. Data obtained from this examination are measured against norms or standards, such as ideal height and weight standards or norms for temperature or blood pressure levels. The data are used to determine the person's general health status.

To conduct the examination, the nurse uses techniques of inspection, auscultation, palpation, and percussion. **Inspection** is visual examination, that is, assessing using the sense of sight. It includes looking with the naked eye and using a lighted instrument such as an otoscope, which assists with visual examination of the ear.

Inspection is an active, not a passive, process, in which the nurse must know what to look for and where. Nurses use inspection frequently to assess color, rashes, scars, body shape, facial expressions that may reflect emotions, and body structures, e.g., the inner eye. Inspection should be systematic, so that no area is missed. Inspection using lighted instruments is discussed in Chapter 35.

Auscultation is the process of listening to sounds produced within the body. Auscultation may be direct or indirect. Direct auscultation is the use of the unaided ear, e.g., to listen to a respiration wheeze or the grating of a moving joint. Indirect auscultation is the use of a stethoscope, which amplifies the sounds and conveys them to the nurse's ears. A stethoscope is used primarily to listen to sounds from within the body, e.g., bowel sounds or valve sounds of the heart.

The stethoscope should be 30 to 25 cm (12 to 14 in) long, with an internal diameter of about 0.3 cm (⅛ in). It should have both a flat-disc and a bell-shaped diaphragm. See Figure 11–2. The flat-disc diaphragm best transmits high-pitched sounds, e.g., bronchial sounds, and the bell-shaped diaphragm best transmits low-pitched sounds, such as some heart sounds.

The earpieces of the stethoscope should fit comfortably into the nurse's ears. The diaphragm of the stethoscope is placed firmly but lightly against the client's skin. If a client is very hairy, it may be necessary to dampen the hairs with a cloth so that they will lie flat against the skin and not cause scratching sounds.

Auscultated sounds are described according to their pitch, intensity, duration, and quality. The **pitch** is the frequency of the vibrations (the number of vibrations per second). Low-pitched sounds, e.g., some heart sounds, have fewer vibrations per second than high-pitched sounds, such as bronchial sounds. The **intensity** (amplitude) refers to the loudness or softness of a sound. Some body sounds are loud, e.g., bronchial sounds heard over the trachea, while others are soft, e.g., normal breath sounds heard

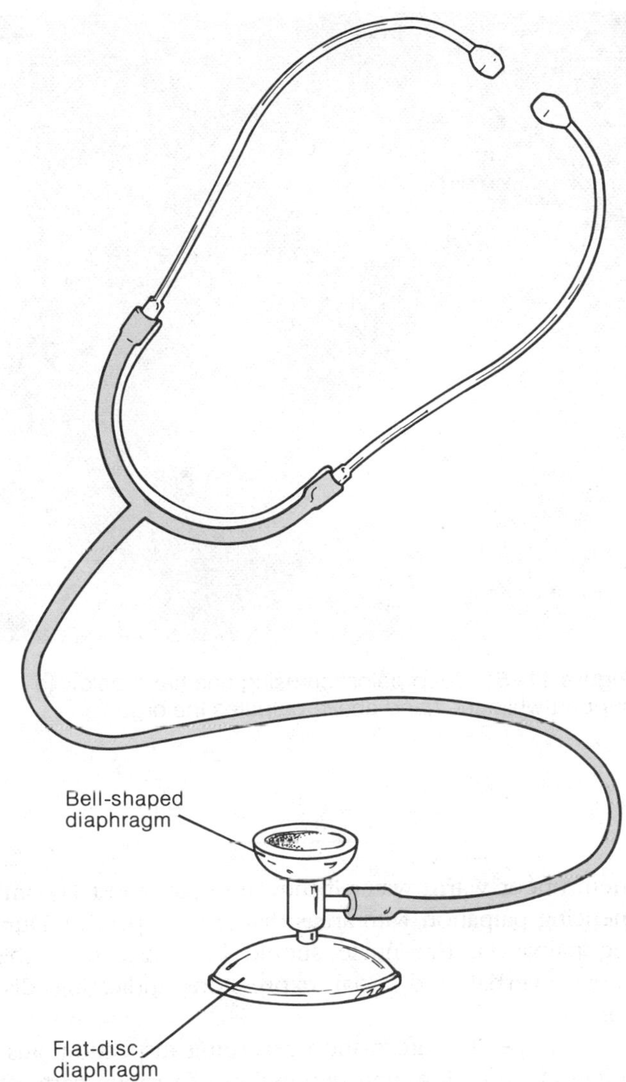

Figure 11–2 A stethoscope with a flat-disc and bell-shaped diaphragm

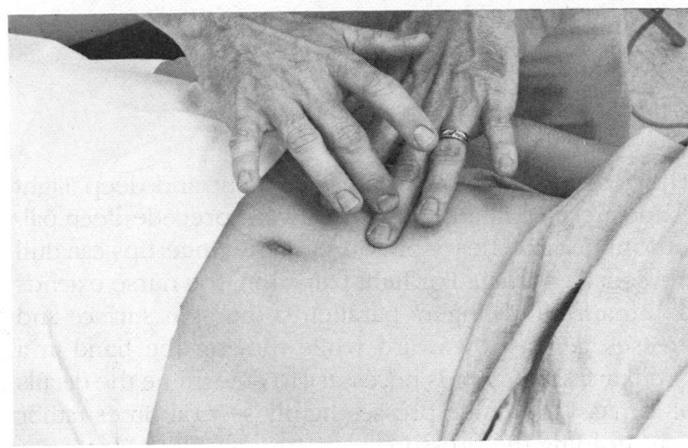

Figure 11–3 The position of the fingers for percussion. Only the middle finger of the nondominant hand is in contact with the skin.

in the lungs. The **duration** of a sound is its length (long or short). The **quality** of sound is a subjective description of a sound, e.g., whistling, gurgling, or snapping.

Percussion is an assessment method in which the body surface is struck to elicit sounds that can be heard or vibrations that can be felt. A commonly used percussion technique is to place the middle finger of the nondominant hand, referred to as the **pleximeter**, on the client's skin. Only the distal phalanx of this finger should be in contact with the skin. Using the tip of the flexed middle finger of the other hand, called the **plexor**, the nurse strikes the pleximeter between the nail and the distal interphalangeal joint. See Figure 11–3. The striking motion should come from the wrist; the forearm remains stationary. The angle between the plexor and the pleximeter should be 90°, and the blows must be firm, rapid, and short to obtain a clear sound.

Percussion is used to determine the size and shape of internal organs by establishing their borders. It indicates whether tissue is fluid-filled, air-filled, or solid. Percussion elicits five types of sound: flatness, dullness, resonance, hyperresonance, and tympany. **Flatness** is an extremely dull sound produced by very dense tissue such as muscle or bone. **Dullness** is a thudlike sound produced by dense tissue such as the liver, spleen, or heart. **Resonance** is a hollow sound such as that produced by lungs filled with air. **Hyperresonance** is not produced in the normal body. It is described as booming and can be heard over an emphysematous lung. **Tympany** is a musical or drumlike sound produced from an air-filled stomach. On a continuum, flatness reflects the most dense tissue (least amount of air) and tympany the least dense tissue (the most amount of air).

A percussion sound, such as resonance, is described according to its intensity, pitch, duration, and quality.

Palpation is the examination of the body using the sense of touch. The pads of the fingers are used because their concentration of nerve endings makes them highly sensitive to tactile discrimination.

Palpation is used to determine:

1. Texture, e.g., of the hair
2. Temperature, e.g., of a skin area
3. Vibration, e.g., of a joint
4. Position, size, consistency, and mobility of organs or masses

5. Distention, e.g., of the urinary bladder
6. Presence and rate of peripheral pulses
7. Tenderness or pain

There are two types of palpation: light and deep. Light (superficial) palpation should always precede deep palpation, because heavy pressure on the fingertips can dull the sense of touch. For light palpation, the nurse extends dominant hand fingers parallel to the skin surface and presses gently downward while moving the hand in a circular fashion. If it is necessary to determine the details of a mass, the nurse presses lightly several times rather than holding the pressure.

Deep palpation is done with two hands (bimanually) or one hand. In deep bimanual palpation, the nurse extends the dominant hand as for light palpation, then places the fingerpads of the nondominant hand on the dorsal surfaces of the distal interphalangeal joint of the middle three fingers of the dominant hand. See Figure 11–4. Pressure is applied by the top hand while the lower hand remains relaxed to perceive the tactile sensations. For deep palpation using one hand, the fingerpads of the dominant hand press over the area to be palpated. Often the other hand is used to support a mass or organ from below. See Figure 11–5.

The effectiveness of palpation depends largely on the client's relaxation. Nurses can assist a client to relax by: (a) gowning and/or draping the client appropriately; (b) positioning the client comfortably; (c) ensuring that their own hands are warm before beginning, e.g., running them under warm water if they are cold; and (d) commencing palpation with areas that are not painful. During palpation, the nurse should be sensitive to the client's verbal and facial expressions indicating discomfort.

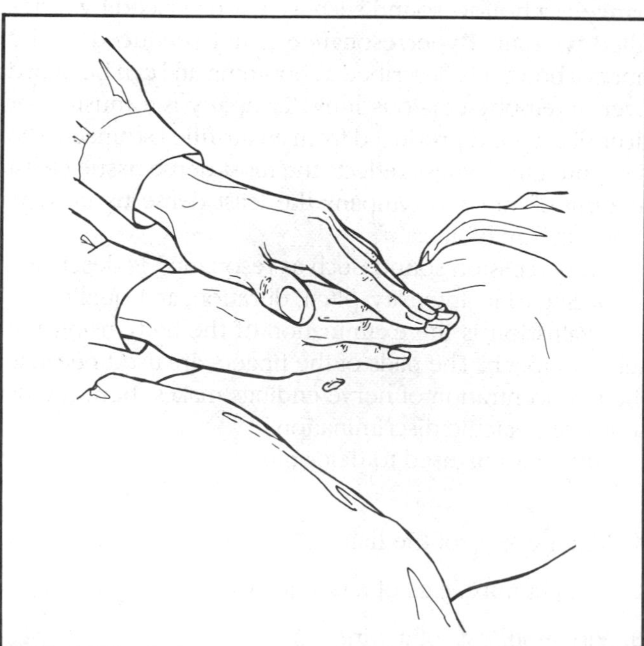

Figure 11–4 The position of the hands for deep bimanual palpation.

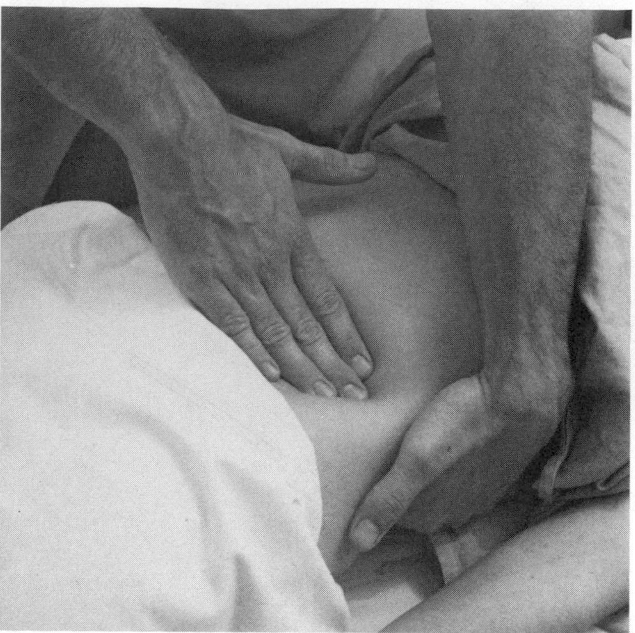

Figure 11–5 Deep palpation using one hand below to support while the hand above palpates the organ.

For specific information regarding inspection, auscultation, palpation, and percussion of various parts of the body, see Chapter 35.

Physical examination is carried out systematically. Generally, the examiner records a general impression about the client's overall appearance and health status, e.g., age, body size, mental and nutritional status, speech, and behavior. Then the examiner takes measurements such as vital signs, height, and weight. Next, the examiner conducts a physical examination beginning at the head and ending at the toes (head-to-toe or **cephalocaudal** examination). See Figure 11–6 for a sample head-to-toe assessment.

Chapter Highlights

- Assessment is the collection, verification, and documentation of data about a client's health status.
- Assessing involves active participation by the client and the nurse.

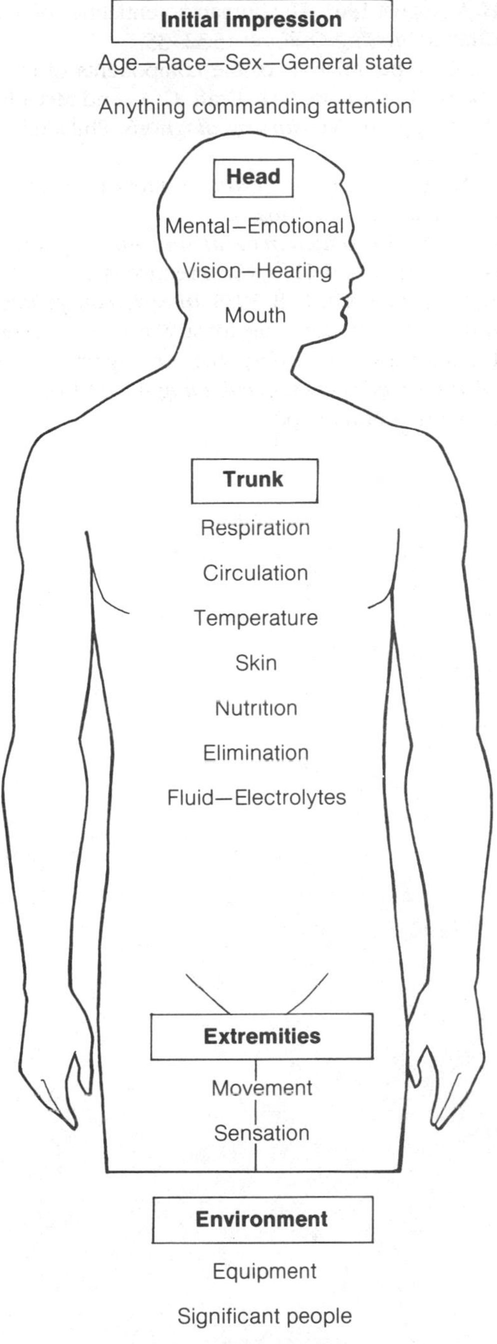

Figure 11–6 A tool for assessment.

Adapted from: H. Wolff and R. Erickson, The assessment man, *Nursing Outlook,* February 1977, 25:103.

- Methods used for data collection are informal conversation, formal interview, nursing assessment (history), physical health examination, and consultation.
- The database should be accurate, complete, and brief.

The nurse needs to use appropriate medical terminology when compiling the database.

- The database should include objective and subjective data.
- Skills required for data collection are communicating, interviewing, observing, and examining.

Suggested Readings

Baer, E. D., McGowan, M. N., and McGivern, D. O. July 1977. How to take a health history. *American Journal of Nursing* 77:1190–93.
The authors discuss a health history with six sections: chief complaint or the client's reason for seeking help, the client profile, family history, past health history, history of present problems, and review of systems.

Jacoby, M. K., and Adams, D. J. April 1981. Teaching assessment of client functioning. *Nursing Outlook* 29:248–50.
The authors present a functional assessment guideline based on Dunn's definition of wellness. Their functional assessment has three main categories: biophysical function, psychosocial function, and spiritual function. They also outline factors that impinge internally and externally upon the client's level of functioning.

Wolff, H., and Erickson, R. February 1977. The assessment man. *Nursing Outlook* 25:103–7.
Nurses can use a simple, practical tool for systematic client assessment. This head-to-toe approach has three major sections: initial impression, the client from head to toe, and the environment.

Selected References

Abdellah, F. G., et al. 1961. *Patient-centered approaches to nursing.* New York: Macmillan Co.

Atkinson, L. D., and Murray, M. E. 1983. *Understanding the nursing process.* 2d ed. New York: Macmillan Co.

Benjamin, A. 1981. *The helping interview.* 3d ed. Boston: Houghton Mifflin Co.

Carnevali, D. L. 1983. *Nursing care planning: Diagnosis and management.* 3d ed. Philadelphia: J. B. Lippincott Co.

Cross, J. R. Betty Newman. In George, J. B., editor. 1985. *Nursing theories: A base for professional practice.* 2d ed., pp. 258–86. Englewood Cliffs, N.J.: Prentice-Hall.

Davis, A. J. 1984. *Listening and responding.* St. Louis: C. V. Mosby Co.

Eggland, E. T. July 1977. How to take a meaningful history. *Nursing 77* 7:22–30.

Fenner, K. 1980. *Ethics and the law in nursing.* New York: D. Van Nostrand Co.

Gordon, M 1982. *Nursing diagnosis process and application.* New York: McGraw-Hill Book Co.

Griffith, J. W., and Christensen, P. J., editors. 1982. *Nursing process: Application of theories, frameworks, and models.* St. Louis: C. V. Mosby Co.

Henderson, V. 1966. *The nature of nursing.* New York: Macmillan Co.

La Monica, E. L. 1985. *The humanistic nursing process.* Monterey, Calif.: Wadsworth Health Sciences.

McCain, R. F. April 1965. Nursing by assessment—not intuition. *American Journal of Nursing* 65:82–84.

McPhetridge, L. M. January 1968. Nursing history: One means to personalize care. *American Journal of Nursing* 68:68–75.

Morreim, H., Donovan, A., Huey, R., Brimigion, J., and Fine, E. May/June 1982. A question of ethics: The patient's right to privacy. *Nursing Life* 2:34–38.

Orem, D. E. 1985. *Nursing: Concepts of practice.* 3rd ed. New York: McGraw-Hill.

Otto, H. A. August 1965. The human potentialities of nurses and patients. *Nursing Outlook* 13:32–35.

Perry, A. G. 1982. Analysis of the components of the nursing process. In Carlson, J. H., Craft, C. A., and McGuire, A. D., editors. pp. 41–54. *Nursing diagnosis.* Philadelphia: W. B. Saunders Co.

Philpott, M. 1985. *Legal liability and the nursing process.* Toronto: W. B. Saunders Co., Canada.

Roy, Sr. C. 1984. *Introduction to nursing: An adaptation model.* 2d ed. Englewood Cliffs, N.J.: Prentice-Hall.

Stewart, C. J., and Cash, W. B. 1985. *Interviewing principles and practices.* 4th ed. Dubuque, Iowa: Wm. C. Brown Publishers.

Yura, H., and Walsh, M. B. 1983. *The nursing process: Assessing, planning, implementing, evaluating.* 4th ed. Norwalk, Conn.: Appleton-Century-Crofts.

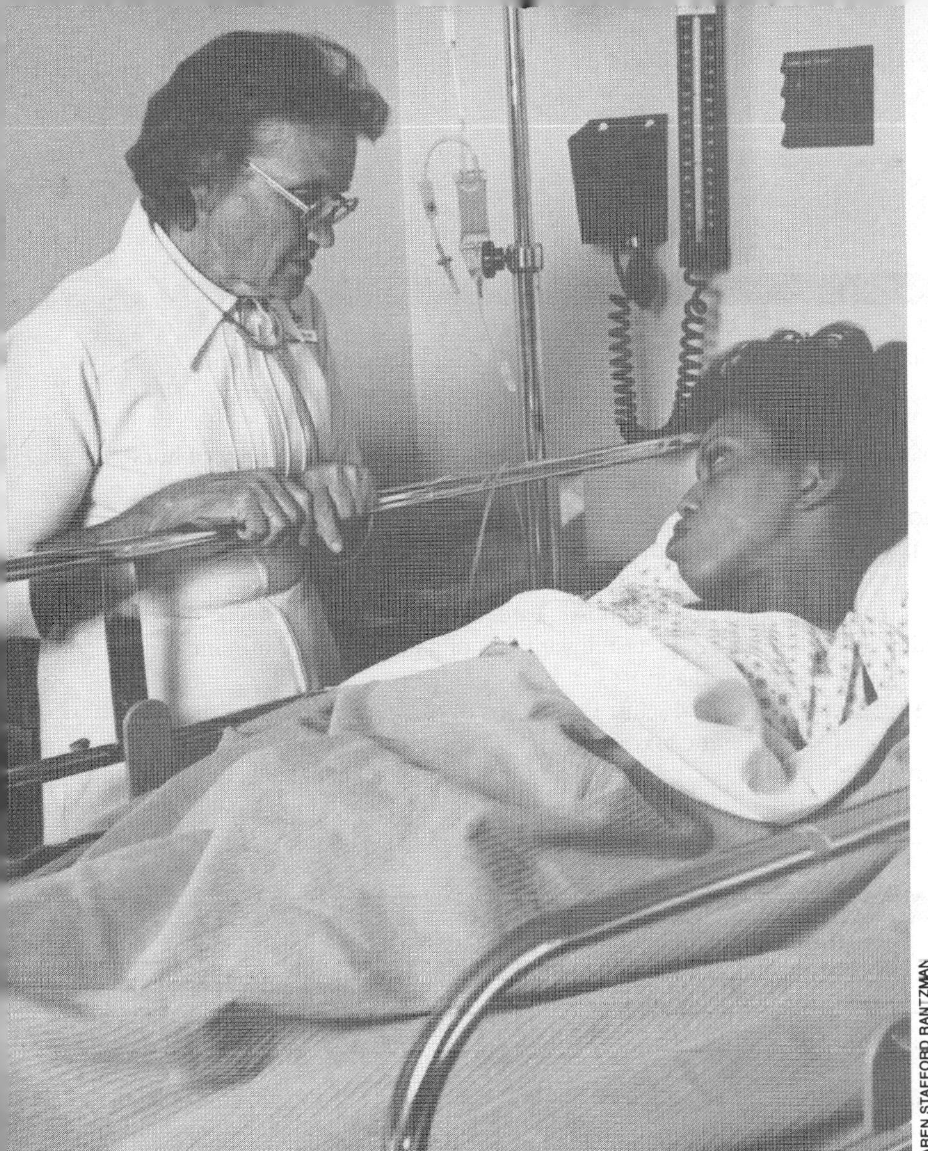
KAREN STAFFORD RANTZMAN

CHAPTER 12

Diagnosing

Contents

12 *Diagnosing*

Objectives

1. Understand essential facts about nursing diagnostic statements and the diagnostic process.
   - **1.1** Define listed terms.
   - **1.2** Describe characteristics of definitions of nursing diagnoses.
   - **1.3** Compare medical and nursing diagnoses.
   - **1.4** Identify basic steps in the diagnostic process.
   - **1.5** Describe the steps involved in data processing.
   - **1.6** Discuss essential aspects of determining the client's health problems and strengths.
   - **1.7** Describe two essential parts of a nursing diagnostic statement.
   - **1.8** Identify essential guidelines for writing diagnostic statements.
   - **1.9** Formulate nursing diagnostic statements.
   - **1.10** Identify advantages of using nursing diagnoses.
2. Appreciate the development of a taxonomy of nursing diagnoses.
   - **2.1** Describe the evolution of a taxonomy of nursing diagnoses.
   - **2.2** Describe three essential components of nursing diagnostic categories.
   - **2.3** List advantages of a taxonomy of nursing diagnoses.
   - **2.4** List limitations of the current nursing diagnostic taxonomy.

Terms

actual health problem
analysis
critical thinking
cue
dependent function
diagnosis
health problem
health status
independent function
inference
nursing diagnosis
objective
peer review
possible nursing diagnosis
potential nursing diagnosis
quality assurance
standard (norm)
synthesis
taxonomy

Nursing Diagnosis

Definitions

The term **diagnosis**, according to the dictionary, is derived from the Greek word *diagignoskein*, which means "to distinguish." Analyzed further, *dia* means "apart" and *gignoskein* means "to know." Definitions include (a) the art of identifying a disease from its signs and symptoms, (b) a statement or conclusion concerning the nature of some phenomenon, and (c) analysis of the course or nature of a condition, situation, or problem. Although the first definition pertains to diagnoses made by physicians, the process of diagnosing is used by several professions to identify aspects of the client's condition that are of concern to that particular profession. In fact, anyone who makes a statement or conclusion about the nature of a condition, situation, or problem is diagnosing. Auto mechanics diagnose the nature or cause of automobile conditions; social workers diagnose economic and social situations; and nurses diagnose the health status of clients requiring nursing care. The term *diagnosis*, therefore, is not restricted to one particular profession and must be qualified by a professional designation, such as medical diagnosis or nursing diagnosis; that is, it is qualified by the subject matter in which the diagnostician is expert.

Several definitions of *nursing diagnosis* have been stated since the early 1950s. Each has different emphases, but all have many similarities. In 1973, the First National Conference on the Classification of Nursing Diagnosis accepted this definition: A **nursing diagnosis** "is the judgment or conclusion [that] occurs as a result of nursing assessment" (Gebbie and Lavin 1975). To Gordon (1976, p. 1299), *nursing diagnoses*, or clinical diagnoses made by professional nurses, describe a combination of signs and symptoms that indicate actual or potential health problems that nurses by virtue of their education and experience are able, licensed, and accountable to treat. To Edel (1982, p. 6), a *nursing diagnosis* is the statement of a potential or actual altered health status of a client, which is derived from nursing assessment and which requires intervention from the domain of nursing. Edel's definition emphasizes that the entity to be diagnosed is *health status,* which avoids the negative connotation of problem and allows for positive diagnoses of clients. **Health status** is the health of a person at a given time. The strength and the problems of the person are considered. To Shoemaker (1984, p. 109), a *nursing diagnosis* is a clinical judgment about an individual family or community that is derived through a deliberate, systematic process of data collection and analysis. The diagnosis is the basis for prescriptions of definitive therapy for which the nurse is accountable. It is expressed concisely and includes the etiology (when known) of the condition.

The trend for nurses to assume more responsibility in overall client care means potential liability may increase accordingly. (Regan 1976, p. 26)

Implied in these definitions are the following characteristics:

1. Professional nurses (registered nurses) are the persons responsible for making nursing diagnoses. Even though other nursing personnel may contribute data to the process of diagnosing and may implement specified nursing care, the formulation of a diagnostic statement lies within the realm of the professional nurse. This restriction is supported by licensing laws and national standards of practice.
2. A **health problem** is any condition or situation in which a client requires help to maintain or regain a state of health or to achieve a peaceful death. It does not always refer to an undesirable state but does refer to a situation for which the client needs nursing assistance.
3. Nursing diagnoses describe (a) **actual health problems** (deviations from health), (b) **potential health problems** (risk factors that predispose persons and families to health problems), and (c) areas of enriched personal growth. Examples of actual health problems are ineffective airway clearance, a fluid volume deficit, or a knowledge deficit. Examples of potential health problems are risk of skin breakdown or a potential sleep pattern disturbance. Examples of areas of enriched personal growth are self-development, health maintenance management, and parenting. In general, these problems encompass "actual or potential disturbances in life processes, patterns, functions, or development, including those occurring secondary to disease" (Gordon 1976, p. 1298).
4. The domain of nursing diagnosis includes only those health states that nurses are able and licensed to treat. For example, nurses are not educated to diagnose or treat diseases such as diabetes mellitus; this task is defined legally as within the practice of medicine. Yet they can diagnose a knowledge deficit, ineffective coping by the individual, alterations in nutrition, and potential for injury, all of which may accompany diabetes mellitus. These problems are within the nurse's capabilities and the scope of the nurse's licensing laws; thus, the nurse is responsible and accountable for the treatment provided for these nursing diagnoses.
5. Nursing diagnosis is a judgment made only after a thorough, systematic process of data collection.

Differences from Medical Diagnoses

Nursing diagnoses differ from medical diagnoses in several ways. For a summary, see Table 12–1. The medical diagnosis describes a specific disease process, which is uniform from one client to the other. It is oriented toward pathology and lasts as long as the client's illness. In contrast, the nursing diagnosis describes a client's *response* to an illness or other situation, which varies among individuals. The nursing diagnosis is oriented to the individual and changes as the client's response changes. For example, in two clients with the medical diagnosis of rheumatoid arthritis, the disease process is quite similar but the responses to it can be very different. A 70-year-old female may respond with acceptance, viewing her condition as part of the aging process. A 20-year-old female may respond with anger and hostility because of the changes this condition will make in her personal identity, body image, role performance, and self-esteem.

Another difference between the diagnoses is that medical diagnoses are described in concise phrases of two or three words and in a universally accepted format. For nursing diagnoses, however, there is no well-developed, universal taxonomy. This results in consid-

Table 12–1 Comparison of Nursing and Medical Diagnoses

Nursing Diagnosis	Medical Diagnosis
Describes an individual's response to a disease process, condition, or situation	Describes a specific disease process
Is oriented to the individual	Is oriented to pathology
Changes as the client's responses change	Remains constant throughout the duration of illness
Guides independent nursing activities: planning, intervening, and evaluating	Guides medical management, some of which may be carried out by the nurse
Is complementary to the medical diagnosis	Is complementary to the nursing diagnosis
Has no universally accepted classification system; such systems are in the process of development	Has a well-developed classification system accepted by the medical profession

erable variation in nursing diagnoses. Some are long and complex. It is doubtful that nursing diagnoses will ever be condensed to the size of medical diagnoses.

A nursing diagnosis may be related to a medical diagnosis, but, just as the medical diagnosis is separate and distinct, so is the nursing diagnosis. A client who has one or more medical diagnoses and medical orders will also have one or more nursing diagnoses and nursing orders. These diagnoses and orders are complementary rather than contradictory. Nursing diagnoses relate to the nurse's **independent functions,** i.e., the areas of health care that are unique to nursing and are separate and distinct from the care included in medical management. Even though the nurse is obligated to carry out medical orders, i.e., **dependent functions,** the nurse is also obligated to diagnose and prescribe within the limits of nurse practice acts.

The Diagnostic Process

Diagnosis is a process of analysis and synthesis. **Analysis** is the separation into components; i.e., breaking down the whole into its parts. **Synthesis** is the opposite; i.e., putting together the parts into the whole.

The cognitive skills required for analysis and synthesis are objectivity, critical thinking, decision making, and inductive and deductive reasoning (Andrews, 1982a, p. 90). Deductive and inductive reasoning and decision making are discussed in Chapter 10. To be objective is to be without bias; i.e., the values and beliefs of the nurse do not affect how data are viewed and analyzed. To be objective, the nurse must be aware of her or his own values and beliefs. Critical thinking is a cognitive process during which data are reviewed and explanations considered before an opinion is formed. In this process, the nurse uses all the data acquired about the client and her or his own knowledge.

The diagnostic process has three main phases:

1. Data processing
2. Determining the client's health problems and strengths (health status)
3. Formulating nursing diagnoses

Data Processing

Data processing, the first aspect of analyzing, is the act of interpreting collected data. It involves organizing the data, comparing data against standards, clustering data, and identifying gaps and inconsistencies in the data. These activities occur continuously rather than sequentially.

Organizing the Data

Once the data are collected, they need to be organized into a usable framework for the nurse and others who may need access to them. One method is to divide the data into five categories (La Monica 1985, p. 105): physiologic factors, psychologic factors, sociologic factors, the medical regimen, and laboratory reports. To illustrate data organization the client example (Joe Smith) given in Chapter 11 will be used (see Figure 11–1 on page 240). A summary of the nursing assessment data for this client using the assessment format is shown on page 254. The organization of these data into the five categories mentioned above is shown on page 255.

Comparing Data against Standards

The nurse compares the client's data to a wide range of standards, such as normal vital signs, laboratory values, basic food groups, growth, and development. The nurse also uses her or his knowledge—e.g., of physiology, psychology, and sociology—as well as past experience when comparing the data.

A **standard** or **norm** is a generally accepted rule, model, pattern, or measure. To be used in comparing, however, a standard must be both relevant and reliable. To be relevant, it must be of the same class as the data to which it is compared. Just as oranges cannot be the standard used to judge apples, the ideal breakfast for a teenager cannot be used as a standard for the breakfast of a person over 65 years. To be reliable, the standard must be based on data from a sufficiently large sample. For example, to determine the average interests of 12-year-olds, one must survey a large number of teenagers, not just three.

When comparing data against standards, the nurse must know the client's view of "normal," which may differ from that of the nurse. For example, a client may think it is perfectly normal to bathe once a month, whereas the nurse may believe once a day is normal. What is considered normal varies according to the client's expectations, culture, values, economics, and knowledge. The nurse must also consider the client's previous condition.

Clustering Data

Clustering or grouping data is a thought process of determining the relatedness of facts and finding patterns in the facts. This is the beginning of synthesis. **Cues** (facts that the nurse acquires by using the five senses) are examined to determine whether any patterns are present, whether the cues are isolated incidents, and whether the cues are significant. The process of data clustering is influenced by the nurse's background of scientific knowledge, past nursing experiences, and concept of nursing. Together, these factors are a mental reference file of facts and principles the nurse uses to verify the significance of the data.

To relate and group data, the nurse must consider nursing diagnostic categories or areas of nursing responsibility. Gordon (1982b, p. 13) states that clustering information involves a search in the nurse's memory stores for previously learned meaningful groups of clinical cues that are associated with a diagnostic category. Gordon believes that clustering occurs in conjunction with data collection and interpretation, as evidenced in remarks or thoughts such as, "I'm getting a picture of . . ." or "This cue doesn't fit the picture." A list of accepted nursing diagnostic categories is shown in Table 12–4 on page 260.

La Monica (1985, p. 103) lists 15 areas of nursing responsibilities:

1. Comfort
2. Nutrition
3. Exercise
4. Personal hygiene
5. Sleep and rest patterns
6. Diversional activities
7. Socializing and privacy
8. Elimination
9. Safety
10. Environmental considerations
11. Teaching
12. Spiritual comfort and/or assistance
13. Prevention of complications
14. Assurance of physiologic status—health maintenance and promotion
15. Emotional support and counseling

Nursing theories and conceptual frameworks are further sources of areas of nursing responsibility.

Data clustering involves making inferences. An **inference** is the nurse's judgment or interpretation of cues. Data clustering or grouping for Mr. Joe Smith is illustrated in Table 12–2 on page 256. The data are clustered according to nursing diagnostic categories.

Identifying Gaps and Inconsistencies in the Data

Gaps are missing information needed to determine a data pattern. For example, during the assessing phase, data about a client's definition of health is essential if the nurse is to understand his statement "I am sick all the time." Data may be completely missing or incomplete. For example, information about a 15-month-old child's mobility may not specify whether she crawls or walks. This information is essential for establishing the child's developmental stage.

Inconsistencies are conflicting data. For example, a nurse may learn from the nursing history that the client reports not seeing a doctor in 15 years, yet during the physical health examination he states, "My doctor takes my blood pressure every week." This inconsistency must be clarified before a valid pattern can be established.

Determining the Client's Health Problems and Strengths

After data are processed, the nurse and the client can together identify strengths and problems. This is primarily a decision-making process.

Health Problems

During data processing, the nurse groups data according to categories, most likely with certain problems in mind. However, for health problems (existing or potential) to have a successful outcome, the client must accept the existence of the problem. The nurse, by contrast, determines whether the client needs help dealing with the problem. The nurse and the client can then make any of the following judgments (Yura and Walsh 1983):

1. No problem exists, and the client's health status is confirmed.
2. No problem exists, but there is a potential problem.
3. A problem exists, but the client is coping effectively.
4. A problem exists, and the client needs help handling it.
5. A problem exists, but the client cannot deal with it at this time.
6. A problem requires further study and diagnosis.
7. A problem is not presently incapacitating but will be at a later date.
8. A problem places heavy demands on the client's ability to cope.
9. A problem is critical to the client.
10. The problem is long term and permanent.

See Table 12–2 for examples of Mr. Joe Smith's problems.

Strengths

At this stage, the nurse and client also establish the client's strengths, resources, and abilities to cope. Generally, people have a clearer perception of their problems or weak-

Summary of Data for Mr. Joe Smith

Health Perception/Health Management

- No energy
- Shortness of breath
- Had left hip replacement 2 years ago
- Eats a good diet
- Does not smoke
- Does not drink

Nutritional/Metabolic

- Has diabetes
- Does not eat sugar
- Lost 5 pounds over past year

Elimination

- Urinates frequently

Activity Exercise

- Lacks energy to do daily ranch chores
- Moves more slowly since hip surgery

Cognitive/Perceptual

- Slightly hard of hearing
- Wears glasses
- Doesn't read much, prefers to be told how to do things

Roles/Relationships

- Lives with wife and 6 of 13 children
- Family "scared" about his illness
- Cattle rancher and farmer

Self-Perception/Self-Concept

- Too weak to do day work on the farm

Coping/Stress

- Usually too busy to worry about things
- Perceives his son Tom as helpful in talking things over
- Wants family to visit

Value/Belief

- Religion/spirituality is important to him
- Wants to see hospital chaplain

Medication/History

- Tolazamide (Tolinase) 250 mg daily
- Furosemide (Lasix) 20 mg daily
- Slow K 20 mEq daily
- Nitroglycerin 1/150 gr p.r.n. for angina

Nursing Physical Assessment

- 81 years old
- Height 171 cm
- Weight 95.3 kg
- TPR 36.5, 80, 16
- Blood pressure 124/80 mm Hg
- Large, slightly obese
- Joint stiffness
- Slight limp
- No pedal edema
- Femoral pulses very strong (R) and bounding (L)
- Popliteal, dorsalis pedis, posterior tibial pulses absent in left leg
- Left leg cooler than right leg
- Heart rhythm is regular
- Loud heart murmur in aortic area
- History of angina (6 months)
- Rales in bases of both lungs cleared by coughing
- Urinary frequency because of Lasix
- No allergies

nesses than of their strengths and assets, which are often taken for granted. By taking an inventory of strengths, the client can develop a more well-rounded self-concept and self-image. Strengths can be an aid to mobilizing health and regenerative processes.

A client's strengths might be that his weight is within the normal range for his age and height, thus enabling him to cope better with surgery. In another instance, a client's strengths might be that she is allergy-free and a nonsmoker. The same client's resources could be a supportive family and an ability to cope. Coping is a learned pattern or response that helps an individual deal with crises and stressful events. Nurses must remember, however, that because of the magnitude of an event, the number of stressful events occurring at one time, or the unfamiliarity of the situation, a client may be unable to cope and require assistance of the nurse.

A client's strengths can be found in the nursing assessment record (health, home life, education, recreation, exercise, work, family and friends, religious beliefs,

Organization of Nursing Assessment Data

Physical

- 81-year-old male
- Slightly hard of hearing
- Wears glasses
- No energy
- Shortness of breath
- Had left hip replacement 2 years ago
- Eats a good diet
- Does not smoke
- Does not drink
- Has diabetes
- Does not eat sugar
- Lost 5 pounds over past year
- Urinates frequently
- Lacks energy to do daily ranch chores
- Moves more slowly since hip surgery
- Height 171 cm
- Weight 95.3 kg
- TPR 36.5, 80, 16
- Blood pressure 124/80 mm Hg
- Large, slightly obese
- Joint stiffness
- Slight limp
- No pedal edema
- Femoral pulses very strong (R) and bounding (L)
- Popliteal, dorsalis pedis, posterior tibial pulses absent in left leg
- Left leg cooler than right leg
- Heart rhythm is regular
- Loud heart murmur in aortic area
- History of angina (6 months)
- Rales in bases of both lungs cleared by coughing
- Urinary frequency because of furosemide (Lasix)
- No allergies

Psychologic

- Alert and oriented
- Views self as too weak to do day work on the farm
- Perceives his son Tom as helpful in talking things over
- Wants family to visit
- Religion/spirituality is important to him
- Wants to see hospital chaplain
- Family "scared" about his illness
- Usually too busy to worry about things
- Doesn't read much, prefers to be told how to do things

Sociologic

- Lives with wife and 6 of 13 children
- Cattle rancher and farmer
- Pleasant but not talkative

Medical Regimen

- Tolazamide (Tolinase) 250 mg daily
- Furosemide (Lasix) 20 mg daily
- Slow K 20 mEq daily
- Nitroglycerin 1/150 gr p.r.n. for angina pain

Laboratory Data

Nil

and sense of humor, for example), the health examination, and the client's records. See Table 12–2 for examples of Mr. Joe Smith's strengths.

Formulating Nursing Diagnoses

At this final stage, the nurse formulates causal relationships between the health problems and the factors related to it. These factors may be, for example, environmental, sociologic, psychologic, physiologic, or spiritual. More than one factor may be related to one health problem. It is also important to determine at this time that the problem can be resolved by independent nursing interventions. If it cannot, the nurse should refer the client to the appropriate health team member. By including the causal factors in diagnostic statements, the nurse can tailor a plan of care for the client. For example, the diagnosis "impaired physical mobility" tells the nurse the problem but does not suggest the direction the nursing intervention should take, whereas "impaired physical mobility related to neu-

Table 12–2 Formulating Nursing Diagnoses for Mr. Joe Smith

Diagnostic Category	Grouping Data	Determining Strengths and Health Problems	Formulating Nursing Diagnostic Statements
Activity intolerance	Shortness of breath Lacks energy to do daily chores Does not smoke	Does not smoke (strength) Activity intolerance (problem)	Activity intolerance related to shortness of breath and lack of energy secondary to decreased strength of cardiac contraction
Ineffective airway clearance	Rales in bases of both lungs relieved by coughing	Able to expel secretions by coughing (strength) Secretions in lung bases (problem)	Potential ineffective airway clearance postoperatively related to chest incision
Potential for injury	Left hip replacement Movement slightly limited Joint stiffness Slight limp	Carries out daily activities independently (strength) Movement slightly limited (problem)	Potential for injury (trauma) related to joint stiffness and limp from hip replacement surgery
Alteration in nutrition	Is diabetic Takes tolazamide (Tolinase) daily "No sugar" in diet "Eats a good diet" Overweight for height Weight loss of 5 pounds in past year	Controls diabetes with Tolinase and "no sugar" (strength) Weight loss of 5 pounds in past year (strength) Overweight (problem)	Alteration in nutrition: more than body requirements related to imbalance of intake versus activity expenditure
Knowledge deficit	Takes furosemide (Lasix) daily Takes Slow K daily Urinates frequently	Complies with medical regime (strength) Does not relate urinary frequency to diuretic (problem)	Knowledge deficit: side-effects of diuretic therapy
Alteration in peripheral tissue perfusion	Vital signs normal Heart rhythm regular Loud heart murmur (aortic area) Femoral pulses stronger than normal Absent pulses (popliteal, dorsalis pedis, posterior tibial) in left leg Left leg cooler than right leg Integument pink and intact	Vital signs within normal range (strength) Skin intact and of good color (strength) Impaired circulation in left leg (problem)	Alteration in peripheral tissue perfusion (left leg) related to impaired arterial circulation
Fear	Hospitalized for cardiac catheterization and possible aortic valve replacement States family "scared" about illness Wants to see chaplain Wants family to visit Perceives son Tom as helpful Says is usually too busy to worry about things	Perceives family as supportive (strength) Says family anxious about illness. Did not indicate own feelings (problem)	Fear related to cardiac catheterization, possible surgery, and its outcome
Comfort	History of angina (6 months) Takes nitroglycerin for angina	Has not needed nitroglycerin for 2 months (strength)	Potential alteration in comfort (angina) related to excessive activity or stress

romuscular impairment" suggests a direction for plans and interventions to deal with the problem. Obviously, the causative factor *neuromuscular impairment* suggests a different direction than the factor *fear of falling* would.

Nurses can refer to a list of accepted nursing diagnoses, discussed later in this chapter, to select a diagnostic category. The causal factors are obtained from the data. If no causal factor appears in the data, the nurse may wish to make a tentative diagnosis based on scientific nursing knowledge and experience. The nurse should then review the database for inconsistencies and gaps and the analysis/synthesis for error. Once the causal relationships have been established, the nurse is ready to write the diagnostic statements. See Table 12–2 for Mr. Joe Smith's nursing diagnostic statements.

Writing a Diagnostic Statement

A nursing diagnostic statement (nursing diagnosis) is a clear statement about a client's actual or potential health problem that is within the scope of independent nursing intervention. It is the outcome of the processes of analysis/synthesis: the second phase in the nursing process.

The nursing diagnostic statement has two parts:

1. Statement of the client's response
2. Factors contributing to or probable causes of the response

The two parts are joined by the words *related to* or *associated with* rather than *due to*. The phrase *due to* implies a cause-and-effect relationship; one clause causes or is responsible for the other clause. By contrast, the phrases *related to* and *associated with* merely imply a relationship, and if one part of the diagnostic statement changes, so may the other part; legal hazards are thus avoided. Examples of nursing diagnoses demonstrating these two parts are:

- Ineffective breathing pattern (response) related to pain (contributing factor)
- Disturbance in self-concept (response) related to loss of arm (contributing factor)
- Grieving (response) related to anticipated loss (contributing factor) secondary to husband's illness

Potential nursing diagnoses are used when a client's responses can be predicted or when health promotion can contribute to well-being. Predictable responses are based on a client's health history, known complications of a disease process, or the nurse's experience. For example, a client who has smoked two packages of cigarettes per day for 40 years may have a potential postoperative nursing diagnosis of "potential alteration to respiratory function related to smoking."

Possible nursing diagnoses are used when evidence about a response is unclear or when the related factors are unknown. The nurse writes the possible nursing diagnosis and collects more data either to support or refute the possible response. For example, an elderly widow who lives alone is admitted to hospital. The nurse notices that she has no visitors and is pleased with attention and conversation from the nursing staff. Until more data are collected, the nurse may write a possible nursing diagnosis of "Social isolation related to unknown etiology."

Characteristics of a Diagnostic Statement

1. A diagnostic statement is clear and concise.
2. It is specific and client centered.
3. It relates to one client problem.
4. It is accurate.
5. It is based on reliable and relevant assessment data.

Guidelines for Writing a Diagnostic Statement

Clear, concise, client-centered nursing diagnoses can be written by following the guidelines presented in Table 12–3. Some common errors in writing diagnostic statements are:

1. Writing the client's response as a need instead of a problem
2. Using judgmental statements
3. Placing the contributing factor before the client's response
4. Using statements that provide no specific direction for planning independent nursing interventions
5. Using medical rather than nursing terminology
6. Starting the diagnosis with a nursing intervention
7. Using a single symptom as the client's response

The accuracy of nursing diagnostic statements also depends on a complete database and appropriate data

Table 12–3 Guidelines for Writing a Nursing Diagnostic Statement

Guideline	Correct Statement	Incorrect and/or Ambiguous Statement
1. State in terms of a problem, not a need.	Actual fluid volume deficit (problem) related to fever	Fluid replacement (need) related to fever
2. State so that it is legally advisable.	Impaired skin integrity related to immobility (legally acceptable)	Impaired skin integrity related to improper positioning (implies legal liability)
3. Use nonjudgmental statements.	Spiritual distress related to inability to attend church services secondary to immobility (nonjudgmental)	Spiritual distress related to strict rules necessitating church attendance (judgmental)
4. Make sure that both elements of the statement do *not* say the same thing.	Potential impairment of skin integrity related to immobility	Potential impairment of skin integrity related to ulceration of sacral area (response and probable cause are the same)
5. Make sure that the client's response precedes the contributing or causal factor.	Noncompliance with diet (response) related to lack of knowledge (contributing factor)	Lack of knowledge (contributing factor) related to noncompliance with diet (response)
6. Use statements that provide guidance for planning independent nursing interventions.	Social isolation related to loss of speech (loss of speech provides direction for planning alternative communication methods)	Social isolation related to laryngectomy (the nurse can do nothing about the laryngectomy)
7. Word diagnosis specifically and precisely to provide direction for planning nursing intervention.	Alteration in respiratory function related to chronic allergy secondary to pollen from roses (specific)	Alteration in respiratory function related to the environment (vague)
8. Use nursing terminology rather than medical terminology to describe the client's response.	Potential ineffective airway clearance (nursing terminology)	Potential pneumonia (medical terminology)
9. Use nursing terminology rather then medical terminology to describe the probable cause of the client's response.	Potential ineffective airway clearance related to accumulation of secretions in lungs (nursing terminology)	Potential ineffective airway clearance related to emphysema (medical terminology)
10. Do not start the nursing diagnosis with a nursing intervention.	Potential alteration in nutrition: less than body requirements related to inadequate intake of protein (directs but does not state nursing intervention)	Provide high-protein diet because of potential alteration in nutrition (starts with nursing intervention)
11. Avoid using a symptom such as nausea as the client's response. A symptom does not reflect a pattern and requires additional data collection	Insufficient data for a diagnosis	Nausea related to medication

processing. If data are omitted, a diagnosis can be missed. If data are not processed properly, e.g., are not clustered appropriately, a diagnosis can be made prematurely, incorrectly, or missed. Gordon (1982, p. 216) categorizes diagnostic errors as (a) errors of omission, i.e., failure to diagnose a problem and (b) errors of commission, i.e., diagnosing a problem when no problem exists. Both errors can occur during data collection, data interpretation, and data clustering.

To avoid such errors during assessment, the nurse needs to ensure that relevant data are not missed and that large quantities of irrelevant data are not obtained. The nurse can prevent data omissions by using an organized assessment plan, striving for accuracy, and drawing on her or his own knowledge. Collecting irrelevant data can be avoided if the nurse asks appropriate questions. An overload of irrelevant data hinders the nurse's capacity to process information.

Data interpretation errors occur when the meaning of cues is misinterpreted. The nurse can avoid inaccurate interpretation of cues by determining how the client perceives the health problem, its probable cause, and actions taken to remedy it. For example, the nurse observes that a client repeatedly gets out of bed after the physician has ordered complete bed rest. The nurse may interpret this behavior as noncompliance. However, the client may be experiencing diarrhea and may be embarrassed to use the bedpan or may be refusing to accept a dependent sick role. Obviously, inaccurate interpretation of cues leads to diagnostic errors. Another source of diagnostic errors in data interpretation is overgeneralization from one isolated observation of client behavior. For example, one episode of angry behavior does not mean that the client is hostile.

A diagnosis may be made prematurely, before all relevant data have been considered or collected. For example, a nurse, learning of a client's history of angina and his prescription for nitroglycerin, may write this diagnostic statement: as "Alteration in comfort: pain." Additional data, however, reveal that angina has not been a problem since the client had cardiac bypass surgery a year ago and that pain is therefore not a current problem.

Incorrect clustering of data also leads to diagnostic errors. For example, by clustering "urinary frequency" and "has diabetes," the nurse could erroneously begin a diagnostic statement for Mr. Joe Smith with "Alteration in urinary elimination." However, clustering other data, such as "takes furosemide (Lasix, a diuretic) daily," "shortness of breath," "no energy," and "aortic valve insufficiency," changes the diagnostic focus from a urinary problem to "Activity intolerance" or "Alteration in cardiac output: decreased."

Advantages of Using Nursing Diagnoses

1. Nursing diagnoses facilitate communication among nurses and with other health team members. A diagnosis identifies a client's health status, strengths, and health problems.
2. They strengthen the nursing process and provide direction for planning independent nursing interventions.
3. They help the nurse focus on independent nursing actions.
4. They help identify the focus of a nursing activity and thus facilitate peer review and quality assurance programs. **Peer review** is the appraisal of a nurse's practice, education, or research by coworkers of equal status. **Quality assurance** is the evaluation of nursing services provided and the results achieved against an established standard.
5. They facilitate nursing intervention when a patient moves from one hospital unit to another or from hospital to home. The nursing diagnoses guide the planning of the nursing interventions that the client requires after discharge.
6. They facilitate comprehensive health care by identifying, validating, and responding to specific health problems (Griffith and Christensen, 1982).

Accepted Taxonomy of Nursing Diagnoses

A **taxonomy** is a classification system or set of categories. Animals and plants, for example, are classified according to their natural relationship, laws, and principles. Nursing diagnoses are classified according to the health responses of clients that nurses are licensed to treat, their etiology, and defining characteristics.

The identification and development of a taxonomy of nursing diagnoses began formally in 1973 when the United States National Conference Group for the Generation and Classification of Nursing Diagnoses was formed. This group originated through the efforts of two faculty members of Saint Louis University, Kristine Gebbie and Mary Ann Lavin, who perceived a need to identify their roles in an ambulatory care setting. The First National Conference held to identify nursing diagnoses was sponsored by the Saint Louis University School of Nursing and Allied Health Professions in 1973. Since that time, national conferences have been held in 1975, 1978, 1980, 1982, 1984 and 1986. Through the efforts of these groups, much progress has been made in defining, classifying, and describing nursing diagnoses. International recognition was shown by the First Canadian Conference, held in Toronto, Ontario, in 1977, and plans for a future international conference have been discussed.

At the first conference in 1973, a national task force was appointed to continue the development of nursing diagnoses. This task force established a Clearinghouse for Nursing Diagnoses in the same year. Its purposes were to maintain a depository of materials on nursing diagnoses, disseminate information about the National Conference Group and other nurses' activities, publish a newsletter, and coordinate arrangements for national conferences. The clearinghouse is established at the Saint Louis University School of Nursing.

Nursing Diagnostic Categories

An outcome of these conferences is an established list of accepted nursing diagnostic categories. See Table 12–4. An accepted nursing diagnosis is a health problem amenable to nursing intervention and sufficiently defined for clinical testing (Gordon 1982a, p. 2). The group that generates these lists is now called the North American Nursing Diagnosis Association (NANDA). The group includes

Table 12–4 List of Accepted Nursing Diagnoses from the Sixth National Conference, 1986

Activity intolerance
Activity intolerance, potential
Airway clearance, ineffective
Anxiety
Bowel elimination, alterations in: constipation
Bowel elimination, alterations in: diarrhea
Bowel elimination, alterations in: incontinence
Breathing pattern, ineffective
Cardiac output, alterations in: decreased
Comfort, alteration in: pain
Communication, impaired verbal
Coping, ineffective individual
Coping, ineffective family: compromised
Coping, ineffective family: disabling
Coping, family: potential for growth
Diversional activity deficit
Family processes, alterations in
Fear (specify)
Fluid volume, alteration in; excess
Fluid volume deficit, actual
Fluid volume deficit, potential
Gas exchange, impaired
Grieving, anticipatory
Grieving, dysfunctional
Health maintenance, alteration in
Home maintenance management, impaired
Injury, potential for (specify)
  Poisoning
  Suffocation
  Trauma
Knowledge deficit (specify)
Mobility, impaired physical
Noncompliance (specify)
Nutrition, alteration in: less than body requirements
Nutrition, alteration in: more than body requirements
Nutrition, alteration in: potential for more than body requirements
Oral mucous membrane, alteration in
Parenting, alteration in: actual
Parenting, alteration in: potential
Powerlessness
Rape-trauma syndrome
Self-care deficit:
  Bathing/hygiene
  Dressing/grooming
  Feeding
  Toileting
Self-concept, disturbance in:
  Body image
  Personal identity
  Role performance
  Self-esteem
Sensory-perceptual alteration:
  Auditory
  Gustatory
  Kinesthetic
  Olfactory
  Tactile
  Visual
Sexual dysfunction
Skin integrity, impairment of: actual
Skin integrity, impairment of: potential
Sleep pattern disturbance
Social isolation
Spiritual distress
Thought processes, alteration in
Tissue perfusion, alteration in:
  Cardiopulmonary
  Cerebral
  Gastrointestinal
  Peripheral
  Renal
Urinary elimination, alteration in pattern
Violence, potential for: self-directed or directed at others

Source: Hurley, M. E., editor. 1986. *Classification of nursing diagnoses. Proceedings of the sixth conference. North American Nursing Diagnosis Association.* St. Louis: The C. V. Mosby Company, pp. 513–514. Used by permission.

staff nurses, clinical specialists, faculty, directors of nursing, deans, theorists, and researchers.

Additional nursing diagnoses accepted at the Seventh National Conference in 1986 are shown on p. 261.

Components of Nursing Diagnostic Categories

There are three essential components of nursing diagnostic categories; they are referred to as the PES format (Gordon 1976, p. 1299). Consideration of these components is essential when developing diagnostic categories. It can also be of benefit to nurses when writing diagnoses for specific clients. The components are:

1. *The terms describing the problem (P).* This component, referred to as the *diagnostic category label* or *title,* is a description of the client's (individual, family, community) health problem (actual or potential) for which nursing therapy is given. The state of the client is described clearly and concisely in a few words. See Table 12–4 for a list of nursing diagnostic categories adopted by the Fifth National Conference on Classifi-

cation of Nursing Diagnoses in 1984. To be clinically useful, category labels need to be specific. Where the word *specify* follows a category label in Table 12–4, the nurse states the area in which the problem occurs. For example, a knowledge deficit may be in the area of medication prescription, dietary adjustments, or disease process and therapy.

2. *The etiology of the problem (E)* or contributing factors. This component identifies one or more probable causes of the health problem and gives direction to the required nursing therapy. Etiology may include behaviors of the client, environmental factors, or interactions of the two. For example, the probable causes of alteration in health maintenance include perceptual or cognitive impairment, lack of gross or fine motor skills, lack of material resources, and ineffective individual coping. See Table 12–5. Differentiating among possible causes in the nursing diagnosis is essential because each may require different nursing therapies.

3. *The defining characteristics or cluster of signs and symptoms (S).* The defining characteristics provide information necessary to arrive at the diagnostic category label (component 1). Each nursing diagnostic category has signs and symptoms that occur as a clinical entity. Nursing diagnostic categories are similar to the medical diagnostic categories. For example, the medical diagnostic category myocardial infarction (heart attack) has a standardized set of signs and symptoms that are universally understood and accepted. Likewise, the nursing diagnostic category alteration in health maintenance has a standardized cluster of signs and symptoms. See Table 12–5.

Nursing Diagnoses Accepted at the Seventh National Conference, 1986

- Impaired adjustment
- Potential alteration in body temperature
- Altered comfort: chronic pain
- Altered growth and development
- Hopelessness
- Hyperthermia
- Hypothermia
- Stress Incontinence
- Reflex Incontinence
- Functional Incontinence
- Total Incontinence
- Urge Incontinence
- Potential for infection
- Unilateral neglect
- Post trauma response
- Altered sexuality patterns
- Impaired social interaction
- Impaired swallowing
- Ineffective thermoregulation
- Impaired tissue integrity
- Urinary retention

Table 12–5 Components of a Nursing Diagnostic Category

Diagnosis	Definition	Etiology	Defining Characteristics
Health maintenance, alteration in	Inability to identify, manage, and/or seek out help to maintain health	Lack of or significant alteration in communication skills (written, verbal, and/or gestural) Lack of ability to make deliberate and thoughtful judgments Perceptual or cognitive impairment Complete or partial lack of gross and/or fine motor skills Ineffective individual coping; dysfunctional grieving Lack of material resources Unachieved developmental tasks Ineffective family coping: disabling spiritual distress	Demonstrated lack of knowledge regarding basic health practices Demonstrated lack of adaptive behaviors to internal or external environmental changes Reported or observed inability to take the responsibility for meeting basic health practices in any or all functional pattern areas History of lack of health-seeking behavior Expressed interest in improving health behaviors Reported or observed lack of equipment, financial, and/or other resources Reported or observed impairment of personal support system

Source: M. J. Kim, G. K. McFarland, and A. M. McLane, editors, *Pocket guide to nursing diagnoses* (St. Louis: C. V. Mosby Co., 1984), pp. 28–29. Used by permission.

Advantages of a Nursing Diagnosis Taxonomy

Many advantages can be derived from a nursing diagnosis taxonomy (Edel 1982, pp. 8–10):

1. It speeds communication among nurses. Instead of relating all pertinent assessment factors to another health care worker, nurses can transmit the same amount of information through a diagnosis. Because a nursing diagnosis consolidates a great deal of information into concise statements and includes assessment parameters, it provides a shorthand method of communication. If a nurse knows that a client has a certain nursing diagnosis, she or he will know the client's problem, causal or contributing factors, and needed nursing actions.
2. It clarifies the independent functions of the nurse and increases nursing accountability. Nursing diagnoses describe and categorize the content of independent nursing practice. Ultimately, specific nursing diagnoses will be associated with prescribed nursing therapies, and the nurse will be accountable for those therapies.
3. It provides a *first* step for building a body of knowledge unique to nursing.
4. It provides an organizing principle and structure for nursing education, practice, and research. Once a taxonomy of nursing diagnoses is developed, educational programs can organize their curricula in relation to the nursing diagnoses and prepare students to develop diagnostic skills. The taxonomy would also provide a focus for nursing practice and research, which in turn would provide feedback for further development of nursing's unique body of knowledge.

Limitations of a Nursing Diagnosis Taxonomy

1. The taxonomy is in early developmental stages and therefore is *not* to be considered a comprehensive guide for nursing practice. Although some nurses feel constrained and frustrated with the existing taxonomy, it is well to remember that disciplines such as medicine with well-established taxonomies have taken over 100 years of development and are still constantly changing. Every NANDA publication emphasizes that the list is a beginning and is not definitive. Gebbie and Lavin (1975, pp. 57–58) state that all categories require further refinement and consideration by nurses at subsequent conferences. A major task of all nurses is to locate diagnoses that are neglected, to test and develop them, and to present them for inclusion in future listings.
2. The relationship between the nursing diagnosis taxonomy and theoretical frameworks for nursing is yet to be demonstrated. The diagnostic focus of proposed conceptual frameworks for nursing depends on the concepts outlined in the nursing theory and therefore do not necessarily fit the taxonomy of nursing diagnoses. This point is illustrated in Table 12–6, which gives examples of the diagnostic focus of three nursing theories. Continued dialogue between nursing practitioners and theorists is essential.
3. The taxonomy needs to be tested for reliability and validity. Although the taxonomy has been approved and accepted by participants in the national conferences, the usefulness of each diagnostic category must still be verified by appropriate research.
4. There is danger of misuse of diagnostic categories by stereotyping, eliminating alternatives, or employing value-laden categories. Hagey and McDonough (1984, pp. 151–56) in discussing the problems presented by professional labeling, (i.e., the use of a formalized list of diagnostic categories) suggest the following problems:
   a. Nursing diagnostic categories do not interpret the client responses in his or her unique sociocultural setting and therefore may deter individualized care.
   b. The use of diagnostic categories curbs the nurse's capacities for inquiry and observation.
   c. Use of the taxonomy makes the nursing process nurse-centered, since the nurse is the one doing the analysis. The client and the nurse may well define problems differently.
   d. Use of the taxonomy can enhance the nurse's authority and power in what should be a reciprocal interaction.

Diagnostic Classification System

The search is underway for a system of classifying nursing diagnoses that will be superior to the alphabetical system now in use. NANDA's fifth national conference, in 1982, generated a taxonomic structure using nine patterns of unitary man. At the sixth national conference (1984) some refinements and revisions were made:

1. The taxonomy was to be called "NANDA Nursing Diagnosis Taxonomy I" to highlight its provisional character. Subsequent taxonomies would be called "Taxonomy II," and so on.
2. The nine patterns were called *human response patterns.* They are:
   a. Exchanging: mutual giving and receiving
   b. Communicating: sending messages
   c. Relating: establishing bonds
   d. Valuing: assigning relative worth
   e. Choosing: selection of alternatives
   f. Moving: activity
   g. Perceiving: reception of information
   h. Knowing: meaning associated with information

Table 12–6 Variations of Diagnostic Focus and Contributing Factors in Selected Conceptual Frameworks for Nursing

Nursing Theory	Diagnostic Focus	Contributing Factors (Etiology)
Orem's self-care agency theory	Actual or potential deficit between the powers of self-care agency and the demands placed on it in relation to three self-care categories: 1. Universal 2. Developmental 3. Health deviation	Lack of knowledge, skills, interest, or motivation; disease process; or type of therapy
Roy's adaptation theory	Actual maladaptation problems or potential adaptation problems in relation to four modes: 1. Physiologic 2. Self-concept 3. Role function 4. Interdependence	Coping activity that is inadequate to maintain integrity in the face of a need deficit or excess
Johnson and Grubb's behavioral system theory	Behavior that does not maintain the equilibrium of eight subsystems in relation to four classifications: 1. Intrasubsystem insufficiency 2. Intrasubsystem discrepancy 3. Intersubsystem incompatibility 4. Intersubsystem dominance	Sources of stress, classified as structural (within a subsystem) or functional (from the environment)

   i. Feeling: subjective awareness of information

3. All accepted nursing diagnoses to date will become subcategories of these nine human response patterns. For example (Kritek 1986, pp. 28–34):

   a. Exchanging includes:
      - Alterations in nutrition
      - Alterations in bowel elimination (constipation, diarrhea, incontinence)
      - Alterations in urinary elimination (incontinence)
      - Alterations in oxygenation (impaired gas exchange, ineffective airway clearance, ineffective breathing)
      - Alterations in circulation (tissue perfusion, fluid volume deficit and excess, decreased cardiac output)
      - Alterations in physical integrity (injury by poisoning, suffocation, or trauma and skin impairment)

   b. Communicating includes:
      - Alterations in communication (verbal, nonverbal)

   c. Relating includes:
      - Alterations in role (role performance, i.e., parenting, sexuality, work)

   d. Valuing includes:
      - Alterations in spiritual state (spiritual distress)

   e. Choosing includes:
      - Alterations in coping (family, individual, community)
      - Alterations in participating (noncompliance)

   f. Moving includes:
      - Alterations in activity (impaired physical mobility, activity intolerance)
      - Alterations in rest (sleep pattern disturbance)
      - Alterations in recreation (diversional activity deficit)
      - Alterations in activities of daily living (home maintenance management)
      - Alterations in self-care (bathing/hygiene, dressing/grooming, feeding, toileting)

   g. Perceiving includes:
      - Alterations in self-concept (body image, self-esteem, personal identity)
      - Sensory/perceptual alteration (visual, auditory, kinesthetic, gustatory, tactile, olfactory)

   h. Knowing includes:
      - Alterations in knowledge (deficit)
      - Alterations in thought processes (confusion)

   i. Feeling includes:
      - Alterations in comfort (pain)
      - Alterations in emotional integrity (anxiety, grieving, violence, fear, rape-trauma syndrome)

   Some diagnoses such as powerlessness, alteration in family processes, alteration in oral mucous membrane, alteration in health maintenance, accepted at the fifth national conference, remain to be categorized.

4. The taxonomy is numerically coded and leveled from the most abstract (Level I) to the most concrete (Level IV or V). Each of the nine human response patterns

will constitute Level I concepts, which are the most abstract. Level II concepts refer to alterations in the human response patterns, and subsequent levels refer to more specific responses. An example of numerical coding and leveling of the fifth human response pattern *choosing* is shown to the right.

One of the major reasons for classifying and coding nursing diagnoses is computer storage and access of information. Kritek (1986, p. 36) states that the *generation* of nursing diagnoses and the *classification* of nursing diagnoses should occur simultaneously. Each process enhances and challenges the other. The classification system indicates areas of strength and weakness. For example, the human response pattern labeled *exchanging* is clearly better developed than any other response pattern. Much work remains to be done in the area of nursing diagnosis.

Numerical Coding and Leveling of the Fifth Human Response Pattern *Choosing*

5. Choosing
    - 5.1 Alterations in Coping
        - 5.1. 1. Family
            - 5.1. 1.1. Ineffective
                - 5.1. 1.1. 1. Disabled
                - 5.1. 1.1. 2. Compromised
            - 5.1. 1.2.
        - 5.1. 2. Individual
            - 5.1. 2.1. Ineffective
            - 5.1. 2.2.
        - 5.1. 3. [Community]
    - 5.2. Alterations in Participating
        - 5.2. 1. Noncompliance
        - 5.2. 2.

(Kritek 1986, p. 33)

Chapter Highlights

- A nursing diagnosis is a statement of an actual or potential health problem amenable to independent nursing intervention.
- The diagnostic process is one of analysis and synthesis.
- The cognitive skills for analysis/synthesis are objectivity, critical thinking, decision making, and deductive and inductive reasoning.
- The three phases of the diagnostic process are data processing, analysis, determination of the client's health problems and strengths, and formulation of nursing diagnoses.
- A nursing diagnostic statement has two parts: statement of the client's response and factors contributing to or probable causes of the response.
- A nursing diagnostic statement should be clear, concise, patient-centered, related to one problem, and based on reliable and relevant assessment data.
- Nursing diagnoses provide direction for planning independent nursing interventions.
- The development of a taxonomy of nursing diagnoses is an ongoing process.

Suggested Readings

Dossey, B., and Guzzetta, C. E. June 1981. Nursing diagnosis. *Nursing 81* 11:34–38.
The authors describe their experiences with nursing diagnosis and how it fits into the nursing process. Included is a suggested three-step process for arriving at a nursing diagnosis, a description of how to write one, and a set of checks on whether it has been written correctly.

Fadden, T. C., and Seiser, G. K. April 1984. Nursing diagnosis: A matter of form. *American Journal of Nursing* 84:470–72.
Staff nurses, who decided that their existing admission profile was not useful in gathering information needed to formulate nursing diagnoses, designed a new nursing history and assessment form. The article includes a completed form and the nursing diagnoses drawn from the data.

Hardy, E. March 1983. The diagnostic wheel: Identifying care that is unique to nursing. *The Canadian Nurse* 79:38–40.
Hardy presents a diagnostic wheel that can be used to collect data about a client and then uses the PES format suggested by NANDA to develop the client's nursing diagnoses.

Leslie, F. M. May 1981. Nursing Diagnosis: Use in long-term care. *American Journal of Nursing* 81:1012–14.
This study determined which nursing diagnoses were useful in describing the problems of long-term patients and found in addition that use of nursing diagnoses had several benefits.

Price, M. R. April 1980. Nursing diagnosis: Making a concept come alive. *American Journal of Nursing* 80:668–71.
Price first defines nursing diagnosis and then describes the diagnostic process. The final section deals with how to use a nursing diagnosis and gives a practical orientation to its use in a clinical area.

Tartaglia, M. J. March 1985. Nursing diagnosis: Keystone of your care plan. *Nursing 85* 15:34–37.
Tartaglia defines nursing diagnosis and then describes how to identify a problem. Writing nursing diagnoses, determining priorities, and writing patient goals and nursing interventions are discussed.

Selected References

Andrews, P. B. Analysis and Synthesis. 1982a. In Griffith, J. W., and Christensen, P. J., editors. pp. 89–110. *Nursing process: Application of theories, frameworks, and models.* St. Louis: C. V. Mosby Co.

———. 1982b. Nursing diagnosis. In Griffith, J. W. and Christensen, P. J., editors. pp. 111–27. *Nursing process: Application of theories, frameworks, and models.* St. Louis: C. V. Mosby Co.

Aspinall, M. J. July 1976. Nursing diagnosis: The weak link. *Nursing Outlook* 24:433–36.

Bircher, A. V. 1975. On the development and classification of diagnoses. *Nursing Forum* 14(1):10–29.

Bockrath, M. March/April 1982. Your patient needs two diagnoses—medical and surgical. *Nursing Life* 2:29–32.

Carlson, J. H., Craft, C. A., and McGuire, A. D. 1982. *Nursing diagnosis.* Philadelphia: W. B. Saunders Co.

Carnevali, D. L. 1983. *Nursing care planning: Diagnosis and management.* 3d ed. Philadelphia: J. B. Lippincott Co.

Carnevali, D. L., Mitchell, P. H., Woods, N. F., and Tanner, C. A. 1984. *Diagnostic reasoning in nursing.* Philadelphia: J. B. Lippincott Co.

Doenges, M. E., Jeffries, M. F., and Moorehouse, M. F. 1984. *Nursing care plans: Nursing diagnoses in planning patient care.* Philadelphia: F. A. Davis Co.

Edel, M. 1982. The nature of nursing diagnosis. In Carlson, J. H., Craft, C. A., and McGuire, A. D. *Nursing diagnosis.* Philadelphia: W. B. Saunders Co.

Fadden, T. C., and Seiser, G. K. April 1984. Nursing diagnosis: A matter of form. *American Journal of Nursing* 84:470–72.

Gebbie, K. M. 1976. *Classification of nursing diagnoses: Summary of the second national conference.* St. Louis: C. V. Mosby Co.

Gebbie, K., and Lavin, M. A. February 1974. Classifying nursing diagnoses. *American Journal of Nursing* 74:250–53. Reprinted in American Journal of Nursing. 1976. *The nursing process in practice.* pp. 188–96. Contemporary nursing series. New York: American Journal of Nursing Co.

———, editors. 1975. *Classification of nursing diagnoses.* Proceedings of the First National Conference. St. Louis: C. V. Mosby Co.

Gordon, M. August 1976. Nursing diagnosis and the diagnostic process. *American Journal of Nursing* 76:1298–300.

———. 1982a. Historical perspective: The National Conference Group for Classification of Nursing Diagnoses. In Kim M. J., and Moritz, D. A. pp. 2–8. *Classification of nursing diagnoses: Proceedings of the Third and Fourth National Conferences.* New York: McGraw-Hill.

———. 1982b. *Nursing diagnosis: Process and application.* New York: McGraw-Hill.

Gordon, M., Sweeny, M. A., and McKeehan, K. April 1980. Nursing diagnosis: Looking at its use in the clinical area. *American Journal of Nursing* 80:672–74.

Griffith, J. W., and Christensen, P. J., editors. 1982. *Nursing process: Application of theories, frameworks, and models.* St. Louis: C. V. Mosby Co.

Hagey, R. S., and McDonough, P. May/June 1984. The problem of professional labeling. *Nursing Outlook* 32:151–57.

Hardy, E. March 1983. The diagnostic wheel: Identifying care that is unique to nursing. *The Canadian Nurse* 79:38–40.

Hurley, M. E., editor. 1986. *Classification of nursing diagnoses. Proceedings of the sixth conference. North American Nursing Diagnosis Association.* St. Louis: The C. V. Mosby Company.

Kim, M. J., McFarland, G. K., and McLane, A. M., editors. 1984. *Pocket guide to nursing diagnoses.* St. Louis: C. V. Mosby Co.

Kim, M. J., and Moritz, D. A., editors. 1982. *Classification of nursing diagnoses: Proceedings of the Third and Fourth National Conferences.* New York: McGraw-Hill.

Kim, M. J., McFarland, G. K., and McLane, A. M., editors. 1984. *Classification of nursing diagnoses: Proceedings of the Fifth National Conference.* St. Louis: C. V. Mosby Co.

Kritek, P. B. 1985. Nursing diagnosis in perspective: Response to a critique. *Image: The Journal of Nursing Scholarship* 17:3–8.

———. 1986. Development of a taxonomic structure for nursing diagnoses: A review and an update. In Hurley, M. E., editor. *Classification of nursing diagnoses. Proceedings of the sixth conference. North American Nursing Diagnosis Association.* St. Louis: The C. V. Mosby Company.

La Monica, E. L. 1985. *The humanistic nursing process.* Belmont, Calif.: Wadsworth Health Sciences.

Lash, A. A. 1978. A re-examination of nursing diagnosis. *Nursing Forum* 17(4):332–43.

Leslie, F. M. May 1981. Nursing diagnosis: Use in long-term care *American Journal of Nursing* 81:1012–14.

Lunney, M. March 1982. Nursing diagnosis: Refining the system. *American Journal of Nursing* 82:456–59.

Mundinger, M. O., and Jauron, G. D. February 1975. Developing a nursing diagnosis. *Nursing Outlook* 23:94–98.

North American Nursing Diagnosis Association. Summer 1986. New diagnoses accepted. *Nursing Diagnosis Newsletter* 13(1):1.

Price, M. R. April 1980. Nursing diagnosis: Making a concept come alive. *American Journal of Nursing* 80:668–71.

Regan, W. A. January 1976. Bicentennial forecast: Nursing and the law. *RN* 39:21,25–27.

Shamansky, S. L., and Yanni, C. R. Spring 1983. In opposition to nursing diagnosis: A minority opinion. *Image: The Journal of Nursing Scholarship* 15:47–50.

Shoemaker, J. 1984. *Essential features of nursing diagnoses.* In Kim, M. J., McFarland, G. K., and McLane, A. M., editors. *Classification of nursing diagnoses: Proceedings of the Fifth National Conference.* St. Louis: C. V. Mosby Co., pp. 104–115.

Stanitis, M. A., and Ryan, J. June 1982. Noncompliance: An unacceptable diagnosis? *American Journal of Nursing* 82:941–42.

Swearingen, P. L. 1986. *Manual of nursing therapeutics: Applying nursing diagnoses to medical disorders.* Menlo Park, Calif.: Addison-Wesley Publishing Co.

Tartaglia, M. J. March 1985. Nursing diagnosis: Keystone of your care plan. *Nursing 85* 5:34–37.

Williams, A. B. 1980. Rethinking nursing diagnosis. *Nursing Forum* 19(4):357–63.

Yura, H., and Walsh, M. B. 1974. The nursing process. In Flynn, J. B., and Heffron, P. B., editors. pp. 141–75. *Nursing: From concept to practice.* Bowie, Md.: Robert J. Brady Co.

———. 1983. *The nursing process: Assessing, planning, implementing, evaluating.* 4th ed. Norwalk, Conn.: Appleton-Century-Crofts.

CHAPTER **13**

Planning

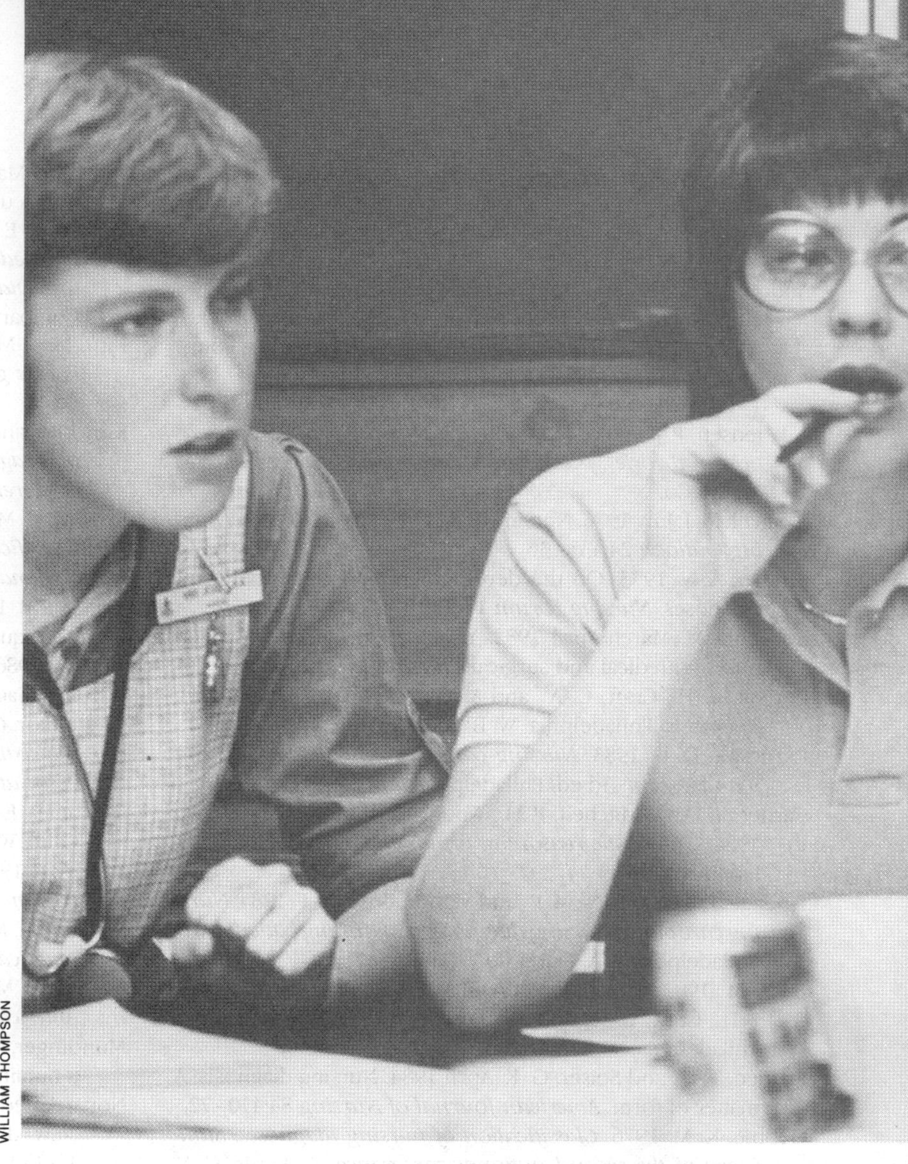

WILLIAM THOMPSON

Contents

Objectives

1. Understand essential aspects of the planning phase of the nursing process.
   1.1 Define listed terms.
   1.2 Identify four components of planning.
   1.3 Identify criteria that assist the nurse and client to set priorities.
   1.4. State the purposes of establishing client goals.
   1.5 Describe the relationship of goals to the nursing diagnoses.
   1.6 Differentiate between goals and outcome criteria.
   1.7 Describe the relationship of outcome criteria to client goals.
   1.8 Identify characteristics of outcome criteria.
   1.9 Describe four components of outcome criteria.
   1.10 Outline essential guidelines for writing goals and outcome criteria.
   1.11 Describe three aspects of planning nursing strategies.
   1.12 Describe three methods commonly used to generate alternative nursing strategies.
2. Understand essential aspects of writing a nursing care plan.
   2.1 Identify major purposes of a written care plan.
   2.2 Identify various formats used for nursing care plans.
   2.3 Describe five components of nursing orders.
   2.4 Identify essential guidelines for writing nursing care plans.

Terms

brainstorming
client goal
criterion
extrapolating
goal
hypothesizing
inference
nursing care plan
nursing order
nursing strategy
outcome criteria
planning
priority setting
prognosis
rationale

Definition and Process

In general, planning is designing or arranging the parts of something to achieve an end or goal. In nursing, planning is the third step of the nursing process. In this context, **planning** is the process of designing the nursing strategies or interventions required to prevent, reduce, or eliminate those client health problems identified during analysis/synthesis. The following people can be involved in planning nursing strategies: one or more nurses; the client, support persons, and/or caregivers; and sometimes members of other health professions. Although the planning process is basically the responsibility of the nurse, input from the client and/or support persons is essential if a plan is to be effective. It is no longer sufficient that nurses plan *for* the client; whenever possible, the client must participate actively.

For a client in a home setting, the home health care nurse needs to involve the client, if his or her health permits, as well as the support persons and/or the caregiver. With the nurse's guidance, these people can implement the plan of care; thus, its effectiveness depends largely on them. They can also provide information about problems previously unknown to the nurse. For example, Mrs. Robson is a 59-year-old woman with impaired mobility because of paralysis of her right side. Her 60-year-old husband cares for her at home. One of the client's health problems is: "Self-care deficit in bathing related to impaired mobility of the right side." Mrs. Robson is developing skin irritations of the groin and inner thighs. One of the alternative nursing strategies could be: "Demonstrate for the husband how to lift Mrs. Robson onto a seat in the bathtub," where thorough washing can be carried out. However, Mr. Robson explains that he is unable to lift or exert himself because of heart disease. It is then necessary to consider alternative ways of washing Mrs. Robson's perineal area or other ways for her to move into the tub. The nurse may have remained unaware of the husband's heart condition had Mr. Robson not been involved in developing nursing strategies to deal with the problem.

Clients and families (support persons) are increasingly better informed about health and illness; cooperative planning is essential because nurses are accountable and responsible for nursing interventions. Including the client in the plan of care is a legal safeguard for the nurse. (Philpott 1985, p. 100)

Planning is a process in which decision making and problem solving are carried out (see Chapter 10). The planning process uses (a) data obtained during assessing and (b) the diagnostic statements that present the client's health problems (potential and actual).

Components of Planning

The four components of planning are:

1. Setting priorities
2. Establishing client goals and outcome criteria
3. Planning nursing strategies
4. Writing a nursing care plan

Setting Priorities

Priority setting is the process of establishing a preferential order for nursing strategies. To set priorities, the nurse and the client first order the nursing diagnoses preferentially, i.e., they decide which deserves attention first, which second, and so on. Diagnoses can be grouped as having high, medium, or low priority. This priority setting, however, does not mean that all the high-priority diagnoses must be resolved before any others are considered. A high-priority diagnosis may be dealt with partially and then a diagnosis of lesser priority may be dealt with. In addition, the nurse may address more than one diagnosis at a time. Because client problems are usually multiple, this is often the case. See Table 13–1 for the assignment of priorities to the diagnostic statements for Mr. Joe Smith.

Setting priorities is made easier by using a framework such as a nursing model or theory. One frequently used framework is Maslow's hierarchy of needs. See Figure 16–1 on page 314. Maslow's physiologic needs, such as air, food, water, etc., are basic to life and receive higher priority than the need for security or activity. Life-threatening problems have the highest priority.

The importance of the client's involvement in setting priorities cannot be overemphasized. Although a nurse may believe she or he knows a client, the client's values may be different than the nurse supposes. Thus, the client may set priorities differently from the nurse. For example, one nursing diagnosis may relate to smoking and another to nutrition. The nurse may give the smoking problem a

Table 13–1 Assigning Priorities to Diagnostic Statements for Mr. Joe Smith (before cardiac catheterization)

Diagnostic Statement List	Priority Rating	Rationale
Activity intolerance related to shortness of breath and lack of energy secondary to decreased strength of cardiac contractions	Medium priority	Lack of energy is the client's stated major concern. Too much activity can create excessive cardiac demands, resulting in further decreased cardiac output with lowered blood pressure and inadequate circulation. However, because Mr. Smith is able to handle basic activities of daily living, strategies to deal with this diagnostic statement can be deferred until after cardiac catheterization and/or cardiac surgery.
Potential ineffective airway clearance postoperatively related to chest incision	Low priority	Until surgery is performed, ineffective airway clearance is not likely since he is currently able to clear his airways by coughing.
Potential for injury (trauma) related to joint stiffness and limp from hip replacement surgery	High priority	The client is independent and moves slowly to accommodate his limitations. However, new surroundings and a sedative given before cardiac catheterization increase his risk of injury.
Knowledge deficit: side-effects of diuretic therapy	Medium priority	Although the client complies with his medical regime, he does not seem to understand the side-effects of the prescribed diuretic, e.g., its relation to increased urination.
Alteration in peripheral tissue perfusion (left leg) related to impaired arterial circulation	High priority	Decreased circulation and tissue perfusion to the client's left leg can result in damage to the tissues of the limb.
Fear related to cardiac catheterization, possible heart surgery, and its outcome	High priority	Extreme fear could impair his coping capacity.
Potential alteration in comfort (angina) related to excessive activity or stress	Medium priority	Angina has not been a problem for 2 months, but it could recur with the stress of hospitalization and planned treatments.

higher priority than the problem of obesity, but the client may see the problem of obesity as more important. Where there is such a difference of opinion, the client and nurse should discuss it openly or resolve the conflict. However, in a life-threatening situation, the nurse needs to take the initiative.

The priorities assigned to problems should not remain fixed. Nursing priorities must change as a client's health problems and therapy change.

The following criteria assist the nurse and the client to set priorities.

Client's Health Values and Beliefs

Values concerning health may be very important to the nurse but not to the client. For example, a client may see attendance at school or being home for the children as more urgent than her or his health.

Client's Priorities

Offering the client the opportunity to set his or her own priorities allows client participation in care planning and enhances cooperation between the nurse and client. Sometimes, however, the client's perception of what is important conflicts with the nurse's knowledge of potential future problems or complications. For example, an elderly female may not regard ambulation or turning and repositioning every 2 hours as important, preferring to be undisturbed. The nurse, however, aware of the potential complications of prolonged bed rest (e.g., muscle weakness and decubitus ulcers), needs to inform the client and implement necessary interventions to prevent such debilitating effects.

Resources Available to the Nurse and Client

If money, equipment, or personnel are scarce, then a health problem may be given a lower priority. Nurses in a home setting, for example, do not have the resources of a hospital; therefore, if the resources needed for specific nursing strategies are not available, solution of that problem might need to be postponed, or the client may need referral.

Client resources, such as finances or coping abilities, may also influence the setting of priorities. For example, a client who is unemployed may defer dental treatment; a client whose husband is terminally ill and dependent on her may consider nutritional guidance directed toward weight loss as too much to handle with her stressful circumstances.

Time Needed for the Nursing Strategies

Each client feels comfortable with a certain pace of action. Some clients may want to discuss the problem with family members or think about it overnight. Others may want "to get on with it." The nurse must allow adequate time for the necessary nursing strategies resulting from the nursing diagnosis.

Urgency of the Health Problem

Life-threatening situations require that the nurse establish priorities quickly. This also applies to situations that affect the integrity of the client, i.e., that could have a negative or destructive effect on the client. Such health problems as drug abuse and radical alteration of self-concept due to amputation can be destructive not only to the individual but also to the family. Such health problems should receive high priority.

Medical Treatment Plan

The priorities for treating health problems must be congruent with treatment by other health professionals. For example, a high priority for the client might be to become ambulatory; however, if the physician's therapeutic regimen calls for extended bed rest, then ambulation must assume a lower priority in the nursing strategy plan. In such a case, however, the nurse can provide or teach exercises to facilitate ambulation later, provided the client's health permits. The diagnostic statement related to ambulation is not ignored; it is merely deferred.

Establishing Client Goals and Outcome Criteria

Goals

A goal is a hoped-for outcome; in terms of the nursing process, a **goal** is the desired outcome of nursing interventions. In the past, nursing goals were often written to direct care. For example, a nursing goal might have been stated as follows: "Increase the client's exercise" or "Increase fiber in diet." From these nursing goals, specific nursing activities were derived, such as ambulating the client at specified intervals, offering instruction about needed dietary adjustments, and ensuring that high-fiber foods were provided. Recently, however, nurses have begun to state goals in terms of desired *client behavior*, not in terms of nursing activities. The term *outcome* means the result of an activity rather than the activity itself.

The concept of goals varies in nursing literature. In nursing education, goals are often referred to as objectives. In nursing process literature, some nurses separate goals from objectives; others use the terms synonymously. Still others use the term *outcomes* or *outcome criteria* synonymously with objectives. In this book, the terms *goal* and *outcome criteria* are differentiated, while *outcome criteria* and *objectives* are used synonymously. Goals are broadly stated and not measurable. Outcome criteria are specific and measurable.

A **client goal,** then, is a broad statement about the expected or desired change in the status of the client after he or she receives nursing interventions. Since goals are broad indicators of performance, the use of such verbs as *increase, decrease, maintain, improve, develop,* and *restore* is appropriate. (See Examples of Client Goals on this page.

The purpose of client goals is to:

1. Provide direction for planning nursing interventions that will achieve the anticipated changes in the client.
2. Provide direction for establishing evaluation criteria to measure the effectiveness of the interventions.

Relationship of goals to the nursing diagnosis Client goals are derived from the first clause of the nursing diagnosis, i.e., from the identified client response. For example, if the first clause of the nursing diagnosis is "Self-care deficit: inability to feed self," the goal might be stated as follows: "Client will demonstrate increased ability to feed self." More specific client outcomes (criteria) are then set from this goal; these criteria form the basis of evaluation. For example, if the goal is "The client will demonstrate increased ability to feed self," two criteria might be, "Will drink from a glass through a straw" and "Will feed self using utensils with sponge-wrapped handles." See the section on outcome criteria next in this chapter.

Long-term and short-term goals Goals may be short term or long term. A short-term goal might be, "Client will raise right arm to shoulder height by Friday." In the same context, a long-term goal might be, "Client will regain full use of right arm." Because a great deal of the nurse's time is focused on the immediate needs of the client, most goals are short term. In addition, the nurse is better able to evaluate the client's progress or lack of it with short-term goals.

Long-term goals are often used for clients living at home and having chronic health problems or clients in nursing homes, extended care facilities, and rehabilitation centers. Short-term goals are useful (a) for clients who require health care for only a short time and (b) for persons who are frustrated by long-term goals that seem difficult to attain and who need the satisfaction of achieving a short-term goal.

Examples of Client Goals

The client will:

- Increase activity tolerance
- Maintain urinary elimination pattern
- Restore fluid volume
- Decrease potential for injury
- Develop coping abilities
- Improve nutritional pattern

Outcome Criteria

Outcome criteria or objectives are needed to add specificity to the broad goal statements. A **criterion** is a standard or model that can be used in judging. **Outcome criteria** are statements that describe specific, observable, and measurable responses of the client. They determine whether the stated goals have been achieved and are therefore essential to the evaluation phase of the nursing process.

Outcome criteria serve four purposes:

1. They provide direction for nursing interventions.
2. They provide a time span for planned activities.
3. They serve as criteria for evaluation of goal achievement.
4. They give the client and nurse a sense of achievement.

Relationship of outcome criteria to client goals Outcome criteria are derived from and relate to the client goals, which in turn are derived from and relate to the nursing diagnosis. For example, if one of the goals for a client confined to bed is, "The client will not develop the preventable complications of imposed immobility," the outcome criteria that might be derived are as follows. The client will:

1. Have intact skin, particularly over bony prominences.
2. Have complete range of motion of the joints in the upper and lower extremities.
3. Have regular bowel evacuation and well-formed stools, but will not be constipated.
4. Drink at least 2500 ml of fluid per day.
5. Void clear amber urine in amounts appropriate to fluid intake.
6. Have normal vital signs.

Generally, three to six outcome criteria are needed for each goal. Some nurses consider outcome criteria to be part of goals and add criteria directly to the goal statement, as follows: "Client's hydration status will be maintained (goal) as evidenced by (outcome criteria): (a) fluid intake of at least 2500 ml daily, (b) urinary output in balance with fluid intake, (c) normal skin turgor, (d) moist oral mucous membranes." Other nurses find this method cumbersome and separate the goal statement from the criteria statements.

Whichever method is used, the process of developing outcome criteria is the same. The nurse needs to ask two questions:

1. How will the client look or behave if the desired goal is achieved?
2. What must the client do and how well must he or she do it before the goal is attained?

Characteristics of outcome criteria These are the characteristics of well-stated criteria:

1. Each outcome criterion relates to the established goal.
2. The outcome stated in the criterion is possible to achieve.
3. Each criterion is a statement of *one* specific outcome.
4. Each criterion is as specific and concrete as possible, to facilitate measurement.
5. Criteria are appraisable or measurable, i.e., the outcome can be seen, heard, felt, or measured by another person.

Components of outcome criteria Outcome criteria generally have all or some of the following four components:

1. *Subject.* The subject, a noun, is the client, any part of the client, or some attribute of the client, such as the client's pulse or urinary output. Often, the subject is omitted in nursing care plan goals; it is assumed that the subject is the client unless indicated otherwise.
2. *Verb.* The verb denotes an action the client is to perform, e.g., what the client is to do, learn, or experience. Verbs that denote directly observable behaviors, such as *administer, demonstrate, show, walk, drink, tell, list, state,* etc., are used.
3. *Conditions or modifiers.* Conditions or modifiers may be added to the verb to explain the circumstances under which the behavior is to be performed. They explain what, where, when, or how. For example:

   Walk *with the help of a walker* (how)

   After attending two group diabetes classes, will list signs and symptoms of diabetes (when)

   When at home will maintain weight at existing level (where)

   Discuss *four food groups and recommended daily servings* (what)

   Conditions need not be included if the standard of performance clearly indicates what is expected.
4. *Criterion of desired performance.* The criterion indicates the standard by which a performance is evaluated or the level at which the client will perform the specified behavior. These criteria may specify time or speed, accuracy, distance, and quality. To establish a time-achievement criterion, the nurse needs to ask "how long?" To establish an accuracy criterion, the nurse asks "how well?" Similarly, the nurse asks "how far?" and "what is the expected standard?" to establish distance and quality criteria, respectively. Examples are:

   Weight 75 kg *by April* (time)

   List *five out of six* signs of diabetes (accuracy)

   Walk *one block per day* (time and distance)

   Administer insulin *using aseptic technique* (quality)

Guidelines for Writing Goals and Outcome Criteria

The following guidelines can help nurses write goals and outcome criteria:

1. Write goal statements and outcome criteria in terms of client behavior. Beginning each outcome criterion with "the client will" helps to focus the statement on the client. Avoid statements that start with *enable, facilitate, allow, let, permit,* or similar verbs followed by the word *client* (Carnevali 1983, p. 191). These verbs indicate what the nurse hopes to accomplish, not what the client will do.
2. Make sure that the goal statement clearly relates to the nursing diagnosis and that the outcome criteria relate to the goal.
3. Make sure that the outcome criteria are realistic for the client's capabilities, internal and external limitations, and designated time span, if it is indicated. *Internal limitations* refer to the person's physical and mental health status and coping mechanisms. *External limitations* refer to finances, equipment, family support, social services, and time. For example, the goal "The client will walk with crutches on level surfaces and on stairs" may be unrealistic for an elderly woman with a heavy leg cast. "The client will walk with crutches from bed to bathroom with assistance" may be more realistic. The goal "Measures insulin accurately" may be unrealistic for a client who has poor vision due to cataracts.
4. Make sure that the client considers the goals important and values them. Discuss the nursing diagnosis and goals with the client to determine if he or she agrees

with the stated problem and goals. Clients are usually motivated and expend the necessary energy to reach a goal if they consider it important.

5. Ensure that the goals and outcome criteria are compatible with the work and therapies of other professionals. The goal "Increase the client's activity tolerance" and the attending criterion "Will increase the time spent out of bed by 15 minutes each day" are not compatible with a physician's prescribed therapy of bed rest for 3 days.
6. Make sure that each *goal* is derived from only one nursing diagnosis. For example, the goal "The client will increase the amount of nutrients ingested and show progress in the ability to feed self" is derived from two nursing diagnoses: "self-care deficit related to inability to feed self" and "Alterations in nutrition related to anorexia." Keeping the goal statement related to only one diagnosis ensures that outcome criteria and planned nursing interventions are clearly related to the diagnosis.
7. When writing *outcome criteria,* use observable, measurable terms; avoid words that are vague and require interpretation or judgment by the observer. For example, such phrases as "increase daily exercise," "increase participation in social activities," and "improve knowledge of nutrition" can mean different things to different people. If used in criteria, these phrases can lead to disagreements about whether the criterion was met. These phrases may be suitable for a broad client goal but are not sufficiently clear and specific for use in outcome criteria used to evaluate the client's response.

Examples of client goals and outcome criteria associated with the diagnostic statements for Mr. Joe Smith are shown in Table 13–2. Note that the diagnostic statements have been reordered according to established priorities.

Planning Nursing Strategies

Nursing strategies are nursing actions designed to achieve established client goals. Selecting nursing strategies is a decision-making process. Planning nursing strategies involves generating a number of alternative nursing actions likely to solve the client's problem, considering the consequences of each alternative action, and choosing one or more nursing strategies.

Generating Alternative Nursing Strategies

The client and nurse can use several methods of generating alternative nursing strategies at this stage: brainstorming, hypothesizing, and extrapolating.

Table 13–2 Goals and Outcome Criteria for Mr. Joe Smith (before cardiac catheterization)

Diagnostic Statement*	Client Goals	Outcome Criteria
1. Fear related to cardiac catheterization, possible heart surgery, and its outcome	Experience increased emotional comfort and feelings of control	Verbalizes specific concerns Communicates thoughts clearly and logically Facial expressions, voice tone, and body posture correspond to verbal expressions of increased emotional comfort or feelings of control After instruction, describes the cardiac catheterization procedure and what is expected of him before and after the procedure
2. Alteration in peripheral tissue perfusion (left leg) related to impaired arterial circulation	Improve circulation to left leg and foot	Skin intact, pink, and moist Skin temperature warm (as other foot) Left dorsalis pedis, posterior tibial, and popliteal pulses palpable and of same strength as corresponding right pulses Verbalizes factors that improve and inhibit peripheral circulation Capillary refill of left toenails within 1 to 3 seconds
3. Potential for injury (trauma) related to joint stiffness and limp from hip replacement surgery	Prevent injury	Moves in and out of bed and ambulates without falling or injuring self
4. Activity intolerance related to shortness of breath and lack of energy secondary to decreased strength of cardiac contraction	Avoid performance of activities causing shortness of breath and excessive cardiac workload	Rests after meals No shortness of breath during activities Pulse and blood pressure remain stable at 80 beats per minute and 124/80 mm Hg

*Note new order of diagnostic statements to reflect highest priorities.

Brainstorming is a technique used by more than one person, usually a group of people. In this process, one person's idea elicits an idea from another, and so forth. The ideas should not be evaluated while they are being generated. An idea is expressed, developed by another, modified by another, etc., until a solution acceptable to all is established. The results of this process are often creative solutions.

Hypothesizing is a technique of predicting which actions will solve a problem or meet a goal. Hypothesized alternatives are the result of knowledge and experience, and each of the proposed alternatives is likely to be effective. Hypothesizing is *not* guessing because the alternatives have been tried successfully in the past.

Extrapolating is inferring facts or data from known facts or data. In this technique, the individual suggests an action because everything that is known about the problem suggests the action will be effective. For example, Mrs. Redden says, "I am unable to sleep at night." Mrs. Redden knows that Miss Hollis in the next bed has a glass of warm milk at 10:00 P.M. and sleeps well at night. Mrs. Redden extrapolates that the warm milk will help her sleep. Therefore, her suggested solution for her insomnia is to take a glass of warm milk at bedtime. If, however, Mrs. Redden knew that she was unable to sleep at night because of the side-effects of a medication, she or the nurse might suggest another solution to the problem.

Extrapolating involves making guesses and inferences. An *inference* is the interpretation of data from knowledge and past experience. When data are incomplete, inferences can be inaccurate, and further data are needed.

Sometimes a nurse, particularly a nurse with limited experience, may wish to generate nursing strategies with other nurses to obtain the best alternatives. The client and/or support persons should be included in this discussion whenever possible. When the conference must take place away from the client, e.g., in an agency conference room when the client is confined to bed at home, the responsible nurse must discuss the alternative strategies with the client, support persons, and the caregiver in the home before definitive decisions are made.

Considering the Consequences of Each Strategy

Often, the nurse and the client can establish a number of nursing strategies for each problem statement. Too many alternatives can be confusing. Usually three to five alternative nursing strategies for each health problem is satisfactory. See Table 13–3. The next step is to consider the consequences of each action, including the risks. Often, each action will have more than one consequence. For example, the strategy "Provide accurate information" could result in the following client behaviors:

Table 13–3 Developing Alternative Nursing Strategies

Diagnostic Statement	Client Goal	Alternative Nursing Strategies
Sleep pattern disturbance related to anxiety	Obtain 6 to 9 hours of sleep	Provide warm milk and a snack in the evening. Provide more activity during daytime. Provide accurate information. Provide soft music. Provide a hypnotic. Encourage verbalization of worries.

1. Increased anxiety
2. Decreased anxiety
3. Wish to talk with the physician
4. Desire to leave hospital
5. Relaxation

Establishing the consequences of each strategy requires nursing knowledge and experience. The nurse's experience may suggest that providing information before the client's bedtime may increase the client's worry and tension and that maintaining the usual rituals before sleep is more effective. Perhaps some alternative nursing actions should be implemented during the day to facilitate sleep at night, e.g., providing accurate information during the day and increasing daytime activity.

Choosing Nursing Strategies

After considering the consequences of the alternative nursing strategies, the nurse chooses one or more that she or he considers likely to be most effective. Although the nurse bases this decision on knowledge and experience, the client's input is very important. For example, a client may say: "I always have a sandwich and glass of milk before going to bed when I am home. I know I'll sleep if I can have that." Maintaining the client's routine may indeed help the client sleep, and this action might be the first choice as a nursing strategy.

The following criteria can help the nurse choose the best nursing strategy. The planned action must be:

1. Safe for the client.
2. Achievable with the resources available (e.g., in the previous example, sandwiches and milk must be available).
3. Congruent with the client's values and beliefs.

4. Congruent with other therapies (e.g., if the client is not permitted food, the strategy of an evening snack must be deferred until health permits).
5. Based on nursing knowledge and experience or knowledge from relevant sciences. Example:

   Client's diagnosis

   Potential impairment of skin integrity related to immobility

   Nursing Strategies

   Assess skin integrity over bony prominences q2h.

   Turn and change position q30 minutes.

   Pad pressure points.

   Use egg crate mattress on bed.

   Rationale

   Continuous pressure on a body area compresses tissue, obstructs blood flow to and from an area, and can result in damaged tissue.
6. Within the stated policy of the agency.

   Many agencies have policies to guide nursing activities and the activities of other health professionals. Policies are usually intended to safeguard clients, e.g., rules for visiting hours, procedures to follow when a client has cardiac arrest, and so on. If a policy does not benefit clients, nurses have a responsibility to bring this to the attention of the appropriate people.
7. Appropriate for the individual's age, health, etc.

Writing the Nursing Care Plan

The **nursing care plan** is a written guide that organizes information about a client's health into a meaningful whole; it focuses on the actions nurses must take to address the client's identified nursing diagnoses and meet the stated goals. It is also referred to as the *client care plan* since its focus is the client.

The responsible nurse (head nurse, primary nurse, or team leader) starts the care plan as soon as a client is admitted to the health care agency. It is constantly updated and revised throughout the client's stay, in response to changes in the client's condition and evaluations of goal achievement.

Purposes

The purposes of a written care plan are:

1. To provide direction for *individualized care* of the client. The plan is organized according to each client's unique nursing care needs. Although many agencies have devised standardized care plans as guides for providing essential nursing care to specified groups of clients, such plans should be used in conjunction with a plan developed for each client. Standardized plans, developed and accepted by the nursing staff of the agency, ensure that the minimally acceptable standards of care are provided. These plans, however, do not ensure individualized care.
2. To provide for *continuity of care*. The written plan is a means of communicating and organizing the actions of a constantly changing nursing staff. The initial plan, updated to show nursing interventions and new assessment data, is often conveyed to all nursing staff at change of shift reports, nursing rounds, and client care conferences.
3. To provide *direction about what needs to be documented* on the client's progress notes. The care plan specifically outlines which observations to make, what nursing actions to carry out, and what instructions the client or family members require. In this way, recording is facilitated.
4. To serve as a *guide for assigning staff* to care for the client. Certain aspects of the client's care may need to be delegated to someone who can make necessary judgments about the client's responses.

Format

Although formats differ from agency to agency, the plan is generally organized into four columns or categories: (a) nursing diagnoses or problem list, (b) goals, (c) nursing strategies/interventions/nursing orders, and (d) outcome or evaluation criteria. Some agencies have a five-column plan that includes a column for assessment data before the nursing diagnoses column. Others use a three-column plan that subsumes the evaluation (outcome criteria) column under the goal column. To help students learn to write care plans and apply their knowledge, educators often modify this plan by adding a column headed "Rationale" after the nursing intervention column. See Table 13–4. A **rationale** is the scientific reason for selecting a specific nursing action. Students may also be required to cite supporting literature for this stated rationale.

Many agencies use a nursing Kardex system for organizing and storing nursing care plans. A nursing *Kardex* is a file of specially designed 6-by-11-inch index cards containing the care plan for a group of clients. Most Kardexes include not only space for the nursing diagnoses, goals, nursing actions, and evaluations but also:

1. A concise profile of the client, with the client's name, medical diagnosis, religion, marital status, occupation, allergies, next of kin, etc.
2. Information about medications the client is receiving, parenteral therapy and other treatments, current operations, and planned laboratory and diagnostic studies.

Table 13–4 Nursing Orders with Rationale for Mr. Joe Smith

Diagnostic Statement	Goals	Nursing Orders	Rationale	Outcome Criteria
1. Fear related to cardiac catheterization, possible heart surgery, and its outcome	Experience increased emotional comfort and feelings of control	Establish a trusting relationship with the client and family	Mistrust in health care providers increases fear	Verbalizes specific concerns
		Encourage client and family to express feelings and concerns	Expression of feelings often relieves tension and enables supportive feedback or correction of misinformation	Communicates thoughts clearly and logically Facial expressions, voice tone, and body posture correspond to verbal expressions of increased emotional comfort or feelings of control
		Discuss the cardiac catheterization procedure and what is expected of him before and after the procedure	Knowledge of the procedure and of what is expected of him will reduce fears of the unknown and feelings of powerlessness	After instruction, describes the cardiac catheterization procedure and what is expected of him before and after the procedure
		Encourage conversation with another client who has recuperated from similar surgery	Another client who has recuperated from heart surgery can provide more hope about the outcome of surgery than the nurse	
2. Alteration in peripheral tissue perfusion (left leg) related to impaired arterial circulation	Improve circulation to left leg and foot	Consult with physician about exercise program, such as walking and range-of-motion exercises to hip, knee, and ankle	Walking and range-of-motion exercises increase peripheral circulation, but because the conditions causing impaired arterial circulation are unknown, the physician must prescribe them	Skin intact, pink, and moist Skin temperature warm (as other foot) Left dorsalis pedis, posterior tibial, and popliteal pulses palpable and of same strength as corresponding right pulses Capillary refill of left toenails within 1 to 3 seconds
		Keep the extremity in a *dependent* position (i.e., lower than the heart)	A dependent position facilitates arterial blood flow by gravity	
		Use Doppler ultrasound stethoscope (DUS) to assess blood flow in left dorsalis pedis, posterior tibial, and popliteal arteries q2h	The DUS detects and indicates movement of blood through arteries by a pulsating sound. When pulses are not palpable, the DUS can determine blood flow	
		Instruct client to keep his legs warm, e.g., wear warm socks but discourage use of external heat sources	Warmth increases circulation; because decreased sensation is often associated with impaired perfusion, external heat may not be perceived and cause burning	
3. Potential for injury (trauma) related to joint stiffness and limp from hip replacement surgery	Prevent injury	Closely assess ambulation and transfers during first few days	Close supervision enables assessment of independence and safety in mobility	Moves in and out of bed and ambulates without falling or injuring self
		Keep bed at lowest level	Low level facilitates safer transfers into and out of bed	
		Encourage to request assistance to ambulate during the night	New surroundings can cause confusion in older people and be the cause of accidents	

(continued)

Table 13–4 *(continued)*

Diagnostic Statement	Goals	Nursing Orders	Rationale	Outcome Criteria
		Closely attend or put side rails up when client is sedated	Sedation can alter perception and impair motor abilities	
4. Activity intolerance related to shortness of breath and lack of energy secondary to decreased strength of cardiac contraction	Avoid performance of activities causing shortness of breath and excessive cardiac workload	Organize client care and provide undisturbed rest periods	A balance of activity and rest is necessary to stabilize cardiac effort	Rests after meals No shortness of breath during activities Pulse and blood pressure remain stable at 80 beats per minute and 124/80 mm Hg
		Discuss energy conservation methods such as taking periodic rest periods	Implementing energy conservation methods reduces the cardiac workload and deleterious effects of reduced cardiac output	
		Tell the client to reduce the intensity, duration, and frequency of activity if he experiences chest pain, shortness of breath, dizziness, or abnormal pulse and blood pressure after activity	These signs indicate inadequate cardiac output	
		Monitor vitals signs q2h and report decreasing blood pressure, increasing heart rate, or increasing respiratory rate	These signs are indicative of additional reduced cardiac output and cardiac failure	

With knowledge of the time and frequency of tests, treatments, and other activities, the nurse can coordinate all care for the client and organize her or his clinical assignment. Coordinating care is essential to preserve the client's energy.

Some health care agencies have adopted 8½-by-11-inch nursing care plan records that correspond to the standard chart size and require that the plan be written in ink so that it can be retained as part of the client's permanent legal record. In other agencies, problem-oriented medical records (POMR) are used; in this situation, the nursing care plan is documented in a SOAP format. See Chapter 30. In still other agencies, medical orders are not included on the Kardex.

Writing Nursing Orders

Carnevali (1983, p. 222) says the term *nursing order* is preferable to the terms *approaches, activities, actions,* and *interventions* because *order* connotes a sense of accountability for the nurse who gives the order and for the nurse who carries it out. **Nursing orders** are the specific actions the nurse takes to help the client meet established health care goals.

As client advocates, nurses must accept the decisions of a client unless the decision may produce harmful results. (Moughton 1982, p. 478)

The degree of detail included in the nursing orders depends to some degree on the health personnel who will carry out the order. It is advisable, however, to be exact in writing orders.

Nursing orders should include five components (Carnevali 1983, p. 222):

1. Date
2. Precise action verb and possibly modifier
3. Content area
4. Time element
5. Signature

Date Nursing orders are dated when they are written and reviewed regularly at intervals that depend on the individual's needs. If a client is acutely ill, in an intensive care unit, for example, the plan of care will be continually monitored and revised. In a community clinic, weekly or biweekly reviews may be indicated.

Action verb The verb starts the order and needs to be precise. For example, "Explain (to the client) the actions of insulin" is a more precise statement than "Teach (the client) about insulin." "Measure and record ankle circumference daily at 0900 hr" is more precise than "Assess edema of left ankle daily." Sometimes a modifier for the verb can make the nursing order more precise. For example, "Apply spiral bandage to left lower leg *firmly*" is more precise than "Apply spiral bandage to left leg." Two examples of imprecise verbs are (Carnevali 1983, p. 223):

1. *Have the client* rather than:
   Ask the client if he will ______
   Request the client to ______
   Remind the client to ______ etc.
2. *Reassure* rather than:
   Listen to him
   Stay with him
   Inform him of ______ etc.

Content area The content is the where and the what of the order. In the above order, "spiral bandage" and "left leg" state the what and the where of the order. The nurse can also clarify in this example whether the foot or toes are to be left exposed.

Time element The time element answers when, how long, or how often the nursing action is to occur. Examples are: "Assist client with tub bath at 0700 daily"; "Immerse client's left arm in sterile saline soak for 1 hr"; or "Assist client to change position every 2 hr between 0700 and 2100 hr."

Signature The signature of the nurse prescribing the order shows the nurse's accountability and has legal significance.

Nursing orders (plans) may be categorized as:

1. Orders for nursing therapy of a problem
2. Orders for collection of additional data to define a problem better or facilitate its management
3. Orders for dissemination of information about the management of a problem

Orders for nursing therapy include those activities that maintain or restore the client's usual patterns, alleviate symptoms, and prevent additional problems. These comprise the majority of orders.

The collection of additional data is often necessary to define a nursing diagnosis better or to learn how to manage a problem. For example, if the nurse notices that a client appears withdrawn, worried, and tense, the nurse needs additional data from the client to clarify the contributing causes of this behavior. The nurse may write a tentative nursing diagnosis of "anxiety" and then write nursing orders that guide interventions toward confirming the cause. For example, a nursing order may state, "Talk with client to determine cause of anxiety."

If the nurse needs information about how to manage a problem, data may be collected from many sources. One example is the order "RN to consult physician about method of cleaning ulcer." In other situations, the nurse may consult with a pharmacist about the side-effects of a medication, a dietitian about the foods allowed on a certain diet, a physical therapist about appropriate exercise, etc.

Nursing orders may specify the need to distribute information about continuing management of a problem to the client's support persons or other health team members. For example, a family member may need to learn how to help the client manage a long-term illness, or a visiting nurse association may need information about follow-up nursing care requirements for a client who is being discharged.

Guidelines for Writing Nursing Care Plans

In addition to following the earlier suggestions for writing nursing orders, the nurse can use the following guidelines when writing nursing care plans:

1. Date and sign the plan. The date the plan is used is essential for evaluation, review, and future planning. The signature of the responsible nurse demonstrates accountability to the client and to the nursing profession, since the effectiveness of nursing actions can be evaluated.
2. Use the category headings "Nursing Diagnoses," "Goals," "Nursing Orders/Interventions," and "Evaluation" and include a date for the evaluation of each goal.
3. Indicate that goals are met or revised by your signature or some other method specified by the agency.
4. List the nursing orders for each goal in order of priority. For example, the nursing orders for a client with a decubitus ulcer might include "Apply an occlusive dressing for 24 hours" and "Clean the ulcer with Betadine Solution daily." The appropriate sequence is to clean the ulcer before applying the dressing, and the orders should be listed in that sequence. An example of priority listing is to explore a client's feelings about administering injectable insulin before demonstrating how to do it.
5. Use standardized medical or English symbols and key words rather than complete sentences to communicate your ideas. For example, write, "Turn and reposition q2h" rather than "Turn and reposition the client every two hours." Or write, "Clean decubitus ulcer c̄ H_2O_2 b.i.d." rather than "Clean the client's decubitus ulcer with hydrogen peroxide twice a day, morning and evening."
6. Do not include all the steps for a procedure on a written plan. Refer personnel to procedure books or other sources for this information. For example, refer

nurses to the procedure book for tracheostomy care or attach a standard nursing plan about such procedures as radiation-implantation care and preoperative or postoperative care. Using these adjuncts for commonalities of care among clients not only saves the nurse time but also focuses the care plan on the unique differences that individualize the care of clients.

7. Tailor the plan to the unique characteristics of the client by ensuring that the client's choices, such as preferences about the times of care and the methods used, are included. This reinforces the client's individuality and sense of control. For example, the written nursing order "Provide warm milk at bedtime rather than prescribed sedative" indicates that the client was given the choice between warm milk and a sedative.
8. Ensure that the nursing care plan incorporates aspects of care that prevent problems and maintain or promote health, as well as those that are restorative. Some nursing orders deal with more than one aspect concurrently. For example, carrying out the order "Provide active-assistance ROM exercises to affected limbs q2h" prevents joint contractures and maintains muscle strength and joint mobility.
9. Include in the plan persons with whom the nurse must collaborate and coordinate activities. For example, the nurse may write orders to ask a nutritionist or physical therapist about specific aspects of the client's care.
10. Include plans for the client's discharge and home care needs. It is often necessary to consult and make arrangements with the community health nurse, social worker, and specific agencies that supply client information and needed equipment.

Chapter Highlights

- Planning is the process of designing nursing strategies required to prevent, reduce, or eliminate a client's health problems.
- Planning can involve the nurse, the client, support persons, and caregivers.
- Nursing strategies are planned around a client's diagnostic statements and goals.
- Four components of planning are setting priorities, establishing client goals, planning nursing strategies, and writing a nursing care plan.
- Nursing diagnoses are assigned high, medium, and low priorities in consultation with the client, if health permits.
- Client goals are used to plan nursing strategies that will achieve anticipated changes in the client.
- Client goals are derived from the first clause of the nursing diagnosis.
- Outcome criteria describe specific and measurable client responses and help the nurse evaluate the effectiveness of the nursing intervention.
- Goal statements and outcome criteria are written in terms of the client's behavior.
- Nursing strategies can be generated by brainstorming, hypothesizing, and extrapolating.
- Establishing the consequences of each nursing strategy requires nursing knowledge and experience.
- The nursing care plan provides direction for individualized care of the client.
- Nursing orders are the specific actions taken by the nurse to help the client meet established health care goals.

Suggested Readings

Forman, M. June 1979. Building a better nursing care plan. *American Journal of Nursing* 79:1086–87.

The author first discusses the semantics of nursing care plans and then describes three questions that help the nurse build a nursing care plan: "What do you mean?"; "How do you know?;" and "What then?" Forman then gives an example of a poor care plan and a better care plan devised by asking these questions.

Vasey, E. K. April 1979. Writing your care plan ... efficiently. *Nursing 79* 9:67–71.

The author explains how care plans help nurses provide care and how to write a care plan. Included are selecting an approach, writing each approach, and revising the plan. Ten rules for writing care plans are also included.

Selected References

Atkinson, L. D., and Murray, M. E. 1983. *Understanding the nursing process.* 2d ed. New York: Macmillan Co.

Bower, F. L. 1981. The process of planning nursing care: A theoretical model. 2d ed. St. Louis: C. V. Mosby Co.

Carnevali, D. L. 1983. *Nursing care planning: Diagnosis and management.* 3d ed. Philadelphia: J. B. Lippincott Co.

Carpenito, L. J. 1983. *Nursing diagnosis: Application to clinical practice.* Philadelphia: J. B. Lippincott Co.

Forman, M. June 1979. Building a better nursing care plan. *American Journal of Nursing* 79:1086–87.

Griffith, J. W., and Christensen, P. J. 1982. *Nursing process: Application of theories, frameworks, and models.* St. Louis: C. V. Mosby Co.

La Monica, E. L. 1985. *The humanistic nursing process.* Monterey, Calif.: Wadsworth Health Sciences.

Lederer, J. et al. 1986. Care planning pocket guide: A nursing diagnosis approach. Menlo Park, Ca.: Addison-Wesley.

Moughton, M. September 1982. The patient: A partner in the health care process. *Nursing Clinics of North America* 17:467–79.

Philpott, M. 1985. *Legal liability and the nursing process.* Toronto: W. B. Saunders Co., Canada.

Roy, C. 1975. A diagnostic classification system for nursing. *Nursing Outlook* 23:90–93.

Vasey, E. K. April 1979. Writing your patient's care plan . . . efficiently. *Nursing 79* 9:67–71.

Yura, H., and Walsh, M. B. 1983. *The nursing process: Assessing, planning, implementing, evaluating.* 4th ed. Norwalk, Conn.: Appleton-Century-Crofts.

CHAPTER 14

Implementing

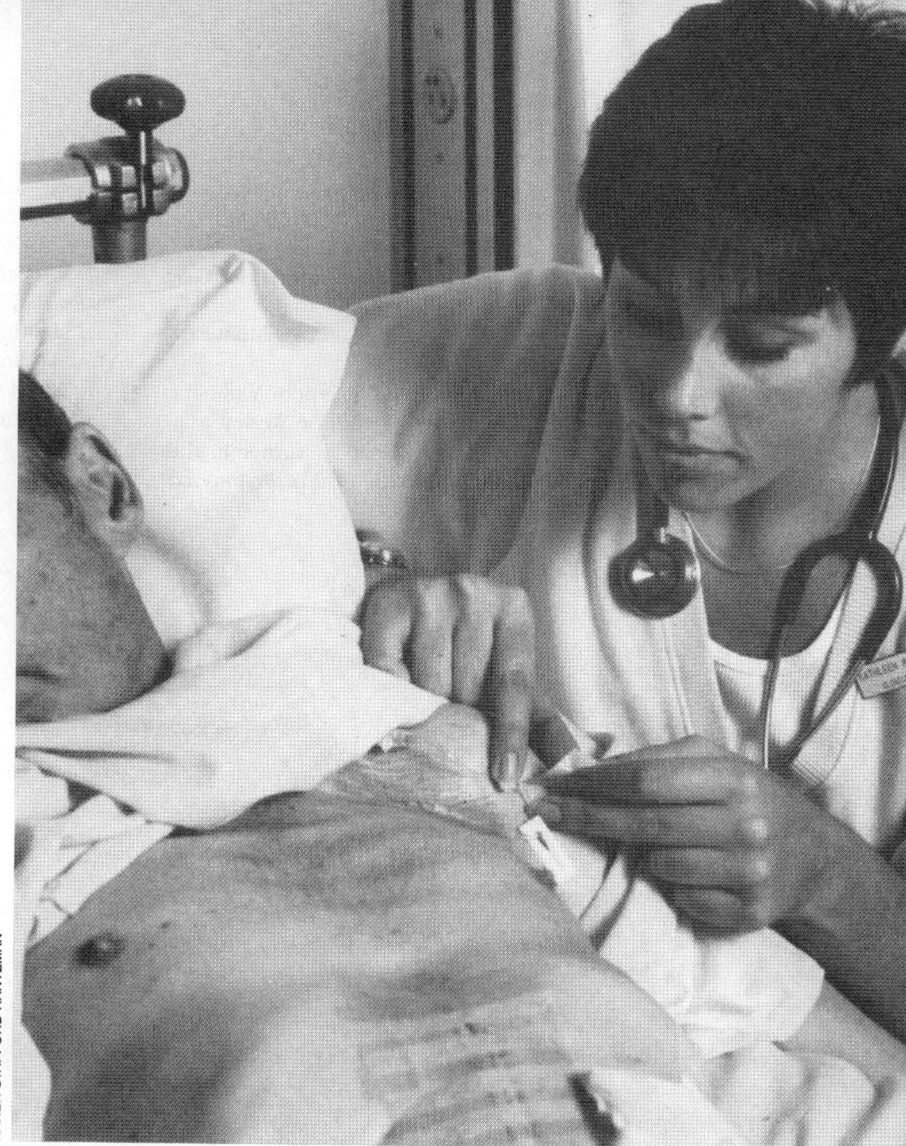

KAREN STAFFORD RANTZMAN

Contents

Objectives

1. Understand essential facts about the implementing phase of the nursing process.
   1.1 Define listed terms.
   1.2 Describe two processes that continuously operate throughout the implementation phase.
   1.3 Describe three categories of skill used to implement nursing strategies.
   1.4 Identify four cognitive skills nurses use when implementing nursing strategies.
   1.5 Identify five essential implementing activities.
   1.6 Give reasons why the need for health teaching by nurses has increased.
   1.7 Describe essential aspects of the counseling process.
   1.8 Identify essential aspects of managing.
   1.9 Identify essential guidelines for implementing nursing strategies.
2. Appreciate the fact that nurses are accountable for all their nursing activities.
   2.1 Discuss the significance of documenting nursing actions accurately.
   2.2 Discuss factors the nurse needs to consider when delegating nursing activities.

Terms

accountability
advocate
associative thinking
authority
change agent
cognitive
collaborative nursing action
concept
counseling
creative thinking
critical thinking
delegation
dependent nursing action
directed thinking
implementing
independent nursing action
interpersonal skills
phenomenal field
protocol
standing order
teaching

Definition

Implementing, also called intervening, is putting the nursing strategies listed in the nursing care plan into action. According to Marriner (1983), implementing involves carrying out nursing orders *and* physician's orders. The client is always the primary participant in implementing the nursing care plan, although the nurse may act on the client's behalf, e.g., referring the client to a community health nurse for home care. The client's degree of participation often depends on his or her health status. For example, because an unconscious man is unable to participate in his care, he needs to have care given to him. By contrast, an ambulatory client may require very little care from the nurse and carry out health care activities independently. The nurse or nurses, other health professionals, support persons, and/or caregivers can all be involved in implementing nursing. Implementing is the nursing action taken to attain the desired outcome or the client's goals.

Types of Nursing Actions

The terms *independent, dependent,* and *collaborative* (interdependent) are often used to describe nursing actions. An action, in this context, is an activity appropriate to a person's role. An **independent nursing action** is an activity that the nurse initiates as a result of her or his own knowledge and skills. Mundinger prefers the term *autonomous nursing practice* to *independent nursing practice.* She states, "knowing why, when, and how to position clients and doing it skillfully makes the function an autonomous therapy (Mundinger 1980, p. 4). In this instance, the nurse determines that the client requires certain nursing interventions, either carries these out or delegates them to other nursing personnel, and is accountable for the decision and the actions. To be *accountable* is to be answerable. An example of an independent action is planning and providing special mouth care to a man after assessing his mouth. Independent nursing actions are receiving increasing attention from nurses today.

Dependent nursing actions are those activities carried out on the order of the physician, under the physician's supervision, or according to specified routines. An example of a dependent action is giving an antibiotic by injection to a client as a result of a physician's written order. The dependent activity in nursing practice is usually directly related to the client's disease, and its importance should not be minimized.

Collaborative nursing actions are those activities performed either jointly with another member of the health care team or as a result of a joint decision by the nurse and another health care team member. Collaborative nursing activities sometimes illustrate the overlapping responsibilities of health personnel and reflect the collegial relationship between health professionals. For example, a nurse and an inhalation therapist together may decide on a schedule of breathing exercises for a woman. The therapist teaches the exercises, and the nurse assists the client in the therapist's absence.

A social policy statement by the American Nurses' Association (ANA) describes collaboration as "true partnership, in which the power on both sides is valued by both, with recognition and acceptance of separate and combined spheres of activity and responsibility, mutual safeguarding of legitimate interests of each party, and a commonality of goals that is recognized by both parties" (ANA 1980, p. 7). To achieve effective collaborative nursing practice, nurses must have clinical competence, feel confident of their knowledge and skills, and assume responsibility for their own actions.

Protocols

A **protocol** is a written plan specifying the procedure to be followed in a particular situation. For example, agencies often have protocols regarding a client's admission and discharge. Nurse practitioners in a community clinic often have protocols about which clients to refer to the physician and which clients to treat directly. Nurses in a home setting usually have protocols about the procedure to follow when a client dies. Nurses in hospitals often have protocols regarding the steps to follow when a postoperative client returns to the unit.

Standing Orders

A **standing order** is a written document about policies, rules, regulations, or orders regarding client care. Standing orders give nurses the authority to carry out specific actions under certain circumstances, often when a physician is not immediately available. In a hospital critical care unit, a common example is the administration of norepinephrine bitartrate when a client's blood pressure falls below a certain point.

In a home care setting, a physician may write a standing order for the administration of epinephrine for a client who becomes excessively dyspneic.

Process of Implementing

The process of implementing normally includes reassessing the client, validating the nursing care plan, determining the need for nursing assistance, implementing the nursing strategies, and communicating the nursing actions. Reassessing the client and validating the nursing care plan are subprocesses that operate continuously throughout the implementing phase.

Reassessing the Client

As was mentioned in Chapter 11 assessing or reassessing is carried out throughout the nursing process, i.e., during assessing, intervening, and evaluating—in fact, whenever the nurse has contact with the client. Nurses must continue to collect data about changes (subtle or acute) in the client's level of wellness, i.e., health problems as well as reactions, feelings, and strengths.

Following an extensive assessment during the first phase of the nursing process, reassessing in later phases usually focuses on more specific needs or responses of the client, i.e., fluid intake, pain, pulse rate, and urine output. Through this mechanism, nurses are able to determine whether planned nursing strategies are currently appropriate for the client.

Although nursing strategies may be independent, collaborative, or dependent, it should never be assumed that once they are established or ordered they must be implemented without assessing the client first (see the next section). For example, Mr. Raymond Ball's nursing diagnosis is: Alteration in bowel elimination: constipation related to prolonged bed rest, decreased fluid intake, and a soft, low-fiber diet. Before administering an enema to Mr. Ball, the nurse establishes that he had a large bowel movement that morning. Therefore, the enema is not needed. However, encouraging Mr. Ball to take fluids and to exercise in bed as his health permits are still appropriate nursing interventions.

New data may, in the nurse's judgment, indicate a need to change the priorities of care or the nursing strategies. For example, a nurse is turning a client, Mr. Dolan, from a supine to left lateral position according to the turning schedule. The nurse observes a reddened area on Mr. Dolan's left hip even though he has not lain on that side for several hours. The nurse decides not to position Mr. Dolan on his left side but turns him to his right side and records the reddened area and the change of nursing strategy. As a further example, a nurse begins to teach a client who has diabetes, Miss Eves, how to give herself insulin injections. Shortly after beginning the teaching, the nurse realizes that Miss Eves is not concentrating on the lesson. Subsequent discussion reveals that she is worried about her eyesight and fears she is going blind. The nurse ends the lesson because the client's level of stress is interfering with her learning and makes arrangement for a physician to examine the client's eyes. The nurse also provides supportive communication to alleviate the client's stress and revises the nursing care plan appropriately.

Validating the Nursing Care Plan

A nursing care plan cannot be fixed; it must be a flexible tool. Once new data are collected, they are compared with the data in the nursing care plan. Sometimes, the new data are incongruent with data in the plan. The nurse must judge the value of the new data and determine whether the nursing care plan is still valid. The nursing care plan is based on the client's goals and the established diagnostic statements. When a client's health status changes, i.e., when physical or psychosocial responses change, the nursing care plan needs to be adjusted.

If the data regarding the client's health status are unchanged, the nurse proceeds with the implementing process. For information on modifying or changing the nursing care plan, see Chapter 15, page 295.

Determining the Need for Assistance

When implementing some nursing strategies, the nurse may require assistance. Assistance is usually required for one of the following reasons: The nurse is unable to implement the nursing strategies safely alone, e.g., turning an obese client in bed; and to reduce stress upon a client, e.g., turning a person who has acute pain when moved. In addition, a nurse should obtain assistance if she or he lacks the knowledge or skills to implement a particular nursing activity. For example, a nurse who is not familiar with a particular model of oxygen mask needs assistance the first time she or he applies it. For additional information about the need for assistance, see the section on delegating, later in this chapter.

Implementing Nursing Strategies

Nursing strategies are implemented to help the client meet his or her health goals. Implementing activities are discussed later in this chapter.

There are four primary areas of nursing practice: health promotion, health maintenance, health restoration, and care of the dying. See Chapter 1, page 16, for additional information. Nursing actions in each of these areas can be independent, dependent, or collaborative.

Six important considerations for implementing nursing strategies are:

1. The client's individuality. Individualized actions are needed, while care is taken not to violate the scientific basis of the activity. For example, a client may prefer to have an oral medication after meals rather than before. However, this might not be justified if the medication will not act in the stomach in the presence of food.
2. The client's need for involvement. Some clients want to be totally involved in their care, while others prefer little involvement. The amount of desired involvement is often related to the client's energy, severity of illness, number of stressors, fear, understanding of the illness, and understanding of the intervention.
3. Prevention of complications. When changing a sterile dressing, for example, the nurse must observe sterile technique to prevent the complication of infection.
4. Preservation of the body's defenses. For example, when turning a client, the nurse protects the client's skin from abrasions, which could permit microorganisms to enter the body and establish an infection.
5. Provision of comfort and support to the client; see "Caring" later in the chapter.
6. Accurate and careful implementation of all nursing activities. The nurse takes care to administer the correct dosage of a medication by the ordered route, for example. See the discussion of implementing activities, later in this chapter.

Communicating Nursing Actions

Nursing actions are communicated in writing and often verbally *after* they have been carried out. Nursing actions must not be recorded in advance because the nurse may determine upon reassessing the client that the action should not or cannot be implemented. For example, a nurse is authorized to inject 10 mg of morphine sulfate subcutaneously to a client, but the nurse finds that the client's respiratory rate is 4 breaths per minute. This finding contraindicates the administration of morphine (a respiratory depressant). The nurse withholds the morphine and reports the client's respiratory rate to the responsible nurse and/or physician. A nurse might also find that a planned nursing action cannot be implemented, e.g., the client objects, the nurse is unable to perforate the skin with a needle, the nurse encounters an obstruction when inserting a rectal tube. Nursing activities, therefore, are always recorded after they are completed, when the nurse can accurately record exactly what occurred.

When documenting a nursing action, the nurse can include data about the effectiveness of the action, i.e., an evaluation of the degree to which the client's goals have been met. Evaluating is included here only in the context of communicating the nursing action. See Chapter 15, "Evaluating," for additional information.

In some instances, it is important to record a nursing action immediately after it is implemented. This is particularly true of medications, treatments, etc., because recorded data about a client must be up to date, accurate, and available to other nurses and health care professionals. Immediate recording helps safeguard the client, for example, from receiving a second dose of medication. The nurse may record such nursing actions as mouth care every 2 hours or turning a client at the end of a shift; in the meantime, the nurse maintains a personal record of these interventions so that they can be accurately recorded later. Many agencies have special forms for this type of recording. See Chapter 30 for additional information regarding recording.

Evaluation data are often recorded at the same time as the nursing action. For example, following a urinary catheterization, the nurse may already have evaluation data regarding the urine obtained and the client's discomfort. In many instances, however, evaluation data are recorded later, e.g., pain relief can be expected roughly 30 minutes after the subcutaneous administration of 10 mg of morphine sulfate.

Nursing actions are often communicated verbally as well as in writing. When a client's health is changing rapidly, the charge nurse and/or the physician may want to be kept up to date with verbal reports. Verbal reports are given to another nurse or other health professionals. Nurses also make verbal reports regarding clients at a change of shift and upon a client's discharge to another unit or health agency. For additional information about assessing the client's response, see Chapter 15; for information on recording and reporting, see Chapter 30.

Implementing Skills

Three skills are needed to implement nursing actions: cognitive, intrapersonal, and technical skills.

Cognitive

The necessary **cognitive** (intellectual) skills for implementing are problem solving, decision making, critical thinking, and creativity. They are crucial to safe, intelligent nursing care. Problem solving and decision making are discussed in Chapter 10.

Critical thinking is a pattern of thinking based on knowledge, experience, and the abilities to conceptualize and analyze relationships. To conceptualize means to form a concept. A **concept** is an abstract idea generalized from particular instances. Critical thinking involves organizing information, picking out relevant information, relating, conceptualizing, and making judgments. Critical thinking enables nurses to make decisions quickly without bias. Critical thinking, like problem solving, is directed thinking in contrast to associative thinking. **Directed thinking** has a goal and is purposeful. A person uses this type of thinking when trying to form a judgment. For example, when determining whether a client would be wise to sit in a chair another 15 minutes, a nurse uses directed thinking. In this example, the goal is a decision about the client, and the data involve relevant information about the client's health and health problems. **Associative thinking**, by contrast, has very little direction and often involves random thoughts. An example is daydreaming.

The ability to think critically is learned. Infants cannot think critically; they do not have the knowledge or experience, and their nervous systems are not sufficiently mature. As people grow and develop, they attempt to deal with new experiences largely through trial and error. As a result, individuals build up a repertoire of thinking skills. With increasing knowledge and experience, individuals enlarge their repertoire and test and modify their skills. The individual learns to think critically.

Creativity, often called creative thinking, is also a form of directed thinking. **Creative thinking** is establishing new relationships and new concepts, solving problems innovatively. When thinking creatively, the individual cannot always weigh alternatives or establish the logic behind all actions. For nurses, planning nursing strategies and changing nursing actions provide opportunities for creative thinking. Creative thinking helps nurses change a nursing activity efficiently.

Interpersonal

Interpersonal skills are all the activities people use when communicating directly with one another. They may be verbal and nonverbal. See Chapter 27. The effectiveness of a nursing action often depends largely on the nurse's ability to communicate with others. Even when giving a medication to a client, the nurse needs to understand the client and in turn to be understood. A nurse who is delegating a nursing action also needs to be understood.

Interpersonal skills are necessary for all nursing activities: caring, comforting, referring, counseling, and supporting are just a few. They include conveying knowledge, attitudes, feelings, interest, and appreciation of the client's cultural values and life-style. Before nurses can be highly skilled in interpersonal relations, they must have self-awareness and sensitivity to others. See Chapter 27.

Technical

Technical skills are "hands-on" skills. Manipulating equipment, giving injections, bandaging, moving, lifting, and repositioning clients all require technical skills. Such skills are also called procedures or psychomotor skills. The term *psychomotor* includes the intrapersonal component, e.g., the communication need of the client. Technical skills require considerable knowledge on the part of the nurse, including the principles behind the steps of the procedure, knowledge about equipment and supplies, and in some instances knowledge as to when the procedure is required. Knowledge of the principles underlying the procedure is of particular importance because it enables the nurse to adapt a procedure to the individual client safely. For example, if a female client cannot turn on her left side for an enema, the nurse can adjust the client's position and still administer the enema effectively if the nurse understands the position of the rectum and large intestine in the body and the flow of fluids by gravity. When the nurse carries out procedures requiring technical skills, it is important that the nurse make significant assessments of the client *before* and *during* the procedure. It is equally important to evaluate the effectiveness of the procedure.

Before a nurse initiates any procedure, it is necessary to relate her or his own knowledge and competence to the needs of the client. Sometimes assistance is necessary to prevent undue stress on the client and to ensure that the procedure is both safe and effective. Technical skills require knowledge and, frequently, manual dexterity.

The number of technical skills expected of a nurse has increased greatly in recent years. Acute care hospitals have become highly technological. Because of the trend toward increased use of technology, humanizing nursing has become a recognized need for clients. See Chapter 2.

The nurse who documents critical observations in the client's record, but who does not communicate verbally to ensure the information is received, will not be insulated against liability in the event that the client suffers harm. (Cushing 1982, p. 1597)

Implementing Activities

To implement nursing care, the nurse generally performs the following activities: communicating, caring, teaching, counseling, managing, and using technical skills. The last is discussed earlier in this chapter.

Communicating

Effective communication is an essential element of all helping professions, including nursing. Communication shapes relationships between nurses and clients, nurses and support persons, and nurses and colleagues. It plays a role in every action the nurse undertakes. The communication process, listening and responding skills, and ways to establish helping relationships are discussed in detail in Chapter 27.

The nurse communicates the nursing strategies planned and implemented for each client to other health care personnel. Planned nursing strategies are written on the client's care plan (see Chapter 13). Once the strategies are implemented, the nurse documents them on the client's record. Assessment findings, procedures implemented, and the client's responses are recorded. Pertinent information is communicated verbally by nurses at change of shift reports, when client's are transferred to another unit, at client rounds, and when clients are discharged to another health care agency. This type of communication needs to be concise, clear, and relevant. See Chapter 30 for details of reporting and recording.

Caring

The terms *nursing care* and *caring* have been used by nurses for more than a century. Leininger (1984, p. 3) states: "Care is the essence and the central, unifying, and dominant domain to characterize nursing: it is an essential human need for the full development, health maintenance, and survival of human beings in all world cultures . . . yet care has not received the same degree of attention by professionals and the public as cure." In an address to the 75th Annual Registered Nurses' Association of Nova Scotia, Benner (1984, p. 3) made this statement: "Caring is often frankly curative because it facilitates healing." Leininger (1984, p. 6) says that there can be no curing without caring, but there may be caring without curing.

Definitions and a clear understanding of the terms *care* and *caring* have been lacking. Systematic research is needed to describe caring behaviors, values, and practices in nursing so that this knowledge can be incorporated into nursing education and practice areas. Some definitions of care and caring are provided in Table 14–1.

In her transcultural care theory, Leininger (1984, pp. 5–6) points out that human caring, although a universal phenomenon, varies among cultures in its expressions, processes, and patterns; it is largely culturally derived. These differences in caring values and behaviors lead to differences in the expectations of those seeking care. For example, cultures that perceive illness primarily as a per-

Table 14–1 Definitions and Descriptions of Care and Caring

Delores Gaut	There is not clear-cut rule for the use of *caring* in common language, but the family of meanings is related to the notion of caring in three senses: (a) attention to or concern about; (b) responsibility for or providing for; and (c) regard or fondness for. The term *caring* in both lay and scholarly literature is found in discussions of: (a) certain feelings or dispositions within a person; (b) the doing of certain activities that seem to identify that person as a caring individual; or (c) a combination of both attitudes and actions in which caring about the other disposes the one to carry out activities for the other. Caring is intentional activity.*
Madeleine Leininger	*Care* in a generic sense refers to those assistive, supportive, or facilitative acts toward or for another individual or group with evident or anticipated needs to ameliorate or improve a human condition or lifeway. *Caring* refers to the direct (or indirect) nurturant and skillful activities, processes, and decisions related to assisting people in such a manner that reflects behavioral attributes which are empathetic, supportive, compassionate, protective, succorant, educational, and others dependent upon the needs, problems, values, and goals of the individual or group being assisted. *Professional caring* embodies the cognitive and deliberate goals, processes, and acts of professional persons or groups providing assistance to others, and expressing attitudes and actions of concern for them, in order to support their well-being, alleviate undue discomforts, and meet obvious or anticipated needs. *Scientific caring* refers to those judgments and acts of helping others based on tested or verified knowledge. *Humanistic caring* refers to the creative, intuitive, or cognitive helping process for individuals or groups based upon philosophic, phenomenologic, and objective and subjective experiential feelings and acts of assisting others.†
M. Mayeroff	We sometimes speak as if caring did not require knowledge, as if caring for someone, for example, were simply a matter of good intentions or warm regard. . . . To care for someone, I must know many things. I must know, for example, who the other is, what his powers and limitations are, what his needs are, and what is conducive to his growth; I must know how to respond to his needs and what my own powers and limitations are. Caring is an important means for self-growth. To help another person grow is at least to help him to care for something or someone apart from himself, and it involves encouraging and assisting him to find and create of his own in which he is able to care. Also, it is to help that other person to come to care for himself, and by becoming responsive to his own needs, to care and to become responsible for his own life.‡
Jean Watson	Human caring in nursing is not just an emotion, concern, attitude, or benevolent desire. Caring connotes a personal response. Human caring involves values, a will and a commitment to care, knowledge, caring actions, and consequences. All of human caring is related to intersubjective human responses to health-illness conditions; a knowledge of health-illness, environmental-personal interactions; a knowledge of the nurse caring process; self-knowledge; [and] knowledge of one's power and transaction limitations. The ideal and value of caring is a starting point, a stance, an attitude, which has to become a will, an intention, a commitment, and a conscious judgment that manifests itself in concrete acts. The most abstract characteristic of a caring person is that he or she is somehow responsive to a person as a unique individual, perceives the other's feelings, and sets apart one person from another from the ordinary. The uncaring person is by contrast insensitive to another person as a unique individual, [not] perceptive of the other's feelings, and does not necessarily distinguish one person from another in any significant way.§

Sources:
*D. Gaut. A theoretic description of caring as action. In M. Leininger, *Care: The essence of nursing and health* (Thorofare, N.J.: Charles B. Slack, 1984) pp. 27–28.
†M. Leininger. *Care: The essence of nursing and health* (Thorofare, N.J.: Charles B. Slack, 1984) pp. 4, 46.
‡M. Mayeroff. *On caring* (New York: Harper and Row, 1971) p. 13.
§J. Watson. *Nursing: Human science and human care—A theory of nursing* (Norwalk, Conn.: Appleton-Century-Crofts, 1985) pp. 29, 31, 32, 34.

sonal and internal body experience—caused by physical, genetic, and intrabody stresses—tend to use more medications and physical techniques than cultures that view illness as an extrapersonal experience.

Leininger identifies many caring and nursing care constructs. Examples are comfort, compassion, concern, coping behaviors, empathy, enabling, involvement, health acts (consultative, instructive, maintenance), love, nurturance, presence, sharing, tenderness, touching, and trust. Each of these constructs has many subdescriptions. Leininger believes the goal of health care personnel should be to work toward an understanding of care and the health of different cultures so that each culture's care, values, beliefs, and life-styles will be the basis for providing culture-specific care.

Caring Factors

Watson (1979, pp. 10–208; 1985, p. 75) identifies ten caring factors in nursing, as follows:

1. Forming a humanistic-altruistic system of values. This factor relates to satisfaction through giving and extending the sense of self. Although the values are learned early in life, they can be greatly influenced by educators.
2. Instilling faith and hope. Feelings of faith and hope promote wellness by helping the client to adopt health-seeking behaviors. By developing an effective nurse-client relationship, the nurse facilitates feelings of optimism, hope, and trust.
3. Cultivating sensitivity to one's self and others. The nurse who is able to recognize and express her or his feelings is better able to allow others to express theirs.
4. Developing a helping-trust (human care) relationship. This kind of relationship involves effective communication, empathy, and nonpossessive warmth. It promotes and accepts the expression of positive and negative feelings.
5. Expressing positive and negative feelings. Sharing feelings of sorrow, love, and pain is a risk-taking experience. The nurse must be prepared for negative feelings.
6. Using a creative problem-solving caring process. Caring linked to the nursing process contributes to a creative problem-solving approach to nursing care.
7. Promoting interpersonal teaching-learning. This factor separates caring from curing and shifts responsibility for wellness to the client.
8. Providing a supportive, protective, or corrective mental, physical, sociocultural, and spiritual environment. Because the client can experience change in any aspect of the internal and external environments, the nurse must assess and facilitate the client's abilities to cope with mental, emotional, and physical changes.
9. Assisting with the gratification of human needs. Caring is conveyed by recognizing and attending to the physical, emotional, social, and spiritual needs of the client.
10. Allowing for existential-phenomenologic-spiritual forces. Phenomenology describes data of the immediate situation that help people understand the phenomena in question. The **phenomenal field** is the individual's frame of reference; this field can be known only to the person. Existential psychology is a science of human existence that employs the method of phenomenologic analysis. Persons possess three spheres of being: mind, body, and soul (Watson 1985, p. 54). Allowing for expression of these forces leads to a better understanding of self and others.

Conditions for Caring

Gaut (1984, pp. 32–36) considers caring as a purposeful human activity requiring an action description. She outlines three conditions for caring. Caring is looked at in the sense of "providing for." The nurse must:

1. Have awareness of a person's need for care and knowledge that certain actions could be taken to improve the situations. To gain awareness, the nurse must demonstrate "wide-awakeness"—an attitude of full attention to life and its requirements (Schutz 1975, p. 69). It is a passive, not an active, attitude that is conveyed by the nurse who fails to notice that something is wrong and performs tasks automatically. The wide-awake nurse watches for and identifies distressing situations requiring interventions.
2. Using that knowledge, choose and implement an action and intend the action to be a means for bringing about a positive change.
3. Judge the positive change solely on the basis of the welfare of the other person, not of self or agency.

Watson (1985, p. 32) adds another condition: There must be an underlying value and moral commitment to care and a willingness to care or act.

The Power of Caring

Benner (1984, pp. 209–15) identifies six different qualities of power associated with caring:

1. Transformative power. With this power, the nurse can help the client to regain a sense of control and to participate actively in situations he or she thought were beyond his or her control. For example, clients often need help to realize that they have a choice and can abandon whatever role they wish.
2. Integrative caring. Caring can also reintegrate the individual into his or her own social world. For example, when prolonged or permanent disability is inevitable, the nurse can help clients to continue with meaningful life activities despite their limitations.
3. Advocacy power. Clients and families frequently need the nurse to act on their behalf. They may be confused

by medical jargon, or their understanding may be hampered by anxiety or fear. The nurse can interpret necessary information to the client and to the physician. Advocacy removes obstacles; it is a standing alongside and enabling of the client.

4. Healing power. To establish a healing relationship and climate, the nurse (a) mobilizes hope in herself or himself, the staff, and the client; (b) finds an interpretation or understanding of the situation (e.g., illness, pain, fear, or other stressful emotion) that is acceptable and clarifying to the client; and (c) helps the client find social, emotional, and spiritual support. A healing relationship helps the client to mobilize internal and external resources by bringing hope, confidence, and trust.

5. Participative/affirmative power. By participating, a nurse finds meanings in specific events. She or he may experience pain but may also experience strength and affirmation. A detached, avoiding approach usually offers only frail protection and develops no positive inner resources.

6. Problem solving. Caring is the prerequisite for creative problem solving. The most difficult problems require perceptual ability as well as conceptual reasoning, and perception requires involvement and attentiveness. Caring provides a sensitivity to cues that allows persons to search for solutions and even makes it possible to recognize solutions when they are not directly sought.

Teaching

Teaching is an interactive process between a teacher and one or more learners in which specific learning objectives or desired behavior changes are achieved (Redman 1984, p. 15). The focus of the behavior change is usually the acquiring of new knowledge or technical skills. The teaching process has four components—assessing, planning, implementing, and evaluating—which can be reviewed as parallel to the parts of the nursing process. In the assessment phase, the nurse determines the client's learning needs and readiness to learn. During planning, specific learning goals and teaching strategies are set. During implementation, teaching strategies are enacted, and, during evaluation, learning is measured. See Chapter 29 for detailed information about the teaching/learning process.

Many factors have increased the need for health teaching by nurses. Today, there is a new emphasis on health maintenance rather than on treatment alone; as a result, people desire and require more knowledge. Shortened hospital stays mean that the clients must be prepared to manage convalescence at home. The increase in long-term illnesses and disabilities often requires that both the client and the family understand the illness and its treatment.

Counseling

Counseling is the process of helping a client to recognize and cope with stressful psychologic or social problems, to develop improved interpersonal relationships, and to promote personal growth. It involves providing emotional, intellectual, and psychologic support. In contrast to the psychotherapist, who counsels individuals with identified problems, the nurse counsels primarily healthy individuals with normal adjustment difficulties. The focus is on helping the person develop new attitudes, feelings, and behaviors rather than on promoting intellectual growth. The client is encouraged to look at alternative behaviors, recognize the choices, and develop a sense of control.

Counseling can be provided on a one-to-one basis or in groups. Often nurses lead group counseling sessions. For example, on the individual level, the nurse counsels clients who need to decrease activity levels, stop smoking, lose weight, accept changes in body image, or cope with impending death. At the group level, the nurse may be a leader, member or resource person in any self-help group in which she or he assumes the role of structuring activities and fostering a climate conducive to group interaction and productive work.

Obviously, counseling requires therapeutic communication skills. In addition, the nurse must be a skilled leader; she or he must be able to analyze a situation, synthesize information and experiences, and evaluate. the progress and productivity of the individual or group. The nurse must also be willing to model and teach desired behaviors, to be genuine in dealing with people, and to demonstrate interest and caring in the welfare of others. The nurse-leader needs an inventive mind, a flexible attitude, and a sense of humor to deal with the varied experiences of people. Essential to leadership abilities is self-awareness, self-assurance, and self-understanding. Group dynamics and leadership are discussed in detail in Chapter 28.

Managing

The nurse manages the nursing care of individuals, families, and communities. The nurse-manager also delegates nursing activities to ancillary workers and other nurses, and supervises and evaluates their performance. Managing requires knowledge about organizational structure and dynamics, authority and accountability, leadership, change theory, advocacy, delegation, and supervision and evaluation.

Organizational Structure

Nurses function in various types of organizations. Some are autocratic; one person has primary knowledge and power, and other persons are subordinate. Some are bureaucratic; the control is through policy, jobs are structured, and actions are compartmentalized. Others decentralize control and emphasize self-direction and self-discipline of members. Still others can be viewed as components of systems that interact interdependently and adapt dynamically to change. This organization is particularly useful for the nurse who manages the care of individuals, families, and communities. On a larger scale, the nurse-manager must work in the organizational framework of the employing agency.

Authority and Accountability

Authority is the right to act and command. It is an integral component of managing. Authority is conveyed through leadership actions; it is determined largely by the situation, and it is always associated with responsibility and accountability.

The basis of accountability is that people with authority must account for how they use it. **Accountability** means being responsible for one's actions and accepting the consequences of one's behavior. Accountability can be viewed within a hierarchical systems framework, starting at the individual level, through the institutional/professional level, and then to the societal level (Sullivan and Decker 1985, p. 18). At the individual or client level, accountability is reflected in the nurse's ethical decision-making processes, competence, commitment, and integrity. At the institutional level, it is reflected in the statement of philosophy and objectives of the nursing department and nursing audits. At the professional level, it is reflected in standards of practice developed by national or provincial nursing associations. At the societal level, it is reflected in legislated nurse practice acts.

Change Agent

As a manager, the nurse acts as a change agent. A **change agent** is any individual or group operating to change the status quo in a system so that the individuals involved must relearn how to perform their role(s) (Zaltman and Duncan 1977, p. 17). By using the nursing process, the nurse promotes change in the health of clients. The nurse as a teacher or counselor facilitates change in the client's knowledge, skill, feelings, and attitudes. On a larger scale, the nurse can be instrumental in promoting change at the institutional, professional, or societal levels. See Chapter 6 for further information.

Client Advocate

An **advocate** is one who pleads the cause of another or argues or pleads for a cause or proposal. The nurse acts as a client advocate by informing clients of their rights, by making sure they have the necessary knowledge to make informed decisions, and by supporting clients in the decisions they make. See Chapter 9 for further information.

Delegating gets the task—but not the responsibility—off your back. The act of delegating creates a responsibility to supervise, even if the person you delegated to would normally be considered your equal. (Rabinow 1982, p. 49)

Delegating

Because it is often impossible to provide all of the nursing care needed by a group of clients, the nurse as a delegator must assign aspects of the client's care to other nursing personnel. Delegation is a major tool in making the most efficient use of time. **Delegation** is the sharing of responsibility and authority with others and holding them accountable for performance (Sullivan and Decker 1985, p. 168). Delegation is a high-level skill. The nurse as a delegator must have the following information:

1. Needs of the client and family
2. Goals of the client
3. Nursing activity that can help the client meet the goals
4. Skills and knowledge of various nursing personnel

The nurse delegator must also determine how many nursing personnel are needed. This information may be indicated on the client's records. Other sources of this information are the client, the charge nurse, other nursing personnel, and the nurse-delegator's own judgment. For example, without help one nurse may not be strong or skillful enough to turn an obese client. Nurses may also require assistance to give clients care quickly in certain situations. Assistance may also be necessary to ensure the client's safety; for example, a nurse administering an intramuscular injection to a 3-year-old might need help to prevent injury to the child. If in doubt, nurses should always obtain aid to safeguard the client.

Once a nurse-delegator establishes that assistance is required, it is important to identify (a) what type of help is needed, e.g., lifting or holding; (b) how long help is required, (c) when it is required, and (d) what assistance is available. The nurse must arrange for assistance, usually by asking the appropriate person on the unit, before commencing the nursing activity.

Delegation does not mean that a nurse-delegator never gets involved in direct client care. Often the nurse-delegator performs nursing activities appropriate to her or his knowledge and skills.

An important aspect of delegation is the development of the potential of nursing personnel. By knowing the backgrounds, experiences, knowledge, skills, and strengths of each person, a nurse can delegate responsibilities that help develop their competencies.

Supervising and Evaluating the Nursing Activities of Others

Nursing personnel to whom aspects of care have been delegated need to be supervised and evaluated. The amount of supervision required is highly variable, depending on the knowledge and skills of each person. The nurse-delegator contributes to this evaluation process, since she or he is the person who assigns the activity and observes the performance. Because individual motivation varies, the nurse-delegator needs to realize that not all persons perform equally. Thus, the nurse should evaluate assigned personnel according to standards of performance stated in job descriptions rather than by comparing one person to another. It is essential, too, that the nurse-delegator realize people require ongoing feedback about the care they give. Feedback should be given in an objective manner and include both positive and negative input.

Guidelines for Implementing Nursing Strategies

1. Nursing actions are related to the knowledge and skill of the nurse. If they are to be safe for the client, nursing activities must be purposeful and have a scientific basis.
2. Nursing actions are adapted to the individual. A client's beliefs, values, age, health status, and environment are factors that can affect a nursing action.
3. Nursing actions should always be safe. Nurses and clients need to take precautions to prevent injury. For example, when changing a sterile dressing, the nurse practices sterile technique to prevent infection; when turning a client, the nurse protects the client's skin from abrasions, which could also lead to infection.
4. Nursing actions often require teaching, supportive, and comfort components. These independent nursing activities can often enhance the effectiveness of a specific nursing action.
5. Nursing actions should always be holistic. The nurse must always view the client as a whole and consider his or her responses in that light.
6. Nursing actions should respect the dignity of the client and enhance his or her self-esteem. Providing privacy and encouraging the client to make his or her own decisions are ways of respecting dignity and enhancing self-esteem.
7. The client's active participation in implementing nursing actions should be encouraged as health permits. Active participation enhances the client's sense of independence and control. Clients vary in the degree of participation they desire. Some clients want total involvement in their care, while others prefer little involvement. The amount of involvement desired is often related to the severity of the illness, the number of stressors, as well as the patient's energy, fear, understanding of the illness, and understanding of the intervention. For instance, a female client with a colostomy who is worried about her appearance may not want to be involved in care of the colostomy right after surgery.
8. Nursing actions resulting from a physician's order (dependent actions) must be carried out accurately unless the nurse believes the order is unsafe for the client. Actions considered unsafe for a client must be discussed with the responsible nurse and/or physician.

Chapter Highlights

- Implementing is putting planned nursing strategies into action.
- The client is always the primary participant in implementing the nursing care plan.
- Reassessing and validating the nursing care plan occur continuously during the implementing phase.
- Cognitive, interpersonal, and technical skills are used to implement nursing strategies.
- Cognitive skills include problem solving, decision making, critical thinking, and creativity.
- Creative thinking helps the nurse and the client to establish innovative nursing actions.
- Implementing activities are communicating, caring, teaching, counseling, managing, and using technical skills.
- Communication is essential for all nursing activities and for establishing relationships.
- The implementing phase of the nursing process is terminated with the documentation of the nursing activities.
- All nursing activities, all assessment data, and all client responses to the nursing activities require documentation.
- Teaching plays an increasing role in most nursing activities.
- Counseling is a helping process designed to promote personal growth and to help the client cope with stress; it requires therapeutic communication skills and leadership skills on the nurse's part.

- Managing nursing interventions requires knowledge of organizational structure, authority, accountability, leadership, change, advocacy, delegation, and supervision and evaluation.
- Nurses are accountable for all their nursing actions.

Suggested Readings

Benner, P. Spring 1983. Uncovering the knowledge embedded in clinical practice. *Image* 2::36–41.
Benner describes a study of the nursing knowledge that accrues over time in clinical nursing practice. The paper examines the difference between practical and theoretical knowledge and provides examples of competence identified from the study of nursing practice. Benner describes aspects of practical knowledge and strategies for preserving and extending practice knowledge.

Cushing, M. October 1982. Failure to communicate. *American Journal of Nursing* 82:1597–98.
Cushing gives examples of clinical situations in which the nurse failed to communicate or delayed communication about essential client findings. As a result, the nurse was held liable.

Rabinow, J. September/October 1982. Delegating safely within the law. *Nursing Life* 2:48–49.
This lawyer says that delegation poses legal risks since law courts look closely not only at what the nurse did but also at what she or he delegated. Rabinow discusses appropriate tasks to delegate, appropriate persons to delegate to, and legal responsibilities after the nurse delegates. A topic box includes what the nurse can safely delegate to a licensed practical nurse (LPN) as well as what the nurse can and cannot delegate in some states and provinces.

Selected References

American Nurses' Association. 1980. Nursing. *A social policy statement.* Kansas City, Mo.: A.N.A. Pub. no. NP–63 35M 12/80.

Benner, P. E. June 5, 1984. *The primacy and power of caring in health promotion and healing.* Lecture given at the 75th Annual Registered Nurses' Association of Nova Scotia.

Bradley, J. C. March/April 1983. Nurses' attitudes toward dimensions of nursing practice. *Nursing Research* 32:110–14.

Carpenito, L. J. 1983. *Nursing diagnosis, application to clinical practice.* Philadelphia: J. B. Lippincott Co.

Cushing, M. October 1982. The legal side: Failure to communicate. *American Journal of Nursing* 82:1597.

DeYoung, L. 1985. *Dynamics of nursing,* 5th ed. St. Louis: C. V. Mosby Co.

Gaut, D. 1984. A theoretic description of caring as action. In Leininger, M. *Care: The essence of nursing and health.* Thorofare, N.J.: Charles B. Slack, pp. 27–44.

La Monica, E. L. 1985. *The humanistic nursing process.* Belmont, Calif.: Wadsworth Health Sciences.

Leddy, S., and Pepper, J. M. 1985. *Conceptual bases of professional nursing.* Philadelphia: J. B. Lippincott Co.

Leininger, M. 1984. *Care: The essence of nursing and health.* Thorofare, N.J.: Charles B. Slack.

Marriner, A. 1983. *The nursing process: A scientific approach to nursing care.* 2d ed. St. Louis: C. V. Mosby Co.

———. 1986. *Nursing theorists and their work.* St. Louis: C. V. Mosby Co.

Mundinger, M. O. 1980. *Autonomy in nursing.* Germantown, Md.: Aspen Systems Corp.

Rabinow, J. September/October 1982. Delegating safely within the law. *Nursing Life* 2:48–49.

Redman, B. K. 1984. *The process of patient education.* 5th ed. St. Louis: C. V. Mosby Co.

Schutz, A. 1975. *On phenomenology and social relations.* Chicago: University of Chicago Press.

Sullivan, E. J., and Decker, P. J. 1985. *Effective management in nursing.* Menlo Park, Calif.: Addison-Wesley Publishing Co.

Watson, J. 1979. *Nursing: The philosophy and science of caring.* Boston: Little, Brown.

———. 1985. *Nursing: Human science and human care—A theory of nursing.* Norwalk, Conn.: Appleton-Century-Crofts.

Yura, H., and Walsh, M. B. 1983. *The nursing process: Assessing, planning, implementing, evaluating.* 4th ed. Norwalk, Conn.: Appleton-Century-Crofts.

Zaltman, G., and Duncan, R. 1977. *Strategies for planned change.* New York: John Wiley and Sons.

CHAPTER 15

Evaluating

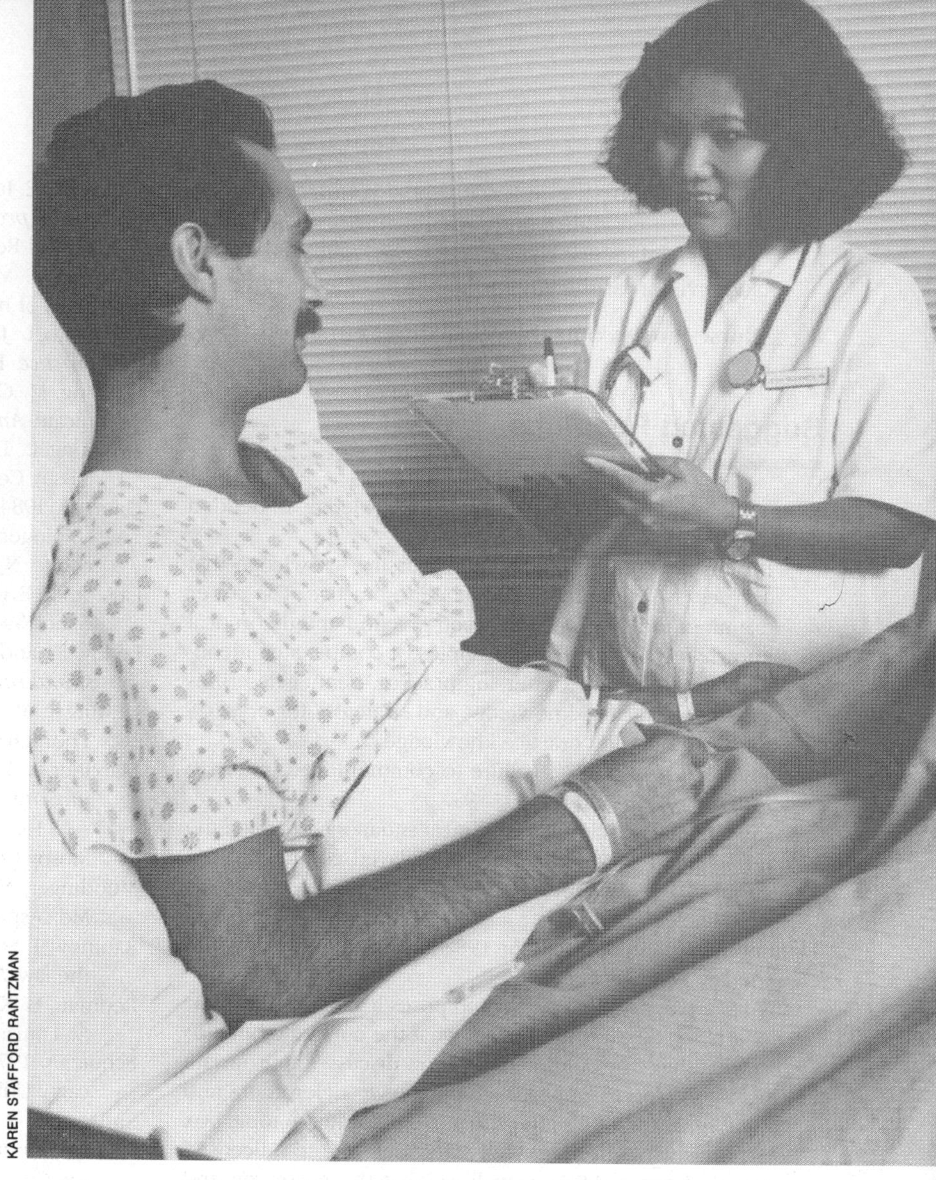

Contents

Objectives

1. Understand essential facts about the evaluation phase of the nursing process.
   1.1 Define listed terms.
   1.2 Describe five components of the evaluation process.
   1.3 Describe the steps involved in reexamining the client's care plan both when goals are met and when they are not met.
2. Appreciate aspects of evaluating the quality of nursing care.
   2.1 Differentiate quality assessment from quality assurance.
   2.2 Describe three approaches to quality evaluation.
   2.3 Identify essential steps in developing tools to evaluate quality care.
   2.4 Identify various methods used to evaluate nursing care.

Terms

audit
concurrent audit
criteria (of nursing care)
evaluate
nursing audit
nursing standards
outcome criteria
peer review
quality assessment
quality assurance
quality assurance criteria
reexamining (reevaluating)
reliable criterion
retrospective audit
standards
valid criterion

Definition of Evaluation

To evaluate is to judge or to appraise. In the context of the nursing process, evaluation is the fifth and last phase. Here, to **evaluate** means to identify whether or to what degree the client's goals have been met. Evaluation is an exceedingly important aspect of the nursing process because conclusions drawn from the evaluation determine whether the nursing interventions can be terminated or must be reviewed or changed.

Evaluating is a concurrent and a terminal process: It is concurrent in that the nurse normally evaluates during the implementing phase of the process. How is the client reacting to this nursing action? Is the reaction expected or unexpected? At this stage, the nurse may change a nursing action to help the client meet his or her goal. It is a terminal process because after the nurse completes the nursing activity, she or he evaluates whether the client's goals have been met. Often the time frame (if stated) in the outcome criteria is used.

Evaluating is a purposeful and organized activity. Through evaluating, nurses accept responsibility for their actions, indicate interest in the results of the nursing actions, and demonstrate a desire not to perpetuate ineffective actions but to adopt more effective ones.

Process of Evaluating

The evaluation process has five components:

1. Identifying the **outcome criteria** (standards for measuring success) that will be used to measure achievement of the goals
2. Gathering data related to the identified criteria
3. Comparing the data collected with the identified criteria and judging whether the goals have been attained
4. Relating nursing actions to the outcomes
5. Reexamining the client's care plan
6. Modifying the care plan

Identifying Outcome Criteria

The identification of outcome criteria used to evaluate the client's response to nursing care is discussed in Chapter 13. See Table 13–2 on page 272. Criteria serve two purposes: They establish the kind of evaluative data that need to be collected, and they provide a standard against which the data are judged. For example, the goal "Client's urinary elimination pattern will be maintained" does not tell the nurse what data to collect while caring for the client. When these criteria are added, however, any nurse caring for the client knows what data to collect:

> Daily fluid intake will be not less than 2500 ml.
>
> Urinary output will be in balance with fluid intake, and residual urine will be less than 100 ml.

Criteria that are clearly stated, precise, and measurable guide the next step of the evaluation process: data collection.

Collecting Data

Data are collected so that conclusions can be drawn about whether goals have been reached. The nurse collects data in relation to the specified criteria, either by observation, direct communication, and purposeful listening or from reports of other health professionals.

Collection of both objective and subjective data may be necessary. Objective, measurable data are preferred for evaluation purposes; for example, "Respirations increased from 12 to 16 breaths per minute, and pulse rate increased from 70 to 90 beats per minute after client walked around the corridor." However, the nurse often needs to collect subjective data and some objective data that require interpretation. Examples of objective data requiring interpretation are the degree of tissue turgor of a dehydrated client or the degree of restlessness of a client with pain. Examples of subjective data include complaints of nausea or pain by the client.

When objective data requires interpretation, the nurse may obtain the views of one or more other nurses to substantiate changes. When subjective data are required, the nurse must rely upon either (a) the client's statements (e.g., "My pain is worse now than it was after breakfast") or (b) objective indicators of the subjective data, even though these indicators may require interpretation (e.g., decreased restlessness, decreased pulse and respiratory rates, and relaxed facial muscles as indicators of pain relief). Data collected must be recorded concisely and accurately to facilitate the third part of the evaluating process. Flowsheets and problem-oriented medical records in the SOAP format (discussed in Chapter 30) are recording aids.

Judging Goal Achievement

If the first two parts of the evaluation process have been carried out effectively, determining whether a goal has been achieved is relatively simple. Both the nurse and the client play active roles in this. The data collected are compared with established criteria. Did the client drink 3000 ml of fluid in 24 hours? Did the client walk unassisted the specified distance per day?

There are three possible outcomes of evaluation:

1. The goal was met; i.e., the client responded as expected.
2. The goal was partially met; i.e., a short-term goal was achieved, but the long-term goal was not.
3. The goal was not met

See Table 15–1 for evaluation examples of Mr. Joe Smith's outcome criteria. For information about the nursing activities related to these outcomes, see the section "Reexamining the Client's Care Plan," later in this chapter.

Relating the Nursing Actions to the Client Outcomes

The fourth aspect of the evaluating process is determining whether the nursing actions had any relation to the outcome. It should never be assumed that a nursing action was the cause of or the only factor in meeting, partially meeting, or not meeting a goal. For example, Mrs. Sophi Ringdale was obese and needed to lose 14 kg (30 lb). When the nurse and client drew up a care plan, one outcome criterion was "Loses 1.3 kg (3 lb) by 4/7/00." A nursing strategy in the care plan was "Explain how to plan and prepare a 900-calorie diet." On 4/7/00, the client weighed herself and had lost 1.8 kg (4 lb). The goal had been met, in fact, exceeded. It is easy to assume that the nursing strategy was highly effective. However, it is important to collect more data before drawing that conclusion. Upon questioning the client, the nurse could find any of the following: (a) the client planned a 900-calorie diet and prepared and ate the food; (b) the client planned a 900-calorie diet but did not prepare the correct food; (c) the client did not understand how to plan a 900-calorie diet, so she did not bother with it. If the first possibility is found to be true, the nurse can safely judge that the nursing strategy "Explain how to plan and prepare a 900-calorie diet" was effective in helping the client lose weight. However, if the nurse learns that either (b) or (c) actually happened, then it must be assumed that the nursing strategy did not affect the outcome. The next step for the nurse is to collect data about what the client actually did to lose weight. The nurse should add these data to the assessment data in the care plan and examine the plan (see the next

---

Nurses are accountable and responsible for their own actions, and legal and moral accountability is an aspect of professional practice. (Leddy and Pepper 1985, p. 44)

---

section). It is important to establish the relationship (or lack thereof) of the nursing actions to the outcomes.

Reexamining the Client's Care Plan

Evaluating goal achievement provides the feedback necessary to determine if the care plan was effective in resolving, reducing, or preventing the client's problems. It is then necessary for the nurse to reexamine all aspects of the care plan, i.e., all aspects of the nursing process, whether or not the goals have been met. Reexamining is a process of reassessing and replanning. See Table 15–1 for an example of evaluating goal achievement for Mr. Joe Smith.

When Goals Are Met

If a goal or goals have been met, one of the following decisions may be made:

1. The nurse may decide that the problem stated in the diagnosis no longer exists. In this instance, the nurse must document that the goal was met and that the care planned to meet this goal is discontinued. For example, a nursing diagnosis of "Activity intolerance related to prolonged bed rest" no longer applies if the client exhibits a decrease in anoxic signs from a specified level of increased activity. As another example, a nursing diagnosis of "Knowledge deficit related to administering insulin" may lead to the criterion "Will independently administer insulin daily using aseptic technique." The diagnosis no longer applies once the client meets this criterion. The nurse documents when goals are met and discontinues related nursing interventions by writing "goal met," dating and signing the care plan, and indicating that the nursing orders related to this problem are discontinued.
2. The nurse may decide that the problem still exists even though the goal was met. For example, if the criterion is "Client will ingest 3000 ml of fluid daily," and the goal is "Client's state of hydration will be maintained," nursing interventions need to continue even though the goal and criterion have been met.

When a long-term goal is met by achieving short-term, progressive goals, the client's problem often remains even though the short-term goals are met. A progressive measurement scale outlined by Inzer and Aspinall (1981, p. 181) illustrates this point:

Goal: To increase range of motion of right arm

Criteria: Can raise arm straight in front
Can raise arm to side
Can raise arm straight overhead
Can raise arm and reach to back

Step 1	Step 2	Step 3	Step 4	Step 5
Does none of above	Does one of above	Does two of above	Does three of above	Does all of above

When Goals are not Met

When goals are not met or only partially met, the nurse needs to reexamine the client's database, nursing diagnoses statements, goal statements, and nursing strategies.

Database The nurse reviews the client's database to ensure it is complete and up to date. An incomplete or incorrect database influences all subsequent steps of the nursing process and care plan. In some instances, new data may invalidate the database, necessitating new nursing diagnoses, new goals, and new nursing actions.

Diagnostic statements If the database is incomplete, new diagnostic statements are required. If the database is complete, the nurse needs to analyze whether the problem was identified correctly and whether the nursing diagnoses are relevant to that database.

Goal statements If the nursing diagnostic statement is inaccurate and requires correcting, it is obvious that the goal statement needs revision. If the nursing diagnostic statement is appropriate, the nurse then checks that the goal statements are realistic and attainable. Unrealistic, unattainable goals require correction. The nurse should also determine whether priorities have changed and whether the client and nurse still agree on the priorities. For example, a priority for the nurse may be to increase the client's fluid intake, but a priority for the client may be to decrease intake because of nausea.

Nursing strategies Last, the nurse investigates whether the nursing strategies are related to the goals and whether the best nursing strategies were selected. If both the diagnoses and goals are appropriate, the nursing strategies selected may not have been the best ones to achieve the goal. Before selecting new strategies, the nurse should check whether the ordered nursing actions have been carried out. Other personnel may not have carried them out, either because the orders were unclear or because the orders were unreasonable in terms of such external constraints as money, staff, and equipment.

Modifying the Care Plan

When it is determined that the care plan needs revising, the nurse follows five steps:

1. Change the data in the assessment column to reflect the more recent findings. The new data should be dated

Table 15–1 Evaluating Goal Achievement for Mr. Joe Smith

Assessment Data	Diagnostic Statement	Goal
Hospitalized for cardiac catheterization and possible aortic valve replacement States family scared about illness Wants to see chaplain Wants family to visit Perceives son Tom as helpful Says is usually too busy to worry about things	Fear related to cardiac catheterization, possible heart surgery, and its outcome	Experience increased emotional comfort and feelings of control
Vital signs normal Heart rhythm regular Loud heart murmur (aortic area) Femoral pulses stronger than normal Absent pulses (popliteal, dorsalis pedis, posterior tibial) in left leg Left leg cooler than right leg Integument pink and intact	Alteration in peripheral tissue perfusion (left leg) related to impaired arterial circulation	Improve circulation to left leg and foot
Left hip replacement Movement slightly limited Joint stiffness Slight limp	Potential for injury (trauma) related to joint stiffness and limp from hip replacement surgery	Prevent injury
Shortness of breath Lacks energy to do daily chores Does not smoke	Activity intolerance related to shortness of breath and lack of energy secondary to decreased strength of cardiac contraction	Avoid performance of activities causing shortness of breath and excessive cardiac workload

Nursing Orders	Outcome Criteria	Evaluation
		Goal met
Establish a trusting relationship with the client and family Encourage client and family to express feelings and concerns Discuss the cardiac catheterization procedure and what is expected of him before and after the procedure Encourage conversation with another client who has recuperated from similar surgery	Verbalizes specific concerns Communicates thoughts clearly and logically Facial expressions, voice tone, and body posture correspond to verbal expressions of increased emotional comfort or feelings of control After instruction, describes the cardiac catheterization procedure and what is expected of him before and after the procedure	Verbalized concerns: "I'm worried about how my wife will support the family especially if anything bad happens during surgery." Asked questions about cardiac catheterization and surgery Nonverbal and verbal communication are congruent Described what to expect and what is expected of him before and after the cardiac catheterization procedure, e.g., "I know I will be taking a pill to help me relax before the procedure."
		Goal partially met
Consult with physician about exercise program, such as walking and range of motion exercises to hip, knee, and ankle Keep the extremity in a dependent position (i.e., lower than the heart) Use Doppler ultrasound stethoscope (DUS) to assess blood flow in left dorsalis pedis, posterior tibial, and popliteal arteries q2h Instruct client to keep his legs warm, e.g., by wearing warm socks, but discourage use of external heat	Skin intact, pink, and moist Skin temperature warm (as other foot) Left dorsalis pedis, posterior tibial, and popliteal pulses palpable and of same strength as corresponding right pulses Capillary refill of left toenails within 1 to 3 seconds	Skin of left foot and ankle intact but pale Skin temperature still cooler in left than right foot Left popliteal pulse palpable but weak Left dorsalis pedis and posterior tibial pulses not palpable Blood flow evident only by DUS Capillary refill in left toenails within 7 seconds
		Goal met
Closely assess ambulation and transfers during first few days Keep bed at lowest level Encourage client to request assistance to ambulate during the night Closely attend client or put side rails up when client is sedated	Gets in and out of bed and ambulates without falling or injuring self	Ambulated and got in and out of bed safely
		Goal met
Organize client care and provide undisturbed rest periods Discuss energy conservation methods, such as taking periodic rests Tell the client to reduce the intensity, duration, and frequency of activity if he experiences chest pain, shortness of breath, dizziness, or abnormal pulse and blood pressure after activity Monitor vitals signs q2h and report decreasing blood pressure, increasing heart rate, or increasing respiratory rate	Rests after meals No shortness of breath during activities Pulse rate and blood pressure remain stable at 80 bpm and 124/80 mm Hg	Rested after meals and activities Experienced no shortness of breath while performing ADL Pulse rate and blood pressure remained stable at 80 bpm and 124/80 mm Hg

and flagged in some way to indicate they are new. Follow agency practice: Some nurses use ink of a different color; others put a colored tab at the edge of the paper.

2. Revise the nursing diagnoses to reflect the new data. The new nursing diagnoses are also dated.
3. Revise the client's priorities, goals, and outcome criteria to reflect the new nursing diagnoses. These are also dated.
4. Establish new nursing strategies to correspond to the new nursing diagnoses. New nursing strategies may reflect increased or decreased need of the client for nursing care, scheduling changes, and rearrangement of nursing activities to group similar activities or to permit longer rest or activity periods for the client. For example, the nurse might assist a male client to walk after a rest period and before a meal so that the client can ambulate when he is rested and sit up for the meal if his health permits.
5. Change the outcome criteria to reflect the other changes in the plan. These changes should project the desired level of wellness indicated by the client. Criteria that apply to outdated nursing diagnoses should be deleted. See Table 15–2 on page 300.

Evaluating the Quality of Nursing Care

Over the past 30 years, there has been considerable work on the evaluation of the quality of nursing care to determine what good care is, whether the care nurses give is appropriate and effective, and whether the quality of care provided is good.

Evaluating the quality of nursing care is an essential part of professional accountability. Other terms used for this measurement are quality assessment and quality assurance. **Quality assessment** is an examination of services only; **quality assurance** implies that efforts are made to evaluate *and* ensure quality health care.

Historical Perspective

Evaluation of the quality of care is not a new concept. Florence Nightingale's *Notes on Hospitals,* published in 1859, included an evaluation of medical and nursing care. Since that time, evaluation has progressed through a number of stages. Initially, it focused on the environment, e.g., whether equipment was available at the time it was needed. Later, organizational standards in agencies were developed. For example, the ratio of nurses to clients was studied and evaluated in terms of clients' needs. From about 1952 on, the Joint Commission on Accreditation of Hospitals (JCAH) has surveyed hospitals. Objective criteria were applied to evaluate a client's record after discharge from the hospital. This was called a **retrospective audit. Retrospective** means relating to a past event, and **audit** means an examination or review of records. A **nursing audit** is a review of clients' charts to evaluate nursing competence or performance. In 1972 and 1973, the JCAH revised its standards to include the requirement that hospitals be subjected to medical and nursing audits before receiving accreditation.

In 1972, the United States government enacted the Bennett Amendment, which created the Professional Standards Review Organization (PSRO). This program was intended to evaluate the quality of health care partially through peer review. A **peer review** is an encounter between two persons equal in education, abilities, and qualifications, during which one person critically reviews the practices that the other has documented in a client's record. Nursing subsequently developed evaluation programs compatible with the PSRO. These evaluative processes may be **concurrent audits**, in that they review present practices.

Approaches to Quality Evaluation

Three aspects of care can be evaluated. Each has advantages and disadvantages.

The Structure in Which Nursing Takes Place

The structural approach focuses on the organization of the client care system, such as administrative and financial procedures that direct the provision of care, staffing patterns, management styles, availability of equipment, and physical facilities. Information about these support structures can be obtained easily. However, proper facilities do not necessarily mean good care.

The Process of Care

The focus of this approach is the nurse's actions, i.e., the performance of the caregiver in relation to the client's needs. This approach may be the most effective in determining the quality of care provided, but it is time-consuming and requires value judgments by appropriate clinical experts.

Outcomes of the Care Received

The focus of this approach is the client's health status, welfare, and satisfaction, or the results of care in terms of changes in the client. Its advantage is that outcomes may be easily observed, especially in relation to medical care, which focuses on disease entities. In nursing, however, outcomes are more difficult to determine since nursing takes a more holistic view of the client than medicine takes. Defining emotional, social, and behavioral outcomes is more complex than defining medical outcomes. In addition, client outcomes cannot be wholly attributed to nursing care. The client's own physical and psychologic mechanisms and contributions by family and other health professionals collectively produce outcomes. Timing can be another confounding factor if the outcome is measured at the time of discharge rather than later.

Tools and Methods for Measuring Quality Care

Measuring the quality of care is a complex task. Development of tools involves a series of steps (Wright 1984, pp. 457–61):

1. Defining and clarifying the nature of nursing.
2. Deciding what approach to take (structure, process, outcome).
3. Developing standards and criteria. **Standards** are optimum levels of care against which actual performance is compared. **Criteria** are indicators of the quality of nursing care or measures by which the nursing care is judged (Gallant and McLane 1979). An example of a standard and its criterion is:
   Standard IV: Each client has a written nursing care plan.
   Criteria: The nursing care plan is: initiated within 24 hours of admission; based on information from the profile and problem-solving plan. . . ; a prescriptive plan of nursing care; and reviewed regularly and modified according to the client's needs (Mackie and Welsh 1982, p. 1757).
   Laing and Nish (1981, p. 23) state that when choosing criteria and standards for outcome, process, and structure, one must ask two questions:

   > "What aspects of care are to be evaluated?"
   >
   > "What is the acceptable level of performance for each aspect of care?"

   For example:
   Criterion: Hydration
   Standard for client outcome
   Retains oral fluid intake of at least 1000 ml per day.
   Standard for nursing processes
   Offers fluids to 1000 ml/day shift, 750 ml/evening shift, 250 ml/night shift.
   Standard for agency structure
   Kind and amount of fluids required are available.

   Note that the terms *criteria* and *standard* are used differently by Laing and Nish; the criterion is like the standard category previously discussed, and the standard is the measurement criterion.
4. Testing the criteria. Criteria must be valid and reliable. A **valid criterion** measures what it is intended to. A **reliable criterion** produces consistent results when used by the same person over time or by a different person.

Several established tools are available for measuring the quality of care. Some are process tools, some are outcome tools, and others are process-outcome tools. Each tool consists of standards and criteria.

Methods of using these tools also vary. Some evaluate by retrospective audits of nursing records using nursing audit committees. Others evaluate using a concurrent audit of process, i.e., direct observation of the nurse or nurses providing the nursing care by educated observers or by peers. Data may also be obtained by questioning and observing clients, questioning the family, and observing the client's environment and the general environment. The time period for measurement also varies. Some tools are designed for use over a 2-hour period; some are designed to evaluate the whole process of care given to the client from admission to discharge.

Scoring systems differ among tools. Levels of care may be rated as *excellent, good, incomplete, poor,* and *unsafe.* Some tools require only simple *yes* or *no* responses. Nurses' performances may be rated on a scale of 5 (best nurse) to 1 (worst nurse). Barba, Bennett, and Shaw (1978) advocate a retrospective audit of nursing care through the use of the American Nurses' Association (ANA) *Standards of Nursing Practice* (1973) using the nursing process. The ANA standards are presented in Table 1–4 on page 20. Assessing includes standards I and II. Planning includes standards III and IV. Implementing includes standards V and VI.

Developing effective quality care evaluation tools is a challenge for the nursing profession. Much work is continuing even on established tools.

Chapter Highlights

- Evaluation determines whether or to what degree the client goals have been met.
- Evaluating is both a concurrent and terminal process.
- Evaluating is purposeful and organized.
- Identifying outcome criteria is the first aspect of evaluating.
- Outcome criteria determine the evaluative data that must be collected to judge whether the goals have been met.

Table 15–2 Modified Care Plan for Mr. Joe Smith after Cardiac Surgery (selected examples only)

Assessment Data	Diagnostic Statement	Goal
Rales in bases of both lungs relieved by coughing before surgery Painful chest incision	Potential ineffective airway clearance related to chest incision	Maintain a clear airway
Aortic valve replacement (7/15) Heart rhythm regular at rest Pulse: 80 beats per minute (bpm) BP: 110/80 mm Hg	Potential alteration in cardiac output related to physical exertion and/or shock	Maintain cardiac output and blood volume
Left dorsalis pedis pulse and posterior tibial artery not palpable Skin of left extremity cool and pale	Alteration in tissue perfusion related to impaired arterial circulation	Improve arterial circulation
Aortic valve replacement (7/15)	Potential activity intolerance related to reduced strength of cardiac contraction	Increase activity tolerance

Nursing Orders	Rationale	Outcome Criteria
Administer analgesics q4h during first 48 hours	Pain relief makes coughing less uncomfortable and more effective	Normal breath sounds auscultated in all areas of both lungs
Splint incision with pillows or hands during coughing	Splinting minimizes pain	
Turn q2h during first 48 hours	Turning prevents the accumulation of secretions in one lung area	
Assist with deep breathing and coughing (DB & C) exercises q2h	DB & C exercises help to move and expel secretions	
Assess vital signs q1h for first 24 hours, q2h if stable for next 48 hours, and q4h thereafter if stable	A lowered blood pressure and rapid pulse indicate lowered blood volume or inadequate cardiac output	Stable vital signs Pulse: 80–100 bpm BP: not less than 110/80 mm Hg Respirations not more than 15 breaths per minute
Assess apical pulse and heart rhythm, not radial pulse		
Report an increase in resting pulse rate above 110 bpm and a BP below 100 mm Hg		
Keep client's legs warm (especially left leg) with blankets or socks	Warmth increases circulation	Left posterior tibial and dorsalis pedis pulses palpable and of same strength as corresponding right pulses
Assess blood flow in left dorsalis pedis artery and posterior tibial artery q2h using DUS	The DUS detects and indicates movement of blood through the arteries	Skin warm, intact, pink Capillary refill of left toenails within 1 to 3 seconds
Keep left leg in dependent position	A dependent position facilitates arterial blood flow by gravity	
Consult physician about a schedule for increasing activity	A gradual increase in activity helps the heart muscle and new valve accommodate increased demands	After activity, heart rate remains below 110 bpm and within 6 bpm of resting pulse after 3 minutes
Monitor and later show the client how to monitor his response to increased activity by: 1. Taking a resting pulse before activity 2. Taking pulse immediately after activity 3. Taking pulse 3 minutes after activity 4. Noting rate decreases, rates about 110, rates not within 6 bpm of resting pulse after 3 minutes	Pulse rate monitoring provides awareness of activities that do not overly exert the heart	
Monitor blood pressure after activity	A drop in blood pressure indicates a reduction in cardiac output	
Starting on 7/19, discuss factors contributing to increased cardiac workload, such as stress, excessive weight, overactivity, large meals	Knowledge of factors contributing to increased cardiac workload may facilitate necessary life-style changes, such as eating smaller meals, losing weight, and altering activity patterns	
Starting on 7/19, discuss the effects of reduced cardiac output such as shortness of breath, pain, fatigue, edema	Knowledge of the effects of reduced cardiac output may motivate him to avoid excessive activity	

- Outcome criteria must be measurable and precise.
- Reexamining the client care plan is a process of reassessing and replanning.
- Evaluating the quality of nursing care is an essential aspect of professional accountability.

Suggested Readings

Horn, B. J. March/April 1980. Establishing valid and reliable criteria: A researcher's perspective. *Nursing Research* 29:88–90.
From Horn's point of view, criteria used to develop measures of nursing care should be (a) based on a conceptual framework; (b) reliable and valid, measuring important aspects of care; (c) relatively simple to obtain; and (d) quantifiable for reporting and comparative purposes.

Hover, J., and Zimmer, M. J. April 1978. Nursing quality assurance: The Wisconsin system. *Nursing Outlook* 26:242–48.
Hover and Zimmer offer an outcome evaluation system with four components: criteria, assessment, standards, and improvement of care. Each must be developed on each implementation. The client outcomes are limited to five sets of criteria: (a) knowledge of illness and its treatment; (b) skills, i.e., ability of the client to conduct technical procedures; (c) knowledge of medications; (d) adaptive behaviors, including activities of daily living, social or productive activities, performance indicative of desired psychologic states, and changes in habits or life-style; and (e) health or physiologic status, including indicators such as skin condition, body temperature, etc. Four figures are included: sample knowledge test, sample outcome and charting guidelines, sample chart-audit worksheet, and sample standards for a chart audit. Even though the focus of this system is quality assurance, Hover and Zimmer provide guidelines for the nurse to write client outcome criteria when using the nursing process.

Inzer, F., and Aspinall, M. J. March 1981. Evaluating patient outcomes. *Nursing Outlook* 29:178–81.
These authors discuss the importance of objective methods of measuring client process. They describe a study in which nurses developed rating scales to measure client progress.

Wright, C., and Wheeler, P. March 1984. Auditing community health nursing. *Nursing Management* 15:40–42.
Wright and Wheeler discuss a computer-assisted audit in which the nursing process is used. An audit form with six standards relating to the nursing process is shown. Audit criteria for each standard are indicated.

Selected References

American Nurses' Association. 1973. *Standards of nursing practice.* New York: ANA.

———. 1975. A plan for implementation of the standards of nursing practice. New York: ANA.

———. 1976. *Guidelines for review of nursing care at the local level.* New York: ANA.

Atwood, J. R. March/April 1980. A research perspective. *Nursing Research* 29:104–8.

Barba, M., Bennett, B., and Shaw, W. J. January 1978. The evaluation of patient care through the use of ANA's standards of nursing practice. *Supervisor Nurse* 9:42, 45–54.

Clinton, J. F., Deynes, M. J., Goodwin, J. O., and Koto, E. M. 1977. Developing criterion measures of nursing care: Case study of a process. *Journal of Nursing Administration* 7:43–45.

Curtis, B. J., and Simpson, L. J. October 1985. Auditing a method for evaluating quality of care. *Journal of Nursing Administration* 15:14–21.

Fawcett, R. January 9, 1985. Management of care quality. Part 2. *Nursing Mirror* 160:29–31.

Gallant, B. W., and McLane, A. M. January 1979. Outcome criteria: A process for validation at the unit level. *Journal of Nursing Administration* 9:14–21.

Hegyvary, S. T., and Haussmann, R. K. D. November 1976a. Monitoring nursing care quality. *Journal of Nursing Administration* 6:3–9.

———. November 1976b. Nursing professional review. *Journal of Nursing Administration* 6:12–18.

———. November 1976c. Relationships of nursing process and patient outcomes. *Journal of Nursing Administration* 6:22–27.

Horn, B. J. March/April 1980. Establishing valid and reliable criteria: A researcher's perspective. *Nursing Research* 29:88–90.

Hover, J., and Zimmer, M. J. April 1978. Nursing quality assurance: The Wisconsin system. *Nursing Outlook* 26:242–48.

Inzer, F., and Aspinall, M. J. March 1981. Evaluating patient outcomes. *Nursing Outlook* 29:178–81.

Jelinek, R. C., Haussmann, R. K. D., Hegyvary, S. T., and Newman, T. F. January 1974. *A methodology for monitoring quality of nursing care.* U.S. Department of Health, Education and Welfare. Publication no. (HRA) 74-25.

Joint Commission on Accreditation of Hospitals. 1975. *Joint commission on accreditation of hospitals.* Chicago: JCAH.

———. 1983. *Manual for hospitals.* Chicago: JCAH.

Laing, M., and Nish, M. November 1981. Eight steps to quality assurance. *The Canadian Nurse* 77:22–25.

Leddy, S., and Pepper, J. M. 1985. *Conceptual base of professional nursing.* Philadelphia: J. B. Lippincott Co.

Lindeman, C. A. June 1976a. Research for nursing. Measuring quality of nursing care. Part 1. *Journal of Nursing Administration* 6:7–9.

———. September 1976b. Research for nursing. Measuring quality of nursing care. Part 2. *Journal of Nursing Administration* 6:16–19.

Maciorowski, L. F., Larson, E., and Keane, A. June 1985. Quality assurance: Evaluate thyself. *The Journal of Nursing Administration* 15:38–42.

Mackie, L. R. C., and Welsh, J. W. October 20, 1982. Quality assurance audit for the nursing process. *Nursing Times* 78:1757–58.

Moore, K. R. April 1979. What nurses learn from nursing audit. *Nursing Outlook* 27:254–58.

Mullins, A. C., Colavecchio, R. E., and Tescher, B. E. December 1979. Peer review: A model for professional accountability. *Journal of Nursing Administration* 9:25–30.

National Center for Health Services. 1978. *Research criterion measures of nursing care quality.* U.S. Department of Health, Education and Welfare. Publication no. (PHS) 78-3187.

Phaneuf, M. C. 1972. *The nursing audit: Profile of excellence.* New York: Meredith Corp.

———. 1976. *The nursing audit: Self-regulation in nursing practice.* New York: Appleton-Century-Crofts.

Phaneuf, M. C., and Wandelt, M. 1974. Quality assurance in nursing. *Nursing Forum* 13(4):328–45.

Quality assurance. May 9–15, 1984. *Nursing Times* 80:56–57.

Risser, N. L. January/February 1975. Development of an instrument to measure patient satisfaction with nurses and nursing care in primary care settings. *Nursing Research* 24:45–51.

Salway, H. December 14, 1983. A valuable estimate: The advantages of continuous assessment. *Nursing Mirror* 157:26–27.

Smith, A. P., editor. 1974. *PEP Workbook for Nurses.* Chicago: Joint Commission on Accreditation of Hospitals.

Sundeen, S. J., Stuart, G. W., Rankin, E. D., and Cohen, S. A. 1985. *Nurse-client interaction: Implementing the nursing process,* 3d ed. St. Louis: C. V. Mosby Co.

Van Maanen, H. M. January 1981. Improvement of quality of nursing care: A goal to challenge in the eighties. *Journal of Advanced Nursing* 6:3–9.

Vengroski, S. M., and Saarmann, L. December 1978. Peer review in quality assurance. *American Journal of Nursing* 78:2094–96.

Wandelt, M. A., and Ager, J. W. 1974. *Quality patient care scale.* New York: Appleton-Century-Crofts.

Wandelt, M. A., and Slater, S. D. 1975. *Slater Nursing Competencies Rating Scale.* New York: Appleton-Century-Crofts.

Wilson-Barnett, J. August 26, 1981. Care evaluation: Sizing up the scores. *Nursing Mirror* 153:31–33.

Wright, D. September 1984. An introduction to the evaluation of nursing care: A review of the literature. *Journal of Advanced Nursing* 9(5):457–67.

Wright, C., and Wheeler, P. March 1984. Auditing community health nursing. *Nursing Management* 15:40–42.

Yura, H., and Walsh, M. B. 1983. *The nursing process: Assessing, planning, implementing, evaluating,* 4th ed. New York: Appleton-Century-Crofts.

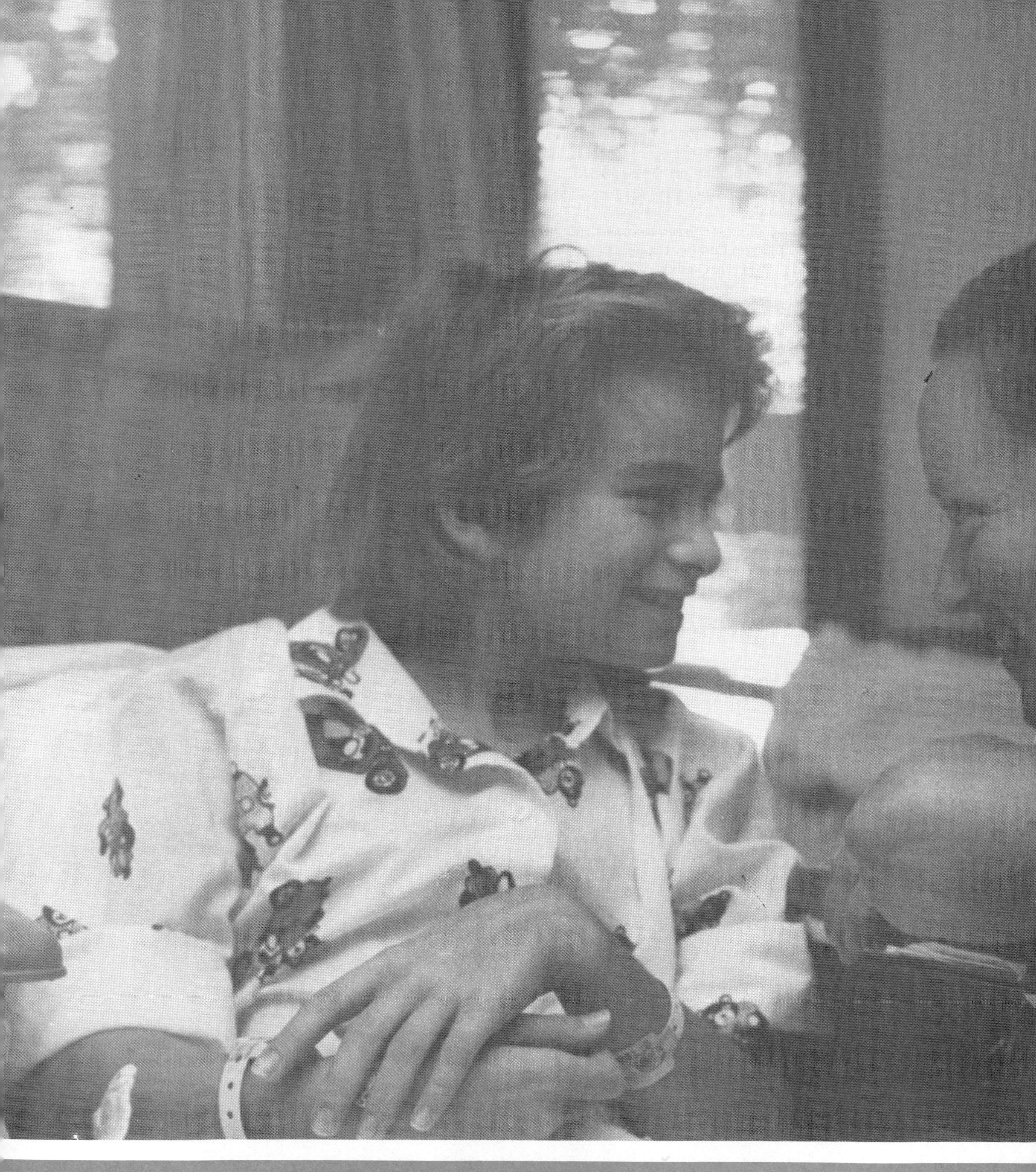

Nursing is caring: both the attitude and the activity. (Margretta M. Styles)

UNIT 4

Concepts About Humans

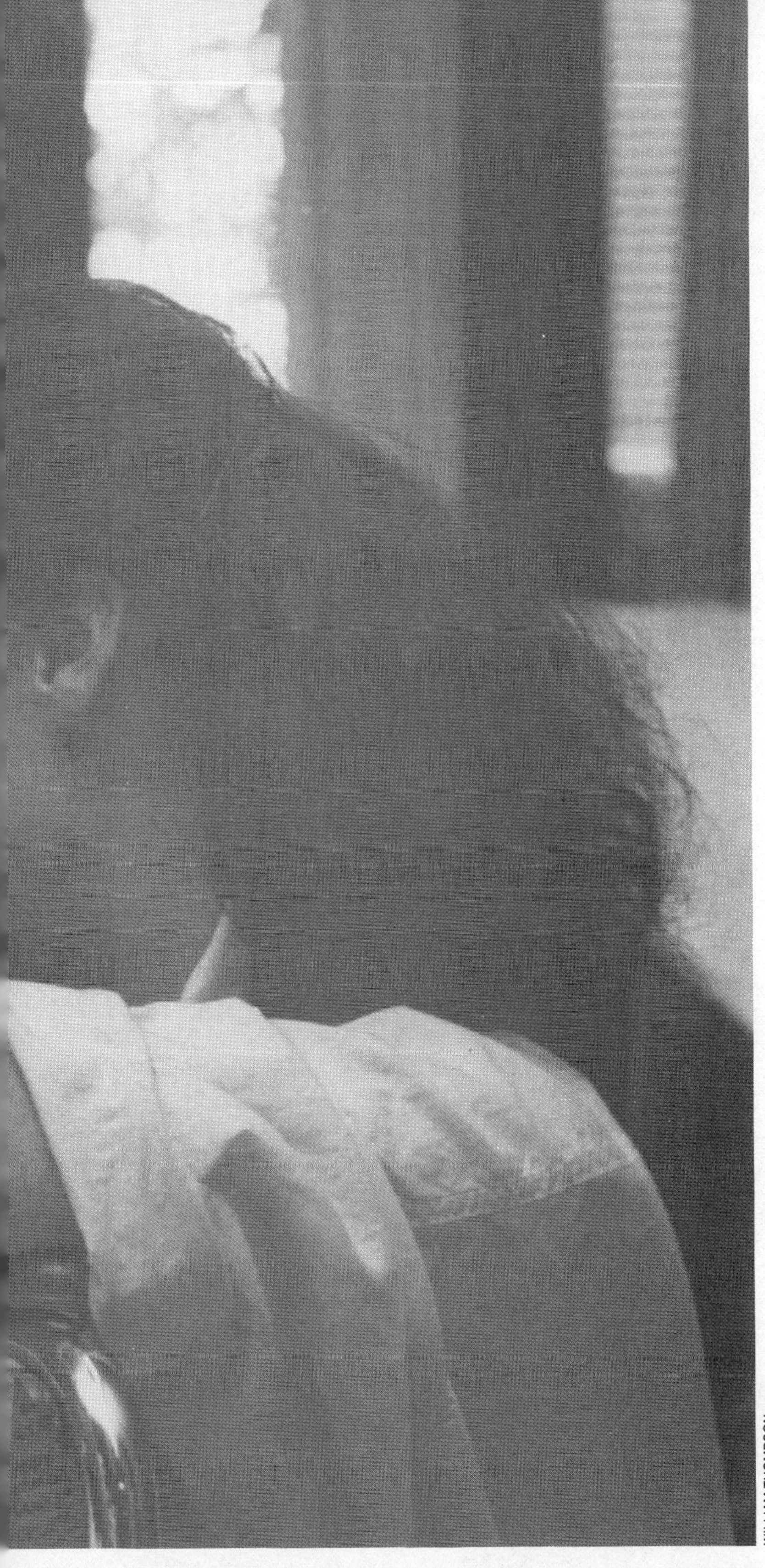

WILLIAM THOMPSON

Contents

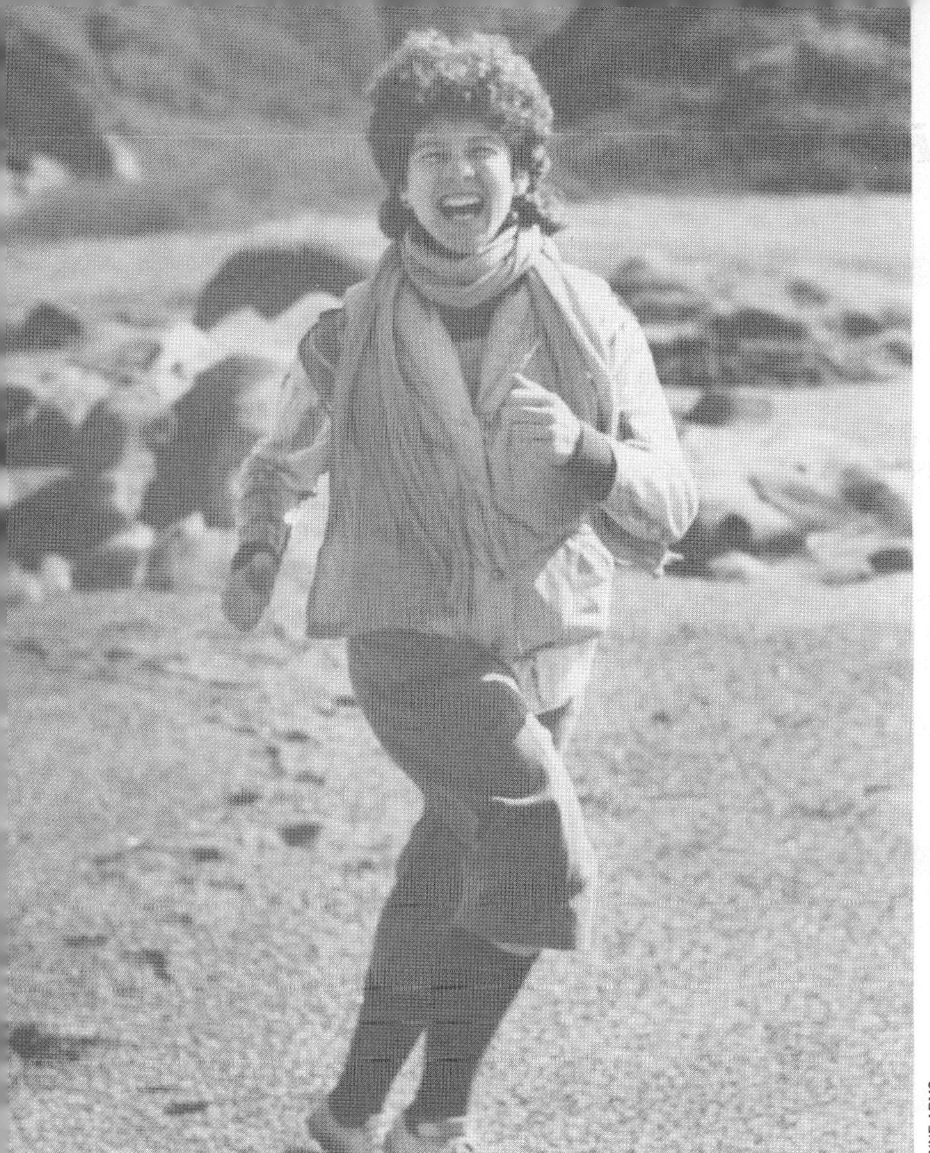

CHAPTER **16**

The Holistic Person

Contents

16 *The Holistic Person*

Objectives

1. Appreciate the concept of holism and various constructs about humans.
   1.1 Describe holism.
   1.2 Explain the relationship of holism to nursing.
   1.3 Describe the concept of the human being as a system.
   1.4 Identify various human subsystems.
2. Understand facts about human needs.
   2.1 Describe Maslow's hierarchy of needs.
   2.2 Describe Kalish's categories of needs.
   2.3 Compare Maslow's hierarchy of needs with Kalish's categories of needs.
   2.4 Give characteristics of the fully self-actualized person.
   2.5 Identify selected characteristics of basic human needs.
   2.6 Identify Maslow's growth needs.
   2.7 Compare Maslow's growth needs and deficiency needs.
   2.8 Describe ways to satisfy needs.
   2.9 Identify factors that affect needs satisfaction.
   2.10 Describe factors influencing priority of needs.
   2.11 Describe ways to apply a knowledge of needs in nursing.

Terms

adaptation
adaptive behavior
being values (metaneeds)
environment
holism
need
self-actualization
system

Holism

Nurses are concerned with the individual as a whole, complete, or holistic person, not as an assembly of parts and processes. The term *holism* was coined by Jan Smuts in his book *Holism and Evolution.* He suggested that evolution demonstrates "underlying patterns that indicated the gradual development and stratification of a progressive series of wholes, stretching from the inorganic beginnings to the highest levels of spiritual creations" (1926, pp. 82–87). This conceptualization was termed **holism**. The terms *holistic* and *holism* are derived from the Greek word meaning "whole."

In holistic theory, all living organisms are seen as interacting, unified wholes that are more than the mere sums of their parts. Viewed in this light, any disturbance in one part is a disturbance of the whole system; in other words, the disturbance affects the whole being.

When applied to humans and health, the concept of holism emphasizes the fact that "nurses must keep the self-identity of the 'whole' person in mind and must strive to understand simultaneously the relationship of the 'part' of the individual under concern to the totality of that individual's interactions and the relationship of the whole to its parts" (Krieger 1981, p. 4). Therefore, when the nurse studies one part of an individual, she or he must consider how that part relates to all others. The nurse must also consider the interaction and relationship of the individual to the external environment and to other related "wholes" (person or systems). For example, a nurse helps a man who is recuperating from a heart attack to consider his life-style and other contributing factors so that he can improve his health in the future. The nurse asks the client why he thinks the attack happened, what stresses he feels in his life, whether he smokes, and how much exercise he normally gets. Using the holistic approach, the nurse considers all contributing factors so that the client can prevent a recurrence.

The ideas of "comprehensive care," "total client care," and "holistic health care" evolved from the concept of holism. Holistic health involves the total person, the whole state of his or her being, and the overall quality of his or her life-style. It includes physical fitness, primary prevention of negative physical and emotional states, stress management, sensitivity to the environment, self-awareness, and spiritual insight (Smith 1984, p. 5). Many holistic health care centers have been established across North America. They help clients to take responsibility for their health, to seek alternative, healthy, self-fulfilling, behaviors, and to mobilize inner healing capacities. Increasing recognition is also being given to therapies other than the traditional medical and nursing therapies. Some of these are acupuncture; biofeedback techniques, which bring normally involuntary body processes under conscious control; acupressure, or massage of acupuncture points; therapeutic touch, or the transfer of energy from the nurse or healer to the patient through the body's energy fields; and homeopathic medicine, which is based primarily on clinical signs and symptoms and remedies derived from naturally occurring substances.

Selected Theoretical Views of Human Beings

The nurse's view of human beings influences the nursing interventions she or he provides. Although most nurses agree that humans are biopsychosocial beings, they differ in how they view human beings as recipients of nursing services.

The Person as a System

General systems theory is discussed in Chapter 10 on page 220. Humans are open **systems** with many interrelated subsystems. Because humans are biopsychosocial beings, their biologic, psychologic, social, and spiritual components can be regarded as systems with hierarchic subsystems.

Biologic System

The biologic system can be subdivided into the neurologic, musculoskeletal, respiratory, circulatory, gastrointestinal, and urinary subsystems, among others. Each subsystem can in turn be subdivided. For example, the urinary system consists of the kidneys, the ureters, and the bladder; the circulatory system consists of the heart and the blood vessels; the neurologic system consists of the brain, the spinal cord, and the nerves. The biologic system can also be subdivided into categories of needs or activities of daily living, such as nutrition and hydration, sleep and rest, exercise, etc. See the section on human needs later in this chapter.

The Psychologic and Social Subsystems

The psychologic and social systems consist of subsystems that include thinking, feeling, and interaction patterns. Names of the psychologic and social subsystems vary considerably. For example, Roy (1980, p. 186) outlines the following psychologic and social subsystems:

1. Self-concept
    a. Physical self
    b. Moral-ethical self
    c. Self-consistency
    d. Self-ideal and expectancy
    e. Self-esteem
2. Role function
3. Interdependence

Johnson (1980, p. 228), who describes the human system in terms of behaviors, lists the following psychologic subsystems:

1. Achievement subsystem, which strives to master or control the self or the environment
2. Aggressive/protective subsystem, which protects the self or others from real or imagined threats
3. Dependency subsystem, which functions to maintain environmental resources needed to obtain help, assistance, attention, permission, reassurance, and security
4. Affiliative subsystem, which strives to relate or belong to something or someone other than oneself

Orem (1980, p. 316) categorizes the psychologic and social systems as follows:

1. Solitude and social interaction, i.e., conditions of being alone or being with people
2. Hazards to life and well-being, i.e., conditions or situations that threaten the life or well-being of individuals or groups
3. Being normal, i.e., efforts to conform to the norm in current fashions, current scientific theories and facts, and cultural beliefs and practices

The Person as an Adaptive System

Adaptation is a process of change allowing the individual to respond to environmental changes yet retain his or her integrity or wholeness (Levine 1969, p. 95). In this sense, **environment** means all the conditions, circumstances, and influences surrounding and affecting the development of an organism or group of organisms. It refers to both the internal and external environments. Levine (1969, p. 95) identifies four levels of physiologic responses that facilitate adaptation: response to fear (the fight-or-flight mechanism), inflammatory response, response to stress, and sensory response (perceptual awareness). Details about adaptive responses are given in Chapter 17.

Roy's concept of adaptation is similar to Levine's (Roy 1976, pp. 12–14). Roy states that the person, as an adaptive system, functions as a totality. **Adaptive behavior** is the behavior of the whole person. Roy identifies two major internal processor subsystems of the adaptive system: the regulator and the cognator (Roy and Roberts 1981, p. 43). The individual uses these subsystems to adapt to or cope with internal and external environmental stimuli. The regulator mechanism has neural, endocrine, and perception-psychomotor components. The cognator mechanism encompasses psychosocial pathways and apparatus for perceptual/information processing, learning, judgment, and emotion. These two mechanisms are linked by the process of perception. For further information, see Chapter 10.

The Person as a Personal, Interpersonal, and Social System

According to King (1976, p. 51) the primary concerns of nursing are human behavior, social interaction, and social movements. Therefore, she includes three dynamic interacting systems in her concept of person:

1. Individuals (personal systems)
2. Groups (interpersonal systems)
3. Society (social systems)

Each of these systems has a set of related concepts.

King sees these concepts as relevant for understanding human beings as persons (i.e., the personal system): (a) perception, (b) self, (c) growth and development, (d) body image, (e) time, and (f) space. Perception is viewed as a process of human interaction with the environment. It is the process of organizing, interpreting, and transforming information from sensory data and memory. King describes these personal concepts as follows:

> An individual's perceptions of self, body image, of time and space influence the way he or she responds to persons, objects, and events in his or her life. As individuals grow and develop through the life span, experiences with changes in structure and function of their bodies over time influence their perceptions of self (King 1981, p. 19).

The interpersonal system involves two, three, or more individuals interacting in a given situation. According to King, concepts that help the nurse understand the interactions of human beings in groups are (a) interaction, (b) role, (c) communication, (d) transaction, and (e) stress (King 1976, p. 54). King believes that the interactions between two or more individuals represent a sequence of goal-directed verbal and nonverbal behaviors. The perceptions, goals, values, and needs of the nurse and the client influence the interactive process. In this process, two or more persons mutually identify goals and the means to achieve them. When they agree about the means of implementing the goals, they move toward transactions, which are defined as goal attainment. Role conflict between the nurse and client leads to stress. Stress is reduced when transactions are made (King 1981, p. 82).

"The social system is an organized boundary system of social roles, behaviors, and practices developed to maintain values and the mechanisms to regulate the practices and rules" (King 1981, p. 115). Social forces in the environment influence perception, interaction, behavior, and health. Examples of social systems are family systems, religious or belief systems, education systems, political systems, and work systems. Selected concepts that help the nurse function in social systems, such as the health care system, are organization, power, authority, decision making, and role.

Other Assumptions

Many other assumptions made about humans influence the focus of nursing interventions. Some examples from various theorists follow. See also Table 16–1 for other concepts and assumptions about human beings by selected nurse theorists.

1. The individual is an organism who lives in an unstable equilibrium and has the ability to learn, develop problem-solving skills, and adapt to the tensions created by his or her needs (Blake 1980, p. 54). This emphasis on learning and developing focuses nursing interventions on education to promote forward movement of the client in the direction of creative, constructive, productive, personal, and community living (Blake 1980, p. 54).

2. The human being is an open system in constant interaction with a changing environment (Roy 1980, p. 180). In other words, the individual engages in a dynamic interchange with the environment, and this interchange is an essential factor of the system's viability, reproductive ability or continuity, and ability to change. Constant input (stimuli) into the system and feedback to it maintain the system in a state of dynamic equilibrium. This premise directs the nurse to look at environmental factors influencing the system and to provide nursing interventions that help the client maintain and achieve a state of dynamic equilibrium.

3. Human beings interact with the environment by adjusting themselves to it or adjusting it to themselves (Neuman 1980, p. 122). This premise directs the nurse to look at ways the client handles changing situations. Does he or she withdraw from the environment, alter the environment, or alter self?

Table 16–1 Selected Nurse Theorists' Concepts and Assumptions about Human Beings

Theorist	Concepts/Assumptions
Dorothy Johnson (1980, pp. 212–14)	The individual is a behavioral system. The behavioral system is comprised of all patterned, repetitive, and purposeful ways of behaving that characterize each person's life. Subsystems carry out specialized tasks to maintain the integrity of the whole behavioral system and manage its relationship to the environment. Subsystems are: 1. Attachment or affiliative 2. Dependency 3. Ingestive 4. Sexual 5. Aggressive 6. Achievement
Imogene King (1981, pp. 143–44)	The individual is a social, sentient, reacting, perceiving, controlling, purposeful, action-oriented, time-oriented being. The individual is conceptualized as a personal system who processes selective inputs from the environment through the senses. The personal system is a unified, complex, whole self who perceives, thinks, desires, imagines, decides, identifies goals, and selects means to achieve them.
Myra E. Levine (1973, pp. 8–10)	The human is a holistic being—a system of systems. The life process of the system is unceasing change that has direction, purpose, and meaning. The change, which is orderly and sequential, occurs through adaptation, which permits the person to protect and maintain his or her integrity as an individual.
Betty Neuman (1974, pp. 101–3; 1980, pp. 119–39)	The total person is a composite of physiologic, psychologic, sociocultural, and developmental variables. Each person has a basic structure or central core of survival factors unique to the individual but in a range common to other humans. The factors include temperature range, genetic response pattern, ego structure, and strengths and weaknesses of body organs. The central core of the person is protected from stressors by concentric rings: 1. A normal line of defense—a normal range of responses or equilibrium state that evolves over time 2. A flexible line of defense—a dynamic, rapidly changing protective buffer that prevents stressors from breaking through the normal line of defense
Dorothea Orem (1980, pp. 41–51, 120)	The person is a unit that can be viewed as functioning biologically, symbolically, and socially. The individual and the environment form an integrated functional whole or system. People have the ability to perform self-care—activities that individuals initiate and perform on their own behalf to maintain life, health, and well-being. The ability to care for oneself is self-care agency; the ability to care for others is dependent-care agency. *Agency* means action. Self- or dependent-care is undertaken to meet three types of self-care requisites: universal, developmental, and health deviation.
Martha E. Rogers (1970, pp. 47–73)	People are unified entities possessing their own integrity and manifesting characteristics that are more than and different from the sum of their parts. The individual and the environment are continually exchanging matter and energy. The life process of human beings evolves irreversibly and unidirectionally along a space-time continuum. Pattern and organization identify individuals and reflect their innovative wholeness. The human being is characterized by the capacity for abstraction and imagery, language and thought, and sensation and emotion.
Sister Callista Roy, in Riehl and Roy (1980, pp. 179–206)	The person is a biopsychosocial being in constant interaction with a changing environment. As an adaptive system, the person functions as a totality; adaptive behavior is behavior of the whole person. The person has four modes of adaptation: physiologic needs, self-concept, role function, and interdependence relations. The person has a great potential for self-actualization. The person is an active participant in his or her own destiny.

4. Human beings maintain varying degrees of harmony and balance between their internal and external environments by a process of interaction and adjustment. Each person evolves a normal range of responses over time (Neuman 1980, p. 122). This premise directs the nurse to consider usual response patterns and the client's strengths and weaknesses in maintaining system balance and in coping with change.

Human Needs

Although each individual has unique characteristics, certain needs are common to all people. Nursing theorists define *need* in various ways. King defines need as "a state of energy exchange within and external to the organism which leads to behavioral responses to situations, events, and persons" (King 1971, p. 80). Roy defines a need as "a requirement within the individual which stimulates a response to maintain integrity" (Roy 1980, p. 184). For the purposes of this book, a **need** is something that is desirable, useful, or necessary. Human need theorists see people as integrated beings (holistic) who are motivated by internal and external needs.

The humanist Abraham Maslow developed his theory of human needs in the 1940s. He defines a need as a satisfaction whose absence causes illness (Maslow 1968, p. 21). According to Maslow, a basic need has the following characteristics:

1. Its absence breeds illness.
2. Its presence prevents illness.
3. Its restoration cures illness.
4. Under certain situations of free choice, it is preferred by a deprived person over other satisfactions.
5. It is found to be inactive or functionally absent in the healthy person.

To Maslow, needs motivate the behavior of the individual.

Maslow's (1970) model of human needs includes both physiologic and psychologic needs, which he ranks according to how critical to survival they are. According to Maslow, the needs at one level must be met before the needs on the next level can be met. Thus, the physiologic needs must be met before the safety needs are met. Throughout life, people strive to meet their needs at each level; however, the dominant needs *within one level* may vary at different times of life. Maslow sees humans as beings who continue to grow and develop from conception until death. Once a need is completely met, Maslow believes, the individual is no longer aware of it. Needs can be completely met, partially met, or not met at all. An individual usually persists in behavior to meet a need until it is met; for example, a thirsty man who cannot find a drinking fountain will search until he finds another source of water.

Maslow also states that an individual who apparently meets all of his or her needs still looks further to self-actualization. Maslow adds two more needs to his list: the need to know and the need to understand. He believes that these needs are always present and permit people to meet the other needs more efficiently.

Maslow's five categories, in order, are (1970, p. 37):

1. Physiologic needs
2. Safety and security needs
3. Love and belonging needs
4. Self-esteem needs
5. Need for self-actualization

According to Maslow, the basic physiologic needs are air, food, water, shelter, rest and sleep, activity, and temperature maintenance. A person who is starving or deprived of fluid for an extended time will center all of his or her activities around meeting that need. After the physiologic needs are met, the need to feel safe in one's environment emerges. This need for safety has both physical and psychologic aspects; the person needs to *be* safe and to *feel* safe, both in the physical environment and in relationships. The third level of needs—for love, affection, and belonging—emerges after the needs for safety are met. According to Maslow, the need for love encompasses both giving and receiving. Belonging needs include attaining a place in a group, e.g., having a family and the feeling of belonging.

The need for esteem is at the fourth level. The individual needs both self-esteem, i.e., feelings of independence, competence, and self-respect, and esteem from others, i.e., recognition, respect, and appreciation. When the need for esteem is satisfied, the individual strives for self-actualization. Maslow's highest level, **self-actualization**, is the apex of the fully developed personality; accordingly, few people are fully self-actualized (Maslow 1968, p. 204).

The fully self-actualized person has realized his or her full potential. Such a person has the ability to connect the past and the future to the present while living fully in the present; that is, he or she is time-competent. The self-actualized person is also inner-directed and autonomous in contrast to being other-directed. To be inner-directed means that the individual is guided by a few basic values and principles, whatever the situation. To be autonomous is to be free from parental and social pressures and to apply these values or principles to behavior in a manner that appears appropriate to the individual. The other-directed individual is influenced by outside pressures, accepts guidance and direction from others, and adheres to this guidance to gain approval.

Not all people become fully self-actualized, and Maslow did not believe that intelligence is required for self-actualization. However, if all the "lower" needs are met, an individual may aspire to become self-fulfilled or self-actualized. Maslow saw self-actualization as a product of maturity that comes about through relating to people in autonomous and time-competent ways.

The fully self-actualized person may not always be happy, successful, or well adjusted. Maslow viewed many of the subjects he believes to be self-actualized as prideful, vain, and possessing doubts and fears. However, they were able to deal positively with their fears, doubts, and failures. See Table 16–2 for the major characteristics of a self-actualized person.

In later research, Maslow identified the growth needs, in contrast to the deficiency needs. He calls the growth needs **Being values** (**metaneeds**, B-values). These being values resemble needs because, when metaneeds are not met, the person has a "sickness of the soul," or **metapathology** (Maslow 1971, p. 43). Maslow believes that for some people being values give meaning to life. There are 14 being values: truth, goodness, beauty, wholeness, aliveness, uniqueness, perfection, completion, justice, simplicity, richness, effortlessness, playfulness, and self-sufficiency. These needs are not ranked (Goble 1970, pp. 47–48).

Richard Kalish (1977, p. 32) has adapted Maslow's hierarchy and suggests an additional category of needs between the physiologic needs and the safety and security needs. This category includes sex, activity, exploration, manipulation, and novelty. See Figure 16–1. Kalish emphasizes that children need to explore and manipulate their environments to achieve optimal growth and development. He notes that adults, too, often seek novel adventures or stimulating experiences before considering their safety or security needs. Maslow, by contrast, includes the pursuit of knowledge and aesthetic needs in the category of self-actualization needs.

Halbert Dunn's (1958) model presents a series of needs that the individual must meet to achieve a state of maximum functioning or high-level wellness. Dunn's basic needs are survival, communication, fellowship, growth, imagination, love, balance, environment, communication with the universe, philosophy of living, dignity, freedom, and space. At any specific time, different needs assume a greater relative importance to the individual.

Jourard (1963) believes that people rank their needs according to their relative importance in their lives. He adds the needs for health (physical and mental), freedom, challenge, cognitive clarity, and varied experience to Maslow's list.

Table 16–2 Maslow's Characteristics of a Self-Actualized Person

1. Is realistic, sees life clearly, and is objective about his or her observations
2. Judges people correctly
3. Has superior perception, is more decisive
4. Has clear notion of right and wrong
5. Is usually accurate in predicting future events
6. Understands art, music, politics, and philosophy
7. Possesses humility, listens to others carefully
8. Is dedicated to some work, task, duty, or vocation
9. Is highly creative, flexible, spontaneous, courageous, and willing to make mistakes
10. Is open to new ideas
11. Is self-confident and has self-respect
12. Has low degree of self-conflict; personality is integrated
13. Respects self, does not need fame, possesses a feeling of self-control
14. Is highly independent, desires privacy
15. Can appear remote and detached
16. Is friendly, loving, and governed more by inner directives than by society
17. Can make decisions contrary to popular opinion
18. Is problem centered rather than self-centered
19. Accepts the world for what it is

Source: Based on Chapter 3, "The Study of Self-Actualization," from *The Third Force, The Psychology of Abraham Maslow,* by Frank Goble. Copyright © 1970 by Thomas Jefferson Research Center. Reprinted by permission of Viking Penguin, Inc.

Characteristics of Basic Needs

1. All people have the same basic needs; however, each person's needs are modified by his or her culture. A person's perception of a need varies according to learning and the standards of the culture. For example, professional achievement may be important in one culture or subculture and unimportant in another.

2. People meet their own needs relative to their own priorities. For example, during a drought, a mother might give up her share of water and die so that her child might have sufficient water to live.

3. Although basic needs generally must be met, some needs can be deferred. An example is the need for independence, which an ill person can defer until well.

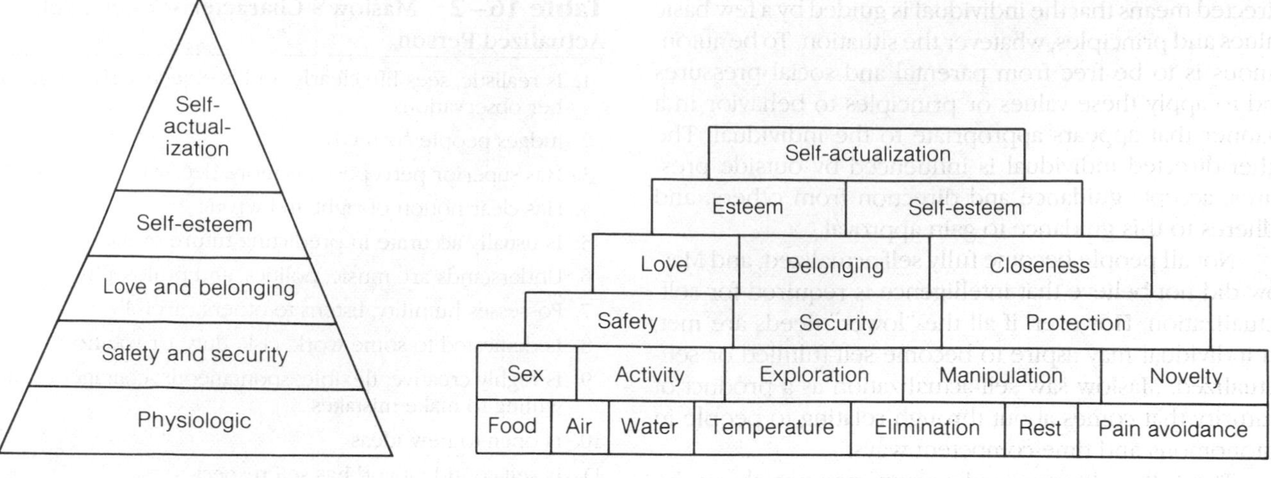

Figure 16–1 Maslow's hierarchy of needs and Maslow's needs as adapted by Kalish.

Source: From *The Psychology of Human Behavior,* 5th ed., by R. A. Kalish. Copyright © 1966, 1970, 1973, 1977, 1983 by Wadsworth, Inc. Reprinted by permission of Brooks/Cole Publishing Company, Monterey, California 93940.

4. Failure to meet needs results in one or more homeostatic imbalances, which can eventually result in illness.

5. A need can make itself felt by either external or internal stimuli. An example is the need for food. A person may experience hunger as a result of thinking about food (internal stimulation) or as a result of seeing a beautiful cake (external stimulation).

6. A person who perceives a need can respond in several ways to meet it. The choice of response is largely a result of learned experiences and the values of the culture. For example, the professional woman who comes home from work feeling tired may meet the need for relaxation by having a cocktail. This response reflects her experience and culture.

7. Needs are interrelated. Some needs cannot be met unless related needs are also met. The need for hydration can be seriously altered if the need for elimination of urine is not also met. Likewise, the need for security can be markedly altered if the need for oxygen is threatened by a respiratory obstruction.

Needs Satisfaction

Needs can be satisfied in healthy and unhealthy ways. An individual can succeed in his or her profession as a way of meeting the needs for belonging and self-esteem. Ways of meeting basic needs are considered healthy when they are not harmful to others or to self, conform to the individual's sociocultural values, and are within the law. Conversely, unhealthy behavior has one or more of the following characteristics: It may be harmful to others or to self, does not conform to the individual's sociocultural values, or is not within the law. Maslow found that people who satisfy their basic needs are healthier, happier, and more effective than those whose needs are frustrated (Goble 1970, p. 50).

Factors Affecting Needs Satisfaction

Gauging whether physiologic needs are met is largely an objective judgment. For example, the nurse can judge whether an individual's need for food has been met by weighing that person, using calipers to measure body fat, or receiving the results of laboratory tests that analyze the metabolic processes of the body. Gauging whether psychologic needs have been met, however, is largely a subjective judgment. If a person believes a psychologic need, e.g., for love, is not satisfied, then for that person it is not met, regardless of how he or she appears to others. Several factors affect people's abilities to satisfy their needs. Four of these are illness, significant relationships, self-concept, and developmental stage.

Illness

Illness frequently interferes with people's abilities to meet their own needs. Nurses can help ill clients to meet their physiological needs on a number of levels. The man recovering from abdominal surgery probably requires oxygen, intravenous fluids, assistance moving, and reassurance immediately after surgery. Each of these interventions helps to meet a different need. As he recovers, his requirements for nursing help will decrease. First he may turn himself without assistance, then take sips of water, and in a short time meet all his physiologic needs independently. As these physiologic needs are met, the client attends to needs at the next level—safety needs, according to Maslow—and so on. Ailing people often direct all their energies to meeting physiologic (survival) needs, and may not identify needs at higher levels until later.

Significant Relationships

A second variable affecting needs satisfaction is significant relationships. It is known that people's ability to meet their needs is greatly influenced by their significant relationships. Often these relationships are with family and support persons. However, nurses frequently establish significant relationships with clients. Nurses are present at critical times in people's lives, and a relationship of trust often develops quickly. In that relationship, nurses can help clients become aware of their needs and establish healthy ways of meeting them.

Self-Concept

A person's self-concept affects not only his or her ability to meet basic needs but also the awareness of whether or not these needs are satisfied. People who feel good about themselves are more likely to change, to recognize needs, and to establish healthy ways of meeting those needs.

Developmental Stage

A fourth variable is an individual's developmental stage. According to Erikson's model of psychosocial human development (see Chapter 22), if an individual satisfactorily achieves the developmental task of learning to trust, then the basic needs of feeling safe and secure are readily resolved. The person who has already learned to trust others transfers those feelings to the health personnel caring for him or her. As another example, if the developmental tasks of establishing identity and intimacy have been achieved, the individual has an increased sense of belonging and being loved at a time of illness.

Assigning Priorities to Needs

Although Maslow's needs are presented in a hierarchy, sometimes clients and nurses must adjust the priority of the needs. People are continually changing and growing; thus, their needs do not stay constant but also continually change. People frequently have many needs at one time. In some instances, the nurse may be able to help a client meet several needs at once, partially meet one need and then go on to another, or deal with one need at a time. Needs related to life-threatening situations, e.g., a suffocating client's need for air, always assume first priority. Nurses have to act quickly in some instances to preserve life.

In many situations, however, one need does not stand out as priority one. In these cases, the client and nurse consider several factors.

Perceptions

A person may not perceive that he or she has a specific need. If so, the nurse may allocate it a low priority, often deferring action until the person is ready. For example, a man who smokes heavily might not see the need to stop.

Health

A client who is recovering from surgery should not be encouraged to participate in strenuous exercise until health permits, even though the client sees exercise as an important need. Similarly, a man whose left side is paralyzed may have to defer a visit to his sister until he is stronger.

Sociocultural Background

Socioeconomic and cultural backgrounds affect how people rank their needs. For example, a man may place his need to return to work ahead of his need to learn exercises. A woman may perceive that getting her husband's breakfast is more important than resting in bed.

Support Persons

Support persons greatly influence in what order and how needs are met. A woman who needs approval and recognition and does not receive them at home may return to work to meet this need. A teenage boy may join a gang because his needs for belonging and esteem are not met in the home.

Applications in Nursing

A knowledge of human needs helps the nurse in several ways. First, by understanding human needs, nurses can understand people's behavior better. Recognizing the causes of certain behavior helps nurses be less judgmental and more objective. In addition, understanding the reason for behavior helps nurses respond therapeutically rather than emotionally. For example, by repeatedly turning on his signal light, a man may be reflecting a need for safety (he feels frightened), a need for belonging or affect, or a need for esteem. The nurse can discuss his feelings to determine what his need is and thus how to respond. If the client is turning on his light because he is frightened, the nurses can employ a variety of methods to reassure him, including explaining about the hospital, answering his call promptly, anticipating some of his needs, and telling him when they will return and returning at that time.

Second, knowledge of basic needs can provide a framework for, and be applied in, the nursing process at the individual and family levels. Human needs can serve as a framework for assessing, assigning priorities to problems, and planning nursing interventions. A client's unmet need for blood can be of high priority and calls for immediate nursing action, whereas the same client's self-esteem needs are of lower priority during that emergency. See Chapters 10 through 15 for additional information about the nursing process.

Third, nurses can apply their knowledge of human needs to relieve distress. Orlando (1961, p. 5) defines a need as "a requirement of the patient which, if supplied, relieves or diminishes his immediate distress or improves his immediate sense of adequacy or well-being." To meet, or help a client meet, unmet needs and thereby alleviate distress, the nurse requires a knowledge not only of needs but also of the situations that bring about these unmet needs and the manner in which the client conveys the need.

Fourth, the nurse can use a knowledge of human needs to help people develop and grow. Sometimes people are unaware or only partially aware of their own needs. Nurses can often help clients move toward self-actualization by helping them to find meaning in their illness experience. To encourage the patient's growth toward self-actualization nurses can help clients to (a) understand what is happening to them, (b) maintain some control over events affecting them, (c) maintain their identities and self-respect, (d) accept inevitable outcomes, and (e) feel good about themselves.

Chapter Highlights

- Nursing involves viewing the individual holistically.
- How nurses view human beings influences how they assess and intervene.
- Humans can be viewed as open systems with many interrelated subsystems.
- Needs are the motivating forces behind behavior.
- Maslow defined a hierarchy of human needs, from physiologic (survival) needs to self-actualization.
- People vary in how they rank their needs at any given moment.
- Needs can be satisfied in healthy and unhealthy ways.
- Needs satisfaction can be altered by illness, significant relationships, self-concept, and developmental levels.
- A knowledge of human needs helps nurses understand behavior and can provide a framework for applying parts of the nursing process.
- A knowledge of human needs can help nurses relieve distress and help people develop and grow.

Suggested Readings

Bulbrook, M. J. December 1984. Health and healing in the future. *The Canadian Nurse* 80:26–29.

Ancient healing traditions are having an impact on how nurses view and administer health care today. Bulbrook says this trend will continue and lead to a different kind of care that will dispel some widely held notions about modern Western medicine. The discussion covers the influence of Eastern philosophy, the concept of energy and therapeutic touch, alternate healing therapies, and guiding principles in the use of healing therapies.

———. December 1984. Bulbrook's model of therapeutic touch: One form of health and healing in the future. *The Canadian Nurse* 80:30–34.

The author describes her experiences with the use of this therapeutic technique originally developed by Dolores Krieger. This technique is becoming a part of the practices of many nurses.

Locheed, T. December 1984. Holistic health: A uniting force for nurses. *The Canadian Nurse* 80:24–25.

Locheed thinks that holistic health may be the uniting force to help nurses form bonds rather than discover new differences. She discusses why nurses should adopt a holistic viewpoint and how to practice nursing holistically.

Selected References

Blake, M. 1980. The Peplau developmental model for nursing practice. In Riehl, J. P., and Roy, C. *Conceptual models for nursing practice.* 2d ed. New York: Appleton-Century-Crofts.

Collins, M. 1983. *Communication in health care: The human connection in the life cycle.* 2d ed. St. Louis: C. V. Mosby Co.

Davis, D. May 16–22, 1984. Holistic health: Homeopathic medicine. Part 7. *Nursing Times* 80:48–50.

Dunn, H. H. November 1958. What high level wellness means. *Canadian Journal of Public Health* 50:447–57.

Fawcett, J. 1984. *Analysis and evaluation of conceptual models of nursing.* Philadelphia: F. A. Davis Co.

Goble, F. G. 1970. *The third force: The psychology of Abraham Maslow.* Richmond Hill, Ontario: Simon and Schuster.

Hazzard, M. E. 1971. An overview of systems theory. *Nursing Clinics of North America* 3:385–93.

Holmes, P. April 18–24, 1984. Holistic nursing. *Nursing Times* 80:28–29.

Johnson, D. E. 1980. The behavioral system model for nursing. In Riehl, J. P., and Roy, C. *Conceptual models for nursing practice.* 2d ed. New York: Appleton-Century-Crofts.

Jourard, S. 1963. *Personality adjustment.* 2d ed. New York: Macmillan Co.

Kalish, R. A. 1977. *The psychology of human behavior.* 4th ed. Belmont, Calif.: Wadsworth Publishing Co.

King, I. M. 1971. *Toward a theory for nursing: General concepts of human behavior.* New York: John Wiley and Sons.

———. 1976. The health care system. Nursing intervention subsystem. In Werley, H.; Zuzich, A.; Zajkowski, M.; and Zagornik, A. D. *Health research: The systems approach.* New York: Springer Publishing Co., Inc.

———. 1981. *A theory for nursing: Systems, concepts, process.* New York: John Wiley and Sons.

Krieger, D. 1981. *Foundations for holistic health nursing practices: The Renaissance nurse.* Philadelphia: J. B. Lippincott Co.

Levine, M. E. January 1969. The pursuit of wholeness. *American Journal of Nursing* 69:93–98.

———. 1973. *Introduction to clinical nursing.* 2d ed. Philadelphia: F. A. Davis Co.

Locheed, T. December 1984. Holistic health: A uniting force for nurses. *The Canadian Nurse* 80:24–25.

Maslow, A. H. 1968. *Toward a psychology of being.* 2d ed. New York: Van Nostrand Reinhold Co.

———. 1970. *Motivation and personality.* 2d ed. New York: Harper and Row.

———. 1971. *The farther reaches of human nature.* New York: Penguin Books.

Neuman, B. 1974. The Betty Neuman health-care systems model: A total person approach to patient problems. In Riehl, J. P., and Roy, C. *Conceptual models for nursing practice.* New York: Appleton-Century-Crofts.

———. 1980. The Betty Neuman health-care systems model: A total person approach to patient problems. In Riehl, J. P., and Roy, C. *Conceptual models for nursing practice.* 2d ed. New York: Appleton-Century-Crofts.

The Nursing Theories Conference Group. George, J. B., Chairperson. 1980. *Nursing theories. The base for professional nursing practice.* Englewood Cliffs, N.J.: Prentice-Hall.

Orem, D. E. 1980. *Nursing: Concepts of practice.* 2d ed. New York: McGraw-Hill.

Orlando, I. J. 1961. *The dynamic nurse-patient relationship: Function, process and principles.* New York: G. P. Putnam's Sons.

Renshaw, J. April 25–May 1, 1984. Holistic health: The power of the will. Part 2. *Nursing Times* 80:38–39.

Riehl, J. P., and Roy, C. 1980. *Conceptual models for nursing practice.* 2d ed. New York: Appleton-Century-Crofts.

Rogers, M. E. 1970. *An introduction to the theoretical base of nursing.* Philadelphia: F. A. Davis.

Roy, C. 1976. *Introduction to nursing: An adaptation model.* Englewood Cliffs, N.J.: Prentice-Hall.

———. 1980. The Roy adaptation model. In Riehl, J. P., and Roy, C. *Conceptual models for nursing practice* (2nd ed.). New York: Appleton-Century-Crofts.

Roy, C., and Roberts, S. L. 1981. *Theory construction in nursing: An adaptation model.* Englewood Cliffs, N.J.: Prentice-Hall.

Ryman, D. May 2–8, 1984. Holistic health: The sweet smell of success . . . aroma therapy. Part 5. *Nursing Times* 80:48–49.

Smith, M. P. August 1984. The new frontier. *RNABC* (Registered Nurses Association of British Columbia) *News* 16:5.

Smuts, J. 1926. *Holism and evolution.* New York: MacMillan Publishing Co., Inc.

Turton, P. May 2–8, 1984. Holistic health: The laying on of hands. Part 4. *Nursing Times* 80:47–48.

CHAPTER 17

Homeostasis, Stress, and Adaptation

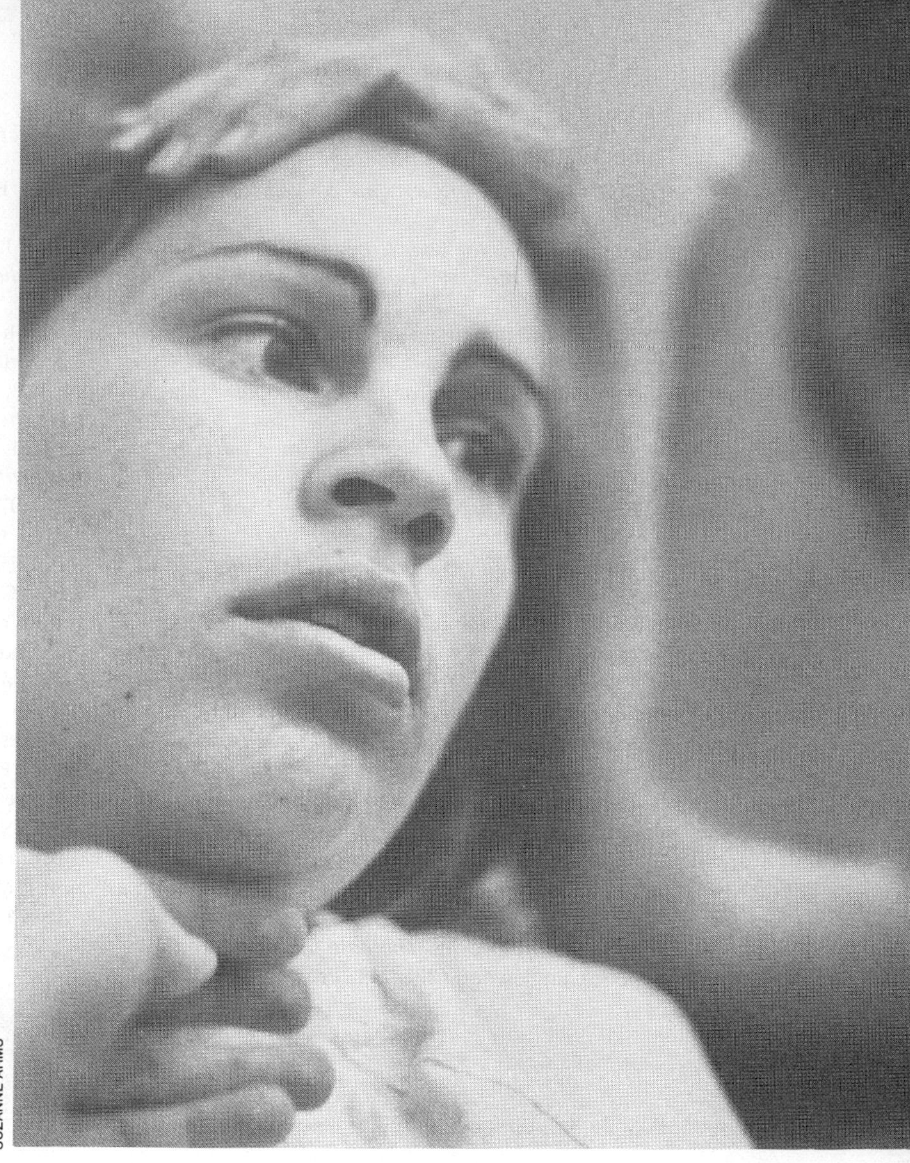

SUZANNE ARMS

Contents

Objectives

1. Understand essential terms and facts about homeostasis.
   1.1 Differentiate homeostasis from homeodynamics.
   1.2 Describe three essential parts of homeostatic mechanisms.
   1.3 Describe four main characteristics of homeostatic mechanisms.
   1.4 Describe how the autonomic nervous system regulates homeostasis.
   1.5 Identify five major glands and two major systems of the body that maintain homeostasis.
   1.6 Name and describe the functions of three homeostatic hormones secreted by the pituitary.
   1.7 Name and describe the functions of two homeostatic hormones secreted by the adrenal medulla.
   1.8 Name and describe the functions of two homeostatic hormones secreted by the adrenal cortex.
   1.9 Identify two body minerals regulated by parathyroid hormone.
   1.10 Describe how the respiratory, cardiovascular renal, and gastrointestinal systems regulate the body's homeostasis.
   1.11 List four prerequisites for the development of psychologic homeostasis.
2. Understand essential terms and facts about stress.
   2.1 Differentiate the concepts of stress as a stimulus, as a response, and as a transaction.
   2.2 Describe the significance of stress-level rating scales outlined in this chapter.
   2.3 Identify Selye's definition of stress.
   2.4 Describe the three stages of Selye's general adaptation syndrome.
   2.5 Describe essential aspects of the Lazarus stress model.
   2.6 Identify the physiologic responses of the body associated with the general adaptation syndrome.
   2.7 Describe Nuernberger's possum response, or general inhibition syndrome.
   2.8 Identify physiologic and psychologic (cognitive, verbal, and motor) manifestations of stress.
   2.9 Identify behaviors related to specific ego defense mechanisms.
   2.10 Differentiate four levels of anxiety.
   2.11 Describe the relationship of anger to anxiety.
   2.12 Describe the sequence of events that occurs in anger.
   2.13 Give examples of constructive and destructive anger.
   2.14 Give examples of seven variables influencing the degree to which stressors affect individuals.
   2.15 Identify characteristics of types A and B personalities and outline how the two types relate to stress.
3. Understand essential terms and facts about adaptation.
   3.1 Define adaptation.
   3.2 Differentiate adaptation from coping.
   3.3 Give examples of four modes of adaptation.
   3.4 Identify characteristics of adaptive responses.
4. Understand essential aspects of applying the nursing process to clients experiencing stress.
   4.1 Describe how to identify a client's stress.
   4.2 Describe ways to assess client coping.
   4.3 Identify examples of nursing diagnoses related to stress.
   4.4 Identify general guidelines to minimize a client's anxiety and stress.
   4.5 Describe interventions to mediate anger.
   4.6 Identify interventions to help clients cope with stress.
   4.7 Describe some advanced stress-reduction techniques.
   4.8 Identify sources of stress in the nurse.
   4.9 Describe common behavioral responses of the nurse to stress.
   4.10 Describe ways that nurses can manage stress.
   4.11 Give examples of evaluative outcome criteria for clients experiencing stress.

Terms

adaptation
aggression
alerting (anger element)
anger
anxiety
biofeedback
chemoreceptor
cognitive appraisal
compensation
conversion
coping
coping strategy
countershock phase
denial
describing (anger element)
disequilibrium
displacement
effector organ
equilibrium
feedback
general adaptation (stress) syndrome (GAS)
general inhibition syndrome (possum response)
glucagon
glucocorticoid
homeodynamics
homeostasis
hostility

identifying (anger element)
local adaptation syndrome (LAS)
meditation
mental (defense) mechanism
negative feedback
positive feedback
projection
proprioceptor
psychologic homeostasis
rationalization
reaction formation
receptor (sensor)
regression
renin
repression
shiatsu
shock phase
stress
stressor
stress syndrome
sublimation
suppression
vasopressor
violence
yoga

Homeostasis

Homeostasis is derived from *homeo,* meaning "similar or like," and *stasis,* meaning "standing or stopping." The concept of homeostasis was first introduced by W. B. Cannon (1939) to describe the relative constancy of the internal processes of the body, such as blood oxygen and carbon dioxide levels, blood pressure, body temperature, blood glucose, and fluid and electrolyte balance. To Cannon, the word *homeostasis* did not imply something stagnant, set, or immobile; it meant a condition that might vary but remained relatively constant. Cannon viewed the human being as separate from his or her external environment and constantly endeavoring to maintain physiologic **equilibrium**, or balance, through adaptation to that environment. **Homeostasis**, then, is the tendency of the body to maintain a state of balance or equilibrium while continually changing. The changes may be minor or major as the body adapts to the internal and external environments.

Today, the concept of homeostasis has broadened to include all physiologic and psychologic processes and the rhythmicity of changes in the internal environment. *Steady state* and *dynamic equilibrium* are other terms often used to denote this balance. *Stability* may also be used to denote mental or emotional balance.

Recently, the term **homeodynamics** has been used by some to replace homeostasis. Homeodynamics implies a continual exchange of energy between human beings and the external environment. Rather than merely adapting to the environment, people interact with the environment and continually change. The concept of homeodynamics was described by Martha Rogers (1970).

Physiologic Homeostasis

Physiologic homeostasis means that the internal environment of the body is relatively stable and constant. All cells of the body require a relatively constant environment to function; thus, the body's internal environment must be maintained within narrow limits. The two major homeostatic regulators are the autonomic nervous system and the endocrine system. In addition, the cardiovascular system, the renal system, the respiratory system, and the gastrointestinal system are important regulators. See Figure 17–1. Although these systems work together to maintain homeostasis, each system is considered separately.

Autonomic Nervous System

The autonomic nervous system operates automatically or without conscious control to regulate visceral activities, i.e., of cardiac muscle, smooth muscle of blood vessels, smooth muscle of the digestive tract, and glands such as sweat glands, digestive organs, pancreas, liver, and glands of the adrenal medulla. The parasympathetic or craniosacral division functions under normal everyday conditions and when the body is at rest. It serves as the main regulator of the heart, stimulates the secretion of digestive juices and insulin, and stimulates the smooth muscle of the digestive tract to increase peristalsis. In short, the parasympathetic division promotes digestion and elimination. The sympathetic and thoracolumbar division functions chiefly as an emergency system. Under stress conditions, this division brings about a group of responses commonly known as the *fight-or-flight response*. Changes for maximum energy expenditure include a faster, stronger heartbeat, dilated blood vessels in skeletal muscles, dilated bronchi, and increased blood sugar level. Not all organs are doubly innervated by both divisions of the autonomic nervous system. For example, the coronary blood vessels, liver, and adrenal medulla are not innervated by parasympathetic fibers. Doubly innervated organs, however, are influenced in opposing or antagonistic ways to maintain stability. For example, the heart continually receives sympathetic impulses that tend to make it beat faster and parasympathetic impulses that tend to slow it down. The ratio between the two determines the actual heartbeat.

Homeostatic mechanisms have four main characteristics:

1. They are self-regulating.
2. They are compensatory.
3. They tend to be regulated by negative feedback systems.
4. They may require several feedback mechanisms to correct only one physiologic imbalance.

Self-regulation means that homeostatic mechanisms come into play automatically in the healthy person. However, if a person is ill, or if a respiratory organ such as a

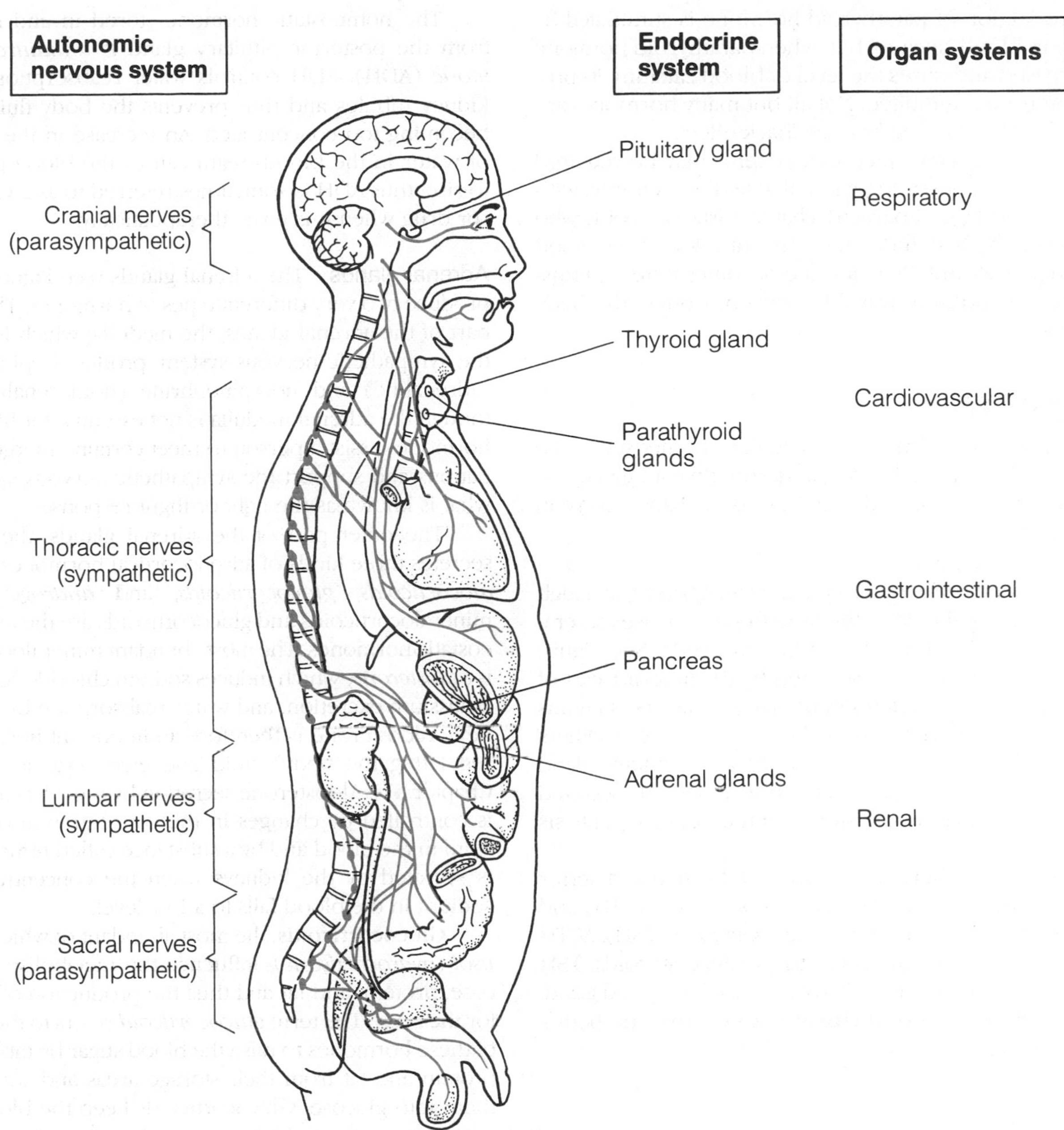

Figure 17–1 The homeostatic regulators of the body: autonomic nervous system, endocrine system, and specific organ systems.

lung is injured, the homeostatic mechanisms may not be able to respond to the stimulus as they would normally.

Homeostatic mechanisms are compensatory (counterbalancing), because they tend to counteract conditions that are abnormal for the person. An example is a sudden drop in temperature. The compensatory mechanisms are that the peripheral blood vessels constrict, thereby diverting most of the blood internally; and increased muscular activity and shivering occur to create heat. Through these mechanisms the body temperature remains stable despite the cold.

Homeostasis mechanisms tend to be regulated by negative feedback mechanisms. **Feedback** is the mechanism by which some of the output of a system is "fed back" into the system as input. This input influences the behavior of the system and its future output. Feedback may be negative or positive. **Negative feedback** inhibits change; **positive feedback** stimulates change. Most biologic systems are controlled by negative feedback to bring the system back to stability. This type of feedback system senses and counteracts any deviations from normal. The deviations may be greater or less than the normal level or range. Negative feedback is a common control mechanism for hormone levels. For example, an increase in the production of parathyroid hormone is stimulated by a drop in blood calcium, but, when parathyroid hormone is increased and raises the level of blood calcium, its production is then inhibited. Not all but many hormones are controlled by this negative feedback effect.

Several negative feedback systems may be required to correct one physiologic imbalance. For example, with hypoxia (shortage of oxygen), characteristic of people who live in very high altitudes, the concentration of red blood cells increases and the heart rate becomes faster to transport the blood and available oxygen around the body adequately.

Endocrine System

Five major endocrine glands regulate homeostasis: the pituitary gland, the adrenal glands, the thyroid gland, the parathyroid glands, and the islands of Langerhans in the pancreas.

Pituitary gland The pituitary gland (*hypophysis*), although only the size of the tip of the little finger, releases several hormones in response to the body's needs. See Figure 17–2. Some of these are secreted by the anterior part of the pituitary gland (*adenohypophysis*) under the stimulus of the *hypothalamus,* a part of the nervous system. Others are stored in the posterior part of the pituitary gland (*neurohypophysis*). These latter hormones are secreted by the hypothalamus and stored in the neurohypophysis until needed.

Two major hormones secreted from the anterior pituitary are *adrenocorticotropic hormone* (ACTH) and *thyrotropic* (or thyroid-stimulating) *hormone* (TSH). ACTH stimulates the adrenal cortex to produce steroids. TSH stimulates the secretion of thyroxin from the thyroid gland. The major function of thyroxin is to control the body's rate of metabolism.

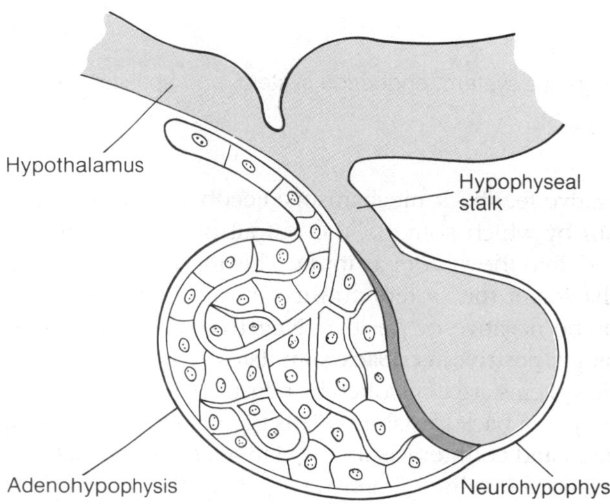

Figure 17–2 The pituitary gland.

The homeostatic hormone stored in and released from the posterior pituitary gland is *antidiuretic hormone* (ADH). ADH controls water reabsorption in the kidney tubules and thus prevents the body fluids from becoming too concentrated. An increase in the amount of water in the bloodstream causes the blood pressure to rise; thus ADH is sometimes referred to as a **vasopressor** drug when it is given therapeutically.

Adrenal glands The adrenal glands (see Figure 17–3) produce two very different types of hormones. The inner part of the adrenal glands, the medulla, which is part of the sympathetic nervous system, produces epinephrine (adrenaline) and norepinephrine (noradrenaline). Although the adrenal medulla is not essential for life, these hormones assist a person to meet certain emergency situations and support the sympathetic nervous system in what is known as the fight-or-flight response.

The outer part of the adrenal glands, the cortex, secretes three kinds of adrenocortical hormones: *mineralocorticoids, glucocorticoids,* and *androgens.* The mineralocorticoids and glucocorticoids are the two homeostatic hormones. The most abundant mineralocorticoid is *aldosterone,* which induces sodium chloride retention, potassium excretion, and water reabsorption by the kidneys. Aldosterone is therefore an important hormone in regulating the body's fluid and electrolyte levels (see Chapter 47). Aldosterone secretion by the adrenal cortex is controlled by changes in the concentration of potassium in the blood and by a substance called **renin,** which is secreted by the kidneys when the concentration of sodium in the blood falls to a low level.

Glucocorticoids, the most abundant of which is *cortisol (hydrocortisone),* influence the metabolism of glucose, protein, and fat and thus the production of energy for the body. The term *glucocorticoid* refers to the ability of these hormones to raise the blood sugar by mobilizing protein and fat from their storage areas and converting them into glucose. Glucocorticoids keep the blood glucose concentration high even during starvation periods and provide essential nutrients for nerve cells, which can use only glucose for energy. Another major function of the glucocorticoids is to increase a person's resistance to such physical stresses as injury, cold, pain, or fright. See the section on the general adaptation syndrome, later in this chapter. Glucocorticoid secretion is controlled by blood levels of pituitary ACTH. A pronounced rise in ACTH blood level is followed by an increase in the secretion of glucocorticoids.

Thyroid gland The thyroid gland, located in the neck below the larynx, consists of two fairly large lateral lobes that are joined by a connecting portion called the isthmus. This gland stores and secretes two homeostatic hormones: *thyroid hormone* (thyroxine and triiodothyronine, TH) and *calcitonin.* The primary physiologic actions of thyroid hormone are to regulate the body's metabolic rate and the processes of growth. Calcitonin decreases the blood's calcium concentration either by promoting the deposit of calcium into bone or by inhibiting bone breakdown, which would release calcium into the blood.

Parathyroid glands The four parathyroid glands located behind the thyroid gland secrete *parathyroid hormone* (parathormone, PTH), which raises plasma calcium levels and lowers plasma phosphate levels. Although knowledge about this hormone and its relationship to calcium and phosphorus metabolism is still incomplete, PTH is considered important for the body's homeostasis. Both calcium and phosphorus are necessary for healthy bones and teeth. Calcium is also necessary for blood coagulation when the body is injured and for proper transmission of nerve impulses.

Secretion of PTH is governed by a negative feedback system. Levels of blood calcium below normal increase the release of the hormone. PTH raises blood calcium primarily by releasing calcium from bone, where most of the body's calcium is found; it also increases the rate of calcium absorption from the intestines and calcium reabsorption by the kidneys. A dramatic example of low calcium levels is tetany, a condition in which the body's skeletal muscles are hyperirritable and in spasm. When spasm of the laryngeal muscles occurs, respiratory obstruction and death can ensue.

Islands of Langerhans The *islands of Langerhans* are clusters of endocrine-secreting cells located in the pancreas. The islands contain two types of cells: alpha cells, which secrete glucagon, and beta cells, which secrete insulin. *Insulin* accelerates the movement of sugar (glucose), protein (amino acids), and fats (fatty acids) out of the blood and into the tissue cells. Insulin, therefore, is a key regulator, since it lowers the blood concentration of these nutrients and promotes their metabolism and use by the cells. **Glucagon,** by contrast, tends to increase blood glucose concentration by stimulating the breakdown of liver glycogen.

Other Regulatory Systems

Cardiovascular-renal systems The kidneys are responsible for excretion and reabsorption of many by-products of metabolism. Their role in maintaining homeostasis of the body's fluids, electrolyte levels, and acid-base balance is vital. The cardiovascular system is the transport system that provides and removes essential elements for all body cells.

Respiratory system The respiratory system regulates intake of oxygen and exhalation of carbon dioxide. Oxygen is essential for metabolism and hence the production of energy. Elimination of carbon dioxide is also essential to maintain the body's acid-base balance, which is a very precise regulatory mechanism. For further discussion, see Chapter 46.

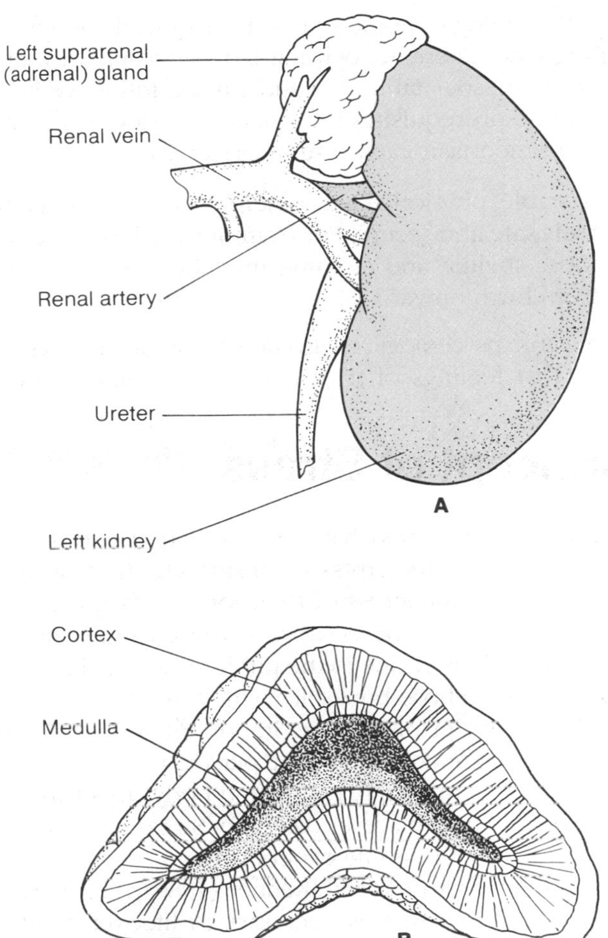

Figure 17–3 The adrenal glands: **A,** position of the gland on the kidney; **B,** cross section of the gland showing the medulla and the cortex.

Gastrointestinal system The gastrointestinal system is normally the only route for intake of fluids and electrolytes. It is thus an important regulator of fluid and electrolyte balance.

Psychologic Homeostasis

The term **psychologic homeostasis** refers to emotional or psychologic balance or a state of mental well-being. It is maintained by a variety of mechanisms. Each person has certain psychologic needs, such as the need for love, security, and self-esteem, that must be met to maintain psychologic homeostasis. When one or more of these needs is not met or is threatened, certain coping mechanisms are activated to protect the person and provide psychologic homeostasis. See the section on psychologic responses to stress, later in this chapter.

Psychologic homeostasis is acquired or learned through the experience of living and interacting with others. In addition, societal norms and culture influence behavior. Some prerequisites for a person to develop psychologic homeostasis can be summarized as:

1. A stable physical environment in which the person feels safe and secure. For example, the basic needs for food, shelter, and clothing must be met consistently from birth onward.
2. A stable psychologic environment from infancy onward, so that feelings of trust and love develop. Growing children and adolescents also need kind but firm and consistent discipline, encouragement, and support to be their own unique selves.
3. A social environment that includes adults who are healthy role models. Children learn the customs and values of society from these individuals.
4. A life experience that provides satisfactions. Throughout life, people encounter many frustrations. People deal with these better if enough satisfying experiences have occurred to counterbalance the frustrating ones.

Concept of Stress

In recent years **stress** has become a household word. Parents refer to the stress of raising children, working people talk of the stress of their jobs. In fact, the 1970s were described as the decade of stress. Familiarity with this word is largely due to the publications of Hans Selye (1974, 1976), whose books are widely read.

The concept of stress is important because it provides a way of understanding the person as a unified being who responds in totality (mind and body) to a variety of changes that take place in daily life. Stress is a universal phenomenon. All people experience it.

In the words of Griffith-Kenney (1986, p. 126), "Stress presents a paradox; it is necessary to life, yet it can be harmful to life." The life of any organism, including humans, is a series of responses to internal and external stress. In humans, these stresses include hunger, thirst, heat, cold, injury, bacterial or viral invasion, danger, joy, the angry remark of a friend, fear of an operation, death of a loved one, an alcoholic spouse, and so on. The more complex the organism, the more complex the stresses to which it is subjected and the more complex the mechanisms by which it responds. Moreover, the capacities of the organism (person) determine whether a given stressor or several stressors will merely challenge it or overwhelm it, and even whether the organism (person) will perceive the situation as a stressor (Griffith-Kenney 1986, p. 127).

Stress can have physical, emotional, intellectual, social, and spiritual consequences. Usually, the effects are mixed because stress affects the whole person. Physically, stress can threaten a person's physiologic homeostasis. Emotionally, stress can produce negative or nonconstructive feelings about self. Intellectually, stress can alter a person's perceptual and problem-solving abilities. Socially, stress can alter a person's relationships with others. Spiritually, stress can change a person's general outlook on life. Many illnesses, including hypertension, duodenal ulcers, bronchial asthma, and coronary heart disease, have been linked to stress.

What is stress? The term *stress* is used in the literature in varying ways. Lyon and Werner (1987) categorized 82 stress-related studies about adults over a 10-year-period (1975 to 1984) into the following theoretical orientations: stress as a stimulus, stress as a response, and stress as a transaction between the person and the environment.

Stress as a Stimulus

Defined as a stimulus, stress is viewed as an event or set of circumstances causing a disrupted response (Lyon and Werner 1987). The event or set of circumstances causing a disrupted response is generally defined as a "life change" or a "life event." The underlying assumption is that too much life change increases vulnerability to illness.

Life Changes and Experiences

The stimulus orientation to stress originated with Holmes and Masuda (1966) and Holmes and Rahe (1967), who developed tools known as the Social Readjustment Rating Scale (SRRS) or Schedule of Recent Experiences or Events (SRE). Holmes and Rahe (1967) assigned a numerical value to 43 life changes or events. The scale of stressful life events is used to document a person's relatively recent experiences, such as divorce, pregnancy, and retirement. In this view both positive and negative events are considered stressful.

Since 1967, similar scales have been developed. Burgess and Lazare (1976, p. 58) caution people in the use of such scales. They emphasize that the degree of stress the event presents can be highly individual. For example, a divorce may be highly traumatic to one person and cause relatively little anxiety to another. What is important is that research has shown that people who have a high level of stress are often more prone to illness and have lowered ability to cope with illness and subsequent stress.

Hospital Stress Rating Scale

Volicer and Burns (1975, p. 358) devised a 49-item hospital stress rating scale to measure client stress. See Table 17–1. The items were ranked by 261 medical and surgical

Table 17–1 The Volicer-Burns Hospital Stress Rating Scale

Assigned Rank	Event	Mean Rank Score
1	Having strangers sleep in the same room with you	13.9
2	Having to eat at different times than you usually do	15.4
3	Having to sleep in a strange bed	15.9
4	Having to wear a hospital gown	16.0
5	Having strange machines around	16.8
6	Being awakened in the night by the nurse	16.9
7	Having to be assisted with bathing	17.0
8	Not being able to get newspapers, radio, or TV when you want them	17.7
9	Having a roommate who has too many visitors	18.1
10	Having to stay in bed or the same room all day	19.1
11	Being aware of unusual smells around you	19.4
12	Having a roommate who is seriously ill or cannot talk with you	21.2
13	Having to be assisted with a bedpan	21.5
14	Having a roommate who is unfriendly	21.6
15	Not having friends visit you	21.7
16	Being in a room that is too cold or too hot	21.7
17	Thinking your appearance might be changed after your hospitalization	22.1
18	Being in the hospital during holidays or special family occasions	22.3
19	Thinking you might have pain because of surgery or test procedures	22.4
20	Worrying about your spouse being away from you	22.7
21	Having to eat cold or tasteless food	23.2
22	Not being able to call family or friends on the phone	23.3
23	Being cared for by an unfamiliar doctor	23.4
24	Being put in the hospital because of an accident	23.6
25	Not knowing when to expect things will be done to you	24.2
26	Having the staff be in too much of a hurry	24.5
27	Thinking about losing income because of your illness	25.9
28	Having medications cause you discomfort	26.0
29	Having nurses or doctors talk too fast or use words you can't understand	26.4
30	Feeling you are getting dependent on medications	26.4
31	Not having family visit you	26.5
32	Knowing you have to have an operation	26.9
33	Being hospitalized far away from home	27.1
34	Having a sudden hospitalization you weren't planning to have	27.2
35	Not having your call light answered	27.3
36	Not having enough insurance to pay for your hospitalization	27.4
37	Not having your questions answered by the staff	27.6
38	Missing your spouse	28.4
39	Being fed through tubes	29.2
40	Not getting relief from pain medications	31.2
41	Not knowing the results or reasons for your treatments	31.9
42	Not getting pain medication when you need it	32.4
43	Not knowing for sure what illness you have	34.0
44	Not being told what your diagnosis is	34.1
45	Thinking you might lose your hearing	34.5
46	Knowing you have a serious illness	34.6
47	Thinking you might lose a kidney or some other organ	35.6
48	Thinking you might have cancer	39.2
49	Thinking you might lose your sight	40.6

Source: B. J. Volicer and M. W. Burns, A hospital stress rating scale, *Nursing Research,* September/October 1975, 24:358. Copyright 1975 American Journal of Nursing Company. Reprinted with permission.

Research Note

Nurses are in an excellent position to educate families about the potential impact of stressful events on a disease process, such as cystic fibrosis. Van Os and colleagues find an important and not surprising relationship between reported parental stress and recurrent illness in children. The researchers do not purport to show whether stressful life events increase the severity of cystic fibrosis, or whether increased life stressors are a response to increased severity of the disease. The researchers support the family-centered approach to client care and suggest further research questions necessary to the development of appropriate strategies for lowering stress levels. (Van Os et al. 1985)

clients. When using the tool, nurses ask clients which events they have experienced since hospitalization. Before administering the tool, the nurse may want to remove the assigned rank numbers. This tool can identify specific stressors of an individual or groups of clients. When stressors are identified, the nurse can then plan nursing interventions to eliminate the stressors. For example, if a client cites item 9, "Having a roommate who has too many visitors," the nurse can limit the visitors or visiting times of the roommate or can perhaps have the client moved to a more private setting. A group of clients or a unit can also be tested. The results can be used to plan nursing interventions. For example, if a large group of clients on the same unit checked item 37, "Not having your questions answered by the staff," and item 42, "Not getting pain medication when you need it," the nursing staff can discuss and develop plans to answer questions and provide pain medication promptly.

Stress as a Response

Stress, as a response, is the disruption caused by a noxious stimulus or stressor (Lyon and Werner in press). It focuses on reactions rather than events. The response view was developed by Hans Selye (1956, 1976). He defined stress as "the nonspecific response of the body to any kind of demand made upon it" (1976, p. 1). Regardless of the cause, situation, or psychologic interpretation of a demanding situation, the stress response to Selye is characterized by the same chain or pattern of physiologic events. This nonspecific response was called the **general adaptation syndrome (GAS)** or **stress syndrome**.

Selye made a number of observations about disease that resulted in his concept of stress. First he noted that, although there were characteristic or different signs and symptoms of numerous diseases, clients all had many signs and symptoms in common (there appeared to be a specific syndrome), which he called stress. Also, there was no common cause (they were nonspecifically induced). To differentiate the cause of stress from the response to stress, Selye created the term **stressor** (1976, p. 51) to denote any factor that produces stress; that is, it is a factor that disturbs the body's equilibrium.

Because stress is a state of the body, it can be observed only by the changes it produces in the body. This response of the body, the **stress syndrome**, causes certain changes in the structure and chemical composition of the body. See the section on the general adaptation syndrome, next. Selye further concluded that these common signs of stress are a part of every disease process.

Some contemporary physiologists use the terms *stress* and *stressor* as Selye did. Others use the term *stress* to mean any stimulus that causes the neurons in the hypothalamus of the brain to release corticotropin-releasing hormone (CRH), which stimulates the many changes in the body that are described in the section on the general adaptation syndrome.

Selye's General Adaptation Syndrome

The general adaptation syndrome is created by the release of certain adaptive hormones within the person's body. The GAS, Selye found, occurred whenever an organism underwent prolonged stress. Body organs affected by stress are the gastrointestinal tract, the adrenals, and the lymphatic structures. The adrenals enlarged considerably; the lymphatic structures, such as the thymus, spleen, and lymph nodes, atrophied (shrank); and deep ulcers appeared in the lining of the stomach. In addition to a general adaptation syndrome, that is, generalized manifestations of stress, it was also proposed that the body can react by a local response. One organ or a part of the body can react alone. This is referred to as the **local adaptation syndrome**, or **LAS**. One example of the LAS is inflammation.

Research Note

A study of hospital stress revealed that clients who entered the hospital with recent experience (within the past 1 to 2 years) of high life stress perceived and reported more changes and problems associated with hospitalization than those with low life stress in the recent past. This finding suggests that life stress prior to hospitalization may be an important factor in the level of stress experienced because of hospitalization itself. This study also indicated correlations between level of hospital stress and (a) age—younger clients reported higher levels of stress than older clients, (b) number of years since last hospitalization—those with recent hospitalization reported more hospital stress than others, (c) seriousness of illness—particularly for surgical clients contrasted to medical clients, and (d) sex—women indicated higher stress levels than men. (Volicer and Burns 1977)

See the section on inflammatory adaptive response in Chapter 32, page 679. Selye proposed that both the GAS and the LAS had three stages (1976, p. 38): (a) alarm reaction, (b) stage of resistance, and (c) stage of exhaustion. See Figure 17–4.

Alarm reaction (AR) The initial reaction of the body is the alarm reaction, which alerts the body's defenses against the stressor, whether the stressor is heat, bacteria, or a verbal or physical attack from someone. The defenses of the whole body are mobilized and prepared to act to protect the body. Selye divided this stage into two parts: the shock phase and the countershock phase.

During the **shock phase**, the stressor may be perceived consciously or unconsciously by the person. In any case, the autonomic nervous system reacts, and large amounts of epinephrine (adrenaline) and cortisone are released into the body. The person is then ready for fight or flight. This primary response is short lived, lasting from 1 minute to 24 hours.

The second part of the alarm reaction is called the **countershock phase**. During this time, the body changes produced during the shock phase are reversed. It is, therefore, during the shock phase of the alarm reaction that a person is best mobilized to react.

Stage of resistance (SR) During the second stage in the GAS and LAS syndromes, the body's adaptation takes place. In other words, the body attempts to cope with the stressor and to limit the stressor to the smallest area of the body that can deal with it. See the section on inflammatory response, Chapter 32, p. 679.

Stage of exhaustion (SE) During the third stage, the adaptation that the body made during the second stage cannot be maintained. This means that the ways used to cope with the stressor have been exhausted. If adaptation has not overcome the stressor, the stress effects may spread to the entire body. At the end of this stage, the body may either rest and return to normal, or death may be the ultimate consequence. The end of this stage depends largely on the adaptive energy resources of the individual, the severity of the stressor, and the external adaptive resources that are provided, such as oxygen administered by mask.

Physiologic responses of the GAS Selye's general adaptation syndrome encompasses a range of physiologic responses to stressors in the body as a whole. See Figure 17–5. Stressors stimulate the sympathetic nervous system, which in turn stimulates the hypothalamus. The hypothalamus releases corticotropin-releasing hormone (CRH), which stimulates the anterior pituitary gland to release adrenocorticotropin (ACTH).

ACTH stimulates the adrenal cortex to produce substances that Selye refers to as *anti-inflammatory corticoids* (A-C). The commonly known A-C is cortisone, which

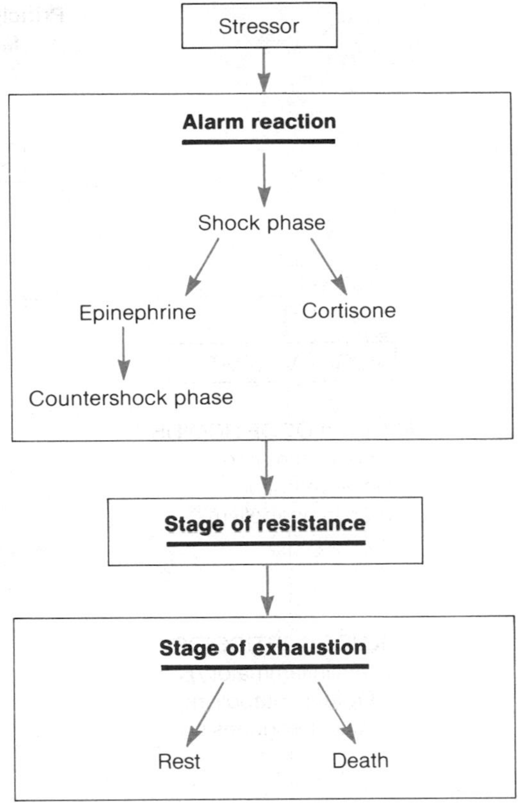

Figure 17–4 The three stages of adaptation to stress: the alarm reaction, the stage of resistance, and the stage of exhaustion.

has been used effectively for clients with rheumatoid arthritis and other inflammatory conditions. Cortisone is also considered a glucocorticoid, since it elevates the blood sugar (glucose) level through increased *gluconeogenesis* (a process by which the liver converts proteins and fats into glucose). *Protein catabolism* also occurs. Catabolism is a process in which complex substances are broken down into simpler substances. Cortisol has the following actions, which are of particular value when there is tissue trauma:

1. *Gluconeogenesis*. It forms glucose from protein and fat compounds, making energy readily available.
2. *Protein mobilization*. It causes the liver to form new proteins that can be used by damaged tissues.
3. *Stabilization of lysosomal membranes*. Lysosomes are the parts of a cell that contain enzymes and thus dissolve or digest most cellular compounds. When cells are damaged and the lysosome membranes are ruptured, the released enzymes cause an inflammatory response. Therefore, cortisol reduces inflammation by strengthening or stabilizing the lysosome membrane.

Mineralocorticoids, which Selye refers to as pro-inflammatory corticoids (P-C), are also released by the

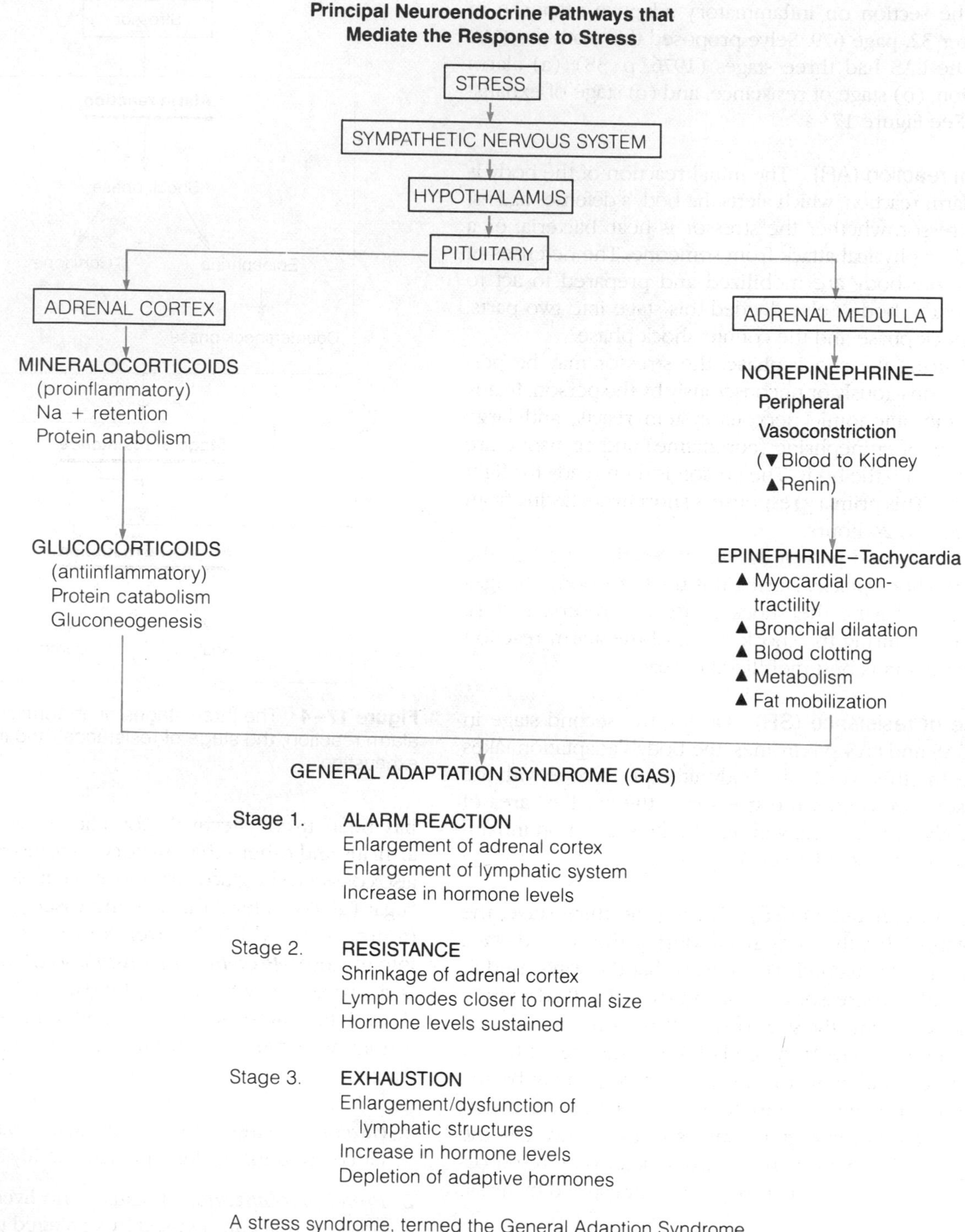

Figure 17–5 Physiologic response to stress: General Adaptation Syndrome

Source: Physiologic responses of the general adaptation syndrome. From Smith, M. J., and Selye, H. November 1979. Stress: Reducing the negative effects of stress *American Journal of Nursing* 79:1954. Used by permission.

adrenal cortex. The principal mineralocorticoid is aldosterone.

Aldosterone regulates the excretion of potassium and absorption of sodium in the kidney tubules. When excessive amounts of aldosterone are secreted, sodium is reabsorbed into the extracellular fluid of the body along with water. This adaptive mechanism conserves water for the body and maintains the blood volume.

Selye believes that the portion between A-Cs and P-Cs is normally maintained in balance. During periods of stress, however, the A-Cs tend to predominate under the influence of ACTH.

During stress the adrenal medulla, which is functionally related to the sympathetic nervous system, secretes *epinephrine* and *norepinephrine* in response to sympathetic stimulation. These hormones are secreted into the circulating bloodstream and distributed to all parts of the body. They have almost the same effects as those caused by direct sympathetic stimulation, except that (a) the effects last longer, since the hormones are released from the blood slowly, and (b) they can stimulate structures of the body that are not innervated by direct sympathetic fibers. The effect of these hormones is often referred to as the fight-or-flight syndrome because the body becomes ready for action as a result. Significant body responses to epinephrine include:

1. Increased myocardial contractility, which increases cardiac output and blood flow to active muscles
2. Broncial dilation, which allows increased oxygen intake
3. Increased blood clotting
4. Increased cellular metabolism
5. Increased fat mobilization to make energy available and to synthesize other compounds needed by the body

The principal effect of norepinephrine is decreased blood to the kidneys and increased secretion of renin. *Renin* is an enzyme that hydrolyzes one of the blood proteins to produce *angiotensin*. Angiotensin tends to increase the blood pressure by constricting arterioles.

The sum of all these adrenal hormonal effects permits the person to perform far more strenuous physical activity than would otherwise be possible.

Stress as a Transaction

Lazarus's Model

Transactional theories of stress are based on the work of Lazarus (1966), who says that neither the stimulus theory nor the response theory of stress considers individual differences. Neither explains which factors lead some persons and not others to respond effectively nor explains why some persons are able to adapt over longer periods than others. In the words of Lazarus, "Stimulus definitions focus on events in the environment such as natural disasters, illness, or termination of employment. This approach assumes that certain situations are normatively stressful but does allow for individual differences in the evaluation of events. Response definitions refer to a state of stress; the person is spoken of as reacting with stress, being under stress, and so on. Stimulus and response definitions have limited utility, because a stimulus gets defined as stressful only in terms of a stress response" (Lazarus and Folkman 1984, p. 21).

Although Lazarus recognizes that certain environmental demands and pressures produce stress in substantial numbers of people, he emphasizes that people and groups differ in their sensitivity and vulnerability to certain types of events, as well as in their interpretations and reactions. For example, in terms of illness, one person may respond with denial, another with anxiety, and still another with depression. In order to understand variations among individuals under comparable conditions, the Lazarus model takes into account cognitive processes that intervene between the encounter and the reaction, and the factors that affect the nature of this mediation. In contrast to Selye, who focused on physiologic responses, Lazarus introduces mental and psychologic components or responses to stress.

The Lazarus transactional stress theory encompasses a set of cognitive, affective, and adaptive (coping) responses that arise out of person-environment transactions. The person and the environment are inseparable; each affects and is affected by the other. *Stress* is defined as a particular relationship between the person and the environment that is appraised by the person as taxing or exceeding his or her resources and endangering his or her well-being (Lazarus and Folkman 1984, p. 19). Stress is viewed as an interactive process between: (a) the individual, (b) the individual's internal and external environments, and (c) the individual's cognitive appraisal of any given stimulus. The individual responds to perceived environmental changes by adaptive or coping responses. **Cognitive appraisal** is an evaluative process that determines why and to what extent a particular transaction or series of transactions between the person and the environment is stressful. **Coping** is the process through which the individual manages the demands of the person-environment relationship that are appraised as stressful and the emotions they generated (Lazarus and Folkman 1984, p. 19).

Cognitive appraisal and coping processes have implications for nurses assisting clients with stress. For example, the nurse using the Lazarus stress model will determine how each client perceives or cognitively appraises a stressful event and assess what coping mechanisms the client uses.

Nuernberger's Model

The general adaptation syndrome emphasizes the response of the sympathetic nervous system to a stressful stimulus.

Nuernberger (1981, p. 69) believes that there is an adaptive pattern of responding beyond the arousal mechanism of the sympathetic nervous system. This other response, based on stimulation of the parasympathetic nervous system, is one of inhibition. He calls this response the **general inhibition syndrome** or **possum response.** To Nuernberger (1981, p. 71), healthy nonstress functioning is represented by a balance between the two parts of the autonomic nervous system: sympathetic and parasympathetic branches. Stress is a state of internal imbalance reflecting the unrelieved dominance of either arousal by the sympathetic nervous system (fight-or-flight response) or inhibition by the parasympathetic nervous system (possum response). The effects of excessive stimulation of or dominance by either of these systems are evinced as a localized response in a specific organ or as a generalized response pattern. Both responses are designed for self-protection.

Nuernberger states that a significant number of people respond to threatening situations with passive withdrawal. Instead of preparing to fight or run away (flight) when faced with a threat, some people "just . . . roll over and play dead." Their response to fear is not arousal but inhibition; it is characterized by extreme parasympathetic dominance that manifests itself in decreased physiologic functioning, loss of skeletal tone, mental lassitude, inactivity, and eventual depression. In contrast to Selye's exhaustion stage in the general adaptation syndrome, during which a person's reserves are depleted, the possum response does not draw on these reserves; they are not depleted. Nuernberger says that the presence of either arousal or inhibition does not in itself constitute stress. Stress occurs only when arousal is not balanced by relaxation or when relaxation (inhibition) is not balanced by activity. Prolonged or intense parasympathetic imbalances are associated with such diseases as asthma or depression. Prolonged sympathetic imbalances are associated with, for example, cardiovascular disease.

Nuernberger (1981, p. 81) believes that the primary source of stress is not the external environment; it is a person's internal state or his or her own mind; it is the emotional and perceptual factors that form a person's basic personality. The greatest source of hypothalamic arousal is the cerebral cortex in response to repetitive thought patterns and apprehensions about unresolved past, present, or future events that people associate with potentially painful or negative consequences in their lives.

To Nuernberger, stress is a physiologic response to one's mental and perceptual activities; the way a person thinks about a situation determines whether or not the person experiences stress. He defines emotional stress as ". . . the result of a mental process: It is a state of autonomic imbalance generated as a reaction to the perception of some kind of threat, pain or discomfort. This perception involves an interpretation of selected sensory stimuli, which is colored, or structured, by memories of past pain. It is also involved with the anticipation that this pain will occur in the future as a consequence of present sensory stimuli and environmental conditions. It is sustained by indecisiveness, the inability to resolve the threat" (Nuernberger 1981, p. 86).

Manifestations of the Stress Experience

Manifestations of the stress experience are viewed by many nurses as coping strategies; the exception is anxiety, which is often considered to be a response to a stressful event.

Coping is the immediate response of a person to a threatening situation, whereas adaptation is the final response or change that occurs. According to Lazarus and Folkman (1984, p. 141), coping refers to constantly changing cognitive and behavioral efforts to manage specific external and/or internal demands that are appraised as taxing or exceeding the resources of a person. Coping may be described as dealing with problems and situations, or contending with them successfully. A **coping strategy** (*coping mechanism*) is an innate or acquired way of responding to a changing environment or specific problem or situation. The term *mechanism* frequently applies to the physiologic or unconscious realm; *strategy,* to the conscious realm. In nursing literature, effective and ineffective coping are often differentiated. *Effective coping* results in adaptation; *ineffective coping* results in maladaptation. Although coping behavior may not always seem appropriate, the nurse needs to remember that coping is always purposeful.

Coping strategies vary among individuals and are often related to the individual's perception of the stressful event. A person's coping strategies often change as she or he appraises and reappraises a situation. There is no one way to cope. Some people choose to avoid the situation; others, to confront a situation as a means of coping. Others seek information or rely on religious beliefs as a means of coping. Bell (1977, p. 137) places coping strategies into two groups: long term and short term. Long-term coping strategies can be constructive and realistic. For example, in certain situations talking with others about the problem and trying to find out more about the situation are long-term strategies.

Short-term coping strategies can reduce stress to a tolerable limit temporarily but are in the long run ineffective ways to deal with reality. They may even have a destructive or detrimental effect on the person (Bell 1977, p. 137). Examples of short-term strategies are using alcoholic beverages or drugs, daydreaming and fantasizing, and relying on the belief that everything will work out.

Physiologic Manifestations

Physiologic manifestations may or may not occur in clients experiencing stress, depending on the way the client perceives the stressful event and on the effectiveness of his or her coping strategies. There is considerable evidence that a person's cognitive coping strategies mediate blood pressure and heart rates. For example, when a person cognitively attends to the stressor or threat, there is a decrease in heart rate. Physiologic manifestations that do occur result from the release of adrenal hormones (discussed earlier in Selye's general adaptation syndrome) and to excessive stimulation and dominance by the sympathetic nervous system or excessive stimulation and dominance by the parasympathetic nervous system. Specific physiologic manifestations are featured nearby.

Psychologic Manifestations

Psychologic manifestations include anxiety, anger, cognitive behaviors, verbal and motor responses, and unconscious ego defense mechanisms. Some of these coping patterns are helpful; others are a hindrance, depending on the situation and the length of time they are used or experienced.

Anxiety **Anxiety**, a common reaction to stress, is a state of mental uneasiness, apprehension, dread, or foreboding or a feeling of helplessness related to an impending or anticipated unidentified threat to self or significant relationships. Anxiety can be experienced at the conscious, subconscious, or unconscious levels. It differs from fear in four ways:

1. Its source is not identifiable; the source of fear is identifiable.
2. It is related to the future, i.e., an anticipated event. Fear is related to the present.
3. It is vague, while fear is definite.
4. It is the result of psychologic or emotional conflict; fear is the result of a discrete physical or psychologic entity.

All people experience anxiety to some degree most of the time. Mild or moderate anxiety is needed to accomplish developmental tasks and motivate goal-directed behavior. For example, mild anxiety motivates students to study. Excessive anxiety, however, has destructive effects.

Anxiety has been classified into four levels. (See also Table 17–2 for signs of these levels.)

Physiologic Manifestations of Stress*

- Pupils dilate to increase visual perception when serious threats to the body arise.
- Sweat production (diaphoresis) is increased to control elevated body heat due to increased metabolism.
- The heart rate increases, which leads to an increased pulse rate to transport nutrients and by-products of metabolism more efficiently.
- Skin is pallid due to constriction of peripheral blood vessels, an effect of norepinephrine.
- Blood pressure is elevated, due to
  a. constriction of vessels in blood reservoirs, such as the skin, kidneys, and most large interior organs.
  b. increased secretion of renin, an effect of norepinephrine.
  c. increased sodium and water retention due to release of mineralocorticoids, which results in increased blood volume.
  d. increased cardiac output.
- The rate and depth of respirations increase due to dilation of the bronchioles, promoting hyperventilation.
- Urinary output is decreased.
- The mouth may be dry.
- Peristalsis of the intestines is decreased, resulting in possible constipation and flatus.
- Mental alertness is improved for serious threats.
- Muscle tension is increased to prepare for rapid motor activity or defense.
- Blood sugar is increased due to release of glucocorticoids and gluconeogenesis.
- Lethargy, mental lassitude, inactivity (parasympathetic dominance) may ensue.
- There may be decreased physiologic functioning and loss of skeletal muscle tone (parasympathetic dominance).

*All signs are the result of increased activity of the sympathetic nervous system unless indicated otherwise.

1. *Mild anxiety* produces a slight arousal state that enhances perception, learning, and productive abilities. Most healthy persons experience mild anxiety, perhaps as a feeling of restlessness that prompts a person to seek information and ask questions.
2. *Moderate anxiety* increases the arousal state to a point where the person expresses feelings of tension, ner-

Table 17–2 Signs of Mild, Moderate, and Severe Anxiety

Sign	Mild	Moderate	Severe (Panic)
Verbalization changes	Expresses feelings of increased arousal and concern Increased questioning or information seeking	Expresses feelings of tension, apprehension, nervousness, or concern Verbalized expectation of danger Voice tremors and pitch changes Increased rate and quantity of verbalization	Expresses feelings of severe dread, apprehension, nervousness, concern, helplessness, and isolation Absence of verbalization Inappropriate verbalization, e.g., false cheerfulness or laughing while discussing a serious subject
Motor activity changes	Mild restlessness	Pacing Hand tremor or shakiness Increased muscle tension	Immobilization Purposeless activity Increased muscle tension Rigid posture Fixed or scattered perceptual focus
Perception and attention changes	Increased awareness Increased attending Ability to focus on most of what is really happening	Narrowed focus of attention Ability to focus on most of what is really happening	Intellectualizing about a subject, e.g., explaining the pathophysiology of leukemia rather than describing own feelings Intent and fearful watching of everything going on Inability to focus on what is really happening Inability to focus on reality, e.g., denial, saying "I don't want to talk about it"
Respiratory and circulatory changes	Nil	Rapid pulse Increased respiratory rate	Tachycardia Palpitations Hyperventilation
Other changes	Nil	Diaphoresis Sleep or eating disturbances, e.g., insomnia, somnolence, overeating, or anorexia Irritability	Diaphoresis Dilated pupils Pallor Clammy hands and skin Dry mouth Sullenness, withdrawal

Source: Compiled from M. Gordon, *Manual of nursing diagnosis* (New York: McGraw-Hill Book Co, 1982), pp. 153–60; and Anxiety: recognition and intervention (programmed instruction) *AJN*, September 1965, 65:129–52.

vousness, or concern. Perceptual abilities are narrowed. Attention is focused more on a particular aspect of a situation than on peripheral activities. The person usually experiences increased muscle tension and elevated respiratory and pulse rates.

3. *Severe anxiety* consumes most of the person's energies and requires intervention. Perception is further decreased. The person, unable to focus on what is really happening, focuses on only one specific detail of the situation generating the anxiety. Learning ability is impaired; the person is able to follow only simple instructions. Increased physical signs—such as palpitations, clammy hands and skin, hyperventilation, and rigid posture—are evident.
4. *Panic* is an overpowering, frightening level of anxiety causing the person to lose control. It is less frequently experienced than other levels of anxiety. The perception of a panicked person can be altered to the point where the person distorts events. Learning ability is absent since the person is intent and fearful. Physical signs may include speechlessness and immobility.

Anxiety is caused by any situation of frustration, conflict, or stress that threatens a person's physical or mental security. Specific examples are countless, including physical and emotional illness and worries about failure, rejection, financial loss, failure to meet a deadline, discovery of a secret, and the opinion of others.

Anger **Anger** is an emotional state consisting of a subjective feeling of animosity or strong displeasure. In North America, the term is unfortunately often used to refer to physical attacks and violence; as a result, any expression of anger may be labeled bad. Many people feel guilty when they feel anger, because they have learned that to feel angry is wrong.

In fact, anger, hostility, violence, and aggression differ. Anger can be expressed in a nonalienating verbal manner; it is then considered a positive emotion and a sign of emotional maturity, since growth and beneficial interactions result from it.

Rothenberg (1971, p. 454) defines the expression of anger as an assertive, altered communicative state that arises as an alternative to, and a defense against, anxiety. Anger is commonly manifested in (a) altered voice tone and (b) a communication to desist from some action or other. Verbal expression of anger can therefore be considered a signal to others of one's internal psychologic discomfort and a call for assistance to deal with perceived stress.

Hostility is usually marked by overt antagonism and harmful or destructive behavior. **Aggression** is usually defined as an unprovoked attack or a hostile, injurious, or destructive action or outlook. **Violence** is the exertion of physical force to injure or abuse. Verbally expressed anger differs from hostility, aggression, and violence, but it can lead to destructiveness and violence if the anger persists unabated.

The state of anger can be viewed as a communication process that involves either a recurring sequence of events with several vicious cycles or a means to achieve closure or completion. See Figure 17–6. The sequence of events, according to Rothenberg (1971, p. 456), is:

1. A threat, need, or obstruction creates a stressful state, which causes anxiety. Anxiety is manifested by undirected, purposeless motor responses (e.g., pacing the floor) or avoidance or escape responses. Anxiety evokes feelings of helplessness and defenselessness.
2. Anxiety develops into anger when motor responses are directed at the real or imagined source of arousal. Anger provides a defense against anxiety and feelings of helplessness, because the person feels more powerful and in control when angry, unless the context makes the anger socially unacceptable. If anger is socially unacceptable, more anxiety is created. If in addition the person has destructive thoughts about the person or object causing the stressful state, guilt feelings often result, which further increase anxiety.
3. Tension is discharged and anger is prolonged or resolved by either:
    a. Fight (attack) or flight responses coupled with noncommunication. These responses prolong tension and lead to potential hostility and violence.
    b. Verbalizing internal experiences clearly or unclearly and avoiding physical attack. When anger is clearly communicated, tension is relieved and anger is dissipated; when it is not clearly communicated, i.e., the communication does not focus on the cause of the anger, the outcome is the same as when no communication has taken place.

People may fail to express anger verbally for several reasons (Rothenberg 1971, p. 456):

1. To be tactful or polite in social situations
2. To avoid loss of power and status or to avoid placing themselves at a disadvantage in conflict relationships
3. For fear of eliciting anger from others
4. For fear of revealing their needs and vulnerability to others in conflict relationships
5. For fear of evoking physical destructiveness in themselves or others
6. For fear of exposing their level of involvement in relationships, e.g., love relationships
7. Because of immediate recognition that they have made an error in perception

Clearly expressed verbal communication of anger is constructive. When the angry person tells the other person about the anger and carefully identifies the source, the anger is constructive. This clarity of communication gets the anger out into the open so that the other person can deal with it and help to alleviate it. The angry person "gets it off his chest" and prevents an emotional buildup. Constructive expressions of anger have three elements: alerting, describing, and identifying (Duldt 1981, p. 516). **Alerting** is the act of engaging another's attention. **Describing** is the process of delineating the source of the angry person's feelings, i.e., what has happened here and now. **Identifying** is the act of seeking a response and support from others. Examples of constructive anger are:

- "Darn! (Alerting.) This electric drill makes me mad! It won't work. (Describing.) What am I doing wrong?" (Identifying.)
- "Robert! (Alerting.) Your going to the football game this afternoon infuriates me. You said yesterday you'd clean the car for me before I have to drive my friends to the church social tonight. (Describing.) Now what am I going to do?" (Identifying.)

Unclear communication of anger is destructive. It is similar to constructive expressions only in the alerting behavior. Then the person fails to describe the source of the feelings adequately and denies any responsibility for the anger by blaming others or by generalizing to other people or past situations. Thus, those in the presence of the angry person are unable to respond helpfully. Examples of unclearly expressed anger are:

- "Darn it! (Alerting.) A woman can never win." (Generalizing.)

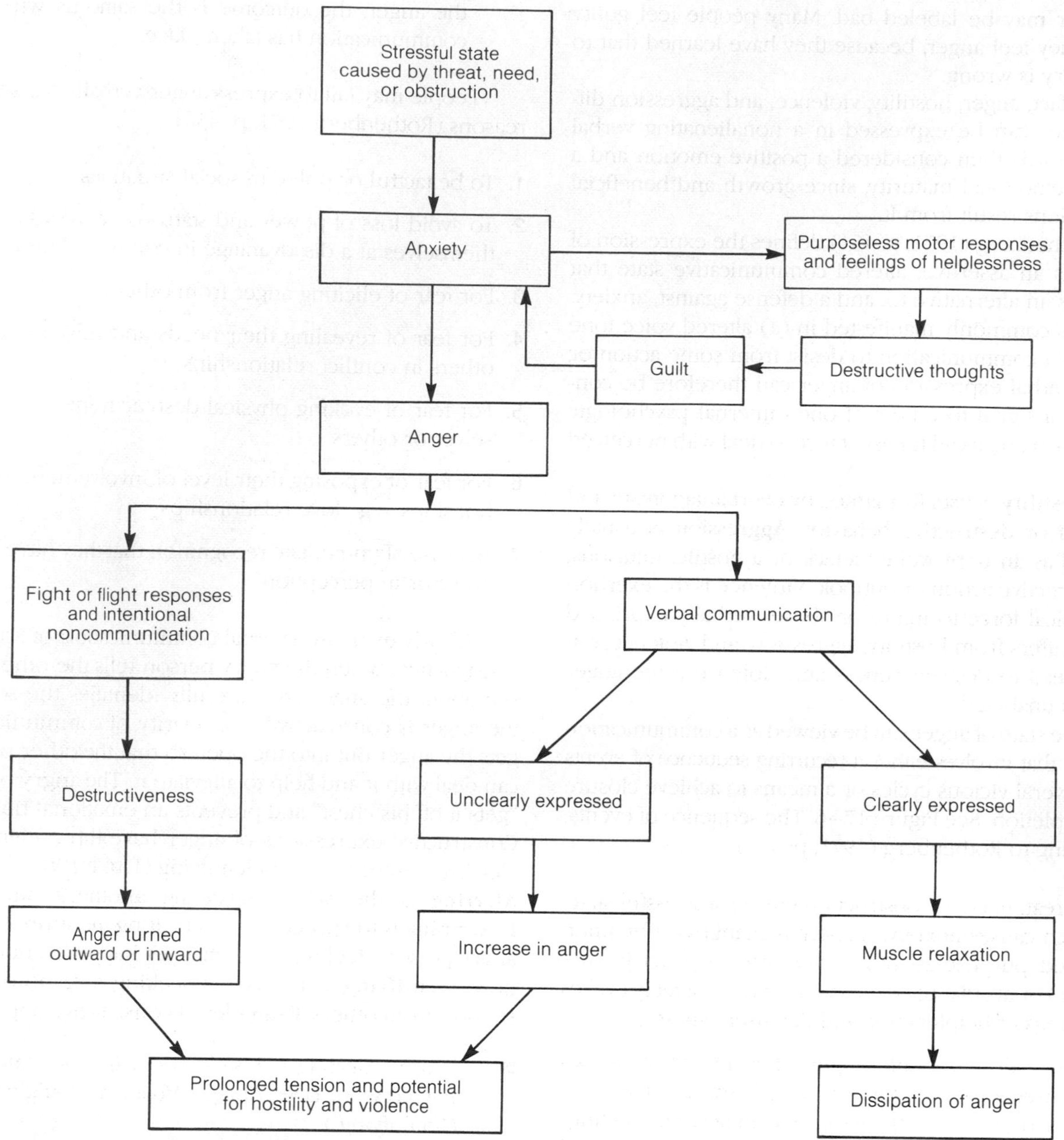

Figure 17–6 Model of anger as a communication process.

Source: Adapted from B. W. Duldt, Anger: An occupational hazard for nurses, *Nursing Outlook,* September 1981, 29:514.

- "You slob! (Alerting.) You're always leaving me in the lurch." (Generalizing, blaming.)

Cognitive Manifestations

Cognitive manifestations are thinking responses that include problem solving, structuring, self-control or self-discipline, suppression, fantasy, and prayer.

1. *Problem solving* involves thinking through the threatening situation, using specific steps similar to those of the nursing process, to arrive at a solution. The person assesses the situation or problem, analyzes or defines it, chooses alternatives, carries out the selected alternative, and evaluates whether the solution was successful. Not all people are adept at problem solving; others who are adept often carry out these steps without conscious awareness. Problem solving is a high-level constructive response. Increased knowledge and growth usually occur with problem solving.
2. *Structuring* is the arrangement or manipulation of a situation so that threatening events do not occur. For example, a nurse can structure or control an interview with a client by asking only direct, closed questions. This strategy avoids information or questions that may be threatening to the nurse's knowledge or values. Similarly, the nurse might follow standardized routines

rather than individualizing care for a client. Structuring, however, can be productive in certain situations. A person who schedules a dental examination semiannually to prevent severe dental disease is using productive structuring. Similarly, the person who plans a travel route to avoid traffic is using productive structuring.

3. *Self-control (discipline)* is assuming a manner and facial expression that convey a sense of being in control or in charge, no matter what the situation is. When self-control prevents panic and harmful or nonproductive actions in a threatening situation, it is a helpful response that conveys strength. Self-control carried to an extreme, however, can delay problem solving and prevent a person from receiving the support of others, who may perceive the person as handling the situation well, cold, or unconcerned.

4. *Suppression* is consciously and willfully putting a thought or feeling out of mind: "I won't deal with that today. I'll do it tomorrow." This response relieves stress temporarily but does not solve the problem. A man who keeps ignoring a toothache, pushing it out of his mind because he fears the pain of having a filling, will not relieve his symptoms or find the solution.

5. *Fantasy* or *daydreaming* is likened to make-believe. Unfulfilled wishes and desires are imagined as fulfilled, or a threatening experience is reworked or replayed so that it ends differently from reality. Experiences can be relived, everyday problems solved, and plans for the future made. Most people have relived a threatening situation in which they replay a part and imagine themselves saying or doing something clever or heroic when in fact they said nothing and were "frozen" and unable to move. The outcome of current problems may also be fantasized. For example, a client who is awaiting the results of a breast biopsy may fantasize the surgeon as saying, "You do not have cancer." Fantasy responses can be helpful if they lead to problem solving. For example, the client awaiting breast biopsy results might say to herself, "The doctor isn't going to say 'You do not have cancer,' but as long as he says I won't need mutilating surgery, I can accept that." Fantasies can be destructive and nonproductive if a person uses them to excess and retreats from reality.

6. *Prayer* often involves identifying and describing the problem, suggesting solutions, and reaching out for support and help. For example, a young woman may pray: "Please help me. The doctor says I have headaches and hypertension because I'm overweight (describing problem). What I need is to discipline myself to exercise more and go on a diet" (suggesting solutions). If these first two problem-solving steps lead to action, prayer can be a constructive response, aside from the support and meaning the person derives from it.

Verbal and Motor Manifestations

The first manifestations of stress may be verbal or motor. These manifestations include:

1. *Crying* releases tension in intense situations perceived as painful, joyful, or sad and when the situation cannot yet be managed cognitively. As a response, crying tends to be more socially acceptable in women and in certain cultures, for instance, among Hispanics or Mediterranean people. People often cry when they perceive that others care. Crying is beneficial as a release of tension and if it is followed by problem solving. It is not helpful without problem solving.

2. *Verbal abuse* is another release mechanism most often expressed toward stress-producing objects and events, such as nonfunctional equipment, misplaced or lost items, and rainy weather. See also the section on anger, earlier in this chapter.

3. *Laughing* is also an anxiety-reducing response that can lead to constructive problem solving. A person may laugh at small incidents and at the way he or she handled a situation. For example, a preoccupied, stressed man whose wife has had an accident may laugh at having put on one black shoe and one brown shoe before rushing to the emergency room.

4. *Screaming* is a response to fear or intense frustration and anger. One may scream in response to a person appearing suddenly out of the dark or in response to a family member who keeps planning other activities to avoid cleaning the garage. Screaming, like other verbal responses, reduces tension but can be harmful if the person is unable to control it and becomes hysterical. The hysterical, frightened person needs to be moved to a quiet place and assured that the threat is over. The hysterical, frustrated person needs assistance to deal with the situation with a more effective coping strategy, e.g., problem solving.

5. *Hitting and kicking* are spontaneous responses to physical threats. Adults who are socialized to control such responses toward people may direct them toward objects by pounding a table with a fist or kicking a wastebasket. Preschoolers, however, have not matured enough to develop control and may, for example, hit or kick a nurse who is administering an injection. Hitting or kicking can be helpful in reducing tension provided the person or object is not damaged and provided they lead toward cognitive coping techniques.

6. *Holding and touching* are often responses to joyful, painful, or sad events. Holding or touching another is a gesture of support and comfort. Holding and touching responses vary considerably, however, among cultures and among individuals in a culture. Vebal communication can also convey caring. "Crisis lines" or

Table 17–3 Unconscious Ego Defense Mechanisms

Mechanism	Description	Adaptive Use	Maladaptive Use
Denial	Blocking painful or anxiety-producing aspects of reality out of consciousness. Reality is either completely disregarded or transformed so that it is no longer threatening.	A man does not acknowledge that he has cancer even though the physician has told him the results of the biopsy. A child insists his mother is not dead, just "out of town for a few days."	A woman who has had a heart attack refuses to acknowledge illness and does not follow prescribed therapy.
Rationalization	Often referred to as the "sour-grapes" or "half-truth" mechanism. Good reasons, acceptable to the conscious mind, are given for behavior or circumstances instead of the real reason. The person often disparages some goal that in reality he or she would like to attain.	A student who fails an examination because she doesn't understand the material says that the teacher did not clarify the material sufficiently or she did not prepare adequately. A client whose work is interrupted by illness prematurely gives up the work and says he wouldn't have been successful in that field anyway.	A man always gives reasons for not attaining his goals and refuses to accept self-responsibility for not achieving them.
Compensation	Substituting an activity for one that the person really would like to do or cannot do.	A short man shows aggressive, dominating traits to suggest strength and authority that his stature does not convey. A boy who cannot participate in athletics studies hard and attains high grades.	A woman abuses alcohol and drugs to make up for feelings of inadequacy.
Repression	Excluding from consciousness desires, impulses, thoughts, memories, and strivings that conflict with self-image or that involve guilt, shame, or lowering of self-esteem. The painful events cannot be recalled or recognized. Repression is the underlying basis of all defense mechanisms.	A woman forgets a repugnant work assignment. A young woman who was raped and was brought to the outpatient clinic by her roommate says she feels very anxious but cannot remember the events of the past few hours.	A woman excludes a number of events from memory (amnesia).
Regression	Adopting behavior that was comforting earlier in life to overcome the discomfort and insecurity of the present situation.	A toilet-trained preschooler begins bed-wetting after his mother returns home with a new baby. A hospitalized elderly woman becomes more dependent on the nurse than is physically warranted.	A teenager assumes the fetal position for prolonged periods or plays with the genitals.
Sublimation	Redirecting libidinal drives (sexual and aggressive) into socially acceptable channels.	A person channels, to a limited degree, a sex drive into athletic activity, work, poetry, or music.	A person has extreme difficulty in communicating with others.

(continued)

close friends often provide meaningful and supportive verbal communication that conveys caring over the telephone or in person.

Unconscious Ego Defense Mechanisms

Psychologic defensive (adaptive) mechanisms, or in the words of Sigmund Freud (1946), **mental mechanisms**, develop as the personality attempts to defend itself, establish compromises among conflicting impulses, and allay inner tensions. Defense mechanisms are the working of the unconscious mind to protect the person from anxiety. They can be considered precursors to conscious cognitive coping mechanisms that will ultimately solve the problem. Like some verbal and motor responses, defense mechanisms release tension. Table 17–3 describes these mechanisms and lists examples of their adaptive and maladaptive use. Adaptive examples are indicative of sporadic use by healthy individuals; maladaptive examples are indicative of consistent use or misuse by unhealthy persons. In all instances, the mechanisms preserve a person's self-concept, self-esteem, and sense of security or psychologic stability.

Table 17–3 *(continued)*

Mechanism	Description	Adaptive Use	Maladaptive Use
		A man who is fired goes to the gym and punches a punching bag to express rage at his boss.	
Identification	Assuming the attitudes, ideas, and behavior patterns of another person or persons; it is an important growth mechanism for children. It is unconscious and differs from imitation, which is conscious.	A teenager changes her hairstyle to that of an idolized movie star. After having surgery, a young boy decides to become a doctor.	A man imitates socially unacceptable or harmful behavior.
Projection	Attributing to others characteristics and feelings that the person does not want to admit are his or her own.	A woman criticizes a neighbor for being a terrible gossip when in fact the woman herself gossips. A wife with illicit sexual wishes claims that all husbands are unfaithful and not to be trusted.	A person fails to take any responsibility for own behavior.
Conversion	Transforming a mental conflict into a physical symptom.	Before taking a math exam, a young girl develops a headache. A woman develops a "lump in her throat" at a sad event.	A man experiences paralysis of his punching arm to avoid letting his anger get out of control and punching his boss. A girl develops an inability to speak in the context of protecting a sexually abusive father. A pregnant woman develops pathologic vomiting to express the forbidden desire not to have the baby.
Displacement	Transferring an emotion or feeling from the actual object to a less dangerous or threatening substitute.	A child directs hostility toward a parent to a teacher. A woman who has had an unpleasant experience with a man with red hair reacts strongly against all men with red hair.	A man is verbally or physically aggressive toward all authority or oppressive figures.
Reaction formation	Acting oppositely to what the person truly feels.	A woman shows great interest and concern for her mother in law, whom she dislikes. A man strongly criticizes pornographic literature when he has a desire to read it.	A young woman is always unnaturally sweet and loving and is unable to consider the possibility of being angry. A person with strong sadistic tendencies becomes an ardent opponent of surgical research on animals.

Source: Adapted from Wilson, H. S., and Kneisl, C. R. 1983. *Psychiatric Nursing,* 2nd ed. Menlo Park, California: Addison-Wesley Publishing Co. pp. 252–57; and Solomon, P., and Patch, V. D. 1974. *Handbook of Psychiatry,* 3rd ed. Los Altos, California: Lange Medical Publications, pp. 500–505.

Factors Influencing the Manifestations of Stress

The degree to which a stressor affects an individual depends on the nature of the stressor, perception of the stressor, number of simultaneous stressors, duration of exposure to the stressor, experiences with a comparable stressor (Byrne and Thompson 1978, p. 3), age, and support people available.

1. *Nature of the stressor.* The nature of the stressor refers to its magnitude. Obviously, a fall from the roof of a building elicits greater stress than a fall from a chair. The pain from a cut on a finger may elicit less stress than pain of unknown cause in the abdomen. Angry remarks from a loved one are more stressful than those from a stranger.

2. *Perception of the stressor.* What the stressor means to the person can be as important as the actual magnitude of the stressor. Because perception is a subjective phe-

Characteristic Behavior Patterns of Type A and Type B Personalities

Type A Behaviors

- Hurried speech
- Constant, rapid movement/eating
- Aggression, ambition, and competitive spirit
- Inability to delegate authority
- Preoccupation with deadlines
- Chronic sense of time urgency
- Impatience with the rate at which things occur and the way others operate
- Career orientation, lack of hobbies
- Little satisfaction with accomplishments
- Restlessness and feelings of guilt during periods of relaxation
- Tendency to think and perform several things at once
- Obsession with money and numbers
- Tendency to dominate conversation, determine topics
- Preoccupation with own thoughts when others are talking
- Overconcern with getting things worth having, less concern with becoming things worth being
- Façade of self-assurance and confidence to hide insecurity about status
- Tendency to measure self-worth by number of achievements
- Nervous gestures: tics, clenched fist or jaw, tooth grinding

Type B Behaviors

- Freedom from all type A traits
- No sense of time urgency
- Ability to relax without guilt
- Ability to work without agitation
- Belief that the purpose of play is fun and relaxation, not to demonstrate superiority
- Tendency to discuss achievements and accomplishments only when situation demands it

Sources: Adapted from M. Friedman and R. Rosenman, *Type A behavior and your heart* (Greenwich, Conn.: Fawcett Publications, 1974) and P. Nuernberger, *Freedom from stress: A holistic approach* (Honesdale, Penn.: The Himalayan International Institute of Yoga Science and Philosophy, 1981).

nomenon, there are wide differences in how people regard a stressor. To one person an inoculation with smallpox vaccine produces a high state of stress, but for another the injection is not a stressor. Being late can create a greater stress response in a punctual person than a nonpunctual person. Some clients associate hospitals solely with dying friends and relatives. To such clients, the act of entering the hospital is particularly stressful, as they worry about whether they will die.

3. *Number of stressors at once.* The number of stressors a person is coping with at one time can greatly affect the response. This often explains why a stressor that the nurse considers small can elicit a disproportionate response. For example, a hospitalized client who is coping with separation from her family, the unknown outcome of her illness, and financial problems can react angrily when the nurse brings her the wrong fruit juice. Normally, this woman would not be upset whichever juice was served; however, she is using up her coping energies on the other problems and has little left to adapt to this incident. This example also shows how a state of high stress can become a stressor itself. A client who reacts angrily feels more stress because of this reaction. Another example is the student who is highly anxious (stressed) about an examination and then gets a cold, an illness he rarely has and would not likely have acquired if he had not been stressed.
4. *Duration of exposure to the stressor.* Nuernberger (1981, p. 80) states that if the external stimulus is brief, and if the person does not extend activation in the cortex by pondering on the threatening event, the associated autonomic response mediated in the hypothalamus will be brief. This response might involve a mild increase in sympathetic discharge (with perhaps some increased adrenal hormone release) but without major activation of the emotions or the hormonal systems associated with the pituitary gland. In such a case, overall functioning can return very quickly to a balanced, relaxed state. If the external stimulus is persistent, however, and if cerebral activation is maintained because one cannot resolve a problem (or through persistent worry), then increasing degrees of sympathetic arousal can result, which involve and reinforce greater degrees of emotional intensity. The pituitary, thyroid, and adrenal cortex responses then become involved.

To Selye, resistance to a stressor is low during the stage of alarm; becomes higher during the resistance stage, when the coping mechanisms are brought into action; and then drops below normal during the stage of exhaustion. Therefore, if the duration of the stressor extends a person's stage of resistance beyond the person's coping powers, he or she becomes exhausted and can eventually die. An example is a man admitted to a hospital with a fractured femur. The client survives the surgery and is healing well but develops an acute pain in the gallbladder, necessitating another operation. By this time, the client's energy reserves have been used up, and, although the operation is successful, the client develops an infection that delays his return home.

5. *Experience with a comparable stressor.* A person who has successfully adjusted to a situation once before is more likely to do so again in a similar situation than a person who is adjusting to the situation for the first time. This person is strengthened by knowledge that he or she handled the situation successfully before. For example, a person who has had one successful job interview is more likely to feel less stress in the next interview than a person who has had an unsuccessful interview. The latter person often feels defeated before the second interview begins. A client who has had an unsuccessful interaction with a physician and other health care personnel once before is more like to experience stress during a second interaction. Determining what a particular event means to a person can assist the nurse in planning care.
6. *Support people available.* Support people can assist a person coping with stress to maintain psychologic and physical integrity. They provide emotional support, often help in decision making, and, by sharing the experience, can relieve the intensity of the stress response.
7. *Age.* The age of the individual affects response and adaptation to stressors. Infants, for example, have poorly developed immune mechanisms and cannot tolerate large fluid losses. Elderly people often have declining physical and mental resources to cope with increased stressors.

Personality Types and Stress

Friedman and Rosenman (1974) identify two personality types: type A and type B. They point out that type A personalities are very prone to cardiovasculoar disease, whereas type B personalities do not usually develop it. The most pervasive cardiovascular disease is hypertension: the higher a person's blood pressure, the higher his or her risk of developing hardening of the arteries, which results in heart attacks and strokes. See the facing page for behavior patterns typical of both personality types.

Type A personalities are under constant pressure to perform and are hurried, impatient, and sometimes hostile. Type B personalities are relaxed, free from the urgencies of time, and able to enjoy work or play. Nuernberger (1981, p. 12) identifies another personality type, called type C, the coping personality. This personality sustains considerable stress but has learned to cope with it. Nuernberger believes many people are type C, since most people share some of the characteristics of types A and B.

Adaptation

Adaptation is the basis of homeostasis and resistance to stress. The word *adapt* is from the Latin *adaptere* meaning "to adjust" and from the French word *adapter* meaning "to fit." To adapt, then, is to modify to meet new, changing, or different conditions. Adaptation is characteristic of all living things; it is one characteristic that differentiates living organisms from inanimate objects. Because it is a phenomenon of all living things, adaptation is studied in many disciplines, such as plant biology, physics, psychology, education (personality adaption), biochemistry, psychiatry, and ecology. These different disciplines have popularized such terms as *accommodation, acclimatization, acculturation, assimilation, equilibrium,* and *stability.* In all disciplines, adaptation or these other similar terms denote interaction and change. The change is viewed as positive, for the better, or healthy.

Modes of Adaptation

Human adaptation occurs in three interrelated modes: physiologic, psychologic, and sociocultural.

Physiologic Mode

Physiologic or biologic adaptation occurs in response to increased or altered demands placed on the body and results in compensatory physical changes. Examples are countless. A few include (1) increased muscle size and strength following prolonged exercise, (2) increased capacity of the heart and lungs after prolonged exercise, and (3) immunity to a specific disease following the invasion of a specific microorganism

Psychologic Mode

Psychologic adaptation involves a change in attitude and behavior, e.g., coping strategies, toward emotionally stressful situations. Examples include (1) changing lifestyle pattern, such as eating a balanced diet, exercising regularly, or balancing leisure time with work, (2) using problem solving in decision making instead of anger or other nonconstructive responses, and (3) stopping smoking.

Adaptation in the psychologic mode may also be maladaptive. For example, abusing alcohol and constantly giving in to others to avoid their anger are maladaptive adaptations.

Sociocultural Mode

Social adaptation involves changes in the person's behavior in accordance with the norms, conventions, and beliefs of various groups, such as family, society, ethnic group, religious group, professional group, and economic group. Examples include (1) becoming socialized into a profession or military group, and (2) living in a new country and learning to speak the language.

Characteristics of Adaptative Responses

All adaptive responses, whether physiologic, psychologic, or sociocultural, have common characteristics:

1. All adaptive responses are attempts to maintain homeostasis. See the section on physiologic homeostasis, earlier in this chapter.
2. Adaptation is a whole body or total organism response. A person experiencing a threat to one body part, e.g., a broken leg, responds as a total organism. Physiologically, the person manifests systemic signs of the general adaptation syndrome. Psychologically, the person responds according to the way he or she perceives the injury to threaten body image, self-concept, or independent functioning.
3. Adaptive responses have limits. Physiologic adaptive responses are more limited than psychologic or social responses. For example, blood oxygen and carbon dioxide levels, blood sugar levels, body temperature, and blood pressure can fluctuate only within relatively narrow limits to maintain life. Psychologic and sociocultural responses, by contrast, have much more creative scope. These responses are limited, however, by the person's intelligence, emotional stability, creativity, past experiences and support, and the confines of human nature.
4. Adaptation requires time. For example, a person can adapt to blood loss from a bleeding ulcer or inadequate cardiac output if these occur gradually over a prolonged time. The bone marrow increases red blood cell production to compensate for the blood loss. The heart compensates for inadequate cardiac output by increasing its pumping rate and the size of the ventricles. In contrast, the body adapts less effectively to rapid blood loss or sudden cardiac failure. Appropriate emergency measures must be initiated to replace rapid blood loss and to maintain cardiac function. In the psychological realm, people are able to think rationally in controlled or expected situations more so than they are in emergency situations.
5. Adaptability varies from person to person. General physical condition and past learning experiences affect the degree and kind of adaptive responses in persons. The person who is physically healthy has greater resources to adapt in times of stress than the unhealthy person. The person who is flexible, responds readily to change, and uses a wide range of coping strategies is more adaptable than the person who does not tolerate change and responds in a limited way.
6. Adaptive responses may be inadequate or excessive. Although the goal of adaptation is homeostasis, this goal is not always achieved without medical assistance. For example, the inflammatory response to bacterial invasion may not be successful in isolating or overpowering the infection unless antibiotic therapy is instituted. Sometimes, inflammation in response to allergies can be excessive and create other problems. For example, the inflammation and bronchial constriction that occur with bronchial asthma seriously impair breathing. In some instances, adaptive responses can hinder medical therapy. For example, the systemic peripheral vasoconstriction that occurs after a severe hemorrhage makes venipuncture difficult and thus hinders blood and fluid replacement.
7. Adaptive responses are egocentric and tiring. Stress and adaptive responses use body energy and tax physical and psychologic resources. Adapting can consume a person's energy to the point that he or she overlooks the needs of others and fails to give the support they require. This failure creates additional stress, which triggers additional coping responses that then can lead to a state of exhaustion.

Assessment

How a person perceives and responds to stressors is highly individual. Vulnerability to stressors is largely related to previous learning, stage of development, life events, health, and coping methods. The nurse can help the client recognize stress and support her or his effective coping strategies, or teach the client new and more effective ways of handling stress.

The key to a person's behavioral response is the individual's perception. If a person perceives (a) that an event is harmful or potentially harmful and (b) that his or her skills to cope with the event are inadequate, then that person experiences stress.

Identifying Stress

Featured nearby is a list that indicates some common areas of stress in a client's life. By asking if anything has happened or is going on that is of concern, the nurse can learn about the client's perceptions of stress.

In some instances a client's perceived stress may result

in an imbalance in the autonomic nervous system, i.e., when coping strategies are inadequate. When the sympathetic nervous system predominates, the fight-or-flight response can occur. When the parasympathetic nervous system predominates, the possum response can occur. See Concepts of Stress earlier in this chapter. Recent research indicates that when a person is stressed, but cognitive coping is effective, clinical signs and symptoms may not occur (Lazarus and Folkman 1984, p. 21).

Developmental transitions occur at critical points in human development. Developmental stages and tasks are outlined in Chapter 22. These developmental transitions are anticipated in a person's life; therefore, the person has the opportunity to prepare for them before they occur. With appropriate support, people are normally able to meet the challenges and turmoils of these transition stages or tasks, and they mature. When support is not available, these transition phases can become crises with negative or destructive effects. Human growth is then stunted, and people may become depressed, withdrawn, or suicidal. Often developmental crises include issues such as dependency, value conflicts, sexual identity, emotional intimacy, power issues, or attaining self-discipline (Burgess and Baldwin 1981, p. 37). See Table 17–4 for selected developmental stressors.

Table 17–4 Selected Stressors Associated with Developmental Stages

Developmental Stage	Stressors
Child	Resolving conflict between independence and dependence
	Beginning school
	Establishing peer relationships and adjustments
	Coping with peer competition
Adolescent	Accepting changing body physique
	Developing heterosexual or other relationships
	Achieving independence
	Choosing a career
Young adult	Getting married
	Leaving home
	Managing a home
	Getting started in an occupation
	Continuing one's education
	Rearing children
Middle adult	Accepting physical changes of aging
	Maintaining social status and standard of living
	Helping teenage children to become independent
	Adjusting to aging parents
Older adult	Accepting decreasing physical abilities and health
	Accepting changes in residence
	Adjusting to retirement and reduced income
	Adjusting to death of spouse and friends

Areas of Stress

- Life-style and recent changes
- Work
- Finance
- Recent or perceived loss of significant other
- Health
- Perceived threats to self-concept
- Family responsibilities and relationships
- Cultural values and conflicts
- Religion
- Relationships with friends or partner

Assessing Client Coping

To date there is no generally accepted way to measure the client's coping abilities. Graydon (1984, pp. 3–12) implemented the following method to measure client coping in a study of 20 hospitalized clients. The method is based on a procedure developed by Weisman and Worden (1976–77).

1. Determine the amount of concern the client is experiencing. A person's coping abilities can be influenced by the problems and concerns the client is having to deal with and by the emotions he or she is experiencing. High concern is associated with less effective coping. See the section on assessing the client's stressors, earlier. See also Meissner (1980) in the Suggested Readings.
2. For each identified problem or concern, determine which coping strategies the client uses and how effective they are. To determine coping strategies, ask "What did you do about it?" or "What are you doing about it?" To determine the effectiveness of strategies, ask "How did it work out?" or "How is it working out?" (Graydon 1984, p. 6). Another method of determining client coping is to have the client self-rate how well he or she is coping in regards to certain events, e.g., hospitalization or illness. A scale of "very well, well, poorly, very poorly" or another similar scale can be used.
3. Determine the client's level of emotional distress. The intensity and quality of emotions a person experiences

are thought to relate directly to the effectiveness of his or her coping. The higher the emotional distress, the poorer the coping. To determine the client's level of emotional distress, ask the client to describe how he or she had been feeling the past few days. Mood state scales can be used to facilitate this procedure.

4. Determine the seriousness of the client's illness. Having a serious illness is thought to be associated with less effective coping. One way to determine the seriousness of illness is to have the client assess his or her symptoms. Ask "How serious do you judge your illness to be?" Although more objective measuring tools have been developed, Graydon (1984, p. 9) believes that the client's subjective appraisal of the seriousness of illness has more influence on coping than an objective appraisal of its seriousness.

Nursing Diagnosis

Examples of nursing diagnoses related to stress are shown to the right.

Examples of Nursing Diagnoses Related to Stress

- Anxiety related to perceived threat to self-concept
- Anxiety related to death of husband
- Ineffective individual coping related to multiple life changes
- Ineffective individual coping related to inadequate support system
- Ineffective family coping related to economic problems
- Ineffective family coping related to prolonged disability

Planning

Planning for stress intervention is based on the assessment data obtained. Interventions are developed in collaboration with the client, and with significant support persons where possible. The client's state of health (e.g., is he or she able to work?), level of anxiety, support resources, coping mechanisms, and sociocultural and religious affiliation are considered. Examples of plans that can be formulated are:

1. Identification of the coping mechanisms most useful to the client
2. Identification of meaningful support persons who can help the client
3. Plans for stress reduction measures such as physical exercise, rest periods, or time management, or referral for advanced stress reduction techniques such as yoga.

Interventions

Stress accompanies every disease and illness. It is therefore important that nurses be able not only to recognize stress but also to assist people to cope with stress.

Stress is highly individual; a situation that to one person is a major stressor may not affect another. Some methods to help reduce stress will be effective for one person; other methods will be appropriate for a different person. A nurse who is sensitive to clients' needs and reactions can choose those methods of intervention that will be most effective for each individual.

Minimizing Anxiety

One way to reduce or perhaps eliminate anxiety is for the nurse and client to establish goals that are attainable.

Clients must first recognize that they are anxious. This recognition is best brought about in an atmosphere of warmth and trust. Sometimes anxious clients react negatively to nurses because of personal frustration. It is important for nurses to understand this response and react to the behavior in a calm, accepting, and confident manner.

After clients realize that they are anxious, it is important to discuss all the possible reasons for their anxiety. Perley (1984, p. 362) categorizes three underlying states of mind associated with anxiety:

1. *A sense of helplessness,* such as that in the person who has recently had a stroke and is unable to perform previous functions.
2. *A sense of isolation,* such as that in the person who believes no one understands how it really feels to have a chronic illness or an adolescent who fears rejection because of a venereal disease.
3. *A sense of insecurity,* such as that in a person who has had mutilating surgery and no longer feels sexually attractive to a partner or who is worried about being unable to earn a living or pay medical bills.

When clients can identify the cause of their anxiety, they find it helpful to explore the cause with the objective of learning better coping strategies. They may see that they have overestimated the threat or that they can reduce the threat by specific action (for example, asking a physician whether a biopsy revealed cancer).

General nursing guidelines to minimize anxiety and stress in clients follow.

1. *Support the client and family at a time of illness.* By conveying caring and understanding, the nurse can help clients reduce their stress. Feeling that someone else helps and cares is a source of support to stressed people. Often families require time to "ventilate" their worries and anxieties, before they can feel assured and less stressed.
2. *Orient the client to the hospital or agency.* The nurse can help both client and family or support persons in their adjustments. In a hospital, the client is assisted in the role change from, for example, independent wage earner to relatively dependent client. Family members are assisted in their adjustment by knowledge of the visiting hours and of what they can do to assist the client.
3. *Give the client in a hospital some way of maintaining identity.* A person's name and clothes are important parts of his or her uniqueness as an individual. Nurses can assist clients by calling them by their correct title and surname, unless otherwise indicated, and by assisting them to wear their own clothes in a hospital setting, when this is possible. In the community, a nurse can help clients maintain their identity by recognizing, for instance, a new shirt or recently styled hair. These actions help people to feel that they are individuals and to maintain their identities.
4. *Provide information when the client has insufficient information.* Fear of the unknown and incorrect information can frequently cause stress. A client who is told a fact may misunderstand it. Additional information or clarification can allay misunderstanding.
5. *Repeat information when the client has difficulty remembering.* Highly stressed individuals frequently have difficulty remembering information and using the information when necessary. Nurses can assist clients by repeating information when it is requested and assisting people to apply it when they so desire. This problem is particularly prevalent among elderly people who are stressed by a change of setting as well as by their illness.
6. *Encourage the client to participate in the plan of care.* Nurses can reduce clients' stress by encouraging their input in planning care and determining what is going to happen. Loss of the right to determine their own destiny can be very stressful to some people, particularly adults who function independently or who assume responsibility for others in their daily lives. Both adults and children can be included in formulating plans for their medical therapy and nursing care. Not only does this activity reduce stress, but also clients then have a greater tendency to comply with their care and feel they are persons of worth, which is important for their self-concept.
7. *Give the client time to express feelings and thoughts.* As part of the plan of care, nurses need to allow time for clients to describe their feelings and worries if they wish. Some people find it relatively easy to talk about their feelings, while others may prove hesitant to do so. The nurse needs to be sensitive to the client's needs and neither probe with questions nor be too busy to listen.
8. *Ensure that expectations are within the client's capabilities.* Whatever the activity, whether an exercise or recreation, the nurse should make sure that it is possible for the client to accomplish it. If an activity is beyond the client's ability, the client is likely to be more stressed by not achieving the goal. Frustration and depression may result. Being able to meet goals helps a client feel personally effective, thus enhancing self-image.
9. *Be sensitive to specific situations and experiences that increase anxiety and stress for clients.* Two examples might be a man who appears highly stressed each time he receives an intramuscular injection and a child who appears frightened and highly stressed when her parents arrive at the hospital to visit her. Often a careful remark by the nurse about the stress will elicit information that the nurse or physician can use to assist the client. In the first example, the client's stress may be reduced by information about the injection and the technique by which it is given. Perhaps this

client has a misconception about the content of the intramuscular syringe, the function of the drug, or the technique of administration. Specific knowledge may allay his apprehension. In the situation of the child, the nurse may learn, after establishing a relationship of trust with the child, that her parents mistreat her at home and neglect her because of their own needs. The nurse can convey this information to the physician, who may request the assistance of a community agency to investigate conditions in the home and help the parents.

10. *Assist a client to make a correct appraisal of a situation.* Sometimes, through a lack of knowledge or misinterpretation of a sequence of events, people draw incorrect conclusions. For example, if the results of a breast biopsy are not back from the hospital laboratory for 2 days, a client may assume that something is seriously wrong. In fact, the test may take 3 days to complete. Knowing this information might relieve the client's stress and restore psychologic balance.

11. *Provide an environment in which a person can function independently to some degree without assistance.* Most adults in North America are accustomed to functioning independently and interdependently, often caring for others at the same time. It is difficult and stressful for an adult to assume the dependent client role even for a short time. By restoring some degree of independent functioning, such as by providing eating utensils adapted so that clients can feed themselves, nurses can lower clients' stress levels. Clients then have an improved self-concept and feel that they are not totally helpless. The feeling of being able to help oneself is important for mental health and morale. Persons are often distressed to feel they are a bother.

12. *Reinforce positive environmental factors and recognize negative ones to help reduce stress.* A nurse can help a client's return to homeostasis by reinforcing factors in the environment that are helpful and by recognizing but not reinforcing factors that are discouraging. Dwelling on problems and difficulties increases stress, but focusing on what can be accomplished positively usually decreases stress.

13. *Arrange for other clients with similar experiences to visit.* Clients with colostomies or similar conditions may be highly stressed and feel that they will never be able to live a normal life again. Meeting another person who has successfully adjusted to a colostomy can lower the stress greatly. Not only are the clients reassured, but they may also gain information that will assist them in rehabilitation.

14. *Bring clients and their families into contact with people in community agencies who can help them make valid plans.* People such as social workers are familiar with planning and arrangements that a client may need to make. Their advice and assistance will enable the client to make plans that are likely to be valid and that can be carried out. Often people are stressed needlessly because they do not know what help is available to them in the community. Plans that have a reasonable chance of success are highly desirable for a stressed person. Disappointment is likely to increase the stress of a client and family.

15. *Communicate competence, understanding, and empathy rather than stress and anxiety.* The client and family or support persons look upon the nurse as a source of knowledge and skill. If a nurse conveys stress or anxiety, the client and family will be stressed about the nurse's competence and ability to function where the client's health and life are involved. To reduce a client's stress, nurses need to know themselves well and be able to function in a nondefensive manner that conveys competence and empathy.

Mediating Anger

Often nurses find clients' anger difficult to handle. Caring for the client who is angry is difficult for two reasons (Gluck 1981, p. 9):

1. Clients rarely state "I feel angry or frustrated" and rarely indicate the reason for their anger. Instead, they may refuse treatment, become verbally abusive or demanding, may threaten violence, or become overly critical. Their complaints rarely reflect the cause of their anger. Anger is the result of the many anxieties the client feels while ill. He or she may feel powerless about his illness and wonder: "Will I be disabled?" "Will I have much pain?" "Will I be able to endure the pain?" "How will this illness affect my life?"

2. Anger from clients often elicits fear and anger in the nurse, who may respond in a manner that intensifies the client's anger even to the point of violence. The majority of nurses respond in a way that reduces their own stress rather than the client's stress (Gluck 1981, p. 11)

Responses whose major purpose is to reduce the nurse's stress include defending, providing reassurance, offering advice or persuading, and retaliating aggressively. For example, this response to a client's demands is defensive: "I can't take care of everyone at once! We've been very busy this evening." This response does not recognize the client's problem and increases the client's tension and anger. A reassuring response, such as "You'll feel better as soon as you are up and about," is a way to recognize the problem and calm the client; however, it does not encourage the person to talk about the problem. Responses meant to offer advice or persuade often begin with the words "Yes, but, . . ." By offering advice or persuading, the nurse focuses on her or his own values and ideas, thus increasing the client's sense of powerlessness. Aggressive responses indicate disapproval of the client's behavior. For example, a nurse might say, "You're spoiled. You could do that yourself." Or a nurse might say, "What do *you* want *now*? Some people here are a lot sicker than you and need my help."

Responses that reduce the client's anger and stress include offering help, apologizing, asking relevant questions, and conveying understanding. These responses focus on helping the client resolve his or her anger. For example, the nurse might respond with understanding to a client who is demanding more attention and care: "I guess it's pretty frustrating being alone and having to wait for others to do things for you." Gluck (1981, p. 10) suggests that nurses wishing to provide understanding responses to clients follow these guidelines:

1. Focus on the feeling words of the client.
2. Note the general content of the message.
3. Restate the feeling and content of what the client has communicated.
4. Observe the client's body language.
5. Ask yourself, "If I were in the client's shoes, what would I be feeling?"

Self and Viau (1980) outline four steps for helping clients to deal with anger:

1. Identify the state of anger.
2. Let the client know that you recognize and accept the anger. Appropriate responses by the nurse include: "You seem to be very upset," and "Many people feel angry when they are hospitalized." It is essential to avoid suppressing the anger by ignoring it, by trying to humor the client out of it, or by smothering the client with kindness.
3. Help the client identify the source of the anger and express feelings. For example, has the client's independence been overly restricted, has a support person disagreed with decisions the client made, or has information been withheld? Knowing the source of his or her anger helps the client to gain some control over the situation. Expression of feelings reduces tension.
4. Help the client to channel the anger constructively by providing increased independence, providing choices about health care as much as possible, and encouraging physical and social activities.

Occasionally, in some hospital settings (e.g., a psychiatric unit), nurses need to handle violent clients. Specific measures include (Anders 1977):

1. Allow some space between the client and the staff and other clients. Ask other clients to leave the room.
2. Do not attempt to take a weapon away from the client.
3. Help the client identify the cause of the anger, and reassure the client that he or she will not be allowed to lose control. The nurse may say, "You seem to be really upset about something, and I'm afraid you might injure someone if you do use that pitcher. I would like to help you control your behavior. I can't allow you to injure yourself or someone else.'"
4. Offer the client alternatives to help regain some self-esteem. The nurse may suggest that the client and the nurse sit down, talk it over, and have a cup of coffee. Generally, this kind of intervention avoids the need for physical restraints. However, restraints must be used as a last resort.

Physical Exercise

Most people agree exercise is necessary to maintain a healthy body and mind. People who exercise consistently are healthier; they have better muscle tone and posture, tend to have fewer frustrations, and usually report greater satisfaction with their lives than those who do not exercise. Stress-related diseases such as obesity, tension headaches, hypertension, coronary-vascular disease, fatigue, and depression are ameliorated by physical exercise programs. See Chapter 37 for additional information about exercise programs. For an exercise program to be effective in altering chronic levels of stress, the person's attention must be on the activity and not on his or her worries. An appropriate mental attitude is necessary. For example, the type A man who is told by his physician to start jogging every day might compulsively set up a schedule and race against the clock to become the best jogger on the block. This attitude will simply add stress to the man's life, and he will not derive the benefits of stress reduction.

Nutrition

People must eat food of good quality and in appropriate quantity to ensure health and to have energy. Nurses need to encourage clients to eat fresh, simple foods; many North Americans eat too much refined sugar and fat. A poorly balanced diet can contribute to lethargy, anxiety, and impaired ability to meet goals and responsibilities. To have a balanced nutritious diet, people need to:

1. Reduce the salt, refined sugar, and animal fat they eat

2. Reduce the red meat they eat
3. Eat more fruit, vegetables, and whole grains

Nutrition is discussed in detail in Chapter 42.

Rest and Sleep

Rest and sleep not only energize the body but also enhance a person's ability to handle daily conflicts and stress. Some clients may need help scheduling regular rest and relaxation or learning relaxation techniques that promote sleep.

Time Management

People who manage their time efficiently generally experience less stress and accomplish more than those who do not. Some time-management techniques include (Bramson and Bramson 1985):

1. Writing a list of tasks to be done and ranking them by importance. Priority lists tell the person what not to do as much as what to do. Knowing and deciding what not to do releases energy to accomplish high-priority tasks. The work-oriented person also learns that it is all right not to do certain tasks.
2. Making sure that all people in the family or other group know who is to do what task. A family group, for example, can collaboratively list tasks to be done by teams, decide on the teams, and agree on when tasks will be done. Contingency plans can be made in the event someone is absent or unable to do the task. Stress is minimized when each person knows what is to be done, by whom, and when.
3. Using memory aids such as telephone message boards, stick-on note pads, and a calendar of events. These devices can help people avoid the stress of forgetting tasks or events and becoming angry with themselves or others.
4. For lengthy complicated projects, making a planning network of all that has to be accomplished. A planning network is essentially a list of tasks scheduled on a calendar to show the sequence in which the tasks are to be done. The purpose of the network is to create time to enjoy leisure activities. The sequence of tasks is also indicated; the network shows which tasks must be done before others can be completed. For example, a woman planning a trip to Europe cannot send an application for a passport until she acquires the forms, passport-sized photographs, and a copy of her birth certificate. The planning network also indicates dates of completion. For example, the woman wishing a passport might learn that it takes 2 weeks to get a copy of her birth certificate and 4 weeks to acquire the passport. Thus, her trip to Europe cannot be scheduled until at least 6 weeks elapse. Planning networks are also valuable tools for group projects. They indicate which tasks need doing and who is responsible for carrying out each step along the way.
5. Learning to delegate tasks and to say no. Effective time management depends on doing tasks that make the best use of one's knowledge, talents, and skills. Tasks that others can accomplish should be delegated. Learning when not to take on certain tasks is also important to avoid disruptions in the current project.

Productive Problem Solving

Some clients may need help learning techniques for solving complicated problems. Some people tend to plunge enthusiastically ahead without a reasoned plan of action. The first step is to help the client identify the problem. Most clients have little difficulty with this step. Many people, however, need help learning the subsequent steps of problem solving, i.e., considering all the possible solutions and their consequences and then deciding on a course of action. See Chapter 10 for additional information on problem solving.

Support Systems

Support systems promote physical and mental well-being and can reduce stress. The nurse may need to help socially isolated clients build support systems. Before encouraging such clients to expand their personal and social contacts, the nurse may need to help the client acquire a more positive self-concept.

Relaxation Techniques

Relaxation techniques reduce anxiety related to stress, promote maximum benefits from rest and sleep periods, and can help people cope with chronic pain. Specific techniques, e.g., progressive relaxation and guided imagery, are discussed in Chapter 41.

Advanced Stress Reduction Techniques

Advanced stress reduction techniques include biofeedback, shiatsu massage, yoga, and meditation. These advanced techniques require advanced education and training. The inexperienced nurse can, however, inform the client about them.

Evaluation

Examples of Outcome Criteria Related to Stress

The client will:

- Verbally recognize own anxiety
- Verbalize effects of own behavior on significant others
- Verbalize feelings related to event or situation
- Identify past and present coping patterns
- Identify consequences of current coping behavior
- Identify personal strengths
- State an increase in psychologic comfort following exercise program
- Use exercise to reduce anxiety
- Ask for help from others
- Make decisions in anxiety-provoking situations and follow through with appropriate actions

Examples of outcome criteria for clients who have stress problems are given to the left.

Specialized Stress Reduction Techniques

Advanced stress reduction techniques include biofeedback, shiatsu massage, yoga, and meditation. These techniques are usually provided by a person who has specialized education. Nurses can inform clients about the availability of community classes in these areas.

Biofeedback

Biofeedback is a technique that brings under conscious control bodily processes normally thought to be beyond voluntary command. In the past, most physiologic processes were considered involuntary. However, it has been discovered that many of these processes are partially subject to voluntary control. Studies show that muscle tension, heartbeat, blood flow, peristalsis, and skin temperature, for example, can be controlled voluntarily. The feedback is usually provided through temperature meters that indicate skin temperature changes or an electromyogram (EMG) that shows the electric potential created by the contraction of muscles. Reduced EMG activity reflects muscle relaxation. Biofeedback teaches clients to achieve a generalized state of relaxation characterized by parasympathetic dominance and antagonistic to the pattern of physiologic arousal manifested in stress-related disorders (Renshaw 1984, p. 38). For additional information on biofeedback see Chapter 41.

Shiatsu Massage

Shiatsu massage is the application of firm, gentle pressure to the acupuncture points of the body and therefore is sometimes referred to as acupressure. Shiatsu aims to restore the balance of true Qi (pronounced "chee"), a balance of the constantly flowing life energy forces of *yang* and *yin*. True Qi circulates around the body through 12 main channels called meridians, which correspond to 12 organs, including the lungs, heart, and stomach. Clients can use shiatsu on themselves to relieve minor ailments. For example, a frontal headache may be relieved by applying firm pressure behind the head at the base of the skull (Box 1984, p. 39).

Yoga

Yoga is a traditional Indian science that helps a person coordinate body and mind more effectively. It promotes tranquillity of mind and increases resistance to stress.

Integrated yoga, described by Patanjali 2500 years ago, incorporated the following methods (Udupa 1983, p. 135):

1. *Yama.* This refers to improvement in social behavior and is achieved by five noble practices: (a) nonviolence (both physical and psychologic), (b) truthfulness, (c) nonstealing, (d) self-restraint in every sphere of life, and (e) nonhoarding.
2. *Niyama.* This refers to improvement in personal behavior and is achieved by (a) maintaining a purity of body and mind, (b) developing a habit of contentment, (c) practicing austerity in every sphere of life, (d) studying relevant literature, and (e) practicing dedication to God daily.
3. *Physical postures.* There are many yoga postures, e.g., cobra posture and plough posture. They are meant to improve the bodily health, especially the functions of various organs, such as the heart, lungs, liver and organs of the gastrointestinal tract, kidneys, and endocrine system. People may assume 10 to 15 yogic postures, including stationary exercises, for all parts of the body for a period of about 15 minutes daily.
4. *Breathing exercises.* In this important part of yogic exercise, one inhales fresh air to the maximum capacity through one nostril, holds the breath for a while, and exhales through the other nostril, practicing deep expiration. Done 20 times or more daily, this exercise improves the oxygenation of all the organs and tissues of the body. Better circulation of oxygenated blood in the body in turn relaxes the person.
5. *Control of the sense organs.* This aspect of yoga involves restraining the activities of all the sense organs with the ultimate goal of restraining the mind. It is achieved by minimizing the stimulation of the sense organs and leading as simple a life as possible.
6. *Concentration of the mind.* Learning to avoid all distractions and concentrate on any object involves tremendous perseverance and willpower. Concentrating on an object of one's choice helps to calm any mental excitement and to induce tranquillity and serenity of the mind.
7. *Meditation.* Research shows that the regular practice of integrated yoga can not only prevent the development of various psychosomatic disorders but also improve a person's resistance and ability to endure stressful situations effectively. Studies on normal individuals indicate that the regular practice of yogic postures leads to psychologic improvement, increased intelligence and memory quotients, and decreased pulse rate, blood pressure, respiration, and body weight (Udupa 1978). See the section immediately following.

Meditation

Meditation is a mental exercise that directs the mind to think inwardly by closing the sense organs to external stimulation. With practice, a person can learn to reduce bodily responses to stimuli voluntarily so that the mind can be directed to perform more useful functions. With meditation, a person can also learn to control the autonomic nervous system and attain a state of superconsciousness, a state of mind beyond the level of self-consciousness.

There are many ways to meditate. One method, transcendental meditation, involves repeating the words of a "mantra" and concentrating on prayer and communication with a deity. Biofeedback devices may be used to measure the degree of psychosomatic changes in the body.

Stress Management for Nurses

Nurses, like clients, are susceptible to experiencing anxiety and crises. In recent years, more attention has been given to the occupational stress of the nurse. Nursing practice involves many stressors related to both clients and the work environment. See Kinzel's stress scale for nurses in Table 17–5 on the following page. Appelbaum (1981, pp. 109–35) cites the following factors that can create stress for the nurse.

1. Incongruence between the nurse's expectations and realities of the job. New graduates in particular have high expectations; such nurses may experience reality shock. Appelbaum (1981, p. 112) emphasizes that although new nursing personnel have different expectations than experienced staff, the value systems of both groups are similar. Values and concerns of both groups include:
   a. Pay
   b. Help and cooperation from coworkers
   c. Opportunity to develop skills and abilities and learn new things
   d. Feeling of really helping the client and family
   e. Stable work schedule
   f. Help and recognition from immediate supervisors
   g. Responsibility
   h. Ability to make independent decisions
   i. Job security
   j. Promotion

   When these values are not realized, both groups of nurses may experience conflict and stress.

Table 17–5 Kinzel's Scale Rating Stress in Nurses

Your Score	Stressful Events		Stress Value
______	Assuming responsibilities you're not trained to handle		67
______	Working with unqualified personnel		64
______	Dealing with nonsupportive supervisors or administrators		61
______	Working with an inadequate staff		58
______	Caring for a patient during a cardiac arrest		55
______	Experiencing conflict with coworkers		52
______	Dealing with the family of a dying patient		49
______	Caring for a dying patient		46
______	Working with broken or faulty equipment		44
______	Working with inadequate supplies		42
______	Working an inconvenient shift or schedule		38
______	Assuming responsibilities without thanks or recognition		36
______	Dealing with a difficult doctor		34
______	Trying to communicate within a bureaucracy		31
______	Discharging a patient inadequately prepared for discharge		28
______	Caring for a seriously ill patient		25
______	Spending long periods of time doing paperwork or phone duties		22
______	Experiencing a problem over salary or promotion		19
______	Working with a demanding or noncompliant patient		16
______	Coordinating ancillary personnel		13
______	YOUR TOTAL	TOTAL POSSIBLE	800

Suggested score interpretation

0–133: The last 24 hours have produced minimal stress, not enough to cause you many problems.

134–266: You're under moderate stress. This is the highest level of stress you should permit on a day-to-day basis.

267–532: You're experiencing high-level stress. You have trouble relaxing and easily become upset. Try relaxation techniques, exercise, and hobbies until you can reduce your stressors.

533–800: You're under extreme stress. Get help fast. You're a prime candidate for burnout.

Source: S. L. Kinzel, What's your stress level? *Nursing Life,* March/April 1982, 2:54–55. Reprinted with permission from the March/April issue of *Nursing Life.*

2. Conflicting loyalties to the professional and bureaucratic systems of the work organization. Organization reward systems contribute to conflict between nurses, who identify with their profession, and supervisors, who identify with the organization. Disproportionate power creates stress. Nurses with a high bureaucratic–low professional orientation tend to be in administratively promoted positions more frequently than those with a high professional orientation. Nurses with a high bureaucratic–high professional orientation tend to be in unusual and clinically oriented positions more often than others. Thus, increased professionalism often means increased conflict and stress unless the bureaucratic structure is flexible enough to deal with the professional modality.
3. Pressures imposed by standards for high-quality medical care and an increasing demand for more humanistic approaches to nurse-client interaction. Nurses use behavioral science and communication skills to develop their professional relationship with clients; physicians employ a clinical, biologic approach. This variance can create stress if (a) the physician expects the nurse to handle the client as the physician does and (b) the physician does not listen to the nurse's concerns and suggestions about the client.
4. Professional socialization and attitudes. Professional attitudes can create conflict. For example, many nursing students have an image of working nurses as dealing with the client from a humanistic, bedside perspective. Many cling strongly to this image of the profession. In the actual work environment, however, nurses are required to carry out the technical, organizational, administrative, and educational duties. In addition, many nurses judge other nurses by their competency in performing diverse and complex technical skills and by their ability to get along with others.

These attitudes may cause conflict for the nurse who is socialized to provide humanistic, interactive client care and sets this as a priority.

5. Increasing professionalism. The role of the professional nurse is changing. Nurses are becoming more involved in planning and organizing health care activities. Today, they are becoming more responsible for delivering total client care services. The nurse's role is becoming one of managing client care activities in general. In this new role, nurses have greater responsibility and accountability and may experience increased stress as a result.
6. Degree of client illness. Providing critical care for acutely ill clients is a source of stress for nurses. A belief common to nurses is that they must preserve life. Failure to preserve life may, therefore, be perceived as failure to do one's job and lead to feelings of anxiety. The impending death of a client can elicit fear about the nurse's own death. The stress responses or behaviors of critically ill clients can also create stress for the nurse. For example, the nurse may have difficulty coping with the anger of a client.
7. Group interaction. Providing effective client care involves teamwork. Because of rapid turnover rates in nursing positions, it is not uncommon for nursing staffs to be integrating a new member into the group almost continually. As a result, group cohesiveness is diminished. Even in a cohesive group, satisfaction for all is not an easily met objective. Tension in a nursing unit can be high when a new member is being assimilated into a group.

Stress Level Scale for Nurses

Kinzel (1982, p. 55) devised a 20-item, 24-hour scale to help nurses measure their stress levels. See Table 17–5. All 20 items fall into five main categories: inadequate knowledge, inadequate support from peers and supervisors, dealing with death, poor communication, and salary and staffing problems. The purpose of such a scale is to make nurses aware of the source of negative feelings and frustration on the job, to help them make adjustments, and to support colleagues.

Stress Manifestations

Physiologic and behavioral manifestations of stress are the same for the nurse as for the client. Janken (1974, p. 18) describes three coping strategies frequently used by nurses: client teaching, withdrawal, and projection. When a client demonstrates behavior that is detrimental to his or her health, the nurse frequently uses client teaching as a coping mechanism. The client's behavior increases the nurse's anxiety since it is contrary to the goal of assisting the client toward optimum health. To decrease anxiety, the nurse tries to change the client's behavior through education. This coping strategy is effective provided the client changes the previous behavior pattern.

Withdrawal, as a coping mechanism, can be helpful in certain situations, (e.g., when the nurse becomes angry with the client), since it allows the nurse time to reassess the situation and plan alternative interventions. Withdrawal may be ineffective in other situations; it may aggravate the problem and cause further anxiety in both the client and the nurse. A nurse, for example, may withdraw from a dying client who makes her feel uncomfortable, yet the nurse realizes that the client is in need of attention.

Projection occurs when the nurse assumes that the client feels as the nurse does about a situation and plans nursing interventions based on that assumption. For example, an unwed pregnant teenager with thrombophlebitis is scheduled to have a therapeutic abortion. The teenager repeatedly refuses her consent to surgery. The nurse believes the baby would be a burden to the teenager, thinks the client should be pleased about the abortion, and believes the client is just being obstinate. The nurse, not realizing the client's true feelings, tries to convince the client to consent to the abortion.

Group responses to stress also occur among nurses, since they work interdependently as a unit (Scully 1980, p. 912). Change in the function of one nurse creates change in the function of the whole team. Scully sees these behaviors as indicators of group stress:

1. Snapping and arguing with others
2. Scapegoating staff members, i.e., blaming another shift or the administration for unit tension
3. Responding to others with sullenness or silence
4. "Busy" behavior
5. Defensiveness
6. Intolerance of others' ideas or behavior
7. Tardiness and absenteeism
8. Rapid staff turnover
9. Errors and inefficiency

Managing Stress

Nurses can manage stress by using all of the techniques discussed for clients. In addition, Hamilton (1984), Scully (1980), and Wilson (1986) suggest the following:

1. First recognize that you are stressed. The identifying process is necessary to help the nurse attune herself or himself to signs of stress. Become attuned to feelings of being overwhelmed, fatigue, angry outbursts, depression, forgetfulness, disorganization, guilt, disil-

lusionment, passivity, and physical illness. Also note increases in smoking, drinking coffee, or other substance abuse and determine whether you are distancing yourself from client interaction.

2. When attuned to your reactions to stress, determine when the reactions occur. For instance, is it when you are caring for a critically ill or dying client, when you witness or have a professional altercation, or when there is lack of staff?
3. When attuned to your stress and when it occurs, determine alternative actions to deal with it constructively. Some suggestions are:
   a. Plan a daily relaxation program with meaningful quiet times to reduce tension. For example, take a walk in the park, listen to music, or take a hot bath.
   b. Establish an activity program to direct energy outward.
   c. Become more assertive to overcome feelings of powerlessness in relationships with others. Learn to say no.
   d. Manage time better by delegating to others and combining tasks.
   e. Take a course in biofeedback, yoga, meditation, or some other advanced relaxation technique.
   f. Learn to accept failures and learn from them.
   g. Learn to ask for help, and share your feelings with colleagues.
   h. Learn to support your colleagues in times of need. Give them a chance to "ventilate" feelings and listen to their concerns.
   i. Learn to handle problems constructively instead of defensively.
   j. Accept what cannot be changed. There are certain limitations in every situation.
   k. If working in an intensive care unit (ICU), establish a structured emotional support group (Skinner 1980, p. 296). Most observers of the intensive care setting recommend that ICU nurses participate in some type of emotional support group. These groups are identified by various names: ventilation groups, discussion forums, or regular staff meetings for the purpose of dealing with feelings and anxieties generated in the work setting.

Chapter Highlights

- Homeostasis is the tendency of the body to maintain a state of relative balance or constancy in response to a changing internal and external environment.
- Physiologic homeostasis is maintained by coordinated functioning of the autonomic nervous, endocrine, respiratory, cardiovascular, renal, and gastrointestinal systems.
- Homeostatic mechanisms regulate hormone secretion, fluid and electrolyte levels, the functions of body viscera, and metabolic processes that provide energy for the body.
- Psychologic homeostasis, or emotional well-being, is acquired or learned through the experience of living and interacting with others.
- Stress is a state of physiologic or psychologic tension that affects the whole person—physically, emotionally, intellectually, socially, and spiritually.
- A person's response to stressors varies according to the way the stressor is perceived, its intensity and duration, the number of stressors, previous experience, coping mechanisms used, support people available, and age.
- Physiologic responses include the fight-flight mechanism, innervated by the sympathetic nervous system; the possum response, innervated by the parasympathetic nervous system; mobilization of glucose reserves for energy; and conservation of water to maintain the blood volume.
- A common psychologic response to stress is anxiety, which is manifested in a variety of cognitive, verbal, and motor responses that reduce tension.
- Unconscious psychologic defense mechanisms, such as denial, rationalization, compensation, and sublimation, also protect the individual from tension.
- Both physiologic and psychologic responses to stressors can be adaptive or maladaptive.
- Prolonged stress can cause illness.
- Adaptation is a process of change that occurs in response to stress. It occurs in three interrelated modes: physiologic, psychologic, and sociocultural.
- Coping is a more immediate response to stress than adaptation.
- Coping strategies can be either effective or ineffective and result in adaptation or maladaptation, respectively.
- The nurse can help clients recognize stress and support clients' effective coping mechanisms.
- Nursing interventions for stress are aimed at reducing anxiety, at promoting clients' physical and mental well-being so that they handle stress more effectively, and at helping clients learn more effective coping mechanisms.
- The nurse, too, is prone to occupational stress and needs to learn effective stress-management techniques.

Suggested Readings

Hamilton, J. M. July/August 1984. Effective ways to relieve stress. *Nursing Life* 4:24–27.
Hamilton describes a number of stressful situations a nurse might encounter. The author provides a number of practical suggestions to reduce the stress of each situation.

Knowles, R. D. January 1981. Dealing with feelings: Managing anxiety. *American Journal of Nursing* 81:110–111.
Knowles points out that anxiety is not a "bad" emotion because it keeps people alert, "urges us to action, and protects us from dangers." An exceptionally high level of anxiety, however, is detrimental because "it narrows perceptions, interferes with learning, [and] produces many unpleasant symptoms." Knowles presents a problem, intervention procedure, rationale, and evaluation format. Three problems are presented: having initial awareness of anxiety, determining the subjective level of anxiety, and dealing with an uncomfortable level of anxiety. The author describes two simple exercises to cope with an uncomfortable level of stress: round breathing and breath holding.

Meissner, J. E. February 1980. Semantic differential scales for assessing patients' feelings. *Nursing 80* 10:70–71.
Meissner presents a semantic differential scale on which the client is asked to check the boxes that most closely describe his or her feelings, e.g., "lonely," "nervous," "indifferent," "calm," and "dejected."

———. May 1980. Uncovering your patient's hidden psychological problems. *Nursing 80* 10:78–79.
The author provides a concise assessment questionnaire for clients to answer so that nurses can plan helpful nursing interventions related to the client's psychosocial needs.

Smitherman, C. October 1981. Your patient's anxious: What should you do? *Nursing 81* 11:72–73. Canadian ed. 11:26–27.
According to Smitherman, nurses can help in a number of ways when anxiety is destructive and makes clients depressed or withdrawn. First, the nurse can help the client recognize the anxiety and focus on specific fears. The nurse can also help the individual identify what helps him or her control anxiety. Staying with an anxious client and touching may help. Smitherman also suggests ways of helping a client feel more secure, including gradual desensitization to a problem. The author includes suggestions for nurses dealing with free-floating anxiety and extreme anxiety.

Storlie, F. J. December 1979. Burnout: The elaboration of a concept. *American Journal of Nursing* 79:2108–11.
Burnout is identified as a disparity between the real and the ideal. Storlie examines why nurses may become automated shells instead of feeling persons.

Selected References

Anders, R. L. July 1977. When a patient becomes violent. *American Journal of Nursing* 77:1144–48.

Appelbaum, S. H. 1981. *Stress management for health care professionals.* Rockville, Md.: Aspen Systems Corporation.

Bell, J. M. March/April 1977. Stressful life events and coping methods in mental-illness and wellness behaviors. *Nursing Research* 26:136–40.

Box, D. April 25, 1984. Holistic health 3: Made in Japan. *Nursing Times* 80:39–40.

Bramson, R. M., and Bramson, S. 1985. *The stressless home: A step-by-step guide to turning your home into the haven you deserve.* Garden City, N.Y.: Doubleday.

Burgess, A. W., and Baldwin, B. A. 1981. *Crisis intervention theory and practice: A clinical handbook.* Englewood Cliffs, N.J.: Prentice-Hall.

Burgess, A. W., and Lazare, A. 1976. *Community mental health: Target populations.* Englewood Cliffs, N.J.: Prentice-Hall.

Byrne, M. L., and Thompson, L. F. 1978. *Key concepts for the study and practice of nursing.* St. Louis: C. V. Mosby Co.

Cannon, W. B. 1939. *The wisdom of the body.* 2d ed. New York: Norton Publishing Co.

Carpenito, L. J. 1983. *Nursing diagnosis: Application to clinical practice.* Philadelphia: J. B. Lippincott Co.

Cohn, L. December 1979. Coping with anxiety: A step-by-step guide. *Nursing 79* 9:34–37.

Detherage, K. S., and Johnson, S. S. 1986. Primary prevention in stress and crisis. In Edelman, C., and Mandle, C. L. *Health promotion throughout the life span.* St. Louis: C. V. Mosby Co.

Dohrenwend, B. S., and Dohrenwend, B. P., editors. 1984. *Stressful life events and their contexts.* Vol. 2 in series. Slaby, A. E., editor. *Psychosocial epidemiology.* Brunswick, N.J.: Rutgers University Press.

Duldt, B. W. September 1981. Anger: An occupational hazard for nurses. *Nursing Outlook* 29:510–18.

Elliott, S. M. October 1980. Denial as an effective mechanism to allay anxiety following a stressful event. *Journal of Psychiatric Nursing and Mental Health Services* 18:11–15.

Freud, S. 1946. *The ego and the mechanisms of defense.* New York: International Universities Press.

Friedman, M., and Rosenman, R. 1974. *Type A behavior and your heart.* Greenwich, Conn.: Fawcett Publications.

Gluck, M. March 1981. Learning a therapeutic verbal response to anger. *Journal of Psychiatric Nursing and Mental Health Services* 19:9–12.

Gordon, M. 1982. *Manual of nursing diagnosis.* New York: McGraw-Hill.

Graydon, J. E. Summer 1984. Measuring patient coping. *Nursing Papers* 16:3–12.

Griffith-Kenney, J. 1986. *Contemporary women's health.* Menlo Park, Calif.: Addison-Wesley Publishing Co.

Guyton, A. C. 1986. *Textbook of medical physiology.* 7th ed. Philadelphia: W. B. Saunders Co.

Hamilton, J. M. July/August 1984. Effective ways to relieve stress. *Nursing Life* 4:24–27.

Holmes, T. H., and Masuda, M. August 1966. Magnitude estimations of social readjustments. *Journal of Psychosomatic Research* 11:219–25.

Holmes, T. H., and Rahe, R. H. August 1967. The social readjustment rating scale. *Journal of Psychosomatic Research* 11:213–18.

Hopping, B. 1980. Physiologic response to stress: A nursing concern. *Nursing Forum* XIX(3):259–69

Janken, J. K. March 1974. The nurse in crisis. *Nursing Clinics of North America* 9:17–26.

Kerr, N. January/February 1978. Anxiety: Theoretical considerations. *Perspectives in Psychiatric Care* 16:36–40, 46.

Kim, M. H., McFarland, G. K., and McLane, A. M. 1984. *Pocket guide to nursing diagnoses.* St. Louis: C. V. Mosby Co.

Kinzel, S. L. March/April 1982. What's your stress level? *Nursing Life* 2:54–55.

Knowles, R. D. November/December 1981. Handling anger: Responding versus reacting. *American Journal of Nursing* 81:2196.

Lathrop, V. G. September/December 1978. Aggression as a response. *Perspectives in Psychiatric Care* 16:202–5.

Lazarus, R. S. 1966. *Psychological stress and the coping process.* New York: McGraw-Hill Book Co.

Lazarus, R., and Folkman, S. 1980. An analysis of coping in a middle-aged community sample. *Journal of Health and Social Behavior* 21:219–39.

Lazarus, R. S., and Folkman, S. 1984. *Stress, appraisal, and coping.* New York: Springer Publishing Co.

Lyon, B. L., and Werner, J. 1987. Stress: Ten years of practice-relevant research. In Werley, H., and Fitzpatrick, J., editors. *Annual Review of Nursing Research.*

Meissner, J. E. August 1980. Measuring patient stress with the hospital stress rating scale. *Nursing 80* 10:24–25.

Nuernberger, P. 1981. *Freedom from stress.* Honesdale, Pa.: The Himalayan International Institute of Yoga Science and Philosophy.

O'Flynn-Comiskey, A. I. November 1979. Stress: The type A individual. *American Journal of Nursing* 79:1956–58.

Perley, N. Z. 1984. Problems in self-consistency: Anxiety. In Roy, C. *Introduction to nursing: An adaptation model.* Englewood, Cliffs, N.J.: Prentice-Hall.

Rahe, R. H. September 1979. Life change events and mental illness: An overview. *Journal of Human Stress* 5:2–10.

Renshaw, J. April 25, 1984. Holistic health 2: The power of the will. *Nursing Times* 80:38–39.

Robinson, K. M.; Bridgewater, S. C.; Molla, P. M.; and Wathen, C. A. July/September 1982. Concepts of stress for nursing. *Issues Mental Health Nursing* 4:167–76.

Rogers, M. E. 1970. *An introduction to the theoretical base of nursing.* Philadelphia: F. A. Davis Co.

Rothenberg, A. October 1971. On anger. *American Journal of Psychiatry* 128:454–60.

Scully, R. May 1980. Stress in the nurse. *American Journal of Nursing* 80:912–14.

Self, P. R., and Viau, J. J. December 1980. Four steps for helping a patient alleviate anger. *Nursing 80* 10:66.

Selye, H. 1956. *The stress of life.* New York: McGraw Hill.

———. 1974. *Stress without distress.* Scarborough, Ontario: New American Library of Canada.

———. 1976. *The stress of life.* Rev. ed. New York: McGraw Hill.

Skinner, K. May 1980. Support group for ICU nurses. *Nursing Outlook* 28:296–99.

Smith, M. J. T., and Selye, H. November 1979. Stress: Reducing the negative effects of stress. *American Journal of Nursing* 79:1953–55.

Smitherman, C. October 1981. Your patient's anxious: What should you do? *Nursing 81* 11:72–73. Canadian ed. 11:26–27.

Solomon, P., and Patch, V. D. 1974. *Handbook of Psychiatry,* 3rd ed. Los Altos, California: Lange Medical Publications.

Taché, J., and Selye, J. 1985. On stress and coping mechanisms. *Issues in Mental Health Nursing* 7:3–24.

Tierney, M. J. G., and Strom, L. M. May 1980. Stress: Type A behavior in the nurse. *American Journal of Nursing* 80:915–18.

Tyrer, P. November 1980. Anxiety states: Easy to recognize—difficult to diagnose—supportive and medical treatment. *Nursing Mirror* 151:36–37.

Udupa, K. N. 1978. *Disorders of stress and their management by yoga.* Varanasi, India: Banaras Hindu University.

———. 1983. Yoga and meditation for mental health. In Bannerman, R. H., Burton, J., and Wen-Chieh, C., editors. *Traditional medicine and health care coverage.* Geneva: World Health Organization.

Van Os, D.; Clark, C.; Turner, C.; and Herbst, J. August 1985. Life stress and cystic fibrosis. *Western Journal of Nursing Research* 7(3):301–15.

Volicer, B. J., and Burns, M. W. September/October 1975. A hospital stress rating scale. *Nursing Research* 24:352–59.

Weisman, A. D., and Worden, J. W. 1976–77. The existential plight in cancer: Significance of the first 100 days. *International Journal of Psychiatry in Medicine* 7:1–15.

———. 1977. *Instructions for scoring the inventory of current concerns.* Unpublished manuscript.

Wilson, H. S., and Kneisl, C. R. 1983. *Psychiatric nursing,* 2nd ed. Menlo Park, California: Addison-Wesley Publishing Co.

Wilson, L. K. May/June 1986. High-gear nursing: How it can run you down and what you can do about it. *Nursing Life* 6:44–47.

Wyler, A. R.; Masuda, M.; and Holmes, T. H. 1968. Seriousness of illness rating scale. *Journal of Psychosomatic Research* 11:363–74.

Volicer, B. J., and Burns, M. W. November-December 1977. Preexisting correlates of hospital stress. *Nursing Research* 26:408–15.

CHAPTER **18**

Ethnicity and Culture

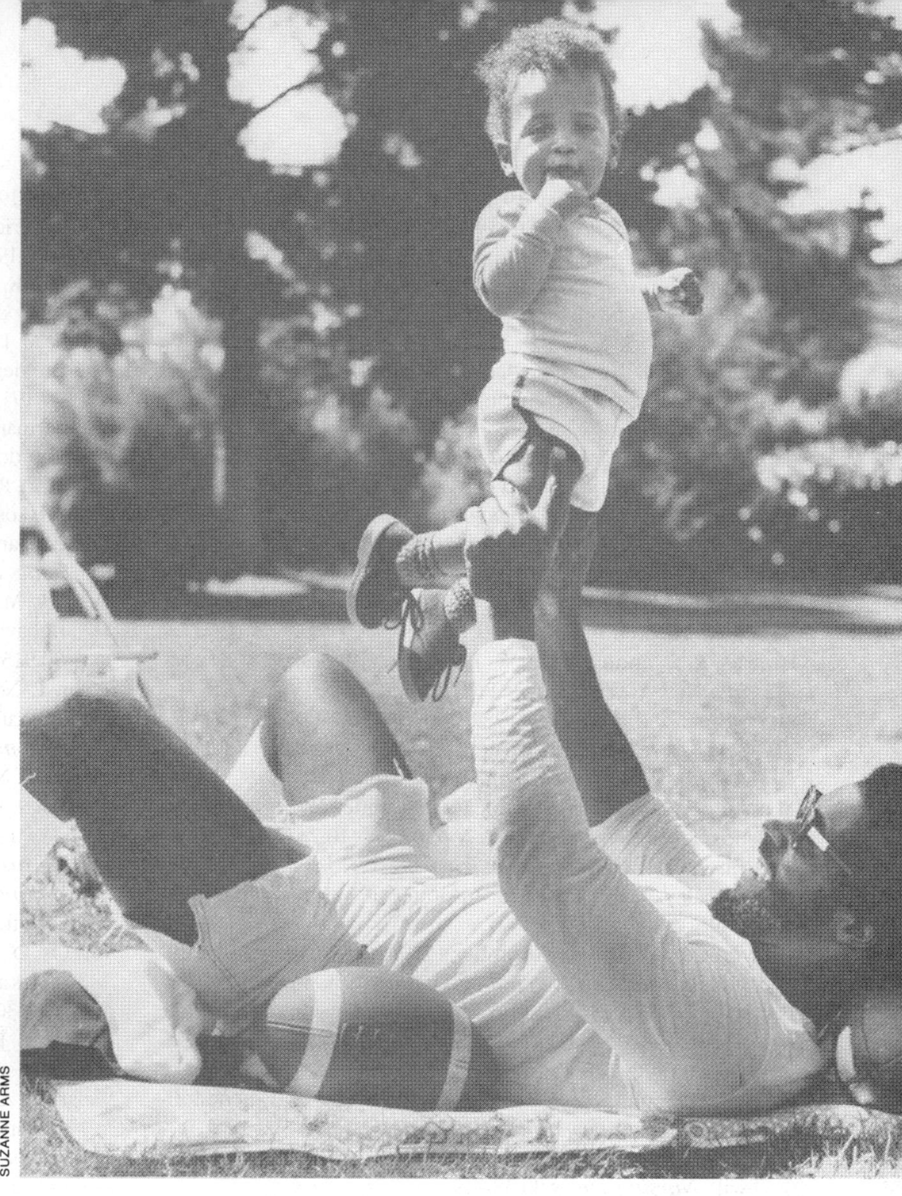

SUZANNE ARMS

Contents

Objectives

1. Know essential facts about culture and ethnicity.
   1.1 Define selected terms.
   1.2 Describe the concept of culture.
   1.3 Identify universal attributes of culture.
   1.4 Identify seven characteristics of culture.
2. Understand aspects of the health needs of multicultural groups.
   2.1 Relate the incidence of specific diseases to certain ethnic groups.
   2.2 Identify problems unique to ethnic minorities in the provision and use of health care services.
   2.3 Identify social characteristics common to all ethnic/cultural groups that require consideration by health care providers.
3. Understand selected essential health-related beliefs and practices of North American cultural groups.
   3.1 Identify unique illness practices of each cultural group.
   3.2 Identify specific characteristics and values of each cultural group that may influence nursing assessment and intervention.
4. Understand essential facts about low- and high-income groups and the health care system as subcultures.
   4.1 Identify health-related beliefs and values of high-income groups.
   4.2 Relate health-related beliefs and practices of low-income groups to the effects of poverty.
   4.3 Contrast the values of the health care culture and minority ethnic cultures.
   4.4 Identify aspects of culture shock.
5. Assess the unique customs, values, and beliefs of an ethnic cultural client.
   5.1 Collect significant data from the client and family.
   5.2 Establish relevant nursing diagnosis.
   5.3 Plan nursing strategies using the data.

Terms

bicultural group
cultural assimilation (acculturation)
culture
culture shock
dominant group
ethnic group
ethnicity
ethnocentrism
ethnoscience
homosexuality
ideational
material culture
meridians (acupuncture)
minority group
nonmaterial culture
personal space
race
racism
stereotyping
territoriality
thanatology

Concepts of Ethnicity and Culture

Definitions

Ethnicity is the condition of belonging to a specific ethnic group. An **ethnic group** is a set of individuals who share a unique cultural and social heritage passed on from one generation to another (Henderson and Primeaux 1981, p. xx). Ethnicity thus differs from race. **Race** denotes a system of classifying humans into subgroups according to specific physical characteristics, including skin pigmentation, stature, facial features, texture of body hair, and head form (Henderson and Primeaux 1981, p. xix). The three racial types that are commonly recognized are Caucasoid, Negroid, and Mongoloid. However, because of the mixture of races, the three groups meld together, and there are many commonalities among groups. See Figure 18–1.

Culture should not be confused with race or ethnic group. **Culture** is the beliefs and practices that are shared by people and passed down from generation to generation. Anthropologists have traditionally divided it into material culture and nonmaterial culture. **Material culture** consists of objects (such as dress, art, religious artifacts, or eating utensils) and the ways these are used. **Nonmaterial culture** consists of beliefs, customs, languages, and social institutions. Races have different ethnic groups, and the ethnic groups have different cultures. It is therefore important to understand that all white or black people do not have the same culture. North America has people of different ethnic groups and different cultures. Their cultural beliefs and practices can affect health and illness and thus become an important consideration for nurses.

Large cultural groups often have cultural subgroups or subsystems. A subculture is usually composed of people who have a distinct identity and yet are also related to a larger cultural group. A subcultural group generally

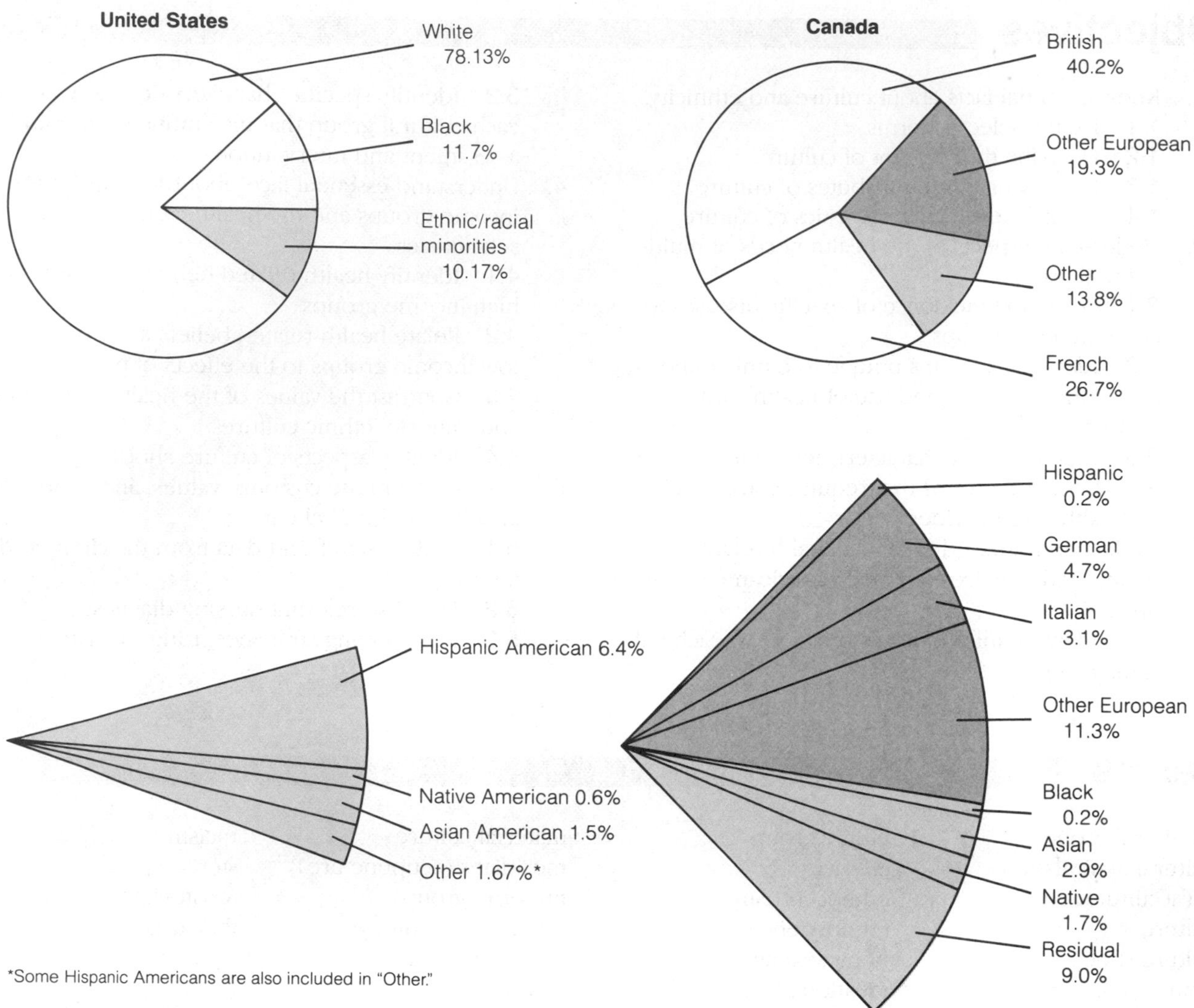

Figure 18–1 Estimates of the distribution of population by ethnic/racial origin based on the United States 1980 census and the Canadian 1981 census.

Sources: U.S. Department of Commerce, Bureau of the Census, *Census of Population, General Population Characteristics United States Survey* (Washington, D.C.: Government Printing Office, April 1984), Table 40; Statistics Canada, *Census of Canada,* Cat. no. 92-911 (Ottawa: Minister of Supplies and Services, 1984), Table 1. Used by permission.

must have reference to the larger cultural group to maintain its existence. A subcultural group may have ethnicity, occupation, or physical characteristics in common with the larger cultural group. Examples of cultural subgroups are occupational groups (e.g., nurses), societal groups (e.g., feminists), and ethnic groups (e.g., Cajuns, who may be black, French, or German but who share French Acadian heritage and customs). A **bicultural group** is a group of people who embrace two cultures, life-styles, and sets of values (Chen-Louie 1980, p. 4).

To clarify the concept of culture, Leininger (1970, pp. 48–49) describes it as having the following characteristics:

1. Culture is a universal experience, yet no two cultures are exactly alike.
2. Culture is stable but also dynamic, manifesting continual change.
3. Culture fills and largely determines the course of our lives, yet people are rarely conscious of it.

Two other terms commonly used with reference to ethnicity and culture are *dominant group* and *minority group*. A **dominant group** is "a collectivity within a society which has a preeminent authority to function as guardians and sustainers of the controlling value system and as prime allocators of rewards in the society" (Schermerhorn 1970, p. 13). A **minority group** or minority is a "group of people who, because of their physical or cultural characteristics, are singled out from the others in the society in which they live for differential and unequal treatment, and who therefore regard themselves as objects of collective discrimination" (Wirth 1945, p. 347). A dominant group is often the largest group in a society, for example, the white middle-class of the United States. However, the dominant group is not always the largest; for example, white South Africans are the dominant group and black South Africans are the minority group, yet the blacks far outnumber the whites.

Not uncommonly, people of a minority group often lose the cultural characteristics that distinguish them from the dominant group. This process is referred to as **cultural assimilation** or **acculturation**. Sometimes mutual cultural assimilation occurs, e.g., Chinese people coming to a North American community learn to speak English, and the people in the community learn to cook Chinese dishes.

Ethnocentrism is the belief that one's own culture is superior to all others, for instance, the comparison of the values and behavior of other cultures to those of one's own culture, which is used as the standard. Although all people are subject to ethnocentrism, it is important for nurses to be consciously aware of ethnic and cultural differences and to accept these as appropriate. These differences should not be viewed as good or bad. Many immigrants to the United States and Canada maintain their ethnic and cultural identities in terms of their dress, language, customs, and rituals; accepting these is basic to accepting the client as an individual.

Stereotyping is assuming that all members of a culture or ethnic group are alike. For example, one may assume that all Italians express pain volubly or that all Chinese people like rice. Stereotyping may be based on generalizations founded in research, or it may be unrelated to reality. For example, research indicates that Italians are likely to express pain verbally; however, a particular Italian client may not verbalize pain. Stereotyping that is unrelated to reality may be positive or negative and is frequently an outcome of racism. **Racism** is the assumption of inherent racial superiority or inferiority and the consequent discrimination against certain races. An example of positive stereotyping is "All Jewish people are very clever. "An example of negative stereotyping is "All Native Americans are alcoholics." Stereotyping can cause problems in nursing practice in that the nurse may plan care based on stereotyping rather than on individual assessment of the client.

Ethnoscience is "the systematic study of the way of life of a designated cultural group with the purpose of obtaining an accurate account of the people's behavior and how they perceive and interpret their universe" (Leininger 1970, p. 168). Anthropologists have for years studied cultural groups' own perceptions of and knowledge about their world. However, ethnoscientists use a more rigorous method of systematic data collection to provide an accurate collection and analysis of data. Ethnoscientists attempt to provide an inside view of a culture from the way the people of the culture talk about it. They study and classify data about a cultural or subcultural group so that their report is meaningful to both people within the culture and people outside the culture who try to understand it. Emphasis is placed on the person's point of view, the person's vision, and the person's world.

Nurses can apply much of the knowledge gained by ethnoscientists, specifically about the health-illness behavior systems of people from cultural backgrounds different from their own. In the past decade or more, the client's personal view of illness has received recognition and emphasis. Nurses have, as a result, implemented methods to discover how well clients understand their illnesses, how clients perceive they can be helped by health personnel, and how illness has affected them and their families. In recent years, cultural views affecting health practices and beliefs have been receiving greater recognition. The fact that health beliefs and practices vary among cultures and the implications of this fact for nursing have also received greater attention. To provide effective nursing services to clients, nurses need data about the client's personal and cultural views regarding health and illness. Nursing care plans need to consider the client's world and daily experiences; to make valid assessments, nurses need to try to see and hear the world as their clients do. Specific cultural data can provide scientific generalizations about health and illness behavior in different cultures. Clients' needs and behaviors can be better understood when particular health norms are identified

Characteristics of Culture

1. *Culture is learned.* It is not instinctive or innate. It is learned through life experiences after birth.

2. *Culture is inculcated.* It is transmitted from parents to children over successive generations. All animals can learn, but only humans can pass culture along. Language is the chief vehicle of culture. Through language, children can learn knowledge in a relatively short time compared to the time it may have taken their forebears to develop it.

3. *Culture is social.* It originates and develops through the interactions of people.

4. *Culture is adaptive.* Cultures tend to adapt to the environment over time. Customs, beliefs, and practices change slowly, but they do adapt to the social environment and to the biologic and psychologic needs of people. As life conditions change, some traditional forms in a culture may cease to provide satisfaction and are eliminated. For example, if it has been customary for family members of different generations to live together (extended family), yet education and employment often require children to leave their parents and move to other parts of the country, the extended family norm may change.

5. *Culture is integrative.* The elements in a culture tend to form a consistent and integrated system. For exam-

ple, religious beliefs and practices influence and are influenced by family organization, economic values, and health practices.

6. *Culture is ideational.* **Ideational** means forming images or objects in the mind. The group habits that are part of culture are to a considerable extent ideal norms or patterns of behavior. People do not always follow those norms. The norms of their culture may in fact be different from the norms of society as a whole.

7. *Culture is satisfying.* Cultural habits persist only as long as they satisfy people's needs. Gratification strengthens habits and beliefs. Once they no longer bring gratification, they may disappear.

Diversity of North American Society

The populations of the United States and Canada are a mixture of many ethnic groups and cultures. In the United States, white Americans make up 76.7% of the total population; minority groups, 23.3%. The minority population can be further broken down as shown in Figure 18–1. In Canada, British Canadians make up 40.2% of the total population; French Canadians, 26.7%. See Figure 18–1.

Grasska and McFarland caution about the use of untrained interpreters: Subtle emotions may be lost when verbal communication is separated from nonverbal communication, the interpreter may not understand medical terminology, and the ethics of confidentiality of information may be violated. Where there is a need for interpretation in a health agency, Grasska and McFarland suggest that the agency hire full-time trained bilingual interpreters who know medical terminology and health information (Grasska and McFarland 1982, pp. 1377–78).

Comparative Ethnic-Cultural Views

The provision of quality nursing care to all North Americans is a desired goal. Because of the multicultural, multiethnic nature of American society, it is essential that consideration be given to the unique needs of ethnic and cultural groups. The following general considerations can help nurses develop an awareness and sensitivity to some of these specific needs.

Male-Female Roles

Most cultures are patriarchal; i.e., the man is the dominant figure. The degree of dominance of men is variable; when men are highly dominant, women are usually passive. An example of a patriarchal society is the Islamic culture of Iran, where women must be veiled in public and all important decisions are left to the men.

In contrast, the Native American culture is matriarchal, i.e., the woman is the dominant person in the family. Knowing who the decision maker or dominant person in a family is helps nurses understand the meaning of illness to a family and its decision-making process relative to health care. In Mexican American families, the father generally holds the primary power, whereas in Jewish American families, the mother is generally "the power behind the throne" (Friedman 1981, p. 271).

Language and Communication Patterns

People of an ethnic or cultural group may speak the language of their group fluently and not the language of the country. This is particularly true of certain women who, because they stay in the home, have limited interaction with people outside the family. Even the mother of a family who has been in the United States for 30 years may know very little English. The degree to which people learn the language of a new country is highly variable. Some people may become fluent in English very quickly, while others may learn only enough English to get along in their daily activities. When people in the latter group become ill, they are frequently unable to describe their symptoms or answer a health questionnaire. If nurses do not establish that there is a language barrier, a client's needs may not be met. Most health agencies have translators to help nurses and clients, or the nurse may require help from a family member who can translate for the nurse.

Language barriers can be particularly frustrating and anxiety producing when a person is ill and can neither state problems nor understand instructions. It is most difficult for people to convey their emotions about threatening situations in a second language, a crucial factor in cases of emotional and psychiatric illness. Language barriers also arise between people using the same language. The idiomatic English of a regional or cultural group may not be readily understood outside the group. For example, *belly* can mean the abdomen or the entire cavity from the nipple line to the pubic area.

Communication patterns also differ among subcultures. For example, Native Americans commonly do not say goodbye before they leave. Swedish people talk more freely over shared food, and most cultures talk more slowly than the dominant American culture (Wold 1981, p. 143).

Territoriality and Personal Space

Territoriality is the pattern of behavior arising from an individual's feeling that certain spaces and objects belong to him or her. **Personal space** is the distance a person prefers to maintain from others when interacting with them. Both territoriality and personal space are influenced by an individual's culture and ethnicity. For example, people of Arabic, Southern European, and African origins frequently sit or stand relatively close to each other when talking, whereas people of Asian, North European, and North American countries are comfortable talking farther apart. For additional information about territoriality and personal space, see Chapter 28.

Time Orientation

The white middle-class group in the United States and in Canada tends to be oriented to the future. People plan for the future, establish long-term goals, and are increasingly concerned about preventing future illness, e.g., by taking calcium to prevent osteoporosis in old age. In daily life, people are oriented to the time of day; meals are taken at a specified time, and clients have appointment times with many health care professionals. The nurse is also highly attuned to time; medications are given at specific times, and work begins and ends at specified times.

However, not all cultures are future oriented. People of other cultures, e.g., Asians, may be oriented to the past. This orientation is illustrated by ancestor worship and the influence that ancient beliefs such as Confucianism have on the present. Other cultures, such as the Native American, are very much oriented to the present. Many Native American homes do not have clocks, and the people live one day at a time with little concern for the future. Some black Americans may appear to have little concern for time. They may be late for appointments because of the relative lack of importance that they ascribe to time. And Hispanic Americans often value relationships with others and the present more than the future and more than time.

Work

The attitude of individuals toward work is highly dependent upon their culture. Middle-class Americans generally believe that everyone should be employed and that work should be pleasurable and of value in itself; this attitude is often referred to as the Protestant work ethic. People in some cultures do not value work as much as the compensation for work, i.e., they view work as a means to an end.

American middle-class society tends to value material possessions, while people of some other cultures value possessions less. People who do not value work or compensation for work may prefer part-time or undemanding employment because of the free time it allows.

Family

The minority client's concept of family can differ from that of white middle-class culture. The minority group family may include the nuclear family plus uncles, aunts, grandparents, cousins, and godparents—the extended family. An associated concept is that family members are most important and must be helped at all costs. When health care is offered to such persons, it is important to consider the needs of the whole family. Sometimes, priorities in such families are detrimental to the health of one of its members. For example, a mother may not think that purchasing elastic stockings for her own ankle edema is as important as purchasing food for an unemployed relative. The home health care nurse in this instance may have to see that the relative's food needs are met before dealing with the mother's health needs.

Cultures that emphasize that the needs of the extended family are as important as personal needs may also hold the belief that personal and family information must stay within the family. Some cultural groups, e.g., the traditional Chinese family, are very reluctant to disclose family information to outsiders, including physicians and nurses. This attitude can present difficulties for psychiatrists and mental health workers who view family interaction patterns as the locus of emotional problems.

Food and Nutritional Practices

The food people eat and the customs associated with food vary widely among subcultures and ethnic groups. For example, the staple food of Asians is rice; of Italians, pasta; and of Europeans, wheat bread. Even families who have been in the United States or Canada for several generations often continue to eat the food of their country (Christian and Greger 1985, p. 213).

Hospitalized clients often have very little choice about the food they are served. The nurse can encourage family members to bring in special meals if the client's condition allows. Instructions about meal planning for clients requiring special diets at home may have to be given to younger family members who are fluent in English or given by a health worker of the same culture, who can act as an interpreter.

When clients are learning about a special diet, nurses must be sensitive to the cultural meanings of food and to the foods a client is accustomed to. For example, it is unwise to recommend a service such as Meals on Wheels if the service is unable to supply the foods to which the client is accustomed, e.g., bean sprouts and vegetables for the Japanese client and fish and rice for the Chinese client.

Susceptibility to Disease

Studies show that some ethnic and cultural groups in American society are more susceptible to certain diseases than the general population is, largely because of genetic and life-style influences. Generally, bicultural groups in a lower socioeconomic area have a higher incidence of acquired diseases, such as infections. The following diseases are more prevalent in certain groups than in the general population:

1. *Sickle-cell* disease affects approximately 50,000 Americans of African and Mediterranean descent. It affects both males and females equally. The most common syndrome is sickle-cell anemia, which affects 1 in 500 black children. Both parents must have the gene for sickling hemoglobin for their children to be affected clinically. It is estimated that between 8% and 10% of the black population in the United States has the sickling trait. The inherited recessive trait is a defect in the hemoglobin molecule. In people with sickle-cell disease, the red blood cells have a 20-day life, in contrast to the normal 120-day life. The symptoms and severity of the disease are variable, depending on the syndrome. Some people are very ill and have a series of crises, while others live fairly long and normal lives (Richardson and Milne 1983, p. 417).
2. *Hypertension* is more prevalent among black and other non-white Americans than white Americans, and the incidence is highest in Taiwan and Japan, two highly industrialized nations. It is also more common in recent immigrants to the United States. The pattern of incidence suggests that stress, obesity, and salt intake are implicated in hypertension (Overfield 1985, p. 114).
3. *Diabetes mellitus* is a major health problem of Native Americans. It occurs at an early age, i.e., teens, and the rate of death from diabetes is 3 to 4 times higher among Native Americans than the general population. It is thought that the incidence of diabetes among Native Americans is related to a diet high in refined carbohydrates and fats and low in traditional foods as well as a sedentary life-style (Overfield 1985, p. 153).
4. A number of *cancers* vary racially in their incidence; however, diet and some other environmental factors appear to be better predictors of cancer than race (Overfield 1985, p. 91). In the United States, white women have a higher incidence of breast cancer than black women. It has also been found that women with dry earwax have a lower incidence of breast cancer than women with wet earwax. Most Asians and Native Americans have dry earwax, and most blacks and whites have wet ear wax. Skin cancers of all types are less common among blacks than whites; this is thought to be due to the added protection dark pigmentation provides against the sun's rays. Although digestive tract cancers show high and low incidences relative to specific geographic areas and racial groups, diet rather than genetic factors are probably the cause (Overfield 1985, pp. 91–93).
5. Differences among races have been found in *alcohol metabolism*. Many Asians and Native Americans convert alcohol into acetaldehyde more rapidly and convert acetaldehyde to acetic acid more slowly than the general population does. Therefore, Asians and Native Americans experience a rapid onset of and prolonged exposure to high blood acetaldehyde levels, which cause many of the symptoms of alcohol intoxication (Overfield 1985, pp. 83–84).
6. Certain *dermatologic conditions* are more common among blacks than whites. Keloid formation, an exaggerated wound healing process of the skin, is commonly found in blacks. Keloids develop following skin trauma, e.g., surgical incision and burns (Bloch 1976, p. 28). A number of other conditions, e.g., acne vulgaris, can cause postinflammatory pigment changes in the skin among blacks. Hypopigmentation (decreased epidermal pigment) is most apparent in black clients. In addition, hyperpigmentation (increased epidermal pigment production) of the oral mucosa occurs in 50% to 90% of blacks by their fourth decade compared to 5% to 10% of whites by age 50 years (*American Journal of Nursing* 1979, p. 1092).
7. *Acquired immune deficiency syndrome* (AIDS) is currently more prevalent in the homosexual community than in the heterosexual community. In 1983, it was reported that 40% of the 2000 Americans who were stricken by AIDS in 1982–83 died (Augusta 1983, p. 49). The majority of AIDS victims are male homosexuals or bisexuals; however, intravenous drug users, Haitian immigrants, the sex partners of people in these groups, and hemophiliacs are also at risk. AIDS clients are particularly susceptible to Kaposi's sarcoma, a rare form of malignancy, and to *Pneumocystis carinii* pneumonia (PCP). Most AIDS victims are between the ages of 25 and 49 years.

Nurses must also be aware of the diseases that new immigrants can bring to North America. It is believed that health problems are linked to socioeconomic problems and that malnutrition or undernutrition is probably the greatest health problem of the developing world (Ohlson and Franklin 1985, pp. 3–4).

Cultural and Ethnic Groups in North America

This section outlines some selected cultural and ethnic characteristics of significance to nurses. It is important to remember, however, that many people in ethnic and cultural subgroups do not conform to all the practices of their group and may be assimilated into the white middle class.

Native Americans

In the United States and Canada, the responsibility for health services for Native Americans rests with the federal government. There are, however, differences in health care among geographic locations in the United States. For example, Native Americans living in the eastern states and in most urban areas are not covered by the services of the Indian Health Service, whereas Native Americans living on reservations in the western states are eligible for such services (Spector 1985, pp. 190–91).

Because about 200 different tribes of Native Americans exist in the United States, each with its own language, folkways, religion, mores, and patterns of interpersonal relationships, caution needs to be taken in generalizing about Native American culture. Moreover, generations of contact with non-Native Americans have diluted each purely Native American ethnic group. In terms of health care, this variability needs to be considered. For example, the Native American who lives in isolation on a reservation may hold to traditional beliefs of cure provided by the tribal medicine man, while the urban Native American who lives away from the reservation may respond more to the values of modern medicine provided by the majority culture. It is not uncommon for Native Americans to accept both kinds of health practices concurrently.

Various tribal groups differ in their traditional values and beliefs. Henderson and Primeaux (1981, pp. 73–74) list the following characteristics, which apply in general to traditional Native Americans:

1. *Oriented to present.* Native Americans tend to live in the present and are not concerned about the future, whereas non-Native Americans tend to be future oriented.
2. *Time conscious.* Native Americans are more concerned about finishing a task rather than about being punctual. In the past, many Native American tribes had no word for time.
3. *Giving.* The Native American who gives to others is highly respected. In some tribes, accumulating goods and saving money are not approved.
4. *Respectful of age.* Leadership positions are often given to the elderly rather than the young.
5. *Cooperative.* A high value is placed upon working together. Among certain Native Americans, inability to achieve a personal goal is often thought to be the result of competition.
6. *Harmonious with nature.* Native Americans believe in living in harmony with nature and taking from it only what one needs to live.
7. *Integrated into extended family.* The Native American extended family may include three generations in one household and includes other households of relatives. The elderly are often the official and symbolic leaders.

Native Americans are sometimes considered unmotivated, uninterested, or shifty-eyed because they may not look directly into the eyes of another person. This practice is based on their respect for the other person's privacy and the other person's soul. Some Native Americans believe that direct eye contact is disrespectful, intrudes on individual privacy, and may even take the other's soul away.

Associated with this belief is the Native American's commitment to autonomy. Each person has the right to speak only for himself or herself, and each person's actions should be self-initiated. Thus, the nurse who tries to obtain a client's history from close family members may have difficulty. Family members may believe they have no right to give personal information about another; they do not mean to be uncooperative but are following an unwritten ethical code.

The quality of life in the here and now is more important than longevity. Native Americans accept that they will die as part of the life cycle and do not worry about how or when or why. They know they will join another world of long-ago ancestors when the Spirit intends. Funerals generally take place in the home and are associated with a large feast and gifts for relatives of the deceased. Burial rituals according to tribal tradition are important to Native Americans.

Associated with burial is the belief of wholeness. Thus, when limbs are amputated, Native Americans may want to reclaim them and retain them for appropriate burial when the person dies. Native Americans also fear the spirits of the dead. It is important to the dying Native American client and his or her family that people, e.g., relatives, be present.

Family

The family, relatives, and friends are important to Native Americans. During illness, the client is comforted by visits from relatives and friends. Visits convey caring and enduring bonds of support. Being present is generally more important than talking, and it is not uncommon for large numbers of people to congregate. Most often, one person likes to remain near the client for long periods. The Native American's kinship system can be confusing to nurses of other cultures. A child, for example, may have several mothers or several sets of brothers or sisters who are not direct relatives but are considered such. These people are all important to the ill client. The aged, particularly, are looked upon for counsel and wisdom. Friendship ties are strong and can be as meaningful as those of the family or extended family in sustaining the client's recuperative powers.

Health Beliefs

Native Americans tend to value harmonious relations with the world around them. Each rock, tree, animal, flower, and person is equally respected, and all are seen to coexist in harmony. A state of health exists when a person is in total harmony with nature. The earth is considered a living organism that has a will and desire to be well, but, just as human beings, may be healthy or less healthy. It is believed that when people harm the earth they harm themselves, and vice versa. Thus, Native Americans believe they should treat the body and the earth with respect.

Many Native Americans view illness as an imbalance between the person who is ill and the natural or supernatural forces around the person, rather than as an altered physiologic state. Causes of illness relate to this concept. Native Americans believe that if one interferes with this harmony by abusing or offending another person or thing, one may become ill. Even bad thoughts or wishes, such as jealousy or anger, may cause illness. In addition, supernatural or spiritual forces may be involved. In the Papago tribe of southern Arizona, for example, many persons believe that ghosts of the dead, returning as owls or other animals of night, bring sickness. All animals are believed to have supernatural powers, which they can use to send sickness (Winn 1976, p. 281).

Native Americans do not relate disease causation to germ theory. A survey of Native American registered nurses from 23 tribes revealed that none of these tribes had a word for *germ* (Henderson and Primeaux 1981, p. 243). This trait makes it difficult for Native Americans to understand the cause of tuberculosis, for example. Some Navajo Native Americans believed that the signs and symptoms caused by tuberculosis were the result of lightning. If lightning struck a tree and a person used the wood from that tree for firewood or other purposes, it would cause abscesses to develop in the lungs (Wauneka 1976, p. 236).

Health Problems

The leading causes of death in the Native American population are accidents, suicide, diabetes, alcoholism, and homicide (Primeaux 1977, pp. 58–59). At least one-third of the Native American population is poverty-stricken. Associated with this income level are poor living conditions, malnutrition, tuberculosis, and high maternal and infant death rates. Native Americans have the highest infant mortality rate in the United States, even though their birth rate is almost twice that of the general population. This rate is attributed to the high incidence of diarrhea in young babies and the harsh environment in which they live (Spector 1985, p. 187).

Health Practices

Various curative and preventive rituals may be conducted to restore balance when illness occurs. Some of these may be carried out by medicine men, others by family members. Sacred foods, such as cornmeal, may be sprinkled on people's shoulders before they enter a home to prevent disease from entering the home. This sacred food or other substance, such as tobacco or feathers, may be sprinkled around an ill person's bed. It is important for nurses to provide privacy for such ceremonies and to inquire about how long the substance is to be left in place, how to dispose of it, and, if it must be disturbed, exactly how and where the nurse may do so. Items such as herbs or mixtures are frequently placed near the client on the bedside stand or on the bed; some may be worn by the client. Nurses need to acquire permission from the client, family, or medicine man, if these have to be removed.

Healing ceremonies, sometimes referred to as *sings* or *prayers,* may be requested. These vary in length from 30 minutes to 9 days. Space and privacy need to be provided for such ceremonies. In the hospital, the sing usually lasts less than 1 hour. A medicine man may also be requested to perform curative rituals, which vary with the signs and symptoms of the client.

Nursing Implications

When caring for Native American clients, nurses need to consider the following:

1. Although most Native Americans recognize the value of Anglo-Western health care, many continue to use traditional medicine and cures either independently or in conjunction with such care.
2. Native Indian medicine and religion cannot be separated. Native Americans make no distinction between physical and mental illness or the mind and the body. They live the concept of wholeness.
3. Tribal healing ceremonies and practices are highly ritualistic, religious ways to deal with sickness and death.
4. Tribal rituals that include extended "family" members are the way that Native Americans share all aspects of life.

5. Each tribe assigns symbolic meanings to foods or other substances.
6. Such characteristics as not looking others in the eye should not be interpreted as disrespect, inattention, lack of interest, or avoidance.
7. Communication with Native Americans needs to include an awareness of the following factors:
   a. The person's custom of speaking only for himself or herself.
   b. Use of extensive questions during history taking may be construed as an intrusion of individual privacy. The history taker may need to rely on observation techniques and make declarative statements to the client such as, "You have an obvious cough that keeps you awake at night."
   c. Note taking may pose a barrier to communication, since Native Americans tend to value conversation, story telling, and listening.
   d. Native Americans often use a very low tone of voice, and the listener is expected to pay attention.

Black Americans

With the arrival of the first African slaves in Jamestown, Virginia, in 1619, a history of deprivation on this continent began for blacks. Even after slavery was abolished, black people endured severe economic and social deprivation. The struggles to overcome these deprivations continue today. However, black American culture now is more similar to white American culture than it was 300 years ago. There is a large black middle class and a large black lower class. United States Census Bureau statistics for 1977 show that the majority of black families/households have incomes of $10,000 or less. There are strong kinship bonds in both low-income and more prosperous black families. These families provide financial support, assist with child care, and serve as buffers against racism and discrimination during children's growing years. A black family may show much cohesion and sharing, particularly in times of trouble.

Often a significant member of a black family must be consulted before important decisions are made. This person may be a father, mother, aunt, son, or grandparent. Nurses need to be sensitive to the fact that a decision may not be made until this person is consulted.

When black Americans who are not familiar with the health care system enter it, they may show defensive behaviors such as hostility and suspicion. These attitudes are often adopted in expectation of being demeaned in some manner. It is important for nurses to recognize the reasons for these responses and learn to relate to all clients as worthy human beings.

Family

Middle-class black households tend to have two parents, and often both parents work to maintain a middle-class life-style. Children of middle-class black families often feel the need to achieve. Many plan to attend college to maintain or advance their position in the community.

Lower-income blacks often live in extended families, i.e., grandparents, aunts, uncles living in the house with the parents and children. Single-parent families in financial difficulty may depend on government programs for income. Black families frequently have extended support systems. LaFargue states that part of the survival strategy of blacks in the urban north is to immerse themselves in a domestic circle of kinfolk who will help them (LaFargue 1980, p. 1637).

Health Beliefs

Black Americans may believe traditionally that health is maintained by proper diet, which includes a hot breakfast. Some believe that laxatives are important to keep the system running and open (Spector 1985, p. 147). A person who is a practicing Black Muslim does not eat pork or pork products.

It is important for nurses to understand the values held by a black client and that person's definition of health. Traditional definitions in black culture stem from the African view of life as a process rather than a state. All things, whether living or dead, were believed to influence each other (Spector 1985, p. 142). Health meant being in harmony with nature; illness was a state of disharmony. Therefore illness could be treated in a number of ways, including reliance on the power of a "healer." These beliefs and practices may or may not apply to a particular black client. However, nurses should be aware of any cultural differences and take these into consideration when planning care. See also Table 18–1. In LaFargue's study, blacks defined illness as "feeling bad" or "inhibition of physical activity" (LaFargue 1972, p. 54).

Health Problems

The major health problems of blacks in the United States are hypertension, sickle cell disease, and cancers of the lungs, oral cavity, larynx, pharynx, esophagus, and urinary bladder. The increase in cancer in these areas is thought to be largely due to the increase in smoking (Orque et al. 1983, p. 106). Poverty among blacks leads to relatively high morbidity and mortality rates among infants and mothers, even though these rates have declined since 1960 (National Center for Health Statistics 1985, p. 2).

Obesity is a greater problem among black women than white women. Approximately 60% of black females 45 to 75 years were overweight in 1975 to 1980 (National Center for Health Statistics 1985, p. 9). Although hypertension is a problem among black adults, the incidence of hypertension decreased from 33.9% in 1971–74 to 28.6% in 1976–80 (National Center for Health Statistics 1985, p. 18).

Table 18–1 Comparison of Health-Related Factors and Subcultures

	Definition of Health	Cause of Illness —Is Prevention Possible; if so, How?	Name of Healer, Healing Practices	Problems of Entry to Health Care System	Communication Patterns	Sexuality and Family Life	Beliefs about Death
Navajo (Native American)	Harmony between individual, earth, and supernatural, as well as the ability to survive difficult circumstances[1,2]	Disease is disharmony and can be caused by violating taboo or attack by witch; illness prevented through elaborate religious rituals; do not believe in germ theory[1,2]	Medicine man, who is more than average human being, is therefore influential figure; medicine man diagnoses and treats problem; treatments include yucca root, massage, herbs, and chanting; his chant states person will get well, and person believes him[1,2]	Language; will first visit medicine man; general beliefs are not compatible with health care system and structure; problems also include money and past experiences of disrespect; fear of spirits of dead may influence decision to leave hospital early[1,2]	Time of silence after each speaker to show respect and reflection on what they said; little eye contact; time orientation not very strict; recording of conversation invasion of privacy[1,2]	Family, extended family, and tribal ties strong; cooperation emphasized; consider children as individuals as soon as they can talk, therefore can make own decisions[1,2]	Fear of spirits of dead; children and family should be with dying person[1]
Hispanic American	Gift from God, also good luck; can tell healthy person by robust appearance and report of feeling well[1,3,4]	Illness is punishment from God for wrongdoing, to be suffered; it can be prevented by eating well, praying, being good, and working; wearing medals may help; physically, illness is an imbalance between "hot" and "cold" properties of body[1,3,4]	Healer called *curandero;* cures hot illness with cold medicine and reverse; classification of hot and cold diseases varies; penicillin is hot medicine; massages and cleanings are common[4]	Language; will first go to woman for advice, then if needed, to "señora," then to curandero, then to physician; many migrant workers are Hispanic, and frequent moves may make access to medical care difficult; belief that hospital is place to go to die causes underuse of system; modesty may result in woman bringing friend to physician with her[1,3,4]	Confidentiality and modesty important; too many questions are insulting; it is more acceptable to make tentative statement to which they can respond; time orientation not strict; politeness essential[1,3–5]	High degree of modesty, may prefer home births for this reason; men are breadwinners, women homemakers; women are healers, men make all decisions[1,3–5]	Afterlife of heaven and hell exists

Traditional black	Harmony with nature, no separation of mind and body[4]	Disease is disharmony caused by spirits and demons; it can be prevented through good diet, rest, cleanliness, and laxatives to clean out system; some use of copper and silver bracelets for prevention	Some belief in voodoo still prevalent; religious healing practiced[4,6]	May seek folk or religious healer first; money and type of service affect decision; emergency room frequent entry point; black women have high "noncompliance" rate[4,6]	Racism toward blacks still prevalent; common names for symptoms should be known by health worker; time orientation not strict	Matriarchy prevalent; almost 30% of black families have woman head of household; therefore women make decisions[4,6]	Death is passage from evils of this world to another state; blacks have shorter life expectancy than national average[6]
Chinese American	Balance of yin and yang (negative and positive energy forces); healthy body is gift from parents and ancestors[4,7,8]	Illness caused by imbalance of yin and yang, which may be due to overexertion or prolonged sitting; disease is prevented through better adaptation to nature[4,7]	Acupuncture and moxibustion (which is a therapeutic application of heat to skin) restore balance of yin and yang; herbal remedies such as ginseng used for many illnesses; healer is called physician[4,7]	Language traditional Chinese physicians were paid to keep their clients well and cared for sick without fees because illness indicated they had failed in their job; Chinese physicians are available in community and may encourage clients to use Western physician; family spokesman may accompany client to Western physician[4,7]	Open expression of emotions not acceptable; therefore might not complain about pain or symptoms; client may smile when he or she does not understand[4,7]	Women subservient to men; patriarchal family; ancestor worship and respect for obedience for parents observed; divorce considered disgrace[1,4,5]	Reincarnation[7]
Low income	Functional definition; if you can work, you are healthy[5,9]	Belief that illness is not preventable; fatalism common; future orientation minimal because present problems are too great[1,5,9]	Will often rely on folk healers and remedies because of belief and problems gaining access to health care system[5]	Use of public funding may limit access and type of care; present time orientation and beliefs about prevention may cause delay in obtaining care; inability to afford health insurance; may lose day's pay to go to physician[5,9]	May use slang and language of subculture; may view providers as authoritarian; time orientation not strict[5]	Many single-parent families with woman head of household[9]	Depends on culture and religion

(continued)

Table 18–1 *(continued)*

	Definition of Health	Cause of Illness—Is Prevention Possible; if so, How?	Name of Healer, Healing Practices	Problems of Entry to Health Care System	Communication Patterns	Sexuality and Family Life	Beliefs about Death
High income	No data available	General belief in prevention of illness through diet, exercise, and good health habits; motivators such as previous experience or family tradition are influential in actual practice of prevention[5]	Combination of traditional practices of religion and culture, frequent use of health care system and self-help information[5]	Access not too difficult, usually through private physician; most have health insurance through employer[5]	Most like health care culture; cannot be expected to understand jargon	Women more likely to have career by choice than financial necessity	Depends on culture and religion
Health care culture	Optimal level of functioning; more than absence of disease; physical, emotional, social, and mental health included[5]	Scientific approach to cause of illness; prevention involves periodic physical examinations, laboratory studies, inoculations, as well as avoiding smoking and overeating[4]	Healing done by physician, usually takes place in office or hospital; treatments based on scientific knowledge and are frequently embarrassing or uncomfortable; often emotional component of disease is ignored[4]	Physician is main access to system; focus is basically curing illness rather than prevention; encouragement given to population to seek care as soon as symptoms appear; consider health care system as only provider	Widespread use of jargon and specialized language; large percentage of workers from middle class; often expect gratitude for care given; time orientation strict; written records kept[4]	Hierarchy, with physicians making decisions	Death usually means workers have failed to do their job; elaborate means are used to keep people alive; ethical and legal questions are being discussed and tested

[1]Data from A. T. Brownlee, *Community, culture, and care: A cross-cultural guide for health workers* (St. Louis: C. V. Mosby Co., 1978).
[2]Data from R. Wood, The American Indian and health. In *Ethnicity and health care* (NLN pub. no. 14–1625, 1976), pp. 29–35.
[3]Data from H. Gonzales, Health care needs of the Mexican American family. In *Ethnicity and health care.* (NLN pub. no. 14–1625, 1976), pp. 21–28.
[4]Data from R. Spector, *Cultural diversity in health and illness* (New York: Appleton-Century-Crofts, 1985).
[5]Data from R. Murray and J. Zentner, *Nursing assessment and health promotion through the life span* (Englewood Cliffs, N.J.: Prentice-Hall, 1975).
[6]Data from B. Martin, Ethnicity and health care: Afro-Americans. In *Ethnicity and health care* (NLN pub. no. 14–1625, 1976), pp. 47–55.
[7]Data from R. Wang, Chinese Americans and health care. In *Ethnicity and health care* (NLN pub. no. 14–1625, 1976), pp. 9–18.
[8]Data from G. Channing, What is a Christian Scientist? In Rosten, L., editor: *A guide to religions of America* (New York: Simon & Schuster, 1955).
[9]Data from M. Fromer, Community health care and the nursing process (St. Louis: C. V. Mosby Co., 1979).

Source: Adapted from Joanne Gingrich-Crass, Structural variables: factors affecting adaptation, in S. J. Wold, *School nursing: A framework for practice* (St. Louis: C. V. Mosby Co.) pp. 136–41.

Health Practices

The poor black client does not seek help until a health problem is serious for many reasons, e.g., "finances, child care problems, fear of hospitals, possibility of becoming a 'guinea pig,' and fear of death" (White 1977, p. 30). Many black families in rural areas of the South continue to use folk health practices (Henderson and Primeaux 1981, p. 210) and home remedies. Voodoo and witchcraft are practiced to a minor extent. Thus the cause of illness may be thought of by a few as the result of a hex. Spiritualists or sorcerers may sometimes be consulted, or clients may vacillate between Western physicians and witch doctors or spiritualists who can remove spells. Historically, churches have been a bulwark of support for blacks, Hence religious practices and Bible reading often continue during hospitalization.

Some black Amcricans find the church a source of refuge from the realities of life. As such, the church helps the poor black person find respect and self-esteem. Often the black clergy can help bridge the gap between the black client and health professionals because they have "the understanding of the rituals, folkways, and mores" of black culture (Smith 1976, p. 12). See Figure 18–2.

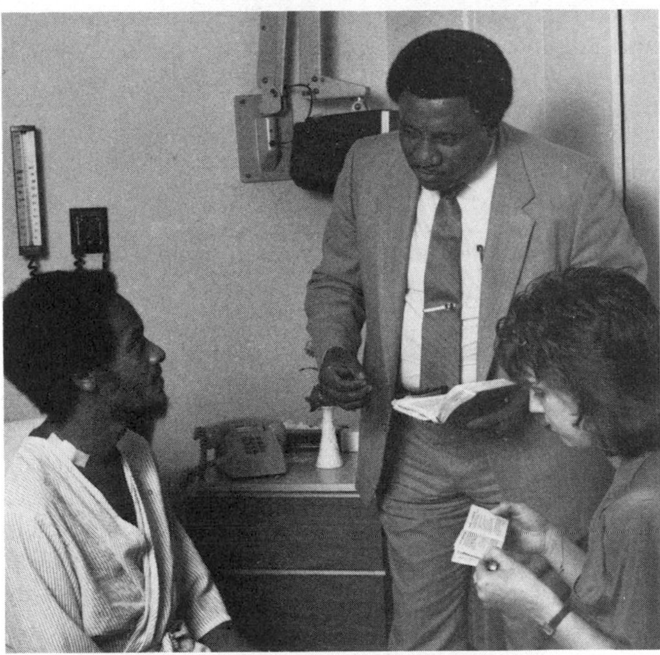

Figure 18–2 Black clergy can often help bridge the gap between the black culture and other cultures, such as the health care culture.

Nursing Implications

Nursing implications relative to the care of the black client include: skin and hair care, assessing skin color, communication, and food preferences. Skin and hair care are discussed in Chapter 36, page 808 and page 810.

Black people are very much aware of any signs of racial discrimination. Talking down to a black client can cause anxiety, which can lead to feelings of suspicion about nurses.

Some black clients speak black English, a highly rhythmical and stylized speech. It differs from standard English in its pronunciation and syntax and in the connotations of some words. Black English has also been called black dialect, black creole, soul talk, Afro-American speech, Ebonics, and Afro (Orque et al. 1983, p. 86). To lessen communication barriers between black clients and nurses, Bigham suggests:

1. Treat blacks as you would others.
2. Use titles such as "Mr.," "Mrs.," and "Miss" unless your acquaintance is on a first-name basis.
3. Do not condescend to a black person because he or she is black.
4. Do not attempt to impress black clients by talking about other blacks you know. (Bigham 1964, p. 115)

Black clients may favor a traditional rural Southern diet, an urban middle-class diet, or a combination of the two. Soul food is the traditional diet of the Southern black. Pork is the chief meat. Hominy grits, black-eyed peas, and mustard and collard greens are also soul food. To these are often added cabbage, rice, white potatoes, okra, macaroni, and noodles (Orque et al. 1983, pp. 95–96). Nurses can often assist blacks who are accustomed to eating soul food to adapt special diets to their tastes.

Asian Americans

The term *Asian American* refers to four primary ethnic groups: Chinese, Japanese, Koreans, and Vietnamese. Recently the term *Pacific Asian* has been used to include people originally from the Pacific islands, such as the Philippines, Samoa, and Guam, as well as the other Asian countries.

It is difficult to classify many Asians because they are of mixed national parentage. For example, the person's parents may be Chinese and Korean or Japanese and Filipino. In addition, most Asians view themselves as belonging to particular subgroups and ethnic groups and generally dislike being viewed as a member of another group. For example, the Chinese Americans and Japanese Americans in Hawaii consider themselves different from the "mainlanders," i.e., those in the United States.

Because of the wide diversity of groups of Asians, full coverage of their views is beyond the scope of this book. This section focuses primarily on Chinese health beliefs and practices, since the traditions of many other Asians derive in part from them. The health beliefs and practices of Japanese Americans, Vietnamese Americans, and Filipino Americans will be considered briefly. First, however, some general traditional Asian values and behaviors are outlined, although the student must recognize that a wide range of behaviors exists among and within groups.

General Traditional Asian Values and Beliefs

Chang (1981, pp. 260–75) outlines the following general Asian values and behaviors:

1. Traditionally, the Asian household consisted of the extended kinship family in which grandparents, parents, siblings, uncles, aunts, and cousins lived together. Although such households are rare in North America today, members of traditional families often maintain strong emotional bonds. It is not unusual, therefore, for hospitalized Asians to have many family members visit them.
2. The traditional Asian family is male dominated. When elderly persons live with the family, they are usually the husband's parents. Asian women historically occupied an inferior position to men, and sons were more welcome in a family than daughters. Even in modern families, sons may receive preferential treatment. It is wise, therefore, for nurses to ascertain the opinion of the father, or in his absence the eldest son, on health care issues requiring decision making.
3. Traditionally, there is unquestioning respect for and deference to authority. It is expected that each individual will maintain filial piety (devotion and loyalty to family authority). Asian families are considered a continuum from past to future. Membership includes not only the present generation but also the ancestors and the unborn. Failure to comply with familial authority, duty, and obligations, to pay obedience to the family, and to engage in behavior that gives the family and the ethnic group a good name results in feelings of shame and guilt.
4. Interactions in the Asian family tend to be less verbal than in the white middle-class family, and praise of self or of members of one's own family is considered bad manners. This behavior of Asians is often misconstrued as lack of self-esteem or as belittling of family members. This does not imply that the nurse should not offer appropriate praise; but she or he should accept a self-deprecating response as a cultural variant.
5. Asians strongly emphasize harmony and avoidance of conflict in groups. In contrast to the behavior of whites, who may consider the individual most important, the behavior of Asians may not benefit the individual but instead be best for the situation and for others in the group. Often behavior is described as quiet, obedient, unassertive, reticent, agreeable, and reserved. For example, an individual may remain quiet or simply nod the head, often to avoid conflicts in ambiguous, embarrassing, or anxiety-producing situations. This behavior may be more apparent in Asian women due to their socialization. Asians avoid direct confrontations in which one of the parties must lose face; to do so, they may blame themselves for a mistake even when facts indicate that it was the other person's error.
6. Asian respect for those in authority positions, such as doctors, teachers, and nurses, often evokes a yes response that is different from the American connotation of the word. Asians tend to answer yes to be polite and to mean, "I don't want to cause embarrassment." For example, in response to a nurse's question, "Is that clear?" an Asian may say yes because it is considered impolite to say "No, it is not clear," since that response may imply that the nurse is either confused or unable to communicate. It is wise, therefore, for nurses to ask questions that require more than a yes-or-no answer.
7. Outward signs of feelings are discouraged. Asians are taught patterns of self-control and bravery even in situations of emotional conflict, hardship, and pain. This has implications for nurses assessing pain in such patients and assisting Asians during emotional crises. Often Asians express feelings of caring by their physical presence and attendance in times of illness rather than by an outward verbal expression of feelings.
8. Asians characteristically avoid attracting special attention to themselves. This inconspicuousness is related to their culture, which emphasizes harmony, consideration of others' rights and feelings, avoidance of behavior that would dishonor the family, and respect for and obedience to those in authority.

Chinese Americans

The Chinese in the United States and Canada are largely concentrated on the west coasts of the countries, on the east coast of the United States, and in large cities such as New York and Chicago. The Chinese population can be considered in three groups: (a) people who were born in rural villages in China and immigrated to North America 40 to 50 years ago; (b) new immigrants who have come within the past 20 years, from several Asian countries and Hong Kong; and (c) Chinese born in North America who are descendants of 19th-century immigrants. Chinese in the first group are still largely oriented to Chinese folk medicine, while those in the third group are oriented to Western medical practices but still may be influenced by their elders in regard to health care. Those in the second group often practice a mixture of Chinese folk and Western medicine.

Family Prior to the revolution in China, the Chinese family was patriarchal and patrilineal. Respect for ancestors and parents was important, and obedience to the family was practiced. The Chinese family was frequently an extended one with several generations living in one household. Family clans were strong social organizations and were formed of people of the same bloodline with the same surnames. People who came to North America 40 to 50 years ago set up the same traditional families, based on associations to which they were accustomed in China.

Following the revolution, traditional family practices and superstitions became less evident in China and among immigrants. Family ties continue to be strong; however, the nuclear family now is seen more commonly in Chinese-American society.

In many Asian families, at least two people are employed full time; they often use their income to support the extended family (Wang 1976, pp. 33–41). The extended family is very important in their lives. The Chinese family is patriarchal, and the wife may not be educated or speak English (White 1977, p. 38).

Health beliefs Campbell and Chang (1973, pp. 245–49) outline the following health beliefs and practices of the Chinese. Chinese folk medicine originated with Taoist philosophy. It proposes that the universe and health are regulated by two forces, the *yin* and the *yang*. The yin is a negative, female force; some of its characteristics are darkness, cold, and emptiness. The yang represents the positive, the male, light, warmth, and fullness. When these two energy forces are in balance, health exists. When a person has too much yin, he or she is nervous and is predisposed to digestive disorders. Too much yang, on the other hand, causes dehydration, fever, and irritability.

The Chinese do not consider their bodies to be personal property. The body is viewed as a gift provided by parents and ancestors, and it thus must be cared for. Various parts of the body are controlled by yin and yang. The inside, front part of the body, and five solid organs (*ts'ang*) that collect and store secretions—i.e., the liver, heart, spleen, lungs, and kidneys—are controlled by yin. The outside, back part of the body, and five hollow organs (*fu*) that excrete—i.e., the gallbladder, stomach, large and small intestines, and bladder—are controlled by yang. Yin stores the vital strength of life; yang protects the body from outside forces. A person who does not balance yin and yang properly will have a short life. Illness occurs when an imbalance of yin and yang exists. The sole cause of disease is considered to be disrupted harmony.

Chinese staples are polished tofu and rice. In addition vegetables such as *bok choy, gai lan,* spinach, Chinese cabbage, and mustard greens are favored. Many Chinese do not tolerate milk or cheese well.

Health problems Specific health problems more prevalent among the Chinese than the general population are eye problems, tuberculosis, dental caries, malnutrition, and mental illness. Some of these are directly related to the poor environmental conditions of North American Chinatowns rather than to an inherited predisposition.

Because of the stress of adjusting to American culture and the lack of family support, mental health problems among aged male Chinese have increased. Another reason for emotional problems is the bicultural conflict between the individual values of freedom, egalitarianism, and individualism and the Chinese values of filial piety, loyalty, and authoritarianism (Orque et al. 1983, p. 196).

Health practices Some clients follow both Western and Chinese medical advice at the same time. This can produce problems if the therapies are not correlated. For example, a client may be receiving the same drug from an herbal pharmacy that is prescribed by the Western physician, thus taking a double dose. Chinese clients should be encouraged to tell a doctor whether they are taking or receiving other therapy.

Folk medicine practices are often carried out during pregnancy. For example, use of soy sauce may be restricted so that the baby's skin will not be very dark, or a mother may refuse to take iron because it will harden the bones and make delivery of the baby difficult.

Following are some differences between Western practice and Chinese folk medicine (see also Table 18–1 on page 364):

1. One dose of an herbal medicine is thought to cure a person or make the person feel better. Thus, the vast number and dosages of medicines prescribed by some Western physicians are puzzling to Chinese clients.
2. Herbs are generally boiled in water for a prescribed time before being ingested rather than prepared as capsules or pills.
3. Chinese clients may change physicians during an illness in order to find the best cure. When they do so, they may not tell the former doctor because they do not want the doctor to lose face.
4. The Chinese do not understand or react well to numerous diagnostic procedures that are painful. They believe that a physician should be able to make a diagnosis solely on the basis of a physical examination. Many may leave the Western system to avoid distasteful procedures.
5. Most Chinese believe that it is best to die with the body intact. This belief originates with Confucius, who taught

that only those shall be truly revered who at the end of their lives return their physical bodies whole and sound. As a result, Chinese clients may refuse surgery and donation of organs after death.

6. Ginseng is a highly valued herb used as a general strength tonic for the pregnant woman (Chung 1977, p. 71).

Chinese folk medicine uses herbs and acupuncture. A folk medicine diagnosis is made chiefly by observation, questioning, listening to the body, and taking the pulse. The prescription is a combination of herbs, which are obtained from a Chinese pharmacy. Acupuncture, or a cold treatment, is used chiefly to treat muscular and skeletal disorders and diseases in which there is excessive yang. Needles are inserted into the body at specific points along certain internal channels, which are called **meridians.** The internal organs are believed to be connected to the skin points and to the meridians; the acupuncture helps to balance the energy that flows within them.

The concept of yin and yang is also involved in a balanced meal. Yin is cold and includes fruits, vegetables, cold drinks, and hot (in temperature) melon soup. Yang is hot and includes, for example, soups containing ginger and scrambled eggs. In Chinese culture the concepts of hot and cold have nothing to do with the temperature of the food. A Chinese patient who is ill with a hot disease, such as an eye infection, may wish to eat cold foods rather than hot foods in order to get well.

Chinese people of the older generations may also believe that their blood is not replaceable. Therefore, they are often very reluctant to give blood even for a blood test. Like many other people, the elderly Chinese often believe that a hospital is a place to go to die rather than to get well.

Nursing implications Implications relative to the care of Chinese clients include:

1. Always convey respect by addressing the client and family members by their given names.
2. Try to provide the Chinese client with the food to which he or she is accustomed. Some communities have hospitals that provide special food for their Chinese clients.
3. Chinese clients are often reluctant to be admitted to hospitals. They believe hospitals are unclean places where people go to die. They may require supportive nursing intervention for reassurance.

Japanese Americans

Japanese Americans often maintain a number of their cultural values while at the same time acculturating to the larger society. Four values of the Japanese are gaman, haji, enryo, and koko. *Gaman* means self-control. A Japanese person who is stoic when experiencing pain is probably practicing gaman. The client will not verbalize the pain and may try to deal with it. Japanese who carry on in spite of adversity are considered strong (Orque et al. 1983, p. 223).

Haji, or shame, is an important cultural concept. Japanese children are taught not to bring shame on themselves or their families by unacceptable behavior. *Enryo* is a type of behavior that encompasses politeness, respect, deference, reserve, and humility. The opposite of enryo is aggressive, boisterous, loud, rude behavior (Orque et al. 1983, p. 224). For example, a Japanese man might not turn on his signal light because he does not want to bother the nurses. *Koko* is filial piety. The Japanese perceive dependence as natural for the elderly and young children. An elderly person who is dependent and has reduced authority still maintains self-esteem. This attitude contrasts to the North American view of dependence as a sign of weakness (Kalish 1967, pp. 65–69).

Japanese Americans consider time valuable and they like to use it well. They will usually follow medication schedules precisely. Some Japanese Americans who were affected by relocation during World War II suffered serious financial and emotional losses and it has taken years for many of them to get over this.

Vietnamese Americans

Thousands of Vietnamese came to the United States following the Vietnamese war. Another, smaller, group came later. South Vietnamese have a family-centered culture in which the children are taught to value the family's interests over their own (Orque et al. 1983, p. 250). Vietnamese value propriety over time and indirectness over confrontation in a disagreement in order to preserve harmony. A Vietnamese client who is embarrassed at a nurse's question may say yes or laugh to lessen his embarrassment.

Filipino Americans

The Filipino culture is diverse. However, its central culture values are shaped by a fatalistic view that God's will and supernatural forces will determine what happens. Filipino culture is family centered, stressing interdependency among members of the family. Filipinos also emphasize achievement and social acceptance. A Filipino client is likely to avoid a disagreement with a nurse and speak evasively. By contrast, the white middle-class American may value an open expression of feelings and honest expression of thoughts. Because of their fatalistic view, Filipinos often show great patience and endurance when faced with illness.

Hispanic Americans

Hispanic Americans have their origins in a number of Spanish-speaking countries: Mexico, Spain, Cuba, Puerto Rico, and the nations of Central and South America. One of the largest groups for whom Spanish is the dominant tongue is the Mexican American population.

Traditional Mexican American foods are beans and tortillas. For clients requiring a special diet, traditional foods can present problems. This situation requires special planning in consultation with dietitians. For example, Hispanics generally prefer rice to potatoes. The manner of preparing the rice is important; it differs from the Asian method. The diet of many low-income Mexican Americans often contains a high proportion of starches: tortillas, beans, corn, and so on. It is usually possible to plan diets to meet clients' preferences and thus increase the chances that the food will be eaten.

Because a full discussion of each Hispanic American culture and its health care implications is beyond the scope of this book, the following pages focus on Mexican American beliefs and practices.

Family

Mexican Americans have extended families that play an important part in their lives. The family is usually large, and life revolves around the home. Often the family's needs take precedence over the individual's needs. At a time of illness, the family will give a great deal of support.

In the Mexican-American family, the woman is the primary caregiver, and often she decides when medical assistance should be sought.

Health Beliefs

Many Mexican Americans entered the United States during the early 1900s and brought with them the values, beliefs, and practices of rural Mexico; others are more recent immigrants. Folk concepts of health and illness continue to affect the thinking of some second- and third-generation Mexican Americans today. See also Table 18–1 on page 364.

Mexican Americans may hold the following health-related beliefs to varying degrees:

1. Certain foods promote good health, while others can produce poor health. An example of the former is tea made from fresh orange leaves; examples of the latter are rice and coffee, which should not be taken during an evening meal.
2. A person must be in tune with God to maintain good health. Thus, a person who is chronically ill is believed to have offended God and is being punished.
3. Health means being free of pain and being robust, even obese, rather than thin.

In addition, health is perceived as the ability to maintain a high level of normal physical activity. Mexican Americans also perceive illness as a state of discomfort. Some Mexican Americans also believe that certain people can use magical powers to make others ill (Abril 1977, pp. 169–70).

Some Mexican Americans believe that illness is due to life-style. They often have precise ideas about the types of rest, activity, recreation, and nutrition that lead to poor and good health (Gonzalez-Swafford and Gutierrez 1983, p. 29).

Illness is seen as an imbalance in the individual's body or as a punishment for wrongdoing. The causes of illness can be grouped into four categories (Spector 1985, p. 161–63):

1. *Imbalance between "hot" and "cold" or "wet" and "dry."* The four humors or body fluids that must be in balance are: blood (hot and wet), phlegm (cold and wet), yellow bile (hot and dry), and black bile (cold and dry). When these fluids are not in balance, illness results. Treatment in hospitals can be based on the principles of hot and cold. For example, illnesses that are classified as hot are treated with food, drugs, and drinks that are classified as cold.
2. *Magic or supernatural forces. Mal de ojo* (evil eye) is disease caused by forces outside the body, such as a person's admiration of part of another person's body, e.g., the hair. The victim can lose the admired part or fall ill. In some places, mal de ojo is thought to be prevented by having the admirer touch the admired person while complimenting him or her, and it is believed to be cured with eggs in a ritual. The symptoms of mal de ojo include headaches, fever, fatigue, and prostration.
3. *"Dislocation" of body parts.* One example of a disease of "dislocation" is *empacho.* This is a disease, primarily seen in children, that produces swelling of the abdomen as a result of intestinal blockage. It is thought to be caused by overeating foods such as soft bread and bananas.
4. *Strong emotional states. Susto* is a disease of emotional origin—fright caused by natural phenomena such as lightning or loud noises. The symptoms have been described as insomnia, restlessness, and nervousness. It is a common folk disease that is difficult to cure, but it can be treated with herbal tea. *Espanto* is a disease with symptoms similar to susto. Its origin is fright caused by seeing supernatural spirits or events and can be likened to being "spooked" in American slang. *Coraje*

is rage, a response to a particular situation. The victim may continually scream, cry, or yell and display hyperactivity.

Many Mexican Americans, when they are ill, may believe a folk medicine diagnosis rather than a Western diagnosis, even though they may also seek help from a Western physician. Healers within the Mexican American community can be either male (a *curandero*) or female (a *curandera*). They offer a number of treatments; one of the most frequently used is herb tea. Mexican Americans have a personal relationship with the curandero, in contrast to the relations in a hospital.

Puerto Rican beliefs about health and illness are not unlike those of Mexican Americans. Their diseases are also classified as hot and cold; however, food and medications are classified as hot (*caliente*), cold (*frio*), and cool (*fresco*) (Spector 1985, p. 167).

Health Problems

Drug addiction is a major health problem among Puerto Ricans. Mexican Americans who are economically deprived may be poorly nourished, e.g., have protein and vitamin deficiencies.

Health Practices

Two symptoms—pain and the appearance of blood—usually indicate that an illness is severe. If it is "natural" for a condition to occur, it is considered harmless. When it is unnatural and folk methods fail, most Mexican Americans seek medical assistance from Western practitioners.

Mexican Americans are generally proud people. Those who are socially and economically deprived may well have low self-esteem and be reluctant to accept care for which they cannot pay. Therefore, Mexican American clients in the hospital may not ask for help when they have pain; a young Mexican-American male may react with hostility rather than passivity in response to nursing intervention to uphold his self-image.

Mexican Americans look upon the hospital as a place to die. Thus, they may avoid hospitals when they can and enter only with great fear, feeling that death is imminent. Illness is generally regarded not as a personal affair but as a family affair. Therefore, when a person is ill, many relatives generally gather around and visit. Restricting visitors can cause mistrust; nurses need to deal with such a requirement in the context of illness and discuss the matter with the entire family. See Figure 18–3.

As a cultural group, Mexican Americans are very modest. Usually they consider bathing, defecating, and urinating to be very personal matters, yet they may be shy about asking a nurse to leave at such times. The sensitive nurse will provide complete privacy when possible.

Hispanic Americans encounter a number of barriers to health care: language, poverty, and time orientation. To Hispanic Americans time is relative; the exact time is not a primary consideration. This hinders effective use of a health care system that values promptness for appointments and mandates specific intervals between doses of medications. Language is another major barrier for many Hispanic Americans seeking help from the health care delivery system. Some do not speak English, and communication is difficult and embarrassing in a system where the English language predominates. In addition, some Hispanic Americans belong to the poverty group in American society. They may not have knowledge of available health resources in the community or the money to use them. See the discussion of low-income groups as a subculture, below.

Nursing Implications

Not all Hispanic Americans identify with their ethnic groups; many identify with white middle-class Americans.

1. The nurse should not stereotype the Hispanic-American client. There are diverse beliefs and practices among various Hispanic-American groups. For example, the majority of Hispanic Americans, though not all, are Roman Catholic (Orque et al. 1983, p. 121).

2. Hispanic Americans value modesty and privacy. The nurse should provide privacy when they must undress for an examination.

3. The man in a Hispanic-American family may find it difficult to depend on other family members or even a nurse to do things for him. He will expect to decide when and how things should be done and should be involved in decisions if health permits.

Appalachians

The 24 million Appalachians in the United States, 6 million of whom live in the Southern Appalachian region, are a subculture in American society (Tripp-Reimer and Friedl 1977, p. 4). A family-oriented group, Appalachians include upper, middle, and poor working classes. The upper and middle classes tend to share many values with the rest of the United States, just as the poverty group does with other poverty groups in America. Much of Appalachia is rural, encompassing parts of the states of New York, Pennsylvania, Ohio, Maryland, West Virginia, Virginia, Kentucky, Tennessee, North Carolina, South Carolina, Georgia, and Alabama (Tripp-Reimer and Friedl 1977, p. 43).

Tripp-Reimer (1982, p. 185) found:

1. Appalachians tend to have large families.
2. Migrants tend to move between urban areas and "the hills."

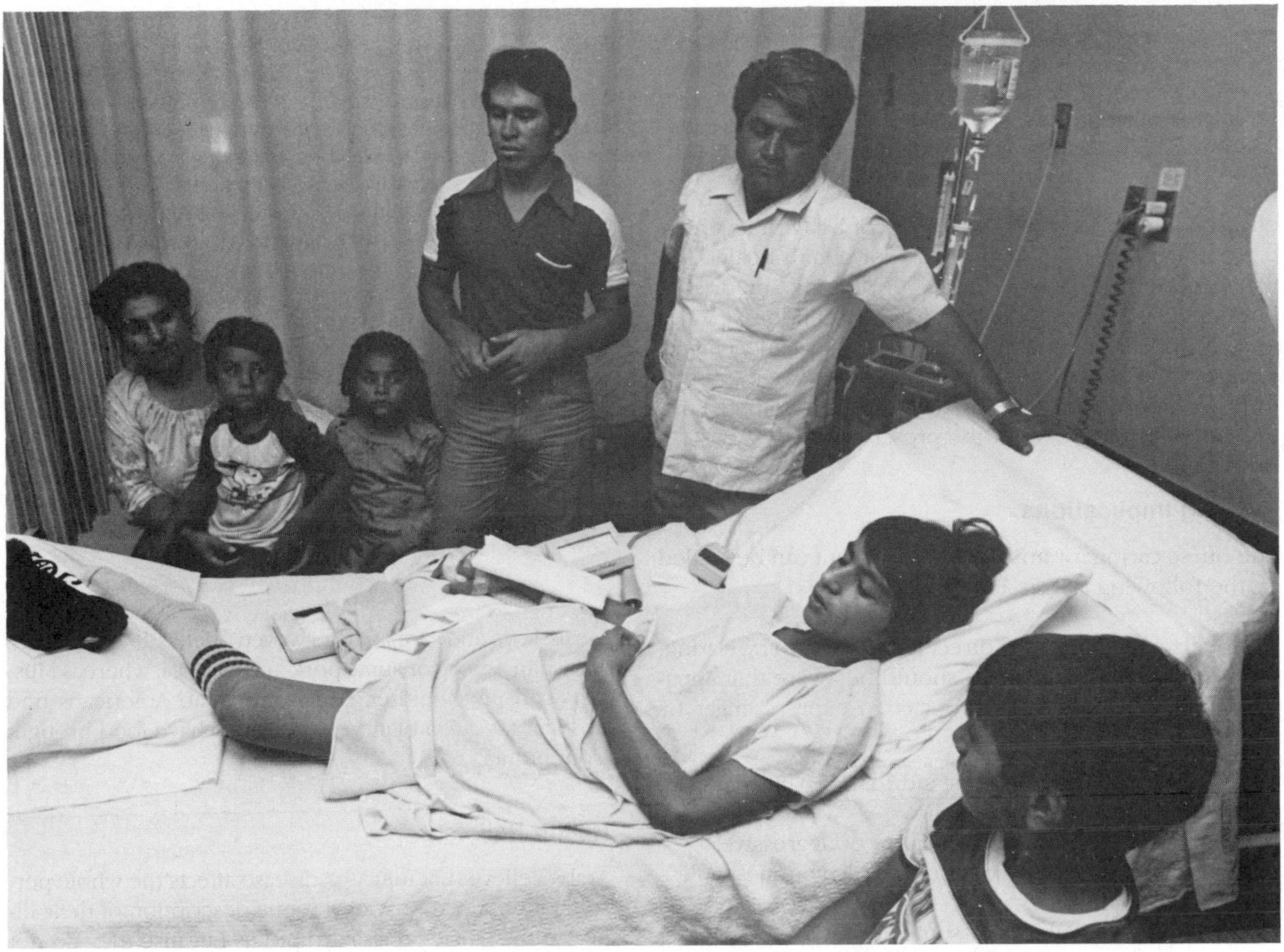

Figure 18–3 Illness is a matter of concern for an entire Hispanic family.

3. Migrants tend to quit school at an early age.
4. Many Appalachians use welfare services.
5. Appalachian migrants tend to be oriented to the present.

The religion of the Appalachians tends to be fundamentalist and fatalistic. Sometimes this fatalism prevents clients from seeking help when they are ill (Lewis et al. 1985, p. 24).

Family

Appalachians value family greatly. The family provides its members with a sense of belonging and a sense of identity. Appalachians value family privacy, a situation that has created some social and cultural isolation. Often many family members accompany a client to a health appointment, and they may wish to stay with the client if he or she is hospitalized. For many Appalachians, socialization begins and ends within the family.

The family is patriarchal, and there are definite divisions between the work of men and women. Family ties are strong, and antagonism against another family may be intense. Time orientation is in the present, and the pressure of finances makes it difficult to plan ahead. Education is usually not stressed.

Health Beliefs

Appalachians tend to define an individual as ill only when the person feels ill. They have a general distrust of health organizations and fear surgery.

Health Problems

The health problems of the Appalachians are largely related to their economic circumstances and to their occupations. Nutritional problems are frequently due to the fact that they cannot afford to buy much meat, and the diet may be deficient in protein and iron. Some Appalachians work in coal mines, and prolonged exposure to coal dust can cause sarcoidosis, a disease of the lungs.

Health Practices

When Appalachians feel ill, they tend to try home remedies, e.g., herb teas and tonics. If these cures are not effective, they may seek the advice of a lay practitioner, e.g., "granny midwife," a herbalist, or a faith healer. It is usual for an Appalachian to seek "orthodox" medical or nursing help in an emergency or during childbirth. When elderly Appalachians go to a physician, they expect immediate help. If the physician prescribes a medicine at that time, the client thinks he or she has been helped; however, the client may reject the prescription.

Nursing Implications

The nurse caring for an Appalachian client can be guided by the following (Hicks 1976):

1. Appalachians consider direct eye contact to be staring, which is impolite. Nurses should be aware that Appalachians use direct eye contact to express anger or aggression.
2. Nurses should also understand that Appalachians follow the "ethic of neutrality."
   a. A person must not be assertive or aggressive.
   b. A person should mind his or her own business unless asked to do otherwise.
   c. A person should not assume authority over others.
   d. Appalachians avoid argument and seek agreement.

Research Note

In a study by Tripp-Reimer, a series of guided interviews revealed important ethnocentric negative biases in health care professionals' attitudes toward their Appalachian clients. The study also showed that health care professionals who were intimately familiar with Appalachian culture made positive interpretations of the same behavior patterns that were seen as negative by the first group. Cultural empathy allowed the Appalachian professionals to be much more generous in the value judgments they placed on clients' behavior.

Tripp-Reimer suggests that consideration be given to hiring professionals whose "perceptual sets" are congruent with those of their clients, but more importantly, that student nurses be taught cultural sensitivity. (Tripp-Reimer 1982)

Arab Americans

The Arab American is a person who speaks Arabic and shares beliefs with the Arabic culture. There are approximately three million Arabs in the United States, including people who are in America temporarily (Meleis 1981, p. 1181). Most Arabs have a common language and share symbols, mores, and beliefs, whether they are Egyptians or Kuwaitis. Arabs are traditionally future oriented and value the use of time to achieve future goals.

Family

The Arab family is traditionally patriarchal and extended. The male of the household is responsible for earning the living outside the home and for making the decisions. Women usually remain at home in the traditional Arab family. Arabs have a need to affiliate with others and use an extensive social network to cope with daily stress (Meleis 1981, p. 1181).

Food plays an important part in Arab family life. When family members assemble, it is often around elaborate meals. Love and care are interwoven (Meleis 1981, p. 1182). Christian Arabs consume pork and alcohol, whereas Muslims consume neither. Sometimes Arab Americans find hospital food too bland and prefer to have food brought from home.

Health Beliefs

Arabs believe that injury or disease affects the whole person. Often Arabs provide a vague description of their illness rather than precise symptoms because they do not have a framework for signs and symptoms. Arabs usually do not refute the germ theory, but they do believe in disease-causing entities such as the evil eye. Arabs also believe that being deprived of food can cause illness.

Health Problems

One health problem that Arabs have in common with people in the Middle East is thalassemia, a genetic condition that results in anemia. It occurs in 7% to 15% of the population in the Middle East (Overfield 1985, p. 85).

Health Practices

Arabs do not believe in sharing a problem or advice until help is offered. The person offering should be able to assess the need without verifying the problem. If a nurse offers an Arab client a choice in care, the client is likely to say "No, thank you." If the nurse accepts this refusal, the client believes the nurse is not interested.

Arabs dislike disclosing information about themselves to strangers and will provide as little information as possible. Arabs also respect authority figures whose expertise is gained through education and experience.

Arabs generally respect Western health care. Intrusive procedures are often highly regarded and thought to offer the greatest chance of cure.

Nursing Implications

1. Nurses must be sensitive to an Arab's dislike of revealing personal information.
2. Many Arabs regard health care as their right, and some may view health care professionals as their employees.
3. Arabs will rely upon others, i.e., the social network, to give advice at times of stress.
4. Sometimes Arabs will defer dealing with a matter until they feel more comfortable sharing information.
5. Deaths are believed to be the result of the will of God and the inadequacy of equipment and medicine.
6. Arab Americans respect expertise, which they regard as knowing about problems, making decisions for others, and being accountable for those decisions (Meleis 1981, p. 1182).
7. Arab Americans may not question caregivers openly because of their respect for authority.
8. Some Arabs wear amulets for protection. Even to say the number "five" is believed to increase protection.

Income Groups

The poor and the rich are viewed by some as subcultures of the dominant society. To describe the lower classes or the upper classes of society as subcultures, one must study both the strengths and the weaknesses of their life situations and behaviors. Unfortunately, many studies dealing with poverty-stricken people tend to focus on only the negative aspects, and little has been written about the health care beliefs, practices, and problems of the rich.

High-Income Groups

Beliefs and behaviors of the rich tend to vary according to whether the persons come from second- or third-generation wealth. Second-generation wealthy persons (new rich) who are close to their parents' value systems tend to value the "work ethic" (Henry and DiGiacomo-Geffers 1980, p. 1426). These persons in their early years had fewer economic advantages and participated in the struggle to get ahead. In contrast, the third-generation rich (older rich) tend not to value work (Henry and DiGiacomo-Geffers 1980, p. 1426). They have been accustomed to wealth from birth, were raised largely by employed help, and grow up expecting great freedom with little discipline. Grinker (1978, p. 913) cites these common characteristics of persons within this group who seek psychotherapy:

- Feelings of emptiness and boredom
- Superficiality; absence of values, goals, ideals
- Low self-awareness; lack of introspection
- Lack of empathy
- Lack of interest in work
- Chronic mild depression
- Intense pursuit of pleasure and excitement
- Belief that they can be happy only with persons like themselves
- Belief that use of their wealth (buying, spending, travel) will solve their emotional problems

Beliefs about health, illness, and death among the rich depend on their specific religion and culture. Generally the rich tend to (a) believe in the prevention of illness through diet, exercise, and good health habits; (b) make frequent use of the health care system and self-help information, and (c) have ready access to the health care system through private physicians. See Table 18–1 on page 364.

Specific problems nurses may encounter with the hospitalized rich are outlined by Henry and DiGiacomo-Geffers (1980, p. 1428):

1. Demands by the client or family members that are not related to health care. Being accustomed to highly responsive employed help, the rich person tends to have the same expectations of nurses, who then feel they are being treated like servants. This behavior is often an attempt to gain attention and to control the unfamiliar, uncertain environment.
2. Restrictions on the times when the nurse can provide care, because of luxuries that the client considers necessities but the nurse often considers unnecessary. For example, some clients routinely have hour-long manicure appointments.
3. A concern with appearance that produces expectations for exceptional treatment. Outward appearance is often of critical importance to nationally known people, who are accustomed to being in the limelight. Prior to surgery, some may refuse to remove make-up or dentures; this necessitates their removal after a general anesthetic is administered.
4. A need to structure the environment and make it more appealing. In some cases, hospital rooms are literally redecorated. Drapes and bedcoverings may be changed, paintings hung on the walls, and the room stocked

with expensive personal supplies such as liqueurs and floral arrangements.

5. Requests for care only by persons of their own ethnic background. The client often abandons such expectations when he or she understands the need for assigning nurses with appropriate skills for the client's care.

Low-Income Groups

The status of being poor is often referred to as the "culture of poverty," a phrase coined by anthropologist Oscar Lewis in the 1960s. Lewis (1966, p. 19) defined the culture of poverty as a subculture of Western society with its own values and behaviors that differ from those of the nonpoor and that are passed on from generation to generation. This subculture transcends ethnic and regional boundaries. Characteristics of the poor include:

- Lack of participation in the larger society
- Hostility toward and mistrust of bureaucratic institutions
- Inadequate use of health services
- Long periods of unemployment
- Use of public assistance
- Authoritarian, mother-centered families that do not value childhood
- Abandonment of mothers and children by fathers
- Lack of privacy
- Disciplining of children by physical violence
- Orientation to the present
- Fatalistic attitudes
- Strong feelings of helplessness, dependence, and inferiority (Lewis 1966, pp. 19–25)

Lewis's portrayal of the poor as a subculture is challenged by other researchers, who believe this cultural viewpoint is negative, makes no attempt to question why these features exist, and fails to recognize the role of the larger society in perpetuating poverty. Some research has shown, for example, that the poor have the same values as the rest of society and that the traits Lewis identified may not be cultural but rather responses to situational circumstances. For example, the negative work behaviors associated with the lower class are not culturally derived but situationally induced. It has been shown that the poor have a strong work ethic, want to work, and do work when given equal opportunity (Mason 1981, p. 83). Lack of societal incentives prevents the poor from obtaining and holding a job. Situational theorists believe, therefore, that if society were rid of poverty, the former poor would demonstrate middle-class attitudes and behaviors.

Still other researchers suggest that all members of a society share general, abstract values but that specific, concrete values differ among subgroups and social classes. This viewpoint combines the cultural and situational perspectives of poverty into an adaptational perspective. In other words, the poor are considered a special subgroup of society in response to social structures that make it impossible for them to actualize the values and behavior forms of the dominant society.

Factors influencing poverty Geographic and social factors influence poverty. *Geographic poverty* refers to the existence of "pockets of poverty." In the United States these pockets occur in dense urban areas (e.g., the ghettos) and in rural regions such as Appalachia, the Deep South, the lower Southwest and northern New England. Unless people move out of such regions of poverty, they are likely to remain destitute, since social mobility, education, and employment opportunities are scarce. In spite of reform efforts, local governments have been ineffective in improving the conditions in such areas. Massive outside assistance is required to upgrade services in education, sanitation, health, employment, job training, transportation, welfare, etc.

Social factors of poverty include demographic characteristics that determine the social position a person occupies. Such characteristics are race, age, family structure and size, education, income, and type of work. Black Americans, Native Americans, and Hispanic Americans are overrepresented in poor populations. For example, in 1979 blacks accounted for 11% of the national population but 29% of the poverty population; whites accounted for only 9.4% of the poor. Statistics for Hispanics showed 23.5% were below the poverty line (Spector 1985, p. 116–23). People over 65 years of age also account for a substantial number of the impoverished, and the number is increasing in direct relationship to inflation. About one-third of the total poverty population is comprised of youths and children due to the poverty of their parents. Families in which the mother provides the major support are generally more poverty-stricken than families in which the father provides the major support, since employment opportunities and incomes for females are substantially less than for males. Large families with set incomes also are more impoverished. Lower educational attainment and lack of educational opportunities contribute to lower employment opportunities and income. The typical low-income person has less than an eighth grade education and, if employed, works at an unskilled occupation.

Health considerations Low-income families often define health in terms of work; if people can work they are healthy. They tend to be fatalistic and believe that illness is not preventable. Because their present problems are so great and all efforts are exerted toward survival, an orientation to the future may be lacking. Most low-income people do not have regular preventive medical checkups, because they cannot afford them. It is more important to them to work than to lose a day's pay visiting a physician. Reliance on public assistance and inability to afford health care insurance limit both the low-income person's access to health care and the type of care available. See also Table 18–1, page 364.

The environmental conditions of poverty-stricken areas also have a bearing on overall health. Slum neighborhoods are overcrowded and in a state of deterioration. Neglect and disorder are common. Sanitation services tend to be inadequate. Many streets are strewn with garbage, and alleys are overrun by rats. Fires and crime are constant threats. Recreational facilities are almost nonexistent, forcing children to play in streets and alleys. Parents who can work usually work long hours and earn barely enough for subsistence. They are often too tired to spend much time with their children, even though they love them. As a result, preschool children often come and go as they please, and elder siblings assume the role of parent for younger children. With all of these problems confronting the poverty-stricken, it is little wonder that frustration tolerance levels are low, physical abuse is used as the form of discipline, and value is placed on children seeking employment rather than completing their educations.

Contrary to the beliefs of some, poverty-stricken clients have the same needs and feelings as other people. They are sensitive, concerned, and easily embarrassed. When admitted to health care agencies, they are often treated in humiliating, condescending, and prejudicial ways by professional caregivers. Because prejudice is usually based on fear of the unknown, and fear is based on insecurity, it is important for nurses to examine their own values and attitudes. Nurses need to become culturally sensitive and to accept and respect the differences in the life-styles of others.

Middle-Class Anglo-Americans

Middle-class Americans are predominantly descendants of immigrants who came to the United States at least two generations ago. The group is composed largely of white, Anglo-Saxon Protestants (WASPs).

Family

Traditionally the white middle-class American family was patriarchal; the father went to work and the mother was the homemaker who raised the children. However, this pattern is changing. The need for extra income, the new assertiveness of women in response to the women's movement, increased awareness of life alternatives, and the rising educational level of women have all influenced this change. In 1960, only 19% of women with young

Research Note

Clinton developed and tested a research tool for the differentiation of health-related beliefs of a group of European Americans, who might have appeared homogeneous under less sensitively devised investigation. A multivariate and computer-assisted approach to the measurement of ethnic data proved useful in isolating cultural differences that persisted through generations of European Americans.

Clinton's study shows that cross-cultural health research is an important source of data, both about the various ethnic groups encountered in nursing practice and about the nature of ethnic bias itself. (Clinton 1982)

children were employed outside the home (Hayghe 1976, pp. 12–19) yet by 1982, 47.8% of women with preschool children were employed (Hayghe 1982, pp. 53–56).

The middle-class American family is generally family oriented. Parents have a strong desire to provide better opportunities for their children than they had and emphasize education. The Protestant work ethic strongly influences the family. A prevailing attitude is that men should work to support their families. Certain work roles are often associated with men and others with women. For example, it is acceptable for women to be secretaries, but it is questioned if men are secretaries.

Middle-class American families are often materialistic. A person measures the success of the neighbors by the car they drive or the size of the house they live in. Middle-class Americans are usually future oriented and as such may be very concerned about the implications of an illness for the future and its immediate effect.

Health Beliefs

Studies have shown that people differ widely in their personal definitions of health and their health beliefs. See Chapter 2. Hautman and Harrison (1982, p. 53) found that many people defined good health as the absence of sickness. Some people stated that their health was good because they could function adequately in spite of the presence of such diseases as a prior heart attack or ongoing diarrhea.

Health Problems

Many of the health problems of middle-class Americans are related to life-style. Despite an increasing awareness of the roles of diet and exercise in disease prevention, many middle-class Americans believe serious illness "happens to others but not to me." Major health problems are discussed in Chapter 2.

Health Practices

Studies show that diagnosis of an individual's illness is usually made by the person, explained within his or her personal or cultural folk model, and usually dealt with by self-care (Hautman and Harrison 1982, p. 51). For additional information on health and illness, see Chapter 2.

Nursing Implications

Because in the American health care system many clients and nurses are middle class, a major danger is that nurses may not allow for individual differences and may expect client values to conform to their own. Other implications are:

1. Consider the cost of health care measures. Many people are conscious of costs, which can affect the degree to which clients follow health care measures.
2. Expect the client to relate illness to the future and want to deal with future implications early in his or her illness.
3. Determine whether or not clients attend church regularly, and whether they may desire to see a clergyman.

The Gay Community

The gay community can be considered a subculture. **Homosexuality** may be defined as repeated and preferential same-sex contacts (Roundtable 1980, p. 69). Gays and lesbians share beliefs, values, and customs of the larger culture; such beliefs are often reflective of their ethnicity, income, or cultural background. However, they may function as members of a gay or lesbian community and as such share values and beliefs common to those communities. One of the most prevalent beliefs of gay and lesbian communities is that sexual and affectional relationships between individuals of the same sex are normal and positive.

Family

Sex roles in the lesbian and gay communities are different than in the nongay community. Both partners often perform all tasks that are normally assigned by gender in the nongay community. For example, both partners may cook, garden, work, and be supportive. These roles may carry over into the health care setting, where a man may comfort another man or a lesbian may deal assertively with a situation as well as be supportive of her partner. Because these sex-role behaviors are not traditional, health care professionals who are not gay may find them upsetting.

Health Practices

Areas of concern to both gays and lesbians include health care issues regarding the genital organs, sexuality, and sexually transmitted diseases. They may also feel concern when revealing information about sexual behavior to health care professionals, or about those professionals' attitudes toward sexuality. For instance, the client may not wish to confide in a health professional who may have a heterosexual bias. For these reasons, some areas of the United States have health clinics especially for gay men and lesbians.

In addition many women, including lesbians, prefer women-centered community health centers because they consider traditional health centers to be both sexist and heterosexual. Another concern of some lesbians is alternative fertilization so that they can bear children without having sexual intercourse with a male.

Health Problems

A major health problem of gay men is acquired immune deficiency syndrome (AIDS), first noted in 1981. By 1985 there were 12,256 known cases of AIDS in the United States (Baumgartener 1985, p. 5).

Nursing Implications

1. It is important for nurses to be informed about homosexuality and to convey an attitude of acceptance toward homosexual clients and their support persons.
2. Nurses need to elicit only that information required for the nursing history.
3. Nurses need to adopt a nonjudgmental tone and attitude.
4. The client needs reassurance that the information he or she gives will be kept confidential and conveyed only to health professionals requiring it.
5. It is important to provide the support persons of a gay or lesbian client with the same support the nurse would provide to support persons of a heterosexual client.

For additional information on sexuality, see Chapter 19.

Health Care System as a Subculture

It is important for nurses to remember that the health care system can be considered a subculture in society. This system has rules, customs, and a language of its own. When individuals obtain an education in health care, they become enculturated into the system. But clients who enter the system may experience culture shock if it is very different from their own. For example, the health care culture values cleanliness; thus, nurses wash their hands often and expect their clients to wash daily. This value may not be shared by all clients, and the practice of washing daily may be new for some people.

The health care culture has its own definition of health; often it is defined as "an optimal level of functioning." See Chapter 2 for additional information. Diagnosis and prescription are usually carried out by physicians, often in offices, clinics, or hospitals. Healing practices are based on scientific knowledge. Treatment procedures are frequently embarrassing or uncomfortable. The emotional component of disease is often ignored (Wold 1981, p. 140).

Jargon is widely used in the system and tends to make clients and support persons feel more like outsiders. Many health care workers are from the middle class; they often expect gratitude for the care they give. Strict time orientation is adhered to and highly valued. This orientation may conflict with the client's. By keeping written records, caregivers may create conflict with patients' cultural beliefs.

Traditionally, health care workers interpreted the death of a client as failure. This belief is currently being reconsidered. Measures were often taken to preserve the lives of clients but seldom to facilitate death. Currently, clinical nurse specialists called **thanatology** *nurses* work with families and clients coping with a terminal illness. See also Table 18-1, page 366.

If nurses recognize that they have been enculturated into the health care system, they can often identify the values of the system that they have adopted. It is then easier to recognize how a client's values differ from those of the system. These differing values may be a source of anxiety or frustration to clients and their support persons. See the next section.

Culture Shock

Culture shock is the reaction of many people to an unfamiliar situation where former patterns of behavior are ineffective. Culture shock can occur when members of one culture are abruptly moved to another culture or setting, for example, when people of Asian background and upbringing suddenly move to the United States, or when clients are abruptly thrust into the health care subculture. When this occurs, a number of stressors impinge on the individual.

Types of Stressors

1. *Communication.* Often there is a change in the system of verbal and nonverbal communication.
2. *Mechanical differences.* These include habits and activities of daily living, which often change with a change in environment. Even tasks such as shopping for food or using the telephone can be unfamiliar.
3. *Isolation.* There appears to be a sense of isolation inherent in any situation totally populated by strangers (Brink 1976, p. 128). When moving from one culture to another, people immediately experience friendlessness and nonrelatedness.
4. *Customs.* Often new customs need to be learned, including systems of etiquette and role behaviors.
5. *Attitudes and beliefs.* Attitudes and values about life and behavior frequently differ from one culture to another. People may find that beliefs they have always taken for granted are radically different in another culture.

Phases of Culture Shock

Brink and Saunders (1976, pp. 129–30) describe four phases of culture shock:

1. *Phase one.* The initial phase is identified as one of excitement and is called the *honeymoon phase.* People are stimulated by being in a new environment. Behavior that indicates this varies with the ethnic origin of the person and the individual personality. Some clients, for example, may express their excitement outwardly, while others are quiet. People try to learn the norms of behavior appropriate for the new environment and often ask questions.
2. *Phase two.* Once the individual feels somewhat comfortable in the new environment, phase two begins. The person then realizes that he or she is actually in the environment. This awareness is often accompanied by feelings of frustration and embarrassment because of errors the individual makes. Accompanying this may be feelings of inadequacy, which can diminish the individual's self-concept and self-esteem. To these feelings is added loneliness. Although many people may be around, there may be no one who enhances the individual's feelings of self-worth. Feelings of anxiety and inadequacy may be expressed through periods of withdrawal or anger.
3. *Phase three.* During the third stage, the individual seeks new patterns of behavior appropriate to the environment. He or she makes friends and can often give newcomers advice. Current friendships take on impor-

tance and occupy much of the individual's conversation. At this time, ties to the old culture become weaker.

4. *Phase four.* In the fourth phase, the individual functions comfortably and effectively. If the person returns to the former culture during this phase, he or she may experience reverse culture shock.

Nursing Implications

Nurses can assist clients and their families who are experiencing culture shock in a number of ways:

1. If there is a language barrier, an interpreter can help with explanations and provide the nurse with information to incorporate into the client's care plan.
2. Nurses can support clients' customs, e.g., the nurse can encourage a Sikh to wear his turban in the hospital, unless this is contraindicated for health reasons. In addition, nurses can offer explanations to other health personnel about values, beliefs, and customs important to the client.
3. Nurses must convey respect for a client's values, beliefs, and customs. The client will interpret an attitude of disdain or amusement as a lack of respect.

Where there is a conflict between, for example, the client's beliefs and the health care system, nurses can try to help the client find a common ground. When the client tries new behavior patterns, nurses can support his or her efforts and provide positive reinforcement. If the client experiences inadequacy or anxiety during culture shock, nurses can help by openly accepting the client and his or her values, beliefs, and customs.

Applying the Nursing Process

To provide meaningful nursing care, nurses must be aware of a client's ethnic and cultural values, beliefs, and practices as they relate to his or her health and health care. Tripp-Reimer et al. (1984) state, "A thorough cultural assessment is not necessary"; however, basic cultural data are required.

Initially the nurse must be aware of her or his own ethnic and cultural values, attitudes, and practices and of their relation to nursing practice. Cultural awareness can be attained by using a values clarification approach discussed in Chapter 8, page 182.

Assessment

A number of assessment guides can assist nurses to gather ethnic cultural data. See Tables 18–2 and 18–3. The purpose of an ethical-cultural assessment is "to identify deviations in cultural parameters with the goal of modifying the client's system or modifying the health care professional's system in order to increase congruence between them" (Tripp-Reimer et al. 1984, p. 81). Tripp-Reimer, Brink, and Saunders propose a two-phase process with substages. See Table 18–2.

Table 18–2 Process of Cultural Assessment

Phase I	Data collection
Stage 1	General assessment
Stage 2	Problem-specific cultural information
Stage 3	Cultural factors that influence nursing intervention
Phase II	Data organization

Source: T. Tripp-Reimer, P. J. Brink, and J. M. Saunders, Cultural assessment: content and process, *Nursing Outlook,* March/April 1984, 32:78–82. Used by permission.

Basic Cultural Data

- Ethnic affiliation
- Religious preference
- Family patterns
- Food patterns
- Ethnic health care practices (Tripp-Reimer et al. 1984, p. 79)

A general assessment of the client identifies significant characteristics and points out areas for in-depth assessment. At this stage, the nurse makes no conclusions but obtains information from the client. The data should be both subjective, preferably in the client's words, and objective. An example of subjective data is this client statement: "I think it is very important to be healthy." An example of objective data is "Attended school to grade 3 in rural Mexico." At this time, it is also important to collect information that would affect the nurse-client interaction, e.g., language, etiquette, style of communication.

The general assessment is then followed by an assessment that is specific to the health care area of concern, e.g., preschool immunizations, diabetic teaching, home care. At this time, the nurse obtains information about the client's own reason for seeking out health care, his or her ideas about the current problem and any previous problems, and the treatment he or she anticipates. For example, the client may say, "I came to the center because I feel ill; the world is moving around me. This

Table 18–3 Bloch's Ethnic/Cultural Assessment Guide

Data Categories	Guideline Questions/Instructions	Data Collected
Cultural		
Ethnic origin	Does the patient identify with a particular ethnic group (e.g., Puerto Rican, African)?	
Race	What is the patient's racial background (e.g., Black, Filipino, American Indian)?	
Place of birth	Where was the patient born?	
Relocations	Where has he lived (country, city)? During what years did patient live there and for how long? Has he moved recently?	
Habits, customs, values, and beliefs	Describe habits, customs, values, and beliefs patient holds or practices that affect his attitude toward birth, life, death, health and illness, time orientation, and health care system and health care providers. What is degree of belief and adherence by patient to his overall cultural system?	
Behaviors valued by culture	How does patient value privacy, courtesy, respect for elders, behaviors related to family roles and sex roles, and work ethics?	
Cultural sanctions and restrictions	*Sanctions*—What is accepted behavior by patient's cultural group regarding expression of emotions and feelings, religious expressions, and response to illness and death?	
	Restrictions—Does patient have any restrictions related to sexual matters, exposure of body parts, certain types of surgery (e.g., hysterectomy), discussion of dead relatives, and discussion of fears related to the unknown?	
Language and communication processes	What are some overall cultural characteristics of patient's language and communication process?	
Language(s) and/or dialect(s) spoken	Which language(s) and/or dialect(s) does patient speak most frequently? Where? At home or at work?	
Language barriers	Which language does patient predominantly use in thinking? Does patient need bilingual interpreter in nurse-patient interactions? Is patient non-English-speaking or limited-English-speaking? Is patient able to read and/or write in English?	
Communication process	What are rules (linguistics) and modes (style) of communication process (e.g., "honorific" concept of showing "respect or deference" to others using words only common to specific ethnic/cultural group)?	
	Is there need for variation in technique of communicating and interviewing to accommodate patient's cultural background (e.g., tempo of conversation, eye-body contact, topic restrictions, norms of confidentiality, and style of explanation)?	
	Are there any conflicts in verbal and nonverbal interactions between patient and nurse?	
	How does patient's nonverbal communication process compare with other ethnic/cultural groups, and how does it affect patient's response to nursing and medical care?	
	Are there any variations between patient's interethnic and interracial communication process or intracultural and intraracial communication process (e.g., ethnic minority patient and white middle-class nurse, ethnic minority patient and ethnic minority nurse; beliefs, attitudes, values, role variations, stereotyping [perception and prejudice])?	
Healing beliefs and practices		
Cultural healing system	What cultural healing system does the patient predominantly adhere to (e.g., Asian healing system, Raza/Latina Curanderismo)? What religious healing system does the patient predominantly adhere to (e.g., Seventh Day Adventist, West African voodoo, Fundamentalist sect, Pentacostal)?	
Cultural health beliefs	Is illness explained by the germ theory or cause-effect relationship, presence of evil spirits, imbalance between "hot" and "cold" (yin and yang in Chinese culture), or disequilibrium between nature and man?	
	Is good health related to success, ability to work or fulfill roles, reward from God, or balance with nature?	
Cultural health practices	What types of cultural healing practices does person from ethnic/cultural group adhere to? Does he use healing remedies to cure *natural* illnesses caused by the external environment (e.g., massage to cure *empacho* [a ball of food clinging to stomach wall], wearing of talismans or charms for protection against illness)?	

(continued)

Table 18–3 *(continued)*

Data Categories	Guideline Questions/Instructions	Data Collected
Cultural healers	Does patient rely on cultural healers (e.g., medicine men for American Indian, Curandero for Raza/Latina, Chinese herbalist, hougan [voodoo priest], spiritualist, or minister for black American)?	
Nutritional variables or factors	What nutritional variables or factors are influenced by the patient's ethnic/cultural background?	
Characteristics of food preparation and consumption	What types of food preferences and restrictions, meaning of foods, style of food preparation and consumption, frequency of eating, time of eating, and eating utensils are culturally determined for patient? Are there any religious influences on food preparation and consumption?	
Influences from external environment	What modifications if any did the ethnic group patient identifies with have to make in its food practices in white dominant American society? Are there any adaptations of food customs and beliefs from rural setting to urban setting?	
Patient education needs	What are some implications of diet planning and teaching to patient who adheres to cultural practices concerning foods?	
Sociological		
Economic status	Who is principal wage earner in patient's family? What is total annual income (approximately) of family? What impact does economic status have on life-style, place of residence, living conditions, and ability to obtain health services?	
Educational status	What is highest educational level obtained? Does patient's educational background influence his ability to understand how to seek health services, literature on health care, patient teaching experiences, and any written material patient is exposed to in health care setting (e.g., admission forms, patient care forms, teaching literature, and lab test forms)? Does patient's educational background cause him to feel inferior or superior to health care personnel in health care setting?	
Social network	What is patient's social network (kinship, peer, and cultural healing networks)? How do they influence health or illness status of patient?	
Family as supportive group	Does patient's family feel need for continuous presence in patient's clinical setting (is this an ethnic/cultural characteristic)? How is family valued during illness or death? How does family participate in patient's nursing care process (e.g., giving baths, feeding, using touch as support [cultural meaning], supportive presence)? How does ethnic/cultural family structure influence patient response to health or illness (e.g., roles, beliefs, strengths, weaknesses, and social class)? Are there any key family roles characteristic of a specific ethnic/cultural group (e.g., grandmother in black and some American Indian families), and can these key persons be a resource for health personnel? What role does family play in health promotion or cause of illness (e.g., would family be intermediary group in patient interactions with health personnel and making decisions regarding his care)?	
Supportive institutions in ethnic/cultural community	What influence do ethnic/cultural institutions have on patient receiving health services (i.e., institutions such as Organization of Migrant Workers, NAACP, Black Political Caucus, churches, school, Urban League, community clinics)?	
Institutional racism	How does institutional racism in health facilities influence patient's response to receiving health care?	
Psychological		
Self-concept (identity)	Does patient show strong racial/cultural identity? How does this compare to that of other racial/cultural groups or to members of dominant society? What factors in patient's development helped to shape his self-concept (e.g., family, peers, society labels, external environment, institutions, racism)? How does patient deal with stereotypical behavior from health professionals? What is impact of racism on patient from distinct ethnic/cultural group (e.g., social anxiety, noncompliance to health care process in clinical settings, avoidance of utilizing or participating in health care institutions)?	

(continued)

Table 18–3 *(continued)*

Data Categories	Guideline Questions/Instructions	Data Collected
	Does ethnic/cultural background have impact on how patient relates to body image change resulting from illness or surgery (e.g., importance of appearance and roles in cultural group)?	
	Any adherence or identification with ethnic/cultural "group identity" (e.g., solidarity, "we" concept)?	
Mental and behavioral processes and characteristics of ethnic/cultural group	How does patient relate to his external environment in clinical setting (e.g., fears, stress, and adaptive mechanisms characteristic of a specific ethnic/cultural group)? Any variations based on the life span?	
	What is patient's ability to relate to persons outside of his ethnic/cultural group (health personnel)? Is he withdrawn, verbally or nonverbally expressive, negative or positive, feeling mentally or physically inferior or superior?	
	How does patient deal with feelings of loss of dignity and respect in clinical setting?	
Religious influences on psychological effects of health/illness	Does patient's religion have a strong impact on how he relates to health/illness influences or outcomes (e.g., death/chronic illness, cause and effect of illness, or adherence to nursing/medical practices)?	
	Do religious beliefs, sacred practices, and talismans play a role in treatment of disease?	
	What is role of significant religious persons during health/illness (e.g., black ministers, Catholic priests, Buddhist monks, Islamic imams)?	
Psychological/cultural response to stress and discomfort of illness	Based on ethnic/cultural background, does patient exhibit any variations in psychological response to pain or physical disability of disease processes?	
Biological/physiological (consideration of *norms* for different ethnic/cultural groups)		
Racial-anatomical characteristics	Does patient have any distinct racial characteristics (e.g., skin color, hair texture and color, color of mucous membranes)? Does patient have any variations in anatomical characteristics (e.g., body structure [height and weight] more prevalent for ethnic/cultural group, skeletal formation [pelvic shape, especially for obstetrical evaluation], facial shape and structure [nose, eye shape, facial contour], upper and lower extremities)?	
	How do patient's racial and anatomical characteristics affect his self-concept and the way others relate to him?	
	Does variation in racial-anatomical characteristics affect physical evaluations and physical care, skin assessment based on color, and variations in hair care and hygienic practices?	
Growth and development patterns	Are there any distinct growth and development characteristics that vary with patient's ethnic/cultural background (e.g., bone density, fatfolds, motor ability)? What factors are important for nutritional assessment, neurological and motor assessment, assessment of bone deterioration in disease process or injury, evaluation of newborns, evaluation of intellectual status, or capacity in relationship to motor/sensory development in children? How do these differ in ethnic/cultural groups?	
Variations in body systems	Are there any variations in body systems for patient from distinct ethnic/cultural group (e.g., gastrointestinal disturbance with lactose intolerance in blacks, nutritional intake of cultural foods causing adverse effects on gastrointestinal tract and fluid and electrolyte system, and variations in chemical and hematological systems [certain blood types prevalent in particular ethnic/cultural groups])?	
Skin and hair physiology, mucous membranes	How does skin color variation influence assessment of skin color changes (e.g., jaundice, cyanosis, ecchymosis, erythema, and its relationship to disease processes)?	
	What are methods of assessing skin color changes (comparing variations and similarities between different ethnic groups)?	
	Are there conditions of hypopigmentation and hyperpigmentation (e.g., vitiligo, mongolian spots, albinism, discoloration caused by trauma)? Why would these be more striking in some ethnic groups?	

(continued)

Table 18–3 *(continued)*

Data Categories	Guideline Questions/Instructions	Data Collected
	Are there any skin conditions more prevalent in a distinct ethnic group (e.g., keloids in blacks)?	
	Is there any correlation between oral and skin pigmentation and their variations among distinct racial groups when doing assessment of oral cavity (e.g., leukoedema is normal occurrence in blacks)?	
	What are variations in hair texture and color among racially different groups? Ask patient about preferred hair care methods or any racial/cultural restrictions (e.g., not washing "hot combed" hair while in clinical setting, not cutting very long hair of Raza/Latina patients).	
	Are there any variations in skin care methods (e.g., using Vaseline on black skin)?	
Diseases more prevalent among ethnic/cultural group	Are there any specific diseases or conditions that are more prevalent for a specific ethnic/cultural group (e.g., hypertension, sickle cell anemia, G6-PD, lactose intolerance)?	
	Does patient have any socioenvironment diseases common among ethnic/cultural groups (e.g., lead paint poisoning, poor nutrition, overcrowding [prone to tuberculosis], alcoholism resulting from psychological despair and alienation from dominant society, rat bites, poor sanitation)?	
Diseases ethnic/cultural group has increased resistance to	Are there any diseases that patient has increased resistance to because of racial/cultural background (e.g., skin cancer in blacks)?	

Source: From M. S. Orque, B. Bloch, and L. S. A. Monrroy, *Ethnic nursing care: A multicultural approach* (St. Louis: C. V. Mosby Co., 1983). Used by permission.

happened once before. The doctor gave me some pills, and it went away."

Some questions that may elicit this information are:

1. What do you think caused your problem?
2. What treatment do you think you need now?
3. What are the chief problems your sickness has caused you? (Kleinman et al. 1977, p. 254).

Nursing Diagnosis

The nursing diagnoses for a client who has special ethnic or cultural needs can relate to any number of factors, such as language and diet. Some examples are listed in Table 18–4.

Planning

When planning nursing goals, the nurse needs to include appropriate cultural factors relative to the client. According to Tripp-Reimer et al. (1984, p. 81), this stage "is directed at cultural factors that may influence nursing strategies." For example, nurses can ask a client:

1. What would you normally eat while you have this condition?
2. What will your family do?
3. Do you think any other measures would help you?

After obtaining this information, a nurse must organize the data. According to Tripp-Reimer et al. (1984, p. 81), "the nurse is interested in the extent to which the client's beliefs, values, and customs are congruent with a trifold set of standards:

- Standards of the client's identified culture or ethnic group
- Standards of the nurse's own culture
- Standards of the health care facility that serves as the setting for the interaction"

A nurse may find that the data are not congruent between the three areas; for example, a client always eats rice as a major part of each meal. The nurse (a) learns that this practice is standard for the client's ethnic group, (b) recognizes that this practice differs from her or his own, and (c) realizes that the health care facility cannot provide rice for each meal. Next, the nurse relates this information by determining whether the client's eating practices are accommodated by the treatment plan. If not, then the nurse can find ways of integrating the client's practice into the nursing care plan, e.g., the client's family might bring cooked rice to the hospital. If, however, rice is contraindicated because of the client's condition, the nurse must establish ways to help the client change if the client is amenable to change or ways to understand the client if the client will not change (Tripp-Reimer et al. 1984, p. 81).

Table 18–4 Examples of Nursing Diagnoses Related to Ethnicity and Culture

Impaired verbal communications related to foreign language barrier
Ineffective individual coping related to change of environment
Ineffective family coping related to absence of extended family
Powerlessness related to inability to communicate verbally
Social isolation related to hospitalization secondary to language barrier

It is often important to include the client's family in the planning of nursing care, particularly if the client is a member of an extended family and if the family is a major support for the client. When planning care strategies, nurses should consider language barriers and assess the need for an interpreter. Sometimes ethnic clients require information to avoid confusion or embarrassment. For example, an ethnic client who is extremely modest may require considerable preparation and support before having an enema.

Intervention

Successful nursing interventions for the ethnic clients require supportive communication by nurses and respect for the client's values, beliefs, and practices. See Table 18–5 for specific nursing guidelines.

Furthermore, White (1977) stresses the importance of being culturally sensitive. Cultural sensitivity includes: feeling respect for individuals, recognizing that people have their own cultural beliefs and practices, being able to act on behalf of the ethnic client who is being denied safe, quality care, and modifying the care plan by incorporating those client beliefs and practices that are not life threatening (Bello 1976, pp. 36–38, 45).

Scott advocates the use of "culture-brokers" to bridge the gap between two people of different cultures, e.g., a black client and an Asian nurse. The culture-broker should be a person with specialized knowledge of the cultures, and the skills to carry out such a function (Scott 1978, p. 62; Powers 1982, p. 44).

Evaluation

To evaluate the effectiveness of nursing care of clients in special ethnic and cultural groups, the nurse determines the extent to which the goals have been met. In these instances, a common goal is reducing social isolation or fear of the health care system.

Nurses must also evaluate their own competence in this area by asking themselves questions such as these: "How well did I communicate?" "How well did I include the client and his or her family in the nursing process?" "How well do I understand the client's values, beliefs, and customs?" "How well did I communicate respect for these?" "Was I able to incorporate any of the client's values, beliefs, and customs into the plan of care?" "How well did I communicate my acceptance of values, beliefs, and customs that differ from mine?" "Am I aware of my values, beliefs, and customs?"

Table 18–5 Guidelines for Nurses Interacting with Clients of Differing Culture or Ethnicity

1. Convey respect for the individual and respect for his or her values, beliefs, and cultural and ethnic practices.
2. Learn about the major ethnic or cultural groups with whom you are likely to have contact.
3. Be aware of your own communication, e.g., facial expression and body language, and how it may be interpreted. See Chapter 27 for additional information.
4. Be aware of differences in ways clients communicate, and do not assume the meaning of a specific behavior, e.g., lack of eye contact, without considering the client's ethnic and cultural background.
5. Be aware of your own biases, prejudices, and stereotypes.
6. When a client describes a belief that differs from your own, e.g., the cause of his swollen feet, try to relate the client's belief to yours, thus conveying interest and respect for the client's beliefs.
7. Recognize that cultural symbols and practices can often bring a client comfort.
8. Support the client's practices and incorporate them into nursing practice whenever it is possible and they are not contraindicated for health reasons, e.g., provide hot tea to a client who drinks hot tea and never drinks cold water.
9. Do not impose a cultural practice on a client without knowing whether it is acceptable, e.g., Puerto Rican clients prefer not to be touched unnecessarily (Shubin 1980, p. 29).
10. Be aware that the color of a client's skin does not always determine his or her culture.
11. Take time to learn how a client views health, illness, grieving, and the health care system.
12. Be aware of your own attitudes and beliefs about health and objectively examine the logic of those attitudes and beliefs and their origins.
13. Be open to learning about different beliefs and values and learn not to be threatened when they differ from your own.

Chapter Highlights

- North Americans come from a variety of ethnic and cultural backgrounds, and many North Americans retain at least some of their traditional values, beliefs, and practices.

- Many minority groups in North America are bicultural in that they embrace two cultures: their original ethnic culture and a North American culture.
- An individual's ethnic and cultural background can influence beliefs, values, and customs.
- Through acculturation, most ethnic and cultural minority groups in North America modify some of their traditional cultural characteristics.
- Individual factors frequently modify an individual's cultural values, beliefs, and customs.
- Incorrect assumptions can result from stereotyping individuals.
- When assessing a client's cultures, the nurse considers values, beliefs, and customs related to health and health care.
- Some health problems are more prevalent in certain ethnic groups than in the general population.
- Nurses must understand their own cultural values, beliefs, and customs in order to provide meaningful nursing care.
- An ethnic and cultural assessment guide can help the nurse gather data about a client.
- People can experience culture shock when they enter an unfamiliar environment where previous patterns of behavior are ineffective.

Suggested Readings

Ellis, D., and Ho, S. L. March 1982. Attitudes of Chinese women towards sexuality and birth control. *Canadian Nurse* 78:28–31.

Focusing on issues of sex and birth control, these authors interviewed a group of Chinese women about menstruation, masturbation, contraception, and coitus during pregnancy.

Hodgson, C. June 1980. Transcultural nursing: The Canadian experience. *Canadian Nurse* 76:23–25.

This author discusses the concepts of transcultural nursing as applied in the Canadian North with traditional Indian and Innuit cultures. She believes that separating culture from illness is like separating mind from body.

Kwok, A. W. H. March 1982. Culture conflict: A study of the problems of Chinese immigrant adolescents in Canada. *Canadian Nurse* 78:32–34.

This author interviewed one Chinese and two Vietnamese adolescents about the conflicts they encounter not only as adolescents but also as individuals having to deal with two cultures. The values of one culture often conflict with those of the other.

Powers, B. A. April 1982. The use of orthodox and black American folk medicine. *Advances in Nursing Science* 4:35–47.

Powers describes the function of healers in black folk culture, including their characteristics and functions. The beliefs and practices of the black folk medical system are explained. The implications for nursing practice include the possible reluctance of clients to admit using folk practices, the need for mutual respect between the nurse and client, and the use of culture brokers.

Primeaux, M. January 1977. Caring for the American Indian patient. *American Journal of Nursing* 77:91–94.

Primeaux describes some common cultural beliefs that pertain to health care for Native Americans. Health rituals, child-rearing practices, and many other specific values and beliefs are discussed.

Tripp-Reimer, T., Brink, P. J., and Saunders, J. M. March/April 1984. Cultural assessment: Content and process. *Nursing Outlook* 32:78–82.

The authors present a process for assessment of a client's ethnic/cultural values, beliefs, and customs. Included is a table comparing the content of nine cultural assessment guides.

White, E. H. March 1977. Giving health care to minority clients. *Nursing Clinics of North America* 12:27–40.

White discusses black, Spanish-speaking, Native-American, and Asian clients in this article. Topics covered include lifestyles, health problems, health practices, and nursing implications.

Selected References

Abril, I. F., May/June 1977. Mexican-American folk beliefs: How they affect health care. *The Journal of Maternal Child Nursing* 2:168–73.

American Journal of Nursing. June 1979. Black skin problems. *American Journal of Nursing* 79:1092–94.

Anderson, A. B., and Frideres, J. S. 1981. *Ethnicity in Canada: Theoretical perspectives.* Toronto: Butterworths.

Augusta, R. September 1983. AIDS. *The Journal of Practical Nursing* 33:48–51.

Backup, R. W. February 1980. Health care of the American Indian patient. *Critical Care Update* 7:16+.

Bannerman, R. H., Burton, J., and Wen-Chieh, C., editors. 1983. *Traditional medicine and health care coverage: A reader for health administrators and practitioners.* Geneva: World Health Organization.

Baumgartener, G. H. 1985. *AIDS: Psychological factors in the acquired immune deficiency syndrome.* Springfield, Ill.: Charles C. Thomas.

Bello, T. A. February 1976. The third dimension: Cultural sensitivity in nursing practice. *Imprint* 23:36–38, 45.

Bhanumathi, P. P. 1977. Nurses' conceptions of "sick role" and "good patient" behavior: A cross-cultural comparison. *International Nursing Review* 24:20–24.

Bigham, G. D. September 1964. To communicate with negro patients. *American Journal of Nursing* 64:113–5.

Bloch, B. 1976. Nursing intervention in black patient care. In Luckraft, D., editor. *Black awareness: Implications for black patient care.* New York: American Journal of Nursing Co.

Brink, P. J., editor. 1976. *Transcultural nursing: A book of readings.* Englewood Cliffs, N.J.: Prentice-Hall.

Brink, P. J., and Saunders, J. M. 1976. Culture shock: Theoretical and applied. Pp. 126–38 in Brink, P. J., editor, 1976. *Transcultural nursing: A book of readings.* Englewood Cliffs, N.J.: Prentice-Hall.

Bush, M. T., Ullom, J. A., and Osborne, O. H. March/April 1975. The meaning of mental health: A report of two ethnoscientific studies. *Nursing Research* 24:130–38.

Campbell, T., and Chang, T. April 1973. Health care of the Chinese in America. *Nursing Outlook* 21:245–49.

———. 1981. Health care of the Chinese in America. In Henderson, G., and Primeaux, M., editors. *Transcultural health care.* Menlo Park, Calif.: Addison-Wesley Publishing Co.

Chang, B. 1981. Asian-American patient care. In Henderson, G., and Primeaux, M., editors. *Transcultural health care.* Menlo Park, Calif.: Addison-Wesley Publishing Co.

Chen-Louie, T. T. 1980. Bicultural experiences, social interactions, and health care implications. In Reinhardt, A. M., and Quinn, M. D. *Family-centered community nursing: A sociocultural framework.* St. Louis: C. V. Mosby Co.

Christian, J. L., and Greger, J. L. 1985. *Nutrition for living.* Menlo Park, Calif.: Benjamin/Cummings Publishing Co.

Chung, H. J. March 1977. Understanding the Oriental maternity patient. *Nursing Clinics of North America* 12:67–75.

Clinton, J. 1982. Ethnicity: The development of an empirical construct for cross-cultural health research. *Western Journal of Nursing Research* 4(3):281–99.

Davis, M., and Yoshida, M. March 1981. A model for cultural assessment of the new immigrant. *Canadian Nurse* 77:22–23.

DeGracia, R. T. August 1979. Cultural influences on Filipino patients. *American Journal of Nursing* 79:1412–14.

———. December 1979. Health care of the American Asian patient. *Critical Care Update* 6:19+.

Drakwlic, L., and Tanaka, W. March 1981. The East Indian family in Canada. *Canadian Nurse* 77:24–26.

Emergency Medicine. October 30, 1983. Aids: Coping with the unknown. *Emergency Medicine* 15:165–68, 173, 176–77.

Falvo, D. et al. September/October 1983. Differences in perception of health status and health needs between refugees and physicians providing care. *Health Values* 7:20–24.

Farris, L. S. March/April 1976. Approaches to caring for the American Indian maternity patient. *American Journal of Maternal Child Nursing* 1:80–87.

Flaskerud, J. H. May/June 1980. Perceptions of problematic behavior by Appalachians, mental health professionals, and lay non-Appalachians. *Nursing Research* 29:140–49.

Friedman, M. M. 1981. *Family nursing theory and assessment.* Norwalk, Conn.: Appleton-Century-Crofts.

Gonzalez-Swafford, M. J., and Gutierrez, M. G. November/December 1983. Ethno-medical beliefs and practices of Mexican-Americans. *Nurse Practitioner* 8:29–30, 32, 34.

Gordon, V. C., Matousek, I. M., and Lang, T. A. November 1980. Southeast Asian refugees: Life in America. *American Journal of Nursing* 80:2031–36.

Grasska, M. A., and McFarland, T. September 1982. Overcoming the language barrier: Problems and solutions. *American Journal of Nursing* 82:1376–79.

Grinker, R. R. August 1978. The poor rich: The children of the super-rich. *American Journal of Psychiatry* 135:913.

Hautman, M. A., and Harrison, J. K. April 1982. Health beliefs and practices in a middle-income Anglo-American neighborhood. *Advances in Nursing Science* 4:49–63.

Hayghe, H. 1976. Families and the rise of working wives: An overview. *Monthly Labor Review* 99:12–19.

———. 1982. Marital and family patterns of worker: An update. *Monthly Labor Review* 105:53–56.

Henderson, G., and Primeaux, M., editors. 1981. *Transcultural health care.* Menlo Park, Calif.: Addison-Wesley Publishing Co.

Henry, B. M., and DiGiacomo-Geffers, E. August 1980. The hospitalized rich and famous. *American Journal of Nursing* 80:1426–29.

Hicks, G. 1976. *Appalachian valley.* New York: Holt, Rinehart and Winston.

James, S. M. November 1978. When your patient is a black West Indian. *American Journal of Nursing* 78:1908–9.

Kalish, R. A. 1967. Of children and grandfather: A speculative essay on dependency. *Gerontologist* 7:65–69.

Kleinman, A. et al. February 1978. Culture, illness, and care: Clinical lessons from anthropologic and cross-cultural research. *Annals of Internal Medicine* 88:251–58.

LaFargue, J. P. 1972. Role of prejudice in rejection of health care. *Nursing Research* 2:53–58.

———. September 1980. A survival strategy: Kinship network. *American Journal of Nursing* 80:1636–40.

Leininger, M. 1970. *Nursing and anthropology: Two worlds to blend.* New York: John Wiley and Sons.

———. 1974. Humanism, health, and cultural values. In Leininger, M., editor. *Health care dimensions.* Philadelphia: F. A. Davis Co.

Lewis, O. October 1966. The culture of poverty. *Scientific American* 215:19–25.

Lewis, S., Messner, R., and McDowel, W. August 1985. An unchanging culture: Caring for Appalachian patients and their families. *Journal of Gerontological Nursing* 11:20–24, 26.

Macdonald, A. C. June 1981. Folk health practices among north coastal Peruvians: Implications for nursing. *Image* 13:51–55.

Martin, B. J. W. Ethnicity and health care: Afro-Americans. In *Ethnicity and health care.* 1976. New York: National League for Nursing.

Mason, D. J. October 1981. Perspectives on poverty. *Image* 13:82–85.

Meleis, A. I. June 1981. The Arab American in the health care system. *American Journal of Nursing* 81:1180–83.

Murillo-Rhode, I. 1976. Unique needs of ethnic minority clients in a multiracial society: A socio-cultural perspective. In *Affirmative action: Toward quality nursing care for a multiracial society.* Pub. no. M-24 2500 5/76. Kansas City, Mo.: American Nurses' Association.

———. May 1980. Health care for the Hispanic patient. *Critical Care Update* 7:29–36.

National Center for Health Statistics. August 1985. *Charting the nation's health trends since 1960.* DHHS pub no. (PHS) 85-1251. U.S. Department of Health and Human Services, Hyattsville, Md.: Public Health Service.

O'Brien, M. E. June 1981. Transcultural nursing research: Alien in an alien land. *Image* 13:37–39.

Ohlson, V. M., and Franklin, M. 1985. *An international perspective on nursing practice.* Pub. no. NP-68F. Kansas City, Mo.: American Nurses' Association.

Orque, M. S., Bloch, B., and Monrroy, L. S. A. 1983. *Ethnic nursing care: A multicultural approach.* St. Louis: C. V. Mosby Co.

Osborne, O. H. 1976. Unique needs of ethnic minority clients in a multiracial society: A psycho-social perspective. In *Affirmative action: Toward quality nursing care for a multiracial society.* Pub. no. M-24 2500 5/76. Kansas City, Mo.: American Nurses' Association.

Overfield, T. March 1977. Biological variation: Concepts from physical anthropology. *Nursing Clinics in North America* 12:19–26.

———. 1985. *Biologic variation in health and illness.* Menlo Park, Calif.: Addison-Wesley Publishing Co.

Parreno, H. 1976. Unique needs of ethnic minority clients in a multiracial society: A biological perspective. In *Affirmative action: Toward quality nursing care for a multiracial society.* Pub. no. M-24 2500 5/76. Kansas City, Mo.: American Nurses' Association.

Powers, B. A. April 1982. The use of orthodox and black American folk medicine. *Advances in Nursing Science* 4:35–47.

Primeaux, M. H. March 1977. American Indian health care practices. *Nursing Clinics of North America* 12:55–65.

Richardson, E. A. W., and Milne, L. S. November/December 1983. Sickle-cell disease and the childbearing family: An update. *American Journal of Maternal/Child Nursing* 8:417–22.

Rotkovitch, R. 1976. Ethnicity and health care: The Jewish heritage. In *Ethnicity and health care.* New York: National League for Nursing.

Roundtable. September 15, 1980. Homosexuality 2: When sexual orientation is in doubt. *Patient Care* 58–59 +.

Schermerhorn, R. A. 1970. *Comparative ethnic relations: A framework for theory and research.* New York: Random House.

Shubin, S. June 1980. Nursing patients from different cultures. *Nursing 80* 10:78–81. Canadian edition 10:26–29.

Smith, J. A. 1976. The role of the black clergy as allied health care professionals in working with black patients. In Luckraft, D., editor. *Black awareness: Implications for black patient care.* New York: American Journal of Nursing Co.

Spector, R. E. 1985. *Cultural diversity in health and illness.* 2d ed. New York: Appleton-Century-Crofts.

Spruce, B. B. 1972. The cultural patterns and values of the American Indian and their relation to health and illness. In *Becoming aware of cultural differences in nursing.* Speeches presented during the 48th annual convention of the ANA. Kansas City, Mo.: American Nurses' Association.

Statistics Canada. 1984. *Census of Canada.* Cat. no. 92-911. Ottawa: Minister of Supplies and Services.

Stein, B. N., and Tomasi, S. M. Spring/Summer 1981. *International Migration Review.* Vol. 15. New York: Center for Migration Studies of New York.

Tripp-Reimer, T. Spring 1982. Barriers to health care: Variations in interpretation of Appalachian client behavior by Appalachian and non-Appalachian health professionals. *Western Journal of Nursing Research* 4:179–91.

Tripp-Reimer, T., and Friedl, M. March 1977. Appalachians: A neglected minority. *Nursing Clinics of North America* 12:41–54.

Tripp-Reimer, T., Brink, P. J., and Saunders, J. M. March/April 1984. Cultural assessment: Content and process. *Nursing Outlook* 32:78–82.

U.S. Department of Commerce. Bureau of the Census. April 1984. *Census of Population, General Population Characteristics United States Survey.* Washington, D.C.: Government Printing Office.

Wang, R. M. 1976. Chinese Americans and health care. In *Ethnicity and health care.* New York: National League for Nursing.

Wauneka, A. D. 1976. Helping a people to understand. In Brink, P. R., editor. *Transcultural nursing: A book of readings.* Englewood Cliffs, N.J.: Prentice-Hall.

West, K., and Kalbsleisch, J. September 1970. Diabetes in Central America. *Diabetes* 19:656–63.

White, E. H. March 1977. Giving health care to minority patients. *Nursing Clinics of North America* 12:27–40.

Winn, M. C. 1976. A proposed tuberculosis program for Papago Indians. In Brink, P. J., editor. *Transcultural nursing: A book of readings.* Englewood Cliffs, N.J.: Prentice-Hall.

Wirth, L. 1945. The problem of minority groups. In Linton, R. *The science of man in the world crisis.* New York: Columbia University Press.

Wold, S. J. 1981. *School nursing: A framework for practice.* St. Louis: C. V. Mosby Co.

Wood, R. 1976. The American Indian and health. In *Ethnicity and health care.* New York: National League for Nursing.

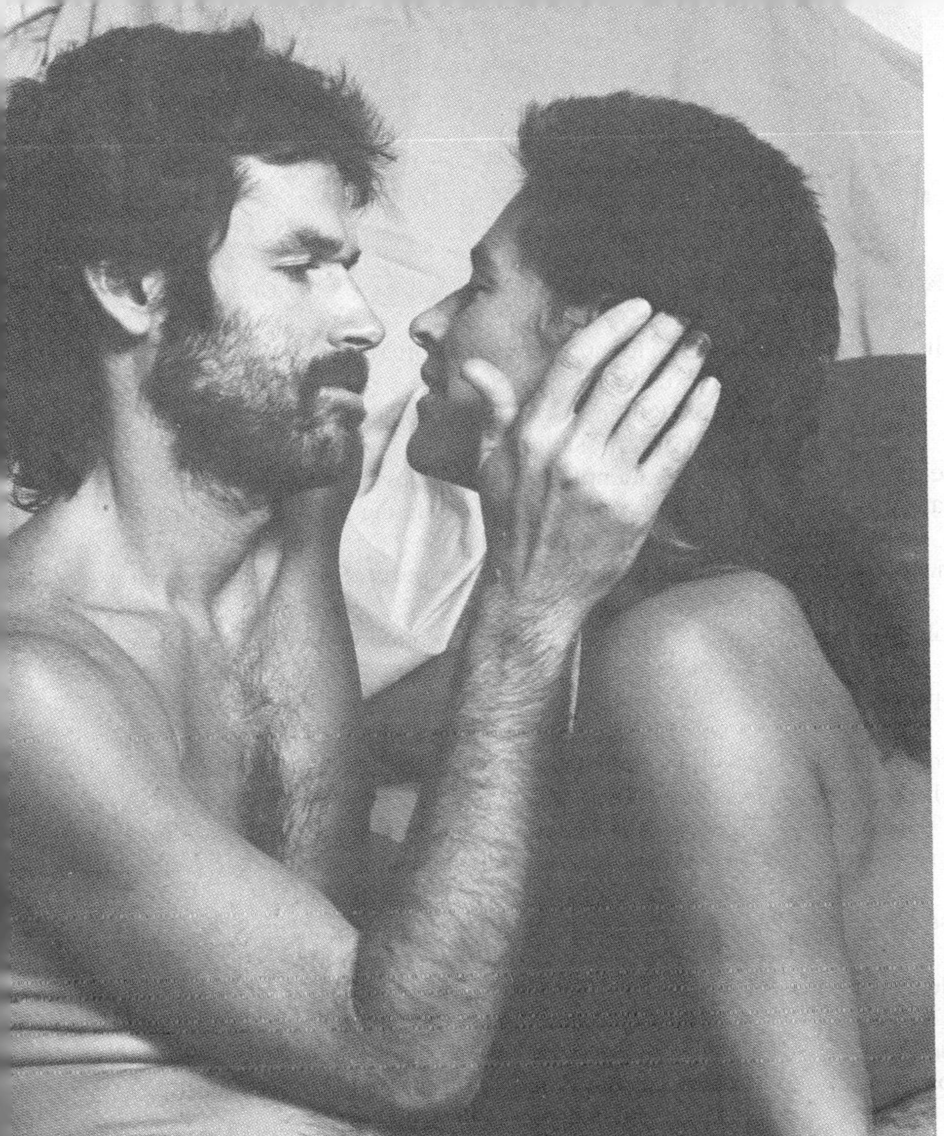

KAREN STAFFORD RANTZMAN

CHAPTER 19

Sexuality

Ross A. Stewart

Contents

19 *Sexuality*

Objectives

1. Know essential facts about sex and sexuality.
   1.1 Define selected terms.
   1.2 Describe the concept of sexuality.
   1.3 Identify components of sexuality.
   1.4 Identify essential aspects of the development of sexuality from the prenatal period to late adulthood.
   1.5 Identify structure and function of male and female genitals.
   1.6 Identify various physical and psychologic sexual stimulation patterns.
   1.7 Identify Masters and Johnson's four phases of sexual response.
   1.8 Identify physiologic changes that occur in males and females during each phase of the sexual response.
2. Know essential information and methods required to assess sexuality.
   2.1 Identify situations in which the nurse assesses sexual function.
   2.2 Identify factors that affect an individual's sexual attitudes and behaviors.
   2.3 Identify sexual aspects of a health history.
3. Know essential facts about nursing diagnoses and common problems related to sexuality.
   3.1 Identify factors contributing to sexual dysfunction.
   3.2 Identify factors that increase and decrease sexual motivation.
   3.3 Identify common problems of genital sexuality and possible causes.
   3.4 Identify common illnesses affecting sexuality.
4. Understand facts about nursing interventions that promote sexual health.
   4.1 Identify essential aspects of developing sexual self-awareness.
   4.2 Identify two intervention models for sexual counseling.
   4.3 Identify essentials of breast and testicular self-examination for health teaching.
   4.4 Identify essentials of various contraceptive methods for health teaching.
5. Apply the nursing process when providing care to selected patients with sexual problems.
   5.1 Obtain necessary assessment data.
   5.2 Analyze and relate assessment data.
   5.3 Write relevant nursing diagnoses.
   5.4 Write relevant nursing goals.
   5.5 Plan appropriate nursing interventions.
   5.6 Implement appropriate nursing interventions.
   5.7 State outcome criteria essential for evaluating client progress.

Terms

adolescence
androgen
androsperm
anilingus
areola
atresia
basalis
biologic sex
bisexual
cervix
chromosomes
clitoris
coitus
condom
contraception
cornification
corpus albicans
corpus luteum
cremaster
cryptorchidism
cunnilingus
detumescence
dildo
diploid number
Doderlein's bacilli
dyspareunia
ectopic pregnancy
ejaculation
ejaculatory ducts
endometrium
epididymis
erection
erotic
estrogen
fallopian tubes
fellatio
follicle stimulating hormone (FSH)
follicular atresia
follicular (preovulatory) stage
foreplay (precoital stimulation)
foreskin (prepuce)
frenulum
functionalis
gender dysphoria
gender identity
gender role
genitals
glans clitoris
glans penis
Graafian follicle
granulosa cells
gynosperm
haploid number
heterosexual
homosexual
hymen
imperforate hymen
impotence
impregnation
interstitial cells of Leydig
intrauterine device (IUD)
labia majora
labia minora
leutenizing hormone (LH)
libido
luteal (postovulatory) stage
mammary glands
masturbation
meiosis
menarche

menopause
menses
mitosis
mons pubis (mons veneris)
myometrium
myotonia
orgasm
orgasmic dysfunction
ovaries
ovarian cortex
ovarian medulla
ovulation
perimetrium
postovulatory stage
preovulatory stage
primordial follicles
progesterone
proliferative (preovulatory) stage
puberty
reflexogenic erection
refractory period
rugae
scrotum
secretory (postovulatory) stage
semen
seminal plasma
seminal vesicles
seminiferous tubules
sex
sex-typed behaviors
sex chromosome pair
sexual differentiation
sexual dysfunction
sexual identity
sexual intercourse
sexuality
sex play
smegma
soixante-neuf
sperm
spermatogenesis
spermicide
testes
testosterone
tubal ligation
tumescent
tunica albuginea
tunica dartos
uterus
vagina
vaginal diaphragm
vaginal orifice
vaginal smear
vaginismus
vas deferens
vasectomy
vestibule
vulva (pudendum)
zygote

Introduction

Sexuality is an integral characteristic of every human being. We are all born with the capacity to function as sexual beings. All clients for whom nurses provide care are sexual beings. They do not leave their sexuality behind when they enter the health care system—their sexuality comes along as part of the whole person. Professional nurses, as health care providers focusing on the holistic nature of care, have a responsibility to provide effective sexual health care for their clients.

A holistic approach to client health care needs indicates that all aspects of being interact. Thus, sexuality influences and is influenced by the biologic, psychologic, sociologic, and spiritual aspects of being. The need to acknowledge and deal with issues of sexuality in health care practice cannot be overemphasized. Until fairly recently, health care has treated sexuality with benign neglect or has actively discouraged it as a focus of interest. Nursing has been as slow as the other health professions to identify sexuality as significant to health care. The difficulty of dealing with sexual issues continues today. (Young 1984; Douglas, Kalman, and Kalman 1985). The evidence reinforces the need for improving nurses' ability to deal with sexual issues.

Nurses practicing in North America in the 1980s (and beyond) are coping with a much more complex world of sexuality than nurses in earlier years. Changes in beliefs, attitudes, and behaviors—and the conflicts thereby engendered—have produced uncertainty and a need to assess nurses' understanding of and attitudes toward the many variations of sexuality. The multicultural nature of North American society has also been a major influence on sexuality, as has the vast increase in mass communication. The impact of influence groups and movements such as the women's movement, gay liberation, handicapped groups, and the "moral majority" has been powerful and is still creating change. The nurse assisting clients to deal with issues of sexual health must be aware of these multiple factors and must integrate them into effective sexual health care plans.

Sex and Sexuality

Definitions Related to Sexuality

The words *sex* and *sexuality* are used interchangeably, and often incorrectly, to define different aspects of sexual being. **Sex** is the term most commonly used to denote biologic male or female status, but it is also used to describe specific sexual behavior, such as sexual intercourse. Examples of such usage include the labelled boxes on questionnaire forms to indicate male or female (M☐, F☐) and the question "How many partners have you had sex with since your last visit?" asked in a sexually transmitted disease clinic.

The more appropriate and descriptive term when dealing with sexual issues is **sexuality**. Because this term is understood to involve all aspects of a person's being, we need a definition or description that reflects the holistic nature of nursing's approach to health. *Sexuality*, then, refers to "the totality of being a person. It includes all of those aspects of the human being that relate specifically to being boy or girl, woman or man, and is an entity subject to life-long dynamic change. Sexuality reflects our human character, not solely our genital nature. As a function of the total personality, it is concerned with the biological, psychological, sociological, spiritual, and cultural variables of life, which, by their effect on personality development and interpersonal relations, can in turn offer social structure" (Sex Information and Education Council of the United States 1980, p. 8).

Components of Sexuality

Although sexuality is an integral part of the whole human being, it can also be categorized and studied according to its major components:

1. Biologic sex
2. Gender identity
3. Gender role

Biologic sex includes all of the human being's genetically determined anatomy and physiology, which is also influenced by intrauterine conditions. The result of genetic plus other prenatal factors usually is clearly developed primary sex characteristics or variations of these characteristics, called ambiguous sex.

Gender identity is the individual's persisting inner sense of being male or female, masculine or feminine. Its development is based on biologic sex and sociocultural reinforcement, which begins at birth with identification of the baby as male or female. Ultimate congruence between biologic sex and learned sense of sexual self is the most common outcome of this developmental process. Variations of this congruence are common, principally at periods of significant change in the life span (e.g., adolescence, menopause, climacteric, old age). The term **sexual identity** is sometimes equivalent to *gender identity* but is more commonly used to indicate sexual orientation (e.g., heterosexual, bisexual, homosexual).

Gender role includes all behaviors reflecting the individual's learned sense of masculinity and femininity, sex behavior, sexual relationships, and sexual dimorphism. The discerning of a person's gender role is based on observation of the person's behavior. The conceptual distinction between gender identity and gender is for descriptive purposes only; in reality, the two are "opposite sides of the same coin" (Money 1980, pp. 11–12).

The Context of Sexuality

As noted in the chapter introduction, sexuality is an integral part of the whole human experience. As such, sexuality must be understood as part of the world with which people interact. Sexuality and the way we respond to it are influenced by a variety of factors; such a view allows us to understand the context of sexuality and sexual being. A review of historical, ethnocultural, religious-ethical, and contemporary perspectives on sexuality will help us see sexuality in the context of the broader human experience.

Historical Perspectives

Sexuality, as a part of the human condition, has been with us since the beginning of time. Humankind's understanding of sexuality has evolved over time, changing to adapt to changes in knowledge, beliefs, and values. Our earliest clear knowledge of sexuality comes from writings, statues, and paintings as old as 10,000 years. Though some of the earlier paintings and sculptures indicate an awareness of sexuality, they give us no clues as to sexual beliefs or practices. The writings, paintings, and sculptures from 5,000 B.C. onward, however, do provide clear information about sexual beliefs, values, laws, and practices; they demonstrate the existence of circumcision, heterosexual genital intercourse, fellatio, anal intercourse, homosexuality, prostitution (male and female), and many other sexual practices. Also indicated is the variation in attitudes towards and laws about those practices.

Historical records from the period known as the "common era" (also known as A.D. in Christian-influenced datings) are much clearer and tell us a great deal about the development of our attitudes, beliefs, and laws relating to sexuality. The historical records from Europe (influenced by the Judeo-Christian tradition), the Middle East (predominately Muslim), India (Hindu), and China (Buddhist and Confucian) show a wide variation in approaches to sexuality. The important message of history is that contemporary approaches to sexuality are part of an ever-evolving process, not something that has always been the same and will always be the same.

Ethnocultural Perspectives

North America is a multicultural, ethnically mixed society. Although the majority of the population traces its roots to Europe, increasingly larger proportions of the population in both Canada and the United States come from non-European roots. Citizenship ceremonies in both countries commonly have participants from up to 50 or more different countries. Native Indians, Afro-Americans, Latin Americans, Chinese, East Indians (including Muslim, Hindu, and Sikh), Japanese, and Southeast Asians exemplify the ethnic groups that make up significant portions of our society. All such groups have their own ethnic and cultural traditions, which influence the ways they view the world and interact with society. Included in these traditions are rules, practices, and values relating to sexuality. Much anthropologic and ethnocultural research indicates that the predominant North American societal approaches to sexuality based on Judeo-Christian traditions are not universal. In North America there are strong negative attitudes about homosexuality; in a number of other societies, however, homosexual behavior is tolerated, and in some instances it has become an integral part of rituals such as coming-of-age. Other differences include attitudes about female sexual behavior, husband / wife roles, childhood sexuality, and nudity.

Because clients (and, often, our colleagues) may differ in their approach to sexuality—based on ethnic or cultural traditions, it is important for nurses to be aware of and be prepared to include ethnocultural issues in their approach to sexual issues in health care. As simple a practice as giving a bed bath can have sexual implications, depending on the cultural traditions of the client and/or nurse.

Religious-Ethical Perspectives

Probably the most obvious influences on our approach to sexuality are religion and ethics. All our dealings with sexuality are affected by beliefs and values that come from either our religious traditions or some other value-developing system. As one of its functions, religion provides adherents with guidelines for the conduct of their human affairs. These guidelines always include sexuality. The most common approach is for a particular religious group or organization to outline acceptable sexual behavior and acceptable circumstances for the behavior, as well as prohibited sexual behavior and the consequences of breaking the sexual rules. The guidelines or rules may be detailed and rigid or broad and flexible. In North America as well as Europe, South America, and other Christian-influenced countries many of the accepted beliefs, values, and laws are based on values from the Jewish and Christian traditions. However, even within the broad Judeo-Christian value system there are variations that, along with beliefs and values from other religious traditions, produce the potential for ongoing societal strain as people attempt to integrate all the differing rules and values.

Although ethics are integral to religion, ethical thought and ethical approaches to sexuality can be viewed separately. Many people and groups have developed written or unwritten codes of conduct based on ethical principles. These principles draw from ethical theories that often cut across religious designations while incorporating important principles from different religious traditions. Again the crucial issue in religious-ethical matters is understanding, respecting, and working with the person's own religious-ethical value system.

Contemporary Perspectives

All of the foregoing comments can be integrated in order to understand the context of sexuality in North America in the 1980s. The ever-evolving nature of our knowledge, beliefs, values, and attitudes about sexuality causes continuing societal stress. It is interesting to note that some groups are pressuring for return to the historically recent times when approaches to sexuality were less ambiguous. Although returning to a different value system may be appealing, those times must also be viewed accurately to understand the influence of the values on all aspects of sexuality and human functioning.

At present one of the major influences on sexual issues is that of particular groups within North American Christian sects. There is increasing pressure to reinforce strict guidelines for sexual behavior based on a specific view of Christian values. These efforts have been aimed not only at the members of those religious sects but at the law, the media, health care agencies, and groups viewed unfavorably. This has created great controversy, since there are many others in our society who are comfortable with and eager to maintain the more flexible values that developed over the last few decades (often labelled the "sexual revolution"). That many in our society accept premarital sex, unwed motherhood, homosexuality, and abortion has produced numerous conflicts, which appear destined to continue in the future.

Another major influence on contemporary sexuality is the information explosion. The media (TV, print, movies, video, computer networks) provide continuous output that has major impact on our views of sexuality. Media stars become the role models for acceptable male or female behavior, at the same time creating potential conflicts. As an example, how does a teenage boy deal with his liking for both the ultra-masculine Arnold Schwarzeneger and the androgynous Boy George? The media also reflect changes in society's attitudes toward sexuality. For instance, at one time (the 1950s and 1960s), television shows always portrayed heterosexual couples as married and sleeping in twin beds. Currently they show same-sex, unmarried and married couples, often in bed together, and—in soap operas—in varying stages of undress.

Specific issues related to sexuality—such as teenage sexuality, contraception, homosexuality, sexually transmitted diseases (including AIDS), abortion, pornography, and sexual abuse—all provoke strong emotions, and they do not respond to simple solutions. These are issues that nurses will confront in their practice. Nurses have a responsibility to be aware of these influences and to utilize this awareness in assisting patients to develop sexual health on their own terms.

Development of Sexuality

The development of sexuality in the human begins with conception and is influenced continuously by many factors throughout the life span. A variety of theories try to explain the development of sexuality, including the interaction of biologic and psychosocial factors. The one currently accepted common understanding is that sexuality as a human experience is complex and multiply influenced. Thus, the psychosocial components described here are to be understood as commonly accepted ways of looking at the interactions that influence the development of sexuality. Every society develops expectations about acceptable ways to be sexual. The components outlined in this section also reflect those societal influences and are organized according to previously identified developmental stages, including Erikson's widely accepted model of human development (see Table 22-6).

Prenatal Period and Infancy

Biologic Components

All cells of the body have 23 pairs of chromosomes, referred to as the **diploid number**. These cells multiply by dividing in half and producing two new cells, each of which contains 23 pairs of chromosomes. Such cell division is called **mitosis**. However, **sperm** cells (*male gametes*, or male reproductive cells) and egg cells (*ova*, or *female gametes*, or female reproductive cells) have only 23 single chromosomes, referred to as the **haploid number**, the result of specialized cell division called **meiosis**. Thus, when a sperm cell fertilizes an egg cell, the cell produced by their union has the required 23 pairs of chromosomes—23 single chromosomes from the female and 23 single chromosomes from the male.

In the developing human fetus, two of these chromosomes make up the **sex chromosome pair**, which determines whether the gonads will develop as testes or ovaries. The female has two identical sex chromosomes, referred to as XX. The male has two different chromosomes, designated XY; thus one chromosome is the same as the female's (X) but the other is different (Y). Sperm are of two types: an X-bearing sperm, called a **gynosperm**, and a Y-bearing sperm, called an **androsperm**. If a gynosperm fertilizes the egg, the fetus develops into a female, but if an androsperm fertilizes the egg, the fetus will be male.

Androsperm are smaller, have longer tails, move or swim faster, and are more susceptible to vaginal pH and other changes in the environment than are gynosperm. It is believed that for a male to be conceived, intercourse must occur very near or at the time of ovulation, when androsperm move toward the egg more quickly than gynosperm. A female is thought to be conceived if intercourse occurs a few days before the egg is ready to be fertilized, at which time gynosperm are thought to move more slowly and withstand the relatively acid vaginal fluids secreted, and then to unite with the egg once it is produced.

The most common outcome of the sex-chromosome influence is an infant with a clearly defined male or female anatomy and physiology. The neurologic, vascular, and other tissues are developed well enough at birth to allow the sexual organs to respond to stimulation. This can produce penile erection in infant boys and vaginal lubrication in infant girls. The infant's behavior in response to stimulation of the genitals (either by the infant or during washing, etc.) indicates pleasure on the part of the infant. It is important to be aware that these small responses are reflexogenic and are not to be confused with postpubertal sexual responses. For the infant this is just another pleasurable feeling.

Psychosocial Components

Much of our understanding of infant development is based on assumptions about the behavior we see. Infants behave in ways that indicate a focus on such basic needs as safety, security, comfort, nutrition, and pleasure. This is the period for development of trust, according to Erikson's model. It is during this period, in response to interactions with parenting figures and others, that infants begin to learn about gender role. From the moment of birth, the approaches and reactions to infants are based, in general terms, on society's guidelines for male and female gender roles. Little boys are talked to differently, handled differently, and expected to react differently than little girls. These adult behaviors are based on what our society believes about male or female gender roles.

There is also evidence, based on observations of behavior, that male and female infants demonstrate **sexual differentiation** in a variety of areas. These include motor activity, musculature, attention span, preference for stimuli, and interactions with parent figures. The origins of these differences are not clearly understood, but their existence demonstrates the complex interaction between biologic and psychosocial components of sexual development.

Early and Late Childhood

Biologic Components

In contrast to the rapid physical growth in other body systems, the anatomic and physiologic components of the sexual self change very little prior to puberty. Structurally, male and female children appear very similar in early childhood, with the genitals being the only obvious difference. Some changes become evident as late childhood progresses, with physical growth occurring fairly rapidly. Boys begin to develop a more solid musculature, and girls generally develop a slighter structure. It also becomes easier to distinguish boys faces from girls faces.

Psychosocial Components

The establishment of gender identity is one of the major issues in early childhood. By the age of 4 or 5 years, the combination of biologic and psychosocial factors has usually produced in the child a clear sense of being male or female. At age 3 years, children are usually able to identify themselves as either boy or girl. This understanding stems from the frequent use of the terms *boy, he, girl*, and *she* in describing the child. At the same time the child is learning a sense of self through interaction with parent figures. This sense of self usually solidifies at about the same age as the sense of being a boy or a girl, 3 years. Other factors influencing the establishment of gender identity include interaction with parent figures, which provides feedback about gender-appropriate behavior, and imitation, which allows the child to mimic and receive reinforcement for same-sex parent behaviors. As with infants, parents and other adults interact differently with boys and girls. Physical as well as interpersonal interactions differ, adding to the development of gender identity.

The development of gender role is another major focus during early and late childhood. This is accomplished through some of the same mechanisms by which gender identity develops. The developmental task of this period is the acquisition of **sex-typed behaviors**, or **gender-appropriate behaviors**, behaviors that also are reinforced by positive responses from parents and later from others in the wider interpersonal world. These gender-appropriate behaviors can include what clothes are worn, games played, playmates chosen, toys played with, and manner of speech, among many others. The nurse needs to be aware that there is in present-day North America a wide variation in sex-typed or gender-appropriate behaviors. Many children will develop a repertoire of behaviors as part of their gender role, including both gender-appropriate and gender-inappropriate behaviors. It is important *not* to label children on the basis of these variations. Only when there is evidence of problems in gender role or gender identity is there a potential for intervention. Such extremes are termed as **gender dysphoria**.

As development progresses, children continue to be curious about their own and others' bodies. Preschool children express this curiosity during bathing, toileting, swimming, and playing. Such curiosity is an important part of learning and should be responded to with factual information in a matter-of-fact manner. As the child learns more socially acceptable ways of expressing curiosity, usually during the early school years, the need for information is expressed as questions. School-age children ask many questions about sex, which again are best responded to with factual, matter-of-fact answers. Their questions arise from observing adults interacting, from reading, from sharing stories with peers, and from fantasies. Children develop the capacity for fantasy after the age of 4 or 5 years.

School-age children also express curiosity about their own and others' bodies. This takes place in individual exploration, in mutual exploration (playing "doctor" or "house"), and by watching adults whenever possible. Mutual exploration involves members of the opposite sex and, because of the sexual separation that occurs in the prepubertal period, members of the same sex. Matter-of-fact, nonjudgmental responses to such behaviors are important in order to avoid the child's adopting negative feelings about his or her own body or sexual interaction.

Puberty and Adolescence

Biologic Components

Changes in sexual anatomy and physiology are more profound during puberty than at any other comparable developmental period. These changes are discussed in Chapter 24. **Puberty** refers to the period of physiologic maturation, and **adolescence** refers to the period of psychosocial maturation.

Psychosocial Components

Changes in the psychosocial component of sexuality during adolescence are also profound. They include dealing with altered body image, dealing with changes in the body's functioning, consolidating gender identity, adjusting gender-role behavior, and learning new social-role behaviors.

Physiologic changes during puberty are relatively rapid and dramatic. The adolescent must deal with a body that is larger and proportioned differently and that requires new skills of coordination. In addition, the growth of secondary sexual characteristics, and the development of physiologic functioning associated with these changes, produces intense psychologic response. Conflicting emotions related to pride, embarrassment, shame, and discomfort require much understanding and explanation by adults. Boys react to the comparison of their own changing body to the idealized male bodies in our culture. Height, weight, muscular development, body hair, and size of penis and testicles are all sources of anxiety as the boy compares himself to the ideal. Analogously for girls, height, weight, body shape, breast size, and menstrual cycles are all influenced by idealized norms. Adolescents need to know that there is a wide variation in healthy anatomy and physiology. This reassurance is particularly needed in response to media depictions of idealized male and female bodies. (Media stars never seem to have pimples, body odor, menstrual cramps, or spontaneous erections.)

The activation of sexual response potential during puberty puts a tremendous strain on the adolescent. Because of the hormonal triggers at work, the male body and female body become susceptible to a wide variety of sexually exciting stimuli. Adolescents respond to this new source of pleasurable sensations by engaging in erotic play, either alone through fantasy and masturbation or with others. Erotic play with a partner may include embracing, kissing, petting, and various methods of genital sexual activity, including mutual masturbation, penile–vaginal intercourse, and oral–genital activity.

Such sexual activity may involve partners of the same sex or the opposite sex. For the majority of adolescents, same-sex erotic play is experimental or exploratory. However, adolescents with a homosexual orientation require acknowledgment of and support for their sexual identity, to avoid anxiety, guilt, and negative self-image. Heterosexual and homosexual adolescents alike need both factual information about their bodies and support and reassurance about emotional and other psychosocial responses to their changing bodies and body functions. All adolescents are engaged in developing a clear sense of when and how to respond to intense sexual impulses.

As well as adapting to a changing body, the adolescent has opportunities to consolidate gender identity through psychosocial interactions. It is important during this period for the adolescent to understand that gender identity allows for wide variation in what constitutes male or female. The distinction between gender identity (maleness / femaleness) and sexual orientation (heterosexual / bisexual / homosexual) must be clarified for the adolescent, particularly in view of the complex signals being received. Gender-role-behavior development also is a source of stress, with frequently conflicting signals about what is gender-appropriate and what is not. There is, as well, an increased expectation for different social-role interactions on the part of the adolescent. The complexity of the influences related to psychosocial development of sexuality makes adolescence a very stressful period of growth and development. All adolescents require a factual, comprehensive knowledge base about biologic and psychosocial factors involved in the development of healthy adult sexuality.

Adulthood and Middle Years

Adulthood is the period when most developmental changes have reached maturity. The adult is both biologically and psychosocially prepared to engage in intimate psychosocial and sexual relationships. Typically, adulthood is seen as a time for developing intimacy with one partner, marrying, and parenting. Currently, a variety of alternatives to this traditional pattern is gaining wider acceptance. Regardless of the pattern of adult interpersonal relationships, sexuality is frequently a crucial component. Society continues to approve the capacity to become involved in a stable, heterosexual relationship as the ideal for adulthood.

Biologic Components

Between the ages of approximately 18 and 30 years, the young adult reaches full anatomic and physiologic maturity. Height, weight, body condition, and secondary sexual characteristics are all at their peak. These years are, for the majority of adults, the prime child-bearing and child-rearing years. The earlier, unpredictable intensity of sexual feelings experienced during adolescence evens out and becomes more predictable.

Development leading to the middle years includes changes in hormone levels in both men and women. For women, development culminates in the cessation of the menstrual cycle and a decrease in estrogens, leading to such changes as the beginning atrophy of breast and vaginal tissue, delay and decrease in vaginal lubrication during sexual arousal, and loss of elasticity of skin and other tissue. For men the changes involve delay in attaining erection, decrease in size and firmness of erection, decrease in expulsive force of ejaculation, and decrease in volume of semen.

Psychosocial Components

Society's expectations for sexual development in adulthood include establishing a permanent intimate relationship with a partner of the opposite sex and bearing and raising children. This expectation may produce stress for many people as individual expectations increasingly differ from this societal "norm." The number of unmarried couples, both heterosexual and homosexual, has increased, as has the number of childless couples. Single parents are becoming more numerous, both as a result of relationship breakups and by choice. These changes in adult role relationships are not universally accepted but must be assessed by the nurse in terms of the overall health of the individual and the relationship.

The establishment of intimate adult relationships produces change in gender-role expectations. Adding to already existing role components are such expectations as partner (husband, wife, spouse, etc.), parent, and lover. These new role components require adjusting to patterns of behavior that are still developing. In addition, individual needs and preferences may encourage individuals to

Research Note

Nurses must meet the challenge of attending to whatever special health care needs their homosexual clients may have; indeed, the alarming rise in the incidence of AIDS brings nurses into increasing contact with the sensitivities, as well as some unusual medical needs, of gay clients.

This study asks and partially answers two questions: (1) How do gay men and lesbians learn they are gay and come to accept their gayness as a positive aspect of self? (2) What health care concerns arise in relation to "coming out" as a homosexual? The author asserts that nurses cannot provide adequate care to gay clients unless they understand this process. The study found distinct differences between gay men and gay women in terms of their childhood upbringing and behavior patterns; the genesis of the homosexual orientation for either sex remained obscure, however. The study also found that coming-out has four distinct stages: (1) identification of self as gay, (2) cognitive changes in previously held negative notions, (3) acceptance of self, and (4) action. Perhaps nurses can help gay people to accept their homosexuality as a positive aspect of self. (Kus 1985)

develop roles and role behaviors that are not congruent with broader societal expectations, for example, the househusband, woman as primary breadwinner, and commuting spouses.

Sexual interaction in adulthood is a major component of being, whether as part of a stable, intimate relationship or as part of a single life-style. The capacity to interact in sexually satisfying ways is influenced by a number of factors. A good knowledge of one's own body and its capabilities, as well as knowledge of the partner, is an essential prerequisite. Open communication about sexuality between partners is also an important factor. Knowledge and communication are frequently described as the most crucial factors determining the health of any sexual relationship. Other factors, such as parenting, role changes, and differences in sexual responsiveness, have less influence when knowledge and communication are effective. Sexuality, like any other part of interpersonal relationships, consists of learned beliefs, attitudes, and behaviors. This learning is best accomplished when it is shared by the partners in a relationship.

Late Adulthood

Biologic Components

The major biologic changes in the older female include a continued atrophy of vaginal and breast tissue (including loss of elasticity), decrease and slowing of vaginal lubrication during arousal, decreased vaginal expansion, diminished orgasmic intensity, and a more rapid resolution. (See the section on "Sexual Stimulation and Response Patterns," later in the chapter.) Older women do retain the capacity for multiple orgasms.

Sexual changes in the older male include lowered sperm production, reduction in the size and firmness of the testicles, delay in achieving erection, greater ejaculatory control, less myotonia, reduced orgasmic intensity, more rapid resolution, and longer refractory period. Many older men also experience enlargement of the prostate gland, which may be benign or malignant.

Psychosocial Components

Major issues influencing sexual development in late adulthood include adjusting to changing body image, adjusting to changes in family or marital status, retirement, change in body function, and decrease in mobility. Despite all these adjustments, the older adult has the capacity to continue with satisfying interpersonal and sexual relationships indefinitely.

Our society places a high value on youth and youthful beauty. The aging person is unable to match such standards and may respond to changes in body image with lowered self-esteem. Widowhood or widowerhood, loss of contact with grown children, and loss of friends have the potential for creating loneliness and depression.

Lowered self-esteem and loneliness, combined with reduced body function and loss of mobility, can lead to social isolation and loss of interaction opportunities. Society has also made it difficult for older adults to interact sexually because of negative attitudes about sexual activity among the aging. The majority of older adults retain the interest and capacity to engage in satisfying sexual relationships, whose nature is frequently more nurturing and caring and less intense sexually than in earlier years. The greatest predictor of sexual interest and activity in the later years is the pattern of sexual activity and interest throughout life, true for married adults, widowed adults, and single adults—whether heterosexual or homosexual.

Patterns of Sexual Functioning

The interaction of contextual and developmental factors results in the capacity to function in reciprocal ways as a sexual being. As noted in the introduction to this chapter, biologic sex, gender identity, and gender role are the major components of individual sexuality. We can understand patterns of sexual functioning by building on our knowledge of these components through discussion of gender-role behavior, sexual structures and function, and sexual stimulation and response patterns.

Gender-role Behavior

Gender-role behavior is the outward expression of a person's sense of maleness or femaleness as well as the expression of what is perceived as gender-appropriate behavior. Expectations regarding gender-appropriate role behavior begin their influence at birth and continue throughout life. Each society or culture, including our own, establishes boundaries for acceptable gender-role behavior. Congruence between an individual's gender identity and expression of role behavior is the ideal, one not always easy to achieve. Physical structure, variations in the internal sense of what is male or female, family values, and cultural values all influence gender-role behavior. The result usually is gender-role behavior that falls within the fairly broad boundaries of what is acceptable in our society. Expected adult male roles (and their accompanying behaviors) include breadwinner, heterosexual lover, father, athlete. Men are expected to wear trousers, demonstrate physical strength, carry themselves in certain ways, and express feelings in a controlled fashion. Women are expected to express their emotions more freely and to be more gentle in their physical responses; they also have a broader choice of clothing than men. These descriptions represent the kinds of gender-role behaviors that are reinforced in our society. However, many individuals today express themselves with gender-role behaviors that do not conform to these stereotypes. This stretching of the boundaries can create stress for the individual and for society.

There have been more and more variations in gender roles and gender-role behavior in recent years, but these variations are still often portrayed as aberrant, humorous, or wrong. In fact, many people are stretching the boundaries of what was once considered the norm. Men sport long hair, earrings, and cosmetics. Women wear construction boots, jeans, and men's suits. Men make loving and sensitive single fathers. Women are bosses—competitive and assertive. Openly gay male and lesbian relationships are on the increase. Sexually active older adults are common. All these are potentially healthy expressions of gender identity and gender role. Such a wide variety of gender-role behaviors represents legitimate expressions of the self as a sexual being. All individuals need sanction of and support for those gender-role behaviors that validate their sense of self. Labeling these behaviors as problematic and intervening for change should rightly occur only when the behaviors create significant problems for the individual and his or her relationship with the world.

Sexual Structures and Function

Male Genitals

The male genitals, which function to produce and transport sperm, include two sperm-producing testes encased in the scrotum, a series of ducts (epididymis and vas deferens) that transport sperm, several glands that secrete fluid (semen) to protect the sperm, and the penis to ejaculate the semen. See Figure 19-1.

Testes The **testes**, or male gonads, are oval organs about 3.75 cm (1½ in) long and 2.5 cm (1 in) wide. Each testis

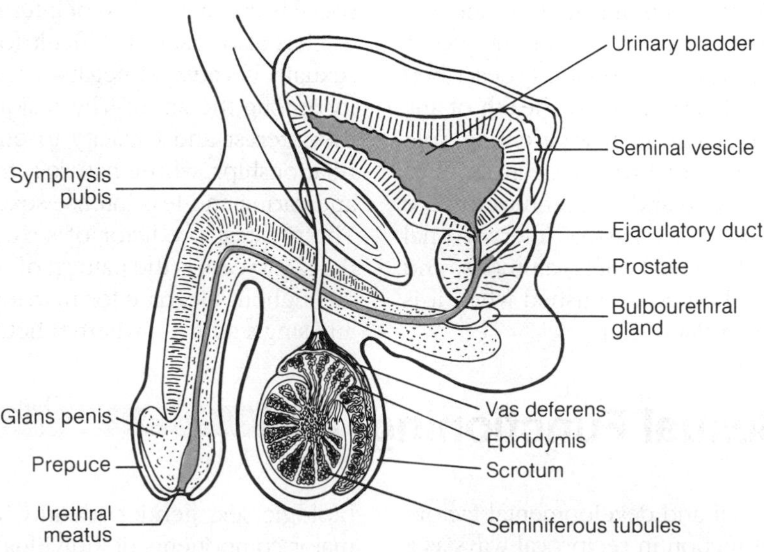

Figure 19–1 The male genitourinary system.

is encased in a dense, white, fibrous capsule called the **tunica albuginea**. Inward extensions (septa) of this capsule divide the testis into 200 or more compartments (lobules). Each compartment contains several highly coiled tubules, called **seminiferous tubules**, that manufacture sperm. Between the seminiferous tubules are clusters of cells, called the **interstitial cells of Leydig**, that secrete male hormones.The two major functions of the testes are **spermatogenesis** (production of the sperm) and the production of sexual hormones.

A sperm consists of a head, neckpiece, midpiece, and tail. The sperm contains **chromosomes**, which transmit inherited characteristics.

The chief testicular hormone is **testosterone**, an androgen, which stimulates genital growth and the development of secondary sexual characteristics, such as a deeper voice, larger musculature, and hair on the face and chest. The testes also produce estrogen and other androgens. **Estrogen**, which is also produced by the adrenal glands, seems to control spermatogenesis.

The male hormones are regulated by the hypothalamus. This organ secretes releasing factors that travel through the bloodstream to the pituitary gland. When stimulated by releasing factors, the pituitary gland secretes **follicle stimulating hormone (FSH)** and **luteinizing hormone (LH)**. LH stimulates the secretion of testosterone, and FSH stimulates spermatogenesis. Both operate via a negative-feedback system.

Scrotum The testes, located outside of the body cavity, are protected from injury by the **scrotum**, the sac that hangs behind the penis. In humans the scrotal sac is located in the groin area and is an outpouching of the abdominal wall. The outer skin layer of the scrotum is wrinkled and relatively hairless. Beneath this layer of skin is a layer of smooth muscle and tough connective tissue called the **tunica dartos** and then another layer of striated muscle and connective tissue called the **cremaster**. Smooth muscles contract involuntarily, whereas striated muscles can contract voluntarily or involuntarily. Within these three layers of tissue the testes lie protected. Usually the left testis hangs lower in the scrotal sac than the right.

In the fetus, the testes are located inside the abdominal cavity, but before birth, male sexual hormones cause the testes to drop into the scrotal sacs. The testes descend through the inguinal canal in the groin, usually before birth.

Failure of one or both testes to descend is called **cryptorchidism**, which in the majority of males is bilateral. During the first year of life, spontaneous descent of the testes may occur. If not, male hormone therapy may be necessary from 1 to 4 years of age to stimulate descent. Surgical intervention to bring the testes into the scrotum is done by 3–4 years of age. If both testes fail to descend by age 5, damage to the testes and sterility result. Although males with undescended testicles produce normal amounts of male sex hormones, they are usually infertile, because the abdominal body temperature is too high for spermatogenesis.

The scrotum not only protects the testes but also helps maintain an appropriate temperature for sperm, as follows:

1. The thin scrotal skin, with little underlying fat, offers little insulation.
2. Many superficial small blood vessels in the scrotum dissipate heat, as necessary.
3. Abundant sweat glands enhance cooling via evaporation.
4. When temperatures are too cool, muscle receptors, particularly in the tunica dartos, contract and push the testes up toward the groin to be warmed.

Athletic supporters and tight garments that squeeze the scrotum up against the groin raise scrotal temperature. Prolonged wear of such garments can reduce sperm production. The cremaster muscle, though not much involved in temperature regulation, also can influence scrotal temperature. Strong contractions of the cremaster muscle brought about by sexual excitement, fear, anxiety, or stimulation of the cremasteric reflex (a response to the stroking of the inner surface of the thighs) increase blood flow from the testes back into the body, thereby decreasing scrotal temperature. However, these contractions are not sustained for long periods.

Epididymis, vas deferens, and ejaculatory ducts The testes contain coiled seminiferous tubules that manufacture sperm. These tubules drain into a highly coiled duct outside of the testis called the **epididymis**. The epididymis then drains into the **vas deferens**, a long tube that extends from the scrotum, curves around the urinary bladder, and empties into the **ejaculatory ducts**. The two ejaculatory ducts, one from each testis, are short, and both connect with the urethra. See Figure 19-1.

The mechanisms by which sperm are transported to the epididymis are not fully understood. Transport may be facilitated by contractions of the seminiferous tubules. Cilia, which line the tubules, also move the sperm toward the epididymis.

The epididymis has the following functions:

1. Maturation of sperm prior to ejaculation
2. Transport from the testis to the exterior
3. Secretion of small amounts of seminal fluid.

The vas deferens serves to store mature sperm between ejaculations. Both the vas deferens and ejaculatory ducts help propel the sperm and semen into the urethra and then out of the body.

Seminal vesicles, prostate gland, and bulbourethral gland The **seminal vesicles**, prostate gland, and bulbourethral glands (see Figure 19-1) produce substances, collectively referred to as **seminal plasma**, that energize the sperm and enhance their transport but are not essential for mature sperm. The bulbourethral glands are also known as Cowper's glands. Seminal plasma combined with sperm is referred to as **semen**. The characteristics of normal semen are:

1. Creamy texture
2. Gray or yellow color
3. Ejaculate volume of 2 to 6 ml
4. 120 million sperm per milliliter of seminal plasma
5. Slightly alkaline pH (7.35 to 7.50)

Primary components of seminal plasma are:

1. Water to transport the sperm
2. Mucus to lubricate the ducts
3. Sugar (fructose) to energize the sperm
4. Salts to maintain isotonicity of the seminal plasma with body fluids
5. Base buffers to neutralize the acidity of the male urethra and subsequently the female vagina
6. Coagulators to clot the semen in the vagina and prevent leakage of sperm from the vagina (Mann 1970, pp. 469–78).

Penis The penis has two parts: the shaft and the **glans penis**. In the uncircumcised penis, the skin of the shaft loosely encloses the glans. This is the **foreskin (prepuce)**. **Smegma**, a cheesy material that is a mixture of glans oil secretions and dead tissue cells, accumulates between the foreskin and the glans, and must be cleaned from the glans at every washing.

Penis shape and size vary considerably, not so much in circumference as in length. Males frequently feel concern about their penis size, relating size directly to their capabilities as lovers. Size, however, is unrelated to capability. Like breast size, penis length has little to do with function. Also, the vagina, mouth, and rectum accommodate different penile circumferences.

The reproductive function of the penis is to transmit semen to the female. This process includes erection of the penis and ejaculation of the semen, after which the penis returns to a flaccid state.

Erection involves the lengthening, widening, and hardening of the penis as it becomes **tumescent** (congested) with blood. Erection is a spinal reflex that is triggered when the erection center, located at the first to fourth sacral segments of the spinal cord, is stimulated. Erection commonly occurs in response to erotic thoughts or other sexual stimuli or to the manipulation (touching) of the penis. However, erections occasionally occur in the absence of apparent sexual stimuli. Such **reflexogenic erections** can be cause for embarrassment. For example, teenagers whose nervous systems are immature often experience unexpected erection when taking a shower following athletic activity. It is not uncommon for nurses to encounter reflexogenic erections in nursing practice, for example, while removing the inguinal sutures of a young teenager. Erection upon awakening is also common among both men and boys. The reason for these erections is not fully understood; they may be due to the pressure of a full bladder, erotic dreams, friction against the sheets, or waking at the end of a paradoxical sleep phase.

Ejaculation, the propulsion of semen out of the penis, is also a spinal reflex. However, the ejaculatory center is higher in the spinal cord than the erection center (from the third lumbar to the twelfth thoracic segment). Ejaculation has two stages: (1) semen is transported to the urethra (emission stage), and (2) the semen is propelled out of the urethra (expulsion stage). The force of expulsion depends on the degree of arousal, the time lapse between ejaculations, age, and other factors. Semen may ooze out over the glans penis or may be projected a certain distance.

Sperm are concentrated in the first third of semen ejaculated. Sperm are also present in secretions from the seminal vesicles, prostate, and bulbourethral glands. These secretions collect at the urethral opening before ejaculation. Thus, pregnancy can occur without ejaculation. Couples who use withdrawal of the penis before ejaculation as a form of contraception need to know this.

After erection the penis returns to a flaccid state. This process, referred to as **detumescence**, occurs whether or not ejaculation has occurred. The penile arteries constrict, thereby reducing the blood flow to the penis, and the venous outflow allows the engorged blood vessels to empty.

Female Genitals

The female genitals include two ovaries, two fallopian tubes, the uterus, the vagina, and the vulva. See Figure 19-2. These structures provide a system for giving sexual pleasure, receiving sperm, producing eggs, housing and nurturing the fertilized egg, and delivering the mature fetus. The mammary glands, although not part of the female genitals, are included in this discussion because they are necessary for suckling the young and give sexual pleasure.

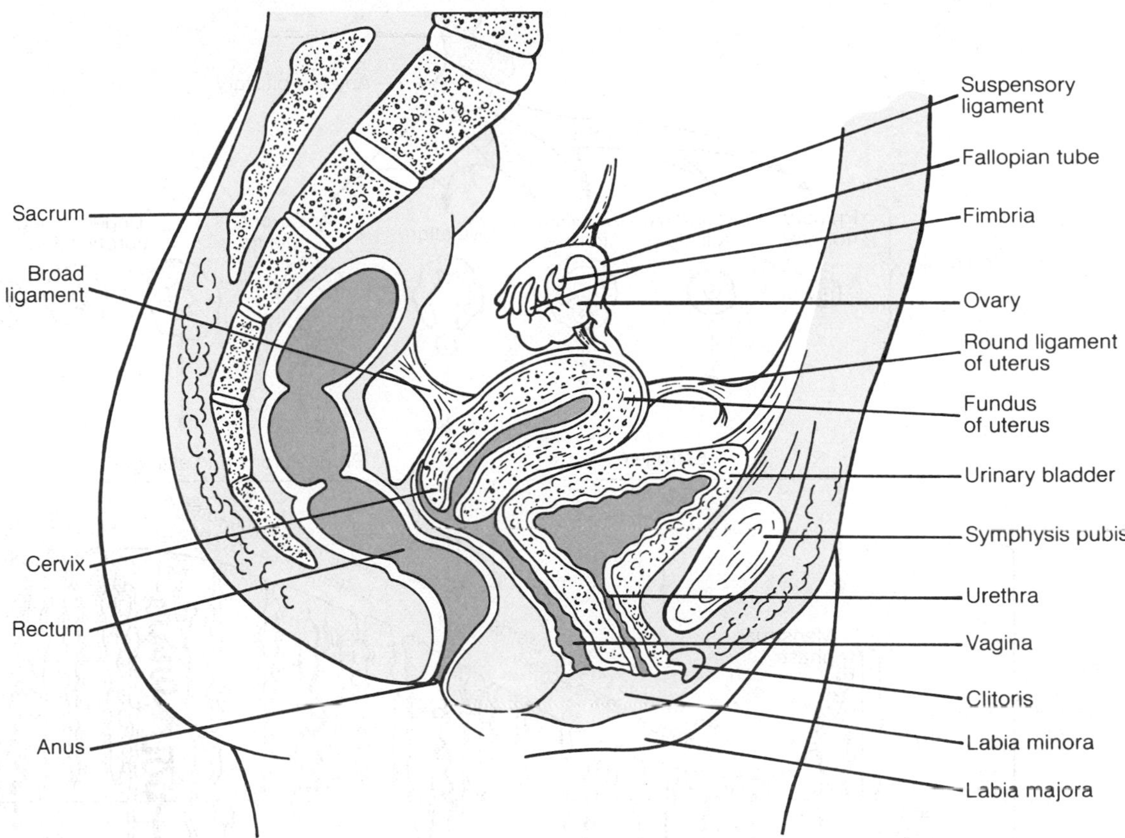

Figure 19–2 The female reproductive tract.

Ovaries The **ovaries**, or female gonads, are analogous to the testes in that they produce reproductive cells (ova, or female gametes) and secrete hormones, but they are located in the pelvic region of the abdominal cavity. Adult ovaries are oval and approximately 2.5 cm (1 in) long. The inner portion of the ovary, called the **ovarian medulla**, consists of spirals or coils of blood vessels and connective tissue. The outer portion, called the **ovarian cortex**, is the site where eggs develop and from which the hormones are secreted.

The ovaries have two primary functions: (a) production and expulsion of ova and (b) production of sexual hormones. In contrast to the testes, which produce sperm throughout life, the ovary contains all the primordial (primitive) ova at birth. These primordial ova originate on the outer surface (germinal layer) of the ovary but move from the outer layer of the cortex during fetal life into the main substance of the cortex, where they then become surrounded by a single layer of **granulosa cells**, and after which time they are referred to as **primordial follicles**. Although at birth about 750,000 primordial follicles are present in the two ovaries, only about 450 of them will develop sufficiently throughout the female reproductive life to expel their ova (Guyton 1981, p. 1005). Primordial follicles degenerate throughout life, a process called **follicular atresia**. By puberty only 400,000 follicles remain, and by **menopause** (the period of natural cessation of menstruation, usually between the ages of 45 and 50) only a few remain (Guyton 1981, p. 1005).

Two female sex hormones are produced by the ovaries: estrogen and progesterone. In addition, some androgens are secreted. **Estrogen** has several effects, including regulating fat distribution and breast development, and neutralizing vaginal pH during ovulation. Its primary control is exerted during the first half of the menstrual cycle. **Progesterone** controls the second half of the menstrual cycle but also influences breast development. It inhibits uterine muscle contractions during pregnancy. The **androgens** are thought to increase sexual motivation.

Like male hormones, female sexual hormones are controlled by homeostatic negative-feedback systems, but they are produced cyclically (hence the female sexual cycle, or monthly menstrual cycle). These feedback systems also involve three different hierarchies of hormones: (a) releasing factors for FSH and LH from the hypothalamus, (b) the pituitary secretions of FSH and LH, and (c) the production of hormones (estrogen and progesterone) from the gonads (ovaries).

Female sexual cycle The female sexual cycle averages about 28 days in length, though it can normally vary between 20 and 35 days. See Figure 19-3. This cycle can be considered in three stages: preovulatory, postovulatory, and menses.

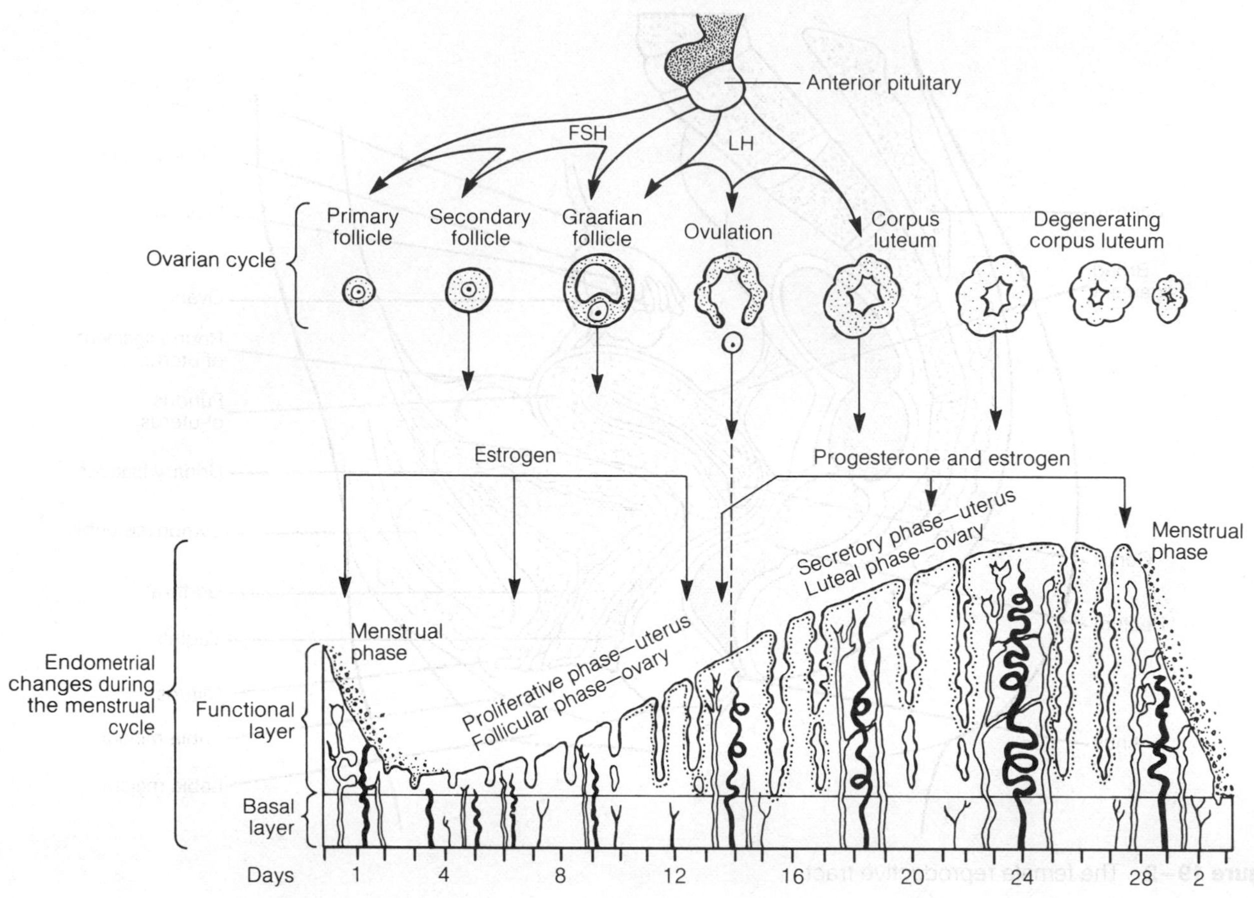

Figure 19–3 Changes in the endometrium and ovary during the menstrual cycle.
Source: S. B. Olds, M. L. London, and P. A. Ladewig, *Maternal newborn nursing,* 2nd ed. (Menlo Park, Calif.: Addison-Wesley, 1984).

Preovulatory stage The **preovulatory stage** (also referred to as the **proliferative** or **follicular stage**) lasts an average of 14 days (plus or minus 3 to 5 days), starting on the first day of menstrual flow and ending with **ovulation** (release of the ovum from the ovary). On the first day of this stage, the follicles begin to grow spontaneously, without hormonal control. Then the pituitary gland, stimulated by the hypothalmic FSH-releasing factor, produces FSH, which stimulates the follicles to enlarge further. One of these follicles, outgrowing the others, becomes large enough to ovulate. The other follicles undergo atresia. The enlarged follicle is called the **Graafian follicle** (maturing follicle). Estrogen secretion is then stimulated by this follicle under the influence of FSH. The effects of estrogen include the buildup of the endometrium (the lining of the uterus) for anticipated conception and the final maturation of the Graafian follicle immediately before ovulation. Once estrogen reaches its peak level in the bloodstream, the production of FSH is decreased by negative feedback. But a sudden surge of LH is then released by the pituitary gland, triggering ovulation.

Postovulatory stage The **postovulatory stage** begins immediately after ovulation and lasts an average of about 13 days in the female whose cycle is 28 days. It ends when the woman begins her menstrual period. This phase is also referred to as the **secretory** or **luteal stage**. The term **secretory** is used because the lining of the uterus secretes a substance (carbohydrate glycogen) to provide nourishment for a fertilized ovum (**zygote**). The term **luteal** stems from the fact that the Graafian follicle, under the influence of LH, undergoes changes, forming a yellowish mass in the ovary known as the **corpus luteum**.

If the ovum is fertilized, the corpus luteum grows and persists for several months. It secretes progesterone as well as estrogen. Progesterone is responsible for keeping the uterine lining receptive for implantation and development of the zygote. Estrogen enhances the action of progesterone. Via negative feedback, progesterone inhibits the production of LH, and estrogen inhibits the production of FSH. These luteal hormones maintain the implanted zygote for about 3 months until the placenta develops. Then the placenta secretes these hormones.

If fertilization does not occur, the corpus luteum gradually degenerates, becoming white and scarred, then being referred to as the **corpus albicans**. Reduction in the production of progesterone and estrogen result, and menstrual flow is induced. Without hormonal stimulation, the endometrial arteries collapse and the endometrium shrinks. The resultant deoxygenation of the endometrium causes the tissue to die. Most of these dead tissues are sloughed off, and bleeding occurs through the weak, collapsed capillaries.

Menses **Menses** (menstruous flow) lasts for 3 to 7 days. Menstruation overlaps with the beginning of the preovulatory phase. The first day of flow is considered the first day of the sexual cycle. The amount of menstrual discharge varies from woman to woman and from cycle to cycle, ranging from 30 to 180 ml (1 to 6 oz) and averaging about 90 ml (3 oz). Women using the combination contraceptive pill tend to have less than the average discharge, whereas women with intrauterine devices (IUDs) often have heavier flows.

Menarche, the first menstrual period, occurs between the ages of 9 and 17 years. For the first few years, ovulation and menses may be somewhat erratic. Eventually a stable rhythm is established, which is maintained until menopause.

Menstrual cramps are common, particularly during the first few days of menstruation because of contractions of the uterus and cervix. Their cause is undetermined.

Moods can change before and during menstruation. A few days before, some women feel tense, anxious, irritable, depressed, or hostile. At menstruation, most of these feelings are eased or disappear. However depression is common until estrogen levels become elevated during the preovulatory stage. By the time of ovulation, when estrogen levels are at their peak, women tend to feel happy and self-confident. Thus mood swings during the female sexual cycle are influenced by the hormonal changes that occur throughout the cycle. Conversely, a woman's emotional state can also influence her hormonal levels. For example, a woman stressed by illness, a work crisis, or a family conflict can experience altered hormonal levels that affect menstruation. Also, a woman may not menstruate during one cycle because of stress.

Fallopian tubes The two **fallopian tubes** (oviducts), which are about 10 cm (4 in) long, extend between the ovaries and uterus but are not attached to the ovaries. Their chief function is to provide an environment appropriate for the transport, in opposite directions, of the ova and sperm and thus for fertilization. Secretory cells in the mucosal lining of the tube are believed to nourish the ovum.

The mechanism by which ova are transported from the ovaries into the fallopian tubes is not fully understood. Because the two structures are unattached, an ovum occasionally is released into the abdominal cavity rather than into a fallopian tube. If this egg is fertilized and implanted in the abdominal cavity, the condition is referred to as an **ectopic pregnancy** (implantation of a zygote outside the uterus). Ectopic pregnancy in the fallopian tube also occurs occasionally.

Fertilization of ova usually occurs in the middle third of a fallopian tube. The transport of the sperm is facilitated by muscle contractions of the tubes and by the sperm's active swimming movements. Transport of the zygote is facilitated by the motion of cilia in the tube, which sweep toward the uterus, and also by tubal muscle contractions. Generally, the zygote is transported to the uterus in about 3 days. However, this rate of transport is influenced by progesterone and estrogen: progesterone retards the rate of transport, whereas estrogen accelerates it. Estrogen can therefore be used to prevent implantation of the zygote. Large doses of estrogen administered after coitus accelerate the transport of the zygote before it is ready for implantation. Estrogen also alters the endometrial lining, making it inappropriate for receiving the zygote.

Uterus The **uterus**, which lies between the rectum and the urinary bladder, is one of the most changeable organs of the body. It is thick-walled and hollow and has three layers: the **perimetrium**, the thin outer layer of serous membrane; the **myometrium**, the thick, middle layer of smooth muscle; and the **endometrium**, the inner mucous membrane lining. The perimetrium covers the entire uterus except for the **cervix** (the neck of the uterus). The myometrium contains many muscle fibers running in different directions. Contractions of these fibers occur during childbirth, sexual tension, and orgasm. During pregnancy the uterus enlarges and the muscle fibers grow longer. Muscular contractions dilate the cervix and help to expel the fetus.

The endometrium has two principal layers: the **functionalis**, the layer shed during menstruation, and the **basalis**, the layer closest to the myometrium. The basalis layer is maintained during menstruation and produces a new functionalis layer after menstruation. The endometrial lining is essential for the reception and maintenance of fertilized egg implantation and for the development of the zygote. The uterine lining of the cervix has glands that produce mucus, which plugs the opening into the uterus. During ovulation, when estrogen levels are high, the characteristics of this mucous plug change. The mucus becomes more copious, thinner, and thus more penetrable by sperm. Examination of the characteristics of the cervical mucous plug can help determine whether a woman is ovulating or infertile.

Vagina The **vagina** has a threefold function. It serves as the lower part of the birth canal, as the passageway for menstrual flow, and as the receptacle for the penis during sexual intercourse. The vaginal organ, a muscular tube lined with mucous membrane, is about 10 cm (4 in) long. The mucosa of the vagina is capable of a great deal of extension because it lies in a series of inwardly directed and transverse folds called **rugae**. The muscular layer of the vagina can also stretch considerably. This distensibility is important during delivery and intercourse.

Large amounts of glycogen (a type of carbohydrate) are produced in the vagina. Glycogen decomposes into lactic acid from the action of normal bacteria of the vagina (**Döderlein's bacilli**). These acids create a low-pH environment, which prevents bacterial and yeast infections in the vagina. Although this acidity is also injurious to sperm cells, the buffering action of semen ensures the sperm's survival. Döderlein's bacilli can be destroyed by antibiotics. Thus it is not uncommon for women taking antibiotics for other infections to get vaginal infections.

Changes in the vaginal mucosa occur in response to estrogen during the menstrual cycle and in response to sexual excitement. Normally, the cells of the vaginal mucosa continually slough off and are replaced by new cells. During the menstrual cycle these cells, under the influence of estrogen, undergo **cornification** (hardening). Such cells can be examined under a microscope, using cells obtained from a vaginal swab and transferred to a glass slide. This examination is commonly called a **vaginal smear**. Examination of vaginal smears taken at the time of ovulation can help diagnose infertility. Estrogen levels at such times are usually high.

During sexual excitement the numerous small blood vessels of the vagina become engorged with blood, giving it a purplish hue. This congestion is also responsible for the lubrication of the vagina when a woman is sexually excited. Initially, small droplets of fluid exude through the blood vessel walls. As sexual excitement increases, these droplets of fluid coalesce to form a shiny layer of lubricant over the mucosa.

At the **vaginal orifice** (the external opening of the vagina) is a thin fold of vascularized mucous membrane called the **hymen**, which forms a border around the orifice and partially closes it. Sometimes the hymen is **imperforate**—that is, it covers the orifice completely. An imperforate hymen warrants medical intervention to permit the passage of menstrual flow.

Vulva The external female genitals are collectively referred to as the **vulva**, or **pudendum**. The structures of the vulva include the mons pubis, two labia majora, two labia minora, the clitoris, and the vestibule.

The **mons pubis**, also referred to as the **mons veneris**, is a pillow of adipose tissue situated over the symphysis pubis and covered by coarse pubic hair. The mons pubis is highly sensitive and contains many touch receptors. Stimulation of the mons during intercourse or masturbation can lead to orgasm.

The **labia majora** ("large lips") are the two longitudinal folds of skin extending downward and backward from the mons pubis. They serve to protect the labia minora and the openings of the vagina and urethra. The labia majora are covered by hair on their upper outer surfaces and contain an abundance of adipose tissue and sebaceous and sweat glands. Usually the labia majora meet in a deep cleft. However, during periods of sexual excitement these lips separate and flatten against the inner thighs to expose the labia minora and vaginal opening.

The **labia minora** lie inside the labia majora. They are devoid of hair and have relatively few sweat glands; however, they do contain numerous sebaceous glands. The labia minora extend upward to unite and form the prepuce (foreskin) of the clitoris and downward to protect the vaginal opening. Because the small lips undergo vivid color changes during sexual excitement, they are often called the "sex skin." The color changes are due to increased influx of blood and vary in proportion to the level of arousal. Pregnancy also contributes to color changes. In the nonpregnant woman the labia minora are normally pale pink, becoming bright red when the woman is sexually excited. In the pregnant woman, the labia minora contain more blood vessels and thus are normally red in color. When a pregnant woman is sexually excited, the labia minora assume a deep wine color. These color changes are positive signs of approaching orgasm.

The **clitoris** is a small round mass of erectile tissue, blood vessels, and nerves located behind the junction of the labia minora (the prepuce). The exposed part of the clitoris is referred to as the **glans clitoris**. The clitoris is capable of enlargement when stimulated and is homologous to the penis. Its principal function is to receive and transmit erotic stimuli during sexual excitement. When a woman is aroused sexually, the glans becomes tumescent and is elevated upward so that it becomes hidden behind the prepuce.

The **vestibule**, the cleft between the labia, contains the vaginal orifice, urethral orifice, hymen, and openings of several ducts. The vaginal orifice occupies the major portion of the vestibule. Above the vaginal orifice and below the clitoris lies the urethral orifice. The ducts of glands that secrete mucus (the lesser **vestibular glands**) are located behind and on either side of the urethra. These lesser vestibular glands are homologous to the prostate. Larger glands (the greater vestibular glands) lie on either side of the vaginal orifice. Their ducts open into the space between the hymen and labia minora. These glands are homologous to the bulbourethral glands and produce a mucous secretion that acts as a lubricant during intercourse.

Mammary glands The **mammary glands** (breasts) not only secrete milk but also respond to stimulation and give sexual pleasure. Each mammary gland consists of lobes (compartments) separated by adipose tissue, which is the primary factor determining the size of the breasts. Each lobe has smaller compartments called lobules, which contain milk-secreting cells, called alveoli, that are clustered in grapelike arrangements. The milk from the alveoli is conveyed into a series of tubules and then into the mammary ducts, the ampullae (expanded sinuses where milk can be stored), and the lactiferous ducts, which terminate in the nipple. Each lactiferous duct conveys the milk from one of the lobes to the nipple. Surrounding the nipple is a circular pigmented area called the **areola**. Because it contains sebaceous glands, the areola is bumpy or rough.

The breasts begin to develop at puberty, under the influence of estrogen produced by the ovaries, progesterone, growth hormone from the pituitary, prolactin from the pituitary, and thyroxine from the thyroid.

Women worry about the size and shape of breasts much as men worry about penis size and shape. Breast size and shape, however, do not affect functioning. Women also may worry about how pregnancy and nursing will affect breast size and shape. During pregnancy the breasts become heavier and some of the supporting ligaments may stretch, causing the breasts to hang slightly lower thereafter. However, nursing does not permanently alter breast size, shape, or "lift."

Sexual Stimulation and Response Patterns

Sexual Stimulation

The sexually functional human body (anatomically and physiologically) is capable of responding to a wide variety of physical and psychologic stimuli. These stimuli, often called **erotic**, may be real or symbolic. In the right circumstances, imagination, sight, hearing, smell, and touch can all invoke sexual arousal.

Physical Stimulation

Physical stimulation involves touch and/or pressure to parts of the body and may be applied by one's self, by another's body contact or by inanimate objects. Nerve receptors then transmit these stimuli to the spinal cord and brain. Examples include kissing, stroking, hugging, squeezing, breast stimulation, manual stimulation of the genitals, oral–genital stimulation, and anal stimulation. Any of these may be engaged in for sexual pleasure on their own or—as is most common in North America—as prelude to genital intercourse. Physical stimulation used as a lead-in to intercourse is called **foreplay** or **precoital stimulation**. Physical stimulation used for sexual pleasure is called **sex play**. Wide variations exist in the amount and types of physical stimulation used by North Americans.

Certain parts of the body are richly supplied with nerve endings and give sexual pleasure when stimulated. These areas are called erogenous zones. There is also a psychological component that involves the linking of particular stimuli to a sexual context. The most common erogenous zones are, of course, the genitals of both sexes. Other areas include the breasts, the mouth, thighs, buttocks, earlobes, neck, and anus; however, stimulation of any body area can become sexually arousing. Erogenous zones adapt rapidly to continuous stimulation by becoming decreasingly responsive. Because touch and pressure receptors respond better to *changes* in stimulation, sexual arousal can be increased by alternating sites of stimulation rather than maintaining continuous contact with one or two areas.

Kissing Kissing, which involves the senses of touch, taste, and smell, is unique to humans as a source of erotic stimulation. This type of sexual stimulation ranges from lip-to-lip kissing to deep tongue kissing.

Stroking, hugging, and squeezing These behaviors vary according to the interests of the individuals involved, extending from light, gentle hugging and stroking, through firm, energetic hugging and stroking, to hard squeezing, pinching, biting, and scratching. These last examples involve some pain, which can be erotically stimulating when engaged in voluntarily by sexual partners.

Breast stimulation Oral or manual stimulation of the female breasts can produce sexual pleasure. Stimulation of the breasts involves release of the pituitary hormone oxytocin, which stimulates milk secretions and smooth muscle contractions in the uterus and related structures. Breast stimulation thus can produce pleasurable, erotically-associated contractions in the pelvic region. These sensations can be a source of sexual satisfaction on their own, including orgasm or as an adjunct to other sexual interaction. They can also be produced in nursing mothers, who may need reassurance that this is a normative, healthy phenomenon. Stimulation of men's nipples may also produce erotic responses. Though this is not as common in men as in women, it is normative and healthy when present.

Manual stimulation of the genitals Manual stimulation may be used to produce orgasm or as part of a range of physical stimulation leading to sexual intercourse. Manual self-stimulation is called **masturbation**. Reciprocal manual stimulation is called **mutual masturbation**. In males, stimulation of the penis produces a more erotic response than stimulation of the scrotum. Firm gripping and stroking of the shaft and glans of the penis is the most common form of masturbation. Light rubbing or tugging at the **frenulum** (the fold of tissue that connects the lower surface of the glans to the prepuce) can also produce sexual excitement. In addition to these more common forms of male masturbation, different men use different variations of stroking, pulling, and rubbing. Whatever method is used, as sexual excitement increases, manipulation often becomes more rapid and intense, until ejaculation occurs. After ejaculation the glans penis is often hypersensitive to touch.

Manipulation of the female genitals is often more variable than that of male genitals. Stimulation of the clitoris is usually a major erotic focus for females. This highly sensitive area rarely requires direct stimulation. Rubbing pressure on the mons pubis, pulling or rubbing the clitoral hood (prepuce), or pulling on the labia will stimulate the clitoral shaft and produce intensely erotic responses. Some women use external manipulation as well as insertion of fingers into the vagina to produce sexual excitement.

Contrary to popular belief, masturbation in itself is neither physically nor mentally harmful. More than 85% of males and 60% of females masturbate, ranging in frequency from several times a day to only occasionally. Most men begin to masturbate earlier in life (often before the age of 20 years) than women, many of whom may not masturbate until adulthood. Some individuals use sexual implements when masturbating, including vibrators, **dildos** (artificial penises), and other genital substitutes.

Oral–genital stimulation There are three forms of oral–genital stimulation. **Cunnilingus** involves oral stimulation (kissing, licking, or sucking) of the female genitals, including the mons pubis, vulva, clitoris, labia, and vagina. **Fellatio** involves oral stimulation of the penis by licking and sucking. **Soixante-neuf** ("69") involves simultaneous oral–genital stimulation by two persons. These practices, like other physical stimulation, may be engaged in for the pleasure they give, including orgasm, or as a component of behaviors around genital intercourse. As with masturbation, there is no evidence that oral–genital contact is harmful. However, some people continue to hold strong negative feelings about these behaviors.

Anal stimulation The anus is richly innervated and can be a source of sexual pleasure. Oral–anal stimulation is called **anilingus**. Stimulation may also be applied by hands or by sex aids such as vibrators or dildos. Because the anus is associated with feces, many people do not include anal stimulation as part of their sexual repertoire.

Psychologic Stimulation

Although the excitatory process involves physiology, erotic stimulation through smell, taste, hearing, sight, or fantasy is considered psychologic because the responses relate to thought processes and feelings. The stimuli evoke pleasant past experiences or hopes and desires.

Odors The odor of bodies, perfumes, certain fabrics (e.g., leather), flowers, etc. can produce erotic responses in sexual situations. Usually, different people associate specific odors with specific situations.

Sights Again because of their specific associations, certain sights can produce erotic responses. The more obvious sights include naked bodies and pictures of naked bodies and sexual acts. Other less obvious sights include romantic photographs, decor, lighting, and colors.

Sounds Sexual excitement is often enhanced by sound. The spoken word and music are frequent adjuncts to sexual activity. "Whispering sweet nothings" and "talking dirty" are examples. Music is frequently associated with specific sexual situations.

Fantasy Most people engage in fantasy in relation to sexuality. The fantasizing usually involves idealized sexual situations but may also include so-called "forbidden" fantasies: mental imagery of unusual or "risqué" activities that are out of bounds in real life. Fantasy is employed both during solo sexual activities (masturbation) and when with a partner.

Sexual Response Patterns

Physiologic responses to sexual stimulation are basically the same for all individuals, male or female. However, such responses are highly variable, with differences occurring between males and females, among members of the same sex, and in the same person at different times.

Genital intercourse The most common form of sexual activity with a partner is heterosexual genital intercourse, also known as **coitus** or **copulation**. Penile–vaginal intercourse can be both physically and emotionally satisfying. There are a variety of positions for this kind of intercourse, the most common being lying down face-to-face (with female or male on top). Side-lying, standing, sitting, and rear-entry are also used. To increase clitoral stimulation, (either by penile contact or manual contact), side-lying, female-on-top, and rear-entry positions are most helpful. An individual's or couple's choice of intercourse positions and activities will depend on physical comfort and beliefs, values, and attitudes about different practices.

The other main form of genital intercourse is **anal intercourse**, which involves insertion of the penis into the anus and rectum of the partner. Anal intercourse is most common in gay male couples but is practiced by heterosexual couples as well. Positions for anal intercourse are similar to those for penile–vaginal intercourse, with minor differences due to the position of the anus. Because anorectal tissue is not self-lubricating, lubrication must be added by the participants. Since normal bacterial flora from the bowel can produce infection in other parts of the body, the penis should be cleaned before being inserted into other body orifices, or a condom should be worn.

Lesbians and gay men, because penile–vaginal intercourse is not the goal of their sexual interactions, engage in a variety of other sexual activities that collectively can be labeled intercourse. Oral sex, manual sex, frottage (body rubbing), and the use of sex aids are all potential parts of the "intercourse" repertoire. There is no evidence that this type of sexual interaction is any less satisfying than heterosexual penile–vaginal intercourse.

Physiology of the Sexual Response Cycle

Two primary physiologic changes occur during sexual arousal: vasocongestion (congestion of the blood vessels) and **myotonia** (increased muscle tension). Physiologic changes have been identified that fall into four phases: excitement, plateau, orgasm, and resolution (Masters and Johnson 1966, p.4). It is important to remember that individual responses will demonstrate variations of this cycle and that such variation falls within the range of the norm.

Excitement phase The *excitement phase* develops from erotic stimuli and involves a gradual increase in the level of sexual arousal. This phase may last minutes to hours. Signs of this stage in the male include:

1. Increased muscle tension
2. Moderate increase in heart rate, respirations, and blood pressure
3. Penile erection
4. Tensing, thickening, and elevation of the scrotum
5. Partial elevation and increase in size of testicles
6. Sex flush (fewer than women)
7. Nipple erection (60% of men)

In the female, the signs of sexual excitement are:

1. Increased muscle tension
2. Moderate increase in heart rate, respirations, and blood pressure
3. Enlargement of the clitoral glans
4. Vaginal lubrication
5. Widening and lengthening of vaginal barrel
6. Separation and flattening of the labia majora
7. Reddening of the labia minora and vaginal wall
8. Nipple erection, breast tumescence, and enlarged areolae
9. Sex flush (75% of women)

Plateau phase The *plateau phase*, the period during which sexual tension increases to levels nearing orgasm, may last from 30 seconds to 3 minutes. Signs of this stage in the male include:

1. Increased voluntary and involuntary myotonia
2. Abdominal, intercostal, anal, and facial muscle contractions
3. Accelerated heart rate and respiratory rate, and increased blood pressure
4. Increase in penile circumference, at the coronal ridge, and deepening of color
5. 50% increase in testicular size, and elevation close to the perineum
6. Appearance of a few drops of mucoid secretions from the bulbourethral glands
7. Appearance of sex flush in some men late in the phase

In the female, signs of this stage include:

1. Increased voluntary and involuntary myotonia
2. Abdominal, intercostal, anal, and facial muscle contractions
3. Accelerated heart rate and respiratory rate and increased blood pressure
4. Retraction of the clitoris, under the hood
5. Appearance of the orgasmic platform, increase in the size of the outer one-third of the vagina and the labia minora
6. Slight increase in the width and depth of the inner two-thirds of the vagina
7. Further reddening of the labia minora
8. Appearance of a few drops of mucoid secretion from the Bartholin's glands
9. Further increase in breast size and areolar enlargement
10. Spread of sex flush over the entire body

Orgasmic phase The *orgasmic phase* is the involuntary climax of sexual tension, accompanied by physiologic and psychologic release. This phase is considered the measurable peak of the sexual experience. Although the entire body is involved, the major focus of the orgasm is felt in the pelvic region. The orgasmic phase is short, lasting 3 to 10 seconds. In the male, physiologic changes include:

1. Involuntary spasms of muscle groups throughout the body
2. Diminished sensory awareness
3. Involuntary contractions of the anal sphincter
4. Peak heart rate, respiratory rate, and blood pressure
5. Rhythmic, expulsive contractions of the penis at 0.8-second intervals

6. Emission of seminal fluid into the prostatic urethra from contraction of the vas deferens and accessory organs (stage 1 of the expulsive process)
7. Ejaculation of semen through the penile urethra and expulsion from the urethral meatus. The force of ejaculation varies from man to man and at different times but diminishes after the first two to three contractions (stage 2 of the expulsive process)

In the female, physiologic changes include:

1. Involuntary spasms of muscle groups throughout the body
2. Diminished sensory awareness
3. Involuntary contractions of the anal sphincter
4. Peak heart rate, respiratory rate, and blood pressure
5. Approximately 5 to 12 contractions in the orgasmic platform at 0.8-second intervals
6. Contraction of the muscles of the pelvic floor and the uterine muscles
7. Varied pattern of orgasms, including minor surges and contractions, multiple orgasms, or a simple intense orgasm similar to that of the male.

Resolution phase The *resolution phase*, the period of return to the unaroused state, may last 10 to 15 minutes after orgasm, or longer if there is no orgasm. The resolution phase involves a reversal of vasocongestion. All signs of myotonia in both men and women are gone within 5 minutes. The genitalia and breasts return to their preexcitement state. The sex flush disappears in reverse order of appearance. Heart rate, respiratory rate, and blood pressure return to normal. Other reactions include sleepiness, relaxation, and emotional outbursts such as crying or laughing.

The major difference in sexual response between men and women occurs during the resolution phase. The *refractory period* in men is a period during which the body will not respond to sexual stimulation. This varies, depending on age and other factors, from a few moments to hours or days.

Assessment of Sexual Health

Information about a client's sexual health status should always be an integral part of a nursing assessment. The amount and kind of data collected will depend on the context of the assessment, that is, the client's reason for seeking health and how his or her sexuality interacts with other problems. The nurse's professional preparation is another factor that influences the level of sexual health assessment. Mims and Swenson (1980) have described a three-level approach to taking a sexual history that provides guidelines useful to the beginning nurse.

Viewing sexuality in its broadest context (see definition at the beginning of the chapter) provides opportunities for the nurse to integrate sexuality into the normative health assessment. It is important for nurses to understand the need to assess sexuality holistically and to integrate this assessment into the nursing history. This can also "normalize" sexuality assessment and reduce client (as well as nurse) discomfort, anxiety, and reluctance to discuss sexuality. A respectful, empathetic, matter-of-fact interview facilitates discussion of sexual issues.

Characteristics of Sexual Health

Lion (1982, pp. 9–10) has described the following characteristics of sexually healthy people:

1. Expression of a positive body image
2. Cognitive knowledge about human sexuality
3. Congruence between biologic sex, gender identity, and gender-role behavior
4. Behavior consistent with self-concept
5. Awareness of own sexual feelings and attributes
6. Capacity for physical and psychosexual responsiveness, which is enhancing to self and others
7. Comfort with a range of sexual behavior and lifestyles
8. Acceptance of responsibility for pleasure and reproduction
9. Ability to create effective interpersonal relationships with both sexes
10. Value system that is developing and usable

These characteristics reflect the integral, holistic nature of sexuality as part of the human experience, and they provide a useful guide for measuring sexual health.

Integrating Sexuality into the Nursing History

Data about sexual health should be an integral part of the nursing history, given that the nursing history is the database for identifying health problems and health strengths. Physiologic assessment should be included in any review of systems, including information on the functioning of the neurologic, cardiovascular, endocrine, and genitourinary systems as well as other systems that interact with sexuality. Data collected should include not only information about direct, sexual functioning but also physiological information that may relate to sexuality. For example, it is certainly important to collect data about erectile functioning in a diabetic male (cardiovascular, neurologic, and genitourinary systems), but it may also be important to note baldness (integumentary system) as a physiologic influence on sexual self-image. To collect such physiologic data for the nursing history does not require extensive or detailed questioning. The screening process of the systems review allows the nurse and client to identify problematic areas. For example, answers to the question "Do you have any concerns about the amount or regularity of your menstrual flow?" can give clues to the presence of problems not otherwise identified. Also, questions asked about the functioning of systems directly related to sexuality often provide clients with an opportunity to give clues to sexual concerns or problems. Informing the client of the need for and use of the data reduces the reluctance of the client to talk about sexual issues. The level of detail of the sexual assessment is directly related to the potential impact of sexuality on the health problem, or vice versa.

Psychosexual assessment should also be a part of the nursing history. Important influences to be cognizant of include development, culture, religion, attitudes, and values. Again, specific, detailed questions about psychosexual issues are not necessary in the usual nursing history unless there are clues that potential or actual problems exist. A useful approach to psychosexual assessment is a review of sexual self-concept (see Table 19–1).

Self-concept is a valid construct that is frequently used by nurses. The self-concept approach also incorporates components of the characteristics of sexual health identified earlier in this section. The listed components of sexual self-concept and the criteria noted for each indicate sexual health. Responses to questions related to these areas will give clues to the existence of sexual concerns.

Table 19-1 Assessment of Sexual Self-concept

Aspect of Self	Assessment Criteria
Sense of being (identity)	Demonstrates a clear sense of self as male or female. Demonstrates comfort with own identity.
Physical self (body image)	Demonstrates a realistic perception of own body. Demonstrates comfort with own body image.
Social self (role behavior)	Demonstrates congruence between identity and behavior. Demonstrates comfort with own role behavior.
Knowledge (self-awareness)	Demonstrates accurate cognitive sexual knowledge. Demonstrates realistic sense of self-congruence with others' view. Demonstrates comfort with self in relation to others.
Expectations (ideal self)	Demonstrates realistic expectations of sexual being congruent with what is possible. Demonstrates comfort with ideal self.
Evaluation (self-esteem)	Demonstrates realistic appraisal of sexual self. Demonstrates growth based on realistic evaluation. Demonstrates overall positive sense of self.

Often, the clues come without direct questioning. Manner of dress, tone of voice, and comments about self and relationships with others can all give the nurse openings to explore issues of sexual self-concept more fully. Because illnesses and other health concerns can have a strong influence on sexual concept, assessment of these areas often provides the first clues to client concerns.

Nursing Diagnoses

Nursing diagnoses for clients with problems related to sexuality fall under the rubric of *altered sexuality patterns*. This is defined as the state in which an individual expresses concern regarding her or his sexuality. **Sexual dysfunction** is defined by The North American Nursing Diagnosis Association as a perceived problem in achieving desired sexual satisfaction. The concept of sexual dysfunction and specific nursing diagnoses for sexual dysfunctions are still being developed.

Factors Influencing Alterations in Sexual Functioning

Current understanding identifies the following as some of the factors contributing to sexual dysfunction (Hurley 1986, p. 540):

1. Ineffectual or absent role models
2. Altered body structure or function due to disease or

trauma, drugs, pregnancy or recent childbirth, or anatomic abnormalities of the genitals

3. Lack of knowledge or misinformation about sexuality
4. Physical abuse (e.g., sexual assault)
5. Psychosocial abuse
6. Value conflict
7. Loss or lack of partner
8. Vulnerability

Nursing Diagnoses for Common Sexual Problems

Examples of existing nursing diagnoses for patients with sexual problems include sexual dysfunctions related to:

- Fear of effects of coitus following heart attack
- Spinal cord injury
- Neurologic changes due to diabetes mellitus
- Negative body image following mastectomy
- Lack of knowledge about sexually transmitted diseases
- Pregnancy and fear of harming fetus by coitus
- Excessive use of alcohol
- Guilt over enjoyment of sexual activities
- Traumatic rape experience
- Fear of inadequate sexual performance
- Lack of knowledge about conception
- Fear of pregnancy and lack of knowledge about contraception
- Painful intercourse from inadequate vaginal lubrication

It is not possible in this chapter to review all nursing diagnoses related to sexual problems or all factors contributing to sexual dysfunction. Examples of common illnesses affecting sexual functioning, changes in sexual motivation, and genital sexual problems will be outlined to illustrate the approach to issues related to sexual problems.

Common Illnesses Affecting Sexuality

Medical Conditions

Included here are conditions that would be categorized as altered body structure or function factors contributing to sexual dysfunction. Heart disease and diabetes mellitus are two common long-term illnesses that frequently influence sexual functioning. Clients with heart disease, particularly those experiencing or at risk for myocardial infarction, are often anxious about or afraid of sexual activity. Concerns about the effect of sexual activity on the heart cause people to restrict or avoid sexual activity. Nursing activities with individuals diagnosed with sexual dysfunction related to fear of effects of coitus following heart attack include assessment of previous sexual activity, identification of desired sexual activity, teaching related to boundaries of physical activity, and teaching related to incorporating sexual activity into postinfarct activities.

Many men with diabetes mellitus develop erectile dysfunction, which is related to developing neuropathy and to a lesser extent vascular changes. Erectile dysfunction related to neurologic changes due to diabetes mellitus is frequently progressive and effects older men more than younger men. Nursing activities can involve teaching about etiology, supportive counseling related to self-image, teaching about continued ability to ejaculate, and providing information about options such as penile prostheses.

Sexual dysfunction related to spinal cord injury is another condition that creates special problems. Because the level of the injury to the spinal cord determines the extent of effects on sexual functioning, individuals may be capable of erection and ejaculation and be fertile, may have psychogenic or reflexogenic genital arousal, or may have no physiologic genital responses. Again, nursing activities will include assessment, teaching, and counseling. Special rehabilitation programs are usually prescribed for such individuals.

Surgical Conditions

All surgical procedures have the potential to alter a person's body image; especially when the surgery involves mutilating, removing, or altering parts of the body. Examples include amputation of a leg, radical neck surgery, and excision of large portions of the lower jaw. Impact is even greater when the surgery alters or removes body parts linked directly with sexual functioning, for instance, mastectomy, hysterectomy, and vaginal excision in women; orchidectomy (removal of the testicles), and penectomy in men; and ostomies in either sex. Feelings of ugliness and loss of masculinity or femininity are common after these surgeries. Nursing activities to assist in postoperative adjustment include teaching about the physiologic effects of the surgery on sexual functioning, counseling related to psychologic adaptation and reintegration of body image, and support for involvement of family, spouse, and significant others.

Changes in Sexual Motivation

The urge or desire for sexual activity is called **libido** (sexual motivation, sex drive). Libido fluctuates within each person and varies from person to person. The range of fluctuation in each individual is broad and is considered a problem only when the client (or those interacting with him or her) identifies it as interfering with the ability to have effective sexual interactions. Many biologic and psychosocial factors affect sexual motivation.

Decreased Sexual Motivation

Factors that may contribute to decreased sexual motivation include the following.

Drugs All central nervous system depressants, such as alcohol, barbiturates, and sedatives, may decrease libido. Morphine, heroin, and methadone (used in the rehabilitation of drug addicts) cause marked reduction of sexual desire. Other libido-inhibiting drugs include estrogens and adrenal steroids in large doses, certain psychotropic drugs, and some antihypertensive agents, e.g., reserpine (Serpasil) and methyldopa (Aldomet).

Depression Depression slows all body functions and lowers libido. Depression in one partner can adversely affect the sexual functioning of the other. Libido generally returns when the depression is relieved.

Disease Libido diminishes with general ill health and chronic diseases that cause debility, pain, or depression, such as arthritis and cancer. Any disorder that causes dyspareunia also lowers libido. This could include vaginitis, genital herpes, and imperforate hymen.

Pregnancy Sexual motivation may decrease during pregnancy, because of physical discomfort, fear of injury to the fetus, or perceived loss of attractiveness. For about 4 weeks following delivery, libido is often reduced due to decreased vaginal lubrication, thinner vaginal walls, and a slower response to stimulation.

Aging Older people vary greatly in their sexual motivation. Psychosocial factors such as beliefs and attitudes about sexual functioning play an important role in this variation. Physical factors such as energy levels, pain, and immobility also have an effect.

Increased Sexual Motivation

Factors contributing to increased sexual motivation include the following.

Puberty and adolescence Both males and females experience increased sexual motivation during puberty and adolescence as a result of hormonal and body changes. This population is at risk of pregnancy and sexually transmitted disease if they do not receive appropriate sex education.

Drugs Amphetamines and cocaine enhance sexual motivation for some people for short periods. Lysergic acid diethylamide (LSD) and marijuana increase libido in some but inhibit it in others.

Problems with Genital Sexual Functioning

The ability to engage in genital intercourse is of great importance to most people. Many people experience transient problems with their ability to respond to sexual stimulation or to maintain the response. Common concerns for the male are being able to achieve and maintain an erection and to develop good partner-related orgasmic timing. For women, common concerns relate to their ability to become and stay aroused and their ability to achieve orgasm.

Erectile Dysfunction

The inability to achieve or maintain an erection sufficient for sexual satisfaction for the self and/or partner is called *erectile dysfunction*. The term **impotence**, also commonly used, is believed by many to be inappropriate, as it has come to be seen as a negative label by the client. Erectile dysfunction is a more specific term.

All men have transient interferences with the ability to attain and maintain erection. Erectile dysfunction becomes a problem when it interferes significantly with the client's ability to achieve sexual satisfaction or to provide satisfaction for his partner. Such interference may occur consistently in all sexual situations, with or without a partner, or it may occur only in certain situations, such as with one partner but not with others or with masturbation.

Erectile dysfunction is classified as primary or secondary. A man with primary erectile dysfunction has never been able to achieve an erection sufficient for intercourse. A man with secondary erectile dysfunction has functioned adequately for some time before developing erectile dysfunction. Both types of erectile dysfunction can be caused by physiologic or psychologic factors, but primary erectile dysfunction is more often associated with psychologic factors. Physiologic factors include:

1. Neurologic disorders created by spinal cord injuries, injury to the genitals or perineal nerves, extensive surgery such as abdominal-perineal bowel resections, radical perineal prostatectomy, and diabetes mellitus
2. Prolonged use of drugs such as sedatives, heroin, antidepressants, and antipsychotics (phenothiazines)
3. Vascular diseases such as sickle cell anemia and leukemia
4. Endocrine disorders such as hypothyroidism and Addison's disease

Psychologic factors may include:

1. Doubts about one's ability to perform or about one's masculinity
2. Fatigue, anger, or stress caused by problems at work, in the family, or in interpersonal relationships
3. Traumatic early sexual experiences (e.g., rejection)
4. Pain, fear, or guilt associated with erection
5. Boredom associated with a specific partner

The treatment for erectile dysfunction depends largely on the cause. Penile implants have been used to treat physiologic erectile dysfunction. Erectile dysfunction of psychologic origin often requires a change in both partners' views of sexuality. Awareness of the cause of the condition and exercises designed to increase sensations are also used.

Premature Ejaculation

Premature ejaculation occurs when a man is unable to delay ejaculation long enough to satisfy his partner. This usually means that ejaculation occurs after only very limited stimulation of the penis. Often the ejaculation occurs either during penetration (of the vagina, mouth, or anus) or immediately following. The condition may relate to conditioning regarding the need for rapid orgasm or performance demands.

Treatment advocated for couples by many sex therapists includes increased sexual communication and responsiveness as well as decreased performance demands. The couple together practice sensate exercises (learning to enjoy the sensation of touch) and then work together to establish satisfying coitus.

Orgasmic Dysfunction

Orgasmic dysfunction, the inability of a woman to achieve orgasm, is of two types: primary and situational. A woman with primary orgasmic dysfunction has never been able to achieve orgasm. A woman with situational dysfunction has experienced at least one orgasm but is at that time nonorgasmic.

Orgasmic dysfunction can be caused by drugs, alcohol, aging, and anatomic abnormalities of the genitals. However, most cases have psychologic causes, including hostility between partners, fear or guilt about enjoying the sexual act, and concern about performance. Therapy usually involves helping both partners to establish new attitudes about sex. Pelvic muscle exercises (Kegel's exercises) can also increase the capacity of women to achieve orgasm by increasing the strength of the pubococcygeal muscle.

Vaginismus

Vaginismus is the irregular and involuntary contraction of the muscles around the outer third of the vagina when coitus is attempted—that is, the vagina closes before penetration. Its cause can be severe sexual inhibition, often associated with early learning. Other causes can be rape, incest, and painful intercourse.

Treatment often involves sensate focus exercises and therapy to bring about psychologic changes. In some instances graduated vaginal dilators are used.

Dyspareunia

Dyspareunia describes the pain experienced by a woman during intercourse, a result of inadequate lubrication, scarring, vaginal infection, or hormonal imbalance. Treatment—such as supplying additional lubrication before intercourse—corrects the underlying cause.

Planning and Intervention for Sexual Health

As in all areas of nursing care, problems related to sexuality require effective planning and intervention. These processes should be based on understanding the nurse's responsibilities, developing self-awareness, selecting appropriate interventions, and incorporating teaching for sexual health.

Responsibilities of the Nurse

The overall nursing goal for clients with sexual problems is to promote sexual health. Nursing subgoals that define nursing responsibilities include:

1. Developing awareness of one's own sexual attitudes, beliefs, and knowledge
2. Providing accurate sexual information and education to patients
3. Identifying sexual problems and providing intervention as appropriate
4. Enhancing the client's body image and self-esteem

Developing Self-Awareness

To be effective in helping clients with sexual problems, the nurse must first have accurate information about sexuality, identify and accept her or his own sexual values and behaviors and those of others, and be comfortable acquiring and disseminating information about sexuality. Results of a study conducted at the School of Nursing, University of Wisconsin at Madison, revealed considerable misinformation and lack of information about sexual matters among graduate and undergraduate nursing students (Mims and Swenson 1978, p. 122). The following *misconceptions*, and their incidence, were reported:

1. Impotence in men over 70 is nearly universal (35%).
2. Certain mental and emotional instabilities are caused by masturbation (10%).
3. Women are not able to respond to further stimulation for a period of time following orgasm (24%).
4. A woman's chances to conceive are greatly enhanced if she has experienced orgasm (16%).
5. Most homosexuals have a distinguishing body build (27%).
6. Exhibitionists are latent homosexuals (32%).

Nurses who hold such misconceptions may be unable to give patients appropriate advice and assistance. Nurses need to become informed about the anatomy and physiology of sexual organs, psychosocial development of sexuality, psychosocial behaviors, sexual variations among people, and diseases and therapies that can alter sexual behavior.

Awareness of one's own attitudes (feelings, values, and beliefs) about sexuality is also essential. Before the nurse can understand clients' sexuality, he or she must develop an awareness and tolerance of his or her own sexuality. This kind of self-awareness can be acquired via values clarification exercises and discussions. Nurses need to consider some of their feelings about the following:

- Masturbation
- Unwanted pregnancy and abortion
- Contraception
- Homosexuality and other sexual variations
- Nudity
- Sterilization
- Various modes of sexual stimulation
- Sexually transmitted diseases
- Premarital intercourse
- Unwed parents
- Cohabitation

When the nurse clarifies her or his own attitudes, she or he gains a greater understanding and tolerance of sexuality in others.

Selecting Appropriate Interventions

Interventions for sexual health problems are many and varied. Major components of any intervention strategy include counseling, education, and referral. Two models of intervention are presented as examples to guide nurses in selecting appropriate interventions.

Frank (1981, p. 64) suggests a three-part program for each sexual counseling session: (a) assessment, (b) information-sharing, and (c) discussion. The *assessment phase* involves asking the patient questions and evaluating his or her answers. Frank suggests that before asking the questions of the client, the nurse should answer this question: "If I were in this client's place, what questions would I ask?" This exercise helps the nurse devise a list of questions and ways to ask them. For example, the nurse might ask a client recuperating from a heart attack the following questions:

> "Now that you're recuperating and you've had some time to sort our your feelings, have you thought about how your heart attack might alter your sex life?"
>
> "Have you and your partner discussed how you both feel about it?"

Information-sharing and discussion should follow each question. In this example, sharing information means the nurse informs the client about how his heart attack might affect his sex life, including the following:

> "Your heart attack will not alter your capacity for sexual response. Most patients can resume intercourse in 4 to 6 weeks, but this should be confirmed by your doctor."
>
> "Many postcoronary patients fear sexual intercourse because of increased heart and respiratory rates associated with it. However, your prescribed program of progressive physical activity will also increase your tolerance for sexual activity."

After sharing information, the nurse should encourage discussion. If the nurse cannot answer the client's questions, the nurse refers the client to someone who can. The nurse may offer helpful suggestions during discussion, for example:

> "Many people express concern about the stress of certain positions for intercourse, but you may use whatever position is comfortable for you and your partner."

Another model to help nurses deliver sexual health care, developed by Mims and Swenson (1978, p. 123), outlines three levels of nursing intervention, all of which require use of the nursing process and communication skills. At the basic level, the nurse helps the client develop awareness of sexuality, which involves his or her knowledge, attitudes, and perceptions. Mims and Swenson believe that all nurses, regardless of educational preparation, should function at this level.

The intermediate level includes giving permission and giving information. This level presupposes teaching skills by the nurse. Giving permission means that the nurse by attitude or word lets the patient know that sexual thoughts, fantasies, and behaviors between informed, consenting adults are sanctioned. Giving permission begins when the nurse acknowledges the client's verbal and nonverbal sexual concerns. For example, an older male with a reduced libido may feel that he cannot discuss sex with the nurse unless the nurse broaches the subject. Other patients may need acknowledgment to feel comfortable about their virginity, homosexual activities, oral–genital sex, or masturbation. Often, many sexual concerns are alleviated when the client receives permission from the nurse to engage or not engage in certain sexual behaviors. Permission giving can be detrimental unless at the same time the nurse provides accurate information. Giving information should include:

1. General information about sexuality, including:
   a. Anatomy and physiology of sexual organs
   b. Stages of sexual development
   c. Sexual response cycles
   d. Coital positions
2. Information specific to the client's needs, which may include:
   a. Alterations in sexuality made necessary by certain disease processes, medication, surgery, or therapies
   b. Alternative modes of sexual expression
   c. Contraception
   d. Sexually transmitted diseases
   e. Pregnancy
   f. Abortion
   g. Infertility

The third level of nursing intervention includes giving suggestions, which involves sexual therapy, educational programs, and research projects. For this level of functioning, the nurse requires advanced and specialized knowledge.

Teaching About Sexual Health

Providing education for sexual health is an important component of nursing intervention. Many sexual problems exist as a result of sexual ignorance; many others can be prevented with effective sexual health teaching. Examples of important areas of teaching include breast and testicular self-examination (see Ch. 25) and contraception.

Contraception

Contraception is the voluntary prevention of conception or **impregnation** (fertilizing or making pregnant). Contraceptive methods include the biologic or ovulation method, coitus interruptus, hormone therapy, and chemical, mechanical, and surgical procedures.

Biologic or ovulation method The biologic method is preferred by people whose religious beliefs conflict with artificial birth control methods and by those who mistrust pharmacologic or mechanical birth control. Basic to this method is the identification of the days of the month when conception could take place and abstinence during that time. Women must learn the following signs of ovulation, since they can conceive when ovulating and must abstain during that time:

1. Changes in vaginal mucus. When the woman is not ovulating, her mucus is thick and yellow or sometimes cloudy. The mucus becomes clearer and thinner near the time of ovulation
2. Breast tenderness
3. Tenderness at either side of the lower abdomen
4. Midcycle spotting of blood
5. Rise in basal temperature. The temperature taken each morning upon arising drops about 0.2°C (0.3°F) 1 or 2 days prior to ovulation and then rises 0.4 to 0.5°C (0.7 to 0.8°F) 1 to 2 days after ovulation. The fertile period around ovulation extends from 1 to 2 days before ovulation to 2 days after.

Economy is one advantage of this method of contraception. Also, no drugs or mechanical devices that interfere with body physiology are used, and the method is readily learned. The disadvantages include abstinence from sexual activity for the period surrounding ovulation, and the fact that cooperation is required of both partners. Between 21 and 40 women out of 100 using one of the biologic methods become pregnant in one year (Hatcher et al. 1980, p. 4).

Coitus interruptus This method of contraception involves the withdrawal of the penis prior to ejaculation and requires considerable self-control. It has two primary disadvantages: Some semen may escape into the vagina prior to ejaculation, and it may decrease sexual gratification. Twenty to twenty-five women out of 100 using this method for one year become pregnant (Hatcher et al. 1980).

Hormone therapy Certain drugs (birth control pills) suppress ovulation and are used as contraceptives. Contraceptive pills usually contain synthetic estrogen and progesterone. Estrogen suppresses ovulation by inhibiting the release of LH and FSH. Progesterone produces changes in the cervical mucus, alters the tubal transport of the ovum, and renders the endometrium less suitable for implantation.

A pill is taken once a day for 20 or 21 days starting on the fifth day of the menstrual cycle. The pill comes in two forms: combined and sequential. In the combined form, each pill contains both estrogen and progesterone. In the sequential form, estrogen only is contained in the first 15 pills and progesterone in the remaining 7 pills. Within 2 or 3 days of stopping the pills, the woman begins menstruation. After the fifth day of menstruation, she begins a new series of pills again. Some pharmaceutical companies manufacture 28-day packets that contain inert tablets for the "off" days. Using this packet, the woman takes a tablet each day. Tablet containers usually allow the woman to see at a glance how many pills she has taken.

Many pill users experience side effects. Minor side effects are nausea, weight gain, breast tenderness, headaches, decreased menstrual flow, spotting, missed periods, vaginal itching, yeast infections, and depression. If these persist, the client should consult her physician. Other symptoms, such as severe headaches, severe abdominal pain, blurred vision, severe leg pain, and chest pain, are warnings of potentially serious problems. These symptoms must be reported to a physician. Birth control pills are contraindicated for clients with cardiac problems, circulatory problems (e.g., thrombophlebitis, thromboembolic disorders, and cerebrovascular disease), severe migraines, liver disease, diabetes mellitus, and known or suspected breast cancer. Four to ten women out of 100

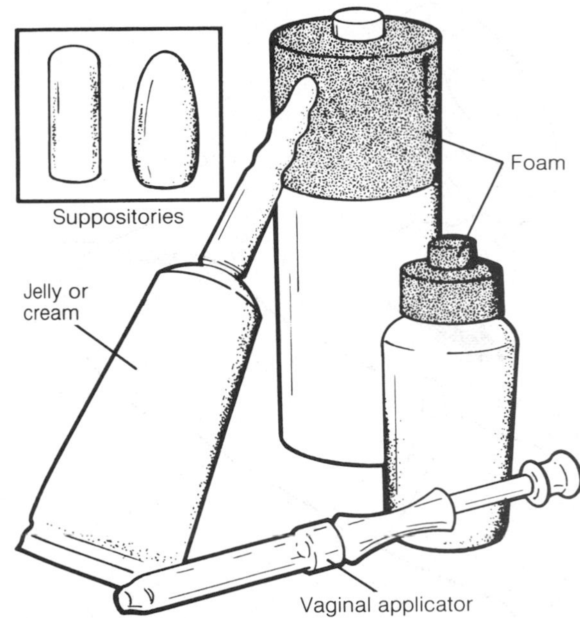

Figure 19–4 Types of spermicides.

Source: S. B. Olds, M. L. London, P. A. Ladewig, and S. V. Davidson, *Obstetric nursing* (Menlo Park, Calif.: Addison-Wesley, 1980), p. 175.

using combined oral contraceptives become pregnant in one year (Hatcher et al. 1980).

Chemical contraception Chemical contraception involves the insertion of foam, jelly, creams, or suppositories into the vagina before intercourse. These products, introduced in the 1950s, form a film of spermicide on the vagina. A **spermicide** destroys sperm.

These products are inserted with an applicator. See Figure 19-4. The woman fills the applicator, inserts it into the vagina, withdraws the applicator about 1¼ cm (½ in) and then depresses the plunger. The substance covers the cervical os (mouth or opening of the cervix), preventing sperm from entering the uterus.

Spermicides that effervesce in a moist environment have an immediate effect, and coitus may take place immediately after insertion. Suppositories do not offer protection until dissolved and may not dissolve for 30 minutes after insertion. The effectiveness of spermicides increases substantially when they are used with a diaphragm or condom. Their chief disadvantages are the difficulty some women have inserting the substance up to the cervical os and leakage from the vagina. Of 100 couples using spermicides alone, 22 to 25 women become pregnant in one year (Hatcher et. al. 1980).

Research Note

We live in a time when the number of unwanted teenage pregnancies is skyrocketing, with disastrous medical, social, and economic consequences. Nurses are often seen as trustworthy, nonthreatening, and knowledgeable adults and may be uniquely positioned to help these adolescents.

This study found that the level of cognitive development in adolescents is the best predictor of their contraceptive decision making, although age and relevant sexual knowledge are also related. Practicing birth control requires repeated, long-range, futuristic thinking, an appreciation of the long-term consequences of behavior; yet this is a cognitive skill not fully developed in many adolescents. The author suggests that nurses assess the level of such thought processes as they also dispense sex education and contraceptive devices. Another idea supported by the study is that actual practice in long-range thinking and decision making be offered as an adjunct to contraceptive instruction. (Sachs 1985)

Mechanical Devices

Condoms The **condom**, or sheath, is a covering placed over the penis prior to intercourse. See Figure 19-5. It must be inspected for holes. The ejaculate is deposited in the condom rather than in the vagina. The man places

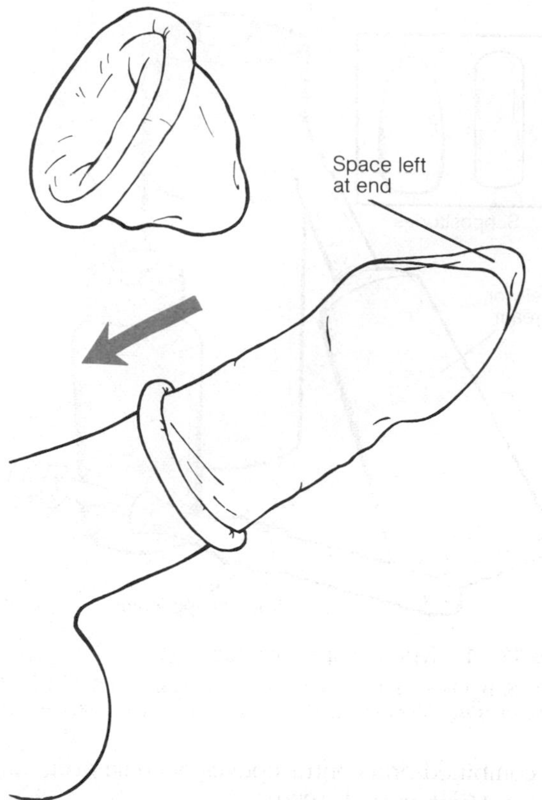

Figure 19–5 **A,** Condom; **B,** condom applied to penis, with space left at end for collection of ejaculate.

Source: S. B. Olds, M. L. London, and P. A. Ladewig, *Maternal newborn nursing,* 2nd ed. (Menlo Park, Calif.: Addison-Wesley, 1984), p. 122.

the condom on the erect penis, rolling the sheath down from the tip to the end of the shaft and leaving a small space at the end of the condom for the ejaculate. This space prevents the condom from breaking at ejaculation. It is important to avoid the use of petroleum-based lubricants, as they damage the condom. After intercourse, when the penis becomes flaccid, the man should hold the edge of the condom while withdrawing from the vagina to prevent the condom from slipping off and spilling semen. Condoms are not a foolproof method of contraception since they may split or be displaced during intercourse. Other disadvantages include expense and the fact that some couples feel condoms dull sexual sensations. Ten women out of 100 whose partners use condoms become pregnant in one year (Hatcher et al. 1980).

Vaginal diaphragms The **vaginal diaphragm** is a round rubber cup inserted into the vagina over the cervix. See Figure 19-6. It offers greater contraceptive protection than the condom, especially when used with spermicide creams. Diaphragms must be properly fitted by trained personnel. They are then inserted by the woman prior to intercourse and must be left in place for 6 hours following intercourse. Diaphragms periodically need to be held up to a light and inspected for holes or tears. Their fit must also be rechecked after each delivery and when there is a weight gain or loss of 20 pounds.

To insert the diaphragm, the woman is instructed to:

1. Apply spermicidal jelly to the diaphragm rim that will face the cervix.
2. Cup the diaphragm between the thumb and fingers and insert it into the vagina, over the cervix.
3. Push the anterior rim of the diaphragm up under the symphysis pubis. (Some women report a popping sensation.)
4. Check its placement by touching the diaphragm with the index finger and feeling the cervix beneath. The cervix is a small rounded structure that feels somewhat like the tip of the nose. The diaphragm should be centered over the cervix.
5. If more than 4 hours elapse before intercourse, additional spermicidal cream should be inserted into the vagina.

Some people feel that having to use a diaphragm inhibits the spontaneity of intercourse. Some women also find insertion and removal of the diaphragm, and the genital manipulation they require, offensive. About 17 women out of 100 become pregnant in one year when using a diaphragm with a spermicide (Hatcher et al. 1980).

Intrauterine devices An **intrauterine device (IUD)** inserted into the uterus is the most effective method of mechanical contraception. IUDs are second in reliability only to oral contraception. When inserted properly they are 95 to 99% effective. IUDs can be nonmedicated or medicated, but all of them, regardless of shape and consistency, create endometrial infiltration by leukocytes, which produces an endometrial exudate. IUDs are therefore thought to serve as a spermicide and inhibit implantation. They have no effect on ovulation, ovarian hormones, or gonadotropins. Nonmedicated IUDs, made of soft plastic, include the Lippes Loop and the Saf-T-Coil. See Figure 19-7. Medicated IUDs, slightly more effective than nonmedicated ones, include the Copper-7, the Copper-T, and Progestasert-T. See Figure 19-8. Copper IUDs have a fine copper wire wrapped around a plastic stem and continually release copper into the endometrium. The Progestasert-T contains the natural hormone progesterone in the shaft of the T. The progesterone released has only a local effect on the endometrium, not a systemic one. IUDs must be inserted by competent trained personnel.

Contraindications to use of IUDs include a history of (a) recurrent or recent pelvic inflammatory disease (PID), (b) valvular heart disease, (c) a previous ectopic pregnancy if the woman desires a future pregnancy, (d) anemia, (e) uterine bleeding, (f) abnormal Pap smear, and (g) pregnancy. IUDs increase the risk of pelvic infection and subsequent loss of fertility.

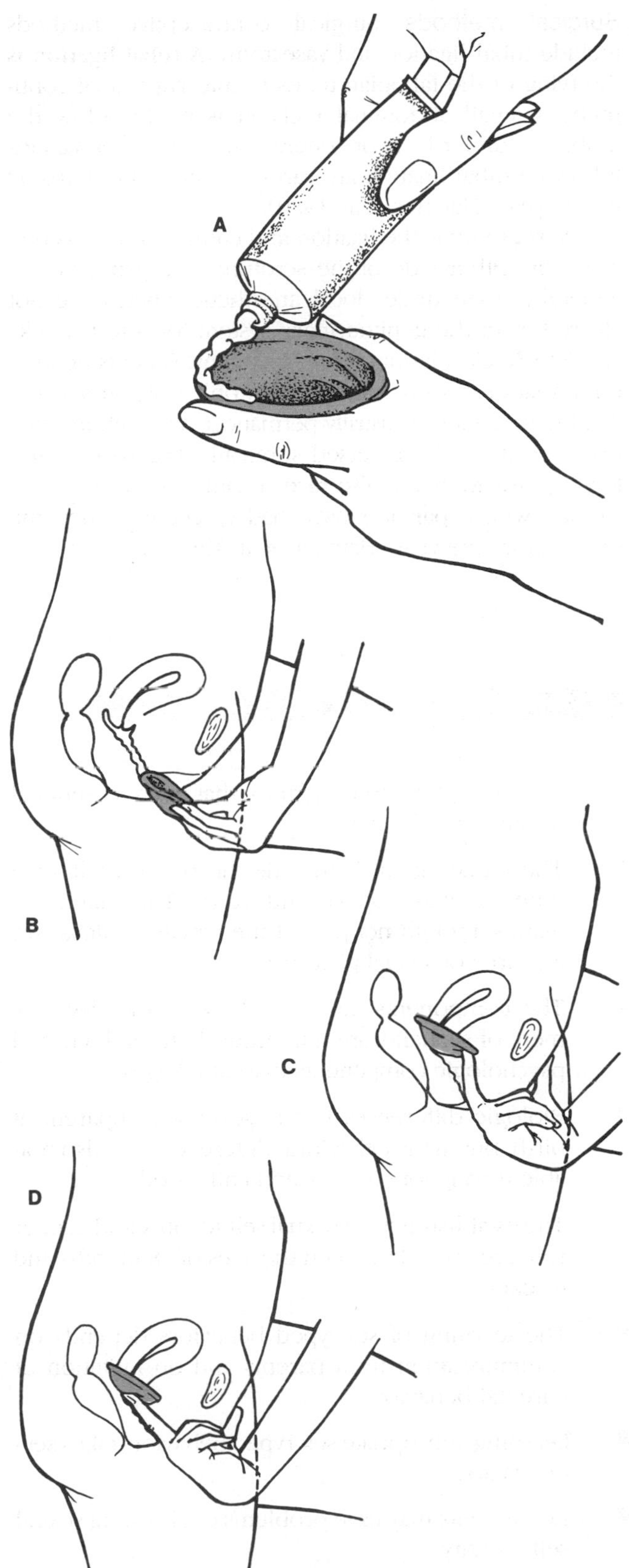

Figure 19–6 **A,** Diaphragm and gel; **B,** insertion of diaphragm; **C,** rim of diaphragm pushed up under the symphysis pubis; **D,** checking placement of diaphragm. The cervix should be felt through the diaphragm.

Source: S. B. Olds, M. L. London, P. A. Ladewig, *Maternal newborn nursing,* 2nd ed. (Menlo Park, Calif.: Addison-Wesley, 1984), p. 123.

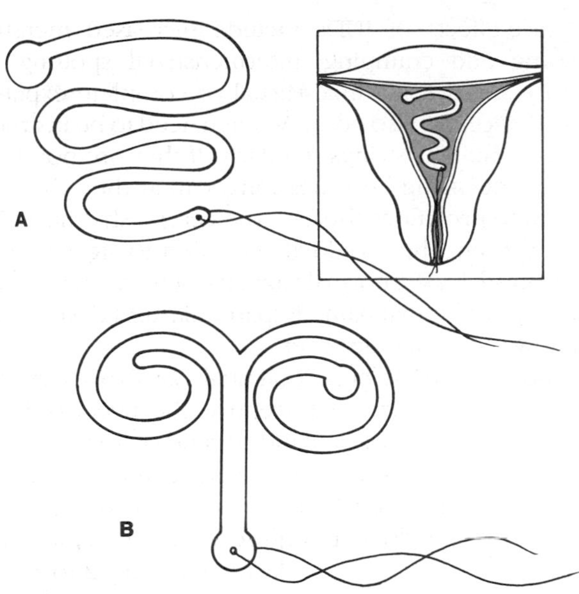

Figure 19–7 Nonmedicated intrauterine devices: **A,** Lippes Loop; **B,** Saf-T-Coil.

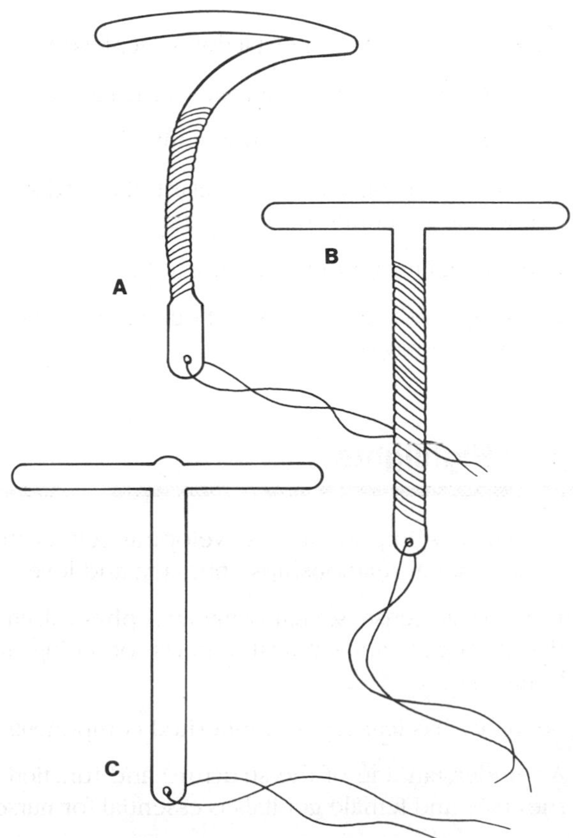

Figure 19–8 Medicated intrauterine devices: **A,** Copper-7; **B,** Copper-T; and **C,** Progestasert-T.

Side-effects of IUDs include increased menstrual bleeding and cramping, intermenstrual spotting, and occasionally dyspareunia. Partial or complete expulsion of the device can also occur. Women need to be instructed to check the IUD strings regularly. If they are not detectable, if one string becomes longer than the other, or if the device protrudes through the cervix, she must notify her physician. She should also be alert to signs of pelvic infection such as abnormal vaginal discharge, fever, chills, pelvic or abdominal pain, dyspareunia, and development of a new menstrual disorder.

Although IUDs pose potential risks to users, their major advantages are contraceptive effectiveness, lack of systemic effects, and lack of interference with intercourse. They are also less expensive than oral contraceptives over time. Nonmedicated IUDs are less expensive than medicated ones and do not require periodic replacement. Medicated IUDs require replacement every 2 to 3 years. About 5 women out of 100 using IUDs become pregnant in one year (Hatcher et al. 1980).

Surgical methods Surgical contraceptive methods include tubal ligation and vasectomy. A **tubal ligation** is the tying of the fallopian tubes to interrupt tubal continuity. A small abdominal incision is made below the umbilicus under local or general anesthetic. Pregnancies following tubal ligation are rare—about 4 out of 10,000 in one year (Hatcher et al. 1980).

Vasectomy is the ligation and cutting of the vas deferens on either side of the scrotum. The procedure is generally done under local anesthetic. Sperm are not cleared from the genitourinary system for 4 to 6 weeks and 6 to 36 ejaculations after vasectomy. Patients need to know that vasectomy affects fertility only, not potency, and that the procedure is usually permanent, although in some instances it can be reversed surgically. Pregnancies following vasectomy are also rare, as only 15 out of 10,000 women whose partners have had vasectomies become pregnant in one year (Hatcher et al. 1980).

Evaluation

The outcome criteria for patients with sexual problems (actual or potential) depend on nursing diagnoses. Some suggested criteria are:

- States desired sexual satisfaction is achieved
- Explains contraception method as instructed
- Verbalizes desired conception control
- Seeks confirmation of sexual desirability and attractiveness less frequently
- Uses sexual terminology as taught
- Expresses positive statements about alternate modes of sexual behavior

Chapter Highlights

- Sexuality is important in developing self-identity, interpersonal relationships, intimacy, and love.
- In its broad sense, sexuality involves physical, emotional, social, and ethical aspects of being and behaving.
- Sexuality has learned and inherited components.
- An understanding of the structure and function of the male and female genitals is essential for nurses.
- The male genitals include the testes and scrotum, a series of ducts (epididymis and vas deferens) that transport the sperm, glands that secrete seminal plasma, and the penis.
- The female genitals include the ovaries, fallopian tubes, uterus, vagina, and vulva. The mammary glands, though not part of the female genitals, are a source of sexual pleasure.
- The components that contribute to the development of sexuality are numerous; both biologic and psychologic components exist at all ages.
- Biologic differences in the sexes are apparent at birth, but many behavioral differences are also notable throughout infancy and childhood.
- The establishment of sexual self-identity and gender role are critical between the ages of 18 months and 4 years.
- The learning of sex-typed behaviors depends on communication from parents and on imitation of parental behavior.
- Learning appropriate sex-typed behaviors takes several years.
- Adolescents may have problems establishing sexual self-identity.
- Adults also often experience sexual problems. A major task of the adult is to develop an intimate relationship with a partner.
- During the middle and later years, there are physical changes in the genitals. However, the desire and

ability to maintain satisfying sexual relationships can remain.

- Assessing actual or potential sexual problems is conducted at four levels. The professional nurse assesses at only the first level. Assessment should be carried out when clients or support persons present cues that problems exist or when an illness could cause sexual problems.
- Nurses assess attitudes toward sexuality, including factors that affect attitudes and behaviors.
- An understanding of sexual stimuli and response patterns can help individuals have satisfying sexual relationships. This understanding is also vital for nurses wishing to help clients with psychologic problems, such as feelings of inadequacy, or medical problems, such as spinal cord injuries or myocardial infarctions.
- Common sexual problems of healthy adults are changes in libido, erectile dysfunction, premature ejaculation, orgasmic dysfunction, vaginismus, and dyspareunia.
- Illnesses that commonly affect sexuality include myocardial infarction and diabetes mellitus. Many surgical procedures also affect sexual abilities and sexual self-image, including mastectomy, hysterectomy, orchiectomy, and enterostomy.
- The nursing diagnosis for clients with sexual problems is "altered sexuality pattern." Many contributing factors exist, including altered body structure or function, lack of knowledge or misinformation about sexual matters, physical or psychologic abuse, value conflicts, and loss or lack of a partner.
- Before assisting clients with sexual problems, the nurse must acquire accurate information about sexuality, identify and accept his or her own sexual values and behaviors as well as those of others, and be comfortable acquiring and disseminating information about sexuality.
- Nursing interventions include helping develop awareness of sexuality, giving permission, giving information, and, at an advanced level, giving suggestions.

Suggested Readings

Assey, J. L., and Herbert, J. M. April 1983. Who is the seductive patient? *American Journal of Nursing* 83:531–32.
Outlines some of the reasons for seductive behavior in clients. Describes the process involved in nurses' responses and methods of constructive response.

Dickerson, J. October 1983. The pill: A close look. *American Journal of Nursing* 83:1392–98.
An extensive review of the risks and benefits of using hormonal contraceptives. Identifies major and minor risks and describes major benefits. Provides lists of types of oral contraceptives available in the U.S.

Divasto, P. February 1985. Measuring the aftermath of rape. *Journal of Psychosocial Nursing and Mental Health Services* 23:33–35.
Describes an interview scale for measuring the severity of postrape symptoms. Outlines symptoms and describes use of the data to guide client care.

Friedman, J. June 1980. Sex education for adults: Use of a sexual knowledge inventory. *Issues in Mental Health Nursing* 2:43–50.
Describes a tool for assessing the sexual knowledge of adults. Identifies ways to use these data to develop sexuality education programs.

Irish, A. August 1983. Straight talk about gay patients. *American Journal of Nursing* 83:1168–70.
Talks about homophobia among nurses and the need to be nonjudgmental about sexual orientation in their professional role. Makes suggestions for effective ways to avoid judgmental responses.

Lutz, R. March 1986. Stopping the spread of sexually transmitted diseases. *Nursing* 16:47–50.
Provides an overview of the most common STD's. Outlines nursing activities in dealing with patients who have an STD and techniques to decrease the spread.

Simmons, K. N. March 1983. Sexuality and the female ostomate. *American Journal of Nursing* 83:409–11.
Provides an excellent overview, by an ostomate, of issues and concerns following ostomies. Provides guidelines for dealing with problems.

Steinke, E. E., and Berger, M. B. June 1986. Sexuality and aging *Journal of Gerontological Nursing* 12:6–10.
Discusses stereotypes of aging and sexuality. Emphasizes need for nurses to examine their own stereotypes to provide effective care to promote sexual health in the elderly. Comprehensive assessment and intervention is emphasized.

Zalar, M. K. September 1982. "Role preparation for nurses in human sexual functioning," in Schuster, E. A., editor, *The Nursing Clinics of North America* 17:351–63.
Reviews the literature to comment on current trends in sexuality education for nurses. Identifies broad areas of knowledge and skills needed for nurses working with sexuality.

Selected References

Allen, M. January 1985. Women, nursing and feminism: An interview with Alice J. Baumgart, R.N., PhD. *Canadian Nurse* 81:20–22.

Bachman, R. February 1981. Homosexuality: The cost of being different. *Canadian Nurse* 77:20–23.

Bailey, C. R., and Miller, N. K. January 1983. Routine circumcision of the male neonate. *Canadian Nurse* 79:28–31.

Barbach, L. G. 1976. *For yourself: The fulfillment of female sexuality.* Garden City, N.Y.: Anchor Books.

Birchell, J. December 1984. Coping with sexuality: In a patient place . . . the mentally handicapped patient . . . masturbation. *Nursing Times* 80:31–34.

Block, G. J., Nolan, J. W., and Dempsey, M. K. 1981. *Health assessment for professional nursing.* New York: Appleton-Century-Crofts.

Boston Women's Health Book Collective. 1984. *The new our bodies, ourselves.* New York: Simon & Schuster.

Boyer, G., and Boyer, J. September 1982. "Sexuality and aging," in Schuster, E. A., editor, *The Nursing Clinics of North America* 17:421–27.

Bullough, B., et al. August 1985. Masculinity and femininity in transvestite, transsexual and gay males. *Western Journal of Nursing Research* 7:317–27.

Carolan, C. September 26–October 2, 1984. Handicap—less important than loving. Part 1. *Nursing Times* 80:28–30.

———. October 3–9, 1984. Sex and disability: Bridging the gap. Part 3. *Nursing Times* 80:49–50.

Chaffee, M. W. November 1984. The missing link in nursing education: Sexuality. *Imprint* 31:43.

Chiarelli, M. January 1985. Women and mental health: A feminist view. *Canadian Nurse* 81:23.

Cochrane, M. September 26–October 2, 1984. Sex and disability: Immaculate Infection . . . those with rheumatoid arthritis. Part 2. *Nursing Times* 80:31–32.

Comfort, A. (ed.). 1972. *The joy of sex.* New York: Simon & Schuster.

Crate, S. September–October 1984. Nurses can help sexual assault victims. *RNABC (Registered Nurses Association of British Columbia) News* 16:30–31.

Crooks, R., and Baur, K. 1987. *Our sexuality.* 3d ed. Menlo Park, Calif.: Benjamin / Cummings.

Davies, M. December 12–18, 1984. Coping with sexuality: Unspoken anxieties. Part 1. *Nursing Times* 80:29–30.

Dawson-Shepherd, R. September 26–October 2, 1984. Sex and disability: Why the carpet is no longer big enough. Part 3. *Nursing Times* 80:33–34.

Dolan, M. B. January 1985. An eternal flame . . . The elderly and sex. *Nursing* (Springhouse) 15:104.

Douglas, C. J., Kalman, C. M., and Kalman, T. P. December 1985. Homophobia among physicians and nurses. *Hospital and Community Psychiatry* 36:1309–11.

Ellis, D., and Ho, M. S. L. March 1982. Attitudes of Chinese women towards sexuality and birth control. *Canadian Nurse* 73:28–30.

Emick-Herring, B. March–April 1985. Sexual changes in patients and partners following stroke. *Rehabilitation Nursing* 10:28–30.

Ford, C. S., and Beach, F. A. 1951. *Patterns of sexual behavior.* New York: Harper & Row.

Francoeur, R. T. 1984. *Becoming a sexual person: A brief edition.* New York: Wiley.

Frank, D. I. January 1981. You don't have to be an expert to give sexual counselling to a mastectomy patient. *Nursing 81* 11:64–67.

Glover, J. January 16, 1985. Family planning and sexual counselling . . . The nurse's role. *Nursing Mirror* 160:28–29.

Gonsiorek, J. C. (ed.). 1982. *Homosexuality and psychotherapy: A practitioner's handbook of affirmative models.* New York: Haworth Press.

Googe, M. C. S., and Mook, T. M. July 1983. The inflatable penile prosthesis: New developments. *American Journal of Nursing* 83:1044–47.

Guyton, A. C. 1981. *Textbook of medical physiology*, 6th ed. Philadelphia: W. B. Saunders Co.

Hacker, S. S. Winter 1984. Students' questions about sexuality: Implications for nurse educators. *Nurse Educator* 9:28–31.

Hatcher, R. A.; Stewart, G. K.; Stewart, F.; Guest, F.; Schwartz, D. W.; and Jones, S. A. 1980. *Contraceptive Technology 1980–81.* 10th ed. New York: Irvington Publishers, Inc.

Heshusius, L. August 1982. Sexuality, intimacy and persons we label mentally retarded. *Mental Retardation* 20:164–168.

Hogan, R. 1980. *Human sexuality, a nursing perspective.* New York: Appleton-Century-Crofts.

———. September 1982. "Influences of culture on sexuality," in Schuster, E. A. (ed.), *The Nursing Clinics of North America* 17:365–376.

Howe, C. L. February 1986. Developmental theory and adolescent sexual behavior. *Nurse Practitioner* 11:65,68,71.

Hurley, M. E. (ed.). 1986. *Classification of Nursing Diagnoses: Proceedings of the Sixth National Conferences.* St. Louis: C. V. Mosby.

Julty, S. 1979. *Men's bodies, men's selves.* New York: Dell Publishing Co.

Kolodny, R. C.; Masters, W. H.; Johnson, V. E.; and Biggs, M. A. 1979. *Textbook of human sexuality for nurses.* Boston: Little, Brown and Co.

Krajicek, M. J. September 1982. "Developmental disability and human sexuality," in Schuster, E. A. (ed.), *The Nursing Clinics of North America.* 17:377–86.

Kus, R. May 1985. Stages of coming out: An ethnographic approach. *Western Journal of Nursing Research* 7(2):177–98.

Lewis, M. November 1984. Sexuality in later life: A challenging issue for nurses. *Imprint* 31:48–49.

Lion, E. M. (ed.). 1982. *Human sexuality in nursing process.* New York: Wiley.

McCormick, G. P., et al. March–April 1986. Coital positioning for stroke-afflicted couples. *Rehabilitation Nursing* 11:17–19.

Malek, C. J., et al. November–December 1984. Rheumatoid arthritis: How does it influence sexuality? *Rehabilitation Nursing* 9:26–28.

Mann, T. 1970. The biochemical characteristics of spermatazoa and seminal plasma. In Rosenberg, E., et al., eds. *The Human Testis.* New York: Plenum Press.

Masters, W. H., and Johnson, V. E. 1966. *Human Sexual Response.* Boston: Little, Brown and Co.

———. 1970. *Human sexual inadequacy.* New York: Bantam Books.

———. 1979. *Homosexuality in perspective.* Boston: Little, Brown and Co.

Mericle, B. P. November 1983. The male as psychiatric nurse. *Journal of Psychosocial Nursing and Mental Health Services* 21:28–34.

Mims, F. H. September 1982. "Sexual stress: Coping and adaptation," in Schuster, E. A. (ed.). *The Nursing Clinics of North America.* 17:395–405.

Mims, F. H., and Swenson, M. February 1978. A model to promote sexual health care. *Nursing Outlook* 26:121–25.

———. 1980. *Sexuality: A nursing perspective.* New York: McGraw-Hill.

Money, J. 1980. *Love and love sickness: The science of sex, gender difference and pair bonding*. Baltimore: Johns Hopkins University Press.

Moses, A. E., and Hawkins, R. O. 1982. *Counselling lesbian women and gay men*. St. Louis: Mosby.

Osis, M. January–February 1986. Sexuality: An interactional perspective . . . Drugs and healthy aging. *Gerontion*. 1:6–8.

Penninger, J. A. April 1985. After the ostomy: Helping the patient reclaim his sexuality . . . a male ostomy patient *R.N.* 48:46–50.

Pollard, M. S., et al. February 1985. Straight talk on sex for the older client. *R.N.* 48:17–18.

Redmond, M. A. September 1982. Couple-directed contraceptive counselling. *Canadian Nurse*. 78:38–39.

Risling, E. October–December 1984. Working with adolescents in sexuality groups. *Canadian Journal of Psychiatric Nursing* 25:9–10.

Rosenbaum, J., and Monahan, M. L. April 1986. A sexuality workshop: Increasing sexual self-awareness. *Canadian Journal of Psychiatric Nursing* 27:8–10.

Sachs, Barbara. 1985. Contraceptive decision-making in urban, black, female adolescents: Its relationship to cognitive development. *International Journal of Nursing Studies* 22(2):116–17.

Schuster, E. A., Unsain, I. C., and Goodwin, M. H. September 1982. "Nursing practice in human sexuality," in Schuster, E. A. (ed.), *The Nursing Clinics of North America*. 17:345–49.

Schwartz Appelbaum, J., et al. November–December 1984 Nursing care plans: Sexuality and treatment of breast cancer. *Oncology Nursing Forum*. 11:16–24.

Selby, J. May 8–14, 1985. Close encounters . . . Nurses in clinical practice . . . Psychosexual counselling. *Nursing Times* 81:31.

Sex Information and Education Council of the United States. 1980. The Siecus / New York University / Uppsala principles basic to education for sexuality. *Seicus Report* 8:8–9.

Sheehan, M. K. et al. January–February, 1986. Perceptions of sexual responsibility: Do young men and women agree? *Pediatric Nursing*. 12:17–21.

Siemens, S., and Brandzel, R. C. 1982. *Sexuality: Nursing assessment and intervention*. Philadelphia: Lippincott.

Silverstein, C., and White, E. 1977. *The joy of gay sex*. New York: Simon & Schuster.

Sisley, E., and Harris, B. 1977. *The joy of lesbian sex*. New York: Crown.

Sorrel, L. J., and Sorrel, P. M. 1979. *Sexual unfolding: Sexual development and sex therapies in late adolescence*. Boston: Little, Brown and Co.

Spennrath, S. July–August, 1982. Understanding the sexual needs of the older patient. *Canadian Nurse*. 78:25–29.

Stuart, G. W., and Sundeen, S. J. 1979. *Principles and Practices of psychiatric nursing*. Toronto: Mosby.

Tannahill, R. 1980. *Sex in history*. New York: Stein and Day.

Unsain, I. C. September 1982. "Diabetes and sexual functioning," in Schuster, E. A. (ed.), *The Nursing Clinics of North America* 17:387–93.

Weinberg, J. S. September, 1982. "Human sexuality and spinal cord injury," in Schuster, E. A. (ed.), *The Nursing Clinics of North America* 17:407–19.

Woods, N. F. 1979. *Human sexuality in health and illness*, 2nd edition. St. Louis: Mosby.

Wright, D. July 31, 1985. *Sex and the elderly*. *Nursing Mirror* 161:18–19.

Young, E. 1984. Patient's plea: Tell us about our sexuality. *Journal of Sex Education and Therapy*. 10:53–56.

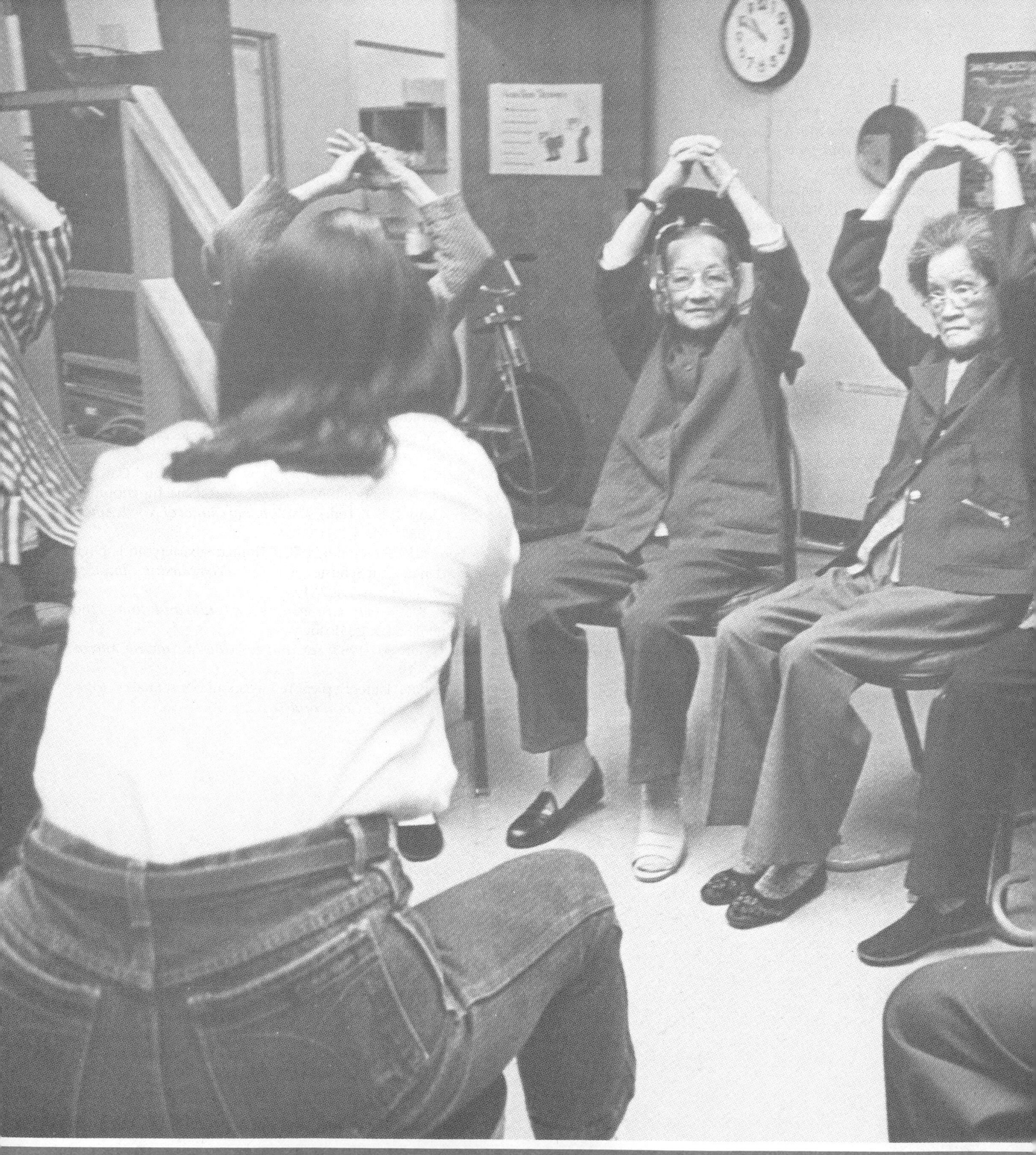

Let us accept the fact that the nurse's place is not necessarily at the bedside, but in the position from which she can assure herself that people in need receive the same kind of care she herself would give . . . . (Veneta Masson)

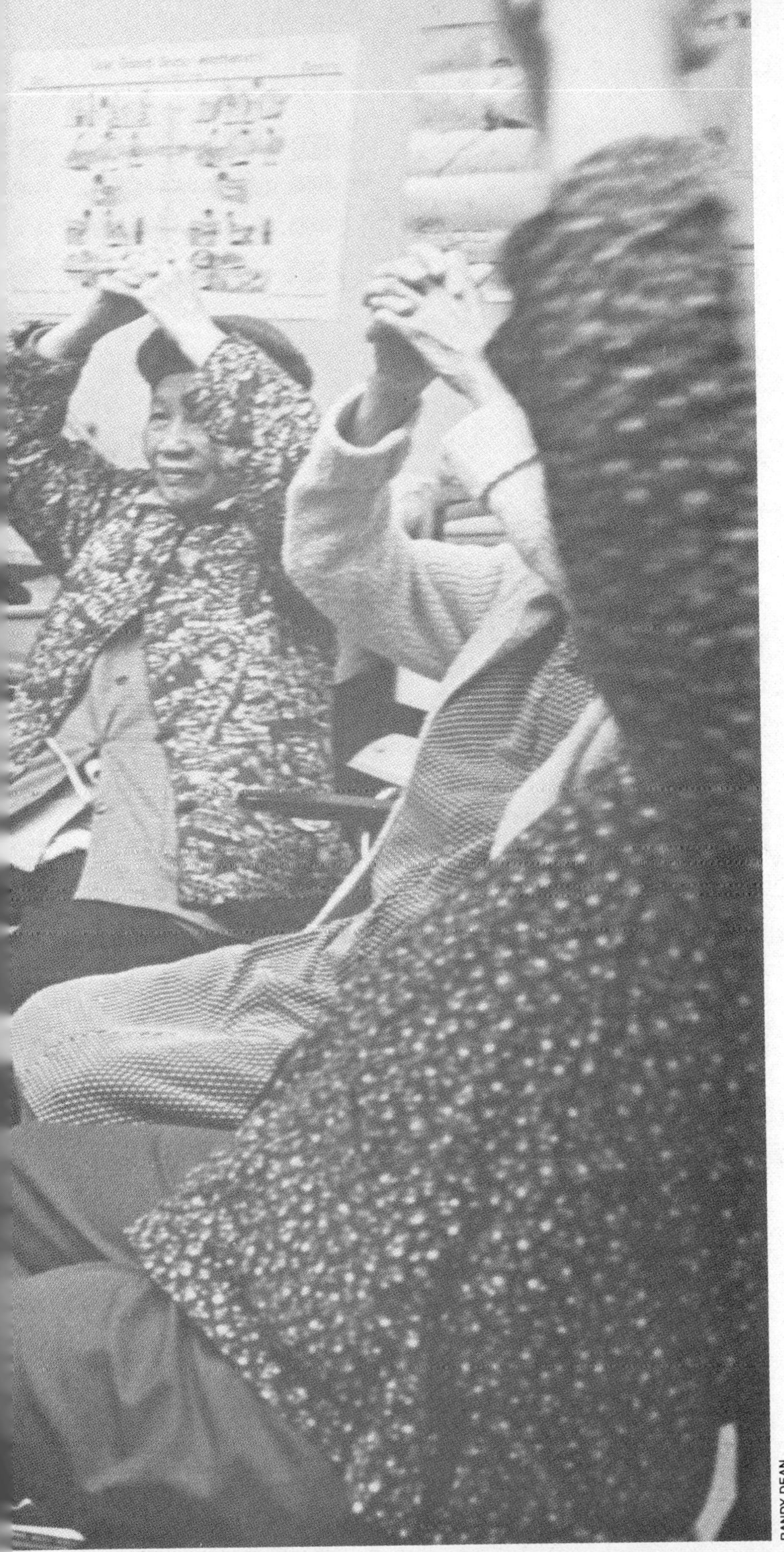

RANDY DEAN

UNIT 5

Health Promotion Through the Life Span

Contents

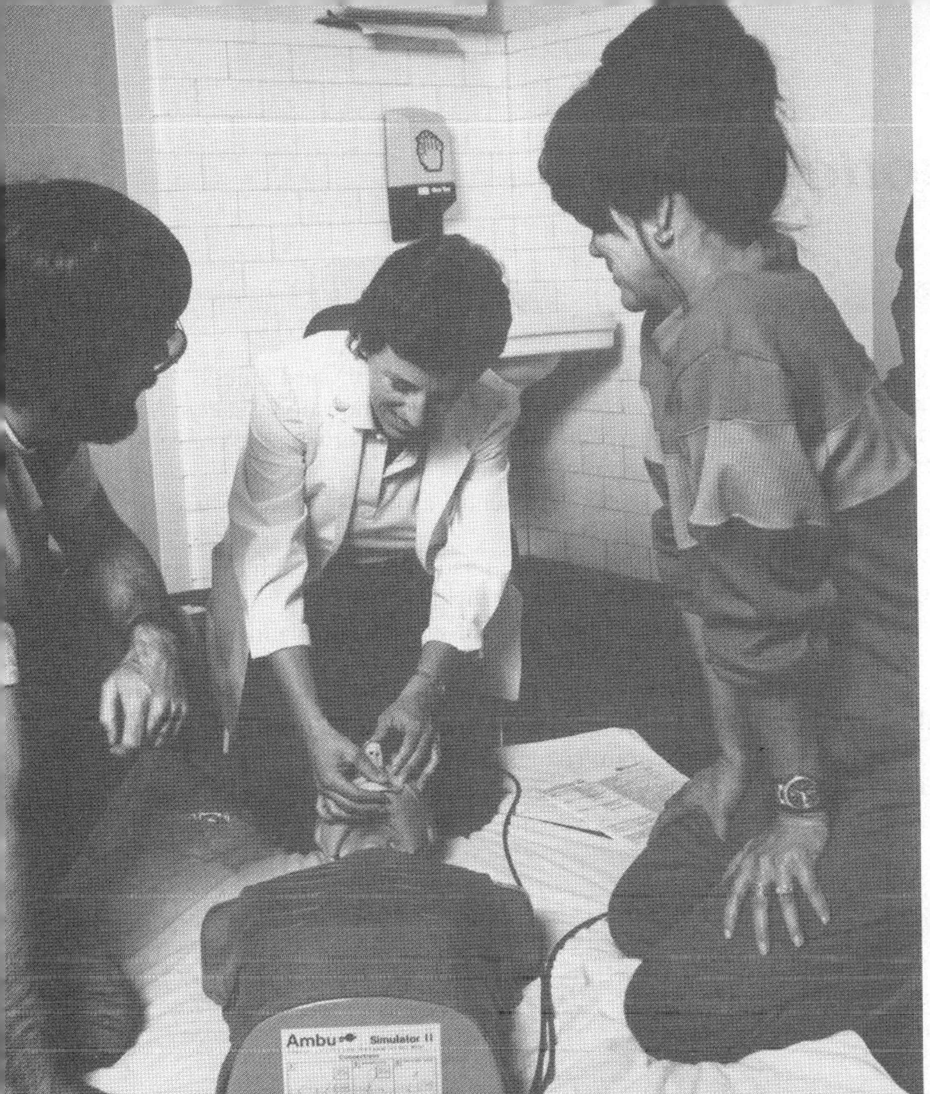

KAREN STAFFORD RANTZMAN

CHAPTER **20**

Health Promotion

Contents

20 *Health Promotion*

Objectives

1. Understand essential facts about health promotion.
   1.1 Define health promotion and wellness.
   1.2 Describe the concept of health promotion.
   1.3 Give examples of various types of health promotion programs.
   1.4 Compare the focus of promoting health and wellness to the focus of traditional health care.
   1.5 Identify outcomes of health promotion interventions.
2. Understand essential aspects of the health promotion process.
   2.1 Identify essential components of health promotion assessment.
   2.2 Describe essential information required for a health history.
   2.3 Describe ways to assess physical fitness.
   2.4 Describe ways to assess nutritional status.
   2.5 Explain the principle underlying the concept of health risk appraisal.
   2.6 Describe essential aspects of life-style assessment tools.
   2.7 Describe the relationship of health care beliefs to health behavior.
   2.8 Identify essential steps in the planning stage of health promotion.
   2.9 Describe ways to support the client.
   2.10 Identify essential aspects of enhancing behavioral change.
   2.11 Explain modeling and the importance of the nurse as a role model.

Terms

at-risk aggregate
behavioral contract
health promotion
health risk appraisal
life-style assessment
modeling
prevention
recovery index
risk factor
traditional health care
wellness

Concept and Scope of Health Promotion

Today, the terms *health; wellness; health maintenance; health promotion; disease prevention; primary, secondary,* and *tertiary health care;* and *prevention* mean different things to different people. These differences are confusing to many clients and professionals. Nursing and other authors also offer different definitions of the concept of health promotion and have different ideas about its application. Brubaker (1983, p. 1) defines **health promotion** as "health care directed toward high-level wellness through processes that encourage alteration of personal habits or the environment in which people live. It occurs after health stability is present and assumes disease prevention and health maintenance as prerequisites or by-products." Opatz (1985, p. 7) defines **wellness** as "the continual process of adapting patterns of behavior that lead to improved health and heightened life satisfaction" and health promotion as "the systematic efforts by an organization to enhance the wellness of its members through education, behavior change, and cultural support." Other definitions of wellness and well-being are provided in Chapter 2 on page 52. Pender (1982, p. 2) defines health promotion as "activities directed toward developing the resources of clients that *maintain or enhance* well-being" and prevention as "activities that seek to protect clients from potential or actual health threats and their harmful consequences."

Other facets of health promotion are the possibility of its occurrence at any point along the continuum of health and illness (see Figure 20–1) and its emphasis on the whole person and self-responsibility for health. The underlying principles of health promotion are twofold.

1. Regardless of a person's health, the quality of life can be increased.
2. Wellness involves all components of life that affect well-being.

Health promotion is a part of primary health care and prevention, since primary prevention takes place before disease or illness occurs. Health promotion activities or strategies however are usually nonspecific; they are geared toward raising the general level of health and well-being of an individual, family, or community. Activities include stress management, nutrition education, weight control, life-style modification, and organized physical activity programs. Other primary prevention strategies

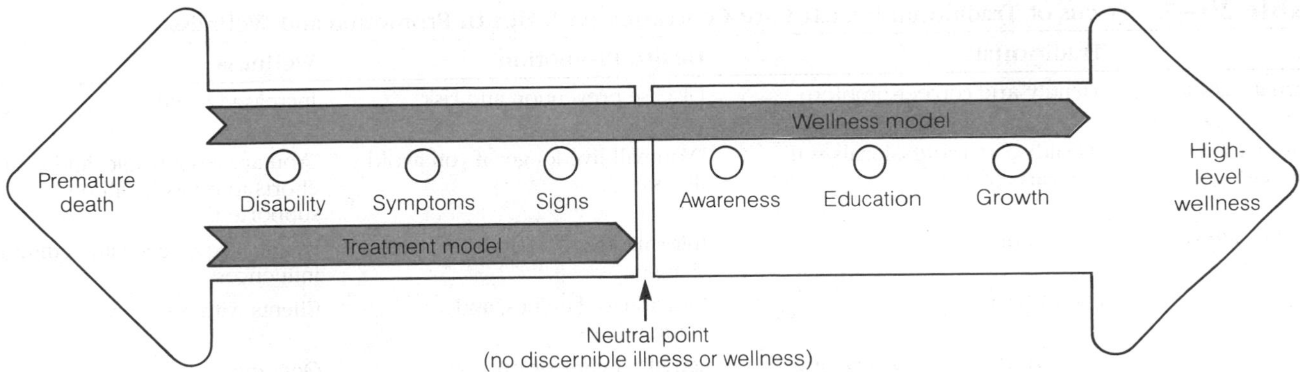

Figure 20–1 Health-illness continuum

Source: From R. S. Ryan and J. W. Travis, *Wellness workbook for health professionals* (Berkeley, Calif.: Ten Speed Press, 1981). Used by permission.

are more specific, i.e., they are directed toward the prevention of a specific disease. The most familiar example of protection against a specific disease is the use of vaccines to produce immunity against certain communicable diseases, such as poliomyelitis. Other specific protection strategies include stop-smoking clinics, purification of public water supplies, and the wearing of helmets by motorcyclists (Moore and Williamson 1984, p. 197).

The goal of health promotion is to raise the client's level of health. Most people equate health promotion and specific protection against disease with primary prevention. Others say that specific prevention is one aspect of health promotion (Spradley 1981).

Health promotion organizations and programs differ from **traditional health care** centers and programs that focus on illness or specific disease entities and health problems. Table 20–1 demonstrates these differences.

Types of Health Promotion Programs

Opatz (1985, p. 59) outlines the following types of health promotion programs:

1. Evaluation/screening programs
   Health risk appraisals
   Wellness inventories
   Breast self-exams
   Fitness evaluations
   Hypertension screening
   Multiphasic screening
   Diet analysis
   Stress evaluation
2. Educational/motivation programs
   Health risk appraisal interpretations
   Health/wellness fairs
   Wellness lectures
   Back education
   Alcohol/drug awareness
   Breast self-exam education
   Nutrition education
   Fitness/weight
3. Behavior change (participatory) programs
   Aerobic exercise
   Running clubs
   Stress management training
   Smoking cessation
   Back strengthening
   Self-care skills
   Blood pressure and pulse monitoring
   Nutrition modification
   Weight reduction
   Career evaluation and goal setting
4. Organizational enhancement programs
   Healthy foods program
   Air quality
   Smoking policies and enforcement
   Personnel policies (e.g., sick leave)
   Professional development
   Worksite stress assessment
   Employee assistance programs

Outcomes of Health Promotion Interventions

The expected outcomes of nursing interventions directed toward promoting health include (Pender 1982, p. 8):

1. Increased levels of health and well-being among individuals, families, and communities
2. Decreased incidence of illness and disability in individuals
3. Increased personal competence to minimize the barriers that prevent personal growth and fulfillment
4. Improvement in the abilities of clients or families to make rational health-related decisions
5. Self-care competence of clients

Table 20–1 Focus of Traditional Health Care Contrasted with Health Promotion and Wellness

	Traditional	Health Promotion	Wellness
Primary goal	Identify and correct problem	Disease prevention and risk reduction	Increased health
Dominant message	"Health care professionals will take care of you."	"You will live longer if you avoid illness."	"You are responsible, and your efforts to be well will be supported."
Change agent	Treatment	Information and behavior change	Positive experience and cultural influences
Target	The problem	Individuals, families, and communities	Clients within cultures
Duration of intervention	Ends when the problems clear up	Length of class or program	Ongoing

Source: Adapted from J. P. Opatz, *A primer of health promotion: Creating healthy organizational cultures* (Washington, D.C.: Oryn Publications, 1985), p. 101.

6. Increased ability of clients to assess personal or family needs for professional health care
7. Judicious use of all types of health care services
8. Greater availability and convenience of health-promoting as opposed to health-damaging options
9. Greater prevalence of health-promoting personal and family life-styles

The outcomes of health promotion are increased levels of health not only among individuals but also among families and communities. In his book about high-level wellness in the individual, Dunn (1973) also explores the concepts of family, community, environmental, and societal wellness. He believes that family wellness enhances wellness in individuals. In a well family that offers trust, love, and support, the individual does not have to expend energy to meet basic needs and can move forward on the wellness continuum. By providing effective sanitation and safe water, disposing of sewage safely, and preserving beauty and wildlife, the community enhances both family and individual wellness. Environmental wellness is related to the premise that humans must be at peace with and guard the environment. Societal wellness is significant because the status of the larger social group affects the status of smaller groups. Dunn believes that social wellness must be considered on a worldwide basis. The steps of the health promotion process are similar to those of the nursing process: health assessment, formulating a nursing diagnosis, development of a health protection/promotion plan, implementation of the plan, and evaluation.

Assessment

A thorough assessment of the client's health status is basic to health promotion. Components of this assessment are the health history and physical examination, physical-fitness assessment, nutrition assessment, health risk appraisal, life-style assessment, health beliefs review, and life-stress review (Pender 1982, p. 79). As nurses move toward greater autonomy in providing client care, expanded assessment skills are essential to provide the meaningful data needed for health planning.

Health History and Physical Examination

The health history and physical examination provide a means for detecting any existing problems. See Chapter 35 for detailed information about the health history and physical examination. Health histories need to include the following information (Edelman and Mandle 1986, p. 52).

1. Demographic data
2. Current and past medical problems
3. Family medical history
4. Surgical and (if appropriate) obstetric history
5. Childhood illnesses
6. Allergies
7. Current medications
8. Psychologic status
9. Social history

10. Environmental background
11. Review of systems

Physical-Fitness Assessment

During an evaluation of physical fitness, the nurse takes girth and skinfold measurements, administers the step test, and assesses strength and endurance of muscles and flexibility of joints.

Girth measurements The nurse measures the girth of the chest, waist, hips, upper arm (biceps), thigh, calf, and ankle. Guidelines for appropriate body proportions are shown in Table 20–2.

Skinfold measurements Skinfold measurements indicate the amount of body fat. To take skinfold measurements, the nurse grasps the skinfold (skin layers and subcutaneous fat) between the thumb and forefinger and measures the skinfold with special calipers. Skinfold sites are the triceps, subscapula, suprailiac, and thigh. See Chapter 42 for further information about skinfold procedures and norms.

The step test For this test, the client steps up and down a 17-inch step for 3 minutes. The following movements constitute one step: left foot up, right foot up, left foot down, right foot down. The rate should be 24 steps per minute for women and 30 steps for men (Getchell 1979, pp. 72–73). After the test, the client sits in a chair while the nurse assesses the pulse rate for 30 seconds at prescribed intervals:

1. 1 to 1½ minutes after the test
2. 2 to 2½ minutes after the test
3. 3 to 3½ minutes after the test

The sum of these three 30-second pulse rates is referred to as the **recovery index.** Normal values for women are 154–170; for men, 149–165 (Getchell 1979, pp. 72–73).

Muscle strength and endurance There are several tests of muscle strength and endurance. One is performing sit-ups with knees bent (bent-knee sit-ups). Women are asked to do these for 1 minute; men, for 2 minutes. The average rate for women is about 20 to 25 sit-ups per minute; for men, 50 to 60 per 2 minutes (Getchell 1979, p. 56).

Joint flexibility Range of motion in joints can be assessed quickly by asking the person to touch his or her toes several times. The average touch point is 1 to 3 inches in front of the toes. See Chapter 37 for detailed discussion of joint range of motion.

Table 20–2 Guidelines for Appropriate Girth Measurements

	Males	Females
Chest or bust	Same size as hips	Same size as hips
Waist	About 13 to 18 cm less than chest	About 25 cm less than bust
Upper arm	Twice the wrist size	Twice the wrist size
Thigh	20 to 25 cm less than abdomen	15 cm less than abdomen
Calf	18 to 20 cm less than thigh	15 to 18 cm less than thigh
Ankle	15 to 18 cm less than calf	13 to 15 cm less than calf

Source: N. J. Pender, *Health promotion in nursing practice* (Norwalk, Conn.: Appleton-Century-Crofts, 1982), p. 87. Used by permission.

Nutritional Assessment

To assess nutritional status, the nurse compares the client's weight to body build and height (see Chapter 35), measures mid-upper arm circumference to determine muscle mass, observes for signs of malnutrition, and takes a dietary history. The latter three are discussed in Chapter 42.

Health Risk Appraisal

A **health risk appraisal** (HRA) or health hazard appraisal (HHA) is an assessment and educational tool that indicates a client's risk of disease or injury over the next 10 years by comparing the client's risk with the mortality risk of his or her age, sex, and racial group. Behavior of the client and his or her demographic data are compared to behaviors of and data about a large national sample. The principle behind risk appraisal is that each person, as a member of a specific group, faces certain quantifiable health hazards and that average risks are applicable to a client if the health professional knows the client's characteristics and the mortality of a large group of cohorts with similar characteristics (Pender 1982, p. 97).

Many HRA instruments are available today. In 1970, Drs. Lewis Robbins and Jack Hall used the medical health model to develop an HRA called Health Hazard Appraisal. Since that time, other health care groups have adapted this tool and marketed it under several names. More recently HRAs have begun to reflect a broader approach to health. The new focus is on the assessment of life-style factors and health behaviors. The objectives of most HRAs are twofold:

1. To assess risk factors that may lead to health problems. A **risk factor** is a phenomenon (e.g., age or life-style behavior) that increases a person's chance of acquiring

a specific disease. The concept of at-risk aggregate is increasingly being used in community nursing practice. An **at-risk aggregate** is a subgroup within the community or population that is at greater risk of illness or poor recovery (Logan and Dawkins 1986, p. 18).

2. To change health behaviors that place the client at risk of developing an illness.

An HRA may have from 25 to 300 or more questions. Clients either score their responses themselves or send them to an organization for computer printouts. Scores are often tabulated according to an overall life-style profile, levels of health risk, and life expectancy.

Risk factors may be categorized according to:

1. Age
2. Genetic factors
3. Biologic characteristics
4. Personal health habits
5. Life-style
6. Environment

Clients cannot control some of the risk factors appraised, such as age, sex, and family history; others, such as blood pressure, stress, and cigarette smoking, can be partially or totally controlled.

Pender (1982, pp. 99–106) developed a comprehensive risk factor assessment tool. She classifies risk factors into five categories:

1. Risk of cardiovascular disease
2. Risk of malignant disease
3. Risk of automobile accidents
4. Risk of suicide
5. Risk of diabetes

Contributing factors, such as family and personal medical history, habits, sex, age, environment, and life-style patterns, are included. See Figure 20–2 for part of Pender's risk appraisal form, i.e., the section related to risk of cardiovascular disease.

A client is usually appraised as being at high risk of developing a specific disease when two or three of the risk factors are at the highest level or four of the risk factors are at the two highest levels. Many computer printout results also predict the person's life expectancy, which is compared to the life expectancy of the average person of the client's age, race, and sex. Most HRA data norms are derived from death rates calculated by the U.S. National Center for Health Statistics. These rates are known as the Geller Mortality Tables. The tables are established for cohorts of 10 years for males and females of black and white races. They list the 10 or 12 leading causes of death in order of decreasing significance for each 10-year chart. The HRA printout also indicates an achievable life expectancy for the client, predicated on the assumption that the client will reduce all possible risk factors. See Figure 20–3 for a sample printout for the Life-Style Assessment (LAQ) Questionnaire, University of Wisconsin-Stevens Point. This LAQ is divided into four sections, the third of which deals with risk factors.

Life-Style Assessment

Life-style assessment focuses on the personal life-style and habits of the client as they affect health. Categories of life-style generally assessed are physical activity, nutritional practices, stress management, and such habits as smoking, alcohol consumption, and drug use. Other categories may be included.

Several tools are available to assess life-style. Pender (1982, pp. 113–18) outlines a comprehensive 10-category tool that includes:

1. Competence in self-care, including dental hygiene, breast self-examination, knowledge about the danger signs of cancer, blood pressure, and other health care practices
2. Nutritional practices
3. Physical or recreational activity
4. Sleep patterns
5. Stress management
6. Self-actualization, including outlook on life and feelings about self, work, and accomplishments
7. Sense of purpose in life and knowledge of what is important in one's life
8. Relationships with others
9. Environmental control to make living areas free of hazards
10. Use of the health care system

The number of statements in each category range from 4 to 16. The reader is referred to Pender 1982 (see Selected References) for detailed information.

Travis (1977) developed a shorter, 16-item life-style assessment form entitled the Wellness Index. This tool may be used for initial assessments when client time is limited. See Figure 20–4.

The goals of life-style assessment tools are:

1. To provide an opportunity for clients to assess the impact of their present life-style on their health
2. To provide a basis for decisions related to desired behavior and life-style change.

In each row, place a check in the box that best describes your current life situation or behavior.

Risk for Cardiovascular Disease

Risk factor:		→ Increasing risk →					
Sex and age:		Female under 40	Female 40–50	Male 25–40	Female after menopause	Male 40–60	Male 61 or over
Family history (mother, father, brothers, sisters)	High blood pressure	No relatives with condition	One relative	Two relatives	Three relatives		
	Heart attack	No relatives with condition	One relative with condition after 60	Two relatives with condition after 60	One relative with condition before 60	Two relatives with condition before 60	
	Diabetes	No relatives with condition	One or more relatives with maturity onset diabetes	One or more relatives with preadolescent or adolescent onset			
Blood pressure*	Systolic	120 or below	121–140	141–160	161–180	181–200	above 200
	Diastolic	70 or below	71–80	81–90	91–100	101–110	above 110

In each row, place a check in the box that best describes your current life situation or behavior.

Risk for Cardiovascular Disease

Sleep patterns*		7 or 8 hr sleep/night	More than 8 hr sleep/night	4–6 hr sleep/night			
Cigarette smoking*	No./day	Nonsmoker	1–10/day	11–20/day	21–30/day	31–40/day	Over 40/day
	No. of yr smoked	Nonsmoker	Less than 10 yr	11–15 yr	16–20 yr	21–30 yr	31 yr or more
Stress*	Domestic	Minimal	Moderate	High	Very high		
	Occupational	Minimal	Moderate	High	Very high		
Behavior pattern* (particularly males)		Type B Relaxed, appropriately assertive, not time dependent, moderate to slow speech	Type A Excessively competitive, aggressive, striving, hyperalert, time dependent, loud, explosive speech				
Air pollution*		Low	Moderate	High			
Use of oral contraceptives* (females)		Do not use oral contraceptives	Under 40 and use oral contraceptives	Over 40 and use oral contraceptives			

*Indicates risk factors that can be fully or partially controlled.
†Serum lipid analysis is also recommended to determine low-density (beta) and high-density (alpha) lipoprotein levels. Evidence suggests that high-density lipoprotein (HDL) carries cholesterol from tissues for metabolism and excretion. An inverse correlation appears to exist between HDL and coronary artery disease.

Figure 20–2 Risk assessment tool for cardiovascular disease (parts 1 and 3 of a 3-part tool)

Source: From N. J. Pender, *Health promotion in nursing practice* (New York: Appleton-Century-Crofts, 1982), pp. 99–101. Used by permission.

SAMPLE PRINTOUTS

UNIVERSITY OF WISCONSIN-STEVENS POINT
LIFESTYLE ASSESSMENT RESULTS

Prepared for 9002 1 000000000

1

WELLNESS INVENTORY

The following scores indicate your wellness compared with average of people taking this survey with you, and averages of all people who have taken the survey.

Category	Your Score	Group Average	Total Average
Physical Exercise	68	73	70
Physical Nutritional	52	67	52
Physical Self Care	46	60	48
Physical Vehicle Safety	47	75	49
Physical Drug Usage	72	95	75
Social Environmental	27	56	32
Emotional Awareness and Acceptance	20	50	24
Emotional Management	47	69	51
Intellectual	68	82	71
Occupational	73	79	73
Spiritual	65	68	66

2

PERSONAL GROWTH SECTION
AUTOMATED REFERRAL

EXERCISE PROGRAMS

A. Media
1. Movies: Coping With Life On the Run—Sports Productions Inc.
   Run Dick, Run Jane—American Heart Association
   The Heart: An Attack—CRM
2. Books: Joy of Running—Kostrubala
   Women's Running—Ullyot
   The Complete Runner—Fixx
   Stretching—Anderson
   Sheehan on Running—George Sheehan
   The Ultimate Athlete—Leonard
   Aerobics—Cooper
   Aerobics for Women—Cooper

B. Community Resources
   YMCA or YWCA programs

3

RISK OF DEATH SECTION

Age 40 Height 73
Race White Weight 222
Sex Male

Life Expectancy Results

1 5 10 15 20 25 30 35 40 45

Average Years of Remaining Life in Your Sex, Age, Race Group 33*********************

Your Expected Yrs. of Remaining Life Based on your Answers 25****************

You can achieve this expected yrs. of remaining life 38***********************

RISK OF DEATH SECTION (Con't.)

Major Hazards to you

Rank Hazard	10 year deaths Per 100,000	Associated risk factors
1. Cirrhosis		
Average	304	Drinking Habits
Your	3800	
Achievable	61	
2. Arteriosclerotic Heart Disease		
Average	1861	Systolic Blood Pressure
Your	2382	Diastolic Blood Pressure
Achievable	447	Cholesterol Level
		Smoking Habits
		Weight
3. Motor Vehicle Accidents		
Average	339	Drinking Habits
Your	1763	Seat Belt Habits
Achievable	203	
4. Cancer of Lungs		
Average	291	Smoking Habits
Your	582	
Achievable	58	

Suggestions For Increasing Your Expected Years Of Remaining Life

1. choosing non-drinking	will add 8.6 exp. years of life
2. choosing non-smoking	will add 2.0 exp. years of life
3. lowering cholesterol level	will add 0.7 exp. years of life
4. lowering diastolic blood pressure	will add 0.6 exp. years of life
5. lowering systolic blood pressure	will add 0.6 exp. years of life
6. losing weight	will add 0.4 exp. years of life
7. always wearing seatbelts	will add 0.1 exp. years of life
8. having annual procto exam	will add 0.1 exp. years of life
Total	13

Remarks:

We have had to make the following assumptions about you:

You have an average blood cholesterol level.

Hazard Summary

Based on the Lifestyle Assessment Questionnaire you have filled out, you have a health age of 48 years. If you follow all the suggestions we have given, you can reduce your health age to 35.

4

ALERT SECTION: Medical/Behavior/Emotional

Significant Past Illnesses
1. Diabetic
2. Physical disability

Immunizations
1. Up-to-date for DPT
2. Up-to-date for polio
3. Rubella status unknown

Allergies
1. Allergic to penicillin

Emotions
1. History compatible with serious depression

Figure 20–3 Sample printout, University of Wisconsin-Stevens Point Life-Style Assessment Results

Source: B. Hettler, Wellness and promotion and risk reduction on a university campus. University of Wisconsin-Stevens Point.

Circle the category that most closely answers the question.

1. I am conscious of the ingredients of the food I eat and their effect on me. Rarely, Sometimes, Very Often (R, S, VO)
2. I avoid overeating and abusing alcohol, caffeine, nicotine, and other drugs. R, S, VO
3. I minimize my intake of refined carbohydrates and fats. R, S, VO
4. My diet contains adequate amounts of vitamins, minerals, and fiber. R, S, VO
5. I am free from physical symptoms. R, S, VO
6. I get aerobic cardiovascular exercise. R, S, VO (Very Often is at least 12–20 minutes 5 times per week vigorously running, swimming, or bike riding)
7. I practice yoga or some other form of limbering/stretching exercise. R, S, VO
8. I nurture myself. R, S, VO (Nurturing means pleasuring and taking care of oneself, for example, massages, long walks, buying presents for self, "doing nothing," sleeping late without feeling guilty, etc.)
9. I pay attention to changes occurring in my life and am aware of them as stress factors. R, S, VO (See Life-Change Index—a score of over 300 is considered very stressful)
10. I practice regular relaxation. R, S, VO (Suggested: 20 minutes a day "centering" or "letting go" of thoughts, worries, etc.)
11. I am without excess muscle tension. R, S, VO
12. My hands are warm and dry. R, S, VO
13. I am both productive and happy. R, S, VO
14. I constructively express my emotions and creativity. R, S, VO
15. I feel a sense of purpose in life and my life has meaning and direction. R, S, VO
16. I believe I am fully responsible for my wellness or illness. R, S, VO

Using your answers above to guide you, you can synthesize a graphic picture of your wellness. Each numbered pie-shaped segment of the circle below corresponds to the same numbered question on the preceding page. (They are divided into quarters representing four major dimensions of wellness.) Color in an amount of each segment corresponding to your answer to the question with the same number. The inner broken circle corresponds to "rarely," the next one to "sometimes," the third to "very often." You don't need to restrict yourself to these categories, however, and can fill in any amount in between. You may use different colors for each section if you like.

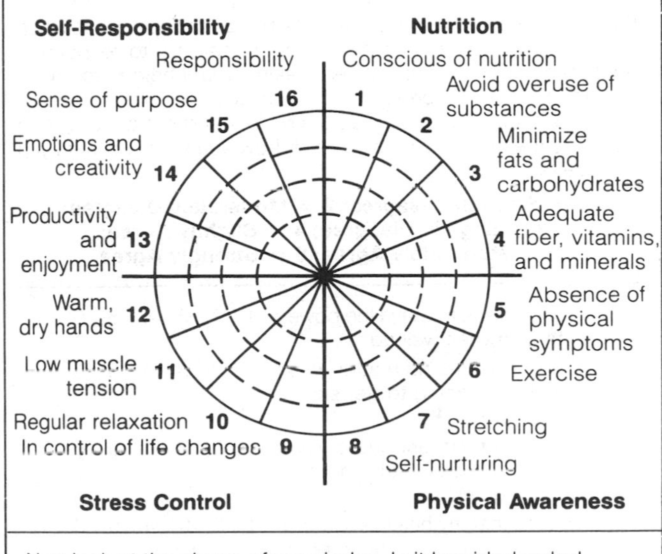

Now look at the shape of your index. Is it lopsided or balanced? This should provide beginning suggestions for improving your lifestyle and health habits.

Figure 20–4 Wellness index

Source: Questions taken from *Wellness Index*. Used with permission, Copyright 1975, 1981, 1986. John W. Travis M.D., Wellness Associates, Box 5433, Mill Valley, CA 94942. Abridged from the *Wellness Workbook*, Ryan & Travis, Ten Speed Press, 1981.

Health Care Beliefs

The client's health care beliefs need to be clarified, particularly those beliefs that determine how he or she perceives control of his or her own health care status. Wallston et al. (1978) developed two Multidimensional Health Locus of Control (MHLC) instruments to assess perceptions of health control. See Figure 20–5 for one such instrument. Assessment of clients' health care beliefs provides the nurse with an indication of how much the clients believe they can influence or control health through personal behaviors.

The Multidimensional Health Locus of Control (MHLC) Scales are derived from the assumptions underlying social learning theory, in which a person's motivation for health behavior is thought to be related to an internal or external orientation toward self and the environment. Persons who are internally controlled are more likely than others to

Research Note

Nurses act as educators and role models for behaviors that promote health and wellness. Laffrey and Isenberg built on other studies of "locus of control" when they measured the relative internality or externality of an individual's locus of control, the importance the subjects assigned to physical exercise, and the amount of physical exercise they engaged in during leisure time. Among the 70 women studied, the importance they assigned to exercise was the key factor determining the amount of exercise they actually undertook. To promote health effectively, then, nurses must understand just how clients view physical exercise. (Laffrey and Isenberg 1983, pp. 187–96)

This questionnaire is designed to determine the way in which different people view certain important health-related issues. Each item is a belief statement with which you may agree or disagree. Beside each statement is a scale that ranges from strongly disagree (1) to strongly agree (6). For each item we would like you to circle the number that represents the extent to which you disagree or agree with the statement. The more strongly you agree with a statement, the higher will be the number you circle. The more strongly you disagree with a statement, the lower will be the number you circle. Please make sure that you answer every item and that you circle *only one* number per item. This is a measure of your personal beliefs; obviously, there are no right or wrong answers.

Please answer these items carefully, but do not spend too much time on any one item. As much as you can, try to respond to each item independently. When making your choice, do not be influenced by your previous choices. It is important that you respond according to your actual beliefs and not according to how you feel you should believe or how you think we want you to believe.

1 = Strongly Disagree; 2 = Moderately Disagree; 3 = Slightly Disagree; 4 = Slightly Agree; 5 = Moderately Agree; 6 = Strongly Agree.

1. If I become sick, I have the power to make myself well again.	1	2	3	4	5	6
2. Often I feel that no matter what I do, if I am going to get sick, I will get sick.	1	2	3	4	5	6
3. If I see an excellent doctor regularly, I am less likely to have health problems.	1	2	3	4	5	6
4. It seems that my health is greatly influenced by accidental happenings.	1	2	3	4	5	6
5. I can only maintain my health by consulting health professionals.	1	2	3	4	5	6
6. I am directly responsible for my health.	1	2	3	4	5	6
7. Other people play a big part in whether I stay healthy or become sick	1	2	3	4	5	6
8. Whatever goes wrong with my health is my own fault.	1	2	3	4	5	6
9. When I am sick, I just have to let nature run its course.	1	2	3	4	5	6
10. Health professionals keep me healthy.	1	2	3	4	5	6
11. When I stay healthy, I'm just plain lucky.	1	2	3	4	5	6
12. My physical well-being depends on how well I take care of myself.	1	2	3	4	5	6
13. When I feel ill, I know it is because I have not been taking care of myself properly.	1	2	3	4	5	6
14. The type of care I receive from other people is what is responsible for how well I recover from an illness.	1	2	3	4	5	6
15. Even when I take care of myself, it's easy to get sick.	1	2	3	4	5	6
16. When I become ill, it's a matter of fate.	1	2	3	4	5	6
17. I can pretty much stay healthy by taking good care of myself.	1	2	3	4	5	6
18. Following doctor's orders to the letter is the best way for me to stay healthy.	1	2	3	4	5	6

Figure 20–5 Multidimensional health locus of control scale (Form B)

Source: From K. A. Wallston, B. S. Wallston, and R. DeVellis, Development of multidimensional health locus of control (MHLC) scales, *Health Education Monographs,* Spring 1978, 6:164–65.

take the initiative in their own health care, be more knowledgeable about their health, and adhere to prescribed health care regimens. Persons who are externally controlled feel that their health can be attributed to luck, fate, or powerful others and thus is beyond their control. The Health Belief Model (HBM) discussed in Chapter 2 on page 59 suggests that the motivation to engage in a behavior is based on the person's belief that (a) one is vulnerable to the health problem, (b) the illness or problem is a threat, (c) the recommended health action will reduce the threat without substantial inconvenience, and (d) people should be generally concerned about health matters and be willing to accept medical advice (Becker et al. 1972, p. 852).

Researchers have not been able to validate a significant association between a person's health beliefs and his or her behaviors (Muhlencamp et al. 1985, p. 327). Cox (1985, p. 178) therefore has developed a new measure of motivation called the Health Self-Determination Index (HSDI). She believes that motivation is multidimensional, i.e., based on many factors. The process of choosing between behaviors is a primary factor.

Cox's HSDI includes a 20-item scale that has four interrelated subscales or factors:

1. *Self-determined health judgments.* Self-determinism in health judgments is assessed by the client's responses to statements such as:

    "Whatever the doctor suggests is OK with me."

    "Only the doctor knows if I am in good health."

    "What the doctor thinks is more important than what I think."

    "I do things to help my health without a doctor's or nurse's input."

2. *Self-determined health behavior.* Self-determinism in health behavior is assessed by the client's responses to statements such as:

    "I know without a doctor's telling me so that I'm doing the right things for my health."

    "I know without someone telling me so when I am in good health."

    "My own ideas are better than the doctor's."

    "I know what I am doing when it comes to taking care of my health."

3. *Perceived competency in health matters.* Perceived competency is determined by the client's responses to statements such as:

"I feel good about how I take care of my health." "I do things to help my health without a doctor's or nurse's input."

"I don't do as well at taking care of my health as others."

4. *Responsiveness to internal and external cues.* Responsiveness is measured by response to statements such as:

"Some people think the doctor should decide about their health, but I think I should."

"I worry about my health."

"I'm never sure I'm doing the right things for my health unless I check with a doctor."

Although this tool has not been tested sufficiently to be used as a diagnostic aid, the data obtained in Cox's study strongly support the multidimensionality of motivation and the contributing roles of judgment, behavior, sense of competency, and responsiveness to internal or external cues. With further refinement and research, the HSDI will enable nurses to (Cox 1985, p. 182):

1. Identify people at risk for decreased health and well-being owing to specific motivational responses.
2. Examine the motivational responses of clients throughout the life span for trends and changes.
3. Evaluate the differential effects of chronic versus acute illness on a person's motivational response.
4. Examine the effectiveness of interventions on specific health outcomes.

Life-Stress Review

There is abundant literature about the impact of stress on mental and physical well-being. Assessment of stressors, signs of anxiety, and stress is discussed in Chapter 17.

Nursing Diagnosis

Nursing diagnoses related to health promotion often involve potential rather than actual health problems. (Examples are shown below.)

Examples of Nursing Diagnoses Related to Health Promotion

- Potential alterations in nutrition (more than body requirements) related to sedentary life-style
- Potential alteration in nutrition (less than body requirements) related to inappropriate eating patterns (e.g., unscheduled meals and eating fast foods)
- Ineffective individual coping related to stress and unsatisfactory support system
- Potential alteration in health maintenance related to substance abuse (tobacco)
- Potential alteration in health maintenance related to lack of appropriate immunization
- Potential alteration in health maintenance related to knowledge deficit about parenting
- Potential alteration in health maintenance related to knowledge deficit about breast self-examination
- Potential for injury related to lack of awareness of environmental hazards and acceptance of declining physical capabilities
- Potential alterations in oral mucous membrane related to inadequate oral hygiene
- Diversional activity deficit related to postretirement inactivity
- Impaired social interaction related to self-concept disturbance secondary to obesity
- Impaired adjustment related to alterations in cardiac function requiring change in lifestyle

Planning

Following assessment, the client and nurse have a great deal of information about the client's health status, health risks, life-style, and health beliefs. Health promotion plans need to be developed according to the desires of the client, who decides on goals, priorities, sequencing, methods, and implementation (Black and McDowell 1984, p. 20). The nurse acts as a resource person rather than as an adviser or counselor. She or he provides information when asked, emphasizes the importance of small steps to behavioral change, and reviews the client's goals and plans to make sure they are realistic, measurable, and acceptable to the client.

Nine Steps in Planning

Pender (1982, p. 178) outlines nine steps in the process of health planning, which is carried out jointly by the nurse and client:

1. *Review and summarize assessment data.* The nurse and client need to consider:
   a. Any existing health problems
   b. The degree of control the client thinks he or she exerts over his or her health status
   c. Level of physical fitness and nutritional status
   d. Illnesses for which the client is at risk
   e. Current positive health practices
   f. Ability to handle stress
   g. Information needed to enhance health care practices

   Nonjudgmental awareness of present attitudes, activities, and behaviors is the first step to behavior change.
2. *Identify health care strengths.* Areas of strength, such as flossing teeth daily, eating breakfast daily, and being able to laugh at oneself, need to be acknowledged and supported. Recognition of strengths enhances self-awareness and self-esteem and makes the client aware of what he or she is controlling.
3. *Identify health care goals and areas for improvement.* Interventions necessary to decrease the risk of developing specific diseases is often a concrete starting point for many clients. Interventions for health promotion, a less tangible concept, are often recognized later, as is the concept of high-level wellness. The client selects two or three top priority goals or areas for improvement. Common goals are to decrease the risk of cardiovascular or other disease, to achieve or maintain a desired weight, to become more physically fit, to cope with stress, to improve relationships with family members or friends, and to manage time more effectively.
4. *Identify possible behavior changes.* For each of the selected goals or areas in step 3, determine what specific behavioral changes are needed to bring about the desired outcome. For example, to reduce the risk of cardiovascular disease, the client may need to change these specific behaviors:
   a. Stop smoking
   b. Lose weight
   c. Increase activity level
   d. Learn to relax
   e. Decrease animal fat in diet
   f. Discontinue use of oral contraceptives
   g. Sleep 7 to 8 hours per night
5. *Assign priorities to behavior changes.* Behavior must be acceptable to the client if it is to be adopted and integrated. From the list of behavior options in step 3, the client selects and assigns priorities to those changes he or she is most willing to try. For example, the client may select increasing activity level, losing weight, and stopping smoking, in that order. It is helpful if the client first selects a behavior change area in which change is most readily perceived as positive. A successful beginning experience is important.
6. *Make a commitment to change behavior.* In the past, commitments to change behavior have usually been verbal. Increasingly, a formal, written **behavioral contract** is being used to motivate the client to follow through with selected actions. Motivation to follow through is provided by a positive reinforcement or reward stated in the contract. Contracting is based on the belief that all persons have the potential for growth and the right of self-determination, even though their choices may be different from the norm. Contracts are of two types: nurse-client contracts or self-contracts. For an example of a nurse-client contract, see the section on health care compliance in Chapter 2, page 65. The self-contract is similar, e.g.,:

   > I, Amy Martin will exercise strenuously for 20 minutes three times per week for a period of 2 weeks and will then buy myself six yellow roses.
   >
   > Amy Martin
   > July 30, 19xx

   To ensure that a contract is explicit and meaningful, Kort (1984, p. 25) recommends that the client review it against the SMART checklist:

   Specific: Do I know how, when, where, with whom, and how long I will do this?

   Measurable: Will I know when it's done?

   Acceptable: Will I feel good about doing this?

Research Note

Behavioral contracts and goal setting for risk reduction have been used to increase client participation and to motivate change in client behavior. Alexy compared the effectiveness of three approaches: client participation (collaborative approach) in goal selection aimed at health risk reduction, selection of goals by the provider, and no selection of goals. No difference in goal attainment was found between the two groups with goals. The group whose goals were set by the provider made significant changes in alcohol intake, seat belt use, and exercise. The group who set goals collaboratively made significant changes in weight reduction and exercise levels. This study suggests that setting goals for risk reduction can be effective in changing behavior, but that client participation in setting goals is not superior to a directive approach. (Alexy 1985)

Realistic: Am I able to do this?

Truthful: Do I really want to?

Before a contract can be made, the client needs to identify actions that will bring about the desired behavior change. If, for example, the behavior change is to increase activity level, the client needs to consider and adopt specific actions. The client may consider swimming for 30 minutes three times a week, walking briskly for 1 hour daily, or some similar activity.

7. *Identify effective reinforcements and rewards.* Rewards tend to provide an incentive for behavior change, more so than individual willpower, provided the reward is meaningful to the client and selected by him or her. Rewards can be objects, experiences, family activities, or praise. Examples of objects used as rewards are books, educational pamphlets, and personal care items. Examples of experiences used as rewards are having a 15-minute talk with a consultant, renting a cassette about a specific health matter, or going to a concert or health spa. Family trips, sports, or picnics are strong reinforcement for some people.
8. *Determine barriers to change.* Some specific barriers to change are:
   a. Lack of support from family members
   b. Lack of space to carry out a certain activity
   c. Inappropriate weather
   d. Lack of motivation
   e. Fatigue or boredom
   f. Strong anxiety
   g. Cost of change
   h. Inconvenience
   i. Lack of time
   j. Culture or peer pressure
9. *Develop a schedule for implementing the behavior change.* Clients need to set up a time frame to make the behavior changes required to meet each goal. Time frames may be several weeks or months. Scheduling short-term goals and rewards can offer encouragement to achieve long-term objectives. Clients may need help to be realistic and to deal with one behavior at a time.

Exploring Available Resources

Another essential aspect of planning is identifying support resources available to the client. These may be community resources, such as a fitness program at a local gymnasium, or educational programs, such as stress management, breast self-examination, nutrition, smoking cessation, and health lectures. The nurse, too, may meet some of the client's educational needs. A major nursing role is to support the client. The nurse can contact the client or be available at specified intervals to review the contract and to assist with problem solving.

Intervention

Implementing is the "doing" part of behavior change. Although self-responsibility is emphasized for implementing the plans, ongoing support from the nurse, family members, and friends is an essential component of health promotion. The nurse also provides information and educational programs as required, assists the client to make and maintain behavior changes (behavior modification), and is a model of good health behaviors.

Providing Support

A vital component of life-style change is ongoing support that focuses on the desired behavior change and is provided in an objective and accepting manner. Support can be offered on an individual basis or in groups. Kort, a coordinator of the Healthstyles Program of the Centertown Community Health Center, Ottawa, outlines five kinds of support the program offers (1984, pp. 24–25). The nurse can implement some or all of these support methods.

1. *Telephone calls.* The Healthstyles staff schedules weekly telephone support calls for at least the first 4 weeks and thereafter on a monthly basis. During these calls, the staff reviews client progress, explores problems with the contract plans, and prepares a contract for the next week. Calls are also an opportunity to reinforce successful behavior changes. The client is asked, "Is your contract working?" "What do you want to do now?" "Continue?" If the contract is not working, the staff member asks, "What would you like to change?" Peer telephone calls are another form of support. These calls continue as long as the clients or participants find them useful.
2. *Follow-up groups.* Group sessions provide an opportunity for participants to learn the experiences of others in changing behavior. Group contact gives individuals a renewed commitment to their goals. Groups can be scheduled at monthly or less frequent intervals for over a year. The Ottawa Healthstyles program offers five sessions at months 1, 3, 7, 12, and 18.
3. *Health awareness sessions.* Community speakers can offer regular workshops on a variety of health-related topics. These sessions are a good way to disseminate information that promotes life-style changes. See the section on health education, next.

4. *Information.* Clients appreciate up-to-date information on community resources that can assist with lifestyle changes. Many community agencies provide programs on nutrition, smoking cessation, weight loss, stress management, and alcohol and drug treatment. Also, many books and articles about health and wellness are available, e.g., books about women's health, parental guidance, and stress reduction.

5. *Individual counseling sessions.* Counseling sessions may be provided if the client encounters insurmountable barriers to change. Clients with long-standing emotional barriers need to be referred to skilled counselors at an appropriate community agency.

Providing Health Education

Health education programs on a variety of topics can be provided to groups, individuals, or communities. Group programs need to be carefully planned before they are implemented. The decision to establish a health promotion program must be based on the assessed health needs of the people; also, specific health promotion goals must be set. After the program is implemented, program outcomes must be evaluated.

Nurses may offer an abundance of information less formally. To do so, however, nurses need up-to-date knowledge, the ability to assess learning needs, and effective teaching skills. See Chapter 29 for detailed information. For example, nurses often disseminate information about parenting, breast and testicular self-examination, prevention of sexually transmitted disease, nutritional needs, and monitoring blood pressure and pulse rates.

Health promotion fairs are a recent method of enhancing the health of the public. See the Suggested Readings at the end of this chapter.

Enhancing Behavior Change

Whether people will make and maintain changes to improve health or prevent disease depends on many interrelated factors. See the section on assessing health care beliefs, earlier in this chapter. Murphy (1982, p. 427) says that the distances between wanting to change, attempting to change, and being able to change can be enormous. She emphasizes this statement by pointing out the difficulty many people have in acquiring regular dental flossing habits. When a client succeeds in making healthy behavior changes because of information the nurse has provided, the nurse feels satisfied and pleased. When, however, the client does not succeed in planned behavioral changes, the nurse tends to feel frustrated and often describes the person as "resistant," "uninterested," "unmotivated," or "noncompliant."

Murphy (1982) says that nurses are erroneously inclined to believe:

1. That change will occur simply by bringing unhealthy behavior to the client's attention
2. That when the client does not change, the desire to change is absent.

The response of the nurse to lack of change in the client is generally to provide more information or to withdraw from the interaction after concluding that there is no point wasting time on people who do not want to change. Both responses deny the client the opportunity to improve his or her health. By providing more information to the client, the nurse assumes that the client lacks knowledge. If, however, the client has understood the information, repeating or amplifying the information more than likely will annoy the client. The nurse has failed to identify the problem clearly. Withdrawal from clients who have difficulty changing implies that the nurse's health promotion efforts will be directed toward persons who readily and willingly comply. Such people, however, are probably the ones who least need the nurse's help.

To help clients succeed in implementing behavior changes, the nurse needs to understand the process of change and the nature of the client's motivation or the client's current situation. An understanding of Lewin's stages of change (Lewin 1951) can help the nurse recognize the client's needs (Murphy 1982, p. 428).

Stage 1 (Unfreezing)

In this stage, the client's motivation to change emerges. The client recognizes the need to change and becomes uneasy about his or her present way of doing things. At this stage, the nurse must help the client feel safe enough to explore and consider alternatives. Murphy says, " 'Unfreezing' " or 'unlearning' old habits is probably the most important stage of change but it is also the most difficult and challenging for the health promoter." The nurse can best help the client by emphasizing what that person values. Loss of an unhealthy behavior may then become tolerable. For example, a client may start to "unfreeze" a habit of eating excessive carbohydrates if emphasis is placed on maximizing energy potential through a balanced food intake rather than just on the components of a healthy diet.

Stage 2 (Moving)

In the second stage, the client is ready to change and develop new responses. Many health promoters tend to focus their efforts on this stage of eliciting new desired responses (Murphy 1982).

Stage 3 (Refreezing)

In this stage, the client internalizes behavior changes and stabilizes a new level of functioning.

To enhance positive behavior changes in clients, the nurse needs to (Murphy 1982, p. 429):

1. Recognize that motivation is the basis of all behavior whether it is healthy or unhealthy, good or bad.
2. Recognize that people are motivated by their needs.
3. Avoid labeling people as unmotivated. The label simply means that the person does not comply with the wishes of the nurse who applies the label.
4. Focus on the sources or factors that motivate the person's behavior rather than on the presence or absence of motivation.
5. Remember that resistance is a normal part of change and a healthy response to a threat.
6. Understand that a client may choose to keep unhealthy habits for many reasons.
   a. The habit may be a culturally learned response. For example, the long-term hazards of cigarette smoking and alcohol consumption have only recently become known and publicized. In North America, these habits were once associated with a glamorous or sophisticated life-style and a certain kind of satisfaction.
   b. The client may be directing all available energies to meet other needs. A person who is grieving the loss of a loved one or a recently divorced person, for example, may not have the energy to follow a weight loss diet.
   c. The conditions required to change may be absent. For example, a client needs help to first "unlearn" or "unfreeze" old habits and recognize the benefits of new habits before he or she can consider or undertake action.
7. Cast aside the idea that the client *must* change. This attitude is not conducive to helping a relationship with the client and does not convey respect for the client. The client who does not change is entitled to the nurse's interest and nonjudgmental response.
8. Measure the nurse's competence in terms of how well the nurse understands the client's needs and implements the client's care rather than by the extent to which a client changes his or her behavior.

Modeling

Modeling consists of observing the behavior of people who have successfully achieved the goal that the client has set for himself or herself (Pender 1982, p. 216). Modeling is not imitating. Through observing a model, the client acquires ideas for behavior and coping strategies for specific problems. The client is not expected to mimic the sequence of actions or behavior patterns of the model.

The nurse and client should mutually select models with whom the client can identify, since the cultural and ethnic backgrounds of the nurse and client often differ. Models should be frequently available during the early learning and change stages of unfreezing and moving. Models should also be people the client respects.

Nurses should serve as models of wellness. Carlin (1982, p. 48) strongly believes that the philosophy nurses manifest in their lives affects their professional effectiveness more than the philosophy they preach. Nurses, therefore, need to assess their own wellness and initiate changes as required before becoming a model for clients. Clients are more likely to respect and trust the nurse who can tell them what worked for her or him.

Evaluation

The process of evaluating involves measurement of the client's progress or lack of progress toward goal achievement. Evaluation is a collaborative effort between the nurse and client. Progress or lack of progress is determined by the goals or outcome criteria specified in the client's contract. It may be necessary to reassess, reorder priorities, set new goals, or revise the contract.

Chapter Highlights

- Health promotion is part of primary health care and prevention.
- Health promotion activities are directed toward developing client resources that maintain or enhance well-being.
- The goal of health promotion is to raise the client's level of health.
- Health promotion can occur at any point along the continuum of health and illness; it emphasizes the whole person and self-responsibility for health.
- Health promotion programs can be categorized as evaluation/screening programs, educational/motivational programs, behavior change (participatory) programs, and organizational enhancement programs.
- A thorough assessment of the client's health status is basic to health promotion.
- Health risk or hazard appraisals provide the data that often spur the client to adopt a healthier life-style.

- Life-style assessment tools give clients the opportunity to assess the impact of their present life-styles on their health and to make decisions about life-style changes.
- The client's health care beliefs provide the nurse with an indication of how much the client believes he or she can influence or control health through personal behaviors.
- To help clients change their life-styles or health behaviors, the nurse provides ongoing support, supplies additional information and education, and explores the motivating sources of the client's behavior.
- By acting as models of wellness, nurses show clients what goals to strive for.

Suggested Readings

Carlin, D. C. March/April 1982. How to assess your wellness—and become a model for your patients. *Nursing Life* 2:48–49.
Carlin outlines essential steps for nurses to promote their health. A self-assessment test and worksheets indicating sample health goals and barriers and strategies are included.

Fuller-Bey, G. April 1983. Antismoking counseling, an important part of cardiac rehabilitation. *The Canadian Nurse* 79:17–20.
Fuller-Bey gives facts about smoking, the physiologic and psychologic cycle of addiction, situations that trigger smoking, and strategies to cope with the events that trigger smoking. To help clients stop smoking, nurses need to show empathy and give support.

Health fairs for older adults. May/June 1982. *Geriatric Nursing* 3:172–76. (Oppeneu, J., and Mundt, M. Steps to the fair, pp. 172–73; Oase, S., and Tracy, J. The big day, pp. 174–75; and LaMonica, G., and Rotherham, D. After the fair is over, p. 176.)
This series of articles describes the steps involved in setting up a health fair that involves client participation and outlines the follow-up steps used to reinforce the advice offered at the fair.

Steckel, S. B. September 1980. Contracting with patient-selected reinforcers. *American Journal of Nursing* 80:1596–99.
Steckel discusses the objectives, principles, process, and benefits of contracts. An essential part of a contract is the reinforcer. Several examples of client-selected reinforcers are included.

Selected References

Alexy, B. September/October 1985. Goal setting and health risk reduction. *Nursing Research* 34:283–88.

Becker, M.; Drachman, R.; and Kirscht, J. 1972. Motivation as predictors of health behavior. *Health Services Reports* 87:852–62.

Black, A., and McDowell, R. April 1984. Health styles: Moving beyond disease prevention. *The Canadian Nurse* 80:18–20.

Brubaker, B. H. April 1983. Health promotion: A linguistic analysis. *Advances in Nursing Science* 5:1–14.

Carlin, D. C. March/April 1982. How to assess your wellness—and become a model for your patients. *Nursing Life* 2:48–49.

Chalmers, K., and Farrell, P. July 1985. Lifestyle counselling: The need for diagnostic clarity. *Journal of Advanced Nursing* 10:311–13.

Chambers, C. C. 1981. *Enhancing wellness.* New York: Springer Publishing Co.

Ciliska, D. April 1983. Lifestyle changes are our business. *The Canadian Nurse* 79:26–27.

Cox, C. L. May/June 1985. The health self-determinism index. *Nursing Research* 34:177–83.

Deci, E. 1975. *Intrinsic motivation.* New York: Plenum Press.

———. 1980. *The psychology of self-determination.* Lexington, Mass.: Lexington Books.

Dunn, H. L. 1973. *High-level wellness.* Arlington, Va.: R. W. Beatty Co.

———. 1975. Points of attack for raising the levels of wellness. *Journal of the National Medical Association* 49:233–35.

Edelman, C., and Mandle, C. L. 1986. *Health promotion throughout the life span.* St. Louis: C. V. Mosby Co.

Faber, M. M., and Reinhardt, A. M. 1982. *Promoting health through risk reduction.* New York: Macmillan Co.

Frachel, R. R. June 1984. Health hazard appraisal: Personal and professional implications. *Journal of Nursing Education* 23:265–67.

Getchell, B. 1979. *Physical fitness: A way of life.* 2d ed. New York: John Wiley and Sons.

Grasser, Sister C., and Craft, B. J. F. June 1984. The patient's approach to wellness. *Nursing Clinics of North America* 19:207–18.

Hettler, B. 1982. Wellness promotion and risk reduction on a university campus. In Faber, M. M., and Reinhardt, A. M. *Promoting health through risk reduction.* New York: Macmillan Co.

Kort, M. April 1984. Support: An important component of health promotion. *The Canadian Nurse* 80:24–26.

Laffrey, S. C., and Isenberg, M. 1983. The relationship of internal locus of control, value placed on health, perceived importance of exercise, and participation in physical activity during leisure. *International Journal of Nursing Studies* 20(3):187–96.

Landry, F., editor. 1983. *Health risk estimation, risk reduction and health promotion: Proceedings of the 18th annual meeting of the Society of Prospective Medicine.* Ottawa: Canadian Public Health Association.

Lewin, K. 1951. *Field theory in social science.* New York: Harper and Row.

Logan, B. B., and Dawkins, C. E. 1986. *Family-centered nursing in the community.* Menlo Park, Calif.: Addison-Wesley.

Logan, M. April 1984. Health contracting: The client's perspective. *The Canadian Nurse* 80:27–29.

Moore, P. V., and Williamson, G. C. June 1984. Health promotion: Evolution of a concept. *Nursing Clinics of North America* 19:195–206.

Muhlenkamp, A. F.; Brown, N. J.; and Sands, D. November/December 1985. Determinants of health promotion activities in nursing clinic clients. *Nursing Research* 34:327–32.

Murphy, M. M. November/December 1982. Why won't they shape up? Resistance to the promotion of health. *Canadian Journal of Public Health* 73:427–30.

Neufeld, A., and Hobbs, H. November/December 1985. Self-care in a high-rise for seniors. *Nursing Outlook* 33:298–301.

Neuman, J.; Sloss, G. S.; and Andersen, S. July/August 1984. Evaluation of a health program. *Geriatric Nursing* 5:234–38.

O'Hagan, M. April 1984. Healthstyles basics: Lifestyle and behavior change. *The Canadian Nurse* 80:21–23.

Olson, E. M. June 1979. Strategies and techniques for the nurse change agent. *Nursing Clinics of North America* 14:323–36.

Opatz, J. P. 1985. *A primer of health promotion: Creating healthy organizational cultures.* Washington, D.C.: Oryn Publications.

Pender, N. J. June 1975. A conceptual model for preventive health behavior. *Nursing Outlook* 23:385–90.

———. 1982. *Health promotion in nursing practice.* Norwalk, Conn.: Appleton-Century-Crofts.

Rosenstock, I. M. 1974. Historical origins of the health belief model. In Becker, M. H., editor. *The health belief model and personal health behavior.* Thorofare, N.J.: Charles B. Slack.

Schlotfeldt, R. M. May 1981. Nursing in the future. *Nursing Outlook* 29:295–301.

Scott, S. September 1983. A hospital-based health promotion program. *The Canadian Nurse* 79:32–33.

Shephard, R. J.; Corey, P.; Renzland, P.; and Cox, M. January/February 1985. The impact of changes in fitness and lifestyle upon health care utilization. *Canadian Journal of Public Health* 74:51–54.

Shultz, C. M. S. June 1984. Lifestyle assessment: A tool for practice. *Nursing Clinics of North America* 19:271–81.

Spradley, B. W. 1981. *Community health nursing: Concepts and practice.* Boston: Little, Brown and Co.

Steckel, S. B. September 1982. Predicting, measuring, implementing and following up on patient compliance. *Nursing Clinics of North America* 17:491–98.

Strickland, B.; Arnn, J.; and Mitchell, J. N. June 1985. Individualizing patient care . . . interpersonal lifestyles. *Journal of Nursing Education* 24:252–55.

Wallston, K. A.; Wallston, B. S.; and DeVellis, R. Spring 1978. Development of the multidimensional health locus of control (MHLC) scales. *Health Education Monograph* 6:164–65.

CHAPTER 21

The Family

Janice Denehy

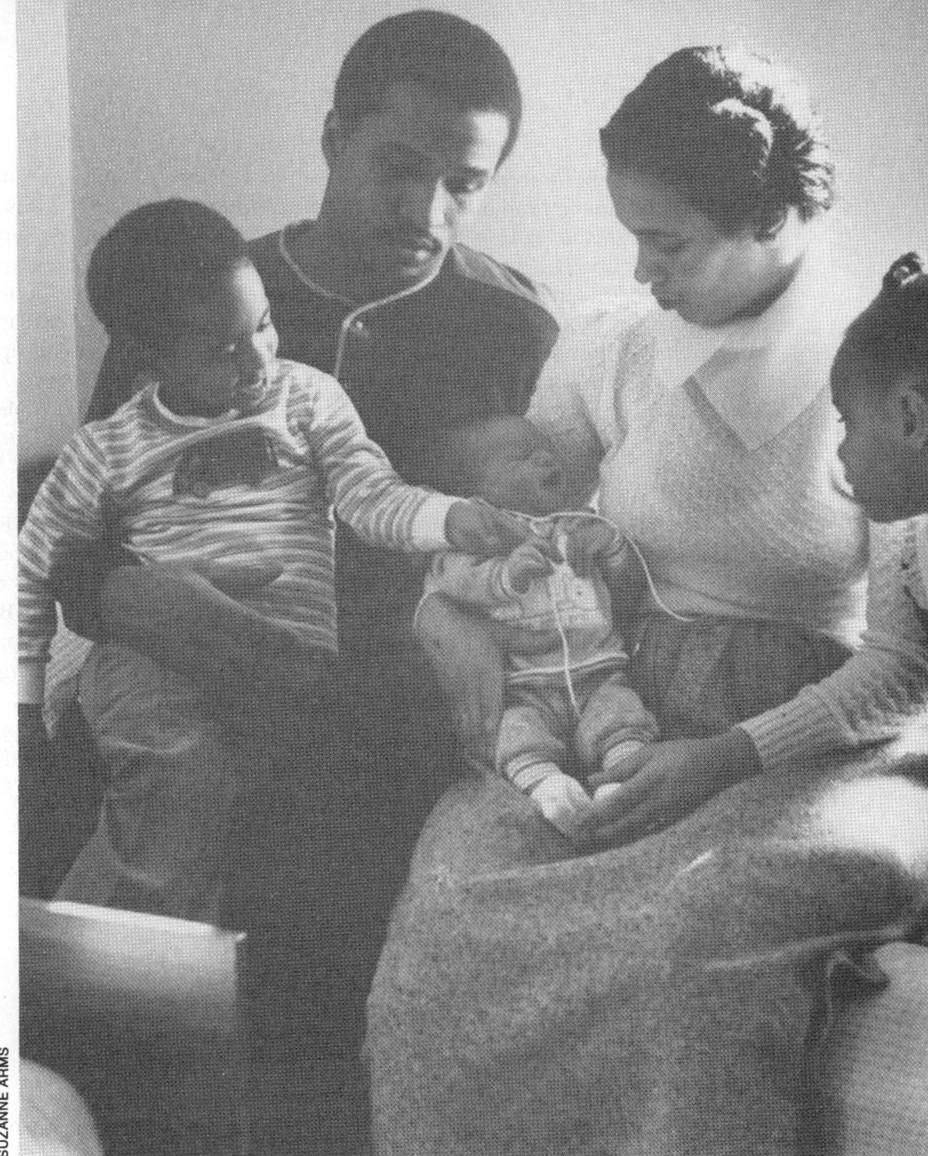
SUZANNE ARMS

Contents

Objectives

1. Define family-centered nursing.
2. Understand how to study the family unit.
   2.1 Differentiate between the traditional definition of the family and the broader definition needed to describe today's families.
   2.2 Describe the role and function of the family.
   2.3 Explain the historical changes that have taken place in the family.
   2.4 Identify three different frameworks used to study the family.
3. Understand the variety of family forms prevalent in today's society.
   3.1 Describe the differences and similarities in these family forms.
   3.2 Describe the special needs of each family form.
4. Know the role of the nurse in assessing and promoting the health of families.
   4.1 Delineate the information included in a health appraisal.
   4.2 Discuss the importance of assessing family health beliefs.
   4.3 Identify family communication patterns.
   4.4 Illustrate the effect of cultural heritage on health beliefs and practices.
   4.5 Identify family risk factors.
   4.6 Outline a plan for health promotion.
5. Understand the impact of illness on the family unit.
   5.1 Describe how family function is altered by the illness of a family member.
   5.2 Discuss coping strategies used by families.
   5.3 Describe the impact of death upon a family.

Terms

adolescent parents
blended family
childbearing family
childrearing family
cohabiting families
contracting family
coping mechanism
cultural heritage
developmental theory
expanding family
extended family
family
family-centered nursing
gay and lesbian families
health appraisal
health beliefs
health promotion
hereditary factors
intrafamily communication
latch-key children
life-style practices
marital family
nuclear family
poverty
reconstituted family
risk assessment
risk reduction
self-care
single-parent family
social support network
structural-functional theory
systems theory
traditional family
two-career family

Introduction

There has been a resurgence of interest in the family unit and its impact on the health, values, and productivity of individual family members. In the nursing profession, this interest in the family as a unit has been expressed by the emergence of **family-centered nursing**: nursing that considers the health of the family as a unit in addition to the health of individual family members. Membership in a family has a tremendous influence on the individual through genetic endowment, ethnicity, and the development of personal, social, moral, and cultural values. Nurses must consider the family's influence on the individual as they assess, diagnose, plan, implement, and evaluate nursing care. This chapter focuses on the evolution of the family and its impact on the health of its members.

Defining the Roles and Functions of the Family

Definitions of *family* are as numerous and different as the many forms of family seen in today's society. When one envisions a family, the first image that comes to mind is a mother and father—the husband and wife—and their children, usually a boy and a girl. A family of parents and their offspring is known as the **nuclear family**. The relatives of nuclear families, such as grandparents or aunts and uncles, comprise the **extended family**. In some families, members of the extended family live with the nuclear family. Such multigenerational families were more common during the last century but are still seen today in many cultures as well as in many American homes. Although members of the extended family may live in different areas, they are a frequent source of support and companionship for the family.

The family is frequently defined as two or more persons who are related through marriage, blood, birth, or adoption (Duvall 1977). Although this definition characterizes a large number of families, it does not adequately describe the membership of many families today. In many family groups, there are no legal or blood relationships among members. As the structure of the family has become more diverse, it has been necessary to define the family more broadly to encompass the wide variety of family forms seen in today's society. To provide flexibility in the study of families, Friedman (1981, p. 8) defines the **family** as follows: "A family is composed of people (two or more) who are emotionally involved with each other and live in close geographical proximity." Emotional involvement is demonstrated through caring and a commitment to a common purpose.

The family is the basic unit of society. Its major roles are to protect and socialize its members. Among the many functions it serves, of prime importance is the role the family plays in providing emotional support and security to its members through love, acceptance, concern, and nurturance. This affective (emotional) component holds families together, gives family members a sense of belonging, and develops a sense of kinship. In addition to providing an emotionally safe environment for members to thrive and grow, the family is also a basic unit of physical protection and safety. This is accomplished by meeting the basic needs of its members: food, clothing, and shelter. Provision of a physically safe environment requires knowledge, skills, and economic resources. In modern society, the economic resources needed by the family are secured by adult members through employment or government programs. The family also protects the physical health of its members by providing adequate nutrition and health care services. Nutritional and life-style practices of the family not only influence the health of family members but also directly affect the developing health attitudes and life-style practices of children.

In addition to providing an environment conducive to physical growth and health, the family creates an atmosphere that influences the cognitive and psychosocial growth of its members. Children and adults in healthy, functional families receive support, understanding, and encouragement as they progress through predictable developmental stages, as they move in or out of the family unit, and as they establish new family units. In families where members are physically and emotionally nurtured, individuals are challenged to achieve their potential in the family unit. As individual needs are met, family members are able to reach out to others in the family and the community, and to society.

The family is a major educator of its members. Parents are often called a child's first teachers. This early learning plays an influential part in the development of a child's attitudes about family, education, health, work, and recreation. These attitudes persist throughout their lives. In addition, families play a major role in the transmission of religious, cultural, and societal values. As the family socializes its new members to the expectations of home, community, and society, it provides a place of warmth, acceptance, and nurturance that insulates its members from the demands of society.

The family is a place of roots, refuge, and rejuvenation. It is a small network where members communicate and work together, delegating roles and responsibilities with a shared purpose: the protection and growth of its members. Through the experiences of family life, the individual learns to participate in and contribute productively to society.

Historical Overview of the Family

Although the evolution of the family is unclear, there is evidence that the family was the center of individual and community life during prehistoric times. As humans developed the knowledge and skills necessary for survival and the development of culture, the structure of the family and the roles its members played changed. Adaptation of the family unit to cultural, political, and economic changes has been demonstrated throughout the centuries into modern times.

Families of yesteryear formed agrarian societies who focused their energy on producing the goods necessary for survival. The industrialization of society had a major impact on the family unit. Family members, who had previously worked together for a singular purpose, left their rural homes for employment in urban factories. Because some family members now worked outside the home, it became necessary to redistribute duties within the family. Out of necessity roles for individual family members became more clearly defined, and many of these roles remain deeply embedded in our culture today. A major change brought on by industrialization was the role children played in the family. Until this time, having a large family was an asset, meaning more hands to help in the fields and in the work of the home. After industrialization, however, goods previously produced at home, such as food and clothing, were purchased. Therefore, families gradually diminished in size because children became an economic burden. The teaching of children, previously done at home, became the responsibility of the school.

The family in today's society continues to be influenced by past traditions and values. As the demands of society have changed, the structure of the family and the roles its members assume have changed. Such changes have been difficult, especially for older family members who see cherished cultural and familial values eroded. Today, however, the trend is to preserve and pass on the cultural heritage and values of the past. Among today's diverse family forms, such preservation gives families a sense of identity and stability in a fast-paced, technical society (Spector 1979).

Frameworks for Studying the Family

There are many ways to look at families. Family theory provides a framework for assessing how families are structured and examining how they function. Family theory also provides information about predictable developmental phases families experience during their lifespan. This information helps the nurse study the family process and the effect of this process on the health of its members.

Systems Theory

According to **systems theory**, a system is a unit composed of interdependent parts. A change in one part of a system influences the system as a whole. Systems are affected by other systems through interaction. The boundaries of a system regulate the amount of input from and output to other systems. An open system allows free interaction with other systems, while a closed system remains impervious to systems outside its boundaries. (See Chapter 10 for a more detailed description of systems theory.)

The family unit can be viewed as a system. Its members are interdependent, working toward specific purposes and goals. Boundaries regulate the input from other systems into the family system; they also regulate output from the family system to other systems in society. Boundaries protect the family from the demands and influences of other systems. Many families are described as open systems because they continually interact with the society surrounding them. Open families are likely to welcome input from without, encouraging members to adapt beliefs and practices to meet the demands of society. Such families seek out health care information and utilize available resources. Family systems also can be described as relatively closed. Closed families are self-contained units resistant to outside interaction or influence. They are less likely to change values and practices; exert more control over the lives of their members; and distrust outsiders. It is more difficult for closed family systems to use community resources or to incorporate new behaviors that may promote a healthier family. Most families, however, have permeable, flexible boundaries and regulate input and output according to family needs, values, and developmental stage.

Structural-Functional Theory

The **structural-functional theory**, as the name implies, focuses on family structure and function. The structural component of the theory addresses the membership of the family and the relationships among family members. Intrafamily relationships are complex because of the numerous relationships that exist in the family: mother-daughter, brother-sister, husband-wife, etc. These relationships are constantly evolving; for example, children mature and leave the nest or adults age and become more dependent on others to meet their daily needs.

The functional aspect of the theory deals with the effects of intrafamily relationships on the family system, as well as their effects on other systems. Some of the main functions of the family include developing a sense of family purpose and affiliation, adding and socializing new members, providing and distributing care and services to members, imparting stability and coping resources during crises, transmitting family values, and reaching out to society as productive citizens. The interaction between family structure and function determines the growth of the family and its subsequent relationship with society.

Developmental Theory

Another method of studying the family is from a developmental framework. **Developmental theories** view families as ever-changing and growing. Crucial, yet predictable, tasks are associated with each level or stage of development. Achievement of tasks appropriate at one level is a prerequisite for entering and successfully achieving the tasks expected at the next level. One of the major tasks of the family, from a developmental perspective, is to create an environment where the family members can master crucial developmental tasks. This ensures orderly progression through the stages of family life.

The use of Duvall's (1977) developmental theory is particularly useful for **childbearing** and **childrearing families.** Duvall describes predictable stages through which families progress, beginning with the formation of a new family unit, the **marital family.** During this first stage, the couple forms a marital relationship, their new roles as husband and wife emerge, and goals for the future are formulated. The family enters the childbearing stage as an infant is added to the family unit. During this phase, the husband and wife take on new roles as parents. Parenthood requires many adaptations in life-style with resultant role changes. The childbearing stage lasts until the child is 30 months old. The family then enters the preschool stage. At this time, emphasis is upon the nurturing of children. When the child is old enough to enter school, at age 5 to 6 years, the family moves into the school-age stage. In this stage, the primary task is the education and socialization of children. During the teenage stage, children begin to move away from the influence and control of the family. Peers become an increasingly significant part of adolescent life. The role of the family during this stage is to provide a sense of equilibrium to the adolescent experiencing physiologic and psychologic changes, conflicting expectations, and pressures to plan and prepare for the future. The family during the childbearing and childrearing years is frequently referred to as the **expanding family.**

As teenagers reach adulthood and begin to leave the family unit, the family moves into the launching stage. At this time, adult family members have time to develop their personal interests and redefine their roles as parents and husbands or wives. After launching is completed, the family enters the middle-age stage, during which role stabilization occurs and the new role of grandparent may be added. Next, the family moves into the aging stage. Aging family members focus their energy on preparing for and experiencing retirement. During this period, family members are likely to experience a decline in health or a major health crisis, which may necessitate a change in life-style or residence. The family during the launching, middle-age, and aging stages has been characterized as the **contracting family.**

Because today's families are having fewer children and adults are enjoying greater health, productivity, and longevity, the middle-age and aging stages occupy an increasing number of years in the life of the family. In the past, more interest was expressed in the early developmental phases of family life—the childbearing and childrearing family. Recently, however, older families, including their unique characteristics and health care needs, have received greater attention, resulting in the growing specialty of geriatrics. As the number of elderly citizens continues to rise, there will be an increased demand for health care services and facilities tailored to the aging population (Ebersole and Hess 1981).

The Family in Today's Society

It is difficult to describe the family of today except as uniquely diverse. Improvements in health care have led to healthier people living longer and more productive lives. The development of reliable contraceptives and the legalization of abortion have resulted in greater control in the planning of families. Today's economic realities, coupled with liberation ideology, have moved many women out of the home and into the workplace, changing traditional family roles. Higher divorce rates and the acceptance of children born to unmarried mothers have led to a dramatic increase in the number of single-parent families. Individuals are also grouping together to form new family units based on sexual preference or economic need.

Traditional Families

The **traditional family** is often viewed as an autonomous unit in which both parents reside in the home with their children, the mother playing the nurturing role and the father providing the necessary economic resources. Although the traditional family is still very much a part of American culture, it is no longer the predominant family form. Although members of the extended family are not likely to live with traditional nuclear families, they remain an important source of information, support, and security to many American families. Contact with members of the extended family is vital to mobile families in times of stress or crisis because contact gives a sense of stability in a complex, impersonal society.

In the modern family, changes are occurring in traditional role patterns. Today's fathers are more involved with their children and family life. Many attend prenatal classes and witness the birth of their infants. In addition, fathers are more involved with household chores as role stereotypes are challenged, even though wives continue to perform a large portion of the housework. Likewise, females are less bound by traditional role patterns in today's society.

Until very recently, the American family commonly portrayed by the print and visual media was the two-parent, white family. Today, however, single-parent families, blended families, minority families, and elderly families are portrayed by the media as well. This trend has given many members of such families a sense of family identity.

Two-Career Families

In **two-career families,** both the husband and wife are employed. Such families have been steadily increasing since the 1960s. The reasons for this trend are many, including the increased educational and career opportunities available to women, a desired increase in standard of living, and economic necessity. Many two-career families are young couples without children who desire to complete and use their education. Other working couples postpone childbearing until they are financially secure, have paid debts, and have purchased some of life's extras. Two-career families may also be parents who have launched their children and find they have many healthy, productive years to spend in the marketplace prior to retirement.

It is estimated that 60% to 70% of working women have children in the home, many of whom are preschoolers. When both parents work, the roles each partner plays in the family need to change. Husbands have become more involved in the care of children and the management of household chores. Time and personal energy constraints also may lead to reevaluation of family activities and goals. Attention must be given to maintaining the husband-wife relationship and individual interests amidst the pressures of juggling family and career commitments.

The increased number of working parents has created a need for quality, affordable child care. Finding such child care is one of the greatest stresses faced by today's working parents. Many children are growing up in day-care homes or child-care centers that expose them at a young age to a host of people with a wide range of ideas and values.

Once children reach school age, parents find that few resources for after-school child care are available. Many school-aged children come home to empty houses or apartments to care for themselves. These **latch-key children**, as they are called because they carry their own house key, may become bored or frightened as they wait for the parents to return from work (McClellan 1984). Parents and professionals are realizing the importance of preparing these children with information about safety and household management to reduce their anxiety and help them make the most of these hours alone. Children of working parents are growing up with new family role models, which will no doubt have an effect on the families of tomorrow.

Single-Parent Families

Today it is estimated that over 50% of North American children live in a **single-parent family**—a home headed by one parent—sometime during their childhood. There are many reasons for single parenthood, including death of a spouse, separation, divorce, birth of a child to an unmarried woman, or adoption of a child by a single man or woman. Single parents frequently express concern about child care, adequate financial resources, social isolation, and lack of adult companionship. Single parents who work experience fatigue and role overload in managing growing children, household tasks, and a job. At times, these concerns seem to occupy their entire lives, leaving little time for personal or recreational activities.

Nearly 90% of single-parent families are headed by a female. Because these women are often young and poorly prepared for the job market, many single-parent families live with financial strain or poverty. In homes where a divorce has occurred, there is frequently a drop in the standard of living. Child support payments dwindle after the first year and in many cases are never received. When families live with inadequate financial resources, the health of the family is likely to suffer from substandard living conditions, poor nutrition, stress, and inadequate health care services. The self-esteem of the family is impaired because members, particularly the head of the household, find it difficult to raise their standard of living due to stigma or lack of skills, time, and energy. Depression and despair are common among women struggling to raise a family (Duffy 1982); these feelings not only affect the woman but also influence the outlook of growing family members, who learn to view society as hostile, not as a place full of challenges and hope for the future.

Single-parent families need to identify a support system. Members of the extended family or friends who are supportive provide an opportunity for mutual caring and sharing of concerns. Such support networks reduce social isolation and provide opportunities for relaxation and recreation. A support system helps the single parent cope with and reduce stress; in addition, it gives the individual a chance to have fun and regain self-esteem. Referral to appropriate community resources helps the single parent locate child care, take advantage of financial or social programs, and develop job skills through education or job-training programs. Continued health supervision is essential to ensure the growth and development of healthy families.

Blended Families

Existing family units who join together to form new family units are known as **blended** or **reconstituted families**. Families with children living with a birth parent and a nonbirth parent are commonly called step families. The blending of two families presents a unique set of challenges to the individuals involved. The joining of two families is often met with hope and anticipation. Each family brings its own history and expectations to the new family constellation. Often expectations for instantaneous adaptation and affection are too high. Children, depending on their ages and past experiences, usually adjust slowly to new patterns of communication and family authority. Family reintegration requires time and effort. Stress occurs as blended families get to know each other, respect differences, and establish new patterns of behavior (Reutter and Strang 1986).

The greatest success in blending or reconstituting families comes when each family member enters the new relationship with realistic expectations and plans to take the time to make the new family unit succeed. Successful parents get along with and enjoy each other, enjoy life, and bring a sense of humor to the challenge of blending the life-styles and values of two families into one.

Adolescent Parents

A disturbing trend is the growing proportion of infants born each year to **adolescent parents**. These young parents, who are still mastering the developmental tasks of childhood, are physically, emotionally, and financially ill prepared to undertake the responsibilities of parenthood. Over 600,000 infants in America are born each year to adolescent mothers (The Adolescent Family 1984, p. 1).

An increasing number of these mothers are 15 years and younger. A disproportionate number of adolescent births are to members of minority racial or ethnic groups. Approximately 95% of infants born to adolescents will be raised by their mothers.

Pregnant adolescents are at greater risk for health problems during pregnancy because of poor nutritional status, physiologic immaturity, and lack of prenatal care. They are more likely to deliver premature infants who are, in turn, at greater risk for subsequent health and developmental problems. In addition, adolescent mothers are more likely to give birth to another infant while still in their teens. Today there is a greater acceptance of unmarried parenthood, and fewer pregnant teens feel pressured to marry the father of the infant or to relinquish the infant for adoption.

Adolescent pregnancy interrupts education and changes the life goals and direction of many young women. The newly formed family unit is often dependent upon others for physical, emotional, and financial assistance. Support systems are crucial to its success. Parenting skills need to be developed, and when possible, the completion of high school education encouraged. While helping the new mother understand the needs of her growing infant is an important intervention for nurses, so is assisting the young mother progress through the developmental tasks of adolescence into adulthood.

The children of adolescent parents are at greater risk for health and social problems as they grow up. These children experience more accidents during their preschool years than their peers, are frequently behind in receiving their childhood immunizations, and are more prone to exhibit learning and behavior problems when they enter school. Raised in poverty, children of adolescent mothers often have few role models to help them break out of the cycle of poverty and subsequent adolescent parenthood.

Cohabiting Families

A current and growing trend in alternate family forms is unrelated individuals or families cohabiting or living under one roof, forming new family units called **cohabiting** or **communal families**. Some individuals join together out of a need for companionship; for example, two widowed adults who share common interests found that living together eliminated previously lonely hours during the evening. Others cohabit to achieve a sense of family or belonging. Many unmarried couples choose to cohabit; some have no desire for a long-term commitment, others wish to test a relationship prior to marriage.

Financial need often leads to the formation of cohabiting families. In these situations, individuals or families share living expenses as well as the responsibilities of household management. Others may cohabit to share services. For example, a single mother moved in with an elderly man who desired to remain in his home but needed help with cooking and cleaning. The single mother was able to provide these services, and she benefited because she and her daughter were now regularly sitting down to nutritious meals, something they rarely experienced previously. An added bonus was the close friendship the elderly man established with her six-year-old daughter. The formation of cohabiting families illustrates the flexibility and creativity of the family unit in adapting to meet individual challenges and responding to changing societal demands.

Gay and Lesbian Families

Of recent interest is the awareness of the number of homosexual adults in today's society who have formed **gay and lesbian families** based on the same goals of caring and commitment seen in heterosexual relationships. While homosexual relationships have been stereotyped as short term and casual, many gay and lesbian relationships are based on long-term mutuality. As the society becomes more educated about homosexuality, it will better understand the complex emotional attachments and affiliation of many homosexual couples and will provide a more accepting atmosphere for these relationships.

Although homosexual marriages are not legally recognized, many homosexual relationships are the basis of new family units. Lesbian women are more likely to live together or cohabit than gay men. Lesbians have fewer sexual partners, are more likely to spend time with their partner, and place a higher value on sexual fidelity than their male counterparts (Williamson 1986). Lesbian women are also more likely to bring children from previous marriages into their partnerships than gay men are. Although many are concerned about the effects of parental homosexuality on the growing child, studies have shown that these children develop sex-role orientations and behaviors similar to children in the general population (Hoeffer 1981). The greatest danger to children reared in gay and lesbian families is the prejudice and ridicule expressed by others in society. For this reason, many homosexual parents keep their sexual preference private to spare their children pain during early childhood, choosing to explain their sexual preference when the children are able to understand homosexuality and emotionally ready to deal with its implications.

Families from Different Cultures

Families from different cultures are an integral part of North America's rich heritage. Each family has values and beliefs (**cultural heritage**) that are unique to their culture of origin and that shape the family's structure, methods of interaction, health care practices, and coping mechanisms. These factors interact to influence the health of families. Families from different cultures may cluster to form mutual support systems and to preserve their heritage; however, this practice may isolate them from the larger society. Children often have greater contact with the world around them than adults; through school, children become more proficient in language and more comfortable with new customs and behaviors. Sometimes children create conflict in the family when they bring home new ideas and values. They want to become part of the culture in which they live and incorporate new practices into existing family customs. In the process, they may reject previously cherished cultural traditions.

Becoming acculturated is a slow, stressful process of learning the language and customs of a new country. Chapter 18 presents information that helps the nurse understand the family traditions, beliefs, and practices of different cultures. This information helps the nurse to provide nursing care that is sensitive to the unique needs of families from different cultural heritages.

Single Adults Living Alone

Although individuals living alone, by definition, are not considered a family unit, in today's society many individuals live by themselves. When society is studied from a family perspective, these individuals are frequently overlooked, yet they represent a significant proportion of the population. Singles may include young, newly emancipated adults who have left the nuclear family and achieved independence. These young adults may have completed their education and entered the job market, becoming self-sufficient and self-supporting. As young adults postpone marriage or choose singleness, living alone will become a more prevalent life-style.

On the other end of the age spectrum is the older adult living alone. Having launched their families, many older adults find themselves single through divorce, separation, or death of a spouse. Some older adults remain in their homes, while others find an apartment more suitable to their changing needs. As they age, and depending on their health status and financial resources, some single adults relocate into retirement homes or extended care facilities. Although many older adults live alone, some have frequent contacts with other family members, especially adult children and grandchildren. As they enter the golden years, their sense of family becomes stronger, and they seek to communicate the history and values of the family to the new generation.

Assessing and Promoting the Health of Families

The importance of family assessment cannot be overemphasized. The information gathered during assessment is the basis for planning and delivering nursing care to family members or to the family as a whole. Numerous family assessment tools are available. The nurse must consider a number of factors in selecting a family assessment tool or in developing a tool that meets the demands of the families served in a particular practice setting. The home care nurse, for instance, may develop a tool to assess the unique needs and problems of a family who has a member with diabetes. A family assessment tool should be holistic, eliciting information about a wide variety of family characteristics, beliefs, and behaviors. The tool should be understandable and acceptable to both the family and the nurse (Speer and Sachs 1985). In other words, the nurse must use terminology comprehensible to a wide range of clients, and the tool should be quickly and easily administered. The instrument should also yield clinically relevant data about the family—information useful in formulating nursing diagnoses and planning nursing interventions that promote the health of families.

The Life-Change Index first introduced in Chapter 17 is an assessment tool designed to measure the amount of change in the life of an individual (Holmes and Rahe 1967). Many of the changes identified in the index affect the entire family, not only one individual. Life changes—even positive ones—are often stressful to the individual or the family. Families who are experiencing a great deal of stress are at higher risk of developing physical illnesses or mental health problems. Therefore, identifying family members who are experiencing stress is an important part of the family assessment process. People perceive and respond to stress differently, so the nurse needs to assess how each family member perceives and copes with stress. Common areas of stress and assessment of client coping are discussed in Chapter 17, page 350.

Health Appraisal

The **health appraisal** begins with a complete health history. The nurse focuses first on the family unit and then on the individuals in that family. The health history is one of the most effective ways of identifying existing or potential health problems. The history is followed by physical assessment of family members. If further evaluation is indicated, referral is made to the appropriate health care professional. Frequently the physical examination focuses on identifying pathological conditions or the potential for them rather than on appraisal of health. When the focus is on health, the appraisal includes information on life-style behaviors and health beliefs. Pender (1982) outlines strategies for assessing physical fitness, body fat, nutritional status, stress, and risk factors (such as age, family history, and life-style practices). The nurse uses data from the health appraisal to formulate a health profile. The health profile provides the data necessary to establish a nursing diagnosis and to plan appropriate nursing interventions to promote optimal health through life-style modification.

Health Beliefs

In addition to appraising health status, the nurse assesses **health beliefs** and values to gain information useful in planning effective nursing interventions. Health beliefs and values develop over a lifetime. They are influenced by culture, family, education, and past experiences with health and illness. Some people feel they have little control over their health status, while others feel that their behaviors have a direct effect on health. To promote health, the nurse must understand the health beliefs of individuals and families and use this information in planning and delivering nursing care.

Health beliefs may reflect a lack of information or misinformation about health or disease. They may also include folklore and practices from different cultures. Because of the many advances in medicine and health care during the last few decades, many clients have outdated information about health, illness, treatment, and prevention. The nurse is frequently in a position to give information or correct misconceptions about health. This function is an important component of the nursing care plan.

Family Communication Patterns

The effectiveness of family communication determines its ability to function as a cooperative, growth-producing unit. Messages are constantly being communicated among family members, both verbally and nonverbally. The information transmitted influences how members work together, fulfill their assigned roles in the family, incorporate family values, and develop skills to function in society. **Intrafamily communication** plays a significant role in the development of self-esteem, which is necessary for the growth of personality.

Families who communicate effectively transmit messages clearly. Members are free to express their feelings without fear of jeopardizing their standing in the family. Family members support one another and have the ability to listen, empathize, and reach out to one another in times of crisis. When the needs of family members are met, they are more able to reach out to meet the needs of others in society.

When patterns of communication among family members are dysfunctional, messages are often communicated unclearly. Verbal communication may be incongruent with nonverbal messages. Power struggles may be evidenced by hostility, anger, or silence. Members may be cautious in expressing their feelings because they cannot predict how others in the family will respond. Many things remain unsaid to preserve family unity and tranquillity. When family communication is impaired, the growth of individual members is stunted. Members often turn to other systems to seek personal validation and gratification.

The nurse needs to observe intrafamily communication patterns closely. Nurses should pay special attention to who does the talking for the family, which members are silent, how disagreements are handled, and how well the members listen to one another and encourage the participation of others. Nonverbal communication is important because it gives valuable clues about what people are feeling.

Family Coping Mechanisms

Family **coping mechanisms** are the behaviors families use to deal with stress or changes. Coping mechanisms can be viewed as an active method of problem solving developed to meet life's challenges. The coping mechanisms families and individuals develop reflect their individual resourcefulness. Freidman (1981) states that families may use the same coping patterns rather consistently over time or may change their coping strategies when new demands are made on the family. Coping is a basic function that helps the family meet demands imposed both from within and without. The success of a family depends on how well it copes with the stresses it experiences.

Nurses working with families realize the importance of assessing coping mechanisms as a way of determining how families relate to stress. Also important are the resources available to the family. Internal resources, such as knowledge, skills, effective communication patterns, and a sense of mutuality and purpose within the family, assist in the problem-solving process. In addition, external support systems promote coping and adaptation. These external systems may be extended family, friends, religious affiliations, health care professionals, or social services. The development of social support systems is particularly valuable today, when many families, due to stress, mobility, or poverty, are isolated from resources that would help them cope.

Cultural Values Related to Health

The nurse who views a client from a holistic perspective must consider the cultural heritage of the family when assessing health beliefs and practices. These cultural values are often important and ingrained in many families, even when several generations have lived away from their country of origin. Understanding and respecting the cultural values of the family are essential in gaining their trust and optimal participation in the health care system. Interventions, whenever possible, should complement existing beliefs. In other cases, existing policies may need to be altered to accommodate the beliefs of families; for instance, allowing special home-cooked foods during the hospitalization of a family member if these foods do not interfere with the medical management of the individual. Chapter 18 describes how culture influences health beliefs and how this information can be applied to the delivery of health care.

Identifying Families at Risk for Health Problems

Risk assessment helps the nurse identify individuals and groups at higher risk than the general population of developing specific health problems, such as stroke, diabetes, and lung cancer. Risk may be related to genetic factors; for example, persons who have a family history of diabetes are at greater risk of developing diabetes than persons with no family history of diabetes. Certain practices also increase the risk of health problems; for instance, cigarette smokers arc at greater risk of developing lung cancer than nonsmokers. Environmental factors, such as air pollution or exposure to toxic chemicals, increase the risk of certain health problems.

Risk reduction among individuals and groups identified as at risk poses a special challenge to health care professionals. Once the individuals or groups are identified, the nurse's role is to plan and implement interventions to reduce health risks when possible or to optimize the current health status of those individuals or groups when risks cannot be reduced. The vulnerability of family units to health problems may be based on family developmental level, age of family members, heredity or genetic factors, sociologic factors, and life-style practices. The goal of the nurse is to promote optimal family health and functioning.

Developmental Factors

Families at both ends of the age continuum are at risk of developing health problems. Newly formed families who are entering the childbearing and childrearing phases of development experience many changes in roles, responsibilities, and expectations. These changes occur when adult family members are attempting to establish financial security. The many, often conflicting, demands on the young family cause stress and fatigue, which may impede growth of family members and the functioning of the group as a unit. Adolescent mothers, because of their developmental level and lack of knowledge about parenthood, and single-parent families, because of role overload experienced by the head of the household, are more likely to develop health problems. The elderly, however, are at risk of developing degenerative and chronic health problems. Because of the emphasis on youth in today's society, many elderly persons feel a lack of purpose and decreased self-esteem. These feelings in turn reduce their motivation to engage in health promoting behaviors, such as exercise or community and family involvement.

Hereditary Factors

Persons born into families with a history of certain diseases, such as diabetes or cardiovascular disease, are at greater risk of developing these conditions. A detailed family health history, including genetically transmitted disorders, is crucial to the identification of persons and families at risk. These data are used not only to monitor the health of individual family members but also to recommend modifications in health practices that potentially reduce the risk, minimize the consequences, or postpone the development of genetically related conditions. For example, **hereditary factors** are important in the health care of Sharon, a young mother of three children. She is concerned about the development of breast cancer because her mother died of this disease when Sharon was 10 years old. Sharon has had two biopsies of benign lumps in her breasts. She performs breast self-examination regularly and is monitored closely by her physician. Sharon is also attempting to reduce the fat in her diet, a factor thought to be associated with breast cancer. These activities are aimed at the prevention and early detection of potential disease made possible through the identification of genetic risk factors.

Other family units or family members may be at risk of developing a disease by reason of sex or race. Males, for example, are at greater risk of having cardiovascular disease at an earlier age than females, and females are at greater risk of developing osteoporosis, particularly after menopause. While at times it is difficult to separate genetic factors from cultural factors, certain risk factors seem to be related to race. Some diseases are more prevalent among whites than blacks and vice versa. Sickle cell anemia, for example, is a hereditary disease limited to blacks of African descent (McFarlane 1977). Native Americans and Asians seem more susceptible to certain diseases and less susceptible to others than the general population.

Life-style Factors

Life-style practices are receiving considerable attention as contributing factors to many diseases. New knowledge and technology have eradicated many diseases that were previously leading causes of death, such as the communicable diseases of childhood. As the understanding of health and illness increases, it has become clear that many diseases are preventable, the effects of some diseases can be minimized, or the onset of disease can be delayed through life-style modification. Cancer, cardiovascular disease, adult-onset diabetes, and tooth decay are among the life-style diseases. The incidence of lung cancer, for example, would be greatly reduced if people stopped smoking. Proper nutrition, good dental hygiene, and use of fluoride—in the water supply, in toothpaste, in topical application, or as supplements—have been shown to reduce dental decay or caries, one of America's most prevalent health problems. Automobile accidents, the leading cause of death among adolescents and young adults, are frequently associated with alcohol consumption and increased risk taking.

In addition to health practices and nutrition, other important life-style considerations are exercise, stress management, and rest. Today, health professionals have the knowledge to prevent or minimize the effects of some of the main causes of disease, disability, and death. Too often, there is little consideration of health until sickness occurs. The challenge is to disseminate information about prevention and to motivate families to make life-style changes prior to the onset of illness. Many demands are made on today's family; an important question is: Will people take the time to be responsible for their own health?

Sociologic Factors

Poverty is a major problem that affects not only the family but also the community and society. Over 35 million people, or nearly one out of every six Americans, live in poverty (Moccia and Mason 1986, p. 20). A disproportionate number of today's poor belong to ethnic or racial minority groups. Poverty is a real concern among the rising number of one-parent families headed by a female, and, as the number of these families increases, poverty will affect a large number of growing children. Because many poor families do not possess the skills or support systems necessary to break out of the cycle of poverty, it is likely that poverty will continue to escalate rapidly in the future.

Poverty has an effect on the health of families. Infant mortality rates are higher among the poor than the general population, and life span is shortened. Even though health care may be available to the poor, many of the poor are unable to gain access to health care services, because of sociologic constraints, such as lack of transportation or language barriers. The poor are less likely than others to take advantage of preventive services; when ill, they are likely to put off seeking services until the illness reaches an advanced state and requires longer or more complex treatment. Even though the Surgeon General has reported that the health of the American people has never been better (U.S. DHEW, 1979), it is clear that this progress has not benefitted all segments of society, particularly the poor.

Health Promotion in the Family

Today's families are concerned about living healthy, productive, fulfilling lives. The media regularly inform the public that many personal behaviors endanger life and health, yet at the same time they accept advertising revenues from products that do not promote health. Much has been learned about the effects of diet, stress, and exercise on health, but changing long-established preferences and practices is difficult. Substance abuse, particularly of tobacco and alcohol, as well as personal and environmental safety hazards have needlessly decreased the productivity and shortened the lives of many persons.

To make changes that improve its own well-being, the family must be aware of potential health problems and their relationship to life-style practices. Information on how to reduce risks within the context of the family's value system is crucial. Support and encouragement of life-style changes help ensure that these changes are not temporary but become an important health value that influences lifelong health practices. The role of health education is to inform, motivate, and facilitate adoption of healthful life-style practices—activities that promote the well-being of individuals and families.

One of the major goals of **health promotion** is to help families take responsibility for their own health through self-care. **Self-care** is defined as activities individuals perform in their own behalf to maintain health and well-being (Orem 1980). Effective self-care requires knowledge and skills relating to health and illness. It includes knowing how to solve health problems of the family, as well as knowing when to seek outside guidance in meeting health problems. Self-care also encompasses health promotion for the family. Through health promotion, families can realize higher levels of wellness, productivity, self-awareness, and personal growth. For a more comprehensive discussion of health promotion, see Chapter 20.

The Family Experiencing a Health Crisis

Illness of a Member

Illness of a family member is a crisis that affects the entire family system. The family is disrupted as members abandon their usual activities and focus their energy on restoring family equilibrium. Roles and responsibilities previously assumed by the ill person are delegated to other family members, or those functions may remain undone during the duration of the illness. The family experiences anxiety because members are concerned about the sick person and the resolution of the illness. This anxiety is compounded by additional responsibilities at a time when there is less time or motivation to complete the normal tasks of daily living. For example, when a young mother is hospitalized, her husband may assume the responsibility for child care and home management. He is also trying to fit in time for hospital visits between work and home obligations. He expends energy worrying about his wife's condition and his added responsibilities. When he arrives home fatigued, he has little interest in housework.

Some of the household tasks may be completed, others may not. He also may be inattentive or short-tempered with the children, who need nurturing, reassurance, and stability during this family crisis.

Many factors determine the impact of illness on the family unit: (a) the nature of the illness, which can range from minor to life-threatening; (b) the duration of the illness, which ranges from short term to long term; (c) the residual effects of the illness, including none to permanent disability; (d) the meaning of the illness to the family and its significance to family systems; (e) the financial impact of the illness, which is influenced by factors such as insurance and ability of the ill member to return to work; and (f) the effect of the illness on future family functioning, for instance, previous patterns may be restored or new patterns may be established. The family's ability to deal with the stress of illness depends on their coping skills. Families with good communication skills are better able to discuss how they feel about the illness and how it affects family functioning. They can plan for the future and are flexible in adapting these plans as the situation changes. An established **social support network** provides strength, encouragement, and services to the family during the illness. During health crises, families need to realize that it is a strength, not a sign of weakness, to turn to others for support. Nurses can be part of the support system for families, or they can identify other sources of support in the community.

During a crisis, families are often drawn together by a common purpose. During this time of closeness, family members have the opportunity to reaffirm personal and family values and their commitment to one another. Indeed, illness may provide a unique opportunity for family growth.

Intervening in Families Experiencing Illness

Nurses committed to family-centered care involve both the ailing individual and the family in the nursing process. Through their interaction with families, nurses can give support and information. Nurses make sure that not only the individual but also each family member understands the disease, its management, and the effect of these two factors on family functioning. The nurse also assesses the family's readiness and ability to provide continued care and supervision at home when warranted. After carefully planned instruction and practice, families are given an opportunity to demonstrate their ability to provide care under the supportive guidance of the nurse. When the care indicated is beyond the capability of the family, nurses work with families to identify available resources that are socially and financially acceptable (McClelland, Kelly, and Buckwater 1985).

In helping families to reintegrate the ill person into the home, nurses use data gathered during family assessment to identify family resources and deficits. By formulating mutually acceptable goals for reintegration, nurses help families cope with the realities of the illness and the changes it may have brought about, which may include new roles and functions of family members or the need to provide continued medical care to the ill or recovering person. Working together, nurses and families can create environments that restore or reorganize family functioning during illness and throughout the recovery process.

Death of a Member

The loss of a member through death has a profound effect on the family. The structure of the family is altered, which may in turn affect how it functions as a unit. Individual members experience a sense of loss. They grieve for the lost person, and they grieve for the family that once was. (See Chapter 50 for a discussion of loss and grieving.) Some of the early stages of grief accompany family disorganization. However, as the family begins to recover, a new sense of normalcy develops, the family reintegrates its roles and functions, and it comes to grips with the reality of the situation. This painful blow takes time to heal. After the death of a member, the family may need counseling to deal with their feelings and to talk about the person who died. They may also want to talk about their fears about and hopes for the future. At this time, families often derive comfort from their religious beliefs and their spiritual adviser. Support groups are also available for families experiencing the pain of death. It is often difficult for nurses to deal with grieving families because the nurses also feel the loss and feel inadequate in knowing what to say or do. By understanding the effect death has on families, nurses can help families resolve their grief and move ahead with life.

Chapter Highlights

- Families are the basic social unit of society.
- The family plays an important role in forming the health beliefs and practices of its members.
- Family-centered nursing addresses the health of the family as a unit, as well as the health of family members.
- Through family assessment, the nurse identifies health beliefs and practices that influence the wellness of the family.
- In working with the wide variety of family forms in today's society, the nurse must be aware of many factors that affect the health of families.
- The nurse must examine her or his own values about family, health, illness, and death to be effective in supporting families in crisis.
- Nurses can help families realize their potential and

their dreams for health and happiness by promoting healthy family functioning.

Suggested Readings

Edelman, C., and Mandle, C. L. 1986. *Health promotion throughout the lifespan.* St. Louis: C. V. Mosby.

Health promotion is discussed and applied to the special needs of individuals at each developmental stage.

Hymovich, D. P., and Barnard, M. U. 1979. *Family health care: General Perspectives.* Vol. 1, 2d ed. New York: McGraw-Hill.

This volume focuses on factors that influence the health of families and interventions designed to promote family adaptation.

———. 1979. *Family health care: Developmental and situational crises.* Vol. 2, 2d ed. New York: McGraw-Hill.

As families expand and contract, the needs and concerns of family members change. The authors present nursing interventions to help families cope with developmental changes as well as unexpected crises.

Jarrett, G. E. March/April 1982. Research: Childrearing patterns of young mothers. *The American Journal of Maternal Child Nursing* 7:119–24.

Education for parenthood is an important role for nurses helping adolescent parents understand and enjoy their infants.

Johnson, S. H. 1986. *Nursing assessment and strategies for the family at high risk: High risk parenting.* 2d ed. Philadelphia: J. B. Lippincott Co.

Identification of and intervention in families at risk are essential to reduce the potential health care problems of these groups.

Logan, B. B., and Dawkins, C. E. 1986. *Family-centered nursing in the community.* Menlo Park, Calif.: Addison-Wesley.

The authors integrate the areas of family and community health into a family-focused community-health nursing text, reflecting contemporary trends and changes in the family, communities, and health policies, and demonstrating the impact of these changes on community health nursing. Contemporary issues discussed include adolescent pregnancy, substance abuse, chronic mental illness, and family violence.

Ludder, P., et al. March/April 1983. Caring for children of divorced families. *The American Journal of Maternal Child Nursing* 8:120–30.

By identifying and counseling the child at risk and providing guidance to the parents, nurses can ease the emotional problems caused by divorce.

Miller, J., and Janosik, E. 1980. *Family-focused care.* New York: McGraw-Hill.

The authors examine the physical and psychosocial stresses experienced by families and outline interventions to promote family health.

Mott, S. R.; Fazekas, N. F.; and James, S. R. 1985. *Nursing care of children and families.* Menlo Park, Calif.: Addison-Wesley Publishing Co.

This comprehensive child health nursing text focuses on the needs of children and their families from a holistic perspective.

Tackett, J., and Hunsberger, M. 1981. *Family-centered care of children and adolescents.* Philadelphia: W. B. Saunders Co.

This basic child health nursing text takes a family-centered approach to the study of children.

Wright, L. M., and Leahey, M. 1984. *Nurses and families: A guide to family assessment and intervention.* Philadelphia: F. A. Davis.

This book illustrates how family theory can be applied to clinical practice and emphasizes the development of interviewing skills with families.

Young, R. K. 1982. *Community nursing workbook: The family as a client.* New York: Appleton-Century-Crofts.

This workbook assists the student in using the nursing process to plan home visits to families.

Selected References

The adolescent family. 1984. Columbus, Ohio: Ross Laboratories.

Duffy, M. A. September/October 1982. When a woman heads a household. *Nursing Outlook* 30:468–73.

Duvall, E. M. 1977. *Marriage and family development.* 5th ed. Philadelphia: J. B. Lippincott Co.

Ebersole, P., and Hess, P. 1981. *Healthy aging.* St. Louis: C.V. Mosby Co.

Friedman, M. 1981. *Family nursing: Theory and assessment.* New York: Appleton-Century-Crofts.

Hoeffer, B. 1981. Children's acquisition of sex-role behavior in lesbian-mother families. *American Journal of Orthopsychiatry* 51:536.

Holmes, T., and Rahe, E. 1967. The social readjustment rating scale. *Journal of psychosomatic research* 11:213.

Knafl, K. May 1985. How families manage a pediatric hospitalization. *Western Journal of Nursing Research* 7(2):151–76.

McClellan, M. A. May/June 1984. On their own: Latchkey children. *Pediatric Nursing* 10:198–204.

McClelland, E.; Kelly, K.; and Buckwalter, K. 1985. *Continuity of care: Advancing the concept of discharge planning.* Orlando: Grune & Stratton, Inc.

McFarlane, J. December 1977. Sickle cell disorders. *American Journal of Nursing* 77:1948–54.

Moccia, P., and Mason, D. J. January/February 1986. Poverty trends: Implications for nursing. *Nursing Outlook* 34(1):20–24.

Orem, D. E. 1980. *Nursing concepts of practice.* 2d ed. New York: McGraw-Hill Book Company.

Pender, N. J. 1982. *Health promotion in nursing practice.* New York: Appleton-Century-Crofts.

Reutter, L., and Strang, V. July/August 1986. Yours, mine, and ours: Step-parents and their children. *The American Journal of Maternal/Child Nursing* 2:264–66.

Spector, R. E. 1979. *Cultural diversity in health and illness.* New York: Appleton-Century-Crofts.

Speer, J. J., and Sachs, B. September/October 1985. Selecting the appropriate family assessment tool. *Pediatric Nursing* 11:349–355.

U.S. Department of Health, Education, and Welfare. 1979. *Healthy people: The Surgeon General's report on health promotion and disease prevention.* DHEW pub. no. 79-55071.

Williamson, M. 1986. Lesbians. In Griffith-Kinney, J., editor. pp. 278–96. *Contemporary women's health.* Menlo Park, Calif.: Addison-Wesley Publishing Co.

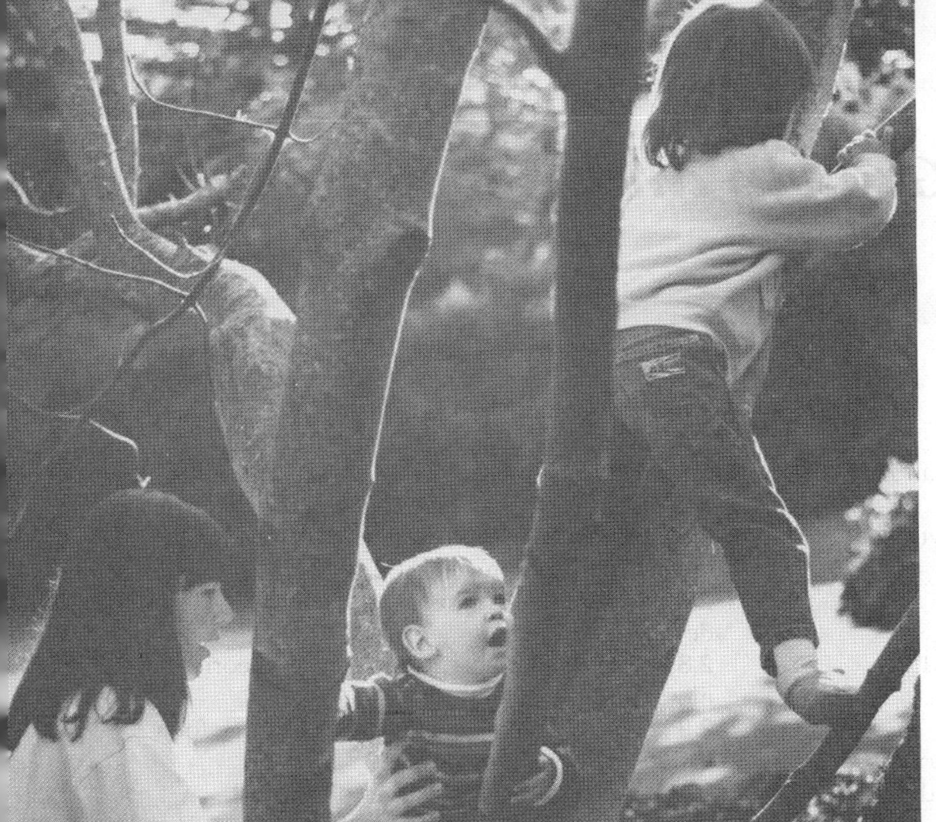

CHAPTER 22

Concepts of Growth and Development

Contents

22 *Concepts of Growth and Development*

Objectives

1. Know essential facts about growth and development.
   1.1 Define selected terms.
   1.2 Differentiate growth, development, and maturation.
   1.3 Describe factors that influence growth and development.
   1.4 Describe the stages of growth and development.
   1.5 Explain the principles of growth and development.
   1.6 Describe specific growth trends.
2. Understand selected theories about development.
   2.1 Explain how Havighurst's theory of development differs from Erikson's.
   2.2 Explain Freud's theory of psychosexual development.
   2.3 Describe Erikson's eight stages of psychosocial development.
   2.4 Compare Mahler's, Sullivan's, and Sears's stages of development.
   2.5 Describe Peek's stages of adult development.
   2.6 Explain how Maslow's theory of development differs from Erikson's.
   2.7 Explain Piaget's theory of cognitive development.
   2.8 Compare Kohlberg's and Peters's theories of moral development.
   2.9 Describe Schulman and Mekler's three foundations of moral development.
   2.10 Describe Fowler's stages of spiritual development.

Terms

accommodation (Piaget)
adaptation (Piaget)
assimilation (Piaget)
defense mechanism (adaptive mechanism)
development
development task (Havighurst)
ego
Electra complex
faith
fixation
growth
habit
id
individuation (Mahler)
libido
malevolent transformation (Sullivan)
maturation
moral
morality
Oedipus complex
separation (Mahler)
superego
unconscious mind

Growth, Development, and Maturation

The terms *growth* and *development* both refer to dynamic processes. Often used interchangeably, these terms have different denotations. **Growth** is physical change and increase in size. Growth can be measured. Indicators of growth include height, weight, bone size, and dentition. **Development** is an increase in the complexity of function and skill progression (Mott et al. 1985, p. 132). It is the capacity and skill of a person to function. Development is the behavioral aspect of growth; for example, a person develops the ability to walk, to talk, and to run. Growth and development are independent, interrelated processes. For example, an infant's muscles, bones, and nervous system must grow to a certain point before the infant can sit up or walk. Growth generally takes place during the first 20 years of life; development continues after that.

Maturation refers to the development of inherited characteristics, such as stature. **Maturation** is the sequence of physical changes that are related to genetic influences (Mott et al. 1985, p. 132). Maturation is independent of the environment, but its timing can be influenced by environmental factors. For example, inadequate nutrition can delay walking and growth.

Stages of Growth and Development

Stages of growth and development correspond to certain developmental changes. See Table 22–1.

The rate of a person's growth and development is highly individual. However, the sequence of growth and development is predictable. The influence of heredity and environment on growth and development is still debatable to some degree. It is generally accepted that those aspects of growth and development that are not determined genetically are influenced by the environment.

Table 22–1 Stages of Growth and Development

Stage	Age	Significant Characteristics	Nursing Implications
Prenatal	Conception to birth	During 9 months, all significant body systems develop. Inherited factors, maternal health and age are significant.	Help mothers develop strategies to establish a suitable environment for healthy fetal growth.
Neonatal	Birth to 28 days	Behavior is largely reflexive and develops to more purposeful behavior.	Assist parents to identify and meet unmet needs.
Infancy	1 month to 1 year	Physical growth is rapid.	Control the infant's environment so that physical and psychosocial needs are met.
Toddlerhood	1 to 3 years	Motor development permits increased physical autonomy. Psychosocial skills increase.	Safety and risk-taking strategies must be balanced to permit growth.
Preschool	3 to 6 years	The preschooler's world is expanding. New experiences and the preschooler's social role are tried during play. Physical growth is slower.	Provide opportunities for play and social activity.
School age	6 to 12 years	Stage includes the preadolescent period (10 to 12 years). Peer group increasingly influences behavior. Physical, cognitive, and social development increases, and the child has increased competence in communication.	Allow time and energy for the school-age child to pursue hobbies and school activities.
Adolescence	12 to 20 years	Self-concept changes with biologic development. Values are tested. Physical growth accelerates. Stress increases, especially in face of conflicts.	Assist adolescents to develop coping behaviors. Help adolescents develop strategies for resolving conflicts.
Young adulthood	20 to 40 years	A personal life-style develops. Person establishes a relationship with a significant other, a commitment to something, and competence (White, 1975).	Accept adult's chosen life-style and assist with necessary adjustments relating to health. Recognize the person's commitment and the function of competence in life. Support change as necessary for health.
Middle adulthood	40 to 65 years	Life-style changes because of other changes, e.g., children leave home, occupational goals change.	Assist clients to plan for anticipated changes in life, to recognize the risk factors related to health, and to focus on strengths rather than weaknesses.
Older adulthood	65 years and over	Adaptation to changing physical abilities is often necessary. Chronic illness may develop.	Assist clients to cope with loss, e.g., hearing, eyesight, death of loved one. Provide necessary safety measures. Assist clients to maintain peer group interactions.

Growth and development occur throughout life, although they are more apparent at certain periods, e.g., during adolescence, than at other times.

Factors Influencing Growth and Development

The factors that influence growth and development are the subject of discussion among developmental theorists. Theorists assign different importance to the respective roles of heredity and environment. Theorists usually hold one of the following beliefs:

1. Heredity determines most if not all growth.
2. The environment is the primary determinant of development.
3. Heredity and environment contribute to development, each affecting the individual to a greater or lesser extent during differing aspects of development.

Heredity

The genetic inheritance of an individual is established at conception. This genetic inheritance remains unchanged throughout life. Genetic inheritance determines such characteristics as sex, physical stature, and race.

Environment

Many environmental factors affect an individual's growth and development. Some of these are family, religion, climate, culture, school, community, and nutrition. For example, a poorly nourished child is more likely to have infections than a well-fed child is and may not attain his or her full height potential.

Principles of Growth and Development

1. Growth is a continuous process determined by many factors. Maturational, environmental, and genetic factors all interact and influence growth and development.
2. All humans follow the same pattern of growth and development. The sequence of each stage is predictable, although the time of onset, the length of the stage, and the effects of each stage vary with the person.
3. Learning can either help or hinder the maturational process, depending on what is learned. Maturation is the growth of the functional aspects of the body. The rate of maturation is determined by heredity. Although the maturational rate is inherited, it can be affected by factors such as nutrition or parental attitudes.
4. Each developmental stage has its own characteristics. For example, Piaget suggests that in the sensorimotor stage (birth to 2 years) children learn to coordinate simple motor tasks.
5. Growth and development occur in a cephalocaudal direction, i.e., starting at the head and moving to the trunk, the legs, and the feet. This pattern is particularly obvious at birth, when the head of an infant is disproportionately large.
6. Growth and development occur in a proximal to distal direction, i.e., from the center of the body outward. For example, infants can roll over before they can grasp an object with the thumb and second finger.
7. Growth and development become increasingly differentiated. An infant's initial response to a stimulus involves his or her total body; a 5-year-old child can respond more specifically with laughter or fear, for example.
8. Certain stages of growth and development are more critical than others. It is known, for example, that the first 10 to 12 weeks after conception are critical. The incidence of congenital anomalies as a result of exposure to certain viruses, chemicals, or drugs is greater during this stage than others (Mott et al. 1985, p. 133).
9. The pace of growth and development is uneven. It is known that growth is greater during infancy than during childhood.

Components of Growth and Development

Growth and development are commonly thought of as having five major components: physiologic, cognitive, psychosocial, moral, and spiritual. The physiologic component refers to an individual's physical size and body functioning. The psychosocial component includes feelings, subjective experiences, and interactions with others. The moral component is the values, attitudes, and beliefs people have about right and wrong. The cognitive component refers to knowledge, reasoning, perceiving, remembering, thinking, abstracting, and generalizing. The spiritual component refers to the relationship individuals understand they have with the universe, and their perceptions about the direction and meaning of life.

Physiologic Growth and Development

The pattern of physiologic growth is similar for all people. However, growth rates vary during different stages of growth and development. See Table 22–1. For example, the growth rate is very rapid during the prenatal, neonatal, infancy, and adolescent stages. The growth rate slows during childhood, and physical growth is minimal during adulthood. Table 22–2 gives an overview of physiologic growth trends from the prenatal stage to elderly adulthood.

Havighurst

Robert Havighurst believes that learning is basic to life and that people continue to learn throughout life. He describes growth and development as occurring during six stages, each associated with from six to ten tasks to be learned. See Table 22–3. Havighurst believes that once a person learns a task, it is mastered for life.

Havighurst promoted the concept of developmental tasks in the 1950s. A **developmental task** is "a task which arises at or about a certain period in the life of an individual, successful achievement of which leads to his happiness and to success with later tasks, while failure leads to unhappiness in the individual, disapproval by society, and difficulty with later tasks" (Havighurst 1972, p. 2).

Nurses can use Havighurst's developmental tasks as a standard against which to compare a person's accomplishments. Therefore, when planning nursing strategies, nurses can incorporate developmental tasks for that age period, thus helping development.

Duvall

Duvall describes developmental tasks as having two primary origins: (a) physical maturation and (b) cultural pressures and privileges. A secondary origin, according to Duvall, is the aspirations and values of the individual, which derive from the two primary origins (Duvall 1977, p. 168). Developmental tasks vary from culture to culture, and even from one region of a country to another.

Duvall sees individuals as assuming developmental tasks in four steps:

1. Perceiving new possibilities for behavior as a result of what is expected by others or as a result of the accomplishments of more mature individuals
2. Forming new concepts of self
3. Coping effectively with conflicting demands
4. Acquiring the motivation to achieve the next developmental steps (Duvall 1977, p. 169)

Duvall lists general categories or tasks common to North American cultures. The tasks for infants through elderly adults are described in subsequent chapters.

Psychosocial Development

Psychosocial development refers to the development of personality. Personality is a complex concept that is difficult to define. It can be considered as the outward (interpersonal) expression of the inner (intrapersonal) self. It encompasses a person's temperament, feelings, character traits, independence, self-esteem, self-concept, behavior, ability to interact with others, and ability to adapt to life changes.

Many theorists attempt to account for psychosocial development in humans. Many of these theories explain the development of a person's personality and the causes of behavior. The theorists discussed in this book are Freud, Sullivan, Erikson, Mahler, Sears, Peck, Maslow, and Havighurst.

Freud

Sigmund Freud, whose writings and research were very popular in the 1930s, introduced a number of concepts about development that are still used today. The concepts of the unconscious mind, defense mechanisms, and the id, ego, and superego are Freud's. The **unconscious mind** is the mental life of a person of which the person is unaware. This concept of the unconscious is one of Freud's major contributions to the field of psychiatry. **Defense mechanisms**, or **adaptive mechanisms** as they are more commonly called today, are the result of conflicts between inner impulses and of the anxiety that attends these conflicts. The **id** is the source of instinctive and unconscious urges, which Freud considers chiefly sexual in nature. The id is also the source of all pleasure and gratification. The **ego** is formed by the person to make effective contact with these social and physical needs. Through the ego, the id impulses are satisfied. The third aspect of the personality, according to Freud, is the **superego**. This is the conscience of the personality, a control on the id. The superego is the source of feelings of guilt, shame, and inhibition. See Chapter 17, pages 346–347, for additional information on adaptive processes and ego defense mechanisms.

Freud proposes that the underlying motivation to human development is an energy form or life instinct, which he calls **libido**.

Each of the stages of development during the first 5 years is associated with a part of the body. See Table 22–4. If the individual does not achieve a satisfactory resolution at each stage, the personality becomes fixated at that stage. **Fixation** is immobilization or the inability of the personality to proceed to the next stage because of anxiety. The first three stages (oral, anal, and phallic) are called the pregenital stages. During the first or *oral stage,* the mouth is the principal source of pleasure, primarily as a result of eating. Feelings of dependence arise in the oral stage, and they tend, according to Freud, to persist throughout life. A person who is fixated at the oral stage may have difficulty trusting others and may demonstrate such behaviors as nail biting, drug abuse, smoking, overeating, alcoholism, argumentativeness, and overdependency. The anal stage occurs when the child is learning toilet training. Fixation at this stage can result in obsessive-compulsive personality traits such as obstinance, stinginess, cruelty, and temper tantrums. During the phallic phase, sexual and aggressive feelings associated with the genitals come into focus. Masturbation offers pleasure at this time, and the child experiences the Oedipus or Electra complex. The **Oedipus complex** refers to the male child's attraction for his mother and his hostile attitudes toward his father. The **Electra complex** is the female child's attraction for her father and her hostility toward her mother. Fixation at the phallic phase can result in such traits as problems with sexual identity and problems with authority. During the latency stage, the sexual impulses tend to be repressed. Unresolved conflict at this stage may be reflected in obsessiveness and lack of self-motivation. Following latency come adolescence and the reactivation of the pregenital impulses. The person usually displaces these impulses and subsequently passes into the final stage of adult maturity, the genital stage. The inability to resolve conflicts during this stage can result in sexual problems, such as frigidity, impotence, and the inability to be satisfied in a heterosexual relationship.

Table 22–2 Growth Trends Throughout Life

Systemic Changes	Prenatal	Neonatal	Infancy	Toddlerhood	Preschool
			Heart and Circulatory System		
During life, the heart is responsive to organ needs and emotional responses.	Heart is formed and begins to beat about third week.		Heart grows more slowly than the rest of the body. —		
	Heart rate is approximately 150 beats/min.		Heart rate falls throughout childhood, is 130 beats/min. in infancy.		
			Urinary System		
Development generally parallels the growth of the body. Proportion of body fluids and solids follows pattern related to growth. Proportion of fluid tends to decrease with age.	Fetus is approximately 90% fluid.	Newborn is 70% fluid.			
	Urinary system begins in the first month.	Renal units are immature. Fluid imbalance occurs readily.	Urinary system is completely developed at end of first year.		
			Gastrointestinal System		
System is responsive to physiologic needs and stress.	Nutrients are supplied through the placental circulation.	Size of stomach increases rapidly during first months. Salivary glands are small.		Stomach size grows steadily throughout childhood. — Salivary glands mature at 2 years.	
			Gastric acidity is low.	Gastric acidity rises in childhood.	
			Senses		
	Senses start to develop at 3 to 6 weeks.	Most senses are well developed at birth.	Eye muscles are fully functioning. Infant perceives simple differences in shape.	Hyperopia increases until eyeball reaches adult size at 8 years.	
			Adipose Tissue		
	Fat accumulates rapidly, peaks at 7 months.	Fat gain increases rapidly during first 6 months.		Fat decreases from age 1 to age 6 or 7. — Tends to be chubby.	
			Lymphoid Tissue		
	Lymphoid tissue begins to grow in ninth month.	Immune system is immature.	System develops rapidly during infancy and childhood. —		
			Respiratory System		
	Air sacs in lungs do not contain air; oxygen supplied through maternal circulation.	Starts breathing at birth. Respiratory rate is high in infancy, slows through childhood. —			
			Skeletal System		
	70% of head growth occurs before birth.		Trunk grows the most rapidly.		There is a rapid growth spurt.

School Age	Adolescence	Young Adulthood	Middle Adulthood	Older Adulthood
		Heart and Circulatory System		
→	There is a growth spurt during prepuberty. Heart reaches mature size by 16 years. Heart rate is approximately 60 beats/min.	Heart weight remains relatively constant throughout life. Cardiac output decreases 30% to 40% between 25 and 65 years. Cardiac power decreases with age. Capacity to increase rate and strength with physical activity decreases with age.		
		Urinary System		
		Adult is 58% fluid. Glomular filtration rate decreases about 47% from age 20 years to 90 years.		
		Gastrointestinal System		
→	Organs have widely varying functional maturity.	Metabolism, enzyme production, HCl production decrease after age 30 years.		Salivation diminishes.
Acidity plateaus at 10 years.	Gastric acidity rises in puberty			
		Senses		
	There is a trend toward myopia until 30 years.		Myopia decreases and hyperopia increases. Lack of normal pain response may occur.	
		Adipose Tissue		
→	→		There is tendency to gain weight in 50s and 60s.	Fat stores often lost during 70s.
		From 25 to 75 years fat increases by 16%, and fluid decreases by 8%.		
		Lymphoid Tissue		
→ Immune system is functionally mature.		Lymphoid tissue mass is smaller in adulthood.		
		Respiratory System		
→	Vital capacity increases with increased stature.			Lung tissue becomes more rigid.
		Skeletal System		
Growth slows. Growth spurt in girls starts at about 10 years; in boys, about 13 years. Growth is greater in boys.		Maximum height is reached by 30s.	Height declines gradually, 1.2 cm every 20 years. Bone mass begins to decrease from age 40 years.	Shortening of spinal column caused by thinning vertebrae.

(continued)

Table 22–2 ***(continued)***

Systemic Changes	Prenatal	Neonatal	Infancy	Toddlerhood	Preschool
Muscular System					
Muscle size varies considerably among individuals.	Muscles begin to assume shape by 2 months.		Muscle size increases rapidly.	Neuromuscular control increases. Abdomen protrudes until abdominal muscles develop.	Muscle size increases slowly.
Reproductive System					
	Genital organs are formed.	Female sex organs are formed. Male sex organs (testes) are formed but dormant.	System is nonfunctional during childhood.		
Nervous System					
	Growth is very rapid.	Temperature regulating system is poorly developed.	Infant has the total number of brain cells by first year. Brain grows rapidly.	Brain cells increase in size and in number and complexity of axons and dendrites.	
Endocrine System					
		System is immature at birth. Adrenal glands decrease in size throughout first year.		Adrenal gland size increases during childhood.	
Integumentary System					
	Hair, skin, and sebaceous glands are fully formed in utero.	Skin contains all structures but is immature in function.		Most children have all deciduous teeth by second year.	Child begins to lose deciduous teeth.
	Lanugo begins to decrease.				
Immune System					
		System is immature at birth.			

Sources: Adapted from D. C. Sutterly and G. F. Donnelly, *Perspectives in human development: Nursing throughout the life cycle* (Philadelphia: J. B. Lipppincott Co., 1973); C. Edelman and C. L. Mandle, *Health promotion throughout the lifespan* (St. Louis: C. V. Mosby, 1986); P. Ebersole and P. Hess, *Toward healthy aging: Human needs and nursing response* (St. Louis: C. V. Mosby Co., 1985); and C. A. Schuster and S. S. Ashburn, *The process of human development: A holistic approach* (Boston: Little, Brown and Co., 1980).

Thus, according to Freud's theory of psychosexual development, the personality develops in five overlapping stages from birth to adulthood. The libido is envisaged as changing its location of emphasis from one stage to another. Therefore, a particular body area has special significance to a client at a particular stage. For example, during the oral phase the mouth is the significant area. Therefore, injury of the mouth has great impact on an infant. Also, nurses can assist an infant's development by making feeding a pleasurable experience. A further example is the 2-year-old who has anal surgery and thus experiences toilet training as unpleasant. A nurse can assist 2-year-olds in their development by making toilet training a positive experience, thereby enhancing their feeling of self-control.

Freud also emphasizes the importance of infant-parent interaction. Therefore, the nurse, as a caregiver, should provide a warm, caring atmosphere for an infant and assist parents to do so also when the infant returns to their care.

Sullivan

Harry Stack Sullivan delineates six stages of interpersonal development. His stages span the period from infancy to adulthood. He sees the growth of the personality from a sociopsychologic viewpoint. Although he does not reject

School Age	Adolescence	Young Adulthood	Middle Adulthood	Older Adulthood
		Muscular System		
→	→	Muscles reach maximum strength between ages 20 and 30 years.	Muscle growth continues in proportion to use.	Atrophy and loss of muscle tone.
Muscle strength at puberty is greater in boys.				
		Reproductive System		
→ System is mature at puberty with menstruation. At puberty, testes and penis increase in size.			Involution occurs after menopause. Uterus reaches maximum weight at age 30 years.	
		Sex drive is active throughout maturity and may subside only during last decade.		
		Nervous System		
→	→	Brain weight decreases with age. →	→	→
Brain reaches 90% adult size by age 7 years.				Myelin sheath decreases.
		Endocrine System		
	There is growth spurt of adrenal glands. Basal metabolic rate increases.	Adrenal glands mature with body.		There is a decrease in function of all endocrine glands.
		Integumentary System		
	There is growth spurt of all structures. Hair distribution changes. Sebaceous gland activity increases.	Skin becomes drier with age.		Skin elasticity and moisture decrease.
		Immune System		
System is functionally mature.				Immune system effectiveness possibly declines.

the role of heredity (biology) in development, he believes that sociologic factors have greater influence. Stack defines interpersonal behavior as "all that can be observed as personality" (Hall and Lindzey 1970, p. 137). He views interpersonal development as a series of stages. In his second stage, for example, he believes that a child develops **malevolent transformation** which is the feeling that one lives among enemies. Sullivan considers his six stages as typical for people in Western European cultures; stages in other cultures may differ. See Table 22–5.

Erikson

Erik H. Erikson adapted and expanded Freud's theory of development. Erikson describes eight stages of development. He believes that the ego is the conscious core of the personality. In his theory, the concept of society is added to his stages of psychosocial development. See Table 22–6.

Life is pictured as a sequence of levels of achievement. Each stage signals a task that must be achieved. The resolution of the task can be complete, partial, or unsuccessful. Erikson believes that the greater the task achievement, the healthier the personality of the person; however, failure to achieve a task influences the person's ability to achieve the next task. These developmental tasks can be viewed as a series of crises, and successful resolution of these crises is supportive to the person's ego; failure to resolve the crises is damaging to the ego.

Erikson further states that, after attaining one stage,

Table 22–3 Havighurst's Age Periods and Developmental Tasks

Infancy and Early Childhood

1. Learning to walk
2. Learning to take solid foods
3. Learning to talk
4. Learning to control the elimination of body wastes
5. Learning sex differences and sexual modesty
6. Achieving psychologic stability
7. Forming simple concepts of social and physical reality
8. Learning to relate emotionally to parents, siblings, and other people
9. Learning to distinguish right from wrong and developing a conscience

Middle Childhood

1. Learning physical skills necessary for ordinary games
2. Building wholesome attitudes toward oneself as a growing organism
3. Learning to get along with age-mates
4. Learning an appropriate masculine or feminine social role
5. Developing fundamental skills in reading, writing, and calculating
6. Developing concepts necessary for everyday living
7. Developing conscience, morality, and a scale of values
8. Achieving personal independence
9. Developing attitudes toward social groups and institutions

Adolescence

1. Achieving new and more mature relations with age-mates of both sexes
2. Achieving a masculine or feminine social role
3. Accepting one's physique and using the body effectively
4. Achieving emotional independence from parents and other adults
5. Achieving assurance of economic independence
6. Selecting and preparing for an occupation
7. Preparing for marriage and family life
8. Developing intellectual skills and concepts necessary for civic competence
9. Desiring and achieving socially responsible behavior
10. Acquiring a set of values and an ethical system as a guide to behavior

Early Adulthood

1. Selecting a mate
2. Learning to live with a partner
3. Starting a family
4. Rearing children
5. Managing a home
6. Getting started in an occupation
7. Taking on civic responsibility
8. Finding a congenial social group

Middle Age

1. Achieving adult civic and social responsibility
2. Establishing and maintaining an economic standard of living
3. Assisting teenage children to become responsible and happy adults
4. Developing adult leisure-time activities
5. Relating oneself to one's spouse as a person
6. Accepting and adjusting to the physiologic changes of middle age
7. Adjusting to aging parents

Later Maturity

1. Adjusting to decreasing physical strength and health
2. Adjusting to retirement and reduced income
3. Adjusting to death of a spouse
4. Establishing an explicit affiliation with one's age group
5. Meeting social and civil obligations
6. Establishing satisfactory physical living arrangements

Source: From *Developmental tasks and education,* 3d ed., by Robert J. Havighurst. Copyright © 1972 by Longman Inc. Reprinted by permission of Longman Inc., New York.

the person may fall back and need to approach it again. Erikson's eight stages reflect both positive and negative aspects of the critical life periods. The resolution of the conflicts at each stage enables the person to function effectively in society.

Erikson expands the work of Freud to include the entire life span. Erikson believes that people continue to develop throughout life. Each phase has its developmental task, and the individual must find a balance between, for example, trust versus mistrust (stage 1) or generativity versus stagnation (stage 7).

When using Erikson's developmental framework, nurses should be aware of indicators of positive and negative resolution of each stage. It is also important to be aware that, according to Erikson, the environment is highly influential in development. Nurses can enhance people's development by being aware of their developmental stage, by providing opportunities for the individual to resolve his or her developmental task, and by helping the person develop coping skills relative to stressors experienced at that level.

Erikson believes that it is important for people to change and adapt their behavior to maintain control over their lives. In his view, no stage in personality development can be bypassed, but people can become fixated at one stage or regress to a previous stage. For example, a middle-aged woman who has never satisfactorily accomplished the task of resolving identity versus role confusion might regress to an earlier stage when stressed by an illness with which she cannot cope.

Table 22–4 Freud's Five Stages of Development

Stage	Age	Characteristics	Implications
Oral	0 to 1 year	Mouth is the center of pleasure.	Feeding produces pleasure and sense of comfort and safety. Feeding should be pleasurable and provided when required.
Anal	2 and 3 years	Anus and rectum are the centers of pleasure.	Controlling and expelling feces provide pleasure and sense of control. Toilet training should be a pleasurable experience, and appropriate praise can result in a personality that is creative and productive.
Phallic	4 and 5 years	The child's genitals are the center of pleasure.	The child identifies with the parent of the opposite sex and later takes on a love relationship outside the family. Encourage identification.
Latency	6 to 12 years	Energy is directed to physical and intellectual activities.	Encourage child with physical and intellectual pursuits.
Genital	13 years and after	Energy is directed toward attaining a mature heterosexual relationship.	Encourage separation from parents, achievement of independence, and making decisions.

Source: Adapted from Patricia H. Miller, *Theories of developmental psychology*. Copyright © 1983 W. H. Freeman and Company. Used by permission.

Nurses should also be aware that, according to Erikson, people continue to change throughout life. Therefore, the client admitted to hospital at age 70 years is not the same client the nurse knew 10 years previously. Nurses can enhance a client's positive resolution of a developmental task by providing the individual with appropriate opportunities and encouragement. For example, a 10-year-old child can be encouraged to be creative, to finish schoolwork, and to learn how to accomplish these tasks within the limitations imposed by health.

Because resolution of developmental tasks is not absolute, a middle-aged man, for example, may feel satisfied about one aspect of life, such as his family, yet be preoccupied about another, perhaps his business. The nurse can help such a man focus on his assets while at the same time recognizing his limitations.

Mahler

Margaret Mahler studied the development of independence in infants from birth to 3 years. To obtain independence, the infant goes through a series of steps in a process called separation-individuation. **Separation** is the development of a picture of self as separate from others. **Individuation** is the development of independent ego functions such as perception or memory. As a result of separation-individuation, the infant attains a personal identity. For example, an infant can separate from his or her mother for a period of time, become absorbed in activities, ask where the mother is, and return to the activity when the mother does not appear. The child is supported by an internalized representation of the mother that exists whether the mother is present or absent (Haber et al. 1982, p. 139).

Table 22–5 Sullivan's Stages of Interpersonal Development

Stage	Age	Selected Characteristics
Infancy	Birth to the appearance of articulate speech	Activity is primarily mouth-centered. Nursing is the infant's first interpersonal experience.
Childhood	Articulate speech to the need for playmates	The child integrates self-esteem and develops **malevolent transformation** (the feeling that one lives among enemies).
Juvenile	First 5 to 6 years	The child becomes social, competitive, and cooperative and learns to supervise own behavior by external controls.
Preadolescence	7 years to adolescence	Child begins to form genuine human relationships. The child forms peer relationships.
Early adolescence	12 to 14 years	The child develops a pattern of heterosexual activity. The erotic need is focused on a member of the opposite sex. The need for intimacy is focused on a member of the same sex.
Late adolescence	15 to 18 years	The person is initiated into the privileges, duties, satisfactions, and responsibilities of social living.

Source: Adapted from C. S. Hall and G. Lindzey, *Theories of personality,* 2d ed. (New York: John Wiley and Sons, 1970). Copyright © 1970 John Wiley & Sons, Inc. Reprinted by permission.

Table 22–6 Erikson's Eight Stages of Development

Stage	Age	Central Task	Indicators of Positive Resolution	Indicators of Negative Resolution
Infancy	Birth to 18 months	Trust versus mistrust	Learning to trust others Sense of trust in self	Mistrust, withdrawal, estrangement
Early childhood	18 months to 3 years	Autonomy versus shame and doubt	Self-control without loss of self-esteem Ability to cooperate and to express oneself	Compulsive self-restraint or compliance Willfulness and defiance
Late childhood	3 to 5 years	Initiative versus guilt	Learning the degree to which assertiveness and purpose influence the environment Beginning ability to evaluate one's own behavior	Lack of self-confidence Pessimism, fear of wrongdoing Overcontrol and overrestriction of own activity
School age	6 to 12 years	Industry versus inferiority	Beginning to create, develop, and manipulate Developing sense of competence and perseverance	Loss of hope, sense of being mediocre Withdrawal from school and peers
Adolescence	12 to 20 years	Identity versus role confusion	Coherent sense of self Plans to actualize one's abilities	Confusion, indecisiveness, and inability to find occupational identity
Young adulthood	18 to 25 years	Intimacy versus isolation	Intimate relationship with another person Commitment to work and relationships	Impersonal relationships Avoidance of relationship, career, or life-style commitments
Adulthood	25 to 65 years	Generativity versus stagnation	Creativity, productivity, concern for others	Self-indulgence, self-concern, lack of interests and commitments
Maturity	65 years to death	Integrity versus despair	Acceptance of worth and uniqueness of one's own life Acceptance of death	Sense of loss, contempt for others

Sources: Adaptation of Erikson's Eight Stages of Development from *Childhood and Society*, 2nd edition, by Erik H. Erikson, by permission of W. W. Norton & Company, Inc. In the British Empire excluding Canada, The Hogarth Press, Ltd., London.

The process of separation-individuation is preceded by two processes and has four subphases. See Table 22–7.

Sears

Robert Richardson Sears tries to reconcile psychoanalytic theory (e.g., that of Freud) with behaviorist theory in his writings about learning theory and development. Sears writes that development is "a continuous, orderly sequence of conditions which creates actions, new motives for actions, and eventual patterns of behavior" (Maier 1965, p. 154). Furthermore, he believes that social conditions dictate the process of development. Sears's phases of development, as described by Maier, are:

1. Phase of rudimentary behavior in early infancy. This phase takes place during the first few months of life when development is related to the infant's basic needs and to his or her attempts to reduce tensions resulting from inner drives. Sears also believes that the social environment, i.e., the parents, greatly influences development in this phase.
2. Phase of secondary motivational systems: family-centered learning. This phase of development is based on family-centered learning. It lasts from about age 6 months to age 6 years. Children use parents as role models during this phase, and children gradually progress from parental control to self-control.
3. Phase of secondary motivational systems: extrafamilial learning. During this phase, wider social factors influence the child's socialization. In this middle childhood period, experience and behavior are increasingly influenced by such people as friends, teachers, peers, and club leaders. Children desire the approval of such people. During this phase, children also acquire more comprehensive internal values as well as social and religious values.

Peck

Theories and models about adult development are relatively recent compared with theories of infant and child development. Research into adult development has been stimulated by a number of factors, including increased longevity and healthier old age. In the past, development was viewed as complete by the time of physical maturity, and aging was considered a decline following maturity. The emphasis was on the decremental aspects rather than

Table 22–7 Mahler's Separation-Individuation Process

Phase	Age	Characteristics
		Preceding the Process
Normal autism	Birth to 1 month	Lacks awareness of others. Is unable to differentiate self from others.
Normal symbiosis	1 to 5 months	Sees caregiver as part of self. Has beginning awareness of not being able to meet own needs.
		Separation-Individuation Process
Differentiation (hatching)	5 to 9 months	Bond between infant and caregiver emerges. Begins to differentiate own body from caregiver's body.
Practicing Early (crawling) Late (walking)	9 to 14 months	Begins to move away physically from caregiver. Is absorbed in own activities, but caregiver must be present to give sense of security.
Reapproachment	14 to 24 months	Recognizes self as physically separate from caregiver. Wants to share new accomplishments with caregiver. Is shy with strangers.
Consolidation	24 to 36 months	Can separate from caregiver without extreme anxiety. Play becomes more purposeful. Able to wait to have needs gratified.

Source: Adapted from *The Psychological Birth of the Human Infant: Symbiosis and Individuation* by Margaret S. Mahler, Fred Pine, and Anni Bergman. Copyright © 1975 by Margaret Mahler. Reprinted by permission of Basic Books, Inc., Publishers. And in the British Empire, Hutchinson Publishing Group, Ltd. London, U.K.

the incremental aspects of aging. However, Peck believes that although physical capabilities and functions decrease with old age, mental and social capacities tend to increase in the latter part of life (Peck 1968).

White identifies three growth trends in young adulthood:

1. Stabilization of identity: Identity is more consistent and resistant to changing influences.
2. Humanization of values: The individual becomes more aware of the personal meaning of values. Values become based on life experiences.
3. Expansion of caring: The person extends the sense of self to the community and becomes more involved in the welfare of others (White 1975).

Robert Peck recognizes four sets of developmental challenges during middle age.

1. The person values wisdom over physical strength and attractiveness. Wisdom, according to Peck, is "effective choices among the alternatives which intellectual perception and imagination present" (Peck 1968, p. 89).
2. Socialization replaces sexuality in male-female relationships. The middle-aged person sees people of the opposite sex as companions and individuals.
3. Experience is used more as a guideline than as a rigid rule for thought and behavior.
4. The person redirects emotional investment to new people, roles, and activities as previous ones become unsatisfactory or change; e.g., as children leave home, parents die, or friends move (Peck 1968).

Peck proposes three developmental tasks during old age, in contrast to Erikson's one (integrity versus despair). Peck believes that the older person must accomplish these three tasks:

1. Ego differentiation versus work-role preoccupation. An adult's identity and feelings of worth are highly dependent on his or her work role. Upon retirement, some people experience feelings of worthlessness unless their sense of identity is derived from a number of roles so that one such role can replace the work role or occupation as a source of self-esteem. For example, a man who likes to garden or golf can obtain ego rewards from those activities, replacing rewards formerly obtained from his occupation.
2. Body transcendence versus body preoccupation. This task calls for the individual to adjust to decreasing physical capacities and at the same time maintain feelings of well-being. Preoccupation with declining body function reduces happiness and satisfaction with life.
3. Ego transcendence versus ego preoccupation. Ego transcendence is the acceptance without fear of one's death as inevitable. This acceptance includes being actively involved in one's own future beyond death. Ego preoccupation, by contrast, results in holding on to life and a preoccupation with self-gratification.

Maslow

In Maslow's theory of motivation, all people have the same basic needs. These needs are established in a hierarchy, with basic physiologic needs forming the base of the pyramid. Successive stages are safety and security, love and belonging, recognition and esteem, and finally, at the point of the pyramid, self-actualization. See Figure 16–1, page 000. In Maslow's needs system, an individual's energy level, not age, is significant. When a person's energy level is sufficient, his or her needs can be met. Maslow believes that energy is the dependent variable, whereas Erikson believes it is age. For additional information about Maslow, see Chapter 16, page 314.

Cognitive Development

Cognitive development refers to the manner in which people learn to think, reason, and use language. It involves a person's intelligence, perceptional ability, and ability to process information. Cognitive development represents a progression of mental abilities from illogical to logical thinking, from simple to complex problem solving, and from understanding concrete ideas to understanding abstract concepts. The most widely known cognitive theorist is Jean Piaget (1896–1980). His theory of cognitive development has contributed to other theories, such as Kohlberg's theory of moral development and Fowler's theory of the development of faith, both discussed in this chapter.

According to Piaget, cognitive development is an orderly, sequential process in which a variety of new experiences (stimuli) must exist before intellectual abilities can develop. Piaget proposes five successive phases. In each phase, the person uses three primary abilities: assimilation, accommodation, and adaptation.

Assimilation is the process through which humans encounter and react to new situations by using the mechanisms they already possess. In this way, people acquire new knowledge and skills as well as insights into the world around them.

Accommodation is a process of change whereby cognitive processes mature sufficiently to allow the person to solve problems that were unsolvable before. This adjustment is possible chiefly because new knowledge has been assimilated.

Adaptation, or coping behavior, is the ability to handle the demands made by the environment.

Piaget's cognitive developmental process is divided into five major phases: the sensorimotor phase, the preconceptual phase, the intuitive phase, the concrete operations phase, and the formal operations phase. A person develops through each of these phases; each phase has its own unique characteristics. See Table 22–8.

Nurses can employ Piaget's theory of cognitive development when developing teaching strategies. For example, a nurse can expect a toddler to be egocentric and literal; therefore, explanations to the toddler should focus on the needs of the toddler rather than on the needs of others. Further, a 13-year-old can be expected to use rational thinking and to reason; therefore, when explaining the need for a medication, a nurse can outline the consequences of taking and not taking the medication, enabling the adolescent to make a rational decision. Nurses must remember, however, that the range of normal cognitive development is very broad, despite the ages arbitrarily associated with each level.

When teaching adults, nurses may become aware that some adults are more comfortable with concrete thought and slower to acquire and apply new information than other adults are.

Moral Development

Moral development is a complex process that is not fully understood. It involves learning what ought to be and what ought to be done. It is more than imprinting parents' rules and virtues or values upon children. The term **moral** means relating to right and wrong. Distinctions need to be made between the terms *morality, moral behavior,* and *moral development.* **Morality** refers to the requirements necessary for people to live together in society; moral behavior is the way a person perceives those requirements and responds to them; moral development is the pattern of changes in moral behavior with age (White 1975).

Freud

Freud (1961) believes that the mechanism for right and wrong within the individual is the superego, or conscience. He hypothesizes that a child internalizes and adopts the moral standards and character or character traits of the model parent through the process of identification during resolution of the Oedipus complex. To Freud, children acquire morals unconsciously from parental standards, specifically from the model parent with whom the child identifies. Freud believes moral behavior results from the strength of the superego, which strives to be "supermoral," in conflict with the ego, which strives to be "moral," and the id, which is totally nonmoral." The strength of the superego depends on the intensity of the child's feelings of aggression and attachment toward the model parent rather than on the actual standards of the parent.

Being a psychoanalyst, Freud focuses on human failings, including moral failure and failure to mature. He notes that some people fixate at a certain level and develop a fixated character. His theory implies that moral development is completed in childhood and focuses on an emotional component. Because, in Freud's view, morals

Table 22–8 Piaget's Phases of Cognitive Development

Phases and Stages	Age	Significant Behavior
Sensorimotor	Birth to 2 years	
Stage 1 Use of reflexes	Birth to 1 month	Most action is reflexive.
Stage 2 Primary circular reaction	1 to 4 months	Perception of events is centered on the body. Objects are extension of self.
Stage 3 Secondary circular reaction	4 to 8 months	Acknowledges the external environment. Actively makes changes in the environment.
Stage 4 Coordination of secondary schemata	8 to 12 months	Can distinguish a goal from a means of attaining it.
Stage 5 Tertiary circular reaction	12 to 18 months	Tries and discovers new goals and ways to attain goals. Rituals are important.
Stage 6 Inventions of new means	18 to 24 months	Interprets the environment by mental image. Uses make-believe and pretend play.
Preconceptual	2 to 4 years	Uses an egocentric approach to accommodate the demands of an environment. Everything is significant and relates to "me." Explores the environment. Language development is rapid. Associates words with objects.
Intuitive thought	4 to 7 years	Egocentric thinking diminishes. Thinks of one idea at a time. Includes others in the environment. Words express thoughts.
Concrete operations	7 to 11 years	Solves concrete problems. Begins to understand relationships such as size. Understands right and left. Cognizant of viewpoints.
Formal operations	11 to 15 years	Uses rational thinking. Reasoning is deductive and futuristic.

Source: Adapted from Jean Piaget, *The Origin of intelligence in children.* International Universities Press, Inc. Copyright © 1966. Used by permission.

develop unconsciously, there is no rational conscious component in moral development. Through feelings of love or affection for the mother or father and identification with that parent's character traits, the child develops feelings of guilt, self-respect, praise, or blame.

Erikson

Erikson's theory of the development of virtues or unifying strengths of the "good man" suggests that moral development continues throughout life. Erikson (1964) believes that if the conflicts of each psychosocial developmental stage are favorably resolved, then an "ego-strength" or virtue emerges. See Table 22–9. This theory of virtues or moral development focuses on goals that can be achieved at various stages of life. It implies that fidelity, love, care, and wisdom are adult phenomena only.

Piaget

Piaget believes that autonomous moral thinking is facilitated through experiencing activities in cooperation with peers and in relationships of mutual respect (Duska and Whelan 1975, p. 13). He emphasizes that learning is an action between the individual and the environment. He believes that moral development, like any other natural growth, follows a certain pattern of invariant stages moving from egocentrism to autonomy. Invariance implies that the individual progresses through hierarchical stages in order; an individual cannot achieve a higher stage without completing the stage preceding it. For additional information about Piaget see the section on cognitive development, earlier in this chapter.

Kohlberg

Kohlberg suggests three levels of moral development that encompass six stages (Berkowitz and Oser 1985, p. 28). Like Piaget, he focuses on the reasons for the making of a decision, not on the morality of the decision itself. At Kohlberg's first level, called the premoral or preconventional level, children are responsive to cultural rules and labels of good and bad, right and wrong. However, children interpret these in terms of the physical consequences of their actions, i.e., punishment or reward. At

Table 22–9 Erikson's Virtues or Ego-Strengths

Stage of Development	Virtue
Trust versus mistrust	*Hope* or *confidence.* Belief that fervent wishes will be attained
Autonomy versus doubt	*Will.* Determination to exercise free choice as well as self-restraint
Initiative versus guilt	*Purpose.* Courage to envisage and pursue valued goals
Industry versus inferiority	*Competence.* Free exercise of dexterity and intelligence in the completion of tasks
Identity versus identity diffusion	*Fidelity.* Ability to sustain loyalties freely pledged in spite of the inevitable contradictions of value systems
Intimacy versus isolation	*Love.* Mutuality of devotion
Generativity versus stagnation or self-absorption	*Care.* Widened concern for what has been generated by love extending to whatever a person generates, creates, produces, or helps to produce
Integrity versus despair	*Wisdom.* Detached concern with life in the face of death

Source: E. H. Erikson, *Insight and responsibility: Lectures on the ethical implications of psychoanalytic insight* (New York: W. W. Norton and Co., 1964). Used by permission.

the second level, the conventional level, the individual is concerned about maintaining the expectations of the family, group, or nation and sees this as right. The emphasis at this level is conformity and loyalty to one's own expectations as well as society's. Level three is called the postconventional, autonomous, or principled level. At this level, people make an effort to define valid values and principles without regard to outside authority or to the expectations of others. For additional information about Kohlberg's levels, see Table 22–10.

With reference to Kohlberg's six stages, Munhall writes that stage four, the "law and order" orientation, is the dominant stage of most adults (Munhall 1982, p. 14). It is recognized that there is a difference in action between nurses who act at the conventional level (level II) and those who act at the postconventional or principled level (level III). As conventional thinkers, nurses base perceptions of moral obligations and rights on the maintenance of the social system and loyalty to established institutions and social groups. However, the postconventional nurse understands that societies and social relationships can be arranged in many ways, and that these different ways can maximize or minimize values (Munhall 1982, p. 13). Therefore, the nurse at level III questions authority and follows social norms as long as they support human values.

Peters

Peters combines aspects of existing theories to arrive at a concept of morality and moral behavior. He proposes a concept of rational morality based on principles. Moral development is usually considered to involve three separate components: moral emotion (what one feels), moral judgment (how one reasons), and moral behavior (how one acts). Various theorists of moral development emphasize one component above the other two. For example, Freud emphasizes the moral emotional component by focusing on the role of one's conscience or ego-strength and feelings such as guilt or self-respect. Piaget and Kohlberg emphasize the moral judgment or reasoning component. They see moral behavior as resulting form either the feelings or reasoning components, or both. Peters (1981, p. 83) states that much of moral philosophy in the past has not addressed *what* is morally important.

Facets of Moral Life

Peters (1981, p. 69) says that morality and moral development are complex phenomena and that at least five facets of moral life must be distinguished:

1. Under the concepts of *good, worthwhile,* and *desirable* fall those activities that are thought to be so important that time must be spent on initiating children into them. Examples are poetry, science, engineering, and a variety of games and pastimes. Most of these activities are intimately connected with possible vocations and ideals of life.
2. Under the concepts of *obligation* and *duty* fall ways of behaving connected with social roles. For example, much of a person's moral life is taken up with his or her station and its duties, for instance, with what is required of that person as a parent, spouse, and citizen.
3. There are those duties, more prominent in an open society, that are not specifically connected with social roles but that relate to the following of general *rules governing conduct* between members of society, e.g., unselfishness, honesty, and fairness. These are personalized as character traits.
4. There are equally wide-ranging goals of life that are personalized in the form of *motives* or *traits of character* thought of as *virtues,* such as honesty, fairness, gratitude, and benevolence, and *vices,* such as meanness, selfishness, greed, and lust. These motives or purposes are not confined to a particular activity or role.
5. Finally, there are those very general traits of character that relate to the *manner in which a person follows rules or pursues purposes,* e.g., integrity, persistence, determination, conscientiousness, and consistency. These are all connected with what people call "the will."

Peters says the reason for spelling out this complexity of moral life is to rid persons of simple-minded views of morality, e.g., morality is just good interpersonal relationships or simply observing rules about stealing, sex,

Table 22–10 Kohlberg's Stages of Moral Development

Level and Stage	Definition	Example
Level I Preconventional		
Stage 1: Punishment and obedience orientation	The activity is wrong if one is punished, and the activity is right if one is not punished.	A nurse follows a physician's order so as not to be fired.
Stage 2: Instrumental-relativist orientation	Action is taken to satisfy one's needs.	A client in hospital agrees to stay in bed if the nurse will buy him a newspaper.
Level II Conventional		
Stage 3: Interpersonal concordance (good boy, nice girl)	Action is taken to please another and gain approval.	A nurse gives elderly clients in hospital sedatives at bedtime because the night nurse wants all clients to sleep at night.
Stage 4: Law and order orientation	Right behavior is obeying the law and following the rules.	A nurse does not permit a worried client to phone home because hospital rules stipulate no phone calls after 9:00 P.M.
Level III Postconventional		
Stage 5: Social contract, legalistic orientation	Standard of behavior is based on adhering to laws that protect the welfare and rights of others. Personal values and opinions are recognized, and violating the rights of others is avoided.	A nurse arranges for an East Indian client to have privacy for prayer each evening.
Stage 6: Universal-ethical principles	Universal moral principles are internalized. Person respects other humans and believes that relationships are based on mutual trust.	A nurse becomes an advocate for a hospitalized client by reporting to the nursing supervisor a conversation in which a physician threatened to withhold assistance unless the client agreed to surgery.

Source: Adapted from *Moral development: A guide to Piaget and Kohlberg* by Ronald Duska and Mariaellen Whelan. Copyright © 1975 by The Missionary Society of St. Paul the Apostle in the State of New York. Used by permission of Paulist Press.

and the like. He believes that getting someone committed to a worthwhile activity is no less a part of morality than is the curbing of selfishness (Peters 1981, p. 70).

Concept of Character

The terms *character* and *character traits,* when applied to humans, denote what is distinctive about people. They usually indicate a manner or style of behaving. The term *character* is commonly used in three ways:

1. *Noncommittal use.* In this use, *character* refers to the sum of a person's character traits. The person has adopted a set of rules that regulate his or her conduct in relation to others and to the pursuit of more personal ends. For example, a person is spoken of exhibiting an amoral, conforming, or altruistic character.
2. *Types of character.* In the second use of *character,* the term means a distinctive style or pattern of traits or some dominant trait. For example, a person's style of life may demonstrate some central trait, such as being careful with money, prudent, honest, or truthful.
3. *Having character.* The third use is illustrated in the sentence "He has character." This statement not only says a great deal about the person but also extols him; it denotes respect and admiration. It means that the person has integrity and strength of character. The speaker attributes no specific traits to the person but rather suggests that the person exhibits control and consistency in manner, is not easily corrupted, does not give way to inclinations, and has developed a distinctive style of rules.

To Peters, the ideal character is an autonomous person who follows rules in a rational and discriminating manner based on the principles of impartiality, consideration of interests, freedom, and respect for others.

Hierarchy of Virtues

Peters's formulations contrast with Kohlberg's, who maintains that character traits such as honesty are comparatively unimportant in morals and that processes of habit formation by which traits are assumed to be established are of secondary importance. Peters, however, believes that the development of character traits or virtues is an essential aspect of moral development. He believes that virtues or character traits can be learned from others and encouraged by the example of others. For example, Peters states that a child develops concern for others much earlier than a sense of justice or honesty; further, concern for others does not require the same level of conceptual development as justice and honesty do. In the early stages of their lives, children cannot grasp the principle of justice.

In addition, Peters believes that some virtues can be described as habits because they are in some sense automatic and therefore are performed habitually. Examples are punctuality, politeness, and honesty (Peters 1981, p. 93). Peters believes that habits need to be established in moral life. A **habit** is a behavior that a person can perform without deliberation or concentration: "Life would be exhausting if, in moral situations, people always had to reflect, deliberate, and make decisions. It would be difficult for people to conduct their social lives if they could not rely on a fair stock of habits such as politeness and punctuality, for example (Peters 1981, p. 98). Kohlberg, by contrast, stresses that the most important features of moral education are cognitive.

Peters categorizes virtues in a hierarchy progressing from type A virtues, which are associated with certain actions and do not require built-in reasons for acting, through type D virtues, which involve self-control. See Table 22–11.

Schulman and Mekler

Schulman and Mekler believe that morality is a measure of how people treat fellow humans and that a moral child is one who strives to be kind and just. Both terms refer to how a person's behavior affects other people. They believe that morality has two components (Schulman and Mekler 1985, p. 6):

1. The intention of the person acting must be good in the sense that the goal of the act is the well-being of one or more people.
2. The person acting must be fair or just in the sense that he or she considers the rights of others without prejudice or favoritism. A person's acts may be moral,

Table 22–11 Peters Hierarchy of Virtues

Type and Examples	Description	Development
Type A virtues Politeness Punctuality Tidiness Thrift Chastity Honesty	These highly specific virtues represent internalized social rules. The virtues are associated with certain acts, are not associated with any innate motivations to act in a certain way, are characterized by automaticity, and can be called habits.	Provide models of expected behavior. Teach children social rules and related concepts. For example, teach the child such associated concepts as property, ownership, lending, borrowing, giving, truth, falsehood, stealing, lying, and cheating. Reinforce appropriate behavior. Draw attention to consequences of wrong action to help children learn the reasons for some rules of behavior.
Type B virtues Compassion Concern for others Caring	Essential to these virtues is affect, i.e., feelings. These feelings are motives for action, and the B virtues cannot be classed as habits. The mind is actively involved in exercising these virtues.	Cultivate appropriate forms of sensitivity. To sensitize children to the suffering of others, expose them a bit to the sight of suffering in others. Encourage concern for interests of others as well as own interests.
Type C virtues Justice Tolerance	These are more artificial virtues that involve more abstract considerations about rights and institutions. Type C virtues cannot be regarded as habits because considerations have to be weighed and assessed.	Teach the child principles of team spirit and fair play. Help the child to adopt a critical attitude toward established rules and standards. Help the child to look at rules and practices from other people's point of view.
Type D virtues Courage Integrity Perseverance Consistency	These virtues of a higher order have to be exercised in the face of counterinclinations and involve development of self-control. Some, e.g., courage, require active attention. Others, e.g., consistency, may become habitual.	Expose children to situations in which they learn to control themselves. For example, do not shield the child from social dangers, such as ridicule, disapproval, or ostracism, and praise the child if he or she maintains self-control. Help the child to cope with typical patterns of response on the part of others, e.g., flattery, bribes, and other social pressures.

Source: R. S. Peters, *Moral development and moral education* (London: Allen and Unwin, Publishers, 1981), pp. 92–110. Used by permission.

immoral, or amoral. An act is considered immoral if through it a person seeks to harm others or gain an unfair advantage over them. An amoral act is not performed specifically to benefit or harm others. Intention is crucial when judging the morality of an act. An act is judged to be well-intentioned when the person performs the act without being threatened or coerced and when the primary reward is the well-being of another. Schulman and Mekler (1985, p. 7) believe that "experiencing gain at someone else's gain is the essence of moral motivation. . . . Without doubt, any normal child has the capacity to find pleasure in the pleasure of others. . . . Caring appears to be as natural to man as aggression."

Schulman and Mekler's (1985, pp. 5–9) theory of moral development is based on three foundations, which they believe can be taught:

1. *Internalizing parental standards of right and wrong.* Children internalize parental standards, such as "Share your toys," "Don't hit," and "Consider other people's feelings." Internalization is more than obeying rules to avoid punishment. It is the learning of standards rather than just rules (Schulman and Mekler 1985, p. 21). The child must "define certain actions as *right* or *wrong* based on the parent's rules and learn to apply to him or herself the same words he or she has heard from the parents on how to behave properly" (Schulman and Mekler 1985, p. 8). The child begins to judge his or her own behavior. Internalization is the first stage of self-control over selfish and aggressive impulses and the first step toward an adult conscience. It is accomplished when the child hears the "inner voice" speaking *before* he or she acts.

   Internalization depends on:
   a. How clearly and consistently the parents state the rules. Rules must be clear and consistent.
   b. What the parents say and do when the child fails to follow the rules. Scolding must be timely and appropriate and followed by guidance for better ways to satisfy needs.
   c. Whether the parents treat the child in ways that foster feelings of love for them. Discipline is more readily accepted from a loving parent.

   Children who are loved anticipate disappointment if rules are broken and feel shame and fear of losing love rather than fear of being caught or being punished. Thus, internalization is based primarily on love for parents and the desire to please them.

2. *Developing empathic reactions.* Children need to learn to react with empathy to someone else's feelings, e.g., feeling good about another person's joy and feeling bad about another person's unhappiness. Schulman and Mekler say that empathy appears to be an inborn capacity and is surprisingly common in children. However, the capacity for empathy varies from person to person. Through empathy, children learn that harming others is bad and comforting them is good.

   Child psychologists have observed empathy in children well before the age of 2 years (Hoffman 1977, pp. 169–218). Schulman and Mekler (1985, p. 53) state the following:
   a. As early as the second day of life, an infant appears to be able to differentiate sad, happy, and surprised expressions on an adult's face.
   b. By 3 months of age, an infant's emotional states are affected by the mood changes of others.
   c. By 2 years of age, children are able to make a connection between people's feelings and the causes of their feelings. This knowledge enables them to act purposefully to make people feel better or worse.
   d. Between 12 and 30 months of age, children seem to be moved spontaneously by the happiness or sadness of others and often try to give comfort to those in distress.
   e. By age 4, children understand emotions sufficiently to playact the circumstances and emotional states of others accurately.
   f. As language skills develop, children are able to feel empathy for others without having to witness an experience but by being told about it.

3. *Acquiring personal standards.* The third foundation of morality is the development of personal standards that guide how a person *should* treat fellow human beings and what kind of person she or he wants to be. When an individual develops personal standards, he or she begins to evaluate parental rules and those of other authorities in relation to the new standards.

   Personal standards are not based on the approval of others. Reliance on them depends on the person's confidence in his or her ability to reason about the long-term consequences of actions. The consequences that keep a person striving to treat others kindly and justly are based on one's personal judgments about whether actions will bring a better world into being. In developing personal moral standards, the child first discerns whether the moral standards acquired from other people, starting with parents, work or not. This process occurs as the child expands relationships and experiences with others. If the moral standards learned earlier seem to bring about a better way of life, the child adopts personal standards learned from others. If the standards do not work, the child formulates new principles and standards.

Gilligan

Carol Gilligan (1982), after more than 10 years research with women subjects, found that women often considered Kohlberg's dilemmas irrelevant. They scored consistently lower on his scale of moral development, in spite of the fact they approached moral dilemmas with considerable sophistication. Gilligan believed that most frameworks do not include the concept of morality in caring and responsibility. Yet it is from these frameworks that most research in moral development is done. The result is that male emphasis upon individualism and autonomy is central to moral development theories.

Gilligan believes women see morality in the integrity of relationships and caring, so that the moral problems they encounter are different from those of men. Men consider what is right to be what is just, whereas for women what is right is taking responsibility for others as a self-chosen decision (Gilligan 1982, p. 140).

Gilligan and Murphy, in their studies of post-college adults, found that these adults began to doubt whether it is possible to construct generalized rules about right and wrong. They found these people evolving a rather new way of thinking in which change and process are primary features of reality. They see contradictions as acceptable, and not needing resolution at all costs (Kegan 1982, p. 229).

Spiritual Development

James Fowler describes the development of faith in people. Fowler believes that faith, or the spiritual dimension, is a force that gives meaning to a person's life. Fowler uses the term *faith* as a form of knowing, a way of being in relation to "an ultimate environment" (Fowler and Keen 1978). To Fowler, **faith** is a relational phenomenon; it is "an active 'made-of-being-in-relation' to another or others in which we invest commitment, belief, love, risk and hope" (Fowler and Keen 1978). Fowler's stages in the development of faith are given in Table 22–12.

Fowler's theory and developmental stages were influenced by the work of Piaget, Kohlberg, and Erikson. Fowler believes that the development of faith is an interactive process between the person and the environment. In each of Fowler's stages, new patterns of thought, values, and beliefs are added to those already held by the individual; therefore the stages must follow in sequence. Faith stages, according to Fowler, are separate from cognitive stages of Piaget. Faith stages evolve from a combination of knowledge and values.

Implications for Nursing Practice

The use of a developmental approach in nursing practice has the following advantages. Such an approach:

1. Helps the nurse and the client plan meaningful nursing interventions. For example, a toddler may prefer to play with toy cars and trucks for diversion, whereas an adolescent may prefer a visit from a peer.
2. Helps provide a framework for the organization of data. No single developmental theory encompasses all nursing practice. However, such an approach does provide a framework for assessing, diagnosing, planning, intervening, and evaluating in relation to developmental stage.
3. Provides guidelines by which nurses can influence

Table 22–12 **Fowler's Stages of Spiritual Development**

Stage	Age	Description
0. Undifferentiated	0 to 3 years	Infant unable to formulate concepts about self or the environment.
1. Intuitive-projective	4 to 6 years	A combination of images and beliefs given by trusted others, mixed with the child's own experience and imagination
2. Mythic-literal	7 to 12 years	Private world of fantasy and wonder; symbols refer to something specific; dramatic stories and myths used to communicate spiritual meanings.
3. Synthetic-conventional	Adolescent or adult	World and ultimate environment structured by the expectations and judgments of others; interpersonal focus.
4. Individuating-reflective	After 18 years	Constructing one's own explicit system; high degree of self-consciousness.
5. Paradoxical-consolidative	After 30 years	Awareness of truth from a variety of viewpoints.
6. Universalizing	Maybe never	Becoming an incarnation of the principles of love and justice.

Source: Adapted from J. Fowler and S. Keen, *Life maps: Conversations in the journey of faith* (Waco, Texas: Word Books, 1978); and A. Hollander, *How to help your child have a spiritual life: A parents' guide to inner development* (New York: A and W Publishers, 1980). Used by permission.

development positively. Nurses can encourage client behaviors that are appropriate to developmental stage. For example, an 18-year-old male can be encouraged to discuss his illness rationally and discouraged from displaying temper tantrums as a means of coping.

4. Helps nurses and clients plan and prepare for anticipated psychosocial and physiologic changes.
5. Assists clients to identify delays or accelerations in growth and development.
6. Helps nurses and clients identify strengths and limitations relative to growth and development.

Chapter Highlights

- Growth and development are independent, interrelated processes.
- Growth is physical change and increase in size. The pattern of physiologic growth is similar for all people.
- Development is an increase in the complexity of function and skill progression.
- Maturation refers to the sequence of physical changes that is primarily related to genetic influences.
- The rate of a person's growth and development is highly individual, but the sequence of growth and development is predictable.
- Heredity and enviroment are the primary factors influencing growth and development.
- Components of growth and development are generally categorized as physiologic, psychosocial, cognitive, moral, and spiritual.
- There are several theories about the various stages and aspects of growth and development, particularly in regard to infant and child development. Theories and models about adult development are more recent.
- Each developmental stage has its own characteristics and unique problems.
- A progression of sequential steps or tasks is proposed in most theories, so that successful achievement of tasks is required in early stages before success can be achieved with later tasks.
- The nurse's major role in relation to growth and development is to assess the client's growth and development using the standards proposed in these theories, and to plan and implement nursing strategies that will maintain or promote the client's development.

Suggested Readings

Erikson, E. H. 1985. *The life cycle completed: A review.* New York: W. W. Norton and Co.

This small book by Erikson describes the relationship of psychoanalytic (Freudian) theory to psychosocial (Eriksonian) theory. Erikson's premise in this book is that all stages are interwoven. In Chapter 3, Erikson discusses the major stages of psychosocial development. The human attributes of hope, will, purpose, competence, fidelity, love, care, and wisdom that emerge from the life stages are explained.

Schulman, M., and Mekler, E. 1985. *Bringing up a moral child: A new approach for teaching your child to be kind, just, and responsible.* Reading, Mass.: Addison-Wesley Publishing Co.

This book written for parents provides practical suggestions for teaching morality to children. It includes what to teach, how to teach, and when to teach. The book is divided into three parts. The first part explains how children actually develop a conscience and how to teach them moral values. The second part includes forces, such as jealousy, anger, and greed, that work against leading a moral life. The third part includes common moral issues and dilemmas that children face at different ages.

Selected References

Berkowitz, M. W., and Oser, F., editors. 1985. *Moral education: Theory and application.* Hillsdale, N.J.: Lawrence Erlbaum.

Betz, C. L. March/April 1981. Faith development in children. *Pediatric Nursing* 7:22–25.

Bloom, M. 1985. *Life span development: Basis for preventive and interventive helping.* 2d ed. New York: Macmillan Co.

Curtin, L. L. 1978. Nursing ethics: theories and pragmatics. *Nursing Forum* 17(1):4–11.

Duska, R., and Whelan, M. 1975. *Moral development: A guide to Piaget and Kohlberg.* New York: Paulist Press.

Duvall, E. 1977. *Family development.* 5th ed. Philadelphia: Lippincott.

Ebersole, P., and Hess, P. 1985. *Toward healthy aging: Human needs and nursing response.* 2d ed. St. Louis: C. V. Mosby Co.

Engel, G. L. 1962. *Psychological development in health and disease.* Philadelphia: W. B. Saunders Co.

Erikson, E. H. 1963. *Childhood and society.* 2d ed. New York: W. W. Norton and Co.

———. 1964. *Insight and responsibility: Lectures on the ethical implications of psychoanalytic insight.* New York: W. W. Norton and Co.

———. 1985. *The life cycle completed: A review.* New York: W. W. Norton and Co.

Fowler, J., and Keen, S. 1978. *Life maps: Conversations in the journey of faith.* Waco, Texas: Word Books.

Freud, S. 1961. *The ego and the id and other works* (Vol. 19, James Strachney, translator). London: Hogarth Press and the Institute of Psychoanalysis.

Gilligan, C. 1982. *In a different voice: Psychological theory and women's development*. Cambridge, Mass.: Harvard University Press.

Gress, L. D., and Bahr, R. T. 1984. *The aging person. A holistic approach*. St. Louis: C. V. Mosby Co.

Grusec, J. E.; Kuczynski, L.; Rushton, J. P.; and Simitis, Z. M. 1978. Modeling, direct instruction, and attributions: Effects on altruism. *Developmental Psychology* 14:51–57.

Haber, J.; Leach, A. M.; Schudy, S. M.; and Sideleau, B. F. 1982. *Comprehensive psychiatric nursing*. 2d ed. New York: McGraw-Hill.

Hall, C. S., and Lindzey, G. 1970. *Theories of personality*. 2d ed. New York: John Wiley and Sons.

Havighurst, R. J. 1972. *Developmental tasks and education*. 3d ed. New York: David McKay Co.

Hersh, R. H.; Paolitto, D. P.; and Reimer, J. 1979. *Promoting moral growth from Piaget to Kohlberg*. New York: Longman.

Hoffman, M. L. 1977. Empathy, its development and prosocial implications. In C. B. Keasey, editor. *Nebraska symposium on motivation*. Vol. 25. Lincoln: University of Nebraska Press.

Hollander, A. 1980. *How to help your child have a spiritual life: A parents' guide to inner development*. New York: A. and W. Publishers.

Kegan, R. 1982. *The evolving self: Problem and process in human development*. Cambridge, Mass.: Harvard University Press.

Maier, H. W. 1965. *Three theories of child development*. New York: Harper and Row.

Miller, D. H. 1983. *Theories of developmental psychology*. San Francisco: W. H. Freeman and Co.

Mott, S. R.; Fazekas, N. F.; and James, S. R. 1985. *Nursing care of children and families*. Menlo Park, Calif.: Addison-Wesley Publishing Co.

Munhall, P. L. June 1982. Moral development: A prerequisite. *Journal of Nursing Education* 21:11–15.

Peck, R. 1968. Psychological developments in the second half of life. In Neugarten, B. L. *Middle age and aging*. Chicago: University of Chicago Press.

Peters, R. S. 1981. *Moral development and moral behavior*. London: George Allen and Unwin, Publishers.

Piaget, J. 1963. *Origins of intelligence in children*. New York: W. W. Norton and Co.

Schulman, M., and Mekler, E. 1985. *Bringing up a moral child: A new approach for teaching your child to be kind, just, and responsible*. Reading, Mass.: Addison-Wesley Publishing Co.

Schuster, C. S., and Ashburn, S. S. 1980. *The process of human development: A holistic approach*. Boston: Little, Brown and Co.

Teung, A. G. 1982. *Growth and development: A self-mastery approach*. Norwalk, Conn.: Appleton-Century-Crofts.

Thompson, H. O., and Thompson, J. B. November 1984. Ethic learning to practice ethically synonymous with being a professional. *AORN Journal*. 40:778, 80, 82.

Watson, J. 1979. *Nursing: The philosophy and science of caring*. Boston: Little, Brown and Co.

Weston, D., and Turiel, E. 1980. Act-rule relations: Childrens concepts of social rules. *Developmental Psychology* 16:417–24.

White, R. 1975. *Lives in progress: A study of the natural growth of personality*. 3d ed. New York: Holt, Rinehart and Winston.

Wilson, J. 1973. *The assessment of morality*. Windsor, Berkshire, Great Britain: NFER Publishing Co.

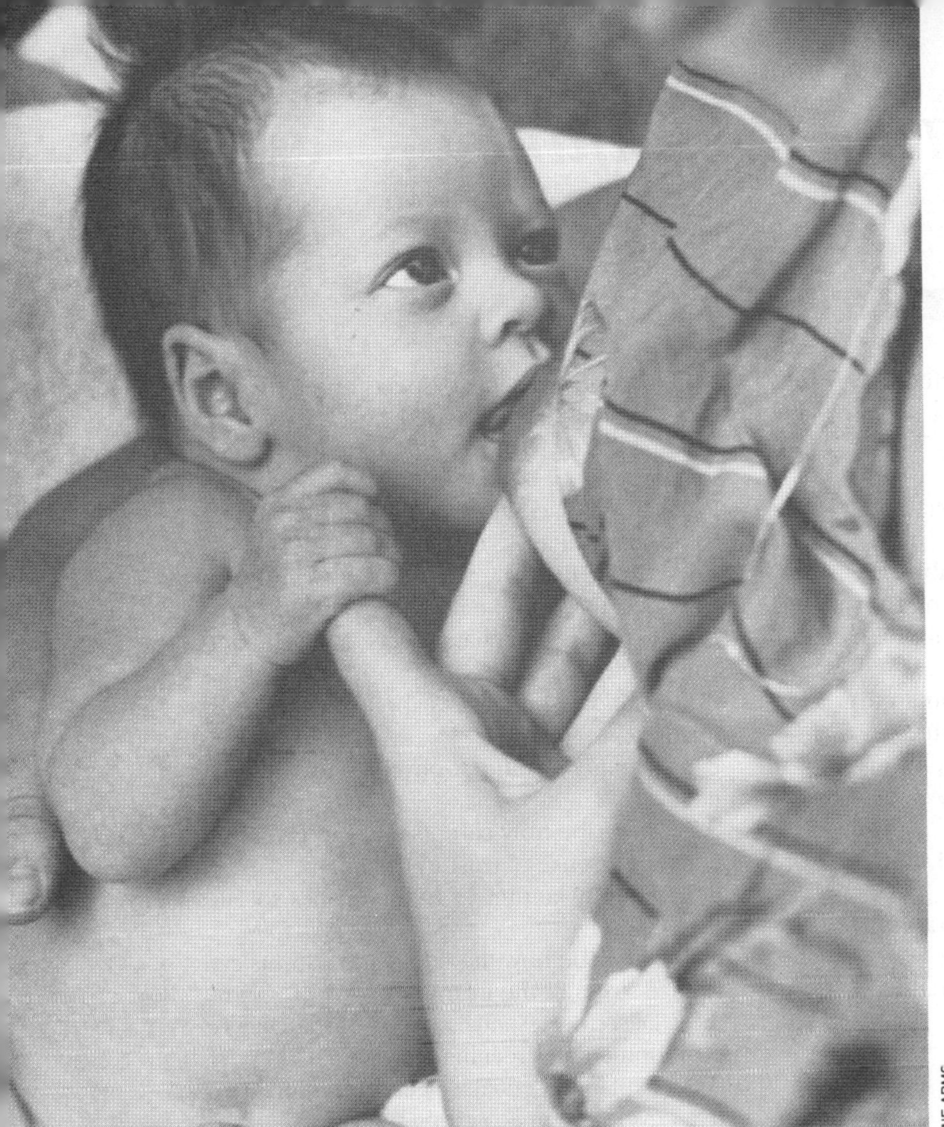

CHAPTER 23

Conception Through Infancy

Contents

23 *Conception Through Infancy*

Objectives

1. Understand essential facts about intrauterine development.
   1.1 Define selected terms.
   1.2 Explain the process of conception.
   1.3 Describe the functions of the placenta and amniotic fluid.
   1.4 Describe essential aspects of the embryonic phase of the intrauterine stage of development.
   1.5 Describe essential aspects of the fetal phase of the intrauterine stage of development.
   1.6 Identify changes in the pregnant woman that help to satisfy the oxygen needs of the fetus.
   1.7 Describe how the nutritional, fluid, elimination, temperature maintenance, and safety needs of the fetus are met.
   1.8 Identify risk factors that threaten the status of the developing fetus.
2. Understand essential facts about neonates and their needs
   2.1 Describe the appearance of the neonate.
   2.2 Explain physiologic jaundice and its treatment.
   2.3 Describe the Apgar scoring system used to assess the neonate's physical status.
   2.4 Identify the normal vital signs, weight, length, and head and chest circumference of the newborn.
   2.5 Identify the average rates of increase in length and weight during the first 6 months.
   2.6 Identify normal times for closure of two prominent skull fontanelles.
   2.7 Identify factors that cause asymmetry of the scalp in the newborn.
   2.8 Describe the neonate's sensory perceptions.
   2.9 Describe ten reflexes normally present at birth.
   2.10 Describe motor abilities of the neonate.
   2.11 Identify essential aspects of the neonate's psychosocial development.
   2.12 Identify ways to begin moral development in the infant.
   2.13 Identify essential aspects of meeting the neonate's physical and safety needs.
   2.14 Describe how a sense of trust and security can be fostered in the newborn.
   2.15 Discuss essential aspects of attachment and engrossment.
3. Understand essential facts about the developing infant.
   3.1 Identify significant physiologic changes in the infant.
   3.2 Describe how parents and caregivers can enhance a sense of trust in the infant.
   3.3 Identify landmarks in the infant's social development.
   3.4 Describe how the nurse and parents can reduce stress in the infant.
   3.5 Describe essential aspects of the Denver developmental screening test.
   3.6 Explain essential aspects of the infant's cognitive development according to Piaget.
   3.7 Describe how moral development can be facilitated.
   3.8 Describe essential aspects of meeting the infant's physical needs.
   3.9 Identify specific safety and protection needs of infants.
   3.10 Discuss how to meet the stimulation needs of infants.
   3.11 Explain the significance of mothering behavior.
   3.12 Describe how to enhance the infant's self-esteem.

Terms

attachment
caput succedaneum
cephalhematoma
ductus arteriosus
ductus venosus
ectoderm
embryo
embryonic phase
endoderm (entoderm)
engrossment
fetus
fontanelle
foramen ovale
hydrocephalus
kernicterus
lanugo
macrocephaly
meconium
mesoderm
microcephaly
milia
miliaria rubra
normocephaly
nystagmus
physiologic jaundice
placenta
strabismus
suture (of skull)
trimester
vernix caseosa
zygote

Intrauterine Development

Intrauterine development lasts approximately 9 calendar months (10 lunar months) or 38 to 40 weeks, depending on the method of calculation. (A lunar month is 28 days.) If the time is calculated from the day of conception, this stage of life is 38 weeks or 9½ lunar months. If the time is calculated from the first day of the last menstrual period, its average length is 10 lunar months or 40 weeks. This time span is not precise, however. Many pregnancies terminate within 1 to 2 weeks before or after the estimated date. To determine an expected day of confinement (EDC) according to Nägele's rule, one counts back 3 calendar months from the 1st day of the last menstrual period and adds 7 days. For example, if the last menstrual period began on April 5, one counts back 3 months to January 5 and adds 7 days. The EDC is then January 12 of the next year.

For conception to take place, the ovum leaves its graafian follicle (ovulation). It is surrounded by a mucopolysaccharide fluid (zona pellucida) and is propelled along the fallopian tube by cilia of the tube. An ovum can be fertilized within 24 to 48 hours after ovulation. During ovulation, the viscosity of the cervical mucus is reduced. Reduced viscosity facilitates the movement of the spermatozoa.

The normal ejaculate of semen contains several million spermatozoa. These spermatozoa are ejaculated at the cervix or move by flagella to the cervix of the uterus within 90 seconds. The spermatozoa cluster around the ovum, and hyaluronidase is released, which dissolves the corona radiata, a sphere of follicle cells surrounding the zona pellucida. One sperm penetrates the cell membrane of the ovum, resulting in conception.

Important in intrauterine development is the formation of the placenta, which normally starts at about the third week. Amniotic fluid surrounds the fetus in utero. A pregnant woman usually has about 30 ml of fluid at 10 weeks and perhaps 1000 ml at 38 weeks, although this amount is variable.

The placenta functions as an endocrine gland and to transport materials between the fetus and the mother. Nutrients as well as oxygen, carbon dioxide, water, and electrolytes move through the placenta. Many drugs, including narcotics and antibiotics, pass through the placenta. Amniotic fluid has a number of functions:

1. It protects the fetus from trauma by equalizing pressures that can occur as a result of a blow to the mother.
2. It permits the fetus to move and thus allows musculoskeletal development.
3. It separates the fetus from the fetal membranes that surround the fetus.
4. It helps even growth of the fetus.
5. It helps maintain a relatively constant fetal temperature.
6. It is a source of oral fluid for the fetus.
7. It functions as a system to collect excretions.

The intrauterine stage of life can be divided into two phases, the embryonic and the fetal (Behrman and Vaughan 1983, p. 11). The **embryonic phase** is the period during which the fertilized ovum develops into an organism with most of the features of the human. This period is considered to extend for either the first 8 weeks, or the first 12 weeks or first trimester of pregnancy. Those authorities who consider the embryonic phase to be 12 weeks believe that some organs develop after 8 weeks.

This embryonic phase derives its name from the Greek word **embryo**, meaning "swell." The fetal phase extends from the first 8 or 12 weeks until birth. The Latin term **fetus** means "young one." From about 20 weeks on, the fetus is considered viable, that is, able or likely to live if born. Before 20 weeks, the fetus is considered previable or unlikely to live if born.

Traditionally, pregnancy has been divided into three periods called **trimesters**, each of which lasts about 3 months. Each trimester marks certain landmarks for developmental changes in the mother and the fetus. The phases of intrauterine life, therefore, can also be considered in trimestral terms. The embryonic phase is the first trimester, and the fetal phase includes the second and third trimesters.

Embryonic Phase

The rapidity of cell division and differentiation of the fertilized ovum (**zygote**) is remarkable. By 12 weeks, the fetus weighs 15 to 20 gm and is about 7.5 to 9.0 cm (3 to 3.5 in) long. It has a sex that can be distinguished, a heartbeat, and a definite human form. The head is very large; the limbs are small with identifiable fingers and toes. Facial features such as nose, mouth, and ears are distinct, and some ossification of the bones has started.

Within the first 3 weeks of life, tissues differentiate into three layers—the **ectoderm** (outer layer), **mesoderm** (inner layer), and **endoderm** or **entoderm** (inner layer). The ectoderm and endoderm are formed in the second week; the mesoderm forms in the third week. From these layers are formed all of the body's complex organs and systems as a series of outpouchings, inpouchings, foldings, and tubular formations. Examples follow:

1. Ectoderm: central and peripheral nervous systems; epithelium of the internal and external ear, nasal cav-

ity, sinuses, mouth, and anal canal; hair follicles; nails and tooth enamel; oral glands; sweat and sebaceous glands

2. Mesoderm: dermis; skeleton; connective tissue (cartilage, bone, and joint cavities); cardiovascular system (blood and bone marrow); genitourinary system (kidneys, ureters, gonads, and genital ducts); muscles; linings of cavities (pericardial, pleural, and peritoneal); teeth except enamel; adrenal cortex; lymphatic tissue
3. Endoderm: epithelial lining of the digestive tract (except portions arising from the ectoderm); epithelial lining of the respiratory tract (larynx, pharynx, trachea, and passages including the alveoli); epithelium of the tongue, tonsils, and auditory tubes; epithelium of the thyroid, parathyroid, and thymus; urethra and the urinary bladder except the trigone; primary tissue of the pancreas and liver; vagina (parts)

Three other events occur concurrently during the first 3 weeks:

1. The embryo is implanted.
2. Placental function starts. The **placenta** is a flat, disc-shaped organ, which is highly vascular. It normally forms in the upper segment of the endometrium of the uterus. Its functions are to exchange nutrients and gases between the fetus and the mother.
3. The fetal membranes differentiate.

Table 23–1 is a summary of this embryonic phase.

Table 23–1 Fetal Development During the First Trimester

Lunar Month	Lunar Week	Developmental Occurrences
1	4	Cells divide actively from zygote.
		The three primary layers (ectoderm, mesoderm, endoderm) form (10th to 14th day).
		Liver function begins.
		Digestive tract begins to form.
		Fetal heartbeats can be heard (7 weeks).
2	8	Heart development is complete (8 weeks).
		Length of fetus is 2.5 to 3 cm crown to rump.
		Digits are formed.
		Optic nerve is formed.
		Eyelids appear but are fused.
		External, middle, and inner ear begin to assume structural form.
		Sex glands begin to differentiate into ovaries and testes.
		Bladder and urethra separate from rectum.
		Diaphragm separates thoracic and abdominal cavities.
3	12	Bones are clearly outlined (12 weeks).
		Some swimming motions occur.
		Nails of fingers and toes begin to grow.
		Fetal circulation develops.
		Bile secretion begins.
		Liver produces red blood cells.
		Lungs acquire shape.
		Skin is pink and delicate.
		External female and male genitals are recognizable.
		Fetus weighs 45 g (12 weeks).
		Length of fetus 8 cm crown to rump.

Source: Adapted from S. B. Olds, M. L. London, and P. A. Ladewig, *Maternal-newborn nursing: A family centered approach.* 2d ed. (Menlo Park, Calif.: Addison-Wesley Publishing Co., 1984, pp. 174–76. Used by permission.

Fetal Phase

This phase of development is characterized by a period of rapid growth in the size of the fetus. Haase's rule offers a guide for estimating the approximate size of the fetus in centimeters each month of the intrauterine life. The length of the fetus during its first 5 months is determined by squaring the number of lunar months. For example, a 3-month fetus is approximately 9 (3 × 3) cm long, and a 5-month fetus is 25 (5 × 5) cm long. After the fifth month, the size of the fetus is estimated by multiplying the month by five. Thus a 7-month fetus is 35 (5 × 7) cm long, and a 9-month fetus is 45 (5 × 9) cm long.

At the end of the second trimester, or 6 lunar months, the fetus resembles a small baby. Because very little fat is present beneath the skin, the skin appears wrinkled, red, and transparent. Underlying vessels are visible. A protective covering called **vernix caseosa** begins to develop over the skin. This is a white cheeselike substance that adheres to the skin and can become ⅛ inch thick by birth. **Lanugo**, a fine downy hair, also covers the body. At about 5 months, the mother first perceives movement by the fetus, and the first fetal heartbeat may be heard. The amount of activity varies among fetuses. There is some evidence that activity may be related to the mother's emotions by the transfer of epinephrine and other hormones through the placenta. Very few fetuses born before or at the end of 6 months survive. See Table 23–2.

At the end of the third trimester (9½ lunar months) the fetus has developed to approximately 50 cm (20 in) and 3.2 to 3.4 kg (7.0 to 7.5 lb). Black, native American Indian, and Oriental newborns often have lower birth weights than Caucasians. The lanugo has disappeared, and the skin is a more normal color and appears less wrin-

Table 23–2 Fetal Development During the Second Trimester

Lunar Month	Lunar Week	Developmental Occurrences
4	16	Hard tissues of teeth and central incisors form.
		Mother can detect fetal movement.
		Intestines begin to collect meconium.
		Eyes, ears, and nose are formed.
		Kidneys are formed.
		Lanugo present on body.
		Sex determination is possible.
		Fetal heart tones may be audible (16 to 20 weeks).
		Blood formation in bone marrow begins.
		Joints develop.
5	20	Fetal antibody levels (IgG type normally) are detectable.
		Fetus actively sucks and swallows amniotic fluid.
		Vernix caseosa begins to form.
		Hair is present on head.
6	24	Brain structure resembles mature brain.
		Respiratory movement may occur.
		Eye structure complete; eyelids open.
		Fetus weighs 650 g.
		Length of fetus is 23 cm crown to rump.

Source: Adapted from S. B. Olds, M. L. London, and P. A. Ladewig, *Maternal-newborn nursing: A family-centered approach,* 2d ed. (Menlo Park, Calif.: Addison-Wesley Publishing Co., 1984), pp. 177–78.

Table 23–3 Fetal Development During the Third Trimester

Lunar Month	Lunar Week	Developmental Occurrences
7	28	Nervous system begins to regulate some body processes.
		Eyebrows and eyelashes are present.
		Testes descend into scrotal sac.
		Fetus can suck.
8	32	More reflexes are present.
		Skin is red and wrinkled.
9	36	Hair is fuzzy or woolly.
		Sebaceous glands are active.
10	40	Moderate to profuse silky hair appears.
		Lanugo present on shoulders, upper back.
		Creases cover soles.
		Fetus weighs 3200 g or more.
		Length of fetus 40 cm crown to rump.

Source: Adapted from S. B. Olds, M. L. London, and P. A. Ladewig, *Maternal-newborn nursing: A family-centered approach,* 2d ed. (Menlo Park, Calif.: Addison-Wesley Publishing Co., 1984), p. 178.

kled. More subcutaneous fat makes the baby look more rotund; the last 2 months in utero are largely devoted to accumulating weight. The fetus born in the last trimester prior to full term has varying chances for survival. Those born at 7 months weigh about 1.1 kg (2.5 lb) and have approximately a 10% chance of survival; at 8 months the fetus weighs about 1.8 kg (4 lb) and has a 75% chance. See Table 23–3.

Health Promotion and Protection

During the intrauterine stage of development, the embryo or fetus relies on the maternal blood flow through the placenta to meet its basic survival needs. The health of the mother is essential for proper growth and development.

Needs

Oxygen To meet the fetal demands for oxygen, the pregnant mother gradually increases her normal blood flow by about one-third, peaking at about 8 months; increases her respiratory rate by about 40%; and increases her cardiac output significantly. Initially, the heart of the embryo lies outside its body but is repositioned in the chest early in the second trimester. Fetal circulation travels from the placenta through one umbilical vein, which carries oxygenated blood to the fetus, and back to the placenta through two umbilical arteries, which carry blood depleted of oxygen away from the fetus. By 20 weeks, the fetal heartbeat is audible through a fetoscope; the heartbeat is audible as early as the tenth week if a Doppler stethoscope with ultrasound is used. These special stethoscopes are described in Chapter 34. Fetal circulation bypasses the fetal lung.

Nutrition and fluids The fetus obtains nourishment from the placental circulation and by swallowing amniotic fluid. Nutritional needs are met when the mother eats a well-balanced diet containing sufficient calories to meet both her needs and those of the fetus.

Rest and activity The fetus sleeps most of the time but does develop a pattern of sleep and wakefulness that can persist after birth. Fetal activity begins about the fourth lunar month of pregnancy.

Elimination Fetal feces are formed from swallowed amniotic fluid throughout pregnancy, but normally no stool is passed until after birth. Inadequate oxygenation of the fetus during the third trimester can result in relaxation of the anal sphincter and passage of feces into the amniotic fluid. Urine normally is excreted into the amniotic fluid when the kidneys mature (16 to 20 weeks).

Temperature maintenance Although amniotic fluid provides a constant temperature for the fetus, significant changes in maternal temperature can alter the temperature of the amniotic fluid and the fetus. Significant temperature rises due to illness, hot whirlpool baths, or saunas can result in birth defects.

Safety A safe environment for the fetus depends on a mother who is free of illness and who ingests no alcohol, addicting drugs, or other medications. See the section on risk factors, next, for further information. Approximate prenatal education and medical care are essential throughout pregnancy.

Risk Factors

Risk factors that threaten the pregnancy must be identified early so that appropriate interventions can be initiated promptly. Risk factors and nursing interventions are shown in Table 23–4.

Neonates (Birth to 28 Days)

The chief task of neonates is to adapt to their new environment. The first step in this process is breathing, an accomplishment that must occur within 30 seconds of birth if asphyxia is to be avoided. Neonates are completely dependent on others; they have no voluntary control over their movements, and their only emotion is a state of excitement. Their lives are dominated chiefly by reflexes.

Physiologic Development

Appearance

A newborn baby (Figure 23–1) usually has puffy eyelids and a flat, broad nose. The lower jaw appears small and the neck very short. The shoulders slope, and the abdomen appears large and rounded with a protruding umbilical stump. The legs are bowed and appear short and out of proportion to the head, which makes up 21% of the total body surface. The arms appear long in proportion to the rest of the body. Lanugo may be apparent, particularly on the shoulders, back, and extremities. The vernix caseosa is obvious in the skin folds but will rub off naturally after a few days.

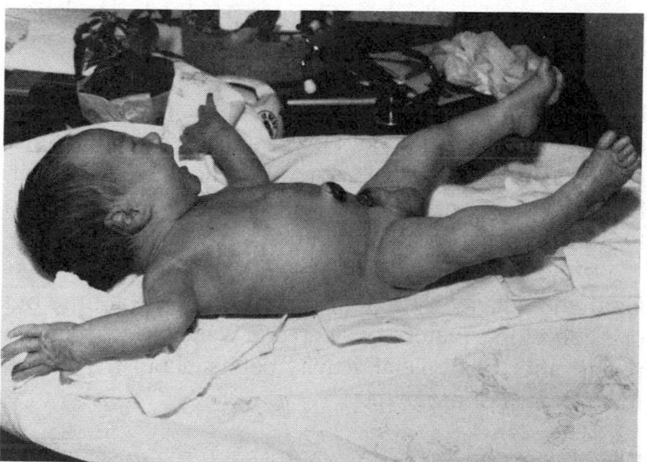

Figure 23–1 A newborn infant showing the short bowed legs, protruding abdomen, and the drying umbilical stump. (Courtesy of the City of Vancouver Health Department.)

The skin of newborns is thin and appears delicate and often pink or reddish in Caucasians. They may have **milia**, which are small white spots on the nose and forehead. These are collections of sebaceous secretions, which usually disappear about 3 weeks after birth. Black, Oriental, and dark-skinned babies usually have bluish brown areas on their lower back called Mongolian spots. These fade without treatment.

Physiologic jaundice of the newborn generally occurs between 3 and 4 days after birth because of excess red blood cells in the baby's blood, which are left over from fetal life and result in elevated bilirubin levels in the blood. This jaundice normally disappears by 2 weeks. Jaundice that occurs within 24 hours of birth, however, must be monitored carefully because it may be caused by an incompatibility between the baby's blood and the mother's blood.

Physiologic jaundice is often treated with phototherapy, which reduces blood bilirubin levels. Excessive bilirubin levels may result in **kernicterus**, a condition in which bilirubin is deposited in brain cells. Kernicterus can lead to varying degrees of mental retardation. Phototherapy involves the use of fluorescent lights, predominantly in the blue spectrum. These lights break down the bilirubin into a form that can be excreted through the intestines. During phototherapy, the neonate's skin is exposed to the lights for about 24 hours. The eyes are covered to protect them from light damage. Physiologic jaundice is a temporary problem due to the newborn's immature liver function.

Newborn babies can be assessed by the Apgar scoring system, which provides a numeric indicator of physical status, that is, of the baby's capacities to adapt to

Table 23–4 Selected Risk Factors During Pregnancy

Risk Factor	Nursing Interventions
Nausea and vomiting that continue beyond the first trimester, predisposing the mother to malnutrition	• Determine severity of symptoms. • Assess emotional stressors. • Notify the physician. • Help client reduce vomiting and maintain adequate food and fluid intake. • Help client reduce stress as needed.
Severe anxiety about pregnancy or labor, predisposing the mother to increased psychologic stress and the fetus to a possible preterm delivery	• Determine reason if possible, e.g., lack of knowledge, misinformation, fear of accepting maternal role. • Provide necessary information and referrals to prenatal classes. • Assist client to develop productive coping strategies. • Encourage client to express feelings.
History of habitual or attempted abortion and stillborn birth before this pregnancy, increasing the risk of another abortion or preterm delivery (stillbirth)	• Encourage client to express feelings about previous and current pregnancy. • Provide information and other support needed to maintain pregnancy. • Inform the physician. • Maintain nonjudgmental attitude about previous abortion attempts.
History of diabetes mellitus, hypertension, renal disease, malnutrition (especially low-protein diet), or obesity, predisposing the client to pregnancy-induced hypertension (PIH) or eclampsia	• Determine presence of these diseases. • Determine previous history of PIH and familial tendency to PIH. • Assess the client for increased blood pressure, increased weight, edema, and protein in the urine. • Monitor client's blood pressure. • Monitor client's weight (a weight gain of 1 kg/week or more in the second trimester of 0.5 kg/week or more in the third trimester is suggestive of PIH) • Test urine for albumin. • Monitor fetal status.
Nonaccepting father, predisposing the mother to increased psychologic distress	• Explore reasons for nonacceptance, e.g., fear of paternal role, misunderstanding of mother's physical and emotional changes during pregnancy, or immaturity. • Identify specific misconceptions. • Provide information and guidance to help the father support the mother.
Excessive alcohol consumption, predisposing the mother to malnutrition and the fetus to alcohol syndrome	• Determine alcohol intake. • Assess nutritional status. • Provide guidance and refer for counseling as needed.
Use of addicting drugs, predisposing the mother to malnutrition and the fetus to congenital anomalies, low birth weight, and neonatal withdrawal	• Determine use of addicting drugs. • Assess nutritional status. • Provide guidance and refer for counseling as needed.
Heavy smoking (one pack per day or more), predisposing the mother to hypertension and cancer and the fetus to low birth weight and reduced placental nourishment	• Determine amount of smoking. • Provide guidance to help reduce smoking.
Age below 16 years, predisposing mother to poor nutrition, poor antenatal care, and increased risk of PIH and the fetus to low birth weight	• Assess the client's nutritional status. • Determine life-style behavior related to diet, exercise, and rest. • Monitor weight and energy level. • Provide information and guidance as needed.
Age above 35 years of age, predisposing the mother to PIH and the fetus to congenital anomalies and chromosomal abberations	• Explore client's feelings and concerns about pregnancy. • Provide information and guidance as needed, e.g., diagnosis of genetic disease by amniocentesis.
Rubella in first or second trimester, predisposing the fetus to congenital heart disease, cataracts, nerve deafness, and bone lesions	• Determine whether mother has immunity to rubella. • Advise client to avoid contact with those who are infected.

Table 23–5 Apgar Scoring System to Assess the Newborn

Sign	Score 0	1	2
1. Heart rate	Absent	Slow (below 100 per minute)	Above 100 per minute
2. Respirations	Absent	Slow, irregular	Regular rate, crying
3. Muscle tone	Flaccid	Some flexion of extremities	Active movements
4. Reflex irritability	None	Grimace	Cries
5. Color	Body pale or cyanotic	Body pink (for black babies, pink mucous membranes), extremities blue	Body completely pink in whites, pink mucous membranes in blacks

extrauterine life. Each of five signs is assigned a maximum score of 2, so that the total score achievable is 10. A score under 7 suggests that the baby is having difficulty, and a score under 4 indicates that the baby's condition is critical. Apgar scoring is usually carried out 60 seconds after birth and is repeated in 5 minutes. Those with very low scores require special resuscitative measures and care. See Table 23–5.

Weight

At birth, most babies weigh between 2.7 to 3.8 kg (6.0 to 8.5 lb). Black infants tend to weigh less than Caucasians. Some of this birth weight (about 10%) is lost the first few days due to fluid loss. Children can be expected to double their weights by 6 months of age and to weigh about 10 kg (22 lb) at 1 year and 13.6 kg (29 lb) at 2 years. A number of factors, such as mother's nutrition, mother's age, and heredity, can affect birth weights.

Just after birth, a baby loses weight due to fluid loss and the excretion of meconium from the intestines. This weight loss is normal, and infants usually regain weight in about 1 week. After the first week, babies usually gain weight at the rate of 5 to 7 ounces weekly for 6 months. Table 23–6 gives average measurements and average vital signs. Chapter 35 describes how infants are weighed.

Table 23–6 Average Normal Vital Signs and Measurements of Newborns

Weight	3.4 kg or 3400 g (7.5 lb)
Length	50 cm (20 in) head to heel
Head circumference	34 to 36 cm (13.5 to 14.5 in)
Pulse	70 to 190 beats per minute at rest (average 125)
Blood pressure	65 to 90 mm Hg systolic 30 to 60 mm Hg diastolic
Temperature	36.1 to 37.7 C (97 to 100 F) by axilla
Respiratory rate	30 to 60 breaths per minute (average 35)

Length

The average Caucasian newborn in the United States is about 50 cm (20 in) long. Black infants tend to be shorter than Caucasians at birth (Clark 1981, p. 81). This range is from 47.5 to 52.5 cm (19 to 21 in). Female babies are on the average smaller than male babies.

Two recumbent lengths are the crown-to-rump length (the sitting length) and the head-to-heel length (from the top of the head to the base of the heels). See Figure 23–2. Normally the crown-to-rump length is approximately the same as the head circumference. During the first 6 months, length increases about 2.5 cm (1 in) per month and 1.25 cm (0.5 in) per month during the next 6 months.

Vital Signs

Newborns have unstable vital signs. Their temperature fluctuates from 36.1 to 37.7 C (97 to 100 F) because their heat-regulating system is not fully developed. The pulse of the baby at birth ranges from 70 to 170 beats per minute at rest. Respirations are irregular, shallow, and quiet, ranging from 40 to 60 breaths per minute. Blood pressure of the newborn normally ranges from 60 to 90 mm Hg (millimeters of mercury) systolic and 30 to 60 mm Hg diastolic (see Table 23–6).

Head Growth

The skull is measured at its greatest diameter from above the eyes to the occipital protuberance. Steel, cloth, or disposable paper tapes can be used. If a cloth tape is used, it should be checked periodically against a metal standard, since cloth tends to stretch with use.

Assessment of skull circumference is of particular importance in infants and children to determine the growth rate of the skull and the brain. An infant's head should be measured at every visit to the physician or nurse until the child is 2 years. Head measurement of infants 3 years or older usually does not need to be done routinely; however, this measurement should be taken during initial examinations of young children. See Figure 23–3.

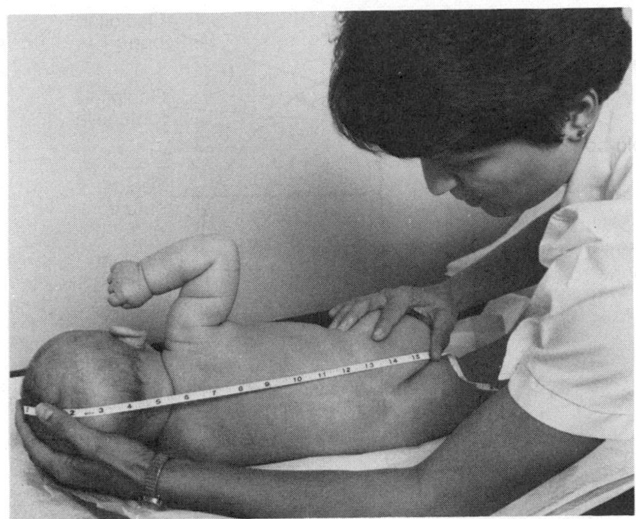

Figure 23–2 Measuring an infant, crown to rump.

Normal head circumference (**normocephaly**) are often related to chest circumferences. At birth, the average infant's head circumference is 35 cm (14 in) and generally varies only 1 or 2 cm (0.5 in). The chest circumference of the newborn is usually less than the head circumference by about 2.5 cm (1 in). As the infant grows, the chest circumference becomes larger than the head circumference. At about 9 or 10 months, the head and chest circumferences are about the same, and after 1 year of age the chest circumference is larger.

Abnormalities in head circumferences are referred to as **macrocephaly** (a large head) or **microcephaly** (a small head). The former is often the result of excessive cerebrospinal fluid within the skull (**hydrocephalus**).

Skull Shape and Fontanelles

Most newborn babies have misshapen heads due to the molding of the head that occurs during vaginal deliveries. Molding of the head is made possible by **fontanelles** (unossified membranous gaps) in the bone structure of the skull and by overriding of the **sutures** (junction lines of the skull bones). Within a week, the newborn's head usually regains its symmetry, a fact that reassures parents.

The eight bones of the cranium are separated by sutures, which gradually ossify during childhood. These bones are the frontal bone, the occipital bone, two parietal and two temporal bones, and the sphenoid and ethmoid bones. See Figure 23–4. Six fontanelles are present at birth, but the two most prominent ones are the frontal (anterior) and the occipital (posterior) ones. The latter is the smaller of the two (1 to 2 cm in diameter) and is generally closed by 4 months. The posterior fontanelle may not be palpated for a few hours after birth because of the overriding of the sutures during delivery. The larger anterior fontanelle (4 to 6 cm in diameter and diamond-shaped) can increase in size for several months after birth. After 6 months, the size gradually decreases until closure occurs between 9 and 18 months (Behrman and Vaughan 1983, p. 16).

Examination of the head of infants for symmetry of shape and for palpation of the fontanelles is best achieved while the infant is sitting comfortably in the mother's lap. Normally, in a crying, coughing, or vomiting infant, the anterior fontanelle has a certain tenseness, fullness, and bulging, indicating increased intracranial pressure. Continual bulging is abnormal and associated with tumors or infections of the brain or hydrocephalus due to obstruction of the cerebrospinal fluid circulation in the ventricles. Depression of the anterior fontanelle generally indicates dehydration.

Asymmetry of the scalp can be caused by a number of factors. Frequently, newborns have disfiguring localized swellings over a portion of the scalp at birth or shortly after birth. **Caput succedaneum** is an edematous swelling of the soft tissues of a part of the scalp that was encircled by the cervix before the latter became fully dilated. This condition commonly occurs over the occipitoparietal region (the presenting part of the fetus) and disappears spontaneously within a few days of birth. Bilateral symmetrical swellings of the scalp can also occur in difficult deliveries that require the use of forceps.

Another type of swelling of the scalp in the newborn is called **cephalhematoma**, which differs from caput succedaneum in that the swelling occurs directly over a bone or portion of it and is not visible until several hours after

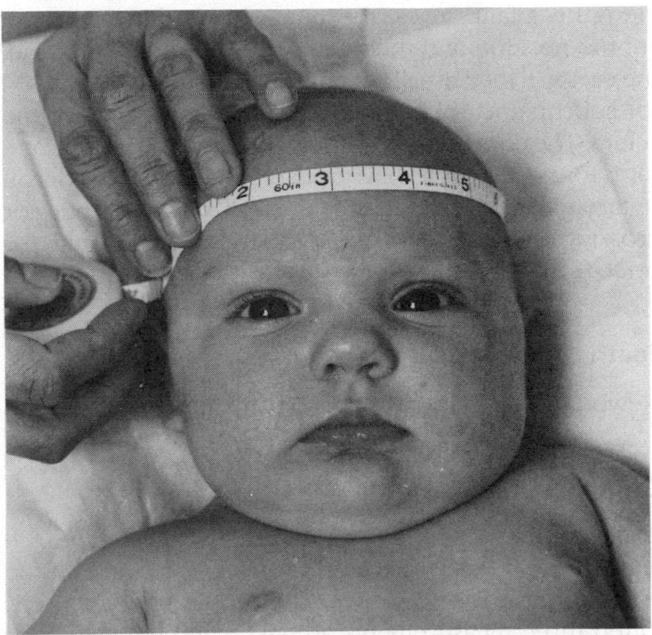

Figure 23–3 An infant's head circumference is measured around the skull, above the eyebrows.

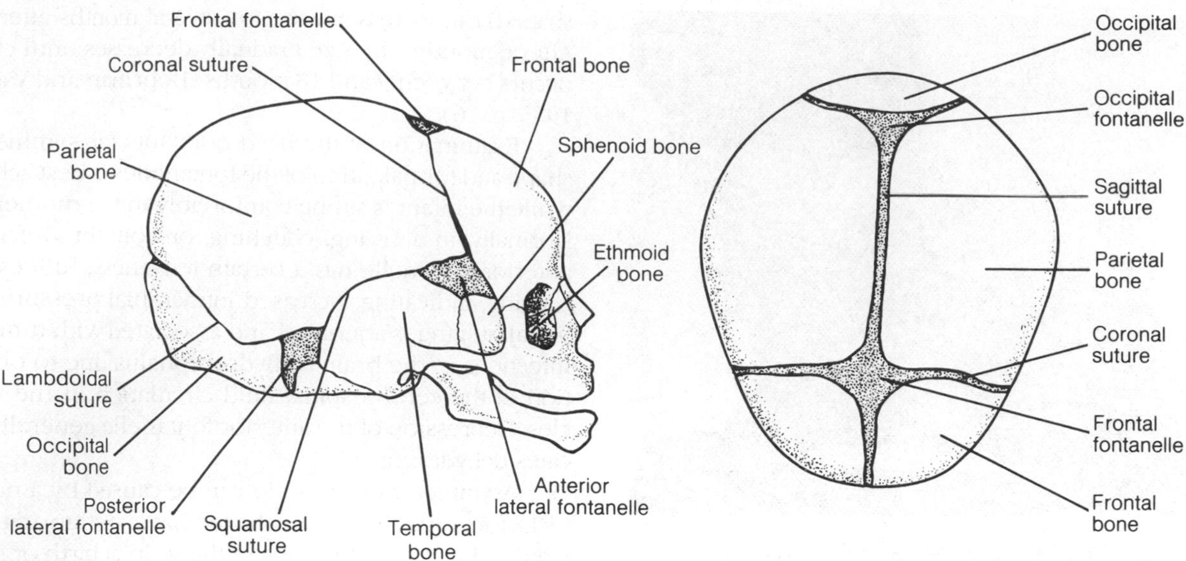

Figure 23–4 The bones of the skull showing the fontanelles and suture lines.

delivery. The cause is an effusion of blood between the periosteum and the bone (subperiosteal); it most commonly occurs over the parietal bones. This hematoma increases gradually in size for about a week and then slowly disappears. Misshaping of the head can also be caused by premature closure of the cranial sutures. Flattening of a part of the scalp frequently occurs in infants who almost always sleep in the same position.

Eyes

The eyes of the newborn are usually tightly closed. To view the infant's eyes, the nurse holds the infant in a supine position and then gently lowers the baby's head; the eyes will then usually open. The eyes should be assessed for subconjunctival hemorrhages that may appear on the sclera. The cornea is examined for clarity. It is not uncommon for newborns to have a searching **nystagmus** (involuntary movement of the eye) or **strabismus** (squinting or crossing of the eyes), which may persist intermittently for up to 4 to 6 months.

Teeth

Newborn babies are normally born without visible teeth.

Chest Circumference

The chest circumference is measured by placing the tape around the chest at the level of the lower aspect of the scapula posteriorly and over the nipple line anteriorly. Often three measurements are taken and the average is recorded. The newborn's chest circumference is normally 30.5 to 33 cm (12 to 13 in).

Senses

The newborn infant is sensitive to touch. Through touch, the newborn perceives warmth, love, and security as well as the opposite of these. The newborn is also sensitive to temperature extremes and pain; however, babies react diffusely and cannot isolate the discomfort. The pain of an open safety pin in the buttock, for example, is not isolated in the buttock.

Visual abilities are present at birth; the newborn can follow large moving objects and can react to changes in the intensity of light. The baby blinks in response to bright light and to sound.

The pupils of the newborn respond slowly, and the eyes cannot focus on close objects. Hearing is indistinct at birth because of the retention of fluid in the middle ear. The newborn does not differentiate sounds for some time but will have a startle reaction (Moro reflex) to a loud noise (see the following section on infant reflexes). The senses of smell and taste are not developed, although the newborn reacts to acid, bitter, salt, and sweet tastes by grimacing.

Reflex Ability

The reflexes of the newborn are unconscious, involuntary responses. They are neither learned nor consciously carried out. They are nervous system reflexes to a number of stimuli. The degree of stimulation that is required to produce a reflex, for example the sucking reflex, varies considerably among newborns. Some newborns respond with vigor to the slightest stimulus, while others respond more slowly.

Ten main reflexes are normally present at birth. They are rooting, sucking, swallowing, Moro, palmar grasp, plantar, tonic neck, placing, stepping, and Babinski. In addition, yawning, stretching, sneezing, burping, and hiccuping are all present at birth.

The *rooting* and *sucking reflexes* are both used in feeding. The former is elicited by touching the baby's cheek, causing the baby's head to turn to the side that was touched. The sucking reflex occurs when the baby's lips are touched. The *swallowing reflex* can be observed when the infant swallows any liquid obtained from sucking.

The *Moro reflex* (startle reflex) is often assessed to estimate the maturity of the central nervous system. A loud noise, a sudden change in position, or an abrupt jarring of the crib elicits this reflex. The infant reacts by extending both arms and legs outward with the fingers spread, then suddenly retracting the limbs. Often the infant cries at the same time.

The *palmar grasp reflex* occurs when a small object is placed against the palm of the hand, causing the fingers to curl around it. The *plantar reflex* is similar in that an object placed just beneath the toes causes them to curl around it.

The *tonic neck reflex* (TNR) or fencing reflex is a postural reflex. When a baby who is lying on his or her back turns the head to the right side, for example, the left side of the body shows a flexing of the left arm and the left leg. This reflex is observed during the first week after birth.

The *placing reflex* is seen when a baby is held vertically with legs separated. When one foot is moved to touch the edge of a table, the baby automatically flexes the knee and hip of the same leg and tries to place the foot on the surface of the table.

The *stepping reflex* (walking or dancing reflex) can be elicited by holding the baby upright so that the feet touch a flat surface. The legs then move up and down as if the baby were walking. This reflex usually disappears at about 2 months.

A newborn baby also has a positive *Babinski reflex.* When the sole of the foot is stroked, the big toe rises and the other toes fan out.

Infant reflexes disappear during the first year of life. After age 1, the infant exhibits a negative Babinski, that is, the toes curl downward; positive Babinski after age 1 indicates brain damage.

Motor Development

Motor development is the development of the baby's ability to move and to control the body. Movement begins before birth at about the third month, when the fetus is able to move arms and legs spontaneously. After birth, activity increases gradually to include sucking, breathing, swallowing, and uncoordinated body movement. At 1 month of age, the infant lifts the head momentarily when prone, turns the head when prone, has a head lag when pulled to a sitting position, holds hands in fists, and fixes the eyes on a bright object and follows it with the eyes when the object moves into the line of vision.

Psychosocial Development

Language and Speech Development

Neonates cry when they are uncomfortable, usually because they are hungry. By 1 month, they begin to make cooing sounds.

Emotional Development

In newborn babies, the capacity to react emotionally is already present. The first sign of emotion is usually that of excitement in response to a strong external stimulus, for example, a loud noise. This response becomes differentiated into a response of pleasure and one of displeasure. Pleasure can be elicited by rocking or patting, while displeasure can be elicited by an abrupt change of position. See also psychosocial development for the infant (1 month to 1 year) on page 491.

Moral Development

Newborns are amoral in that their behavior is neither guided nor influenced by moral considerations. Making the infant feel loved is crucial for moral development. Children who feel secure in their parents' love tend to give love back, develop friendships more readily, and are more inclined to like people and to be liked in return (Schulman and Mekler 1985, p. 215). Love can be communicated to the infant through smiling, caressing, and talking in pleasant tones.

Health Promotion and Protection

Health promotion and protection activities of the neonate include attention to the neonate's basic needs and parental guidance.

Needs

Oxygen Within 1 minute after birth, neonates usually establish independent respirations at the rate of 30 to 60 breaths per minute. Because neonates are nose-breathers, nasal passages must always be kept clear. Before the first breath, the nurse applies suction to the neonate's nasal passages and mouth to clear them of fluids and repeats suctioning as necessary. The first breath occurs when the respiratory center in the medulla is stimulated by a rising blood carbon dioxide level, a decreasing blood oxygen level, a decreasing (acidic) blood pH, and the sudden release in external pressure exerted by the vaginal canal on the chest.

After birth, the neonate's blood must circulate through the lungs rather than bypassing them. In fetal circulation, blood bypasses the lungs by moving through the **foramen ovale**, an opening between the right and left atrium of the heart. After birth, the foramen ovale closes. The **ductus arteriosus**, a fetal blood vessel connecting the pulmonary artery directly to the descending aorta, also closes within 1 day of birth. In fetal circulation, this duct allows blood to bypass the lungs and move directly from the pulmonary artery into the aorta. The **ductus venosus**, the vessel connecting the umbilical cord to the fetal venous blood system, also closes at birth. Failure to establish lung circulation is a serious problem for the neonate and requires prompt, specialized care.

Temperature maintenance Immediately after birth, the baby's body temperature drops, usually because the temperature of the delivery room is lower than the temperature inside the uterus. Failure to provide warmth at this time can lead to increased metabolic rate, which, if prolonged, can result in an increased consumption of glucose, subsequent hypoglycemia, and consequent brain damage. Wrapping the newborn in a warm blanket or using radiant infant warmers or incubators helps newborns establish a normal temperature. They continue to require protection from abrupt temperature changes because their temperature regulation is poorly developed. A draft-free room at a temperature of between 20.0 to 24.4 C (60 to 76 F) is considered appropriate.

New parents often need guidance about dressing infants appropriately. **Miliaria rubra** (prickly heat rash) occurs on the face, neck, trunk, and diapered areas when the infant is overly dressed.

Nutrition and fluids The neonate's fluid and nutritional needs are met by breast milk or formulas. Water or other supplements are unnecessary, although water may be prescribed for neonates who perspire excessively in very warm environments. Newborn babies may become hungry shortly after they are born, or they may not develop an appetite for 1 or 2 days. Behavior such as restlessness, crying, and moving the head can indicate hunger. The neonate requires abut 80 to 100 ml of milk or formula per kilogram of body weight per day. For added information on infant feeding, see Chapter 42. New mothers, in particular, need guidance about breast-feeding or safe methods to prepare formulas.

Elimination Newborn babies cannot control defecation and urination. **Meconium** is the first fecal material passed by the newborn, normally up to 24 hours after birth. It is black, tarry, odorless, and sticky. Transitional stools, which follow for about a week, are generally greenish-yellow; they contain mucus and are loose.

The neonate passes stool frequently, often after each feeding. Because the intestine is immature, water is not well absorbed, and so the stool is soft, liquid, and frequent. When the intestine matures, bacterial flora increase. After solid foods are introduced, the stool becomes less frequent and firmer. Breast-fed babies have orange to yellow stool that is lighter in color, less firm, and less malodorous than the stool of bottle-fed babies. In later months, before the breast-fed baby is introduced to solid food, the baby may not have a bowel movement for several days. Parents need to be informed that this is normal as long as the infant's behavior and feeding and sleeping patterns are unchanged. New parents may also need guidance in diapering if disposable diapers are not used. See Chapter 36 for diapering methods.

Urine output varies according to fluid intake but usually is about 15 to 60 ml per day after birth, increasing to 250 to 400 ml per day by 1 month of age.

Sleep Newborns can be expected to sleep from 18 to 22 hours a day and 15 to 18 hours by 1 month of age. It is normal for them to suck and move their arms during sleep. At first, they usually awaken every 3 or 4 hours, eat, and then go back to sleep. At about age 4 weeks, they may take three or four naps during the day and sleep for longer periods at night. Parents may need instruction in the proper handling and positioning of the baby. See Chapter 40.

Safety Although newborns receive some antibodies from their mothers, they have very little resistance to infection. For this reason nurses wash their hands before handling a baby and, in some settings, wear masks and sterile gloves. Persons with respiratory or skin infections normally avoid contact with a newborn baby.

To protect the infant against trauma, vitamin K is often administered into the vastus lateralis muscle. See Chapter 51 on intramuscular injections. Vitamin K, necessary for clotting, is not produced by bacteria in the intestines for several days until bacteria start to colonize the area.

The eyes are also checked for infection and trauma. It is legally required in most places to treat newborns' eyes with a germicide that destroys the gonorrhea organism, which can be present if the mother is infected. The usual germicide is a 1% solution of silver nitrate, two drops in each eye. A few minutes after the drops are inserted, the eyes are irrigated with warm distilled water. Today, penicillin is also used. It is administered as an ophthalmic ointment or intramuscularly. It is important to record the administration of the medication on the appropriate record.

During a baby's first 24 hours of life, the umbilical cord stump needs to be observed for bleeding. The cord usually heals in about 1 week by dry healing. It is customary to clean the cord daily, usually after bathing the baby, with a 60% alcohol solution to facilitate drying and a povidone-iodine (Betadine) solution to prevent infection. The stump must be observed closely for any signs of infection. Washing it with mild soap and water and thorough drying help prevent infection.

Accident prevention is essential. To prevent falls, the nurse never leaves the neonate unattended. To prevent burns, the nurse teaches parents to test the bath water temperature before putting the infant in, to avoid the handling of hot liquids near the neonate, and to protect the neonate from the sun. The parents need to acquire an approved infant car seat. Some agencies do not allow the parents to take the infant home until they obtain an appropriate seat.

Security Feelings of security and trust are fostered when the mother promptly, lovingly, and consistently attends to the newborn's physical needs. Lack of attention and inconsistent attention cause tension in the newborn and convey the sense that the environment is unpredicable and disorganized. This sense fosters fear, anger, insecurity, and mistrust. The quality of the mother's response is also important. Newborns and infants can discern whether or not the mother derives pleasure from caring for them.

Sexuality Newborn males on the average have more muscle mass and are larger at birth than females. Breast enlargement, due to the presence of maternal hormones, may be observed in newborns; the breasts decrease to normal several days following birth. Female newborns have thick vaginal secretions that decrease during the first week of life. Vaginal secretions are also related to maternal hormone levels during gestation. Male newborns may have erections, and parents need to be informed that these are normal. Routine circumcision of male newborns is not usually recommended by pediatricians today but is performed if parents desire it for religious or cultural reasons.

The sex of the newborn often influences parental relationships and expectations. A new mother may be disappointed if her baby is a girl and she knows the father wanted a son. Disappointment can delay the development of a close attachment and affect the way the child is raised. Some parents may find fault and blame the infant for not meeting expectations. Combined with other factors, this disappointment can place the infant at risk for child abuse.

Stimulation Although not fully developed, all of the senses are functioning at birth, and the infant can be stimulated in a variety of ways. Handling and environmental stimulation are required for optimal development. The baby can perceive color, shape, and motion, and hanging toys placed above the crib can stimulate the baby's senses. However, newborns spend a great deal of time looking at the human face and respond positively to soothing tones of voice. Touching, stroking, and rocking are also soothing to newborns.

Love and belonging The establishment of an emotional bond between the mother and her newborn is called **attachment.** Attachment is crucial for optimum physical and emotional development of the neonate and infant; it is the basis for the interdependence needed for development. Maternal behaviors indicating attachment include:

1. Touching proceeding from fingertip exploration of the baby's extremities to enfolding the baby in the hands and arms
2. Direct face-to-face and eye-to-eye contact
3. Rubbing the cheek with the fingertip
4. Responding verbally to the baby's cries, coughs, and sneezes
5. Verbally expressing the connectedness between the baby and the rest of the family, e.g., "He's got your strong chin, Daddy."
6. Responding early to the newborn's needs
7. Smiling and providing soothing and comforting behaviors

Because attachment is a reciprocal interaction, the newborn also perceives and communicates. The baby lies quietly with eyes open, looks about, moves limbs occasionally, makes sucking motions, and attempts to put a hand in the mouth. When placed close to the mother, the baby focuses briefly on the mother's face, attends to her voice, and often moves in reaction to changes in the mother's voice.

Attachment by the mother is influenced by many factors. Some of these are the kind of mothering the mother received as an infant, the concept of motherhood she has developed, her overall self-concept as a person, her relationship with the father, her knowledge about children and childrearing, her capacity for enjoying herself, and her expectations of the newborn.

The process of bonding is also necessary for fathers. This process, called **engrossment**, has these major characteristics (Greenberg and Morris 1974, p. 520):

1. Visual awareness of the newborn
2. Desire to hold the newborn
3. Perception of the newborn's distinct features, especially those that resemble the father's
4. Perception of the baby as perfect
5. Attraction that results in intense focusing of attention
6. Elation
7. Deep satisfaction and self-esteem.

Engrossment is often enhanced by the father's witnessing of the birth.

Infants (1 Month to 1 Year)

An infant's basic task is survival, which requires breathing, sleeping, sucking, eating, swallowing, digesting, and eliminating. This stage in development is called the oral stage because many of the infant's activities and pleasures are mouth-centered. See Table 22–4 on page 465.

Physiologic Growth and Development

Duvall outlines a number of developmental tasks for infants of this age (see below). Nurses can assist parents to help the infant accomplish these developmental tasks by:

1. Discussing the importance of environmental stimulation. Lourie believes that external stimulation appears to influence internal, anatomic, and maturation processes by:
   a. Influencing the progressive formation of the dendrites of the nervous system.
   b. Increasing the formation of blood vessels of specific structures in the brain, e.g., the centers associated with vision.
   c. Increasing myelinization. Myelinization is closely related to the development of some body functions. The myelin sheath coats the nerves and brain (Lourie 1981, p. 7).
2. Explaining the various stimuli, e.g., auditory, visual, and tactile, suitable for an infant.

Developmental Tasks of Infancy

- Establishing oneself as a very dependent being
- Beginning the establishment of self-awareness
- Developing a feeling for affection
- Becoming aware of the alive as against the inanimate, and the familiar as against the unfamiliar
- Developing rudimentary social interaction
- Beginning to adjust to the expectations of others
- Adjusting to adult feeding demands
- Adjusting to adult cleanliness demands
- Adjusting to adult attitudes toward genital manipulation
- Developing physiologic equilibrium
- Developing eye-hand coordination
- Establishing satisfactory rhythms of rest and activity
- Exploring the physical world
- Developing preverbal communication
- Developing verbal communication
- Forming rudimentary concepts

From Table 8–4 in *Marriage and Family Development*, Fifth Edition by Evelyn Millis Duvall (J. B. Lippincott).

Infants undergo significant physiologic change in these areas:

Weight

Infants are twice their birth weight by 6 months and three times their birth weight by 12 months.

Height

By 6 months, they gain another 13.75 cm (5.5 in). By 12 months, they add another 7.5 cm (3 in). Rate of increase is largely influenced by the baby's size at birth and by nutrition.

Vital Signs

Pulse averages 120 beats per minute between 1 month and 11 months. Respirations are 20 to 40 breaths per minute at 1 year. Temperature at 1 year is 37.7 C (99.7 F). The mean blood pressure at 1 year is 96 mm Hg systolic and 65 mm Hg diastolic.

Head Growth

By 12 months, head circumference has increased about 33% over the birth size.

The posterior fontanelle between the parietal bones and the occipital bone closes from 4 to 8 weeks after birth. The anterior fontanelle (between the frontal and parietal bones) closes between 10 and 18 months.

Vision

By 3 months, vision develops so that both eyes are coordinated both horizontally and vertically. At 4 months, the infant recognizes familiar objects and follows moving objects.

Teeth

At about 5 to 6 months, the infant's first teeth appear.

Motor Development

By 2 months, infants can raise the head from a prone position, and by 6 months they can sit without support.

See Figure 23–5. At 12 months, they can turn the pages of a book, walk with help, and help to dress themselves. See Table 23–7.

Psychosocial Development

According to Erikson, the central crisis at this stage is trust versus mistrust. Resolution of this stage determines how the person approaches subsequent developmental stages. An infant first learns trust from the parent or caregiver and then from others in the environment. Parents and caregivers can enhance a sense of trust by:

1. Responding consistently to an infant's needs
2. Providing a predictable environment in which routines are established
3. Being sensitive to the infant's needs and meeting these skillfully and promptly

Emotional Development

At 1 month, the emotional response of infants is generally restricted to tension and occasional panics. The latter are exhibited by crying, arching the back, and flexing and extending the extremities. Infants also experience satisfaction chiefly from being fed, cuddled, held, and rocked. At 3 months, they need to suck to meet emotional needs, and by 6 months other members of the family are important in meeting their emotional needs. At 6 months, infants smile at the mother and family members, and they are able to wait a short time when they are hungry. By 6 months, infants have a beginning sense of self and, for instance, may pull at their toes as they learn to associate parts of the body with the concept of self.

Learning Adaptive Responses

Initially, an infant has few psychologic adaptive responses. Infants have no understanding of waiting and no time frame by which to measure waiting. The initial reaction of an infant to stress is crying, and crying is the infant's way of communicating distress. Infants learn gradually to tolerate stress. Nurses and parents can reduce the stress of an infant by:

1. Permitting an infant who is or will be distressed to keep a favorite toy nearby
2. Maintaining the infant's routine as much as possible
3. Establishing a relationship of trust with the infant
4. Limiting to the minimum the number of strangers interacting with the infant
5. Providing a warm, accepting environment for the infant

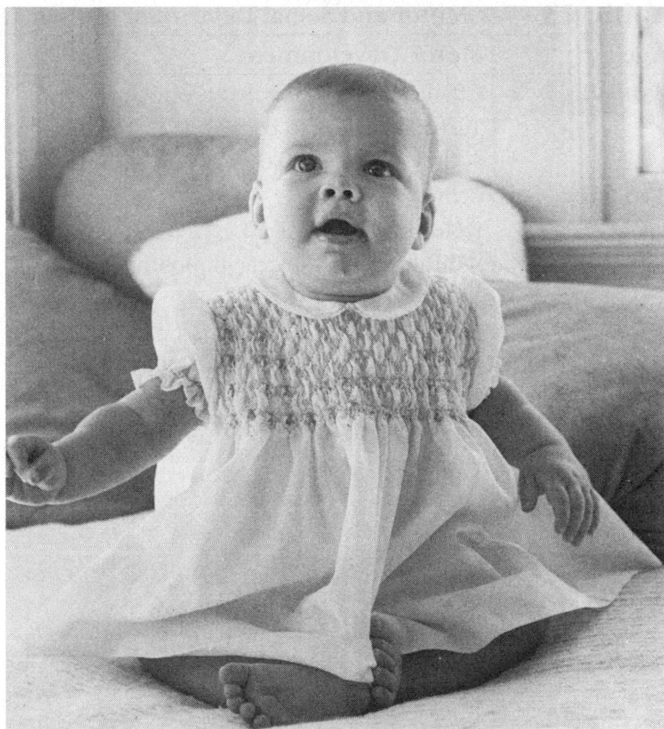

Figure 23–5 An infant sits without support at 6 months of age.

Language Development

By 1 month, infants coo with pleasure and start to babble a little by the second or third month. By 6 months, they chatter in nonsense syllables and continue to do so into the second year. By 12 months, some children can say a few words they have heard, such as *Mummy* and *Daddy*.

Social Development

By the second month, infants enjoy playing with objects and with people. They vocalize in response to the parents' voices. By 7 months, infants begin to perceive strangers, and by 9 months they wave "bye-bye." By 12 months, they recognize the meaning of *yes* and *no*. Infants are still egocentric, concerned only with themselves. See Table 23–7.

Developmental Screening

Psychosocial development can be assessed by observing the infant's behavior and by using standardized tests such as the Denver Developmental Screening Test (DDST). Nurses usually have many opportunities to observe clients interacting with others, e.g., children at play; clients with friends, family, and other clients; and clients interacting with nurses.

Developmental screening tests, such as the Revised DDST, are standardized screening tools used to assess

Table 23–7 Motor and Social Development in Infancy

Age	Motor Development	Social Development
2 months	Lifts head off table when prone	Recognizes familiar face
	Turns from side to back	Attends to speaking voice
	Follows moving object with eyes	Social smile appears
3 months	Actively holds rattle	Laughs aloud
	Holds head erect	Shows pleasure in vocalization
	Willfully places objects in mouth	Smiles in response to mother's face
		Makes prelanguage vocalizations: coos and babbles
4 months	Holds head steady in sitting position	Reaches out to people
	Rolls from back to side and abdomen to back	Squeals
	Grasps objects in two hands	
5 months	Grasps objects with whole hand	Discriminates between strangers and family
	Plays with toes	Vocalizes displeasure when a desired object is removed
	Rolls from stomach to back or vice versa	Smiles at image in mirror
6 months	Lifts cup by handle	Starts to imitate sounds
	Sits without support	Vocalizes one syllable sounds: *ma ma,da da*
		Plays peek-a-boo
7 months	Able to bear weight when held in standing position	Shows fear of strangers
	Bangs objects together	Imitates simple acts
	Grasps toys with one hand	
8 months	Feeds self with fingers	Is bashful and nervous with strangers
	Pulls toys	Opens arms to be picked up
		Responds to *no*
9 months	Creeps and crawls	Cries when scolded
	Sucks, chews, and bites objects	Complies to simple verbal requests
	Handles cup or glass with help	Displays fear of being alone, e.g., going to bed
	Pulls self to standing position	Waves bye-bye
	Uses pincer grasp with thumb and forefinger	
10 months	Sits by falling	Aware of own name
	Picks up objects	Presents toy to another person but will not release it
	Pulls self to standing position	
	Stands if holding onto support	
11 months	Pushes toys	Imitates speech sounds
	Puts objects into container	
	Tries to walk unsupported	
	Tries to hold spoon	
12 months	Hand dominance manifested	Knows own name
	Walks with help	Shakes head for *no*
	Uses spoon to feed self	Does things to attract attention

Source: Adapted from C. Edelman and C. L. Mandle, *Health promotion throughout the life span* (St. Louis: C. V. Mosby Co., 1986), pp. 318–19. Reproduced by permission of the C. V. Mosby Co.

developmental delays in children. See Figure 23–6. The DDST is used to screen children from birth to 6 years of age. The test is intended to estimate the abilities of a child compared to those of an average group of children of the same age. The DDST does not provide diagnostic information about a child's problem, does not predict how a child will develop, and should not be used to assign a child to a developmental age group. Four main areas of development are screened: personal-social, fine motor adaptive, language, and gross motor. For each behavior, an age range is given that indicates whether 25%, 50%, 75%, or 90% of the children perform the task.

DDST manuals, kits, and scoring forms include directions for administering the test. The test is intended to be administered by professionals, such as nurses or psychologists. Usually, the child is asked to perform tasks of increasing difficulty. The child's performance is then scored according to the instructions.

Another screening tool, the Denver Prescreening Developmental Questionnaire (PDQ), is completed by parents when the DDST cannot be administered. It consists of 97 questions grouped according to the child's age. The parents need to answer only 10 questions.

There are many other screening tests, for example, the Brazelton Neonatal Behavioral Assessment Scale, which focuses on neonatal behavior, and the Washington Guide to Promoting Development in Young Children.

Cognitive Development

Cognitive refers to such processes as remembering, thinking, perceiving, abstracting, and generalizing. It is the development of a logical method of looking at the world and utilizing perceptual and conceptual abilities. *Intelligence,* by contrast, is the ability to learn. *To learn* is to acquire and retain knowledge, to respond to new situations, and to solve problems.

According to Piaget, cognitive development is a result of interaction between an individual and the environment. Piaget refers to the initial period of cognitive development as the sensorimotor phase. See Table 22–8, page 469. This phase has six stages, three of which take place during the first year. From 4 to 8 months, infants begin to have perceptual recognition. By 6 months, they respond to new stimuli, and they remember certain objects and look for them for a short time. By 12 months, infants have a concept of both space and time. They experiment to reach a goal, such as a toy on a chair.

An infant's cognitive development also proceeds from reflexive ability of the newborn to using one or two actions to attain a goal by the age of 1 year. Nurses can encourage an infant's cognitive development by providing a variety of sensory and motor stimuli. In addition, nurses can help parents understand an infant's future needs and what and how an infant communicates.

Moral and Spiritual Development

At this early stage of development, children associate right and wrong with pleasure and pain. What gives them pleasure is right, since they are too young to reason otherwise. When infants receive abundant positive responses from the parent such as smiles, caresses, and voice tones of approval in these early months, they learn that certain behaviors are wrong or good and that pain or pleasure is the consequence. In later months and years, the child can tell easily and quickly by changes in parental facial expressions and voice tones that his or her behavior is either approved or disapproved. The less pleasure and more frustration the infant experiences in interactions with parents, the more important other sources of pleasure become. The child is then liable to risk parental anger and do things he or she likes and desires even though others disapprove.

An infant's stage of spiritual development is undifferentiated, i.e., the infant is unable to formulate or communicate concepts. Fowler describes this as stage 0 (Undifferentiated). See Table 22–12, page 474.

Health Promotion and Protection

During the first year, the infant's physical, psychosocial, and cognitive growth proceed at a rapid pace, although more slowly than during the first 28 days of life. During the first year, the infant depends completely on others to meet all needs. The nurse's role, therefore, is largely teaching parents or caregivers what the infant's needs are, how the infant communicates them, and how to meet them.

Nutrition and Fluid

Because of the infant's rapid growth, food and fluid are extremely important during this stage. The brain and nervous system develop rapidly and may suffer because of inadequate nutrition, although research has not yet proven this (Satter 1983, pp. 90–91).

An important aspect of infant nutrition is providing sufficient calories for growth but not so many that the infant becomes obese. Recommended intake during the first 6 months is usually 115 kcal per kilogram of body weight per day and 2 g of protein per kilogram of body weight per day (National Academy of Sciences 1980, pp. 23, 47). During the second 6 months of life, the infant requires slightly fewer calories and less protein: 105 kcal and 2 g of protein per kilogram of body weight per day.

Infants receive only liquid nourishment until about 4 months of age, when solid foods are introduced. The nutritional needs of infants are initially met by breast milk or formula.

The fluid needs of infants are proportionately greater than those of adults due to a higher metabolic rate, immature kidneys, and greater water losses through the skin and the lungs. The last is largely due to the rapid respirations. Therefore, fluid balance is a critical factor. A general rule for the water an infant requires is 1.5 ml/kcal per day (National Academy of Sciences 1980, p. 168). See Chapter 42 for additional information.

Body Temperature Regulation

Infants have immature temperature regulating systems: They perspire minimally, and shivering starts at a lower temperature than it does in adults; therefore, they lose more heat before shivering begins. In addition, because the infant's body surface area is very large in relation to body mass, the body loses heat readily (Guyton 1986, p. 1003). Parents and caregivers must be aware of an infant's

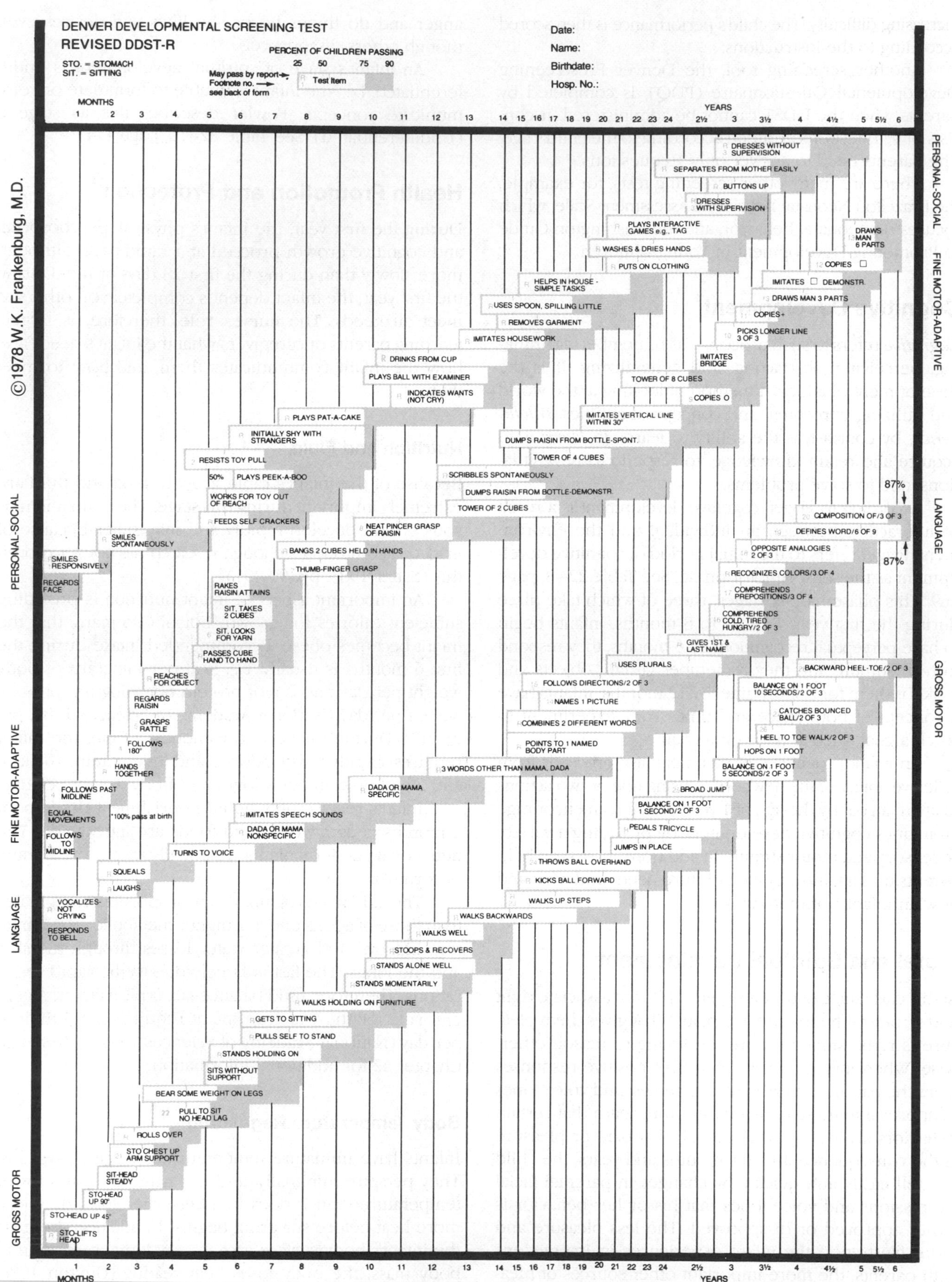

Figure 23–6 The Revised Denver Developmental Screening Test. **A,** Screening Form. **B,** Test Instructions.
(Reprinted with permission of W. K. Frankenburg, University of Colorado Medical Center.)

1. Try to get child to smile by smiling, talking or waving to him. Do not touch him.
2. When child is playing with toy, pull it away from him. Pass if he resists.
3. Child does not have to be able to tie shoes or button in the back.
4. Move yarn slowly in an arc from one side to the other, about 6" above child's face. Pass if eyes follow 90° to midline. (Past midline; 180°)
5. Pass if child grasps rattle when it is touched to the backs or tips of fingers.
6. Pass if child continues to look where yarn disappeared or tries to see where it went. Yarn should be dropped quickly from sight from tester's hand without arm movement.
7. Pass if child picks up raisin with any part of thumb and a finger.
8. Pass if child picks up raisin with the ends of thumb and index finger using an over hand approach.

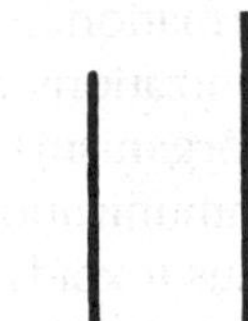
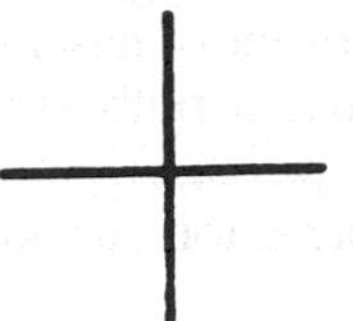
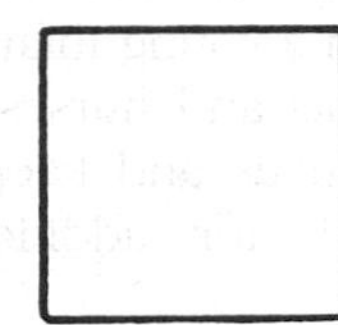

9. Pass any enclosed form. Fail continuous round motions.

10. Which line is longer? (Not bigger.) Turn paper upside down and repeat. (3/3 or 5/6)

11. Pass any crossing lines.

12. Have child copy first. If failed, demonstrate

When giving items 9, 11 and 12, do not name the forms. Do not demonstrate 9 and 11.

13. When scoring, each pair (2 arms, 2 legs, etc.) counts as one part.
14. Point to picture and have child name it. (No credit is given for sounds only.)

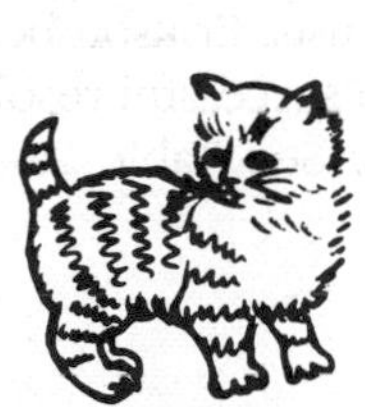
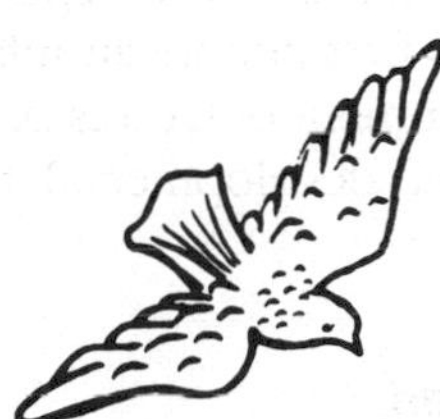
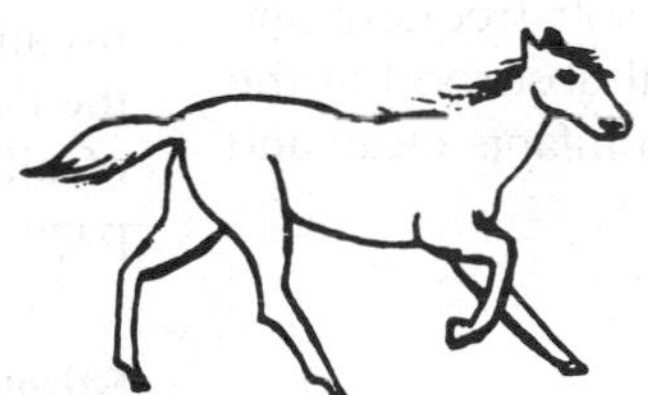
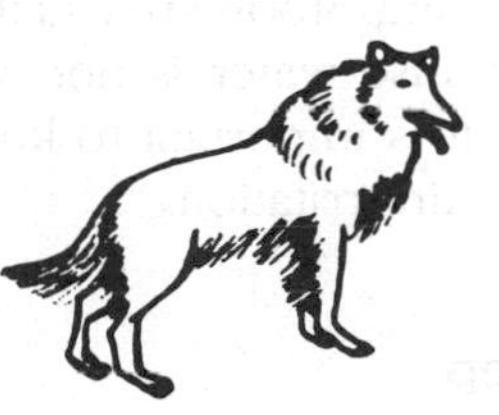
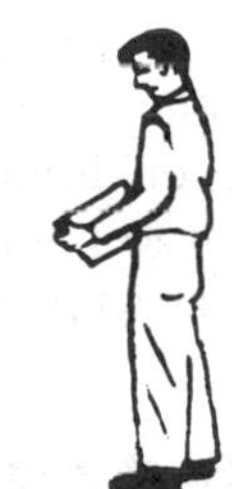

15. Tell child to: Give block to Mommie; put block on table; put block on floor. Pass 2 of 3. (Do not help child by pointing, moving head or eyes.)
16. Ask child: What do you do when you are cold? ..hungry? ..tired? Pass 2 of 3.
17. Tell child to: Put block <u>on</u> table; <u>under</u> table; <u>in</u> <u>front</u> of chair, <u>behind</u> chair. Pass 3 of 4. (Do not help child by pointing, moving head or eyes.)
18. Ask child: If fire is hot, ice is ?; Mother is a woman, Dad is a ?; a horse is big, a mouse is ?. Pass 2 of 3.
19. Ask child: What is a ball? ..lake? ..desk? ..house? ..banana? ..curtain? ..ceiling? ..hedge? ..pavement? Pass if defined in terms of use, shape, what it is made of or general category (such as banana is fruit, not just yellow). Pass 6 of 9.
20. Ask child: What is a spoon made of? ..a shoe made of? ..a door made of? (No other objects may be substituted.) Pass 3 of 3.
21. When placed on stomach, child lifts chest off table with support of forearms and/or hands.
22. When child is on back, grasp his hands and pull him to sitting. Pass if head does not hang back.
23. Child may use wall or rail only, not person. May not crawl.
24. Child must throw ball overhand 3 feet to within arm's reach of tester.
25. Child must perform standing broad jump over width of test sheet. (8-1/2 inches)
26. Tell child to walk forward, ⊂⊃⊂⊃⊂⊃⊂⊃→ heel within 1 inch of toe. Tester may demonstrate. Child must walk 4 consecutive steps, 2 out of 3 trials.
27. Bounce ball to child who should stand 3 feet away from tester. Child must catch ball with hands, not arms, 2 out of 3 trials.
28. Tell child to walk backward, ←⊂⊃⊂⊃⊂⊃⊂⊃ toe within 1 inch of heel. Tester may demonstrate. Child must walk 4 consecutive steps, 2 out of 3 trials.

<u>DATE AND BEHAVIORAL OBSERVATIONS</u> (how child feels at time of test, relation to tester, attention span, verbal behavior, self-confidence, etc,):

Figure 23–6 *(continued)*

response to changes in environmental temperatures. Infants must be dressed warmly in cold environments and lightly in hot ones. See Chapter 34 for additional information.

Oxygen

Infants are obligatory nose-breathers until about 3 to 4 months of age, when they learn to breathe through their mouths. Therefore, an occluded nasal passage is a serious problem in a young infant. In the event of nasal congestion, parents and nurses should use a bulb syringe to remove mucus and keep the air passages patent. See Chapter 45 for additional information about bulb suctioning.

Elimination

Infants usually cannot control the elimination of urine or feces during the first year. Control is not established until the neuromuscular systems are sufficiently developed. Infants normally excrete 250 to 500 ml per day in increasing amounts during the first year. An infant may urinate as often as 20 times a day.

A young infant will pass many stools in 24 hours, often after a feeding. Stools are usually soft, frequent, and even liquid because water is not well absorbed in the large intestine. It is important to keep infants clean and dry to prevent skin irritation.

Rest and Sleep

Infants have longer periods of wakefulness than neonates do. Newborns usually sleep 17 hours daily, but periods of wakefulness gradually increase by the end of the first months.

In infants of 2 months, a nurse may note a preference for one sleeping position, but this preference may have been present at birth. By 3 months, the infant exhibits routines before sleeping, such as crying, sucking on fingers or toys, or shifting positions repeatedly. By 4 months, most infants sleep through the night and establish a pattern of daytime naps that varies among individuals. They generally awaken early in the morning, however. At the end of the first year, an infant usually takes one or two naps per day and sleeps about 14 of every 24 hours. The infant also begins to show fear of being left alone.

Pain Avoidance

When infants experience pain, they communicate their discomfort by crying. Crying due to pain has a different quality from crying due to hunger. Infants who perceive pain do not know the exact location of the pain, but they may try to pull away from it.

Safety and Security Needs

Accidents are the leading cause of morbidity and mortality among infants. Drowning, poisoning, suffocation, and falls are the most common accidents. For example, an unwatched baby may roll off a table; thus infants need careful watching even during ordinary activities. Parents often require assistance in identifying potential dangers in the home, and nurses in hospitals need to be actively involved in accident prevention. See Chapter 33 for additional information.

Immunizations are needed to protect infants from the microorganisms causing diphtheria, pertussis, and tetanus. Immunization is provided in a combined diphtheria, tetanus toxoids, and pertussis (DTP) vaccine. Infants also require the orally administered poliomyelitis vaccine. In the United States and Canada, infants usually receive DTP and poliomyelitis vaccines at approximately 2, 4, and 6 months. Measles-rubella vaccine or a combined measles-mumps-rubella vaccine is recommended at age 1 year, as well as a tuberculin test to determine exposure to the tuberculosis bacillus. In some areas, smallpox vaccine is also given between the third and twelfth months. See Chapter 33 for further information.

Security needs of the infant are related to the development of trust. The parents or primary caregivers are usually the first people an infant trusts. Erikson believes the development of trust is basic to successful resolution of all other developmental crises. See Table 22–6 on page 466.

Stimulation

Initially, the newborn's actions are reflexive; however, actions become more purposeful with maturation. Infants learn from stimuli in the environment. They experience auditory, visual, and other stimuli and eventually learn to manipulate objects in the environment. Initially the infant learns to roll over, sit, crawl, stand, and then walk, often all in 12 months. Infants play with their toes and hands and assume many positions. Colorful hanging toys, particularly toys that move, are important from birth to about 3 months. After that, infants require toys they can grasp and put into the mouth but cannot swallow, e.g., large wooden spoons, stuffed toys, and small plastic animals. By age 1, they like building blocks and other toys they can pull apart and move. They also enjoy playing in sand; they fill pails and dump small loads of sand. When infants begin to walk, they like push-and-pull toys, such as wagons, and pounding toys, such as drums.

An environment with a variety of sights, sounds, smells, tastes, and textures stimulates an infant's development. Speech development is enhanced by stimuli. Initially the infant coos, laughs, and imitates sounds. By 1 year, an infant usually can name some objects in the environment, such as "dada" or "doggie."

Sexuality

A young infant is not aware of his or her sex. Freud refers to this stage of psychosexual developmental as the oral phase. Freud believes that the newborn infant has "germs of sexual feelings" but that these feelings differ from those of an adult (Freud 1930, pp. 35–45).

The parents' attitudes toward the sex of the child can affect their relationship with the infant. For example, parents who hoped for a girl but had a boy may find attachment and engrossment more difficult.

Love and Belonging

Close bonding with parents or a caregiver is essential for healthy psychosocial development. This attachment is demonstrated by mothering behaviors such as loving care, handling, stroking, and cuddling. From months 3 to 15, mothering behavior is essential for both physical and intellectual growth. Infants deprived of mothering in this stage of development will not learn to form significant relationships or to trust others.

Infants who fail to establish a loving, responsive relationship with an adult often fail to develop normally. The disturbed parent-child relationship can result in the failure-to-thrive syndrome. The infants show delayed development without any physical cause. They are often malnourished and fail to gain weight and grow normally. Another problem that can result from a disturbed parent-infant relationship is infant or child abuse. Abusing parents were often abused themselves as children.

Research Note

Mercer researched the process by which mothers achieve competence in their role and come to identify themselves as mothers. Three age groups were studied: teenage mothers, 20- to 29-year-old mothers, and 30- to 42-year-old mothers. Role strain and self-image as mothers did not differ among the age groups; teenage mothers, however, were less competent in their mothering behaviors and experienced particular strain around the time of the infants' individuation strivings at 8 months. The study supports the idea that competency in role behaviors increases with age. Age was not a factor, however, in mothers' feelings of gratification about their babies. Nurses who work with first-time mothers clearly need to assist them in anticipating and preparing for the realities of the maternal role, including the fact that one's mothering skills do not necessarily increase with experience, because the child presents different challenges at each developmental stage. (Mercer 1985)

Self-Esteem

By 1 year of age, infants have learned to distinguish self from the environment. Piaget believes that from 1 to 4 months of age, infants perceive objects as extensions of self, by 8 months they acknowledge the external environment as separate from self, and by 12 months they can distinguish goals as separate from the means of attaining them. See Table 22–8 on page 468. Mahler refers to the individuation process as starting at about 5 months, when the infant differentiates between the body of the caregiver and his or her own body (see Table 22–7, page 467).

Infants need to be able to manipulate the environment. Sullivan believes that early infant-parent experiences mold a child's self-concept. Infants need to do some things independently; receiving positive feedback from a significant person can enhance a sense of pride and sense of self.

Chapter Highlights

- The intrauterine period of development is one of phenomenal growth and change.
- Fetal heartbeats can be heard in the first trimester.
- In the second trimester, the mother can detect fetal movement, and the fetus assumes the form of a small baby although it is thin and wrinkled.
- In the third trimester, the nervous system starts to regulate some body processes, and the fetus acquires subcutaneous fat and increases in size and weight.
- A fetus born before term has varying chances of survival; at 6 months, chances for survival are minimal; at 7 months, 10%; at 8 months, 75%.
- The health of the mother is basic to the growth and development of the embryo and fetus; appropriate nutrition, rest, exercise, and prenatal care are essential.
- Maternal consumption of alcohol, excessive smoking, use of addictive drugs or medications, stress, and disease have harmful effects on the fetus.
- The newborn's first essential task is to accomplish independent respiration; the nurse helps by suctioning the newborn's nasal passages and mouth.
- An essential nursing function is assessment of the newborn's physical status by the Apgar scoring system.
- Measurements of length, weight, head and chest circumferences, fontanelle size and status, reflex abilities, and motor development are important indicators of the newborn's growth and health.

- A sense of trust and security in the newborn is essential for subsequent development; the infant derives this sense from parental love, warmth, and prompt attention to physical needs.
- Attachment between the mother and newborn and engrossment between the father and newborn are basic to optimal development of the infant.
- Infants from 1 month to 1 year reveal marked growth in size and stature with appropriate nutrition and care: birth weight is doubled by 6 months and tripled by 12 months.
- During infancy, motor development is notable; at 3 months, infants can raise their heads from the prone position, at 6 months, they can sit unsupported, and at 12 months, they can stand momentarily and walk with help.
- Continuing, sensitive, loving, and consistent attention to the infant's needs must be maintained to develop a sense of trust and security.
- Language and social development begin in infancy.
- Although infants are largely egocentric, they recognize the meaning of *yes* and *no*.
- To develop cognitively, the infant needs a variety of sensory and motor stimuli.
- The nurse can assess the psychosocial and motor development of infants by using the Denver Developmental Screening Test and similar tests.
- To promote and protect the health of the infant, caregivers must provide appropriate nutrition, maintain body temperature, ensure adequate rest and sleep, protect the infant from accidents, immunize the infant, and teach parents to give appropriate stimulation and love.
- When infants' needs are met and they receive positive feedback for their achievements, they begin to develop a sense of pride, sense of self, and self-esteem.

Suggested Readings

Sande, D. R., and Billingsley, C. S. September 1985. Language development in infants and toddlers. *Nurse Practitioner* 10:39–41, 44, 47.

The authors discuss the significance of language development, the growth and development of language, language and communication, the use of objects in interaction, and the evaluation of speech and language problems by selected screening tests. Also included is a list of questions nurses can ask parents to gain information about linguistic and auditory milestones. Sections on promoting normal development and finding resources for help conclude the article.

Scharping, E. M. January/February 1983. Physiological measurements of the neonate. *American Journal of Maternal Child Nursing* 8:70–73.

Scharping discusses monitoring neonatal temperature, pulse, respiration, and blood pressure. Changes in a sick infant's body temperature are highly significant. Brachial and femoral pulses are valuable for monitoring an infant's pulse. Scharping presents a four-point scale for evaluating the quality of an infant's pulse.

Yoos, L. January/February 1984. Taking another look at failure. *Maternal Child Nursing* 9:32–36.

Yoos discusses the "failure-to-thrive" syndrome. The most commonly accepted cause of nonorganic failure to thrive is a disturbance in the interactions between mother and child. Such mothers exhibit behaviors that differ from those of women whose children do thrive. The behaviors of mothers of nonthriving infants are lack of affection, and infrequent holding, cuddling, talking to, or playing with the infant. Yoos gives an outline by which to assess risk of the failure-to-thrive syndrome. Early nursing interventions include changes in diet and feeding schedule and support for family members. Hospitalization should be a last resort. Yoos also includes some nursing interventions for the failure-to-thrive infant admitted to hospital.

Selected References

Behrman, R. E., and Vaughan, V. C., III. 1983. In W. E. Nelson, editor. *Nelson textbook of pediatrics.* 12th ed. Philadelphia: W. B. Saunders Co.

Clark, A. L. 1981. *Culture and childrearing.* Philadelphia: F. A. Davis Co.

Committee on Dietary Allowances, National Research Council. 1980. *Recommended Dietary Allowances.* 9th ed. Washington, D.C. National Academy of Sciences.

Duvall, E. M. 1977. *Marriage and family development.* 5th ed. New York: J. B. Lippincott.

Edelman, C., and Mandle, C. L. 1986. *Health promotion throughout the life span.* St. Louis: C. V. Mosby Co.

Endres, J. B., and Rockwell, R. E. 1980. *Food, nutrition, and the young child.* St. Louis: C. V. Mosby Co.

Engel, G. L. 1962. *Psychological development in health and disease.* Philadelphia: W. B. Saunders Co.

Erikson, E. H. 1963. *Childhood and society.* 2d ed. New York: W. W. Norton and Co.

Fong, B. C., and Resnick, M. R. 1980. *The child: Development through adolescence.* Menlo Park, Calif.: Benjamin/Cummings Publishing Co.

Freud, S. 1930. *Three contributions to the theory of sex.* 4th ed. New York: Nervous and Mental Disease Publishing.

Greenberg, M., and Morris, N. April 1974. Engrossment: The newborn's impact upon the father. *American Journal of Orthopsychiatry* 44:520.

Guyton, A. C. 1986. *Textbook of medical physiology.* 7th ed. Philadelphia: W. B. Saunders Co.

Havighurst, R. J. 1972. *Developmental tasks and education.* 3d ed. New York: David McKay Co.

Hogan, R. 1985. *Human sexuality: A nursing perspective.* 2d ed. Norwalk, Conn.: Appleton-Century-Crofts.

Klaus, M. H., and Kennell, J. H. 1983. *Bonding: The beginnings of parent-infant attachment.* St. Louis: C. V. Mosby Co.

Lourie, R. S. July/August 1981. Primary prevention in infancy. *Children To-day* 10:6–9.

Mercer, R. July/August 1985. The process of maternal role attainment over the first year. *Nursing Research* 34(4):198–203.

Mott, S. R.; Fazekas, N. F.; and James, S. R. 1985. *Nursing care of children and families: A holistic approach.* Menlo Park, Calif.: Addison-Wesley Publishing Co.

Murray, R. B., and Zentner, J. P. 1985. *Nursing assessment and health promotion through the life span.* 3d ed. Englewood Cliffs, N.J.: Prentice-Hall.

Olds, S. B.; London, M. L.; and Ladewig, P. A. 1984. *Maternal-newborn nursing: A family-centered approach.* 2d ed. Menlo Park, Calif.: Addison-Wesley Publishing Co.

Piaget, J. 1963. *Origins of intelligence in children.* New York: W. W. Norton and Co.

Pipes, P. L. 1981. *Nutrition in infancy and childhood.* St. Louis: C. V. Mosby Co.

Sahler, O. J. Z., and McAnarney, E. R. 1981. *The child from three to eighteen.* St. Louis: C. V. Mosby Co.

Sande, D. R., and Billingsley, C. S. September 1985. Language development in infants and toddlers. *Nurse Practitioner* 10:39–41, 44, 47.

Satter, E. 1983. *Child of mine: Feeding with love and good sense.* Palo Alto, Calif.: Bull Publishing Co.

Scharping, E. M. January/February 1983. Physiologic measurements of the neonate. *American Journal of Maternal Child Nursing* 8:70–73.

Schulman, M., and Mekler, E. 1985. *Bringing up a moral child: A new approach for teaching your child to be kind, just, and responsible.* Reading, Mass.: Addison-Wesley Publishing Co.

Yoos, L. January/February 1984. Taking another look at failure. *Maternal Child Nursing* 9:32–36.

CHAPTER 24

Childhood Through Adolescence

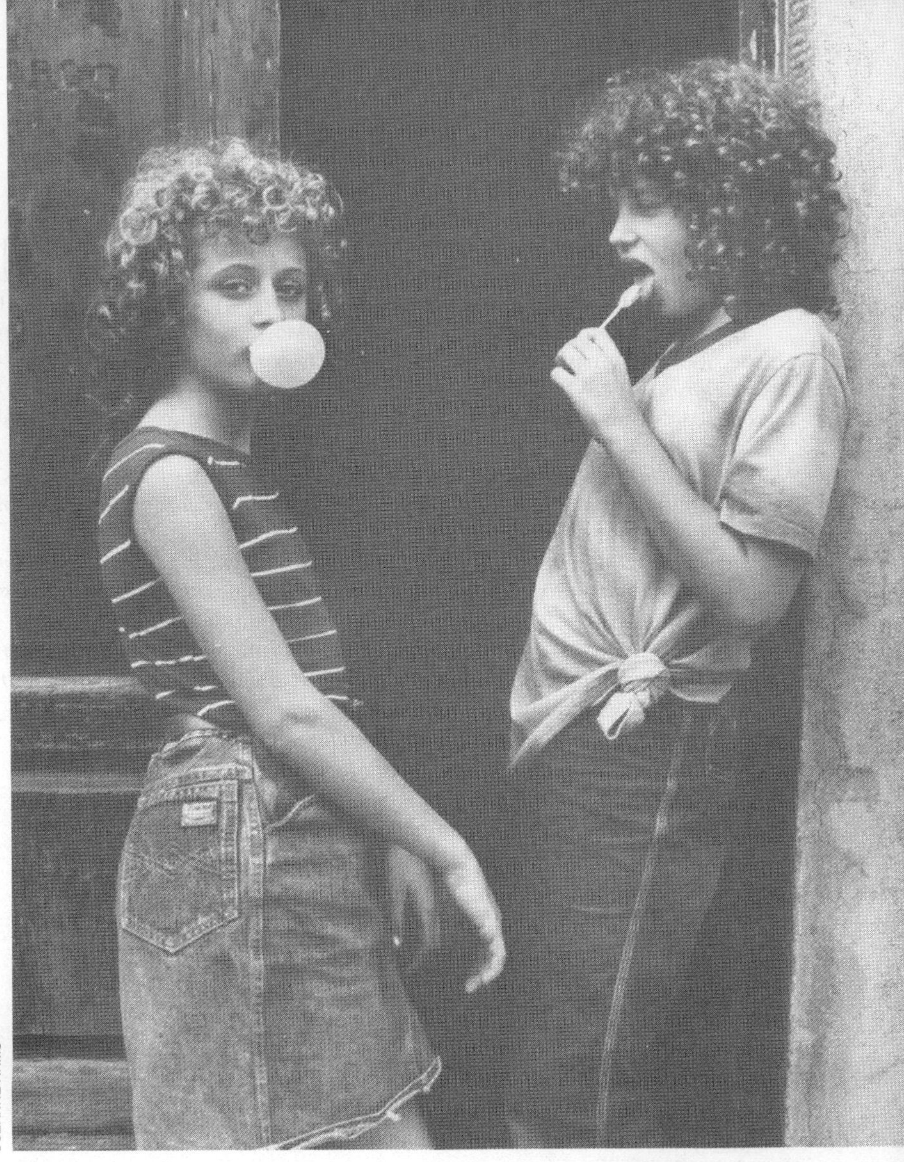

SUZANNE ARMS

Contents

Objectives

1. Understand essential facts about the development of toddlers, school-age children, and adolescents.
   1.1 Identify developmental tasks at different stages of development during childhood and adolescence.
   1.2 Identify essential aspects of physical development throughout childhood and adolescence.
   1.3 Describe psychosocial development according to Erikson throughout childhood and adolescence.
   1.4 Describe changes in cognitive development according to Piaget throughout childhood and adolescence.
   1.5 Describe moral development according to Kohlberg throughout childhood and adolescence.
   1.6 Describe spiritual development according to Fowler throughout childhood and adolescence.
2. Understand essential aspects of health promotion and protection for children and adolescents.
   2.1 Identify essential assessment data for toddlers, preschoolers, school-age children, and adolescents.
   2.2 Identify essential health promotion and protection activities to meet the needs of toddlers, preschoolers, school-age children, and adolescents.

Terms

adolescence
anorexia nervosa
apocrine glands
areola
breast bud
bulimia
dysmenorrhea
eccrine glands
ejaculation
identification
imagination
introjection
malingering
menarche
nocturnal emission
papule
primary sexual characteristics
puberty
pustule
rationalization
regression
repression
ritualistic behavior
sebaceous glands
sebum
secondary sexual characteristics

Toddlers (1 to 3 Years)

Toddlers develop from having no voluntary control to being able both to walk and speak. They also learn to control their bladder and bowels, and they acquire all kinds of information about their environment. Developmental tasks for the toddler are shown to the right.

Physical Development

Appearance

Two-year-old children lose the baby look. Toddlers are usually chubby with relatively short legs and a large head. See Figure 24–1. The face appears small in comparison to the skull; but as the toddler grows, the face seems to grow from under the skull and appears better proportioned.

Weight

Two-year-olds can be expected to weigh approximately four times their birth weight. The weight gain is about 2 kg (5 lb) between 1 year and 2 years and about 1 to 2 kg (2 to 5 lb) between 2 and 3 years. The 3-year-old weighs about 13.6 kg (30 lb).

Height or Length

A toddler's height can be measured as height or length. Height is measured while the toddler stands, and length is measured while the toddler is in a recumbent position. Although the measurements differ slightly, nurses must specify which measurement is used to avoid confusion.

Between ages 1 and 2 years the average growth in

Developmental Tasks of the Toddler (1 to 3 Years)

Erikson's stage: Autonomy versus shame and doubt

- Achieving physiologic stability
- Learning to become physically independent while remaining emotionally dependent
- Expanding verbal communication
- Learning to control the elimination of body wastes
- Learning to coordinate large muscles and small muscles

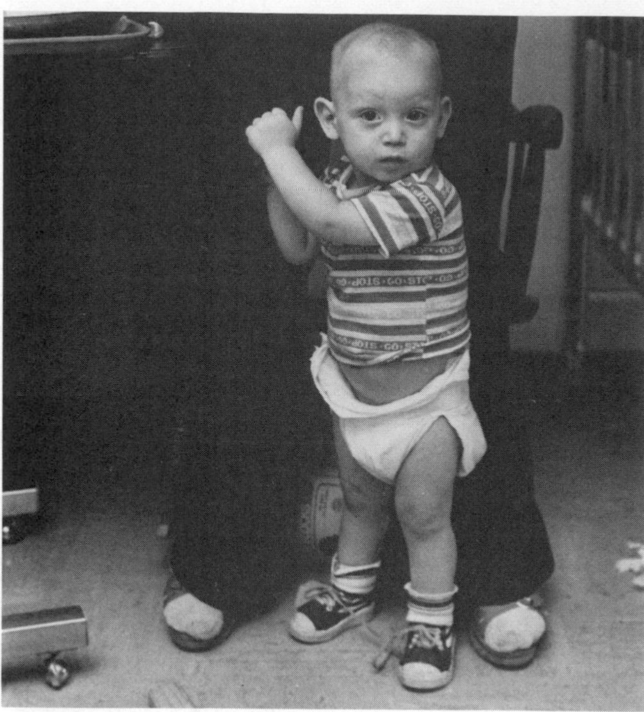

Figure 24–1 The toddler appears chubby with relatively short legs and a large head.

height is 10 to 12 cm (4 to 5 in) and between ages 2 to 3 years it slows to 6 to 8 cm (2½ to 3½ in).

Head

The head circumference of the toddler increases on an average about 2.5 cm (1 in), and by 24 months the head is four-fifths of the average adult size. The brain is 70% of its adult size by the time the infant is 2 years old.

Teeth

Toddlers are likely to have between 16 and 20 (all) of their deciduous teeth at 2 years of age. It is also during this period that the permanent teeth, with the exception of the second and third molars, begin to calcify.

Senses

Visual acuity is fairly well established by 1 year; however, it is continually refined until the age of 6 years, when it becomes 20/20. Full binocular vision is usually established by 1 year. The senses of hearing, taste, smell, and touch become increasingly developed and associated with each other.

Touch is a very important sense to the toddler. He or she is often soothed by tactile sensations. When toddlers are hospitalized or ill, it is often the nurse's function to cuddle, hold, or rock them.

Posture

Toddlers have a pronounced lumbar lordosis and a protruding abdomen. The abdominal muscles develop gradually as the toddler grows, and the abdomen flattens.

Motor Development

At the age of 18 months, babies can pick up small beads and place them in a receptacle. They can also hold a spoon and a cup and walk upstairs with assistance. They will probably crawl down the stairs.

At 2 years, toddlers can hold a spoon and put it into the mouth correctly. They are able to run; their gait is steady; and they can balance on one foot and ride a tricycle.

By 3 years, most children are toilet trained, although they still may have the occasional accident when playing or during the night.

Psychosocial Development

According to Freud, the ages of 2 and 3 years represent the anal phase of development, when the rectum and anus are the specially significant areas of the body. Erikson sees the period from 18 months to 3 years as the time when the central developmental task is autonomy versus shame and doubt (see Table 22–6 on page 466).

Mahler describes the process of attainment of separateness that continues in toddlerhood as part of the separation-individuation process. These years roughly correspond to Mahler's third subphase: the period of reapproachment. See Table 22–7 on page 467. Mahler also describes the final subphase, consolidation of individuality and the beginning of emotional constancy (Haber et al. 1982, p. 147).

Nurses can assist parents and caregivers to help a toddler's development by:

1. Providing toys suitable for the toddler, including some challenging toys. However, do not set up situations in which the toddler will fail, as this will intensify feelings of self-doubt and shame.
2. Making positive suggestions rather than commanding. Avoid an emotional climate of negativism, blame, and punishment.
3. Giving the toddler choices, all of which are safe; however, limit the child's autonomy.
4. If the toddler has a temper tantrum, make sure the toddler is safe and then leave.
5. Help the toddler to develop inner control by setting and enforcing consistent, reasonable limits.
6. Praise the toddler's accomplishments.

Emotional Development

At 18 months, toddlers imitate their parents and play games. They indicate displeasure over a wet diaper. By 2 years, routine is very important; toddlers find change disturbing and often cry when routine is changed. Toddlers' emotions of love and hate are often extreme.

Toddlers begin to develop their sense of autonomy by asserting themselves with the frequent use of the word *no*. They are often frustrated by restraints to their behavior; between ages 1 and 3 children may have temper tantrums. However, they slowly gain control over their emotions, usually with the guidance of their parents.

The period of the development of a sense of autonomy (1 to 3 years) is a time of expanding social contacts. Toddlers are curious and ask many questions. Children at this age are often creative, although the products of this activity may not be perfect.

Learning Adaptive Responses

The toddler will likely continue to use the adaptive responses he learned as an infant, although the toddler can begin to use basic problem solving. Common responses to stress are separation anxiety and regression. For example, toddlers who are stressed may become highly anxious when separated from their parents and admitted to hospital. Regression or reverting to an earlier developmental stage may be indicated by bed wetting or using baby talk. Nurses can assist parents by helping them understand that this behavior is normal and indicates that the toddler is trying to establish his or her position in the family. Toddlers are asserting their independence by saying no or by dawdling.

Language and Speech

Most children learn to imitate words in the second year, when sufficient cortical maturity has taken place. By 2 years, they usually can arrange several words into a sentence. Three-year-olds speak almost constantly. They practice speaking in bed and during play. They imitate adults and can express feelings, thoughts, desires, and problems in words. Logic is elusive, so not all their words at any one time relate to the same activity.

Social Development

At 2 years, children are very possessive of their toys. They are dependent on their parents and react strongly to separation from them. By age 3, toddlers are learning to play with their peers.

Cognitive Development

According to Piaget, the toddler completes the 5th and 6th stages of the sensorimotor phase and starts the preconceptual phase at about 2 years of age. See Table 22–8 on page 469. In the fifth stage, the toddler solves problems by a trial-and-error process. By stage 6, toddlers can solve problems mentally. For example, when given a new toy, the toddler will not immediately handle the toy to see how it works but will look at it carefully to think about how it works.

During Piaget's preconceptual phase, toddlers develop considerable cognitive and intellectual skills. They learn about the sequence of time. They have some symbolic thought; for example, a chair may represent a place of safety, while a blanket may symbolize comfort. Concepts start to form in late toddlerhood. A concept develops when the child learns words to represent classes of objects or thoughts. An example of a concrete concept is *table,* representing a number of articles of furniture, which are all different but all tables.

Moral Development

According to Kohlberg, the first level of moral development is the preconventional when children respond to labels of "good" or "bad" (see Table 22–10, page 471). During the second year of life, children begin to know that some activities elicit affection and approval. They also recognize that certain rituals, such as repeating phrases from prayers, also elicit approval. This provides children with feelings of security. By 2 years of age, toddlers are learning what attitudes their parents hold about moral matters.

Spiritual Development

According to Fowler, the toddler's stage of spiritual development is undifferentiated (see Table 22–12, page 472). Toddlers may be aware of some religious practices, but they are primarily involved in learning knowledge and emotional reactions rather than establishing spiritual beliefs. A toddler may repeat short prayers at bedtime, conforming to a ritual, because praise and affection result. This parental response enhances the toddler's sense of security.

Health Promotion and Protection

During their second and third years, toddlers require preventive health care. The American Academy of Pediatrics recommends regular health care visits during this period at 18, 21, 24, 30, and 36 months of age (American Academy of Pediatrics 1972).

Assessing Growth and Development

Assessment guidelines for growth and development of the toddler are shown on the next page. Parents need reassurance that there are wide ranges of "normal" standards.

Nursing Assessment Guidelines for the Toddler

Does the toddler:

- Indicate physical development within normal range?
- Eat and drink appropriately?
- Feed self?
- Start to develop bowel and bladder control?
- Exhibit physical skills appropriate for his or her age?
- Express likes and dislikes or exhibit any other autonomous behavior?
- Imitate simple words and arrange several words into a sentence?
- Venture away from the mother?
- Begin to play and communicate with children and others outside the immediate family?
- Display curiosity and ask many questions?
- Imitate religious rituals of the family?

Nutrition and Fluid

Because of a maturing gastrointestinal tract, toddlers can eat most foods and adjust to three meals each day. In addition, by age 3, when most of the deciduous teeth have emerged, the toddler is able to bite and chew adult table food. Toddler's manipulative skills are sufficiently well developed for them to learn how to feed themselves. Before the age of 20 months, most toddlers require help with glasses and cups because their wrist control is limited.

The daily diet of a toddler must be nutritious, although their daily requirement may be only 1000 to 1500 kcal because of their slowed growth rate. Developing independence may be exhibited through the toddler's refusal of certain foods. Meals should be short because of the toddler's brief attention span and environmental distractions. Parents and caregivers should be taught about nutritional needs of the toddler, eating patterns, and sizes of servings. (See Chapter 42 for further information.) A hospitalized toddler may regress for a period of time and want to be fed.

Often toddlers display their liking of rituals by eating foods in a certain order, cutting foods a specific way, or accompanying certain foods with a particular drink. Entering hospital can disrupt a toddler's rituals and affect eating; therefore, nurses should consult with the parents to adapt to the toddler's food habits whenever possible.

The toddler is less likely to have fluid imbalances than the infant. Toddlers' gastrointestinal function is more mature, and the percent of fluid body weight is lower. A healthy toddler needs about 100 to 125 ml of liquid per kilogram of body weight per day (Smith et al. 1982, p. 211).

Elimination

During the toddler's second or third year, bowel control becomes possible as the muscles and nervous system mature. Feces are firmer as a result of a more mature large intestine and increased fluid absorption from the intestinal contents into the bloodstream. Stools are less frequent than during infancy, and timing of defecation is evident.

The bladder grows larger throughout toddlerhood; the average bladder of a 2-year-old holds about 80 ml (2¾ oz) of urine (Shuster and Ashburn 1980, p. 234). Increasingly, the toddler can remain dry during the day, thus facilitating toilet training. The urethra of female toddlers is less than 2 cm (0.8 in) long, predisposing them to urinary infections.

Toddlers need help with toilet training. Usually, daytime control can be attained during this time; however, total urinary control at night may not be achieved until preschool years. Toddlers admitted to hospital may regress in toilet training due to the stress of illness and hospitalization, the change in routine, and the unfamiliar environment, e.g., an unfamiliar potty chair. Nurses should consult with parents about the words a toddler uses to indicate the need to void or defecate and the routine used at home. Because of the possibility of urinary infections as well as skin irritation, toddlers should be kept clean and dry.

Sleep and Rest

The sleep requirements of toddlers decrease to 10 to 14 hours per day. Most toddlers still need an afternoon nap, but the need for midmorning naps gradually decreases. Some toddlers have nightmares and need to be comforted and helped to differentiate between dreams and reality. Favorite toys can give toddlers a feeling of security, particularly at night.

Protection

Accidents are a leading cause of morbidity and mortality of toddlers. Drowning, poisoning, suffocation, and falls are the most common accidents. For example, a toddler may swallow liquid household cleaners if they are left in reach.

Precautions need to be taken to keep medicines, cleaners, and the like out of the reach of toddlers. Parents may need to learn to lock cupboards or to place dangerous substances out of reach. See Chapter 33 for additional information.

Immunizations continue to be an important aspect of safety. The toddler's immune system is now functioning and producing antibodies in response to various microorganisms in the environment. At 15 months, toddlers should receive rubeola, rubella, and mumps (MMR) vaccine; at 18 months, diphtheria, tetanus toxoids, and pertussis (DTP) vaccine as well as oral attenuated poliomyelitis virus (OPV) vaccine. For immunization schedules, see Chapter 33, pages 752 and 753.

During early childhood, body temperature appears to be more labile than it is later, hence toddlers are likely to have very high fevers, e.g., 40 C (104 F), due to infections. The toddler, however, can respond to changes to the environmental temperature far better than the infant can, largely because of the growth and maturation of the blood capillaries. In response to changing temperatures, the toddler's body can increase or decrease the blood flow to surface capillaries, thereby increasing or decreasing heat loss (Guyton 1986, p. 854). A toddler with an infection or fever should be closely monitored for extreme fluctuations, which should be reported immediately to a nurse or physician.

Stimulation

Play is stimulating to toddlers, and they take play very seriously. Play serves a number of purposes: It improves coordination and dexterity, helps develop spatial and sensory perception, helps the toddler learn to socialize, and releases emotional tension (Murray and Zentner 1985, p. 164). When toddlers reach the age of 2 or 2½ years, it is evident that boys are more aggressive than girls both physically and verbally (Maccoby and Jacklin 1985, p. 166).

Play for the toddler is solitary and parallel. The toddler plays alone or beside others, but not with others. Nurses can help parents understand the importance of play to the toddler and the safety aspects of toys and play.

Sexuality

Parents' attitudes toward the sex of the toddler influence both skills and attitudes. Parents usually encourage more independent behavior in boys; therefore, boys often venture farther and explore more than girls do. Boys are usually expected to achieve more than girls do. By 2 years, toddlers can categorize others as boys or girls and often have some awareness of physical differences.

Nurses can assist parents to understand the sexuality of their child and to be comfortable with their own sexual identities. In this way, parents can demonstrate affection and easily answer their child's questions. Parents need to learn that play can often help children learn adult roles.

Love and Belonging

Toddlers still need a close, loving relationship with their parents. Abandonment is their greatest fear. Although they like to explore, they always need the security of having a significant person nearby. Toddlers can be loving and cuddly one moment and energetic, exploring. and self-absorbed the next.

Nurses may need to explain to parents the toddler's need for approval and attention. Parents should attend to the toddler, but not to the degree that the child is encouraged to show off.

Self-Esteem

The toddler is vaguely aware of self. As the sense of autonomy develops, the toddler is increasingly aware of the physical self and of emotions. The child does need some limits on activities for safety. Toddlers develop feelings of self-worth as a result of how others appraise their behavior. Children who constantly get negative feedback see themselves as bad. This perception is the basis of a negative self-concept.

Parents can provide a safe environment in which the toddler can practice skills such as playing or running. They also need to give toddlers positive input so that they develop a positive and emotionally healthy self-image. With a healthy sense of self-esteem and security, the toddler is able to deal with periodic failures later in life without damaging his or her self-esteem.

Preschoolers (4 and 5 Years)

During this period, physical growth slows, but control of the body and coordination increase greatly. The preschooler's world gets larger as he or she meets relatives, friends, and neighbors. Developmental tasks for the preschooler are shown on the next page.

Physical Development

Appearance

By the time children are 4 or 5 years old, they appear taller and thinner than toddlers because children tend to grow more in height than in weight. The preschooler's brain reaches almost its adult size by 5 years. The extremities of the body grow more quickly than the body trunk, making the child's body appear somewhat out of proportion. The posture of preschoolers gradually changes as the pelvis is straightened and the abdominal muscles become stronger. Thus the preschooler appears slender with erect posture.

Weight

Weight gain in preschool children is generally slow. By 5 years, they have added only another 3 to 5 kg (7 to 12 lb) to their 3-year-old weight, increasing it to somewhere between 18.1 and 20.4 kg (40 and 45 lb).

Developmental Tasks of the Preschooler (4 and 5 Years)

Erikson's stage: Initiative versus guilt

- Learning sex differences and developing sex modesty
- Learning to give affection and to share affection
- Beginning to interact with age-mates
- Relating emotionally to parents, siblings, and others
- Learning to identify with male and female adult roles
- Learning simple concepts about the social and physical world
- Learning to distinguish right and wrong, being obedient, and developing a conscience

Height

Preschool children grow about 5 to 6.25 cm (2.0 to 2.5 in) each year. Thus by 5 years of age, they double the birth length and measure 100 cm (40 in).

Vision

Preschool children are generally hyperopic (farsighted). As the eye grows in length, it becomes emmetropic (it refracts light normally). If the eyes become too long, the child becomes myopic (nearsighted).

Motor Development

By 5 years of age, children are able to wash their hands and face and brush their teeth. They are self-conscious about exposing their body and go to the bathroom without telling others.

Typically, preschool children run with increasing skill each year. By 5 years of age, they run skillfully and can jump three steps. Preschoolers can balance on their toes and dress themselves without assistance.

Psychosocial Development

Erikson writes that the major developmental crisis of the preschooler is initiative versus guilt. See Table 22–6 on page 466. Preschoolers must solve problems in accordance with their consciences. Their personalities develop. Erikson views the crises at this time as important for the development of the individual's self-concept.

Parents and caregivers can enhance the development of the preschoolers by:

1. Praising effort at new activities
2. Providing opportunities to repeat new activities until they are mastered

Emotional Development

According to Erikson, preschoolers must learn what they can do. As a result, preschoolers imitate behavior, and their imagination and creativity become lively.

Preschoolers also become increasingly aware of themselves. They play with their bodies largely out of curiosity. They know where the body begins and ends as well as the correct names for the different parts. By 5 years of age, they are able to draw a person including all the features. Preschoolers also learn about their feelings; they know the words *cry, sad, laugh* and the feelings related to them. They also begin to learn how to control their feelings and behavior.

Learning Adaptive Mechanisms

The preschooler uses the same types of coping mechanisms in response to stress as the toddler does, although protest behavior (kicking, screaming) is less likely to occur in the older preschooler. Preschoolers usually have greater ability to verbalize stress.

During the preschool years, four adaptive mechanisms are learned: identification, introjection, imagination, and repression. **Identification** occurs when the child perceives the self as similar to another person and behaves like that person. For example, a boy may internalize the attitudes and gender behavior of his father. **Introjection** is similar to identification. It is the assimilation of the attributes of others. When preschoolers observe their parents, they assimilate many of their values and attitudes. **Imagination** is an important part of preschoolers' life. The preschooler has an active imagination and fantasizes in play; for example, a chair becomes a beautiful throne to a girl, and she is the ruler. **Repression** is removing experiences, thoughts, and impulses from awareness. The preschooler generally represses thoughts related to the Oedipus or Electra complex.

Language and Speech

By 4 years of age, children tend to believe that what they know is right. They tend to be dogmatic in their speech. Four-year-olds love nonsense words such as *jump-jump* and can string them together much to an adult's exasperation. At 4, children are aggressive in their speech and capable of long conversations, often mixing fact and fiction.

By 5 years of age, speaking skills are well developed. Children use words purposefully and ask questions to acquire information. They do not merely practice speaking as 3- and 4-year-olds do, but speak as a means of social interaction. Exaggeration is common among 4- and 5-year-olds.

Social Development

Preschool children gradually emerge as social beings. At the age of 3 or 4, they learn to play with a small number of their peers. They gradually learn to play with more people as they grow older.

Relationships

Preschoolers participate more in the family than they did previously; however, they also start to play with their peers. In associations with neighbors, family guests, and babysitters, too, they learn about relationships.

The phase of close emotional relationship with both parents changes to the phase Freud referred to as the Electra or Oedipus complex (Engel 1962, pp. 90–104). At this time, the child focuses feelings of love chiefly on the parent of the opposite sex, and the parent of the same sex may receive some hostile feelings. At this time, the child begins to develop sexual interests. The child becomes interested in clothes and hair styles.

Cognitive Development

The preschooler's cognitive development, according to Piaget, is the phase of intuitive thought. This phase is an extension of the preconceptual phase. The child is still egocentric, but egocentrism gradually subsides as he or she encounters wider experiences. Preschoolers learn through trial and error, and they think of only one idea at a time. They do not understand relationships such as those between mother and father or sister and brother. Children start to form concepts in late toddlerhood or the early preschool years. Preschoolers become concerned about death as something inevitable, but they do not explain it. They also associate death with others rather than themselves.

Most children at the age of 5 years can count pennies; however, the opportunity to spend money usually does not occur until they attend school. Reading skills also start to develop at this age. Young children like fairy tales and books about animals and other children.

At this age, the preschooler may experience conflict with the introduction of a new baby into the family. Parents' time and affection are now shared, and the preschooler may react jealously.

Moral Development

Preschoolers are capable of prosocial behavior, i.e., any action that a person takes to benefit someone else. See Figure 24–2. The term *prosocial* is synonymous with *kind* and connotes sharing, helping, protecting, giving aid, befriending, showing affection, and giving encouragement (Schulman and Mekler 1985, p. 232).

At this stage of development, preschoolers do not have fully formed consciences; however, they do develop some internal controls. Moral behavior is largely learned by modeling, initially after parents and later after significant others. The preschooler usually behaves well in social settings.

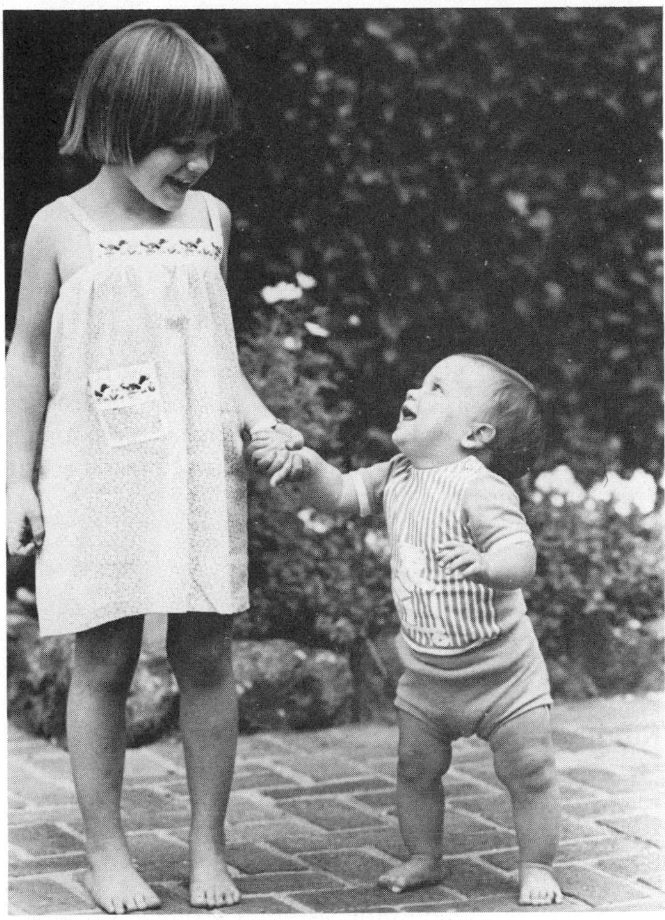

Figure 24–2 Preschoolers are capable of deriving pleasure from helping and encouraging others.

Children who perceive their parents as strict may become resentful or overly obedient. Preschoolers usually control their behavior because they want love and approval from their parents. Moral behavior to a preschooler may mean taking turns at play or sharing.

Nurses can assist parents by discussing moral development and encouraging parents to give preschoolers recognition for actions such as sharing. It is also important for parents to answer a preschooler's "why" questions and discuss values with them.

Spiritual Development

Many preschoolers enroll in Sunday school or faith-oriented classes. The preschooler usually enjoys the social interaction of these classes. According to Fowler, children between the ages of 4 to 6 years are at the intuitive-projective stage of spiritual development. See Table 22–12 on page 474.

Faith at this stage is primarily a result of the teaching of significant others, e.g., parents and teachers. Children learn to imitate religious behavior, e.g., bowing the head in prayer, although they don't understand the meaning of the behavior. Preschoolers require simple explanations, like those in picture books, of spiritual matters. Children at this age use their imaginations to envision such ideas as angels or the devil.

Health Promotion and Protection

Health promotion and protection during the preschool years center on accident prevention, nutrition, dental care, play, and guidance. Therefore, the nurse's role is largely related to detecting children at risk and counseling children and their parents about health.

Assessing Growth and Development

Assessment guidelines for growth and development of the preschooler are shown below.

Nutrition and Fluid

Preschool children still need milk in addition to a balanced diet of fruit, vegetables, bread, cereals, and meat or fish daily. Children eat much like adults except that they need smaller quantities. Generally, a preschooler's age is a good guide to the size of a serving: 4-year-olds eat 4 Tbsp servings of foods from each group at each meal; 5-year-olds eat 5 Tbsp servings.

Preschoolers also require sufficient protein for the growth of new tissues. A child who weighs 13.6 kg (30 lb) requires 37 gm of protein daily as well as 30 mg of vitamin C. The latter is found in fruits, fruit juices, and some vegetables. One medium orange contains 55 mg of vitamin C.

Preschool children also require snacks, usually in the morning, afternoon, and evening. A snack might be a glass of milk and a sandwich. They usually eat one food at a time and often dislike coarse-textured and strong-tasting foods.

Nurses caring for hospitalized or ill children need to be aware of children's special nutritional requirements.

The preschooler is even less susceptible to fluid imbalances than the toddler. The average 5-year-old weighing 20 kg (44 lb) requires at least 45 ml of liquid per kilogram of body weight per day or 900 ml every 24 hours (Mott et al. 1985, p. 1754). The water requirements are generally estimated to be 1 liter per 1000 kcal of food intake. See Chapter 42.

Nursing Assessment Guidelines for the Preschooler

Does the preschooler:

- Indicate physical development within a normal range?
- Possess physical skills appropriate for the age?
- Demonstrate that he or she is toilet trained?
- Perform simple hygiene measures and dress and undress self?
- Play cooperatively with peers?
- Display imagination and creativity?
- Exhibit appropriate emotional expressions in different situations?
- Understand right and wrong, and respond to others' expectations about behavior?
- Ask questions and exhibit increasing vocabulary?
- Appear eager to do things and to please others?
- Identify with people of own sex?

Elimination

The preschooler's elimination control should be complete at this age. The bladder capacity is between 600 to 750 ml. With a change of environment, e.g., due to hospitalization, the preschooler may be incontinent. Incontinence is usually very distressing to the child. Nurses can assist hospitalized preschoolers by learning about their elimination habits at home and continuing these as much as possible. If a preschooler has an "accident," he or she should not be punished or ridiculed.

Protection

Accidents continue to be the major cause of mortality among preschool children. These children are active and often clumsy and are therefore susceptible to injury. Accidents can be prevented in two ways: control of the environment and education of the child. Parents may need to learn to control the environment, for instance, by keeping matches out of the child's reach, teaching the child to put toys away when they are not being used, and safeguarding swimming pools and other potentially dangerous areas. The education of the preschooler may involve learning how to cross streets, what traffic signals mean, and how to ride a bicycle safely.

Preschoolers who have not yet been immunized may need to be so before they can enter school. Regular dental examinations are essential at this age; caries develop quickly in young children. Examinations usually are initiated at about 2½ years. It has been estimated that 80% of children have some tooth decay. Deciduous teeth guide the entrance of permanent teeth; therefore, abnormally placed or lost deciduous teeth can cause the misalignment of permanent teeth. Dental care also involves teaching children to brush after each meal and before retiring. For additional information on dental care, see Chapter 36.

Stimulation

Preschoolers spend most of the day playing. Play serves a number of purposes:

1. Children learn to cooperate with others.
2. Focus changes from family to peers.
3. Children develop strength and coordination.
4. Abundant energy is dispersed.
5. Children have an avenue to express initiative and imagination.

Play is also fun. Preschoolers take it seriously but express joy and pleasure during play. Play at this age is loosely organized. Preschoolers who are hospitalized can frequently have play time included in their nursing plans.

Sexuality

Preschoolers are very much aware of their sexual identity. They often imitate sexual stereotypes. Because boys are traditionally permitted to take more risks than girls, they have a higher incidence of accidents. In contemporary American society, boys and girls participate in many of the same activities.

Preschoolers are aware of the two sexes and identify with the correct sex. Preschoolers are very curious about others' bodies and sexual function. Questions about others' bodies should be answered simply and truthfully.

Love and Belonging

Preschoolers need to feel they are a part of the family, particularly if a new baby arrives. Jealous of the baby, the preschooler needs additional attention and time to adjust to the new infant.

Guidance is an essential need of preschoolers. Guidance and discipline should be consistent and fair. Through guidance, they gain a sense of security and the feeling that their parents care about them. It is important that parents follow through with a punishment once it is imposed; a child confined to his or her room for 1 hour should stay the full hour. In a hospital setting, nurses often must provide the guidance normally given by parents.

Self-Esteem

The preschooler emerges from toddlerhood with a sense of self which he or she continues to develop and refine. The successful accomplishment of tasks builds self-esteem. Acceptance in new social roles, e.g., brother, son, or daughter, also enhances self-esteem.

School-Age Children (6 to 12 Years)

The school-age period starts when children are about 6 years of age, when the deciduous teeth are shed. This period includes the preadolescent (prepuberty) period. It ends at about 12 years, with the onset of puberty. Puberty is the age when the reproductive organs become functional and secondary sex characteristics develop. Because the average age of onset of puberty is 10 for girls and 12 for boys, some people define the school-age years as 6 to 10 for girls and 6 to 12 for boys. Skills learned during this stage are particularly important in relation to work later in life and willingness to try new tasks.

Starting school is significant for a number of reasons; for one, children are able to compare their skills to those of their peers. They also receive impressions of how their skills are perceived by others: the teacher, the school nurse, and their peers. These perceptions can bolster a child's self-image or can weaken feelings of self-worth. In general, the period from 6 to 12 years is one of rapid and dramatic change. The developmental tasks of this period are shown to the right.

Developmental Tasks of School-Age Children (6 to 12)

Erikson's stage: Industry versus inferiority

- Building a wholesome attitude toward oneself
- Developing and refining skills in the use of small muscles
- Learning to form friendships with peers
- Learning to give as much love as one receives
- Learning appropriate behaviors for the masculine and feminine role and identifying with contemporaries of the same sex
- Learning to use language to exchange ideas or to influence listeners
- Learning more rules and developing a beginning scale of values, inner moral control, and respect for moral rules

Physical Development

Appearance

School-age children at 7 years gain weight rapidly and thus appear less thin than previously. Individual differences due to genetic influences and environment are generally obvious at this time.

Weight

At 6 years, boys tend to weigh about 21 kg (46 lb), about 1 kg (2 lb) more than girls. The weight gain of school children from 6 to 12 years of age averages about 3.2 kg (7 lb) per year, but the major weight gains occur from age 10 to 12 for boys and from age 9 to 12 for girls. By 12 years of age, boys and girls weigh on the average 40 to 42 kg (88 to 95 lb); girls are usually heavier.

Height

At 6 years, both boys and girls are about the same height, 115 cm (46 in). They are about 150 cm (60 in) by 12 years. Before puberty, children of both sexes have a growth spurt, girls between 10 and 12 years and boys between 12 and 14 years. Thus, girls may well be taller than boys at 12 years, although the boys are usually stronger. The extremities tend to grow more quickly than the trunk, thus school-age children's bodies appear somewhat ill-proportioned.

Vision

The depth and distance perception of children 6 to 8 years of age is accurate. By age 6, children have full binocular vision: The eye muscles are well developed and coordinated, and both eyes can focus on one object at the same time. Because the shape of the eye changes during growth, the farsightedness of the preschool years gradually changes to 20/20 vision during the school-age years; 20/20 vision is usually well established between 9 and 11 years of age. In later childhood, myopia is not uncommon; that is, the child is able to see clearly only objects that are close. This problem is generally corrected by eyeglasses.

Teeth

Permanent teeth start to appear between 6 and 7 years of age, and dental caries also can appear. Thus regular dental checkups are needed. By the age 13 or 14, children have most of their permanent teeth with the exception of their third molars (wisdom teeth), which erupt between 17 and 24 years of age.

Posture

By 6 years, the thoracic curvature starts to develop, and the lordosis disappears. Full adult posture is not assumed, however, until after the complete development of the skeletal musculature during the adolescent period.

Reproductive and Endocrine Changes

Very little change takes place in the reproductive and endocrine systems until the prepuberty period. During prepuberty, at about ages 9 to 13, endocrine functions slowly increase. This change in endocrine function can result in increased perspiration and more active sebaceous glands. As a result, acne may develop, particularly on the face, neck, and back.

Certain physical changes occur in both boys and girls during prepuberty. Some of the changes in approximate sequence are as follows:

For the boy:

1. The testes and scrotum increase in size.
2. The skin over the scrotum changes color; it becomes reddened and stippled.
3. The breasts may enlarge slightly, but this growth disappears in a few months.
4. Sparse, downey pubic hair grows at the base of the penis.
5. The penis gradually becomes wider and longer. Development of the genitals to adult size takes about 5 to 6 years.
6. The boy grows taller, and his shoulders widen.
7. Axillary sweating begins.

For the girl:

1. The pelvis and hips broaden.
2. The breast tissues develop and may be tender. At first the nipple is slightly elevated, at 7½ to 8 years of age. The areolae become somewhat protuberant and enlarged between the ages of 9 and 11 years.
3. Axillary sweating begins.
4. The initial growth of pubic hair occurs at 8 to 14 years.
5. Vaginal secretions become milky and change from an alkaline to an acid pH, and vaginal flora change from mixed to Döderlein's lactic acid–producing bacilli (Murray and Zentner 1985, pp. 253–54).

Motor Development

During the middle years (6 to 10), children perfect their muscular skills and coordination. By 9 years, most children are becoming skilled in games of interest, such as football or baseball. These skills are often associated with school, and many of them are learned there. By 9 years most children have sufficient fine motor control for such activities as building models or sewing.

Psychosocial Development

According to Erikson, the central task of school-age children is industry versus inferiority. At this time children begin to create and develop a sense of competence and perseverance. School-age children are motivated by activities that provide a sense of worth. They concentrate on mastering skills that will help them function in the adult world. Although children of this age work hard to succeed, they are always faced with the possibility of failure, which can lead to a sense of inferiority. If children have been successful in previous stages, they are motivated to be industrious and to cooperate with others toward a common goal (Erikson 1963).

Sullivan refers to this period (7 years to adolescence) as the preadolescent stage, during which genuine human relationships develop. Sullivan believes that peer relationships are highly significant at this time (Hall and Lindzey 1970, p. 148).

Parents and caregivers can assist school-age children to develop psychosocially by:

1. Recognizing success and providing praise for achievements
2. Guiding the child to perform tasks in which he or she is likely to succeed
3. Guiding the child to complete the task
4. Teaching the child how to get along with peers by collaborating, compromising, cooperating, and competing
5. Teaching the child how to get along with adults

Emotional Development

In school, children have the restraints of the school system imposed on their behavior and learn to develop controls. Children compare their skills with those of their peers in a number of areas, including motor development, social development, and language. This comparison assists in the development of self-concept. Schoolchildren can sometimes be cruel in their honesty, and teachers often need to intercede to assist children who have limitations.

Learning Adaptive Mechanisms

The schoolchild develops a number of adaptive mechanisms. Four of these are regression, malingering, rationalization, and ritualistic behavior.

Regression is returning to a form of behavior that was suitable at an earlier age. For example, the child who is anxious about starting school may start bedwetting at night or perhaps revert to baby talk. **Malingering** is a familiar mechanism to schoolchildren. It is pretending to be ill rather than facing something unpleasant; the child who feels sick the morning before a test may be malingering.

Rationalization is an attempt to justify behavior by logical reason and explanation. A girl who does not make the swimming team may rationalize to her parents by saying she really did not try because she doesn't want swimming to interfere with her piano lessons.

Ritualistic behavior is demonstrated by schoolchildren in many settings. For example, a child may walk down the sidewalk without stepping on a crack. Clubs and gangs often have rituals of membership. These rituals become very important to schoolchildren even though they usually do not persist for a long time. For example, the boy who must have a shower every morning may forget this ritual after a few weeks.

Language and Speech

The average length of sentences spoken by children increases until the age of 9½, at which time sentence length stabilizes or decreases slightly. Boys tend to lag behind girls in speech development. They usually speak with shorter sentences, and their grammar is less correct. Children between 8 and 12 years often boast to win peer approval. Children between 8 and 12 also engage in name calling; frequently, it is done to gain attention.

Social Development

As they grow older, schoolchildren learn to play with more children at one time. Usually the 6- or 7-year-old is a member of a peer group. This group can be a greater influence than the family in teaching attitudes. During late childhood, children join a gang, a small group of peers, which is formed by the children themselves. It is usually informal and transitory, and the leadership changes from time to time. During this period of socialization with others, children gradually become less self-centered and selfish and more cooperative and conscious of the group.

Cognitive Development

According to Piaget, the ages 7 to 11 years mark the phase of concrete operations. See Table 22–8 on page 469. During this stage, the child changes from egocentric interactions to cooperative interactions. See Figure 24–3. School-age children also develop an increased understanding of concepts that are associated with specific objects, for example, environmental conservation or wildlife preservation. Children at this time also develop logical reasoning from intuitive reasoning. For example, they learn to add and subtract to obtain an answer to a problem.

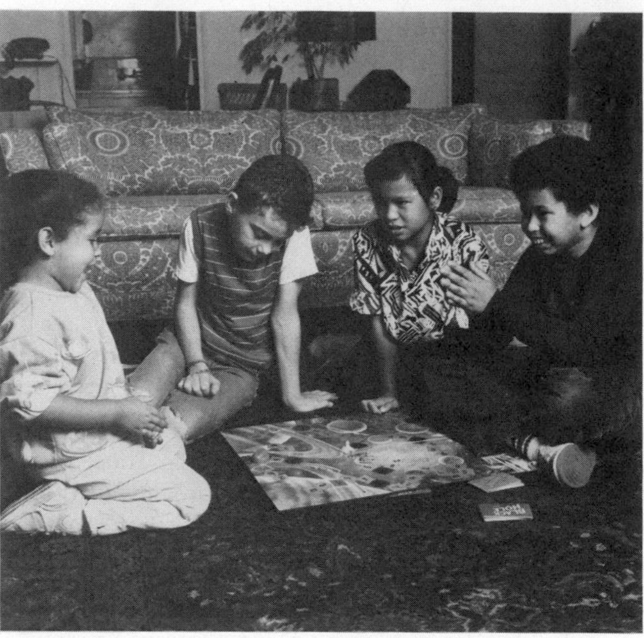

Figure 24–3 The expanding cognitive skills of school-age children enable cooperative interactions of an increasingly complex nature, as shown by the children playing this board game.

Children also learn about cause-and-effect relationships at this age, e.g., they know that a stone will not float because it is heavier than water.

Money is a concept that gains meaning for children when they start school. By the time they are 7 or 8 years old, children usually know the value of most coins.

The concept of time is also learned at this age. By 6 years of age, children enter school; the schedule in school helps them to learn time periods, but it is not until 9 or 10 years of age that children are able to understand the long periods of time in the past. Knowing the time of day and the day of the week are relatively easy for children because they relate time to routine activities. For example, a girl may go to school Monday through Friday, play on Saturday, go to Sunday school on Sunday morning, and go out with her father Sunday afternoon. Children are beginning to read a clock by the time they are 6 years old.

Later in childhood reading skills are usually well developed, and what a child reads is largely influenced by the family. By 9 years of age, most children are self-motivated. They compete with themselves, and they like to plan in advance. By 12 years, they are motivated by inner drive rather than by competition with peers. They like to talk, to discuss different subjects, and to debate.

Moral Development

Some school-age children are at Kohlberg's stage 1 of the preconventional level (punishment and obedience), i.e., they act to avoid being punished. Some school-age children, however, are at stage 2 (instrumental-relativist orientation). These children do things to benefit themselves. Fairness, e.g., everyone getting a fair share or chance, becomes important. Later in childhood, most children progress to the conventional level. This level has two stages: Stage 3 is the "good boy–nice girl" stage, and stage 4 is the law and order orientation. See Table 22–10 on page 471. Children usually reach the conventional level between the ages of 10 and 13. The child shifts from the concrete interests of individuals to the interests of groups. The motivation for moral action at this stage is to live up to what significant others think of the child (Hersh et al. 1979, pp. 71–74).

Spiritual Development

According to Fowler, the school-age child is at stage 2 in spiritual development, the mythical-literal stage. Children learn to distinguish fantasy from fact. Spiritual facts are those beliefs that are accepted by a religious group, whereas fantasy is thoughts and images formed in the child's mind. Parents and the minister, rabbi, or priest help the child distinguish fact from fantasy. These people still influence the child more than peers in spiritual matters.

When the child does not understand events such as the creation of the world, he or she uses fantasy to explain them. The school-age child needs to have concepts such as prayer presented in concrete terms. For example, the child thinks of God as having human qualities, e.g., as a kind old man or a person who punishes when behavior does not meet his standards.

School-age children may ask many questions about God and religion in these years and will generally believe that God is good and always present to help. Just before puberty, children become aware that their prayers are not always answered and become disappointed. At this age, some children reject religion, while others continue to accept it. This decision is largely influenced by the parents. If a child continues religious training, the child is ready to apply reason rather than blind belief in most situations.

Health Promotion and Protection

The school-age child understands what health and illness are even though their ideas may differ from those of adults. Wood found that school-age children believed illness was caused by germs, self, or an outside force, e.g., the rain or an accident (Wood 1983, pp. 103–4).

School-age children are usually taught preventive health practices such as dental hygiene and good nutrition by their parents. Most children still need supervision carrying out these practices.

Assessing Growth and Development

Assessment guidelines for growth and development of the school-aged child are shown on the facing page.

Nursing Assessment Guidelines for the School-Age Child

Does the school-age child:

- Indicate physical development within normal range?
- Possess coordinated fine motor skills?
- Read, write, and manipulate numbers?
- Develop a concept of money and its value?
- Apply himself or herself to given physical or mental tasks?
- Begin to solve problems?
- Interact well with parents?
- Interact well with peers?
- Become less dependent on family and venture away from them?
- Control strong and impulsive feelings?
- Begin to understand the importance of sharing with family and peers?
- Like to help others?
- Think of self as likeable and healthy?

Nutrition and Fluid

Most school-age children require a balanced diet including 2400 kcal per day. School-age children eat four or five times a day, including a snack after school. Children need a protein-rich food at breakfast to sustain the prolonged physical and mental effort required at school. Studies reveal that children who eat well-balanced breakfasts have better attitudes and school records than those who skip breakfast (Pipes 1981, p. 173). Undernourished children become fatigued easily and face a greater risk of infection, resulting in frequent absences from school.

The average school-age child generally requires:

1. 4 servings per day of milk or milk products (1 serving equals 1 cup).
2. 2 or more servings per day of meat (1 serving equals 6 to 8 Tbsp).
3. 4 or more servings per day of cereals and breads (1 serving equals ½ to 1 cup or 1 to 2 slices).
4. 4 or more servings per day of green or yellow vegetables and fruits (1 serving equals ⅓ to ½ cup).

Fluid requirements of school-age children vary according to age, activity level, and environmental temperatures. The average healthy 10-year-old schoolchild requires about 2000 to 2500 ml of fluid daily or about 70 to 85 ml of fluid per kilogram of body weight per day (Pipes 1981, p. 73).

Nurses may need to counsel children and their parents about preventing obesity. Obesity in school-age children tends to result in decreased activity as well as psychosocial problems. Obese children may be ridiculed by their peers and discriminated against by peers and adults. Such behavior reinforces an already low self-esteem. Counseling should include:

1. Reviewing the child's eating habits, including snacks
2. Altering meal content
3. Using rewards other than food
4. Regular exercise

Respiration and Circulation

The respiratory and circulatory systems grow as the child grows. The child's gas exchange becomes more efficient, and vital capacity continues to increase.

The heart is still small in proportion to the rest of the body and continues to grow slowly. Since the heart must supply the circulatory needs of the body, sustained physical activity is not desirable because of the strain on the heart. The heart reaches its adult size at puberty.

Protection

By the time children attend school, they are learning to think before they act. They often prefer adult equipment to toys. They want to be active with other children in such activities as bicycling, hiking, swimming, and boating.

Nurses need to teach safety, as follows:

1. Teach school-age children safe ways to use the stove, garden tools, and other equipment.
2. Teach them traffic rules for bicycling.
3. Teach them safety rules for swimming, boating, skateboarding, and other recreations.
4. Supervise them when they use saws, electric appliances and tools, and other potentially dangerous equipment.
5. Teach them not to play with fireworks, gunpowder, and firearms.

During the school-age years, children need boosters for those immunizations given in infancy. Generally, they are given against tetanus, diphtheria, and poliomyelitis. Local health departments have their own recommended schedules, which are revised regularly in light of medical advances. See the schedules in Chapter 33.

Some physicians recommend that girls receive the rubella vaccine before puberty to prevent the possibility of rubella during pregnancy and subsequent congenital defects. Boys need to be protected against mumps, thus preventing subsequent sterility, which can occur as a result of contracting mumps later in life.

Regular dental checkups every 6 months are required during these years. Permanent teeth begin to appear about 7 years and are usually all in place except for the third molars (wisdom teeth) by 12 years of age. Nurses may need to teach children and their parents about regular dental hygiene. See Chapter 36 for additional information.

Stimulation

Play is stimulating to school-age children. They have more friends than preschoolers. In early school years, they like to playact familiar roles, such as police officer or teacher. By the age of 9 or 10 years, they become more interested in skill games, such as football or baseball. Boys and girls of this age separate for play activities and form preadolescent gangs. Membership in the gang is strictly regulated. Often membership in a gang or club is predicated on a skill, such as tying knots, or a ritual, such as making a finger bleed without acknowledging pain. At this age, most children have a best friend, usually someone of the same sex; the child shares feelings, thoughts, and activities with the friend.

Sexuality

The sexual identity of school-age children changes during these years. Both boys and girls are independent and dependent. Sex education should begin for both sexes at this time. Children have many questions, which should be answered truthfully and simply to meet the child's needs. It is also important not to give the child too much information at one time. Parents should be as comfortable as possible giving this information.

During the school-age years, the child learns to identify with the parent of the same sex and learns the behaviors associated with the role of that parent. At this time, the child probably has some conflict with siblings, although this conflict is less severe than it is for the preschooler. Again, the school-age child may resent a new baby, although this is less likely than in preschool years. School-age children may resent the freedom given older brothers and sisters. Parents who compare siblings' accomplishments and talents can cause resentment and rivalry.

Love and Belonging

School-age children begin to enjoy other adults as well as their parents. They want approval from their parents and other significant adults, e.g., teachers. Schoolchildren can discuss matters of discipline with their parents. They may need several alternative courses of action and probably more guidance than discipline. It is important not to embarrass children by disciplining them in front of others. Children also may be confused if a parent provides two messages at once. For example, when a father tells his son that he should not lie, but then tells a lie in front of the child, the child receives two messages.

Self-Esteem

The schoolchild's self-concept continues to mature. Children recognize similarities and differences between themselves and others. The school-age child compares self with others and obtains feedback from teachers and peers. The child who is successful and receives recognition for his or her efforts feels competent and in control of self and of the environment. Children who feel unaccepted by their peers or who receive negative feedback and little recognition can feel inferior and worthless.

Adolescence

Adolescence is a critical period in development. Its length is culturally determined to some extent. In North America, adolescence is longer than in some cultures, extending to 18 years of age for girls and to 20 years for boys. **Adolescence** is the period during which the person becomes physically and psychologically mature and acquires a personal identity. At the end of adolescence, the person is ready to enter adulthood and assume its responsibilities.

Puberty is the first stage of adolescence in which sexual organs begin to grow and mature. **Menarche** (onset of menstruation) begins in girls. **Ejaculation** (expulsion of semen) occurs in boys. For girls, puberty normally starts between 10 and 14 years; for boys, between 12 and 16 years. The adolescent period is often subdivided into three stages: early adolescence lasts from ages 12 and 13; middle adolescence extends from 14 to 16 years; and late adolescence extends from 17 to 18 or 20 years. Late adolescence is a more stable stage than the other two. In the late period, adolescents are involved mostly with planning their future and economic independence. Developmental tasks that should be met by the end of adolescence are shown on the facing page.

Physical Development

During puberty, growth is markedly accelerated compared to the slow, steady growth of the child. This period, marked by sudden and dramatic physical changes, is referred to as the adolescent growth spurt. In boys, the growth spurt usually begins between ages 12 and 16; in girls, it begins earlier, usually between ages 10 and 14. Because the growth spurt begins earlier in girls, many girls surpass boys in height at this time.

Musculoskeletal Changes

Growth is noted first in the musculoskeletal system. This growth follows a sequential pattern: The head, hands, and feet are the first to grow to adult status. Next, the extremities reach their adult size. Because the extremities grow before the trunk, the adolescent looks leggy, awkward, and uncoordinated. After the trunk grows to full size, the shoulders, chest, and hips grow. Skull and facial bones also change proportions: The forehead becomes more prominent, and the jawbones develop.

Physical growth continues throughout adolescence. Growth is fastest for boys at about 14 years, and the maximum height is often reached at about 18 or 19 years. Some men add another 1 or 2 cm to their height during their 20s, as the vertebral column gradually continues to grow. During the period of 10 to 18 years of age, the average American male doubles his weight, gaining about 30 kg (67 lb) and grows about 34 cm (13½ in) (Suitor and Hunter 1980, p. 95).

The fastest rate of growth in girls occurs at about age 12; they reach their maximum heights at about 15 to 16 years. During ages 10 to 18, the average American female gains about 22 kg (49 lb) and grows about 24 cm (9 in) (Suitor and Hunter 1980, p. 95).

Physical growth during adolescence is greatly influenced by a number of factors. Some of these are heredity, nutrition, medical care, illness, physical and emotional environment, family size, and culture. Generally, people in the United States have grown taller in recent years. This increase in average height is thought to be due largely to many of the above factors.

Poor posture is a common problem during adolescence. The risk for postural problems increases among this age group because weight gains may precede a corresponding strengthening of postural muscles.

Organs and Glands

Internal organs also undergo changes. The heart grows larger and stronger, and the heart rate decreases to adult levels. Blood volume and blood pressure increase. The liver, kidney, spleen, and digestive tract enlarge, even though these organs developed functional maturity in the early school years.

The eccrine and apocrine glands increase their secretions and become fully functional during puberty. The **eccrine glands**, found over most of the body, produce sweat. The **apocrine glands** develop in the axillae, anal and genital areas, external auditory canals and around the umbilicus and the areola of the breasts. Apocrine sweat is released onto the skin in response to emotional stimuli only.

Developmental Tasks of Adolescents

Erikson's stage: Self-identity versus role confusion

- Accepting changing body size, shape, and function in relation to others and understanding the meaning of sexual and physical maturity.
- Achieving a socially accepted and satisfying masculine or feminine role and recognizing the distinctions and similarities in each.
- Achieving new and more adult relationships with peers of both sexes.
- Selecting and preparing for an occupation and economic independence.
- Desiring and achieving socially responsible behavior.
- Developing a workable set of values, ideals, and standards as a guide for behavior.

Sebaceous glands also become active under the influence of androgens in both males and females. The sebaceous glands, which secrete **sebum**, become most active on the face, neck, shoulder, upper back, chest, and genitals. When these glands become plugged and inflamed, the result is acne, a condition common in adolescence. Noninflammatory acne appears as open and closed whiteheads and blackheads. Inflammatory acne appears as inflamed skin together with pustules and papules. A **pustule** is a visible collection of pus within the epidermis. A **papule** is a superficial, circumscribed elevation of the skin. Inflammatory acne may cause scarring.

Thorough cleansing of the skin is important in the treatment of acne. A well-balanced diet and avoidance of fatigue, stress, and excessive perspiration are also desirable. Teenagers who find acne a problem should consult a physician.

Sexual Development

During puberty, both primary and secondary sex characteristics develop. **Primary sexual characteristics** relate to the organs necessary for reproduction, such as the testes, penis, vagina, and uterus. **Secondary sexual characteristics** differentiate the male from the female but do not relate directly to reproduction. Examples are pubic hair growth, breast development, and voice changes.

In boys, development of secondary sexual characteristics proceeds in the following order, starting at about 12 years of age:

1. Beginning enlargement of the testes and scrotum, reddening of the scrotal skin, and appearance of long, straight hair at the base of the penis.

2. Enlargement of the penis and appearance of hair over the entire pubic area. At this time, facial hair also appears and the voice deepens.
3. Further growth of the glans penis and further spread of pubic hair, not yet extending to the thighs. This occurs about age 14, when height growth peaks. Axillary hair also begins to grow.

Often, the first noticeable sign that puberty has begun in males is the appearance of pubic hair. The milestone of male puberty is considered to be the first ejaculation, which commonly occurs at about 14 years of age. Fertility follows several months later. Sexual maturity is achieved by age 18.

In girls, development of secondary sexual characteristics proceeds in the following order, starting at about age 11:

1. Increased pigmentation of the nipple.
2. Enlargement in the diameter of the **areola** (darkened area around the nipple) and a small area of elevation around the nipple. This occurs about the age of 12, when height growth peaks. Long, straight, downy hair appears along the labia.
3. Further elevation and enlargement of the breasts and areolas, appearance of hair over entire pubic area, and the onset of menarche at about age 12.
4. Projection of areolas and nipple, further spread of pubic hair, and appearance of axillary hair.
5. Recession of areolas into general breast contour by about age 14 or 15.

Often the first noticeable sign of puberty in females is the appearance of the **breast bud**, although the appearance of hair along the labia may precede this. The milestone of female puberty is the menarche, which occurs about 2 years after the breast bud appears. At first, menstrual periods are scanty and irregular and may occur without ovulation. Ovulation is usually established 1 to 2 years after menarche. Female internal reproductive organs reach adult size about age 18 to 20.

Vital Signs

During adolescence, the pulse rate drops about 10 beats per minute in both boys and girls. The usual pulse rate for boys of 14 years is about 80 beats per minute; by age 18, the pulse drops to about 70 beats per minute. The usual pulse rate for girls of 14 years is 85 beats per minute; it drops to about 75 (Whaley and Wong 1933, inside cover) per minute by age 18.

Adolescents' blood pressure increases until age 14 or 15, when it levels off. At that age, systolic values are about 118 mm Hg, and diastolic values are about 60 mm Hg (Mott et al. 1985, p. 1745).

Psychosocial Development

Self-Identity/Concept

According to Erikson (1963, p. 261), the adolescent seeks answers to "Who am I?" and "What am I to be?" The psychosocial task of the adolescent is the establishment of identity. The danger of this stage is role confusion.

The inability to settle on an occupational identity commonly disturbs the adolescent. Less commonly, doubts arise about sexual identity. Because of the adolescent's dramatic body changes, the development of a stable identity is difficult. Erikson says that adolescents help one another through this identity crises by forming cliques and a separate youth culture. These cliques exclude all those who are "different" in skin color, cultural background, aspects of dress, gestures, and tastes.

Adolescents are usually concerned about their bodies, their appearances, and their physical abilities. Hair styling, skin care, and clothes become very important. Ingroupers of an adolescent clique can be excessively clannish and cruel in excluding out-groupers; this intolerance is a temporary defense against identity confusion (Erikson 1963, p. 236).

In their search for a new identity, adolescents have to refight the battles of many of the previous stages of development. The task of developing trust in self and others is again encountered when the adolescent looks for ideal persons whom he or she can trust and with whom he or she can prove trustworthy. Development of autonomy is restaged in the adolescent's search for ways to express his or her right to choose freely. The search for an occupational role that allows expression of an autonomous, freely chosen direction is one example. Free choice and autonomy present conflicts to the adolescent. Conflict arises between behaving well in the eyes of the parents and behaving in a manner that may expose them to the ridicule of their peers. The sense of initiative is also restaged. The adolescent has unlimited imagination and ambition and aspires to great accomplishments. The sense of industry is reenacted when the adolescent chooses a career. The extent to which these tasks were achieved earlier influences the adolescent's ability to achieve a healthy self-concept and self-identity.

The adolescent needs to establish a self-concept that accepts both personal strengths and weaknesses. Adolescents need to learn to build on their strengths and not be preoccupied by such defects as acne. They gain self-concepts largely from the impressions that others have of them. If others accept defects—e.g., a lost finger—adolescents accept those defects more readily.

Sexual Role Identity

Although sexual identification begins at about 3 or 4 years of age, it is established during adolescence. The adolescent male strives to achieve a masculine sexual identity; the adolescent female, a feminine sexual identity. Because sex roles are becoming less defined in North American society, adopting masculine and feminine roles is increasingly confusing to today's adolescent. Job and family roles are less traditional and sex-specific. In forming a sexual identity, adolescents first fantasize the male or female role and then enact various aspects of that imagined role. In response to their own feelings and that of others, aspects of the role are either adopted or rejected. Later, adolescents begin to establish intimacy with a partner or partners. This intimacy lays the groundwork for the commitments of adulthood. Sexual experimentation is not part of true intimacy, but once intimacy is achieved, sexual activity is included.

Adolescents are sexually active and may engage in masturbation as well as heterosexual and homosexual activity. Homosexual activity during adolescence is not necessarily an indicator of sexual preference, since both gay and nongay adolescents may experiment sexually with persons of the same and opposite sex. Boys have a greater sex drive than girls in late adolescence and therefore often become more experienced. Premarital intercourse and pregnancies are on the rise among adolescents. In one report from Hawaii, 25% of the 400 women who had abortions were adolescents (Gedan 1974, p. 1856).

Adolescence is also a time for forming ideas about what qualities are desired in a life partner. During this time, young people choose the criteria they use later in the selection process.

Family Relationships

About the age of 15 years, many adolescents gradually draw away from the family and gain independence. This need for independence and the need for family support sometime create conflict within the adolescent and between the adolescent and the family. The young person may appear hostile or depressed at times during this painful process.

At this age, adolescents prefer to be with their peers rather than their parents and may seek advice from adults other than their parents. Parents sometimes are bewildered by this stage of development; instead of reducing controls, they increase them, which causes the adolescent to rebel.

Adolescents also have to resolve their ambivalent feelings toward the parent of the opposite sex. As part of resolution, adolescents may develop brief crushes on adults outside the family—teachers or neighbors, for example. Adolescents sometimes adopt some of the attributes of the adults with whom they are infatuated. This modeling can be helpful in the maturing process.

Some of the discord in the family at this time is due to the generation gap. The values of the adolescent may differ from those of the parents. This difference may be difficult for the parents to understand and to accept.

Adolescents still need guidance from their parents, although they appear neither to want it nor to need it. However, adolescents need to know that their parents care about them and that their parents still want to help them. Restrictions and guidance need to be presented in a manner that makes adolescents feel loved. They need consistency in guidance and fewer restrictions than previously. They should have the independence they can handle yet know that their parents will assist them when they need help.

Peer Group Relationships

During adolescence, peer groups assume great importance. See Figure 24–4. The peer group has a number of functions. It provides a sense of belonging, pride, social learning, and sexual roles. Most peer groups have well defined, sex-specific modes of acceptable behavior. In adolescence, the peer groups change with age. They start as single-sex groups, evolve to mixed groups, and finally narrow to couples who share activities.

Dating helps prepare adolescents for marriage by teaching them how to act with members of the opposite sex. In the United States, dating starts early, often by 11

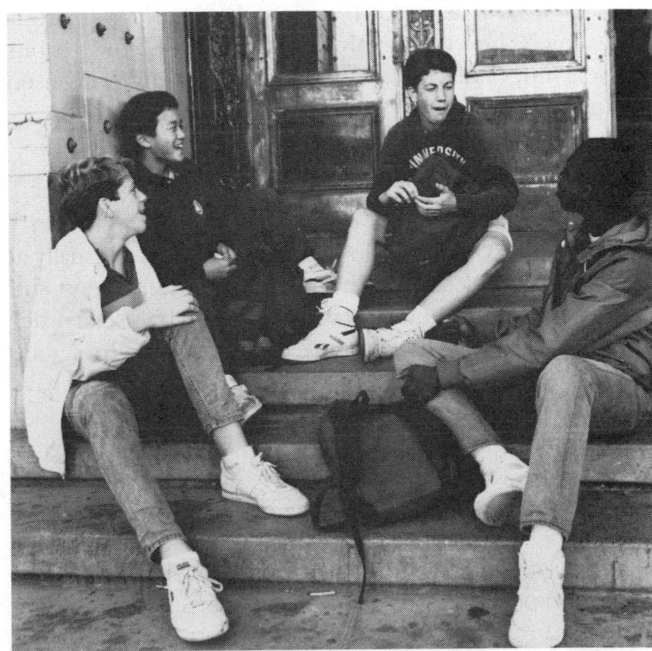

Figure 24–4 Adolescent peer group relationships enhance a sense of belonging, self-esteem, and self-identity.

years for girls and later, perhaps 15, for boys, although dating ages vary with culture, social class, and pressures from society. Some adolescents initially date in groups of couples and eventually progress to going on dates alone.

Not all adolescents, however, are heterosexual. For homosexuals, adolescence is a difficult time. Because peer acceptance is crucial to self-acceptance, lesbian and gay adolescents usually conform to the heterosexual codes and behaviors of their peer groups even though these do not feel natural or correct. Conforming may exact a great personal cost. Adolescents who choose to be openly gay or lesbian face not only the ostracism of their peers but also the misunderstanding and hostility of parents, teachers, and other important adults.

Cognitive Development

Cognitive abilities mature during adolescence. Between the ages of 11 and 15, the adolescent begins Piaget's formal operations stage of cognitive development. The main feature of this stage is that people can think beyond the present and beyond the world of reality. Adolescents are highly imaginative and idealistic. They consider things that do not exist but that might be and consider ways things could be or ought to be. This type of thinking requires logic, organization, and consistency.

The adolescent becomes more informed about the world and environment. Adolescents use new information to solve everyday problems and can communicate with adults on most subjects. The adolescent's capacity to absorb and use knowledge is great. Adolescents usually select their own areas for learning; they explore interests from which they may evolve a career plan. Study habits and learning skills developed in adolescence are used throughout life.

Moral Development

According to Kohlberg, the young adolescent is usually at the conventional level of moral development. Most still accept the Golden Rule and want to abide by social order and existing laws. Adolescents examine their values, standards, and morals. They may discard the values they have adopted from parents in favor of values they consider more suitable.

When adolescents move into the postconventional or principled level, they start to question the rules and laws of society. Right thinking and right action become a matter of personal values and opinions, which may conflict with societal laws. Adolescents consider the possibility of rationally changing the law and emphasize individual rights. Not all adolescents or even adults proceed to this postconventional level. See Kohlberg's stages of moral development in Table 22–10 on page 471.

Spiritual Development

According to Fowler, the adolescent or young adult reaches the synthetic-conventional stage of spiritual development (see Table 22–12 on page 474). As adolescents encounter different groups in society, they are exposed to a wide variety of opinions, beliefs, and behaviors regarding religious matters. The adolescent may reconcile the differences in one of the following ways:

1. Deciding any differences are wrong
2. Compartmentalizing the differences (For example, a friend may not be able to go to dances on Friday evenings because of religious observances, but the friend can share activities on other days.)
3. Obtaining advice from a significant other, e.g., a parent or a minister

Often the adolescent believes that various religious beliefs and practices have more similarities than differences. At this stage, the adolescent's focus is on interpersonal rather than conceptual matters.

Nursing interventions relative to this stage of spiritual development include:

1. Present an open, accepting attitude to adolescents' questions and statements regarding spiritual matters and their implications to health.
2. Arrange for the adolescent to see a member of his or her religious faith if this is desired. An adolescent may want to talk with members of his or her church peer group for support.
3. Provide a comfortable environment in which the adolescent can practice the rituals of his or her faith.

Health Promotion and Protection

Assessing Growth and Development

Assessment guidelines for growth and development of the adolescent are shown on the facing page.

Nutrition

Because of the growth spurt, adolescents have increased nutritional needs to support growth. Adolescents have tremendous appetites; a boy between the ages of 11 and 14 needs 60 kcal per kilogram of body weight per day, decreasing to 42 kcal per kilogram by age 15 to 18; a girl between the ages of 10 and 14 needs 48 kcal per kilogram of body weight per day, thereafter decreasing to 39 kcal per kilogram per day (Howard and Herbold 1982, pp. 280–81).

Nursing Assessment Guidelines for the Adolescent

Does the adolescent:

- Indicate physical and sexual development consistent with standards?
- Interact well with parents, peers, siblings, and persons in authority?
- Like himself or herself?
- Make educational or career plans?
- Have a set of moral values to guide behavior?
- Consider factors contributing to religious beliefs and practices?
- Seek help from appropriate persons about his or her problems?
- Exhibit healthy life-style practices?

The need for protein, calcium, and vitamin D increases during adolescence. An adequate diet for an adolescent is 1 quart of milk per day as well as appropriate amounts of meat, vegetables, fruits, breads, and cereals. See Chapter 42 for further information. Even when adolescents eat nutritionally balanced meals and meet their needs for specific nutrients, they may still require extra calories. This need prompts frequent snacking of high-calorie foods such as cookies, doughnuts, and soft drinks. Parents and nurses can promote better lifelong eating habits by encouraging teenagers to eat healthful snacks.

Common problems related to nutrition and self-esteem among adolescents include obesity, anorexia nervosa, and bulimia.

Obesity Obesity is a common problem of the preadolescent period and continues to be a problem in the adolescent period. It is estimated that 10% to 16% of people between the ages of 10 and 19 years are obese.

Obese adolescents are frequently discriminated against in many ways. They are usually rejected by their peers, badgered by their parents, and ridiculed on television and in the movies. Many feel ugly and socially unacceptable. Depression is not unusual among obese adolescents.

Treatment of obesity in this age group includes education on nutrition as well as assessment of psychosocial problems that may produce overeating.

Anorexia nervosa Under social pressure to be slim, some adolescents severely limit their food intake to a level significantly below that required to meet the demands of normal growth. **Anorexia nervosa** is a severe psychophysiologic condition usually seen in adolescent girls and young women. It is characterized by a prolonged inability or refusal to eat and rapid weight loss in persons who believe they are fat even though they are emaciated. Anorexics may also induce vomiting and use laxatives and diuretics to remain thin. This illness is most effectively treated in the early stages by psychotherapy that also involves the parents. Hospitalization may be necessary when the effects of starvation become life-threatening.

Bulimia An increasing problem among teenagers, **bulimia** is an uncontrollable compulsion to consume enormous amounts of food and then expel it by self-induced vomiting or by taking laxatives. For example, the afflicted person may consume a whole cake, a dozen doughnuts, and a half dozen apple turnovers before inducing vomiting. After prolonged periods of alternately gorging and vomiting, the person no longer needs to induce vomiting; it becomes an uncontrollable reflex. Voluntary organizations are established in some regions to assist individuals with bulimia.

Rest and Sleep

Most adolescents require 8 to 10 hours of sleep each night to prevent undue fatigue and susceptibility to infections. A change in sleep pattern is common in adolescence. Children who once were early risers begin to sleep late in the mornings and occasionally take afternoon naps. The reason for daytime sleeping is not fully understood, but it is possibly a result of physical maturity and reduced nocturnal sleep.

During adolescence boys begin to experience **nocturnal emissions** (orgasm and emission of semen during sleep), known as "wet dreams," several times each month. Boys need to be informed about this normal development to prevent embarrassment and fear.

Sexuality

Adolescents want to know about sex but are often uneasy discussing sexual concerns with their parents. Accurate information needs to be provided by the family, schools, and nurses. One study of 417 high school students assessed what teenagers believed their needs were and what knowledge they already possessed. Most of the students had obtained their first information about sex from friends or from reading while in grade school. The family and school were the other major sources of information (Inman 1975, pp. 217–19).

Some teenagers wanted sex information from both parents, and some wanted the church to be involved. White students had more formal knowledge than nonwhite students, and Protestants and boys had more informal knowledge than Catholic students and girls.

The subjects teenagers wanted included in sex education classes were:

1. Sexually transmitted disease
2. Biology of sexes and reproduction
3. Pregnancy
4. Birth control (requested by boys)
5. What boys think of girls and development of a sexual code of conduct (requested by girls)

Major sexual problems of adolescents are unplanned pregnancies, sexually transmitted diseases, and dysmenorrhea.

Unplanned pregnancies Unplanned pregnancies during adolescence are not uncommon. Adolescents need education about sexuality, sexual actions and consequences, the individual's right to make a decision about ways to express himself or herself sexually, and contraceptive measures. Pills, diaphragms, intrauterine devices (IUDs), the rhythm method, and condoms are discussed in Chapter 19. The incidence of abortion is notable among this group, and those who choose to carry their pregnancies to term have unique needs and problems. Adolescents are high-risk mothers, physiologically and emotionally. Rearing a child as an unwed single parent or placing a child for adoption can precipitate an emotional crisis.

Sexually transmitted disease Sexually transmitted diseases (STDs) are the most common bacterial infections among adolescents. STDs, formerly called veneral diseases, include syphilis, gonorrhea, genital warts, genital herpes virus type 2, chlamydial urethritis or nongonococcal urethritis (NGU), *Trichomonas* and *Candida* infections, and Acquired Immune Deficiency Syndrome (AIDS). *Trichomonas* and *Candida* infections can also be acquired nonsexually. Increases in these diseases are due to two factors: changing sexual mores of the young, which permit increased sexual activity, and an increase in the number of sexual partners. Because the term *sexually transmitted disease* elicits feelings of guilt, shame, and fear, adolescents frequently do not seek medical help as early as they should. Adolescents need education about these diseases, preventive measures, and early treatment. Table 24–1 lists common signs of STDs for which teenagers should seek medical care.

Dysmenorrhea **Dysmenorrhea** (painful menstruation) is prevalent among adolescent females and causes much short-term absenteeism. Cramping, lower abdominal pain radiating to the back and upper thighs, nausea, vomiting, diarrhea, and headaches may occur for a few hours up to 3 days. Dysmenorrhea results from powerful uterine contractions, which cause ischemia and in turn cramping pain. Dysmenorrhea is associated with the release of prostaglandins through the activity of progesterone. Traditional treatments for the symptoms of dysmenorrhea have been bed rest, administration of simple analgesics such as aspirin, application of heat to the abdomen, and certain exercises. Today, treatment with antiprostaglandins such as ibuprofen (Motrin or Advil) and naproxen (Naprosyn) helps many. These drugs, however, should be administered under medical supervision and have potentially toxic effects. Aspirin itself is a mild antiprostaglandin. More recent, nondrug approaches, such as biofeedback, are being used. See Chapter 41 for further information about biofeedback.

Protection

The adolescent needs to be safeguarded from accidents and injury. Accidents are the leading cause of death and injury among adolescents. Motor-vehicle accidents and sports injuries are the most common accidents. Obtaining a driver's license is an important event in the life of an adolescent in the United States and Canada, but the privilege is not always wisely handled. Head injuries and fractures are frequent outcomes of automobile and motorcycle accidents. Adolescents need appropriate instruction about the safe handling of motor vehicles. Parents often need guidance in setting limits on the use of motor vehicles by their teenage children. Limits should be negotiated by the parents and the teenager and periodically reviewed and revised according to the teenager's safety record. Teenagers may use driving as an outlet for stress, as a way to assert independence, or as a way to impress peers. When setting limits on automobile use, parents need to assess the teenager's level of responsibility, common sense, and ability to resist peer pressure. The age of the teenager alone does not determine readiness to handle this responsibility.

Adolescents are at risk for sports injuries because their coordination skills are not fully developed. However, sports activities are important to the adolescent's self-esteem and overall development. In addition to providing beneficial exercise, sports activities enhance social and personal development. They help the adolescent experience competition, teamwork, and conflict resolution. The nurse can help adolescents prevent sports injuries by encouraging:

1. The use of proper safety equipment
2. Appropriate physical examinations before participating in sports
3. Enforcement of regulations that prevent an injured player from further participation in sports activities until a physician advises it

Table 24–1 Clinical Signs of Sexually Transmitted Diseases

Disease	Male	Female
Gonorrhea	Painful urination; urethritis with watery white discharge, which may become purulent.	May be asymptomatic; or vaginal discharge, pain, and urinary frequency.
Syphilis	Chancre, usually on glans penis, which is painless and heals in 4 to 6 weeks; secondary symptoms—skin eruptions, low-grade fever, inflammation of lymph glands—in 6 weeks to 6 months after chancre heals.	Chancre on cervis or other genital areas, which heals in 4 to 6 weeks; symptoms same as for male.
Genital warts (condyloma acuminatum)	Single lesions or clusters of lesions growing beneath or on the foreskin, at external meatus, or on the glans penis. On dry skin areas, lesions are hard and yellow-gray. On moist areas, lesions are pink or red and soft with a cauliflowerlike appearance.	Lesions appear at the bottom part of the vaginal opening, on the perineum, the vaginal lips, inner walls of the vagina, and the cervix.
Herpes genitalis (*Herpes simplex* of the genitals)	Primary herpes involves the presence of painful sores or large, discrete vesicles that last for weeks; vesicles rupture. Recurrent herpes is itchy rather than painful; it lasts for a few hours to 10 days.	Same as for males.
Chalmydial urethritis	Urinary frequency; watery, mucoid urethral discharge.	Commonly a carrier; vaginal discharge, dysuria, urinary frequency.
Trichomonas vaginalis	Slight itching; moisture on tip of penis; slight, early morning urethral discharge. Many males are asymptomatic.	Itching and redness of vulva and skin inside thighs; copious watery, frothy vaginal discharge.
Candida albicans	Itching, irritation, discharge, plaque of cheesy material under foreskin.	Red and excoriated vulva; intense itching of vaginal and vulvar tissues; think, white, cheesy or curdlike discharge.
Acquired Immune Deficiency Syndrome (AIDS)	Symptoms can appear anytime from several months to several years after acquiring the virus. The person has reduced immunity to other diseases. Symptoms include any of the following for which there is no other explanation: persistent heavy night sweats; extreme fatigue; severe weight loss; enlarged lymph glands in neck, axillae, or groin; persistent diarrhea; skin rashes; blurred vision or chronic headache; harsh dry cough; thick gray-white coating on tongue or throat.	

Self-Esteem

Faced with dramatic changes in body structure and function and greater expectations to assume responsibilities, many adolescents experience temporary difficulty in developing a positive self-image. Adolescents who are accepted, loved, and valued by family and peers generally tend to gain confidence and feel good about themselves. Adolescents who have difficulty forming relationships or who are perceived by peers as too different and not included in adolescent cliques may develop less favorable self-images and have low self-esteem. Teenagers with physical handicaps or illnesses are particularly vulnerable to peer rejection. Nurses and educators can promote peer understanding and acceptance by discussing the individual's specific problems with the peer group. Establishing groups of peers who have similar problems can provide an opportunity for the individual to develop close relationships with others and feel valued and accepted.

Common teenage problems related to self-esteem and self-concept include drug abuse, suicide, and homicide, although they can also be considered protection needs.

Drug abuse Drug and substance abuse, including alcohol abuse, is on the rise among teenagers, especially among those with emotional problems. Many adolescents take drugs to have a new experience, to feel they belong to the group and thus relieve loneliness, or to prove they are courageous. This experimental use of drugs is a one-time or infrequent occurrence. Some teenagers, however, use drugs regularly. Compulsive users become dependent on drugs. Some drugs abused by teenagers are alcohol, glue and similar substances, barbiturates and amphetamines, hallucinogens, marijuana, and cocaine.

Teenagers who use drugs habitually create problems for themselves and for the people with whom they associate. These teenagers may need help from physicians and other professionals, such as psychiatrists who specialize in adolescent problems.

Adolescent health promotion programs provided by nurses should include the following information:

1. The underlying reasons for drug use and more positive coping mechanisms to deal with stress
2. The hazards of drug misuse and abuse

3. Responsible ways to make decisions about drug use before experimentation and ways to handle peer pressure

The nurse should also be alert for signs that a teenager is misusing drugs. Some of these are a drop in school achievement, mood swings, sleepiness or fatigue, and personality changes, such as withdrawal or boisterous behavior.

Suicide and homicide Suicide and homicide are two of the leading causes of death among teenagers. Adolescent males are more likely to commit suicide than adolescent females, and blacks are more likely to commit homicide than whites. Suicides by firearms, drugs, and automobile exhaust gases are the most common.

Most suicidal persons give verbal or behavioral warnings prior to suicide, and certain tendencies or behaviors are suspect. For example, most people who commit suicide have made previous attempts, are severely depressed, and are at odds with themselves and those close to them. Such individuals need to be referred to professional help.

Homicide is more common among the poor than other economic classes, and both killers and their victims are more likely to be men than women. Often homicide is associated with alcohol abuse and occurs most frequently at night and on weekends. Factors influencing the high homicide rate include economic deprivation, family breakup, and the availability of firearms, which are the most frequently used weapons. Cutting or stabbing tools are the next most frequently used weapons.

Health promotion programs for adolescents need to include information about suicide, alternatives to suicide, and ways to deal with a peer who might be suicidal.

Chapter Highlights

- Early childhood spans the period from 1 to 6 years and is subdivided into two groups: the toddler group, ages 1 to 3, and the preschool group, ages 4 and 5.
- During childhood, dramatic changes occur in physical, psychologic, and cognitive development; the child moves from being a dependent person to becoming an independent person entering school.
- As the nervous system develops, body systems mature to the point where the child can control his or her body, achieve finer muscle control, and perform all the activities of daily living, such as washing and dressing.
- The child also develops a unique personality and way of behaving.
- From age 2 onward, peers play an important role during play.
- Investigation of sexual differences among peers is common during childhood.
- Critical to psychosocial development during childhood is the development of a sense of autonomy and initiative.
- By the end of early childhood, the child has reached the phase of intuitive thought in cognitive development, has developed some internal moral controls, and is at the undifferentiated level of spiritual development.
- The school-age period of development begins at age 6 and ends with the onset of puberty.
- School-age children perfect their muscular skills and coordination and develop a sense of competence, perseverance, and self-worth.
- During emotional development, school-age children face the conflict of industry versus inferiority.
- Peers are very important to school-age children; same-sex friendships develop.
- School-age children begin to understand relationships and change from being egocentric to having cooperative interactions; according to Piaget, they are in the concrete operations phase of cognitive development.
- Most school-age children progress to the conventional level of moral development and to the mythical-literal stage of spiritual development.
- Adolescence is a critical period of development extending from the onset of puberty to age 18 or 20.
- Rapid growth in height, development of secondary sexual characteristics, sexual maturity, and increasing independence from the family are major landmarks of adolescence.
- The dramatic physical changes of early adolescence require major adjustments in body image.
- Peer groups assume great importance during adolescence; they provide a sense of belonging and self-esteem and facilitate the development of a positive self-concept.
- Late adolescence is a more stable stage, during which the adolescent is mostly involved with planning a future and economic independence.
- Adolescents between the ages of 11 to 15 begin the formal operations stage of cognitive development; they are able to think logically, rationally, and futur-

istically and can conceptualize things as they could be rather than as they are.

- The adolescent is at Kohlberg's conventional level of moral development, and some proceed to the postconventional or principled level.
- Adolescents are at Fowler's synthetic-conventional stage of spiritual development.
- The nurse plays a major role in assessing the growth and development of children and adolescents.
- Because accidents are the leading cause of morbidity and mortality among toddlers, preschoolers, and school-age children, parental guidance about accident prevention is essential.
- Major problems of adolescents that require primary preventive interventions are obesity, anorexia nervosa, bulimia, sexually transmitted disease, unplanned pregnancy, motor vehicle accidents, sports injuries, drug abuse, and suicide.

Suggested Readings

Betz, C. L. March/April 1981. Faith development in children. *Pediatric Nursing* 7:22–25.
Betz examines the transformation in the content of beliefs during childhood and adolescence. She gives nursing interventions for each of five stages of faith.

Boyle, M. P.; Koff, E.; and Gudas, L. J. November/December 1981. Assessment and management of anorexia nervosa. *American Journal of Maternal Child Nursing* 6:412–18.
The authors discuss the disease process and the cause of anorexia nervosa and give a profile of an anorexic adolescent. Common fantasies and family dynamics are included as well as the nursing interventions often required.

Campbell, C. E., and Herten, R. J. September 1981. VD to STD: Redefining venereal disease. *American Journal of Nursing* 81:1629–35.
Campbell and Herten redefine venereal disease (VD) as sexually transmitted disease (STD). They describe a variety of diseases that fall into this category, including herpes progenitalis, trichomoniasis, and nonspecific urethritis. Included is a table of diseases and colored photographs of the organisms and the clinical pictures the diseases present.

Canum, C. August 1984. Developing a peer-helping program for adolescents. *The Canadian Nurse* 81:41–44.
This expert in the field of adolescence outlines eight steps that those developing a peer-helping program need to take. Adolescents who could benefit from a peer helper include pregnant teenagers who refuse to go to prenatal classes, heavy marijuana users who continue their habit despite counseling, overweight teenagers who won't stick to a diet, and diabetics who are unwilling to test their urine.

Parker, K., January 1986. Health works: An adolescent assessment tool. *The Canadian Nurse* 82:28–31.
The House in Toronto, Canada, offers confidential and nonjudgmental help to teenagers about sexuality, substance abuse, and emotional upsets—topics that adolescents say they will probably not discuss with their family physician. Four to six questions are used to assess such areas of functioning as school and work, recreation, tobacco and toxins, sexuality, friends, emotional health, and family. Examples of assessment questions are provided.

Rice, M. A., and Kibbee, P. E. March/April 1983. Review: Identifying the adolescent substance abuser. *American Journal of Maternal Child Nursing.* 8:139–42.
Psychoactive substances make the world seem more bearable to some adolescents. Using alcohol or drugs places the adolescent at high risk for long-term substance abuse. The telltale signs of substance abuse are outlined.

Sande, D. R., and Billingsley, C. S. September 1985. Language development in infants and toddlers. *Nurse Practitioner* 10:39–41, 44–45.
These authors say that nurse practitioners are in a unique position to observe the language development of a young child and the social-communicative interaction between parent and child. A table outlines early milestones in language development that the nurse can use to identify problems.

Webster-Stratton, C. September/October 1983. Recognizing and assessing conduct disorders in children. *American Journal of Maternal and Child Nursing.* 8:330–35.
Nurses can play a vital role in helping parents identify and correct their child's behavioral problems. An outline for a behavioral interview and a parent-child observational assessment tool are presented.

Selected References

Adams, B. N. June 1983. Adolescent health care: Needs, priorities, and services. *Nursing Clinics of North America* 18:237–48.

American Academy of Pediatrics, Committee on Standards of Health Care. 1972. Standards of child health care. In Edleman, C., and Mandle, C. 1986. *Health promotion throughout the life span.* St. Louis: C. V. Mosby Co.

Berzonsky, M. D. 1981. *Adolescent development.* New York: Macmillan.

Betz, C. L. March/April 1981. Faith development in children. *Pediatric Nursing* 7:22–25.

Duvall, E. M. 1977. *Marriage and family development.* 5th ed. New York: J. B. Lippincott.

Engel, G. L. 1962. *Psychological development in health and disease.* Philadelphia: W. B. Saunders Co.

Erikson, E. H. 1963. *Childhood and society.* 2d ed. New York: W. W. Norton and Co.

Fong, B. C., and Resnick, M. R. 1980. *The child: Development through adolescence.* Menlo Park, Calif.: Addison-Wesley Publishing Co.

Gedan, S. October 1974. Abortion counseling with adolescents. *American Journal of Nursing* 74:1856–58.

Griffith-Kenney, J. 1986. *Contemporary women's health: A nursing advocacy approach.* Menlo Park, Calif.: Addison-Wesley Publishing Co.

Guyton, A. C. 1986. *Textbook of medical physiology.* 7th ed. Philadelphia: W. B. Saunders Co.

Haber, J.; Leach, A. M.; Schudy, S. M.; and Sideleau, B. F. 1982. *Comprehensive psychiatric nursing.* 2d ed. New York: McGraw-Hill.

Hall, C. S., and Lindzey, G. 1970. *Theories of personality.* 2d ed. New York: John Wiley and Sons.

Havighurst, R. J. 1952. *Developmental tasks and education.* 2d ed. New York: David McKay Co.

Hersh, R. H.; Paolitto, D. P.; and Reimer, J. 1979. *Promoting moral growth from Piaget to Kohlberg.* New York: Longman.

Howard, R. M., and Herbold, N. H. 1982. *Nutrition in clinical care.* New York: McGraw-Hill.

Inman, M. 1975. What teen-agers want in sex education. Reprinted in O'Connor, A. B., editor. *Contemporary nursing series: Nursing of children and adolescents.* New York: American Journal of Nursing Co.

Kaluger, G., and Kaluger, M. F. 1979. *Human development: The span of life.* 2d ed. St. Louis: C. V. Mosby Co.

Kandell, N. December 1979. The unwed adolescent pregnancy: An accident? *American Journal of Nursing* 79:2112–14.

Maccoby, E. E., and Jacklin, C. N. 1985. The psychology of sex differences (summary and commentary). In Bloom, M. *Life span development: Bases for preventive and interventive helping.* 2d ed. New York: Macmillan.

Mott, S. R.; Fazekas, N. F.; and James, S. R. 1985. *Nursing care of children and families: A holistic approach.* Menlo Park, Calif.: Addison-Wesley Publishing Co.

Murray, R. B., and Zentner, J. P. 1985. *Nursing assessment and health promotion through the life span.* 3d ed. Englewood Cliffs, N.J.: Prentice-Hall.

Nelms, B. C. November/December 1981. What is a normal adolescent? *American Journal of Maternal Child Nursing* 6:402–5.

Pipes, P. L. 1981. *Nutrition in infancy and childhood.* 2d ed. St. Louis: C. V. Mosby Company.

Schulman, M., and Mekler, E. 1985. *Bringing up a moral child: A new approach for teaching your child to be kind, just, and responsible.* Reading, Mass.: Addison-Wesley Publishing Co.

Schuster, C. S., and Ashburn, S. S. 1980. *The process of human development: A holistic approach.* Boston: Little, Brown and Co.

Smith, M. J.; Goodman, J. A.; Ramsey, N. L.; and Pasternack, S. B. 1982. *Child and family: Concepts of nursing practice.* New York: McGraw-Hill.

Suitor, C. W., and Hunter, M. F. 1980. *Nutrition: Principles and application in health promotion.* Philadelphia:: J. B. Lippincott Co.

Whaley, L. F., and Wong, D. L. 1983. *Nursing care of infants and children.* St. Louis: C. V. Mosby Co.

Wood, S. P. March/April 1983. School-aged children's perceptions of the cause of illness. *Pediatric Nursing* 9:101–4.

Zborowski, M. April 1982. Cultural components in response to pain. *Journal of Social Issues* 8:16–30.

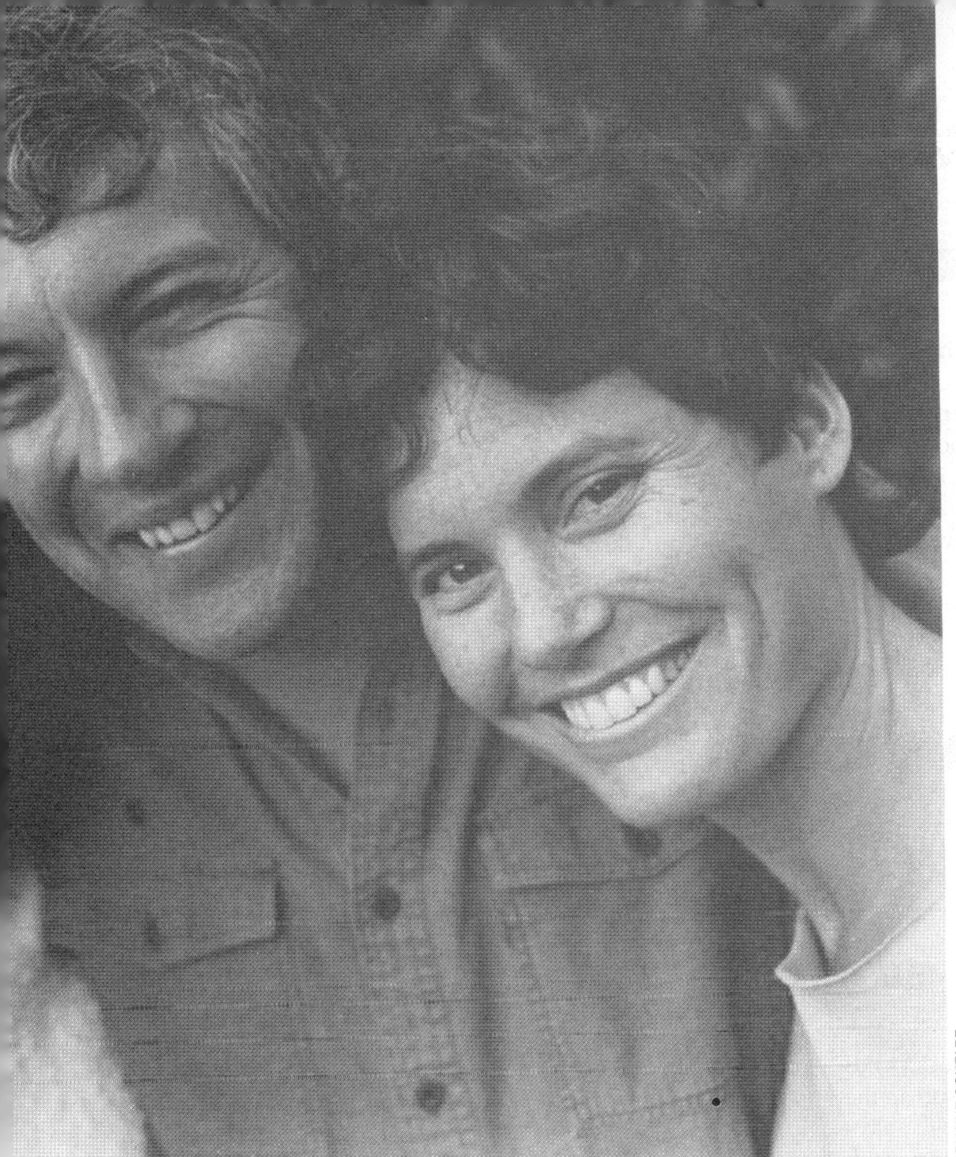
MARIANNE GONTARZ

CHAPTER 25

Young Through Middle Adulthood

Contents

25 *Young Through Middle Adulthood*

Objectives

1. Understand essential facts about development of the young and middle-aged adult.
   1.1 Describe physical changes that occur from young adulthood through middle adulthood.
   1.2 Explain essential aspects of psychosocial development according to Erikson.
   1.3 Describe essential aspects of cognitive development according to Piaget.
   1.4 Explain essential aspects of moral development according to Kohlberg.
   1.5 Explain essential aspects of spiritual development according to Fowler.
2. Understand essential facts about health promotion and protection for the young adult and middle-aged adult.
   2.1 Identify common health hazards of the young and middle-aged adult.
   2.2 Discuss nursing implications related to common health hazards.

Terms

chronic disease
climacteric
generativity
maturity
menopause
principled reasoning

Adulthood and Maturity

The age at which a person is considered an adult depends on how adulthood is described. Legally, a person in the United States can vote at 18 years. The legal age for alcohol consumption outside the home varies among states from 18 years to 21 years.

Another criterion of adulthood is financial independence, which is also highly variable. Some adolescents support themselves as early as 16 years of age, usually because of family circumstances. By contrast, some adults are financially dependent on their families for many years, as for example, during prolonged education.

Adulthood may also be indicated by moving away from home and establishing one's own living arrangements. Yet this independence is also highly variable. Some adolescents leave home perhaps because of family problems, whereas some people in their 20s remain at home because they are unable to obtain work. The latter is not unusual during periods of economic depression.

Maturity is the state of maximal function and integration or a state of being fully developed. Maturity in the adult can be described by the following:

1. The individual has developed a system of internal and external behavior controls that are acceptable on the adult level. In other words, the person can control emotions and behavior in a way acceptable to society.
2. The individual has developed a value-judgment system that enables him or her to live acceptably in a social group. This system reflects a personal philosophy of what is important and unimportant, good and evil, desirable and undesirable. The value system helps people makes choices (Kaluger and Kaluger 1979, p. 372).

Mature people have a number of traits. Kaluger and Kaluger (1979, pp. 372–74) describe a mature person as one whose behavior reflects a balance of intellectual insight, emotion, and imagination. The person learns to live with problems that cannot be solved and looks for solutions to problems that can be solved. Mature people have some knowledge of the requirements for living in society, take responsibility for their own behavior, and do not expect others to make decisions for them.

Many other traits are generally recognized as representative of maturity. Mature individuals are judiciously realistic with a reflective sense of values, guided by an underlying philosophy of life that they maintain with integrity, and open to new experiences and continued growth. In addition, mature people adapt to others and can tolerate and control most stresses; they have warmth, compassion, and respect for others. They are also integrated, accepting of themselves, self-reliant, capable of loving relationships, and creative (Heath 1965).

Young Adults

The adult phase of development encompasses the years from the end of adolescence to death. Because the developmental tasks of young adults differ from those of older adults, adulthood is often divided in three phases—the young adult phase, the middle-aged adult phase, and the elderly adult phase. In this book young adults are defined as people 20 to 40 years old; middle-aged adults, as 40 to 65; and elderly adults, over 65.

During young adulthood, people have a number of developmental tasks. See below. They become independent of their families, establish careers, often establish a close relationship with a significant other, and decide whether to have children. The young adult is typically a busy person who faces many challenges.

Physical Development

Persons in their early 20s are in their prime years physically. The musculoskeletal system is well developed and coordinated. This is the period when athletic endeavors reach their peak. Indeed, after 40 years, most athletes are considered old.

All other systems of the body are also functioning at peak efficiency. The circulatory system is well developed. Pregnant women, for example, are able to provide additional blood supplies to the placenta. The reproductive system is fully developed. The woman's menstrual cycle is regular, and sexual organs are sufficiently mature to cope with childbearing. The man's sexual maturity, reached in adolescence, remains at a peak so that the sexual urge remains high throughout this phase. In summary, physical change is minimal during this phase; psychosocial development, by contrast, is great.

Psychosocial Development

According to Erikson, the central task of the young adult is intimacy versus isolation. Young adults are viewed as developing an intimate, lasting relationship with another person or a cause, institution, or creative effort (Erikson 1963, p. 263). The basic strength that evolves from this relationship is love, the outcome of negative resolution is exclusivity (Erikson 1982, p. 33).

Peck identifies three growth trends during young adulthood: stabilization of identity, humanization of values, and expansion of caring (White 1975). See Chapter 22, page 477.

Gould also studied adult development. He believes that transformation is a central theme during adulthood: "Adults continue to change over the period of time considered to be adulthood and ... developmental phases may be found during the adult span of life" (Gould 1972, p. 33). The group Gould studied is divided into seven different age groups:

1. The first group, 16 to 18 years, repeated the theme "We have to get away from our parents." They considered themselves to be part of the family rather than individuals.
2. The second group, 18 to 22 years, felt their autonomy was established but in jeopardy. They felt that they could be pulled back into the family.
3. The third group studied, 22 to 28 years, felt quite established as adults and autonomous from their families. They saw the self as well defined but felt they still had to prove their competence as adults to their parents. They repeated the theme "Now is the time for living as well as growing and building for the future." They also felt their lives were on the right course.
4. In the fourth group studied, ages 29 to 34 years, marriage and career lines were well established, but they questioned what life is all about. They no longer saw the necessity of proving themselves and wanted to be accepted as they are.
5. The next group, ages 35 to 43 years, continually looked within and questioned themselves, their values, and life itself. They had the sense that they had very little time left to shape the behavior of adolescent sons and daughters. In general, they saw time as finite.
6. In the next age period, 43 to 50 years, people were resigned to time as finite and felt their personalities were set. They had a special interest in social activities, friends, and spouse. They actively looked for sympathy and affection from their spouses.

Developmental Tasks of Early Adulthood

Erikson's stage: Intimacy versus isolation

- Select a life partner
- Choose an occupation or career
- Establish independence from parents and financial self-sufficiency
- Establish intimate relationships
- Establish a social network
- Form a personal philosophy and ethical structure

7. In the seventh group, ages 50 to 60, there was decreasing negativism and increasing mellowing and warming. The spouse was seen as a valuable source of companionship. In this period of transformation, there was a realization of mortality and a concern for health (Gould 1972, pp. 525–27).

Young adults face a number of new experiences and changes in life-style. They must make decisions for themselves, and many of the decisions made now influence the person's life-style in years to come. The expectations of the young adult are often taken for granted, since they are well defined in most cultures. Choices must be made about education and employment, about whether to marry or remain single, about starting a home, and about rearing children. Social responsibilities include forming new friendships and assuming some community activities.

Selecting Education and Employment

Today, education is more important than ever. It enhances employment opportunities, enriches leisure time, and ensures economic survival. Occupational choice and education are largely inseparable. Education influences occupational opportunities; conversely, an occupation, once chosen, can determine the education needed and sought.

In the past, young men were encouraged more than young women to pursue advanced education, particularly college education. Traditionally, education was deemed unnecessary for women in the roles of wife and mother. This notion has changed and the role of women has changed. Many now choose to assume active careers and civic roles in society.

Staying Single

Remaining single is becoming the life-style of more and more North Americans. Many people choose to remain single, perhaps to pursue an education and then to have the freedom to pursue their chosen vocations.

Some unmarried individuals choose to live with another person of the opposite or same sex and share living arrangements and certain expenses. Some unmarried people are gay or lesbian and live with or are involved with a partner to whom they are committed.

Nurses should not assume that an unmarried person has no partner. Discrete, sensitive, and unprejudiced questioning of a client can often elicit information about a friend or support person who is especially significant to the client.

Because single adults may live alone or with other adults who are employed, problems can arise when single persons are ill. Finding someone to drive them to a hospital or to help with shopping and meals during recuperation can be major challenges. A support system for a single adult may take more organization than the support system of a married person.

Choosing a Life Partner

Deciding on a life partner is a difficult task. It is in many ways more complex and confusing than other tasks required of the young adult. In North America, there is emphasis on falling in love as a basis for mate selection. However, the multiple aspects of love make it difficult for some people to recognize and to know the meaning of love. Numerous definitions of love are available in literature, but the one important aspect of love is that it is lasting. Love survives times of frustration, strained relationships, and sadness, as well as times of happiness and achievement. It evolves out of interaction and requires adjustments and readjustments of the personalities of the people involved. There is a desire to do all one can to make the other person's life meaningful. In contrast, infatuation is sexually stimulating and exciting, but it is too shallow to nurture total personal growth of either partner and lasts only a short time.

Cognitive Development

Piaget believes that cognitive structures are complete during the formal operations period, from roughly 11 to 15 years. From that time, formal operations (for example, generating hypotheses) characterize thinking throughout adulthood and are applied to more areas. Egocentrism continues to decline; however, according to Piaget, these changes do not involve a change in the structure of thought, only a change in its content and stability (Miller 1983, pp. 62–65).

Moral Development

Young adults who have mastered the previous stages of Kohlberg's theory of moral development now enter the postconventional level. See Table 22–10 on page 471. At this time, the person is able to separate self from the expectations and rules of others and to define morality in terms of personal principles. When individuals perceive a conflict between society's rules or laws, they judge according to their own principles. For example, a person may intentionally break the law and join a protest group to stop hunters from killing wild animals, believing that the principle of conservation of wildlife justifies the protest action. This type of reasoning is called **principled reasoning.**

Spiritual Development

According to Fowler, the individual enters the individuating-reflective period sometime after 18 years of age. During this period, the individual focuses on reality. A

27-year-old adult may ask philosophic questions regarding spirituality and may be self-conscious about spiritual matters.

Health Promotion and Protection

Common health hazards during young adulthood include accidents, infections, suicide and homicide, drug abuse, obesity, and hypertension.

Assessing Growth and Development

Assessment guidelines for growth and development of the young adult are shown below.

Nursing Assessment Guidelines for the Early Adult

Does the young adult:

- Feel independent from parents?
- Have a realistic self-concept?
- Like self and the direction in which life is going?
- Interact well with family and friends?
- Have an enriching intimate relationship?
- Have a meaningful social life?
- Have a well-established career or occupation?
- Demonstrate emotional, social, and economic responsibility for own life?
- Have a set of values that guides behavior?
- Have a healthy life-style?

Accidents

Accidents are a leading cause of death. In 1977, motor vehicle accidents were the leading cause of mortality among people 15 to 24 years old (U.S. DHHS 1984, p. 19). Alcohol consumption was associated with 60% of these fatalities.

Nursing has a preventive function in this regard, in particular relative to changing attitudes that allow people to drive recklessly and while intoxicated.

Infections

Sexually transmitted diseases (STD) such as genital herpes, syphilis, and gonorrhea are the most common bacterial infections in young adults. Nursing functions are largely educational. The use of condoms greatly reduces the transfer of infectious microorganisms from one partner to another. Knowledge about the symptoms of these diseases can help the client obtain early treatment. In dealing with clients with STD, the nurse must be nonjudgmental and accepting of the client's life-style and treat any information obtained as confidential.

Upper respiratory tract infections also occur frequently in young adults. Nursing function is largely preventive: reducing the individual's susceptibility by supporting body defenses through adequate nutrition, rest, liquids, and exercise. Part of prevention is reducing susceptibility by teaching the dangers of alcohol, cigarettes, and contaminants. When ill, the young adult should be encouraged to obtain medical treatment rather than risk chronic respiratory problems later in life.

Suicide and Homicide

Suicide is the third leading cause of death among teenagers and young adults. Homicide accounts for 10% of all deaths among teenagers and young adults: 7% of all deaths among whites and nearly 30% among blacks in this age group (U.S. DHEW 1984, p. 19). Measures to prevent suicide include (Murray and Zentner 1985, p. 460):

1. Educating the public about the early signs of suicide
2. Establishing significant relationships for high-risk people
3. Encouraging young adults to participate in social activ ities thus preventing isolation

Nursing counseling services and crisis facilities can often assist young adults at times of high stress to make important decisions and constructive adaptations to their environments, thereby decreasing the incidence of suicide and homicide.

Drug Abuse

Drug abuse is a major threat to the health of young adults. Alcohol, marijuana, amphetamines, and cocaine, for example, can bring about feelings of well-being that may be highly valued by people with adjustment problems. Prolonged use can lead to physical and psychologic dependency and subsequent health problems. For example, drug abuse during pregnancy can lead to fetal damage. Prolonged use of alcohol can lead to such diseases as cirrhosis of the liver and cancer of the esophagus.

Nursing strategies related to drug abuse include teaching about the complications of their use, changing individual attitudes toward drug abuse, and counseling regarding problems that lead to drug abuse.

Smoking is another type of drug abuse that can lead to such diseases as cancer of the lung and cardiovascular disease. The nurse's role regarding smoking is to (a) serve as a role model by not smoking; (b) provide educational information regarding the dangers of smoking; (c) help make smoking socially unacceptable, e.g., by posting "no smoking" signs in client lounges and offices; and (d) suggest resources, e.g., hypnosis, life-style training, and behavior modification, to clients who desire to stop smoking.

Obesity

Physical growth is completed during adolescence or early adulthood. Caloric needs are highly individual, depending primarily on the physical activity of the individual, the climate, and body size. Most people require fewer calories than they did during adolescence because of the cessation of growth. The average 25-year-old woman needs 2000 kcal per day; the average man, 2700 kcal per day (National Academy of Sciences 1980, p. 23).

Young adults usually lead busy lives, and fast foods may make up much of their diets. Nurses can counsel clients about the need for a balanced, nourishing diet that includes fruits and vegetables. Exercise should also be encouraged, because people who exercise regularly are less likely to overeat.

Hypertension

High blood pressure is a major cause of illness in young adults. In the United States, 13% to 17% of whites and 26% to 28% of blacks age 20 and older have both high blood pressure and weight problems (Edelman and Mandle 1986, p. 491). Nursing strategies to prevent and treat hypertension are largely educational. Clients must reduce the intake of foods that are high in cholesterol, fat, and salt.

Breast and Testicular Self-Examination

Of all cancers among women, cancer of the breast is the most frequent cause of death. The peak incidence of breast cancer is during middle age. However, the young woman needs to form the habit of examining the breasts regularly. The effectiveness of treatment increases significantly the earlier a breast lump is discovered.

Testicular cancer accounts for approximately 1% of all the cancer in men and often occurs in men in their early 30s (Crooks and Baur 1983, p. 129). It is most commonly found on the anterior and lateral surfaces of the testes. See Figure 25–1. This cancer is often serious and requires extensive surgery if discovered in the later stages. In the early stages, the cancer is asymptomatic except for a mass within the testicle. The lump often feels hard and bumpy and can usually be differentiated from tissue around it. The patient may also experience a feeling of heaviness in the scrotum.

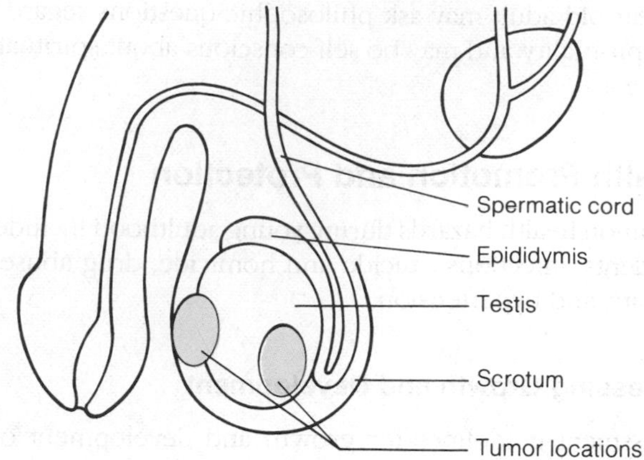

Figure 25–1 Common tumor locations of the testes.

Breast self-examination Breast self-examination (BSE) should be conducted once a month. A regular time is best, such as immediately following menstrual flow or on the first day of the month.

Women who examine themselves regularly become familiar with the shape and texture of their breasts. Any changes must be reported immediately to a physician for accurate diagnosis. Before beginning to teach BSE to a client, the nurse needs to identify the client's attitudes toward this procedure. Some women are reluctant to conduct BSE because they fear what they might find. The nurse needs to explore these fears with the client. Women often offer these reasons for avoiding BSE: "I don't have time" and "I just don't think of doing it." The nurse also needs to explore these reasons with the client with particular reference to her self-esteem (see Chapter 48) and her need to spend time on herself.

Another reason for not conducting BSE is a reluctance to handle the breasts. Manipulation may be associated with fondling and masturbation. This reason often goes unexpressed among older women and some religious and cultural groups. Changing such attitudes frequently requires in-depth counseling as well as accurate information about BSE. A woman may accept information only after attitudes have changed.

BSE has three stages: the first takes place in the bath or shower; the second takes place while the client sits in front of a mirror; and the third takes place while the client lies down. During a bath or shower, the woman checks for any lumps or thickenings by moving flat fingers over every part of each breast. Fingers glide easily over wet skin. The right hand is used to examine the left breast, and the left hand is used to examine the right breast.

In the second stage, the woman sits before a mirror with hands first at the sides and then clasped over the head. Each breast is observed in both positions for:

1. Indentations, rippling, puckering, or dimpling
2. Asymmetry of the nipples; e.g., a nipple pulled to one side

3. Discoloration
4. Discharge from the nipple
5. Any change in the size or shape of the breasts

Dimpling can be caused by scar tissue formation or a lesion. See Figure 25–2. Show the client how to accentuate any retraction by raising her arms above her head, pushing her hands together with elbows flexed (see Figure 25–3, *A*), or pressing her hands down on her hips (see Figure 25–3, *B*).

The client conducts the last part of the examination while lying in bed and palpating the breasts. Instruct the client to palpate the breast as follows:

1. To examine the right breast, place a pillow or folded towel under the right shoulder and the right hand behind the head. This position distributes breast tissue more evenly on the breast.
2. With the left hand:
   a. Press the palmar surfaces of the middle three fingers on the skin surface, starting in the upper lateral quadrant, i.e., the outermost top of the breast.
   b. Use a gentle rotating motion to press the breast tissue against the chest wall.
   c. Palpate from the periphery to the areola.
   d. Move the peripheral starting point around the breast clockwise. See Figure 25–4.
   e. Finally, squeeze the nipple of each breast gently between the thumb and index finger. Note any clear or bloody discharge.
3. Repeat the above for the left breast with a pillow under the left shoulder and the left hand behind the head.
4. Report a lump or nipple discharge to the physician immediately. A ridge of firm tissue in the curve of each breast is normal.

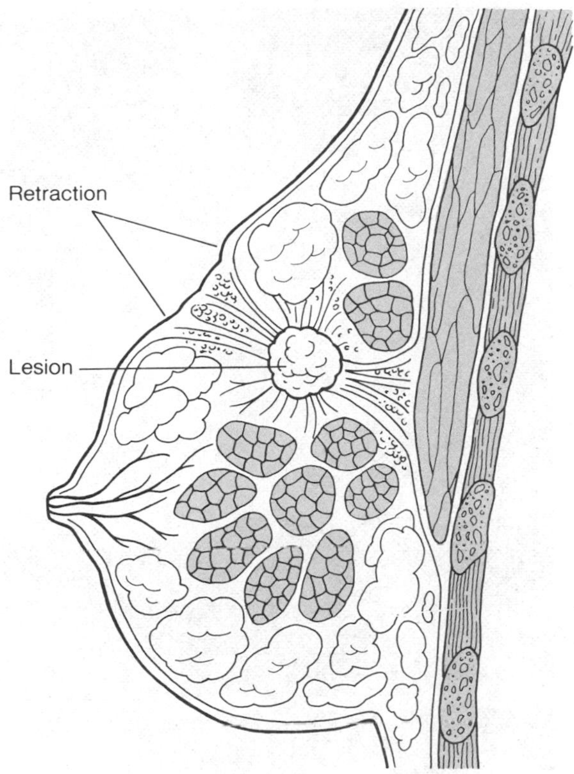

Figure 25–2 A breast lesion can cause retraction or dimpling of breast tissue.

Testicular self-examination Testicular self-examination should be conducted monthly. The client can examine the testicles while he sits, stands, or lies down. A good time for this exploration is after a hot bath or shower since the heat causes the scrotal skin to relax and the testes to descend. Instruct the man to:

1. Examine the testicles one at a time.
2. Use the fingertips to gently probe the surface as if examining an egg for imperfections. The surface should be smooth and fairly firm.
3. Using the thumb and fingers of both hands and placing one hand under the scrotum and the other over the scrotum, palpate the testicle. It normally feels rubbery, smooth, and free of lumps.
4. After palpating both testicles, compare the weights of the testicles.
5. Then palpate the epididymis, which is at the top of the testicle and extends behind it. It should feel soft and slightly tender.
6. Last, locate the spermatic cord, which ascends from the epididymis behind the testicle. It normally feels firm and smooth (Murray and Wilcox 1978, p. 2074).

Middle-Aged Adults

The middle years, from 40 to 65, have been called the years of stability and consolidation. For most people, it is a time when children have grown and moved away or are moving away from home. Thus, partners generally have more time for and with each other and time to pursue interests they may have deferred for years. Middle adulthood has a number of broad developmental tasks. See page 533.

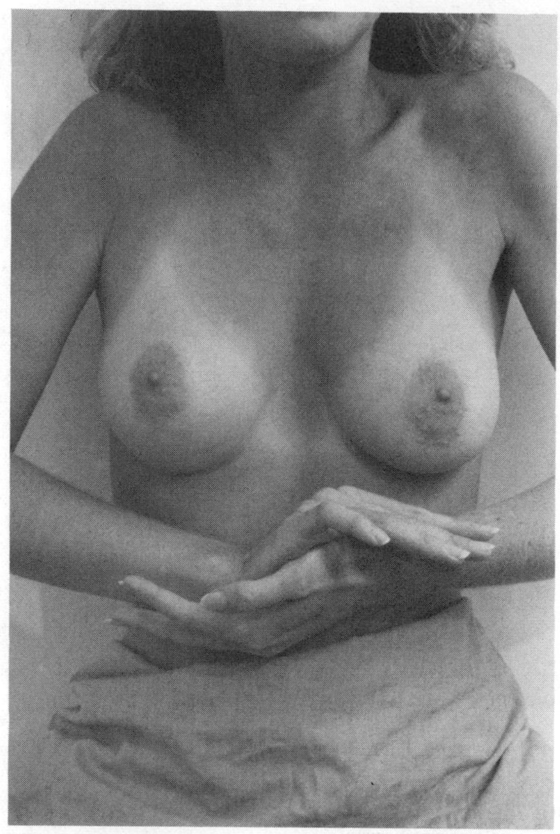

A

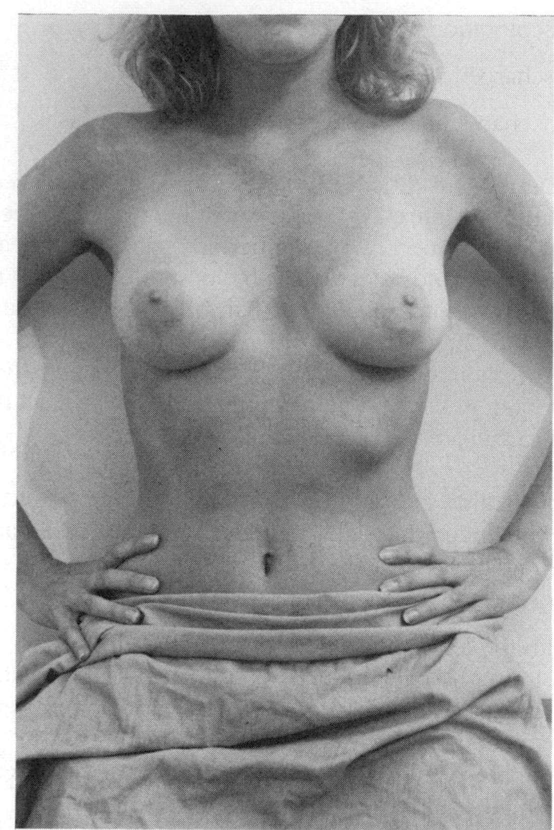

B

Figure 25–3 Retraction of breast tissue can be accentuated by **A,** pressing the hands together, or **B,** pressing the hands down on the hips.

Physical Development

A number of changes take place during the middle years. At 40, most adults can function as effectively as they did in their 20s. However, during ages 40 to 65, physical changes do take place. Some of these are as follows:

1. Gray hair appears.
2. Crease lines appear at the lateral aspects of the eyes (laugh lines).
3. Fatty tissue is redistributed in men and women; men tend to develop fat on their abdomens, and women also deposit fat around the middle of the body.
4. Energy is more slowly recovered and more quickly expended. Vigor and endurance start to deplete at about 40 years.
5. Hearing acuity decreases and sight diminishes; reading glasses or bifocals may be needed.
6. Skeletal muscle bulk decreases at about 60 years.
7. General slowing of metabolism results in weight gain.
8. Hormonal changes take place in both men and women (see following section).

Hormonal Changes

Both men and women experience decreasing hormonal production during the middle years. The **menopause** refers to the so-called change of life in women, when menstruation ceases. The **climacteric** (andropause) refers to the change of life in men, when sexual activity decreases. Sometimes *climacteric* is also used to refer to that time in the life of women when conception is no longer possible.

The menopause usually occurs anywhere between ages 40 and 55. The average is about 47 years. At this time, the ovaries decrease in activity until ovulation ceases. A number of menstrual patterns can signal the menopause. Four of these are:

1. Periods remain regular, but menstrual flow decreases.
2. Periods occur irregularly, and some periods are missed.
3. Menstrual flow ceases abruptly.
4. Menstrual flow occurs irregularly, with irregular amount of menses.

During this time, the ovaries decrease in size, and the uterus becomes smaller and firmer. Progesterone is not produced, and the estrogen levels fall. Although the pituitary gland continues to produce the luteinizing hormone (LH) and the follicle-stimulating hormone (FSH), the ovaries do not respond. As a result of the lack of feedback, the pituitary gland increases the production of the gonadotropins, in particular FSH. This disturbed endocrine balance accounts for some of the symptoms of the menopause. Common symptoms are hot flashes, chilliness, a tendency of the breasts to become smaller and flabby, and a tendency to become obese. Insomnia and headaches also occur with relative frequency. Psychologically, the menopause can be an anxiety-producing time, especially if the ability to bear children is an integral part of the woman's self-concept.

In men, there is not a change comparable to the menopause in women. Androgen levels decrease very slowly; however, men can father children even in late life. The psychologic problems that men experience are generally related to the fear of getting old and to retirement, boredom, and finances.

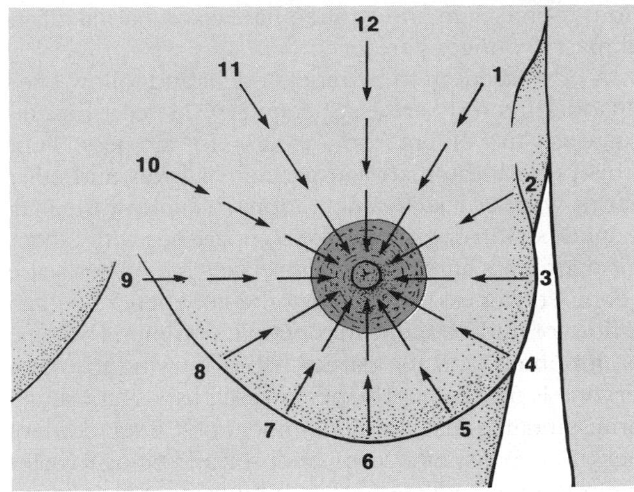

Figure 25–4 This clockwise palpation method for breast self-examination ensures that all parts of the breast are examined.

Psychosocial Development

Until recently, the developmental tasks of middle-aged adults have received little attention. Erik Erikson (1963, p. 266) viewed the developmental choice of the middle-aged adult as generativity versus stagnation. **Generativity** is defined as the concern for establishing and guiding the next generation. In other words, there is concern about providing for the welfare of humankind that is equal to the concern of providing for self. People in their 20s and 30s tend to be self- and family-centered. In middle age, the self seems more altruistic, and concepts of service to others and love and compassion gain prominence. These concepts motivate charitable and altruistic actions, such as church work, social work, political work, community fund-raising drives, and cultural endeavors. Marriage partners have more time for companionship and recreation; thus, marriage can be more satisfying in the middle years of life. There is time to work together in volunteer activities. There is time for one partner to go out for lunch and for the other to go fishing. Generative middle-aged persons are able to feel a sense of comfort in their lifestyle and receive gratification from charitable endeavors. Erikson believes that persons who are unable to expand their interests at this time and who do not assume the responsibility of middle age suffer a sense of boredom and impoverishment, i.e., stagnation. These persons have difficulty accepting their aging bodies and become withdrawn and isolated. They are preoccupied with self and unable to give to others. Some may regress to younger patterns of behavior, e.g., adolescent behavior. At this time, adults usually face a number of adjustments in relation to their relationships and activities. Husbands and wives generally have more time for leisure activities. Relationships with families change. Children move away and marry and have children of their own. Parents are elderly and often have additional needs. Thus people in their 40s and 50s often find themselves grandparents, enjoying their grandchildren but having few responsibilities for them, and at the same time assisting with the care of their own elderly parents. At this time people often face the death of a parent and as a result come to terms with their own aging and inevitable death.

Developmental Tasks of Middle Adulthood

Erikson's stage: Generativity versus stagnation

- Accepting the changes of middle age
- Investing in a new generation
- Adjusting to the needs of aging parents
- Reevaluating life's goals and accomplishments

For adults who are career oriented, these years often represent the peak professional and occupational performance. Adults have many experiences behind them, which, together with intellectual skills, permit them to be effective in many areas, such as financial and career endeavors.

Retirement plans are also essential for middle-aged people. It is important that feelings about retirement be considered and that thought be given to ways in which increased leisure time is used. Middle-aged people who plan ahead for the financial needs of retirement and establish new ways to keep active often adapt to the retirement situation more effectively than those who do not.

Changing Self-Image and Self-Concept

The middle-aged person looks older and feels older. People usually accept the fact that they are aging; however, a few try to defy the years by their dress and even their actions. Some men and women have extramarital affairs and marry younger partners.

A new freedom to be independent and follow one's individual interests arises. Sheehy (1977) describes this change as a movement from "us-ness" to "me-ness." Prior to this period, the marriage partner or lover and other persons were crucial to a definition of self. Now the middle-aged person does not make comparisons with others, no longer fears aging or death, relaxes his or her sense of competitiveness, and enjoys the independence and freedom of middle age. Other people's opinions become less important, and the earlier habit of trying to please everyone is overcome. The person establishes ethical and moral standards that are independent of the standards of others. The focus shifts from inner self and being to outer self and doing. Religious and philosophical concerns become important.

Developing Alternative Abilities

The stereotyped image of women at mid-life as lonely, depressed, and clinging pathetically to the past—"the empty nest syndrome"—is a fallacy, according to a study by Rubin. Almost all of the women she spoke with responded to the pending or actual departure of their children with a decided sense of relief (Rubin 1969, p. 15). Even women who were divorced were relieved to be freed of the responsibilities of mothering and happy to be able to call their lives their own.

In middle age, the interests set aside in favor of family and career can be renewed and developed. Hobbies such as photography, collecting antiques, or painting may develop into serious work. Some people who deferred education now pursue it or take refresher and other courses to keep abreast of changes. Some women enter the work force. Many middle-aged people feel a mixture of excitement and fear about these new undertakings.

Midlife Crisis

Gail Sheehy (1977) suggests that the transition into middle life is as critical as adolescence. She outlines characteristics of the midlife crisis and calls the decade between the ages of 35 to 45 the "deadline decade."

According to Sheehy, most women pass through the midlife crisis between 35 and 40; most men, between 40 and 45. This crisis occurs when a person recognizes he or she has reached the halfway mark of life. Although people of these ages are reaching their prime, there is a beginning recognition that time is at a premium and that life is finite. Youthfulness and physical strength can no longer be taken for granted.

Sheehy (1977, p. 44) describes this midlife crisis as an "inner crossroads" or "footbridge" leading to the second half of life. It is an "authenticity" crisis in which people face the discrepancy between their youthful ambitions and their actual attainment. To overcome this crisis, people need to reexamine their purposes and reevaluate ways to use their abilities and energies from now on. In Sheehy's words, it is a time when people ask, "Why am I doing all this? What do I really believe in? Is this all there is?" The parts of self that have been previously suppressed now need to be expressed. Both men and women in midlife crises sense a feeling of urgency and perhaps despair when they look at those options they have set aside and realize that aging and ill health may soon hinder such opportunities.

Lillian Rubin (1979, p. 6), in her study of 160 women between the ages of 35 and 54 and from all walks of life, describes midlife for women as a time of endings and also a time of beginnings. The words of one woman (a 44-year-old student and homemaker married 22 years to a businessman) clearly express this beginning and ending and her strong desire to change her primary tasks of marriage and motherhood to something more, something new: "Twenty years of kids and doctors and chauffeuring and PTA and bridge and all that talk, talk, talk about nothing is enough. I got so I knew I couldn't stand another afternoon of that kind of talk. Enough! There's got to be more to life than hot flashes and headaches" (Rubin 1979, p. 155). Rubin does not define midlife for women as a stage tied to a chronological age. Rather, it is that point in the life cycle of the family when the children are grown and gone, or nearly so, and when perhaps for the first time in her adult life a woman can attend to her own needs, desires, and development as a separate and autonomous being (Rubin 1979, p. 7).

Women often respond to a midlife crisis by entering the job market or attending college. Men may respond by seeking second careers, by seeking promotions into management, by departing from well-established base lines (such as marriage), or by becoming more interested in developing themselves personally. Some people become self-destructive. When people confront the midlife crises constructively, they can feel revitalized; the middle years of life can be the happiest years of one's life. When people do not make changes through this transition stage, they experience a sense of staleness and feelings of resignation.

Some characteristics of the midlife crisis include:

1. Feeling bored, burdened, restless, and unappreciated
2. Dissatisfaction with the way one's life has developed
3. Ambivalence and uncertainty about the future
4. Dismay about signs of aging
5. Fear that time will be insufficient to accomplish goals
6. Feelings of self-doubt
7. Need to search for self, i.e., establish a true identity
8. Worry about health
9. Feelings of sadness, loneliness, or depression

Cognitive Development

The middle-aged adult's cognitive and intellectual abilities change very little. Cognitive processes include reaction time, memory, perception, learning, problem solving, and creativity. According to Murray and Zentner, reaction time during the middle years stays much the same or diminishes during the later part of the middle years. Memory and problem solving are maintained through middle adulthood. Learning continues and can be enhanced by increased motivation at this time in life. Middle-aged adults are able to carry out all the strategies of Piaget's phase of formal operations, see Chapter 22, page 468. The middle-aged person can "reflect on the past and current experience and can imagine, anticipate, plan and hope" (Murray and Zentner 1985, pp. 515–17.

Moral Development

According to Kohlberg, the adult can move beyond the conventional level to the postconventional level. Kohlberg believes that extensive experience of personal moral choice and responsibility is required before people can reach the postconventional level. Kohlberg found that few of his subjects achieved the highest level of moral reasoning. To move from stage 4, a law and order orientation, to stage 5, a social contract orientation, requires that the individual move to a stage in which rights of others take precedence. People in stage 5 take steps to support another's rights.

Spiritual Development

Not all adults progress through Fowler's stages to the fifth, called the paradoxical-consolidative stage. At this stage, the individual can view "truth" from a number of viewpoints. Fowler's fifth stage corresponds to Kohlberg's fifth stage of moral development. Fowler believes that only some individuals after the age of 30 years reach this stage.

In middle age, people tend to be less dogmatic about religious beliefs, and religion often offers more comfort to the middle-aged person than it did previously. People in this age group often rely on spiritual beliefs to help them deal with illness, death, and tragedy.

Health Promotion and Protection

Common health hazards during middle adulthood include: obesity, chronic diseases, smoking, excessive use of alcohol, neoplasms, and sexually transmitted diseases (STD).

Assessing Growth and Development

Assessment guidelines for growth and development of the middle-aged adult are shown on this page.

Nursing Assessment Guidelines for Middle Adulthood

Does the middle-aged adult:

- Accept aging body?
- Feel comfortable with and respect self?
- Adjust to increasing independence of children?
- Adjust to increasing dependence of parents?
- Enjoy new freedom to be independent?
- Feel a sense of comfort in his or her career and life-style?
- Interact well and share companionable activities with life partner?
- Expand or renew previous interests?
- Pursue charitable and altruistic activities?
- Consider plans for retirement?
- Have a meaningful philosophy of life?
- Follow preventive health care practices?

Obesity

Obesity, which remains a problem in middle age, is associated with such disorders as diabetes and cardiovascular problems. Weight tends to increase with age. Decreased metabolism together with decreased activity mean a decreased need for calories. For each decade after 25 years, there should be a 7.5% reduction in total calories consumed (Williams 1981, p. 474).

Nurses often need to counsel people in this age group to prevent or reduce obesity by reducing caloric intake and increasing exercise, which together help the client attain and maintain weight loss (Overfield 1980, p. 26).

Chronic Diseases

A **chronic disease** is a condition that lasts for longer than 3 months (Edelman and Mandle 1986, p. 526). Chronic diseases common in middle age are heart disease, osteoarthritis, cancer, pulmonary disease, glaucoma, and diabetes. The nurse can assist clients by advising regular screening for these diseases and encouraging the individual to attain and maintain an optimum level of health. See Chapter 20.

Smoking

Heavy smoking increases the risk of pulmonary cancer, cardiovascular disease, and chronic obstructive lung disease. See the section on drug abuse earlier in the chapter for additional information.

Excessive Use of Alcohol

The excessive use of alcohol is a multifaceted problem for the individual and society. Use of the drug is part of the life-style of many Americans and Canadians. Excessive use can result in unemployment, disrupted homes, accidents, and diseases. It is estimated that four million people in the United States are dependent on alcohol and can be considered alcoholics.

Nurses can help clients by providing information about the dangers of excessive alcohol use, by helping the individual clarify values about health, and by referring the client to special groups such as Alcoholics Anonymous.

Neoplasms

Cancer accounts for considerable mortality and morbidity in both men and women. It is the second leading cause of death among people between the ages of 25 and 64 in the United States. The patterns of cancer types and incidences for men and women have changed over the past several decades. Over one-third of the deaths due to cancer occur between the ages of 35 to 64. Men have a higher incidence of cancer of the lung and bladder than women. In women, breast cancer is highest in incidence followed by cancer of the colon and rectum, uterus, and lung. See Figure 25–5.

Female clients should learn to make monthly breast self-examinations and male clients should palpate their testicles monthly in order to detect growths. See the section on self-examination earlier in this chapter. Postmenopausal women should report any vaginal bleeding. For information on sexually transmitted diseases, see the section on infections earlier in this chapter.

Chapter Highlights

- An adult reaches maturity when he or she has developed a system of internal and external controls and a value-judgment system that enables the person to live acceptably within a social group.
- The mature person takes responsibility for his or her own behavior and does not expect others to make his or her decisions.
- The young adult is in essentially a stable period physically but psychosocial change is great.
- Cognitive development continues throughout adulthood.
- Some young adults enter Kohlberg's postconventional level of moral development and develop principled reasoning.

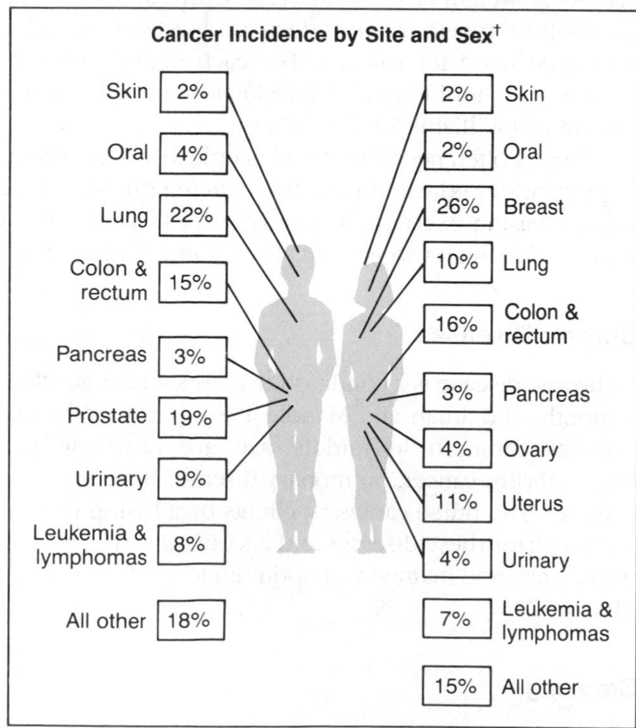

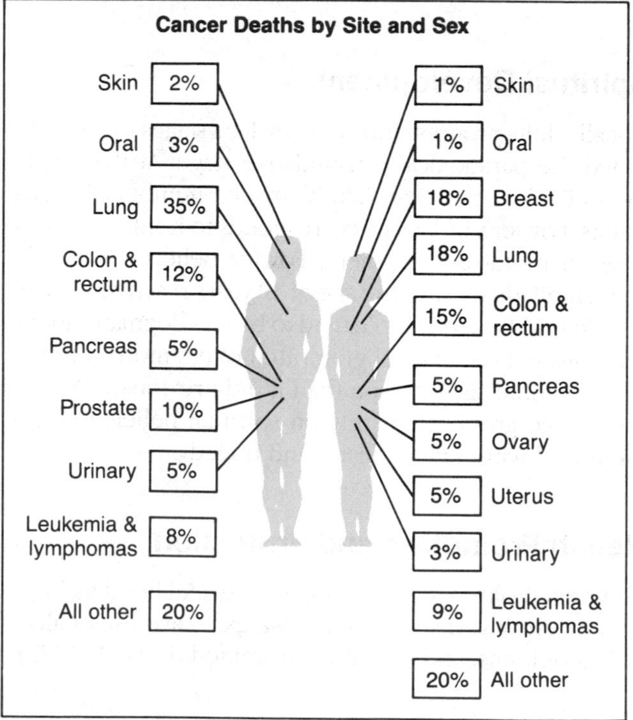

†Excluding nonmelanoma skin cancer and carcinoma in situ.

Figure 25–5 Estimates of cancer incidence and deaths by site and sex, 1985.
Source: American Cancer Society, *Cancer facts and figures* (New York: American Cancer Society, 1985). Courtesy American Cancer Society.

- Spiritual development of young adults continues into Fowler's paradoxical-consolidative stage; young adults often feel self-conscious about spiritual matters.
- Hazards to the health of young adults include accidents, infections, suicide and homicide, drug abuse, obesity, and hypertension.
- Nurses can assist clients to decrease the impact of these hazards.
- The middle-aged adult needs to adjust to an aging body, the increasing dependence of parents, and the increasing independence of children; however, new independent interests can be pursued.
- Both middle-aged men and women enter a midlife crisis in which they need to reexamine their purpose and reevaluate ways to use their energies and abilities.
- Common health hazards of middle-aged adults include obesity, chronic diseases, smoking, excessive use of alcohol, neoplasms, and sexually transmitted diseases.
- Positive health practices can protect and promote health.

Suggested Readings

Diekelmann, N. L. June 1975. Emotional tasks of the middle adult. *American Journal of Nursing* 75:997–1001.
The article outlines four areas in which middle-aged adults become more self-oriented. Specific examples of how several couples and singles view these years enhance the content.

———. August 1976. The young adult: The choice is health or illness. *American Journal of Nursing* 76:1272–77.
Nurses can help young adults to recognize the importance of health maintenance and promotion by encouraging them to develop proper sleeping, eating, and exercising habits and fulfilling emotional tasks. Many problems can occur in later life if attention to health is lacking between the ages of 20 and 35.

Diekelmann, N. L., and Galloway, K. June 1975. A time of change. *American Journal of Nursing* 75:994–96.
Psychologic, physical, environmental, value, and social changes occur in the middle-aged adult. The nurse's role in teaching and preparing families for these changes is outlined.

Galloway, K. June 1975. The change of life. *American Journal of Nursing* 75:1006–11.
The problems and concerns of both men and women at the change of life are outlined as well as the nurse's role in helping people cope with these changes.

Johnson, L. June 1975. Living sensibly. *American Journal of Nursing* 75:1012–16.

Changes in patterns of diet and exercise are required of the middle-aged adult. Routine preventive care, in addition, can promote healthier and happier people.

Selected References

Crooks, R., and Baur, K. 1983. *Our sexuality.* 2d ed. Menlo Park, Calif.: Benjamin/Cummings Publishing Co.

Diekelman, N. L. 1976. The young adult: The choice is health or illness. *American Journal of Nursing* 76:1276.

———. 1977. *Primary health care of the well adult.* New York: McGraw-Hill.

Edelman, C., and Mandle, C. L. 1986. *Health promotion throughout the life span.* St. Louis: C. V. Mosby Co.

Erikson, E. H. 1982. *The life cycle completed: A review.* New York: W. W. Norton and Co.

Golan, N. 1981. *Passing through transitions. A guide for practitioners.* New York: The Free Press.

Gould, R. L. November 1972. The phases of adult life: A study in developmental psychology. *American Journal of Psychiatry* 129:33–43.

Heath, D. 1965. *Explorations of maturity.* New York: Appleton-Century-Crofts. Cited in Kaluger, G., and Kaluger, M. F. 1979. *Human development: The life span.* 2d ed. St. Louis: C. V. Mosby Co.

Kaluger, G., and Kaluger, M. F. 1979. *Human development: The life span.* 2d ed. St. Louis: C. V. Mosby Co.

Miller, P. H. 1983. *Theories of developmental psychology.* San Francisco: W. H. Freeman and Co.

Murray, B. L. S., and Wilcox, L. J. December 1978. Testicular self-examination. *American Journal of Nursing* 78:2074–75.

Murray, R. B., and Zentner, J. P. 1985. *Nursing assessment and health promotion throughout the life span.* 3d ed. Englewood Cliffs, N.J.: Prentice-Hall.

National Academy of Sciences. 1980. *Recommended dietary allowances.* 9th ed. Washington, D.C.: National Academy Press.

Overfield, T. September/October 1980. Obesity: Prevention is easier than cure. *Nurse Practitioner* 5:25–26, 33, 62.

Peck, R. 1955. Psychological developments in the second half of life. In Anderson, J., editor. *Psychological aspects of aging.* Washington, D.C.: American Psychological Association.

Rubin, L. B. 1979. *Women of a certain age: The midlife search for self.* New York: Harper and Row.

Sheehy, G. 1977. *Passages: Predictable crises of adult life.* New York: E. P. Dutton and Co.

Stevens-Long, J. 1984. *Adult life.* 2d ed. Palo Alto, Calif.: Mayfield Publishing Co.

U.S. Department of Health and Human Services. December 20, 1984. *Monthly vital statistics report.* Hyattsville, Md.: National Center for Health Statistics.

———. December 1985. *Health United States 1985.* U.S. DHHS No. (PHS) 86-1232. Hyattsville, Md.: Public Health Service.

White, R. 1975. *Lives in progress: A study of the natural growth of personality.* 3d ed. New York: Holt, Rinehart and Winston.

Williams, S. R. 1981. *Nutrition and diet therapy.* 4th ed. St. Louis: C. V. Mosby Co.

CHAPTER **26**

Late Adulthood

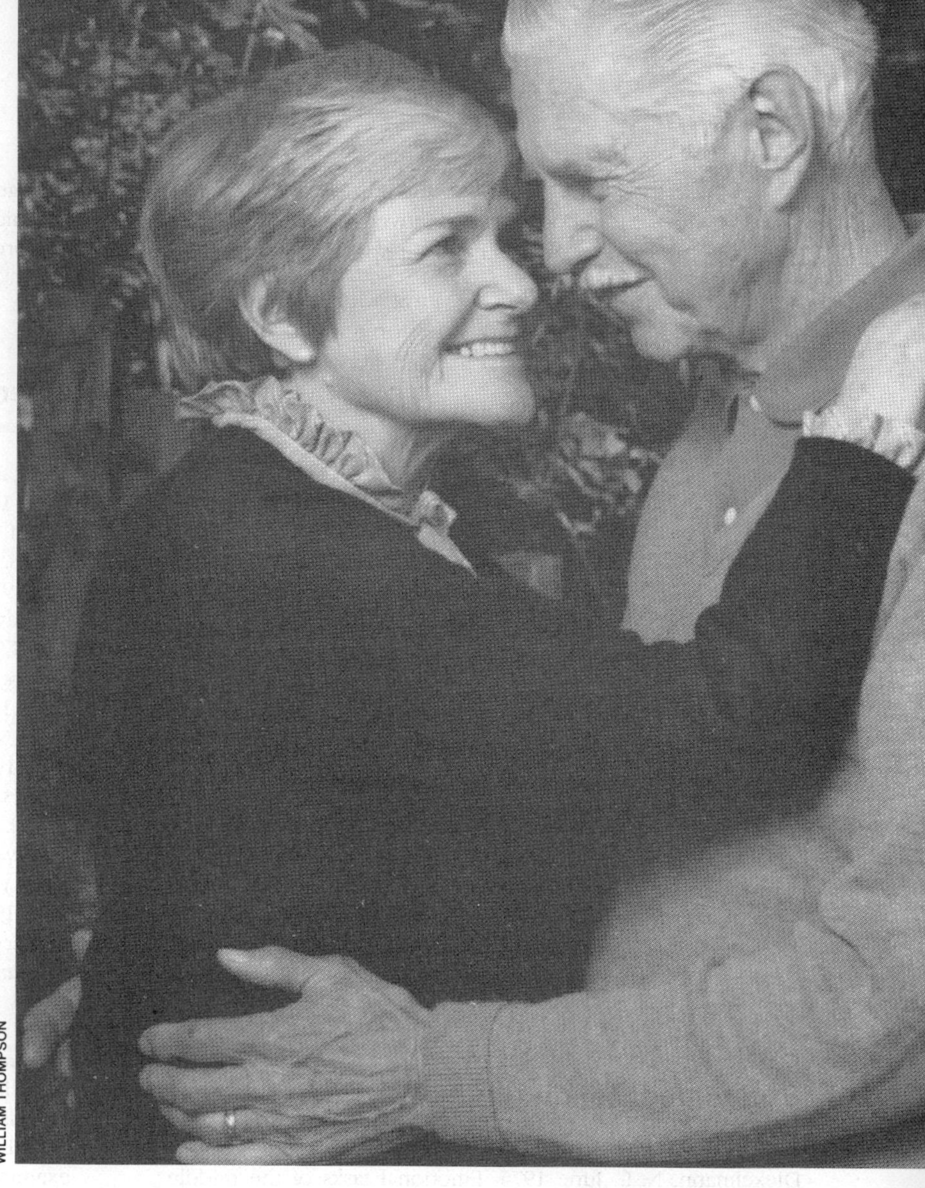

WILLIAM THOMPSON

Contents

Objectives

1. Understand essential facts about the development of the older adult.
   1.1 Describe the physical changes that occur from middle adulthood through old age.
   1.2 Explain essential aspects of psychosocial changes.
   1.3 Describe essential aspects of cognitive changes.
   1.4 Explain essential aspects of moral development.
   1.5 Explain essential aspects of spiritual development.
2. Understand essential facts about health promotion in and protection of elderly adults.
   2.1 Identify common health hazards and problems among elderly adults.
   2.2 Discuss nursing implications related to the health hazards and problems.

Terms

activity theory
cataracts
continuity theory
cystocele
disengagement theory
dyspneic
extrinsic
geriatric nursing
gerontic nursing
gerontologic nursing
gerontology
intrinsic
kyphosis
malignant
neuritic plaque
neurofibrillary tangle
osteoporosis
premalignant (precancerous)
presbycusis
presbyopia
primary memory (PM)
rectocele
secondary memory (SM)
senescence

Late Adulthood Defined

Late adulthood, for the purposes of this book, is the years after 65. Sometimes it is referred to as **senescence** or old age. Because of advances in medical and related sciences and health promotion and protection, an increasing number of people are living to an advanced age. In 1960, life expectancy at birth was about 70 years, i.e., the average person born in 1960 could expect to live about 70 years. By 1983, life expectancy had increased to 75 years (U.S. DHHS 1985, p. 1).

Gerontology is the study of all aspects of aging. **Geriatric nursing** is practice involving the diseases of aging. **Gerontologic nursing** deals with the scientific study and care of the elderly. Ebersole and Hess use the term **gerontic nursing**, which they describe as "nursing of older persons [which is not] limited to illness or scientific principles but rather encompasses both and includes the art and intuition of caring for and maintaining the well elderly" (Ebersole and Hess 1985, p. 4).

The person reaching late adulthood must accomplish a number of broad developmental tasks. These are listed below.

Developmental Tasks of Late Adulthood

Erikson's stage: Integrity versus despair

- Accepting diminishing abilities and limitations
- Adjusting to retirement
- Adjusting to reorganized life patterns
- Accepting loss and death with serenity

Theories of Aging

Although researchers have investigated how, for example, the muscles and nervous system age, knowledge about the aging process is largely theoretical. A number of theories explain physiologic aging. Table 26–1 lists some well-known theories. Biologic theories are either intrinsic or extrinsic. Extrinsic theory encompasses factors in the environment; intrinsic theory addresses factors within the body.

Table 26–1 Biologic Theories of Aging

Biologic Theory	Description
Genetic theory	Aging results from biochemical changes programmed into the DNA molecule in each cell.
Immunologic slow virus theory	The immune system becomes less effective with age, and viruses that have incubated in the body become able to damage body organs.
Autoimmune theory	The production of autoimmune antibodies increases, and they attack the body cells.
Cross-link theory	As cells age, chemical reactions create strong bonds, especially in collagen tissues. These bonds cause loss of elasticity, stiffness, and eventual loss of function.
Stress theory	Aging results from cellular loss due to wear and tear on the body. Regeneration of body tissues eventually cannot keep pace with wear and tear, and the body is unable to maintain a stable internal environment.
Free-radical theory	Unstable free radicals (groups of atoms) result from the oxidation of organic materials, such as carbohydrates and proteins. These radicals cause biochemical changes in the cells, and the cells cannot regenerate themselves.
Program theory	The organism is capable of a predetermined number of cell divisions, after which the cells die.

A number of theories explain psychosocial aging as well. According to **disengagement theory**, aging involves mutual withdrawal (disengagement) between the older person and others in the elderly person's environment. This withdrawal relieves the elderly person of some of society's pressures and gradually reduces the number of people with whom the elderly person interacts. According to **activity theory**, the best way to age is to stay active physically and mentally, and according to **continuity theory**, people maintain their values, habits, and behavior in old age. A person who is accustomed to having people around will continue to do so, and the person who prefers not to be involved with others will more likely disengage. This theory accounts for the great variety of behavior seen in elderly people.

Physical Changes

See Table 26–2.

Integumentary System

Obvious changes occur in the integument (skin, hair, nails) with age. These changes cause concerns in relation to self-image more than they cause acute physical problems. These changes include wrinkles, dryness, loss of fullness, itching, and baldness or thinning and graying hair. The skin also becomes paler and blotchy and loses its elasticity. Fingernails and toenails become thickened and brittle, and in women over 60 years, facial hair increases.

These skin changes accompany progressive losses of underlying adipose and muscle tissue and loss of elastic fiber. Initially adipose tissue is redistributed from the extremities to the hips and abdomen in middle age. Generalized loss of adipose tissue progresses along with muscle atrophy, creating a wrinkled and wasted appearance. Bony prominences become visible, a double chin develops, and lower eyelids appear puffy. In elderly women, the breasts become smaller and may sag, if large and pendulous, causing chafing where the skin surfaces touch. Loss of subcutaneous fat also decreases the elderly person's tolerance of cold.

Itching increases due to dryness of the skin and to deterioration of the nerve fibers and sensory endings. Decreased blood flow to the skin causes pallor and blotchiness. Baldness is thought to be due to decreased blood flow to the skin. The loss of hair color is due to a decrease in the number of functioning pigment-producing cells.

The ways people respond to these changes varies among individuals and cultures. For example, one person may feel distinguished with gray hair, while another may feel embarrassed by it. Most women dislike their facial hair because hirsute women do not conform to the feminine cultural ideal of North Americans.

Nursing interventions in this area include teaching the client how to protect the skin from bruising and injury. Inspect the skin regularly for damage and changes in pigmentation. Some skin lesions can reflect circulatory, neurologic, hormone, or metabolic problems. Skin lesions can be premalignant or malignant, and the client needs to be referred to a physican. **Premalignant** (or precancerous) means possessing the potential of becoming malignant. **Malignant** means possessing the tendency to grow and invade other tissues. Elderly people with dry skin should bathe less often than before and decrease or eliminate the use of soap, which dries the skin.

Body Temperature

Body temperature is lower in the elderly adult due to a decrease in the metabolic rate. It is not uncommon for an elderly adult to have a temperature of 35 C (95 F), particularly in the early morning when the body's metabolism is low. This fact has implications for nurses assessing the elderly adult for fever. For example, a temperature of 37.5 C (99.5 F) can represent a marked fever in some elderly people, although it represents only a mild fever in most young adults. It is important that the normal temperature of each individual person be known as a baseline for assessing changes.

One of the body's normal compensating reactions to a fall in heat production is the contraction of the surface blood vessels and shivering. Because elderly adults have a diminished shivering reflex and do not produce as much body heat from metabolic processes, they tolerate prolonged exposure to cold poorly. At the other extreme, the body compensates for higher temperatures by slowing down muscular activity to produce less heat and by dilating surface blood vessels and sweating to increase losses of body heat. Older people, however, often have sluggish sweating and circulatory mechanisms and therefore cannot cope with heat as well as younger people. For example, they do not tolerate working in moderately high temperatures for prolonged periods. It is therefore important for the elderly adult to have a constant, comfortable environmental temperature. Nurses often need to provide extra clothes to elderly persons who feel cold in rooms with a "normal" temperature.

Table 26–2 Normal Physiologic Aging

1. Decreased immune system function, which may be related to the increased incidence of infection, cancer, and autoimmune diseases
2. Decreased production of saliva
3. Decreased production of hydrochloric acid and pepsin in the stomach
4. Decrease in kidney mass; 33% to 50% decrease in the number of nephrons
5. Decreased concentrating and diluting ability of the kidney
6. Gradual decline in male reproduction
7. Cessation of ovum production at menopause
8. Slowing of motor neuron transmission
9. Decline in the function of the autonomic nervous system
10. Progressive decrease in sleep stages 3 and 4 (deep sleep)
11. Decline in the visual fields of the eye and hearing ability
12. Decline in sensitivity to the four tastes—salt, sweet, sour, and bitter—after age 50
13. Progressive increase in threshold for deep pain after age 60
14. Decreased ability of the body to adapt to stress

Source: F. C. Gioiella and C. W. Bevil, *Nursing care of the aging client: Promoting healthy adaptation* (Norwalk, Conn.: Appleton-Century-Crofts, 1985). Used by permission.

Skeletal System

Slight loss in overall stature occurs with age due to atrophy of the discs between the spinal vertebrae. This can be exaggerated by muscular weakness resulting in a stooping posture and **kyphosis** (humpback of the upper spine). **Osteoporosis**, a decrease in bone density, along with increased brittleness of bone, makes the elderly adult prone to serious fractures, some of which are spontaneous. Since the incidence of osteoporosis is higher in elderly women, the effects of the menopause on the skeleton are being investigated. Causes of osteoporosis are thought to be lack of activity and inadequate calcium intake or inability to metabolize calcium.

Some degenerative joint changes occur, which make movement stiffer and more restricted. Stiffness is aggravated by inactivity; for example, if persons sit too long, their joints become stiff and they have difficulty standing and walking. Although these skeletal changes do restrict the activity of the elderly adult, prevention of severe disability is possible. Nursing interventions should include counseling clients to take adequate exercise and include adequate amounts of protein and calcium in the diet.

Muscular System

With aging there is a gradual reduction in the speed and power of skeletal or voluntary muscle contractions. The capacity for sustained muscular effort is also decreased. Great individual differences in muscular efficiency are apparent throughout life. Exercise can strengthen weakened muscles, and up to about age 50 the skeletal muscles can increase in bulk and density. After that time, there is a steady decrease in muscle fibers, ultimately leading to the typical wasted appearance of the very old person. Thus, elderly adults often complain about their lack of strength and how quickly they tire. Activities can still be carried out, but at a slower pace. Often balance is impaired with age. Prolonged muscular efforts may be sustained by older people provided they take judicious rest pauses and avoid capacity or peak performance.

The effects of age on the smooth or involuntary muscles such as the stomach, the colon, the respiratory tubes, and the bladder are small in contrast to the effects on the skeletal muscles, with the exception of the blood vessels. These muscles function relatively normally until late senescence.

Nurses can advise clients about safety measures, such as using hand rails to prevent falls, removing small rugs to prevent slips, and putting away items over which an elderly person could trip. Clients may also need to learn to limit their activity to a level they tolerate well.

Senses

Vision Obvious changes around the eye are the shrunken appearance of the eyes due to loss of orbital fat, the slowed blink reflex, and the looseness of the eyelids, particularly the lower lid, because of poorer muscle tone. Other changes result in loss of visual acuity, less power of accommodation to darkness and dim light, loss of peripheral vision, and difficulty in discriminating similar colors. The degenerative change in the eyes leading to the relative inflexibility of the lens is called **presbyopia**.

As the lens of the eye ages, it becomes more opaque and less elastic. By the age of 80 all elderly people have some lens opacity (**cataracts**) that reduces visual acuity. Surgical removal of cataracts is common at this age. Accompanying this are changes in the ciliary muscles, which control the shape of the lens. These changes reduce the power of the lens to adjust to near and far vision. It is thought that changes in the nervous system play a part in reducing the diameter of the pupil, thereby restricting the amount of light entering the eye. This slows the reaction time to decreases in light or illumination, a problem compounded at night with driving. Reduced blood supply due to arteriosclerosis can diminish retinal function. Reduced peripheral vision also is thought to be a result of arteriosclerosis.

Many elderly adults require eyeglasses for close work. It is not uncommon for elderly people to buy inexpensive magnifying eyeglasses from department stores. Nurses should encourage elderly adults to have routine eye examinations by a physician and use appropriate eyeglasses. Many places now offer free eye examinations and eyeglasses to elderly people.

Elderly people may need a night light to get to the bathroom on their own; at night their vision is often diminished. Nurses can encourage elderly people to move slowly and carefully in the dark.

Hearing The loss of hearing due to senescent change is called **presbycusis**. Presbycusis comes about through changes in the structure of the inner ear: changes in nerve tissues in the inner ear and a thickening of the eardrum. Gradual loss of hearing is usual among the aging and more common among men than women, perhaps because men are more frequently in noisy work environments. Hearing loss is usually greater in the left ear than the right and greater in the higher frequencies than the lower. Thus, elderly adults with hearing loss usually hear speakers with low, distinct voices best. Elderly adults have more difficulty compensating for hearing loss than the young, who pay closer attention to the lip movements of the speaker.

Nurses can assist elderly people who are hard of hearing by the following measures:

1. Speaking more loudly and in a lower tone
2. Speaking slowly and sometimes using alternative words
3. Using facial expressions that convey moods and feelings, thus helping comprehension
4. Encouraging clients to use hearing aids when appropriate
5. Speaking clearly and facing the person, but not shouting
6. Not covering the face or mouth while talking to an elderly person
7. Assisting the elderly person to learn ways to ask others to repeat their words or speak more clearly.

Taste and smell Older persons have a poorer sense of taste and smell and are less stimulated by food than the young. The number of taste buds in the tongue grows smaller, and the olfactory bulb (responsible for smell perception) at the base of the brain atrophies.

Voice

Changes in the voice occur throughout life as a result of hardening and decreased elasticity of the laryngeal cartilages. These processes are completed by middle age. With age, the laryngeal muscles atrophy, and the vocal cords slacken. The voice becomes higher pitched, less powerful, and restricted in range. These changes are generally unnoticed unless greater demands on capacity, such as singing or public speaking, are made. Noticeable changes, such as slower speech and eventual slurring, are the result of central nervous system changes rather than local mechanisms.

Respiratory System

Respiratory efficiency is reduced with age. The person inhales a smaller volume of air due to the musculoskeletal changes in the chest wall that reduce the size of the chest. There is a greater volume of residual air left in the lungs after expiration and a decreased capacity to cough efficiently because of weaker expiratory muscles. Mucous secretions tend to collect more readily in the respiratory tree due to decreased ciliary activity. Thus, susceptibility to respiratory infections is notable in elderly adults.

Dyspnea occurs frequently with increased activity, such as running for a bus or carrying heavy parcels up stairs. This dyspnea occurs in response to an oxygen debt in the muscles. Intense exercise is followed by short, heavy, rapid breathing, which is an attempt to repay this oxygen debt in the muscles. Although this response is normal, it occurs more quickly in the aged because delivery and diffusion of oxygen to tissues is often diminished by changes in both respiratory and vascular tissues.

Nursing interventions include teaching the client deep breathing and coughing (see Chapters 45 and 53) and prompt treatment at the first sign of a respiratory infection. Also, the client needs to learn how to control activities so as not to become **dypsneic** (short of breath).

Cardiovascular System

The working capacity of the heart is diminished with age. This is particularly evident when increased demands are made on the heart muscles, such as during periods of exercise or emotional stress. The valves of the heart tend to become harder and less pliable, resulting in reduced filling and emptying abilities. In addition, the pumping action of the heart is reduced due to changes in the coronary (cardiac) arteries, which supply progressively smaller amounts of blood to the heart muscle. These changes are evidenced by shortness of breath on exertion and pooling of blood in the systemic veins.

Changes in the arteries occur concurrently. The elasticity of smaller arteries is reduced by the thickening of their walls and increased calcium deposits in the muscular layer. Reduced arterial elasticity often results in diminished blood supply to, for instance, the legs and the brain, resulting in pain on exertion in the calf muscles and dizziness, respectively.

Blood pressure measurements often indicate increases in both systolic and diastolic pressures, partly as a result of the inelasticity of the systemic arteries. Variations in the pulse rate of the aged also occur. A rate of 70 to 80 beats per minute is quite usual.

Nursing interventions include teaching the client to move more slowly so as to avoid dyspnea and cardiac discomfort. Encourage clients to seek medical advice if they experience dyspnea or chest pain.

Gastrointestinal System

The digestive system is significantly less impaired by aging than other body systems are. Previously mentioned was the diminished ability to taste and smell, which contributes in part to a lack of appetite. Gradual decreases in digestive enzymes occur; examples are ptyalin in salivary secretions, which converts starch; pepsin and trypsin, which digest protein; and lipase, a fat-splitting enzyme. Yet digestive functioning and absorption of food are relatively unimpaired. The common complaints of heartburn, gas, and indigestion are largely due to other disease processes or to dietary excesses, such as highly spiced or fried foods.

The majority of elderly adults have poor teeth or wear dentures and therefore may have difficulties masticating food. Foods that require extensive chewing, such as meat and fresh vegetables or fruit, may as a result be avoided, leading to nutritional deficiencies.

Constipation is a common complaint of older people. However, the aging process has little if any effect on the bowels, which retain their ability to function normally. Thus, constipation is usually a result of poor fluid intake, inadequate roughage in the diet, and insufficient exercise.

Urinary System

The excretory function of the kidney diminishes with age, but usually not significantly below normal levels unless a disease process intervenes. Blood flow can be reduced by arteriosclerotic changes, impairing renal function. With age, the number of functioning nephrons (the basic functional units of the kidney) is reduced to some degree, thus impairing the kidney's filtering abilities.

More noticeable changes are those related to the bladder. Complaints of urinary urgency and frequency are common. In men, these changes are often due to an enlarged prostate gland and in women to weakened muscles supporting the bladder or weakness of the urethral sphincter. The capacity of the bladder and its ability to empty completely diminish with age. This explains the need for elderly adults to arise during the night to void (nocturnal frequency) and the retention of residual urine, predisposing the elderly adult to bladder infections.

Reproductive System

In men, degenerative changes in the gonads are very gradual. The testes can produce sperm well into old age, although there is a gradual decrease in the number of sperm produced. In women the degenerative changes in the ovaries are noticed by the abrupt cessation of menses in middle age, during the menopause.

Changes in the gonads of elderly women result from diminished secretion of the ovarian hormones. Some changes, such as the shrinking of the uterus and ovaries, go unnoticed. Other changes are obvious. The breasts atrophy, and lubricating vaginal secretions are reduced. Reduced natural lubrication is the cause of painful intercourse, which often necessitates the use of lubricating jellies.

Sexual drives persist into the 70s, 80s, and 90s, provided health is good and there is an available and interested partner. However, sexual activity does become less frequent with age. Sometimes a chronic cardiac or respiratory illness saps sexual energy. Nurses may need to teach a couple to adjust the time and technique of sexual activity to accommodate such factors as fatigue and arthritic joints.

Nervous System

The person's reaction time is slowed with age because of the diminished conduction speed of nerve fibers. Reaction time can be delayed further by decreased muscle tone as a result of diminished physical activity. Elderly people compensate for this reaction difference by being exceptionally cautious, for instance, in their driving habits, which exasperate some impatient young drivers. Because sensory nerve endings in the skin also change with age, old people are less sensitive to touch, and safety precautions are necessary, for example, when a hot-water bottle is applied.

Experts do not agree whether the brain decreases in weight with age, although it is thought that the brain may lose about 10% to 12% of its mass by very old age (Gioiella and Bevil 1985, p. 76). It is believed, however, that there is a progressive loss of neurons with age. Neurofibrillary tangles have also been found in the hippocampal cortex, the area of the brain concerned with memory. A **neuro-**

fibrillary tangle is an abnormal mass of fibrillar material found in the cytoplasm. Neuritic plaques are also found in the aging brain. A **neuritic plaque** is a structure composed of amyloid material surrounded by abnormal neural structures. Neurofibrillary tangles and neuritic plaques could account for some of the functional changes found in normal aging people.

Elderly people can be taught to take precautions because of their slower reaction times, and they can learn to assist their memories, for example, by writing lists. Nurses may also need to teach aging people how to protect themselves from burns because they often have a diminished perception of heat.

Alzheimer's Disease (AD) One of the most tragic conditions to strike the elderly, this progressive degenerative disorder affects more than 2.5 million Americans. Characterized by *dementia,* the deterioration of intellectual capacity, it is the fifth leading cause of total disability in the United States and the fourth leading cause of death among the elderly. Each year 120,000 Americans die from AD. Experts predict that in the next century, it will be the leading cause of death (Schneider and Emr, 1985).

The cause of AD is unknown; however, in late 1986, researchers identified an abnormal protein, A-68, that appears in the brain of AD victims and also in the spinal fluid of living persons thought to have the disease. While it is not known whether A-68 is a causative factor, the protein is unique to AD. Depending on further studies, a routine laboratory test could be developed that would make possible early and accurate diagnosis. Until such a test is developed, definitive diagnosis can only be made at autopsy. Such a test would not only aid in diagnosing the disease when it is still reversible, but it would also identify those persons who are misdiagnosed with AD. These are persons whose apparent confusion and memory loss may be due to depression, malnutrition, or other treatable disorder.

No means of prevention or treatment is yet available for AD. In late 1986, however, early results of a study showed some success with the drug *tetrahydroaminoacridine* (THA) in helping to restore some cognitive function (Davis and Mohs, 1986). Further drug trials are underway.

The Federal Government spends $36 million annually on research related to AD; the care of AD patients costs $28 billion annually. Neither of these figures, however, reflects the cost in human terms to persons affected and their families. Witnessing the steady deterioration of a loved one and trying to cope with the increasing disability can have devastating effects on family members, particularly an aging spouse. Thus a large part of the nurse's role is to teach and role model the following concepts for families (Gioiella and Bevil, 1985): structured environment; safety; activity; respite; and support. In addition, the nurse can perform important counseling, advocacy and referral functions.

Symptoms of Alzheimer's have been grouped into four stages (Cutler and Narang, 1985). In a period of 2 to 15 years, the person with AD gradually slides into a child-like dependency.

Psychosocial Development

Elderly people must adapt to many psychosocial changes, for example, the death of a life partner, retirement, or reduced income. According to Erikson, the developmental task at this time is ego integrity versus self-despair. See Table 22–6 on page 466. People who attain ego integrity view life with a sense of wholeness and satisfaction with past accomplishments. They view death as an acceptable completion of life. According to Erikson, people who develop integrity accept "one's one and only life cycle" (Erikson 1963, p.263). By contrast, people who despair often believe they have made poor choices during life and wish they could live life over. Robert Butler sees integrity as bringing serenity and wisdom, and despair as resulting in the inability to accept one's fate. Despair gives rise to feelings of frustration, discouragement, and a sense that one's life has been worthless (Butler 1963, p. 65).

Kart and associates, by contrast, discuss three tasks described by Peck (1955) as paramount in old age: First, elderly people must establish new activities so that the loss of accustomed roles is less keenly felt. Second, they must select activities compatible with the physical limitations of old age. Third, individuals may make contributions that extend beyond their own lifetimes, thereby providing a meaning for life (Kart et al., 1978, p. 180).

Housing for Elderly People

According to a Chinese saying, the house with an old grandparent harbors a jewel. However, in North American society, most aging people live apart. Most think it unwise to live with married sons and daughters, since overcrowded, tense situations can arise. It is also difficult for some elderly people to assume a new role while living with their children—relinquishing the authority they had, allowing their children to be independent.

Nurses must be sensitive to the stress that the presence of an elderly person in the home of a child may cause for all family members, including the older person. An ill elderly person often requires considerable care, and the primary caregiver may be one of the family. This living arrangement can often involve adjustments in lifestyle for all concerned. Nurses can assist people in their adjustments and at the same time be supportive and caring.

Only a small percentage of elderly adults live in nursing homes. However, an increasing number of nursing home residents are over the age of 85 years (U.S. DHHS

1985, p. 11). These lodgings vary in many ways and offer varying degrees of independence to the residents. All provide meals but vary in giving other services, such as assistance with hygiene and dressing, physical therapy or exercise, recreational activities, transportation services, and medical and nursing supervision.

Nurses in hospitals should find out whether a client is being discharged to a nursing home or to home. Many nursing homes provide nursing services to clients and require appropriate information to provide for continuity of care. Clients returning home, however, may require the assistance of a home care nurse. See Chapter 4 for additional information about home health care.

Retirement

Today, a majority of the people over 65 are unemployed, a sharp contrast from the early 1900s, when the majority lived in rural areas and continued to work. Most industries and professions make retirement mandatory, although this policy is currently being questioned. Some who are self-employed continue to work as long as they are healthy. Work offers these people a better income, a sense of self-worth, and the chance to continue long-established routines. Some need to work for economic reasons.

Retirement can be a time when projects or recreational activities deferred for a long time can be pursued. See Figure 26–1. Older retired people are no longer governed by an alarm clock and can get up when they please. The enjoyment of staying up later is another luxury. Few elderly people, however, spend much time resting or sleeping. Being accustomed to activity most of their lives, most elderly find many outlets: jobs, community projects, volunteer services, intellectual or recreational pursuits, or hobbies such as stamp collecting or fishing. Travel opportunities are expanding.

The life-style of later years is to a large degree formulated in youth. This fact was recognized by Robert Browning: "Grow old along with me! / The best is yet to be, / The last of life, for which the first was made." People who attempt suddenly to refocus and enrich their lives at retirement usually have difficulty. Those who learned early in life to live well-balanced and fulfilling lives are generally more successful in retirement. The woman who

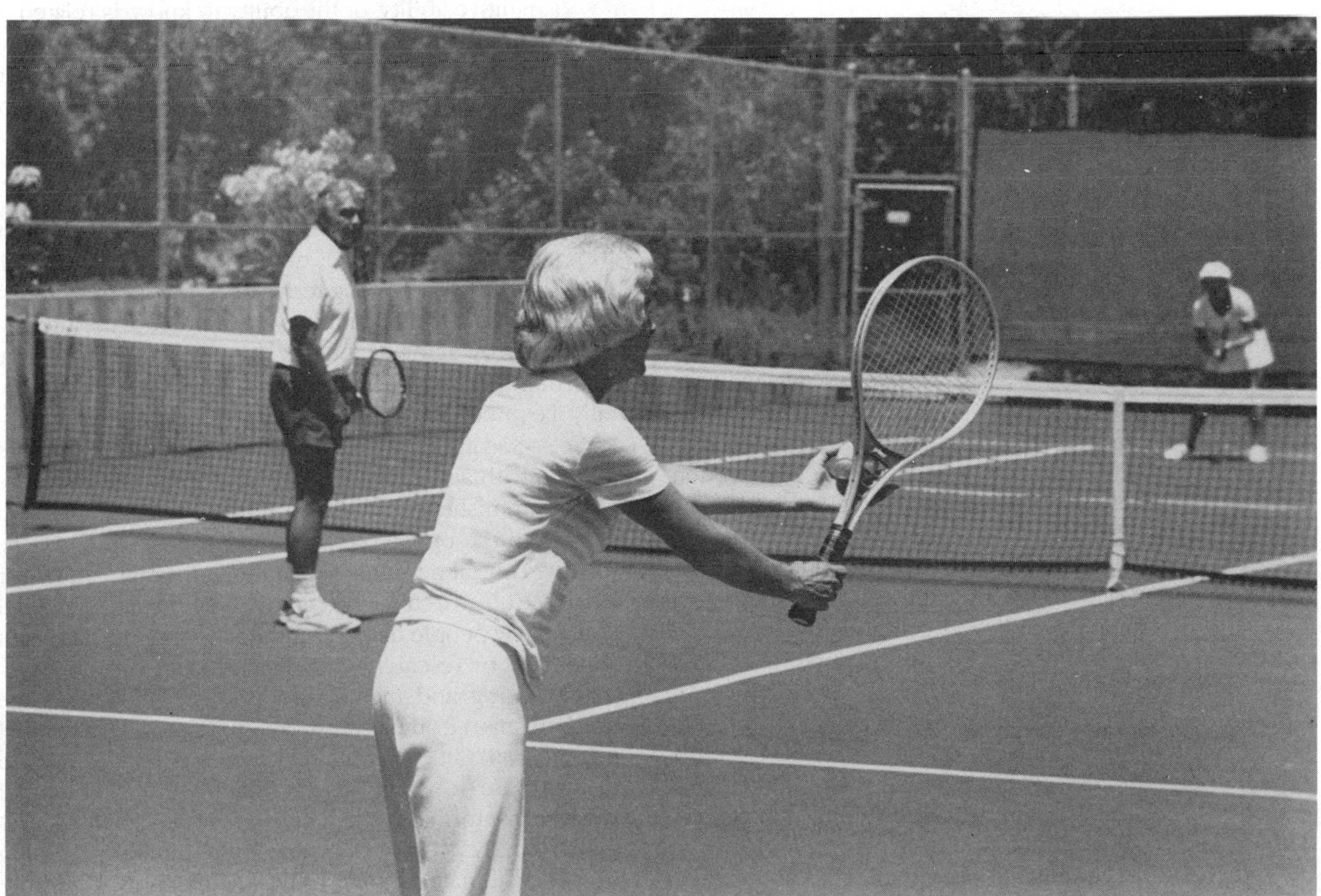

Figure 26–1 Retirement allows older people to persue interests that were previously put aside for child rearing and work.

has been concerned only with the accomplishments of her children or the man who has been concerned only with the paycheck and his job status can be left with a feeling of emptiness when children leave and the job no longer exists. The later years can foster a sense of integrity and continuity, or they can be years of despair.

Lowered Income

Some of the financial needs of elderly people diminish considerably. Though they need less money for clothing, entertainment, and work, and may own their homes outright, costs continue to rise, making it difficult for some. For some people, food and medical costs alone are a financial burden. When older people speak about their greatest need, often it is not happiness or health, but money. Money allows them to be independent and look after themselves.

Nurses should be aware of the costs of health care. For example, while assisting a client to plan a diet, the nurse must consider which foods the client can afford to buy. In addition, the supplies used in a client's care should be as economical as possible.

Facing Bereavement and Dying

Well-adjusted aging couples usually thrive on companionship. Many couples rely increasingly on their mates for this company and may have few outside friends. Great bonds of affection and closeness can develop during this period of aging together and nurturing each other.

When a mate dies, the remaining partner inevitably experiences feelings of loss, emptiness, and loneliness. Many are capable and manage to live alone; however, reliance on younger family members increases as age advances and ill health occurs. Some widows and widowers remarry, particularly the latter, because widowers are less inclined than widows to maintain a household.

Women face bereavement and solitude more often than men, since women usually live longer. The brevity of life is constantly reinforced by the death of friends. It is a time when one's life is reviewed with happiness or regret. Feelings of serenity or guilt and inadequacy can arise. Independence established prior to loss of a mate makes this adjustment period easier. A person who has some meaningful friendships, economic security, ongoing interests in the community, or private hobbies and a peaceful philosophy of life copes more easily with bereavement. Successful relationships with children and grandchildren are also of inestimable value. Facing death is discussed in Chapter 50.

Nurses can sometimes help clients who are alone a great deal to adjust their living arrangements or life-style so that they have more companionship. Moving to a retirement home that has other people in similar circumstances and organized social activities is one example. Many communities provide social centers for the elderly, for example, drop-in centers or community centers that offer day trips for seniors. Nurses can refer clients to services and encourage them to obtain companionship.

Cognitive Development

Piaget's phases of cognitive development end with the formal operations phase. However, there is currently considerable research on cognitive abilities and aging. Researchers generally believe that there is minimal change in intellectual capacity of the healthy aging person (Gress and Bahr 1984, p. 72).

Intellectual capacity includes perception, cognitive ability, and learning. Perception, or the ability to interpret the environment, depends on the acuteness of the senses. If the aging person's senses are impaired, the ability to perceive the environment and react appropriately is diminished. Perceptual capacity may be affected by changes in the nervous system as well. See the section on physical changes, earlier in this chapter.

Cognitive ability, or the ability to know, is related to perceptual ability. An older man, for example, may know that he will be retiring next year but be unable to plan for retirement. He cannot accept the knowledge psychologically because his work provides his sense of worth, self-esteem, and identity.

Memory is also a component of intellectual capacity and is closely related to learning. Memory, or the ability to retain information, is of two types: short-term or primary memory and long-term or secondary memory. According to Gress and Bahr, primary memory is affected minimally by aging as long as the person perceives the information adequately and need not reorganize it mentally, i.e., need not reintegrate it to fit changing circumstances. Secondary memory, however, has been found to decline with aging. The ability to recall declines because aging diminishes the ability to retrieve information from storage in the brain. The reason for this decline may be that the central nervous system functions more slowly or because the search within the brain is longer. The belief that elderly people have intact long-term memories is not supported by research (Gioiella and Bevil 1985, p. 38).

Learning and memory involve some of the same mechanisms, i.e., the acquisition, storage, and retrieval of information. Older people usually require more time to demonstrate learning, largely due to the problem of retrieving information. Motivation is important for learning in elderly people. They have more difficulty learning nonsensical material than young people; however, if the material is meaningful, retention is equal to that of younge people (Gioiella and Bevil 1985, p. 38).

Moral Development

According to Kohlberg, moral development is completed in the early adult years. Most old people stay at Kohlberg's conventional level of moral development (see Table 22–10 on page 471), and some are at the preconventional level. An elderly person at the preconventional level obeys rules to avoid pain and the displeasure of others. At stage 1, a person defines good and bad in relation to self, whereas an older person at stage 2 may act to meet another's needs as well as his or her own. Elderly people at the conventional level follow society's rules of conduct in response to the expectations of others. They value conformity, loyalty, and social order (Edelman and Mandle 1986, p. 548).

Rybash, Roodin, and Hoyer studied the kinds of moral problems elderly people face. These researchers found that the moral concerns of the elderly are more interpersonal than social or legalistic. For example, an elderly man is more likely to be concerned with the moral problems involving a member of his family than with the moral problems posed by his occupation or a friend's extramarital affair (Rybash et al. 1983, p. 253).

Spiritual Development

According to Maslow, religious experiences integrate life experiences. These "plateau experiences" are more frequent in old age. They are less intense than "peak experiences," are felt as joy or happiness, and can endure for long periods (Maslow 1970). Also see the discussion of Maslow in Chapter 16.

Murray and Zentner (1985, p. 584) write that the elderly person with a mature religious outlook strives to incorporate views of theology and religious action into thinking. Elderly people can contemplate new religious and philosophical views and try to understand ideas missed previously or interpreted differently. The elderly person also derives a sense of worth by sharing experiences or views. In contrast, the elderly person who has not matured spiritually may feel impoverishment or despair as the drive for economic and professional success wanes.

The older person's knowledge becomes wisdom, an inner resource for dealing with both positive and negative life experiences. Spiritual development adds joy and meaning to life in later years (Gress and Bahr 1984, p. 85).

According to Fowler (1978), some people enter the sixth stage of spiritual development, universalizing. See Table 22–12 on page 474. People whose spiritual development reaches this level think and act in a way that exemplifies love and justice.

Nursing Assessment Guidelines for the Older Adult

Does the older adult:

- Enjoy retirement?
- Have a social network of friends and support persons?
- View life as worthwhile?
- Have high self-esteem?
- Have the abilities to care for self or to secure appropriate help?
- Gain support from value system or spiritual philosophy?
- Adapt life-style to diminishing energy and ability?
- Cope constructively with loss?

Health Promotion and Protection

Areas of concern for the older adult include safety, nutrition, elimination, exercise and rest, sexuality, independence, respect, and isolation. Chronic health problems, such as altered thought processes, hypertension, cancer, and arthritis, are also common in old age.

Assessing Growth and Development

Guidelines for assessment of growth and development of the elderly adult are shown on this page.

Accidents

Accident prevention is a major concern for elderly people. Because vision is limited, reflexes are slowed, and bones are brittle, climbing stairs, driving a car, and even walking require caution. Safety precautions in homes of the elderly are discussed on pages 748–750.

Driving, particularly night driving, requires caution because accommodation of the eye to light is impaired and peripheral vision is diminished. Older persons need to learn to turn the head before changing lanes and should not rely on side vision, for example, when crossing a street. Driving in fog or other hazardous conditions should be avoided.

Fires are a hazard for the elderly person with a failing memory. The older person may forget that the iron or stove is left on or may not extinguish a cigarette completely.

Because of reduced sensitivity to pain and heat, care must be taken to prevent burns when the person bathes or uses heating devices. Elderly people do not tolerate cold well and need warm clothing and often a blanket over their extremities. At night, woolen socks are safer for cold feet than hot-water bottles.

Because older clients who take analgesics or sedatives may become lethargic or confused, they should be monitored regularly and closely. Other measures should be used whenever possible. For example, if an elderly client who lives at home cannot sleep at night without a sedative, a nurse should assess the sleeping environment for noise and light. A light snack before bedtime, e.g., warm milk and a cookie, or soothing music may help the client to sleep.

Nurses can help elderly clients make the home environment safe. Specific hazards can be identified and corrected, e.g., stair handrails can be installed. The nurse teaches the importance of taking only prescribed medications and contacting a health professional at the first indication of intolerance to them.

Nutrition

Elderly adults need well-balanced diets. However, smaller servings with fewer calories are appropriate because of the reduction in metabolic rate and exercise. A diet high in protein, moderate in carbohydrates, and low in fat is recommended. Malnutrition is not uncommon in elderly people because many have bad teeth, many cannot afford the cost of food (particularly protein), and many eat alone. Also, appetite can be reduced by a dulled sense of taste and smell.

In addition, some elderly people's diets are deficient in iron and vitamins A, C, and B. Nurses need to determine whether the client's nutritional status is adequate and if not why not. Perhaps artificial teeth need adjusting or the client needs help shopping.

Constipation

Constipation is not infrequent among the elderly. A cup of hot water or tea taken at a regular hour in the morning is helpful for some. For most, an assessment of fluid intake, exercise, and diet will help in deciding on a remedy. Adequate roughage in the diet, adequate exercise, and six to eight glasses of fluid daily are essential preventive measures for constipation.

Urinary Problems

Many older people learn to deal with nocturnal frequency by restricting their fluid intake in the latter part of the evening, particularly those fluids that stimulate voiding, such as coffee or alcohol. Eventually most men require prostatic surgery to relieve increasing urinary frequency throughout the day, and some women require vaginal surgery for cystoceles or rectoceles. A **cystocele** is a protrusion of the urinary bladder through the vaginal wall. A **rectocele** is the protrusion of part of the rectum through the vaginal wall. Both of these conditions produce pressure and reduce bladder capacity, thereby creating urinary urgency and frequency.

Research Note

It is essential for nurses to understand which factors affect a client's compliance with health care regimens and how these factors interact to produce eventual adherence or nonadherence. Chang et al. studied 268 older women (ages 58 to 89), and found that characteristics most closely correlated with compliance were widowed status, preexisting satisfaction with health care, a well-developed social network, and perception of the examination as important.

This study brings much needed clarity to the body of literature on adherence, or compliance. Most salient among its findings is that the personal characteristics of the client are much more powerful determinants of health-seeking and health-maintaining behaviors than are such factors as the technical quality of care, the amount of attention paid by nurses to psychosocial issues, or the extent of client participation in formulating the health care regimen.

(Chang et al. 1985)

Nursing interventions include encouraging the client to drink an adequate amount of fluid, e.g., 3000 ml per day if health permits. Also advise the client to seek medical advice at the first sign of an infection, urinary frequency, or urinary retention. See Chapter 44 for further information.

Inadequate Exercise and Rest

A regular program of moderate exercise is recommended for elderly adults. Walking, golfing, gardening, bowling, and bicycling are common activities. These can be performed at a leisurely pace. It is important that exercise not be too strenuous and that rest periods be taken as needed. Rapid breathing and accelerated heartbeat should disappear within a few minutes after exercise; exercise should refresh rather than fatigue. People who are too disabled to engage in active exercise can implement a program of isometric exercises to maintain joint mobility and muscle tone. Exercise is also essential to maintain bone calcification. See Chapter 37.

Older people require more rest than before because they tire more easily. Often sleep habits change. Naps taken frequently throughout the day can cause difficulty sleeping at night. Measures to promote rest are discussed in Chapter 40. Moderate exercise often helps the client to sleep at night.

Sexuality

Certain aspects of sexuality persist into later life. Grooming as part of sexual identity is one. For instance, a woman might care greatly about her appearance, e.g., her clothes or her hair. A man, too, might place great value on a neat appearance, close shave, and trimmed hair.

An important aspect of sexual relations is intimacy. The closeness and love manifested as sexuality can provide a sense of belonging and worth. The loss of a partner is a crisis for the older person. Sometimes the survivor feels that it will be impossible to be close to another person. With time, however, a new significant relationship can be formed, although it may differ from the previous relationship. The elderly often find companionship and affection in seniors centers and volunteer societies. Nurses can provide information about such agencies.

Nurses may also need to teach clients about the physical sexual changes that take place with advanced age. Women, for example, may need to learn how to insert lubricating vaginal suppositories.

Independence

Most elderly people thrive on independence. It is important to them to be able to look after themselves even if they have to struggle to do so. Although it may be difficult for younger family members to watch the oldster completing tasks in a slow, determined way, the aging need this sense of accomplishment. Children might notice that the aging father or mother with failing vision cannot keep the kitchen as clean as before. The aging father and mother may be slower and less meticulous in carpentry tasks or gardening. To maintain the elderly adult's sense of self-respect, nurses and family members need to encourage them to do as much as possible for themselves. Many young people err in thinking that they are helpful to older people when they take over for them and do the job much faster and more efficiently. See Figure 26–2.

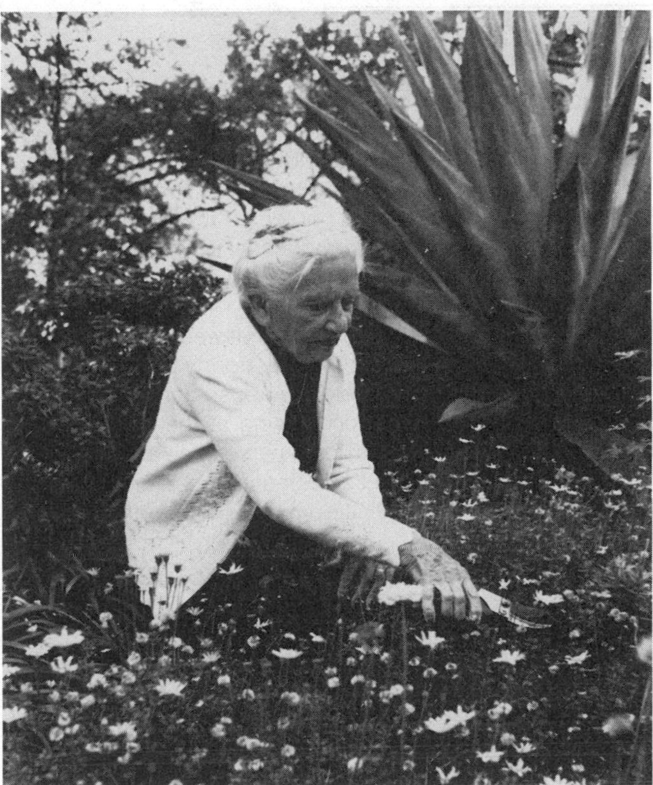

Figure 26–2 Independence fosters self-respect.

Some older people who are ill appear to enjoy the dependent role of being waited on and attended to. Nurses need to show an interest in such people as persons and set realistic, achievable goals. Praise and recognition for each accomplishment, no matter how small, are important. Success at getting out of bed independently or feeding oneself, if recognized by the nurse, can encourage people to achieve more and more. Some people may be afraid that they are not going to get better; others may feel that dependence brings them more recognition and importance. The nurse needs to understand each person's feelings and concerns before helping the older person toward independence. If clients know, for example, that an increasing level of wellness is possible and that the nurse will pay as much attention to them when they attempt tasks independently as when they are dependent, they probably will feel better about their progress.

Respect

Aging people need to be recognized for their unique individual characteristics. It can be difficult to recognize these differences, since elderly people have less energy than the young to show how they are different. Perhaps this is one reason elderly people tend to talk about past accomplishments, jobs, deeds, and experiences.

Nurses need to acknowledge the elderly client's ability to think, reason, and make decisions. Most elderly people are willing to listen to suggestions and advice, but they do not need to be ordered around. The nurse can support a decision by an elderly client even if eventually the decision is reversed because of failing health.

Older people appreciate thoughtfulness, consideration, and acceptance of their waning abilities. For example, having dinner out in a well-lighted restaurant or not expecting grandmother to babysit for too many hours, if at all, are actions that recognize the diminishing vision and energy of older people.

The values and standards held by older people need to be accepted, whether they are related to ethical, religious, or household matters. For example, it is wise to respect an older person's decision to hang the laundry outside rather than to use a dryer, or to cook on a wood stove.

Chronic Health Problems

Chronic health problems, such as impaired vision or hearing, osteoporosis, hypertension, and depression, must be monitored and treated. Perhaps the elderly person needs assistance and encouragement to seek health care.

Research Note

Although the focus of a study by Phillips and Rempusheski is on the decision-making processes of professionals who work with the frail elderly, there is a secondary, more clinical focus. The data presented here suggest that the detection of abuse and neglect of the elderly is often difficult and that decisions about how to ameliorate these situations are frought with conflict, ambivalence, and "postdecisional regret."

Phillips and Rempusheski interviewed 29 professionals who provide health care to the elderly to find out how the professionals defined elderly abuse and neglect and what values they applied in arriving at that definition. A clear finding is that professional nurses use complex and highly subjective criteria to diagnose abuse or neglect in an elderly population. (Phillips and Rempusheski 1985)

Programs in the community are directed toward (a) early detection of illness; (b) services such as dietary counseling, eye care, foot care, and routine medical care; and (c) activities that encourage exercise and social interaction to help prevent social isolation.

Nurses can assist elderly people to maintain maximum independent function. Elderly clients can learn new skills to help them function as fully as possible within any limitations. In some cases, episodes of acute illness or injury, e.g., influenza, burns, and falls, can be prevented.

Chapter Highlights

- The life expectancy of North Americans is increasing.
- A number of theories strive to account for the biologic aging process.
- Psychosocial theories about aging include the disengagement, activity, and continuity theories.
- Certain physical changes in most body systems are associated with aging.
- The elderly person usually has to adjust to many psychosocial changes.
- There is minimal change in the intellectual abilities of the healthy elderly person.
- Of the two types of memory, primary and secondary, secondary memory has been found to decline with aging.
- In learning, the elderly person has problems retrieving information in the brain.
- The moral concerns of elderly people tend to be interpersonal rather than social or legalistic.
- Spiritual maturity can provide the elderly person with inner resources for dealing with life experiences.

Suggested Readings

Hirst, S. P., and Metcalf, B. J. February 1984. Promoting self-esteem. *Journal of Gerontological Nursing* 10:72–77.
Hirst and Metcalf describe the importance of self-esteem. The components of self-esteem—roles, touch, meaningful relationships, sexuality, independence, and space—are explained in relation to the needs of the elderly. The authors identify a number of problems that result when the components of self-esteem are not acknowledged. The article also includes nursing interventions that can foster self-esteem.

Mace, N., and Rabins, P. 1981. The 36-hour day: A family guide to caring for persons with Alzheimer's disease, related dementing illnesses and memory loss in later life. Baltimore: Johns Hopkins University Press.

Ravish, T. October 1985. Prevent social isolation before it starts. *Journal of Gerontological Nursing*. 11:10–13.
Ravish discusses social isolation and the reasons for isolation among the elderly. Ravish points out that disengagement does not mean isolation but merely the self-determined narrowing of one's social circle. Stereotyping of the aging contributes to social isolation. Ravish emphasizes that the elderly client should not be compared to the hospitalized client. It is possible to assess the vulnerability of the elderly to social isolation, which can be conceptualized as a hierarchy.

Tavon, E. January/February 1984. Tips to trigger memory. *Geriatric Nursing* 5:26–27.
According to Tavon, memory loss is the biggest single impediment to the independent living of a group of clients at the Geriatric Day Care Center at the Jewish Home and Hospital for the Aged in New York. These clients were reluctant to admit memory loss. Tavon discusses classes that help the elderly sharpen memory and gives tips to help the clients remember the placement of such items as keys and eyeglasses. The article also includes methods nurses can use to help their clients keep their homes safe.

Selected References

Boettcher, E. G. March 1985. Linking the aged to support systems: Aging. *Journal of Gerontological Nursing* 11:27–33.

Butler, R. 1963. The life review: An interpretation of reminiscence in the aged. *Psychiatry* 26:65.

Butler, R. N., and Lewis, M. I. 1981. *Aging and mental health*. 3d ed. St. Louis: C. V. Mosby Co.

Carnevali, D. L., and Patrick, M., editors. 1986. *Nursing management for the elderly*. 2d ed. Philadelphia: J. B. Lippincott.

Chang, B.; Uman, G.; Linn, L.; Ware, J.; and Kane, R. January/February 1985. Adherence to health care regimens among elderly women. *Nursing Research* 34(1):27–31.

Clites, J. August 1984. Maximizing memory retention in the aged. *Journal of Gerontological Nursing* 10:34–35, 38–39.

Cutler, N. R., and Narang, P. K. May–June, 1985. Drug Therapies (Alzheimer's Disease). Geriatric Nursing 6:160–163.

Davis, K. L., and Mohs, R. C. November 13, 1986. Cholinergic drugs in Alzheimer's disease. New England Journal of Medicine, 315:1286.

Ebersole, P., and Hess, P. 1985. *Toward healthy aging: Human needs and nursing response.* 2d ed. St. Louis: C. V. Mosby Co.

Edelman, C., and Mandle, C. L. 1986. *Health promotion throughout the life span.* St. Louis: C. V. Mosby Co.

Erikson, E. H. 1963. *Childhood and society.* 2d ed. New York: W. W. Norton and Co.

Ferguson, D., and Beck, C. September/October 1983. H.A.L.F.—A tool to assess elder abuse within the family. *Geriatric Nursing* 4:301–4.

Fowler, J., and Keen, S. 1978, 1985. *Life maps: Conversations in the journey of faith.* Waco, Texas: Word Books.

Gioiella, E. C., and Bevil, C. W. 1985. *Nursing care of the aging client: Promoting healthy adaptation.* Norwalk, Conn.: Appleton-Century-Crofts.

Gress, L. D., and Bahr, R. T. 1984. *The aging person: A holistic perspective.* St. Louis: C. V. Mosby Co.

Kart, C. S.; Metress, E. S.; and Metress, J. F. 1978. *Aging and health: Biologic and social perspectives.* Menlo Park, Calif.: Addison-Wesley Publishing Co.

King, F. E.; Figge, J.; and Harpman, P. January 1986. The elderly coping at home: A study of continuity of nursing care. *Journal of Advanced Nursing* 11:41–46.

Kohlberg, L. 1971. *Recent research in moral development.* New York: Holt, Rinehart and Winston.

Maslow, A. 1970. *Religions, values, and peak-experiences.* New York: Viking Press.

Murray, R. B., and Zentner, J. P. 1985. *Nursing assessment and health promotion through the life span.* 3d ed. Englewood Cliffs, N.J.: Prentice-Hall.

Peck, R. 1955. Psychological developments in the second half of life. In Anderson, J., editor. *Psychological aspects of aging.* Washington, D.C.: American Psychological Association.

Phillips, L., and Rempusheski, V. May/June 1985. A decision-making model for diagnosing and intervening in elder abuse and neglect. *Nursing Research* 34(3):134–39.

Powell, L., and Courtice, K. 1983. Alzheimer's Disease: A Guide for Families. Reading, MA: Addison-Wesley.

Prehn, R. A., et al. January 1984. Can you assess the total population? . . . Assessing the elderly. *Journal of Gerontological Nursing* 10:8–13.

Rybash, J. M.; Roodin, P. A.; and Hoyer, W. J. 1983. Expressions of moral thought in later adulthood. *Gerontologist* 23:254–59.

Schneider, E. L., and Emr, M. May–June, 1985. Alzheimer's Disease: Research Highlights. *Geriatric Nursing* 6:135–138.

Stevens-Long, J. 1984. *Adult life developmental processes.* 2d ed. Palo Alto, Calif.: Mayfield Publishing Co.

United States Department of Health and Human Services. August 1985. *Charting the nation's health trends since 1960.* DHHS Pub. no. (PHS) 85-1251. Hyattsville, Md.: Public Health Service.

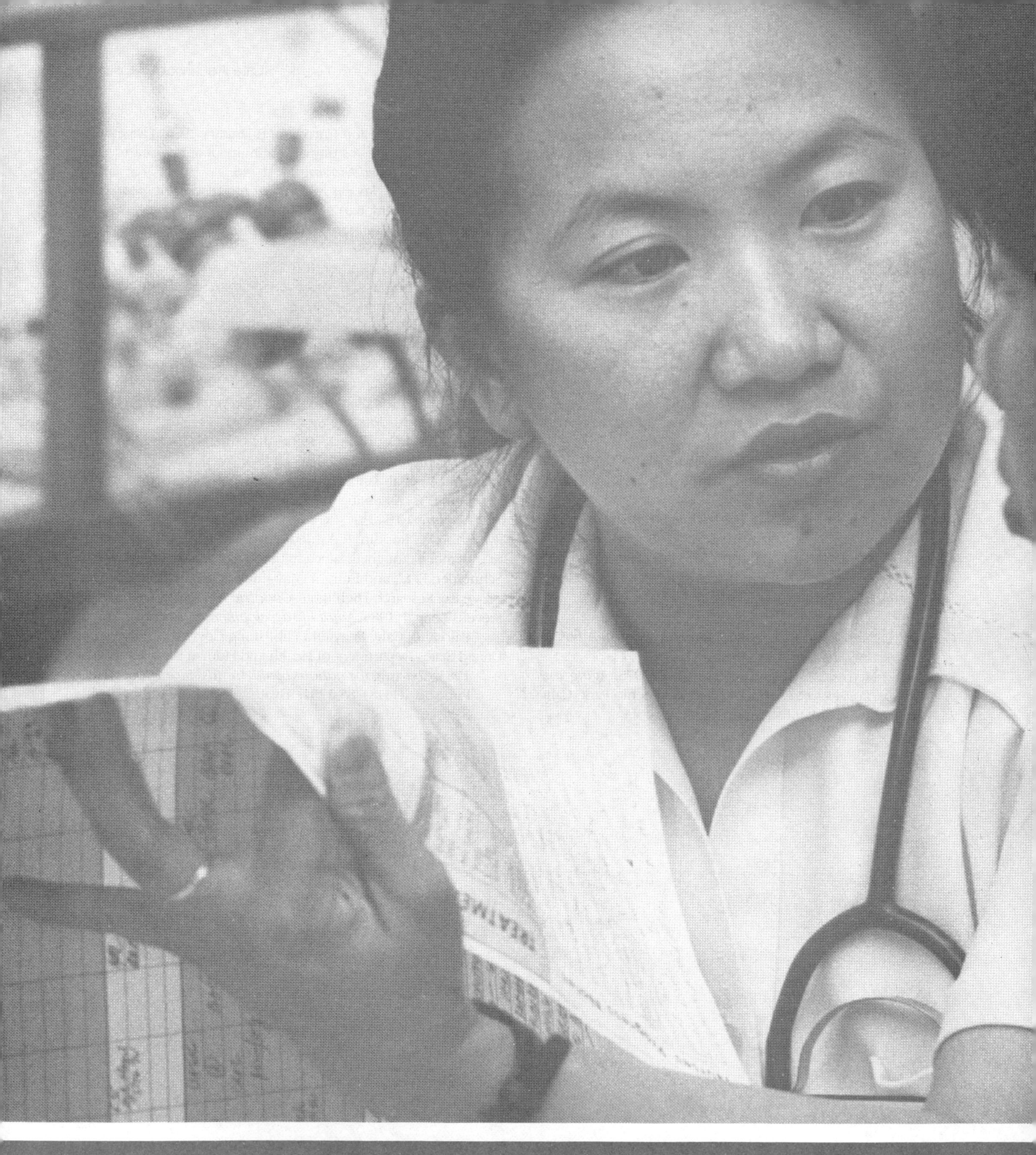

The nursing craft speaks in a language of its own—the silent language of human exchange which is eloquent and exciting without words.
(Myra Estrin Levine)

UNIT **6**

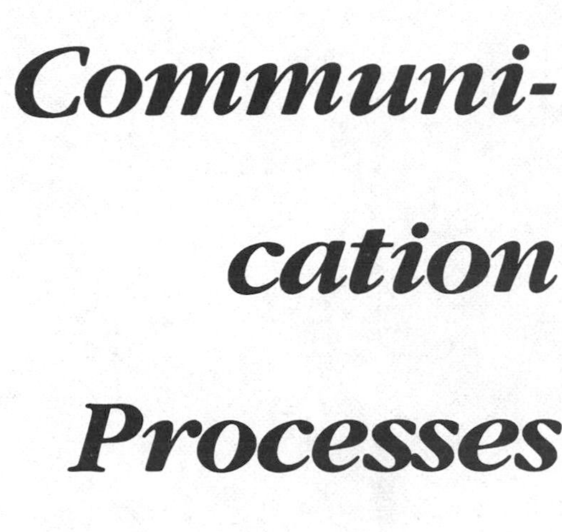

Communication Processes

Contents

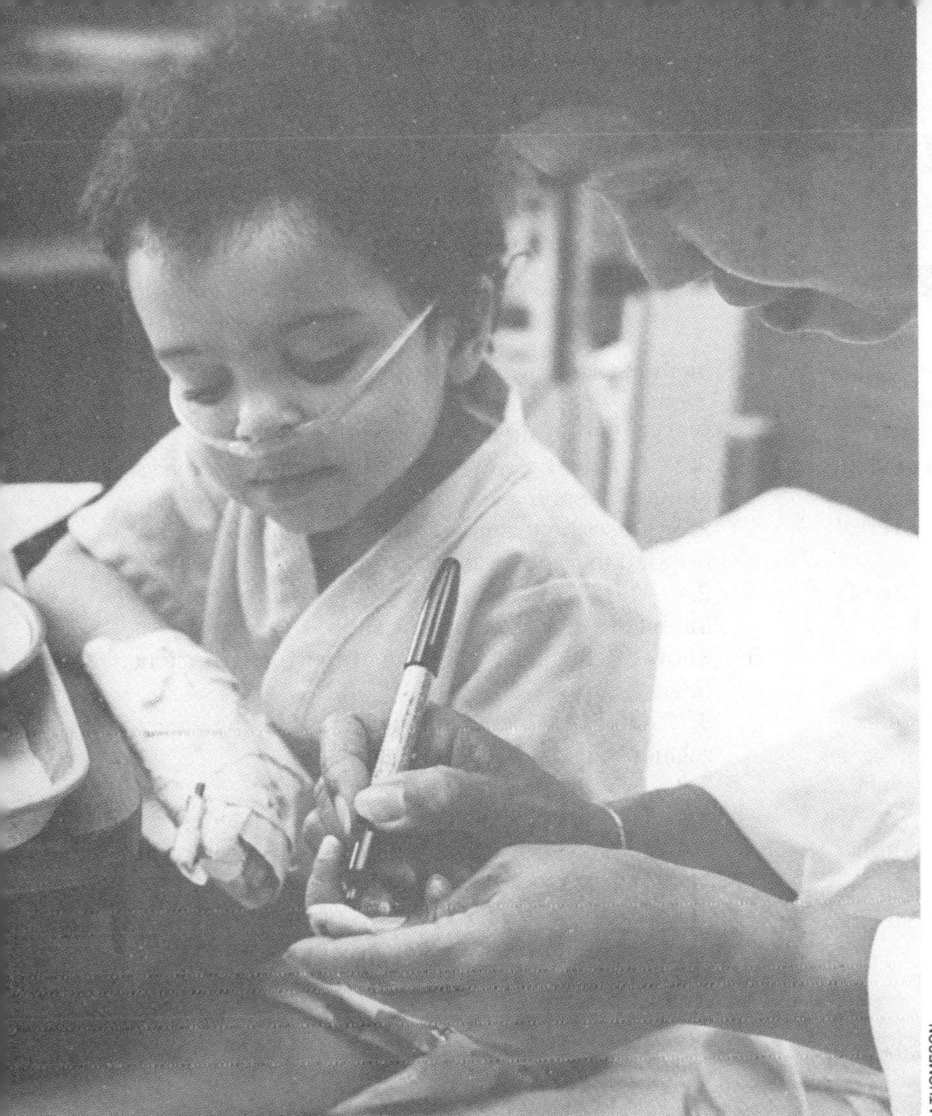

WILLIAM THOMPSON

CHAPTER 27

Communicating

Contents

27 *Communicating*

Objectives

1. Understand essential facts about communication, the communication process, and language development
   1.1 Differentiate between verbal and nonverbal communication
   1.2 Identify five characteristics of effective verbal messages
   1.3 Identify various attributes and limitations of nonverbal communication
   1.4 Identify aspects of nonverbal behavior that need to be assessed
   1.5 Explain the four elements of the communication process outlined in this chapter
   1.6 Identify ways in which selected factors influence the communication process
   1.7 Describe essential aspects of neurolinguistic programming
   1.8 Outline aspects of communication (language) development
   1.9 Identify factors that influence language development
   1.10 Identify ways in which language development can be stimulated
2. Know essential facts about effective and ineffective methods used by nurses when communicating with clients
   2.1 Describe attentive (active) listening.
   2.2 Outline five ways in which the nurse conveys physical attending
   2.3 Describe techniques the nurse can use to respond therapeutically to the client
   2.4 Describe responses the nurse may give that inhibit the client's communication
3. Know essential facts about an effective nurse–client relationship
   3.1 Outline general guidelines for helping relationships
   3.2 Describe empathy
   3.3 List behaviors associated with genuineness
   3.4 Identify four phases of the nurse–client relationship
   3.5 Identify essential elements of each phase of the nurse–client relationship
4. Evaluate the nurse–client communication interaction
   4.1 Write a process recording of an interaction with a selected client
   4.2 Analyze the interaction

Terms

babbling
communication
congruence
decode
echolalia
egocentric speech
empathy
encoding
feedback (in communication)
holophrastic speech
lalling
mirroring
monologue
neurolinguistic programming
nonverbal communication
paraphrasing
perception checking
personal space
probing
process recording
proxemics
reflexive vocalization
semantics
socialized speech
territoriality
verbal communication

Kinds of Communication

The term **communication** has various meanings, depending on the context in which it is used. To some, communication is the interchange of information between two or more people; in other words, the exchange of ideas or thoughts. This kind of communication uses methods such as talking and listening or writing and reading. However, it can also use painting, dancing, and story telling. Thoughts are conveyed to others not only by spoken or written words but also by gestures or body actions.

Communication may have a more personal connotation than the interchange of ideas or thoughts. It can be a transmission of feelings, or a more personal and social interaction between people. In this context, communication often is synonymous with relating. Frequently one member of a couple comments that the other is not communicating. Some teenagers complain about a generation gap—being unable to communicate with understanding or feeling to a parent or authority figure. Sometimes a nurse is said to be efficient but lacking in something called *bedside manner.* For the purpose of this text, *communication* is any means of exchanging information or feelings between two or more people. It is a basic component of human relationships.

The intent of any communication is to elicit a response. Thus, communication is a process. It includes all the techniques by which an individual affects another. It has two main purposes: to influence others and to obtain information. Whether verbal or nonverbal, communication can be described as helpful (therapeutic) or unhelpful (nontherapeutic). The former encourages a sharing of information, thoughts, or feelings between two or more people. The latter hinders or blocks the transfer of information and feelings.

To communicate effectively with clients and their support persons, nurses need to become skilled in therapeutic communication techniques and in developing helping relationships.

Communication is generally categorized into two basic kinds, verbal and nonverbal. **Verbal communication** uses the spoken or written word; **nonverbal communication** uses other forms, such as gestures or facial expressions. Although both kinds of communication occur concurrently, the majority of communication (some say 80 to 90%) is nonverbal. This may be surprising to those who associate communication with only verbal expression. Learning about nonverbal communication is thus an important consideration for nurses in developing effective communication patterns and relationships with clients.

Verbal Communication

Verbal communication is largely a conscious effort in that people choose the words they use. The words used vary among individuals according to culture, socioeconomic background, age, and education. As a result, countless possibilities exist in the way ideas are exchanged. An abundance of words can be used to form messages. In addition, a wide variety of feelings can be conveyed when talking. The intonation of the voice can express animation, enthusiasm, sadness, annoyance, or amusement, to name some examples. The number of different intonations heard when people say "hello" or "good morning" illustrates the variety that is possible. The pacing or rhythm of a person's communication is another variable. Monotonous rhythms or very rapid rhythms can be products of lack of energy or interest or of anxiety or fear.

Characteristics of Effective Verbal Messages

When choosing words to say or to write, nurses need to consider several criteria of effective communication. These include (a) simplicity, (b) clarity, (c) timing and relevance, (d) adaptability, and (e) credibility.

Simplicity The best teachers can state complex ideas in simple words. The same holds true for persons communicating everyday concerns. Simplicity includes the use of commonly understood words, brevity, and completeness.

Many people have a tendency to overcommunicate. Their messages are wordy, contain too many extraneous explanations, or use words that are highly academic, technical, or slangy. In the world of nursing, many complex technical terms become natural to nurses. However, these terms can often be misunderstood even by informed laypeople. Words such as *discombobulate* or *cholecystectomy* may be meaningful to the speaker and easy to use but are ill-advised when communicating with most clients. Nurses need to learn to select simple words intentionally even though effort is required to do so. For example, instead of saying to a client, "The nurse will be catheterizing you tomorrow for a urine specimen," it is better to say, "Tomorrow a sample of your urine is needed, and it will be necessary to collect it by putting a tube into your bladder." The latter statement is likely to produce a response from the client about why it is needed and whether it will hurt or be uncomfortable. The former statement may simply make the client wonder what the nurse means.

Another consideration related to simplicity is brevity. Most people have heard others give lengthy explanations of events, to which they respond, "Get to the point." By using short sentences and avoiding unnecessary material, the speaker or writer can achieve brevity. This is of particular importance in writing. Busy people do not have the time to read several pages before discovering the main issue or recommendations. Reports or memos need to be concise and should be condensed into a single paragraph or page, if possible.

The opposite of overcommunicating is undercommunicating. Shortcuts for the sake of simplicity can lead

Research Note

Some nurses think that today's clients are better informed than clients of years ago because they receive better health education and watch more television. However, in a research study of 100 randomly selected clients, Aina Apse found that many are bewildered by 41 commonly used clinical terms: Not one of the research subjects could correctly define all of the terms. The results ranged from one client who understood only 4% of the terms to another who understood 97%. Most of the clients understood between 51% and 75% of the terms.

The least understood terms included *N.P.O.*, *ambulate*, and *impaction*. Surprisingly, 63% didn't understand the term *blood pressure;* and 29% didn't understand *malignant*. Some clients thought *dilate* means "smaller," *orally* means "every hour," *P.O.* means "afternoon." This research demonstrates how important it is for the nurse to find out which terms a particular client understands and then to avoid using potentially confusing terms. (Apse 1985)

to incomplete or unclear communication. For example, initials or abbreviations such as b.i.d. (twice a day) or ICU (intensive care unit) should be avoided unless the nurse is certain that the initials will be readily understood. Because clarification is required, abbreviations can waste the listener's or reader's time. At the first use, names should be expressed in full; later they can be shortened when the nurse is sure that the client or reader knows the meanings.

Clarity *Clarity* means saying exactly what is meant. It also is aligned with meaning what is said. The latter involves a blending of the speaker's behavior (nonverbal communication) with the words that are spoken. When the words and the behavior blend together or are unified, the communication is regarded as consistent or congruent.

The goal of clarity is to communicate so that people know the what, how, why (if necessary), when, who, and where of any specific event. Without these, people are left to make assumptions. To ensure clarity in communication, the nurse also needs to speak slowly and enunciate words well. It may be helpful to repeat the message and to reduce distractions such as surrounding noises.

Some common pitfalls that can produce unclear communications are ambiguous statements, generalizations, and opinions. For example, "Men are stronger than women" is both a generalization and an opinion, and the term *stronger* is open to several interpretations. Another example is a nurse's statement to a client, "Mrs. Smith, you need to keep busy today." The specific actions Mrs. Smith is expected to carry out and the reasons for them are open to many interpretations.

Timing and relevance No matter how clearly or simply words are stated or written, the timing needs to be appropriate to ensure that words are heard. Moreover, the messages need to relate to the person or to the person's interests and concerns. Consider the woman whose children are crying and whose doorbell is ringing while she is on the telephone. This is not the best time for the person on the other end of the telephone to try to make a sale, even if the woman is interested.

Nurses need to be aware of both relevance and timing when communicating with clients. This involves being sensitive to the client's needs and concerns. For example, if a female client is enmeshed in fear of cancer, she may not hear the nurse's explanations about the expected procedures before and after her gallbladder surgery. In this situation it is better for the nurse first to encourage the client to express her concerns, and to then deal with those concerns; at another time the necessary explanations can be provided.

Another pitfall is to ask several questions at once. For example, a nurse enters a client's room and says in one breath, "Good morning, Mrs. Brody. How are you this morning? Did you sleep well last night? Your husband is coming to see you before your surgery, isn't he?" The client no doubt would feel bombarded and confused and wonder which question to answer first, if any. A related pattern of poor timing is to ask a question and then not wait for an answer before making another comment. To Mr. Ramirez the nurse says, "How is that swollen leg this morning? I'm getting your bath water now before the doctor comes."

Adaptability Spoken messages need to be altered in accordance with behavioral cues from the receiver. This adjustment is referred to as *adaptability.* Moods and behavior may change minute by minute, hour by hour, or from day to day. In this sense the nurse needs to avoid routine or automatic speech. What the nurse says and how it is said must be individualized and carefully considered. This requires astute assessment and sensitivity on the part of the nurse. For example, a nurse who usually smiles, appears cheerful, and greets her client every afternoon with an enthusiastic "Hi, Mr. Brown!" notices that he is not smiling and appears distressed when she appears. In response to the client's cues, the nurse adapts her usual greeting and tones down her cheery manner. She may say "Hi" in a much softer and caring manner and express concern in her facial expression while she moves toward him.

Credibility *Credibility* means worthy of belief, trustworthy, reliable. Credibility may be the most important criterion of effective communication. A nurse's credibility to clients depends in part on the opinion of others. If other health workers and clients regard the nurse as trustworthy, then so will the client. Developing trust is discussed later in this chapter in the section on "Developing helping relationships."

To become credible, the nurse needs to be knowledgeable about the subject matter being discussed and to have accurate information. The nurse also needs to convey confidence and certainty in what she or he is saying. This is often referred to as *positivism.* People tend to perceive confidence, which is dynamic and emphatic, as more credible than hesitance or uncertainty, which is less forceful and less active. However, care needs to be taken not to sound overconfident or authoritarian. This can be prevented by stating messages in a constructive way focused on being helpful to clients.

Reliability, the third aspect of credibility, is developed by being consistent, dependable, and honest. People value the nurse who acknowledges limitations and can say, "I don't know the answer to that, but I'll find someone who does, and you can talk to that person."

Nonverbal Communication

Nonverbal communication is sometimes called *body language.* It includes gestures, body movements, and physical appearance, including adornment. The majority of communication is nonverbal. Nonverbal communication often tells others more about what a person is feeling than what is actually said, because nonverbal behavior is controlled less consciously than verbal behavior. As a result, listeners tend to rely on body language more than on words. Nonverbal communication either reinforces or contradicts what is said verbally. For example, a nurse may say to a client, "I'd be happy to sit here and talk to you for a while," yet if she glances nervously at her watch every few seconds, the actions contradict the verbal message. The nonverbal behavior, suggesting "I am very busy," is more likely to be believed.

Certain limitations exist in nonverbal communication. Observers cannot always be sure of the feelings being expressed by nonverbal behavior. On the one hand, the same feeling can be expressed nonverbally in more than one way. For example, anger may be communicated by aggressive or excessive body motion, or it may be communicated by a frozen stillness. On the other hand, a variety of feelings, such as embarrassment, pleasure, or anger, can be expressed by a single nonverbal cue, such as blushing.

Observing and interpreting the client's nonverbal behavior are essential skills for nurses. Observational skills use the senses of seeing, hearing, touching, and smelling. Interpreting the observations requires validation with the client, using specific communication techniques discussed subsequently in this chapter.

The nurse's own nonverbal behavior is under constant scrutiny by clients. It is therefore necessary for nurses to gain awareness of their actions and to learn to convey understanding, respect, and acceptance to clients.

Assessing Nonverbal Behavior

To observe nonverbal behavior efficiently requires a systematic approach. Generally the nurse assesses the person's overall physical appearance, including adornments, posture, and gait, and then assesses specific parts of the body, such as the face and the hands.

Physical appearance The person's appearance includes physical characteristics and manner of dress. Physical characteristics can denote the person's state of health. Skin color and texture, length of fingernails, weight, and deformities causing physical limitations are a few examples. The skin may appear dry, mottled, or pale. Weight may indicate malnourishment. Nails may be well manicured or extremely short. Whatever is observed, the nurse needs to exercise caution in interpretation. For example, pale skin may be normal for that person. Nails may be short because they were bitten nervously or because they were broken by hard manual labor.

Clothing and adornments are sometimes rich sources of information about a person. Choice of apparel is highly personal. Clothing may convey social and financial status, culture, religion, group association, and self-concept. Adornments such as jewelry, perfume, and cosmetics reveal additional information.

How a person dresses is often an indicator of how the person feels. People who are tired or ill may not have the energy or the desire to maintain their normal grooming. The nurse also needs to be alert to sudden changes in a person's dress. When a person known for immaculate grooming becomes lax about appearance and stays in nightclothes all day, this may suggest a loss of self-esteem or a physical illness. Hair care and nail care may be lacking, and dress may be inappropriate. Appropriateness of dress also depends on context. A swimsuit worn to a beach party is appropriate, whereas a swimsuit worn to a formal dinner party is not.

In acute general hospital settings, indications that a client is feeling better often relate to dress, particularly personal adornment. A male client may request a shave, or a female client may request a mirror and her lipstick.

Posture and gait The ways people walk and carry themselves often are a reliable indicator of self-concept, current mood, and health. Erect posture and an active, purposeful stride suggest a feeling of well-being. Slouched posture and a slow, shuffling gait suggest dejection or physical discomfort. Tense posture and a rapid, determined gait suggest anxiety or anger. Likewise, the sitting or lying postures of clients can communicate feelings.

Facial expression No part of the body is as expressive as the face. See Figure 27–1. Feelings of joy, sadness, fear, surprise, anger, and disgust can be conveyed by facial expressions. The muscles around the eyes and the mouth are particularly expressive. Although actors learn to control these muscles to convey emotions to audiences, facial expressions generally are not consciously controlled.

Clients are quick to notice the nurse's facial expression, particularly when the clients feel unsure or uncomfortable. The client who questions the nurse about a feared diagnostic result will watch the nurse to see whether the nurse looks at him or her to answer or whether the nurse looks away. The client who has disfigurement will examine the nurse's face for signs of disgust. Nurses, like actors, need to be aware of their facial expressions and what they are communicating to clients. Although it is impossible to control all facial expressions, the nurse must learn to control feelings such as fear and disgust in certain situations.

Many facial expressions convey a universal meaning. The smile conveys happiness. Contempt is conveyed by the mouth turned down, the head tilted back, and the eyes directed down the nose. No single expression can be interpreted accurately, however, without considering (a) other reinforcing physical cues, (b) the setting in which it occurs, and (c) the expression of others in the same

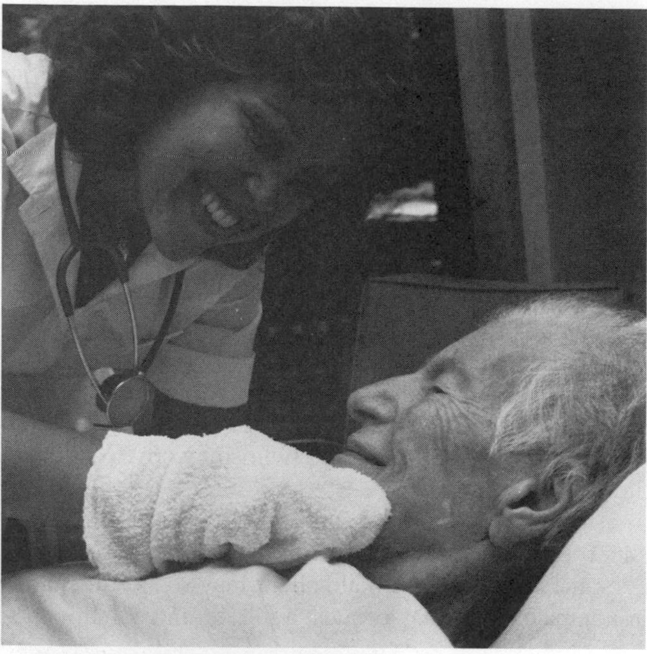

Figure 27–1 The nurse's facial expression communicates warmth and caring.

setting. For instance, when a person is smiling at others who are intently watching an accident victim on the street, the smile could convey contempt.

Eye contact is another essential element of facial communication. Mutual eye contact acknowledges recognition of the other person and a willingness to maintain communication. Often the eye initiates contact with another person with a glance, capturing the person's attention prior to communicating. Eye contact is generally averted or avoided when a person feels weak or defenseless. The communication received may be too embarrassing or too dominating. Animals are known to succumb to dominance by averting first their eyes and then their presence. See also the discussion of eye contact in Native American cultures, on page 371.

Hand movements and gestures Like faces, hands are expressive. They can communicate feelings at any given moment. Envision a relative waiting for word about a client in surgery. Anxious people may wring their hands or pick their nails; relaxed persons may interlock their fingers over their laps or allow their hands to fall over the ends of armrests. Hands also communicate by touch: Hitting someone in the face or caressing another person communicates obvious feelings.

Hands are frequently involved in gestures. The handshake, the victory sign, the wave good-bye, the hand motion to ask a visitor to sit down are gestures that have relatively univeral meanings. Some gestures, however, are socially accepted in one culture but not in another. European women walk together holding hands as a sign of friendship; in North American society, for two women to hold hands is usually regarded as unacceptable. Even the same gesture can have different meanings in different cultures. The North American gesture of the hands that means "shoo away" or "go away" means "come here" or "come back" in some Japanese cultures.

Hands are also very expressive in illustrating or stylizing verbal communication. The French and Italian cultures are noted for using their hands in this manner. Instead of using words alone to describe the shape and size of an object, the hands are manipulated to reinforce the verbal message.

For people with special communication problems, such as the deaf, the hands are invaluable in communication. Many deaf people learn sign language. Ill persons who are unable to reply verbally can similarly devise a unique communication system using the hands. The client may be able to raise an index finger once for "yes" and twice for "no." Other signals can often be devised by the client and the nurse to denote other meanings.

Gestures often involve body parts other than the hands. In some cultures a gentleman may bow before a lady; two European men greet each other by embracing and touching opposite cheeks alternately; men and women kiss to say hello or goodbye.

The Communication Process

A number of models have been used to explain the communication process. The purpose of a model is to break down the process of communication into its essential components so that it can be better understood. A communication model has two main parts: people and messages. In face-to-face communication there is a sender, a message, a receiver, and a response (feedback). See Figure 27–2. In its simplest form, communication is a two-way process involving the sending and the receiving of a message. Since the intent of communication is to elicit a response, the process is ongoing; the receiver of the message then becomes the sender of a response message, and the original sender then becomes the receiver. Several sequential models have been proposed for the communication process, incorporating from four to six elements, but sender, message receiver, and response are essential to all models.

Sender

The sender, a person or group who wishes to convey a message to another, is sometimes called the *source-encoder.*

This term includes the concept that the person or group sending the message first must have an idea or reason for communicating (source) and second must put the idea or feeling into a form that can be transmitted. **Encoding** involves the selection of specific signs or symbols (codes) to transmit the message, such as the use of English or French words, the specific arrangement of the words, and the tone of voice and gestures to use. For example, if the receiver speaks English, English words will usually be selected. If the message is "No, Johnny, you may not have any more cookies before dinner!" the tone of voice selected will be one of firmness, and a shake of the head or a pointing index finger can reinforce it. In addition, the nurse must not only consider dialects and foreign languages but also must cope with two language levels—the layman's and the health professional's.

Message

The second component of the communication process is the message itself—what is actually said or written, the body language that accompanies the words, and how the message is transmitted. Various channels can be used to convey messages, and frequently combinations are used. It is important that the channel be appropriate for the message and make the intent of the message clear.

Talking face-to-face with a person may be more effective in some instances than telephoning or writing a message. Recording messages on tape or communicating by radio or television may be more appropriate for larger audiences. Written communication is often appropriate for long explanations or for a communication that needs to be preserved. The nonverbal channel of touch is often highly effective.

Receiver

The receiver, the third component of the communication process, is the listener, who must be listening, observing, and attending. This person, sometimes called the *decoder,* must perceive what the sender intended (sensation) and then analyze the information received (interpretation). Perception involves use of all the senses to receive all verbal and nonverbal messages. To **decode** means to relate the message perceived to the receiver's storehouse of knowledge and experience and to sort out the meaning of the message. Whether the message is decoded accurately by the receiver, according to the sender's intent, depends largely on their similarities in knowledge and experience. For example, Johnny may perceive the message accurately—"No more cookies for me right now." However, if experience has taught him that he can help himself to the cookie jar without punishment, he will interpret the message differently from the way his mother intended it.

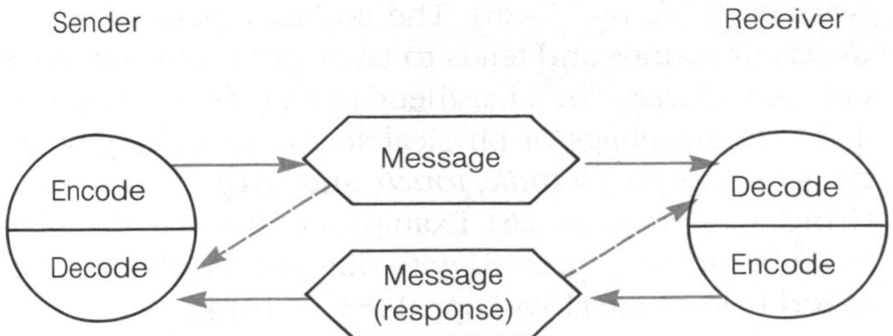

Figure 27–2 The communication process. The dashed arrows indicate internal feedback from the sender of the message (or response).

Response

The fourth component of the communication process, the response, is the message that the receiver returns to the sender. It is also called **feedback.** Feedback can be either positive or negative. Nonverbal examples are a nod of the head or a yawn. Either way, feedback allows the sender to correct or reword a message. In the case of Johnny, the receiver may cry or move away from the cookie jar or say, "Well, Judy had three cookies and I only had two." The sender then knows the message was interpreted accurately. However, now the original sender becomes the receiver, who is required to decode and respond.

The receiver is not the sole source of feedback. Communicators constantly receive *internal feedback* from themselves. Internal feedback is often used for written messages. For example, after composing a letter, a person will read it silently or out loud to see how it sounds; or a person who makes a social blunder (faux pas) may instantly realize the mistake and say, "That isn't what I really meant" or "I didn't mean it that way."

Neurolinguistic Programming (NLP)

Neurolinguistic programming (NLP) is an approach to the process of human communication recently developed by Bandler and Grinder (1975; 1976). It looks at the manner in which a person accesses (takes in) and processes (makes sense of) information. In this culture three modalities, referred to as *representational systems,* are most often used to access and process information: the visual mode, the auditory mode, and the kinesthetic mode (Bandler and Grinder 1975, p. 6). Even though people use all three modalities to some extent, a person tends to favor one mode over the others. The most effective communicators move from one mode to another willfully and easily.

Visually oriented persons are more receptive to information that is pictorially represented and they process information using internal pictures. They choose verbs, adjectives, and adverbs (predicates) that reflect a visual orientation, such as *see, illustrate,* and *clear* (Bandler and

Grinder 1976, pp. 3–26). The auditory person prefers words or sounds and tends to favor predicates like *hear, say,* and *discuss.* The kinesthetic person favors messages that reflect feelings or physical action, preferring predicates such as *feel, handle, touch,* and *grasp* (Bandler and Grinder 1976, pp. 3–26). Examples of the way the same thought can be expressed with different predicates (italicized below) are (Brockopp 1983, p. 1014):

> *Visual:* "Yes, I can *see* that you are much better. You *look* good, your eyes are *clear,* your *appearance* has certainly changed."
>
> *Auditory:* "Yes, I can *hear* from the *sound* of your voice that you are better. *Talking* with you today is quite different from yesterday."
>
> *Kinesthetic:* "Yes, you do seem to be *feeling* much better today. You're *holding* your head up, and your *grasp* is certainly *firmer* than yesterday."

Bandler and Grinder carefully observed outstanding communicators (such as Virginia Satir, a family therapist, and Fritz Perls, the developer of Gestalt therapy) to discover what made them such effective communicators. They noticed that such people instinctively listened to the client's choice of predicates and adapted themselves to or matched the client's representational system.

Nurses who use NLP techniques can learn to identify, improve, and expand their communication methods and become more effective communicators. Knowles (1983, p. 1011) says that nurses who identify their client's representational system can enhance their ability to get on the client's wavelength and to establish rapport. To determine whether the client's orientation is visual, auditory, or kinesthetic, the nurse observes the client's choice of predicates, eye cues, gross hand movements, breathing patterns, and speech patterns or tones. See Table 27–1. The nurse then attempts to comfortably reflect or mirror what is familiar to the other person—e.g., match the client's body position, breathing pattern, and use of predicates. **Mirroring** (matching the client's experience) is thought to reassure clients and make them feel secure, since they are observing something familiar to them. Mirroring takes considerable practice and must be done gradually to appear natural and respectful of the client. Knowles says that when nurses "try on" clients' styles, they increase their ability to "feel" with them.

Factors Influencing the Communication Process

In addition to the factors mentioned previously, such as variations in a person's sociocultural background, language, age, and education, and the limitations and attributes of nonverbal communication, the following factors affect the communication process: ability of the communicator; perceptions; personal space; territoriality; roles, relationships, and purposes; time and place; attitudes; and emotions and self-esteem.

Ability of the Communicator

The person's abilities to speak, hear, see, and comprehend stimuli influence the communication process. People who are hard of hearing may require messages that are short, loud, and clear. Those who are unable to read or write will be unable to comprehend written information. Some, because of disease processes, are unable to see or to speak, and individual methods for communication need to be devised with them.

The receiver of a message also needs to be able to interpret the message. Mental faculties can be impaired for such reasons as brain damage or use of sedative drugs or alcohol.

Even if a client is free of physical impairments, the nurse needs to determine how many stimuli the client is

Table 27–1 Selected Determinants of Neurolinguistic (NLP) Representational Systems

Determinant	Visual Accessing	Auditory Accessing	Kinesthetic Accessing
Preferred predicates	See, illustrate, imagine, view, notice, recognize, observe.	Hear, say, discuss, listen, hearsay, gripe, eavesdrop.	Handle, touch, grasp, feel, shudder, excite, thrill.
Eye cues	When visualizing, the eyes are turned upward or defocused straight ahead.	When processing auditory information, such as on a telephone, the eyes move from side to side or focus on the nondominant hand.	When thinking about experiences or feelings, the eyes focus on the dominant hand.
Gross hand movements	Often points toward the eye.	Often points toward the ear.	Often points to the chest or heart.
Breathing pattern	Shallow thoracic breathing.	Even breathing, or prolonged expiration.	Deep abdominal breathing.
Speech patterns and tones	Quick bursts of words; high-pitched, nasal tone.	Clear mid-range voice tone, or rhythmic tempo with well-enunciated words	Slow voice with a low volume, or deep tone or breathing tone with long pauses.

capable of receiving in a given time frame. Frequently the receiver is expected to assimilate too much information. The nurse may be talking too quickly or presenting too many ideas at once. This is of particular importance when offering health instruction.

Perceptions

Because each person has unique personality traits, values, and life experiences, each will perceive and interpret messages differently. For example, the nurse may draw the curtains around a crying woman and leave her alone. The woman may interpret this as "The nurse thinks I shouldn't cry and will upset the other clients" or "The nurse doesn't like crying" or "The nurse respects my need to be alone." It is important in many situations to validate or correct the perceptions of the receiver.

Personal Space

Personal space is the distance people prefer in interactions with others. **Proxemics** is the study of distance between people in their interactions. Middle-class North Americans use definite distances in various interpersonal relationships, along with specific voice tones and body language. Communication thus alters in accordance with four distances, each with a close and a far phase, that have been described by Hall (1969, p. 45):

1. Intimate: Physical contact to 1½ feet
2. Personal: 1½–4 feet
3. Social: 4–12 feet
4. Public: 12 feet and beyond

Intimate distance communication is characterized by body contact, heightened sensations of body heat and smell, and vocalizations that are low. Vision is intense, restricted to a small body part, and may be distorted. Intimate distance is frequently used by nurses. Examples occur in cuddling a baby, touching the sightless client, positioning clients, observing an incision, and restraining a toddler for an injection. It is a natural protective instinct for people to maintain a certain amount of space immediately around them, and the amount varies with individuals. When someone who wants to communicate steps too close, the receiver automatically steps back a pace or two. In their therapeutic roles, nurses often are required to violate this personal space. However, it is important for them to be aware of when it will occur and to forewarn the client, if possible. In many instances, the nurse can respect (not come as close as) a person's intimate distance. In other instances, the nurse may come within intimate distance to communicate warmth and caring.

Personal distance is less overwhelming than intimate distance. Voice tones are moderate, and body heat and smell are noticed less. Physical contact such as a handshake or touching a shoulder is possible. More of the person is perceived at a personal distance, so that nonverbal behaviors such as body stance or full facial expressions are seen with less distortion. Much communication between nurses and clients occurs at this distance. Examples occur when nurses are sitting with a client, giving medications, or establishing an intravenous infusion. Communication at a close personal distance can convey involvement by facilitating the sharing of thoughts and feelings. At the outer extreme of 4 ft, however, less involvement is conveyed. Bantering and some social conversations are usual at this distance.

Social distance is characterized by a clear visual perception of the whole person. Body heat and odor are imperceptible, eye contact is increased, and vocalizations are loud enough to be overheard by others. Communication is therefore more formal and is limited to seeing and hearing. The person is protected and out of reach for touch or personal sharing of thoughts or feelings. Social distance allows more activity and movement back and forth. It is expedient in communicating with several people at the same time or within a short time. Examples occur when nurses make rounds or wave a greeting to someone. Social distance is important in accomplishing the business of the day. However, it is frequently misused. For example, the nurse who stands in the doorway and asks a client "How are you today?" will receive a more noncommittal reply than the nurse who moves to personal distance to inquire.

Public distance requires loud, clear vocalizations with careful enunciation. Although the faces and forms of people are seen at public distance, individuality is lost. Instead, a general notion is perceived about a group of people or a community.

Territoriality

Territoriality is a concept of the space and things that an individual considers as belonging to him or her. Territories marked off by people may be visible to others. For example, a client in a hospital often considers his or her territory as bounded by the curtains around the bed unit or by the walls of a private room. This human tendency to claim territory must be recognized by all health care workers. Clients often feel the need to defend their territory when it is invaded by others; for example, when a visitor removes a chair to use at another bed, the visitor has inadvertently violated the territoriality of the client whose chair was moved.

The way in which territoriality affects the communication process is seen in the following example. Mrs. Brown, an elderly woman, had been hospitalized in an extended care unit for 3 months. A nurse removed the overbed cradle from her bed, because, in the nurse's opinion, Mrs. Brown no longer had a need for it, and it was needed for a newly admitted client's bed. Mrs. Brown got angry with the nurse and voiced loudly, "That's mine and belongs on my bed. If you take it away I'll report you to the administrator." The nurse continued to transfer the cradle and responded, "You can't report me, and you don't need this." The outcome was that Mrs. Brown's anger toward the nurse increased; she became distrustful and withdrew from further interactions with that nurse.

Roles, Relationships, and Purposes

The roles and the relationship between sender and receiver affect the communication process. Roles such as nursing student and instructor, client and physician, or parent and child will affect the content and responses in the communication process. Choice of words, sentence structure, and tone of voice vary considerably from role to role. In addition, the specific relationship between the communicators is significant. The nurse who meets with a client for the first time will communicate differently from the nurse who has previously developed a relationship with that client.

The intended purpose of a communication also alters interactions with others. For example, if the purpose is to acknowledge another's presence, the nurse may say, "Hello, how goes it today?" But if the purpose is to assess the person's pain and the effect of an analgesic, several more specific questions and responses are necessary.

Time and Setting

The time factor in communication includes what precedes and follows the interaction. The setting of the interaction is a related factor. The hospitalized client who is anticipating surgery or who has just received news that a spouse has lost a job will not be very receptive to information. A client who has had to wait for some time to express needs may respond quite differently from one who has endured no waiting period. The setting also influences communication. If the room lacks privacy or is hot, noisy, or crowded, the communication process can break down.

Nurses' use of time can facilitate or inhibit a client's communication. The nurse who tells a client "I'll be back in a moment" while delivering medications is likely to convey "I haven't time now" or "I've got work to do." This inhibits client communications. Some clients learn that requests need to be made as soon as the nurse appears. Often their request is accompanied by an apology for taking the nurse's time. However, if this nurse says to the client, "Would you tell me now what your concern is about, and then when I've finished delivering medications I'll come back and help you with it," the communication process is facilitated.

The concept of time also has cultural connotations. Caucasians, for example, tend to emphasize punctuality and think in terms of the hour, the day, the week, or the month. American Indians, on the other hand, are governed more by events of nature, such as the season. Appointments for child care or health screening programs will usually be kept by Caucasians. American Indians, however, may well defer appointments when nature beckons, regardless of how well in advance the communication was offered. Priority for them may be that "the salmon are running" or "the geese are flying."

Attitudes

Attitudes convey beliefs, thoughts, and feelings about people and events. They are communicated convincingly and rapidly to others. Attitudes such as caring, warmth, respect, and acceptance facilitate communication, whereas condescension, lack of interest, and coldness inhibit communication.

Caring and *warmth* are terms frequently used to describe the attitudes of people. They convey a feeling of emotional closeness, in contrast to impersonal distance. Caring is more enduring and intense than warmth. It conveys deep and genuine concern for the person. Warmth, on the other hand, conveys friendliness and consideration, shown by acts of smiling and attention to physical comforts (Brammer 1985, p. 34). Caring involves giving feelings, thoughts, skill, and knowledge. It requires psychologic energy and the risk of little in return, yet it usually reaps the benefits of greater communication and understanding.

Respect is an attitude that emphasizes the other person's worth and individuality. It conveys that the person's hopes and feelings are special and unique even though similar to others in many ways. People have a need to be different from others and at the same time to be similar to others. Being too different can be isolating and threatening. Respect is conveyed by listening open-mindedly to what the other person is saying, even if the nurse disagrees. Nurses can learn new ways of approaching situations when they conscientiously listen to another person's perspective.

Acceptance emphasizes neither approval nor disapproval. The nurse willingly receives client's honest feelings and actions without judgment. An accepting attitude allows clients to express personal feelings freely and to be themselves. The nurse may find that acceptance has to be restricted in situations where the client's actions are personally harmful or harmful to others.

In contrast, *condescension* is an attitude that conveys superiority over the other person. It magnifies the client's differences and inequality. Clients who feel helpless often perceive nurses to be in an elevated position with their knowledge and skill as helpers. In these instances, the nurse may convey condescension by an air of superiority and intellectualism. One common condescending act by nurses is to call clients "honey" or "dear" whether they are male or female, young or old. This makes the nurse a superior mother and the client an inferior child. Another is to pat an elderly client on the head.

Lack of interest also inhibits communication by saying "I'm not concerned" or "What you say is not important." This attitude is conveyed when the nurse forgets part of the client's conversation or does not concentrate on it sufficiently to respond. The nurse may be tired after a long day's work or in a hurry to complete tasks.

Coldness is the opposite of caring and warmth. This attitude can be conveyed to clients by nurses who appear more interested in the technical and procedural aspects of nursing than in the concerns of the person receiving the therapy. For example, the nurse who is more concerned about the neatness of the client's bed than about the client's restlessness, or one who focuses more on the efficient functioning of a cardiac monitor than on the client's anxiety conveys an attitude of coldness. A rigid body posture, the nurse's tone of voice, and the *way* things are said (in contrast to *what* is said) can also convey a nurse's lack of genuine concern for the client.

Emotions and Self-esteem

All kinds of emotions can influence a person's ability to communicate. Most people have experienced overwhelming joy or sorrow that is difficult to express in words. Anger may produce loud, profane vocalizations or controlled speechlessness. Fright may produce screams of terror or paralyzed silence.

Emotions also affect a person's ability to interpret messages. Large parts of a message may not be heard, or the message may be misinterpreted when the receiver is experiencing strong emotion. This situation occurs frequently in nursing. For example, the client feeling great fear may not remember all the preoperative instructions offered by a nurse.

Self-esteem also influences communication patterns. People whose self-esteem is high communicate honestly, with confidence, and with **congruence** (agreement or coinciding) between verbal and nonverbal messages. For example, a nurse explaining the importance of preoperative exercises would present a sincere and serious facial expression. Those with low self-esteem or under high stress tend to give double messages; that is, their verbal and nonverbal messages are incongruent (lack consistency). For example, while explaining about a client's colostomy to the client's family, a nurse laughs. Many patterns of communication are used to alleviate feelings of low self-esteem.

Development of Communication

The development of communication, from the cry of the infant to the verbal fluency of the adult, is a complex process. The art of language is learned by sharing ideas and feelings with others. The precise ways by which children learn socialized speech are not fully understood. Various theories of language development have been proposed; they are beyond the scope of this book. This section describes the various sounds and phases of children's language development.

Phases of Development

Prelinguistic Phase

The first sound of a newborn is the birth cry as air moves across the vocal cords. This is a reflexive response associated with the air pressure and the temperature changes of extrauterine life. Although infants are speechless for almost 1 year, they do communicate their needs. Within 2–3 weeks after birth, parents can describe notable differences in the cries of their infant. Babies cry in one way when they are hungry and in a different way when they are wet, tired, in pain, or wanting attention. The hunger cry may start out in a plaintive way and become increasingly demanding. The cry of pain is usually a sudden yell, because the baby is startled about what is happening. The cry of discomfort or the need for attention may sound like complaining, because it goes on and on. Some babies will cry jerkily when they are put down to sleep. Some become loudly demanding, but when a parent does not appear they settle down with progressively fading crying spurts. Each mother and father soon learns to communicate in response to the child's unique sounds. Infants also make comfort sounds. Smiling is noted in a number of infants as early as the second week of life. Soon after, some begin small, throaty, cooing sounds while feeding or bathing. Babies usually make these comfort sounds when they are contented, for example, when they are cuddled or when others talk to them.

Until the age of 10 months to 1 year the infant's sounds are not related to language and therefore are considered *prelinguistic*. These early sounds are actually exercise for the vocal cords. The first sounds are vowels or gurglings from the throat. When the mouth is opened, air is exhaled, resulting in various happy noises such as "uuuuuuu" or "eeeeeeeee." To produce consonant sounds such as "b" or "k," infants need sufficient motor development to manipulate their lips, tongue, throat, and voice at the same time. These sounds therefore appear less frequently and later than vowel sounds. The consonants are then combined into syllables with the vowel sounds. Such sounds as "da" and "ge" are then heard.

The prelinguistic phase includes reflexive vocalization, babbling, and echolalia. **Reflexive vocalization** is a term for the nondescriptive sounds infants make in response to various stimuli and environmental conditions. These are the discomfort cries and the comfort coos.

Babbling begins when infants become aware that they are making noises. They delight in producing and repeating sounds, particularly when they are enjoying themselves. They spend more time making noises and will talk to themselves when alone. Babbling often occurs just after waking up or before going to sleep. It is as if they are practicing self-produced sounds. By about 7 months, babbling includes some sounds infants have picked up from their environment. Hearing and the sounds they produce are now associated. This is referred to as **lalling:** Infants are repeating sounds they have heard.

Echolalia is the repetition of sounds just spoken by another. This involves definite acoustic awareness. Whole sequences of the sound may be strung together, such as "dadadadada." At this point there is no meaning associated with the infant's sounds, but they have learned to manipulate their tongue, lips, and throat and to imitate sounds spoken by others. Language and speech development proceed at a faster pace if the parent at this time repeats the baby's sounds. The baby in turn echoes the parent's sounds.

First Words

The first word of the infant is a notable event for proud parents. By about 10 to 12 months of age children develop a *passive* understanding of the language. They will respond to a few familiar words, such as "no," and familiar names—their own and those of family members and household pets. Even when family members are not present, children will turn to look for them when their names are mentioned.

Active use of language follows. The first words that children use may be unrecognized by parents, since children often invent their own first words. A word such as "nenene" may mean many things to a child. It may mean comfort when spoken softly, or it may mean a scolding or wrongdoing when spoken sharply. The word "mama" may mean food, comfort, warmth, and love. To understand this early language, it is necessary to listen to what children say in relation to what they are doing and their situation. Whole messages can be involved in one word, depending on the tone or manner of voice. This is not surprising, since babies respond to their mother's tone of voice as early as 4 or 5 weeks after birth, when they are comforted by soothing, soft tones. Although they do not understand the words, it is known that at the age of 4 to 5 months babies respond differently to the same word said with different intonations.

True speech begins at 12 to 18 months of age, when the child correctly uses a conventional word or facsimile of the word. It is used with intent, and a response is anticipated; a child may bang a cup on the high chair and say "wawa" (water). This type of speech is referred to as **holophrastic speech** (one word expresses a whole sentence). "Wawa" means "I want some water." "Bath" means "I want to take a bath now." Generally children can say about four words at 15 months, about ten words at 18 months, and about 50 words by 2 years. The vocabulary that children understand is much larger. They can respond to commands such as "Give that to me" and "Touch your nose."

First Sentences

By 2 years of age children learn to put words together. This period is considered the beginning of complete speech, the use of different word combinations in grammatical form.

In the beginning, only two words are combined; later three-word and four-word sentences appear, until full adultlike sentences are constructed. The child's sentences, like the first words, have personal meanings and do not follow the rules of grammar. Examples are: "See plane," "Kitty sleep," "Dat mine." Some peculiar combinations can be made up, such as "Bye-bye shoe." Regardless of the combinations, a certain order exists in the child's language. Some words will always appear at the beginning of a phrase and others at the end. "See" is usually at the beginning and "it" is usually at the end.

Learning to use the past tense and to create questions is more complex. Most of the early phrases spoken use the present tense. When learning the past tense, children provide much amusement for adults. They initially put an "ed" on every verb, saying things like "Dolly eated" or "Mommy boughted it." As the child grows older, questions are formulated. Three stages are involved in transferring a statement into a question (Bee 1985, p. 281). These can be exemplified using the statement "Daddy is driving a blue car." Although we could use any of dozens of words to phrase a question, the word "why" will be used to illustrate the three changes:

1. The word "why" must be added: "Daddy is driving a blue car why?"
2. The word "why" then needs to be moved to the beginning of the statement: "Why daddy is driving a blue car?"
3. Then the verb "is" needs to be moved to follow the word "why": "Why is daddy driving a blue car?"

The earliest questions of a child do not change the sentence structure. Instead inflections are used at the end of a phrase, such as "See tree?" raising the voice as the child says "tree." Then questions will occur without verbs, such as "Where my coat?" followed by ones with verbs but not subjects, such as "Why can't do it?"

Children also have various ways of dealing with some consonants. One child who could not pronounce "f" to say her uncle Fred's name constructed the name "Pete" to avoid her difficulty. Another child pronounced Valerie as "Bralerie."

Egocentric and Socialized Speech

The French psychologist Jean Piaget (1952) categorized the conversation of children from ages 4 to 11 into egocentric and socialized speech. **Egocentric speech** is self-centered, noncommunicative speech. Children talk merely to please themselves or to please anyone who happens to be there to hear. Although the conversation is not directed at anyone in particular, the talking is about the child's thoughts and activity of the moment. The child is thinking out loud. Three categories of egocentric speech are repetition, monologue, and collective monologue.

An example of *repetitive speech* is provided by 4-year-olds in a nursery school:

Judy: I've got a red block.

Tracey: I've got a red block.

Judy: I've got a red block.

Tracey: I've got a red block.

The **monologue** refers to a long speech that occurs when there is no listener. For example, the preschooler who is building a castle with blocks will mutter, "This big red block goes here . . . that's good . . . and now this green block goes there . . . uh . . . let's see, I'll put it this way . . . now, where's the bridge? That will keep the bad guys out." In contrast, the *collective monologue* involves the presence of others. Children speak with awareness of another child's presence, but they are indifferent to what others are saying.

In contrast to Piaget, the Russian psychologist Lev Vygotsky (1962, pp. 16–17) proposed that egocentric speech is a form of self-guidance and assists the child in problem-solving situations. He believes that egocentric speech is both goal oriented and communicative. It is the state between external speech and what he refers to as "silent inner speech" (Vygotsky 1962, p. 149). Egocentric or external speech goes underground and becomes internalized as thought processes.

Socialized speech refers to the exchange of thoughts with others. It includes questions, answers, commands, and criticism of others. In school-age children the use of egocentric speech gradually diminishes, and communicating thoughts to other people becomes predominant.

Semantic Development

Semantics is the study of the meanings of words in a given language. Increasing attention has been given to semantic development in recent years. The words children use do not always indicate their meaning to adults. A preschooler said before his birthday that he did not want his birthday in January. After his parents explored what bothered him about having his birthday in January, his response was, "I want my birthday here at home on the farm." Although the child had the vocabulary, his personalized meaning referred to a place.

Children learn the meanings of concrete words and their categories first; later, abstract words and their categories are understood. A child learns "chair" and "table" before learning the meaning of the category "furniture," or learns "apple" and "orange" before learning the category "fruit." Abstract words such as "quality" or "relation" are learned primarily after the preschool years.

Words in the English language that have double meanings are also difficult for preschoolers. Such words as "sweet" and "crooked" can have either a physical or psychologic meaning. They are not fully comprehended until about age 10. See Table 27–2 for a summary of language development.

Factors Influencing Language Development

Growth in language development is affected by a number of factors: intelligence, sex, bilingualism, status as a single

Table 27–2 Language Development

Stage	Normal Behavior
Newborn	At birth—cries as air passes over vocal cords. Within 2 to 3 weeks—cries becomes differentiated.
Infant	At 2 to 3 months—babbling begins. At 7 months—repeats sounds heard from environment. At 10 to 12 months—responds to few familiar words; single words are pronounced. At 15 months—can say about four words.
Toddler	At 2 years—initially has over 50-word vocabulary; this increases progressively to about 800–1000 words by 3 years. Associates symbols with form, e.g., words, pictures. Grammatical errors are common.
Preschooler	At 4 years—vocabulary has grown to about 1600 words. Sentences are complete. By 5 to 6 years—most infantile pronunciations have disappeared.
School-age child	At 6 years—has command of most sentence structures. Speech is less egocentric. Vocabulary continues to increase; comprehension exceeds use. Slang and swear words become part of vocabulary. At 8 to 12 years—boasting commonly occurs.
Adolescent	Uses language of subgroup. Speech reflects consideration of hypotheses.
Adulthood	Has full speech skills. Language often reflects specialized education.

child or twin, parental stimulation, and socioeconomic components.

Intelligence

Brighter children begin to talk earlier than those with lower intelligence. Vocabulary development of intelligent children occurs more rapidly, and they articulate better and use sentences that are longer and grammatically more correct. Mentally defective children show notable lags in vocabulary growth.

Sex

During the first year there is not much difference in the sounds produced by boys and girls. After this time girls tend to be superior in both the rate of vocabulary development and articulation. In later school years boys tend to equal girls in reading abilities and be superior in use of certain words. Females on the whole exceed males in grammatical word usage and spelling tests.

Bilingualism

Research has contradicted the belief that a child of a bilingual home is hindered in language development. Lambert and Tucker (1972) found that language development was not retarded in bilingual children over a 7-year period. The bilingual children also scored high on tests of creativity.

Status as a Single Child or Twin

Evidence suggests that twins and triplets exhibit certain aspects of retarded language development, particularly during the preschool years. It is thought that (a) twins may receive less verbal stimulation from parents, (b) they grow up so close together that they understand each other's speech patterns early, and (c) they lack the motivation to verbalize with others. The school years are apparently instrumental in resolving these problems (Helms and Turner 1976, p. 164.).

Parental Stimulation

Vocabulary growth occurs at a more rapid pace in children who are spoken to more frequently by their parents. Less rapid growth has been noted in children who spend most of their time with other children and who watch a great deal of television. The kind of stimulation offered by parents is significant (Bee 1985, p. 298). An only child may show rapid growth of communication skills largely due to interaction with the parents, whereas the youngest of six children may have less communication with parents and hence develop communication skills more slowly. Children who have mothers described as "object oriented and noncritical" acquire language more rapidly. These mothers tend to talk and ask questions about the child's toys rather than criticizing what the child is doing with the toys. In contrast, children who have mothers described as "critical and intrusive" display inhibited language development. These mothers focus on giving their children directions (commands and demands) about what to do with their toys. Vocabulary is enhanced in children who travel away from their homes and who have contact with several different adults.

Socioeconomic Components

The social and economic family setting in which the child is reared affects language development. Children from upper-class families, such as those whose parents are lawyers and doctors, use many more words even by age 3 than children from lower social classes, where the parents are unskilled workers. The caliber of conversation overheard by youngsters is an influencing factor in their choice of vocabulary and sentence structure. Middle-class and upper-class families tend to discourage the use of profane language or slang; instead, proper word usage and grammar are encouraged and often rewarded by praise. Homes that expose their children to a variety of educational aids also enhance the child's language development. Lack of development is noted in homes without magazines, books, newspapers, encyclopedias, radios, or a television set.

Although language development differs among social classes, lower-class children should not be regarded as inferior. These children possess a fully developed language that is similar to a dialect. They are able to articulate well in their own cultural setting but not as well with middle-class or upper-class children. The converse also applies. Upper- and middle-class children have difficulty articulating in dialects from outside their own cultural settings.

Stimulating Children's Language Development

Nurses can be instrumental in assisting parents to become active stimulants in language development and helping children when they are hospitalized. The following interventions are suggested:

1. *Improve the parental model.* Parents can be encouraged to provide the best possible instruction and to become good models. Some parents may need to attend English classes; others may need encouragement to acquire educational aids such as storybooks.
2. *Encourage verbal and nonverbal means of communication.* Children need different verbal experiences, such as rhyming games, reading aloud, and songs, with accompanying nonverbal gestures, such as smiling and laughing. See Figure 27–3. Expanding on the child's

remarks, drawing, painting, and musical endeavors also is a vital part of learning the communication process.

3. *Provide experiences to talk about.* Children talk when they have something to talk about. Whenever possible, parents and/or nurses need to provide pets, toys, picture books, numbers, and colors that the child can experiment with and talk about.

4. *Encourage listening.* Articulation skills of children can be enhanced by teaching them to pay attention and to listen to sounds. Parents can encourage these skills by having children listen to and repeat nursery rhymes or jingles or asking questions such as "What was that sound?"

5. *Encourage speech as a substitute for action.* Children's ability to express themselves verbally can be enhanced when parents, rather than responding to physical action, direct them to say what they want. The child who tugs at a playmate's tricycle can be instructed by the parent to express a want verbally by the remark "Tell him what you want; perhaps he will let you have it."

6. *Use exact terms.* Children learn to distinguish color, size, shape, position, and ownership of objects when exact terms are used. Parents can be encouraged to say, "Bring the big red ball from the playroom table," rather than "Bring that thing from over there—you know what I mean." Asking a child to "Put away your toys" instead of "the toys" can clarify property problems.

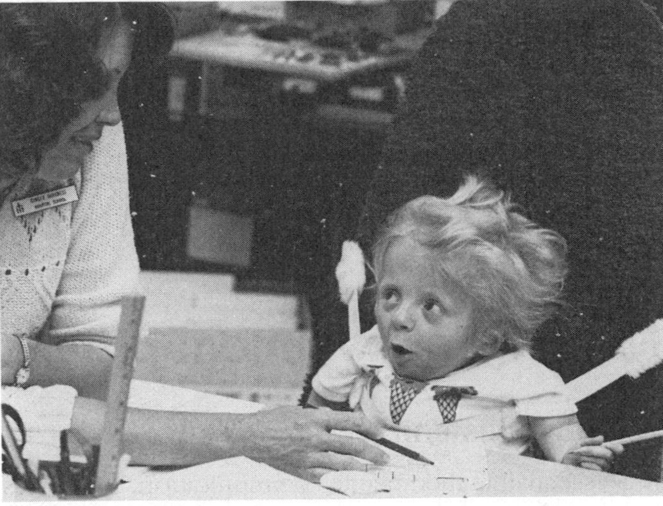

Figure 27–3 Development of a child's language is stimulated by reading together.

Assessing Communication

When nurses assess the communication of clients, they need to include language development, nonverbal behavior, and communication style.

Language Development

The nurse assesses the following aspects of language development:

1. The language skills presented by the client, compared to the language skills normally expected.
2. Adequacy of the language skills in relation to the individual's need.
3. The chief method of communicating, e.g., words or gestures.
4. Obstacles to language development, such as deafness or absence of environmental stimuli.
5. Specific forms of language impairment, e.g., a school-age child's inability to write or lack of abstractions in the language of an adult.
6. Cultural influences on language development, e.g., the language used in the home or customs about when and how to speak.

Nonverbal Behavior

In assessing nonverbal communication, the nurse considers:

1. Gestures used by the individual.
2. Posture and facial expressions employed.
3. Use of touch as a means of communication. See the discussion of "Using touch" later in this chapter.
4. The interpersonal distance with which the person feels comfortable, e.g., whether the person assumes an intimate distance for most discussions.
5. The grooming and appearance of the individual. These may affect the communication process, e.g., when dress is inconsistent with a setting or presents a stereotype that may evoke biases.

Style of Communication

A person's style of communiation is often affected by such factors as his or her health, culture, education, stress level, fatigue, and cognitive ability. In assessing communication style, the nurse considers the following:

1. The vocabulary of the individual, particularly any changes from the vocabulary normally used. For exam-

ple, if a person who normally never swears starts using swear words, this may indicate an increased stress level, illness, etc.

2. The use of symbols and gestures to communicate. Some uses of symbols and gestures are culturally determined; for example, a Puerto Rican girl may be taught not to look an adult in the eyes, as a sign of respect and obedience, not as a sign of guilt.
3. The presence of characteristics such as hostility, aggression, assertiveness, reticence, hesitance, anxiety, or loquaciousness in the communication.
4. Difficulties with verbal communication, such as stuttering, inability to pronounce a particular sound, or lack of clarity in enunciation.

Nursing Intervention: Listening and Responding

Attentive Listening

It is essential, in therapeutic communication, that nurses listen and respond to clients purposefully and deliberately. Attentive listening is listening actively, using all the senses, as opposed to listening passively with just the ear. It is probably the most important technique of all. Attentive listening is an active process that requires energy and concentration. It involves paying attention to the total message, both verbal messages and nonverbal messages that can modify what is spoken, and noting whether these communications are congruent. Attentive listening absorbs both the content and the feeling the person is conveying, without selectivity. This means that the listener does not select or listen to solely what he or she wants to hear; the nurse does not focus on her or his own needs but rather on the client's needs. Attentive listening conveys an attitude of caring and interest, thereby encouraging the client to talk. In summary, attentive listening is a highly developed skill, but fortunately it is one that can be learned with practice.

How attentive a nurse is in listening to clients can be conveyed in various ways. Common responses are a nod of the head, uttering "uh huh" or "mmm," repeating the words that the patient has used, or saying "I see what you mean." Each nurse will have characteristic ways of responding. Caution needs to be taken not to sound insincere or phony.

Gerard Egan (1982, pp. 60–61) has outlined five specific ways to convey physical attending. Egan defines physical attending as the manner of being present to another or being with another. Listening, in his frame of reference, is what a person does while attending. The five actions of physical attending, which convey a "posture of involvement," are:

1. *Face the other person squarely.* This position says, "I am available to you." Moving to the side lessens the degree of involvement.
2. *Maintain good eye contact.* This was discussed earlier in the section on "Facial expression." Mutual eye contact, preferably at the same level, recognizes the other person and denotes a willingness to maintain communication. Eye contact neither glares at nor stares down another but is natural.
3. *Lean toward the other.* People move naturally toward one another when they want to say or hear something—by moving to the front of a class, by moving a chair nearer a friend, or by leaning across a table with arms propped in front. Whispering a secret into someone's ear is an extreme example. Likewise, the nurse conveys involvement when he or she leans forward, closer to the client.
4. *Maintain an open posture.* The nondefensive position is one in which neither arms nor legs are crossed. It conveys that the person wishes to encourage the passage of communication, as the open door of a home or an office does.
5. *Remain relatively relaxed.* Total relaxation is not feasible when the nurse is listening with intensity. The term *relative* acknowledges that the nurse can show relaxation by taking time in responding, allowing pauses

Research Note

Does attending behavior influence performance of the elderly? The hypothesis of Rosendahl's and Ross's study was that the elderly who receive attending behavior while answering the Goldfarb Mental Status Questionnaire would have higher performance ratings on that questionnaire than the elderly who received no attending behavior. Attending behavior consisted of looking directly at the subject at eye level, maintaining a comfortable posture and natural movements, asking about the subject's comfort, permitting reconsideration of a response, and using comments following topics the subject introduced. The findings indicated that subjects who received attending behavior scored significantly higher on the questionnaire than those who did not receive attending behavior. Use of attending behavior by the nurse practitioner may therefore serve to enhance the performance of an elderly client (Rosendahl and Ross 1982).

as needed, balancing periods of tension with relaxation, and using gestures that are natural. See Figure 27–4. The nurse who feels tight and tense will generally offer responses too quickly to the client and prevent a free flow of thoughts and feelings.

These five attending postures need to be adapted to the specific needs of clients in a given situation. For example, leaning forward may not be appropriate at the beginning of an interview. It may be reserved until a closer relationship grows between the nurse and the client. The same applies to eye contact, which is generally uninterrupted when the communicators are very involved in the interaction. At times, however, eye contact may need to be interrupted.

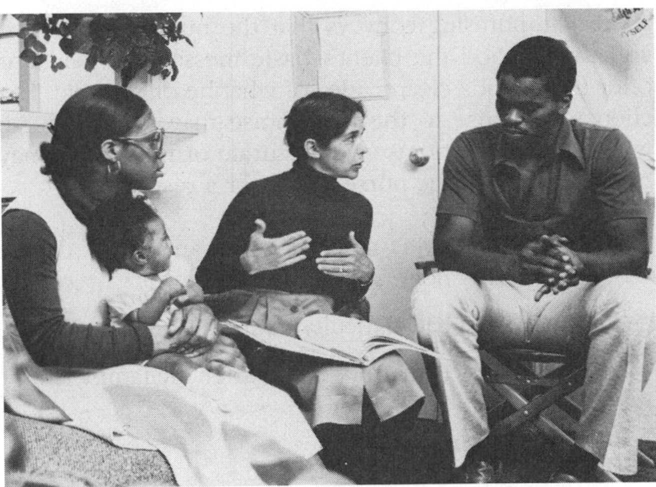

Figure 27–4 The nurse conveys attentive listening through a posture of involvement.

Responding

Nurses can learn much by examining and becoming aware of their own reactions (feelings) and responses. Although it is difficult for nurses to see their own nonverbal communication other than by videotape feedback, much can be learned by reflecting on what was heard, what the nurse said, and when and how it was said. Methods such as role playing, process recordings, and audiotapes can be useful.

Nurses need to respond not only to the content of a client's verbal message but also to the feelings expressed. It is important to understand how the client views the situation and feels about it, before responding. This understanding, called *empathy,* is discussed later, in the section on "Developing helping relationships."

The content of the client's communication is the words or thoughts, as distinct from the feelings. Sometimes people can convey a thought in words while their emotions contradict the words; i.e., words and feelings are incongruent. For example, a client says, "I am glad he has left me; he was very cruel." However, the nurse observes that the client has tears in her eyes as she says this. To respond to the client's *words,* the nurse might simply rephrase, saying "You are pleased that he has left you." To respond to the client's *feelings,* the nurse would need to acknowledge the tears in the client's eyes, saying, for example, "You seem saddened by all this." Such a response helps the client to focus on her feelings. In some instances, the nurse may need to know more about the client and her resources for coping with these feelings.

Sometimes clients need time to deal with their feelings. Strong emotions are often draining to a person. Yet feelings usually need to be dealt with before a person can cope with other matters, such as learning new skills or planning for the future. This is most evident in hospitals when clients learn that they have a terminal illness. Some require hours, days, or even weeks before they are ready to start other tasks. The degree of assistance that clients require varies considerably. Some need only time to themselves, others need someone to listen, others need assistance identifying and verbalizing feelings, and others need assistance making decisions about future courses of action. A number of techniques are used to help clients. These are discussed in the next section.

Techniques for Responding Therapeutically

Several techniques can be used to facilitate therapeutic communication that promotes understanding by both the sender and the receiver. These techniques also assist in the formation of a constructive relationship between the nurse and the client, although use of the techniques is no guarantee of effective communication. So many factors are involved in communication that the nurse will be ill-advised to rely solely on any one technique or even several techniques. Not all people feel comfortable with all techniques, and skill in using them appropriately is essential. It is important that the nurse be comfortable with the technique used and convey sincerity to the client. A phony or false response is usually quickly identified by clients and hinders the development of an effective relationship.

Paraphrasing

Paraphrasing, also called *restating,* involves listening for the client's basic message and then repeating those thoughts and/or feelings in similar words. Usually fewer words are used. Paraphrasing conveys that the nurse has listened and understood the client's basic message. It may also offer the client a clearer idea of what he or she said. The client's response to the paraphrase may tell the nurse whether the paraphrase was accurate or helpful. (It may be necessary for the nurse to ask for a response.)

> Client: I couldn't manage to eat any of my dinner last night—not even the dessert.
>
> Nurse: You had difficulty eating yesterday.
>
> Client: Yes, I was very upset after my family left.

Clarifying

Clarifying is a method of making the client's message more understandable. It is used when paraphrasing is difficult, when the communication has been rambling or garbled. To clarify the message the nurse can (a) make a guess and restate the basic message, or (b) confess confusion and ask the client to repeat or restate the message (Davis 1984, p. 9). In the former situation, if the client says, "I didn't sleep at all last night," the nurse might say, "You didn't sleep at all last night." In the latter instance the nurse might say, "I'm puzzled" or "I'm not sure I understand that" and "Would you please say that again?" or "Would you tell me more?"

If the reason for not understanding the message was the nurse's inattention, it is best to admit it and apologize. "I'm sorry, I was distracted by . . ." or "I was thinking about . . ." When possible, the nurse should discuss the distraction with the client.

Nurses sometimes need to clarify their own messages to clients. The need to do so is generally discovered from the client's nonverbal feedback. Then the nurse might ask a question or say, "It seems to me I didn't make that clear" and repeat or rephrase the message. Sometimes only one word or phrase in a message needs clarifying.

Clarifying also includes *verifying what is implied.* In this instance, the client implies or hints at something without actually saying it. The nurse then tries to clarify the client's statement without interpreting it.

> Client: There is no point in asking for a pain pill.
>
> Nurse: Are you saying that no one gives you an analgesic when you have pain?
>
> or
>
> Nurse: Are you saying that your pills are not helping your pain?

Another clarifying technique is **perception checking,** or *consensual validation.* This verifies the accuracy of the nurse's listening skills by giving and receiving feedback about what was communicated. It involves paraphrasing what the nurse thinks she or he heard and asking the client for confirmation. It is important to allow the client to correct inaccurate perceptions. The advantage of frequent perception checking is that inaccurate perceptions are corrected before communications become confused and misunderstandings arise. Examples of perception checking are: "You sound annoyed with me—is that correct?" or "You seem to have some doubts about the decision you made, and I'd like to see if what I'm hearing is accurate."

Clarifying Reality, Time, or Sequence

Sometimes it is important for nurses to clarify reality when a client has misrepresented it. This assists the client to differentiate the real from the unreal.

> Client: Someone took my magazine last night.
> Nurse: Your magazine is here in your drawer.
>
> Client: There is a dead mouse in that corner.
> Nurse: It is a discarded washcloth, not a mouse.

It may also be necessary to clarify a sequence of events or a time period:

> Client: I vomited this morning.
> Nurse: Was that after breakfast?
>
> Client: I feel that I have been asleep for weeks.
> Nurse: You had your operation Monday, and today is Tuesday.

Using Open-ended Questions and Statements

An *open-ended question* is one that leads or invites clients to explore (elaborate, clarify, or illustrate) their thoughts or feelings. It allows clients the freedom to talk about what they wish. It also places responsibility on clients to explore and to understand themselves, in contrast to receiving advice from another (Stewart and Cash 1985, p. 79). Examples of open-ended questions are: "How did you feel in that situation?" "What do you think she meant by that remark?" "Would you describe more about how you relate to your child?" "What would you like to talk about today?" Examples of open-ended statements are "I'd like to hear more about that" and "Tell me about . . ."

These questions or statements require more than a "yes" or "no" or other short response, such as "yesterday" or "I don't know." They encourage clients to discover what their thoughts and feelings truly are. Such questions usually begin with "what" or "how." Questions that begin with "when," "where," "who," "do (did, does)" or "is (are, was)" tend to produce short answers that impede self-exploration. However, nurses need to use this latter type of question in situations that require information gathering, such as taking a nursing history.

Focusing

Focusing is used when the client's communication is vague, when the client is rambling, or when the client seems to be talking about numerous things. Focusing can be compared to using a telephoto lens, which focuses sharply on a certain aspect of a view; similarly the nurse assists or leads the client to focus on one specific aspect of a communication. It is important for the nurse to wait until the client thinks he or she has talked about the main concerns before attempting to focus. The focus may be an idea or a feeling; however, a feeling is often emphasized, to help the client recognize an emotion disguised behind words.

> Client: My wife says she will look after me but I don't think she can, what with the children to take care of, and they're always after her about something—clothes, homework, what's for dinner that night.
>
> Nurse: You are worried about how well she can manage.

Being Specific, Tentative, and Informative

When responding to another person's comments, it is helpful to make statements that are (a) specific rather than general, (b) tentative rather than absolute, and (c) informative rather than authoritarian. Examples are: "You scratched my arm" (specific statement); "You're as clumsy as an ox" (general statement); "You seemed unconcerned about Mary" (tentative statement); "You don't give a damn about Mary and you never will" (absolute statement); "I haven't finished yet" (informative statement); "Stop interrupting!" (authoritarian statement).

In being informative, the nurse needs to present facts or specific information simply and directly. If the nurse does not know some fact, this is also stated simply, together with a suggestion about where or how the information can be obtained.

> Client: I don't know the visiting hours.
> Nurse: The visiting hours are 9 A.M. to 9 P.M. each day.
>
> Client: When will my doctor be in?
> Nurse: I don't know. But Ms. Lu, the charge nurse, will be here in a few minutes, and she may know.

Another way to be informative is to make an observation. This indicates that the nurse has noticed a change of behavior but is not placing a value judgment on it. For example: "You have washed your hair" (neutral observation); "Your hair looks better now that you have washed it" (value judgment); "You are holding your arm carefully; is it painful?" (observation; verifying implication).

Using Touch

Certain forms of touching indicate affection. For example, cheek patting, hand patting, and putting an arm over the person's shoulder are valued forms of affection in North America. The "laying on of hands" is a common expression indicating curative and comforting actions. This expression is often attributed to individuals in the healing professions such as religion, medicine, and nursing. Tactile contacts vary considerably among individuals, families, and cultures. Some families have a great deal of tactile contact among members. Other families, even within the same culture, have minimal contact. Appropriate forms of touch can be helpful in reinforcing caring feelings by the nurse. See Figure 27–5. The use of touch alone often says much more than words for clients, such as for those who are terminally ill or who are unable to speak, for whatever reason. It is important, however, for the nurse to be sensitive to the differences in attitudes and practices

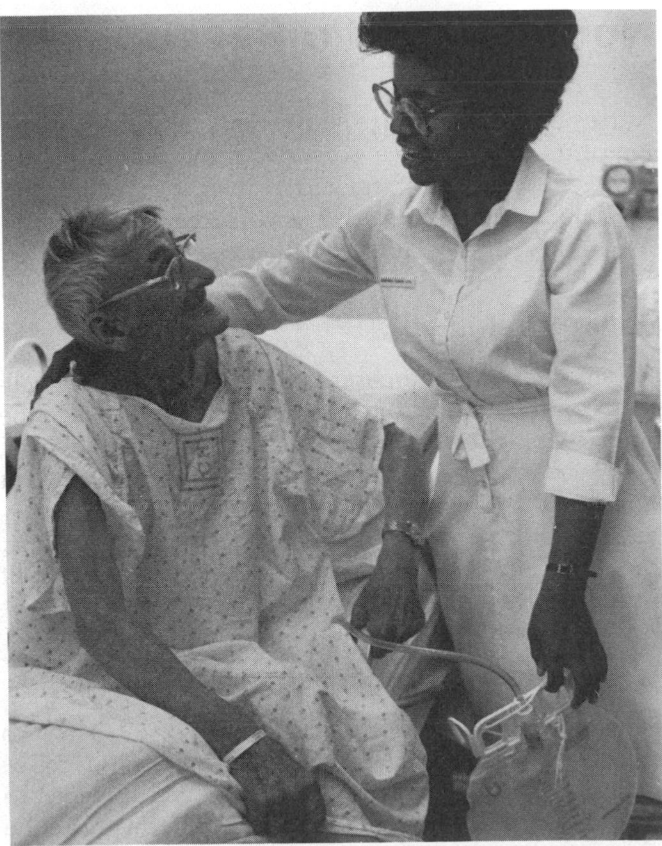

Figure 27–5 Appropriate forms of touch can communicate caring.

related to touch among individuals, including the nurse's own attitudes.

Using Silence

In everyday conversations natural pauses or silences are often accepted without thought. The listener attentively waits until the talker resumes conversation. These natural pauses are generally used to recall a name or event or to put thoughts or feelings into the most accurate words possible. Pauses or silences that extend for several seconds or minutes, however, make some listeners extremely uncomfortable. The listener often interjects with thoughts, questions, or explanations to reduce the discomfort. This puts words into the other person's mouth, so to speak. The unfortunate result is that self-expression is blocked for the initial communicator.

When people are ill, communication about how they feel is often difficult for them. Many prefer to remain stoically silent until they are sure that the nurse is interested or to be trusted. Once communication is initiated, it may be expressed awkwardly, with many pauses. The nurse needs to learn to be silent in these situations and to wait patiently until the person is able to put thoughts and feelings into words.

Providing General Leads

By providing a general lead, the nurse encourages the client to verbalize and at the same time choose the topic of conversation.

> Client: I am sure glad yesterday is over.
>
> Nurse: Perhaps you would like to talk about it.
>
> or
>
> Nurse: Would it help you to discuss your feelings?

Summarizing

Summarizing the main points of a discussion is a useful technique near the end of an interview, after a significant discussion, or to review a health-teaching session. It clarifies for both the nurse and the client the relevant points discussed and often acts as an introduction to future care planning. For example, the nurse might say, "During the past half hour we have talked about. . . . Tomorrow afternoon we may explore this further" or "In a few days, I'll review what you have learned about the actions and effects of your insulin." A word of caution about summarizing: No new material should be added.

Nontherapeutic Responses

Nurses need to recognize nontherapeutic techniques that interfere with effective communication. These include failing to listen; unwarranted reassurance; using judgmental responses; being defensive; agreeing or disagreeing; and probing, testing or challenging.

Failing to Listen

Because listening is the most effective technique to facilitate communication, the opposite, failure to listen, is the primary inhibitor to communication. It says to the client, "I'm not interested" or "I'm bored" or "You are not important." It suggests that the nurse needs to be entertained, that the nurse's needs require attention, or that the nurse prefers to discuss topics that concern herself or himself.

Unwarranted Reassurance

Statements such as "You'll feel better soon," "I'm sure everything will turn out all right," "Don't worry," and "You're looking better each day" are futuristic and intended to provide hope for the client. However, they disregard the client's feelings of the moment and in many instances are said when there is no hope of improvement. The client who fears death, for example, needs to express these concerns rather than have them dismissed with false reassurance. The nurse who offers reassurance in this manner needs to examine her or his own feelings and recognize that this type of response is of more help to the nurse than to the client.

Judgmental Responses

Passing judgment on the client implies that the client *must* think as the nurse thinks—the client's values must be the same as the nurse's—if the client is to be accepted. Several responses that fall into this category are discussed in the next sections.

Approval and Disapproval

Approving or disapproving responses, such as "That's good (bad)," "You shouldn't do that," and "That's not good enough," tell clients they must measure up to the nurse's standards rather than to their own goals. Perhaps what the nurse considers "bad" the client considers "good."

Approving or disapproving responses can also be nonverbal. For example, a client may have managed to bathe herself completely without the nurse's assistance for the first time. Although this activity took time and effort, she is feeling pleased. The nurse, who thinks she took too long, says nothing but hurriedly makes her bed.

Common Advice

Giving common advice removes decision-making control from the client to the nurse. It suggests that the client is inferior and less wise than the nurse. Moreover, it fosters dependence, and often the advice is not followed. Note that *common,* not *expert,* advice is spoken of here. This differentiation is significant, since giving expert advice can be therapeutic. Brammer (1985, p. 7) writes:

> Advice can be helpful if it is given by trusted persons with expert opinions based on solid knowledge of a supporting field such as law, medicine, or child rearing. Sometimes . . . clients need a recommended course of action supported by wide experience and . . . facts.

Common advice, on the other hand, refers to matters dealing with individual choice. For example, when clients ask, "Should I move from my home to a nursing home?" "I'm separated from my wife. Do you think I should have sexual relations with another woman?" "Do you think I should have an abortion?" or "Should I give up my baby to an adoption agency?" offering advice such as "If I were you . . ." is unwise for the nurse. The client needs support to make his or her own decisions.

Stereotypes

Stereotyping responses place the client into categories that negate his or her uniqueness as an individual. *Stereotypes* are generalized and oversimplified beliefs we hold about various groups of people, which are based upon experiences too limited to be valid. The less one knows about a person, the more the tendency to stereotype. Examples of stereotyping statements are: "Two-year-olds are brats," "Women are complainers," and "Men don't cry." Communication between nurse and client can be inhibited, depending on how emotionally charged the stereotype is for the nurse. For example, if the nurse is not deeply committed to the "brat" theory, the communication pattern with a 2-year-old who is cooperative may be only temporarily affected. On the other hand, the nurse who has marked feelings about men who cry will probably ignore the individualism of a male client who expresses his grief.

Another common error is to offer meaningless stereotyped responses to clients:

> Client: I'm sure having a lot of pain.
>
> Nurse: Really? Most people don't have pain after this type of surgery.
>
> Client: I don't have the energy I'd like to have.
>
> Nurse: Rome wasn't built in a day.

Research Note

Client self-exploration is one goal of helping. In a study of 30 post-RN students, Forrest analyzed the nurses' verbal behavior with patients, particularly the verbal communication techniques that foster self-exploration. For the analysis, nine facilitating verbal behaviors and nine blocking verbal behaviors were identified and defined. The findings revealed that 45% of all verbal behavior of the 30 nurses consisted of a general lead such as "Go on" or "uh-huh," which, though a facilitating response, represented a low level of verbal communication skill. Few reflecting statements (3%) were used. The most frequent blocking response by the nurses was closed questioning. One blocking behavior, defending, was not used by any of the nurses. (Forrest 1983)

Defensive Responses

Many clients offer opinions or comments about their care, directed toward the nurse, the nurse's colleagues, or the institution. Feeling threatened or attacked, the nurse may become defensive and prevent the client from expressing feelings. Following are two examples:

> Client: The food here is lousy.
>
> Nurse: It's a lot better here than in the county hospital. You should consider yourself lucky.
>
> Client: Those night nurses must just sit around and talk all night. They didn't answer my light for over an hour.
>
> Nurse: I'll have you know we literally run around on nights. You're not the only client, you know.

These responses prevent the client from expressing true concerns. The nurse is saying, "You have no right to complain." Defensive responses protect the nurse from admitting weaknesses in the health care services, including personal weaknesses.

Agreement and Disagreement

Agreeing and disagreeing imply that the client is either right or wrong and that the nurse is in a position to judge this. They can deter the client from thinking through his or her position. Disagreement sometimes causes the client to defend a position.

> Client: I don't think Dr. Broad is a very good doctor. He doesn't seem interested in his patients.
>
> Nurse: Dr. Broad is head of the Department of Surgery and is an excellent surgeon.

Probing, Testing, and Challenging Responses

Probing, testing, and challenging are often considered hostile responses. **Probing** is asking for information chiefly out of curiosity rather than with the intent to assist the client. Usually probing is considered prying, and the client feels that his or her privacy is not being respected. Often asking "why" is probing and can place the client in a defensive posture:

> Client: I was speeding along the street and didn't see the stop sign.
>
> Nurse: Why were you speeding?
>
> Client: I didn't ask the doctor when he was here.
>
> Nurse: Why didn't you?

Testing is questioning by nurses to make clients admit to something. With testing, the nurse usually asks a question that permits the client only limited answers. Testing often meets the nurse's need rather than the client's. Examples of testing questions are: "Who do you think you are?" which forces the client to admit that his or her status in the health care agency is that of "only a client," and "Do you think I am not busy?" which forces the client to admit that the nurse really *is* busy.

Challenging is giving a response that makes a client prove his or her statement or point of view. Usually the client's feelings are not considered, and he or she feels the necessity to defend a position. Challenging a client's perceptions rarely changes them; often it strengthens them, because the client feels forced to find proof to support the position.

> Client: I felt nauseated after that red pill.
>
> Nurse: Surely you don't think I gave you the wrong pill?
>
> Client: I feel as if I am dying.
>
> Nurse: How can you feel that way when your pulse is 60?
>
> Client: I believe my husband doesn't love me.
>
> Nurse: You can't say that; why, he visits you every day.

Nurse–Client Relationships

Nurse–client relationships are referred to by some as *interpersonal relationships,* by others as *therapeutic relationships* and by still others as *helping relationships.* Helping is a growth-facilitating process in which one person assists another to solve problems and to face crises in the direction the assisted person chooses (Brammer 1985, p. 5). Several terms are used to describe the persons involved in a helping relationship: *helper* and *helpee; giver* and *receiver;* and *counselor* and *client.* For purposes of consistency, in this text the term *nurse* or *helper* will refer to the person who gives the help, and the term *client* will denote the person receiving the help. However, we recognize that various people in all walks of life act as helpers and receivers of help.

Imogene King (1981) uses the term *nurse/client interaction* rather than *interpersonal relationship.* According to King (1981, p. 60), "The process of *interactions* between two or more individuals represents a sequence of verbal and nonverbal behaviors that are goal directed." In King's theory, *interpersonal relationships* are a subconcept of the *interaction.* She points out that in many nurse practice settings, such as critical care, where the nurse only has time to attend to physiologic variables that are life-threatening, interpersonal relationships cannot be established. In the interactive process, two individuals mutually identify goals and the means to achieve them. When they agree on the means to implement the goals, they move toward transactions. *Transaction* is defined as goal attainment (King 1981, p. 61). Communication is involved in this transactional process. King (1981) later defines *transaction* as "a process of interaction in which human beings communicate with the environment to achieve goals that are valued" (King 1981, p. 82).

Whatever the practice setting, the nurse establishes some sort of helping relationship in which mutual goals are set with the client, or with support persons if the client is unable to participate. The following sections on helping relationships show how the nurse applies to various situations some or all of the actions just discussed.

Developing Helping Relationships

Although special training in counseling techniques and psychiatry is advantageous for nurses to become effective helpers, there are many ways of helping clients that do not require special training. Shanken and Shanken (1976, pp. 24–27) have outlined 11 of these:

1. Listen actively.
2. Help to identify what the person is feeling.
3. Put yourself in the other person's shoes.
4. Be honest.

5. Do not tell a person not to feel.
6. Do not tell a person what he or she should feel.
7. Do not make excuses for the other person.
8. Be personal.
9. Use your ingenuity.
10. Try to summarize to the person at the end of the interview.
11. Know your role and your limitations.

Active listening, discussed previously, involves being attentive, clarifying, paraphrasing, and asking questions to understand the other person accurately.

Helping clients to identify their feelings requires feedback from the nurse about how the client appears. Often clients who are troubled are unable to identify or to label their feelings and consequently have difficulty working them out or talking about them. Responses by the nurse such as "You seem angry about taking orders from your boss" or "You sound as if you've been lonely since your wife died" can assist clients to recognize what they are feeling and to talk about it.

Putting oneself into another person's shoes is referred to as **empathy**. According to Egan (1975, p. 76), empathy involves the ability to:

> (1) *discriminate:* get inside the other person, look at the world through the frame of reference of the other person and get a feeling for what the other's world is like; and (2) *communicate* to the other this understanding in a way that shows the other that the helper has picked up both his *feelings,* and the *behavior* and *experience* underlying these feelings.

Empathy therefore requires more than sharing past similar feelings and events that people have all experienced, such as fright or depression. The nurse needs to understand the client's world as if the nurse were inside it, to see it through the client's eyes, and to feel as the client feels. Empathy is valuable in supporting clients to explore their situation and to move toward resolution of their problems. Feelings of closeness and understanding gradually evolve between client and nurse. Neither person, however, loses a sense of self.

Four steps have been identified in the process of empathy (Ehmann 1971, pp. 77–78). All the steps occur rapidly and tend to overlap.

1. *Identification.* To understand the feelings and situation of another, the helper must first lose consciousness of self and become engrossed in the personality and situation of the other person (identification). The nurse needs to relinquish a certain amount of self-control to achieve this.
2. *Incorporation.* At a step beyond identification, the experiences of the other person are taken into the helper's self (incorporation). The experience, however, is still recognized as belonging to the client.
3. *Reverberation.* The next step involves understanding the feelings of the other. There is interaction between the nurse's feelings from past experience and the experience incorporated from the client. Because all humans have the same potential for feelings, the experiences people share need not be identical for them to understand associated feelings.
4. *Detachment.* In the last step the nurse returns to her or his own identity. The results of the three preceding steps are then combined with other knowledge about the client, and all information is used collectively as a basis for responding to the client.

The value of *honesty* was previously mentioned as an aspect of credibility. In effective relationships nurses honestly recognize any lack of knowledge by saying, "I don't know the answer to that right now"; openly discuss their own discomfort by saying, for example, "I feel uncomfortable about this discussion"; and admit tactfully that problems do exist, when a client says such things as "I'm a mess, aren't I?"

Nurses *should not tell a client not to feel.* Feelings expressed by clients often create discomfort for nurses. Common examples occur when the client expresses anger or worry or cries. When the nurse is uncomfortable, a common response is "Don't worry about it, everything will be fine" or "Please don't cry." Such a response inhibits the client's expression of feelings. Unless feelings are extremely inappropriate, it is best to encourage ventilation (voicing) of them. This allows them to be expressed in words and examined objectively. Indirectly it tells clients "Your feelings are not that awful, since I am not bothered by them."

Nurses *need to avoid telling clients what they should feel.* Statements that indicate to clients how they should feel, rather than how they actually do feel, in essence deny clients' true feelings and suggest that they are inappropriate. Examples are: "You shouldn't complain about pain; many others have gone through this same experience stoically," and "You should be glad that you are alive and not worry about the loss of your arm."

It is *not helpful to make excuses for the other person.* When a person reacts with an intense feeling such as anger or grief and seems to have lost control of behavior to the astonishment or discomfort of others, a common error is to explain the behavior by offering excuses. Examples are: "Well, Mr. Brown, you're upset about not finishing your lunch, but the dietitian and I gave you too much," and "I guess you've had a tough session in physical therapy." These responses discourage and divert the person from discussing feelings of anger or inadequacy. The helper has made assumptions about the reasons for the client's behavior and therefore inhibits exploration of what is really being experienced and felt by the client.

Not all people feel comfortable about *offering personal statements* about themselves to strangers or to those they do not know well. Used with discretion, however, personal statements can be helpful in solidifying the rapport between the nurse and the client. The nurse might offer such comments as "I recall when I was in (a similar situation) and I felt angry about being put down." Egan (1982, p. 128) states that the helper "must be spontaneous, open. He can't hide behind the role of counselor. He must be a human being to the human being before him." Egan refers to this as *genuineness* and outlines five behaviors that are components of it (Egan 1982, pp. 127–31):

1. The genuine helper does not take refuge in or overemphasize the role of counselor.
2. The genuine person is spontaneous.
3. The genuine person is nondefensive.
4. The genuine person displays few discrepancies—that is, the person is consistent and does not think or feel one thing but say another.
5. The genuine person is capable of deep self-disclosure (self-sharing) when it is appropriate.

Caution needs to be exercised by nurses when making references about themselves. These statements must be used with discretion. The extreme of matching each of the client's problems with a better story of the nurse's own is of little value to the client.

Nurses can *use their ingenuity to help identify options* for clients. There are always many courses of action to consider in handling problems. Whatever course is chosen needs to achieve the client's goals, be compatible with the client's value system, and offer the probability of success. These actions are not explored until the relationship is well established (see "Phases of the Helping Relationship," next) and the exploration is done jointly by client and nurse. The client needs to choose the ways to achieve goals; however, the nurse can assist in identifying options. For example, a widower may ask for help because he is depressed and anxious about retirement. The nurse could suggest that he:

- Read books and articles on retirement
- Consider working part-time at his former employment
- Talk to other senior citizens about retirement
- Move in to live with a child and grandchildren
- Join a senior citizens' club
- Renew old hobbies, such as gardening or golf
- Join a counseling group
- Move from his house to an apartment
- Remarry
- Move into a senior citizens' lodge
- Join a volunteer service group
- Increase church activities
- Get involved in politics
- Write articles for the local newspaper
- Make plans to travel more extensively

The ingenious nurse will help the client select acceptable alternatives. For example, if this man loves animals, young children, and story telling, the nurse might direct his thoughts toward activities such as acquiring a puppy, writing children's stories, and volunteering at the public library.

Summarizing at the end of a discussion or interview is the process of tying together several thoughts and feelings into one or two statements. It is broader than paraphrasing and includes both what was said and how it was said. Several purposes are achieved by summarizing: (a) it helps to terminate the interview, (b) it reassures the client that the nurse has listened, (c) it checks the accuracy of the nurse's perceptions, (d) it clears the way for new ideas, and (e) it assists the client to note progress and forward direction (Brammer 1985, p. 74). Sometimes clients may spontaneously offer a summary; at other times the nurse must initiate it or ask the client to do so. The nurse may say, "Let's look at what has happened in this interview. What do you think has been accomplished?"

Every person has unique strengths and problems. It is important for nurses to *recognize their role and their limitations* and to be as open about them as necessary. When the nurse feels unable to handle some problems, the client should be informed and referred to the appropriate health professional.

Phases of the Helping Relationship

The relationship process can be described in terms of four sequential phases, each of which is characterized by identifiable tasks and skills. Progression through the stages must occur in succession, as each builds on the one before. Nurses can identify the progress of a relationship by understanding these phases: preinteraction phase, introductory phase, working (maintaining) phase, and termination phase.

Preinteraction Phase

In most situations the nurse has information about the client before the first face-to-face meeting. Such information may include the client's name, address, age, medical history, and/or social history. Tasks of this phase for the nurse include reviewing pertinent knowledge, considering potential areas of concern, and developing plans for the initial interaction. For example, prior to meeting a young pregnant woman in her home, a nursing student may need to review the normal physical changes that occur with pregnancy and related needs and discomforts. If the woman is in the first trimester of pregnancy, the nurse may anticipate areas of concern about urinary frequency, nausea, fatigue, or feelings of ambivalence, which are common discomforts during this period. Planning for the initial visit may generate some anxious feelings in the nurse. By recognizing these feelings and identifying specific information to be discussed, positive outcomes will evolve. It is wise for the nurse to recognize limitations at this stage and to seek assistance as required.

Introductory Phase

The introductory phase is also referred to as the *orientation phase* or the *prehelping phase.* The tone is set during this phase for the rest of the relationship phases. Some of the tasks of this phase were discussed in Chapter 11 for the nursing assessment interview. Three stages of this introductory phase are: (a) entry—preparing the client and opening the relationship; (b) clarification—stating the problem or concern and reasons for seeking help; and (c) structure—formulating the contract and the structure (Brammer 1985, p. 47).

Other important tasks of the introductory phase include getting to know each other and developing a degree of trust.

Opening the relationship Initially the nurse and the client need to identify each other by name as a friendly gesture and to open the relationship. When the nurse initiates the relationship, it is important to explain her or his role to give the client an idea of what to expect. When the client initiates the relationship, the nurse needs to help the client express concerns and reasons for seeking help. Vague, open-ended questions such as "What's on your mind today?" are helpful at this stage. The nurse needs to be aware that it is not easy for all clients to receive help. Thus, a relaxed, attending attitude on the part of the nurse is important. Providing a setting with minimal distractions and disturbances is also helpful.

Clarifying the problem Initially the client may not see the problem clearly. To clarify the problem, the nurse needs to use such techniques as attentive listening, paraphrasing, and clarifying, discussed previously in this chapter. A common error at this stage is to ask too many questions of the client.

Structuring and formulating the contract A contract includes the obligations to be met by both the nurse and the client. These commitments are agreed on verbally and need to evolve naturally. Contracts need to cover:

1. Location, frequency, and length of meetings.
2. Overall purpose of the relationship.
3. How confidential material will be handled.
4. Duration and indications for termination of the relationship.

The first three points are described in Chapter 11 (see "Formal Interview"). Determining the duration of the relationship and indications for termination depends in part on conditions outside the relationship. For example, many relationships are terminated when the client is discharged from the hospital or when the nursing student ends clinical rotation. In these situations the nurse and the client need to discuss these limits. When outside controls do not exist, both participants need to agree on indications for termination. These are largely determined by the purpose of the relationship. An example is the nurse who terminates the relationship after the client has learned how to care for his colostomy and is able to resume a life-style acceptable to himself.

Developing trust During the initial parts of the introductory phase, the client may display some resistive behaviors and some testing behaviors. *Resistive behaviors* are those that inhibit involvement, cooperation, or change. Three major reasons for their occurrence are (a) difficulty in acknowledging the need for help and thus a dependent role, (b) fear of exposing and facing feelings, and (c) anxiety about the discomfort involved in changing problem-causing behavior patterns. *Testing behaviors* are those that examine the nurse's interest and sincerity. For example, a client may refuse to talk, to test whether the nurse will stay with her for the prescribed period of time.

By the end of the introductory phase, the client begins to develop trust in the nurse. Both participants also begin to view each other as unique individuals. Characteristics of trusting individuals include (a) a feeling of comfort with growth in self-awareness, (b) an ability to share this awareness with others, (c) acceptance of others as they are without needing to change them, (d) openness to new experiences, (e) consistency between words and actions, (f) openness and honesty about motives, (g) willingness to confide, offer information and opinions, and (h) ability to delay gratification (Thomas 1970, p. 118; and Kaul and Schmidt 1971, p. 542).

Working Phase

When the nurse and the client begin to view each other as unique individuals, they begin to appreciate this uniqueness and care about each other. *Caring* is sharing deep and genuine concern about the welfare of another person. Once caring develops, the potential for empathy increases. The purpose of the working phase is to accomplish the tasks that have been outlined in the introductory phase.

The working phase has three successive stages: (a) responding and exploring, (b) integrative understanding and dynamic self-understanding, and (c) facilitating and taking action (Egan 1975, pp. 34–40). A summary of these stages and the specific skills required by both participants follows. Each stage builds on the previous one; therefore, they must occur in succession.

Responding and exploring During the introductory phase, emphasis is placed on the listening or attending skills of the nurse. These skills must be continued in the working phase of the relationship, but in addition the nurse now must respond to the client in ways that assist the client to explore thoughts, feelings, and actions.

The nurse requires four skills for this first stage:

1. *First-level empathy.* The nurse must communicate (respond) in ways that indicate she or he has listened to what was said and understands how the client feels. The nurse responds to content or feelings or both, as appropriate.

   The nurse's nonverbal behaviors are also important. In a study of five nurses and five clients, Hardin and Halaris (1983, p. 15) found that nonverbal communication and specific nonverbal behaviors may be linked to empathy. They observed the engaging and defensive nonverbal behaviors of clients and nurses, and compared nurses whom the clients rated as either highly empathetic or not empathetic. Nonverbal engaging behaviors included direct gaze, slight smile, laugh, forward torso, gestures, head nods, and leg position. Defensive behaviors included crossed arms and crossed legs. Their findings indicated that high-empathy nurses employed moderate head nodding, a steady gaze, moderate gesturing, and little activity or body movement. The low-empathy nurse used frequent head nodding and gesturing, laughed more than the high-empathy nurse, and displayed more eye movement, leg movement, and torso movement.

2. *Respect.* The nurse must show respect for the client, willingness to be available, and desire to work with the client.

3. *Genuineness.* This was discussed earlier in the chapter.

4. *Concreteness.* The nurse must assist the client to be concrete and specific rather than to speak in generalities. When the client says, "I'm stupid and clumsy," the nurse narrows the topic to the specific by pointing out, "You tripped on that scatter rug."

In self-exploration, the client explores feelings and actions associated with problems. This is also referred to as *self-disclosure.*

During this first stage of the working phase, trust and rapport are enhanced. The intensity of interaction increases, and feelings such as anger, shame, or self-consciousness may be expressed. If the nurse is skilled in this stage and if the client is willing to pursue self-exploration, the outcome is a beginning understanding on the part of the client about behavior and feelings.

Integrative understanding and dynamic self-understanding In this second working stage, clients achieve an objective understanding of themselves and their world (dynamic self-understanding). This ultimately enables clients to change and to take action. More self-exploration occurs, and more information is produced. As a result of this, isolated pieces of information can now be integrated into larger contexts that reveal behavior patterns or themes.

To acquire integrative understanding about the client, the nurse needs the following skills in addition to those of the first stage:

1. *Advanced-level empathy.* The nurse responds in ways that indicate an understanding not only of what is said but also of what is hinted at or implied nonverbally. Isolated statements become connected.

2. *Self-disclosure.* The nurse willingly but discreetly shares personal experiences.

3. *Confrontation.* The nurse points out discrepancies between thoughts, feelings, and actions that inhibit the client's self-understanding or exploration of specific areas. This is done empathetically, not judgmentally.

The skills required by the client include:

1. *Nondefensive listening.* The client, with support from the nurse, develops the skill of listening.

2. *Dynamic self-understanding.* The client gains insight into personal behavior, and this understanding forms the basis for changing behavior.

Facilitating and taking action Ultimately the client must make decisions and take action to become more effective. The responsibility for action belongs to the client. The nurse, however, collaborates in these decisions and may offer options or information.

When planning action programs, the client needs to learn to take risks, that is, to accept that either failure or success may be the outcome. Whatever action is taken needs to fall within the client's capabilities.

Short-term and long-term goals are considered, and it is essential that the nurse offer support at this time.

Successes need to be reinforced, and failures need to be recognized realistically. The fact that new problems may arise during this period also needs consideration. Often solving one problem raises new ones. Each new problem then needs to be dealt with by beginning at the first stage of the working phase (responding and exploring).

Termination Phase

Terminating the relationship is often expected to be difficult and filled with ambivalence. However, if the previous phases have evolved effectively, the client can accept this phase of the relationship without feelings of anxiety or dependence. The client generally has a positive outlook and feels able to handle problems independently. However, because caring attitudes have developed, it is natural to expect some feelings of loss, and each person needs to develop a way of saying good-bye.

Many methods can be used to terminate relationships. Summarizing or reviewing the process can produce a sense of accomplishment. This may include sharing reminiscences of how things were at the beginning of the relationship, compared to now. It is also helpful for both the nurse and the client to express their feelings about termination openly and honestly. Thus termination discussions need to start in advance of the termination interview. This allows time for the client to adjust to independence. In some situations referrals are necessary, or it is appropriate to offer an occasional standby meeting to give support as needed.

Evaluating Communication

Techniques that enhance or interfere with therapeutic communication were discussed earlier in this chapter. For nurses to evaluate the effectiveness of their own communications with clients, process recordings are frequently used. A **process recording** is a verbatim (word-for-word) account of a conversation. It can be taped or written, and it includes all verbal and nonverbal interactions.

One method of writing a process recording is to make three columns on a page. The first column lists what the client said and did, the second what the nurse said and did, and the third contains interpretive comments about the nurse's responses. See Table 27–3.

Once a process recording has been completed, it should be analyzed in terms of (a) the direction and development of the interaction (process), and (b) the content. The nurse's interaction can be analyzed for process according to a number of questions:

1. Was the client's verbal and nonverbal behavior really heard and seen?
2. Were any cues missed?
3. Were the nurse's verbal responses and behavior congruent?
4. Did the client respond to the nurse or independently of the nurse?
5. Did the communication process flow smoothly?
6. Were the nurse's responses consistent with what the nurse observed and heard? Or were they unrelated, exaggerated, or underresponsive?
7. Were the nurses's responses therapeutic or nontherapeutic? See the previous sections on responding therapeutically or nontherapeutically.

Each response can also be analyzed for content in terms of facilitating or inhibiting communication. See Table 27–3 for a sample analysis.

Chapter Highlights

- Communication incorporates all means of exchanging information between two or more people and is a basic component of human relationships and nurse–client relationships.
- Communication is usually categorized as verbal or nonverbal.
- Verbal communication is effective when the criteria of simplicity, clarity, timing, relevance, adaptability, and credibility are met.
- Nonverbal communication often reveals more about a person's thoughts and feelings than verbal communication; it includes physical appearance, posture and gait, facial expressions, hand movements, and other gestures.
- When assessing nonverbal behaviors, the nurse needs to consider cultural influences and be aware that a variety of feelings can be expressed by a single nonverbal expression.
- When communication is effective, verbal and nonverbal expressions are congruent.
- Communication is a two-way process involving the sender of the message and the receiver of the message.
- Because the sender must encode the message and determine the appropriate channels for conveying it, and because the receiver must perceive the message, decode it, and then respond, the communication process includes four elements: (a) sender, (b) message, (c) receiver, and (d) feedback.

Table 27–3 Sample Process Recording

Mary Jane Adams, a nursing aide, reports to Irene Olsen, the staff nurse, that Sandra Barrett, the client in room 815, had finished only her orange juice when Ms. Adams collected the breakfast trays. Mrs. Barrett had been admitted two days earlier for diagnostic studies. Concerned about her client, Miss Olsen walks down the corridor to room 815, knocks, and enters. Mrs. Barrett turns away from the window, tears in her eyes, as Miss Olsen enters.

Client	Nurse	Comments
	Good morning, Mrs. Barrett.	Acknowledging.
Hello.		
	I understand you didn't eat your breakfast.	Making a specific statement, but ignoring the nonverbal.
I wasn't hungry.		
	Is something wrong?	Asking a closed-ended question that fails to facilitate exploration.
No. (Eyes fill with tears.)		
	You look sad; as if you're about to cry.	Giving feedback.
(Cries.)		
	I'll sit here a while with you. (Sits down.)	Offering self.
(Continues to cry.)	(After a 30-second pause): Sometimes it's hard to share the things you're concerned about with someone you don't know well. I'd like to be able to help.	Empathizing. Supporting. Offering self.
(Angrily): You can help me by telling me the truth.		
	(Leans forward and maintains eye contact.)	Actively listening and demonstrating interest.
Everyone beats around the bush when I ask them what's wrong with me. The head nurse said, "What do *you* think is wrong?" That kind of put-off drives me up the wall!		
	You're angry because you're not getting any answers. It seems as if the staff knows something about your condition and they're keeping it from you.	Paraphrasing.
They all seem to be in cahoots. Nobody tells me anything. (Pause.) (Softly): If the news was good, they wouldn't beat around the bush.		
	I'm wondering if you're worried that because people haven't answered your question it means that you have a serious illness?	Paraphrasing.
Good news is always easy to give.		
	Yes, people do seem to be able to deliver good news easier and faster. I also know that we don't have any news—good or bad—to give you because none of the laboratory or x-ray results are back yet. I know that doesn't help answer your questions, but I hope it relieves you a bit from worrying that there is some bad news that's being withheld.	Giving information. Supporting.
Well, when my father-in-law had surgery for a bleeding ulcer, the x-ray and laboratory results were available immediately.		
	When there's a question of emergency surgery being needed, then tests results are asked for immediately. Usually, though, it's preferable to wait for an accurate reading and a thorough written report.	Giving information.

Table 27–3 *(continued)*

Client	Nurse	Comments
Are you absolutely sure?		
	You don't sound convinced.	Acknowledging the implied.
Listen, I don't mean to give you a hard time. It's just that . . . it may not seem like an emergency to my doctor or the lab people, but it sure is to me. I can't stand not knowing. I don't know the results of the tests I had yesterday. I don't know how many more tests I have to have. Will I have to have surgery? When can I go home?		
	The problem you need help with now is finding out the answers to four questions: What are the results of yesterday's tests? Is your doctor considering any other tests for you, and if so what are they? Is surgery being planned? And when can you go home? Let's try to figure out how you can get the answers to these questions.	Summarizing. Encouraging problem-solving.
Well, I can't call my doctor on the phone. All his receptionist will do is take the message. And, anyway, I'm afraid that he'll be offended if he thinks I'm complaining about him. You won't tell him, will you?		
	No, not unless you and I decide together that it would be the best solution.	Encouraging collaboration.
I suppose I could just try to forget about it and be patient, just like everyone tells me to.		
	You've tried that, but you're still worried, fearful, and angry. Let's think of some other possibilities.	Encouraging further exploration.
Maybe you could call his office for me! Since you're a nurse, they'll probably put your call right through.		
	So far there are three possible solutions—calling his office yourself, waiting until he comes to visit you later this afternoon, or having me call his office. Are there any other possible solutions that we haven't considered?	Focusing on solutions.
I can't think of any others.		
	Okay, then, which do you think would be best?	Demonstrating respect for the client.
I guess I'd feel better if you called his office. I just don't want him to think that I'm criticizing him.		
	You're concerned about what he might think of you because of this phone call. Let's discuss how I should handle the call and what I should say.	Paraphrasing. Encouraging collaboration and problem-solving.

After a few minutes they develop a plan for calling Mrs. Barrett's physician, and Miss Olsen makes the call. The physician has decided to call both the laboratory and the X-ray department for the results of Mrs. Barrett's tests and promises to phone her as soon as he learns the results. They will discuss further possible tests and treatment plans that afternoon when he makes his hospital rounds. Mrs. Barrett asks Miss Olsen to stay with her while she receives the physician's telephone call about the test results.

Courtesy of Carol Ren Kneisl, Associate Clinical Professor, School of Nursing, State University of New York at Buffalo.

- Many factors influence the communication process: the ability of the communicator, perceptions, personal space (intimate, personal, social, and public distance), territoriality, roles and relationships, purposes, time and setting, attitudes, emotions, and self-esteem.
- The development of communication is a complex process; the nurse needs to be familiar with the phases of language development for assessment purposes.
- Factors that influence language development are intelligence, sex, bilingualism, single child versus twin status, parental stimulation, and socioeconomic components.
- Nurses can assist parents in stimulating the language development of children by encouraging verbal and nonverbal communication, listening, using speech as a substitute for action, and using precise terminology.
- There are three broad areas for assessing communication: language development, nonverbal behavior, and style of communication.
- Many techniques facilitate therapeutic communication: attentive listening; paraphrasing; clarifying; using open-ended questions and statements; focusing; being specific; using touch and silence; clarifying reality, time, or sequence; providing general leads; and summarizing.
- Techniques that inhibit communication include offering unvalidated reassurance, stating approval or disapproval, giving common (not expert) advice, stereotyping, and being defensive.
- The effective nurse–client relationship is a growth-facilitating process.
- Four phases of the helping relationship include the preinteraction phase, the introductory phase, the working phase, and the termination phase; each has a specific purpose or goal and requires specific skills of the nurse.
- Process recordings are frequently made by nurses to evaluate their own communication. With them, nurses can analyze both the process and the content of the communication.

Suggested Readings

Bigham, G. D. September 1964. To communicate with Negro patients. *American Journal of Nursing* 64:113–15.
This public health supervisor, writing from the standpoint of a black, a nurse, and an occasional patient, describes some of the subtleties in black–white client–nurse communication. In addition to nurses treating blacks the same way they would treat all persons, several other concrete and specific suggestions applicable to today are offered.

Goodykoontz, L. 1979. Touch: Attitudes and practice. *Nursing Forum* 18(1):4–17.
Communicating through touch, procedural touch, and nonprocedural touch are described. Factors that influence touch and the approaches to using touch are presented.

MacDonald, M. R. June 1977. How do men and women students rate empathy? *American Journal of Nursing* 77:998.
This article reveals the empathy ratings of men and women in nursing contrasted to those of men and women not in nursing. The results are contrary to what many would think.

Seaman, L. May/June 1982. Affective nursing touch. *Geriatric Nursing* 3:162–64.
The need to be touched continues throughout life and may even be intensified by the sensory and personal losses that occur with aging. The author discusses why touch is important and implications for nursing touch, including appropriate ways of touching.

Stillman, M. J. October 1978. Territoriality and personal space. *American Journal of Nursing* 78:1670–72.
Territoriality and personal space are explained, with some applications to patients in hospitals.

Travelbee, J. February 1963. What do we mean by rapport? *American Journal of Nursing* 63:70–72.
The basic ingredients of rapport are outlined in this article. Nurses are constantly reminded that they need to develop rapport with patients but often are unable to explain its meaning.

Whaley, L. F., and Wong, D. L. November/December 1985. Effective communication strategies for pediatric practice. *Pediatric Nursing* 11:429–32.
A variety of unconventional communication techniques can be used to help nurses elicit children's feelings. The authors describe techniques such as the third-person, storytelling, three wishes, rating game, pros and cons, bibliotherapy, writing, drawing, and play.

Selected References

Almore, M. G. June 1979. Dyadic communication. *American Journal of Nursing* 79:1076–78.

Allekian, C. I. May/June 1973. Intrusions of territory and personal space: An anxiety-inducing factor for hospitalized persons—an exploratory study. *Nursing Research* 22:236–41.

Apse, A. December 1985. Avoiding terms of bewilderment. *Nursing 85* 15:42–43.

Bandler, R., and Grinder, J. 1975. *The structure of magic,* Volume 1. Palo Alto, Calif.: Science and Behavior Books.

Bandler, R., and Grinder, J. 1976. *The structure of magic,* Volume 2. Palo Alto, Calif.: Science and Behavior Books.

Bee, H. 1985. *The developing child,* 4th ed. New York: Harper & Row.

Benjamin, A. 1981. *The helping interview,* 3rd ed. Boston: Houghton Mifflin Co.

Brammer, L. M. 1985. *The helping relationship: Process and skills,* 3d ed. Englewood Cliffs, N.J.: Prentice-Hall.

Brockopp, D. Y. July 1983. What is NLP? *American Journal of Nursing* 83:1012–14.

Brown, B. G. July 1972. The language of space: A silent component of the therapeutic process. *Nursing Papers* (School for Graduate Nurses, McGill University, Montreal)4:29–34.

Collins, M. 1981. *Communication in health care: Understanding and implementing effective human relationships.* 2d ed. St. Louis: C. V. Mosby Co.

Collins, M. 1983. *Communication in health care. The human connection in the life style.* St. Louis: C. V. Mosby Co.

Cooper, J. April 1979. Actions really do speak louder than words. *Nursing 79* 9:29–32 (United States ed. 9:113–16).

Cosper, B. December 1977. How well do your patients understand hospital jargon? *American Journal of Nursing* 77:1932–34.

Davis, A. J. 1981. *Please see my need.* Charles City, Iowa: Satellite Books.

Davis, A. J. 1984. *Listening and responding.* St. Louis: C. V. Mosby Co.

Devillers, L. March 1982. What to do when you just can't communicate. *Nursing Life* 2:34–39.

Egan, G. 1975. *The skilled helper: A model for systematic helping and interpersonal relating.* Monterey, Calif.: Brooks/Cole Publishing Co.

Egan, G. 1982. *The skilled helper. Model, skills, and methods for effective helping,* 2d ed. Monterey, Calif.: Brooks/Cole Publishing Co.

Ehmann, V. 1971. Empathy: Its origin, characteristics and process. *Perspectives in Psychiatric Care* 9(2):72–80.

Ernst, P., and Shaw, J. September/October 1980. Touching is not taboo. *Geriatric Nursing* 1:193–95.

Forrest, D. Autumn 1982. Analysis of nurses' verbal communication with patients. *Nursing Papers* 15:48–56.

Hall, E. T. 1969. *The hidden dimension.* Garden City, N.Y.: Doubleday and Co.

Hardin, S. B., and Halaris, A. L. January 1983. Nonverbal communication of patients and high- and low-empathy nurses. *Journal of Psychosocial Nursing and Mental Health Services* 21:15–20.

Helms, D. B., and Turner, J. S. 1976. *Exploring child behavior.* Philadelphia: W. B. Saunders Co.

Herth, K. June 1974. Beyond the curtain of silence. *American Journal of Nursing* 74:1060–61.

Hurst, J. B., and Keenan, M. January 1986. Do you have any other ideas for improvement? *Nursing Success Today* 3:1–29.

Iveson-Iveson, J. February 2, 1983. The art of communication . . . how nurses communicate with their patients and colleagues and the skills needed. *Nursing Mirror* 156:47–48.

Jungman, L. B. June 1979. When your feelings get in the way. *American Journal of Nursing* 79:1074–75.

Kaul, T., and Schmidt, L. 1971. Dimensions of interviewer trustworthiness. *Journal of Counseling Psychology* 34:134–39.

King, I. M. 1981. *A theory for nursing. Systems, concepts, process.* New York: John Wiley & Sons.

Knowles, R. D. July 1983. Building rapport. Through neuro-linguistic programming. *American Journal of Nursing* 83:1011–14.

Kramer, M., and Schmalenberg, C. November 1977. Constructive feedback: Are you and your coworkers getting the message? *Nursing 77* 7:20–21 (United States ed. 7:102).

Lambert, W. E., and Tucker, G. R. 1972. *Bilingual education of children: The St. Lambert experiment.* Boston: Newbury House.

Lancaster, J. September 1983. Communication: The anatomy of messages. *Nursing Management* 14:42–45.

Leonard, R. November 1985. Speak for yourself. *Nursing 85* 15:30–31.

Long, L., and Prophit, P. 1981. *Understanding/responding: A communication manual for nurses.* Belmont, Calif.: Wadsworth Publishing Co.

Lynch, J. J. June 1978. The simple act of touching, *Nursing 78* 8:32–36.

MacKinnon, J. R. February 1984. Health professionals' patterns of communication: Gross purpose or problem solving? *Journal of Allied Health* 13:3–12.

Macrae, J. April 1979. Therapeutic touch in practice. *American Journal of Nursing* 79:664–65.

Mitchell, A. C. February 1978. Barriers to therapeutic communication with black clients. *Nursing Outlook* 26:109–12.

Morgan, B. S., and Barden, M. E. September 1985. Nurse–patient interaction in the home setting. *Public Health Nursing* 2:159–67.

Muldary, T. W. 1983. *Interpersonal relations for health professionals. A social skills approach.* New York: Macmillan Publishing Co.

Piaget, J. 1952. *The language and thought of the child.* London: Routledge and Kegan Paul.

Purtilo, R. 1978. *Health professional/patient interaction,* 2d ed. Philadelphia: W. B. Saunders Co.

Ramaekers, M. J. June 1979. Communication blocks revisited. *American Journal of Nursing* 79:1079–81.

Rawnsley, M. M. April 1980. Toward a conceptual base for affective nursing. *Nursing Outlook* 28:244–47.

Rosendahl, P. B., and Ross, V. October 1982. Does your behavior affect your patient's response? *Journal of Gerontological Nursing* 8:572–75.

Schulman, L. 1984. *The skills of helping individuals and groups,* 2d ed. Itasca, Ill.: F. E. Peacock Publishers.

Seaman, L. May/June 1982. Affective nursing touch. *Geriatric Nursing* 3:162–64.

Shanken, J., and Shanken, P. February 1976. How to be a helping person. *Journal of Psychiatric Nursing and Mental Health Services* 14:24–28.

Shubin, S. November 1976. Familiarity: Therapeutic? Harmful? When? *Nursing 76* 6:18–24.

Stewart, C. J., and Cash, W. B. 1985. *Interviewing principles and practices,* 4th ed. Dubuque, Iowa: Wm. C. Brown Publishers.

Sundeen, S. J., et al. 1981. *Nurse-client interaction: Implementing the nursing process,* 2d ed. St. Louis: C. V. Mosby Co.

Thomas, M. 1970. Trust in the nurse-patient relationship. In Carlson, Carolyn E., editor. *Behavioral concepts and nursing intervention.* Philadelphia: J. B. Lippincott Co.

Ujhely, G. B. 1979. Touch: Reflections and perceptions. *Nursing Forum* 18(1):18–32.

Veninga, R. November 1978. Are you a successful communicator? *Canadian Nurse* 74:34–37.

Vygotsky, L. S. 1962. *Thought and language.* Cambridge, Mass.: MIT Press.

Wilkinson, R. April 1986. Communication: Learning from the market. *Nursing Management* 17:42J, 42L.

CHAPTER 28

Functioning in Groups

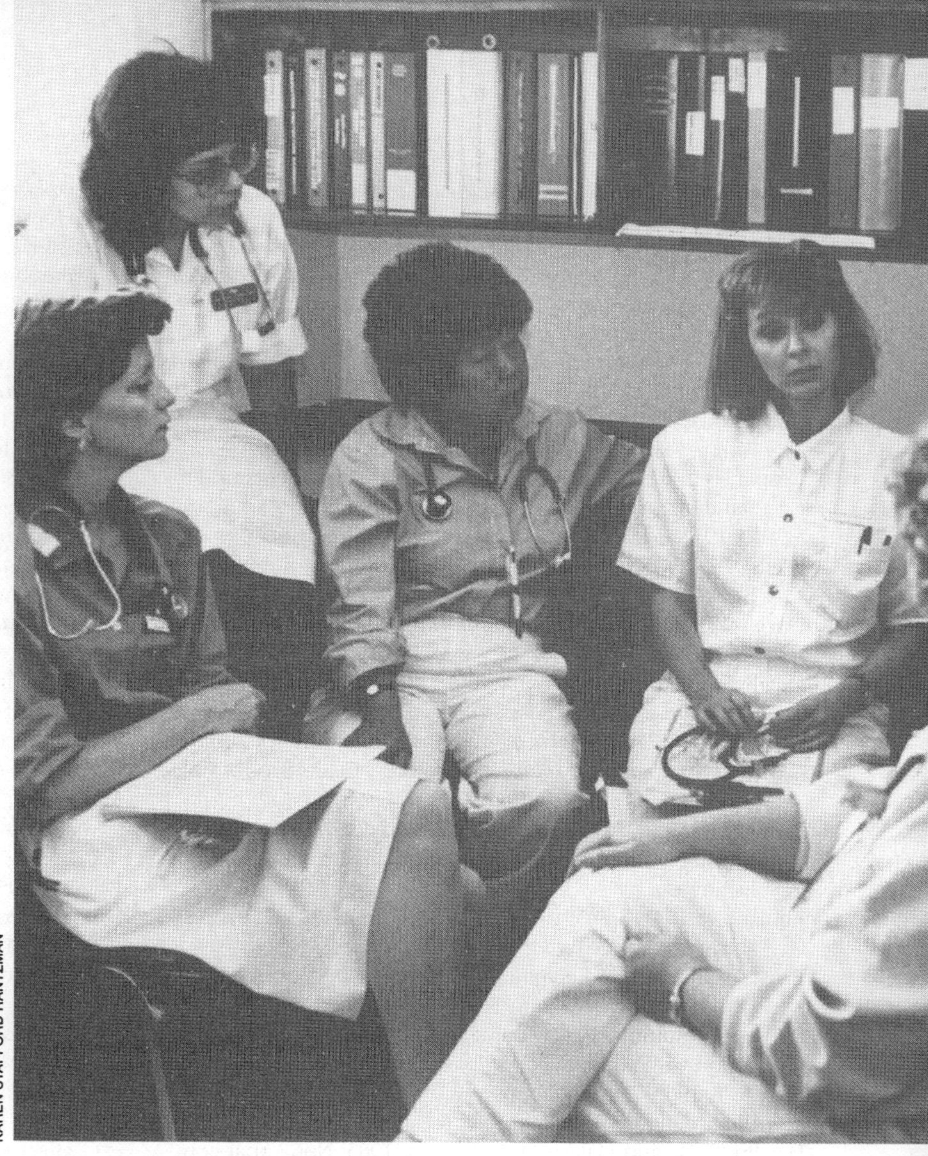

KAREN STAFFORD RANTZMAN

Contents

Objectives

1. Know essential facts about groups.
   1.1 Define selected terms.
   1.2 Identify differences between primary and secondary groups.
   1.3 Identify features of formal, semiformal, and informal groups.
   1.4 Identify structural and functional characteristics of groups.
   1.5 Describe three stages of group development.
   1.6 Identify features of effective groups.
2. Understand essential facts about forces influencing group dynamics (process).
   2.1 Identify forces that influence group dynamics.
   2.2 Outline attitudes and behaviors indicating group commitment.
   2.3 Identify advantages and disadvantages of three leadership styles.
   2.4 Explain the concept of diffused leadership.
   2.5 Identify behaviors of an effective leader.
   2.6 Identify five methods of decision making.
   2.7 Identify ways in which effective decisions are made.
   2.8 Identify three categories of functional roles of group members.
   2.9 Identify behaviors associated with member roles.
   2.10 Explain how the sociogram can be used to ascertain group interaction patterns.
   2.11 Outline attitudes and behaviors indicating group cohesiveness.
   2.12 Explain the concept of power.
   2.13 Identify some kinds of power.
3. Understand essential factors about common group problems and interventions to handle them.
   3.1 Differentiate between productive and nonproductive conflict.
   3.2 State reasons for nonproductive conflict.
   3.3 Identify ways the group leader can resolve productive conflict.
   3.4 Identify ways the group leader can handle nonproductive conflict.
   3.5 Identify indications of inadequate group decision making.
   3.6 Identify common causes of group apathy.
   3.7 Identify ways the group leader may deal with group apathy.
   3.8 Identify ways the group leader may intervene when a member monopolizes the group.
4. Know essential facts about group self-evaluation.
   4.1 Identify the purpose of feedback.
   4.2 Identify essential feedback information.
   4.3 Describe the role of a group productivity observer.
5. Understand essential facts about self-help groups.
   5.1 Explain the eight characteristics of self-help groups.
   5.2 Identify the six unique aspects of a self-help group.
   5.3 Explain the nurse's role relative to self-help groups.

Terms

apathy
assimilation
authority
cohesiveness
commitment
conformity
dyad
group
group dynamics (group process)
homogeneity
influence
mores
norms
polarization
power
primary group
role
sanctions
secondary group
self-help group
sociogram
tone

Groups

People are born into a group (i.e., the family) and interact with others at all stages of their lives in various groups: peer groups, work groups, recreational groups, religious groups, etc. A **group** is defined as two or more persons who have shared needs and goals, who take each other into account in their actions, and who thus are held together and set apart from others by virtue of their interactions.

Much of a nurse's professional life is spent in a wide variety of groups, ranging from **dyads** (two-person groups) to large professional organizations. As a participant in a group, the nurse may be required to fulfill different roles: member or leader, teacher or learner, adviser or advisee, etc.

Groups exist to help people achieve goals that would be unattainable by individual effort alone. For example, groups can often solve problems more effectively than one person, by pooling the ideas and expertise of several individuals; and information can be disseminated to groups more quickly than to individuals. In addition, groups often take greater risks than do individuals. Just as responsibilities for actions are shared by group members, so are the consequences of actions. The overall effectiveness of groups in attaining goals depends on many factors, discussed in this chapter.

Types of Groups

Groups are classified as either primary or secondary, according to their structure and type of interaction. A **primary group** is a small, intimate group in which the relationships among members are personal, spontaneous, sentimental, cooperative, and inclusive. Examples are the family, a play group of children, informal work groups, and friendship groups. Members of a primary group communicate with each other largely in face-to-face interactions and develop a strong sense of unity or "oneness." What belongs to one person is often seen as belonging to the group. For example, a success achieved by one member is shared by all and is seen as a success of the group.

Primary groups set standards of behavior for the members but also support and sustain each member in stresses he or she would otherwise not be able to withstand. Expectations are informally administered and involve primarily internal constraints imposed by the group itself. To its members, the primary group has a value in itself, not merely as a means to some other goal. The group has a sense of "we" and "our" to it, in contrast to "I" and "mine." Affective relationships are stressed.

The role of the primary group, particularly the family, in health care is increasingly recognized. It is to the primary group that people turn for help and support when they have health problems. Treatment and health care of individuals therefore are developing an expanded focus that includes the family.

A **secondary group** is generally larger, more impersonal, and less sentimental than a primary group. Examples are professional associations, task groups, ad hoc committees, political parties, and business groups. Members view these groups simply as means of getting things done. Interactions do not necessarily occur in face-to-face contact and do not require that the members know each other in any inclusive sense. Thus, there is little sentiment attached to such relationships. Expectations of members are formally administered through impersonal controls and external restraints imposed by designated enforcement officials. Once the goals of the group are achieved or change, the interaction is discontinued.

Levels of Group Formality

Formal Groups

Groups may be classified as formal, semiformal, or informal. The most common example of the formal group is the work organization. People become familiar with many different formal work groups during their lifetimes and spend a major part of their working hours in such groups. Formal groups usually exist to carry out a task or goal rather than to meet the needs of group members. Traditional features of formal groups include:

1. Authority is imposed from above.
2. Leadership selection is assigned from above and made by an authoritative and often arbitrary order or decree (fiat).
3. Managers are symbols of power and authority.
4. The goals of the formal group are normally imposed at a much higher level than the direct leadership of the group.
5. Fiscal goals have little meaning to the members of the group.
6. Management is endangered by its aloofness from the members of the work group.
7. Behavioral **norms** (expected standards of behavior), regulations, and rules are usually superimposed. The larger the turnover rate of members, the greater the structuring of rules.
8. Membership in the group is only partly voluntary.
9. Rigidity of purpose is often a necessity for protection of the formal group in the pursuit of its objectives.
10. Interactions within the group as a whole are limited, but informal subgroups are generally formed.

Semiformal Groups

Some examples of semiformal groups are churches, lodges, social clubs, PTAs, and some labor unions. Many of a person's social needs and ego needs are satisfied by membership in these groups. The groups are similar in form to formal groups, but exhibit slight differences. Features of semiformal groups include:

1. The structure is formal.
2. The hierarchy is carefully delineated.
3. Membership is voluntary but selective and difficult to achieve.
4. Prestige and status are often accrued from membership.
5. Structured, deliberate activities absorb a large part of the group's meeting time.
6. Objectives and goals are rigid; change is not recognized as desirable.
7. In many cases, the leader has direct control over the choice of a successor.
8. The day-to-day operating standards and methods (group

norms) are negotiable. Because most people become bored at quibbling about norms, leaders can often "railroad" acceptance of a list of norms they desire.

Informal Groups

All people, from childhood on, have membership in numerous informal groups. These groups provide much of a person's education and develop most cultural values. Five types of groups are representative of the numerous informal groups in existence:

Friendship groups. The first groups formed in life are friendship groups. They are often formed on the basis of common interests. Many arise out of semiformal group interactions or are formed spontaneously from work organization.

Hobby groups. Hobby groups bring together a wide variety of people from all walks of life. The differences in members' personalities and backgrounds are largely ignored in the interests of the hobby itself.

Convenience groups. Many examples of convenience groups are found both in and out of the work setting. Two examples are the car pool and the child-care group organized by mothers.

Work groups. Informal work groups can make or break an organization. Managers need to be sensitive to such groups and cultivate their cooperation and good will. Friendships often arise out of such groups between a new member and the first person who makes him or her feel a welcome addition to the group.

Self-protective groups. Self-protective groups can be found anywhere but are particularly common in work organizations. They arise spontaneously out of a real or perceived threat. For example, a supervisor may approach a worker too strongly and find a group of workers organizing a united front against the threat. Such groups dissipate as soon as the threat has subsided.

Features of informal groups include:

1. The group is not bound by any set of written rules or regulations.
2. Usually there is a set of unwritten laws and a strong code of ethics.
3. The group is purely functional and has easily recognized basic objectives.
4. Rotational leadership is common. The group recognizes that only rarely are all leadership characteristics found in one person.
5. The group assigns duties to the members best qualified for certain functions. For example, the member who is recognized as being effective during times of stress will be called upon for guidance when threats or problems arise; the person who is recognized as outgoing and sociable will be assigned responsibilities for planning parties, etc.
6. Judgments about the group's leader are made quickly and surely. The leader is replaced when he or she makes one or more mistakes or does not get the job done efficiently.
7. The group is an ideal testing ground for new leadership techniques, but there is no guarantee that such techniques can be transferred effectively to a large, formal organization. For example, management by committee originated in small, informal group structures.
8. Behavioral norms are developed either by group effort or by the leader and adopted by the group.
9. Deviance by one member from the group's behavioral norms is more threatening to the perpetuation of small, informal groups than to large, formal, heterogeneous groups. Conformity and group solidarity are important for the protection and preservation of small groups.
10. Group norms are enforced by **sanctions** (punishments) imposed by the group of those who violate a norm. Examples are the withholding of privileges or isolation of the offender from the group. Different values are placed on norms, however, in accordance with the values of the leader. One leader may regard an action as a gross violation, whereas another leader may find it quite acceptable.
11. Interpersonal interactions are spontaneous.

Characteristics of Groups

Many characteristics of groups are associated with the type and level of formality of the specific group, as discussed earlier in this chapter. Groups of all kinds, however, have certain structural and functional characteristics that need to be understood before the nurse can gain a perspective on the interactions that occur between individual members and the group. These characteristics are outlined and described in Table 28–1.

Structural properties refer to the ways in which persons in a group are involved in (a) ordered arrangements, (b) that define and regulate their behavior, and (c) that provide a patterned constancy and stability to their behavior together. Structural properties of a group are defined independently of the particular persons who are members. Thus a change in group membership does not create a change in group structure. For example, a hospital has ordered arrangements of personnel whose behavior is

Table 28–1 Characteristics of Groups

Characteristic	Description	Characteristic	Description
Structural		*Functional*	
Size	Number of members. Ranges from two members to infinity. The smaller the group, the less formal the relationship.	Norms	Expected standards of behavior based on the group **mores** (values). May be established by: (a) tradition, (b) imposition by the highest authority or immediate supervisor of the group, (c) cooperation between the leader and the group, or (d) group action.
Membership methods	How people become members of the group. May be ascribed or assigned. *Ascribed* membership means voluntary choice, e.g., membership in a hobby club. *Assigned* membership means involuntary draft, e.g., membership in the armed forces. Permeability (access to membership in the group by outsiders) varies from highly selective to highly permissive.	Homogeneity	Degree of likeness of attitudes and beliefs among members.
Relationship to other groups	Whether the group functions autonomously from or in concert with other groups; whether it is a separate organization or a subgroup of a larger structure.	Sanctions	Measures used to enforce normative behavior. Range from light censure to expulsion from the group.
Stability	The degree of permanence of a group and the sense of continuity felt by the group.	Tone	Pleasant or unpleasant atmosphere sensed in a group.
		Cohesiveness	Degree of group unity (oneness); sense of members being "we." Forces that tend to hold the group together include: (a) perceived threats from outside, (b) leadership that communicates and reinforces group objectives, (c) homogeneity, and (d) member identification with the group's objectives.
		Climate	Unwritten traditions, habits, relationships, practices, rules, beliefs, and attitudes that become characteristic of a group.
		Conformity	Actions in accordance with specified standards of authority or of the group.

defined and regulated in prescribed role and power structures. Even when personnel change, the structure remains the same or similar.

Functional properties relate to operational and procedural methods of functioning and to group process or dynamics as determined by group norms, climate, tone, etc.

Stages of Group Development

There are three stages of group development: the initiation, functional, and dissolution stages. The *initiation stage,* when a group first forms, involves interactions in which members become familiar with one another, determine a method of operation, and establish their roles within the group. Tasks predominate, and behavior is tested. The group is viewed more as a series of individuals than as a unified whole, and differences among individuals are more evident than similarities. People seek a place in the group in relation to others in various ways: some hang back as observers; others are highly extroverted, relating with excessive good humor and amicability. As the group forms, a testing process begins in which people gradually increase their personal exchanges and contacts and try to find out about one another's attitudes, values, and readiness to be contacted. At this stage the group may appear to be acting effectively. It is progressing with its tasks, and there appears to be a friendly comradeship among members. However, this condition is only superficial, arising from experiences established before the group was formed.

The *functional stage* occurs when the members feel comfortable with one another. It is during this phase that group properties such as **tone**, **homogeneity**, **cohesiveness**, and **conformity** develop and increase. See Table 28–1 for definitions. Group goals are established, and **polarization** (movement by members toward a common goal) occurs. Individual behavior is less obvious, due to the process of **assimilation** (the blending of attitudes and beliefs among members); a group unified in approach becomes evident. The tasks to be achieved are also evident.

The *dissolution stage* occurs when group members no longer see a need for the group. Group goals may or may not have been attained, and group properties such as cohesiveness and assimilation may not have been achieved. Members may feel a sense of relief or frustration about dissolution. Relief may be felt if (a) the degree of members' dependence on the group for meeting their needs is low, (b) the potency (importance) of the group for its members is minimal, (c) the climate of the group has been tense, and (d) group cohesion has not occurred. Frustration or anxiety will be felt if dependence on and potency of the group were high and if the climate and group cohesion were pleasant and agreeable.

Features of Effective Groups

To be effective, a group must achieve three main functions:

1. Accomplish its goals
2. Maintain its cohesion
3. Develop and modify its structure to improve its effectiveness

Fisher (1985, p. 6) describes ten characteristics of an effectively functioning group:

1. The tasks and goals are clear and are understood and accepted by the group members.
2. The group members listen to one another. Every idea that affects the group is considered.
3. The group accepts disagreement and uses differing ideas to come up with creative solutions.
4. Decisions are clear-cut and made in such a way that all members of the group are in general agreement and willing to support them.
5. Feedback is constructive, and the members are comfortable with feedback.
6. Group members express their feelings and their ideas about problems and interpersonal issues.
7. Following decisions, clear assignments are made and accepted.
8. Leadership shifts from time to time, and the designated leader does not dominate the group. The main issue is not who controls the group but how to do the job.
9. Group members have a sense of loyalty to and dependency on each other.
10. The group has the ability to examine its own process.

The many factors that influence the effectiveness of a group are further amplified in Table 28–2.

Assessing Group Dynamics (Process)

During recent years the terms *group dynamics* and *group process* have frequently appeared in literature and discussions among group workers, educators, and professional organizations. **Group dynamics** (or **group process**) are forces in the group situation that determine the behavior of the group and its members (Jenkins 1974, p. 5). They are a way of looking at groups. Every group has its own unique dynamics and constantly changing pattern of forces, just as each individual has unique forces from within that shape the person's character. To study the dynamics of a group, several factors, in addition to group structure and organization, may be analyzed: (a) commitment, (b) leadership style, (c) diffused leadership function, (d) decision-making methods, (e) member behaviors, (f) interaction patterns, (g) group cohesiveness, and (h) power.

Commitment

The members of effective groups have a **commitment** (agreement, pledge, or obligation to do something) to the goals and output of the group. Because groups demand time and attention, members must give up some autonomy and self-interest. Inevitably conflicts arise between the interests of individual members and those of the group. However, members who are committed to the group feel close to each other and willingly put themselves out for the group. Some indications of group commitment are:

1. Members feel a strong sense of belonging.
2. Members enjoy each other.
3. Members seek each other for counsel and support.

Table 28–2 Comparative Features of Effective and Ineffective Groups

Factor	Effective Groups	Ineffective Groups
Atmosphere	Informal, comfortable, and relaxed. It is a working atmosphere in which people demonstrate their interest and involvement.	Obviously tense. Signs of boredom may appear.
Goal setting	Goals, tasks, and objectives are clarified, understood, and modified so that members of the group can commit themselves to cooperatively structured goals.	Unclear, misunderstood, or imposed goals may be accepted by members. The goals are competitively structured.
Leadership and member participation	Shift from time to time, depending on the circumstances. Different members assume leadership at various times, because of their knowledge or experience.	Delegated and based on authority. The chairperson may dominate the group, or the members may defer unduly. Members participation is unequal, with high-authority members dominating.
Goal emphasis	All three functions of groups are emphasized—goal accomplishment, internal maintenance, and developmental change.	One or more functions may not be emphasized.
Communication	Open and two-way. Ideas and feelings are encouraged, both about the problem and about the group's operation.	Closed or one-way. Only the production of ideas is encouraged. Feelings are ignored or taboo. Members may be tentative or reluctant to be open and may have "hidden agendas" (personal goals at cross-purposes with group goals).
Decision making	By consensus, although various decision-making procedures appropriate to the situation may be instituted.	By the highest authority in the group, with minimal involvement by members; or an inflexible style is imposed.
Cohesion	Facilitated through high levels of inclusion, trust, liking, and support.	Either ignored or used as a means of controlling members, thus promoting rigid conformity.
Conflict tolerance	High. The reasons for disagreements or conflicts are carefully examined, and the group seeks to resolve them. The group accepts unresolvable basic disagreements and lives with them.	Low. Attempts may be made to ignore, deny, avoid, suppress, or override controversy by premature group action.
Power	Determined by the members' abilities and the information they possess. Power is shared. The issue is how to get the job done.	Determined by position in the group. Obedience to authority is strong. The issue is who controls.
Problem solving	High. Constructive criticism is frequent, frank, relatively comfortable, and oriented toward removing an obstacle to problem solving.	Low. Criticism may be destructive, taking the form of either overt or covert personal attacks. It prevents the group from getting the job done.
Self-evaluation as a group	Frequent. All members participate in evaluation and decisions about how to improve the group's functioning.	Minimal. What little evaluation there is may be done by the highest authority in the group rather than by the membership as a whole.
Creativity	Encouraged. There is room within the group for members to become self-actualized and interpersonally effective.	Discouraged. People are afraid of appearing foolish if they put forth a creative thought.

From H. S. Wilson and C. R. Kneisl, *Psychiatric nursing,* 2d ed. (Menlo Park, Calif.: Addison-Wesley Publishing Co., 1982), p. 221. Used by permission.

4. Members support each other in difficulty.
5. Members value the contributions of other members.
6. Members are motivated by working in the group and want to do their tasks well.
7. Members express good feelings openly and identify positive contributions.
8. Members feel that the goals of the group are achievable and important.

Leadership Style

Three leadership styles have been described: autocratic, democratic, and laissez-faire. The three are often blended in a selective combination to fit the situation, the needs of the leader, and the needs of the group, rather than being implemented continuously in pure form.

Autocratic Leadership

In autocratic leadership the leader makes the decisions for the group. This style is likened to dictatorship and presupposes that the group is incapable of making its own decisions. The leader determines policies and gives orders and directions to the members. Autocratic leadership generally has negative connotations and often makes group members dissatisfied. It may, however, be a necessary style of leadership when urgent decision making is required, or when group members do not wish to participate in making a decision.

Democratic Leadership

In democratic leadership the leader participates as a facilitator, encouraging group discussion and decision making. This supportive style increases group productivity and satisfaction. It presupposes that group members are capable of making decisions, are motivated to do so, and value independence. Democratic leadership generally has positive connotations, but it requires time for consultation and collaboration. It may not always be the most effective method.

Laissez-faire Leadership

In laissez-faire leadership the leader participates minimally and often only on request of the members. This style is described as a "hands-off" approach. It recognizes the group's need for autonomy and self-regulation. It is most effective after a group has made a decision, is committed to it, and has the expertise to implement it. The leader acts as a resource person and consultant.

Diffused Leadership

Diffused leadership can be described as an approach to group leadership in which functions are distributed. This concept recognizes that the leadership function is not held irrevocably by one person but rather is distributed among the group members. To clarify this concept, Francis and Young (1979, p. 63) distinguish the roles of group manager (the formal head of the group) from those of group leader. Managers have special responsibilities and functions recognized by the organization and vital to the group's performance as an energizing and creative force. However, group leadership is a broad function. Different members come to the fore in their areas of strength to suit the tasks at hand. To determine which group members carry out leadership functions, the following questions may be asked:

1. Who starts the meeting or the work?
2. Who contributes additional information to help the group carry out its functions?
3. Who represents the group with other groups?
4. Who encourages contributions from group members?
5. Who provides support to members with difficult situations?
6. Who clarifies thoughts expressed in discussions?
7. Who keeps the discussions relevant?

Effective Leadership

Much has been written about effective leadership and style. Listed below are some descriptive statements. Effective leaders:

- Use a leadership style that is natural to them.
- Use a leadership style appropriate to the task and the members.
- Assess the effects of their behavior on others and the effects of others' behavior on themselves.
- Are sensitive to forces acting for and against change.
- Express an optimistic view about human nature.
- Are energetic.
- Are open and encourage openness, so that real issues are confronted.
- Facilitate personal relationships.
- Plan and organize activities of the group.
- Are consistent in behavior toward group members.
- Delegate tasks and responsibilities to develop members' abilities, not merely to get tasks performed.
- Involve members in all decisions.
- Value and use group members' contributions.
- Encourage creativity.
- Encourage feedback about their leadership style.

Decision-making Methods

Five methods of decision making have been identified:

Individual or authority-rule decisions. The designated leader of the group makes the decision, and group members or others involved in the decision are expected to abide by it. Authority-rule decisions may be made without discussion or consultation with the group or may be made after discussing the issue and eliciting the group's ideas and views. Decisions made without discussion are often advantageous for simple, routine matters. Those made after discussion are advantageous in that they use the resources of the group and gain the benefits of discussion. However, this type of decision making does not develop a commitment in members to implement the decision, and it fails to resolve controversies among members.

Minority decisions. A few group members meet to discuss an issue and make a decision that is binding for all. This method of decision making is advantageous when the total group is unable to meet together due to time pressures. It is useful for routine decisions. Its limitations are similar to those of decision making by authority rule. Often, executive committees of large groups exercise minority control in decision making.

Majority decisions. More than half of those involved make the decision. This method is commonly used in large groups when complete member commitment is unnecessary. It is an effective method to close a discussion on issues that are not highly important for the group and when sufficient time is lacking for a decision by consensus.

Consensus decisions. Each group member expresses an opinion, and a decision is made by which members can abide, if not in whole, at least in part. This type of decision making takes a great deal of time and energy and therefore is not effective when time pressures are great or when an emergency is in progress. It is useful, however, when important and complex decisions requiring commitment from all members need to be made. This method has several advantages: (a) it produces creative, high-quality decisions, (b) it elicits commitment by all members and responsibility for implementing action, (c) it uses the resources of all members, and (d) it enhances the future decision-making ability of the group.

Unanimous decisions. Every group member agrees on the decision and can support the action to be taken. This method is commonly used for issues that are highly important to the group and require complete member commitment. Unanimous decisions are not practical for simple, routine matters or controversial issues, however.

Effective Decisions

Making sound decisions is essential to effective group functioning. Effective decisions are made when:

1. The group determines which decision method to adopt.
2. The group listens to all the ideas of members.
3. Members feel satisfied with their participation.
4. The expertise of group members is well used.
5. The problem-solving ability of the group is facilitated.
6. The group atmosphere is positive.
7. Time is used well; i.e., the discussion focuses on the decision to be made.
8. Members feel committed to the decision and responsible for its implementation.

Member Behaviors

The degree of input by members into goal setting, decision making, problem solving, group evaluation, etc. is due in part to the group structure and leadership style, but members, too, have responsibilities for group behavior and participation. Each member participates in a wide range of **roles** (assigned or assumed functions) during group interactions. These roles have been categorized as (a) task roles, (b) maintenance or building roles, and (c) self-serving roles.

Task Roles

A task role is related to the task of the group. Its purpose is to enhance and coordinate the group's movement toward achievement of its goals. Task roles and the behaviors associated with them include (Wilson and Kneisl 1979, p. 444):

Information and opinion giver: offers facts, opinions, ideas, suggestions, and relevant information to help group discussion

Information and opinion seeker: asks for facts, information, opinions, ideas, and feelings from other members, to help group discussion

Starter: proposes goals and tasks to initiate action within the group

Direction giver: develops plans on how to proceed, and focuses attention on the task to be done

Summarizer: pulls together related ideas or suggestions; restates and summarizes the major points discussed

Coordinator: shows relationships among various ideas; harmonizes activities of various subgroups and members

Diagnoser: identifies sources of difficulties the group has in working effectively and blocks to progress in accomplishing the group's goals

Energizer: stimulates a higher quality of work from the group

Reality tester: examines the practicality and workability of ideas; evaluates alternative solutions, and applies them to real situations to see how they will work

Evaluator: compares group decisions and accomplishments with group standards and goals

Maintenance or Building Roles

The maintenance role is related to maintaining or building the group's continuity, cohesion, and stability. Roles and behaviors associated with this include (Wilson and Kneisl 1979, p. 444):

Encourager of participation: warmly encourages everyone to participate, giving recognition for contributions, demonstrating acceptance and openness to the ideas of others; is friendly and responsive to group members

Harmonizer and compromiser: persuades members to analyze their differences of opinion constructively, searches for common elements in conflicts, and tries to reconcile disagreements

Tension reliever: eases tensions and increases the enjoyment of group members by joking, suggesting breaks, and proposing approaches to group work that will be fun

Communication helper: shows good communication skills and makes sure that each group member understands what other members are saying

Active listener: listens and serves as an interested audience for other members; is receptive to others' ideas; goes along with the group when not in disagreement

Trust builder: accepts and supports the openness of other group members, reinforces risk taking, and encourages individuality

Self-serving Roles

Self-serving roles often present obstacles to effective group functioning. The self-serving role is aimed at satisfying the individual's needs and does not enhance group effectiveness. Examples of self-serving roles and behaviors are (Wilson and Kneisl 1979, p. 444):

Aggressor: deflates the status of others by expressing disapproval of their values, acts, or feelings, by attacking the group or the problem it is working on, or by joking aggressively

Blocker: tends to be negative and stubbornly resistant; attempts to maintain or bring back issues after group has rejected or bypassed them

Recognition seeker: calls attention to self through boasting, reporting on personal achievements, acting in unusual ways, or struggling not to be placed in an "inferior" position

Dominator: tries to assert authority or superiority by engaging in flattery, claiming a superior status or the right to attention, giving directions authoritatively, and interrupting the contributions of others

Interaction Patterns

Interaction patterns can be observed and ascertained by a **sociogram**, a diagram of the flow of verbal communication within a group during a specified period, e.g., 5 or 15 minutes. This diagram indicates who speaks to whom and who initiates the remarks. Ideally the interaction patterns of a small group would indicate verbal interaction from all members of the group to all members of the group. See Figure 28–1. In reality, however, such an interaction pattern does not occur. See Figure 28–2. This second diagram illustrates that not all communication is a two-way process. The lines with arrowheads at each end indicate that the statement made by one person was responded to by the recipient; a short cross-line drawn near one of the arrowheads indicates who initiated the remark. One-way communication is indicated by lines with an arrowhead at only one end. Remarks made to the group as a whole are indicated by arrows drawn to only the middle of the circle. By using a sociogram, nurses can analyze strengths and weaknesses in a group's interaction patterns. Used in conjunction with member behavior tools, this can offer considerable data about the group's dynamics.

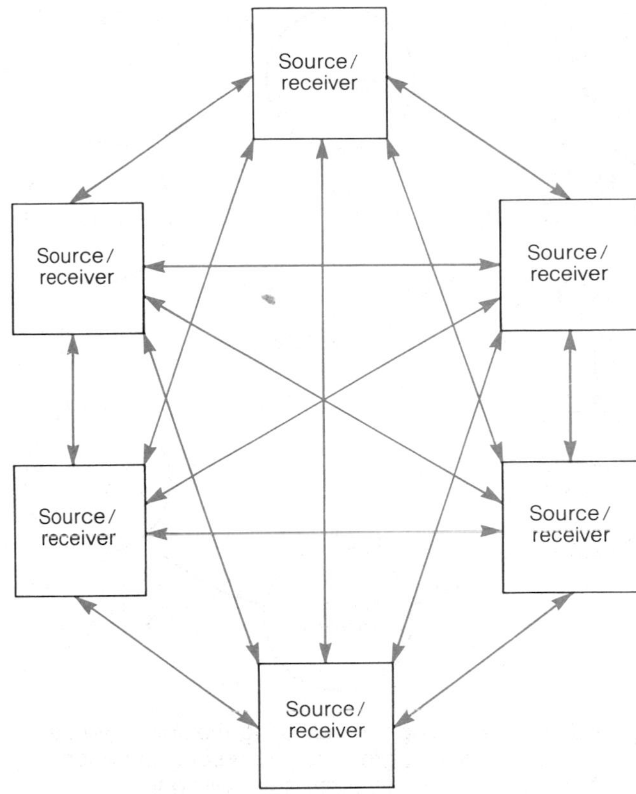

Figure 28–1 An ideal small-group interaction pattern. All members interact with all other members.

Cohesiveness

Cohesive groups possess a certain group spirit, a sense of being "we," and a common purpose. Groups lacking in cohesiveness are unstable and prone to disintegration. The following membership attitudes and behaviors and group properties characterize high-cohesion groups (Wilson and Kneisl 1982, p. 229):

Membership attitudes and behaviors

1. Members like each other, trust one another, and are friendly and willing to interact.

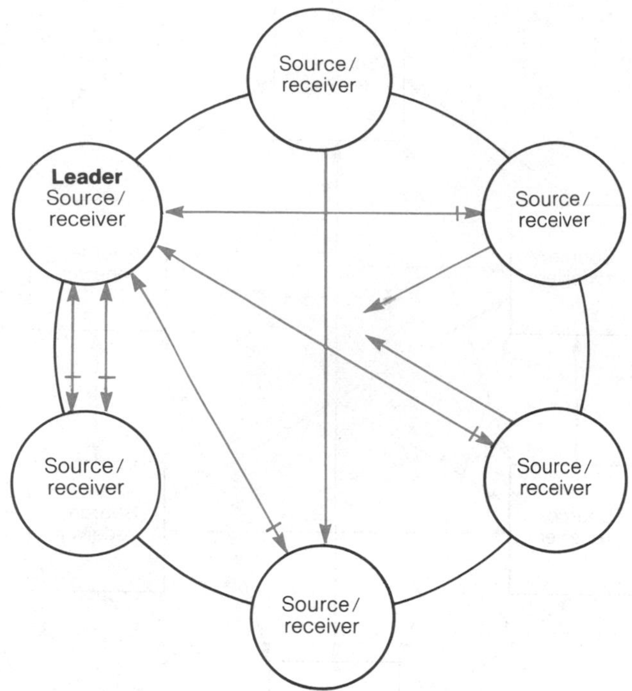

Figure 28–2 A sociogram indicating the flow of verbal communication within a group during a specific period. Note that five questions or comments calling for a response were directed at the leader.

2. Members receive support from the group and praise one another for accomplishments.
3. Members have similar attitudes and beliefs.
4. Members are loyal to the group and defend it against outside criticism.
5. Members readily accept assigned roles and tasks.
6. Members influence each other and value being influenced by others.
7. Members feel satisfied and secure.
8. Members stay in the group and value group goals.

Group properties

1. Group goals are valued and are consistent with the goals of individuals.
2. Group activities are handled by group action.
3. Group actions are interdependent and cooperative.
4. Group goals that are difficult to achieve are met by persistent efforts.
5. Participation is high.
6. Commitment is high.
7. Communication is high.
8. "We" is frequently heard in discussions.
9. Group productivity is high.
10. Group norms are adhered to and protected.

Power

Patterns of behavior in groups are greatly influenced by the force of power. **Power** can be defined as the ability to influence another person in some way or the ability to do something, whether it is to decide the fate of a nation or to decide that a certain change in policy or practice is necessary. Claus and Bailey (1977, p. 17) define power in terms of three interrelated elements: *ability* (based on strength of the person), *willingness* (based on positive energy), and *results,* such as affecting the behavior of others (produced by action). The relationship of the three is pyramidal: *strength* (the basis of ability) supports *energy* (the basis of willingness to use the ability), which in turn supports *action* (the basis of results). See Figure 28–3.

Many people have a negative concept of power, likening it to control, domination, and even coercion of others by muscle and clout. However, power can be viewed as a vital, positive force that moves people toward the attainment of individual or group goals. The overall purpose of power is to encourage cooperation and collaboration in accomplishing a task.

Power versus Influence and Authority

Often the terms *power, influence,* and *authority* are used interchangeably, but they need to be differentiated. **Power** is the source of influence, whereas **influence** is the result of proper use of power. **Authority** is the official or legitimized right to use a given amount or type of power, i.e., the right to act and the right to command (Claus and

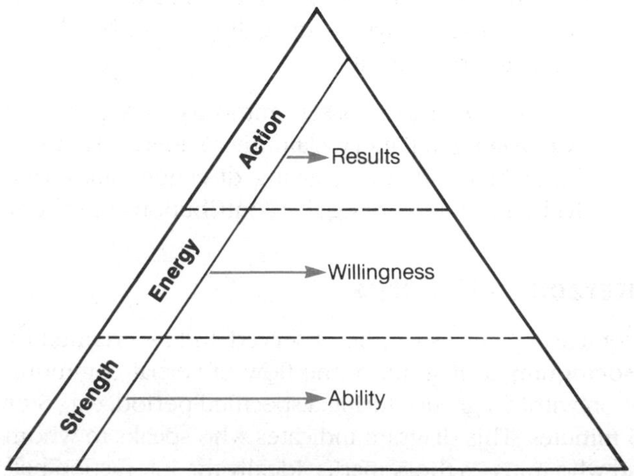

Figure 28–3 The tripartite and pyramidal nature of power according to Claus and Bailey (1977)

Table 28–3 Stages of Power Orientation and Development

Stage	Object of Power	Source of Power	Characteristics
1	Self: to feel stronger	External phenomena (God, mother, leader) strengthen self	Desire to talk, to share, and to nurture
2	Self: to strengthen, control, direct self	Self; internal phenomena (autonomy, will power) strengthen self	Desire for knowledge of how to control things better; emphasis on outward control of expressions of anger; attempts to be independent
3	Others: to influence others	Self; internal phenomena (assertiveness, desire to experience power) strengthen self	Concern with prestige and possessions; having a goal of power rather than achievement
4	Others: to serve or influence others	External phenomena (religion, law, group values) strengthen self	View of power-related actions in terms of duty or responsibility to a higher authority; development of loyalty

From D. C. McClelland, *Power: The inner experience* (New York: Irvington Publishers, 1975). Used by permission.

Bailey 1977, p. 21). Authority may be either delegated or acquired.

Stages of Power Orientation and Development

Four stages of power orientation and development are categorized by McClelland (1975, p. 14). See Table 28–3.

For information on the kinds of power, see Chapter 6, pages 139–42.

Dimensions and Levels of Power

Rollo May (1972, p. 99) defines power as the ability to cause or prevent change and asserts that it has two dimensions: *potentiality* (latent power) and *actuality.* Latent power is power that has not yet developed fully but has the ability to cause a change at some future time.

Five levels of power are categorized by May (1972, p. 99):

1. The power to be
2. Self-affirmation
3. Self-assertion
4. Aggression
5. Violence

When lower levels of power are ineffective for attaining goals or needs, a person feels powerless and moves to a higher, more destructive level of power, such as aggression and violence.

Common Group Problems

Conflict

Conflict, a normal stage of the life of most groups, refers to disagreement, impatience, and argument among members. It can be either productive or nonproductive, and group leaders need to distinguish destructive conflict from constructive conflict by making observations and interpretations (diagnoses).

Productive Conflict

Conflict is productive and beneficial when members feel involved, when the issue being discussed is important to them, and when they are working intensively on a problem. Productive conflict contributes to problem solving as long as the goal is clearly understood. Observations that indicate a conflict is productive, according to Sampson and Marthas (1977, p. 269), include:

1. Members have an agreed-upon goal in mind and are working toward it.
2. Members make comments that are relevant to the task.
3. Members encourage all to participate, even those with different points of view.
4. Members listen to and hear others even though they may be impatient with one another and disagree with the suggestions made.
5. The bases for disagreements are examined and evaluated openly and critically.

6. Problems are solved by rational discussion and compromise and do not tend to recur.

Nonproductive Conflict

Conflict that is nonproductive leads the group astray and hinders the achievement of group goals. Three common reasons (or diagnoses) for this type of conflict, identified by Bradford, Stock, and Horwitz (1974, p. 38), are:

1. The group has been given an impossible task or the task is not clear, and members are frustrated because they feel unable to meet the demands on them.
2. The main concern of members is to find status in the group and to deal with their personal and individual tasks rather than the group problem.
3. Members are operating from unique, unshared points of view and may have competing loyalties to and conflicting interests in outside groups.

Each of these diagnoses for nonproductive conflict has typical signs. See Table 28–4.

Interventions

Conflict-handling interventions depend on both the who and the what of the conflict, the group climate, and whether the conflict is perceived as productive or nonproductive. Interventions that occur within a climate of group cohesion and trust are most effective. Where such a climate does not exist, the leader first needs to facilitate its development. Early diagnosis of conflict and early intervention are also essential. Early intervention can thwart an escalating cycle of nonproductive conflict and form a basis for using constructive conflict effectively in the future.

1. *Productive conflict resolution.* According to Sampson and Marthas (1977, p. 272), the group leader has three tasks in resolving productive conflict:
   a. *Supporting and legitimizing disagreement and conflict.* Supporting disagreement helps members realize that they can disagree without losing their integrity and that the disagreement can be useful for problem solving. The leader may say, for example, "I think there are disagreements being expressed on this problem, and I consider it a sign of a healthy group."
   b. *Clarifying the basis and the meaning of the conflict.* In this step the leader assists members to focus on the basis of their disagreement. For example, the leader may say, "I realize the two of you are disagreeing, but I'm not exactly sure what the disagreement is about. Could each of you take a minute to say what your position is?" Once the basis of the conflict is identified, all members are encouraged to discuss it further.
   c. *Negotiating a compromise.* After the basis of the conflict is identified, the group leader and members are ready to examine acceptable solutions. It is helpful to focus first on the commonalities members share rather than emphasizing ways in which they differ. A compromise is then developed for the opposing perspectives. For example, if two members feel that they are both overloaded and unable to give anyone more time, a compromise may be reached in which one person is given some assistance for the overload, thus freeing that person to provide assistance to the other.
2. *Nonproductive conflict resolution.* Resolving nonproductive conflicts is more complex. In some instances, the conflict needs to be avoided or played down rather

Table 28–4 Diagnoses and Indications of Nonproductive Group Conflict

Diagnosis	Indications
The group has been given an impossible task.	Every suggestion made seems impossible. Some members feel the group is too small. Members think the group does not have the knowledge or experience to get anywhere. Members feel pushed for time. Members are impatient with one another. Members have different ideas about what the group is supposed to do.
The main concern of members is in finding status in the group.	Members take sides and refuse to compromise. Ideas are attacked before they are completely expressed. There are subtle attacks on leadership and personal attacks on members. There is much clique formation. There is no concern about finding a goal or sticking to a point.
Members operate from unshared points of view and may have competing loyalties to outside groups.	Members take sides and refuse to compromise on general terms. Members do not listen to one another. The group goal is stated in very general terms. Each member pushes his or her own plan. Members disagree on suggestions and do not build on previous suggestions.

From L. P. Bradford, *Group Development* (La Jolla, Calif.: University Associates, 1974), pp. 38–40. Used by permission.

than confronted. This is a matter of careful judgment on the part of the group leader. Strategies that can be employed if the leader decides it is more beneficial for the group to face the issue directly (Sampson and Marthas 1977, p. 271) include:

a. *Interpreting.* The leader explains her or his view of the problem. For example, the leader might say, "I think the group is having trouble making a decision because there are some distinct conflicts among several members. Before we try to accomplish any other task I think we had better take some time and look at those conflicts."
b. *Reflecting.* With this strategy, the leader points out certain behaviors of the members or points out his or her own feelings. To *reflect behavior* the leader may say, "I've noticed that several persons have been very quiet for some time, that others are talking a great deal but usually at cross-purposes, and that as a group we seem unable to focus our efforts on any thing except diagreeing." To *reflect feeling* the leader may say, "I'm not sure how anyone else feels, but I'm feeling frustrated and annoyed over the constant bickering. I know we have a job to do, and I'd like to get on with it."
c. *Confronting.* With this strategy, the leader calls the group's attention to what she or he perceives is taking place with one or more members. For example, the leader may say, "Mrs. Purple, I think you are angry because . . . , and you seem to feel . . . . Is that why you are so distressed?" or "I think that Mr. Black and Ms. White are each trying to gain some points in this discussion, but this is not helping us deal with the task at hand. I wonder if you two could either cool it for a while or let us all explore your behavior with you?"

Inadequate Decision Making

Inefficient decision making generally arises if (a) the decision is threatening to the group because of unclear consequences, fear of reactions of other groups, or fear of failure by the members, or (b) the decision is too difficult or has been requested prematurely and the group lacks faith in itself. According to Bradford, Stock, and Horwitz (1974, p. 44), indications that group decision making is inadequate include:

1. There is continued effort to leave the decision making to others, i.e., the leader, a subgroup, or an outside source.
2. Group members refuse responsibility.
3. A decision is challenged after it is made.
4. The group is divided and unclear about what the decision is.
5. The group almost makes decisions but retreats at the last minute.
6. Members frequently ask for definition and redefinition of minute points.
7. Members vacillate between making decisions too rapidly and not deciding anything.
8. Group discussion wanders, often into abstraction.

Apathy

Apathy (nonparticipation or silence) varies from complete indifference to the group task and signs of boredom to lack of genuine enthusiasm, inability to mobilize much energy, lack of persistence, and being satisfied with poor work. Apathy can affect either an individual or the group as a whole. An apathetic group may be the result of an autocratic leadership style or several other factors, discussed in the next session.

Indications of apathy, familiar to most people, include:

1. Members arrive late and are frequently absent.
2. The participation level is low; conversation drags.
3. Members yawn, doze, slouch, and are restless.
4. The concentration level is low, and often the point of the discussion is lost.
5. Decisions are made too quickly, and there is failure to follow through on decisions.
6. Members are reluctant to assume additional responsibility.
7. Suggestions for adjournment are abundant, and arrangements for the next meeting are neglected.

Causes

Some common causes of apathy identified by Bradford, Stock, and Horwitz (1974, p. 44) are:

1. *The task facing the group does not seem important to members,* even though it is important to someone, e.g., the group leader or the larger organization of which the group is a part. In this situation, members may raise questions about what their job really is, what "they" (others) want the group to do, and what the reason for doing the task is. Suggestions may be made that the group work on something else.
2. *The group has inadequate problem-solving procedures or capabilities.* This situation is revealed when:
   a. No one can suggest the first step in getting started on the task.
   b. Members are unable to stay on a given point.
   c. The same points are made over and over.

d. Little attention is given to fact-finding or use of special resources.
e. Minimal consideration is given to evaluating the possible consequences of decisions reached.
f. Private discussions are held in subgroups.
g. Members feel their abilities are inadequate to carry out the task.

3. *Members feel powerless about influencing final decisions.* This situation is indicated when:
   a. Members express the view that someone with more authority and power should be at the meeting.
   b. Members feel that decisions arrived at will be "meaningless," group efforts will just be wasted, and someone outside the group will not really listen to the ideas of the group.
   c. Members try to get the group leader to understand and listen rather than try to reach a consensus decision by the group.
   d. Members feel that the management of the organization is pretending to be democratic by asking for their participation.
   e. Discussions arise about power structures either inside the group (i.e., the leader or a subgroup) or outside the group.
4. *A conflict among a few members dominates the group.* In this situation a few members control the conversation but never agree, and they appeal to others for support, while the less dominant members withdraw from participation and become apathetic.

Interventions

Nonparticipation or apathy of one or a few members is sometimes best handled by nonintervention. Sometimes such silences are not a reflection of something in the immediate group setting but rather of some past traumatic experience in the person's life. For example, after expressing an idea previously, this person may have been told, "That was a stupid thing to say," or "You should know better than that." Having been hurt once in a group, such persons feel insecure about their views and are reluctant to express themselves again in groups.

Continued nonparticipation or apathy, however, needs to be dealt with by the leader, after a careful assessment of whether the apathy is a reflection of leadership style, task issues, or interpersonal conflicts. Sampson and Marthas (1977, p. 259) offer the following suggestions for dealing with apathy:

1. For apathy reflecting the members' opinion that the task is unimportant, the leader may suggest, "I think there is general boredom with today's task. Do people feel that what we are doing is not really relevant or important?" After members have responded, the leader needs to ask, "What things would you prefer the group to do?"
2. For apathy due to members' feelings of inadequacy about handling the task or lack of the structure and organization needed for problem solving, the leader may ask, "Are people feeling generally that the group is not up to handling the task we are facing?" or "I think, because we're not really sure of what to do or how to go about dealing with the task facing us, that it may be helpful if we break up the task into smaller parts, decide what the important issues are, and develop a method for dealing with each part."
3. For apathy based on an interpersonal issue such as anger or fear and expressed by silence, the leader needs to decide whether to let the silence simply pass or to intervene. If generally responsive group members suddenly become silent, it is important to note which issue or topic immediately preceded the silence. Sometimes a conflict among a few members has been uncovered or the group has been pushed into discussing a topic considered irrelevant or threatening. In this situation the leader may say, "I am wondering whether people are angry at what I've done," or "Are some of you anxious about bringing up that topic, since it may bring out bad feelings?"
4. For apathy due to an autocratic leadership style, the leader must implement measures to change the style and assist the group to work through and change their relationship with him or her.

Monopolizing Member

Because most group meetings have time restraints, domination of the discussion by one member seriously deprives others of their chances to participate. A sense of injustice develops, and ultimately the frustration and anger of members may be directed toward the group leader, who in the members' opinion should be doing something to stop that person's behavior.

Indications

Signs of monopolization include:

1. Compulsive, incessant talking
2. Interruption of others who start to talk
3. Tendency to complete others' sentences
4. Inability to listen
5. Inability to keep still
6. Apparent belief that the act of talking is more important than what is said

7. Responses of restlessness, inattentiveness, and anger deflected to the leader by other members

There may be several reasons for monopolizing behavior (e.g., anxiety or a need for attention, recognition, and approval). Whatever the reason, the goal of the leader is to assist the person to moderate his or her participation in the group. Often, compulsive talkers are unaware of their behavior and its effect on others and need help to look at what they are doing and the consequences.

Interventions

The following intervention strategies for groups in general are suggested by Sampson and Marthas (1977, p. 254):

1. *Interrupt simply, directly, and supportively.* This strategy is an initial attempt to get the person to hear others. The leader may say, "Thank you very much, David; I don't like to cut you off right now, since that is an interesting and valuable idea, but I feel it is important for us to hear from everyone about this issue. Perhaps after the others have had a chance to convey their thoughts, we can return to you."
2. *Reflect the person's behavior.* This strategy is an attempt to help the person become aware of the monopolizing behavior. The leader may say, "Lisa, we are really having difficulty hearing from everyone today because you are using up considerable time talking. I wonder if you are aware of this?"
3. *Reflect the group's feelings.* This strategy is an attempt to help the person become aware of the effects of his or her behavior on others. The leader may say, "Todd, I've noticed that you have been talking so much today that few others have been able to participate. I've also realized that I am getting frustrated and bored, I haven't kept up with what you are saying, and I finally stopped listening. I really do want to hear what you have to say, as well as what others have to say, and I wonder if other people are having the same trouble?"
4. *Confront the person and/or the group.* This strategy can be directed toward the individual, or toward the group to help members realize their own responsibility for the problem. To confront the individual, the leader may say, "Mary, could you please be quiet for a few minutes and let other people have the floor?" To confront the group, the leader may say, "I've noticed that Mary is talking so much that none of you others have had a chance to participate. I am wondering why all of you have allowed Mary to dominate this discussion and whether you want to take more responsibility for working in this group?"

Group Self-Evaluation

Groups need to set up mechanisms for feedback of information to the members about their method of operation. Only when a group acquires information about itself can it make adjustments to improve its efficiency. Several mechanisms can be set up for group feedback and self-evaluation: use of a group-productivity observer, use of a group self-evaluation guide, general open discussion initiated by the group leader prior to the end of the meeting, or combinations of these.

Some groups establish a rotating position for a group-productivity observer, just as positions are established for a recorder; others acquire the assistance of an outsider specially trained in this area. The responsibility of this person is to observe the group during its discussions, rather than participate, and to provide feedback to the group about perceptions of the group's behavior. The observer notes the general atmosphere of the group, leadership techniques, orientation of the group, participation by members, and any factor considered to affect the productivity of the group. See Table 28–5 for a sample group self-evaluation guide that can be used by the observer.

The provision of feedback requires skill by the observer in presenting comments. It is helpful to present objective data first and then phrase comments in the form of tentative hypotheses, alternative solutions, or expressions of the observer's feelings. This allows group members the chance to reject a comment if they are not ready to handle it. The observer can be viewed as "in error." For example, the observer of the group meeting evaluated in Table 28–5 might comment (Jenkins 1974, p. 82):

> *Objective data:* During the time we were trying to suggest solutions to problems, two of us seemed impatient to tear a new idea apart. Out of five suggestions made, four were immediately criticized. Right after that, suggestions for solutions lagged.
>
> *Alternative solution:* I was wondering at the time whether more and better ideas might have emerged if we had withheld our critical comments until after most of the ideas about solutions were on the blackboard.

Open discussion needs to follow such comments.

Table 28–5 Example of Group Self-Evaluation Guide

Criteria	Comments
A. Group direction and orientation	
1. How much was achieved?	1. Only one-third of agenda covered. Too much time spent on irrelevant material
2. How clear are goals and purposes?	2. A few members not clear about purposes.
3. How clear is procedure to achieve goals?	3. No discussion about how to try to achieve task.
4. Was sufficient relevant information available?	4. Yes
B. Group motivation and unity	
5. What degree of interest is there in task?	5. A few do not think problem is important.
6. Was interest maintained throughout?	6. Interest lagged when one member made lengthy lecture.
7. Is group united in purpose?	7. Feelings of unity not evident in two members.
C. Group atmosphere	
8. Formal?	
9. Informal?	9. Yes
10. Permissive?	10. Yes
11. Inhibited?	
12. Cooperative?	12. Yes
13. Competitive?	
14. Friendly?	14. Yes
15. Hostile?	
D. Member contributions	
16. What is degree of participation by members?	16. All participated. Some monopolization by one member.
17. Were contributions relevant, factual, and problem-centered?	17. Most were.
18. Were members listening to what others said?	18. A few were not, at point of high interest in discussion.
19. How did special members serve group?	
a. Leader	19. a. Facilitated discussion. Could have handled dominating member better. Let group wander too much.
b. Recorder	b. Asked for clarification of some points. Assisted group to focus on issue.
c. Resource person	c. Provided essential clarifying information.
d. Others	d. Two members criticized four out of five ideas while they were being suggested. After that, fewer suggestions were offered.
20. How did majority of members feel about meeting?	
a. Poor	
b. Mediocre	20b. Yes
c. Okay	
d. Good	
e. Excellent	

Adapted from David H. Jenkins, "Feedback and group self-evaluation" from the *Journal of Social Issues*, Vol IV, No. 2, pp. 50–60. Reprinted by permission of The Society for the Psychological Study of Social Issues, Ann Arbor, MI.

Self-Help Groups

A **self-help group,** also called a self-care or self-health group, is a group of laypersons who act on their own behalf to deal with health matters. Jerston (1975, p. 144) defined self-help groups as "small groups of people with common problems who work together to achieve specific behavioral, attitudinal, or cognitive goals." These groups often address specific problems, such as drug addiction or spinal cord injury. Self-help groups may deal with an ongoing problem, e.g., the members all have a colostomy, or they may aim to prevent problems, e.g., child abuse.

Self-help groups have existed for many years. Some researchers trace the origins to the time of the British industrial revolution and the friendly societies and unions (Katz and Bender 1976, p. 265). In recent times they have grown enormously. Katz estimated that more than one million people in the United States are involved in self-help groups (Katz 1970, p. 58).

Characteristics

According to Katz (1970, p. 58), self-help groups have eight characteristics:

1. They are similar to small autonomous groups and form along the lines of friendship networks.

2. They are problem-centered and organized with reference to a specific problem or problems.
3. Members of the group tend to be peers. The role of a "professional" is unclear in a self-help group. Many groups prohibit membership of a professional. Others allow professionals as members, but the professional is seen as a peer rather than as an authority figure.
4. The members of the group have common goals and the group's goals are formed by the group.
5. The action of the group is group action. According to Corbin (1983, p. 12), "this is one of the main reasons for joining a group rather than 'going it alone.' "
6. A norm of the group is helping others. Riessman (1976, p. 42) lists three reasons why people who help others obtain special benefits:
   a. The helper is less dependent.
   b. In struggling with another's problems that are like his/her own, the helper has an opportunity to view his/her problem from a distance.
   c. The helper attains a feeling of social usefulness.
7. Power and leadership are on a peer basis. Leaders evolve from the group over a period of time.

Program

The program of a self-help group has several aspects: First, the members should gain confidence in their abilities to handle their problems. Second, a member's failure to deal with a problem should afford an opportunity for that person to learn how to deal with the failure. Third, peers in self-help groups need to balance support with critical feedback. Peers in a self-help group are generally judgmental, critical, active, and supportive, whereas a therapist in an orthodox psychotherapy group is usually noncritical, nonjudgmental, and neutral. Fourth, peers in a self-help group serve as role models; therefore they act as reminders to the other members that "it can be done." Fifth, a self-help group helps the members assume a "wellness role" rather than a "sickness role" in which one is dependent and helpless. Finally, the emphasis in these groups is on self-control or will power. The locus of control is within, not external to, the member.

Nursing Implications

Nurses have two major functions in relation to self-help groups. First, nurses can inform clients and their support persons about community resources that are available to assist them. Some self-help groups are organized nationally, for instance, Alcoholics Anonymous (alcoholism), Weight Watchers (obesity), and United Ostomy Association (any ostomy). Community service organizations and social work agencies can usually provide the names of local self-help groups. Second, the nurse can be a participating member of a self-help group when this is appropriate. For example, a nurse in a nursing home might participate in a self-help group of elderly clients, or a nurse could be a member of a self-help group in the larger community.

Chapter Highlights

- Groups can be classified as primary or secondary, according to their structure or according to their type of interaction.
- In small, primary groups, relationships are spontaneous, personal, and sentimental. In larger, secondary groups, relationships are impersonal and less sentimental.
- Groups develop in three stages: initiation stage, functional stage, and dissolution stage.
- Effective groups produce outstanding results, succeed in spite of difficulties, and have members who feel responsible for the output of the group.
- Group self-evaluation is essential to improving the efficiency of a group.
- Self-help groups are groups of laypeople who act on their own behalf to deal with health matters.
- Self-help groups are problem-centered, and members of such groups tend to be peers.
- Self-help groups assist members to assume a "wellness" role.

Suggested Readings

Huber, K., and Miller, P. March/April 1984. Reminiscence with the elderly—Do it. *Geriatric Nursing* 5:84–87.
The authors describe their study of a group of elderly people in a long-term-care facility involving clients who require total assistance. The goals for the group and the leader's goals are described. The group's meetings led to a number of changes, including some clients becoming more interested in others, and a decrease in one client's depression.

Kron, T. October 1976. How to become a better leader. *Nursing 76* 6:67–68 (Canadian ed. 6:6–7).
Tips on how to improve leadership ability are provided. Techniques, qualities, and rules for leadership are included.

Larson, M. L., and Williams, R. A. August 1978. How to become a better group leader? Learn to recognize the strange things that happen to some people in groups. *Nursing 78* 8:65–72 (Canadian ed. 8:12–15).
These authors outline several nonfunctional or problem behaviors of group members: deserter, nontalker, interrogator, smoke-screener, rescuer, scapegoat, seducer, and angry

aggressor. Effective ways for the group leader to deal with them are outlined.

McConnell, E. A. October 1978. What kind of delegator are you? *Nursing 78* 8:105–6 (Canadian ed. 8:12–14).
Five ineffective delegators and four nondelegators are described.

Small, L. L. July 1980. Finding your leadership style in groups. *American Journal of Nursing* 80:1301–3.
This author analyzes and critiques her experiences as a group leader.

Selected References

Alberti, R. E., and Emmons, M. L. 1974. *Your perfect right.* 2d ed. San Luis Obispo, Calif.: Impact Publishing Co.

Benne, K. D., and Sheats, P. 1974. Functional roles of group members. In Bradford, L. P., editor. *Group development.* La Jolla, Calif.: University Associates.

Bradford, L. P., editor. 1974. *Group development.* La Jolla, Calif.: University Associates.

Bradford, L. P.; Stock, D.; and Horwitz, M. 1974. How to diagnose group problems. In Bradford, L. P., editor. *Group development.* La Jolla, Calif.: University Associates.

Browne, S. E. March 1980. Group leadership experiences for students. *Nursing Outlook* 28:166–69.

Claus, K. E., and Bailey, J. T. 1977. *Power and influence in health care: A new approach to leadership.* St. Louis: C. V. Mosby Co.

Cohen, R. G., and Lipkin, G. B. 1979. *Therapeutic group work for health professionals.* New York: Springer Publishing Co.

Corbin, D. E. May/June 1983. Self-help groups: What the health educator should know. *Health Values* 7:10–14.

Donnelly, G. F.; Mengel, A.; and Sutterley, D. C. 1980. *The nursing system: Issues, ethics, and politics.* New York: John Wiley and Sons.

Fisher, D. W. January 1985. Guidelines to effective group functioning. *Point View* 22:6–8.

Francis, D., and Young, D. 1979. *Improving work groups: A practical manual for team building.* San Diego, Calif.: University Associates.

Hamm, S. R. December 1980. The influence of formal and informal organization within a modern hospital. *Supervisor Nurse* 11:38–40.

Hill, K. 1983. Helping you helps me. *A guide book for self-help groups.* Ottawa: Canada Council on Social Development Pub. No. ISBN: 0-88810-336-0.

Jenkins, David H. 1974. Feedback and group self-evaluation. In Bradford, L. P., editor. *Group development.* La Jolla, Calif.: University Associates.

Jerston, J. M. February 1975. Self-help groups. *Social Work* 20:144–45.

Katz, A. H. January 1970. Self-help organizations and volunteer participation in social welfare. *Social Work* 15:57–60.

Katz, A. H., and Bender, E. I. March 1976. Self-help groups in Western society: History and prospects. *Journal of Behavioral Science* 12:265–82.

McClelland, D. C. 1975. *Power: The inner experience.* New York: Irvington Publishers.

Marley, M. S. May 1980. The making of a group. *Journal of Gerontological Nursing* 6:275–79.

May, Rollo. 1972. *Power and innocence: A search for the sources of violence.* New York: W. W. Norton and Co.

Moniz, D. October 1978. Putting assertiveness techniques into practice. *American Journal of Nursing* 78:1713.

Reeves, Elton T. 1970. *The dynamics of group behavior.* New York: American Management Association.

Riessman, F. 1976. How does self-help work? *Social Policy* 7:41–45.

Sampson, E. E., and Marthas, M. S. 1977. *Group process for the health professions.* New York: John Wiley and Sons.

Shotman, L. 1984. *The skills of helping individuals and groups.* 2d ed. Itasca, Ill.: F. E. Peacock Publishers.

Wilson, H. S., and Kneisl, C. R. 1979. *Psychiatric nursing.* Menlo Park, Calif.: Addison-Wesley Publishing Co.

Wilson, H. S., and Kneisl, C. R. 1982. *Psychiatric nursing.* 2d ed. Menlo Park, Calif.: Addison-Wesley Publishing Co.

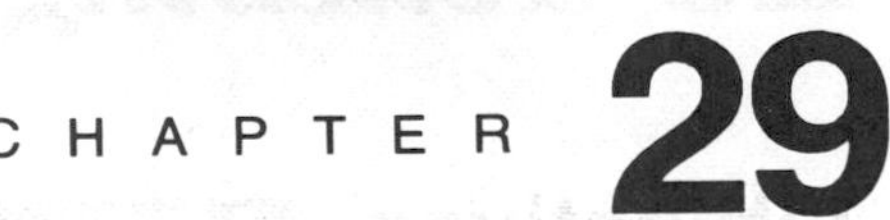

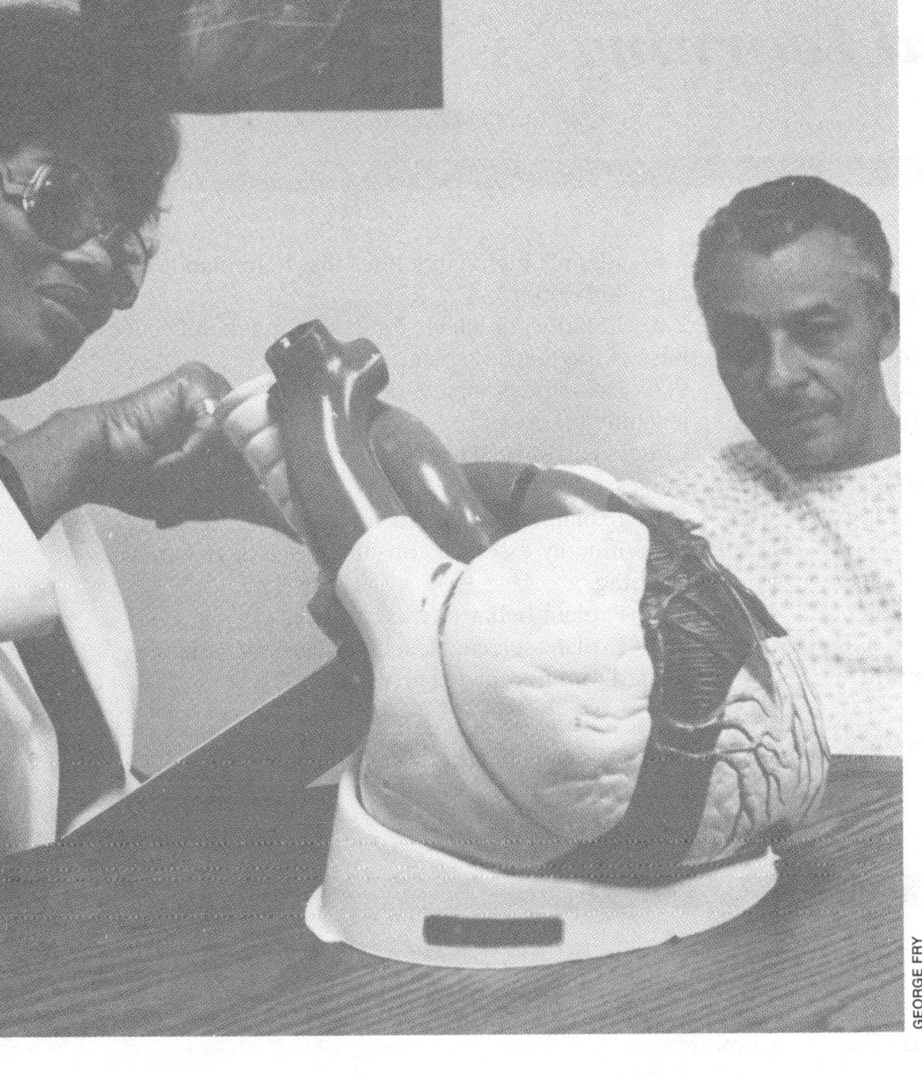

CHAPTER **29**

Teaching and Learning

Contents

29 *Teaching and Learning*

Objectives

1. Know essential facts about learning and teaching.
   1.1 Define terms commonly used in the learning and teaching context.
   1.2 Describe Bloom's three domains of nursing.
   1.3 Describe the factors that facilitate learning.
   1.4 Describe the factors that inhibit learning.
   1.5 Outline five principles of teaching.
2. Understand essential factors about the nursing process as it is applied to the learning/teaching process.
   2.1 Identify the sources of the client's learning needs.
   2.2 Explain relevant client data.
   2.3 Explain the essential aspects of planning teaching.
   2.4 Identify four guidelines for ordering the learning experiences.
   2.5 Identify eight guidelines that help plan teaching intervention.
   2.6 Identify guidelines for evaluating the effectiveness of the teaching plan.
   2.7 Describe complete documentation of the teaching process.
3. Understand special teaching strategies required by nurses.
   3.1 Explain client contracting.
   3.2 Identify essential considerations of group teaching.
   3.3 Explain behavior modification.
   3.4 Explain selected teaching/learning variables related to different age groups.

Terms

adaptation
analysis
application
characterization
complex overt response
compliance
comprehension
evaluation
guided response
knowledge
learning
learning need
mechanism
modeling
motivation
organization
origination
perception
receiving
responding
set
synthesis
teaching
valuing

Client Education

Client education is a major aspect of nursing practice.

Client education is multifaceted. According to DeHaes (1982, pp. 95–96), it includes four broad areas:

1. Client education in primary care. This may relate to areas such as the physician–patient relationship, to medications, to client information, and to therapy compliance.
2. Client education in a hospital. This includes communication about examinations, surgery, responses to client questions, and information required by the client following discharge, e.g., care of an ostomy, use of oxygen at home.
3. Client education concerned with revalidation, e.g., how the client should live with residual defects, how the client can augment the healing process and increase self-acceptance and self-esteem, or how the client can cope with dying.
4. Client education about chronic illness, e.g., self-management and adaptation to changing health.

In 1972 the American Hospital Association passed the Patients' Bill of Rights mandating client education as a right of all clients. In addition, legislation relating to nursing frequently has included client teaching as a function of nursing, thereby making teaching a legal and professional responsibility. (Phillips and Heckelman 1983, pp. 42–46)

Client teaching is also related to promoting and protecting health. Nursing practice in this area involves teaching about reducing health risk factors and increasing a person's level of wellness, and employing specific protective health measures. See Chapter 20 for additional information.

Clients have a variety of learning needs. A **learning need** is a need to change behavior. **Learning** is a change in human disposition or capability that persists over a period of time and that cannot be solely accounted for by growth. Learning is represented by a change in behavior (Gagne 1977).

An important aspect of learning is the individual's desire to learn and to act on the learning. This is referred to as **compliance**. Compliance is best illustrated when the person recognizes and accepts the need to learn, willingly expends the energy required to learn, and then follows through with the appropriate behaviors that reflect the learning. For example, a male client diagnosed as having diabetes willingly learns about the special diet he needs and then plans and follows the learned diet. For additional information about compliance see Chapter 2, page 65.

Research Note

Woody et al. set out to determine if nurses were efficiently performing at least the first stage in facilitating client learning. They predicated that if clients learn what nurses say they have taught them, then the nurse's role as teacher is valid. Sixteen LPNs and 17 RNs participated in the study. No statistical difference was found between what the nurses taught and what the clients learned. The authors concluded that client teaching is a viable nursing role for all types of nurses. (Woody, et al. 1984.)

Domains of Learning

Bloom (1956) has identified three domains or areas of learning: cognitive, affective, and psychomotor. The *cognitive domain* includes intellectual skills such as thinking, knowing and understanding. The *affective domain* includes feelings, emotions, interests, attitudes, and appreciations. The *psychomotor domain* includes motor skills such as giving an injection. Nurses should include each of these three domains in client teaching plans. For example, when a nurse teaches a client how to irrigate a colostomy, this is the psychomotor domain. An important part of such a teaching plan is to teach the client why a specific amount of fluid is used and when the irrigation should be carried out; this is the cognitive domain. Helping the client accept the colostomy and maintain self-esteem is the affective domain.

Each of these domains has a developed hierarchical classification system; i.e., the behaviors in each category are arranged from the simplest to the most complex.

Cognitive Domain

Bloom established six categories in the cognitive domain, from the simplest, the acquisition of knowledge, to the most complex, evaluation (Bloom 1956, pp. 201–207).

1. **Knowledge**, the remembering of previously learned material, is the simplest and most basic level of the cognitive domain. It includes acquiring facts and being able to recall them. For example, a client learning to change a surgical dressing recalls that the incision is cleaned from the top toward the bottom and from the center toward the outside.
2. **Comprehension** is the ability to grasp the meaning of learned material. For example, a client explains, in his own words, how his wound should be cleaned.
3. **Application** is the ability to use newly learned material in new, concrete situations. For example, when one client explains to another client how to clean his surgical wound, he is applying the principles behind the cleaning technique.
4. **Analysis** involves breaking down information into its component parts and determining the relationship between the parts. For example, a client distinguishes between information that is relevant to cleaning his incision and information that is irrelevant.
5. **Synthesis** is the ability to put parts together to form a new whole. For example, a nurse adapts knowledge about the nursing process to the teaching process.
6. **Evaluation** involves the ability to judge the value of material for a given purpose. For example, a nurse and client evaluate how effectively the client goals have been met, relating the client behaviors to the stated goals. Nurses are expected to synthesize and evaluate; clients, however may not need to do this.

Affective Domain

The affective domain emphasizes feelings, emotions, or a degree of acceptance or rejection. This domain also relates to ethics and moral behavior (Krathwohl et al. 1964, p. 7).

1. **Receiving** is the willingness to give attention to certain stimuli, including being sensitive to another's words and listening attentively. For example, a client listens carefully to a nurse's explanation about presurgical preparation.
2. **Responding** is active participation, that is, not only listening (level 1) but also responding in some way. For example, the presurgical client questions the nurse about information the nurse has provided.
3. **Valuing** is the attaching of value or worth to some object or behavior, as expressed by the valuer's own behavior. For example, a person who values healthy teeth goes to a dentist regularly.
4. **Organization** is the bringing together of different values, resolving conflicts among them, and thus building a consistent value system. A client at this level of the affective domain would, for example, plan life relative to his or her abilities, interests, and beliefs; thus a man who has lost the ability to walk plans and adjusts his life relative to health.
5. **Characterization** means that the individuals' value system has controlled his or her behavior long enough that he or she has a consistent and predictable life-style that reflects the value system. The person at this highest level of the affective domain displays consistent behavior, and any learning outcomes should be consistent with his or her life-style.

Psychomotor Domain

There are a number of models that classify psychomotor behavior. The one used here (Simpson 1972) has seven levels.

1. **Perception**, the first level of the psychomotor domain, involves the use of the sense organs to obtain cues that guide motor activity. For example, a person tastes food and, recognizing the need for seasoning, reaches for the salt shaker.
2. **Set**, the readiness to take a particular action, includes mental set (mental readiness), physical set (physical readiness), and emotional set (emotional readiness or willingness) to act. That is, the individual perceives cues and then acts. For example, a client demonstrates correct body stance when given a set of crutches, or holds a cane correctly.
3. **Guided response** involves the early stages of learning a complex skill. For example, a client repeats an act demonstrated by the nurse. This category also includes trial and error; for example, the client tries several ways to fold a gauze dressing until a correct fold is obtained.
4. **Mechanism** refers to performing acts that have become habitual and can be carried out with some degree of proficiency. An example is a client who quickly and confidently sets up a colostomy irrigation set.
5. **Complex overt response** is the skillful performance of complex motor acts with movements that are quick, smooth, and accurate and that require minimal energy. For example, a client draws up and administers insulin by syringe. This level of psychomotor skill requires highly coordinated motor activities.
6. **Adaptation** involves skills that are so well developed they can be modified to fit special circumstances. For example, when a nurse inserts a urinary catheter into a female client whose hips and knees are fixed in an acutely flexed position, the nurse is adapting the catheterization procedure to the client's leg position.
7. **Origination** is creating new movement patterns to suit a particular situation or problem. This creative level of psychomotor skill is exemplified by the nurse who originates a new method for providing oral care to an unconscious client.

Principles of Learning

Learning involves the entire person, and it can affect the person's life-style, methods of handling problems, attitudes, and knowledge. To learn requires energy and the ability to concentrate. Teachers, to be effective, must understand those factors that facilitate learning and those that inhibit it.

Factors Facilitating Learning

Genuine motivation **Motivation** to learn is the desire to learn. Such motivation is generally greatest when a person recognizes a need and believes the need will be met through learning. It is not enough for the need to be identified and verbalized by the nurse; it must be experienced by the client. Often the nurse's task is to assist the client to personally work through the problem and identify the need. Sometimes clients or families need help identifying relevant situational elements before they can see a need. For instance, clients with heart disease may need to know the effects of smoking and being overweight before they recognize the need to stop smoking or adopt a weight-reduction diet. Or adolescents may need to know the consequences of an untreated sexually transmitted disease before they see the need for treatment.

Physical and emotional readiness *Readiness* involves two facets: emotional, or motivational, and experiential. *Emotional readiness* determines the person's willingness to put forth the effort needed to learn. *Experiential readiness* involves the person's background of experiences, skills, and attitudes, and his or her ability to learn (Redman 1984, p. 21).

Active involvement Active involvement in the learning process makes learning more meaningful. For example, if the learner actively participates in planning and discussion, learning is faster and retention is better. See Figure 29–1. Passive learning, such as listening to a lecture or watching a film, does not foster optimal learning.

Successful learning Once learners have succeeded in accomplishing a task or understanding a concept, they gain self-confidence in their ability to learn. This reduces their anxiety about failure and can motivate greater learning. Successful learners have increased confidence with which to accept failure.

Accepting, nonjudgmental environment People learn best when they believe they are accepted and will not be judged. The person who expects to be judged as a "poor" or "good" client will not learn as well as the person who feels no such threat.

Feedback *Feedback* is information relating a person's performance to a desired goal. It has to be meaningful to the learner. Feedback that accompanies practice of psychomotor skills helps the person to learn those skills. Support of desired behavior through praise, positively worded corrections, and suggestions of alternative methods are ways of providing positive feedback. Negative feedback such as ridicule, anger, or sarcasm can lead people to withdraw from learning. Such feedback, viewed as a type of punishment, may cause the client to avoid the teacher in order to avoid punishment.

Simple to complex Learning is facilitated by material that is logically organized and proceeds from the simple to the complex. Such organization enables the learner to comprehend new information, assimilate it with previous learning, and form new understandings. Of course, *simple* and *complex* are relative terms, depending on the level at which the person is learning—what is simple for one person may be complex for another.

Repetition. Repetition of key concepts and facts facilitates retention of newly learned material. Practice of psychomotor skills improves performance of those skills and facilitates their transfer to another setting.

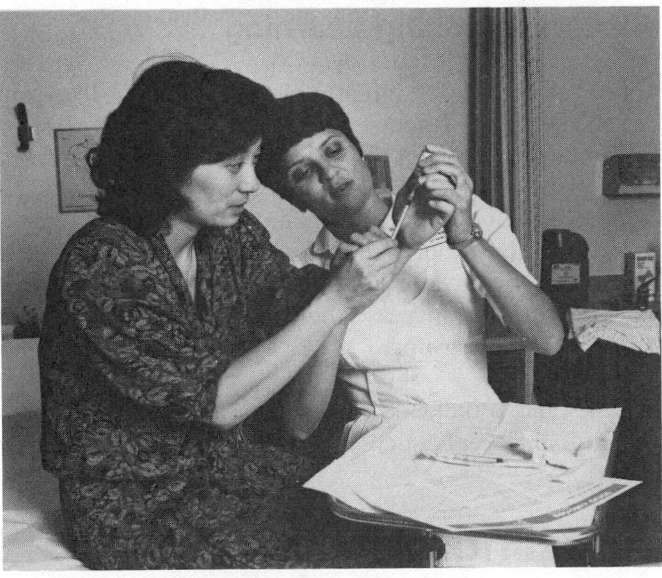

Figure 29–1 Learning is facilitated when the client is interested and actively involved.

Relevance When a person appreciates the relevance of specific material, then learning is facilitated. For example, the client who understands the relevance to his health of a special diet is better able to learn about the diet than a person who sees no such connection.

Using knowledge and skills People retain information and psychomotor skills best when the time between learning and use is short; the longer the time interval, the more that is forgotten. For example, a man may be taught how to administer his own intravenous insulin, but if he is not permitted to do so for several weeks after discharge from hospital, then it is unlikely that he will remember much of what he learned. However, if he is allowed to give his own injections while in hospital, then his learning will be enhanced.

Comfortable environment Environmental factors include heat, light, temperature, ventilation, noise, and supports such as chairs and tables. An optimal learning environment has adequate lighting that is free from glare, a comfortable room temperature, and good ventilation. Most students know what it is like to try to learn in a hot, stuffy room; the subsequent drowsiness interferes with concentration. Noise can also distract—loud voices, interruptions, and outside traffic can all interfere with listening and thinking. For the best learning in a hospital setting, nurses may choose a time when there are no visitors present and interruptions are unlikely. Privacy is essential for some learning. For example, when a client is learning to irrigate a colostomy, the presence of others can be embarrassing and thus interfere with learning.

Factors Inhibiting Learning

Extreme anxiety A greatly elevated anxiety level can impede learning. Clients or families who are very worried may not hear spoken words or may retain only part of the communication. Extreme anxiety might be reduced by medications or by information that relieves uncertainty. On the other hand, clients who appear disinterested and unconcerned may need to be told about potential problems, to increase their anxiety slightly and thus facilitate their learning.

Physiologic processes Learning can be inhibited by physiologic events such as a critical illness or pain or impaired hearing. Because of the client's inability to concentrate and apply energy to learning, the learning itself is impaired.

Cultural barriers There are also cultural barriers to learning, such as language or values. Obviously the client who does not understand the nurse's language will find learning seriously impaired. When client values differ from those of the health team, it can also impede learning. For example, a client who does not value being thin may have difficulty learning about a reducing diet.

Teaching

Teaching is a system of activities intended to produce learning. The teaching process is intentionally designed to produce specific learning. Teaching is considered one of the functions of nursing. In some states in the United States teaching is included in the legal definition of nursing, making it a required function under the law.

The teaching/learning process involves dynamic interaction between teacher and learner. Each participant in the process communicates information, emotions, perceptions, and attitudes to the other. The teaching process and the nursing process are very much alike. See Table 29–1.

Teaching also involves a type of communication for which there are specific goals. For example, clients who need to administer their own eye drops or to change an incision dressing share these goals with the nurse. Another aspect of teaching is the relationship between the teacher and the learner. It is essentially one of trust and respect. The learner trusts that the teacher has the knowledge and skill to teach, and the teacher respects the learner's ability to attain the recognized goals. Once a nurse starts to instruct a client and/or support persons, it is important that the teaching process continue until the participants reach the goals, change the goals, or decide that the goals will not help meet the learning objectives.

Principles of Teaching

The following principles may be helpful to nursing students:

1. Teaching activities should help the learner meet individual learning objectives. If certain activities do not assist the learner, these need to be reassessed; perhaps other activities can replace them. For example, explanation alone may not be able to teach a client to handle a syringe. Actually handling the syringe may be more effective.
2. Rapport between teacher and learner is essential. A relationship that is both accepting and constructive will best assist learning.
3. The teacher who can use the client's previous learnings in the present situation encourages the client and facilitates the learning of new skills. For example, a person who already knows how to cook can use this knowledge when learning about a special diet.
4. A teacher must be able to communicate clearly and concisely. The words the teacher uses need to have the same meaning to the learner as to the teacher. For example, a client who is taught not to put water on an area of the skin may think a wet washcloth is permissible for washing the area. In effect, the nurse needs to explain that no water or moisture should touch the area.

Table 29–1 Comparison of the Teaching Process and the Nursing Process

Step	Teaching Process	Nursing Process
1	Collect data; analyze client's learning strengths and deficits.	Collect data; analyze client's strengths and deficits.
2	Make educational diagnoses.	Make nursing diagnoses.
3	Prepare teaching plan.	Plan nursing intervention.
4	Implement teaching plan.	Implement nursing strategies.
5	Evaluate client learning (effectiveness of teaching plan)	Evaluate effectiveness of nursing interventions.

5. The teaching activities need to be oriented around the learning objectives. Thus information and skills not related to the learner's objectives need to be eliminated from the teaching process. If they remain, they may confuse the learner or be a distraction from effective learning.

Assessment

Assessing for teaching essentially has two foci: the identification of the client's learning needs and the assessment of relevant data about the client.

Identifying Client Learning Needs

Smitherman (1981, pp. 125–28) describes three sources for identifying learning needs.

1. *The client.* The client's learning needs may be identified by the client him- or herself. A client aware of a learning need may ask pertinent questions or seek out the needed information in some other way.
2. *The client's behavior.* Learning needs are not always easily detected; frequently, consultation with the client is necessary to confirm or deny the existence of these needs. For example, a client who appears angry may be insecure or worried because he does not understand what is happening, and only after discussion with the client can the nurse be sure that he has a need for information.
3. *Health care professionals.* Anticipatory learning needs related to the client's health problem often are known by health professionals. For example, a client anticipating surgery will probably need to learn about deep breathing and leg exercises. Or a client receiving oxygen who is being discharged from hospital will need to know how to operate the oxygen equipment and the appropriate safety measures to employ while at home.

Relevant Client Data

Particular client data that need to be collected and examined include client readiness, client motivation, and personal characteristics such as age and education.

Readiness

Clients who are ready to learn often behave differently from those who are not. A client who is ready may search out information, for instance, by asking questions, reading books or articles, talking to others, and generally showing interest. The person unready to learn is more likely to avoid the subject or situation and hope or believe that someone else will take care of the problem (Smitherman 1981, pp. 126–27). In addition, the unready client may change the subject when it is brought up by the nurse. For example, the nurse might say, "I was wondering about a good time to show you how to change your dressing," and the client responds, "What did you think of the ball game last night?" Or clients having surgery may have somatic symptoms (such as headaches, upset stomach, or gas pains) that make it difficult for them to pay attention (Laird 1975, p. 1340).

Tyson (1984) points out that in assessing readiness there are two major factors: emotional and experiential. Emotional factors affecting readiness include anxiety. If the anxiety level of the client is high, perceptions are narrowed and thus interfere with learning. Experiential factors include occupational status, client capabilities, and educational level.

Nurses can sometimes facilitate a client's readiness by tactfully calling attention to a learning need (for example, "Have you thought about learning to change your dressing?"). Two other ways to facilitate readiness are by giving the client information to read and by pointing out an opportunity to learn (for instance, "There is a baby bath demonstration at 3 P.M. today in the next room").

Motivation

As discussed earlier, motivation relates to whether the client wants to learn, and it is usually greatest when the client is ready, the learning need is recognized, and the content is meaningful to the client (Smitherman 1981, p. 127).

There are two types of motivation: internal and external. *Internal* motivation arises from within the individual. Sometimes clients may even be unaware of their motivation or unwilling to share it. For example, a client may be motivated to learn in order to gain the nurse's approval or in order to return to work. Why a person is motivated is often not clear, and it is unwise to assume a reason. *External* motivation comes from outside the client, such as praise from a support person.

Nurses can often determine whether a client's motivation is internal or external: An internally motivated person often takes the initiative in learning and usually does more than is required. Many externally motivated learners seek frequent feedback and may need to tell others about their learning. Both internal and external motivation are influenced by a person's physical and emotional needs. When clients are tired, worried, or in pain, for example, most of their energy is devoted to those problems and motivation is usually low.

Nurses can positively influence a client's internal motivation in three ways:

1. By relating the learning to something the client values and helping the client see the relevance of the learning
2. By helping the client to make the learning situation pleasant
3. By encouraging self-direction

To influence the externally motivated learner a nurse can use *positive reinforcement*, which involves rewarding the learner for achievements, e.g., giving praise, or reading a bedtime story to a child. Reinforcement is most effective when given immediately after the desired response. Negative reinforcement, or punishment for undesirable responses, is considered less motivating than positive reinforcement. However, negative reinforcement can be motivating if it is accompanied by encouragement and an explanation of how to correct the response (for instance: "I agree that looks right, but if you place the tube like this the urine should flow more readily").

Sociocultural Factors

Many ethnic/cultural groups have their own beliefs and practices, a number of them related to diet, health, illness, and life-style. It is therefore important to know whether any of the beliefs and values held by the client impinge on their learning needs. Although a nurse may be inclined to assume that because a client belongs to a specific racial or cultural group he or she will follow the norms of the group, this is not always the case. Thus, nurses should avoid stereotyping and should determine the relevant beliefs and values of each client. For example, although the diet of some Jews excludes pork, other Jews have no objection to eating pork.

Folk beliefs of certain groups in North America, e.g., low-income Hispanics, may also affect learning. Although the client may readily understand the health care information being taught, this learning may not be implemented in the home, where folk medical practices prevail. See Chapter 18 for additional information.

Age

Age provides information on the person's developmental status. Simple questions to school-age children and adolescents will elicit information on what they know. Observing children in play provides information about their motor and intellectual development as well as relationships with other children. For the elderly person, conversation and questioning may reveal slow recall or limited psychomotor skills and learning difficulties. For additional information, see "Specific Teaching Strategies" later in this chapter.

Health Beliefs and Practices

A client's health beliefs and practices are important to consider in any teaching plan. The health belief model described in Chapter 1, page 58, provides a predictor of preventive health behavior. However, even if a nurse is convinced that a client's health beliefs should be changed, this may not be possible because so many factors are involved in a person's health beliefs (Redman 1984, p. 27).

Intelligence

Clients' intelligence will probably influence their present knowledge as well as the teaching method that is most effective. Although some research indicates that education does not always affect learning (Nickerson 1972, p. 938), whether a client can read or write does affect the teaching style.

Nursing Diagnosis

Nursing diagnoses pertinent to a client's learning needs are all grouped under the heading "Knowledge deficit." Examples are shown below.

Examples of Nursing Diagnoses Related to Learning

- Knowledge deficit: low-calorie diet related to newly ordered therapy
- Knowledge deficit: diabetic diet related to prescribed treatment
- Knowledge deficit: preoperative care related to impending surgical procedure
- Knowledge deficit: medications related to language differences
- Knowledge deficit: home safety hazards related to denial of declining health
- Knowledge deficit: substance abuse related to lack of motivation to acquire information

Planning

The planning of teaching is accomplished in a series of steps. Involving the client at this time facilitates the formation of a meaningful teaching plan and stimulates client motivation.

Determining Teaching Priorities

Priorities must be established among the client's learning needs. The client and the nurse should do this together, with the client's priorities always being considered. Once a client's priorities have been dealt with, the client often is more motivated to concentrate on other identified learning needs. For example, a client who wants to know all about diabetes mellitus may not be ready to learn how to give himself injections until his own knowledge needs are met. Nurses can also use theoretical frameworks to establish priorities, such as Maslow's hierarchy of needs. See Chapter 16, page 312.

Developing Objectives

The terms *goals* and *objectives* are used interchangeably by some educators and distinguished by others. Used interchangeably, they can be considered as both immediate and long-term aims to be accomplished in a learning situation. However, *goal* is often the more general term, describing a general, long-range intended outcome of learning, whereas *objective* is used to mean a specific, immediate, short-range intended outcome of a learning situation.

The setting of goals and objectives is done by the client (or support persons) and the nurse. Objectives relate to immediate client needs, such as perineal care after birth of a baby. Goals relate to long-term needs, such as an obese new mother's need to lose weight (in which case the goal may be a specific weight loss through diet and exercise). The client (or family) and the nurse should set the learning objectives together because the learner who is actively involved in planning at this stage is more likely to follow through in meeting the objectives. In some instances, the client might be grateful to the nurse for doing most of the planning, for example, when the client is very weak but still needs to learn. If a client wants and needs to learn about medications yet has difficulty concentrating on the subject, it will often be helpful to have a written plan that can be discussed in several short sessions.

The objectives for learning should be both specific and observable in terms of behavior. A specific objective might be "to take 60 mg furosemide (Lasix) upon identifying ankle edema." An objective needs to be stated in terms of client behavior, not nurse behavior. For example, "Will write his own diets as instructed" (client behavior), not "To teach the client about his diet" (nurse behavior). Objectives should contain three types of information: performance, conditions, and criteria (Mager 1975, p. 21).

Performance

Performance, or behavior, describes what the learner will be able to do after mastering the objective. The objective must reflect an observable activity. The performance may be visible, e.g., walking, or invisible, e.g., adding a column of figures. However, it is necessary to be able to deduce whether an unobservable activity has been mastered from some performance that represents the activity. Therefore, the performance of an objective might be written: "Writes the total for a column of figures in the indicated space" (observable), not "Adds a column of figures" (unobservable).

Conditions

In some instances it is necessary to state the conditions under which a performance is to be carried out so that the objective is clear. For example, "Walks to the end of the hall and back without crutches" describes a performance clearly; "without crutches" is a condition of the objective.

Nurses always need to determine the conditions in which an activity will be carried out. Then the objectives for the learning plan can reflect those conditions. For example, if a client lives alone and must irrigate his own colostomy, then "Irrigate his colostomy *independently* as taught" would be correct.

Criteria

Criteria state the standards of performance that are considered acceptable. Each objective should specify a standard against which the performance can be measured. Examples include speed, quality, and accuracy.

For clients, quality is often used in the objective. For example, "as instructed," "as listed," "as described" all refer to quality as determined by someone. Learners need to understand the criteria so that they can evaluate their

When instructions to clients and their support persons are complex or extensive, formal written instructions may be essential. Written instructions should supplement, not replace, verbal explanations and discussions. (Cushing 1984)

performance validly. Sometimes it is necessary to clarify criteria for them. For additional information on objectives and criteria, see Chapter 13.

Choosing Content

The content to be taught is determined by the objectives. For instance, "Identify appropriate sites for insulin injections" means the nurse must include content about the body sites suitable for insulin injections.

There are many sources for content information. Nurses will have some knowledge as a result of their own education. Pamphlets, books, and journals can also assist nurses and clients. In addition, clients can learn a great deal from peers. For example, the client who has recently had a colostomy often can learn a great deal from a person who has had a colostomy for several years. Self-help groups function on this premise. See chapter 28 for additional information about self-help groups.

Audiovisual aids often are helpful for client learning, e.g., film strips, films, posters, line drawings. It is important, however, that the nurse review these aids before presenting them to clients, for sometimes they are out of date, or they differ in content from other materials (even minimal differences can be confusing to clients).

Selecting Teaching Strategies

The method of teaching chosen by the nurse should be suited to the individual, to the material to be learned, and to the teacher. For example: the person who cannot read needs material presented in other ways; a discussion is usually not the best strategy for learning to give an injection; and a teacher should be competent as a group leader in order to use group discussion for teaching. See Table 29–2 for selected teaching strategies.

The following guidelines can assist the nurse in selecting the best teaching technique.

1. The teaching method should suit the type of learning, i.e., cognitive, affective, or psychomotor.
2. The method should encourage client involvement, i.e., discussion rather than lecture.
3. The method should be congruent with the client's learning style.
4. The method should facilitate the transfer of the learning to other settings and circumstances.

Research Note

In a descriptive survey of the opinions of 21 vascular surgery clients about a booklet used for preoperative teaching, 95% said they would recommend the booklet to a friend. Further implications: clients have different learning needs, and the booklet alone cannot be assumed to provide comprehensive preoperative teaching—nurses must also make time to discuss the booklet with each client. (Parrinello 1984.)

Cognitive Learning

Cognitive learning involves the acquisition of knowledge, i.e., theoretical content. The content can be presented formally or informally. An example of informal teaching strategy, and one that involves active participation by both nurse and client, is a conversation in which the nurse provides information, the client asks questions and responds, and the nurse also responds.

A number of teaching strategies are appropriate for the cognitive domain: discussion (small or large group), lecture, audiovisual materials, and printed materials.

Affective Learning

Learning affective content, such as attitudinal change, usually requires an interactive process with one or even several people. This kind of learning takes considerable time. Attitudinal learning may be conscious or unconscious. For example, a woman can learn attitudes about the surgical removal of her breast from the attitudes a nurse conveys while changing her dressing or discussing the surgery. Participants in group discussions can change their attitudes in many areas.

Values, another area of affective learning, can be taught through modeling. **Modeling** is setting an example. For instance, a nurse who values health would look healthy and act healthy.

Psychomotor Learning

To learn psychomotor skills, such as administering insulin using a syringe, usually involves four phases:

1. Teaching in relation to fear, anxiety, etc., if this is present. Often this phase requires considerable client interaction with the nurse and/or discussions in a small supportive group.
2. Teaching the cognitive basis for the skill. The nurse may do this through discussions, furnishing reading materials, showing films, etc.
3. Demonstration of the psychomotor skill by the nurse. This may be done for a group or an individual.
4. Repeated practice of the skill by the learner, with feedback from the nurse.

Table 29–2 Selected Teaching Strategies

Strategy	Major Type of Learning	Characteristics
Explanation or description (e.g., lecture)	Cognitive	Teacher controls content and pace. Feedback is determined by teacher. May be given to individual or group. Encourages retention of facts.
One-to-one discussion	Affective, cognitive	Encourages participation by learner. Permits reinforcement and repetition at learner's level. Permits introduction of sensitive subjects.
Answering questions	Cognitive	Teacher controls most of content and pace. Teacher must understand question and what it means to learner. Can be used with individuals and groups. Teacher sometimes needs to confirm whether question has been answered by asking learner, e.g., "Does that answer your question?"
Demonstration	Psychomotor	Often used with explanation. Can be used with individuals, small or large groups. Does not permit use of equipment by learners.
Group discussion	Affective, cognitive	Learner can obtain assistance from supportive group. Group members learn from one another.
Practice	Psychomotor	Allows repetition and immediate feedback. Permits "hands-on" experience.
Printed and audiovisual materials	Cognitive	Forms include books, pamphlets, films, programmed instruction, and computer learning. Learners can proceed at their own speed. Nurse can act as resource person, need not be present during learning.
Role playing	Affective, cognitive	Permits expression of attitudes, values, and emotions. Can assist in development of communication skills. Involves active participation by learner.
Modeling	Affective, psychomotor	Nurse sets example by attitude, psychomotor skill.

Some people learn best through seeing—they are visually oriented; others learn best through hearing—having the skill explained. This attribute of the client should be considered during the planning phase. If it is not identified until the teaching plan has been implemented, it may be a reason to revise the plan.

Ordering the Learning Experiences

There are a number of guidelines to help the nurse order the learning experiences:

1. Attend to those experiences directly related to needs identified by the client. The teacher can start with something the learner is concerned about, e.g., before learning how to administer insulin to himself, an adolescent wants to know how he can adjust his life-style and still play football.
2. Start with what the learner knows and proceed to the unknown. This gives the learner confidence. Sometimes a nurse does not know the client's knowledge or skill base and needs to elicit this information initially, usually by asking questions. Sometimes the nurse can have the client fill out a form, such as a pretest, to ascertain needed information.
3. Any area of learning that is anxiety provoking should be taught first. A high level of anxiety can impair concentration in other areas. For example, a woman highly anxious about turning her husband in bed might not be able to learn about bathing him until she has successfully learned to turn him.
4. Teach the basics first, then proceed to the variations or adjustments. It is very confusing to learners to have to consider every possible adjustment and variation before the basic concepts are understood. For example, when teaching a female client how to insert a retention catheter, it would be best to teach the basic procedure before teaching any adjustments that might be needed if the catheter stops draining post-insertion.

Writing a Teaching Plan

Preparing a written teaching plan serves several purposes:

1. It facilitates communication by providing a written record for other health professionals.

2. It assists in identifying any inconsistencies in the plan.
3. It provides a legal record of the planned teaching actions and the client's responses.

Some institutions provide a form on which to write the teaching plan. There are many formats in existence today. Figure 29–2 shows one such form. It is important for nurses to remember that although a teaching plan is written, it must be changed as needed, such as when the client's needs change, or when the planned teaching strategies prove ineffective.

Some health agencies have also developed teaching guides for lessons that nurses commonly give. These guides save nurses time in constructing their own guides. They also standardize content and assist staff in remembering it (Redman 1984, p. 194).

Intervention

The teaching plan is implemented by executing the planned strategies. See the earlier section on teaching methods.

It is important for the nurse to be flexible in implementing any teaching plan, for, as just mentioned, it may be necessary to revise the plan, such as when the client tires sooner than anticipated or is faced with too much information too quickly, or because the client's needs change or external factors intervene. For instance, the nurse and the client may have planned for the client to learn to administer his own insulin at a particular time, but when the time comes the nurse finds that the client wants additional information before actually giving himself the insulin. So the nurse alters the teaching plan and discusses the desired information, provides written information, and defers teaching the psychomotor skill until the next day.

It is also important for nurses to use teaching techniques that enhance learning and to consider any barriers to learning. See Table 29–3 for barriers to learning.

When implementing a teaching plan, the nurse may find the following guidelines helpful.

1. The timing, pace, and length of each teaching session can affect learning. The exact time for each session will depend largely on the particular learner. Some people, for example, learn best at the beginning of the day, when they are most rested; others prefer late afternoon, when no other activities are scheduled. This attention to a client's biorhythms can help learning by capitalizing on the client's mood and performance peaks (Murdaugh 1982, p. 33–34).

   The pace of each teaching session also will vary. Nurses should be sensitive to any signs that the pace is too fast or too slow. A client who appears confused or does not comprehend material when questioned may be finding the pace too fast. When the client appears bored and loses interest, the pace may be too slow or the learning period may be too long and the client tired. Sessions can sometimes be lengthened by changing the type of teaching during the session. For example, the first part of the teaching session could be discussion, followed by a demonstration and some practice. The client should set the pace. The nurse should also be prepared for wide variations in pace by arranging for subdivision of the content into "essential" and "desirable" portions so that the quick-paced client can move on to "desirable" content and the slower-paced client can end a session at the end of the "essential" material.

2. An environment can detract or assist learning; e.g., noise or interruptions usually interfere with concentration, whereas a comfortable environment helps learning. Environmental characteristics that should be considered are: lighting, temperature, sound, ventilation, visibility, and a chair or support for the learner. A good environment for learning is quiet and free of interruptions, is well ventilated and free of odors, and has a comfortable temperature, good lighting, and comfortable seating for the client.

3. The presence of teaching aids in the environment can assist learning. Posters and displays, for example, can help focus a learner's attention. It is also important to use the type of supplies or equipment that the client will eventually use, because this will assist the transfer of learning to another environment.

4. Learning is more effective when the learners *discover* the content for themselves. Teaching that stimulates the client's participation and interest facilitates learning and promotes independent learning activities. Ways to increase learning include stimulating motivation and stimulating self-direction (Redman 1984, p. 90). This can be done by providing specific objectives, providing feedback, and assisting the learner to obtain satisfaction from learning. Nurses can maximize the latter by setting realistic goals with the learner (Redman 1984, p. 90).

5. It is important to establish an atmosphere conducive to learning. Smitherman (1981, p. 139) describes six characteristics of a teacher that promote such an atmosphere:

   - well informed and interested in the subject
   - in tune with learners, with accurate perceptions about their behavior

Teaching Plan

Home IV Antibiotic Administration

Equipment: Alcohol swabs
Needles
IV tubing & add-a-line connector
IV antibiotics
Heparin lock solution
Metal/plastic disposal container

Goal	Behaviors	Comments about practice sessions
1. Knows the principles of sterile technique	1.1 Washes hands before initiating intermittent IV antibiotic infusion. 1.2 Stabilizes arm that holds heparin lock to prevent contamination (using Velcro apparatus). 1.3 Does not touch needle when removing cover sheath before hooking up line to heparin lock. 1.4 Wipes heparin lock plug with alcohol wipe before inserting needle. 1.5 Checks needle hub connection to prevent leaking and maintain a closed system. 1.6 Demonstrates ability to insert needle into stabilized heparin lock without contaminating either surface.	
2. Identifies signs and symptoms of IV site infiltration	2.1 Checks heparin lock site before each IV dose and observes for redness, swelling, tenderness, or leakage during or after each infusion. 2.2 Observes rate of infusion to verify potency of infusion system.	

(continued)

Figure 29–2 Sample teaching plan for home use
Source: Courtesy of the Department of Nursing, University of British Columbia Health Sciences Centre Hospital.

3. Follows procedure to change heparin lock if IV site is interstitial	3.1 Stops infusion if signs and symptoms in 2.1 are observed. 3.2 Discontinues antibiotic drip; caps needle using sterile technique. 3.3 Reports to emergency department for a change of site.
4. Initiates infusion of IV antibiotic independently	4.1 Sets up IV flush solution (D_5W bag) and add-a-line tubing with IV antibiotic using sterile technique (see 1.1–1.6). Priming the tubing and drip chambers to prevent air emboli: 4.2 Ensures antibiotic mini-bag is elevated higher than flush bag. 4.3 Flushes IV tubing with flush D_5W solution. 4.4 Stabilizes arm holding heparin lock with Velcro apparatus. 4.5 Inserts needle into heparin lock using sterile technique, and begins to check the site for signs of infiltration (see 2.1–2.2). Tapes into place. 4.6 Proceeds to flush with D_5W solution by opening IV control 1/4 way. If heparin lock site is clear and pain-free, switches open the IV antibiotic tubing line control knob. 4.7 Observes IV drip chamber, and adjusts to run for 15-20 mins. 4.8 When IV antibiotic mini-bag is empty, the IV flush bag should automatically begin to drip.

	4.9 Checks to confirm that medication is completely absorbed. Flushes tubing with D_5W solution. Closes control knob on IV tubing.	
Terminates infusion of IV antibiotic	4.10 Removes needle from heparin lock plug using sterile technique; caps the needle.	
5. Knows how to store IV antibiotics to maintain sterile technique	5.1 Keeps IV antibiotic mini-bags refrigerated in separate plastic container with seal-tight lid. 5.2 Checks label on IV mini-bag for correct drug, dosage, and expiration date.	
6. Knows how to handle and dispose of equipment to promote safety	6.1 Uses a new IV tubing and add-a-line q 2 days. 6.2 Uses a new needle for each IV antibiotic dose following sterile technique. 6.3 Disposes of needles in a metal/plastic container.	
7. Identifies support systems in the community	7.1 Knows when public health nurse will visit. 7.2 Knows telephone numbers of emergency department and physician. 7.3 Knows how to contact family members in case of problems with care.	
8. Knows emergency procedure if heparin lock becomes dislodged	8.1 Applies clean gauze to site. 8.2 Applies pressure to site. 8.3 Calls for assistance and reports to emergency department to replace IV heparin lock.	T. Savage H. Lobo M. Pringle G. Gleason 2A June 1986

Table 29–3 Barriers to Learning

Barrier	Explanation
Acute illness	Requires all resources for survival.
Pain or discomfort	Decreases ability to learn.
Restlessness	Due to stressors such as electrolyte imbalances, can alter orientation, memory, intellectual capacity, judgment, mood, perceptions, motor control, level of consciousness, and concentration.
Age	Vision or hearing can be impaired in the elderly.
Prognosis	Receptivity to learning can be negatively affected when prognosis is poor.
Biorhythms	Mental and physical performances have a circadian rhythm.
Anxiety, denial, hostility, depression, fear, regression, etc.	Such behavioral responses to acute illness can impair learning.
Language, ethnic background, etc.	Can prevent learning.
Iatrogenic barriers	Barriers set up by the nurse, such as talking down to clients, hurried and fragmented teaching, ignoring client cues.

Adapted from Murdaugh, C. L. November / December 1982. Barriers to patient education in the coronary care unit. *Cardiovascular Nursing* 18:33–35. Used by permission of the American Heart Association, Inc.

- aware of own behavior and motives
- understands how people learn
- uses effective teaching methods
- uses "self" as part of the teaching method

6. Using repetition can strengthen learning. There are a number of ways to do this, e.g., summarizing content, rephrasing (using other words), and approaching the material from another point of view. An example of the latter technique: After discussing the kinds of foods that can be included in a diet, the nurse describes the foods again, but in the context of the three meals for a day's diet.
7. It is helpful to employ "advanced organizers" to introduce material to be learned and to present it at a higher level of abstraction, generality, or inclusiveness (Redman 1984, p. 91). Advanced organizers provide a means of relating unknown material to known material and generating logical relationships among material. For example: "You understand how urine flows down a catheter from the bladder. Now I will show you how to inject fluid so it will flow up the catheter into the bladder." The details that follow such an introduction are then seen within its framework, thereby giving the details added meaning.
8. Using a layperson's vocabulary enhances communication. So often nurses use terms and abbreviations that have meaning to other health professionals but limited or no meaning to clients. Even words such as "urine" or "feces" may be unfamiliar to clients; and abbreviations such as "RR" or "PAR" are often misunderstood.

Evaluation

Evaluation is an ongoing and terminal process in which the client, the nurse, and often the support persons determine what has been learned. Both short-term objectives and long-term goals need to be evaluated. Learning is measured against the predetermined objectives. Thus, the objectives serve not only to direct the teaching plan but they also provide criteria for evaluation. For example, the objective "Selects foods that are low in carbohydrates" can be evaluated by asking the client to name such foods or to select low-carbohydrate foods from a list.

The best method for evaluating depends to some degree on the type of learning. In cognitive learning, asking questions of the client is one way to determine what has been learned. Observing client behaviors that reflect knowledge is another method; e.g., can the client select foods low in sodium while shopping? The acquisition of psychomotor skills is best evaluated by observing the client carry out a procedure, such as changing a dressing or carrying out a urinary self-catheterization. Affective learning is more difficult to evaluate. Whether attitudes or values have been learned may be inferred by listening to the client's responses to questions and by the way the client speaks about relevant subjects and by observing the client's behavior. For example, has an obese client learned to value health sufficiently to follow a reducing diet? Does a client who states that he values health actually stop smoking?

Following evaluation, the nurse may find it necessary to modify or repeat the teaching plan if the objectives have not been met or met only partially. For the hospitalized client, follow-up teaching in the home may be needed.

It is important for the nurse to evaluate her or his own teaching. This should include a consideration of all factors—the timing, the teaching strategies, the amount of information, whether it was helpful, etc. The nurse may find, for example, that the client was overwhelmed with too much information, was bored, or was motivated to learn more.

The following guidelines (Smitherman 1981, pp. 141–44) can assist nurses in the evaluative process:

1. Forgetting is normal and should be anticipated. Nurses can suggest to clients that they write down information they might forget. Often, clients are provided printed instructions, because such information may be easily forgotten.
2. Both the client and the teacher should evaluate the learning experience. The learner may tell the nurse what was helpful, interesting, etc. Questionnaires and videotapes of the learning sessions can also be helpful.
3. Behavior change does not always take place immediately after learning. Often the person will accept change intellectually first, and then may change his or her behavior only periodically (e.g., the person who knows that he or she must lose weight may diet and exercise off and on). If the new behavior is to replace old behavior it must emerge gradually, otherwise the old behavior may prevail. Nurses can assist clients with behavior change by allowing for client vacillation and by providing encouragement.

Documentation

Documentation of the teaching process is essential, for this provides a legal record that the teaching took place and communicates the teaching to other health professionals. The record should include the client's achievements. A specific client teaching record or the nurse's notes can be used. The client's reaction to the teaching should also be included, and this reaction should be incorporated into further planning. Documentation of the responses of support persons are also important to include.

The record of the teaching process should include written teaching plans, nursing Kardexes (see Chapter 30, page 641), and planning sessions with other health team members. Documentation of the teaching/learning process serves several other functions as well: reference for client learning and support-person learning; reevaluation of the teaching plan; reinforcement of identified areas of learning need; and revision of the teaching strategies (Corkadel and McGlashan 1983, pp. 14–15).

Specific Teaching Strategies

There are a number of special strategies that nurses can use in teaching: client contracting, group teaching, behavior modification, and various accelerated strategies.

Client Contracting

Client contracting involves establishing a contract with a client that specifies certain objectives and when they are to be met. The contract, drawn up and signed by the client and the nurse, specifies not only the learning objectives but also the responsibilities of the client and the nurse, and the teaching plan. The agreement allows for freedom, mutual respect, and mutual responsibility. For additional information about client contracting see Chapter 2, page 67, and Chapter 20, page 446.

Group Teaching

Group instruction is economical, and it provides members with an opportunity to share with and learn from others. A small group allows for discussion in which everyone can participate. A large group often necessitates a lecture technique.

It is important that all members involved in group instruction have a need in common, e.g., prenatal health, diabetic instruction. It is also important that sociocultural factors be considered in the formation of a group. Whereas middle-class Americans may value sharing experiences with others, people from a culture such as Japan may consider it inappropriate to reveal their thoughts and feelings.

Behavior Modification

The behavior modification system for changing behavior has as its basic assumptions that human behaviors are learned and can be selectively strengthened, weakened, eliminated, or replaced and that a person's behavior is under conscious control. Under this system, desirable behavior is rewarded and undesirable behavior is ignored.

The client's response is the key to behavior change. For example, clients trying to quit smoking are not criticized when they smoke, but they are praised or rewarded when they go without a cigarette for a certain period of time. For some people a learning contract is combined with behavior modification.

Some pertinent features of behavior modification are:

1. Positive reinforcement—e.g., praise—is used.
2. The client participates in the development of the learning plan.
3. Undesirable behavior is ignored, not criticized.
4. The expectation of the client and the nurse is that the task will be mastered, i.e., the behavior will change.
5. Success is maximized through positive reinforcement; failure and the threat of failure are minimized.

Infants and Toddlers

The primary caregiver, i.e., the parent, is the best person to teach the infant or toddler. Infants learn by exploring their environment with their senses. An infant's routines normally should not be changed, unless they involve something that is making the infant ill. Predictable routines help infants feel secure. When teaching toddlers before surgery, the nurse should make sure they are able to hold the mask or the equipment with which they will come into contact later. Toddlers like to explore, e.g., handle equipment. They also need to be reassured that their parents have seen the room in which they will "wake up," because then the children know their parents will be able to find them.

Toddlers who reply "no" when they are being taught a new activity such as brushing their teeth are asserting their independence; this does not mean they will not learn. Better results will usually be produced if the nurse postpones the teaching to another time and repeats the lesson rather than arguing with the toddler.

Preschoolers

Most preschoolers want to learn. They have limited verbal abilities, and they like to explore, just as toddlers do. Most preschoolers like to practice procedures such as bandaging; such activity helps them deal with their fears.

Preschoolers like to ask questions, but the nurse's answers should be short and at a level that can be understood. Preschoolers like explanations, and they worry about such things as providing a blood specimen because the nurse "may take all my blood." The nurse should emphasize that treatment is not punishment.

School-Age Children

School-age children know more about their bodies than do preschoolers. Since their attention span is short, they learn best in brief stages. They usually like to handle objects and to draw pictures and color in books. Although their vocabulary is limited, they are learning new things. A school-age child's day is often filled with short projects.

School-age children love to ask why. They require explanations that meet their needs and that use words they understand. Children at this age should be encouraged to express their feelings, including fears about dying. School-age children love to do things the "right way," and any changes they consider as not "right" they often do not accept.

Peers become increasingly important during the school years. School-age children usually have busy schedules, so teaching plans must take into consideration their interests and activities and fit into their school and social schedules.

Adolescents

Adolescents may prefer to learn in the absence of their parents. Although they do have knowledge about their bodies, some of it may be incorrect. Adolescents learn best when they see immediate benefit to themselves. For example, an adolescent who understands that taking his medicine regularly will permit him to continue playing football is more likely to follow through than if he is told the medication will prevent heart problems when he is in his forties.

Adolescents assume more responsibility for their own health, and they usually want to be in control. Therefore a problem-solving approach is more likely to be successful with an adolescent than an authoritarian approach. For example, a nurse teaching an adolescent to take a medication regularly is more likely to succeed by explaining the alternatives and their possible consequences than by simply telling the adolescent that he or she must take the medicine.

Young and Middle-Age Adults

Young adults often take health for granted ("It won't happen to me"), and they may not be interested in learning about other people's problems. However, when young adults understand how something affects them, learning is facilitated. Young adults not living at home may find it unacceptable to be dependent on parents for health matters, and they may prefer a friend or the nurse to help them through a health problem.

Middle-age adults are usually aware of the problems that can result from unhealthy life-styles. This is the period when changes in life-style are often indicated. Some middle-age people change despite difficulty, and others still believe "it won't happen to me." Adults should be self-directed learners (Robinson 1986, p. 49).

Elderly Adults

Healthy elderly adults can learn new techniques and procedures and usually desire to do so if it will mean their continued health and independence. Recent research has shown that there is no general decline in intelligence with age. However, learning and problem-solving performance do decline later in life, though retention of *meaningful* learning equals that of young adults (Gioiella and Bevil 1985, p. 38). Nurses may need to adjust teaching methods to account for diminished hearing or vision or other physical limitations in the elderly person.

Check and Wurzbach (1984, p. 39) list the following guidelines regarding teaching the elderly:

1. Be cognizant of ill health and sensory deficits on the elderly person's learning.
2. Elderly people tend to be solitary learners.
3. Arrange groups or networks where the elderly can share ideas, experiences, and similar concerns.
4. Creatively generate interest in learning.
5. The ability to learn is affected by loneliness, loss, and death of significant others.
6. Along with the acquisition of skills and exposure to new ideas, emphasize the emotional and personal values in learning.

Chapter Highlights

- Learning is represented by a change in behavior.
- Bloom identified three learning domains: cognitive, affective, and psychomotor.
- A number of factors facilitate learning, including motivation, readiness, active involvement, and success at learning.
- Factors such as extreme anxiety, certain physiologic processes, and cultural barriers impede learning.
- Teaching is a system of activities intended to produce learning.
- Rapport between the teacher and the learner is essential for effective teaching.
- Assessment relative to the preparation of a teaching plan must include identification of the client's learning needs and relevant client data.
- Readiness is an important aspect of assessment *prior* to teaching.
- Teaching priorities must always be established and must take into consideration the client's priorities.
- Learning objectives guide the content of the teaching plan and are written in terms of client behavior.
- Teaching strategies should be suited to the client, the material to be learned, and the teacher.
- A teaching plan is a written plan and must be revised when the client's needs change or the teaching strategies prove ineffective.
- Evaluation of the teaching/learning process is an ongoing and terminal process.

Suggested Readings

Check, J. F., and Wurzbach, M. E. January/February 1984. How elders view learning. *Geriatric Nursing* 5:37–39.
The authors first describe the findings from their study of 30 elderly subjects. They then provide 11 recommendations for supporting the elderly person's learning, which should be very helpful to nurses teaching elderly clients.

Corkadel, L., and McGlashan, R. January/February 1983. A practical approach to patient teaching. *The Journal of Continuing Education in Nursing* 14:9–15.
This overview of client teaching includes an explanation of selected barriers to effective teaching and how to minimize those barriers.

Robinson, Y. K. January 1986. Teaching adults: Some issues in adult education for health education. *Physiotherapy* 72:49–52.
Discusses adults as learners, including a list of ten beliefs about an andragogical humanistic approach to adult learning. The author sees learning as a cooperative effort on the part of the teacher and the learner, and describes participatory and group learning as well as individual differences and cognitive style and change.

Selected References

Alford, D. M. September/October 1982. Tips for teaching elderly adults. *Nursing Life* 2:60–63.

Allendorf, E. E., and Keegan, M. H. July 1975. Teaching patients about nitroglycerin. *American Journal of Nursing* 75:1168–70.

American Public Health Association. 1983. Reimbursement for patient education services. *American Journal of Public Health* 73:339–40.

Bigge, M. L. 1976. *Learning theories for teachers.* 3d ed. New York: Harper & Row.

Bille, D. A. March/April 1983. Process-oriented patient education. *Dimensions of Critical Care Nursing* 2:108–15.

Bloom, B. S. (ed.). 1956. *Taxonomy of educational objectives.* Book 1, *Cognitive domain.* New York: Longman, Inc.

Check, J. F., and Wurzbach, M. E. January/February 1984. How elders view learning. *Geriatric Nursing* 5:37–39.

Corkadel, L., and McGlashan, R. January/February 1983. A practical approach to patient teaching. *The Journal of Continuing Education in Nursing* 14:9–15.

Cushing, M. June 1984. Legal lessons on patient teaching. *American Journal of Nursing* 84:721–22.

DeHaes, W. F. M. 1982. Patient education: A component of health education. *Patient Counseling and Health Education* 4(2):95–102.

Frank-Stromborg, M. January/February 1985. Evaluating patient education material. *Oncology Nursing Forum* 12:65–67.

Frisbie, D. A. November 1984. Looking at teaching through the nursing process. *Journal of Nursing Education* 23:401–403.

Gagne, R. M. 1977. *The conditions of learning.* 3rd ed. New York: Holt, Rinehart and Winston.

Gioiella, E. C., and Bevil, C. W. 1985. *Nursing care of the aging client. Promoting healthy adaptation.* Norwalk, Conn.: Appleton-Century-Crofts.

Gronlund, N. E. 1978. *Stating objectives for classroom instruction.* 2d ed. New York: Macmillan Publishing Co.

Huckabay, L.M.D. 1980. *Condition of learning and instruction in nursing.* St. Louis: C. V. Mosby Co.

Krathwohl, D. R.; Bloom, B. S.; and Masia, B. B. 1964. *Taxonomy of educational objectives.* Book 2, *Affective domain.* New York: Longman, Inc.

Laird, M. August 1975. Techniques for teaching pre- and post-operative patients. *American Journal of Nursing* 75:1338–40.

Lewis, S. J. May 1984. Teaching patient groups. *Nursing Management* 15:49–50, 52, 54–56.

Mager, R. F. 1975. *Preparing instructional objectives.* 2d ed. Belmont, California: Fearon Publishers, Inc.

Murdaugh, C. L. November/December 1982. Barriers to patient education in the coronary care unit. *Cardiovascular Nursing* 18:31–35.

Parrinello, K. 1984. Patient's evaluation of a teaching booklet for arterial bypass surgery. *Patient Education and Counselling* 5:183–88.

Phillips, J. A., and Hekelman, F. P. September/October 1983. The role of the nurse as a teacher: A position paper. *Nephrology Nurse* 5:42–46.

Redman, B. K. 1984. *The process of patient education.* 5th ed. St. Louis: C. V. Mosby Co.

Robinson, Y. K. January 1986. Teaching adults: Some issues in adult education for health education. *Physiotherapy* 72:49–52.

Simpson, E. J. 1972. The classification of educational objectives in the psychomotor domain. *The psychomotor domain*, Vol. 3. Washington, D.C.: Gryphon House.

Smitherman, C. 1981. *Nursing actions for health promotion.* Philadelphia: F. A. Davis Co.

Taylor, P. November/December 1982. Patient teaching: Keys to more success more often. *Nursing Life* 2:25–32.

Tiche, S.; Dobson, J.; and Olker, L. April 1984. Pediatric teaching. The small hospital. *American Operating Room Nurses Journal* 39:793–97.

Tyson, J. 1984. Before we educate. *Diabetes Educator* (special issue) 10:23–24.

Woody, A. F., et al. December 1984. Do patients learn what nurses say they teach? *Nursing Management* 15:26–29.

Zangari, M. E., and Duffy, P. March 1980. Contracting with patients in day-to-day practice. *American Journal of Nursing* 80:451–55.

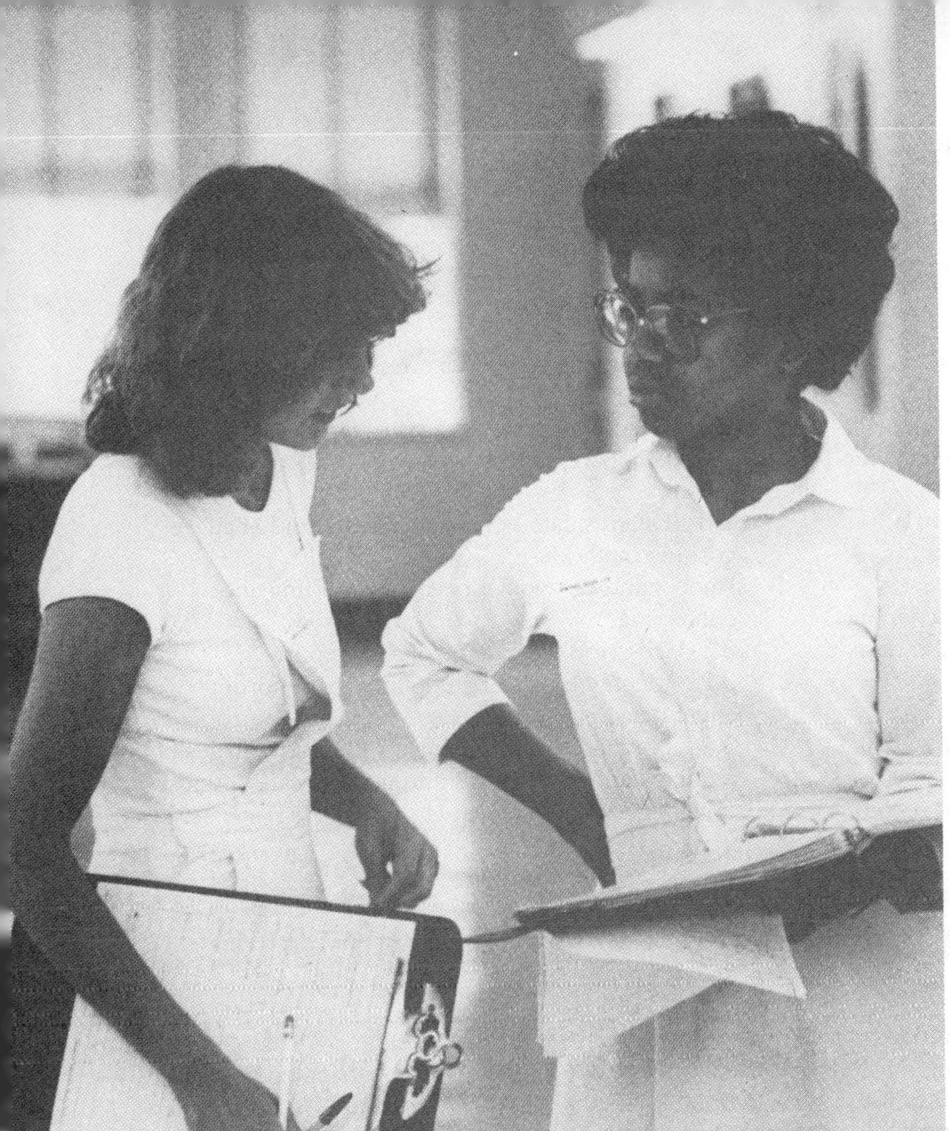

CHAPTER 30

Recording and Reporting

Contents

30 *Recording and Reporting*

Objectives

1. Know essential terms and facts about recording.
   1.1 Identify seven purposes of client records.
   1.2 Describe the components of source-oriented medical records and problem-oriented medical records (POMR).
   1.3 Describe three types of progress records.
   1.4 Identify abbreviations commonly used for charting.
   1.5 Identify symbols commonly used for charting.
   1.6 Identify medical terms used to describe data about clients.
2. Understand facts about recording.
   2.1 Identify measures used to maintain the confidentiality of client records.
   2.2 Identify measures used to ensure that recording meets legal standards.
   2.3 Identify essential data required on selected nursing records.
   2.4 Describe the advantages of flowsheets.
   2.5 Compare various acronyms used to record in POMR.
   2.6 Differentiate between narrative and SOAP recording methods.
3. Understand essential aspects of reporting and conferring.
   3.1 Describe the change-of-shift report.
   3.2 Identify essential guidelines for reporting client data.
   3.3 Compare the advantages and disadvantages of nursing care conferences and nursing care rounds.

Terms

audit
confer
database
flowsheet
Kardex
medical record (chart)
narrative charting
nursing care conference
nursing care rounds
objective data
problem-oriented medical record (POMR; POR)
recording (charting)
SOAP
source-oriented medical record
subjective data

Importance of Communication Among Health Team Members

Written and verbal communication among health team members is vital to the quality of client care. Generally, health team members communicate through discussions, reports, and records. A discussion is an informal oral consideration of a subject by two or more members of the health team, often leading to a decision. A report is an oral or written account by one member to others in the health team; for instance, nurses always report on clients at the end of a hospital work shift. A record is always written; it is a formal, legal documentation of a client's progress and treatment.

Accurate, complete communication serves several purposes:

1. It helps coordinate care given by several people.
2. It prevents the client from having to repeat information to each health team member.
3. It promotes accuracy in the provision of care and lessens the possibility of error.
4. It helps health personnel make the best use of their time by avoiding overlapping of activities.

Purposes of Client Records

Traditionally, written records have been an important aspect of care. All health agencies keep written records, although the form of the record may vary considerably from place to place.

A client's **medical record**, or **chart**, is an account of the client's health history, current health status, treatment, and progress. It is a highly confidential, legal document by means of which physicians, nurses, social workers, and other health team members communicate about that client. When a client goes to a physician's office or enters a hospital, a record is usually started. Records are generally kept in folders, in binders, or on clipboards, and they are updated continually while clients attend the health care facility. When clients are discharged, their records are stored for future reference in the medical records department of the agency.

Although the forms of client records may vary considerably from place to place, nurses are universally required to make entries about clients' health, including, for example, all assessments and interventions. The process of making entries on client records is called **recording** (or **charting**).

Client records are kept for a number of purposes: communication, legal documentation, research, statistics, education, audit, and planning client care.

Communication

The record serves as the vehicle by which different members of the health team communicate with each other. Although these members also communicate verbally, the record is an efficient and effective method of sharing information. It also allows health team members on different shifts to convey meaningful data about the client to one another. An accurate record can prevent errors such as duplication of a medication.

Legal Documentation

The client's record is a legal document and is admissible in court as evidence. In some jurisdictions, however, the record is considered inadmissible as evidence when the client objects, because information the client gives to the physician is confidential.

A record is usually considered the property of the agency, although there is increasing belief that the client has a right to the information in the record upon request. See "Client's Rights" in Chapter 9. Legal decisions have recognized this right (Creighton 1981, p. 329). Some agencies, however, do not permit clients access to their records; thus the nurse needs to be guided by the agency's policy.

Research

The information contained in a record can be a valuable source of data for research. The treatment plans for a number of clients with the same illness can yield information helpful in treating a particular client.

A record made years earlier may also assist members of the health team with a current problem. A client's memory of an illness may provide limited data, but a record of that illness will generally reveal additional and accurate data. Records are also very important documents when experimental drugs and treatments are being used.

Statistics

Statistical information from client records can help an agency anticipate and plan for people's future needs. For example, the number of births or kinds of illnesses can be obtained from records. Some statistics, such as records of births and deaths, are required by law. They are filed with a government agency and become a part of the local, national, and international statistics.

Education

Students in health disciplines often use client records as educational tools. A record can frequently provide a comprehensive view of the client, the illness, and the kinds of assistance given. In this context, records are used by nursing students, medical students, dietitians, and other health team members.

Audit

The client's record is used to monitor the care the client is receiving and the competence of the people giving that care. A nursing **audit**, for example, monitors the nursing interventions and measures them against established standards. Often the audit is a retrospective audit, in that the care has already been given.

When a nursing audit is carried out by other nurses, it is sometimes referred to as a *peer review*. Many agencies have audit committees that monitor the practice of individual nurses. Audits are also carried out by outside groups for approval and accreditation purposes.

Various aspects of care are assessed in nursing audits: the database, the identification of health problems, the goals of nursing interventions, the choice of nursing interventions, and the level of goal attainment. The nurse's skills, judgment, and knowledge are audited.

Planning Client Care

The entire health team uses data from the client's record to plan care for that client. A physician, for example, may order a specific antibiotic after establishing that the client's temperature is steadily rising and that laboratory tests reveal the presence of a certain microorganism. Nurses use data from the history they took on the client's admission to establish an individual nursing care plan. The social worker's data about the client's home environment can assist the nurse in developing an appropriate discharge teaching plan. Data from the physical therapist help the nurse to implement specific physical exercises for the client.

Types of Records

There are two types of medical records: the *traditional* or *source-oriented medical record* and the *problem-oriented medical record* (POMR or POR). The POR is also referred to as the *Weed system,* after its originator, L. L. Weed.

Source-Oriented Medical Records

In the traditional client record, or *source-oriented medical record,* each person or department has a record or records for notations. For example, the admission department has an admission sheet; the physician has a doctor's order sheet, a doctor's history sheet, and progress notes; nurses have records that are sometimes called the nurse's notes; and other departments or personnel have their own records. In this type of record, information about a particular problem is distributed throughout the record. For example, if a client had left hemiplegia (paralysis of the left side of the body), data about this problem might be found in the doctor's history sheet, on the doctor's order sheet, in the nurse's notes, in the physical therapist's record, and in the social service record.

Components

Source-oriented client records generally have five components: admission sheet, physician's order sheet, history sheet, the nurse's notes, and special records and reports.

1. The *admission sheet* is a part of the record in most agencies. It generally contains demographic data about the client, including an identification number. In hospitals, admission sheets usually set forth the client's full name, address, date of birth, name of attending physician, sex, marital status, nearest relative, occupation and employer, financial status for hospital payments, religious preference, date and hour of admission to the hospital, hospital unit or agency of admission, previous hospital admission, admitting diagnosis or problem, and identification number. Often this sheet contains a list of allergies presented by the client.

2. The *physician's order sheet* is a written record of orders. The physician is expected to write the date with the order and sign each order (or sign for several orders written at once). Often agencies have a method of flagging a client's chart to indicate to the nurse or clerk that there is a new order.

   When the doctor phones in orders about a client, these are written on the physician's sheet by the recipient of the call and signed by that person, indicating a telephone order. Often the physician is expected to countersign the telephone order within 24 or 48 hours of the call. Before a nurse can accept a verbal order from a physician, however, agency policies and procedures must be checked. Usually, nursing students are not allowed to take verbal orders.

3. The *history sheet* is a record of the client's health history, written by the physician. The physician may also use this sheet to record progress notes on the client and future plans, although some agencies have separate records for progress notes.

4. The *nurse's notes* are a record of the nursing interventions carried out, assessments of the client, and evaluations of the effectiveness of the interventions. In general, nurses' notes record the following kinds of information:
   a. Assessments of the client by various nursing personnel, e.g., pale or flushed skin color or the aroma of urine
   b. Dependent nursing interventions, such as medications or treatments ordered by a physician
   c. Independent nursing interventions, such as special skin care or health teaching, carried out on the nurses' judgment
   d. Evaluation of the effectiveness of each nursing intervention
   e. Measures carried out by the physician, for example, shortening a drain in an incision
   f. Visits by members of the health team, such as a consulting physician, social worker, or chaplain

5. *Special records and reports* also become part of the client's permanent record. These include roentgenographic reports, laboratory findings, reports of surgery, anesthesia records, physical therapy records, occupational therapy records, and social service records. In addition, special flowsheets are often used to record certain data about the client. These include graphic records for vital signs, fluid intake and output, and medications. The flowsheets are not to be confused with worksheets used at the client's bedside. Worksheets are used to collect data that are later transferred to the client's permanent record. A common example is the daily bedside fluid intake and output worksheet.

Problem-Oriented Medical Records

In a **problem-oriented medical record (POMR or POR)**, data about the client are recorded and arranged according to the problems the client has, rather than according to the source of the information. The record integrates all data about a problem, whether gathered by physicians, nurses, or others involved in the client's care. Then plans for each active problem are drawn up, and progress notes are recorded for each problem. Unlike the traditional record, which separates the medical data on a problem from the nursing data and other data into different sections of the record, the POR coordinates the care given by all health team members and focuses on the client and her or his health problems.

Components

The POR has four basic components:

1. The defined database
2. The problem list
3. The initial list of orders or care plans
4. Progress notes

The defined database The defined **database** consists of all information known about the client when the client first entered the health care agency. It includes the nursing assessment (history) (see Chapter 11), the physician's history, and the physical health examination (see Chapter 35). To this are added social and family data from other sources, such as the social worker, and baseline laboratory and roentgenographic data. The chief complaint of the client is an important datum. In most agencies a standardized form is used, to help team members obtain a complete database.

The problem list The problem list is a carefully drawn-up list of the problems that is compiled once the databases have been collected and analyzed. Some problems are obvious on initial contact with the client; others are established as additional data are gathered. Problems are essentially needs that the client is unable to meet without assistance from members of the health care team.

The initial problem list is usually made either by the first health care worker to encounter the client or by the person who assumes primary responsibility for the client's care. Subsequent contributions are made by other members of the health team.

To be complete, the problem list should include socioeconomic, demographic, psychologic, and physiologic problems. The list is attached to the front of the client's record. Each problem is labeled and numbered so that it can be identified throughout the record. This list has been likened to an index or table of contents. See Figure 30–1. Problems are usually categorized as active or inactive.

A problem that is potential rather than actual is generally entered on the progress notes rather than the problem list. Only when a problem actually becomes active is it added to the list.

Traditionally problems were classified as:

- A sign or symptom, such as edema, vomiting, pain, or fatigue.
- An abnormal diagnostic measure, such as positive urine culture, low hemoglobin, or elevated blood pH.
- An established diagnosis with manifestations, such as congestive heart failure with bilateral ankle edema.
- A behavioral disturbance, such as hitting others or taking drugs.
- A risk factor, such as a strongly positive family history of heart disease.

Signs, symptoms, and abnormal diagnostic measures, if used, are usually considered as temporary labels until a diagnosis is established. With the development of nursing diagnoses, many nurses are now using the NANDA taxonomy of nursing diagnoses to state nursing problems.

Problems statements must refer to only one problem, must be written unambiguously (so no interpretation is required), must be written in behavioral terms when appropriate, and should provide direction for client care.

When several problems have a common etiology or cause, two methods are used to relate the problems: sublisting and cross-referencing.

1. *Sublisting.* A sublist is a group of all manifestations of a major problem that require separate management. Manifestations may be either behavioral or clinical indicators of the same problem. Example (See Figure 30–1):

No.	Client Problem
1	Multiple CVAs resulting in Rt hemiplegia and left-sided weakness
1A	Self-care deficit (hygiene, toileting, grooming, feeding)
1B	Impaired physical mobility
1C	Alteration in urinary elimination: incontinence
1D	Progressive dysphasia

When a major problem and a manifestation do *not* require separate management they are grouped together. Example: Congestive heart failure resulting in bilateral pitting ankle edema.

2. *Cross-referencing.* The cross-referencing method lists all problems separately, using consecutive numbers. A "Related to" column to the right of the "Client Prob-

No.	Date Entered	Date Inactive	Client Problem	Related to
#1	Mar 9/86		Multiple CVAs resulting in Rt hemiplegia and left-sided weakness. Redefined Feb 7/88	
#1a	Mar 9/86		Selfcare deficit (hygiene, toileting, grooming, feeding)	
#1B	Mar 9/86		Impaired physical mobility. Redefined Feb 7/88	
#1C	Mar 9/86		Alteration in urinary elimination: incontinence. Redefined Nov 10/87	
#1D	Mar 9/86		Progressive dysphasia	
#2	Mar 9/86		Alteration in bowel elimination: constipation. Redefined Nov 10/87	
#3	Mar 9/86		History of depression	
#4	Mar 9/86		Essential hypertension	
#5	June 6/86	Nov 86	Altered comfort: pruritus	
#2	Nov 10/87		Potential for constipation	
#1C	Nov 10/87		Nocturnal urinary incontinence	
#1	Feb 7/87		Cerebral vascular disease (multiple CVAs) resulting in bilateral hemiplegia	
#1B	Feb 7/87		Needs major assist. to transfer/unable to walk	

Figure 30–1 A client's problem list using the sublisting method to relate problems. Note that problems 1, 1B, 1C, and 2 were redefined on the dates indicated and listed subsequently.

Source: Courtesy of the University of British Columbia Health Sciences Centre Hospital, Extended Care Unit.

lem" column lists the number of the major problem to which the manifestations are related. Example:

No.	Client Problem	Related to:
1	Multiple CVAs resulting in Rt hemiplegia and left-sided weakness	
2	Self-care deficit (hygiene, toileting, grooming, feeding)	#1
3	Impaired physical mobility	#1
4	Alteration in urinary elimination: incontinence	#1
5	Progressive dysphasia	#1

Major problems can also be cross-referenced to other major problems. Example:

No.	Client Problem	Related to:
1	Cerebral vascular disease	#4
4	Essential hypertension	#1

"Redefinition" of problems is often necessary to reflect a change in the client's problem or to increase understanding of the problem. Redefining does *not* involve changing the stated nature of the problem; it involves changing the wording of the problem to reflect a change in its frequency or intensity, or increased knowledge. The problem retains the same number. Example (See Figure 30–1):

No.	Client Problem
1C	Alteration in urinary elimination: incontinence REDEFINED NOV 10/87
1C	Nocturnal urinary incontinence

The initial list of care plans Initial care plans are made with reference to the active problems. Care plans or orders are generated by the person who lists the problems. Physicians write physician's orders or medical care plans; nurses write nursing orders or nursing care plans. The written plan in the record is listed under each problem in the progress notes (discussed next) and is not isolated as a separate list of orders or in a separate Kardex.

The plan generated by the physician focuses on three aspects:

1. In the *diagnostic workup* the physician indicates what needs to be done first. Setting priorities helps to prevent duplication, may eliminate some distress for the client, and often saves time and money. Included in the diagnostic workup may be plans to collect further data to establish a medical diagnosis or to assist in therapeutic management of the client.
2. The *therapy* aspect of the plan presents the physician's orders, often including drug therapy and specific treatments. Each order is numbered to correspond to the problem with which it deals. This organization gives the reader (the nurse) considerable information about the plan, including the reason for each order.
3. The *patient education* aspect of the plan describes the client's needs for skills and information that will assist in the management of the problem.

Nurse-generated plans focus more on how the client's *activities* are to be observed, modified, or assisted. Nurses make many decisions dealing with activity, diet, observation of the client behavior (such as vital signs, wound healing, and emotional responses), client education, and other aspects of care. Plans should outline *actions* related to client activity, observations, diagnostic studies, therapy, and client education (Yarnall and Atwood 1974, p. 223). See Figure 30–2 on page 632.

Progress notes Progress notes in the POR are made by all members of the health team involved in a client's care: nurse, occupational therapist, dietitian, physician, social worker, and others. All members of the health team add progress notes on the same type of sheet. Progress notes are numbered to correspond to the problems on the problem list.

One systematic format for writing progress notes is referred to as the **SOAP**, an acronym for subjective data, objective data, assessment, and planning. The acronyms SOAPIE and SOAPIER refer to formats that add implementation, evaluation, and revision. Many agencies use only the SOAP. A more recent format is the APIE (assessment, plan, implementation, and evaluation), which condenses the client data into fewer statements (Groah and Reed 1983, p. 1184). In APIE the assessment combines the subjective and objective data with the nursing diagnosis, the plan combines the nursing actions with the expected outcomes, and the implementation and evaluation are the same. See Figure 30–9 later in this chapter for an example of a nurse's progress notes using the SOAP, SOAPIER, and APIE formats.

1. **Subjective data** report what the client perceives and the way the client expresses it.
2. **Objective data** include measurements such as vital signs, observations made by health team members using their senses, laboratory and roentgenographic findings, and client responses to diagnostic and therapeutic measures such as medications. Examples of subjective and objective data are provided in Chapter 11.
3. In the *assessment* stage, the observer makes interpretations and draws conclusions from the subjective and objective data. Again all team members have made assessments, using the knowledge in their possession.

THE UNIVERSITY OF BRITISH COLUMBIA
HEALTH SCIENCES CENTRE HOSPITAL
EXTENDED CARE UNIT

FLOW SHEET

Miss Ann Smith

DATE: January, 1986

PARAMETER/PROCEDURE	TIME	17	18	19	20	21	22	23	24	25	26	27	28	29	30	31
B.P. 92 days weekly	1000				180/88			162/90				160/98			160/90	
(Tues/Fri)																
Weekly diabetic testing																
for G/A																
(at lunch)	1200			N/N							+1/N					
Wash perineal area -																
daily and prn																
Heat lamp to area																
X10-15 mins	1000	JD	JD	JD	CR	CR	CR	CR	YC	YC	YC	PD	PD	PD	ST	PD
Describe skin condition		Red			Red				Less red			Less red			Area	
		excoriated			open area 2 cm				open area			open area			clear	
					no drainage				crusted			healed				
		open area 2.5 cm														
		small amt														
		drainage														

Figure 30–2 A flowsheet on which the parameter or procedures to be measured are written by the nurse.
Source: Courtesy of the University of British Columbia Health Sciences Centre Hospital, Extended Care Unit.

At this point the nurse writes a nursing diagnostic statement in accordance with the guidelines discussed in Chapter 12.

4. The *plan* is a plan for action based on the above data. The initial plan is written by the person who enters the problem into the record. All subsequent plans, considered revisions, also are entered into the progress notes. Plans may include:
   a. Termination of certain activities if the problem is resolved
   b. Initiation of new actions if the problem is unchanged
   c. Activities being done to resolve a particular problem
5. *Implementation,* or *intervention,* is documentation of activities in the plan that were actually done for the client. These entries are very specific.
6. *Evaluation* is documentation of the client's response to the plan, stated in terms of client behavior, e.g., what the client did or said. The question asked at this stage is "Does the client's behavior indicate that the plan was unsuccessful in lessening or alleviating the identified problem?"
7. *Revision,* or *reassessment,* refers to changes that must be made in the initial or original plan. Based on the evaluation notes and decision, the condition of the client may have improved or deteriorated. New data may now be available.

Some portions of the SOAPIER format may not be included in a recording. Some agencies recommend that a notation be made explaining why a portion is missing.

Types of Progress Records

Three kinds of progress notes are generally recognized: narrative notes, flowsheets, and discharge notes. These are used in both source-oriented and problem-oriented medical records.

Narrative Notes

Narrative notes record the client's progress descriptively, on a day-to-day basis. They are keyed to client problems and therapy and are filled out by all members of the health team. If there is no additional information to record on a particular day, the nurse need only enter "as above." Narrative notes are further discussed later in this chapter. In POMRs, narrative notes are always written in the SOAP format. In some hospitals, because of DRGs, a note *must* be written every 24 hours.

Flowsheets

When specific client variables such as pulse, blood pressure, medications, and progress in learning a new skill need to be recorded accurately, narrative notes are often too long. Instead the **flowsheet**, a graphic record, is used to quickly reflect the client's condition. See Figure 30–2. A common example is the vital signs graphic sheet shown in Figure 30–6 later in this chapter.

The time parameters for flowsheets can vary from minutes to months. In a hospital intensive care unit, a client's blood pressure may be monitored by the minute, whereas in an ambulatory clinic, a client's blood glucose level may be recorded once a month.

Flowsheets are also often used in POMRs to record the daily nursing care provided. See Figure 30–3.

Discharge Notes

A discharge note may be written by the physician or another member of the health team, depending on the health care agency. In a home visiting service or community clinic, it may be written by the nurse. The discharge note refers to the client problems identified earlier and describes the degree to which each problem has been resolved. If the client has been referred to another agency, this is also noted. Figure 30–4 shows a nursing discharge summary.

Computer Records

Since about 1968, a number of health institutions have introduced computers. Early installations were primarily in hospital business offices. However, increasing numbers of computers are being used in health care planning and delivery as well as in laboratories and physicians' clinics. For further information see Chapter 31.

Guidelines About Recording

Because the client's record is a legal document and may be used to provide evidence in court, many factors are considered in recording. Health care personnel not only maintain the confidentiality of the client's record but also meet legal standards in the process of recording. Some of these factors are described in the sections

NURSING CARE FLOW SHEET

IMPORTANT CONSIDERATIONS

1. The assigned R.N. is responsible for the documentation of all nursing care. Charting for acute care patients is completed on the Nurses' Notes at least every 24 hrs. Nurses' Notes are completed for long term care patients at least weekly.
2. The initialling of the flow sheet indicates that the required hourly observations of the patient's well-being by nursing staff members have been conducted (including functioning of all equipment, e.g. I.V. infusions).
3. Charting in the Nurses' Notes is necessary when the flow sheet does not adequately reflect the patient's status. [NN] indicates documentation on Nurses' Notes.
4. Complete all boxes. Use a circle [O] for areas that are not applicable.
5. Select the abbreviation that most accurately reflects the patient's condition. Place a tick [✓] e.g. eating well [✓] if the statement reflects the patient's condition.
6. Do not chart pedal pulses or dressings on this flow sheet.

IDENTIFYING INFORMATION

Date	– Insert new date at 0730. This date is for the time frame 0730-0730.
Time Period	– Maximum time period is 12 hours [0730 / 1930] Start a new column for shorter time periods that correspond to changes in patient status (e.g. pre-post op).
Initials	– Assigned nurse inserts initials and completes the Nurses' Signature Record with a full legible signature.

INSTRUCTION FOR COMPLETION OF SUB-SYSTEMS

Urine	– Insert [QS] if patient voiding adequate amounts. – Insert [HNV] if patient has not voided. – Insert amount if measuring urine (ml.) – Insert [FB] if recording amount on Fluid Balance Record.
Stool	– Record number with [0] [1] [SC] – Stool Chart.
Diet	– Insert [T] if patient is on a therapeutic diet. Chart in Nurses' Notes when therapeutic diet is initiated or changed.
Turns	– Record frequency e.g. q2h etc.
Bedrails	– Indicate if one [x1] or, if both, [x2] are raised.
Mobility	– Record highest level of activity achieved. Indicate [WC] under chair, if using wheelchair.

INSERT ONLY THESE ITEMS INTO BLANK SPACES

Blank spaces are provided for recording other routine nursing care not requiring Nurses' Notes.

1. Heparin Lock Intact.
2. I.V. Intact.
3. TPN Intact.
4. Telemetry Intact.
5. Holter Monitor Intact.
6. Urine Strained.
7. Catheter Care.
8. Calorie Count.

Use a [✓] if no problem observed. Chart in Nurses' Notes [NN] where a problem exists.

9. Extremity Check: (CWMS) colour/warmth, movement, sensation of area (identify) and side, e.g. CWMS rt. foot. } Use a [✓] if no problems observed. Document in Nurses' Notes [NN] if problem observed.

10. Eye Patch Intact. } (Identify side)
11. Eye Shield Intact. }
12. Tensor Bandage Intact (Identify side and area).

} Use a [✓] if no problems observed. Document in Nurses' Notes [NN] if problem observed.

13. Oral Intake.
14. Davol Drain.
15. Penrose Drain.
16. Heyer Drain.

} Insert measured amount. Use the FLUID BALANCE RECORD if patient has an I.V. or a 24 hr. fluid balance is necessary.

17. Cardiac Activity Level.
18. Seizure Level.

} Insert number that indicates assigned level. Indicate measurement in box.

19. Abdominal Girth. (Centimeter, Time)

Figure 30–3 A nursing care flow sheet used in conjunction with the problem-oriented record.

Source: Courtesy of the University of British Columbia Health Sciences Centre Hospital.

UBC HEALTH SCIENCES CENTRE HOSPITAL

NURSING CARE FLOW SHEET

Legend:
I – Independent
S – Supervised
Ⓐ – Assisted
T – Total Care
NN – Refer to Nurses' Notes

Section	Legend	Item								
		Date 86	10/2							
	Time Period		0730 1930							
	Initials of nurse assigned to patient		BKE							
EXCRETORY	CT – Catheter CM – Condom I – Incontinent	Urine	CT 750ml							
		Stool (#)	1							
INGESTIVE	N – Normal B – Blenderized MS – Mechanical Soft FF – Fluid CF -- Clear Fluid P – Pureed NPO	Diet (T – Therapeutic)	NPO							
		Eating Poorly								
		Eating Well								
		Weight (kg.)								
PROTECTIVE	HYGIENE	Sponge Bath	✓							
		Tub Bath								
		Shower								
		Mouth Care	q6h							
	SKIN INTEGRITY	Intact								
		Turns	q2h							
	SAFETY P – Posey W – Wrist M – Mitts LT – Lap Tray LR – Lap Restraint	Restraint	M							
		Bed Rails Up (x1) (x2)	x2							
REPARATIVE	MOBILITY AIDS C – Cane CR – Crutches W – Walker WC – Wheelchair	Bedrest (+D = Dangle)	✓+D							
		B.R.P.								
		Chair								
		Walking								
	REST DURING NIGHT	Slept Poorly	✓							
		Slept Well								
	Catheter Care		x1							
	I. V. Intact		✓							

KN 109-1-85 Rev. 1

Figure 30–3 *(continued)*

THE UNIVERSITY OF BRITISH COLUMBIA
HEALTH SCIENCES CENTRE
EXTENDED CARE UNIT

NURSING SUMMARY

MISS ANN SMITH
Age 82 years BD: 1 Aug. 98
Admitted: March 5, 1986

DISCHARGE SUMMARY

Admitted March 5, 1986 from Victoria General Hospital in Victoria, B.C.

Problems

1. Multiple CVAs with bilateral hemiplegia resulting in need for assistance with ADLs and mobility/transfers--needs 2-person assist to transfer, needs maximum assist with ADLs; dressing, washing and bathing done by staff. She is concerned about her appearance.
2. Continent of urine if routinely toileted during the day--occasionally incontinent of urine at night.
3. Prone to constipation--has soft, formed BM q 2-3 days when toileted--needs occasional glycerine suppository and receives Metamucil 15cc daily.
4. Essential hypertension--B.P. ranges from 150/90 to 184/108--monitored 2 days weekly (Tues & Fri.). Receives Nadolol 80 mg daily.
5. Has a history of depression--has become lethargic, withdrawn and weepy at times. Minimal response to antidepressant drugs (Amitriptyline 25 mg ghs - was D/C May 19/87). Involved in numerous social groups and 1-1 interaction--responded well to both. Family visited frequently and very supportive.
6. Diet--minced--has occasional difficulty with swallowing and tongue mobility due to dysarthria.
7. Progressive dysphasia--speech slurred--difficult to understand; very slow to respond; appreciates help from staff.

Next of Kin

Ray Smith--phone 123-4567 (brother)
Sue Brown--phone 261-0941 (niece)

Medication regimen

Metamucil 15 cc daily
Nadolol 80 mg daily
Brandy 30 cc q h.s. prn

Allergies

--elastoplast--suffered period of general pruritus but was unable to relate to specific drugs or food--spontaneously resolved.

Safety Needs

Vision--good/able to read clock on wall and small print
Hearing--able to hear normal conversation
Mechanical aids--side rails and support in chair with pillows and belt restraints
--trunk balance poor
Orientation--well oriented to time, place, person despite deterioration in physical condition

Strengths and Resources

Miss Smith has a very supportive family. She is concerned about her appearance and feels comfortable letting staff know what her needs are.

Resident and family wish Miss Smith to move to LTC facility (X-E.C.U) in South Vancouver as it is much closer for family to visit--family visits 2-3 x weekly.

June 10, 1987
Date

J. Doe, R.N.
Signature

Figure 30–4 A nursing discharge summary.

Source: Courtesy of the University of British Columbia Health Sciences Centre Hospital.

that follow. They apply to either type of recording system.

Restricted Access

The client's record is protected legally as a private record of the client's care. Thus, access to the record is restricted to health workers involved in giving care to the client. Insurance companies, for example, have no legal right to demand access to medical records, even though they may be determining compensation to the client. On the other hand, a client who is making a claim for compensation may ask to have the medical history used as evidence. In this instance, the client must sign an authorization for review, copying, or release of information from the record. This form clearly indicates what information is to be released and to whom. In no instance may a nurse allow access to a client's record by family members or any person other than a caregiver.

For purposes of education and research, most agencies allow student and graduate health professionals access to client records. The records are used in client conferences, clinics, rounds, and written papers or client studies. The student or graduate is bound by a strict ethical code to hold all information in confidence. Some agencies code medical records when they are filed, so that the names of clients are removed. This allows records to be used without identifying individuals. When this is not the practice, it is the responsibility of the student or health care professional to protect the client's privacy by not using a name or any statements in the notations that would identify the client. Many agencies also require documentation from the student or health professional wishing to use medical records of discharged clients. A permission note from the student's instructor will confirm the person's status as a student at a particular school.

Use of Ink

All entries on the client's record are made in black or dark blue ink so that the record is permanent and changes can be identified. Dark-colored ink is generally required because it reproduces well on microfilm and in duplication processes. Entries need to be legible. Hand printing or easily understood handwriting is permissible.

Signature

Each recording on the nursing notes is signed by the nurse making it. The signature consists of the first name, middle initial, legal last name, and the nurse's title or position, abbreviated—for example, "Susan J. Green, RN." The following title abbreviations are often used, but nurses are advised to check the practice in their agencies.

RN registered nurse

LVN licensed vocational nurse

LPN licensed practical nurse

NA nursing assistant

NS nursing student

SN student nurse

Errors

If an error is made, a line is drawn through it, and the word "error" is written above it, with the nurse's initials or name (depending on agency policy). Errors should not be erased or blotted out, so there is no doubt about the nursing care given or the charting error made.

Sample Recording

Date	Time	Notes
Dec 10/87	0100	error A.J.R Pulse ~~180 beats/minute~~ 108 beats/minute.- ———————— Abby J. Roberts, NS

In the above example, the nature of the error is also clear. When it is not, many attorneys feel it is helpful and legally acceptable to indicate what the error was, in order to protect the client and the nurse. An example might be, "Charted for wrong client." The policy of the agency, however, needs to be checked.

Blanks

If a blank appears in a notation, a line is drawn through the blank space and it is signed.

Sample Recording

Date	Time	Notes
Nov 7/87	0730	Urine appears cloudy, light brown with dark flecks. No odor.———Lin I. Ma, NS C/o burning pain in pubic region prior to voiding.————————Lin I. Ma, NS

Accuracy

It is essential that notations on records be accurate and correct. To keep them accurate, notations are written to consist of facts or exact observations, rather than opinions or interpretations of an observation. It is more accurate, for example, to write that the client "refused medication" (fact) than to write that the client "was uncooperative" (opinion); to write that a client "was crying" (observation) is preferable to noting that the client "was depressed" (interpretation). Opinions or interpretations may or may not be accurate. Similarly, when a client expresses worry about the diagnosis or problem, this should be quoted directly on the record: "Stated: 'I'm worried about my leg.' " Nurses should record what they hear as well as what they observe.

Correct spelling is essential for accuracy in recording. If unsure how to spell a word, the nurse looks it up in a dictionary. Most agency units have one available for this purpose. Two decidedly different medications may have similar spellings—for example, digitoxin and digoxin.

Appropriateness

Only information that pertains to the client's health problems and care is recorded. Any other personal information that the client conveys to the nurse is inappropriate for the record. If irrelevant information is recorded, it can be considered an invasion of the client's privacy and/or libelous. A client's disclosure that she or he was a prostitute and has smoked marijuana, for example, would *not* be recorded on the client's medical record unless it had a direct bearing on the client's health problem.

Completeness

Not all data that a nurse obtains about a client can be recorded. However, the information that is recorded needs to be complete and helpful to the client, physicians, other nurses, and participating health care workers. Incomplete records could be used as evidence in court to show that the client did not receive the quality of care considered to meet generally accepted standards. For example, if a diabetic client's record does not indicate that insulin was given and that the urine was tested, the record could be used as evidence of negligence on the part of the nurse responsible for providing this care. Of course, other examples and evidence would be needed to support a finding of negligence by the nurse. However, the client's record can be used to indicate the kind of care given. A complete notation for a client who has vomited, for example, includes the time, the amount, the color, the odor, and any other data about the client (e.g., pain).

Sample Recording

Date	Time	Notes
Aug 12/87	1410	Vomited approx 500 ml of black liquid with foul fecal odor. C/o cramplike pain in epigastric region immediately prior to vomiting.———— Nancy R. Long, NS

The following guide may assist nurses in selecting essential and complete information to record about clients. Note that the emphasis is on facts that denote a change in the client's health status or behavior or that indicate a deviation from what is usually expected. Essential information includes:

1. Any behavior changes, for example:
   a. Indications of strong emotions, such as anxiety or fear
   b. Marked changes in mood
   c. A change in level of consciousness, such as stupor
   d. Regression in relationships with family or friends
2. Any changes in physical function, such as:
   a. Loss of balance
   b. Loss of strength
   c. Difficulty hearing or seeing
3. Any physical sign or symptom that:
   a. Is severe, such as severe pain
   b. Tends to recur or persist
   c. Is not normal, such as elevated body temperature
   d. Gets worse, such as gradual weight loss
   e. Indicates a complication, such as inability to void following surgery

In a legal battle, incomplete medical records may present difficulties that cannot be overcome. Courts take a dim view of evidence based on recall unsupported by written documentation, especially when a great deal of time has elapsed between the events and the trial.

A plaintiff's attorney will never lose an opportunity to draw it to the attention of the jury when an important event went unrecorded by the providers of care. Some courts have held that lack of exactitude in documentation implies lack of attention. In extreme cases, lack of documentation could be considered evidence of negligence. (Cushing 1982)

Research Note

Coronary care nurses have become one of the most highly trained groups within the nursing profession. An important function performed by coronary care nurses is arrhythmia (abnormal heart rhythm) detection. In a study that evaluated the efficiency in arrhythmia detection of the staff of a coronary care unit at a large university hospital by measuring efficiency rate under two different systems of documentation (the only variable manipulated), it was found that the efficiency (speed and accuracy) rate improved with an increase in the quality and quantity of documentation of arrhythmias. Quite simply, when the nurses made more frequent and longer observations of the heart tracings of patients, they were able to pick up a much higher percentage of rhythm changes. This illustrates a fact that cuts across nursing disciplines—the benefit received by a patient is in direct proportion to the actual amount of time and attention the nurse gives to the patient. (Breu and Gowlinski 1981)

f. Is not relieved by prescribed measures, such as continued failure to defecate or to sleep
g. Indicates faulty health habits, such as lice on the scalp
h. Is a known danger signal, such as a lump in the breast

4. Any nursing interventions provided, such as:
   a. Medications administered
   b. Therapies
   c. Activities of daily living, if agency policy dictates
   d. Teaching clients self-care
5. Visits by a physician or other members of the health team

Standard Abbreviations, Symbols, and Terms

The nurse needs to use only commonly accepted abbreviations, symbols, and terms that are specified by the agency. Then, if the record is used in court as evidence, other professionals responsible for interpreting the data can do so correctly. Many abbreviations are standard and used universally; others are confined to certain geographic areas. Some agencies supply a list of the abbreviations they accept. When in doubt about whether to use an abbreviation, the nurse writes the term out in full, until certain about the abbreviation. Table 30–1 lists some commonly used abbreviations (except those used for medications, which are described in Chapter 51). Table 30–2 indicates commonly accepted symbols.

Medical terminology is generally made up of root words, prefixes, and suffixes. A root word may be derived from Latin or Greek. A prefix is a sequence of letters that comes before the word and often describes a variation of the normal. A suffix is a sequence of letters that occurs at the end of the word; it often describes a condition of or act performed on the root word. Root words, suffixes, and prefixes are provided in Appendix B. Further terms are given in the glossary at the end of the book.

Dates and Times

Documentation of the date and time of each notation is essential not only for legal reasons but also for safe care.

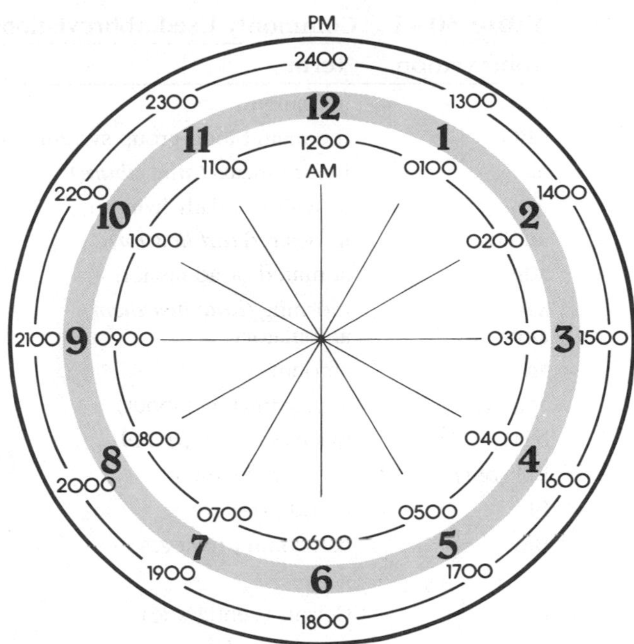

Figure 30–5 The 24-hour clock.

For example, the time at which a narcotic was administered to a client needs to be determined before the next one can safely be given. Time can be recorded in the conventional manner, i.e., 9 A.M. or 3:20 P.M., or according to the 24-hour clock (military clock), which avoids confusion about whether a time was A.M. or P.M. See Figure 30–5.

Brevity

Recordings need to be brief as well as complete, to save time in communication. The client's name and the word "client" are omitted, as it is obvious about whom the nurse is charting. Each thought or sentence is terminated with a period.

Sample Recording

Date	Time	Notes
Aug 21/87	0900	Perspiring profusely. Respirations shallow, wet, 28/min.———Julia L. Cardoza, NS

Records the Nurse Commonly Uses

Client records on which nurses commonly make notations include:

1. The nursing history
2. Flowsheets
3. The nurse's notes (nursing progress notes)
4. The problem list record, in the POR (in source-oriented medical records, the nurse lists the client's problems on the client's nursing care plan)
5. The Kardex and/or nursing care plan
6. The discharge note or summary
7. Consents and releases

Table 30–1 Commonly Used Abbreviations

Abbreviation	Term
abd	abdomen
ABO	the main blood group system
a.c.	before meals *(ante cibum)*
ADL	activities of daily living
ad lib	as desired *(ad libitum)*
adm	admitted or admission
A.M.	morning *(ante meridiem)*
amb	ambulatory
amt	amount
approx	approximately (about)
b.i.d.	twice daily *(bis in die)*
BM (bm)	bowel movement
BP	blood pressure
BRP	bathroom privileges
c̄ (C)	with
C	Celsius (centigrade)
CBC	complete blood count
CBR	complete bed rest
c/o	complains of
DAT	diet as tolerated
dc (disc)	discontinue
drsg	dressing
Dx	diagnosis
ECG (EKG)	electrocardiogram
F	Fahrenheit
fld	fluid
GI	gastrointestinal
GP	general practitioner
gtt	drops *(guttae)*
h. (hr)	hour *(hora)*
H_2O	water
h.s.	at bedtime *(hora somni)*
I & O	intake and output
IV	intravenous
Lab	laboratory
liq	liquid
LMP	last menstrual period
lt (L)	left
meds	medications
ml (mL)	milliliter
mod	moderate
neg	negative
nil (ō)	none
no. (#)	number
NPO (NBM)	nothing by mouth *(per ora)*
NS (N/S)	normal saline
O_2	oxygen
od	daily *(omni die)*
OD	right eye *(oculus dexter);* overdose
OOB	out of bed
os	mouth
OS	left eye *(oculus sinister)*
p.c.	after meals *(post cibum)*
PE (PX)	physical examination
per	by or though
P.M.	afternoon *(post meridiem)*
p.o.	by mouth *(per os)*
postop	postoperative(ly)
preop	preoperative(ly)
prep	preparation
p.r.n.	when necessary *(pro re nata)*
pr (Pt)	patient
q.	every *(quaque)*
q.d.	every day *(quaque die)*
q.h. (q.1h.)	every hour *(quaque hora)*
q.2h., q.3h., etc	every two hours, three hours, etc
q.h.s.	every night at bedtime *(quaque hora somni)*
q.i.d.	four times a day *(quater in die)*
req	requisition
Rt (rt, R)	right
S (s̄)	without *(sine)*
SI	seriously ill
spec	specimen
stat	at once, immediately *(statim)*
t.i.d.	three times a day *(ter in die)*
TL	team leader
TLC	tender loving care
TPR	temperature, pulse, respirations
Tr.	tincture
VO	verbal order
VS (vs)	vital signs
WNL	within normal limits
wt	weight

Nursing Assessment (History)

Nursing assessment forms vary considerably among agencies. Even within an agency, forms may differ among nursing units—for example, an adult medical-surgical unit, an obstetric unit, a pediatric unit, and a psychiatric unit may want different nursing histories. Figure 11–1 on page 240 shows a sample for an adult in a medical-surgical unit.

Histories are usually completed when the client is admitted to the agency. For additional information about nursing histories, see Chapter 11, page 237.

Table 30–2 Commonly Used Symbols

Symbol	Term	Symbol	Number
>	greater than	$\bar{o}$	0
<	less than	$\overline{ss}$	½
=	equal to	$\dot{t}$	1
↑	increased	$\dot{t}\dot{t}$	2
↓	decreased	$\dot{t}\dot{t}\dot{t}$	3
♀	female	$\dot{t}v$	4
♂	male	$\bar{v}$	5
°	degree	$v\dot{t}$	6
#	number; fracture	$v\dot{t}\dot{t}$	7
ʒ	dram	$v\dot{t}\dot{t}\dot{t}$	8
℥	ounce	$\dot{t}x$	9
×	times	$\bar{x}$	10
@	at		

Flowsheets

Flowsheets commonly used are the clinical record, the medication record, the fluid intake and output record, and daily nursing care records such as the one shown in Figure 30–3 on page 634.

Clinical Record

The clinical record (also called the graphic chart or graphic observation record) indicates:

1. Body temperature
2. Pulse rate
3. Respiratory rate
4. Blood pressure readings
5. Weight

Some agencies also show special medications (such as dicumarol), central venous pressure (CVP), 24-hour fluid intake and output, weight, bowel movement, glucose and acetone in the urine, etc. See Figure 30–6.

24-Hour Fluid Balance Record

Before notations are made on a 24-hour fluid balance record, the nurse records the amount of the client's fluid intake and output on a form kept at the client's bedside. The client and support persons should be taught to use this record. It documents intake and output for the duration of one shift only (8 or 12 hours). The totals for each shift are then recorded on the 24-hour fluid balance record. In the sample shown in Figure 30–7, the totals for each 8-hour shift (days, evenings, and nights), are recorded, and then the 24-hour totals are calculated.

All routes of fluid intake must be measured and recorded: oral, intravenous, and gavage (tube feedings into the stomach). Similarly, all routes of fluid loss or output are measured and recorded: urine, emesis (vomitus), diarrhea, and drainage from any tube (such as a T-tube, Levin (nasogastric) tube, suprapubic drain, wound suction, or bladder or ureteral catheter). When heavy perspiration occurs, this also needs to be estimated. More information about ways to measure and record specific amounts of fluid intake and output are described in Chapter 46.

Nurse's Notes

Nurse's notes (also called the *nursing progress notes* or *record*) and the manner of recording vary, depending on whether a source-oriented medical record or POR is used.

In source-oriented medical records, the nursing notes consist of both narrative and chronological charting. **Narrative charting** is a description (narration) of information, and *chronological charting* records data in sequence as time moves forward. The minimum number of words and many abbreviations are used, to keep the information concise. (See "Guidelines about Recording" earlier in this chapter.) Figure 30–8 shows a narrative type of nurse's notes. The forms used for the nurse's notes may vary from place to place. Some agencies have separate columns for treatments, nursing observations, and comments.

The major disadvantage of narrative charting is that it is difficult for a reader to find all the data about a specific problem without examining all of the recorded information. For this reason, specific flow records are often used for certain information.

In the POR, the nurse's progress notes are written in relation to a specific problem identified on the problem list. Graphic records and flowsheets are used to provide other routine or necessary information. When entering nurse's notes in the POR, the SOAP, SOAPIER, or APIE format is used. See Figure 30–9.

Kardex and Nursing Care Plan

The **Kardex** (see Figure 30–10) is a widely used, concise method of organizing and recording data about a client, making information quickly accessible to all members of the health team. The system consists of a series of cards kept in a portable index file. The card for a particular client can be quickly turned up to reveal specific data. Often Kardex data are recorded in pencil so that they can be changed and kept up to date. The information on Kardexes may be organized into sections, for example:

1. Pertinent information about the client, such as name, room number, age, religion, marital status, admission date, doctor's name, diagnosis, type of surgery and date, occupation, and next of kin
2. List of medications, with the date of order and the times of administration for each

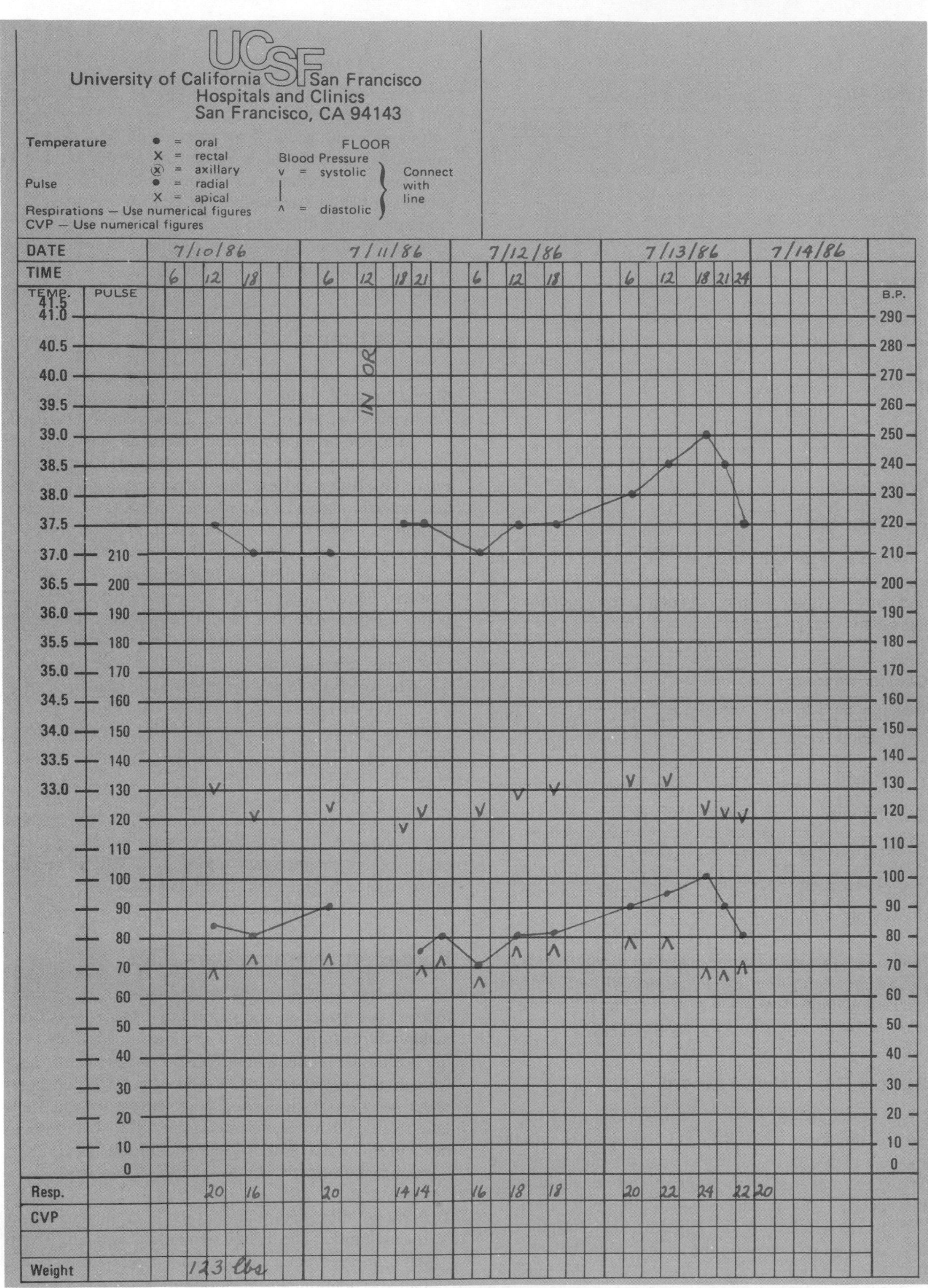

Figure 30–6 A clinical/graph record

Source: Courtesy of the Department of Nursing at the Medical Center, University of California, San Francisco.

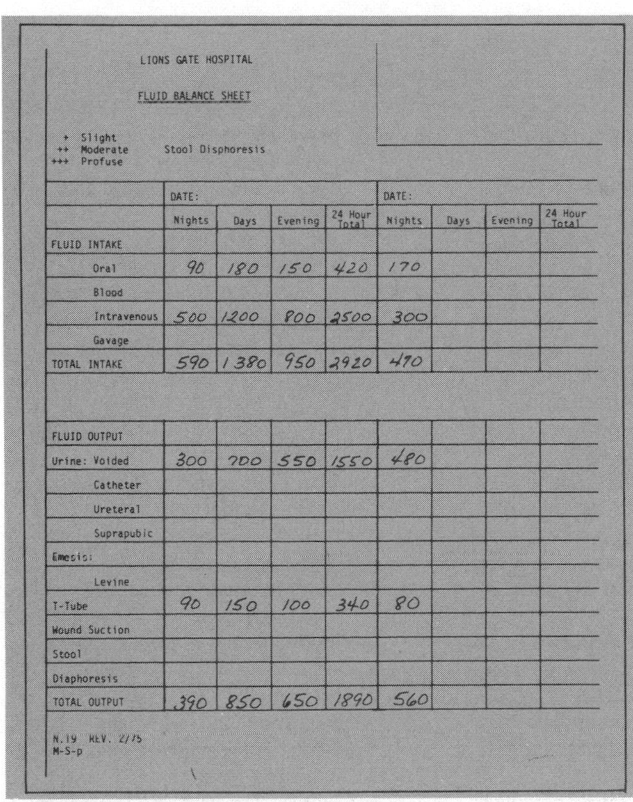

LIONS GATE HOSPITAL

FLUID BALANCE SHEET

\+ Slight
++ Moderate
+++ Profuse

Stool Disphoresis

	DATE:				DATE:			
	Nights	Days	Evening	24 Hour Total	Nights	Days	Evening	24 Hour Total
FLUID INTAKE								
Oral	90	180	150	420	170			
Blood								
Intravenous	500	1200	800	2500	300			
Gavage								
TOTAL INTAKE	590	1380	950	2920	470			
FLUID OUTPUT								
Urine: Voided	300	700	550	1550	480			
Catheter								
Ureteral								
Suprapubic								
Emesis:								
Levine								
T-Tube	90	150	100	340	80			
Wound Suction								
Stool								
Diaphoresis								
TOTAL OUTPUT	390	850	650	1890	560			

N.19 REV. 2/75
M-S-p

Figure 30–7 A sample 24-hour fluid intake and output record.

Source: Courtesy of Lion's Gate Hospital, North Vancouver, British Columbia.

3. List of intravenous fluids, with dates of infusions
4. List of daily treatments and procedures, such as irrigations, dressing changes, postural drainage, or measurement of vital signs
5. List of diagnostic procedures ordered, such as roentgenography or laboratory tests
6. Allergies
7. Specific data on how the client's physical needs are to be met, such as type of diet, assistance needed with feeding, elimination devices, activity, hygienic needs, and safety precautions (use of side rails, etc.)
8. A problem list, stated goals, and a list of nursing approaches to meet the goals and relieve the problems

Although much of the information on the Kardex may be recorded by the responsible nurse or a delegate (e.g., the ward clerk), any nurse who cares for the client plays a key role in initiating the record and keeping the data current. When caring for the client, a nurse has the best opportunity to assess and reassess with the client the accuracy of the information and the effectiveness of treatment.

Discharge Note and Referral Summary

An example of a nursing discharge note was shown earlier in Figure 30–4.

NURSING NOTES

Date	Time	
2/13/87	1400	Passive ROM exercises provided for R arm and leg. Active assistive exercises to L arm and leg. Has scratch marks on L and R forearms. States, "My skin on my back and arms has been itchy for a week." Rash not evident. No previous history of pruritus. Is allergic to elastoplast but has not been in contact. Dr. J. Wong notified.—
	1430	Applied calamine lotion to back and arms.— Incontinent of urine. Is restless.—Tom Ritchie, R.N.

Figure 30–8 An example of narrative nurse's notes.

SOAP Format

2/13/87 #5 Generalized pruritus
1400 S—"My skin is itchy on my back and arms and it's been like this for a week."
O—Skin appears clear—no rash or irritations noted. Marks where client has scratched noted on left and right forearms. Allergic to elastoplast but has not been in contact.
No previous history of pruritus.
A—Alteration in comfort (pruritus): cause unknown
P—Instructed to not scratch skin
—Applied calamine lotion to back and arms at 1430 hrs.
—Cut fingernails
—Assess further to determine if recurrence associated with specific drugs or foods
—Refer to physician and pharmacist for assessment
Tom Ritchie, R.N.

SOAPIER Format

2/13/87 #5 Generalized pruritus
1400 S—"My skin is itchy on my back and arms and it's been like this for a week."
O—Skin appears clear—no rash or irritation noted. Marks where client has scratched noted on left and right forearms. Allergic to elastoplast but has not been in contact.
No previous history of pruritus.
A—Alteration in comfort (pruritus):
P—Instruct not to scratch skin
—Apply calamine lotion as necessary
—Cut nails to avoid scratches
—Assess further to determine if recurrence associated with specific drugs or foods
—Refer to physician and pharmacist for assessment
I —Instructed not to scratch skin
Applied calamine lotion to back and arms at 1430 hrs.
Assisted to cut fingernails
Notified physician and pharmacist of problem
1600 E—States "I'm still itchy. That lotion didn't help."
R—Remove calamine lotion and apply hydrocortisone ungt. as ordered.
Tom Ritchie, R.N.

APIE Format

2/13/87 #5 Generalized pruritus
1400 A—Alteration in comfort; cause unknown. States "My skin is itchy on my back and arms and it's been like this for a week." Skin appears clear
—No rash or irritations noted. Marks where client has scratched noted on left and right forearms. Allergic to elastoplast but has not been in contact. No previous history of pruritus.
P—Instruct to not scratch skin
—Apply calamine lotion as necessary
—Cut nails to avoid scratches
—Assess further to determine if recurrence associated with specific drugs or foods
—Refer to doctor and pharmacist for assessment
I —Instructed not to scratch skin
Applied calamine lotion to back and arms at 1430 hrs.
Assisted to cut fingernails
Notified physician and pharmacist of problem
E—States, "I'm still itchy. That lotion didn't help."
Tom Ritchie, R.N.

Figure 30–9 Examples of nursing progress notes using the SOAP, SOAPIER, and APIE formats.

A referral summary is completed when the client is being discharged and transferred to another institution or to a home setting where a visit by a public health nurse is required. Referral summaries usually include:

1. Any active health problems
2. Current medications
3. Current treatments that are to be continued
4. Eating and sleeping habits
5. Self-care abilities
6. Support networks
7. Life-style patterns
8. Religious preferences

This exchange of information ensures continuity of health care for the client.

Consents and Releases

Unless the client gives consent, certain kinds of care could be considered assault or battery and thus cannot be given (see "Informed Consent" in Chapter 7). It is important for nurses to ensure that the proper consent forms are signed and made part of the client's record. A common form gives consent for treatment and operation. See Figure 53–2.

Release of a client from the hospital without the doctor's consent also necessitates a signed form from the client, to absolve the physician and the hospital of neglect. The nurse often is the one who obtains the client's signature in this less frequent situation.

Reporting

Reports can be either oral or written. The purpose of reporting, in general, is to communicate specific information to a person or group of people. A report should be concise. A good report includes pertinent information, but not extraneous detail.

Two common types of reports are the change-of-shift

NURSING CARE PLAN

KN22-8-80

NAME Mrs. M. Brown

DATE	#	PROBLEM	GOAL	EVALUATION DATE	NURSING INTERVENTIONS	INITIAL	DATE RESOLVED
M-23	1	Anxiety related to SOB secondary to emphysema and respiratory failure	Will have normal skin color and temperature	ongoing	1.1 Keep head of bed at 45° when supine, 20-30° when side-lying		
				daily	1.2 Give O_2 as ordered		
				q shift	1.3 Assess respirations & auscultate chest at least q 8h		
					1.4 Stay with ct. & reassure when she has SOB		
					1.5 Give bronchodilator as ordered		
				ongoing	1.6 Encourage frequent rest periods	JM	
M-23	2	Urinary incontinence related to aging and health status	Will maintain skin integrity	q shift	2.1 Assist onto bedpan or commode q 2h & prn		
					2.2 Provide pericare q 2-4h & prn		
					2.3 Use Attends at night—Pericare each time changed		
					2.4 Turn side to side q 3h & massage bony prominences	JM	
J-17	3	Poor nutritional intake related to extreme SOB	Will eat at least ½ of each meal	q meals	3-1 Feed ct. pureed diet slowly		
					3-2 Feed ct intermittently as tolerated by SOB		
				ongoing	3-3 Ensure adequate fluid intake		
					3-4 Offer some fluid whenever in room	JM	
J-22	4	Nosebleeds related to unknown cause	Will experience no further nosebleeds	q shift	4-1 Assess condition of nares q shift		
					4-2 Lubricate nares c̄ water-soluble lubricators		
				ongoing	4-3 Report all nosebleeds to physician	JM	

DATE	DISCHARGE PLAN	INITIAL	CONSULTATIONS
M-22	Lives in basement apartment of daughter's home		
	Has home O_2, homemaker, and homecare nurse		
M-25	S. W. consult to arrange for extended care		

Figure 30–10 An example of a nursing Kardex. *(continued)*

Source: Courtesy of the University of British Columbia Health Sciences Centre Hospital.

DATE	
May 23/86	No Code Blue In case of decease – forms are stamped and on back of chart (see letter from daughter)
May 25/86	Secretion precautions – sputum

DATE	TREATMENTS
June 20	Continuous O_2 @ 4 l/min nasal prongs
June 22	May get up for walks c̄ portable O_2
Nights	Change O_2 bottle, tubing, and Ventolin tubing and mask q 2 d June 2, 4, 6, 8, 10, 12
June 2/86	No I.V. infusion unless daughter notified first – Family request

DATE TO BE DONE	LABORATORY TESTS	FAST	DONE
Aug 7/86	Swab Lt forearm C & S		✓
Aug 14/86	Swab Rt eye C & S		✓
Aug 20/86	Discontinue all blood tests		✓

WEIGHT

DIET — ASSIST ☐

May 22/86	Reg. — pureed diet Needs to be fed

ACTIVITY AND HYGIENE — L.B.M. June 22

June 28/86	Toilet program q 2 h

DIAGNOSTIC PROCEDURES

INTRAVENOUS

None

SURGICAL PROCEDURES

REFERRALS

May 22/86	Chest physio & mobilization
May 22/86	Dietary consult

DIAGNOSIS AND PERTINENT HISTORY

Emphysema & respiratory failure

ALLERGIES None known.

INTAKE ☐ OUTPUT ☐

VITAL SIGNS daily

NEXT OF KIN Mrs. C. Smith

RELATIONSHIP daughter

TELEPHONE 555-5555 (home) 555-1111 (work)

BED NO.	NAME	AGE	ADMITTING DOCTOR	RESIDENT
218D	Mrs. M. Brown	79.	Dr. Imrie	None

KN21-8-80

Figure 30–10 *(continued)*

report and the incident report. The incident report is discussed in Chapter 7 on page 164.

Change-of-Shift Report

A *change-of-shift report* is an oral report usually given by the on-duty charge nurse to all nursing personnel coming on duty. Variations occur, however. In units where primary nursing is employed the report may be given from one RN to another; in units where team nursing is practiced the report may be given from one team leader to another. Change-of-shift reports may be given either in a face-to-face exchange or by audiotape recording. The face-to-face report allows the listener to ask questions during the report, although if given to all on-coming nurses it can be time-consuming. On-coming nurses, for example, are required to listen to the report on all clients, including many not under their care. The tape-recorded report is often briefer and less time-consuming. It allows the charge nurse to finish last-minute responsibilities before going off duty.

Guidelines that can help nurses prepare and present reports about clients include (Hesse 1983 and Smith 1986):

1. Follow a particular order when reporting about a series of clients. For example, follow room numbers in a hospital or times of appointments in a community clinic.
2. Identify the client by name, room number, and bed designation. For example, Mrs. Jessie Jones, 702, Bed D. This enables the listeners, especially float nurses or those returning from days off or vacation, to immediately relate subsequent information to this client's case.
3. Depending on the type of unit, provide the reason for admission, that is, the client's medical diagnosis or original complaint. This information may not be necessary in long-term geriatric units or newborn nurseries; in acute-care settings, however, it is often necessary because of multiple tests, consultations, and transfers.
4. Include diagnostic tests and/or results and other therapies performed in the past 24 hours, such as blood transfusions, surgery, initiation of intravenous therapy, narcotics administered, blood gas levels, and group therapy data.
5. Note any significant changes in the client's condition. On-coming nurses must know about changes for the worse to monitor the client's condition appropriately. Significant improvements toward goal attainment should also be noted so the nurse can provide positive feedback to the client.
6. When reporting about changes, present the pertinent information in this order: assessment, nursing diagnoses (if appropriate), planning, intervention, and evaluation. For example, "Mr. Ronald Oakes said he had an aching pain in his left calf at 1400 hours. Inspection revealed no other signs. Calf pain is related to altered blood circulation. Rest and elevation of his legs on a footstool for 30 minutes provided relief."
7. Provide exact information, such as "Ms. Jessie Jones received Demerol 100 mg intramuscularly at 2000 hours (8 P.M.)," not "Ms. Jessie Jones received some Demerol during the evening."
8. Do not include unremarkable measurements such as normal temperature, pulse, and blood pressure unless a desired change is involved. For example, a normal body temperature for a client who has had an elevated temperature should be reported.
9. Report the client's emotional responses that need attention before other interventions can be implemented. For example, a client who has just learned his biopsy results revealed malignancy and who is now scheduled for a laryngectomy needs time to discuss his feelings before the nurse commences preoperative teaching.

Conferring

To **confer** is to consult another person or persons for advice, information, ideas, or instructions. Nurses confer with colleagues and other health professionals about some aspect of client care or to elicit or validate data needed to plan nursing care. Two ways nurses share information are through the nursing care conference and nursing care rounds.

Nursing Care Conferences

A **nursing-care conference** is a meeting of a group of nurses to discuss possible solutions to certain problems of a client, such as inability to cope with an event or lack of progress toward goal attainment. Examples: a middle-age woman is so distressed about her body image after mastectomy that she is not perceiving her husband's love and not performing her arm exercises; an adolescent boy with severe diabetes is not following his diet but is eating chocolate bars and milk shakes that he has enticed his friends to bring into the hospital for him. The nursing care conference allows each nurse an opportunity to offer an opinion about possible solutions to the problem. Other health practitioners or nurse-clinicians may be invited to attend the conference to offer their expertise; for example, a nurse-clinician may discuss the emotional problems of a severely burned child and his responses, or a dietitian may discuss dietary problems.

Nursing care conferences are most effective when there is a climate of respect—i.e., nonjudgmental acceptance of others even though their values, opinions, and beliefs may seem different. The nurse needs to accept and respect each person's contributions, listening with an open mind to what others are saying even when the nurse disagrees. Everyone can learn new ways of approaching situations when they conscientiously listen to another perspective.

Nursing Care Rounds

Nursing care rounds refers to a procedure in which a group of nurses visit all or selected clients at each client's bedside to:

1. Obtain information that will help plan nursing care
2. Provide the client the opportunity to discuss his or her care
3. Evaluate the nursing care the client has received

During rounds the nurse assigned to the client provides a brief summary of the client's nursing needs and the interventions being implemented. The advantage of nursing rounds for the clients is that they can participate in the discussions; the advantage for the nurses is that they can see the client being discussed. To facilitate client participation in nursing care rounds, nurses need to use terms that the client can understand. Medical terminology excludes the client from discussion.

Chapter Highlights

- Health team members must communicate among themselves effectively to provide coordinated, high-quality care.
- When there is accurate communication, all health team members become informed about client needs, and overlapping of activities is avoided.
- Written records serve several purposes. They ensure transmission of information to all health workers caring for the client, are a source of research, educational, and statistical data, and allow the audit of client care standards.
- Client records are admissible as evidence in a court of law.
- The problem-oriented medical record (POMR or POR) (Weed system) is increasingly recognized as a method that provides a client-centered problem-solving approach to care.
- The POR has four basic components: a defined database, a complete problem list, an initial plan for each identified problem, and progress notes.
- Progress notes follow the systematic SOAP format and include narrative notes, flowsheets, and discharge notes.
- Traditional client records are source-oriented records, in that each category of health worker keeps separate records.
- Traditional records generally have six parts: admission sheet, face sheet, physician's order sheet, medical history sheet, nurses' notes, and other special records such as the laboratory records.
- The Kardex record is widely used for quick access to current data about clients.
- Computerized information systems are being used increasingly in health care agencies.
- Record entries should be brief, accurate, legible, chronological, made on consecutive lines, and appropriately signed.
- Record entries are made after nursing interventions and usually when the client is admitted or transferred.
- Because the record is a legal document, nurses sign their full legal names and use standard terms and abbreviations.
- Erasures on the client record are not permitted.
- Reports about clients need to be concise and pertinent and must include significant changes in the client's condition and therapy.
- Two ways in which nurses share information needed to plan nursing care are the nursing care conference and nursing rounds.

Suggested Readings

Eggland, E. T. February 1980. Charting: How and why to document your care daily—and fully. *Nursing 80* 10:38–43.
Eggland explains the purposes of daily charting and the mechanics and ways to chart in specific instances, for example, when the client refuses a treatment. Eggland also gives information about nurses' notes and errors and a list of do's and don'ts of daily charting.

King, I. M. April 1984. Effectiveness of nursing care: Use of a goal-oriented nursing record in end stage renal disease. *The American Association of Nephrology Nurses and Technicians Journal* 1:11–17, 60.
King's theory of goal attainment provides the basis for this goal-oriented nursing record (GONR). The GONR system, a modification of the problem-oriented medical record designed for physicians, was designed for nurses to gather

data in a systematic way, to record data, to identify nursing problems, make a nursing diagnosis, construct a goal list, write orders for nursing care, and report the effectiveness of nursing care through goal attainment. In this article King discusses the seven elements of GONR: database, problem list, goal list, nursing orders, flowsheets, progress notes, and discharge summary and applies them to a client with end-stage renal disease (ESRD).

McKiel, R. E., and Rogers, C. A. March/April 1986. The chart critique: A learning activity for nursing students. *Nurse Educator* 11:23–24.

This article describes the chart critique, a written assignment designed to help students develop skill in using a client's chart as one resource for identifying actual and potential problems and planning nursing care. The chart critique questionnaire is provided.

Rutkowski, B. October 1985. How D.R.G.s are changing your charting. *Nursing 85* 15:49–51.

Because of DRGs, peer review organizations and hospital administrators are looking at nursing notes more thoroughly than ever before. Nursing notes therefore must be more concise, specific, and complete. The SOAP format is discussed as one way to meet the current need.

Simpson, K. June 1985. Using Kardex cards to improve the quality of patient care. *The Canadian Nurse* 81:37–40.

While serving as a medical-surgical clinical specialist in an acute-care hospital in San Francisco, Simpson developed a new Kardex design. Samples of the four cards are shown. Of note is a client-teaching card that includes the client's previous education, barriers to learning, check list of education completed, and discharge planning.

Selected References

Bell, E. A. March 1981. Charting: How to get out of a rut. *Nursing 81* 11:43.

Bergerson, S. R. July/August 1982. Charting with a jury in mind. *Nursing Life* 2:30–33.

Blount, M., et al. September 1978. Documenting with the problem-oriented record system. *American Journal of Nursing* 78:1539–42.

Breu, C., and Gowlinski, A. November/December 1981. A comparative study of the effects of documentation on arrhythmia detection efficiency. *Heart and Lung* 10(6):1058–62.

Costello, S., and Summers, B. Y. June 1985. Documenting patient care: Getting it all together. *Nursing Management* 16:31–34.

Creighton, H. 1981. *Law every nurse should know.* 4th ed. Philadelphia: W. B. Saunders Co.

Cushing, M. December 1982. The legal side. Gaps in documentation. *American Journal of Nursing* 82:1899–1900.

Donaghue, A. M., and Reiley, P. J. November 1981. Some do's and don'ts for giving report. *Nursing 81* 11:117.

Eggland, E. T. February 1980. Charting: How and why to document your care daily—and fully. *Nursing 80* 10:38–43.

Gay, P. March 1983. Get it in writing. *Nursing Management* 14:32–35.

Glover, J. C. December 1981. Reducing discharge planning paperwork with a pocket-size discharge planning record. *Nursing 81* 11:50–51.

Greenlaw, J. September 1982. Documentation of patient care: An often underestimated responsibility. *Law, Medicine and Health Care* 10:172–74.

Groah, L., and Reed, E. A. May 1983. Your responsibility in documenting care. *Association of Operating Room Nurses Journal* 37:1174, 1176–77, 1180–85.

Hesse, G. February 1983. A better shift report means better nursing care. *Nursing 83* 13:65. Canadian ed. 13:17.

Johnson, I., and Stegen, A. January/February 1982. Will the computer be the new "nurses" aid? *Registered Nurses Association of British Columbia News* 14:8–9.

Katz, B. F. April 1983. Reporting and review of patient care: The nurse's responsibility. *Law, Medicine and Health Care* 11:76–79.

Kunkel, J. March/April 1983. Charting: Some pointers for doing it better. *Nursing Life* 3:57–64.

Memorial Hospital of Burlington County, Mt. Holly, N.J. September/October 1985. Cut documentation time by 50%. *Nursing Life* 5:30–32.

Mezzanotte, E. J. April 1976. Getting it together for end-of-shift reports. *Nursing 76* 6:21–22.

Pepper, G. A. June 1978. Bedside report: Would it work for you? *Nursing 78* 8:73–74.

Regan, W. A. July 1980. Legally speaking: Verbal orders: Invitations to disaster. *RN* 43:61–62.

Rich, P. L. March 1983. Make the most of your charting time. *Nursing 83* 13:34–39.

——— July 1985. With this flow sheet less is more. *Nursing 85* 15:25–29.

Sklar, C. L. March 1978. Legal significance of charting. *The Canadian Nurse* 74:10–11.

——— February 1981. You and the law: When nurses fail to communicate. *The Canadian Nurse* 77:47–48.

——— May 1984. The patient's record, an invaluable communication tool. *The Canadian Nurse* 80:50, 52.

Smith, C. E. February 1986. Upgrade your shift reports with the three R's. *Nursing 86* 16:63–64.

Weed, L. L. 1971. *Medical records, medical education and patient care: The Problem-oriented record as a basic tool.* Cleveland: Case Western Reserve University Press.

Yarnall, S. R., and Atwood, J. June 1974. Problem-oriented practice for nurses and physicians. General concepts. *Nursing Clinics of North America* 9(2):215–28.

CHAPTER **31**

Computers in Nursing and Health

Rita Olivieri

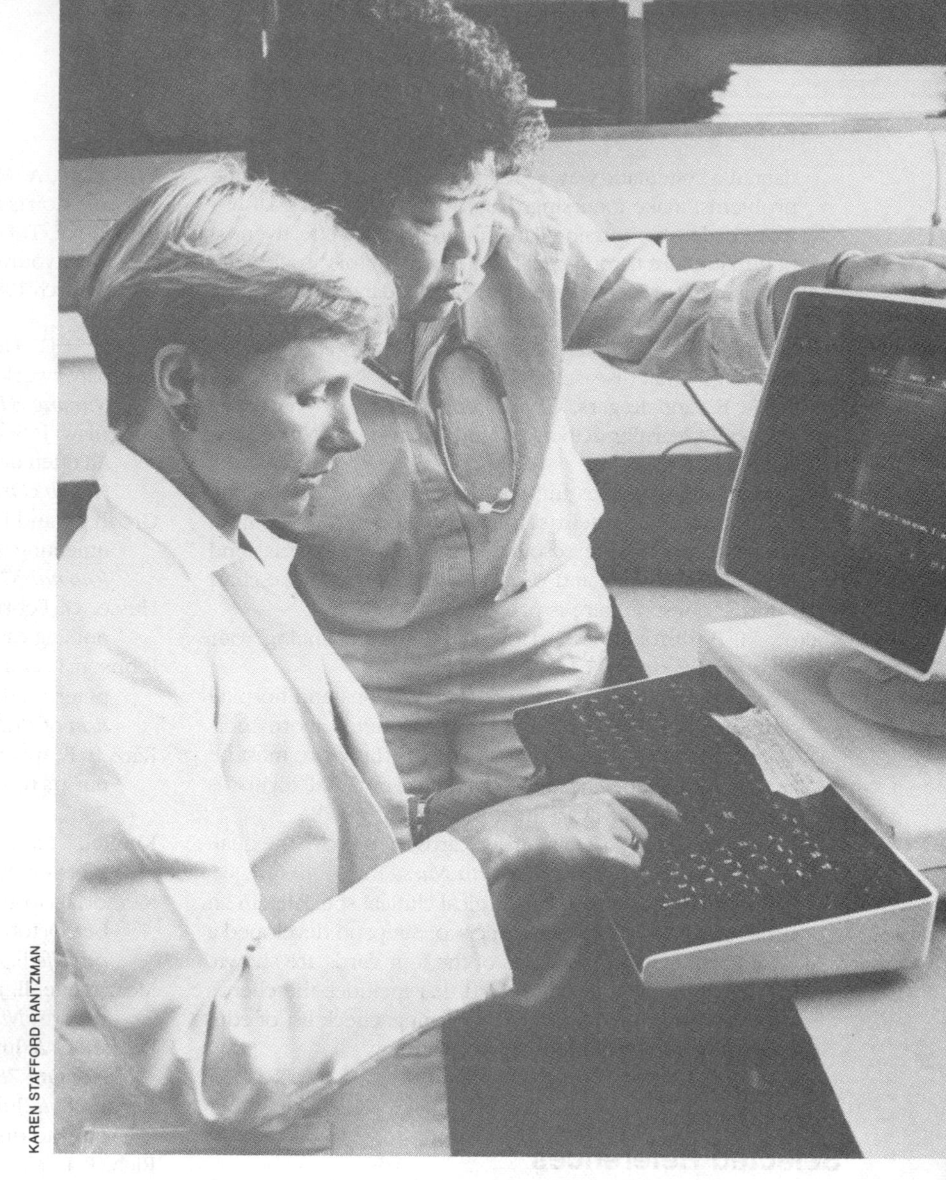

KAREN STAFFORD RANTZMAN

Contents

Objectives

1. Appreciate the current applications of the computer in nursing.
   1.1 Describe the features of an automated client care system.
   1.2 Identify ways in which the nurse can use the computer to organize client care.
   1.3 Describe the benefits of an automated client care planning system.
   1.4 Explain the concept of an expert system.
   1.5 Describe the advantages of a computerized client discharge summary.
   1.6 Identify the role of the computer in nursing research.
   1.7 Identify the role of the computer in nursing management.
   1.8 List some currently available computer applications in classroom education.
   1.9 Identify how the computer is used in client education in the clinical and community settings.
   1.10 Give some examples of computer-based client monitoring systems.
2. Understand the computer concepts that are necessary for the nurse to know.
   2.1 List the advantages of word processing.
   2.2 Identify a spreadsheet application.
   2.3 Explain the concept of a database management system.
   2.4 Identify the advantages of a telecommunications system.
   2.5 Differentiate between computer devices used for input, processing, and output.
   2.6 List three ways that computer output can be displayed.
   2.7 Compare a microcomputer with a mainframe computer.
   2.8 Describe three ways to input information into a computer.
3. Indicate the computer applications likely to affect nurses during the next decade.
   3.1 List some of the future computer applications in the health care setting.
   3.2 Explain some technologic developments expected in the future.
   3.3 Describe some of the possible changes in information storage and retrieval.
4. Explain some important issues in computing and how they relate to the role of the nurse.
   4.1 Describe the threats to client privacy posed by computer systems.
   4.2 List some reasons why client records are accessed.
   4.3 Explain the role of the nurse in the design of computerized hospital information systems.
   4.4 Explain the possible effects of ignoring the nurse's role when a computer system is designed.
5. List the avenues by which to obtain additional information about computers.
   5.1 Describe the resources nurses can use to enhance their computer knowledge.

Terms

artificial intelligence	field	mainframe	records
CD ROMs	file	microcomputer	software
CPU	graphics	minicomputer	spreadsheet
database	hardware	modem	storage devices
disk (diskette)	input	mouse	telecommunications
disk drive	laser printer	output	terminals
dot-matrix printer	letter-quality printer	processing	touch screen
expert system	light pen	programs	word processing

Current Applications of Computers in Nursing and Health Care

By the turn of the century, most nurses will use computers in many aspects of their professional practice. Already, "user friendly" machines are of great help to the nurse in assessing, planning, implementing, and evaluating nursing care. The nurse educator and the nurse manager have also discovered the usefulness of computers in managing staffing, budgeting, producing grade reports, writing papers, and improving productivity. In fact, computer skills and knowledge will soon be expected and perhaps required for a great many positions. Those who ignore this technologic revolution may be left behind.

The nurse is clearly the manager of client care. Hospital information flows to and through nursing departments. Nurses who allow computer systems to design their practice may find themselves both frustrated and victimized. Instead, they must take an active role in the design, development, and implementation of any such systems. Those professional nurses who understand the conceptual framework of computer applications will find computers to be an extraordinarily useful tool in their professional practice.

Nursing Practice

Nursing Care Plans

In the past, hospital computer applications have been administrative. Tasks such as patient billing, maintaining financial records, and long-term planning are necessary aspects in support of the business side of the hospital. As computers get smaller, less costly, more powerful, and easier to use, they will be used increasingly in other areas of the health care system as well. Today, it is common to find a microcomputer system or computer terminal in the nurse's station. It is likely that such machines will become a more integral part of the nurse's activities during the next decade. Some examples of existing computer systems illustrate this point clearly.

An automated client care planning system has been designed on the premise that nurses, "besides directly caring for patients according to the principles of the nursing process, actually should organize and manage the patient's hospital care" (Albrecht and Lieske 1985).

This client care system allows an "on line" (i.e., directly connected to the computer) use of standardized nursing care plans (see Figure 31–1). These care plans are categorized according to the taxonomy of the North American Nursing Diagnosis Association (NANDA). Nursing staff are thus able to create a care plan easily, customize it for each client, type in additions as needed, evaluate and update information at any time, and retrieve data appropriate to a specific nursing diagnosis.

One such system provides work lists, as needed, directly from the computer. In this way, lists generated for treatments, procedures, and medications can always be kept up to date. Such an application eliminates the need for the Kardex (a card filing system) and the treatment sheets, since all of the same information is available both in the computer and on computer-printed update forms (McNeill 1979).

A management information system (MIS) containing patient data can provide many benefits to the nurses, staff, and administrators at a client care facility. One such system has been in existence for about 10 years and its use has resulted in (a) significant reduction of written documentation, (b) simpler entry and retrieval of client information, (c) improved communication, and (4) better legibility, accuracy, and quality of the information being maintained (Romano et al. 1985).

Specific ways in which an automated client care plan can facilitate the role of the nurse include the following:

1. Entry of nursing assessments is simplified; e.g., the nurse can touch a computer screen display of possibilities.
2. Laboratory data can be ordered by entering a request at a computer workstation.
3. Laboratory results can be retrieved in a shorter time with less paperwork.
4. The system facilitates complete and legible medication orders.
5. The system promotes consistent doctor's orders (verbal orders are not accepted).
6. The nursing implications of a doctor's order can be sent to the nurse. Client preparation needs for a particular test can be listed automatically in the client's nursing care plan.
7. The use of nursing diagnosis is facilitated; a common format can be used.
8. Current information can be updated easily. Discontinued medication orders can be deleted easily, making all information timely, legible, and complete.

Research Note

A study by Ball, Snelbecker, and Schecter sought to find out how nurses view the influence of computer technology on nursing and nurses' roles, and how their views changed following a presentation and discussion of computer uses in nursing. The investigators found that most nurses reacted favorably to the idea of incorporating computers into their work; in addition, 58% of the reactions to certain statements about computers were more favorable after the presentation. The authors conclude that employers should do preliminary assessments of the attitudes of their employees and be prepared to offer computer literacy coursework specifically geared to the work at hand. (Ball et al. 1985)

Expert Systems

The term *expert system* will no doubt become familiar to those in the health care professions over the next decade. An **expert system** is a computer-based model (using some

Client name :	Martha Johnson	**Rm number**	403
Admission date :	05/25/87		
Sex :	F	**Religion :**	Catholic
Age :	54	**Date of birth :**	03/13/33
Admitting physician :	Dr. Raymond Atkins		
Medical diagnosis :	Diabetes		
Primary nurse :	Judy Foster, R.N.		
Allergies :	Penicillin	**Diet :**	1500 c ADA
Risk factors :	Hearing aid	**Vital signs :**	T.I.D.
Nursing diagnosis :	Impairment of skin integrity related to pruritus.		
Long-term goals :	Client will experience improved skin integrity within 48 hours.		

Short-term goals	Nursing interventions	Evaluation
Givcn thc prcscribed care, client will experience descreased itching sensation.	1. Infrequent baths. 2. Use cool water. 3. Soap substitute. 4. Blot skin dry. DO NOT RUB! 5. Lubricate skin with lotion after bath.	
Client will understand and implement health teaching.	1. Explain phenomenon of itching. 2. Teach avoidance of excessive warmth. 3. Teach need for increased humidity.	

Figure 31–1 Computer-generated nursing care plan

of the principles of an exciting area of computer science called **artificial intelligence**) that strives to simulate the way human experts in a particular discipline gather data and make decisions. The human expert is an important part of the design of these systems. Although many exciting applications of such systems are not yet developed, some are currently being used.

COMMES (Creighton On-Line Multiple Modular Expert Systems) is an artificial intelligence system that can simulate a consultation with a professional nurse. To do so, the system must have a current knowledge base and be able to mimic professional decision-making skills while avoiding the risk of providing incorrect or inappropriate data (Ryan 1985).

The COMMES system provides several options within its "consultant" framework. By using the Educational (BSN) consultant, the staff nurse enters keywords (e.g., *emphysema* and *rehabilitation*) that define information needed to resolve client care problems. The computer system then provides recommendations in the form of goals and suggests specific reading material to provide further information. An audio-visual database consultant component, in a similar way, refers the nurse to those resources that are available in the local audio-visual department.

These applications are only just beginning to fulfill the promise of expert systems. Some are, in many ways, just computer databases that allow retrieval of data in various ways. It is quite likely that, in the near future, expert systems will not only contain the information of a human considered an expert in a particular field but also the logical analysis capability of that human expert and his or her decision-making capability. In this way, the "system" can begin to provide assistance in educational settings, hospital settings, and emergency settings and facilitate client care of consistent quality.

Some such expert systems already exist. The INTERNIST system accepts data (e.g., the results of tests, a client history, etc.), questions the physician for additional symptoms, and then offers possible diagnoses based upon the responses of the physician, the specific client information, and the knowledge base in the computer (Pople 1977).

Other such systems include:

MYCIN provides advice in the diagnosis and treatment of infections.

IRIS tracks associations between glaucoma and disease processes.

CASNET offers glaucoma medical diagnosis by computer.

EXPERT provides advice in rheumatology, ophthalmology, and endocrinology.

Some of these expert systems not only assist in diagnosis but also provide guidelines for treatment and predict the course of the disease.

Discharge Summaries

With access to a completely automated care plan, the nurse can prepare client discharge summaries that include information from the time of admission. These summaries are important in determining the appropriate follow-up care for the client in the home, the outpatient setting, or the doctor's office. These reports can include all current unresolved nursing diagnoses and the relevant interventions. Computer-generated reports can include relevant information for teaching the client, including instructions about the use of drugs, details of a required diet, activity restrictions, and the date of the next visit to return to the physician's office.

Nursing Research

Computers have facilitated research in many ways. As more nurses become familiar with computer use, their ability to access timely and relevant information increases greatly. **Databases** are collections of information on particular topics. These repositories of information are generally kept in a computer and accessed via a computer/telephone link. Services such as Med-line allow the researcher to enter a few keywords on a particular topic. The computer can then be directed to search through all of the entries in a database and select all references that contain those keywords. Depending upon the length and extent of the resulting entries, one can either look at the selections immediately or have them forwarded by surface mail in the next day or two. Since many databases contain several years of citations, this process can save the nurse researcher an enormous amount of time.

Nursing research is also made easier by the computer's ability to access information in client records. Many hospitals maintain extensive computerized records. If access to these data is allowed, the nurse researcher can gather information that may be important in a particular study or project. For example, a researcher interested in determining what interventions were most successful in caring for clients with the nursing diagnosis "Alteration in skin integrity" can retrieve the care plans containing this information from the computer-based record. In addition, other key variables, such as the client's age, background, sex, etc., can be obtained and used to facilitate the analysis of the research problem. Collecting these data manually (if they were available at all) would take a long time.

Nursing Management

The particular needs of the nursing administrator or manager can often be met by a hospital's computer system. The director of nurses or the division head of client services in a hospital needs data related to staffing, nurse scheduling, budgeting, and the evaluation of client services. If the appropriate information is stored in a computer-based information system, the manager can generate reports on the acuity levels of clients on each unit. These can be used to devise a formula for determining both the appropriate skill levels and the number of nurses required per shift and per floor. In addition, the scheduling of personnel is often made difficult by changing shifts, different skill levels, vacations, weekends, legal coverage requirements, and so on. Computer-based scheduling models can save much time and provide options that can be difficult to discover if the information is handled manually.

Nursing Education

In the educational setting, the computer is becoming increasingly important, both as a teaching tool and as a resource for improving faculty and student productivity. It is likely that the use of the computer in these ways will increase dramatically over the next few years as these machines become easier to use.

At present, the literature search is a popular and useful feature. It is now quite common to find very large bibliographic databases of nursing, medical, and health care information. Access to this information by nursing students and faculty is critical to getting timely and relevant information.

In the training labs, the "medical dummy" is, in many ways, a robot. Depending on the sophistication of the device, such mannequins can simulate many of the circumstances that affect real clients. These teaching tools are effective because they add realism to the learning experience.

Finally, many computer programs have been written in support of the teaching environment. These applications vary considerably in terms of their quality and effectiveness. However, as more applications are developed by members of the health care community, both the quantity and the quality of computer applications in nursing education are likely to increase.

Table 31–1 shows some educational applications that are currently available. Although brief, the list in the table illustrates the variety of computer applications available in health education.

Client education has also been furthered by the computer. Computers are an effective tool in this regard because they allow "customized" instruction, client interaction, immediate feedback, and a private (often motivating) learning environment. Some research studies have shown that clients often prefer such instruction (Ellis et al. 1982). In addition, it has been shown that computer-based models of instruction are effective, save time, and are well received by students in an academic setting (Bitzer and Boudroux 1980).

It is equally important to consider the impact that such systems can have on primary prevention. For example, Ellis and Raines (1981, p. 81) found that "health fair participants waited in lines for up to 30 minutes for a chance to use microcomputers that were running computer programs related to good health habits."

It is quite likely that the microcomputer will become even more pervasive as a resource for educators and students. Additional computer applications programs in nursing and health care will be developed, machines will become easier to use, and professional and academic organizations will begin to require graduates to have some familiarity with them.

Other Areas of the Health Care System

Nurses, in their day-to-day activities, are likely to come in contact with a wide variety of computer-based systems and equipment. It is useful to give a brief list of some of the major ones. This list gives some insight into the technology in the health care disciplines.

Computer-Based Scanning Systems

The CAT (computerized axial tomography) scanner is a computer-controlled device that combines x-ray machinery with computers to produce detailed pictures of slices of the human body.

The PET (positron emission tomography) scanner can map brain activity and help determine if a client is suffering from abnormal metabolism, epilepsy, schizophrenia, and a variety of other health problems.

Table 31–1 Selected Computer Applications Available in Health Education

Computer Program	What It Does	Audience
Calculate with Care	Tutorial for mathematics	Beginning students
NURSESTAR	Review of nursing	RN students
TESTSTAR	Test construction	Nursing faculty
Build Medical Vocabulary	Tutorial/drill	Beginning students
Cardiac Arrest Simulation	Tutorial and simulation	Nurses and physicians
Hemodynamic Management	Clinical simulation	Critical care RNs
Clinical Nursing	Computer simulations	Advanced nursing students
Drug Interactions	Database of interactions	Nursing students
Nasogastric Suction	Client care simulations	Nursing students
Chest Suction	Client care simulations	Nursing students
Sugar	Hyperglycemia	Nursing students
Pre-lab Testing	30 pre-lab nursing test	Beginning students
Dosages and Solutions	Medication dosage math	Beginning students
Health History	Taking health histories	Beginning students
Genetic Training	Basic human genetics	Nurses
Drug Therapy	Tutorial	Nursing students
CPR Certification	CPR exam	Nurses, students
Gross Anatomy	Tutorials	Nursing students
Automated Nurse Staffing	Staffing application	Administrators

Client Monitoring Systems

The monitoring of clients in clinical practice includes monitoring and recording a client's vital signs, electrocardiograph (EKG) recording, and a variety of other physiologic parameters. More sophisticated systems feature automated blood and fluid infusion and pulmonary monitoring systems that detect errors and provide corrective action (Martin 1982; Johnson et al. 1980).

Major Application Areas

Computers are useful only because people enter instructions that direct the machine to perform certain tasks. The machine can do nothing without instructions. When these instructions are put together to solve a problem, they are referred to as computer **programs**, which are also called applications programs, or simply **software**. Most users of programs never have to write them; most users are content to use programs developed by others. The following sections address areas where computers are now being routinely applied. For purposes of consistency, all such applications programs will be called software.

Word Processing

The ability to manipulate words entered into a computer's memory can save both time and effort. For example, to prepare an extensive clinical report for an instructor, nursing students must laboriously gather the data, write a rough draft by hand, and then spend several hours typing the final version. The following day, the student hands in a 20-page masterpiece to the instructor, who reviews it and suggests several additions and deletions. The student who used a traditional typewriter has only one choice: Make the corrections and retype the entire report. A more common alternative is to use a word processor.

Word processing refers to the process of using a computer to prepare papers and reports. The advantages of using a computer are many. They include:

1. The paper, once typed, can be saved on a storage device, for instance, a **disk**. Thus, any changes, additions, or deletions can be made quickly without retyping the entire paper.
2. The computer can be told how to format the paper before final printing. That is, the user can specify the margins, the position and sequence of all page numbers, the type of paper to be used (e.g., letterhead or continuous form paper), the number of copies to be printed, and so on.
3. Of particular importance is the fact that the computer reorganizes (retypes) the paper to accommodate additions or deletions.
4. Many word processing software packages come with spelling checkers. These are additional programs that compare the words the user types against a "dictionary" of thousands of words in the computer's memory. This can be of particular help in the medical and health professions since the user can add words to these dictionaries. Thus, frequently used or misspelled terms can be checked for accuracy.
5. When one original document is to be sent to several people, it is often desirable to customize each letter by including some information that applies only to the intended recipient. Word processing packages usually supply such a feature, often called "mail merge" or "print merge." It allows the user to create one master letter and a second document that contains all of the individualized information. The two are then merged by the word processing software, and separate customized letters are printed.

Most word processing packages have options for enhancing the quality of the finished report. These enhancements include:

1. Various sizes of type
2. A variety of type fonts
3. Printing in *italics,* **bold**, and outline form

Word processing not only saves time but also can be used to create reports and letters, keep notes, prepare mailing labels, and design forms. Today's technology has made using a word processor simpler than using a typewriter. The quality of printers range from dot-matrix printers (that print characters made up of small dots) to laser printers (that prints type simulating typeset copy). Once users become familiar with using modern word processing systems, they find it difficult to return to the traditional methods of preparing written material.

Spreadsheets

Spreadsheets manipulate numbers much as word processing packages manipulate words. Their use is perhaps best demonstrated by an example. A supervisor calls a nurse into the office late Friday and asks the nurse to prepare a budget or staffing plan over the weekend. There are 100 budget categories and data collected over 18 months. The nurse takes the data home over the weekend and spreads a sheet of paper out on the table. After entering all of the row and column headings, the nurse laboriously writes in the appropriate numbers. Next comes the hard part. With a calculator, the nurse adds all of the rows and all of the columns.

Late Sunday night, the supervisor calls to say that by accident the nurse worked with the wrong data for months 10 and 11 and also the wrong figures for budget categories 60 through 70! The nurse now must enter the new information and then add all the rows and columns again.

A spreadsheet software package eliminates most of the drudgery involved in budgeting and similar applications. With a spreadsheet, the user can direct the computer to add all the rows and columns in the table. Then, when changes have to be made, the computer automatically recalculates all of the row and column totals.

The intersection of a spreadsheet row and column is called a cell. See Figure 31–2. The number in a cell can be the result of applying a formula; for instance, the number in one cell might be the result of multiplying the numbers in two other cells. When those numbers change, the cell containing the product is recalculated automatically.

Spreadsheet software packages are very popular. There are hundreds of books available that are filled with sample uses. Some spreadsheets can calculate budgets, predict the future value of investments, schedule personnel, calculate tax liabilities, prepare invoices, perform statistical analyses, and so on.

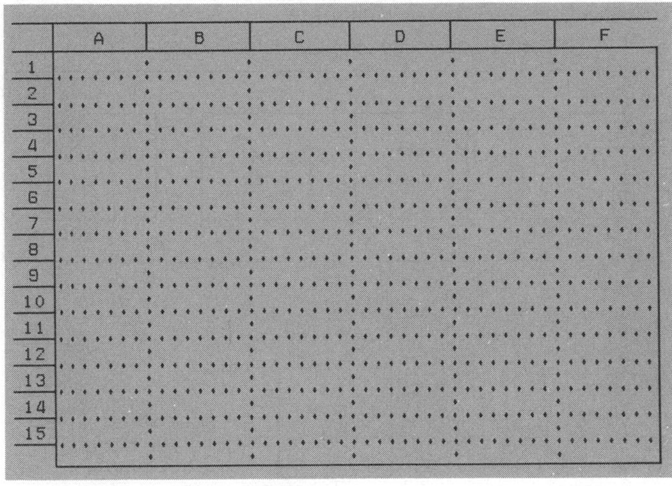

Figure 31–2 Spreadsheet

Database Management Systems

We live in an information-oriented society. Data are everywhere. The ability to retrieve data rapidly, in a variety of formats, is especially important in the medical and health care fields. Database management software packages give users the ability to create their own magnetic "file cabinets" of information.

A **database** is a collection of related information. A **file** is a specialized collection of data about one area. A **record** contains the information about one file member. A **field** is one piece of information from a record. These ideas are best illustrated by example. If the organization is a hospital, then Figure 31–3 shows how we might interpret the contents of the hospital's database.

All database software packages must provide the user with the following capabilities:

1. Creating a new database from scratch
2. Changing the contents of any field of information in the database
3. Adding new records to the database
4. Deleting records from the database
5. Searching for and locating any information of special interest
6. Printing detailed and summary reports

The more easily that these tasks can be accomplished, the more likely it is that the database will be put to use. Here are some examples of databases that might be useful to those in the medical professions:

1. A collection of all articles from a particular discipline
2. Nursing student clinical records
3. In-service education programs
4. Client records
5. Hospital inventories
6. Pharmacy inventories

Since we are in an information-oriented society (and profession), the ability to retrieve and manipulate information can be critical to success. Database management software packages provide many of the tools that make this possible.

A well-designed database system can make the entry and retrieval of information a relatively easy task for the nurses who use it. Figure 31–4 is an illustration of how a portion of a client's record might appear on the computer screen. The nurse enters the appropriate information into the form by typing it on the computer's keyboard. Changes can be made easily to update this record. Later, as the needs of the nurse dictate, information about a particular client, diagnosis, or physician can be recalled to the screen.

Graphics

Pictures often make a point more effectively than numbers in a table. For example, Table 31–2 summarizes information about the incidence of a certain disease in the population at large over several years. The data are fictitious and used for illustrative purposes only.

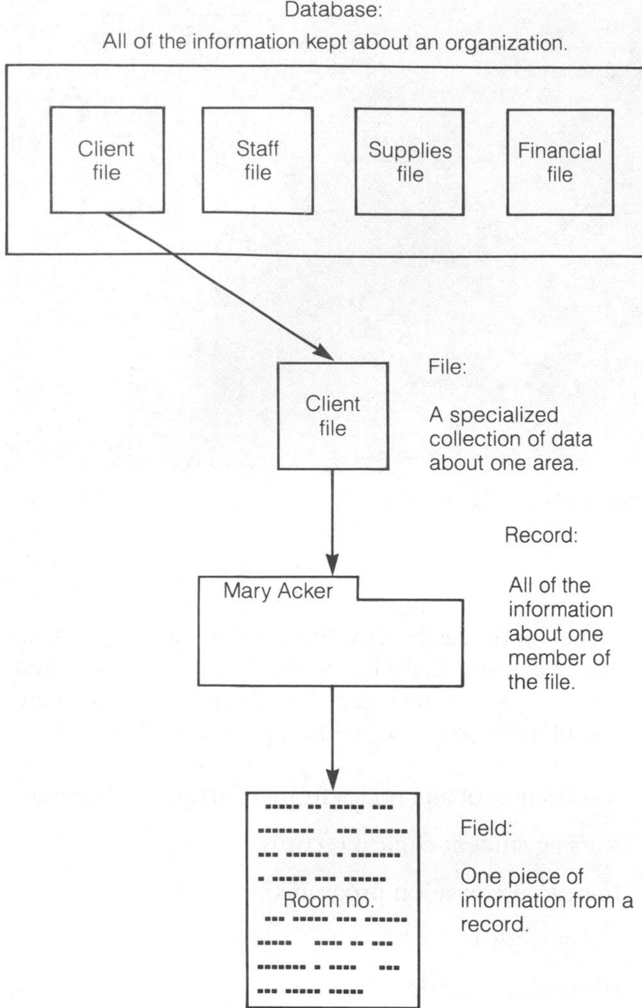

Figure 31–3 Hospital database

Client Information File

Client name
Street
City
State Zip
Sex
Date of birth
Health plan
Physician
Diagnosis

Figure 31–4 Segment of a client's database

It is difficult to extract information from the table. For example, in which age group is the disease most prevalent? In which group is the incidence increasing most rapidly? Least rapidly? Have any unusual trends occurred over the years? If this same information is displayed as a graph, it is easier not only to answer these questions but also to see some relationships that were impossible to detect simply by examining the numbers in the table. This same information is depicted graphically in Figure 31–5.

Current graphics software packages allow the user to type in the data and then simply specify the kind of graph to be drawn. The computer does the rest. In fact, several packages automatically take the data from a spreadsheet or a database management system and then draw the graph of the user's choice.

Table 31–2 A Computer-Generated Table

	DISEASE STATISTICS BY AGE					
YEAR	UNDER 18	18–24	25–34	35–44	45–54	OVER 54
72	567	703	806	818	329	626
73	653	749	833	869	343	668
74	789	881	875	911	357	696
75	961	959	858	877	644	364
76	1074	1050	891	917	670	421
77	1149	1089	858	857	641	413
78	1340	1274	928	882	667	426
79	1457	1372	931	828	627	401
80	1500	1514	990	823	635	398
81	1661	1785	1128	887	685	425
82	1797	1935	1203	900	697	430
83	1794	1958	1270	884	681	413
84	1717	1869	1179	768	597	360
85	1683	1886	1140	664	500	299

Telecommunications

If one computer can "talk to" another computer, then each machine's power is significantly enhanced. Software programs that allow this information exchange are called **telecommunications** packages. With such software, users can connect several machines in a hospital to share programs and data. Moreover, small, local microcomputers can communicate with larger computers that are more powerful and contain more extensive libraries of data than smaller machines can hold. In addition, if one computer can communicate with another, it becomes possible to access bibliographic or medical information databases over the telephone and copy information of interest to one's local environment.

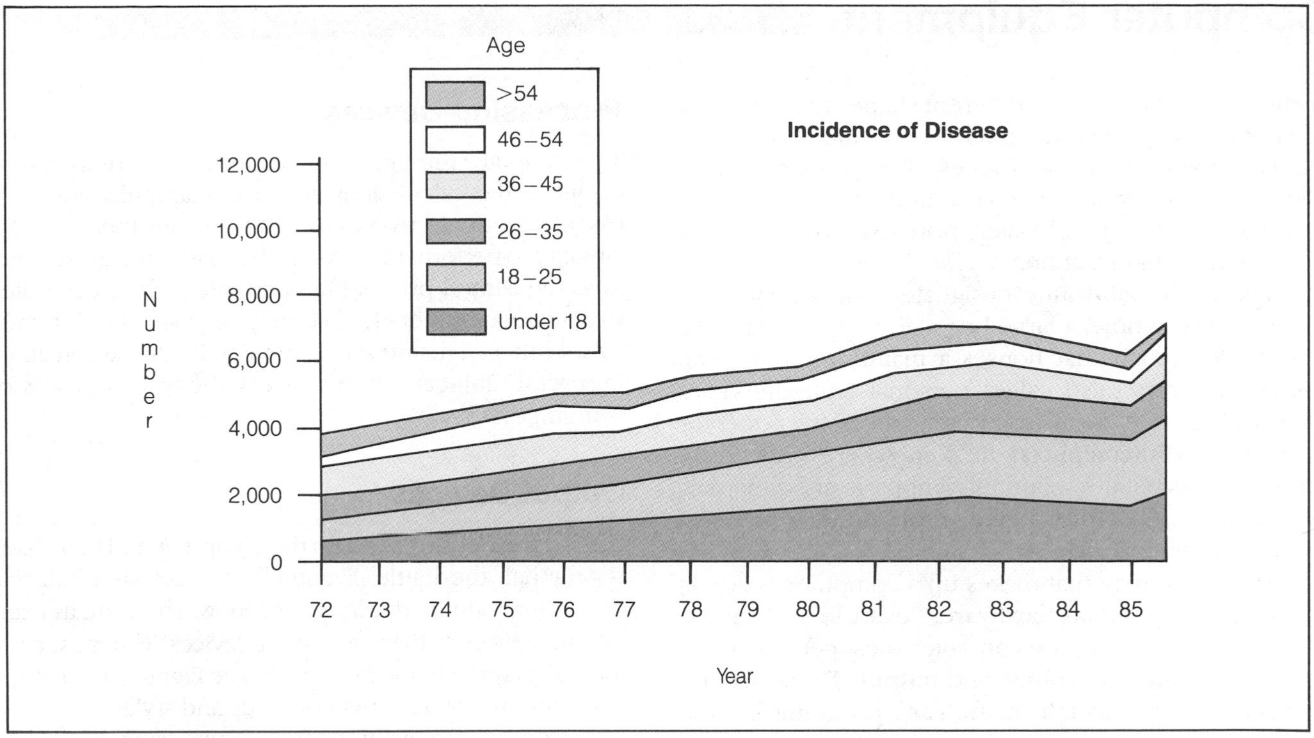

Figure 31–5 Computer-generated graph

Software alone is not enough, however. It is necessary to add a modem. Essentially, a **modem** is a small box that translates the digital signals that a computer sends into modulated signals that the telephone accepts, making it possible to send and receive data over the telephone. Their costs depend primarily on how fast they facilitate the transfer of data. The faster the transfer, the less computer and telephone time is used. These data transfer speeds range up to thousands of characters per second. Of course, the faster the transmission speed, the more expensive the modem is. Costs can range from $100 to $600 just for the equipment.

Customized Medical Applications

All of the applications mentioned so far are general ones. For instance, the user can design a variety of applications with one spreadsheet software package. Databases are as varied as the data they contain. Such generalized packages are very popular because users can adapt the package to their own needs and easily create a customized application.

Every field has its own established set of applications already designed by someone else. If these particular applications meet the user's needs, then they may be the best choice. Instead of taking the time and effort to design a system, the user can buy one that has already been designed by an expert. Of course, it is necessary to determine if the package was actually designed by someone knowledgeable in the field. The user has to judge whether such a package is cost-effective. Ready-made applications can be very expensive.

Table 31–3 shows a sampling of some commercially available packages. A quick scan of the table demonstrates the pervasive influence of the computer on the health professions.

Table 31–3 Selected Software Used in the Health Sciences

Medical Practice Management System
Client Medical Billing System
Health Encounter System
Clinical Data Processing System
Mental Health Administration
Medical Staff Affairs System
Medical History
Blood Bank System
Prenatal Baby Care System
Clinical Research System
Nutritional Analysis
Psychiatric Illness Screening
Computerized Health Appraisals
Fitness Profile
Dementia Database
General Neurology Database
Drugs

Source: Adapted from J. S. Lewis and R. Cromartie, editors, ***The software catalog: Health professions*** (New York: Elsevier, 1985).

Computer Equipment

Computers come in many different shapes and sizes. The most commonly used designations are microcomputers, minicomputers, and mainframes. The primary distinctions among them are size, cost, and speed. The larger machines are, in general, faster, more expensive, and able to store more information.

The term **mainframe** designates a large computer system. For example, a large hospital complex may have a computer center that houses a mainframe computer. **Microcomputers** (also called personal computers) are small and provide "local" computer processing power for their users. **Minicomputers** lie somewhere in between. Some analysts believe that minicomputers are disappearing because they are being replaced by powerful microcomputers.

The equipment that makes up a computer system is normally referred to as **hardware**. Regardless of the system being considered, the computer must perform three functions: **input**, **processing**, and **output**. There must be an input device to get information and programs into the computer. There must also be processing devices that somehow manipulate the information to achieve the desired objective. Finally, an output device must display the results in some meaningful format. All computers, large or small, must have these components.

Input Devices

The input device is most usually a keyboard. However, there are a variety of input devices. Some computers accept one or more of the following as legitimate ways to input information:

1. Touching a certain point on the computer display screen with a finger (a **touch screen**)
2. Using a **light pen** to touch the screen at a certain location (see Figure 31–6)
3. Optically scanning printed material with a TV-like camera
4. Recognizing signals from biologic feedback devices
5. Scanning a printed code with a wand (as in the supermarket)
6. Accepting audio input (voice, cassette recorder, etc.)
7. Using a mouse (A **mouse** is a small device with a button. The user rolls the mouse on a desktop. As the mouse moves, an arrow moves correspondingly on the screen. Pressing the button selects what the arrow is pointing at.)
8. Using pressure-sensitive devices that accept handwritten material (e.g., nurse's notes, a signature, etc.)

Processing Devices

The computer must contain the electronics equipment to do all of the calculations and data manipulations. It is, essentially, an electronic chip that contains the necessary circuitry to perform these tasks. This chip is usually referred to as the central processing unit (**CPU**) of the computer. In a microcomputer, the CPU may be as small as a thumbnail, while in a mainframe computer, it may be contained in several cabinets. For most users, the type of processor is unimportant.

Output Devices

Getting the information into the computer and processed is only half the battle. Eventually, the results of all that processing must be displayed somehow. There are as many output devices as there are input devices. The most common display device is the printer (see Figure 31–7). Printers come in a wide variety of types and styles.

A **dot-matrix printer** forms letters from small dots; these characters made up of dots are often associated with computer printing. **Letter-quality printers** form characters by pressing a wheel of characters against the paper. The resulting printing is exactly like that produced by a high-quality electric typewriter. **Laser printers** are more expensive but provide output that is very attractive and of nearly the same quality as typeset material.

Printers are not the only output devices. Computers can generate output in all the following ways:

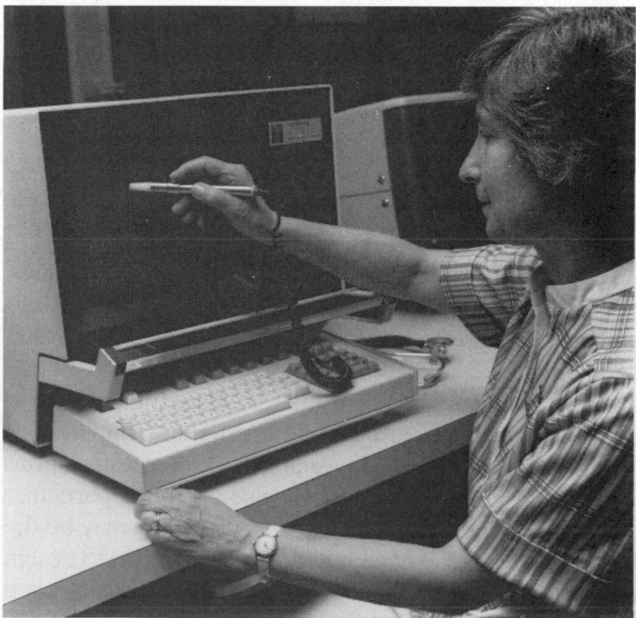

Figure 31–6 An input device

1. On a television or monitor
2. On microfilm or microfiche
3. In audio form
4. To control devices (lights, heating, monitoring equipment, controlling devices, etc.)
5. On cassette tape
6. On a diskette
7. Via a graphics plotting device

Other Computer Equipment

The nurse may encounter a variety of other hardware devices in the course of a work day. The most commonly used device is a computer **terminal**, which is simply an input and output device combined. The terminal is not a computer itself but is simply connected to some other machine, usually a mainframe. It is not uncommon to find computer terminals located at a nurse's workstation.

Storage devices provide ways to keep reports, databases, spreadsheets, and the like for later use. These devices are usually either tape drives or, more commonly, disk drives. **Disk drives** are units that "record or play back" information from a recordlike device called a **disk** or **diskette**. Some diskettes are referred to as "floppies" or "floppy disks" because they are not rigid like a phonograph record.

Diskettes for microcomputers are relatively inexpensive, costing about five dollars. These can store from 120,000 to 800,000 characters of information. Larger disk units for mainframe computers are considerably more expensive and can store up to 400 million characters of information.

Video disks will certainly provide some exciting applications in the medical and health professions. The idea is to connect a microcomputer to a video disk recorder. Video disks can store up to 50,000 frames of graphic/picture information or billions of characters of data. The combination of video and data allows for a wide variety of innovative applications.

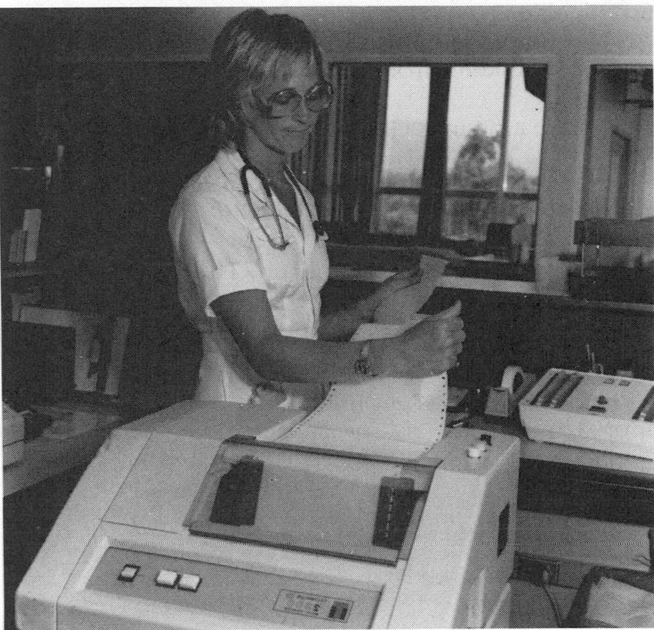

Figure 31–7 An output device

For example, in such a training program, the student nurse might sit down at a microcomputer and start an application designed to teach the appropriate activities associated with a tour in the emergency room. As the exercise begins, the student views a moving picture on the screen depicting a client being wheeled into the emergency room from an ambulance. The video stops, and the student is asked to choose from among a list of alternative actions. When the student selects one, for instance, "Take an x-ray film," the video continues, showing the client being wheeled to the radiology department. Thus, the application allows the student to choose from alternative courses of action and immediately see the results of those choices, right or wrong.

Frequently Asked Questions

Do I have to be a mathematician to use computers effectively?

No! Today, manufacturers have been concentrating on making computers as easy to use as possible. It is becoming clear that one does not need to be a computer scientist, engineer, or mathematician to use these machines effectively. All that is needed is some common sense and a bit of confidence in one's ability.

How might a nurse use a computer on a day-to-day basis?

The answer to this question depends a good deal on the nurse's work environment. If it is a modern hospital facility, then the nurse may use a computer often. In some environments, however, the computer does not play a major role.

Here are some possible uses for computers in health care settings:

1. Assessing client information
2. Recording client information
3. Preparing nurse's notes
4. Preparing a nursing care plan

5. Calculating appropriate dosages, IV drip rates, etc.
6. Ordering items from the pharmacy
7. Participating in self-paced continuing education

Can I accidentally erase client information stored in the computer?

Accidental erasure is unlikely. The designers of the computer software programs that are used to retrieve and display client data have included controls to prevent the accidental erasure or changing of information. Of course, if the designers are not professional or thorough in their approach, then the risk of damaging the data is greater. Generally, it is difficult for a user to accidentally erase data.

Are any health problems associated with the use of computers?

This frequently asked question has been addressed in a variety of articles. To date, the consensus seems to be that no specific health problems are associated with the continued use of a computer. Of course, in individual instances, extended use might cause eye strain, back strain, and similar problems, but these problems are associated with the extended use of any machinery.

Should a nurse take a computer programming course?

Generally, no. Most computer programming courses have two objectives. The first is to acquaint the student with the ways in which the computer does its magic. The second is to teach students how to write computer programs. (However, to become competent at programming takes more than a single course.) In most cases, the nurse will use neither of these two skills. A better choice might be to take an applications-oriented course that centers on the use of some software packages currently available on microcomputers (e.g., spreadsheets and databases).

Future Expectations

We are in the midst of a technologic revolution brought on by computers. The next few decades are likely to give the ordinary person computer resources that were unimaginable a short time ago. Encyclopedias the size of a watch, robots that perform many redundant tasks, and expert systems that mimic the decisions made by professionals are all very real possibilities. Those in the medical and health professions are likely to be among the first to feel the impact of these changes.

A speculative list of what is in store over the next two decades includes:

1. Robots that help teach medical students. These robots might be humanlike in appearance and function. Under computer control, they might exhibit a wide variety of symptoms and have an epileptic attack, myocardial infarction, or other medical crisis.
2. Expert systems are computer systems that can provide intelligent answers similar to those a human expert might give in a similar situation. Several such medical diagnosis systems have already been built.
3. Increased computer-aided help, perhaps implants, for the handicapped. These would include vision systems for the blind, computer-controlled prosthetics for amputees, specialized computer input devices for the multiply handicapped, voice synthesizers for those who cannot speak, artificial body parts, and much more.
4. Computer-assisted medicine will be available via computer/telephone link to the typical home. Most homes will have computers and the communication of data will exceed that of voice communications.
5. CD ROMs, or compact disks with read-only memory with massive storage capacities, will be commonplace. Compact disks are a bit like 45 rpm phonograph records in appearance but store millions and millions of characters of information instead of songs. When CD ROMs are combined with a computer chip, information can be quickly accessed and reviewed by someone with a disk player. Such compact disks will contain encyclopedias, medical references, huge databases and cost about as much as a household television set.
6. Computers will be smaller, have very large storage capacities, and be available at low cost. For example, it is possible, at present, to purchase a $99 watch that can be loaded with 2000 characters of information from a microcomputer. This information can be recalled at the touch of a button on the watch. In the future, a nurse might wear a wrist watch that contains all of the vital information about all of the clients on her or his duty station.
7. Perhaps the most exciting area under development is that of artificial intelligence. Researchers in this field have been studying how to make machines exhibit intelligent behavior. Obviously, such developments would have significant moral, ethical, medical, philosophic, and social ramifications. Does such a machine have feelings?

Issues of Relevance to the Nurse

Confidentiality of Client Records

Nurses are bound by their professional ethics to maintain a client's privacy. This means that information about a client cannot be disseminated outside of the realm of the caregivers. The use of computer-based informations systems to store client data has increased the risk of an accidental or intentional violation of a client's rights. Just as computers are becoming easier to use, they are becoming easier to abuse.

Clients have a right to privacy and confidentiality even where computer-based information systems are used. Nurses should not give their signature codes to anyone or let anyone without an access code use the computer.

In today's information age, health care providers tend to collect more data, share more databases, and access more client information than in earlier days. Client records are queried for insurance claims, during audits of the nursing (as well as some other) departments, and sometimes on the demand of the courts.

There has not been a similar growth in the sophistication of the security systems (both manual and computerized) that are used to limit access to these data. Passwords limiting access to data can often be guessed; disgruntled employees may change, delete, or disseminate data; computer "enthusiasts" may deem it a challenge to "break into" a hospital's computer information system.

Nurses must be aware of these problems and risks if they are to fulfill their responsibility to the client. The specific role of the nurse (or student, educator, researcher, manager) does not absolve them from the accountability for ensuring a client's right to privacy.

The Nurse's Role in the Design and Development of Applications

Nurses can play many roles to integrate the computer into their environment. One method is to become more comfortable with, knowledgeable about, and an advocate of the use of microcomputers. In addition (and perhaps more important), nurses need to become involved with the planning, design, and implementation of any computer systems that have an effect on their profession. In most cases, health care applications are designed by persons or groups with computer expertise. They often lack the skills and knowledge of the application area in which they plan to put the computer to use. Sometimes, these developers seek out the active participation of those who will use the implemented system every day. Many times, no such attempt is made. It is essential that nurses demand involvement in the design of any systems that will eventually affect them and/or their clients. Otherwise, they run the risk of having to work with a computer system designed by someone unfamiliar with their needs. The probability of such systems being successful without this involvement is, indeed, remote.

Keeping Up To Date

In the fields of nursing and technology, it is absolutely essential to stay relevant and up to date. The interested nurse can keep abreast of what is taking place in the computer field in several ways.

1. Most major cities have computer user groups. These groups began to form as microcomputers found their way into homes and small businesses. In most cases, special interest groups (SIGs) form to pursue areas of interest to particular members. It is not uncommon to find groups oriented toward computer applications in medicine and the health professions.
2. A wide variety of popular magazines cover, in a non-technical way, what is taking place in the world of computers. Stopping by a local magazine store and examining the contents of current issues is an excellent way to determine which publications might be appropriate. Check the local (and/or university) library also. Many times, a magazine has a special issue (e.g., computers in nursing) that may provide a great deal of relevant information. Some suggested publications are listed at the end of this chapter.
3. Professional journals in the computer sciences may be too technical or too specialized to be of interest. However, some publications are available to the medical and health professions. These are included at the end of this chapter under "Suggested Readings."
4. A wide variety of educational programs are available to those who wish to pursue an interest in computers.

These might be offered by a local college or university, an in-service education program, or even a private organization.

Chapter Highlights

- Computers will play an ever-increasing role in the activities of tomorrow's professional nurse. Their effects will be particularly strong in nursing practice, where automated client care planning systems will greatly facilitate the role of the practicing nurse. Expert systems will be developed to aid in diagnosis and client care.
- The research efforts of nurses will be greatly enhanced by the ability to access data, bibliographic references, and powerful analysis procedures.
- The education of the student nurse and of clients in the hospital will also be affected by this technology. Computers will provide very powerful ways to learn and communicate.
- Nurse managers will appreciate the increase in productivity and the savings in time that computers will bring about. The staffing of nurses, access to information, and budgeting will be facilitated by these machines.
- The application areas of most interest to nurses at present are word processing, spreadsheets, database management systems, graphics, and telecommunications.
- Essentially, computer systems are made up of input devices, processing devices, and output devices. The options available in each of these areas are quite varied and depend to a great extent on the particular application being used.
- Nurses need to become comfortable with and knowledgeable about the use of the computer.
- Nurses must plan an active role in the design, development, and implementation of any computer systems that affect the role of the nurse.
- Nurses should be concerned with the ethical implications of using computers to maintain client information.
- Nurses must keep up to date with the advances in technology and their impact on the nursing profession.

Suggested Readings

Ball, M. J., and Hannah, K. 1984. *Using computers in nursing.* Reston, VA: Reston Publishing Co.

This text is a very thorough resource for information about how the computer is used in nursing. Each chapter includes a list of nursing experts in the particular application presented.

Computers in Nursing, a bimonthly publication prepared by J. B. Lippincott Co.

Contains articles describing the relevant research going on in this area, software reviews, and reference lists of what computer-based software is currently available.

Deitel, H., and Deitel, B. 1985. *Computers and data processing.* Orlando, FL: Academic Press.

This nontechnical book covers a wide variety of topics in the computer field. It is an excellent reference and learning guide for those with an interest in computers.

Grobe, S. 1984. *A computer-based resource guide for nurses.* Philadelphia: J. B. Lippincott Co.

This is an excellent introductory-level book for the nurse. It is easy to read and contains computer applications that are relevant both for nursing practice and for nursing education.

Lewis, J., editor. 1985. *The software catalog: Health professions.* New York: Elsevier Publishing Co.

This publication contains a list of all the currently available software oriented to those in the health professions.

Scholes, M., et al., editors. 1983. *The impact of computers on nursing.* New York: Elsevier Publishing Co.

This book contains the proceedings from an international conference jointly sponsored by the International Medical Informatics Association and the International Federation for Information Processing. Topics covering both education and client care are included in the publication.

Werley, H., and Grier, M., editors. 1981. *Nursing information systems.* New York: Springer Publishing Co.

This text contains a variety of articles on nursing information systems. Topics include the identification of the appropriate data to collect, experiences with the process of using a computer, and the evaluation of informations systems.

Selected References

Albrecht, C., and Lieske, A. M. 1985. Automating patient care planning. *Nursing Management* 16(7):21–26.

Andreoli, K., and Musser, L. A. January/February 1985. Computers in nursing care: The state of the art. *Nursing Outlook* 33:16–21.

Ball, M. J.; Snelbecker, G. E.; and Schecter, S. L. January/February 1985. Nurses' perceptions concerning computer uses before and after a computer literacy lecture. *Computers in Nursing* 3(1):23–32.

Bitzer, M., and Boudreaux, M. 1969. Using a computer to teach nursing. *Nursing Forum* 8(3):234–54.

Ellis, L., and Raines, J. 1981. Health education using microcomputers. *Preventive Medicine* 10(1):77–84.

Ellis, L.; Raines, J.; and Hakanson, N. 1982. Health education using microcomputers II: One year in the clinic. *Preventive Medicine* 11:212–24.

Johnson, D. S.; Ranzenberger, J.; Herbert, R. D.; Gardner, R. M.; and Clemmer, T. P. June 1980. A computerized alert program for acutely ill patients. *Journal of Nursing Administration* 10:26–35.

McNeill, D. G. November 1979. Developing the complete computer-based information system. *Journal of Nursing Administration* 9:34–46.

Martin, M. 1982. Computers: Help or hindrance to the clinical nurse? In M. Scholes (editor), *The impact of computers on nursing*. New York: Elsevier Publishing Co.

Pople, H. 1977. The formation of composite hypotheses in diagnostic problem-solving: An exercise in synthetic reasoning. *Proceedings of the Fifth International Joint Conference on AI*.

Romano, C.; Ryan, L.; Harris, J.; Boykin, P.; and Power, M. March/April 1985. A decade of decisions: Four perspectives on computerization in nursing practice. *Computers in Nursing* 3(2):64–76.

Ryan, S. A. March/April 1985. An expert system for nursing practice: Clinical decision support. *Computers in Nursing* 3(2):77–84.

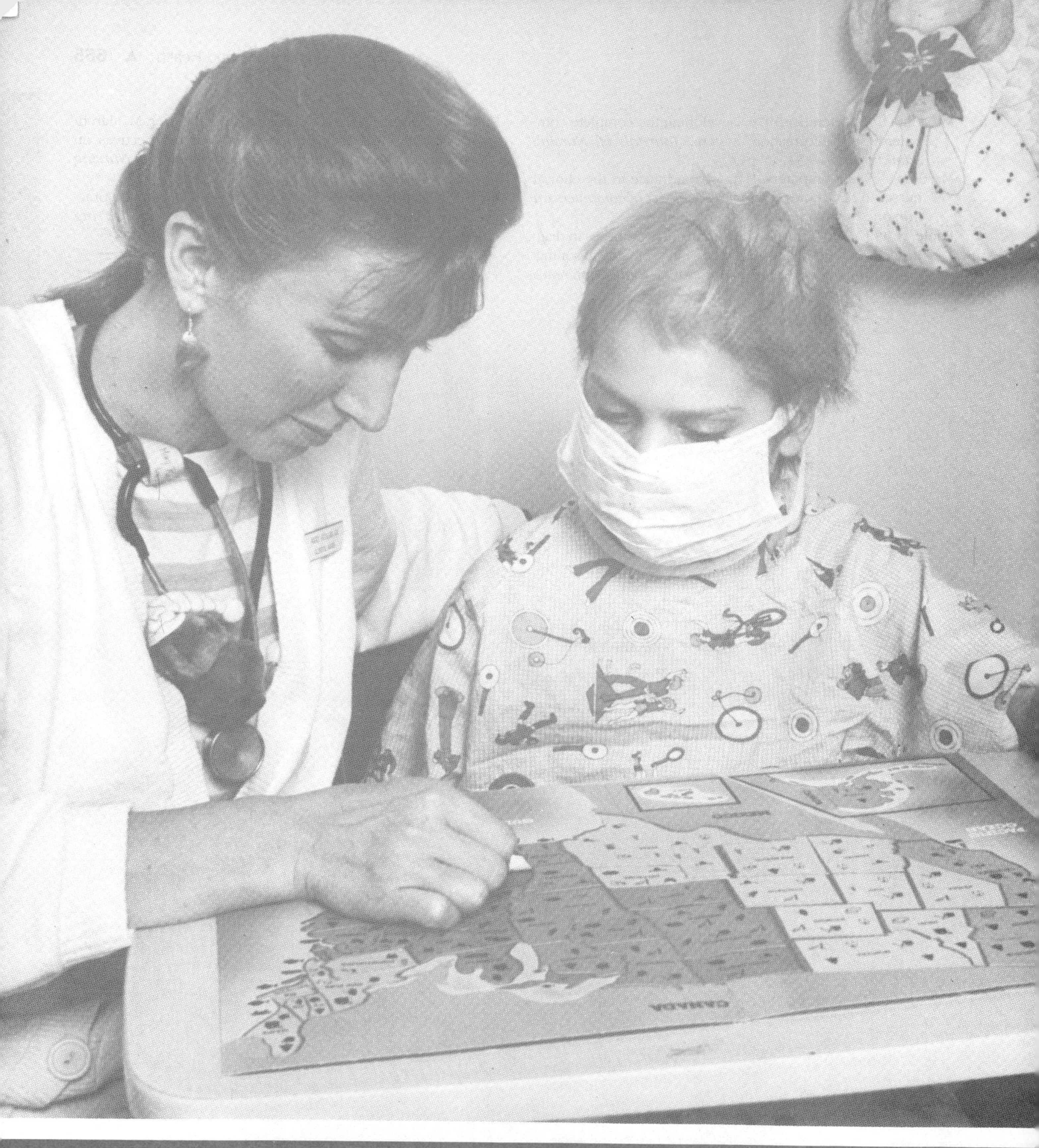

[The nurse] is temporarily the consciousness of the unconscious . . . the leg of the amputee, the eyes of the newly blind, the means of locomotion of the infant . . . , and the mouthpiece for those too weak or withdrawn to speak. (Virginia Henderson)

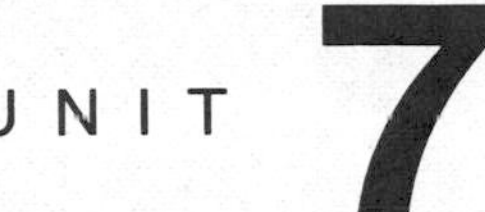

UNIT 7

Health Protection

KAREN STAFFORD RANTZMAN

Contents

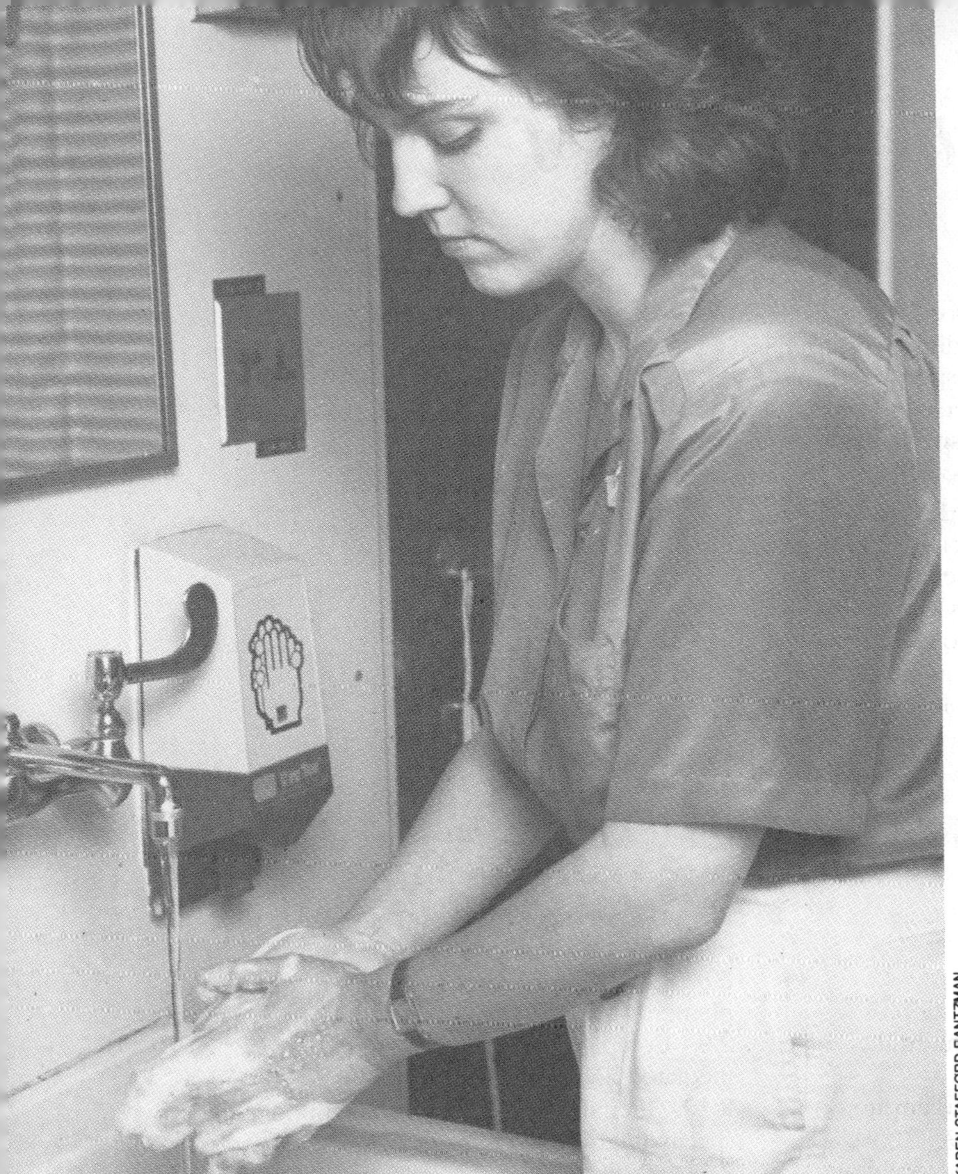
KAREN STAFFORD FANTZMAN

CHAPTER 32

Preventing the Transfer of Microorganisms

Contents

(continued)

32 *Preventing the Transfer of Microorganisms*

Contents *(continued)*

Objectives

1. Understand terms and facts about the infectious process and nosocomial infections.
   1.1 Define listed terms.
   1.2 Identity six links in the chain of infection.
   1.3 Identify measures that break each link in the chain of infection.
   1.4 Identify factors influencing a microorganism's capability to produce an infectious process.
   1.5 Describe environmental conditions favorable to the growth of microorganisms.
   1.6 Identify ways microorganisms exit from six parts of the body.
   1.7 Describe various modes of transmission of microorganisms.
   1.8 Describe four stages of an infectious process.
   1.9 Identify causal factors of nosocomial infections.
   1.10 Identify people at risk of acquiring an infection.
2. Understand essential facts about normal body defenses.
   2.1 Describe the difference between nonspecific and specific defenses of the body.
   2.2 Describe the difference between resident flora, transient flora, and colonization.
   2.3 Identify anatomic and physiologic barriers that defend the body against microorganisms.
   2.4 Describe vascular and cellular responses that occur in the inflammatory process.
   2.5 Identify types of inflammatory exudates and give examples of each.
   2.6 Differentiate between the healing processes of regeneration and replacement with fibrous tissue.
   2.7 Describe the origin and purpose of interferon.
   2.8 Compare the properidin system and the complement system.
   2.9 Compare antibody-mediated and cell-mediated body defenses.
   2.10 Identify the five classes of antibodies and specify their known functions.
   2.11 Differentiate between natural and acquired types of immunity.
   2.12 Identify the four divisions of acquired immunity in terms of their antigen-antibody sources and the durations of immunity attained.
3. Understand methods required to assess a client's susceptibility to infection or to assess a client with an infection.
   3.1 Identify nursing history data required to determine whether the client is at risk of acquiring an infection.
   3.2 Identify nursing history data required to determine the presence of an infection.
   3.3 Identify signs of localized infection.
   3.4 Identify signs of systemic infection.
   3.5 Identify laboratory data indicating the presence of an infection.
4. Understand essential facts about nursing interventions that prevent and control infections.
   4.1 Explain the concepts of medical and surgical asepsis.
   4.2 Identify interventions to prevent infections.
   4.3 Identify interventions to protect body defenses.
   4.4 Identify essentials of hand washing.

4.5 Identify essential steps in cleaning articles soiled with organic material.
4.6 Identify appropriate methods of disinfecting and sterilizing selected objects.
4.7 Identify seven types of protective asepsis (isolation) precautions.
4.8 Identify precautions taken in each type of protective asepsis.
4.9 Identify psychologic problems associated with protective asepsis.
4.10 Relate basic practices of surgical asepsis to the principles of surgical asepsis.
4.11 Demonstrate correct methods of performing aseptic procedures.
4.12 Explain the reasons for selected steps of aseptic procedures.

Terms

acquired immunity
antibody (immunoglobulin)
antigen
antiseptic
asepsis
autoantigen
bactericidal
bacteriocin
bacteriostatic
barrier drape
carrier
cellular immunity
chemotaxis
cicatrix
clean
colonization
colonized person
communicable disease
contact transmission
contaminated
convalescent period
culture
diapedesis
disease
disinfectant
disinfection
emigration
enanthema
endogenous
erythrocyte sedimentation rate
etiology
exanthema
exogenous
exudate
fibrinogen
fibrous tissue
flora
granulation tissue
humoral immunity
hyperemia
iatrogenic
illness period
immunity
incubation period
infection
inflammation
interferon
lactoferrin
leukocyte
leukocytosis
localized symptoms
lymphocyte
lymphokine
lysozyme
macrophage
margination
medical asepsis
monocyte
natural immunity
nonspecific defenses
nosocomial infection
obligate aerobe
obligate anaerobe
opportunistic pathogen
parasite
parenchyma
pathogenicity
phagocyte
phagocytosis
primary immune response
prodromal period
purulent exudate
pyogenic bacteria
regeneration
reservoir
resident flora
sanguineous (hemorrhagic) exudate
secondary immune response
serous exudate
specific (immune) defenses
spore
sterile field
sterilization
stroma
suppuration
surgical asepsis
susceptible (compromised) host
systemic symptoms
transient flora
trauma
vector
vehicle
virulence

Importance of Biologic Safety

Nurses are directly involved in providing a biologically safe environment and promoting health. Microorganisms exist everywhere in the environment: in water, soil, and within and on the body. The number of microbial colonists on and in the body exceeds the number of body cells by 10 to 1 (Norton 1981, p. 580). Most microorganisms are harmless, and some are even beneficial in that they perform essential functions in the body. Some microorganisms found in the intestines, i.e., enterobacteria, produce substances called bacteriocins, which are lethal to related strains of bacteria. Others produce antibioticlike substances and toxic metabolites that repress the growth of other microorganisms. Some microorganisms are normal in one part of the body and produce infection in another, e.g, *Escherichia coli* is a normal inhabitant of the large intestine but a common cause of infection of the urinary tract.

An **infection** is an invasion of body tissue by microorganisms and their proliferation there. Such a microorganism is called an infectious agent. If the microorganism produces no significant damage, the infection is called asymptomatic or subclinical. A detectable alteration in normal tissue function, however, is called **disease**.

Microorganisms vary in their **virulence**; i.e., their ability to produce disease. In the environment, five groups of microorganisms normally can cause d
viruses, fungi, protozoa, and Rickettsia. M
also vary in the severity of the diseases the
their degree of communicability. For exa
mon cold virus is more readily transmitted

lus that causes leprosy (*Mycobacterium leprae*). If the infectious agent can be transmitted directly from one person to another, the infectious process is called a **communicable disease.**

Trauma is injury to the body. Trauma can be physical, such as a cut by a piece of glass; trauma also describes injury caused by invading microorganisms. Thus, an infectious process can be described as trauma. Often, the trauma of infection follows physical trauma, as when a cut becomes infected.

Pathogenicity means the ability to produce disease; thus, a pathogen is a microorganism that causes disease. No microorganism produces disease 100% of the time (Norton 1981, p. 34). However, many microorganisms that are normally harmless can cause disease under certain circumstances. A "true" pathogen causes disease or infection in a healthy individual. An **opportunistic pathogen** causes disease only in a susceptible individual.

Etiology is the study of causes; the etiology of an infectious process is the identification of the invading microorganisms. The control of the spread of microorganisms and the protection of people from communicable diseases and infections are practiced on four levels: international, national, community, and individual.

An example of infectious disease control at the international level is the required immunization people must have against certain diseases, such as cholera, before traveling to certain countries. Similarly, international health regulations govern the immunizations required of American and Canadian citizens returning home.

National regulations govern, for example, the interstate and interprovincial transportation of food. These regulations protect people from receiving contaminated food. Also, national regulations attempt to control pollution of water, the air, and the environment, subjects currently receiving much publicity.

Communities regulate the disposal of sewage and the purity of drinking water, for example. Such community regulations protect people from infectious disease.

Protection from infection is also an individual responsibility. Individuals protect themselves not only by practicing good hygiene (see Chapter 36, "Personal Hygiene") but also by eating a balanced diet and taking exercise.

Asepsis

Asepsis is the freedom from infection or infectious material. Hands washed with a disinfectant can be considered aseptic; i.e., free from infectious organisms. However, some microorganisms in all probability are still present on washed hands.

There are two types of asepsis: medical and surgical. **Medical asepsis** refers to those practices that limit the number of microorganisms and their growth and spread. Medical asepsis includes all practices intended to confine a specific microorganism to a specific area. In medical asepsis, objects are often referred to as clean or dirty. **Clean** denotes the presence of some microorganisms but the absence of infectious agents. **Contaminated** (dirty) denotes the presence of disease-producing microorganisms. Aseptic measures are protective in that they are meant to prevent infections or the spread of infections.

Surgical asepsis, or sterile technique, refers to those practices that keep an area or objects free of all microorganisms; it includes practices that destroy all microorganisms and spores. (A **spore** is a round or oval structure enclosed in a tough capsule. Some microorganisms assume this structure in response to adverse conditions; in this form, they are highly resistant to destruction.) An example of surgical aseptic practice is the technique used to clean and dress a surgical wound to prevent microorganisms from entering through the incision.

Chain of Infection

There are six links in the chain of infection:

1. Etiologic agent, or microorganism
2. Source (**reservoir**)
3. Portal of exit from the source
4. Method (mode) of transmission
5. Portal of entry
6. Susceptibility of the person (host) (See Figure 32–1.)

Etiologic Agent

Microorganisms and parasites are the sources of infection. A **parasite** is an animal or plant that lives in or on another and obtains its nourishment from it. Some microorganisms, such as the gonococcus bacillus, are parasites. The extent to which any microorganism or parasite is capable of producing an infectious process depends on these factors:

1. Number of organisms
2. Virulence and potency of the organisms

3. Their ability to enter the body
4. The susceptibility of the host
5. Their ability to live in the body

Some microorganisms, such as the smallpox virus, have the ability to infect almost anyone on first contact. By contrast, microorganisms such as the tuberculosis bacillus attack a relatively small number of the population who are particularly susceptible, often people who are poorly nourished and living in unsanitary conditions. Some animals and humans are **carriers**, i.e., they carry disease-producing organisms in their bodies although they are not ill themselves. Carriers can pass the microorganisms along to other people. For example, some persons harbor the typhoid bacillus in the gallbladder, excrete it in feces, but manifest no symptoms of the disease.

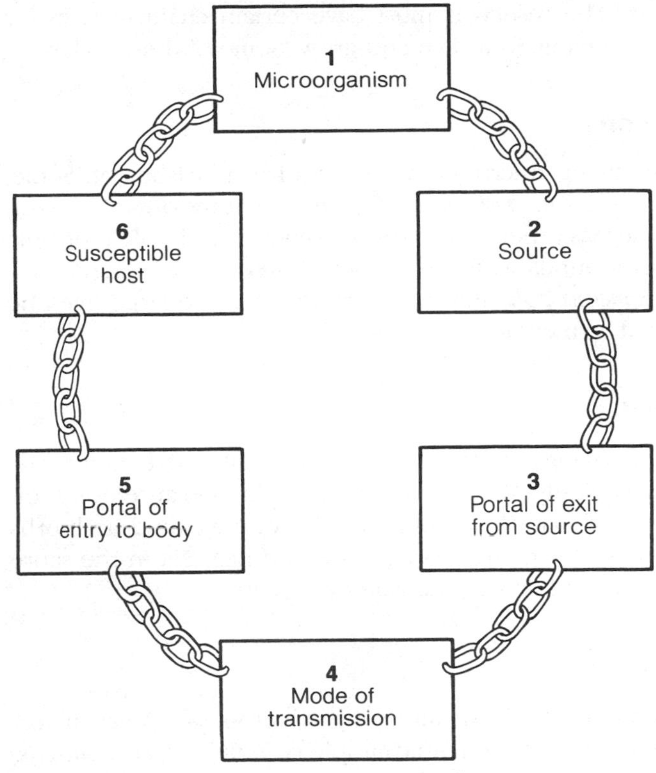

Figure 32–1 The chain of infection

Source

There are many sources or reservoirs of microorganisms. Common sources are other humans, the client's own microorganisms, plants, animals, or the general environment. See Table 32–1. Quite commonly people are the source of infection for others and for themselves. The person with, for example, an influenza virus frequently spreads it to others. When resistance is lowered by fatigue and other factors, an infection emerges. See "Patients at Risk of Acquiring an Infection," later in this chapter.

Insects, birds, and other animals are common sources of infection. The *Anopheles* mosquito carries the malaria parasite. Food, water, milk, and feces also can be reservoirs. An example is contaminated chicken at a club luncheon.

Table 32–1 Human Source and Method of Transmission of Common Microorganisms

Body Area (Source)	Transport Vehicle	Common Infectious Organisms
Respiratory tract	Droplets expelled while sneezing and coughing	Parainfluenza virus *Klebsiella* species *Staphylococcus aureus*
Gastrointestinal tract	Emesis, feces, drainage (such as from the gallbladder), saliva	Viral hepatitis A *Shigella* species *Salmonella enteritidis*
Urinary tract	Urine	*Escherichia coli* enterococci *Pseudomonas aeruginosa*
Reproductive tract (including genitals)	Urine and semen	*Neisseria gonorrhoeae* *Treponema pallidum* Herpes simplex virus type 2 Viral hepatitis B
Blood	Blood sample, needle used for venipuncture	*Escherichia coli* *Staphylococcus aureus* *Klebsiella* species *Staphylococcus epidermidis*
Tissue	Drainage from a cut or wound	*Staphylococcus aureus* *Escherichia coli* enterococci *Proteus* species

The reservoir must have certain characteristics for the organisms to live and grow. Some of these follow.

Food

All living microorganisms require nourishment. Some, such as *Clostridium perfringens*, require organic matter, whereas others use carbon dioxide and simple inorganic compounds as foods. Others, such as the anaerobe *Escherichia coli*, attack food residues in the large intestine by a fermentation process.

Water

Most living organisms require water, although their needs vary widely. Water is important to life because it is a solvent of many compounds, it is cohesive, and it absorbs and stores energy as heat. Certain bacteria in the spore form can live without water for years.

Oxygen

Some microorganisms (**obligate aerobes**) require molecular (free) oxygen. An example is *Staphylococcus aureus*. Others, such as the tetanus bacillus (*Clostridium tetani*), cannot live in the presence of molecular oxygen. These are referred to as **obligate anaerobes**. *Obligate* means "obliged."

Temperature

Organisms thrive only in certain temperature ranges, and most die if the temperature rises above or falls below the boundaries of that range. Temperature is an important factor in asepsis. Some viruses, e.g., Hepatitis B virus and spore-forming bacteria, are not destroyed by boiling. Cold tends to be more bacteriostatic than bacteriocidal. (**Bacteriostatic** means preventing the growth and reproduction of bacteria. **Bactericidal** means destroying bacteria.)

pH

Microorganisms are sensitive to changes in pH. Most grow best in an alkaline environment, between pH 6 and 8. The stomach is generally thought to be relatively free of bacteria because the fasting pH drops to about 2. Although some acid-tolerant bacteria are attached to the gastric mucosa, their activity is considered insignificant.

Light

Most microorganisms thrive in environments without light, e.g., the urinary bladder, under dressings, in the ear canal, and under the female breast. Ultraviolet rays generally inhibit or kill microorganisms. Sunlight is the best source of ultraviolet light.

Portal of Exit

Before an infection can establish itself in a host, the microorganisms must leave the source. If the reservoir is within a human, the microorganisms have a number of exits, depending on the site of the reservoir.

Respiratory Tract

The respiratory tract is one of the most common exit routes for pathogens. Microorganisms can leave the tract through the nose and the mouth when a person sneezes, coughs, breathes, and talks. In clients with tracheostomies or endotracheal tubes, the microorganisms can leave by that route.

Gastrointestinal Tract

The gastrointestinal tract is another site of exit. Pathogens can be expelled in feces; through drainage, such as gallbladder drainage; and even in vomitus. One example is the typhoid bacillus, which some clients carry in the gallbladder and/or the large intestine and expel in feces. Saliva can also be the means of exit for microorganisms in the mouth.

Urinary Tract

The urinary tract (the kidneys, the bladder, and the urethra) are normally sterile. There are usually organisms at the entry of the urethra. Persons with a urinary tract infection can expel microorganisms in the urine. The portals of exit can be the urethral meatus and urinary diversion ostomies.

Reproductive Tract

Microorganisms in the reproductive tract of women exit by the vagina. In men, they exit through the urinary meatus. Microorganisms living in the reproductive tract may exit in urine, semen, and vaginal discharges.

Blood

Blood normally does not contain microorganisms. However, circulating blood may be a reservoir of microorganisms, such as the virus that causes hepatitis B. Any escape of blood from the circulatory system, e.g., as a result of a needle puncture, provides an exit for such microorganisms.

Skin and Mucous Membranes

The tissues of the body also can be a reservoir, and thus any opening into the tissues through the skin or mucous membranes can serve as the exit. For example, surgical wounds can become infected and produce drainage that contains a high concentration of microorganisms.

Method of Transmission

Microorganisms are transmitted by a number of routes, and the same microorganisms can be transmitted by more than one route. For example, the varicella virus can be transmitted by droplet contact (through the air) and by direct contact. There are four main routes of transmission: contact, vehicle, airborne, and vector-borne.

Contact Transmission

Contact transmission is the most important and frequent means of transmission of microorganism (Williams 1983, p. 341). There are three types of contact transmission: direct contact, indirect contact, and droplet contact.

Direct contact transmission Direct contact transmission is direct physical transfer between an infected or colonized person and a susceptible person. A **colonized person** is one who has a strain of bacteria that have become a part of the person's normal flora. Direct contact transmission can occur when nurses change dressings, give baths, or have any physical contact with infected material.

Transmission can occur between any two people. For example, the virus causing acquired immune deficiency syndrome (AIDS) can be transmitted through sexual intercourse and through direct contact with the infected person's blood.

Indirect contact transmission In indirect contact transmission, a susceptible host comes in contact with a contaminated object. The object could be a stethoscope, any equipment, soiled tissues, etc. Respiratory equipment that is taken from client to client can be a source if it is not cleaned appropriately after use.

Droplet contact transmission Infectious microorganisms can come in contact with a susceptible person's mouth, nose, or conjunctivae when an infected person sneezes or coughs. Droplets are usually sprayed no further than 90 cm (3 ft). Thus, one is in close contact if one is within 90 cm (3 ft) of another person.

Vehicle Transmission

A **vehicle** is a transporting agent or medium. Food, water or blood can be vehicles. For example, the virus causing hepatitis A may be transmitted through water. Municipal laws in the United States and Canada protect the public from contaminated food and water. However, in remote areas of the country, contaminated water is still a threat.

Airborne Transmission

Airborne transmission occurs by dissemination of droplet nuclei or dust particles that contain microorganisms and remain in the air. The microorganisms are then inhaled or deposited on a susceptible host. Microorganisms that attach themselves to dust particles in the air can be carried quickly to other people, even over some distance.

Vector-Borne Transmission

A **vector** is an animal that transfers microorganisms from a reservoir to a host. Insects and other animals can spread such organisms as certain *Salmonella* species, which are part of the normal flora of some domestic animals but cause gastroenteritis in humans. Because flies carry microorganisms also, they can contaminate food and fluids on contact. A fly, for example, may pick up microorganisms from soiled diapers and then transmit them to various exposed foods.

Portal of Entry

Before a person can become infected, microorganisms must enter the body. The skin is a barrier to infectious agents; however, any break in the skin can readily serve as a portal of entry. Microorganisms can enter the body through the same routes they use to leave the body. Often, microorganisms enter the body by the same route they used to leave the source.

Susceptible Host

A **susceptible** (or **compromised**) **host** is an individual who for one or more reasons is more likely than others to acquire an infection. Susceptible hosts are also called persons "at risk." Impairment of the body's natural defenses and a number of other factors can affect susceptibility to infection. See "Factors Affecting Risk of Infection," later in this chapter.

Breaking the Chain of Infection

Various practices break the chain of infection, thus preventing its occurrence and spread. For example, the first link in the chain—the etiologic agent—is interrupted by the use of antiseptics and disinfectants and by sterilization. See "Cleaning, Disinfecting, and Sterilizing," later in this chapter.

Nurses carry out practices that break other links in the chain. See Table 32–2. The aim of most hospital precautions is breaking the chain during the mode of transmission phase of the cycle, because the factors involving the infectious agent and the host are more difficult to control (Williams 1983, p. 341).

Table 32–2 Nursing Interventions That Break the Chain of Infection

Link	Interventions	Rationale
Etiologic agent	Ensure articles are properly cleaned and disinfected or sterilized before use.	Proper cleaning, disinfecting, and sterilizing reduce or eliminate microorganisms.
	Educate clients and family members about appropriate methods to clean, disinfect, and sterilize articles.	Knowledge of ways to reduce or eliminate microorganisms reduces the numbers of microorganisms present and the likelihood of disease.
Source	Change dressings and bandages when they are soiled or wet.	Moist dressings are ideal environments for microorganisms to grow and multiply.
	Assist clients to carry out appropriate skin and oral hygiene.	Hygienic measures reduce the numbers of resident and transient microorganisms and the likelihood of infection.
	Dispose of damp, soiled linens appropriately.	Damp, soiled linens harbor more microorganisms than dry linens.
	Dispose of feces and urine appropriately.	Urine and feces, in particular, contain many microorganisms. Feces may also be the source of certain virulent microorganisms, such as the hepatitis A virus in asymptomatic carriers.
	Ensure that all fluid containers, such as bedside water jugs and suction and drainage bottles, are covered or capped.	Prolonged exposure increases the risk of contamination and promotes microbial growth.
	Empty suction and drainage bottles at the end of each shift.	Drainage harbors microorganisms that, if left for prolonged periods, proliferate.
Portal of exit	Avoid talking, coughing, or sneezing over open wounds or sterile fields and cover the mouth and nose when coughing and sneezing.	These measures limit the number of microorganisms that escape from the respiratory tract.
Mode of transmission	Wash hands between client contacts, after touching infectious material, and before performing invasive procedures or touching open wounds. Instruct clients and family members to wash hands before handling food or eating, before and after eliminating, and after touching infectious material.	Hand washing is the most effective means of controlling and preventing the spread of microorganisms.
	Place discarded soiled materials in moisture-proof refuse bags.	Moisture-proof bags contain the spread of microorganisms to others.
	Handle bedpans with caution.	Urine and feces in particular contain many microorganisms.
	Initiate and implement aseptic precautions for infected clients.	Controlling the mode of transmission of specific microorganisms prevents their spread.
	Wear masks when in close contact with clients who have infections transmitted by droplets from the respiratory tract.	Masks prevent the transmission of airborne microorganisms.
	Wear gloves when handling infectious secretions and excretions. Wear gowns if there is danger of soiling clothing with infectious material.	Gloves and gowns prevent soiling of the hands and clothing.
Portal of entry	Use sterile technique for invasive procedures such as injections and catheterizations.	Invasive procedures penetrate the body's natural protective barriers to microorganisms.
	Use sterile technique when exposing open wounds or handling dressings.	Open wounds are vulnerable to microbial infection.
	Handle needles and syringes with caution.	Injuries from needles contaminated by blood or body fluids from an infected client or carrier are a primary cause of serum hepatitis.
	Provide each client with his or her own personal care items.	People have less resistance to another person's microorganisms than to their own.
Susceptible host	Maintain the integrity of the client's skin and mucous membranes.	Intact skin and mucous membranes protect against invasion by microorganisms.
	Ensure that the client receives a balanced diet.	A balanced diet supplies essential proteins and vitamins necessary to build or maintain body tissues.
	Educate the public about the importance of immunizations.	Immunizations protect people against virulent infectious diseases.

Stages of an Infectious Process

The course of an infection has four stages: the incubation period, the prodromal period, the illness period, and the convalescent period.

Incubation Period

The **incubation period** is the time between the entry of the microorganisms into the body and the onset of the symptoms. During this time, the organism adapts to the person and multiplies sufficiently to produce an infection. The length of incubation varies greatly, depending on the microorganism. For example, rubella (measles) develops in 10 to 14 days, whereas tetanus (lockjaw) takes from 4 to 21 days to develop. An average incubation period is 7 to 10 days.

Prodromal Period

The **prodromal period** is the time from the onset of nonspecific symptoms, e.g., fatigue, malaise, elevated temperature, and irritability, until the specific symptoms of the infection appear. Infected persons are most infectious and most likely to spread the infecting organisms during this stage. Because the symptoms are general, precautions to prevent spread are often not taken at this time. A prodromal stage usually lasts a short time, hours or days at the most.

Illness Period

During the **illness period**, specific symptoms develop and become evident. The symptoms of most infectious processes are manifested both in the affected body organ or area and in the entire body. The latter are called **systemic symptoms**; the symptoms manifested in a discrete area are called **localized symptoms**. During this period, the person often has fever and headache and feels fatigued. Sometimes a skin rash (**exanthema**) or a rash of the mucous membrane (**enanthema**) appears at this stage. The severity of the symptoms and the length of the illness vary with the susceptibility of the person and the pathogenicity of the microorganism.

Convalescent Period

The **convalescent period** extends from the time the symptoms start to abate until the person returns to a normal state of health. Depending on the severity of the illness and the person's general health, convalescence can last from a few days to months. Often it is longer than the person expects.

Normal Body Defenses

The human normally has microbial flora that reside in and outside the body, e.g., on the skin, on mucous membranes, inside the respiratory passages, and inside the gastrointestinal tract. These microorganisms are called **resident flora** because they are always present, usually in numbers compatible with the individual's health. See Table 32–3. **Flora** are the collective vegetation in a given area. In contrast to resident flora, **transient flora** are microorganisms that come and go; they are normally not carried by the individual. **Colonization** is the process by which strains of bacteria become resident flora.

Individuals normally have defenses that protect the body from infection. These defenses can be categorized as nonspecific and specific. **Nonspecific defenses** protect the person against all microorganisms, regardless of prior exposure. **Specific** (or **immune**) **defenses**, by contrast, are directed against specific bacteria, viruses, fungi, or other infectious agents. They require the formation of specifically programmed **lymphocytes**.

Nonspecific Defenses

Anatomic and Physiologic Barriers

Intact skin and mucous membranes are the body's first line of defense against microorganisms. Unless the skin and mucosa become cracked and broken, they are an effective barrier against bacteria. Fungi can live on the skin, but they cannot penetrate it. The dryness of the skin also is a deterrent to bacteria; they are most plentiful in moist areas, e.g., perineum and axillae. Another deterrent is sebum, which contains an unsaturated fatty acid that kills some bacteria. Resident bacteria of the skin also prevent other bacteria from multiplying. They use up the available nourishment, and the end products of their metabolism inhibit other bacteria. Normal secretions make the skin slightly acidic; acidity also inhibits bacterial growth.

The nasal passages have a defensive function. As entering air follows the tortuous route of the passage, it comes in contact with moist mucous membranes and small hairlike projections called cilia. These trap microorgan-

Table 32–3 Common Resident Bacteria of the Body

Body Area	Bacteria	Comment
Skin	*Staphylococcus epidermidis*	Normally nonpathogenic
	Propionibacterium acnes	Uses skin fat and oil for growth
	Staphylococcus aureus	Potential pathogen
	Corynebacterium xerosis	Most numerous in axilla
	Pityrosporum oxale (yeast)	Found on scalp and oily skin
Nasal passages	*Staphylococcus aureus*	Potential pathogen
	Staphylococcus epidermidis	
Oropharynx	*Streptococcus pneumoniae*	Potential pathogen
Bronchi, lungs	None	
Mouth	*Streptococcus*	Adhere to tooth enamel
		Component of plague
	Lactobacillus	Involved in tooth decay
	Neisseria	
	Branhamella	
	Bacteroides	Increased with gum disease
	Actinomycetales	May cause deposition of calcium salts in plaque
Stomach	None	
Esophagus	None	
Small intestine	(See large intestine)	Fewer microorganisms than in large intestine
Large intestine	*Bacteroides*	Ferment food residues
	Fusobacterium	
	Eubacterium	
	Lactobacillus	Produce lactic acid
	Streptococcus	Low pathogenicity
	Enterobacteriaceae	Produce bacteriocins
	Vibrio	
	Escherichia coli	
Urethral orifice	*Staphylococcus epidermidis*	
Uretha	None	
Bladder	None	
Ureters	None	
Kidneys	None	
Vagina	*Lactobacillus*	Balance can be upset by antibiotics
	Bacteroides	
	Clostridium	
Nervous system	None	
Blood, lymph system	None	

isms, dust, and foreign materials. The lungs have alveolar **macrophages** (large **phagocytes**) that ingest foreign particles, including microorganisms. Healthy lungs are free of microorganisms. The central nervous system is protected by the skull and spinal column, which prevent microbial entry.

Each body orifice also has protective mechanisms. The oral cavity regularly sheds mucosal epithelium to rid the mouth of colonizers. The flow of saliva and its partially buffering action help prevent infections. Saliva contains microbial inhibitors, e.g., lactoferrin, lysozyme, and secretory IgA. **Lactoferrin** is an iron-binding protein that inhibits the growth of invading microorganisms by making iron unavailable to them. The enzyme **lysozyme**, present in saliva and tears, functions as an antibacterial agent. Secretory IgA (SIGA) is an immunoglobulin that coats bacteria and thus prevents their attachment to the oral epithelium and to the teeth.

The eye is protected from infection by tears, which continually wash microorganisms away and contain inhibiting lysozyme. The gastrointestinal tract also has defenses against infection. The high acidity of the stomach normally prevents microbial growth. The role that the normal microorganisms of the small intestine play in the body's defense is unknown. However, the resident flora of the large intestine help prevent the establishment of disease-producing microorganisms. Many enterobacteria produce bacteriocins that are lethal to closely related bacterial strains. (A **bacteriocin** is a substance released by bacteria that kills other bacteria.) Some enterobacteria release an antibioticlike substance that kills or inhibits the growth of some bacteria.

The vagina also has natural defenses against infection. When a girl reaches puberty, lactobacilli ferment sugars in the vaginal secretions, creating a vaginal pH of 3.5–4.5. This low pH inhibits the growth of many disease-producing microorganisms. A reasonably healthy female normally has a relatively constant number of these lactobacilli in the vagina. However, antibiotic therapy can upset the bacterial balance because the lactobacilli are highly susceptible to antibiotics. Colonization by *Candida albicans* (yeast) often results.

The entrance to the urethra normally harbors many microorganisms, e.g., *Staphylococcus epidermidis* (from the skin) and *Escherichia coli* (from feces). It is believed that the urine has a flushing and bacteriostatic action that keeps the bacteria from ascending the urethra.

Inflammatory Response

Inflammation is the response of the tissues to injury or infection. It is an adaptive mechanism that destroys or dilutes the injurious agent, prevents further spread of the injury, and promotes the repair of damaged tissue. It is characterized by five signs: pain, swelling, redness, heat, and impaired function of the part if the injury is severe. Commonly, words with the suffix *-itis* describe an inflammatory process. For example, *appendicitis* means inflammation of the appendix; *gastritis* means inflammation of the stomach. Inflammation is a local and nonspecific defensive response. It is important to remember that not all inflammations are the result of infections.

Injurious stressors (inflammatory agents) to body tissues can be categorized as physical agents, chemical agents, and microorganisms. Physical agents include mechanical objects causing trauma to tissues, excessive heat or cold (causing burns or frostbite), and radiation. Chemical agents include external irritants—such as strong acids, alkalis, poisons, and irritating gases—and internal irritants (substances manufactured within the body)—such as excessive hydrochloric acid in the stomach due to altered function. Microorganisms include the broad groups of bacteria, viruses, fungi, protozoa, and Rickettsia.

The inflammatory response involves a series of dynamic events, or defenses of the tissues, not yet completely understood:

1. Vascular and cellular responses
2. Formation of inflammatory exudate
3. Repair of tissues

Vascular and cellular responses In the first stage of inflammation, constriction of the blood vessels occurs at the site of injury, lasting only a few moments. This momentary response is followed by (a) dilation of small blood vessels, (b) increased permeability of the blood vessel walls, (c) slowing of blood flow, and (d) mobilization of leukocytes.

Dilation of small local blood vessels occurs as a result of histamine released by the injured cells. Thus, more blood flows to the injured area, bringing with it large numbers of leukocytes. This marked increase in blood supply is referred to as **hyperemia** and is responsible for the characteristic signs of redness and heat.

Vascular permeability is increased simultaneously at the injured site. This is thought to occur in response to tissue necrosis, the release of chemical mediators, such as bradykinin, serotonin, and prostoglandin, and the release of histamine. The result of this altered permeability is an outpouring of fluid, proteins, and leukocytes into the interstitial spaces. This stage is responsible for the characteristic sign of swelling (edema) and for the associated pain of inflammation. The pain is caused by the pressure of accumulating fluid on local nerve endings and the chemical mediators, which are thought to irritate the nerve endings. Too much fluid pouring into areas such as the plural or pericardial cavity can seriously affect organ function. In other areas, such as joints, mobility is impaired.

Blood flow slows in the dilated vessels. This altered rate of flow facilitates the mobilization of leukocytes and their movement into the tissue spaces along with other substances.

Mobilization of leukocytes includes the two processes of margination and emigration. Normally blood cells (erythrocytes, leukocytes, and platelets) flow along the center of a blood vessel, while a cell-less stream of plasma flows around them against the walls of the blood vessel. When the blood flow slows, **leukocytes** (white blood cells) aggregate or line up along this inner surface of the blood vessels. This process is known as **margination.** Leukocytes then move through the blood vessel wall into the affected tissue spaces, a process called **emigration.** The actual passage of blood corpuscles through the blood vessel wall is referred to as **diapedesis.** The reason leukocytes are attracted to injured cells has been described by the term positive **chemotaxis.** The action of chemotaxis is not fully understood, but basically leukocytes are drawn toward the source of chemicals released in the injured cells (positive chemotaxis), or they are propelled away from the chemical (negative chemotaxis). Leukotaxine released by injured cells is thought to have positive chemotaxic properties.

In response to the exit of leukocytes from the blood vessels, the bone marrow produces large numbers of leukocytes and releases them into the bloodstream (**leukocytosis**). The exact mechanism stimulating this increase is unknown, but it is another cardinal sign of inflammation. A normal leukocyte count of 4500 to 11,000 per cubic millimeter of blood can rise to 20,000 or more.

Having gained entrance to the tissue spaces, the leukocytes attack the injurious agent by **phagocytosis**—a process during which the leukocytes engulf microorganisms, dead cells, or other foreign particles. Neutrophils, one type of white blood cells, are the first to arrive at the injured site. They act easily in the inflammatory process but tend to die rapidly. **Monocytes**, another type of white blood cells, follow; they have greater phagocytic properties than neutrophils. Macrophages (reticuloendothelial cells) present in the tissue spaces assist the leukocytes in phagocytosis. Antibodies from plasma also come to the site. Their function is discussed in more detail later in this chapter. During the inflammatory response, antibodies can make the inflammatory agent more susceptible to phagocytosis.

Formation of the inflammatory exudate In the second stage of inflammation, fluid that escaped from the blood vessels, dead phagocytic cells, as well as dead tissue cells and products that they release produce the inflammatory **exudate.** A plasma protein called **fibrinogen** (which is converted to fibrin when it is released into the tissues), thromboplastin (a product released by injured tissue cells), and platelets together form an interlacing network to form a barrier, wall off the area, and prevent its spread. This network also provides the framework for the reparative stage.

During the second stage, the injurious agent is overcome and the exudate is cleared away by lymphatic drainage. When this is achieved, the reparative (third phase) begins.

The nature and amount of exudate vary in accordance with the tissue involved and the intensity and duration of the inflammation. The major types of exudate are serous, purulent, and hemorrhagic (sanguineous).

A **serous exudate** is comprised chiefly of serum (the clear portion of the blood) derived from the blood and serous membranes of the body, such as the peritoneum, pleura, pericardium, and meninges. It is watery in appearance and has few cells. An example is the fluid in a blister from a burn.

A **purulent exudate** is thicker than serous exudate due to the presence of pus. It consists of leukocytes, liquefied dead tissue debris, and dead and living bacteria. The process of pus formation is referred to as **suppuration**, and the bacteria that produce pus are called **pyogenic bacteria.** Not all microorganisms are pyogenic. Purulent exudates vary in color, some acquiring tinges of blue, green, or yellow. The color may depend on the causative organism.

A **sanguineous**, or **hemorrhagic**, **exudate** consists of large amounts of red blood cells, indicating damage to capillaries that is severe enough to allow the escape of red blood cells from plasma. This type of exudate is frequently seen in open wounds. Nurses often need to distinguish whether the sanguineous exudate is dark or bright. A bright sanguineous exudate indicates fresh bleeding, whereas dark sanguineous exudate denotes older bleeding.

Mixed types of exudates are often observed. A serosanguineous exudate is commonly seen in surgical incisions; it consists of serous and sanguineous drainage.

Repair of tissues (healing) Injured tissues can be repaired by (a) regeneration or (b) replacement with fibrous tissue (scar) formation.

Regeneration is the replacement of destroyed tissue cells by cells that are identical or similar in structure and function. It involves not only replacement of damaged cells one by one but also organization of these cells so that the architectural pattern of the tissue and function are restored.

The **stroma** is the tissue that forms the framework (connective tissue) or ground substance of an organ. The **parenchyma** is the essential functional elements of an organ. Functional cells must have proper relationships between stroma and parenchyma, and among their blood vessels, lymph vessels, nerves, and ducts. All must regenerate concurrently. If one component lags behind the others, a normal product will not be formed. The villain of this scenario, fibrous (scar) tissue, frequently wins, since it has the capacity to proliferate under the unusual conditions of ischemia and altered pH.

The ability to reproduce cells varies considerably from one type of tissue to another. For example, epithelial tissues of the skin and of the digestive and respiratory tracts have a good regenerative capacity, provided that their underlying support structures are intact. The same holds true for osseous, lymphoid, and bone marrow tissues. Tissues that have little regenerative capacity include nervous, muscular, and elastic tissues. These are highly specialized tissues that cannot be replaced by identically organized cells, but rather are replaced by scar tissue. Unfortunate examples are the damage to the brain from a stroke and the damage to the heart muscle from a cardiac incident. These tissues cannot be replaced.

When regeneration is not possible, repair occurs by **fibrous tissue** formation. The inflammatory exudate with its interlacing network of fibrin provides the framework for this tissue to develop. Damaged tissues are replaced with the connective tissue elements of collagen, blood capillaries, lymphatics, and other tissue ground substances. In the early stages of this process, the tissue is called **granulation tissue**. It is a fragile, gelatinous tissue, appearing pink or red because of the many newly formed capillaries. Later in the process, the tissue shrinks (the capillaries are constricted, even obliterated) and the collagen fibers contract, so that a firmer fibrous tissue remains. This is called a **cicatrix** or scar.

Although scar tissue has the positive attribute of repairing the injured area, it also can present problems. It can reduce the functional capacity of the tissue or organ. For example, scar tissue in cardiac muscle renders that area weaker. Mechanical obstructions can also arise, for example, in the healing of a duodenal ulcer. Sometimes the pyloric sphincter becomes stenosed as granulation tissue contracts into scar tissue.

Interferon

Interferon is a protein produced by cells that are infected by a virus; it binds to the surface of uninvolved cells, stimulating them to produce antiviral proteins that prevent the virus from multiplying. Interferon is active against many viruses but is host-cell-specific, i.e., effective in only the human or animal species that produces it.

Properidin System

The properidin system consists of a group of three serum proteins. It stimulates the inflammatory response, destroys certain bacteria, enhances phagocytosis, and activates the complement system.

Complement System

The complement system functions to complete certain immune reactions that involve antibodies. The system consists of a group of eleven inactive proteins called complement in normal blood serum. They are designated as C1 to C9 (C1 consists of three proteins). When stimulated by the presence of a foreign substance, these proteins become active and participate in the release of histamines, in chemotaxis, and in the release of substances that facilitate phagocytosis. In these activities, the complement system is considered a nonspecific defense. The function of the system as a specific defense is discussed subsequently.

Specific Defenses

Specific defenses of the body involve the immune system. It responds to foreign protein in the body—e.g., bacteria or transplanted tissues—or, in some cases, even the body's own proteins. Foreign proteins in the body are called **antigens** and are considered invaders. If the proteins originate in a person's own body, the antigen is called an **autoantigen**.

The immune response has two components: antibody-mediated defenses and cell-mediated defenses. These two systems provide distinct but overlapping protection. Both defenses are thought of as specific because (a) they recognize, remember, and respond to unique pattern configurations on the surfaces of antigens, and (b) they respond only to one specific antigenic configuration.

Antibody-Mediated Defense

This defense is also referred to as **humoral** (circulating) **immunity**, since it resides ultimately in the blood serum, or the B-cell system. It is mediated by antibodies produced by B cells. **Antibodies**, also called **immunoglobulins**, are part of the body's plasma proteins, specifically, the gammaglobulins. B cells are one type of lymphocyte; they comprise 30% of blood lymphocytes and are short-lived, having a life span of 15 days. The antibody-mediated response defends primarily against the extracellular phases of bacterial and viral infections.

B cells are activated when they recognize a foreign invader, an antigen. They then differentiate into plasma cells, which secrete antibodies, and serum proteins, which bind specifically to the foreign substance and initiate a variety of elimination responses.

Types of antibodies The B-cell response to an antigen may produce antibody molecules of five classes of immunoglobulins designated by the letters G, A, M, D, and E, and usually written as follows: IgG, IgA, IgM, IgD, and IgE. Each of the five has a unique structure and function (see Table 32–4). IgG is the most abundant immunoglobulin, constituting about 75% of the immunoglobulins in plasma. IgA and IgM constitute about 25%, and IgD and IgE comprise less than 1%. Note that IgM is involved in blood transfusion reactions (see Chapter 46). Before an antibody response, the phagocytic cells of the blood bind and ingest foreign substances. However, the rate of binding and phagocytosis increases if the foreign substance is coated with IgG antibodies.

The first interaction between an antigen and antibody is known as the **primary immune response**. The principal characteristics of this response are (a) a latent period before the appearance of an antibody; (b) the production of only a small amount of antibody, chiefly IgM, and (c) most importantly, the creation of a large number of memory cells capable of responding to the same antigen in the future. The **secondary immune** (or booster) **response** takes place on subsequent encounters with the same antigen. The principal characteristics of this response are: (a) rapid proliferation of B cells; (b) rapid differentiation of B cells into plasma cells that promptly produce large quantities of antibody, chiefly class IgG; and (c) release of antibody into the blood and other body tissues, where it can react with the antigen.

Table 32–4 Antibodies and Their Functions

Antibody	Description	Function
IgM	Principally an antibody of the blood; the first antibody produced in response to an antigen	Provides an early immune response Activates the complement system Stimulates ingestion by macrophages Serves as A, B, and O blood groups' isoantibodies and antibodies to serious infections, such as by Gram-negative microorganisms Responds to artificial immunization
IgG	The most prevalent antibody in the blood and a major antibody in tissue spaces; produced later in the immune response than IgM	Triggers complement fixation Activates macrophage ingestion The only antibody to cross the placental barrier Neutralizes microbial toxins and has antiviral and some antibacterial actions
IgA	Resides under the epithelial mucosal cells, especially of the gastrointestinal tract, but also found in tears, saliva, sweat, colostrum, and breast milk; also produced later in the immune response than IgM	Acts as a protective barrier against microorganisms at several points of entrance Easily crosses cell barriers Protects the mucous membranes of the gastrointestinal and the respiratory tracts Because it is a major antibody of milk and colostrum, may function to protect the gastrointestinal tracts of nursing infants
IgD	Normally present in only minute concentrations in the blood	Unknown
IgE	Normally present in only minute concentrations in the blood	Responds primarily to allergic reactions

Types of immunity **Immunity** is the specific resistance of the body to infection (pathogens or their toxins). There are two major types of immunity: natural or innate, and acquired.

Natural immunity is inherited resistance to infection. It is present at birth and depends largely on the nonspecific defenses of the host. This immunity may occur at the individual, species, and racial levels. Some species are more resistant than others to specific microorganisms. Humans, for instance, are resistant to distemper virus, a morbid invader of cats and dogs. Racial differences also exist. For example, blacks are more resistant to malaria than whites. Observations indicate that even at the individual level some persons are more resistant to certain infections, such as the influenza virus, than others.

Acquired immunity occurs only after a person has been exposed to a disease agent. It is obtained during life and results from the production of antibodies. It can be an active or passive process of the body, and in either case it may be naturally or artifically induced. Thus, there are four divisions of acquired immunity. See Table 32–5.

Cell-Mediated Defense

This defense is also referred to as **cellular immunity**, since it resides in cells of the lymphoid system or the T-cell system. T cells are a second type of lymphocyte that are present in the thymus gland at birth; they are therefore thymic-lymphoid cells. These cells leave the thymus to circulate in the blood as long-lived lymphocytes with a life span of up to 5 years. Some settle in lymph nodes and the spleen. T cells comprise 70% of circulating blood

Table 32–5 Types of Acquired Immunity

Type	Antigen or Antibody Source	Duration
1. Active	Antibodies are produced by the body in response to infection	Long
a. Natural	Antibodies are formed in the presence of active infection in the body	Lifelong
b. Artificial	Antigens (vaccines or toxoids) are administered to the person to stimulate antibody production	Many years; the immunity must be reinforced by booster inoculations
2. Passive	Antibodies are produced by another source, animal or human	Short
a. Natural	Antibodies are transferred naturally from an immune mother to her baby through the placenta or in colostrum	6 months to 1 year
b. Artificial	Immune serum (antibody) from an animal or another human is injected	2 to 3 weeks

lymphocytes. This cell-mediated response defends against viral infection, fungal infection, some bacterial infections, and malignant cells. Malignant cells are thought to arise from changes in normal body cells and therefore are regarded as foreign cells. The response is also responsible for graft rejection.

There are three types of T cells:

1. T helper (Th) cells. These enhance the production of antibodies by the B cells, specifically IgG, IgA, and IgE responses. Most IgM responses are T helper cell independent.
2. T suppressor (Ts) cells. These inhibit antibody production by the B cells.
3. T cytolytic (Tc) cells. These are cell-destroying cells, some of which are now called killer T cells.

The helper-suppressor function of T cells is not fully understood. The cytolytic cells, however, travel to the invading antigen, where they produce a variety of powerful chemicals or factors called **lymphokines.** The types and functions of some T-cell lymphokines are shown in Table 32–6. Like the B cells, T cells function as memory cells and thus greatly enhance the defense reaction to a second invasion by the same antigen.

Table 32–6 Types and Functions of Some T-Cell Lymphokines

Lymphokine	Functions
Chemotactic factor (CF)	Attracts macrophages and monocytes to the antigen site
Migration inhibition factor (MIF)	Prevents departure of macrophages from the site
Macrophage activation or aggregation factor (MAF)	Increases phagocytosis of macrophages and agglutinates (clumps) them
Lymphotoxin factor (LT)	Acts as a cytotoxin and directly destroys microorganisms
Transfer factor	Causes nonsensitized lymphocytes at the site to act as a sensitized cell
Interferon (also produced by cells other than lymphocytes)	Blocks viral infection of tissue cells

Factors Affecting Risk of Infection

Whether a microorganism causes an infection depends on a number of factors already mentioned. One of the most important factors is susceptibility, which is affected by (a) age, (b) heredity, (c) level of stress, (d) nutritional status, (e) immunization status, (f) current medical therapy, and (g) preexisting disease processes.

Age

Newborns and elderly people have reduced defenses against infection. Infections are a major cause of death of newborns, who have immature immune systems and are protected only for the first 2 or 3 months by IgG type immunoglobulins received from the mother. At birth, infants can manufacture significant amounts of IgM but begin producing IgA only within the first month. Between 1 to 3 months of age, infants begin to synthesize their own immunoglobulins; about 40% of adult levels are reached by 1 year of age (Whaley and Wong 1983, p. 421). Immunizations against diphtheria, tetanus, and pertussis are usually started at 2 months, when the infant's immune system can respond. See Table 32–4 for information about immunoglobulins.

As the immune system matures in growing children, immunoglobulins normally develop. However, young children are still susceptible to colds; common infectious diseases, such as measles, mumps, and chicken pox; and intestinal infections. An only child may experience these chiefly upon entering nursery school, while a child with older brothers and sisters acquires these infections earlier. Young and middle-aged adults have well-developed body defenses to infection. Viral infections are most common in this age group. With advancing age, the immune responses again become weak. The immune response (cell-mediated immunity) is reduced. Lymphocytes become more diverse with age, and there is a progressive loss of cellular regulation in the body. Although there is still much to learn about aging, it is known that immunity to infection decreases with advancing age.

Heredity

Some people have a genetic susceptibility to certain infections. For example, some people may be deficient in serum immunoglobulins, which play a significant role in the internal defense mechanism of the body.

Onset of infections before age 6 months suggests a cell-mediated immune defect; onset after age 6 months, a humoral immune defect.

Stress

The nature, number, and duration of physical and emotional stressors can influence susceptibility to infection. Stressors elevate blood cortisone. Prolonged elevation of blood cortisone decreases antiinflammatory responses, depletes energy stores, leads to a state of exhaustion, and decreases resistance to infection. For example, a person recovering from a major operation or traumatic injury is more likely to develop an infection than a healthy person who has not had surgery or injury. Similarly, a person who is anxious about the outcome of an illness, is worried about financial problems, and is coping with separation from family members or a recent loss may have little energy left for coping with invading organisms.

Nutritional Status

It is generally accepted that resistance to infection depends on adequate nutritional status. Exactly how adequate nutrition provides the body with sufficient defenses is not known. Because antibodies are proteins, the ability of the body to synthesize antibodies may be impaired by inadequate nutrition, especially when protein reserves are depleted (e.g., as a result of traumatic injury, surgery, or debilitating diseases such as cancer).

Immunization Status

Active and passive immunization are needed to combat infections. Childhood immunization is discussed in Chapter 33. Because of the prevalence of influenza and its potential for causing death, immunization against influenza is recommended for the elderly and for persons with chronic cardiac, respiratory, metabolic, and renal disease. Immunization is usually provided in early October or November; annual boosters are required to maintain immunity.

Current Medical Therapy

Some medical therapies predispose a person to infection. For example, radiation treatments for cancer destroy not only cancerous cells but also some normal cells, thereby rendering them more vulnerable to infection. Certain medications also increase susceptibility to infection. Antineoplastic (anticancer) medications may depress bone marrow function, resulting in inadequate production of white blood cells and lymphocytes necessary to combat infections. Antiinflammatory medications, such as adrenal corticosteroids, inhibit the inflammatory response, an essential defense against infection. Even some antibiotics used to treat infections can have adverse effects. Antibiotics may kill resident flora, allowing the proliferation of strains that would not grow and multiply in the body under normal conditions.

Some diagnostic procedures also predispose the client to an infection, especially when the skin is broken or sterile body cavities are penetrated during the procedure.

Existing Disease

Any disease that lessens the body's defenses against infection places the client at risk. Examples are chronic pulmonary disease, which impairs ciliary action and weakens the mucous barrier; peripheral vascular disease, which inhibits blood flow; burns, which prejudice skin integrity, chronic or debilitating diseases, which deplete protein reserves; and such immune system diseases as leukemia and aplastic anemia, which alter the production rate of white blood cells.

Nosocomial Infections

Nosocomial infections originate in a hospital or other medical facility. They include infections clients acquire during their stay in a facility or manifest after discharge and infections occurring among health personnel working in the facility. These infections have received increasing attention in recent years. They are considered more difficult to prevent and treat, more unpredictable, and more resistant to cure than infections contracted in the community (Norton 1981, p. 813).

Incidence

U.S. surveys reveal that nosocomial infections occur in about 5% of all persons admitted to acute care hospitals and in about 8% of persons in long-term care facilities (Norton 1981, p. 815). In a survey in the United Kingdom, Meers (1982, p. 146) found that of 400 hospitalized clients, 19.1% had active infections. Of these, 9.9% were community acquired infections (CAI) and 9.2% were hospital acquired (HAI). In a national survey in the United States, Palmer reported 44,785 nosocomial infections occurring in 1,362,342 clients hospitalized and discharged in 1979. The mean nosocomial infection rate was 3.3% of discharged acute care clients (Palmer 1984, p. 4). Clients undergoing surgical procedures have a higher incidence of nosocomial infections than others. One survey indicated that about 70% of all nosocomial infections in a hospital developed in postoperative clients (Simmons 1983, p. 133).

Brem and Torok analyzed the data about the nosocomial infections occurring in a community hospital during 1 year. They found that people under the age of 65 years had an infection rate of 2.1%, while people over 65 years had a rate of 10%, i.e., a rate five times greater (Brem and Torok 1979, p. 42). Other researchers conducted a study of nosocomial infections in a long-term care facility with 460 clients whose median age was 76.9 years. The infection rate was 12% (Setia et al. 1985, p. 57). In addition, they found that the most common sites were skin (5.6%), urinary tract (4.7%), lower respiratory tract (2.3%), and sepsis (0.2%) (Setia et al. 1985, pp. 58–59). The study further revealed that 21.5% of all clients who developed infections acquired them during the first year of hospitalization (Setia et al. 1985, p. 59).

Etiology

The source of microorganisms that cause nosocomial infections can be the clients themselves (an endogenous source) or the hospital environment and hospital personnel (exogenous sources). Most infections appear to have endogenous sources (Simmons 1983, p. 134). The National Nosocomial Infections study, conducted between 1979 and 1983, found that *Escherichia coli* was the most common infecting organism, followed by *Staphylococcus aureus* and enterococci (Pickering and DuPont 1986, p. 28).

Contributing Factors

A number of factors contribute to nosocomial infections:

1. Medical therapy. Illness due to any aspect of medical therapy is called **iatrogenic**. Iatrogenic infections are as a direct result of a diagnostic or therapeutic procedure. An example of an iatrogenic infection is bacteremia caused by inserting an unsterile heart valve into a client. Not all nosocomial infections—for example, the development of a respiratory infection in an immobilized elderly female—are iatrogenic.
2. The presence of many susceptible persons, i.e., clients whose normal defenses have been lowered by surgery or illness. See the section on clients "at risk."
3. Insufficient hand washing by personnel after handling clients or infected materials. Personnel can acquire microorganisms from colonized clients and pass them on to other clients. The hands of personnel are a common vehicle for the spread of microorganisms.

Economic Implications

The cost of nosocomial infections to the client, the facility, and funding bodies (e.g., insurance companies and provincial governments in Canada) is very great. Nosocomial infections extend hospitalization time, increase clients' time away from work, cause disability and discomfort, and even result in loss of life. The Centers for Disease Control (CDC) estimate that up to $6 billion are spent yearly because of nosocomial infections and that at least $1 billion could be saved through reduction of preventable infections (Reinarz 1978, p. 31). Freeman et al (1979, p. 732) found that clients who acquired one nosocomial infection had their hospital stays extended by an average of 13 days and that clients with two nosocomial infections had their stays extended by an average of 35.4 days.

In the United Kingdom, the costs of nosocomial infections in acute bed hospitals in 1981 were £30 million and in Germany in 1980 they were DM3200 million. Losos and Trotman (1984, p. 249) estimate that the annual costs in Canada due to a nosocomial infection rate of 7% in 1984 were $Cdn1,019,544,636.

Assessment

The nurse assesses (a) the degree to which a client is at risk of acquiring an infection and (b) the presence of clinical signs of an existing infectious process.

Nursing History Data

Determining Clients at Risk

The nurse elicits the following data:

1. History of immunizations
2. History of recurrent acute or chronic infections. If the client has had such infections, the nurse elicits a specific description of the infection, the related signs and symptoms, the frequency and duration of the infection, and the mode of treatment.
3. The medications or therapies the client is receiving, noting particularly corticosteroids, antineoplastic drugs, and radiotherapy.
4. The client's existing disease processes. These data may also be obtained from the client's medical record. Determine particularly chronic diseases that affect the respiratory and circulatory systems; debilitating diseases that deplete protein reserves; and traumatic disorders, such as surgery or burns, that alter skin integrity.
5. The nature, number, and duration of current emotional stressors. To determine emotional stressors, the nurse:
   a. Observes verbal and nonverbal clues. Lack of communication or excessive communication, a "poker face," poor grooming, complaints of stress-related symptoms such as headache, change in appetite, backache, or fatigue may suggest emotional stress.
   b. May ask broad, indirect questions, such as "How would you describe your current life situation?"
   c. Acquires a history of life-style.
6. Nutritional status. Assessment of nutritional status is discussed in Chapter 42.

Determining the Presence of an Infection

An interview reveals the client's chief complaints, i.e., loss of energy, loss of appetite, nausea, headache, or other signs associated with specific body systems. For example, the client may complain of vomiting or diarrhea if there is a gastrointestinal infection, productive cough if there is a respiratory infection, or pain and difficulty urinating if there is a urinary infection. Clinical signs of infection are discussed next.

Physical Health Data

During the physical examination, the nurse inspects the client for local and systemic signs of infection. Signs of a local infection are caused by the inflammatory response and include:

1. Swelling
2. Redness
3. Pain or tenderness with palpation or movement
4. Palpable heat at the infected area
5. Loss of function of the body part affected, depending on the site and extent of involvement

The involved area may also have various colored drainages if there is an open wound. For additional information regarding localized responses and description of exudate, see the section on inflammatory adaptive responses earlier in this chapter.

Signs of a systemic infection include:

1. Fever
2. Increased pulse and respiratory rate, if the fever is high
3. Lassitude, malaise, and loss of energy
4. Anorexia and, in some situations, nausea and vomiting
5. Headache
6. Enlargement and tenderness of lymph nodes that drain the area of infection

Laboratory Data

Laboratory data that indicate the presence of an infection include:

1. Elevated leukocyte (white blood) cell (WBC) count (4500 to 11,000/cu mm is normal).
2. Increases in specific types of leukocytes as revealed in the differential white blood cell count. Specific types of white blood cells are increased or decreased in certain infections. Normal values are cited for the adult.
   a. Neutrophils are increased in acute suppurative infections but may be decreased in acute bacterial infection, especially in older people. Normal range is 54 to 75%.
   b. Lymphocytes are increased in chronic bacterial and viral infections. Normal is 25 to 40%.
   c. Monocytes are increased in some protozoal and Rickettsial infections and in tuberculosis. Normal is 2 to 8%.
   d. Eosinophils are generally unaltered in an infectious process. Normal is 1 to 4%.
   e. Basophils are generally unaltered in an infectious process. Normal is 0 to 1% (Byrne et al. 1986, p. 78).
3. Elevated **erythrocyte sedimentation rate** (ESR), commonly referred to as sedimentation rate. The ESR is a measure of the speed with which red blood cells in anticoagulated whole blood settle to the bottom of a calibrated tube. Sedimentation normally takes place slowly, but the rate increases in the presence of an inflammatory process.
4. Urine, blood, sputum, or other drainage cultures that indicate the presence of microorganisms.

Nursing Diagnosis and Planning

Nursing diagnoses for clients with an infection or at risk for acquiring infection may include potential for infection, potential social isolation, potential diversional activity deficit, and disturbance in self-concept. Examples of nursing diagnoses are shown on page 687. Nurses, however, formulate diagnoses from the assessment data obtained for each client. After deriving pertinent causative factors from the database, nurses individualize interventions for the client.

Overall nursing responsibilities for clients at risk of acquiring an infection or for those with infections include the following:

1. Prevent the spread of an infection.
2. Maintain and/or restore the client's body defenses.
3. Reduce or alleviate problems associated with the infection.

Planned nursing interventions to prevent the spread of an infection include use of meticulous medical and surgical aseptic techniques—especially for required invasive procedures, such as injections, intravenous therapy, or urinary catheterization; initiation of appropriate protective aseptic (isolation) precautions; and client education about immunization, hygiene, sanitation, and appro-

Examples of Nursing Diagnoses Related to Infection

- Potential for infection related to knowledge deficit about required immunization
- Potential for infection related to altered skin integrity
- Potential for infection related to change in pH of vaginal secretions
- Potential for infection related to decreased ciliary action
- Potential for infection related to suppressed inflammatory response secondary to cortisone therapy
- Potential for infection related to immunosuppression secondary to chemotherapy
- Social isolation related to misinformation by others about transmission of Acquired Immune Deficiency Syndrome
- Potential diversional activity deficit related to strict protective aseptic (isolation) precautions
- Potential disturbance in self-concept related to acquisition of sexually transmitted disease

priate food handling practices. The latter are discussed in Chapter 33. Interventions to maintain or restore the client's body defenses include the provision of adequate fluids and nutrition, rest, administering and monitoring prescribed antimicrobial therapy.

Because malaise, fever, pain, and dehydration from fluid loss are often associated with an infection, plans need also to incorporate interventions that promote comfort and reduce or prevent these discomforts.

Interventions to Prevent Infections

1. Wash hands before and after any direct client contact, before any invasive procedure (e.g., urinary catheterization), before contact with clients who have immunodeficiencies, and after contact with any infectious materials (e.g., feces, urine, wound drainage, etc.).

Nurses are accountable for their own aseptic practices, and any errors in practice must be reported to the responsible nurse or corrected by the nurse. Because microorganisms cannot be seen, only the nurse carrying out a particular aseptic practice knows when a break in asepsis occurs.

2. Employ practices to reduce the number of organisms in the environment, e.g., change bed linens regularly and change moist dressings frequently, as permitted. Drainage on dressings often has a heavy concentration of microorganisms.
3. Dispose of materials—e.g., tissues, needles, dressings, etc.—that are known to be contaminated in moisture-resistant containers for appropriate disposal.
4. Handle needles and syringes carefully to avoid needle-prick injuries.
5. Take special precautions when performing invasive techniques, such as intravenous therapy or urinary catheterization. Use strict aseptic technique when inserting any intravenous needle or catheter, change intravenous tubing and solution containers according to hospital policy (e.g., every 24 hours), and check intravenous solutions for expiration date and clarity. See Chapter 46 for further information. To prevent urinary infections, use strict aseptic technique when inserting the catheter, use a closed drainage system, do not irrigate a catheter unless ordered to do so, provide regular catheter care, and keep the drainage bag and spout off the floor. See Chapter 44 for further information.
6. Prevent respiratory infections by encouraging the client to move, cough, and breathe deeply at least every 2 hours. Assess the client's breath sounds, obtain sputum cultures as required, use aseptic technique when suctioning clients, use sterile water in oxygen humidifiers, change the humidifier water at least every 24 hours, and use only clean inhalation equipment for each client. See Chapter 45 for further information.
7. Prevent wound infections by using aseptic technique when changing dressings, detecting signs of infection early, and using local antimicrobial agents as ordered. See Chapter 52 for further information.
8. Educate the public about preventive measures for common communicable diseases. See Table 32–7 on pages 688–91 and recommended immunization schedules in Chapter 33.
9. Take appropriate protective aseptic precautions for infectious clients to safeguard other clients and self. See Table 32–11 later in this chapter.
10. Be aware of clients who are at risk of infection and take measures to prevent infection and enhance the body's defenses. See "Protecting Body Defenses," later in the chapter.
11. Assess clients consistently and frequently for early signs of an infection.
12. Educate individuals about the importance of seeking medical advice if they have a fever or skin eruption.

Table 32–7 Overview of Selected Infectious Diseases

Disease	Infectious Organism	Sources	Method of Spread	Entry Site	Prevention
AIDS (Acquired immune deficiency syndrome)	HTLV-III (Human T cell leukemia virus)	Blood and body fluids of infected person	Sexual contact (predominantly homosexual intercourse), unclean I.V. needles, transfusion of blood or blood products, transplacental transfer	Intravenously, urethra, vagina, rectum, mouth	Avoid sexual contact, especially anal intercourse, with infected person Avoid needle-stick injuries Wear gloves when handling blood or body fluids of infected person Avoid having multiple sexual partners to lessen probability of exposure Refrain from accepting blood or plasma donations from high-risk groups Screening of plasma or blood by manufacturers and collection agencies to protect recipients
Chickenpox (varicella)	Virus	Infected human	Respiratory droplets, direct contact with lesion secretions until crusted, indirect contact with articles soiled by infectious material	Most likely the nasopharynx	Keep children home from school until lesions are dry Follow strict isolation precautions for infected persons in hospital Isolate exposed susceptible patients
German measles (rubella)	Virus	Infected human	Most likely respiratory droplets Articles soiled with discharges from nose and throat, blood, urine, or feces		Give rubella virus vaccine Ensure pregnant females, especially those in the first trimester, avoid contact Wear a mask when in close contact with the client Avoid contact with infectious secretions Keep children home from school and adults from work for 7 days after onset of rash
Gonorrhea	*Neisseria gonorrhoeae*	Human urethral and vaginal secretions	Sexual contact	Urethra or vagina	Early case-finding and treatment of infected persons Avoid sexual contact with infected persons until posttreatment cultures are free of gonococci Disinfect articles contaminated by infectious secretions

Table 32–7 ***(continued)***

Disease	Infectious Organism	Sources	Method of Spread	Entry Site	Prevention
Type A hepatitis	Hepatitis A virus (HAV)	Principally contaminated water or food and feces of asymptomatic carriers	Person-to-person by fecal-oral route	Gastrointestinal tract	Educate public about sanitary disposal of feces and careful handwashing after diaper changing and before eating Apply enteric aseptic precautions during the first 2 weeks of illness or 1 week after onset of jaundice Wear gloves when handling infectious material
Type B hepatitis	Hepatitis B virus (HBV)	Principally the blood of infected persons but also in saliva, semen, and vaginal fluids	Primarily contaminated blood (and serum-derived) transfusions and contaminated needles, syringes, and other intravenous equipment, especially among drug addicts. Also sexual contact	Parenteral routes and open cuts in skin	Immunize contacts with HB vaccine Screen blood donors Avoid needle-prick injuries Strict discipline in blood banks, i.e., testing of all donated blood for presence of HBV Initiate and maintain blood and body fluid precautions for infected persons Wear gloves when handling blood and blood-soiled articles
Infectious mononucleosis	Virus	Infected humans	Oropharyngeal route via saliva; kissing facilitates spread among adults; hands or toys infected by saliva facilitates spread among children	Oral mucous membrane	None
Influenza	Virus	Infected humans, animal sources are suspected	Respiratory droplets	Respiratory tract	Specific flu virus vaccine
Measles (rubeola)	Virus	Infected humans	Droplet spread or direct contact with nasopharyngeal secretions	Respiratory tract	Measles vaccine Keep children home from school for at least 4 days after appearance of rash If susceptible wear mask when in close contact with the infected person
Mumps	Virus	Infected humans	Respiratory droplets and direct contact with saliva	Upper respiratory tract	Immunization with mumps vaccine If susceptible wear mask when in close contact with the client Disinfect articles soiled with nose and throat secretions

(continued)

Table 32–7 *(continued)*

Disease	Infectious Organism	Sources	Method of Spread	Entry Site	Prevention
Pediculosis	*Pediculosis corporis* (body) caused by *Pediculus humanus corporis* *Pediculosis capitis* (head) caused by *Pediculus humanis capitis* *Pediculosis pubis* (genital) caused by *Phthirus pubis*	Infected persons	For head and body lice, direct contact with infested person and indirect contact with personal clothing For crab lice, sexual contact	External hairy parts of body	Contact isolation until 24 hours after application of effective pesticide, e.g., Kwell, Gamene Disinfect clothing and bedding Examine household members and other close personal contacts
Pneumococcal pneumonia	*Pneumococcus*	Pharynx of self or human carrier	Respiratory droplets up to 24 hours after start of antibiotic therapy	Respiratory tract	Assess and control respiratory infections early
Poliomyelitis	Virus	Infected humans	Fecal-oral route	Gastrointestinal tract	Administer Salk (parenteral) and Sabin (oral) vaccines Isolate infected person (enteric precautions)
Syphilis	*Treponema pallidum*	Infected body fluids and secretions (saliva, semen, blood, vaginal discharges) and secretions for 24 hours after start of effective therapy	Sexual intercourse; transplacental transfer; blood transfusions if donor is in early stages of disease	Mucosal surfaces of external genitals; cervix; placenta; and skin lesions	Educate the public about symptoms of sexually transmitted disease (STD) and modes of spread Discourage sexual promiscuity Refrain from sexual intercourse with infected person until lesions are healed Screen blood donors Early case finding, diagnosis, and treatment of infected persons Serologic examination in both early and late pregnancy and treatment of positive reactors to prevent congenital syphilis For hospitalized clients, avoid direct contact with infected secretions; implement drainage/secretions and blood/body fluid precautions
Tetanus (lockjaw)	*Clostridium tetani*	Intestines of animals, including humans, in which the organism is a harmless, normal inhabitant; soil contami-	Introduction of spores through open wounds by contact with contaminated soil, street dust, or animal feces	Contaminated puncture wound, laceration or burns and injected, contaminated street drugs	Active immunization with tetanus toxoid Proper wound management, i.e., cleaning, debridement if needed, appropriate antibiotic therapy, and passive immunization with tetanus immune

Table 32–7 (*continued*)

Disease	Infectious Organism	Sources	Method of Spread	Entry Site	Prevention
		nated with animal feces; rarely, human feces			globulin (TIG) if necessary
Tuberculosis	*Mycobacterium tuberculosis*	Infected humans; in some areas, diseased cattle	Respiratory droplets from infected sputum; ingestion of raw unpasteurized milk or dairy products	Respiratory tract or gastrointestinal tract if from ingesting diseased cattle products	Improve social conditions, such as overcrowding, that increase risk Educate the public in mode of spread and methods of control Early assessment and treatment of infected persons Home supervision and follow-up to encourage infected persons to carry out therapy Tuberculin testing and BCG vaccination for uninfected persons at high risk of becoming infected Use of pasteurized milk When around hospitalized clients, wear a mask if the infected person does not reliably cover the mouth when coughing
Typhoid fever	*Salmonella typhi*	Contaminated water and food; carriers with infected urine and feces (fecal carriers most common)	Food or water contaminated by the urine or feces of a carrier; flies	Gastrointestinal tract; ingestion of infectious material	Sanitary water supply Sanitary disposal of human feces Control of flies Pasteurize milk and dairy products Treatment and control of carrier Vaccination in regions with contaminated water supplies Emphasize hand washing after urinating and defecating and before food preparation Implement enteric precautions for hospitalized clients
Whooping cough (pertussis)	*Bordetella pertussis*	Infected bronchial secretions of humans	Respiratory droplets	Respiratory tract	Active immunization with pertussis vaccine Wear mask when in close contact with hospitalized, infected clients Keep infected children away from day-care centers, schools, and public places until they have received 5 days of antibiotic therapy

Interventions for Clients with Infections

Nursing interventions for clients with infections include:

1. Assist in identifying the causative microorganism and medical diagnosis by:
   a. Obtaining specimens of feces, urine, sputum, blood, nose and throat secretions, and wound exudates for bacterial culture and sensitivity tests. Collection of these specimens is discussed in Chapters 43 (feces), 44 (urine), 45 (sputum, nose and throat secretions), 46 (blood), and 52 (wound exudate). A culture and sensitivity test, commonly referred to as a C&S, involves **culture** (incubation) of the contaminated material in the laboratory to identify the microorganisms and exposure of the culture growth to antibiotic discs to determine which drug or drugs most effectively inhibit growth, i.e., to which antibiotics the microorganisms are sensitive. The laboratory culture and sensitivity report indicates the causative microorganisms and their relative sensitivity to various antibiotics.
   b. Assisting the physician to aspirate body fluids or tissues, such as spinal or pleural fluid, bone marrow, or liver tissues. Chapter 54 discusses these special procedures.
   c. Assisting with or obtaining blood specimens for differential white blood cell counts or serum immunoglobulins.
   d. Performing intradermal skin tests for diagnostic reactions as directed by the physician. See Chapter 51.

2. Initiate and maintain protective aseptic precautions specific to the infecting organism and its mode of transmission. Types of protective aseptic (isolation) precautions are discussed later in this chapter.

Employees are bound under legal concept of duty to care for persons who are admitted for treatment. If a person employed by a facility refuses to care for a client, the facility has the right to terminate that employee. (Parent 1985, p. 279)

3. Assist in controlling the client's infection by:
   a. Administering prescribed antimicrobial medications.
   b. Observing the client's response to antimicrobial therapy.
   c. Administering specific immune therapies ordered by the physician such as vaccines, antitoxins or toxoids, and immune antiserums.

4. Implement interventions to alleviate or reduce the client's problems, e.g.:
   a. Fever. Nursing interventions for a client with a fever are discussed in Chapter 34.
   b. Cough. Provide a humidifier to moisten and loosen respiratory secretions and soothe respiratory membranes. Administer expectorants or cough suppressants as prescribed.
   c. Malaise and generalized aches. Limit the client's physical activity and keep the client comfortable.
   d. Pain. Immobilize painful body parts, provide relaxation and comfort measures, and administer prescribed analgesics.
   e. Fluid loss through excessive perspiration, diarrhea, or vomiting. Encourage an appropriate fluid intake and monitor the client's urinary output to ensure it is appropriate for the intake.
   f. Lack of stimulation and social contact if isolated. Ensure that the client has books, magazines, radio or television available and increase interactions between the nursing staff and the client.

5. Measure and record the client's vital signs regularly to determine the extent to which the client's body defenses are coping with the infectious agent and with the therapy. Assess breath sounds if the client has a respiratory infection.

6. Take periodic sputum, wound, blood, urine, or fecal cultures to determine the effectiveness of antimicrobial and other therapies.

7. Encourage an adequate nutritional intake, especially of proteins and vitamins, to promote healing of injured tissues.

8. Always use sterile technique when performing invasive procedures or when changing dressings of open wounds.

9. Educate the client and family members about the infectious organism, its mode of transmission, and ways to control and prevent its spread. Education must stress the need for meticulous hand washing after contact with infectious material, keeping hands away from drainage areas, and disposing of infectious materials properly. Some clients may need to learn how to take body temperature to monitor a fever; others, how to apply hot or cold compresses to localized infections.

Protecting Body Defenses

The normal defenses of the body are described earlier in this chapter. The nurse can enhance these defenses in a variety of ways.

Maintaining the intactness of the skin and mucous membranes is an important and pervasive nursing function. During many nursing activities, e.g., turning and positioning clients, the nurse must protect these barriers. Chapter 37 discusses methods of preventing skin breakdown of clients with impaired mobility. In addition, regular and thorough hygienic practices by or for the client remove transient microorganisms, thereby decreasing the likelihood of infection.

1. Hand washing. Washing one's hands after urination and defecation removes microorganisms acquired from the perineum and feces, thus preventing their spread to objects and food. Hand washing before handling food also prevents contamination of the food and subsequent ingestion of the organisms by others. See the section on hand washing in this chapter.
2. Perineal care. Females should clean the rectum and perineum after elimination by wiping from the area of least contamination (the urinary meatus) to the area of greatest contamination (the anus). This method of wiping helps to prevent the spread of microorganisms to the genitourinary tract and reduces the risk of genitourinary infections. See the section on perineal and genital care in Chapter 36.
3. Regular bathing. Bathing removes transient microorganisms from the skin and helps prevent infections. See Chapter 36.
4. Brushing and flossing teeth regularly. See the section on oral hygiene in Chapter 36. Regular brushing and flossing remove catatonic salivary proteins mechanically from the teeth, thereby preventing the adherence of endogenous oral microorganisms, such as lactobacilli. **Endogenous** means originating within, e.g., the mouth, in this instance. **Exogenous** means originating from the outside. Good oral hygiene prevents excessive accumulation of these microorganisms in the mouth. Brushing and flossing also prevent the plaque build-up and oral infections, e.g., gingivitis and periodontitis.
5. Blowing the nose. Blowing the nose and sneezing clear microorganisms from the upper respiratory tract and help remove microorganisms and dust caught in the cilia. Children need to be taught not to pick their noses. This practice contaminates the hands and may damage the nasal mucous membrane, permitting microorganisms to establish themselves in the tissue.
6. Coughing. Coughing helps remove microorganisms and dust from the lower portions of the respiratory tract. When coughing, people should cover their mouths with tissues to avoid spraying droplets into the air. Microorganisms in droplets can come into contact with the conjunctivae, nose, or mouth of a susceptible person.
7. Nail care. Carefully cutting the nails and not the adjacent tissue maintains the integrity of the nail-skin barrier and so prevents the entry of organisms. The tissue around nails may also need regular lubrication with oil to prevent drying and cracking.
8. Eyes. Tears are a natural defense, and an impaired flow places the eyes at risk of infection. In such cases, cleaning around the eyes to prevent the spread of microorganisms into the eyes is important. In addition, it may be necessary to administer eye drops to serve the function of the tears. In most settings, eye drops are ordered by a physician.
9. Vaginal hygiene. Special hygiene measures are normally not required to maintain the natural defenses of the vagina. When, however, the balance of the vaginal flora is disturbed, e.g., by antibiotic therapy, yeast infection can result. Preventing this problem involves teaching clients to use antibiotics only when necessary and only after consulting a physician.

In addition to enhancing these nonspecific body defenses, nurses can strengthen the body's defenses by interventions in the areas of immunization, nutrition, rest and sleep, and stress.

1. Immunization. The immunologic system is the body's major defense against infections. The body gradually builds up natural defenses against pathogens with which it comes in contact; immunizations give additional protection.
2. Nutrition. A balanced diet enhances the health of all body tissues. Proper diet helps keep the skin intact and promotes its ability to repel microorganisms. Adequate nutrition enables tissues to maintain and rebuild themselves and helps keep the reticuloendothelial system functioning well. This is the system of connective tissue cells (**phagocytes**) that combat and prevent infections by ingesting microorganisms, other cells, and foreign matter. There are three types of phagocytes: reticuloendothelial cells, which line the liver, spleen, and bone marrow; macrophages, which wander in the tissues; and microglia, which are located in the central nervous system.
3. Rest and sleep. Adequate rest and sleep are essential

to health and to one's ability to perform usual activities. See Chapter 40 for additional information.

4. Stress. Stress predisposes a person to infection. A balance, for example, between work and recreation is important. See the section on psychologic homeostasis in Chapter 17, page 333.

Cleaning, Disinfecting, and Sterilizing

The removal and destruction of microorganisms is accomplished by cleaning, disinfecting, and sterilizing.

Cleaning

Cleanliness inhibits the growth of microorganisms. An object that is not free of infectious or potentially infectious agents is considered contaminated or dirty. When cleaning infected objects, nurses must always wear gloves to avoid direct contact with infectious microorganisms. Increasingly, disposable equipment and supplies, e.g., catheters, gloves, syringes, forceps, etc., are used in client care. After using such articles, the nurse does not clean them. They are bagged, labeled, and disposed of for incineration. Most objects used in the care of clients, whether artery forceps or drawsheets, can be cleaned by rinsing them in cold water to remove any organic material, washing them with hot soapy water, then rinsing them again to remove the soap. The following steps should be followed when cleaning objects in a hospital or in a home where infectious agents exist.

1. Rinse the article with cold water to remove organic material. Hot water coagulates the protein of organic material and tends to make it adhere. Examples of organic material are blood and pus.
2. Wash the article in hot water and soap. The emulsifying action of soap reduces surface tension and facilitates the removal of dirt. Washing dislodges the emulsified dirt.
3. Use an abrasive, such as a stiff-bristled brush, to clean equipment with grooves and corners. Friction helps dislodge foreign material.
4. Rinse the article well with warm-hot water.
5. Dry the article; it is now considered clean.
6. Clean the brush, gloves, and sink. These are considered soiled until they are cleaned appropriately, usually with a disinfectant.

Disinfecting and Sterilizing

Disinfection is the removal or destruction of infectious microorganisms that do not form spores. Noninfectious organisms may or may not be completely eliminated. A **disinfectant** is a chemical preparation, e.g., phenol or iodine compounds, used to treat inanimate objects. Disinfectants are frequently caustic and toxic to tissues. An **antiseptic** is a chemical preparation used on skin or tissue. Disinfectants and antiseptics are often the same chemical preparation, but the disinfectant is a more concentrated solution. See Table 32–8 for commonly used antiseptics.

Both antiseptics and disinfectants are said to have bactericidal or bacteriostatic properties. A bactericidal preparation destroys bacteria, whereas a bacteriostatic preparation prevents the growth and reproduction of some bacteria.

Sterilization is a process that destroys *all* microorganisms, including spores and viruses. Before choosing a method for disinfecting or sterilizing it is important to consider:

1. The type and number of infectious organisms. Some microorganisms are readily destroyed, while others require longer contact with the disinfectant. Also, a large number of organisms requires a proportionately longer disinfecting time.
2. The recommended concentration of the disinfectant and the duration of contact. A lesser concentration or shorter exposure could be ineffective.

Table 32–8 Commonly Used Antiseptics

Solution	Action
Isopropyl alcohol	Bactericide
Ethyl alcohol	Bactericide, unreliable fungicide, virucide, inactive against dried spores. Acts as a disinfectant also but can damage plastic.
Silver nitrate	Astringent and caustic.
Benzalkonium chloride (Zephiran, Bactine)	Antibacterial, low toxicity.
Hydrogen peroxide	Bactericide; oxidizing agent.
Antiseptics	
Povidone-iodine (Betadine, Povadyne)	Broad-spectrum microcidal effect. Applied topically as spray, gargle, shampoo, surgical scrub, vaginal douche, ointment, solution.
Hexachlorophene (pHisoHex)	Bacteriostatic. Absorbed from intact skin. Do not use with infants; may be neurotoxic.

3. The temperature of the environment. Most disinfectants are intended for use at room temperature. In lower temperatures, the exposure must usually be increased.
4. The presence of soap. Some disinfectants are ineffective in the presence of soap or detergent. Such disinfectants are cationic and react with the anions in the soap rather than the bacterial membrane.
5. The presence of organic materials. The presence of saliva, blood, pus, or excretions can readily inactivate many disinfectants. The disinfectant acts on the nonmicrobial organic matter, reducing its antimicrobial action. It is therefore important to wash off the organic material before disinfecting.
6. The limitations of the available methods.
7. The surface areas to be treated. The sterilizing or disinfecting agent must come into contact with all surfaces and areas.

The following are common methods of disinfecting and sterilizing.

Moist Heat

For sterilizing, moist heat (steam) can be employed in two ways: as steam under pressure or as free steam. Steam under pressure attains temperatures higher than the boiling point. Autoclaves supply steam under pressures of 15 to 17 pounds and temperatures of 121 to 123 C (250 to 254 F). The time required to ensure sterilization depends on how the autoclave is packed, how the pressure and temperature are maintained, how the articles are wrapped, and what equipment, e.g., glass, cloth, etc., is being sterilized. Autoclaving is used to sterilize surgical dressings, surgical linens, parenteral solutions, and metal and glass objects.

Free steam, 100 C (212 F), is used to sterilize objects that would be destroyed at the higher temperature and pressure of the autoclave. Usually, it is necessary to steam the article for 30 minutes on 3 consecutive days. The intervals are required so that unkilled spores will return to their vegetative state and again become vulnerable to the heat.

One example of free steam used in a hospital is the bedpan flusher. Because the temperature of the flusher never exceeds 100 C, it does not really sterilize bedpans but washes away some microorganisms. Some viruses, e.g., the virus that causes hepatitis A, can survive this free steam application.

Boiling Water

This is the most practical and inexpensive method for sterilizing in the home. The main disadvantage is that spores and some viruses are not killed by this method. The water temperature rises no higher than 100 C (212 F). Boiling a minimum of 15 minutes is advised for disinfection of articles in the home.

Dry Heat

Dry heat is no longer used in health facilities. As a method of sterilization it is unreliable because the heat is not proven to penetrate sufficiently to kill all microorganisms. However, dry heat is still used to disinfect articles at home.

Radiation

Both ionizing and nonionizing radiation can be used for disinfection and sterilization. Ultraviolet light, a type of nonionizing radiation, can be used for disinfection. Its main drawback is that the ultraviolet rays do not penetrate deeply. Ionizing radiation is used effectively in industry to sterilize foods, drugs, and other items that are sensitive to heat. Its main advantage is that it is effective for items difficult to sterilize; its chief disadvantage is that the equipment is very expensive.

Chemicals

There are many disinfectants and antiseptics on the market today, and new ones are added daily. The characteristics of a desirable disinfectant are:

1. Destroys infectious agents in a reasonable time
2. Is readily soluble, penetrates cracks, and coats surfaces
3. Is nontoxic to humans
4. Is noncorrosive to metal, rubber, and plastics
5. Is inexpensive
6. Is not inactivated by dilution with fluids or contact with organic substances

Table 32–9 lists some commonly used disinfecting agents for selected equipment.

Ethylene Oxide Gas

This gas destroys microorganisms by interfering with their metabolic processes. It is also effective against spores. It is effective at a relatively low temperature 54.4 to 65.5 C (130 to 150 F) when humidity is 30% to 60%. Its advantages are good penetration and effectiveness for heat-sensitive items. Its major disadvantage is its toxicity to humans. See Table 32–10 for common methods of sterilizing equipment.

Table 32–9 Disinfecting Agents for Selected Equipment

Kind of Equipment	Examples of Equipment	Agent	Time (Min) Low Level*
Smooth, hard-surfaced objects	Metal forceps	Ethyl alcohol 70%–90%	10
		Formaldehyde 8% + alcohol 70% solution	5
		Phenolic solutions 1% Ag	10
Rubber tubing (filled)	Catheters	Phenolic solutions 1% Ag	15
		Iodophor-100 ppm** available iodine	10
Polyethylene tubing (filled)	Catheters	Iodophor-100 ppm** available iodine	10
		Ethyl or isopropyl alcohol 70%–90%	10
		Phenolic solutions 1% Ag	10
Lensed instruments	Otoscopes, endoscopes	Iodophor-100 ppm** available iodine	10
		Phenolic solutions 1% Ag	10
		Quaternary ammonium solutions 1:500 Ag	10
Thermometers	Client thermometers (thoroughly wiped)	Ethyl or isopropyl alcohol 70%–90% + 0.2% iodine	10
Hinged instruments	Forceps	Ethyl or isopropyl alcohol 70%–90%	15
		Formaldehyde 8% + alcohol 70% solution	10
Inhalation equipment	Mouth pieces of respiratory equipment	Ethyl or isopropyl alcohol 70%–90%	15
Floors, furniture, walls, etc.	Metal beds	Quaternary ammonium solution 1:500 Ag	—

*Kills vegetative bacteria, fungi, and influenza viruses but *not* tuberculosis bacilli, enteroviruses, bacterial and fungal spores, hepatitis viruses.
**ppm = parts per million

Table 32–10 Common Methods of Sterilizing Equipment

Method	Action	Types of Objects
Steam under pressure	Sterilization by coagulation of protoplasm	Smooth, hard surfaces: instruments, forceps
Dry heat	Sterilization by oxidizing the protein of microorganisms	Glassware, sharp instruments, special needles, powders, oils, creams
Irradiation using cobalt 60	Sterilization by altering the metabolic processes of microorganisms	Many commercially packaged items, e.g., syringes, needles, catheterization sets
Ethylene oxide	Sterilization by interfering with the metabolic processes of microorganisms	Rubber, plastic, paper items

Hand Washing

Hand washing is important in every setting where people are ill, including hospitals. It is considered one of the most effective infection control measures. The goal of hand washing is to remove microorganisms that might be transmitted to clients, visitors, or other health care personnel.

Any client may harbor microorganisms that are currently harmless to the client yet potentially harmful to another person or to the same client if they find a portal of entry. It is important that hands be washed at the following times to prevent the spread of these microorganisms.

For clients

1. Before eating
2. After using the bedpan or toilet
3. After the hands have come in contact with any known infectious material, such as sputum or drainage from a wound

For nurses and health personnel

The hands should be washed before and after any direct client contact. The CDC recommends:

1. Before performing invasive procedures, whether or not sterile gloves are used
2. Before and after contact with wounds, whether surgical, traumatic, or associated with an invasive device (e.g., intravenous catheter)
3. Before contact with particularly susceptible clients
4. After contact with a source that is likely to be contaminated with virulent microorganisms or hospital pathogens, e.g., an infected client or an object contaminated with secretions or excretions
5. Between contact with different clients in special care units, e.g., newborn nursery.

During routine client care, the CDC recommends a vigorous hand washing under a stream of water for at least 10 seconds using bar soap, granule soap, soap-filled tissues, or nonmicrobial liquid soap (Garner and Favero 1985, p. 7). The CDC recommends antiseptic hand washing agents:

> When dealing with clients in isolation (see Protective Asepsis (Isolation Precautions) later in this chapter)
>
> When there are known multiple resistant bacteria
>
> Before invasive procedures
>
> In special care units

These agents can be any chemical germicides listed with the EPA (Environmental Protection Agency) (Garner and Simmons 1983, p. 5).

Garner and Favero write that superficial contact with an object not visibly soiled or suspected of being contaminated does not require hand washing. However, prolonged contact with a client should be followed by hand washing. In addition, hand washing is indicated: *before* invasive procedures, e.g., urinary catheterization, *before* contact with a susceptible client, e.g,. newborn, *before* and *after* touching wounds and after hands have touched contaminated sources, e.g., secretions or excretions, even when gloves have been used (Garner and Favero 1985, p. 7).

There is controversy about the best position for the hands during washing. Some authorities believe that when the hands are contaminated and during routine hand washing, most microorganisms are on the hands. Therefore, the hands are held downward to wash the microorganisms into the sink. However, when washing before any sterile procedure or for a surgical scrub, the nurse holds the hands upward to remove as many microorganisms as possible.

Other authorities, however, believe that the hands should be held downward for all hand washing except surgical scrubs because the intention is to remove only transient microorganisms, leaving the resident microorganisms on the hands. Yet others believe that the hands should be held upward for all handwashing, thereby avoiding the confusion of two positions (Palmer 1984, p. 50).

This book recommends that the hands be held down (below the elbows) when washing off infectious materials and during routine hand washing so that the microorganisms are washed directly into the sink. When washing before sterile techniques, it is recommended that the hands be held above the elbows so that the water runs from the cleanest to least clean area, although it has not been proved that this position results in cleaner hands during hand washing, as distinct from the surgical scrub. When the hands are contaminated, the hands should not be held higher than the elbows because the infectious agents are washed onto the arms, where they may remain.

Procedure 32–1 ▲ Hand Washing

Equipment

1. Soap. Most hospitals supply soaps that contain a germicide. Liquid soaps are frequently supplied in dispensers at the sink.
2. Warm running water.
3. Towels. Nurses usually dry their hands with paper towels; they discard the towels in the appropriate container immediately after use.

Intervention

1. File the nails short.

   Rationale Short nails are less likely to harbor microorganisms or scratch a client. Long nails are hard to clean.
2. Remove jewelry, except a plain band, from the hands and arms. Some nurses slide their watches up above their elbows. Others pin the watch to the uniform so that it can still be used.

Research Note

Hand washing is considered one of the best ways to prevent the spread of infection. Larson (1982) conducted a study to assess the presence of bacteria on the hands of hospital staff; 103 hospital personnel and 50 controls participated over a 35-day period. Twenty-one percent of the 103 staff were found to carry one or more of 22 species of Gram-negative bacteria. "Persons who washed hands less than eight times per day were significantly more likely to persistently carry the same species than those who washed more than eight times per day" (p. 122). Of the 541 nosocomial infections in the institution over 7 months, 21% were caused by the same species found on the hands. The study indicates that hand washing reduced the number of organisms without changing the ecologic balance. (Larson 1982)

Rationale Microorganisms can lodge in the settings of jewelry. Removal facilitates proper cleaning of the hands and arms.

3. Check hands for breaks in the skin, such as hangnails or cuts. Report cuts to the instructor or responsible nurse before beginning work, or check agency policy about cuts. Use lotions to prevent hangnails and cracked, dry skin. A nurse who has open sores may have to change work assignments or wear gloves to avoid contact with clients' body substances.

4. Stand in front of the sink. Do not lean on the sink or splash water on your uniform. Flex your knees slightly if the sink is low.

   Rationale Microorganisms thrive in moisture. Dampness can contribute to contamination of the uniform. Flexing the knees keeps the nurse's waist below the level of the sink.

5. Turn on the water. There are four types of faucet controls:
   a. Hand-operated handles. Use paper towels to turn these. Some agencies use paper towels only to turn the faucets on, others to turn faucets off, others at both times, and some in neither instance. See Figure 32–2.

      Rationale Towels protect the hands from possible contamination.
   b. Knee levers. Move these with knee to regulate flow and temperature. See Figure 32–3.
   c. Foot pedals. Press these with the foot to regulate flow and temperature. See Figure 32–4.
   d. Elbow controls. Move these with the elbows, instead of the hands. This type of handle is most frequently used for surgical asepsis.

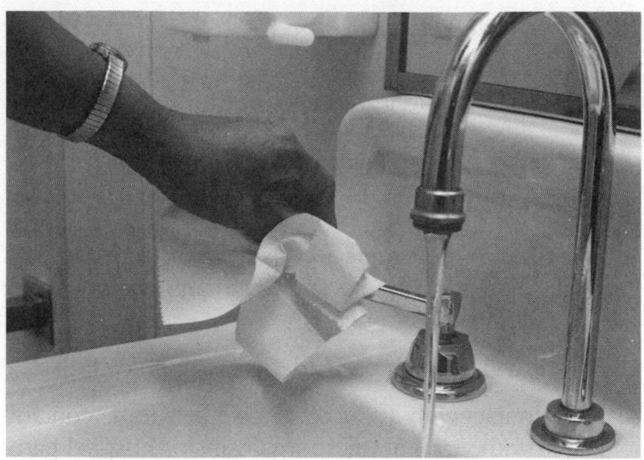

Figure 32–2

6. Adjust the flow so that the water is warm.

   Rationale Warm water removes less of the protective oil of the skin than hot water.

7. Wet the hands and lower arms thoroughly by holding them under the running water. Hold the hands lower than the elbows so that the water flows from the arms to the fingertips.

   Rationale The water should flow from the least contaminated to the most contaminated area, and the hands are more contaminated than the lower arms.

8. Apply soap to the hands. If the soap is liquid, apply 2 to 4 ml (1 tsp). If it is bar soap, rub it firmly between the hands, and rinse the bar before returning it to the dish.

   Rationale Rinsing the bar removes microorganisms.

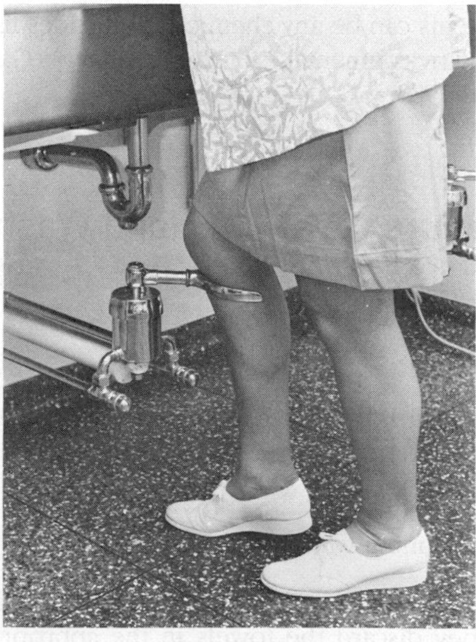

Figure 32–3

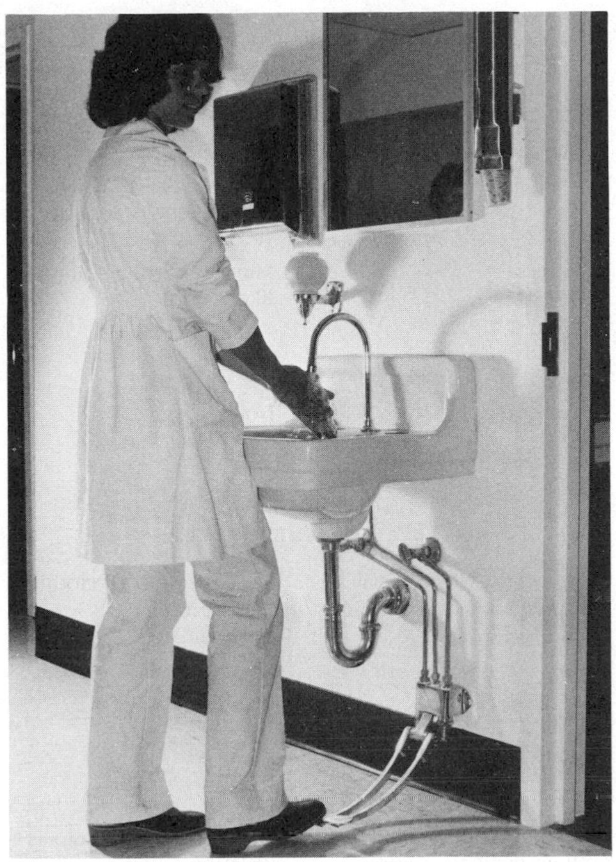

Figure 32–4

9. Use firm, rubbing, circular movements to wash the palm, back, and wrist of each hand. Interlace the fingers and thumbs, and move the hands back and forth. See Figure 32–5. Continue this motion for 10 to 15 seconds.

   Rationale The circular action helps remove microorganisms. Interlacing the fingers and thumbs cleans the interdigital spaces.

10. Rinse the hands.

11. For a 1-minute hand wash, repeat steps 7 through 9. For 2- and 3-minute hand washes, repeat steps 7 through 9 but extend the washing time.

12. Dry the hands and arms thoroughly with the paper towel. Discard it in the appropriate container.

    Rationale Moist skin becomes chapped readily; chapping produces lesions.

13. Turn off the water. Use paper towels to grasp hand-operated control.

    Rationale The towel prevents contact with microorganisms on the faucet knobs.

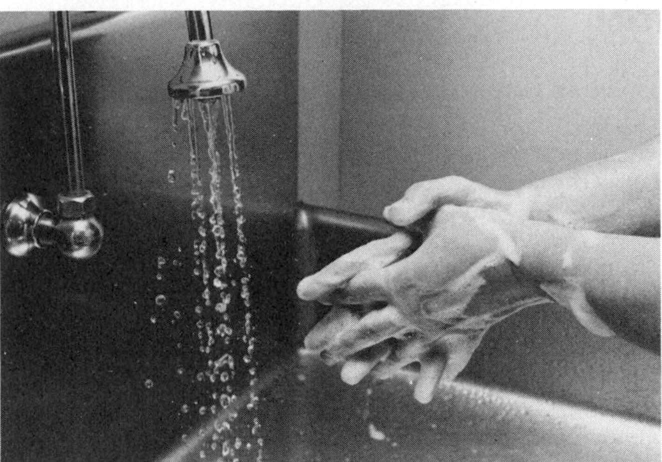

Figure 32–5

Variation: Hand Washing Before Sterile Techniques

Hold the hands higher than the elbows during this hand wash. Wet the hands and forearms under the running water, letting it run from the fingertips to the elbows, so that the hands become cleaner than the elbows. See Figure 32–6. In this way, the water runs from the area with the fewest microorganisms to areas with a relatively greater number. Apply the soap and wash as in Procedure 32–1, maintaining the hands uppermost. After washing and rinsing, use a towel to dry one hand thoroughly from the fingers to the elbow in a rotating motion. Use a clean towel to dry the other hand and arms. A clean towel prevents the transfer of microorganisms from one elbow (least clean area) to the other hand (cleanest area).

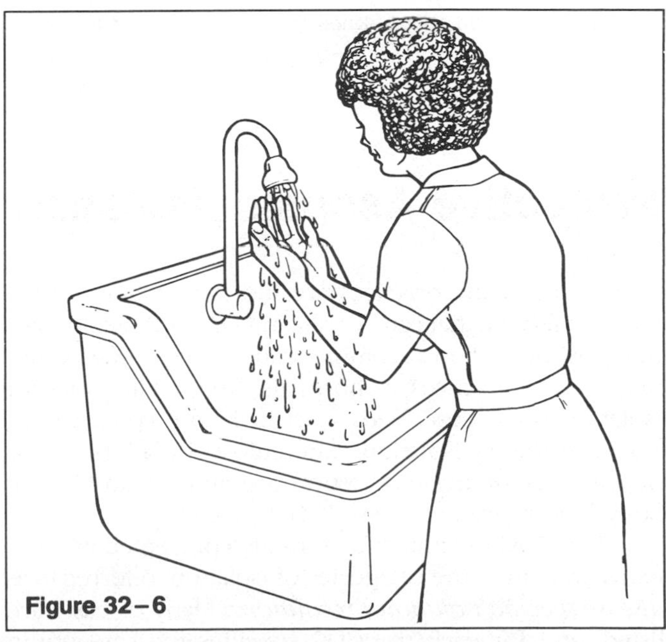

Figure 32–6

Table 32–11 Category-Specific Protective Asepsis (Isolation)

Isolation Category	Purpose	Private Room	Gowns
Strict isolation, e.g., for diphtheria pneumonic plague, smallpox, varicella (chickenpox), zoster	To prevent airborne or contact transmission of highly contagious or virulent microorganisms	Necessary; door must be kept closed	Must be worn by all persons entering room; for smallpox, coverings for cap and shoes are also recommended
Contact isolation, e.g., for acute respiratory infections and influenza in children, pediculosis, wound infections, herpes simplex, impetigo, rubella, scabies	To prevent highly transmissible infections not requiring strict isolation but spread by close or direct contact	Necessary	Must be worn if soiling is likely
Respiratory isolation, e.g., for epiglottitis, measles, meningitis, mumps, pertussis, pneumonia in children	To prevent infections spread by contaminated articles (e.g., tissues) and respiratory droplets that are coughed, sneezed, or exhaled	Necessary	Not necessary
Tuberculosis isolation (AFB isolation) for pulmonary tuberculosis when clients have positive sputum smear or suggestive chest x-ray film	To prevent spread of acid-fast bacilli (AFB)	Necessary, with special ventilation	Necessary only if clothing may become contaminated
Enteric precautions, e.g., for hepatitis A, some gastroenteritis, typhoid fever, cholera, diarrhea with suspected infectious etiology, encephalitis, meningitis	To prevent infections spread through direct or indirect contact with feces	Necessary if client hygiene is poor, e.g., client is incontinent	Same as for tuberculosis isolation
Drainage/secretion precautions, e.g., for any draining lesion, abscess, infected burn, infected skin, decubitis ulcer, conjunctivitis)	To prevent infections, spread through direct or indirect contact with material or drainage from body site	Not necessary unless client hygiene is poor	Same as for tuberculosis isolation
Blood/body fluid precautions, e.g., for hepatitis B, syphilis, AIDS, malaria	To prevent infections spread through direct or indirect contact with infected blood or body fluids	Necessary if patient hygiene is poor	Same as for tuberculosis isolation

Source: CDC guidelines for isolation precautions in hospitals.

Protective Asepsis (Isolation Precautions)

Protective aseptic practices are indicated when a client has an infection that can be transmitted to others. In 1983, the CDC published recommendations regarding protective asepsis practices in hospitals. Seven categories for isolation were described: strict isolation, contact isolation, respiratory isolation, tuberculosis isolation, enteric precautions, drainage/secretion precautions, and blood/body fluid precautions (see Table 32–11).

The CDC recommendations also presented an alternative system to the categories of isolation, referred to as *disease-specific isolation precautions.* Many diseases are listed, and for each the CDC specifies the category in which the disease falls, the type of infectious material present, and the time during which precautions need to be taken. In addition, it recommends that modified isolation precautions be taken in intensive care units, in newborn and infant nurseries, and in the care of the severely compromised and of clients with burns. Agencies may also develop their own systems (Garner and Simmons 1983, pp. 258–261).

The CDC guidelines are designed (a) to establish a balance between ideal and practical isolation precautions, (b) to eliminate practices that are not based on scientific data, and (c) to establish effective precautions that isolate the disease but not the client.

Masks	Gloves	Hand Washing	Disposal of Contaminated Articles
Must be worn by all persons entering room	Must be worn by all persons entering room	Necessary after touching client or potentially contaminated articles and before caring for another client	Discard in plastic-lined container or bag and label before sending for decontamination and reprocessing
Must be worn if person comes near client	Worn if touching infected material	Same as for strict isolation	Same as for strict isolation
Must be worn by all persons in close contact	Not necessary	Same as for strict isolation	Same as for strict isolation
Necessary if client is coughing and does not always cover mouth	Not necessary	Same as for strict isolation	Clean and disinfect, although these articles rarely transmit disease
Not necessary	Necessary if touching infected material	Same as for strict isolation	Same as for strict isolation
Not necessary	Same as for enteric precautions	Same as for strict isolation	Same as for strict isolation
Not necessary	Necessary if touching infected blood or body fluid	Necessary if hands can become contaminated and before caring for another client	Same as for strict isolation; used needles must be placed in puncture-proof container for disposal

Guidelines for Protective Asepsis

1. Hand washing is the single most important means of preventing the spread of infection (Garner and Favero 1985, p. 7). See Procedure 32–1 in the previous section.

2. A private room reduces the spread of microorganisms by separating the infected client from susceptible clients. Visitors and personnel are reminded to wash their hands before leaving the room. The private room should have hand-washing and toilet facilities. In some instances, e.g., tuberculosis isolation, the room also needs special ventilation. The air pressure in the room is kept lower than the air pressure in the connecting room or hall so that the air does not move readily out of the room; instead, it is discharged outdoors or into special vents that filter out any microorganisms.

   A private room is recommended for clients placed on strict, contact, respiratory, and tuberculosis isolation. Private rooms are not necessary for clients placed on enteric, drainage/secretion, or blood/body fluid precautions provided the client can understand and carry out the necessary precautions. If the client is an infant, young child, or adult with altered mental status and cannot carry out the precautions, a private room is necessary. Such clients might not wash their hands after touching infectious material and thus contaminate the environment.

   An anteroom between the room and hall is also recommended. Supplies are stored in this room, and it lessens the airborne spread of infectious agents into the corridor when the door of the room is opened. An anteroom is particularly important for clients who have highly infectious diseases transmitted by droplets in the air.

When there is a shortage of private rooms, a client may share a room with someone infected by the same microorganism or with a noninfected client who is resistant or not at risk. For example, infants with the same respiratory infection, e.g., croup, may share rooms, or a client with an enteric infection may share a room with a noninfected client provided the infected person washes his or her hands carefully and health care personnel take appropriate precautions. In no instance should an infected client be placed in a room with a client who is at risk of acquiring an infection.

3. Masks prevent the transmission of microorganisms through the air. Masks should be used only once and discarded in the appropriate receptacle when they become moist.
4. Gowns are worn when it is possible that clothes will become contaminated. Gowns should be worn only once and then discarded. Contaminated gowns must not be worn outside the room because they may contaminate other people or objects.
5. Gloves are used for several purposes: to protect the nurse from microorganisms; to reduce the likelihood that the nurse may transmit microorganisms to the client; and to reduce the possibility that the nurse may acquire microorganisms that can be transmitted to others. Disposable gloves should be used only once and then discarded in the appropriate receptacle.
6. Soiled articles are bagged and labeled before being removed from the room. A single bag that is impervious and sturdy can be used, as long as the outside of the bag is unsoiled.
7. Use of disposable equipment reduces the possibility of transferring microorganisms if the equipment is discarded correctly.
8. Contaminated reusable equipment is bagged, labeled, and decontaminated and/or sterilized.
9. Used needles are not recapped but placed in labeled, puncture-proof containers for disposal. Reusable syringes are bagged and labeled for decontamination and reprocessing.
10. Soiled linen is handled minimally. It is bagged and labeled before being sent for decontamination. Handling is reduced by placing contaminated linen in hot-water-soluble laundry bags, which can be put directly into the washing machine. Hot-water-soluble bags may need to be double-bagged, however, because they are more easily torn than standard laundry bags and dissolve when wet.
11. Dishes normally do not require special precautions unless they are visibly contaminated. Disposable contaminated drinking cups or glasses are discarded in the same way as disposable contaminated equipment. Reusable contaminated dishes may be bagged, labeled, and sent to the hospital kitchen for decontamination. Fluid containers and glasses are handled in the same way as dishes.
12. Dressings, paper tissues, and contaminated disposable items are bagged, labeled, and discarded according to the agency's policy for disposal of contaminated wastes.
13. Urine and feces are normally flushed down the toilet. Urinals and bedpans are decontaminated or sterilized before use by another client.
14. When nurses collect specimens, care is taken to keep the outside of the container uncontaminated. If it comes in contact with infectious material, it is disinfected, placed in an impervious bag, and labeled for transport to the laboratory.
15. Visitors are given information about the precautions they need to take when visiting a client on medical aseptic precautions. They may need help with gowns, masks, etc., depending on the client's illness.
16. When clients are transported from their rooms, barriers are set up to prevent the transmission of microorganisms to others. For example, if the client is on respiratory isolation, both the client and transport personnel should wear masks during transport; a client with an infected draining wound requires a moisture-proof dressing.
17. The client's chart is not allowed to come into contact with infectious objects or material.
18. Books and toys that become visibly contaminated are disinfected or destroyed.
19. In terminal cleaning, all items that have come in direct contact with the client or infectious secretions are decontaminated.
20. Nurses caring for a client on medical aseptic precautions are constantly aware of their hands. Once contaminated, the hands do not touch any clean objects, e.g., the nurse's hair or watch or the medication tray.
21. Any cut or scratch on the nurse's hands is covered with an occlusive bandage impervious to moisture, because the abrasion can become the portal of entry for microorganisms. The nurse may need to wear gloves while giving care.

Psychologic Problems of Protective Asepsis

Clients on protective aseptic precautions can develop several problems as a result of the separation from others and of the special precautions taken in their care. Two of the most common are sensory deprivation and feelings of inferiority. Sensory deprivation occurs when the environment lacks normal stimuli for the client, e.g., frequent communications with others. The client is usually in a private room and thus has no contact with other clients. Because support persons may need to put on gowns before entering the room, they may not visit as often as usual. Visits by other clients are usually discouraged. Nurses should therefore be alert to common clinical signs of sensory deprivation: boredom, inactivity, slowness of thought, daydreaming, increased sleeping, thought disorganization, anxiety, panic, and hallucinations.

A client's feeling of inferiority can be due to the infection itself or to the precautions. In North America, many people place a high value on cleanliness, and the idea of being "contaminated" or "dirty" can give clients the feeling that they are at fault and substandard. While this is obviously not true, the infected persons may feel "not as good" as others and blame themselves.

Nurses need to provide care that prevents these two problems and/or deals with them positively. Nursing interventions include:

1. Assessment of the individual's need for stimulation.
2. Measures to help meet the need, including regular communication with the client's diversionary activities, e.g., toys for a child and books, television, or radio for an adult; stimulation of the sense of taste with a variety of foods; stimulation of the visual sense by providing a view or an activity to watch.
3. Explanation of the infection and the associated procedures, to help clients and their support persons understand and accept the situation.
4. Warm, accepting behavior. This is particularly important for clients on protective asepsis. The nurse needs to make efforts not to convey to the client any sense of annoyance about the precautions or any feelings of revulsion about the infection.

Initiating Protective Asepsis

The nurse first confirms the precautions that are appropriate for the client and determines the type of protective asepsis required and the reason. At some hospitals, precautions must be ordered by the physician; in other agencies placement on protective asepsis may be a nursing decision or specified by agency policy.

The equipment required depends primarily on the type of protection and the physical arrangement of the agency. Practices vary, and thus the necessary equipment and supplies also vary. For example, masks are advised for nurses caring for clients on respiratory protective asepsis, but they are not required by nurses caring for clients on enteric precautions. Some clients cooperate with the precautions, whereas others, e.g., a confused adult, cannot. A nurse may not need to don a gown before measuring the blood pressure of a rational, cooperative client, whereas gowning is essential before taking the pressure of a confused client who is likely to contaminate the nurse's uniform.

Physical arrangements also affect the equipment and supplies required. Some hospitals have specially designed rooms for protective asepsis with an anteroom on the nursing unit. Most necessary equipment is stored in this anteroom, and so very little setting up is required. Generally, a private room is highly desirable to prevent the transmission of microorganisms.

Assessing the Client

The assessment practices described below are not always carried out before a unit is set up; some practices may be appropriate at that time, and others when protective asepsis is being implemented.

1. Assess the client's ability to understand and to cooperate with the practices.
2. Assess the client's understanding of the procedures and need for information.
3. Continually assess the client's need for stimulation. Be aware of the clinical signs of sensory deprivation: boredom, inactivity, slowness of thought, daydreaming, increased sleeping, thought disorganization, anxiety, panic, and hallucinations.
4. Assess the amount, color, consistency, and odor of body drainage, excreta, or secretions pertinent to the client's condition.

Preparing the Client and Support Persons

Explain the practices and the reasons for them to the client. If appropriate, provide explanations and demonstrations after the client is moved to the unit or after the equipment has been set up. Explain in clear simple language what substances are presumed to be infectious and what precautions are necessary.

Be reassuring and supportive. If the client is to be moved to a protective asepsis unit, assist him or her to gather clothing and personal effects.

Explain the practices that support persons need to carry out, e.g., gowning. Demonstrating procedures is often helpful. Arrange diversionary activities for the client as appropriate and a teaching plan as needed for the client and support persons.

Assembling the Equipment

The equipment required depends on the type of protective asepsis. The following equipment is usually needed:

1. A sink with liquid germicidal soap for washing hands and cleaning used articles.

2. Paper towels near the sink.
3. At least one waste container with a moisture-proof liner.
4. A laundry hamper to collect used linen. Some agencies use hampers specially marked with red or the word *isolation*.
5. A table on which to place supplies, e.g., a stethoscope and thermometer.
6. A toilet for the disposal of excreta. Some agencies also dispose of waste food in the toilet. Others provide a hopper in addition to a toilet for the disposal of waste products.
7. A tub or shower for the client.
8. Bedside supplies for the client, e.g., tissues, drinking water, and a cup.
9. Clean supplies such as gowns, plastic bags, isolation tags, disinfectant solutions, masks, plastic disposal bags, plastic gloves, moisture-proof bags, as needed by the client.
10. A sign to place on the outside of the door, indicating the type of precautions to be taken, with the message "Visitors inquire at the desk."

Donning and Removing Face Masks

Masks are worn to prevent the airborne transmission of microorganisms. They protect the wearer from inhaling microorganisms and protect others from the microorganisms the wearer exhales. The CDC recommends that masks be worn (Garner and Simmons 1983, p. 254):

1. Only by those close to the client if the infection, e.g., acute respiratory diseases in children, measles, and mumps, is transmitted by large-particle aerosols (droplets). Large-particle aerosols are transmitted by close contact and generally travel short distances (about 1 m, or 3 ft).
2. By all persons entering the room if the infection (e.g., diphtheria) is transmitted by small-particle aerosols (droplet nuclei). Small-particle aerosols remain suspended in the air and thus travel greater distances by air.

Masks are worn by nurses in close contact with clients who require (a) contact isolation, (b) respiratory isolation, and (c) tuberculosis isolation when the client is coughing and does not cover her or his mouth. They are worn by all persons entering the rooms of clients who require strict isolation. They are also worn during certain techniques requiring surgical asepsis. During a procedure requiring sterile technique, masks are worn to prevent the airborne transmission of exhaled microorganisms to the sterile field or to a client's open wound.

If masks are made of cotton or similar material, they are washed and reused; if made of less durable material, they are discarded after use. High-efficiency, disposable masks are being used increasingly. Masks may have upper and lower strings or elasticized side loops that slip over the ears. Disposable side-loop masks are often used in general-care areas, since they can be rapidly donned and removed. Some masks have a metal strip that molds the mask over the bridge of the nose. When this strip is fitted snugly over the nose, very little air escapes around the edges of the mask. This mask is particularly suited to people who wear eyeglasses, since it prevents the glasses from fogging.

Masks must cover the nose and mouth (see Figure 32–7). To don a mask, first hold it by the top strings or loops, position the mask over the bridge of the nose, and tie the upper strings at the top back of the head so that the ties lie above the ears. If glasses are worn, fit the top edge of the mask under the glasses to minimize fogging of the glasses. Then make sure the lower part of the mask is well under the chin, and tie the lower ties at the nape of the neck. If the mask has a metal strip, adjust it firmly over the bridge of the nose. While wearing the mask, avoid talking as much as possible to keep respiratory airflow at a minimum. Masks become moist and ineffective after a few hours. For this reason, masks should be worn only once and disposed of appropriately. If a mask becomes moist during a lengthy procedure, e.g., an operation, it may be necessary to have another nurse who is not gowned and gloved put a clean, dry mask over the one being worn. Before removing a mask, remove gloves, if used, or wash the hands if they have been in contact with infectious material. After removing the mask, fold it in half with the moist inner surfaces together to contain the

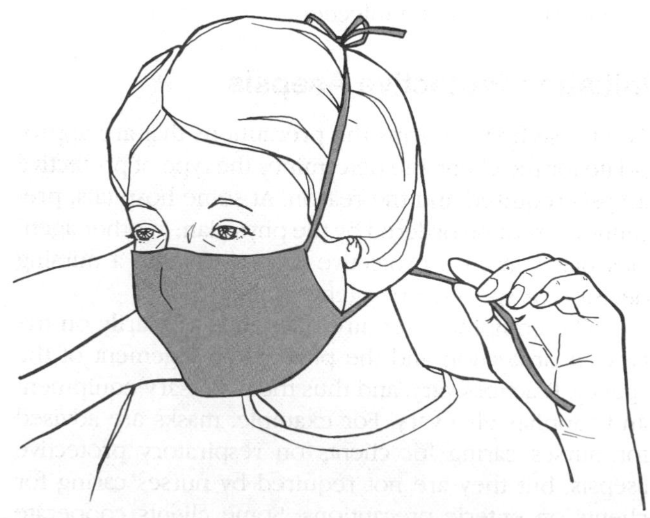

Figure 32–7 A face mask covering the nose and mouth

microorganisms. Dispose of the mask in the appropriate waste or laundry container.

Gowning for Protective Asepsis

Clean or disposable gowns are worn for protective asepsis when the nurse's uniform is likely to become contaminated, e.g., when a client's excreta or secretions may come in contact with the nurse's clothes. Examples are the respiratory secretions of an infant and the fecal material of an incontinent client. Gowns are also required when persons enter the room of a client who has an infection, for example, varicella (chicken pox), that could cause serious illness if spread to others, even though soiling of the clothing is not likely (Garner and Simmons 1983, p. 254). Sterile gowns may be indicated when the nurse is changing the dressings of a client with extensive wounds, e.g., burns. It is recommended that a clean gown be used only once and then discarded in the receptacle designated for the purpose. Gowns may be disposable or reusable after laundering.

Before donning a gown, the nurse washes the hands thoroughly and dons a face mask, if required. When donning the gown the nurse fastens the ties at the neck, overlaps the gown at the back as much as possible, and fastens the waist ties. Overlapping securely covers the uniform at the back. See Figure 32–8. No special precautions are necessary when removing a gown unless the gown is soiled with infectious materials.

When a gown is soiled with infectious material, the nurse removes the gown so that it does not contaminate the uniform by following these steps.

1. Remove disposable gloves if worn, and dispose of them in the appropriate container. See "Donning and Removing Disposable Gloves." The gloves are likely to be more contaminated than the waist ties and are therefore removed first.
2. Untie the waist belt or ties, and let the ends hang freely at the sides.
3. Untie the neck ties, and bring them forward until the gown is partially off the shoulders. Avoid touching soiled parts on the outside of the gown if possible. For instance, the top part of the gown may be soiled after a nurse holds an infant with a respiratory infection.
4. Working from the inside of the gown, slide the gown down the arms and over the hands. See Figure 32–9.
5. Holding the gown away from the body, grasp the gown with both hands at the inside shoulder seams. Bring the hands together. See Figure 32–10. Invert onc shoulder over the other so that the clean inside surface is outermost.
6. Roll the gown up inside out, and discard it in the appropriate container.
7. Wash the hands if they are soiled with infectious material.

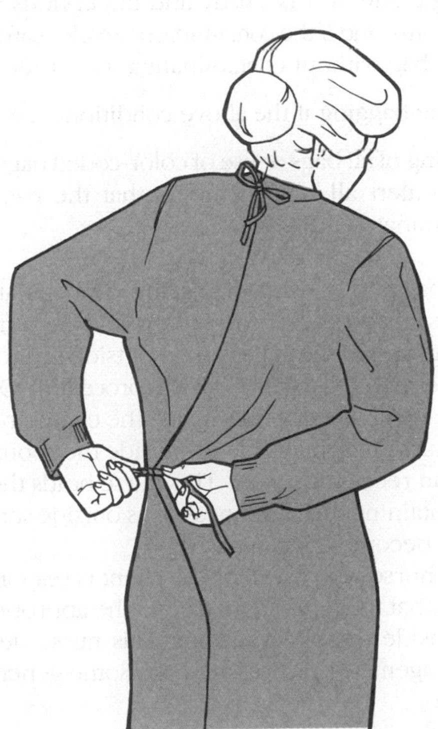

Figure 32–8 Overlapping the gown at the back to cover the nurse's uniform

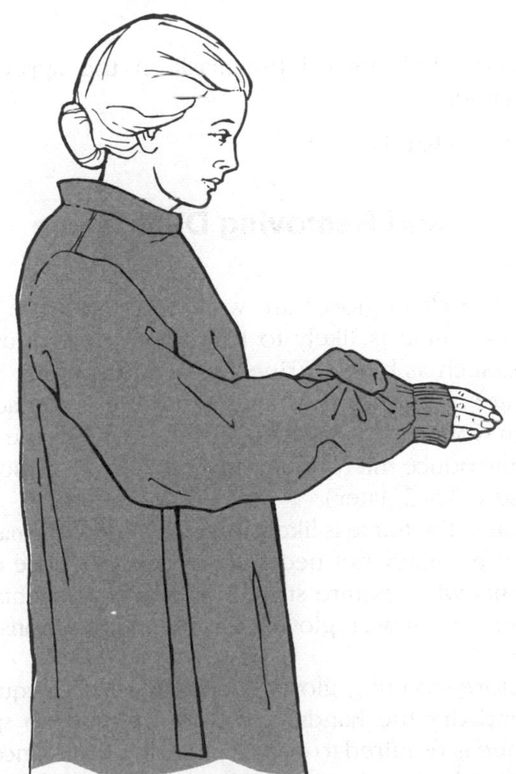

Figure 32–9 Pulling a soiled gown down the arms by working from the inside of the gown

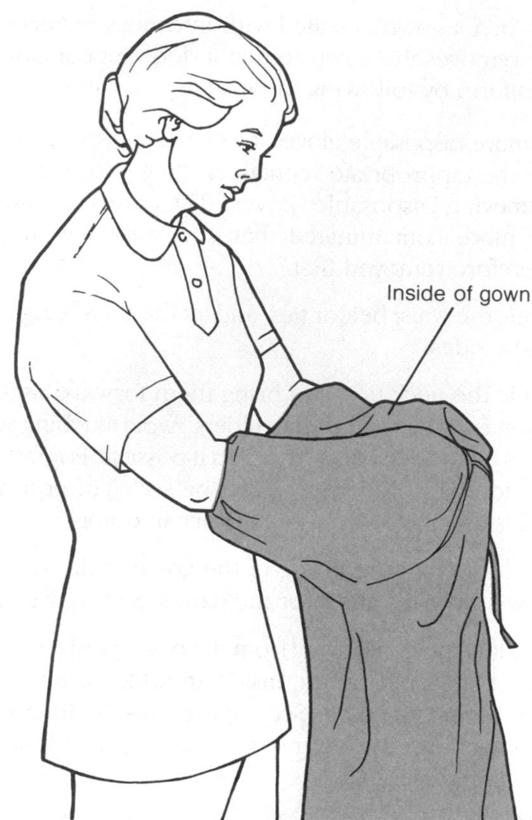

Figure 32–10 Rolling a soiled gown up with the inside outermost

8. Remove and discard the mask in the appropriate container.
9. Wash the hands.

Donning and Removing Disposable Gloves

Disposable clean gloves are worn to protect the hands when the nurse is likely to handle any infectious substances, such as blood, urine, feces, and sputum. Sterile gloves are used when the hands will come in contact with an open wound or mucous membrane or when the hands might introduce microorganisms into a body orifice (see Procedure 32–3, later).

Unless the nurse is likely to touch infectious material, gloves are usually not necessary. However, those caring for clients who require strict isolation, e.g., clients with diphtheria, must wear gloves (Garner and Simmons 1983, p. 258).

Before donning gloves, don a mask (if required), wash and dry the hands, and don a gown. No special technique is required to don disposable gloves since they are relatively shapeless and either glove fits either hand. They need to be donned carefully, however, so that they do not tear. If a gown is worn, pull up the gloves to cover the cuffs of the gown. If a gown is not worn, pull up the cuffs to cover the wrists.

To remove soiled gloves without contaminating the hands, grasp the first glove to be removed on its palmar surface just below the cuff, taking care that only glove touches glove and not the skin of the wrist or hand, which is considered clean. See Figure 32–11. Pull the first glove completely off by inverting or rolling the glove inside out. Continue to hold the inverted removed glove with the fingers of the gloved hand. Then place the first two fingers of the bare hand inside the cuff of the second glove and pull the second glove off to the fingers by turning it inside out. This action pulls the first glove inside the second. See Figure 32–12. Using the bare hand, continue to remove the gloves, which are now inside out, and put them in the refuse container. See Figure 32–13. The bare hands, which are considered clean, touch only the insides of the gloves, which are also considered clean. Wash the hands well. Even though gloves were worn, it is safe practice to wash the hands after handling contaminated material.

Bagging Articles

Articles contaminated with infectious material must be bagged before they are removed from the room or unit of a client who requires protective asepsis. Only articles that are contaminated or likely to be contaminated with infectious material need to be bagged. The 1983 CDC guidelines recommend the following methods:

1. A single bag, if it is sturdy and impervious to microorganisms, and if the contaminated articles can be placed in the bag without contaminating its outside.
2. Double-bagging if the above conditions are not met.
3. Labeling of all bags or use of color-coded bags or markers to alert all staff members that the bags contain contaminated articles.

Double-bagging consists of placing contaminated items into bags inside the client's room and in turn placing those bags inside clean bags held outside the room. Two nurses are required to carry out this procedure. One nurse, who may be gowned, works inside the client's room. The second nurse may be inside or outside the room and acts as a "clean receiving nurse." This nurse holds the outside bag, maintaining the cleanliness of its outside surface, and does not become contaminated.

The nurse who cares for the client is responsible for ensuring that all items are placed in the appropriate containers inside the client's room. This nurse determines what the agency's practices are first. Some general guidelines are:

1. Handle soiled linen as little as possible and with the least agitation possible, to prevent gross microbial con-

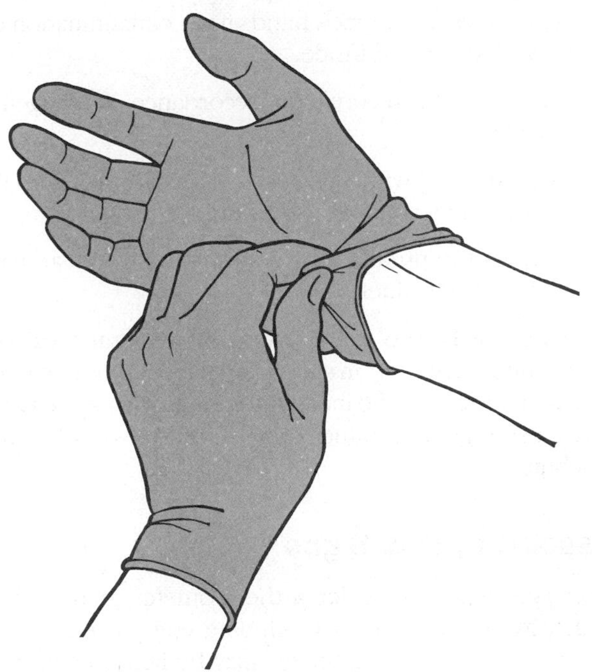

Figure 32–11 Removing the first soiled disposable glove

tamination of the air and/or persons handling the linen. Place soiled linen in the linen hamper in the infected client's room or unit. Some agencies use hot-water-soluble bags, which can be placed directly into the washing machine. In this way, laundry workers need not sort the linen before it is laundered. Such bags may require double-bagging, however, because they are generally easily torn or punctured and dissolve when wet.

2. Place garbage and contaminated *disposable* equipment in the plastic bag that lines the waste container. Some agencies separate dry and wet waste material and incinerate dry items, e.g., paper towels and disposable items. They place other waste materials in a central garbage chute or storage area.
3. Place glass bottles or jars in separate plastic or paper containers.
4. Place leftover food in the wet garbage container or flush it down the toilet.
5. Food trays and dishes do not require special precautions unless they are visibly contaminated with infectious material. If the client's hygienic practices are unsafe, use disposable dishes and discard them in the appropriate waste receptacle in the client's unit. Bag and label contaminated nondisposable (reusable) dishes, utensils, and trays before sending them to the food service department.
6. Place dressings in either the wet or the dry waste container, depending on how soiled they are.
7. Place special *nondisposable* equipment in a separate bag to be sent to the central supply area. Place glass and metal equipment in separate bags from rubber and plastic items. Glass and metal can be sterilized in an autoclave, but rubber and plastic are damaged by

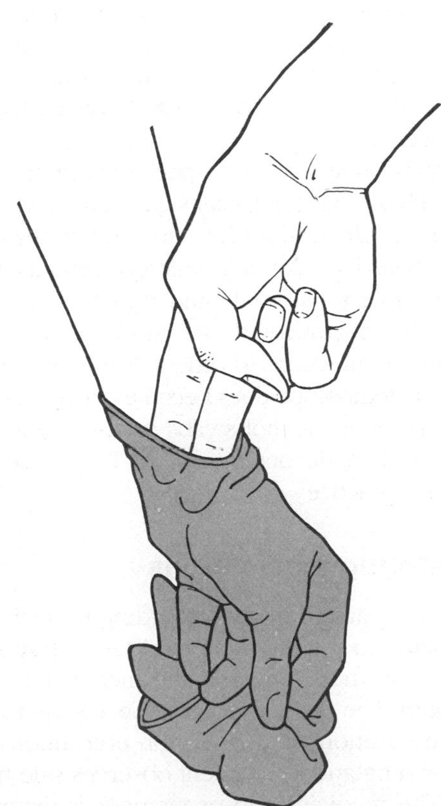

Figure 32–12 Removing the second soiled disposable glove

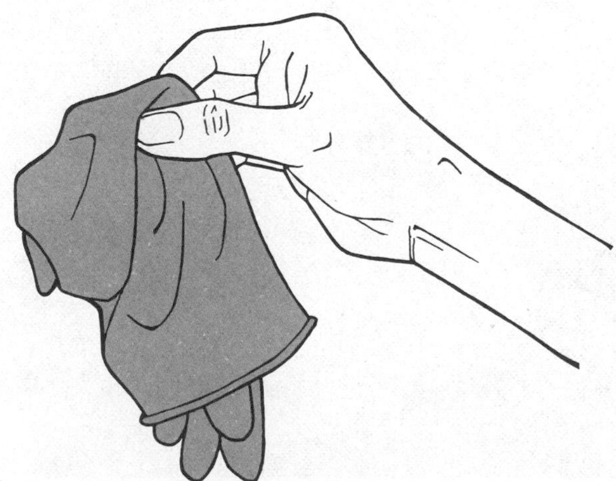

Figure 32–13 Holding soiled disposable gloves with the inside outermost

this process and must be cleaned by other methods, e.g., gas sterilization.

8. Disassemble special procedure trays into component parts. Some components can be discarded; others need to be sent to the laundry or central services for cleaning and decontaminating.

To double-bag articles the first nurse:

1. Seals all bags securely to ensure that microorganisms are confined to the bag.
2. Places the bag or bags in an appropriate clean bag opened by the nurse at the room entrance.

The second nurse:

1. Makes a cuff on the bag and holds the bag wide open or places it on a frame while the first nurse places the sealed bag into it. See Figure 32–14. The cuff on the bag protects the nurse's hands from contamination by the articles placed inside.
2. Seals the bag securely in accordance with agency practice.
3. Labels the bag with a protective asepsis (isolation) tag and marks its contents as required.
4. Provides the nurse in the room with new clean bags for refuse and linen.
5. Takes the bag to the appropriate disposal area. For example, dressing materials or paper goods may be taken directly to the incinerator. Laundry may be taken to a storage area rather than placed down a laundry chute.

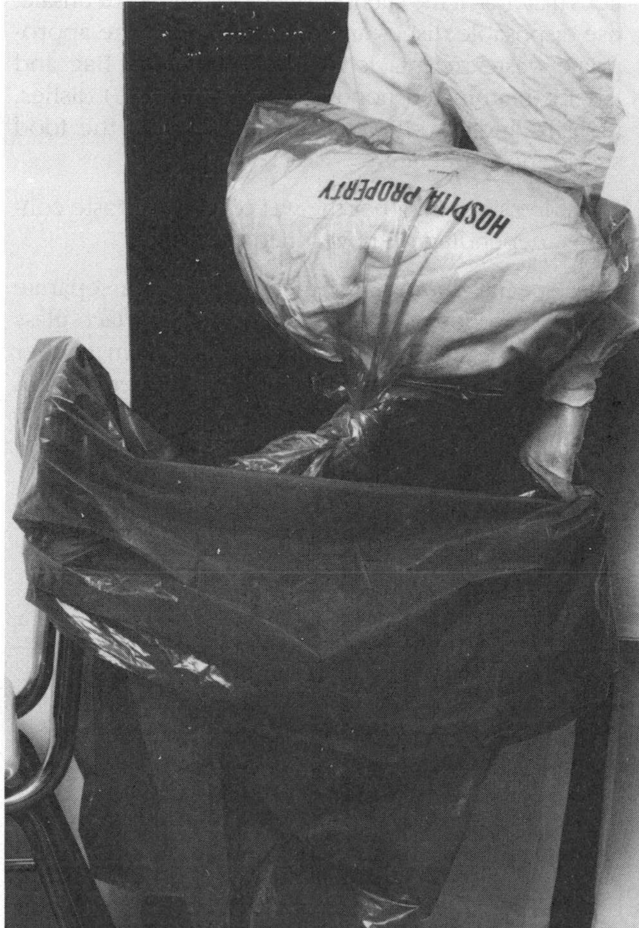

COURTESY SWEARINGEN PHOTO-ATLAS

Figure 32–14 Double-bagging contaminated articles

Assessing Vital Signs

Most agencies arrange for a thermometer, stethoscope, and sphygmomanometer (including cuff) to be kept at the bedside. The thermometer may be kept in a tube of disinfectant solution that is changed daily. Many agencies use disposable or electronic thermometers to measure a client's temperature. When using an electronic thermometer, discard the protective cover in the client's wastebasket. If there is no sphygmomanometer or stethoscope for the client's use only, no special precautions are indicated unless the equipment is contaminated or is likely to be contaminated with infectious material. (The nurse should ensure that the client's arm is clean and dry before using the shygmomanometer.) Contaminated equipment must be bagged, labeled, and/or disinfected in accordance with agency practice.

The nurse need take no special precautions when using a watch, stethoscope, vital signs notebook or worksheet, and pencil, unless they are contaminated with infectious material. Although microorganisms may be present on table tops, walls, and floors, such surfaces, unless visibly contaminated, are rarely associated with transmission of infections to others. If the nurse's watch, notebook, or stethoscope does become contaminated with infectious material, alcohol swabs or spray disinfectants are often used to decontaminate it. The nurse should check agency practice.

Administering Medications

All medications are prepared according to agency practices and taken to the unit. The medication tray and cart are left outside the room, and the medication is taken into the room. The nurse need not don a gown to administer oral medications if the isolation precautions do not warrant gowning and if the client observes safe hygienic practices. The medicine cup or wrapper is discarded in the wastebasket or client's bedside paper bag. The nurse washes hands prior to leaving the room and then charts the medications.

To administer injectable drugs, the nurse dons a gown only when the client is in strict isolation and when there is danger of being contaminated by infectious secretions. Only the prepared syringe and needle are taken into the room. Use of disposable needles and syringes is preferred, especially if the client's blood is known to be infected. Syringes and needles should be handled with caution at all times since it is not always known which clients carry the hepatitis virus or other microorganisms in the blood. Used syringes and needles are not put into wastebaskets in the client's room but are usually placed in specially provided, puncture-proof containers in the client's room. If containers are not available in the room, the used syringe and needle may be wrapped in clean paper towels and taken to the nursing station for disposal. This practice poses a greater risk for microbe transfer, however. To avoid needle punctures, the nurse should avoid recapping, bending, or breaking used needles. Most punctures occur during recapping.

Collecting Specimens

All specimens should be put into impervious containers with secure lids to prevent leakage during transport to the laboratory. The outside of the container should be disinfected if it is visibly contaminated. Whether the specimen is bagged before removal from the client's room and transport to the laboratory depends on what the specimen is and how it is collected, handled, and transported to the laboratory. Check agency practices. Bagging prevents inadvertent exposure of transport and laboratory personnel and contamination of the environment.

Disposing of Urine and Feces

Urine and feces are flushed down the toilet, since infectious microorganisms are destroyed by sewage treatment systems. Bedpans, urinals, or bedside commodes should be rinsed and dried with paper towels. Microbial growth is less likely in dry articles.

Handling Personal Effects

Clothing soiled with infectious material should be double-bagged and sent to the client's home. A family member should be instructed to place the clothing directly into the washing machine and to wash it in hot water with a laundry detergent and bleach. Hand-washable items should be soaked for at least 10 minutes in hot water with laundry detergent and 1 ounce of household bleach per gallon of water.

Toys, books, and magazines require no special precautions unless they are visibly contaminated with infectious material; if so, they should be disinfected or destroyed. The same precautions apply to money or outgoing mail.

Transporting Clients

Clients requiring protective asepsis are transported from their rooms only as necessary to diagnostic areas or to the operating room. Both the client and the transport person need to take necessary precautions during transport. The transport person should also alert personnel in the destination area about needed precautions and instruct the client about ways he or she can help prevent the transmission of infectious microorganisms to others. For example, a client requiring respiratory asepsis should be given some tissues and a bag so that he or she can follow proper tissue technique, and the transport nurse and receiving personnel should wear masks when in close contact with the client. A client with wound drainage should have an occlusive dressing applied. Gowns must be worn by all persons if soiling is likely. The transport vehicle must be disinfected if it becomes contaminated during use.

Reverse Protective Asepsis

In reverse protective asepsis (also called barrier technique or reverse isolation), the client must be protected from microorganisms transmitted by health care personnel and in the environment. Such clients are severely compromised and highly susceptible to infection. They include clients who:

1. Have certain diseases, such as leukemia or an immune deficiency
2. Have extensive skin impairments, such as severe dermatitis or major burns, that cannot be effectively covered with dressings
3. Are receiving certain therapies, such as steroid or antimetabolite therapy or total body irradiation

The 1983 CDC guidelines state that barrier technique "does not appear to reduce the risk of infection for severely compromised patients any more than strong emphasis on appropriate hand washing during patient care" (Garner and Simmons 1983, p. 325). Compromised clients are often infected (a) by their own microorganisms, (b) by microorganisms on the inadequately washed hands of health personnel, and (c) by nonsterile items (food, water, air, and client care equipment).

The 1983 CDC guidelines recommend the following for severely compromised clients (Garner and Simmons 1983, p. 254):

1. Frequent and appropriate hand washing by all personnel before, during, and after client care

2. Private rooms whenever possible
3. Use of sterile gloves, sterile gowns, and masks by people caring for clients with major wounds or burns that cannot be enclosed by dressings.

Some agencies also require that sterile linens be used and that nurses wear caps. Proper technique for donning sterile gloves and sterile gowns is discussed in Procedures 32–3 and 32–4.

Invasive Procedures and Wound Protection

The CDC has established guidelines for providing infusion therapy safely and for preventing catheter-associated infections of the urinary tract, respiratory tract infections, and wound infections. These guidelines are discussed in Chapters 44, 45, 46, and 52.

Surgical Asepsis

Surgical asepsis, or sterile technique, goes one step beyond medical asepsis in that it controls the transmission of all microorganisms, including spores. An object is sterile only when it is free of all microorganisms. It is well known that sterile techniques are carried out in operating rooms, labor and delivery rooms, and special diagnostic areas. Less known perhaps is that sterile technique is also employed for many procedures in general care areas—procedures such as administering injections, changing wound dressings, performing urinary catheterizations, and administering intravenous therapy. In these situations, all of the principles of surgical asepsis are applied as in the operating or delivery room; however, not all of the sterile techniques that follow are always required. For example, before an operating room procedure, the nurse generally puts on a mask and cap, performs a surgical hand scrub, and then dons a sterile gown and gloves. In a general care area, the nurse may only perform a hand wash and don sterile gloves.

Sterile technique is indicated in the following instances:

1. Whenever the client's skin is intentionally perforated for therapeutic reasons, e.g., when giving a hypodermic injection or making a surgical incision
2. Whenever the skin is diseased or injured, e.g., a burn or ulceration
3. Whenever a catheter or surgical instrument is inserted into a body cavity that is considered sterile, e.g., the urinary bladder

Principles and Practices of Surgical Asepsis

The nine basic principles of surgical asepsis, and practices that relate to each principle, follow:

1. All objects used in a sterile field must be sterile.
   a. All articles are sterilized appropriately by dry or moist heat, chemicals, or radiation before use.
   b. Sterile articles can be stored for only a prescribed time; after that, they are considered unsterile.
   c. Always check a package containing a sterile object for intactness and dryness. Any package that appears already open, torn, punctured, or wet is considered unsterile. Never assume an item is sterile.
   d. Storage areas should be clean and dry.
   e. Always check the sterilization dates and periods on the labels of wrapped items before using the items.
   f. Always check chemical indicators of sterilization before using a package. The indicator is often a tape used to fasten the package or contained inside the package. The indicator changes color during sterilization, indicating that the contents are sterile. If the color change is not evident, the package is considered unsterile. Commercially prepared sterile packages may not have indicators but are marked with the word *sterile.*
2. Sterile objects become unsterile when touched by unsterile objects.
   a. Handle sterile objects that will touch open wounds or enter body cavities only with sterile forceps or sterile gloved hands.
   b. Discard or resterilize objects that come into contact with unsterile objects.
   c. Whenever the sterility of an object is questionable, assume the article is unsterile.
3. Sterile items that are out of vision or below the waist level of the nurse are considered unsterile.
   a. Once left unattended, a sterile field is considered unsterile.
   b. Sterile objects are always kept in view. Nurses do not turn their backs on a sterile field.
   c. Only the front part of a sterile gown (from the waist to the shoulder) and the front part of the sleeves are considered sterile.
   d. Always keep sterile gloved hands in sight and above waist level; touch only objects that are sterile.
   e. Once a sterile field becomes unsterile, it must be set up again before proceeding.
4. Sterile objects can become unsterile by prolonged exposure to air.
   a. Areas in which sterile procedures are carried out

are kept as clean as possible by frequent damp cleaning with detergent germicides.

b. The nurse's uniform is kept clean and dry.
c. The nurse's hair is kept clean and short or enclosed in a net to prevent hair from falling on sterile objects. Microorganisms on the hair can make a sterile field unsterile.
d. Surgical caps are worn in operating rooms and delivery rooms.
e. Sneezing or coughing over a sterile field can make it unsterile because droplets containing microorganisms from the respiratory tract can travel 3 feet. Some nurses believe that masks covering the mouth and the nose should be worn by anyone working over a sterile field or an open wound.
f. Nurses with mild upper respiratory tract infections refrain from carrying out sterile procedures or wear masks.
g. Anyone working over a sterile field keeps talking to a minimum. The nurse averts the head from the field if talking is necessary.
h. The nurse refrains from reaching over a sterile field and from moving unsterile objects over a sterile field because microorganisms can fall onto it. Always reach around a sterile field or carefully turn it by reaching under the wrapper or by touching the wrapper edges.
i. Sterile objects are moved as little as possible within the sterile field to minimize the danger of contact with unsterile objects.
j. Doors are closed and traffic is kept to a minimum in areas where a sterile procedure is being performed because moving air can carry dust and microorganisms.
k. Sterile draped tables in the operating room or elsewhere are considered sterile only at surface level.
l. Any article that falls outside the edges of a sterile field is considered unsterile.
m. Sterile packages are opened by grasping only the outer edges or corners of the coverings.

5. Fluids flow in the direction of gravity.
   a. Wet forceps are always held with the tips below the handles. When the tips are held higher than the handles, fluid can flow onto the handle and become contaminated by the hands. When the forceps are again pointed downward, the fluid flows back down and contaminates the tips.
   b. During a surgical hand wash, the hands are held higher than the elbows to prevent contaminants from the forearms from reaching the hands.

6. Moisture that passes through a sterile object draws microorganisms from unsterile surfaces above or below to the sterile surface by capillary action.
   a. Sterile waterproof barriers are used beneath sterile objects. Liquids (sterile saline or antiseptics) are frequently poured into containers on a sterile field. If they are spilled onto it, the barrier keeps the liquid from seeping beneath the sterile field.
   b. The sterile covers on sterile equipment are kept dry. Damp surfaces can attract microorganisms in the air.
   c. When pouring sterile solutions into sterile containers, care is taken to avoid dampening the sterile field.
   d. Sterile drapes that do not have a sterile barrier underneath and that become moist are replaced.

7. The edges of a sterile field are considered unsterile.
   a. A 2.5 cm (1 in) margin at each edge of an opened drape is considered unsterile, since the edges are in contact with unsterile surfaces.
   b. All sterile objects are placed more than 2.5 cm (1 in) inside the edges of a sterile field.

8. The skin cannot be sterilized and is unsterile.
   a. Sterile gloves are worn and/or sterile forceps are used to handle sterile items.
   b. Prior to a surgical aseptic procedure, the hands are washed to reduce the number of microorganisms on them.

9. Conscientiousness, alertness, and honesty are essential qualities in maintaining surgical asepsis.
   a. When a sterile object becomes unsterile, it does not necessarily change in appearance.
   b. The person who sees a sterile object become contaminated must correct the situation.

Assessing Prior to Sterile Procedures

Nurses frequently carry out procedures requiring sterile technique on clinical units, e.g., urinary catheterizations and surgical dressing changes. Before any such procedures, the nurse assesses what the client needs to know about sterile technique and what precautions need to be taken to prevent contamination during the procedure.

Knowledge Needs

Clients often need to be taught how to maintain sterile technique during specific procedures. For example, they may need to learn the following:

1. To refrain from coughing, sneezing, and talking near a sterile field. These actions can transmit microorganisms from the respiratory tract and thus contaminate the sterile field.

2. To refrain from touching sterile supplies or a sterile field, thus making it unsterile.

3. To avoid sudden movement of body parts covered by sterile drapes. The sterile drapes or equipment

could become unsterile upon contact with the bedding, table, etc.

Client Precautions

The nurse needs to assess the comfort needs of the client before the procedure so that equipment and supplies will remain sterile. For example, some clients may need to urinate, defecate, or take an analgesic for pain before the procedure. Others may need assistance from another nurse to maintain the appropriate position during the procedure.

Opening Sterile Wrapped Packages

Equipment is wrapped in a variety of materials to maintain its sterility. Commercially prepared items are frequently wrapped in plastic, paper, glass, or plastic and paper. Commercially prepared sterile liquids for both internal and external use are often supplied in plastic or glass containers. Plastics are often pliable, usually transparent, impervious to dust, and relatively resistant to tearing. Intravenous solutions are commonly packaged in plastic bags. Liquid medications are sterilized in glass containers. Liquids used in hospitals may be prepared commercially or in the hospital. In the past it was not unusual for sterile liquids, e.g., sterile water for irrigations, to be supplied in large glass containers and used many times. This practice is considered undesirable today because once a container has been opened, there can be no assurance that it is sterile. Liquids are preferably packaged in amounts adequate for one use only. Any leftover liquid is discarded. Hospital-packaged liquids are often sterilized in reusable containers; commercially packaged liquids are supplied in disposable containers. These containers normally have a seal over the cap, and often the word *sterile* is clearly marked on the top. If the cap has been tampered with or if the seal is broken, the liquid is considered unsterile.

Other sterile supplies are frequently wrapped in disposable or reusable paper. Laminated paper wrappers are sturdier than paper. Paper wrappers have the advantage of being relatively cheap, impervious to dust, and permeable to steam, hence allowing steam sterilization. The disadvantages are that paper can be torn or punctured, making the items within unsterile, and that the paper is not flexible (a disadvantage if one wishes to use it as a sterile field). Hospital packs are usually wrapped in muslin; two or four layers of good quality, 140-thread count muslin should be used. The American Hospital Association (AHA) recommends using four layers of muslin or a nonwoven, single-use fabric (AHA 1979). Reusable muslin must be laundered before being resterilized to avoid fiber damage (Ryan 1976, p. 984).

Commercially prepared packages are generally heat sealed. Usually they are opened by pulling tabs or flaps while maintaining the sterility of the items inside. The area inside the heat seal line is considered sterile. Items are also wrapped "envelope style." Packages sterilized in the institution are usually wrapped in this manner. The inner aspect of the wrapper to within 2.5 cm (1 in) of the edge is considered contaminated.

Opening a Wrapped Package on a Flat Surface

Before one opens a sterile package, it is important to place it above waist level on a clean, dry surface. This surface should be away from any infectious material and air currents. The package is placed in the center of the work area so that the top flap opens away from the nurse. The flap farthest from the nurse is opened first, but the nurse takes care not to reach over the sterile field. See Figure 32–15. The nurse holds the arm out at the side or lateral to the package. Then the side flaps are opened (Figure 32–16), and the flap nearest the nurse is opened last (Figure 32–17). When opening the flaps, the nurse takes care not to touch the inside of the wrapper. Usually the corners are turned outward so that the nurse can grasp them easily and avoid touching the inside. When opening the last flap, the nurse stands well back from the package—15 to 30 cm (6 to 12 in)—to avoid contamination from the nurse's uniform. If space on the table is limited, it may

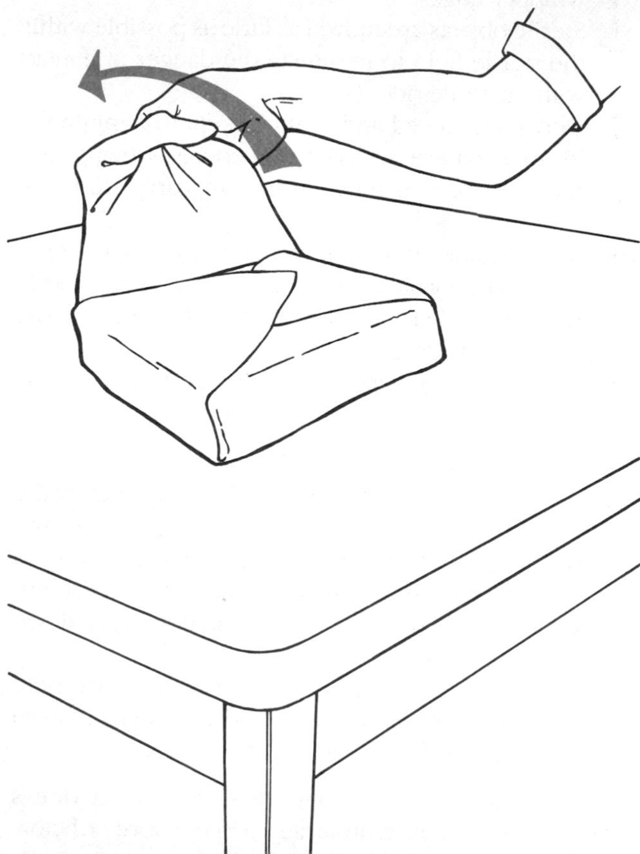

Figure 32–15 Opening the first flap of a sterile wrapped package

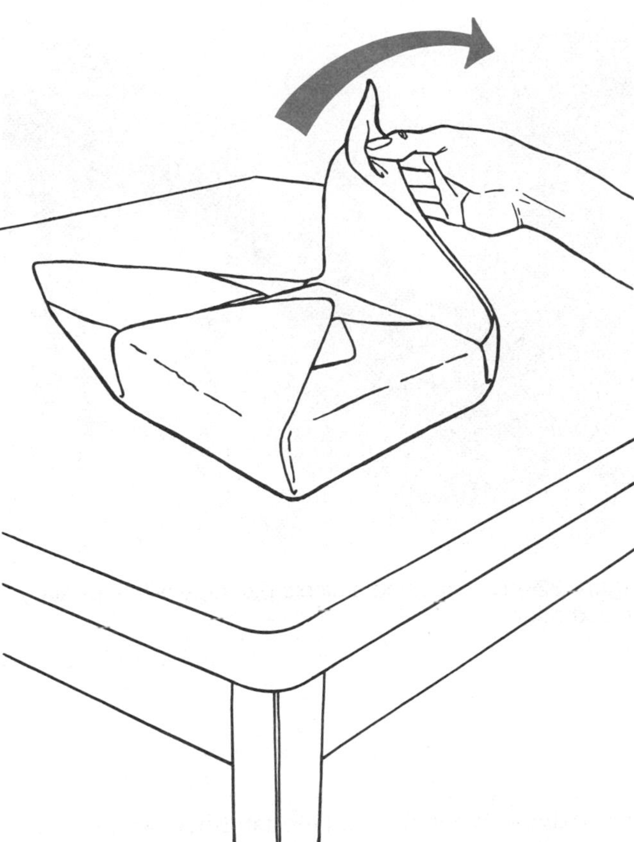

Figure 32–16 Opening the second flap to the side

be necessary to fan fold this flap so that it remains above the waist level of the nurse. Some sterile sets have an inner wrapping as well. This wrapping is opened in similar fashion, but sterile forceps are used.

In some situations, it may be necessary to close or loosely wrap a sterile package for a few minutes. For example, after solutions have been added to a dressing set, the set may need to be rewrapped for transport to the bedside. However, a sterile package can be rewrapped only if the inside of the wrapper has remained sterile, i.e., if the nurse has touched only the tabs or the outside of the wrapper. Rewrapping is done in the *reverse* order to unwrapping. The proximal flap is closed first to prevent reaching across the sterile field, the side flaps next, and the distal flap last.

Opening a Wrapped Package While Holding It

The package is held in one hand with the top flap opening away from the nurse. Using the other hand, the nurse opens the package as described above, pulling the corners of the flaps well back. See Figure 32–18. Because the hands are considered contaminated, they should not touch the contents of the package at any time. The sterile item is now exposed so that it can be transferred to a sterile field or handed to another person who is wearing sterile gloves. See "Establishing a Sterile Field," next.

Opening Commercially Prepared Packages

Manufacturers usually supply directions for opening commercially prepared sterile packages and containers. The container is held in one hand, and the flap or tab is pulled back with the other hand. See Figure 32–19. If the package has two flaps, both flaps are grasped, one with each hand, and pulled apart gently. See Figure 32–20.

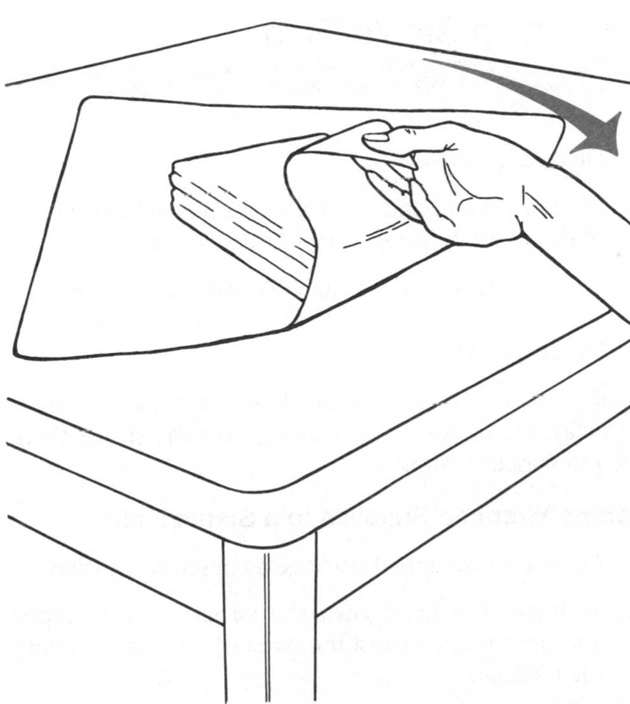

Figure 32–17 Pulling the last flap toward the nurse by grasping the corner

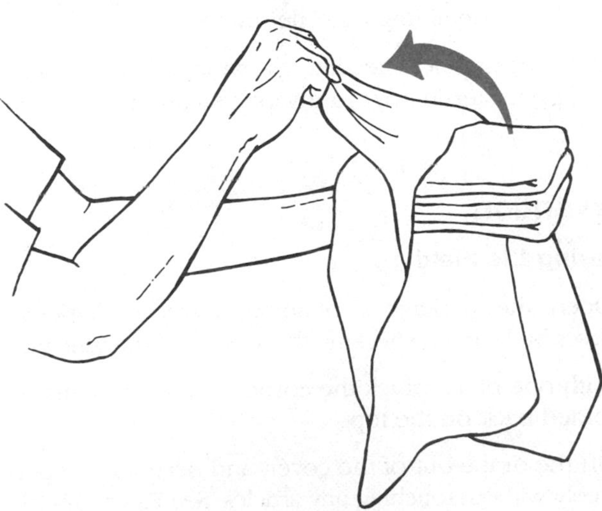

Figure 32–18 Opening a wrapped package while holding it

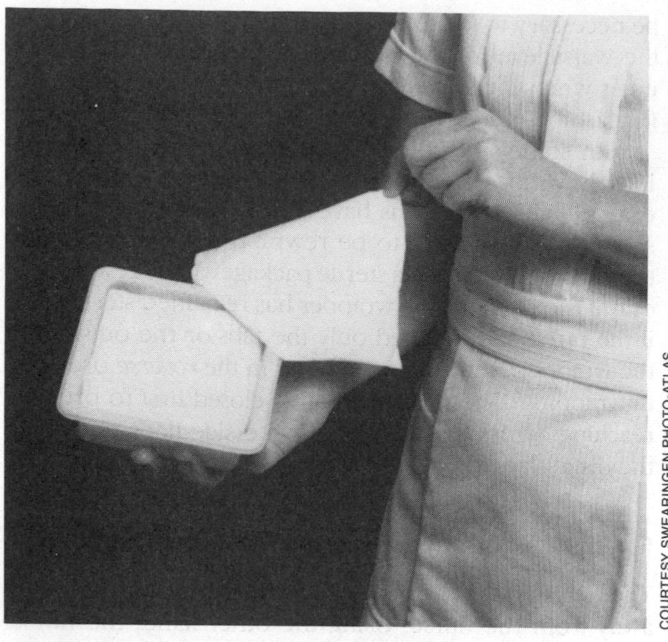

Figure 32–19 Opening a sterile package with an unsealed corner

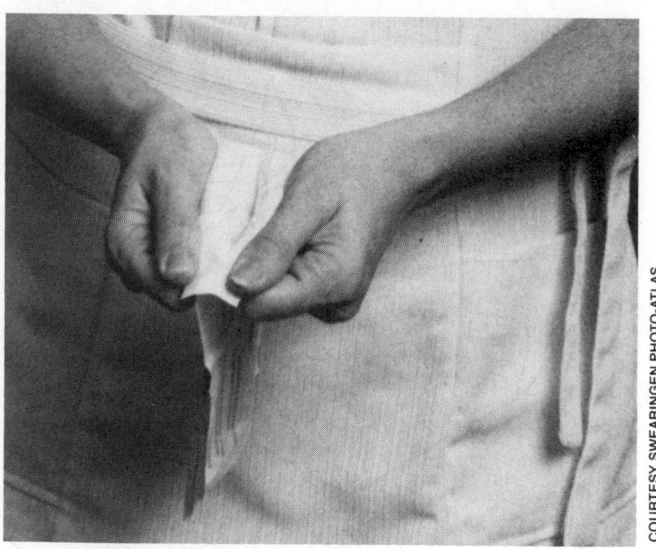

Figure 32–20 Opening a sterile package with a partially sealed edge

Establishing a Sterile Field

A **sterile field** is a microorganism-free area that can receive sterile supplies. It is often established by using the innermost side of a sterile wrapper or by using a wrapped sterile drape. When the field is established, wrapped supplies and sterile solutions can be placed on it. Sterile forceps are used in many instances to handle and transfer the sterile supplies (see the next section).

Procedure 32–2 ▲ Establishing and Maintaining a Sterile Field

Equipment

1. A package containing a sterile drape
2. Sterile equipment as needed, e.g., wrapped sterile gauze, a wrapped sterile bowl, antiseptic solution.

Intervention

Preparing the Field

1. Open the package containing a sterile drape as described earlier, checking the sterility of the contents.
2. With one hand, pluck the corner of the drape that is folded back on the top.
3. Lift the drape out of the cover, and permit it to open freely without touching any articles. See Figure 32–21.

   Rationale If the drape touches the outside of the package, the nurse's uniform, or any unsterile surface, it is considered contaminated.
4. Discard the cover.
5. With the other hand, carefully pick up another corner of the drape holding it well away from yourself.
6. Lay the drape on a clean, dry surface, placing the bottom, freely hanging side farthest from you. See Figure 32–22.

   Rationale By placing the lowermost side farthest away, the nurse avoids leaning over the sterile field and contaminating it.

Adding Wrapped Supplies to a Sterile Field

7. Open each wrapped package as described earlier.
8. With your free hand, grasp the corners of the wrapper and hold them against the wrist of the hand holding the package.

   Rationale The hand is now covered by the sterile wrapper and rendered sterile.
9. Place the sterile bowl, drape, etc., on the sterile field

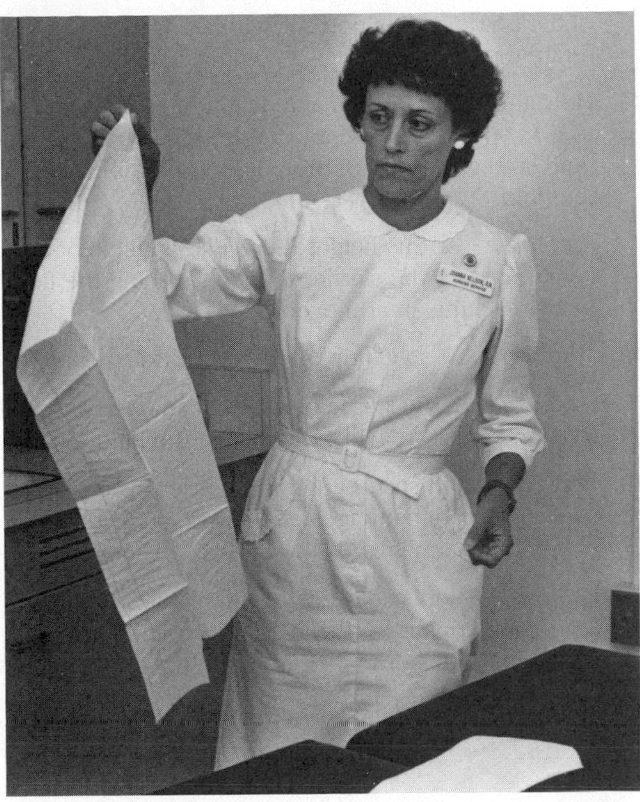

Figure 32–21

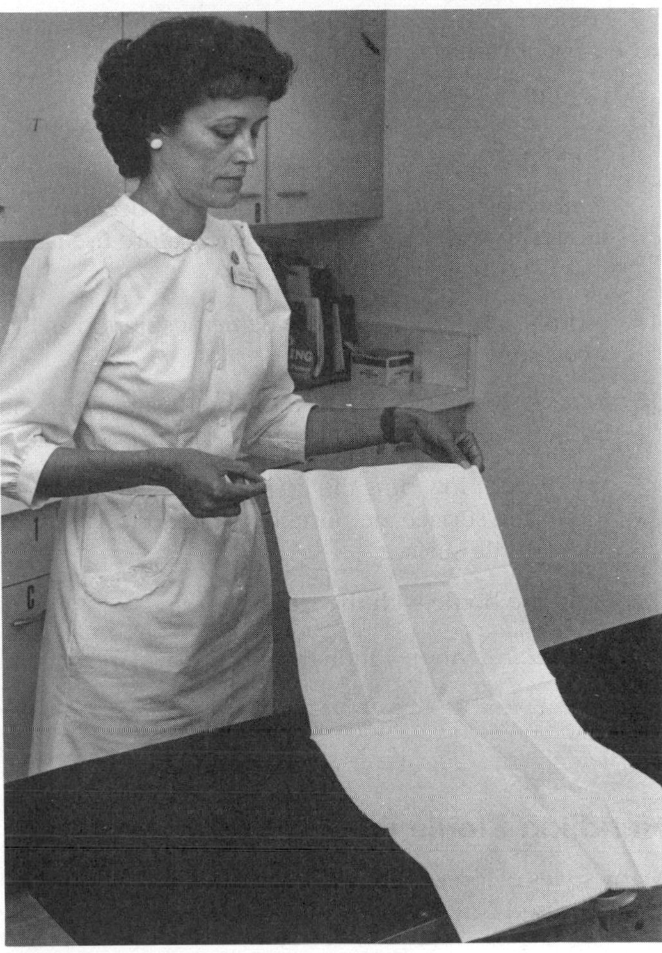

Figure 32–22

approaching from an angle rather than holding your arm over the field.

10. Discard the wrapper.

Adding Commercially Packaged Supplies to a Sterile Field

11. Open each package as described earlier.
12. Hold the package 15 cm (6 in) above the field, and permit the contents to drop onto the field. See Figure 32–23. Keep in mind that 2.5 cm (1 in) around the edge of the field is considered contaminated.

    Rationale At a height of 15 cm (6 in), the outside of the package is not likely to touch and contaminate the sterile field.

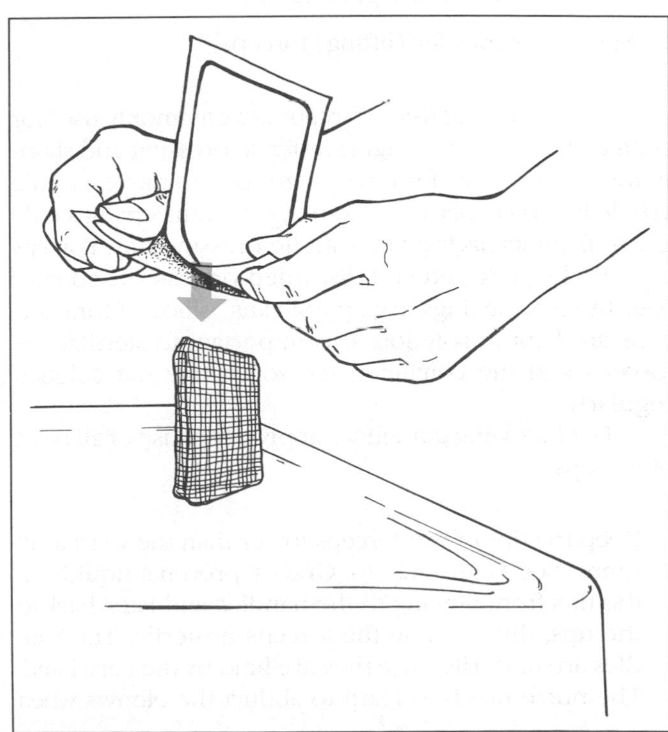

Figure 32–23

Adding Sterile Solution to a Sterile Bowl

Sterile liquids (e.g., normal saline) frequently need to be poured into metal or nonabsorbent containers within a sterile field. Bottles or flasks that contain sterile solutions are considered sterile on the inside and contaminated on the outside, since the bottle may have been handled. Bottles used in an operating room may be sterilized on the outside as well as the inside, however, and these are handled with sterile gloves.

Before pouring any liquid, read the label three times to ensure it is the correct solution.

13. Obtain a container with the exact amount of solution, if possible.

    Rationale Once a sterile container has been opened, its sterility cannot be ensured for a future use unless it is used again immediately.

14. From the label, confirm the name of solution and its strength.

15. Remove the lid or cap from the bottle and invert the lid before placing it on a surface that is not sterile.

    Rationale Inverting the lid maintains the sterility of the inside surface, because it is not allowed to touch an unsterile surface.

16. Hold the bottle with the label uppermost.

    Rationale Any solution that flows down the outside of the bottle during pouring will not damage or obliterate the label.

17. Hold the bottle of fluid at a height of 10 to 15 cm (4 to 6 in) over the bowl and to the side of the sterile field so that as little of the bottle as possible is over the field.

    Rationale At this height there is less likelihood of contaminating the sterile field by touching the field or by reaching an arm over it.

18. Pour the solution gently so as not to splash the liquid.

    Rationale If the sterile drape is on an unsterile surface, any moisture will contaminate the field.

19. Replace the lid securely on the bottle if you plan to use it again. In many agencies, any opened container of sterile solution is used only once and then discarded.

    Rationale Replacing the lid immediately prevents accidental contact with the lid or solution, thereby rendering it unsterile.

Handling Sterile Forceps

Many styles of forceps are used to handle sterile supplies. Forceps used commonly by nurses are:

1. Hemostat or artery forceps. See Figure 32–24.
2. Tissue forceps. See Figure 32–25.
3. Sponge or transfer (lifting) forceps.

Hemostats and tissue forceps are commonly used for such techniques as changing a sterile dressing and shortening a drain. Transfer forceps are used to move a sterile article from one place to another, e.g., transferring sterile gauze from its package to a sterile dressing tray. Forceps are usually packaged and discarded or resterilized after use. In some settings, e.g., physicians' offices, lifting forceps are kept in solution. It is important to sterilize the forceps and the container and to change the solution regularly.

The following guidelines apply to the use of all types of forceps.

1. Keep the tips of wet forceps lower than the wrist at all times. See Figure 32–26. Gravity prevents liquids on the tips from flowing to the handles and later back to the tips, thus making the forceps unsterile. The handles are unsterile once they are held by the bare hand. The nurse needs to learn to abduct the elbows when handling forceps. This abduction keeps forceps tips in the downward position.
2. Hold sterile forceps above waist level. There is less danger of contamination if the forceps are held nearer to eye level.
3. Hold sterile forceps within sight. While out of sight,

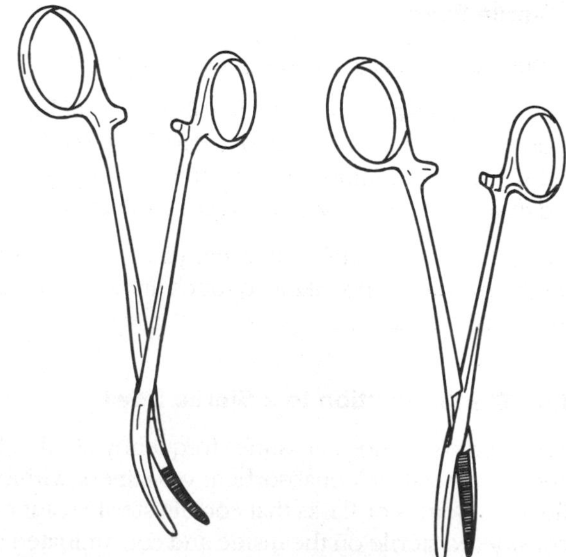

Figure 32–24 Hemostat forceps (curved and straight)

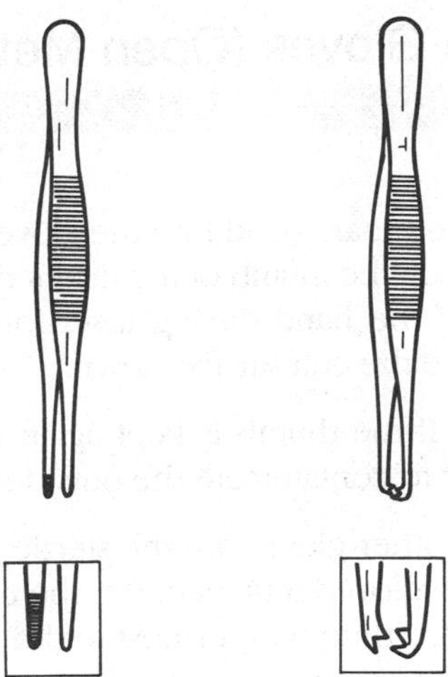

Figure 32–25 Tissue forceps (plain and toothed)

forceps may inadvertently become unsterile. Any such forceps should be considered unsterile.

4. Remove transfer forceps from their package or a solution container by lifting the forcep directly upward. Make sure that the forceps do not touch the edge or inside of the container or the outside of the wrapper. These areas are not sterile.

5. When using forceps to lift sterile supplies out of a commercially prepared package, be sure that the forceps do not touch the edges or outside of the wrapper. The edges and outside of the package are handled, and are thus unsterile.

6. When placing forceps whose handles were in contact with the bare hand on a sterile field, position the handles outside the sterile area. The handles of these forceps harbor microorganisms from the nurse's hand unless the nurse was wearing sterile gloves.

7. Deposit a sterile item on a sterile field without permitting moist forceps to touch the sterile field when the surface under the absorbent sterile field is unsterile and a barrier drape is not used. A **barrier drape** is resistant to moisture, e.g., blood and antiseptics, and should be used whenever a procedure involves the use of liquids. Made of chemically treated cotton or synthetic materials, barrier drapes prevent a sterile field from becoming unsterile when the drape becomes wet. It is known that a sterile cloth becomes unsterile when dampened (even with sterile water) if it is on an unsterile surface or has contact with any unsterile object (LeMaitre and Finnegan 1980, p. 103). Microorganisms can move through a damp sterile cloth from an unsterile surface, contaminating the field. If the underlying surface is sterile (e.g., a plastic container) the field will not become unsterile when moist.

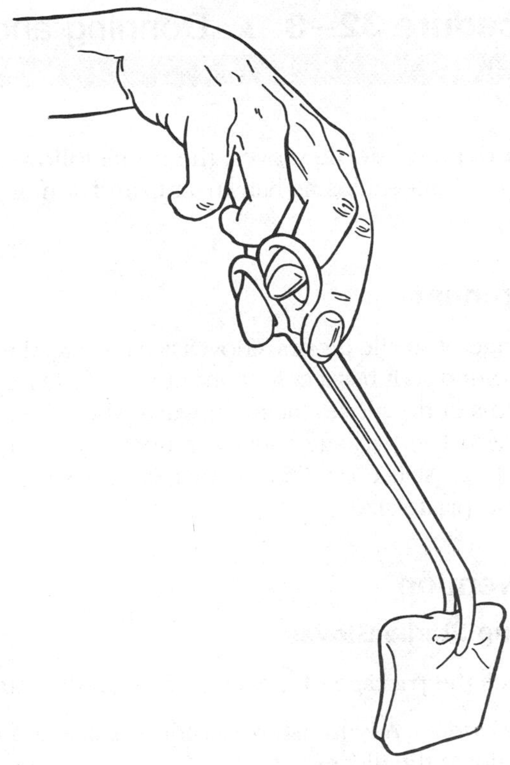

Figure 32–26 Holding forceps with tips lower than the hand

8. Discard disposable transfer forceps after use or send reusable transfer forceps for repackaging and sterilization. If sterilizing contaminated transfer forceps by immersing them in solution, indicate on the container when they will be sterilized. Others will consider the forceps in solution sterile unless notified. The length of time they will remain unsterile depends upon the type and strength of the solution.

Donning Sterile Gloves (Open Method)

Sterile gloves may be donned by the open method or the closed method. The open method is most frequently used outside the operating room, since the closed method requires that the nurse wear a sterile gown.

Gloves are worn during many sterile procedures to maintain the sterility of equipment and protect a client's open wound. Gloves may or may not be used with sterile forceps. For example, when inserting a catheter, the nurse generally wears gloves and uses sterile forceps; when changing a dressing, the nurse uses sterile forceps but may not wear gloves.

Procedure 32–3 ▲ Donning and Removing Sterile Gloves (Open Method)

Before donning sterile gloves, the nurse follows agency practices about enclosing hair in a cap and donning a face mask.

Equipment

A package of sterile gloves. Gloves are packaged with the glove folded so it has a cuff of about 5 cm (2 in) and with the palms of the gloves facing upward when the package is opened. The package usually indicates the size of the gloves (e.g., size 6 or 7½), so that the nurse can select the appropriate size.

Intervention

Donning Sterile Gloves

1. Place the package of gloves on a clean dry surface.

   Rationale Any moisture on the surface could contaminate the gloves.

2. Some gloves are packed in an inner as well as an outer package. Open the outer package without contaminating the gloves or the inner package. See "Opening Sterile Wrapped Packages," earlier in this chapter. Remove the inner package from the outer package.

3. Open the inner package as above or according to the manufacturer's directions. Some manufacturers specify a numbered sequence for opening the flaps and provide folded tabs to grasp when opening the flaps. If no tabs are provided, pluck the flap so that the fingers do not touch the inner surfaces.

   Rationale The inner surfaces, which are next to the sterile gloves, will remain sterile.

4. If the gloves are packaged so they lie side by side, grasp the glove for your dominant hand by its cuff (on the palmar side) with the thumb and first finger of the nondominant hand. Touch only the inside of the cuff. See Figure 32–27.

   or

   If the gloves are packaged one on top of the other, grasp the cuff of the top glove as above, using the opposite hand.

   Rationale The hands are not sterile. By touching only the inside of the glove, the nurse avoids contaminating the outside.

5. Insert the dominant hand into the glove and pull the glove on. Keep the thumb of the inserted hand against the palm of the hand during insertion. See Figure 32–28. Leave the cuff turned down.

   Rationale If the thumb is kept against the palm, it is less likely to contaminate the outside of the glove.

6. Pick up the other glove with the sterile gloved hand, inserting the gloved fingers under the cuff and holding the gloved thumb outermost to the gloved palm. See Figure 32–29.

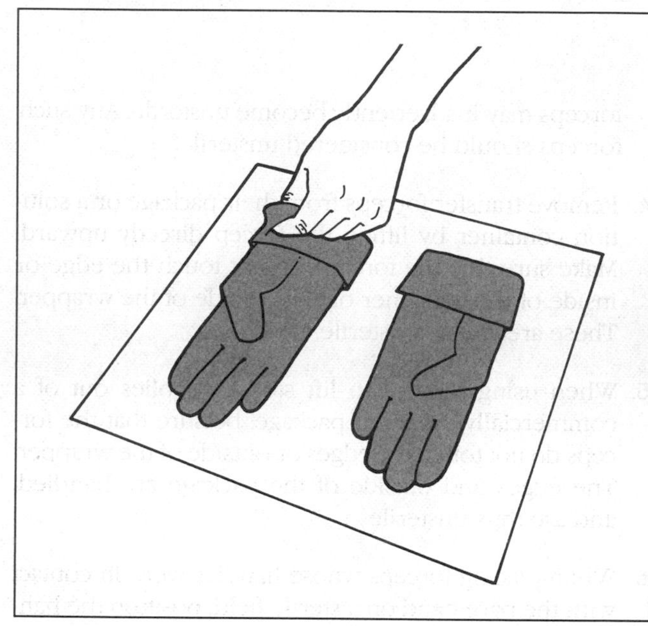

Figure 32–27

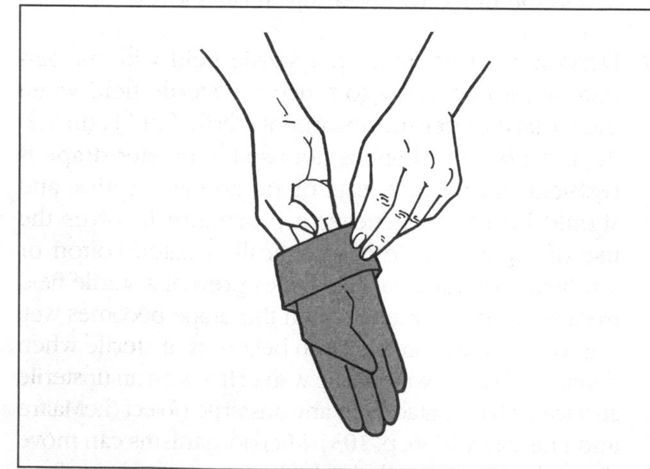

Figure 32–28

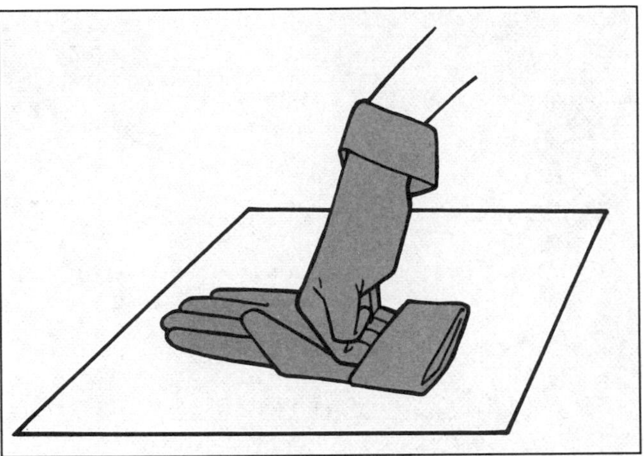

Figure 32–29

Rationale This helps prevent accidental contamination of the glove by the bare hand.

7. Pull on the second glove carefully. Hold the thumb of the gloved first hand outermost. See Figure 32–30.

   Rationale In this position, the thumb is less likely to touch the arm and become contaminated.

8. Adjust each glove so that it fits smoothly, and carefully pull the cuffs up by sliding the fingers under the cuffs.

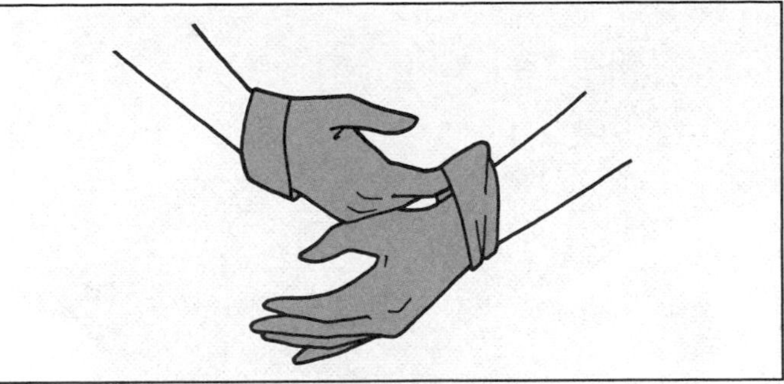

Figure 32–30

Removing Used Gloves

9. Pluck either glove near the cuff end and pull the glove over the hand so that the glove inverts itself, with the contaminated surface inside.

   Rationale Sterile gloves are considered contaminated once they have been used.

10. Slide two fingers of the bare hand against the wrist under the cuff of the other glove and slide the second glove off, inverting it over itself and the first glove. Discard the gloves in the designated container.

Donning a Sterile Gown and Sterile Gloves (Closed Method)

Sterile gowning and closed gloving are chiefly carried out in operating or delivery rooms, where surgical asepsis is necessary. The closed method of gloving can be used only when a sterile gown is worn because the gloves are handled through the sleeves of the gown. Prior to these techniques, the nurse dons a hair cover and a mask, and performs a surgical hand wash.

Procedure 32–4 ▲ Donning a Sterile Gown and Gloves (Closed Method)

Equipment

A sterile pack containing a sterile gown and sterile gloves. In some agencies the gloves are provided in a separate package.

Intervention

Donning a Sterile Gown

1. Open the sterile pack.
2. Remove the outer wrap from the sterile gloves, and drop the gloves in their inner sterile wrap on the sterile field established by the sterile outer wrapper. See Procedure 32–3, steps 7–10.
3. Carry out a surgical hand wash for the length of time required by the agency. Before procedures in areas such as the operating room, the washing time required is commonly longer than before procedures in clinical areas, e.g., 10 minutes, and washing includes scrubbing with a stiff-bristled brush.
4. Grasp the sterile gown at the crease near the neck, and let it unfold freely without touching anything, including the uniform.

   Rationale The gown will be unsterile if its outer surface touches any unsterile articles.

5. Put the hands inside the shoulders of the gown and work the arms partway into the sleeves without touching the outside of the gown. See Figure 32–31.

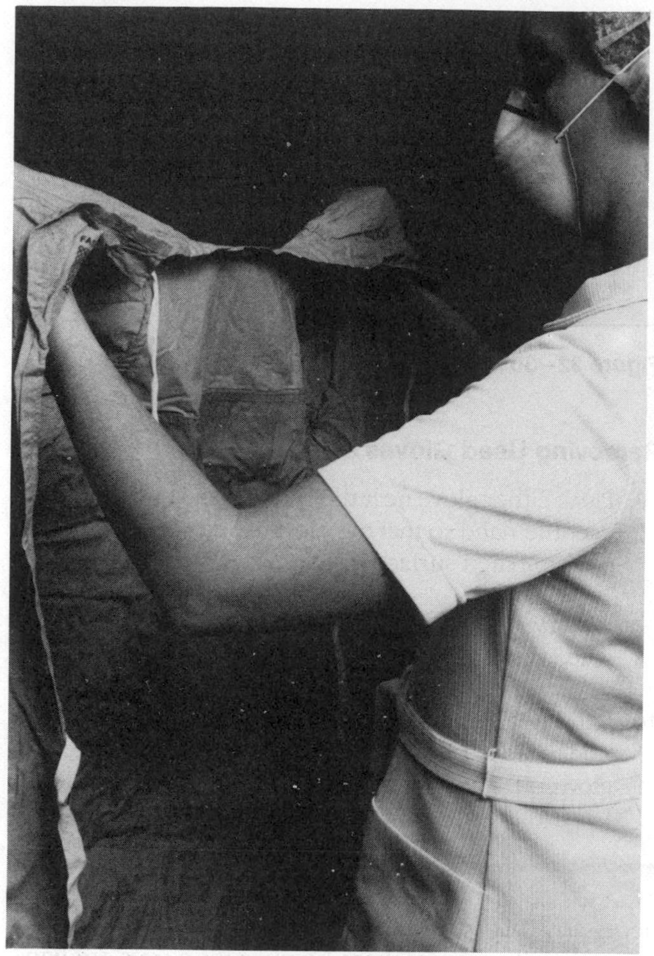

COURTESY SWEARINGEN PHOTO-ATLAS

Figure 32–31

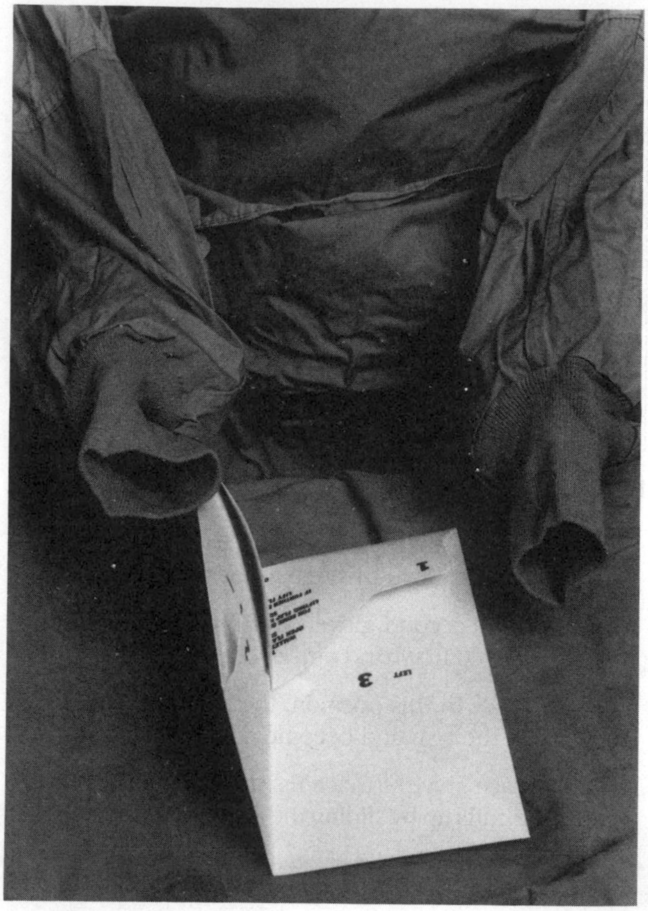

COURTESY SWEARINGEN PHOTO-ATLAS

Figure 32–32

6. Work the hands down the sleeves only to the proximal edge of the cuff, if donning sterile gloves using the closed method (see steps 8–16 below).

   or

   Work the hands down the sleeves and through the cuffs if donning sterile gloves using the open method.
7. A coworker wearing a hair cover and mask grasps the neck ties without touching the outside of the gown and pulls the gown upward to cover the neckline of the uniform in front and back. The coworker ties the neck ties. Gowning continues at step 17.

Donning Sterile Gloves (Closed Method)

8. While the hands are still covered by the sleeves, open the inner sterile wrapper containing the sterile gloves. See Figure 32–32.
9. Pick up the opposite glove with the thumb and index finger of the dominant hand, handling the glove through the sleeve.
10. Lay the glove on the sleeve cuff of the opposite arm, thumb side down, with the glove opening positioned toward the fingers. See Figure 32–33. Position the palm of the nondominant hand upward inside the sleeve.
11. With the nondominant hand, grasp the cuff of the glove through the gown cuff and firmly anchor it.
12. With the dominant hand still inside the sleeve, grasp the upper side of the glove's cuff and stretch it over the cuff of the gown.
13. Pull the sleeve up to draw the cuff over the wrist and extend the fingers of the nondominant hand into the glove's fingers. See Figure 32–34.
14. To don the second glove, place the fingers of the gloved hand under the cuff of the remaining glove. See Figure 32–35.
15. Place the glove over the cuff of the second sleeve.
16. Extend the fingers into the glove as you pull the glove up over the cuff. See Figure 32–36.

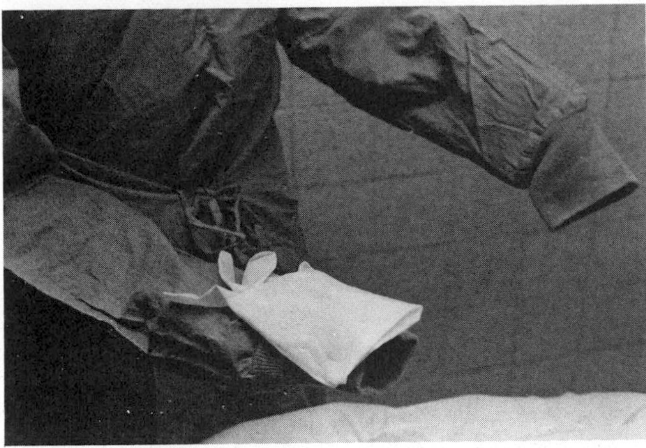

Figure 32–33

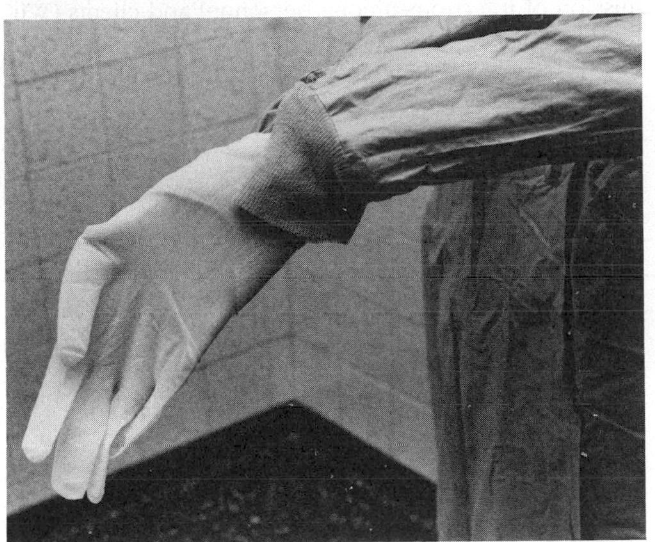

Figure 32–34

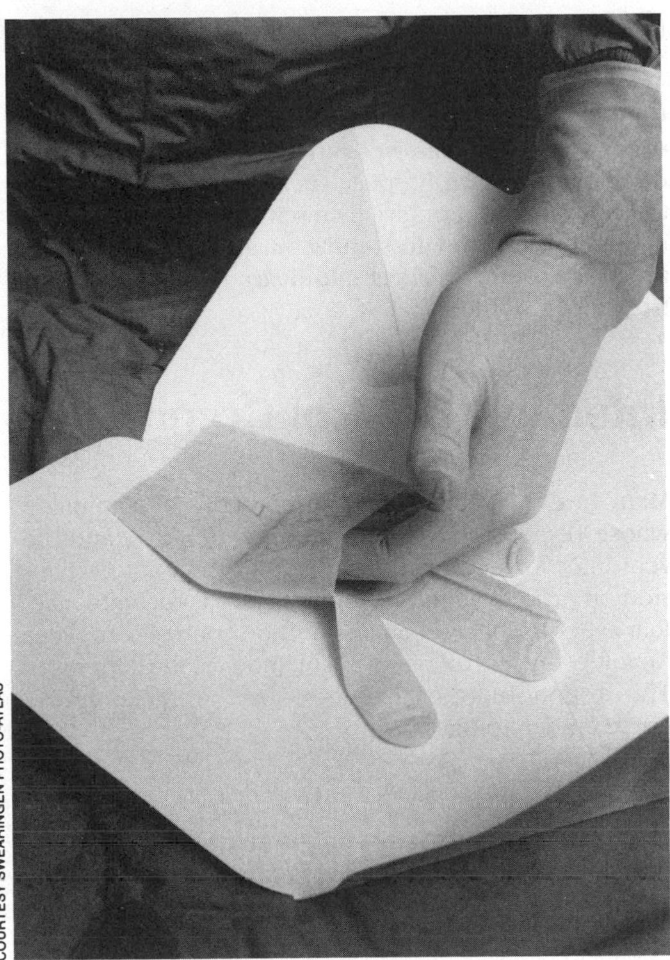

COURTESY SWEARINGEN PHOTO-ATLAS

Figure 32–35

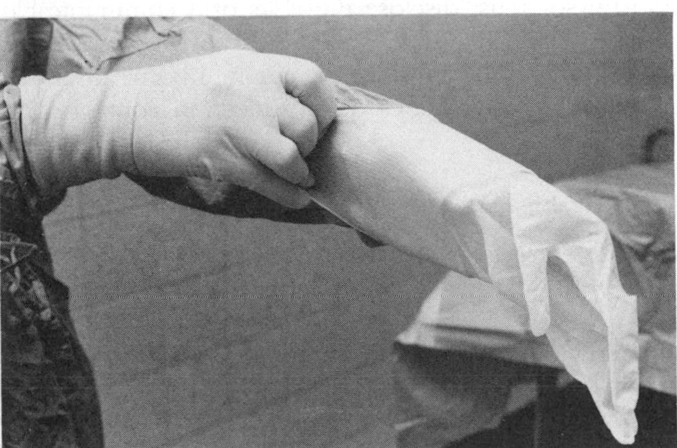

Figure 32–36

Completion of Gowning

17. A coworker who is masked and whose hair is covered holds the waist tie of the gown, using sterile gloves or a sterile wrapper or drape.

    Rationale The tie remains sterile.

18. Make a three-quarter turn, then take the tie and secure it in front of the gown.

    or

    A coworker wearing sterile gloves takes the two ties at each side of the gown and ties them at the back of the gown, making sure that the uniform is completely covered.

    Rationale In both methods, the back of the gown remains sterile.

Client Education

Clients and support persons must often learn aseptic practices to protect themselves and others. For instance, after discharge from the hospital, clients may need to change their own dressing or give themselves injections. A mother needs to learn how to sterilize an infant's formula, and after a colostomy, a client must learn to dispose of feces from a colostomy safely.

Clients and support persons have diverse educational needs in relation to asepsis. Often nurses need to demonstrate specific techniques, and clients need to practice the technique until they can carry out the practices safely.

Infection Control Committees

Many health facilities have infection control committees whose responsibility is to investigate, control, and prevent infections in the facility. In 1958, the Joint Commission on Accreditation of Hospitals (JCAH) recommended that every hospital set up an infection control committee. An infection control nurse is a member of the committee. The responsibility of this nurse, often referred to as a nurse epidemiologist, is to:

1. Promote personnel behaviors that help control infection
2. Provide facts and statistical data regarding epidemiologic investigations
3. Supervise the hospital infection control program

Whether clients must be informed of the possibility of a nosocomial infection before any treatment presents an ethical/legal dilemma. The law states that physicians and nurses must disclose the risks of a communicable disease (Parent 1985, p. 278). However, not everyone agrees that a nosocomial infection is a communicable disease.

The responsibilities of the infection control committee are:

1. To establish a system for reporting infections
2. To keep records of infections
3. To review the hospital's bacteriologic services
4. To review and make recommendations about the hospital's aseptic practices
5. To undertake an educational program for hospital employees

Control of Infections Among Hospital Personnel

In the United States, about 5 million people work in hospitals. Workers who acquire infections from infected clients or from people in the community can pass the infection along to susceptible clients, other hospital personnel, members of their households, or others in the community. The CDC made recommendations to minimize transmission of infections among personnel and clients (Williams 1983).

The recommendations of the CDC are (Williams 1983, pp. 342–343):

1. Appropriate staff placement. Personnel should be evaluated before they are placed in certain hospital areas to minimize the risk of infection to themselves, other personnel, clients, and visitors (Williams 1984, pp. 34–35). For example, a health inventory of workers should elicit any history of measles, tuberculosis and dermatologic conditions.
2. Staff education program on infection control.
3. Immunizations for hospital personnel. The U.S. Public Health Service Immunization Practices Advisory Committee (ACIP) recommends:
   a. Rubella immunization for all personnel who are likely to have contact with pregnant clients or clients who have rubella
   b. Hepatitis B immunizations for personnel likely to have contact with clients who have hepatitis B or for personnel who are particularly susceptible
   c. Measles immunization for all susceptible personnel and all personnel likely to be in contact with clients who have measles
   d. Primary immunization and inactivated poliomyelitis vaccine (IPV) for personnel who have direct contact with clients who may be excreting the poliomyelitis virus
   e. Influenza immunization for all hospital personnel
4. Prompt diagnosis and management of job-related illness. Personnel who have contact with a serious infection that is transmissible or are exposed to such an infection may be excluded from direct contact with clients.
5. Access to health counseling about illnesses that personnel may acquire from or transmit to others. Pregnant personnel should be aware that infection by cyto-

megalovirus, hepatitis B, and rubella poses a threat to the fetus.

6. Coordinated planning between the infection control program, the personnel health service, and various hospital departments.
7. Maintenance of health records for all personnel.

Implicit in these recommendations are the responsibilities of the hospital and the responsibilities of the personnel.

Protecting Self from Infection

Nurses have a responsibility to make the environment of clients, support persons, and health personnel (including themselves) as free as possible of infectious agents. It is known that the incidence of disease after exposure to an infectious agent depends on: (a) the mechanism of transmission and the contagious potential of the infected person, e.g., a client who has pulmonary tuberculosis but does not cough is a minimal threat; (b) the type and duration of the contact; (c) the susceptibility of the host; and (d) the degree to which suggested precautions are taken (Williams 1983, p. 341). In view of these factors, nurses have responsibilities in all four areas for preventing the acquisition of infections. First, nurses can teach clients how to minimize the spread of microorganisms, e.g., by covering the mouth when coughing. Second, nurses can take appropriate precautions when in contact with infectious clients. Third, nurses must employ appropriate aseptic practices while providing nursing care. Fourth, nurses are responsible for implementing measures to prevent, assess, and manage infections. The nurse has responsibilities toward clients, support persons, other nurses and health personnel to teach sound aseptic practices. It is sometimes necessary to remind others about appropriate aseptic practices.

Because they often have prolonged contact with clients, nurses are at particular risk of acquiring infections and transmitting microorganisms to susceptible persons. Nurses need to maintain their own body defenses and good general health. Any break in the nurse's body defenses, e.g., a cut or break in the nurse's skin, must be reported to the responsible nurse. In such a case, the nurse takes appropriate measures to ensure that infectious microorganisms do not enter through the cut, for instance, the nurse may wear gloves or assume duties that do not involve direct client contact. Most health facilities have policies and practices to be followed in these instances.

Function of the Infection Control Nurse (Practitioner)

The function of the infection control nurse varies from agency to agency. The following are common responsibilities:

1. To convey and support positive attitudes toward infection control
2. To report relevant information to the hospital infection control committee, e.g., problems with implementing specific control measures
3. To initiate and present proposals regarding infection control to the committee
4. To carry out an infection control education program for staff
5. To collect data regarding hospital infections among clients and staff
6. To teach clients, support persons, and staff specific protective measures for clients
7. To keep statistics regarding the incidence of infections
8. To coordinate the hospital program with the community program

---

The infection control practitioner has a moral responsibility to inform the infection control committee and hospital administration of all information about infections because of potential corporate liability. The courts state that nurses are responsible for reporting negligence regarding aseptic precautions through appropriate channels. (Parent 1985, p. 279)

Chapter Highlights

- Microorganisms are everywhere. Most are harmless and some are beneficial; however, many can cause infection in susceptible persons.
- Effective control of infectious disease is an international, national, community, and individual responsibility.
- Asepsis is the freedom from infection or infectious material.
- Medical aseptic practices limit the number, growth, and spread of microorganisms.
- Surgical aseptic practices keep an area or objects free of all microorganisms.
- An infection can develop if the six links in the chain of infection—infectious agent, reservoir, portal of exit, mode of transmission, portal of entry, and susceptible host—are not interrupted.
- Aseptic practices can be used to break any of the six links in the chain of infection.

- Humans have both nonspecific and specific defenses that combat infectious agents.
- Intact skin and mucous membranes are the body's first line of defense against microorganisms.
- Some normal body flora release bacteriocins and antibiotic-like substances that inhibit microbial growth and destroy foreign bacteria.
- Some body secretions (e.g., saliva and tears) contain enzymes that act as antibacterial agents.
- The inflammatory response limits physical, chemical, and microbial injury and promotes repair of injured tissue.
- Interferon, the properidin system, and the complement system support the inflammatory process.
- The immune defense responds to specific antigens; it is mediated either by antibodies produced by lymphoid B cells circulating in blood serum or by lymphoid T cells residing in cells of the lymphoid system.
- Both B cells and T cells are memory cells that defend against invasions by the same antigen.
- Immunity is the specific resistance of the body to infectious agents and may be natural or acquired.
- Acquired immunity is active or passive and in either case may be naturally or artificially induced.
- Especially at risk of acquiring an infection are the very young or old; those with poor nutritional status, a deficiency of serum immunoglobulins, multiple stressors, insufficient immunizations, or an existing disease process; and those receiving certain medical therapies.
- The incidence of nosocomial infections is significant. Major sites for these infections are the respiratory and urinary tracts, the bloodstream, and surgical or open wounds.
- Factors that contribute to nosocomial infections are invasive procedures, medical therapies, the existence of a large number of susceptible persons, and insufficient hand washing after client contact and after contact with infected materials.
- Preventing infections in healthy or ill persons and preventing the spread of microorganisms from infected clients to others are major nursing functions.
- The nurse must be knowledgeable about sources and modes of transmission of microorganisms.
- Microorganisms are invisible, and nurses have an ethical obligation to ensure that appropriate aseptic measures are taken to protect clients, support persons, and health personnel, including themselves.

Suggested Readings

Hargiss, C. O., and Larson, E. December 1981. Guidelines for prevention of hospital acquired infections. *American Journal of Nursing* 81:2175–83.

The authors describe many nosocomial infections and methods for reducing the incidence of these infections, surgical wounds, respiratory tract infections, and bacteremia. A table of common skin-cleaning agents is included.

Jones, I. April 1985. You can drive back infection . . . if you know where to make your stand. *Nursing 85* 15:50–52.

Jones discusses the process by which an infection takes hold. Colonization by the microorganism, the barriers to infection, two methods of transmission, and the targets of infection are explained. Included is a chart indicating the normal flora of each system, common signs and symptoms of an infection of each system, laboratory data, and special nursing considerations.

Stark, J. L., and Hunt, V. January 1985. Don't let nosocomial infections get your patients down. *Nursing 85* 15:10–11.

The authors describe some of the measures nurses can take to prevent nosocomial infections in intensive care clients whose normal defenses are severely compromised. The information appears to be appropriate for clients in general care units and includes the four main types of infection, causes, signs and symptoms, preventive measures, and nursing management.

Selected References

American Hospital Association. 1979. *Infection control in hospitals*. 4th ed. Chicago: American Hospital Association.

Aspinall, M. J. October 1978. Scoring against nosocomial infections. *American Journal of Nursing* 78:1704–7.

Axnick, K. J., and Yarbrough, M., editors. 1984. *Infection control: An integrated approach*. St. Louis: C. V. Mosby Co.

Benenson, A. S., editor. 1985. *Control of communicable diseases in man*. 14th ed. An official report of the American Public Health Association. Washington, D.C.: The American Public Health Association.

Berger, S. A., editor: 1982. *Clinical manual of infectious diseases*. Menlo Park, Calif.: Addison-Wesley Publishing Co.

Brandt, S. L., and Benner, P. March 1980. Infection control in hospitals: What are the challenges? *American Journal of Nursing* 80:432–34.

Brem, A. M., and Torok, E. M. December 1979. Nosocomial infections in the elderly. *Hospital Topics* 57:10, 40–43.

Byrne, J. C.; Saxton, D. F.; Pelikan, P. K.; and Nugent, P. M. 1986. *Laboratory tests: Implications for nursing care*. Menlo Park, Calif.: Addison-Wesley Publishing Co.

Centers for Disease Control. 1980. "Antiseptics, handwashing and handwashing facilities." In *Guidelines for the prevention and control of nosocomial infections*. Atlanta: Centers for Disease Control.

Freeman, J.; Rosner, B. A.; and McGowan Jr., J. E. Adverse effects of nosocomial infection. *The Journal of Infectious Diseases* 140:732–40.

Garner, J. S., and Favero, M. S. 1985. *Guideline for handwashing and hospital environmental control 1985*. U.S. Government Printing Office.

Garner, J. S., and Simmons, B. P. July/August 1983. CDC guidelines for isolation precautions in hospitals. *Infection Control* 4:245–325. Special Supplements.

Hargiss, C. O., and Larson, E. December 1981. Infection control: How to collect specimens and evaluate results. *American Journal of Nursing* 81:2166–74.

Jackson, M. M., and Lynch, P. February 1984. Infection control: Too much or too little? *American Journal of Nursing* 84:208–10.

Jones, I. April 1985. You can drive back infection . . . if you know where to make your stand. *Nursing 85* 15:50–52.

Kneedler, J. A., and Dodge, G. H. 1983. *Perioperative patient care: The nursing perspective.* Boston: Blackwell Scientific Publications.

Kolff, C. A., and Sanchez, R. 1979. *Handbook for infectious disease management.* Menlo Park, Calif.: Addison-Wesley Publishing Co.

Larson, E. March/April 1982: Persistent carriage of gram negative bacteria on the hands. *Nursing Research* 31:121–22.

LeMaitre, G. D., and Finnegan, J. A. 1980. *The patient in surgery: A guide for nurses.* 4th ed. Philadelphia: W. B. Saunders Co.

Losos, J., and Trotman, M. May/June 1984. Estimated economic burden of nosocomial infection. *Canadian Journal of Public Health* 75:248–50.

Mallison, G. F., and Standard, P. G. 1974. Safe storage times for sterile packs. *Hospitals* 48(20):77–78, 80.

Meers, P. D. March 10, 1982. Infection in hospitals. *Nursing Times* 16:146.

Moree, N. A., and Garner, J. S. (consultant). February 1984. New infection control guidelines. *American Journal of Nursing* 84:210–11.

Nadolny, M. D. March 1980. What does the infection control nurse do? *American Journal of Nursing* 80:430–1.

Norton, C. F. 1981. *Microbiology.* Reading, Mass.: Addison-Wesley Publishing Co.

Palmer, M. B. 1984. *Infection control: A policy and procedure manual.* Philadelphia: W. B. Saunders Co.

Parent, B. December 1985. Moral, ethical, and legal aspects of infection control. *American Journal of Infection Control* 13:278–80.

Pickering, L. K., and DuPont, H. L. 1986. *Infectious diseases of children and adults: A step-by-step approach to diagnosis and treatment.* Menlo Park, Calif.: Addison-Wesley Publishing Co.

Reinarz, J. A. 1978. Nosocomial infections. *Clinical Symposia* 30(6):2–32.

Ryan, P. May 1976. Inhospital packaging rationale. *AORN Journal* 23:980–88.

Setia, U.; Serventi, I.; and Lorenzo, P. April 1985. Nosocomial infection among patients in a long-term care facility: Spectrum, prevalence, and risk factors. *American Journal of Infection Control* 13:57–62.

Simmons, B. P. August 1983. CDC guidelines for the prevention and control of nosocomial infections. Guidelines for prevention of surgical wound infections. *American Journal of Infection Control* 11:133–41.

Spradley, B. W. 1981. *Community health nursing.* Boston: Little, Brown and Co.

Stark, J. L., and Hunt, V. January 1985. Don't let nosocomial infections get your patients down. *Nursing 85* 15:10–11.

Taylor, L. J. J. January 19, 1978. An evaluation of handwashing techniques—2. *Nursing Times* 74:108–110.

Weissman, I. L.; Hood, L. E.; and Wood, W. B. 1978. *Essential concepts in immunology.* Menlo Park, Calif.: Benjamin/Cummings Publishing Co.

Whaley, L. F., and Wong, D. L. 1983. *Nursing care of infants and children.* 2d ed. St. Louis: The C.V. Mosby Co.

William, A. R. October 1985. Cost-effective application of the Centers for Disease Control guideline for handwashing and hospital environmental control. *American Journal of Infection Control.* 13:218–23.

Williams, P., and Bierer, B. March/April 1984. Wash your hands! *Geriatric Nursing* 5:103–4.

Williams, W. W. July/August 1983. CDC guideline for infection control in hospital personnel. *Infection Control* 4:326–49.

———. February 1984. CDC guidelines for the prevention and control of nosocomial infections: Guideline for infection control in hospital personnel. *American Journal of Infection Control* 12:34–57.

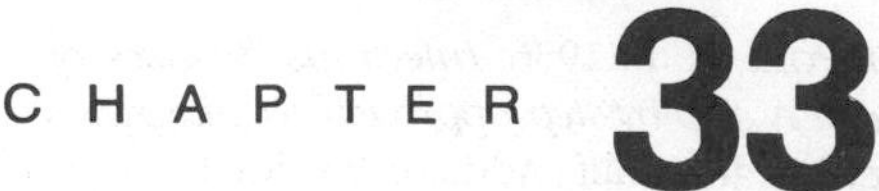

CHAPTER 33

Reducing Environmental Hazards

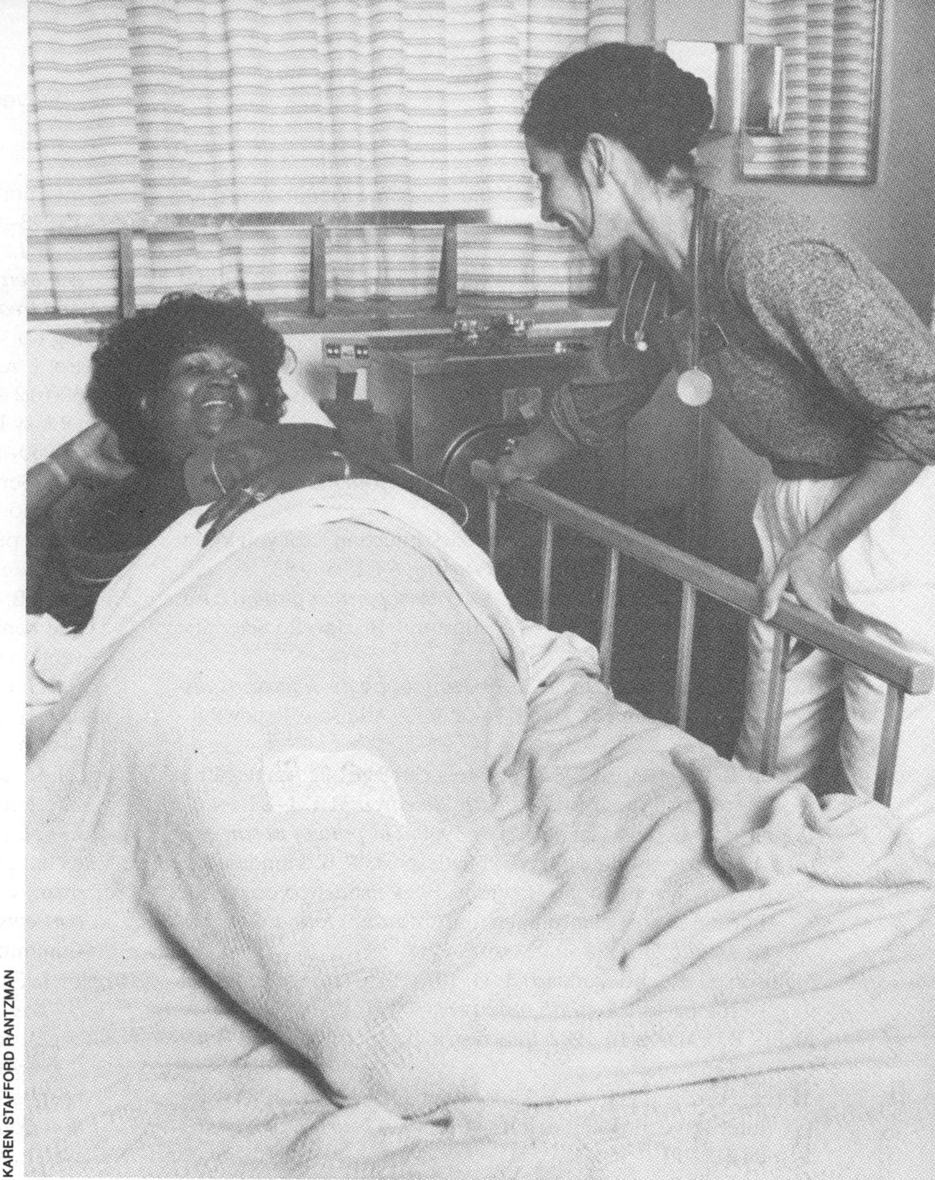

KAREN STAFFORD RANTZMAN

Contents

Objectives

1. Understand health protection strategies to prevent accidents.
   - 1.1 Identify major causes of accidental death.
   - 1.2 Identify clients at risk of physical injury.
   - 1.3 Give example of nursing diagnoses for clients at risk of accidental injury.
   - 1.4 Identify four classes of fires.
   - 1.5 Identify types of fire extinguishers appropriate for class A, B, C, and D fires.
   - 1.6 Describe practices to prevent fires.
   - 1.7 Identify essential steps to take in the event of a fire.
   - 1.8 Describe six carries used to evacuate clients in the event of a fire.
   - 1.9 Identify essential precautions to prevent falls of hospitalized clients.
   - 1.10 Identify legal implications of restraints.
   - 1.11 Identify situations in which restraints are warranted.
   - 1.12 Identify various types of restraints.
   - 1.13 Outline guidelines for selecting and applying restraints.
   - 1.14 Outline essential precautions to prevent suffocation.
   - 1.15 Outline essential precautions to prevent poisoning in children.
   - 1.16 Describe essential steps to take in the event of poisoning.
   - 1.17 Identify measures to reduce electrical hazards.
   - 1.18 Identify measures to minimize noise.
   - 1.19 Identify precautions to prevent exposure to radiation.
   - 1.20 Identify essential safety precautions for each developmental stage.
2. Understand health protection strategies implemented to prevent infectious disease.
   - 2.1 Identify immunization requirements for clients of various ages.
   - 2.2 Describe selected tests for immunity.
   - 2.3 Describe immunization and testing procedures that may be administered to hospital personnel.
   - 2.4 Describe seven environmental sanitation and control measures.

Terms

asphyxiation
burn
communicable disease
dynamic electricity
electron
epidemic
epidemiology
grounding
immunization
induration
orthostatic hypotension
pandemic
poison
restraint
scald
static electricity
suffocation
toxoid
vaccine
vector

Health Protection Strategies

Health protection strategies are designed to protect both individuals and the general population. These strategies prevent dental disease, infectious diseases, and injury as a result of accidents. Common accidents include falls, poisoning, suffocation, burns, and electric shock. Other health protection strategies include water supply protection—through chlorination, pollution control, and control of animals that carry diseases—and public health policies such as food sanitation and pasteurization of milk.

Education is a major factor in preventing accidents and infectious disease. It is directed toward helping people identify environmental hazards and changing their health practices and habits.

The environment contains many hazards, both seen and unseen. The automobile, which may run down a pedestrian, is an obvious hazard. Microorganisms and radiation are unseen hazards.

The need for a safe environment is a national, community, and individual concern. Nurses are voicing their thoughts individually and collectively about such issues as air and water pollution and the safety of foods, cosmetics, and medications. The need for safety on the highways is underscored by newspaper reports of morbidity and mortality from automobile accidents. Increasingly, governments are being pressed to take action and legislate in these areas to make the environment safer. In addition, people are also becoming aware of safety hazards in their communities. Regulations to control the speed of boats on lakes used for swimming, local ordinances curbing the burning of refuse, and stricter local regulation of industrial pollution are all indications of increasing awareness of the need for safety in the environment.

Traditionally, nurses have thought of safety in relation to a client's immediate environment, and this awareness is no less important today in spite of the broader focus on human protection. A primary concern of nurses is awareness of what constitutes a safe environment for a particular person and how this environment can be achieved. The blind person may need railings; the crawling baby, a protective gate at the head of the stairs; and the elderly person, secure footing and an uncluttered floor. Nurses thus focus attention on preventing accidents and injury as well as on assisting the injured.

Preventing Accidents

In 1982, accidents were the third leading cause of death among the total deaths from all causes (94,082) in the United States (*Accident Facts* 1985, p. 7). Accidents are, however, the leading cause of death of infants, children, adolescents, and young adults. Major causes of accidental death among children and adults are listed in order of prevalence in Table 33–1.

Assessing Potential for Injury

The ability of people to protect themselves from injury is affected by a number of factors. Nurses need to assess each of these factors when they plan care or teach clients to protect themselves.

Age

Age is an important factor affecting people's ability to protect themselves. Through knowledge and accurate assessment of the environment, people learn to protect themselves from many injuries. Children walking to school learn to stop before crossing the street and wait for oncoming traffic. They also learn not to touch a hot stove. For the very young, learning about the environment is essential. Only through knowledge and experience do children learn what is potentially harmful.

Parents normally attach a great deal of importance to teaching children what is potentially dangerous and at the same time childproofing the home environment. Safety precautions adequate for an older child or an adult are not adequate for a young child. For example, the young child who cannot read is likely to mistake lye or medications for candy. Accordingly, it is most important to place these hazards out of reach of the young child.

Elderly people also can have special problems protecting themselves from injury. Often the balance of elderly people is impaired by their flexed posture, which places their center of gravity forward. Once balance is lost, it is not readily regained. An elderly person may need to learn to stand up slowly, thus avoiding the fall that can result from a quick, sudden movement. Slowness of movement and diminished sensual acuity also contribute to the likelihood of injury. Elderly persons may neither see nor hear an oncoming car. They may not see a footstool. They may also be unable to pull themselves out of a bathtub safely.

Life-Style

Life-style is a significant factor affecting safety. Fifty percent of deaths are due to unhealthy behavior or life-style. See Chapter 2. Factors that place people at risk are: unsafe work environments, where workers are in danger from machinery, industrial belts and pulleys, and chemicals; residence in neighborhoods with high crime rates; access to guns and ammunition; insufficient income to buy safety equipment or make necessary repairs; and access to illicit drugs, which may also be contaminated by harmful additives. Risk-taking behavior is a factor in accidents. For example, some people disregard safety recommendations by driving automobiles at high speeds and refusing to wear seat belts in automobiles, headgear on motorcycles, or flotation jackets in boats.

Sensory Perception

Accurate preception of environmental stimuli is vital to safety. These stimuli, which are received by sensory receptors of the body, travel through the nerves to the central nervous system. In a reflex action, such as jerking the hand away from a hot object, some of the impulses travel directly to motor neurons, which then convey the impulses to the muscles that cause the sudden, quick withdrawing of the hand. At the same time, other sensory impulses travel to the cerebral cortex; and the person, now aware of the stimulus, initiates further impulses that result in voluntary muscle movement. Impairment of any

Table 33–1 Major Causes of Accidental Death, United States, 1982

Type	Number
Motor vehicle	45779
Falls	12077
Drowning	6351
Fire and flames	5210
Poisoning (by solids and liquids)	3474
Suffocation (by ingested objects)	3254
Firearms	1756

Source: From *Accident Facts*, 1985 edition (Chicago, Illinois: National Safety Council), p. 12. Used by permission.

of these areas—the sensory receptors, sensory pathways, the internuncial neurons that transmit the impulse from the sensory pathways to the motor pathways, the motor pathways, or the cerebral cortex—can diminish ability to respond normally to environmental stimuli.

People with impaired touch perception, hearing, taste, smell, and vision are highly susceptible to injury. A person who does not see well may trip over a toy or not see a signal cord at a hospital bed unit. Deaf persons do not hear a siren in traffic, and persons with impaired olfactory sense may not smell burning food or escaping gas. Paralysis and other neurologic impairments diminish touch perceptions. A paralyzed person may not feel a burn from a burning hot-water bottle, and a person whose sense of taste is impaired may not detect contaminated food.

Awareness

Clients with impaired awareness include:

1. Persons lacking in sleep. A fatigued driver may fail to see a sign on the side of the highway, or a tired parent may forget to place cleaning solution out of the reach of a toddler.
2. Unconscious or semiconscious persons. There are varying levels of consciousness, that is, levels of lack of response to environmental stimuli. One unconscious client, for example, may respond to painful stimuli, whereas another may not. See Table 35–29 on page 897.
3. Disoriented persons, who may not understand where they are or what to do to help themselves.
4. Persons who perceive stimuli that do not exist. For example, during alcohol withdrawal, a person may believe worms are crawling on the bed.
5. Persons whose judgment is altered by medications, such as narcotics, tranquilizers, hypnotics, and sedatives.

Mobility

Persons who have paralysis, muscle weakness, and poor balance or coordination are obviously prone to injury. Clients with spinal cord injury and paralysis of both legs may be unable to move even when they perceive discomfort. Hemiplegic clients or clients with leg casts often have poor balance and fall easily. Clients weakened by illness or surgery are not always fully aware of their condition. It is not uncommon for clients to believe themselves able to walk and fall while trying. Nurses need to consider mobility when assessing a client's potential for injury. Mobility increases the possibility of injury. For example, a slippery floor does not threaten the bedridden client's safety as it does the ambulatory client's.

Emotional State

Extreme emotional states can alter ability to perceive environmental hazards. The acutely anxious or angry person has reduced perceptual awareness. Depressed persons may think and react to environmental stimuli more slowly than usual. People worried about their own or loved ones' illnesses are less aware than usual of potential dangers in the environment, such as a street curb or an oncoming automobile.

Ability to Communicate

Obviously, people with diminished ability to receive and convey information are at risk. Aphasic clients, people with language barriers, and those unable to read are among them. For example, the person unable to interpret the sign "No smoking–oxygen in use" may cause a fire.

Previous Accidents

It has been recognized for some time that some people are accident prone. These people have accidents more frequently than the average person. Some children cut themselves and fracture bones more often than their peers. Some adults drive a car for 15 years without an accident, while others have at least one accident each year.

Predisposition to accidents is thought to have an emotional basis. One theory is that emotional tension impairs a person's perceptions and judgments, thus making that person more likely to have an accident. Some propose that accidents may fulfill masochistic and hostile needs or fulfill desires to be cared for by others.

Safety Knowledge

Information is crucial to safety. Clients in hospitals and other unfamiliar environments frequently need specific safety information. Unfamiliar equipment, such as oxygen tanks, intravenous tubing, and hot packs, is a potential hazard. Nurses need to teach clients what safety precautions to take when oxygen is in use and how to maintain intravenous infusions. See Chapters 45 and 46. Knowledge and use of safety precautions are essential in daily living. Specific precautions for various age levels are listed later in this chapter.

Nursing Diagnosis

Accepted nursing diagnoses for clients at risk of accidental injury are (Kim et al. 1984, pp. 30–36):

1. Potential for trauma (physical injury)
2. Potential for poisoning
3. Potential for suffocation

Many factors—some internal (individual) and some external (environmental)—contribute to these potentials. Examples of nursing diagnoses are shown on page 732. Nurses, however, formulate diagnoses from the assessment data obtained for each client. After deriving pertinent causative factors from the data base, nurses individualize interventions for the client.

Planning

The nurse planning health protective measures must consider the age, knowledge, and sensory deficits of the client. The nursing care plan should include two aspects: educating clients about preventive actions and modifying the environment to make it safe. The latter can involve not only arranging the environment but also limiting the environment in some ways.

The overall client goal is to prevent injury and illness by helping the client to identify hazards and to take related safety measures. Outcome criteria are discussed later in this chapter. See the section on evaluation.

Interventions for Specific Hazards

Fire

Fire is a constant danger in homes and hospitals. Common causes of home fires are smoking in bed, failure to extinguish cigarette butts before placing them in waste containers, accumulated grease on stoves, and faulty electrical equipment. Common causes of hospital fires are smoking in bed and faulty electrical equipment. Hospital fires are particularly hazardous to clients who are incapacitated and unable to leave the building without assistance.

Kinds of Fires

Fires are categorized into four classes depending on the type of material that is burning:

1. Class A fires are those involving paper, wood, cloth (e.g., drapes and upholstery), and similar solid combustible materials (e.g., rubbish).
2. Class B fires involve flammable liquids and gases, such as fuel oil, gasoline, paint, tar, grease in a frying pan, solvents, and, in hospitals, anesthetic agents.
3. Class C fires involve electrical equipment, such as wiring, fuse boxes, switchboards, conductors, motors, and other electrical sources.
4. Class D fires involve combustible metals such as certain chips, shavings.

A fire can burn only if three elements are present: sufficient heat to start the fire, a combustible material, and sufficient oxygen to support the fire.

Types of Fire Extinguishers

Several types of fire extinguishers are in use today. The right type of extinguisher must be used to fight a fire. It is dangerous to use a water extinguisher, for example, on grease or electrical fires. See Table 33–2 for various types of extinguishers and indications for their use. It is now common for fire extinguishers to be labeled with picture symbols showing on which fires they should and should not be used. Directions for use are also attached to the extinguisher.

Table 33–2 Types of Extinguishers: Indications and Procedures for Use

Type of Extinguisher	Class and Kind of Fire	Procedure	Comments
Water: a) Stored pressure type b) Gas cartridge type c) pump type d) Soda acid type	Class A: paper, wood, draperies, upholstery, and ordinary rubbish	Stored Pressure Type: Pull locking pin, then squeeze handle. Gas Cartridge Type: Pull locking pin, then squeeze handle (or) turn unit upside down. Pump Type: Release lock latch if present, then pump plunger rapidly. Soda Acid Type: Turn unit upside down to mix chemicals. (Do *not* invert extinguisher until *ready* to use.) - Direct water stream at the base of the fire, not at the smoke. - Use side-to-side sweeping motions to wet all surfaces.	- Water soaks and cools the burning material below its ignition temperature. - Do not use on electrical or flammable liquid fires (e.g., grease); water conducts electricity and causes grease to splatter, thus spreading the fire. - For home use this type of extinguisher could be placed in a living room, den, or office.
Carbon dioxide (CO_2)	Classes B and C: flammable liquids and gases and electrical fires	Self-Expellant Type: Pull locking pin, then squeeze the operating handle. Avoid touching the discharge horn since it gets very cold and may accumulate static electricity. - For *flammable liquid fires* get close to the fire, point the nozzle at the near edge, and slowly sweep the nozzle side to side. - When the fire is out, continue the extinguisher discharge to prevent reflash of flames. - For *electrical fires* first shut off power to remove possible fire source.	- Carbon dioxide smothers flames and cuts off the oxygen supply to the fire. - Because it has a limited range, the extinguisher must be used close to the flames. - For home use this type of extinguisher should be placed in the kitchen.
Regular dry chemical: a) Stored pressure type b) Gas cartridge type	Classes B and C: flammable liquid and gases and electrical fires	Stored Pressure Type: Pull locking pin, then squeeze handle. Gas Cartridge Type: Pull locking pin and press cartridge puncture lever. Then squeeze operating handle. - Stand relatively far away and direct the discharge of dry chemical accross the entire fire front. - Move toward the fire and use quick side-to-side motions. - When the fire is out, continue the extinguisher discharge to prevent reflash of flames - For an *electrical fire,* shut off the power as soon as possible to remove potential fire source.	- Regular dry chemical extinguishers interrupt and smother the flames. - Starting far enough away avoids splashing and allows the discharge stream to flare out. - For home use, see comment about CO_2 extinguisher.
Multipurpose dry chemical: a) Stored pressure type b) Gas cartridge type	Classes A, B and C: paper, wood, cloth, flammable liquids, and electrical equipment	- As above for regular dry chemical. - Use the same as the regular dry chemical extinguishers on class B and class C fires. - On class A fires, coat all exposed surfaces and wet thoroughly to prevent rekindling.	- Multiple-purpose dry chemicals interrupt and smother the flames, cutting off the oxygen supply. - These extinguishers are good anywhere in the home since they put out most types of fires.
Foam	Class B: flammable liquid fires only	- Operate like the soda-acid water extinguisher. Turn the unit upside down to operate. (Do *not* invert unit until *ready* to use.)	- Foam smothers and cools the fire. - For home use this type of extinguisher could be placed in a garage or basement.

(continued)

Table 33–2 *(continued)*

Type of Extinguisher	Class and Kind of Fire	Procedure	Comments
		- To avoid splashing, curve the stream upward so foam falls lightly, *or* direct the foam at the floor to spread it. - For *fires in containers,* direct the stream at the back wall so that the foam flows forward.	
Special dry powder extinguishants	Class D: metal	Used for designated metals. May be applied by scoop, shovel, or extinguisher.	Special dry powder extinguishants absorb heat.
Loaded stream	Classes A and B	Follow instructions on device.	Uses a water-chemical mixture.
Liquefied gas	Classes B and C	Follow instructions on device.	Chemical turns to gas when discharged.

Protective Practices

Most health care agencies establish procedures to be followed in an emergency or during a fire. Nurses need to become familiar with the practices of their employing agency. General protective practices include:

1. Making sure the telephone numbers of emergency services are displayed on all telephones
2. Knowing the location of fire exits
3. Knowing the location and types of fire extinguishers and learning to operate them
4. Learning the agency's fire drill or fire evacuation procedure
5. Keeping access to firehoses clear at all times
6. Keeping hallways free of unnecessary furniture and equipment
7. Posting signs on elevator doors so that people will know to use the stairs in the event of fire
8. Making sure the location of fire exits is clearly marked

When a fire occurs, the nurse has two major goals:

1. To protect clients from injury
2. To contain and put out the fire

See page 733 for the steps the nurse should follow when she or he notices a fire. Nurses should carry out these steps regardless of how small the fire is initially. A small fire in a wastebasket can quickly become a larger fire. Before evacuating clients with chest tubes, the nurse needs to clamp and cut the tubes. Clients on respirators need to be manually resuscitated with Ambu bags (see Chapter 45).

Evacuating clients

There are six methods of carrying persons from the scene of a fire. Generally, nurses use these carries for clients when they cannot wheel out bedridden clients in their beds or transfer them out on stretchers.

Examples of Nursing Diagnoses Related to Potential for Injury

- Potential for falling related to impaired balance associated with decreased gross muscle coordination
- Potential for burns related to decreased temperature and tactile sensation associated with paralysis
- Potential for electric shock related to inability to pay for repair of faulty wiring
- Potential for trauma related to failure to use headgear when cycling
- Potential for burns related to smoking in bed
- Potential for injury related to exposure to dangerous machines
- Potential for overdose of prescribed medications related to disorientation and failing memory
- Potential for child poisoning related to improper storage of medicines and other household toxic substances
- Potential for poisoning related to lack of knowledge of poisonous vegetation
- Potential for child suffocation related to lack of water safety precautions
- Potential for suffocation related to nonvented, fuel-burning heaters
- Potential for injury related to lack of awareness of environmental hazards

Steps to Follow in the Event of Fire

1. Evacuate clients who are in immediate danger. First direct ambulatory clients to a safe area or enlist their help in moving clients in wheelchairs. This clears the area for the evacuation of nonambulatory clients, who can be moved in a stretcher or bed, carried, or dragged on sheets and blankets.
2. Activate the fire alarm if one is nearby.
3. Notify the hospital switchboard of the location of the fire.
4. If the fire is small, use the fire extinguisher on the fire.
5. Close windows and doors in the area of the fire to reduce ventilation.
6. Turn off oxygen and any electrical appliances in the vicinity of the fire.
7. Clear fire exits, if necessary.
8. Contain smoke as necessary by placing damp cloths or blankets around the outside edges of doors.
9. Protect clients from smoke inhalation by giving them wet washcloths through which to breathe.

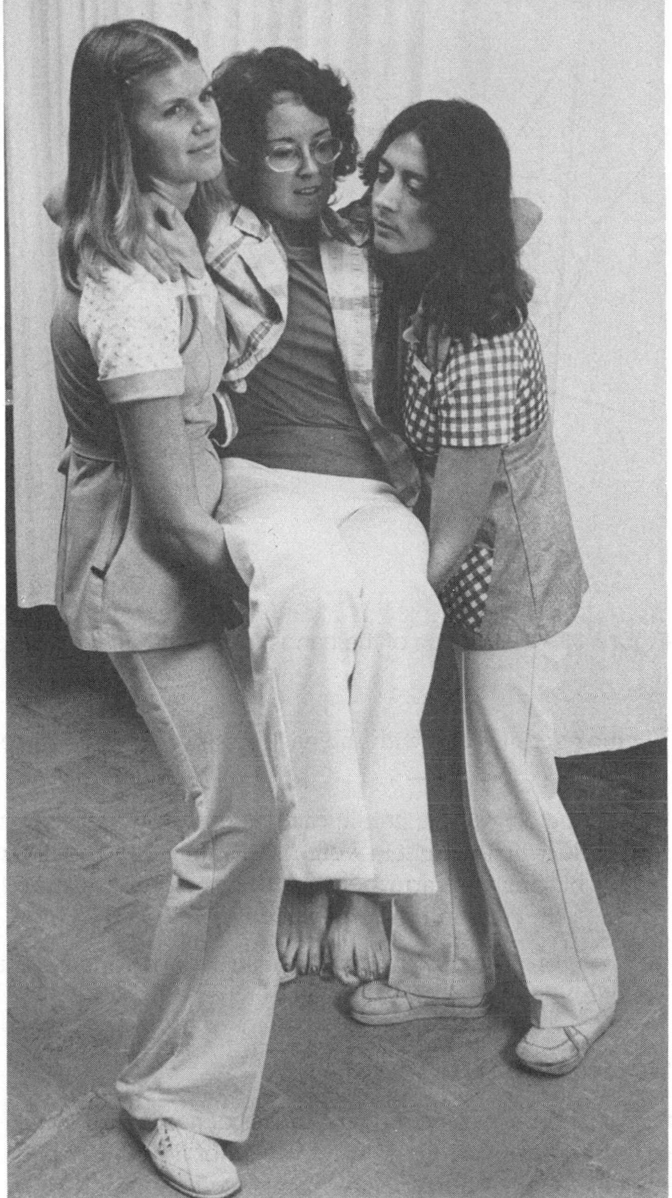

Figure 33–1 The swing carry

1. *Swing carry.* The swing is a two-person carry used for heavy clients. The client, in a sitting position, places the arms around each nurse's shoulders. Each nurse holds the client's wrists, which are over each nurse's shoulders, to support the client. Each nurse then reaches behind the client and grasps the other nurse's shoulder or upper arm. The nurses then release the client's wrists, reach under the client's thighs, and grasp each other's wrists. They lift and carry the client in this sitting position. See Figure 33–1. This carry is sometimes referred to as the two-handed seat, in which a hand-forearm interlock is used. A variation is the four-handed seat, used for clients who are able to sit up with less support. See Figure 33–2.
2. *Pack strap carry.* The pack strap is a one-person carry. The nurse faces the seated client and grasps the wrists. The nurse's right hand grasps the client's left wrist; the left hand grasps the client's right wrist. The nurse then pivots and slips under one of the client's arms so that the nurse's back is to the client and the client's arms are crossed in front of the nurse. The nurse assumes a broad stance, one leg in front of the other, and rolls the client onto her or his back. See Figure 33–3.
3. *Hip carry.* The client lies laterally at the side of the bed facing the nurse. The nurse faces the head of the bed. The nurse places the arm nearest the client over the client's back and under the lower axilla. The nurse then turns away from the client and places the second arm around and under the thighs. Assuming a broad stance for balance, the nurse then draws the client onto the nurse's hips so that the client's abdomen is over the nurse's hips. See Figure 33–4.
4. *Piggy-back carry.* This carry is used for clients who are conscious and have some strength to help. The client sits at the edge of the bed. The nurse stands in front of the client with her or his back toward the client. The client reaches over the nurse's shoulders and clasps his or her hands in front of the nurse while the nurse grasps the backs of the client's legs above the knees. With this carry, the nurse can support the client's weight

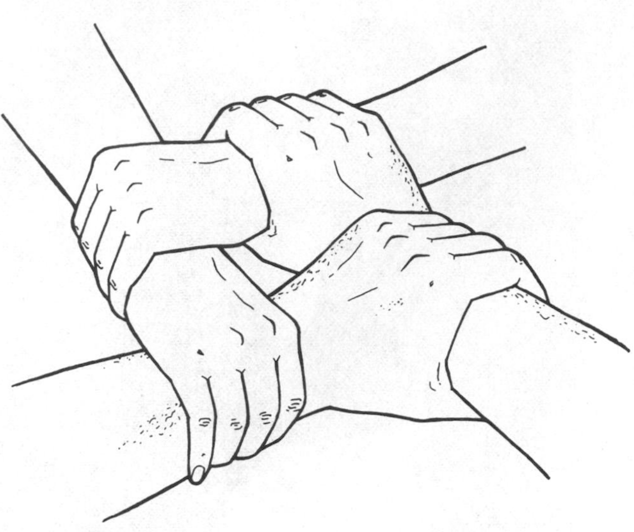

Figure 33–2 Position of the hands for a four-handed seat

more easily than with the pack strap carry. See Figure 33–5.

5. *Cradle carry.* The cradle carry is used for children or adults who are light in weight. The nurse lifts the client by placing one arm beneath the person's knees and the other around the back. See Figure 33–6.
6. *Three-person carry.* See the instructions for lifting a client between a bed and a stretcher, Chapter 39.

Scalds and Burns

Scalds and burns are frequent causes of accidental injury in the home. A **scald** is a burn from a hot liquid or vapor, such as steam. A **burn** results from excessive exposure to thermal, chemical, electrical, or radioactive agents.

Common hazards causing scalds are:

1. Pot handles that protrude over the edge of a stove
2. Electrical appliances used to heat liquids or oils, especially those that have dangling cords within reach of crawling infants and young children
3. Excessively hot bath water
4. Excessively hot coffee or other beverages that are accidentally spilled

Burns are usually caused by:

1. Improper use of matches
2. Cigarettes

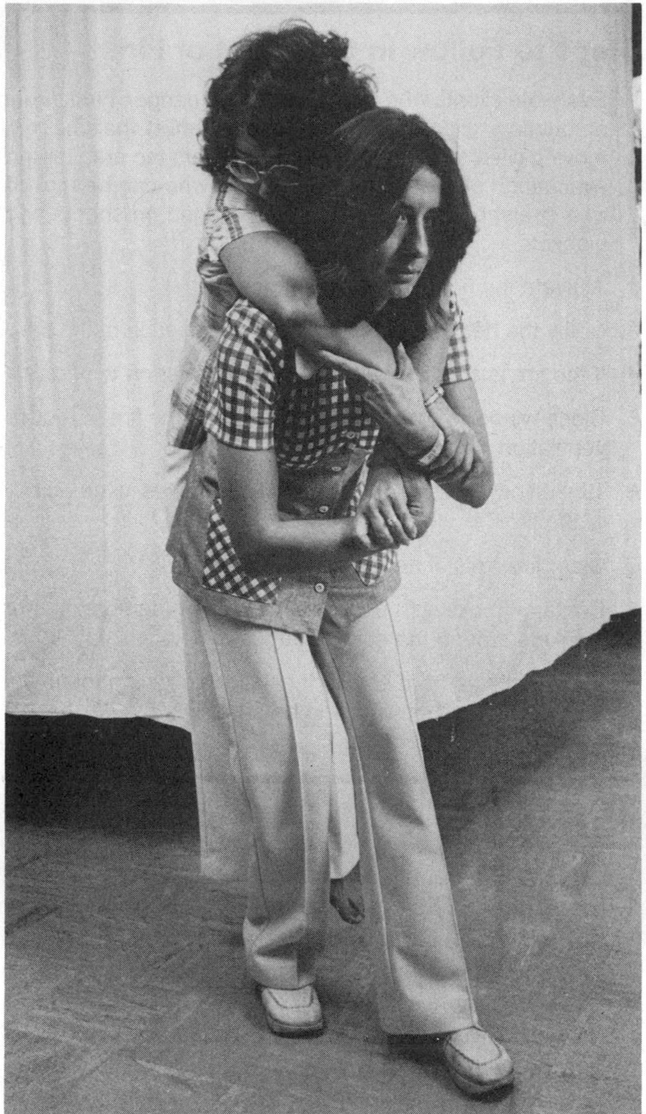

Figure 33–3 The pack strap carry

3. Improper use of gasoline or lighter fluid in barbecue grills
4. Uncontrolled fires in fireplaces
5. Faulty electrical wiring
6. Excessively hot heating pads

In health care agencies, the risk of scalds and burns is greater for clients with impaired skin sensitivity to temperature. Scalds can occur from overly hot bath water or from overly hot moist dressings. Heat lamps can cause burns. (The therapeutic application of heat is discussed in Chapter 52.) It is important for the nurse to assess how well clients can protect themselves and what special precautions, if any, need to be taken.

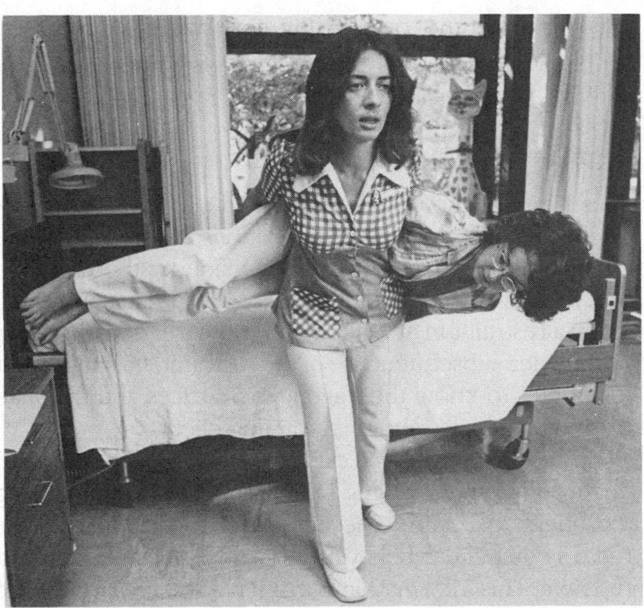

Figure 33–4 The hip carry

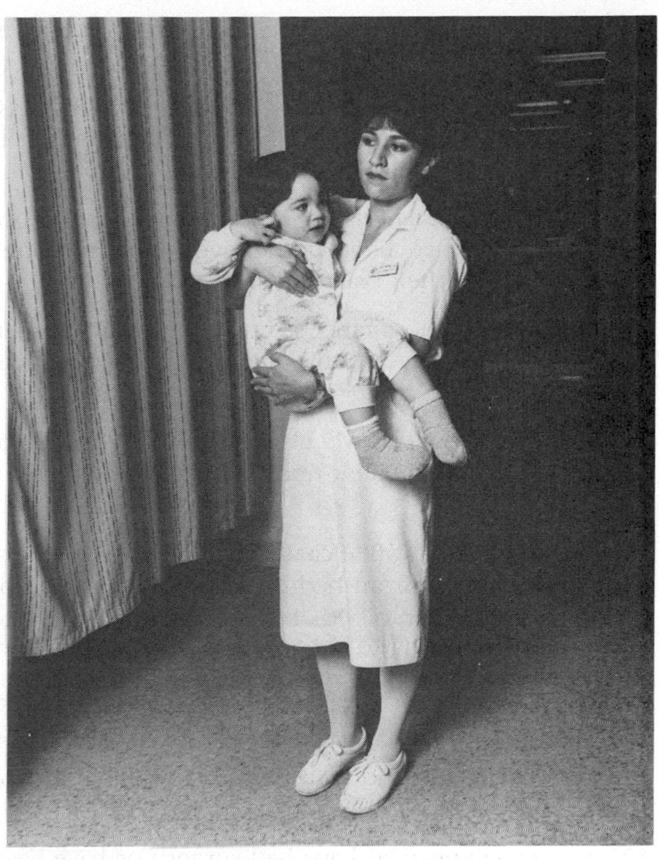

Figure 33–6 The cradle carry

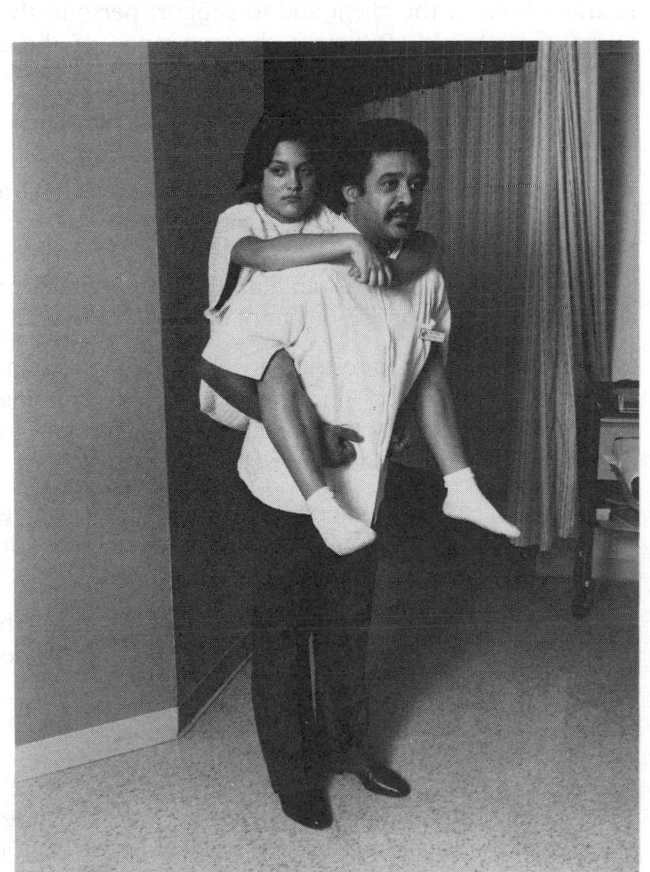

Figure 33–5 The piggy-back carry

Falls

Falls are common not only among the very young and the elderly but also among the ill or injured, who are weakened and frequently lose their balance. Seventy-five percent of all fatal falls in the United States involve people 65 or older (Louis 1983, p. 142). Actions to prevent falls of infants and young children are shown in Tables 33–3 and 33–4, pages 746 and 747. Actions to prevent falls among the elderly are shown on page 750. This section deals with interventions to prevent falls and self-inflicted injury of hospitalized clients.

To prevent falls of hospitalized clients, the nurse:

1. Orients clients on admission to their surroundings and explains the call system.
2. Carefully assesses the client's ability to ambulate and transfer. The nurse provides walking aids and assistance as required. See Chapter 39.
3. Closely supervises the client during the first few days, especially at night. Unfamiliar surroundings can confuse clients, especially older clients, and contribute to accidents.

4. Encourages the client to use night lights and request assistance.
5. Makes sure that the client's call bell is within easy reach and that ambulatory clients are informed about call bells installed in bathrooms.
6. Places bedside tables and overbed tables near the bed or chair so that clients do not overreach and consequently lose their balance.
7. Always keeps hospital beds in the low position when not providing care so that clients can move in or out of bed easily.
8. Makes sure the bed wheels are locked. Movement of the bed when a client transfers is a major cause of falls.
9. Makes sure that wheelchairs are locked when transferring a client from bed or toilet to wheelchair or from wheelchair to bed or toilet. The nurse needs to teach the client how to lock and unlock wheels.
10. Encourages clients to use grab bars mounted in toilet and bathing areas and railings along corridors.
11. Makes sure nonskid bath mats are available in tubs and showers.
12. Advises clients who have had surgery or have been in bed for some time to accept assistance when first getting out of bed.
13. Encourages the client to wear nonskid footwear.
14. Keeps the environment tidy, especially keeping light cords from underfoot and furniture out of the way.
15. Attaches side rails to the bed of confused, sedated, restless, and unconscious clients and keeps the rails in place when the client is unattended. Side rails are discussed in Chapter 36.

Use of Restraints

Restraints are protective devices used to limit the physical activity of the client or a part of the body. They are applied to safeguard the client against injury, e.g., from falling, or to prevent movements that would disrupt therapy to a limb connected to tubes or appliances. Because people tend to resist restraint of any kind and consider it a violation of their right to move about freely, nurses need to ensure that clients understand the reason for using a restraint. Clients need to know that it is a protective device and understand why the body part has to be kept relatively still.

Recently, there has been a shift toward means other than restraints to protect clients. Restrained clients often become restless and anxious as a result of the loss of self-control. Sometimes nurses can remain with the restrained client and speak quietly to give reassurance and allay distress.

Legal Implications of Restraints

Because restraints restrict an individual's ability to move freely, their use has legal implications. In some settings, the decision to use a restraint is made by the nurse; in others, it must be made by a physician. Often a nurse can apply a restraint in an emergency; however, the physician must order subsequent use of the restraint. It is important for nurses to know their agency's practices and the state or provincial laws about restraining clients.

Before restraining a client, a nurse needs to try (and document) other nursing interventions, e.g., reorienting the client to reality. The nurse has to describe in the record what client behavior led to the decision to use a restraint. This information documents that restraints were applied for the client's safety, not for the nurse's convenience.

The nurse must document the type of restraint used, the exact times the restraint was applied and removed, the client's behavior before and with the restraint, care given while the restraint was applied, and notification of the physician. It is important to explain the need for the restraint both to the client and to support persons; the nurse also should document the substance of these explanations.

When to Use a Restraint

Restraints are used in a number of situations to limit a client's movement. Some of these are:

1. To prevent a client (e.g., an elderly confused person) from falling out of bed or out of a chair
2. To remind clients to restrict movement (e.g., restraining an arm while an intravenous infusion is running or limiting the movement of clients who are likely to fall if they get out of bed alone)
3. To prevent confused clients or children from harming themselves (e.g., by pulling out urinary catheters or pulling off surgical dressings)
4. To prevent clients from harming others through aggressive actions (e.g., placing mitts on clients who hit out at others)

Kinds of Restraints

Jacket Restraint While jacket restraints vary, they are all essentially sleeveless jackets (vests) with straps (tails) that can be tied to the bed frame under the mattress or to the legs of a chair. The jacket may be put on with the ties at the front or at the back, depending on the type.

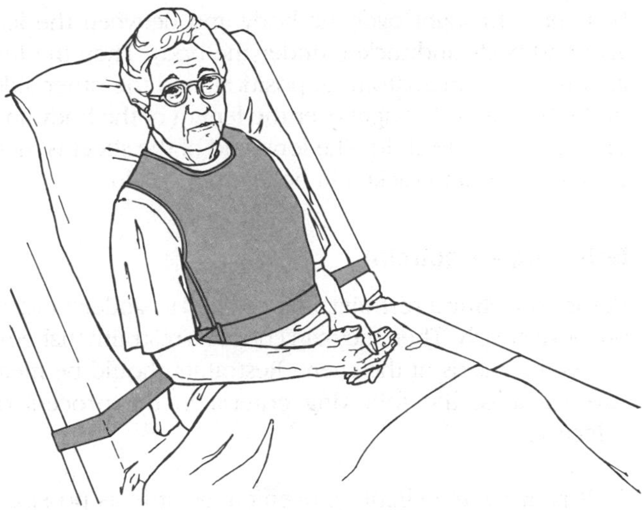

Figure 33–7 Poncho-type jacket restraint

See Figure 33–7. These body restraints are used for confused or sedated clients to prevent them from falling out of a bed or chair.

Belt Restraint Belt or safety strap body restraints are used to ensure the safety of all clients who are being moved on stretchers or in wheelchairs. They may also be used for certain clients lying in bed or sitting in a chair.

Mitt or Hand Restraints A mitt or hand restraint is used to prevent confused clients from using their hands or fingers to scratch and injure themselves. For example, a confused client may need to be prevented from pulling at intravenous tubing or a head bandage following brain surgery. Hand or mitt restraints allow the client to be ambulatory and/or to move the arm freely rather than be confined to a bed or a chair. Mitt restraints are commercially available. See Figure 33–8.

Hand restraints can also be made using large dressings and stockinette. The nurse asks the client to grasp a small pad, so that the hand assumes a natural position. The client's wrist is padded with large dressings to prevent skin abrasions, and all skin surfaces are carefully separated, also to prevent abrasions. The nurse then places two large dressings over the hand, one from side to side and the other from the ventral surface to the dorsal surface. The dressings are secured with gauze bandage and adhesive tape. See the section on bandaging turns in Chapter 52. Stockinette is then put over the hand and secured just above the wrist pad with adhesive tape.

Mittens need to be removed at least once in 24 hours to permit the client to wash and exercise the hands. If the client reports discomfort, the nurse needs to take off the mitten and check the circulation to the hand.

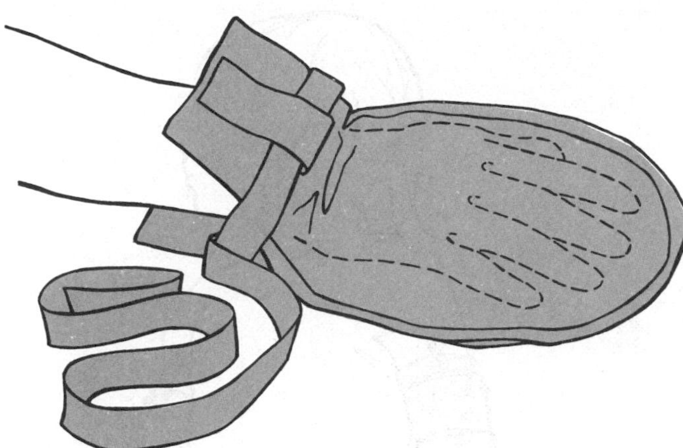

Figure 33–8 A commercially made mitt restraint

Wrist or Ankle Restraint Wrist and ankle restraints, generally made of cloth, are also referred to as limb-holder restraints, since they are used to immobilize a limb, primarily for therapeutic reasons (e.g., to maintain an intravenous infusion). Some commercially prepared restraints are available. A restraint can also be improvised from padded dressings and gauze. See Figure 33–10, later in this chapter.

Crib Net A crib net is simply a net placed over the top of a crib to prevent active young children from climbing out of the crib. At the same time, it allows them freedom to move about in the crib.

Elbow Restraint Elbow restraints are used to prevent infants or small children from flexing their elbows to

Research Note

After analyzing 2000 incident reports over a 4½-year period, Lynn concludes that 2% of all clients admitted to hospital are going to fall. Most incidents occur between 0830 and 1300 hours.

In 1 year, 73 clients fell from bed: 30% of the clients fell when they climbed over the side rail, and 11% fell after they had unlatched the rail. Thus, in 41% of falls, use of the side rail neither kept the client in bed nor prevented the tumble. To anyone intent on getting out of bed, side rails are not a deterrent; they are, at best, only a reminder. (Lynn 1980)

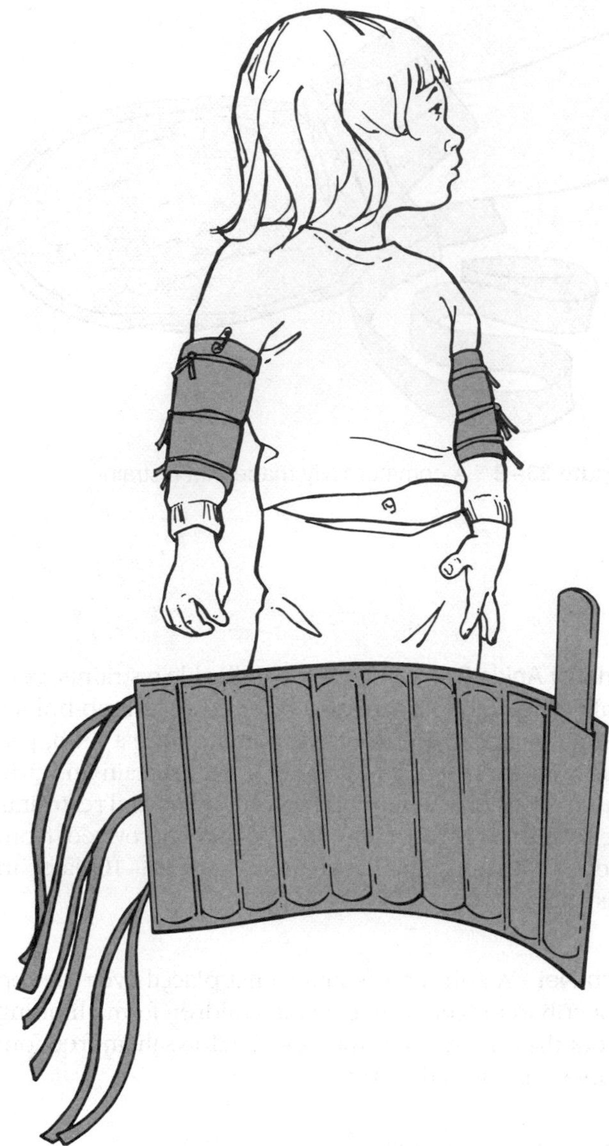

Figure 33–9 An elbow restraint for a young child

touch or scratch a surgical incision or skin lesion, e.g., eczema. See Figure 33–9. This restraint consists of a piece of material with pockets into which plastic or wooden tongue depressors are inserted to provide rigidity. After the restraint is applied, it is sometimes pinned to the child's shirt to prevent it from sliding down the arm.

Mummy Restraint The mummy restraint is a special folding of a blanket or sheet around the child to prevent movement during a procedure such as gastric washing, eye irrigation, or collection of a blood specimen. The child lies supine on a blanket with the upper edge of the blanket slightly above the shoulders and the lower edge at least 10 to 12 inches below the feet. The child's right arm is placed at his or her side, then one side of the blanket is brought over the body and between the left arm and body and tucked under the body. Then the left arm is placed in anatomical position, and the other side of the blanket is brought over the length of the body and tucked under the child. The long end of the sheet is then brought over and tucked in beneath the child.

Selecting a Restraint

Before selecting a restraint, nurses need to understand its purpose clearly. Then they can choose a restraint that best meets the needs of the client. Restraints should be measured against the following criteria in the process of selection:

1. It restricts the client's movement as little as possible. If a client needs to have one arm restrained, do not restrain his or her entire body.
2. It is the least obvious to others. Both clients and visitors are often embarrassed by a restraint, even though they understand why it is being used. The less obvious the restraint, the more comfortable people feel. A crossover jacket restraint may be less conspicuous than arm and leg restraints.
3. It does not interfere with the client's treatment or health problem. If a client has poor blood circulation to the hands, apply a restraint that will not aggravate that circulatory problem.
4. It is readily changeable. Restraints need to be changed frequently (see the next session), and more often if they become soiled. Keeping other guidelines in mind, choose a restraint that can be changed with minimal disturbance to the client.
5. It is safe for the particular client. Choose a restraint with which the client cannot self-inflict injury. For example, a physically active child could incur injury trying to climb out of a crib if one wrist is tied to the side of the crib. A jacket restraint would restrain the child more safely.

Guidelines for Use of Restraints

1. Explain the restraint and the reasons for its use to the client and the client's support persons. Often people are very disturbed when they visit a hospital and find "grandfather tied down." A simple explanation and assurance that the restraint is temporary, that it is a protection for the client rather than a punishment, are usually sufficient. A restraint must never be applied as punishment for any behavior or merely for the nurse's convenience.
2. Apply the restraint in such a way that the client can move as freely as possible without defeating the pur-

pose of the restraint. For example, a jacket restraint need not pin the client against the bed. It may permit some movement, such as bending forward or turning slightly to one side, while still preventing the client from falling out of bed.

3. Ensure that limb restraints are applied securely but not so tightly that they impede blood circulation to any body area or extremity.

4. Pad bony prominences (e.g., wrists and ankles) before applying a restraint over them. The movement of a restraint without padding over such prominences can quickly abrade the skin (damage it by friction).

5. Always tie a limb restraint with a knot that will not tighten when pulled. For example, a clove hitch applied to a wrist will stay secure, while a slip knot will tighten with pulling. The clove hitch is shown in Figure 33–10.

6. Tie the ends of a body restraint to the part of the bed that moves when the head is elevated. Never tie the ends to a side rail or to the fixed frame of the bed if the bed position is to be changed. The client could be injured if the restraint is pulled tight when the side rail or bed part is moved.

7. Remove most limb restraints at least every 4 hours, and provide range-of-motion (ROM) exercises (see Chapter 37) and skin care (see Chapter 36). For elderly clients, restraints may need to be removed more often, e.g., every 2 hours, to maintain blood circulation and mobility of the joints.

8. When a restraint is temporarily removed, do not leave the client unattended.

9. Immediately report to the responsible nurse and record on the client's chart any persistent reddened or broken skin areas under the restraint.

10. At the first indication of cyanosis or pallor, coldness of a skin area, or a client's complaint of a tingling sensation, pain, or numbness, loosen the restraint and exercise the limb. Impaired blood circulation can cause these symptoms.

11. Apply a restraint in such a way that it can be released quickly in case of an emergency. For example, secure a body restraint to a place on the bed that is easily reached.

12. Apply a restraint so that the body part can assume a normal anatomic position, e.g., the elbow is slightly flexed.

13. Provide emotional support verbally and through touch for the client. Being restrained causes a great deal of anxiety in some people, and they can exhaust themselves fighting the restraint. Stay with the client as required.

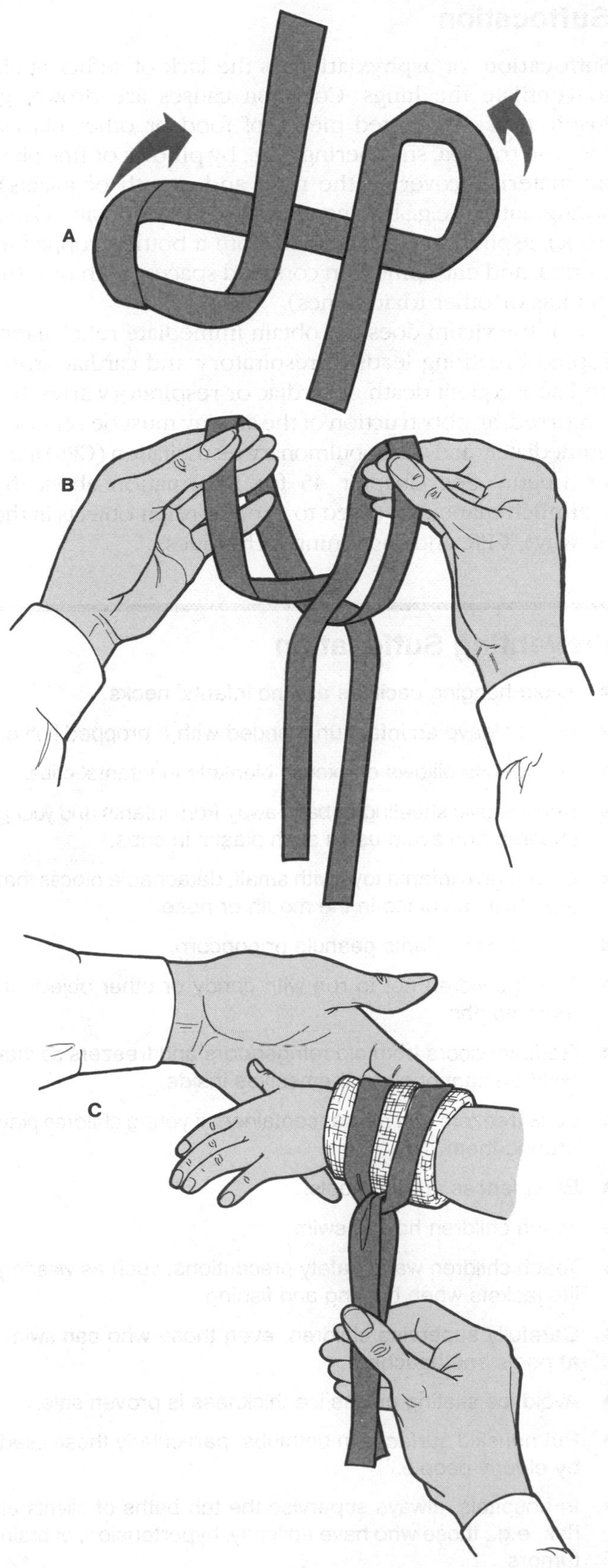

Figure 33–10 To make a clove hitch: **A,** Make a figure-eight; **B,** pick up the loops; **C,** put the limb through the loops and secure it.

Suffocation

Suffocation, or **asphyxiation**, is the lack of sufficient air to ventilate the lungs. Common causes are drowning, inspiration of ingested pieces of food or other objects into the trachea, smothering (e.g., by pillows or fine plastic materials covering the nose and mouth of infants), strangulation (e.g., by a pacifier placed around an infant's neck), aspiration (e.g., of milk from a bottle propped in a crib), and entrapment in confined spaces (with or without gas or other toxic fumes).

If the victim does not obtain immediate relief, interrupted breathing leads to respiratory and cardiac arrest and subsequent death. If cardiac or respiratory arrest has occurred, any obstruction of the airway must be removed immediately and cardiopulmonary resuscitation (CPR) must be begun. See Chapter 45 for information about the Heimlich maneuver (used to expel foreign objects in the airway), CPR, and suctioning techniques.

Preventing Suffocation

- Avoid hanging pacifiers around infants' necks.
- Do not leave an infant unattended with a propped bottle.
- Do not use pillows or excess blankets in infants' cribs.
- Keep plastic sheeting or bags away from infants and young children and avoid using such plastic in cribs.
- Do not give infants toys with small, detachable pieces that the child can place in the mouth or nose.
- Do not give infants peanuts or popcorn.
- Teach children not to run with candy or other objects in their mouths.
- Remove doors from old refrigerators and freezers so that children cannot close themselves inside.
- Lock freezers and similar containers if young children play around them.
- Build fences around pools.
- Teach children how to swim.
- Teach children water safety precautions, such as wearing life jackets when boating and fishing.
- Carefully supervise children, even those who can swim, at pools and beaches.
- Avoid ice skating unless ice thickness is proven safe.
- Put nonskid surfaces in bathtubs, particularly those used by elderly people.
- In hospitals, always supervise the tub baths of clients at risk, e.g., those who have epilepsy, hypertension, or brain tumors.
- Keep suction equipment at the bedsides of clients who might choke, such as clients who have difficulty swallowing.

Most incidents of asphyxiation in the community and hospital are preventable. Education of the public about accident prevention is important. See the preventive actions listed to the left.

Poisoning

A **poison** is any substance that injures or kills through its chemical action when inhaled, injected, applied, or absorbed in relatively small amounts. Poisons can impair the function of many body systems: respiratory, circulatory, gastrointestinal, renal, hepatic, and central nervous systems. For certain poisons, specific antidotes or treatments are available; for many, there is no specific therapy.

In response to the ever-increasing number of poison hazards, many countries have established poison centers. The American and Canadian Association of Poison Control Centers is a nationwide network of poison control centers and concerned individuals, who work together and with government and industry to make life safer from the hazards of poisons. Poison control centers provide accurate, up-to-date information about potential hazards and recommend treatment as needed.

Emergency information is usually provided 24 hours a day, 7 days a week. The centers supply physicians and hospitals specific information to assist with medical care. Educational materials and prevention programs are also available. Nurses need to encourage people to call poison control centers before attempting home remedies, which may intensify the problem. For example, inducing vomiting after poisoning by corrosive substances (e.g., drain or oven cleaners, chlorine bleach, electric dishwasher granules, and household ammonia) only causes further burns of the esophagus and throat.

Ingestion of poisonous or toxic agents is very common in children 5 years or younger, particularly in 2-year-olds, whose curiosity and independence prompt them to investigate objects, often by tasting them. Almost all nonfood substances, including many house plants, are potentially harmful to children. Selected poisonous plants and household chemicals are shown on pages 741 and 742. Additional information is available from poison control centers.

The major reasons for poisoning in children are inadequate supervision and improper storage of many household toxic substances (over 500 in the average home). Adolescent and adult poisonings are usually caused by insect or snake bites and drugs used for recreation or in suicide attempts. Poisoning in elderly people usually is a result of accidental ingestion of a toxic substance due to failing eyesight or an overdose of a prescribed medication due to impaired memory.

Prevention

Teach clients to:

1. Place potentially toxic agents out of reach of crawling infants.

Selected Poisonous and Nonpoisonous Plants

Poisonous*		Nonpoisonous†	
Avocado (leaves)	Morning glory	African violet	Honeysuckle
Azaleas	Mushrooms	Aster	Impatiens
Buttercups	Narcissus	Baby's tears	Jade plant
Cherries (pits)	Oleander	Bamboo	Lipstick plant
Crocus, autumn	Philodendron	Begonia	Magnolia
Daffodil	Poison hemlock	California poppy	Marigold
English ivy	Poison ivy	Camellia	Orchid
Foxglove	Poison oak	Christmas cactus	Petunia
Holly berries	Poppy (California poppy excepted)	Chrysanthemum (dermatitis)	Piggy-back plant
Horsetail reed	Potato (sprouts)	Crabapples	Prayer plant
Hyacinth	Rhododendron	Dahlia	Rose
Hydrangea	Rhubarb (leaves)	Daisies	Rubber plant (dermatitis)
Iris	Tobacco	Dandelion	Umbrella tree
Ivy (Boston, English, and others)	Tomato (except fruit)	Easter lily	Wandering jew
Larkspur	Tulip	Eucalyptus (caution)	Weeping fig
Lily-of-the-valley	Wisteria	Gardenia	Yucca
Lobelia	Yew berries	Gloxinia	Zebra plant
Mistletoe		Hibiscus	

*These plants are considered poisonous and possibly dangerous. They contain a wide variety of poisons, and symptoms of ingestion may vary from a mild stomachache, skin rash, and swelling of the mouth and throat to involvement of the heart, kidneys, or other organs. Many plants are not toxic unless ingested in very large amounts.

†These plants are considered essentially safe, not poisonous. It is unlikely that an individual will develop symptoms from eating or handling these plants, but any plant may cause an unexpected reaction in certain individuals.

Source: British Columbia Poison Control Centre and Province of British Columbia Ministry of Health.

2. Put all drugs (prescription and nonprescription) in a locked cabinet. Even though legislation mandates child-guard tops on prescription drugs, many 4-year olds can manipulate these.
3. Lock cleaning agents in a cupboard or attach special plastic hooks to the inside of cabinet doors to keep them securely closed. Unlatching these hooks, obtainable at most hardware stores, requires firmer thumb pressure than small children can usually exert.
4. Avoid keeping a large surplus of cleaning agents, laundry additives, furniture polish, insecticides, paints, and solvents.
5. Avoid storing toxic liquids or solids in food containers, such as soft drink bottles, peanut butter jars, or milk cartons. Even though the containers are well labeled, the child who cannot read associates them with food.
6. Do not remove container labels or reuse empty containers to store different substances. Laws mandate that the labels of all poisons specify antidotes. Removing labels or changing the contents thus negates this safety measure.
7. Keep poisonous house plants out of reach of young children. Store bulbs and seeds out of sight and out of reach.
8. Learn to identify the poisonous plants in your neighborhood.
9. Do not assume a plant is not poisonous because birds or other wildlife eat it.
10. Do not rely on cooking to destroy toxic chemicals in plants. Never use anything prepared from nature as a medicine or "tea."
11. When children are old enough to learn, teach them the difference between food and those substances that must never be ingested or tasted. Teach them never to eat any part of an unknown plant or mushroom and to never put leaves, stems, bark, seeds, nuts, or berries from any plant into their mouths.

Figure 33–11 The "Mr. Yuk" poison label

12. Place poison warning stickers designed for children on containers of bleach, lye, kerosene, solvent, and other toxic substances. See Figure 33–11. Teach children that the Mr. Yuk label means danger.
13. Do not take medications in front of children. They may imitate you.

Poisonous Household Chemicals

Ammonia	Model cement
Antifreeze	Nail polish
Ant syrup or paste	Nail polish remover
Automotive products	Oven cleaner
Bathroom bowl cleaner	Paint
Bleach	Paint remover
Boric acid	Paint thinner
Charcoal lighter	Perfume
Cleaning fluid	Permanent wave solutions
Cologne	Pesticides
Copper and brass cleaners	Pine oil
Detergents	Rat poisons
Dishwasher detergents	Rubbing alcohol
Disinfectants	Shaving lotion
Drain cleaners	Silver polish
Epoxy glue	Snail bait
Furniture polish	Spot removers
Garden sprays	Sulfuric acid
Gasoline	Super glue
Gun cleaners	Turpentine
Hair dyes	Veterinary products
Insecticides	Weed killers
Kerosene	Window wash solvent
Lighter fluid	

14. Never call medicine candy when giving medications to children. They may generalize that all medicine is candy.
15. Read and follow label directions on all products before using them.
16. Purchase syrup of ipecac from a local drug store and keep it on hand at all times. Syrup of ipecac is a nonprescription emetic available in single-dose 15 ml vials in all drugstores. Use it only after advice from the local poison control center or the family physician.
17. Make sure babysitters, friends, and relatives know the number of the poison control center.
18. Display the phone number of the poison control center near or on all telephones in the home.

Intervention for Accidental Poisoning

People need to be prepared to deal with poisoning. Nurses can intervene by educating the public about what to do in the event of poisoning. Recommended information and actions follow.

1. Identify the specific poison by searching for an opened container, empty bottle, or other evidence. This information helps to determine the type and amount of antidote needed.
2. Contact the poison control center, indicate the exact quantity of poison the person ingested, and state the person's age and apparent symptoms.
3. If instructed to induce vomiting:
   a. Administer 10 to 15 ml (2 to 3 tsp) of syrup of ipecac followed by one or two cups of water. Syrup of ipecac causes vomiting and emptying of the stomach. It is not recommended for children under 1 year of age.
   b. If vomiting does not occur in 15 to 20 minutes, administer a second dose of ipecac. Proper use and dosage of ipecac syrup are essential. Overdoses have occurred due to multiple doses of syrup or to the use of fluid extract of ipecac, 14 times more potent than the syrup.
   c. If ipecac is not available or if the victim is an infant, administer one or two glasses of warm water and tickle the back of the victim's throat with a spoon or other blunt instrument.
4. Keep the victim as quiet as possible and position the victim on one side or with head placed between the legs to prevent aspiration of vomitus.
5. If so instructed by the poison control center, take all evidence of the poison, such as urine, vomitus, and substance container, to the poison control center, or call an ambulance to take the person to an emergency room.

First Aid for Poisoning

SWALLOWED POISONS

Medicine: Do not give anything by mouth until you call for advice.

Household products or chemicals: Unless the person is unconscious, having convulsions, or cannot swallow, give milk or water immediately and then call the poison control center about whether you should make the victim vomit or not. Use syrup of ipecac only on the advice of the poison control center, emergency department, or physician.

POISON IN THE EYE

Flood the eye with lukewarm (not hot) water poured from a jug or large glass 2 or 3 inches from the eye. Repeat for 15 minutes. Have the person blink as much as possible while flooding the eye. Do not force the eyelid open.

POISONS ON THE SKIN

Flood the skin with water for 10 minutes. Remove contaminated clothing. Then wash gently with soap and water and rinse.

INHALED POISONS

Immediately get the person to fresh air. Avoid breathing fumes. Open the doors and windows wide. If the person is not breathing, start artificial respiration.

Source: British Columbia Poison Centre in cooperation with the Province of British Columbia Ministry of Health.

Inducing vomiting is contraindicated (a) when the client is unconscious or convulsing because of the risk of aspirating emesis into the lungs or (b) when the poison is one of the following:

1. A strong corrosive (acid or alkali), such as lye (drain or oven cleaners), chlorine bleach, electric dishwasher granules, and household ammonia, which burn the esophagus and throat.
2. A petroleum distillate, such as kerosene, turpentine, cleaning fluid, lighter fluid, furniture polish, metal polish, and some insecticides, which can be readily aspirated.

Electric Shock

Electricity is used extensively in homes and health care agencies. An essential nursing function is to keep clients safe from electrical hazards in health care and other settings.

There are two types of electricity: **dynamic** (moving electric charges) and **static** (stationary electric charges). Dynamic electricity poses a danger in that a current can pass through the body to the ground, giving the individual a shock or a macroshock. Nurses need to use electrical equipment that is properly **grounded** (that transmits an electric current from an object or surface to the ground). The electrical plug of grounded equipment has three prongs. The two short prongs transmit the power to the equipment. The third, longer prong is the grounding device, which carries short circuits or stray electric current to the ground. See Figure 33–12. Grounding prongs offer a path of least resistance to stray electric currents. (A phenomenon of electricity is that it follows the path of least resistance.)

Dynamic electricity operates most equipment. If the equipment is faulty, e.g., if a cord is frayed, there is a danger of electric shock. Also, faulty electrical equipment can start fires. For example, an electric spark near certain anesthetic gases or a high concentration of oxygen may cause a serious fire.

If an individual receives a macroshock, it is important not to touch that person until the electricity is shut off and the person is safely away from the electric current. A macroshock can cause both superficial and deep burns, muscle contractions, and cardiac and respiratory arrest. Macroshock is prevented by using machines in good repair, wearing shoes with rubber shoes, standing on a nonconductive floor, and using nonconductive gloves.

Static electricity builds up on the surface of the body and of certain materials. It is caused by the transfer of **electrons** (negatively charged electric particles) from one surface to another. Lightning is the most powerful form of static electricity.

Static electricity is a danger in hospital operating rooms, where the building up and sparking of static charges near anesthetic agents could cause an explosion. To prevent explosion, operating room personnel do not use nylon, dacron, and other materials that tend to build up static charges. Because dry air is conducive to the buildup of static electric charges, the air is humidified, and antistatic sprays are used in areas where explosion is a danger. Actions to reduce electrical hazards are shown on page 744.

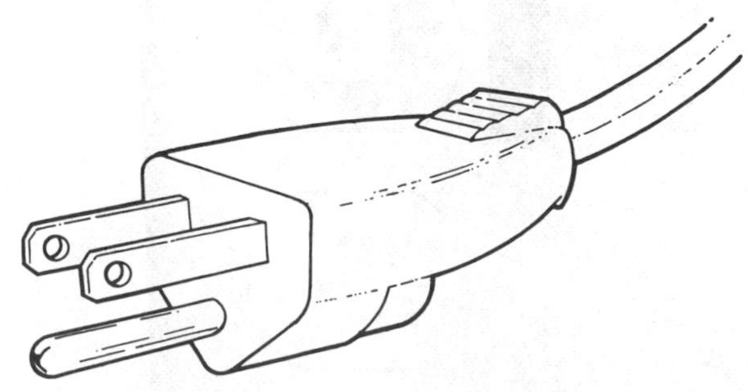

Figure 33–12 Three-pronged ground plug

Reducing Electrical Hazards

Teach clients to:

- Check cords for fraying or other signs of damage before using an appliance. Do not use if damage is apparent.
- Avoid overloading outlets and fuse boxes with too many appliances.
- Use only grounded outlets and plugs.
- Always pull a plug from the wall outlet by firmly grasping the plug and pulling it straight out. Pulling a plug by its cord can damage the cord and plug unit.
- Never use electrical appliances near sinks, bathtubs, showers, or other wet areas since water readily conducts electricity.
- Keep electrical cords and appliances out of the reach of young children.
- Place protective covers over wall outlets to protect young children (See Figure 33–13).
- Have all noninsulated wiring in the home altered to meet safety standards.
- Carefully read instructions before operating electrical equipment. Clients who do not understand how to operate the equipment should seek advice.
- Always disconnect appliances before cleaning or repairing them.
- Unplug any appliance that has given a tingling sensation or shock and have an electrician evaluate it for stray current.
- Keep electrical cords coiled or taped to the ground away from areas of traffic to prevent others from damaging the cord or tripping over it.

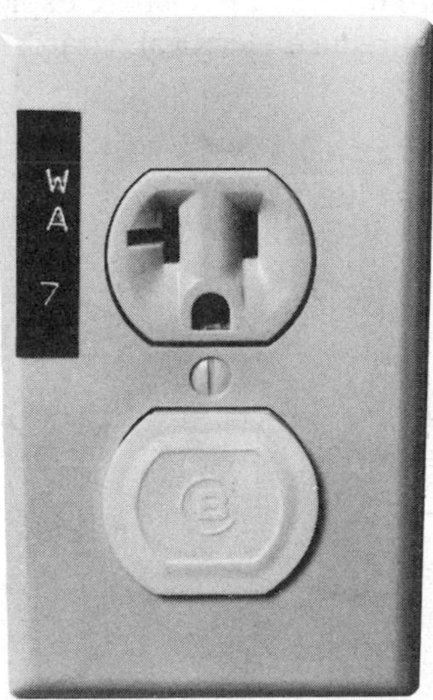

Figure 33–13 Safety cover for an electrical outlet

Noise

Excessive noise is a health hazard that can cause hearing loss, depending on (a) the overall level of noise, (b) the frequency range of the noise, and (c) the duration of exposure and individual susceptibility. Sound levels above 120 decibels (units of loudness) are painful and may cause hearing damage even if a person is exposed for only a short period. Exposure to 85 to 95 decibels for several hours a day can lead to progressive or permanent hearing loss. Noise levels below 85 decibels usually do not affect hearing.

Tolerance of noise is largely individual. The rural dweller may find the city noisy, whereas the city dweller may be oblivious to urban sounds. Adults often find teenager's music uncomfortably loud. Noise has psychosocial effects, such as feelings of annoyance, disrupted sleep and relaxation, and interruption of thought and conversation patterns. Noise can also interfere with job performance and safety.

The ill and injured are frequently sensitive to noises that normally would not disturb them. Loud voices, the clatter of dishes, and even a nearby television can disturb clients, some of whom react angrily.

Physiologic effects of noise include increased heart and respiratory rates, increased muscular activity, nausea, and, if the noise is sufficiently loud, hearing loss. The exact mechanism by which noise causes hearing loss has not been determined. It is thought that excessive noise levels overstimulate the hair cells within the inner ear, resulting in degeneration of the organ of Corti. When this happens, some sound waves are no longer converted into nerve impulses to the brain, and there is hearing loss. People with noise-induced hearing loss tend not to hear high-frequency consonants, such as *sh* or *ch*. Further, people with such hearing loss are usually not aware of it until the exposure to noise affects sounds in the frequency range of speech.

Noise can be minimized in several ways. Acoustic tile on ceilings, walls, and floors as well as drapes and carpeting absorb sound. Background music can mask noise and have a calming effect on some people. It is important for nurses to encourage clients to protect their hearing as much as possible.

Radiation

Radiation as a health hazard is a recent source of concern. Nurses are concerned specifically with those radioactive materials used in diagnostic and therapeutic practices. Radiation injury can occur from overexposure or from exposure to radiation that treats specific tissues and at the same time injures other tissues.

Radioactive materials are used in diagnostic procedures such as radiography, fluoroscopy, and nuclear medicine. In nuclear medicine, radioactive isotopes that have an affinity for specific tissues are given by mouth or intravenously. Isotopes of these elements are used: calcium, which has an affinity for bones; iodine, which is attracted to the thyroid gland; and phosphorus, which is attracted to blood. See the section on radiography and nuclear medicine in Chapter 54.

Radioactive materials are provided in sealed sources and unsealed liquid sources. For example, cobalt implants are sealed; iodine 131 and phosphorus 32 are unsealed liquids.

Principles governing the degree of exposure to radiation are as follows:

1. The longer the time in the presence of radiation, the greater the exposure
2. The closer a person is to the radioactive source, the greater the exposure
3. The more extensive the use of lead and other radiation shields, the greater the protection against radiation.

Often nurses help care for clients treated or diagnosed with radioactive substances. The client diagnosed through radiography or fluoroscopy generally receives minimal exposure, and few precautions are necessary. The nurse restraining a small child during radiography needs to wear a lead apron. Clients with radioactive implants are a source of radiation to the immediate environment. The nurse who is in close contact with such clients also needs to wear a lead apron.

It is important to deal safely with radioactive body discharges. Nurses wear rubber gloves and in some instances may place excreta in containers for special disposal. It is also important that the nurse's gloved hands be washed well before the gloves are removed and that contaminated materials be placed in a special container for disposal.

Hospitals in which radioactive materials are used usually have a radioisotope committee. This committee establishes policies and procedures to be used in the care of clients who receive radioactive materials. It is important that nurses be cognizant of these policies.

One important aspect of caring for clients receiving radiation treatment is making sure they understand the treatment and the precautions they need to take. Often such clients are restricted to bed or to a confined area to protect others. Like clients who are on protective asepsis, these clients need emotional support to deal with the precautions. They accept treatments and precautions better when they know what will happen, when, and why.

Intervention for Particular Age Groups

Accidental hazards vary among different age groups. The nurse needs to be aware of hazards specific to clients of different ages and to educate people about safety precautions. Most accidents are due to negligence and are preventable.

Infants

Although infants are completely dependent on others for care, they soon learn to roll from side to side, put objects in their mouths, and crawl. They are oblivious to such dangers as falling or ingesting harmful substances. Infants need constant surveillance by adults, who must provide protective measures. Potential hazards to infants and preventive actions are shown in Table 33–3.

Toddlers

Toddlers are curious and like to feel and taste everything. Young toddlers (12 to 18 months) can walk alone, although unsteadily, and would rather run than walk. They like to stop and retrieve, climb, and explore. Older toddlers (2 to 3 years) can jump, stand on one foot, and enjoy riding toys and imitating adults. Because toddlers are curious and fascinated by such potential dangers as garden pools and busy streets, they need constant supervision and protection. Training in safety should begin when the child is a toddler. Potential hazards to toddlers and preventive actions are shown in Table 33–4.

Preschoolers

It is important to teach preschoolers accident prevention and safety rules, particularly since at this age they become increasingly independent. Preschoolers have well-developed gross motor coordination and are very active; they run, climb, and often act before they think. They like to imitate their parents, and adults can teach safety through example. Potential hazards to preschoolers and preventive actions are shown in Table 33–5.

School-Age Children

By the time children attend school, they are learning to think before they act. They often prefer adult equipment to toys. They want to be active with other children in such activities as bicycling, hiking, swimming, and boating. Although sensitive to peer pressure, the school-age child responds to rules. Children of this age engage in fantasy and magical thinking. They often imitate actions of parents and superheroes with whom they identify. Potential hazards to preschoolers and preventive actions are outlined in Table 33–6.

Adolescents

Adolescents spend much of their time away from home with their peers. However, they still need guidance from parents. The accident rate among adolescents is high. Most of these accidents are associated with automobiles. In

Table 33–3 **Potential Hazards and Preventive Actions for Infants (Birth to 1 Year)**

Potential Hazard	Preventive Actions
Suffocation in crib	Do not put pillows, excess blankets, plastic, or anything that might suffocate a baby in the crib.
Strangulation by objects hung around the neck	Do not suspend a pacifier or anything that might cause strangulation around the infant's neck.
Choking from aspirated milk or ingested objects	Hold the infant at feeding time. Do not leave the infant alone with a propped bottle.
	Provide only soft, large toys that do not have parts the infant can remove, swallow, and aspirate.
	Cut solid foods into small pieces, and do not feed the child peanuts or popcorn.
	Do not leave the infant unattended while he or she is eating.
	Hold the infant relatively upright while he or she is nursing or feeding from a bottle and have older infants eat only when sitting.
	Keep pins, needles, buttons, and nails out of reach of the baby. It is natural for infants to put such objects in their mouths.
Falling	Do not leave a baby alone in the bath, at the bed or table, or anywhere the infant may roll off or fall. Always keep a hand on the infant.
	Always keep the sides of the crib up when not handling the baby.
	On stairs, hold the baby with two hands.
	When the infant begins to crawl, place guard rails at the top and bottom of stairs and put screens on windows.
	Supervise the child constantly when he or she is in a walker, jumper, swing, or high chair.
Automobile accidents	Use approved infant car seats to restrain infants in automobile (see Figure 33–14).
	Place the infant in the back seat.
Burns	Always test bath water before immersing the infant.
	Remove potential hazards such as hot coffee while the baby is sitting in your lap.
	Turn pot handles toward the back of the stove and use back burners.
	Remove stove burner dials if they are within the infant's reach.
	Fence off wood-burning stoves and portable heaters.
	Protect the baby from sunburn.
Cuts, puncture wounds, bruises, and other injury	Place bumpers in the crib to prevent the infant from putting his or her head between the crib slats; slats should be no more than $2\frac{3}{8}$ inches apart.
	Stuff towels between loose-fitting mattress and the sides of the crib to prevent infants from catching their arms or fingers between them.
	Keep the sharp points of diaper pins away from the baby's skin.
	Cut the baby's fingernails while the baby sleeps; sharp fingernails can scratch the infant.
	Use only plastic bottles and feeding cups; broken glass is a hazard.
	Make sure that toys have no sharp edges.
	Keep hazardous equipment such as fans and humidifiers off the floor and out of the infant's reach, and remove dangerous objects from counters and tables.
	Raise the sides of playpens and use corrals with net siding.
Electrical shock	Cover electrical outlets (see Figure 33–13 earlier in this chapter). Coil the cords on appliances to keep them out of reach.
Poisoning	Place plants, household cleaners, and wastebaskets out of the infant's reach.
	Lock cabinets that contain such potential poisons as medicines, paint, and gasoline.
	Store formula in a cool, dry place to prevent it from spoiling.

addition, adolescents are at risk of injury when riding motorcycles, snowmobiles, and minibikes. Wounds from firearms and drowning are other causes of death among adolescents. Adults can help the adolescent minimize risks by setting an example of appropriate behavior and by teaching the responsibilities that accompany independence and adult activities. Potential hazards to adolescents and safety measures are outlined in Table 33–7.

Young and Middle-Aged Adults

Accidents rank fourth as the cause of death among middle-aged adults. Alcohol and stress are significant factors in many of these accidents. Adults need to learn not to drink if they are driving motor vehicles, boating, or swimming and to learn stress management techniques (see Chapter 17).

Table 33–4 Potential Hazards and Preventive Actions for Toddlers (1 to 3 Years)

Potential Hazard	Preventive Actions
Physical trauma from falling, banging into objects, or getting cut by sharp objects	Because accidents occur most frequently when parents are preoccupied, such as at mealtimes, parents need to share responsibility for preparing meals and supervising children.
	If the child still sleeps in a crib, lower the sides while the child sleeps. Obtain a bed.
	Keep the house free of clutter.
	Keep furniture with sharp edges (e.g., glass-topped tables) out of the child's way.
	Place knives and other sharp tools out of reach.
	Make sure that windows and balconies are made safe, for instance, sturdily screened.
	Make children wear seat belts and sit in the back seat while they are in the car.
	Make sure that pull-toy strings are no longer than 12 inches. Toys with longer strings can be lost from sight and pulled over hazardous objects.
	Teach the child not to ride a tricycle in the streets or behind cars.
Burns	Teach the words *no* and *don't.* Make the child understand that these words often signify danger and must be obeyed.
Burns (*continued*)	Keep matches safely out of reach.
	Place hot pots on the back burners, away from the toddler's reach.
	Test bath water before allowing the child to get in the tub.
	Teach the dangers of charcoal fires.
Poisoning	Keep cleaning solutions, insecticides, and medicines in locked cupboards.
	Teach children not to put objects in their mouths. Especially warn against vegetation (e.g., leaves and berries), peeling paint, plaster, or objects picked up from the floor or street.
	Teach the child never to take pills unless they are given by a parent, nurse, or trusted adult.
Drowning	Do not leave toddlers unattended in bath tubs or pools.
	Do not overfill the bathtub.
	Do not let toddlers play near deep ditches and wells.
	Teach the child to swim but never leave the child unsupervised at a pool or beach.
	Fence in pools.
Electrical shock	Ensure that the toddler is protected from electrical outlets and equipment.

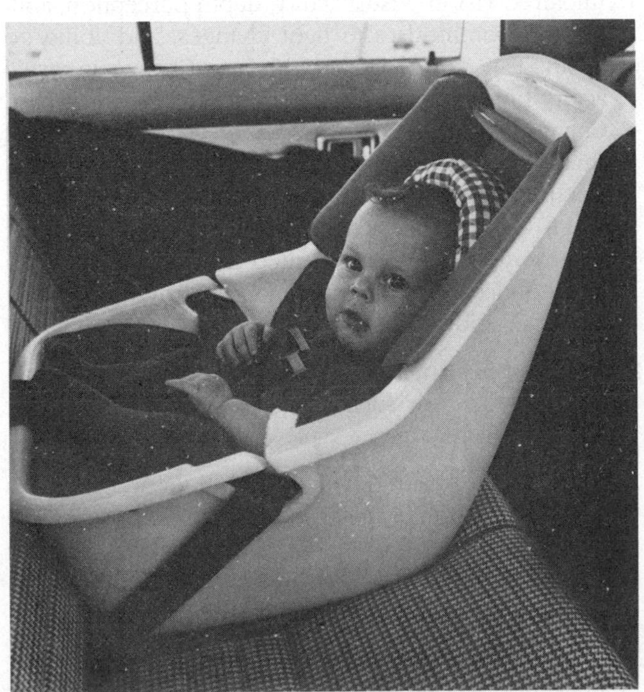

Figure 33–14 An infant carrier for the infant from birth to about 12 months of age

Research Note

Ford studied use of crash-tested and approved restraining devices for infants in relationship to parents' locus of control, knowledge scores, and demographic data. Of 66 mothers who provided complete data, 19 (29%) owned and made proper use of the devices. Thirty-four mothers (52%) owned devices but did not use them properly. Nonwhite parents, those from lower socioeconomic groups, those with only a high school education or less, and unmarried parents were least likely to own or use restraints. Nursing implications are that nurses should (a) discuss the existence of child restraints and the advantages of consistently using them with all mothers or mothers-to-be in office, clinic, or hospital visits or in prenatal and postpartum classes and (b) provide information to parents about which restraints are most adequate and how to use the restraint properly. (Ford 1980)

Table 33–5 Potential Hazards and Preventive Actions for Preschoolers (3 to 5 Years)

Potential Hazards	Preventive Actions
Choking, suffocation, and obstruction of the airway and ear canal by foreign objects	Do not allow the child to run while he or she has candy or other objects in the mouth.
	Teach children not to put small objects in the mouth, nose, and ears.
	Remove doors from unused equipment such as refrigerators, which can entrap and asphyxiate the child who hides in them.
Injury from traffic, playground equipment, and other objects	Teach preschoolers to cross streets safely and to obey traffic signals.
	Teach them to play on sidewalks or grass rather than in driveways, in the street, or on railroad tracks.
	Teach them not to walk in front of swings and not to push others off playground equipment.
	Encourage them to put their toys away so that people will not trip over them.
Poisoning	Check Halloween treats before allowing the child to eat them; discard any loose or open candy.
	Reinforce that they should not eat any vegetation or objects from the street.
	Reinforce that they should not take pills without the parent's consent.
Drowning	Same as for the toddler, Table 33–4.
Fire and burns	Teach the preschooler the dangers of playing with matches and near charcoal or other controlled fires and heating appliances.
Harm from other people or animals	Teach the child to avoid strangers and to keep parents informed of his or her whereabouts.
	Teach children to walk quietly near animals and to avoid approaching them if a trusted adult is not present.

Accident prevention starts with education about precautions such as these:

1. Store combustibles and corrosives, for example, oily rags and lye, in appropriate places.
2. Ensure that electrical plugs, wires, and appliances are in good repair.
3. Anchor small rugs securely.
4. Clean up litter or spills on the floor immediately.
5. Keep stairs and walkways free from obstructions, snow, and ice.
6. Avoid using unsteady ladders or chairs.
7. Screen fires and heaters.
8. Avoid wearing plastic aprons or loose clothing around open flames.
9. Do not smoke in bed.
10. Put nonskid material in bathtubs and shower stalls.
11. Ensure that automobiles are mechanically sound.
12. Do not work on a running automobile in a non-ventilated area.
13. Wear safety belts when driving, and make sure that windshields, side mirrors, and rearview mirrors are clean.

Older Adults

Older adults are particularly prone to accidents because of the following factors:

1. Impaired vision. Visual acuity, depth perception, ability to accommodate to light changes, and ability to distinguish color decline with age. Change in visual acuity hinders the person's ability to discern danger. Changes in depth perception increase the chance of stumbling when stepping off curbs or negotiating stairs. Declining ability to accommodate to changes in light and to discern colors makes driving more hazardous. For example, the glare created by automobile headlights and street lights can momentarily incapacitate the older adult.
2. Impaired hearing. Older adults with hearing loss are less likely to hear such danger warnings as sirens or honking horns.
3. Changes in posture and mobility. Older adults have a stooped posture, broad-based gait, shuffling walk, and the tendency to sway and lose balance. Thus they are at increased risk of falling and less able to avoid hazards.
4. Diminished ability to sense temperature and smell. Impaired skin sensitivity to temperature makes the older adult more prone to burns. Impaired ability to smell may prevent the older person from sensing a fire.

Table 33–6 Potential Hazards and Preventive Actions for School-Age Children (6 to 12 Years)

Potential Hazards	Preventive Actions
Sports injuries	Teach the child safety rules for swimming, boating, ice skating and other recreations, e.g., "Never swim or skate alone. Always wear a life jacket when you are in a boat and do not skate unless the ice is proven safe or without my consent."
	Teach them to wear protective helmets, knee pads and elbow pads when appropriate.
	Carefully supervise any sport (e.g., archery) in which the child aims at a target, and place targets in isolated areas against walls.
	Teach the child not to throw objects at people or moving vehicles.
Traffic accidents	Teach the child traffic rules for bicycling.
	Caution the child to follow traffic safety rules when he or she is roller skating or skateboarding.
	Teach the child not to play or hide near cars.
	Make sure children wear seat belts at all times when they are in automobiles.
	Teach the child to wear light-colored clothing and reflective material when walking or cycling at night.
Tools and machinery	Teach the child safe ways to use the stove, garden tools, and other equipment.
	Supervise children when they use saws, electric appliances and tools, and other potentially dangerous equipment.
	Teach the child to avoid excavations, quarries, and vacant buildings and not to play around heavy machinery.
Firearms	Teach the child not to play with fireworks, gunpowder, and firearms.
	Keep firearms unloaded, locked up, and out of reach.
Substance abuse	Teach the child the effects of drugs and alcohol on judgment and coordination.

Table 33–7 Potential Hazards and Preventive Actions for Adolescents (12 to 18 Years)

Potential Hazards	Preventive Actions
Vehicle accidents	Have adolescents complete a driver's education course, and take practice drives with them in various kinds of weather.
	Reinforce the importance of wearing seat belts when driving and when riding as a passenger.
	Teach them to wear safety helmets when riding motorcycles, scooters, and the like.
	Set firm limits on automobile use, e.g., "Never drive after drinking or taking mind-altering drugs, and never ride with a driver who has done so."
	Encourage them to call home for a ride if they have been drinking by assuring them that they can do so without a reprimand.
Recreational accidents no longer under parental supervision	Encourage the adolescent to swim, jog, or go boating in groups so others can obtain help in case of an accident.
	Reinforce water safety rules.
Firearms	Teach rules for hunting and proper use and care of firearms.
	Keep firearms unloaded and locked up.
Substance abuse	Inform the adolescent of the dangers of drugs and alcohol.
	Be alert to changes in the adolescent's mood and behavior.
	Listen to and maintain open communication with the adolescent. Open communication between parents and children is a powerful preventive measure.
	Set a good example of behavior that the adolescent can follow.

5. Decreased sensitivity to light touch, vibration, and deep pressure. Older adults may not realize that they have bumped into an object.
6. Physical disorders that impair mobility or cause dizziness. One example is **orthostatic hypotension**. When persons with orthostatic hypotension change position suddenly, their vasoactive reflexes may not be rapid enough to prevent a significant drop in blood pressure. As a result, they may faint, fall, and injure themselves.
7. Certain prescribed medications or combinations of prescribed medications. Narcotics and tranquilizers can impair alertness and judgment. Diuretics, antidepressants, barbiturates, antihistamines, levodopa, and diazepam contribute to postural hypotension. A combination of diuretics, tranquilizers, and narcotics can alter level of consciousness, muscle strength, and coordination (Gray-Vickrey 1984, p. 180).

Most injuries of older adults are due to falls, burns, and pedestrian and automobile accidents. See below for strategies to minimize these potential hazards to older adults.

Accident Prevention for the Older Adult

PREVENTING FALLS

- Make sure all rooms, hallways, and stairwells are adequately lit.
- Have an easily accessible light switch next to the bed.
- Leave a night light on in the hallway or bathroom.
- Get out of bed slowly, i.e., sit before standing and stand briefly before walking, to prevent dizziness from orthostatic hypotension.
- Install grab bars in the bathroom near the toilet and tub.
- Make sure rugs and carpets are firmly attached to floors and stairs.
- Make sure that electrical cords are secured against baseboards to prevent tripping.
- Keep indoor and outdoor walkways and stairs in good repair.
- Install sturdy slip-resistant hand railings along stairs.

PREVENTING BURNS

- Check the temperature of bath water and heating pads. Run cold water before hot water.
- Lower thermostats of water heaters to provide warm rather than very hot water.
- Avoid smoking in bed or when sleepy.
- Install smoke alarms.
- Place a hand fire extinguisher in a convenient area of the home, e.g., the kitchen.
- Smother kitchen grease fires with a large lid or baking soda.
- Avoid wearing loose-fitting clothing when cooking.
- Do not overload electric circuits and keep electrical appliances in good repair.
- Keep passageways to outside doors unobstructed.

PREVENTING PEDESTRIAN ACCIDENTS

- Wear reflective or light-colored clothing at night.
- Cross streets at intersections with cross walks and traffic lights when possible; do not cross major streets in the middle of the block.
- Be sure to look both ways before stepping from the curb.

PREVENTING AUTOMOBILE ACCIDENTS

- Have regular eye examinations to assess vision, acquire appropriate refractive corrections, and detect other problems early.
- Wear good-quality gray or green sunglasses during daytime driving to reduce glare.
- Keep car windows clean and windshield wipers in good condition.
- Place mirrors on both sides of the car and always check rearview and side mirrors before changing lanes.
- Always look behind your vehicle for people or obstacles before backing up.
- Avoid smoking when driving, especially at night. Smoke can reduce visibility.
- Follow your physician's restrictions, if any, about when and where to drive.
- Learn the effects of prescribed medications on driving ability.
- Do not drink and drive.
- Stop periodically to stretch your muscles and rest your eyes.
- Leave car windows partially open and set the radio and fans low so that you can hear sirens and horns.
- Have your ability to drive periodically reevaluated.
- Keep your automobile in good repair and keep headlights, tail lights, and turn signals clean so they are visible to others.

Evaluation

Examples of outcome criteria for clients with potential for injury include:

The client will:

1. Identify potential environmental hazards.
2. Identify preventive measures for fire, and/or electric shock, and/or falls, and/or suffocation, and/or burns.
3. Identify safety adaptations required in the home.
4. Implement safety measures to prevent trauma, and/or poisoning, and/or suffocation.
5. Teach children safety practices.

Preventing Infectious Disease

An infectious, contagious, or **communicable disease** is any disease transmitted from one person to another. Modes of transmission include (a) direct contact, such as contact with excreta or discharges from open sores; (b) indirect contact, such as contact with contaminated drinking glasses, clothing, toys, or other objects; and (c) **vectors** (carriers), such as flies, mosquitoes, or other animals that spread the disease. Infections and infection control are discussed in Chapter 32.

Immunization is the process of producing or augmenting resistance to an infectious disease by introducing an antigen or antibody. The immune response and the various types of immunity—natural or acquired, and passive or active—are described in Chapter 32, page 682. The goal of immunization is to prevent the occurrence of an infectious or communicable disease.

Communicable diseases against which North Americans are commonly immunized include:

1. Poliomyelitis
2. Diphtheria
3. Pertussis (whooping cough)
4. Tetanus
5. Rubella (German or three-day measles)
6. Rubeola (measles)
7. Mumps

Epidemiology is the study of the occurrence, causes, and distribution of infectious disease as it occurs in humans. **Epidemic** describes the occurrence of disease in many people at the same time or in rapid succession in an area. **Pandemic** describes widespread occurrence of a disease in many parts of the world at the same time. Immunizations have greatly reduced pandemic incidence of disease. Smallpox and diphtheria, for example, have been virtually eliminated as a result of vigorous immunization programs. The incidence of poliomyelitis, rubella, and rubeola has decreased markedly since the development of vaccines.

Assessment and Nursing Diagnosis

Assessment of clients at risk of acquiring an infectious disease and nursing diagnoses for such clients are discussed in Chapter 32 on pages 685 and 686.

Intervention

Immunization

Immunization against communicable diseases is a preventive health measure advocated by government agencies in the United States and Canada.

Newborn infants have limited ability to produce antibodies until they are about 3 months of age. However, during the last months of pregnancy, certain maternal antibodies pass through the placenta, thus providing the baby with some passive immunity. This immunity is temporary; so it is vital to practice good hygiene around infants, sterilize their formulas, and not expose them to people who have infections.

At 2 or 3 months of age, children should receive their first immunizations. Antigens in the form of **vaccines** (living or dead microorganisms) or **toxoids** (detoxified toxins) are administered to induce active immunity. Tables 33–8 and 33–9 show the immunizations advised in the United States and Canada. In addition, rubella (German measles) vaccine is recommended for (a) all susceptible children between the ages of 15 months and 12 years and (b) female adolescents and women of childbearing age who are not protected against the disease. Rubella contracted during the first trimester of pregnancy may cause birth defects of the eyes, heart, and brain.

Immunizations are normally not given to persons with elevated temperatures, but mild infections, such as a cold without a fever, do not contraindicate immunizations. The most frequent reaction to an immunization is slightly elevated temperature; occasionally a reaction can be more severe—high temperature, sleepiness, or even convulsion. Physicians need to be consulted if the immunized person has a severe reaction or continues to feel ill 48 hours after the immunization.

Table 33–8 Recommended Schedule for Active Immunization of Normal Infants and Children

Recommended Age*	Vaccine(s)	Comments
2 months	DTP-1‡, OPV-1§	Can be given earlier in areas of high endemicity
4 months	DTP-2, OPV-2	6-week to 2-month interval desired between OPV doses to avoid interference
6 months	DTP-3	Additional dose of OPV at this time optional for use in areas with a high risk of polio exposure
15 months¶	MMR**	
18 months¶	DTP-4, OPV-3	Completion of primary series
4–6 years††	DTP-5, OPV-4	Preferably at or before school entry
14–16 years	Td§§	Repeat every 10 years throughout life

*These recommended ages should not be construed as absolute; that is, 2 months can be 6–10 weeks, etc.

†For all products used, consult manufacturer's package enclosure for instructions for storage, handling, and administration. Immunobiologics prepared by different manufacturers might vary, and those of the same manufacturer might change from time to time. The package insert should be followed for a specific product.

‡DTP—Diphtheria and tetanus toxoids and pertussis vaccine.

§OPV—Oral, attenuated poliovirus vaccine contains poliovirus types 1, 2, and 3.

¶Simultaneous administration of MMR, DTP, and OPV is appropriate for clients whose compliance with medical care recommendations cannot be assured.

**MMR—Live measles, mumps, and rubella viruses in a combined vaccine.

††Up to the seventh birthday.

§§Td—Adult tetanus toxoid and diphtheria toxoid in combination, which contains the same dose of tetanus toxoid as DTP or DT and a reduced dose of diphtheria toxoid.

Source: New immunization guidelines issued by the CDC, *Hospital Practice,* (March) 1983, 18:1000.

Risks Associated with Immunization

The risks of immunization include potential side-effects and complications, contamination of the serum with microorganisms other than the desired antigens, worsening of a natural disease, and failure to protect against the disease. Vaccinating a person whose resistance to infection is decreased or who is allergic to the vaccine could result in death. Nurses who administer immunizations must be knowledgeable about the indications, storage, dosage, preparation, and contraindications for each of the vaccines to be administered. Specific immunization guidelines and precautions are available from national public health service departments.

Tests for Immunity

It is sometimes advisable for the nurse to test clients for antibodies to a disease before giving the toxoid or vaccine. Examples of tests for immunity are:

1. Schick test for diphtheria
2. Moloney test for diphtheria
3. Dick test for scarlet fever
4. Tuberculin test for tuberculosis

Table 33–10 provides details about these tests.

Immunization and Testing for Hospital Personnel

Because they come in contact with clients with infections, hospital personnel are at risk of exposure to and transmission of vaccine-preventable diseases. Maintenance of immunity is therefore an essential part of a hospital's personnel health and infection control program. Immunization recommendations are made by the U.S. Public Health Service Immunization Practices Advisory Committee (ACIP). Each hospital usually develops its own specific immunization strategy because risks vary among different segments of the population and in different localities. Nurses who work in intensive care units, for example, may receive hepatitis B vaccine because they frequently administer blood, or they may be given immune globulins for hepatitis B soon after a needle-stick injury. Nurses who work in an obstetric unit may be immunized against rubella to protect pregnant clients. Serologic screening tests for susceptibility to either hepatitis B virus (HBV) or rubella may be conducted to determine the need for immunization of personnel before they enter a high-risk area.

Bacillus Calmette-Guérin (BCG) vaccination is available for personnel at risk of acquiring tuberculosis. Risk varies in accordance with local epidemiologic data. A screening tuberculin skin test is first carried out to determine need for the vaccine. Persons with negative reactions (see Table 33–10) are given the BCG vaccine. Initial

Table 33–9 Recommended Routine Immunization Schedules—Canada

Age	Agent	Description
2 months	DPT 0.5 ml	Combined diphtheria toxoid, pertussis vaccine, and tetanus toxoid
	TOPV (Sabin) 3 gtt	Trivalent oral polio vaccine
4 months	DPT 0.5 ml TOPV 3 gtt	
6 months	DPT 0.5 ml TOPV 3 gtt[1]	
12 months	MMR 0.5 ml[2]	Combined measles, mumps, and rubella vaccine (see note for rubella vaccine)
18 months	DPT 0.5 ml TOPV 3 gtt	
4–6 years	DPT 0.5 ml TOPV 3 gtt	
14–16 years	Td 0.5 ml TOPV 3 gtt[1]	Combined diphtheria and tetanus toxoid (weaker than DT, the diphtheria and tetanus toxoid used for the very young) given to persons 7 years and older
Adults	Tetanus toxoid every 10 years	

[1]These doses may be omitted if live (oral) polio vaccine is being used.

[2]Rubella vaccine is also indicated for all girls and women of childbearing age who lack proof of immunity. At all medical visits the opportunity should be taken to check whether girls and women of childbearing age have received rubella vaccine. A rubella titer test may be done. If the results are negative, immunization is given.

Source: From *A Guide to Immunization for Canadians,* 2d ed., 1984, National Advisory Committee on Immunization, Canada. Catalog No. H49-8/1984E (Ottawa: Minister of Supply and Services, Canada Health Protection Branch, Laboratory Centre for Disease Control), pp. 19–20.

chest radiography is recommended for persons with positive skin-test reactions to determine development of the disease.

Serologic screening tests can also be used to assess a person's susceptibility to the varicella-zoster virus (VZV). Varicella is the etiologic agent of varicella (chickenpox) and zoster (shingles). Personnel who lack immunity to varicella should not be assigned to employment areas where VZV is present.

Environmental Sanitation and Control

Sanitation has a direct effect on health. Contaminated food or water can cause widespread illness. Some environmental sanitation concerns follow.

Water Purification

Nearly all water is polluted while falling as rain or running over the surface of the ground or through the soil. Pollution by wastes further contaminates many water supplies. The most significant diseases spread by contaminated water are typhoid fever, dysentery, paratyphoids, infectious hepatitis, and cholera. The incidence of these diseases has declined in recent years, primarily due to (a) water treatment including filtration and chlorination, (b) protection of water supplies, (c) improved waste disposal methods, and (d) immunizations during epidemics.

The presence of fluoride in the water in minute quantities (0.6–1.7 mg/liter) has been found to reduce the incidence of dental caries significantly.

The U.S. Public Health Service has established purity standards for drinking water; these are enforced by state departments of health.

Pollution Control

Air pollution is the presence in the outdoor atmosphere of contaminants such as dust, fumes, gas, mist, odor, smoke, or vapor in sufficient quantities and of sufficient duration to be harmful to humans, plants, or animals. Air pollution is an increasing problem in all countries where urban

Research Note

A survey of 1473 nursing and medical personnel employed in two hospitals in a large metropolitan area was conducted to determine perceptions and beliefs about needle-handling practices and needle-stick injuries. Additional questions focused on responsibility for discarding needles and syringes and the correct practice for disposal of needles and syringes. Analyses were based on 488 responses (33%). Nurses at the 437-bed University Hospital handled more needles and experienced more needle-stick injuries than did nurses at the 300-bed Community Hospital. Needle-handling and needle-stick injuries among medical personnel at the two hospitals were similar, although University Hospital interns and residents and University Hospital fourth-year medical students handled more needles than did the medical staff at either hospital. A total of 164 (33.6%) respondents reported receiving one or more needle-stick injuries during 1983. A large proportion of respondents in each group reported that they did nothing about the needle-stick injuries they experienced. Carelessness was perceived by all groups to be the most common reason for needle-stick injuries. Most respondents reported some knowledge of proper needle disposal techniques and perceived lack of knowledge as the least important reason for needle-stick injuries. (Jackson et al. 1986)

Table 33–10 Selected Tests for Immunity

Test	Description	Reaction Indicating Lack of or No Immunity	Reaction Indicating Immunity
Schick test for diphtheria	A specified amount of diphtheria toxin is given intracutaneously.	A positive reaction (i.e., no antitoxin present) is indicated by reddening at the site of inoculation and **induration** (hardness) of 10 mm or more diameter in 24 to 48 hours.	A negative reaction, i.e., no redness or induration, indicates immunity.
Moloney test for diphtheria	A specified amount of diphtheria toxoid is given by intradermal injection.	A negative reaction indicates absence of antibodies (antitoxin).	A positive reaction i.e., an area of redness and induration of 10 mm or more in diameter in 12 to 24 hours, indicates immunity.
Dick test for scarlet fever	A specified amount of group A beta hemolytic streptococcus toxin is injected intracutaneously.	A positive reaction, i.e., redness of 1 cm or more in diameter at the inoculation site, indicates no immunity.	A negative reaction indicates previous exposure and neutralization of toxin and immunity.
Tuberculin (Mantoux) test for tuberculosis	A specified amount of tuberculin purified protein derivative (PPD) is given intradermally.	A negative reaction (no redness) indicates lack of exposure and immunity.	A positive reaction (area of redness) indicates previous exposure and immunity.

growth has meant industrial development and greater numbers of automobiles.

Health problems associated with air pollution include respiratory disease and eye, nose, and throat irritations.

Smoking is also generally recognized as a health hazard. The incidence of lung cancer and heart disease is higher in smokers than nonsmokers. Some people believe that cigarette smoke is also a health hazard even when not directly inhaled but merely in the environment. Nonsmokers are often segregated from smokers in theaters, restaurants, trains, and airplanes. Increasingly, smoking is being banned in areas of employment, such as offices and health care facilities.

Pollution of the environment is an increasingly acknowledged problem. The inappropriate disposal of industrial and nuclear wastes endangers the lives and health of people, animals, and plants. In all industrialized societies, waste disposal is a major problem that requires careful planning.

Disposal of Human Wastes

A very important aspect of environmental sanitation is disposal of human wastes. Sewage contains microorganisms, such as *Escherichia coli* (*E. coli*), which normally inhabits the intestines of humans, and *Aerobacter aerogenes* and *A. cloacae,* also found in feces and in soils. Diseases transmitted through sewage include typhoid fever, paratyphoid, poliomyelitis, and hepatitis.

In rural areas, sewage is usually disposed of in cesspools and septic tanks. Filtration, dilution, or activated sludge are three commonly used methods. The purposes of sewage treatment are (a) to make the sewage inoffensive, (b) to eliminate the danger of contaminating water and bathing areas, and (c) to prevent the destruction of fish and wildlife.

Milk Pasteurization

Pasteurization is the application of heat to milk to destroy disease-producing microorganisms. Unpasteurized milk can spread tuberculosis, diphtheria, dysentery, streptococcal infections, and Q fever. Milk must be not only free of disease, but also clean, with relatively few bacteria. To be safe and clean, milk must be given by healthy cows in clean barns, handled by clean, healthy workers working in clean surroundings with clean utensils, processed in separate milk rooms, and pasteurized.

Food Sanitation

Contaminated food can cause serious illness and death. The five types of contaminants are as follows:

1. Animal parasites, such as tapeworms, that may infest meat or fish
2. Microorganisms, such as the bacteria that cause typhoid fever and dysentery
3. Toxins, which are produced by certain bacteria in food, for example, *Clostridium botulinum*
4. Poisonous plants, such as toadstools
5. Poisonous sprays

Laws govern the preparation, storage, transportation, and sale of food, including the sanitation of eating and drinking establishments.

Insect and Rodent Control

Insects are significant transmitters of disease. Some significant vectors are mosquitoes, which pass on malaria, encephalitis, and yellow fever; flies, which carry bacteria from excreta to food; and cockroaches, which can contaminate food with bacteria from sewage. Fleas and lice that harbor microorganisms also can transmit disease, such as typhus.

There has been a worldwide effort to control the mosquito that transmits malaria. The incidence of malaria in the United States is low because of protection of rural homes from mosquitoes, drainage of swamp waters where mosquitoes breed, mass medication, and spraying. Other insects are also controlled by sprays.

Rats and other rodents are also a potential source of disease, such as hemorrhagic jaundice and amebic dysentery. It is estimated that the rat population in the United States equals the human population. Rats can be controlled in two ways: adequate garbage disposal to limit their food supply, and poisons, such as the coumarin anticoagulant, Warfarin sodium.

Chapter Highlights

- The provision of a safe external environment is a constant concern of the nurse.
- Education is a major health protection strategy in preventing accidents and infectious disease.
- When planning to meet safety needs of clients, nurses need to consider physical factors in the environment and the psychologic and physiologic state of the individual.
- Accidents are a major cause of death among individuals of all ages in the United States and Canada.
- The seven major causes of accidental deaths in the United States are motor vehicle accidents, falls, fires, drowning, poisoning, suffocation, and firearms.
- Most accidents are due to negligence and are preventable.
- Nursing assessment of the clients at risk includes assessment of age, life-style, sensory-perceptual alterations, level of awareness, mobility, emotional state, language barriers, history of previous accidents, and knowledge and use of safety precautions.
- Nursing diagnoses for clients at risk of accidental injury can be categorized as potential for trauma, for poisoning, and for suffocation.
- Nursing intervention must include education in accident prevention and modification of the environment to make it safe.
- Nurses must be familiar with the fire procedures in their employing agency.
- In the event of a fire, the nurse must protect clients from injury and contain and put out the fire.
- Falls are a common cause of injury among the very young, the elderly, and the ill or injured.
- To prevent falls, the nurse must provide constant surveillance for infants and young children and carefully assess older clients' safety needs.
- Side rails and handrails protect hospitalized clients from falls; restraints keep clients from falling and from inflicting injuries on themselves and others.
- Because restraints restrict a client's basic freedom to move, careful assessment and accurate, complete documentation are important when restraints are used.
- Poisoning from numerous plants, household chemicals, and medications is a major threat to young curious children.
- Major reasons for poisoning in children are inadequate supervision and improper storage of household toxic substances.
- Faulty electrical equipment and improper grounding pose health hazards in the hospital and the home.
- Electrical accidents can be prevented by using grounded outlets and plugs, putting protective covers over outlets, keeping appliances in good repair, and making sure that electrical wiring and circuits meet safety standards.
- Prolonged exposure to excessive noise can produce hearing loss.
- In hospitals, radioactive substances are used for both diagnostic and treatment purposes; agency policy should be followed to safeguard clients and staff from inadvertent exposure.
- Infants are completely dependent on parents to protect them from all environmental hazards.
- Protective measures for infants include putting guard rails at the top and bottom of stairs, covering electrical wall outlets, giving the child large soft toys that do not have parts the infant can remove and swallow, using only cribs with closely spaced slats, and constantly observing the child during feeding and bathing.
- Toddlers are curious and must be protected from such hazards as medicines, sharp tools, and cleaning solutions. Fences should enclose pools or ditches and the play area. Teaching toddlers that *no* and *don't* are spoken at times of risk is essential.

- Preschoolers can be taught to observe and to act safely. They should be taught to observe traffic safety, to play in safe areas, to swim, and to keep toys from underfoot. Preschoolers imitate the behavior of parents, who can use this trait to teach safe behavior.
- School-age children prefer grown-up equipment to toys and need instruction in safe use of such equipment.
- Adolescents need water safety instruction and information about the hazards of motor vehicles, firearms, and drugs and alcohol.
- Because of their diminished sensory acuity and balance, elderly people need to make the home safe. They also need education about ways to prevent automobile and pedestrian accidents.
- Immunization of infants, children, and health personnel working in high-risk areas is vital to prevent the spread of communicable disease.
- Environmental sanitation has a direct effect on health. Areas of concern include water purification, environmental pollution, disposal of human wastes, milk pasteurization, food sanitation, and the control of insects and rodents.

Suggested Readings

Berger, M. E., and Hubner, K. F. August 1983. Hospital hazards: Diagnostic radiation. *American Journal of Nursing.* 83:1155–59.

This guide to radiation management looks at the pros and cons of portable radiography and fluoroscopy. It includes some of the reasons for radiation mismanagement.

DiFabio, S. May 1981. Nurses' reactions to restraining patients. *American Journal of Nursing* 81:973–75.

DiFabio interviewed 15 nurses in a psychiatric nursing unit where clients had to be put in restraints. Twenty-eight different responses were categorized, including fear, guilt, anxiety, and inadequacy.

Hernandez, M., and Miller, J. March/April 1986. How to reduce falls. *Geriatric Nursing* 7:97–102.

Hernandez and Miller collected data on falls on a geropsychiatric unit to identify precipitants and predictors of falls, to develop and test levels of all precautions, and to decrease the incidence of falls. Findings are shown in a Falls Assessment Tool. Included are risk factors identified, a comparison of nonfallers and fallers, precautions to prevent falls, and recommendations for nurse administrators and staff.

Rice, M. A., and Kibbee, P. E. March/April 1983. Review: Identifying the adolescent substance abuser. *The American Journal of Maternal Child Nursing* 8:139–42.

Commonly used depressants (downers) and stimulants (uppers) and their effects are described. The telltale clues and causes of abuse of each are shown in a table.

Valenti, W. M., and Anarella, J. P. April 1986. Brief reports: Survey of hospital personnel on the understanding of the acquired immune deficiency syndrome. *American Journal of Infection Control* 14:60–63.

The recent spread of the acquired immune deficiency syndrome (AIDS) has generated a significant amount of media coverage, much of which creates confusion and alarm instead of disseminating information. Valenti and Anarella devised a tool to measure the respondents' understanding of the disease and to determine how concerned they were about dealing with persons with AIDS, what sources of information were available, and what additional information employees wanted about AIDS. This article includes the true-false questionnaire used and the results of the survey.

Widder, B. September/October 1985. A new device to decrease falls. *Geriatric Nursing* 6:287–88.

A new device called the Ambularm, developed by the associate director of medicine at the Saint Vincent Hospital and Medical Center in Portland, Oregon, and a colleague, summons help when the client is in the act of arising. It has reduced falls by 45%.

Selected References

Accident facts. 1985. Chicago: National Safety Council.

Barbieri, E. B. March 1983. Patient falls are not patient accidents. *Journal of Gerontological Nursing* 9:164–73.

Bozian, M. W., and Clark, H. M. March 1980. Counteracting sensory changes in the aging. *American Journal of Nursing* 80:473–76.

Breeding, M. A., and Wollin, M. May 1976. Working safely around implanted radiation sources. *Nursing 76* 6:58–63.

Burnside, I. M. 1981. Falls: A common problem in the elderly. In Burnside, I. M., editor. *Nursing and the aged.* 2d ed. New York: McGraw-Hill.

Campbell, E. B.; Williams, M. A.; and Mlynarczyk, S. M. February 1986. After the fall: Confusion. *American Journal of Nursing* 86:151–53.

Carmack, B. J. August 1981. Fighting fire: Your role in hospital fire safety. *Nursing 81* 11:61–63.

Chipman, C. September 1981. What does it mean when a patient falls? Part I. Pinpointing the cause. *Geriatrics* 36:83–85.

Consultation: Promoting electric safety. May 1983. *Nursing 83* 13:129 (Horsham edition).

Cooper, S. July/August 1981. Accidents and older adults. *Geriatric Nursing* 2:287–90.

DeSwarte J. January/February 1984. Nursing's responsibility in promoting the use of car safety seats for children. *Home Health Care Nurse* 2:23–25.

Ford, A. H. September/October 1980. Use of automobile restraining devices for infants. *Nursing Research* 29:281–84.

Friedman, F. B. January 1983. Restraints: When all else fails, there still are alternatives. *RN* 46:79–80, 82, 84.

Gray-Vickrey, M. May/June 1984. Education to prevent falls. *Geriatric Nursing* 5:179–83.

Hernandez, M., and Miller, J. March/April 1986. How to reduce falls. *Geriatric Nursing* 7:97–102.

Hyams, P. J.; Marge, C. S.; Stuewe, R. N.; and Heitzer, V. February

1984. Herpes zoster causing varicella (chickenpox) in hospital employees: Cost of a casual attitude. *American Journal of Infection Control* 12:2–5.

Jackson, M. M.; Dechairo, D. C.; and Gardner, D. F. February 1986. Perceptions and beliefs of nursing and medical personnel about needle-handling practices and needle-stick injuries. *American Journal of Infection Control* 14:1–10.

James, S. M.; Skolnick, R. B.; Habel, L.; and Agee, B. A. February 1985. A survey of hepatitis B vaccination programs for hospital employees. *American Journal of Infection Control* 13:32–34.

Kim, M. J.; McFarland, G. K.; and McLane, A. M. 1984. *Pocket guide to nursing diagnoses.* St. Louis: C. V. Mosby Co.

Kohl, H. W. June 1985. Rubella screening and vaccination follow-up by a hospital employee health office. *American Journal of Infection Control* 13:124–27.

Lee, P. S., and Pash, B. J. February 1983. Preventing patient falls. *Nursing 83* 13:118, 120 (Canadian edition, pp. 14–15).

Louis, M. March 1983. Falls and their causes. *Journal of Gerontological Nursing* 9:142–56.

Lynn, F. H. June 1980. Incidents: Need they be accidents? *American Journal of Nursing* 80:1098–1101.

MacLean, J.; Shamian, J.; Butcher, P.; et al. June 1982. Restraining the elderly agitated patient. *Canadian Nurse* 78:44–46.

Marcus, D. F. May/June 1981. Child car seats: A must for safety. *Pediatric Nursing* 7:13–17.

Meth, I. M. July 1980. Electrical safety in the hospital. *American Journal of Nursing* 80:1344–48.

Misik, I. August 1981. About using restraints—with restraint. *Nursing 81* 11:50–55.

Mott, S. R.; Fazckas, N. F.; and James, S. R. 1985. *Nursing care of children and families.* Menlo Park, Calif.: Addison-Wesley Publishing Co.

Nursing guidelines for the use of restraints in nonpsychiatric settings. March 1983. *Journal of Gerontological Nursing* 9:180–81.

Riffle, K. L. May/June 1982. Falls: Kinds, causes, and prevention. *Geriatric Nursing* 3:165–69.

Rumack, B. H. October 1980. The poison control center: Answers not antidotes. *Hospital Practice* 15:123–29.

Snider, D. E., and Cauthen, G. M. December 1984. Tuberculin skin testing of hospital employees: Infection, "boosting," and two-step testing. *American Journal of Infection Control* 12:305–11.

Sumner, S. M. July 1985. Action STAT! Electric shock. *Nursing 85* 15:43.

Trefler, E. September 1982. Arm restraints during functional activities. *American Journal of Occupational Therapy* 36:599–600.

Witte, N. S. November 1979. Why the elderly fall. *American Journal of Nursing* 79:1950–52.

Williams, B. G., and Pruitt, B. October 1984. Natural and induced immunity to hepatitis B virus among the staff of a pediatric oncology center. *American Journal of Infection Control* 12:261–65.

Williams, M. V. February 1986. Infection control and the pregnant health care worker. *American Journal of Infection Control* 14:20–27.

Williams, W. W. February 1984. CDC guidelines for the prevention and control of nosocomial infections: Guideline for infection control in hospital personnel. *American Journal of Infection Control* 12:34–57.

Wyatt, D. M. February 1985. Are you prepared for a hospital fire? *Nursing 85* 15:51.

Yarmesch, M., and Sheafor, M. July/August 1984. The decision to restrain. *Geriatric Nursing* 5:242–44.

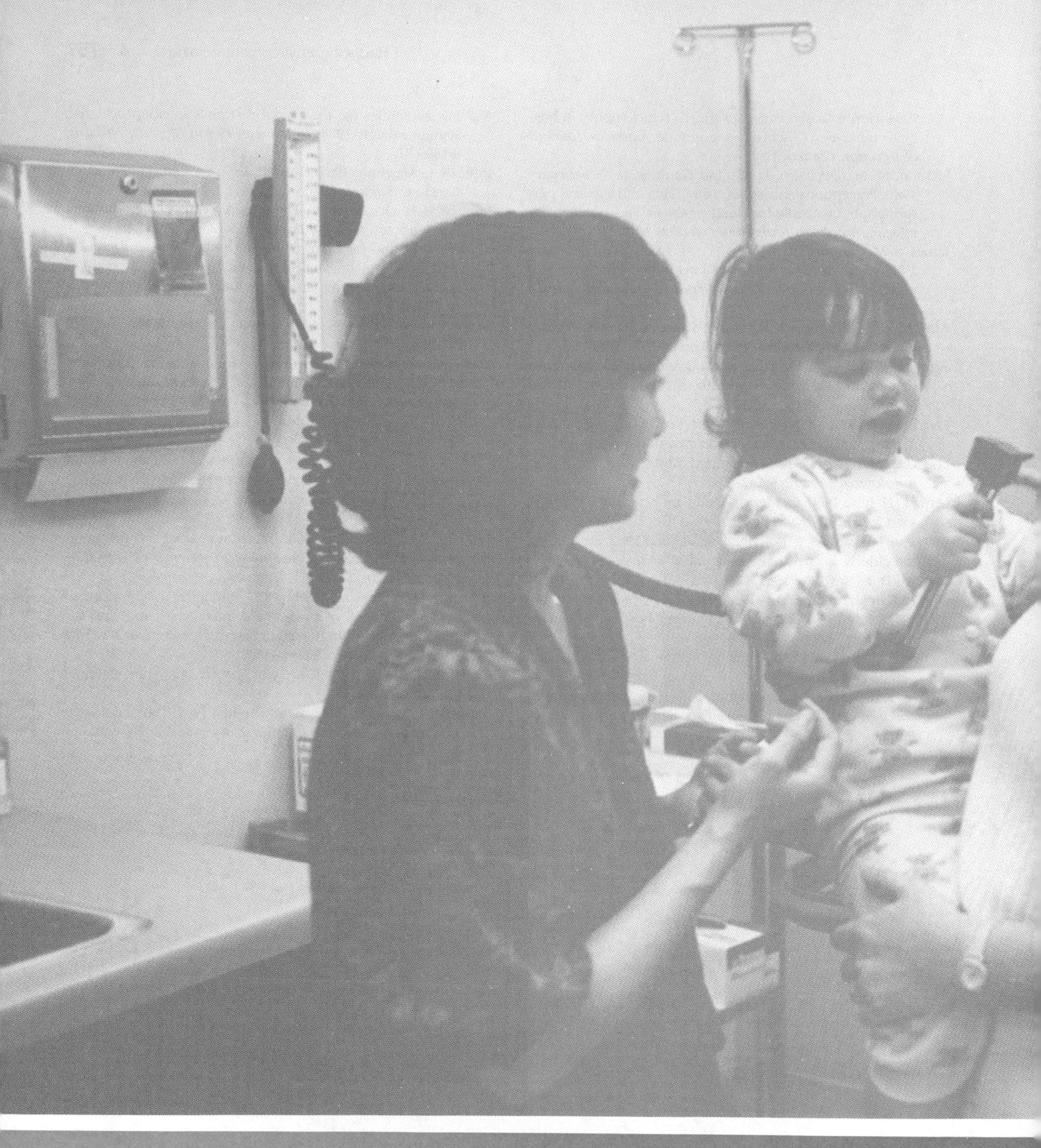

If nurses are to succeed, they must believe in the value of their services and in their own ability to perform them. (Leah Curtin)

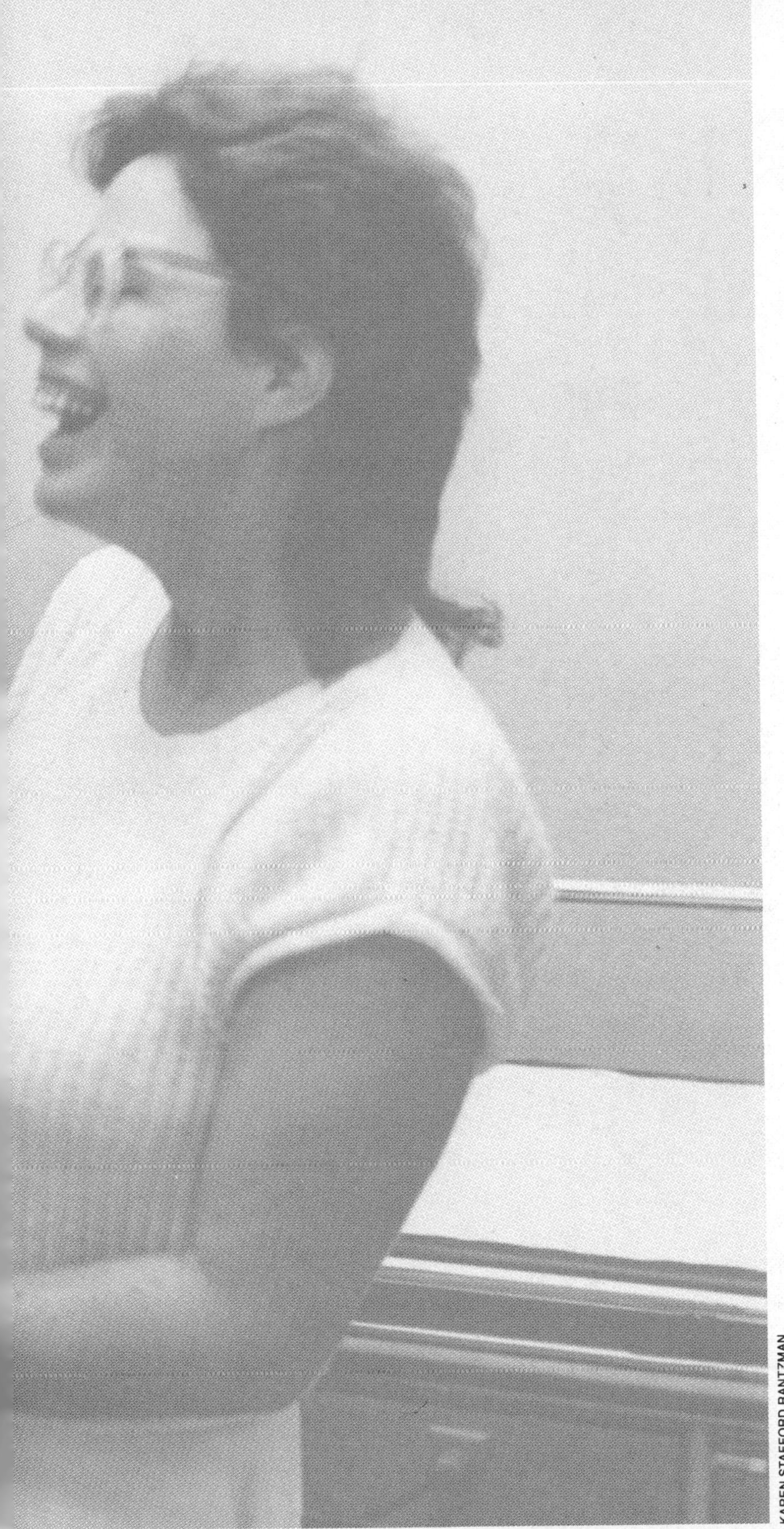
KAREN STAFFORD RANTZMAN

UNIT **8**

Health Assessment

Contents

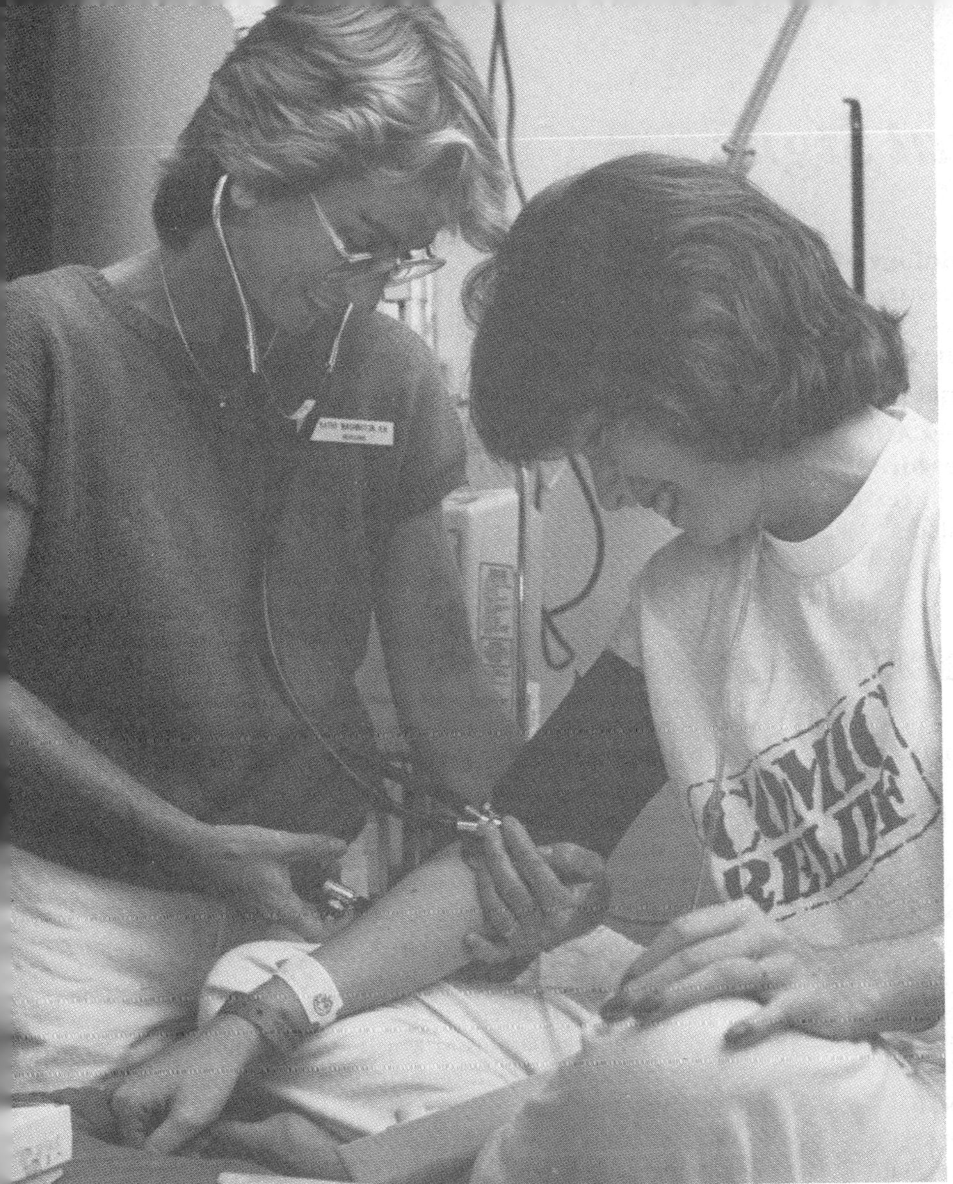

WILLIAM THOMPSON

CHAPTER 34

Assessing Vital Signs

Contents

(continued)

34 *Assessing Vital Signs*

Contents *(continued)*

Objectives

1. Understand essential facts about body temperature, pulse, respiration, and blood pressure.
   1.1 Define selected terms associated with the vital signs.
   1.2 Identify appropriate times to assess vital signs.
   1.3 Describe the core-shell concept of body temperature.
   1.4 Describe five factors influencing the body's heat production.
   1.5 Identify four ways in which the body loses heat.
   1.6 Describe the system that regulates body temperature.
   1.7 Identify the changes that occur in the vital signs as age increases.
   1.8 Differentiate stroke volume output from cardiac output.
   1.9 Identify nine pulse sites commonly used to assess the pulse and reasons for their use.
   1.10 Differentiate internal from external respiration.
   1.11 Differentiate thoracic from abdominal breathing.
   1.12 Describe the mechanics of breathing.
   1.13 Describe mechanisms that control respirations.
   1.14 Differentiate systolic from diastolic blood pressure.
   1.15 Identify some major factors that affect body temperature, pulse, respirations, and blood pressure.
2. Understand essential facts about fever, hypothermia, and related thermal disorders.
   2.1 Describe the mechanism of a fever.
   2.2 Identify three types of fevers.
   2.3 Identify appropriate nursing interventions for the chilling phase of a fever.
   2.4 Identify appropriate nursing interventions for the flush phase of a fever.
   2.5 Describe three types of hypothermia.
   2.6 Differentiate heat stroke from heat cramps and heat exhaustion.
   2.7 Identify clinical signs of fever, hypothermia, heat stroke, heat cramp, and heat exhaustion.
3. Understand essential facts related to assessment methods used to measure vital signs.
   3.1 Contrast oral, rectal, and axillary measurements of body temperature.
   3.2 Identify situations in which measurements of body temperature by mouth, rectum, and axilla are indicated and contraindicated.
   3.3 Identify recommended intervals between placing a thermometer and obtaining a temperature reading.
   3.4 Identify alternative methods of measuring body temperature.
   3.5 Identify qualitative data needed to assess pulse and respirations.
   3.6 Explain how to locate the apex of the heart.
   3.7 Describe various methods and sites used to measure blood pressure.
   3.8 Give reasons for selected steps of vital signs procedures.
4. Demonstrate skill in performing procedures for assessing the vital signs of clients of all ages.
   4.1 Assemble all necessary equipment before the procedure.
   4.2 Carry out essential medical aseptic practices such as hand washing and appropriate cleaning and disinfection of equipment.
   4.3 Prepare the client, physically and psychologically.
   4.4 Implement steps to acquire the vital signs measurements accurately and safely.
   4.5 Record the vital signs measurements accurately.

Terms

accidental hypothermia
apical pulse
apnea
apneustic breathing
arrhythmia
arterial blood pressure
arteriosclerosis
basal metabolic rate
Biot's respirations
bladder (of a cuff)
blood pressure cuff
body temperature
bradycardia
bradypnea
brown fat
cardiac output
chemical thermogenesis
Cheyne-Stokes respiration
circadian rhythm
compliance
conduction
convection
core temperature
costal (thoracic) breathing
diaphoresus
diaphragmatic (abdominal) breathing
diastole
diastolic pressure
diurnal cycle
dyspnea
eupnea
exhalation (expiration)
external respiration
fever (pyrexia)
forced convection
frostbite
gluconeogenesis
glycolysis
heat balance
heat cramps
heat exhaustion
heat stroke
hematocrit
hyperpyrexia
hypertension
hyperventilation
hypotension
hypothermia
hypoventilation
induced hypothermia
inhalation (inspiration)
insensible vaporization
intermittent (quotidian) fever
internal respiration
Korotkoff's sounds
Kussmaul's breathing
lumen
mean blood pressure
meniscus
metabolic rate
metabolism
natural convection
obligatory heat
orthostatic hypotension
peripheral pulse
pulse
pulse pressure
pulse rhythm
pulse volume
pulsus regularis
pyrogen
radiation
rales (rhonchi)
relapsing fever
remittent fever
respiration
shivering
sphygmomanometer (aneroid and mercury)
stethoscope
stridor
stroke volume output
surface temperature
systole
systolic pressure
tachycardia
tachypnea
tidal volume
vaporization
ventilation
viscosity
vital capacity
vital (cardinal) signs

Vital Signs

The **vital** or **cardinal signs** are body temperature, pulse, respirations, and blood pressure. These signs, which should be looked at in total, are used to monitor the functions of the body. The signs reflect changes in function that otherwise might not be observed.

Monitoring a client's vital signs should not be an automatic or routine procedure; it should be a thoughtful, scientific assessment. When and how often to assess a specific client's vital signs are chiefly nursing judgments determined by the client's health status. Some hospitals have policies about taking clients' temperature, for example, and physicians may order assessment of a vital sign, e.g., "Blood pressure q2h." Ordered assessments should be considered minimal, and nurses should measure a client's vital signs more often if his or her health status requires it. For times to assess vital signs, see list to the right.

Times to Assess Vital Signs

- When a client has a change in health status or reports symptoms such as feeling hot or faint
- Upon admission to a health care agency
- According to a nursing or medical order
- Before and after surgery or an invasive diagnostic procedure
- Before and after the administration of a medication that could affect the respiratory or cardiovascular systems; for example, before giving a digitalis preparation that affects the heart
- Before and after any nursing intervention, e.g., ambulating a client who has been on bed rest, that could affect any of the vital signs

Body Temperature

Body temperature is the balance between the heat produced by the body and the heat lost from the body. There are two kinds of body temperature: core temperature and surface temperature. **Core temperature** is the temperature of the deep tissues of the body. It remains relatively constant and varies as little as ±1 F except when a person

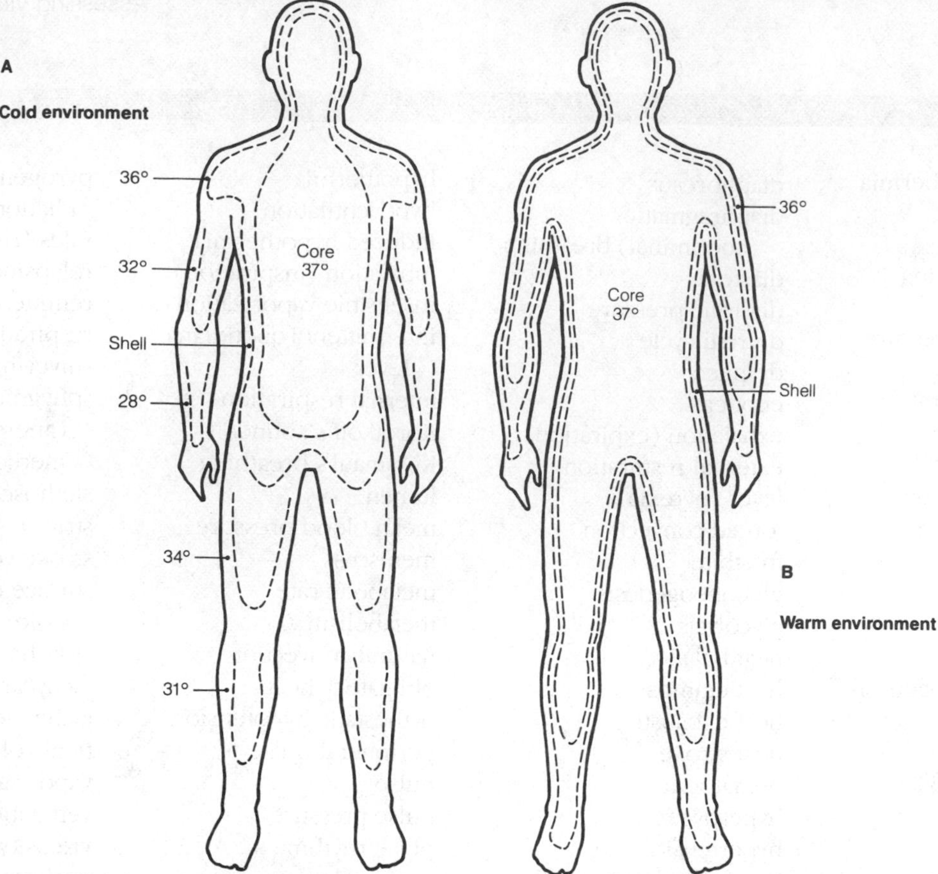

Figure 34–1 Core-shell concept in the human body. The temperature of the core is kept constant over a wide range of ambient temperatures. The temperature of the surface and underlying areas (shell) varies with the ambient temperature. The shell is "thicker" in a cold environment (A) and "thinner" in a warm environment (B).

Source: Redrawn, with permission, from J. Aschoff and R. Wever, *Naturwissenschaften,* 1958, 45:477.

has a fever. The **surface temperature**, by contrast, rises and falls in response to the environment (Guyton 1986, p. 849).

Core-Shell Concept

The core-shell concept is a physiologic paradigm of the body's heat sources and heat loss. See Figure 34–1. The body is visualized as having a core and shell. The core consists of the cranium, thorax, abdominal cavity, and pelvic cavity. The shell is the skin, the subcutaneous tissues, and fat. Fat is an insulator in that it conducts heat only one-third as readily as other body tissues (Guyton 1986, p. 849). In a healthy person, the core temperature is relatively constant (37 C, 98.6 F) while the shell temperature varies with the ambient temperature. During heat loss, heat is transferred from the core to the shell by the circulating blood. When warm blood is brought to the surface, the shell becomes "thinner." When the body is in a cold environment, the ratio of core to shell decreases, and the temperature of the shell decreases.

The core is the major source of heat in a person at rest. Thus, the cranium, thorax, abdomen, and pelvis are the body's "hot spots" (Vick 1984, p. 890). When a person exercises, the skeletal muscles become sources of heat.

Normal Body Temperature

The normal core body temperature is not an exact point on a scale but a range of temperatures. When measured orally, the average body temperature of an adult is between 36.7 C (98 F) and 37 C (98.6 F). See Figure 34–2 for the normal ranges of body temperature.

Balance Between Heat Production and Heat Loss

The body continually produces heat as a by-product of metabolism. Carbohydrates, fats, and proteins are used to synthesize large quantities of adenosine triphosphate (ATP), which in turn is used as source of energy by body cells. However, about 50% of the energy in food becomes heat rather than ATP, and further heat is produced as the food is changed to ATP (Guyton 1986, p. 844). When the amount of heat produced by the body exactly equals the amount of heat lost, the person is in **heat balance**.

Heat Production

Metabolism is all the chemical reactions of the cells of the body. The **metabolic rate** is the rate of heat production during the chemical reactions. The **basal metabolic rate** is the rate of energy utilization in the body during wakeful and absolute rest. The basal metabolic rate, therefore, is a measure of the activity of the body tissues independent of exercise and digestion.

A number of factors affect the body's heat production. The most important are as follows:

Basal metabolic rate A person's basal metabolic rate (BMR) is usually determined by placing the person in basal conditions. (See below.) The rate of oxygen use is then measured, and the BMR is calculated from the oxygen used and expressed in kilocalories. The kilocalories are then expressed in terms of the individual's body surface area ($kcal/m^2$), e.g., BMR = 70 $kcal/kg^{0.75}$/day (Vick 1984, p. 909). BMR is normally expressed as a percentage above or below normal.

BMRs vary with sex and age. After the age of 2 years, a female's BMR is usually about 5% to 10% less than a male's of the same age and sizc. The greatest difference between sexes (18% to 27%) occurs during adolescence (Vick 1984, p. 909). Metabolic rates decrease with age. From birth to about 20 years of age, the decline is rapid, after which it slows considerably (Vick 1984, p. 910).

Muscle activity Muscle activity, including shivering, can greatly increase metabolic rate. For example, maximum muscle exercise can increase heat production to about 50 times normal (Guyton 1986, p. 845). A person doing heavy work, e.g., mining, can use as much as 6000 to 7000 kcal, or 3.5 times the BMR (Guyton 1986, p. 846).

Shivering is skeletal muscle contraction, which increases heat production. The center for shivering is located in the dorsomedial portion of the posterior hypothalamus. This center is usually inhibited by signals from the heat center in the preoptic thermostatic arca; however, it is excited by cold signals from the skin and spinal cord. Once the center is stimulated, signals travel through the bilateral tracts, down the brain stem, into the lateral columns of the spinal cord, and to the anterior motor neurons. From there, the signals travel to the skeletal muscles throughout the body increasing muscle tone and heat production. During maximal shivering, body heat production can be increased four to five times normal (Guyton 1986, p. 855).

Nurses must be aware that muscle activity increases heat production, particularly when caring for clients who already have elevated temperatures. Even walking down a hall or moving from a bed to a chair can increase heat production and thus body temperature. Also, shivering can be brought about by a lowered surface temperature even when the core temperature is elevated, further increasing the client's core temperature.

Thyroxine output In response to stimulation of the preoptic area, the hypothalamus increases the production of the neurosecretory hormone thyrotropin-releasing hormone. This hormone is carried to the anterior pituitary gland, where it stimulates the secretion of thyroid-stimulating hormone. This thyroid-stimulating hormone stimulates the thyroid gland to secrete thyroxine.

The increased thyroxine output increases the rate of cellular metabolism throughout the body. This effect is called **chemical thermogenesis**: the stimulation of heat production in the body through increased cellular metabolism.

Thyroid hormone (TH) in normal amounts assists in the synthesis of protein, which is reflected in a positive nitrogen balance. For more information on nitrogen bal-

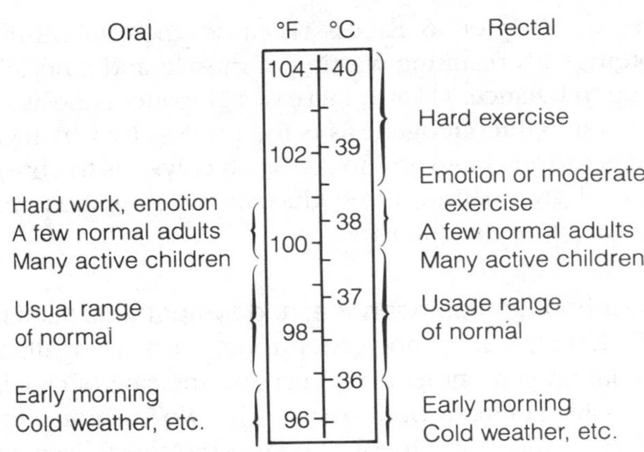

Figure 34–2 Estimated ranges of body temperatures in normal persons

Source: From E. F. DuBois, *Fever and the regulation of body temperature* (Springfield, Ill.: Charles C. Thomas, 1948). Courtesy of Charles C. Thomas, Publisher, Springfield, Illinois.

Basal Conditions for Measuring Metabolic Rate

- No food for at least 12 hours: Food increases the metabolic rate.
- A restful night's sleep: Rest reduces sympathetic nervous system activity and metabolic activity.
- No strenuous exercise after sleeping and at least 30 minutes rest in a reclining position.
- As little psychologic and physical stimulation as possible.
- Air temperature between 20 to 26.6 C (68 to 80 F): Below 20 C (68 F), sympathetic nervous system activity increases; above 26.6 C (80 F), discomfort and sweating, for example, increase metabolic rate. (Guyton 1986, p. 847)

ance, see Chapter 46. Excess TH causes the catabolism of protein, with resulting wasting of muscle and a negative nitrogen balance. TH also increases gluconeogenesis and glycolysis. **Gluconeogenesis** is the process by which glucose is formed from amino acids. **Glycolysis** is the breakdown of glycogen into free glucose, which is then available for rapid metabolism.

Epinephrine, norepinephrine, and sympathetic stimulation Epinephrine, norepinephrine, and sympathetic stimulation can immediately increase the rate of cellular metabolism in many body tissues. The two hormones epinephrine and norepinephrine directly affect liver and muscle cells, thereby increasing cellular activity. Of more importance is sympathetic stimulation of **brown fat**. When the cells of this fat are stimulated, they produce a large amount of heat. The newborn infant has a large number of these fat cells, and maximum sympathetic stimulation can increase the infant's metabolism more than 100% (Guyton 1986, p. 846).

Increased temperature of body cells Increased body temperature (fever) also increases the cellular metabolic rate, due to the fact that chemical reactions increase an average of about 120% for every 10 C rise in temperature (Guyton 1986, p. 846). Although this mechanism is mediated somewhat by the body's temperature control system (see later in this chapter) the presence of fever acts to increase the body's temperature further.

Heat Loss

Heat is lost from the body through radiation, conduction, convection, and vaporization. See Figure 34–3. Sweating, panting, lowering the environmental temperature, and wearing less clothing all promote heat loss through one or more of these methods.

Radiation **Radiation** is a method of transfer of heat from the surface of one object to the surface of another without contact between the two objects. One object contains more heat than the other; the former loses heat through radiation. For example, a nude person standing in a room at normal room temperature loses about 60% of her or his total heat loss through radiation (Guyton 1986, p. 850). Most heat loss through radiation is in the form of infrared rays.

Conduction **Conduction** is the transfer of heat from one molecule to another. Again, a temperature gradient is implied: The heat transfers to a molecule of lower temperature. Conductive transfer cannot take place without contact between the molecules and normally accounts for minimal heat loss except, for example, when a body is immersed in ice water. The amount of heat transferred depends on the temperature difference and the amount and duration of contact.

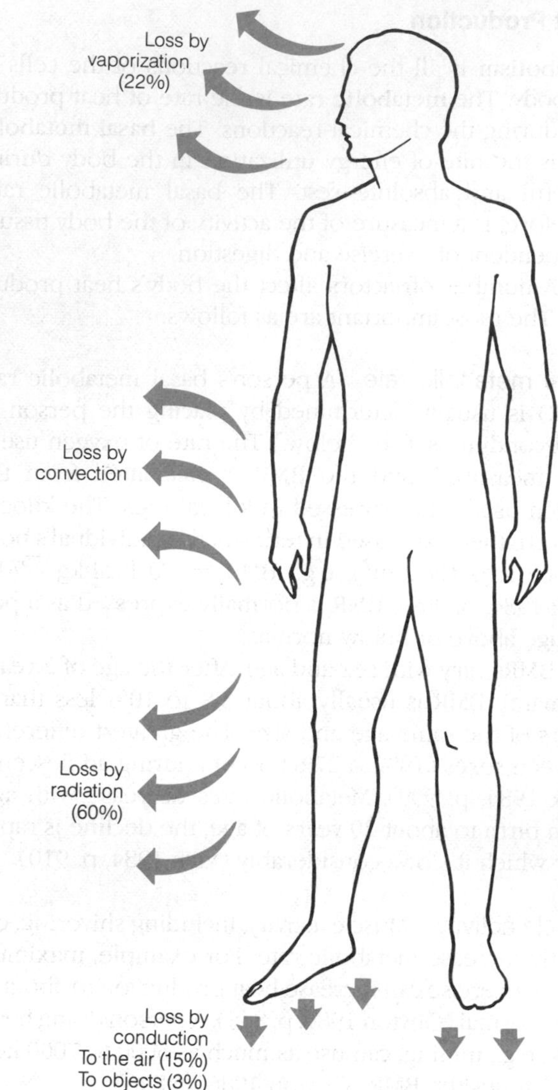

Figure 34–3 Sources of heat loss from the body

Convection **Convection** is the dispersion of heat by air currents. There is usually a small amount of warm air adjacent to the body. This warm air rises and is replaced by cooler air, so people always lose a small amount of heat loss through convection. This type of convection is called **natural convection**. The precise mechanism of such heat loss is that the heat is first conducted to the air and dissipated by convection. In **forced convection**, air is moved artificially, for example, by a fan. The layer of warm air adjacent to the body moves away more quickly than it normally does, and the heat loss is accordingly greater.

Vaporization **Vaporization** or evaporation is the fourth method of heat loss. Vaporization occurs continuously from the respiratory tract and from the mucosa of the mouth. This is called **insensible vaporization**, and accounts for 20% to 25% of the heat lost from the body (Vick 1984, p. 892). Body sweating increases heat loss by this method, providing that the surrounding air is not saturated (unable to hold more water vapor). Vaporization is a highly variable method of heat loss. It depends upon the relative humidity of the surrounding air. See Chapter 46 for more information about the electrolytes in sweat.

Regulation of Body Temperature

The system that regulates body temperature has three main parts: sensors in the shell and in the core, an integrator in the hypothalamus, and effector system that adjust the production and loss of heat.

Sensors

Most sensors or sensory receptors are in the skin, which is a major part of the shell. There are fewer receptors in the tongue, respiratory tract, and viscera. The skin has receptors of both cold and warmth; however, far more receptors detect cold than warmth (Guyton 1986, p. 854). Therefore, cold is more efficiently detected than warmth by skin sensors.

When the skin becomes chilled over the entire body, three physiologic processes take place to increase the body temperature:

1. Shivering increases heat production.
2. Sweating is inhibited to decrease heat loss.
3. Vasoconstriction decreases heat loss.

The receptors in the body's core, i.e., in the abdominal viscera, in the spinal cord, and in or around the large veins, respond only to the body's core temperature, not to the body's surface temperature. They also detect mainly cold rather than warmth. Thermoreceptors in the hypothalamus are also sensitive to the core temperature.

Hypothalamic Integrator

The preoptic area of the hypothalamus contains a center that controls the core temperature. Some sensors are sensitive to heat, and some are sensitive to cold. Neurons transmit signals in response to signals from the sensors in the body shell.

When the sensors in the hypothalamus detect heat, they send out signals intended to reduce the temperature, i.e., decrease heat production and increase heat loss. When the cold sensors are stimulated, signals are sent out to increase heat production and decrease heat loss.

Effector System

The signals from the cold-sensitive receptors of the hypothalamus initiate vasoconstriction, shivering, and the release of epinephrine, which increases cellular metabolism and hence heat production. Stimuli also suppress the release of thyroxine by the thyroid gland. When the warmth-sensitive receptors in the hypothalamus are stimulated, they send out signals that initiate sweating and peripheral vasodilation.

In addition, the somatic nervous system is stimulated so that the person consciously makes appropriate adjustments, such as putting on additional clothing in response to cold or turning on a fan in response to heat.

Factors Affecting Body Temperature

Nurses should be aware of the factors that can affect a client's body temperature so that they can recognize normal temperature variations and understand the significance of body temperature measurements that deviate from normal.

1. *Age.* Age affects core body temperature to some degree. See Table 34–1. A newborn's body temperature mechanism is imperfect. As a result, the infant is greatly influenced by the temperature of the environment and must be protected from extreme changes. In the newborn, the normal body temperature measured by axilla fluctuates between 36.1 and 37.7 C (97 and 100 F). In fact, a child's temperature continues to be more labile than an adult's until puberty. A 2-year-old's body temperature is about 37.2 C (98.9 F); a 12-year-old's, an average of 37 C (98.6 F), the same as an adult's.

   In elderly adults, body temperature drops to an average of 36 C (96.8 F). Thus, elderly people have less heat to lose than younger adults before reaching hypothermia (very low temperature levels). Kurtz found that a group of elderly people had a mean temperature (orally measured) of 36.2 C (97.2 F) (Kurtz 1982, p. 85). Studies by Kolanowski and Gunter indicate that many elderly people, particularly those over 75 years, are at risk of hypothermia (in this case temperatures

Table 34–1 Variations in Vital Signs by Age

Age	Average Temperature	Pulse Rate at Rest/Min Average	Pulse Rate at Rest/Min Range	Respiratory Rate/Min	Mean Blood Pressure
Newborn	36.1–37.7 C 97.0–100.0 F (axilla)	125	70–190	30–80	78 systolic 42 diastolic by flush technique: 30–60
1 year	37.7 C 99.7 F	120	80–160	20–40	96 systolic 65 diastolic
2 years	37.2 C 98.9 F	110	80–130	20–30	100 systolic 63 diastolic
4 years		100	80–120	20–30	97 systolic 64 diastolic
6 years	37.0 C 98.6 F (oral)	100	75–115	20–25	98 systolic 65 diastolic
8 years		90	70–110		106 systolic 70 diastolic
10 years		90	70–110	17–22	110 systolic 72 diastolic
12 years		Male: 85 Female: 90	65–105 70–110	17–22	116 systolic 74 diastolic
14 years		Male: 80 Female: 85	60–100 65–105		120 systolic 76 diastolic
16 years		Male: 75 Female: 80	55–95 60–100	15–20	123 systolic 76 diastolic
18 years		Male: 70 Female: 75	50–90 55–95	15–20	126 systolic 79 diastolic
Adult		Same as 18 years		15–20	120 systolic 80 diastolic
Elderly (over 70 years)	36.0 C 96.8 F	Same as 18 years		15–20	Diastolic pressure may increase

Sources: Pulse rates: R.E. Behrman and V.C. Vaughan, III, editors, *Nelson textbook of pediatrics*, 12th ed. (Philadelphia: W. B. Saunders, 1983), p. 1100. G. H. Lowrey, *Growth and Development of Children*, 7th ed. Year Book, 1978, p. 450. For newborn and 1 year ages, National Heart, Lung, and Blood Institute, Task Force on Blood Pressure Control in Children: Report of the Task Force on Blood Pressure Control in Children, *Pediatrics* (May) 1977, 39(Suppl):819–20.

below 36 C, or 96.8 F) for a variety of reasons, such as lack of central heating, inadequate diet, loss of subcutaneous fat, lack of activity, and reduced thermoregulatory efficiency. Elderly people are also particularly sensitive to extremes in the environmental temperature due to decreased thermoregulatory controls (Kolanowski and Gunter 1981, p. 362).

2. *Diurnal variations.* Body temperatures normally change throughout the day. The 24-hour cycle is called the **circadian rhythm** or **diurnal cycle.** It is observable in the body temperature, which can vary as much as 2 C (1.8 F) between the early morning and the late afternoon. The point of highest body temperature is usually reached between 2000 and 2400 hours (8:00 P.M. and midnight), and the lowest point is reached during sleep between 0400 and 0600 hours (4:00 and 6:00 A.M.) (Vick 1984, p. 890). See Figure 34–4.

   The variation was thought to be due to variations in muscular activity and digestive processes, which are at a minimum in the early morning, while people are sleeping. However, research has shown no simple relationship between circadian rhythms and body temperatures; in nocturnal creatures and in some humans, the cycle is reversed, and body temperatures increase at night and decrease during the daytime (Vick 1984, p. 889).

3. *Exercise.* Exercise increases heat production. Hard work or strenuous exercise can increase body temperature to as high as 38.3 to 40 C (101 to 104 F) measured rectally.

4. *Hormones.* Hormone secretion also affects body temperature. In women, progesterone secretion at the time of ovulation raises body temperature by 0.3 to 0.6 C

(0.5 to 1 F) above basal temperature (Olds et al. 1984, p. 115). Just before this, as ovulation approaches, the production of estrogen increases and at its peak may decrease basal temperature slightly. Thyroxine, norepinephrine, and epinephrine also affect body temperature. See the section on heat production earlier in this chapter.

5. *Stress.* Physiologic and psychologic stress can also raise body temperature. Stimulation of the sympathetic nervous system can increase the production of epinephrine and norepinephrine, thereby increasing metabolic activity and heat production. See the section on heat production earlier in this chapter. Nurses may anticipate that a highly stressed or anxious client could have an elevated body temperature for that reason.

6. *Environment.* Extremes in environmental temperatures can affect a person's temperature regulatory systems. Factors such as humidity are discussed earlier in this chapter. However, when environmental temperatures reach about 33 C (91.4 F), the ability of the body to adjust is impaired (Vick 1984, p. 895). When the core temperature falls to about 25 C (77 F), death can occur.

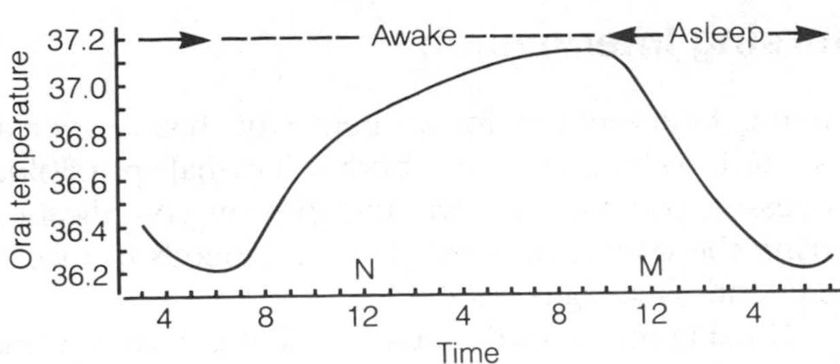

Figure 34–4 Range of oral temperature during 24 hours for a healthy young adult.

Fever

A body temperature above the usual range is called **fever** or **pyrexia.** A very high fever—40.5 C (105 F) or more—is called *hyperpyrexia.*

Mechanism of a Fever

The core temperature of the body is 37.1 C (98.7 F), and the mechanisms of heat production and heat loss are continually adjusted to maintain this temperature. For example, when a person exercises strenuously, mechanisms such as sweating are set in motion to increase heat loss and thereby maintain the core temperature at 37.1 C. This temperature is called the set-point of the temperature control mechanism. The hypothalamus controls this set-point.

An individual's set-point can be reset by pyrogens. A **pyrogen** is a substance, e.g., a protein or a lipopolysaccharide, secreted by bacteria or released by degenerating tissue. When a person's set-point is suddenly changed from the normal level, the body takes several hours to reach the new temperature set-point (Guyton 1986, p. 858). During this time, the person's blood temperature is lower than the new set-point. As a result, the body responds by increasing heat production. The person shivers and feels cold and the skin feels cold because of vasoconstriction even though the body temperature is above normal. The chills continue until the core temperature reaches the new set-point temperature. Once the body temperature reaches the new set-point, the chills stop and the person feels neither hot nor cold. However, once the reason for the new set-point is removed, e.g., the infectious bacteria are destroyed, the set-point is suddenly reduced. At this time, the body temperature is still elevated, e.g., 39.4 C (103 F), but the hypothalamus is trying to regulate the temperature at 37.1 C (98.7 F). As a result, mechanisms such as sweating and vasodilation are put in motion to reduce the body temperature. This sudden change is called a crisis.

Three common types of fevers are intermittent, remittent, and relapsing. During an **intermittent** or **quotidian fever**, the body temperature is elevated but returns to normal sometime in a 24-hour period. It is not unusual for an intermittent fever to be highest in the later afternoon or evening and lowest in the early morning. During a **remittent fever**, there is a wide range of temperatures over the 24-hour period, all of which are above normal. In a **relapsing fever**, short febrile periods of a few days are interspersed with periods of 1 or 2 days of normal temperature.

Nursing Assessment

Nursing assessment related to the presence of a fever includes identifying clients who are most at risk of developing an elevated body temperature as well as assessing the presence of any clinical signs of a fever. People at risk are those who have an infection or who may acquire an infection, e.g., postsurgical clients. The clinical signs of a fever are given on page 770.

Nursing Diagnosis

Examples of nursing diagnoses related to a fever are given on page 770.

Nursing Intervention

Nursing interventions for a client who has a fever are designed to support the body's normal physiologic processes, provide comfort, and prevent complications. During the course of fever, the nurse needs to monitor the client's vital signs closely.

Nursing measures during the chill phase are designed to help the client's body increase heat production and decrease heat loss. At this time, the body's physiologic processes are attempting to raise the core temperature to

Clinical Signs of a Fever

Onset (cold or chill stage)

- Increased heart rate
- Increased respiratory rate and depth
- Shivering due to increased skeletal muscle tension and contractions
- Pallid, cold skin due to vasoconstriction
- Cyanotic nail beds due to vasoconstriction
- Complaints of feeling cold
- "Gooseflesh" appearance of the skin due to contraction of the arrector pili muscles
- Cessation of sweating
- Rise in body temperature

Course

- Skin that feels warm and appears flushed due to vasodilation
- Complaints of feeling warm or neither hot nor cold
- Increased pulse and respiratory rates
- Increased thirst
- Mild to severe dehydration
- Simple drowsiness, restlessness, or delirium and convulsions due to irritation of the nerve cells
- Herpetic lesions of the mouth
- Loss of appetite with prolonged fever
- Malaise, weakness, and aching muscles due to protein catabolism

Defervescence (fever abatement)

- Skin that appears flushed and feels warm
- Sweating
- Decreased shivering
- Possible dehydration

Examples of Nursing Diagnoses Related to Hyperthermia

- Hyperthermia related to exposure to an excessively hot environment
- Hyperthermia related to increased metabolic activity and dehydration
- Hyperthermia related to decreased ability to perspire

Nursing Interventions During the Chill Phase

- Provide adequate nourishment to meet the body's needs because of the increased metabolic rate.
- Provide additional oxygen because of the increased metabolic rate if the client's health so indicates. For example, a client with respiratory or cardiovascular problems may need supplemental oxygen.
- Provide extra warmth, e.g., blankets, when the client feels chilled, but remove blankets when he or she feels warm.
- Provide additional fluids as the client's health permits to meet the needs of the body's increased metabolic rate.
- Reduce physical activity to limit the body's increased need for oxygen.

Nursing Interventions During the Flush Phase

- Remove excess blankets when the client feels warm.
- Provide fluids, e.g., 3000 ml per 24 hours, if the client's health permits. Clients who sweat profusely can become dehydrated.
- Provide oral hygiene to keep the mucous membranes moist. They can become dry and cracked as a result of excessive fluid loss.
- Provide a tepid sponge bath to increase heat loss through conduction.
- Provide cool circulating air to increase heat loss through convection.
- Provide dry clothing and bed linens to increase heat loss through conduction.
- Reduce physical activity to limit heat production.

the new set-point temperature. See page 770 for specific nursing interventions.

During the flush or crisis phase, the body processes are attempting to lower the core temperature to the reduced or normal temperature set-point. At this time, nursing measures are designed to increase heat loss and decrease heat production.

Hypothermia

Hypothermia is a core temperature that remains consistently below normal. When people without protection are exposed to a cold environment, the rate of heat loss can exceed that of heat production, thereby resulting in hypothermia. Once the core temperature drops to about 33 C (91.4 F), the ability of the body to compensate is impaired; once it has dropped to 29 to 31 C (84.2 to 87.8 F), its ability is lost (Vick 1984, p. 895), due to the reduced metabolic rate of the cells. Loss of consciousness occurs at about 30 C (86 F). Death can occur when the core temperature drops to 25 C (77 F).

There are three types of hypothermia: mild, moderate, and deep or severe. Mild hypothermia occurs when the core temperature reaches just below normal, i.e., 35 to 32 C (95 to 89.6 F). Moderate hypothermia occurs at temperatures between 26 to 32 C (78.8 to 89.6 F), and severe or deep hypothermia occurs below 26 C (78.8 F). The three physiologic mechanisms of hypothermia are: (a) excessive heat loss, (b) inadequate heat production to counteract the heat loss, and (c) impaired hypothalamic thermoregulation. See below for the major clinical signs of hypothermia.

Hypothermia may be accidental or induced. **Accidental hypothermia** can occur as a result of exposure to a cold environment, i.e., below 16 C (60.8 F) or from immersion in cold water. In elderly people, the problem can be compounded by a decreased metabolic rate and the use of sedatives, which depress the metabolic rate further. Management includes removing the client from the cold and rewarming the client's body. Methods of rewarming include the application of blankets for mild hypothermia and the application of a hyperthermia blanket and warm intravenous fluids when the client has severe hypothermia.

Induced hypothermia is the deliberate lowering of the body temperature to a range of 25 to 21 C (77 to 69.9 F) to decrease the need for oxygen by the body tissues. Induced hypothermia can involve the whole body or a body part. It is sometimes indicated prior to surgery, e.g., cardiac and brain surgery.

Major Clinical Signs of Hypothermia

- Decreased body temperature
- Severe shivering
- Feelings of cold and being chilled
- Pale, cool, waxy skin
- Hypotension
- Decreased urinary output
- Lack of muscle coordination
- Disorientation
- Drowsiness progressing to coma

Nursing Assessment

Nursing assessment should include identifying people who are at risk of hypothermia as well as identifying the clinical signs of hypothermia. People at risk of developing hypothermia are: people who participate in cold-weather sports, e.g., skiing and mountain climbing; infants and children whose thermoregulatory systems are immature; elderly people who have insufficient food, clothing, or fuel; people who have neurologic deficits and are unable to identify or respond to cold; alcoholics who have extreme heat loss secondary to vasodilation; and "street people" who lack adequate clothing and shelter.

All people who may be hypothermic, whether the hypothermia is induced or accidental, should be assessed carefully. All hypothermia is potentially dangerous. See significant clinical signs of hypothermia listed in the left-hand column.

Nursing Diagnosis

Some common nursing diagnoses related to hypothermia are listed on page 772.

Nursing Intervention

Nursing interventions for hypothermia are designed to increase heat production and decrease heat loss. For clients with mild hypothermia, providing blankets or warm clothes is frequently sufficient to rewarm the body. A client with severe hypothermia is placed on a hyperthermia blanket and given warm intravenous fluids. A hyperthermia blanket is electronically controlled to provide a specified temperature. Because rapid rewarming can cause vasodilation and subsequent additional heat loss, the client should be monitored closely, usually in an intensive care unit.

Preventive measures for hypothermia include teaching people to be aware of the temperature of their dwellings, to dress warmly in a cold environment, and to keep their clothing dry. Wet clothing fails to prevent heat loss because of the high conductivity of water. In a person wearing wet clothes, the rate of heat loss increases as much as 20-fold (Guyton 1986, p. 852).

Other preventive measures include providing adequate fluid and food to maintain body metabolism and undertaking an appropriate exercise program to stimulate heat production.

Examples of Nursing Diagnoses Related to Hypothermia

- Hypothermia related to exposure to a cold environment
- Hypothermia related to excessive evaporation from the skin secondary to consumption of alcohol
- Hypothermia related to aging

Related Thermal Disorders

A number of disorders are related to thermoregulation. Disorders of hyperthermia include heat stroke, heat cramps, and heat exhaustion. Disorders related to hypothermia include frostbite and accidental hypothermia.

Heat Stroke

Heat stroke occurs when the body temperature rises above 41.1 to 42.2 C (106 to 108 F). At those temperatures, the cells are damaged. The clinical signs of heat stroke include dizziness, abdominal distress, sometimes delirium, and eventual loss of consciousness.

A heat stroke is a medical emergency that often occurs quickly. The physiologic mechanism causing heat stroke is thought to be failure of the thermoregulatory mechanisms of the body. The person should be removed from the heat immediately, vital signs should be monitored, and treatment should be given to increase heat loss. Some medical authorities recommend that the client be placed in ice water, however; such immersion can induce vasoconstriction and shivering, which increase heat production (Guyton 1986, p. 859). Therefore, it has been suggested that the person's skin be sprayed or sponged with cool water to decrease the body's core temperature. In addition, ice packs can be placed on the head, axillae, and groin.

Heat Cramps

Heat cramps are painful, intermittent spasms of the skeletal muscles. People who exercise vigorously, sweat profusely, and then replace lost fluid with water can lower their serum sodium. This low serum sodium probably causes the cramps. Intervention should include telling the person to stop exercising and to replace the lost sodium with sodium tablets or fluids, such as tomato juice, that contain sodium.

Heat Exhaustion

Heat exhaustion or prostration is caused by severe fluid volume depletion, often as a result of exposure to an extremely hot environment. The person experiences low blood pressure, tachycardia, and faintness, and the skin is cold, pale, and clammy. The body temperature can be below normal. Management of a person who has heat exhaustion includes placing the person in a dorsal recumbent position, administering slightly salty fluids, and monitoring vital signs.

Frostbite

Frostbite is the localized freezing of areas of tissue due to exposure to cold. Frostbite is most common in the earlobes, fingers, and toes. In frostbite, the peripheral blood vessels constrict for a long period of time, resulting in tissue damage. The clinical signs of frostbite are given below.

Nursing intervention includes removing the client from the cold environment, warming the area (for example, by soaking it in tepid water), supporting the client if he or she is experiencing pain, and covering the area following warming to prevent infection.

Clinical Signs of Frostbite

- The afflicted area feels hard and cold upon palpation.
- The area feels numb and becomes painful upon rewarming.
- The skin is unusually pale or white, turning blotchy and red on rewarming.
- Swelling, necrosis, and gangrene can ensue.

Advising people how to prevent frostbite is also important. Preventive measures include wearing adequate, dry clothing, using protective creams, avoiding excessive fatigue, and avoiding smoking because nicotine is a vasoconstrictor.

Body Temperature Measurement

Sites

Body heat is produced in the body's core. As heat moves to the surface of the body, it dissipates; therefore, the surface of the body is cooler than the core. Among the common ways to assess temperature, the most accurate is by rectum, i.e., a thermometer is placed 5 to 8 cm (1.9 to 3.1 in) inside the adult rectum. In a resting adult, rectal temperature is slightly higher than the temperature of the arterial blood, about the same as the temperature of the liver, and slightly lower than that of the brain. When measured in the axilla or orally (by mouth), the temperature is about 0.65 C (1 F) less than the rectal temperature (Vick 1984, p. 888). Each of the sites—oral, rectal, and axillary—has advantages and disadvantages. See Table 34–2.

Oral

The body temperature is usually measured by mouth (per os, abbreviated po). This method reflects changing body temperature more quickly than the rectal method (Blainey 1974, p. 1861). Traditionally, the oral method was not used for clients receiving oxygen, since the accuracy of the measurement was considered questionable. Recent evidence, however, suggests that oral readings are accurate in clients receiving oxygen by nasal cannula, aerosol mask, Venturi mask, and nasal prongs (Graas 1974, p. 1863; Hasler and Cohen 1982, p. 265).

Before taking a temperature orally, nurses should wait 30 minutes if a client has been taking cold or hot food or fluids or smoking to make sure that the temperature of the mouth is not affected by the temperature of the food, fluid, or warm smoke (Erikson 1980, p. 164).

Rectal

Rectal temperature readings are considered to be the most accurate. In some agencies, taking temperatures rectally is contraindicated for clients with myocardial infarction. It is believed that inserting a rectal thermometer can produce vagal stimulation, which in turn can cause myocardial damage. Recent research, however, indicates that the rectal method has no deleterious effects on the heart (Creative Care Unit 1977, p. 997).

Blainey (1974, pp. 1860–61) points out several disadvantages of taking temperature by rectum:

1. Placement of the rectal thermometer at different sites within the rectum yields different temperatures, yet placement at the same site each time is difficult.
2. A rectal thermometer does not respond to changes in arterial temperatures as quickly as an oral thermometer, a fact that may be potentially dangerous for febrile clients, since misleading information may be acquired.
3. The presence of stool may interfere with thermometer placement. If the stool is soft, the thermometer may be embedded in stool rather than against the wall of the rectum. If the stool is impacted, the depth of thermometer insertion may be insufficient.

Table 34–2 Advantages and Disadvantages of Three Sites for Body Temperature Measurement

Site	Advantages	Disadvantages
Oral	Most accessible and convenient	Mercury-in-glass thermometers can be broken if bitten, thereby injuring the client. Therefore, it is contraindicated for infants, children under 6 years, and clients who are confused or who have convulsive disorders. Inaccurate if client has just eaten very hot or cold food or fluid. Inaccurate if client breathes through her or his mouth, therefore contraindicated for clients who have nasal surgery and must breathe through their mouths. Could injury the mouth following oral surgery.
Rectal	Most reliable measurement	Inconvenient and more unpleasant for clients; difficult for client who cannot turn to her or his side. Could injure the rectum following rectal surgery.
Axillary	Safest and most noninvasive	

4. In newborns and infants, insertion of the rectal thermometer has resulted in tragic ulcerations and rectal perforations. Many agencies advise against using rectal thermometers on neonates.

Axillary

Although the axillary temperature was considered less accurate than the rectal or oral method, studies now indicate that there is no clinically important difference in accuracy between axillary and rectal temperatures (Eoff and Joyce 1981, p. 1011; Axillary temps safer 1978, p. 1081; Schiffman 1982, p. 274). The axilla is therefore the preferred site for temperature measurements in children, not only because it is easily accessible but also because there is less likelihood of (a) spreading infection and (b) rectal perforation and subsequent peritonitis (Eoff and Joyce 1981, p. 1010; Axillary temps safer 1978, p. 1081).

Clients requiring this method of assessment include:

1. Newborns and infants
2. Toddlers and preschoolers
3. Clients with oral inflammation or wired jaws and clients recovering from oral surgery
4. Clients who are breathing through their mouths, e.g., following nasal surgery
5. Irrational clients
6. Clients for whom oral and rectal temperatures are contraindicated

Types of Thermometers

Traditionally, body temperatures have been measured using mercury-in-glass thermometers. Oral thermometers may have long slender tips, short rounded tips, or pear-shaped

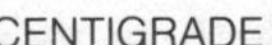

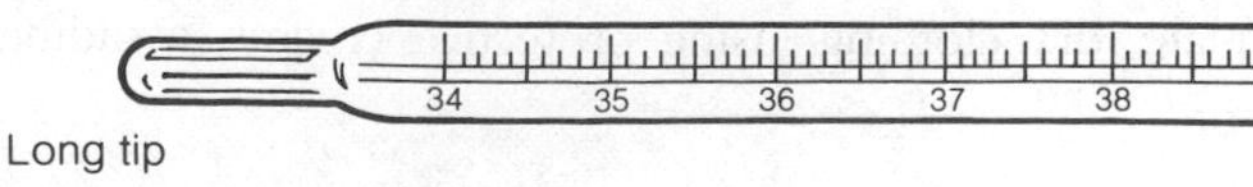

Long tip

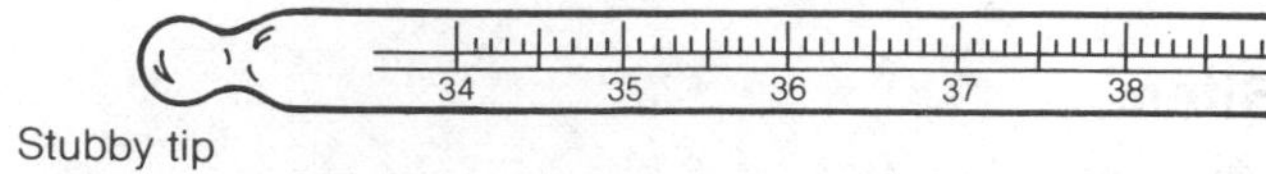

Stubby tip

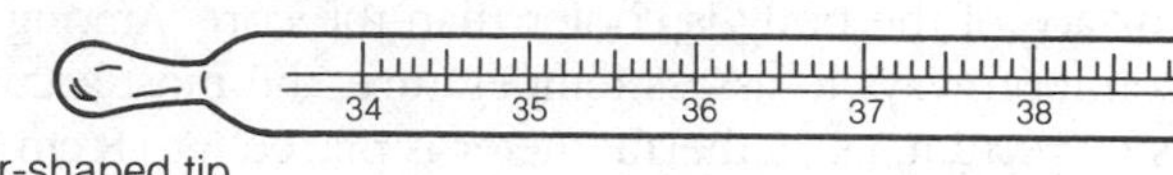

Pear-shaped tip

Figure 34–5 Three types of thermometer tips.

tips. See Figure 34–5. The rounded thermometer can be used at the rectal as well as other sites. In some agencies thermometers may be color coded; for example, blue-colored thermometers may be used for rectal temperatures, and silver-colored ones for oral and axillary temperatures. Disposable thermometers are also manufactured; these are used only once.

Electronic thermometers offer another method of assessing body temperatures. They can provide a reading in only 2 to 60 seconds, depending on the model. The equipment consists of a battery-operated portable electronic unit, a probe that the nurse attaches to the unit, and a probe cover, which is usually disposable. See Figure 34–6. Some models have a different circuit for each method of measurement, and the nurse needs to make sure that the correct circuit is switched on before taking the temperature.

Chemical disposable thermometers are also used to measure body temperatures. They come in individual cases

Research Note

Graves and Markarian studied whether plastic-sheathed thermometers recorded temperatures as accurately as unsheathed thermometers. During a period of 5 months, 90 nursing students were tested with sheathed and unsheathed thermometers. The results indicated that the unsheathed thermometers consistently showed higher readings than sheathed thermometers; however, the difference was less than 0.2 F. The study also showed that a 3-minute time interval for assessing oral temperatures was sufficient when using sheathed and unsheathed thermometers. (Graves and Markarian 1980)

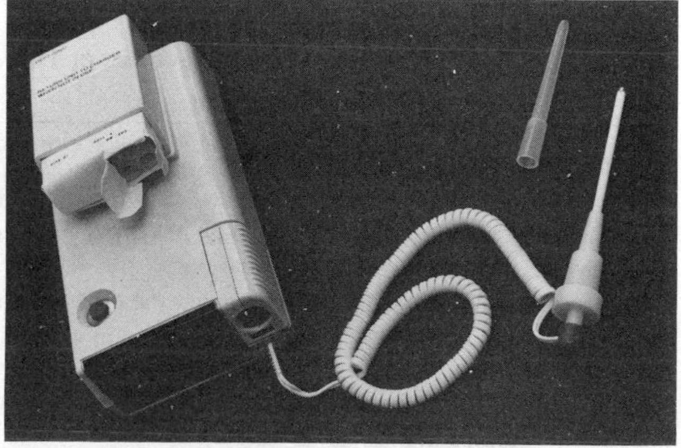

Figure 34–6 An electronic thermometer. Note the probe and the probe cover beside it.

and are discarded after use. One type has small chemical dots at one end that respond to body heat by changing color, thereby providing a reading of the body temperature. The thermometer comes in a plastic case. To activate the chemicals, the nurse holds the thermometer with the handle toward herself or himself, moves the handle up and down, and then pulls the plastic straight off the thermometer.

The thermometer is inserted under the client's tongue, the same as a glass thermometer, and left in place for the time recommended by the manufacturer (e.g., 45 seconds). After it is removed, the dots are observed for a change in color. The dot that has changed in color and represents the highest reading indicates the temperature measurement. See Figure 34–7. The chemical thermometer is discarded after use.

Temperature-sensitive tape is used to obtain a general indication of body surface temperature. When applied to the skin, usually of the forehead or abdomen, the tape responds by changing color. The skin area should be dry. After the length of time specified by the manufacturer (e.g., 15 seconds), a color appears on the tape. On one brand, a green N indicates a normal temperature, a brownish NF indicates a transition phase, and a blue-green F indicates an elevated temperature. The transition phase reflects the onset of a high temperature in the area where the tape was placed—for example, a sunburn on the forehead. Because infants under 2 years of age generally have an immature temperature-regulating system, any variation from the normal in an infant should be confirmed by a regular thermometer. The tape is removed and discarded after the color has been noted. This method is particularly useful at home and for infants whose temperatures are to be monitored for any reason.

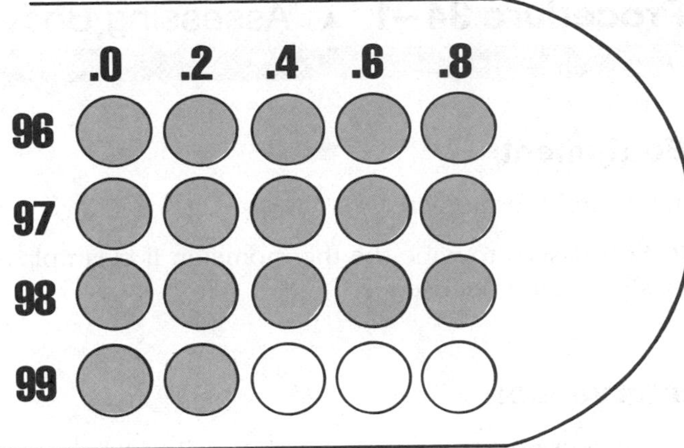

Figure 34–7 A chemical thermometer showing a reading of 99.2 F.

Temperature Scales

The body temperature is measured in degrees on two scales: centrigrade and Fahrenheit. The thermometer is the tool generally used to measure body temperature. The most common type is a glass tube with a column of mercury inside it. Heat expands the mercury, thus extending the column along the tube, where it can be measured against marked calibrations. The centrigrade scale normally extends from 34.00 to 42.0 C. The Fahrenheit scale usually extends from 94 to 108 F. See Figure 34–8. Body temperatures rarely extend beyond these scales.

Sometimes a nurse needs to convert a centigrade reading to Fahrenheit or vice versa. To convert from Fahrenheit to centigrade, deduct 32 from the Fahrenheit reading and then multiply by the fraction 5/9; that is:

$$C = (\text{Fahrenheit temperature} - 32) \times 5/9$$

For example, when the Fahrenheit reading is 100:

$$\begin{aligned} C &= (100 - 32) \times 5/9 \\ &= (68) \times 5/9 \\ &= 37.7\ C \end{aligned}$$

To convert from centigrade to Fahrenheit, multiply the centigrade reading by the fraction 9/5 and then add 32, that is:

$$F = (\text{centigrade temperature} \times 9/5) + 32$$

For example, when the centigrade reading is 40:

$$\begin{aligned} F &= (40 \times 9/5) + 32 \\ &= 72 + 32 \\ &= 104\ F \end{aligned}$$

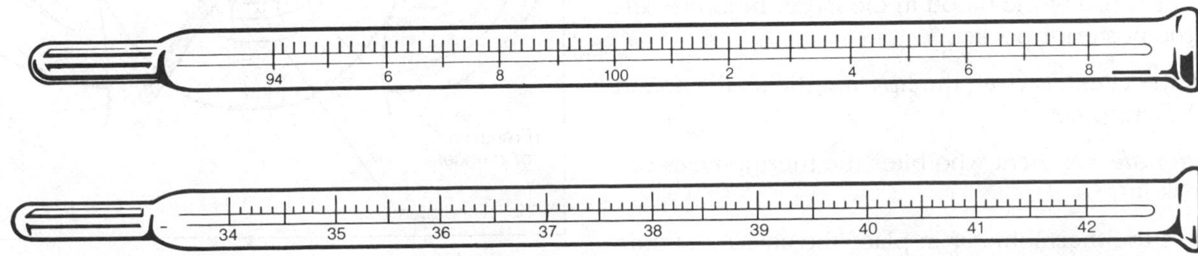

Figure 34–8 Thermometers. The upper one shows the Fahrenheit scale; the lower one, the centigrade scale.

Procedure 34–1 ▲ Assessing Body Temperature by Mouth

Equipment

1. An oral thermometer
2. Soft tissues to wipe the thermometer, if clean plastic sheaths are not used

Intervention

1. a. If using a mercury thermometer: Remove the thermometer from its container. If the thermometer is stored in disinfectant, wipe the solution from the thermometer with a soft tissue or rinse it under cold water. Wipe from the bulb end to fingers in a rotating fashion. Discard the tissue.

   Rationale Disinfectant can irritate the mucous membrane and taste unpleasant. Cold water is used because hot water causes the mercury to expand and can break the thermometer. The thermometer is wiped from the cleanest to the least clean area. Rotating ensures that all sides are wiped.

   b. If using an electronic thermometer: Gather the kit and disposable probe covers. Attach the probe to the unit, being sure to attach it to the appropriate circuit (oral, rectal, or axillary) in models that have separate circuits for each. Place a cover on the probe. Warm up the machine by switching it on, if not kept on.

2. Check the temperature reading on the thermometer. If necessary, shake down a mercury thermometer by holding it between the thumb and forefinger at the end farthest from the bulb. See Figure 34–9. Sharply snap the wrist downward. Repeat until the mercury is below 35 C (95 F).

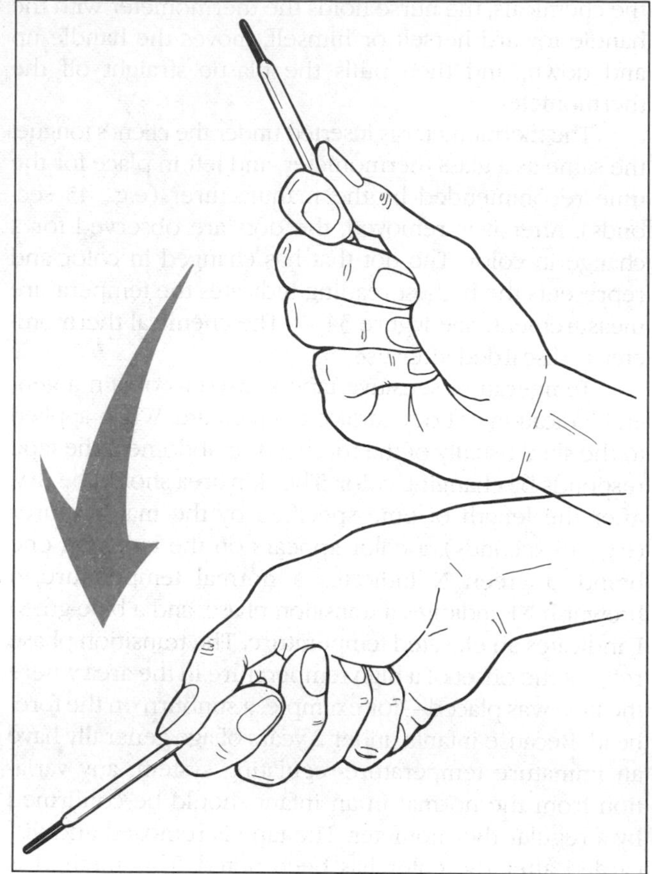

Figure 34–9

3. Ask the client to open his or her mouth, and place the thermometer or probe at the base of the tongue to the right or left of the frenulum (posterior sublingual pocket). See Figure 34–10.

   Rationale The thermometer needs to reflect the core temperature of the blood in the larger blood vessels of the posterior pocket.

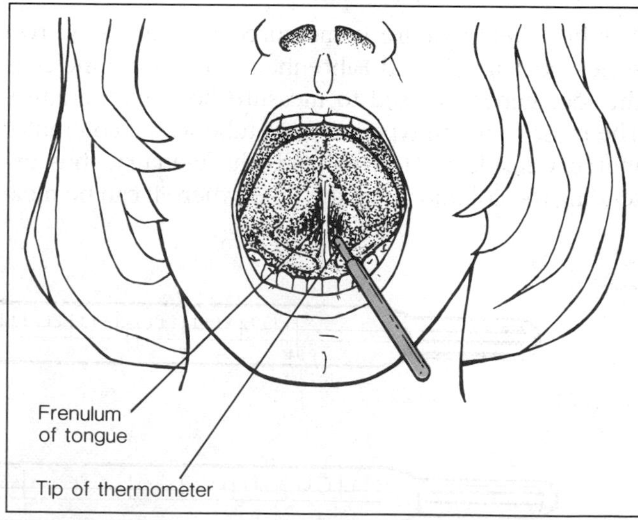

Figure 34–10

4. Ask the client to close the lips, not the teeth, around the thermometer.

   Rationale A client who bites the thermometer can break it.

5. Leave the thermometer in place the amount of time necessary for an accurate reading.

Rationale The nurse must allow sufficient time for the temperature to register. The recommended time is 2 minutes (Baker et al. 1984, p. 111) or 3 minutes (Graves and Markarian 1980, p. 323). If an electronic oral thermometer is used, the client holds the thermometer under the tongue 10 to 20 seconds or until it completes registering.

6. If using an electronic thermometer, read the temperature on the dial or readout.

7. Remove the thermometer. Remove the plastic sheath or wipe the thermometer with a tissue. Start at the end you are holding, and wipe in a rotating manner toward the bulb. Discard the tissue. If using an electronic thermometer, remove and discard the probe cover.

   Rationale The thermometer is wiped from the area of least contamination to that of greatest contamination.

8. Read the temperature, if using a mercury thermometer. Hold it at eye level, and rotate it until the mercury column is clearly visible. The upper end of the mercury column registers the client's body temperature. On the Fahrenheit thermometer, each long line reflects 1 degree and each short line 0.2 degree. On the centigrade thermometer, each long line reflects 0.5 degree and each short line 0.1 degree.

9. Wash the mercury thermometer in tepid soapy water, rinse it in cold water, dry it, and then disinfect it.

   Rationale Organic material such as mucus must be removed before the thermometer is placed in disinfectant. Organic materials on the thermometer can inhibit the action of the disinfectant solution. Effective disinfectants are ethyl alcohol 70% and synthetic phenols.

10. Shake down the thermometer and return it to its container. Many agencies store the thermometer in a small container of disinfectant at the bedside; others place it in a large container in the utility area. Some agencies also have special equipment for spinning down the mercury levels.

11. Record the temperature to the nearest indicated tenth (e.g., 98.4 F, 37.1 C) on the book, record, or worksheet.

Procedure 34–2 ▲ Assessing Body Temperature by Axilla

Equipment

1. An axillary thermometer. Oral thermometers are usually used in most agencies.
2. Soft tissues to wipe the thermometer.
3. A towel to remove perspiration from the axilla.

Intervention

1. Follow steps 1–2 in Procedure 34–1.
2. Expose the client's axilla. If the axilla is moist, dry it with the towel, using a patting motion.

   Rationale Friction created by rubbing can raise the temperature of the axilla.

3. Place the thermometer in the client's axilla.
4. Assist the client to place the arm tightly across the chest. See Figure 34–11.

   Rationale This position keeps the thermometer in place.

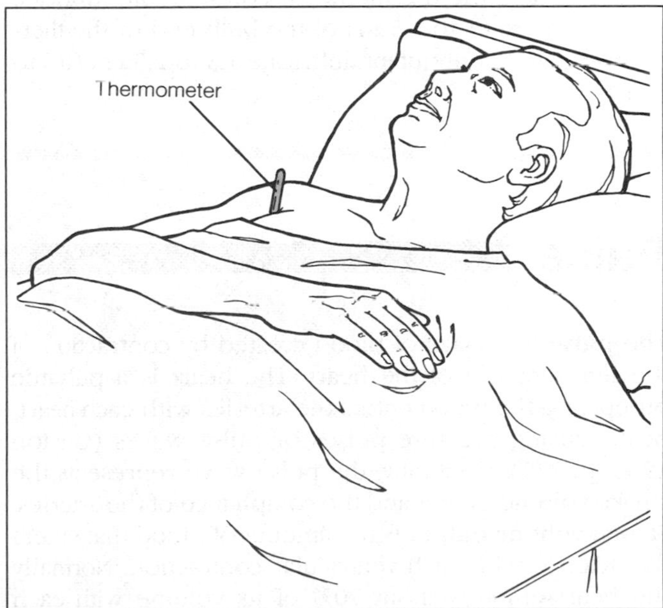

Figure 34–11

5. Leave the thermometer in place for 9 minutes (Nichols et al. 1966, p. 310), or as recommended by agency policy. Remain with the client and hold the thermometer in place, if the client is irrational or very young. For infants and children, leave the thermometer in place 5 minutes (Eoff and Joyce 1981, p. 1011).
6. Follow steps 6–11 in Procedure 34–1.

Procedure 34–3 ▲ Assessing Body Temperature by Rectum

Equipment

1. A rectal thermometer
2. Soft tissues to wipe the thermometer
3. Lubricant to apply to the thermometer to ease insertion into the rectum

Intervention

1. Follow steps 1–2 in Procedure 34–1 on page 776.
2. Assist the client to assume a lateral position. A newborn may be placed in a lateral or prone position (Axillary temps safer 1978, p. 1081). Provide privacy before folding the bedclothes back to expose the buttocks.

   Rationale Privacy is essential since exposure of the buttocks embarrasses most people.
3. Place some lubricant on a piece of tissue. Then apply lubricant to the thermometer. For an adult, lubricate 2.5 to 4 cm (1 to 1.5 in) of the bulb end of the thermometer. For an infant, lubricate 1.5 to 2.5 cm (0.5 to 1 in).

   Rationale The lubricant facilitates insertion of the thermometer without irritating the mucous membrane.
4. With one hand, raise the client's upper buttock to expose the anus.
5. Ask the client to take a deep breath, and insert the thermometer into the anus anywhere from 1.5 to 4 cm (0.5 to 1.5 in), depending on the age and size of the client (for example, 1.5 cm for an infant, 4 cm for a large adult). *Do not force insertion of the thermometer.*

   Rationale Having the client take a deep breath relaxes the external sphincter muscle, thus easing insertion. Inability to insert the thermometer into a newborn could indicate the rectum is not patent. The end of the thermometer should not be embedded in feces or the temperature measurement will not be accurate.
6. Hold the thermometer in place for 2 minutes (Nichols 1972) or for the length of time recommended by the agency. For neonates, hold the thermometer in place for 5 minutes (Schiffman 1982, p. 276), or as recommended by agency policy. Hold an electronic thermometer in place for 10 to 20 seconds.
7. Follow steps 6–11 in Procedure 34–1.

Pulse

The **pulse** is a wave of blood created by contraction of the left ventricle of the heart. The heart is a pulsatile pump, and the blood enters the arteries with each heartbeat, causing pressure pulses or pulse waves (Guyton 1986, p. 225). Generally, the pulse wave represents the stroke volume output and the compliance of the arteries. **Stroke volume output** is the amount of blood that enters the arteries with each ventricular contraction. Normally the heart empties about 70% of its volume with each contraction, i.e., about 70 ml of blood in a healthy adult (Guyton 1986, p. 155). Compliance of the arteries is the distensibility of the arteries, i.e., their ability to contract and expand. When a person's arteries lose their distensibility, as can happen in old age, greater pressure is required to pump the blood into the arteries.

When an adult is resting, the heart pumps 4 to 6 liters of blood each minute. This volume is called the **cardiac output.** The cardiac output (CO) is the result of the stroke volume (SV) and the heart rate (HR) per minute.

In a healthy person, the pulse reflects the heartbeat, i.e., the pulse rate is the same as the rate of the ventricular contractions of the heart. However, in some types of cardiovascular disease the heartbeat and pulse rates can differ. For example, a client's heart may produce very weak or small pulse waves that are not detectable in a peripheral pulse. In these instances, the nurse should assess the heartbeat *and* the peripheral pulse. See the section on assessing the apical pulse, later in this chapter.

A **peripheral pulse** is a pulse located in the periphery of the body, e.g., in the foot, hand, or neck. The **apical pulse**, in contrast, is a central pulse, i.e., it is located at the apex of the heart.

Factors Affecting Pulse Rate

The rate of the pulse is expressed in beats per minute. A pulse rate varies according to a number of factors: age, sex, exercise, emotions, heat, and body position, for example.

1. *Age.* The pulse of a newborn baby averages 125 beats per minute with a wide range of variability from 70 to 190. As age increases, the pulse rate gradually decreases to its adult rate of about 70 to 75 beats per minute. Unless a disease process exists, the pulse rate is stabilized at the adult level for the rest of a person's life. Refer to Table 34–1 for specific variations in pulse rates from birth to adulthood.
2. *Sex.* The pulse rate tends to vary somewhat between men and women of similar ages. After puberty, the average male's pulse rate is slightly lower than the female's.
3. *Exercise.* The pulse rate normally increases with activity. Increased metabolism of the muscles during exercise results in a vasodilation and increased need for oxygen and nutrients. The rate of increase in the professional athlete is often less than in the average person because of greater cardiac size, strength, and efficiency.
4. *Fever.* Fever also can accelerate the heart (pulse) rate. The pulse rate increases in response to the lowered blood pressure, which in turn is a result of a peripheral vasodilation response to the heat.
5. *Medications.* Some medications decrease the pulse rate and others increase it. For example, digitalis preparations decrease the heart rate, whereas epinephrine increases the pulse rate.
6. *Hemorrhage.* The loss of blood from the vascular system (hemorrhage) normally increases pulse rate. The loss of a small amount of blood, e.g., 500 ml, as after a blood donation, results in a temporary adjustment of the heart rate as the body makes up for the lost blood volume. An adult has about 5 liters of blood in her or his system and can lose up to 10% without adverse effects (Vick 1984, p. 346).
7. *Stress.* In response to stress, sympathetic nervous stimulation increases the overall activity of the heart. Stress increases the rate as well as the force of the heartbeat. Emotions such as fear and anxiety as well as the perception of severe pain stimulate the sympathetic system.
8. *Position changes.* When a person assumes a sitting or standing position, blood usually pools in the vessels of the dependent venous system. Pooling results in a transient decrease in the venous blood return to the heart and a subsequent reduction in blood pressure. These changes are primarily mediated through the sympathetic nervous system, increasing cardiac rate, force of the ventricular contractions, and tone of the veins and arteries.

Pulse Sites

Nine of the sites where a pulse is commonly taken (see Figure 34–12) are:

1. *Temporal:* where the temporal artery passes over the temporal bone of the head. The site is superior (above) and lateral (away from the midline) to the eye.
2. *Carotid:* at the side of the neck below the lobe of the ear where the carotid artery runs between the trachea and the sternocleidomastoid muscle.
3. *Apical:* at the apex of the heart. In an adult this is located on the left side of the chest, no more than 8 cm (3 in) to the left of the sternum (breastbone) and under the fourth, fifth, or sixth intercostal space (area between the ribs). Another way to locate the apex is to find the midclavicular line (MCL), an imaginary line dropping straight down from the center of the clavicle (collarbone). See Figure 34–13. Normally, the apex lies inside or on the MCL at the fourth, fifth, or sixth intercostal space. In men, the MCL usually passes through the nipple area. To locate the center of the clavicle, first feel for the medial end of this bone where it joins the sternum. This joint can be felt more readily by having the client move the shoulder forward. Next, locate the lateral end of the clavicle, where it joins the shoulder, by feeling along the front edge of the clavicle until a bony prominence or notch is felt at the shoulder. Midway between these identified points at the sternum and the shoulder is the center of the clavicle.

   For a child 7 to 9 years of age, the apical pulse is located between the fourth and fifth intercostal spaces. Before 4 years of age it is left of the MCL, between 4 and 6 years it is at the MCL. See Figure 34–13.
4. *Brachial:* at the inner aspect of the biceps muscle of the arm or medially in the antecubital space (elbow crease).
5. *Radial:* where the radial artery runs along the radial bone, on the thumb side of the inner aspect of the wrist.
6. *Femoral:* where the femoral artery passes alongside the inguinal ligament.
7. *Popliteal:* where the popliteal artery passes behind the knee. This point is difficult to find, but it can be palpated if the client flexes the knee slightly.

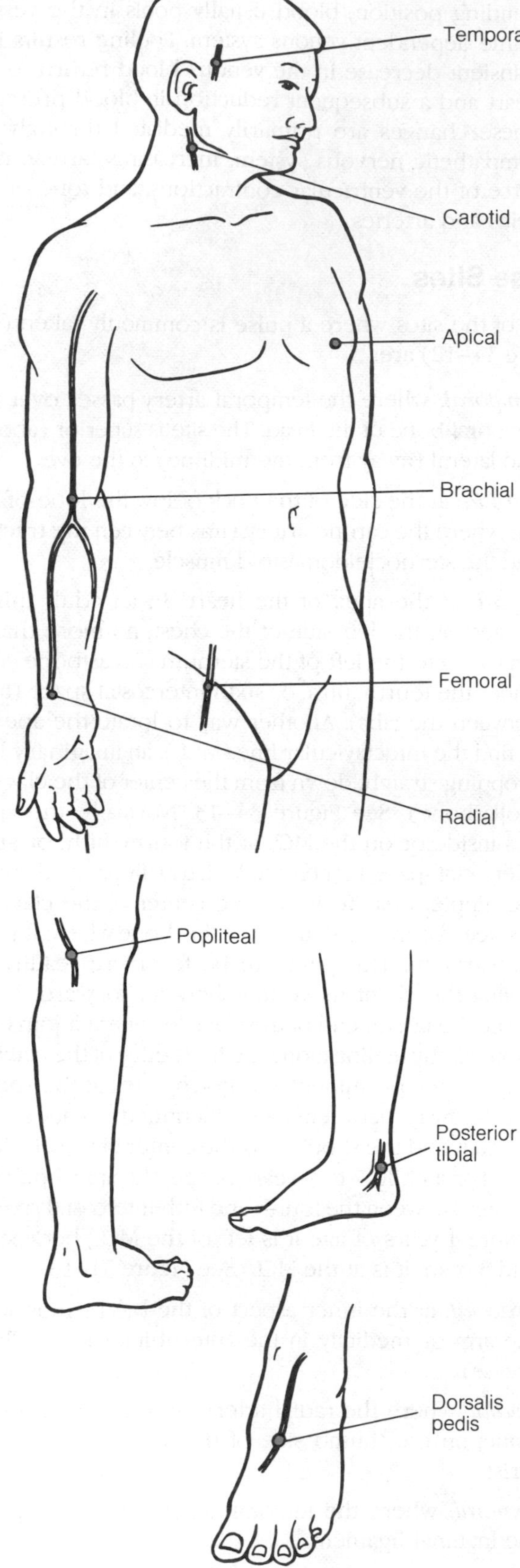

Figure 34–12 Nine sites commonly used for assessing a pulse.

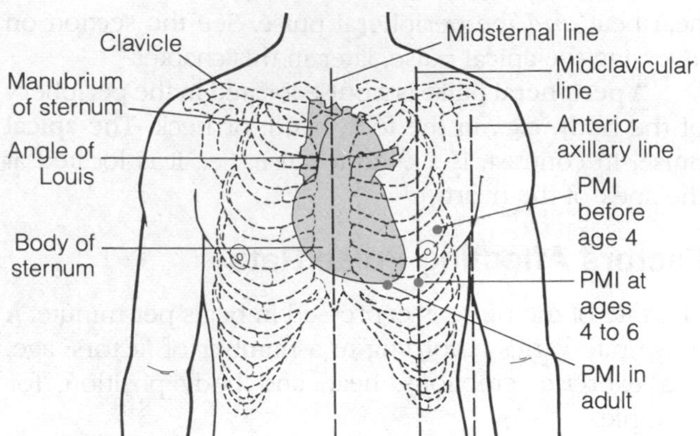

Figure 34–13 Location of the apical pulse for a child under 4 years, a child 4 to 6 years, and an adult.

8. *Posterior tibial:* on the medial surface of the ankle where the posterior tibial artery passes behind the medial malleolus.
9. *Pedal (dorsalis pedis):* where the dorsalis pedis artery passes over the bones of the foot. This artery can be palpated by feeling the dorsum (upper surface) of the foot on an imaginary line drawn from the middle of the ankle to the space between the big and second toes.

The reasons for use of each site are given in Table 34–3. The radial site is most commonly used. It is readily found in most people and accessible.

Table 34–3 Reasons for Using Specific Pulse Sites

Pulse Site	Reasons for Use
Radial	Readily accessible and routinely used
Temporal	Used when radial pulse is not accessible
Carotid	Used for infants
	Used in cases of cardiac arrest
	Used to determine circulation to the brain
Apical	Routinely used for infants and children up to 3 years of age
	Used to determine discrepancies with radial pulse
	Used in conjunction with some medications
Brachial	Used to measure blood pressure
	Used during cardiac arrest for infants
Femoral	Used in cases of cardiac arrest
	Used for infants and children
	Used to determine circulation to a leg
Popliteal	Used to determine circulation to the lower leg
	Used to determine leg blood pressure
Posterior tibial	Used to determine circulation to the foot
Pedal	Used to determine circulation to the foot

Pulse Assessment

A pulse is normally palpated by applying moderate pressure with the three middle fingers of the hand. The pads on the most distal aspects of the finger are the most sensitive areas for detecting a pulse. With excessive pressure, one can obliterate a pulse, whereas with too little pressure, the pulse may not be detectable.

Pulse Rate

Before the nurse assesses the pulse rate, the client should assume a comfortable position. The nurse should also be aware of:

1. Any medication, e.g., digitalis, that could interfere with the heart rate.
2. Whether the client has been physically active. If so, the nurse should wait 10 to 15 minutes until the client has rested and the pulse has slowed to its usual rate.
3. Whether the client needs to assume a particular position, e.g., sitting, before the pulse rate is assessed. Some nurse practitioners prefer a particular position, e.g., sitting, lying, or standing, because the rate can vary with the position due to changes in blood flow volume and autonomic nervous system activity.
4. Any baseline data about the normal heart rate for the client. For example, a physically fit athlete may have a heart rate below 60 beats per minute.

The pulse rate is regulated by the autonomic nervous system (ANS). Impulses pass through the parasympathetic branch to the sinoatrial node (SA node), which is the pacemaker of the heart. These impulses decrease the heart rate. When body demands indicate a need for an increased heart rate, the impulses of the parasympathetic system are inhibited and the impulses of the sympathetic system increase.

The normal pulse rates are shown in Table 34–1. An excessively fast heart rate, e.g., over 100 beats per minute in an adult, is referred to as **tachycardia**. A heart rate in an adult of 60 beats per minute or less is called **bradycardia**. If a client has either tachycardia or bradycardia, the apical pulse should be assessed.

Pulse Rhythm

The **pulse rhythm** is the pattern of the beats and the intervals between the beats. Equal time elapses between beats of a normal pulse; this steady beat is called **pulsus regularis**. A pulse with an irregular rhythm is referred to as an **arrhythmia**.

Arrhythmia may be characterized by random, irregular beats or by a predictable pattern of irregular beats. When assessing a pulse rhythm, the nurse should carefully attend to the time between each beat. Usually, when an arrhythmia is detected, the apical pulse should also be assessed. An electrocardiogram (ECG or EKG) is necessary to define an arrhythmia further. See Chapter 54.

Pulse Volume

Pulse volume, also called the pulse strength or quality, refers to the force of blood with each beat. Usually, pulse volume is the same with each beat. It can range from absent to bounding. A normal pulse can be felt with moderate pressure of the fingers, and it can be obliterated with greater pressure. A forceful or full blood volume that is obliterated only with difficulty is called a *full* or *bounding* pulse. A pulse that is readily obliterated with pressure from the fingers is referred to as *weak, feeble,* or *thready.* A pulse volume is usually measured on a scale of 0 to 4. See Table 34–4.

Arterial Wall Elasticity

The elasticity of the arterial wall reflects its expansibility or its deformities. A healthy, normal artery feels straight, smooth, soft, and pliable. Elderly people often have inelastic arteries that feel twisted (tortuous) and irregular upon palpation. The elasticity of the arteries may not affect the pulse rate, rhythm, or volume but it does reflect the status of the client's vascular system.

Bilateral Equality

When assessing a peripheral pulse to determine the adequacy of blood flow to a particular area of the body, the nurse should also assess the corresponding pulse on the other side of the body. This second assessment gives the nurse data with which to compare the pulses. For example, when assessing the blood flow to the right foot, the nurse assesses the right dorsalis pedis pulse and then the left dorsalis pedis pulse.

Table 34–4 Scale for Measuring a Pulse Volume

Scale	Description of Pulse
0	Absent
1	Thready or weak
2	Obliterated with pressure
3	Normal, detected readily
4	Bounding, difficult to obliterate

Peripheral Pulse Assessment

A pulse is commonly measured by palpation (feeling) or auscultation (hearing). The middle three fingertips are used for palpating all pulse sites except the apex of the heart. A stethoscope is used for assessing apical pulses and fetal heart tones. Increasingly ultrasound (Doppler) equipment is being used to assess pulses that are difficult to assess. See Procedure 34–4, step 3.

Occasionally, a radial pulse and an apical pulse are taken simultaneously by two persons. This is called an apical-radial pulse. Differences between the two rates can indicate cardiovascular disorders.

The cardiac monitoring machine is another device for assessing the apical pulse. It indicates the rate on a screen or readout graph. However, this method is beyond the scope of this chapter.

A peripheral pulse, usually the radial pulse, is assessed by palpation for all individuals *except:*

1. Newborns and children up to 2 or 3 years. Apical pulses are assessed in these clients.
2. Very obese or elderly clients, whose radial pulse may be difficult to palpate. Doppler equipment may be used for these clients, or the apical pulse is assessed.
3. Individuals with a heart disease, who require apical pulse assessment.
4. Individuals in whom the circulation to a specific body part must be assessed, e.g., following leg surgery the pedal (dorsalis pedis) pulse is assessed.

Procedure 34–4 ▲ Assessing a Peripheral Pulse

Equipment

1. A watch with a second hand or indicator to count the pulse rate
2. If a Doppler ultrasound stethoscope (DUS) will be used, the transducer in the DUS probe (a device resembling a small transistor radio), a stethoscope headset, and transmission gel. See Figure 34–14. Do not use K-Y jelly, which contains probe-damaging salts. The DUS headset has earpieces similar to standard stethoscope earpieces but it has a long cord attached to a volume-controlled audio unit and an ultrasound transducer. The DUS detects *movement* of red blood cells through a blood vessel. In contrast, the conventional stethoscope amplifies only *sound,* not movement. The DUS can detect blood flow if the blood cells are moving faster than 6 cm per second and at a depth of about 5 cm (Hudson 1983, p. 55). It cannot detect blood flow in deep vessels or in those underlying bone, such as the vessels in the abdomen, thorax, or skull. The DUS is battery operated, and batteries need replacement about every 6 months. Many agencies write the date of battery installation on a small adhesive label and attach it to the case as a reminder to replace the battery.

Intervention

1. Select the pulse point. Normally, the radial pulse is taken, unless it cannot be exposed or circulation to another body area is to be assessed.
2. Assist the client to a comfortable resting position. When the radial pulse is assessed, the arm can rest alongside the client with the palm facing downward, or the forearm can rest at a 90° angle across the chest with the palm downward. For the client who can sit, the forearm can rest across the thigh with the palm of the hand facing downward or inward.
3. a. When palpating the pulse, place three middle fingertips lightly and squarely over the pulse point. See Figure 34–15.

   Rationale Using the thumb is contraindicated because the thumb has a pulse that the nurse could mistake for the client's pulse.

   b. For using a Doppler ultrasound device, Hudson (1983, p. 56) outlines the following steps:

   - Plug the stethoscope headset into one of the two output jacks located next to the volume control.

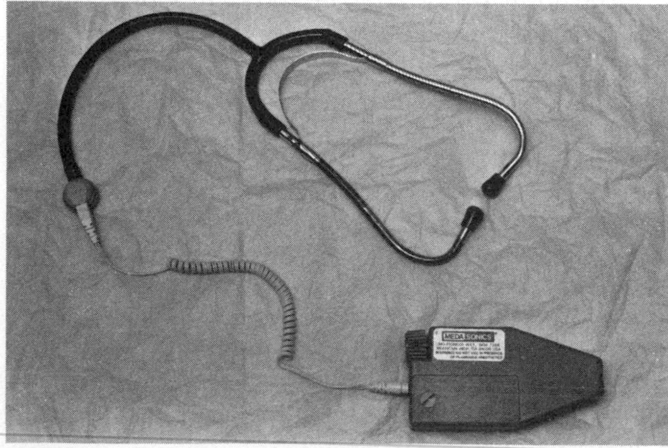

Figure 34–14 An ultrasound (Doppler) stethoscope.

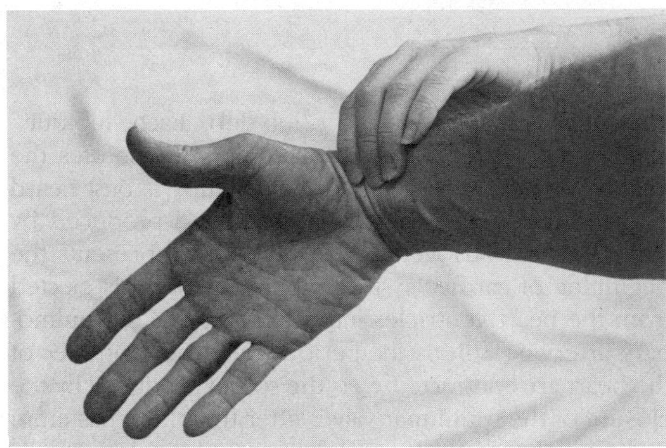

Figure 34–15

DUS units have jacks for two headpieces and accessory loudspeakers so that another person can listen to the signals.

- Apply transmission gel either to the probe, at the narrowed end of the plastic case housing the transducer, or to the client's skin.

  Rationale Ultrasound beams do not travel well through air. The gel makes an airtight seal, which promotes optimal ultrasound wave transmission.
- Press the "on" button.
- Hold the probe at a 45° angle against the skin over the pulse site. Use a light pressure, and keep the probe in contact with the skin.

  Rationale Too much pressure can stop the blood flow and obliterate the signal.
- Distinguish between artery and vein sounds. The artery sound (signal) is distinctively pulsating and has a pumping quality. The venous sound is like the wind, is intermittent, and varies with respirations.

  Rationale Both artery and vein sounds are heard simultaneously through the DUS, since major arteries and veins are situated close together throughout the body.
- If you have difficulty hearing arterial sounds, reposition the probe.

4. Count the pulse for 30 seconds and multiply by 2 if the pulse is regular. If it is irregular, count for 1 full minute.

   Rationale An irregular pulse requires a full minute's count for a correct assessment.
5. Assess the pulse rhythm by noting the pattern of intervals between the beats. A normal pulse has equal time periods between beats. If this is an initial assessment, assess for 1 full minute.

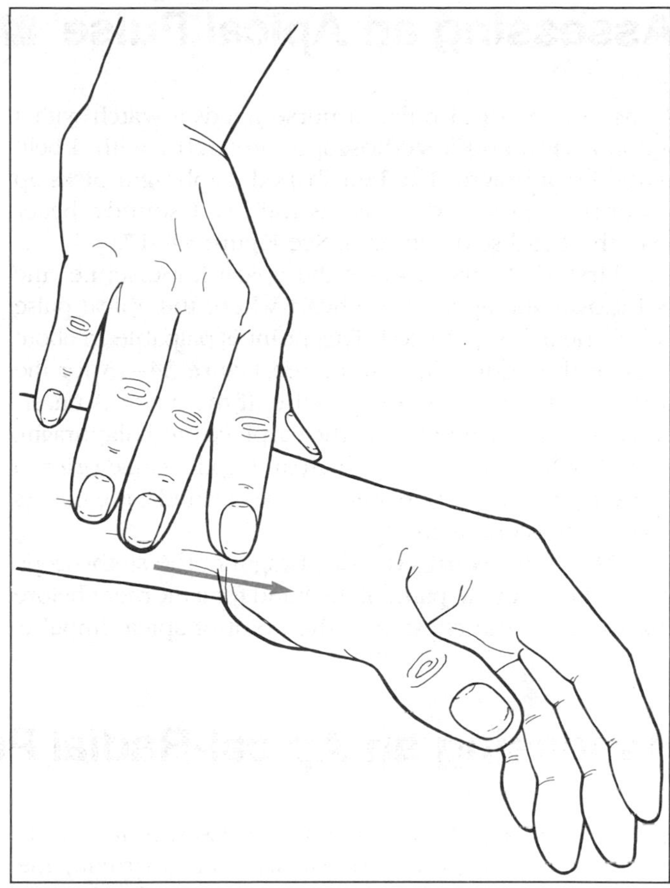

Figure 34–16

6. Assess the pulse volume. A normal pulse can be felt with moderate pressure, and the pressure is equal with each beat. Relate the volume to the scale in Table 34–4.
7. To assess the arterial wall, compress the artery firmly and run a finger distal to the heart along the artery. See Figure 34–16. A normal arterial wall is smooth and straight.
8. Record the pulse rate, rhythm, and volume, and the condition of the arterial wall.

Sample Recording

Date	Time	Notes
5/8/87	0900	Pale and listless. Pulse 116, regular, volume #1. Reported above to Ms. N. McNamara. ——— ——— Sally M. Sahara, NS

9. After using the DUS, remove all the gel from the probe to prevent damage to its surface. Clean the transducer with aqueous solutions.

   Rationale Alcohol or other disinfectants may damage the face of the transducer.

Assessing an Apical Pulse

To assess an apical pulse, a nurse needs a watch with a second hand and a stethoscope, preferably with a bell-shaped diaphragm. The bell-shaped diaphragm picks up lower-pitched sounds, such as the heart sounds, better than the flat-disc diaphragm. See Figure 34–17.

First, the nurse locates the apical impulse, i.e., the point over the apex of the heart where the apical pulse is best heard or palpated. This point is palpable in about 50% of the adult population. See Figure 34–13 for the usual positions of the apical pulse. If the nurse is uncertain about the cleanliness of the earpieces and diaphragm, they should be cleaned with an antiseptic gauze prior to use. Only the diaphragm needs to be cleaned if the nurse's own stethoscope is used.

The nurse warms the diaphragm of the stethoscope by holding it in the palm of the hand for a moment before placing it on the chest over the point of apical impulse. The apical pulse sounds like a "lub dub." Each "lub-dub" counts as one heartbeat. The "lub-dub" constitutes the heart sounds called S_1 and S_2. S_1, or "lub," is best heard at the apex of the heart; it is the sound produced by closure of the atrioventricular valves. S_1 represents the beginning of cardiac systole, when the blood is ejected from the heart ventricles into the aorta and the pulmonary artery. **Systole** is the period when the ventricles of the heart are contracted. S_2 is the sound produced by the closure of the semilunar valves after the blood has emptied from the ventricles and the ventricles relax. The S_2 sound, then, indicates the beginning of diastole. **Diastole** is the period when the ventricles of the heart are relaxed. Usually, S_1 and S_2 are very brief, and systole and diastole are longer. For more information about assessment of the heart, see Chapter 35.

Assessing an Apical-Radial Pulse

An apical-radial pulse may need to be assessed for clients who have certain cardiovascular disorders. Normally, the apical and radial rates are identical. An apical pulse rate greater than a radial pulse rate can indicate that the thrust of the blood from the heart is too feeble for the wave to be felt at the peripheral pulse site, or it can indicate that vascular disease is preventing impulses from being transmitted. Any discrepancy between the two pulse rates needs to be reported promptly. In no instance is the radial pulse greater than the apical pulse.

An apical-radial pulse can be taken by two nurses or one nurse, although the one-nurse technique may not be as accurate. In the two-nurse technique, one nurse counts the radial pulse at exactly the same time as the other nurse counts the apical beat. The nurse who is assessing the radial pulse often holds the watch and indicates when they should start counting.

Respirations

Respiration is the act of breathing; it includes the intake of oxygen and the output of carbon dioxide. Reference is often made to **external respiration** and **internal respiration**. The former refers to the interchange of oxygen and carbon dioxide between the alveoli of the lungs and the pulmonary blood. Internal respiration, by contrast, takes place throughout the body; it is the interchange of these same gases between the circulating blood and the cells of the body tissues.

The term **inhalation** or **inspiration** refers to the intake of air into the lungs. **Exhalation** or **expiration** refers to breathing out or the movement of gases from the lungs to the atmosphere. **Ventilation** is another word that is used to refer to the movement of air in and out of the lungs. **Hyperventilation** refers to very deep, rapid respirations; **hypoventilation** refers to very shallow respirations.

There are basically two types of breathing that nurses observe, **costal** or thoracic breathing and **diaphragmatic** or abdominal breathing. Costal breathing involves chiefly the external intercostal muscles and other accessory muscles, such as the sternocleidomastoid muscles. It can be observed by the movement of the chest upward and outward. By contrast, diaphragmatic breathing chiefly involves the contraction and relaxation of the diaphragm, and it is observed by the movement of the abdomen, which occurs as a result of the diaphragm's contraction and downward movement.

Mechanics of Breathing

Respiration includes the intake of oxygen and the output of carbon dioxide. Respirations are generally described as deep or shallow. In deep respirations, a large volume of air is inhaled and exhaled. In shallow respirations, the volume of air moved is small.

During inhalation the following processes normally occur (see Figure 34–18):

1. The diaphragm contracts (flattens).
2. The ribs move upward and outward.
3. The sternum moves outward.
4. The thorax enlarges, and thus the lungs expand.

During exhalation (see Figure 34–19):

1. The diaphragm relaxes (its curvature increases).
2. The ribs move downward and inward.
3. The sternum moves inward.
4. The thorax decreases in size, and thus the lungs are compressed.

For additional information see Chapter 45.

Normal respirations are quiet and effortless. Normal breathing is called **eupnea**. An inspiration normally lasts 1 to 1.5 seconds, and an expiration lasts 2 to 3 seconds.

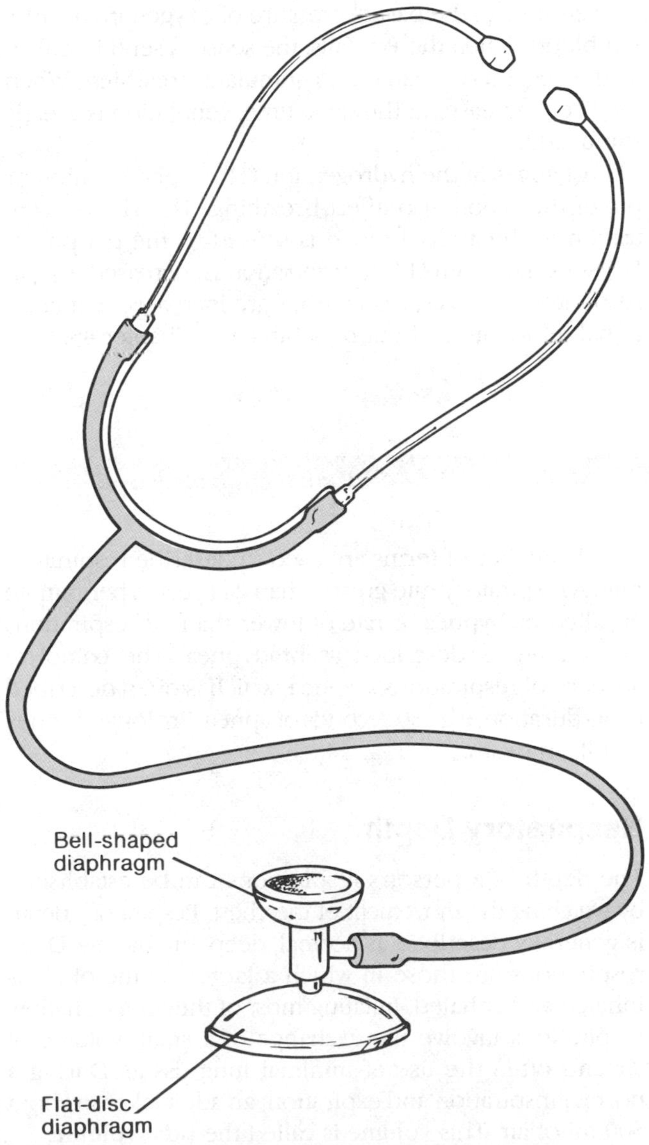

Figure 34–17 A stethoscope with a bell-shaped diaphragm and a flat-disc diaphragm.

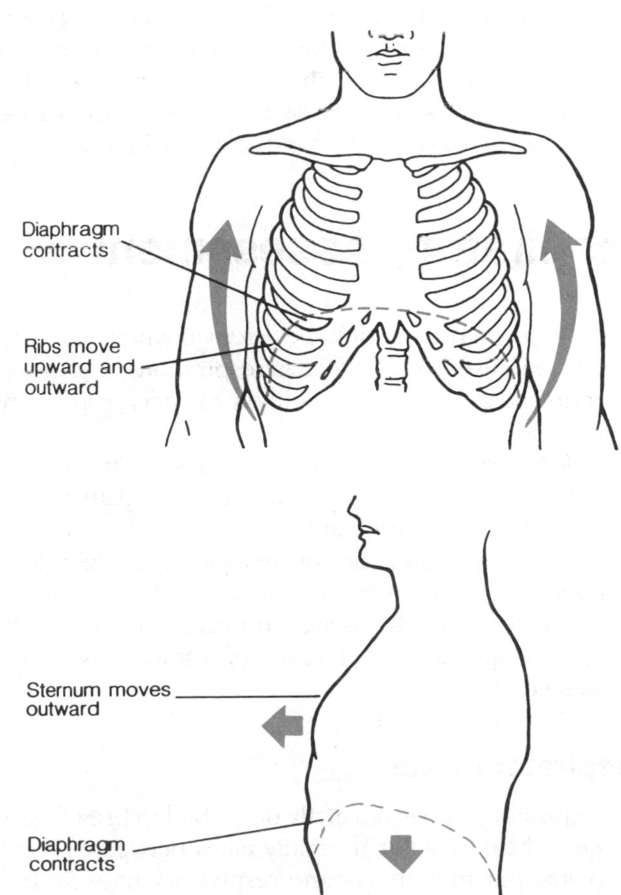

Figure 34–18 Respiratory inhalation: anterior and lateral views.

Control of Respirations

Breathing is normally carried out without effort and automatically. Respiration is controlled by respiratory centers in the brain, sensors, and the mechanisms of response.

Respiratory Centers

The medulla oblongata contains one center that controls inspiration and another that controls expiration. The apneustic center in the pons prolongs inspiration when not inhibited by impulses carried by the vagus nerve. The pneumotaxic center, in the upper area of the pons, receives impulses from the other respiratory center and is thought to "fine tune" the pattern of breathing (Vick 1984, p. 449).

Sensors

Ventilation is regulated by the concentrations of oxygen (O_2), carbon dioxide (CO_2) and hydrogen (H^+) in the arterial blood. Certain sensors (also called chemoreceptors), located centrally and peripherally, respond to these concentrations. The central sensors are located in the upper medulla, near the medullary respiratory centers. The peripheral sensors are located in the carotid bodies just above the bifurcation of the common carotid arteries. These sensors are stimulated by a decrease in the partial pressure of the oxygen (Po_2) in the arterial blood.

Mechanisms of Response

There are three mechanisms of response: to CO_2, O_2, and H^+. The mechanism of response to CO_2 affects alveolar ventilation directly. The normal partial pressure of CO_2 (Pco_2) is 40 mm Hg. An increase in the Pco_2 stimulates the respiratory centers to increase respirations. A concentration of about 10% CO_2 in the inspired air stimulates ventilation maximally (Vick 1984, p. 451). A decrease in the Pco_2 in the alveoli enhances the ventilatory response. Therefore, the partial pressure of carbon dioxide (Pco_2) in the arterial blood is the most important factor controlling ventilation.

The peripheral sensors, mainly in the carotid bodies, are sensitive to the partial pressure of oxygen in the arterial blood. When the Po_2 falls, the sensors send impulses to the respiratory centers to stimulate breathing. When the Pco_2 increases at the same time, ventilation is greatly stimulated.

Changes in the hydrogen ion (H^+) concentration or pH of the blood also affect breathing. The H^+ concentration in the arterial blood is sensed by the peripheral H^+ sensors. When H^+ concentration is increased, e.g., in respiratory acidosis, respirations are increased. For additional information about breathing, see Chapter 45.

Respiratory Assessment

A client's respirations should be assessed when he or she is at rest because exercise affects respirations, increasing their rate and depth. Anxiety is likely to affect respiratory rate and depth as well.

Before assessing a client's respirations, a nurse should be aware of the client's normal breathing pattern, the influence of the client's health problems on his or her respirations, any medications or therapies that might affect respirations, and the relationship of the client's respirations to his or her cardiovascular function. The rate, depth, rhythm, and special characteristics of respirations should be assessed.

Respiratory Rate

The respiratory rate is normally described in breaths per minute. A healthy adult normally takes between 15 and 20 breaths per minute. For the respiratory rates for different age groups, see Table 34–1. Several factors influence respiratory rate. Some factors are listed in Table 34–5.

A number of terms are used to describe respiratory rate. A respiratory rate greater than 24 breaths per minute is called **tachypnea.** A rate of fewer than 10 respirations per minute is described as **bradypnea.** The complete absence of respirations is **apnea,** which is often described by its duration, e.g., 30 seconds of apnea. Prolonged apnea results in death.

Respiratory Depth

The depth of a person's respirations can be established by watching the movement of the chest. Respiratory depth is generally described as normal, deep, or shallow. Deep respirations are those in which a large volume of air is inhaled and exhaled, inflating most of the lungs. Shallow respirations involve the exchange of a small volume of air and often the use of minimal lung tissue. During a normal inspiration and expiration, an adult takes in about 500 ml of air. This volume is called the **tidal volume.**

The depth of respirations can also be measured accurately by the use of pulmonary equipment. See the discussion of pulmonary capacities in Chapter 45. It is also sometimes necessary to assess the symmetry of chest expansion by palpation. This technique is described in Chapter 35.

The capacity of the lungs varies with sex, age, stature, physical development, and body position. Men generally have a greater lung capacity than women of the same age. Variance by age is obvious: Babies have less vital capacity than children, children less than adolescents, and adolescents less than adults. However, elderly people usually have less vital capacity than young adults. Stature affects lung volume: Tall, thin people usually have a greater vital capacity than obese people. The athlete in top condition usually has a vital capacity that is above normal. (**Vital capacity** is the total of the tidal volume plus the inspiratory reserve volume plus the expiratory reserve volume. For further discussion of these volumes see Chapter 45.)

Body position also affects the amount of air that can be inhaled. People in a supine position experience two physiologic processes that suppress respiration: an increase in the volume of the intrathoracic blood and compression of the chest. Consequently, clients in a supine position have poorer lung aeration, which can predispose to the stasis of fluids and subsequent infection.

Certain medications also affect the respiratory depth. For example, such barbiturates as secobarbital sodium, when taken in large doses, depress the respiratory centers in the brain, thereby depressing the respiratory rate and depth.

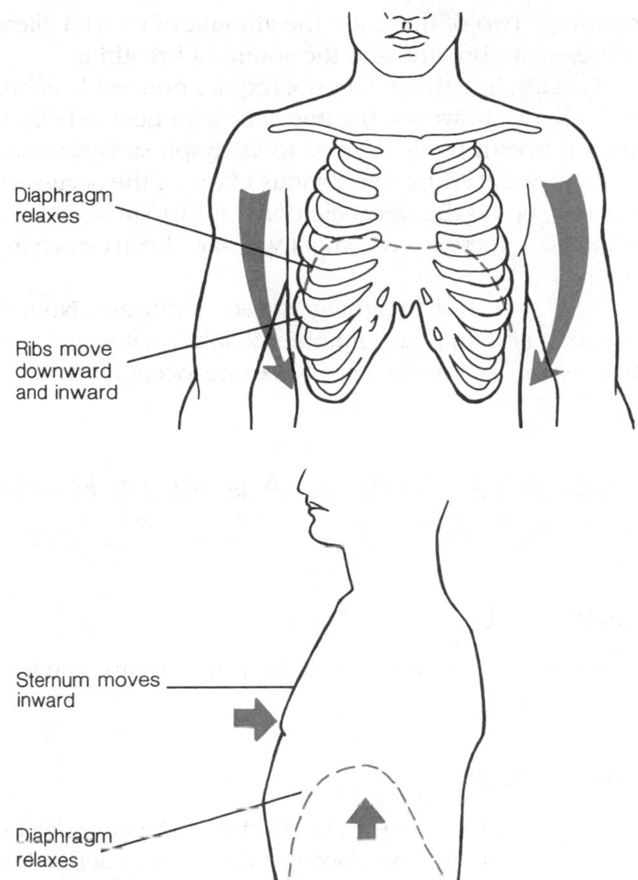

Figure 34–19 Respiratory exhalation: anterior and lateral views.

Respiratory Rhythm

Respiratory rhythm or pattern refers to the regularity of the expirations and the inspirations. Normally, respirations are evenly spaced. Respiratory rhythm can be described as regular or irregular. An infant's respiratory rhythm may be less regular than an adult's.

Some disease conditions affect a person's respiratory rhythm. Four abnormal respiratory rhythms are:

1. **Cheyne-Stokes respiration** is marked rhythmic waxing and waning of respirations from very deep to very shallow breathing and temporary apnea (cessation of breathing). The common causes of Cheyne-Stokes breathing are congestive heart failure, increased intracranial pressure, and drug overdose.
2. **Kussmaul's breathing**, also called air hunger or hyperventilation, is characterized by an increased rate and depth. Often, the rate exceeds 20 breaths per minute. It is seen in metabolic acidosis and renal failure.
3. **Apneustic breathing** is characterized by a prolonged gasping inspiration followed by a very short expiration. The expiration is usually inefficient. Apneustic breathing is seen in clients with central nervous system disorders.
4. **Biot's respirations** are shallow breaths interrupted by apnea. They are seen in healthy people and in clients with central nervous system disorders.

Table 34–5 **Major Factors Influencing Respiratory Rate**

Factor	Influence
Exercise: increases metabolism	Increase
Stress: readies the body for "fight or flight"	Increase
Environment: increased temperature	Increase
Increased altitude: lower oxygen concentration	Increase
Certain medications, e.g., morphine	Decrease

Respiratory Quality

The quality of respiration refers to those aspects of breathing that are different from normal, effortless breathing. Two of these are the amount of effort a client must exert to breathe and the sound of breathing.

Usually, breathing does not require noticeable effort; some clients, however, breathe only with decided effort. Difficult breathing is referred to as **dyspnea**. Dyspnea is usually evidenced by the obvious effort of the accessory muscles, such as the sternocleidomastoid, to maintain respirations. Sometimes the client will say, "I can't catch my breath."

The sound of breathing is also significant. Normal breathing is silent, but a number of abnormal sounds are obvious to the nurse's ear. Wheezing occurs when the airway is constricted; wheezing is usually more apparent on expiration than inspiration. Acute constriction of the trachea produces a harsh crowing sound on inspiration called **stridor**. This usually reflects respiratory distress. **Rales** or **rhonchi** are bubbling or crackling sounds that are evident with respirations. These sounds occur as a result of the presence of fluid in the lungs and are most clearly heard with a stethoscope. See Chapter 35, pages 844–47, for auscultation and percussion methods used to assess lung sounds and Chapter 35, page 847, for further information about abnormal breath sounds.

Procedure 34–5 ▲ Assessing Respirations

Equipment

A watch with a second hand or indicator to time the respiratory rate.

Intervention

1. Place a hand against the client's chest to feel the client's chest movements or place the client's arm across his or her chest and/or observe the chest movements while supposedly taking the radial pulse.

   Rationale An explanation about assessing respirations could cause the client to alter his or her respiratory pattern.

2. Count the respirations for 30 seconds if they are regular. Count for 1 minute if they are irregular. An inhalation and an exhalation count as one respiration. For an infant or young child, count the respirations for a full minute. If the respiratory rate is abnormally slow or fast, count for a full minute.

3. Observe the depth of respirations by watching the movement of the chest. During deep respirations, a large volume of air is exchanged; during shallow respirations, a small volume is exchanged.

4. Observe the respirations for regular or irregular rhythm. Normally, respirations are evenly spaced. If the respirations are irregular, observe them for a full minute.

5. Observe the quality of respirations—the sound they produce and the effort they require. Normally, respirations are silent and effortless.

6. Record the respiratory rate, depth, rhythm, and quality on the appropriate record.

Sample Recording

Date	Time	Notes
Jun/20/87	0900	R 38 and shallow. Dyspneic when talking. Dr. Woo notified.——————John P. Brown, NS

Blood Pressure

Arterial blood pressure is a measure of the pressure exerted by the blood as it pulsates through the arteries. Because the blood moves in waves, there are two blood pressure measures: the **systolic pressure**, which is the pressure of the blood as a result of contraction of the ventricles, i.e., the pressure at the height of the blood wave; and the **diastolic pressure**, which is the pressure when the ventricles are at rest. Diastolic pressure, then, is the lower pressure, present at all times within the arteries. The difference between the diastolic and the systolic pressures is called the **pulse pressure**.

Blood pressure is measured in millimeters of mercury (mm Hg). This measurement registers on a sphygmomanometer, which reflects the pressure of air in a rubber cuff wrapped around a client's extremity, e.g., the upper arm.

Physiology of Arterial Blood Pressure

The arterial blood pressure is the result of the cardiac output times the resistance the blood encounters while it flows, i.e., the peripheral vascular resistance.

A person's blood pressure is directly affected by the volume of blood in the systemic circulation. The human body normally has about 5 liters of blood. Of this 5 liters, about 80% to 90% is in the systemic circulation and 10% to 20% is in the pulmonary circulation. Of the blood in the systemic circulation, about 75% is in the veins, about 20% is in the arteries, and about 5% is in the capillaries (Vick 1984, p. 197). The amount of blood in the veins can vary considerably. When a person hemorrhages, the loss of blood volume is made up by decreased venous vascular tone, i.e., the venous volume becomes smaller.

Blood flows in the vascular system along a pressure gradient. The blood pressure of the blood in the aorta, for example, is higher than the pressure in the arterioles, and in the arterioles it is higher than in the capillaries. See Figure 34–20.

Cardiac Output

Cardiac output increases with fever and exercise, and the systolic pressure may increase as a result. However, cardiac output can be decreased as a result of heart disease, and the systolic pressure may then be low.

Peripheral Vascular Resistance

Peripheral resistance can increase blood pressure, especially diastolic pressure. Some factors that create resistance in the arterial system are the size of the arterioles and capillaries, the compliance of the arteries, and the viscosity of the blood.

Size of the Arterioles and Capillaries

The size of the arterioles and the capillaries determines in great part the peripheral resistance to the blood in the body. A **lumen** (plural: lumina) is a channel within a tube: the smaller the lumina the greater the resistance. Normally, the arterioles are in a state of partial constriction. Increased vasoconstriction raises the blood pressure, whereas decreased vasoconstriction lowers the blood pressure.

Compliance of the Blood Vessels

The arteries contain smooth muscles that permit them to contract, thus decreasing their **compliance** (distensibility). Arteries normally yield somewhat during systole and retract during diastole. The arteries account for most of the peripheral resistance (Vick 1984, p. 199).

The major factor reducing arterial compliance is the pathologic changes that affect the arterial walls. In old age, the elastic and muscular tissues of the arteries are replaced with fibrous tissue; thus, the arteries lose much of their compliance. The condition is known as **arteriosclerosis**.

Viscosity of the Blood

The viscosity of the blood is its "thickness." **Viscosity** is a physical property that results from friction among its molecules. In a viscous fluid, there is a great deal of friction among the molecules as they slide by each other. The blood pressure is higher when the blood is highly viscous, i.e., when the proportion of red blood cells to the blood plasma is high. This ratio is referred to as the **hematocrit**. The viscosity increases markedly when the hematocrit is more than 60% to 65% (Vick 1984, p. 204).

Normal Blood Pressure

The average blood pressure of a healthy young adult is 120/80 mm Hg. A number of conditions influence blood pressure. The most common is **hypertension**, an abnormally high blood pressure of 140 mm Hg systolic and/or 90 mm Hg diastolic when these are confirmed during a minimum of two consecutive visits by a client (National Heart, Lung, and Blood Institute 1984, p. 1045). **Hypotension,** or an abnormally low blood pressure, is a pressure below 100 mm Hg systolic.

Because blood pressure can vary considerably among individuals, it is important for the nurse to know a specific client's usual blood pressure. For example, if a client's usual blood pressure is 180/100 mm Hg and it is assessed following surgery to be 120/80 mm Hg, this drop in pressure must be reported to the charge nurse or physician. A number of conditions affect blood pressure. Some of these are listed in Table 34–6.

Factors Affecting Blood Pressure

Among the factors influencing blood pressure are age, exercise, stress, race, sex, medications, and diurnal variations.

1. *Age.* Blood pressure increases with age. See Table 34–1. In elderly people, the diastolic pressure often increases as a result of the reduced compliance of the arteries.
2. *Exercise.* Exercise increases the cardiac output and hence the blood pressure. Therefore, a client should be rested when blood pressure is taken if the reading is to be reliable. Usually, a rest of 20 to 30 minutes following exercise is indicated before the blood pressure can be assessed.
3. *Stress.* Stress due to anxiety, fear, and moderate pain can also increase the blood pressure. Stimulation of the sympathetic nervous system increases cardiac output and vasoconstriction of the arterioles. However, severe pain can decrease blood pressure greatly and cause shock. In this case, the vasomotor center is inhibited, and vasodilation takes place.
4. *Race.* Blood pressure varies with race. Black males over 35 years have higher blood pressures than white males of the same age. This is a complex problem often related to body weight. Blood pressure is consistently higher in overweight and obese people than in people of normal weight (Overfield 1985, p. 46).
5. *Sex.* There is no difference in the blood pressures of preadolescent girls and boys. After puberty, however, females usually have lower blood pressures than males of the same age. This difference is thought to be due to hormonal variations. After menopause, women generally have higher blood pressures than before.
6. *Medications.* Some medications such as clonidine hydrochloride, an agent that depresses the sympathetic nervous system, decrease the blood pressure, while other medications, such as epinephrine bitartrate (Primatene Mist), increase the blood pressure by stimulating the sympathetic nervous system.
7. *Diurnal variations.* The blood pressures of individuals usually vary with the time of day. Usually, pressure is lowest early in the morning, when the metabolic rate is lowest. The blood pressure then rises throughout the day and peaks in the late afternoon or early evening.

Blood Pressure Assessment

Blood pressure can be assessed directly or indirectly. Direct measurement involves the insertion of a catheter into the brachial, radial, or femoral artery. Arterial pressure is represented as wavelike forms displayed on an oscilloscope. Generally, physicians insert the catheters, and nurses monitor the pressure readings. This pressure reading is highly accurate.

There are three methods of measuring blood pressure indirectly: the auscultatory, palpatory, and flush methods.

Table 34–6 Selected Conditions Affecting Blood Pressure

Condition	Effect	Cause
Fever	Increase	Increases metabolic rate
Stress	Increase	Increases heart rate
Arteriosclerosis	Increase	Decreases artery compliance
Obesity	Increase	Increases peripheral resistance
Hemorrhage	Decrease	Decreases blood volume
Low hematocrit	Decrease	Decreases blood viscosity
External heat	Decrease	Increases vasodilation and thus decreases peripheral vascular resistance
Exposure to cold	Increase	Causes vasoconstriction and thus increases peripheral vascular resistance

Auscultatory Method

The auscultatory is the method of assessing blood pressure most commonly used in hospitals, clinics, and homes. Required equipment is a sphygmomanometer, cuff, and a stethoscope (see "Blood Pressure Equipment," later in this chapter). External pressure is applied to a superficial artery, and the nurse reads the pressure from the sphygmomanometer when the blood flow is first heard through a stethoscope. This method is described in detail in Procedure 34–6. When carried out correctly, the auscultatory method is relatively accurate.

Palpatory Method

The palpatory method is sometimes used when **Korotkoff's sounds** (the sounds heard over an artery when blood pressure is determined by the auscultatory method) cannot be heard and electronic equipment to amplify the sounds is not available. Instead of listening for the blood flow sounds, the nurse palpates the pulsations of the artery as the pressure in the cuff is released. The systolic pressure is read from the sphygmomanometer when the first pulsation is felt. A single whiplike vibration, felt in addition to the pulsations, identifies the point at which the pressure in the cuff nears the diastolic pressure (Enselberg 1961, p. 273). This vibration is no longer felt when the cuff pressure is below the diastolic pressure. To palpate the diastolic pressure, the nurse applies light to moderate pressure over the pulse point.

Flush Method

The flush method for determining blood pressure is used on infants when Korotkoff's sounds cannot be heard by auscultation and electronic equipment is not available. The measurement is determined by a change in skin color when blood flow to an extremity resumes, i.e., when the extremity is no longer extremely pale but becomes reddened (vascular flush). The cuff is applied to the infant's arm and the limb is wrapped in a bandage distally to proximally to force venous blood out of and restrict arterial flow into the extremity. The cuff is then inflated and the bandage is removed. The cuff pressure is released, and the nurse reads the pressure from the sphygmomanometer when the extremity flushes. This reading is the **mean blood pressure**, the midway point between the systolic and diastolic pressures.

Blood Pressure Assessment Sites

Upper Arm

The upper arm is usually used for assessing a client's blood pressure. The client should be seated comfortably with the whole forearm supported at heart level. The forearm should be horizontal at the level of the fourth intercostal space (at the heart level) (American Heart Association 1980, p. 12). Raising the arm above that level lowers the blood pressure, and lowering the arm below it increases the blood pressure. The brachial pulse is used to auscultate the blood pressure.

Thigh

The thigh is the indicated site when the arm cannot be used because of injury or when the blood pressure in one thigh is to be compared with the pressure in the other thigh. The client assumes a prone or a supine position with the knee slightly flexed. A thigh blood pressure cuff is wrapped around the thigh, and the pulsations of the blood are auscultated above the popliteal artery.

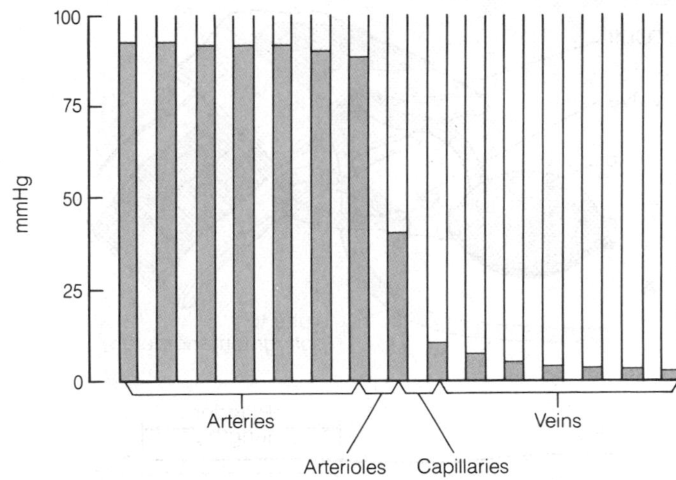

Figure 34–20 The mean blood pressure in the different parts of the vascular system

Source: Adapted from R. L. Vick, *Contemporary medical physiology* (Menlo Park, Calif.: Addison-Wesley Publishing Co., 1984), p. 198.

Leg

The leg is the indicated site when the other areas are not available or when it is necessary to obtain a leg pressure, e.g., when the client has peripheral vascular disease.

To obtain the blood pressure, the nurse applies a leg cuff to the lower leg. The distal border of the cuff should be at the malleoli. The sounds are auscultated at the posterior tibial or dorsalis pedis pulse sites.

Forearm

When the upper arms and thighs cannot be used for some reason, the forearm can be used. A cuff of appropriate size is placed around the forearm, with the proximal border 13 cm (5.1 in) below the elbow. Korotkoff's sounds are auscultated at the radial pulse.

Blood Pressure Equipment

Blood pressure is measured with a **blood pressure cuff**, a **sphygmomanometer**, and a **stethoscope**. The blood pressure cuff consists of a rubber bag that can be inflated with air. It is called the **bladder**. See Figure 34–21. It is usually covered with cloth and has two tubes attached to it. One tube connects to a rubber bulb that inflates the bladder. When turned counterclockwise, a small valve on the side of this bulb releases the air in the bladder. When the valve is tightened (turned clockwise), air pumped into the bladder remains there. The other tube is attached to a sphygmomanometer.

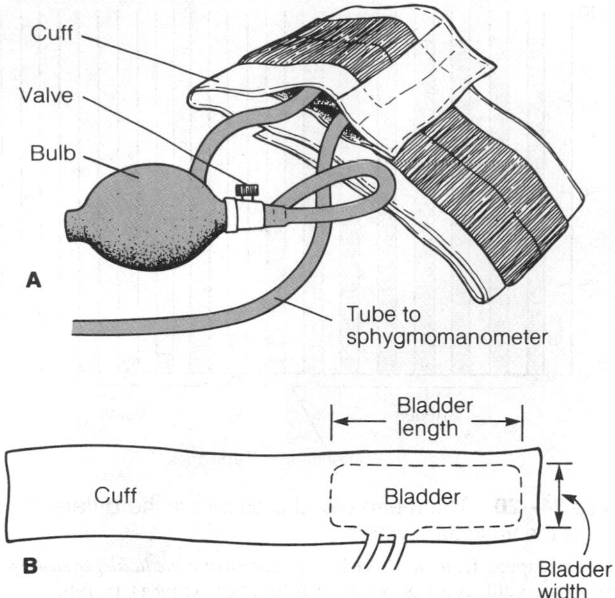

Figure 34–21 **A,** A blood pressure cuff and bulb; **B,** the bladder inside the cuff.

The sphygmomanometer indicates the pressure of the air within the bladder. There are two types of sphygmomanometers: **aneroid** and **mercury**. See Figure 34–22. The aneroid sphygmomanometer is a calibrated dial with a needle that points to the calibrations. The mercury sphygmomanometer is a calibrated cylinder filled with mercury. The pressure is indicated at the point to which the **meniscus** of the mercury (the crescent-shaped top surface of the column) rises. It is important to view the meniscus at eye level to avoid distortions in the reading.

Some agencies use electronic sphygmomanometers, which eliminate the need to listen to the sounds of the client's systolic and diastolic blood pressures through a stethoscope. With some electronic sphygmomanometers, as the pressure in the cuff is lowered, a light flashes to indicate the systolic and diastolic pressures.

Ultrasound (Doppler) stethoscopes are also used to assess blood pressure. See Figure 34–14, earlier. These are of particular value when Korotkoff's sounds are difficult to hear, e.g., in infants, obese clients, and clients in shock. Transmission gel is applied to a transducer probe, which is placed over the pulse point, and the blood pressure is measured. A systolic blood pressure assessed with a Doppler stethoscope is recorded with a large D, e.g., 85D. Systolic pressure may be the only blood pressure obtainable with some ultrasound models.

Blood pressure cuffs come in various sizes, since the bladder must be the correct width and length for the client's arm. If the bladder is too narrow, the blood pressure reading will be erroneously elevated; if it is too wide, the reading will be erroneously low. The width should be 40% of the circumference, or 20% wider than the

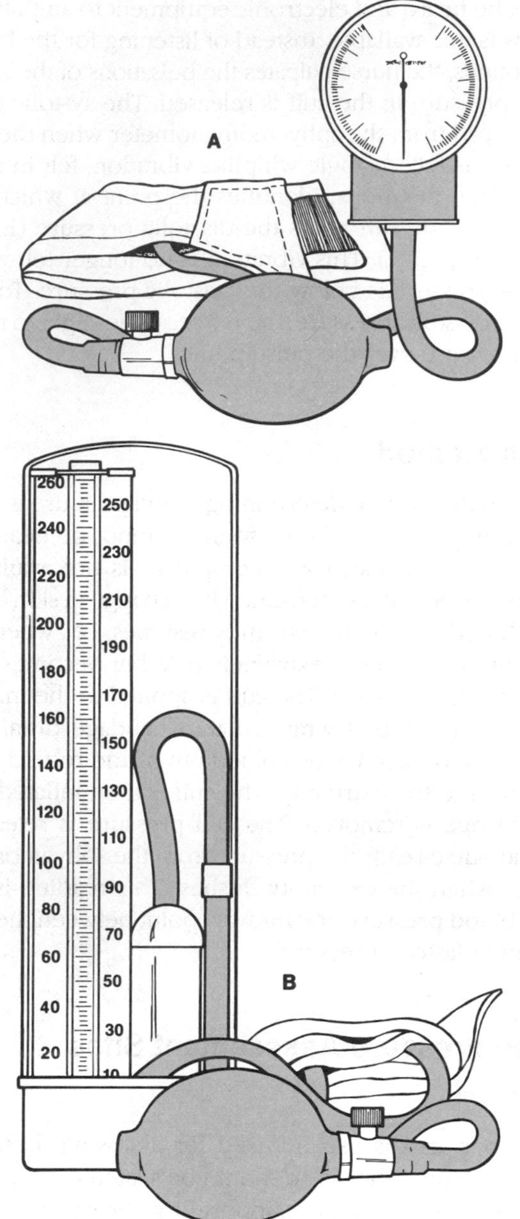

Figure 34–22 Blood pressure equipment: **A,** an aneroid manometer and cuff; **B,** a mercury manometer and cuff.

diameter of the midpoint of the limb on which it is used (American Heart Association 1980, p. 4). To determine whether the width of a blood pressure cuff is appropriate, lay the cuff lengthwise at the midpoint of the upper arm. Hold the outermost side of the bladder edge laterally on the arm. With the other hand, wrap the width of the cuff around the arm and determine whether the width is 40% of the arm circumference. See Figure 34–23.

The length of the bladder also affects the accuracy of measurement. The bladder should be sufficiently long to almost encircle the limb and cover from 60% to 100% of its circumference, preferably 80%, i.e., twice the rec-

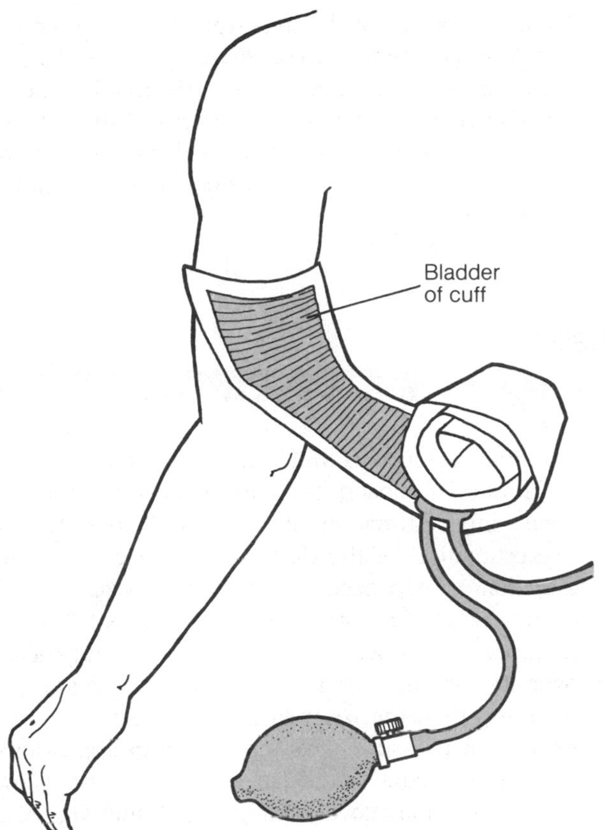

Figure 34–23 Determining if a blood pressure cuff is the correct width.

ommended width (American Heart Association 1980, pp. 4, 5). The bladder dimensions of various cuff sizes, which are given age group names, are shown in Table 34–7; the arm circumference, not the age of the client, should always determine bladder size.

Blood pressure cuffs are made of nondistensible material so that an even pressure is exerted around the limb. Most cuffs are held in place by hooks, snaps, or Velcro. Others have a cloth bandage that is long enough to encircle the limb several times; this type is closed by tucking the end of the bandage into one of the bandage folds.

Korotkoff's Sounds

When taking a blood pressure using a stethoscope, the nurse identifies five phases in the series of sounds called Korotkoff's sounds. First the nurse pumps the cuff up to about 30 mm Hg above the point where the last sound is heard; that is the point when the blood flow in the artery is stopped. Then the pressure is released slowly (2 to 3 mm Hg per sound), while the nurse observes the pressure readings on the manometer and relates them to the sounds heard through the stethoscope. Five phases occur (American Heart Association 1980, p. 11):

Table 34–7 Recommended Blood Pressure Cuff Bladder Dimensions by Arm Circumference

Adult Size	Arm Circumference Range (cm)	Bladder Width (cm)
Adult (Regular)	26-33*	12
Adult (Large)	33-41	15
Thigh	41	18

*Range by Canadian Heart Foundation is 22-33 cm.

Source: American Heart Association. *Recommendations for human blood pressure determination by sphygmo-manometers,* Pub No. 701005. American Heart Association, 1987 p. 10 and Canadian Heart Foundation: *Know your blood pressure by heart: professional guide,* Pub No. 87-09-4.5M. Canadian Heart Foundation, 1987, p. 3.

Phase 1. The period initiated by the first faint clear tapping sounds. These sounds gradually become more intense. To ensure that they are not extraneous sounds, the nurse should identify at least two consecutive tapping sounds.

Phase 2. The period during which the sounds have a swishing quality.

Phase 3. The period during which the sounds are crisper and more intense.

Phase 4. The period during which the sounds become muffled and have a soft, blowing quality.

Phase 5. The point where the sounds disappear.

When Korotkoff's sounds are difficult to hear, the nurse can augment them. See below.

The American Heart Association (AHA) recommends that the systolic pressure be considered the point where

To Augment Korotkoff's Sounds:

- Apply the cuff correctly.
- Raise the arm over head.
- Inflate the cuff quickly.
- Lower arm so that the cuff is at heart level.
- Take the blood pressure reading. (Hill 1980, pp. 942–945)

the first tapping sound is heard (Phase 1). In adults, the diastolic pressure is the point where the sounds become inaudible (Phase 5). In children, however, the AHA recommends that diastolic pressure be considered to be the onset of Phase 4, where the sounds become muffled. In agencies where the fourth phase is considered the diastolic pressure of adults, three measures are recommended (systolic pressure, diastolic pressure, and Phase 5). These may be referred to as systolic, first diastolic, and second diastolic pressures. The Phase 5 (second diastolic pressure) reading may be zero; that is, the muffled sounds are heard even when there is no air pressure in the blood pressure cuff. In some instances, muffled sounds are never heard, in which case a dash is inserted where the reading would normally be recorded.

Procedure 34–6 ▲ Assessing Blood Pressure

Equipment

1. A stethoscope. Clean the ear attachments with disinfectant, if others have worn it.
   or
   An ultrasound (Doppler) stethoscope (see Figure 34–14, earlier).
2. A blood pressure cuff of the appropriate size (newborn, infant, child, small adult, adult, large adult, thigh).
3. A sphygmomanometer.

Intervention

1. Help the client to assume the appropriate position. A sitting position is normally used unless otherwise specified. The arm should be slightly flexed with the palm of the hand facing up and the forearm supported at heart level. Readings in any other position should be specified.

   Rationale The blood pressure is normally similar in sitting, standing, and lying positions, but it can vary significantly by position in certain persons. There is an increase in the blood pressure when the arm is below heart level and a decrease when it is above heart level (AHA 1980, p. 12).

2. Expose the upper arm.
3. Wrap the deflated cuff evenly around the upper arm so that the center of the bladder is applied directly over the medial aspect of the arm. To take an adult's blood pressure, place the lower border of the cuff about 2.5 cm (1 in) above the antecubital space. The lower edge can be nearer the antecubital space of an infant.

   Rationale The bladder inside the cuff must be directly over the artery to be compressed if the reading is to be accurate.

4. If this is the client's initial examination, perform a preliminary palpatory determination of systolic pressure.

   Rationale The initial estimate tells the nurse the maximal pressure to which the manometer needs to be elevated in subsequent determinations. It also prevents underestimation of the systolic pressure or overestimation of the diastolic pressure should an auscultatory gap occur. An auscultatory gap, which occurs particularly in hypertensive clients, is the temporary disappearance of sounds normally heard over the brachial artery when the cuff pressure is high and then the reappearance of the sounds at a lower cuff pressure. This temporary disappearance of sounds occurs in the latter part of Phase 1 and Phase 2 and may cover a range of 40 mm Hg (AHA 1980, p. 11).

   a. Palpate the brachial artery with the fingertips. The brachial artery is normally found medially in the antecubital space. See Figure 34–24.
   b. Close the valve on the pump by turning the knob clockwise.
   c. Pump up the cuff until you no longer feel the brachial pulse.

      Rationale At that pressure the blood cannot flow through the artery.

   d. Note the pressure on the sphygmomanometer at which the pulse is no longer felt.

      Rationale This gives an estimate of the maximum pressure required to measure the systolic pressure.

   e. Release the pressure completely in the cuff and wait 1 to 2 minutes before making further measurements.

      Rationale A waiting period gives the blood trapped in the veins time to be released.

5. Insert the ear attachments of the stethoscope in your ears so that they tilt slightly forward.

   Rationale Sounds are sharper when the ear attachments follow the direction of the ear canal.

6. Ensure that the stethoscope hangs freely from the ears to the diaphragm.

Rationale Rubbing the stethoscope against an object can obliterate Korotkoff's sounds.

7. Place the diaphragm of the stethoscope over the brachial pulse. Use the bell-shaped diaphragm of the stethoscope (see Figure 34–17, earlier) (AHA 1980, p. 7). Hold the diaphragm with the thumb and index finger.
8. Pump up the cuff until the sphygmomanometer registers about 30 mm Hg above the point where the brachial pulse disappears.
9. Release the valve on the cuff carefully so that the pressure decreases at the rate of 2 to 3 mm Hg per second.

   Rationale If the rate is faster or slower, an error in measurement may occur (AHA 1980, p. 11).
10. As the pressure falls, identify the manometer reading at each of the five phases.
11. Deflate the cuff rapidly and completely and wait 1 to 2 minutes before repeating.

    Rationale This wait permits blood trapped in the veins to be released.
12. Repeat steps 8–11 once or twice as necessary to confirm the accuracy of the reading.
13. Remove the cuff from the client's arm.
14. If this is the client's initial examination, repeat the procedure on his or her other arm. The arm found to have the higher pressure should be used for subsequent examinations (AHA 1980, p. 10).
15. Record the blood pressure according to agency policy. Record two pressures in the form "130/80" where "130" is the systolic (Phase 1) and "80" is the diastolic (Phase 5) pressure. Record three pressures in the form "130/110/90" where "130" is the systolic, 110 is the first diastolic (Phase 4), and "90" is the second diastolic (Phase 5) pressure. If agency policy permits, use abbreviations RA for right arm and LA for left arm.
16. Report any significant change in the client's blood pressure to the responsible nurse.

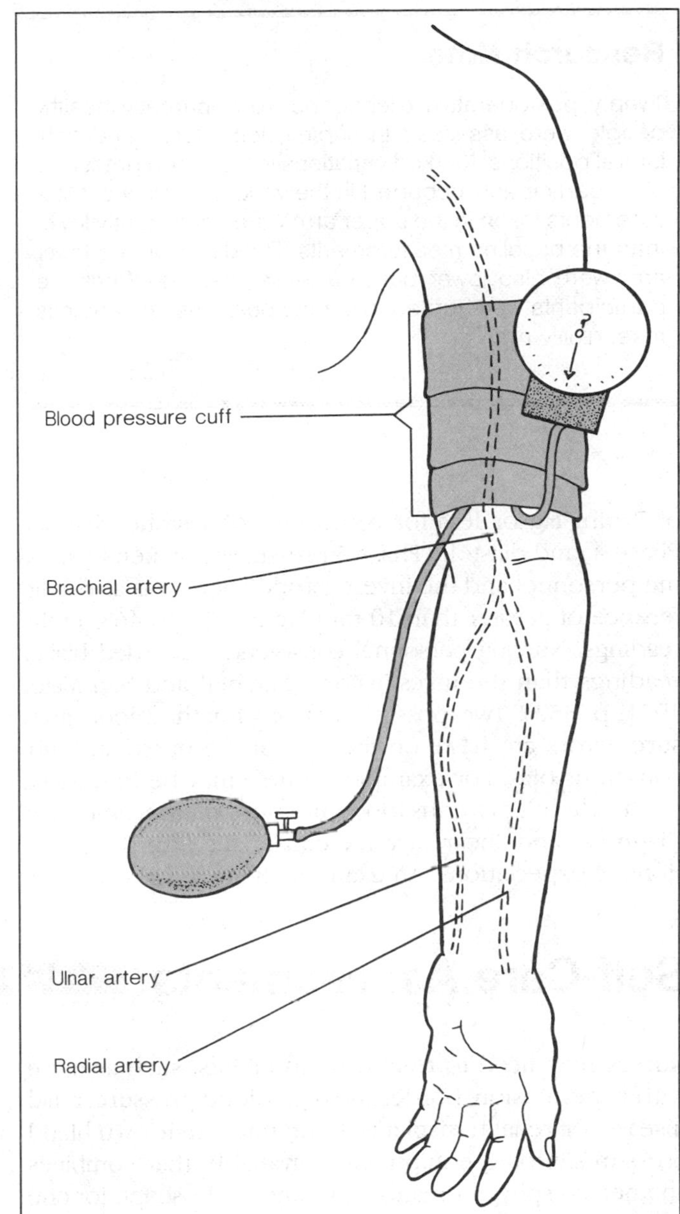

Figure 34–24

Sample Recording

Date	Time	Notes
May/14/87	1300	BP 130/90 in RA in bed-sitting position. Color pale. ——— Ruth P. O'Shea, SN

Blood Pressure Measurement Errors

The importance of the accuracy of blood pressure assessments cannot be overemphasized. Many judgments about a client's health are made as a result of his or her blood pressure. It is an important indicator of the client's condition and is used extensively as a basis for nursing interventions. Mitchell and Van Meter found a mean difference

Research Note

Twenty postoperative clients and 40 apparently healthy people were assessed in supine, left lateral, and right lateral positions. Marked variations in the blood pressures of all participants occurred in the various positions. Measurements taken in the upper arm were consistently lower than the baseline measurements. Readings on the lower arm were also lower but to a lesser degree. When the participants were turned to supine positions, all readings rose. (Foley 1971)

of 7 mm Hg or less for recordings of systolic, diastolic Phase 4, and diastolic Phase 5 pressures as taken by nursing personnel and the investigators. There was also a difference of greater than 10 mm Hg in 37% to 46% of the readings. Nursing personnel consistently recorded higher readings than the investigators (Mitchell and Van Meter 1971, p. 352). Two possible reasons for the blood pressure errors are haste on the part of the nurse and subconscious bias. For example, a nurse may be influenced by the client's previous blood pressure measurements or diagnosis and "hear" a value consonant with the practitioner's expectations. An example of such a bias is "digit preference," a predilection for pressures ending with zero, e.g., 130 systolic, 70 diastolic, more often than would be expected (AHA 1980, p. 21). Some reasons for erroneous blood pressure readings are given in Table 34–8.

Table 34–8 Sources of Error in Blood Pressure Assessment

Error	Effect
Bladder cuff too narrow	Erroneously high
Bladder cuff too wide	Erroneously low
Arm unsupported	Erroneously high
Insufficient rest before the assessment	Erroneously high
Repeating assessment too quickly	Erroneously high systolic or low diastolic readings
Cuff wrapped too loosely or unevenly	Erroneously high
Deflating cuff too quickly	Erroneously low systolic and high diastolic readings
Deflating cuff too slowly	Erroneously high
Failure to use the same arm consistently	Inconsistent measurements
Arm above level of the heart	Erroneously low
Assessing immediately after a meal or while client smokes or has pain	Erroneously high
Failure to identify auscultatory gap	Erroneously low

Self-Care Assessments

Nurses may need to teach certain clients, such as those with hypertension, borderline high blood pressure, renal disease, or renal transplants, to monitor their own blood pressures. Home equipment is available that combines an aneroid sphygmomanometer and stethoscope for one person to use. The advantages of self-monitoring include:

1. Increased motivation to follow a therapeutic regime such as taking antihypertension medication
2. Increased involvement of the family in the client's treatment program
3. Reinforcement of the importance of frequent blood pressure measurement
4. Provision of a record of daily blood pressure by which caregivers can assess the effects of prescribed therapy.

When teaching clients self-monitoring, the nurse needs to check the client's equipment for accuracy, ascertain the client's understanding of the procedure, and assess the client's ability to perform the technique correctly. Teaching can be enhanced by the use of visual aids available from the AHA.

Coin-operated blood pressure machines are now available in many public places. The client sits facing the machine and rests his or her arm inside an inflatable cuff that contains a pressure sensor. A visual display panel shows the blood pressure within 60 to 90 seconds. Nurses should inform clients about possible inaccuracies in measurements obtained from such machines. Computer function can be altered by nearby noise, and often the cuff is improperly placed. Clients who report high readings on such machines, however, should be advised to see their physicians. A problem with coin-operated machines is the lack of educational material to support the information they impart. People need explanations about the meaning and implications of the measurements.

Chapter Highlights

- Vital signs reflect changes in body function that otherwise might not be observed.
- The nurse uses her or his own judgment to determine the frequency of vital signs assessment.

- Vital signs are assessed when a client is admitted to a health care agency to establish baseline data and when there is a change or possibility of a change in the client's condition.
- Data obtained from vital signs measurements are used to plan and implement appropriate nursing interventions.
- Vital signs measurements are also used to evaluate a client's response to nursing interventions or prescribed medical therapy.
- Knowledge of the normal ranges of vital signs and of the factors that regulate and influence vital signs helps the nurse interpret the measurements that deviate from normal.
- Body temperature is the balance between heat produced by the body and heat lost from the body.
- Heat is produced by the body's metabolic processes, which can be accelerated by muscle activity, thyroxine output, and stimulation of the sympathetic nervous system.
- Heat is lost from the body by radiation, conduction, convection, and vaporization.
- Knowledge of factors affecting heat production and heat loss helps the nurse to implement appropriate interventions when the client has a fever, hypothermia, or other related disorders, such as heat stroke.
- Pulse rate and volume reflect the stroke volume output, the compliance of the client's arteries, and the adequacy of blood flow.
- Normally, a peripheral pulse reflects the client's heartbeat, but it may differ from the heartbeat in clients with certain cardiovascular diseases; in these instances, the nurse takes an apical pulse and compares it to the peripheral pulse.
- Respirations are normally quiet, effortless, and automatic and are assessed by observing respiratory movements.
- Blood pressure reflects cardiac output and peripheral vascular resistance; peripheral vascular resistance varies according to the size of the arterioles and capillaries, compliance of the arteries, and blood viscosity.
- Various sites and methods can be used to assess vital signs.
- The nurse selects the site and method that is safe for the client and that will provide the most accurate measurement possible.
- The most accurate values are obtained when the client is at rest and comfortable.
- Change in one vital sign can trigger changes in other vital signs.

Suggested Readings

Adelman, E. M. February 1980. When the patient's blood pressure falls ... What does it mean? What should you do? *Nursing 80* 10:26–33.
Adelman discusses causes of hypotension and provides guidelines for the nurse to follow when hypotension is suspected. In addition, six mistakes that produce abnormally low blood pressure readings are listed.

Blainey, C. G. October 1974. Site selection in taking body temperature. *American Journal of Nursing* 74:1859–61.
Blainey discusses rectal temperatures and their advantages and disadvantages as well as oral and other temperatures. The author concludes that the sublingual site provides the most accurate reflection of body temperature under normal conditions.

Castle, M., and Watkins, J. February 1979. Fever: Understanding a sinister sign. *Nursing 79* 9:26–33.
The authors include case examples of remittent and constant fever, intermittent fever, and relapsing fever. The nurse's role in caring for the client with a fever is outlined.

Hill, M. N. May 1980. Hypertension: What can go wrong when you measure blood pressure. *American Journal of Nursing* 80:942–45.
Hill gives a nine-step procedure for taking the blood pressure. Rationales for each step are provided. Also included is a description of each phase of Korotkoff's sounds.

Jarvis, C. M. April 1976. Vital signs: How to take them more accurately and understand them more fully. *Nursing 76* 6:31–37.
Jarvis gives in-depth meanings of the vital signs.

Seaman, D. January 1985. Should you trust automatic blood pressure monitors? *Nursing 85* 15:54–57.
Seaman describes the basic features of automatic blood pressure monitors and how they work. Advantages and tips to prevent inaccurate readings are included.

Tate, G. V., et al. September 1970. Correct use of electric thermometers. *American Journal of Nursing* 70:1898–99.
The authors point out that distrust of the electric thermometer may be related to the nurse's insecurity in using it or to the sensitivity of the instrument itself. Correct ways to operate the thermometer are discussed.

Selected References

Abbey, J. C., et al. August 1978. How long is that thermometer accurate? *American Journal of Nursing* 78:1375–76.

American Heart Association. 1980. *Recommendations for human blood pressure determination by sphygmomanometers.* Pub No. 70-019-B, 80-100M, 9-81-100M. American Heart Association.

Axillary temps safer in infants. June 1978. (Medical Highlights.) *American Journal of Nursing* 78:1081.

Baker, N. C.; Cerone, S. B.; Gaze, N.; and Knapp, T. R. March/April 1984. The effect of thermometer and length of time inserted on oral temperature measurements of afebrile subjects. *Nursing Research* 33:109–11.

Behrman, R. E., and Vaughan, V. C. III, editors. 1983. *Nelson textbook of pediatrics.* 12th ed. Philadelphia: W. B. Saunders.

Blainey, C. G. October 1974. Site selection in taking body temperature. *American Journal of Nursing* 74:1859–61.

Canetto, V. November 1964. T.P.R. q.4h. ad infinitum? *American Journal of Nursing* 64:132.

Correcting common errors in blood pressure measurements: Programmed instruction. October 1965. *American Journal of Nursing* 65:133–64.

Creative Care Unit. June 1977. Turnabout: Rectal temperatures for postcoronary patients. *American Journal of Nursing* 77:997.

Davis-Sharts, J. November 1978. Mechanisms and manifestations of fever. *American Journal of Nursing* 78:1874–77.

DuBois, E. F. 1948. *Fever and the regulation of body temperature.* Springfield, Ill.: Charles C. Thomas.

Enselberg, C. D. 1961. Measurement of diastolic blood pressure by palpation. *New England Journal of Medicine* 265:272–74.

Eoff, M. J., and Joyce, B. May 1981. Temperature measurement in children. *American Journal of Nursing* 81:1010–11.

Eoff, M. J.; Meier, R. S.; and Miller, C. November/December 1974. Temperature measurement in infants. *Nursing Research* 23:457–60.

Erickson, R. May/June 1980. Oral temperature differences in relation to thermometer and technique. *Nursing Research* 29:157–64.

Evans, M. J. March 1983. Tips for taking a child's blood pressure quickly. *Nursing 83* 13:61.

Felton, G. January/February 1970. Effect of time cycle change on blood pressure and temperature in young women. *Nursing Research* 19:48–58.

Foley, M. F. January/February 1971. Variations in blood pressure in the lateral recumbent position. *Nursing Research* 20:64–69.

Graas, S. October 1974. Thermometer sites and oxygen. *American Journal of Nursing* 74:1862–63.

Graves, R. D., and Markarian, M. F. September/October 1980. Three-minute intervals when using an oral mercury-in-glass thermometer without J-temperature sheaths. *Nursing Research* 29:323–24.

Guyton, A. C. 1986. *Textbook of medical physiology.* 7th ed. Philadelphia: W. B. Saunders Co.

Hasler, M. E., and Cohen, J. A. September/October 1982. The effect of oxygen administration on temperature assessment. *Nursing Research* 31:265–68.

Hudson, B. May 1983. Sharpen your vascular skills with the Doppler ultrasound stethoscope. *Nursing 83* 13:55–57.

Jarvis, C. M. April 1976. Vital signs: How to take them more accurately and understand them more fully. *Nursing 76* 6:31–37.

Kolanowski, A., and Gunter, L. September/October 1981. Hypothermia in the elderly. *Geriatric Nursing* 2:362–65.

Kurtz, K. J. January 1982. Hypothermia in the elderly: The cold facts. *Geriatrics* 37:85.

Lim-Levy, F. May/June 1982. The effect of oxygen inhalation on oral temperature. *Nursing Research* 31:150–52.

Mitchell, P. W., and Van Meter, M. J. July/August 1971. Reproducibility of blood pressure recorded on patients' records by nursing personnel. *Nursing Research* 20:348–52.

National Heart, Lung, and Blood Institute. May 1977. Report of the Task Force on Blood Pressure Control in Children. *Pediatrics* 59(Suppl):819–20.

———. May 1984. *The 1984 report of the Joint National Committee on Detection, Evaluation, and Treatment of High Blood Pressure.* U.S. Department of Health and Human Services, Public Health Service, National Institutes of Health. Reprinted in *Archives of Internal Medicine* 144:1045–57.

Nichols, G. A. June 1972. Taking adult temperatures: Rectal measurement. *American Journal of Nursing* 72:1092–93.

Nichols, G. A., and Kucha, D. H. June 1972. Taking adult temperatures: Oral measurement. *American Journal of Nursing* 72:1090–92.

Nichols, G. A., and Verhonick, P. J. November 1967. Time and temperature. *American Journal of Nursing* 67:2304–6.

Nichols, G. A., et al. Fall 1966. Oral, axillary, and rectal temperature determinations and relationships. *Nursing Research* 15:307–10.

Olds, S. B.; London, M. L.; and Ladewig, P. A. 1984. *Maternal-newborn nursing: A family-centered approach.* Menlo Park, Calif.: Addison-Wesley Publishing Co.

Overfield, T. 1985. *Biologic variation in health and illness.* Menlo Park, Calif.: Addison-Wesley Publishing Co.

Patient assessment: Pulses, programmed instruction. January 1979. *American Journal of Nursing* 79:115–32.

Perfecting your blood pressure technique. June 1984. *Nursing 84* (Canadian ed.) 14:17.

Purintun, L. R., and Bishop, B. E. January 1969. How accurate are clinical thermometers? *American Journal of Nursing* 69:99–100.

Putt, A. M. Winter 1966. A comparison of blood pressure readings by auscultation and palpation. *Nursing Research* 15:311–16.

Scharping, E. M. January/February 1983. Physiologic measurements of the neonate. *Maternal and Child Nursing* 8:70–73.

Schiffman, R. F. September/October 1982. Temperature monitoring in the neonate: A comparison of axillary and rectal temperatures. *Nursing Research* 31:274–77.

Takacs, K. M., and Valenti, W. M. June 1981. For the research record: Perforation of the plastic thermometer sheaths. *American Journal of Nursing* 81:1198.

———. November/December 1982. Temperature measurement in a clinical setting. *Nursing Research* 31:368–70.

Thompson, L. R. February 1963. Thermometer disinfection. *American Journal of Nursing* 63:113–15.

Vick, R. L. 1984. *Contemporary medical physiology.* Menlo Park, Calif.: Addison-Wesley Publishing Co.

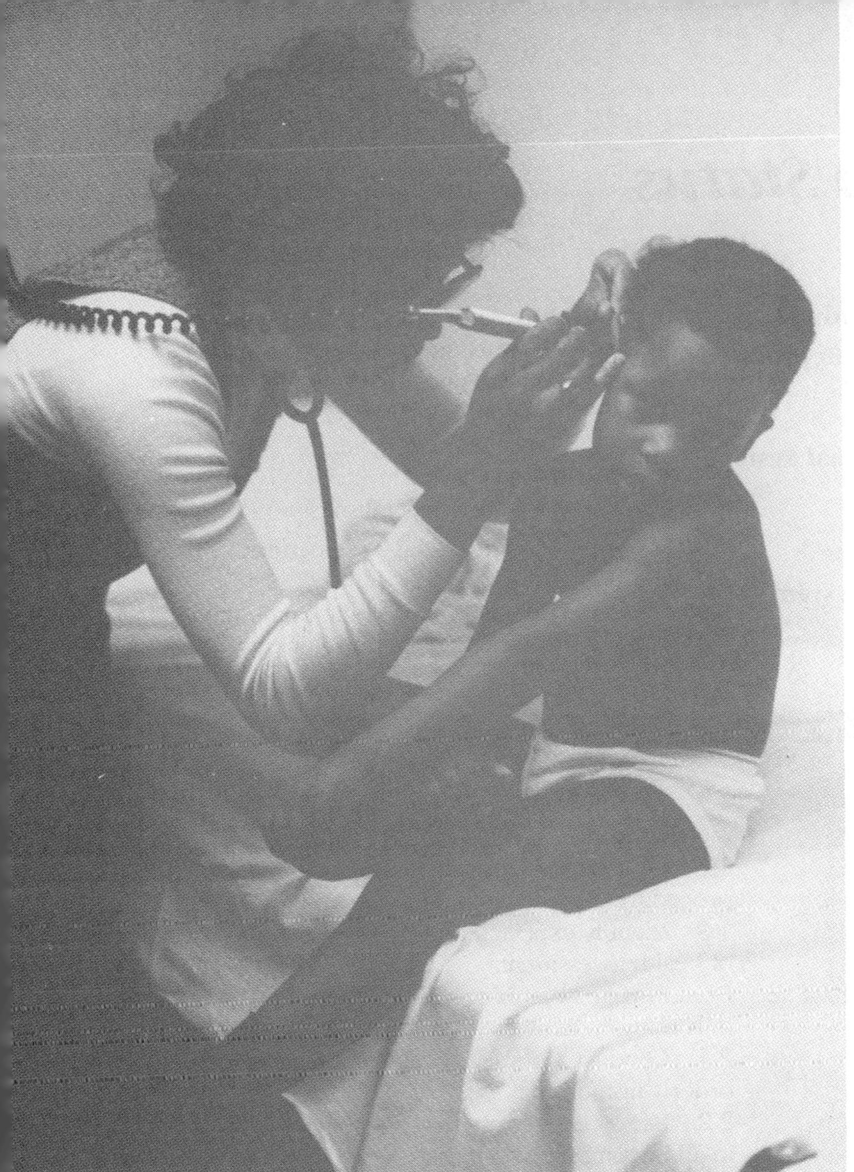

DAVID BARNETT

CHAPTER 35

Assessing Health Status

Contents

(continued)

35 *Assessing Health Status*

Contents *(continued)*

Objectives

1. Know essential terms and facts related to health assessment.
   1.1 Define terms associated with health assessment.
   1.2 Identify purposes of physical health assessment.
   1.3 Describe essential preparation for performing a physical health assessment.
   1.4 Describe specific positions clients assume during each phase of assessment.
   1.5 Identify various ways to drape clients during assessment.
   1.6 Identify equipment and supplies required during each phase of assessment.
   1.7 Identify the various steps in selected assessment procedures.
   1.8 Give reasons for selected steps in assessment procedures.
   1.9 Identify expected and unexpected outcomes of health assessment.
2. Demonstrate beginning skill in assessment of various body systems.
   2.1 Conduct a physical health assessment in an orderly fashion.
   2.2 Use aspects of physical assessment procedures in all nursing interventions.

Terms

abrasion
acromegaly
affect
alopecia
anesthesia
aneurysm
anisocoria
aphasia
astigmatism
ataxia
atrophy
barrel chest
blanch test
borborygmi
bromhidrosis
bruit
Buerger's test
cataract
conduction hearing loss
conjunctivitis
contusion (hematoma)
crepitation
Cushing's syndrome
cystocele
dacryocystitis
delusion
dullness (of sound)
ectropion
edema
emmetropia
emphysema
enterocele
entropion
epispadius
excoriation
extinction
fasciculation
fenestrated drape
flaccidity
fremitus
funnel chest
glaucoma
goniometer
graphesthesia
hallucination
hirsutism
Homans' sign
hordeolum
hyperesthesia
hyperhidrosis
hyperopia
hypertrophy
hypoesthesia
hypospadius
illusion
intention tremor
iritis
koilonychia
kyphosis
miosis
mixed hearing loss
mood
moon face
murmur (cardiac)
mydriasis
myopia
myxedema facies
nasal speculum
nystagmus
one- and two-point discrimination

osteitis deformans (Paget's disease)
otitis externa
otitis media
otoscope
paraphasia
paresthesia
paronychia
perseveration
petechiae
photophobia
pigeon chest
point of maximal impulse (PMI)
presbyopia
ptosis
rectocele
reflex
resting tremor
Romberg's sign
scoliosis
sensorineural hearing loss
serous otitis
spasticity
stereognosis
strabismus
thrill
tonicity
turgor
tympany
vitiligo

Physical Health Examination

Assessment of a client's health status encompasses both physical and psychosocial aspects. It is also adjusted to the client's needs. A health assessment may be (a) a complete assessment, e.g., on admission to a health agency; (b) an assessment of a body system, e.g., the cardiovascular system; (c) an assessment of a body part, e.g., the lungs when difficulty breathing is observed. This chapter concerns health assessment techniques applied primarily to adults.

A complete health assessment is generally conducted from the head to the toes; however, the procedure can vary in many ways according to the age of the individual, the severity of the illness, the preferences of the nurse, and the agency's priorities and procedures. Regardless of what procedure is used, the client's energy and time need to be considered. The health assessment is therefore conducted in a systematic and efficient manner that requires the fewest position changes for the client.

Because assessment is an integral part of the nursing process, aspects of specific assessment techniques should be used in the assessment, intervention, and evaluation phases of the nursing process. For example, nurses inspect clients' skin as a matter of course when they bathe clients. The assessment required by an individual at a given time is a nursing judgment based upon knowledge and the client's needs.

Purposes

Purposes of the physical health examination include:

1. To obtain baseline data about the client's functional abilities
2. To supplement, confirm, or refute data obtained in the nursing history
3. To obtain data that will help the nurse establish nursing diagnoses and plan the client's care
4. To evaluate the physiologic outcomes of health care and thus the progress of a client's health problem

Methods of Physical Assessment

The physical assessment methods of inspection, palpation, percussion, and auscultation are discussed in detail in Chapter 11.

Client Preparation

Most people need an explanation about the physical health examination. The nurse should explain when and where the examination will take place, why it is necessary, who will conduct it, and what will happen during the examination. Children need explanations that address their concerns. Generally, the nurse needs to tell the child that the examination will not hurt (since most examinations are not painful), how the child can assist, whether a parent can accompany the child, and that a nurse will be there to help.

Special circumstances—for instance, the need to go to a different room or assume a special position, such as a lithotomy position—should be explained. The client should also be told that appropriate draping will be provided so that his or her body will not be unnecessarily exposed.

Most clients should empty their bladders before the examination. This helps them feel more relaxed and facilitates palpation of the abdomen and pubic area. Since an empty rectum facilitates rectal examination, the client should be encouraged to defecate before such an examination. If a urinalysis is required, the urine should be collected in a container for that purpose.

Enemas or medications may be required before special examinations such as sigmoidoscopy. Special procedures and examinations are discussed in Chapter 54.

Equipment for an Examination

All equipment required for an examination should be arranged so that it is readily available to the examiner. It is usually arranged on a tray or table in the order in which it will be used. In some agencies, trays or carts are set up for health examinations. Figure 35–1 shows examination equipment arranged in order for use. Equipment commonly used during a physical health examination is listed in Table 35–1.

Positions and Draping

Clients frequently need to assume one or more positions during a health examination. Some of these may be uncomfortable. The nurse indicates specific positions for the client at the time needed. Clients who are assessed while in bed or on a stretcher can assume only some of the positions. Many hospitals, offices, and clinics have special examination tables, usually with extendable leaves for the supine and Sims's positions, stirrups for the lithotomy position (see Figure 35–2), and a platform for the genupectoral position.

Clients need to be draped appropriately during an examination to prevent unnecessary exposure, chilling, and embarrassment. An embarrassed or chilled client is usually tense, and tenseness can limit the effectiveness of some aspects of the examination.

Drapes are made of cloth or paper. Bedding (bath blankets, sheets, and drawsheets) can also be used for draping. Some drapes are specially made, e.g., circumcision drapes or special socks to cover the client's feet and legs. A drape with one or more round or rectangular openings is referred to as a **fenestrated** (window) **drape**.

Dorsal Recumbent (Supine) Position

During the health examination, the client usually assumes a dorsal recumbent position. Some practitioners differentiate between the horizontal recumbent position and the dorsal recumbent position. The horizontal recumbent position is a flat back-lying position. To assume the dorsal recumbent position, the client flexes the knees and rotates the hips externally.

The appropriate drapes for a client in this position usually include:

1. A hospital gown or bath towel for the chest
2. A bath blanket or sheet to cover the remainder of the body from the waist to the toes

The bath towel is placed across the chest, and the bath blanket or sheet is placed diagonally over the person. If the client's perineal area is to be examined, opposite corners of the sheet are wrapped around the feet to cover the legs. The corner between the client's legs can be raised

Table 35–1 Equipment Used for a Health Examination

Equipment	Purpose
Drapes	To cover the client (The number and type needed depends on the specific examination.)
Head mirror	To direct light to a specific body area, e.g., the pharynx
Flashlight	To assist viewing the pharynx and cervix or to determine the reactions of the pupils of the eye
Sphygmomanometer and cuff	To measure the blood pressure
Stethoscope	To auscultate body sounds, e.g., blood pressure, chest, bowel sounds
Thermometer	To assess body temperature
Laryngeal or dental mirror	To assess the pharynx
Tongue depressors	To depress the tongue to assess the mouth and pharynx
Ophthalmoscope	A lighted instrument to help visualize the interior of the eye
Otoscope	A lighted instrument to help visualize the eardrum and external auditory canal (A nasal speculum may be attached to the otoscope to inspect the nasal cavities.)
Percussion hammer	To test reflexes
Tape measure	To measure a body part, e.g., skull of an infant or an edematous leg
Tuning fork	To test hearing acuity and vibratory sense
Clean disposable gloves	To examine the vagina and the rectum
Lubricant	To apply to gloved fingers or to a vaginal speculum to ease insertion
Vaginal speculum of the needed size	To assess the cervix and the vagina
Waste container, e.g., plastic bag	To collect disposable used supplies
Sterile, cotton-tipped applicators	To obtain specimen of secretions as needed
Ayre spatula	To obtain a cervical scrape
Assorted containers and slides	For specimens, e.g., urine

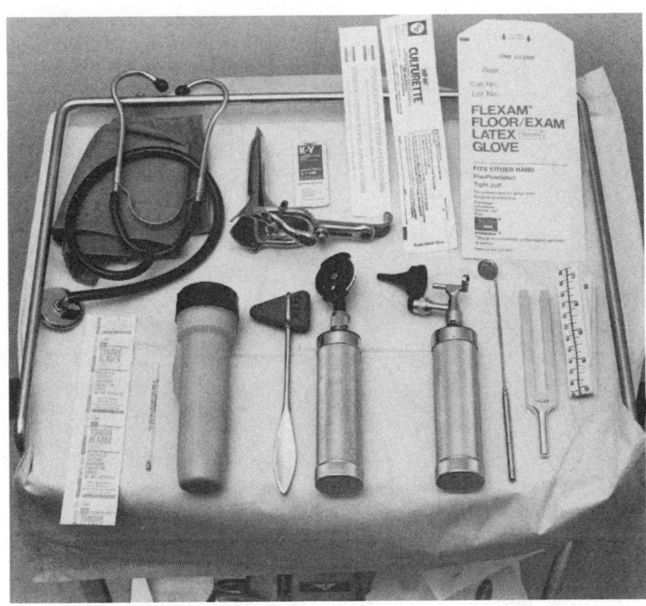

Figure 35–1 Equipment used for a physical health examination

to expose the perineum at the appropriate time. See Figure 35–3.

Genupectoral (Knee-Chest) Position

This position is used to view the rectal and sometimes the vaginal areas. The client kneels, using knees and chest to bear the body's weight. The back is straight and the body is at a 90° angle to the hips. The head is turned to one side and the arms are held above the head. Some

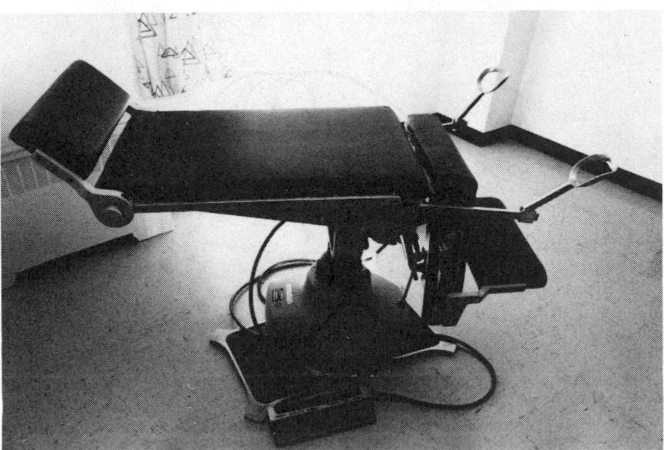

Figure 35–2 An electrically operated examination table

agencies provide a special table, which supports the client in this position.

The drapes often used for a client in this position are:

1. A hospital gown to cover the upper body.
2. A fenestrated drape to cover the client's back, buttocks, and thighs. The hole in the drape exposes only the area to be examined. See Figure 35–4. If a fenestrated drape is not available, a rectangular drape can be used. The two lateral corners are tucked around the client's thighs. The corner between the thighs can then be lifted up to expose the area to be examined, e.g., the anus. See Figure 35–5.
3. Socks to cover the feet and lower legs (optional).

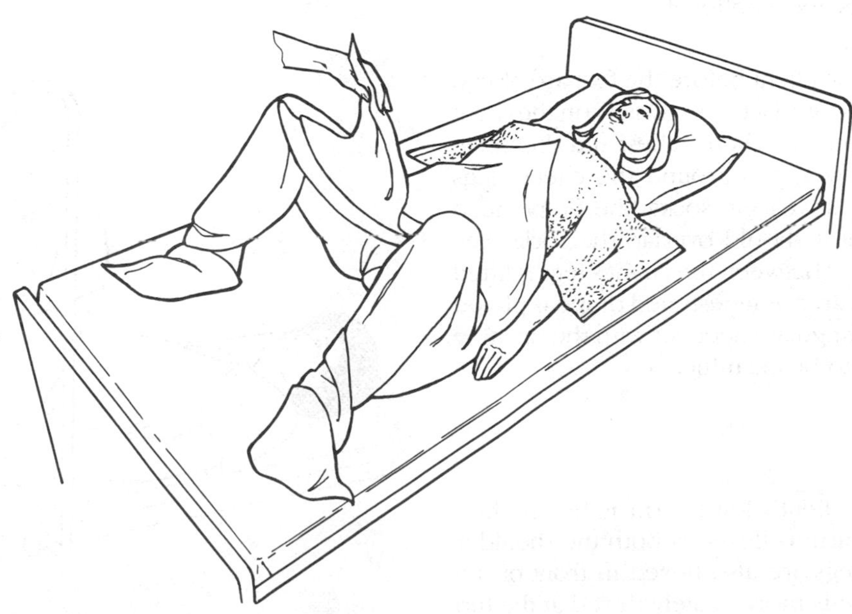

Figure 35–3 A client draped in a dorsal recumbent position

Figure 35–4 A fenestrated drape exposes only the anal area of a client in the genupectoral position.

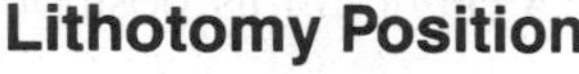

Lithotomy Position

The lithotomy position is frequently used for examinations of the vagina, and sometimes for urinary catheterizations in women. The client assumes a back-lying position, and the feet are held in supports called **stirrups**. The knees are flexed, and the hips are externally rotated. The client's hips are usually brought down to the bottom edge of the examining table, to expose the perineal area.

For the lithotomy position, the drapes usually used are:

1. A gown for the upper body (optional)
2. A rectangular sheet or a fenestrated sheet
3. Socks for the clients' feet (optional)

The socks are put on the client before the feet are placed in the stirrups. The sheet is placed diagonally on the client so that the top part covers the client's chest and abdomen. The side corners are wrapped around the client's legs and feet. If the client is wearing socks, the drape need not cover the feet, but it should overlap the socks. See Figure 35–6. The corner between the client's legs is lifted to expose the perineal area. A fenestrated drape is placed the same way as a rectangular sheet but with the opening directly over the area to be examined.

Sims' Position

In Sims' position, the client's lower arm is behind him or her, and the upper arm is flexed at both the shoulder and the elbow. Both legs are also flexed in front of the person. The upper one is more acutely flexed at the hip and the knee than the lower one.

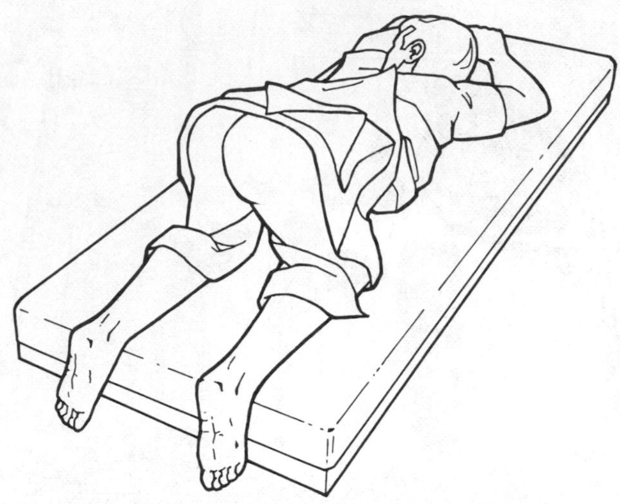

Figure 35–5 A client draped in the genupectoral position

Sims' position is usually assumed for examinations of the rectum and/or vagina. The drape is usually one rectangular sheet, placed diagonally on the client. See Figure 35–7. At the time of examination, the corner is folded back to expose the area. Because this position can be difficult for some clients to assume, particularly the elderly and the obese, it is normally not assumed until immediately before the examination. For additional information, see Chapter 38, page 1047.

Additional positions used during the health examination include sitting, back-lying, and face-lying positions. For information about these positions, see Table 35–2 and Chapter 38.

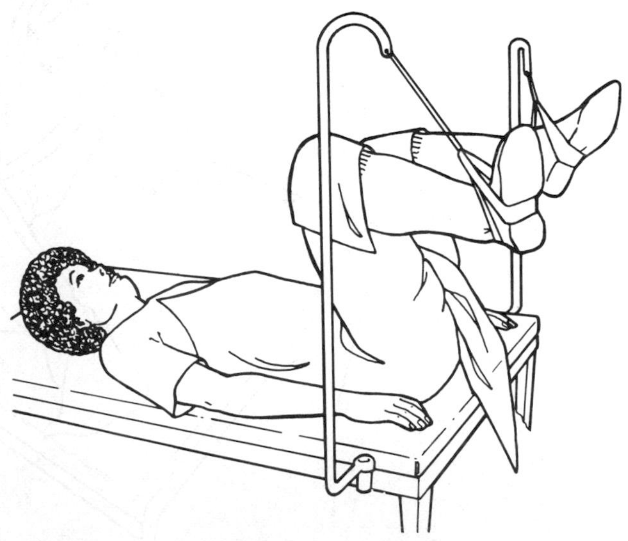

Figure 35–6 A client draped in the lithotomy position

General Appearance and Behavior

The general appearance and behavior of an individual must be assessed in terms of culture, educational level, socioeconomic status, and current circumstances. An individual who has recently experienced a personal loss may naturally appear depressed. An individual who has had an accident while working may be dressed in workclothes that he or she would not normally wear when seeing a nurse or physician.

Assessment should be carried out systematically. Most data about the client's general appearance and behavior are obtained during the nursing assessment or nursing health history (see Chapter 11, page 237). Data include the client's sex, race, body build, posture and gait, hygiene and grooming, dress, body odor, distress, overall health, attitude, mood, speech, self-concept, thought sequence and clarity, and orientation. During this general survey, the nurse also determines the client's vital signs, height, and weight. Head and chest circumferences of infants are also taken.

General Appearance

Points to consider when observing the client's general appearance include:

1. *Sex and race.* Observe the client's sex and race. Subsequent assessment findings should be considered in light of these, since the client's sex, race, and cultural beliefs can affect the meaning of specific assessment data.
2. *Body build.* Observe body build, height, and weight in relation to the client's age, life-style, and health. Note whether the client is excessively thin, obese, or muscular.
3. *Posture and gait.* Observe the client's posture standing, sitting, and walking as well as his or her gait. Note whether the client (a) is relaxed or tense; (b) has an erect, slouched, or bent posture, and (c) has coordinated or uncoordinated movements or tremors. Posture can indicate mood. For example, a slumped position may reflect depression; too rigid and upright a position, anxiety.
4. *Hygiene and grooming.* Observe the client's overall hygiene and grooming; then assess these factors from head to toe. Include cleanliness of the hair and nails. Does the client appear clean and neat or dirty and unkempt? Relate your findings to the person's activities prior to the assessment.
5. *Dress.* Observe the client's dress in relation to his or her age, life-style, climate, socioeconomic status, and culture.
6. *Body odor.* Assess the client's body and breath odor. Relate these to the client's activity. People who have been exercising may have a normal body odor. A foul breath may indicate poor oral hygiene.
7. *Distress.* Observe for signs of distress, such as wincing or labored breathing, in posture, behavior, and facial expression. The behavior of the client, e.g., wringing the hands or continual shifting of the feet, may reflect nervousness. Any obvious, unusual behavior is observed as part of the general impression; perhaps the client paces the room or verbalizes anger or fear about illness. Facial expressions may reveal clients' attitudes to their illnesses. Expressions can reflect anxiety, pain, anger, or disinterest. Question the client about any pain. Observe for signs of pain, e.g., a person may hold or rub a painful limb in a protective manner, bend over because of abdominal pain, or hold a painful side.
8. *Health.* Observe for obvious signs of health or illness, e.g., in color or breathing.
9. *Attitude.* Observe the client's attitude as reflected in appearance, speech, and behavior. Note whether the client is cooperative, withdrawn, negative, or hostile.
10. *Affect/mood.* **Affect** is the emotional state as it appears to others. **Mood** is the emotional state as described

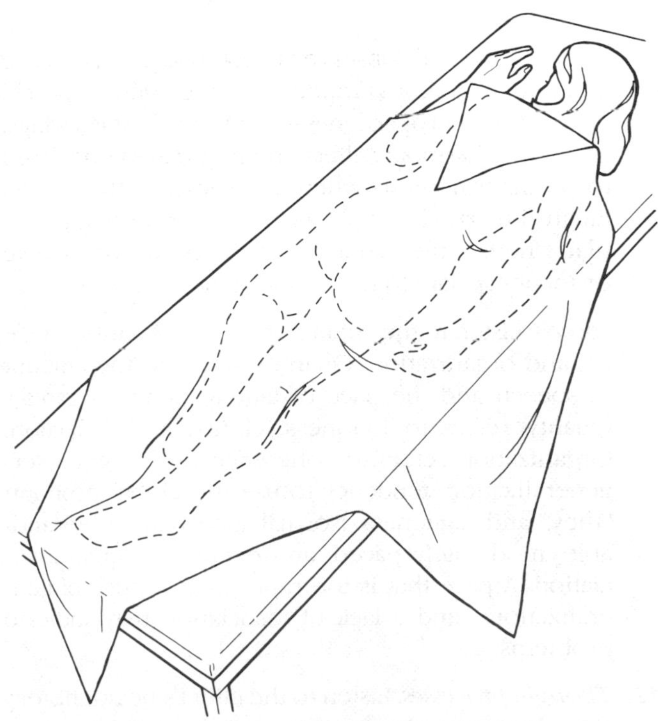

Figure 35–7 A client draped in the Sims' position

Table 35–2 Client Positions and Body Areas Examined

Position	Description	Areas examined	Cautions
Dorsal recumbent	Back-lying position with knees flexed and hips externally rotated; small pillow under the head	Head and neck, axillae, anterior thorax, lungs, breasts, heart, abdomen, extremities, peripheral pulses, vital signs, and vagina	May be difficult for elderly clients to assume
Horizontal recumbent	Back-lying position with legs extended; small pillow under the head	Head, neck, axillae, anterior thorax, lungs, breasts, heart, extremities, peripheral pulses	Not used for abdominal assessment because of the increased tension of abdominal muscles
Dorsal (supine)	Back-lying position without a pillow	As for horizontal recumbent	Tolerated poorly by clients with cardiovascular and respiratory problems
Sitting	A seated position, back unsupported and legs hanging freely	Head, neck, posterior and anterior thorax, lungs, breasts, axillae, heart, vital signs, upper and lower extremities, reflexes	Elderly and weak clients may require support
Lithotomy	Back-lying position with feet supported in stirrups	Female genitals, rectum, and female genital reproductive tract	May be difficult and tiring for elderly people
Genupectoral	Kneeling position with body at a 90° angle to hips	Rectum	Uncomfortable position tolerated poorly by clients who have respiratory problems
Sims's	Side-lying position with lowermost arm behind the body and uppermost leg flexed (See Chapter 38)	Rectum, vagina	Difficult for the elderly and people with limited joint movement
Prone	Face-lying position, with or without a small pillow	Posterior thorax, hip movement	Often not tolerated by the elderly and people with cardiovascular and respiratory problems

by the individual. Observe affect through appearance and behavior. Assess mood from the client's speech. Assess for appropriateness of mood, mood swings, and mood harmony. Affect and mood are considered to be inharmonious when, for instance, the person laughs but says he or she is sad. Determine in particular whether the client's affect/mood is appropriate or inappropriate to the circumstances.

11. *Speech.* Listen to the client's speech for quantity, quality, and organization. Quantity refers to the amount of speech and the pace of talking (slow or rapid). Quality refers to loudness, clarity, and inflection. Organization refers to coherence of thought, overgeneralization, tendency to use the global pronoun "they," and vagueness. Normal speech is understandable, moderately paced, and exhibits thought association. A pace that is too rapid or slow, use of generalizations, and a lack of association may indicate problems.

12. *Thought processes.* Listen to the client's health history for relevance and organization of the thoughts. Does the thought flow logically and make sense, or does it indicate an illogical sequence, flight of ideas, and confusion? Is the client in contact with reality, or is he or she experiencing delusions or hallucinations? A **delusion** is a false belief, one not based upon fact. An **illusion** is the false perception of a stimulus, e.g., a shadow that the client sees as a large ant is a visual illusion. A **hallucination** is a false perception having no relation to reality. It cannot be accounted for by any external stimuli. It can be visual, auditory, or olfactory.

Vital Signs

Vital signs are usually measured before assessment of various body parts and systems, since movement required during the examination can alter the measurements. Some nurses, however, prefer to assess only the body temperature and blood pressure during this initial part of the examination. The pulse is then assessed during examination of the heart and peripheral pulses, and respirations are assessed during examination of the thorax and lungs. See Chapter 34 for procedures used to determine vital signs.

Height and Weight

In adults, the ratio of weight to height provides a general measure of health. In infants and growing children, these measurements are an index of normal or abnormal growth and are essential in calculating body surface area to determine safe dosages of medications. See Chapter 51. Before measuring the client's height and weight, the nurse should ask the client what he or she weighs and how tall he or she is. This gives the nurse an idea of how the client perceives himself or herself. Excessive discrepancies between the client's responses and the measurements obtained by the nurse provide clues to a possible problem in self-image (Block et al. 1981, p. 59). The nurse should also ask the client about any recent weight gains or losses. The nurse determines how much weight the client gained or lost, during what period it occurred, and whether the gain or loss has occurred before. Associated data, such as fatigue or weakness and past and present stressors, should also be explored.

Height

Height is measured with a measuring stick attached to weight scales or to a wall. The client removes his or her shoes and stands erect with heels together, buttocks and head against the measuring stick, and eyes looking straight ahead. See Figure 35–8. The nurse raises the L-shaped sliding arm on the weight scale until it rests on top of the client's head or places a small flat object, such as a ruler or book, on the client's head. The edge of the ruler should abut the measuring guide.

To measure the recumbent length of an infant who cannot stand, the nurse places the baby supine on a hard surface and supports the soles of the baby's feet in an upright position. The nurse extends the baby's knees and measures the length from the soles of the feet to the vertex of the head. See Figure 35–9.

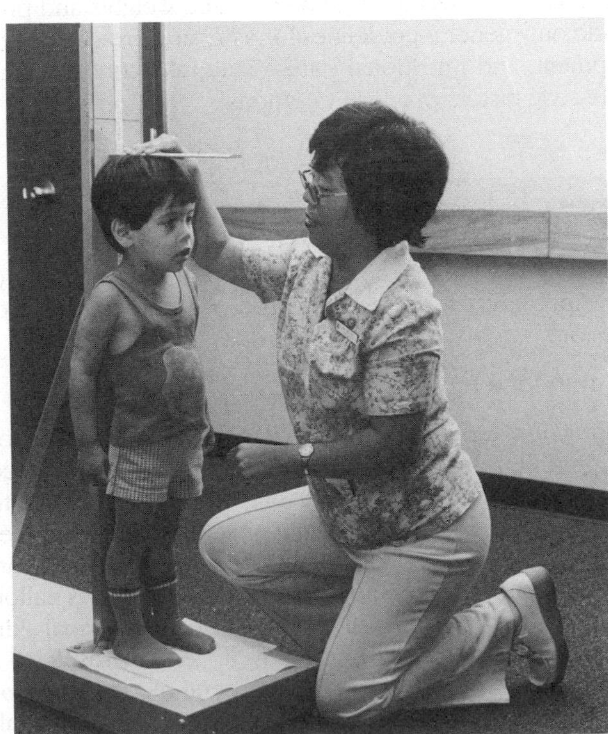

Figure 35–8 Measuring the height of a child

Weight

Weight is often measured when a client is admitted to a health agency. The weight of some clients is measured regularly, e.g., each morning before breakfast. This regular weighing is usually done for obese clients on reducing diets or for clients who retain excess fluid. When accuracy is essential, an effort should be made to use the same scale each time, since every scale weighs differently. Measurements should also be taken at the same time each day. The client should wear the same kind of clothing and no shoes. Clients who can stand are weighed on various types of standing scales. The client stands on a platform, and the weight is read from a digital display panel or a balancing arm. Clients who cannot stand are weighed on bed and chair scales. See Figures 35–10 and 35–11. The bed scales have canvas straps or a stretcherlike apparatus. A machine lifts the client above the bed, and the weight is reflected either on a digital display panel or on a balance arm like that of a standing scale.

Several types of scales are used to weigh babies. Many hospitals use scales with a container in which the baby is placed to be weighed. Some scales are portable. It is important to weigh a baby unclothed or to weigh the clothes separately and subtract their weight.

Before placing an infant on a scale, the nurse drapes the scale to prevent cross-infection. Some agencies use a

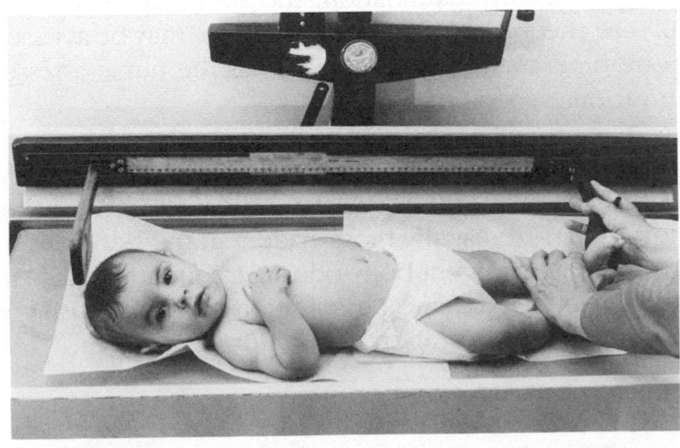

Figure 35–9 Measuring the recumbent length of an infant

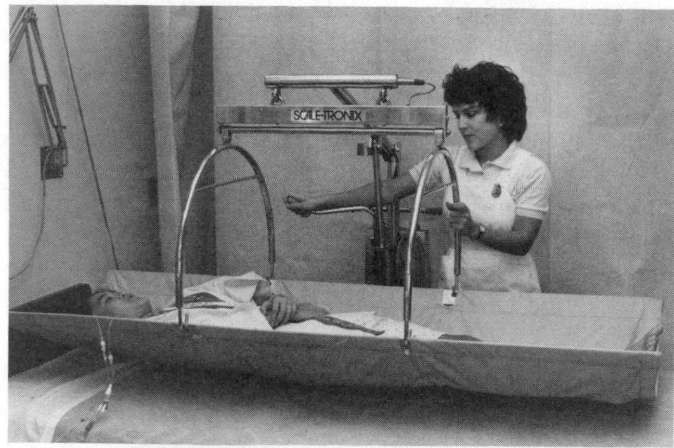

Figure 35–10 A bed scale

special sterile paper that prevents urine and other fluids from seeping through and contaminating the scale. The nurse balances the draped scale, if necessary, and places the unclothed infant on the tray. Holding one hand about 2.5 cm (1 in) over the baby, the nurse uses the other hand to adjust the scale. The weighed infant is returned to the crib and covered.

Standardized Charts

Standardized charts reflect average heights and weights of children and adults. To date, most of these charts are based on Caucasian standards. Studies indicate that black children tend to be taller and heavier at all ages than whites (Robson et al. 1975, pp. 1017–18). For information about recommended weights of adults, see Table 35–3. It is important for the nurse to remember that standardized charts reflect average heights and weights and provide only general guidelines for assessing growth, development, and nutritional status. Cultural, economic, and life-style factors produce variations.

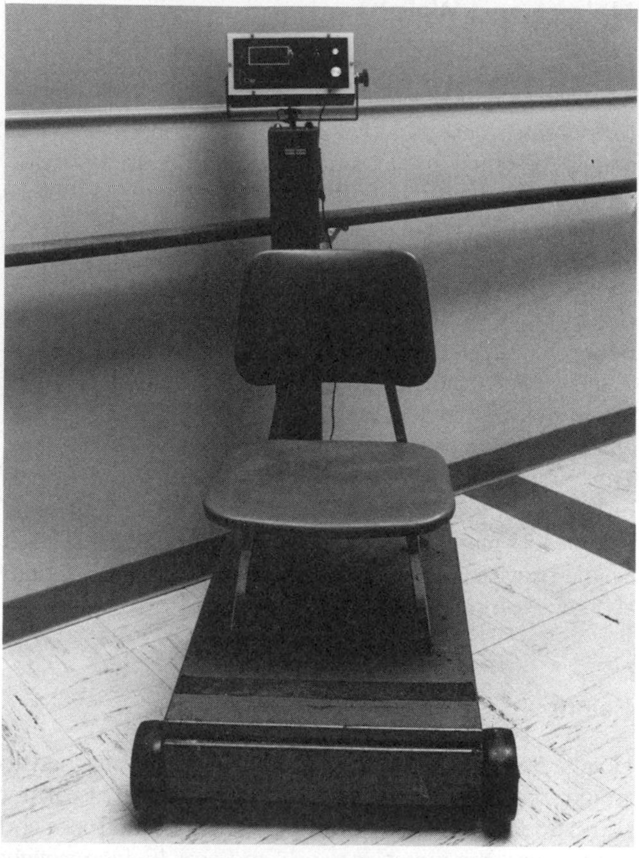

Figure 35–11 A chair scale

The Integument

The **integument** is the covering of the body, i.e., the skin. During a health examination, the skin, hair, scalp, and nails are checked. The entire skin surface may be assessed at one time, or it may be assessed as the nurse assesses the various aspects of the body.

Assessment of the skin usually involves inspection and palpation. In some instances, the nurse may also need to use her or his olfactory sense to detect unusual skin odors; these are usually most evident in the skin folds or in the axillae. Pungent body odor is frequently related to poor hygiene, excessive perspiration (**hyperhidrosis**) or foul-smelling perspiration (**bromhidrosis**).

Skin

Nursing history data relative to the skin are outlined on page 809. The skin should be assessed for color, tone, uniformity of color, moisture, surface temperature, vascularity and edema, pigmented areas, turgor and elasticity, mobility, texture and thickness, and the presence of lesions.

Color Tone

Skin color varies over the body; therefore, the skin color should be assessed in areas that have not been exposed to the sun. Normal skin pigmentation varies from light to deep brown, ruddy pink to light pink, or yellow overtones to olive. Skin color depends on the client's race. In particular, nurses should be aware of findings such as pallor, cyanosis, or jaundice. Pallor, the absence of normal skin color reflected in a whitish-gray tinge, is a result of a decreased blood flow to the peripheral blood vessels or of decreased hemoglobin in the blood. Pallor is difficult to detect in clients with dark skin. In these clients, pallor is most readily seen in the buccal mucosa. Pallor in people with light skins may also be evident in the face, the con-

Table 35–3 1983 Metropolitan Height and Weight Tables, Men and Women, Ages 25 to 59

Men

Height	Weight (lb) Small frame	Medium frame	Large frame
5′ 2″	128–134	131–141	138–150
5′ 3″	130–136	133–143	140–153
5′ 4″	132–138	135–145	142–156
5′ 5″	134–140	137–148	144–160
5′ 6″	136–142	139–151	146–164
5′ 7″	138–145	142–154	149–168
5′ 8″	140–148	145–157	152–172
5′ 9″	142–151	148–160	155–176
5′10″	144–154	151–163	158–180
5′11″	146–157	154–166	161–184
6′ 0″	149–160	157–170	164–188
6′ 1″	152–164	160–174	168–192
6′ 2″	155–168	164–178	172–197
6′ 3″	158–172	167–182	176–202
6′ 4″	162–176	171–187	181–207

Women

Height	Weight (lb) Small frame	Medium frame	Large frame
4′10″	102–111	109–121	118–131
4′11″	103–113	111–123	120–134
5′ 0″	104–115	113–126	122–137
5′ 1″	106–118	115–129	125–140
5′ 2″	108–121	118–132	128–143
5′ 3″	111–124	121–135	131–147
5′ 4″	114–127	124–138	134–151
5′ 5″	117–130	127–141	137–155
5′ 6″	120–133	130–144	140–159
5′ 7″	123–136	133–147	143–163
5′ 8″	126–139	136–150	146–167
5′ 9″	129–142	139–153	149–170
5′10″	132–145	142–156	152–173
5′11″	135–148	145–159	155–176
6′ 0″	138–151	148–162	158–179

Weights at ages 25–59 based on lowest mortality.
Weight in indoor clothing weighing 5 lb for men, 3 lb for women; height in shoes with 1″ heels.

Source of basic data: 1979 Build Study, Society of Actuaries and Association of Life Insurance Medical Directors of America, 1980. Courtesy Metropolitan Life Insurance Company.

junctiva of the eyes, and the nails. Cyanosis, a blue tinge to the skin, is caused by decreased oxyhemoglobin binding in the blood or by decreased oxygenation of the blood. Cyanosis is most evident in the nail beds, lips, and buccal mucosa. Jaundice, seen as a yellow or green hue to the skin, occurs when tissue bilirubin is increased. In adults, jaundice may first be evident in the sclera of the eyes and then in the mucous membranes and the skin. Nurses should take care not to confuse jaundice with the normal yellow pigmentation in the sclera of a dark-skinned or black client.

The nurse assesses other generalized color changes of the skin, e.g., redness due to fever or sunburn. Localized color changes, such as localized pallor, can reflect impaired blood circulation to a specific area, e.g., as a result of edema.

Uniformity of Color

The color of the skin is generally uniform over the body except in areas exposed to the sun. Dark-skinned clients have areas of lighter pigmentation, such as the palms, lips, and nail beds. Areas of hyperpigmentation (increased pigmentation) and hypopigmentation (decreased pigmentation) may also occur. An example of hyperpigmentation in a defined area is a birthmark; an example of hypopigmentation is vitiligo. **Vitiligo**, seen as patches of hypopigmented skin, is caused by the destruction of melanocytes in the area.

Moisture

Assess moisture of the skin visually and by palpation. It varies from one area of the body to another. Moisture refers both to wetness and oiliness. The skin folds and axillae are normally moist. The moisture varies according to environmental temperature and humidity, muscular activity, and body temperature. Skin is often dry when environmental temperature and humidity are low, and often moist when they are elevated. The elderly often have dry skin. Excessive oiliness may occur during adolescence.

Nursing History Data: Skin

Determine:

- Presence of pain or itching
- Presence and spread of any lesions, bruises, abrasions, pigmented spots
- Previous experience with skin problems
- Associated clinical signs
- Family history
- Presence of problems in other family members
- Related systemic conditions
- Use of medications, lotions, home remedies
- Relative dryness or moisture of the skin
- History of easy bruising
- Possible relation of a problem to season of year, stress, occupation, medications, recent travel, housing, personal contact, etc.
- Any recent contact with allergens, e.g., metal paint

Temperature

The skin temperature depends on the peripheral vascular circulation to the skin, which can reflect the client's cardiovascular status. The nurse palpates the skin over the whole body to assess temperature. It may be the same throughout the body or higher or lower in one area, e.g., a foot. When one area is cooler, the nurse palpates the corresponding area on the other side of the body to gain comparative data. Skin temperature should always be assessed when there is concern about the blood circulation to a body part. Normally, a person's skin temperature is relatively uniform over the body.

Vascularity and Edema

Vascularity refers to the blood circulation to the skin. **Edema** is the presence of excess interstitial fluid. Abnormal vascularity can be seen by the presence of petechiae or bruises, for example. **Petechiae** are pinpoint red spots in the skin. An area of edema appears swollen, shiny, and taut. The location, color, temperature, and shape of edematous skin, and the degree to which it remains indented when pressed by a finger, should be assessed. See this page for a scale describing degrees of edema. Edema is most often an indication of impaired venous circulation and in some cases reflects cardiac dysfunction or vein abnormalities.

Turgor

Turgor means fullness or elasticity. Skin or tissue turgor refers to the normal skin fullness, or the capacity of the skin and underlying tissue to return to their prior condition after being lifted and pinched. If skin turgor is poor, e.g., in a dehydrated client, the skin returns to its original shape slowly, remaining pinched or tented after it is released. Loss of skin turgor is often related to advanced age, when the skin becomes lax and wrinkled.

Mobility

Skin mobility refers to the normal ability of the skin to move freely back and forth over the underlying structures. Lack of skin mobility is seen when edema or a malignant lesion are present.

Texture

Although there is some variation in the texture of normal skin, it is usually smooth, soft, and flexible. The thickness of the skin is widely variable: thicker in areas that are exposed to pressure, friction, or other types of irritation. The skin is often thicker on the soles of the feet and the palms of the hands. Skin textures can become dry and rough as a result of certain diseases, such as hypothyroidism.

Lesions

Normal skin does not have lesions. Table 35–4 lists some common lesions. The nurse's main responsibility is to describe lesions accurately, including (a) distribution and location, (b) size, (c) contour, and (d) consistency.

Excoriations and Abrasions

An **excoriation** is the loss of superficial layers of the skin. For example, a nurse with long fingernails may scratch a client when palpating him or her, causing an excoriation. An **abrasion** is the wearing away of a structure, such as the skin or teeth, often by friction (e.g., when a client is dragged instead of rolled across a bed).

Hair

Hair grows on the whole body surface except on the palms of the hands, the soles of the feet, the dorsal surfaces of terminal phalanges, and parts of the genitals (the inner surface of the labia and inner surface of the prepuce of the glans penis).

Surface hair is of two types: the vellus, which is the fine, nonpigmented hair covering large areas of the body, and terminal hair, which is longer, coarser, and pigmented. Hair grows at varying rates and is shed at varying times. The scalp of the average person loses between 20 and 100 hairs per day. Body hair is shed in 3 to 4 months, whereas hair in beards lasts 3 or 4 years (Brown et al. 1973, p. 39).

The visible part of a hair is called the hair shaft. The root is in a tube known as a hair follicle. Muscles known as arrector pili muscles are attached to the hair follicles. See Figure 35–12. When these contract, the skin assumes a gooseflesh appearance. Sebaceous glands, which secrete sebum, grow from the walls of hair follicles. Sebum is produced in greater quantities on the scalp and the face than elsewhere on the body.

Assessment of an individual's hair includes inspection of the hair, consideration of developmental changes, and determination of the individual's hair care practices and the factors influencing them. Much of the information about hair can be obtained by questioning the client. See page 811.

Scale for Describing Edema

- 1+ Barely detectable
- 2+ Indentation of less than 5 mm
- 3+ Indentation of 5 to 10 mm
- 4+ Indentation of more than 10 mm

Table 35–4 Skin Lesions

Type of lesion	Description	Examples
	Primary	
Macula	A flat, circumscribed area of color with no elevation of its surface; 1 mm to 1 cm	Freckles, flat nevi
Papule	A circumscribed solid elevation of skin; less than 1 cm	Warts, acne, pimples, flat nevi
Nodule	A solid mass extending deeper into dermis than a papule	Pigmented nevi
Tumor	A solid mass larger than a nodule	Epitheliomas
Cyst	An encapsulated, fluid-filled mass in dermis or subcutaneous tissue	Epidermoid cysts
Wheal	A relatively reddened, flat, localized collection of edema fluid	Mosquito bites, hives
Vesicle	A circumscribed elevation containing serous fluid or blood	Herpes, chickenpox
Bulla	A larger fluid-filled vesicle	Second degree burns
Pustule	A vesicle or bulla filled with pus	Acne vulgaris
	Secondary	
Scale	Thickened epidermal cells that flake off	Dandruff
Fissure	A linear crack	Athlete's foot
Erosion	Loss of epidermis that does not extend deeper	Abrasions
Atrophy	A decrease in the volume of epidermis	Striae
Scar	A formation of connective tissue	Keloid
Ulcer	An excavation extending into the dermis or below	Stasis ulcer
Crust	Dried serum on the skin surface	Infected dermatitis

Nursing History Data: Hair

Determine:

- Recent use of hair dyes, rinses, or curling or straightening preparations
- Recent chemotherapy (if alopecia is present)
- Presence of disease, such as hypothyroidism, which can be associated with dry, brittle hair

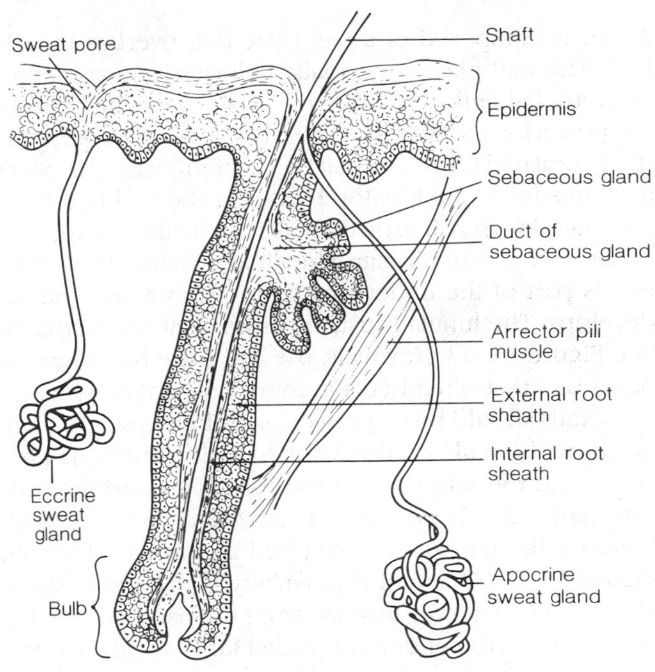

Figure 35–12 The parts of a hair follicle

Normal, natural hair is black, brown, red, yellow, or shades of these colors. Hair fibers vary in shape—they may be straight, spiral, wavy, or helical. This variation makes the texture of the hair straight, wavy, kinky, or woolly. Hair also varies from fine to coarse. Black-skinned people often have thicker, drier, curlier hair than white-skinned people.

Normal hair has resilience and is evenly distributed. People with severe protein deficiency (kwashiorkor) have faded hair colors that appear reddish or bleached and coarse, dry hair texture. Some therapies for cancer cause **alopecia** (baldness), and some disease conditions affect the coarseness of hair.

Hair is assessed for:

1. The evenness of growth over the scalp and, in particular, any patchy loss of hair.
2. Texture, i.e., whether it is coarse or silky.
3. Oiliness, i.e., whether it is dry or greasy.
4. Thickness or thinness.
5. Presence of infections or infestations on the scalp, including flaking, sores, lice, nits (louse eggs), and ringworm.
6. Presence on the body. **Hirsutism** is the presence of unusually dark, thick hair on the body. It has little significance in men but should be noted in children and women.

Nails

A nail is composed of a nail plate that overlies the nail bed. The nail plate is normally colorless and composed of epithelial cells. Covering the base of the nail plate is the posterior nail fold; the lateral borders are covered by the lateral nail folds. The nail bed is highly vascular, which accounts for its pink color. However, the nail bed is not associated with nail growth or nail formation. At the base of the nail is a semilunar whitish area called the lunula; this is part of the underlying tissue from which the nail develops. The lunula is usually prominent on the thumb. See Figure 35–13. Normally, the nail plate has longitudinal ridges that often become more prominent with age.

Nails should be inspected for nail plate shape, angle between the nail and the nail bed, nail texture, nail bed color, and the intactness of the tissues around the nails. The nail plate is normally a convex curve. The angle between the nail and the nail bed is normally 160°. See Figure 35–14. One nail abnormality is the spoon shape. Here, the nail curves upward from the nail bed. See Figure 35–15. This condition is called **koilonychia** and may be seen in clients with iron deficiency anemia.

Clubbing is a condition in which the angle between the nail and the nail bed is 180° or greater. It may be caused by long-term oxygen lack and is seen in the elderly. See Figure 35–16.

Nail texture is normally smooth. Excessively thick nails can appear in the elderly, and excessively thin nails or the presence of grooves or furrows can reflect prolonged iron-deficiency anemia. Beau's lines are horizontal depressions in the nail that can result from injury or severe illness. See Figure 35–17. The nail bed color in Caucasians is pink; in blacks, brown or black pigmentation in longitudinal streaks or along the edge of the nail may normally be present. A bluish or purplish tint to the nail bed may reflect cyanosis, and pallor may reflect poor arterial circulation.

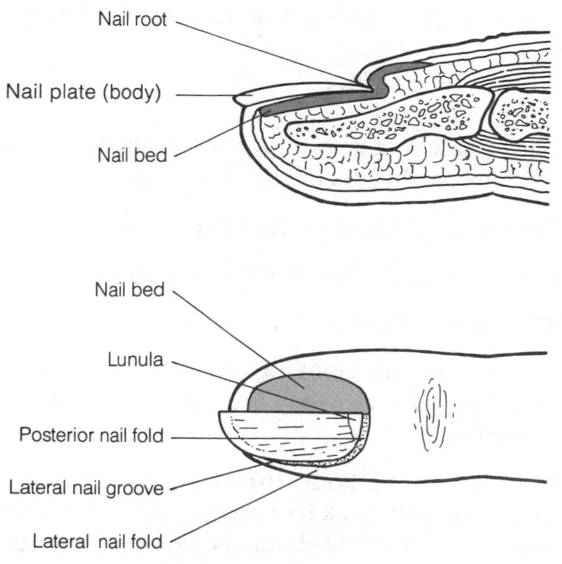

Figure 35–13 The parts of a nail

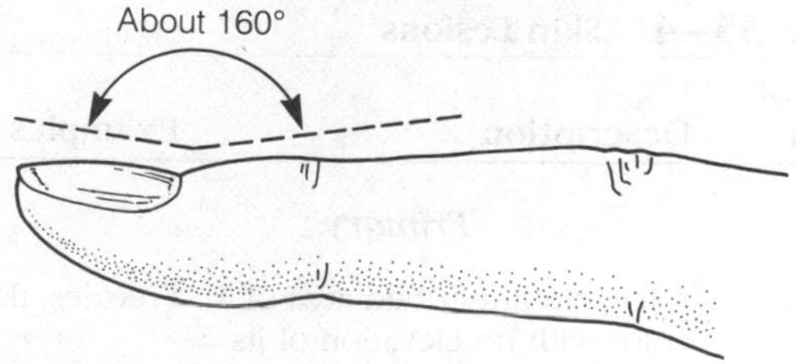

Figure 35–14 A normal nail, showing the convex shape and a nail plate angle of about 160°

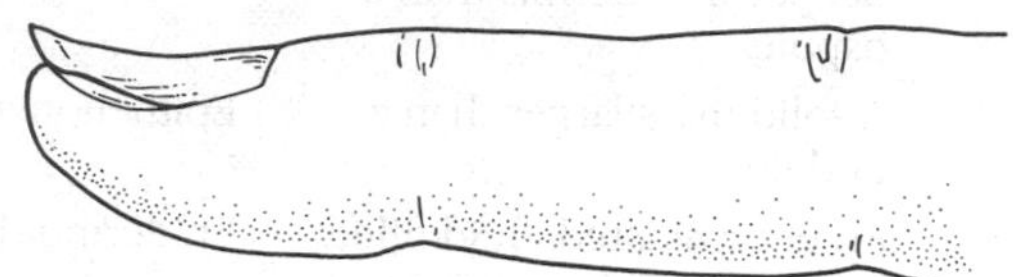

Figure 35–15 A spoon-shaped nail

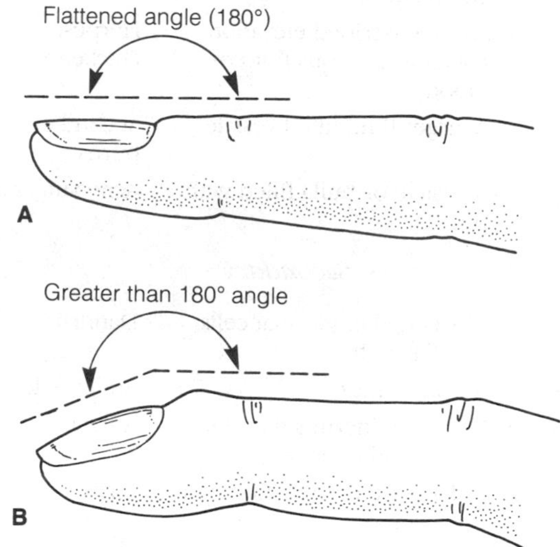

Figure 35–16 **A,** Early clubbing; **B,** late clubbing

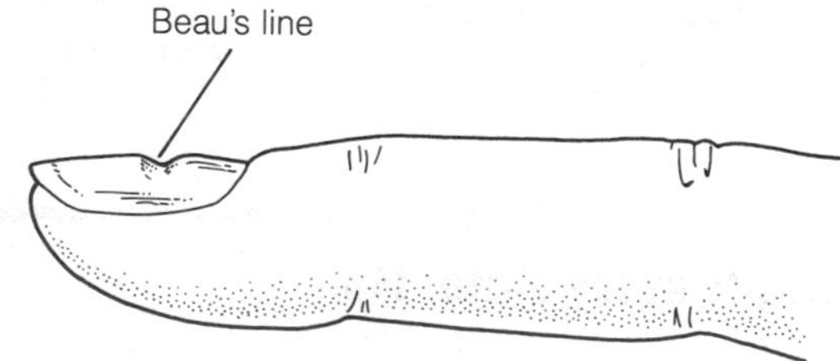

Figure 35–17 Beau's line on a nail

The tissue surrounding the nails is normally intact epidermis. **Paronychia** is an inflammation of the tissues surrounding a nail. The tissues appear inflamed and swollen, and tenderness is usually present.

A **blanch test** can be carried out to test the capillary refill, i.e., peripheral circulation. Normal nail bed capillaries blanch when pressed but quickly turn pink (in Caucasians) or their usual color when pressure is released. In dark-skinned people, the nail may be pigmented along the edges or in lines along the nail, and the rate of return of nail bed color may be more significant than the color. A slow rate of capillary refill may indicate circulatory problems. See the section on peripheral vascular assessment, later in this chapter.

Head and Neck

During an examination of the head and neck, the nurse often uses inspection and palpation simultaneously, and auscultation. The nurse examines the head, face, neck muscles, trachea, thyroid gland, and lymph nodes. Areas to be included in the nursing history are shown below. Required equipment includes a good light source, a glass of water, and a stethoscope.

Head

Although there is a large range of normal shapes of skulls, inspect the head at all angles for size, shape, and symmetry. Areas of the head are named from underlying bones: frontal, parietal, occipital, mastoid process, mandible, maxilla, and zygomatic. See Figure 35–18. Note particularly areas of local trauma, lumps or bumps, and overall size. In adults, a large head may result from osteitis deformans or acromegaly. **Osteitis deformans** (Paget's disease) is a disorder in which bony thickness increases. The skull, spine, pelvis, and femur are the usual sites of involvement. When the skull is involved, it appears enlarged, with prominent superficial veins, and often there is hearing impairment. **Acromegaly** is a disorder caused by excessive secretion of growth hormone. The skull becomes thickened and enlarged, mandible length increases, the nose and forehead become more prominent, and the facial features look coarsened. Associated signs include changes in the skin, which becomes thickened, coarse, leathery, and oily and develops thick folds, and similar bone and skin changes in the hands and feet.

Palpate the skull for nodules or masses. Use a gentle rotating motion with the fingertips. Begin at the front and palpate down the midline; then palpate each side of the head. In the occipital region, palpate the occipital lymph nodes. See "Lymph Nodes," later in this section.

Palpation may detect sebaceous cysts, local deformities resulting from trauma, or enlarged lymph nodes. Sebaceous cysts result from occlusion of the sebaceous gland ducts; they feel smooth, rounded, and nodular. Auscultate over the occipital, temporal, and orbital regions for bruits. See Figure 35–19. Bruits are discussed in the section on carotid artery assessment, later in this chapter.

Nursing History Data: Head and Neck

Determine:

- Any past problems with lumps or bumps, neck pain, stiffness, itching, scaling, or dandruff
- Any history of loss of consciousness, dizziness, seizures, headache, facial pain, or injury
- The cause of any lumps and time elapsed since the lumps occurred
- Duration of any other problem
- Any known cause of problem
- Associated symptoms, treatment, and recurrences
- Any previous diagnosis of thyroid problem, including whether thyroid was over- or underfunctioning, what tests were taken, what the test results were, whether and what medications were ordered, what amounts were taken, whether still being taken, and whether other treatments (e.g., surgery, radiation) were provided

Face

Inspect the facial skin for color, the hair distribution and condition, and the facial structures (eyebrows, eyes, nose, mouth, and ears) for size and symmetry. Many disorders cause a change in facial shape or condition. Kidney or cardiac disease can cause edema of the eyelids. Thyroid overactivity (hyperthyroidism) can cause protrusion of the eyeballs with elevation of the upper eyelids, resulting in a startled or staring expression. Thyroid underactivity (hypothyroidism or myxedema) can cause a dry, puffy face with dry skin and coarse features, referred to as **myxedema facies**, and thinning of scalp hair and eyebrows. **Cushing's syndrome**, a disorder in which there is increased adrenal hormone production, can cause a round face with reddened cheeks, referred to as "**moon face**," and excessive hair growth on the upper lips, chin, and sideburn areas. Intake of synthetic adrenal hormones also produces these changes. Prolonged illness, starvation, and dehydration can result in sunken eyes, cheeks, and temples.

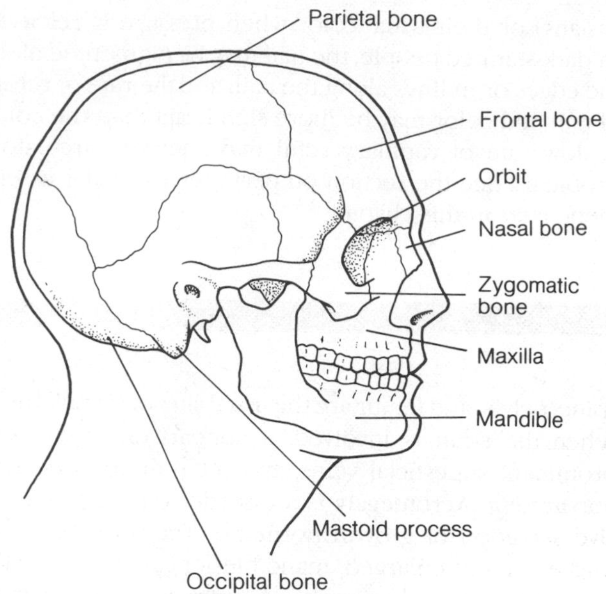

Figure 35–18 The bones of the head

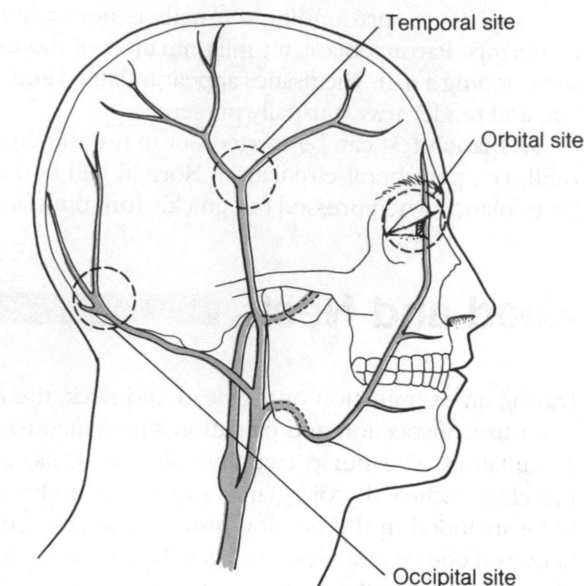

Figure 35–19 Auscultation sites for bruits

Ask the client to elevate the eyebrows, frown or lower the eyebrows, close the eyes tightly, puff the cheeks, and smile and show the teeth. These movements determine the function of the muscles of facial expression and the seventh cranial (facial) nerve. (Sensation of the face, supplied by the fifth cranial [trigeminal] nerve, is tested as part of the neurologic examination, discussed later in this chapter.

Palpate the facial sinuses. See "Nose and Sinuses," later in this chapter.

Neck

Have the client hold his or her head erect, and inspect the neck muscles (sternocleidomastoid and trapezius) for abnormal swellings or masses. Each sternocleidomastoid muscle extends from the upper sternum and the medial third of the clavicle to the mastoid process of the temporal bone behind the ear. See Figure 35–20. These muscles turn and laterally flex the head. Each trapezius muscle extends from the occipital bone of the skull to the lateral third of the clavicle. These muscles draw the head to the side and back, elevate the chin, and elevate the shoulders to shrug them. Areas of the neck are defined by the sternocleidomastoid muscles, which divide each side of the neck into two triangles: the anterior and posterior triangles. See Figure 35–20. The trachea, thyroid gland, anterior cervical nodes, and carotid artery lie within the anterior triangle (the carotid artery runs parallel and anterior to the sternocleidomastoid muscle); the posterior lymph nodes lie within the posterior triangle. See Figure 35–21.

Instruct the client to:

1. Move the chin to the chest (head flexion). This determines function of the sternocleidomastoid muscle.
2. Move the head back so that the chin points upward (head hyperextension). This determines function of the trapezius muscle.
3. Move the head so that the ear is moved toward the shoulder (lateral flexion) on each side. This determines function of the sternocleidomastoid muscle.

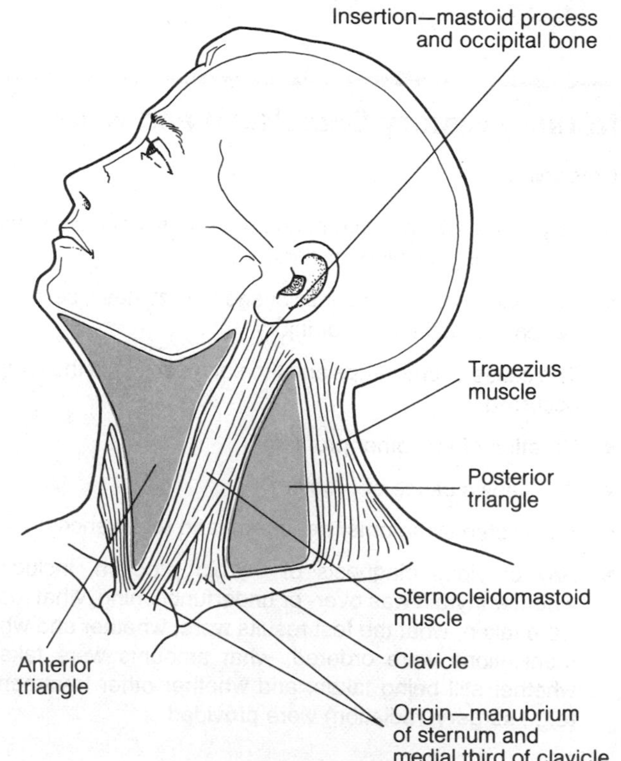

Figure 35–20 Major muscles of the neck

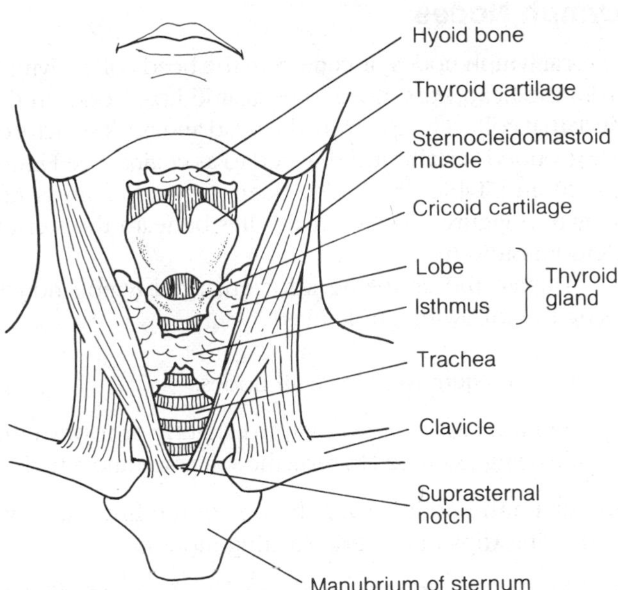

Figure 35–21 Structures of the neck

4. Turn the head to the right and to the left (lateral rotation). This determines function of the sternocleidomastoid muscle.

Have the client turn the head to one side against the resistance of your hand. Repeat with the other side. This determines the strength of the sternocleidomastoid muscle. Ask the client to shrug his or her shoulders against the resistance of your hands. This determines the strength of the trapezius muscles.

Trachea

Palpate the trachea for lateral deviation. Place a fingertip or a fingertip and thumb on the trachea in the suprasternal notch (see Figure 35–22) and then move the finger(s) laterally to the left and the right in the spaces bordered by the clavicle, the anterior aspect of the sternocleidomastoid muscle, and the trachea. These spaces are normally equal on both sides, and the trachea is centrally placed.

Thyroid Gland

Inspect the thyroid gland:

1. Stand in front of the client.
2. Observe the lower half of the neck overlying the thyroid gland for symmetry and visible masses.
3. Have the client hyperextend the head and swallow. If necessary offer a glass of water to make it easier for the client to swallow. This determines how the thyroid and cricoid cartilages (see Figure 35–21) move and whether swallowing causes a bulging of the gland.

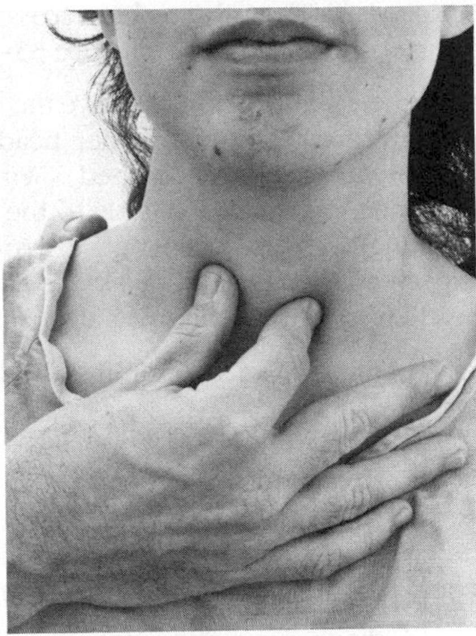

Figure 35–22 Palpating the trachea for lateral deviation

Normally the thyroid gland ascends during swallowing and is not visible.

To palpate the thyroid gland, stand either in front of or behind the client and have the client lower the chin slightly. Lowering the chin relaxes the neck muscles, facilitating palpation.

For the posterior approach:

1. Place your hands around the clients' neck with your fingertips on the lower half of the neck over the trachea. See Figure 35–23.
2. Have the client swallow (using a sip of water, if necessary), and feel for any enlargement of the thyroid

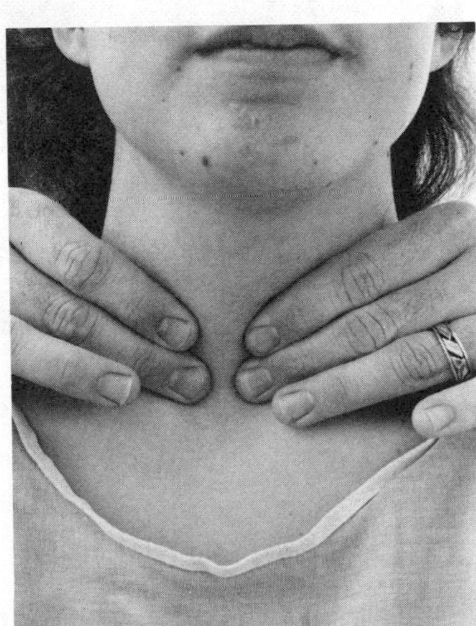

Figure 35–23 Palpating the thyroid: posterior approach

isthmus, as it rises. The isthmus lies across the trachea below the cricoid cartilage. See Figure 35–21, earlier.

3. To examine the right thyroid lobe, have the client lower the chin slightly and turn his or her head slightly to the right (the side being examined). With your left fingers displace the trachea slightly to the right. With your right fingers palpate the right thyroid lobe for any enlargement, masses, or nodules. See Figure 35–24. Have the client swallow while you are palpating.
4. Repeat step 3 in reverse to examine the left thyroid lobe.

For the anterior approach:

1. Place the tips of your index and middle fingers over the trachea, and palpate the thyroid isthmus as the client swallows.
2. To examine the right thyroid lobe, have the client lower the chin slightly and turn his or her head slightly to the right. With your right fingers, displace the trachea slightly to the client's right (your left). With your left fingers, palpate the right thyroid lobe. See Figure 35–25.
3. To examine the left thyroid lobe, repeat step 2 in reverse.

If enlargement of the gland is suspected, auscultate over the thyroid area for a bruit. Use the bell-shaped diaphragm of the stethoscope. In an enlarged hyperactive thyroid gland, blood flow through the thyroid arteries is increased and produces vibrations that may be heard as a soft rushing sound (bruit). See "Carotid Arteries," later in this chapter, for further discussion of bruits.

Lymph Nodes

Several lymph nodes or centers in the head collect lymph from the head, ears, nose, cheeks, and lips. Nodes in the neck that collect lymph from the head and neck structures are grouped serially and referred to as chains. See Figure 35–26 and Table 35–5. The deep cervical chain is not shown in Figure 35–26, since it lies beneath the sternocleidomastoid muscle.

Palpate the entire neck for enlarged lymph nodes, using the following guidelines:

1. Face the client to palpate all nodes.
2. Bend the client's head forward slightly or toward the side being examined to relax the soft tissue and muscles.
3. Palpate the nodes using the tips of the fingers. Move the fintertips in a gentle rotating motion.
4. When examining the submental and submandibular nodes, place the fingertips under the mandible on the side nearest the palpating hand, and pull the skin and subcutaneous tissue laterally over the mandibular surface so that the tissue rolls over the nodes.
5. When palpating the supraclavicular nodes, have the client bend his or her head forward to relax the tissues of the anterior neck and to relax the shoulders so that the clavicles are dropped. Use your hand nearest the side to be examined when facing the client, i.e., your left hand for the client's right nodes. Use your free hand to flex the client's head forward if necessary. Hook your index and third fingers over the clavicle

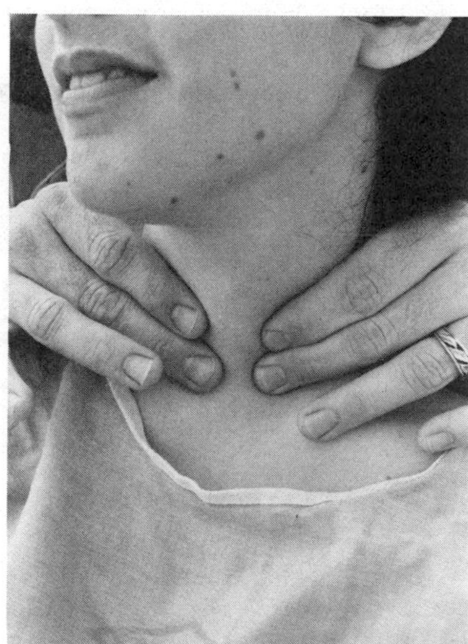

Figure 35–24 Palpating the right thyroid lobe: posterior approach

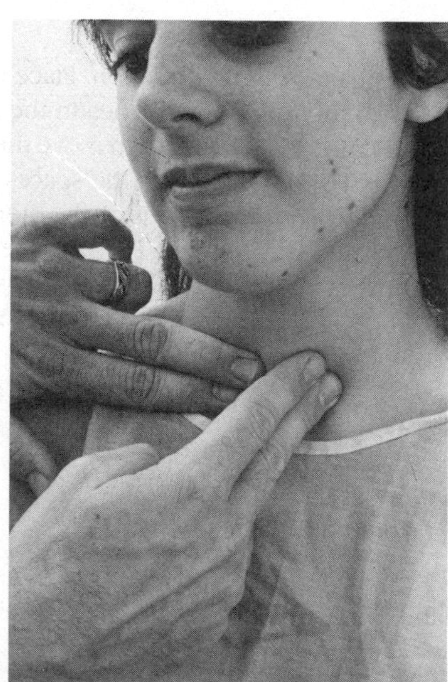

Figure 35–25 Palpating the right thyroid lobe: anterior approach

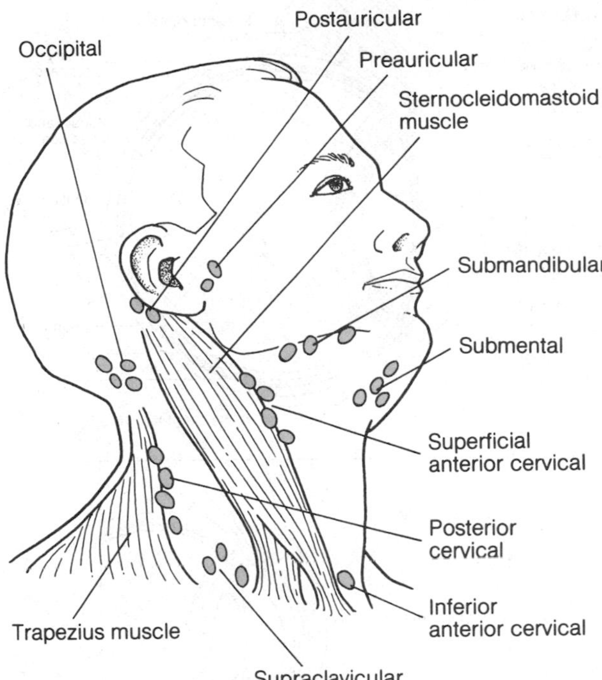

Figure 35–26 Lymph nodes of the neck

lateral to the sternocleidomastoid muscle. See Figure 35–27.

6. When palpating the anterior cervical nodes and posterior cervical nodes, move your fingertips slowly in a forward circular motion against the sternocleidomastoid and trapezius muscles, respectively.
7. To palpate the deep cervical nodes, bend or hook your fingers around the sternocleidomastoid muscle.

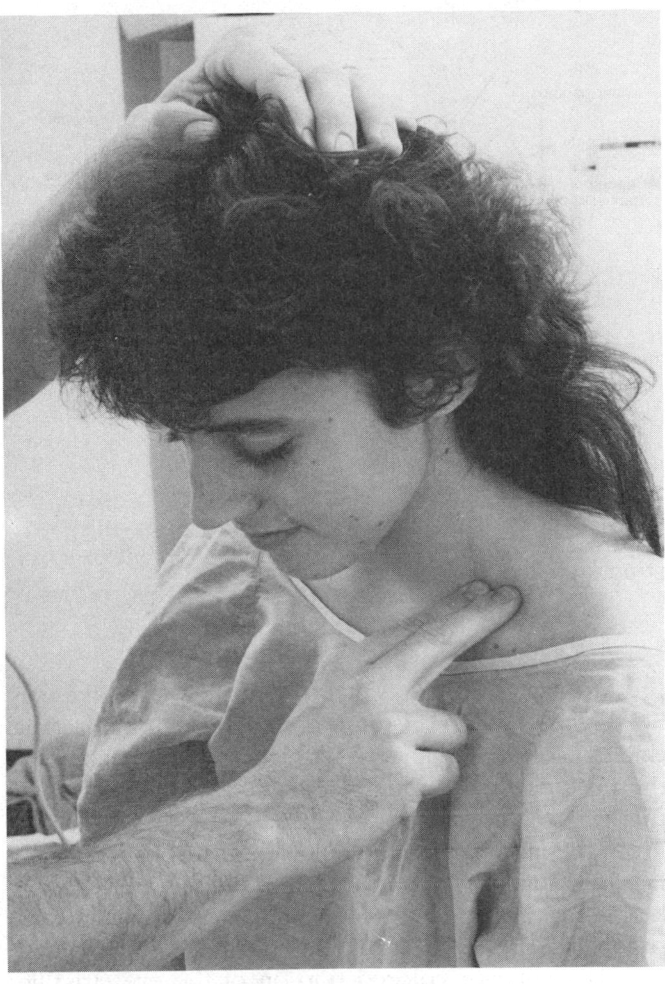

Figure 35–27 Palpating the supraclavicular lymph nodes

Eyes and Vision

Vision is considered by many people the most important sense, since it allows them to interact freely with their environment and enjoy the beauty of life around them. To maintain optimum vision, the eyes need to be examined throughout the life cycle. It is recommended that people under age 40 have their eyes tested every 3 to 5 years, or more frequently if there is a family history of diabetes, hypertension, blood dyscrasia, or eye disease (e.g., glaucoma). After age 40, an eye examination is recommended every 2 years, to rule out the possibility of glaucoma.

An eye assessment should be carried out as part of the client's initial physical examination; periodic reassessments need to be made for long-term care clients. Examination of the eyes includes assessment of visual acuity, ocular movement, visual fields, external structures, and the fundus. Most eye assessment procedures involve inspection. Consideration is also given to developmental changes and to individual hygienic practices, if the client wears contact lenses or an artificial eye.

The purposes of eye assessments are:

1. To obtain baseline data on the client's vision, eye mobility, and health status of the external and internal eye structures
2. To screen for specific eye problems

Nursing history data taken in conjunction with assessment of the eyes are shown on page 819.

For the anatomic structures of the eye, see Figures 35–28 and 35–29.

The lacrimal glands, situated in a depression in the frontal bone at the upper outer angle of the eye orbit,

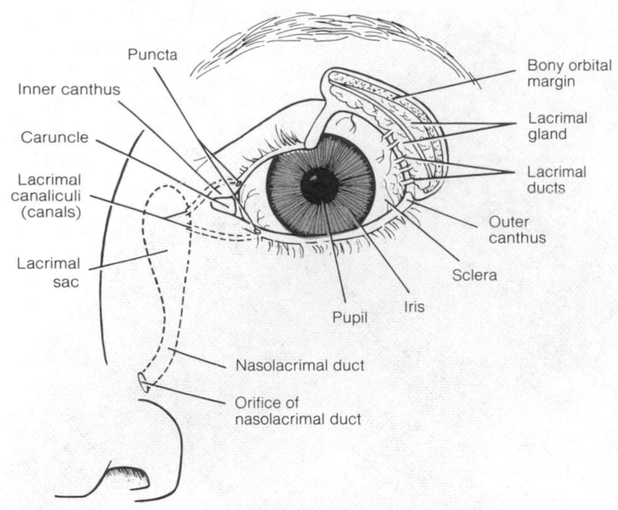

Figure 35–28 The left eye showing the external structures and the lacrimal apparatus

produce lacrimal fluid, which continually washes the eyes. See Figure 35–28. This fluid drains through the lacrimal ducts onto the conjunctiva at the upper outer corner of the eye and then through lacrimal canaliculi (canals) to the lacrimal sac, which is situated in the inner canthus. From the lacrimal sac, the fluid drains through the nasolacrimal duct to the inferior meatus of the nose. The fluid keeps the eyeball moist and helps wash away foreign particles. Excessive lacrimal fluid forms tears.

The anterior colored portion of the eye (iris) lies within the anterior chamber and is covered by the cornea, which joins the sclera, or white of the eye. See Figure 35–29. The sclera forms the support for the eyeball; it extends posteriorly to cover about 75% of the eyeball. The cornea acts to refract the light rays entering the eye. The iris regulates the amount of light permitted through the pupil.

Developmental Variables

Visual abilities are present at birth; the newborn can follow large moving objects, is attracted to black-white contrast, can fixate on certain stimuli for 4–10 seconds, and can react to changes in the intensity of light. The pupils of the newborn respond slowly, however, and the eyes cannot focus on close objects. By 3 months of age, the infant can coordinate both eyes horizontally and vertically. By 4 months, the infant recognizes familiar objects and follows moving objects. At 6 years of age, the child has visual acuity comparable to that of an adult. Preschool children are generally farsighted until their eyes grow in length and become **emmetropic** (refracting normally and focusing objects on the retina).

Loss of visual acuity occurs in elderly people as the lens of the eye ages, becomes more opaque, and loses

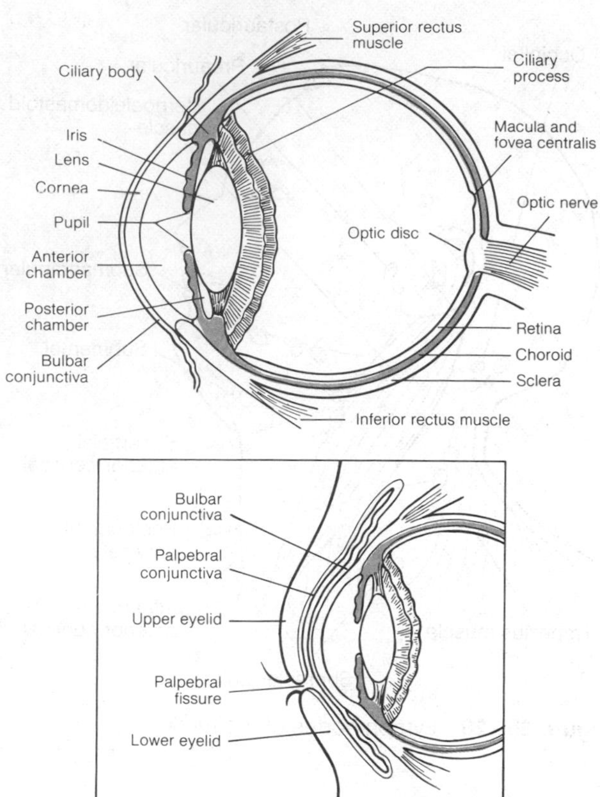

Figure 35–29 Anatomic structures of the right eye, lateral view

elasticity. Other changes include loss of ability of the iris to accommodate to darkness and dim light, loss of peripheral vision, and difficulty in distinguishing similar colors.

Common Problems

In children, **strabismus** is the most common congenital problem. The muscles of the two eyes are not coordinated, and, when the child has one eye directed straight ahead, the other eye may be directed inward, outward, or upward. The eyes appear crossed. Eyeglasses may be used to correct strabismus; in some cases, surgery is performed on the eye muscles.

Eyeglasses and contact lenses are worn by many children and adults to correct common refractive errors of the lens of the eye. These errors include **myopia** (nearsightedness), **hyperopia** (farsightedness), and **presbyopia** (loss of elasticity of the lens and thus loss of ability to accommodate to close objects). Presbyopia begins at about 45 years of age. People notice that they have difficulty reading newsprint. Often two corrective lenses (bifocals) are required—one for near vision or reading, and the other for far vision.

Astigmatism, an uneven curvature of the cornea that prevents horizontal and vertical rays from focusing on the retina, is a common problem that may occur in conjunction with myopia and hyperopia.

Table 35–5 Lymph Nodes of the Head and Neck

Node center	Location	Area drained
	Head	
Occipital	At the posterior base of the skull	The occipital region of the scalp and the deep structures of the back of the neck
Postauricular (mastoid)	Behind the auricle of the ear over or in front of the mastoid process	The parietal region of the head and part of the ear
Preauricular	In front of the tragus of the ear	The forehead and upper face
	Floor of mouth	
Submandibular (submaxillary)	Along the medial border of the lower jaw, halfway between the angle of the jaw and the chin	The chin, upper lip, cheek, nose, teeth, eyelids, part of the tongue and of the floor of the mouth
Submental	Behind the tip of the mandible, in the midline, under the chin	The anterior third of the tongue, gums, and floor of the mouth
	Neck	
Superficial (anterior) cervical chain	Along and anterior to the sternocleidomastoid muscle	The skin and neck
Posterior cervical chain	Along the anterior aspect of the trapezius muscle	The posterior and lateral regions of the neck, occiput, and mastoid
Deep cervical chain	Under the sternocleidomastoid muscle	The larynx, thyroid gland, trachea, and upper part of the esophagus
Supraclavicular	Above the clavicle, in the angle between the clavicle and the sternocleidomastoid muscle	The lateral regions of the neck and lungs

Common inflammatory problems that nurses may encounter in clients at any age include conjunctivitis, dacryocystitis, hordeolum, iritis, and contusions or hematomas of the eyelids and surrounding structures. **Conjunctivitis** (inflammation of the bulbar and palpebral conjunctiva) may result from foreign bodies, chemicals, allergenic agents, bacteria, or viruses. Redness, itching, tearing, and mucopurulent discharge occur. After sleep, the eyelids may be encrusted and matted together. **Dacryocystitis** (inflammation of the lacrimal sac) is manifested by tearing and a discharge from the nasolacrimal duct. **Hordeolum** (sty) is a redness, swelling, and tenderness of the hair follicle and glands that empty at the edge of the eyelids. **Iritis** (inflammation of the iris) may be caused by local or systemic infections and results in pain, tearing, and **photophobia** (sensitivity to light). **Contusions** or **hematomas** are "black eyes" resulting from injury.

Cataracts tend to occur in those over 65 years old. This opacity of the lens or its capsule, which blocks light rays, is frequently corrected by surgery. Cataracts may also occur in infants due to a malformation of the lens if the mother contracted rubella in the first trimester of pregnancy.

Glaucoma (a disturbance in the circulation of aqueous fluid, which causes an increase in intraocular pressure) is the greatest cause of blindness in people over 40. It can be controlled if diagnosed early. Danger signs of glaucoma include blurred or foggy vision, loss of peripheral vision, difficulty focusing on close objects, difficulty adjusting to dark rooms, and seeing rainbow-colored rings around lights.

Nursing History Data: Eyes

Determine:

- When the client last visited an ophthalmologist
- Whether there is a family history of diabetes; hypertension; blood dyscrasia; or eye disease, injury, or surgery
- Whether the client is currently taking eye medications
- Whether the client wears contact lenses or eyeglasses
- What hygienic practices the client uses for corrective lenses
- Whether there are current symptoms of eye problems, such as changes in visual acuity, blurring of vision, tearing, spots or floaters, photophobia, burning, itching, pain, diplopia, flashing lights, or halos around lights

Visual Acuity

The child acquires normal 20/20 vision by 6 years of age. Persons with denominators of 40 or more on the Snellen chart with or without corrective lenses need to be referred to an ophthalmologist. Procedure 35–1 outlines the steps to follow to assess a client's near vision, far vision, and functional vision.

Procedure 35–1 ▲ Assessing Visual Acuity

Equipment

1. Newsprint for testing near vision.
2. A Snellen eye chart; for a person unable to read, a Snellen E chart; for a child of 3 years, a chart with identifiable pictures. See Figure 35–30.
3. An eye cover or opaque index card.
4. A penlight.

Intervention

1. *Near vision.* Provide adequate lighting and have the client read from a magazine or newspaper held at a distance of 36 cm (14 in). If the client normally wears corrective lenses, the glasses or lenses should be worn as she or he reads.
2. *Distance vision.* Have the client wear her or his corrective lenses, unless they are used for reading only, i.e., for distances of only 30 to 36 cm (12 to 14 in). Have the client stand or sit 6 m (20 ft) from a Snellen chart. Take three readings as follows:
   a. Have the client cover the eye not being tested (left eye) and identify the letters on the Snellen chart, starting at the line he or she can most comfortably read and continuing to lower lines. If the client is unable to read, use the Snellen E chart, and ask him or her to say in which direction the E is pointing.

   Rationale The right eye is usually tested first. It is wise to get in the habit of starting with the right eye, to prevent inadvertent errors in documenting data about each eye.

   b. Have the client cover the right eye, and identify the letters with the left eye.
   c. Have the client read the Snellen chart with both eyes *uncovered.*
   d. Record the readings of each eye and both eyes, i.e., the smallest line from which the client is able to read one half or more of the letters. The Snellen chart has standardized numbers (fractions) at the end of each line of the chart. For the top line it is 20/200. The numerator (top number) is always 20, the distance the client stands from the chart. The denominator (bottom number) is the distance from which the normal eye can read the chart. Therefore, if a client has 20/40 vision, he or she can see at 20 feet from the chart what a normal-sighted person can see at 40 feet from the chart. Visual acuity is recorded as s̄c (without correction), or c̄c (with correction). You can also indicate how many letters were misread in the line, e.g., "visual acuity 20/40 – 2 c̄c" indicates that two letters were misread in the 20/40 line by a client wearing corrective lenses.
3. *Functional vision.* If the client is unable to see the top line (20/200) of the Snellen chart, perform functional vision tests (Boyd-Monk 1980, p. 63):
   a. *Light perception* (LP). Shine a penlight into the client's eye from a lateral position and then turn the light off. Ask the client to tell you when the light is on or off. If the client knows when the light is on and off, he or she has light perception, and the vision is recorded as LP.
   b. *Hand movements* (H/M). Hold your hand 30 cm (1 ft) from the client's face and move it slowly back and forth, stopping periodically. Ask the client to tell you when your hand stops moving. If the client

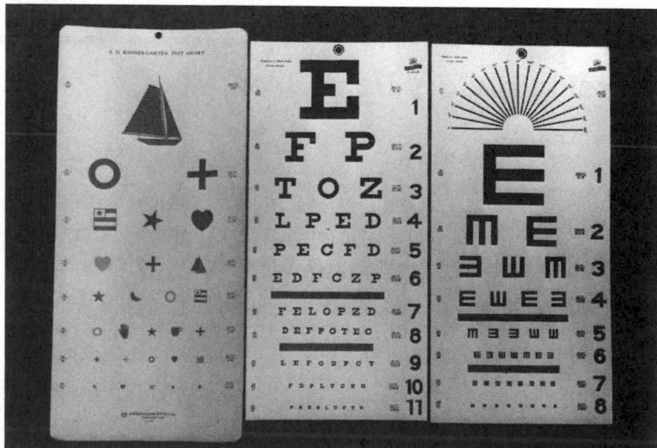

Figure 35–30 Three types of eye charts: the preschool children's chart (left), Snellen standard chart (center), and Snellen E chart for clients unable to read (right)

knows when your hand stops moving, record the vision as H/M 1 ft.

c. *Counting fingers* (C/F). Hold up some of your fingers 30 cm (1 ft) from the client's face, and ask him or her to count your fingers. If the client can do so, note on the vision record C/F 1 ft.

Rationale Clients who can pass these three functional tests are able to manage fairly well independently. If the person is unable to perform them in either eye, he or she is blind. Legal blindness is a visual acuity of 20/200 or less in both eyes with corrective lenses.

Extraocular Movements (EOM)

Three tests can be performed on clients over 6 months of age: the six cardinal fields of gaze, the cover-uncover patch test, and the corneal light reflex test.

Six Cardinal Fields of Gaze

This test determines eye coordination and alignment. To perform the test:

1. Stand directly in front of the client and hold a penlight at a comfortable distance, e.g., 30 cm (1 ft) in front of the client's eyes.
2. Ask the client to hold his or her head in a fixed position facing you and to follow the movements of the penlight with the *eyes only.*
3. Move the penlight in a slow, orderly manner through the six cardinal fields of gaze: from the center of the eye along the lines of the arrows in Figure 35–31 and back to the center.

   These six positions are used because six muscles guide the movement of each eye. Four rectus muscles (superior, inferior, lateral, and medial) move the eye in the directions indicated. Two oblique muscles (superior and inferior) rotate the eyeball on its axis. Cranial nerves III (oculomotor), IV (trochlear), and VI (abducens) innervate these muscles. The six positions can identify a nonfunctioning muscle or associated cranial nerve.
4. Stop the movement of the penlight periodically. This enables the nurse to detect **nystagmus** (an involuntary rapid movement of the eyeball). Slight nystagmus on the extreme lateral gaze (end-point nystagmus) occurs normally in many people. Other nystagmus is abnormal.

Normally, both eyes are coordinated, move in unison, and have parallel alignment. There may also be end-point nystagmus. Eye movements that are not coordinated or parallel, failure of one or both eyes to follow the penlight in specific directions, and nystagmus other than end-point are abnormal.

Cover-Uncover Patch Test

This test determines eye alignment. To perform the test:

1. Ask the client to stare straight ahead at a fixed point, e.g., at a penlight held 15 cm (6 in) in front of the eyes.
2. Cover one of the client's eyes with an eye cover or index card while observing the uncovered eye. If well aligned, the uncovered eye should not move from the fixed point when the other eye is covered. If it does move, to focus on the fixed point, it was *not* well aligned before the other eye was covered; it is shifting from a medial or lateral to central gaze.

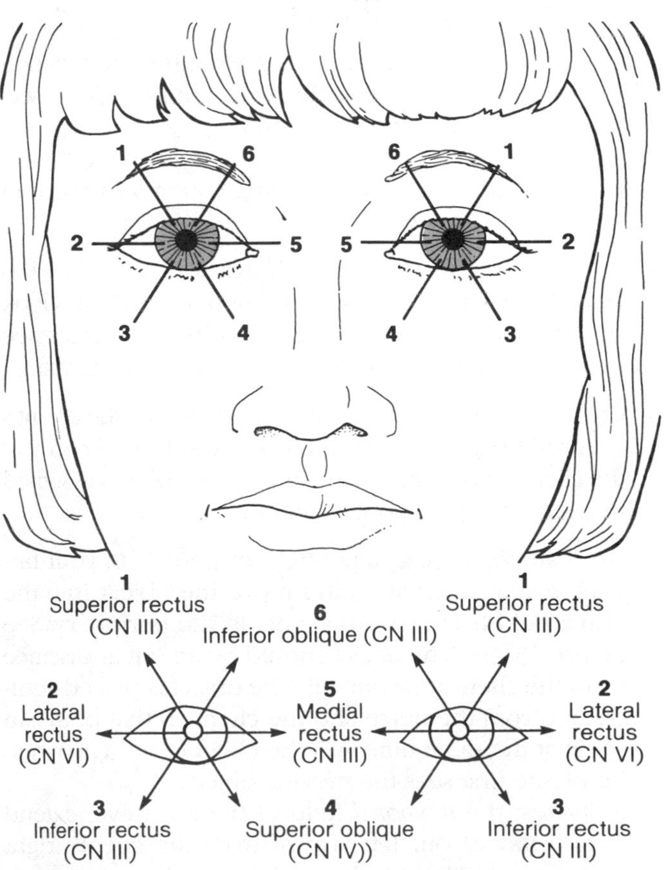

Figure 35–31 The six cardinal fields of gaze

3. Remove the eye cover, and observe the newly uncovered eye for movement. The newly uncovered eye, if well aligned, should not move. If it does move to focus on the fixed point when uncovered, it was *not* well aligned when covered. Muscle weakness is apparent when the eye turns inward or outward while covered. As the eye is uncovered, a quick inward or outward movement occurs to bring it back to alignment.
4. Repeat steps 1–4 for the other eye.
5. Test each eye several times to confirm your findings.

Corneal Light Reflex Test

This test also determines eye alignment. To perform this test:

1. Darken the room.
2. Ask the client to stare straight ahead.
3. Shine a penlight on the bridge of the nose.
4. Observe the light reflection in both corneas. Light reflection is normally situated in the same spot on both eyes.

Peripheral Visual Fields

Testing of peripheral visual fields determines the function of retina, neuronal visual pathway to the brain, and second (optic) cranial nerve function.

1. Have the client sit directly facing you at a distance of 60 to 90 cm (2 to 3 ft).
2. Ask the client to cover the left eye with a card and to look directly at your nose. The client must always look straight ahead in order to test what he or she can see in all areas away from the centralmost point of vision.
3. Cover or close your eye directly opposite the client's covered eye (i.e., your right eye), and look directly at the client's nose. The nurse acts as a control. It is assumed that she or he has good visual fields.
4. Hold an object (e.g., a penlight or pencil) in your fingers, extend your arm, and move the object into the visual field from various points in the periphery. See Figure 35–32. The object should be an equal distance from the client and yourself. The object is placed equidistant from the nurse and the client so that both can see it at the same time. Ask the client to tell you when he or she first sees the moving object.
   a. To test the *temporal* field of the right eye, extend and move your left arm in from the client's right periphery. Temporally, peripheral objects can normally be seen at right angles (90°) to the central point of vision.

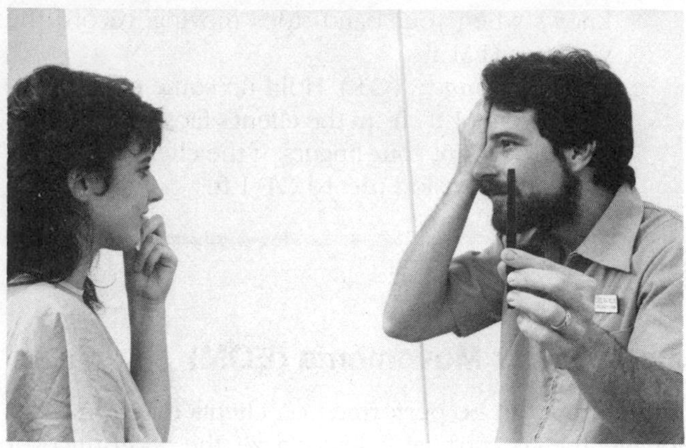

Figure 35–32 Testing peripheral visual fields

   b. To test the *upward* field of the right eye, extend and move the left arm down from the upward periphery. The upward field of vision is normally only 50° since the orbital ridge is in the way.
   c. To test the *downward* field of the right eye, extend and move the left arm up from the lower periphery. The downward field of vision is normally 70° since the cheekbone is in the way.
   d. To test the *nasal* field of the right eye, extend and move your right arm in from the periphery. The nasal field of vision is normally 50° away from the central point of vision since the nose is in the way.
5. Repeat the above steps for the left eye, reversing the process.

External Eye Structures

To assess the external eye structures, have the client sit at eye level directly in front of you. Inspect the external ocular structures in the order described.

Eyebrows

Inspect the eyebrows for hair distribution and alignment, skin quality, and movement. Ask the client to raise and lower the eyebrows. Note loss of hair, and scaling or flakiness of the skin.

Eyelashes

Inspect the eyelashes for evenness of distribution and direction of curl. Normally, eyelashes are equally distributed and curled slightly outward. Inward turning of the eyelashes occurs with inversion of the eyelid.

Eyelids

Inspect the eyelids for surface characteristics, (e.g., skin quality and texture), position, ability to close, ability to blink, and frequency of blinking.

1. To inspect the upper lids, have the client close the eyes. Elevate the eyebrows with your thumb and index finger. Elevation stretches the skin folds for proper visual examination. See Figure 35–33. Note skin color, skin texture, and eyelid closure. The skin should be intact, there should be no discharge or discoloration, and the eyelids should close symmetrically. Document any redness, swelling, flaking, crusting, plaques, discharge, nodules, or lesions.

2. To inspect the lower lids, have the client open the eyes. Note the characteristics listed for the upper lids, ability to blink, frequency of blinking, and the position of the eyelids in relation to the cornea. Normally, there are approximately 15 to 20 involuntary blinks per minute, blinking is bilateral, and there is no visible sclera above corneas when the lids open. The upper and lower borders of the cornea are slightly covered. A visible rim of sclera between the lid and the iris is often associated with hyperthyroidism. Asymmetric lid closure; incomplete or painful closure; and blinking that is rapid, monocular, absent, or infrequent must be reported.

Eyelids that lie at or below the pupil margin are referred to as **ptosis** and are usually associated with aging, edema from drug allergy or systemic disease (e.g., kidney disease), congenital lid muscle dysfunction, neuromuscular disease (e.g., myasthenia gravis), and third cranial nerve impairment.

Eversion, an outturning of the eyelid, is called **ectropion**; inversion, an inturning of the lid, is called **entropion**. These abnormalities are often associated with scarring injuries or the aging process.

Lacrimal Apparatus

See Figure 35–28 on page 818.

1. Inspect and palpate the lacrimal gland. See Figure 35–34. Note any edema or tenderness.

2. Inspect and palpate the lacrimal sac and nasolacrimal duct. See Figure 35–35. Observe for edema between the lower lid and the nose and for evidence of increased tearing. Using the tip of your index finger, palpate inside the lower orbital rim near the inner canthus, not on the side of the nose. Regurgitation of fluid on palpation of lacrimal sac is abnormal.

Bulbar Conjunctiva

1. Retract the client's eyelids with your thumb and index finger, exerting pressure over the upper and lower bony orbits.

2. Ask the client to look up, down, and from side to side.

3. Inspect the conjunctiva for color, texture, and presence of lesions.

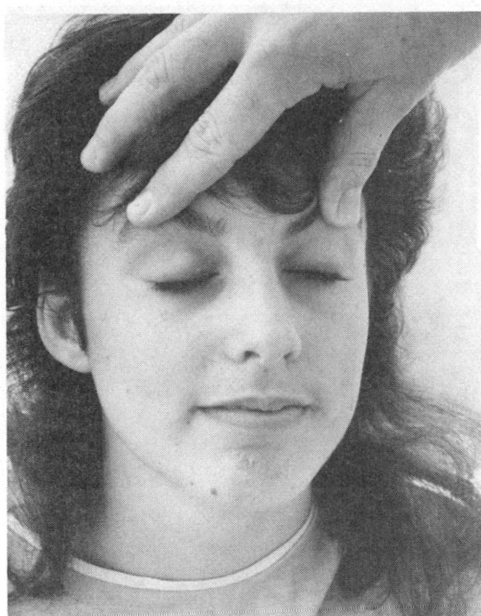

Figure 35–33 Inspecting the upper eye lids

The conjunctiva should be transparent, although capillaries are sometimes evident. The sclera should appear white or slight yellow in blacks. Sclera that appear jaundiced, excessively pale, or reddened are not normal and may indicate biliary obstruction; anemia; or damage by mechanical, clinical, allergenic, or bacterial agents. Any lesions or nodules must also be reported.

Palpebral Conjunctiva

Assessment of the palpebral conjunctiva requires eversion of the eyelids.

1. Evert both *lower* lids. Ask the client to look up, and gently retract the lower lids with your index fingers.

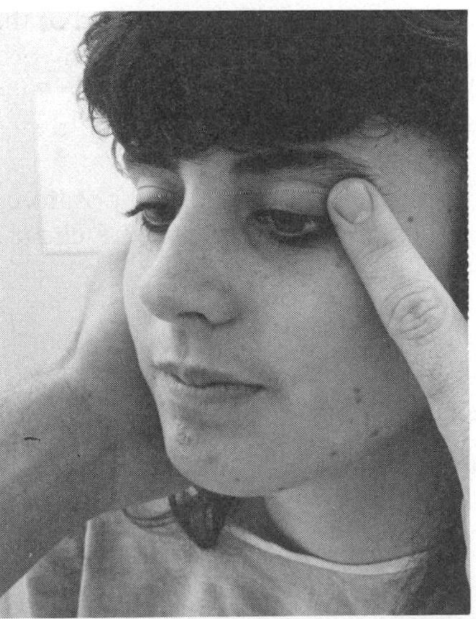

Figure 35–34 Palpating the lacrimal gland

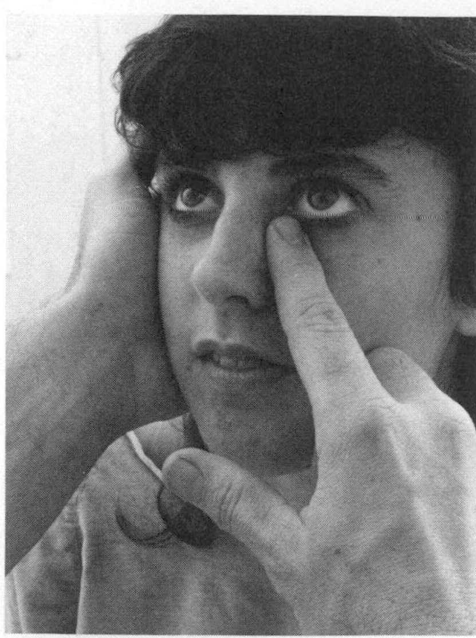

Figure 35–35 Palpating the lacrimal sac and nasolacrimal duct

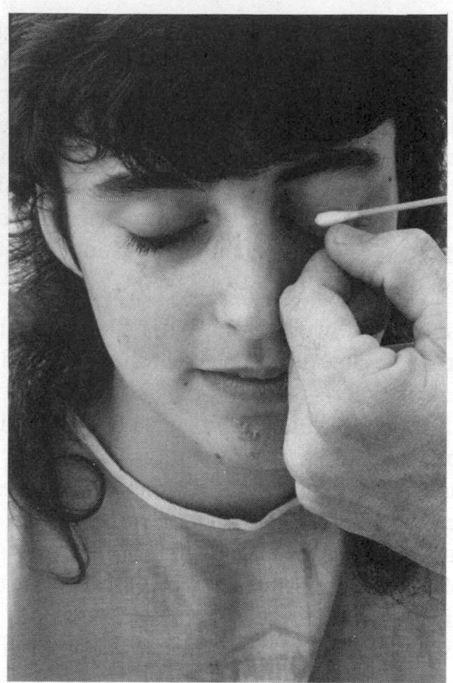

Figure 35–36 Everting the upper eyelid

Inspect the conjunctiva for color, texture, and presence of lesions. It normally appears pink and smooth.

2. Evert the *upper* lids *only if a problem is suspected.*
   a. Ask the client to look down and to keep the eyes slightly open. Closing the eyelids contracts the orbicular muscle, which prevents lid eversion.
   b. Gently grasp the eyelashes with your thumb and index finger. Pull the lashes gently downward. Upward or outward pulling on the eyelashes causes muscle contraction.
   c. Place a cotton-tipped applicator stick about 1 cm above the lid margin, and push it gently downward while still holding the eyelashes. See Figure 35–36. These actions evert the lid, i.e., flip the lower part of the lid over on top of itself.
   d. Hold the margin of the everted lid or the eyelashes against the ridge of the upper bony orbit with the applicator stick or your thumb. See Figure 35–37.
   e. Inspect the conjunctiva for color, texture, lesions, and foreign bodies.
   f. To return the lid to its normal position, gently pull the lashes forward, and ask the client to look up and to blink.

Cornea

1. Ask the client to look straight ahead.
2. Hold a penlight at an oblique angle to the eye, and move the light slowly across the corneal surface.
3. Inspect the cornea for clarity and texture.

Normally, the cornea is transparent, shiny, and smooth. Details of the iris are visible. In older people, a thin, grayish-white ring around the margin, called arcus senilis, may be evident. Arcus senilis in clients under age 40 is abnormal. An opaque or uneven surface of the cornea may be the result of trauma or an abrasion.

The corneal sensitivity (reflex) test determines the function of the fifth (trigeminal) cranial nerve.

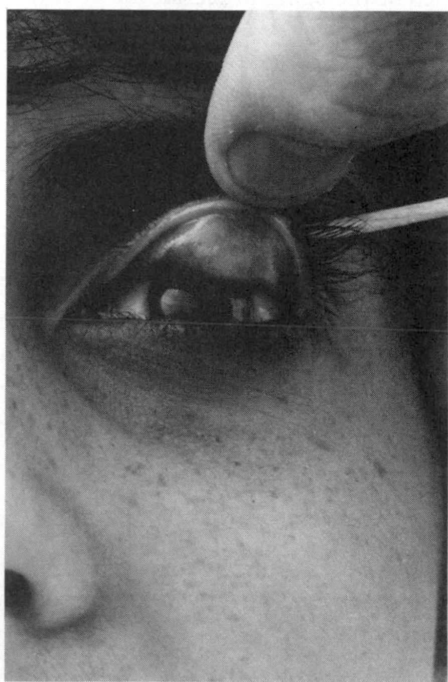

Figure 35–37 Holding the margin of the everted upper eye lid

Assessing the Pupil

1. Ask the client to look straight ahead.
2. Inspect the pupils for color, shape, and symmetry of size. Pupil charts are available in some agencies. See Figure 35–38 for variations in pupil diameters in millimeters.
3. Assess each pupil's direct and consensual reaction to light to determine the function of the third (oculomotor) cranial nerve.
   a. Partially darken the room.
   b. Ask the client to look straight ahead.
   c. Using a penlight and approaching from the side, shine a light on the pupil.
   d. Observe the response of the illuminated pupil. It should constrict (direct response).
   e. Again shine the light on the pupil, and observe the response of the other pupil. It should also constrict (consensual response).
4. Assess each pupil's reaction to accommodation.
   a. Hold an object (a penlight or pencil) about 10 cm (4 in) from the bridge of the client's nose.
   b. Ask the client to look first at the top of the object and then at a distant object (e.g., the far wall) behind the penlight. Alternate the gaze from the near to the far object.
   c. Observe the pupil response. The pupils should constrict when looking at the near object and dilate when looking at the far object.
   d. Next move the penlight or pencil toward the client's nose. The pupils should converge.
5. To record normal assessment of the pupils, use the abbreviation PERRLA (pupils equally round and react to light and accommodation).

1. Ask the client to keep both eyes open and look straight ahead.
2. With a wisp of cotton, approach from behind and beside the client and lightly touch the cornea with the cotton wisp. The blink response normally occurs when the cornea is touched, indicating that the trigeminal nerve is intact.

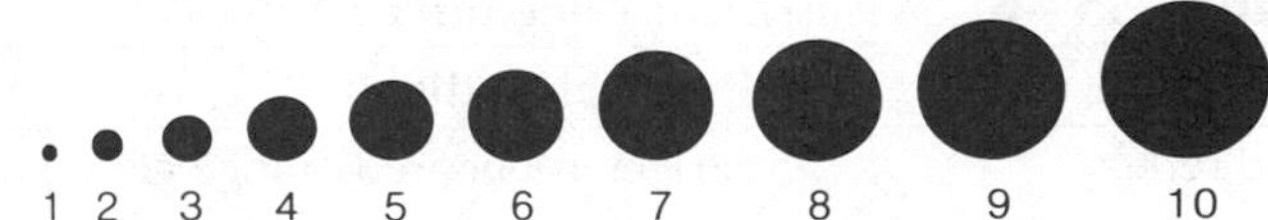

Figure 35–38 Variations in pupil diameters in millimeters

Anterior Chamber

1. Use the same oblique lighting technique used to test the cornea.
2. Inspect the anterior chamber for transparency and depth. Normally, the anterior chamber is transparent and not cloudy. No shadows of light should appear on the iris. A crescent-shaped shadow on the far side of the iris indicates a bulging iris, a shallow anterior chamber, and a predisposition to glaucoma. The anterior chamber normally has a depth of about 3 mm. Deep chambers are indicative of glaucoma.

Pupil and Iris

Pupils are normally black, are equal in size, (about 3 to 7 mm in diameter), and have round, smooth borders. Cloudy pupils are often indicative of cataracts. Enlarged pupils (**mydriasis**) may indicate injury, glaucoma, or be the result of certain drugs (e.g., atropine). Constricted pupils (**miosis**) may indicate an inflammation of the iris or be the result of such drugs as morphine or pilocarpine. Unequal pupils (**anisocoria**) are usually the result of a central nervous system disorder. Steps in assessing the pupil are shown to the left.

The iris is normally flat and round. A bulging toward the cornea can indicate increased intraocular pressure.

Internal Eye Structures

The internal part of the eye posterior to the lens, visible through the pupil by an ophthalmoscope, is called the fundus of the eye. Structures of the fundus include the retina, choroid, fovea, macula, disc, and retinal vessels. Ophthalmic or funduscopic examination of the eye requires practice and skill. See Procedure 35–2.

Procedure 35–2 ▲ Assessing the Internal Eye Structures

In some practice settings the nurse does not perform ophthalmic examination of the eye.

Equipment

An ophthalmoscope. See Figure 35–39.

Intervention

See Table 35–6 for normal and abnormal findings.

Funduscopic examinations of infants may be deterred until age 2 to 6 months unless other assessments, such as the neurologic examination, suggest pathologic condi-

Table 35–6 Assessment Data: Internal Eye

Structure test	Normal findings	Abnormal findings
Red reflex	Bright, round, red-orange glow through pupil	Decreased redness or roundness Opacities
Optic disc and cup	Yellowish or creamy pink, almost round disc; lighter than retina	Pale disc
	Distinct regular outline (nasal edge less distinct than temporal edge)	Blurred disc margins and reddened disc
	About 1.5 mm in diameter but appears larger with magnification × 15	Discs unequal size and shape
	Physiologic cup occupies one-third to one-half of disc area	Cup extends to disc border, is asymmetrical
	Cups equal in size	Cups unequal in size
	Cup paler than disc (yellow-white)	
Retinal vessels	Arteries	
	Light red color	Copper or silver color Pale or white vessel
	Narrow band of light in center (arteriolar light reflex) about one-fourth diameter of blood column	Narrowed light reflex
	Arteries two-thirds to four-fifths diameter of veins	
	Regular caliber, decreasing in size toward periphery	Irregularities in caliber (dilations or constrictions)
	Veins	
	Larger than arteries Darker color than arteries No prominent light reflex	Dilated and tortuous veins
	Arteriovenous crossings	
	Caliber of underlying vessel; not indented, pinched, or displaced	
Retinal background (periphery)	Uniform orange-pink color; lighter in fair people, darker in black people	Pallor Linear, or large or small dark or red patches Discrete tiny red dots Fuzzy white patches
Macula and fovea	Slightly darker than retina Tiny capillaries may be evident on surface Fovea seen as tiny bright light in center	Same as for retinal background, above

tions. For proper visualization a mydriatic is required. Generally, the drops are instilled three times before the test at 15-minute intervals. The baby can lie supine on the examining table or be held on an adult's lap or upright over one shoulder. The optic disc of infants is paler than that of adults, and edema of the optic disc is rare even with increased intracranial pressure, since the sutures and fontanelles are not ossified and will permit fluid collection.

1. Red reflex through pupil
   a. Assemble the ophthalmoscope. Align the base of the head with lugs on the top of the handle. Push the head down and rotate it, until you hear it click into place.
   b. Darken the room to dilate the pupils.
   c. Have the client remove his or her eyeglasses. Contact lenses may be left in, although removal can decrease light reflection.
   d. Have the client sit or stand in front of you.
   e. Adjust the aperture selection dial on the back of the ophthalmoscope head, to regulate the amount of light. Use the largest round light at first.
   f. Select the appropriate lens by adjusting the lens selection wheel on the side of the ophthalmoscope head. To begin, you may set the lens wheel at the 0 setting.
   g. To examine the right eye, hold the ophthalmoscope comfortably against your right eye with your right hand. Reverse the position to examine the left eye.

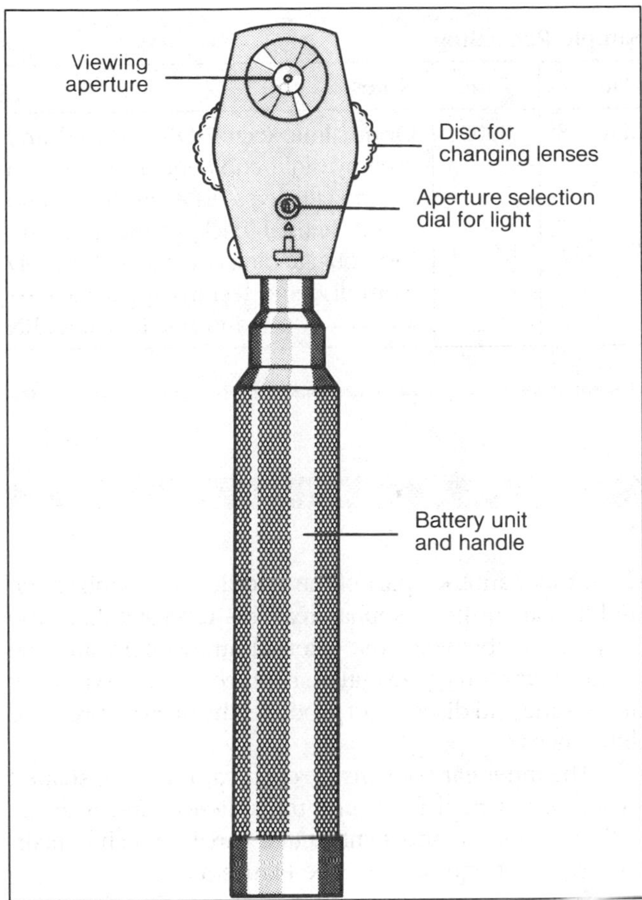

Figure 35–39 An ophthalmoscope, used to examine the interior of the eye

h. Hold the ophthalmoscope at least 30 cm (1 ft) from the client's pupil and at an angle of about 25° lateral to the client's line of central vision.
i. Ask the client to keep both eyes open and to focus on a distant object.
j. Shine the light on the client's pupil.
k. Observe the bright round orange glow through the pupil (the red reflex). In dark-skinned persons, the fundus may appear brown or purplish. Grayish-white opacities of the lens (cataracts) may impair visualization of the retina.

2. Optic disc and cup
   a. Keeping the red reflex in sight, slowly move the ophthalmoscope close to the client's pupil.

      Rationale Slow movement promotes dilation of the pupil and prevents eye movement.

   b. Locate some retinal structure, such as a blood vessel, and focus the image. Adjust the lens until the margins of the structure appear sharp.
   c. Locate the optic disc by following the blood vessels toward the midline. See Figure 35–40.

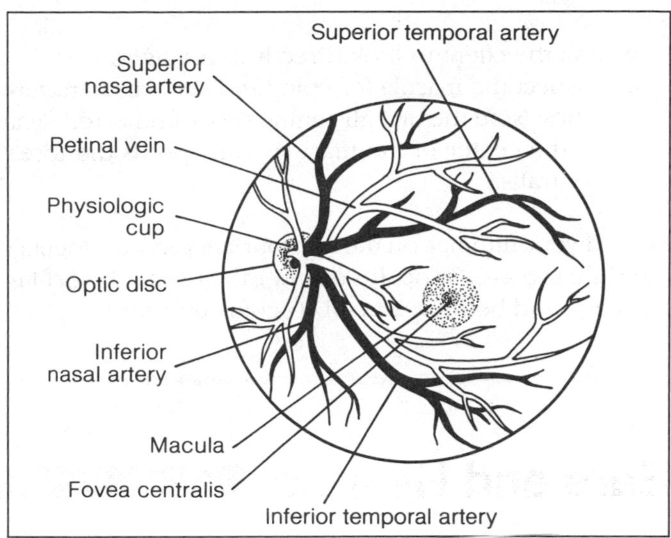

Figure 35–40 The fundus of the left eye

   d. Note the color, size, and shape of the disc, the distinctness of its margins, and its physiologic cup (the depressed central area of the disc).

3. Retinal blood vessels
   a. Follow the blood vessels peripherally in each of four quadrants: superior temporal, inferior temporal, superior nasal, and inferior nasal.

      Rationale The central retinal artery arises from the depth of the optic disc and divides into four main branches, which supply each retinal quadrant. The central retinal vein leaves the disc in company with the central artery and has similar branches in each quadrant. The four quadrants are scanned, since blood vessel abnormalities are not evenly distributed.

   b. Inspect the vessels for size, color, pattern, and arteriovenous crossings. See Table 35–6 earlier for normal and abnormal findings.

4. Retinal background (periphery)
   a. Ask the client to look upward, downward, and from side to side.
   b. Inspect the retinal background of the four quadrants.
   c. Note color and surface characteristics.

5. Macula and fovea centralis
   a. Avoid directing light on the macula for long periods.

      Rationale The macula is the center of most acute vision and is sensitive. Prolonging the time the light is on the macula can cause the client discomfort.

   b. Locate the macula by first locating the optic disc and then looking two disc diameters (DD) away toward the client's temple. It is a small circular structure 1 DD in size.

or

c. Ask the client to look directly at the light.
d. Inspect the macula for color and surface characteristics. Note the tiny glistening spot of reflected light in the center of the macula. This spot is the fovea centralis.

Record your findings on the appropriate records. Identify the right eye as OD (oculus dexter), the left as OS (oculus sinister), and both eyes as OU (oculus uterque).

Sample Recording

Date	Time	Notes
May/7/88	0900	Ophthalmic exam: Discs round and creamy pink; cups equal in size and color. Retinal vessels even caliber and intact. Retinal background has uniform orange-pink color. Maculae 2 DD from discs; no lesions apparent. —————— Simone L. White, RN

Ears and Hearing

The ear is divided into three parts: external ear, middle ear, and inner ear. The external ear includes the auricle or pinna, the external auditory canal, and the tympanic membrane (eardrum). See Figure 35–41. Landmarks of the auricle include the lobule (earlobe), helix, anthelix, tragus, triangular fossa, and external auditory meatus. Although not part of the ear, the mastoid, a bony prominence behind the ear, is another important landmark. See Figure 35–42. The external ear canal is curved, is about 2.5 cm (1 in) long in the adult, and ends at the tympanic membrane. It is covered with skin that has many fine hairs, glands, and nerve endings. The glands secrete cerumen (earwax), which lubricates and protects the canal.

The middle ear is an air-filled cavity that starts at the tympanic membrane and contains three ossicles (bones of sound transmission): the malleus (the most easily seen), the incus, and the stapes. See Figure 35–41. The eustachian tube, another part of the middle ear, connects the middle ear to the nasopharynx. This tube stabilizes the air pressure between the external atmosphere and the middle ear, thus preventing rupture of the tympanic membrane and discomfort produced by marked pressure differences.

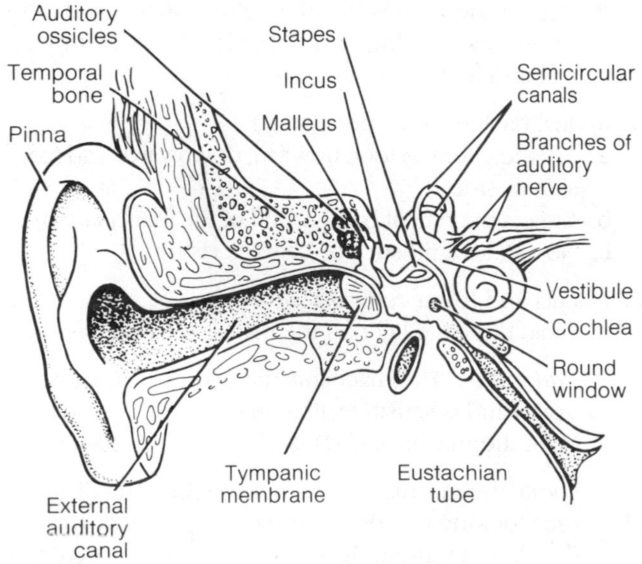

The inner ear contains the cochlea, a seashell-shaped structure essential for sound transmission and hearing, and the vestibule and semicircular canals, which contain the organs of equilibrium. See Figure 35–41.

Sound transmission and hearing are complex processes. In brief, sound can be transmitted by air conduction or bone conduction. Air-conducted transmission occurs when:

1. A sound stimulus enters the external canal and reaches the tympanic membrane.
2. The sound waves cross the tympanic membrane and reach the ossicles.
3. The sound waves travel from the ossicles to the opening in the inner ear (oval window).
4. The cochlea receives the sound vibrations.
5. The stimulus travels to the auditory nerve (the eighth cranial nerve) in the cerebral cortex.

Bone-conducted sound transmission occurs when skull bones transport the sound directly to the auditory nerve.

Figure 35–41 Anatomic structures of the external, middle, and inner ear

Developmental Variables

The curvature of the external ear canal differs with age. In the infant and toddler, the canal has an upward curvature. By age 3, the ear canal assumes the more downward curvature of adulthood.

Audiometric evaluations, which measure hearing at various decibels, are recommended for the elderly. A common hearing deficit with age is loss of ability to hear

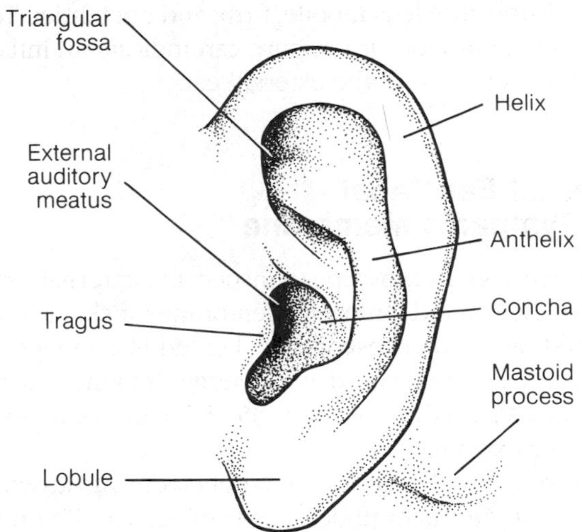

Figure 35–42 Landmarks of the external ear

Nursing History Data: Ears

Determine:

- Family history of hearing problems or loss
- Recent complaints of ear problems such as pain, itching, discharge, tinnitus (ringing in the ears)
- Any hearing difficulty, its onset, factors contributing to it, and its interference with activities of daily living
- Use of a corrective hearing device, duration of use, and supplier
- Medication history, especially if there are complaints of ringing in the ears
- Presence of high noise levels in the work environment

high-frequency sounds, such as *f*, *s*, *sh*, and *ph*. Because this deficit can distort normal conversation, older people may display inappropriate or confused behaviors sometimes. This neurosensory hearing deficit does not respond well to use of a hearing aid.

Common Problems

Localized infections of the external ear canal (**otitis externa**), the middle ear (**otitis media**), and the eustachian tube (**serous otitis**) are most common in children but also occur in adults. The client with external otitis may experience pain when touching or pressing the tragus or the auricle, and the canal is inflamed. Otitis media is manifested by redness and bulging of the tympanic membrane, and pus or blood in the ear canal. Serous otitis is often associated with otitis media and upper respiratory infections. An amber-colored fluid is usually seen through the eardrum and the client complains of "ear popping."

Mechanical blockages of the external ear canal most commonly arise from a buildup of cerumen or from foreign bodies lodged in the canal. Children are notorious for inserting small objects in their ears. Signs of blockage are pain and some loss of hearing.

The most common traumatic stress to the eardrum involves exposure to loud noises. Frequent, close exposure to loud music or machines is associated with a high potential for hearing loss.

Neurologic disorders that are congenital, inherited, or acquired are responsible for varying degrees of hearing loss. Congenital hearing losses are commonly seen in children who were exposed before birth to rubella, especially in the early months of pregnancy. Most inherited hearing losses do not manifest themselves until adulthood. Acquired hearing losses can occur as a result of mumps, meningitis, or severe reactions to some drugs, e.g., streptomycin. Some hearing loss often occurs with the normal aging process.

Assessment of the ear includes direct inspection and palpation of the external ear, inspection of the remaining parts of the ear by an otoscope, and determination of auditory acuity. The ear is usually assessed during an initial physical examination; periodic reassessments may be necessary for long-term clients or those who have hearing problems.

Nursing history data to be obtained during assessment of the ear are shown above.

Auricles

The auricles are inspected and palpated.

1. Assist the client to a comfortable sitting position.
2. Inspect the auricles for color and texture. Normally, the auricles are the same color as the facial skin. Excessive redness may be associated with fever; bluish earlobes, with cyanosis; and extreme pallor, with frostbite. Normal texture is smooth. Note flaky, scaly skin, cysts, or other lesions.
3. Inspect the auricles for symmetry of size, position, and angle. To inspect position, note the level at which the superior aspect of the auricle attaches to the head. Relate this point to the position of the eye. One should be able to visualize an imaginary straight line from the lateral angle of the eye to the point where the superior aspect of the auricle joins the head. Low-set ears are indicative of a congenital abnormality, e.g., mongolism. An imaginary line drawn from the top to the bottom of the ear should not vary more than 10° from the vertical. See Figure 35–43.

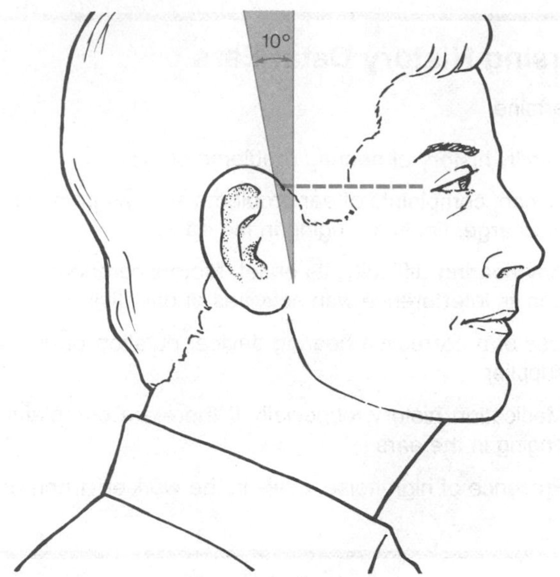

Figure 35–43 Normal ear alignment and ear angle

4. Palpate the auricle for texture, elasticity, and areas of tenderness.
   a. Pull the auricle upward, downward, and backward.
   b. Fold the pinna forward (it should recoil).
   c. Push in on the tragus.
   d. Apply pressure to the mastoid process.

Normally the auricle is mobile, firm, and not tender. Tenderness with motion or pressure can indicate an inflammation or infection of the external ear.

External Ear Canal and Tympanic Membrane

The nurse uses an otoscope to inspect the external structures of the ear and tympanic membrane for skin lesions, pus, and blood. An **otoscope** is a lighted instrument that has a funnel-shaped part that is inserted into the external auditory canal. See Procedure 35–3 for the steps in an otoscopic examination.

A child must be carefully restrained during otoscopic assessment. An infant under 1 year of age can lie on his or her back on the examining table with the head turned to one side and the arms over the head. An adult holds the infant's arms securely at the elbows. The nurse then leans over the infant's chest and uses both hands when examining the ear. A young child sits on an adult's lap. The adult restrains the child's legs between the adult's knees and restrains the child's arms against the child's chest. The adult uses the free hand to hold the child's head against the adult's chest. Older children generally cooperate when standing or sitting.

Procedure 35–3 ▲ Assessing the External Ear Canal and Tympanic Membrane

In some practice settings, the nurse does not perform otoscopic examinations.

Equipment

An otoscope with several sizes of ear specula and an air insufflator (optional). See Figure 35–44. The air insufflator (at the left) may be used to test tympanic membrane movement.

Intervention

See Table 35–7 for normal and abnormal findings.

External Ear Canal

1. Attach a speculum to the otoscope. Use the largest diameter that will fit the ear canal without causing discomfort.

   Rationale Maximum vision of the tympanic membrane is achieved.

2. Hold the otoscope either:
   a. Right side up with your fingers between the otoscope handle and the client's head.

      or

   b. Upside down with your fingers and the ulnar surface of your hand against the client's head. See Figure 35–45.

   Rationale Holding the fingers and/or ulnar surface of the hand between the otoscope and the client's head stabilizes the head and protects the eardrum and canal from injury if a quick head movement occurs.

3. Tip the client's head away from you and straighten the ear canal.
   a. For an adult, straighten the ear canal by pulling the pinna up and back. See Figure 35–46.
   b. For a child under 3 years of age, pull the pinna down and back. See Figure 35–47.

   Rationale Both of these actions facilitate vision of the tympanic membrane.

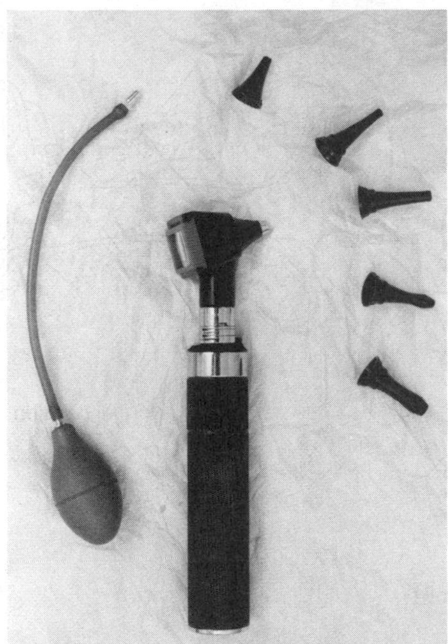

Figure 35–44 An otoscope with ear specula and an air insufflator

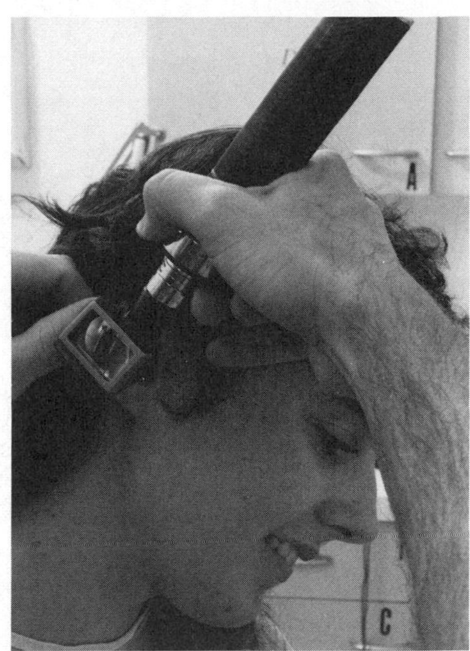

Figure 35–45 Inserting an otoscope

4. Gently insert the tip of the otoscope into the ear canal.

   Rationale The inner-two thirds of the ear canal is bony; if the speculum is pressed against either side, the client will experience pain.

5. Inspect the ear canal for cerumen, inflammation, scaling, foreign bodies, or other lesions.

6. If there is excessive cerumen in the canal, remove it. Dry cerumen is best removed by an irrigation. Wet and

Table 35–7 Assessment Data: External Ear Canal and Tympanic Membrane

Structure	Normal findings	Abnormal findings	Possible health problems
External ear canal	Distal third contains hair follicles and glands	Redness and discharge	Inflammation, infection
		Scaling	
	Dry cerumen, grayish-tan in color; or wet cerumen, sticky and various shades of brown	Excessive cerumen obstructing canal	
Tympanic membrane	Pearly gray color, semitransparent	Pink to red, some opacity	Inflammation
		Yellow-amber	Serum in middle ear
		White	Pus
		Blue or deep red	Blood in middle ear
		Dull surface	Fibrosis
	Superior aspect is more anterior than lower rim; dimension is slightly conical	Loss of conical dimension and convex bulging	Inflammation, serum, pus, or blood in middle ear
	Fluctuates (vibrates) slightly when client swallows	Membrane fixed, does not fluctuate	Inflammation, serum, pus, or blood in middle ear; obstructed eustachian tube; perforation of eardrum
	Light reflex (cone of light) bright to dim	Light reflex dimmed or absent	Inflammation; infection in middle ear
	Malleus is dense whitish streak	Malleus poorly defined or not visible	Inflammation; infection
	Umbo appears regressed	Umbo not visible	Inflammation; infection
	Annulus is defined and whitish-gray	Annulus poorly defined or not visible	Inflammation; infection

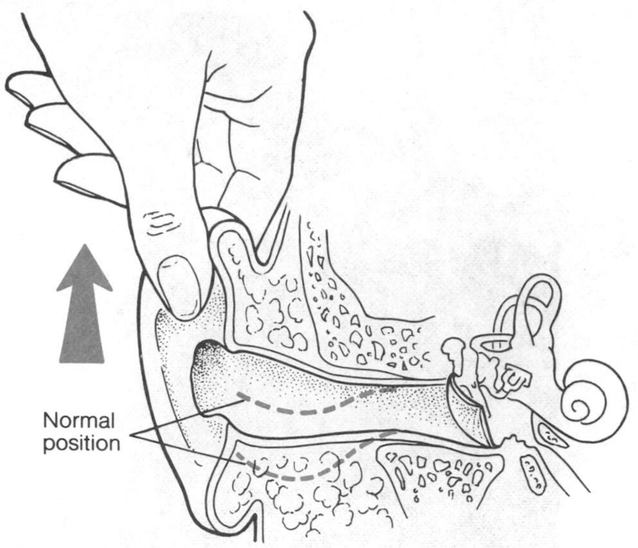

Figure 35–46

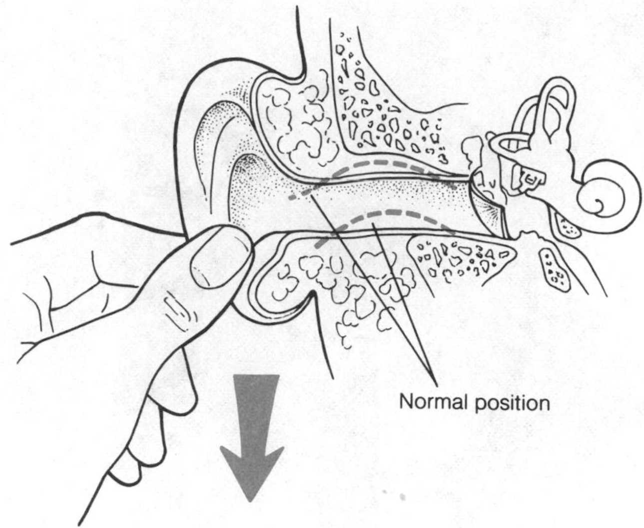

Figure 35–47

waxy cerumen can be removed with a curette (cerumen spoon) or a cotton-tipped applicator. Use of a curette, however, requires special skill.

Rationale Removal of cerumen is essential for proper visualization of the canal and tympanic membrane.

Tympanic Membrane

7. Locate the tympanic membrane. If you have difficulty seeing it, try repositioning the client's head and pulling the pinna in a slightly different direction.
8. Inspect it for color and gloss, position, movement, and appearance of specific landmarks: the umbo, the annulus, the malleus, and the light reflex (cone of light). Skill is necessary for observing the normal landmarks. The membrane is systematically inspected in four quadrants: anterior superior, anterior inferior, posterior superior, and posterior inferior. The anterior-posterior division is a hypothetical straight line running through the handle of the malleus. See Figure 35–48. The tympanic membrane is nearly oval, measuring about 9 to 10 mm in its downward and forward diameter, and 8 to 9 mm in its shorter diameter. The greater part of its circumference is thickened, forming a fibrocartilaginous ring (*tympanic ring* or *annulus*). Inside the ring, a triangular part of the tympanic membrane, located at the top between two folds (anterior and posterior malleolar folds), is lax and thin; it is referred to as the pars flaccida. The remainder of the membrane is taut and is referred to as the pars tensa. The malleus (hammer) originates in the anterior superior quadrant of the membrane and extends approximately to its center. The handle of the malleus is firmly attached to the inner surface of the tympanic membrane as far as its center, which projects inward toward the tympanic cavity, making the inner surface of the membrane convex. The point of greatest convexity is called the umbo. The light reflex (a cone of light) is seen in the anterior inferior quadrant. Its point is directed toward the umbo and its broad base is at the periphery of the tympanic annulus. See Table 35–7 for normal and abnormal findings.
9. Optional. Test the mobility of the tympanic membrane (pneumatic otoscopy).

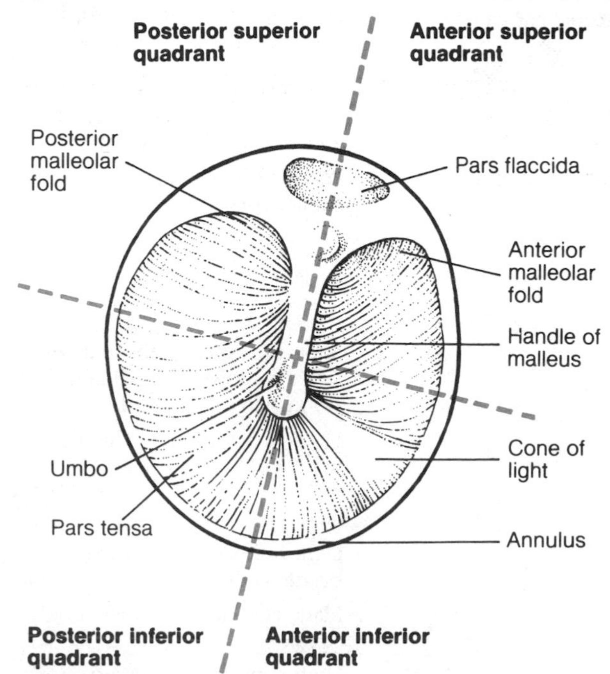

Figure 35–48

a. Attach the rubber bulb and connecting tube to the otoscope.
b. Alternately squeeze and release the bulb a few times while observing the tympanic membrane.

Rationale Squeezing the bulb pushes air into the canal, causing the membrane to move inward. Releasing the bulb removes air, causing the membrane to move outward. No movement or jerky movement of the tympanic membrane suggests a middle ear disorder or an obstructed eustachian tube.

Hearing Acuity

Gross Hearing Acuity Tests

Gross hearing acuity can be assessed by the client's response to voice tones, i.e., normal voice tones and whispered voice tones, and the ticking of a watch. First note generally how well the client hears your voice. If the client has difficulty, assess the client's response to the whispered voice. Requesting the nurse repeat words or statements, leaning toward the speaker, turning the head, cupping the ears, and speaking in a loud or unvaried tone of voice all suggest hearing problems.

To test the client's response to the whispered voice:

1. Stand 30 to 60 cm (1 to 2 ft) from the client in a position where the client cannot read your lips. Ask the client to occlude one ear by putting his or her finger in it.
2. Whisper some nonconsecutive numbers and have the client tell you what he or she heard. Whisper nonconsecutive numbers so that the client cannot anticipate the sequence of numbers. Increase the loudness of the whisper until the client can identify at least 50% of the numbers. Repeat the process with the other ear. This test is used only for screening, since it is difficult to maintain consistency in the whispered voice.

Another screening test is the watch tick test. The ticking of a watch has a higher pitch than the human voice. For this test:

1. Have the client occlude one ear. Out of the client's sight, place a ticking watch 2 to 5 cm (1 to 2 in) from the unoccluded ear.
2. Ask the client whether he or she can hear it. Repeat with the other ear.

Tuning Fork Tests

Tuning fork tests are used to assess whether the client's hearing loss is a conduction, sensorineural, or mixed problem. **Conduction hearing loss** is the result of interrupted transmission of sound waves through the outer and middle ear structures. Possible causes are a tear in the tympanic membrane or an obstruction, due to swelling or other causes, in the auditory canal. **Sensorineural hearing loss** is the result of damage to the inner ear, the auditory nerve, or the hearing center in the brain. **Mixed hearing loss** is a combination of conduction and sensorineural loss.

Weber's, Rinne, and Schwabach tests differentiate between conductive and sensorineural hearing loss. Tuning fork tests are described in Procedure 35–4.

Procedure 35–4 ▲ Tuning Fork Tests

Weber's Test

This test assesses bone conduction by testing the lateralization (sideward transmission) of sounds.

1. Hold the tuning fork at its base. Activate it by tapping the fork gently against the back of your hand near the knuckles or by stroking the fork between your thumb and index fingers. It should be made to ring softly.

   Rationale If the tone is too loud, you must wait a long while for it to quiet. A quiet tone is needed.

2. Place the base of the vibrating fork on top of the client's head (see Figure 35–49) and ask the client where he or she hears the noise. Normally the sound is heard in both ears or localized at the center of the head (Weber negative). Clients with a conductive hearing loss hear the sound better in the poor or damaged ear. Clients with a sensorineural loss hear the sound better in the ear without a problem. Record positive findings as Weber right or Weber left.

Rinne Test

This test compares air conduction to bone conduction.

3. Have the client intermittently block the hearing in one ear by moving a fingertip in and out of the ear canal.

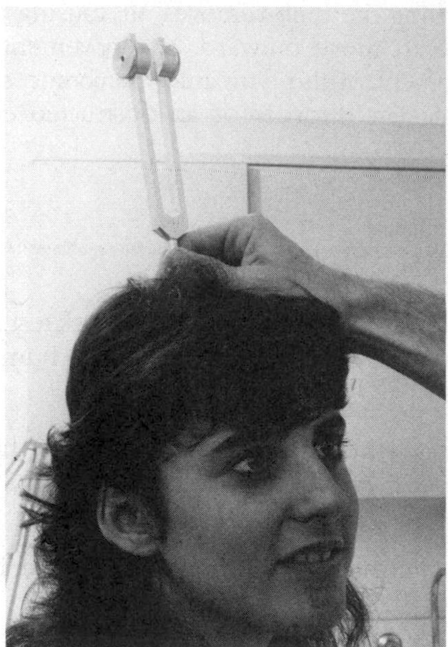

Figure 35–49

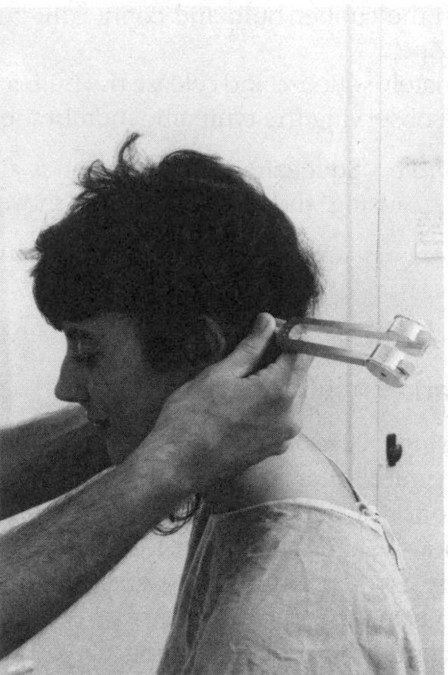

Figure 35–50

4. Hold the *handle* of the activated tuning fork on the mastoid process of one ear (see Figure 35–50) until the client tells you he or she can no longer hear the vibrations.
5. Then immediately hold the still vibrating fork *prongs* in front of the client's ear canal. Push aside the client's hair if necessary. See Figure 35–51. Ask whether the client now hears it again.

   Rationale Sound conducted by air is heard more readily than sound conducted by bone. The tuning fork vibrations conducted by air are therefore heard longer.
6. Repeat the procedure with the other ear. When air-conducted hearing is greater than bone-conducted hearing, the Rinne test is normal and is said to be positive, i.e., AC > BC. When there is a conductive loss, the bone conduction time is equal to or longer than the air conduction time, i.e., negative Rinne test, BC = AC or BC > AC.

Schwabach Test

This test compares the client's bone conduction to the nurse's. The nurse is presumed to have normal hearing.

7. Place the handle of a vibrating tuning fork alternately on the client's and examiner's mastoid process.
8. Ask the client to indicate when he or she no longer hears the vibrations.
9. Repeat the procedure with the client's other ear. Normally, the client and nurse hear the vibrations for the same length of time. The client with conductive hearing loss hears the tones longer than the nurse; the client with sensorineural hearing loss does not hear the tones as long.
10. Record your findings on the appropriate record.

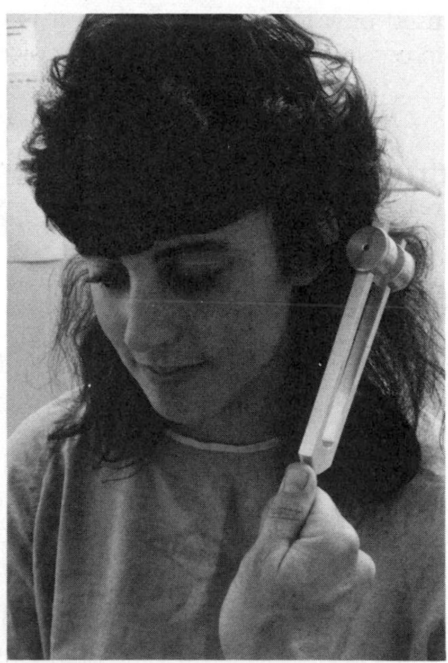

Figure 35–51

Nose and Sinuses

A nurse can inspect the nasal passages very simply with a flashlight. However, a **nasal speculum**, which is a lighted instrument, facilitates examination of the nasal chambers. See page 836 for suggestions to help the nurse obtain data about a client's nose and sinuses.

Nose

Palpate the external nose lightly for tenderness. Inspect both nares (nasal chambers) using a lighted nasal speculum. The nares open externally via the anterior nares and internally through the posterior nares into the nasopharynx. See Figure 35–52. Normally, the nares are patent; the external nose is symmetrical, straight, and not tender; and there is no discharge. Air should move freely as the client breathes through her or his nares. To assess the nares:

1. Inspect the lining of the nares (mucosa) and the coarse hairs that filter the air. Observe the presence of redness, swelling, growths, and discharge. The mucosa is usually pink with clear watery discharge.
2. Inspect the position of the nasal septum between the nasal chambers, in particular any deviation to right or left. The nasal septum is normally intact and in the midline.
3. Inspect the inferior and middle turbinates. The superior turbinate is difficult to inspect because of its position. See Figure 35–52. These bones increase the surface of the mucous membrane in the nares. The mucous membranes warm and moisten the inspired air. The clefts between the turbinates are called meati. Each meatus is named for the adjacent turbinate, e.g., the inferior meatus is near the inferior turbinate.
4. Inspect the mucous membranes for purulent drainage and nasal polyps. These are an abnormal finding.

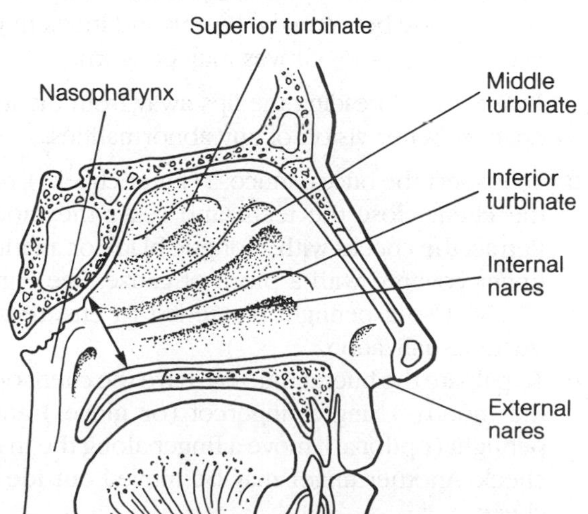

Figure 35–52 Major structures of the nose

Sinuses

Palpate the maxillary and frontal sinuses. See Figure 35–53. Palpation can reveal tenderness. Normally, the sinuses are not tender. Transilluminate the frontal sinuses by placing a penlight against the inner aspect of the supraorbital ridge of the frontal bone (see Figure 35–53). This is best done in a darkened room. Normally, the light shines through the bone and outlines the sinus. Transillumination can reveal the presence of air or fluid in the sinuses. Normally, the sinuses contain air; they appear darker when fluid is present. Transilluminate the maxillary sinuses by placing a penlight in the client's mouth and shining it to the left and to the right. The sinuses should light up equally.

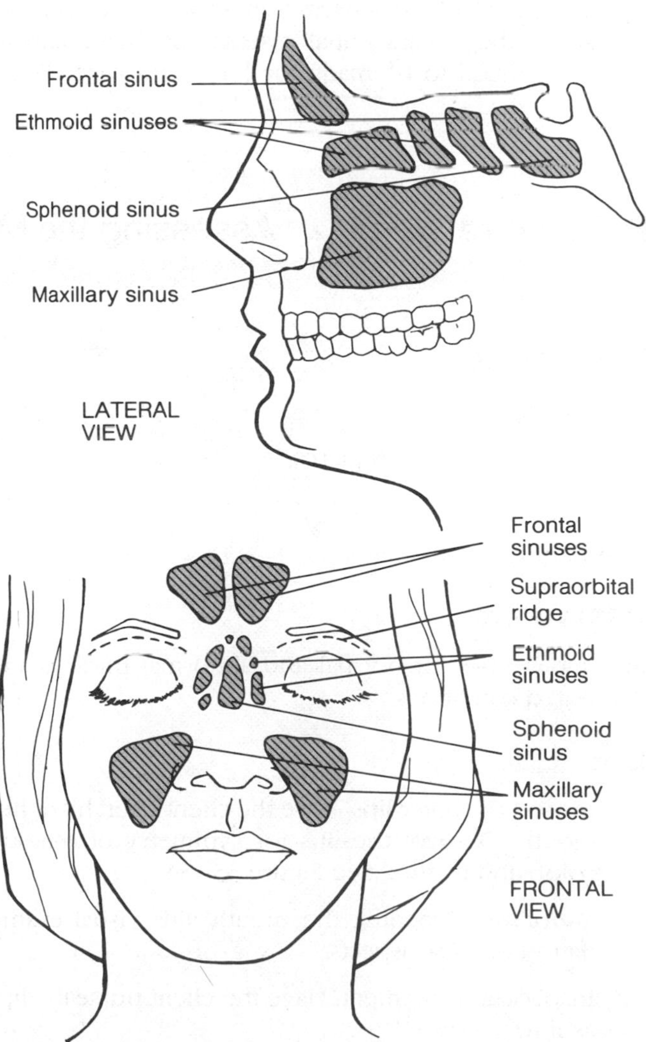

Figure 35–53 The facial sinuses

Nursing History Data: Nose and Sinuses

Determine:

- Whether the client has history of allergies, difficulty breathing through the nose, sinus infections, injuries to nose or face, or nosebleeds
- Whether the client takes any medications
- Whether the client has experienced any changes in sense of smell

Nursing History Data: Mouth

Determine:

- Routine pattern of dental care
- The date of the last visit to the dentist
- Length of time ulcers or other lesions have been present
- The presence of dentures and any associated discomfort
- Any medications the client is receiving

Mouth

Assessment of an individual's mouth includes examination of its physical characteristics, consideration of developmental changes, and determination of the person's hygienic practices. Oral assessment should be carried out as part of the client's initial assessment. Periodic reassessments need to be made for long-term care clients.

Physical examination of the mouth includes inspection and palpation techniques. The status of the lips, mucous membranes, teeth, gingiva (gums), tongue, palates, and uvula is assessed. See above for data to be obtained during nursing history.

Procedure 35–5 ▲ Assessing the Mouth

Equipment

1. A tongue blade
2. Some 2 × 2 gauze squares
3. A fingercot or disposable glove
4. A penlight or flashlight

Intervention

See Table 35–8 for normal and abnormal findings and associated conditions.

Lips

1. Inspect the outer lips. Have the client open his or her mouth. Observe the lips for symmetry of contour, color, and texture. See Figure 35–54.

   Rationale Opening the mouth aids visual examination of these aspects.

2. Inspect lip movement. Have the client purse the lips as if to whistle.

   Rationale Inability to purse the lips can indicate damage to the facial (seventh cranial) nerve.

Inner Lips and Buccal Mucosa

3. Inspect and palpate the inner lips and buccal mucosa for color, moisture, and texture.
   a. To inspect the inner lip mucosa of the bottom and top lips, have the client relax the mouth and pull the lip outward away from the teeth. Grasp the lip on each side between the thumb and index finger. See Figure 35–55. Gloves may be worn.

      Rationale Spreading the lips away from the teeth enables better vision of any abnormalities.

   b. To inspect the buccal mucosa (inner cheeks), have the client close the teeth and relax the mouth. Retract the cheeks with a tongue blade or an index finger covered with a piece of gauze. See Figure 35–56. Use a penlight if needed to ensure adequate visualization.
   c. To palpate the buccal mucosa, have the client open the mouth. Using a fingercot (or gloves) and a penlight (optional), move a finger along the inside cheek. Another finger may be moved outside the cheek.

      Rationale Palpation can determine the presence of nodules, ulcerations, or cysts.

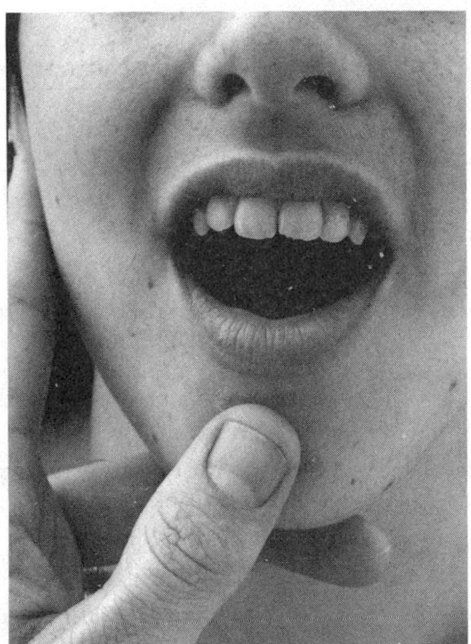

Figure 35–54

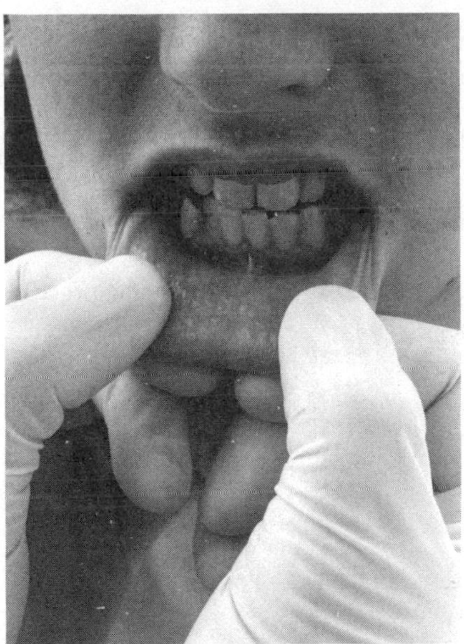

Figure 35–55

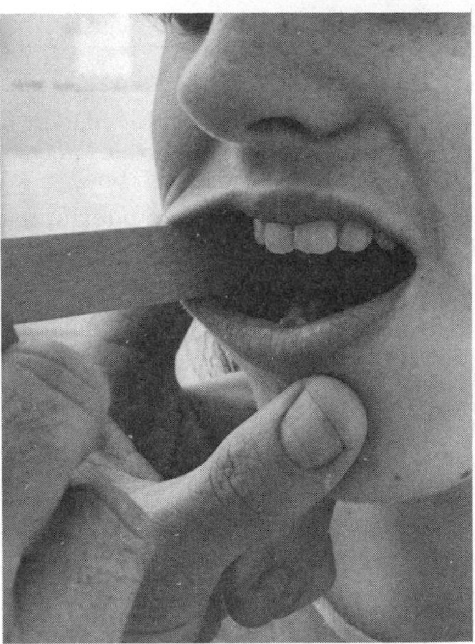

Figure 35–56

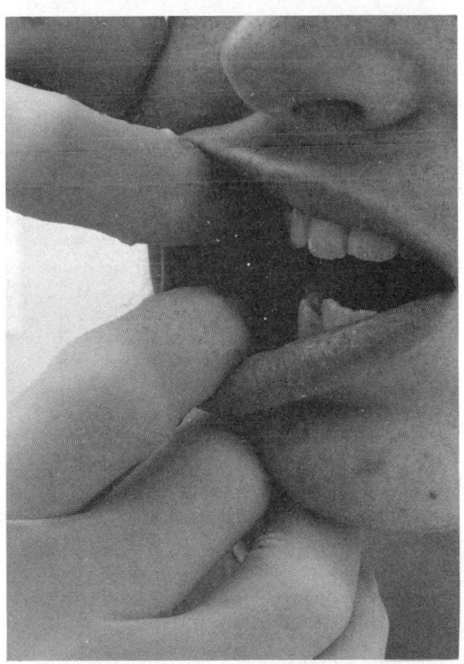

Figure 35–57

Teeth and Gums

4. Inspect the teeth and gums while examining the inner lips and buccal mucosa.
   a. Examine the back teeth while examining the buccal mucosa. Use the index fingers of both hands to retract the cheek if necessary. See Figure 35–57. Have the client relax the lips and first close the teeth, then open them. Observe the number of teeth, teeth color, the state of fillings, the presence of partial or complete dentures, and the fit of dentures, if any. By age 25, most people have 32 permanent teeth. See Figures 36–10 and 36–11 on page 808.

      Rationale Adequate retraction of the cheeks is necessary for proper visualization of the molars. Closed teeth assist in observation of the tooth alignment and loss of teeth; opened teeth assist in observation of dental fillings and caries.
   b. Assess the gums around the molars while examining the buccal mucosa. Observe the color and moisture of the gums. Assess the texture of the gums by gently pressing the gum tissue with a tongue blade.
   c. Inspect the front teeth and gums while examining

Table 35–8 Assessment Data: Mouth

Structure	Normal findings	Abnormal findings	Possible health problems
Lips	Uniform pink color (darker in Mediterranean groups and blacks, e.g., bluish hue)	Pallor	Anemia
	Soft, moist, smooth texture	Bluish discoloration	Cyanosis
	Symmetry of contour	Blisters	Herpes simplex
	Ability to purse lips	Generalized swelling	Allergic reaction
		Localized swelling	Trauma
		Fissures, crusts, scales	Excessive moisture; nutritional deficiency; fluid deficit
		Inability to purse lips	Facial nerve damage
Inner lips and buccal mucosa	Uniform pink color (brown freckled pigmentation in blacks)	Pallor	Anemia
		White patches (leukoplakia)	Early oral cancer; heavy smoking and drinking
	Moist, smooth, soft and elastic texture (drier oral mucosa in elderly due to decreased salivation)	Excessive dryness	Dehydration
		Mucosal cysts	Glandular irritation
		Irritations	Infections; ill-fitting dentures
		Abrasions	Trauma
		Ulcerations, nodules	Possible carcinoma
Teeth	32 adult teeth	Missing teeth, bridges, full or partial dentures	Trauma; dental disease
		Dental caries	Poor oral hygiene
	Smooth, white tooth enamel	Discoloration of enamel	Excessive use of tobacco; certain medications (e.g., iron)
Gums	Pink color (bluish or dark patches in blacks)	Excessive redness	Ill-fitting dentures; periodontal disease
	Moist, firm texture	Spongy texture, bleeding, tenderness	Periodontal disease
	No retraction (pulling away from the teeth)	Receding atrophied gums	Normal aging process
		Swelling that partially covers the teeth	Dilantin therapy; leukemia
Tongue	Central position	Deviated from center	Damage to hypoglossal (12th cranial) nerve
	Pink color (some brown pigmentation on tongue borders in blacks), moist, slightly rough, thin whitish coating	Dry, furry	Fluid deficit
		Smooth and red	Iron, vitamin B_{12}, or Vitamin B_3 deficiency
	Moves freely	Nodes, ulcerations, discolorations, restricted mobility	Possible carcinoma
	Smooth tongue base with prominent veins	Varicosities (tiny bluish-black or purple swollen areas)	Normal aging process
Palates	Light pink, smooth, soft palate	Discolorations	Jaundice
	Lighter pink hard palate, more irregular texture	Palates the same color	Anemia
		Irritations	Ill-fitting dentures
Uvula	Positioned in midline of soft palate	Deviation to one side	Tumor; trauma
		Immobility	Damage to trigeminal (fifth cranial) nerve or vagus (tenth cranial) nerve
Oropharynx and tonsils	Pink and smooth posterior wall	Reddened, lesions, plaques	Pharyngitis
	Tonsils pink and normal size	Tonsillar crypts inflamed, filled with exudate, swollen	Tonsillitis

the inner lip mucosa. Have the client "grit" the teeth and retract the lips, or follow step 3a on page 836.

d. If the client has complete or partial dentures, ask him or her to remove them. Inspect the condition, e.g., broken parts, of the dentures.

Tongue

5. Inspect and palpate the tongue for color, texture, position, and mobility.
   a. To inspect the surface of the tongue, have the client protrude the tongue. Observe it for position, color, and texture.
   b. To inspect tongue movement, have the client roll the tongue upward and move it from side to side.
   c. To inspect the base of the tongue, the mouth floor, and the frenulum, have the client place the tip of the tongue against the roof of the mouth.
   d. To palpate the tongue, grasp its tip, using a piece of gauze, and with the index finger of the other hand, palpate the back of it, its borders, and its base. See Figure 35–58.

   Rationale Grasping the tongue stabilizes it for proper palpation.

Palate and Uvula

6. Inspect the hard and soft palate for color and texture. Have the client tilt back the head and open the mouth widely. Depress the tongue with a tongue blade. Use a penlight for better vision.
7. While examining the palates, inspect the uvula for position and mobility.

Oropharynx and Tonsils

8. Inspect the oropharynx one side at a time to avoid eliciting the gag reflex. The oropharynx is that area of the pharynx behind the mouth and tongue.
   a. With a tongue depressor, press the tongue to one side while the client is sticking the tongue out. Use a penlight to view the oropharynx, if needed.
   b. Repeat for the other side of the oropharynx.
9. Inspect the tonsils behind the fauces for color and size. The tonsils are oval-shaped lymphoid tissues situated on each side of the fauces. The fauces is the passage from the mouth to the oropharynx. See Figure 35–59. The tonsils may be normally enlarged in the young child.
10. Elicit the gag reflex by pressing the posterior tongue with the tongue depressor.

    Rationale Lack of the gag reflex can indicate problems with the glossopharyngeal or vagus nerves.
11. Record your findings on the appropriate records.

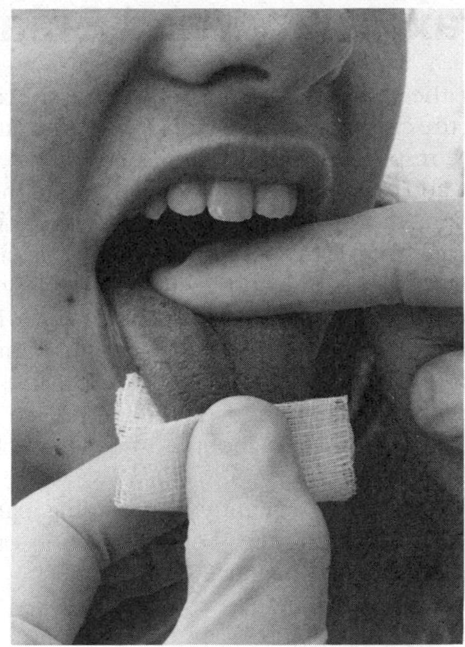

Figure 35–58

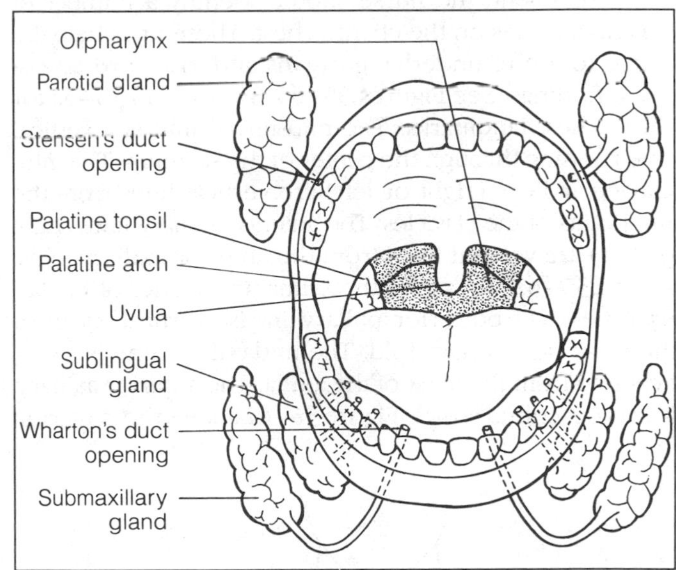

Figure 35–59 Anatomic structures of the mouth

Sample Recording

Date	Time	Notes
Apr/7/87	1500	C/o discomfort from ill-fitting upper dentures and difficulty chewing. Refuses to wear dentures. Oral cavity assessed. Left superior buccal mucosa reddened. Hard palate swollen and reddened, is tender to touch. Dr. Woo notified. ———— ———— Susan M. Maraket, SN

Thorax, Lungs, and Breasts

Assessing the thorax and lungs is frequently critical to assessing the client's aeration status. Two of the chief functions of the respiratory system are to maintain the exchange of oxygen and carbon dioxide in the lungs and the tissues and to maintain acid-base balance in the body. Changes in the respiratory system can come about slowly or quickly. In clients with chronic obstructive pulmonary disease (COPD), changes are frequently gradual; however, in clients who are acutely ill, e.g., those who have a pneumothorax (accumulation of gas or fluid in the pleural cavity), changes occur quickly, and death can result if immediate action is not taken. For information about the mechanics of breathing see Chapter 34, page 785.

The breasts are frequently examined as part of the female reproductive system. For information on breast self-examination, see Chapter 25 page 540.

Thorax

To assess a client's thorax, the nurse uses the examination techniques of inspection and palpation. Before beginning the assessment, the nurse should identify a number of imaginary lines on the client's chest. These lines help the nurse to locate underlying organs and to record assessment findings. See Figures 35–60, 35–61, and 35–62 for these chest landmarks. The midsternal line is a vertical line running through the center of the sternum. The midclavicular lines (right or left) are vertical lines from the midpoints of the clavicles. The anterior axillary lines (right or left) are vertical lines from the anterior axillary folds. Figure 35–61 shows the three imaginary lines of the lateral chest. The posterior axillary line is a vertical line from the posterior axillary fold. The midaxillary line is a vertical line from the apex of the axilla. The anterior axillary line is described above. Figure 35–62 shows the posterior chest landmarks. The vertebral line is a vertical line along the spinous processes. The scapular lines (right or left) are vertical lines from the inferior angles of the scapulae.

Posture

The client's posture is important to note. Some people with chronic respiratory problems tend to bend forward or even prop their arms on a support to elevate their clavicles. This posture is an attempt to expand the chest fully and thus breathe with less effort.

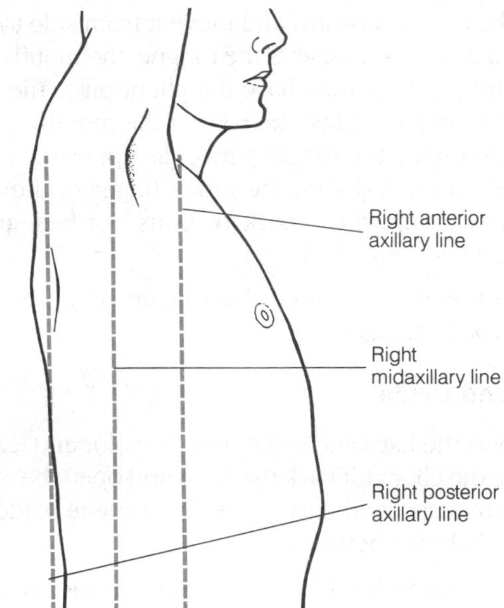

Figure 35–61 Lateral chest landmarks

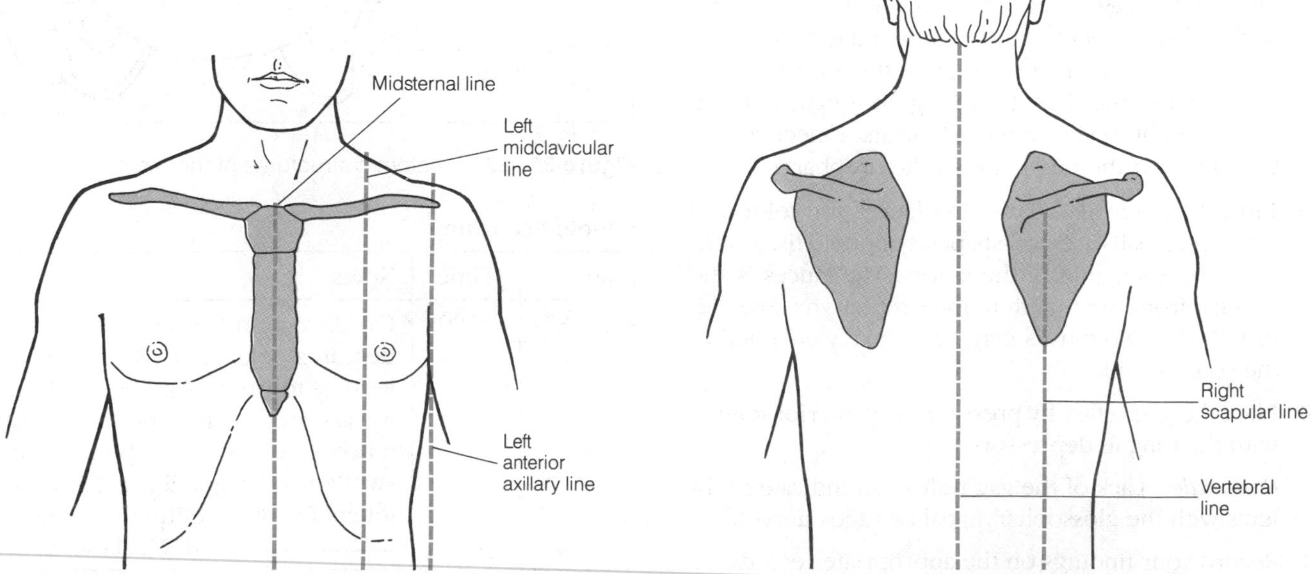

Figure 35–60 Anterior chest landmarks

Figure 35–62 Posterior chest landmarks

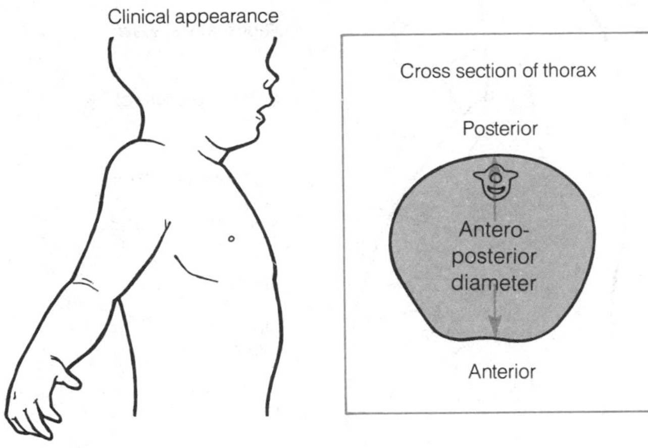

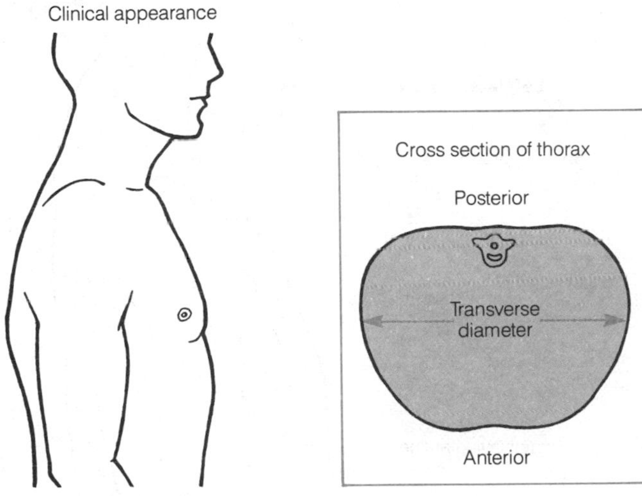

Figure 35–63 Configurations of the thorax showing anteroposterior diameter and transverse diameter: **A,** infant; **B,** adult

Shape

In the infant, the thorax is rounded; that is, the diameter from the front to the back (anteroposterior) is equal to the transverse diameter. It is also cylindrical, having a nearly equal diameter at the top and the base. When a child reaches 6 years, the anteroposterior diameter has decreased in proportion to the transverse one. In adults, the thorax is oval. Its anteroposterior diameter is two times smaller than its transverse diameter. See Figure 35–63. The overall shape of the thorax is elliptical; i.e., its diameter is smaller at the top than at the base. In the elderly, kyphosis and osteoporosis alter the size of the chest cavity as the ribs move downward and forward.

The shape of the chest is assessed from the front, sides, and back. There are several deformities of the chest.

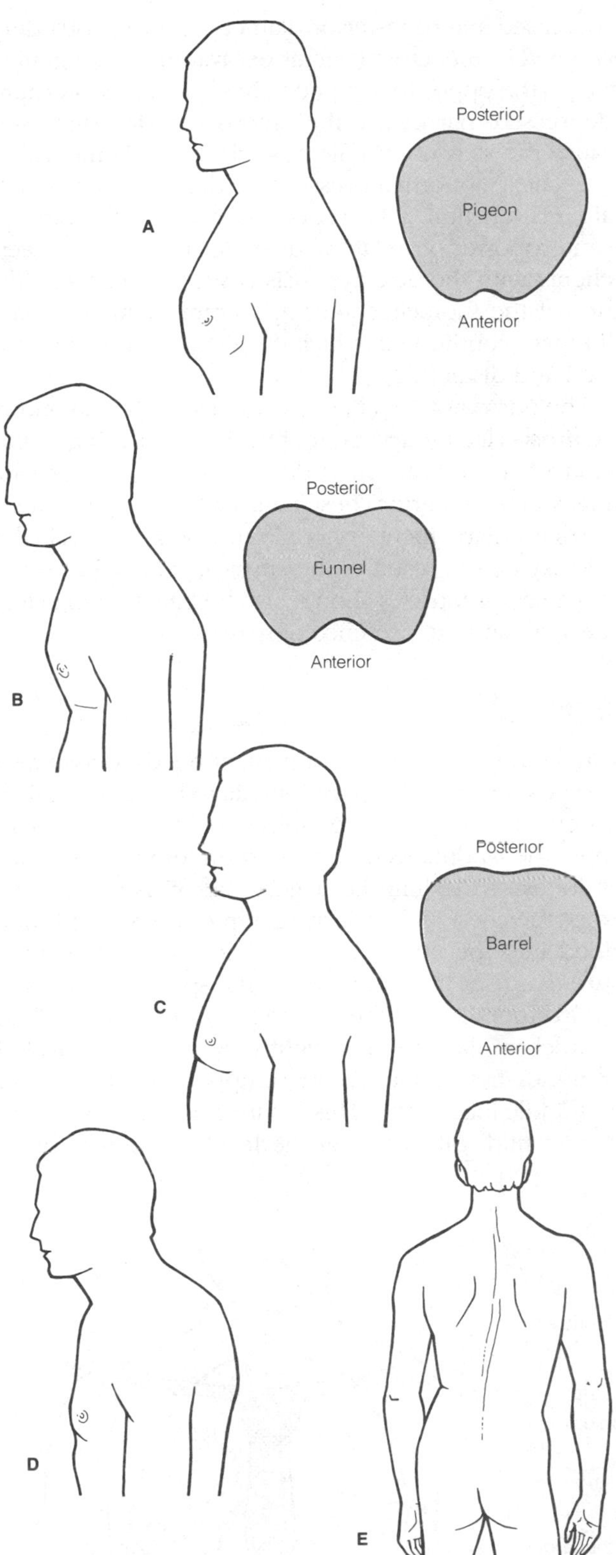

Figure 35–64 Chest shapes: **A,** pigeon chest; **B,** funnel chest; **C,** barrel chest; **D,** kyphosis; **E,** scoliosis

See Figure 35–64. **Pigeon chest** (pectus carinatum), a permanent deformity, may be caused by rickets. Pigeon chest is characterized by a narrow transverse diameter, an increased anteroposterior diameter, and a protruding sternum. A **funnel chest** (pectus excavatum), a congenital defect, is the opposite of pigeon chest in that the sternum is depressed, narrowing the anteroposterior diameter. Because the sternum points posteriorly in clients with a funnel chest, abnormal pressure on the heart may result in altered function. A **barrel chest**, in which the ratio of the anteroposterior to lateral diameter is 1 to 1, are seen in clients with thoracic **kyphosis** (excessive convex curvature of the thoracic spine) and **emphysema** (chronic pulmonary condition in which the air sacs, or alveoli, are dilated and distended).

The nurse notes spinal deformities, such as kyphosis or **scoliosis** (lateral deviation of the spine), during examination of the thorax. In addition, the nurse looks for changes in the exterior chest wall, such as bulges caused by cardiac enlargement or neoplasms. Depressions in the chest may be the result of the surgical removal of some ribs. The chest muscles should also be palpated to detect tenderness and the presence of masses.

Lungs

During a lung examination, the client needs to assume a sitting position. See this page for data to be obtained during a nursing history of the lungs. First the nurse should identify the landmarks on the chest under which the various lobes of the lung lie. Figure 35–65 is an anterior view of the chest and underlying lungs. Each lung is first divided into the upper and lower lobes by an oblique fissure that runs from the level of the spinous process of the third thoracic vertebra to the level of the sixth rib at the midclavicular line. The right lung is further divided by a minor fissure into the right upper lobe (RUL) and right middle lobe (RML). This fissure runs anteriorly from the right midaxillary line at the level of the fifth rib to

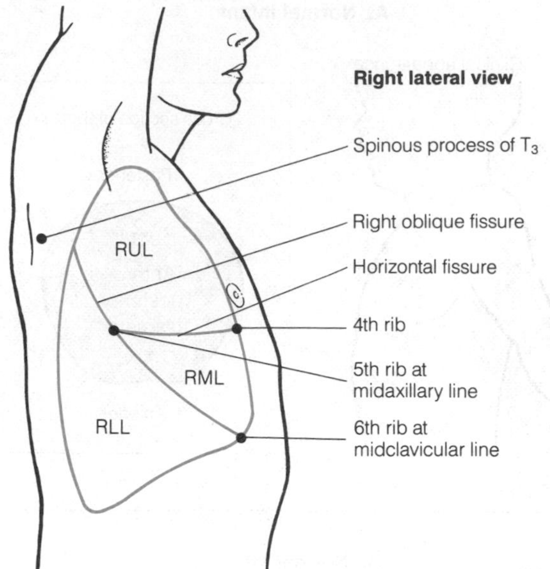

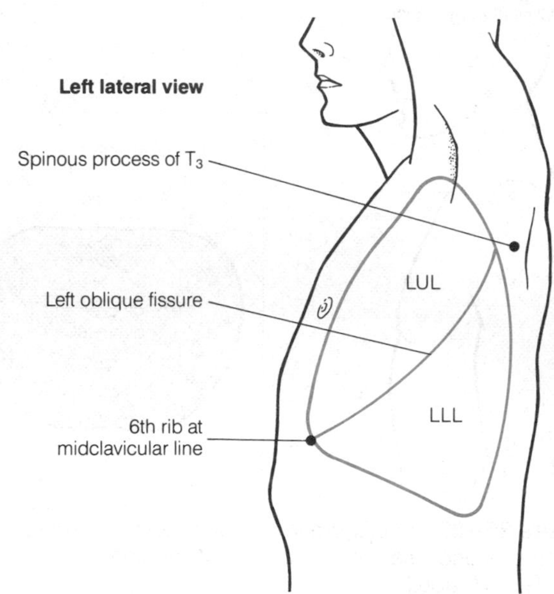

Figure 35–66 Lateral chest landmarks and underlying lungs

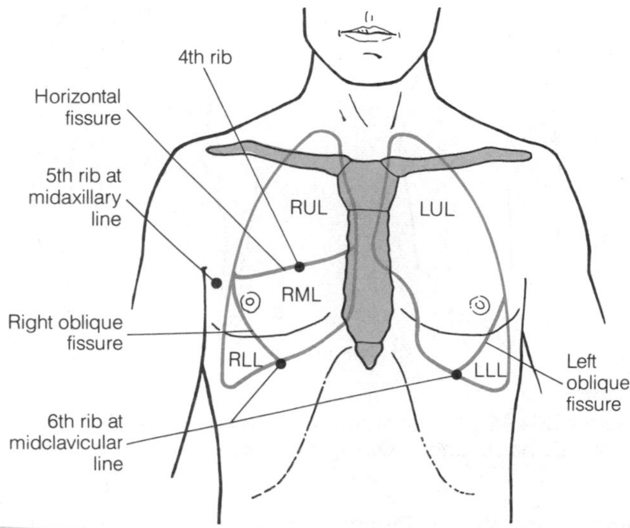

Figure 35–65 Anterior chest landmarks and underlying lungs

Nursing History Data: Lungs

Determine:

- Family history of illness, including cancer, allergies, tuberculosis
- Life-style, including smoking and occupational hazards, e.g., inhaling fumes
- Any medications the client is currently taking
- Current problems, e.g., swelling, cough, wheezing, pain

Abbreviations Commonly Used in Lung Assessment

- T_3: Third Thoracic vertebra
- RUL: Right upper lobe
- RML: Right middle lobe
- RLL: Right lower lobe
- LUL: Left upper lobe
- LLL: Left lower lobe

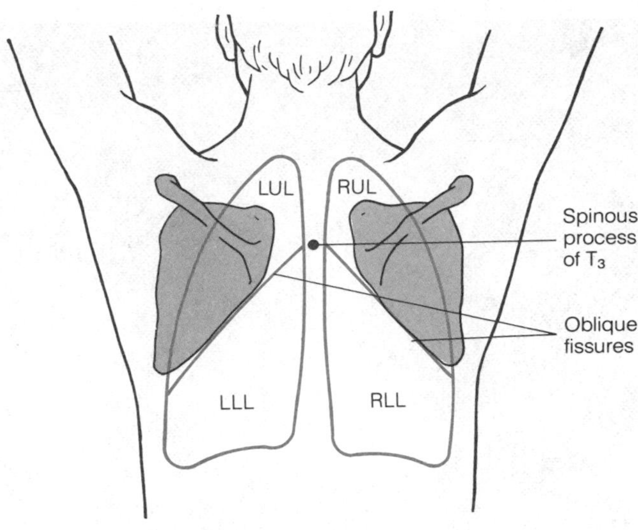

Figure 35–67 Posterior chest landmarks and underlying lungs

the level of the fourth rib. The lateral views show the three lobes of the right lung and the two lobes of the left lung. See Figure 35–66. The posterior view shows the upper and lower lobes of each lung. See Figure 35–67. Commonly used abbreviations are shown above.

Procedure 35–6 ▲ Assessing the Lungs

Equipment

1. A stethoscope
2. A plumb line (a line or string with a weight at one end)
3. A marking pencil

Intervention

See Table 35–9 for normal and abnormal findings.

1. Assess the rate, depth, and type of respirations. See chapter 34, page 786.

Palpation

2. Palpate the posterior chest for respiratory excursion (expansion). Place the palms of both hands over the lower thorax with the thumbs adjacent to the spine and the fingers stretched laterally. See Figure 35–68. Ask the client to take a deep breath while you observe the movement of your hands and any lag in movement.

   Rationale When the client takes a deep breath, the nurse's thumbs should move apart an equal distance and at the same time, reflecting chest expansion.

3. Palpate the anterior chest as in step 2, placing the palms of both hands on the lower thorax with the fingers laterally along the lower rib cage and the thumbs along the costal margins. See Figure 35–69.

4. Palpate the lungs for vocal (tactile) **fremitus**, the vibration felt through the chest wall when the client speaks.
   a. Place the palms of your hands on the posterior chest near the apex of the lungs, position *A* in Figure 35–70.

Table 35–9 Assessment Data: Lungs

Normal findings	Abnormal findings
Respiratory rate 16–20/min and regular (adult)	Increased or decreased rate Irregular pattern Retraction or bulging of intercostal muscles
Respiratory excursion is full and symmetrical	Impairment in movement
Vocal fremitus is symmetrical bilaterally	Decreased or increased fremitus
Percussion notes resonant except over liver, heart, sternum, scapula, and stomach	Asymmetry in percussion Areas of dullness Areas of hyperresonance
Auscultated vesicular breath sounds (see Table 35–11)	Auscultated adventitious breath sounds (see Table 35–12) Rales Rhonchi Wheeze Friction rub

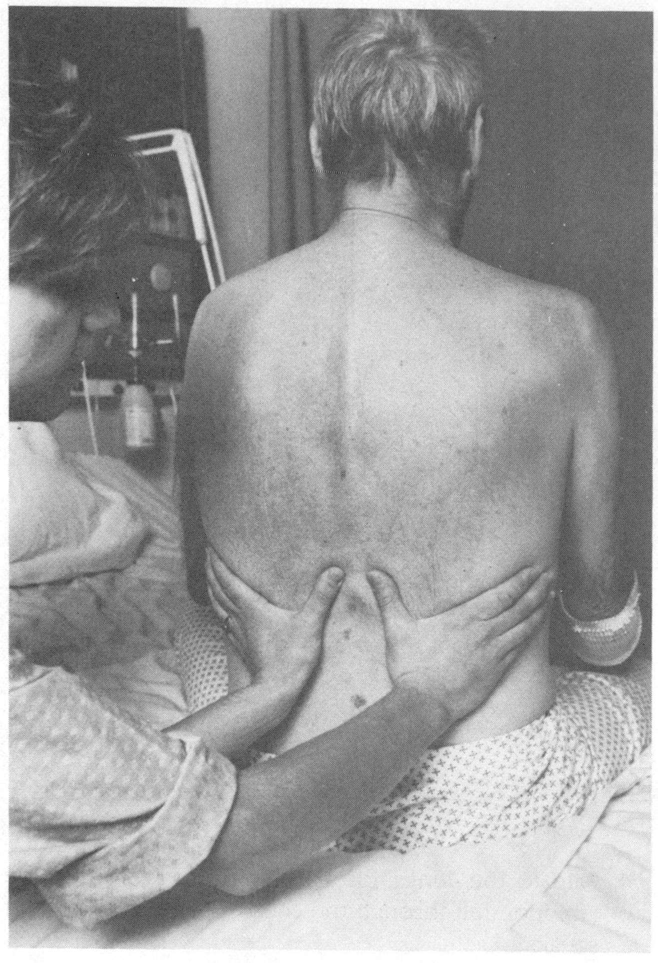

Figure 35–68

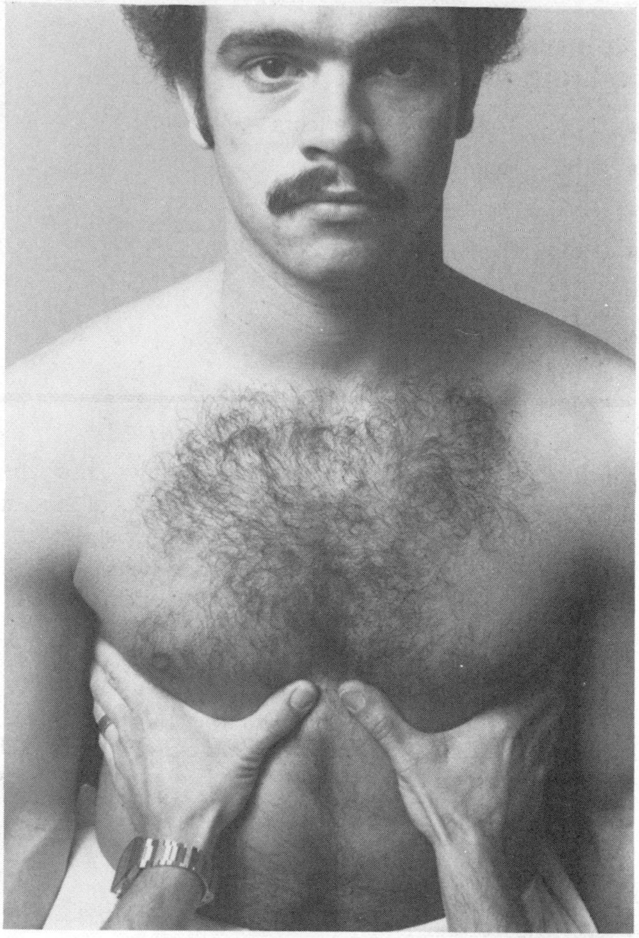

COURTESY SWEARINGEN PHOTO-ATLAS

Figure 35–69

b. Ask the client to repeat words such as "blue moon" or "one, two, three."
c. Repeat steps a and b with the hands moving sequentially to the base of the lungs, through positions *B–E* in Figure 35–70.
d. Compare the fremitus on both lungs and between the apex and the base of each lung. Increased fremitus occurs with consolidated lung tissue as in pneumonia, and decreased or absent fremitus occurs in pneumothorax.

5. Repeat steps 4a–d for the anterior chest. See Figure 35–71, positions *A–E*.

   Rationale The vibrations from speaking are normally transmitted through the chest wall. They are felt most clearly at the apex of the lungs. Low-pitched voices of males are more readily palpated than the higher pitches of females.

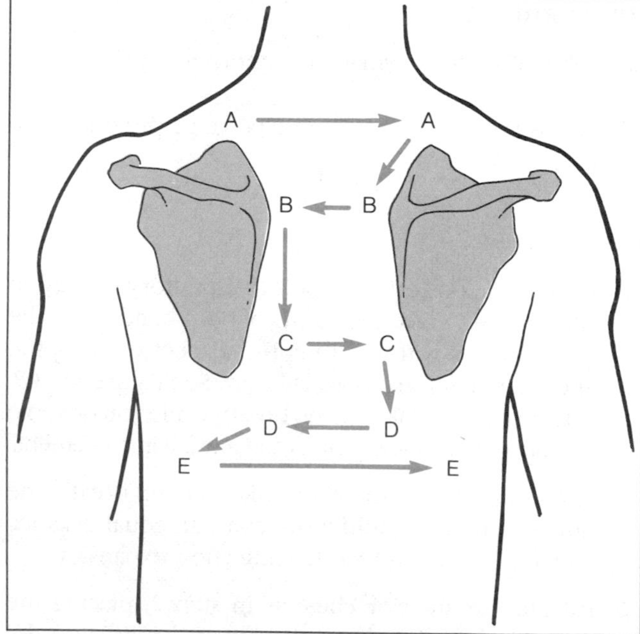

Figure 35–70

Percussion

6. Percuss the anterior surface of the chest. See the description of percussion in Chapter 11, page 245.

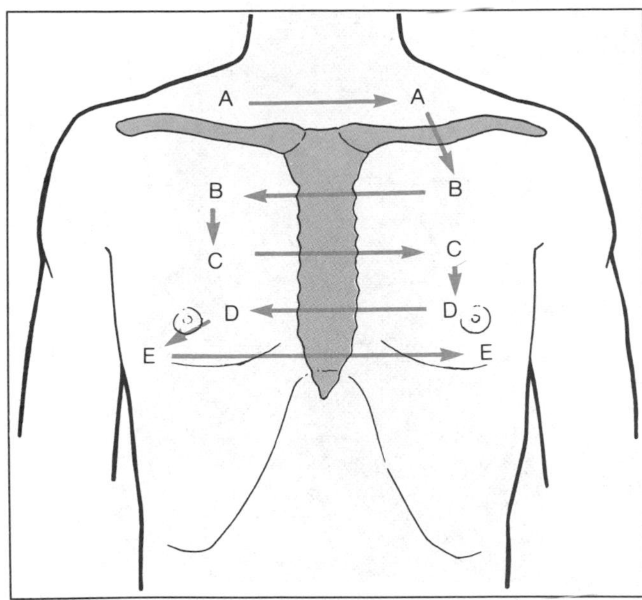

Figure 35–71

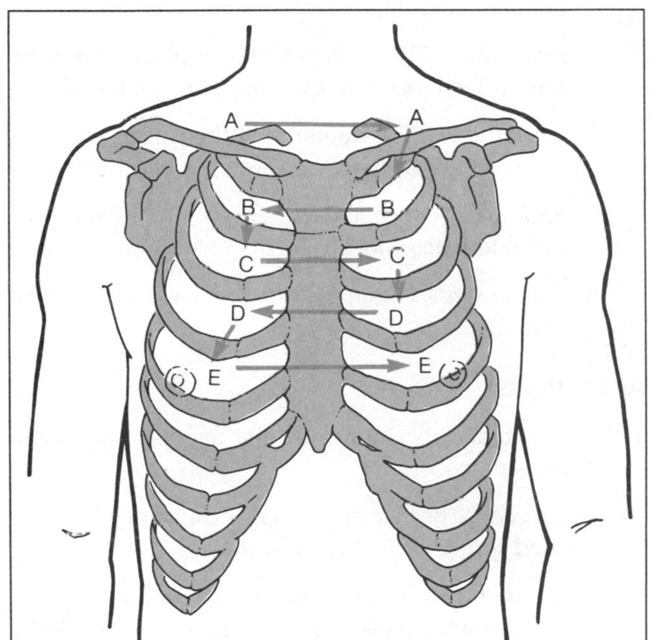

Figure 35–72

a. Percuss in the intercostal spaces in a systematic sequence, beginning above the clavicles in the supraclavicular space, and proceeding downward to the diaphragm. See Figure 35–72.

Rationale Percussion on a rib normally elicits dullness. The lowest point where resonance can normally be detected is at the diaphragm, i.e., at the level of the eighth to tenth rib.

b. Compare one side of the chest with the other. For each percussion, note the intensity, pitch, and duration. See Table 35–10.

7. Percuss the lateral chest wall, starting at the axilla and working down to the tenth rib. Percuss every few inches. Repeat for the other side.

8. Percuss the posterior chest wall while the client leans forward, neck flexed. Start at the apex of each lung and proceed downward to the diaphragm. See Figure 35–73. Compare one side of the chest to the other.

Rationale Percussion sounds are loudest where the chest wall is thinnest. For normal percussion sounds, see Figure 35–74.

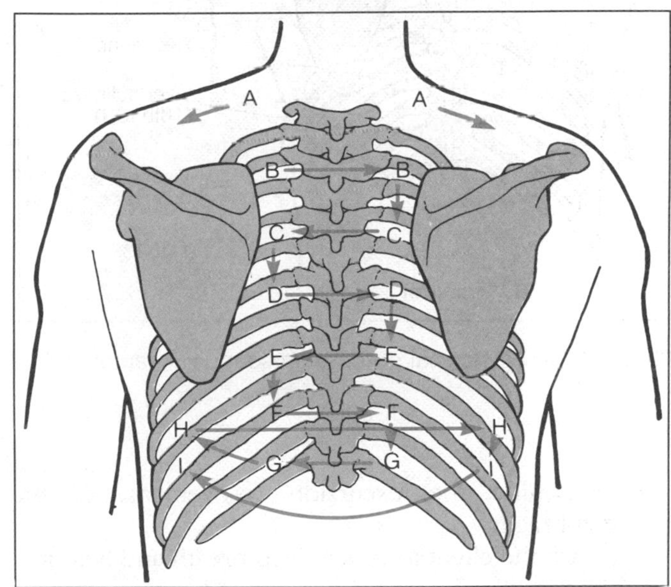

Figure 35–73

Table 35–10 Percussion Sounds

Sound	Intensity	Pitch	Duration	Quality	Example of location
Flatness	Soft	High	Short	Extremely dull	Muscle, bone
Dullness	Medium	Medium	Moderate	Thudlike	Liver, heart
Resonance	Loud	Low	Long	Hollow	Lung
Hyperresonance	Very loud	Very low	Very long	Booming	Emphysematous lung
Tympany	Loud	High (distinguished mainly by musical timbre)	Moderate	Musical	Stomach filled with gas (air)

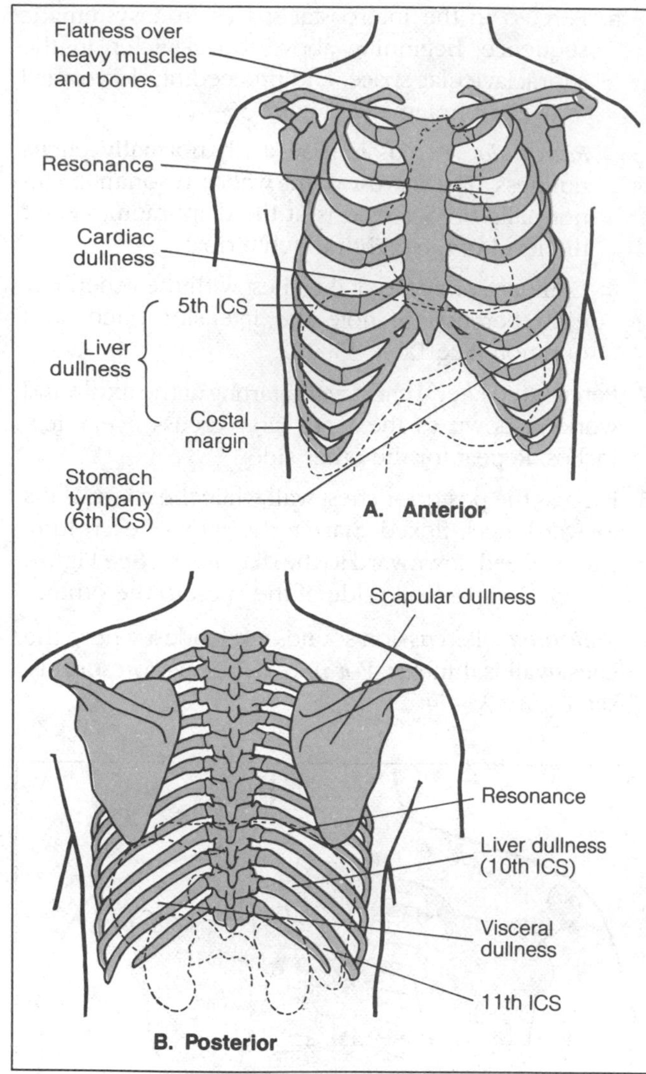

Figure 35–74 Normal percussion sounds: A, anterior; B, posterior

9. Determine the excursion (movement) of the diaphragm.
   a. Ask the client to take a deep breath and hold it.

      Rationale On inspiration, the diaphragm normally moves downward.

   b. Percuss downward on one side of the posterior chest until dullness is produced.

      Rationale The dullness indicates the level of the diaphragm.

   c. With a marking pencil place a mark on the skin at the level of dullness.
   d. Ask the client to expel the breath completely and hold it.

      Rationale Upon expiration, the diaphragm normally moves upward.

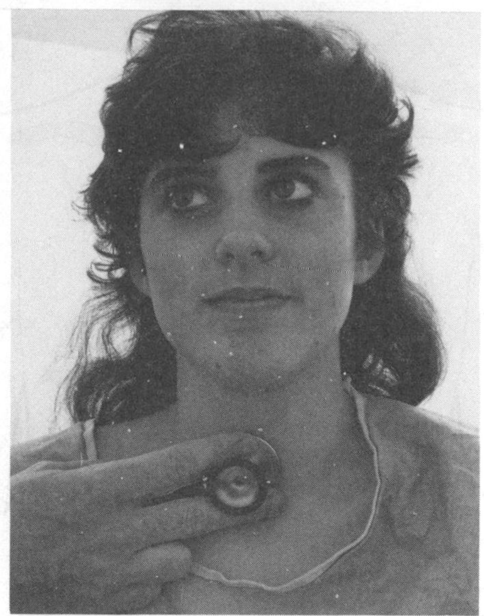

Figure 35–75

   e. Percuss as in step b for the level of dullness.

      Rationale The level normally is above the inspiratory level, because the lungs have deflated.

   f. Mark the level of dullness on the skin.
   g. Measure the distance between the two marks.

      Rationale Normal excursion is 3 to 5 cm (1 to 2 in) in females and 5 to 6 cm (2 to 2.3 in) in males.

   h. Repeat steps a–g on the other side of the posterior cest.

Auscultation

10. To auscultate the lungs, use the flat-disc diaphragm of the stethoscope.

    Rationale The flat diaphragm best transmits high-pitched sounds, e.g., breath sounds.

    a. Facing the client, place the diaphragm firmly against the skin starting over the trachea. See Figure 35–75.
    b. Ask the client to breathe normally.
    c. Proceed in the sequence shown in Figure 35–72, earlier, first auscultating over the bronchi between the sternum and the clavicles, then following the sequence for percussion in Figure 35–72.
    d. Listen for normal and adventitious breath sounds at each point on the chest. See Tables 35–11 and 35–12.

       Rationale Breath sounds occur as a result of the movement of the air through the trachea, bronchi, and alveoli.

    e. Repeat for the lateral chest and the posterior chest. Follow the percussion sequence described in steps 7–8 and shown in Figure 35–73.

Table 35–11 Normal Breath Sounds

Type	Description	Location	Characteristics
Vesicular	Soft, low-pitched, "gentle sighing"	Over bronchioles and alveoli; best heard at base of lungs	Best heard on inspiration
Bronchial (tracheal)	Moderately high-pitched, "harsh"	Over trachea; not normally heard over lung tissue	Louder than vesicular sounds; long inspiratory phase and short expiratory phase
Bronchovesicular	Moderate intensity	Over bronchioles lateral to the sternum at the first and second intercostal spaces and between the scapulae	Equal inspiratory and expiratory phases

Table 35–12 Adventitious Breath Sounds

Name	Description	Characteristics
Rales	Fine crackling sounds; alveolar rales are high-pitched; bronchial rales are lower-pitched	Best heard on inspiration
Rhonchi	Coarse, gurgling, harsh, louder sounds as air passes through bronchi filled with fluid	Best heard on expiration
Wheeze	Squeaky musical sounds often indicative of bronchial constriction	Best heard on expiration
Friction (pleural rub)	Rubbing of the pulmonary and visceral pleura; grating sound	Best heard over the lower anterior and lateral chest

11. When abnormal breath or percussion sounds—bronchophony, whispered pectoriloquy (exaggerated bronchophony), and egophony—are discovered, carry out further investigation.

    Rationale Fluid or consolidated tissue transmits vibrations of the spoken or whispered voice through the chest wall.

    a. Bronchophony and whispered pectoriloquy. Using a stethoscope, listen to the chest, using the sequence described for assessing vocal fremitus. See Figures 35–70 and 35–71, earlier. Have the client softly repeat "one, two, three."

       Rationale With tissue consolidation, the words may be clearly heard in the periphery of the lung.

    b. Egophony. Listen to the chest while the client repeats the sound of a long *e*, as in "she."

       Rationale Fluid in the lungs alters the sound from an *e* to an *ay*, as in "say," when heard through the stethoscope.

Breasts

The breasts of men, women, and children need to be examined. Men and children have some glandular tissue beneath each nipple, while mature women have glandular tissue throughout the breast. The breasts of newborns may be slightly enlarged due to maternal hormones. This usually disappears in a few days. During adolescence, asymmetrical development is not unusual, and boys may have some breast development in early adolescence.

During pregnancy, both breasts become enlarged. In the second month, the areolae normally become raised, pigmented, and edematous. It is not unusual for some colostrum to be expressed from the breasts during the third month. During a breast examination, the nipples are observed for discharge, crusting, edema, retraction, and disease. Although retraction is not necessarily indicative of any disease process, it needs to be noted.

The breasts are observed for size, shape, and position, and then the two breasts are compared according to these criteria. Size varies according to age, heredity, endocrine functions, and amount of adipose tissue. See page 850 for data to be obtained during a nursing history of the breasts.

Breasts must also be palpated for masses. Women today are encouraged to palpate their own breasts regularly. See the section on breast self-examination in Chapter 25, page 530.

The axillae are usually examined for enlarged lymph nodes, infections, and bulges. To palpate the axillae, the nurse helps the client relax the arm, perhaps by resting it on a table. The nurse presses the fingers as far up toward the apex of the axilla as possible and brings them downward, pressing against the chest wall. Nodes in the central area of the axilla and toward the thorax may be palpated in this manner. The central nodes are the most readily palpable. If the thoracic nodes are palpable and/or either group of nodes feels enlarged, this finding is reported. The procedure is then repeated on the other axilla.

Procedure 35–7 ▲ Assessing the Breasts

Intervention

See Table 35–13 for normal and abnormal findings and possible health problems.

1. Ask the client to assume a sitting position, and assess the breasts.
   a. Inspect the size, shape, and symmetry of the breasts. Breasts are normally round and fairly symmetric, and may be described as small, medium, or large.
   b. Inspect the skin for lesions, increased vascular patterns, edema, and "pig skin" or a pitted appearance.

      Rationale Pitting of the skin can be the result of lymphatic edema.
   c. Inspect the color of the areolae. They are normally darker in brunettes and pregnant women than in fair-haired women.
   d. Inspect the breasts and nipples for any dimpling or retraction, which can be the result of scar tissue formation or can be caused by the presence of a lesion. See Figure 35–76. In front of a mirror, show the client how to accentuate any retraction by raising her arms above her head, pushing her hands together with elbows flexed (see Figure 35–77), or pressing her hands down on her hips (see Figure 35–78).
   e. Inspect the nipples for any discharge, ulceration, inversion, crusting, or scaling. Note the position of

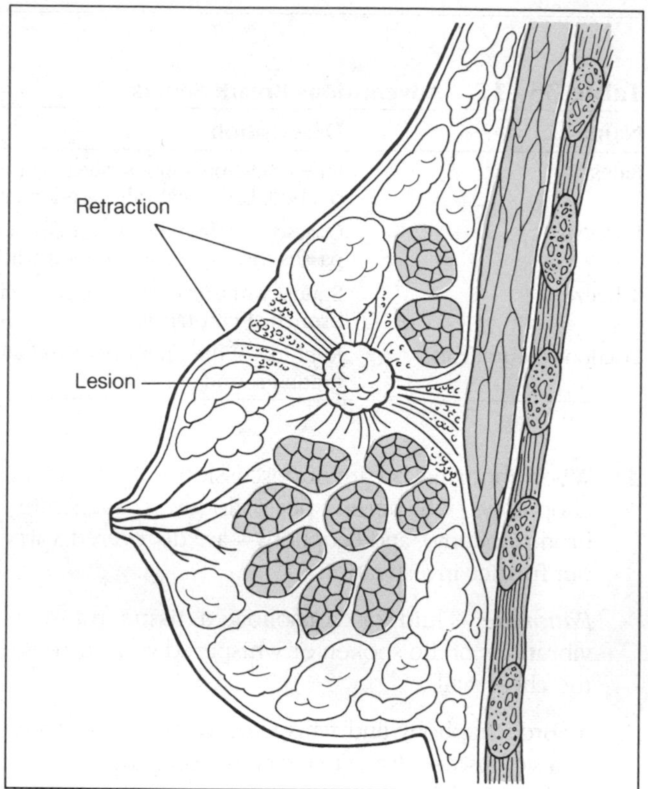

Figure 35–76 Breast tissue and a lesion that causes retraction of the skin

Table 35–13 Assessment Data: Breasts

Normal findings	Abnormal findings	Possible health problems
Rounded shape; small, medium, or large size	Change in breast size; swellings	Inflammation
Symmetrical	Marked asymmetry	
Skin smooth, intact	Dimpling, redness, vascularities, edema	
	Retraction	Scarring, carcinoma
Nipples everted, no discharge or lesions	Nipples inverted, crusting, ulcers, cracks, discharge	Inflammation; abscess; malignancy
No swelling in axillae	Swelling, tenderness in axillae	Malignancy
No tenderness, masses, or nodules on palpation	Tenderness, masses, or nodules (note location, client's position, size, mobility, consistency, surface, tenderness, and shape)	Tumor; abscess

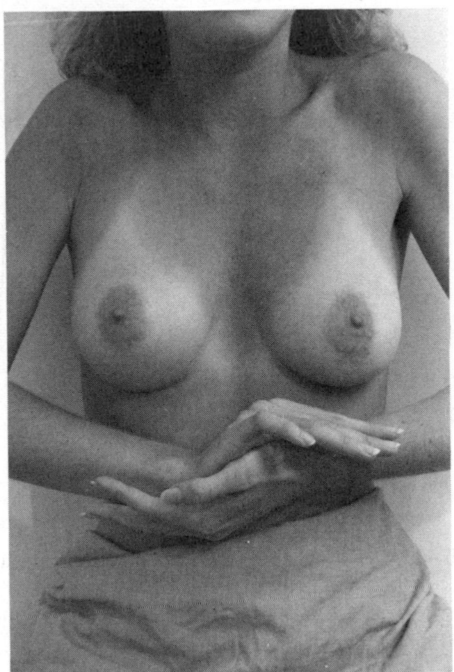

Figure 35–77

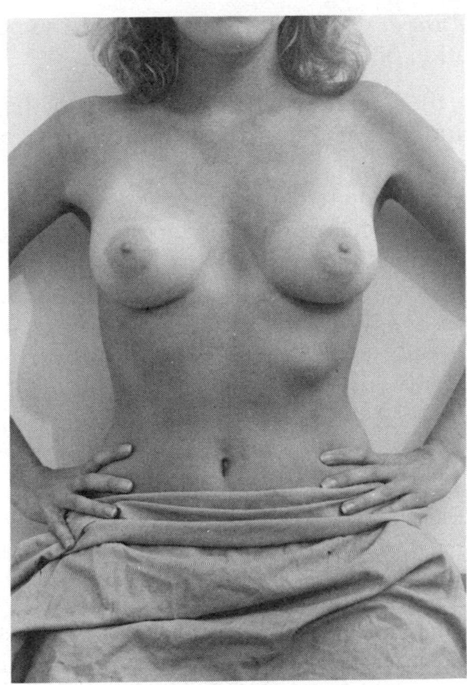

Figure 35–78

the nipples. Both nipples normally point in the same direction.

2. Inspect the axilla and clavicular areas for any swelling or redness.

3. Palpate around the nipple to check for discharge. If discharge is present, strip the breast by compressing the breast tissue between the thumb and index finger while moving the fingers toward the nipple. Strip one lobe at a time to identify the source of the discharge.
   a. Observe any discharge for amount, color, consistency, and odor.
   b. Note any tenderness upon palpation.

4. Palpate the clavicular and axillary regions while the client is sitting, arms at her sides.

   Rationale These areas contain lymph nodes that drain the breasts. See Figure 35–79.

5. Lightly palpate each breast. A bimanual technique is often preferred, particularly for large breasts. The nondominant hand is placed under the breast, and the dominant hand palpates the breast.

   Rationale A bimanual technique can be most effective in detecting small deep masses.

   a. Press the palmar surfaces of the middle three fingers on the skin surface starting in the upper lateral quadrant.
   b. Use a gentle rotary motion pressing the breast tissue against the other hand (bimanual) or against the chest wall.

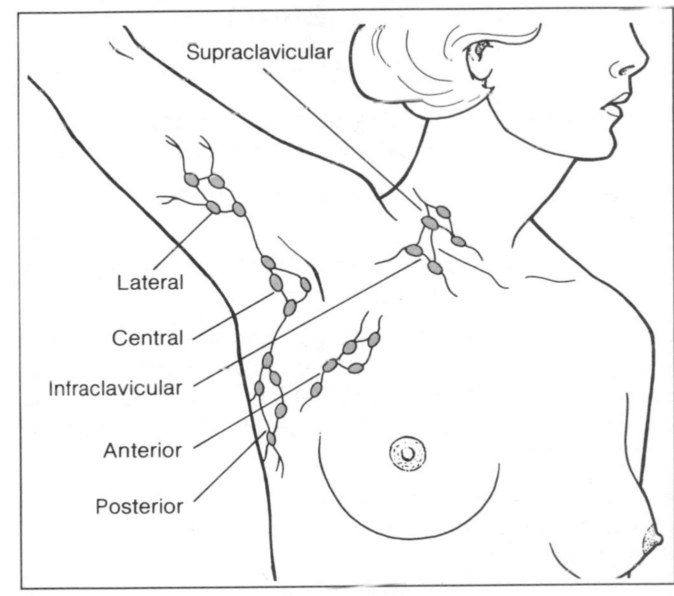

Figure 35–79

   c. Palpate from the periphery to the areola.
   d. Move your peripheral starting point around the breast clockwise. See Figure 35–80.

6. Record the following data about any masses:
   a. *Location:* the exact location relative to the clock (as in Figure 35–80) and the distance from the nipple in centimeters.
   b. *Client's position:* whether the arms were raised or lowered, the client was sitting or supine.

Rationale The position can change the perceived location of the mass.

c. *Size:* the length, width, and thickness of the mass in centimeters. If you are unable to determine the discrete edges, record this fact.
d. *Mobility:* whether the mass is movable or fixed. If it is fixed, determine whether it is firmly or moderately fixed, if possible.
e. *Consistency:* whether the mass is hard or soft.
f. *Surface:* whether the surface is smooth or irregular.
g. *Tenderness:* whether palpation is painful to the client.
h. *Shape:* whether the mass is round, discoid, regular, or irregular.

7. Repeat steps 5–6 for the other breast.
8. Assist the client to a supine position, with a small pillow or towel under the shoulder of the side to be palpated. Repeat steps 5–6 for each breast.

Rationale Slightly raising the shoulder helps spread the breast tissue over the chest wall, facilitating palpation.

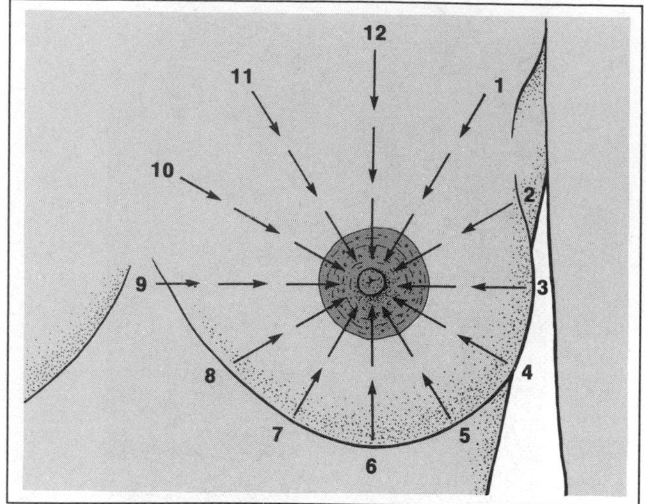

Figure 35–80 Pattern for palpating a breast and using the clock to describe the location of any masses

Nursing History Data: Breast

Determine:

- In both males and females, past history of breast masses, nipple discharge, areolar rash, breast pain, and tenderness.
- Relation of pain or tenderness, if experienced, to the menstrual cycle.
- Family history of breast cancer, particularly of the client's mother, sister, aunt, or grandmother before menopause.
- Age at menarche, at menopause, and at time of first pregnancy; there is a higher incidence of breast cancer among women who had an early menarche (before age 13), who had a late menopause (after age 50), and who had the first child after age 35.
- Racial background. Incidence of breast cancer is higher among white women than among Japanese or Chinese women.
- Frequency of breast self-examination, technique used, and time performed in relation to the menstrual cycle (see breast self-examination in Chapter 25).
- Normal breast changes for young adolescent females (see Chapter 24).
- Breast enlargement in young adolescent males; 50% of young adolescent males have enlargement of one or both breasts due to the hormonal changes of puberty. It is usually resolved in 1 or 2 years but is abnormal in adult males.
- Breast changes in pregnant women. Normal changes include tingling or tenderness, enlargement, prominent veins, and erect nipples. In later pregnancy, the aerolae darken and a thick yellowish fluid can be extracted from the nipples.
- Normal decreasing breast size and firmness in menopausal women.
- Currently prescribed medications. Oral contraceptives, digitalis, diuretics, and steroids can alter hormone balance and cause nipple discharge. Estrogens may cause cystic breast changes.

Heart

Heart function can be assessed to a large degree by findings in the history, by symptoms such as shortness of breath, by the client's general appearance (e.g., cyanosis and edema of the legs suggest impaired function), and by pulse rate, rhythm, and quality. Direct examination of the heart, however, offers more specific information, including the heart sounds, the heart size, and findings such as lifts, heaves, or murmurs. Nurses assess heart

Nursing History Data: Heart

Determine:

- Family history (include age of onset) of heart disease, high cholesterol levels, high blood pressure, stroke, obesity, congenital heart disease, and rheumatic fever
- Client's past history of heart problems, e.g., rheumatic fever, heart murmur, heart attack, or heart failure
- Life-style habits (e.g., smoking, alcohol intake, eating habits, exercise patterns, and areas and degree of stress perceived) that place the client at risk of cardiac disease
- Present symptoms (e.g., fatigue, dyspnea, orthopnea, edema, cough, chest pain, palpitations, syncope, hypertension, or wheezing) indicative of heart disease
- Presence of diseases (e.g., obesity, diabetes, lung disease, endocrine disorders) that affect the heart

functions through observations (inspection), palpation, and auscultation, in that sequence. Auscultation is more meaningful when other data are obtained first. The heart is usually assessed during an initial physical examination; periodic reassessments may be necessary for long-term or at-risk clients or those who have cardiac problems.

Nursing history data taken in conjunction with physical assessment are shown above. Purposes of assessing the heart are:

1. To determine baseline data about the client's cardiac function
2. To detect cardiac problems
3. To identify potential risk factors for cardiac disease

To perform cardiac assessment, the nurse must first know the exact location of the heart. In the average adult, most of the heart lies behind and to the left of the sternum. A small portion (the right atrium) extends to the right of the sternum. The upper portion of the heart (both atria), referred to as its base, lies toward the back. The lower portion (the ventricles), referred to as its apex, points forward. The apex of the left ventricle actually touches the anterior chest wall at or medial to the left midclavicular line (MCL) and at or near the fifth left intercostal space (LICS), which is slightly below the left nipple. See Figure 34–13 on page 780. This point where the apex touches the anterior chest wall is known as the **point of maximal impulse** (PMI). In infants and small children, because their hearts are positioned more horizontally, the PMI is located at the third or fourth LICS just to the left of the MCL. By the age of 7, however, a child's PMI is found in the same location as the adult's.

Inspection and Palpation

The precordium, the area of the chest overlying the heart, is inspected and palpated simultaneously for the presence of abnormal pulsations or lifts or heaves. It is inspected in a systematic manner at the following anatomic sites: aortic area, pulmonic area, tricuspid (or right ventricular) area, apical (or mitral) area, and epigastric area. See Figure 35–81. All pulsations are described by their location in an intercostal space and their distance from the midsternal, midclavicular, or axillary line. Inspect and palpate the precordium as follows:

1. Assist the client to a supine position with head elevated 30° to 45°, and stand at the client's right side. This position facilitates palpation of the cardiac area and allows for optimal inspection.
2. Locate the angle of Louis, the angle between the manubrium and the body of the sternum. It is felt as a prominence on the sternum.
3. Move your fingertips down each side of the angle until you can feel the second intercostal spaces. The client's *right* second intercostal space is the aortic area, and the *left* second intercostal space is the pulmonic area.
4. Inspect and palpate the aortic and pulmonic areas, observing them at an angle and to the side, to note the presence or absence of pulsations. Observing these areas at an angle increases the likelihood of seeing pulsations. Normally, these areas do not have pulsations, although some individuals may have aortic pulsations.
5. From the pulmonic area, move your fingertips down three left intercostal spaces along the side of the sternum. The left fifth intercostal space close to the sternum is the tricuspid or right ventricular area. Inspect and palpate the tricuspid area for pulsations and heaves

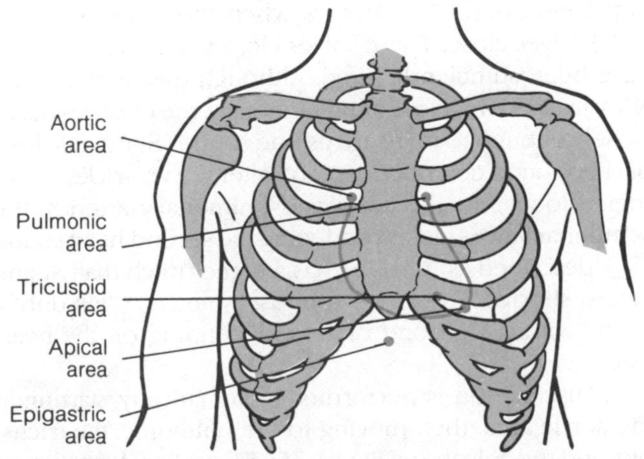

Figure 35–81 Anatomic sites of the precordium

or lifts. Normally pulsations, lifts, and heaves are absent. The terms *lift* and *heave,* often used interchangeably, refer to a rising along the sternal border with each heartbeat. A lift occurs when cardiac action is very forceful (overactive). It should be confirmed by palpation with the palm of the hand. Enlargement or overactivity of the left ventricle produces a heave lateral to the apex, while enlargement of the right ventricle produces a heave at or near the sternum.

6. From the tricuspid area, move your fingertips laterally 5 to 7 cm (2 to 3 in) to the left midclavicular line (LMCL). This is the apical or mitral area, or PMI.
7. Inspect and palpate the apical area for pulsation, noting its specific location (it may be displaced laterally or lower) and diameter. An apical impulse can be seen in about 50% of the adult population and is palpable in most people. The apical impulse is a good index of cardiac size. If the heart is enlarged, this impulse is lateral to the MCL and may be lower. Record the distance between the apex and the MCL in centimeters. If the apical beat cannot be observed, the apex may be located by palpation, but not always. If you have difficulty locating the PMI, have the client roll onto the left side, thus moving the apex closer to the chest wall. Normally, no lifts or heaves are visible or palpable in this area. Diffuse lifts or heaves lateral to the apex indicate enlargement or overactivity of the left ventricle.
8. Inspect and palpate the epigastric area at the base of the sternum for abdominal aortic pulsations. Pulsations are normally felt in this area; however, bounding pulsations are abnormal.

Auscultation

Several heart sounds can be heard by auscultation. Only the first and second heart sounds (S_1 and S_2) will be emphasized in this book. The normal first two heart sounds are produced by closure of the valves of the heart. The first heart sound (S_1) occurs when the atrioventricular (A-V) valves close. These valves close when the ventricles have been sufficiently filled. Although the right and left A-V valves do not close simultaneously, the closures occur closely enough to be heard as one sound (S_1), a dull, low-pitched sound described as "lub." After the ventricles empty their blood into the aorta and pulmonary arteries, the semilunar valves close, producing the second heart sound (S_2), described as "dub." S_2 has a higher pitch than S_1 and is also shorter. These two sounds, S_1 and S_2 ("lub-dub"), occur within 1 second or less, depending on the heart rate.

Auscultation is performed systematically, starting at the aortic area, then moving to the pulmonic, the tricuspid, and the apical. See Figure 35–81, earlier. Auscultation need not be limited to these areas, however. First locate these areas, and then move the stethoscope to find the most audible sounds for each particular client. The two heart sounds are audible anywhere on the precordial area, but they are best heard over these areas. Each area is associated with the closure of heart valves: the aortic area with the aortic valve (inside the aorta as it arises from the left ventricle); the pulmonic area with the pulmonic valve (inside the pulmonary artery as it arises from the right ventricle); the tricuspid area with the tricuspid valve (between the right atrium and ventricle); and the apical (mitral) area with the mitral valve (between the left atrium and ventricle).

Associated with these sounds are systole and diastole. Systole is the period in which the ventricles are contracted. It begins with the first heart sound and ends at the second heart sound. Systole is usually shorter than diastole. Diastole is the period in which the ventricles are relaxed. It starts with the second sound and ends at the subsequent first sound. Normally no sounds are audible during these periods. See Figure 35–82. The experienced nurse, however, may perceive extra heart sounds (S_3 and S_4) during diastole. Both sounds are low in pitch and heard best at the apical site, with the bell of the stethoscope, and with the client lying on the left side. S_3 occurs early in diastole right after S_2 and sounds like "lub-dub-*ee*" (S_1, S_2, S_3) or "Ken-tuc-*ky*." It often disappears when the client sits up. S_3 is normal in children and young adults. In older adults it may indicate heart failure. S_4 is rarely heard in normal clients. It occurs near the very end of diastole just beore S_1 and creates the sound of "*dee*-lub-dub" (S_4, S_1, S_2) or "*Ten*-nes-see." S_4 may be heard in many elderly clients and can be a sign of hypertension. Normal heart sounds are summarized in Table 35–14. See Procedure 35–8 for the steps of heart auscultation.

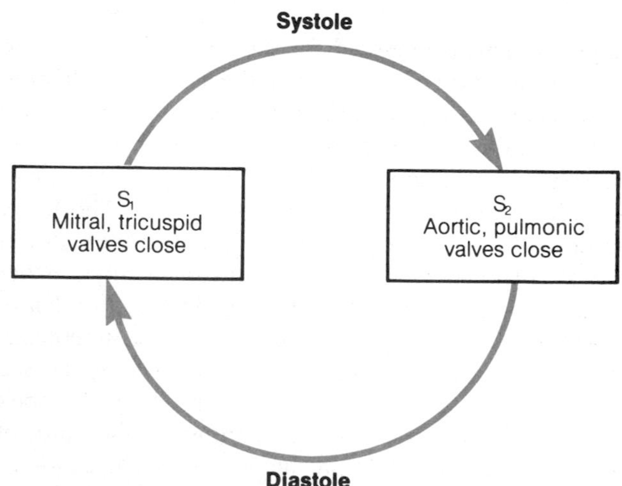

Figure 35–82 Relationship of heart sounds to systole and diastole

Table 35–14 Assessment Data: Normal Heart Sounds

Sound or phase	Description	Area: Aortic	Pulmonic	Tricuspid	Apical
S_1	Dull, low-pitched, and longer than S_2; sounds like "lub"	Less intensity than S_2	Less intensity than S_2	Louder than or equal to S_2	Louder than or equal to S_2
S_2	High-pitched, snappy, and shorter than S_1; creates sound of "dub"	Louder than S_1	Louder than S_1; abnormal if louder than the aortic S_2 in adults over 40	Less intensity than or equal to S_1	Less intensity than or equal to S_1
Systole	Normally silent interval between S_1 and S_2				
Diastole	Normally silent interval between S_2 and next S_1				

Procedure 35–8 ▲ Auscultating the Heart

Equipment

A stethoscope with a bell-shaped and flat-disc diaphragm. The bell transmits lower-pitched sounds best, while the flat disc transmits higher pitched sounds best.

Intervention

1. Eliminate all sources of room noise.

   Rationale Heart sounds are of low intensity, and other noise lowers the nurse's ability to hear them.

2. Assist the client to a supine position with head elevated 30° to 45°, and stand at the client's right side. Later reexamine the heart while the client is in the upright sitting position.

   Rationale Certain sounds are more audible in certain positions.

3. Auscultate the heart in the following manner using both the flat-disc diaphragm and the bell to listen to all areas. See Table 35–14 for descriptions of normal heart sounds. See Table 35–15 for normal and abnormal findings. In every area of auscultation, both S_1 and S_2 need to be distinguished. When auscultating, concentrate on one particular sound at a time in each area; the first heart sound, followed by systole, then the second heart sound, then diastole. Systole and diastole are normally silent intervals.
   a. Locate and auscultate the aortic area using the flat diaphragm and bell attachment of the stethoscope. Listen for both sounds and for systole and diastole. S_2 is loudest in this area, louder than S_1.

      Rationale The higher-pitched sounds of S_1 and S_2 are transmitted better through the flat diaphragm of the stethoscope. The lower-pitched sounds of S_3 and S_4 are best transmitted through the bell of the stethoscope.

   b. Locate and auscultate the pulmonic area as in step a. S_2 is normally louder than S_1 in this area.
   c. Compare the loudness of S_2 between the aortic and pulmonic areas.

      Rationale The loudness of S_2 in the pulmonic area relates to the blood pressure in the pulmonary artery, while the loudness of S_2 in the aortic area relates to the arterial blood pressure in the systemic circulation. Thus, when the pulmonary artery pressure increases, e.g., in clients with some chronic obstructive lung diseases, the loudness of pulmonic S_2 also increases. In contrast, the aortic S_2 is louder than normal in clients with hypertensive disease. When the pulmonic S_2 is louder than the aortic S_2 in adults over age 40, the finding is abnormal.

   d. Locate and auscultate the tricuspid area as in step a. S_2 is normally louder than or equal to S_1 in this area.

   e. Locate and auscultate the apical (mitral) area as in step a. S_2 is normally louder than or equal to S_1 in this area.

Table 35–15 Assessment Data: Heart Auscultation

Auscultation sound	Normal findings	Abnormal findings	Possible health problem
S_1	Usually heard at all sites	Increased or decreased intensity	
	Usually louder at apical area	Varying intensity with different beats	Complete heart block
S_2	Usually heard at all sites	Increased intensity at aortic area	Arterial hypertension
	Usually louder at base of heart	Increaed intensity at pulmonic area	Pulmonary hypertension
Systole	Silent interval	Sharp-sounding ejection clicks	Valvular deformities
	Slightly shorter duration than diastole at normal heart rate (60 to 90 beats/min)		
Diastole	Silent interval	S_3 in older adults	Heart failure
	Slightly longer duration than systole at normal heart rates		
	S_3 in children and young adults		
	S_4 in older adults		

f. Assess the heart rate and rhythm at the apical area as described in Chapter 34 on page 780. Note irregularities in rhythm, and note murmurs. **Murmurs** result when blood flow becomes turbulent within the heart due to valve defects or abnormal openings between the compartments of the heart. Not all murmurs indicate cardiac disease. Murmurs are described in terms of their location of maximum intensity, quality (e.g., loud, harsh, rumbling), and timing in relation to the phases of the cardiac cycle. Diastolic murmurs are usually considered abnormal. Murmurs relating to the valves are usually heard over the valvular areas. To increase your ability to hear an S_3 sound or a mitral murmur, have the client lie on the left side. Using the bell of your stethoscope, listen carefully in and around the apical area.

g. Record your assessment findings. Describe the intensity or loudness of the sounds as normal, absent, diminished, or accentuated, and the quality of sounds as sharp, full, booming, or snapping.

Peripheral Vascular System

Assessment of the peripheral vascular system includes measurement of the blood pressure; palpation of peripheral pulses; inspection, palpation, and auscultation of the carotid pulse; inspection of the jugular and peripheral veins; and inspection of the skin and tissues to determine perfusion to the extremities. Certain aspects of peripheral vascular assessment are often incorporated into other parts of the assessment procedure. For example, blood pressure is usually measured at the beginning of the physical examination; the nurse observes signs of impaired peripheral perfusion during inspection of the skin; and the nurse may palpate the carotid artery and observe the jugular veins when palpating lymph nodes in the neck.

Nursing history data taken in conjunction with assessment of the peripheral vascular system are shown on page 855.

Blood Pressure

Blood pressure measurement is discussed in detail in Procedure 34–6 on page 794. The client's blood pressure is an indication of the overall functioning of the heart and arterial system. Specifically, it indicates the adequacy of cardiac output and the condition of the arteries. Insufficient cardiac output decreases the blood pressure; inelastic, narrowed arteries elevate the blood pressure.

Peripheral Pulses

Pulse sites and pulse assessments are described in Chapter 34. To assess the client's peripheral pulses:

1. Palpate the peripheral pulses (except the carotid pulse) on both sides of the client's body simultaneously and

Nursing History Data: Peripheral Vascular System

Determine:

- Past history of heart disorders, phlebitis, varicosities, arterial disease, and hypertension
- Life-style, specifically exercise patterns, activity patterns and tolerance, smoking habits, and use of alcohol
- Presence of signs indicative of peripheral vascular disease in one or more extremities, such as pain or cramping, numbness, tingling, burning, edema, enlarged or bulging leg veins, and changes in temperature and color
- The relation of pain or cramping to activity and the effectiveness of rest in relieving them

systematically. This determines the symmetry of pulse volume. Inequality may indicate arterial disease.

a. Start at the head, and assess the temporal and facial pulses.
b. Move to the arms, and assess the brachial, radial, and ulnar pulses. See Figure 35–82A.
c. Move to the legs, and assess the femoral, popliteal, posterior tibial, and pedal pulses.
d. Note whether each pulse volume is (a) absent, (b) weak, thready, or decreased, (c) normal, or (d) increased and bounding. Normal findings are symmetric pulse volumes and easily palpable full pulsations. A scale for grading pulse volumes is shown below. Asymmetric volumes indicate impaired circulation; absent pulsations indicate arterial spasm or occlusion. Decreased, weak, thready pulsations indicate impaired cardiac output, and increased pulse volumes may indicate hypertension, high cardiac output, or circulatory overload.

Scale for Grading Pulse Volumes

0: No pulse.
1: Pulse is thready, weak, and difficult to palpate; it may fade in and out and is easily obliterated with pressure.
2: Pulse is difficult to palpate and may be obliterated with pressure; thus, light palpation is necessary. Once located, pulse is stronger than scale 1 pulse.
3: Pulse is easily palpable, does not fade in and out, and is not easily obliterated by pressure (normal pulse).
4.: Pulse is strong or bounding, easily palpated, and not obliterated with pressure; in some cases, e.g., in cases of aortic regurgitation, scale 4 pulse may indicate disease.
(Miller 1978, p. 1674)

2. If you have difficulty palpating some peripheral pulses, use a Doppler ultrasound probe, if available. See Procedure 34–4 on page 782.
   a. Lubricate the transducer with transmission gel.
   b. Position the earpieces (if present) in your ears.
   c. Place the probe over the pulse site. See Figure 35–83, which shows the probe over the client's brachial pulse site.
   d. Listen for wavelike "whooshing" sounds, which indicate blood flow.
   e. Record either the presence or absence of pulsations, their rate, and their intensity.

Carotid Arteries

The carotid arteries supply oxygenated blood to the head and neck. See Figure 35–84. Since they are the only source of blood to the brain, prolonged occlusion of one of these arteries can result in serious brain damage. The carotid pulses correlate with central aortic pressure, thus reflecting cardiac function better than the peripheral pulses. When cardiac output is diminished, the peripheral pulses may be difficult or impossible to feel, but the carotid pulse should be felt easily. The carotid arteries are inspected, palpated, and auscultated as follows:

1. With the client in a sitting position, inspect the carotid arteries for obvious pulsations; sometimes a wave can be seen.
2. **Extreme caution is required when palpating the carotid artery. Generally, carotid artery palpation is done only by highly experienced practitioners on clients who have specific cardiac conditions.** To palpate the carotid arteries, have the client turn his or her head slightly toward the side being examined, to make the artery more accessible, and place your index and middle fingers around the medial side of the sternocleidomastoid muscle.
   a. Palpate *one* carotid artery at a time. This ensures adequate cerebral blood flow through the other and prevents possible cerebral ischemia.
   b. Avoid exerting too much pressure and massaging the area. Pressure can occlude the artery, and carotid sinus massage can precipitate bradycardia. The carotid sinus is a small dilation at the beginning of the internal carotid artery just above the bifurcation of the common carotid artery, in the upper third of the neck.
   c. Note the rate, rhythm, and volume of each carotid pulse and the condition of the artery wall. Compare their equality. Normal pulse volumes are symmetric, full, and thrusting. The thrusting quality remains the same when the client inhales or exhales, turns the head, and changes from a sitting to a supine

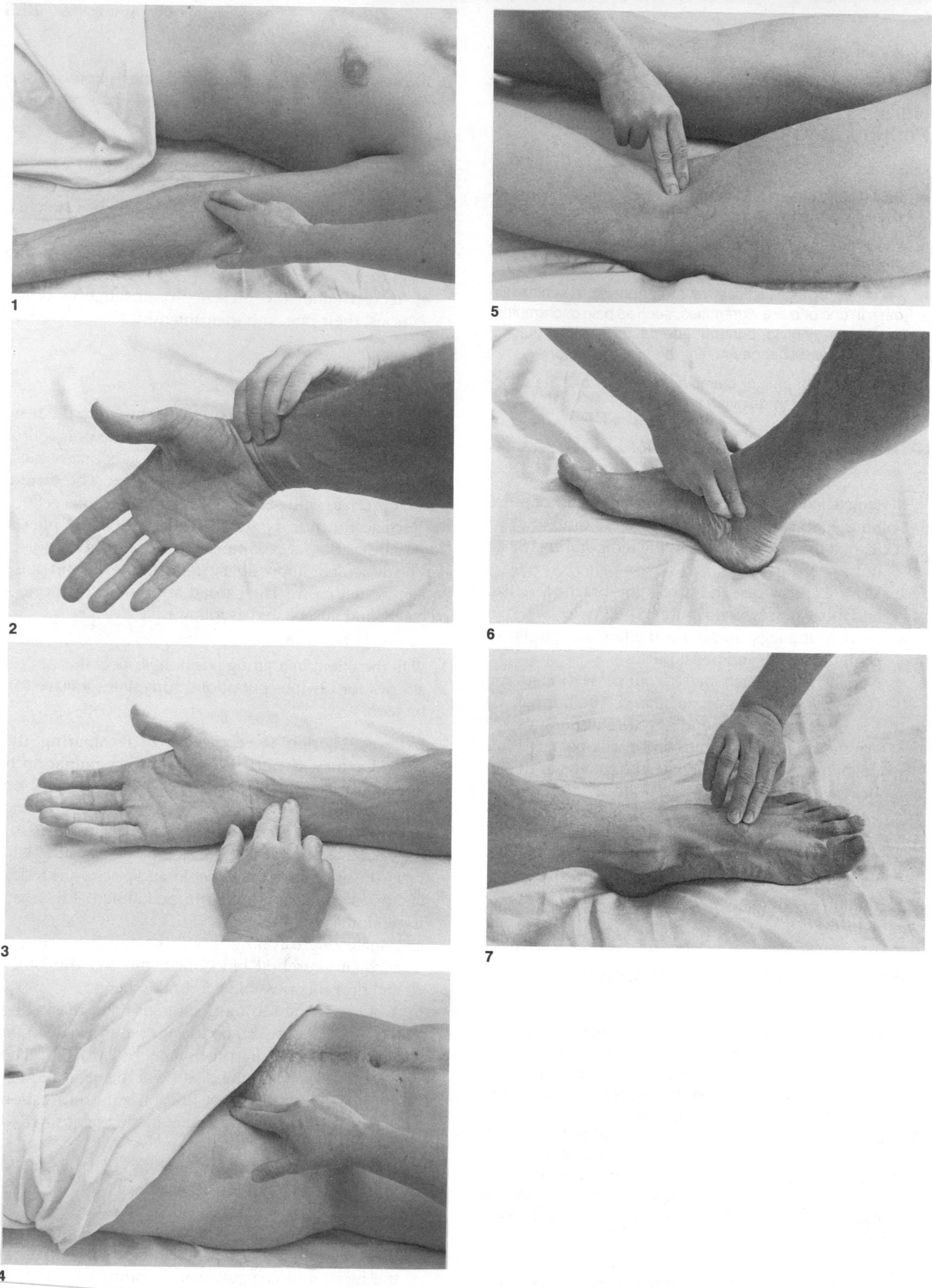

Figure 35–82A Assessing the pulses: **1,** brachial; **2,** radial; **3,** ulnar; **4,** femoral; **5,** popliteal; **6,** posterior tibial; **7,** pedal

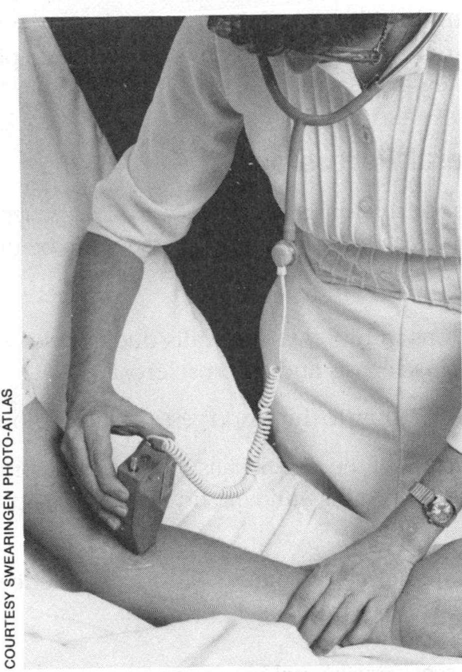

Figure 35–83 Assessing a brachial pulse using a Doppler ultrasound stethoscope

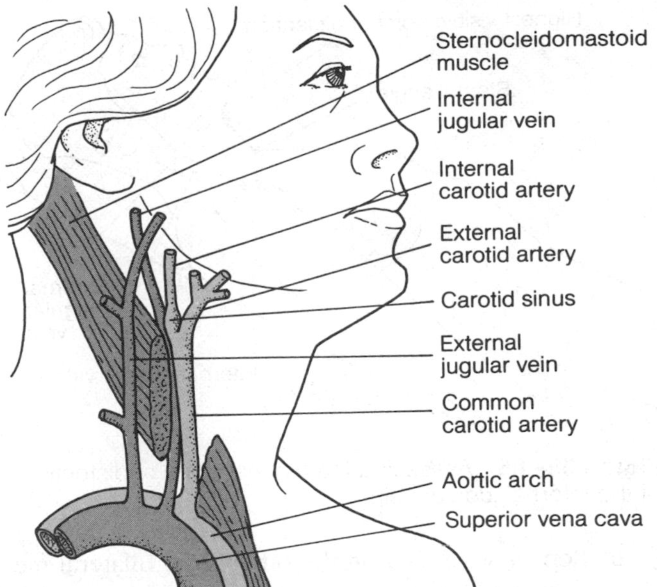

Figure 35–84 Arteries and veins of the right side of the neck

position. The arterial wall normally feels elastic. Asymmetric volumes or decreased pulsations may indicate carotid artery stenosis or thrombosis, or inadequate left cardiac output. Thickened, hard, rigid, beaded, inelastic walls are indicative of arteriosclerosis.

3. To auscultate the carotid artery, turn the client's head slightly away from the side being examined to facilitate placement of the stethoscope. Auscultate the carotid artery on one side and then the other.
   a. Listen for the presence of a **bruit** (a blowing or swishing sound) created by turbulence of blood flow due either to a narrowed arterial lumen (a common development in older people) or to a condition, such as anemia or hyperthyroidism, that elevates cardiac output. Normally no sound is heard by auscultation.
   b. If you hear a bruit, gently palpate the artery to determine the presence of a thrill, which frequently accompanies a bruit. A **thrill** is a vibrating sensation like the purring of a cat or water running through a hose. It, too, indicates turbulent blood flow due to arterial obstruction.

Jugular Veins

The jugular veins drain blood from the head and neck directly into the superior vena cava and right side of the heart. See Figure 35–84. The external jugular veins are superficial and may be visible above the clavicle. The internal jugular veins lie deeper along the carotid artery and may transmit pulsations onto the skin of the neck. Normally, external neck veins are distended and visible when a person lies down; they are flat and not as visible when a person stands up, since gravity encourages venous drainage. By inspecting the jugular veins for pulsations and distention, the nurse can assess the adequacy of function of the right side of the heart and venous pressure.

1. Remove clothing around the client's neck and thorax, and assist the client to a semi-Fowler's position with the head supported on a small pillow. Clothing is removed to prevent constriction. Semi-Fowler's position is used, since at a 30° to 45° angle, neck veins should not be prominent if the right side of the client's heart is functioning normally. A small pillow aligns the head sufficiently to prevent neck hyperextension; a large pillow would create neck flexion.
2. If jugular distention is present, assess the jugular venous pressure (JVP) as follows:
   a. Locate the highest visible point of distention of the internal jugular vein. Although either the internal or the external jugular vein can be used, the internal jugular vein is more reliable. The external jugular vein is more easily affected by obstruction or kinking at the base of the neck.
   b. Measure the vertical height of this point in centimeters from the sternal angle or suprasternal notch (the point at which the clavicles meet). See Figure 35–85.

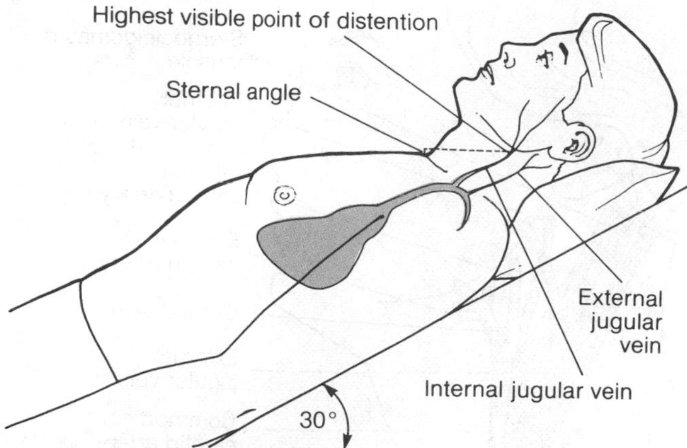

Figure 35–85 Assessing the highest point of distention of the internal jugular vein

c. Repeat steps a–b on the other side. Bilateral measurements above 3 cm are considered elevated and may indicate right-sided heart failure. Unilateral distention may be caused by local obstruction.
d. Note whether other veins in the neck, shoulder, and upper chest are distended.

Peripheral Veins

Peripheral veins in the arms and legs are inspected for the presence and/or appearance of superficial veins when limbs are dependent and when limbs are elevated. When the limb is dependent, distention and nodular bulges in the calf veins are common, especially in older people. Distended veins in the anteromedial part of the thigh and/or lower leg or in the posterolateral part of the calf from the knee to the ankle are abnormal. When the legs are elevated, the veins normally collapse.

The nurse also assesses the peripheral leg veins for signs of phlebitis, as follows:

1. Inspect the calves for redness and swelling over vein sites. These may be indicative of phlebitis.
2. Palpate the calves for firmness or tension of the muscles, the presence of edema over the dorsum of the foot, and areas of localized warmth. Palpation augments inspection findings, particularly when the client is highly pigmented and redness may not be visible.
3. Push the calves from side to side to test for tenderness.
4. Firmly dorsiflex the foot while supporting the entire leg extension or have the person stand or walk. If forceful dorsiflexion of the foot produces pain in the calf muscles (positive **Homans's sign**), a deep phlebitis of the leg is present.

Peripheral Perfusion

Peripheral perfusion is blood flow to the tissues in the extremities. Perfusion of peripheral tissues can be impaired by:

1. Alterations in blood vessel walls due to diseases such as arteriosclerosis and atherosclerosis
2. Obstructed flow to the blood vessels due to blood clots
3. Constriction of the vessel walls due to edema or devices (e.g. casts, dressings, and elastic bandages) applied too tightly
4. Severe depletions of blood volume experienced with hemorrhage and shock

To assess peripheral perfusion:

1. Inspect the skin of the hands and feet for color, temperature, edema, and skin changes.
2. Assess the adequacy of arterial flow if arterial insufficiency is suspected.
   a. Assist the client to a supine position. Have him or her raise one leg or one arm about 30 cm (1 ft) above heart level, move the foot or hand briskly up and down for about 1 minute, and then sit up and dangle the leg or arm. This procedure is called **Buerger's test**, or the arterial adequacy test.
   b. Observe the time elapsed until return of original color and vein filling. Original color normally returns in 10 seconds, and the veins fill in about 15 seconds. Delayed color return indicates arterial insufficiency.
3. Test capillary refill:
   a. Squeeze a fingernail and a toenail between your fingers sufficiently to cause blanching.
   b. Release the pressure and observe how quickly normal color returns. Color normally returns immediately.
4. Inspect the fingernails for changes indicative of circulatory impairment. See the section on assessment of nails, earlier in this chapter. See Table 35–16 for clinical signs of adequate and inadequate tissue perfusion.

Abdomen

Description of abdominal findings is facilitated by two commonly used methods of subdivision: quadrants and nine regions. To divide the abdomen into quadrants, the nurse imagines two lines: a vertical line from the xiphoid process to the pubic symphysis, and a horizontal line across the umbilicus. See Figure 35–86. These quadrants

Table 35–16 Clinical Signs of Adequate and Inadequate Tissue Perfusion

Assessment criterion	Normal findings	Abnormal findings	Possible health problem
Skin color	Pink	Cyanotic	Venous insufficiency
		Pallor that increases with limb elevation	Arterial insufficiency
		Dusky red color when limb lowered	Arterial insufficiency
		Brown pigmentation around ankles	Arterial insufficiency
Skin temperature	Skin not excessively warm or cold	Skin cool	Arterial insufficiency
Edema	Absent	Marked edema	Venous insufficiency
		Mild or absent	Arterial insufficiency
Skin texture	Skin resilient, moist	Skin thin and shiny or thick, waxy, shiny, and fragile, with reduced hair and ulceration	Venous or arterial insufficiency
Arterial adequacy test	Original color returns in 10 seconds; veins in feet or hands fill in about 15 seconds	Delayed color return or mottled appearance; delayed venous filling; marked redness of arms or legs	Arterial insufficiency
Capillary refill test	Immediate return of color	Delayed return of color	Arterial insufficiency
Peripheral pulse	Easily palpable	No pulse, decreased or absent	Arterial insufficiency

are labeled upper right quadrant, (*1*), upper left quadrant (*2*), lower right quadrant (*3*), and lower left quadrant (*4*). Using the second method, division into nine regions, the nurse imagines two vertical lines, which extend superiorly from the midpoints of the inguinal ligaments, and two horizontal lines, one at the level of the edge of the lower ribs and the other at the level of the iliac crests. See Figure 35–87. Specific organs or parts of organs lie in each abdominal region. See Tables 35–17 and 35–18.

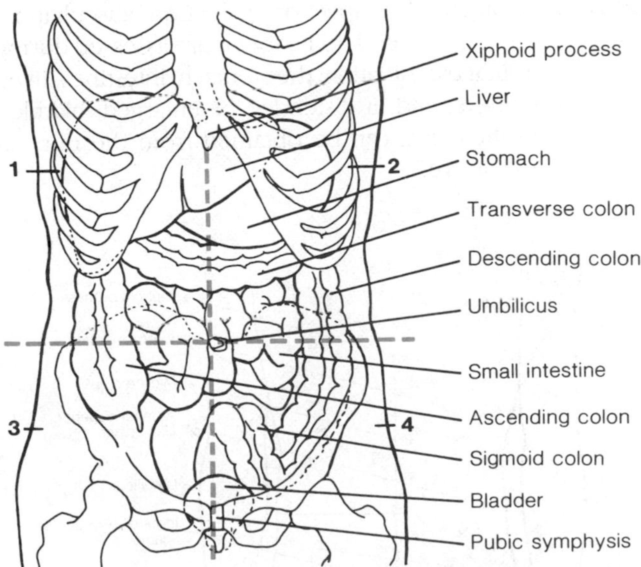

Figure 35–86 The four abdominal regions and the underlying organs: **1,** right upper quadrant; **2,** left upper quadrant; **3,** right lower quadrant; **4,** left lower quadrant

Table 35–17 Organs in the Four Abdominal Quadrants

Upper right quadrant	*Upper left quadrant*
Liver	Left lobe of liver
Gallbladder	Stomach
Duodenum	Spleen
Head of pancreas	Upper lobe of left kidney
Right adrenal gland	Pancreas
Upper lobe of right kidney	Left adrenal gland
Hepatic flexure of colon	Splenic flexure of colon
Section of ascending colon	Section of transverse colon
Section of transverse colon	Section of descending colon
Lower right quadrant	***Lower left quadrant***
Lower lobe of right kidney	Lower lobe of left kidney
Cecum	Sigmoid colon
Appendix	Section of descending colon
Section of ascending colon	Left ovary
Right ovary	Left fallopian tube
Right fallopian tube	Left ureter
Right ureter	Left spermatic cord
Right spermatic cord	Part of uterus (if enlarged)
Part of uterus (if enlarged)	

Midline

Uterus
Bladder

Table 35–18 Organs in the Nine Abdominal Regions

Right hypochondriac	*Epigastric*	*Left hypochondriac*
Right lobe of liver Gallbladder Part of duodenum Hepatic flexure of colon Upper half of right kidney Suprarenal gland	Aorta Pyloric end of stomach Part of duodenum Pancreas Part of liver	Stomach Spleen Tail of pancreas Splenic flexture of colon Upper half of left kidney Suprarenal gland
Right lumbar	*Umbilical*	*Left lumbar*
Ascending colon Lower half of right kidney Part of duodenum and jejunum	Omentum Mesentery Lower part of duodenum Part of jejunum and ileum	Descending colon Lower half of left kidney Part of jejunum and ileum
Right inguinal	*Hypogastric (pubic)*	*Left inguinal*
Cecum Appendix Lower end of ileum Right ureter Right spermatic cord Right ovary	Ileum Bladder (if enlarged) Uterus (if enlarged)	Sigmoid colon Left ureter Left spermatic cord Left ovary

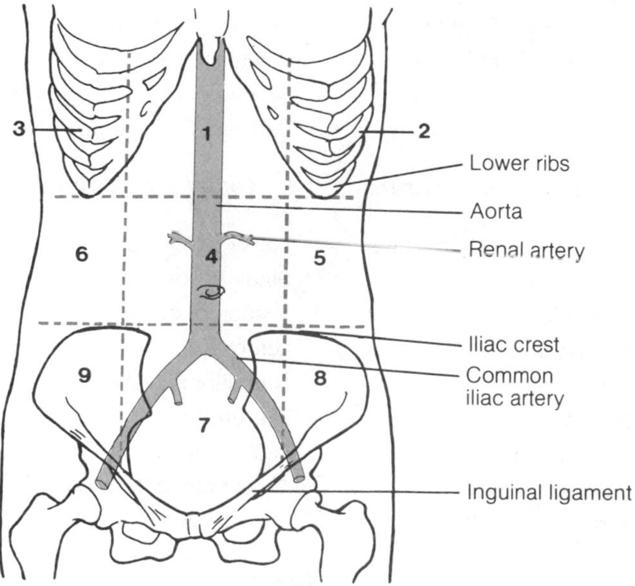

Figure 35–87 The nine abdominal regions: **1,** epigastric; **2, 3,** left and right hypochondriac; **4,** umbilical; **5, 6,** left and right lumbar; **7,** suprapubic and hypogastric; **8, 9,** left and right inguinal or iliac

Nursing History Data: Abdomen

Determine:

- Incidence of abdominal pain, its location, onset, sequence, and chronology
- Its quality (description)
- Its frequency
- Associated symptoms, e.g., nausea, vomiting, diarrhea
- Bowel habits
- Incidence of constipation or diarrhea (have client describe what he or she means by these terms)
- Change in appetite, food intolerances, and foods ingested in last 24 hours
- Specific signs and symptoms, e.g., heartburn, flatulence and/or belching, difficulty swallowing, hematemesis, blood or mucus in stools, and aggravating and alleviating factors
- Previous problems and treatment, e.g., stomach ulcer, gallbladder surgery, history of jaundice

In addition, certain landmarks are often used to facilitate the location of abdominal signs and symptoms. These are the xiphoid process of the sternum, the costal margins, the midline (a line drawn from the tip of the sternum through the umbilicus to the pubic symphysis), the anterosuperior iliac spine, the inguinal ligaments (Poupart's ligaments), and the superior margin of the pubic symphysis. See Figure 35–88.

Assessment of the abdomen involves all four methods of examination (inspection, palpation, auscultation, and percussion). Several body organs are assessed during the abdominal examination: the stomach, intestines, liver, spleen, kidneys, and, if distended or enlarged, bladder. More revealing data can be obtained from the nursing history. See above.

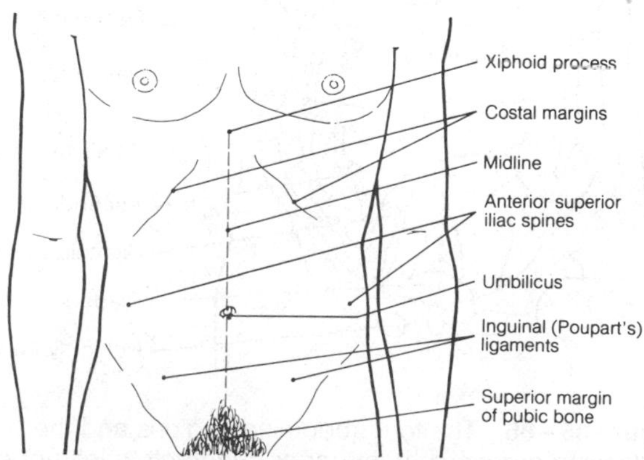

Figure 35–88 Landmarks commonly used.to identify abdominal areas

Procedure 35–9 ▲ Assessing the Abdomen

Equipment

1. A stethoscope
2. A tape measure (metal or unstretchable cloth)
3. A skin-marking pencil
4. An examining light

Intervention

See Table 35–19 for normal and abnormal findings. When assessing the abdomen, inspection is done first, followed by auscultation, palpation, and/or percussion. Auscultation is done before palpation and percussion since movement or stimulation of the bowel caused by palpation and percussion can increase bowel motility and thus heighten bowel sounds, creating false results.

1. Ensure that the client has recently urinated. Assist the client to a supine position with the arms placed comfortably at the sides. Place small pillows beneath the knees and the head.

   Rationale This position and an empty bladder prevent tension in the abdominal muscles. By contrast, the abdominal muscles tense when the client is sitting or supine with knees and arms extended and with hands clasped behind the head.

2. Ensure that the room is warm, and expose only the client's abdomen from chest line to the pubic area.

   Rationale Chilling and shivering can tense the abdominal muscles.

Inspection

3. Direct the examining light over the abdomen, and inspect the abdominal surface, with your head only slightly higher than the client's abdomen. Note surface characteristics, distention, masses, visible peristaltic waves or pulsations, movements with respiration, abdominal and umbilical contours, and presence of scars or rashes. Abdominal contour is the profile line from the rib margin to the pubic bone viewed by the examiner at a right angle to the umbilicus when the client is supine. Abdominal contour is described as flat, rounded, or scaphoid. The flat contour lies in an approximately horizontal plane from the rib cage to the pubic area; the rounded contour is convex to the horizontal plane; and the scaphoid is concave to the horizontal plane.

4. Instruct the client to take a deep breath and to hold it. Inspect the abdominal contour.

   Rationale A deep breath forces the diaphragm downward, thus decreasing the size of the abdominal cavity and making masses such as an enlarged liver or spleen more obvious.

5. Instruct the client to raise his or her head and shoulders without using the arms for support. Again inspect the abdominal contour, and observe the rectus abdominus muscles for separation (diastasis recti abdominis). See Figure 35–89.

   Rationale Separation of the rectus abdominis muscles can be observed as a ridge or bulge between the muscles when intraabdominal pressure is increased by raising the head and shoulders. This defect does not seriously affect the functions of abdominal organs.

6. Move to the foot of the bed or examining table, and inspect the contour of the abdomen for symmetry.

   Rationale Asymmetry of the abdominal contour is more readily assessed from this position.

Auscultation

Listen for two abdominal sounds: bowel or peristaltic sounds caused by gas and food moving along the intestines, and vascular sounds. In the pregnant woman, fetal heart sounds are also assessed.

7. Warm your hands and the stethoscope diaphragms.

   Rationale Cold hands and a cold stethoscope may cause the client to contract the abdominal muscles, and these contractions may be heard during auscultation.

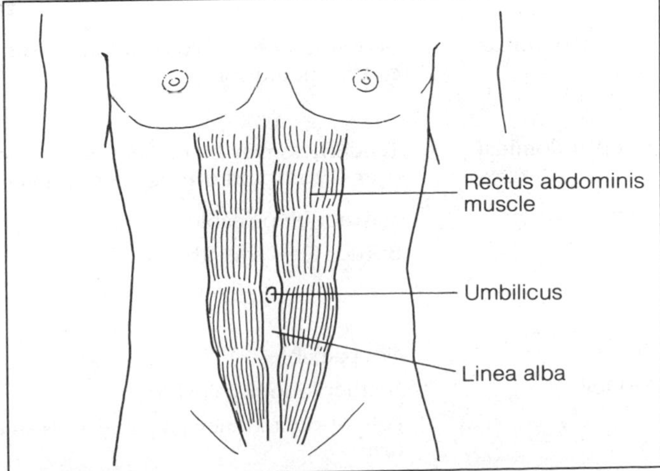

Figure 35–89

Table 35–19 Assessment Data: Abdomen

Method and structure	Normal findings	Abnormal findings
	Inspection	
Abdomen	Smooth, soft; flat, rounded, or scaphoid contour	Tense, glistening skin Distention Visible peristalsis Visible midline pulsations
	Symmetrical contour	Asymmetrical contour, e.g., localized protrusions around umbilicus, around inguinal ligaments, or near scars
	Silver-white striae or surgical scars	Purple striae
	Unblemished skin	Rash or other skin lesions
	After deep breath, smooth, even, symmetrical movements	After deep breath, bulges or masses appear After deep breath, abdominal movement is restricted
	After raising head and shoulders, little or no midline bulge	After raising head and shoulders, marked ridge or bulge
	Auscultation	
Abdomen	Audible bowel sounds	Absent or hypoactive bowel sounds Hyperactive bowel sounds
	Absence of arterial bruits	Loud bruit over aortic area Bruit over renal or iliac arteries
	Absence of venous hum	Medium-pitched hum in periumbilical region Friction rub
	Percussion	
Abdomen	Predominantly tympanic percussion sound; suprapubic dullness over distended bladder	Dullness in localized area
Liver	Span of 6–12 cm at midclavicular line and 4–8 cm at midsternal line	Span exceeding 12 cm at midclavicular line and 8 cm at midsternal line Midsternal line span is equal to midclavicular line span Lower liver border displaced inferiorly Lower liver border displaced superiorly
Spleen	Span of about 7 cm at left midaxillary line between sixth and tenth ribs	Span exceeds 7 cm
Shifting dullness test		Change in first and second demarcation lines (between tympany and dullness)
Fist percussion	No tenderness of liver or kidney	Tenderness of liver Tenderness of kidney
	Palpation	
Light abdominal	No tenderness; relaxed abdomen with smooth, consistent tension	Tenderness and hypersensitivity Superficial masses Localized areas of increased tension
Deep abdominal	Tenderness may be present near xiphoid process, over cecum, and over sigmoid colon	Generalized or localized areas of tenderness Mobile or fixed masses
Liver	May not be palpable Border feels smooth	Enlarged but smooth and not tender Smooth but tender Nodular Hard
Spleen	Not palpable	Palpated
Kidney	Neither kidney palpable	Either or both kidneys palpable
	Pole of right kidney palpable, feels smooth and firm	Enlarged, hard, tender, or nodular
Bladder	Not palpable	Distended and palpable as smooth, round, tense mass

8. Applying only light pressure with the stethoscope, use the flat-disc diaphragm to listen to the abdominal intestinal sounds, and use the bell-shaped diaphragm to detect arterial and venous sounds.

   Rationale Light pressure is adequate to detect the sounds. Intestinal sounds are relatively high-pitched and best accentuated by the flat diaphragm; arterial and venous sounds are lower-pitched and best accentuated by the bell.

9. Ask when the client last ate.

   Rationale Shortly after or long after eating, bowel sounds may be normally increased. They are loudest when a meal is long overdue. Four to 7 hours after a meal, bowel sounds may be heard continuously over the ileocecal valve area, while the digestive contents from the small intestine empty through the valve into the large intestine.

10. Place the flat diaphragm of the stethoscope in each of the four quadrants of the abdomen, and listen for active bowel sounds—irregular gurgling noises occurring about every 5 to 20 seconds. The duration of a single sound may range from less than a second to more than several seconds. The frequency of sounds relates to the state of digestion or the presence of food in the gastrointestinal tract. Normal bowel sounds are described as audible. Alterations in sounds are described as (a) absent or hypoactive, i.e., extremely soft and infrequent (e.g., one per minute), and (b) hyperactive or increased (**borborygmi**), i.e., high-pitched, loud, rushing sounds that occur frequently (e.g., every 3 seconds).

11. If bowel sounds appear to be absent, listen for 3 to 5 minutes before concluding that they are absent. Listen over all the auscultatory sites shown in Figure 35–90.

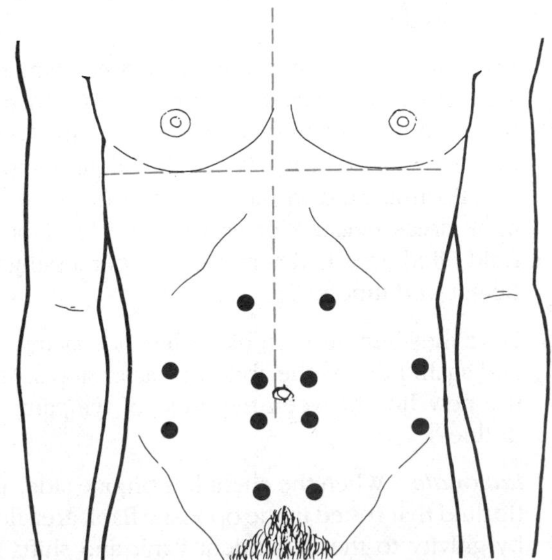

Figure 35–90

   Rationale Because bowel sounds are so irregular, a longer time and more sites are used to confirm absence of sounds.

12. Place the bell of the stethoscope over the aorta, renal arteries, and iliac arteries, and listen for arterial sounds (bruits).
    a. Auscultate the aorta superior to the umbilicus.
    b. Auscultate the renal arteries at or to the left and right of the upper abdominal midline or further toward the flank.
    c. Auscultate the iliac arteries to the left and right of the abdominal midline below the umbilicus. See Figure 35–87, earlier, to locate these areas.

13. Place the bell of the stethoscope over the periumbilical (around the umbilicus) region and listen for a venous hum, rarely heard in the abdomen.

14. At the various auscultating sites, especially above the liver and spleen, listen for peritoneal friction rubs that sound like two pieces of leather rubbing together.

    Rationale The liver and spleen have large surface areas in contact with the peritoneum; thus they are most frequently the beginning sites for friction rubs.

    a. To auscultate the splenic site, place the stethoscope over the left lower rib cage in the anterior axillary line and have the client take a deep breath.

       Rationale A deep breath may accentuate the sound of a friction rub area.

    b. To auscultate the liver site, place the stethoscope over the lower right rib cage.

Percussion

Percussion is used to detect gas, fluid, and/or masses within the abdomen as well as the position and size of the liver and spleen.

15. Lightly percuss the entire abdomen in a systematic manner:
    a. Move from the right upper quadrant in a clockwise direction from the client's perspective (counterclockwise from your perspective). See Figure 35–91.
    b. If the client is experiencing pain or tenderness in a specific area, percuss that area last.

       Rationale Pain felt early in the percussion sequence might cause the client to tense the abdominal muscles, making evaluation of percussion sounds more difficult.

    c. Percuss for areas of tympany and dullness, noting specifically areas of dullness. **Tympany** is a bell-like, musical percussion sound of somewhat higher pitch than resonance. It is characteristic of a gas-filled cavity or organ. Tympanic sounds predominate in the abdomen due to the presence of gas

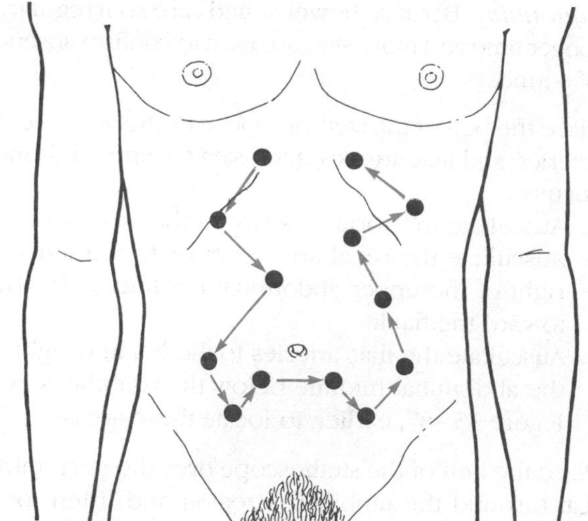

Figure 35–91

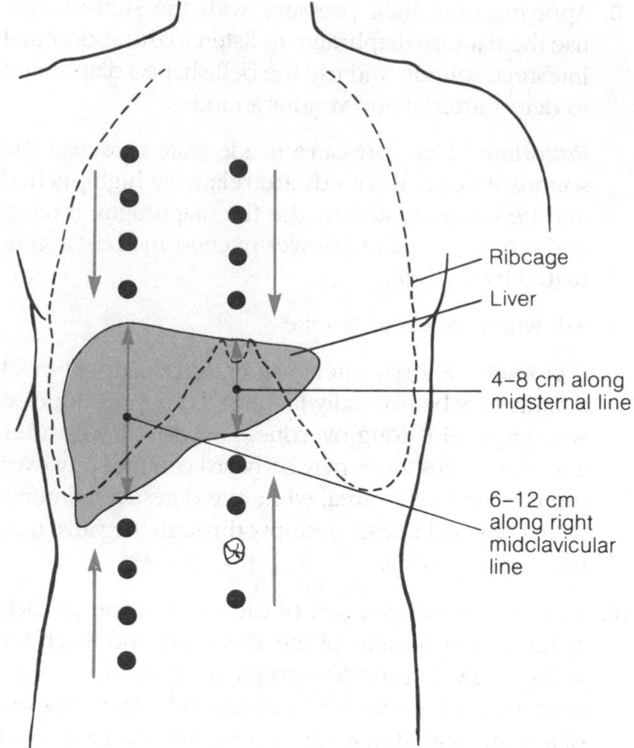

Figure 35–92

in the stomach and intestines. **Dullness** is a decrease, absence, or flatness of resonance. Dullness is heard over solid masses such as ascites, a distended bladder, a sigmoid colon filled with stool, enlarged organs such as the liver or spleen, and tumors.

16. *Liver size and position.*
    a. Begin percussion in the right midclavicular line at or below the level of the umbilicus, and percuss upward over tympanic areas until a dull percussion sound indicates the lower liver border. Mark this site with a skin-marking pencil. See Figure 35–92.
    b. Then percuss downward at the right midclavicular line beginning from an area of lung resonance and progressing downward until a dull percussion sound indicates the upper liver border. Mark this site.
    c. Measure the distance between the two marks (upper and lower liver border) in centimeters, to establish the liver span or size. Normally, the range of liver span in the midclavicular line is 6 to 12 cm (2.3 to 4.7 in), and the lower liver border is at or just below the rib cage.
    d. Repeat steps a–c at the midsternal line. Normally, the range of liver span at the midsternal line is 4 to 8 cm (1.5 to 3.1 in).
17. *Liver descent.*
    a. Have the client take a deep breath and hold it.
    b. Again percuss upward in the midclavicular line.
    c. Estimate liver descent in centimeters.

    Rationale On inspiration, the diaphragm moves downward and shifts the span of liver dullness downward 2 to 3 cm (0.7 to 1.2 in).
18. *Spleen size and position.* The spleen is most easily percussed when it is enlarged. Percuss upward and downward along the left midaxillary line and note where a dull tone is heard. Normally, a dullness is heard between the sixth and tenth ribs for a span of about 7 cm (2.7 in).
19. *Shifting dullness test.* This test is used to detect free-floating intraabdominal fluid (ascites) in the peritoneal cavity.
    a. While the client is supine, percuss the abdomen, progressing laterally from the umbilicus toward the flank. Mark the point where dullness is first percussed.

    Rationale From the umbilical area, tympanic sounds will be elicited over gas-filled structures until the area of fluid is reached; at this point, dullness will be heard. When the client is supine, free-floating fluid in the abdomen moves to the flank areas because of gravity. The level of the fluid-filled area is determined by percussing the height of dullness.

    b. Have the client turn on his or her side facing you, and again percuss the abdomen as in step a. Mark the new line between the areas of tympany and dullness.

    Rationale When the client lies on one side, ascitic fluid that rested in the opposite flank area flows by gravity to the dependent flank and shifts the line of dullness closer to the umbilicus. If the area of dullness does not shift significantly, the fluid is not free-floating and may be confined within the bowel, cysts, or the abdominal wall. This technique also helps the nurse to make a rough estimate of fluid volume.

20. *Fist percussion.* Fist percussion is used to detect areas of tenderness over regions of dullness of the liver and kidney. Two methods are used to apply fist percussion: direct and indirect. In the indirect method, the palm of the nondominant hand is placed over the specific region, e.g., the liver, and is then struck with a light blow by the fisted dominant hand. In the direct method, the side of the fisted hand is applied directly to the specific region, e.g., the kidney. Do not apply fist percussion until the end of the examination, since it may produce discomfort and tenderness. You will assess the tenderness by the client's reaction. Always alert the client before fist percussion. Otherwise, although the client's reaction may simply indicate surprise, you may interpret it as an indication of tenderness.
    a. For the liver, apply only indirect fist percussion. Place the palm of your nondominant hand parallel to and below the right costal margin and strike it with the back of the fist of the other hand. See Figure 35–93. Note if tenderness occurs.
    b. For the kidney, apply either direct or indirect fist percussion while the client is sitting upright or lying on his or her side. Place the palm of your nondominant hand or the back of your clenched fist over the costovertebral angle between the spine and the twelfth rib. See Figure 35–94.

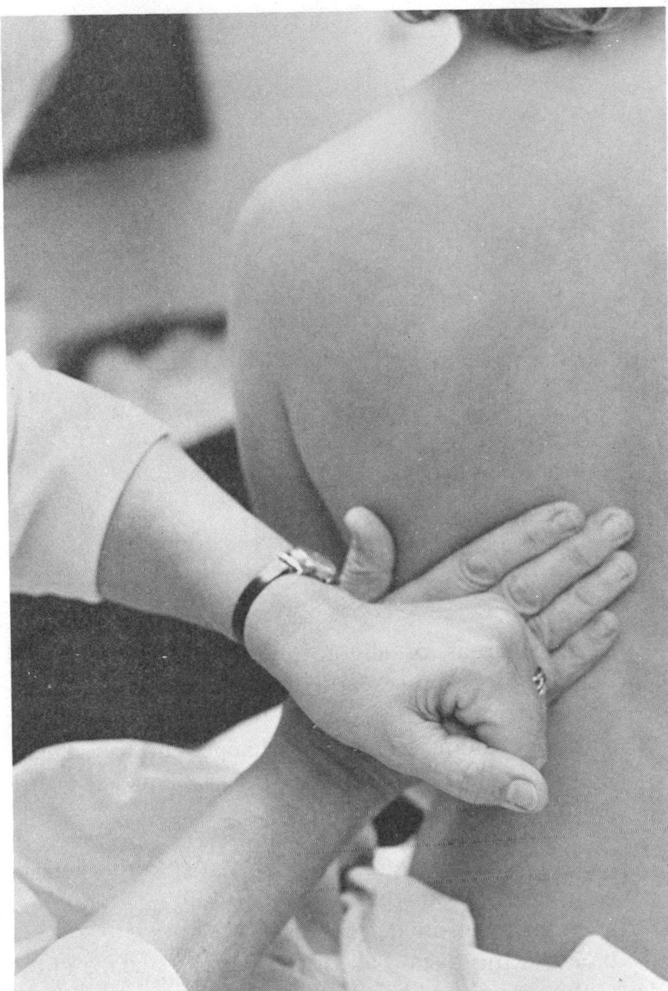

Figure 35–94

Palpation

Palpation is used to detect tenderness, the outline and position of abdominal organs (e.g., the liver, spleen, and kidneys), and the presence of masses or distention. Two types of palpation are used: light and deep.

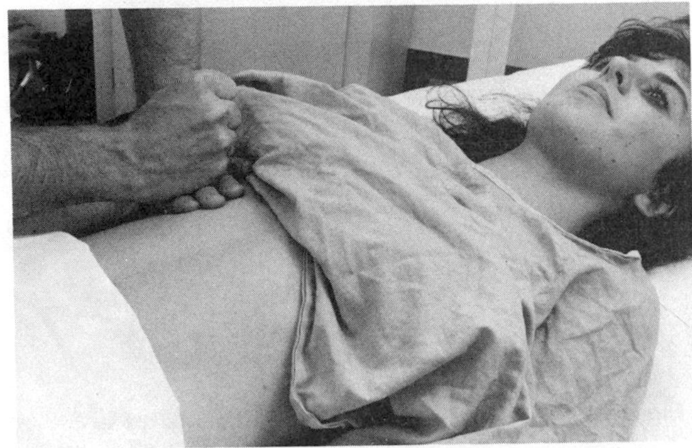

Figure 35–93

21. Warm your hands.

    Rationale Cold hands can elicit muscle tension that impedes palpatory evaluation.

22. *Light palpation.* Perform light palpation first, and systematically explore all four abdominal quadrants.

    Rationale Light palpation alerts the nurse to areas of tenderness and/or muscle guarding (stiffening) before more vigorous palpation is performed.

    a. Hold the palm of your hand slightly above the client's abdomen with your fingers parallel to the abdomen.
    b. Depress the abdominal wall lightly, about 1 cm or to the depth of the subcutaneous tissue, with the pads of the fingers. See Figure 35–95.
    c. Move the finger pads in a slight circular motion.
    d. If the client is extremely ticklish, place his or her hand under or over your own hand.

    Rationale This decreases the degree of ticklishness and resulting muscle tenseness.

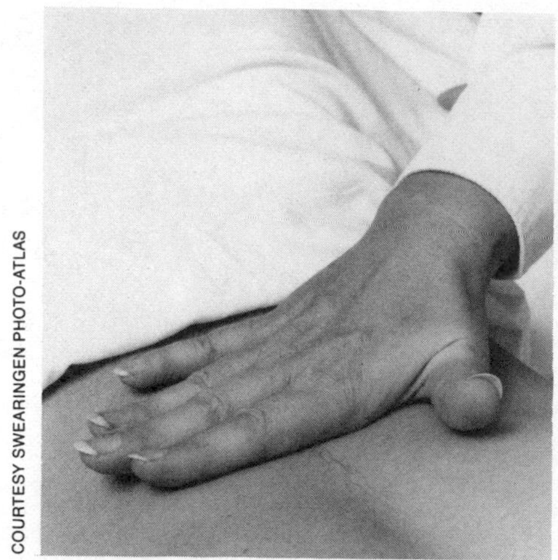

COURTESY SWEARINGEN PHOTO-ATLAS

Figure 35–95

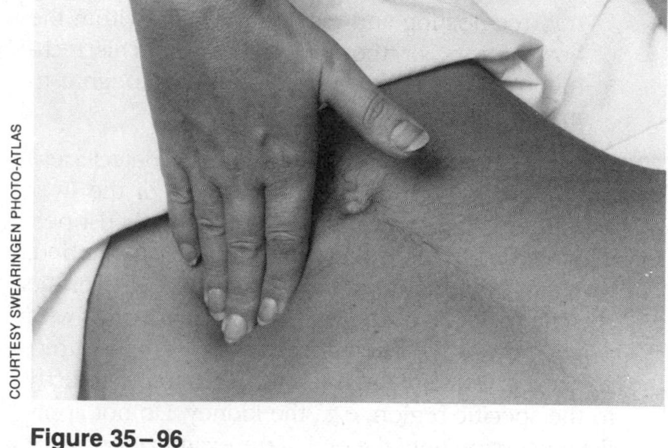

COURTESY SWEARINGEN PHOTO-ATLAS

Figure 35–96

e. Note areas of slight tenderness or superficial pain, large masses, and muscle guarding. To determine areas of tenderness, have the client tell you about them, watch for changes in the client's facial expressions, and note areas of muscle guarding.

23. *Deep palpation.* Perform deep palpation systematically over all four quadrants.
    a. Palpate sensitive areas last.
    b. Press the distal half of the palmar surface of the fingers of one hand into the abdominal wall.

       or

       Use the bimanual method of palpation discussed earlier in Chapter 11, page 246.
    c. Depress the abdominal wall about 4 to 5 cm (1.5 to 2.0 in) or an appropriate distance beyond subcutaneous tissue. See Figure 35–96.
    d. Note masses and the structure of underlying contents. If a mass is present, determine its size, location, mobility, contour, consistency, and tenderness. Normal abdominal structures that may be mistaken for masses include: the lateral borders of the rectus abdominis muscles; the feces-filled ascending, descending, or sigmoid colon; the aorta; the uterus; the common iliac artery; and the sacral promontory.

24. *Liver palpation.* The liver is palpated to detect enlargement and tenderness. Two bimanual approaches are used.
    a. Stand on the client's right side.
    b. Place your left hand on the posterior thorax at about the eleventh or twelfth rib.
    c. Push upward with the left hand.

       Rationale This hand braces the subsequent anterior palpation.
    d. Place your right hand along the rib cage at about a 45° angle to the right of the rectus abdominis muscle or parallel to the rectus muscle with the fingers pointing toward the rib cage. See Figure 35–97.
    e. While the client exhales, exert a gradual and gentle downward and forward pressure beneath the cos-

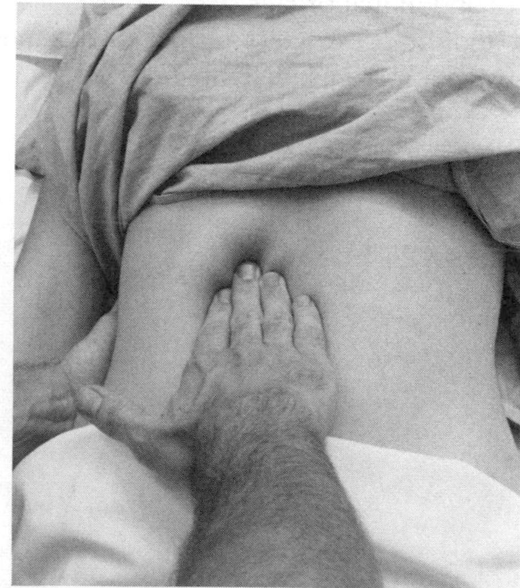

Figure 35–97

tal margin until a depth of 4 to 5 cm (1.5 to 2.0 in) is reached.

Rationale During expiration, the abdominal wall is relaxed, facilitating deep palpation.

f. Maintain your hand position, and ask the client to inhale deeply.

Rationale Inspiration makes the liver border descend and moves the liver into a palpable position.

g. While the client inhales, feel the liver border move against your hand. It should feel firm and have a regular contour. If the liver is not palpated initially, have the client take two or three more deep breaths, while you maintain or apply slightly more palpation pressure. Livers are difficult to palpate in obese, tense, or very physically fit people.

h. If the liver is enlarged, i.e., palpable below the costal margin, measure the number of centimeters it extends below the costal region. The second method is the bimanual palpation method discussed on page 246, in which one hand is superimposed on the other. The techniques and principles used in steps d–h apply to that method as well.

25. *Spleen palpation.* Although the spleen is not palpable in the normal adult, the splenic area is palpated in the same manner as the liver.

a. Have the client turn onto his or her right side.

Rationale This position brings the spleen forward and down by gravity and closer to the abdominal wall.

b. Palpate at the left costal margin.

26. *Kidney palpation.* The upper lobes of both kidneys touch the diaphragm, and the kidneys descend upon inhalation. The right kidney is normally more easily palpated than the left, because the right one lies a little lower than the left. The right kidney lies in line with the twelfth rib; the left kidney, with the eleventh rib. See Figure 35–98, *A,* for the anterior view, and 35–98, *B,* for the posterior view. The adult kidney is normally smooth, solid, firm, and shaped like a lima bean. It is generally about 11 cm (4.5 in) long, 5 to 7 cm (2 to 3 in) wide, and 2.5 cm (1 in) thick. To palpate the kidneys, have the client lie supine. The nurse stands at the client's right side while assessing either kidney.

a. To palpate the right kidney, place your left hand under the client's flank to elevate the kidney anteriorly.

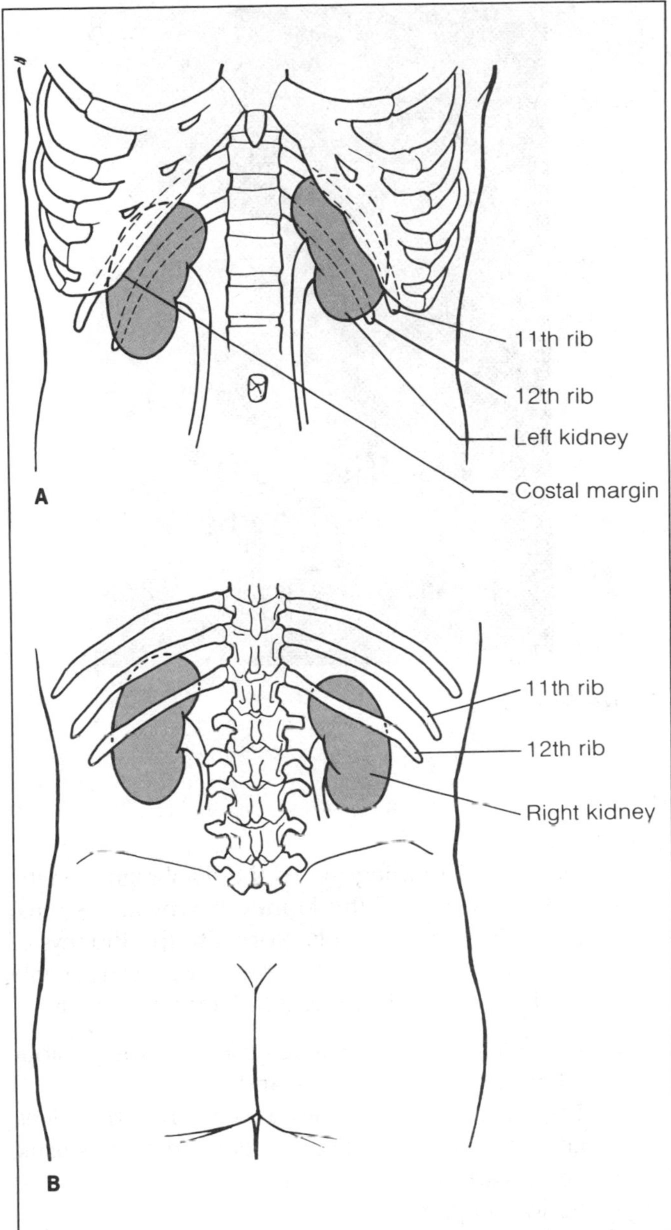

Figure 35–98 Normal position of the kidneys: A, anterior view; B, posterior view

b. Place your right hand on the anterior abdominal wall at the midclavicular line and at the inferior edge of the costal margin.

c. Press directly upward beneath the costal margin while the client takes a deep breath. See Figure 35–99.

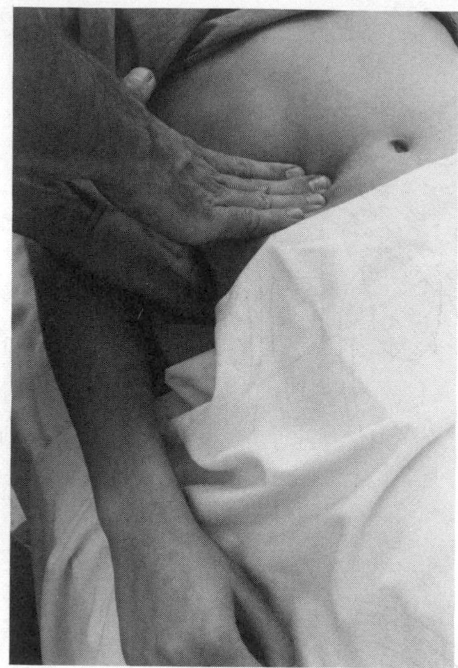

Figure 35–99

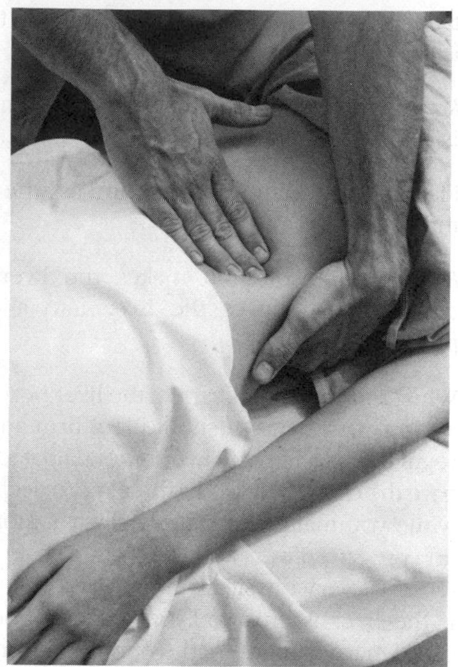

Figure 35–100

Rationale Inhaling moves the diaphragm and the inferior aspect of the kidney downward, so that the kidney may be felt. Normally the kidneys of the adult are not palpable, but in very thin people the lower part of the right kidney may be felt.

d. If the kidney is palpable, check it for contour (shape), size, tenderness, and lumps.
e. To palpate the left kidney, reach across the client, and place your left hand under the client's flank. See Figure 35–100.
f. Follow steps b–d.

27. *Bladder palpation.* With one or two hands, palpate the area above the symphysis pubis. See Figure 35–101. The bladder is palpable only when distended with urine. If it is distended, percuss the area for level of dullness.

28. Record your findings on the appropriate record.

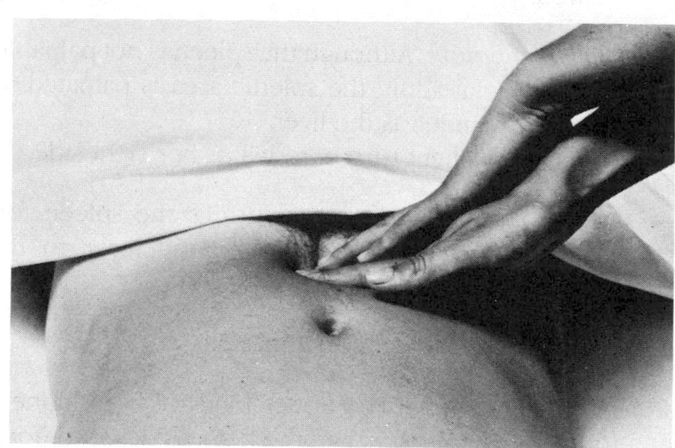

Figure 35–101

Rectum and Anus

The anal canal is the most distal portion of the gastrointestinal tract. At the point where it joins the rectum, the skin lining the anal canal changes to mucous membrane lining the rectum. In an adult, the anal canal is about 4 cm (1.5 in) long, and the rectum is about 12 cm (8 in) long. On its proximal end, the rectum joins the sigmoid colon. Distally it opens onto the body surface; the orifice is called the anus. See Figure 35–102. The anus has many somatic nerve endings and thus is highly sensitive to discomfort. The rectum is innervated by the vagus nerve; care *must* be taken not to overstimulate this nerve, because of the danger of causing a decreased heart rate, since the vagus nerve also innervates the heart.

The lumen of the rectum has three folds, called Houston's valves, which extend across the rectum and help hold feces in the rectum. The most inferior fold, which projects posteriorly, can sometimes be felt digitally. There are also several folds that extend vertically. Each of the vertical folds contains a vein and an artery. When the veins become distended, as can occur with repeated pressure, a condition known as hemorrhoids occurs. An enlargement of the rectum just proximal to the anal canal is called the ampulla of the rectum. It serves as a temporary storage place for feces, although the main reservoir for feces is the sigmoid colon.

The anal canal is bound by an internal and an external sphincter muscle. See Figure 35–102. The internal sphincter is under involuntary control, and the external sphincter normally is voluntarily controlled. The external sphincter's action is augmented by the levator ani muscle of the pelvic floor. The internal sphincter muscle is innervated by the autonomic nervous system; the external sphincter is innervated by the somatic nervous system. The mucosa of the anal canal has vertical folds called the anal columns of morgagni, which form pockets called anal sinuses.

Nursing history data taken in conjunction with assessment of the rectum and anus are shown on page 870. **Completeness of assessment of the rectum and anus depends on the needs and problems of the individual client. In many practice settings the nurse performs only inspection of the anus.**

To examine the rectum and anal canal, a nurse will require a drape to avoid unnecessary exposure of the client, a disposable examining glove, and a lubricant. The nurse assists the female client to a dorsal recumbent position with hips externally rotated and knees flexed or to Sims's position. The male client can assume a lateral (side-lying) position with the upper leg acutely flexed. Drape the client appropriately. See the section on positions and draping, earlier in this chapter.

Spread the buttocks and ask the client to bear down while observing the anus. Bearing down normally causes the anal sphincter to contract, and the nurse can thus determine whether the nerves to the area are intact. Also inspect the anus for protruding hemorrhoids (distended veins that appear as red bodies), fissures, cracks, and redness. Normally, the skin is intact, and there are no hemorrhoids, lesions, or reddened areas.

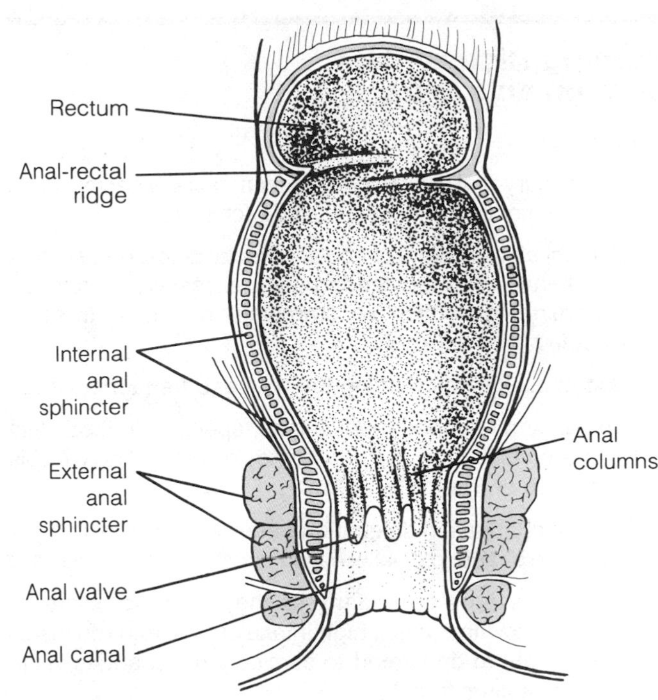

Figure 35–102 Interior view of the rectum and anal canal

If allowed by agency policy, the nurse then dons a glove, lubricates the index finger, and slowly inserts the finger into the anus and into the rectum. If the finger is inserted slowly, the anal sphincter muscles will relax, permitting the finger to extend into the rectum. The nurse then palpates the rectal walls with the pad of the index finger, feeling for nodules, masses, and tenderness. Normally, the wall is smooth and not tender. Note the location on the rectum, e.g., anterior wall, 2 cm proximal to the internal anal sphincter, of any palpated mass.

In the male, the prostate gland can be palpated through the anterior wall of the rectum. See Figure 35–103. The nurse should be able to feel the median sulcus, which divides the gland into two lobes. The prostate should be about 4 cm (1.5 in) in diameter, firm and rubbery, with discrete edges, smooth, and mobile. The client does not normally experience tenderness during the exam.

In the female, the cervix of the uterus can be palpated through the anterior rectal wall. See Figure 35–104. The cervix normally feels smooth, round, firm, and movable. It is not normally tender.

Nursing History Data: Rectum and Anus

Determine:

- Past history of diarrhea, constipation, rectal bleeding, black or tarry stools, rectal pain, itching, or spasm
- Current clinical signs of bowel or rectal disorders, such as abdominal pain or tenderness, excessive flatulence, abdominal distention or cramping, painful defecation, bleeding, and diarrhea
- Use of laxatives, including the type and frequency of use
- Currently prescribed medications, specifically those that cause constipation (e.g., codeine) or black, tarry stools (e.g., iron or Pepto-Bismol)
- Recent changes in defecation patterns and stool consistency and shape, e.g., alternating constipation and diarrhea
- Dietary patterns particularly as they relate to colorectal cancer (Low-fiber diets, high intake of fats, and red meats are thought to be related to carcinogenic changes in the gastrointestinal tract.)
- Family history of inflammatory or carcinogenic bowel disease

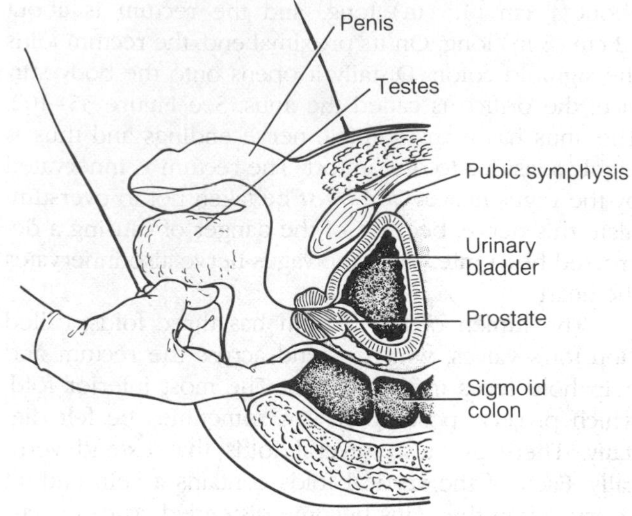

Figure 35–103 Palpating the prostate gland through the anterior wall of the rectum

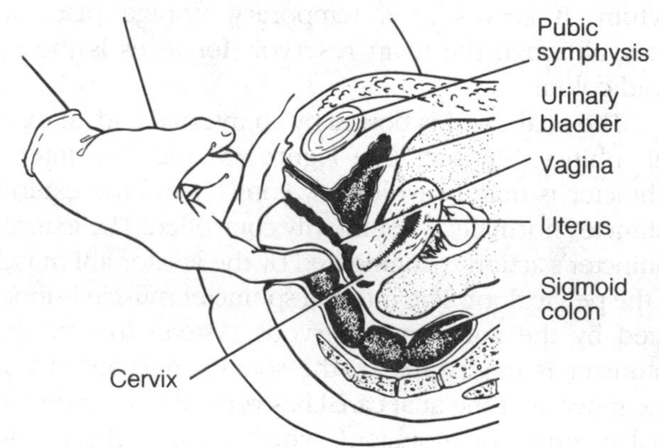

Figure 35–104 Palpating the cervix through the anterior rectal wall

Upon withdrawing the finger from the rectum and anus, observe it for feces. Feces are normally brown. Observe the feces for the presence of any mucus or blood. Record the color of the feces, and send a sample to the laboratory to test for occult blood. Record your findings on the appropriate record.

Genitals and Reproductive Tract

Nurses assess the genitals of newborns for normalcy. Nurses examine newborn boys to check that a urinary meatus is on the glans penis and that the meatus is patent. The testes are also palpated within the scrotum. Undescended testes are noted. Normally, both testes have descended at birth. The vaginal orifice of newborn girls is also inspected. Any discharge is noted and recorded, although a reddish discharge may be normal. The first rectal temperature is taken with particular care in case the anus is closed (imperforate anus).

Nurses need to pay close attention to problems involving the genitals of children. Bed wetting may be the result of a urinary infection or anxiety. Young boys' scrotums are palpated to check for descended testicles. The external genitals of the female child are usually inspected, but a pelvic examination is usually not performed.

During assessment of male adolescents it is most important to establish the descent of the testicles into the scrotum; undescended testes are noted. Assessment of adolescent girls is limited to an inspection of the external genitalia unless the girl is sexually active. If so, a Papanicolaou test (Pap test) is advised once a year to detect cancer of the cervix and uterus. See the following section for information about taking a specimen for a Papanicolaou test. If the adolescent is sexually active and has an increased or abnormal vaginal discharge, specimens should be taken to check for sexually transmitted disease.

Female Genitals

In adult females, examination of the genitals and reproductive tract includes assessment of the inguinal lymph nodes, external genitals, vagina and cervix, uterus, ovaries, and cervix. Listed to the right are data to be collected during a nursing history.

Completeness of assessment of the genitals and reproductive tract depends on the needs and problems of the individual client. ***In many practice settings*** **nurses will perform** ***only*** **inspection of the external genitalia.**

Nursing History Data: Female Genitals

Determine:

- Age of onset of menstruation, last menstrual period (LMP), regularity of cycle, duration, amount of daily flow, and presence of painful menstruation
- Incidence of pain during intercourse
- Vaginal discharge
- Number of pregnancies, number of live births, labor or delivery complications
- Frequency, urgency, frequency of urination at night, blood in urine, painful urination, incontinence
- History of sexually transmitted disease, past and present

Procedure 35–10 ▲ Assessing the Female Genitals

Equipment

1. Good lighting. A flashlight may be necessary to view the cervix.
2. Drapes to avoid undue exposure of the client.
3. An examining table on which the client can assume the lithotomy position.
4. Disposable gloves.
5. A vaginal speculum of the correct size. A virgin or an elderly woman will probably require a small speculum. The size of the speculum required otherwise depends on the individual's sexual and obstetric history. See Figure 35–105.
6. Warm water to lubricate the speculum.
7. Lubricant.
8. Supplies for cytology studies: cotton applicators, normal saline solution, an Ayre spatula (for a cervical scrape), slides, and fixative spray or solution for the specimen.

Intervention

See Table 35–20 for normal and abnormal findings.

Inguinal Lymph Nodes

There are two groups of superficial lymph nodes in the inguinal area: the superior (horizontal) group, and the inferior (vertical) group. See Figure 35–106. The superior group drain the skin of the abdominal wall, below the external genitals, anal canal, and lower vagina. The inferior group receives lymph from the medial aspect of the leg and foot.

1. Assist the client to a back-lying position and drape her appropriately (see the section on positioning and draping, earlier in this chapter).

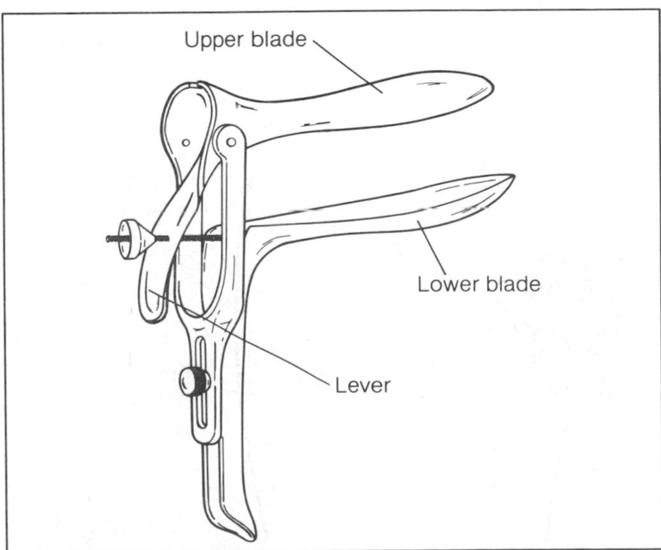

Figure 35–105 A vaginal speculum

Table 35–20 Assessment Data: Female Genitals

Structure	Normal findings	Abnormal findings
External genitals	Normal pubic hair pattern and amount	Scant pubic hair except in elderly clients
	Labia majora and minora intact	
	Absence of lesions, scars, fissures, swelling, or erythema	
	No urethral dischage	Urethral discharge
	Skene's and Bartholin's glands not tender or inflamed	Inflamed Bartholin's glands
Vagina	Walls intact	Cystocele, rectocele, enterocele
	Pelvic musculature has good tone	
	Mucosa pink, no discharge	Vaginal discharge, mucosa inflamed
Cervix	Positioned posteriorly	
	Smooth, mobile, not tender	Nodular, tender
	Size 2–3 cm (0.7–1 in) in diameter	Lacerations, erosions, masses, discharge, polyps, cysts
	Nulliparous os is round or oval	
	Parous os is slitlike	
Uterus	About fist size	
	Freely movable	Not movable, tender
	Positioned anteriorly, firm, smooth surface	
Ovaries	Slightly tender	Acute discomfort
	Less than 4 cm (1.5 in)	
	Smooth, mobile	Nodular surface, fixed
Rectovaginal wall	Smooth, thin, and pliable	Bulging, inflamed
	Posterior surface of uterus smooth	Surface nodular

2. Palpate the groin area for the lymph nodes indicated in Figure 35–106, using the pads of your fingers in a rotary motion.
3. Assess the lymph nodes for enlargement and tenderness.

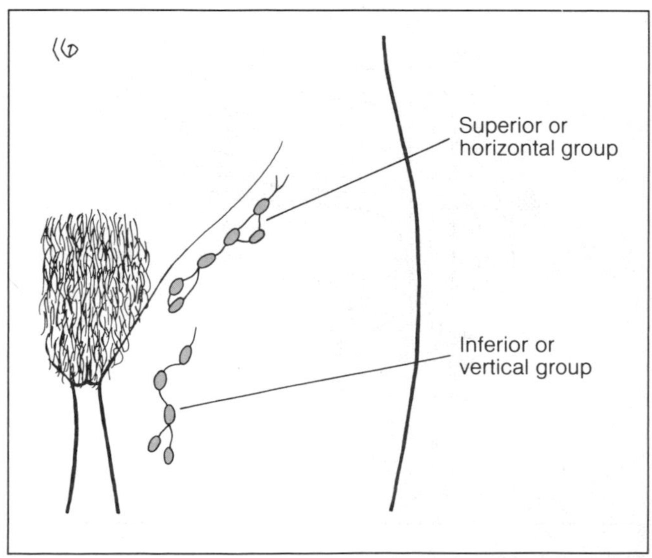

Figure 35–106 Lymph nodes of the groin area

External Genitals

4. Ask the client to empty her bladder before the pelvic examination. A urine specimen may or may not be sent for urinalysis.

   Rationale The client will feel more comfortable during the examination. Relaxation of the abdominal muscles is important for successful assessment.

5. Assist the client to a lithotomy position, and drape her appropriately.
6. Inspect the distribution and amount of pubic hair. There are wide variations. Generally, the pubic hair of menstruating adults is kinky; after menopause, it is thinner and straighter.
7. Inspect the skin in the pubic area for lice, lesions, erythema, leukoplakia, fissures, and excoriations.
8. Separate the labia majora, and inspect the interior of the labia majora and the labia minora for the problems noted in step 7.
9. Inspect the clitoris for size and lesions. The normal clitoris is about 0.5 cm (0.2 in) in diameter.
10. Inspect the urethral meatus for signs of inflammation.

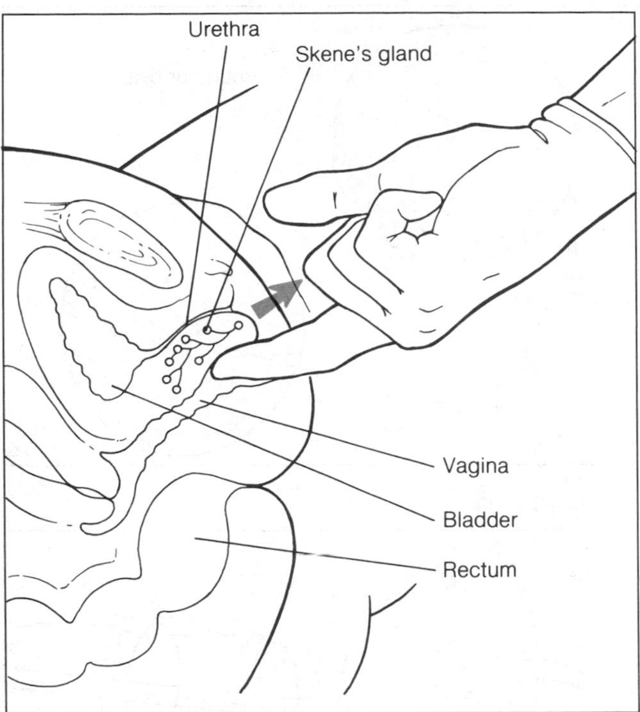

Figure 35–107 Palpating the Skene's glands

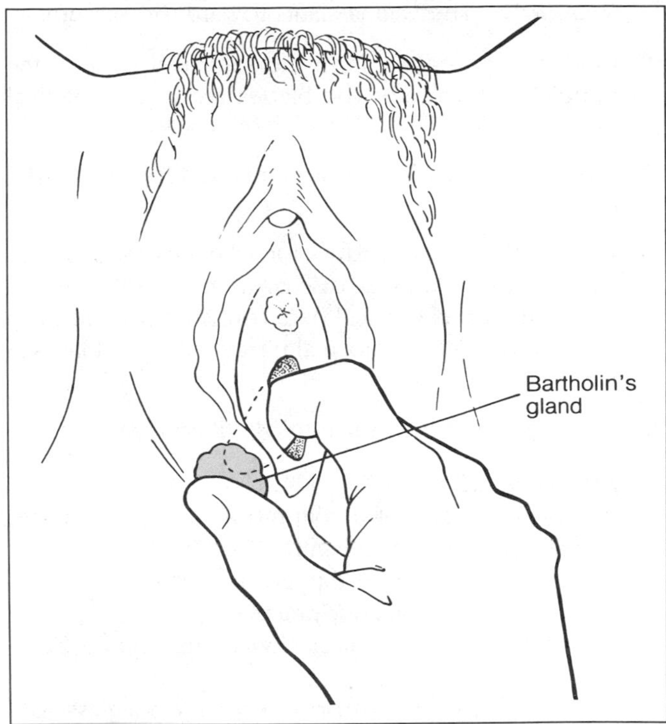

Figure 35–108 Palpating Bartholin's gland

11. Palpate the Skene's (paraurethral) glands at the urethral meatus. These are located on either side of the urethral orifice. They are not normally palpable. See Figure 35–107.
    a. Insert a gloved index finger, palm uppermost, into the entrance of the vagina about 2.5 cm (1 in).
    b. While pressing gently upward, palpate for the Skene's glands, then draw the finger outward.

    Rationale This action will milk the urethra of any discharge.

    c. Observe for any discharge.
12. Palpate the Bartholin's glands, which are normally located on the posterior aspect of the vaginal orifice. See Figure 35–108.
    a. Insert a gloved finger into the entrance of the vagina.
    b. Move the finger to the side and posterior aspect of the vagina.
    c. Palpate against the thumb at the posterior aspect of the labia majora.
    d. Repeat for the other side.

    Rationale The Bartholin's glands are not normally tender or palpable.
13. While the gloved finger is in the vaginal orifice, assess the pelvic musculature.
    a. Ask the client to constrict her vaginal orifice. A nulliparous female will probably have a high degree of muscle tone, while a multiparous female will have less tone.
    b. Ask the client to bear down while the fingers spread the vaginal wall laterally. Observe the vaginal wall for bulges. A **cystocele** is a bulging of the anterior vaginal wall as a result of a prolapse of the anterior wall and the bladder. A **rectocele** is a bulging of the posterior vaginal wall as a result of a prolapse of the posterior wall and the rectum. An **enterocele** is a bulging from the posterior fornix as a result of prolapse of the pouch of Douglas into the vagina.

Vagina and Cervix

Nurses do not perform vaginal examinations in some practice settings.

14. Lubricate the vaginal speculum. Use warm water rather than lubricating jelly if a specimen is to be taken.

    Rationale Lubricants can interfere with cytologic studies.
15. With two fingers just inside the vaginal entrance, press gently down on the posterior wall.
16. Make sure that there is no pubic hair at the vaginal entrance.

    Rationale The hair can get caught in the speculum and be pulled, causing discomfort.
17. Insert the speculum at a 45° angle with slight pressure toward the posterior wall.

Rationale The vagina slants toward the sacrum.

18. Once the speculum is in the vagina, turn it so the handle is down, i.e., the blades are in a horizontal position.
19. Open the blades, locate the cervix, and lock the blades open.
20. Inspect the cervix and os for size, lacerations, erosions, nodules, masses, discharge, and color. The normal nulliparous cervical os is round or oval (see Figure 35–109, *A*), the normal parous os is slitlike (see Figure 35–109, *B*).
21. Acquire a specimen for cytology, if indicated.

    Endocervical smear

    a. Insert the end of a cotton-tipped applicator into the cervical os. See Figure 35–110. The applicator may or may not be dipped first in normal saline, depending on agency practice.
    b. Rotate the applicator clockwise and counterclockwise in the os.
    c. Remove the applicator, and roll it on a glass slide (numbered 1).
    d. Fix the specimen with a fixative spray or solution.

    Cervical scrape

    e. Insert an Ayre spatula with the longer end extending into the cervical os. See Figure 35–111.
    f. Rotate the spatula a full circle.
    g. Place the scrapings on a glass slide (numbered 2).
    h. Fix the specimen with a fixative.

    Vaginal smear

    1. Insert a cotton-tipped applicator to a position below the cervix. See Figure 35–112. The applicator may be dipped in normal saline, particularly if the vaginal mucosa is dry.
    j. Roll the applicator on the vaginal wall below the cervix.
    k. Place the smear on a glass slide (numbered 3).
    l. Fix the specimen with a fixative.

22. Withdraw the speculum slowly while observing the vagina.
23. When the speculum is clear of the cervix, release the screws, and close the speculum as it is withdrawn from the vaginal entrance.
24. Insert your index and middle fingers or just your index finger, gloved and lubricated, into the vagina. Abduct your thumb, and flex your other fingers into the palm of the hand. See Figure 35–113.

    Rationale The number of fingers inserted depends on the size of the vagina.

25. Press the other hand downward about halfway betwen the umbilicus and the symphysis pubis.

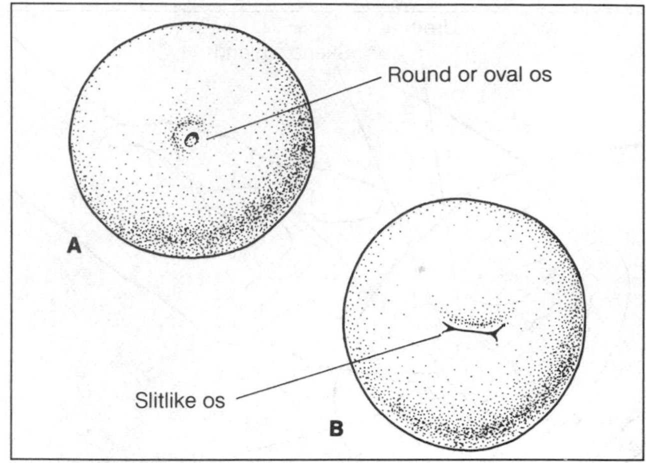

Figure 35–109

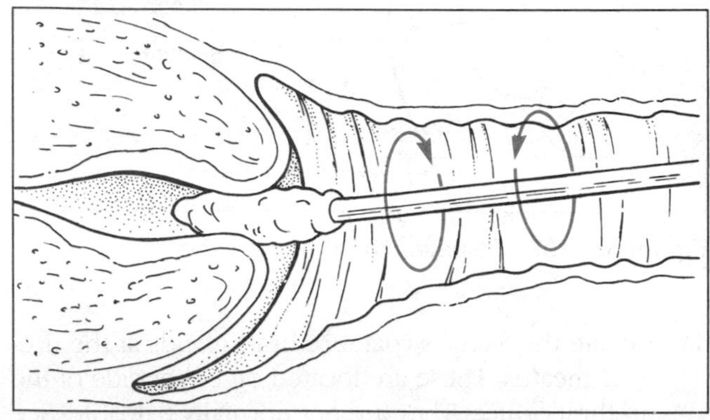

Figure 35–110

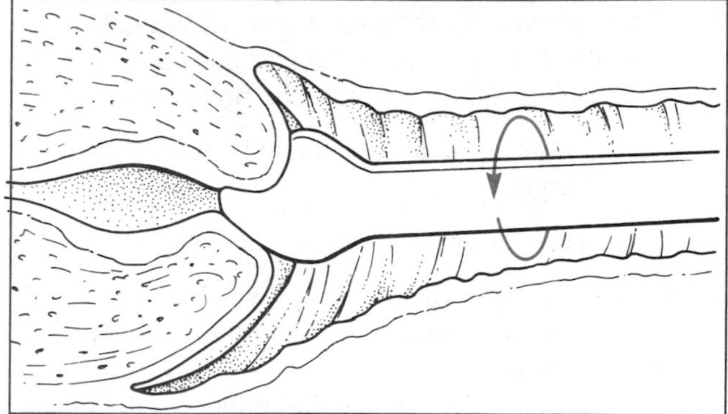

Figure 35–111

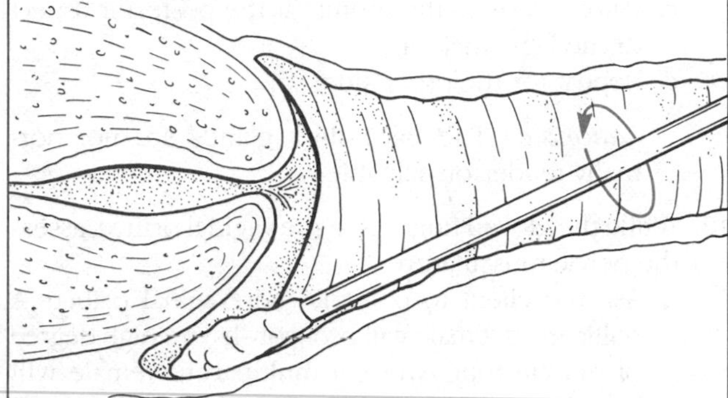

Figure 35–112

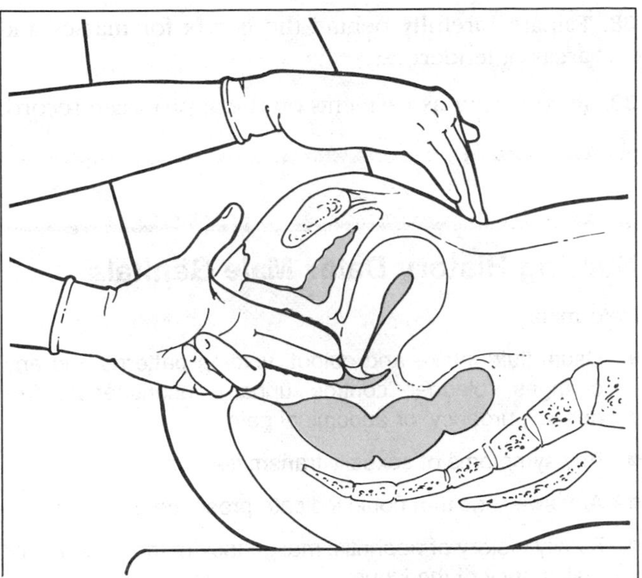

Figure 35–113

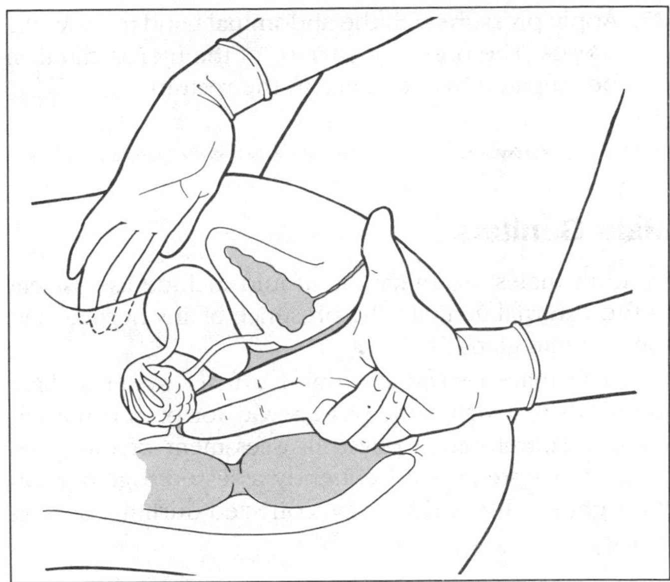

Figure 35–114

Rationale The second hand stabilizes the uterus.

26. Palpate the cervix for smoothness, size, mobility, and tenderness.

Uterus

27. Place the fingers of the hand on either side of the cervix, palm facing upward.

    Rationale This placement of the hand stabilizes the uterus.

28. Press down with the hand on the abdomen and locate the uterus between the two hands.
29. Palpate the uterus for size, shape, consistency, and mobility. Determine if there are any masses or areas of tenderness.

Ovaries

30. Place the fingers in the right lateral fornix (to the right of the cervix). See Figure 35–114.
31. Press the abdominal hand down firmly but gently in the lower right quadrant.
32. Palpate the right ovary between the two hands. The fallopian tube is not normally palpated.
33. Palpate the ovary for size, mobility, shape, consistency, and tenderness. Normally, 5 years after menopause, the ovaries cannot be palpated because of atrophy.
34. Repeat steps 30–33 for the left ovary, with the vaginal hand in the left lateral fornix and the abdominal hand pressed downward in the left lower quadrant.

Rectovaginal-Abdominal Palpation

35. Don clean gloves, and lubricate the index and middle fingers.

    Rationale Clean gloves will prevent cross contamination between the vagina and the rectum.

36. Insert the index finger into the vagina and the middle finger into the rectum. See Figure 35–115. The client may feel that her bowels will move.

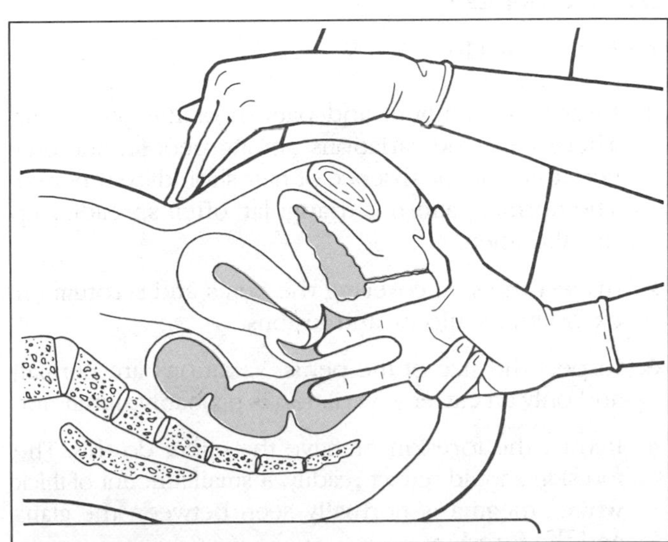

Figure 35–115

37. Apply pressure with the abdominal hand to move the uterus. The posterior surface of the uterus can then be palpated by the finger in the rectum.

38. Palpate carefully behind the cervix for masses and areas of tenderness.

39. Record your assessments on the appropriate record.

Male Genitals

In adult males, examination should include assessment of the external genitals, the presence of any hernias, and the prostate gland.

The male reproductive and urinary systems share the urethra, which is the passageway for both urine and semen. Therefore, in physical assessment of the male, these two systems are frequently assessed together. On the right is a list of data to be collected during a nursing history.

Nursing History Data: Male Genitals

Determine:

- Usual fluid intake and output, voiding patterns and any changes, bladder control, urinary incontinence, frequency, urgency, or abdominal pain
- Any symptoms of sexually transmitted disease
- Any swellings that could indicate presence of hernia
- Family history of nephritis, malignancy of the prostate, or malignancy of the kidney.

Procedure 35–11 ▲ Assessing the Male Genitals

Equipment

1. A flashlight
2. A disposable glove
3. Lubricant

Intervention

See Table 35–21 for normal and abnormal findings.

External Genitals

See Figure 35–116.

1. Inspect the amount and pattern of the pubic hair. There are wide variations among people, and only very thin hair or absence of hair should be reported. The normal pattern is triangular, often spreading up the abdomen.
2. Inspect the skin covering the penis and scrotum for excoriations, ulcers, and lesions.
3. Inspect the size of the penis. Variations are normal, and only an extreme variation is probably significant.
4. Retract the foreskin or have the client do this. The foreskin should retract readily. A small amount of thick white smegma is normally seen between the glans and the foreskin.
5. Palpate the penile shaft for tenderness, thickening, and nodules.
6. Locate the site of the urethral meatus, which is normally at the tip of the penis. Variations in its location are: **hypospadius**, on the underside of the penile shaft, and **epispadius**, on the upper side of the penile shaft.
7. Inspect the urethral meatus and the glans for ulcers, scars, nodules, inflammation, and discharge. Compress the glans slightly to open the urethral meatus

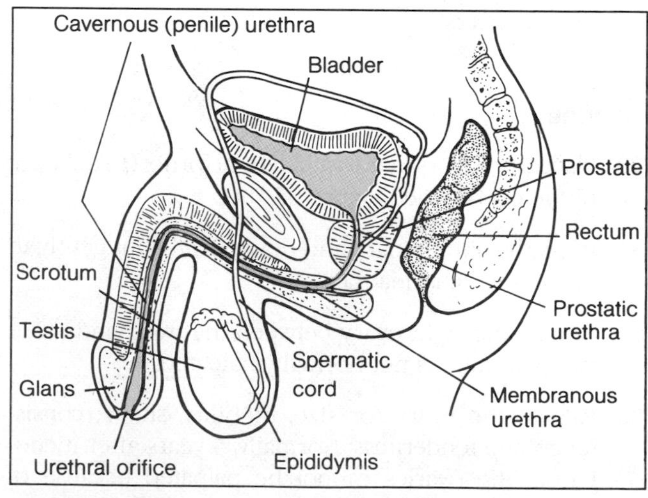

Figure 35–116

Table 35–21 Assessment Data: Male Genitals

Structure	Normal findings	Abnormal findings
Pubic hair	Usually triangular pattern	Scant amount
Skin over penis and scrotum	Intact	Excoriations, ulcers, lesions
Penis	Normal size	Extremely large or small
	Foreskin retracts	Foreskin does not retract
	Absence of tenderness, thickening, or nodules	
	Urethral meatus at tip	Meatus on underside of penis
		Meatus on upper side of penis
	Urethral meatus has no discharge, swelling, ulcers, scars, nodules, or inflammation	Discharge
	No discomfort voiding, good urinary stream	Dysuria, poor or recently changed urinary stream
Scrotum	Skin intact, no inflammation	Ulcers, swellings, excoriations, nodules
	Testicles rubbery, smooth, free of nodules and masses	Testicles enlarged, uneven surface
	Testis about 2 × 4 cm (0.7 × 1.5 in)	Testis has swelling that transilluminates
Epididymis	Tender, softer than the spermatic cord	
Spermatic cord	Firm	
Inguinal and femoral areas	No swellings or bulges	Swelling or bulge
Prostate gland	Size 4 cm (1.5 in) in diameter, firm, rubbery, smooth, movable, with discrete borders	Enlarged, not movable, nodular surface, tender

to inspect it for discharge. If the client has pain on voiding (dysuria) or a poor urinary stream, assess for a urethral stricture or prostatic hyperplasia.

8. Inspect the scrotum for redness, swelling, ulcers, excoriations, or nodules. Lift the scrotum to inspect the posterior aspect.

9. Palpate the scrotum and testicles. Using your index finger and thumb, palpate each testis for size, consistency, shape, smoothness, and masses. The testicle normally feels rubbery and smooth and is free of nodules or masses. Each testis is normally about 2 × 4 cm (0.7 × 1.5 in).

10. Palpate the epididymis between your thumb and index finger. It is located at the top of the testis and extends behind it. The epididymis is normally tender.

11. Palpate the spermatic cord between thumb and index finger. It is usually found at the top lateral portion of the scrotum and feels harder than the epididymis.

12. Inspect any swelling of the scrotum by transillumination.
    a. Darken the room.
    b. Shine the flashlight from behind the scrotum through the mass. Serous fluid causes the light to show with a red glow; tissue or blood does not transilluminate.

Hernias

13. Inspect the inguinal and femoral areas for swellings. See Figure 35–117.

14. Palpate for an inguinal hernia.
    a. Ask the client to stand, with the leg on the side to be examined slightly flexed.
    b. Using your right hand for the client's right side or left hand for the client's left side, insert your index finger into the loose scrotal skin.
    c. Advance your finger up to the external inguinal ring. See Figure 35–118.

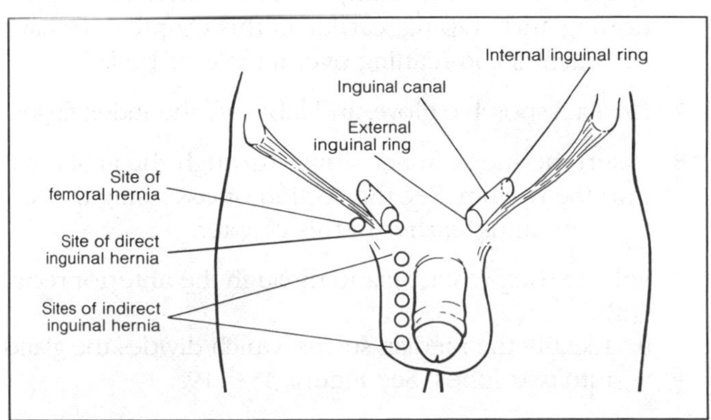

Figure 35–117 Site of hernias

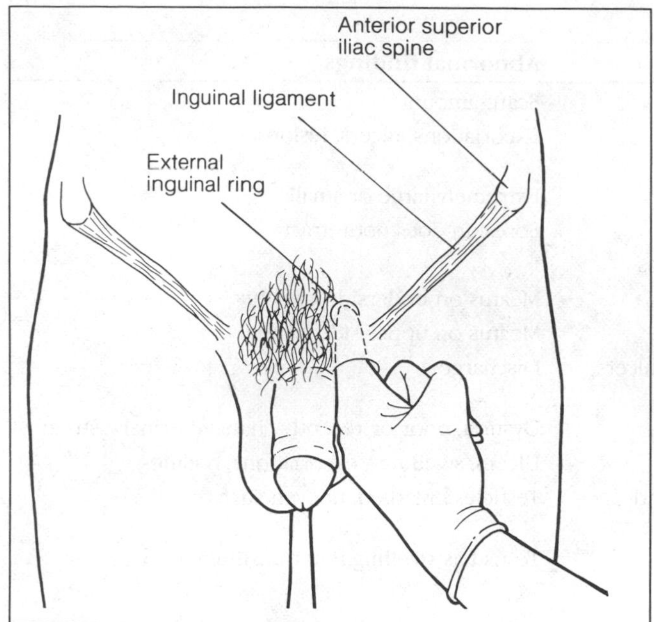

Figure 35–118

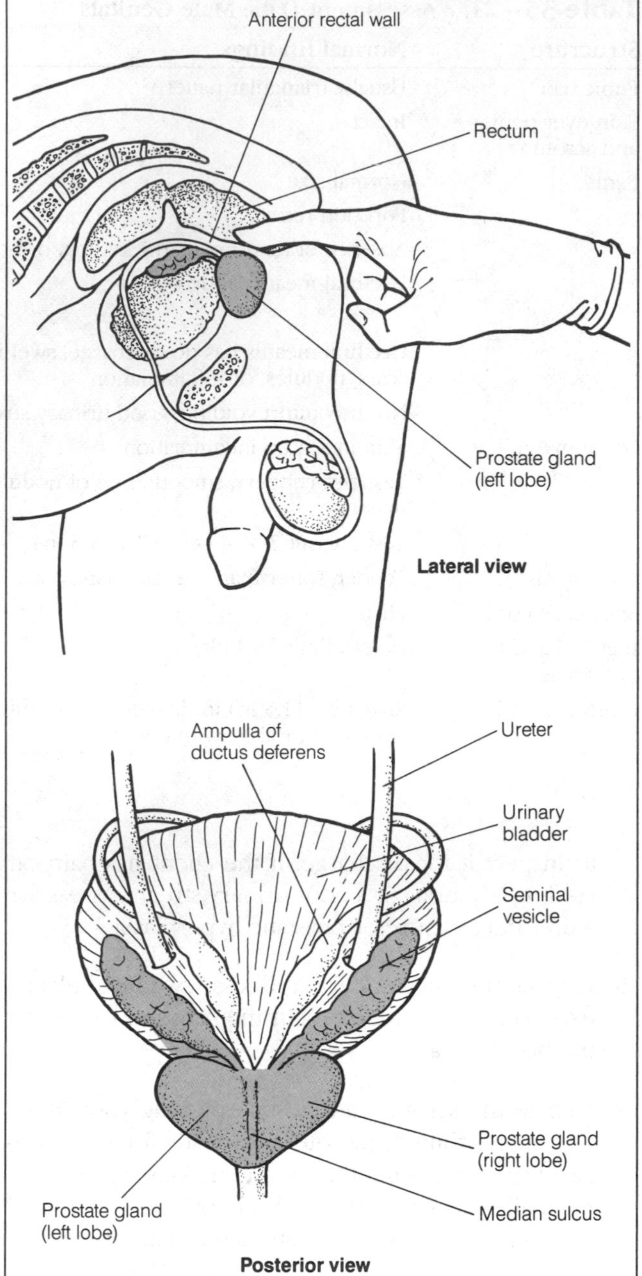

Figure 35–119

d. If the ring is enlarged, extend your finger through the ring.
e. Ask the client to bear down or cough; an inguinal hernia may touch your finger.

15. Palpate the anterior thigh in the area of the femoral canal for a femoral hernia.
    a. Ask the client to cough or strain during palpation.
    b. Note any bulging, swelling, or tenderness in the area.
    c. Ask the client to lie down. Often a hernia returns to the abdomen.

Prostate Gland

Nurses do not perform rectal examination of the prostate gland in some practice settings.

16. Assist the client to a lateral or Sims' position, and drape him appropriately (see the section on positioning and draping, earlier in this chapter), or have the client stand leaning over a table or bed.
17. Don a disposable glove, and lubricate the index finger.
18. Insert the index finger slowly through the anal canal into the rectum. See the section on assessing the rectum and anus, earlier in this chapter.
19. Palpate the prostate gland through the anterior rectal wall.
    a. Identify the median sulcus, which divides the gland into two lobes. See Figure 35–119.
    b. Palpate the prostate for size, consistency, smoothness, mobility, and discrete borders. The prostate is normally firm and rubbery, about 4 cm (1.5 in) in diameter, smooth, with discrete borders, movable, and not tender.
20. Record your findings on the appropriate record.

Musculoskeletal System

The musculoskeletal system encompasses the muscles, bones, and joints. The completeness of an assessment of this system depends largely on the needs and problems of the individual client.

The nurse assesses the musculoskeletal system for muscle strength, tone, and size and symmetry of muscle development. Bones are assessed for normalcy of form. Joints are assessed for tenderness, swelling, thickening, crepitation, presence of nodules, and range of motion. Body posture is assessed for normalcy in standing and sitting positions. For information about body posture see Chapter 38. Nursing history data taken in conjunction with musculoskeletal assessment are shown on this page.

Muscles

Inspect the muscles for size. Compare the muscle on one side of the body, e.g., arm, thigh, calf, to the same muscle on the other side. Determine if there is any atrophy or hypertrophy. **Atrophy** is a decrease in size or wasting away. **Hypertrophy** is an increase in size. If there appears to be a discrepancy between the sides, measure the muscles with a tape.

Observe muscles and tendons for contractures. These can be indicated by malposition of a body part, e.g., a foot fixed in dorsiflexion. Also, observe muscles for fasciculations and tremors. A **fasciculation** is an abnormal contraction (shortening) of a bundle of muscle fibers. A **tremor** is an involuntary trembling of a limb or body part. Tremors may involve large groups of muscle fibers or small bundles of muscle fibers. An **intention tremor** becomes more apparent when an individual attempts a voluntary movement, e.g., holding a cup of coffee. A **resting tremor** is more apparent when the client is at rest and diminishes with activity.

Inspect any tremors of the hands and arms by having the client hold his or her arms out in front of the body. Palpate muscles at rest to determine muscle tonicity. Muscle **tonicity** is the normal condition of tension (tone) of a muscle at rest. Muscles are normally firm. Palpate muscles while the client is active and passive (see Chapter 19) for flaccidity, spasticity, and smoothness of movement. **Flaccidity** is weakness or laxness. **Spasticity** is a sudden involuntary muscle contraction.

Tests for muscle strength are shown in Table 35–22. Compare the right side with the left side. See Figure 35–120. An individual normally has equal strength on each body side. Muscle strength is graded from zero (complete paralysis) to five (normal). See Table 35–23.

Bones

Inspect the skeleton for normal structure and deformities. See Chapter 38 for information about body alignment. Palpate the bones to locate any areas of edema or tenderness. The client's facial or verbal expressions are good indicators of discomfort. Tenderness can reflect such conditions as fractures, neoplasms, and osteoporosis. Then inspect the bones for bruising and swelling, which can indicate fractures.

Joints

A joint is the functional unit of the musculoskeletal system. It is where the bones of the skeleton articulate. Most of the skeletal muscles attach to the two bones at the joint. These muscles are categorized according to the type of joint movement they produce upon contraction. Muscles are therefore called flexors, extensors, internal rotators, etc. The flexor muscles are stronger than the extensor muscles. Thus, when a person is inactive, the joints are pulled into a flexed (bent) position. If this is not counteracted with exercise and position changes, permanent

---

Nursing History Data: Musculoskeletal System

Determine:

- Family history of arthritis (type), gout, congenital defects, cardiovascular or neurologic disorders, cancer.
- Previous history of musculoskeletal problems, e.g., fractures, muscle strains or sprains, joint swelling, sports or other injuries, muscle weakness.
- History of current pain or loss of function. If pain exists, ask: When did the pain occur? What precipitated it? Exactly where is the pain? (Does it radiate?) What is the nature of the pain? (Aching, burning, sharp, stabbing, throbbing, or other?) Does the pain come and go, or is it constant? What makes the pain increase? What relieves or aggravates the pain? How does it affect your daily activities?
- Loss of function. If there is loss, ask: When did it occur? What precipitated it? What is the extent of it? How does it affect your daily activities?
- Associated phenomena such as headache, fever, weakness, numbness, tingling, redness and/or swelling of joints, and weight loss.

Table 35–22 Testing Muscle Strength

Muscle	Client/examiner activity
Deltoid	Client holds arm up and resists while examiner tries to push it down.
Biceps	Client fully extends each arm and then tries to flex it while examiner attempts to hold arm in extension.
Triceps	Client flexes each arm and then tries to extend it against the examiner's attempt to keep arm in flexion.
Wrist and finger muscles	Client spreads the fingers and then resists as examiner attempts to push the fingers together.
Grip strength	Client grasps the index and middle fingers of the examiner while the examiner tries to pull the fingers out.
Hip muscles	Client is supine, both legs extended; client raises one leg at a time while the examiner attempts to hold it down.
Hip abduction	Client is supine, both legs extended. Examiner's hands are on the lateral surface of each knee; client is asked to spread the legs apart against the examiner's resistance.
Hip adduction	Client is in same position as for hip abduction; the examiner's hands are now placed between the knees; client is asked to bring the legs together against the examiner's resistance.
Hamstrings	Client is supine with both knees bent. Client resists while examiner attempts to straighten them.
Quadriceps	Client is supine with knee partially extended; client resists while examiner attempts to flex the knee.
Muscles of the ankles and feet	Client resists while examiner attempts to dorsiflex the foot and again resists while examiner attempts to flex the foot.

Source: From C. R. Kneisl and S. W. Ames, *Adult health nursing: A biopsychosocial approach* (Menlo Park, Calif.: Addison-Wesley Publishing Co., 1986), p. 174. Reprinted with permission.

shortening of the muscles develops, and the joint becomes fixed in a flexed position.

Inspect each joint for swelling, which might indicate arthritis. Palpate each joint for tenderness, smoothness of movement, swelling, **crepitation** (a crackling, grating sound), and the presence of nodules. Normally, joints are not tender, move smoothly, and have no swelling, crepitation, or nodules.

Establish the range of motion of the body joints, as needed. The range of motion of a joint is the maximum movement that joint allows. Each person's range of motion is determined by genetic makeup, developmental patterns, the presence or absence of disease, and that person's degree of physical activity. Table 35–24 gives the types of joint movements. The types of synovial joints are described in Chapter 37, page 967.

When assessing joint movement, ask the client to move selected body parts as shown in Table 35–25. The amount of movement can be measured by a **goniometer**, a device that measures the angle of the joint in degrees. See Figure 35–121.

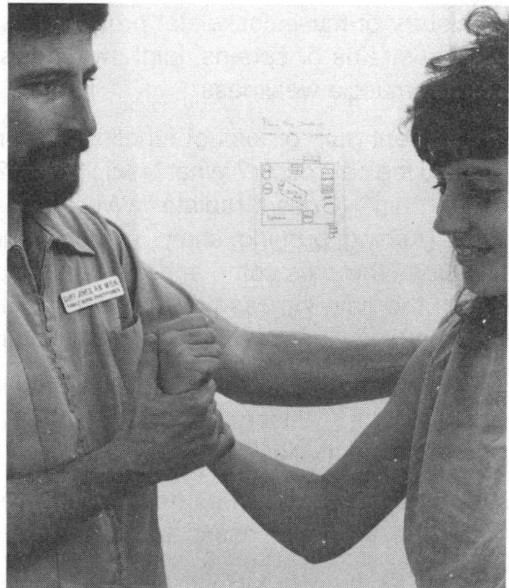

Figure 35–120 Testing muscle strength by providing resistance

Table 35–23 Grading Muscle Strength

Scale	Percentage of normal strength	Characteristics
0	0	Complete paralysis
1	10	No movement
		Contraction of muscle is palpable or visible
2	25	Full muscle movement against gravity, with support
3	50	Normal movement against gravity
4	75	Normal full movement against gravity and against minimal resistance
5	100	Normal strength
		Normal full movement against gravity and against full resistance

Table 35–24 Types of Synovial Joint Movements

Movement	Action
Flexion	Decreasing the angle of the joint (e.g., bending the elbow)
Extension	Increasing the angle of the joint (e.g., straightening the arm at the elbow)
Hyperextension	Further extension or straightening of a joint (e.g., bending the head backward)
Abduction	Movement of the bone away from the midline of the body
Adduction	Movement of the bone toward the midline of the body
Rotation	Movement of the bone around its central axis
Circumduction	Movement of the distal part of the bone in a circle while the proximal end remains fixed
Eversion	Turning the sole of the foot outward by moving the ankle joint
Inversion	Turning the sole of the foot inward by moving the ankle joint
Pronation	Moving the bones of the forearm so that the palm of the hand faces downward when held in front of the body
Supination	Moving the bones of the forearm so that the palm of the hand faces upward when held in front of the body
Protraction	Moving a part of the body forward in the same plane parallel to the ground
Retraction	Moving a part of the body backward in the same plane parallel to the ground

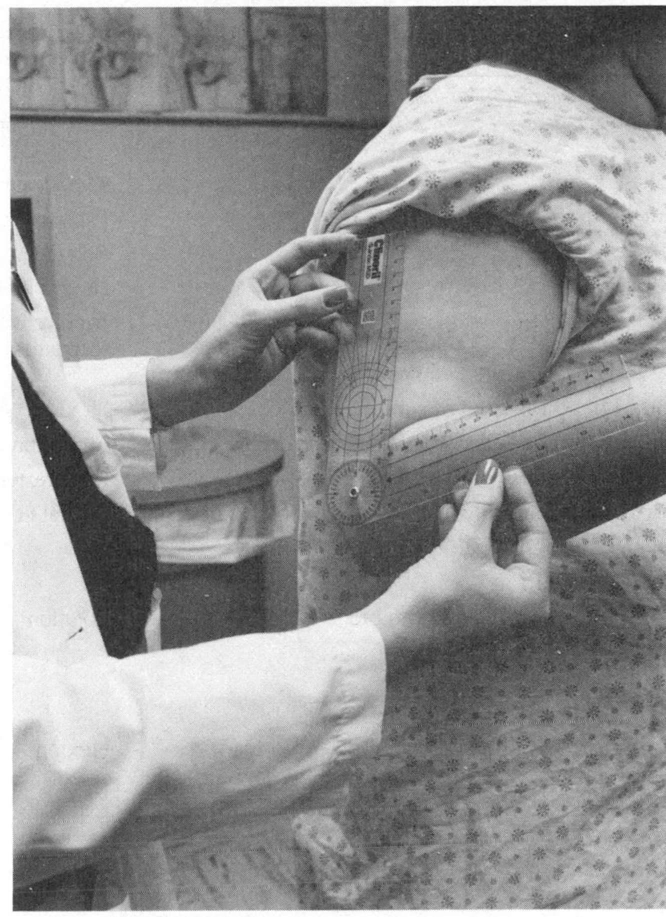

Figure 35–121 A goniometer used to measure joint range of motion

Neurologic System

The nervous system integrates all other body systems, but it is also dependent upon the appropriate functioning of peripheral organs from which it receives internal and external environmental stimuli. A thorough neurologic examination may take 1 to 3 hours; however, routine screening tests are usually done first, and if the result of these tests are questionable, then more extensive evaluations are made. Three major considerations determine the extent of a neurologic exam: (a) the client's chief complaints, (b) the client's physical condition (e.g., level of consciousness and ability to ambulate), since many parts of the exam require movement and coordination of the extremities, and (c) the client's willingness to participate and cooperate.

Examination of the neurologic system includes assessment of the cranial nerves, the proprioception and cerebellar function, the motor system, the sensory system, reflexes, mental status, and levels of consciousness. Nursing history data are shown on page 882.

Cranial Nerves

Assessment of the functions of the 12 pairs of cranial nerves is included to a large degree in an examination of the head and neck. A neurologist usually conducts specific examinations of these nerves, if needed; however, the routine neurologic assessment of a basic physical examination includes assessment of some of them. For the specific functions and assessment methods of each cranial nerve, see Table 35–26. The nurse needs to be aware of these functions to detect abnormalities. (The names and order of the cranial nerves can be recalled by remembering this sentence: "On old Olympus's treeless top, a Finn and German viewed a hop." The first letter of each word in the phrase is the same as the first letter of the names of the cranial nerves.)

The sense of smell (cranial nerve I) and the sense of taste (cranial nerves VII and IX) are not routinely tested. Vision and eye movements have been previously dis-

Table 35–25 Joint Movement

Instruction*	Movement	Normal range
Temporomandibular joint (TMJ)		
Open mouth.	TMJ opening	3 to 6 cm (1 to 2.3 in)
Close mouth.	TMJ closure	Complete closure
Jut out jaw.	Protrusion	
Tuck chin in.	Retrusion	
Move jaw from side to side.	Lateral motion	Distance 1 to 2 cm from midline
Sternoclavicular joint	Involved in shoulder movement	
Neck joint		
Bend head forward so chin rests on chest.	Flexion	45° from midline
Move head back to upright position.	Extension	45° from flexed position
Move head backward as far as possible.	Hyperextension	10° from upright position
Move head laterally as if to lay ear on shoulder:	Lateral flexion	
■ to the right		40° from midline
■ to the left		40° from midline
Turn head to as far as possible:	Rotation	
■ to the right		70° from midline
■ to the left		70° from midline
Shoulder joint		
Raise arm from position by side of body forward and upward to beside head.	Flexion	180° from side of body
Lower arm from beside head forward to side of body.	Extension	180° from vertical position beside head
Move arm from side of body backward behind body.	Hyperextension	50° from side position
Move arm laterally from side position to above head, palm facing outermost	Abduction	180° from side position.
Move arm from beside head to the side and in front of body as far as possible.	Anterior abduction	230°
Move arm from beside head to the side and then behind body as far as possible	Posterior abduction	230°
Hold arm in front of body at shoulder height then move across front of body as far as possible.	Horizontal flexion	130 to 135°
Hold arm to the side at shoulder height and move behind body as far as possible.	Horizontal extension	45°
Move each arm in a full circle: forward, up, back, and down.	Circumduction	360°
Hold arm to the side at shoulder level, elbow bent and fingers pointing downward. Move arm so fingers point upward.	External rotation	90°
Hold arm to the side at shoulder level, elbow bent, fingers pointing upward. Bring arm forward and down so fingers point downward.	Internal rotation	90°
Repeat all motions, using other arm.		
Elbow joint		
Bring lower arm forward and upward toward shoulder.	Flexion	150°
Bring lower arm forward and downward, straightening arm.	Extension	150°
Move lower arm backward from the straightened position.	Hyperextension	0 to 15°
Holding arm in front of the body, elbow bent, turn each hand and forearm so that palm faces upward.	Supination	70 to 90°

Table 35–25 *(continued)*

Instruction*	Movement	Normal range
Holding arm in front of body, elbow bent, turn hand so that palm faces downward.	Pronation	70 to 90°
Repeat all motions, using other arm.		
Wrist joint		
Bring fingers of hand toward inner part of forearm	Flexion	80 to 90°
Straighten wrist from flexed position.	Extension	80 to 90°
Bend finger of hand backward as far as wrist permits.	Hyperextension	70 to 90°
Bend wrist to the thumb side while palm faces upward.	Radial flexion (abduction)	0 to 20°
Bend wrist toward the fifth finger side while palm faces upward.	Ulnar flexion, Adduction	30 to 50°
Repeat all motions, using other hand.		
Hand and finger joints		
Make a fist of one hand.	Flexion	90°
Straighten fingers of one hand.	Extension	90°
Bend fingers of hand back as far as possible	Hyperextension	30°
Spread fingers of one hand apart as far as possible.	Abduction	20°
Bring fingers together from abducted position.	Adduction	20°
Repeat all motions, using other hand and fingers.		
Thumb joint		
Move thumb across the palm of hand toward fifth finger.	Flexion	90°
With palm uppermost, move thumb away from palm toward self.	Extension	90°
Move thumb as far as possible to the side.	Abduction	30°
Move thumb from abducted position toward hand.	Adduction	30°
Touch the tip of each finger with thumb of same hand.	Opposition	
Repeat all motions, using other thumb.		
Hip joint		
Move leg forward with knee:	Flexion	
■ straight		90°
■ bent		120°
Move leg from flexed position back to other leg.	Extension	90 to 120°
Move leg back behind the body.	Hyperextension	30 to 50°
Move leg out to the side as far as possible.	Abduction	45 to 50°
Move leg from abducted position back to other leg and in front of it as far as possible.	Adduction	20 to 30° beyond second leg
Move leg backward, up, to the side, and down, making a circle.	Circumduction	360°
Turn foot and leg inward toward other leg as far as possible.	Internal rotation	90°
Turn foot and leg outward from other leg as far as possible.	External rotation	90°
Repeat all motions, using other leg.		
Knee joint		
Bend leg as far as possible bringing heel toward back of thigh.	Flexion	120 to 130°
Straighten leg from flexed position.	Extension	12 to 130°

(continued)

Table 35–25 *(continued)*

Instruction*	Movement	Normal range
Straighten knee beyond extended position	Hyperextension	0 to 10°
Repeat all motions, using other knee.		
Ankle joint		
Point toes of foot downward as far as possible.	Extension (plantar flexion)	45 to 50°
From normal ankle position point toes of foot upward as far as possible.	Flexion (dorsiflexion)	20°
Repeat both motions, using other ankle.		
Foot and toe joints		
Turn sole of foot to the side as far as possible.	Eversion	5°
Turn sole of foot from normal position toward other foot.	Inversion	5°
Curve toes downward.	Flexion	35 to 65°
Straighten toes.	Extension	35 to 65°
Spread toes apart as far as possible.	Abduction	0 to 15°
Bring toes together from abducted position.	Adduction	0 to 15°
Repeat all motions, using other foot.		
Vertebral joints		
Bend trunk toward toes.	Flexion	70 to 90°
Straighten trunk from flexed position.	Extension	70 to 90°
Bend trunk backward as far as possible.	Hyperextension	20 to 30°
Bend trunk to the right side as far as possible and then to the left side.	Lateral flexion	35° from the midline to each side
Turn the upper part of body as far as possible to the right and then to the left.	Rotation	30 to 45° from the midline to each side

*For illustrations of each movement and the muscles involved, see Chapter 37.

Nursing History Data: Neurologic System

Determine:

- History of loss of consciousness, convulsions, fainting, tingling or numbness, tremors or tics, clumsiness, paralysis, limps, loss of memory, speech impairments, disorientation, mood swings, nervousness, anxiety, phobias, or depression
- Onset of above symptoms, cause, treatment, and outcomes of the treatment
- Current signs of the above
- Changes in vision, hearing, smell, taste, or touch
- Current symptoms, e.g., numbness and tingling, paresthesia, dizziness, falling, uncontrolled muscle movements, tics, tremors, or speech changes
- Decrease in memory
- Muscle weakness or paralysis

cussed; these activities involve cranial nerves II, III, IV, and VI. The cranial nerves V (trigeminal) and VII (facial) are not routinely tested other than by observing facial expression and the symmetry of the face, both moving and at rest. Any facial weakness may be made more obvious by having the client close the eyes tightly, wrinkle the forehead, and show the teeth. Only the cochlear branch of nerve VIII, responsible for hearing ability, is routinely tested. The vestibular branch of nerve VIII is concerned with balance and is tested with cerebellar functions. Swallowing, the gag reflex, tongue movement, and phonation, which involve cranial nerves IX, X, and XII, are routinely tested in the examination of the mouth. Nerves IX and X are tested together. Each side of the pharynx is touched with a tongue blade, which normally elicits the gag reflex (contraction of the pharyngeal muscles). Another test is to have the client say "ah." The soft palate normally moves; imperfect movement suggests difficulty with nerves IX and X. Nerve XII (hypoglossal) can be readily examined by having the client protrude the tongue as far as possible. Deviation of the tongue toward either side suggests paralysis. Cranial nerve XI (accessory), which is the motor nerve of the sternocleidomastoid muscle, can be tested

Table 35–26 Cranial Nerve Functions and Assessment Methods

Cranial nerve	Name	Type	Function	Assessment methods
I	Olfactory	Sensory	Smell	Ask client to close eyes and identify different mild aromas, such as coffee, tobacco, vanilla, oil of cloves, peanut butter, orange, lemon, lime, chocolate.
II	Optic	Sensory	Vision and visual fields	Ask client to read Snellen chart; check visual fields by confrontation; and conduct an ophthalmoscopic examination (see pages 825 to 828).
III	Oculomotor	Motor	Extraocular eye movement (EOM); movement of sphincter of pupil; movement of ciliary muscles of lens	Assess directions of gaze and pupil reaction (see pages 821 and 825).
IV	Trochlear	Motor	EOM, specifically moves eyeball downward and laterally	Assess directions of gaze.
V	Trigeminal			
	Ophthalmic branch	Sensory	Sensation of cornea, skin of face, and nasal mucosa	While client looks upward, lightly touch lateral sclera of eye to elicit blink reflex; to test light sensation, have client close eyes, wipe a wisp of cotton over client's forehead and paranasal sinuses; to test deep sensation, use alternating blunt and sharp ends of a safety pin over same areas.
	Maxillary branch	Sensory	Sensation of skin of face and anterior oral cavity (tongue and teeth)	Assess skin sensation as for ophthalmic branch above.
	Mandibular branch	Motor and sensory	Muscles of mastication; sensation of skin of face	Ask client to clench teeth.
VI	Abducens	Motor	EOM; moves eyeball laterally	Assess directions of gaze.
VII	Facial	Motor and sensory	Facial expression; taste (anterior two thirds of tongue)	Ask client to smile, raise the eyebrows, frown, puff out cheeks, close eyes tightly; ask client to identify various tastes placed on tip and sides of tongue: sugar (sweet), salt, lemon juice (sour), and quinine (bitter); identify areas of taste.
VIII	Auditory			
	Vestibular branch	Sensory	Equilibrium	Assessment methods are discussed with cerebellar functions (in next section).
	Cochlear branch	Sensory	Hearing	Assess client's ability to hear spoken word and vibrations of tuning fork (see page 833).
IX	Glossopharyngeal	Motor and sensory	Swallowing ability and gag reflex, tongue movement, taste (posterior tongue)	Use tongue blade on posterior tongue while client says "ah" to elicit gag

(continued)

Table 35–26 *(continued)*

Cranial nerve	Name	Type	Function	Assessment methods
				reflex; apply tastes on posterior tongue for identification; ask client to move tongue from side to side and up and down.
X	Vagus	Motor and sensory	Sensation of pharynx and larynx; swallowing; vocal cord movement	Assessed with cranial nerve IX; assess client's speech for hoarseness.
XI	Accessory	Motor	Head movement; shrugging of shoulders	Ask client to shrug shoulders against resistance from your hands and turn head to side against resistance from your hand (repeat for other side).
XII	Hypoglossal	Motor	Protrusion of tongue	Ask client to protrude tongue at midline, then move it side to side.

by having the client attempt to shrug the shoulders while the nurse presses down on them with the hands. Any weakness is noted.

Proprioception and Cerebellar Function

Examination of proprioception and cerebellar function includes assessment of the proprioceptive system. Structures involved in proprioception are the proprioceptors, the posterior columns of the spinal cord, the cerebellum, and the vestibular apparatus (which is innervated by cranial nerve VIII) in the labyrinth of the internal ear.

Proprioceptors are sensory nerve terminals, occurring chiefly in the muscles, tendons, joints, and the internal ear, that give information about movements and position of the body. Stimuli from the proprioceptors travel through the posterior columns of the spinal cord. Deficits of function of the posterior columns of the spinal cord result in impairment of muscle and position sense. A client with such an impairment often must watch his or her own arm and leg movements to ascertain the position of the limbs. The posterior columns also carry nerve fibers for tactile discrimination.

The cerebellum performs three general functions below the level of consciousness:

1. It helps to control posture.
2. It acts with the cerebral cortex to produce skilled movements by coordinating the activities of groups of muscles. It therefore makes body movements smooth, steady, efficient, and coordinated instead of jerky, trembling, ineffective, awkward, and uncoordinated.
3. It controls skeletal muscles to maintain equilibrium. Afferent (sensory) impulses from the vestibular apparatus of the labyrinth of the ear travel to the cerebellum, where connections are made with the proper efferent (motor) fibers for contraction of the necessary muscles to maintain bodily equilibrium. Vestibular dysfunction is characterized by vertigo, nausea, and vomiting.

Cerebellar disorders cause certain characteristics and common symptoms: **ataxia**, impairment of position sense, lack of muscle coordination, hypotonia, tremors, disturbance of equilibrium, disturbance in the timing of movements, and disturbance of gait. An example of ataxia is overshooting a mark or stopping before reaching it when trying to touch a given point on the body. Tremors are especially pronounced toward the end of movements. Clients with cerebellar disease also have difficulty performing rapid skilled movements, alternating movements such as supinating and pronating the arms or hands, and starting and stopping motions and replacing them with a movement in the opposite direction. The cerebellar gait, although it may vary, is commonly characterized by a wide base of support; a rigid head, trunk, and arms; lurching or staggering; legs bending at the hips; arm movements not coordinated with stride; a clumsy manner of raising the foot too high and bringing it down with a clap; and frequent falling. Paralysis does not occur with cerebellar disorders.

Gross Motor and Balance Tests

There are several gross motor function and balance tests. The nurse needs to use only two of the following tests:

1. Have the client walk across the room and back, and assess his or her gait.
2. Romberg test: Ask the client to stand with feet together and arms resting at the sides, first with eyes open, then closed. Stand close during this test to prevent the client from falling. A positive **Romberg's sign** is indicated by excessive swaying or an inability to maintain the stance

without widening the foot base (with eyes open or shut). If the client has trouble maintaining his or her balance with the eyes shut, he or she has a loss of position sense referred to as sensory ataxia. If balance cannot be maintained whether the eyes are open or shut, the condition is referred to as cerebellar ataxia.

3. Have the client close his or her eyes and stand on one foot and then the other.
4. Ask the client to walk a straight line, placing the heel of one foot directly in front of the toes of the other foot.
5. Have the client walk several steps on the toes and then on the heels.
6. Instruct the client to hop in place on one foot and then the other. A certain amount of muscle strength is required for this test and is not indicated for a frail or elderly client.
7. Ask the client to stretch the arms forward (in front of the body at shoulder level) and then do several knee bends. This test also requires muscle strength and is not indicated for weak clients. See Table 35–27 for normal and abnormal findings.

Table 35–27 Assessment Data: Proprioception and Cerebellum

Test	Normal findings	Abnormal findings
	Gross motor function and balance	
Walking gait	Has upright posture and steady gait with opposing arm swing; walks unaided maintaining balance	Has poor posture and unsteady, irregular, staggering gait with wide stance; bends legs only from hips; has rigid or no arm movements
Romberg test	May sway slightly but is able to maintain upright posture and foot stance	Cannot maintain foot stance; moves the feet apart to maintain stance
Standing on one foot with eyes closed	Maintains stance for at least 5 seconds	Cannot maintain stance for 5 seconds
Heel-toe walking	Maintains heel-toe walking along a straight line	Assumes a wider foot gait to stay upright
Toe or heel walking	Able to walk several steps on toes or heels	Cannot maintain balance on toes or heels
Hopping in place	Has adequate muscle strength to hop on one foot	Cannot hop or maintain single leg balance
Knee bends	Has adequate balance and muscle strength to perform knee bends	Does not have adequate balance or muscle strength to perform knee bends
	Fine motor function: upper extremities	
Finger-to-nose test	Repeatedly and rhythmically touches the nose	Misses the nose or gives lazy response
Alternating supination and pronation of hands on knees	Can alternately supinate and pronate hands at rapid pace	Performs with slow, clumsy movements and irregular timing, has difficulty alternating from supination to pronation
Finger to nose and to examiner's finger	Performs with coordination and rapidity	Misses the finger and moves slowly
Fingers to fingers	As above	Moves slowly and is unable to touch fingers consistently
Fingers to thumb (same hand)	Rapidly touches each finger to thumb with each hand	Cannot coordinate this fine discrete movement with either one or both hands
Patting and polishing the examiner's hand	Performs these maneuvers smoothly and rapidly	Performs with clumsy movements and irregular timing
	Fine motor function: lower extremities	
Heel down opposite shin	Demonstrates bilateral equal coordination	Has tremors, is awkward, heel moves off shin
Toe or ball of foot to examiner's finger	Moves smoothly, with coordination	Misses the examiner's finger, is unable to coordinate movement
Figure-eight	Can perform this test	Unable to perform the test

Fine Motor Tests for the Upper Extremities

Only two of the following tests are needed to screen for fine motor function of the upper extremities. The client may be seated for these tests. Have the client:

1. Abduct and extend the arms at shoulder height and rapidly touch the nose alternately with one index finger and then the other. The client repeats the test with the eyes closed if the test is performed easily. In abnormal responses, the client misses the nose and may bring the finger beyond the nose (past-pointing). See Figure 35–122.
2. Alternately pat both knees with the palms of both hands and then with the backs of the hands at an ever-increasing rate. See Figure 35–123.
3. Touch his or her nose and then the nurse's index finger, held at a distance of about 45 cm (18 in), at a rapid and increasing rate.
4. Spread the arms broadly at shoulder height and then bring the fingers together at the midline, first with the eyes open and then closed, first slowly and then rapidly.
5. Touch each finger of one hand to the thumb of the same hand as rapidly as possible. See Figure 35–124.
6. Pat the back of the nurse's hand with increasing speed; then use a circular motion on the back of the examiner's hand with increasing speed.

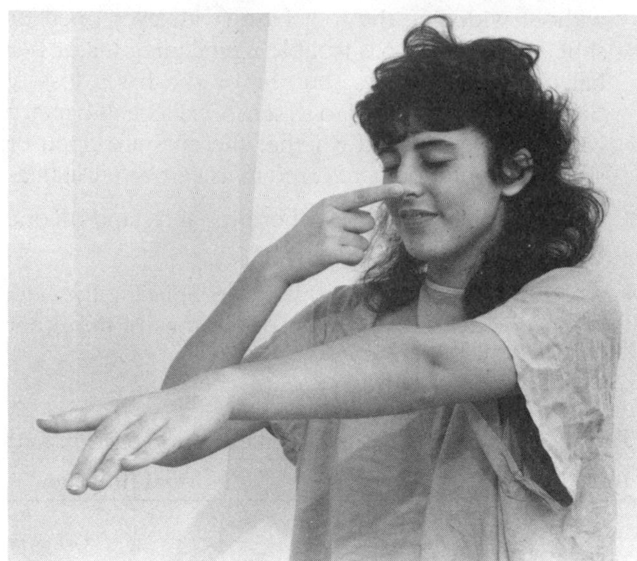

Figure 35–122 A test of fine motor coordination: touching the nose

Fine Motor Tests for the Lower Extremities

Only two of the following tests are needed to screen for fine motor function of the lower extremities. Have the client lie supine and:

1. Place the heel of one foot just below the opposite knee and run the heel down the shin to the foot. Repeat with the other foot. See Figure 35–125. (The client may also use a sitting position for this test.)
2. Touch the nurse's finger with the large toe of each foot. See Figure 35–126.
3. Touch the nurse's finger with the ball of each foot.
4. Draw a figure-eight in the air.

Motor Function

Assessment of muscle size, strength, and tone and of involuntary movements are discussed on page 879.

Sensory Function

Sensory functions include touch, pain, vibration, position, temperature, and tactile discrimination. The first three are routinely tested in a few locations. Vibration is tested

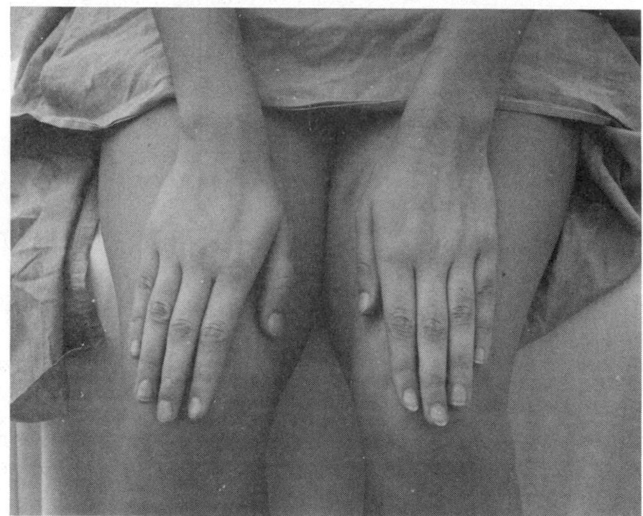

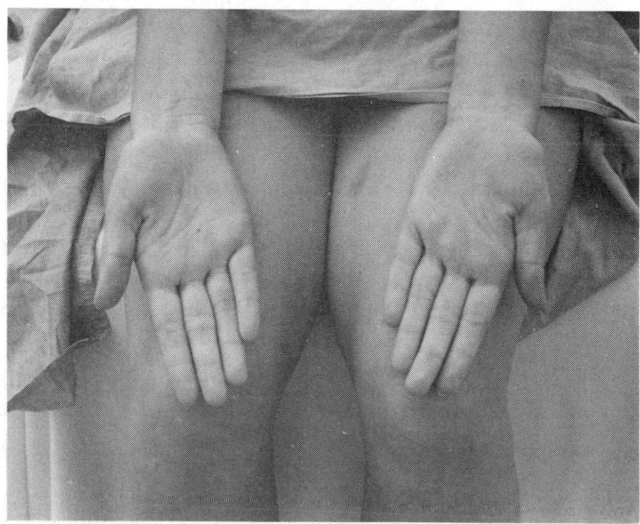

Figure 35–123 A test of fine motor coordination: supinating and pronating hands

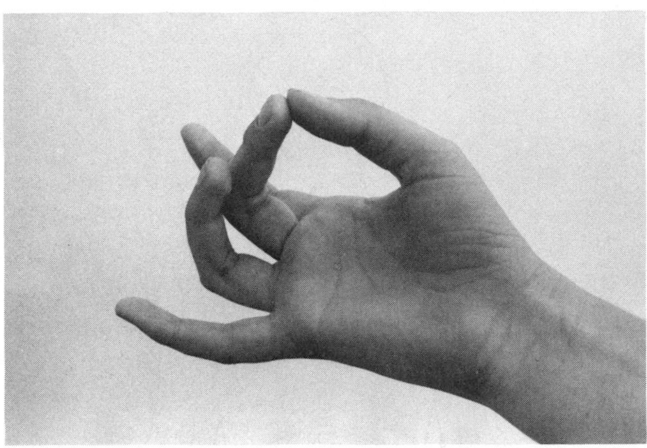

Figure 35–124 A test of fine motor coordination: touching the tip of each finger with the thumb

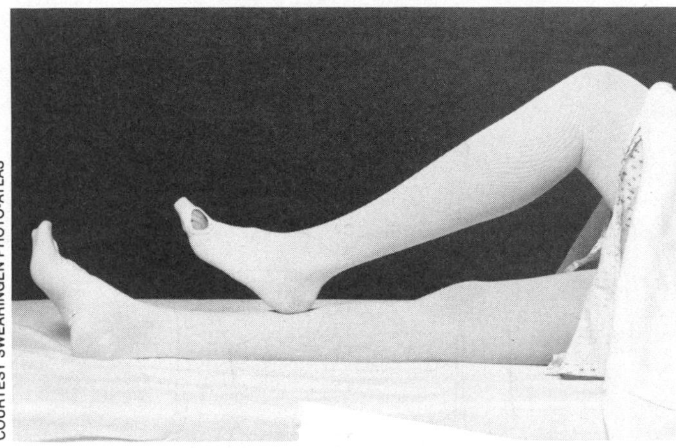

COURTESY SWEARINGEN PHOTO-ATLAS

Figure 35–125 Running the heel down the shin to the foot

at the wrists, elbows, knees, and ankles. Generally the face, arms, legs, hands, and feet are tested for touch and pain, although all parts of the body can be tested. If the client complains of numbness, peculiar sensations, or paralysis, sensation should be checked more carefully over flexor and extensor surfaces of limbs. Abnormality of touch or pain should then be mapped out clearly by examining responses in the area about every 2 cm (1 in). This is a lengthy procedure. A more detailed neurologic examination includes position sense, temperature sense, and tactile discrimination.

Sensory function of neurologically impaired clients can be evaluated by the use of dermatome zones, or segmented skin bands, that compare anatomically to the innervation by a dorsal root cutaneous nerve. See Figure 35–127. These nerves deliver the sensations of pain, temperature, touch, and vibration to the spinal cord and, ultimately, to the brain. The spinothalmic tract transmits the sensations of pain, temperature, and crude touch; the dorsal column tract transmits the perceptions of light touch and vibrations. Even though there is usually a great deal of overlap in nerve distribution, a knowledge of the dermatome zones can help you locate the approximate level of the neurologic lesion or injury. For example, a diminished or heightened response at the client's thumb can alert you to a potential disorder at level C-6 of the spinal cord.

To assess sensory function, the nurse needs the following equipment:

1. Wisps of cotton to assess light touch sensation
2. Sterile safety pin or sterile hypodermic needle to assess pain sensation
3. Large tuning fork to assess vibratory sense
4. Test tubes of hot and cold water for skin temperature assessment (optional)

Assessing Light Touch Sensation

1. Ask the client to close the eyes and to respond by saying "yes" or "now" whenever he or she feels the cotton wisp touching the skin.
2. With a wisp of cotton, lightly touch one specific spot and then the same spot on the other side of the body. See Figure 35–128. Normally, a light tickling or touch sensation occurs. Sensitivity to touch varies with different skin areas, so it is important to compare the sensation of symmetrical areas of the body.
3. Test areas on the forehead, cheek, hand, lower arm, abdomen, foot, and lower leg. This ensures assessment of the major dermatome zones and peripheral nerves. A specific area of the limb is checked first (e.g., the hand before the arm and the foot before the leg), since the sensory nerve may be assumed to be intact if sensation is felt at its most peripheral part.

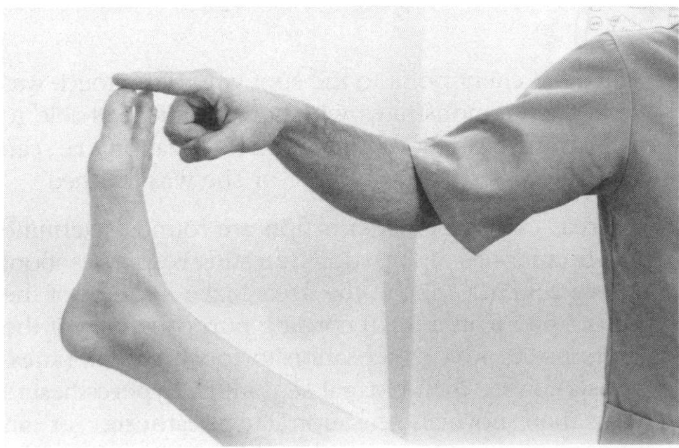

Figure 35–126 Touching the toes to the nurse's finger

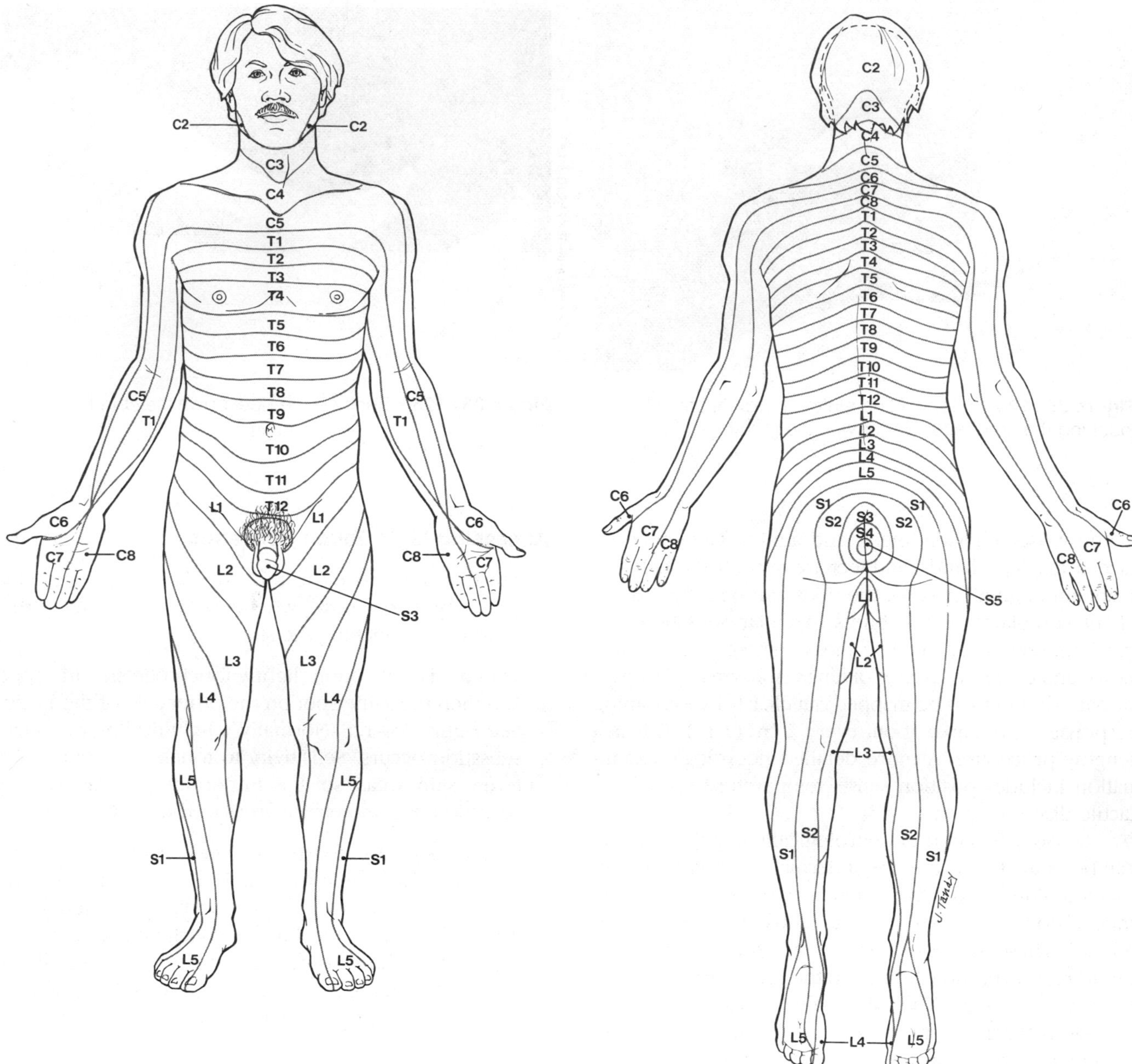

Figure 35–127 Sensory dermatome zones

4. Have the client point to the spot where the touch was felt. This demonstrates whether the client is able to determine tactile location (point localization), i.e., can accurately perceive where he or she was touched.

5. If areas of sensory dysfunction are found, determine the boundaries of sensation by testing responses about every 2.5 cm (1 in) in the area. Make a sketch of the sensory loss area for recording purposes. Note if the response is loss of sensation to touch stimuli (**anesthesia**); more than normal sensation (**hyperesthesia**); less than normal sensation (**hypoesthesia**); or an abnormal sensation such as burning, pain, or the feel of an electric shock (**paresthesia**).

Assessing Pain Sensation

1. Ask the client to close his or her eyes and to say "sharp," "dull," or "don't know" when the sharp or dull end of the safety pin or needle is felt.

2. Alternately use the sharp and dull end of the sterile pin or needle to lightly prick designated anatomic areas at random, e.g., hand, forearm, foot, lower leg, abdomen. The face is not tested in this manner. See Figure 35–129. Alternating the sharp and dull ends of the instrument more accurately evaluates the client's response. A sterile safety pin or needle is used to avoid the risk of infection.

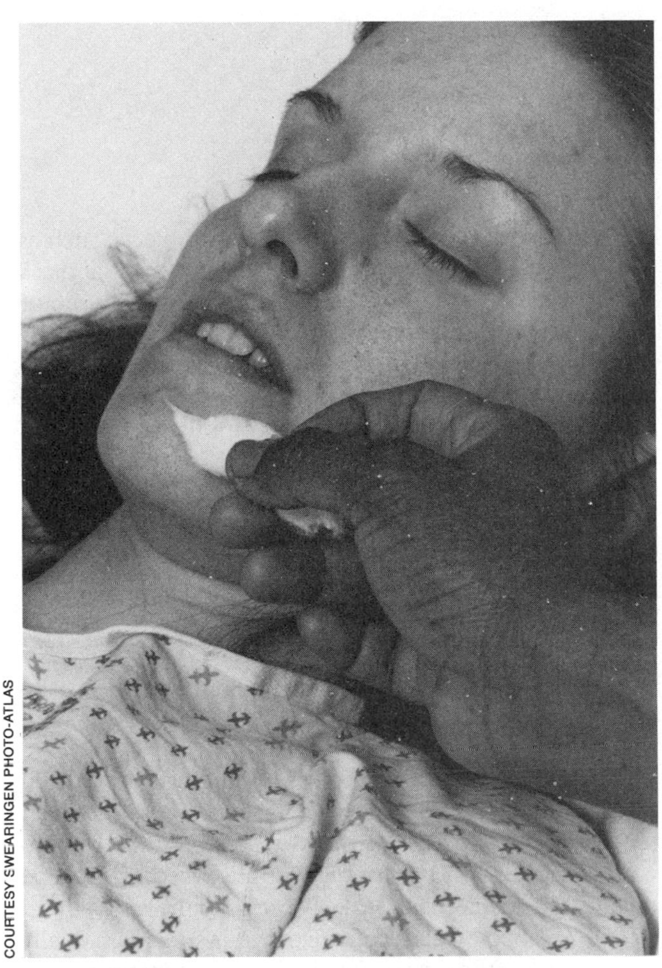

Figure 35–128 Assessing light touch sensation with a cotton wisp

3. Allow at least 2 seconds between each test to prevent summation effects of stimuli, i.e., several successive stimuli perceived as one stimulus.
4. Note areas of reduced, heightened, or absent sensation, and map them out for recording purposes.
5. If pain sensation is dulled or lost, assess temperature sensation in these areas. When sensations of pain are dulled, temperature sense is usually also impaired because distribution of these nerves over the body is similar.

Assessing Temperature Sensation

Temperature sensation is not routinely tested if pain sensation is found to be within normal limits. If pain sensation is not normal or is absent, testing sensitivity to temperature may prove more reliable.

1. Touch skin areas with test tubes filled with hot or cold water.

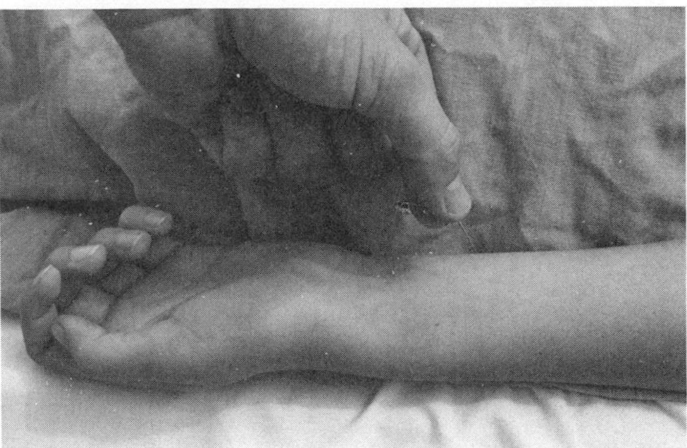

Figure 35–129 Assessing pain sensation with a pin

2. Have the client respond by saying "hot," "cold," or "don't know."

Assessing Vibration Sense

The vibratory sense is tested with a vibrating tuning fork held firmly against a bone. Bones commonly used arc in the ankle, the knee, the thumb side of the wrist, and the outside of the elbow. Routinely, the distal bones of an extremity are tested first. If some impairment is noted, the more proximal bones are also tested. The nurse may test other bones, such as fingers, toes, the sternum, the clavicle, the spinous processes, and the iliac crests. A person normally perceives the vibration as a buzzing or tingling sensation. In older persons (over 65 years of age), vibratory sensation may be diminished, particularly in the extremities. A large tuning fork is recommended because vibration cycles decline more slowly in a larger instrument.

1. Ask the client to close his or her eyes and to tell you (a) when vibrations are first felt by indicating "yes" or "now" and (b) when vibrations stop by indicating "not now" or "gone."
2. Apply the vibrating tuning fork to the designated area. See Figure 35–130.
3. Stop the vibrations between successive tests to facilitate more rapid assessment.
4. Compare the client's response to your own to confirm a normal response.
5. Compare the vibratory sensations felt on symmetrical sides of the body.
6. If you believe the client is confusing the pressure of the fork against the skin with its vibrations, strike the tuning fork but place it on the client only after the vibrations stop; the client then should not report vibrations.

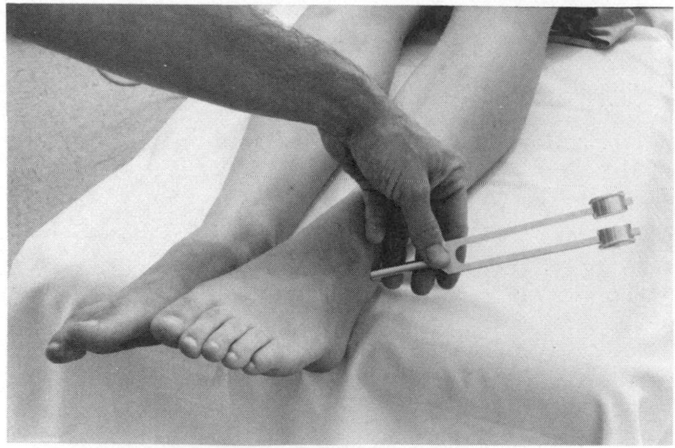

Figure 35–130 Assessing the vibratory sense

Assessing Position or Kinesthetic Sensation

Commonly, the middle fingers and the large toes are tested for the sense of position.

1. To test the fingers, support the client's arm with one hand and hold the client's palm in the other; to test the toes, place the client's heels on the examining table.
2. Have the client close his or her eyes.
3. Grasp a middle finger or big toe firmly between your thumb and index finger and exert the same pressure on both sides of the finger or toe while moving it.
4. Move the finger or toe until it is up, down, or straight out, and ask the client to identify the position.
5. Use a series of brisk up-and-down movements before coming to rest suddenly in one of the three positions. Normal persons can readily determine the position of their fingers and toes.

Assessing Tactile Discrimination

Three types of tactile discrimination are generally tested: **one- and two-point discrimination**, the ability to sense whether one or two areas of the skin are being stimulated by pressure; **stereognosis**, the act of recognizing objects by touching and manipulating them; and **extinction**, the failure to perceive touch on one side of the body when two symmetrical areas of the body are touched simultaneously. For all tests, the client's eyes need to be closed.

1. To assess one- and two-point discrimination, alternately stimulate the skin with two pins simultaneously and then with one pin. Ask the client if he or she feels one or two pinpricks. Wide perceptual variability occurs in adults over different parts of the body. Normally, a person can distinguish between a one- and two-point stimulus within the following minimum distances:
   a. Fingertips, 2.8 mm
   b. Palms of hands, 8 to 12 mm
   c. Chest, forearm, 40 mm
   d. Back, 50 to 70 mm
   e. Upper arm, thigh, 75 mm
   f. Toes, 3 to 8 mm
2. To assess stereognosis, place familiar objects, such as a key, paper clip, or coin, in the client's hand and ask her or him to identify them. If the client has a motor impairment of the hand and is unable to voluntarily manipulate an object, write a number or letter on the client's palm, using a blunt instrument, and ask the client to identify it. Recognition of a figure drawn on the hand is called **graphesthesia**.
3. To assess the extinction phenomenon, simultaneously stimulate two symmetrical areas of the body, such as the thighs, the cheeks, or the hands. Normally, both points of stimulus are felt. Extinction is frequently noted in clients with lesions of the sensory cortex.

Deep Tendon Reflexes

A **reflex** is an automatic response of the body to a stimulus. It is not voluntarily learned or conscious. The deep tendon reflex (DTR) is activated when a tendon is stimulated (tapped) and its associated muscle contracts. The quality of a reflex response varies among individuals and by age. As a person ages and the nervous system gradually deteriorates, reflex responses become less intense.

Reflexes are tested using a percussion hammer. The response is described on a scale of 0 to +4 (+ + + +). See Table 35–28. Experience is necessary to determine appropriate scoring for an individual. It is important to compare one side of the body with the other when assessing reflexes to evaluate the symmetry of response.

Several reflexes are normally tested during a physical examination. These are (a) the biceps reflex, (b) the triceps reflex, (c) the bradioradialis reflex, (d) the patellar reflex, (e) the Achilles reflex, and (f) the plantar reflex.

Biceps Reflex

This reflex tests the spinal cord level C-5, C-6.

1. Partially flex the client's arm at the elbow, and rest the forearm over his or her thighs, placing the palm of the hand down.
2. Place the thumb of your nondominant hand horizontally over the biceps tendon.
3. With your other hand, hold the percussion hammer between thumb and index finger.
4. Deliver a blow (slight downward thrust) with the percussion hammer to your thumb.

Table 35–28 Grading Reflex Responses

Scale	Response
0	No reflex response
+1	Minimal activity (hypoactive)
+2	Normal response
+3	More active than normal
+4	Maximum activity (hyperactive)

5. Observe the normal slight flexion of the elbow and feel the bicep's contraction through your thumb. See Figure 35–131.

Triceps Reflex

This reflex tests the spinal cord level C-7, C-8.

1. Flex the client's arm at the elbow and support it in the palm of your nondominant hand.
2. Palpate the triceps tendon about 2 to 5 cm (1 to 2 in) above the elbow.
3. Deliver a blow with the percussion hammer directly to the tendon. See Figure 35–132.
4. Observe the normal slight extension of the elbow.

Brachioradialis Reflex

This reflex tests the spinal cord level C-3, C-6.

1. Rest the client's arm in a relaxed position on your forearm or on the client's own leg.
2. Deliver a blow with the percussion hammer directly on the radius 2 to 5 cm (1 to 2 in) above the wrist or the styloid process (bony prominence on the thumb side of the wrist). See Figure 35–133.

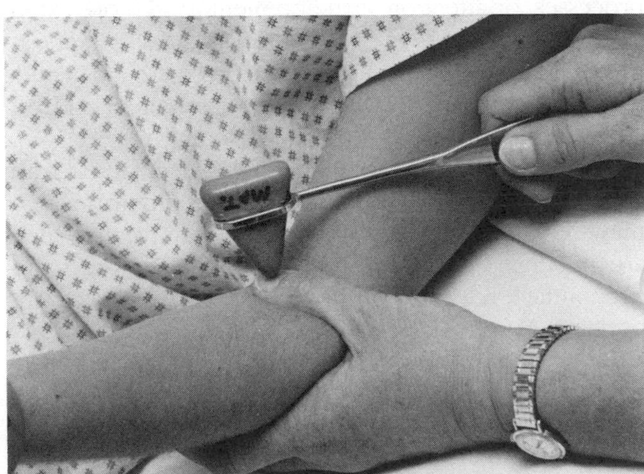

Figure 35–131 Assessing the biceps reflex

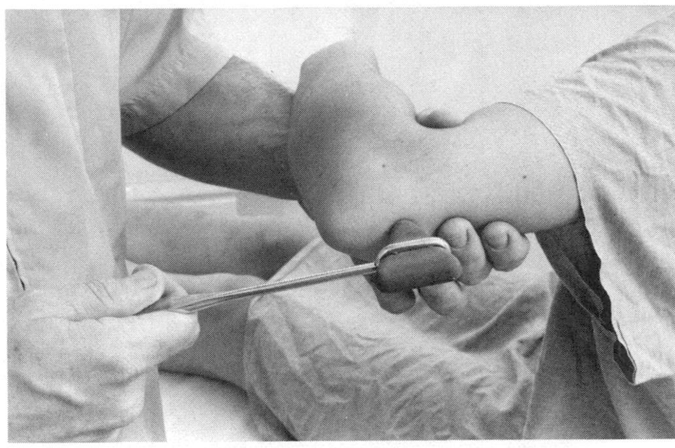

Figure 35–132 Assessing the triceps reflex

3. Observe the normal flexion and supination of the forearm. The fingers of the hand may also extend slightly.

Patellar Reflex

This reflex tests the spinal cord level L-2, L-3, L-4.

1. Have the client sit on the edge of the examining table so that the legs hang freely.
2. Locate the patellar tendon directly below the patella (kneecap).
3. Deliver a blow with the percussion hammer directly to the tendon. See Figure 35–134.

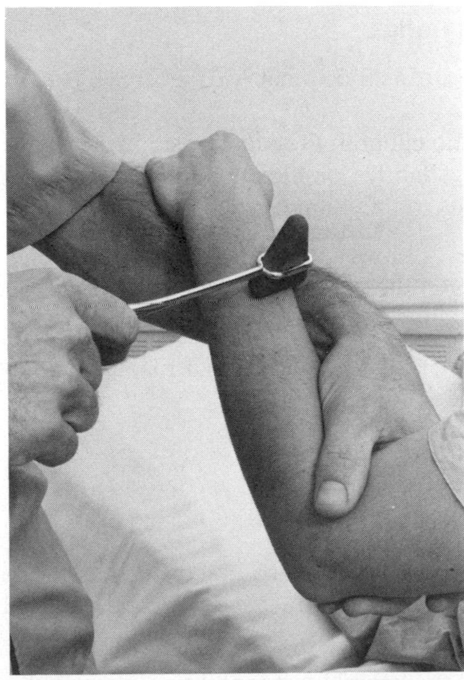

Figure 35–133 Assessing the brachioradialis reflex

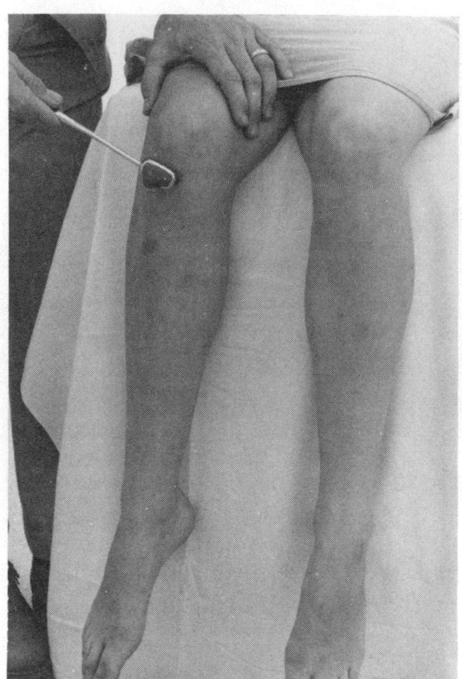

Figure 35–134 Assessing the patellar reflex

4. Observe the normal extension or kicking out of the leg as the quadriceps muscle contracts.
5. If no response is obtained and you suspect the client is not relaxed, ask him or her to interlock his or her fingers and pull. This action often enhances relaxation so that a more accurate response is obtained.

Achilles Reflex

This reflex tests the spinal cord level S-1, S-2.

1. With the client in the same position as for the patellar reflex, slightly dorsiflex the client's ankle by grasping the toes in the palm of your hand.
2. Deliver a blow with the percussion hammer directly to the Achilles tendon just above the heel. See Figure 35–135.
3. Observe and feel the normal plantar flexion (downward jerk) of the foot.

Plantar (Babinski) Reflex

This reflex is superficial.

1. Use a moderately sharp object such as the handle of the percussion hammer, a key, or the dull end of a pin or applicator stick.
2. Stroke the lateral border of the sole of the client's foot, starting at the heel, continuing to the ball of the foot, and then proceeding across the ball of the foot toward the big toe. See Figure 35–136.
3. Observe the response. Normally, all five toes bend downward; this reaction is negative Babinski. In an abnormal response, positive Babinski, the toes spread outward and the big toe moves upward. Positive Babinski is abnormal after the child ambulates.

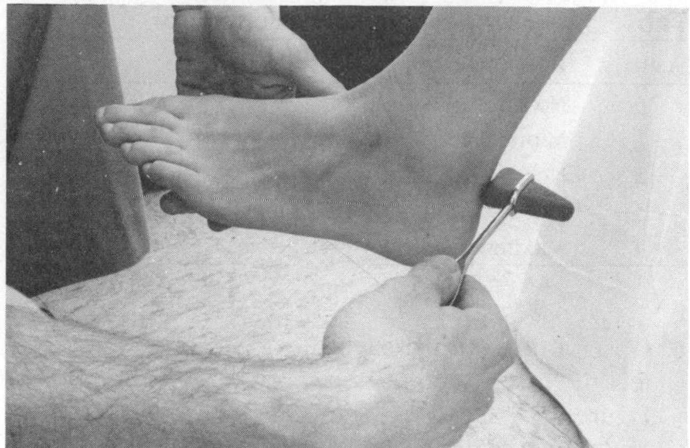

Figure 35–135 Assessing the Achilles reflex

Mental Status

Assessment of mental status reveals the client's general cerebral function. The highest functions of the nervous system are carried out in the brain. These functions include intellectual (cognitive) as well as emotional (affective) functions. This section addresses the cognitive functions. See the section on psychosocial assessment, next, for the affective functions.

A large part of the mental status assessment is performed during the taking of the history and when observing the client's general appearance. If problems are noted with use of language, memory, concentration, thought processes, or attention span and memory, a more extensive examination is required during neurologic assessment. Major areas of mental status assessment include language, orientation, memory, attention span and calculation, judgment, and abstract reasoning.

Assessing and interpreting a client's mental status are more difficult than obtaining objective physical assessment data. The perceptions of both the nurse and client are influenced by educational background, culture, socioeconomic level, values and beliefs, race, sex, age, and previous life experiences.

Language

Any defects in or loss of the power to express oneself by speech, writing, or signs or to comprehend spoken or written language due to disease or injury of the cerebral cortex is called **aphasia.** Aphasias can be categorized as sensory or receptive aphasia and motor or expressive aphasia.

Sensory/receptive aphasia is the loss of the ability to comprehend written or spoken words. Two types of sensory aphasia are auditory or acoustic aphasia, in which clients have difficulty understanding what is being said even though they hear the sounds, and visual aphasia, in which clients cannot read words even though they can see them. Such clients are neither deaf nor blind. They have lost the ability to understand the symbolic content associated with sounds (auditory aphasia) or with printed or written figures (visual aphasia).

Motor/expressive aphasia involves loss of the power to express oneself by writing, making signs, or speaking. Clients may find that even though they can recall words, they have lost the ability to combine speech sounds into words. The most common aphasias involve partial sensory and motor losses. Because speech is a complex act involving the tongue, mouth, palate, larynx, respiratory system, and cerebrum, the nurse must keep in mind that disturbances of speech may or may not relate to the nervous system.

To assess language deficits related to aphasia:

1. Point to common objects and ask the client to name them.
2. Ask the client to read some words and to match the printed and written words with pictures.
3. Ask the client to respond to simple verbal and written commands, e.g., "point to your toes" or "raise your left arm."
4. Note particulars about the client's speech patterns. Various types of aphasia are reflected in characteristic speech patterns. A pattern of repeating the same response as different questions are asked (**perseveration**) is common in all forms of aphasia. The speech of clients with auditory receptive aphasia is abundant and appropriately expressive but contains many incorrect words (**paraphasia**). Clients with motor aphasia have painfully slow speech, poor articulation, and a tendency to delete prepositions and pronouns (Kneisl and Ames 1986, p. 171).

Orientation

As the nurse takes the nursing history, the client's responses to questions about dates, places, and persons indicate whether a more detailed assessment is required during neurologic assessment. The client's orientation to time, place, and person is determined by tactful questioning. Orientation is easily assessed by asking the client the city and state of residence, time of day, date, day of the week, duration of illness, and names of family members. More direct questioning may be necessary for some people, e.g., "Where are you now?" "What day is it today?" "What is your name?" Most people readily accept these questions if initially the nurse asks, "Do you get confused at times?"

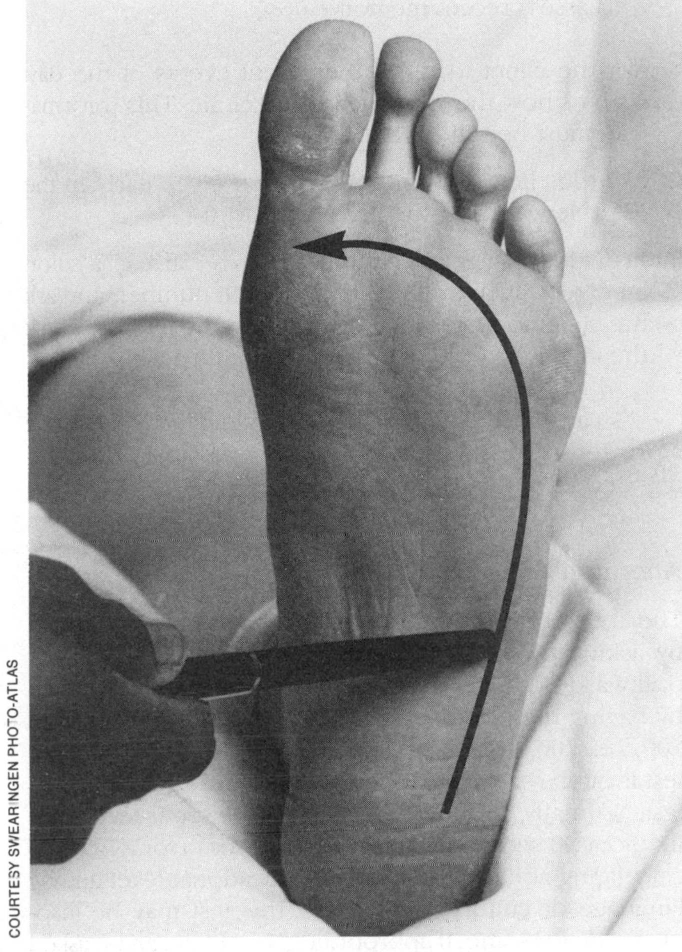

Figure 35–136 Assessing the plantar (Babinski) reflex

Memory

Listen for lapses in memory. First, ask the client about difficulty with memory. If problems are apparent, three categories of memory are tested: immediate recall, recent memory, and remote memory.

To assess immediate recall:

1. Ask the client to repeat a series of three digits, e.g., 7-4-3, spoken slowly.
2. Gradually increase the number of digits, e.g., 7-4-3-5, 7-4-3-5-6, and 7-4-3-5-6-7-2, until the client fails to repeat the series correctly.
3. Start again with a series of three digits but this time ask the client to repeat them backward. The average person can repeat a series of five to eight digits in sequence and four to six digits in reverse order.

To assess recent memory:

1. Ask the client to recall the recent events of the day, such as how the client got to the clinic. This information must be validated, however.
2. Ask the client to recall information given early in the interview, such as the name of a doctor.
3. Provide the client with three facts to recall, e.g., a color, an object, an address, or a three-digit number, and ask the client to repeat all three. Later in the interview, ask the client to recall all three items.

To assess remote memory, ask the client to describe a previous illness or surgery, e.g., 5 years ago, or a birthday or anniversary.

Attention Span and Calculation

The ability to concentrate or attention span can be tested by asking the client to recite the alphabet or to count backward from 100. The ability to calculate can be tested by having the patient subtract 7 or 3 progressively from 100; i.e., 100, 93, 86, 79, or 100, 97, 94, 91. This standard test is often referred to as the serial sevens or serial threes test. Normally, an adult can complete the serial sevens test in about 90 seconds with three or fewer errors. Because calculating ability is affected by educational level and by language or cultural differences, this test may be inappropriate for some. If appropriate, the client can be asked to add or to subtract small numbers.

Judgment

To test judgment, the nurse asks relatively simple questions and judges the response, always considering the person's cultural background.

1. Ask direct questions about what a person would do in certain situations, e.g., What would you do if a policeman pulled you over for not observing a stop sign? If you broke a shovel you had borrowed from your neighbor? If you found a wallet with money and owner identification in it?
2. Have the person pick from a series a word that does not relate to the others. For example, large, small, and red; or up, left, and down.

Abstract Reasoning

To assess abstract reasoning:

1. Give the client a proverb to interpret, e.g., "A stitch in time saves nine" or "People who live in glass houses should not throw stones."
2. Ask the client to explain how two words, e.g., "climate and season" or "orange and apple," differ or relate. Normally, an abstract or semiabstract response is expected. Concrete interpretations may indicate a problem or may indicate level of education.

Level of Consciousness

The state of consciousness or level of alertness is often determined at the beginning of the physical examination. Level can vary from a state of alertness to coma. These levels are assessed by describing the client's response to various verbal and physical stimuli. See Table 35–29 and Figure 35–137.

To assess level of consciousness:

1. Speak to the client to arouse her or him if necessary.
2. If the client cannot be aroused verbally, press your fingernail into the client's nail or press a skinfold with your fingers.

Psychosocial Assessment

Psychosocial assessment is an ongoing process begun in the initial contact with the client. It requires the collection of data about the client's:

1. Psychologic patterns or nonphysical components, such as emotional state, thoughts, feelings, motivations, and perception of self.
2. Interactions with other people, e.g., cultural, economic, ethnic, and family factors, especially as they relate to health.

Psychologic and social components of assessment are closely interrelated; each realm affects the other and both are functionally indivisible from the person's physical self. Mind and body are inseparable to those who take a holistic approach.

Psychosocial assessment is more difficult than physical assessment, since psychosocial data are much less precise—less classifiable as normal or abnormal—than physical data. Many factors influence both the client's and nurse's perception and interpretation of data. How the nurse and client view phenomena and interpret events is influenced by personal values, culture, age, sex, and such factors as anxiety, fear, and pain or discomfort. Effective communication skills are needed for psychosocial assessment (see Chapter 27). Communication skills help the nurse to make the client feel comfortable and respected. A nonthreatened client discloses data of a personal nature more readily.

Purposes

The purposes of psychosocial assessment are:

1. To obtain data that help the nurse understand and appreciate the client's life experiences
2. To obtain data that assist the nurse to provide more complete and appropriate care to the client
3. To initiate a nonjudgmental, trusting interpersonal relationship with the client
4. In collaboration with the client, to identify problems affecting the client's health and to plan suitable approaches

Psychosocial assessment is made by observing, questioning, and listening to the client. It starts as the nurse takes the nursing history and observes the client's general appearance and behavior.

Selected Psychologic Components

See also assessment of general appearance and behavior on page 805 for data about the client's attitude, affect/mood, signs of distress, speech, posture, and other factors that contribute to the nurse's overall impression of the client's psychologic state.

1. *Major Stressors.* Determine major stressors the client has experienced in the past year and his or her perception of them.
2. *Normal coping pattern.* Ask the client what he or she normally does to cope with a serious problem or a high level of stress. See the section on assessing client coping in Chapter 17 page 351.
3. *Changes in psychophysiologic functions.* Determine changes in the client's sleep patterns, appetite, bowel functioning, energy levels, and sexual functioning.
4. *Communication style.* Observe the client's nonverbal communication and ability to verbalize appropriate emotion. Nonverbal communication—e.g., eye movements, gestures, use of touch, and posture—and the client's interactions with support persons can reveal anxiety, suspicion, withdrawal, anger, or other feelings. Note particularly the congruence of nonverbal behavior and verbal expression. Examples of incongruent expresson are being overly cheerful in response to bad news, laughing while discussing a serious topic, or crying when talking about a pleasant topic.

Table 35–29 Levels of Consciousness: Glasgow Coma Scale

Faculty Measured	Response	Score
Eye opening	Spontaneous	4
	To verbal command	3
	To pain	2
	No response	1
Motor response	To verbal command	6
	To painful stimuli:	
	• Localizes pain	5
	• Flexes and withdraws	4
	• Assumes decorticate posture	3
	• Assumes decerebrate posture	2
	• No response	1
Verbal response (arouse client with painful stimuli, if necessary)	Oriented, converses	5
	Disoriented, converses	4
	Uses inappropriate words	3
	Makes incomprehensible sounds	2
	No response	1

Coma is defined as a score of 7 or less. A score of 3 or 4 indicates an 85% chance of dying or remaining vegetative. A score of 11 or more suggest an 85% chance of moderate disability or good recovery.

SOURCE: Adapted from Teasdale G. Bennet B: Assessment of coma and impaired consciousness: A practical scale. *Lancet* 1974; 2(7872):81.

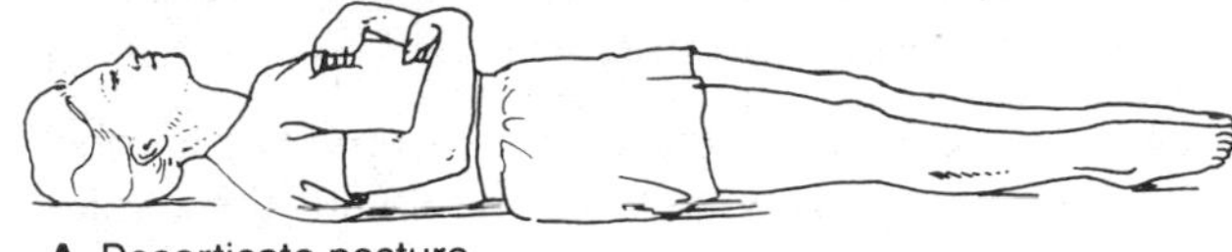

A. Decorticate posture

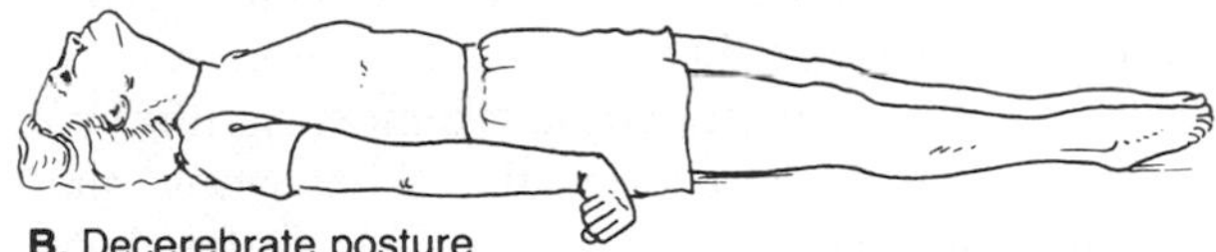

B. Decerebrate posture

Figure 35–137 Decorticate and decerebrate posturing. **A.** *Decorticate* posture (indicating damage to the internal capsule and corticospinal tracts above the brain stem): the client's arms are adducted with elbows and wrists in rigid flexion, the hands rotated internally and fingers flexed; the lower extremities are hyperextended. **B.** *Decerebrate* posture (indicating midbrain damage): the client has hyperextended upper and lower extremities; **opisthotonos** (head extended, body arched) is an exaggerated decerebrate posture seen in tetanus, when the body may be supported on the back of the head and the feet during a convulsion.

5. *Self-concept.* Ask the client, "What do you like or dislike about yourself?" or "How would you describe yourself?" Have the client describe his or her physical self, e.g., personal perceptions of his or her shape, size, and appearance. Note whether the client establishes eye

contact. Feelings of anxiety, guilt, anger, and powerlessness can indicate low self-esteem.

6. *Mood.* The nurse may need to question the client about mood if he or she appears underactive (flat or unresponsive). Ask if the client sleeps well at night, gets discouraged, feels down, or cries frequently. The client's answers help the nurse determine whether the client is depressed. The nurse can then ask other questions to probe the depth of a depression. For example, a nurse may ask whether the client ever feels life is not worth living or whether things are getting too bad for the client to cope. Affirmative answers to these questions warrant other questions: "Have you ever thought of killing yourself or tried to kill yourself?" "How did you do it or how did you plan to do it?" By gradually leading up to questions of suicide, the nurse can gauge the depth of depression.

Selected Social Components

1. *Socioeconomic factors.* Ask the client about:
   a. Economic factors: income and living arrangements and their effects on life-style, sense of adequacy, and self-worth
   b. Employment and attitudes about it
   c. Racial, cultural, and ethnic identification and sense of belonging
   d. Religious identification and link to significant value systems, norms, and practices
2. *Social roles.* Determine the client's assumed or ascribed roles and perceived competence in fulfilling these roles.
3. *Social network*
   a. Observe who accompanies the person to and from the health care facility.
   b. Ask the client which people are most significant to him or her. Do not judge the client whose most significant person is of the same sex as the client.
   c. Determine the client's dominant network, e.g., kinship or friendship.
   d. Determine the names of persons to contact in case of an emergency.
   e. Determine if hospitalized clients want restrictions placed on visitors.

Chapter Highlights

- The physical health examination is conducted to assess the function and integrity of the client's body parts.
- It may entail a complete head-to-toe assessment or assessment of a body system or body part.
- The health assessment is conducted in a systematic manner that requires the fewest position changes for the client.
- Aspects of physical assessment procedures should be incorporated in the assessment, intervention, and evaluation phases of the nursing process.
- Data obtained in the physical health examination supplement, confirm, or refute data obtained during the nursing history.
- Nursing history data help the nurse focus on specific aspects of the physical health examination.
- Data obtained in the physical health examination help the nurse establish nursing diagnoses, plan the client's care, and evaluate the outcomes of nursing care.
- Initial assessment findings provide baseline data about the client's functional abilities against which subsequent assessment findings are compared.
- Skills in inspection, palpation, percussion, and auscultation are required for the physical health examination; these skills are used in that order throughout the examination except during abdominal assessment, when auscultation follows inspection.
- Knowledge of the normal structure and function of body parts and systems is an essential requisite to conducting physical assessment.

Suggested Readings

Farrell, J. April 1980. The human side of assessment. *Nursing 80* 10:74–75.
Farrell presents guidelines to help nurses maintain their "humanness" and not become automatic assessment machines. These guidelines are: look beyond the obvious, don't be pat in your assessment, take your client's complaints seriously, don't be overzealous, assess the whole client, listen for what your client really thinks and feels, and stick your neck out.

Hudson, M. F. November 1983. Safeguard your elderly patient's health through accurate physical assessment. *Nursing 83* 13:58–61, 63–64.
Hudson makes the point that not all functional changes identified in the elderly are related to disease. Hudson then proceeds to explain changes that take place in the various body systems because of aging.

Performing palpation. January 1983. *Nursing 83* 13:24–25.
This article is a reprint from the *Nurses' Reference Library Series: Assessment.* It describes both light and deep palpation. Light palpation probes to a depth of about 1 to 2 cm (½ to ¾ inch); deep palpation, to 4 to 5 cm (1½ to 2 inches). Photographs clarify palpation techniques.

Performing percussion. February 1983. *Nursing 83* 13:63–64.
This article is a reprint from the *Nurses' Reference Library Series: Assessment.* Three methods of percussion are described: mediate, immediate, and fist. Photographs of the hand positions for each technique are included, together with a chart describing the sounds that can be elicited through percussion.

Smith, C. E. December 1984. With good assessment skills you can construct a solid framework for patient care. *Nursing 84* 14:26–31.
Smith describes the right environment for assessment and provides some suggestions for taking a nursing history. The author then goes on to explain palpation, percussion, and auscultation, including practical suggestions to make these techniques more effective.

Selected References

Alexander, M. M., and Brown, M. S. Physical examination series. Parts 1–18. *Nursing 73, 74, 75,* and *76.*

Bates, B. 1983. *A guide to physical examination.* 3d ed. Philadelphia: J. B. Lippincott.

Behrman, R. E., and Vaughan, V. C. III. 1983. *Nelson textbook of pediatrics.* 12th ed. Philadelphia, W. B. Saunders Co.

Bellack, J. P., and Bamford, P. A. 1984. *Nursing assessment: A multidimensional approach.* Monterey, Calif.: Wadsworth Health Sciences Division.

Block, G. J., Nolan, J. W., and Dempsey, M. K. 1981. *Health assessment for professional nursing: A developmental approach.* New York: Appleton-Century-Crofts.

Bowers, A. C., and Thompson, J. M. 1984. *Clinical manual of health assessment.* 2d ed. St. Louis. C. V. Mosby Co.

Boyd-Monk, H. May 1980. Examining the external eye: Testing visual acuity. *Nursing 80* 10:58–63.

Brown, M. S. September 1973. Physical examination. Part 3. Examining the skin. *Nursing 73* 3:39–51.

Burns, K. R., and Johnson, P. J. 1980. *Health assessment in clinical practice.* Englewood Cliffs, N.J.: Prentice-Hall.

Derbes, V. J. March 1973. Rashes: Recognition and management. *Nursing 73* 3:44–49.

Gillies, D. A., and Alyn, I. B. 1976. *Patient assessment and management by the nurse practitioner.* Philadelphia: W. B. Saunders Co.

Grimes, J., and Iannopollo, E. 1982. *Health assessment in nursing practice.* Monterey, Calif.: Wadsworth Health Sciences Division.

Hagerty, B. K. 1984. *Psychiatric-mental health assessment.* St. Louis: C. V. Mosby Co.

Humbrecht, B., and VanParys, E. April 1982. From assessment to intervention: How to use heart and breath sounds as part of your nursing care plan. *Nursing 82* 12:34–41.

Jarvis, C. M. May 1977. Perfecting physical assessment. Part 1. *Nursing 77* 7:28–37. June 1977. Part 2. 7:38–45. July 1977. Part 3. 7:44–53.

King, P. A. October 1980. Foot problems and assessment. *Geriatric Nursing* 1:182–86.

Kneisl, C. R., and Ames, S. W. 1986. *Adult health nursing: A biopsychosocial approach.* Menlo Park, Calif.: Addison-Wesley Publishing Co.

Malasanos, L.; Barkauskas, V.; Moss, M.; and Stoltenberg-Allen, K. 1986. *Health assessment.* 3d ed. St. Louis: C. V. Mosby Co.

McFarlane, J. December 1974. Pediatric assessment and intervention. Some simple how-to's for ambulatory settings. *Nursing 74* 4:66–68.

Miller, K. M. October 1978. Assessing peripheral perfusion. *American Journal of Nursing* 78:1673–74.

Nurses' Reference Library Series. 1982. *Assessment.* Horsham, Pa.: Intermed Communications.

Nursing 80 Photobook Series. 1980. *Assessing your patients.* Horsham, Pa.: Intermed Communications.

Peterson, F. Y. November 1983. Assessing peripheral vascular disease at the bedside. *American Journal of Nursing* 83:1549–51.

Roach, L. B. November 1972. Color changes in dark skins. *Nursing 72* 2:19–22.

Robson, J. K.; Larkin, F.; Bursick, J. H.; and Perri, K. P. December 1975. Growth standards for infants and children: A cross-sectional study. *Pediatrics* 56:1017–18.

Saul, L. December 1983. Heart sounds and common murmurs. *American Journal of Nursing* 83:1679–89.

Slessor, G. April 1973. Auscultation of the chest: A clinical nursing skill. *Canadian Nurse* 69:40–43.

Smith, C. E. April 1984. Assessment under pressure: When your patient says "my chest hurts." *Nursing 84* 14:34–39.

Taylor, D. L. January 1985. Clinical applications: Assessing heart sounds. *Nursing 85* 15:51–53.

——— March 1985. Clinical applications: Assessing breath sounds. *Nursing 85* 15:60–62.

Visich, M. A. November 1981. Knowing what you hear: A guide to assessing breath and heart sounds. *Nursing 81* 11:16–28.

Westra, B. May 1984. Assessment under pressure: When your patient says "I can't breathe." *Nursing 84* 14:34–39.

White, J. H., and Schroeder, M. A. March 1981. When your client has a weight problem: Nursing assessment. *American Journal of Nursing* 81:550–52.

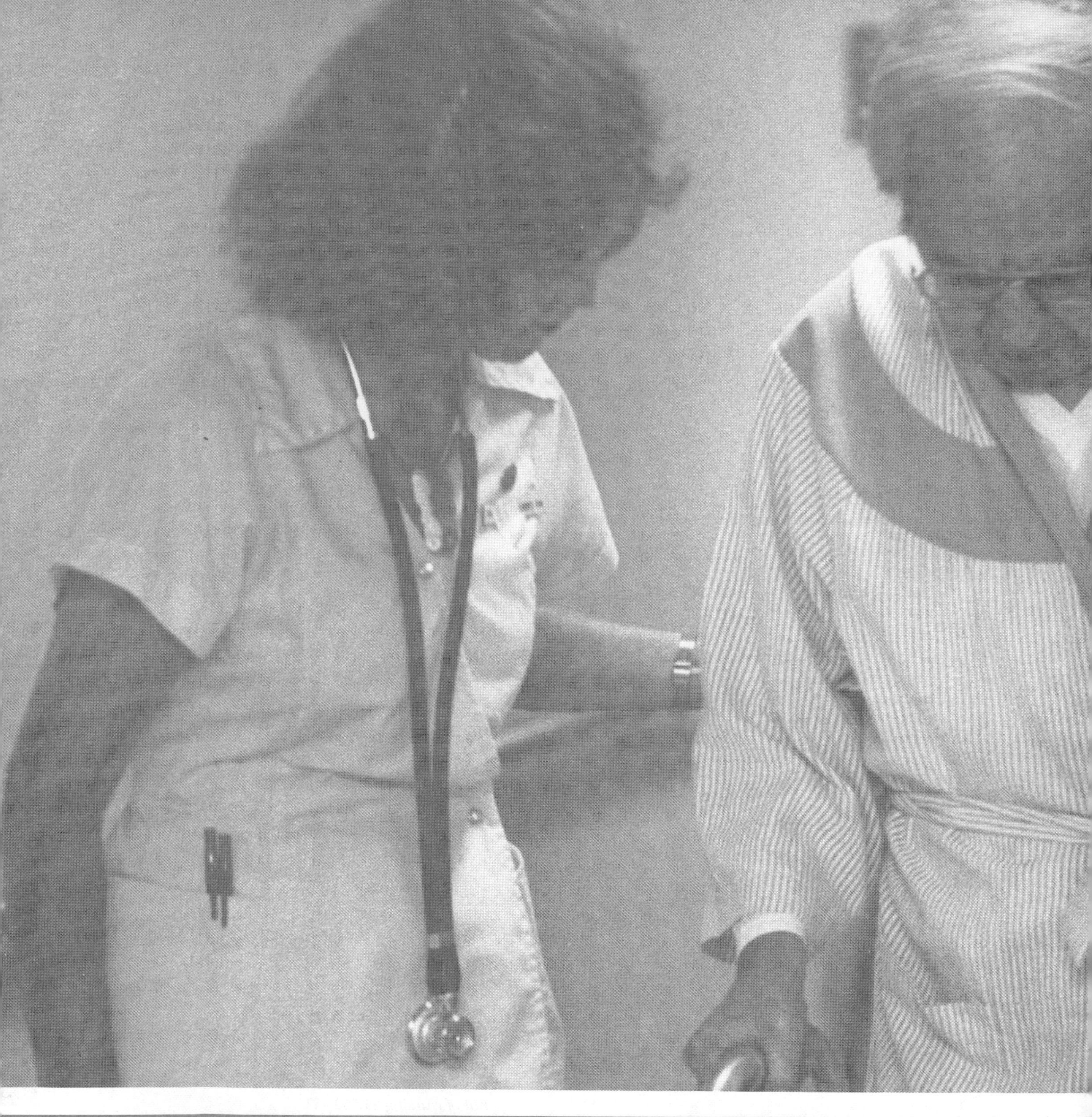

We are accountable professionals, being recognized for our knowledge as well as our skills. We have clinical competence that is unique, that is not substitutable... (Thelman Schorr)

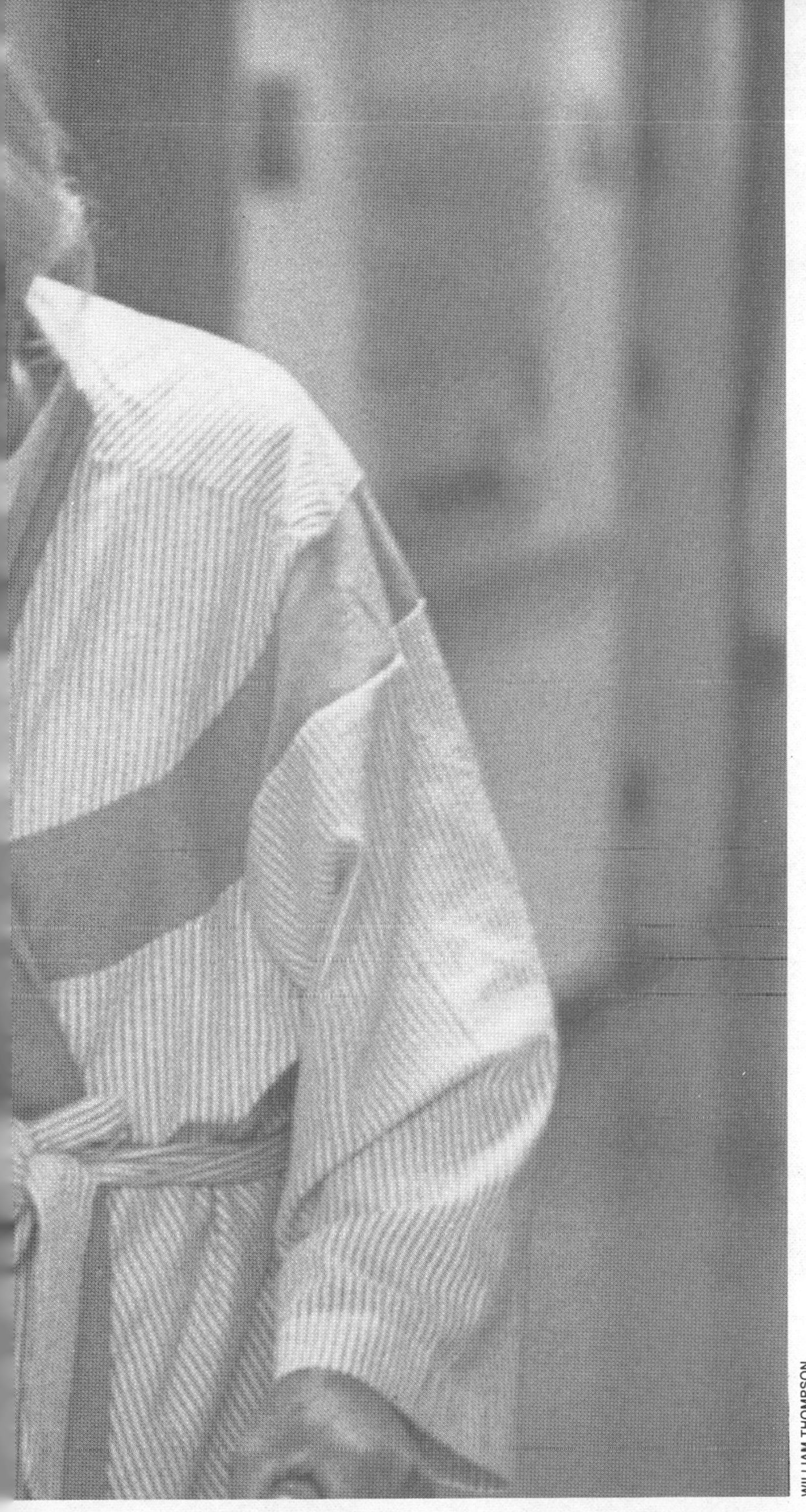

UNIT **9**

Physiologic Concepts

Contents

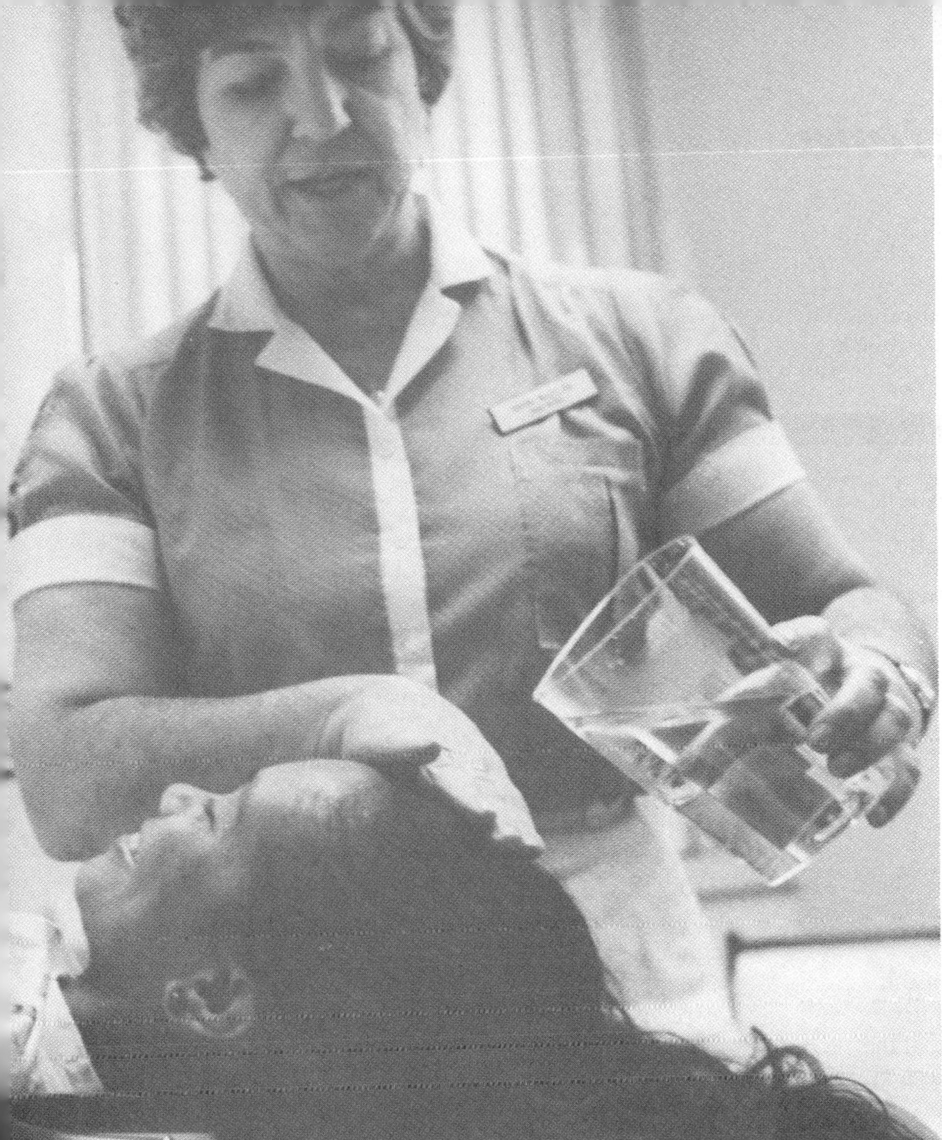

GEORGE FRY

CHAPTER 36

Personal Hygiene

Contents

(continued)

36 *Personal Hygiene*

Contents *(continued)*

Objectives

1. Understand essential facts about hygiene and the skin, feet, nails, mouth, hair, eyes, ears, and nose.
   1.1 Define selected terms.
   1.2 Identify factors influencing personal hygiene.
   1.3 Describe kinds of hygienic care nurses provide to clients.
   1.4 Identify layers and functions of skin.
   1.5 Identify four major functions of mucous membrane.
   1.6 Identify structures of a tooth.
   1.7 Identify structures of the mouth.
   1.8 Identify structures of hair.
2. Know essential facts about assessment of the skin, mouth, hair, nails, eyes, ears, and nose.
   2.1 Identify normal and abnormal findings obtained during inspection and palpation of the skin, feet, nails, mouth, hair, eyes, ears, and nose.
   2.2 Describe variations in the appearance of the skin, nails, and mucous membranes of white and black clients.
   2.3 Identify developmental changes in the skin, teeth, hair, feet, and nails.
3. Know facts about common problems and nursing diagnoses about the skin, feet, nails, mouth, hair, eyes, ears, and nose.
   3.1 Identify common problems of the skin and formulate related nursing diagnoses.
   3.2 Identify factors that render a person susceptible to skin breakdown.
   3.3 Identify common problems of the feet and nails and formulate related nursing diagnoses.
   3.4 Identify common problems of the mouth and formulate related nursing diagnoses.
   3.5 Identify common problems of the hair and scalp and formulate related nursing diagnoses.
   3.6 Identify common problems of the external eye structures.
   3.7 Identify common problems of the external ear.
4. Understand essential factors about planning and implementing nursing interventions for the skin, feet, nails, mouth, hair, eyes, ears, and nose.
   4.1 Identify outcome criteria for evaluating nursing interventions.
   4.2 Identify guidelines for interventions related to the skin.
   4.3 Identify the purposes of bathing.
   4.4 Describe various types of baths.
   4.5 State the rationale for essential steps in the procedure for bathing an adult in bed.
   4.6 Identify essential aspects of skin care for newborns and infants.
   4.7 Describe essential steps in perineal and genital care.
   4.8 Explain five techniques used in back rubs.
   4.9 Identify measures to prevent foot problems.
   4.10 Describe essential steps in nail care.
   4.11 Identify essential steps in brushing and flossing teeth.
   4.12 Explain specific ways in which nurses help hospitalized clients with oral hygiene.
   4.13 Describe safety measures involved in denture care.
   4.14 Identify essential steps in brushing, combing, and shampooing hair.
   4.15 Identify essential aspects of eye care.
   4.16 Identify essential steps in applying and removing contact lenses.
   4.17 Describe essential steps in inserting and removing hearing aids.
   4.18 Identify essential aspects of nose care.
   4.19 Identify safety and comfort measures underlying bed-making procedures.
5. Demonstrate beginning skill in assisting clients with hygiene.
   5.1 Assist clients with bathing.
   5.2 Provide back rubs.
   5.3 Assist clients with perineal and genital care.
   5.4 Assist clients with foot care.
   5.5 Provide nail care.
   5.6 Assist clients with oral hygiene.
   5.7 Clean dentures.
   5.8 Give special mouth care.
   5.9 Apply and remove clients' contact lenses.
   5.10 Insert and remove clients' hearing aids.
   5.11 Assist clients with hair care.
   5.12 Give clients shampoos.
   5.13 Make occupied and unoccupied beds.

Terms

apocrine gland
body image
callus
cementum
cerumen
corn
crown (of tooth)
dentin
dentures
dermis
eccrine gland
effleurage
emaciation
enamel (of tooth)
epidermis
frenulum
friction stroke
gingiva
gingivitis
glossitis
halitosis
hallux valgus (bunion)
hammer toe
hirsutism
hygiene
hypodermis
ischemia
keratized cells
lanugo
mastication
melanin
mucous membrane
necrosis
palate
parotitis
petrissage
plantar wart
pulp cavity
sebaceous gland
sebum
smegma
sordes
stasis dermatitis
stomatitis
sudoriferous (sweat) gland
sulcular technique
tapotement
three-handed effleurage
tinea pedis
uvula
vernix caseosa

Hygiene

Hygiene is the science of health and its maintenance. Personal hygiene is the self-care by which people maintain health. Mental, oral, sexual, and social hygiene are just a few of the subdivisions described in the literature.

Hygiene is a highly personal matter determined by individual values and practices. It is influenced by cultural, social, familial, and individual factors, as well as by the person's knowledge of health and hygiene and perceptions of personal comfort and needs. People may or may not be aware of their individual needs. A person with particularly malodorous feet is likely to be aware of this problem; however, people with underarm perspiration odors may need assistance, for example, from a nurse, to cope with the problem.

When people are ill, hygienic practices frequently become secondary to other functions, such as breathing, which in health are taken for granted. One sign that a formerly ill or depressed client is feeling better is an interest in shaving, hair care, or make-up.

Hygiene involves care of the skin, hair, nails, teeth, oral and nasal cavities, eyes, ears, and perineal and genital areas.

Factors Influencing Hygiene

Each individual has unique hygiene practices. These practices are influenced by the individual's body image, sociocultural factors, the expectations of the person's social group, and the person's knowledge level, developmental status, personal preferences, and health.

Body Image

Body image is the continually changing perception that an individual has of his or her own body. One man may view his body as trim, clean, and neatly groomed, whereas another sees himself as untidy and ungroomed. The view affects the hygiene of the individual. People who see themselves as clean and neatly groomed are likely to have established practices to support this view.

Sociocultural Factors

Many sociocultural factors affect hygiene. The individual's economic resources affect such practices as the use of cosmetics. Cultural patterns influence the frequency of bathing. For example, in some European cultures a full tub bath is normally not taken more than once a week, whereas in North America people may bathe once a day if water and facilities are available.

Expectations of the Person's Social Group

A number of social groups, e.g., family, work groups, and friends, may affect a person's hygiene. Early in life, children learn practices from their parents, and these are often continued in adult life. Some practices relate to physical conditions, such as the availability of hot water and the number of people in the family, as well as to family customs. Perhaps a father believes the use of deodorant is unmanly. His sons may adopt this attitude or, on the contrary, use deodorants because of other influences. Teenagers who want to be accepted by their peers may wash frequently and use advertised deodorants and hair creams. If the school football hero uses a particular toothpaste, boys who admire him may use it. A person's colleagues at work often have expectations that affect hygiene practices. Nurses usually expect other nurses to be clean and without body odor, whereas members of a male logging crew may consider body odor masculine and the use of deodorants effeminate.

Knowledge Level

The information an individual possesses about hygiene affects his or her practices. Knowledge about the effect of personal appearance on others, the various methods to maintain hygiene, and the implications of hygienic practices for health can alter a person's practices.

Developmental Status

Hygiene practices vary with an individual's stage of development. Many adolescents spend considerable time on their appearance, reflecting the values of their peer group. A 4-year-old, in contrast, may enjoy being dirty and resist parents' efforts to encourage washing.

Personal Preferences

Preferences often reflect a person's values and are highly individual. They can dictate the brand of soap used, the frequency of bathing, and the choice of a bath rather than a shower. For some people, relaxing in a tub of water is a luxury to be enjoyed after a day of work; to others, it is a waste of time that could be used to better advantage. Nurses' own personal preferences should not affect their assessment of appropriate behavior for clients. For example, a nurse may believe that daily bathing is appropriate, while a client may be accustomed to bathing once a week. If bathing once a week does not affect the client's health adversely, the nurse should not try to change the pattern. The nurse needs to intervene if a client's hygiene practices warrant change for health reasons. A female client, for example, who repeatedly has infections in the skin creases of the groin and under the breasts needs to learn to wash and thoroughly dry those areas each day, rather than once a week.

Health State

People who are very ill often are unable or lack the energy to bathe or brush their teeth, for example. They require assistance to carry out many hygienic activities. It is important for nurses to know exactly how much a client can safely do and how much assistance is required.

Purposes of Hygiene

Hygiene serves a number of purposes:

1. Promotes cleanliness, e.g., removes transient microorganisms and body secretions and excretions.
2. Provides comfort and relaxation, refreshes the client, and relaxes tired, tense muscles.
3. Improves self-image by improving appearance and eliminating offensive odors.
4. Conditions skin, e.g., a warm bath causes peripheral vasodilation and thus increases the blood circulation to the skin.

Kinds of Hygiene Care

Nurses commonly use the following terms to describe hygiene care:

Early Morning Care

Care is provided to clients as they awaken in the morning. In a hospital, nurses on the night shift may provide early morning care. This care helps clients ready themselves for breakfast or for early diagnostic tests. Usually, it consists of providing a urinal or bedpan to the client confined to bed, washing the face and hands, and giving oral care.

Morning Care

Morning care is provided after clients have breakfast. It usually includes the provision of a urinal or bedpan (to clients who are not ambulatory), a bath or shower, perineal care, back massage, and oral, nail, and hair care. Making the client's bed is part of morning care.

Afternoon Care

Clients often require additional care in the afternoon, e.g., when they return from physiotherapy or diagnostic tests. Providing a bedpan or urinal, washing the hands and face, and assisting with oral care refresh clients.

Hour of Sleep (HS Care)

This care is provided to clients before they retire for the night. It usually involves providing for elimination needs, washing face and hands, giving oral care, and giving a back massage.

In addition, clients may require care at other times: after urinating or defecating, after vomiting, and whenever they become soiled, e.g., from wound drainage or from profuse perspiration. Nurses must keep the hygiene needs of clients in mind and assist them whenever indicated.

Skin

The skin covers the entire surface of the body and thus is the largest organ of the body. At body orifices such as the ears, eyes, nose, rectum, and vagina, the skin is continuous with the mucous membrane that lines these orifices. Skin varies in thickness from about 0.5 mm over the ear lobes to 1.5 mm on the palms of the hands and soles of the feet.

Composition

The skin is made up of three layers: the epidermis (outer layer), the dermis or corium, and the subcutaneous tissue or hypodermis. The **epidermis** is made up of five layers in most areas of the body, none of which has blood vessels in it. The outermost layer of the epidermis is the stratum corneum or horny layer, which is continually being shed. It consists of dead cells referred to as **keratized cells**, because they are converted to protein before being shed. The other layers of the epidermis are the stratum lucidum, stratum granulosum, stratum spinosum, and the deepest layer, the stratum germinativum. It is in this last layer that new cells are formed and start to move toward the surface; it is also here that **melanin** is formed, which gives skin its dark pigment. Exposure to the sunlight stimulates melanocytes to produce melanin, which gives some people a tan. Certain races have more active melanocytes and hence darker pigmentation of the skin than others. The distribution of pigmentation in dark-skinned people varies considerably. People from the Mediterranean area tend to have blue lips. Blacks usually have a bluish pigmentation of the gums, either evenly distributed or in patches. The observable portion of the sclera of the eyes may also have melanin deposits.

The **dermis** is situated under the epidermis. It is a tough, elastic, flexible tissue, which is highly vascular and contains nerves and nerve endings. The pink tint of skin is due to blood vessels in the dermis. Hair follicles, sweat glands, and oil-supplying glands (**sebaceous glands**) are situated in this layer of the skin. The sebaceous glands secrete **sebum**, an oily substance that lubricates the skin.

Below the dermis is the **hypodermis.** It is a loosely knit connective tissue containing blood and lymph vessels, nerves, and fat globules. It serves to anchor the other skin layers and provides the springy base for the skin.

The normal skin of a healthy person has transient microorganisms that are not usually harmful. Adults usually have some resident micrococci, bacteria of the genera *Corynebacterium* and *Propionibacterium,* and a genus of fungi, *Pityrosporon.* Children also have gram-positive, spore-forming rods and *Neisseria* bacteria.

Transient microorganisms vary considerably from one person to another. They do not maintain themselves on the skin. Normally the skin can rid itself of these microorganisms in three general ways: (a) the drying and (b) the chemical effects of the fatty acids in the sebum, and (c) the normal skin pH of 5 to 6, which is too acidic for many microorganisms.

Functions

The skin serves four major functions:

1. It regulates the body temperature.
2. It protects underlying tissues from drying and injury by preventing the passage of microorganisms. The skin and mucous membrane are considered the body's first line of defense.
3. It secretes sebum, which has antibacterial and antifungal properties.
4. It transmits sensations through nerve receptors, which are sensitive to pain, temperature, touch, and pressure.

Sweat Glands

Sudoriferous (sweat) glands are on all body surfaces except the lips and parts of the genitals. The body has from two to five million, which are all present at birth. They are most numerous on the palms of the hands and the soles of the feet. Sweat glands are classified as apocrine and eccrine. The **apocrine glands**, located in the axillae and pubic areas, are of little use. Bacteria act upon the sweat produced by these glands, causing odor. The **eccrine glands** are important physiologically. The sweat they produce cools the body through evaporation. Sweat is made of up of water, sodium, potassium, chloride, glucose, urea, and lactate.

Developmental Changes

In early embryonic life, the skin is a single layer of cells. Other layers develop quickly. The fetus's skin is covered by a substance called **vernix caseosa**, a whitish, cheesy material seen on newborns. It usually disappears in the first day. The skin of an infant is thinner than an adult's, it is usually mottled, and in whites it varies from pink to red and becomes ruddy when the baby cries. Babies who are genetically dark-skinned are lightly pigmented at birth. Skin pigmentation gradually increases until about 6 or 8 weeks. Sweat glands of babies begin to function at about 1 month of age.

In adolescence, the sebaceous glands increase in activity as a result of increased levels of hormones (andro-

Examples of Nursing Diagnoses Related to Skin Problems

- Potential impairment of skin integrity related to edema
- Potential impairment of skin integrity related to emaciation
- Potential impairment of skin integrity related to peripheral vascular alterations
- Potential impairment of skin integrity related to radiation
- Potential impairment of skin integrity related to urinary incontinence
- Potential impairment of skin integrity related to imposed immobility
- Potential impairment of skin integrity related to reduced sensation in lower extremities
- Potential impairment of skin integrity related to wound drainage
- Actual impairment of skin integrity related to immobility decubitus ulcer
- Actual impairment of skin integrity (dry, cracked skin) related to fever and dehydration
- Actual impairment of skin integrity related to pruritus and scratching
- Actual impairment of skin integrity (stasis ulcer of left leg) related to impaired venous circulation

gens). This is thought to be one factor responsible for the development of acne, a common skin problem of adolescents.

The older adult also experiences skin changes. The skin tends to be thinner, drier, somewhat inelastic, and thus subject to fine wrinkling. This process begins any time after age 40. The elderly person's skin typically shows wrinkles, sagging, pigmentations, and keratotic spots, usually on areas exposed to the sun. The skin is less resilient, i.e., when pinched, it returns to place more slowly than the skin of a younger person does.

Assessment

Assessing a client's skin includes inspecting and palpating the skin, observing developmental changes, and determining the client's skin care practices and the factors influencing them.

Physical Examination

Normal skin:

1. Exhibits variations of pigment or color
2. Has good tissue turgor (firmness and elasticity) and is smooth, soft, and flexible
3. Has a variety of pigmented spots
4. Shows no evidence of cyanosis, jaundice, or pallor
5. Feels warm to the touch
6. Is intact, i.e., has no abrasions or excoriations

For information about skin assessment see Chapter 35, pages 808 to 810. Common skin problems are outlined in Table 36–1.

Skin Care Practices

Hygiene practices vary greatly among people. Sometimes, because of health problems, clients need to learn new hygiene practices, e.g., to prevent infection or skin breakdown. See factors affecting hygiene practices, earlier in this chapter.

Clients at Risk

A number of conditions place clients at risk of developing skin impairments. Seven of these are:

1. *Alterations in nutritional status,* such as emaciation and insufficient protein intake. **Emaciation** is a wasted appearance due to extreme weight loss. In emaciated individuals, subcutaneous fat is insufficient to provide padding or support over bony prominences to withstand normal stress or pressure. Individuals with inadequate protein intake are also prone to skin breakdown, since protein is essential for the building, maintenance, and repair of all body tissues.
2. *Immobility.* Normally, people change position frequently, even during sleep. When position cannot be altered, e.g., if the person is paralyzed or unconscious, or when it is not altered for prolonged periods (1 or 2 hours), blood circulation, which carries essential nutrients to the skin, is reduced. Without essential nutrients, tissues of the skin are ultimately destroyed.
3. *Altered hydration.* In dehydrated individuals, the skin becomes excessively dry, and skin turgor is diminished. Both conditions make the skin less resistant to injury.
4. *Altered sensation.* Loss of sensation in a body area may be the result of paralysis or other neurologic disease. Loss of sensation reduces a person's ability to discern injurious heat and cold and to feel the tingling (pins and needles) that signals loss of circulation. This loss makes the person prone to skin damage.
5. *Presence of secretions or excretions on the skin.* An accumulation of secretions, such as perspiration and sebum, or excretions, such as urine or feces, is irritat-

Table 36–1 Common Skin Problems

Problem and Appearance	Nursing Implications
Abrasion Superficial layers of the skin are scraped or rubbed away. Area is reddened and may have localized bleeding or serous weeping.	1. Prone to infection; therefore, wound should be kept clean and dry. 2. Do not wear rings or jewelry when providing care to avoid causing abrasions to clients. 3. Lift, do not pull, a client across a bed. See Chapter 38.
Excessive dryness Skin can appear flaky and rough.	1. Prone to infection if the skin cracks; therefore, provide lotions to moisturize the skin and prevent cracking. 2. Bathe client less frequently and use no soap or limit use of nonirritating soap. Rinse skin thoroughly because soap can be irritating and drying. 3. Encourage increased fluid intake if health permits to prevent dehydration.
Ammonia dermatitis (diaper rash) Caused by skin bacteria reacting with urea in the urine. The skin becomes reddened and is sore.	1. Keep skin dry and clean by applying protective ointments containing zinc oxide to areas at risk, e.g., buttocks and perineum. 2. Treat by exposing area to the warmth of a 40-watt gooseneck lamp, placed 30 cm (12 inches) away for 30 minutes, three times a day. This warmth helps to dry the rash. 3. Boil an infant's diapers or wash them with an antibacterial detergent to prevent infection. Rinse diapers well, because detergent is irritating to an infant's skin.
Acne Inflammatory condition with papules and pustules.	1. Keep the skin clean to prevent secondary infection. 2. Treatment varies widely.
Erythema Redness associated with a variety of conditions: e.g., rashes, exposure to sun, elevated body temperature.	1. Wash area carefully to remove excess microorganisms. 2. Apply antiseptic spray or lotion to prevent itching, promote healing, and prevent skin breakdown.
Hirsutism Excessive hair on a person's body and face, particularly in women.	1. Remove unwanted hair by using depilatories, shaving, electrolysis, or tweezing. 2. Enhance client's self-concept. See Chapter 48.

ing to the skin, harbors microorganisms, and makes an individual prone to skin breakdown and infection.

6. *Mechanical devices.* The presence of restraints, casts, or braces that create pressure or a shearing force can alter skin integrity considerably.

7. *Altered venous circulation.* Stasis of venous blood in the lower extremities, which is associated with varicose veins, can cause **stasis dermatitis** (inflammation of the skin) on the feet and around the ankles. This dermatitis is characterized by redness, dryness, itching, and swelling. Ultimately, skin tissues become **ischemic** (deficient of blood) and **necrotic** (dying), and ulcerations form. See Chapter 37, page 1014.

Nursing Diagnoses

Assessment data indicate whether or not a client has an actual or potential alteration in skin integrity. Examples of nursing diagnoses related to skin problems are shown on page 911.

Planning

Planning for assisting a client with personal hygiene includes consideration of: the client's personal preferences, health, and limitations; the time; and the equipment, facilities, and personnel available. Clients' personal preferences—about when and how they bathe, for example—should be followed as long as they are compatible with their health, the equipment available, etc. Nurses need to provide whatever assistance the client requires because of individual limitations. The nurse may provide help directly or delegate this task to other nursing personnel. In some instances, clients say they can perform activities, e.g., shaving, that they should not or cannot do. Nurses need to be guided by the health needs of the client, which are often specified on the nursing care plan.

Planning involves establishing outcome criteria. For suggestions, see page 922.

Intervention

General Guidelines

1. *An intact, healthy skin is the body's first line of defense.* It protects the body from invasion by microorganisms and from harmful agents such as chemicals. Nurses need to ensure that all skin care measures prevent injury and irritation. Scratching the skin with jewelry or long, sharp fingernails is avoided. Harsh rubbing or use of rough towels and washcloths can cause tissue damage, particularly when the skin is irritated or when circulation or sensation is diminished. Bottom bedsheets are kept taut and free from wrinkles to reduce friction and abrasion to the skin. Top bed linens are arranged to prevent undue pressure on the toes. When necessary, bed cradles or footboards are used to keep bedclothes off the feet.

2. *The degree to which the skin protects the underlying tissues from injury depends on the general health of the cells, the amount of subcutaneous tissue, and the dryness of the skin.* Skin that is poorly nourished and dry has less ability to protect and is more vulnerable to injury. When the skin is dry, lotions or creams with lanolin are applied, and bathing is limited to once or twice a week. For back rubs, lotion is used rather than alcohol. The greater the amount of subcutaneous tissue, the more padding there is, particularly over bony prominences. Nurses also assess the client's nutritional and fluid intake. When either one is deficient, measures are taken to improve it.

3. *Moisture in contact with the skin for a period of time can result in increased bacterial growth and irritation.* After a bath, the client's skin is dried carefully. Particular attention is paid to areas such as the axillae, the groin, beneath the breasts, and between the toes, where the potential for irritation is greatest. A nonirritating dusting powder, such as cornstarch, tends to reduce moisture and can be applied to these areas after they are dried. If clients are incontinent of urine or feces or if they perspire excessively, immediate cleaning is provided to prevent skin irritation.

4. *Body odors are caused by resident skin bacteria acting on body secretions.* Cleanliness is the best deodorant. Commercial deodorants and antiperspirants can be applied only after the skin is cleaned. Deodorants diminish odors, whereas antiperspirants reduce the amount of perspiration. Neither is applied immediately after shaving, because of the possibility of skin irritation. They are also not used on skin that is already irritated.

5. *Skin sensitivity to irritation and injury varies among individuals and in accordance with their health.* Generally speaking, skin sensitivity is greater in infants, very young children, and the elderly. A person's nutritional status also affects sensitivity. Emaciated or obese persons tend to experience more skin irritation and injury. The same tendency is seen in individuals with poor dietary habits and insufficient fluid intake. Even in healthy persons, skin sensitivity is highly variable. Some people's skin is sensitive to chemicals in skin care agents and cosmetics. Hypoallergenic cosmetics and soaps or soap substitutes are now available for these people. The nurse needs to ascertain whether the client has any sensitivities and what agents are appropriate to use.

6. *Agents used for skin care have selective actions and purposes.* Commonly used agents are described in Table 36–2.

Bathing and Skin Care

Purposes of bathing Bathing has a number of functions. The skin is bathed continuously in sebum and perspiration from the sebaceous and sudoriferous glands, respectively. Sebum and perspiration have protective functions: Sebum prevents dryness, and perspiration provides a slightly acid medium, which discourages bacterial

Table 36–2 Agents Commonly Used on the Skin

Type	Description
Soap	Lowers surface tension, and thus helps in cleaning. Some soaps contain antibacterial agents, which can change the natural flora of the skin.
Detergent	Used instead of soap for cleaning. Some people who are allergic to soaps may not be allergic to detergents, and vice versa.
Bath oil	Used in bath water; provides an oily film on the skin that softens and prevents chapping.
Skin cream, lotion	Provides a film on the skin that prevents evaporation and therefore chapping.
Powder	Can be used to absorb water and prevent friction. For example, powder under the breasts can prevent skin irritation. Some powders are antibacterial.
Deodorant	Masks or diminishes body odors.
Antiperspirant	Reduces the amount of perspiration.

growth. These two processes, however, can be injurious or disadvantageous if bathing is not carried out regularly, so that perspiration, sebum, and dead skin cells accumulate. Excessive perspiration interacts with bacteria on the skin, causing body odor, considered offensive in some cultures. An accumulation of sebum on the skin can be irritating in itself, since it promotes the growth of bacteria. Large numbers of bacteria on the skin can cause problems, particularly when the skin integrity is interrupted, for example, by a cut. Dead skin cells also harbor bacteria. Bathing, then, removes accumulated oil, perspiration, dead skin cells, and some bacteria. The quantity of oil and dead skin cells produced can be appreciated when nurses observe the skin of a person after the removal of a cast that has been on for 6 weeks. The skin is crusty, flaky, and dry underneath the cast. Applications of oil over several days are usually necessary to remove the debris.

Excessive bathing, however, can interfere with the intended lubricating effect of the sebum, causing dryness of the skin. This is an important consideration for people who produce limited sebum.

In addition to its cleaning value, bathing also stimulates circulation. A warm or hot bath dilates superficial arterioles, bringing more blood and nourishment to the skin. Vigorous rubbing has the same effect. Rubbing with long smooth strokes from the distal to proximal parts of extremities (from the point farthest from the body to the point closest) is particularly effective in facilitating venous blood flow.

Bathing also produces a sense of well-being. It is refreshing and relaxing and frequently improves morale, appearance, and self-respect. Some people take a morning shower for its refreshing, stimulating effect. Others prefer an evening bath because it is relaxing. These effects are more evident when a person is ill. For example, it is not uncommon for clients who have had a restless or sleepless night to feel relaxed, comfortable, and sleepy after a morning bath.

The effectiveness of bathing in eliminating some body odors can also be important. The apocrine glands, which produce sweat, are situated in the axillae and pubic areas and appear at puberty. Their secretions are decomposed by bacterial action, resulting in a noticeable odor that is often distasteful to others. Apocrine glands are thought to secrete less after menopause and to enlarge and become more active before and after monthly menses. The use of antiperspirants to control perspiration and odor from the axillae is prevalent in North America. On occasion, the nurse may recommend its use to persons with problem perspiration.

The bathing procedure can offer opportunities for the nurse to assess ill clients. The nurse can observe the condition of the client's skin and physical conditions such as sacral edema or rashes. The skin is said to mirror health, but it is not always an accurate index. While assisting a client with a bath, the nurse can also assess the client's psychosocial needs, e.g., orientation to time and ability to cope with the illness. Learning needs, such as a diabetic client's need to learn foot care, can also be assessed.

There are generally two categories of baths given to clients: cleaning and therapeutic. Cleaning baths are given chiefly for hygienic purposes, whereas therapeutic baths are given for a physical effect, such as to soothe irritated skin or to treat an area (e.g., the perineum).

Cleaning baths

1. *Complete bed bath.* The nurse washes the entire body of a dependent client in bed.

2. *Self-help bed bath.* A client confined to bed is able to bathe himself or herself with help from the nurse for washing the back and perhaps the feet.

3. *Partial bath (abbreviated bath).* Only the parts of the client's body that might cause discomfort or odor, if neglected, are washed: the face, hands, axillae, perineal area, and back. Omitted are the arms, chest, abdomen, legs, and feet. The nurse provides this care for dependent clients and assists self-sufficient clients confined to bed by washing their backs. Some ambulatory clients prefer to take a partial bath at the sink. The nurse can assist them by washing their backs.

4. *Tub bath.* Tub baths are preferred to bed baths, since washing and rinsing are easier in a tub. Tubs are also used for therapeutic baths. The amount of assistance offered by the nurse depends on the abilities of the client. Many agencies have specially designed tubs for dependent clients. These tubs greatly reduce the work of the nurse in lifting clients in and out of the tub and have greater benefits than a sponge bath in bed.

5. *Shower.* Many ambulatory clients are able to use shower facilities and require only minimal assistance from the nurse.

Therapeutic baths A therapeutic bath is usually ordered by a physician. Medications may be placed in the water. A therapeutic bath is generally taken in a tub one-third or one-half full, about 114 liters (30 gal). The client remains in the bath for a designated time, often 20 to 30 minutes. If the client's back, chest, and arms are to be treated, these areas need to be immersed in the solution. The bath temperature is generally included in the order; 37.7 to 46 C (100 to 115 F) may be ordered for adults and 40.5 C (105 F) is usually ordered for infants. See Table 36–3 for types of therapeutic baths.

Table 36–3 Types of Therapeutic Baths

Bath Solution	Directions	Uses
Saline	4 ml (1 tsp) sodium chloride (NaCl) to 500 ml (1 pt) water.	Has a cooling effect. Cleans. Decreases skin irritation.
Oatmeal or Aveeno	720 ml (3 cups) cooked oatmeal in a cheesecloth bag. Tie the bag securely and twirl it in the tub until the water is opalescent.	Soothes skin irritations. Softens and lubricates dry, scaly skin.
Cornstarch	0.45 kg (1 lb) cornstarch in sufficient cold water to dissolve it; then add boiling water until the mixture is thick. Add to the tub water.	Soothes skin irritation.
Sodium bicarbonate	4 ml (1 tsp) sodium bicarbonate to 500 ml (1 pt) water, or 120–360 ml (4–12 oz) to 120 liters (30 gal).	Has a cooling effect. Relieves skin irritation.
Potassium permanganate ($KMnO_4$)	Available in tablets, which are crushed, dissolved in a little water, and added to the bath.	Cleans and disinfects. Treats infected skin areas.

Procedure 36–1 ▲ Bathing an Adult

Equipment

1. Two bath towels, one for the face and one for the remainder of the body.
2. A washcloth.
3. Soap in a soap dish.
4. A basin for the wash water (for a partial or complete bed bath).
5. Hygienic supplies such as lotion, powder, and deodorant.
6. A bath blanket to cover the client during the bath (for a partial or complete bed bath).
7. Water between 43 and 46 C (110 and 115 F) for adults. The water should feel comfortably warm to the client. People vary in their sensitivity to heat. Most clients will verify a suitable temperature. The water for a bed bath should be changed at least once.
8. A clean gown or pajamas as needed.
9. Additional bed linen and towels, if required.
10. A bedpan or urinal.

Intervention

1. Explain what you plan to do. Adjust the explanation to the client's needs.

   Rationale This interaction reassures the client by providing knowledge of what will happen, identifies the client, and allows the nurse to assess whether any special equipment, e.g., a razor, is needed.

2. Close the windows and doors to make sure that the room is free from drafts.

   Rationale Air currents increase loss of heat from the body by convection.

3. Provide privacy by drawing the curtains or closing the door. Some agencies provide signs indicating the need for privacy.

   Rationale Hygiene is a personal matter.

4. Offer the client a bedpan or urinal or ask whether the client wishes to use the toilet or commode.

   Rationale The client will be more comfortable after voiding, and voiding is advisable before cleaning the perineum.

For a Bed Bath

5. Place the bed in the high position.

   Rationale This avoids undue strain on the nurse's back.

6. Remove the top bed linen, and replace it with the bath blanket. If the bed linen is to be reused, place it over the bedside chair. If it is to be changed, place it in the linen hamper.
7. Assist the client to move near you.

   Rationale This facilitates access without undue reaching and straining.

8. Remove the client's gown.
9. Make a bath mitt with the washcloth (see Figure 36–1):
   a. Triangular method: (1) Lay your hand on the washcloth; (2) fold the top corner over your hand; (3, 4) fold the side corners over the hand; (5) tuck the second corner under the cloth on the palmar side to secure the mitt.

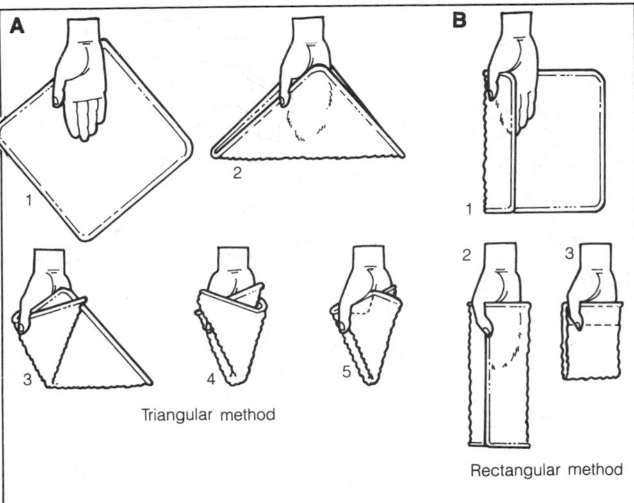

Figure 36–1

b. Rectangular method: (1) Lay your hand on the washcloth, and fold one side over your hand; (2) fold the second side over your hand; (3) fold the top of the cloth down, and tuck it under the folded side against your palm to secure the mitt.

Rationale A bath mitt retains water and heat better than a cloth loosely held.

10. Place one towel across the client's chest.

11. Wash the client's eyes with water only, and dry them well. Use a separate corner of the washcloth for each eye, and wipe from the inner to the outer canthus.

Rationale Using separate corners prevents transmitting microorganisms from one eye to the other. Cleaning from the inner to the outer canthus prevents secretions from entering the nasolacrimal ducts.

12. Ask whether the client wants soap used on the face. Wash, rinse, and dry the client's face, neck, and ears.

Rationale Soap has a drying effect, and the face, which is exposed to the air more than other body parts, tends to be drier.

13. Place the bath towel lengthwise under the client's arm. Wash, rinse, and dry the arm, using long, firm strokes from distal to proximal areas (from the point farthest from the body to the point closest). Wash the axilla well. Repeat for the other arm. (Omit the arms for a partial bath.) Exercise caution if an intravenous infusion is present, and check its flow after moving the arm.

Rationale The bath towel protects the bed from becoming wet. Firm strokes from distal to proximal areas increase venous blood return.

14. Place a towel directly on the bed and put the basin on it. Place the client's hands in the basin. Assist the client to wash, rinse, and dry them, paying particular attention to the spaces between the fingers.

Rationale Many clients enjoy immersing their hands in the basin and washing themselves.

15. Fold the bath blanket down to the client's pubic area and place the towel alongside the chest and abdomen. Wash, rinse, and dry the client's chest and abdomen, giving special attention to the skin fold under the breasts. Keep the client's chest and abdomen covered with the towel between the wash and the rinse. Replace the bath blanket when the areas have been dried. (Do not wash the chest and abdomen during a partial bath. However, the creases under a woman's breasts may require bathing if they are irritated.) Avoid undue exposure when washing the client's chest and abdomen. For some clients, it may be preferable to wash the chest and the abdomen separately. In that case, the bath towel is placed horizontally across the abdomen first and then across the chest.

16. Wrap one of the client's legs and feet with the bath blanket, ensuring that the pubic area is well covered. See Figure 36–2. Place the bath towel lengthwise under the other leg, and wash that leg. Use long, smooth, firm strokes, washing from the ankle to the knee and from the knee to the thigh. Rinse and dry that leg, reverse the coverings, and repeat for the other leg. (Omit this step for a partial bath.)

Rationale Washing from distal to proximal areas stimulates venous blood flow.

17. Wash the feet by placing them in the basin of water. Dry each foot. Pay particular attention to the spaces between the toes. If you prefer, wash one foot after that leg, before washing the other leg. (Omit this step for a partial bath.)

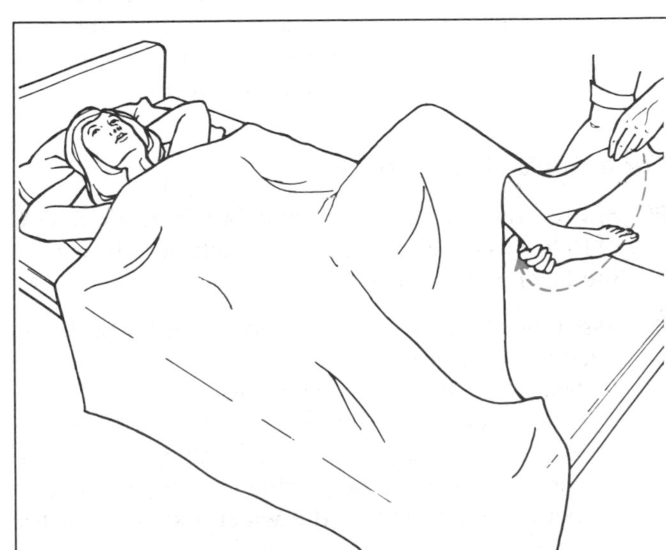

Figure 36–2

18. Obtain fresh, warm bath water now or when necessary.

    Rationale The temperature of the water in the basin cools relatively rapidly, and the water becomes soapy. It needs to be changed often.

19. Assist the client to turn to a prone position or side-lying position facing away from you. Place the bath towel lengthwise alongside the client's back and buttocks. Wash and dry the back, buttocks, and upper thighs, paying particular attention to the gluteal folds. Give a back rub. See Procedure 36–3. Avoid undue exposure of the client, as for the abdomen and chest. See step 15.

20. Assist the client to the supine position, and determine whether the client can wash the genital-perineal area independently. Say, for example, "I have washed all but your genital area. Would you like to complete your bath?" If the client cannot do so, drape the client as shown in Figure 36–3, and wash the area. See Procedure 36–3.

    Rationale Many clients prefer to clean their own perineums, if they are able, because it is embarrassing to have this done by another person.

21. Assist the client to use any hygenic aids desired, such as powder, lotion, or deodorant. Use powder sparingly, because it tends to accumulate.

22. Help the client to put on a clean gown or pajamas. If intravenous apparatus is attached, place the sleeve of the gown over the infusion bottle first.

23. Assist the client with hair, mouth, and nail care. See later sections of this chapter. Some clients prefer or need mouth care prior to the bath.

24. Record on the chart significant assessments made during the bath (such as excoriation in the folds beneath the breasts or reddened areas over bony prominences) and progress in relief of previous problems. Bathing is not normally recorded.

For a Tub Bath or Shower

25. Fill the tub about halfway with water at 43 to 46 C (110 to 115 F). For a therapeutic bath, add the correct medication. See Table 36–3.

26. Assist the client to the tub or shower and provide any needed assistance.
    a. Many clients can manage a tub bath or shower independently. Others require assistance only to wash their backs. The client taking a standing shower may need help initially to adjust the temperature and flow of the water. Explain how the client can signal for help, and then leave the client for 2 to 5 minutes.
    b. If the client requires considerable assistance, a second nurse may be needed to help the client into and out of the tub and/or to hold the client in a sitting position throughout the bath. When assisting clients into and out of tubs, take safety measures to prevent the client from falling or slipping. For example, if the client can step into the tub, he or she should hold the handbar while you support the client's upper trunk under the axillae. To provide support as the client sits down in the tub, fold a towel lengthwise and place it around the client's chest, under both axillae; then hold the ends securely at the back of the client as the client sits.
    c. Other clients may need to sit on the edge of the tub or on a chair beside the tub before transferring into the tub. Some tubs have a nonskid surface to prevent the client's feet from slipping. A rubber mat or a towel placed in the bottom of the tub can provide a secure base for the client's feet.

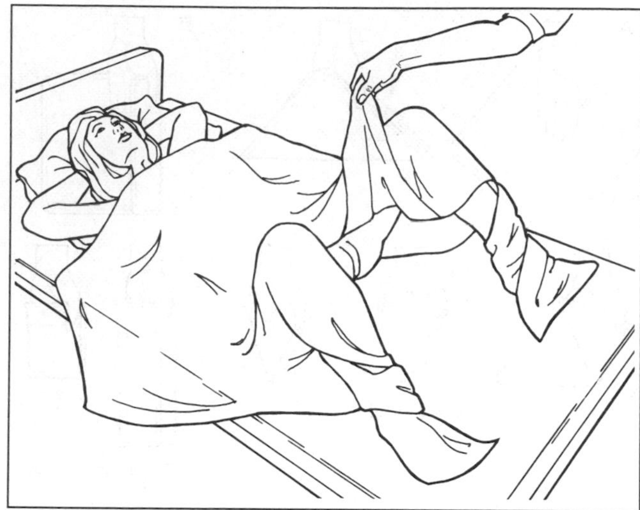

Figure 36–3

27. Wash the client's back, if necessary, and assist the client out of the tub.

28. Assist the client as necessary to dry and to don a clean gown or pajamas.

29. Assist the client back to the room, and provide a back rub if the client is spending long periods in bed. See Procedure 36–3.

30. Clean the tub or shower in accordance with agency practice, discard used linen in the laundry hamper, and place the "unoccupied" sign on the door.

31. Follow steps 21, 23, and 24.

Skin Care for the Newborn

Practices in skin care of the newborn vary. When the baby is first admitted to the nursery, some nurses give an admission bath; others remove any blood or vernix caseosa from the infant's face for aesthetic reasons only, then diaper and wrap the baby loosely in a blanket. The newborn's temperature-regulating mechanisms are undeveloped, so measures to avoid chilling are important. Hexachlorophene soap was previously used for admission baths to prevent *Staphylococcus* infections in nurseries. However, its use has been largely discontinued, since it was suggested that central nervous system damage follows repeated use. After the newborn's status is stabilized, daily hygienic care includes a sponge bath (optional) until the cord falls off, cleaning the genitals and buttocks during diaper changes, cord care, and, for some male infants, circumcision care. If sponging is done, small soft washcloths or cotton balls should be used. The vernix caseosa usually disappears in about 24 hours. If it persists in creases and folds, it can become an irritant and needs to be removed with gentle wiping with a cotton ball moistened with warm water.

The cord falls off spontaneously, usually in 5 to 8 days, but it may remain up to 2 weeks. Attempts should *not* be made to remove it. To encourage drying of the cord and to discourage infection, the nurse may wipe the base of the cord once a day with alcohol. In most nurseries, the cord is left exposed to the air; however, in some agencies a small gauze dressing is applied. This dressing needs to be changed when soiled.

If a baby is circumcised, the penis must be inspected for bleeding, although most incisions heal rapidly. If the baby is diapered lightly over the penis, any bleeding is noticeable on the diaper. Immediately after a circumcision, the area is covered with sterile gauze saturated with petroleum jelly. This gauze may be left on until it falls off spontaneously or it may be removed when the infant voids; the area is then cleaned gently with moistened cotton balls, and a new dressing is applied each time the diaper is changed.

Smegma, a curdlike secretion, may collect under the prepuce of the glans in male babies and between the labia in female babies. Smegma can be removed with a moistened cotton ball. For females one swab should be used for each stroke, and the nurse should wipe from the front of the body toward the back.

Babies usually wear a shirt and a diaper, although the shirt may not be necessary, depending on the temperature of the environment. Babies do not perspire for the first month nor do they respond with gooseflesh; therefore, the nurse must use judgment about clothing babies appropriately. If they are too hot, they develop miliaria rubra (prickly heat, a rash) on the face, neck, and/or places where skin surfaces rub together.

Infant Bathing

Sponge baths are given to infants until the cord stump disappears and the umbilicus is well healed. Then tub baths may be given. The general bathing measures previously discussed should be employed for the infant's bath, but the nurse must pay particular attention to preventing undue exposure.

Sponge bath The equipment required for sponging the baby depends on agency facilities and policies. Generally included are a shirt, a diaper, safety pins, a soft washcloth, cotton balls, a towel, a moisture-resistant bag for soiled cotton balls, facial tissue or toilet tissue to remove feces, a mild, nonperfumed soap, and a basin of water at 38 to 40.5 C (100 to 105 F). The water should feel slightly warm to the nurse's wrist or the elbow. Optional materials include alcohol to apply at the base of the cord stump and mild lotion or baby oil if needed for dry skin. If used, soap should be used sparingly, since it can dry a baby's skin. Cotton-tipped applicators are contraindicated, because they can break when the baby moves, causing injury to the mucous membranes of the nose or to an eardrum. Powders are also avoided, since the baby may inhale them while they are being shaken from the container. Powders also tend to cake with moisture and cause skin irritation.

The infant's face, neck, ears, and scalp are cleaned before the baby is undressed. The nurse wipes the baby's eyes, behind the ears, and neck creases with a cotton ball. The nurse wipes the eyes from the inner canthus to the outer canthus using only water and one cotton ball for each stroke. The inside of the ears can be cleaned with a rolled wisp of cotton, dampened and rotated gently in the ear. To clean the baby's scalp, the nurse slides one hand under the baby until the baby's head is well supported in the palm, and picks up the baby securely. The baby's head is held over the basin, and the scalp is soaped, rinsed, and dried thoroughly.

The infant's shirt is then removed, and the trunk, arms, and legs are washed. The infant is turned to wash the back. Alcohol may be applied at the base of the cord stump before putting the shirt back on. To put on an open-fronted shirt, the nurse lays the baby in the shirt and then reaches through a sleeve and grasps the baby's arm to pull it through the sleeve. To put a pullover shirt on the baby, the nurse pulls the neck opening rapidly over the baby's head and then pulls the arms through the sleeves.

The baby's buttocks and perineum are cleaned last. First, excess feces are removed with facial tissue or toilet tissue. The genital area is cleaned from front to back. The circumcised area should not require special care, and the trend is *not* to retract the foreskin of uncircumcised male infants. The folds between the labia and around the scrotum should receive particular attention and be dried thoroughly. A baby's perineum usually does not need oil.

However, if the skin is excessively dry, moisturizing lotions or baby oil can offer protection.

Tub bath Infants can be given tub baths when the umbilicus is well healed, usually within the first 2 weeks of life. This can be a pleasurable experience for the baby. Preparation of the environment and of supplies is the same as for the sponge bath. It is important to keep safety pins out of the infant's reach and to have all supplies available. Infants must never be left alone in a bassinet even for a few seconds, because they do move and can fall.

Before putting the baby into the bath, the nurse washes the baby's face, neck, eyes, and scalp as for the infant sponge bath. The baby is then undressed and excess feces wiped away.

The baby is submerged gradually in the tub and held firmly with one hand. Using the free hand, the nurse soaps and rinses the baby. If the baby appears to be enjoying the experience, the bath can be leisurely. When removed from the tub, the baby is wrapped completely in a towel and gently patted dry. Special attention is given to drying body creases. The baby is then dressed.

Perineal-Genital Care

Perineal-genital care is also referred to as perineal care on peri-care. Some nurses use these terms only for special perineal care provided at prescribed times other than during a bed bath. For example, peri-care is a nursing order commonly prescribed for postdelivery clients, whose perineal area must be irrigated or cleaned after each defecation and urination. Because postdelivery clients often have swollen perineal tissues, vaginal discharge of blood, mucus, and tissue from the uterus (lochia), and in some cases an incision of the perineum (episiotomy), frequent cleaning of the perineum is essential to prevent infection.

Perineal care is a part of the bed bath. It is an embarrassing procedure for most clients. Nurses also may find it embarrassing initially, particularly when the client is of the opposite sex. Most clients who require a bed bath from the nurse are able to clean their own genital areas with minimal assistance. The nurse may need to hand a moistened washcloth and soap to the client, rinse the washcloth, and provide a towel.

Because some clients are unfamiliar with terminology for the genitals and perineum, it may be difficult for nurses to explain what is expected. Most clients, however, understand what is meant if the nurse simply says, "I'll give you a washcloth to finish your bath." Elderly patients may be familiar with the term *private parts*. Whatever expression the nurse uses, it needs to be one that the client understands and one that is comfortable for the nurse to use.

The nurse needs to provide perineal care efficiently and matter-of-factly. Some nurses wear gloves while providing this care for the comfort of the client and to protect the nurse from infection.

Procedure 36–2 ▲ Perineal-Genital Care

Equipment

When perineal-genital care is provided in conjunction with the bed bath, the following bed bath equipment is used:

1. A bath basin two-thirds filled with water at 43 to 46 C (110 to 115 F)
2. Soap in a soap dish
3. A washcloth
4. A bath towel
5. A bath blanket
6. Powder or protective ointment as required

When special perineal-genital care is provided other than during the bath, the equipment listed below may be needed. Some agencies have special peri-trays for postdelivery clients.

1. A bath towel
2. A bath blanket
3. Disposable gloves
4. Cotton balls or swabs
5. A solution bottle, pitcher, or container filled with warm water or a prescribed solution
6. A bedpan to receive the rinse water
7. A moisture-resistant bag or receptacle for used cotton swabs
8. A perineal pad

Intervention

1. Offer an appropriate explanation, being particularly sensitive to any client expressions of embarrassment.

2. Fold the top bed linen to the foot of the bed, and fold the client's gown up to expose the genital area.
3. Place a bath towel under the client's hips so that the lower end can be used to dry the anterior perineum, while the upper end can dry the rectal area.

   Rationale The bath towel prevents the bed from becoming soiled.

For Females

4. Position the client in a back-lying position with the knees flexed and spread well apart (abducted).
5. Cover the client's body and legs with the bath blanket. Drape the client's legs by tucking the bottom corners of the bath blanket under the inner sides of the legs. See Figure 36–2, earlier. The middle portion of the base of the blanket is then brought up over the pubic area. See Figure 36–3, earlier.

   Rationale Minimum exposure lessens the client's embarrassment and prevents chills.
6. Wash and dry the upper inner thighs.
7. Clean the labia majora. Then spread the labia to wash the folds between the labia majora and the labia minora. See Figure 36–4. Use separate corners of the washcloth for each fold, and wipe from the pubis to the rectum. For menstruating women and clients with indwelling catheters, use cotton balls or gauze. Use a clean ball for each stroke.

   Rationale Smegma, which tends to collect around the labia minora, promotes bacterial growth. Using separate corners of the washcloth or new cotton balls or gauzes prevents the transmission of microorganisms from one area to the other. Wiping is done from the area of least contamination (the pubis) to the area of greatest contamination (the rectum).

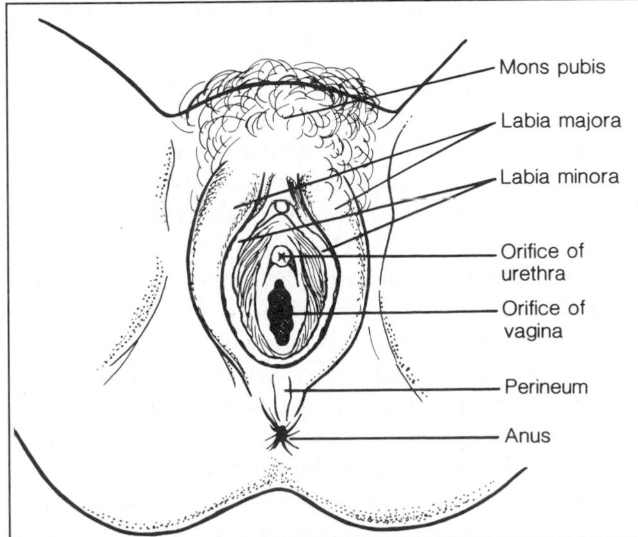

Figure 36–4 Female genitalia

8. Rinse the area well. You may place the client on a bedpan and pour a pitcher of warm water over the area.
9. Dry the perineum thoroughly, paying particular attention to the folds between the labia.

   Rationale Moisture supports the growth of many microorganisms.
10. Inspect the labia and perineal orifices for intactness. Inspect particularly around the urethra of clients with indwelling catheters. Apply a protective ointment if necessary.

    Rationale A catheter may cause excoriation around the urethra.
11. To clean between the buttocks, assist the client to turn on her side facing away from you. Pay particular attention to the anal area. Clean the anus with toilet tissue before washing it, if necessary. Dry the area well.
12. Apply powder or protective ointments, such as petroleum jelly, if necessary.

    Rationale Powder tends to absorb moisture. Petroleum jelly can protect excoriated areas.
13. For postdelivery clients, apply a perineal pad from front to back.

    Rationale This prevents contamination of the vagina and urethra by organisms from the anal area.
14. Record on the client's chart any significant observations, such as redness, swelling, or discharge.

For Males

15. Position the client in a supine position with knees slightly flexed and hips slightly rotated externally.
16. Wash and dry the upper inner thighs.
17. Put on gloves (optional). Wash and dry the penis using firm strokes. If the client is uncircumcised, retract the prepuce (foreskin) to expose the glans penis (the tip of the penis) for cleaning. Push the foreskin over the glans after cleaning the glans penis. See Figure 36–5.

    Rationale By handling the penis firmly, the nurse may prevent an erection. Having the nurse wear gloves may also be more comfortable for the client. Retracting the foreskin is necessary to remove the smegma that collects under the foreskin and promotes bacterial growth.

18. Wash and dry the scrotum. The posterior folds of the scrotum may need to be cleaned when the buttocks are cleaned.

    Rationale The scrotum tends to be more soiled than the penis because of its proximity to the rectum; thus it is usually cleaned after the penis.

19. Clean the buttocks in the manner described for female clients (steps 11–12 above).

20. Record on the client's chart any significant observations, such as redness, swelling, or discharge.

Sample Recording

Date	Time	Notes
July 10/87	0900	Perineal care given. Circular reddened area about 2.5 cm diameter to left of urethral orifice. No discharge apparent. ——————— ——— Patricia L. Snow, SN

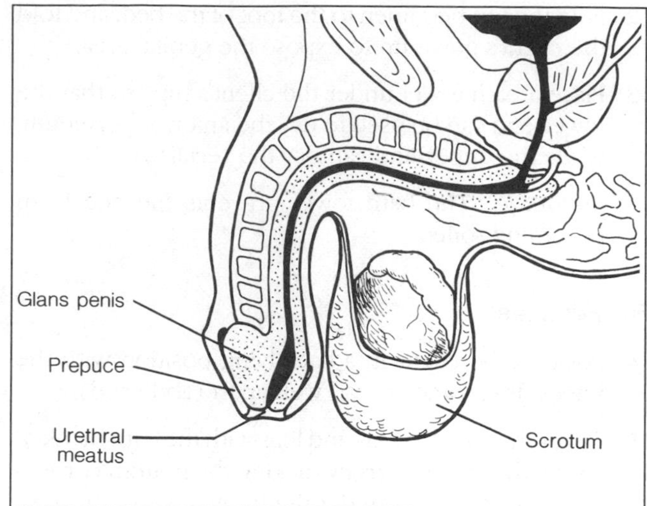

Figure 36–5 Male genitalia

Back Rubs

Back rubs, or massage of the back, have two chief objectives: to relax and relieve tension (sedative effect), and to stimulate blood circulation to the tissues and the muscles. Friction from the rubbing produces heat at the skin surface. Heat dilates the peripheral blood vessels in the area, thus increasing the blood supply to the area. Because tissues are under pressure when a client is in bed and muscles are usually relaxed, stimulation of the circulation is essential so that the tissues obtain nutrients and oxygen.

Five massage methods can be used to rub the back and the bony prominences of the body:

1. In the **tapotement**, the little-finger side of each hand is used in a sharp, hacking movement on the back. Care must be taken not to bruise the client. This method is not advised for elderly, debilitated clients, or clients who have disease conditions of the back.

2. The **petrissage** is a kneading or large, quick pinch of the skin, subcutaneous tissue, and muscle. Pinches are taken first up the vertebral column and then over the entire back. The tapotement and the petrissage are primarily stimulating, especially if done quickly and with firm pressure.

3. The **friction stroke** is a circular stroke accomplished with both thumbs. The nurse massages the back from the buttocks to the shoulders, using smooth, tiny circles.

4. The **effleurage** is a smooth, long stroke: a moving of the hands up and down the back. The hands move lightly down the sides of the back, maintaining contact with the skin, but move firmly up the back. This rub has a relaxing, sedative effect if slow movement and light pressure are used.

5. The **three-handed effleurage** is a smooth, stroking motion that gives the client an impression of being rubbed by three hands. The nurse starts with one hand at the base of the client's neck and moves the hand to the lateral aspect of the shoulder. The nurse then makes the same movement with the other hand, moving it to the other shoulder before removing the first hand from the shoulder and returning it to the base of the neck. This rub is particularly effective in relieving tension of the neck muscles.

Effleurage with circular motions is the method that nurses usually use to rub hospitalized clients.

In addition to using the four types of rubs described, the nurse can apply long, smooth strokes up and down the back combined with circular motions over the bony prominences to relax the client and stimulate blood circulation to the tissues and muscles in the area. The hands and lotion are warmed first. Then, with lotion on both hands, the nurse begins rubbing with circular motions over the sacrum. The nurse moves the hands up the center of the back and, using circular motions, massages the skin over the scapulae. The nurse continues these circular motions as she or he moves the hands down the back on the lateral aspects and massages the right and left iliac crest areas. This pattern is repeated for 3 to 5 minutes, depending on the client's needs.

Other pressure points on the body that generally benefit from massage and the application of lotions are the elbows, knees, and heels. Sometimes massage of the anterior aspects of both iliac crests of very thin clients is also indicated.

During the back rub, the nurse observes any reddened areas that do not disappear after a few minutes of massage, any breaks in the skin, and any bruises. They should be reported and recorded. Often, these conditions predispose to decubitus ulcers.

Nurses are advised not to rub tender, reddened areas on the lower legs of clients, particularly the calves. Redness, tenderness, and heat, particularly along the course of a vein, may indicate a thrombus (blood clot) in the area. Massage might dislodge the clot, which could travel to the heart or the lung, causing a myocardial or pulmonary embolus. This can present a very serious problem.

Emolient creams and lotions are frequently used to lubricate the skin during back rubs. Alcohol preparations are cooling, but they are used infrequently today. They are refreshing, and they toughen skin by hardening the skin protein, but they tend to dry the skin, and very dry skin is likely to crack. Alcohol preparations are particularly undesirable for use on elderly clients, whose skin is usually dry. Dehydrated and poorly nourished clients may also not benefit from an alcohol back rub.

The position of choice for a back rub is the prone position (lying on the stomach). The second preferred position is the side-lying position; its disadvantage is the difficulty of massaging the lateral aspect of the hip on which the client is lying, and the client must be turned to the other side.

Procedure 36–3 ▲ Giving a Back Rub

Equipment

1. Lotion, alcohol, or powder depending on the client's preference. Often clients have a container of back rub solution at the bedside. Unless another agent is specifically ordered by the physician, lotion is preferred because of its lubricating action on the skin. Alcohol has a cooling, refreshing effect, but it tends to be drying and is therefore not indicated for people with dry skin, particularly the elderly.
2. A towel to remove excess moisture.

Intervention

1. Assist the client to move to the near side of the bed within your reach.
2. Establish which position the client prefers. The prone position is recommended for a back rub. If the client cannot assume this position, a side-lying position is used, although that makes it difficult to massage the lateral aspect of the hip on which the client is lying. The client will need to turn to the other side for you to complete that part of the back rub.
3. Expose the client's back from the shoulders to the inferior sacral area.
4. Pour a small amount of lotion onto the palms of your hands and hold it for a minute, or place the container in a bath basin filled with warm water.

   Rationale Back rub preparations tend to feel uncomfortably cold to clients. Holding warms the solution slightly, so that it will be more comfortable.
5. Rub in a circular motion over the sacral area.
6. Move your hands up the center of the back and then over both scapulae.
7. Massage in a circular motion over the scapulae.
8. Move your hands down the sides of the back.
9. Massage the areas over the right and left iliac crests. See Figure 36–6.
10. Repeat steps 5–9 for 3 to 5 minutes. Repeat step 4 as necessary.
11. While massaging the client's skin, watch for:
    a. Whitish or reddened skin areas that do not disappear after rubbing.
    b. Broken or raw skin, especially on the elbows or heels.
12. Massage pressure areas gently and only if there is no evidence of underlying tissue damage.

    Rationale Vigorous massage over bony prominences can increase damage in nutrient-deprived tissues.
13. Pat dry any excess solution with a towel.
14. Record on the client's chart any redness, broken skin areas, and bruises.

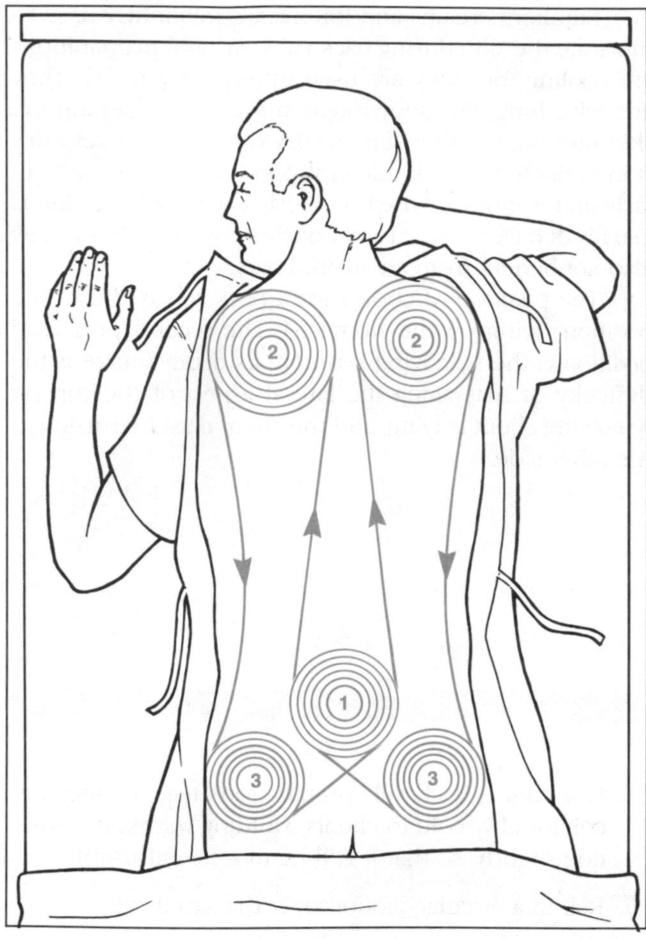

Figure 36–6

Evaluation

Examples of outcome criteria for clients with skin problems are outlined on page 922. See also the section on decubitus ulcers in Chapter 37, page 1012.

Feet

The feet are essential for ambulation and merit attention even when clients are confined to bed. Each foot contains 26 bones, 107 ligaments, and 19 muscles. These structures function together when the client stands or walks.

During childhood, the bony structure and the small muscles of the feet are easily damaged by tight, binding stockings and ill-fitting shoes. For normal development, it is important that the arches be supported and that the bony structure and the feet be allowed to grow with no external restraints.

Developmental Variations

At birth, a baby's foot is relatively unformed. The arches are supported by fatty pads and do not take their full shape until 5 or 6 years of age. Feet are not fully grown until about age 20. Healthy feet remain relatively unchanged during life. However, the feet of elderly people often require special attention. Reduced blood supply and accompanying arteriosclerosis, for example, can predispose the foot to infection following trauma.

Assessment

Each foot is inspected for shape, size, and the number of toes present and palpated to assess areas of tenderness, edema, and circulatory status. Normally, the toes are straight and flat. The plantar surface of each foot should have the following landmarks: the medial longitudinal arch, an apparent heel, and an apparent ball of the foot (metatar-

Table 36–4 Assessment Data: Feet

Physical Assessment	Data	Method	Normal Findings	Abnormal Findings
Inspection	1. Skin surfaces, for cleanliness, odor, dryness, inflammation, swelling, abrasions, or other lesions	Carefully check all skin surfaces, paying particular attention to areas between toes.	Intact skin Absence of swelling or inflammation	Excessive dryness Areas of inflammation or swelling, e.g., corns, calluses Fissures Scaling and cracking of skin, e.g., athlete's foot Plantar warts
	2. Status of toenails		See next section, "Nails"	
	3. Toe contour	Observe toe profile.	Toes extended (straight and flat)	Bunion (hallux valgus) Hammer toe Claw toe
	4. Longitudinal foot arch	Observe medial foot profile when client is standing.	Presence of medial longitudinal arch, i.e., medial concavity, with prominent heel and ball of foot	Flat foot (pes planus) High arch (pes cavus)
	5. Foot alignment	Observe alignment of foot to ankle and tibia, and metatarsal alignment (alignment of forefoot to heel).	Foot in straight alignment	Toeing-in (pes vargus) Toeing-out (pes valgus) Abduction of forefoot (metatarsus varus) Adduction of forefoot (metatarsus valgus) Clubfoot
	6. Ability to stand, walk, and perform range-of-motion exercises with each ankle and set of toes	See Chapters 37 and 39.	Full range of motion	Deformity (e.g., foot drop) Impaired range of motion in ankle or toes
Palpation	7. Areas of tenderness on body or muscular structures or on plantar surface	Palpate bony and muscular structures of foot and plantar surface to locate points of tenderness.	Absence of tenderness and nodules Smooth, firm, fleshy plantar surface	Tenderness in certain areas, related to arthritic changes, muscle strain, or lesions, e.g., plantar warts or bunions
	8. Ankle edema	Palpate anterior and posterior surfaces of ankle.	No swelling	Swelling or pitting edema
	9. Circulatory status	Palpate dorsalis pedis pulse on dorsal surface of foot just above longitudinal arch. Compare skin temperatures of two feet.	Strong, regular pulses in both feet Warm skin temperature	Weak or absent pulses Cool skin temperature in one or both feet

sophalangeal joints). See Table 36–4 for physical assessment methods and normal and abnormal findings. The nurse also determines the client's history of diabetes mellitus and peripheral circulatory disease, which place the client at risk of foot problems; foot discomfort and its onset and location; and any perceived problems with foot mobility.

Common foot problems include calluses, corns, unpleasant odors, plantar warts, fissure between the toes, fungal infections such as athlete's foot, and deviations in toe contour.

Epidermal Problems

A **callus** is a thickened portion of epidermis, a mass of keratotic material. Calluses are flat and usually found on the bottom or side of the foot over a bony prominence. Calluses are usually caused by pressure from shoes. They can be softened by soaking the foot in warm water with Epsom salts, and they can be abraded by pumice stones or similar abrasives. Creams with lanolin help to keep the skin soft and prevent the formation of calluses.

A **corn** is a keratosis caused by friction and pressure from a shoe. It commonly occurs on a toe, usually the

Outcome Criteria: Skin

The client will:

- Have intact, pink, smooth, soft, and hydrated skin
- Have good tissue turgor
- Have warm skin
- Experience less discomfort
- Describe factors, when known, that contribute to skin alterations
- Demonstrate evidence of healing (e.g., reduced size of impairment or amount of drainage)
- Describe hygienic and other interventions to maintain skin integrity
- Describe interventions to prevent specific skin problems
- Express positive statements about sense of well-being
- Participate in prescribed treatment plan to promote wound healing

fourth or fifth toe, and usually on a bony prominence such as a joint. Corns are usually conical (circular and raised). The base is the surface of the corn and the apex is in deeper tissues, sometimes even attached to bone. Corns are generally removed surgically. They are prevented from reforming by relieving the pressure on the area and massaging the tissue to promote circulation.

Unpleasant odors occur as a result of perspiration and its interaction with microorganisms. Regular and frequent washing of the feet and wearing clean hosiery help to minimize odor. Foot powders and deodorants also help to prevent this problem.

Plantar warts appear on the sole of the foot. These warts are caused by the virus papovavirus hominis. They are moderately contagious. The warts are frequently painful and often make walking difficult. The treatment ordered by a physician may be curettage, freezing with solid carbon dioxide several times, or repeated applications of salicylic acid.

Fissures between the toes occur frequently as a result of dryness and cracking of the skin. A fissure is a deep groove. The treatment of choice is good foot hygiene and application of an antiseptic to prevent infection. Often a small piece of gauze is inserted between the toes in applying the antiseptic and left in place to assist healing by allowing air to reach the area.

Athlete's foot or **tinea pedia** (ringworm of the foot) is caused by a fungus. The symptoms are scaling and cracking of the skin, particularly between the toes. Sometimes small blisters form, containing a thin fluid. In severe cases the lesions may also appear on other parts of the body, particularly the hands. Treatments vary from potassium permanganate soaks, using a 1:8000 solution, to application of commercial antifungal ointments or powders. Prevention is important. Common preventive measures are keeping the feet well ventilated, wearing clean socks or stockings, and not going barefoot in public showers.

Toe Contour Deviations

Common deviations in toe contour include hallux valgus and hammer toe. **Hallux valgus** (bunion) is a lateral deviation of the big toe at its metatarsophalangeal joint, with enlargement and development of a bursa or callus over the area, which constitutes the bunion. See Figure 36–7, *A*. If the deviation is severe, the great toe may overlap the second toe. Displacement may cause the second toe to develop hammer toe. A familial tendency toward hallux valgus is apparent, and it is more common in females than in males. Contributing causes include poorly fitted shoes, flat feet, and degenerative arthritic changes. Conservative treatment consists of well-fitted shoes with ample room for the forefoot and use of bunion pads to relieve

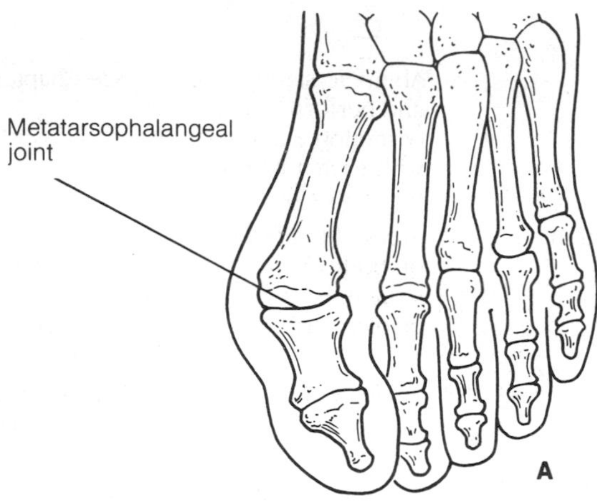

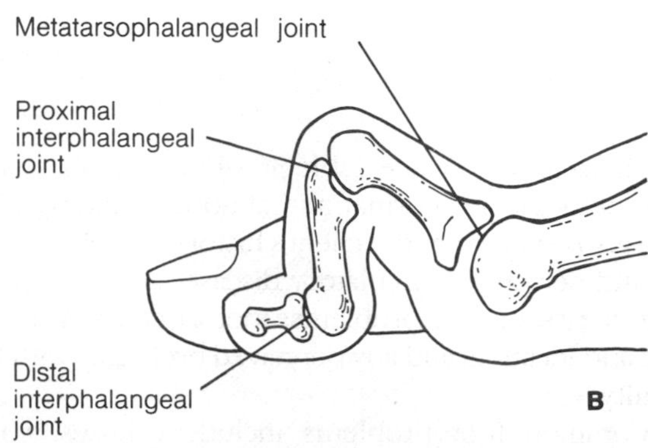

Figure 36–7 Toe deviations: **A,** hallux valgus; **B,** hammer toe

Examples of Nursing Diagnoses Related to Foot Problems

- Potential impairment of skin integrity related to reduced peripheral tissue perfusion associated with edema
- Potential impairment of skin integrity related to reduced tissue perfusion associated with inadequate arterial circulation
- Potential for infection related to broken or traumatized skin
- Potential for infection related to impaired tissue perfusion
- Actual impairment of skin integrity related to excessive perspiration and ineffective hygiene practices
- Actual impairment of skin integrity related to reduced peripheral tissue perfusion
- Impaired mobility related to painful foot lesion (e.g., corn, ingrown toenail, or plantar wart)
- Impaired mobility related to altered foot alignment (e.g., foot drop)

Outcome Criteria: Feet

The client will:

- Have intact, pink, smooth, soft, and hydrated skin
- Have warm skin
- Experience less pain or discomfort
- Have intact cuticles and skin surrounding nails
- Have quick return of nail bed color after blanch test
- Wear shoes and walk without discomfort
- Describe hygienic and other interventions to maintain skin integrity and peripheral tissue perfusion
- Describe interventions to prevent specific foot problems

shoe pressure. A severe, painful bursitis may require incising and applying hot, moist compresses. Surgical correction is sometimes necessary. Intraarticular injections of corticosteroids may be given if there is osteoarthritic joint involvement.

Hammer toe is characterized by hyperextension of the metatarsophalangeal joint, flexion of the proximal interphalangeal joint, and hyperextension of the distal interphalangeal joint. See Figure 36–7, *B*. The second toe is most frequently involved, often bilaterally, and it may be associated with hallux valgus. Painful calluses often develop over the proximal interphalangeal joint. Hammer toes may be congenital, linked to a familial tendency, or acquired. If acquired, they are caused most frequently by poorly fitted shoes that force the involved toe into a flexion deformity. Conservative treatment for hammer toe includes passive stretching exercises and well-fitted shoes, perhaps with padding and inserts to decrease pressure over the proximal interphalangeal joint. Surgery to correct the flexion of the joint and splinting are sometimes necessary.

Nursing Diagnoses

Examples of nursing diagnoses related to foot problems are shown on this page.

Intervention

Care of the foot is described in Procedure 36–4.

Procedure 36–4 ▲ Foot Care

Equipment

1. A washbasin
2. Soap
3. A washcloth
4. Towels
5. A moisture-resistant disposable pad
6. Lotion
7. Toenail cleaning and trimming equipment (see next section)

Intervention

1. Fill the washbasin with water at 40 C (105 F).

   Rationale Warm water promotes circulation, is comforting, and is refreshing.

2. Assist the ambulatory client to a sitting position in a chair, or the bed client to a supine or semi-Fowler's position.

3. Place a pillow under the bed client's knees.

   Rationale The pillow provides support and prevents muscle fatigue.

4. Place the washbasin on the moisture-resistant pad at the foot of the bed for a bed client or on the floor in front of the chair for an ambulatory client.
5. For a bed client, pad the rim of the washbasin with a towel.

   Rationale The towel prevents undue pressure on the skin.
6. Place one of the client's feet in the basin.
7. Allow the client's foot to soak for at least 10 minutes. Rewarm the water as needed.

   Rationale Soaking softens the skin and nails and loosens debris under the toenails.
8. Wash the foot with soap, and rinse it. Rub callused areas of the foot with the washcloth.

   Rationale Friction created by rubbing removes dead skin layers.
9. Remove the foot from the basin and place it on the towel.
10. Blot the foot gently with the towel to dry it thoroughly, particularly between the toes.

    Rationale Harsh rubbing can damage the skin. Thorough drying reduces the risk of infection.
11. Apply lotion to the foot.

    Rationale Lotion moistens dry skin.
12. Assess the foot for any problems.
13. Empty the washbasin, refill it with water, and soak and clean the other foot.
14. While the second foot is soaking, clean and trim the toenails of the first foot (see next section), if agency policy permits. In many agencies, toenail trimming is contraindicated for clients with diabetes mellitus, toe infections, and peripheral vascular disease, unless performed by a podiatrist or general practice physician.
15. Record any foot problems observed. Foot care is not generally recorded unless problems are noted.
16. Instruct the client with diabetes mellitus or peripheral vascular disease about appropriate foot care. Many foot problems can be prevented by having the client follow simple guidelines:
    a. Wash the feet daily, and dry them well, especially between the toes.
    b. Use creams or lotions to moisten the skin or soak the feet in warm water with Epsom salts to avoid excessive drying of the skin of the feet. Lotion will also soften calluses, which can then be removed with an abrasive such as pumice stone. A lotion that reduces dryness effectively is a mixture of lanolin and mineral oil.
    c. To prevent or control an unpleasant odor due to excessive foot perspiration, wash the feet frequently and change socks and shoes at least daily. Special deodorant sprays are also helpful.
    d. File the toenails rather than cutting them to avoid skin injury. File the nails straight across the ends of the toes. If the nails are too thick or misshapen to file, consult a podiatrist.
    e. To prevent burns, check the water temperature before immersing the feet.
    f. Wear clean stockings or socks daily. Avoid socks with holes or darns that can cause pressure areas.
    g. Wear correctly fitting shoes that neither restrict the foot nor rub on any area; rubbing can cause corns and calluses. For the elderly, a supportive, laced shoe (e.g., an oxford), or slip-on style with a flexible nonskid sole and 2.5 to 5 cm (1 to 2 in) heels is advised. Check worn shoes for rough spots in the lining. Break in new shoes gradually by increasing the wearing time 30 to 60 minutes each day.
    h. Avoid walking barefoot, since injury and infection may result. Wear slippers in public showers and change areas to avoid contracting athlete's foot or other infections.
    i. Avoid wearing constricting garments such as knee-high elastic stockings or garters or sitting with the legs crossed at the knees, which may decrease circulation.
    j. When the feet are cold, use extra blankets and wear warm socks rather than using heating pads or hot water bottles, which may cause burns.
    k. Several times each day, exercise the feet to promote circulation. Point the feet upward, point them downward, and move them in circles.
    l. When washing, check the skin of the feet for breaks or red or swollen areas.
    m. Wash any cut on the foot thoroughly, apply a mild antiseptic, and notify the physician.
    n. Avoid self-treatment for corns or calluses. Pumice stones and some callus and corn applications are injurious to the skin. Consult a podiatrist.

Evaluation

Examples of outcome criteria to evaluate the achievement of goals and effectiveness of nursing intervention are shown on page 923.

Nails

The fingernails and toenails are epidermal appendages. Like the hair, they are made of epidermal cells that have been changed to keratin. Nails usually grow regularly, about 1 mm per week, but this growth may stop at times of severe stress or illness. See the discussion of Beau's line on page 812. The nail is surrounded by a cuticle, which tends to grow over the nail and thus regularly requires pushing back. A lost fingernail takes 3½ to 5½ months to regenerate, and a toenail takes 6 to 8 months.

Developmental Variations

Nails are normally present at birth. They continue to grow throughout life, and they change very little until people are old. At that time the nails tend to be tougher, more brittle, and in some cases thicker. The nails of an elderly person normally grow less quickly than those of a younger person, and they may be ridged and have grooves.

Assessment

For information about assessing the nails and common problems, see Chapter 35, pages 812 and 813.

Nursing Diagnosis

Examples of nursing diagnoses related to the nails are shown below.

Intervention

When a client requires help with nail care, the nurse needs a nail cutter or sharp scissors, a nail file, an orange stick to push back the cuticle, hand lotion or mineral oil to lubricate any dry tissue around the nails, and a wash basin with water to soak the nails if they are particularly thick or hard.

One hand or foot is soaked, if needed, and dried; then the nail is cut or filed straight across beyond the end of the finger or toe. See Figure 36—8. Clients who have diabetes or circulatory problems should have their nails filed, rather than cut. After the initial cut or filing, the nail is filed to round the corners, and the nurse cleans under the nail. The nurse then gently pushes back the cuticle, taking care not to injure it. The next finger or toe is cared for in the same manner. Any abnormalities, such as an infected cuticle or inflammation of the tissue around the nail, are recorded and reported.

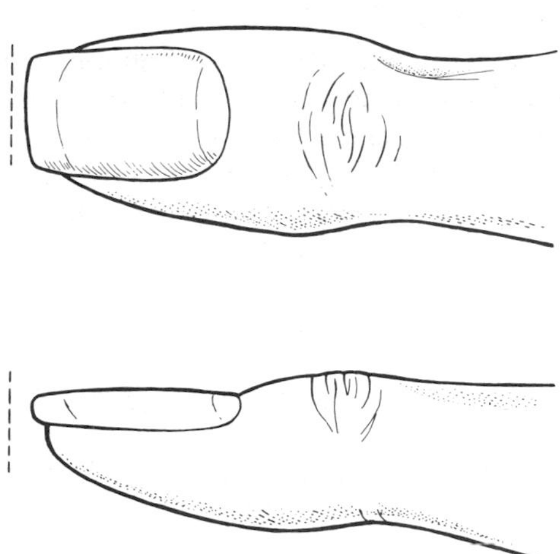

Figure 36–8 Nails are trimmed straight across.

Examples of Nursing Diagnoses Related to Nail Problems

- Potential for infection around the nail bed related to altered peripheral circulation
- Self-care deficit (grooming) related to impaired vision
- Self-care deficit (grooming) related to impaired coordination

Evaluation

Outcome criteria to evaluate the achievement of client goals or the effectiveness of nursing interventions are shown below.

Outcome Criteria: Nails

The client will:

- Have smooth, convex nails
- Have pink nail beds
- Have intact cuticles and hydrated surrounding skin
- Have quick return of nail bed color after the blanch test
- Experience less or no pain and inflammation
- Have short nails with smooth edges
- Describe factors contributing to the nail problem
- Describe preventive interventions for the specific nail problem

Mouth

Mucous membrane, which is continuous with the skin, lines the digestive, urinary, reproductive, and respiratory tracts and the conjunctiva of the eye. It is an epithelial tissue, and it forms mucus, concentrates bile, and secretes or excretes enzymes, for example, in the digestive tract. It serves four general functions:

1. Protection
2. Support for associated structures
3. Absorption of nutrients into the body (in the digestive tract)
4. Secretion of mucus, enzymes, and salts

The mouth (oral cavity) is bordered by the lips anteriorly, the cheeks laterally, and the pharynx posteriorly. The cheeks contain several accessory muscles of **mastication** (chewing), which keep food from escaping the masticating motions of the teeth. The tongue, containing numerous taste buds, extends from the floor of the mouth and is attached to it by a fold of mucous membrane called the **frenulum**. The tongue helps to mix saliva, keeps food pressed between the teeth for chewing, and pushes food into the pharynx for swallowing. The **palate** (roof of the mouth) has two parts: the anterior portion (hard palate) and the posterior portion (soft palate), which ends in a free projection called the **uvula** that marks the opening of the mouth into the pharynx.

The mouth contains two sets of **dentures** (teeth), which are discussed under "Developmental Variations." Teeth are necessary to masticate food so that it can be swallowed and digested in the stomach. Each tooth has a number of parts: the crown, the root, and the pulp cavity. The **crown** is the exposed part of the tooth, which is outside the gum. It is covered with a hard substance called **enamel**. The ivory-colored internal part of the crown below the enamel is the **dentin**. See Figure 36–9. The root of a tooth is embedded in the jaw and covered by a bony tissue called **cementum**. The **pulp cavity** in the center of the tooth contains the blood vessels and nerves.

Assessment of the mouth is covered in Chapter 35, pages 836 to 839.

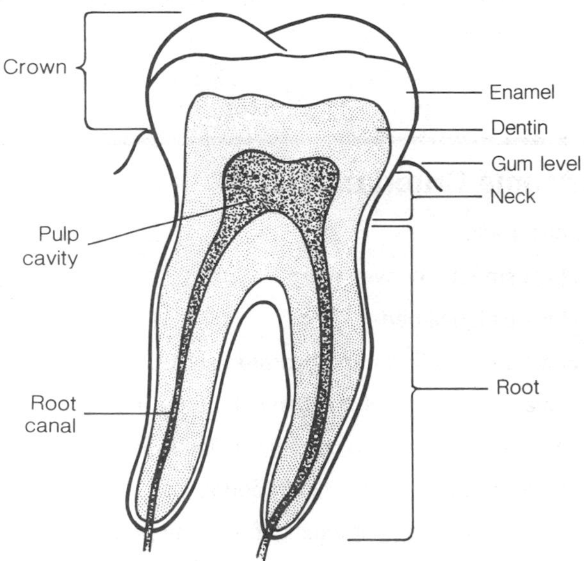

Figure 36–9 The anatomic parts of a tooth

Developmental Variations

Teeth usually appear 5 to 8 months after birth. By the time children are 2 years old, they usually have all 20 of their temporary teeth. See Figure 36–10. At about age 6

Examples of Nursing Diagnoses Related to Problems of the Mouth

- Alteration in oral mucous membranes related to ineffective oral hygiene
- Alteration in oral mucous membranes related to dehydration
- Alteration in oral mucous membranes related to radiation therapy
- Alteration in oral mucous membranes related to ill-fitting dentures
- Potential alteration in oral mucous membranes related to unconscious state
- Alteration in comfort related to painful, inflamed gums
- Self-care deficit (oral hygiene) related to neuromuscular impairment
- Potential alteration in nutrition (less than body requirements) related to absence of teeth
- Potential alteration in nutrition (less than body requirements) related to sore, inflamed buccal cavity
- Disturbance in self-concept (altered body image) related to absence of teeth

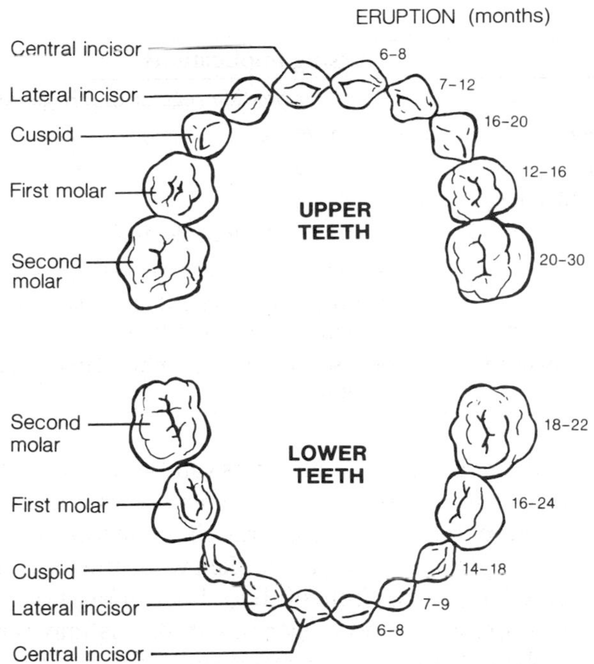

Figure 36–10 Temporary teeth and their times of eruption (stated in months)

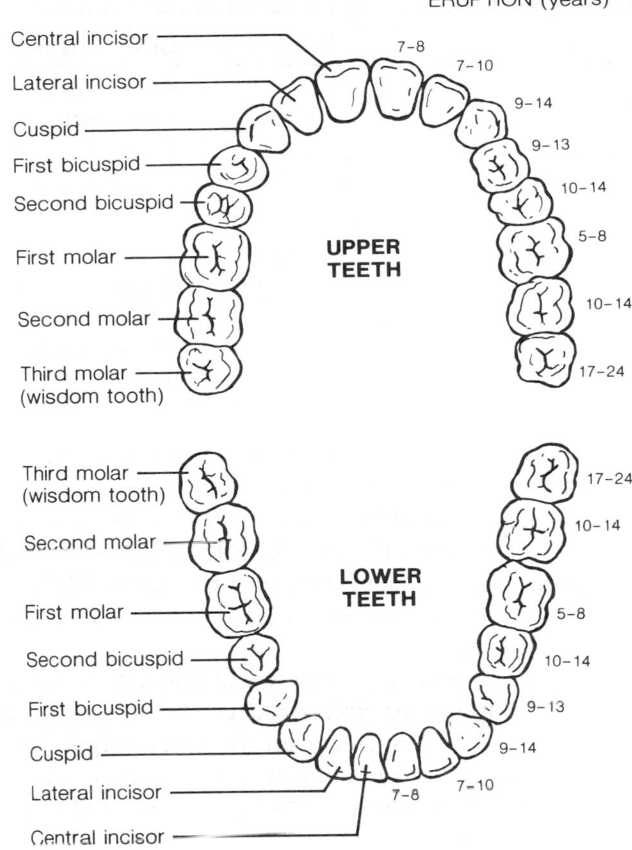

Figure 36–11 Permanent teeth and their times of eruption (stated in years)

or 7, children start losing their deciduous teeth, and these are gradually replaced by the 32 permanent teeth. See Figure 36–11. By age 25, most people have all their permanent teeth.

The incidence of periodontal disease increases during pregnancy, since an increase in female hormones affects gingival tissue and increases its reaction to bacterial plaque. Many pregnant women manifest increased bleeding from the gingival sulcus during brushing and increased redness and swelling of the gums. These gingival changes heighten the pregnant woman's chances of acquiring periodontal disease (Martin and Reeb 1982, p. 391).

Elderly people may have few permanent teeth left, and many have dentures. Most people have lost all their own teeth by age 70, mainly because of periodontal disease rather than dental caries; however, caries are also common in the middle-aged adult. Preventive dental care is important.

Some receding of the gums and a brownish pigmentation of the gums occur with age. Because saliva production decreases with age, dryness of the oral mucosa is a common finding in older people. A dry mouth can be aggravated by poor fluid intake, heavy smoking, alcohol use, high salt intake, anxiety, and many medications. Medications that can cause a dryness of the mouth include diuretics; laxatives, if used excessively; all major tranquilizers, e.g., chlorpromazine (Thorazine); some minor tranquilizers, e.g., diazepam (Valium), chlordiazepoxide (Librium); some antidepressants, e.g., amitriptyline (Elavil), imipramine (Tofranil); some antihypertensives, e.g., trimethaphan (Arfonad); some antispasmodics, e.g., propanthaline (Pro-Banthīne); and antihistamines used in cold and cough remedies and in analgesics (Todd 1982, p. 122).

Clients at Risk

Certain clients are prone to oral problems often because of lack of knowledge or the inability to maintain oral hygiene. Among these are seriously ill, confused, and dehydrated clients. In addition, persons with nasogastric tubes or receiving oxygen are likely to develop dry oral mucous membranes, especially if they breathe through their mouths. Clients who have had oral or jaw surgery must have meticulous oral hygiene care to prevent the development of infections.

Assessment

For information about mouth assessment, see Chapter 35, pages 836 to 839. See also Table 36–5 for common problems of the mouth.

Table 36–5 Common Problems of the Mouth

Problem	Description	Nursing Implications
Halitosis	Bad breath	Teach or provide regular oral hygiene.
Glossitis	Inflammation of the tongue	As above
Gingivitis	Inflammation of the gums	As above
Periodontal disease	Gums appear spongy and bleeding	As above
Reddened or excoriated mucosa		Check for ill-fitting dentures.
Excessive dryness of the buccal mucosa		Increase fluid intake as health permits.
Chilosis	Cracking of lips	Lubricate lips, use antimicrobial ointment to prevent infection.
Dental caries	Teeth have darkened areas, may be painful	Advise client to see a physician and/or dentist.

Dental caries and periodontal disease are the two problems that most frequently affect the teeth. Periodontal disease (pyorrhea) is characterized by red, swollen gingiva and bleeding. Inflammation of the gums is referred to as **gingivitis**. Another common problem is **halitosis** (bad breath), which may be caused by poor oral hygiene or a disease process.

Other problems nurses may see in hospitalized clients are **glossitis**, **stomatitis**, and **parotitis**. The accumulation of foul matter (food, microorganisms, and epithelial elements) on the teeth and gums is *sordes*. See also Table 35–8 on page 839 for assessment of the mouth and related health problems.

Nursing Diagnosis

See page 926 for examples of nursing diagnoses related to problems of the mouth.

Intervention

Oral Hygiene

Good oral hygiene includes daily stimulation of the gums, mechanical scrubbing of the teeth, and flushing of the mouth. Checkups by a dentist every 6 months are also recommended. The nurse is often in a position to help people, young or old, ill or well, to maintain oral hygiene by helping or teaching them to clean the teeth and oral cavity, by inspecting whether clients (especially children) have done so, or by actually providing mouth care to clients who are ill or incapacitated. The nurse can also be instrumental in identifying and referring problems that require the intervention of a dentist.

Teaching situations regarding oral hygienic practices Oral hygienic practices include brushing teeth or cleaning dentures, flossing teeth, and using fluoride. When assessing a client's practices, the nurse determines the frequency of cleaning and the methods used. Examples of learning needs are:

1. In areas where the water is not fluoridated, nurses may recommend that parents obtain fluoride supplements for their children. Supplements can be started in the first month of a baby's life. If given regularly, they help to prevent but do not necessarily eliminate tooth decay. The supplements need to be taken while the teeth are being formed, i.e., from birth to about 14 years of age. Prescriptions are no longer required. It is important to take only the recommended amount and to take it with water, milk, or juice. Recommended dosages are:
   - Under 1 year, 2 drops daily
   - 1–4 years, 4 drops daily
   - 4–8 years, 6 drops daily
   - Over 8 years, 8 drops or 1 tablet
2. Parents may need guidance when their baby starts teething at about 6 to 8 months of age. Teething is often accompanied by sore gums, drooling, and fretfulness. Teething babies want to put everything into their mouths, so their safety must be monitored. To relieve the baby's sore gums, parents can allow babies to chew on rubber or plastic toys, teething rings, and teething biscuits. Slightly chilled strained or chopped fruit can also make the mouth feel better. Teething powders or syrups should be avoided unless prescribed by a physician. If the baby becomes too fretful and feverish, the physician should be consulted about a soothing medication that will relieve the gum irritation.
3. The brushing of teeth needs to be demonstrated to children as soon as their teeth appear. Until the child can manipulate the toothbrush effectively, parents need to help the child brush after each meal and before going to bed.
4. A child's first visit to the dentist should occur at about age 2½ or 3, so that the child learns not to fear such visits. Preventive measures such as topical fluoride applications can be started, and any defects can be corrected. Primary teeth can decay very rapidly. Dental examinations are needed every 6 months. Some people mistakenly believe that it is not necessary to fill primary teeth, since they will inevitably be replaced. The nurse can be instrumental in teaching the facts in this situation. It is important that primary teeth be looked after, since some must last up to 12 years. Primary teeth

are needed as guides for permanent tooth eruption, for stimulating natural growth of the jaws, for an attractive appearance, and for normal speech development. The early loss of primary teeth can cause permanent teeth to erupt out of line. Once a tooth is lost, adjacent teeth drift over to close the space, and they may interfere with eruption of the underlying permanent tooth. When the space for the new permanent tooth is narrowed, that tooth is forced to grow either in toward the tongue or out toward the cheek. The dentist can insert a temporary device to maintain the space until the permanent tooth erupts, to prevent malalignment.

5. Clients of all ages may need reinforcement to practice good oral hygiene to prevent dental caries and periodontal disease. The following measures combat tooth decay:
   a. Brush the teeth thoroughly after meals and at bedtime. Assist children or inspect their mouths to be sure the teeth are clean.
   b. Floss the teeth daily.
   c. Ensure an adequate intake of nutrients, particularly calcium, phosphorus, vitamins A, C, and D, and fluoride.
   d. Avoid sweet foods and drinks between meals. Take them in moderation at meals.
   e. Eat coarse, fibrous foods (cleansing foods), such as fresh fruits and raw vegetables.
   f. Take a fluoride supplement daily until age 14 or 16 unless the drinking water is fluoridated.
   g. Have topical fluoride applications as prescribed by the dentist.
   h. Have a checkup by a dentist every 6 months.

Brushing teeth Thorough brushing of the teeth is important in preventing tooth decay. Teeth should be brushed at least four times a day: after meals and at bedtime. Use of a medium or soft multibristled brush is advised, since it minimizes the chance of trauma to the gums. The mechanical action of brushing removes food particles that can harbor and incubate bacteria. It also stimulates circulation in the gums, thus maintaining their healthy firmness.

The technique most recently recommended for brushing teeth is called the **sulcular technique**, which removes plaque and cleans under the gingival margins. A soft-bristled, small toothbrush is required. See Procedure 36–5.

Many toothpastes are marketed, any of which can be used. They are flavored and scented to make them pleasant tasting. However, an effective dentifrice can be made by combining two parts of table salt to one part of baking soda.

After the teeth are brushed, the mouth is rinsed with water to remove dislodged food particles and excess dentifrice. Many antiseptic mouthwashes are marketed, and some people prefer these for rinsing. If the teeth cannot be brushed after eating, vigorous rinsing of the mouth with water is recommended.

Children should be taught the habit of brushing their teeth by age 2, when the teeth appear. Because children cannot manage this independently for several years, parents are advised to do the brushing for them. A small stool to help the child reach the basin and a special place for the child's toothbrush can enhance positive attitudes about this habit.

Dental flossing Daily flossing of the teeth is advised. It is especially beneficial in preventing the formation of plaque and removing it from the teeth, particularly at the gum line. A method for flossing is described in Procedure 36–5.

Procedure 36–5 ▲ Brushing and Flossing Teeth

Equipment

Many clients have these supplies at the bedside; if not, they can be assembled by the nurse.

1. A dentifrice. Most clients have a flavor preference and have their own dentifrice. The client who does not have dentifrice and cannot purchase any can use a mixture of table salt and baking soda.

2. A curved basin that fits snugly under the client's chin, such as a kidney basin, to receive the rinse water. A client who can brush and floss teeth at a sink does not require a basin.

3. A toothbrush. Small toothbrushes are available for children. A soft toothbrush is recommended when using the sulcular technique of cleaning, described in the Intervention, step 5.

4. A cup of tepid water.

5. A towel to protect the client and the bedclothes.

6. Dental floss, at least two pieces 20 cm (8 in) in length. Waxed floss is less likely to fray than unwaxed floss; particles between the teeth attach more readily to unwaxed floss than to waxed floss. Some believe that waxed floss leaves a residue to which plaque adheres (Gannon and Kadezabek 1980, p. 16).

7. A floss holder (optional).

8. A mouthwash to rinse the mouth after brushing the teeth. Normally, a slightly antiseptic solution is used.

Most clients have their own commercial mouthwash. Some hospitals supply a mouthwash. The National Formulary lists the official mouthwash as a preparation of potassium, bicarbonate, sodium borate, thymol, eucalyptol, methyl salicylate, amaranth solution, alcohol, glycerin, and purified water. A mouth rinse of normal saline or diluted hydrogen peroxide can be an effective cleaner and moisturizer.

Intervention

1. Assist the client to a sitting position in bed, if this is permitted. If the client cannot sit, assist him or her to a side-lying position with the head on a pillow so that the client can spit out the rinse water.
2. Place the towel under the client's chin.
3. Moisten the bristles of the toothbrush with tepid water, and apply the dentifrice.

   Rationale Tepid water is to be used because hot water softens the brush.
4. Place or hold the curved basin under the client's chin, fitting the small curve around the chin or neck.
5. Hand the toothbrush to the client, or brush the client's teeth as follows:
   a. Hold the brush against the teeth with the bristles at a 45° angle. See Figure 36–12. The tips of the outer bristles should rest against and penetrate under the gingival sulcus. See Figure 36–13. The brush will clean under the sulcus of two or three teeth at one time.

      Rationale This sulcular technique removes plaque and cleans under the gingival margins.

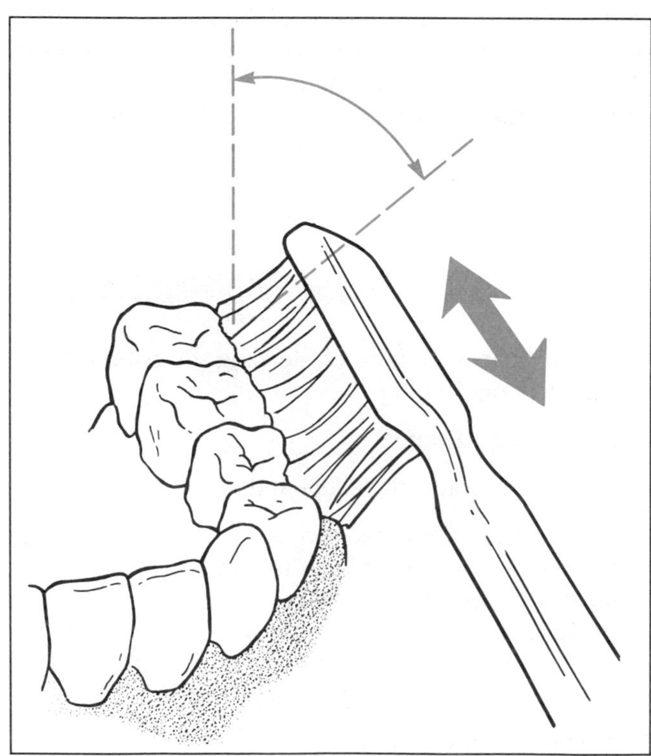

Figure 36–12

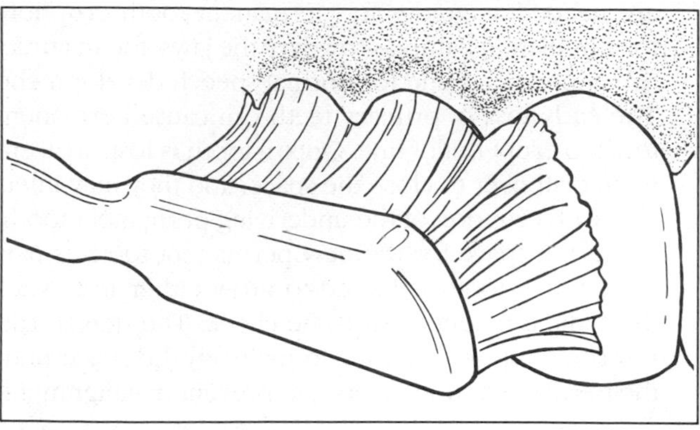

Figure 36–13

   b. Move the bristles back and forth using a vibrating or jiggling motion, from the sulcus to the crowns of the teeth.
   c. Repeat until all outer and inner surfaces of the teeth and sulci of the gums are cleaned.
   d. Clean the biting surfaces by moving the brush back and forth over them in short strokes.
   e. If the tongue is coated, brush it gently with the toothbrush.

      Rationale Brushing removes accumulated materials and coatings. A coated tongue may be caused by poor oral hygiene and low fluid intake. Brushing gently and carefully prevents the client from gagging or vomiting.
6. Hand the client the water cup or mouthwash to rinse the mouth vigorously. Have the client spit the water and excess dentifrice into the basin.

   Rationale Vigorous rinsing loosens food particles and washes out already loosened particles.
7. Repeat step 6 until the client's mouth is free of dentifrice and food particles.
8. Remove the curved basin, and help the client wipe his or her mouth.
9. Wash your hands before putting them inside the client's mouth, or assist the client to wash hands before commencing to floss independently.
10. Wrap one end of floss around the third finger of each hand. See Figure 36–14.
11. To floss the upper teeth, use your thumb and index finger to stretch the floss. See Figure 36–15. Move the floss up and down between the teeth from the tops

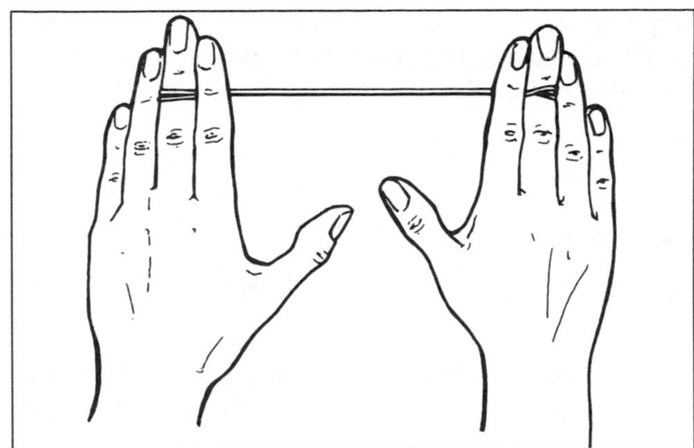

Figure 36–14

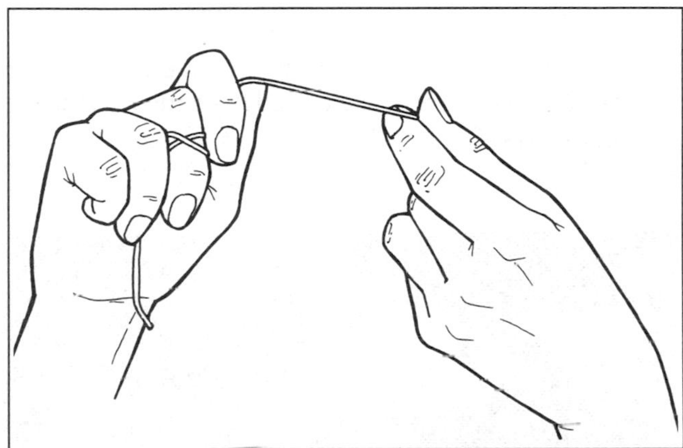

Figure 36–15

of the crowns to the gum and along the gum lines as far as possible. Make a figure "C" with the floss around the tooth edge being flossed. Start at the back on the right side and work around to the back of the left side, or work from the center teeth to the back of the jaw on either side.

12. To floss the lower teeth, use your index fingers to stretch the floss. See Figure 36–16.
13. Give the client tepid water or mouthwash to rinse the mouth and a curved basin in which to spit the water.
14. Remove the curved basin and assist the client to wipe his or her mouth.
15. Record any problems of the teeth, tongue, gums, and oral mucosa, such as sordes or inflammation and swelling of the gums. Brushing and flossing teeth are not usually recorded.

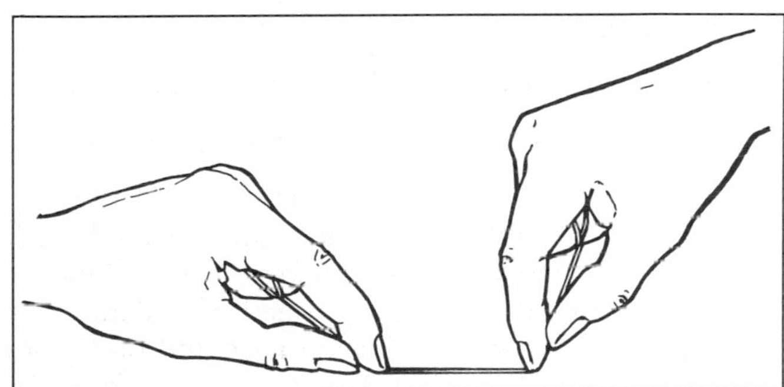

Figure 36–16

Care of dentures Most clients in a hospital can clean their own dentures. However, if the client is incapacitated, elderly, confused, or confined to bed, care of dentures becomes the nurse's responsibility.

To remove upper dentures, the nurse grasps them at the front with the thumb and index finger, using a piece of tissue or gauze. They may need to be moved slightly up and down to overcome the suction on the roof of the mouth. Lower dentures are readily removed by retracting the cheek, turning them slightly, and pulling them out between the lips on one side and then the other. Partial plates and removable bridges may also need to be taken out by the nurse. Dentures must be handled carefully, since they can break if dropped or knocked against metal water taps.

Dentures are cleaned with a toothbrush or special stiff-bristled brush, a dentrifice, and tepid water. Hot water is not used because heat can change the shape of some dentures. The dentures are rinsed well and replaced in the client's mouth.

Special Mouth Care

Some clients, e.g., the clients who are unconscious or have excessive dryness, sordes, or irritations of the mouth, require special mouth care. Practices differ in regard to special mouth care and the frequency with which it is provided. Depending on the state of the client's mouth, special care may be needed every 2 to 8 hours. The following procedure focuses on oral care for the unconscious client but may be adapted for conscious clients who are seriously ill or have mouth problems.

Mouth care for unconscious clients is very important, since their mouths tend to become dry and consequently susceptible to infections. Dryness occurs because:

1. The client cannot take fluids by mouth.
2. The client often breathes through the mouth.
3. The client may be receiving oxygen, which tends to dry the mucous membranes.

The dentures of unconscious clients are normally kept in water in a denture cup labeled with the client's name and identification number, in the bedside table drawer. In some agencies, dentures are soaked in a commercially prepared solution. The dentures are always cleaned before they are put into the denture cup.

Procedure 36–6 ▲ Providing Special Oral Care

Equipment

1. Dentifrice or denture cleaner.
2. A toothbrush.
3. A cup of tepid water.
4. A curved basin, such as a kidney basin.
5. A towel.
6. Mouthwash.
7. A denture container for the client with dentures.
8. A tissue or piece of gauze to remove dentures.
9. Applicators and cleaning solution for cleaning the mucous membranes. Commercially prepared applicators of lemon juice and oil can be used. If these are not available, a gauze square rolled around the index finger and dipped into lemon juice and oil or into mouthwash solution usually suffices. Applicator swabs or tongue blades covered with gauze may also be used. Mineral oil is generally contraindicated, because if it is aspirated it can initiate an infection (lipid pneumonia).
10. A rubber-tipped bulb syringe to apply the rinse solution to the mouth.
11. Petroleum jelly (Vaseline) or cold cream to lubricate the lips.
12. A cleaning agent such as hydrogen peroxide for use prior to the lemon juice and oil, if necessary. This agent is effective in removing encrustations that coat the tongue. It should be diluted with water. See Intervention, step 8.
13. A bite-block to hold the mouth open and teeth apart (optional).

Intervention

1. Position the unconscious client on his or her side with the head of the bed lowered, so that the saliva automatically runs out by gravity rather than being aspirated into the lungs. This position is the one of choice for the unconscious client receiving mouth care. If the client's head cannot be lowered, turn it to one side so that fluid will readily run out of the mouth or pool in the side of the mouth where it can be suctioned.
2. Place the towel under the client's chin.

   Rationale The towel protects the client and the bedclothes.
3. Place the curved basin against the client's chin and lower cheek to receive the fluid from the mouth. See Figure 36–17.

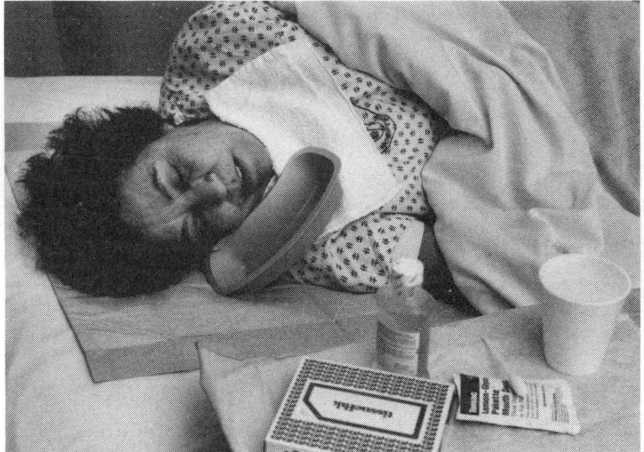

Figure 36–17

4. If the patient has natural teeth, brush the teeth as in Procedure 36–5 on page 929. Brush gently and carefully to avoid injuring the gums. If the client has artificial teeth, clean them as described earlier.
5. Rinse the client's mouth by drawing about 30 ml (1 (one) oz) of water or mouthwash into the syringe and injecting it gently into each side of the mouth.

   Rationale If the solution is injected with force, some of it may flow down the client's throat and be aspirated into the lungs.
6. Watch carefully to make sure that all the rinsing solution has run out of the mouth into the basin. If not, suction the fluid from the mouth. See the section on oropharyngeal suctioning in Chapter 45.

Rationale Fluid remaining in the mouth may be aspirated into the lungs.

7. Repeat the rinsing until the mouth is free of dentifrice, if used.

8. Inspect the client's mouth. If the tissues appear dry or unclean, clean them with the applicators or gauze and cleaning solution. If hydrogen peroxide is used, dilute it 1:1 with water, and rinse thoroughly before applying oil and lemon juice.

   Rationale The gums and mucosa can become spongy from prolonged action of hydrogen peroxide.

9. Picking up one oil applicator, wipe the mucous membrane of one cheek. In the absence of commercially prepared applicators, wrap a small gauze square around your index finger, and moisten it with oil and lemon solution. Discard the applicator or gauze in a waste container, and with a fresh one clean the next area. Clean in an orderly progression around the mouth, using a fresh applicator or gauze once the previous one becomes soiled or dry.

   Rationale Using separate applicators for each area of the mouth prevents the transfer of microorganisms from one area to another.

10. Clean all the mouth tissues: the cheeks, roof of the mouth, base of the mouth, and tongue. Observe the tissues closely for inflammation and dryness.

11. Rinse the client's mouth, repeating steps 5–7.

12. Remove the basin, and dry around the client's mouth with the towel. Replace artificial dentures if indicated.

13. Lubricate the client's lips with petroleum jelly or cold cream.

    Rationale Lubrication prevents cracking and subsequent infection.

14. Record special oral hygiene and pertinent observations. Report problems to the responsible nurse.

    Sample Recording

Date	Time	Notes
April 7/87	1500	Special mouth care using oil and lemon q1h. Outer aspect of lower right gum remains reddened and swollen. ——— ———Sally R. Nolan, SN

15. Establish a plan for the frequency of special mouth care and any specific methods to be used. Record these on the client's nursing care plan.

Evaluation

Outcome criteria to evaluate the achievement of client goals or the effectiveness of nursing intervention are shown below.

Outcome Criteria: Mouth

The client will:

- Have an intact, smooth, well-hydrated oral mucosa of uniform color
- Have no inflammation of the oral mucosa
- Have firm, well-hydrated, nonbleeding gums of uniform color
- Have a well-hydrated tongue without inflammation
- Have smooth and well-hydrated lips
- Experience no oral discomfort
- Have teeth free of food particles and plaque
- Demonstrate appropriate brushing and flossing techniques
- Describe interventions that prevent tooth decay and dental plaque
- Express positive feelings about sense of well-being and appearance

Hair

The appearance of a person's hair often reflects his or her feelings of well-being. A person who feels ill may not groom hair as before. The hair may also reflect state of health, e.g., endocrine changes can affect the pattern of hair growth, and color changes may reflect aging. In addition, hair texture can also reflect health status, e.g., excessive coarseness and dryness may be associated with endocrine disorders such as hypothyroidism. For information about the anatomy of hair and hair assessment, see Chapter 35, page 811.

Developmental Changes

Newborns may have **lanugo** (the fine hair on the body of the fetus, also referred to as *down* or *woolly hair*) over their shoulders, back, and sacrum. This generally disappears, and the hair distribution becomes noticeable on the eyebrows, head, and eyelashes of young children. Some newborns have hair on their scalps; others are free of hair at birth but grow hair over the scalp during the first year of life.

Pubic hair usually appears in early puberty followed in about 6 months by the growth of axillary hair. Boys develop facial hair in later puberty.

In adolescence, the sebaceous glands increase in activity as a result of increased hormone levels. As a result, hair follicle openings enlarge to accommodate the increased amount of sebum, and the adolescent's hair may become more oily.

In elderly people, the hair is generally thinner, grows more slowly, and loses its color as a result of aging tissues and diminishing circulation. Men often lose their scalp hair and may become completely bald. Even relatively young men may be bald. The older person's hair also tends to be drier than normal. With age, axillary and pubic hair becomes finer and scanter, in contrast to the eyebrows, which become bristly and coarse. Most women develop hair on their faces, which some view as a problem.

Factors Affecting Hair Care

Each person has particular ways of caring for hair, influenced by a number of factors. Some shampoo it daily; others shampoo once a week or even less often. Black-skinned people often need to oil their hair daily because it tends to be dry. Oil prevents the hair from breaking and the scalp from drying. A wide-toothed comb is usually used, because finer combs pull and break the hair. Some people brush their hair vigorously before retiring, others comb their hair frequently.

Assessment

Assessment of the hair is dicussed in Chapter 35, page 811. Problems associated with the hair include ticks, lice, dandruff, and hirsutism.

Ticks

Ticks are small parasites that bite into tissue and suck blood. They take many forms and can adapt themselves to various conditions. The genera *Ornithodoros* and *Dermacentor* are found in North America. They can attach to human beings and are found frequently in the hair. They can be as large as 1.3 cm (0.5 in) and appear gray-brown. They attach to a person with the apparatus by which they suck blood and should not be torn off, because the sucking apparatus may be left in the skin and become infected. Pouring oil on the tick causes it to lose its hold, because it is deprived of oxygen, and it withdraws its sucker.

Ticks transmit several diseases to people, in particular, Rocky Mountain spotted fever and tularemia.

Lice

Lice are parasitic insects that infest mammals. Hundreds of varieties of lice infest humans. Three common kinds are *Pediculus capitis* or the head louse, *Pediculus corporis* or the body louse, and *Pediculus pubis* or the crab louse.

Pediculus capitis is found on the scalp and tends to stay hidden in the hairs; similarly, *Pediculus pubis* stays in pubic hair. *Pediculus corporis* tends to cling to clothing, so that, when a client undresses, the lice may not be in evidence on the body; these lice suck blood from the person and lay their eggs on the clothing. The nurse can suspect their presence in the clothing if (a) the person habitually scratches, (b) there are scratches on the skin, and (c) there are hemorrhagic spots on the skin where the lice have sucked blood.

Head and pubic lice lay their eggs on the hairs; the eggs look like oval particles, similar to dandruff, clinging to the hair. Bites and pustular eruptions may also be noticed at the hair lines and behind the ears.

Lice are very small, grayish white, and difficult to see. The crab louse in the pubic area has red legs. Lice may be contracted from infested clothes and direct contact with an infested person.

The treatment now used in most areas is gamma benzene hexachloride (Kwell), available as a cream, a lotion, and a shampoo. If the client has head lice, the hair is washed with the shampoo and the bed linens are changed. This treatment is repeated 12 to 24 hours later if needed. A client with pubic or body lice takes a bath or shower, dries, and applies the lotion or cream—to the entire body surface for body lice, and to the pubic area and adjacent areas for pubic lice. After 12 to 24 hours, the lotion is washed off, and clean clothing and linens are supplied.

Dandruff

Dandruff appears as a diffuse scaling of the scalp often accompanied by itching. In severe cases it involves the auditory canals and the eyebrows. Mild cases of dandruff can usually be treated effectively with a commercial shampoo specifically recommended for dandruff. In severe or persistent cases, the client may need the advice of a physician.

Hirsutism

Hirsutism is the growth of excessive body hair. The acceptance of body hair in the axillae and on the legs is largely dictated by culture. In North America, the well-groomed woman, as depicted in magazines, has no hair on her legs or under her axillae (although this idea is changing). In many European cultures, it is not customary for well-groomed women to remove this hair.

Excessive facial hair on a woman is thought unattractive in most Western and Oriental cultures. For example, some Japanese brides follow the custom of shaving their faces the day before the wedding.

The cause of excessive body hair is not always known. Elderly women may have some on their faces, and women during menopause may also experience the growth of facial hair. These conditions may be due to the action of the endocrine system. It is also thought that heredity influences both the pattern of hair distribution and the production of androgens by the adrenal glands.

There are a number of ways of removing hair: waxing, pulling with tweezers, shaving with a razor, applying depilatory lotions, and electrolysis. In the waxing process, warm wax is poured on the area and allowed to harden. The hairs become embedded in the wax and come away from the skin when the wax is removed. Tweezers are commonly used to remove excess hair from the eyebrows and the face. This can be a time-consuming project if there is a great deal of hair, and it needs to be repeated when the hair grows back, often in 2 to 3 weeks. Shaving with a razor is done frequently for leg and axilla hair. It is an inexpensive and effective method, but it must be repeated frequently. Depilatory creams and lotions destroy the hair shaft through a chemical action, so that the hair wipes away easily. This method of hair removal is expensive compared to shaving. In the initial use of a product, it is important to assess the amount of skin irritation it causes. It is advisable to put lotion on a small area initially and observe for signs of irritation. Electrolysis is the only permanent way of removing hair. The hair follicle is destroyed by means of an electric current. Usually, repeated treatments are needed before a follicle is completely destroyed. This method of treatment is relatively expensive.

Nursing Diagnosis

For examples of nursing diagnoses relative to hair and scalp problems, see next column.

Planning

Planning for assisting a client with hair care includes consideration of his or her personal preferences, health, and energy resources and the time, equipment, and personnel available. Often, clients like to have hair care following a bath, before receiving visitors, and/or before retiring. At some agencies shampoos can be given to clients only after a physician's order.

Planning involves establishing outcome criteria. For suggestions, see the section on evaluation, later in this chapter.

Examples of Nursing Diagnoses Related to Hair and Scalp Problems

- Potential for infection related to ticks on scalp
- Potential for disturbance in self-concept (body image) related to loss of hair associated with chemotherapy
- Self-care deficit in grooming related to pain associated with surgery of right upper extremity

Intervention

Hair Care

Brushing and combing To be healthy, hair needs to be brushed daily. Brushing has three major functions: It stimulates the circulation of blood in the scalp, it distributes the oil along the hair shaft, and it helps to arrange the hair, although most people use a comb for this.

Long hair may present a problem when clients are unable to go to a hairdresser for a long period. To prevent hair from matting, the client or nurse needs to comb it at least daily. Some clients are pleased to have it tied neatly in the back or braided until other assistance is available or until they feel better and can look after it. Black-skinned people often have thicker, drier, curlier hair than white-skinned people. Spiraled or very curly hair usually stands out from the scalp. Although the shafts of spiraled hair look strong and wiry, they have less strength than straight hair shafts and are easily broken.

Some blacks have their spiraled hair straightened. Even if straightened, the hair tends to tangle and mat easily, especially at the back and the sides if the client is confined to bed. Other blacks style their hair in cornrows. See Figure 36–18. These cornrows do not have to be unbraided before shampooing and washing. The nurse should obtain the client's permission before any such unbraiding.

To comb "natural" (Afro) hairstyles, apply a lubricant as the client indicates or as needed. Then, using a large open-toothed comb, start at the neckline and lift and fluff the hair outward, moving upward toward the forehead. Continue to fluff the hair outward and upward until all of the hair is combed on one half of the head. Then repeat for the other half of the head. To remove tangles:

1. After the hair is lubricated, weave and lift your open fingers through the hair to ease the tangles free.

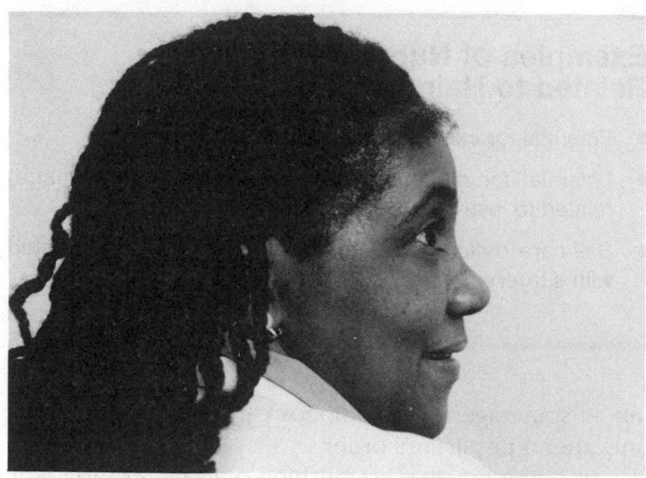

Figure 36–18 A black person's hair styled with cornrow braids

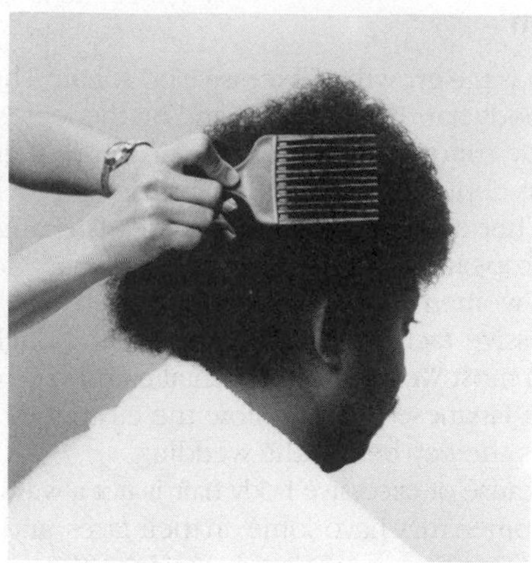

Figure 36–19 Removing tangles with a long-toothed comb

or

2. Support the hair securely at the base of the scalp, if possible, to prevent pulling and discomfort. Insert a long-toothed comb into the ends of the hair and carefully comb out the ends of the tangles. See Figure 36–19. Repeat this step, each time working the comb farther up the hair shaft toward the scalp, until the hair is untangled.

Shampooing Among both men and women, the cleanliness and grooming of hair frequently reflects their sense of well-being. Often after clients begin to feel better, having their hair done is a boost to morale and leads to positive feelings about their appearance.

How often a person needs a shampoo is highly individual, depending to a large degree on the person's activities and the amount of sebum secreted by the scalp. Oily hair tends to look stringy and dirty, and it feels unclean to the person.

There are a wide variety of shampoos, and most clients have their own favorite brands. If a person's hair tends to tangle after it is washed, a cream rinse after the shampoo may be needed. A black-skinned person's hair needs to be combed with a wide-toothed comb before it dries so that the hair will not tangle. Following a shampoo, many women and some men like to have their hair rolled on curlers and styled. Some hospitals also provide hair driers.

There are several ways to shampoo clients' hair, depending on their health, strength, and age. The client who is well enough to take a shower can shampoo while in the shower. The client who is unable to shower may be given a shampoo while sitting on a chair in front of a sink. The back-lying client who can move to a stretcher can be given a shampoo on a stretcher wheeled to a sink. The client who must remain in bed can be given a shampoo with water brought to the bedside. This method is the least convenient, but it allows the person who is confined to bed to receive a shampoo.

A nurse who assists a client with a shampoo should wet the hair with warm water, apply the shampoo, and make a good lather while massaging the scalp with the pads of the fingertips. Massaging stimulates the blood circulation in the scalp. The pads of the fingers are used so as not to scratch the scalp with the fingernails. The nurse then rinses the hair thoroughly, making sure no shampoo remains in the hair to dry and irritate the scalp. The hair is then dried thoroughly, often with a hair drier.

Shaving

Male clients often shave or are shaved after a bath. Female clients may prefer to shave the hair of the axillae and legs during a bath. Frequently clients supply their own electric or safety razors. When using a safety razor to shave a client's beard, apply shaving cream or shaving soap and water first to soften the bristles and make the skin more pliable. Hold the razor so that the blade is at a 45° angle to the skin and shave in short, firm strokes in the direction of hair growth. Hold the skin tautly, particularly around creases, to prevent cutting the skin. After shaving the entire area, wipe the client's face with a wet washcloth to remove any remaining shaving cream and hair. Dry the face well, then apply after-shave lotion or powder as the client prefers. To prevent irritating the skin, pat on the lotion with the fingers and avoid rubbing the face.

Beard Care

Beards and mustaches also require daily care. The most important aspect of the care is to keep them clean. Food particles tend to collect in beards and mustaches, and they need washing and combing periodically. Clients may also wish a beard or mustache trim to maintain a well-groomed appearance. A beard or mustache should not be shaved off without the client's consent.

Evaluation

Outcome criteria to evaluate the achievement of client goals or the effectiveness of nursing intervention are shown to the right.

Outcome Criteria: Hair

The client will:

- Have even hair growth
- Have resilient hair with a healthy sheen
- Have reduced or absent scalp lesions or infestations
- Describe contributing factors and interventions for dandruff (or other hair problem)
- Express positive statements about sense of well-being

Eyes

Normally, eyes require no special hygiene since lacrimal fluid continually washes the eyes, and the eyelids and lashes prevent the entrance of foreign particles. Special interventions are needed, however, for unconscious clients and for clients recovering from eye surgery or having eye injuries, irritations, or infections. In unconscious clients, the blink reflex may be absent, and excessive drainage may accumulate along eyelid margins. In clients with eye trauma or eye infections, excessive discharge or drainage is common. Excessive secretions on the lashes need to be removed before they dry on the lashes as crusts. Clients who wear eyeglasses, contact lenses, or an artificial eye also may require instruction from and care by the nurse.

Assessment

All external eye structures are inspected for signs of inflammation, excessive drainage, encrustations, or other obvious abnormalities. Inspection of the external eye structures is discussed in Chapter 35.

Ask the following questions of all clients who wear eyeglasses or contact lenses:

1. When were the glasses/lenses prescribed?
2. When did you last visit an ophthalmologist?
3. What is your vision like with and without the corrective device?

If a client wears contact lenses, ask these additional questions:

1. Have you had any problems with either or both eyes or eyelids, such as excessive tearing, burning, redness, sensitivity to light, swelling, or feelings of dryness? (Have the client describe them.)
2. Are you using any eyedrops or ointments? (These medications can combine chemically with *soft* lenses and cause lens damage and eye irritation.)
3. How often do you wear the lenses? Daily? On special occasions?
4. What is your lens-wearing time in a given day, including sleep time?
5. Do you wear lenses alternately with eyeglasses?
6. Do you remove the lenses for certain activities, e.g., contact sports or swimming?
7. Do you have any problems with the lenses, e.g., cleaning, insertion, removal, damage?
8. Do you carry an emergency identification label to alert others to remove the lenses and ensure appropriate care in an emergency? (If not, advise the client to acquire one.)
9. What are your insertion and removal procedures?
10. What are your cleaning and storage procedures?

Nursing Diagnoses

Nursing diagnoses related to eye problems are shown on the next page.

Intervention

Newborn Care

The eyes of newborns are treated soon after birth to prevent ophthalmia neonatorum (gonorrheal conjunctivitis). Penicillin and silver nitrate are the drugs used. Treatment is mandatory by law in all states in the United States. The method of instilling the drops is the same for babies as for children and adults. See Chapter 51.

Nursing Diagnoses Related to Eye Problems

- Potential for infection related to improperly cleaned contact lenses
- Potential for infection related to possible accumulation of excessive secretions on eyelids
- Potential for impaired tissue integrity (cornea) related to absence of blink reflex associated with unconsciousness
- Self-care deficit (contact lenses removal, cleaning and insertion) related to lack of coordination associated with aging
- Potential for impaired tissue integrity (cornea) related to wearing contact lenses for prolonged periods
- Disturbance in self-concept related to altered body image associated with eye prosthesis

Cleaning the Eyes

Washing the eyelids is discussed in the section on bathing. If dried secretions accumulate on the lashes, they need to be softened and wiped away. Hospital nurses soften dried secretions by placing a sterile cotton ball moistened with sterile water or normal saline over the lid margins. The nurse then wipes the loosened secretions from the inner canthus of the eye to the outer canthus, to prevent the particles and fluid from draining into the lacrimal sac and nasolacrimal duct. In the home, it is usually not necessary for the fluid to be sterile, and the excess fluid is usually wiped away with a soft tissue.

If the client is unconscious and lacks a blink reflex or cannot close the eyelids completely, drying and irritation of the cornea must be prevented. Lubricating eye drops may be administered if ordered by the physician. An eye patch may also be placed over the affected eye or eyes.

Eyeglass Care

Caution is essential when cleaning eyeglasses to prevent breaking or scratching the lenses. Glass lenses can be cleaned with warm water and dried with a soft tissue that will not scratch the lenses. Plastic lenses are easily scratched and require special cleaning solutions and drying tissues. When not being worn, all glasses should be placed in a case and stored in the client's bedside table drawer.

Contact Lens Care

Contact lenses, thin curved discs of hard or soft plastic, fit on the cornea of the eye directly over the pupil. They float on the tear layer of the eye. Advantages of contact lenses over eyeglasses for some people are:

1. They cannot be seen and thus have cosmetic value.
2. They are highly effective in correcting some astigmatisms.
3. They are safer than glasses for some physical activities.
4. They do not fog, as eyeglasses do.
5. They provide better vision in many cases.

Contact lenses may be either hard or soft or a compromise between the two—gas permeables. Hard contact lenses, introduced in the 1940s, cover part of the cornea and can endure up to 20 years of use. They are made of a rigid, unwettable, airtight plastic that does not absorb water or saline solutions. The portion of the eye beneath the hard lens is lubricated and oxygenated by tears. Disadvantages are that they restrict oxygen supply to the cornea, usually cannot be worn for more than 12 to 14 hours, and are rarely recommended for first-time wearers.

Soft contact lenses, introduced in the early 1970s, cover the entire cornea. Being more pliable and soft, they mold to the eye for a firmer fit. They are composed of polymers that absorb water, allow through-the-lens oxygen transmission, and are easier on the eyes. There are many varieties: bifocal, toric (for high astigmatism), tinted (to enhance eye color), and extended-wear. The duration of extended wear varies by brand from 1 to 30 days or more. Eye specialists and Health and Welfare Canada recommend that long-wear brands be removed and cleaned at least once a week. Extended-wear soft lenses that are ultrathin are comfortable but very flimsy and difficult to keep clean. Disadvantages of soft lenses are that they do not provide vision as crisp as the hard lenses, are more prone to bacterial buildup, are easily ripped, and need to be replaced every year or so. They require scrupulous care and handling.

Gas permeables, introduced in the late 1970s, are rigid enough to provide clear vision but are more flexible than the traditional hard lens. They permit oxygen to reach the cornea, thus providing greater comfort, and will not cause serious damage to the eye if left in place for several days.

Most clients normally care for their own contact lenses. There are a number of ways to place contact lenses on the eyes and to remove them. Clients learn the method that best suits them from their eye specialists. In certain cases or emergencies, the nurse may need to remove a client's lenses. A hard contact lens wearer who is unconscious and unable to blink can develop corneal abrasions from lack of tears for lubrication. Clients with impaired judgment, e.g., due to psychiatric illness or substance abuse, are prone to eye damage from prolonged lens wearing. Proper handling of the lenses by the nurse is essential.

Procedure 36–7 outlines the steps involved in removing, cleaning, and inserting contact lenses.

Contact lenses need to be cleaned in a sterile, nonirritating wetting solution before they are inserted. The wetting solution helps the lens to glide over the cornea, thus reducing the risk of injury. Some clients use their saliva to wet their lenses. This practice needs to be discouraged, since contaminants in saliva can cause bacterial buildup on the lens and infection.

Lenses are cleaned relatively easily with chemical lens-cleaning solutions. Sot lenses can also be cleaned by electric heat disinfecting units. In addition to regular heat disinfection, weekly cleaning with an enzymatic solution that dissolves protein deposits is necessary. Proper storage of lenses is essential. Soft lenses can become dry, brittle, and permanently damaged if left exposed to the air for an hour or less. Sterile saline is the preferred storage solution. Unsterile solutions promote bacterial growth, and the minerals in tap water can damage a soft lens.

Procedure 36–7 ▲ Removing, Cleaning, and Inserting Contact Lenses

Equipment

For Removal

1. A lens storage case. Most users have a special container for their lenses. In some, the lenses are stored in a solution; in others, the lenses are stored dry. Each case has two labeled slots indicating which lens should be stored there. It is essential to store each lens in the appropriate slot, since each lens is ground for a specific eye. The case is placed on the bedside table within easy reach.

   or

2. If a lens storage case is not available, two small medicine cups or specimen containers partially filled with normal saline solution. Mark one cup "L lens"; the other, "R lens."
3. A flashlight (optional) to help locate the lens.
4. A cotton applicator dipped in saline (optional) to reposition a lens.

For Cleaning

1. The client's lens storage case and lenses.

For hard lenses

2. Contact lens cleaner. This is usually a sterile, antiseptic, nonirritating solution labeled lens cleaner.
3. An absorbent applicator or cotton balls for spreading the cleaning solution (optional).
4. Warm water.
5. Soaking solution (optional).

For soft lenses: Heat disinfection

6. A heat disinfecting case.
7. Saline solution (a salt tablet and distilled water).
8. Cleaning solution (an enzyme tablet and distilled water).

For soft lenses: Chemical disinfection

9. Lens cleaning solution.
10. Rinsing solution.
11. Disinfection and storage solution.

For Insertion

1. The client's lens storage case.
2. A wetting agent to lubricate the lenses. Solutions of methyl cellulose or polyvinyl alcohol are frequently used.

Intervention

To Remove a Hard Lens

1. Assist the client to a supine position or a sitting position with the head tilted back.

   Rationale This position prevents the lens from falling onto the floor.

2. Locate the position of the lens:
   a. Retract the client's upper eyelid with your index finger and ask him or her to look up, down, and from side to side.
   b. Retract the lower eyelid with your index finger and have the client look up and down and from side to side.
   c. Use a flashlight if necessary.

   Rationale Some colorless soft lenses are difficult to see. The lens must be positioned directly over the cornea for proper removal.

3. If the lens is displaced:
   a. Ask the client to look straight ahead.
   b. Using your index fingers, gently exert pressure on the inner margins of the upper and lower lids, and move the lens back onto the cornea.

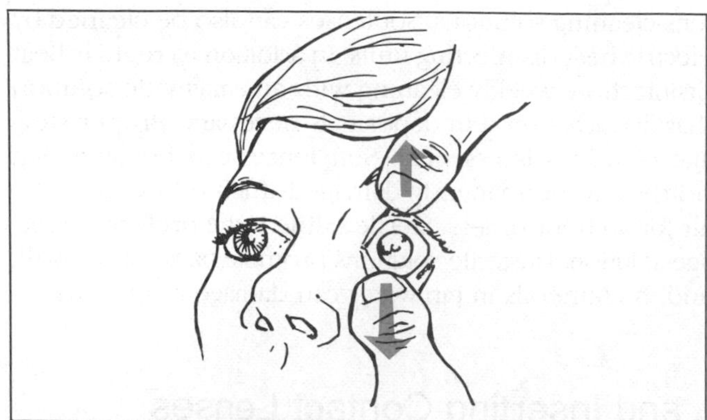

Figure 36–20

or

c. Using a cotton-tipped applicator dipped in saline, gently move the lens into place.

4. Using both thumbs or index fingers, separate the upper and lower eyelids of one eye until they are beyond the edges of the lens. See Figure 36–20. Exert pressure toward the bony orbit above and below the eye.

   Rationale A two-handed method may be needed for clients unable to cooperate. Retraction of the eyelids against the bony orbit prevents direct pressure, discomfort, and injury to the eyeball.

   or

   Use the middle finger to retract the upper eyelid and the thumb of the same hand to retract the lower lid.

   Rationale Using one hand for retraction keeps the other hand free to receive the lens.

5. Gently move the margins of both the lower eyelid and the upper eyelid toward the lens.

   Rationale The margins of the lids trap the edges of the lens.

6. Hold the top eyelid stationary, and lift the bottom edge of the contact lens by pressing the lower lid at its margin firmly under the lens. See Figure 36–21.

   Rationale Pressure exerted under the edge of the lens overcomes the suction of the lens on the cornea. The lens then tips forward at the top edge.

7. Slide the lens off and out of the eye by moving both eyelids toward each other.

8. Grasp the lens with your index finger and thumb and place it in the palm of your hand.

9. Place the lens in the correct slot in its storage case. The slots are labeled for right and left lenses.

10. Repeat steps 4–9 for the other lens.

11. Be sure each lens is centered well in the storage case. Tighten or close the cover. Proceed to step 21.

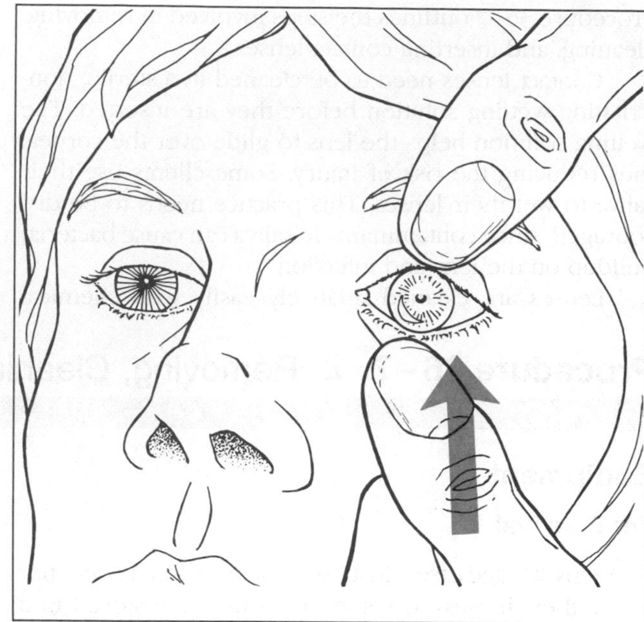

Figure 36–21

Rationale If the lens is not centered, it may crack, chip, or tear.

To Remove a Soft Lens

12. Ask the client to look upward at the ceiling and keep the eye opened wide.

13. Retract the lower or upper lid with one or two fingers of your nondominant hand.

14. Using the index finger of your dominant hand, move the lens down to the inferior part of the sclera. See Figure 36–22.

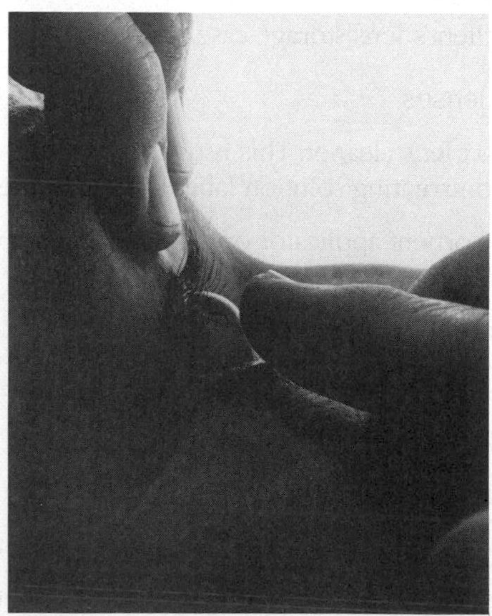

Figure 36–22

Rationale Moving the lens onto the sclera reduces the risk of damage to the cornea.

15. Gently pinch the lens between the pads of the thumb and index finger of your dominant hand, and remove the lens. See Figure 36–23.

    Rationale Pinching causes the lens to double up, so that air enters underneath the lens, overcoming the suction and allowing removal. The pads of the fingers are used to prevent scratching the eye or the lens with the fingernails.

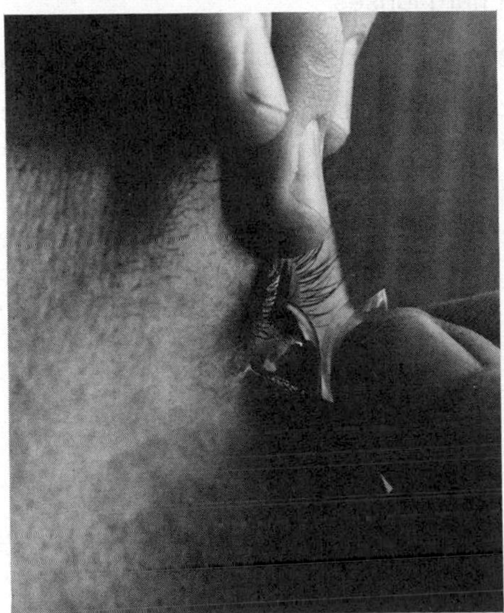

Figure 36–23

16. Place the lens in the palm of your hand.
17. For *ultrathin* lenses, slide the lens open with the thumb and index finger *immediately* upon removal.

    Rationale It is important to keep the edges from sticking together.

18. Place the lens in the correct slot in its storage case. The slots are labeled for right and left lenses.
19. Repeat steps 12–18 for the other lens.
20. Be sure each lens is centered well in the storage case. Tighten or close the cover.

    Rationale If the lens is not centered, it may crack or tear.

21. Place the contact lens container in the drawer of the bedside table.

    Rationale The lenses and the case should never be exposed to direct sunlight or extreme heat, which can dry or warp them.

22. Record removal of the lenses prior to surgery or when this is a nursing responsibility. Record any problems observed, such as redness of the conjunctiva, and report problems to the responsible nurse.

Sample Recording

Date	Time	Notes
Mar 22/87	2100	Contact lenses removed. No redness of the conjunctiva noted. ——— ——Anita R. Rodriguez, SN

Cleaning Contact Lenses (Hard and Soft)

1. Open the lens container carefully.

   Rationale Soft contact lenses tend to pop out unexpectedly when the case is opened quickly.

2. Pick up one lens from the container.

   Rationale The lenses are cleaned one at a time to make sure they are not put in the wrong slot or wrong eye.

3. Assess the lenses for scratches or tears.

To clean hard lenses

4. Place a few drops of lens cleaner on both sides of the lens.
5. Spread the solution on both surfaces with the thumb and index finger or an absorbent applicator, or place the lens in the palm of your hand and spread the solution with your index finger.

   Rationale The solution removes dirt and film.

6. Position the lens on the palm side of the index or middle finger.
7. Rinse the lens with warm tap water that feels comfortable to the fingers. If the tap water contains excessive chlorine or minerals, use distilled or purified water. If rinsing the lens over a sink, be sure the sink drain is closed.

   Rationale Hot water is contraindicated because it may warp the lens. The closer the lens is to body temperature the more comfortable it will feel on insertion. While rinsing removes dirt, it is not necessary to rinse away all of the lens cleaner since this agent has beneficial sterilizing and wetting properties.

8. Place the lens in a soaking solution or store it dry in accordance with the recommendations of the client's physician.
9. Follow steps 4–8 to clean the second lens.

To clean soft lenses by chemical disinfection

10. Place a few drops of lens cleaner on both sides of the lens and spread it as described in step 5.
11. Position the lens as described in step 6.
12. Rinse the lens thoroughly with rinsing solution.

13. Place the lens in the correct slot of the storage area.
14. Fill the slot with storage and disinfectant solution and tightly close the cap.
15. Follow steps 10–14 for the other lens.
16. Store both lenses for at least 4 hours.
17. Clean and rinse the lenses before insertion. Follow steps 10–12.
18. Clean the storage slots by emptying the solution and rinsing them with hot water and rinsing solution. Allow them to air dry.

To clean soft lenses by heat disinfection

19. Put a few drops of normal saline solution on each lens and spread it on the lens as described in step 5.
20. Rinse the lenses thoroughly with tap water.
21. Place each lens in the appropriate slot of the heat disinfecting unit, and fill the slots with normal saline solution.
22. Make sure the disinfecting unit is placed on a heat-resistant surface. Plug the unit into an electric outlet, and turn it on. The unit will turn off automatically after disinfection is completed.

To clean soft lenses with an enzymatic solution (weekly)

23. Rinse and fill the plastic or glass wells of the lens storage case with distilled water.
24. Place an enzymatic cleaning tablet in each well.
25. Place one lens in each well and securely close the caps.
26. Shake the wells to dissolve the tablets.
27. Soak the lenses for 6 to 12 hours or overnight.
28. Remove the lenses, and thoroughly rinse them with saline solution.
29. Place the lenses in the heat disinfecting unit and follow steps 21–22.
30. Rinse the storage wells with tap water, and allow them to air dry.
31. Record cleaning of the lenses with removal or insertion of the lenses.

Inserting Contact Lenses

Seriously ill clients who have had their contact lenses removed will not need them reinserted until they become more active in their care and require their lenses to see properly.

1. Ensure that the lenses are clean.

   Rationale This reduces the chance of introducing an infection to the eye.

2. Ensure that the correct lens is selected for the eye. It is wise always to start with the right eye.

   Rationale Each lens is ground to fit the individual eye and correct its visual defect. Getting into the habit of always starting with the right eye reduces the risk of inserting the wrong lens.

To insert hard lenses

3. Put a few drops of wetting solution on the right lens.

   Rationale Wetting solution lubricates the lens, facilitates insertion, and lessens the chance of damage to the eye.

4. Spread the wetting solution on both surfaces of the lens using your thumb and index finger, or place the lens in the palm of your hand and spread the solution with your index finger.
5. Place the lens convex side down on the tip of your dominant index finger. See Figure 36–24.

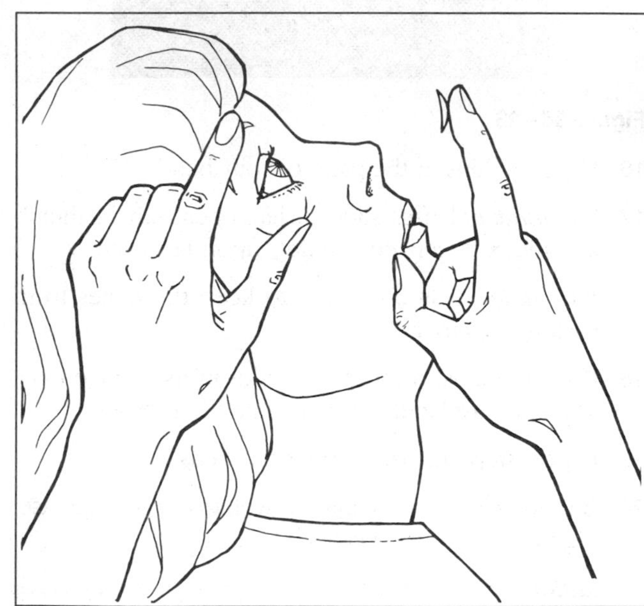

Figure 36–24

6. Ask the client to bend his or her head backward.
7. Separate the upper and lower eyelids of the client's right eye with the thumb and index finger of your nondominant hand. See Figure 36–24. Place your thumb on the skin over the infraorbital bone and

your index finger on the skin over the supraorbital bone.

Rationale Retraction of the eyelids against the bony orbit prevents direct pressure, discomfort, and injury to the eyeball.

8. Place the lens as gently as possible on the cornea directly over the iris and pupil.
9. Ask whether the client's vision is blurred following insertion.

   Rationale If vision is blurred, the lens may be off center.

10. If so, center the lens as follows:
    a. Separate the eyelids, using the index or middle finger of the left hand to lift the upper lid and the index or middle finger of the right hand to depress the lower lid. See Figure 36–25.
    b. Locate the lens, and have the client gaze in the opposite direction. See Figure 36–25.
    c. Gently push the lens in the direction of the cornea, using a finger or the eyelid margins.

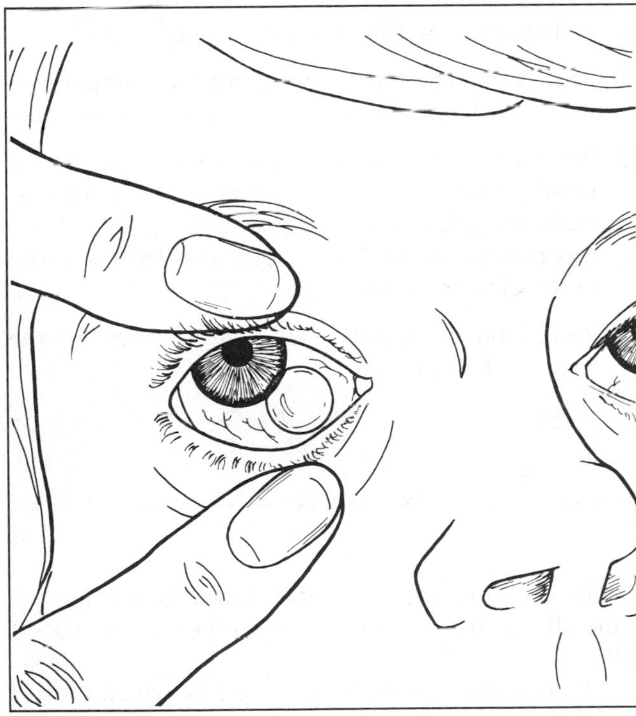

Figure 36–25

    d. Ask the client to look slowly toward the lens. The lens will slide easily onto the cornea as the client looks toward it.

11. Repeat steps 3–10 for the left lens. Then proceed to step 22.

To insert soft lenses

12. Remove the lens from its saline-filled storage case with your nondominant hand. If the lens is ultrathin allow it to air dry for a few seconds.

    Rationale The dominant fingers must be kept dry for inserting the lens.

13. Position a regular (not ultrathin) lens correctly for insertion:
    a. Hold the lens at the edge between your thumb and index finger. See Figure 36–26.

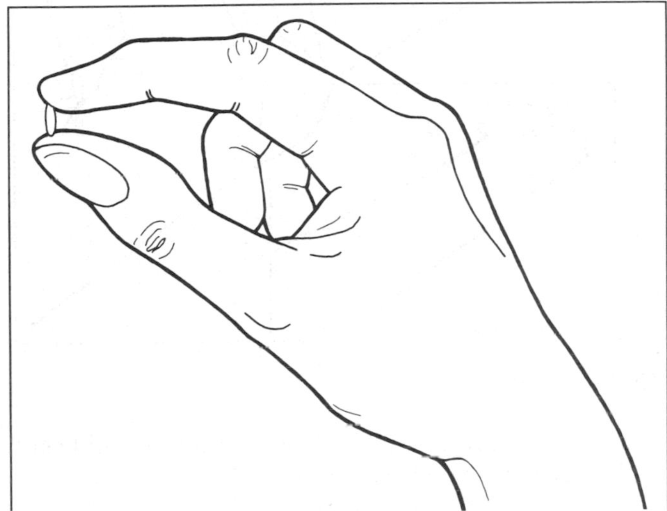

Figure 36–26

    b. Flex the lens slightly. The lens is in the correct position if the edges point inward. It is in the wrong position (i.e., inside-out) and must be reversed if the edges point outward. See Figure 36–27.

    Rationale A lens placed on the eye inside-out is less comfortable, tends to fold on the eye, can drop to a lower position on the eye, and may move excessively on blinking.

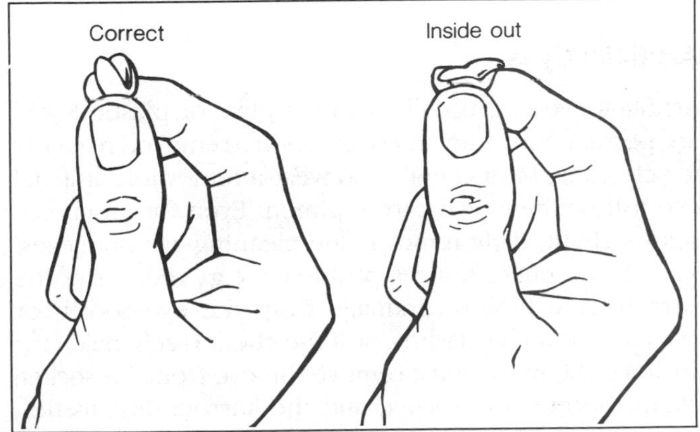

Figure 36–27

14. Do *not* flex the lens if it is *ultrathin*. Instead, put the lens on your placement finger and allow it to dry slightly for a few seconds. Closely inspect the lens to see if the edges turn upward. See Figure 36–28, *A*. If they turn downward, the lens is inside-out and must be reversed. See Figure 36–28, *B*.

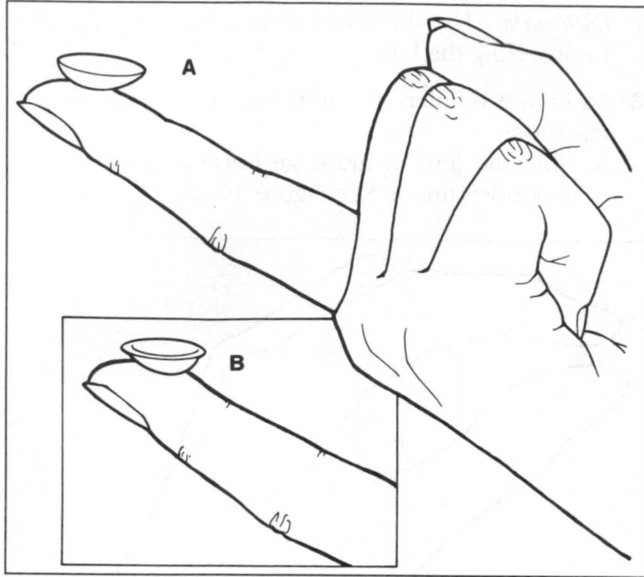

Figure 36–28

Rationale Flexing an ultrathin lens may cause the lens to fold and stick together.

15. Wet the lens with saline solution as described in step 4, using your nondominant fingers.

16. Ensure that your placement finger is dry. This is particularly important for ultrathin soft lenses.

    Rationale "Water-loving" soft contact lenses have a natural attraction to wet surfaces. The lens adheres more readily to the moist eye if the finger is dry.

17. Place the lens convex side down on the tip of your dominant index finger.

    Rationale The concave side of the lens rests against the cornea.

18. Keep the lens parallel with the fingertip, with all edges up and toward the eye. See Figure 36–28, *A*.

    Rationale Balancing the lens in an upright position facilitates insertion. It is difficult to insert a lens that rocks forward or sideways with one edge touching the fingertip.

19. If the lens curls and the edges stick together, place the lens in the palm of your hand, wet it thoroughly with saline solution, and gently move the edges apart by rubbing the lens between your thumb and index finger, or soak the lens in saline solution.

20. If the lens flattens or drapes across the finger, move the lens to the palm of your nondominant hand, dry the placement finger, and allow the lens to air dry for a few seconds.

    Rationale The placement finger on the lens may be too wet.

21. Follow steps 6–8 above for insertion.

22. Replace the client's lens container, lens cleaner, and wetting solution in the drawer of the bedside table.

23. Record insertion of the contact lenses if a nurse is required to remove them; otherwise, this is not normally recorded (consult agency policy). Record and report to the responsible nurse any problems observed in the eyes or the lenses.

24. Record on the nursing care plan the time for the lenses to be removed.

Artificial Eyes

Artificial eyes are usually made of glass or plastic. Some are permanently implanted; others are removed regularly for cleaning. Most clients who wear a removable artificial eye follow their own care regimen. Even for an unconscious client, daily removal and cleaning are not necessary. If the nurse notices problems, e.g., redness of the surrounding tissues, drainage from the eye socket, or crusting on the eyelashes, or if the client is scheduled for surgery, the nurse must remove the eye from the socket; clean the eye, the socket, and the surrounding tissues; and then reinsert the eye. Clients whose mobility is impaired by injury or paralysis may also require assistance. In addition, the nurse must determine the client's routine eye care practices so that these can be followed. Some clients may remove and clean the eye and socket daily.

To remove an artificial eye, pull the client's lower eyelid down over the infraorbital bone with your dominant thumb, and exert slight pressure below the eyelid to overcome the suction. See Figure 36–29. An alternate method is to compress a small rubber bulb and apply the tip directly to the eye. As the nurse gradually releases the finger pressure on the bulb, the suction of the bulb counteracts the suction holding the eye in the socket and draws the eye out of the socket.

Clean the eye with warm normal saline. If the eye is not to be reinserted, place it in a container filled with

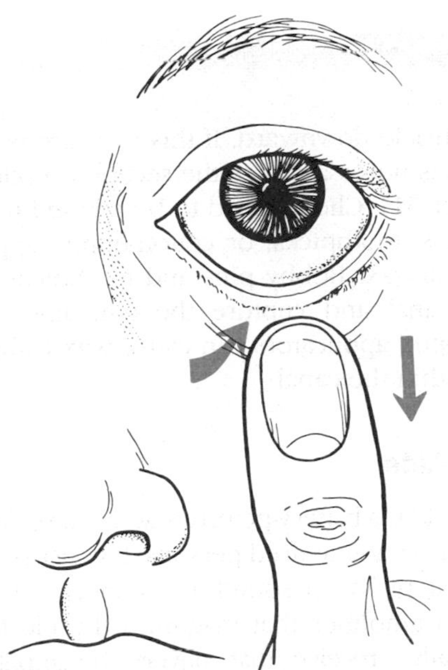

Figure 36–29 When removing an artificial eye, the nurse retracts the lower eyelid and exerts slight pressure below the eyelid.

water or saline solution, close the lid, label the container with the client's name and room number, and place it in the drawer of the bedside table. The nurse should also clean the socket and tissues around the eye with soft gauze or cotton wipes and normal saline or warm tap water. After inspecting these tissues, the nurse must report and record any abnormal findings. To insert the eye, retract the eyelids with your thumb and index fingers of one hand, exerting pressure on the supraorbital and infraorbital bones. Holding the eye between the thumb and index fingers of the other hand, slip the eye gently into the socket. See Figure 36–30.

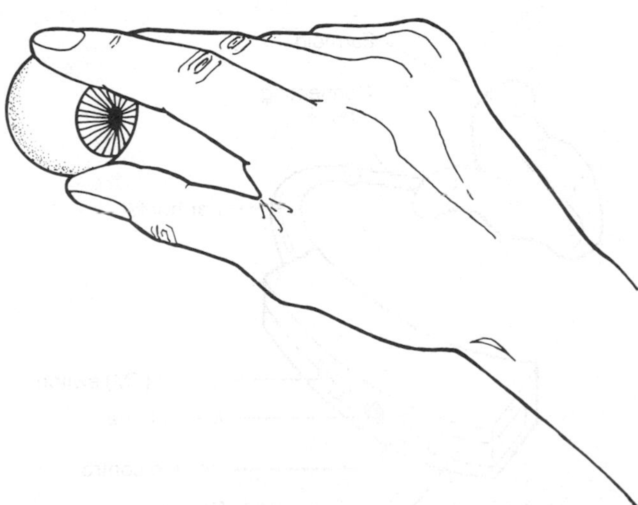

Figure 36–30 An artificial eye is held between the thumb and index finger for insertion.

Teaching Situations Regarding Eye Care

1. Parents may need to learn facts about eye care for their children. Children need to have their eyes examined when they are old enough to walk and again when they begin school. Crossed eyes need to be treated, usually with proper eyeglasses and muscle exercises. By school age, children may need glasses for persistent hyperopia or newly developed myopia or astigmatism. Parents may suspect eye problems if a child is unusually clumsy when playing or holds objects close to the eyes to see them.
2. People may need to be encouraged to avoid home remedies for eye problems. Eye irritations or injuries at any age need to be treated medically and immediately. If dirt or dust gets into the eyes, copious cleaning with clean, tepid water can be used as an emergency treatment.
3. Nurses may need to reinforce good visual hygiene measures to prevent eyestrain and protect vision. Among them are use of adequate lighting for reading and appropriate use of glasses when prescribed. Shatterproof lenses are recommended.
4. Middle-aged and older adults may need to be reminded of the importance of regular eye examinations to detect glaucoma or cataracts. Nurses may also remind them of health insurance benefits they may receive for prescribed treatments for visual impairments or problems.

Evaluation

Examples of outcome criteria to evaluate the achievement of client goals or the effectiveness of nursing intervention are shown below.

Outcome Criteria: Eyes

The client will:

- Have clear conjunctiva and white sclera without inflammation
- Have reduced secretions on eyelids
- Experience no tearing
- Experience no eye discomfort
- Express positive feelings about appearance with eye prostheses
- Demonstrate appropriate methods of caring for contact lenses
- Describe interventions to prevent eye injury and infection

Ears

Normal ears require minimal hygiene. Clients who have excessive **cerumen** (earwax) and dependent clients who have hearing aids may require assistance from the nurse.

Assessment

The nurse inspects external ear structures for signs of inflammation, excessive drainage, discomfort, or other obvious abnormalities. Inspection of the external ear structures is discussed in Chapter 35.

If a client wears a hearing aid, the nurse determines:

1. When and where the hearing aid was obtained and from whom
2. How the client maintains and cleans the hearing aid
3. Whether the client experiences problems with the hearing aid
4. What ear problems, if any, the client experiences

Nursing Diagnosis

Nursing diagnoses related to ear problems are shown below.

Intervention

Cleaning the Ears

The auricles of the ear are cleaned during the bed bath. The nurse or client must remove excessive cerum that is visible or that causes discomfort or hearing difficulty. Visible cerumen may be loosened and removed by retracting the auricle downward. If this measure is ineffective, irrigation is necessary (see the section on otic irrigation in Chapter 51). Clients need to be advised never to use bobby pins, toothpicks, or cotton-tipped applicators to remove earwax. Bobby pins and toothpicks can injure the ear canal and rupture the tympanic membrane; cotton-tipped applicators can cause wax to become impacted within the canal.

Hearing Aids

A hearing aid is a battery-powered, sound-amplifying device used by hearing-impaired persons. It consists of a microphone that picks up sound and converts it to electric energy, an amplifier that magnifies the electric energy electronically, a receiver that converts the amplified energy back to sound energy, and an earmold that directs the sound into the ear. There are several types of hearing aids:

1. *Behind-the-ear aid.* This is the most widely used type, since it fits snugly over the ear. The hearing aid case, which holds the microphone, amplifier, and receiver, is attached to the earmold by a plastic tube. See Figure 36–31.
2. *In-the-ear aid.* This one-piece aid is the most compact hearing aid. All its components are housed in the earmold. See Figure 36–32.
3. *Eyeglasses aid.* This is similar to the behind-the-ear aid except that the components are housed in the temple of the eyeglasses. A hearing aid can be in one or both temples of the glasses. See Figure 36–33.

Nursing Diagnoses Related to Ear Problems

- Potential for injury related to methods used to remove cerumen
- Potential for infection related to ineffective practices for cleaning of hearing aid
- Potential for impaired verbal communication related to refusal to wear hearing aid
- Self-care deficit (hearing aid removal, cleaning, and inserting) related to neuromuscular impairment
- Potential for disturbance in self-concept associated with need to wear hearing aid

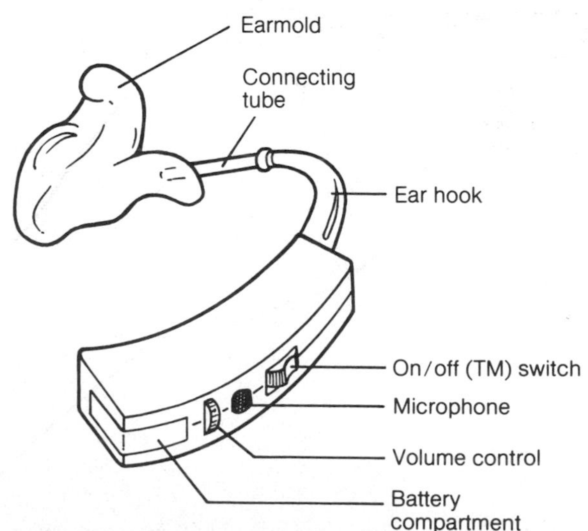

Figure 36–31 A behind-the-ear hearing aid

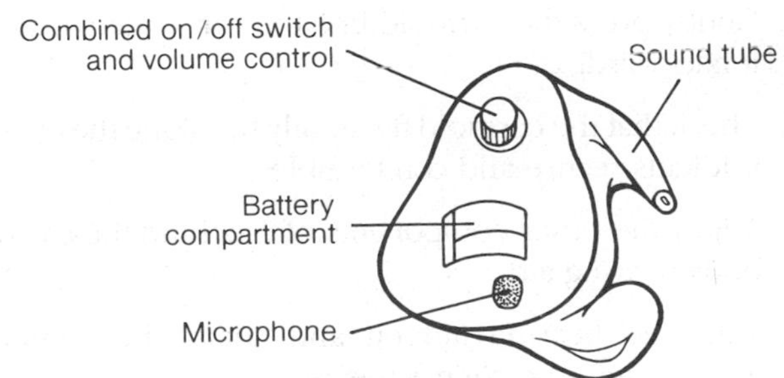

Figure 36–32 An in-the-ear hearing aid

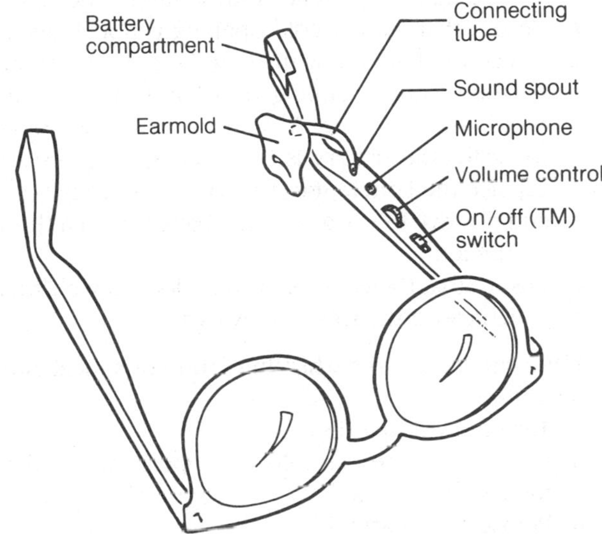

Figure 36–33 An eyeglasses hearing aid

4. *Body hearing aid.* This pocket-sized aid, used for more severe hearing losses, clips onto an undergarment, shirt pocket, or harness carrier supplied by the manufacturer. See Figure 36–34. The case, containing the microphone and amplifier, is connected by a cord to the receiver, which snaps into the earpiece.

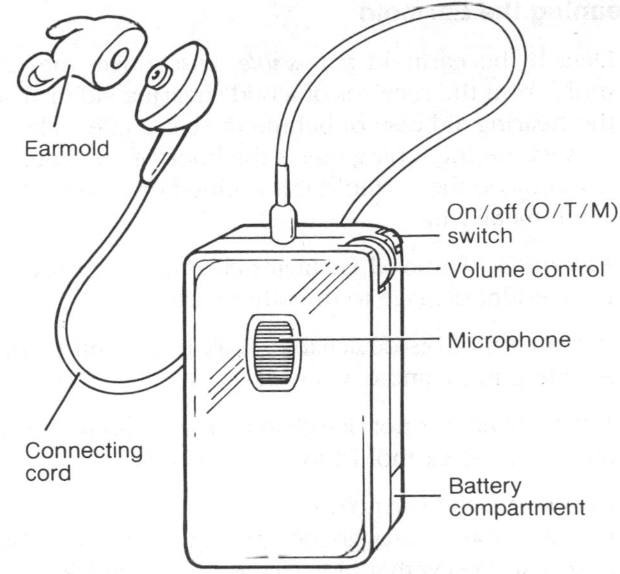

Figure 36–34 A body hearing aid

To ensure proper functioning, the wearer must handle the hearing aid appropriately during insertion and removal, clean the earmold regularly, and replace dead batteries. Although most clients can look after their hearing aids themselves, some debilitated clients may require assistance. Hearing aids must be removed before surgery. Procedure 36–8 outlines the steps involved in removing, cleaning, and inserting a hearing aid.

Procedure 36–8 ▲ Removing, Cleaning, and Inserting a Hearing Aid

Equipment

1. The client's hearing aid
2. A new battery (if needed)
3. A pipe cleaner or toothpick (optional)
4. Soap, water, and towels or a damp cloth

Intervention

Removing a Hearing Aid

1. Turn the hearing aid off and lower the volume. The on/off switch may be labeled "O" (off), "M" microphone, "T" (telephone), or "TM" (telephone/microphone).

   Rationale The batteries continue to be used if the aid is not turned off.

2. Remove the earmold by rotating it slightly forward and pulling it outward.
3. If the aid is not to be used for several days, remove the battery.

   Rationale Removal prevents corrosion of the aid from battery leakage.

4. Store the hearing aid in a safe place. Avoid exposure to heat and moisture.

   Rationale Proper storage prevents loss or damage.

Cleaning the Earmold

5. Detach the earmold *if possible*. Disconnect the earmold from the receiver of a body hearing aid or from the hearing aid case of behind-the-ear and eyeglasses aids where the tubing meets the hook of the case. Do not remove the earmold if it is glued or secured by a small metal ring.

   Rationale Removal facilitates cleaning and prevents inadvertent damage to the other parts.

6. If the earmold is detachable, soak it in a mild soapy solution. Rinse and dry it well.
7. If the earmold is not detachable or is for an in-the-ear aid, wipe the earmold with a damp cloth.
8. Check that the earmold opening is patent. Blow any excess moisture through the opening or remove debris (e.g., earwax) with a pipe cleaner or toothpick.
9. Reattach the earmold if it was detached from the rest of the hearing aid.

Inserting the Hearing Aid

1. Determine from the client whether the earmold is for the left or the right ear.
2. Check that the battery is inserted in the hearing aid. Turn off the hearing aid, and make sure the volume is turned all the way down.
3. Inspect the earmold to identify the ear canal portion.

   Rationale Some earmolds are fitted for only the ear canal and concha; others are fitted for all the contours of the ear. The canal portion, common to all, can be used as a guide for correct insertion.

4. Line up the parts of the earmold with the corresponding parts of the client's ear.
5. Rotate the earmold slightly forward and insert the ear canal portion.
6. Gently press the earmold into the ear while rotating it backward.
7. Check that the earmold fits snugly by asking the client if it feels secure and comfortable.
8. Adjust the other components of a behind-the-ear or body hearing aid.
9. Turn the hearing aid on and adjust the volume according to the client's needs.
10. If the hearing aid is not functioning properly, i.e., if the sound is weak or there is no sound:
    a. Ensure that the volume is turned high enough.
    b. Ensure that the earmold opening is not clogged.
    c. Check the battery, by turning the aid on, turning up the volume, cupping your hand over the earmold, and listening. A constant whistling sound indicates the battery is functioning. If necessary, replace the battery. Be sure that the negative (−) and positive (+) signs on the battery match those on the aid.
    d. Ensure that the ear canal is not blocked with wax, which can obstruct sound waves.
11. If the client reports a whistling sound or squeal after insertion:
    a. Turn the volume down.
    b. Ensure that the earmold is properly attached to the receiver.
    c. Reinsert the earmold.
12. When communicating with the client, be sure to face the client, and talk distinctly in natural tones. Do not shout.

    Rationale Facing the client directly facilitates lip reading by some clients. Natural tones are more easily amplified.

13. Report and record any problems the client has with the hearing aid. Removal and insertion of a hearing aid are not normally recorded.

Evaluation

Examples of outcome criteria to evaluate the achievement of client goals or the effectiveness of nursing interventions are shown to the right.

Outcome Criteria: Ears

The client will:

- Describe measures to prevent ear injury and infection
- Demonstrate appropriate methods of caring for a hearing aid
- Experience no ear discomfort
- Wear a hearing aid throughout the day
- Express positive feelings about wearing a hearing aid

Nose

Nurses usually need not provide special care for the nose because clients can ordinarily clear nasal secretions by blowing into a soft tissue. However, clients with tubes that exit from the nares or those whose excessive secretions impair breathing may require special assistance.

Assessment

Assessment of the nares is discussed in Chapter 35. If a client has a nasogastric tube or any tube exiting from the nares, the nurse inspects the nares, particularly the surfaces in contact with the tube, for signs of inflammation, tenderness, bleeding, and sloughing. Pressure and movement of these tubes can cause tissue irritation and damage.

Nursing Diagnosis

Nursing diagnoses related to nose problems are shown below.

Nursing Diagnoses Related to Nose Problems

- Impaired tissue Integrity related to nasogastric tube
- Ineffective breathing pattern related to excessive secretions in nasopharynx
- Potential for infection related to impaired integrity of nasal mucous membrane secondary to nasogastric tube

Intervention

Excessive nasal secretions can be removed by inserting a cotton-tipped applicator moistened with water or normal saline or by applying suction. A cotton-tipped applicator should not be inserted beyond the length of the cotton tip. Suctioning of the nares is discussed in Chapter 45.

The nares of clients with nasal tubes should be cleaned with a moistened, cotton-tipped applicator to prevent the accumulation of secretions around the tubing. The tape that anchors the tube should be changed when it becomes moist to prevent maceration of the skin and mucous membrane. Methods of taping tubes to minimize their movement are discussed in Chapter 53.

Evaluation

Outcome criteria for problems related to the nose are shown below.

Outcome Criteria: Nose

The client will:

- Have intact nasal mucous membranes
- Have pink nasal mucosa with clear watery discharge
- Experience no tenderness
- Have patent nares

Beds

Ill persons are frequently confined to bed, sometimes for weeks or months. The bed then becomes an important piece of furniture, and the client's ability to rest and sleep depends on how comfortable he or she feels in bed.

There are different types of beds. People who are ill at home may find their own beds quite satisfactory as long as the periods of illness are brief. A hospital bed has characteristics particularly suited to people who are in bed continuously or for a long time:

1. Hospital beds can be adjusted to a variety of positions (see the discussion later in this chapter). Most hospitals use Gatch beds. When the gatches, or joints, are flexed, the client is raised to a sitting position with the knees elevated. The cranks that operate the gatches are usually at the bottom or side of the bed. When not in use, manual cranks are left in the retracted position under the bed. Otherwise, people walking by the bed might easily hit their legs against the cranks. Some hospital beds have electric motors to operate the gatches. The motor is activated by pressing a button or moving a small lever, located either at the side of the bed or on a small panel separate from the bed but attached to it by a cable.
2. Hospital beds are usually 66 cm (26 in) high. (Long-term care facilities for ambulatory clients usually have low beds to facilitate movement in and out of bed.) Some hospital beds have "high" and "low" positions that can be adjusted either mechanically by a crank at the center of the foot of the bed or electrically by a button or lever on the same panel as the gatch controls. The high position permits the nurse to reach the

client without undue stretching or stooping. The low position allows the client to step easily to the floor.

3. A hospital bed is normally 0.9 m (3 ft) wide, narrower than the usual bed, so that the nurse can reach the client from either side of the bed without undue stretching. The length is usually 1.9 m (6.5 ft). Some beds can be extended in length, if required.
4. Most hospital beds have casters and can be moved easily and quietly.

Standard Equipment

Mattresses

Most mattresses used in hospitals have innersprings, which give even support to the body. When changing a bed, nurses need to note any unevenness of the mattress surface, which might indicate a broken spring. Mattresses are usually covered with a water-repellent material that resists soiling and can be cleaned easily. Most mattresses have handles on the sides called lugs by which the mattress can be removed.

Foam rubber egg crate mattresses are also used in hospitals. They provide support and have the advantage of relieving pressure on the body's bony prominences, such as the heels. Foam mattresses are particularly helpful for clients confined to bed for a long time.

Another option is the air mattress, which is attached to a motor that lowers or raises the air pressure inside the mattress. It is also called the alternating pressure mattress.

The water mattress is a plastic bag filled with water. This mattress employs the principle of weight displacement. If the body displaces 9 kg (20 lb) of water, there is 9 kg less pressure on the weight-bearing areas.

The surfaces of air and water mattresses must be intact so that the air or water will not escape. It is therefore inadvisable to use pins on the sheets covering these mattresses. Special mattresses are placed atop the standard bed mattress, although the water mattress may be placed on the base springs.

Bed Boards

A bed board, or fracture board as it is sometimes called, is a board placed directly under a mattress to give added support. Physicians often order bed boards for clients with back injuries.

The bed board is usually the size of the mattress. Some are plain flat boards, while others are hinged so that the head of the bed, and sometimes the foot of the bed, can be elevated.

Side Rails

Side rails, or safety sides, are used on both hospital beds and stretchers. They are of various shapes and sizes and are usually made of metal. Devices to raise and lower them differ. Often one or two knobs are pulled to release the side and permit it to be moved.

Side rails have a number of functions:

1. To prevent clients from rolling or falling out of bed. This is a danger particularly for the elderly, young children, restless clients, and unconscious clients.
2. To give some clients, especially the elderly, the blind, and the sedated, a sense of security.
3. To provide a hand hold so that a client can move up in bed or turn over.
4. If they are half rails, to provide support for a client who is getting out of bed.

When side rails are being used, it is important that the nurse never leave the bedside while the rail is lowered. Some side rails have two positions: up and down. Others have three: high, intermediate, and low. The down and low positions are employed when a side rail is not needed. With some models, the bed foundation must be raised before the side rail can be put in the low position; otherwise, the side rail might hit the floor and be damaged. The intermediate position is used when the bed is in the low position and the nurse is present. The up or high side rail position is used when a client is in bed and requires protection from falling.

Footboards

A footboard is a flat panel, often made of wood or plastic, placed at the foot of a bed. It serves three purposes:

1. To provide support for the client's feet and maintain a natural foot position while the client is in bed. See Figure 36–35.
2. To keep the top bed covers off the client's feet, relieving the pressure of the weight of the covers.
3. To make the foot comfortable (for example, when a client has a painful foot).

Without the support of a footboard, a client's feet drop from their normal right angle to the legs and assume a plantar flexion position with the toes pointing toward the foot of the bed. See Figure 36–36. Prolonged assumption of this position results in permanent shortening of the muscles and tendons at the back of the legs. When that

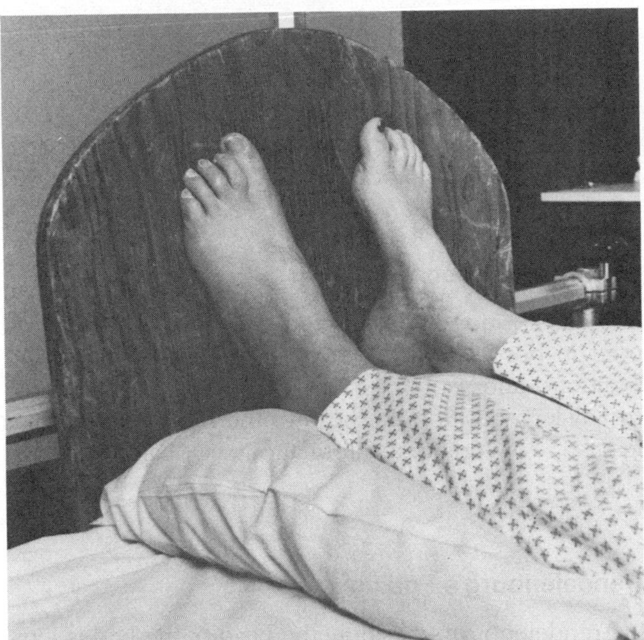

Figure 36–35 A footboard maintains dorsiflexion.

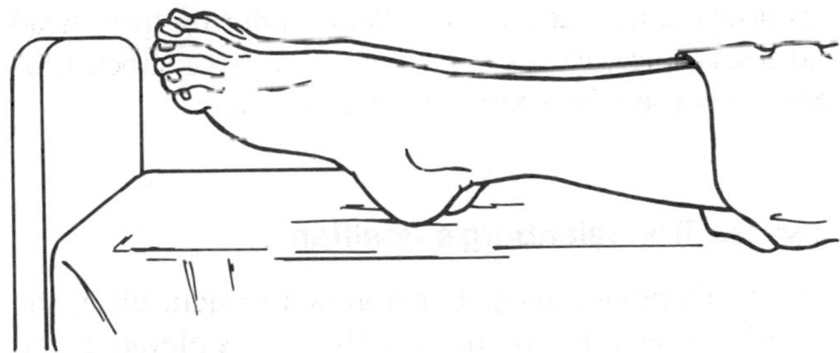

Figure 36–36 Feet in plantar flexion

happens, the client is unable to stand flat-footed on the floor, and walking is seriously impaired.

Footboards are often made in an **L** shape so that the base of the **L** fits under the foot of the mattress. Some footboards can be moved along the mattress to adjust to the client's height. If a board cannot be adjusted, sandbags and rolled pillows or blankets can be used to fill the space between the client's feet and the board.

Bed Cradles

A bed cradle, sometimes called an Anderson frame, is a device designed to keep the top bedclothes off the feet, legs, and even abdomen of a client. The bedclothes are arranged over the device and may be pinned in place.

There are several types of bed cradles. One of the most common is a curved metal rod that fits over the bed. Part of the cradle fits under the mattress, and small metal brackets press down on each side of the mattress to keep the cradle in place. The frame of some cradles extends over only half of the bed, above only one leg.

Intravenous Rods

Intravenous rods (poles, stands, standards), usually made of metal, support intravenous (IV) infusion containers while fluid is being administered to a client. These rods were traditionally freestanding on the floor beside the bed. Now, intravenous rods are often attached to the hospital beds. Some hospital units have overhead hanging rods on a track for IVs.

Bedside Tables

A small table placed beside the bed frequently has a drawer for the client's personal articles and below that a cupboard containing a washbasin, soap dish and soap, mouthwash container, and emesis or kidney basin. Some bedside tables also have a place for a bedpan or urinal and a rod at the back for washcloths and towels.

Overbed Tables

The overbed table stands on the floor but fits over the client's bed. It is usually on casters, so it can be easily moved. It can be raised or lowered to suit the client, usually by turning a handle at the side. Some overbed tables have a mirror and a small compartment for personal articles beneath the table top. Overbed tables are often used for the client's meal tray. A client who can assume a sitting position in bed can eat from that table in relative comfort. Nurses also use these tables for sterile supplies.

Chairs

Most bed units have chairs for client and visitor use. Often a chair without arms is kept near the bed. There may also be an easy chair that is more comfortable to sit in for long periods.

Clothing Storage Spaces

Hospital bed units generally contain a locker or closet for the storage of clothes. These facilities are usually larger in a long-term care unit than in an acute care setting. Some units also have a chest of drawers or other drawer space for clothing.

Lights

Each bed unit has one or more lights. At the head of the bed, there is often a movable light with an extendable neck. Some rooms have overhead lights as well. Most bed units also have a signal light. When a client pulls a switch or presses a button, a light goes on, for instance, at the nurses' station or a service area. Clients generally turn on their signal lights when they require assistance. It is important for nurses to be aware of the signal light areas, so that they can note when a light goes on and respond quickly. Some acute hospitals are equipped with intercoms that permit a nurse at the nursing station to talk with the client before going to the bedside. Intercom signal lights can also be turned off from the nurse's station. Nursing units generally have subdued night lighting. Some also have emergency signal lights.

Other Equipment

Hospitals vary in the equipment provided as part of the bed unit. Long-term care facilities may have very little additional equipment, whereas an acute facility may have several commonly used devices built into each unit. Three types of equipment are often installed on the wall at the head of the bed: a suction outlet for several kinds of suction, an oxygen outlet for most oxygen equipment, and a sphygmomanometer to measure the client's blood pressure.

Some long-term care agencies also permit clients to have personal equipment, such as a television, a chair, and lamps, at the bedside.

Specialized Beds

Whenever a client's body alignment must be strictly maintained, a specially designed bed that rotates on an axis is used to turn the client from the supine to the prone position and vice versa. Two such beds are the Stryker wedge frame and the CircOlectric bed. The Stryker wedge frame, which is manually operated by the nurse, turns the client laterally through the side-lying position. The CircOlectric bed, which is operated electrically by the nurse using a push button, rotates the client vertically through the standing position. These turning frames are used for clients with certain types of spinal injuries, e.g., extensive burns, arthritis, and pressure sores, who require position changes that cannot be effectively managed in the standard bed.

Bed Positions

The Flat Position

In the flat position, the mattress is completely horizontal. Pillows may or may not be used.

Fowler's Position

Fowler's position is a semisitting bed position frequently used in hospitals. It gives clients relief from the lying positions and is convenient for eating and reading. In Fowler's position the head of the bed is raised to at least 45°. For additional information, see Chapter 38, page 1040.

Trendelenburg's Position

In Trendelenburg's position, the head of the bed is lowered and the foot of the bed is elevated in a straight incline. See Figure 36–37. If the foundation cannot be raised mechanically, this position may be obtained by placing blocks or special pins under the foot of the bed. The blocks are often referred to as shock blocks, because this position was used some years ago for clients in shock. It is now contraindicated for clients suffering from head injuries, respiratory distress, chest injuries, or shock. Currently it is used for some postural drainage.

Reverse Trendelenburg's Position

Reverse Trendelenburg's position is a straight tilt in the opposite direction: The head of the bed is elevated, and the foot of the bed is lowered. Sometimes the legs at the head of the bed are raised by blocks or by pins if the foundation cannot be raised mechanically. This position

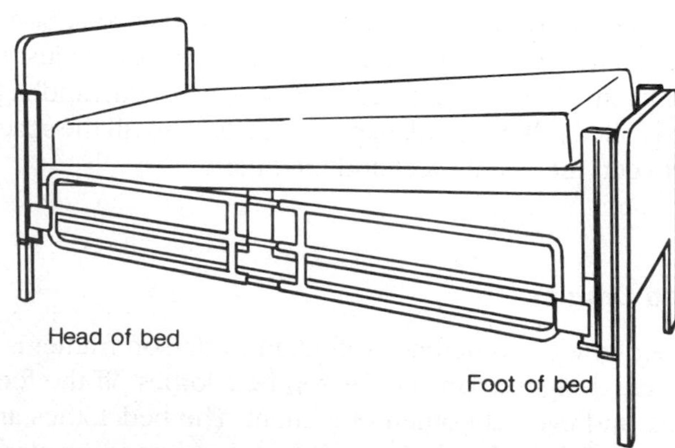

Figure 36–37 A bed in Trendelenburg's position

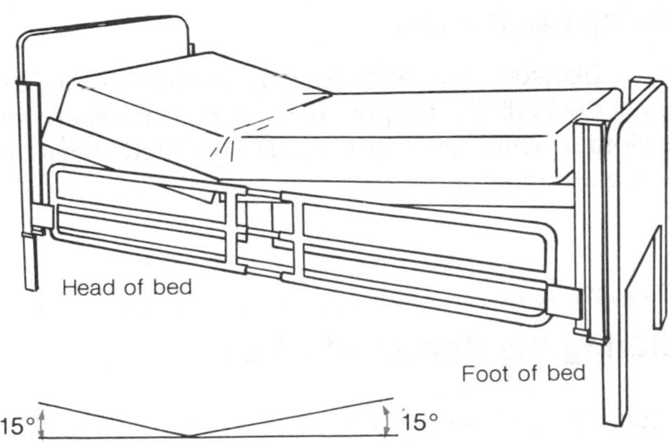

Figure 36–38 A bed in contour position

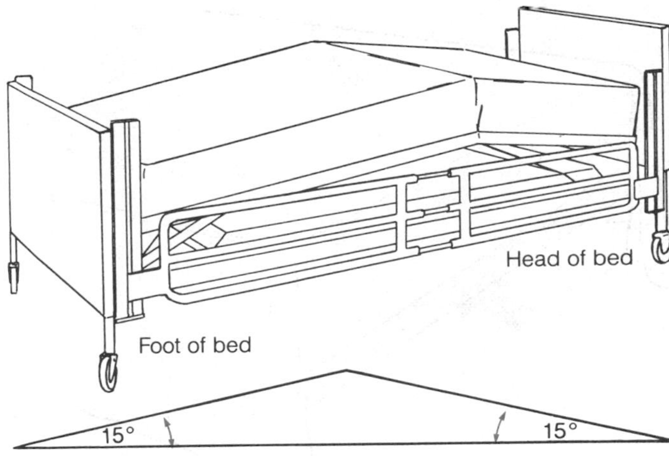

Figure 36–39 A bed in hyperextension position

may be used for clients experiencing problems with arterial circulation to the legs.

The Contour Position

In the contour bed position, both the head and foot of the bed are elevated about 15°. See Figure 36–38. It is necessary to raise both the knee and the foot sections of some hospital beds to obtain this position.

The Hyperextension Position

For the hyperextension bed position, both the head and the foot sections are lowered 15°. See Figure 36–39. This position is sometimes used for clients with spinal fractures. It should be used only with specific orders and continuous nursing assessment of the client is important. Not all hospital beds assume this position.

Making Beds

Nurses need to be able to prepare hospital beds in different ways for specific purposes. In most instances, beds are made after the client receives certain care and when beds are unoccupied. At times, however, nurses need to make an occupied bed or prepare a bed for a client who is having surgery (an anesthetic, postoperative, or surgical bed).

Concepts Basic to Bed Making

1. Linens and equipment that have been soiled with secretions and excretions harbor microorganisms that can be transmitted to others directly or by the nurse's hands or uniform. Therefore, nurses must wash hands thoroughly after handling a client's bed linen. They also hold soiled linen away from their uniforms.

2. Clean linen intended for one client is never momentarily placed on another client's bed, and one client's soiled linen is never placed on another client's bed. Even seemingly clean linen on a made bed can harbor microorganisms. In addition, soiled linen is never shaken in the air, because shaking can disseminate microorganisms.

3. Soiled linen is placed directly in a portable linen hamper or tucked in at the end of the bed before it is gathered up for disposal in the linen hamper or linen chute.

4. When stripping and making a bed, nurses conserve time and energy by making up one side as completely as possible before making up the other side.

5. To avoid unnecessary trips to the linen supply area, nurses gather all needed linen before starting to strip a bed.

Open and Closed Beds

An unoccupied bed can be either closed or open. Generally the top covers of an open bed are folded back (open bed) to make it easier for a client to get in. Open and closed beds are made the same way, except that the top sheet, blanket, and bedspread of a closed bed are drawn up to the top of the bed and under the pillows.

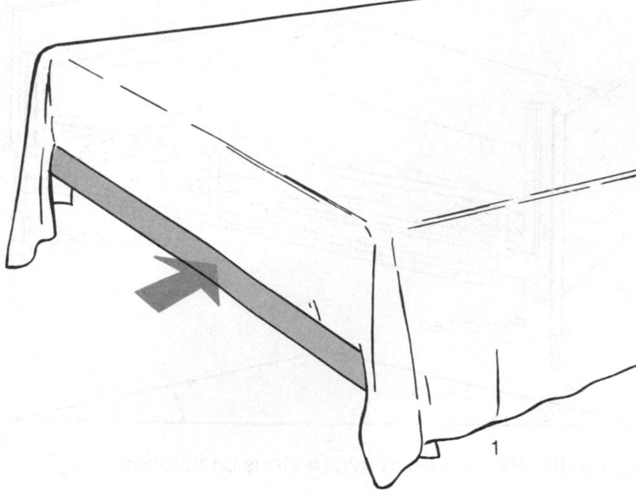

Figure 36–40

Mitering Bed Corners

Sheets, blankets, and bedspread are mitered at the corners of the bed. The purpose of mitering is to secure the bedclothes while the bed is occupied. Fitted sheets do not require mitering.

Mitering the Corner of a Bed

1. Tuck the bedcover (sheet, blanket, and/or spread) in firmly under the mattress at the bottom or top of the bed. See Figure 36–40.
2. Lift the bedcover at point 1 so that it forms a triangle with the side edge of the bed, and the edge of the bedcover is parallel to the end of the bed. See Figure 36–41.
3. Tuck the part of the cover that hangs below the mattress under the mattress (see Figure 36–42) while holding the cover at point 1 against the mattress.
4. Bring point 1 down toward the floor while the other hand holds the fold of the cover against the side of the mattress. See Figure 36–43.
5. Remove the hand, and tuck the remainder of the cover under the mattress, if appropriate. See Figure 36–44. The sides of the top sheet, blanket, and bedspread may be left hanging freely rather than tucked in. The bedspread is mitered separately and left hanging freely if the top sheet and blanket are tucked in.

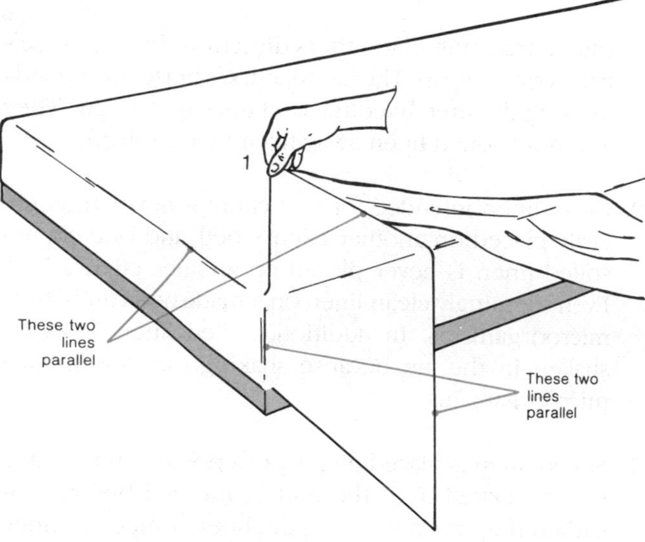

Figure 36–41

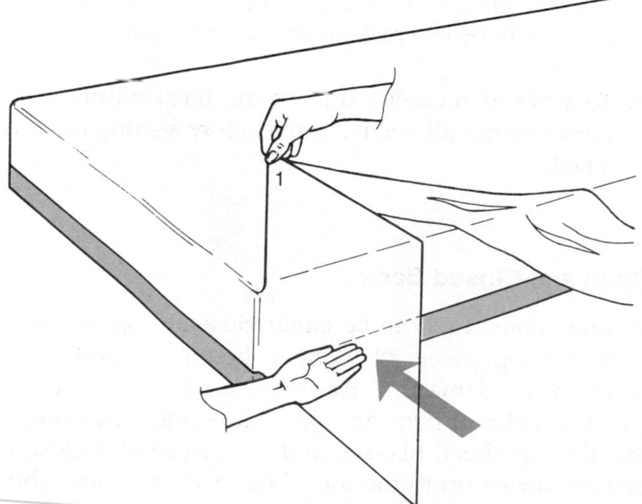

Figure 36–42

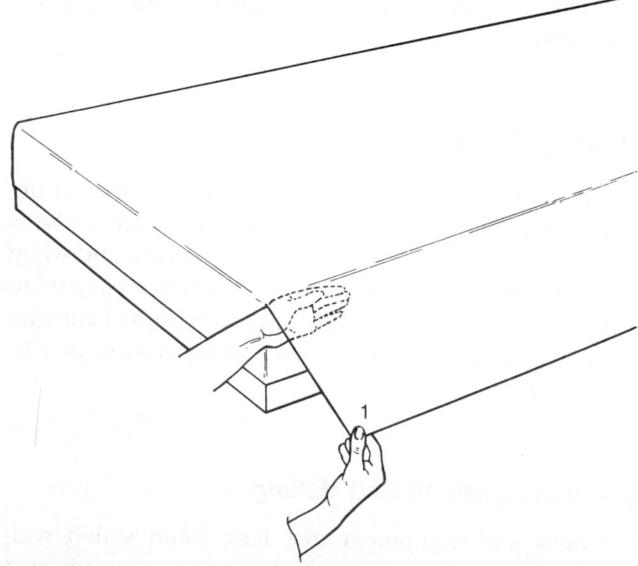

Figure 36–43

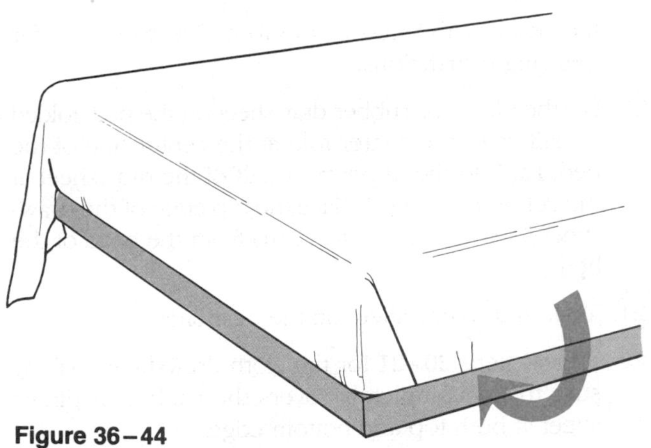

Figure 36–44

Procedure 36–9 ▲ Changing an Unoccupied Bed

Equipment

1. A mattress pad, if used. Some agencies do not use pads, so check agency practice. Some mattress pads are attached to the bed by elastic or ties at the corners. Some lie freely on the mattress.
2. Two large sheets. Fitted sheets, which do not require mitering, are being used increasingly in hospitals.
3. A plastic or rubber drawsheet, if required, to place across the center of the bed to protect the bottom sheet from drainage, urine, or feces. In some agencies, drawsheets are used only when the nurse decides it is necessary.
4. A cloth drawsheet to be placed over the plastic or rubber drawsheet, if required.
5. One blanket.
6. One bedspread.
7. Two pillowcases for the two head pillows. Additional pillowcases may be needed if additional pillows are used.
8. Portable linen hamper, if available, for the soiled linen.

Intervention

1. Place the fresh linen on the client's chair or overbed table; do not place it on another client's bed.

   Rationale It is important to prevent cross-contamination (the movement of microorganisms from one client to another) via soiled linen.
2. Make sure that this is an appropriate and convenient time for the client to be out of bed.
3. Assist the client to a comfortable chair.

Stripping the Bed

4. Starting at the head of the bed, on the side nearer the clean linen, loosen the bedding, including the foundation, moving down the bed, working around the foot, and moving up to the other side of the head. Remove the call signal, if it is attached to the linen.
5. Return to the first side.
6. Remove the pillowcases, if soiled, and place the pillows on the bedside chair near the foot of the bed.

   Rationale The bedside chair can be used to hold bedding that can be reused.
7. Using both hands, grasp the top edge of the spread, one hand at the center, the other at the mattress edge. Fold it in half by bringing the top edge even with the bottom edge.

   Rationale Linens folded this way are readily reapplied to the bed later.

   If the spread is soiled, place it in the linen hamper, if the agency has portable linen hampers that can be taken to the bed unit. If the agency has a central disposal chute for linen, tuck in the soiled spread at the foot of the bed, and collect all the soiled linen here to take to the chute. Take care to prevent soiled bed linen from touching your uniform.

   Rationale A soiled uniform can transmit microorganisms to other clients.

   or
8. If the spread is not soiled, pick it up carefully by grasping it at the center of the middle fold and the bottom edges.

Rationale It is useful to fold the spread in such a way that it can be readily reapplied.

9. Lay the spread over the back of the bedside chair if it is to be reused.
10. Repeat steps 7–9, first for the blanket and then for the top sheet.
11. Pick up the cotton drawsheet at the center of the top and bottom edges, and lay it over the back of the bedside chair or, if the sheet is soiled, discard it in the hamper.
12. Repeat step 11 for the plastic or rubber drawsheet.
13. Repeat steps 7–9 for the bottom sheet if it is to be changed.
14. Grasp the mattress lugs and, using good body mechanics, move the mattress up to the head of the bed. If there are no lugs, grasp the lower edge of the mattress.

Making the Bed

15. Standing at the same side of the bed as the linen supply, place the mattress pad on the bed.
16. Smooth the mattress pad so that it is free of wrinkles.

    Rationale Wrinkles can irritate the client's skin and cause discomfort.

17. Working from the foot of the bed, place the bottom sheet, folded into four layers, on the bed so that the vertical center fold of the sheet is at the center line of the mattress and the bottom edge of the sheet extends about 2.5 cm (1 in) over the end of the mattress.

    Rationale Unless a contour sheet is used, the sheet is not tucked in at the foot of the bed so that it can be changed without removing the top bedcovers.

    Make sure that the hem of the sheet is facing down.

    Rationale The hem edge can irritate the client's skin.

    Open the sheet across the bottom of the bed, and then pull the top layer up to the top of the bed so that the sheet is fully spread. (Agency practice may vary on methods of folding and spreading sheets on beds. This is one common method. In some agencies, the sheet is spread over only one side of the bed at a time.)

18. Move to the head of the bed on the same side. Tuck the excess sheet under the mattress at the near side of the head of the bed. If a contour sheet is used, fit it under the corner of the mattress.
19. Miter the sheet at the top corner on that side, and tuck the sheet under the mattress side, working from the head of the bed to the foot. See page 954 for mitering instructions.
20. Lay the plastic or rubber drawsheet on the bed, folded in half, with the center fold at the center line of the bed. Fanfold the uppermost half of the drawsheet at the center of the bed. Place the top edge of the drawsheet 30 to 37 cm (12 to 15 in) from the head of the bed.
21. Tuck in the drawsheet on the near side.
22. Repeat steps 20–21 for the cloth drawsheet, making sure that it completely covers the rubber or plastic sheet at both top and bottom edges.

    Rationale Any exposed plastic or rubber can irritate the client's skin.

23. Move to the opposite side of the bed.
24. Starting at the head of the bed, tuck the excess bottom sheet under the head of the mattress.
25. Pulling the sheet firmly, miter the side corner at the head of the bed or fit a contour sheet under the mattress corner.
26. Tuck in the bottom sheet, working toward the foot of the bed. Pull the sheet firmly so that there are no wrinkles in it.
27. Pull the plastic or rubber drawsheet over firmly, and tuck it in at the side.
28. Repeat step 27 for the cotton drawsheet.
29. Return to the first side of the bed. The foundation of the bed is now complete.
30. Place the top sheet on the bed so that the vertical center fold is at the center line of the bed, the top edge is even with the top edge of the mattress, and the hems of the sheet will face up when unfolded.

    Rationale With the hems facing up, the edges of the sheet will not rub against the client's skin.

31. Spread the sheet over the bed as described in step 17 or according to agency practice.
32. Tuck in the sheet at the bottom of the bed on the near half (optional).
33. Make either a vertical or a horizontal toe pleat in the sheet.
    a. Vertical toe pleat: Standing at the foot of the bed, make a fold in the sheet 5 to 10 cm (2 to 4 in), perpendicular to the foot of the bed. See Figure 36–45. Tuck in the end of the sheet at the foot of the bed. See Figure 36–46.
    b. Horizontal toe pleat: Make a fold in the sheet 5 to 10 cm (2 to 4 in), across the bed, 15 to 20 cm (6 to 8 in) from the foot. Tuck in the sheet at the foot. See Figure 36–47.

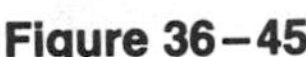

Figure 36–45

Rationale A toe pleat provides additional room for the client's feet. It is an optional comfort measure. Additional toe space can also be provided by loosening the top covers around the feet after the client is in bed.

34. Place the blanket on the bed so that the top edge is about 15 cm (6 in) from the head of the bed and the center fold is at the center of the bed.

    Rationale This allows a cuff of sheet to be folded over the blanket and spread.

35. Tuck in the blanket at the foot of the bed on the near side. Make a toe pleat if needed. See step 33.

36. Put the bedspread on the bed so that the center fold is at the center of the bed and the top edge extends about 2.5 cm (1 in) beyond the blanket. Tuck the top edge of the spread under the top edge of the blanket.

37. Fold the top of the top sheet down over the spread, providing a cuff of about 15 cm (6 in). Smooth the spread, working from the top to the foot of the bed.

    Rationale The cuff of sheet protects the client's face from rubbing against the blanket or bedspread, thus preventing skin irritation.

38. Tuck in the spread at the foot of the bed on the near side.

39. Miter all three layers of linen (top sheet, blanket, and spread) at the bottom corner of the bed. Leave the sides of the top sheet, blanket, and spread hanging freely.

    Rationale Mitering makes the corner of the bedclothes secure even though they are left hanging freely to permit easy access by the client.

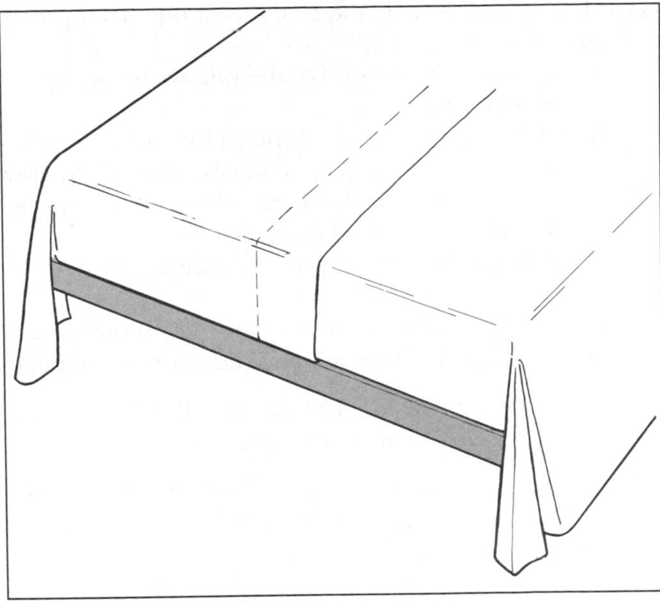

Figure 36–46

40. Walk around the foot of the bed to the far side, pulling the blanket and spread over the bed. Work toward the head of the bed on the second side.

41. Fold the remainder of the spread under the top of the blanket. Fold the remainder of the top sheet over the spread to make a cuff.

42. Going to the foot of the bed, tuck in the top sheet, blanket, and spread at the bottom of the bed on the second side. Maintain the toe pleat if one was made.

43. Miter this corner as in step 39.

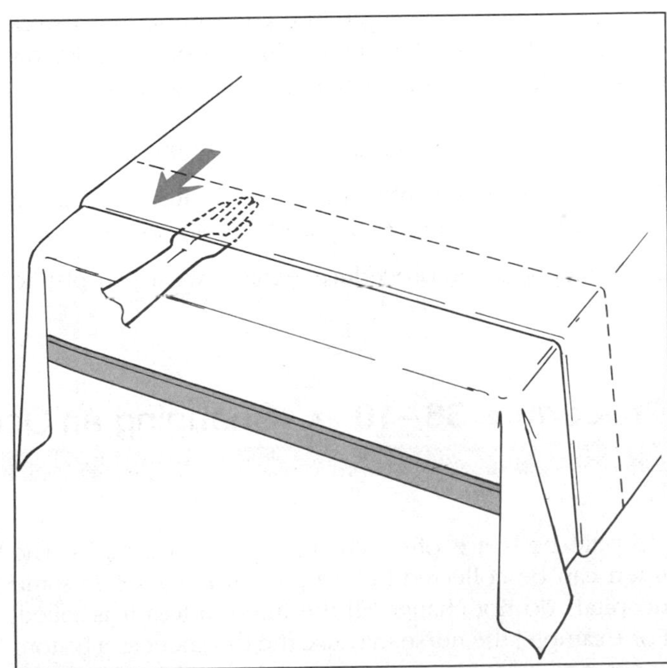

Figure 36–47

44. Moving to the first side of the bed put clean pillowcases on the pillows:
    a. Grasp the closed end of the pillowcase at the center with one hand.
    b. Gather up the sides of the pillowcase, and place them over the hand grasping the case. Then grasp the center of one short side of the pillow through the pillowcase. See Figure 36–48.
    c. With the free hand, pull the pillowcase over the pillow.
    d. Adjust the pillowcase so that the pillow fits into the corners of the case and the seams are straight.

    Rationale A smoothly fitting pillowcase is more comfortable than a wrinkled one.

45. Place the pillows at the head of the bed in the center, with the open ends of the pillowcases facing away from the door of the room.

    Rationale This provides a neat appearance.

46. Attach the signal cord so that the client can conveniently use it. Some cords have clamps that attach to the sheet or pillowcase. Others are attached by a safety pin.
47. If the bed is currently being used by a client, either fold back the top covers at one side or fanfold them down to the center of the bed.

    Rationale This makes it easier for the client to get into the bed.

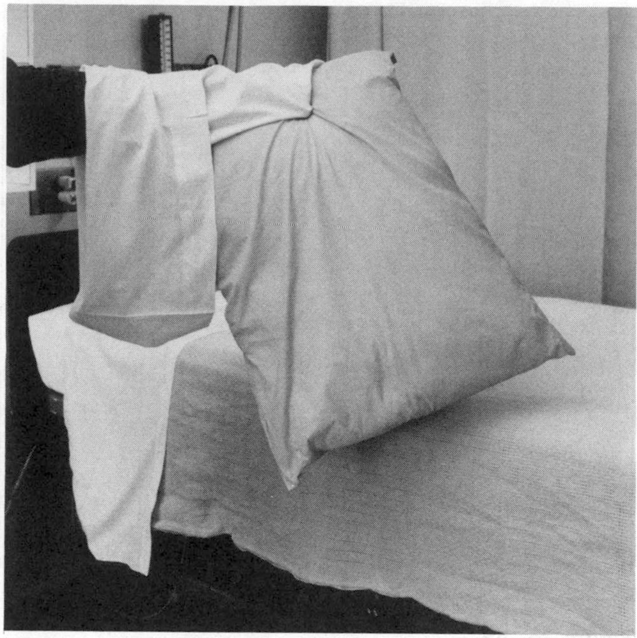

Figure 36–48

48. Put the bedside table and the overbed table where they are available to the client.
49. Put the bed in the low position. (Place the bed in the high position if the client is returning by stretcher.)

Changing an Occupied Bed

When changing an occupied bed, the nurse must work quickly and disturb the client as little as possible. Follow these guidelines when changing an occupied bed:

1. Maintain the client in good body alignment.
2. Move the client gently and smoothly. Rough handling can cause the client discomfort and abrade the skin.
3. Throughout the procedure, explain what you plan to do before you do it. Use terms that the client can understand.
4. Never move or position a client in a manner that is contraindicated by his or her health. For example, a dyspneic client should be maintained in Fowler's position and not placed in a supine position.
5. Use the bed-making time, like the bed bath time, to assess and meet the client's needs (e.g., the need for information about a forthcoming operation).

Procedure 36–10 ▲ Changing an Occupied Bed

Hospital beds are often changed after bed baths. The linen can be collected before the bath. Nurses in some hospitals do not change all the linen unless it is soiled. For example, the nurse may use the top sheet as a bottom sheet and provide a clean top sheet, drawsheet, and pillowcases.

The following equipment is usually required for a complete bed change:

1. A mattress pad, if necessary
2. Two large sheets

3. A bedspread
4. A plastic or rubber drawsheet (optional)
5. A cloth drawsheet
6. Two pillowcases
7. Bath blanket (optional)

Intervention

1. Place the fresh linen on the bedside chair or overbed table within easy reach and in order of use.
2. Remove any equipment attached to the bed linen, such as a call light.

Removing the Top Bedding

3. Loosen all the top linen at the foot of the bed.
4. Using both hands, grasp the top edge of the spread, one hand at the center, the other at the mattress edge. Fold it in half by bringing the top edge even with the bottom edge.

   Rationale Linens folded this way are readily reapplied to the bed later.

5. Pick up the spread carefully by grasping it at the center of the middle fold and the bottom edges.
6. If the spread is soiled, place it in the linen hamper or tuck it in at the bottom of the bed. Some agencies have portable linen hampers that can be taken to the bed unit. If the agency has a central disposal chute for linen, collect all the soiled linen at the foot of the bed to take to the chute later. Take care to prevent the soiled linen from touching your uniform.

   Rationale Soiled uniforms can transmit microorganisms to other clients.

7. If the spread is not soiled and is to be reused, lay it over the back of the bedside chair.
8. Repeat steps 4–7 for the blanket.
9. Leave the top sheet over the client (the top sheet can remain over the client if it is being discarded and if it will provide sufficient warmth) *or* replace it with a bath blanket as follows:
   a. Spread the bath blanket over the top sheet.
   b. Ask the client to hold the top edge of the blanket.
   c. Reaching under the blanket from the side, grasp the top edge of the sheet and draw it down to the foot of the bed, leaving the blanket in place.
   d. Remove the sheet from the bed and place it with the soiled linen.

Moving the Mattress Up on the Bed

10. Place the bed in the flat position if the client can tolerate this.
11. Loosen the bedclothes on the near side to expose the mattress.
12. Grasp the mattress lugs and, using good body mechanics, move the mattress up to the head of the bed. Have the client assist, if able, by grasping the head of the bed and pulling as you push. If the client is very heavy, you may need help from another nurse.

    Rationale When the head of the bed is raised, the mattress tends to slide toward the foot of the bed, thus moving the client toward the foot of the bed.

Changing the Foundation of the Bed

13. Assist the client to turn on his or her side facing away from the linen supply and on the far side of the bed. Raise the side rail on the far side.

    Rationale This leaves the near half of the foundation free to be changed. The raised side rail protects the client from falling. If there is no side rail, have another nurse support the client at the edge of the bed.

14. Returning to the first side of the bed, loosen the foundation linen at the side. Fanfold the two drawsheets and the bottom sheet at the center of the bed, as close to the client as possible.

    Rationale Close fanfolding makes room for the new linen.

15. Smooth the mattress pad, if it is to be retained. If not, fanfold it, and place a new pad on the bed, with the center fold at the center of the bed and the uppermost half fanfolded at the center.

    Rationale Smoothing removes wrinkles that could irritate the client's skin.

16. Place the new bottom sheet on the bed so that the lower edge extends slightly, e.g., 2.5 cm (1 in), over the end of the mattress. Make sure that the hem of the sheet is facing down.

    Rationale The hem edge can irritate the client's skin.

17. Moving from the foot to the head, open the sheet lengthwise.
18. Fanfold the uppermost half of the clean bottom sheet vertically at the center of the bed.
19. Tuck the sheet under the near half of the head of the bed. Miter the sheet at the top corner of the side of the bed or fit the corner of a contour sheet under the mattress. See page 954 for mitering instructions.

    Rationale A mitered corner holds the sheet firmly in place.

20. Moving toward the foot of the bed, tuck the bottom sheet under the side of the mattress, smoothing the sheet at the same time.

Rationale Wrinkles could irritate the client's skin.

21. Pull the plastic or rubber drawsheet from the center of the bed where it was fanfolded. Tuck it under the side of the mattress. If a clean plastic drawsheet is to be used:
    a. Lay it on the bed with the center fold at the center of the bed. The drawsheet should extend from midway down the client's back to midway down the thighs.
    b. Fanfold the uppermost half vertically at the center of the bed.
    c. Tuck the near side edge under the side of the mattress.
22. Repeat step 21 for the cloth drawsheet, making sure that it covers the plastic or rubber drawsheet at the top and bottom edges.

    Rationale Exposed plastic or rubber can irritate the client's skin.
23. Assist the client to roll over toward you onto the clean side of the bed. The client rolls over the fanfolded linen at the center of the bed.
24. Move the pillows to the clean side for the client's use.

    Rationale Pillows provide comfort.
25. Raise the side rail, if necessary, before leaving the side of the bed.

    Rationale The side rail provides safety and a sense of security for the client.
26. Move to the other side of the bed and lower the side rail if it was raised.
27. Loosen the foundation linen on that side. Fanfold the drawsheets if they are being reused, and remove the soiled bottom sheet. Remove the drawsheets with the bottom sheet if they are being changed. Roll the linens so that the client does not see the soiled parts.

    Rationale Sight of the soil might be embarrassing to the client.
28. Place the soiled linen at the foot of the bed or in the portable linen hamper.

    Rationale This helps to prevent the spread of microorganisms in linens soiled with excretions or other body discharges.
29. Smooth out the mattress cover to remove any wrinkles.
30. Unfold the fanfolded bottom sheet from the center of the bed.
31. Tuck the top of the sheet under the near half of the head of the bed. Miter the sheet at the top corner of the side of the bed.

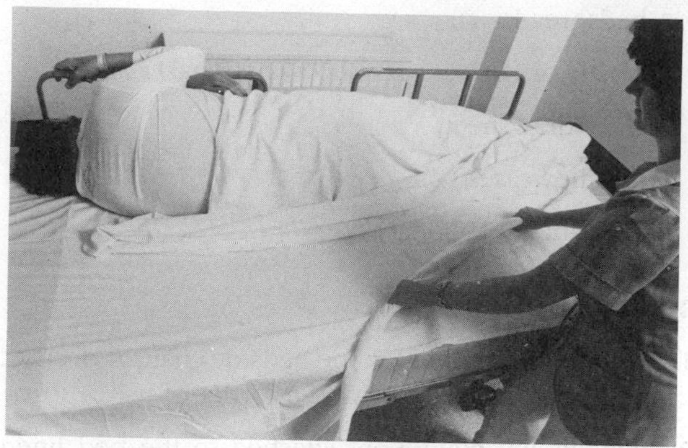

32. Facing the side of the bed, use both hands to pull the bottom sheet so that it is smooth, and tuck the excess under the side of the mattress. See Figure 36–49.

    Rationale Pulling at an angle removes wrinkles.
33. Unfold the plastic or rubber drawsheet fanfolded at the center of the bed, and pull it tightly with both hands. Pull the sheet in three sections: Face the side of the bed to pull the middle section, face the far top corner to pull the bottom section, and face the far bottom corner to pull the top section. Tuck the excess sheet under the side of the mattress.
34. Repeat step 33 for the cloth drawsheet.
35. Reposition the pillows at the center of the bed. If a pillowcase is soiled, remove it and place it with the soiled linen. Put on a clean pillowcase as follows:
    a. Grasp the closed end of the pillowcase at the center with one hand.
    b. Gather up the sides of the pillowcase, and place them over the hand grasping the case. Then grasp the center of one short side of the pillow through the pillowcase.
    c. With the free hand, pull the pillowcase over the pillow.
    d. Adjust the pillowcase so that the pillow fits into the corners of the case and the seams are straight.

    Rationale A smoothly fitting pillowcase is more comfortable than a wrinkled one.
36. Assist the client to the center of the bed. Determine what position the client requires or prefers, and assist him or her to that position.
37. Raise the side rail on the second side of the bed, if required, and return to the first side. Lower the side rail on the first side. Repeat steps 37 through 46 (pages 957–958) to complete the procedure.

Changing a Crib

Cribs are changed much as beds are. The major difference is that no drawsheets are used, because most crib mattresses have plastic covers and the undersheet is easily changed. The sides of an occupied crib are kept in the raised position when the nurse is not actually working at that side.

Making a Surgical Bed

A surgical bed is made for clients who are having surgical or diagnostics procedures that require use of an anesthetic agent. See Chapter 53 for information about how to prepare a surgical bed.

Nursing Care Plan

Assessment Data

Nursing Assessment

Mrs. Ann Rodgers is a 55-year-old sales clerk who has been admitted to Fairfax County Hospital for treatment of a leg ulcer. She is married and has six children. Her full-time position entails standing for long periods of time. She is always well groomed and meticulous about her appearance. She has a history of varicose veins and venous problems, and last week, while at work, she accidentally struck her leg against the sales counter. A leg ulcer began to develop at the site of the injury, and yesterday she saw her physician, who suggested hospitalization for the treatment of the ulcer. Now that she is in the hospital, her physician has written orders for bedrest and Betadine soaks to be applied three times a day.

Physical Examination

Height: 167.6 cm (5′6″)
Weight: 61.2 kg (135 lb)
Temperature: 37.5 C (97.5)
Pulse rate: 90 BPM
Respirations: 20 per minute at rest
Blood pressure: 132/82 mm Hg
Left ankle edematous with a 5.5 cm ulcer present above the medial malleolus
Veins of both legs dilated and visible
Skin from ankles to mid calf area, scaly, dry, pigmented

Diagnostic Data

Chest x-ray film: Negative
WBC: 11,500 cu mm
Urine: Negative

Nursing Diagnosis	Client Goals and Outcome Criteria	Nursing Interventions and Rationales	Evaluation
Impaired skin integrity related to altered venous circulation resulting in destruction of skin layers by ulceration, edema, redness.	Client Goals: Improved venous circulation. Healed ulcer. Outcome Criteria: Reduced size of impairment is noted by day 7. Skin temperature of both feet is warm to touch. Skin is intact, pink and moist by day 21. Client has no complaint of ulcer pain by day 5. Temperature is 37 C by day 3.	Apply wet to dry dressings to keep ulcer moist. *Rationale:* Extensive wounds need moisture to heal. Cleanse ulcer daily at 1000 hrs with Betadine solution. *Rationale:* Betadine is an antiseptic that is effective for cleaning ulcers and removing dead tissue. Assess nutritional status and encourage intake of foods high in protein and vitamin C. *Rationale:* Good nutrition is essential to promote healing. Change dressings 4 times daily employing sterile technique. *Rationale:* Sterile technique prevents infection and wet to dry dressings entrap infected and necrotic material. Keep affected leg above heart level whenever possible. *Rationale:* Facilitates venous circulation and decreases edema formation. Instruct client on care of ulcer. *Rationale:* Instruction will prevent complications of skin disruption.	Skin temperature of both feet was warm to touch by day 3. The circumference of both ankles was equal—20 cm by week's end. Mrs. Rodgers was pain free by day 5. Her temperature was 36.5 C by day 4. The size of the ulcer was reduced by 3 cm.

(continued)

Nursing Diagnosis	Client Goals and Outcome Criteria	Nursing Interventions and Rationales	Evaluation
Self-care deficit related to impaired mobility status, resulting in inability to get to bathroom, to bathe and dress independently; feelings of depression and anxiety.	Client Goal: Client cares for self as much as possible. Outcome Criteria: States feeling of comfort and satisfaction with body cleanliness. Demonstrates coping ability with inability to toilet self. Uses bedpan after each meal. Assists with daily grooming.	Involve client in plan of care. *Rationale:* Enhances sense of control. Encourage self-care in bathing. *Rationale:* Enhances feeling of self-worth. Change client's position every 2 hours. *Rationale:* Body surfaces will bear weight alternately. Keep client's skin clean and dry. *Rationale:* Prevents skin breakdown. Offer toileting devices as necessary. *Rationale:* Prevents constipation and urinary retention. Provide privacy. *Rationale:* Important to self-esteem.	Client participates in partial bed bath daily. States she feels comfortable and refreshed after bathing. Has adjusted to use of bedpan and voids several times each day. Has a daily bowel movement.

Chapter Highlights

- Clients' hygiene is influenced to a large degree by their sociocultural background.
- When people become ill, hygiene is often of secondary importance to vital body needs, such as breathing and rest.
- When a client cannot meet his or her hygiene needs, the nurse usually assumes them.
- The major functions of the skin are to help regulate body temperature, to protect underlying tissues, to secrete sebum, to contain nerve receptors that act in sensory perception.
- While assisting a client with hygiene measures, the nurse has an opportunity to assess the client's health.
- While planning hygiene care, the nurse must take the client's preferences into consideration.
- The back rub is an essential part of hygiene care for clients confined to bed.
- Nurses provide perineal-genital care for clients who are unable to do so for themselves.
- Nurses can often teach clients how to prevent foot problems.
- Oral hygiene should include daily dental flossing and mechanical brushing of the teeth.
- Regular dental checkups and fluoride supplements are recommended to maintain healthy teeth.
- Nurses provide special oral care to clients who are helpless, e.g., unconscious, and who have oral problems.
- Hair care includes daily combing and brushing and regular shampooing.
- A black person's hair may require special care.
- Nurses may need to assist helpless clients with their artificial eyes, eyeglasses, and contact lenses.
- The deaf client may require nursing assistance with his or her hearing aid.
- Changing beds is a part of maintaining hygiene.
- It is important to keep beds clean and comfortable for clients.

Suggested Readings

Davis, M. April 1977. Getting to the root of the problem. *Nursing 77* 7:60–65.
Davis describes hair care for a black client. It is important to select the right comb and learn some basic grooming techniques. Removing tangles and preventing matting are discussed.

Gannon, E. P., and Kadezabek, E. March 1980. Giving your patients meticulous mouth care. *Nursing 80* 10:14–19.
The authors describe examining the mouth and throat, helping with mouth care, providing mouth care to unconscious clients, removing and cleaning dentures, and using special aids. Photographs clarify the content.

MacMillan, K. March 1981. New goals for oral hygiene. *Canadian Nurse* 77:40–43.
Problems of the mouth commonly associated with hospitalized clients are described. Good oral hygiene and nursing measures for mouth care are discussed.

Michelsen, D. July 1978. Giving a great back rub. *American Journal of Nursing* 78:1197–99.
The author describes a 15-step technique, referred to as a *back massage,* that stimulates circulation and relieves muscle tension. Photographs illustrate the steps of the technique.

Schaeffer, A. M. May/June 1982. Nursing measures to maintain foot health. *Geriatric Nursing* 3:182–83.
Schaeffer discusses early clues to decreased foot circulation and what to do about them.

Smiler, I. May/June 1982. Foot problems of elderly diabetics. *Geriatric Nursing* 3:177–81.
Conserving the feet of the person who has diabetes mellitus is an important goal of the nurse. Smiler discusses ulcers of the foot, vascular impairment, foot health rules, orthotics, and various types of shoes that decrease pressure on the foot.

Wells, R., and Trostle, K. January 1984. Creative hairwashing techniques for immobilized patients. *Nursing 84* 14:47–51.
These authors include photographs that illustrate inventive ways to wash the hair of clients, including those confined to bed; those wearing cervical collars, braces, or halo vests; and those on Stryker frames.

Selected References

Barnhill, S. E., and Chenoweth, E. E. March 1966. Cleansing the perineum. *American Journal of Nursing* 66:566.

Bates, B. 1983. *A guide to physical examination.* 3d ed. Philadelphia: J. B. Lippincott Co.

Block, P. L. July 1976. Dental health in hospitalized patients. *American Journal of Nursing* 76:1162–64.

Bowers, A. C., and Thompson, J. M. 1984. *Clinical manual of health assessment.* 2d ed. St. Louis: C. V. Mosby Co.

Brown, M. S., et al. September 1973. Physical examination. Part 3: Examining the skin. *Nursing 73* 3:39–43.

Burns, K. R., and Johnson, P. J. 1980. *Health assessment in clinical practice.* Englewood Cliffs, N.J.: Prentice-Hall.

Cahn, M. M. July 1960. The skin from infancy to old age. *American Journal of Nursing* 60:993–96.

Carney, R. G. June 1963. The aging skin. *American Journal of Nursing* 63:110–12.

Davis, E. D. November 1970. Give a bath? *American Journal of Nursing* 70:2366–67.

Dyer, E. D., et al. July 1976. Dental health in adults. *American Journal of Nursing* 76:1156–59.

Eliopoulos, C., editor. 1984. *Health assessment of the older adult.* Menlo Park, Calif.: Addison-Wesley Publishing Co.

Gannon, E. D., and Kadezabek, E. March 1980. Giving your patients meticulous mouth care. *Nursing 80* 10(3):14–19.

Gibbs, G. E. January 1969. Perineal care of the incapacitated patient. *American Journal of Nursing* 69:124–25.

Giles, S. F. 1972. Hair, the nursing process and the black patient. *Nursing Forum* 11(1):78–88.

Holder, L. April 1982. Hearing aids: Handle with care. *Nursing 82* 12:64–67.

Kamenir, S., and Fothergill, R. December 1982. Hands-on skills for dealing with hearing aids. *Canadian Nurse* 78(11):44–45.

King, P. A. September/October 1980. Foot problems and assessment. *Geriatric Nursing* 1:182–86.

Martin, B. J., and Reeb, R. M. November/December 1982. Oral health during pregnancy: A neglected nursing area. *American Journal of Maternal and Child Nursing* 7:391–92.

Meissner, J. E. April 1980. A simple guide for assessing oral health. *Nursing 80* 10:70–75 (Canadian ed., pp. 24–25).

Norman, S. April 1982. The pupil check. *American Journal of Nursing* 82:588–91.

Osguthorpe, N. C. October 1984. If your patient has contact lenses. *American Journal of Nursing* 84:1255–56.

Roach, L. B. November 1972. Assessment of color changes in dark skins. *Nursing 72* 2:19–22.

———. March 1974. Assessing skin changes: The subtle and the obvious. *Nursing 74* 4:64–67.

———. January 1977. Color changes in dark skin. *Nursing 77* 7:48–51.

Schweiger, J. L., Lang, J. W., and Schweiger, J. W. April 1980. Oral assessment: How to do it. *American Journal of Nursing* 80:654–57.

Slattery, J. July 1976. Dental health in children. *American Journal of Nursing* 76:1159–61.

Temple, K. D. October 1967. The back rub. *American Journal of Nursing* 67:2102–3.

Todd, B. March/April 1982. Drugs and the elderly: Dry mouth—causes and cures. *Geriatric Nursing* 3(2):122–23.

Zucnick, M. M. May 1975. Care of an artificial eye. *American Journal of Nursing* 75:835.

CHAPTER 37

Mobility and Immobility

Mary Kelly Memmer
Barbara Kozier

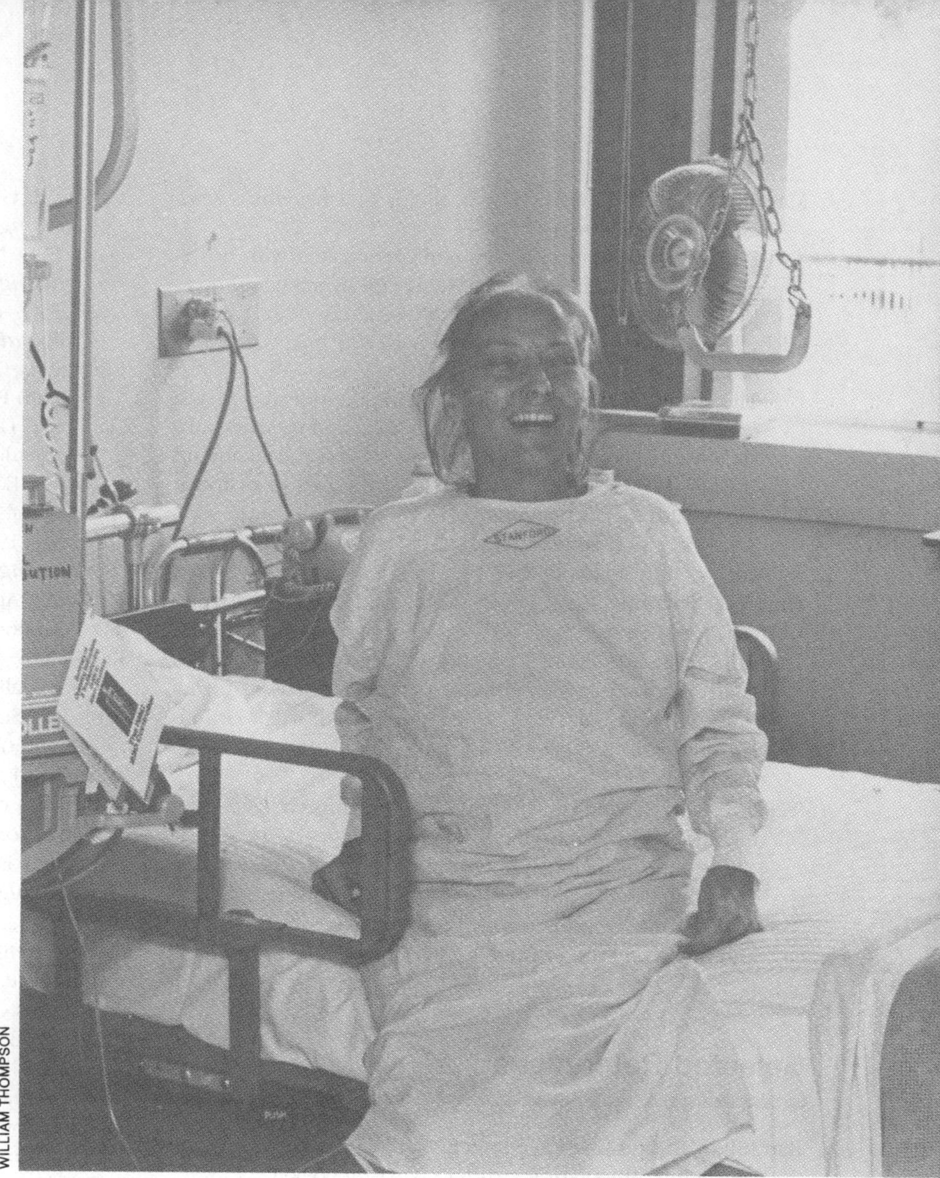

WILLIAM THOMPSON

Contents

(continued)

Contents *(continued)*

Objectives

1. Understand essential factors about mobility and immobility.
   1.1 Define selected terms.
   1.2 Describe the concepts of mobility and immobility.
   1.3 Describe the physiologic and psychosocial benefits of mobility.
   1.4 Identify the factors that affect a person's mobility.
   1.5 Describe the etiology and pathogenesis of pressure sores.
2. Know essential facts about assessment of client's mobility and immobility.
   2.1 Discuss problems of immobility.
   2.2 Describe assessing joint range of motion.
   2.3 Discuss assessing activities of daily living.
   2.4 Describe assessing activity tolerance.
3. Understand essential factors about planning and implementing regarding client mobility.
   3.1 Discuss the essential elements in an exercise program for adults.
   3.2 Describe the nurse's responsibility for promoting mobility.
4. Understand essential factors about planning and implementing nursing interventions to minimize the negative effects of immobility and to restore mobility.
   4.1 Describe guidelines for nursing interventions to prevent problems related to mobility.
   4.2 Describe physiologic and psychosocial nursing interventions to prevent immobility and restore mobility.
   4.3 Describe nursing interventions for clients who are at risk of having or have pressure sores.

Terms

abduction
abrasion
active-assistive exercises
active range-of-motion exercises
activities of daily living (ADLs)
adduction
aerobic exercise
anabolism
anaerobic exercise
ankylosis (of joint)
anorexia
atelectasis
atrophy
bed rest
catabolism
circumduction
contracture
debridement
deep ulcers
demineralization
disability
disuse osteoporosis
disuse phenomena
diuresis
dyspnea
dysuria
eversion
excoriation
extension
flexion
fibrosis
frequency (urination)
frontal plane
hypercalcuria
hyperextension
hypoproteinemia
hypostatic pneumonia
incompetent valves
incontinence (of urine)
inversion
isometric exercise
isotonic exercise
Krebs cycle
ligament
natriuresis
orthostatic (postural) hypotension
passive range-of-motion exercises
physical fitness
pressure sore (decubitus ulcer)
pronation
protaction
pyrexia
range-of-motion (ROM) movements
reactive hyperemia
resistive exercises
retraction
rotation
sagittal plane
superficial ulcers
supination
synovial joint
thrombophlebitis
transverse plane
turgor (of skin)
urinary reflux
urinary stasis
Valsalva maneuver
Virchow's triad

Concepts Related to Mobility

The ability to move freely, easily, rhythmically, and purposefully in the environment is an essential part of living. People must move to obtain food and water, to protect themselves from trauma, and to meet other basic needs. Mobility is vital to independence; a fully immobilized person is as vulnerable and dependent as an infant.

People often define their health and physical fitness by their ability to move, since mental well-being and the effectiveness of body functioning depend largely on their mobility status. For example, when a person is upright, the lungs expand more easily, intestinal activity (peristalsis) is more effective, and the kidneys are able to empty completely. In addition, motion is essential for proper functioning of bones and muscles.

The ability to move also influences a person's self-esteem and body image, both components of self-concept. For most people, self-esteem depends on a sense of independence and a feeling of usefulness or being needed. People with mobility impairments may feel helpless and burdensome to others. Body image can be altered by paralysis, amputations, or any motor impairment. A man may dissociate himself from a paralyzed limb by calling it "Oscar," suggesting that it is not part of his body. The reaction of others to impaired mobility can also significantly alter self-esteem and body image.

Physical fitness is a state of purposeful, active, physical conditioning. Physical fitness is essential to living a dynamic, satisfying, and productive life. Regular activity to promote physical fitness improves health, enhances wellness, prevents disability, and slows the onset of degenerative diseases that may accompany the aging process.

Joint Mobility

A joint is the functional unit of the musculoskeletal system. The bones of the skeleton articulate at the joints. Most of the skeletal muscles attach to the two bones at the joint. These muscles are categorized according to the type of joint movement they produce upon contraction. Muscles are therefore called flexors, extensors, internal rotators, and the like. The flexor muscles are stronger than the extensor muscles. Thus, when a person is inactive, the joints are pulled into a flexed (bent) position. If this tendency is not counteracted with exercise and position changes, the muscles are permanently shortened, and the joint becomes fixed in a flexed position.

Range of Motion

The range of motion of a joint is the maximum movement that is possible for that joint. Joint range of motion varies from individual to individual and is determined by genetic makeup, developmental patterns, the presence or absence of disease, and the amount of physical activity in which the person normally engages.

Types of Synovial Joints

A **synovial joint** is freely movable and characteristically has a cavity enclosed by a capsule. Within this capsule is a lining of synovial membrane, which secretes synovial fluid to lubricate the joint. Cartilage provides a smooth surface upon which the bone glides during movement. Thick bands of collagenous fibers extending from one bone to another are called **ligaments**. Ligaments strengthen the joint, and they are usually stretched taut when the joint is in the position of greatest stability. The muscles surrounding the joint provide the most stability for the joint. The primary functions of synovial joints are to bear weight and to allow movement. There are six types of synovial joints, and only certain movements are normally possible for each type. See also Table 37–1.

1. *Ball-and-socket.* In ball-and-socket joints, the ball-shaped head of one bone fits into the concave socket of another bone or bones. This type of joint provides for the greatest movement in all planes. Examples are the hip and shoulder joints.
2. *Hinge.* In the hinge joint, a bone with a convex surface fits into one with a concave surface. The motion of this type of joint is limited to flexion and extension. Examples are the elbow and knee joints.
3. *Pivot.* The pivot joint is made up of a process that rotates within a bony fossa around a longitudinal axis. The motion of this joint is limited to rotation. Examples are the axis and atlas joints of the vertebral column.
4. *Condyloid.* In the condyloid joint, an oval-shaped bony projection fits into an elliptical cavity. This kind of joint does not permit rotation; it permits movement in only two planes. An example is the wrist, which permits flexion, extension, and hyperextension in one plane, and abduction and adduction in the second plane, but not rotation.
5. *Saddle.* The saddle joint has convex and concave surfaces so that the two bones fit together. This kind of joint does not permit rotation, but movement is possible in the two planes at right angles to each other. For example, the carpometacarpal joint of the thumb and the hand permits flexion and extension, abduction and adduction.
6. *Gliding.* The gliding joint is formed when the two bone surfaces are flat or when one is slightly convex and the other is slightly concave, so that they glide over each other. Examples are the joint between the tibia and fibula and the intervertebral joints.

Body Planes

These three planes correspond to the three dimensions in space and are used to describe body movement.

Table 37–1 Types of Synovial Joints

Type	Description	Examples	Movement
Ball-and-socket	The ball-shaped head of one bone fits into the concave socket of another bone.	The hip and shoulder joints	Movement in three planes. Greatest range of all joints: flexion and extension; abduction and adduction; rotation.
Hinge	The convex, spool-shaped end of one bone fits into the concave surface of another bone.	The elbow, knee, ankle, finger, and toe joints	Movement in one plane. Flexion and extension.
Pivot	An arch-shaped surface rotates in a rounded or longitudinal axis.	The axis and atlas joints of the vertebral column, the joints between the radius and the ulna	Movement in one plane. Rotation only.
Condyloid (ovoid)	The oval-shaped part of one bone fits into an elliptical cavity.	The wrist joints	Movement in two planes at right angles to each other. Flexion and extension; abduction and adduction.
Saddle	Two bones have opposite concave-convex surfaces that fit together.	The base of the thumb only	Same movements as for condyloid joints but freer.
Gliding	Two flat bone surfaces glide over each other.	The carpal bones, the tarsal bones, the medial end of the clavicle with the sternum, the ribs with the bodies of the vertebrae, the sacrum and the ilia, the fibula with the tibia	Gliding only.

1. **Sagittal plane.** Movement occurs directly in front of the body or directly in back of it. Flexion, hyperextension, and extension movements occur in this plane.
2. **Frontal plane.** Movement occurs laterally to the sides of the body. Abduction, adduction, and lateral flexion movements occur in this plane.
3. **Transverse plane.** One part of the body rotates while the second part remains stable. Rotation movements occur in this plane.

See Figure 37–1 and Table 37–2.

Synovial Joint Movements

The following are movements of synovial joints:

1. **Flexion** is decreasing the angle between two bones, i.e., bending the joint (e.g., bending the arm at the elbow joint).
2. **Extension** is increasing the angle between two bones, i.e., straightening the joint (e.g., straightening the arm at the elbow joint).
3. **Hyperextension** is further extension between two bones or stretching out a joint (e.g., bending the head backward).
4. **Abduction** is movement of the bone away from the midline of the body (e.g., raising the arm at the shoulder joint laterally).
5. **Adduction** is movement of the bone toward the midline of the body (e.g., lowering the arm held laterally toward the side of the body).
6. **Rotation** is movement of the bone around its central axis (e.g., turning the head as if to look over the shoulder). Internal rotation is turning toward the midline, external rotation is turning away from the midline. An example of these kinds of rotation occurs at the hip joint. When a person assumes the back-

Table 37–2 The Three Body Planes and Joint Movements

Plane	Joint Movement	Example
Transverse	Pronation	Elbow
	Supination	Elbow
	Internal rotation	Hip, shoulder
	External rotation	Hip, shoulder
	Flexion (dorsiflexion)	Ankle
	Extension (plantar flexion)	Ankle
Sagittal	Flexion	Hip, knee
	Extension	Hand, elbow
	Hyperextension	Hip, neck
Frontal (coronal)	Abduction	Wrist, shoulder
	Adduction	Wrist, shoulder
	Inversion	Foot
	Eversion	Foot

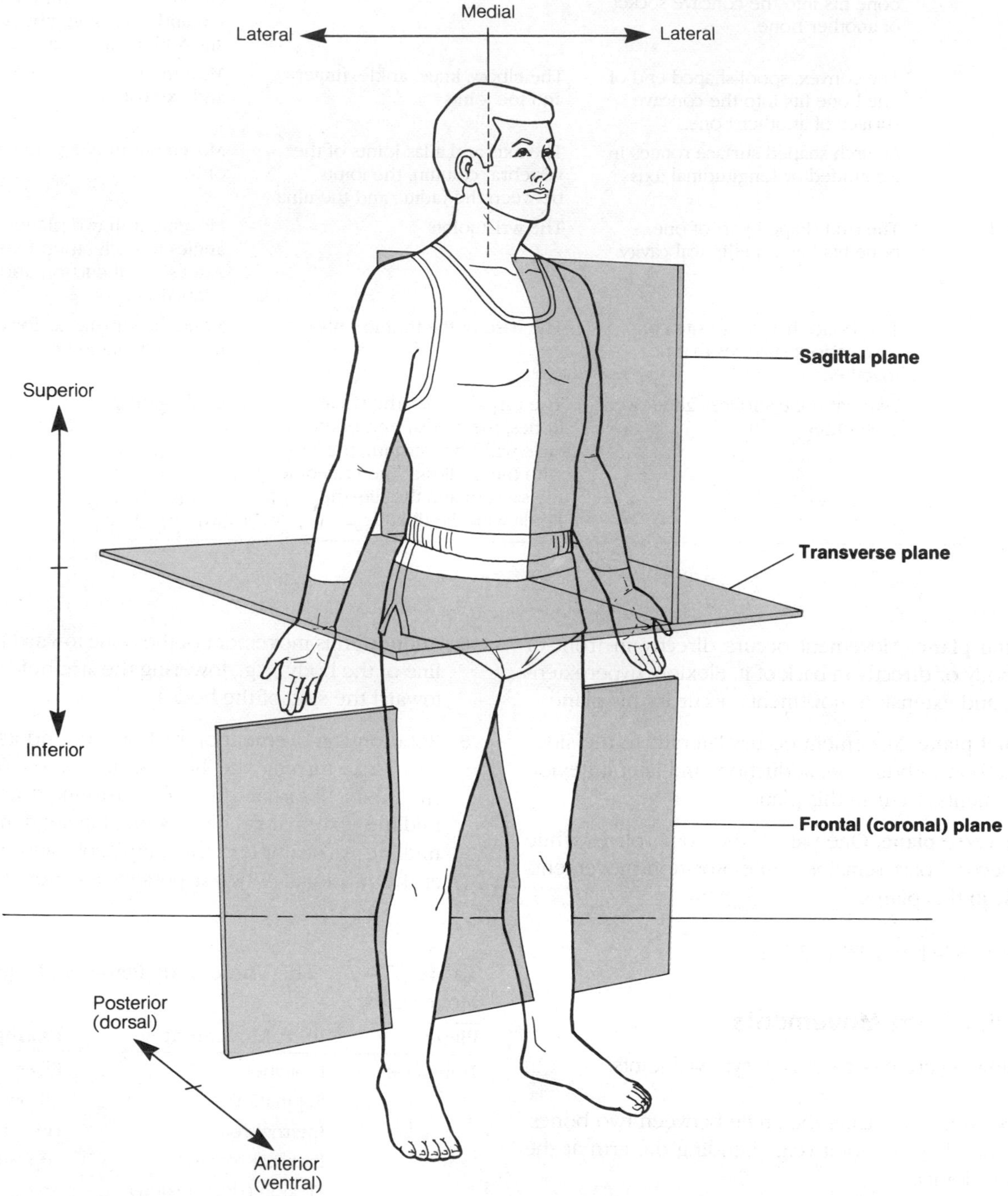

Figure 37–1 Planes of the body

lying position, the leg normally rotates externally at the hip.

7. **Circumduction** is movement of the distal part of the bone in a circle while the proximal end remains fixed (e.g., describing a circle with the arm, moving the shoulder joint).
8. **Eversion** is turning the sole of the foot outward by moving the ankle joint.
9. **Inversion** is turning the sole of the foot inward by moving the ankle joint.
10. **Pronation** is moving the bones of the forearm so that the palm of the hand moves from an anterior to a

posterior anatomic position (so that the thumb rotates toward the body).

11. **Supination** is moving the bones of the forearm so that the palm of the hand moves from a posterior to an anterior anatomic position (so that the thumb rotates away from the body).

12. **Protraction** is moving a part of the body forward in the plane parallel to the ground (e.g., pushing the lower jaw outward).

13. **Retraction** is moving a part of the body backward in the plane parallel to the ground (e.g., pulling the lower jaw inward).

Factors Affecting Mobility

A person's mobility depends to a large degree on habits developed throughout life and on the importance the individual attaches to activity as a means of maintaining health. Mobility is affected by life-style, primary disability, individual energy level, and age.

Life-Style

People learn early in life, often from their families, the value of activity in relation to health. Some children are encouraged to play out of doors, while others spend much of their time watching television. Some people participate in physical activity regularly in an effort to maintain or improve their health.

Some cultures value physical activity more than others do. The boy who lives in a small town in France walks to and from school each day, while the North American boy living in a middle-class suburb rides to and from school. Adults in North America often watch sports activities, while adults in less industrialized nations often participate in such activities.

Primary Disability

A **disability** is a persistent mental or physical dysfunction or weakness that prevents a person from carrying out the normal activities of life and work. Disabilities are of two types:

1. Primary disabilities, e.g., paralysis due to a spinal cord injury, are a direct result of disease or trauma.
2. Secondary disabilities, e.g., muscle weakness and bedsores,do not exist at the onset of the primary disability but develop later as a result of the disorder causing the primary disability.

Disuse phenomenon is often used as a synonym for secondary disability due to immobility. **Disuse phenomena** are physiologic and psychologic dysfunctions that occur in all body organs and systems as a result of immobility and lack of use. Each of these pathologic changes begins with the onset of immobility (Kottke et al. 1982, p. 209). Primary disabilities, such as multiple sclerosis and injuries to the spinal cord, can seriously restrict an individual's mobility.

Mobility can also be limited because of fear and/or pain. A client recovering from surgery may be reluctant to move for fear of opening the incision or because of the pain experienced with movement.

A person who has a disease or is injured is often restricted in activity. Bed rest is commonly advised in illness. It usually has two purposes: (a) to conserve energy so that a diseased or injured part of the body will heal, and (b) to prevent further damage to a body part. A person who has had a myocardial infarction usually requires bed rest for both purposes. A person with a fractured hip may be confined to bed with the leg in traction while healing takes place. See below for the major reasons for client immobility.

Energy Level

Energy levels vary greatly among individuals. Also, one individual demonstrates different energy levels at different times. Sometimes people voluntarily restrict activity without always knowing why or without feeling ill. The reason is generally that the person needs to withdraw from physical and psychologic stressors to maintain physical and psychologic equilibrium. A student, after final examinations, may want only to go to bed and sleep, to regain energy and stability.

Age

Age greatly affects activity levels. Generally, people slow down as they grow older. Assessment information for developmental levels from birth to age 5 is presented in Chapters 23 through 26.

Major Reasons for Client Immobility

- Severe pain
- Impairment of the musculoskeletal or nervous systems
- Generalized weakness
- Psychosocial problems, e.g., depression
- Infectious processes

Immobility

There are three reasons for immobility:

1. Therapeutic restrictions to movement, e.g., following injury to a limb or surgery
2. Unavoidable restrictions because of a primary disability, e.g., multiple sclerosis or paralysis following a cerebrovascular accident
3. Voluntary restrictions due to life-style

Degrees of Immobility

There are varying degrees of immobility. The unconscious client is often completely immobilized. Immobility is sometimes partial, as in a client with a fractured leg. In addition, some clients restrict activity for health reasons. For example, a client who is short of breath may be advised not to walk up stairs.

Bed Rest

Nurses use the term **bed rest** to describe a client's degree of immobility. The term has different meanings in different nursing settings. For example, in some settings, "complete bed rest" means that the client never moves from the bed and does not go to the bathroom or sit in a chair. "Bed rest," in contrast, may mean that the client stays in bed except when he or she uses a bedside commode or goes to the bathroom. Nurses should be familiar with the meaning of such terms in their practice setting. See above for some of the common benefits of bed rest.

Whether bed rest causes any problems often depends on the duration of the bed rest, the client's health, and the client's sensory awareness. When confined to bed, many clients are aware of pressure on their bodies and can change position slightly to relieve this pressure. Such clients are less susceptible than others to decubitus ulcers and other problems. Clients on bed rest, like clients immobilized in other ways, must be continually assessed for problems.

Benefits of Bed Rest

- Reduces the needs of the body cells for oxygen because of reduced metabolism secondary to reduced activity
- Directs energy resources toward the healing process rather than toward activity
- Reduces pain in some instances, thereby decreasing the need for analgesics

Clients at Risk

Certain clients are more at risk than others of developing problems as a result of being immobilized. One factor to consider is how great a body area is affected: the larger the body area immobilized, the greater likelihood of problems. For example, a client who is immobilized from the waist down is more likely to develop problems than a client with an immobilized ankle. A second factor is the duration of the immobility: A person immobilized for 2 days is less likely to develop problems than one immobilized for 1 month. Other clients at risk include the elderly and people who experience pain upon movement. Clients at risk are listed on the facing page.

Physiologic Responses to Immobility

Many body systems respond physiologically to immobility. The degree of change depends largely on the risk factors mentioned earlier.

Musculoskeletal Changes

The most obvious signs of prolonged immobility are often manifested in the musculoskeletal system. The client experiences a significant decrease in muscular strength whenever he or she does not maintain a moderate amount of physical activity. The studies of Hettinger and Mueller demonstrate that as much as 20% of muscle strength may be lost after 1 week of bed rest, and as much as another 20% may be lost with each succeeding week of bed rest (Hettinger and Mueller 1953, pp. 111–26). A decrease in physical endurance is a direct result of decreased muscle strength and occurs at a similar rate (Kottke et al. 1982, p. 967). A decrease in the muscle mass, or muscle **atrophy**, occurs when the muscle fibers do not contract as much as they would during normal physical activity. Muscle atrophy is the cause of decreased muscle strength and endurance.

Muscular dysfunction due to immobility is, in turn, the primary cause of skeletal dysfunction. In a mobile person, there is a balance between the forming and breaking down of bone tissue. This balance is brought about primarily by the daily stresses of the tendons pulling on the bones and of gravity pulling on the weight-bearing structures as the client stands and moves. Prolonged immobilization in a horizontal position causes dramatic changes in the bones and joints.

Disuse osteoporosis is a result of lack of weight-bearing, decreased muscular activity, and complex endocrine and metabolic disturbances that accompany bed rest. During immobility, increased amounts of calcium are extracted from the bone, resulting in a significant decrease in bone mass. Studies demonstrate that bone **demineralization** starts in the second or third day of immobilization; there is measurable calcium loss from bone after 2 weeks of bed rest (Mitchell and Laustau 1981, p. 355). The bone becomes porous and brittle and can fracture easily. Demineralization occurs regardless of the amount of calcium in the person's diet.

Bone demineralization in turn affects other body systems, primarily because the excessive amounts of calcium extracted from the bones (which may be further added to by dietary supplements of calcium) produce slight hypercalcemia, significant hypercalcuria, and frequently deposition of calcium in injured soft tissues (Kottke et al. 1982, p. 968).

Fibrosis (an increase in the amount of fibrous connective tissue) and **ankylosis** (fixation) of joint structures occur whenever joints are not moved normally. The flexor muscles of an immobilized person, because they are strong, often remain contracted for long periods, and the weaker extensors are not used. In turn, the fibrous muscle tissue that covers the joint is gradually replaced by connective tissue, and the joint becomes increasingly stiff and painful. The problem may be exacerbated by the deposition of excessive amounts of calcium in the soft tissues around the joint. In time, the joint may become irreversibly deformed and ankylosed, and the muscles that cover the joint may permanently shorten into a **contracture**. The most common are flexion contractures of the lower extremities: hips, knees, and the plantar flexors of the ankles. The position that the client most consistently assumes in bed and wheelchair is mirrored when the person eventually is able to stand and walk. The result is a stooped "wheelchair" posture: The client's heels cannot rest flat on the floor, making ambulation difficult or impossible.

Muscle atrophy, decreased muscle strength, and limited endurance can impair muscle coordination in both upper and lower extremities. Lack of coordination hinders the client's ability to perform normal daily activities and impairs his or her balance and ability to stand and walk.

Clients at Risk

The following factors increase the risk of problems due to immobilization:

- A large body area is immobilized.
- The immobilization lasts for a long period.
- The immobilized client is elderly.
- The client experiences pain or muscle spasms.
- The client's sensitivity to temperature, pain, or pressure is decreased.
- The client is poorly nourished.
- The client is unable to learn how to prevent problems.
- The client is immobilized in one position for a long time.

Cardiovascular Changes

Prolonged immobility weakens the cardiovascular system, which cannot respond adequately to meet the demands placed on it. Decreased mobility creates an imbalance in the autonomic nervous system, resulting in a preponderance of sympathetic activity over cholinergic activity that increases heart rate. Resting heart rate increases approximately 0.5 beats/minute per each day of immobilization (Kottke et al. 1982, p. 210).

In a mobile, active person with a slow heart rate, the diastolic phase of the cardiac cycle is longer than the systolic phase. Since blood flow through coronary vessels occurs primarily during the diastolic phase, there is sufficient time for adequate blood flow through the coronary arteries. During immobility, however, the rapid heart rate reduces diastolic pressure, coronary blood flow, stroke volume, and the capacity of the heart to respond to any metabolic demands above basal levels. Due to this diminished cardiac reserve, the immobilized person may experience tachycardia and angina with even minimal exertion. Bedfast clients tend to use the **Valsalva maneuver**, during which the person takes a deep breath and strains against a closed glottis as he or she turns and moves about in bed (see Chapter 45). The Valsalva maneuver markedly increases intrathoracic pressure, which is followed by a marked increase in the volume of blood within the heart and possible arrhythmias when the glottis is again opened. When the heart has marginal reserves, the client may have difficulty coping with this additional stress.

Osthostatic (postural) hypotension is a common sequel of immobilization. Due to sympathetic nervous system activity, automatic vasoconstriction occurs in the blood vessels in the lower half of the body when a mobile person changes from a horizontal to a vertical posture. Vasoconstriction prevents pooling of the blood in the legs and effectively maintains central blood pressure to ensure adequate perfusion of the heart and brain. During prolonged immobility, this reflex becomes dormant. When the immobilized person attempts to sit or stand, this reconstricting mechanism fails to function properly in spite of increased adrenalin output. The blood pools in the lower extremities, and central blood pressure drops. Cerebral perfusion is seriously compromised, and the person feels dizzy or lightheaded and may even faint. This sequence is usually accompanied by a sudden and marked increase in heart rate, the body's effort to protect the brain from an inadequate blood supply.

The skeletal muscles of an active person contract with each movement, compressing the blood vessels in those muscles and helping to pump the blood back to the heart against gravity. The tiny valves in the leg veins, which remain constricted, aid in venous return to the heart by preventing backward flow of blood and pooling. In an immobilized person, the skeletal muscles do not contract sufficiently, and the muscles atrophy. The skeletal muscles can no longer assist in pumping blood back to the heart against gravity. Blood pools in the leg veins, causing vasodilation and engorgement. The valves in the veins can no longer work effectively to prevent backward flow of blood and pooling (see Figure 37–2). This phenomenon is known as **incompetent valves.** As the blood continues to pool in the veins, its greater volume increases venous blood pressure, which can become much higher than that exerted by the tissues surrounding the vessel. When the venous pressure is sufficiently great, some of the serous part of the blood is forced out of the blood vessel into the interstitial spaces surrounding the vessel, causing edema. Edema is most common in parts of the body positioned below heart level and maintained in that position. Dependent edema is most likely to occur around the sacrum or heels of a client who sits up in bed or in the feet and lower legs of a client who sits on the side of the bed. Edema further impedes venous return of blood to the heart, causing more pooling and more edema. Edematous tissue is uncomfortable and more susceptible to injury than normal tissue.

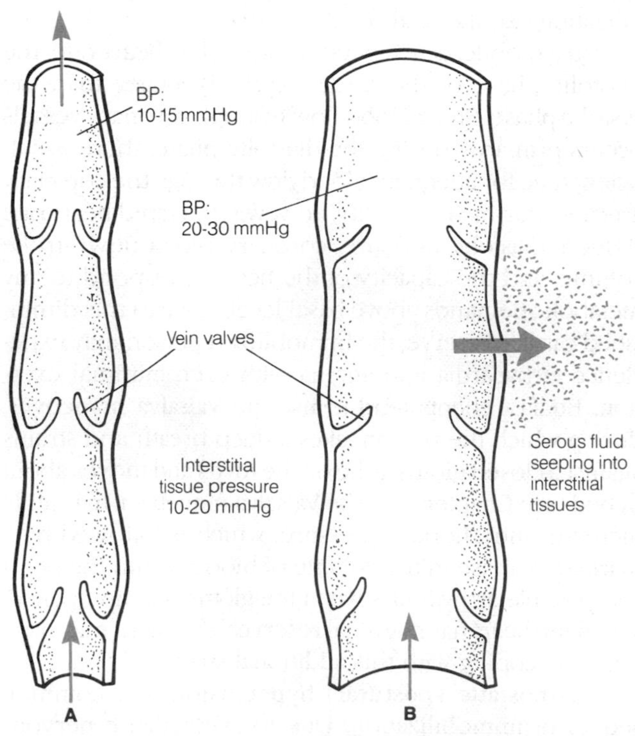

Figure 37–2 Leg veins: **A**, in a mobile person, and **B**, in an immobilized person

Three factors, known as **Virchow's triad,** collectively predispose a client to the formation of a **thrombophlebitis** (a clot that is loosely attached to an inflamed vein wall). These are impaired venous return to the heart, hypercoagulability of the blood, and injury to a vessel wall.

Although prolonged immobility has not clearly been shown to slow venous return in most persons, it is a significant factor in the immobile elderly who are paralyzed, have heart disease, or have had recent surgery (Kottke et al. 1982, p. 969; Patrick et al. 1986, p. 623). Hypercoagulability due to a disturbance in the clotting mechanism or to decreased blood volume may be a factor in immobilized persons as it is in postoperative clients. Injury to vein walls can occur as a result of (a) atherosclerotic plaque formation due to aging or (b) sustained pressure against a leg due to improper body alignment and immobility.

A thrombus is particularly dangerous if it breaks loose from the vein wall to enter the general circulation as an embolus. At least 15% of deep vein thrombi do migrate (Fahey 1984, p. 36). Large emboli that enter the pulmonary circulation may occlude the vessels that nourish the lungs to cause an infarcted (dead) area of the lung. If the infarcted area is large, pulmonary function may be seriously compromised, or death may ensue. Emboli traveling to the coronary vessels or brain can produce a similarly dangerous outcome.

Respiratory Changes

An upright, mobile person has no impediments against the chest wall to restrict respiratory movement. During normal activity, the person periodically sighs, maximally inhaling or forcefully exhaling to expand the alveoli fully and allow effective gaseous exchange. Mucus, normally present in the respiratory tract, is loosened by movement and removed from the bronchi by ciliary action and coughing.

In a recumbent, immobilized client, ventilation of the lungs is passively altered. The rigid bed presses against the body and curtails chest movement. The abdominal organs push against the diaphragm, further restricting chest movement and making it difficult to expand the lungs fully. An immobilized, recumbent person rarely sighs, partly because overall muscle atrophy also affects the respiratory muscles and partly because there is no need to do so without the stimulus of activity. Without these periodic stretching movements, the cartilaginous intercostal joints may become fixed in an expiratory phase of respiration, further restricting the potential for maximal ventilation (Kottke et al. 1982, p. 970). These changes produce shallow respirations and reduce vital capacity significantly. An immobilized, paralyzed client can lose as much as 25% to 50% of normal vital capacity (Kottke et al. 1982, p. 970).

Blood flow through the lungs is also passively altered by the client's horizontal position, due primarily to the effects of gravity. The dependent parts of the lung, tightly sandwiched between the bed with the body's weight on top, expand less effectively with each respiration. These dependent areas are least effectively ventilated, yet blood tends to pool there. The result is reduced gaseous exchange. Poor oxygenation and retention of carbon dioxide in the blood can, if allowed to continue, predispose the person to respiratory acidosis, a potentially lethal disorder. See Figure 37–3.

Mucous secretions are affected by gravity and inactivity. The secretions tend to accumulate in the dependent areas of the alveoli. In immobilized persons, these secretions become more viscous and stick to the lining of the respiratory tract. Due to weakened thoracic muscles, the inability to inhale maximally, and decreased ciliary movement, the coughing mechanism is impaired and the client cannot effectively clear the bronchi of the mucus.

When ventilation is decreased, these secretions may accumulate in a dependent area of a bronchiole and effectively block it. Due to changes in regional blood flow, bed rest decreases the amount of surfactants produced. (Surfactants enable the alveoli to remain open.) The combination of decreased surfactants and blockage of a bronchiole with mucus can cause **atelectasis** (the collapse of a lobe or of an entire lung) distal to the mucous blockage. Immobilized, elderly, postoperative clients are at greatest risk of atelectasis.

Static mucus is an excellent medium for bacterial growth. Under these conditions, a minor upper respiratory infection can evolve rapidly into a severe infection of the lower respiratory tract. **Hypostatic pneumonia** caused by static respiratory secretions can severely impair oxygen-carbon dioxide exchange in the alveoli and is a fairly common cause of death among weakened, elderly, immobilized individuals.

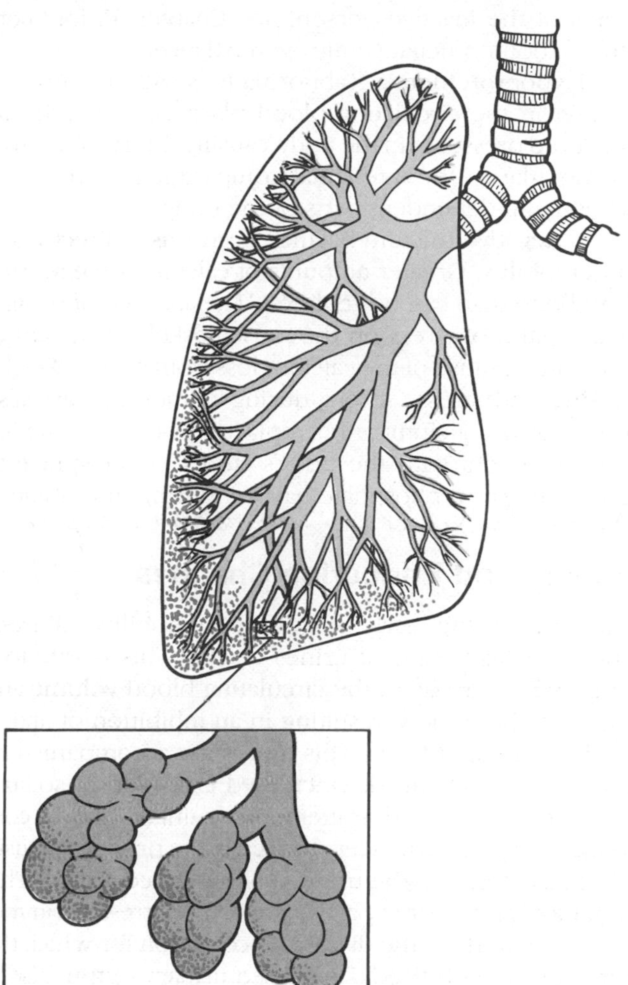

Figure 37–3 Pooling of secretions in the lungs of an immobilized person

Metabolic and Nutritional Changes

In immobilized clients, the basal metabolic rate decreases as the energy requirements of the body decrease. Gastrointestinal motility and secretions of various digestive glands are also reduced.

In an active person, there is a balance between protein synthesis (**anabolism**) and protein breakdown (**catabolism**). Immobility creates a marked imbalance, and the catabolic processes exceed the anabolic processes. Over time, more nitrogen is excreted than is ingested, producing a negative nitrogen balance. Catabolized muscle mass is the source of this excreted nitrogen. Excessive amounts are excreted in the urine, reaching peak levels at about the sixth to tenth day of immobilization (Kottke et al. 1982, p. 210). The negative nitrogen balance represents a depletion of protein stores that are essential for building muscle tissue and for wound healing. The problem is further compounded by **anorexia** (lack of appetite), common among immobilized persons. The anorexic client may reduce his or her intake of protein and calories. If protein intake is reduced, the nitrogen imbalance may become more pronounced, sometimes so severely that malnutrition ensues. Reduced caloric intake is usually a response to the decreased energy requirements of the inactive person. See Chapter 42 for more information on negative nitrogen balance.

Hypoproteinemia (abnormally small amounts of protein in the circulating blood plasma), if severe, can alter fluid pressures in the body, causing fluid to shift from the vascular to the interstitial compartments. The result is edema in dependent parts of the body.

A negative calcium balance occurs as a direct result of immobility. Greater amounts of calcium are extracted from bone than can be replaced. The absence of weight-bearing and of stress on the musculoskeletal structures is the direct cause of the calcium loss from bones. Weight-bearing and stress, absent during immobility, are also required for calcium to be replaced in bone. A similar process occurs with the body's stores of phosphate to cause a negative phosphate balance during immobility.

Urinary and Endocrine Changes

Primarily in the early stages of immobility, **diuresis** (increased excretion of urine) occurs. This is due to a temporary increase in the circulating blood volume and the renal blood flow, resulting in an inhibition of antidiuretic hormone (ADH). This diuresis is accompanied by a temporary **natriuresis** (increased excretion of sodium in the urine), the body's attempt to maintain plasma concentrations at a normal level. Later, urine production usually decreases, and the urine is more concentrated. This condition is probably partly due to the stress of immobility and partly to the disease or condition for which the person is immobilized. Decreased urinary output also is an attempt by the body to compensate for the decreased blood volume. As a result, fluid-retaining hormones—ADH, aldosterone, and cortisol—may be secreted in excessive amounts (Kottke et al. 1982, p. 971).

Gravity plays an important role in the emptying of the kidneys and the bladder in mobile persons. The shape and position of the kidneys and active kidney contractions are important in completely emptying the urine from the calyces, renal pelvis, and ureters. See Figure 37–4, *A*. The shape and position of the urinary bladder (the detrusor muscle), and active bladder contractions are also important in achieving complete emptying. See Figure 37–5, *A*.

When the person remains in a horizontal position, gravity impedes the emptying of urine from the kidneys and the urinary bladder. When the person is supine (in a back-lying position), urine must be pushed upward, against gravity, to be removed from the kidney or bladder. See Figures 37–4, *B* and 37–5, *B*. The renal pelvis may fill with urine before any of it is pushed into the ureters. Emptying is not as complete, and **urinary stasis** (stagnation) occurs after only a few days of bed rest. Due to the overall decrease in muscle tone during immobilization, including the tone of the detrusor muscle, bladder emptying is further compromised.

In a mobile person, calcium in the urine remains dissolved due to a balance of calcium and citric acid in an appropriately acid urine. With immobility and the resulting excessive amounts of calcium (and phosphate) in the urine, this balance is no longer maintained. The urine becomes more alkaline, and the calcium salts precipitate out as crystals to form renal calculi (stones) (Mitchell and Laustau 1981, p. 364). In an immobile person in a horizontal position, the renal pelvis filled with stagnant, alkaline urine is an ideal location for calculi to form. The stones usually develop in the renal pelvis and pass through the ureters into the bladder. As the stones pass along the long, narrow ureters, they cause extreme pain and bleeding and can sometimes obstruct the urinary tract. Some researchers suggest that 15% to 30% of persons who have been immobilized for prolonged periods develop renal stones (Mitchell and Laustau 1981, p. 365).

The immobile person may suffer from urinary retention, bladder distention, and occasionally urinary **incontinence** (involuntary urination). The decreased muscle tone of the urinary bladder inhibits its ability to empty completely, and the immobilized person is unable to relax the perineal muscles sufficiently to urinate. The discomfort of using a bedpan or urinal, the embarrassment and lack of privacy associated with this function, and the unnatural position for urination combine to make it difficult for the client to relax the perineal muscles sufficiently to urinate while lying in bed.

When urination is not possible, the bladder gradually becomes distended with urine. The bladder may stretch excessively, eventually inhibiting the urge to void. When bladder distention is considerable, some involuntary urinary "dribbling" may occur. This does not relieve the urinary distention because most of the stagnant urine remains in the bladder.

Static urine provides an excellent medium for bacterial growth. The flushing action of normal, frequent urination is absent, and urinary distention often causes minute tears in the bladder mucosa, allowing infectious organisms to enter. The increased alkalinity of the urine caused by the hypercalcuria supports bacterial growth.

The organism most commonly causing urinary tract infections is *Escherichia coli,* which normally resides in the colon. See Chapter 32 for additional information. The normally sterile urinary tract may be contaminated by improper perineal care, the use of an indwelling urinary catheter, or occasionally **urinary reflux** (backward flow). During reflux, contaminated urine from an overly distended bladder backs up into the renal pelvis to contaminate the kidney pelvis as well.

Bowel Elimination Changes

Constipation is a frequent problem for immobilized persons. Due to increased adrenalin production, peristalsis and colon motility are decreased, and the sphincters are

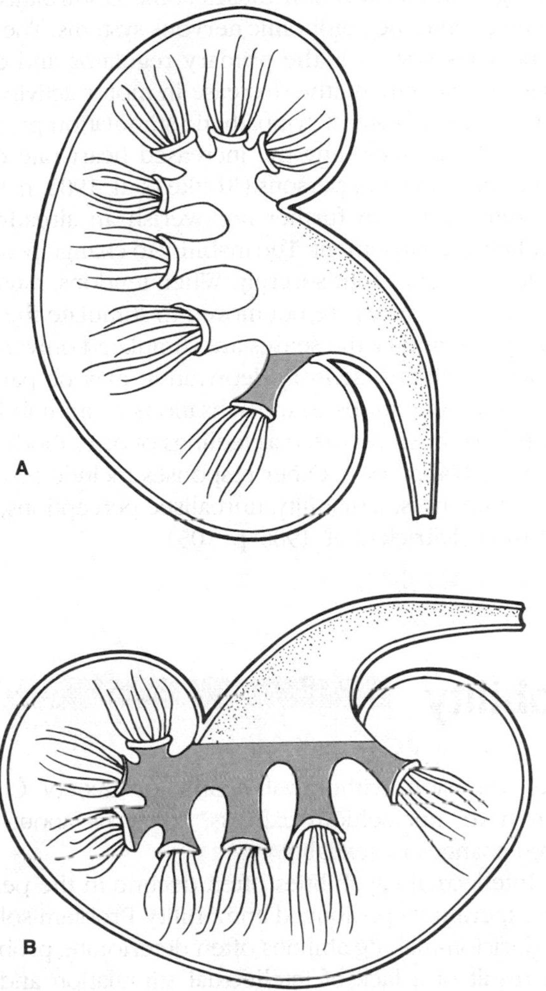

Figure 37–4 Pooling of urine in the kidney. **A**, The client is in an upright position. **B**, The client is in a back-lying position.

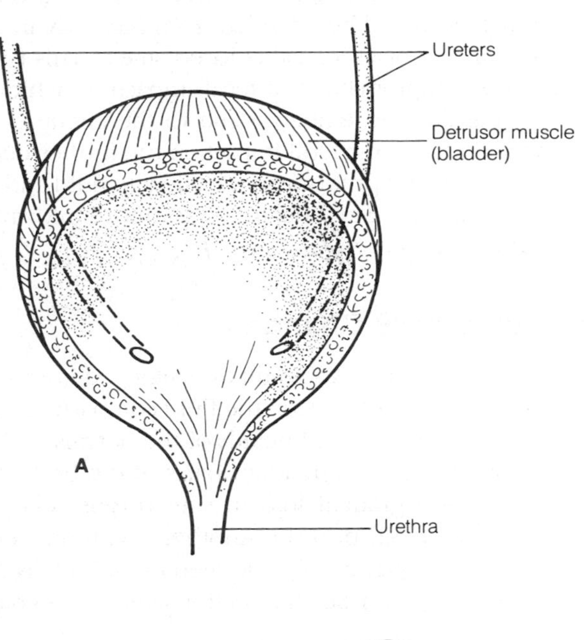

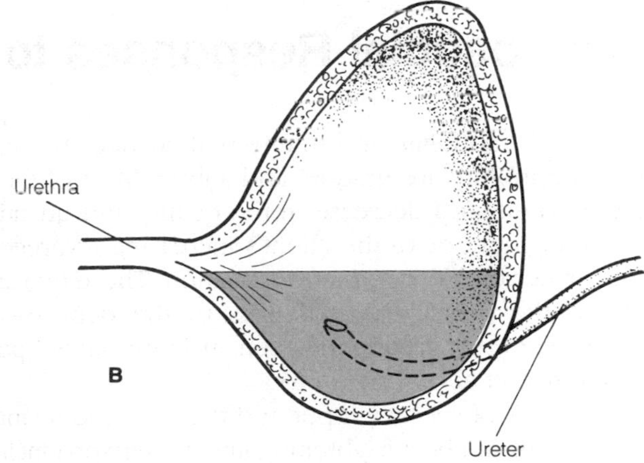

Figure 37–5 Pooling of urine in the urinary bladder. **A**, The client is in an upright position. **B**, The client is in a back-lying position.

more tightly constricted (Kottke et al. 1982, p. 971). The overall skeletal muscle weakness affects the abdominal and perineal muscles used in defecation. When the stool becomes very hard, more strength is required to expel it. The immobilized person may lack this strength.

The bedfast person's unnatural and uncomfortable position on the bedpan does not facilitate elimination. The backward-leaning posture does not promote effective use of the muscles used in defecation. Some persons are reluctant to use the bedpan in the presence of others. The embarrassment, lack of privacy, dependence on others to assist with the bedpan, and disruption of normal bowel habits may cause the individual to postpone or ignore the urge for elimination. Repeated postponement eventually suppresses the urge and weakens the defecation reflex.

The longer the fecal mass remains in the colon, the more water is extracted from it, making the stool increasingly hard, dry, and difficult to expel. The situation may be exacerbated by a decreased intake of food, including fibrous foods. If the person also decreases his or her intake of fluid or is dehydrated, the body may compensate by extracting more fluid from the colon. Severe constipation is often accompanied by headache, abdominal distention and discomfort, malaise, nausea, and dizziness, all of which further decrease appetite. Some persons may make excessive use of the Valsalva maneuver by straining at stool in an attempt to expel the hard stool, dangerously increasing intraabdominal and intrathoracic pressures and placing undue stress on the heart and circulatory system.

When repeated attempts to evacuate the hard stool are unsuccessful, a fecal impaction may develop. The rock-hard stool is pushed distally as the newer, softer stool collects behind it, to create a partial or complete mechanical colon obstruction. The intraluminal pressures created by colonic contractions can be so great that the fluid part of the softer stool may be forced around the hard, unyielding stool and be expelled from the body in a ribbon of diarrhea or as a fecal-colored smear. This type of diarrhea is symptomatic of a fecal impaction, which can be very painful and embarrassing to the client to have removed. If severe, the fecal impaction can further depress colon function and predispose the client to fluid and electrolyte imbalances. See Chapter 43 for more information on fecal impaction.

Integumentary Changes

The skin can atrophy as a result of prolonged immobility. Shifts in body fluids between the fluid compartments can affect the consistency and health of the dermis and subcutaneous tissues in dependent parts of the body, eventually causing a gradual loss in skin **turgor** (elasticity) (Kottke et al. 1982, p. 971). Another common but not inevitable consequence of prolonged immobility is decubitus ulcer formation. See the section later in this chapter.

Neurosensory Changes

Prolonged immobilization causes some disturbances in the central and the autonomic nervous systems. The central nervous system is the primary regulator and coordinator of movement; the decrease in motor activity and the hyperactive state of sympathetic stimulation produce several effects, including the increased heart rate often seen in immobilized persons (Kottke et al. 1982, p. 966).

Immobility can further impoverish an already unstimulating environment. The inability to change position restricts sensory input severely. When tendons, muscles, and other structures are not moved to stimulate the proprioceptors, and tactile senses are stimulated only by the bed and its linens, sensory deprivation may be particularly acute. Alterations in the sensations of immobilized clients have been reported as feelings of disembodiment (Downs 1974, p. 436). Other responses include restlessness, drowsiness, irritability, unrealistic perceptions, and confusion (Patrick et al. 1986, p. 105).

Psychosocial Responses to Immobility

The social, emotional, and intellectual changes brought on by immobility are gradual and subtle. Most of these are due to either a decrease in the quality and quantity of sensory input or to the client's increasing awareness of his or her own unproductive situation. These two factors are the primary contributors to the depression-anxiety syndrome frequently seen in immobilized persons (Kottke et al. 1982, p. 966).

The lack of sensory input and the new and strange environment can be a frightening and anxiety-producing experience for the client. Significant changes in self-concept and role perception often occur as the person recognizes his or her dependence and observes the effect that his or her illness and immobility have on the family. Financial and work concerns often cause considerable worry and anxiety. The client may have unwarranted feelings of personal worthlessness, hopelessness, and emptiness, which he or she may express as hostility, belligerence, confusion, withdrawal, apathy, or anxiety. Clients often have, but seldom express, concerns about perceived changes in sexuality.

Intellectual capabilities often decline in the person who experiences prolonged immobility. Problem-solving and decision-making abilities often deteriorate, probably as a result of a lack of intellectual stimulation and the stress of the illness and immobility. This decline is often accompanied by diminished ability to concentrate, exaggeration of the person's usual defense mechanisms, and decreased ability to cope with problems effectively.

Immobility affects children, especially those not yet of school age, and the elderly most significantly. Immobilization can slow the intellectual and social development of young children and retard the development of motor skills. Immobilization of the elderly can increase their dependence on others.

Assessment: Mobility and Immobility

It is extremely important to obtain and record baseline assessment data soon after the client is first immobilized. These baseline data serve as the standard against which all data collected throughout the period of immobilization are compared. As with any assessment, it is just as important to obtain and record normal as abnormal data, in order to analyze the changes and progress of the client accurately.

Assessing Problems of Immobility

Specific criteria for assessment of immobility are outlined, and abnormal assessment findings related to the complications of immobility are indicated. These assessment criteria are summarized in Table 37–3.

Musculoskeletal System

Muscle mass can be assessed by measuring the circumference of the upper arm or the calf with a tape measure. It is important to position the tape at the same place—at the mid-upper arm or 10 cm below the knee—during each successive measurement. Decreased circumference in both arms or legs suggests muscle atrophy.

It is not possible to measure bone demineralization accurately. Observation of laboratory tests can, however, suggest that bone catabolism is greater than anabolism. Excessive catabolism is reflected in decreased serum protein levels, increased serum calcium and phosphate levels, and significantly increased urine calcium and phosphate levels.

Changes in joint structures are assessed by observing and palpating for stiffness or pain with movement and by observing for painful deposits of calcium around the joints. Changes in joints and the structures that move the joints can be measured with a goniometer, an instrument that measures the degree of joint mobility. Decreasing goniometric measurements and decreasing ability to extend a joint fully suggest that fibrosis and ankylosis of the joint and muscle contracture are beginning to occur.

Decreased muscle strength and impaired coordination can be assessed subjectively through careful observation.

Cardiovascular System

Changes in the heart muscle are assessed by auscultating the heart rate and blood pressure. Several abnormal findings serve as a warning that the heart is becoming less able to respond adequately to the metabolic demands placed upon it. A gradually increasing heart rate, either when the client is at rest or after very mild exertion (and particularly when accompanied by chest pain), indicates that the heart is overly stressed by its workload. Pulse pressure, the difference between the systolic and diastolic blood pressures, is roughly equal to stroke volume. A narrowed pulse pressure reflects a smaller stroke volume and a diminished cardiac reserve.

Additional changes in heart sounds and function may signal impending cardiac failure as a result of the workload placed on the heart during immobility. One of the first indications of impending failure may be the presence of a third sound heard at the heart apex in persons over age 30 (Patrick et al. 1986, p. 480). Dependent peripheral edema in the sacrum, feet, or legs may suggest impending cardiac failure.

The effectiveness of the sympathetic nervous system in achieving vasoconstriction of the peripheral blood vessels with postural changes is assessed in several ways. A sudden, marked fall in blood pressure accompanied by a sudden, marked increase in heart rate when a person changes position from a supine to a vertical posture indicates acute orthostatic hypotension. When dizziness, or less frequently, lightheadedness and dimming of vision are also experienced, the client may be in danger of fainting (Robertson and Robertson 1985, p. 1).

Peripheral vascular function is assessed for possible abnormalities caused by immobility. Peripheral vascular function is assessed for possible abnormalities caused by immobility. Peripheral venous engorgement and dilation; peripheral edema, particularly in dependent areas; decreasing strength of peripheral pulses; and cooler skin temperature in hands and feet suggest impaired peripheral circulation.

While many clients who have a thrombosis experience no signs or symptoms, edema in the affected leg is common (Fahey 1984, p. 36). Additionally, the client may experience pain in the area of the thrombus with movement or when the calf is quickly squeezed front to back or side to side. The circumference of the affected thigh or calf is often slightly greater than that of the uninvolved leg, due to the edema associated with the thrombus.

Respiratory System

Changes in the respiratory system caused by immobility are assessed in several ways. Although shallow respirations are common in immobilized persons, all chest areas over the lungs should be carefully auscultated every few hours to detect diminished breath sounds as a result of impaired ventilation. It is especially important to auscultate dependent lung areas, where secretions or blood may pool and impair diffusion of gases. Analysis of blood laboratory tests may demonstrate poor blood oxygenation, reflected in a decreased Po_2, and retention of carbon dioxide in the blood, reflected in an increased Pco_2. Careful observation is essential to halt this potentially dangerous situation before it gets out of hand. Moist lung sounds or wheezes may be caused by pooled secretions or suggest the presence of hypostatic pneumonia. Chest wall movements should be carefully assessed during several full cycles of inspiration and expiration. When atelectasis occurs, movements of different sides of the chest may appear asymmetrical or unequal.

The presence of a moist, productive cough with thick, sticky, greenish-yellow mucus suggests hypostatic pneumonia. It is usually accompanied by fever, pain with each respiration, and increasing **dyspnea** (difficult, labored respirations).

Metabolism and Nutrition

Assessment of the adequacy of body protein stores and of caloric intake is particularly important in analyzing the metabolic-nutritional status of immobilized clients. Height and weight measurements should be obtained every week or two and compared with accepted standards to observe for possible weight loss due to anorexia. To determine the adequacy of protein and calorie intake, the nurse assesses the amount and kind of food that the client ingests.

Further analysis of body protein stores is accomplished by review of serum protein levels and of the blood

Table 37–3 Assessing the Complications of Immobility

Assessment Technique	Abnormal Findings Related to Immobility
Musculoskeletal system	
Measure arm and leg circumferences	Decreased circumference
Observe lab tests	Decreased serum protein levels
	Increased serum calcium and phosphate levels
	Increased urine calcium and phosphate levels
Palpate, observe	Stiffness or pain in joints
	Painful calcium deposits in soft tissue around joints
Take goniometric measurements of joint ROM	Inability to extend joints, especially of lower extremities, fully
	Decreased ROM of joints
Observe	Poorly coordinated movements of upper and lower extremities
Cardiovascular system	
Auscultate	Increased resting heart rate
	Increased heart rate with chest pain after minimal exertion
Auscultate, palpate	Narrow pulse pressure
Auscultate	Presence of a third heart sound at heart apex
Palpate, observe	Peripheral dependent edema at sacrum, legs, feet
Auscultate, palpate, observe	Sudden decrease in blood pressure, sudden increase in heart rate, dizziness upon change from supine to vertical position
Palpate, observe	Increased peripheral vein engorgement, dilation, and edema that make palpation of peripheral pulses difficult
Palpate	Cold feet and hands
Observe, palpate	Thigh or calf tenderness, edema in affected leg, pain with movement, pain when area quickly squeezed front to back or side to side
Measure thigh and calf circumferences	Increased circumference of thigh or calf
Respiratory system	
Observe	Shallow respirations
Auscultate	Diminished breath sounds in portion of lung
Observe lab tests	Increased P_{CO_2} level and decreased P_{O_2} level in blood
Auscultate	Moist lung sounds or wheezes
Observe	Asymmetrical chest wall movement with full inspiration and expiration
	Moist, productive cough with thick, sticky greenish-yellow mucus
	Pain with respirations, labored respirations
Measure body temperature	Fever
Metabolism and nutrition	
Measure height and weight	Weight loss due to decreased food intake and muscle atrophy
Observe	Decreased intake of protein and calories
Observe lab tests	Decreased serum protein levels
	Increased blood urea nitrogen (BUN)
Observe, palpate	Peripheral dependent edema
Observe	Slow wound healing
Observe lab test	Increased serum calcium and phosphate
Urinary and endocrine systems	
Measure 24-hour input and output	Dehydration
Measure body weight	Weight loss due to dehydration
Observe lab tests	Increased specific gravity of urine, increased BUN, increased serum hematocrit

Table 37–3 *(continued)*

Assessment Technique	Abnormal Findings Related to Immobility
Observe, palpate	Restlessness; decreased urinary output; lower abdominal discomfort; or hard, distended bladder: urine retention
	Voiding very small amounts of urine or "dribbling" urine: retention with overflow or incontinence
Observe lab tests	Increased serum calcium and phosphate and significantly increased urine calcium and phosphate levels
	Increased urine pH (alkalinity)
	Increased white blood cell count
	Increased urine cloudiness, turbidity
	Urine specimen with more than 100,000 colonies of bacteria per ml urine (unsterile specimen); positive urine culture for *E. coli* or other organisms
Observe	Restlessness, frequent urination of small amounts, burning with urination, fever, malaise
Observe	Abdominal cramping or pain, blood or stones in urine
Bowel elimination	
Measure 24-hour input and output	Dehydration
Observe lab tests	Increased specific gravity of urine, increased BUN, increased hematocrit
Observe	Decreased dietary intake and decreased intake of high-fiber foods
	More time elapsed since last bowel movement than usual
	Stool is unusually hard, dry, small, or difficult or painful to expel
	Lower abdominal discomfort, abdominal distention, nausea, malaise, headache, dizziness
	Increased use of Valsalva maneuver to expel stool
Observe, palpate	Rock-hard mass felt in lower abdomen; fecal-colored smear or ribbon of diarrhea (impaction)
Integumentary system	
Measure 24-hour input and output	Dehydration
Observe lab tests	Increased specific gravity of urine, increased BUN, increased hematocrit
Observe	Dependent, peripheral edema in sacrum, legs, feet
Palpate, observe	More than 5 seconds for skin to return to position after a gentle pinch: decreased skin turgor
Neurosensory system	
Auscultate	Increased heart rate
Observe	Overall decrease in motor activity
	Comments about unrealistic perceptions, including feelings of disembodiment
	Restlessness, drowsiness, irritability, or confusion
Social, emotional, and intellectual considerations	
Observe	Behaviors that suggest anxiety, hostility, belligerence, or confusion
	Behaviors that suggest depression: unwarranted feelings of personal worthlessness, hopelessness, emptiness, apathy, or withdrawal
	Behaviors that suggest alterations in self-concept, independent-dependent status, role in family or work group
	Concerns about finances
	Concerns about sexuality
	Behaviors that suggest diminished ability to concentrate, make decisions, or cope

urea nitrogen (BUN). A decrease in serum protein and an increase in BUN suggest that catabolism is exceeding anabolism, leaving inadequate stores of body proteins. Peripheral dependent edema may be caused by decreased serum proteins, and slow progress in wound healing may be due to insufficient protein for tissue repair.

Increases in serum calcium and phosphate levels reflect loss of these minerals from bone as a result of immobility.

Urinary and Endocrine Systems

Assessment of hydration status is important in analyzing overall urinary function in immobilized clients. Careful measurement and analysis of 24-hour intake and output records and periodic measurements of body weight are necessary in assessing for potential dehydration. Dehydration increases the risk of urinary tract infections and formation of renal calculi. A 24-hour fluid intake of less than 1500 ml, greater output than intake, and weight loss suggest dehydration. Analysis of laboratory tests provides additional assessment data: An elevated urine specific gravity, BUN, and serum hematocrit suggest dehydration.

The potential for urinary retention is assessed by observing the volume of recent voidings. Urinary retention is probable if the client has not voided more than about 100 ml in the past 6 to 8 hours; has a hard, distended bladder that can be palpated just above the symphysis pubis; complains of lower abdominal discomfort; and is restless.

Increased levels of serum calcium and phosphate and significant increases in urinary calcium and phosphate as a result of bone demineralization are readily assessed through analysis of laboratory reports. When urinary calcium and phosphate are elevated, the urine pH is probably also elevated. Highly alkaline urine, like dehydration, predisposes the client to urinary tract infections and to the formation of renal calculi.

The possibility of urinary tract infections is readily assessed in laboratory reports. An increased white blood cell count, cloudy urine showing more than 100,000 colonies of bacteria in 1 ml of urine (unsterile specimen), and a urine culture that is positive for *Escherichia coli* or other organisms all indicate infection. Client complaints of **frequency** (frequent voidings of small amounts), **dysuria** (burning with urination), fever, and malaise are additional evidence of a urinary tract infection.

The presence of urinary calculi is assessed by observing for client complaints of abdominal cramping or pain, blood in the urine, or the appearance of renal calculi in the voided urine.

Bowel Elimination

An analysis of hydration status (see the preceding section on "Metabolism and Nutrition") is also important in assessing the immobilized client's bowel elimination status. Analysis of the 24-hour intake and output records and laboratory tests is necessary in assessing potential dehydration. Analysis of fluid intake patterns over the past 4 or 5 days to observe for a decrease in overall intake in food volume (bulk), including fibrous foods, helps the nurse assess constipation.

Analysis of bowel elimination records to assess the client's normal and current pattern of bowel elimination is especially useful. Constipation is probable (a) if more time than usual has elapsed since the client's last bowel movement; (b) if the stool passed is unusually hard, dry, compact, or difficult or painful to expel; (c) if the client complains of lower abdominal discomfort, abdominal distention, nausea, malaise, headaches, or dizziness; or (d) if the client uses the Valsalva maneuver excessively to expel the stool.

When these signs and symptoms of constipation become more exaggerated and a rock-hard mass can be palpated in the lower abdomen, a fecal impaction can be anticipated. A fecal-colored smear of stool or a ribbon of diarrhea usually confirms this suspicion.

Integumentary System

An analysis of hydration status (see the section on "Metabolism and Nutrition") is also important in assessing the immobilized client's integumentary status, since dehydration increases the skin's vulnerability to injury and breakdown. It is also important to assess for indications of peripheral dependent edema, which eventually decreases skin turgor (elasticity) and makes the skin more vulnerable to injury and breakdown. Skin turgor can be crudely assessed by gently pinching the skin over the scapula. Healthy, elastic skin quickly returns to its normal position; atrophied skin usually requires more than 5 seconds to return to its normal position, except in elderly clients. See also the section on pressure sores later in this chapter.

Neurosensory System

Nervous system changes as a result of immobility are closely allied to the cardiovascular and motor changes brought about by immobility. These are readily assessed by observing the client's gradually increasing heart rate and the gradual overall decrease in motor activity. Sensory and perceptual changes are more subtle but may be reflected in client comments that suggest unrealistic perceptions. The client may complain of "feelings of disembodiment" or exhibit restless, drowsy, irritable, or confused behavior.

Social, Emotional, and Intellectual Considerations

Social, emotional, and intellectual changes in a client occur gradually and insidiously. Adequate assessment requires careful, perceptive observations over a period of time by the same nurse. Emotional changes that suggest anxiety include hostile, belligerent, or confused behavior. Although everyone experiences peaks and valleys, real clinical depression is entirely different. Emotional changes that suggest clinical depression include such behaviors as unwarranted feelings of personal worthlessness, hopelessness, emptiness, apathy, or withdrawal.

Other behaviors by the immobilized client may reflect alterations in the client's self-concept or his or her perception of independent-dependent status and work or family roles. The client may express concern about the cost of the illness or about sexuality. Diminishing intellectual capacity may be exhibited as an inability to concentrate, make decisions, or cope with the numerous stresses and changes brought on by the immobilization.

Assessing Body Alignment

Body alignment is the geometric arrangement of body parts in relation to each other. Good alignment promotes optimal balance and body function in whatever position the client assumes: standing, sitting, or lying down. The specific criteria for assessing alignment in each of these positions are outlined in Chapter 38, page 1030.

Assessing Body Mechanics

Good body mechanics is the efficient, coordinated, and safe use of the body to produce motion and maintain balance during activity. Assessing body mechanics is discussed in Chapter 39.

Assessing Ambulation

Assessing ambulation and balance and safety is discussed in Chapter 39.

Assessing Joint Range of Motion

In **range-of-motion movements**, each joint in the body moves through the complete range of all movements normally possible. It is important to determine the complete, maximal range of movement possible: the greater the degree of movement, the more flexible the joint; the smaller the degree of movement the more inflexible and ankylosed the joint. The maximal amount of movement possible can be accurately measured with an instrument called a goniometer (see Chapter 35). Joint movements are described in relation to the body's planes. See the description of body planes earlier in the chapter and Table 37–2.

Procedure 37–1 ▲ Assessing Joint Mobility (Range of Motion)

Equipment

The amount of movement of a joint can be measured by a goniometer, a device that measures the angle of the joint in degrees. See Figure 35–121, on page 881.

Assessment

1. While the client performs the range-of-motion exercises described for each joint, assess:
   a. The degree of movement of the joint
   b. Any discomfort experienced by the client
   c. Any joint swelling or redness, which could indicate the presence of an injury or an inflammation
   d. The muscle development associated with each joint and the relative size of the muscles on each side of the body
   e. The client's tolerance of the exercise

   Assessment of range-of-motion should not be unduly fatiguing.

2. Assist the client to either a standing or a supine position, with the heels parallel and the arms placed along the sides.

   Rationale Assessment of joint range-of-motion can be carried out in either position. When the client is lying down, the prone or lateral position is required for hyperextension of the neck, hips, and shoulders.

3. Make sure that the client is not wearing clothing that restricts movement.

   Rationale The clothing will not limit the joint movement, and the joint motion can be clearly observed.

4. Ask the client to perform the motions smoothly, slowly, and rhythmically and not to force any joint.

   Rationale Uneven, jerky movement and forcing can injure the joint and the muscles and ligaments surrounding it.

Neck—Pivot Joint

5. Flexion occurs in the sagittal plane. Move the head from the upright midline position forward, so that the chin rests on the chest. See Figure 37–6. Normal range: 45° from midline. Major muscle: sternocleidomastoideus.

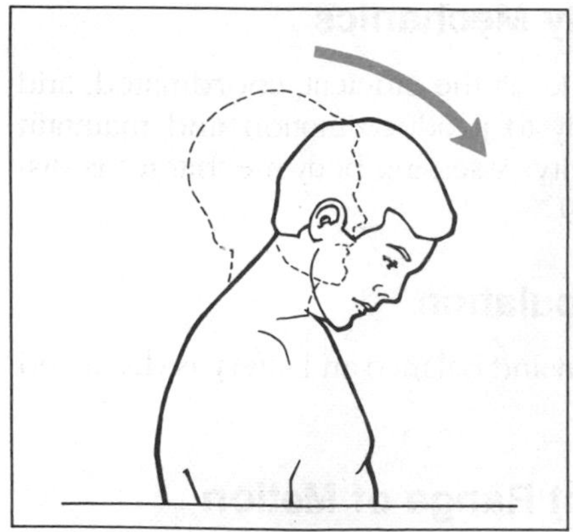

Figure 37–6

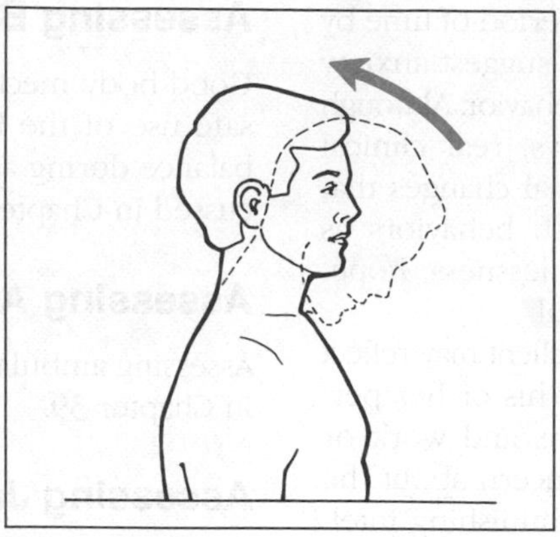

Figure 37–7

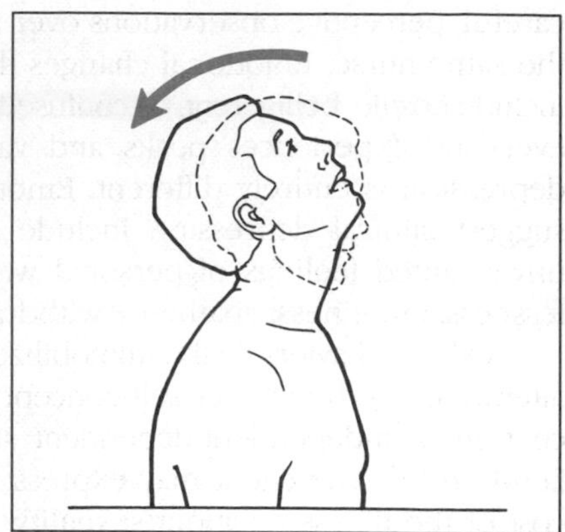

Figure 37–8

6. Extension occurs in the sagittal plane. Move the head from the flexed position to the upright position. See Figure 37–7. Normal range: 45° from the midline. Major muscle: trapezius.

7. Hyperextension occurs in the sagittal plane. Move the head from the upright position back as far as possible. See Figure 37–8. Normal range: 10°. Major muscle: trapezius.

8. Lateral flexion occurs in the frontal plane. Move the head laterally to the right and left shoulders, while facing front. See Figure 37–9. Normal range: 40° from the midline. Major muscle: sternocleidomastoideus.

9. Rotation occurs in the transverse plane. Turn the face as far as possible to the right and left. See Figure 37–10. Normal range: 70° from the midline. Major muscles: sternocleidomastoideus and trapezius.

Shoulder—Ball-and-Socket Joint

10. Flexion occurs in the sagittal plane. Raise each arm from a position by the side forward and upward to a position beside the head. See Figure 37–11. Normal range: 180‘ from the side. Major muscles: pectoralis major, coracobrachialis, and deltoideus.

11. Extension occurs in the sagittal plane. Move each arm from a vertical position beside the head forward and down to a resting position at the side of the body. See Figure 37–12. Normal range: 180° from a vertical position beside the head. Major muscles: latissimus dorsi, deltoideus, and teres major.

12. Hyperextension occurs in the sagittal plane. Move each arm from a resting side position to behind the body. See Figure 37–13. Normal range: 50° from side position. Major muscles: latissimus dorsi, deltoideus, and teres major.

13. Abduction occurs in the frontal plane. Move each arm laterally from a resting position at the sides to a side position above the head, palm of the hand away from the head. See Figure 37–14. Normal range: 180°. Major muscles: deltoideus and supraspinatus.

14. Adduction occurs in the frontal plane. Move each arm from a position beside the head downward laterally

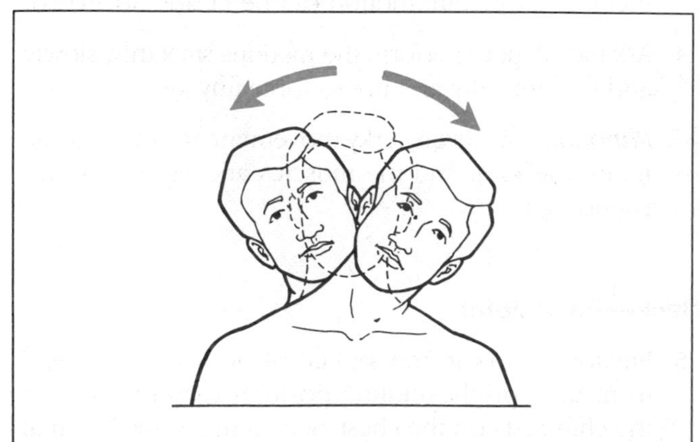

Figure 37–9

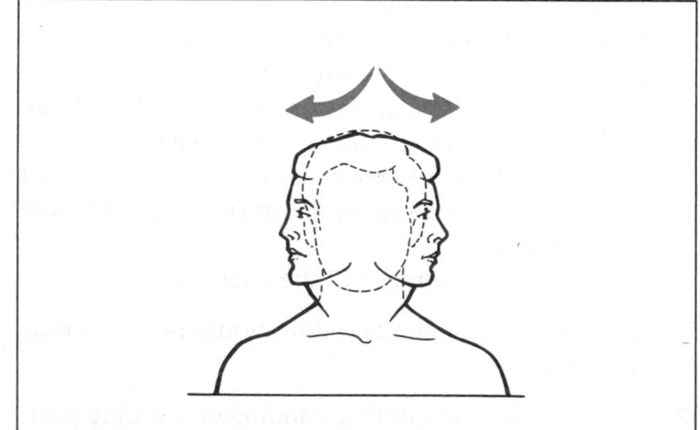

Figure 37–10

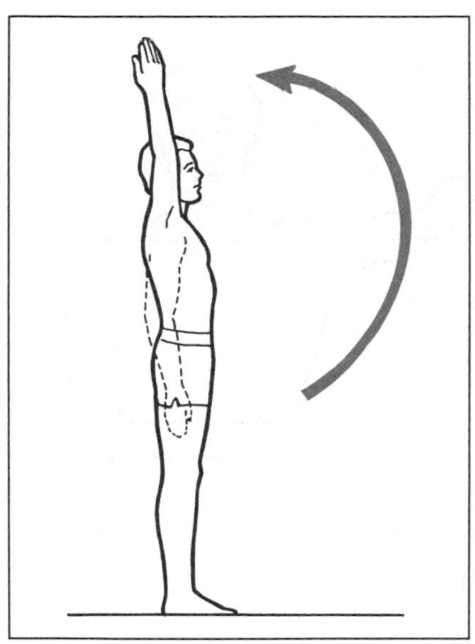

Figure 37–11

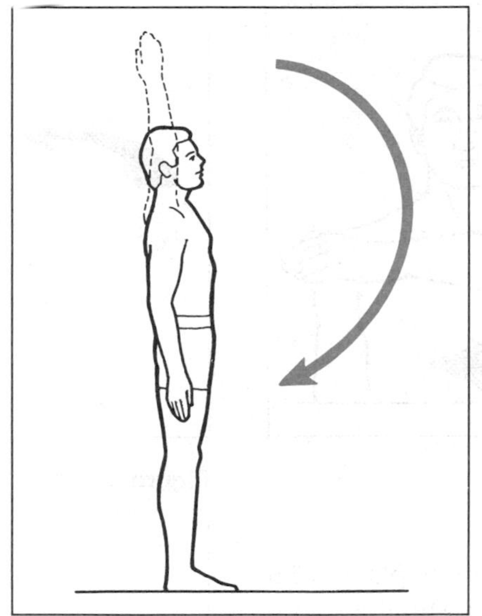

Figure 37–12

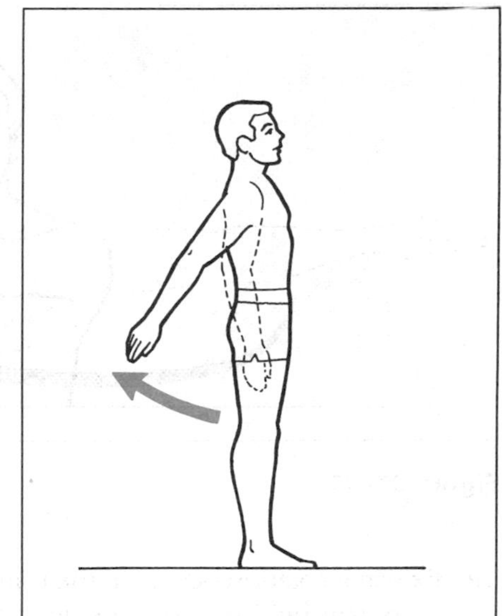

Figure 37–13

and across the front of the body as far as possible. See Figure 37–15. Normal range: 230°. Major muscles: pectoralis major and teres major.

15. Posterior adduction occurs in the frontal plane. Move each arm from a position beside the head downward laterally and across behind the body as far as possible. See Figure 37–16. Normal range: 230°. Major muscles: latissimus dorsi and teres major.

16. Horizontal flexion (anterior adduction) occurs in the frontal plane. Extend each arm laterally at shoulder height and move it through a horizontal plane across the front of the body as far as possible. See Figure 37–17. Normal range: 130°–135°. Major muscles: pectoralis major and coracobrachialis.

17. Anterior abduction occurs in the frontal plane. Extend each arm laterally at shoulder height and move it through a horizontal plane as far behind the body as possible. See Figure 37–18. Normal range: 45°. Major muscles: latissimus dorsi, teres major, and deltoideus.

18. Circumduction occurs in the sagittal plane. Move each arm forward, up, back, and down in a full circle. See Figure 37–19. Normal range: 360°. Major muscles: deltoideus, coracobrachialis, latissimus dorsi, and teres major.

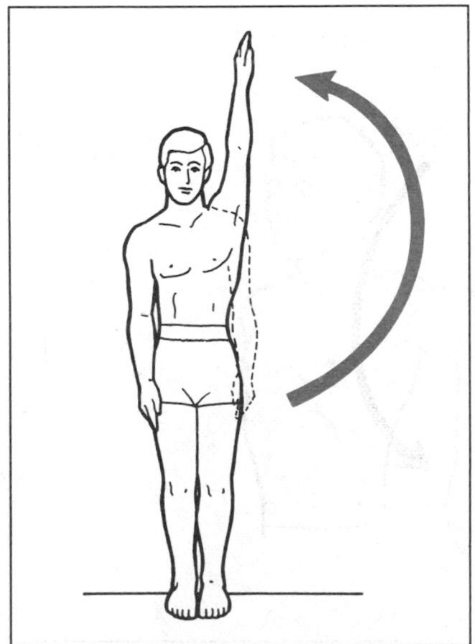

Figure 37–14

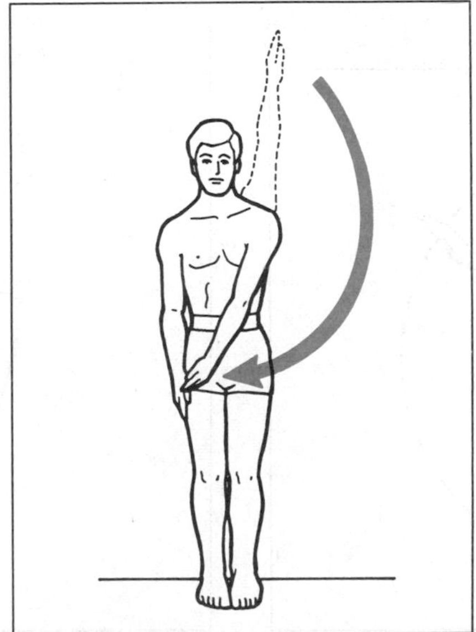

Figure 37–15

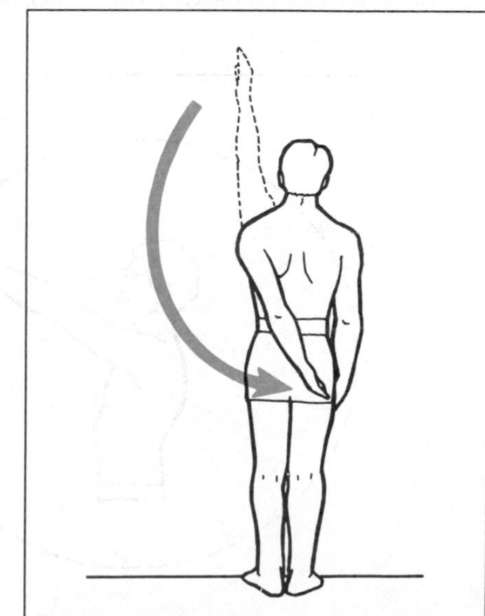

Figure 37–16

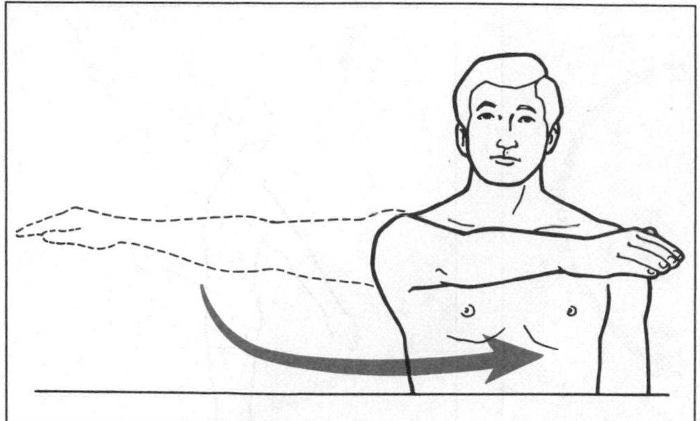

Figure 37–17

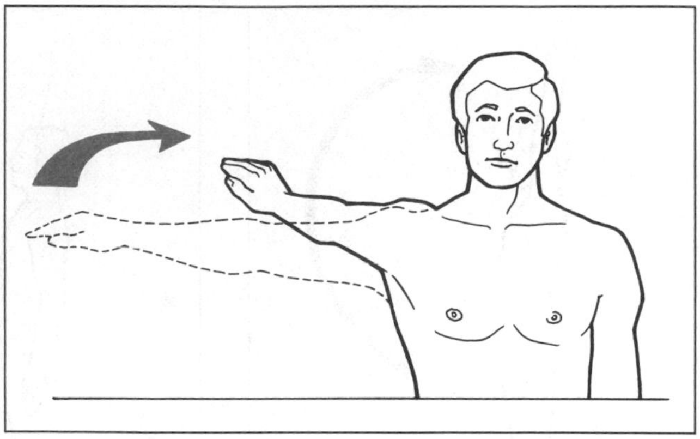

19. External rotation occurs in the transverse plane. With each arm held out to the side at the shoulder level and the elbow bent to a right angle, fingers pointing down, move the arm upward so that the fingers point up. See Figure 37–20. Normal range: 90°. Major muscles: infraspinatus and teres minor.
20. Internal rotation occurs in the transverse plane. With each arm held out to the side at shoulder level and the elbow bent to a right angle, fingers pointing up, bring the arm forward and down so that the fingers point down. See Figure 37–21. Major muscles: subscapularis, pectoralis major, latissimus dorsi, and teres major.

Elbow—Hinge Joint

21. Flexion occurs in the sagittal plane. Bring each lower arm forward and upward so that the hand is at the shoulder. See Figure 37–22. Normal range: 150°. Major muscles: biceps brachii, brachialis, and brachioradialis.

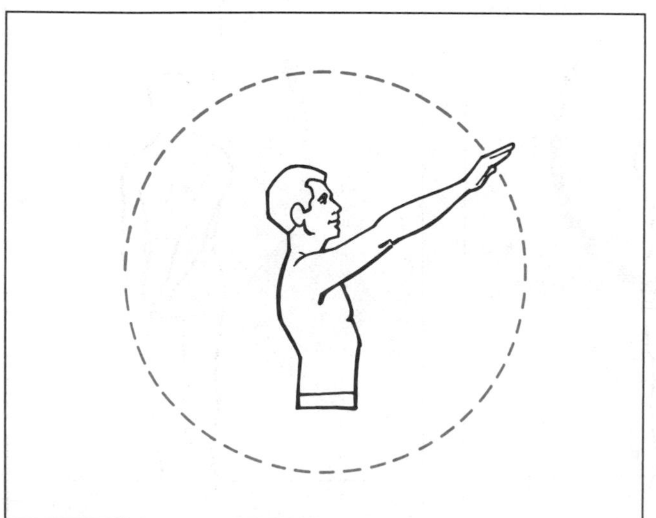

Figure 37–19

Figure 37–18

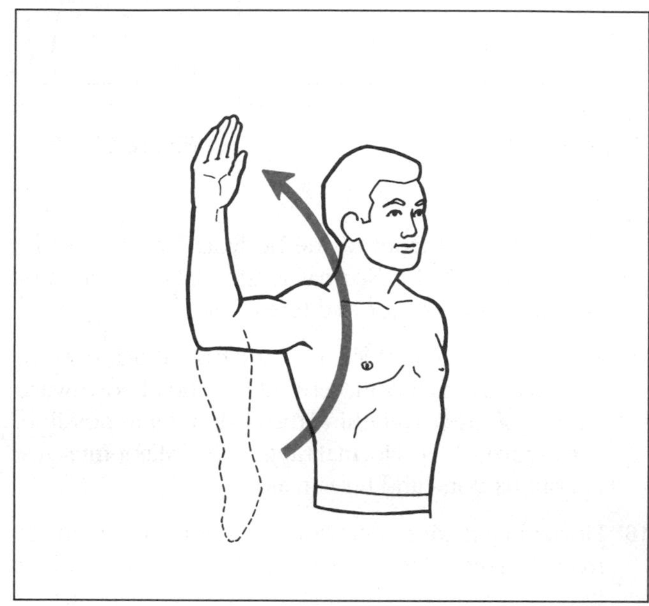

Figure 37–20

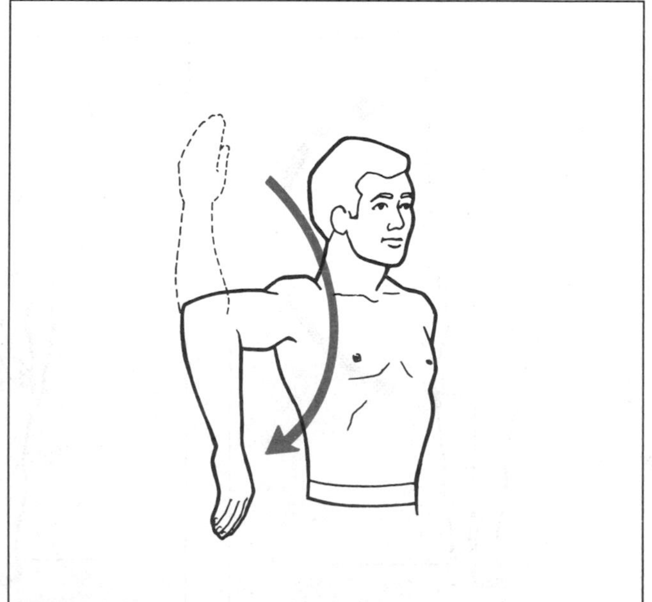

Figure 37–21

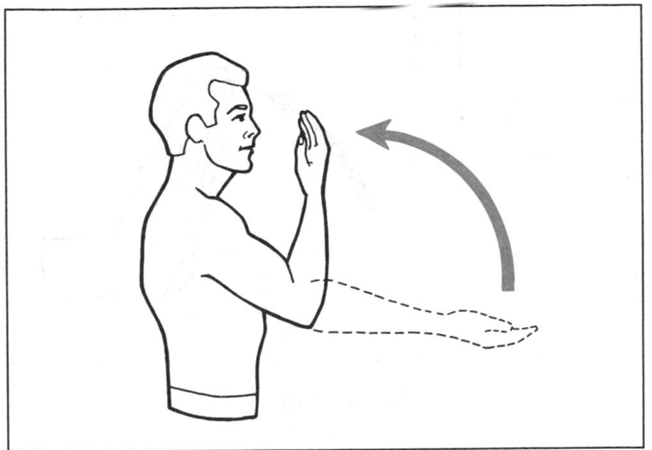

Figure 37–22

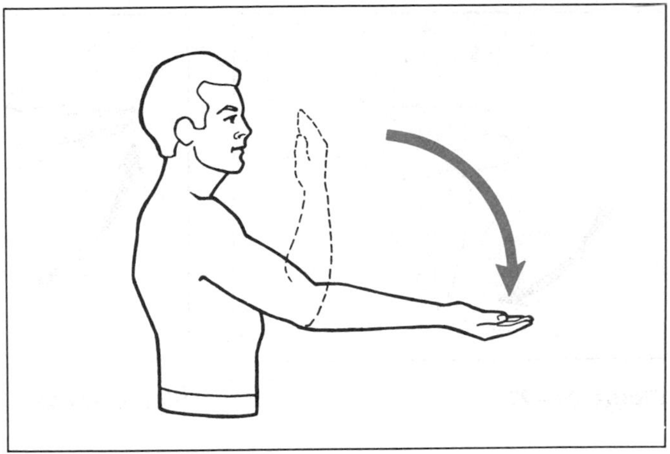

Figure 37–23

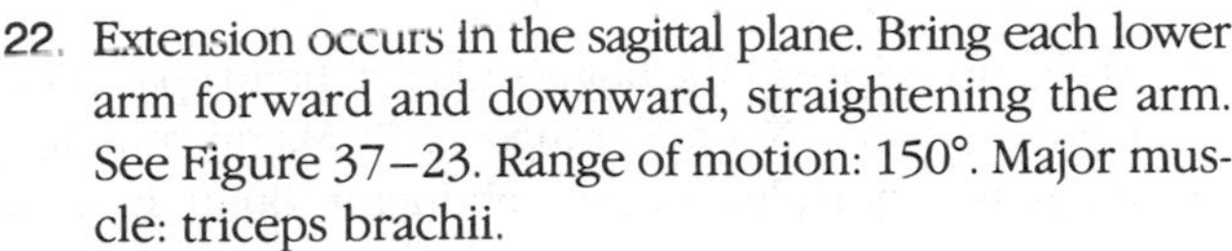

22. Extension occurs in the sagittal plane. Bring each lower arm forward and downward, straightening the arm. See Figure 37–23. Range of motion: 150°. Major muscle: triceps brachii.

23. Rotation for supination occurs in the frontal plane. Turn each hand and forearm so that the palm is facing upward. See Figure 37–25. Normal range: 70°–90°. Major muscles: biceps brachii and supinator.

24. Rotation for pronation occurs in the frontal plane. Turn each hand and forearm so that the palm is facing downward. See Figure 37–26. Normal range: 70°–90°. Major muscles: pronator teres and pronator quadratus.

Wrist—Condyloid Joint

25. Flexion occurs in the sagittal plane. Bring the fingers of each hand toward the inner aspect of the forearm. See Figure 37–27. Normal range: 80°–90°. Major muscles: flexor carpi radialis and flexor carpi ulnaris.

26. Extension occurs in the sagittal plane. Straighten each hand to the same plane as the arm. See Figure 37–28. Normal range: 80°–90°. Major muscles: extensor carpi radialis longus, extensor carpi radialis brevis, and extensor carpi ulnaris.

27. Hyperextension occurs in the sagittal plane. Bend the fingers of each hand back as far as possible. See Fig-

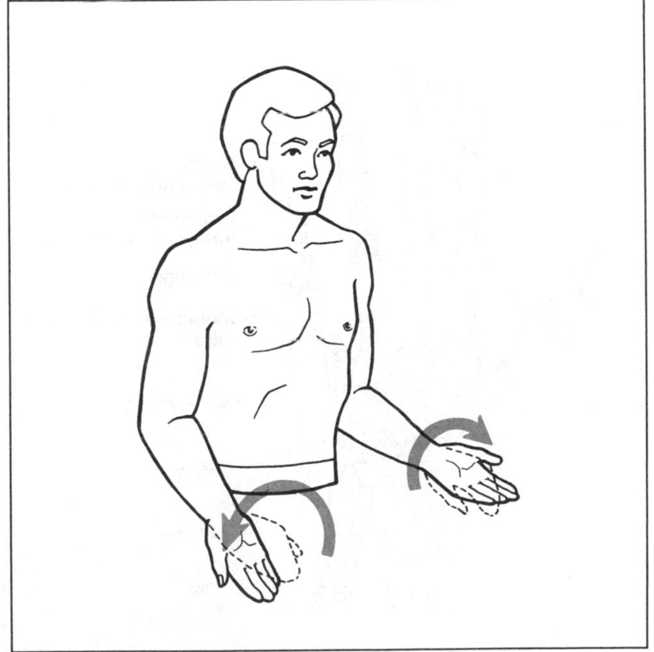

Figure 37–25

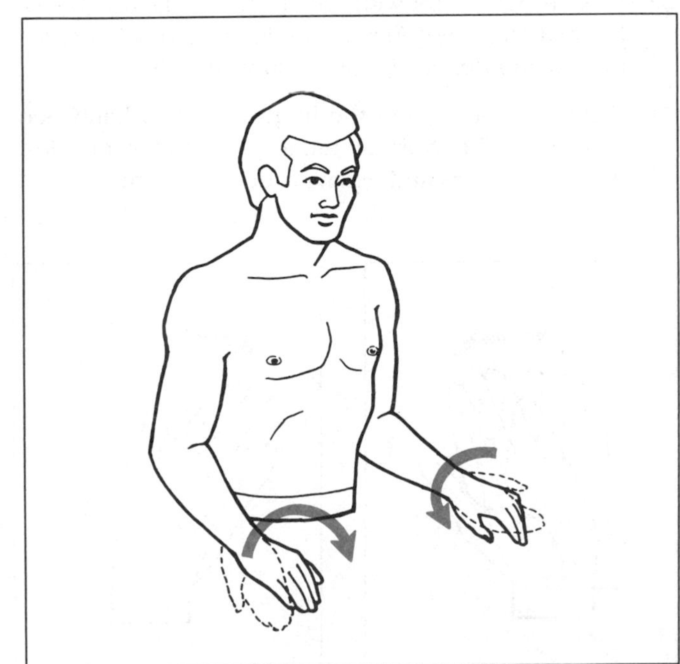

Figure 37–26

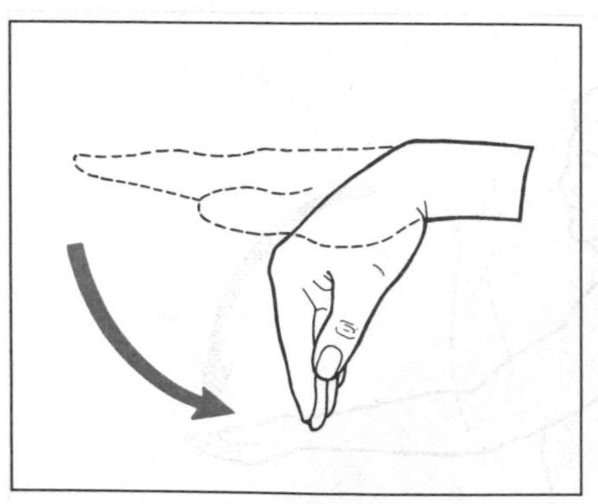

Figure 37–27

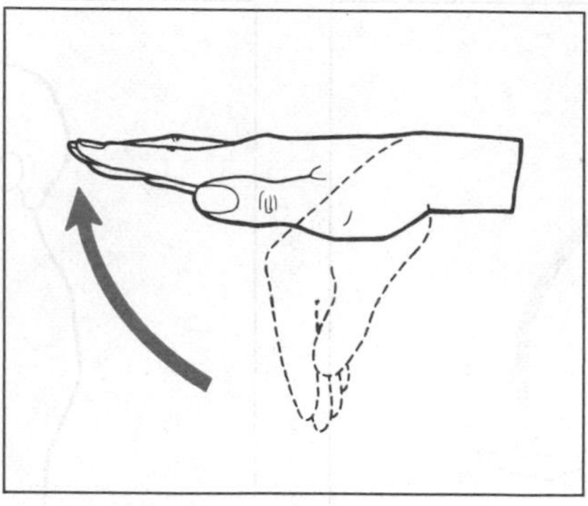

Figure 37–28

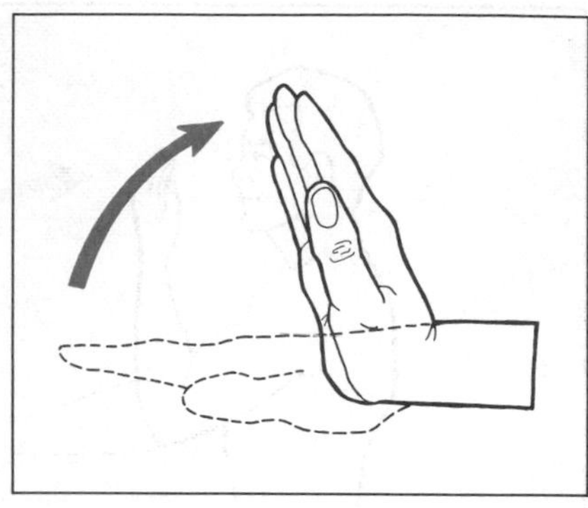

Figure 37–29

ure 37–29. Normal range: 70°–90°. Major muscles: extensor carpi radialis longus, extensor carpi radialis brevis, and extensor carpi ulnaris.

28. Radial flexion occurs in the transverse plane. Bend each wrist laterally toward the thumb side with hand supinated. See Figure 37–30. Normal range: 0°–20°. Major muscle: extensor carpi radialis longus.

29. Ulnar flexion occurs in the transverse plane. Bend each wrist laterally toward the fifth finger with the hand supinated. See Figure 37–31. Normal range: 30°–50°. Major muscle: extensor carpi ulnaris.

Hand and Fingers: Metacarpophalangeal Joints—Condyloid; Interphalangeal Joints—Hinge

See Figure 37–32.

30. Flexion: Make a fist with each hand. See Figure 37–33. Normal range: 90°. Major muscles: interossei dorsales manus and flexor digitorum superficialis.

31. Extension: Straighten the fingers of each hand. See Figure 37–34. Normal range: 90°. Major muscles: extensor indicis and extensor digiti minimi.

32. Hyperextension: Bend the fingers of each hand back as far as possible. See Figure 37–35. Normal range: 30°. Major muscles: extensor indicis and extensor digiti minimi.

33. Abduction: Spread the fingers of each hand apart. See Figure 37–36. Normal range: 20°. Major muscles: interossei dorsales manus, abductor digiti minimi manus, and opponens digiti minimi.

34. Adduction: Bring the fingers of each hand together. See Figure 37–37. Normal range: 20°. Major muscle: interrossei palmares.

Thumb—Saddle Joint

35. Flexion: Move each thumb across the palmar surface of the hand toward the fifth finger. See Figure 37–38.

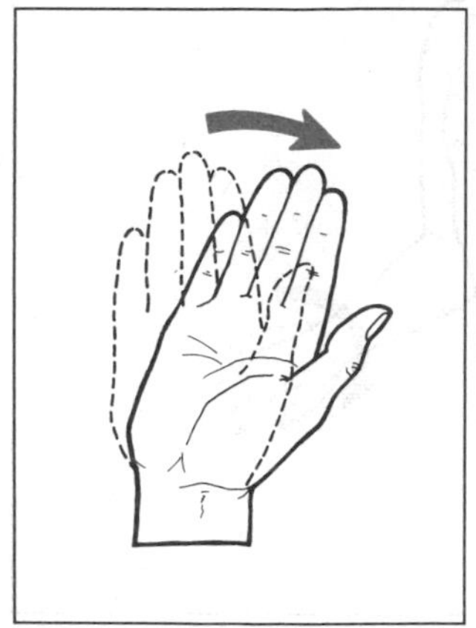

Figure 37–30

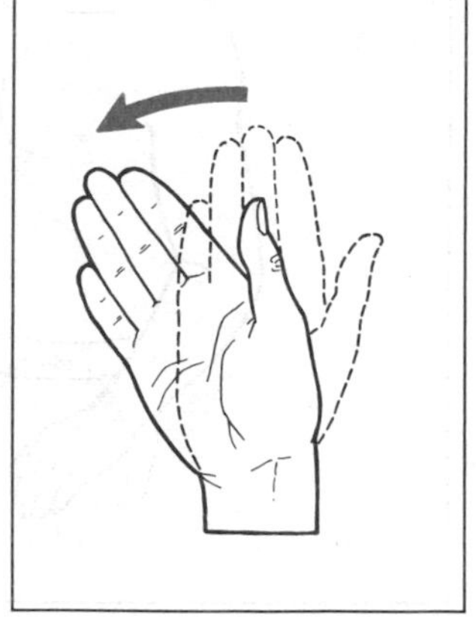

Figure 37–31

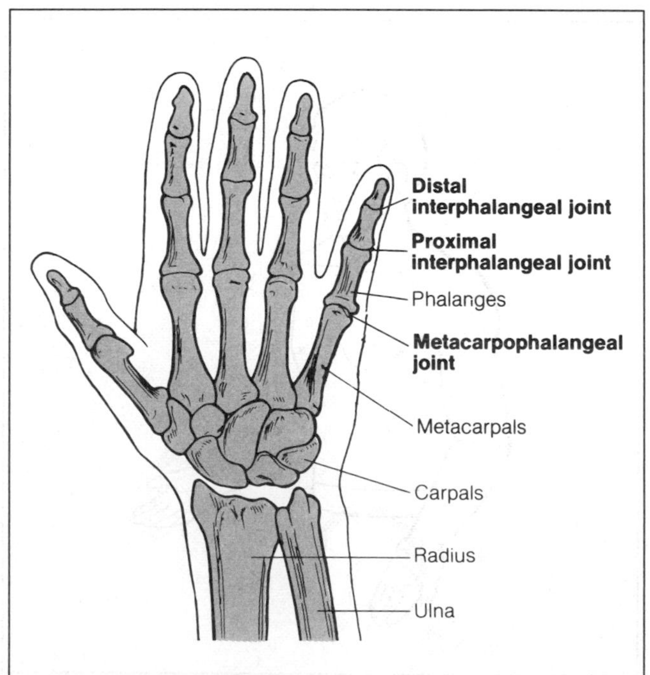

Figure 37–32

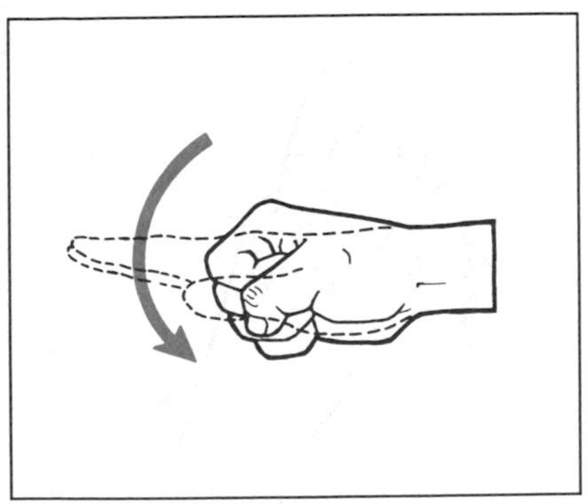

Figure 37–33

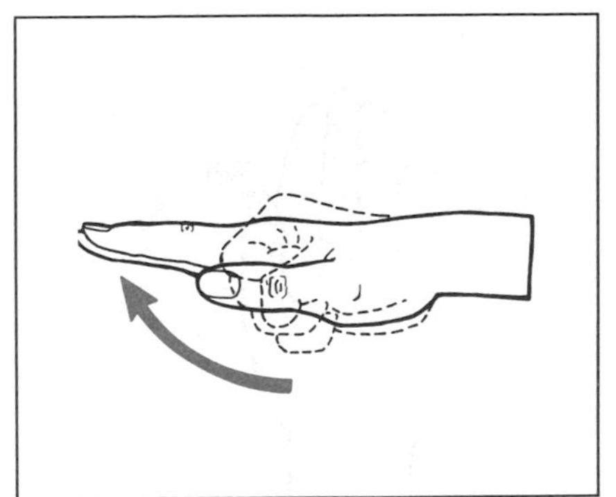

Figure 37–34

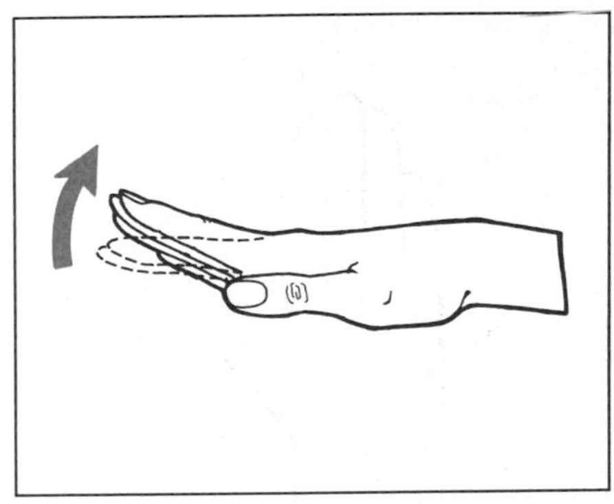

Figure 37–35

Normal range: 90°. Major muscles: flexor pollicis brevis and opponens pollicis.

36. Extension: Move each thumb away from the hand. See Figure 37–39. Normal range: 90°. Major muscles: extensor pollicis brevis and extensor pollicis longus.

37. Abduction: Extend each thumb laterally. See Figure 37–40. Normal range: 30°. Major muscles: abductor pollicis brevis and abductor pollicis longus.

38. Adduction: Move each thumb back to the hand. See Figure 37–41. Normal range: 30°. Major muscle: adductor pollicis.

39. Opposition: Touch each thumb to the tip of each finger of the same hand. The thumb joint movements involved are: adduction, rotation, and flexion. See Figure 37–42. Major muscles: opponens pollicis and flexor pollicis brevis.

Hip—Ball-and-Socket Joint

40. Flexion occurs in the sagittal plane. Move each leg forward and upward. The knee may be extended or flexed. See Figure 37–43. Normal range: knee extended, 90°; knee flexed, 120°. Major muscles: psoas major and iliacus.

41. Extension occurs in the sagittal plane. Move each leg back beside the other leg. See Figure 37–44. Normal range: 90°–120°. Major muscles: gluteus maximus, adductor magnus, semitendinosus, and semimembranosus.

42. Hyperextension occurs in the sagittal plane. Move each leg back behind the body. See Figure 37–45. Normal range: 30°–50°. Major muscles: gluteus maximus, semitendinosus, and semimembranosus.

43. Abduction occurs in the frontal plane. Move each leg out to the side. See Figure 37–46. Normal range: 45°–50°. Major muscles: gluteus medius and gluteus minimus.

44. Adduction occurs in the frontal plane. Move each leg back to the other leg and beyond in front of it. See Figure 37–47. Normal range: 20°–30° beyond the other leg. Major muscles: adductor magnus, adductor brevis, and adductor longus.

45. Circumduction occurs in the transverse plane. Move each leg backward, up, to the side, and down in a circle. See Figure 37–48. Normal range: 360°. Major muscles: psoas major, gluteus maximus, gluteus medius, and adductor magnus.

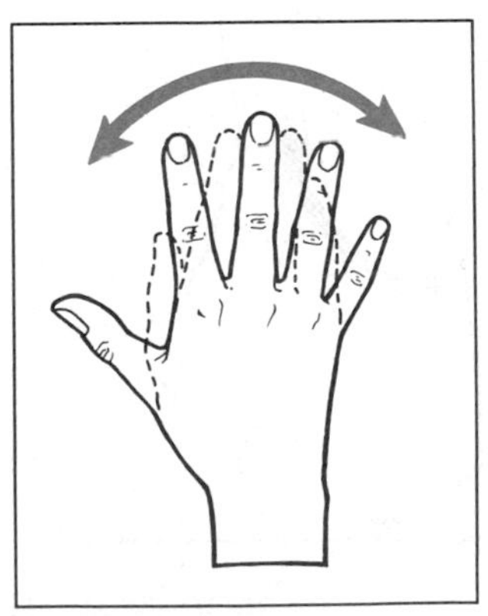

Figure 37–36

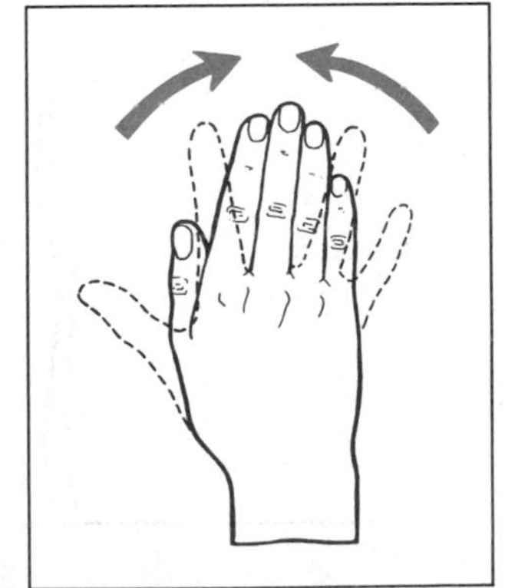

Figure 37–37

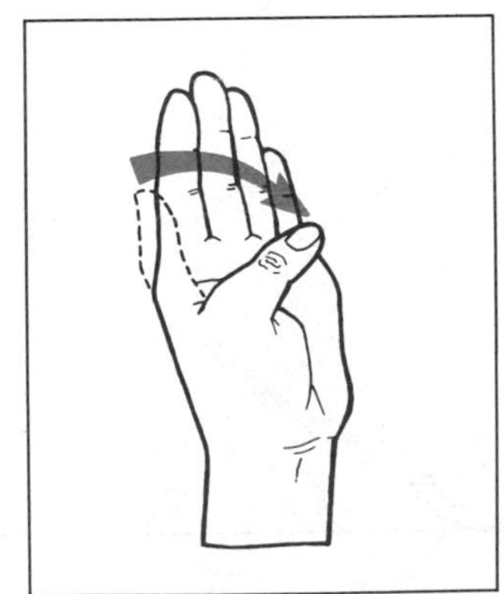

Figure 37–38

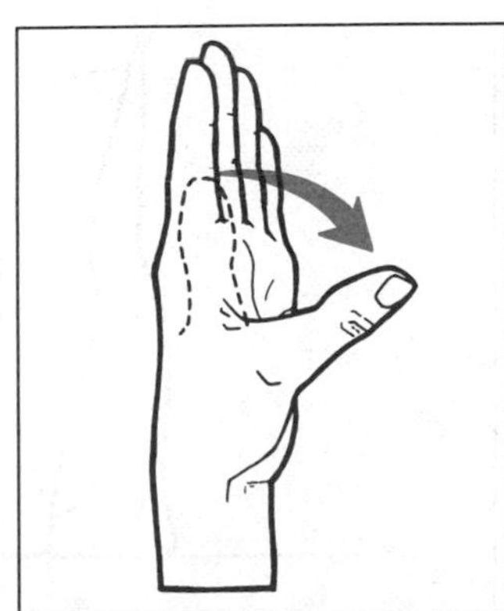

Figure 37–39

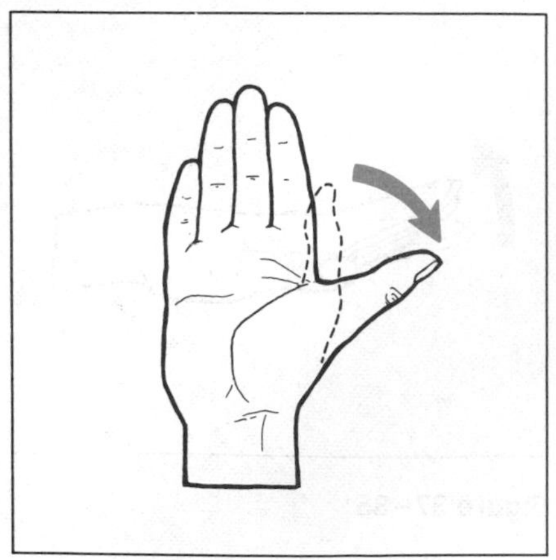

Figure 37–40

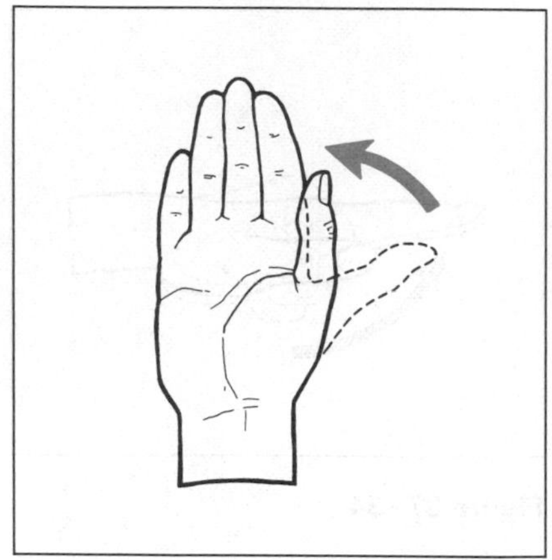

Figure 37–41

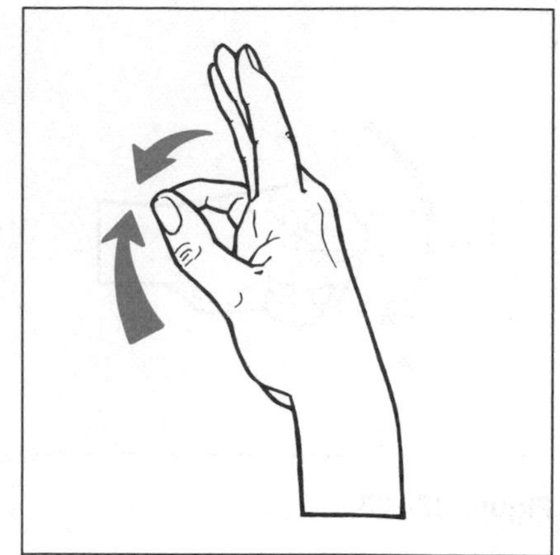

Figure 37–42

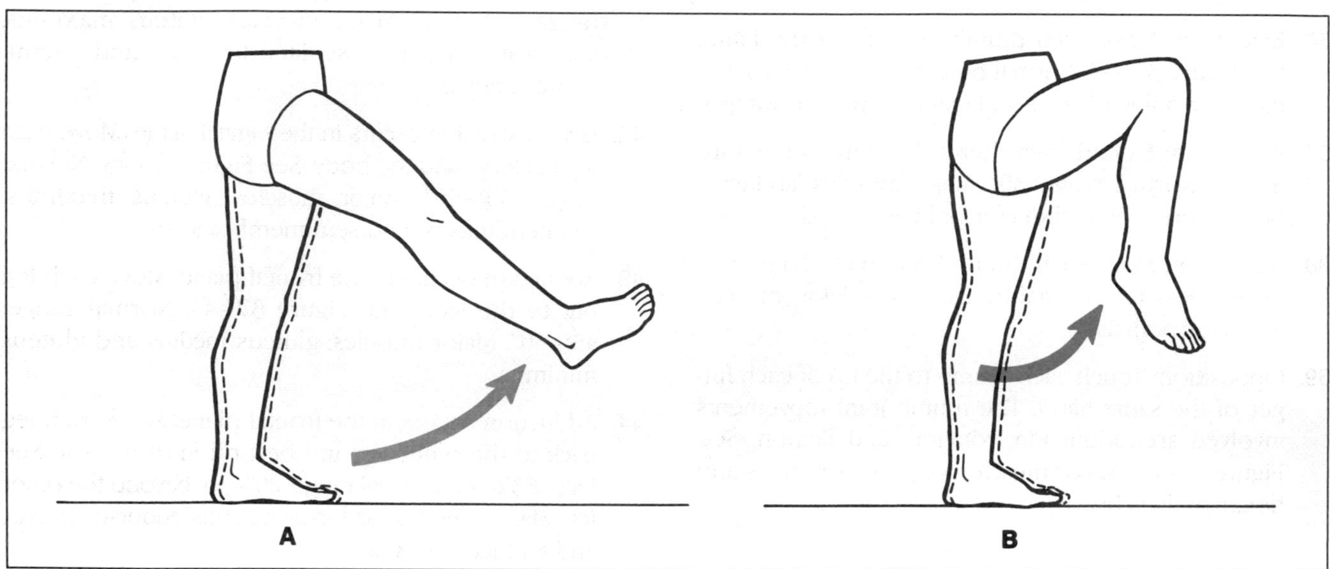

Figure 37–43

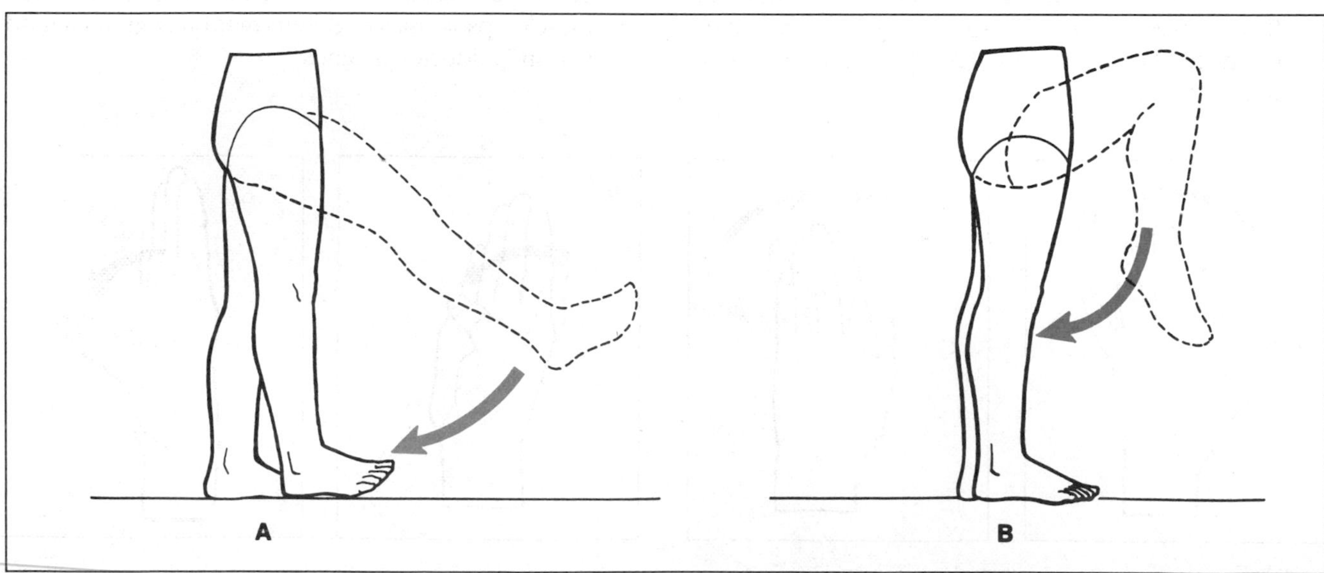

Figure 37–44

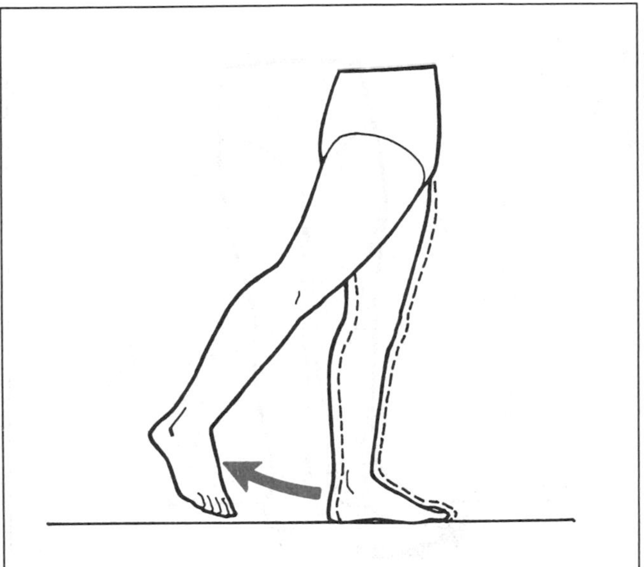

Figure 37–45

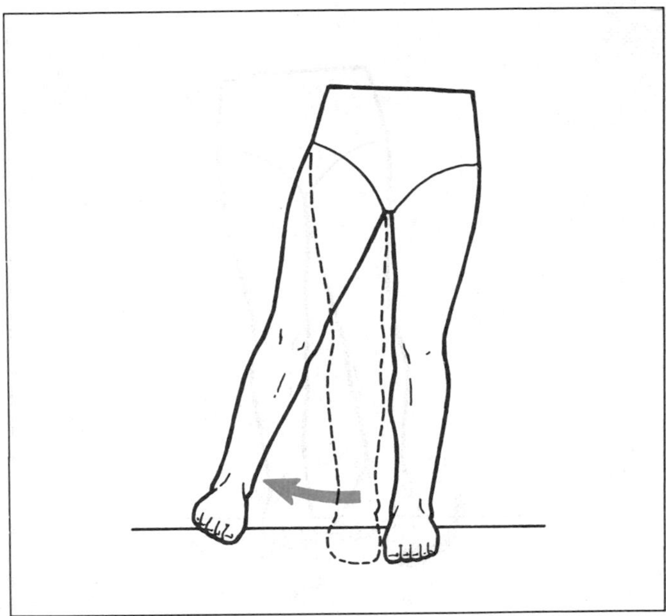

Figure 37–46

46. Internal rotation occurs in the transverse plane. Turn each foot and leg inward so that the toes point as far as possible toward the other leg. See Figure 37–49. Normal range: 90°. Major muscles: gluteus minimus and tensor fasciae latae.

47. External rotation occurs in the transverse plane. Turn each foot and leg outward so that the toes point as far as possible away from the other leg. See Figure 37–50. Normal range: 90°. Major muscles: obturator externus, obturator internus, and quadratus femoris.

Knee—Hinge Joint

48. Flexion occurs in the sagittal plane. Bend each leg, bringing the heel toward the back of the thigh. See Figure 37–51. Normal range: 120°–130°. Major muscles: biceps femoris, semitendinosus, semimembranosus, and popliteus.

49. Extension occurs in the sagittal plane. Straighten each leg, returning the foot to its position beside the other foot. See Figure 37–52. Normal range: 120°–130°. Major

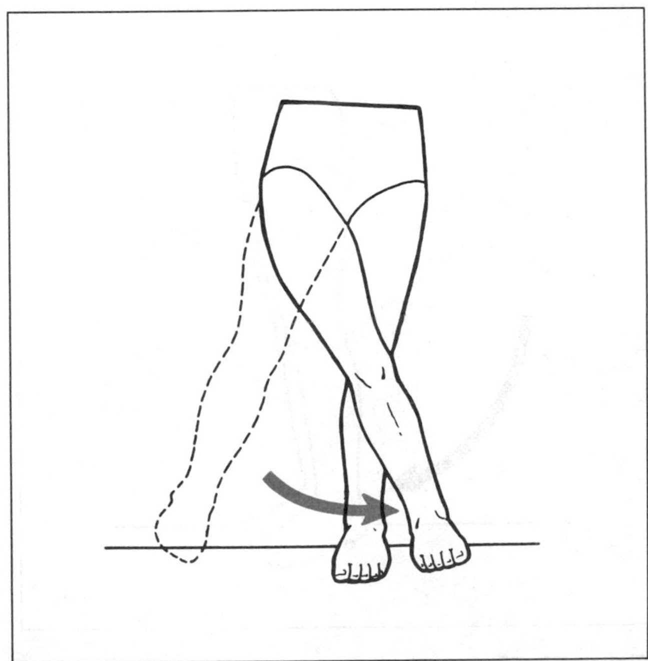

Figure 37–47

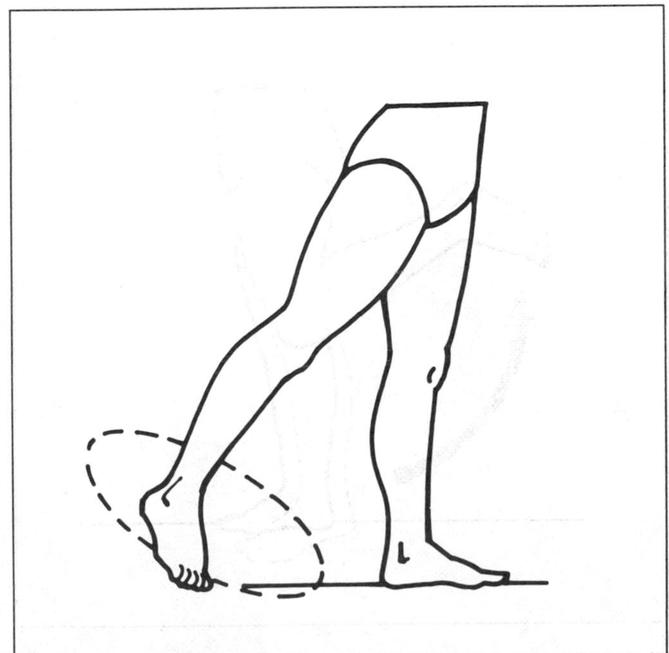

Figure 37–48

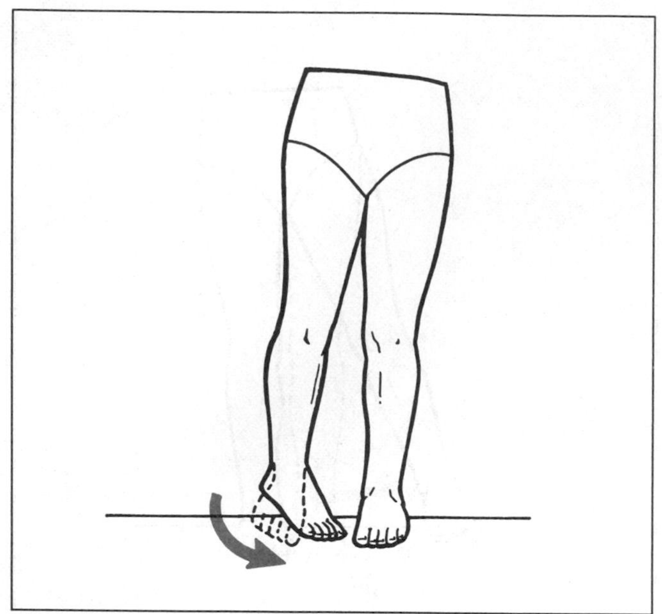

Figure 37–49

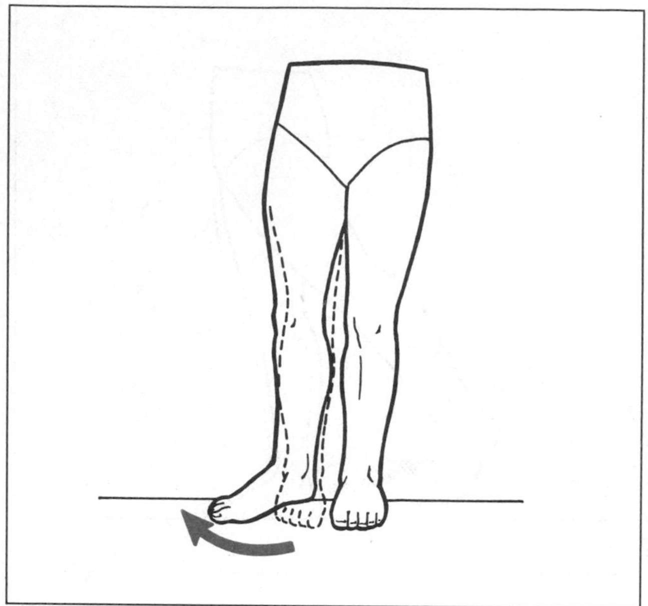

Figure 37–50

muscles: rectus femoris, vastus lateralis, vastus medialis, and vastus intermedius.

Ankle—Hinge Joint

50. Extension (plantar flexion) occurs in the sagittal plane. Point the toes of each foot downward. See Figure 37–54. Normal range: 45°–50°. Major muscles: gastrocnemius and soleus.
51. Flexion (dorsiflexion) occurs in the sagittal plane. Point the toes of each foot upward. See Figure 37–55. Normal range: 20°. Major muscles: peroneus tertius, tibialis anterior.

Foot and Toes: Interphalangeal Joint—Hinge; Metatarsophalangeal Joint—Hinge; Intertarsal Joint—Gliding

See Figure 37–56.

52. Eversion occurs in the frontal plane. Turn the sole of each foot laterally. See Figure 37–57. Normal range:

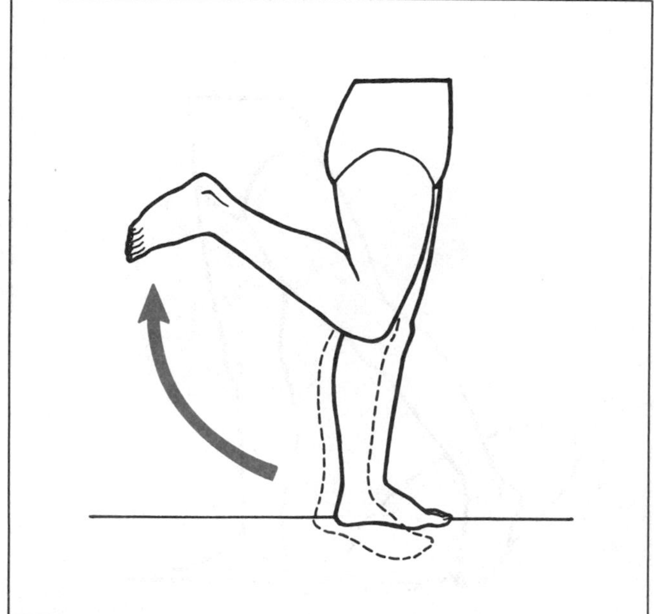

Figure 37–51

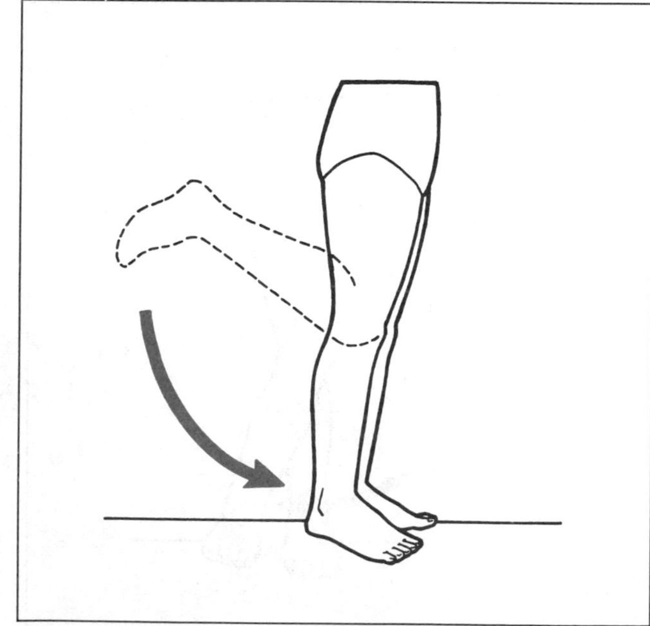

Figure 37–52

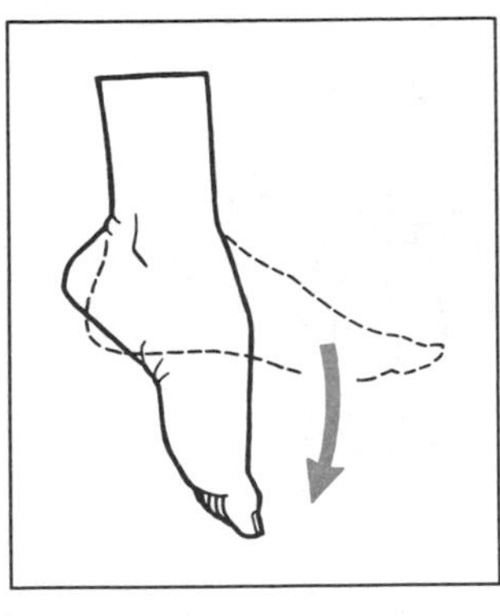

Figure 37–54

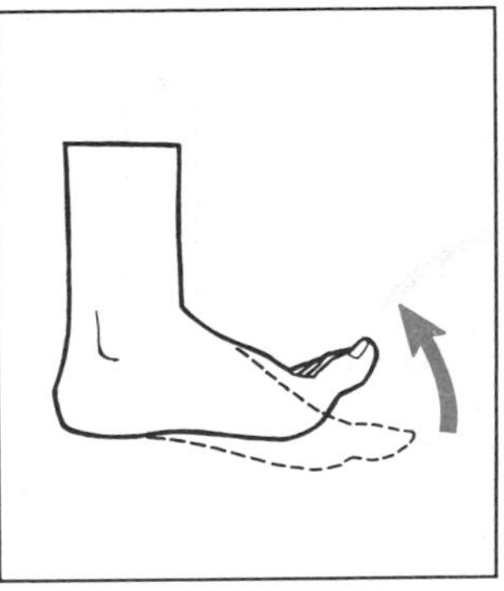
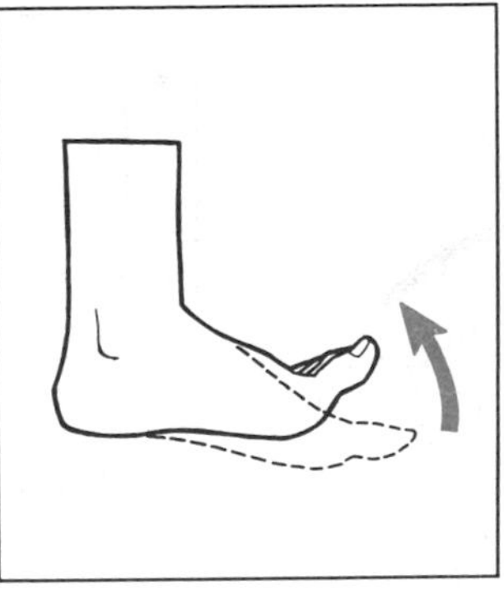

Figure 37–55

5°. Major muscles: peroneus longus and peroneus brevis.

53. Inversion occurs in the frontal plane. Turn the sole of each foot medially. See Figure 37–58. Normal range: 5°. Major muscles: tibialis posterior and tibialis anterior.

54. Flexion occurs in the sagittal plane. Curve the toe joints of each foot downward. See Figure 37–59. Normal range: 35°–60°. Major muscles: flexor hallucis brevis, lumbricales pedis, and flexor digitorum brevis.

55. Extension occurs in the sagittal plane. Straighten the toes of each foot. See Figure 37–60. Normal range: 35°–60°. Major muscles: extensor digitorum longus, extensor digitorum brevis, and extensor hallucis longus.

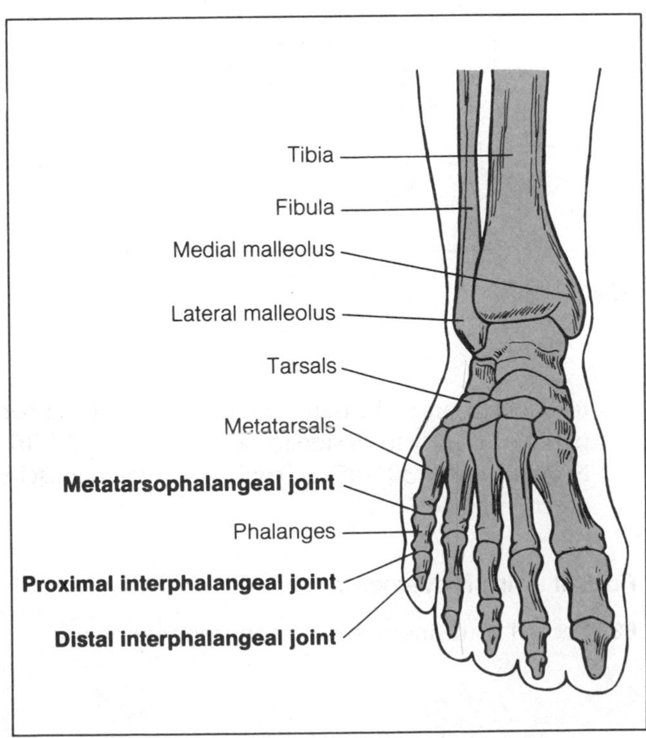

Figure 37–56

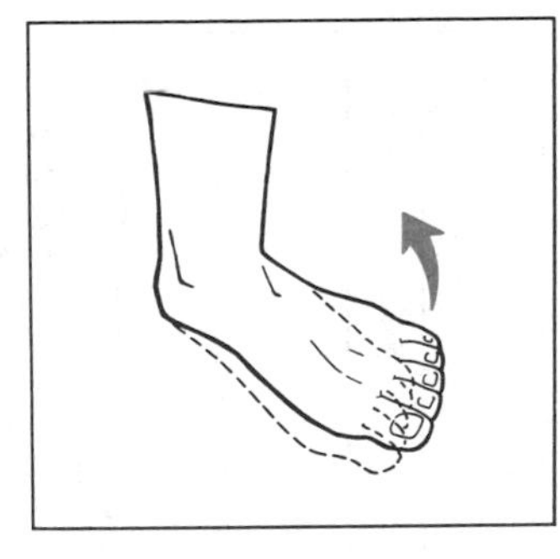

Figure 37–57

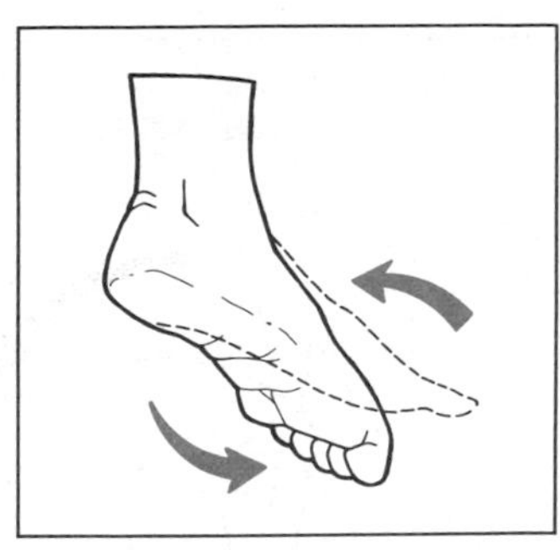

Figure 37–58

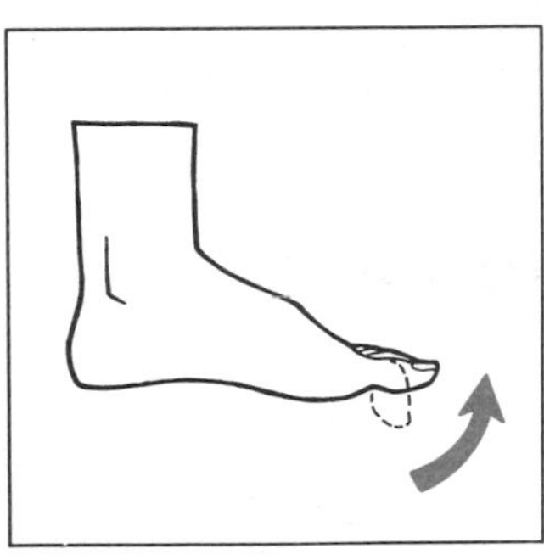

Figure 37–59

Figure 37–60

56. Abduction occurs in the frontal plane. Spread the toes of each foot apart. See Figure 37–61. Normal range: 0°–15°. Major muscles: interossei dorsales pedis and abductor hallucis.

57. Adduction occurs in the frontal plane. Bring the toes of each foot together. See Figure 37–62. Normal range: 0°–15°. Major muscles: adductor hallucis, interossei plantares.

Trunk—Gliding Joint

58. Flexion occurs in the sagittal plane. Bend the trunk toward the toes. See Figure 37–63. Normal range: 70°–90°. Major muscles: rectus abdominis, psoas major, and psoas minor.

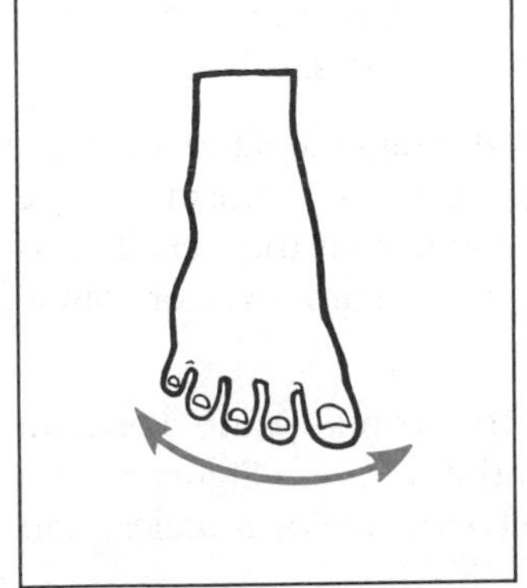

Figure 37–61

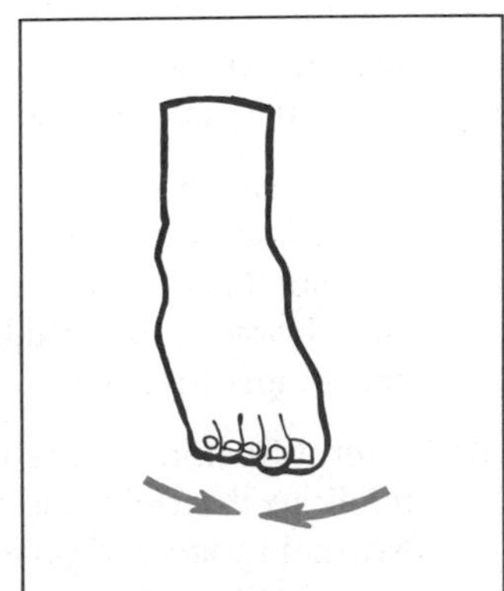

Figure 37–62

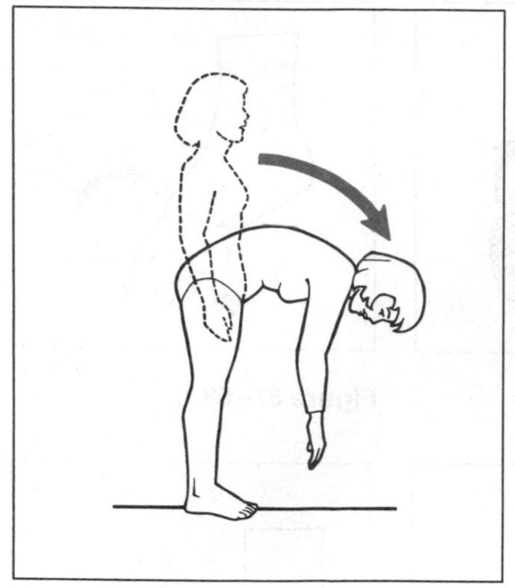

Figure 37–63

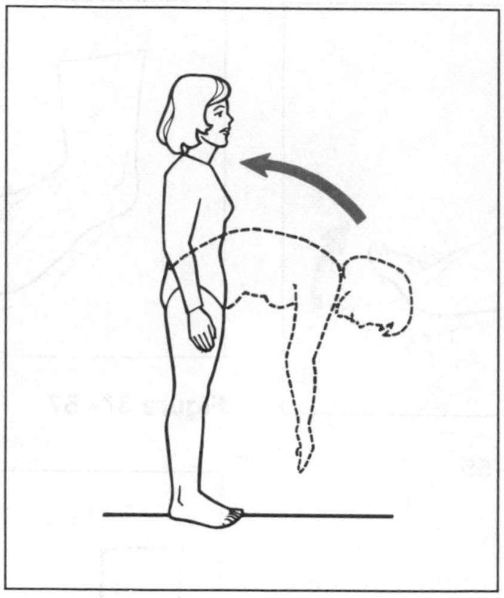

Figure 37–64

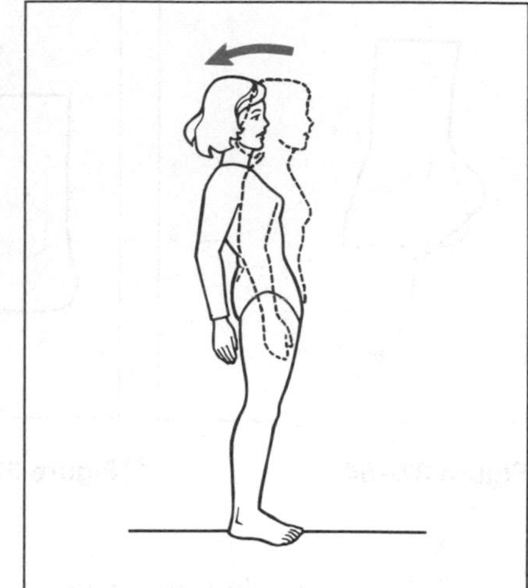

Figure 37–65

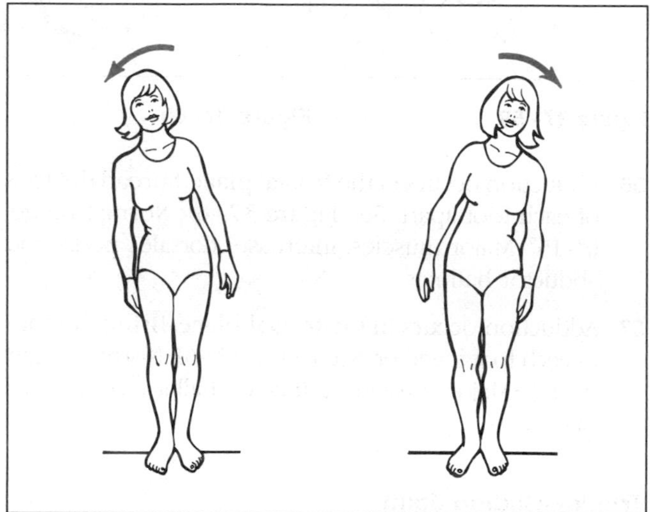

Figure 37–66

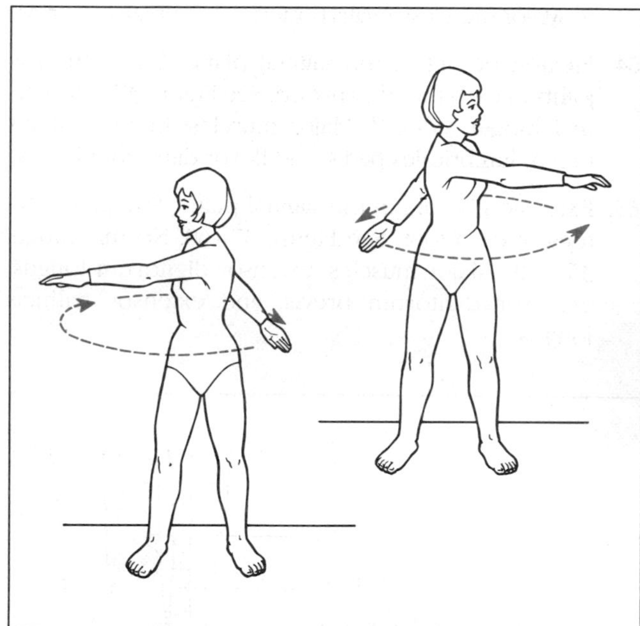

Figure 37–67

59. Extension occurs in the sagittal plane. Straighten the trunk from a flexed position. See Figure 37–64. Normal range: 70°–90°. Major muscles: longissimus thoracis, iliocostalis thoracis, iliocostalis lumborum, erector spinae, and longissimus cervicis.

60. Hyperextension occurs in the sagittal plane. Bend the trunk backward. See Figure 37–65. Normal range: 20°–30°. Major muscles: longissimus thoracis, iliocostalis thoracis, iliocostalis lumborum, erector spinae, and longissimus cervicis.

61. Lateral flexion occurs in the frontal plane. Bend the trunk to the right and to the left. See Figure 37–66. Normal range: 35° on each side. Major muscle: quadratus lumborum.

62. Rotation occurs in the transverse plane. Turn the upper part of the body from side to side. See Figure 37–67. Normal range: 30°–45° to each side. Major muscle: erector spinae.

For All Joint Movements

63. Record your findings on the appropriate record.

Assessing Activities of Daily Living

Activities of daily living (ADLs) are the tasks of daily life, e.g., feeding oneself, bathing and dressing oneself, and taking care of one's toileting needs. Children develop independence in these skills in a set order, beginning with learning to feed themselves and moving up the hierarchy to learning to bathe themselves. There seems to be an equally orderly regression when one loses independence in these skills as the result of aging, illness, or disability. See the hierarchy of independence on the right. Disabled clients regain their independence in a pattern similar to the one of childhood. For example, a disabled woman won't be able to dress herself independently until she regains the ability to accomplish toileting tasks independently (Meissner 1980, pp. 72–73).

Several different rating scales help the nurse to assess a client's capabilities and define the degree of the client's current functional abilities in each of the six areas. This assessment enables the nurse to know how much and what kind of assistance the client needs to maintain or improve functional capability. In this way, the nurse can avoid assisting the client with ADLs that the client can perform independently. At the same time, the nurse knows which tasks the client cannot perform and so provides appropriate help. The rating scale also promotes clear communication of the client's self-care capabilities to others.

Hierarchy of Independence in Activities of Daily Living

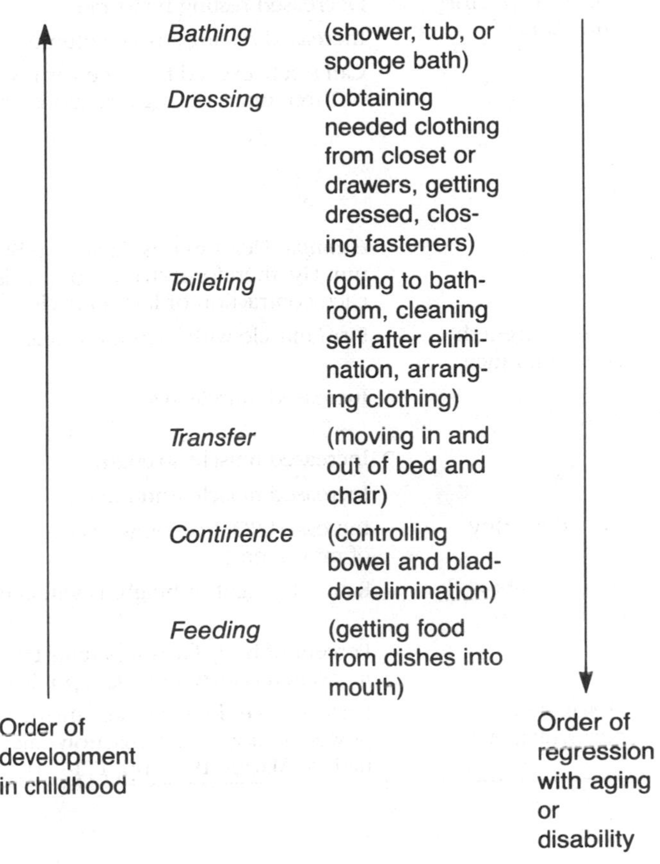

Assessing Physical Fitness

There are five components of physical fitness:

1. *Cardiorespiratory endurance* is the capability of the heart, blood vessels, and lungs to deliver nutrients and oxygen to muscles and remove carbon dioxide and wastes from muscles. Cardiorespiratory efficiency is best measured by assessing maximal oxygen consumption during activity to determine how effectively muscle extracts oxygen from the blood that nourishes it. When this assessment tool is not available, assessment of heart rate and stroke volume, at rest and with maximal activity, provides useful data for determining the fitness of an individual.

2. *Muscular strength and endurance* is the capability of working muscles to maintain maximal force for an extended time. This, in turn, is dependent on the muscle's ability to consume oxygen efficiently. Assessment of muscle tone, mass (size), strength, and endurance is important in determining degree of fitness.

3. *Joint flexibility* is the capability to achieve maximum range of motion (ROM) in each joint. The flexibility of a joint is limited by the size and strength of the muscles that move it and by the fitness of the ligaments and tendons used in movement. Joint flexibility is assessed by the range of motion that the person exhibits. (Range-of-motion assessment is discussed earlier.)

4. *Body weight and composition.* The ratio of weight to height determines whether a person is underweight, overweight, or of normal weight. Body composition refers to the ratio of lean muscle tissue to body fat or adipose tissue. There is a strong relationship between cardiorespiratory fitness and relative lack of body fat. Assessment is accomplished by measuring skinfold thickness with special calipers to determine the percent of body fat (Marley 1982, p. 120). See Chapter 42.

5. *Motor skill performance* is the individual's ability to demonstrate balance, power, agility, speed, fast reaction time, and coordination in the performance of motor skills (Marley 1982, pp. 171–72). Table 37–4 describes criteria for discriminating between the physically fit and the physically unfit individual.

Assessing Activity Tolerance

By determining an appropriate activity level for a client, the nurse can predict whether a client has the strength and endurance to participate in activities that require sim-

Table 37–4 Criteria for Discriminating between the Physically Fit and the Physically Unfit Person

Criterion	Physically Fit Person	Physically Unfit Person
1. Cardiorespiratory endurance	Decreased resting heart rate	Increased resting heart rate
	Increased resting stroke volume	Decreased resting stroke volume
	Can safely exceed baseline resting heart rate two or three times during strenuous exercise	No cardiorespiratory reserve with exercise; may overtax heart; danger of irregular heart rate with exercise
		Shortness of breath, chest pain, and skeletal muscle pain indicate inadequate perfusion of heart muscle and working skeletal muscle
	Example Heart rate is 72 at rest; BP is 120/60 mm Hg; therefore, stroke volume is 60 ml with each contraction of left ventricle	*Example* Heart rate is 94 at rest; BP is 120/90 mm Hg; therefore, stroke volume is 30 ml with each contraction of left ventricle
2. Muscle strength and endurance	Firm muscle with increased tone	Flabby muscle with decreased tone
	Increased muscle size	Tone or muscle too tightly contracted, tight ligaments; decreased muscle size
	Increased muscle strength	Decreased muscle strength
	Increased muscle endurance	Decreased muscle endurance
3. Joint flexibility	Increased ROM of joints (as measured in degrees of movement)	Decreased ROM of joints (as measured in degrees of movement)
4. Body weight and composition	Ratio of weight to height is within normal limits	Ratio of weight to height is above normal limits (overweight)
	Percent of body fat is less than 15% in men, 25% in women (Heywood 1984, pp. 101–2)	Percent of body fat is more than 16% in men, 26% in women (Heywood 1984, pp. 101–2)
5. Motor skill performance	Performance demonstrates increased balance, power, agility, speed, reaction time, and coordination (Marley 1982, pp. 171–74)	Performance demonstrates decreased balance, power, agility, speed, reaction time, and coordination (Marley 1982, pp. 171–74)

ilar expenditures of energy. This assessment is useful in encouraging increasing independence in a disabled person and is especially important for the client who has a cardiovascular or respiratory disability or who has been completely immobilized for a prolonged period.

The most useful measures in predicting activity tolerance are heart rate, strength, and rhythm, particularly for those clients with heart problems. Blood pressure readings are also useful. Assessment data are collected by measuring heart rate:

1. Before the activity starts (baseline data)
2. During the activity
3. Immediately after the activity stops, and
4. At intervals of 3, 5, and 10 minutes after the activity has stopped (Gordon 1976, p. 73)

The activity should be stopped immediately if any of the following changes occur:

1. The heart rate exceeds 20 beats per minute above baseline levels (cardiac client only).
2. The heart rhythm changes from regular to irregular.
3. The pulse weakens.
4. Chest pain occurs.

These warning signals indicate that the activity is too strenuous or prolonged for the client and that the client's health status needs to be reassessed before he or she attempts any other activity (Gordon 1976, p. 73).

If, however, the client tolerates the activity well, and if the client's heart rate returns to baseline levels within 5 minutes after the activity ceases, the activity is considered safe. This activity, then, can serve as a standard for predicting the client's tolerance for similar activities (Gordon 1976, p. 73).

The most useful measures in predicting the activity tolerance of clients with respiratory problems are measurements of respiratory rate, depth, and rhythm, at 3-, 5-, and 10-minute intervals. Dyspnea (difficult breathing), a decreased respiratory rate, or an irregular respiratory rhythm during the activity indicate that the activity should be stopped immediately (Gordon 1976, p. 74). If the client's respiratory rate returns to baseline levels within 3 or 4 minutes after the activity ceases, the activity is considered to be within safe limits.

Other, more subjective measures of activity tolerance are useful when combined with the measures described.

The nurse may need to determine whether client complaints of fatigue during an activity are due to decreased activity tolerance, to anxiety about his or her condition, or to decreased motivation (Gordon 1976, p. 75).

Accomplishment of ADLs places demands on the client's tolerance for activity. The energy costs of some common ADLs are shown in Table 37–5. Note especially the greater energy levels required to get onto and off a bedpan in bed than are required to get out of bed to use a bedside commode.

Nursing Diagnosis

Assessment data indicate whether a client has an actual or potential problem with mobility. See page 996 for examples of nursing diagnoses related to mobility problems.

Planning and Implementing

Client Goals

The overall goals of physical fitness include:

1. Improved cardiovascular endurance
2. Improved respiratory function
3. Improved muscular strength and endurance
4. Improved joint flexibility
5. Improved motor skill performance
6. Maintenance of appropriate body weight with decreases in the ratio of adipose tissue to lean muscle tissue
7. Improved gastrointestinal function preventing constipation
8. Improved emotional outlook
9. Improved productivity
10. Greater energy levels
11. Slowing of the aging process
12. Prolonging of life expectancy

Guidelines for Planning Exercise for Healthy Adults

1. It is important to select an exercise program that the client enjoys and that is appropriate to the client's physical capabilities and health limitations. If not, the client usually discontinues the program soon after starting it.
2. The exercise should be regular and systematically integrated into the person's daily life. The exercise should be performed for 30 to 60 minutes, 4 or 5 days a week, but daily exercise is optimal (Pender 1982, p. 240). People may overrate the benefits of sporadic bursts of exercise; a once-a-month vigorous game of tennis may, in fact, overtax the cardiovascular system dangerously.
3. The client should exercise vigorously enough to expend a minimum of 400 calories. An expenditure of 3500 calories a week is optimal. This can be accomplished by doing 6 to 8 hours of strenuous exercise each week or walking 30 to 35 miles a week (De Witt 1986, p. 66).
4. The target heart rate should be achieved and sustained for 20 to 30 minutes at each exercise session (Pender 1982, p. 233). The target heart rate depends on the person's age, maximum safe heart rate, and fitness level. Target heart rates for adults are shown in Table 37–6. The safe heart rate is determined by subtracting the person's age from 220. The target heart rate is 60% to 75% of the safe heart rate. After 6 months or more of regular exercise, the target heart rate can be gradually increased up to 85% of the safe heart rate (American Heart Association 1984, p. 2).

Table 37–5 Energy Costs of Activities of Daily Living

Activity	Number of Calories used per Minute
Resting, back-lying bed position	1.0
Sitting	1.2
Standing, relaxed	1.4
Eating	1.4
Conversing	1.4
Dressing/undressing	2.3
Washing hands and face	2.5
Using bedside commode	3.6
Walking 2.5 mph	3.6
Showering	4.2
Using bedpan	4.7
Walking downstairs	5.2
Walking 3.75 mph	5.6

Source: Adapted from M. A. Levin, Bed exercises for acute cardiac patients, *American Journal of Nursing,* July 1973, 73:1227.

Table 37–6 Target and Maximum Heart Rates by Age

Age	Target Heart rate	Maximum Heart rate
20	120–150	200
25	117–146	195
30	114–142	190
35	111–138	185
40	108–135	180
45	105–131	175
50	102–127	170
55	99–123	165
60	96–120	160
65	93–116	155
70	90–113	150

Source: The American Heart Association, Exercise diary (Dallas: The Association, 1984), p. 3.

5. Each exercise session should be started with a 5 to 10 minute warm-up before strenuous exercise. The exercise session should conclude with a 5 to 10 minute cooling-down period.
6. The exercises should be rhythmic movements during which muscles alternately contract and relax. Most authorities feel that jogging or running, swimming, bicycling, and walking are the most effective exercise forms involving the entire body.
7. People need to adhere to an effective exercise program throughout their lives. The need for exercise does not diminish with increasing age. Table 37–7 lists the benefits of physical exercise.

Preparations for Exercise

If not accustomed to regular exercise, a male older than 45 years or a female older than 50 years should have a complete physical examination before starting an exercise program. This examination should include a personal and family history of risk factors for exercise, a blood-lipid profile, resting heart rate and blood pressure, and a resting and exercise 12-lead electrocardiogram. A treadmill stress test or bicycle ergometer test is recommended (Pender 1982, p. 239).

The following people should consult a physician before starting an exercise program:

1. People with a personal or family history of cardiovascular disease or signs and symptoms of cardiovascular disease
2. People who experience pain in the chest, neck, shoulder, or arm after exercise
3. Those who do not know what their blood pressure is or who have uncontrolled high blood pressure
4. People who experience dyspnea after mild exertion
5. People with joint or bone problems
6. People who have episodes of dizziness or fainting
7. Insulin-dependent diabetics (American Heart Association 1984, pp. 3–4).

Other preparations for exercise are shown in Table 37–8.

Exercising

Each exercise session should start with a 5 to 10 minute warm-up period immediately before the period of strenuous exercise. The warm-up gradually increases blood

Examples of Nursing Diagnoses Related to Mobility

Metabolic

Actual fluid volume deficit related to anorexia secondary to immobility

Cardiovascular

Alterations in cardiac output related to immobility

Musculoskeletal

Activity intolerance related to sedentary life-style

Impaired physical mobility related to pain secondary to surgery

Impaired physical mobility related to trauma to the spinal cord

Integumentary

See examples on page 1018

Elimination—Urine

Altered pattern of urinary elimination related to dysuria secondary to renal calculi and prolonged immobility

Functional incontinence related to impaired physical mobility

Elimination—Feces

Alterations in bowel elimination: constipation related to immobility

Alterations in bowel elimination: constipation related to insufficient fluid and fiber in diet secondary to anorexia

Psychosocial

Ineffective individual coping related to immobility of lower legs

Anxiety related to threat to self-concept secondary to immobility

Table 37–7 Benefits of Physical Exercise

Musculoskeletal system	*Metabolism and nutrition*
Increased muscle strength	Decreased serum triglyceride levels
Increased muscle tone	Decreased serum cholesterol levels
Muscle hypertrophy (increased muscle mass)	Increased glucose tolerance
Increased muscular endurance	Improved perfusion of nutrients into body tissues and removal of metabolic wastes from body tissues
Increased muscular coordination and balance	Overall decrease in body fat and improved long-term control of body fat
Overall increase in lean muscle tissue	
Increased joint mobility/flexibility	*Urinary and endocrine systems*
Bone density maintained or increased	Decreased potential for neuroendocrine overreaction
	Increased tolerance for stress
Cardiovascular system	
Decreased heart rate during rest and during exertion	*Bowel elimination*
Faster recovery of heart rate following exertion	Increased motility of gastrointestinal tract, decreasing the potential for constipation
Increased size of heart muscle, especially of left ventricle	
Increased strength of heart muscle contraction	*Neurosensory system*
Increased stroke volume with each heartbeat	Decreased potential for neuroendocrine overreaction
Increased collateral blood supply to heart muscle and to lungs	Decreased sympathetic nervous system tone
Increased blood volume	Increased motor activity
Decreased systolic and diastolic blood pressure, especially if previously elevated	
Increased efficiency of peripheral circulation, especially venous	*Social, emotional, intellectual, and developmental considerations*
Decreased platelet stickiness	Decreased nervous tension related to psychologic stress
Decreased potential for cardiac arrythmia	Increased ability to cope with stress
	Improved self-concept
Respiratory system	Increased sense of well-being
Increased vital capacity and functional capacity at rest and with exertion	Increased energy levels
Increased diffusion/perfusion of oxygen and carbon dioxide, increasing oxygenation of blood and decreasing retention of carbon dioxide	Decreased tendency toward depression and anxiety reactions
Increased maximal oxygen consumption (increased effectiveness of muscle tissue in extracting oxygen from the blood)	Decreased tendency toward addictive behaviors (e.g., smoking or alcohol and drug abuse)
Decreased susceptibility to upper respiratory infections	Improved work performance
	Improved quality of sleep
	Increased achievement of developmental tasks

Source: Adapted from N. J. Pender, *Health promotion in nursing practice* (Norwalk, Conn.: Appleton-Century-Crofts, 1982), pp. 234–35, and R. C. Cantu, editor, *Health maintenance through physical conditioning* (Littleton, Mass.: PSG Publishing Co., 1981), pp. 24–26.

flow to the heart and muscles and increases oxygen consumption before strenuous exercise. Warm-up exercises can include brisk walking or slow running for 1 or 2 minutes, jumping rope, or similar exercise. Stretching exercises should be avoided during the warm-up.

During the period of strenuous exercise, the target heart rate should be achieved and sustained for at least 20 to 30 minutes. Brisk walking is a safe and appropriate activity during this period for people of all ages. Jogging, running, swimming, cycling, and innumerable other vigorous exercises are appropriate. Stretching exercises are less likely to produce injury when they are performed after the period of strenuous exercise.

Each exercise session should conclude with a 5- to 10-minute cooling-down period. During this recovery period, circulation and other functions gradually return to normal levels. Not including this period in an exercise program can cause pooling of blood in leg muscles and possible fainting, nausea, and muscle soreness. Stretching exercises or brisk walking with deep breathing are appropriate during this period. Stretching exercises should be done slowly. The client should adopt a position and hold it for a few seconds before continuing. At the completion of the cooling-down period, the heart rate should be below 100 beats per minute (Pender 1982, p. 236).

Preventing Injuries

There is always some risk of injury during vigorous exercise, even for the physically fit. The risk, however, is greater for the physically unfit person. Injuries are more common when:

1. Exercise is irregular.
2. The exercise is not compatible with the person's health status.
3. The warm-up or cool-down period is omitted.
4. The person exceeds his or her target heart rate.
5. The person increases the target heart rate goal too soon after starting a program of regular exercise.

Musculoskeletal injuries, especially of the knee and ankle joints and the ligaments of the feet, and gynecologic injury, especially involving the uterus, are most common in older persons who jog, run, or do stretching or aerobic exercises. Back injury from exercises that involve back flexion and twisting are also fairly common.

Nursing Interventions to Prevent Problems from Immobility

Musculoskeletal System

The following interventions help to prevent the musculoskeletal complications of immobility or to restore musculoskeletal function following a period of disabling immobility:

1. Body repositioning
2. Weight-bearing activity
3. Independence in ADLs
4. Aerobic, isotonic, and isometric exercises
5. Exercise

These activities are most useful when initiated as soon as possible after the client is immobilized.

Body repositioning Correct body alignment in each position is essential. Interventions to promote correct body alignment in standing, sitting, and bed-lying positions are outlined in Chapter 38. Improper body positioning can exacerbate many of the complications of immobility. The nurse and client should plan daily and full extensions of the hips and knees, which are especially vulnerable to flexion contractures.

Normally, an individual adjusts his or her position automatically every few minutes in response to increasing pressure sensed in a body area. The immobilized person who is unable to sense this pressure or who is unable to move is highly vulnerable to deterioration of the musculoskeletal and other systems. A schedule for position changes, at least every 2 hours and preferably every hour, should be planned with the client and posted in the nursing care plan or in the client's room. If possible, standing, sitting, and all bed-lying positions should be included. A sample position change schedule is shown in Table 37–9.

Nurses should teach clients to shift, adjust, or change their positions frequently. Clients can learn to use their

Table 37–8 Preparations for Exercise

Preparation	Reason
Wear comfortable support shoes and well-fitting socks.	Proper footgear prevents blisters and injury.
Avoid running or walking on hard surfaces or in hilly areas.	Running on hard surfaces can jar the joints.
Avoid exercising on the hottest or most humid days.	Body temperature may become overly elevated.
Wait 1½ to 2½ hours after a meal.	Blood flow will be directed to the muscles rather than the alimentary tract.
Ingest increased amounts of glucose 1½ or 2½ hours before exercising.	Glucose provides energy for exercise.
Ingest adequate salt and potassium before exercising.	Salt and potassium prevent muscle cramps during exercise.
Drink ample fluid before exercising.	Adequate intake prevents dehydration due to fluid lost as perspiration.

Table 37–9 Sample Schedule of Position Changes during a 24-Hour Period

0200	Supine position in bed
0400	Left lateral position in bed
0600	Right lateral position in bed
0800	Up in wheelchair (W/C) for breakfast; encourage client to shift weight in W/C every 15 minutes
0900	Left lateral position in bed
1000	Supine position in bed
1100	Right, lateral position in bed
1200	Stand with legs fully extended for 2 to 3 minutes; walk two or three steps to W/C; then, up in W/C for lunch; encourage client to shift weight in W/C every 15 minutes
1400	Left lateral position in bed, encourage client to shift weight backward or forward using side rail and trapeze
1600	Right lateral position in bed, encourage to shift weight backward or forward using side rail or trapeze
1700	Stand with legs fully extended for 2 to 3 minutes; walk two or three steps to W/C; then up in W/C for dinner; encourage to shift weight in W/C every 15 minutes
1900	Prone position in bed with legs fully extended
2000	Fowler's position in bed
2200	Left lateral position in bed
2400	Right lateral position in bed

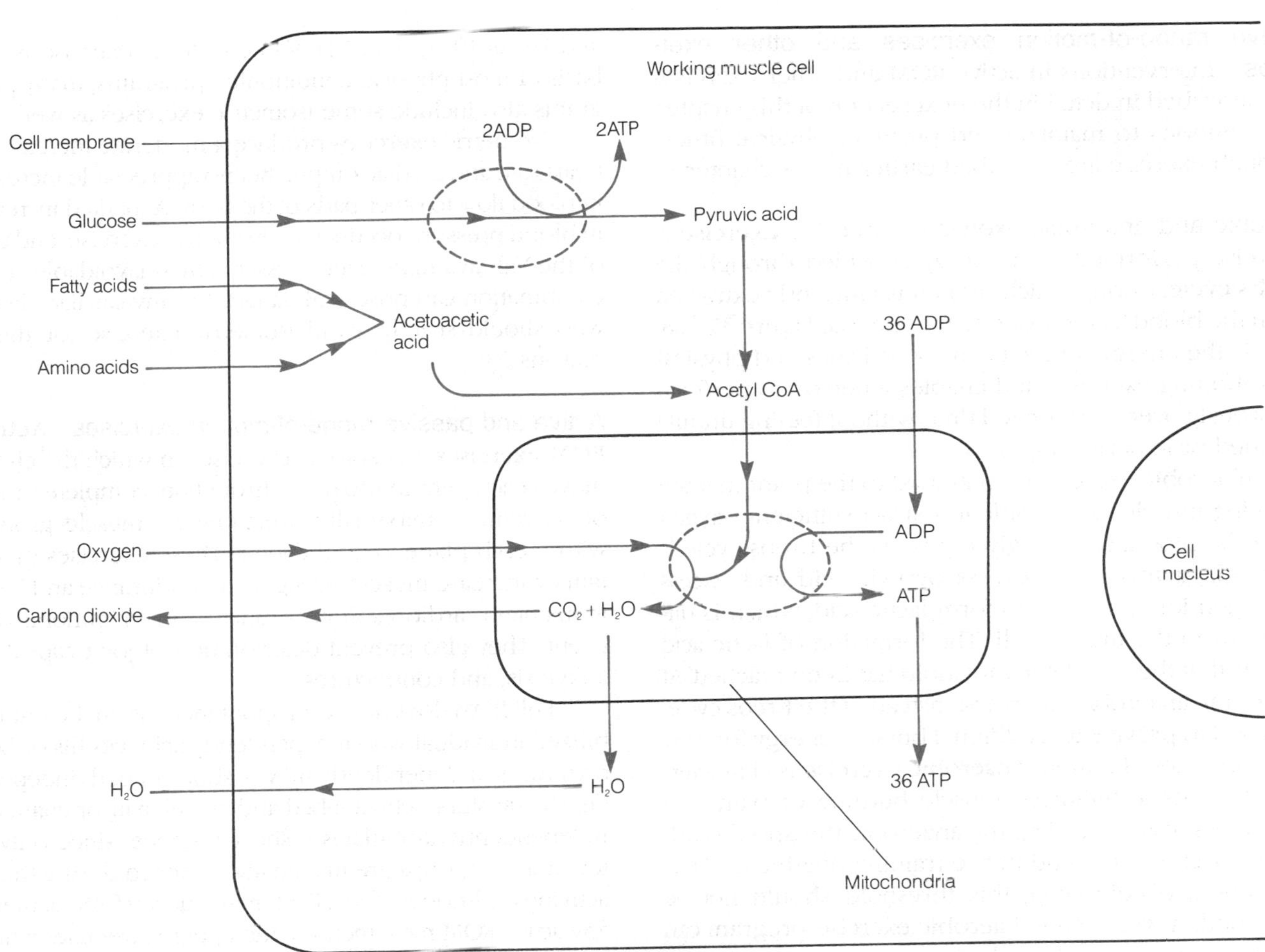

Figure 37–68 The Krebs Cycle: The formation of adenosine triphosphate (ATP), the energy used to produce muscle work in aerobic exercise

Source: Adapted from A. C. Guyton, *Textbook of medical physiology*, 7th ed. (Philadelphia: W. B. Saunders Co.), p. 22.

feet and legs to turn and position themselves in bed and to use the side rails or an overhead trapeze to become more independent in these activities. Clients in wheelchairs should be taught to shift their weight from one ischial tuberosity to the other every 15 minutes or so to relieve pressure. The top bed linens over the foot of the bed should be loose so that they do not restrict leg and foot movement, and unnecessary pillows or other encumbrances on the bed should be removed, as they may restrict movement.

Weight-bearing activity Interventions for assisting clients to ambulate with or without devices to aid them are outlined in Chapter 39. Early ambulation is practiced almost universally today. In other words, the client is helped to get out of bed and assisted to walk as soon as possible after surgery or any period of immobility. First the client sits up in bed, then on the side of the bed. Then the client is assisted out of bed to stand and move into a chair. Finally, the client is made to walk with assistance. Distances are gradually increased. Many postoperative clients are ambulatory on the day of surgery or the day after surgery.

Standing and walking not only fully extend the hip and knee joints but also produce the stress of weight-bearing to halt calcium loss from bone. Clients who do not have the strength or balance to stand and walk can be assisted to achieve passive weight-bearing through the use of a tilt table or CircOlectric bed. Clients are strapped into these special beds, which are then tilted to a vertical position, allowing the client to stand and bear weight.

Independence in activities of daily living Clients need to be encouraged to become as independent as possible as soon as possible without being made to face the frustration of attempting ADLs they cannot yet handle successfully.

Carefully assessing for activity intolerance during the client's performance of ADLs is useful for encouraging steady progress toward greater independence. Nurses need to teach clients to monitor their heart rates before, during, and after an activity. The client should be taught the signs and symptoms of activity intolerance (fatigue, dizziness, chest pain, shortness of breath, or profuse perspiration) and be warned to stop activity if these signs and symptoms occur.

Active range-of-motion exercises and other exercises Interventions in active ROM and other exercises are described in detail in the next section of this chapter. Interventions to maintain and promote physical fitness through exercise are described earlier in this chapter.

Aerobic and anaerobic exercises **Aerobic exercise** is exercise performed with energy provided through the **Krebs cycle**, during which oxygen is efficiently extracted from the blood by the working muscle. See Figure 37–68. This is the energy source for most activities and physical conditioning exercises and enables a person to perform vigorously over a prolonged time without feeling unduly fatigued or experiencing pain.

If aerobic exercise is continued to the point that the working muscles are unable to extract sufficient oxygen from the blood, aerobic glycolysis via the Krebs cycle is stopped. At this point, excess pyruvic acid and excess hydrogen ions combine to form lactic acid, which is diffused from the muscle cell. The formation of lactic acid signals that the anaerobic threshold has been reached. At this point, anaerobic pathways, instead of the Krebs cycle, are used to provide an additional burst of energy for only a few minutes' duration. **Anaerobic exercise** is characterized by muscle tightness, muscle burning or pain, and breathlessness. Exceeding the anaerobic threshold is primarily useful in the endurance training of athletes. During fitness conditioning, this threshold should not be exceeded. A well-planned aerobic exercise program can improve a person's maximal oxygen uptake, an important measure of physical fitness, by 20% to 30% (Pender 1982, p. 234).

Isotonic and isometric exercises **Isotonic** (dynamic) **exercises** are those in which muscle tension is constant and the muscle shortens to produce muscle contraction and movement. Most physical conditioning exercises—running, walking, swimming, cycling, and other activities—are isotonic, as are ADLs and active ROM exercises.

Isotonic exercises increase muscle strength and endurance and can improve cardiorespiratory function. During isotonic exercise, both heart rate and cardiac output quicken to increase blood flow to all parts of the body. Little or no change in blood pressure occurs.

Isometric (static or setting) **exercises** are those in which there is a change in muscle tension but no change in muscle length. No muscle or joint movement occurs. These exercises are useful for strengthening abdominal, gluteal, and leg muscles. When an immobilized client's leg is confined in a cast or traction, isometric exercises may help to maintain muscle strength in the affected limb. Isometric exercises may be useful for strengthening arm muscles in preparation for crutch-walking. These exercises are most effective in increasing muscle strength when five maximal tensions are achieved in succession, each lasting 5 seconds with 2 minutes rest in between (Brower and Hicks 1972, p. 1252). While isotonic exercise is the basis of most physical conditioning programs, many programs also include some isometric exercises as well.

Isometric exercises produce a moderate increase in heart rate and cardiac output, but no appreciable increase in blood flow to other parts of the body. A marked increase in blood pressure occurs with isometric exercise, and use of the Valsalva maneuver is essentially unavoidable. This combination can pose real danger for any cardiac client, who should strictly avoid isometric exercise for these reasons.

Active and passive range-of-motion exercises **Active ROM exercises** are isotonic exercises in which the client moves each joint in the body through its complete range of movement, maximally stretching all muscle groups within each plane, over the joint. These exercises maintain or increase muscle strength and endurance and help to maintain cardiorespiratory function in an immobilized client. They also prevent deterioration of joint capsules, ankylosis, and contractures.

Full ROM does not occur spontaneously in the immobilized individual who independently achieves his or her own ADLs, independently moves about in bed, independently transfers between bed and wheelchair or chair, or independently ambulates a short distance, since only a few muscle groups are maximally stretched during these activities. Although the client may successfully achieve few active ROM movements of the upper extremities while combing the hair, bathing, and dressing, the immobilized client is very unlikely to achieve any active ROM movements of the lower extremities when these are not used in their normal functions of standing and walking about. For this reason, most wheelchair and many ambulatory clients need active ROM exercises until they regain their normal activity levels (Kelly 1966, p. 2212).

A physician's order for ROM exercises is usually required if a client has an abnormal or injured musculoskeletal part or if the client's overall condition could be compromised by exercise. A nursing order is expected before beginning preventive exercises involving an otherwise normal musculoskeletal system that is suffering from the consequences of immobility.

The nurse encourages the client to perform each ROM exercise to the point of slight resistance, but not beyond, and never to the point of discomfort. The client should perform the movements systematically, using the same sequence during each session.

At first, the nurse may need to help the client perform the needed ROM exercises; eventually, the client may be able to accomplish these independently, with only periodic guidance from the nurse.

During **passive ROM exercises**, another person moves each of the client's joints through their complete range of movement, maximally stretching all muscle groups within each plane over each joint. Since the client does

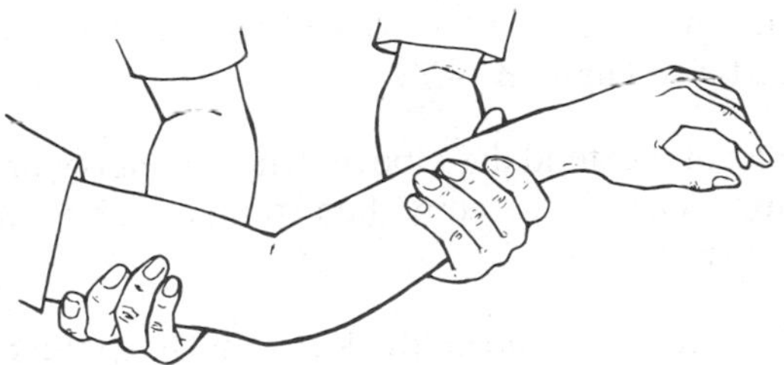

Figure 37–69 Supporting a limb above and below the joint, for passive exercise

not contract the muscle, passive ROM exercises are of no value in maintaining muscle strength but are useful in maintaining joint flexibility (Brower and Hicks 1972, p. 1253). For this reason, passive ROM exercises should be performed only when the client is unable to accomplish the movements actively.

Passive ROM exercises should be accomplished for each movement of the arms, legs, and neck that the client is unable to achieve actively. As with active ROM exercises, passive ROM exercises should be accomplished to the point of slight resistance, but not beyond, and never to the point of discomfort. The movements should be systematic, and the same sequence should be followed during each exercise session. Each exercise should consist of three repetitions, and the series of exercises should be done twice daily (Kottke 1982, p. 398). Performing one series of exercises along with the bath is helpful.

Passive ROM exercises are accomplished most effectively when the client lies on his or her back in bed. The client should wear a loose gown and be covered with a bath blanket. The bed should be at an appropriate height for the nurse. The nurse supports the client's limbs below the joints (see Figure 37–69) or supports them by cupping and cradling (see Figure 37–70). Neck hyperextension movements should be avoided in the elderly immobilized person, as they can cause painful nerve damage (Hogan and Beland 1976, p. 1106). To hyperextend the client's shoulder and hip, the nurse turns the client onto his or her side, facing away from the nurse. The shoulder or hip is then moved backward, directly toward the nurse. See Procedure 37–2. The needed passive ROM exercises should be incorporated into the client's plan of care.

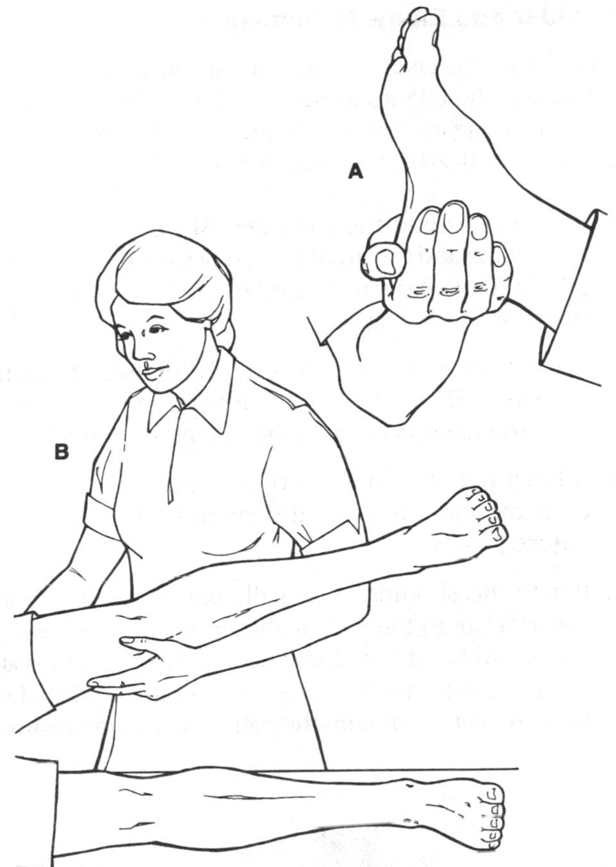

Figure 37–70 Holding limbs for support during passive exercise: **A**, cupping; **B**, cradling

If muscle spasms occur during passive ROM, the movement should be stopped temporarily. Continuous gentle pressure should be applied until the muscle relaxes and movement can slowly proceed. Consultation with a physical therapist is especially useful for nurses working with clients who have such spasms.

An automatic passive ROM machine is occasionally used for clients recovering from knee surgery. The machine provides continuous exercise and is set to move the knee to a prescribed degree over a prescribed time.

Procedure 37–2 ▲ Providing Passive Range-of-Motion Exercises

Intervention

1. Assist the client to a supine position on your side of the bed, and expose the body parts requiring exercise. Place the client's feet together, place the arms at the sides, and leave space around the head and the feet.

   Rationale Positioning the client close to the nurse prevents excessive reaching.

2. Return to the starting position after each motion. Repeat each motion five times.

Shoulder and Elbow Movement

Begin each exercise with the client's arm at his or her side. Grasp the client's arm beneath the elbow with one hand and beneath the wrist with the other hand unless otherwise indicated. See Figure 37–71.

3. Flex and extend the shoulder: Move the arm up to the ceiling and toward the head of the bed. See Figure 37–72. The elbow may need to be flexed if the headboard is in the way.
4. Abduct the shoulder: Move the arm away from the body (see Figure 37–73) and toward the client's head until the hand is over the head (see Figure 37–74).
5. Adduct the shoulder: Move the arm over the body until the hand touches the client's other hand. See Figure 37–75.
6. Rotate the shoulder internally and externally: Place the arm out to the side at shoulder level (90° abduction), and bend the elbow so that the forearm is at a right angle to the mattress. See Figure 37–76. Move the forearm down until the palm touches the mattress and then up until the back of the hand touches the bed. See Figure 37–77.
7. Flex and extend the elbow: Bend the elbow until the fingers touch the chin, then straighten the arm. See Figure 37–78.
8. Pronate and supinate the forearm: Grasp the client's hand as for a handshake and turn the palm upward (see Figure 37–79) and downward (see Figure 37–80), ensuring that only the forearm, not the shoulder, moves.

Wrist and Hand Movement

For wrist and hand exercises, flex the client's arm at the elbow until the forearm is at a right angle to the mattress. Support the wrist joint with one hand while your other hand manipulates the joint and the fingers. See Figure 37–81.

9. Hyperextend the wrist, and flex the fingers: Bend the wrist backward and at the same time flex the fingers,

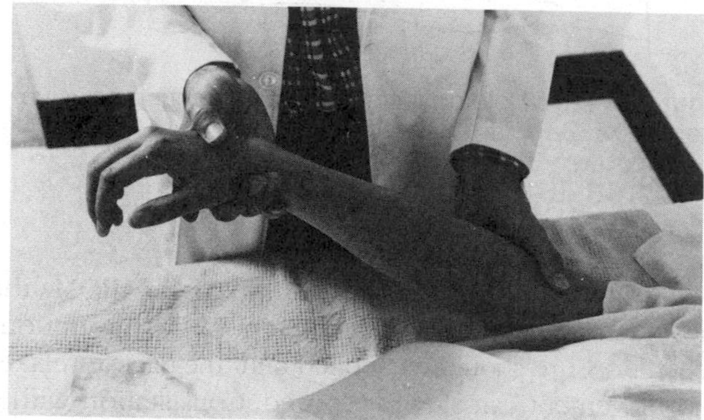

Figure 37–71

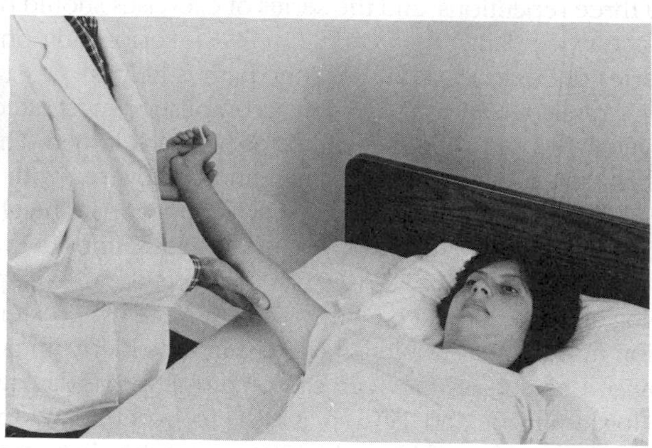

Figure 37–73

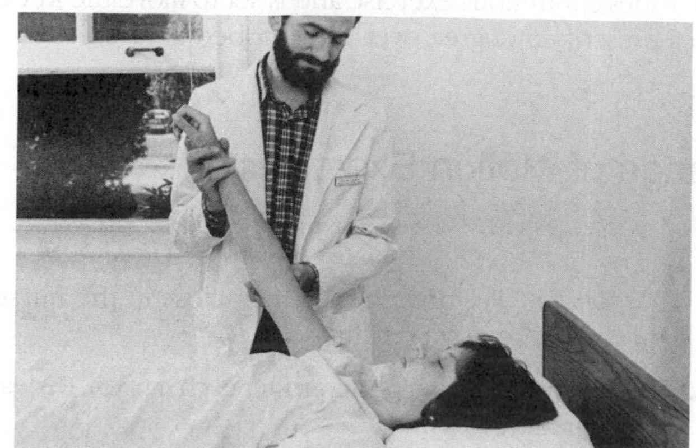

Figure 37–72

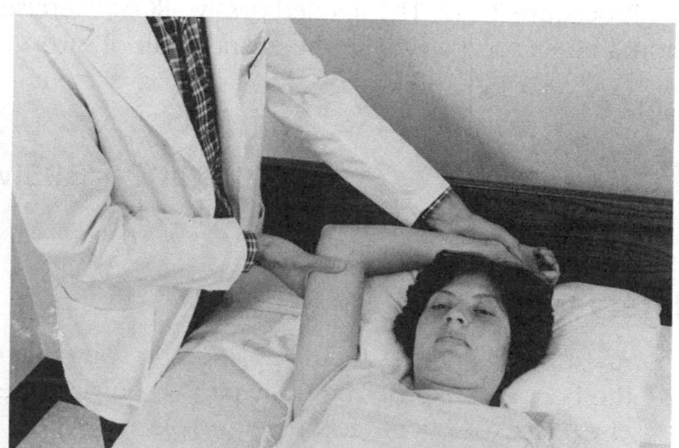

Figure 37–74

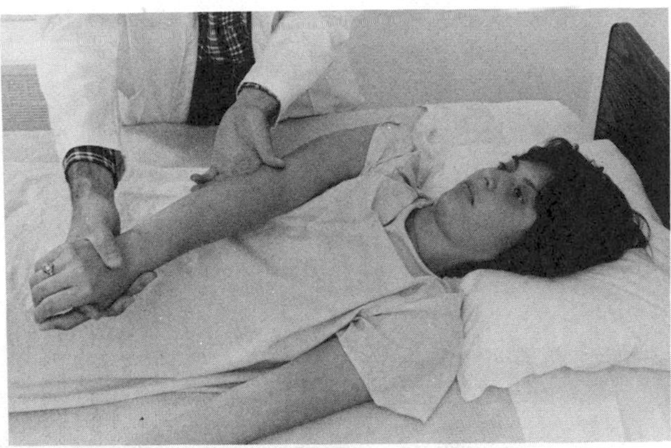

Figure 37–75

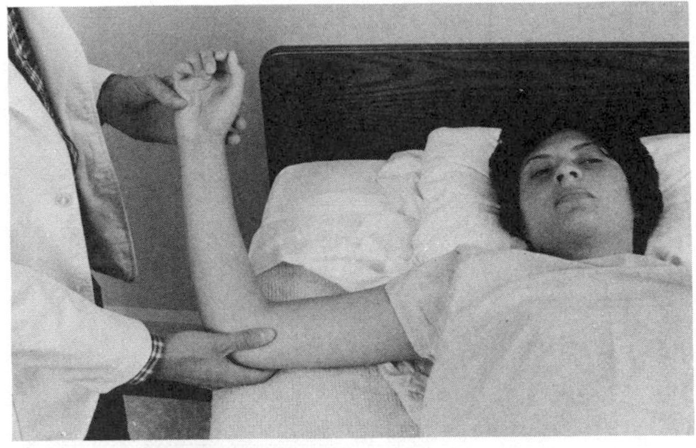

Figure 37–77

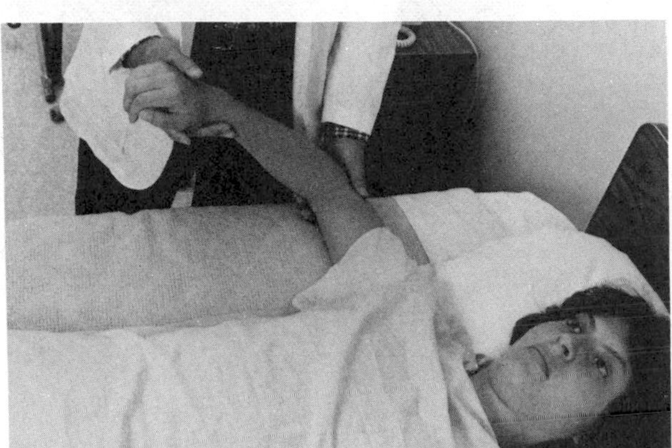

Figure 37–76

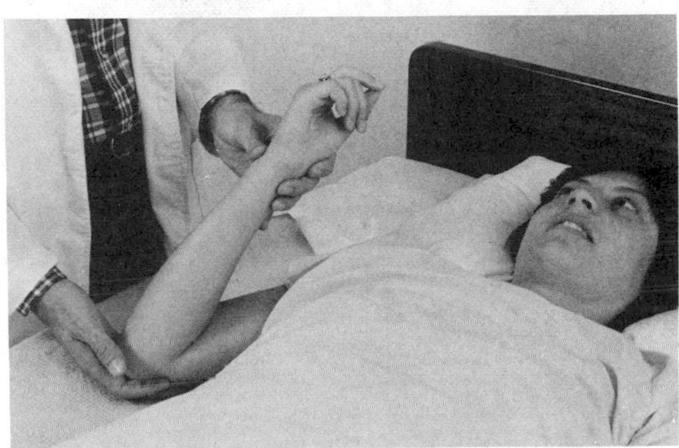

Figure 37–78

moving the tips of the fingers to the palm of the hand. See Figure 37–82. Align the wrist in a straight line with the arm and place your fingers over the client's fingers to make a fist. Then, with the wrist straight, flex it laterally toward the thumb side and then to the opposite side.

10. Flex the wrist and extend the fingers: Bend the wrist forward and at the same time extend the fingers. See Figure 37–83.

11. Abduct and oppose the thumb: Move the thumb away from the fingers and then across the hand toward the base of the little finger. See Figure 37–84.

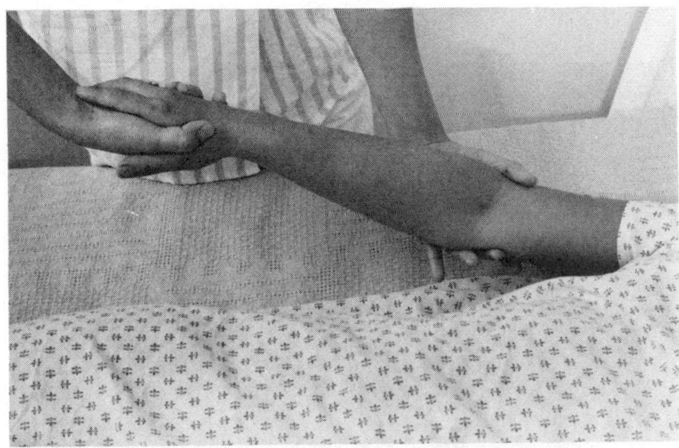

Figure 37–79

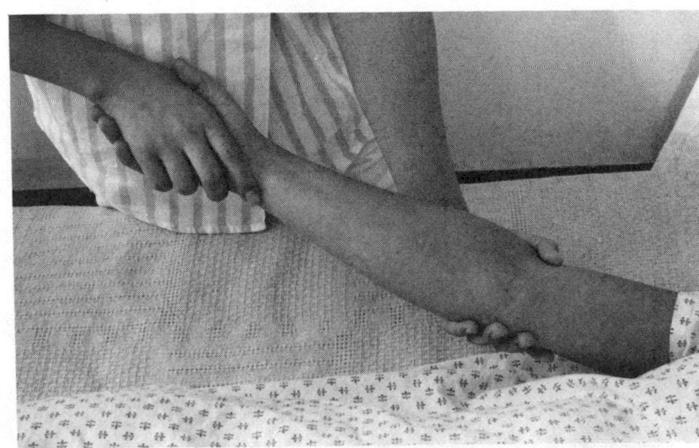

Figure 37–80

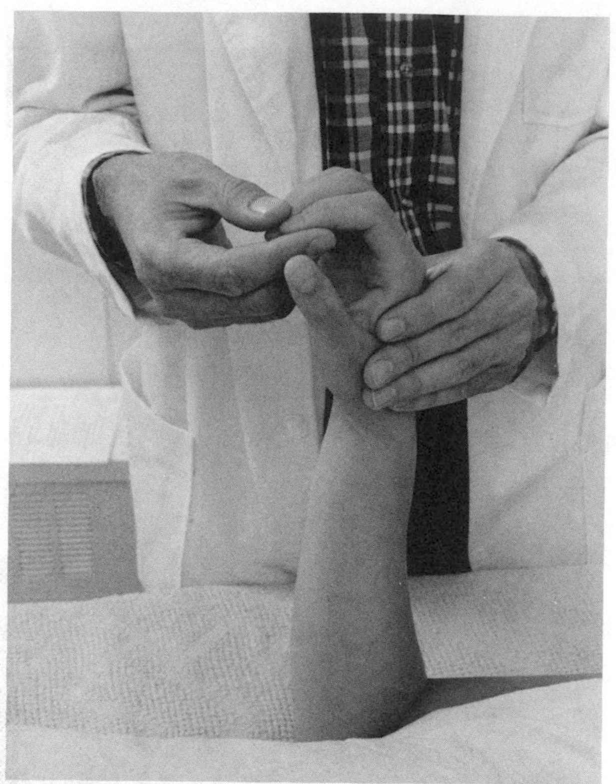

Figure 37–81

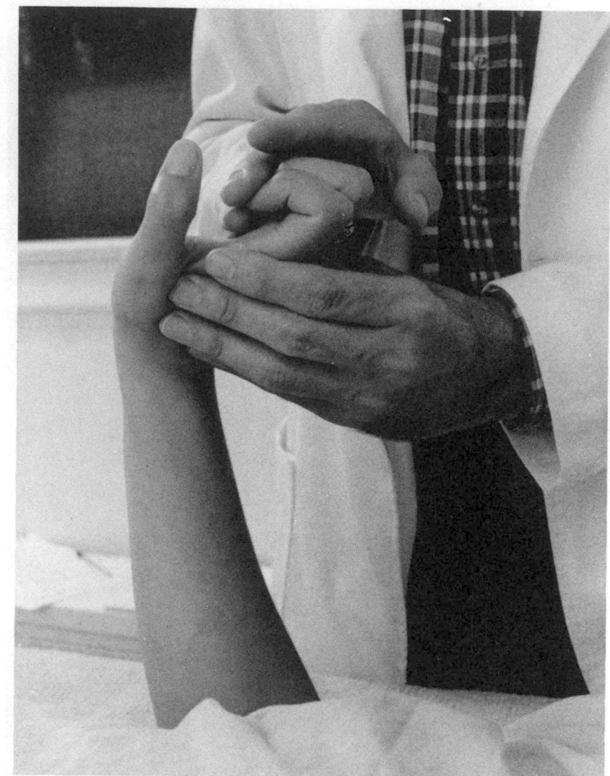

Figure 37–82

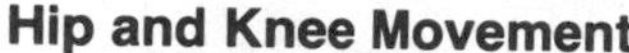

Hip and Knee Movement

To carry out hip and knee exercises, place one hand under the client's knee and the other under the ankle. See Figure 37–85.

12. Flex and extend the hip and knee: Lift the leg and bend the knee, moving the knee up toward the chest as far as possible. Bring the leg down, straighten the knee, and lower the leg to the bed. See Figure 37–86.

13. Abduct and adduct the hip: Move the leg to the side, away from the client (see Figure 37–87) and back across in front of the other leg (see Figure 37–88).

14. Rotate the hip internally and externally: Roll the leg inward (see Figure 37–89), then outward (see Figure 37–90).

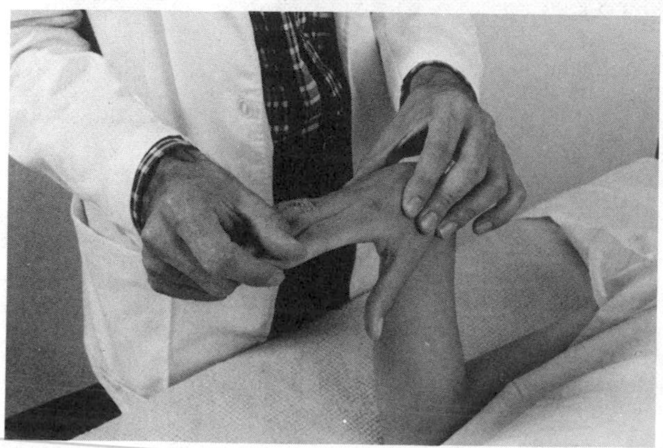

Figure 37–83

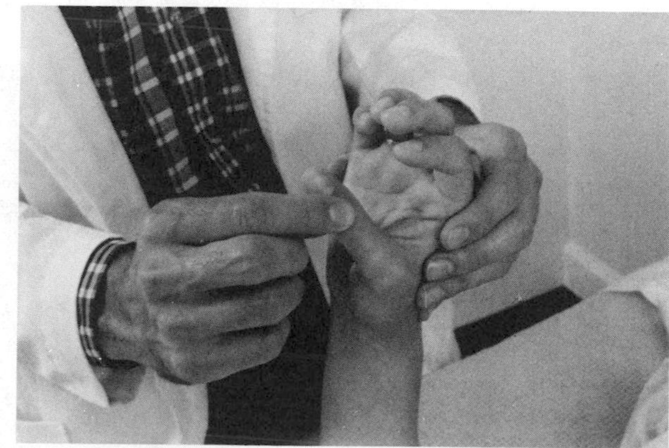

Figure 37–84

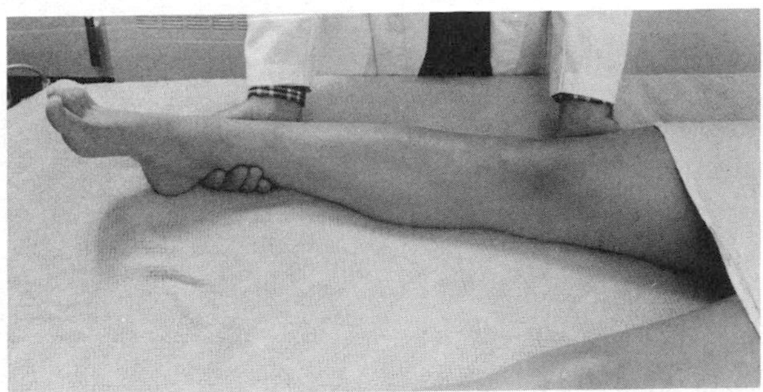

Figure 37–85

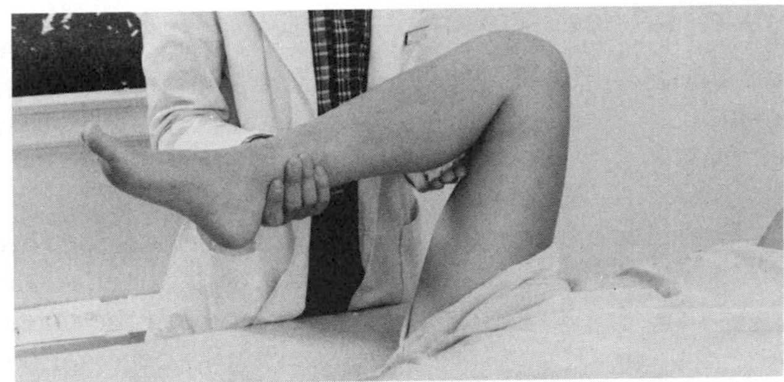

Figure 37–86

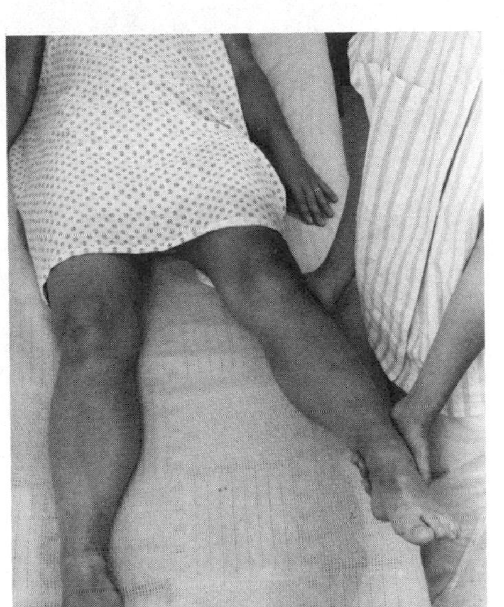

Figure 37–87

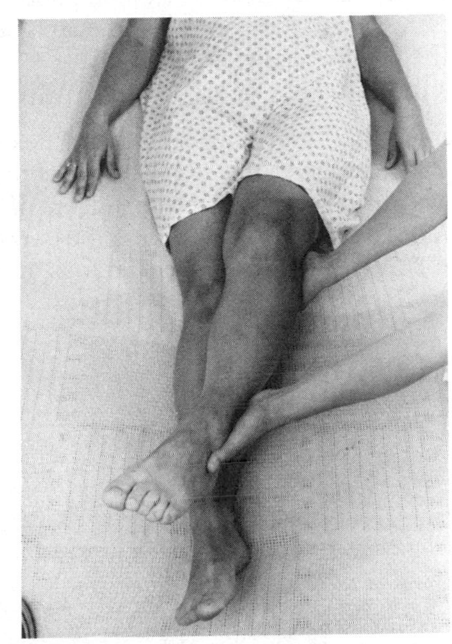

Figure 37–88

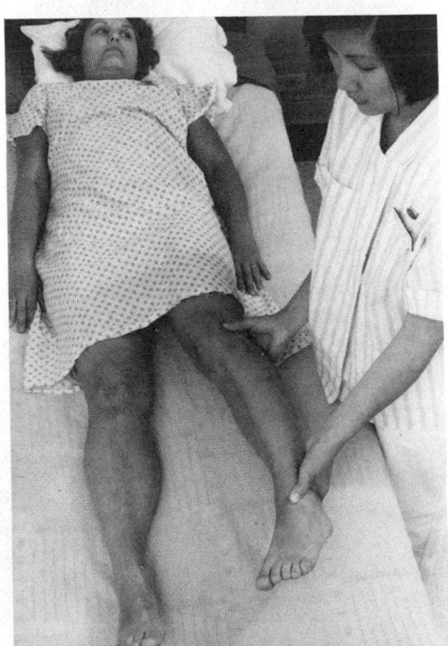

Figure 37–89

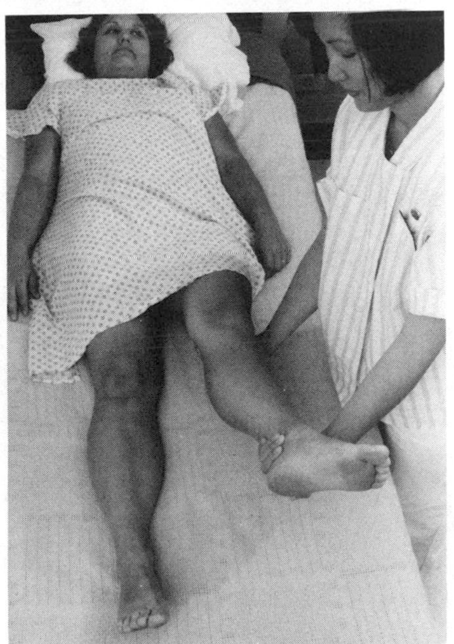

Figure 37–90

Ankle and Foot Movement

For ankle and foot exercises, place your hands in the positions described, depending on the motion to be achieved.

15. Dorsiflex the foot and stretch the Achilles tendon (heel cord): Place one hand under the client's heel, resting your inner forearm against the bottom of the client's foot. Place the other hand under the knee to support it. Press your forearm against the foot to move it upward toward the leg. See Figure 37–91.
16. Invert and evert the foot: Place one hand under the client's ankle and the other over the arch of the foot. Turn the whole foot inward (see Figure 37–92), then turn it outward (see Figure 37–93).
17. Plantar flex the foot and extend and flex the toes: Place one hand over the arch of the foot to push the foot away from the leg. Place the fingers of the other hand under the toes, to bend the toes upward (see Figure 37–94), and then over the toes, to push the toes downward (see Figure 37–95).

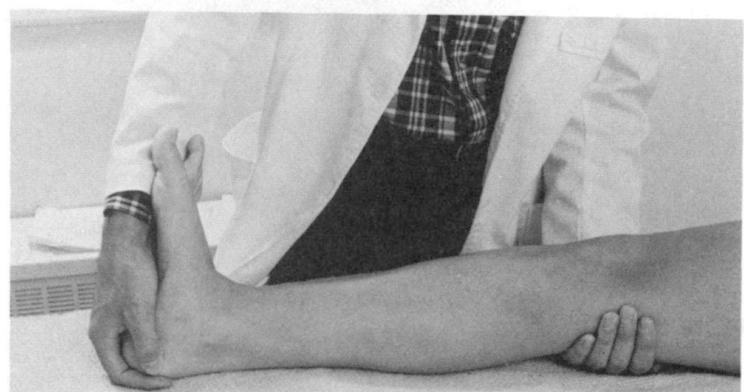

Figure 37–91

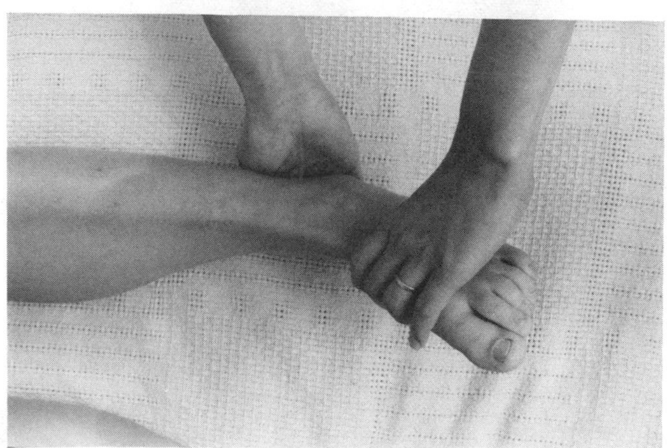

Figure 37–92

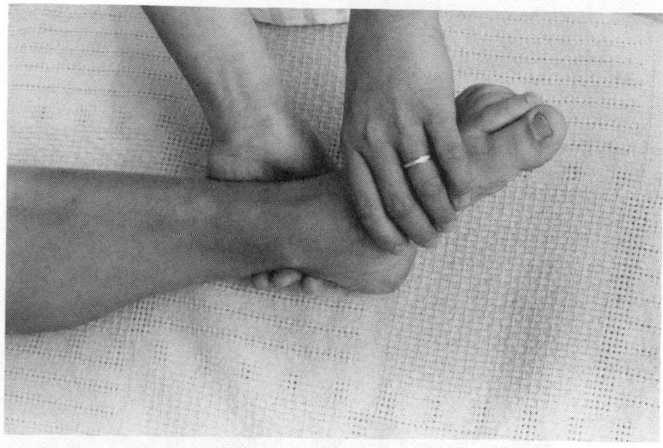

Figure 37–93

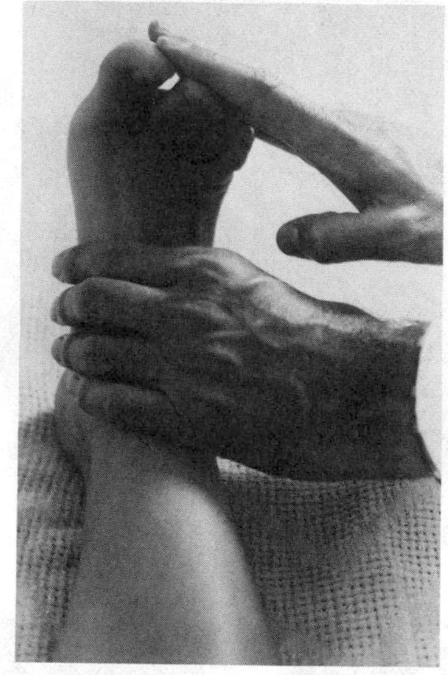

Figure 37–94

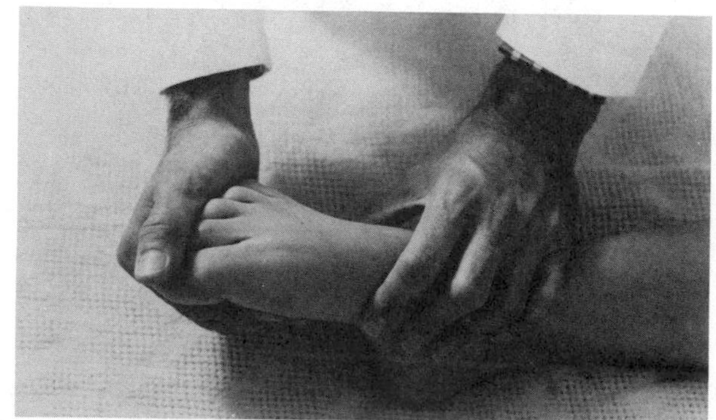

Figure 37–95

Neck Movement

Remove the client's pillow.

18. Flex and extend the neck: Place the palm of one hand under the client's head and the palm of the other hand on the client's chin. Move the head forward until the chin rests on the chest, then back to the resting supine position without the head pillow. See Figure 37–96.
19. Rotate the neck: Place the heels of the hands on each side of the client's cheeks. Move the top of the head to the right and to the left. See Figure 37–97.

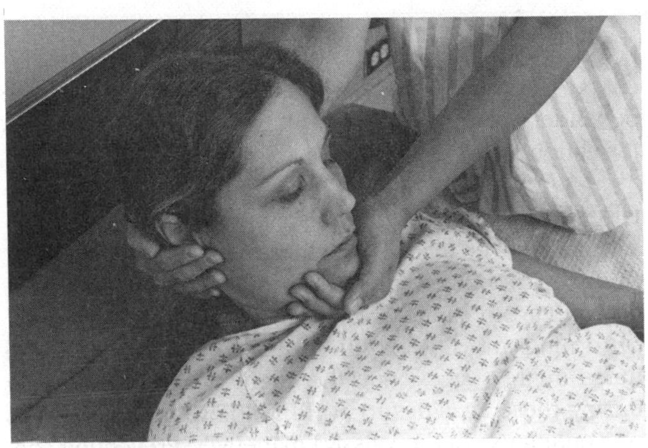

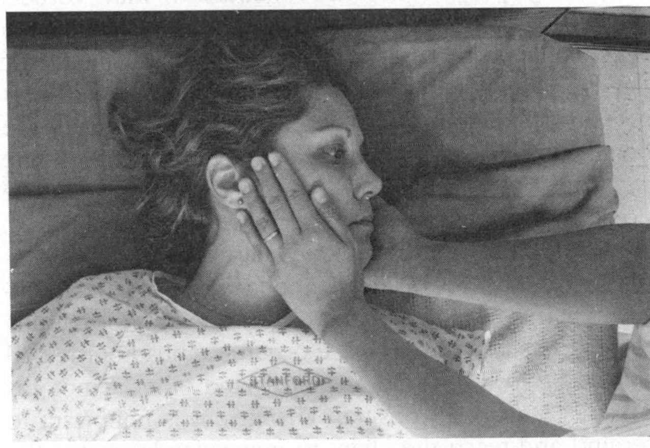

Hyperextension Movements

20. Assist the client to a prone or lateral position on your side of the bed.
21. Hyperextend the shoulder: Place one hand on the shoulder to keep it from lifting off the bed and the other under the client's elbow. Pull the upper arm up and backward. See Figure 37–98.

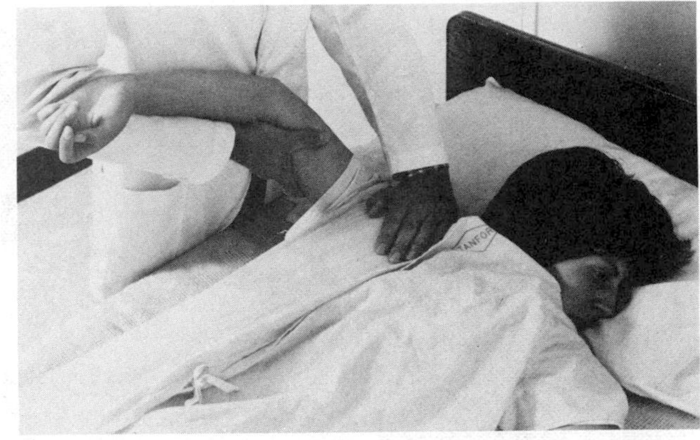

Figure 37–98

22. Hyperextend the hip: Place one hand on the hip to stabilize it and keep it from lifting off the bed. With the other arm and hand, cradle the lower leg over the forearm, and cup the knee joint with the hand. Move the leg backward from the hip joint. See Figure 37–99.
23. Hyperextend the neck: Remove the pillow. With the client's face down, place one hand on the forehead and the other on the back of the skull. Move the head backward. See Figure 37–100.

Following the Exercises

24. Take the client's pulse rate to assess his or her endurance of the exercise.
25. Report to the responsible nurse unusual problems or notable changes in the client's movements, e.g., rigidity or contractures.

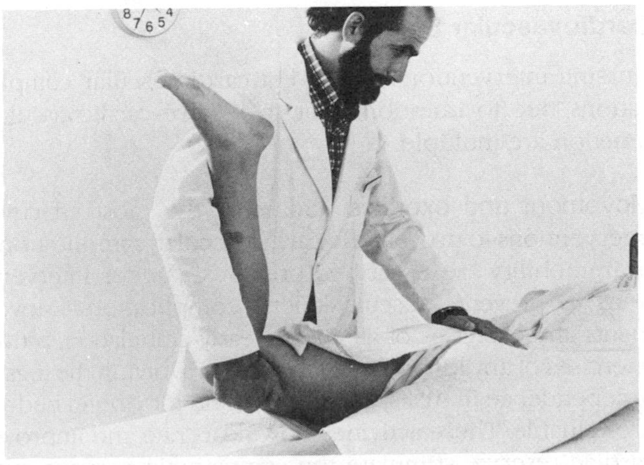

Figure 37–99

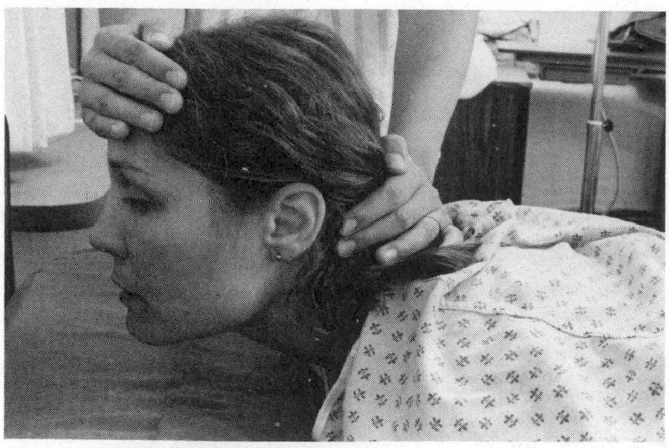

26. Record appreciable changes or difficulties in the client's movements.

Sample Recording

Date	Time	Notes
June 14/87	1100	Passive exercises provided to R leg and foot. Full ROM in hip, knee, and ankle.——— ————Sally S. Ames, SN

♦ **Figure 37–100**

Active-assistive range-of-motion exercises During **active-assistive ROM exercises**, the client uses a stronger, opposite arm or leg to move each of the joints of a limb incapable of active motion. The client learns to support and move the weak arm or leg with the strong arm or leg as far as possible. Then the nurse continues the movement passively to its maximal degree. This activity increases active movement on the strong side of the client's body and maintains joint flexibility on the weak side. Such exercise is especially useful for stroke victims who are hemiplegic (paralyzed on one half of the body). Some clients who begin with passive ROM exercises after a disability progressively improve to use active-assistive ROM exercises, and finally active ROM exercises.

Resistive exercises **Resistive exercises** are a form of either isotonic or isometric exercise during which the client moves (isotonic) or tenses (isometric) against resistance. Resistive exercise is used in physical conditioning. Helping clients to push their feet against a footboard placed in the bed, lift weights, or use an overhead trapeze to lift themselves up toward the head of the bed are examples.

Cardiovascular System

Nursing interventions to prevent cardiovascular complications due to immobility or to restore cardiovascular function are multiple.

Movement and exercise Some of the most effective interventions to prevent the cardiovascular complications of immobility are described previously under interventions to prevent musculoskeletal complications. Movements and exercises of all kinds—early ambulation, active exercises of any kind (especially those involving the legs), independence in ADLs, and turning and moving in bed—are valuable. These activities slow heart rate and improve cardiac reserve, stimulate the sympathetic nervous system to restore peripheral vasoconstriction with postural changes, improve muscle tone and thus prevent or reduce dependent edema, and prevent thrombus and embolus formation.

Discouraging use of the Valsalva maneuver The Valsalva maneuver increases the stress placed on the heart of the immobilized client. The nurse should teach the client to avoid taking a deep breath and holding it prior to turning, moving, or lifting in bed. For instance, the nurse might suggest that the client count or even sing during these activities to avoid holding the breath, thus preventing use of the Valsalva maneuver. Preventing constipation reduces straining at stool and decreases the potential for use of the Valsalva maneuver.

Regaining peripheral vasoconstriction with vertical postures The period of immobility gives the nurse an opportunity to promote the recovery of the sympathetic nervous system and to assess its recovery before the client gets out of bed for the first time. Gradually increasing the height of the head of the bed for longer periods of time stimulates the peripheral vasoconstrictors. Meanwhile, the nurse carefully assesses for a decrease in blood pressure, a sudden or marked increase in heart rate, or client complaints of dizziness or lightheadedness, all of which indicate that the sympathetic nervous system has not yet fully regained its function. If these occur, the head of the bed should be lowered until dizziness and other symptoms subside. During all position changes, it is important to remind and teach the client to move slowly so that the sympathetic nervous system can adjust to the new posture.

Before the client gets out of bed the first time after a period of immobility, and while the client is still lying flat in bed, the nurse should measure and record baseline blood pressure and heart rate. These should again be measured after the client has been slowly moved into a high Fowler's position. If the client's heart rate and blood pressure remain stable when compared with baseline levels, and if the client does not complain of dizziness or lightheadedness in this position, the nurse helps the client to pivot slowly and sit on the edge of the bed with the feet supported on the floor. While the client sits in this "dangle" position, the nurse should again measure heart rate and blood pressure and compare them against baseline levels. The client is helped into his or her robe and slippers, and a transfer belt is placed around the client's waist. The belt provides a safe means for the nurse to control the client's movements and prevent injury if the client should faint.

Next, the nurse helps the client to stand at the bedside, where heart rate and blood pressure are again measured and compared to baseline levels. If the client's cardiovascular system seems stable, the client is then assisted to ambulate under the close supervision of the nurse, who holds onto the transfer belt and is prepared to take quick action if the client becomes lightheaded or dizzy. During the client's first experience out of bed after a period of immobility, it is prudent to have an assistant follow with a wheelchair in case the client experiences signs of orthostatic hypotension. In this event, the nurse quickly helps the client to sit down and place his or her head between the knees to relieve cerebral ischemia (lack of circulation to the brain), thus preventing a potentially dangerous fall. The nurse and client together should determine the duration and distance of this first ambulation.

When the client completes the ambulation and returns to bed, the nurse again measures heart rate and blood pressure and compares them to baseline levels. This measurement helps the nurse assess activity tolerance. These data are the basis for determining the duration and distance of the client's next ambulatory session.

Elastic stockings Elastic stockings or elastic bandages help to prevent orthostatic hypotension, pooling of blood in the leg veins causing vein dilation and engorgement, incompetent valves in the leg veins, and dependent edema and thrombus formation while improving venous return of blood to the heart. See Chapter 53, page 1625. The custom-fitted stockings are available in toe-to-knee length and in toe-to-mid-thigh length. They should be put on the legs after the client has been lying flat in bed with legs slightly elevated for 20 minutes. The stockings are removed twice daily for 20 to 30 minutes while skin care is given.

Automatic "pulsating" (pneumatic compression) stockings are occasionally used for very high-risk immobilized clients following certain kinds of surgery. The stockings exert continuous pressure against the leg, and a motor creates an additional pulsating, compressing movement that stimulates the leg muscles to contract, thus increasing venous return to the heart.

Protective leg positioning Proper alignment in standing, sitting, and bed-lying positions is described in Chapter 38. It is important to prevent undue pressure to the intimal lining of the veins since this pressure may cause injury, and thrombi often begin at the roughened, inflamed, and healing sites where injury has occurred. Improper positioning can create the pressure that causes intimal damage. Examples are positioning one leg directly on top of the other in the lateral (side-lying) position, placing undue pressure at the popliteal space behind the knee or intense point pressure anywhere along the calf, or sitting in one position or with the legs crossed for a prolonged time. Improper positioning can also impede venous circulation in the legs and impair venous return to the heart. The client should be taught to avoid garters or knee-high socks for similar reasons.

Immobilized persons should be encouraged to elevate their legs several times each day for 20 minutes to improve peripheral venous circulation and should be warned not to massage their calves. If a thrombus is present, massaging could dislodge it.

A thrombus suspected in a client's leg must be reported immediately. The client's leg should be elevated and the client prevented from ambulating, exercising, or massaging the leg. These activities could dislodge the thrombus, enabling it to migrate upward in the circulation.

Respiratory System

Nursing interventions for the respiratory system focus on increasing alveolar expansion, preventing stasis of respiratory secretions, maintaining a patent airway, and promoting adequate exchange of gases in the alveoli.

Deep-breathing and coughing exercises Performing deep-breathing and coughing exercises is an effective way to achieve all four goals for the respiratory system. See Chapter 45.

Diaphragmatic-abdominal breathing exercises Abdominal-diaphragmatic breathing exercises help decrease the amount of trapped, stagnant air in the alveoli and reduce the effort of breathing. While lying on the back, the client watches the abdomen, rather than the chest, rise with deep inspirations, and fall with slow, forceful contractions of the abdominal muscles. For additional information, see Chapter 45.

Turning, positioning, and exercise Changing the client's position allows previously dependent lung areas to expand and to drain by gravity. Pulmonary secretions in the alveoli, bronchi, and trachea are moved along the respiratory tract to a point where coughing can effectively expel them, reducing the potential for bacterial growth and hypostatic pneumonia. In addition, blood that has pooled in the dependent part of the lung can circulate after the client changes position, reducing the potential for vascular complications. To achieve these results, the client should change position every 1 to 2 hours. Any exercise that moves the chest from one position to another enhances these effects.

Postural drainage, a technique in which the client assumes a variety of postures to promote drainage by gravity from each lobe of each lung, promotes the drainage of respiratory secretions. In addition, the techniques of chest percussion and vibration, which require special skills, may be performed while the client assumes the positions for postural drainage. These techniques help to dislodge respiratory secretions and move them along the respiratory tract to a point where they can be removed by coughing. See Chapter 45.

Metabolism and Nutrition

Diet The immobilized client needs a diet that is high in protein, calories, and fiber. Protein is necessary to replace depleted body protein stores and to repair damaged tissue. Calories provide the fuel needed for energy and tissue repair; energy stores have been depleted by anorexia and by immobility itself. Fiber is needed to prevent or correct the constipation that often accompanies immobility.

Encouraging an anorexic client to eat is a challenge for the nurse. It is important to include (a) easily chewed and swallowed foods so that eating will not tire the client and (b) foods that the client especially enjoys. Favorite items prepared by family members or friends may improve both food intake and morale. Flavorful high-protein, high-calorie dietary supplements between meals are often useful.

Vitamin and mineral supplements Due to the decrease in overall food intake, the immobilized client often has reduced vitamin and mineral stores. The client needs mineral and vitamin supplements, especially those containing vitamin C, to help replace protein stores. It is important not to include excess calcium (and phosphate) because the body will not use this mineral to replace calcium lost from bone unless weight-bearing occurs. Instead, the excess calcium circulates in the blood and is excreted in the urine, increasing the complications caused by calcium loss from bone. Sources of vitamins and minerals include food given at meals, dietary supplements (many high-protein, high-calorie dietary supplements are also high in vitamins and minerals), and multivitamin with mineral tablets ordered by the physician.

Weight-bearing and exercise Weight-bearing is essential for replacing calcium and phosphate in bone. If possible, the nursing plan should include some weight-bearing activity for a few minutes each day. Any form of exercise helps to prevent muscle atrophy and protein loss.

Parenteral and enteral dietary supplements When the client is unable to eat, total parenteral nutrition (TPN), in which nutritional supplements are delivered through a central intravenous catheter, or nasogastric tube feeding, in which nutritional supplements are delivered directly into the gastrointestinal tract, may be necessary to prevent further debilitation and to restore energy levels so that the client can again eat.

Urinary and Endocrine Systems

Turning, repositioning, and exercise Frequent turning and repositioning reduce the amount of stagnant urine in the kidneys and bladder and help to achieve complete kidney and bladder emptying with each urination. Assisting the client to assume an upright sitting or, if possible, standing position several times each day is especially important to counteract the urinary stagnation and incomplete emptying. Exercise enhances this process and strengthens the muscles that control urination.

Improving hydration Improved hydration is especially important in preventing or reducing the effects of immobility on the urinary tract. Unless the client has a disease process that could be exacerbated by increased fluid intake, he or she should be encouraged to drink 2000 ml or more of fluid each day. Adequate intake increases the volume of urine flushing through the kidneys and bladder, reduces urinary stagnation, and lessens the risk of renal calculi formation and urinary tract infections.

Increased fluid intake, however, can increase the possibility of urinary retention and bladder distention. It is prudent to measure fluid intake and urinary output as well as the frequency and amount of urinations to assess for this potential complication.

If the immobilized client is incontinent, increased intake can make incontinent episodes more frequent. This, in turn, can increase the possibility for skin breakdown in the perineal area. If the client is incontinent, meticulous perineal care is essential to prevent skin breakdown and decubitus ulcer formation.

Perineal hygiene In any immobilized client, careful perineal hygiene is important in preventing urinary tract infections. Careful cleaning of the perineal area from front to back after each urination and scrupulous personal hygiene with soap and water at least twice daily reduce the likelihood of bladder infection.

Acidifying the urine Acidifying the urine reduces the potential for both renal calculi formation and urinary tract infections. One can lower urine pH by eating meat, eggs, cheese, whole grains, cranberries, prunes, and plums. Cranberry juice, readily available in most agencies, is effective in lowering urine pH. Foods that increase urine pH, such as carbonated drinks, foods containing baking powder or soda, and fruit juices, should be avoided. The physician may prescribe high doses of ascorbic acid, ammonium chloride, or aspirin to lower urine pH.

Position and relaxation for urination Nursing measures to facilitate urination, prevent urinary retention and bladder distention, and prevent urinary reflux from a distended bladder are essential in reducing the potential for urinary tract infections. An upright, natural posture during urination is especially important in achieving a normal urination pattern and complete bladder emptying. Enhancing relaxation and providing privacy during urination are also important.

Urinary catheterization When normal urination is not possible and the client's bladder is distended, catheterization is necessary before distention becomes so pronounced that bladder injury occurs. See Chapter 44.

Preventing urinary incontinence Urinary incontinence often occurs in immobilized, elderly clients who are dependent on others for assistance with toileting. Incontinence is more likely among clients who do not receive sufficient assistance with urination at sufficiently frequent intervals. Immobilized clients are more likely to be incontinent at night, when they are drowsy and haven't urinated for 4 or 5 hours. Providing sufficient fluid throughout the day so that fluids can be somewhat restricted after the evening meal helps reduce clients' need to urinate at night. Scheduling times for assistance with toileting every 2 hours (somewhat less frequently at night) reduces the incidence of incontinence. See Chapter 44.

Bowel Elimination

Some of the nursing interventions effective in facilitating urinary elimination are also effective in facilitating bowel elimination.

Movement and exercise Movement and exercise improve the tone and strength of the abdominal and perineal muscles used in defecation. Movement and exercise improve smooth muscle tone to enhance peristalsis. See Chapter 43 for further interventions to promote bowel evacuation.

Integumentary System

See the section on pressure sores later in this chapter.

Neurosensory System

Turning, repositioning, and exercise All movement increases motor activity and stimulates the proprioceptive sense organs.

Increasing tactile stimuli Any activity that increases stimulation and use of the tactile sensory organs is useful in preventing sensory deterioration or reducing its severity. Increasing client independence in ADLs and encouraging recreational and social activities that provide tactile stimulation are especially useful.

Social, Emotional, Intellectual, and Developmental Considerations

The social, emotional, intellectual, and developmental problems associated with immobility usually occur gradually and subtly. The skills of a perceptive, sensitive, knowledgeable, and caring nurse are needed to prevent or minimize their consequences.

Social considerations Social stimulation and interaction help to prevent withdrawal of the immobilized client. If possible, an immobilized client should share a room with a mobile, active person who has a similar life-style and values. If possible, the same group of nurses should be assigned to care for the client throughout his or her stay. Nurses and roommates who are honestly interested in the client as a person foster positive social interaction.

It is important, however, to promote positive relationships with family members, friends, coworkers, or others whose social contact the client values. The nurse encourages visits by the client's clergy or employer and, when possible, by the client's children or pets. Such visits reassure the client and reinforce a positive perception of his or her role in the family and work group. When visitors arrive, it is important to make them feel welcome. Chairs and privacy should be graciously provided. The nurse may also supply a telephone and letter-writing materials.

Emotional considerations Nurses strive to maintain client orientation and prevent disorientation, especially when the immobilized client is elderly. A clock with a large dial, a calendar marked so that the client can immediately determine the correct day, and a daily newspaper are useful in preventing disorientation related to time, day, or date. To prevent disorientation of person or place, the nurse frequently addresses the client by name, consistently reorients the client to the names of staff, and provides explanations about impending nursing activities, meal times, and other activities. Encouraging the client to wear a hearing aid, glasses, or contact lenses, if needed, helps to reduce sensory distortions.

Frequent interruptions in normal sleep patterns are tiring and predispose the immobilized client to anxiety, depression, or disorientation. It is important to plan nursing activities to minimize the interruption of sleep during the night.

Assisting an immobilized client to maintain his or her self-image as a worthwhile, independent, and productive individual is important. When possible, clients should be encouraged to attend to their own hygiene and wear their house clothes rather than institutional clothing, night clothes, or a bathrobe. Such clothing fosters a dependent, sick-role image. Attention to appearance—e.g., dentures, shaving, or wearing cosmetics—enhances self-image. It is especially important to encourage the client to become as independent in ADLs as possible. Placing toilet and personal items within easy reach increases the client's sense of independence. Demonstrating respect for the client's privacy and belongings helps to promote the client's self-image as a worthwhile person.

When the client provides cues of potential problems, the nurse should, in a nonjudgmental, accepting, and supportive manner, encourage the client to express feelings and concerns about his or her immobility, disease, dependent status, finances, work, family, and sexuality. The nurse must be a good listener. The nurse should also encourage the client to discuss these feelings with family members, close friends, or others whose judgment the client values. If cues suggest that the client is experiencing difficulty in coping with his or her situation, outside professional assistance and referral may be needed.

Intellectual concerns Helping the immobilized client to set realistic short- and long-term goals for recovery and to make rational plans for working toward these goals is a useful way to bolster the client's self-image and feelings of personal worth. The nurse should provide opportunities for the client to make choices and decisions about his or her own care and to solve problems and make plans for his or her own future during recovery.

Magazines, newspapers, books, television, and radio help the immobile client to maintain his or her intellectual capabilities. A project from home or work that requires the client's attention not only stimulates intellectual activity but also helps the client to achieve worthwhile, productive tasks that improve the client's sense of independence and self-worth.

Developmental concerns It is probably unrealistic to expect anyone of any age to continue making progress toward their developmental tasks during a period of immobility. This seems especially true of the immobilized elderly client.

With children, it is especially important to stimulate social and intellectual development as much as possible so that they will not lose ground in achievements made prior to the period of immobility. When possible, the nurse should place the immobilized child with more active children of the same age or provide opportunities to socialize with other children. Play activities sharpen fine motor and intellectual skills. Family members can help by providing favorite games, toys, and books. The nurse can encourage visits from the child's teacher or friends, and, if the child's health permits, the teacher can assign schoolwork. Of course, every opportunity for visits from the child's parents must be provided. Involving the child in decisions about his or her own care also helps to maintain intellectual skills.

After a period of immobility, elderly individuals often do not fully regain their former level of functional ability. For this reason, nurses should make every effort to help elderly clients maintain their previous level of independence during the period of immobility.

Evaluation

Examples of outcome criteria for clients with mobility problems are on the right.

Examples of Outcome Criteria for Clients with Mobility Problems

The client will:

- Have normal range of motion in right shoulder
- Have no skin problems as a result of immobilization
- Have less discomfort
- Express positive statements about sense of well-being

Pressure Sores

Pressure sores, also called decubitus ulcers (decubiti), bedsores, or distortion sores, are reddened areas, sores, or ulcers of the skin occurring over bony prominences. They are due to interruption of the blood circulation to the tissue, resulting in a localized ischemia. The tissue is caught between two hard surfaces, usually the surface of the bed and the bony skeleton. The localized ischemia means that the cells are deprived of oxygen and nutrients, and the waste products of metabolism accumulate in the cells. The tissue dies because of the resulting anoxia. Prolonged, unrelieved pressure also damages the small blood vessels. This appears to be the most significant injury caused by pressure (Torrance 1981a).

Etiology of Pressure Sores

Shannon (1984) describes three causes of pressure sores: pressure, friction, and shearing force. Usually, two causes must be present before a pressure sore develops.

Pressure

Pressure is the perpendicular force exerted on the skin by gravity. Lindan et al. (1965) found that for a person of ideal weight, the points of highest pressure in the supine position are the sacrum, buttocks, and heels. These areas support pressure of 40 to 60 mm Hg. Clients in the prone position have fewer areas of high pressure and more areas of low pressure than clients in the supine position do. The knees were found to support pressures up to 50 mm Hg. Clients in the sitting position experience the greatest pressure over the ischial tuberosities. These pressures range up to 75 mm Hg (Lindan et al. 1965). Husian (1953) found that evenly distributed pressure over a larger area is less injurious than localized pressure to a very small area and that low pressure over a long period is more damaging than high pressure for a short period. Because the normal hydrostatic pressure of blood in the capillaries is 32 mm Hg at the arteriole end and 15 mm Hg at the venous end, the pressure placed on the skin exceeds these pressures, obstructing the capillaries.

After the skin has been compressed, it appears white, as if the blood had been squeezed out of it. A white person's skin loses its pink color in the affected area, and a black person's skin is also less pink, although the change is more difficult to see.

When pressure is relieved, the skin takes on a bright red flush, called **reactive hyperemia**, which is the body's mechanism for preventing pressure ulcers. The flush is due to vasodilation; extra blood floods to the area to compensate for the preceding period of impeded blood flow. The blood carries oxygen and removes the accumulated metabolic wastes. Reactive hyperemia is effective only if the pressure is relieved before irreversible changes occur in the tissues and blood vessels. The hyperemia is also thought to reduce the risk of microvascular thrombosis (Smith 1978) and to increase the sensitivity of the nerve endings in the area so that further injury to the area can be avoided or reduced (Lowthian 1982).

Reactive hyperemia usually lasts one half to three quarters as long as the duration of impeded blood flow to the area (Shannon 1984). If the redness disappears in that time, no tissue damage can be anticipated. If, however, the redness does not disappear, then tissue damage has occurred.

Friction

Friction is a force acting parallel to the skin. For example, when a client pulls up in bed, the skin rubbing against the sheet creates friction. Friction can abrade the skin, i.e., remove the superficial layers, making it more prone to breakdown.

Shearing Force

Shearing force is a combination of friction and pressure. It occurs commonly when a client assumes a Fowler's position in bed. In this position, the body tends to slide downward toward the foot of the bed. This downward movement is transmitted to the sacral bone and the deep tissues. At the same time, the skin over the sacrum tends not to move because of the friction between the skin and the bedsheets. The skin and superficial tissues are thus relatively unmoving in relation to the bed surface, whereas the deeper tissues are firmly attached to the skeleton and move downward. This causes a shearing force in the area where the deeper tissues and the superficial tissues meet. The force damages the blood vessels and tissues in this area.

Pathogenesis of Pressure Sores

Pressure sores can be categorized as superficial or deep (Ahmed 1980). **Superficial ulcers** start at the skin with excoriation. If left untreated, superficial ulcers can penetrate to deeper tissue layers. **Deep ulcers** start in underlying tissues over a bony prominence and extend upward to the surface. Initially, deep ulcers may not be obvious except as a dusky redness even though the destruction of underlying tissue may be extensive. It may take several days before the pressure is apparent (Norton 1975). See Figure 37–101.

Guttmann (1955) proposes six stages in the development of pressure sores.

1. Transient circulatory disturbance. This stage is reversible: the reddening of the skin when the pressure is relieved. See the discussion of reactive hyperemia in the section "Etiology of Pressure Sores."
2. Permanent damage to superficial blood vessels and tissue. Redness and congestion of the area do not disappear with relief of the pressure. The superficial skin layers may be blistered or excoriated. If the deeper tissues are involved, superficial necrosis and ulcers may result.
3. Deep penetrating necrosis. Destruction extends to subcutaneous tissue, including fascia, muscle, and bone.

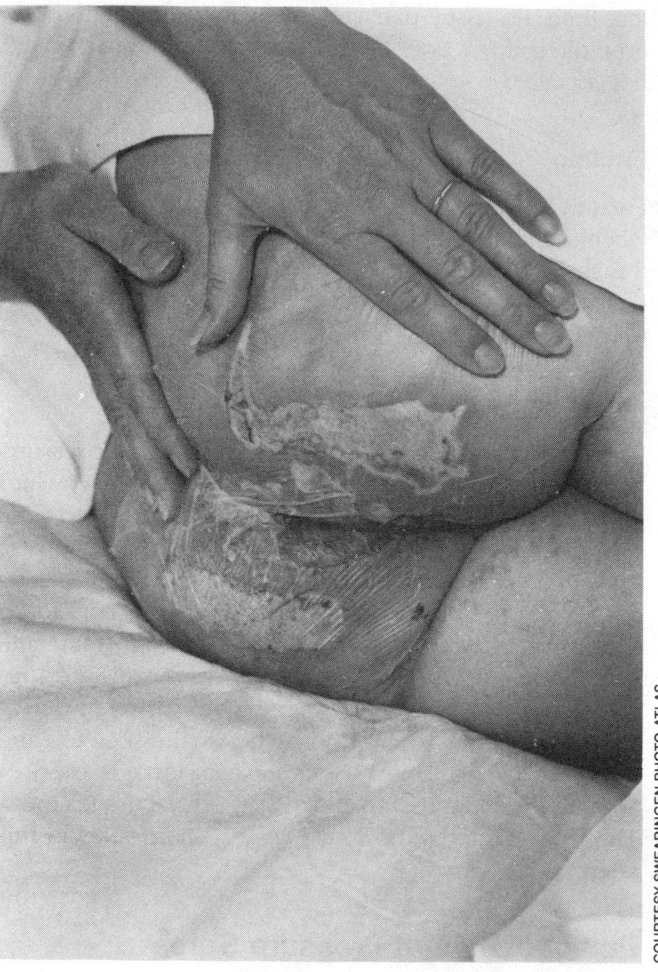

COURTESY SWEARINGEN PHOTO-ATLAS

Figure 37–101 The decubitus ulcers on the buttocks of this patient are covered with a transparent protective dressing.

This stage usually develops over the sacrum and trochanters.

4. Infection of the pressure sore. Mixed infections are common with microorganisms such as *Staphylococcus aureus,* beta hemolytic *Streptococcus, Proteus,* and *Escherichia coli.*
5. Closed ischial bursa. The skin over the bursa becomes ischemic and necrotic, and a sinus sore develops.
6. Cancerous degeneration of the sore. This is a rare complication of a pressure sore.

Of Guttmann's six stages, the last three are in effect complications of a pressure sore.

Byrne and Feld (1984) define four stages of decubitus ulcers:

1. Pinkish-red mottled skin that does not return to normal color after the pressure is relieved
2. Cracked, blistered, broken skin; shallow to full-thickness skin injury
3. Broken skin with tissue involvement, exudate (usually), and a distinct ulcer
4. Extensive ulceration with penetration to the muscle and bone; necrotic tissue and profuse drainage usually present

Factors Affecting the Formation of Pressure Sores

Six factors affect the formation of decubitus ulcers: moisture, hygiene, nutrition, body heat, anemia, and mobility.

Moisture

Moisture due to urine, feces, drainage, and perspiration reduces the resistance of the skin to other forces, such as friction. The presence of moisture, e.g., due to incontinence, was found to be the single most reliable indicator of future development of a pressure sore (Exton-Smith et al. 1962).

Hygiene

Good hygiene reduces the number of microorganisms present on the skin. Bacteria localize in ischemic tissue, which is a good medium for their growth, and the presence of bacteria increases the severity of the sore and its rate of development (Berecek 1975).

Nutrition

Nutritional factors are crucial in the development of decubitus ulcers. Generally, prolonged inadequate nutrition causes weight loss, muscle atrophy, and the loss of subcutaneous tissue. These three occurrences reduce the amount of padding between the skin and the bones, thereby increasing the risk of pressure sore development. More specifically, hypoproteinemia (abnormally low protein content in the blood), either due to inadequate intake or abnormal loss, results in negative nitrogen balance, which predisposes the client to dependent edema. The presence of edema makes skin more prone to injury by decreasing its elasticity, resilience, and vitality. Edema also slows the diffusion of oxygen to the tissue cells and metabolites away from the cells because of the increased distance between the capillaries and the cells. Vitamin C is essential for healing tissue damage due to pressure.

Body Heat

Body heat is a factor in the development of pressure sores. **Pyrexia** (elevated body temperature) increases the body's metabolic rate, thus increasing the need of the cells for oxygen. This increased need is reflected in the cells of the area under pressure, which is already oxygen deficient. Therefore, severe infections with accompanying elevated body temperatures can affect the body's ability to deal with the effects of tissue compression.

Anemia

Anemia or anoxemia results in the decreased delivery of oxygen to the body cells. This is due to a decrease in the amount of hemoglobin present in the blood, since hemoglobin carries oxygen to the cells. Therefore, decreased hemoglobin exacerbates the oxygen deficiency already present in the tissues because of tissue compression.

Mobility

Normally, people move when they experience discomfort due to pressure on an area of the body. Healthy people rarely exceed their tolerance to pressure. However, paralysis, sensory disturbances, extreme weakness, apathy, and clouding of consciousness may diminish the ill person's response to tissue compression.

Other factors contributing to the formation of pressure sores are poor lifting techniques, incorrect positioning, repeated injections in the same area, hard support surfaces, and incorrect application of pressure-relieving devices. See Figure 37–102 for pressure areas in selected positions.

Clients at Risk

The following conditions can put people at risk of developing pressure sores (Berecek 1975):

1. Poor nutrition associated with anemia, hypoproteinemia, and vitamin deficiencies
2. Aging process associated with arteriosclerotic changes, loss of subcutaneous tissue, loss of tissue elasticity, and clouding of the sensorium
3. Motor paralysis
4. Superficial sensory loss
5. Disturbed autonomic function

Norton et al. (1962) published a pressure area risk assessment form that includes five categories: physical condition, mental condition, activity, mobility, and incontinence. See Table 37–10. Their study showed that only 5% of clients in good general condition developed pressure sores. In contrast, Torrance (1981b) found that 48% of those in poor general condition developed pressure sores. In a study of the clients with a score of 12 and below, almost 50% developed pressure sores (Norton 1975).

Kerr et al. (1981, p. 27) devised a pressure assessment scale with five categories: physical condition, mental condition, activity, mobility, and continence. This scale needs to be used weekly or whenever there is a change in the client's condition or situation. Clients at risk include:

1. Those with paralysis from either brain or spinal cord injury. Incidence rates for these people are as high as 80%, due to their extensive loss of sensory and motor function.
2. Those with a reduced level of awareness, e.g., unconscious or heavily sedated clients (those taking analgesics, barbiturates, or tranquilizers). In these clients, the usual perceptions stimulating changes of position are reduced or absent.
3. Those who are malnourished and whose diet is insufficient in protein and vitamin C. Good nutrition promotes normal tissue maintenance and healing.
4. Those who are over age 85. These clients have problems with mobility and incontinence and are generally lean. The circulatory system of aging clients is less able to carry essential nutrients to the skin.
5. Those who are confined to bed or to a wheelchair, particularly if they are dependent on others for movement.

Shannon (1984) published a scoring system for identifying clients at risk. This form has eight categories. See Table 37–11. Clients with a score of 16 or less are at significant risk of developing pressure sores.

Table 37–10 **Breakdown of Pressure Areas: Risk Assessment Form (Scoring System)**

A		B		C		D		E	
General Physical Condition		**Mental State**		**Activity**		**Mobility**		**Incontinence**	
Good	4	Alert	4	Ambulatory	4	Full	4	Absent	4
Fair	3	Apathetic	3	Walks with help	3	Slightly limited	3	Occasional	3
Poor	2	Confused	2	Chairbound	2	Very limited	2	Usually urinary	2
Very bad	1	Stuporous	1	Bedfast	1	Immobile	1	Double	1

Source: D. Norton, R. McLaren, and A. N. Exton-Smith, *An investigation of geriatric nursing problems in hospital* (Edinburgh: Churchill Livingstone, 1962). Reissued, 1975. Used by permission.

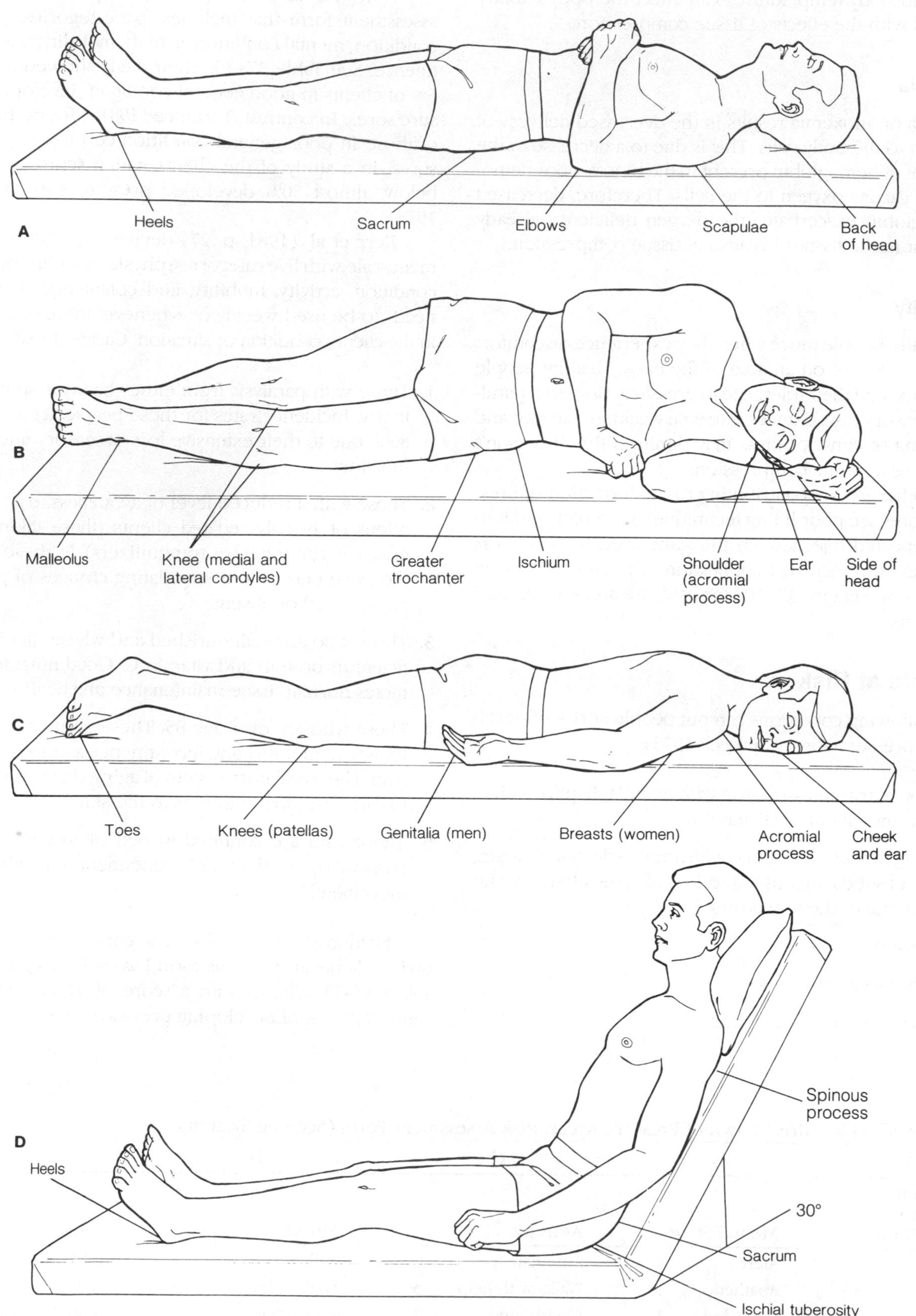

Figure 37–102 Body pressure areas in **A**, supine position; **B**, lateral position; **C**, prone position; **D**, Fowler's position

Table 37–11 Determining Clients at Risk of Developing Pressure Sores*

	Mental Status	Continence	Mobility	Activity	Nutrition	Circulation	Temperature	Medications
4	Alert	Continent	Fully mobile	Ambulatory	Good	Immediate capillary refill	36.6–37.2 C (98–99 F)	No analgesics, tranquilizers, or steroids
3	Apathetic	Incontinent of urine (without catheter)	Slightly limited	Walks with assistance	Fair	Delayed capillary refill	37.2–37.7 C (99–100 F)	One of the above
2	Confused	Incontinent of feces	Very limited	Confined to wheelchair	Poor	Mild edema	37.7–38.3 C (100–101 F)	Two of the above
1	Stuporous or comatose	Incontinent of urine and feces	Immobile	Bedridden	Cachectic	Moderate to severe edema	>38.3 C (>101 F)	All of the above

*Evaluate clients for each of the above categories, then assign appropriate score. Clients with a score of 16 or less on this assessment scale are at significant risk of developing pressure sores.

Source: Reprinted, with permission, from M. L. Shannon, Five famous fallacies about pressure sores, *Nursing 84,* October 1984, 14:37.

Procedure 37–3 ▲ Assessing Pressure Areas

Equipment

1. A good light, preferably natural or fluorescent, since incandescent lights can create a transilluminating effect.
2. A room that is not too hot or too cold. Heat can cause the skin to flush; cold can cause the skin to blanch or become cyanotic.

Assessment

1. Inspect the pressure areas (see Figure 37–102, earlier) for any whitish or reddened spots.

   Rationale This discoloration can be caused by impaired blood circulation to the area. It should disappear in a few minutes when rubbing restores circulation.

2. Inspect the pressure areas for abrasions and excoriations.

   Rationale An **abrasion** (wearing away of the skin) can occur when skin rubs against a sheet, e.g., when the client is pulled. **Excoriations** (loss of superficial layers of the skin) can occur when the skin has prolonged contact with body secretions or excretions or with dampness in skin folds.

3. Identify the stage of any cell damage. See page 1013 for stages of decubitus ulcers.
4. Inspect the pressure sore for amount, color, consistency, and odor of drainage.

   Rationale If the sore is infected, the drainage may be abnormal, e.g., thick white drainage with a putrid odor.

5. With warm hands, palpate the surface temperature of the skin over the pressure areas. Normally, the temperature is the same as that of the surrounding skin. Increased temperature is abnormal.

   Rationale Warm hands are more pleasant for the client than cold hands. Elevated temperature may be due to inflammation or blood trapped in the area.

6. With warm hands, palpate over bony prominences and dependent body areas for the presence of edema, which feels spongy upon palpation.

Nursing Diagnosis

For examples of nursing diagnoses relevant to pressure sores see page 1018.

Planning

When planning nursing strategies, the nurse considers two aspects of pressure sore care: prevention strategies

Examples of Nursing Diagnoses Related to Skin Integrity

- Potential impairment of skin integrity related to immobility, poor nutrition, and incontinence
- Impairment of skin integrity related to pressure ulcer

and strategies to treat existing pressure sores. The plan should include criteria by which to evaluate the client's response to the nursing interventions. See the examples of outcome criteria on page 1022.

Preventive Nursing Interventions

1. Change the client's position at least every 15 minutes to 2 hours, depending on the client's need, even when a special support mattress is used, so that another body surface bears the weight. Six body positions can usually be used: prone, supine, right and left lateral (side-lying), and right and left Sims's positions.
2. Provide good nutrition, particularly a diet high in protein and vitamin C. Elderly people have increased protein requirements (up to 0.6 g per kg of body weight) to maintain proper nitrogen balance (Kerr et al. 1981, p. 26).
3. Keep the client's skin clean and dry, and protect damaged skin from irritation and maceration by urine, feces, sweat, incomplete drying after a bath, soap, and alcohol.
4. Apply powders (rather than astringents, such as alcohol or witch hazel) on tissues with limited blood flow. Astringents constrict the blood vessels and thus inhibit the supply of blood and essential nutrients to the skin.
5. Lubricate dry skin areas to prevent cracking. Superfatted soaps and oils may be used.
6. Avoid massaging bony prominences with soap. The alkalis in soap produce swelling, drying, and loss of natural oils of the skin, thus promoting skin damage. In addition, prolonged exposure to soap alters the pH of the skin, one of its natural defense barriers (Kerr et al. 1981, p. 25). Vigorous massage over bony prominences is avoided, since it increases tissue damage in deep ulcers that are not apparent to the eye (Kerr et al. 1981, p. 24).
7. Provide a smooth, firm, wrinkle-free foundation on which the client can lie.
8. Use foam rubber pads and artificial sheepskins under pressure areas, such as the sacrum and heels, and elevate the heels above the bed surface. Urine passes through artificial sheepskins, whereas real sheepskins retain urine. Thus, artificial sheepskins are preferred, especially for incontinent clients.
9. Avoid the use of rubber rings. Doughnut-shaped, inflated rubber rings were traditionally placed around actual or potential pressure areas to prevent pressure over bony prominences or actual decubitus ulcers. These rings exert great pressure on areas of contact, however, and restrict blood flow in both direct contact areas and the enclosed area. Sheets of polyurethane foam stacked in a pyramid fashion and with a hole cut out over the pressure point can be used with greater safety.
10. Use a special mattress, such as an alternating pressure, egg crate, or flotation mattress, to decrease pressure on body parts. See Table 37–12.
11. Teach clients to be aware of discolored areas and of sensations such as tingling, which can indicate pressure.
12. Be alert to early symptoms of pressure sores, particularly over bony prominences. These symptoms include localized redness or pallor, tenderness, an unpleasant sensation frequently described as burning, coldness, and localized edema.
13. Massage pressure areas gently and only if there is no evidence of underlying tissue damage.
14. Reduce friction by applying a thin layer of cornstarch to the bedsheet or wheelchair seat cover.

Research Note

A comparative study was conducted at Stanford University Medical Center for 1 year to determine a standardized nursing care plan for the treatment of decubitus ulcers. This plan focused on client comfort, rapid healing of the decubitus ulcer, and cost containment.

Two nursing care plans—one using Opsite and the other a traditional method of decubitus care—were devised. Opsite is a self-adhesive transparent polyurethane dressing that seals in the body's normal leukocytes, plasma, and fibrin to promote natural healing. Although the Opsite did not improve healing time, it did significantly reduce the average nursing time required to care for decubitus ulcers and was found to be cost effective.

Decubitus ulcers are a major problem for both clients and nursing staff because they are painful and time consuming to care for. Preventive measures such as egg crate mattresses, frequent position changes, massage, and adequate nutrition are mandatory for clients confined to bed. When decubitus ulcers occur, these measures, along with Opsite, maintain client comfort and promote healing. (Howard-Kurzuk et al. 1985)

Table 37–12 Mechanical Devices for Preventing and Treating Pressure Sores

Device	Description
Alternating pressure mattress	Composed of a number of cells in which the pressure alternately increases and decreases; utilizes a pump
Foam mattress	Foam molds to the body
Air-fluidized bed	Provides uniform support; controls temperature and humidity
Low air loss (LAL) bed	Supports the client and reduces amount of air required; utilizes a pump; provides very low pressure; controls temperature
Water bed	Special mattress filled with water; controls temperature of water
Egg crate mattress	Polyurethane foam mattress resembling an egg crate; some types are flammable
Gel flotation pads	Polyvinyl, silicone, or silastic pads filled with a gelatinous substance similar to fat
Sheepskins (natural and artificial)	Some manufacturers produce mixed natural and synthetic pads; artificial pads are less likely to be damaged by washing but are more likely to make the client hot than natural skins
Air or foam rings	Limit blood supply to the area
Cushions (foam, gel and air, foam and fluid)	Some have cutouts for the pressure points
Heel protectors (sheepskin boots, padded splints, foam wedges)	Limit pressure on heels when client is in bed

15. Teach the client to change his or her position frequently, even if only slightly, to change the pressure point.
16. Reduce the shearing force by elevating the head of the bed no more than 30° if the client's condition permits.
17. Encourage exercise and ambulation whenever possible to stimulate blood circulation.

Interventions for Existing Pressure Sores

1. Clean the pressure sore daily by placing the client in a whirlpool bath containing povidone-iodine (Betadine) if his or her condition permits (Shannon 1984). The warmth and mechanical action of the whirlpool promotes circulation, decreases pressure on soft tissues, and helps debride the ulcer.
2. Clean and dress the sore using sterile technique. Clean the sore with an antiseptic, e.g., povidone-iodine solution. Refrain from using antiseptics, such as alcohol, which are vasoconstrictors and reduce blood flow to the area. If the pressure sore is not infected, cover it with an occlusive dressing, e.g., Opsite, and leave the wound undisturbed for several days. Covering the sore with an occlusive dressing prevents microorganisms from entering it, and leaving the sore undisturbed promotes healing. If the pressure sore is infected, obtain a sample of the drainage for culture and sensitivity to antiseptic agents.
3. Minimize direct pressure on the sore. Reposition the client at least every 2 hours. Make a schedule for the position changes. See Table 37–9 on page 998.
4. Reduce friction by applying a small amount of cornstarch to the bedsheet.
5. Reduce shearing force by not elevating the head of the bed higher than 30° if the client's condition permits.
6. If the client cannot keep his or her weight off the pressure sore, use a gel flotation mattress or pad. See Table 37–12 for other mechanical devices.
7. Teach the client to move, if only slightly, to relieve pressure.
8. Encourage ambulation or sitting in a wheelchair if the client's condition permits. See Chapter 39. Ambulation stimulates circulation. Moving out of the bed can enhance feelings of self-esteem and provide diversion.
9. Provide ROM exercises as the client's condition permits. ROM exercises help maintain joint mobility and stimulate circulation.

Overview of Pressure Sore Treatment

Pressure sores are a challenge for nurses because of the number of variables involved (e.g., risk factors, types of ulcers, and degrees of impairment) and because numerous treatment measures are advocated. Interventions need to be selected from the following:

1. Take a wound culture as soon as the ulcer is noticed to ascertain the specific invading organisms, and then weekly or whenever increases in drainage appear or healing is delayed. If infection is present, antiseptics are preferred to local or systemic antibiotics. Locally applied antibiotics have not proved effective (Morley 1981, p. 29; Ahmed 1980, p. 115), and systemic anti-

Research Note

Many agents have been used in the treatment of decubitus ulcers. Diekmann carried out a pilot study to determine if a dental irrigating device could be successfully employed to treat ulcers. Sixteen patients participated in the study: eight in the experimental group and eight in the routine care group. The ulcers were situated in various locations: trochanter, buttock, coccyx, gluteal fold, calf, foot, and heel. Clients in the experimental group had their ulcers irrigated with 200 cc sterile normal saline at room temperature, delivered at the lowest pressure on the irrigating device, twice a day for 2 weeks. The pressure sores were not dressed after the irrigation. The decubitus ulcers of both groups were measured before and after the test. Diekmann found that the data did not support the hypothesis; however, the use of irrigating devices can debride ulcers and stimulate local circulation without harm to the client. (Diekmann 1984)

biotics do not reach the desired site of action because the blood supply to the ulcer is disrupted (Ahmed 1980, p. 115). Antiseptics are discussed subsequently.

2. **Debride** (remove foreign and contaminated or devitalized material from) deep ulcers to remove necrotic tissue, which impedes healing and provides an excellent culture medium for bacteria. Debridement may be achieved by chemical or surgical means:
   a. Enzyme ointments such as collagenase (Santyl), fibrinolysin and desoxyribonuclease (Elase), and sutilains (Travase) are used in chemical debridement. Use of enzymes requires a physician's order. Collagenase, an enzyme that digests collagen, may be more effective than Elase or Travase, since 79% of the necrotic and living tissue is collagen, and, in the normal healing process, a small amount of collagenase is produced. Thus, collagenase ointment seems to simulate and enhance the body's normal self-debridement process for healing wounds (Barrett and Klibanski 1973, p. 849; Ahmed 1980, p. 114). Because enzymes do not penetrate thick hard eschar, either the eschar is softened for several days or weeks with continuous saline soaks or the eschar is surgically scored or crosshatched to permit the enzyme to penetrate. Once the eschar is softened, it is removed with forceps or scissors. Generally, collagenase dressings are changed daily or whenever soiled; Elase twice daily; and Travase up to four times daily (Judd 1981, p. 33). Before applying enzymes, the nurse cleans the ulcer with normal saline or hydrogen peroxide to remove old ointment and digested material. The enzyme ointment is applied to only the ulcerated area, since it can irritate normal skin and damage new granulation tissue. Surrounding skin may be protected with zinc oxide, karaya paste, or petroleum jelly. Generally, a moist gauze dressing is applied over the area and covered with a waterproof (e.g., plastic) pad. Ahmed (1980, p. 114) cautions that antiseptics or detergents containing metal ions or acidic substances should not be used in conjunction with enzymes. Tincture of iodine, Merthiolate, nitrofurazone (Furacin), and hexachlorophene inactivate collagenase, and Burow's solution inhibits enzyme action by altering the pH. When debridement is complete (i.e., the wound appears clean), the enzyme ointment is discontinued, and other measures to promote healing (discussed subsequently) are initiated.
   b. Surgical debridement is performed by a physician. It may be done with or without anesthetic agents. The wound is surgically excised with a scalpel blade. This procedure may have to be repeated several times until the wound remains clean. Surgical debridement has the disadvantage of increasing ulcer size and increasing the client's risk of infection and hemorrhage. Following debridement, the ulcer should appear clean and pink and reveal evidence of healing by secondary union (see Chapter 52). Because the ulcer is susceptible to infection, every effort is then made to keep the wound clean and promote healing. In some instances, surgical closure using skin grafts may be necessary.

3. Promote healing by keeping the ulcer moist and preventing infection. Wounds needs moisture to heal; thus, dehydrating solutions, such as liquid antacids, are avoided (Ahmed 1980, p. 114). Heat lamps and hair driers were erroneously recommended in previous years to dry the surface of the ulcer; they are contraindicated. Various measures are advocated:
   a. Saline or povidone-iodine soaks may be applied to a superficial ulcer to keep the wound moist (Ahmed 1980, p. 114).
   b. Opsite, a commercially prepared, transparent, self-adhesive film, may be applied to superficial ulcers and some deep, draining, or necrotic ulcers (Chrisp 1977, p. 1202; Ahmed 1980, p. 117). This preparation acts like skin in that it isolates the ulcer from contaminants and keeps it moist. It is also permeable to air, is waterproof (it can be washed if soiled), and allows freedom of movement. Before Opsite is applied, the wound and surrounding skin are cleaned with saline solution or water and thoroughly dried to ensure proper adhesion. The Opsite is applied without tension over the ulcer and at least 2.5 cm (1 in) over the surrounding skin. It is left in place

5 to 7 days or until seepage or an odor is detected. The application is repeated until the ulcer has healed. When removing the Opsite, the nurse takes care to remove only the nonadherent portion, since an attempt to remove adherent portions may tear the skin. In some instances, the nurse may need to cut a hole in the center and apply the new piece over it.

c. Gelfoam (absorbable gelatin sterile) powder and sponges, applied with a dressing, are effective for small or medium-sized clean ulcers but not for draining or hard, necrotic ulcers. Draining or necrotic wounds must be cleaned or debrided before Gelfoam is applied. Gelfoam powder seems more advantageous for healing than Gelfoam sponge, since it adheres well to the ulcer. Some authorities recommend changing the Gelfoam dressing daily; others, every 3 to 7 days (Ahmed 1980, p. 116; Lang and McGrath 1974, p. 461). If the dressing is changed every 3 to 7 days, the ulcer must be inspected daily to ensure that it is free of drainage.
d. Silver nitrate 1:400 dressings, covered with a plastic wrap and secured with nonallergenic tape, can be used for superficial ulcers involving only the epidermis. Higher strengths of silver nitrate may cause bleeding (Morley 1981, p. 30).
e. Karaya powder (a vegetable gum) is advocated for clean or draining superficial and deep ulcers but not for hard, leathery eschar. The procedure outlined by Wallace and Hayter (1974, p. 1094) is: (1) irrigate the ulcer with saline or 3% hydrogen peroxide solution (any karaya adhering is left in place), (2) encircle the wound with a karaya gum ring, and (3) cover the ulcer and karaya ring with a plastic wrap, like Saran wrap. The wrap is opened every 8 hours to add more karaya powder, and the entire procedure is repeated daily.
f. Stomahesive, another vegetable gum, may be used for clean and draining superficial and deep ulcers and is effective in debriding hard, necrotic eschar (Ryan 1976, p. 299). This preparation is similar to Opsite but thicker, and it is applied in the same way.
g. Debrisan (molecular chains of dextran beads) is a product used for infected, draining ulcers only. The dry, porous beads absorb bacteria, proteins, fibrin, and toxins. When drainage stops, the ulcer may be grafted or other therapies that promote healing initiated (Ahmed 1980, p. 116).
h. Antiseptics such as povidone-iodine in ointment or solution form, merbromin (Mercurochrome) in 5% or 10% solutions, Helafoam, an aerosol foam of povidone-iodine, and sodium hypochlorite solution (Hygeol) are effective for draining infected or clean ulcers. They do not, however, penetrate hard eschar. Povidone-iodine can be applied at any stage of the healing process (even prior to debridement), since its antiseptic properties are effective in the presence of pus, necrotic tissue, serum, or blood. Often the ulcer is cleaned with povidone-iodine solution and then packed with gauze impregnated with povidone-iodine ointment. If only solution is used, dressings are changed twice daily; if ointment is used, dressings are changed daily (Judd 1981, p. 33). Clients need to be watched for allergy to iodine prior to the use of povidone-iodine. Mercurochrome solution can also be applied at any stage of the healing process, but is not as strong as povidone-iodine. It is said to stimulate the formation of granulation tissue, however (Judd 1981, p. 33). Helafoam requires less frequent application than Betadine and other forms of povidone-iodine. Helafoam is advocated in conjunction with Betadine Viscous Formula Antiseptic Gauze Pads, which prolong the foam's action (Ahmed 1980, p. 116). Hygeol solution (1:12 to 1:20 dilution) is effective for dermal ulcers only. It may be caustic to some persons and must be used with caution on soft tissue where bleeding is suspected (Judd 1981, p. 33).

Many other measures have been used to treat decubitus ulcers, but their therapeutic value is questionable or not established, and they therefore should be avoided. These include applications of granulated sugar, sugar and egg white mixture, and insulin. The therapeutic value of granulated sugar is unknown. A sugar and egg white mixture has been found to have no therapeutic value and may even retard normal healing (Ahmed 1980, p. 118). However, a paste of powdered cane sugar, lanolin, and compound benzoin tincture in specified amounts may have some therapeutic value when used to treat clean ulcers (Ahmed 1980, p. 118). The effectiveness of insulin (10 I.U. of regular insulin) applied topically is highly questionable. Moreover, insulin can be absorbed through the ulcer, causing hypoglycemic (low blood sugar) reactions (Gerber and Van Ort 1981, p. 1159).

Clearly, treatment of decubitus ulcers is a complex matter. It requires strict sterile technique (see Chapter 52). Very superficial ulcers may heal within a few days; deep, necrotic ulcers may take several months. The nurse must set specific outcome criteria to evaluate the effects of therapy. If after a specified period of time (e.g., 14 or 21 days) the criteria have not been met, the therapy must be reevaluated.

Evaluation

See page 1022 for examples of outcome criteria related to skin integrity.

Outcome Criteria

The client will:

- Have intact, well-hydrated skin
- Describe factors that contribute to alterations of the skin
- Describe interventions to maintain skin integrity
- Participate in a prescribed treatment to promote wound healing

Nursing Care Plan

Assessment Data

Nursing Assessment

Several weeks ago, Kevin Andrews, a 17-year-old high school gymnast, fell from the parallel bars and fractured his left femur. Kevin has been on bedrest in skeletal traction since the accident. He is quite depressed and bored with the hospital routine of care. Because of painful muscle spasms, he often refuses to be turned or to move voluntarily. His appetite is poor, and he often refuses his hospital meals. He needs encouragement from the nursing staff to cough and deep breathe.

Physical Examination

Height: 175.3 cm (5′9″)
Weight: 70 kg (155 lb) on admission
Temperature: 37 C (98.6 F)
Pulse rate: 80 BPM
Respirations: 16 per minute
Blood pressure: 114/70 mm Hg

Diagnostic Data

Chest x-ray film: Negative
Urine: Negative
Hemoglobin: 12.2
Hematocrit: 37%

Nursing Diagnosis	Client Goals and Outcome Criteria	Nursing Interventions and Rationales	Evaluation
Impaired physical mobility, related to left fractured femur/ skeletal traction resulting in decreased muscle strength, weakness, pain, and limitations in range of motion.	Client Goal: Client will regain use and strength of upper and lower limb musculature. Outcome Criteria: Range-of-motion (ROM) exercises of upper limbs and unaffected lower limb are performed by client 3× daily. Overhead trapeze is used q3 hrs to strengthen muscles in upper limbs by day 3. Supplemental feedings, e.g., milk shakes and eggnogs, are taken 1× daily. Performs activities of daily living within limitation of skeletal traction.	Assist client with full range of motion to all unaffected joints of extremities 3 or 4 times daily. *Rationale:* ROM exercises help maintain muscle tone and mobility. Teach the client isometric exercises for left lower limb. *Rationale:* Isometric exercises cause muscles to contract without involving joints and help maintain muscle strength and mass. Permit client to participate in activities of daily living as much as possible. *Rationale:* Independence enhances client's self-esteem and increases muscular activity and strength. Offer client supplemental feedings high in protein and vitamins. *Rationale:* Proteins and vitamins are necessary for bone healing and positive nitrogen balance.	Performs active ROM exercises of upper limbs and unaffected lower limb daily before breakfast, lunch, and dinner. Uses overhead trapeze to strengthen upper limbs at least 5× daily. Drinks 4 oz of milkshake or eggnog each day after lunch or at bedtime. Participates in his bath each morning and feeds himself 3× a day.

(continued)

Nursing Diagnosis	Client Goals and Outcome Criteria	Nursing Interventions and Rationales	Evaluation
Potential for injury, infection, thrombus formation, and nerve damage related to skeletal traction and immobility resulting in odors, redness, pain, numbness, and elevated temperature and WBC.	Client Goal: Infection and thrombophlebitis do not occur. Outcome Criteria: Temperature remains normal. Traction site remains free of drainage and odor. Homans' sign remains negative.	Inspect pin insertion site for signs of inflammation. *Rationale:* Skin infection may lead to bone infection. Instruct client not to touch pin insertion sites. *Rationale:* Reduces chance of infection. Use sterile technique when doing site care. *Rationale:* Reduces chance of infection to skin and/or bone. Assess for Homans' sign frequently. *Rationale:* A positive Homans' sign is evidence of a thrombus. Encourage ROM and involvement with ADLs. *Rationale:* Exercise prevents complications of immobility.	Temperature remains at 37 C. Skin surrounding pin insertion site remains odorless, dry, and intact. Homans' sign is negative.

Chapter Highlights

- Physical fitness affects almost every body organ and system favorably and has psychosocial benefits.
- Immobility affects almost every body organ and system adversely; complications include psychosocial problems.
- Factors influencing mobility include life-style, disease process or injury, understanding of health and physical fitness, motivation and attitudes toward health, and age.
- Specific criteria for assessing mobility-immobility status include physical fitness, complications of immobility, body alignment, body mechanics, ambulation, joint range-of-motion movements, independence in activities of daily living, and activity tolerance.
- The nurse has responsibilities to prevent deterioration in the fitness levels of clients, prevent the complications of immobility, reduce the severity of any problems resulting from immobility, and help clients improve their fitness.
- Pressure sores are thought to be the result of pressure, friction, and shearing forces.
- There are four stages in the formation of pressure sores.
- Clients at risk of developing pressure sores include: the poorly nourished, the elderly, and people with superficial sensory loss, motor paralysis, or disturbances in autonomic nervous system function.
- Nursing interventions can help prevent and heal pressure sores.

Suggested Readings

Hirschberg, G. G.; Lewis, L.; and Vaugh, P. May 1977. Promoting patient mobility. *Nursing 77* 7:42–47.
The authors describe common disuse syndromes and a variety of nursing interventions to prevent the complications of immobility or restore mobility.

Rameizl, P. November/December 1983. CADET: A self-care assessment tool. *Geriatric Nursing* 4:377–78.
CADET, a self-care assessment tool, is an acronym for communication, ambulation, daily activities, excretion, and transfer functions. A technique for scoring each category is included.

Shannon, M. L. October 1984. Five famous fallacies about pressure sores. *Nursing 84* 14:34–41.
Shannon discusses common misconceptions nurses have about pressure sores and gives facts and realistic interventions. Two tables are included: one about determining clients at risk and the other about the effects of nursing interventions on the causes of pressure sores.

Sivarajan, E. S., and Halpenny, C. J. December 1979. Exercise testing. *American Journal of Nursing* 79:2162–70.
The authors describe and interpret several cardiovascular tests that are used to determine the exercise capacity of an individual and to prescribe a safe exercise program for that person.

Selected References

Ahmed, M. C. December 1980. Special report: Choosing the best method to manage pressure ulcers. *Nurses' Drug Alert* 4(15):113–20.

American Heart Association. 1984. Exercise diary. Dallas, Texas: The Association.

Arnell, I. June 1983. Treating decubitus ulcers: Two methods that work. *Nursing 83* 13:50–55.

Barrett, D., and Klibanski, A. May 1973. Collagenase debridement. *American Journal of Nursing* 73:849–51.

Bassett, C.; McClamrock, E.; and Schmelzer, M. March/April 1982. A 10-week exercise program for senior citizens. *Geriatric Nursing* 3:103–5.

Baum, L. March 1985. Heed the early warning signs of peripheral vascular disease. *Nursing 85* 15:50–58.

Beller, L. C., and Neunaber, K. L. April 1986. The "simple" Valsalva. *American Journal of Nursing* 86:398–99.

Berecek, K. March 1975. Treatment of decubitus ulcers. *Nursing Clinics of North America* 10:171–210.

Blom, M. F. March/April 1985. Dramatic decrease in decubitus ulcers. *Geriatric Nursing* 6:84–87.

Brower, P., and Hicks, D. July 1972. Maintaining muscle function in patients on bedrest. *American Journal of Nursing* 72:1250–53.

Byrne, N., and Feld, M. April 1984. Preventing and treating decubitus ulcers. *Nursing 84* 14:55–57.

Byrne, C. J.; Saxton, D. F.; Pelikan, P. K.; and Nugent, P. M. 1986. *Laboratory tests: Implications for nursing care* 2d ed. Menlo Park, Calif.: Addison-Wesley Publishing Co.

Cantu, R. C., editor. 1981. *Health maintenance through physical conditioning.* Littleton, Mass.: PSG Publishing Co.

Chrisp, M. August 4, 1977. New treatment for pressure sores. *Nursing Times* 73:1202–5.

Ciuca, R.; Bradish, J.; and Trombly, S. August 1978. Active range-of-motion exercises. *Nursing 78* 8:45–49.

Clark, M. O., et al. March 2, 1978. Pressure sores. *Nursing Times* 74:363–66.

Cohen, S., and Villion, G. April 1981. Patient assessment: Examining joints of the upper and lower extremities. *American Journal of Nursing* 81:763–86.

Dehn, M. M. March 1980. The effects of exercise. *American Journal of Nursing* 81:435–40.

De Hoff, V. December 1983. Motivating patients to do what's good for them: The exercise contest. *Nursing 83* 13:31.

De Witt, P. E. March 17, 1986. Extra years for extra effort. *Time,* p. 66.

Diekmann, J. M. September/October 1984. Use of dental irrigating device in treatment of decubitus ulcers. *Nursing Research* 33:303–5.

Downs, F. March 1974. Bed rest and sensory disturbances. *American Journal of Nursing* 74:434–38.

Dyson, R. June 15, 1978. Bed sores: The injuries hospital staff inflict on patients. *Nursing Mirror* 146:30–32.

Exton-Smith, A. N., et al. 1963. A study of factors concerned in the production of pressure sores and their prevention. In *Investigation of geriatric nursing problems in hospitals.* London: The National Corporation for Care of Old People.

Fahey, V. March 1984. An in-depth look at deep-vein thrombosis. *Nursing 84* 14:35–41.

Frankel, L. J., and Richard, B. B. December 1977. Exercise to help the elderly—to live longer, stay healthier, and be happier. *Nursing 77* 7:58–63.

Friedman, F. B., editor. February 1982. An innovation in decubitus treatment sparks debate. *RN* 45:46–47, 118.

Gerber, R. M., and Van Ort, S. R. June 1981. Topical application of insulin to pressure sores: A questionable therapy. *American Journal of Nursing* 81:1159.

Gordon, M. January 1976. Assessing activity tolerance. *American Journal of Nursing* 76:72–75.

Griffin, W.; Anderson, S.; and Possos, J. September 1971. Group exercise for patients with limited mobility. *American Journal of Nursing* 71:1742–43.

Guttmann, L. 1955. The problem of treatment of pressure sores in patients with spinal paraplegia. *British Journal of Plastic Surgery* 8:196.

Guyton, A. C. 1986. *Textbook of medical physiology.* 7th ed. Philadelphia: W. B. Saunders Co.

Harrin, J., and Hargest, T. March 1970. The air-fluidized bed: A new concept in the treatment of decubitus ulcers. *Nursing Clinics of North America* 5:181–87.

Hettinger, T., and Mueller, S. A. 1953. Muskelleistung und Muskeltraining. *Arbeitsphysiologie* 15:111–26.

Heywood, V. H. 1984. *Designs for fitness.* Minneapolis: Burgess Publishing Co.

Hirschberg, G. G.; Lewis, L.; and Vaugh, P. May 1977. Promoting patient mobility. *Nursing 77* 7:42–47.

Hogan, L., and Beland, I. July 1976. Cervical neck syndrome. *American Journal of Nursing* 76:1104–7.

Horpfel-Harris, J. A. March 1980. Improving compliance with an exercise program. *Nursing 80* 10:449–50.

Howard-Kurzuk, G.; Simpson, L.; and Palmeri, A. 1985. Decubitus ulcer care: A comparative study. *Western Journal of Nursing Research* 7(1):58–79.

Husian, T. 1953. An experimental study of some pressure effects on tissues, with references to the bed-sore problem. *Journal of Pathology and Bacteriology* 66:347–58.

Judd, C. O. July/August 1981. The prevention and treatment of pressure sores. *Canadian Nurse* 77:32–33.

Jungreis, S. W. August 1977. Exercises for expediting mobility in bedridden patients. *Nursing 77* 7:47–51.

Kelly, M. M. October 1966. Exercises for bedfast patients. *American Journal of Nursing* 66:2209–13.

Kerr, J. C.; Stinson, S. M.; and Shannon, M. L. July/August 1981. Pressure sores: Distinguishing fact from fiction. *Canadian Nurse* 77:23–28.

Kottke, F. G.; Stillwell, G. K.; and Lehmann, J. F., editors. 1982. *Krusen's handbook of physical medicine and rehabilitation.* 3d ed. Philadelphia: W. B. Saunders Co.

Lane, L. D., and Gaffney, F. A. June 1985. Overcautious use of the bedpan. *American Journal of Nursing* 85:642–44.

Lang, C., and McGrath, A. March 1974. Gelfoam for decubitus ulcers. *American Journal of Nursing* 74:460–61.

Levin, M. A. July 1973. Bed exercises for acute cardiac patients. *American Journal of Nursing* 73:1226–27.

Lindan, O.; Greenway, R. M.; and Piazza, J. M. 1965. Pressure distribution on the surface of the human body, evaluation in lying and sitting positions using a bed of springs and nails. *Archives of Physical Medicine and Rehabilitation* 46:378–85.

Lowthian, P. January 20, 1982. A review of pressure sore pathogenesis. *Nursing Times* 78:117–21.

Marley, W. P. 1982. *Health and physical fitness.* Philadelphia: Saunders College Publishing.

Meissner, J. E. September 1980. Evaluate your patient's level of independence. *Nursing 80* 10:72–73.

Milazzo, V. October 1981. An exercise class for patients in traction. *American Journal of Nursing* 81:1842–44.

Mitchell, P. H., and Laustau, A. 1981. *Concepts basic to nursing.* 3d ed. New York: McGraw-Hill Book Co.

Morley, M. H. October 1973. Decubitus ulcer management: A team approach. *Canadian Nurse* 69:41–43.

———. July/August 1981. Sixteen steps to better decubitus ulcer care. *Canadian Nurse* 77:29–31.

Norton, D. February 13, 1975. Research and the problem of pressure sores. *Nursing Mirror* 140:65–67.

Norton, D.; McLaren, R.; and Exton-Smith, A. N. 1962. An investigation of geriatric nursing problems in hospital. Edinburgh: Churchill and Livingstone.

Patrick, M. I., et al., editors. 1986. *Medical-surgical nursing: Pathophysiological concepts.* Philadelphia: J. B. Lippincott Co.

Pender, N. J. 1982. *Health promotion in nursing practice.* Norwalk, Conn.: Appleton-Century-Crofts.

Peterson, F. November 1983. Assessing peripheral vascular disease. *American Journal of Nursing* 83:1549–51.

Reeder, J. M. November 1984. Help your disabled patient be more independent. *Nursing 84* 14:43.

Robertson, D., and Robertson, R. February 1985. Orthostatic hypotension: Diagnosis and therapy. *Modern concepts of cardiovascular disease* 54:1–14.

Rodts, M. F. May 1983. An orthopedic assessment you can do in 15 minutes. *Nursing 83* 13:65–73.

Ryan, D. M. February 26, 1976. Pressure sores: Treatment using stomahesive. Part 5. *Nursing Times* 72:299–300.

Smith, B. April 20, 1983. Danger: Points under pressure. *Nursing Mirror* 156:24–27.

Smith, S. E. 1978. Prostaglandins. *Nursing Times* 74(6):231–33.

Torrance, C. January 15, 1981a. Pressure sores. Part 1. Pathogenesis. *Nursing Times* 77:center pages.

———. February 19, 1981b. Pressure sores. Part 2. Predisposing factors: The "at-risk" patient. *Nursing Times* 77:5–8.

———. March 19, 1981c. Pressure sores. Part 3. Medical management and surgical intervention. *Nursing Times* 77:9–12.

———. April 16, 1981d. Pressure sores. Part 4. Mechanical devices. *Nursing Times* 77:13–16.

———. May 7, 1981e. Pressure sores. Part 5. Topical applications and wound agents. *Nursing Times* 77:17–20.

———. June 18, 1981f. Pressure sores. Part 6. Physical methods. *Nursing Times* 77:21–24.

Tyler, M. L. May 1984. The respiratory effects of body positioning and immobilization. *Respiratory Care* 29:472–83.

Van Ort, S. R., and Gerber, R. M. January/February 1976. Topical application of insulin in the treatment of decubitus ulcers: A pilot study. *Nursing Research* 25:9–12.

Verhonick, P. J. August 1961. A preliminary report of a study of decubitus ulcer care. *American Journal of Nursing* 61:68–69.

Vivens, S., and Woolfork, C. November/December 1983. Nursing home admissions made more rational. *Geriatric Nursing* 4:361–64.

Wade, D. July 1982. Teaching patients to live with chronic orthostatic hypotension. *Nursing 82* 12:64–65.

Walker, J. M., et al. June 1984. Active mobility of the extremities in older subjects. *Physical Therapy* 64:919–23.

Winslow, E. H., and Weber, T. M. March 1980. Progressive exercises to combat the hazards of bedrest. *American Journal of Nursing* 80:440–45.

Wallace, G., and Hayter, J. June 1974. Karaya for chronic skin ulcers. *American Journal of Nursing* 74:1094–98.

Young, C. March 1975. Exercise: How to use it to decrease complications in immobilized patients. *Nursing 75* 5:81–83.

Ziegler, J. C. August 1980. Physical reconditioning—for the convalescent patient. *Nursing 80* 10:67–69.

CHAPTER **38**

Body Alignment

Mary Kelly Memmer

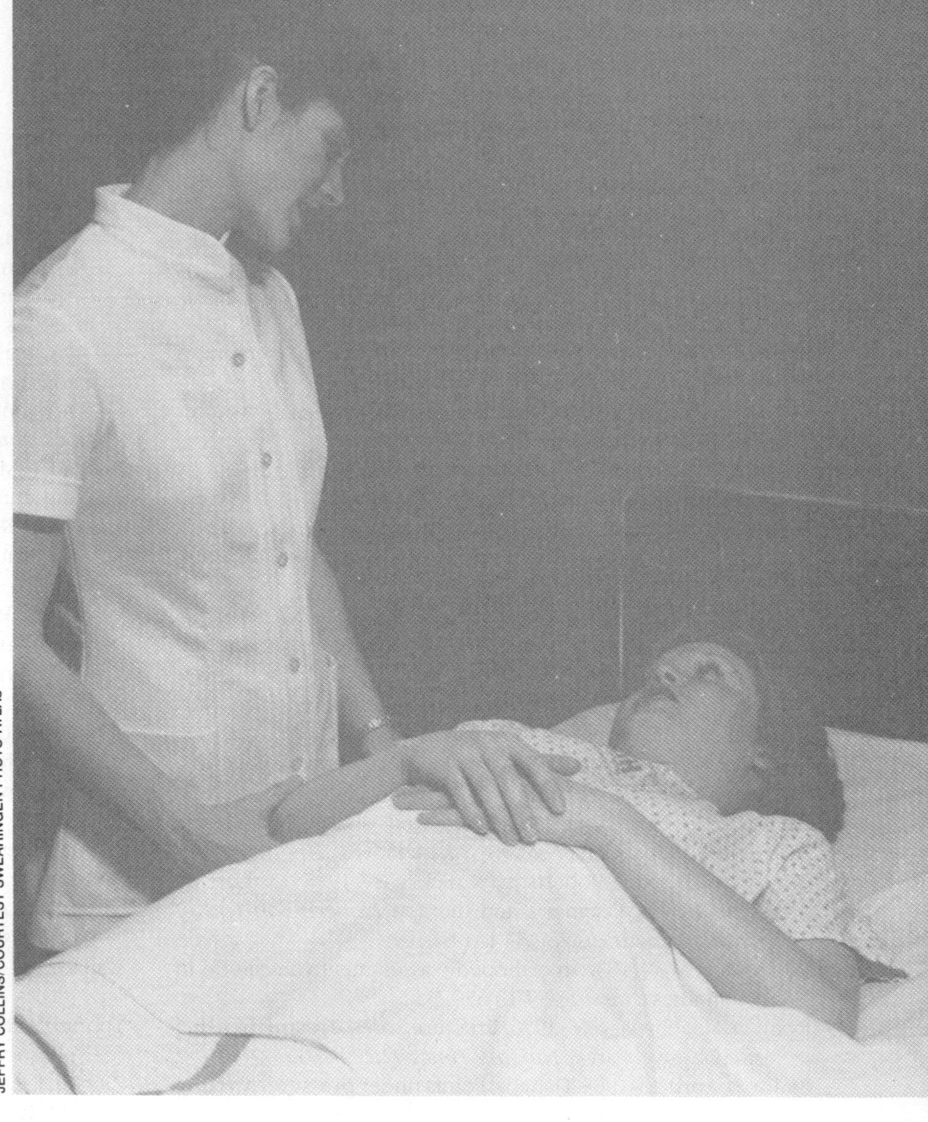

JEFFRY COLLINS/COURTESY SWEARINGEN PHOTO-ATLAS

Contents

Objectives

1. Understand facts and principles of body alignment
   1.1 Define listed terms.
   1.2 Describe the importance of good body alignment for clients and nurses.
   1.3 Describe four principles of body alignment.
   1.4 Describe six postural reflexes.
2. Understand the assessment process in body alignment.
   2.1 Describe assessment criteria for the alignment of adults in standing, sitting, and various bed-lying positions.
   2.2 Describe standing postural variations among different age groups.
   2.3 Identify factors that influence body alignment.
   2.4 Differentiate correct from incorrect alignment in persons in standing, sitting, and various bed-lying positions.
   2.5 Describe potential alignment problems inherent in standing, sitting, and lying positions.
   2.6 Describe what assessment data about alignment the nurse must look for in the client's records.
3. Understand the nursing diagnosis and planning processes as they relate to body alignment.
   3.1 Describe the overall goals of good alignment.
   3.2 Describe the consequences of poor body alignment.
   3.3 Describe common structural abnormalities that affect body alignment.
   3.4 Describe the nurse's responsibility for client alignment.
   3.5 Identify nursing diagnoses related to common body alignment problems.
4. Identify nursing interventions to maintain, promote, or restore good body alignment, and use the evaluation process to assess their effectiveness.
   4.1 Identify principles of positioning clients in bed.
   4.2 Describe guidelines for positioning clients.
   4.3 Describe specific interventions to help a client assume well-aligned standing, sitting, and lying positions.
   4.4 Specify how the nurse can teach clients and caregivers to improve body alignment and prevent alignment problems.
   4.5 Identify outcome criteria to evaluate the effectiveness of nursing interventions to maintain, promote, or restore good body alignment.

Terms

balance
base of support
body alignment
center of gravity
contracture
cupula
dorsal recumbent (back-lying) position
dowager's hump
eversion
extension
external rotation (of hip)
femoral anteversion
Fowler's position
gravity
high-Fowler's position
hyperphosphatemia
hypocalcemia
hypophosphatemia
internal girdle
inversion
kyphosis
lateral (side-lying) position
line of gravity
long midriff
lordosis
low-Fowler's position
metatarsus adductus
orthopneic position
osteomalacia
osteoporosis
pelvic tilt
postural tonus
posture
prone position
rickets
righting reflexes
scoliosis
semi-Fowler's position
Sims' (semiprone) position
supine (dorsal) position
tonus
trochanter roll

The Importance of Good Body Alignment

Body alignment is the geometric arrangement of body parts in relation to each other. Good alignment promotes optimal balance and maximal body function in whatever position the client assumes: standing, sitting, or lying down. Good body alignment and good **posture** are synonymous terms. When the body is well aligned, balance is achieved without undue strain on the joints, muscles, tendons, or ligaments. Muscles are usually in a state of slight tension (**tonus**) when the body is healthy and well aligned. This state requires minimal muscular force and yet supports the internal framework and organs.

Balance is a state of equipoise in which opposing forces counteract each other. Good body alignment is essential to body balance. It is difficult to differentiate balance from body alignment, although balance is the result of proper alignment. Both are results of the principles discussed in the next section.

A person's posture is one criterion for assessing his or her general health, physical fitness, and attractiveness. Posture reflects the mood, self-esteem, and personality of an individual. Proper body alignment promotes proper body function of musculoskeletal structures, reducing the amount of energy required to maintain balance and therefore minimizing fatigue. Proper body alignment enhances lung expansion and promotes efficient circulatory, renal, and gastrointestinal functions. Conversely, poor body alignment detracts from a pleasing appearance and affects an individual's health adversely.

The nurse is an important role model in teaching good health habits, including good posture. The nurse with poor posture cannot expect clients to learn good posture from the negative example he or she portrays.

Many clients depend on nurses for assistance in body alignment. The discomfort and potentially disabling complications of prolonged poor body alignment are a real concern for clients. Clients often evaluate the quality of the nursing care they receive by how comfortable they feel, and proper alignment is crucial to comfort.

Principles of Body Alignment

Good body alignment and balance require integrated functioning of the musculoskeletal and nervous systems. Adequate muscle tone, coordinated movements of opposing muscle groups, and neuromuscular reflexes (including the vestibular and proprioceptive reflexes) are essential to body alignment and balance. The following influence body alignment: gravity, postural reflexes and opposing muscle groups, changes in posture, and individual differences in structural anatomy.

Gravity

The following definitions help the nurse understand alignment:

1. **Gravity** is the mutual attraction between an object and the earth.
2. The **center of gravity** is the point at which all of the mass of an object is centered. The center of gravity of a standing adult is located slightly anterior to the upper part of the sacrum. See Figure 38–1.
3. The **line of gravity** is an imaginary vertical line drawn through an object's center of gravity.
4. The **base of support** is the foundation on which an object rests. In an adult standing with the feet together, the center of the base of support is just over the instep of the foot. See Figure 38–1.

Standing posture can be unstable because of the narrow base of support, the high center of gravity, and a constantly shifting line of gravity. For greatest balance and stability, a standing adult must center body weight symmetrically along the line of gravity. A person maintains balance as long as the line of gravity passes through the center of gravity and the base of support: the broader the base of support and the lower the center of gravity, the greater the stability and balance. Whenever the line of gravity and the center of gravity lie outside the base of support, the body is unbalanced and unstable. When a person rests in a chair or bed, the feet of the chair or bed form a considerably wider base of support. The center of gravity is lower and the line of gravity is less mobile. Thus, a person in a sitting or lying position has greater stability and balance than in a standing position. See Figure 38–2.

Postural Reflexes and Opposing Muscle Groups

Continuous action of postural muscles sustains humans in an upright position against the force of gravity. The extensor muscles, often referred to as the antigravity muscles, carry the major load. Sustained contraction of the muscles supporting this upright position is called **postural tonus.** Numerous postural or **righting reflexes** stimulate and maintain postural tonus:

1. *Labyrinthine sense.* Sensory organs of the inner ear stimulate postural tonus through impulses that arise when the head is moved. To maintain balance, the body responds to changes of head position through information received by the cerebellum from receptors in the ampullae of the three semicircular ducts of the inner ear. Each duct contains endolymph, and the three are arranged at right angles to one another. Any body movement is relayed by the endolymph in these ducts to sensory hair cells embedded in a gelatinous, dome-shaped structure called the **cupula.** Stimulation of the hair cells produces nerve impulses that flow along the nerve fibers of the vestibular division of the vestibulocochlear nerve to the brain. See Figure 38–3.
2. *Tonic neck-righting reflexes.* Movement of the head from side to side affects tonic neck reflexes as well as labyrinthine reflexes. Tonus of the neck muscles seems most affected when the head is thrown backward.
3. *Visual or optic reflexes.* Visual impressions are important in maintaining erect posture. Visual sensations help

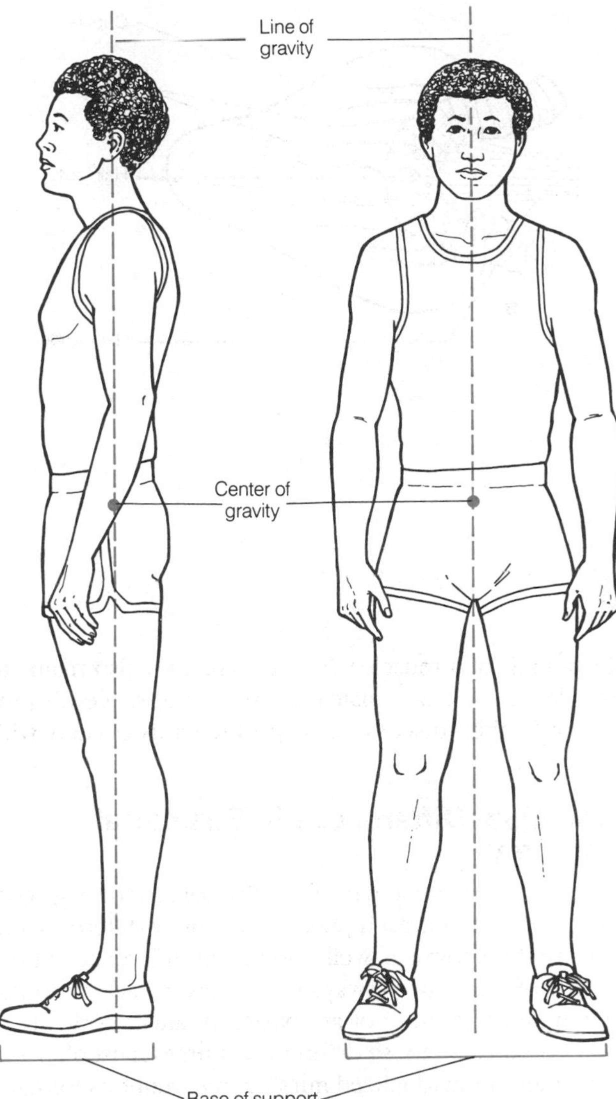

Figure 38–1 Gravity influences standing alignment.

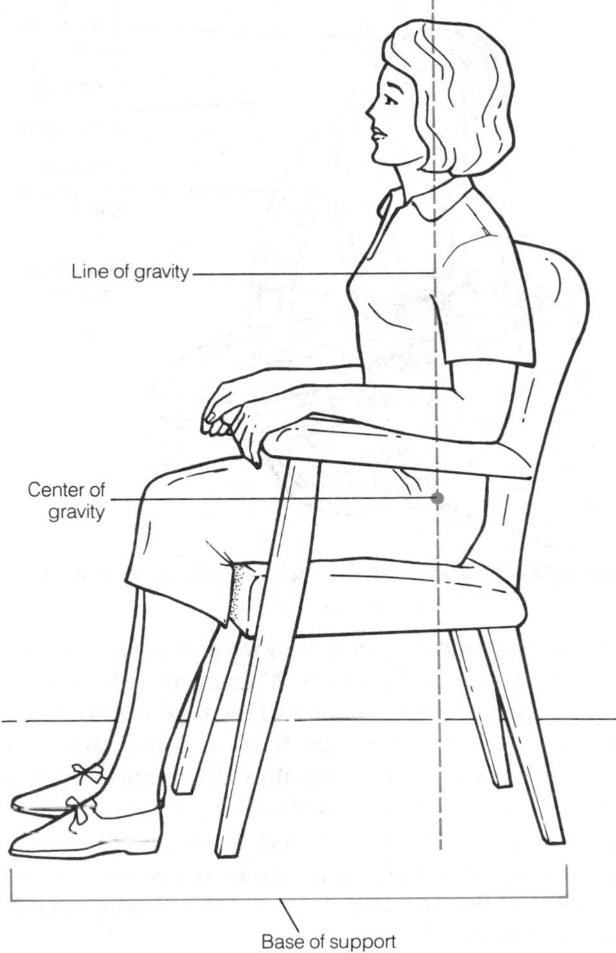

Figure 38–2 Gravity influences sitting alignment.

the person establish spatial relationships to objects in the environment.

4. *Proprioceptor or kinesthetic sense.* The kinesthetic sense, sometimes referred to as the sixth sense, is activated when nerve endings in muscles, tendons, and fascia are stimulated by movements of joints. The individual becomes aware of his or her position when the brain is informed of the location of a limb or body part at any given moment.

5. *Extensor or antigravity (stretch) reflexes.* One of the basic elements of posture is the so-called stretch reflex. This reflex is best developed in the extensor muscles, which counteract the tendency of the body flex at the hip and the knees because of its own weight. If, for example, the knees begin to buckle under the influence of gravity, the extensor muscles of the knee joint are stretched, and their muscle spindles are stimulated. Stimulation results in a reflex contraction of the extensor muscles, which straightens the knee joint and maintains upright posture. Extensor muscles involved in posture include the extensors of the lower extremities, the abdominal muscles, the adductors of the scapulae, and the extensors of the spinal column. Extensors of the spinal column are the site of the spinal stretch reflex.

6. *Plantar reflexes.* Pressure against the sole of the foot by the ground elicits a reflexive contraction of the extensor muscles of the lower legs.

Structures in the cerebral cortex, midbrain, brain stem, cerebellum, and spinal cord regulate and control these reflexes. Postural reflexes enable opposing muscle groups to work together automatically to coordinate the delicate muscle movements required to maintain upright posture, body alignment, and balance. When the flexors contract to bend a joint, the extensors relax; when the extensors contract to straighten a joint, the flexors relax.

Whenever the line of gravity moves away from the center of the base of support, muscles on the side of the

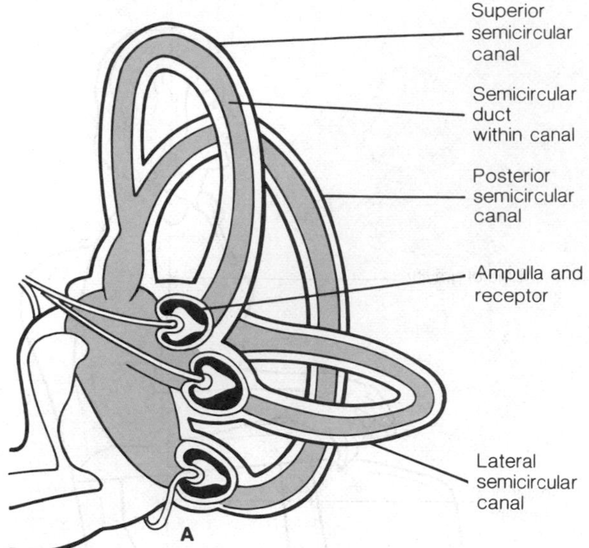

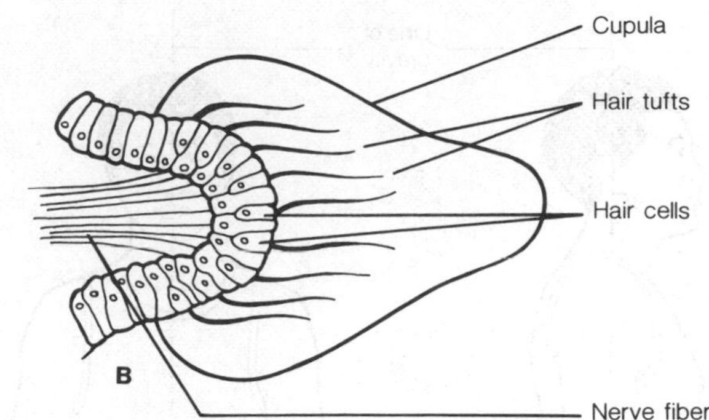

Figure 38–3 The inner ear: **A**, semicircular canals; **B**, cupula

body opposite the direction of movement contract to bring the body back into alignment. Whenever the line of gravity shifts away from the center of the base of support, the energy required to maintain balance is increased. Constant muscle activity to maintain balance and to prevent instability and falling contributes to increased energy expenditure and muscle fatigue. Good posture reduces the number of muscle contractions needed to maintain balance by dividing the work evenly among opposing muscle groups.

Change in Posture

Any position, correct or incorrect, can be detrimental if maintained for a prolonged period. Frequent change of position helps to prevent muscle discomfort, undue pressure resulting in decubitus ulcers, damage to superficial nerves and blood vessels, and **contractures** (permanent shortening of a muscle). Position changes also maintain muscle tone and stimulate postural reflexes. See Chapter 37 for further discussion of problems associated with immobility.

Individual Differences in Structural Anatomy

Since each person has a highly individual pattern of growth and development, each person has minor differences in structural anatomy as well. Individual differences in the degree of curvature (sway) in the lower back or in the length and flexibility of an extremity affect body alignment. Because of these differences, nurses must plan and implement individualized nursing interventions for each client. See a later section of this chapter.

The principles of body alignment are summarized on the facing page.

Assessment

Assessment of body alignment includes an inspection of the client while standing, sitting, or lying. The nurse must also consider developmental and other factors that influence body alignment. A review of the client's health records is essential to determine past and current medical and nursing problems. Alignment criteria for the standing and sitting positions are presented next. Alignment of the client in various supported lying positions is discussed in later sections. The purpose of body alignment assessment is to determine normal changes resulting from growth and development; to identify poor posture and learning needs to maintain good posture; to identify factors contributing to poor posture, such as fatigue or low self-esteem; and to identify muscle weakness or other motor impairments.

Criteria for Assessing Standing Alignment

To assess standing alignment, the nurse must view the client from anterior, lateral, and posterior perspectives. Unnatural or rigid positions can be avoided by ensuring the client is at ease.

When Viewed Anteriorly

See Figure 38–1, earlier.

1. A vertical line from the body's center of gravity (located on the midline halfway between the umbilicus and the symphysis pubis) falls between the feet (the

body's base of support) and extends upward through the middle of the forehead.

2. The head is erect and midline, i.e., not flexed laterally.
3. The shoulders are level, slightly abducted from the sides of the body, and relaxed, neither pulled upward nor downward.
4. The arms are relaxed at the sides, and the elbows are slightly flexed.
5. The hands are positioned midway between pronation and supination. The wrists are extended.
6. The fingers are slightly flexed.
7. A line drawn through the patella and the middle of the ankle ends at the second or third toe.
8. The patellae face straight ahead.
9. The toes point forward.
10. The feet are apart, and one foot is slightly in front of the other to broaden the base of support.

When Viewed Laterally

1. The chin is held in at a 90° angle to the body.
2. The head is erect, neither flexed forward nor extended backward.
3. The shoulders are relaxed, neither pulled forward nor backward.
4. The rib cage is positioned upward and forward to allow increased chest expansion and freer action of the diaphragm.
5. The vertebral curves are normal:
   a. The lumbar curve is anteriorly convex (rounded).
   b. The thoracic curve is posteriorly convex.
   c. The cervical curve is anteriorly convex.
6. The abdomen is pulled in and up.
7. The hips are extended.
8. The knees are slightly flexed.
9. The ankles are dorsiflexed to maintain the feet at right angles to the lower leg.
10. The line of gravity passes over the meatus of the ear canal, the acromial process of the shoulder, the trochanter of the hip, slightly anterior to the center of the knee joint, and anterior to the ankle. See Figure 38–1, earlier.
11. The person appears to be stretched fully but is relaxed and poised with minimal muscle strain.

Principles of Body Alignment

- Balance is maintained when the line of gravity passes through the center of gravity and the base of support.
- The broader the base of support and the lower the center of gravity, the greater the stability in balance.
- When the line of gravity shifts outside the center of the base of support, more energy is required to maintain balance.
- A broad base of support and good alignment of body parts conserve energy and prevent muscle fatigue.
- Change in body position helps to prevent muscle discomfort.
- Prolonged poor body alignment contributes to pain, muscle fatigue, and contractures.
- Because of individual differences in structural anatomy, nursing interventions must be individualized to meet the client's needs.
- Strengthening weak muscle groups helps prevent muscle and ligament strain when poor body alignment is temporarily or inadvertently used.

When Viewed Posteriorly

1. The shoulders are level.
2. The hips are level.
3. The spine is straight, not curved to either side.
4. The main body weight is borne well forward on the outer sides of the feet.

Good body alignment enables the weight-bearing joints to function effectively, prevents damage to ligaments and other joint structures, and elongates the lumbar spine. This elongation flattens the abdomen and prevents an exaggerated lumbar curvature. By using good body alignment, a person can stand for long periods without experiencing undue muscle discomfort or back pain.

Common Problems in Standing Alignment

When the pelvis is well aligned, i.e., "tucked under" (see Figure 38–4, *A*), the lumbar spine is elongated. This alignment flattens the abdomen and prevents an exaggerated lumbar curvature of the spine. A tensed trunk alignment in which the pelvis is tucked under is referred to as the **pelvic tilt**, using a **long midriff**, or putting on an **internal girdle**. The pelvic tilt is absent when alignment is poor.

The "slumped" posture (see Figure 38–4, *B*) is the most common problem that occurs when people stand.

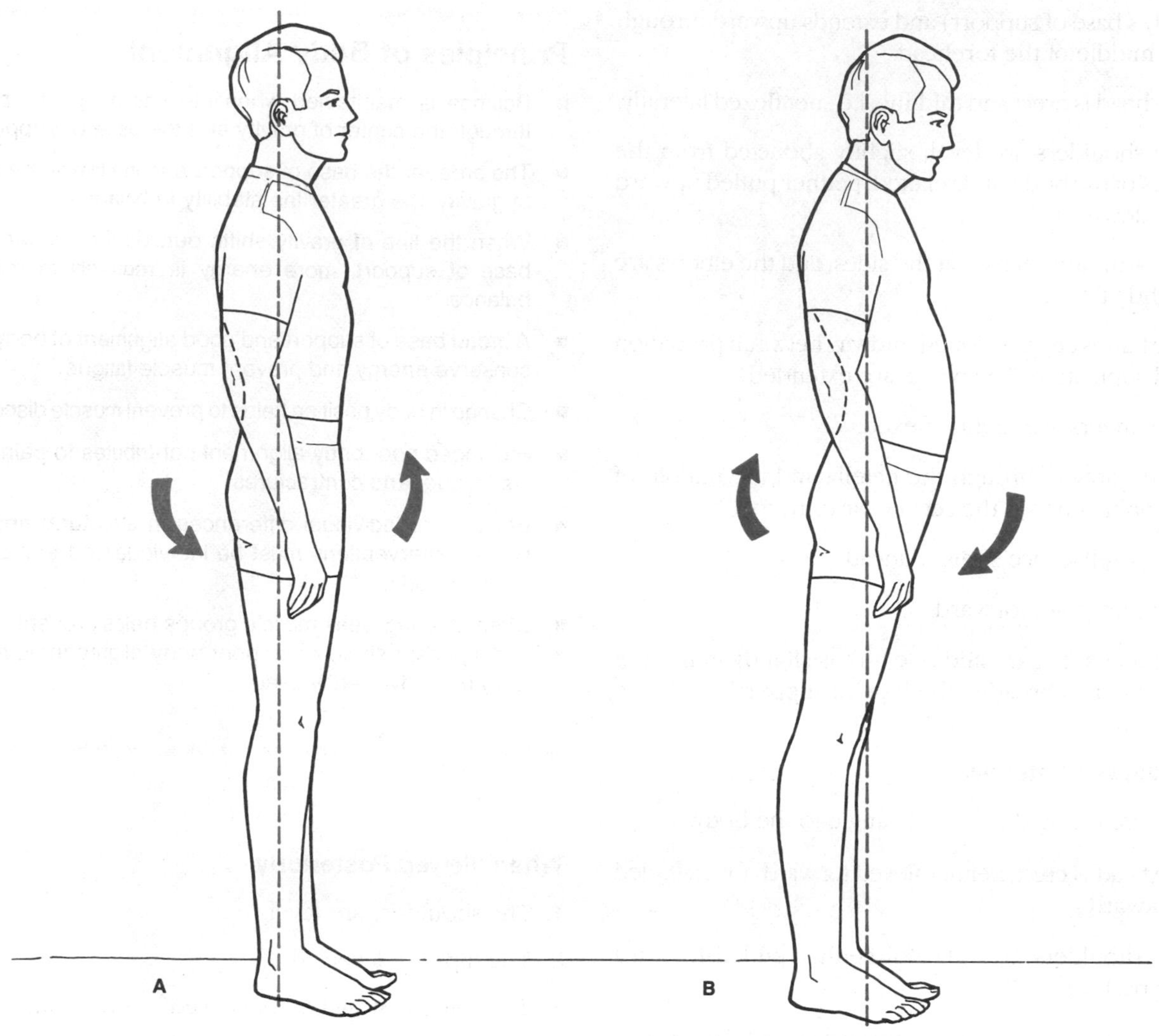

Figure 38–4 A standing person with: **A,** good trunk alignment; **B,** poor trunk alignment. The arrows indicate the direction in which the pelvis is tilted.

Source: Adapted from D. Drapeau, Getting back into good posture, *Nursing 75,* 5:63. Used by permission.

The neck is flexed far forward, the abdomen protrudes, the pelvis is thrust forward to create an exaggerated curvature of the lumbar spine (**lordosis**), and the knees are markedly hyperextended. Lower back pain and fatigue occur quickly in people with poor posture. When one segment of the body deviates from proper alignment, compensatory deviations occur in other body segments; the result is strain and damage to the malaligned ligaments and joint structures supporting body weight (Foss 1973, p. 25).

Criteria for Assessing Sitting Alignment

To assess sitting alignment, the nurse views the client from a lateral perspective. In an adult assuming a well-aligned sitting position, the head and trunk are the same as in the standing position.

1. The head is erect, neither flexed forward nor extended backward.
2. The chin is held in.
3. The rib cage is positioned upward and forward.
4. The cervical and thoracic curves are the same as when standing.
5. The lumbar curve is less anteriorly convex due to hip flexion.
6. The abdomen is pulled up and in.

7. The hips are flexed at right angles to the trunk so that the thighs are horizontal.
8. The knees are flexed at an angle dependent on the position of the feet.
9. The popliteal spaces are at least 2.5 cm (1 in) away from the edge of the chair to avoid pressure on the blood circulation and the nerves of the legs.
10. Both feet are on the floor, and one foot is in front of the other.
11. The weight of the body from the head to the buttocks is centered on the buttocks and thighs.
12. The forearms are supported on the lap, chair armrests, or a table in front. Figure 38–2 on page 1029 shows a person in the well-aligned sitting position. If the arms are supported on armrests:
    a. The forearms and hands are supported up to the elbow so as to prevent upward or downward pulling of the shoulder girdle.
    b. The elbows do not rest on the chair arm to prevent pressure on the bony prominences of the elbows.

Common Problems in Sitting Alignment

Sitting with one leg crossed over the other creates a C shape, or postural **scoliosis**, of the lumbar-thoracic spine. It may be relaxing to assume this position for short periods, but care must be taken not to exert undue pressure against the delicate nerves and blood vessels in the popliteal area. Persons who have peripheral vascular problems should avoid crossing the legs for this reason. Habitually sitting with the same leg crossed over the other can eventually contribute to permanent postural scoliosis. Slouching while sitting may be relaxing for short periods, but habitual slouching can contribute to permanent postural abnormalities.

Developmental Variations in Body Alignment

Body alignment or posture changes significantly during growth and with age. An understanding of the normal variations is helpful for the nurse in promoting good posture, in assessing postural faults, and in helping others correct them. The following sections describe normal developmental postural variations.

Newborns and Infants

In the newborn, the spine is straight and lacks the anteroposterior curves of the adult, but it can be flexed. The abdomen is rounded and prominent. All extremities are generally flexed, but they can be passively moved through a full range of motion. The feet may normally turn inward (**inversion**) but can be passively turned outward (**eversion**). It is normal for young infants to have the toes point in, or be pigeon-toed. This is due to internal tibial torsion or inward rotation of the lower legs. However, if the lower legs are straight and toeing-in occurs in early infancy, it can be due to an abnormal congenital condition called **metatarsus adductus**, which warrants treatment. Toeing-in can also be caused by an internal rotation of the hip, which rotates the entire limb. Internal hip rotation extending beyond the normal position of the hip is called **femoral anteversion.**

The appearance of flat-footedness due to a fat pad in the instep is normal in infants and may occur in toddlers with knock-knees to a mild degree. In most cases, tibial torsion, femoral anteversion, and mild metatarsus adductus tend to disappear without treatment as the child grows.

When infants learn to stand at about 1 year of age, they stand with legs slightly bowed, feet far apart, toes turned outward, and knees hyperextended. The head and upper part of the trunk are carried forward, and the arms are abducted to enhance balance. Their balance is rather precarious, and, when they fall, they usually fall backward. A "pot belly" and exaggerated lumbar curvature are characteristic at this age.

Toddlers

Toddlers have a marked lumbar lordosis (swayback or marked anterior concavity in the lumbar spinal curvature) and a protruding abdomen. The pelvis tilts forward, and there is only a slight convex curvature of the thoracic spine. Some toeing-out and a wide stance may occur normally in 2-year-olds due to a slight outward rotation of the hips. The feet are typically everted. Growth, with its functional stresses, eventually produces an inward rotation of the hips, which results in disappearance of the foot eversion.

Children

From 3 to 5 years of age, children become slimmer, taller, and more solid looking. They assume the so-called little adult appearance: The protrusion of the abdomen is less exaggerated, and the arms and legs grow longer. They are more steady and evenly balanced on their feet. They no longer widely abduct their arms for balance. They may normally have a very mild degree of knock-knees and pigeon toes (Brower 1979, p. 60).

By age 7 or 8, the child's legs have straightened out and the toes point straight ahead. Children of this age usually have excellent posture by any standards, often the best that they will have at any time during their lives.

Adolescents

Significant changes in body proportions and contours occur during adolescence. In early adolescence, ages 11 to 13, a boy's form is characterized by straight leg lines, narrow hips, wide shoulders, a broad chest, and noticeable muscular development in the shoulders, arms, and thighs. In contrast, a young adolescent girl has curved leg lines; her hips become wider, and her breasts develop. Fat is deposited in the buttocks, thighs, and upper arms.

Motor awkwardness is common at this age because of the rapid and uneven growth of the muscles and bones. For example, when the bones grow more quickly than the muscles, the muscles become tight and respond in quick, jerky motions. If, however, the muscles grow more quickly than the bones, the muscles are loose and sluggish, resulting in clumsy movements. This awkwardness of leg and arm movements disappears once growth of the bones and muscles stabilizes.

Postural problems often occur at this age because of the discrepancies in weight and height between girls and boys. Because the growth spurt in girls occurs between 8½ and 11½ years of age, while for boys it happens from 10½ to 14½ years of age, it is not uncommon for girls to tower above their male partners on a dance floor. Posture may suffer as a consequence. By late adolescence, the gawky look and awkward movements of early adolescence disappear.

The posture of adolescents is highly individual and determined to a large extent by the person's self-image. Poor posture is, unfortunately, very common. A habitual stooped posture is not considered appropriate. The posture of adolescents is assessed by the same criteria used to assess the posture of the young adult. The postural habits formed during adolescence often persist into adulthood. Slight flexion contractures of the neck are common by late adolescence.

Adults

Body alignment and posture of adults are described earlier in this chapter.

Older Adults

The aging person tends to have some contraction in all flexor muscles. Postural **kyphosis** (humpback) is quite common as the neck and shoulder girdles become more flexed and stooped with advancing age. Any lumbar lordosis that the person may have had earlier in life disappears as kyphosis progresses. The hips and knees may have slight flexion contractures, causing the person to take short, shuffling steps. Deterioration of postural reflexes gradually increases instability, causing the person to use a wider base of support with toes pointing outward slightly to achieve balance (Witte 1979, p. 1952).

Osteoporosis, a condition in which the bones become increasingly brittle and fragile due to depletion of calcium, is common among older women. Osteoporosis primarily affects the weight-bearing joints of the lower extremities and back. It can cause compression fractures of the vertebrae, resulting in a forward-leaning stooped posture, sometimes called **dowager's hump**, and a significant loss in body height.

Persons who wear bifocals may hyperextend the head so that they can see where they are going. Hyperextension of the cervical spine can potentially injure ligaments and joint structures in this area, which may already be damaged due to the degenerative effects of aging and disease (Hogan and Beland 1976, p. 1106).

Factors That Influence Body Alignment

General Health

Illness, disability, immobility, inactivity, poor physical fitness, and chronic fatigue have adverse effects on musculoskeletal function and posture.

Nutrition

Adequate nutrition supplies vitamins and minerals essential for normal bone and muscle function. It also supplies glucose, the energy source that powers muscle. Poor nutrition may cause muscle weakness and fatigue. An inadequate calcium intake by elderly women places them at risk of postural problems due to osteoporosis. An inadequate intake of vitamin D in infancy and childhood can cause **rickets**, a disease marked by bending and distortion of the bones. Obesity distorts alignment, and obese persons must expend more energy to maintain balance.

Emotions

Security, joy, confidence, and self-esteem are reflected in good posture. Worry, discouragement, insecurity, and a sense of inferiority are often reflected in a slumped posture. Causes of these attitudes need to be sought before posture correction can be effective.

Situational Factors

People can develop poor posture due to situational causes, such as:

1. Soft beds with sagging springs, which disrupt the appropriate distribution of weight
2. Chairs not adjusted to body height and build
3. Tables, desks, and working equipment placed so that the person must strain to work at them

4. Tight clothing that restricts freedom of movement and hinders normal muscular function
5. Shoes that are worn down at the heels and tilt the body out of line
6. Constant wearing of high-heeled shoes, which exaggerate the forward tilt of the body
7. Bifocal eyeglasses, because the person may need to make abnormal adjustments in head alignment to see clearly.

Life-Style

An individual's life-style can affect posture. Postures repeatedly assumed during work can result in permanent postural defects; for example, a mail carrier may walk for years leaning to one side from carrying a heavy bag, or an assembly line worker may sit for hours hunched over a bench. Repeated physical activity, e.g., by a weight lifter, can produce muscle hypertrophy and concomitant alignment changes to accommodate the hypertrophy. Continual inactivity and resulting poor physical fitness can produce muscle atrophy and concomitant alignment changes to accommodate the atrophy.

Attitudes and Values

Personal values about body alignment are important influences. The tall adolescent may slouch because he or she does not value being taller than peers. Some people value good posture and intentionally try to maintain body alignment for reasons of health or appearance.

Level of Understanding About Body Alignment

An understanding of the elements of good alignment is conducive to good posture. Unfortunately, many individuals either have no opportunity to learn about good body alignment or are misinformed.

Neuromuscular and Skeletal Impairments

Disease processes and injuries that affect the neuromuscular or skeletal systems can severely hinder body alignment and result in functional disabilities. Genetically transmitted muscle-wasting diseases, disorders causing sensory or motor impairment, inflammatory conditions, injuries, and pain can severely impair body alignment.

Review of Records

When assessing body alignment, the nurse reviews information in the client's records so as to plan appropriate nursing interventions. The physician's physical examination and history are important sources of information about disabilities affecting the musculoskeletal system, e.g., contractures, edema, pain in the extremities, or generalized fatigue, that affect the planning of nursing interventions for that client. A review of the recent nurses' notes is also useful.

Diagnostic tests chiefly used to assess the integrity of the musculoskeletal and neuromuscular systems involve roentgenography (x-ray examination) to determine the size and shape of bones or areas of variable density. Blood tests for serum calcium levels can detect some types of bone pathology. Normal serum calcium is 5 mEq/liter (Byrne et al. 1986, p. 273). Calcium deficiency can result in rickets (decalcification of bone) when found in children and **osteomalacia** in adults. Serum phosphate and inorganic phosphorus (normal adult level, 1.8–2.6 mEq/liter; child, as high as 4.1 mEq/liter) have a function in maintaining serum calcium concentrations. Phosphate is needed for the generation of bone. Phosphate levels are always in inverse proportion to calcium levels in the blood.

Increased phosphorus levels (**hyperphosphatemia**) are often found with kidney dysfunction. They are also associated with bone tumors and **hypocalcemia** (calcium deficiency). Phosphorus deficiency (**hypophosphatemia**) is found in rickets and osteomalacia.

Nursing Diagnosis

The Consequences of Poor Body Alignment

The consequences of poor body alignment are multiple. The individual who exhibits poor posture not only presents a poor physical appearance but also reflects an unfavorable self-image to others.

The musculoskeletal system is particularly affected by poor alignment. Fatigue and muscle strain occur when the work of maintaining balance is not evenly divided among opposing muscle groups. Contractures brought about by using poor alignment over a prolonged time may eventually develop into permanent disabilities. Muscles, ligaments, and joint structures in the back may be weakened and permanently damaged when not aligned correctly over time. Poor posture also contributes to instability, which may in turn predispose the client to accidents.

Poor alignment can affect the function of other body systems as well. Poor alignment can reduce chest expansion. Undue or prolonged pressure brought about by improper body alignment may impede blood flow, damage superficial nerves, and contribute to the formation of decubitus ulcers. When the abdominal muscles are weakened and the spinal column is not properly aligned, gastrointestional function can be compromised, predisposing the person to a variety of problems, including constipation (Memmer 1974, pp. 16–17). All of these consequences of poor body alignment can be prevented.

Structural Abnormalities Affecting Alignment

Structural impairments in body alignment are usually caused by congenital abnormalities, developmental abnormalities, or abnormal intrauterine positions before birth. Several common abnormalities are listed in Table 38–1. Of course, functional abnormalities, such as poor posture during the growing years or improper alignment during illness, can also cause these abnormalities.

Nursing Diagnosis

Examples of nursing diagnoses related to problems with body alignment are shown on the right.

Examples of Nursing Diagnoses Related to Altered Body Alignment

- Potential for injury related to poor standing and sitting alignment secondary to wearing of long leg cast
- Potential for injury related to impaired standing and sitting alignment secondary to left-sided paralysis
- Potential for impaired mobility related to foot drop and knee and hip contractures, secondary to imposed bed rest
- Potential alteration in comfort related to poor standing alignment secondary to constant wearing of high-heeled shoes
- Alteration in comfort related to kyphosis secondary to tuberculosis of the spine
- Alteration in comfort related to impaired standing alignment secondary to pregnancy
- Potential for injury related to difficulty with alignment and balance associated with neurologic impairment and muscle weakness

Planning

Goals

The nursing assessment and nursing diagnoses help the nurse identify goals for care and design an individualized plan of nursing intervention for the client. Overall goals for clients with potential or actual body alignment problems include:

1. Maintain proper body alignment
2. In persons who have poor body alignment:
   a. Restore body alignment to an optimal level
   b. Prevent muscle shortening (contractures), reduced chest expansion, and other complications of poor alignment

The Nurse's Responsibility for Client Alignment

The nurse is responsible for identifying those clients who need assistance with body alignment and determining the degree of assistance they need. The nurse must be sensitive to the client's need to function as independently

Table 38–1 Common Structural Abnormalities that Affect Alignment

Deviation	Description	Cause	Treatment
Scoliosis	Lateral curvature of the spine, which increases during active growth periods	May be secondary to other deformities, such as a discrepancy in leg lengths, or defects of spinal supporting tissues (a functional scoliosis); the most common cause of structural scoliosis is heredity, which produces an idiopathic structural scoliosis, a condition occurring five times more often in females than males, between the ages of 8 and 15	Treatment of underlying cause or application of a brace or cast from occiput to pelvis; surgical fusion of the spinal vertebrae may be necessary
Kyphosis (roundback or humpback)	A fixed flexion deformity of the thoracic spine	Congenital—rickets, tuberculosis of spine	Exercises to extend the thoracic spine; sleeping without a pillow; occasionally bracing or spinal fusion may be required
Lordosis (swayback)	A fixed hyperextension deformity of the lumbar spine	Congenital, most often secondary to other abnormalities such as kyphosis or muscular dystrophy	The underlying disease is treated

as he or she can yet provide assistance when the client needs it.

Clients who are mobile and completely capable of helping themselves may not require nursing interventions to maintain proper body alignment. Some may require guidance and assistance to correct poor postural habits or to prevent further postural deviations. At the other extreme are clients who are not very mobile, can help themselves only minimally, and have low energy levels. They are at high risk of developing contractures and other complications of immobility outlined in Chapter 37. These persons are totally dependent on caregivers and must be instructed to achieve and maintain correct body alignment. Most clients fall somewhere in between these two extremes. They require varying kinds and degrees of nursing guidance and assistance to learn about, achieve, and maintain proper alignment. Most clients will benefit from at least some of the specific nursing interventions outlined in the next section.

Planning nursing care for clients with altered body alignment is usually an independent nursing function. The physician usually orders specific body positions only after surgery, anesthesia, or trauma involving the nervous and musculoskeletal systems. The client's current "activity order" contains data essential for planning nursing interventions for body alignment. All clients should have an activity order written by their physician when they are admitted to the agency for care. Examples of common activity orders are shown above.

Planning also involves the writing of outcome criteria. See "Evaluation," later in this chapter.

Examples of Activity Orders

- **BR (bed rest) or SCB (strictly confined to bed). This order indicates that the client is not to get out of bed for any reason.**
- **BRP (bathroom privileges) c̄ assistance. This order indicates that the client is not to get out of bed except to urinate or defecate. A caregiver must always accompany the client to the bathroom.**
- **Up ad lib. This order indicates that the client may be in and out of bed as he or she wishes.**
- **HOB 30 continuously. This order indicates that the head of the bed is to be elevated 30° (in Fowler's position) both day and night.**

Intervention

For Standing Alignment Problems

A frequent postural problem in the standing client is a forward thrusting of the neck, which produces a stooped position (see Figure 38–4, *B*). Slight flexion contractures of the neck, preventing appropriate neck extension, are common by late adolescence and are usually due to poor posture. If the client has a flexion contracture of the cervical spine, the nurse should make every effort to prevent further contractures and, if possible, to reduce the contracture already present. If the client has no neck flexion contracture, the nurse makes every effort to prevent it. The client should make a conscious effort to prevent neck flexion when standing and walking. Proper sitting and sleeping postures (see later sections) alleviate this problem.

Another frequent postural problem in the standing client is an exaggerated curvature, or lordosis, of the lumbar spine (see Figure 38–4, *B*). The lordosis is usually accompanied by an abnormally protruding abdomen. Conscientious use of the pelvic tilt, shown in Figure 38–4, *A*, flattens the abdomen and prevents lordosis of the lumbar spine. Exercises to strengthen and protect the back muscles that support the lumbar spine and the abdominal muscles help prevent or reduce postural lordosis. For specific exercises, see Owen (1980) in the "Suggested Readings" at the end of this chapter. Note that as the client performs exercises that strengthen the back, he or she should keep the hips and knees flexed, not straight. Persons with a history of back problems should follow an exercise program prescribed by a physician. Any program of exercise should be started slowly and intensified gradually.

Flexion of the hip and knee straightens the lumbar spine and reduces lordosis. Clients should avoid prolonged standing; however, if prolonged standing is unavoidable, the client should elevate one foot onto a support to straighten the spine. Periodically changing the foot that is elevated prevents undue strain to one side of the spinal column at the expense of the other (Ishmael and Shorbe 1969, p. 7).

General exercise promotes good standing alignment. Walking and swimming, which maintain overall muscle tone, are especially useful. Postural habits tend to deteriorate in people who are chronically overtired. Thus, chronic fatigue should be avoided.

Conscientious and continuous awareness of and effort to improve posture in everyday activities are important in achieving and maintaining good posture. To put forth this effort, the client must be motivated; motivation is in turn usually dependent on self-image. The nurse who practices good postural habits can be a significant role model and motivator. No amount of verbal instruction and encouragement will influence clients to use good posture as strongly as the example of a nurse who "practices what she or he preaches" (Memmer 1974, p. 28).

For Sitting Alignment Problems

Nursing interventions to promote good sitting alignment apply whether the client is sitting in a chair, in a wheelchair, or on the side of the bed. In the sitting client, alignment problems frequently affect not only the back, but also the top extremities. Alignment problems are often due to the size and shape of the object on which the person is sitting; the chair or wheelchair may simply not fit the person.

Chair Seats and Backs

A chair seat that is too high creates undue pressure against the thighs, especially in the popliteal area behind the knees, since the lower legs and feet are unsupported. Prolonged pressure can damage the delicate nerves and blood vessels in the popliteal area. Fatigue and discomfort can ensue rapidly. A firm footrest of an appropriate height improves alignment and comfort. A chair seat that is too low causes no alignment problems of the back but, unless the thighs are supported, exerts undue pressure on the ischial tuberosities, due to the narrow base of support for the trunk. If too low, the seat may be difficult to get into and, especially, out of. Pillows placed on the chair seat support the thighs and improve alignment. A chair seat that is too deep produces undue flexion of the thoracolumbar spine. The weight of the body does not rest on the ischial tuberosities, and the lower back is not supported properly by the chair back. This position can be quite uncomfortable. Pillows placed between the chair back and the person's back improve alignment.

If the chair back is too low or if there is no chair back, there is no effect on alignment, but most persons find that a higher back supports the spinal column and prevents fatigue.

In all instances, proper alignment in the sitting client is best promoted by a chair seat that allows the knees to be slightly higher than the hips and supports the full length of the thighs (see Figure 38–2) and by a chair back that supports the entire back.

Armrests

When the arms of a chair are too high, the person's shoulder girdle may be forced upward into an uncomfortable position. In this case, placing pillows on the chair seat to elevate the body improves alignment. When the arms of the chair are too low, the person's shoulder girdle is pulled downward, causing the shoulders and back to slump when the person attempts to rest his or her arms on the chair arms. Padding to raise the level of the chair arms improves alignment. When the arms of the chair are too far apart, the person may have to stretch to rest his or her arms on the chair arms. Such stretching may cause back discomfort. Supports placed between the chair arms and the person, on one or both sides of the body, can substitute for chair arms and improve alignment.

Whenever possible, the elbow should not lean on the hard chair arm. Undue pressure over this bony prominence can produce discomfort. The client who leans the elbows on the arms of a wheelchair or other chair for prolonged periods is at risk of developing a pressure sore.

Both people and chairs come in a variety of sizes and shapes. No chair is conducive to the proper alignment of everyone who sits in it. Many alignment problems, however, can be prevented or corrected when the chair is specifically adapted to fit the person who uses it (Memmer 1974, p. 28).

Principles of Positioning Clients

Principles of positioning clients are outlined on page 1039.

Guidelines for Positioning Clients in Bed

1. Make sure the mattress is firm and level yet has enough give to fill in and support natural body curvatures. A properly filled water bed can provide good support. Poor alignment is inevitable when the client rests on a sagging mattress, a mattress that is too soft, or an underfilled water bed. Mattresses such as these, when used over a prolonged period, can contribute to the development of hip flexion contractures and low back strain and pain.

   Bed boards made of plywood and placed beneath a sagging mattress are increasingly recommended for clients who have back problems or are prone to them. Some bed boards are hinged across the middle so that they will bend as the head of the bed is raised.

2. Ensure the best possible body alignment to prevent stress on the client's muscles and joints. This is achieved by placing support devices (e.g., pillows, rolled towels, foam rubber supports) in specified areas according to the client's position. Common alignment problems are:
   a. Flexion of the neck
   b. Internal rotation of the shoulder
   c. Adduction of the shoulder
   d. Flexion of the wrist
   e. Anterior convexity of the lumbar spine
   f. External rotation of the hips
   g. Hyperextension of the knees
   h. Plantar flexion of the ankle

3. Not all clients require identical supports. Adapt support devices to the individual's body and physical ability. A client who is muscular and has adequate adipose tissue in the lumbar region may not require support in this area while sitting or lying. A person with a paralyzed leg will require a support against the

Principles of Positioning Clients

- The lower the degree of mobility, the capacity for self-care, and the energy level, the greater the need for careful alignment.
- Postural lordosis, kyphosis, and scoliosis created by malpositioning contribute to back and neck pain and to the development of contractures.
- When poor body alignment is prolonged, temporary postural contractures may develop into permanent contractures.
- In the immobilized client, the most frequently occurring contractures are flexion contractures of the hips, knees, and plantar flexors of the ankles. Flexion contractures of the cervical spine and shoulders are also common.
- Body parts aligned in a functional position of comfort, as close to anatomic position as possible, ensure the least stress on muscles and joints and the greatest comfort for the client.
- Gravity pulls unsupported body parts downward. Support devices (e.g., bedboards, pillows, trochanter rolls, sandbags, footboards, and hand-wrist splints) counteract the pull of gravity.
- Flexion of the hip and knee straightens the lumbar spine, reducing postural lordosis.
- All sitting and most bed lying positions, if assumed for prolonged periods, promote flexion contractures of the hips and knees.
- Use of too many pillows beneath the head of a client lying in bed promotes flexion contractures of the neck.
- Disuse atrophy can occur rapidly when the client does not use the lower extremities to support total body weight during standing and walking.
- Dorsiflexor muscles of the ankle deteriorate rapidly when not used for standing and walking. Plantar flexor muscles of the ankles are stronger than dorsiflexor muscles.
- Devices that provide a broad base of support pose the least risk of focal pressure areas. Devices with a narrow base of support can cause discomfort to the area and undue pressure against tissues, blood vessels, and nerves.

Source: Adapted from M. K. Memmer, *Posture and alignment* (Los Angeles: The Intercampus Nursing Project, California State University and College System, 1974), pp. 21–23.

thigh and hip when lying to prevent external rotation. A client with a paralyzed arm may require a wrist and hand splint to prevent flexion of the wrist.

4. Plan a systematic 24-hour schedule for position changes. See the next column. Frequent position changes are essential to prevent decubitus ulcers in immobilized clients. Usually, such clients are repositioned every 2 hours throughout the day and night and more frequently when there is concern about skin breakdown. This schedule is usually outlined on the client's nursing care plan.

Sample Schedule for Position Changes

Time		Position
10:00 A.M.	(1000 hr)	Left lateral
Noon	(1200 hr)	Fowler's or chair
2:00 P.M.	(1400 hr)	Right lateral
4:00 P.M.	(1600 hr)	Right Sims'
6:00 P.M.	(1800 hr)	Fowler's or chair
8:00 P.M.	(2000 hr)	Left lateral
10:00 P.M.	(2200 hr)	Left Sims'
Midnight	(2400 hr)	Supine
2:00 A.M.	(0200 hr)	Right lateral
4:00 A.M.	(0400 hr)	Right Sims'
6:00 A.M.	(0600 hr)	Supine
8:00 A.M.	(0800 hr)	Fowler's

5. Provide support devices for pressure areas created by the former position. The bony prominences that bore the body weight can be gently massaged with lotion, although some authorities question the value of this except as a comfort measure (Shannon 1984).
6. Ensure that the foundation of the bed is firm, clean, and dry. Wrinkled or damp sheets increase the risk of decubitus ulcer formation.
7. Make sure extremities can move freely whenever possible. For example, the top bedclothes need to be loose enough for the client to move the feet.
8. Ensure that elbows, hips, and knees are slightly flexed to maintain natural body alignment.
9. Support natural body curvatures of the body resting against the bed and unnatural hollows created by physical deformities, such as contractures. Appropriate supports prevent muscle strain and discomfort.
10. Avoid placing one body part, particularly one with bony prominences, directly on top of another body part. Excessive pressure can damage veins and predispose the client to thrombus formation.
11. Avoid excessive pressure against the popliteal space to prevent damage to nerves and blood vessels in this area.

12. Use only those support devices needed to maintain alignment. If the person is capable of movement, too many devices limit mobility and increase potential for muscle weakness and atrophy.
13. Before changing a client's position, assess the client's ability to move and obtain assistance as required. The risk of muscle strain and body injury, to both the client and nurse, is lowered when appropriate assistance is provided.
14. Encourage or provide range of motion (ROM) exercises for the client's major joints, unless contraindicated, each time the position is changed. ROM exercises prevent the formation of contractures. These exercises may be contraindicated if the client cannot tolerate the movement, e.g., if the client has an acute illness or an extensive malignancy. See Chapter 37 for information about ROM exercises.
15. Schedule periods throughout the day during which the client assumes positions that provide full extension of the neck, hips, and knees to prevent flexion contractures of these joints.
16. Use appropriate methods to lift and move the client's extremities. Detailed information about these methods is provided in Chapter 37.
17. Always elicit information from the client to determine which position is most comfortable and appropriate. Seeking information from the client about what feels best to him or her is a useful guide when aligning persons and is an essential aspect of evaluating the effectiveness of an alignment intervention. Sometimes a person who appears well aligned may be experiencing real discomfort. Both appearance, in relation to alignment criteria, and comfort are important in achieving effective alignment.
18. Whenever positioning a client in bed, the alignment criteria for standing alignment outlined in this chapter and in Table 38–2, p. 1049, must be followed as closely as possible. These criteria serve as the basis for guiding nurses' interventions in positioning clients in bed and for evaluating the interventions achieved.

Criteria for Selecting Support Devices

1. *The client's adipose tissue.* A client who has ample adipose tissue generally requires less support and cushioning than the emaciated client while in a back-lying position, but greater support to maintain a lateral position.
2. *The client's skeletal structure.* Both the amount and the type of support needed vary according to the individual's skeletal structure. A client with a marked lumbar lordosis requires more lumbar support than one with a slight lumbar curvature.
3. *The client's state of health.* A client with a paralyzed arm or leg requires more support to maintain body alignment than the client who can move his or her limbs.
4. *The client's discomfort.* A client who experiences pain when he or she moves requires more support to prevent movement than one who can move without pain.
5. *The condition of the client's skin.* Clients with nutritional problems and/or impaired circulation require more cushioning of the pressure points to prevent skin breakdown than do healthy persons.
6. *The client's ability to move.* A client who can move in bed can change position frequently. The client who is unable to move requires considerable support so that muscles do not become strained because of immobility.
7. *The client's hydration.* Dehydrated clients are at greater risk of decubitus ulcer formation than well-hydrated clients and therefore need more support under pressure areas.

Fowler's Position

Fowler's position, or semisitting position, is a bed position in which the head and trunk are raised 45° to 90°. See Figure 38–5. In **low-Fowler's**, or **semi-Fowler's, position**, the head and trunk are raised 15° to 45°; in **high-Fowler's position**, the head and trunk are raised 90°. In this position, the knees may or may not be flexed. Nurses need to clarify the meaning of the term *Fowler's position* in a particular agency. In some hospitals, *Fowler's position* refers to elevation of the upper part of the body without knee flexion, and the term *semi-Fowler's* is used to refer to the sitting position with knee flexion.

Fowler's position is the position of choice for people who have difficulty breathing and for some people with heart problems. When the client is in this position, gravity pulls the diaphragm downward, allowing greater lung expansion. Clients confined to bed but capable of eating, reading, watching television, or visiting find this position comfortable.

Malalignments associated with an *unsupported* Fowler's position are:

1. Hyperextension of the neck
2. Flexion of the lumbar curvature
3. Hyperextension of the knees
4. External rotation of the hips
5. Plantar flexion

In clients who lack arm movement, shoulder muscle strain, edema of the hands and arms, and wrist flexion are added problems.

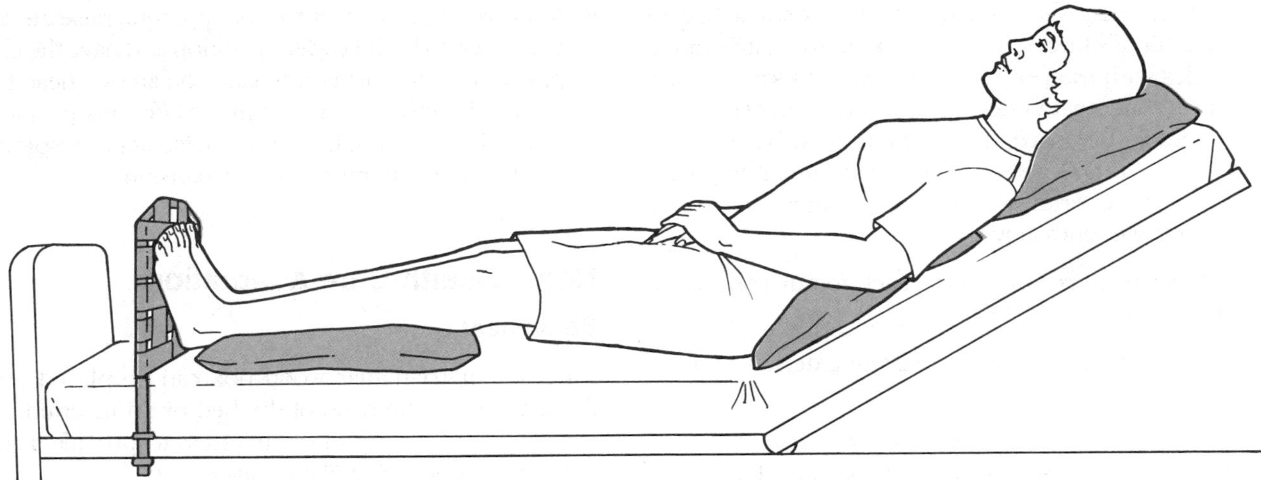

Figure 38–5 Fowler's position (supported)

A common error nurses make when aligning clients in Fowler's position is placing an overly large pillow or more than one pillow behind the client's head. These errors promote the development of neck flexion contractures. If a client desires several head pillows, the nurse should encourage the client to rest without a pillow for several hours each day to extend the neck fully and counteract the effects of poor neck alignment.

Procedure 38–1 ▲ Supporting a Client in Fowler's Position

Equipment

1. Up to 6 small pillows, depending on client need
2. Trochanter roll (optional)
3. Footboard

Intervention

Using the alignment criteria as a guide:

1. Have the client flex the knees slightly before raising the head of the bed. Be certain the client's hips are positioned directly over the point where the bed will bend when the head is raised.

   Rationale Slight knee flexion prevents the person from sliding toward the foot of the bed as the bed is raised. The hip position ensures that the client will be sitting on the ischial tuberositis when the head of the bed is raised.

2. Raise the head of the bed to 30°, 45°, or the angle required by or ordered for the client.
3. Place a small pillow or roll under the lumbar region of the back if you feel a space in the lumbar curvature.

   Rationale This pillow supports the natural lumbar curvature and prevents flexion of the lumbar spine.

4. Place a small pillow under the client's head or have the client rest his or her head against the mattress.

   Rationale This pillow supports the cervical curvature of the vertebral column. Too many pillows beneath the head can cause neck flexion contracture.

5. Place one or two pillows under the lower legs from below the knees to the ankles. Make sure that no pressure is exerted on the popliteal space and that the knees are flexed.

   Rationale This pillow provides a broad base of support that is soft and flexible and causes no localized pressure areas in the lower legs. The pillow prevents uncomfortable hyperextension of the knees and reduces pressure on the heels. Keeping the knees slightly flexed also prevents the person from sliding down in the bed. Pressure against the popliteal space is avoided, since it can damage nerves and vein walls, predisposing the client to thrombus formation.

Avoid using the knee gatch of a hospital bed to flex the client's knees. The position of the gatch rarely coincides with the position of the client's knees. Even when the knee gatch does bend at the client's knees, considerable pressure, due to the narrow base of support beneath the knees and the firm, unyielding mattress, can be exerted against the popliteal space and beneath the client's calves.

6. Put a trochanter roll lateral to each femur (optional). See Procedure 38–2.

   Rationale Trochanter rolls prevent external rotation of the hips.

7. Support the client's feet with a footboard that protrudes several inches above the toes. See Chapter 36. Place the footboard about 1 inch away from the client's heels.

   Rationale The footboard prevents plantar flexion. Placing it 1 inch away from the heels prevents undue pull on the Achilles tendon and discomfort. A footboard that protrudes above the toes protects them from pressure exerted by the top bedding.

8. Place pillows to support both arms and hands if the client does not have normal use of them. Pillows should support only the forearms and hands, up to the elbow, in this way supporting the shoulder girdle.

   Rationale These pillows prevent shoulder and muscle strain from the effects of downward gravitational pull, dislocation of the shoulder in paralyzed persons, edema of the hands and arms, and flexion contracture of the wrist.

9. If severe respiratory distress is apparent, raise the head of the bed to high-Fowler's position and have the client position the forearms and hands on an overhead table placed directly in front of him or her. This position is called the **orthopneic position.** It facilitates respiration by allowing maximum chest expansion.

Home Health-Care Adaptation

Equipment

A bolster or triangular wood box can be placed under the mattress at the head of the bed or an inverted chair can be placed on top of the mattress to provide a semi-Fowler's position. See Figure 38–6.

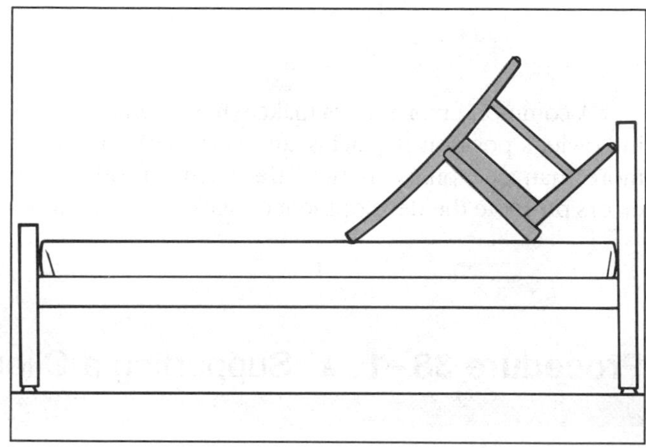

Figure 38–6

Trochanter Rolls

A **trochanter roll** is a roll of cloth, frequently a towel, placed against the greater trochanter of the femur to prevent external rotation of the hip. The greater trochanter is palpated and the middle of the roll is placed against it. Trochanter rolls need not extend more than 8 to 10 inches on either side of the trochanter, since leg rotation occurs at the hip joint. Firm support by the trochanter roll inhibits its outward rotation. Trochanter rolls are made commercially or can be constructed as described in Procedure 38–2. A commercial roll needs only to be covered before it is used. Covered sandbags are commonly used.

Procedure 38–2 ▲ Making and Applying a Trochanter Roll

Equipment

A towel or towel-sized cloth

Intervention

1. Fold the towel in half lengthwise. See Figure 38–7, *A*.

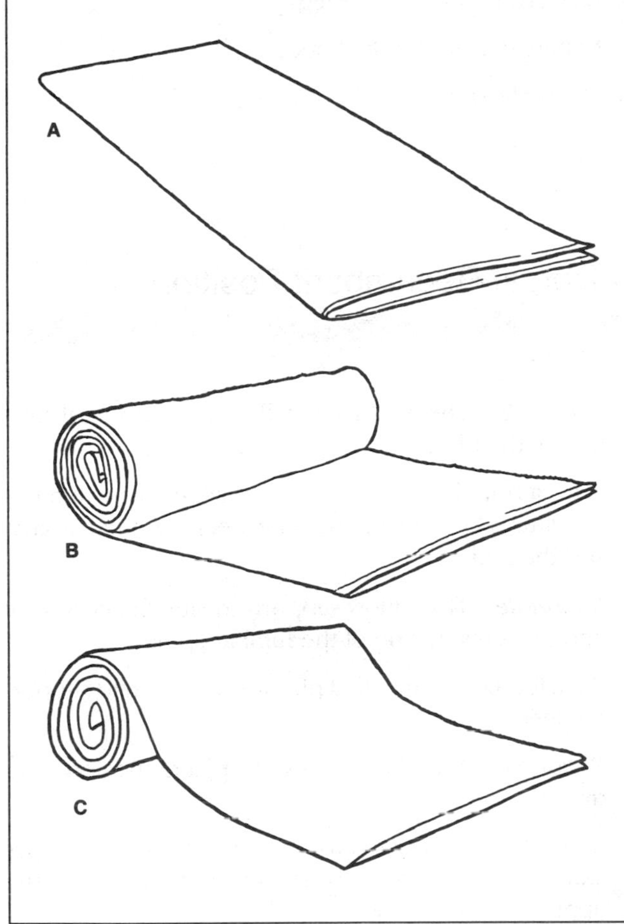

Figure 38–7

Figure 38–8

2. Roll the towel tightly, starting at one narrow edge and rolling to within about 30 cm (1 ft) of the other edge. See Figure 38–7, *B*.
3. Invert the roll. See Figure 38–7, *C*.
4. Place the flat part of the towel under the client's hip. See Figure 38–8.
5. Turn the roll under and position it tightly against the greater trochanter until the client's toes point directly upward, i.e., until the hip is neither externally nor internally rotated.
6. Repeat for the other leg if required.

Dorsal Recumbent Position

In the **dorsal recumbent (back-lying) position**, the client's head and shoulders are slightly elevated on a small pillow. Although in some agencies the terms *dorsal recumbent* and *supine* are used interchangeably, strictly speaking, in the **supine** or **dorsal position** the head and shoulders are not elevated. In both, the client's forearms may be elevated on pillows or placed at the client's sides. Supports are similar in both positions, except for the head pillow. See Figure 38–9.

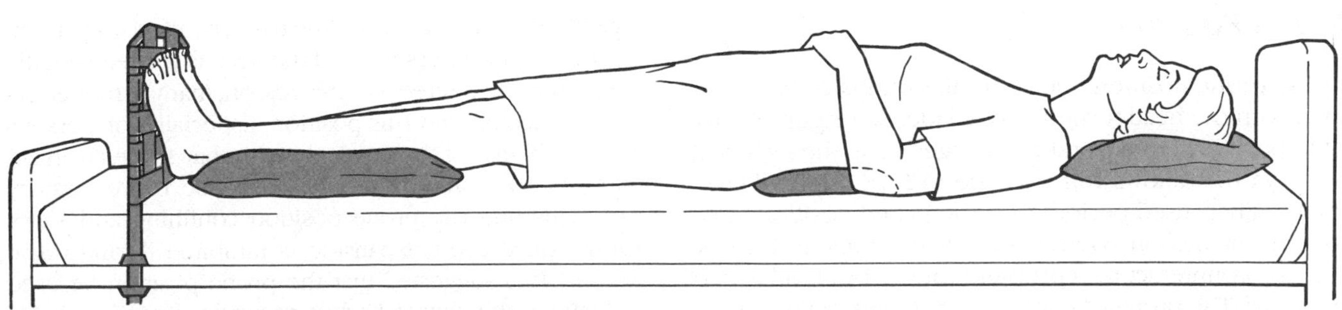

Figure 38–9 Dorsal recumbent position (supported)

Malalignments associated with an *unsupported* dorsal recumbent position are:

1. Hyperextension of the neck
2. Flexion of the lumbar curvature
3. External rotation of the legs
4. Hyperextension of the knees
5. Plantar flexion

Procedure 38–3 ▲ Supporting a Client in Dorsal Recumbent Position

Equipment

1. Up to 6 small pillows, depending on client need
2. 2 trochanter rolls (optional)
3. Footboard
4. Handrolls or wrist splints, if needed

Intervention

Using the alignment criteria as a guide:

1. Assist the client to a supine position.
2. Place a pillow of suitable thickness under the client's head and shoulders as needed.

   Rationale The pillow prevents hyperextension of the neck. Too many pillows beneath the head may cause or worsen neck flexion contracture.

3. Place a pillow under the lower legs from below the knees to the ankles.

   Rationale This pillow causes the client to flex the knees slightly and prevents hyperextension of the knees. It also keeps the heels off the bed surface and reduces lumbar lordosis.

4. Place trochanter rolls laterally against the femurs (optional).

   Rationale The trochanter rolls prevent external rotation of the hips.

5. Place a rolled towel or small pillow under the lumbar curvature if you feel a space between the lumbar area and the bed.

   Rationale This pillow supports the lumbar curvature and prevents flexion of the lumbar spine.

6. Put a footboard or rolled pillow on the bed to support the feet.

   Rationale A footboard prevents plantar flexion (foot drop).

7. If the client is unconscious or has paralysis of the upper extremities, elevate the forearms and hands, *not* the upper arm, on pillows.

   Rationale This position promotes comfort and prevents edema. Pillows are not placed under the upper arms to prevent shoulder flexion (Memmer 1974, p. 28).

8. If the client has actual or potential finger and wrist flexion deformities, use handrolls or wrist/hand splints. Handrolls, having a circumference of 5 to 6 inches, exert even pressure over the entire flexor surface of the palm and fingers. Evidence suggests that a firm, unyielding handroll made of cardboard is more useful than a soft, pliable roll in preventing flexion contractures of the fingers (Dayhoff 1975, p. 1143).

Prone Position

In the **prone position**, the client lies on his or her abdomen with the head turned to one side. See Figure 38–10. This position has several advantages. It is the only bed position that allows full extension of the hip and knee joints. When used periodically, the prone position helps to prevent flexion contractures of the hips and knees, thereby counteracting a problem caused by all other bed positions. The prone position also promotes drainage from the mouth and is especially useful for clients recovering from surgery of the mouth or throat.

The prone position poses some distinct disadvantages. The pull of gravity on the trunk produces a marked lordosis in most persons, and the neck is rotated laterally to a significant degree. For this reason, many orthopedists do not recommend this position, especially for persons with problems of the cervical or lumbar spine (Ishmael 1969, p. 9). Some clients with cardiac or respiratory problems find the prone position confining and suffocating, since chest expansion is inhibited during respirations. It is suggested that the prone position be used only when the client's back is properly aligned, only for short periods, and only for persons with no evidence of spinal abnormalities. This position also causes plantar flexion.

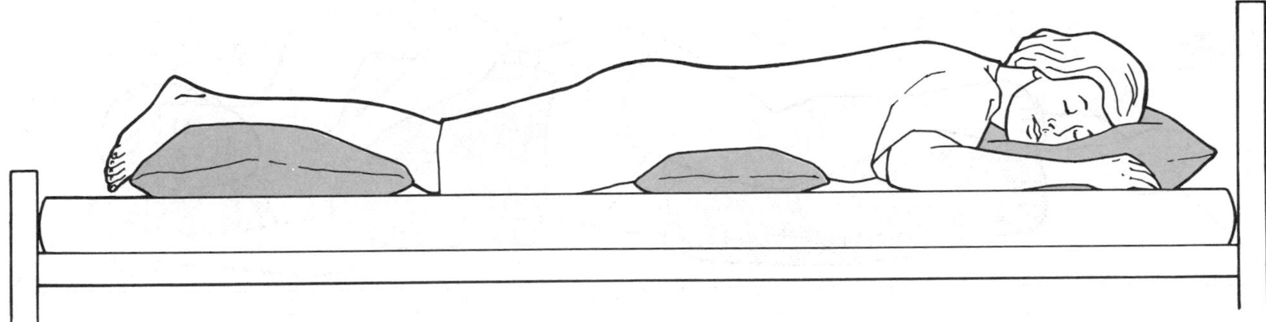

Figure 38–10 Prone position (supported)

Procedure 38–4 ▲ Supporting a Client in Prone Position

Equipment

3 pillows

Intervention

Using the alignment criteria as a guide:

1. Assist the client to a prone position.
2. Turn the client's head to one side and either omit the pillow entirely or place a small pillow under the head (unless contraindicated, e.g., if the pillow will impede the drainage of mucus) to align the head with the trunk. Avoid placing the pillow under the shoulders.

   Rationale The absence of a pillow prevents flexion of the neck laterally. A pillow placed under the shoulders increases lumbar lordosis.
3. Place a small pillow or roll under the abdomen in the space between the diaphragm (or the breasts of a woman) and the iliac crests.

   Rationale This pillow prevents hyperextension of the lumbar curvature, difficulty breathing, and pressure on some women's breasts. Supports placed too high impede respirations. Supports placed too low can increase lumbar lordosis and pressure on bony prominences.
4. Place a pillow under the lower legs from below the knees to just above the ankles, or position the client on the bed so that the feet extend in a normal anatomic position over the lower edge of the mattress. There should be no pressure on the toes.

   Rationale The pillow raises the toes off the bed surface, flexes the knees slightly for comfort, and prevents excessive pressure on the patellae. It also reduces plantar flexion.

Lateral Position

In the **lateral** or **side-lying position**, the person lies on one side of the body. See Figure 38–11. By having the client flex the top hip and knee and placing this leg in front of the body, a wider, triangular base of support is created, and greater stability is achieved. The greater the flexion on the top hip and knee, the greater the stability and balance in this position.

This flexion reduces lordosis and promotes good back alignment. For this reason, the lateral position is good for resting and sleeping clients. The lateral position helps to relieve pressure on the sacrum and heels in persons who sit for much of the day or who are confined to bed and rest in Fowler's or dorsal recumbent positions much of the time. In the lateral position, most of the body's weight is borne by the lateral aspect of the lower scapula, the lateral aspect of the ilium, and the greater trochanter of the femur. Persons who have sensory or motor deficits on one side of the body usually find that lying on the uninvolved side is more comfortable.

Malalignments associated with the *unsupported* lateral position include:

1. Lateral neck flexion

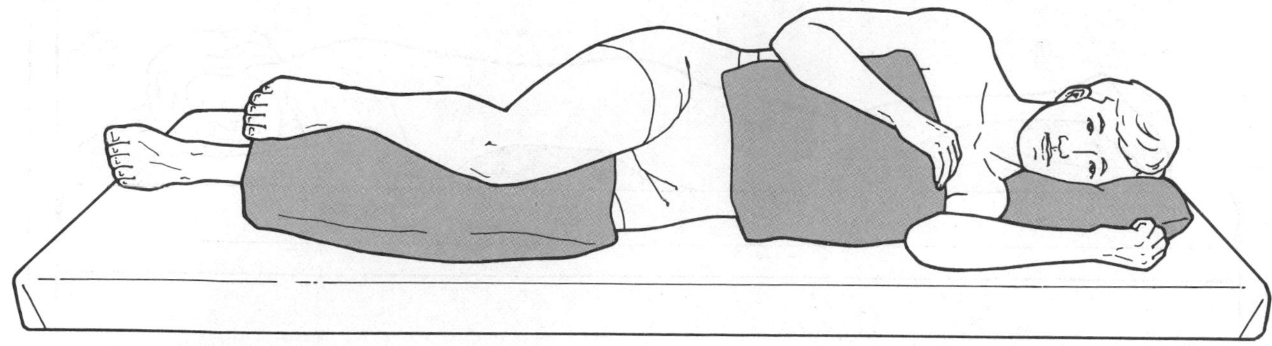

Figure 38–11 Lateral position (supported)

2. Internal rotation and adduction of the upper shoulder
3. Internal rotation and adduction of the upper thigh
4. Tendency for the spine to curve laterally toward the bed at the waist (postural scoliosis)
5. Twisting of the lumbar spine with the shoulders pulled forward or backward into a different plane than the hips
6. Plantar flexion—usually unavoidable (Memmer 1974, p. 28)

Procedure 38–5 ▲ Supporting a Client in Lateral Position

Equipment

1. Up to 5 small pillows
2. A folded towel (optional)

Intervention

Using the alignment criteria as a guide:

1. Assist the client to a lateral position.
2. Place a pillow under the client's head to align the head and neck with the trunk.

   Rationale This pillow prevents lateral flexion and discomfort of the major neck muscles, the sternocleidomastoid muscles.

3. Have the client flex the lower shoulder, position it forward so that the body does not rest on it, and rotate it into any position of comfort so that circulation is not disrupted.
4. Place a pillow under the upper arm.

   Rationale This pillow prevents internal rotation and adduction of the shoulder and downward pressure on the chest that could interfere with chest expansion during respiration. If the client has respiratory difficulty, increase the shoulder flexion and position the upper arm in front of the body off the chest.

5. Place two or more pillows under the upper leg and thigh so that the extremity lies in a plane parallel to the surface of the bed.

   Rationale A position parallel to the bed most closely approximates correct standing alignment and prevents internal rotation of the thigh and adduction of the leg. The pillow also prevents pressure caused by the weight of the top leg resting on the lower leg. Such pressure can damage the vein walls in the lower leg and predispose the client to thrombus formation.

6. Ensure that the two shoulders are aligned in the same plane as the two hips. If they are not, pull one shoulder or hip forward or backward until all four joints are aligned in the same plane.

   Rationale Proper alignment prevents twisting of the spine.

7. Place a folded towel under the natural hollow at the waistline. Take care to fill in only the space at the waistline (optional).

Rationale A folded towel prevents postural scoliosis of the lumbar spine. A towel support that extends too high or too low creates undue pressure against the rib cage or iliac crests.

8. Place a rolled pillow at the client's back to stabilize the position (optional). This pillow is not usually needed when the client's upper hip and knee are appropriately flexed.

Sims' Position

In the **Sims'** or **semiprone position**, the client assumes a posture halfway between the lateral and the prone positions. See Figure 38–12. In Sims' position, the client's lower arm is positioned behind him or her, and the upper arm is flexed at the shoulder and the elbow. Both legs are flexed in front of the client. The upper leg is more acutely flexed at both the hip and the knee than the lower one is.

Sims' position is occasionally used for unconscious clients because it facilitates drainage from the mouth. It is also used for paralyzed (paraplegic or hemiplegic) clients because it reduces pressure over the sacrum and greater trochanter of the hip. It is often used for clients receiving enemas and occasionally for clients undergoing examinations or treatments of the perineal area. Many people, especially pregnant women, find Sims' position comfortable for sleeping. Persons with sensory or motor deficits on one side of the body usually find that lying on the uninvolved side is more comfortable.

Malalignments associated with the *unsupported* Sims' position include:

1. Lateral flexion of the head
2. Internal rotation and adduction of the upper arm
3. Internal rotation and adduction of the upper leg
4. Potential twisting of the thoracolumbar spine if the shoulders are rotated in one direction and the hips in another
5. Lumbar lordosis
6. Plantar flexion

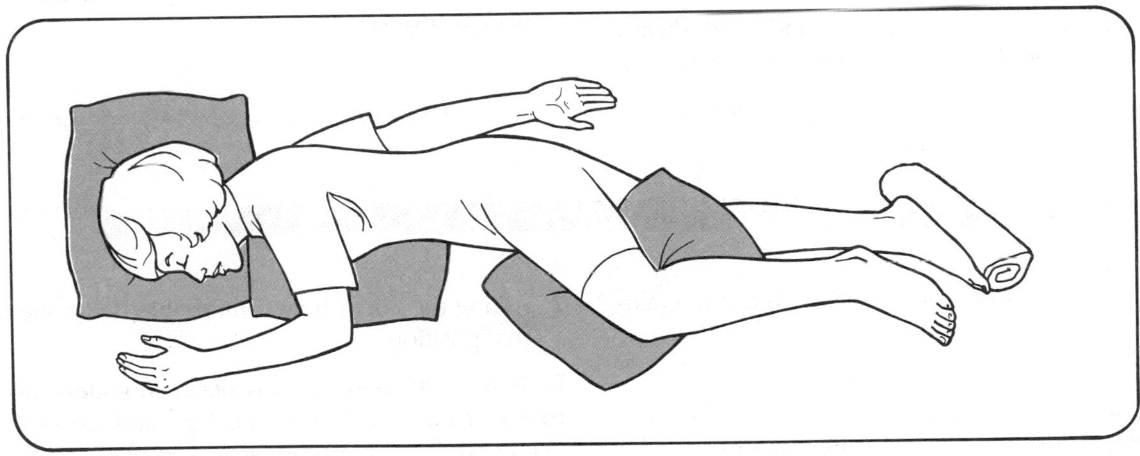

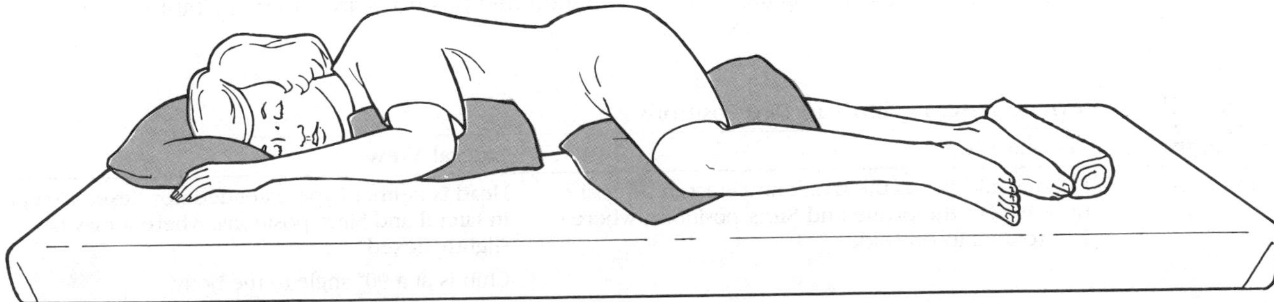

Figure 38–12 Sims' position (supported)

Procedure 38–6 ▲ Supporting a Client in Sims' Position

Equipment

1. 3 small pillows
2. Sandbag or rolled towel

Intervention

Using the alignment criteria as a guide:

1. Turn the client as for a prone position.
2. Place a small pillow under the client's head, unless drainage from the mouth is being encouraged.

   Rationale This pillow prevents lateral flexion of the neck and cushions the cranial and facial bones and the ear. It is contraindicated if drainage of mucus is required. Too large a pillow produces an uncomfortable lateral flexion of the neck.
3. Place the lower arm behind and away from the client's body in a position that is comfortable and does not disrupt circulation.

   Rationale This position prevents damage to nerves and blood vessels in the axillae.
4. Position the shoulder so that it is abducted slightly from the body and the shoulder and elbow are flexed. Use a pillow to support the space between the chest and abdomen and the upper arm and bed.

   Rationale This position prevents internal shoulder rotation and adduction and maintains alignment of the upper trunk.
5. Use a pillow to support the space between abdomen and pelvis and the upper thigh and bed.

   Rationale This position prevents internal rotation and adduction of the hip and also reduces lumbar lordosis.
6. Ensure that the two shoulders are aligned in the same plane as the two hips. If they are not, pull one shoulder or hip forward or backward until all four joints are aligned in the same plane.

   Rationale Proper alignment prevents twisting of the spine.
7. Place a support device, e.g., a sandbag or rolled towel, against the lower foot.

   Rationale This device may prevent foot drop. Efforts to correct plantar flexion in this position, however, are usually unsuccessful.

Evaluation

Body alignment can most easily be observed and evaluated by:

1. Standing directly in front of the person to evaluate the frontal plane of standing and sitting positions, or by standing at the foot of the bed to evaluate the bed positions.
2. Standing laterally to the client to view the sagittal plane.
3. Asking the client how comfortable he or she feels in that position.

Each body area—head and neck, shoulders, arms and hands, trunk, and finally hips, legs, and feet—is viewed from both frontal and lateral perspectives.

For examples of outcome criteria for evaluating standing and sitting body alignment, see the assessment section earlier in this chapter. Criteria for clients in well-aligned bed positions are shown in Table 38–2.

Table 38–2 Criteria to Assess Clients in Bed Positions

Body Region	Frontal View	Lateral View
Head and neck	Head is midline to the trunk and erect in all positions except the prone and Sims' positions, where it is rotated to one side.	Head is neither hyperextended nor flexed except in lateral and Sims' positions, where it may be slightly flexed. Chin is at a 90° angle to the body.

(continued)

Table 38–2 *(continued)*

Body Region	Frontal View	Lateral View
Shoulders and arms	Shoulders are level in all positions.	
	Shoulder girdle is relaxed, neither pulled upward or downward.	Shoulder girdle is relaxed, pulled neither forward nor backward.
	Shoulders are slightly abducted from body except in the lateral position, where only the upper shoulder is abducted.	In lateral and Sims' positions, the upper shoulder and arm are slightly flexed. In lateral position, the lower shoulder and elbow are flexed in front of the body. In Sims' position, the lower shoulder is extended, and the elbow is flexed behind the body.
	Arms are relaxed at sides with: hands in lap (Fowler's position), hands on abdomen or above head (dorsal recumbent position), one or both hands near head (prone position).	
Wrists and hands	Wrists are extended, and fingers are flexed in all positions.	
Trunk	Trunk is straight and not curved to either side in all positions.	Slight lumbar curvature occurs in all positions.
Hips and legs	Hips are level in all bed positions.	Hips are in the same plane as the shoulders. Hips are flexed in varying degrees in all positions except the prone position, where they are extended.
	Hips are slightly abducted from each other.	The upper hip and knee are more acutely flexed than the lower leg in lateral and Sims' positions. In the lateral position, the upper knee and ankle are in a horizontal plane with the hip and parallel to the bed. Knees are slightly flexed in all positions.
	Patellae face: upward in Fowler's and dorsal recumbent positions, downward in prone position, and laterally in lateral position. In Sims' position, the patellae lie at a point halfway between lateral and downward.	
Ankles and feet	Toes point: upward in Fowler's and dorsal recumbent positions, downward in prone position, laterally in lateral position, and halfway between the lateral and downward plane in Sims' position.	Ankles are dorsiflexed as much as possible in all positions. Toes and heels are kept off the bed surface in prone, dorsal recumbent, and Fowler's positions.

Nursing Care Plan

Assessment Data

Nursing Assessment

Mrs. Ruth Harris is a 72-year-old widow who lives with her son. Six weeks ago there was a house fire, and she suffered full thickness burns to her chest, abdomen, thighs, and knees. She has been receiving burn treatment for her wounds in the burn unit at the local hospital for the past 6 weeks. Bedrest has been prescribed, and she has been immobile and has become progressively weaker. Her ankles have been in a plantar flexion position. Dorsiflexion exercises and a footboard have not been implemented as part of her therapy. Mrs. Harris is unable to plantarflex or dorsiflex her ankles without a great deal of discomfort.

Physical Examination

Height: 157.5 cm (5′2″)
Weight: 55.8 kg (123 lb)
Temperature: 36.2 C (97.2 F)
Pulse rate: 86 BPM
Respirations: 22 per minute at rest
Blood pressure: 128/84 mm Hg
Full thickness (3rd degree) burns and eschar to chest, abdomen, thighs, and knees
R&L ankles in plantarflexed position with no actual movement possible.

Diagnostic Data

Chest x-ray film: Minimal lobar scattered infiltration
WBC: 12,500
RBC: 10.8

Nursing Diagnosis	Client Goals and Outcome Criteria	Nursing Interventions and Rationales	Evaluation
Posttrauma response: footdrop related to full thickness burns and 6 weeks' bedrest resulting in plantar flexion of both ankles, inability to bear weight on feet, and ankle discomfort.	Client Goal: Weight bearing of lower extremities and ambulation. Outcome Criteria: Dorsiflexes both ankles q1–2 hrs by day 5. Describes rationale for dorsiflexion of ankles by day 3. Uses footboard effectively when in dorsal recumbent position. Wears soft-soled shoes as a splint a minimum of 4 hrs each day.	Perform five repetitions of active ROM dorsiflexion exercises to both ankles q.i.d. *Rationale:* Prevents contractures, which are more apt to occur over joints. Assist with active-resistive exercises to both ankles against a footboard q.i.d. *Rationale:* Maintains functional positioning of ankles. Apply hightop soft-soled shoes to function as splints for at least two hours each day. *Rationale:* Maintains functional positioning of ankles. Instruct client to point toes and knees toward ceiling when in dorsal recumbent position. *Rationale:* Assures a more normal body alignment for ambulation. Explain need for frequent dorsiflexion of ankles. *Rationale:* Client will be more likely to cooperate if she understands the rationale for exercises. Reposition client in good alignment q2 hrs with dorsiflexion to both ankles. *Rationale:* Prevents problems as a result of immobility and reduces chances of ankle contractures.	Dorsiflexes both ankles 5× with nurse's assistance 4× daily. Keeps both feet positioned on footboard with toes pointed toward ceiling for 45–60 minutes between exercise sessions. Wears soft-soled shoes as splints 2 hrs each day. States, "I must exercise my ankles even though it's painful so that I'll be able to walk again when my burns heal."
Knowledge deficit regarding rehabilitation and contractures resulting in questioning need for exercises, repositioning, and treatments that cause pain and discomfort.	Client Goal: Understanding of need for participation in rehabilitation activities. Outcome Criteria: Participates in active and passive exercises 3× daily by day 5. Describes footdrop and how to prevent it by day 3.	Assess client's level of understanding regarding need for daily ankle exercises. *Rationale:* This is necessary in order to elicit client cooperation. Explain exercise routine carefully before initiating exercises. *Rationale:* Telling the client what to expect reduces her fear and increases cooperation. Teach client exercises that prevent ankle contractures. *Rationale:* If client is instructed properly, exercises will be performed correctly. Instruct client to keep toes pointed to ceiling when in dorsal recumbent position. *Rationale:* Client will be more mindful of proper positioning to prevent contractures.	Participates in passive ROM exercises 4× daily despite some discomfort. States, "I must allow the nurse to bend my ankles several times a day so that I'll be able to walk again." Reminds son and nurses to "keep my toes pointed to the ceiling."

Chapter Highlights

- Good body alignment is essential for good body functioning and for preventing injury to body structures, discomfort, and fatigue.
- The nurse acts as a role model and teacher of good body alignment.
- Factors influencing body alignment include general health, nutrition, emotions, environment, life-style, attitudes and values, level of understanding, and neuromuscular or skeletal impairments.
- The principles of body alignment and balance guide the nursing assessment process.
- Specific assessment criteria for standing, sitting, and lying positions guide the nurse's assessment of body alignment.
- Postural variations occur among different age groups.
- The nurse identifies nursing diagnoses and goals related to impairments or potential impairments in body alignment.
- The nurse is responsible for assisting clients to achieve proper body alignment.
- The principles of body alignment and the guidelines for positioning clients help the nurse to plan individualized interventions.
- The nurse uses specific outcome criteria to evaluate the effectiveness of the nursing interventions implemented.

Suggested Readings

Drapeau, D. September 1975. Getting back into good posture: How to ease your lumbar aches. *Nursing 75* 5:63–65.
Drapeau describes the relationship between poor posture and low back pain in a group of nurses. The article illustrates some ways to enhance use of the pelvic tilt and shows some exercises for strengthening back and abdominal muscles.

Owen, D. M. May 1980. How to avoid that aching back. *American Journal of Nursing* 80:894–97.
Owen describes how to assess standing and sitting postures and illustrates some exercises for strengthening back and abdominal muscles.

Selected References

Bilger, A. J., and Greene, E. H., editors. 1973. *Winter's protective body mechanics.* New York: Springer Publishing Co.

Broer, M. A., and Zernicke, R. A. 1979. *Efficiency of human movement.* 4th ed. Philadelphia: W. B. Saunders Co.

Brower, E. W., and Nash, C. L. April 1979. Evaluating growth and posture in school-age children. *Nursing 79* 9:58–63.

Byrne, C. J.; Saxton, D. F.; Pelikan, P. K.; and Nugent, P. M. 1986. *Laboratory tests: Implications for nursing care.* 2d ed. Menlo Park, Calif.: Addison-Wesley Publishing Co.

Dayhoff, N. July 1975. Soft or hard devices to position hands? *American Journal of Nursing* 75:1142–44.

deToledo, C. H. September 1979. The patient with scoliosis: The defect—classification and detection. *American Journal of Nursing* 79:1588–1591.

Foss, G. May 1973. Use your head and save your back: Body mechanics. *Nursing 73* 3:25–32.

Hirschberg, G.; Lewis, L.; and Vaughn, P. May 1977. Promoting patient mobility and other ways to prevent secondary disabilities. *Nursing 77* 7:42–47.

Hogan, L., and Beland, I. July 1976. Cervical neck syndrome. *American Journal of Nursing* 76:1104–7.

Howden, L. July/August 1981. Basic back care: It doesn't have to hurt. *Canadian Nurse* 77:46–50.

Ishmael, W., and Shorbe, H. 1969. *Care of the back.* 2d ed. Philadelphia: J. B. Lippincott Co.

Kottke, F.; Stillwell, G.; and Lehmann, J., editors. 1982. *Krusen's handbook of physical medicine and rehabilitation.* 3d ed. Philadelphia: W. B. Saunders Co.

Memmer, M. K. 1974. *Posture and alignment.* Los Angeles: The Intercampus Nursing Project, California State University and College System.

Mitchell, P., and Houston, A. 1981. *Concepts basic to nursing.* 3d ed. New York: McGraw-Hill.

Owen, B. May 1980. How to avoid that aching back. *American Journal of Nursing* 80:894–97.

Shannon, M. L. October 1984. Five famous fallacies about pressure sores. *Nursing 84* 14:34–41.

Witte, N. S. November 1979. Why the elderly fall. *American Journal of Nursing* 79:1950–52.

CHAPTER **39**

Body Mechanics and Ambulation

Mary Kelly Memmer

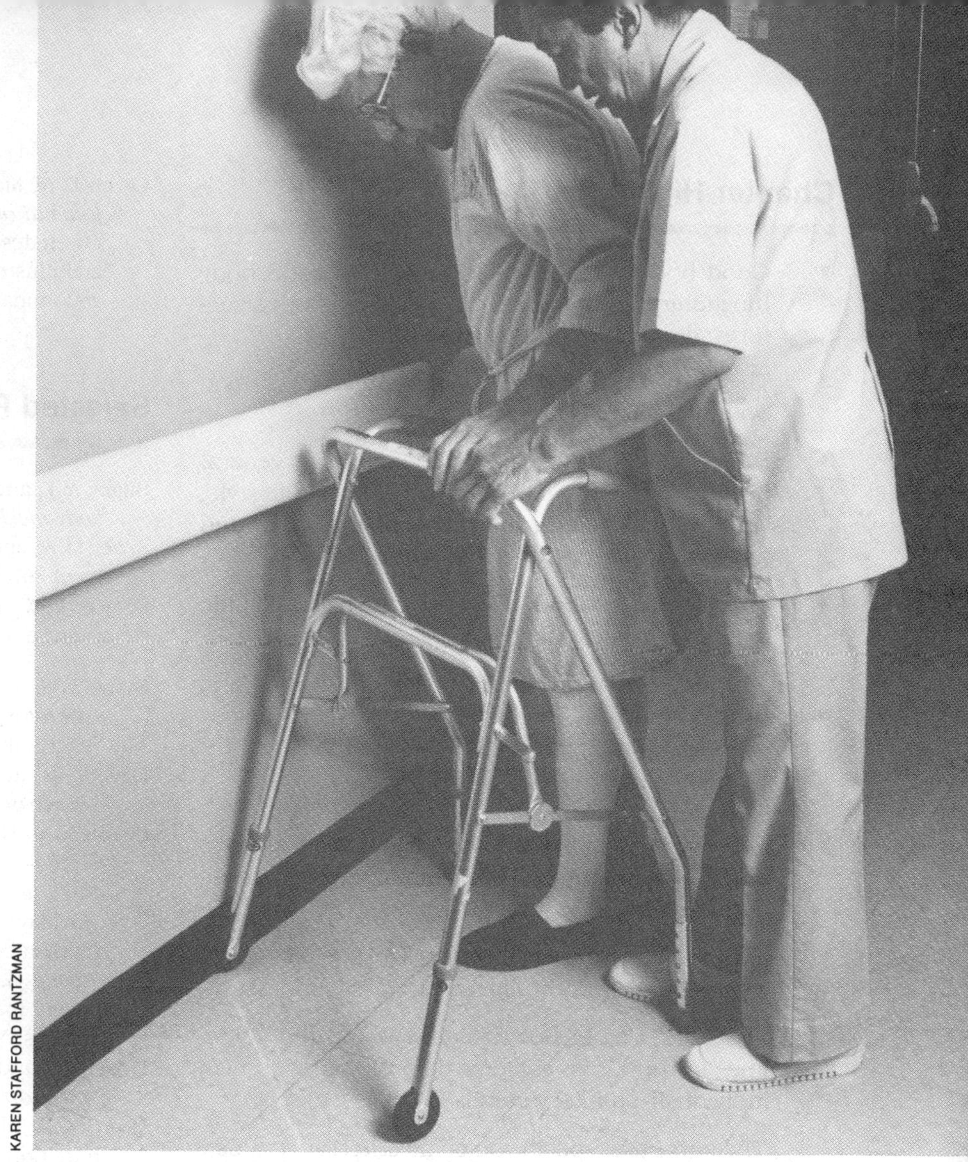
KAREN STAFFORD RANTZMAN

Contents

Contents *(continued)*

Objectives

1. Understand essential concepts about body mechanics and ambulation.
   1.1 Define selected terms.
   1.2 Discuss the importance of good body mechanics.
   1.3 Describe how gravity, weight, and balance affect movement.
   1.4 Describe how friction, force, inertia, and leverage affect movement.
   1.5 Describe how musculoskeletal function and voluntary and involuntary muscle and reflex activity affect movement.
   1.6 State specific principles of body mechanics.
   1.7 Describe essential aspects of fine basic movements used in body mechanics.
   1.8 Identify factors that influence body mechanics.
   1.9 Describe long-term effects of body mechanics.
   1.10 Identify occupational groups at risk of back injury.
   1.11 Identify ways to prevent back injury.
   1.12 Identify the consequences of poor ambulation.
   1.13 Identify structural abnormalities that affect body mechanics and ambulation.
2. Know information required and methods used to assess a client's body mechanics and ambulation.
   2.1 Identify criteria used to assess body mechanics.
   2.2 Identify ways to determine the client's capabilities and limitations for movement.
   2.3 Identify criteria used to assess a client's gait.
3. Understand essential aspects of developing nursing diagnoses and planning care for clients with impaired mobility.
   3.1 State nursing diagnoses for clients with body mechanics and ambulation problems.
   3.2 Identify client goals.
4. Understand essential facts about nursing interventions to maintain, promote, or restore normal body mechanics and ambulation.
   4.1 Identify information required before assisting clients to move.
   4.2 Identify essential steps of procedures to move and turn clients in bed and to transfer clients from bed to chair or stretchers.
   4.3 State outcome criteria essential for evaluating the nursing interventions.

Terms

ankylosing spondylitis
atrophy
body mechanics
compression fracture
elbow extensor (Canadian) crutch
flaccid (muscle)
force
friction
fulcrum
gait
inertia
insertion (of muscle
lever
Lofstrand crutch
origin (of muscle)
osteoarthritis
osteomyelitis
osteoporosis
pace
paresis
rheumatoid arthritis
scoliosis
spastic (muscle)
sprain
stance
strain
swing phase (of walking)
tripod (triangle) position
underarm (axillary) crutch
weight-bearing phase (of walking)

The Importance of Good Body Mechanics

Good **body mechanics** is the efficient, coordinated, and safe use of the body to produce motion and maintain balance during activity. Proper movement promotes proper body functioning of musculoskeletal structures, reducing the energy required to move and maintain balance and therefore reducing fatigue.

People often define their health status by their ability to move about, maintain their independence, and feel useful. Movement is necessary to sustain life, obtain food and water, meet basic needs, and protect oneself from injury. People whose movement is impaired may feel helpless and dependent on others to meet their basic needs. Good body mechanics is important because it promotes and preserves mobility and independence.

Falls are a major cause of accidental injury to hospitalized clients, especially elderly clients. Nurses are legally and ethically responsible for preventing client falls. Teaching correct body mechanics helps prevent falls.

Nurses themselves are at high risk of back injuries because they regularly move and lift clients. Good posture, physical fitness, and use of good body mechanics can prevent back injury. The nurse is an important role model in teaching good body mechanics to others. A nurse who uses poor body mechanics in daily activities and whose back hurts as a result cannot teach health promotion and prevention of disability as effectively as a nurse who uses good body mechanics.

Principles of Body Mechanics

Gravity, Weight, and Balance

Gravity as an influence in static body alignment is discussed in Chapter 38. Gravity as an influence on movement is discussed here.

In a well-aligned standing person, the center of gravity remains fairly stable, slightly anterior to the upper sacrum. When the person moves, however, the center of gravity shifts continuously in the direction of the moving body parts. Balance depends on the interrelationship of the center of gravity, the line of gravity, and the base of support. When a person moves, the closer the line of gravity is to the center of the base of support, the greater his or her stability is. See Figure 39–1, *A*. Conversely, the closer the line of gravity is to the edge of the base of

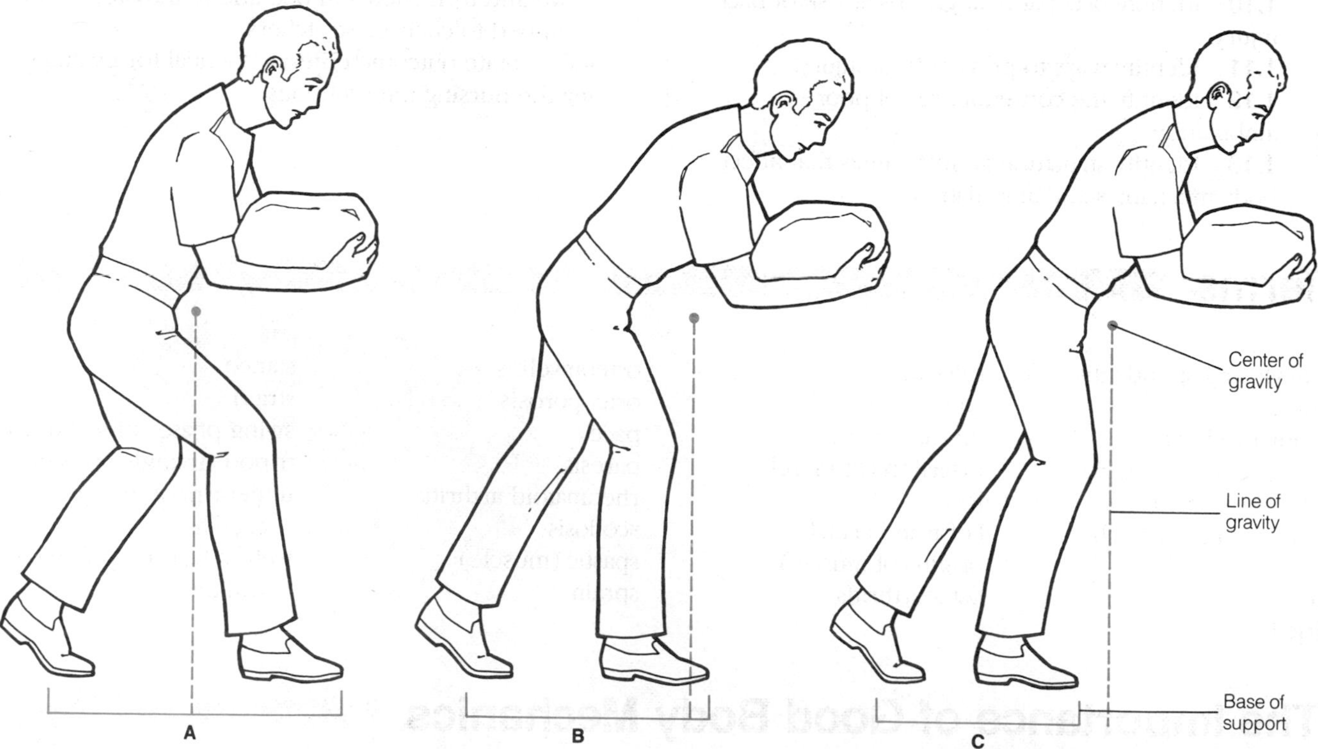

Figure 39–1 **A,** Balance is maintained when the line of gravity falls close to the base of support. **B,** Balance is precarious when the line of gravity falls at the edge of the base of support. **C,** Balance cannot be maintained when the line of gravity falls outside the base of support.

support, the more precarious the balance is. See Figure 39–1, *B*. If the line of gravity falls outside the base of support, the person falls. See Figure 39–1, *C*. For this reason, the base of support should be large enough so that the constantly shifting center of gravity does not cause the line of gravity to fall outside the base of support. A lower center of gravity also produces greater stability (Broer and Zernicke 1979, p. 50). The base of support is easily widened by spreading the feet farther apart. The center of gravity is readily lowered by flexing the hips and knees until a squatting position is achieved. The importance of these compensations cannot be overemphasized.

When pulling or pushing an object, a person maintains balance with least effort when the base of support is enlarged in the direction in which the movement is to be produced or opposed. For example, when pushing an object, a person can enlarge the base of support by moving the front foot forward. When pulling an object, a person can enlarge the base of support by (a) moving the rear leg back if the person is facing the object; or (b) moving the front foot forward if the person is facing away from the object. It is easier and safer to pull an object toward one's own center of gravity than to push it away, as the person can exert more control of the object's movement when pulling it.

Moving an object on a level surface requires less energy than moving that same object up an inclined surface against the pull of gravity. It takes less energy to work with materials that rest on a surface as close to the person's center of gravity as possible than to lift the materials above this working surface. It takes less energy to slide an object along a surface than to lift the object, since lifting requires moving the weight of the object against the pull of gravity. Consequently, rolling, turning, and pivoting require much less energy expenditure than lifting does.

When a person lifts or carries an object, the weight of the object becomes part of the person's body weight. This weight affects the location of the person's center of gravity, which is displaced in the direction of the added weight. To counteract this potential imbalance, body parts move in a direction away from the weight. In this way, the center of gravity is maintained over the same point in the base of support. See Figure 39–2. By holding the center of gravity of the lifted object as close as possible to his or her center of gravity, the lifter avoids undue displacement of the center of gravity and achieves greater stability (Broer and Zernicke 1979, p. 53).

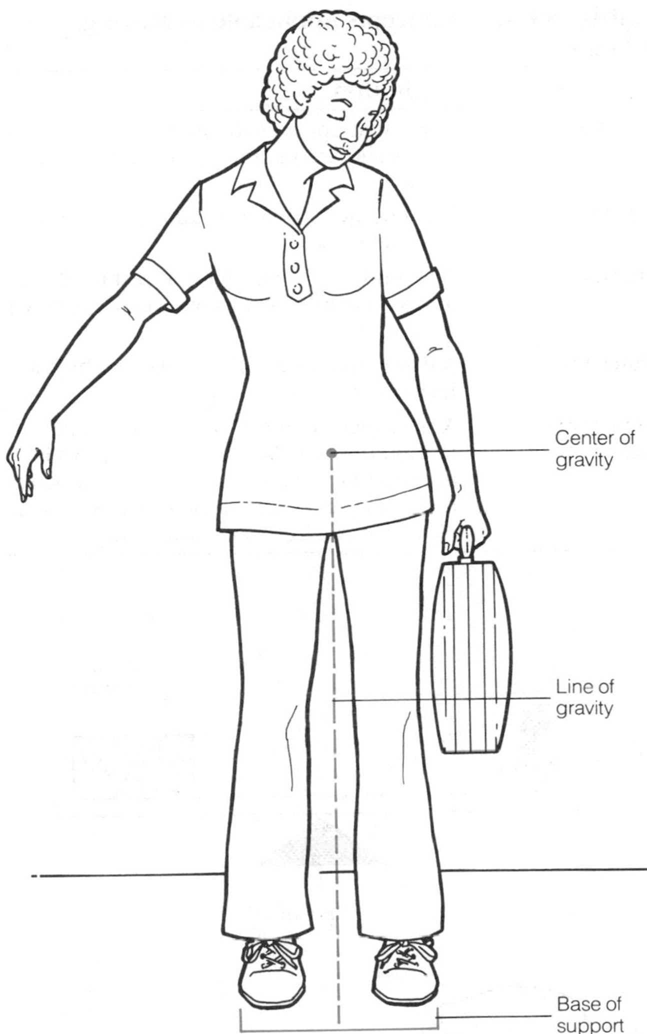

Figure 39–2 Body parts move in the direction opposite the weight to compensate for it and maintain the center of gravity over the base of support.

Friction, Force, Inertia, and Leverage

Friction, force, inertia, and leverage are four concepts applicable to pushing, pulling, and lifting clients. They are thus directly relevant to the work of nurses. These terms are defined in Table 39–1.

The heavier an object and the greater the friction against the surface beneath it, the greater the force required to move the object. Friction can be reduced by sliding the object on a smooth, clean, dry, firm surface, in contrast to a rough, wet, or soiled surface. To reduce friction when moving (sliding) a client up in bed, for example, the nurse provides a smooth, dry, firm bed foundation.

It is preferable to pull rather than push a client along the surface of a bed because pushing compresses the client's vertebrae and creates discomfort (Broer and Zernicke 1979, p. 231). Also, pulling creates less friction than pushing, since the nurse must pull at an upward angle

Table 39–1 Concepts Applicable to Moving Clients

Concept	Definition
Friction	Force that opposes the motion of an object as it is slid across the surface of another object.
Force	The energy or power required to accomplish movement.
Inertia	The tendency of an object at rest to remain at rest and an object in motion to remain in motion.
Fulcrum	A fixed point (e.g., elbow) about which a lever moves.
Lever (first class)	A rigid piece that transmits or modifies motion or force. When force (energy) is applied to the rigid arm with a fixed point (fulcrum), an object at the other end of the rigid arm can be lifted more easily.

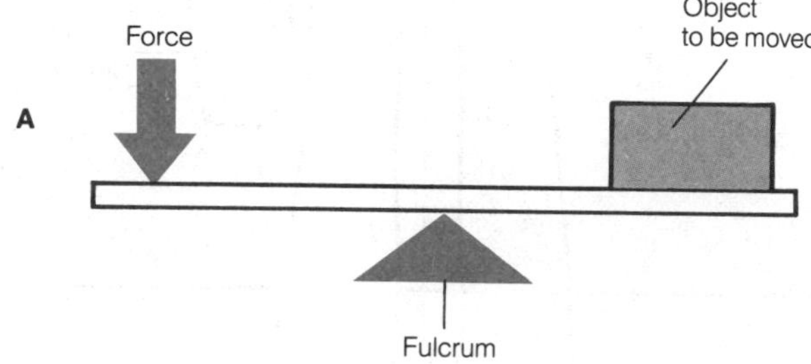

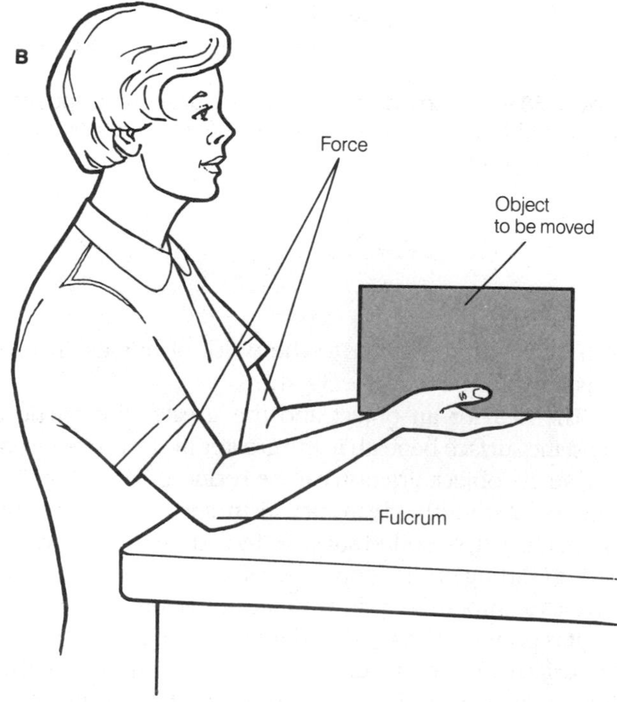

Figure 39–3 **A,** A first class lever; **B,** using the arm as a lever

that reduces friction between the client and the bed (Broer and Zernicke 1979, pp. 228–30). Friction can be further avoided by rolling, rather than pushing or pulling, the person.

Due to inertia, one must use more force to put an object into motion than to keep it in motion. The heavier the object, the greater the force required to put it into motion. To move an object efficiently, one applies force directly toward or against the object's center of gravity and in the direction in which the movement is to occur. A person can use his or her body weight in a rocking motion to apply additional force or leverage, thus counteracting the object's inertia and reducing the energy required to start the pulling, pushing, or lifting movement (Broer and Zernicke 1979, pp. 74–75).

Although there are three types of levers, the type nurses use most frequently in lifting is the first class lever. See Figure 39–3, *A*. When the nurse lifts objects, the resisting force or weight is held in the hands or on the forearms, the fulcrum is the elbow, and the force is applied by contraction of the biceps (flexor) muscles of the arm. See Figure 39–3, *B*. The lifting power is increased when the elbow (fulcrum) is supported on a bed surface or a countertop. People can lift more weight when they use this lever than when they do not (Broer and Zernicke 1979, pp. 80–101). Women's arm muscles have much less strength for lifting than men's (Hayne 1981). The ordinary person can lift only about 20 pounds of weight without danger of back strain when a lever is not used. When the weight to be lifted exceeds 35% of body weight, the lifter must use mechanical devices or seek the assistance of other persons (Owen 1980, p. 896).

Musculoskeletal Function

Body mechanics involves the integrated functioning of the musculoskeletal and nervous systems. Muscle tone, the coordinated movements of opposing voluntary muscle groups (the antagonistic, synergistic, and antigravity muscles), and the neuromuscular reflexes (including the visual and proprioceptive reflexes) play important roles in producing balanced, smooth, purposeful movement.

The bones of the skeleton are linked at joints by ligaments: broad, fibrous bands of tissue that provide support, strength, and flexibility to the skeleton. The cartilage between bones provides a smooth surface over which the bones glide. This cartilage also absorbs shock from sudden movement or injury. The tendons are fibrous cords that attach muscles to the bones.

Moving bones act as levers. The skeletal muscles provide the energy that moves the lever. A muscle attaches to two bones. One end of the muscle attaches to a bone that is relatively stationary. This is the *origin* of the muscle. The other end of the muscle attaches to the more moveable bone. This is the *insertion* of the muscle. This muscle shortens as it contracts (flexes), decreasing the angle between the two bones to which it is attached. As the muscle relaxes (extends), it lengthens, increasing the angle between the two bones to which it is attached. The working of opposing voluntary skeletal muscle groups to provide balance and coordinated movement is discussed in Chapter 38. Coordinated movement conserves energy.

Voluntary Muscle Activity

The cerebellum coordinates all voluntary muscle activity, especially that involved in the complex movements. Skeletal muscle activity is initiated in the cerebral cortex. Most motor nerves descend and cross over in the area of the medulla to the spinal cord, traveling through efferent pathways to the muscles, where purposeful movement is produced. These muscles remain in a constant state of slight tension (tonus), which requires minimal energy expenditure yet maintains adequate support and alignment for body parts.

Most skeletal muscle movement is a combination of isotonic and isometric contraction (see Chapter 37). At the initiation of movement, an isometric contraction occurs. When enough tension is achieved, an isotonic contraction occurs to produce movement. The preparatory isometric contraction, during which muscle tension is greatly increased, is especially important prior to lifting. The greater this preparatory isometric tensing, the less the energy required to lift an object.

The larger muscles of the lower extremities and the muscles of the abdomen and back all produce movement by leverage and synchronized action. The flexors of the legs, and to a lesser degree the leg extensors, are the largest and strongest muscles in the body. Exercise and consistent use of the weaker lumbar muscle groups and the abdominal muscles maintain their tone and strength, and protect them from injury. One can increase overall muscle strength by synchronized use of as many muscle groups as possible during an activity. For instance, when the arms are used in an activity, dividing the work between the arms and legs helps to prevent back strain. Exercise and use increase the mass and strength of skeletal muscles, increasing their capacity for work and protecting them from injury.

Two movements to avoid because of their potential for causing back injury are twisting (rotation) of the lumbarthoracic spine and acute flexion of the back with hips and knees straight. Undesirable twisting of the back can be prevented by squarely facing the direction of movement, whether pushing, pulling, or sliding, and moving the object directly toward or away from one's center of gravity.

Overactivity can produce muscle fatigue. Prolonged, strenuous overexertion can result in overstretching and tearing of muscle fibers, muscle strain, and damage. One can prevent muscle fatigue by alternating periods of rest and activity. A change in activity or in the position in which the activity is performed helps to prevent muscle fatigue as well. Any accommodation to improve stability in balance, create better alignment of body parts, and reduce energy expenditure during an activity reduces muscle fatigue.

Involuntary Reflex Activity

Involuntary reflexes also play an important role in balance and coordination. See Chapter 38.

Five Basic Movements Used in Body Mechanics

Five movements—walking (ambulating), squatting, pulling, lifting and pivoting—are basic to all nursing interventions that require moving and transferring clients. These five movements are also basic to appropriate movement in daily life. The mechanics of each of these five movements is discussed in the following sections.

Ambulating

A walking person's balance is more unstable than a standing person's balance. Like standing stability, walking stability is directly related to the size of the base of support. When a person walks, the base of support shifts from side to side, and the center of gravity shifts to a position above the supporting foot with each step. This shifting of weight produces a slight swaying motion with each step.

There are two distinct phases in walking: the weight-bearing phase and the swing phase. Each leg alternates between these two phases to produce a smooth, rhythmic motion. The **weight-bearing**, **double-stance**, or **support phase** is initiated when the heel strikes the ground. This slows the forward momentum of the body slightly. The body weight is spread over this supporting foot until the weight reaches the toes. At this point, the ball of the foot and the extended toes, now behind the body, push off with force to propel the body forward. See Figure 39–4, *A*.

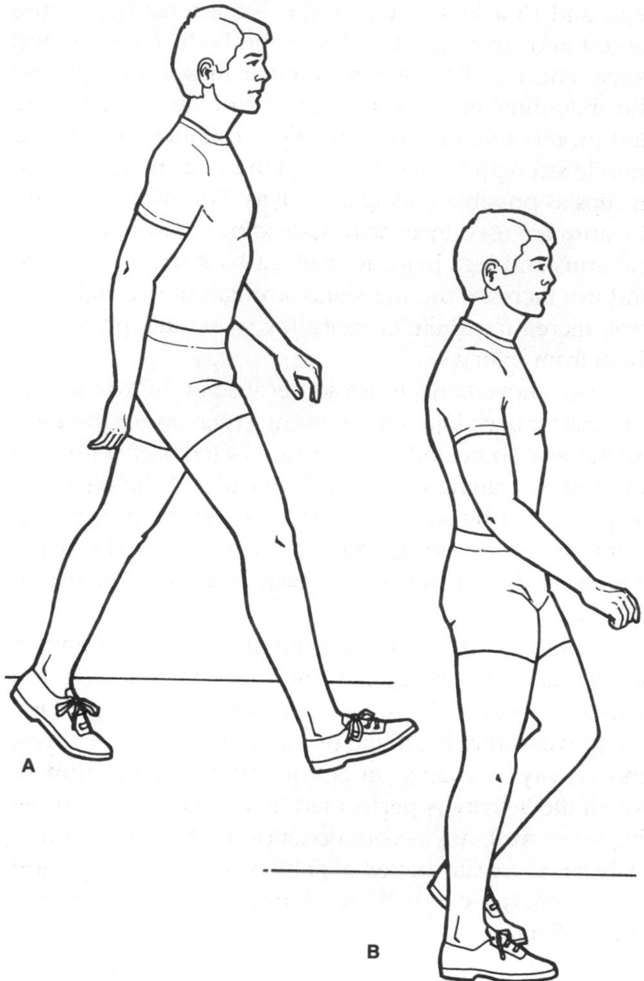

Figure 39–4 Phases in walking: **A,** weight-bearing phase; **B,** beginning of swing phase

Source: Adapted from L. Daniels and C. Worthingham, *Therapeutic exercise,* 2d ed. (Philadelphia: W. B. Saunders Co., 1977), p. 35. Used by permission.

The **swing phase** is initiated as the hip joint flexes to lift the toes from the ground. Then the knee and ankle flex as the leg and foot are swung forward. As the leg begins to swing in front of the body, the hip begins to extend. The swing phase is ended as the heel strikes the ground to initiate the weight-bearing phase (Broer and Zernicke 1979, p. 137). See Figure 39–4, *B.*

As a person walks, there is a short period of double support, when the toe of one foot and the heel of the other foot are both on the ground. The rolling of the weight over the foot from the posterior aspect to the anterior, spreading equally to both sides of the foot, absorbs and reduces the impact of the heel striking the ground. For this reason, there is a slight up-and-down motion of the body with each step.

Foot position is important in walking. As a person walks, the inner borders of the feet should move along a path where the line of gravity would naturally fall. The toes should point straight ahead. This pattern of ambulation produces minimal body sway from side to side and directs the force of movement straight ahead. See Figure 39–5. This action enhances balance and prevents wasted energy in movement (Broer and Zernicke 1979, pp. 176–77).

As a person walks, the arms should swing in opposition to the leg movements to counteract the tendency of the body to rotate as a result of the off-center application of force with each step. The reflexive arm swing helps to propel the body forward without wasted energy (Broer and Zernicke 1979, p. 178).

Stance is the manner in which a person stands. **Gait** is the characteristic pattern of the person's walk. Gait can be assessed not only by observing a person walk but also by observing the pattern of wear on the soles and heels of the shoes.

Pace is the number of steps taken per minute. A normal walking pace is 70 to 100 steps per minute. A fast pace is 120 steps per minute. The pace of an elderly person may slow to about 40 steps per minute. A person can increase pace by moving the center of gravity slightly forward, lengthening the stride, and increasing the pushing force of the toes at the end of each weight-bearing phase of a step (Broer and Zernicke 1979, p. 175).

Squatting

Squatting, in contrast to stooping, is a means of lowering the center of gravity to bring it closer to the base of support. Squatting enhances body balance when a person lifts objects that lie below the body's center of gravity. See Figure 39–6. When lifting an object from the floor, a person can assume the squatting position not only to bring his or her center of gravity closer to the object's center of gravity but also to use the major leg extensor muscles rather than the muscles of the back.

Effective squatting and lifting are achieved as follows:

1. Start in correct standing alignment.
2. Move as close as possible to the load to be lifted, and make sure the load is directly in front of the body. See Figure 39–7, *A.*
3. Lean slightly forward by flexing the hips and place one foot forward slightly to enlarge the base of support in the direction in which the movement is to occur. See Figure 39–7, *B.*
4. Contract stabilizing muscles of the body.
5. Keep the back straight and distribute the body weight on both feet while flexing the hips, knees, and ankles to lower the body. See Figure 39–7, *C.*

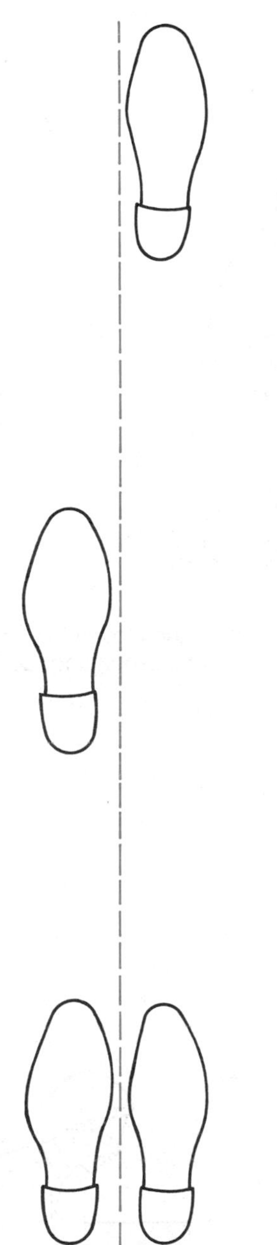

Figure 39–5 Normal foot position of a walking person

Source: Adapted from M. R. Broer and R. F. Zernicke, *Efficiency of human movement,* 4th ed. (Philadelphia: W. B. Saunders Co., 1979), p. 176. Used by permission.

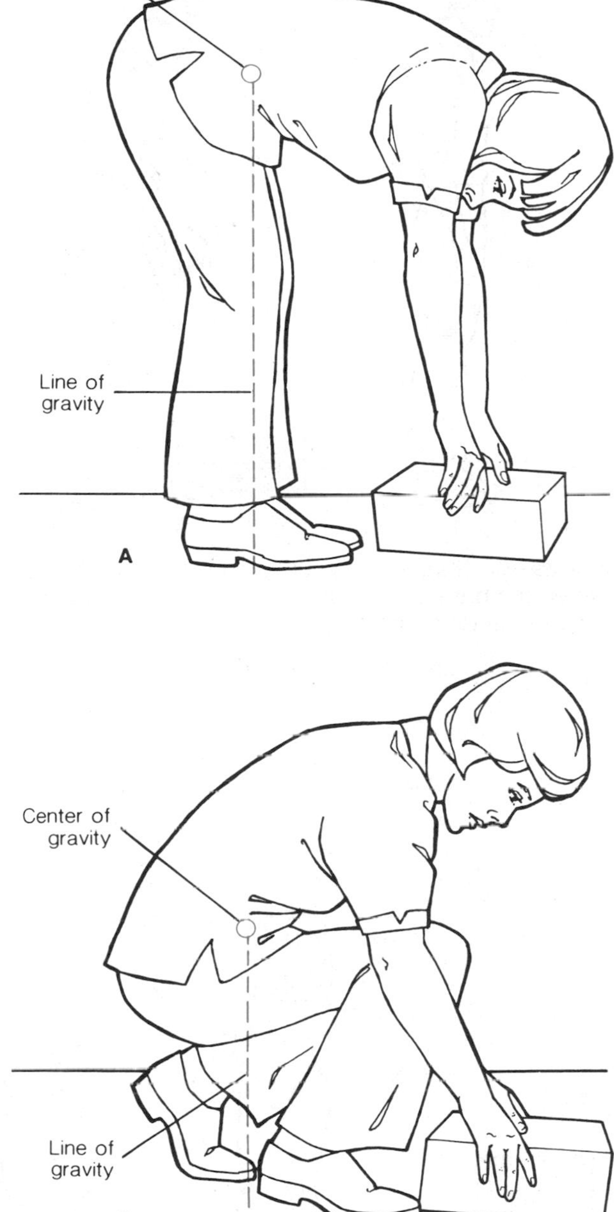

Figure 39–6 The center of gravity **A,** remains high during stooping and **B,** is lowered by squatting.

6. Pull the load toward the body and lift it by extending the knees and hips and flexing the elbows. See Figure 39–7, *D*.

Pulling

To pull objects or clients using good body alignment, the nurse carries out the following steps:

1. Make sure the object or client is at an appropriate height. Elevate the client's bed if necessary so that the client is as close as possible. See Figure 39–8, *A*.
2. Make sure the client's bed surface is flat if health permits.
3. Move as close to the load to be pulled as possible.
4. Make sure the load to be pulled is directly in front of the body.

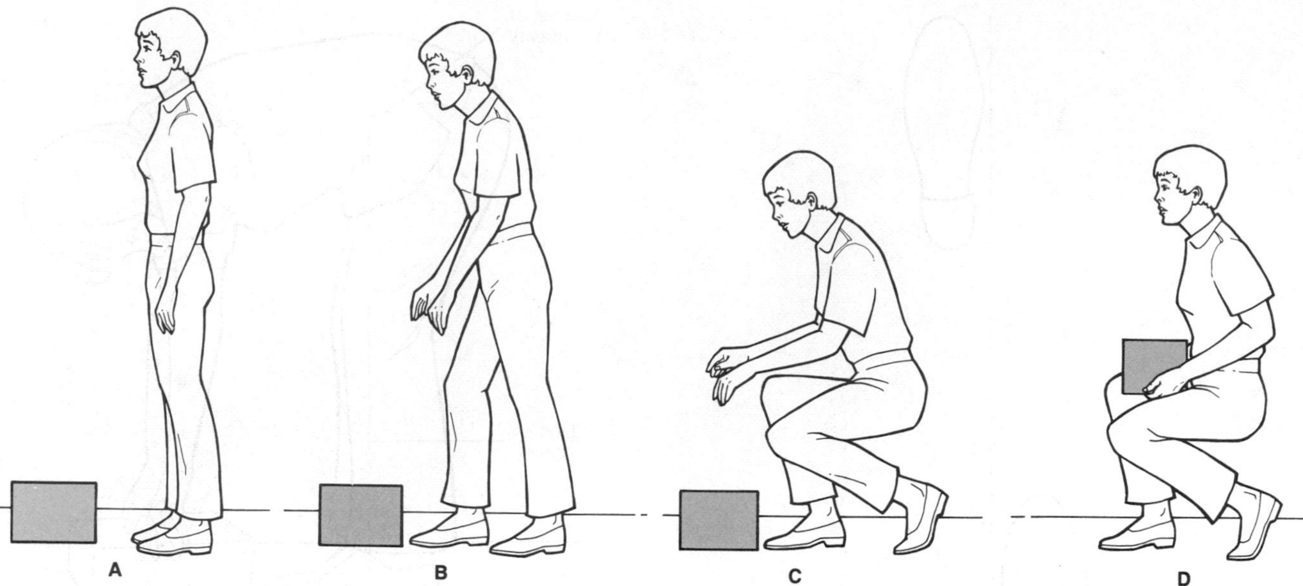

Figure 39–7 Stages in squatting and lifting: **A,** Start with the body correctly aligned and move close to the object. **B,** Widen the base of support and lean toward the object. **C,** Keep the back straight while squatting. **D,** Pull the load toward the body's center of gravity.

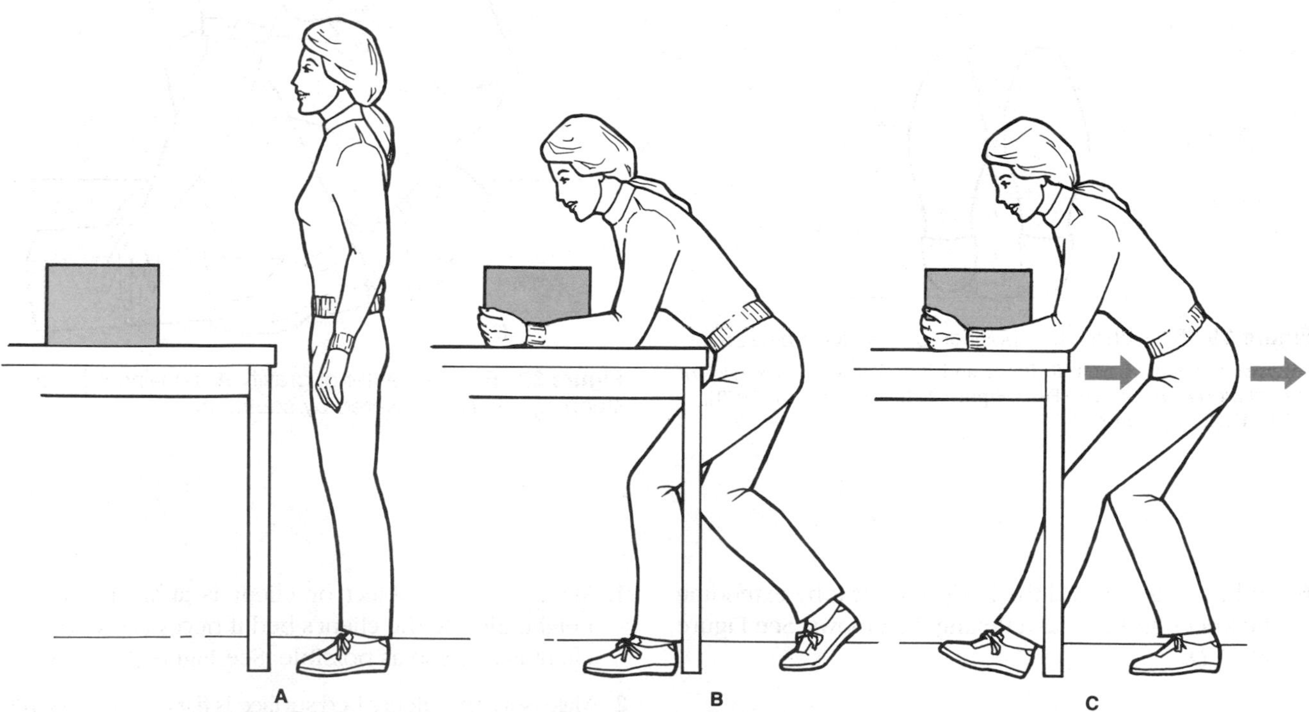

Figure 39–8 Schematic of good body mechanics: **A,** Load to be pulled rests on a surface about as high as the person's center of gravity. **B,** The base of support is enlarged, the body is flexed, and the muscles are tensed for action. **C,** The weight is shifted toward the rear leg as the load is pulled toward the person.

5. Place one foot forward and put the body weight on the forward foot.
6. Prepare to pull by:
    a. Inclining trunk forward from the hips.
    b. Placing forearms and palms-up hands beneath the client's center of gravity.
    c. Resting forearms and elbows on surface of bed.
    d. Flexing hips, knees, and ankles.
    e. Contracting stabilizing muscles of the body. See Figure 39–8, *B*.
7. Pull the object/client toward yourself by:
    a. Pushing with the forward foot and extending the forward leg.
    b. Shifting your weight to the backward foot in a rocking motion.
    c. Pulling directly toward your body and using extra force at the beginning of the pull to overcome friction and inertia. See Figure 39–8, *C*.

Lifting

Because lifting involves movement against gravity, the nurse must use major muscle groups of the thighs, knees, upper and lower arms, abdomen, and pelvis to prevent back strain. The initial steps involved in lifting are the same as for pulling, steps 1 to 6. Instead of pulling the client toward the nurse's center of gravity, however, the nurse uses the arms as levers to lift the client. (See Figure 39–3, earlier.) The elbows are used as fulcrums, the force is supplied by the biceps muscles, and the weight of the client is supported in the palms of the hands and wrists. See Figure 39–9, *A*. Lifting power is further enhanced by using the nurse's body weight to counteract the client's weight. The nurse increases hip and knee flexion to lower the center of gravity. As she or he does so, the forearms and hands supporting the client automatically rise. See Figure 39–9, *B*.

Use of the arms as levers is often applied in clinical practice when the nurse needs to raise the buttocks of a client in bed, e.g., to assist the client onto a bedpan or to give back care to a client in traction. Figures 39–9, *C* and 39–9, *D* illustrate this lifting technique.

Pivoting

Pivoting is a technique in which the body is turned in a way that avoids twisting of the spine. To pivot, place one foot ahead of the other, raise the heels very slightly, and put the body weight on the balls of the feet. When the weight is off the heels, the frictional surface is decreased and the knees are not twisted when turning. Keeping the body aligned, turn (pivot) about 90° in the desired direction. The foot that was forward will now be behind.

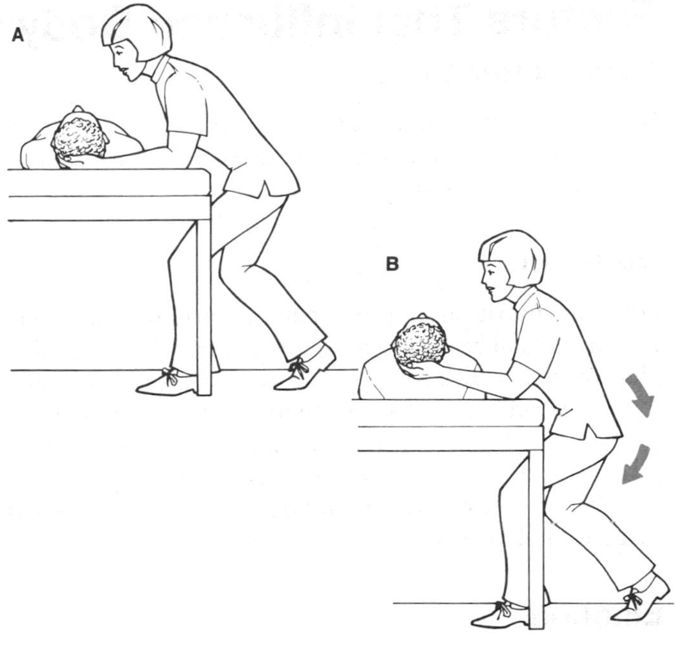

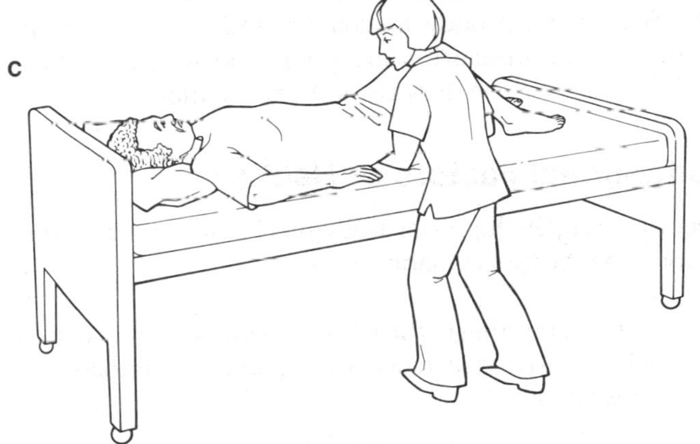

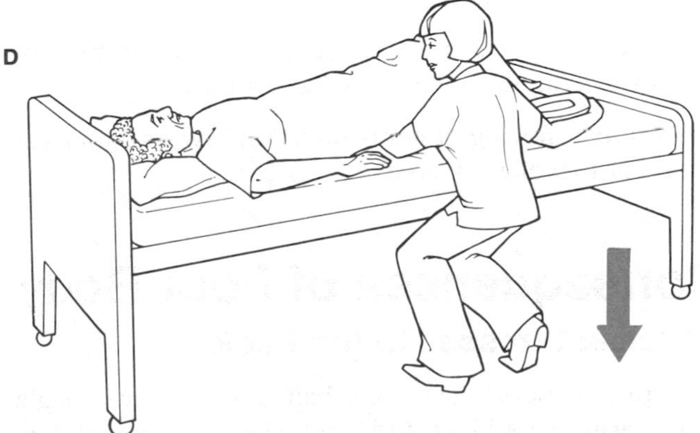

Figure 39–9 This nurse uses her arms as levers and employs her body weight to lift a client. **A,** Position before lifting; **B,** Position after lifting; **C and D,** The nurse uses positions A and B to lift a client's buttocks.

Factors That Influence Body Mechanics and Ambulation

General Health

Illness, disability, immobility, inactivity, poor physical fitness, and chronic fatigue have unfavorable effects on musculoskeletal function.

Nutrition

Adequate nutrition supplies vitamins and minerals essential for normal bone and muscle function. It also supplies glucose that powers muscle. Poor nutrition may cause muscle weakness and fatigue. An inadequate calcium intake places older women at risk of painful compression fractures of the vertebrae. Obesity distorts movement, and the obese person must expend extra energy to move and maintain balance.

Emotions

Security, joy, confidence, and self-esteem are reflected in the use of good body mechanics and gait. Worry, discouragement, insecurity, and poor self-esteem are often reflected in the use of poor body mechanics.

Situational Factors or Habits

People can develop poor body mechanics and gait from situational factors or habits, such as:

1. Frequent twisting of the back in work or daily activities, such as driving a truck or loading or unloading a dishwasher
2. Frequent lifting of heavy loads in work or daily activities, such as stocking shelves or carrying small children
3. Frequent stooping in work or daily activities, such as housework or gardening
4. Frequent pulling or pushing of heavy loads in work or daily activities, such as moving furniture
5. Frequent moving of items stored in low or high areas to waist-level work areas
6. Walking on slick or uneven surfaces, which predispose the person to falls
7. Wearing tight clothing that restricts freedom of movement
8. Wearing shoes with uneven or slick soles or high heels, which predispose the wearer to falls

Life-Style

An individual's life-style can affect body mechanics. Repeatedly performed movements, especially twisting or bending of the back, can result in permanent disability. Repeatedly walking on slippery or uneven surfaces can result in disabling falls. The person who leads an overly busy, stressful, and active life can become careless and is at risk of injury. Continued inactivity and poor physical fitness can predispose the individual to back injury.

Attitudes and Values

Personal values about body mechanics are important influences. Persons who value their appearance and health are more likely to practice good body mechanics and gait to protect their backs and prevent falls.

Level of Understanding

An understanding of the elements of good body mechanics usually encourages its use. Unfortunately, many individuals have no opportunity to learn these elements, are misinformed, or have forgotten them.

Neuromuscular and Skeletal Impairments

Diseases and injuries that affect the neuromuscular or skeletal systems can severely hinder movement. Genetically transmitted muscle-wasting diseases, disorders causing sensory or motor impairment, inflammatory conditions, injuries, and pain can severely impair movement.

Consequences of Poor Body Mechanics

Physical Stresses to the Back

The spine supports over one half of the body's weight (chest, arms, shoulders, and head) (Donaldson and Hoover, p. 42). In a person with good standing alignment, the lumbar spine is somewhat curved. See Chapter 38. In a person with poor standing alignment, the lumbar curvature is exaggerated and the spine cannot support the weight that a well-aligned column can support.

The muscles of the lumbar spine support and protect the spinal vertebrae, which in turn protect the delicate spinal cord. The abdominal muscles also support the back structures. Lumbar muscles are not strong enough, by themselves, to lift the upper body against gravity when it is bent forward with a load. A person can lift such a load only if the lumbar muscles are strong and if they work in synchrony with other strong muscle groups.

When a person bends forward only 20 degrees with knees extended, pressure on the lower back is 50% greater than in a person standing erect. If, in addition, the forward-leaning person is carrying a 44-pound load, the pressure on the lower back is more than 100% greater than in a person standing erect. Bending forward while keeping knees straight lifting a load, and twisting the spine is the worst possible combination of events predisposing to back injury (Donaldson and Hoover 1982, pp. 142–44).

Long-Term Effects

A strong and healthy back, undamaged by disease or previous injury, can usually handle the sequence of events just described. Not all backs, however, are strong and healthy. Most lower back problems are the result of a series of minor injuries and strains over many years. Each additional insult further damages the vertebrae and discs or the muscles and ligaments that support them. These minor injuries have a cumulative effect and often lead to more serious and painful disease or injury of the back. Most of these back problems occur in the lower back, just below the waist, at lumbar vertebrae 4 and 5 (L4-L5).

Lower back problems usually first occur in the young adult and persist for years, flaring up from time to time and just as spontaneously subsiding. Most frequently the cause is a **strain** (an overstretching of a muscle or ligament often due to overexertion) or, less frequently, a **sprain** (a partial tearing of a muscle or ligament usually due to injury).

These injuries usually become more serious with each additional insult to the back. The discomfort usually reaches a peak during middle age (30 to 55 years), and the person seeks medical advice. The most effective treatment for long-term back problems is prevention: taking care of the back all one's life.

Occupational Groups at Risk of Back Injury

Studies demonstrate that in all occupational groups backaches are second only to upper respiratory infections as a cause of absence from work. Most back problems are a result of lifting a heavy load from floor or knee level to waist level (Owen 1980, p. 894). A significant proportion of all compensation paid for disability injuries in recent years has been for back injuries. Workers who lift and transfer heavy loads, especially furniture movers, warehouse and storeroom workers, truck drivers, housekeepers, mothers of small children who lift and carry them about, and nurses and other caregivers, are at risk of back injury. Harber et al. (1986) list the five most common causes of work-related back injury among hospital nurses as lifting a client in bed (48%), helping a client out of bed (30%), moving the bed itself (27%), lifting a client to a stretcher (22%), and carrying equipment weighing more than 30 pounds (10%). Fifty-two percent of the nurses in this study experienced work-related back pain within a 6-month period (Harber et al. 1986, p. 118). Nurses therefore are at risk of back pain and injury.

Many factors increase the potential for lower back injuries. A major contributor is habitually poor standing and sitting posture, which produces an exaggerated lumbar lordosis. Overweight individuals who carry their extra weight over their abdomen, pregnant women, and women who consistently wear high-heeled shoes are at risk because of the exaggerated lumbar lordosis these situations produce. Persons who sit long hours at their work, are sedentary, or take little exercise are at greater risk because of weak back and abdominal muscles. There seems to be a higher incidence among persons who were gymnasts, acrobatic or ballet dancers, or equestrians in their younger years. The extreme flexing and twisting of the spine or compression of vertebrae may have produced permanent damage. One study of nurses, 80% of whom experienced occasional back problems, indicates that most had lax postural, exercise, and activity habits (Drapeau 1975, p. 63). Another study indicates that most of the nurses who experienced back problems did not remember how to use the pelvic tilt or proper lifting techniques that they learned in their nursing programs and were not using these in their work (Hoover 1973, p. 2079). Clearly, lower back injuries are preventable. Guidelines to prevent back injuries are summarized on page 1064.

The Consequences of Poor Ambulation

Falls are, by far, the most common serious consequence of ambulation dysfunction. Falls are the second leading cause of accidental death in the United States, and almost 25% of these occur among the elderly (Witte 1979, p. 1950). The elderly are most susceptible to falls, and the consequences of falling are far more serious for the elderly than for younger persons. About 6% of all falls among the elderly result in a fractured bone, and as many as 17% of those with broken bones die as a result of complications of the fracture (Hogue 1982, pp. 185–86). Although many elderly persons fall in their homes, the incidence of falls among the elderly rises significantly when they are hospitalized.

There are many reasons for the elderly person's susceptibility to falls. All are associated with the normal processes of aging. The most significant are poor vision, dizziness, and "drop attacks." There is a high incidence of dizziness among elderly persons, and some clouding

Guidelines for Preventing Back Injuries

- Become consciously aware of your posture and body mechanics.
- Make a conscious effort to improve your posture and body mechanics. Seek assistance if you need it.
- Minimize lumbar lordosis as much as possible:

    1. When standing for a period of time, periodically flex one hip and knee and rest your foot on an object if possible.
    2. When sitting, keep your knees slightly higher than your hips.
    3. Unless you have a pillow or other support beneath your abdomen, avoid sleeping in the prone position.

- Use a firm mattress that provides good body support at natural body curvatures.
- Exercise regularly to maintain overall physical condition.
- Practice exercises that strengthen the pelvic, abdominal, and lumbar muscles.
- Avoid exercises that require spinal flexion with straight legs (e.g., toe-touching and sit-ups) or spinal rotation (twisting).
- Unless physically fit, avoid activities that require an excessive arching of the spine (e.g., hockey) and spinal rotation (e.g., golf or tennis).
- Avoid exercises that cause pain.
- Apply principles of body mechanics continuously in your work and daily life.
- Rearrange storage areas at work and at home so that frequently used items are at least 2 feet above the floor. Lifting from this height to waist level minimizes back strain.
- Avoid lifting above waist level when possible. Lifting a load above this level places strain on the lower back.
- Avoid catching a heavy, falling object.
- Avoid lifting more than 20 pounds of weight alone. A load that exceeds 35% of body weight is considered excessively heavy.
- When lifting a load with another person, coordinate your efforts and use smooth, rhythmic movements. Choose a leader so that you can lift simultaneously.
- Size up a load to be lifted or moved. Determine whether you need assistance. If you need it, get it.
- Plan ahead how you will move a load and where you will move it. Make sure the area is free of obstructions.
- Do not force yourself to go on with an activity when you become tired.
- Maintain good general health.
- Control your weight.
- Wear clothing that allows you to use good body mechanics (e.g., avoid wearing a short, tight skirt).
- Wear comfortable shoes that provide good foot support and will not cause you to slip, stumble, or turn your ankle. Choose shoes with low heels.
- See your physician if you have persistent back pain.

Source: Adapted from M. Memmer, *Body mechanics* (Los Angeles: Intercampus Nursing Project, California State University and College System, 1974), pp. 16–17.

of the ocular lenses occurs in almost everyone by age 65. A drop attack is a fall caused by sudden loss of muscle tone in the legs, without warning but with no loss of consciousness. Several hours may elapse before the person regains muscle tone and can get up alone or with assistance. While the cause is unknown, drop attacks seem to occur exclusively among the elderly and account for about 25% of falls among this group (Hogue 1982, p. 185). Other factors include declining postural and movement reflexes resulting in unstable posture and gait, increased body sway with gait, and increased difficulty regaining balance when it becomes unstable.

When an elderly person is hospitalized, additional factors increase his or her potential for a fall:

1. Unfamiliarity with the surroundings
2. Strangeness of the diagnostic tests and surgery
3. Immobilization and the weakness it causes
4. Pain
5. Loss of independence and control over one's own activities
6. Drugs that contribute to dizziness, sedation, and confusion, especially diazepam (Valium), furosemide (Lasix), and antidepressants
7. Elimination dysfunction, which often intensifies with hospitalization
8. Confusion.

After surgery, the elderly person is much more likely to be confused than a younger person and much more likely to attempt to get out of bed without help.

Recent studies of elderly, hospitalized clients who have fallen suggest a profile of a person who is at high risk of falling. The typical client is a woman, over age 60, who has a history of falls at home or during previous hospitalizations. Due to unsteady ambulation, she used a wheelchair or other aid for ambulation at home, has had urinary dysfunction involving frequency and nocturia for several years, and has cataracts (lens clouding). She has been hospitalized for less than 1 week, has had surgery, and has been fairly immobile since then. Since the surgery, she has been somewhat disoriented and confused, especially at night. She is taking Valium and Lasix. This typical client usually falls at her bedside as she attempts to get out of bed at night (11:30 P.M. to 7:30 A.M.), unassisted, to go to the bathroom (Lee and Pash 1983, p. 120). Contusions, minor abrasions, and a loss of confidence in her ability to walk without falling often result.

Primarily due to the effects of osteoporosis, an older person is much more likely to fracture a bone during a fall than a younger person is. The most common fractures in elderly people who fall are hip fractures, Colles's (wrist) fractures, and compression fractures of vertebrae. When an elderly person breaks a bone, the complications of immobility are more dangerous than the fracture itself.

Structural Abnormalities That Affect Body Mechanics and Ambulation

Damage from injury or disease to any part of the neuromuscular or skeletal systems increases the risk of potential or actual impairment of movement. Many disorders produce pain, often severe, that further limits movement.

Many disorders of the skeletal system can impair movement. **Osteoporosis**, a condition in which the bones become brittle and fragile due to calcium depletion, is common in older women and primarily affects the weight-bearing joints of the lower extremities and the back. Weaknesses of the vertebrae may cause one vertebra to collapse under the weight of the upper body and crush down upon the anterior surface of the vertebra below it. This **compression fracture** of the vertebrae produces pain and nerve damage. When this type of fracture occurs, the spine bends sharply forward, producing a kyphosis (humpback) and an overall reduction in the person's height (Donaldson and Hoover 1982, pp. 73–74). Fractures of bones or joints in any part of the body can severely limit movement.

Degenerative arthritis (**osteoarthritis**) is another common cause of damage to the skeletal system. This disorder, common among the elderly, also affects the weight-bearing joints of the lower extremities and the back. Frequently, the knee and hip joints degenerate or develop bony spurs that cause pain upon movement. In the back, degeneration of the vertebrae may produce painful narrow disc spaces or bony spurs on the edges of a vertebra.

A prolapsed or ruptured disc between the vertebrae is less common but usually the final stage in a long series of insults to the back over many years. It often produces severe pain and markedly reduces mobility. Other and less common skeletal abnormalities that can limit movement include **osteomyelitis** (inflammation of the bone), **ankylosing spondylitis** (inflammation of the vertebrae), **rheumatoid arthritis** (inflammation of the joints), malignant tumors of the bone, and structural **scoliosis** (a lateral curvature of the spine).

Many foot problems severely hamper movement due to pain. Corns, bunions, hammer toes, and overgrown, horny toenails are almost universal among the elderly (Witte 1979, p. 1951). A number of disorders of the muscles and related structures can impair movement. Immobility can decrease muscle strength and mass markedly, often causing profound generalized muscle weakness. Muscle **atrophy** (a reduction in the size of a muscle) and joint stiffness can readily occur with disuse. Less frequently, strains and sprains, damage to cartilage, joint dislocations, or damage as a result of injury can impair movement. Muscle-wasting diseases, such as muscular dystrophy, can also take their toll.

Disorders of the nervous system that impair movement occur less frequently but are often more serious. Inner ear infections and dizziness can impair balance with movement. Parkinson's disease, multiple sclerosis, central nervous system tumors, cerebral vascular accidents (strokes), and spinal cord injuries can leave muscle groups weakened, paralyzed, **spastic** (with too much muscle tone), or **flaccid** (without muscle tone).

Assessment

Assessment of the client's problems related to immobility, joint range of motion, activities of daily living, and activity tolerance is discussed in Chapter 37. Assessment of body alignment is discussed in Chapter 38. A discussion of assessment of body mechanics and ambulation follows.

To assess the client's body mechanics and ambulation, the nurse collects information from the client, from other nurses, and from the client's records. The nurse needs to know the client's health status and its effect on his or her movement. The nurse determines how weak the client is, how well he or she tolerates movement, and whether he or she is hampered by pain, obesity, age, poor vision, or the side-effects of medication. The nurse needs to anticipate the client's potential for postural (orthostatic) hypotension (see Chapter 37) during movement and to be aware of the encumbrances to the client's movement, e.g., an IV in place or a heavy cast on one leg. The nurse also needs to anticipate how much assistance the client will require in moving, recognize environmental hazards that might endanger the client as he or she moves, and assess the client's ability to follow directions and recognize his or her capabilities and limitations.

Capabilities and Limitations for Movement

To determine the client's capabilities and limitations for movement, the nurse assesses the client while the client is:

1. Rising from a lying position to a sitting position on the edge of the bed. The client can normally rise without support from the arms; however, a client with muscle weakness may roll to the side and push with the arms or pull with the arms on side rails or nearby furniture to rise.
2. Rising from a chair to a standing position. Normally this can be done without pushing with the arms; however, a person with weak muscles may use the arms to push upward and may thrust the upper body forward before rising.
3. Moving in the bed. Specifically observe the amount of assistance required for turning:
   a. From a supine position to a lateral position
   b. From a lateral position on one side to a lateral position on the other
   c. From a supine position to a prone position
   d. From a supine position to a sitting position in bed

Body Mechanics

Criteria the nurse can use to assess a client's body mechanics are outlined on the facing page. These criteria are derived from the principles of body mechanics discussed earlier in this chapter. The nurse can observe a client's body mechanics in a home or work setting or whenever the client performs incidental movements.

Ambulation (Gait)

To assess the client's gait, the nurse asks the client to walk down a corridor and observes whether the client's:

1. Trunk is steady and upright
2. Arms swing appropriately
3. Gait is free and easy or unsteady
4. Legs follow through in the swing phase
5. Steps are appropriate or too small
6. Instep falls along the line of gravity or whether the feet are spread apart
7. Feet are dorsiflexed in the swing phase
8. Gait starts and stops with ease

Normal gait and common abnormalities of gait are described in Table 39–2.

Nursing Diagnosis

Nursing idagnoses related to the client's body mechanics and gait may include impaired physical mobility, potential for injury, fear, self-care deficit, and knowledge deficit. Examples of nursing diagnoses are shown opposite.

Planning

Client Goals

The nurse uses assessment data and nursing diagnoses to identify goals for care and design an individualized plan of nursing interventions. The overall goals of body mechanics and ambulation include:

1. Improved use of body mechanics in work and in daily life
2. Restored or improved ambulatory capability
3. Prevention of back injuries and falls

Nursing Responsibilities

Each nurse has the responsibility to use proper body mechanics to prevent back injury. As a role model, the nurse continuously teaches clients through the body

Table 39–2 Assessing Gait

Normal Findings	Abnormal Findings	Some Associated Conditions
Head is erect, and vertebral column straight	Body is rigid and bent forward.	Parkinsonism
Gaze is straight ahead.	Gaze is toward ground.	Fear of falling
Toes point forward.	Toes are everted.	Flat-footedness
Kneecaps point forward.	Legs are knock-kneed with feet apart (normal until age 3 or 4).	Rickets; congenital bone disorders
	Legs are bowlegged with feet together (normal until age 2 or 2½).	Rickets; congenital bone disorders
Elbows are slightly flexed.	One elbow is flexed and held close to body.	Hemiplegia
Foot is dorsiflexed in swing phase.	One foot is plantar flexed and drags.	Hemiplegia
Arm opposite swing-through foot moves forward at same time.	Arms swing forward and do not swing with steps.	Parkinsonism
Steps are smooth, coordinated, and rhythmic.	Steps are weaving, uncoordinated, and uneven.	Alcohol or barbiturate intoxication; cerebellar disorder
	Steps are short, shuffling, and often on tiptoe	Parkinsonism
	Gait starts slowly, gradually increases, and may be difficult to stop.	Parkinsonism
	Steps are stiff, jerking, and uncoordinated, with legs held stiffly together.	Spastic paraplegia; multiple sclerosis; spinal cord tumor
	Exaggerated lateral leaning accompanies steps.	Hip disorder

Criteria to Assess Body Mechanics

The client:

- Uses a wide base of support when moving objects
- Enlarges his or her base of support by placing feet appropriately in the direction in which the movement occurs
- Keeps objects to be moved close to his or her body (center of gravity)
- Pushes, pulls, rolls, or slides objects rather than lifting them whenever possible
- Avoids twisting the spine by pushing or pulling objects directly away from or toward the body and squarely facing the direction of movement
- Squats rather than stoops to pick up heavy objects from the floor and uses large muscle groups of the body
- Uses his or her body weight to counteract the weight of the object when pushing or pulling objects
- Tenses stabilizing muscles before moving objects
- Maintains muscle mass and strength through exercise

Examples of Nursing Diagnoses Related to Body Mechanics and Gait

- Impaired physical mobility related to musculoskeletal spasms in lower extremities
- Impaired physical mobility related to painful, inflamed joints
- Impaired physical mobility related to long leg cast
- Potential for injury related to left-sided paralysis
- Potential for injury related to unsteady gait
- Potential for injury from falling related to altered judgment and drowsiness associated with medication (Elavil)
- Potential for injury from falling related to confusion at night
- Potential for injury related to improper use of crutches
- Potential for back injury related to use of improper body mechanics
- Fear of falling related to unsteady gait and muscle weakness
- Self-care deficit (toileting) related to impaired physical mobility secondary to joint pain
- Knowledge deficit (body mechanics) of unknown etiology

mechanics she or he uses. A serious back injury could prevent a nurse from continuing professional practice.

The nurse is expected to protect the client from harm, since client safety is a major nursing responsibility. The nurse is responsible for anticipating safety risks for the client, protecting the client from unsafe practices, providing proper supervision during activities that pose potential risks, and protecting clients from falls in all situations. The more vulnerable the client, the greater the nurse's responsibility to protect him or her from harm (Cushing 1985, p. 138).

The nurse is responsible for teaching clients proper body mechanics. For example, a postoperative cataract client needs to learn how to squat rather than stoop to avoid increased intraocular pressure, a client with a back injury needs to learn how to get out of bed safely and comfortably, a client with an injured leg needs to learn how to transfer from bed to wheelchair safely, and a client with a newly acquired walker needs to learn how to use it safely. Nurses often need to assist family members or caregivers in the home to learn safe moving, lifting, and transfer techniques. Nurses who practice in hospitals and nursing homes have a responsibility to teach nursing assistants how to protect their backs from injury as they move, lift, and transfer clients.

Providing proper body mechanics and ambulatory care to clients is almost always an independent nursing function. Although certain activity orders are medically prescribed (see Chapter 38, page 1037), the physician rarely writes specific directions to indicate how the order is to be accomplished.

Planning also involves the designing of outcome criteria. See the section on evaluation, later in this chapter.

Intervention

Moving and Turning Clients

Clients require varying degrees of assistance to move while they are in bed. Some are completely helpless and require the assistance of nurses to make the smallest change in position. Those who are weak or very ill frequently require assistance from a nurse, although they may be able to help themselves a little.

Before nurses assist any client to move, they need to be aware of the following information:

1. How the client's illness influences his or her ability to move. Unconscious clients and those with generalized muscular weakness, loss of or injury to one or both lower extremities, acute spinal cord injury, paralysis of one or both lower extremities, or paralysis of one or both upper extremities need assistance by one, two, or more nurses.
2. Whether the client's illness contraindicates exertion. Clients with severe cardiac or respiratory impairments often cannot tolerate what would be minor exertion to most people.
3. The client's mental status, i.e., ability to comprehend instructions and to participate in the move. Obviously, unconscious clients are unable to participate and to assist the nurse. Clients, for example, who are medicated for pain postoperatively or who have experienced brain changes associated with age or disease may be too lethargic or mentally impaired to understand instructions.
4. The client's degree of comfort. Clients who have severe discomfort when moving, such as those with painful burns, acute inflammatory disease of the joints (e.g., arthritis), or recent surgery, require more help. These clients may require an analgesic at least 30 minutes before they are moved, to help them relax and move with minimal discomfort.
5. The position that the client needs to assume and the degree to which the client can tolerate another position. The client who has a respiratory pathologic condition may require a Fowler's position to breathe satisfactorily. This client may not be able to tolerate lying flat on the back even for a few minutes.
6. The amount of force required to move the client, i.e., the client's weight. If the nurse requires assistance, the second lifter needs to know the position to which the client will move. Sometimes mechanical lifters can help nurses move clients. See Procedure 39–7.

In all cases where the client is not able to assist, the preferred method is to use two or more nurses to move or turn the client.

Procedure 39–1 ▲ Moving a Client Up in Bed

Clients who have slid down in bed from the Fowler's position or been pulled down by traction need assistance to move up in bed. Whenever the client is capable of accomplishing this movement independently, he or she should be encouraged to do so.

There are a number of alternatives for the nurse who

is assisting a client to move up in bed. Some of these are not yet widely accepted. New research and new methods for performing basic nursing procedures more safely and effectively are being developed and refined constantly. Underlying all of them are the same basic principles of body mechanics, and the same concern for safety already discussed. These concerns and principles apply to both client and nurse.

Intervention

1. Adjust the head of the bed to a flat position or as low as the client can tolerate.

   Rationale Moving the client upward against gravity requires more force and can cause back strain.

2. Raise the bed to the height of the nurse's center of gravity and lock the wheels on the bed. Raise the rail on the side of the bed opposite the nurse.

3. Remove all pillows, then place one against the head of the bed to protect the client's head during the upward move.

4. Ask the client to flex his or her hips and knees and position the feet so that they can be used effectively for pushing.

   Rationale Flexing the hips and knees keeps the entire lower leg off the bed surface, preventing friction during movement. Flexing the hips and knees ensures use of the large muscle groups in the client's legs when pushing and increases the force of movement. The client is encouraged to assist as much as possible with movement to lessen the workload of the nurse.

5. If the client can assist with the move, ask the client to:

   a. Grasp the head of the bed with both hands and pull during the move.

   or

   b. Raise the upper part of the body on the elbows and push with the hands and forearms during the move.

   or

   c. Grasp the overhead trapeze with both hands and lift and pull during the move.

   Rationale Client assistance provides additional power to overcome friction during the move. These actions also keep the client's arms partially off the bed surface, reducing friction during movement, and make use of the large muscle groups of the client's arms to increase the force during movement. When the client requires minimal help, the nurse assists with the move by facing the direction of movement, placing the near arm under the client's thighs, and pushing down on the mattress with the far arm. During the move, the nurse rocks forward and shifts her or his weight from the rear to the forward foot. See Figure 39–10.

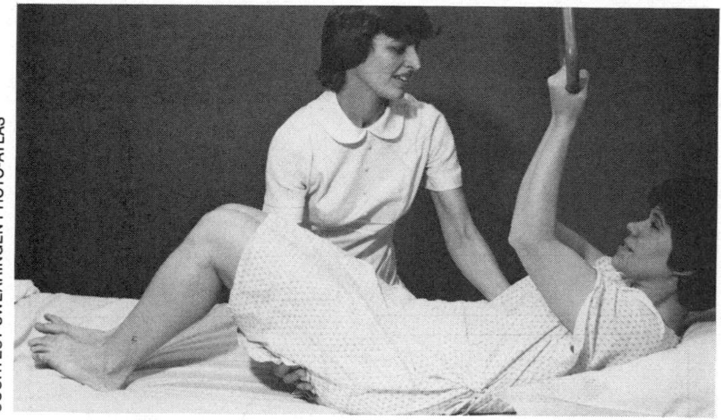

Figure 39–10

6. If the client has limited mobility or strength of the upper extremities and cannot assist with the move, place his or her arms across the chest.

   Rationale Keeping the client's arms off the bed surface prevents friction during movement.

7. Ask the client to flex the neck during the move.

   Rationale Flexing the neck keeps the head off the bed surface and prevents friction during movement.

8. Incline the trunk forward from the hips. Flex the hips, knees, and ankles. Assume a broad stance with the foot nearest the bed backward and the weight on the forward foot.

   Rationale The broad stance provides balance. Flexing the joints of the lower extremities lowers the center of gravity, increases stability, and ensures use of the large muscle groups in the legs during movement.

9. Place one arm under the client's back and shoulders and the other arm under the client's thighs. See Figure 39–11.

   Rationale This placement of the arms distributes the client's weight and supports the heaviest part of the body (the buttocks).

10. Tighten your gluteal, abdominal, leg, and arm muscles.

    Rationale Isometric contraction of stabilizing muscles helps to prevent musculoskeletal strain and injury.

11. Rock from the back leg to the front leg and back again; then shift weight to the front leg as the client pushes with the heels and pulls with the arms, moving the client toward the head of the bed.

    Rationale Rocking helps to attain a balanced, smooth motion and to overcome inertia. The nurse's weight shift helps to counteract the client's weight.

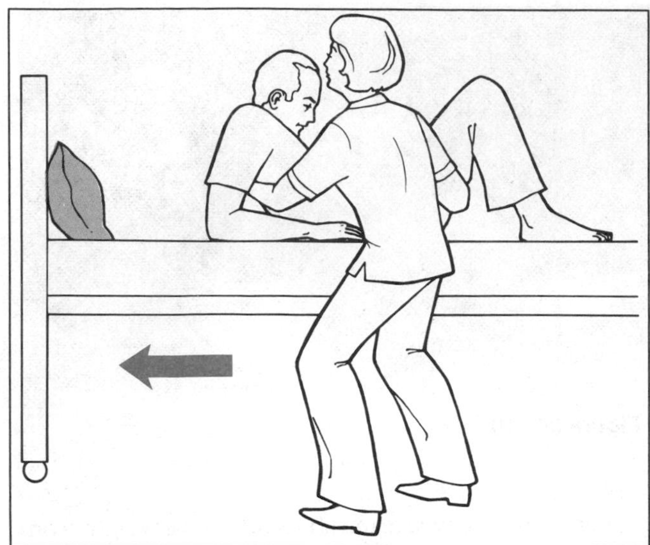

Figure 39–11

12. Elevate the head of the bed. Provide appropriate support devices for the client's new position. See the sections on positioning clients in Chapter 38.

Variation: Pulling a Client Up in Bed

This method emphasizes pulling the client up toward the head of the bed rather than lifting the client. It is designed to create less back strain for the nurse than a method that utilizes lifting.

The steps are:

1. Follow steps 1–3 as described above.
2. Move the client to the edge of the bed closest to the nurse's body. (Procedure 39–2 describes how to perform this action.)
3. Follow steps 4 and 5 as described above.

   Rationale Client assistance provides additional power to overcome friction during the move. These actions keep the client's arms partially off the bed surface, reducing friction during movement, and make use of the large muscle groups of the client's arms to increase the force during movement.

4. Follow steps 6–8 as described above.
5. Facing the foot of the bed, place both hands together beneath the client's coccyx. The nurse's elbow closest to the client will be beneath the client's upper back. Both elbows should rest on the surface of the bed. Align your body so that it is directly in line with your hands.

   Rationale This placement of the arms, beneath the heaviest part of the client's body, enables the nurse to pull the client directly toward the nurse's center of gravity, preventing spinal twisting. Placement of the nurse's hands focuses and increases the force needed for movement and reduces the friction of the client's body against the bed surface. Resting the elbows on the bed surface prevents inadvertent lifting by the nurse. Pulling rather than pushing can be more comfortable for the client and is safer for the nurse, since she or he retains greater control over the movement.

6. Follow step 10 as described above.
7. Coordinating your efforts with those of the client, rock backward and shift weight from the forward to the backward foot, pulling the client directly toward you while the client pushes with the heels and pulls with the arms. The hip closest to the bed should slide along the side of the mattress. Your elbows should slide along the bed surface.

   Rationale Rocking backward uses the nurse's body weight to increase the force of movement in the direction of the pull and helps to overcome inertia. Pulling from the client's center of gravity directly toward the nurse's own center of gravity requires less force than lifting and prevents spinal twisting. Keeping elbows on the bed surface also prevents inadvertent lifting by the nurse.

8. Raise the side rail and move to the opposite side of the bed. Move or pull the client as above, and move again to the opposite side of the bed. Move or pull the client back to the center of the bed. (Procedure 29–2 describes the pulling movement used in this last step.) Raise rail.

   Rationale A raised side rail is essential in preventing the client from falling out of bed.

Variation: Two Nurses Using a Hand–Forearm Interlock

Two people are required to move a client who is unable to assist because of his or her health or weight. Using the technique described above, with the second nurse on the opposite side of the bed, the two nurses interlock their forearms under the client's thighs and shoulders. See Figure 39–12.

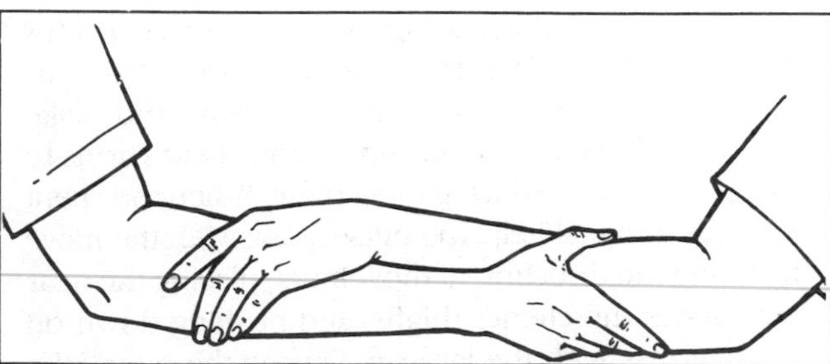

Figure 39–12

Variation: Two Nurses Using a Turn Sheet

Two nurses can use a turn sheet to move a client up in the bed. A turn sheet distributes the client's weight more evenly, decreases friction, and exerts a more even force on the client during the move. In addition, it prevents injury to the client's skin, since the friction created between two sheets when the client is moved is less than that created by the client's body moving over the sheet.

A drawsheet or a full sheet folded in half is placed under the client, extending from the shoulders to the thighs.

Each nurse rolls up or fanfolds the turn sheet close to the client's body on either side. The nurses then grasp the sheet close to the shoulders and buttocks of the client. This draws the weight closer to the nurses' base of support and increases the nurses' balance and stability, permitting a smoother movement. The method described in steps 8, 10, and 11 is then used to move the client up in the bed.

Procedure 39–2 ▲ Moving a Client to the Side of the Bed in Segments

This movement is used in preparation for moving the client onto a stretcher, in preparation for turning the client to the lateral (side-lying) position, or when changing the client's bed. Whenever the client is capable of assisting with this movement, he or she should be encouraged to lift his or her body by holding onto the raised side rail or by using the overhead trapeze. In this movement, the nurse's weight is used to counteract the client's weight; the nurse's arms serve as connecting bars between the client and the nurse.

Intervention

1. Stand as close as possible at the side of the bed toward which the client will be moved and opposite the client's chest.

   Rationale The nurse avoids spinal twisting by placing her or his center of gravity as close as possible to the client's center of gravity and squarely facing the direction of movement. This position also reassures the client that he or she will not fall.

2. Place the client's near arm across his or her chest.

   Rationale Placing the client's arm across the chest avoids friction and resistance to movement and prevents injury to the arm.

3. Incline your trunk forward from the hips. Flex your hips, knees, and ankles. Assume a broad stance, with one foot forward and the weight placed upon this forward foot.

   Rationale The broad stance provides balance. Flexing the joints of the lower extremities lowers the center of gravity, increasing stability, and ensures use of the large muscle groups in the legs during movement.

4. Place your arms and hands with palms facing upward close together beneath the client's scapulae. (If the client cannot support his or her head during the movement, position your arm which is nearest the head of the bed so that it cradles the client's head.) Flex your fingers around the client's far shoulder and rest your elbows on the surface of the bed.

   Rationale Placing the arms and hands beneath the heaviest part of the client's upper trunk focuses and increases the force for movement. Placing the arms close together reduces the friction of the client's body against the bed, making the pull easier. The hand and finger positions increase the force of movement. The elbow position prevents inadvertent lifting by the nurse.

5. Tighten your gluteal, abdominal, leg, and arm muscles.

   Rationale Isometric contraction of stabilizing muscles helps to prevent musculoskeletal strain and injury.

6. Rock backward, shifting your weight from the forward to the backward foot, pulling the client's shoulders directly toward you.

   Rationale Pulling requires less energy than lifting. Rocking backward uses the nurse's body weight to assist with the pull. The enlarged base of support enhances stability. Pulling the client's upper body directly toward one's center of gravity requires less force and prevents spinal twisting.

7. To move the client's buttocks, place your arms and hands close together beneath the client's buttocks. Repeat steps 5 and 6, pulling the buttocks to the side of the bed.

8. To move the client's legs and feet, place your hands close together beneath the client's ankles. Repeat steps 5 and 6, pulling the client's legs and feet to the side of the bed.

9. Elevate the side rail next to the client.

   Rationale The side rail is essential to prevent the client from falling off the bed.

Variation: Using a Pull Sheet

A pull sheet beneath the client's trunk and thighs can be used to pull the client to the side of the bed. The nurse rolls up the sheet as close as possible to the client's body and first pulls the client's shoulders, then the buttocks, to the side of the bed. The legs and feet are moved as described in step 8, above.

Procedure 39–3 ▲ Turning a Client to a Lateral or Prone Position in Bed

Movement to a lateral (side-lying) position may be necessary when placing a bedpan beneath the client, when changing the client's bed linen, or when repositioning the client.

Intervention

1. Before moving a client to a lateral position, move the client closer to the side of the bed opposite the side the client will face when turned. See Procedure 39–2.

   Rationale This ensures that the client will be positioned safely in the center of the bed after turning.

2. While standing on the side of the bed nearest the client, place the client's near arm across his or her chest. Abduct the client's far shoulder slightly from the side of the body.

   Rationale Pulling the one arm forward facilitates the turning motion. Pulling the other arm away from the body prevents that arm from being caught beneath the client's body when he or she is rolled onto that side.

3. Place the client's near ankle and foot across the far ankle and foot. Raise the side rail next to the client before going to the other side of the bed.

   Rationale Placing the near ankle and foot forward facilitates the turning motion. Making these preparations on the side of the bed closest to the client helps the nurse prevent unnecessary reaching. The raised side rail prevents the client who is close to the edge of the mattress from falling out of the bed.

4. Position yourself on the side of the bed toward which the client will turn, directly in line with the client's waistline and as close to the bed as possible.

   Rationale The nurse avoids spinal twisting by placing her or his center of gravity as close as possible to the client's center of gravity and squarely facing the direction of movement.

5. Incline your trunk forward from the hips. Flex your hips, knees, and ankles. Assume a broad stance with one foot forward and the weight placed upon this forward foot.

   Rationale The broad stance provides balance. Flexing the joints of the lower extremities lowers the center of gravity, increasing stability, and ensures use of the large leg muscles during movement.

6. Place one hand on the client's far hip and the other hand on the client's far shoulder. See Figure 39–14.

   Rationale This position of the hands supports the client at the two heaviest parts of his or her body, providing greater control in movement during the roll.

7. Tighten your gluteal, abdominal, leg, and arm muscles.

   Rationale Isometric contraction of stabilizing muscles helps to prevent musculoskeletal strain and injury.

8. Rock backward, shifting your weight from the forward to the backward foot, and roll the client onto his or her side to face you. See Figure 39–15.

   Rationale Pulling requires less energy than lifting. Rocking backward uses the nurse's body weight to assist with the pull. The enlarged base of support enhances stability. Pulling the client's body directly toward your own center of gravity requires less force and prevents spinal twisting.

Variation: Turning the Client to a Prone Position

To turn a client to the prone position, the nurse follows all of the above steps with two exceptions:

1. Instead of abducting the far arm, the client's arm is kept alongside the body for the client to roll over.

   Rationale Keeping the arm alongside the body prevents it from being pinned under the client when he or she is rolled.

2. The client is rolled completely onto his or her abdomen. It is essential to move the client as close as possible to the bed edge before the turn so that he or she will be lying in the center of the bed after rolling. A client should never be pulled across the bed while in the prone position because doing so can injure the breasts of a woman or the genitals of a man.

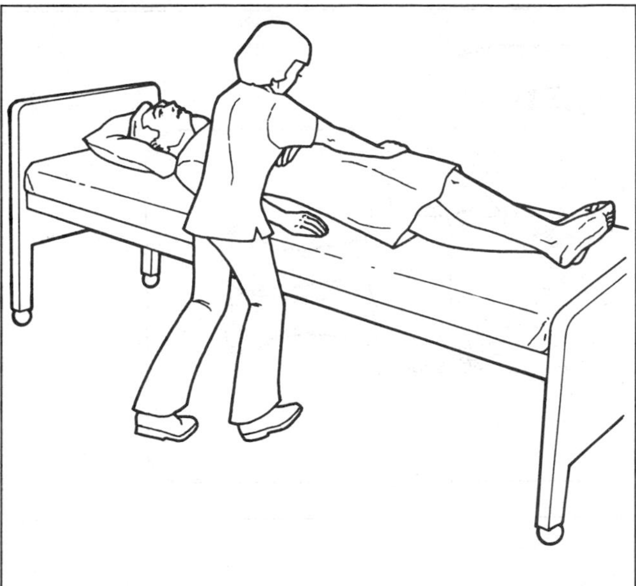

Figure 39–14

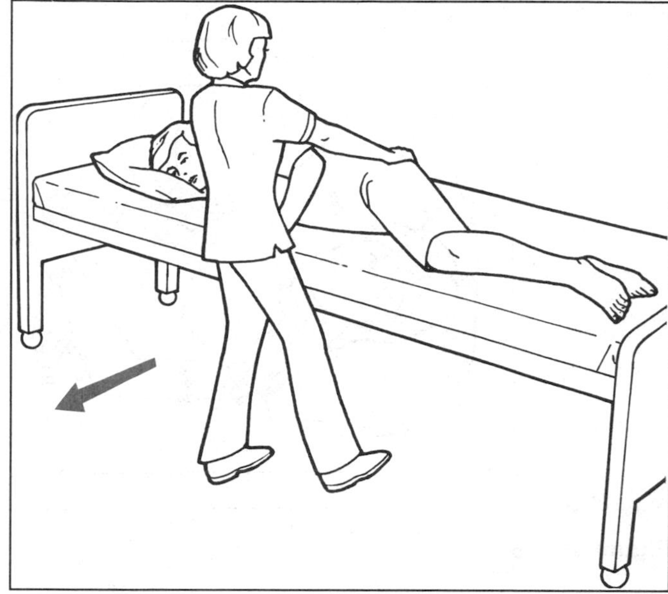

Figure 39–15

Procedure 39–4 ▲ Logrolling a Client

Logrolling is a technique used to turn a client whose body must at all times be kept in straight alignment (like a log). An example is the client who has a spinal injury. Considerable care must be taken to prevent additional injury. This technique requires two nurses or, if the client is large, three nurses.

Intervention

1. The nurses stand on the same side of the bed and assume a broad stance with one foot ahead of the other.

   Rationale A broad stance enhances balance.

2. Place the client's arms across his or her chest.

   Rationale The client's arms then will not be injured or become trapped under him or her.

3. Incline your trunk and flex your hips, knees, and ankles.

   Rationale Flexing these joints ensures use of the large muscle groups in the legs when moving and lowers the center of gravity, enhancing stability.

4. Place your arms under the client as shown in Figure 39–16 or Figure 39–17, depending upon the client's size.

   Rationale Each nurse then has a major weight area of the client centered between the arms.

5. Tighten your gluteal, abdominal, leg, and arm muscles.

   Rationale Isometric contraction of these muscles prepares them for action and prevents injury.

6. One nurse counts "one, two, three, go." Then, at the same time, all nurses pull the client to the side of the bed by shifting weight to the back foot and flexing the knees.

   Rationale Moving the client in unison maintains the client's body alignment.

7. Elevate the side rail on this side of the bed.

   Rationale Elevating the side rail prevents the client from falling while lying so close to the edge of the bed.

8. All nurses move to the other side of the bed.

9. Place a pillow where it will support the client's head after he or she is turned.

   Rationale The pillow prevents lateral flexion of the neck and ensures alignment of the cervical spine.

10. Place one or two pillows between the client's legs to support the upper leg when the client is turned.

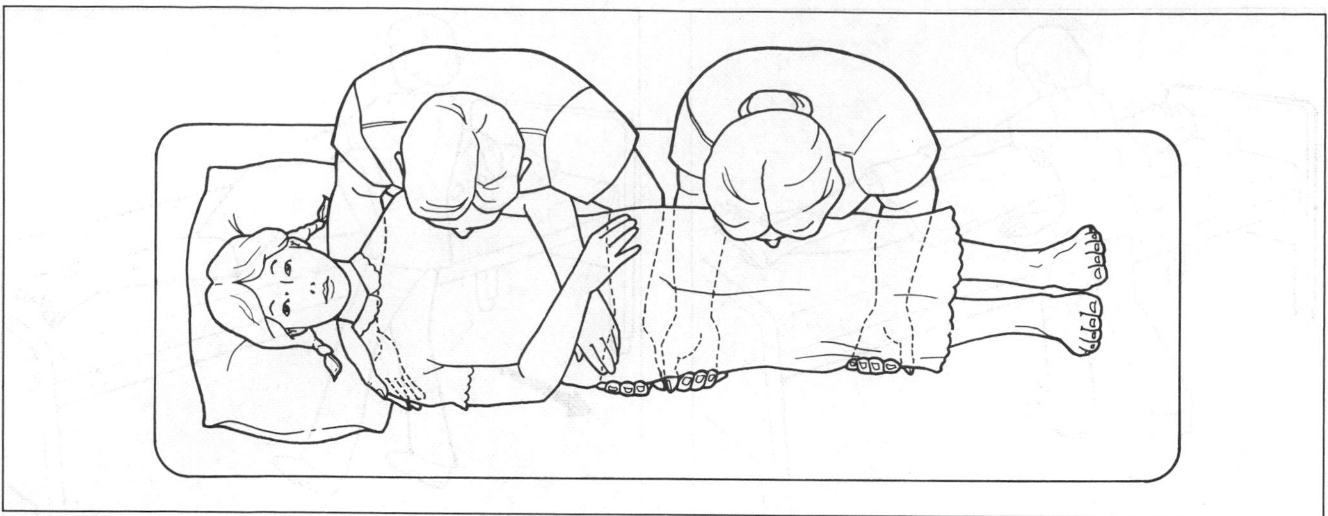

Figure 39–16

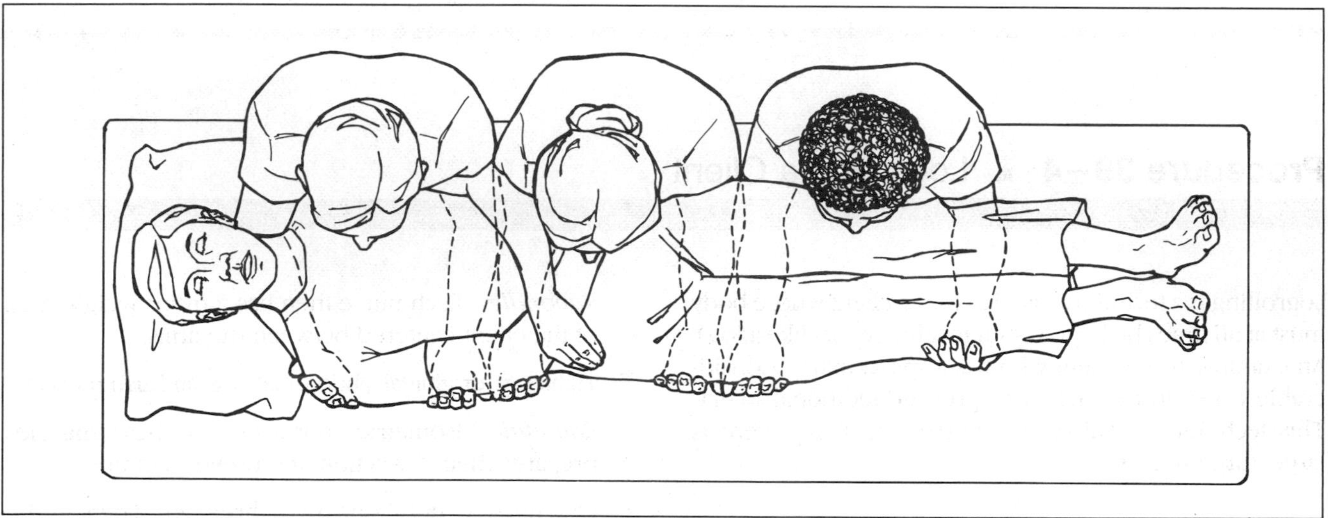

Figure 39–17

Rationale The pillow between the client's legs prevents adduction of the upper leg and keeps the legs parallel and aligned.

11. All nurses flex the hips, knees, and ankles and assume a broad stance with one foot forward.
12. All nurses reach over the client and place hands as shown in Figure 39–18.

    Rationale This centers a major weight area of the client between each nurse's arms.
13. One nurse counts "one, two, three, go." Then, at the same time, all nurses roll the client to a lateral position.
14. Place pillows to maintain the client's lateral position. See the discussion of the lateral position in Chapter 38.

Variation: Using a turn sheet

Logrolling can be facilitated with the use of a turn sheet. The client is first moved to the side of the bed by two nurses who stand on the same side of the bed. Each nurse assumes a broad stance with one foot forward and grasps half of the fanfolded or rolled edge of the turn sheet. On a signal, the nurses pull the client toward them. See Figure 39–19.

Before the client is turned, pillow supports are placed for the head and the legs, as described in steps 9 and 10, to maintain the client's alignment when turning. One nurse then goes to the other side of the bed (farthest from the client) and assumes a stable stance. Reaching over the client, this nurse grasps the far edges of the turn sheet and rolls the client toward her or him. See Figure 39–20. The second nurse (behind the client) helps to turn the

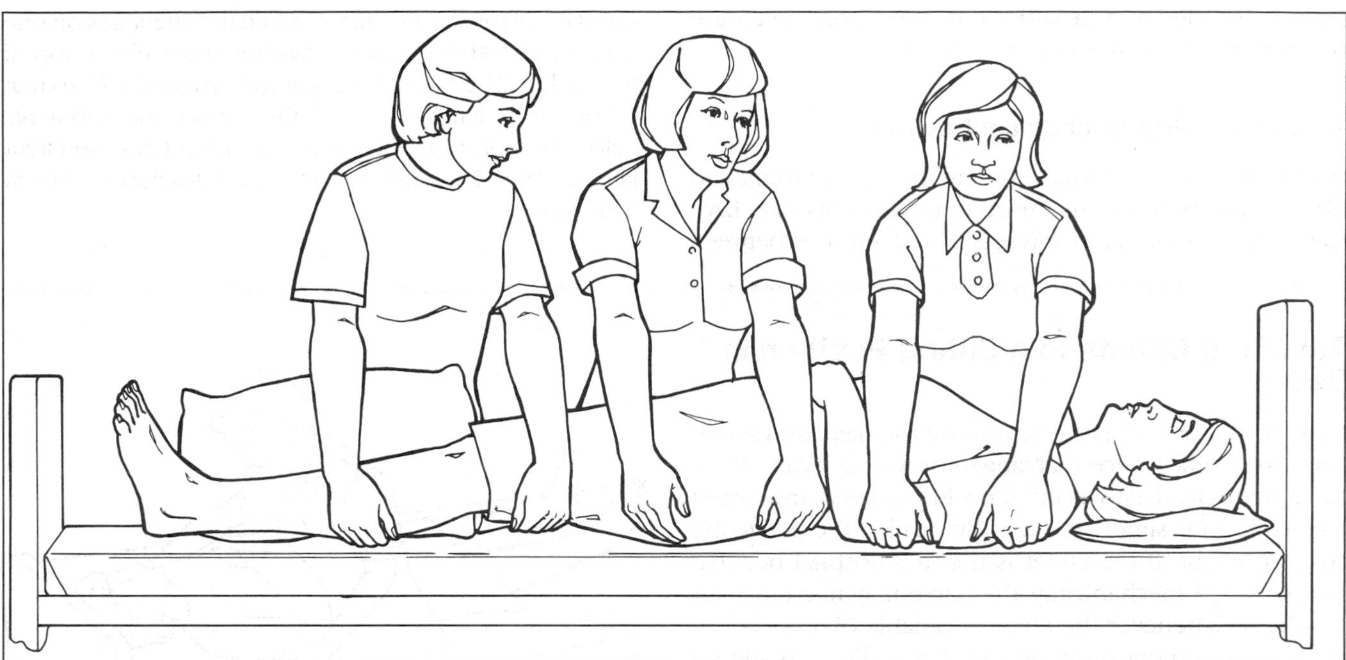

Figure 39–18

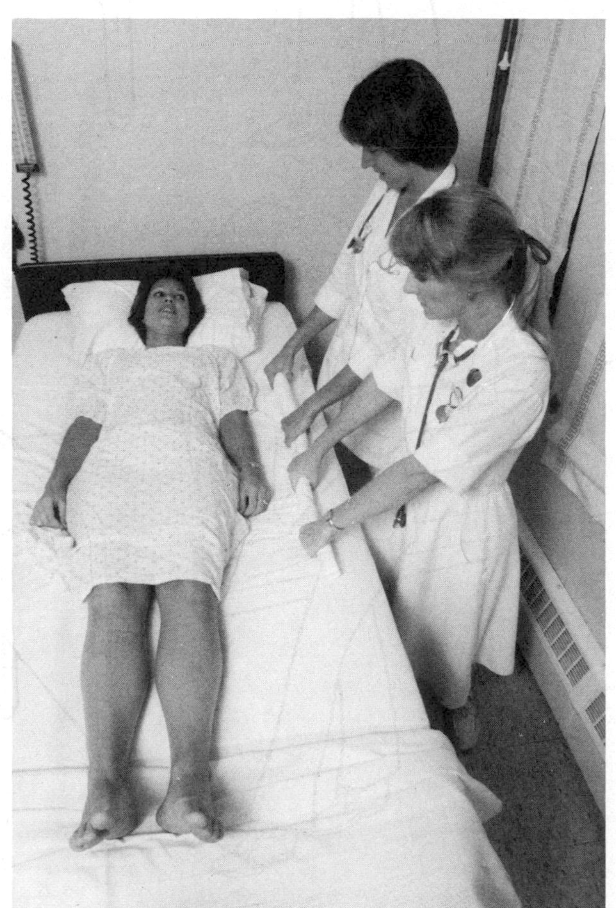

Figure 39–19

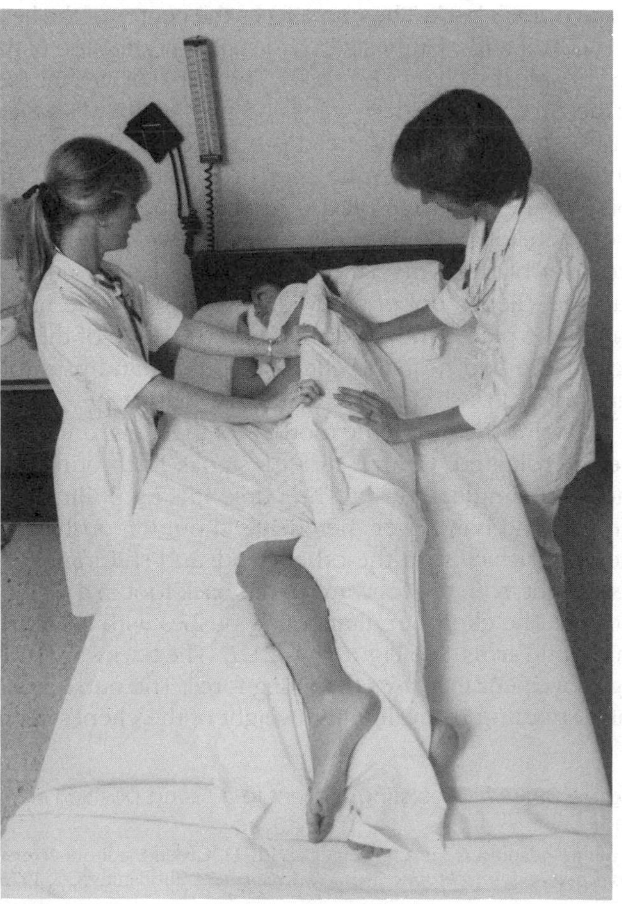

Figure 39–20

client as needed and provides pillow supports to ensure good alignment in the lateral position.

Variation: Using Mechanical Devices

Several mechanical devices, such as the Stryker frame and CircOlectric bed, are also used to turn clients who have spinal injuries or are paralyzed. The client lies between two flat, narrow bed surfaces. While the client lies on one surface, the other surface is fastened securely on top of him or her. Then the client is quickly rotated 180° so that he or she is lying on top of the surface that moments before was on top. The Stryker frame rotates the client laterally 180°. The CircOlectric bed rotates the client from head to toe.

Assisting Clients to a Sitting Position in Bed

A client may need assistance to raise the head and shoulders while pillows are rearranged or for back care. If the client needs to rise to a sitting position in bed, the easiest way to do so is simply to raise the head of the bed to the desired height. If the client is not in a hospital bed that can be raised mechanically, the nurse may need to assist the client. Whenever the client is capable of accomplishing this movement independently, the client should be encouraged to do so.

When the client needs assistance, the nurse first asks the client to place the arms at the sides with the palms of the hands ready to push against the surface of the bed. Client assistance provides additional power during the movement and reduces the potential for strain and injury to the nurse's back. The nurse faces the center of the head of the bed and assumes a broad stance at the side of the bed beside the client's buttocks. The nurse places the foot farthest from the bed forward and puts her or his weight on this foot. Facing the head of the bed at the angle in which the movement will occur prevents twisting of the spine. The nurse then places the hand nearest the client over the client's far shoulder to rest between the client's shoulder blades. This hand position enables the nurse to pull the client's upper body directly toward the nurse. The nurse places the other hand on the edge of the surface of the bed near the client's shoulder and uses it to support and push during the lift. See Figure 39–21, *A*.

During the move, the motions of the nurse and client are coordinated. On the nurse's signal, both nurse and client lift simultaneously. The nurse lifts by pulling with the arm and hand over the client's shoulder, pushing on the bed surface with the other hand, and shifting her or his weight from the forward to the back foot in a rocking motion. The client simultaneously pushes with his or her hands and arms. See Figure 39–21, *B*. The backward rocking movement increases the lifting force. The nurse avoids spinal twisting by pulling the weight of the client's upper

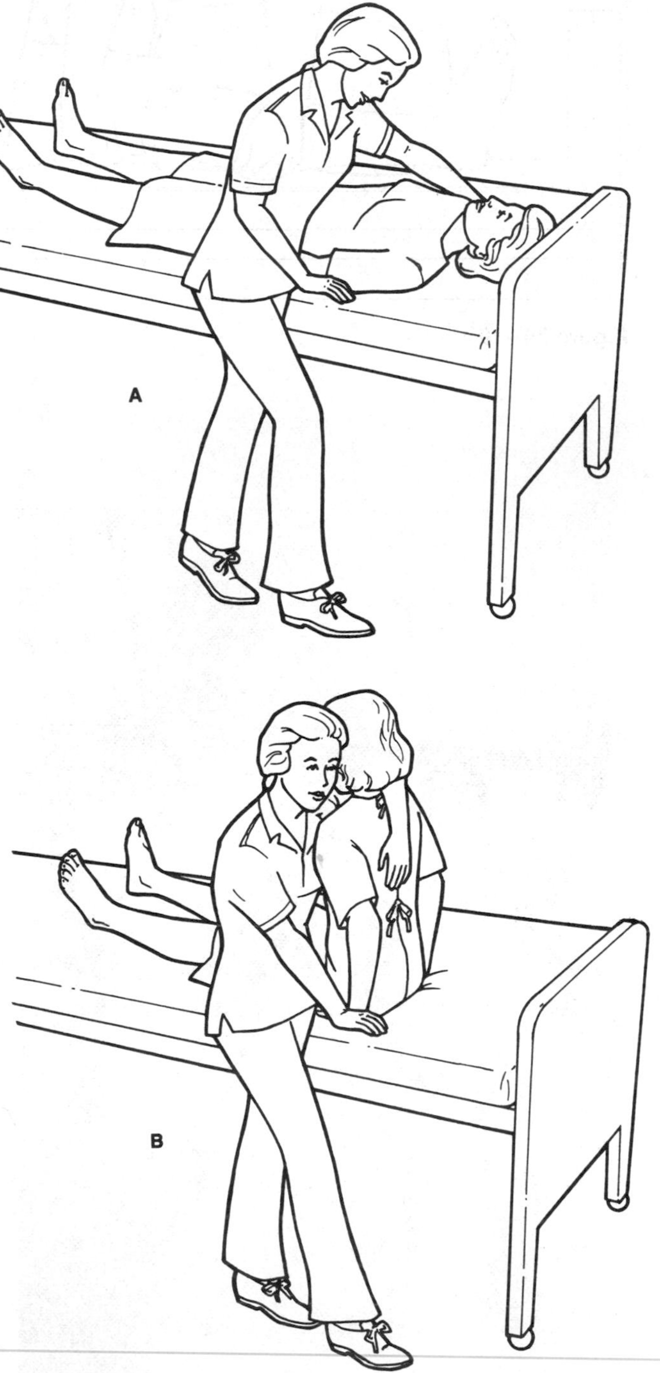

Figure 39–21 Assisting a client to a sitting position in bed

Source: Adapted from A. J. Belger and E. H. Greene, editors, *Winter's protective body mechanics* (New York: Springer Publishing Co., 1973), p. 35.

body directly toward the nurse's center of gravity and in the direction of the movement. Pushing with the muscles of one arm while pulling with the muscles of the other arm distributes the work load and increases lifting power. The client's pushing motion provides additional power for the lift.

Procedure 39–5 ▲ Moving a Client to a Sitting Position on the Edge of the Bed

The client assumes a sitting postion on the edge of the bed before walking, moving to a chair or wheelchair, eating, or performing other activities.

Intervention

1. Assist the client to a lateral position facing the nurse. See Procedure 39–3.
2. Raise the head of the bed slowly as high as it will go.

   Rationale This decreases the distance that the client needs to move to sit up on the side of the bed.
3. Position the client's feet and lower legs just over the edge of the bed.

   Rationale This enables the client's feet to move easily off the bed during the movement, and the client is aided by gravity into a sitting position.
4. Stand beside the client's hips and face the far corner of the bottom of the bed. Assume a broad stance, placing the foot nearest the client forward. Incline your trunk forward from the hips. Flex your hips, knees, and ankles. See Figure 39–22.

   Rationale The broad stance provides balance. Flexing the joints of the lower extremities lowers the center of gravity, increases stability, and ensures use of the large leg muscles during movement. The nurse avoids twisting of the spine by facing the foot of the bed at the angle in which the movement will occur.
5. Place one arm around the client's shoulders and the other arm beneath both of the client's thighs near the knees. See Figure 39–22.

   Rationale Supporting the client's shoulders prevents the client from falling backward during movement. Supporting the client's thighs reduces friction of the thighs against the bed surface during the move and increases the force of the movement.
6. Tighten your gluteal, abdominal, leg, and arm muscles.

   Rationale Isometric contraction of stabilizing muscles helps to prevent musculoskeletal strain and injury.
7. Lift the client's thighs slightly. Pivot on the balls of your feet toward the rear leg while pulling the client's feet and legs off the bed. See Figure 39–23.

   Rationale Raising the thighs off the bed reduces the friction of the client's thighs and the nurse's arm against the bed surface. Pivoting prevents twisting of the nurse's spine. The weight of the client's legs swinging downward increases downward movement of the lower body and helps make the client's upper body vertical.
8. Keep supporting the client until he or she is balanced and comfortable.

   Rationale This movement may cause some clients to feel faint.

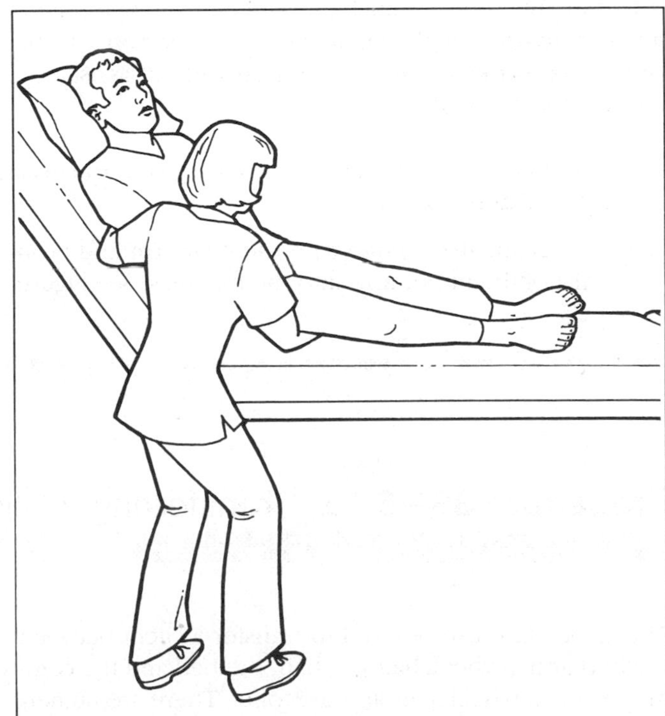

Figure 39–22

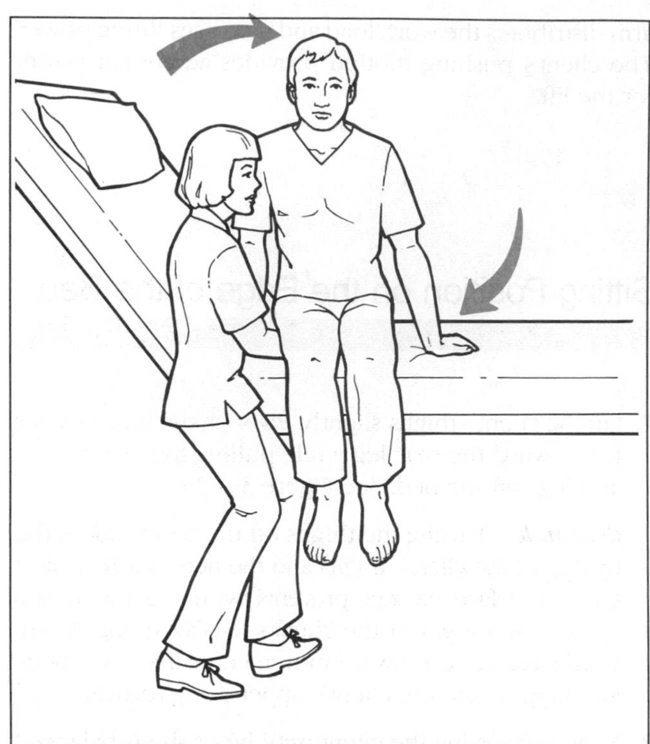

Figure 39–23

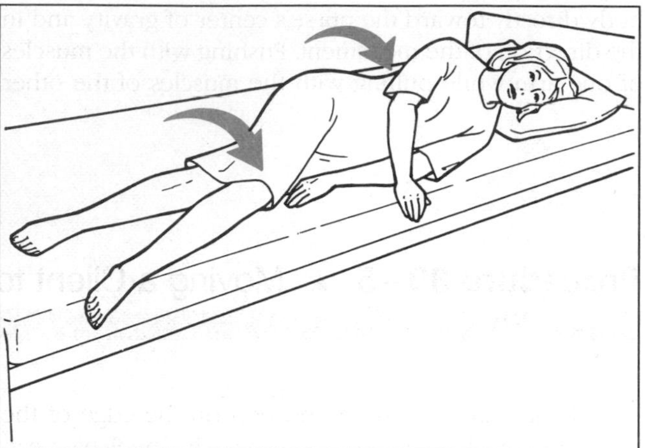

Figure 39–24

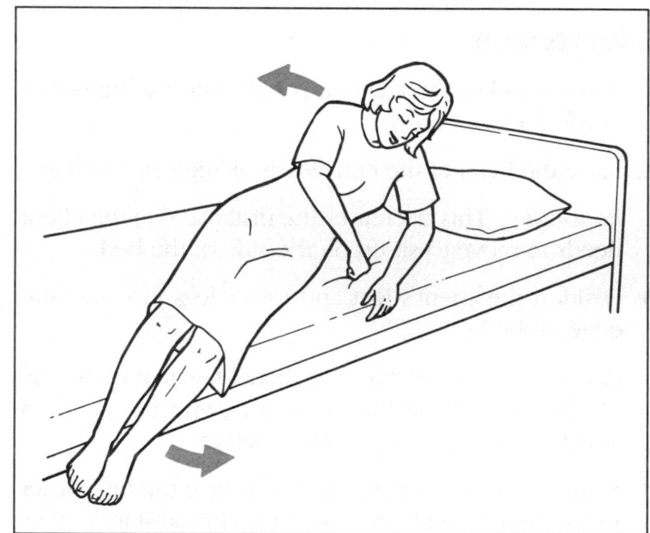

Figure 39–25

Variation: Teaching a Client How to Sit on the Side of the Bed Independently

A client who has had recent abdominal surgery or who is weak may have too much abdominal pain or too little strength to sit straight up in bed. This person can be taught to assume a "dangle" position without assistance. Instruct the client to:

1. Roll to his or her side and lift the far leg over the near leg. See Figure 39–24.
2. Grasp the mattress edge with the near arm and push the fist of the upper arm into the mattress. See Figure 39–25.
3. Push up with the arms as the heels and legs slide over the mattress edge. See Figure 39–25.
4. Maintain sitting position by pushing both fists into the mattress behind and to the sides of the buttocks.

Procedure 39–6 ▲ Transferring a Client Between a Bed and a Wheelchair

This procedure can be used to transfer a client between the bed and a wheelchair or chair, the bed and the commode, and a wheelchair and the toilet. There are numerous variations of this transfer technique; several are described in this procedure. Which variation the nurse selects depends on a number of factors: the client's disabilities and body size, the technique with which the client is familiar, the space in which the transfer is maneuvered (bathrooms, for instance, are usually cramped), the number of assistants (1 or 2) needed to accomplish the transfer safely, and the skill and strength of the nurse(s). For these reasons, it is useful to know how to use several different transfer methods safely.

Transfer belts provide the greatest safety. See Figure 39–26. This belt has a handle that allows the nurse to control movement of the client during the transfer. An increasing number of hospitals and nursing homes are requiring that personnel use the transfer belt to transfer clients.

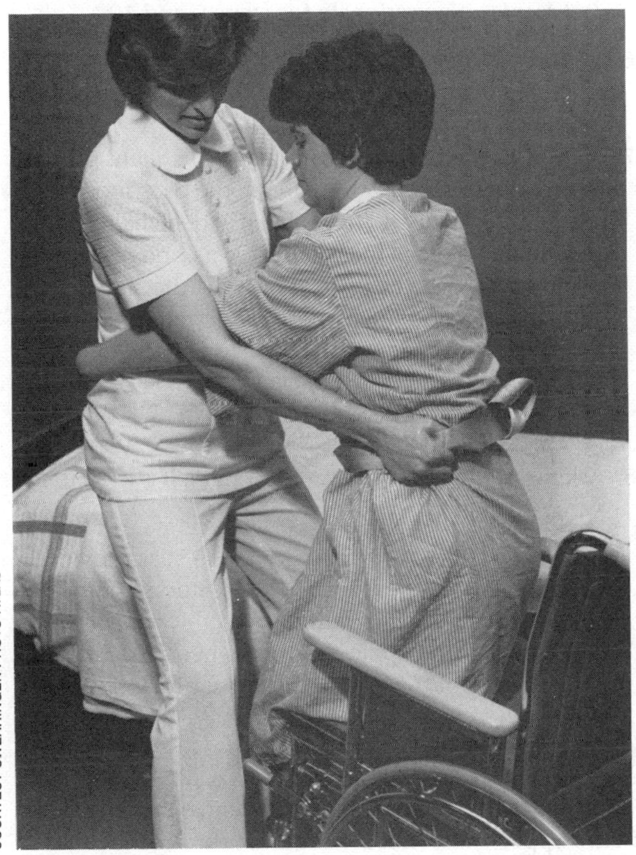

Figure 39–26

Intervention

1. Assist the client to a sitting position on the side of the bed. See Procedure 39–5.
2. Assist the client to put on a bathrobe and nonskid slippers or shoes.
3. Place a transfer belt snugly around the client's waist. Check to be certain that the belt is securely fastened.
4. Lower the bed to its lowest position so that the client's feet rest flat on the floor. Lock the wheels of the bed.
5. Assess the client for orthostatic hypotension (see Chapter 37, page 977) prior to moving him or her from the bed.
6. Place the wheelchair at a right angle to the bed, and as close to the bed as possible, as shown in Figure 39–27. Lock the wheels of the wheelchair.

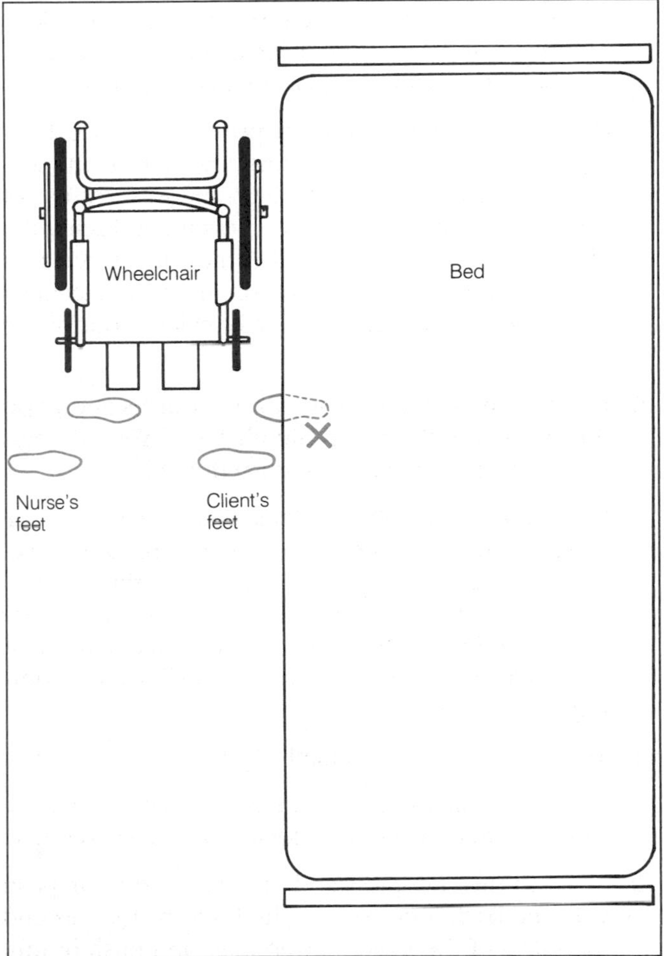

Figure 39–27

7. Ask the client to: move forward to sit on the edge of the bed, lean forward slightly from the hips, place the foot of the stronger leg beneath him or her, and put the other foot forward.

   Rationale These actions bring the client's center of gravity closer to the nurse's and more directly over the client's base of support as the weight is shifted forward during the transfer. By placing the stronger foot and leg in this way, the client can use the stronger leg muscles to stand and power the movement. A broader base of support makes the client more stable during the transfer.
8. Ask the client to place his or her hands on the bed surface or on the nurse's shoulders so that he or she can push while standing. The client should not grasp the nurse's neck for support because doing so can injure the nurse.

Rationale Use of the client's arm muscles provides additional force for the movement and reduces the potential for strain on the nurse's back.

9. Stand directly in front of the client. Incline the trunk forward from the hips. Flex the hips, knees, and ankles. Assume a broad stance, placing one foot forward and one back, mirroring the placement of the client's feet.

   Rationale The broad stance provides balance. Flexing the joints of the lower extremities lowers the center of gravity, increases stability, and ensures use of the large leg muscles during movement. Facing the client in the direction of the movement prevents twisting of the spine. The complementary placement of the feet helps to prevent loss of balance during the transfer.

10. Encircle the client's waist with your arms and grasp the transfer belt at the client's back. Your thumbs should point down as you grasp the belt.

    Rationale The belt provides a secure handle for holding onto the client and controlling the movement. The downward placement of the thumbs prevents potential wrist injury as the nurse lifts (Leinweber 1978). By encircling the client in this manner, the nurse keeps the client from tilting backward during the transfer.

11. Tighten your gluteal, abdominal, leg, and arm muscles.

    Rationale Isometric contraction of stabilizing muscles helps to prevent musculoskeletal strain and injury.

12. To assist the client to stand: (a) Have the client push with the back foot, rock to the forward foot, extend the joints of the lower extremities, and push or pull up with the hands while (b) the nurse pushes with the forward foot, rocks to the back foot, extends the joints of the lower extremities, and pulls the client into a standing position.

    Rationale The broad stance promotes stability for both nurse and client. Client assistance provides additional power for movement and reduces the potential for strain and injury to the nurse's back. Pulling the client directly toward the nurse's center of gravity prevents spinal twisting.

13. Support the client in an upright standing position for a few moments. Then, both client and nurse pivot or take a few steps together toward the wheelchair. Ask the client to back up to the wheelchair, placing his or her legs against the seat.

    Rationale Standing upright for a few moments extends the joints and provides an opportunity to ensure that the client is all right before moving away from the bed. Having the client place his or her legs against the wheelchair seat minimizes the risk of the client's falling when sitting down.

14. Ask the client to place the foot of the stronger leg slightly behind the other; to keep the other foot, with the weight upon it, forward; and to place both hands on the wheelchair arms or on the nurse's shoulders.

    Rationale See rationale for steps 7 and 8.

15. Stand directly in front of the client. Place one foot forward and one back to mirror the placement of the client's feet, as before. Tighten your grasp on the transfer belt.

    Rationale See rationale for steps 9 and 10.

16. Tighten your gluteal, abdominal, leg, and arm muscles.

    Rationale See rationale for step 11.

17. To assist the client to sit: (a) Have the client shift his or her body weight by rocking to the back foot, lower the body onto the edge of the wheelchair seat by flexing the joints of the legs and arms, and place some body weight on the arms while (b) the nurse shifts her or his body weight by rocking to the forward foot and flexes the hips and knees to lower and guide the client onto the wheelchair seat.

    Rationale See rationale for step 12.

18. Ask the client to push himself or herself back into the wheelchair seat.

    Rationale Sitting well back on the seat provides a broader base of support and greater stability and minimizes the risk of falling from the wheelchair. A wheelchair can topple forward when the client sits on the edge of the seat and leans far forward.

Variation: Transferring Without a Belt

The nurse places his or her hands against the side of the client's upper chest (not at the axilla) during the transfer. See Figure 39–28. The other steps are the same as described previously.

Variation: Transferring with a Belt and Two Nurses

When the client is able to stand, the nurses position themselves on both sides of the client, facing the same direction as the client. The nurses flex their hips, knees, and ankles; grasp the client's transfer belt with the hand closest to the client; and with the other hand support the client's elbows. Coordinating their efforts, all three stand simultaneously, pivot, and move to the wheelchair where the process is reversed to lower the client onto the wheelchair seat.

Variation: Transferring a Client with an Injured Lower Extremity

When the client has an injured lower extremity, movement should always occur toward the client's unaffected

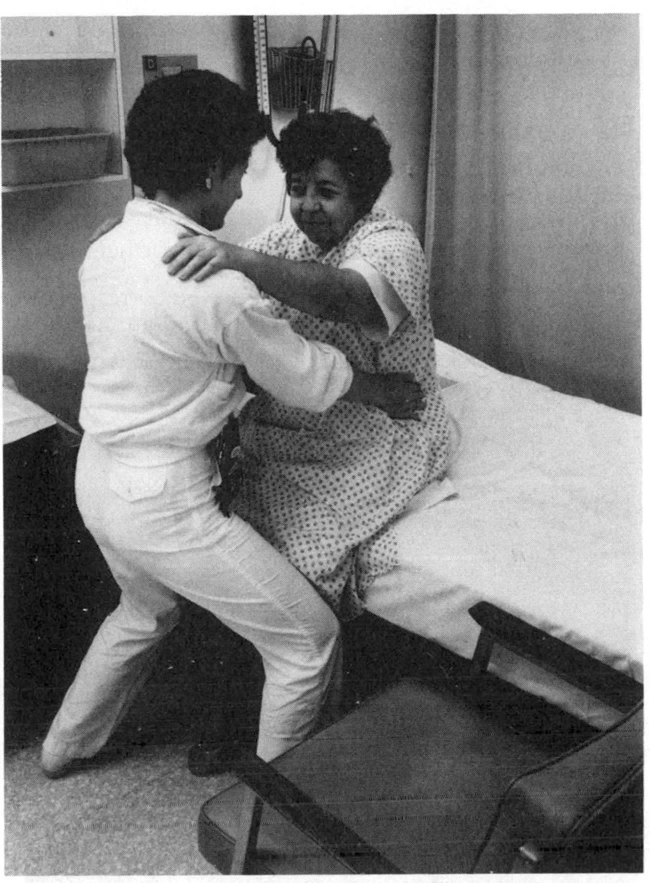

Figure 39–28

(strong) side. For example, if the client's right leg is injured and he or she is sitting on the edge of the bed preparing to transfer to a wheelchair, the nurse positions the wheelchair on the client's left side so that the client can use the left leg most effectively and safely.

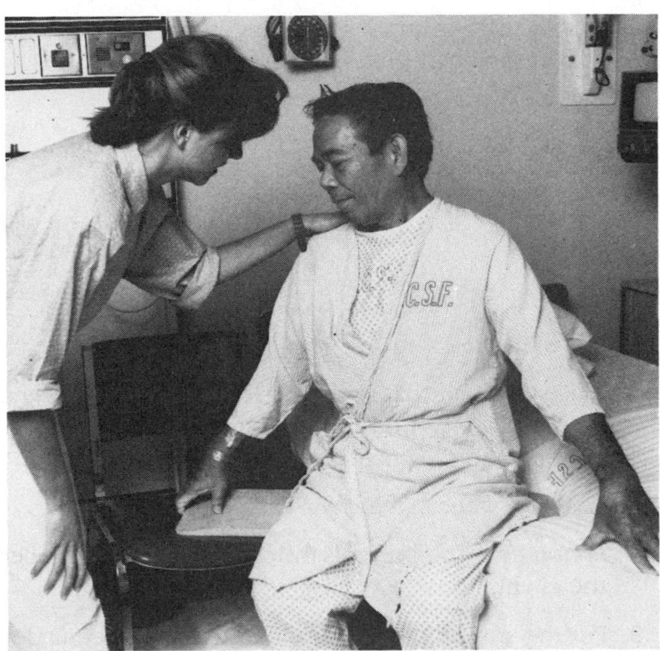

Figure 39–29

Variation: Using a sliding board

Clients who cannot stand can use a sliding board to move without nursing assistance. This method not only promotes the client's sense of independence but preserves the nurse's energy. See Figure 39–29.

Wheelchair Safety Guidelines

Wheelchairs, like stretchers, are unstable and can predispose the client to falls and injury. Always lock the brakes on both wheels of the wheelchair when the client transfers in or out of it. Use seat belts that fasten behind the wheelchair to protect confused clients from falls. Back the wheelchair into or out of an elevator, rear large wheels first. When on an incline, place your body between the wheelchair and the bottom of the incline.

Procedure 39–7 ▲ Transferring a Client to a Chair Using a Mechanical Lifter

Mechanical lifters are used primarily for clients who cannot help themselves or who are too heavy for others to lift safely. Transfers may be made between the bed and a wheelchair, the bed and the bathtub, and the bed and a stretcher. Various types of mechanical lifters are used to lift and move clients. It is important that nurses be familiar with the model used and the practices that accompany use. Before using the lifter, the nurse ensures that it is in working order and that the hooks, chains, straps, and canvas seat are in good repair. Most agencies recommend that two nurses operate a lifter. Agency policy should be checked in this regard.

Before lifting the client, the nurse explains the procedure and demonstrates the lifter. Some clients are afraid of being lifted and will be reassured by a demonstration.

The lifter may have a one-piece or two-piece canvas seat. The one-piece seat stretches from the client's head to the knees. The two-piece seat has one canvas strap to support the client's buttocks and thighs and a second strap to support the back, extending up to the axillae.

Equipment

1. A mechanical lifter
2. A chair

Intervention

1. Place the chair that is to receive the client beside the bed. Allow room for the lifter and the client to clear the bed and the chair.
2. Lock the wheels, if a chair with wheels is used.

   Rationale This prevents the chair from moving under the client.

3. Put the canvas seat or straps exactly in place under the client. See Figure 39–30.

   Rationale Correct placement permits the client to be lifted evenly with minimal shifting.

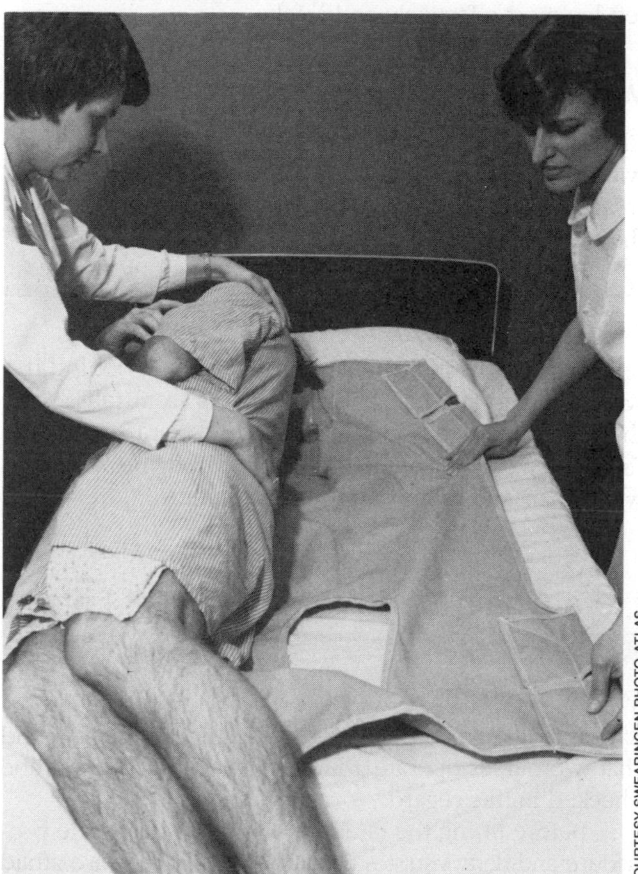

Figure 39–30

4. Wheel the lifter into position at a right angle to the side of the bed, with the footbars under the bed. Lock the wheels of the lifter and the bed.
5. Ask the client to remove his or her glasses, and put them in a safe place.

   Rationale The client should not wear glasses because the swivel bar may come close to his or her face.

6. Attach the lifter straps or hooks to the corresponding openings in the canvas seat. See Figure 39–31. Check that the hooks are correctly placed and that matching straps or chains are of equal length.

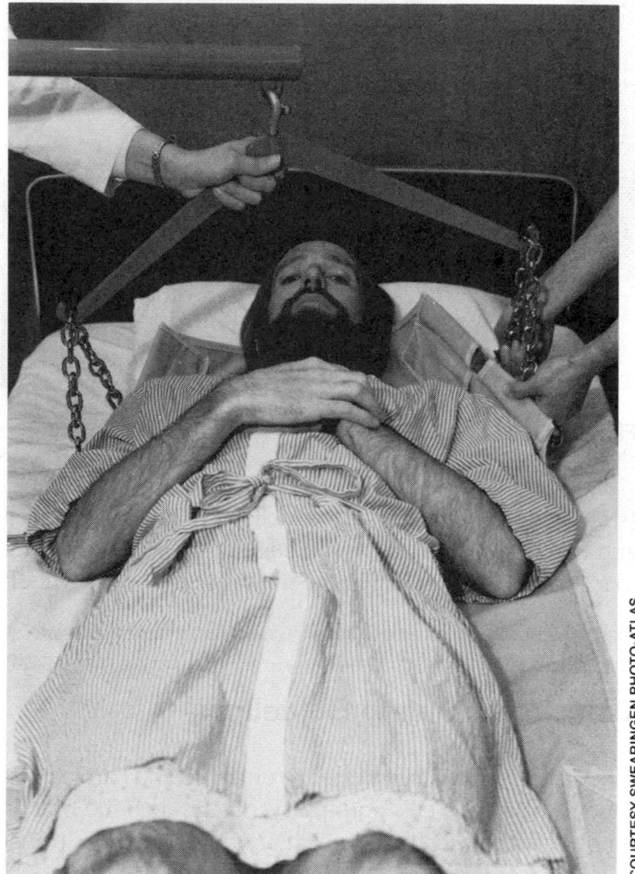

Figure 39–31

7. a. Nurse 1: Close the pressure valve, and gradually pump up the lift until the client is above the bed surface.

   Rationale Gradual elevation of the lift is less frightening to the client than a rapid rise.

   b. Nurse 2: Assume a broad stance and tighten your abdominal and pelvic muscles. Guide the client with your hands as he or she is lifted.

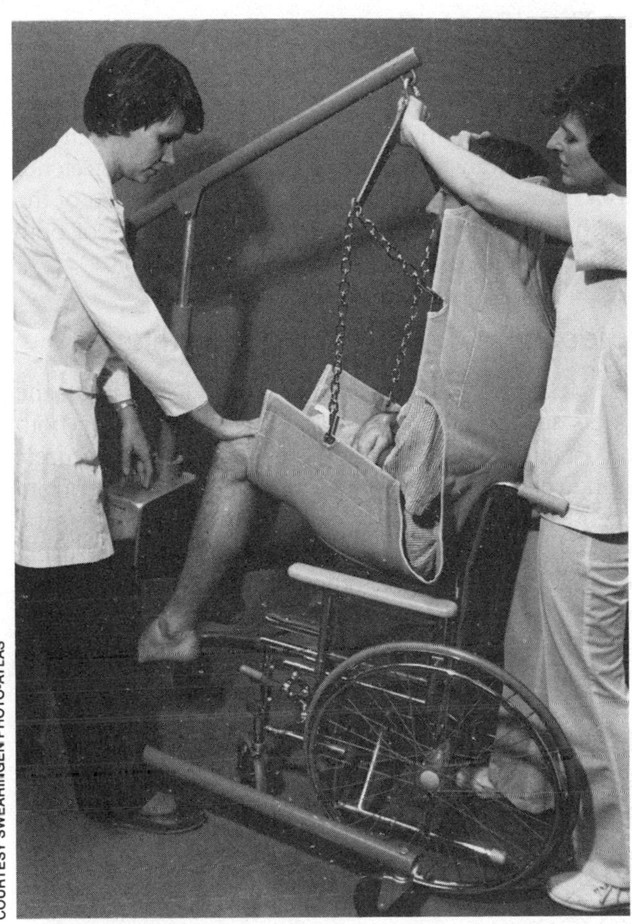
COURTESY SWEARINGEN PHOTO-ATLAS

Rationale The nurse prepares to hold the client and provide control during the movement.

8. a. Nurse 1: With the pressure valve securely closed, slowly roll the lifter until the client is over the chair.

   b. Nurse 2: Guide the client by hand until he or she is directly over the chair. See Figure 39–32.

   Rationale Slow movement decreases swaying and is less frightening. Guidance also decreases swaying and gives a sense of security.

9. a. Nurse 1: Release the pressure valve very gradually.

   b. Nurse 2: Guide the client into the chair.

   Rationale Gradual release lowers the client slowly and is less frightening than a quick descent.

10. Remove the hooks from the canvas seat. Leave the seat in place.

    Rationale The seat is left in place in preparation for the lift back to bed.

11. Align the client appropriately in a sitting position. See section on the adult sitting position in Chapter 38. Give the client his or her glasses if appropriate.

Figure 39–32

Transferring Clients Between a Bed and a Stretcher

The stretcher, or guerney, is used to transfer supine clients from one location to another. Whenever the client is capable of accomplishing the transfer from bed to stretcher independently, either by lifting onto it or by rolling onto it, the client should be encouraged to do so. If the client cannot move onto the stretcher independently, at least two nurses are needed to assist with the transfer; more are needed if the client is totally helpless or heavy. In preparation for the transfer, the nurses lower the head of the bed until it is flat or as low as the client can tolerate. The bed is raised so that it is slightly *higher* than the surface of the stretcher, and the wheels on the bed are locked. The drawsheet is pulled out from both sides of the bed and rolled as close to the client's sides as possible. The client is then pulled to the edge of the bed where the stretcher will be positioned. A sheet or bath blanket is used to cover the client. The stretcher is placed parallel to the bed, next to the client. The stretcher wheels are locked. The gap between the bed and the stretcher can be filled loosely with bath blankets or pillows.

Considerable care must be taken to prevent the client from falling between the bed and the stretcher during the transfer. The nurses press their bodies tightly against the stretcher to prevent its movement, flex their hips, and pull the client on the pull sheet directly toward themselves and onto the stretcher. The client flexes his or her neck during the move, if possible, and places the arms across the chest to prevent injury to these body parts.

Because the nurses must keep their bodies tightly pressed against the stretcher to prevent its movement during the transfer, the usual pulling technique is not possible. As a result, more of the pulling force is transferred to the nurses' arms and back. Nurses can help to protect themselves, however, by keeping their backs straight, not lifting the client during the transfer, and securing a sufficient number of persons to assist with the transfer. Better control over client movement is achieved when the pull sheet is tightly rolled against the client. Also, pulling downward is easier and requires less force than pulling along a flat surface.

After making the client comfortable, the stretcher wheels are unlocked and the stretcher is moved away from the bed. The nurse immediately raises the stretcher side rails and/or fastens the safety straps across the client. Because the stretcher is high and narrow, the client is in danger of falling unless these safety precautions are taken.

Using Three or More Assistants to Transfer the Client

If three or more assistants are needed to transfer the client onto the stretcher, the additional assistants should stabilize the stretcher tightly against the bed so that it does not roll during the transfer or assist in pulling the client onto the stretcher with the pull sheet. No one should attempt to assist from the opposite side of the bed, as this inevitably puts strain on that person's back as she or he attempts to lift the client onto the stretcher.

Using a Roller Bar During the Transfer

A roller bar is a metal frame covered with longitudinal rollers. The bar is placed over the gap between the bed and the stretcher. The client is pulled on a pull sheet onto the roller bars and rolled easily onto the stretcher.

The Three-Person Carry

Lifting and carrying the client from bed to stretcher should be avoided except in emergencies, because of the potential for strain and injury to the nurses' backs. When it is necessary to transfer a client in this manner, the stretcher is placed at right angles to the bed, with the head of the stretcher near the foot of the bed. The wheels of both stretcher and bed are locked. See Figure 39–33.

Guidelines for Safe Use of Stretchers

Never leave a client unattended on a stretcher unless the wheels are locked and the side rails are raised on both sides of the stretcher and/or the safety straps are securely fastened across the client. Always push the stretcher from the end above the client's head. This position protects the client's head in the event of a collision. Most stretchers have four swivel wheels; others have two swivel wheels and two stationary wheels. When this latter type of stretcher is used, always position the client's head at the end with the stationary wheels. The stretcher is more easily maneuvered when pushed from the end with the stationary wheels.

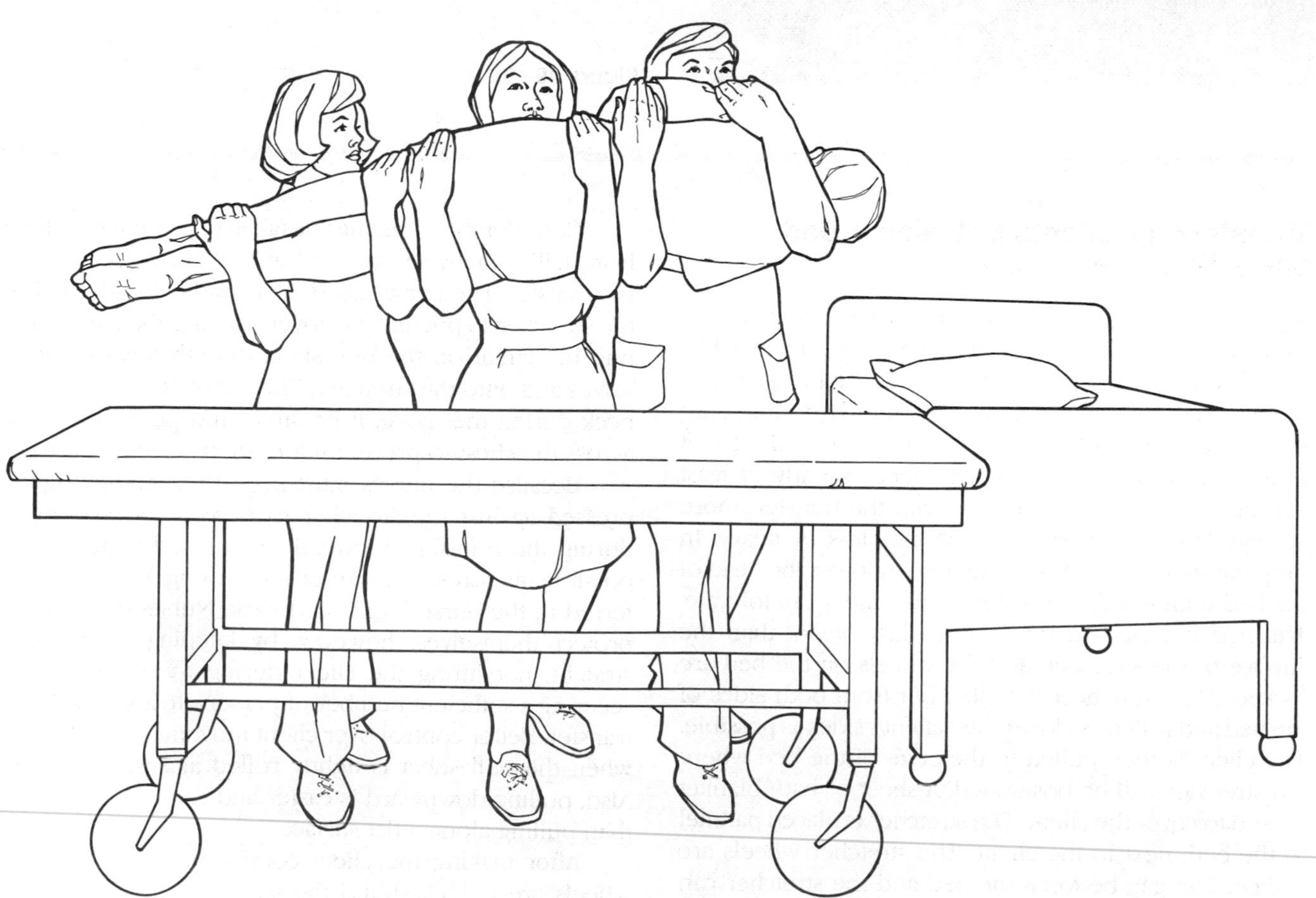

Figure 39–33 The three-person carry should be used only in emergencies.

Assisting Clients to Ambulate

Most people who are ill require only a brief period of rest before they begin to walk and gradually increase their activity. The more physically fit the person is before becoming ill or immobilized, the sooner the person's return to health.

Even 1 or 2 days of bedrest can make a person feel weak, unsteady, and shaky when first getting out of bed. A client who has had surgery, is elderly, or has been immobilized for a longer time will feel more pronounced weakness. The potential problems of immobility are far less likely to occur when clients become ambulatory as soon as possible. The nurse can assist clients to prepare for ambulation by helping them become as independent as possible while in bed. Nurses should encourage clients to perform activities of daily living, maintain good body alignment, perform orthostatic tension stimulating exercises, and carry out active range-of-motion exercises to the maximum degree possible yet within the limitations imposed by their illness and recovery program. See Chapters 37 and 38 for information about these interventions.

Preambulatory Exercises

Clients who have been in bed for long periods often need a plan of muscle tone exercises to strengthen the muscles used for walking before attempting to walk. One of the most important muscle groups is the quadriceps femoris, which extends the knee and flexes the thigh. This group is also important for elevating the legs, e.g., for walking upstairs. To strengthen these muscles, the client consciously tenses them, drawing the kneecap upward and inward. The client pushes the popliteal space behind the knee against the bed surface, raising the heels off the bed surface. See Figure 39–34. On the count of 1, the muscles are tensed; they are held during the counts of 2, 3, 4; and they are relaxed at the count of 5. The exercise should be done within the client's tolerance, i.e., without fatiguing the muscles. Carried out several times an hour during waking hours, this simple exercise significantly strengthens the muscles used for walking.

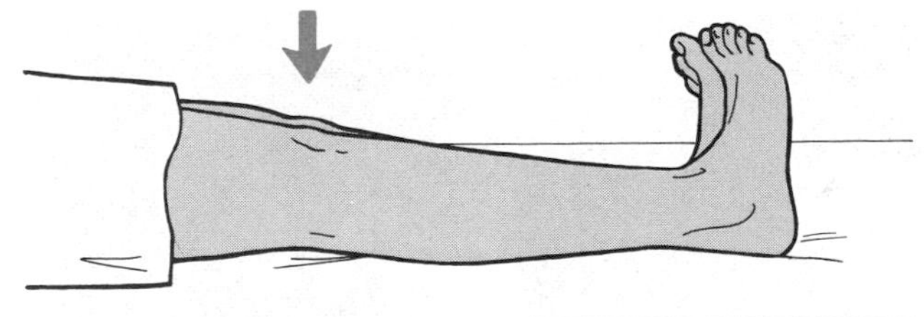

Figure 39–34 Tensing the quadriceps femoris before ambulation

Ambulation Guidelines

1. Use ambulating techniques that facilitate a normal walking gait yet provide the support needed.
2. Carefully assess the client for signs and symptoms of orthostatic hypotension (dizziness, lightheadedness, or a sudden increase in heart rate) prior to leaving the bedside and periodically during the ambulatory experience.
3. If it is the client's first time out of bed following surgery, injury, or an extended period of immobility or if the client is quite weak or unstable, have an assistant follow the nurse and client with a wheelchair in the event that it is needed quickly.
4. Have the client wear comfortable shoes with nonskid soles when walking.
5. Continually encourage the client to stand up straight and look straight ahead when walking to prevent instability.
6. Remain physically close to the client in case assistance is needed.
7. Assess the amount of support the client requires from the nurse. Too much physical support can inhibit client independence and prevent the client from gaining strength. Too little physical support can predispose the client to an injurious fall.
   a. If the client can ambulate independently, encourage the client to do so but walk beside him or her.
   b. If the client is slightly weak and unstable, use a transfer or walking belt. Make sure the belt is pulled snugly around the client's waist and fastened securely. Grasp the belt at the client's back and walk behind and slightly to one side of the client. See Figure 39–35.
   c. If the client is moderately weak and unstable, interlock your forearm with the client's closest forearm and walk on the client's weaker side. Encourage the client to press his or her forearm against your hip or waist for stability if desired. In addition, have the client wear a transfer or walking belt so that you can quickly grab the belt and prevent a fall if he or she feels faint.
   d. If the client is very weak and unstable, place your near arm around the client's waist and with your other arm support the client's near arm at the elbow. Walk on the client's stronger side. Again, have the client wear a transfer or walking belt in case of an emergency.

Two nurses can assist with any of these ambulation techniques, one on each side of the client.

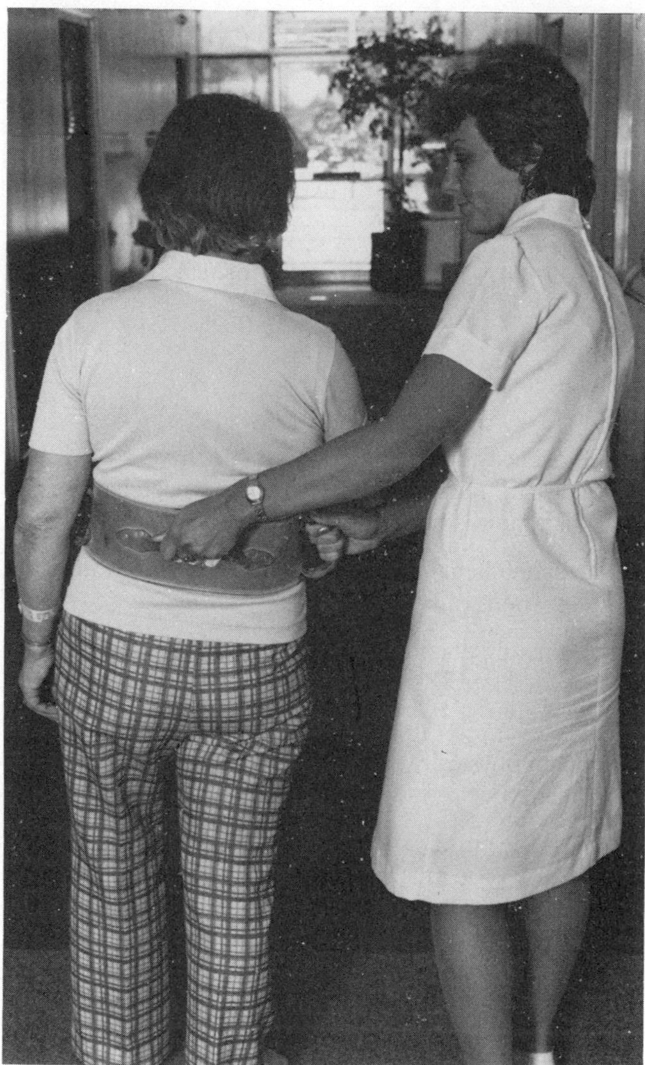

Figure 39–35 A walking belt

Protecting a Client Who Begins to Fall While Ambulating

If a client begins to experience the signs and symptoms of orthostatic hypotension or extreme weakness, he or she should be quickly assisted into the nearby wheelchair or other chair and helped to lower his or her head between the knees. The nurse must stay with the client. If the client faints while in this position, he or she could fall, head first, out of the chair. When the client feels better, he or she can be wheeled back to bed.

If a wheelchair or chair is not close by, the client should be assisted to a horizontal position on the floor before fainting occurs, since a vertical position may increase feelings of faintness. Clients who do faint or start to fall and cannot regain their strength or balance usually drop straight downward or pitch slightly forward due to the momentum of ambulating; thus, their head, hips, and knees are most vulnerable to injury. In this situation a nurse assumes a broad stance with one foot in front of the other and brings the client backward so that he or she is supported by the nurse's body. The nurse then allows the client to slide down the nurse's leg and lowers the client gently to the floor, making sure that the client's head does not hit any objects. See Figure 39–36. The nurse's broad stance widens the base of support for stability. Placing one foot behind the other allows the nurse to rock backward and use the femoral muscles when supporting the client's weight and lowering his or her center of gravity, thus preventing back strain. Bringing the client's weight backward against the nurse's body allows gradual movement to the floor without injury to the client.

If the client who is ambulating with two nurses starts to fall, the two nurses slip their arms under the client's axillae, grasp the client's hands, and lower the client gently to the floor or to a nearby chair.

Mechanical Aids for Walking

Cane Three types of canes are used today: the simple straight-legged cane; the tripod or crab cane, which has three feet; and the quad cane, which has four feet and provides the most support. See Figure 39–37. Cane tips should have rubber caps to improve traction and prevent

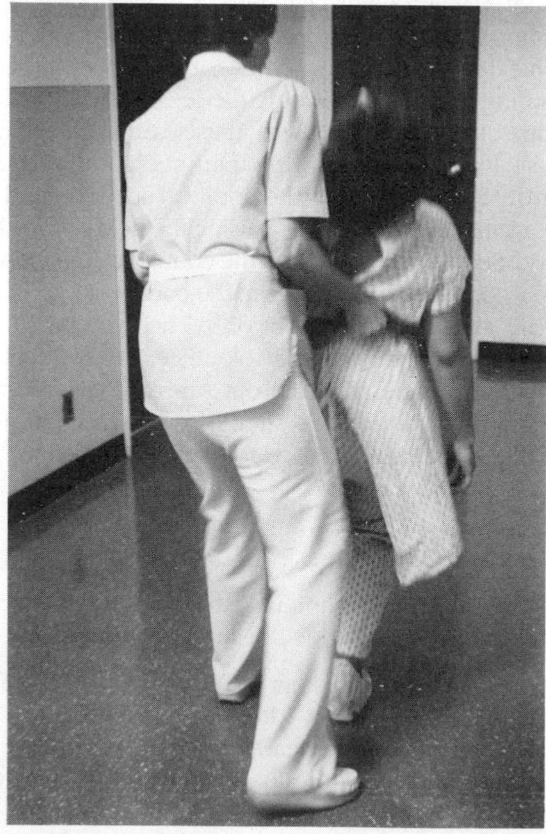

Figure 39–36 A client who has fainted is lowered to the floor.

slipping. The quad cane may have two tips and two wheels, permitting the client to keep it in contact with the ground all the time. The client tilts the cane toward the body, lifting the tips while the wheels remain on the ground, and then pushes the cane forward. The standard cane is 91 cm (36 in) long; some aluminum canes can be adjusted from 56 to 97 cm (22 to 38 inches). Clients may use either one or two canes, depending on how much support they require.

The client should hold a cane with the hand on the stronger side of the body to provide maximum support and appropriate body alignment when walking. The tip of the cane is positioned about 15 cm (6 in) to the side and 15 cm (6 in) in front of the near foot so that the elbow is slightly flexed.

When maximum support is required, the client (a) moves the cane forward about 30 cm (1 ft), or a distance that is comfortable while the body weight is borne by both legs, (b) moves the affected (weak) leg forward to the cane while the weight is borne by the cane and stronger leg, (c) moves the unaffected (stronger) leg forward ahead of the cane and weak leg while the weight is borne by the cane and weak leg, and (d) repeats steps (a)–(c). This pattern of moving provides at least two points of support on the floor at all times.

As the client becomes stronger and less support is required, the client can (a) move the cane and weak leg forward at the same time, while the weight is borne by the stronger leg, and (b) move the stronger leg forward, while the weight is borne by the cane and the weak leg.

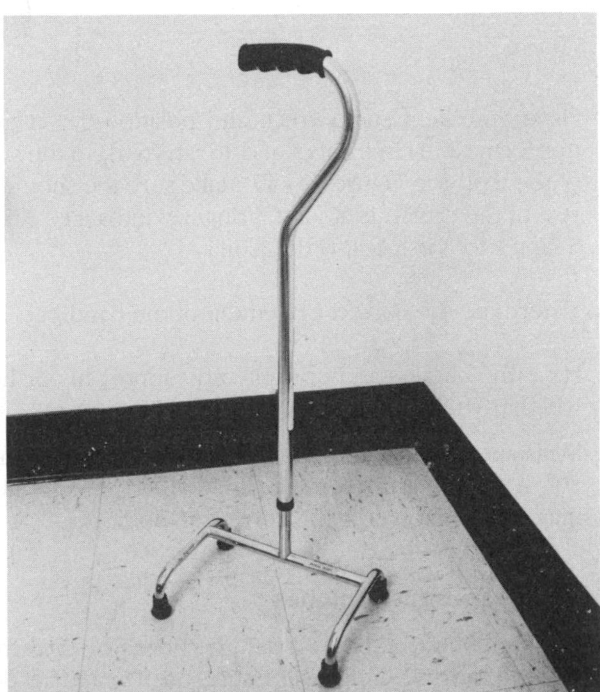

Figure 39–37 A quad cane

Walker Walkers are mechanical devices for ambulatory clients who need more support than a cane provides. There are many types of walkers of different shapes and sizes, with devices suited to individual needs. The standard type is made of polished aluminum. It has four legs with rubber tips and plastic hand grips. See Figure 39–38. Many walkers have adjustable legs.

The standard walker needs to be picked up to be used. The client therefore requires partial strength in both hands and wrists, strong elbow extensors, such as the triceps brachii, and strong shoulder depressors, such as the pectoralis minor. The client also needs the ability to bear at least partial weight on both legs. Four-wheeled models of walkers (roller walkers) do not need to be picked up to be moved, but they are less stable than the standard walker. They are used by clients who are too weak or unstable to pick up and move the walker with each step. Some roller walkers have a seat at the back so the client can sit down to rest when desired. The nurse may need to adjust the height of a client's walker so that the hand bar is just below the client's waist and the client's elbows are slightly flexed. This position helps the client assume a more normal stance. A walker that is too low causes the client to stoop; one that is too high makes the client stretch and reach.

When maximum support is required, the client:

1. Moves the walker ahead about 15 cm (6 in) while body weight is borne by both legs

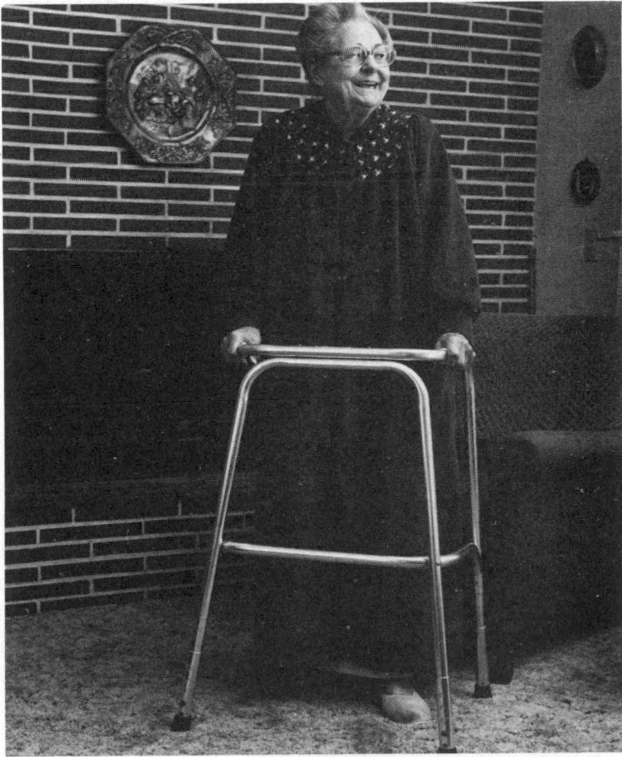

Figure 39–38 A standard walker

2. Moves the right foot up to the walker while body weight is borne by the left leg and both arms
3. Moves the left foot up to the right foot while body weight is borne by the right leg and both arms

If the client has one weaker leg, the client:

1. Moves the walker and the weak leg ahead together about 15 cm (6 in) while the weight is borne by the stronger leg
2. Moves the stronger leg ahead while the weight is borne by the affected leg and both arms

Crutches Crutches may be a temporary need for some people and a permanent one for others. Crutches should enable a person to ambulate independently; therefore, it is important to learn to use them properly.

There are several kinds of crutches. The most frequently used are the **underarm** or **axillary crutch** with hand bars and the **Lofstrand crutch**, which extends only to the forearm. The underarm crutch can be extended. It has double uprights, an underarm bar, and a hand bar. See Figure 39–39, *A*. The Lofstrand crutch is a single adjustable tube of aluminum to which are attached a curved piece of steel, a rubber-covered hand bar, and a metal forearm cuff. See Figure 39–39, *B*. This type of crutch is most useful as a substitute for a cane. The metal cuff around the forearm and the metal bar stabilize the wrists and thus make walking safer and easier. The person can release the hand bar to use his or her hand, and the metal cuff will hold the crutch in place, while a cane would fall.

The **Canadian** or **elbow extensor crutch** is like the Lofstrand in that it is made of a single tube of aluminum with lateral attachments, a hand bar, and a cuff for the forearm, but it also has a cuff for the upper arm. See Figure 39–39, *C*. This crutch is usually used by clients who require support for weak extensor muscles of the forearm and trunk (e.g., weak triceps brachii).

All crutches require suction tips, which are usually made of rubber. The tips help prevent the crutches from slipping on a floor surface.

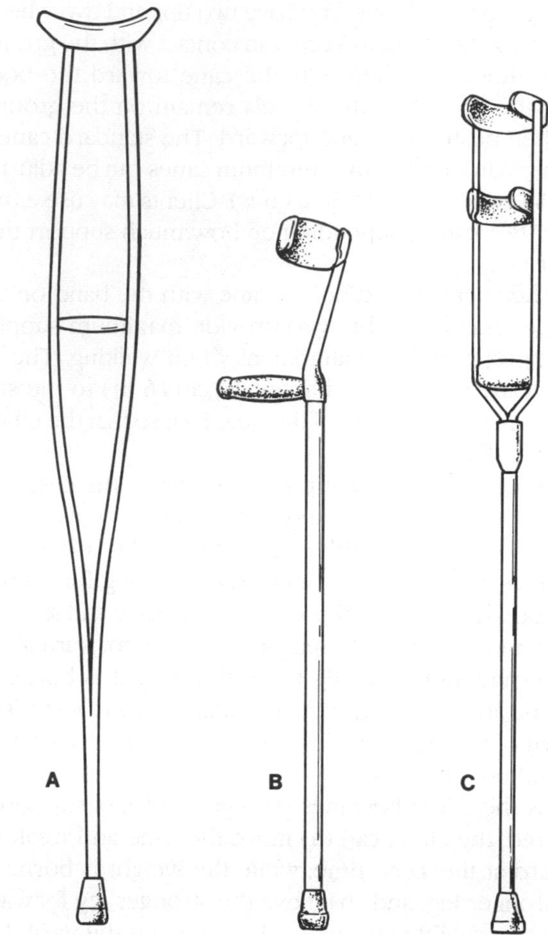

Figure 39–39 Three types of crutches: **A,** axillary crutch; **B,** Lofstrand crutch; **C,** Canadian or elbow extensor crutch

Measuring Clients for Crutches

When nurses measure clients for axillary crutches, it is most important to obtain the correct length for the crutches and the correct placement of the hand piece. If the crutches are too long, the shoulders are forced upward, and the client cannot push his or her body off the ground. If the crutches are too short, the client hunches over uncomfortably and has poor body alignment. There are two methods of measuring crutch length:

1. Have the client lie supine, and measure from the anterior fold of the axilla to a point 10 cm (4 in) lateral from the heel of the foot.
2. Have the client stand erect, and position the crutch tips 5 cm (2 in) in front of and 15 cm (6 in) to the side of the feet. See Figure 39–40. Make sure the shoulder rest of the crutch is at least 3 finger widths, i.e., 2.5 to 5 cm (1 to 2 in), below the axilla.

To determine the correct placement of the hand bar:

1. Have the client stand upright and support his or her weight by the hand grips of the crutches.
2. Measure the angle of elbow flexion. It should be about 30°. A goniometer (see Figure 35–121 on page 881) may be used to verify the correct angle.

Guidelines About Crutches

1. The weight of the body should be borne by the arms rather than the axillae. Pressure on the axillae can injure the radial nerve and eventually cause crutch palsy, a **paresis** (weakness of the muscles) of the forearm, wrist, and hand.

2. The client should maintain erect posture to prevent strain on muscles and joints and to maintain balance.
3. The shoulder rests of axillary crutches can be slightly padded for comfort, but the padding must not press against the axillae.
4. Each step taken with crutches should be a comfortable distance for the client. It is wise to start with a small rather than a large step.
5. Crutches should have rubber (suction) tips to prevent slipping.
6. Crutch tips should be inspected regularly and replaced if worn.
7. Crutch tips should be kept dry to maintain their surface friction. If they become wet, the client should dry them well before use.

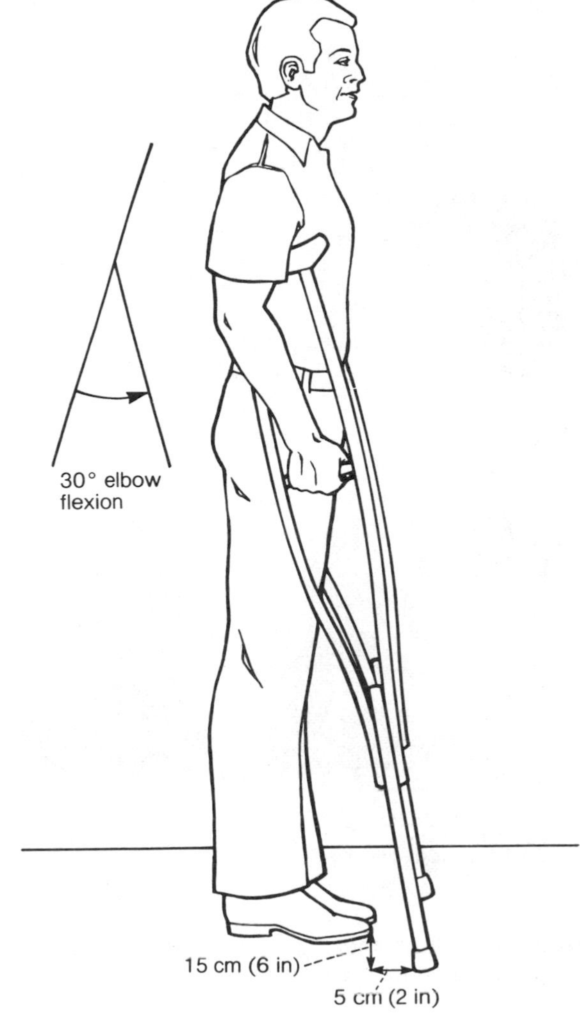

Figure 39–40 The standing position to measure the correct length of crutches

Exercises for Crutch Walking

In crutch walking, the client's weight is borne by the muscles of the shoulder girdle and the upper extremities. Five major muscle groups are used:

1. The flexor muscles of the arms (e.g., the pectoralis major and brachialis) move the crutches forward.
2. The extensor muscles of the forearms (e.g., the triceps brachii) hold the elbows up at an angle while the body weight is raised off the ground.
3. The finger and thumb flexors (e.g., the flexor pollicis brevis) allow the hands to grasp the hand bars.
4. The muscles that dorsiflex the wrists (e.g., the flexor carpi radialis) maintain the hands in the correct position on the hand bars.
5. The shoulder girdle depressors and the downward rotators (e.g., the pectoralis minor) support the body weight off the floor.

Before beginning crutch walking, the client should exercise to develop and strengthen these muscle groups. A plan of exercises should be developed for each client. The following exercises are recommended:

1. The client flexes and extends the arms in several directions.
2. The client comes from a supine position to a sitting position by flexing the elbows and pushing the hands against the bed surface. This exercise strengthens the flexor and extensor muscles of the arms and the muscles that dorsiflex the wrist.
3. The client pushes his or her body off the bed surface by pushing down with the hands and extending the elbows. See Figure 39–41. This exercise is particularly useful in strengthening the extensor muscles of the arms.
4. The client squeezes a rubber ball or a gripper with the hands. This exercise strengthens the flexor muscles of the fingers.

Crutch Gaits

The crutch gait is the gait a person assumes on crutches by alternating his or her weight on one or both legs and the crutches. Five standard crutch gaits are the four-point gait, three-point gait, two-point gait, swing-to gait, and swing-through gait. The gait used depends on the following individual factors:

1. Ability to take steps
2. Ability to bear weight and keep balance in a standing position on both legs or only one

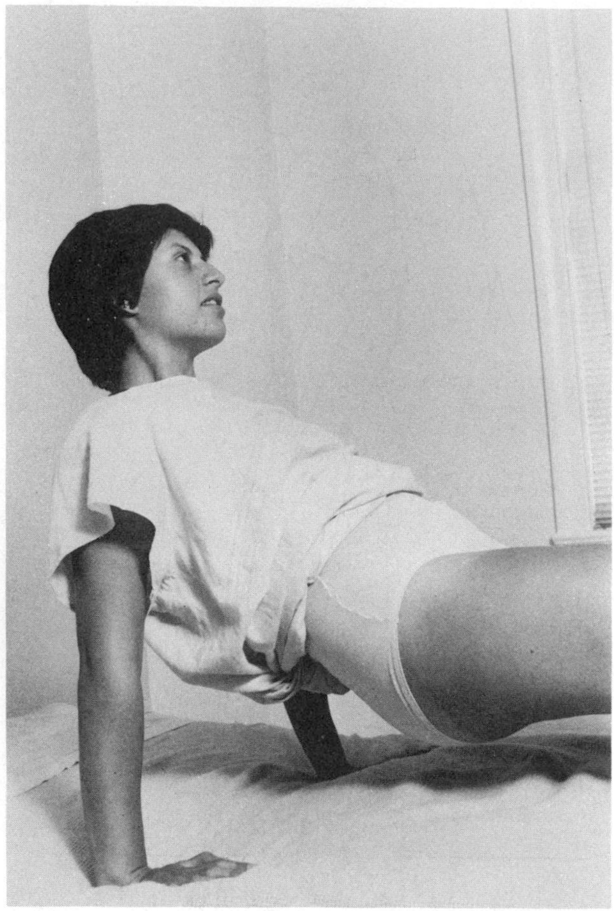

Figure 39–41 Strengthening the extensor muscles of the arms in preparation for crutch walking

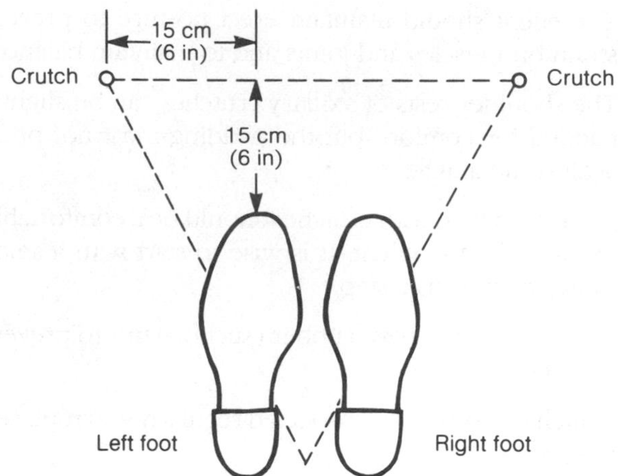

Figure 39–42 The tripod position

3. Ability to bear weight and keep balance with the upper body, e.g., to push off from a chair or bed by using the crutches
4. Ability to hold the body erect

A physiotherapist or a physician usually decides which crutch gait is best for a particular client. Nurses are increasingly involved in these decisions, however. Often, a physiotherapist teaches the crutch gait initially, but nurses give follow-through lessons. In some instances, nurses alone teach the client the technique.

Clients also need instruction about how to get into and out of chairs and go up and down stairs safely. All of these crutch skills are best taught before the client is discharged and preferably before the client has surgery.

Crutch stance (tripod position) Before a client attempts crutch walking, he or she needs to learn facts about posture and balance. The proper standing position with crutches is called the **tripod (triangle) position.** See Figure 39–42. The crutches are placed about 15 cm (6 in) in front of the feet and out laterally about 15 cm (6 in), creating a wide base of support. The feet are slightly apart. A tall person requires a wider base than a short person. Hips and knees are extended, the back is straight, and the head is held straight and high. There should be no hunch to the shoulders and thus no weight borne by the axillae. The palms are positioned lateral to the feet, and the elbows are extended sufficiently to allow weight bearing on the hands. If the client is unsteady, place a walking belt around his or her waist; grasp it from above, not from below. A fall can be prevented more effectively if the belt is held from above.

Sometimes clients are discouraged when they attempt crutch walking. Clients confined to bed are often unaware of weakness that becomes apparent when they try to stand or walk. Clients realize that they can no longer take balance for granted when they must cope with the weight of a heavy cast or a paralyzed limb. Frequently, progress may be slower than the client anticipated. Thus encouragement from the nurse and the setting of realistic goals are especially important.

Four-point alternate gait This is the most elementary and safest gait, providing at least three points of support at each time, but it requires coordination. Clients can use it when walking in crowds because it does not require much space. To use this gait, the client needs to be able to bear weight on both legs. See Figure 39–43 (reading from bottom to top). The client:

1. Moves the right crutch ahead a suitable distance, e.g., 10 to 15 cm (4 to 6 in).
2. Moves the left front foot forward, preferably to the level of the left crutch.
3. Moves the left crutch forward.
4. Moves the right foot forward.

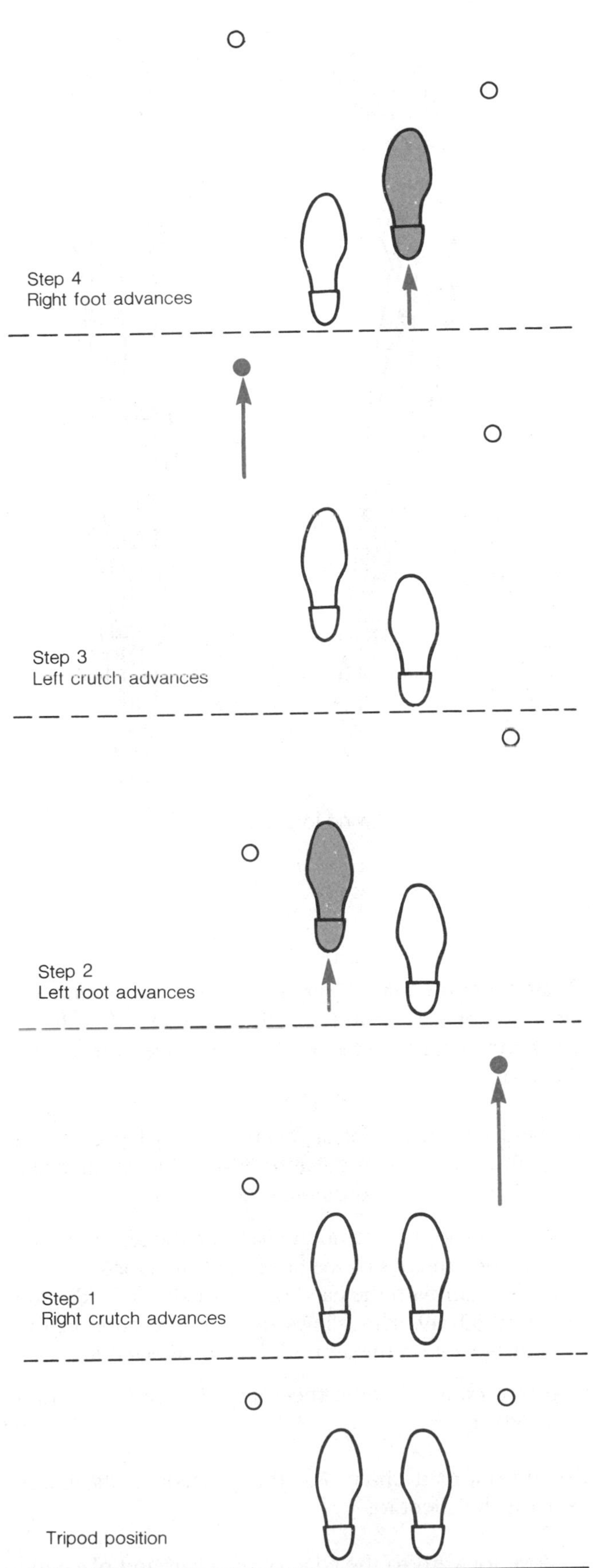

Figure 39–43 The four-point alternate gait

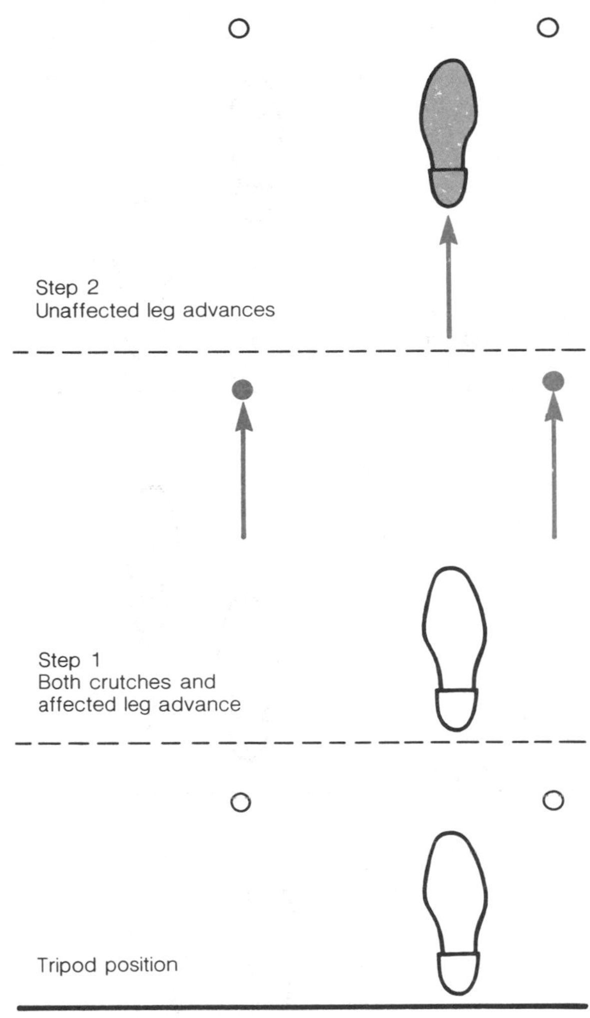

Figure 39–44 The three-point crutch gait

Three-point gait To use this gait, the client must be able to bear her or his entire weight on the unaffected leg. The two crutches and the unaffected leg bear weight alternately. See Figure 39–44 (reading from bottom to top). The client:

1. Moves both crutches and the weaker leg forward.
2. Moves the stronger leg forward.

Two-point alternate gait This gait is faster than the four-point gait. It requires more balance, because only two points support the body at one time; it also requires at least partial weight bearing on each foot. In this gait, arm movements with the crutches are similar to the arm movements during normal walking. See Figure 39–45 (reading from bottom to top). The client:

1. Moves the left crutch and the right foot forward together.
2. Moves the right crutch and the left foot ahead together.

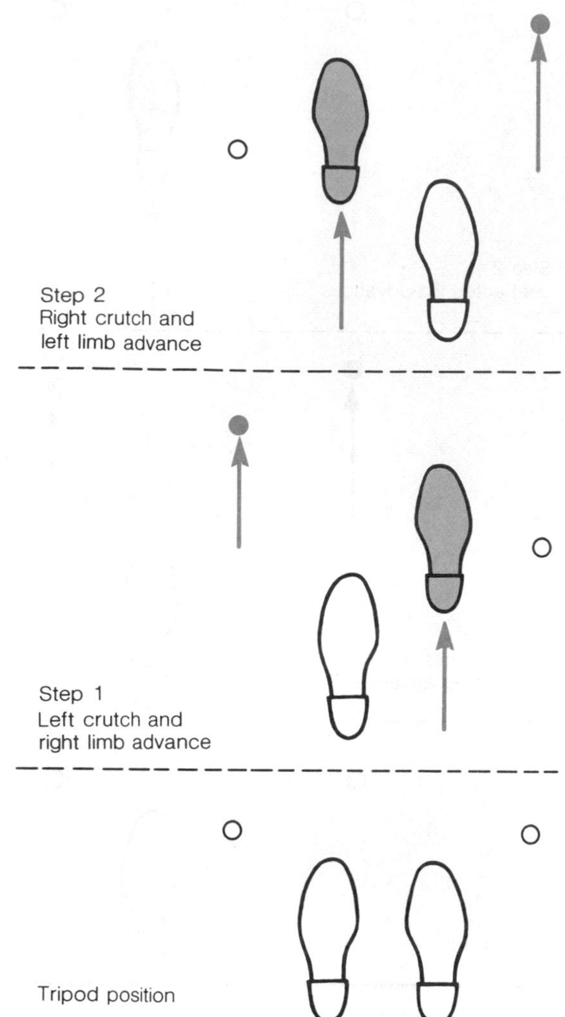

Figure 39–45 The two-point alternate gait

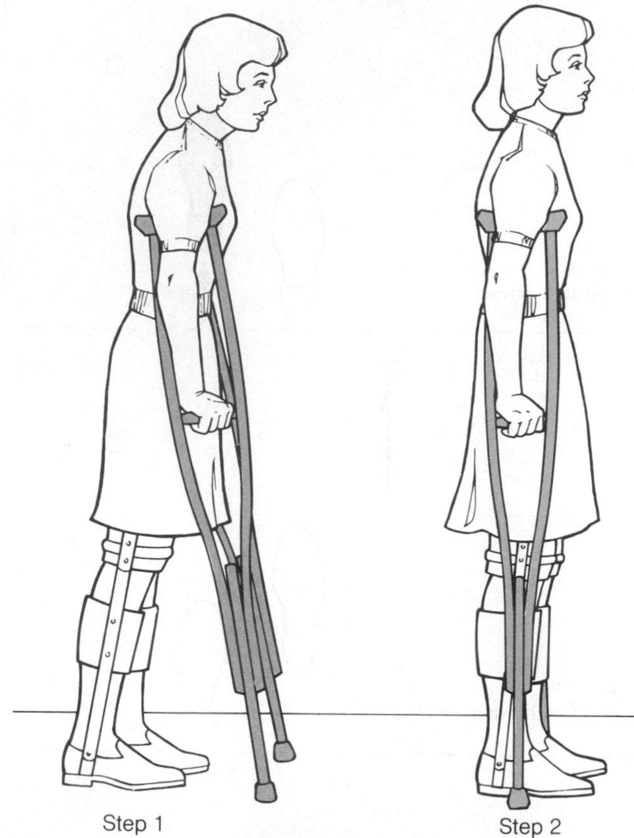

Figure 39–46 The swing-to gait

Swing-to gait The swing gaits are used by clients with paralysis of the legs and hips. Prolonged use of these gaits results in atrophy of the unused muscles. The swing-to gait is the easier of these two gaits. See Figure 39–46. The client:

1. Moves both crutches ahead together.
2. Lifts his or her weight by the arms and swings to the crutches.

Swing-through gait This gait requires considerable skill, strength, and coordination. See Figure 39–47. The client:

1. Moves both crutches forward together.
2. Lifts his or her weight by the arms and swings through and beyond the crutches.

Getting into a chair Chairs that have armrests and are secure or braced against a wall are essential for clients using crutches. For this procedure the nurse instructs the client to:

1. Stand with the back of the unaffected leg centered against the chair. See Figure 39–48. The chair helps support the client during the next steps.
2. Transfer the crutches to the hand on the affected side, hold the crutches by the hand bars and grasp the arm of the chair with the hand on the unaffected side. See Figure 39–49. This allows the client to support the body weight on the arms and the unaffected leg.
3. Lean forward, flex the knees and hips, and lower into the chair.

Getting out of a chair For this procedure, the nurse instructs the client to:

1. Move forward to the edge of the chair and place the unaffected leg slightly under or at the edge of the chair. This position helps the client stand up from the chair

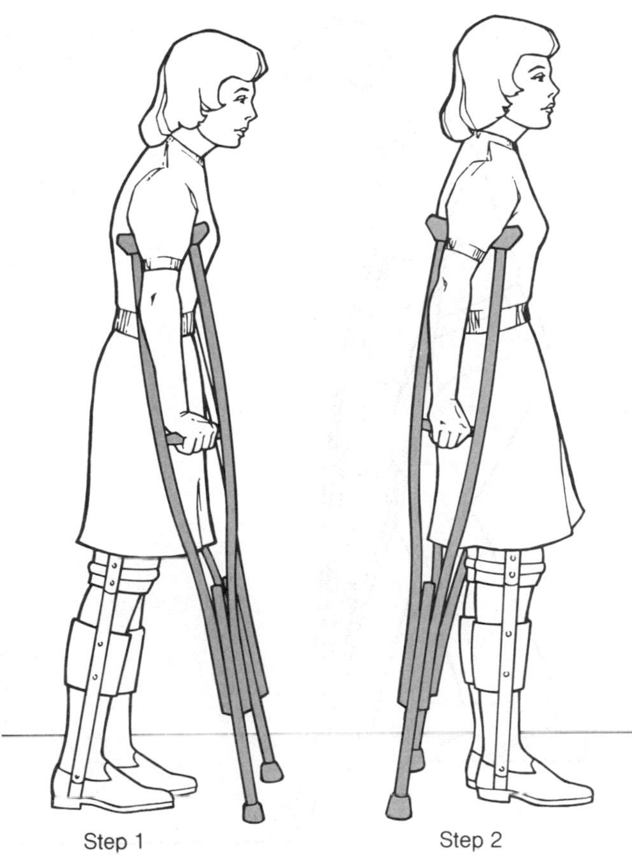

Figure 39–47 The swing-through gait

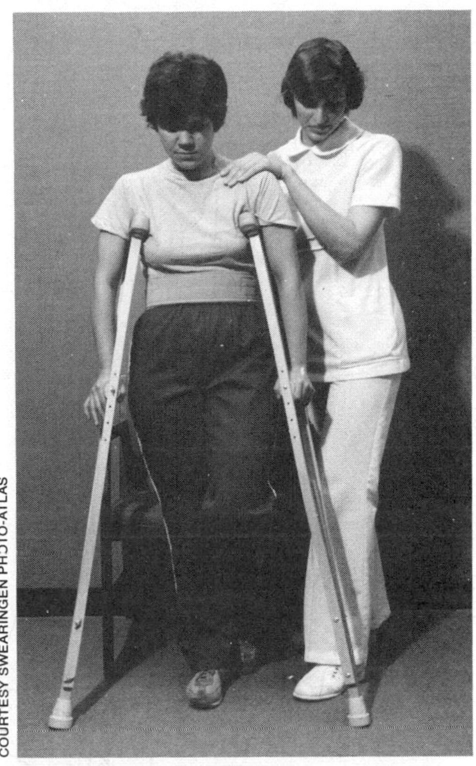

Figure 39–48 The client positions the back of the unaffected leg against the chair before sitting.

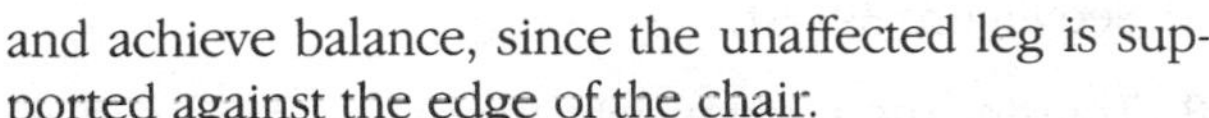

and achieve balance, since the unaffected leg is supported against the edge of the chair.

2. Grasp the crutches by the hand bars in the hand on the affected side, and grasp the arm of the chair by the hand on the unaffected side. The body weight is placed on the crutches and the hand on the armrest to support the unaffected leg when the client rises to stand.
3. Push down on the crutches and the chair armrest while elevating his or her body out of the chair.
4. Assume the tripod position before moving.

Going up stairs For this procedure, the nurse stands behind the client and slightly to the affected side. Instruct the client to:

1. Assume the tripod position at the bottom of the stairs.
2. Transfer the body weight to the crutches and move the unaffected leg onto the step. See Figure 39–50.
3. Transfer the body weight to the unaffected leg on the step and move the crutches and affected leg up to the

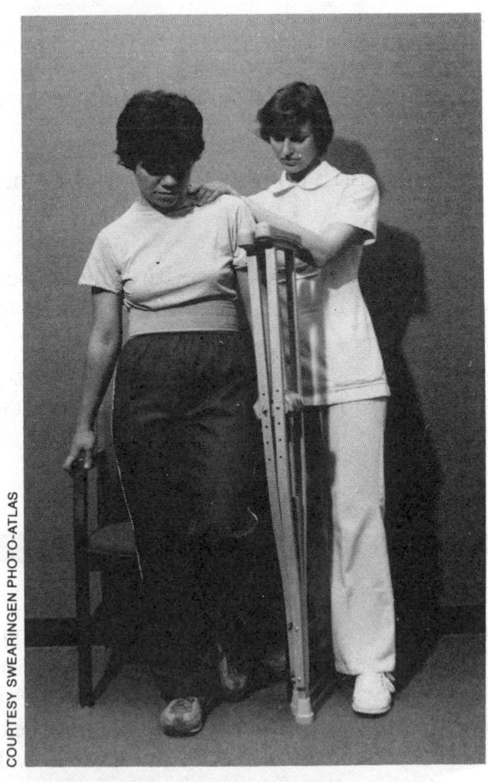

Figure 39–49 After transferring the crutches to one hand, the client supports the body weight on the arms and the unaffected leg before sitting.

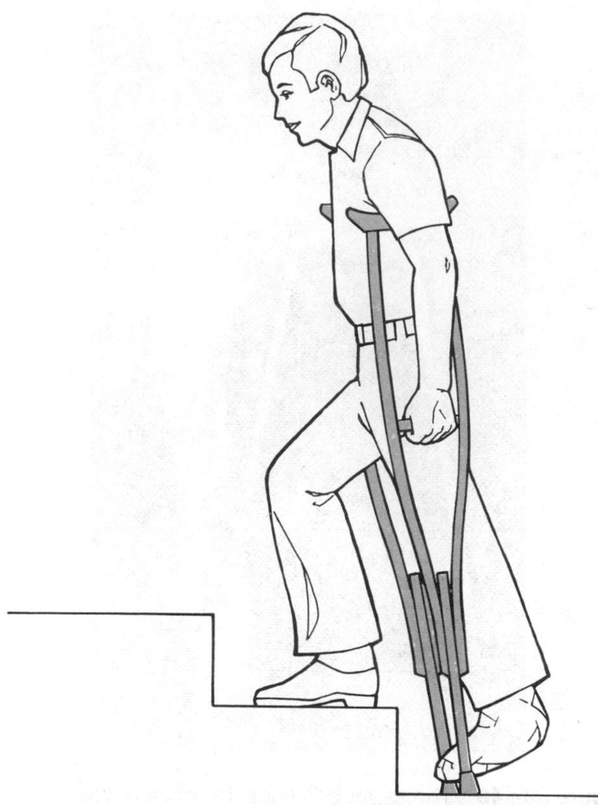

Figure 39–50 When climbing stairs, the client places weight on the crutches while moving the unaffected leg onto a step.

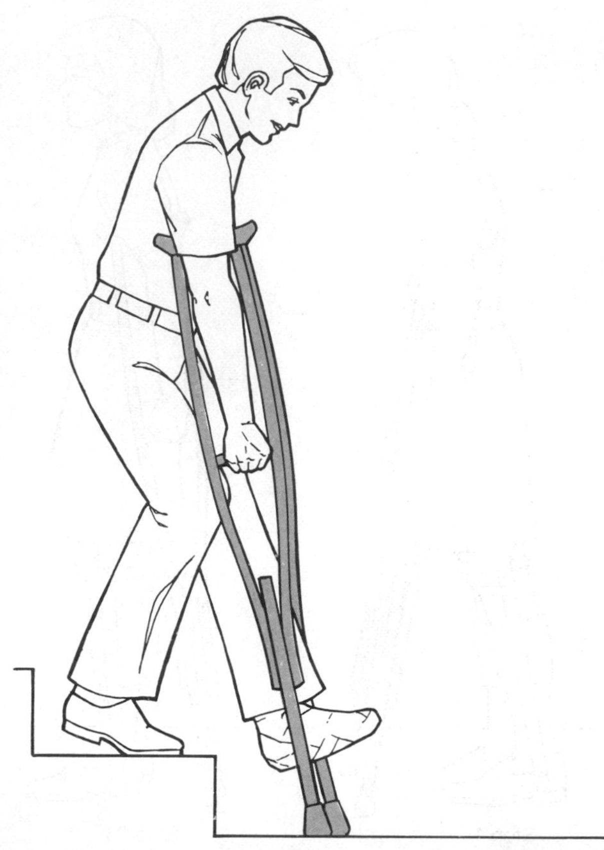

Figure 39–51 When descending stairs, the client places weight on the crutches while moving the unaffected leg onto a step.

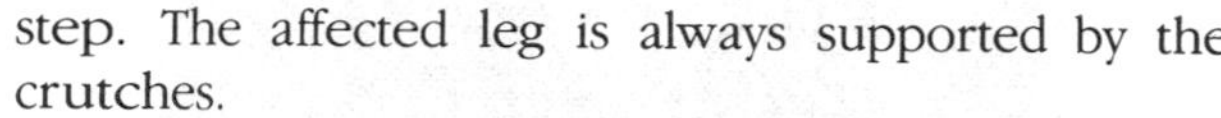

step. The affected leg is always supported by the crutches.

4. Repeat steps 2 and 3 until the client reaches the top of the stairs.

Going down stairs For this procedure, the nurse stands one step below the client on the affected side. Instruct the client to:

1. Assume the tripod position at the top of the stairs.
2. Shift the body weight to the unaffected leg, and move the crutches and affected leg down onto the next step. See Figure 39–51.
3. Transfer the body weight to the crutches, and move the unaffected leg to that step. The affected leg is always supported by the crutches.
4. Repeat steps 2 and 3 until the client reaches the bottom of the stairs.

Evaluation

The principles of body mechanics and ambulation, used previously as assessment criteria, are also used as outcome criteria to evaluate the effectiveness of the nurse's interventions in moving and transferring clients. The quality ...one's body mechanics in daily activities is evaluated ...iow well the person conforms to the prin- ...y mechanics and prevents back injury. The ...yone's ambulation is evaluated according to how well he or she conforms to the principles of ambulation and achieves stability in gait without falling.

Examples of outcome criteria to measure the client's goal achievement and the effectiveness of nursing interventions are shown on the next page. Criteria used to evaluate body mechanics were shown earlier on page 1067; criteria to evaluate gait were shown earlier in Table 39–2.

Examples of Outcome Criteria Related to Body Mechanics and Ambulation

The client will:

- Demonstrate use of good body mechanics when lifting and pulling objects.
- Identify factors contributing to back strain.
- Experience no back pain or muscle fatigue.
- Stand erect when walking.
- Use a walker to move independently from the bed to the nursing station three times a day.
- Demonstrate correct use of 4-point crutch gait.
- Demonstrate correct methods of getting into and out of a chair and ascending and descending stairs with crutches.

Nursing Care Plan

Assessment Data

Nursing Assessment

Miss Harriet Longstreet is a 69-year-old retired crossing-guard. She suffers from osteoarthritis and has bilateral cataracts. As of late she has experienced "drop attacks." She uses a cane when walking. Ten days ago she suffered back strain when attempting to move an old trunk. She was admitted to the hospital for treatment of back strain. She has been on bedrest with a firm mattress for support and in Fowler's position with the knees flexed. She has B.R.P. She has been receiving pain medications for her back pain and also hypnotics whenever necessary at bedtime. On occasion, she becomes slightly disoriented and confused at night and has attempted to get out of bed unassisted.

Physical Examination

Height: 160 cm (5′3″)
Weight: 61.3 kg (135 lb)
Temperature: 36.0 C (98.6 F)
Pulse rate: 82 BPM
Respirations: 20 per minute at rest
Blood pressure: 156/88 mm Hg
Heberden's nodes at distal interphalangeal joints of fingers

Diagnostic Data

Chest x-ray film: Negative
Knee x-ray film: Bony hypertrophy with spur formation
Spinal column x-ray film: Evidence of degenerative joint disease and spurs

Nursing Diagnosis	Client Goals and Outcome Criteria	Nursing Interventions and Rationales	Evaluation
Potential for injury related to impaired vision and limited movement possibly resulting in falls, fracture, contusions, and abrasions.	Client Goal: Ambulates independently without falling. Outcome Criteria: Uses call system before attempting to get out of bed 1 to 2× each night. Verbalizes helpfulness of night light and is oriented to placement of room furnishings.	Orient client to surroundings and system. *Rationale:* Provides for greater comfort and decreases disorientation. Encourage client to request assistance during the night by using call system. *Rationale:* Decreases chance of client falling while attempting to get out of bed without assistance. Keep bed in low position at all times. *Rationale:* Increases safety of client by decreasing chance of falling from a height. Turn on night light each night. *Rationale:* Decreases risk of falling. Observe for signs of disorientation in the evening. *Rationale:* Disorientation may occur in the evening, especially if client is sedated. Keep side rails up at all times. *Rationale:* Decreases risk of falling.	Client has attempted to get out of bed without assistance only once in 3 nights and has used call system appropriately on all other occasions. States night light is helpful to see where things are in this room: "I use one at home all the time."

(continued)

Nursing Diagnosis	Client Goals and Outcome Criteria	Nursing Interventions and Rationales	Evaluation
Knowledge deficit of disease process and body mechanics resulting in questioning etiology of low back pain, need for proper body mechanics, and possibility of paralysis.	Client Goals: Uses good body mechanics. Outcome Criteria: Identifies cause of low back pain. Identifies proper body mechanics to be utilized when moving heavy objects by day 3. Identifies proper posture for standing and sitting by day 3. Identifies proper sleeping position by day 2.	Assess client's learning needs regarding etiology of low back pain. *Rationale:* Can build upon knowledge client already has regarding causes of back pain. Allow adequate time for discussing problem, giving and reinforcing information. *Rationale:* Adequate time is necessary to help the client develop understanding of disease and its treatment. Instruct client regarding sleep patterns, e.g., to avoid prone position and to sleep on side with knees flexed. *Rationale:* Understanding and then practicing proper sleep positions will decrease back strain. Discuss importance of proper body mechanics, e.g., keep the back straight and the knees bent when lifting and do not lift above the elbows. *Rationale:* Understanding and practicing good body mechanics will decrease chances of back pain. Instruct client about proper standing and sitting positions. *Rationale:* Knowledge of proper posture positions will help to decrease back strain.	Client is able to discuss but not demonstrate proper body mechanics for pulling, pushing, and lifting heavy objects. States, "I should not sleep on my stomach because it'll give me a backache." Knows to use footstool when sitting and watching TV.

Chapter Highlights

- Good body mechanics is the efficient, coordinated, and safe use of the body to produce motion and maintain balance during activity.
- Proper movement promotes proper body functioning of musculoskeletal structures, reducing the energy required to move and maintain balance and therefore reducing fatigue.
- Good body mechanics and ambulation promote good body functioning and prevent back injury in nurses and falls in clients.
- An understanding of the laws of gravity, friction, force, inertia, and leverage help the nurse to use good body mechanics.
- The nurse acts as a role model and teacher of good body mechanics.
- The five basic movements of body mechanics are walking, squatting, pulling, lifting, and pivoting.
- A number of factors influence body mechanics and ambulation: general health, nutrition, emotions, environment, life-style, attitudes and values, level of understanding, and neuromuscular or skeletal impairments.
- Assessment of body mechanics and ambulation includes identification of the client's capabilities and limitations for movement, use of body mechanics, and gait.
- Nursing diagnoses related to the client's body mechanics and gait may include impaired physical mobility, potential for injury, fear, self-care deficit, and knowledge deficit.
- The nurse uses assessment data and nursing diagnoses to identify goals for care and design an individualized plan of nursing interventions.
- Overall client goals include improved use of proper body mechanics in work and in daily life, restored or improved ambulatory capability, and prevention of back injuries and falls.
- Before moving or turning a client, the nurse must consider the client's health and mental status, degree of exertion permitted, degree of discomfort, position required, and amount of force required.

- Assistance from others or the use of mechanical lifting aids is essential when clients are too heavy for the nurse to move or lift safely.
- Ambulating techniques that facilitate normal walking gait yet provide the support needed are most effective.
- The nurse can assist clients to prepare for ambulation by helping them become as independent as possible while in bed and encouraging them to perform orthostatic tension.
- Preambulatory exercises that strengthen the muscles for walking are essential for clients who have been immobilized for prolonged periods.
- Clients need specific instructions about appropriate use of canes, walkers, and crutches.
- Safety precautions and use of appropriate body mechanics are essential whenever assisting others to move to prevent client injury from falls and to prevent back strain of the nurse.

Suggested Readings

Cushing, M. February 1985. First, anticipate the harm. *American Journal of Nursing* 85:137–38.

This nurse-attorney discusses some legal implications that client falls pose for nurses.

Harber, P., et al. July 1985. Occupational low-back pain in hospital nurses. *Journal of Occupational Medicine* 27:518–24. Abstract in February 1986. Oh, my aching back. *American Journal of Nursing* 86:118.

This research report outlines the incidence, causes, and outcomes of back ache among a large group of hospital nurses.

Selected References

Axe, J. C.; Zeimelis, M. R.; and Zink, M. R. September 1980. Turning your patients mechanically. *RN* 43:47–49.

Bilger, A. J., and Greene, E. H., editors. 1973. *Winter's protective body mechanics.* New York: Springer Publishing Co.

Broer, M. R., and Zernicke, R. F. 1979. *Efficiency of human movement.* 4th ed. Philadelphia: W. B. Saunders Co.

Campbell, E. B.; Williams, M. A.; and Mlynarczyk, S. M. February 1986. After the fall—confusion. *American Journal of Nursing* 86:151–54.

Cohen, S., and Viellion, G. June 1979. Teaching a patient how to use crutches. *American Journal of Nursing* 79:1111–26.

Cushing, M. February 1985. First, anticipate the harm. *American Journal of Nursing* 85:137–38.

Daniels, L., and Worthingham, C. 1977. *Therapeutic exercise.* 2d ed. Philadelphia: W. B. Saunders Co.

Donaldson, W. F., and Hoover, N. W. 1982. *The American Medical Association book of back care.* New York: Random House.

Drapeau, J. September 1975. Getting back into good posture: How to ease your lumbar aches. *Nursing 75* 5:63–65.

Eliopoulos, C., editor. 1984. *Health assessment of the older adult.* Menlo Park, Calif.: Addison-Wesley Publishing Co.

Ford, J. R., and Duckworth, B. February 1976. Moving a dependent patient safely. *Nursing 76* 3:25–32.

Foss, G. May 1973. Use your head and save your back: Body mechanics. *Nursing 73* 3:25–32.

———. January/February 1984. Nonenvironmental causes of falls in a nursing home. *Geriatric Medicine Currents.* Ross Laboratories.

Gordon, J. E. February 1977. CircOlectric beds: Circumventing the trauma of positioning. *Nursing 77.* 7:42–47.

Harber, P., et al. July 1985. Occupational low-back pain in hospital nurses. *Journal of Occupational Medicine* 27:518–24. Abstract in February 1986. Oh, my aching back. *American Journal of Nursing* 86:118.

Hayne, C. R. August 1981. Manual transport of loads by women. *Physiotherapy* 67:226–31.

Hefferin, E. A., and Hill, B. J. June 1976. Analyzing nursing's work-related injuries. *American Journal of Nursing* 76:924–27.

Hogue, Carol. March 1982. Injury in late life. Part I: Epidemiology. *American Geriatric Society* 30: 183–89.

Hoover, S. December 1973. Job-related back injuries in a hospital. *American Journal of Nursing* 73:2078–79.

Howden, L. July/August 1981. Back care: It doesn't have to hurt. *Canadian Nurse* 77:46–50.

Jacobs, B., and Young, M. August 1981. Transferring patients safely and efficiently. *Nursing 81* 11:64–67.

Klabek, L. February 1978. Getting a grip on the transfer belt technique. *Nursing 78* 8:10.

Lee, P. S., and Pash, B. J. February 1983. Preventing patient falls. *Nursing 83* 13:118–20.

Leinweber, E. December 1978. Belts to make moves smoother. *American Journal of Nursing* 78:2080–81.

Long, B. C., and Buergin, P. S. June 1977. The pivot transfer. *American Journal of Nursing* 77:980–82.

Marino, N. M. April 1985. After the fall: An analysis. *American Journal of Nursing* 95:362.

Memmer, M. K. 1974a. *Body Mechanics.* Los Angeles: Intercampus Nursing Project, California State University and College System.

———. 1974b. *Introduction to alignment, body mechanics, and exercise.* Los Angeles: Intercampus Nursing Project, California State University and College System.

Owen, B. D. May 1980. How to avoid that aching back. *American Journal of Nursing* 80:894–97.

Potter, P., and Perry, A. 1985. *Fundamentals of nursing: Concepts, process, and practice.* St. Louis: C. V. Mosby Co.

Raistrick, A. May 14, 1981. Nurses with back pain: Can the problem be prevented? *Nursing Times* 77:853–56.

Snyder, M., and Baum, R. July 1974. Assessing station and gait. *American Journal of Nursing* 74:1256–57.

Witte, N. S. November 1979. Why the elderly fall. *American Journal of Nursing* 79:1950–52.

Works, F. F. February 1972. Hints on lifting and pulling. *American Journal of Nursing* 27:260–61.

CHAPTER **40**

Rest and Sleep

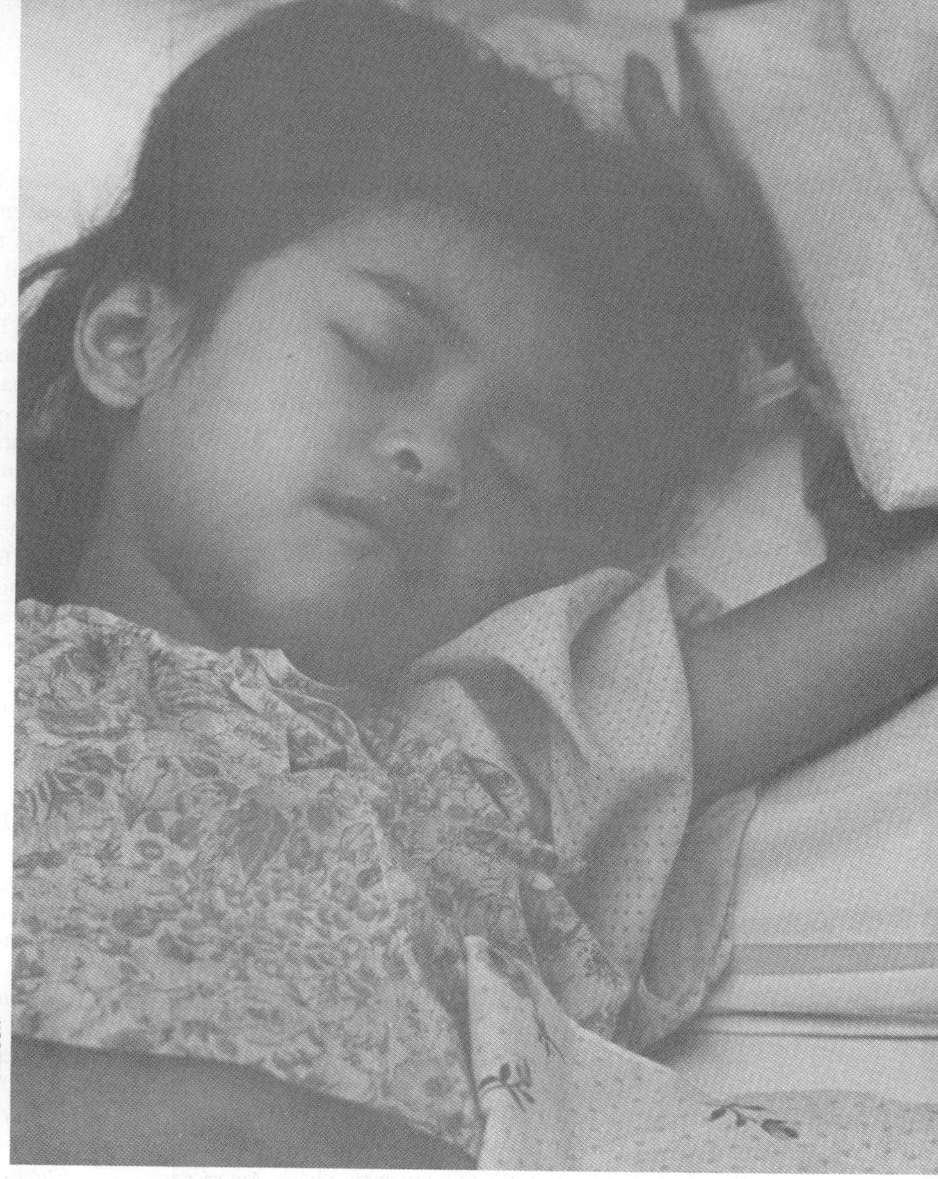

WILLIAM THOMPSON

Contents

Objectives

1. Understand essential facts about rest and sleep.
   - 1.1 Define selected terms.
   - 1.2 Identify six conditions necessary to promote rest.
   - 1.3 Compare three common human biorhythmic cycles.
   - 1.4 Identify characteristics of NREM and REM sleep.
   - 1.5 Identify four stages of NREM sleep.
2. Know information required to assess a person's sleep and rest patterns.
   - 2.1 Identify required information to assess sleep habits.
   - 2.2 Identify clinical signs and symptoms indicative of insufficient rest and sleep.
   - 2.3 Identify developmental variations in rest and sleep patterns.
   - 2.4 Identify factors influencing rest and sleep.
3. Know essential facts about common rest and sleep disorders and nursing diagnoses.
   - 3.1 Define terms related to common rest and sleep disorders.
   - 3.2 Identify three types of insomnia.
   - 3.3 Identify factors contributing to selected sleep disorders.
   - 3.4 Identify data indicative of common rest and sleep disorders.
4. Understand facts about nursing interventions required to maintain, promote, and restore normal rest and sleep patterns.
   - 4.1 Identify interventions that promote sleep and rest in newborns and infants, toddlers, preschoolers, school-age children, adolescents, and adults.
   - 4.2 State the rationale for selected interventions that promote sleep.
   - 4.3 Identify interventions that restore appropriate sleep and rest patterns for selected disorders.
5. Apply the nursing process to promote rest and sleep in selected clients.
   - 5.1 Obtain necessary assessment data.
   - 5.2 Analyze and relate assessment data.
   - 5.3 Write relevant nursing diagnoses.
   - 5.4 Plan appropriate nursing interventions.
   - 5.5 Implement appropriate nursing interventions.
   - 5.6 State outcome criteria against which to evaluate a client's response.

Terms

biorhythm
brain waves
cataplexy
circadian rhythm
electroencephalogram
hypersomnia
infradian rhythm
insomnia
narcolepsy
night terrors
nocturnal enuresis
NREM (slow-wave) sleep
parasomnias
REM sleep
rest
sleep
sleep apnea
somnambulism
ultradian rhythm

Purposes of Rest and Sleep

Rest and sleep are essential for health. Everyone needs rest and sleep to function at an optimal level. During sleep, the body repairs itself for the next day. People who are ill frequently require more rest and sleep than normal. Often, debilitated people expend unusual amounts of energy just to regain health or maintain the activities of daily living. As a result, such people experience increased and frequent fatigue and thus need more rest and sleep than usual. In addition, the ill person's normal sleep schedule usually becomes altered, and nursing intervention may be needed to promote the required sleep.

Rest

The ill and injured need rest. Rest, however, is not mere inactivity, and distraught clients may find rest difficult. **Rest** implies calmness, relaxation without emotional stress, and freedom from anxiety. Therefore, rest does not always imply inactivity; in fact, some people find some activities restful. For example, a student studying for examinations may find it restful to walk in the fresh air. The meaning of rest and the need for rest vary among individuals. Providing a restful environment for clients is an important function of nurses. To assess the client's need for rest and to evaluate how effectively this need is met, nurses need to consider conditions that promote rest.

Narrow (1967, p. 1645) outlines six characteristics that most people associate with rest. These summarize the meaning of rest and guide the nurse in assessing and promoting rest for clients.

Most people can rest when they:

1. Feel that things are under control
2. Feel accepted

3. Feel that they understand what is going on
4. Are free from irritation and discomfort
5. Have a satisfying amount of purposeful activity
6. Know they will receive help when it is needed

To rest, the client needs to feel both that his or her personal life is under control and that he or she is receiving competent health care. By providing competent care, the nurse gives peace of mind and allows the client to relax. A nurse often can promote rest by listening carefully to clients' personal concerns and alleviating them when possible. For example, a man taken to an emergency ward may be unable to relax until a nurse telephones his wife to inform her. A busy lawyer who suffers a heart attack may be more worried about whether certain papers were delivered to a client than about pain and discomfort.

Even when the person comes prepared for hospitalization, the nurse must consider the client's personal concerns and worries. For example, if a client admitted for elective diagnostic cystoscopy is also recovering successfully from a fractured hip and routinely walks prescribed distances each day, the client may worry that recovery from the fracture will be slowed by this interruption in exercise. Many clients experience discomfort or anxiety when well-established routines are interrupted. The routine might be reading oneself to sleep, drinking hot milk each evening, or following certain religious practices. Children often have security rituals before sleeping. Clients hospitalized for long periods may need the routine of sleeping in on a Saturday or Sunday morning or scheduled daily quiet or privacy. Most people need some time to themselves.

Rest is impossible for clients who do not feel accepted. Clients need to feel acceptable to themselves and to others. Grooming is often one important aspect of self-acceptance. Women may be concerned about the growth of body hair on their legs or the need for a shampoo or manicure; men may be concerned about an untrimmed beard or mustache. The nurse needs to be sensitive to and attend to these aspects of care. Acceptance by the staff is also important to the client. Acceptance can be conveyed, for instance, by recognizing both client limitations and client progress and recognizing individual differences.

A client's understanding of what is happening is another condition essential for rest. The unknown generates varying degrees of anxiety and interferes with rest. The nurse can help by offering explanations about diagnostic tests, surgery, agency policies or routines, and the client's progress. When information is given freely, clients do not feel the tension associated with having to ask questions.

Irritation and discomfort have both physical and emotional aspects. Generally, the nurse can easily detect physical discomforts, such as pain, insufficient supports for body positions, damp bedclothes, and loud noise. Emotional discomforts include having too many or too few visitors, feeling a lack of privacy, being hurried, having to wait long periods, being alone, or being concerned about the life problems of self or others.

Purposeful activity can be relaxing and often provides a sense of self-worth. The grandparent who knits a scarf for a grandchild, the person who helps make the bed, the adolescent who makes a wallet for her father, or the child who makes a toy puppet generally have a sense of contentment and accomplishment. Such activity often promotes rest throughout the day and undisturbed sleep at night.

The last prerequisite for rest is the security of knowing help is available when needed. The client who feels isolated and helpless cannot rest properly. Friends and family members can promote rest by helping the client with daily tasks and difficult decisions. Nurses can help by anticipating and meeting clients' needs. Knowing that the call bell will be answered, for example, can be exceedingly important to a client. Also, the support and understanding of the nurse can help clients facing major decisions, such as "Shall I place the baby for adoption?" or "Shall I move to a nursing home?" Although such decisions are the client's alone, nurses can be instrumental in helping the client clarify issues—for example, by offering additional information about referral agencies or by helping the client to express feelings.

Sleep

Sleep, a basic physiologic need, is defined as a state of unconsciousness from which a person can be aroused by appropriate sensory or other stimuli (Guyton 1986, p. 670). Sleep is characterized by minimal physical activity, variable levels of consciousness, changes in the body's physiologic processes, and decreased responsiveness to external stimuli (Hayter 1980, p. 457).

Functions of Sleep

Sleep is known to have a restorative function. During non-REM sleep the stress on the pulmonary, cardiovascular, nervous, endocrine, and excretory systems decreases. For example, the normal heart rate of a healthy adult decreases from a rate of 70 to 80 beats per minute during wakefulness to 60 or fewer beats per minute during sleep.

Also, energy is conserved during sleep. The skeletal muscles are relaxed; thus energy is redirected to more essential cellular functions. In addition, sympathetic activity decreases and parasympathetic activity occasionally increases (Guyton 1986, p. 674). Other body changes during sleep are shown to the right.

Sleep is believed to mediate stress, anxiety, and tension and to help the person regain energy for concentrating, coping, and maintaining interest in daily activities.

Sleep does not appear to be necessary to recharge energy lost during the day. If that were the case, the relative durations of wakefulness and sleep would remain constant, and they do not. For example, when people are deliberately kept awake for 3 to 10 days, they sleep for less than a day after the enforced wakefulness. Conversely, when people are immobilized for long periods, they still sleep and apparently need to. Sleep is also unnecessary for body organ function, although physiologic changes occur during sleep (Guyton 1986, p. 674).

Physiologic Changes During Sleep

- Arterial blood pressure falls.
- Pulse rate decreases.
- Peripheral blood vessels dilate.
- Activity of the gastrointestinal tract occasionally increases.
- Skeletal muscles relax.
- Basal metabolic rate decreases 10% to 30%.

(Guyton 1986, p. 674)

Biorhythms

Biorhythmology, the study of the biologic rhythms of the body, is receiving increasing attention from biologists and health professionals. **Biorhythms** (rhythmic biologic clocks) exist in plants, animals, and humans. In humans, these are controlled from within the body and synchronized with environmental factors, such as light and darkness, gravity, and electromagnetic stimuli. Human rhythms are demonstrated biologically and behaviorally. Examples of biologic rhythms in humans are the repetitive rhythmic contractions of the heart muscle, the waking and sleeping cycles, and regular temperature fluctuations. Each biorhythmic cycle has peaks and troughs. These cycles vary somewhat among individuals. For example, most adults sleep at night, and most sleep about 8 hours. However, some people, referred to as "night owls," seem to be more alert during the late evening hours and retire late. Others, referred to as "early birds," prefer to retire early and perform well in the early hours of the morning. Some people need only 4 hours of sleep daily.

Biorhythms are classified according to the length of the cycle. The most common cycle is the **circadian rhythm**, a 1-day cycle. The term *circadian* is from the Latin *circa dies,* meaning "about a day." A second rhythm is the **infradian rhythm**, a monthly cycle. An example is the menstrual cycle. A third rhythm is the **ultradian rhythm**, consisting of cycles completed in minutes or hours. An example is the rapid eye movement (REM) cycle of sleep. Biorhythms are not altered by changes in the environment. They are *endogenous,* that is, arising from within the human body and persisting regardless of environmental influences (Deters 1980, p. 250).

Circadian regularity approaching that of adults begins by the 3rd week of life and may be inherited. Babies are awake most often in the early morning and the late afternoon. After 4 months of age, babies enter a 24-hour cycle in which they sleep mostly during the night. By the end of the 5th or 6th month, babies' sleep–wakefulness patterns are almost like those of adults.

Kinds of Sleep

The **electroencephalogram** (EEG) provides a good picture of what occurs during sleep. Electrodes are placed on various parts of the sleeper's scalp. The electrodes transmit electric energy from the cerebral cortex to pens that record the fluctuations in energy (**brain waves**) on graph paper. Each pen of the electroencephalogram corresponds to an electrode, moving up when the electric charge is negative and down when it is positive.

There are two kinds of sleep: **REM** (rapid eye movement) **sleep** and **NREM** (non-REM, or **slow-wave**) **sleep**. REM sleep is not a passive state but a relatively active state; so REM sleep is also referred to as *paradoxical sleep*. The characteristics of REM sleep are listed below.

The sympathetic nervous system dominates during REM sleep. REM sleep is thought to restore a person mentally—that is, for learning, psychologic adaptation, and memory (Hayter 1980, p. 458). During REM sleep, the

Characteristics of REM Sleep

- Active dreaming occurs.
- The sleeper is more difficult to arouse than during NREM (slow-wave) sleep.
- Muscle tone is depressed.
- Heart rate and respiratory rate often are irregular.
- A few irregular muscle movements occur—in particular, rapid eye movements.

sleeper reviews the day's events and processes and stores the information. The sleeper gains perspective on problems and may resolve some problems. Thus, there is wisdom in the traditional advice to "sleep on" a problem or big decision.

NREM sleep is also referred to as deep, restful sleep or slow-wave sleep, because the brain waves of a sleeper during NREM sleep are slower than the alpha and beta waves of a person who is awake or alert. See Figure 40–1. Characteristics of NREM sleep include:

- Dreamlessness
- Profound restfulness
- Decreased blood pressure
- Decreased respiratory rate
- Decreased metabolic rate
- Slow and rolling eye movements

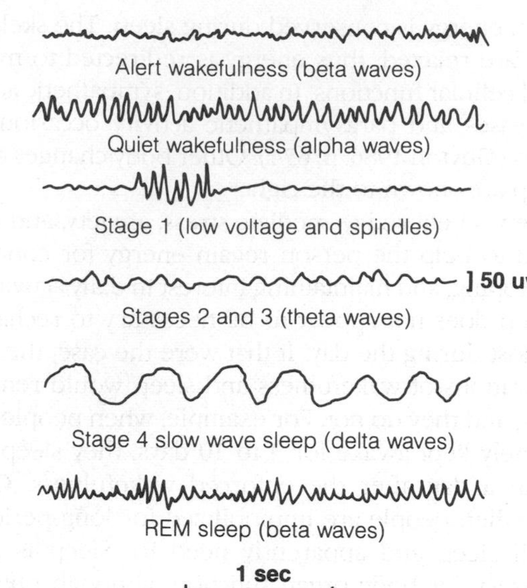

Figure 40–1 Characteristic brain waves during waking, the four stages of NREM sleep, and REM sleep.

Source: From A. C. Guyton, *Textbook of medical physiology,* 7th ed. (Philadelphia: W. B. Saunders Co., 1986), p. 671. Used by permission.

Stages of NREM (Slow-Wave) Sleep

An electroencephalogram shows different brain waves during the different stages of sleep. See Figure 40–1. Slow-wave sleep is generally divided into four stages. Before sleeping a person shows the high-frequency beta waves of alert wakefulness. This is followed by quiet wakefulness, when alpha waves appear.

Stage I

This is the stage of very light sleep. The brain waves are of low voltage, though broken periodically by *sleep spindles* (short, spindle-shaped bursts of alpha waves). During Stage I the person feels drowsy and relaxed, the eyes roll from side to side, and the heart and respiratory rates drop slightly. The sleeper can be readily awakened during this stage.

Stage II

Stage II is the stage of light sleep during which body processes continue to slow down. The eyes are generally still, the heart and respiratory rates decrease slightly, and body temperature falls. The brain waves during Stages II and III are theta waves. Stage II lasts only about 10 to 15 minutes.

Stage III

During stage III, the heart and respiratory rates as well as other body processes slow further, due to domination of the parasympathetic nervous system. The sleeper becomes more difficult to arouse. The brain waves become more regular. Slow delta waves are added to the stage II theta wave pattern.

Stage IV

Stage IV signals deep sleep, during which delta waves predominate and become even slower. The sleeper's heart and respiratory rates drop 20% to 30% below those exhibited during waking hours. The sleeper is very relaxed, rarely moves, and is difficult to arouse. Stage IV is thought to physically restore the body. Physical exercise 2 hours before bedtime promotes stage IV sleep (Hayter 1980, p. 457).

Physiology of Sleep

Control of the cyclic nature of sleep is centered in two specialized areas of the brain stem: the reticular activating system (RAS) and the bulbar synchronizing region (BSR) in the medulla. There are two theories about sleep, the passive theory and the active theory. The passive theory holds that the reticular activating system of the brain simply fatigues and therefore becomes inactive. The active theory, which is more widely accepted today, proposes some sort of center or centers that cause sleep by inhibiting other parts of the brain (Guyton 1986, p. 672).

The two systems, RAS and BSR, are thought to intermittently activate and then suppress the brain centers. The RAS is associated with the body's state of alertness and receives sensory input, i.e., auditory, visual, pain, and tactile stimuli. These sensory stimuli maintain a person's sense of wakefulness and alertness. During sleep the body sends fewer stimuli from the cerebral cortex or the peripheral sensory receptors to the RAS. The person awakens from sleep when there is an increase in such stimuli. There is less known about the BSR; however, it is known that its activity increases with sleep.

Sleep Cycle

Sleep is cyclic. The usual sleeper experiences four to six cycles of sleep during 7 to 8 hours. Each cycle lasts about 90 minutes. The cycle is made up of most, if not all, of the four stages of NREM (slow-wave) sleep and the final stage—REM sleep. See Figure 40–2. A sleeper passes from stage I NREM sleep through stages II and III to stage IV in about 20 to 30 minutes. Stage IV may last about 30 minutes. The process is then reversed, and the sleeper ascends through stages III and II, after which REM sleep occurs. REM sleep completes the first cycle, and the cycle then repeats. The sleeper who is awakened during any stage must begin anew at Stage I NREM sleep and proceed through all the stages to REM sleep.

The duration of NREM stages and REM sleep varies throughout the 8-hour sleep period. As the night progresses, the sleeper becomes less tired and spends less time in Stages III and IV of NREM sleep. REM sleep increases, and dreams tend to lengthen. See Figure 40–2. If the sleeper is very tired, REM cycles are often short—for example, 5 minutes instead of 20—during the early portion of sleep. Before sleep ends, periods of near wakefulness occur, and Stages I and II NREM sleep and REM sleep predominate.

The ratio of NREM to REM sleep varies with age. See Figure 40–2.

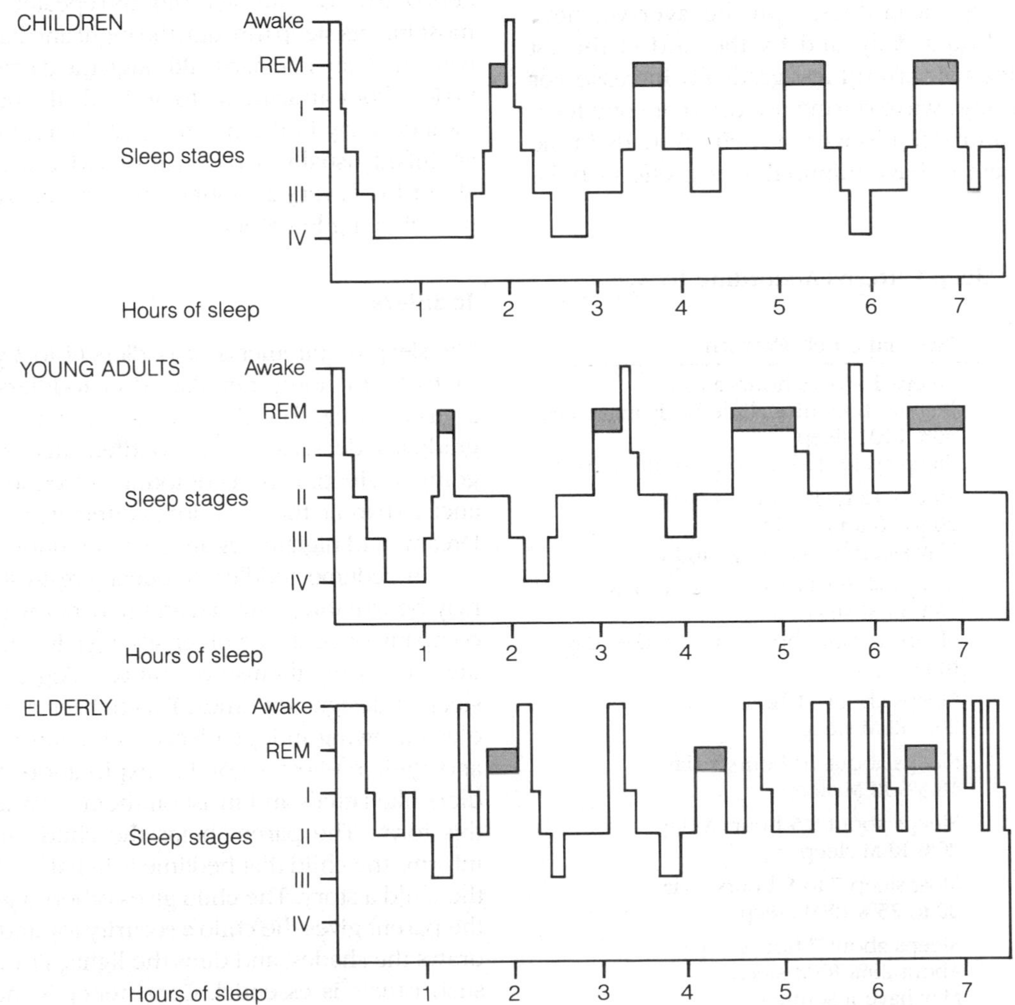

Figure 40–2 Normal sleep cycles of children, young adults, and elderly adults. The sleep of children and young adults shows early preponderance of NREM Stages III and IV, progressive lengthening of the first three REM periods, and infrequent awakenings. In elderly adults there is little or no NREM Stage IV sleep, REM periods are fairly uniform in length, and awakenings are frequent and often lengthy.

Source: A. Kales, Sleep and dreams: Recent research in clinical aspects, *Annals of Internal Medicine,* May 1968, 68:1078. Reprinted with permission.

Sleep Requirements

The amount of sleep individuals require decreases not only with age but also as the growth rate decreases. See Table 40–1.

Age-Related Needs

Newborns and Infants

The newborn, regardless of gestational age or type of delivery, is awake, alert, and active during the transition from intrauterine to extrauterine life. This activity lasts only for about 90 minutes, however, and a sleep of 4 to 8 hours follows, depending on the stresses of birth. After this initial phase, periods of wakefulness stabilize, occurring every 3 or 4 hours. For the first few weeks, the infant's wakefulness is dictated largely by hunger. Later, the need to socialize affects wakefulness. On the average, newborns sleep 17 hours daily, and by the end of the 1st month, the periods of wakefulness gradually increase. For example, some stay awake during the day from one feeding to another and sleep longer at night. Sounds in the environment seem to have minimal, if any, effect on the newborn's sleep. This fact can be observed in nurseries, where often one newborn cries loudly in one crib while another sleeps soundly in an adjacent crib.

Newborns usually can be aroused easily from sleep, and they return to sleep just as easily, provided they are comfortable. Frequent body movements and facial grimaces are normal during sleep and indicate REM sleep. When newborns do not sleep well and cry or fuss for long periods, they are usually hungry, wet, hot, or cold. If comfort measures offer no relief, illness may be the cause.

In infants of 2 months, the observer may note a preference for one sleeping position, a preference that may have been present at birth. By 3 months, the infant exhibits routines before sleeping, such as crying, sucking on fingers or toys, or shifting positions repeatedly. By 4 months, most infants sleep through the night and have a scheduled pattern of daytime naps. Although the daytime nap pattern varies from individual to individual, infants generally awaken early in the morning. At the end of the 1st year, an infant usually naps once or twice a day and sleeps about 14 of every 24 hours. The infant also begins to show fear of being left alone.

Table 40–1 Sleep Patterns According to Age

Developmental Level	Normal Sleep Pattern
Newborn	Sleeps 14 to 18 hours a day Regular breathing, little body movement 50% REM sleep Sleep cycles last 45 to 60 minutes each
Infant	Sleeps 12 to 14 hours a day 20 to 30% REM sleep May sleep through the night
Toddler	Sleeps about 11 to 12 hours a day 25% REM sleep Sleeps during the night and takes daytime naps
Preschooler	Sleeps about 11 hours a day 20% REM sleep
School-age child	Sleeps about 10 hours a day 18.5% REM sleep
Adolescent	Sleeps about 8.5 hours a day 20% REM sleep
Young adult	Most sleep 7 to 8 hours a day 20 to 25% REM sleep
Middle-age adult	Sleeps about 7 hours a day About 20% REM sleep May have insomnia
Elderly adult	Sleeps about 6 hours a day 20 to 25% REM sleep May have insomnia

Adapted from L. Malasanos, V. Barkauskas, M. Moss, and K. Stoltenberg-Allen, *Health assessment,* 3d ed. (St. Louis: C. V. Mosby Co., 1977), pp. 122–23.

Toddlers

The sleep requirements of toddlers (1 to 3 years) decrease to 10 to 14 hours per day. Most toddlers still need an afternoon nap, but the necessity for mid-morning naps gradually decreases. Still, toddlers may have problems going to sleep. Parents of toddlers frequently seek guidance to handle their children's difficulty in going to sleep. Dreams and nightmares are common during toddlerhood.

At bedtime, toddlers frequently resist sleep, feel tense, may be irritable, may cry, and may not want to leave the company of adults or older siblings. It is normal for toddlers to assert themselves by refusing to nap or go to sleep at designated times. This behavior reflects the toddler's growing independence, self-control, and curiosity and their endless vigor for exploration. However, toddlers like rituals and insist on them. A typical ritual takes this form: The parent helps the child into bedclothes, informs the child that bedtime is in half an hour, and tells the child a story. The child gives others a goodnight hug; the parent gives the child a security toy and glass of juice, draws the shades, and dims the lights. Firm adherence to such rituals is essential. Consistency is more important than the form of the ritual.

Toddlers often develop their own ways of going to sleep. They may talk to themselves for a while, roll their heads, rock in bed, or play with a toy. These behaviors are normal and relieve tension. Similar behavior is observed before daytime naps; prenap rituals also should be consistent. Often, mothers of toddlers require an afternoon nap, which can be scheduled to coincide with the toddler's.

Preschoolers

Preschoolers (3 to 6 years), like toddlers, are unaware of their need for rest or sleep. Preschoolers are more interested in what is happening around them and also may resist sleep. The difference is that the preschooler requires more privacy, not only for sleep but also for fantasy, sexual exploration, enjoyment of possessions, or for intervals to deal with disappointments and hurts. Preschoolers need a room or portion of a room to themselves for such private activities.

Three-year-olds frequently have nightmares that are associated with real or imaginary fears. Sometimes it is difficult for them to differentiate between what is real and what is not. It is not unusual for preschoolers to wander into their parents' bedroom, wanting to sleep with them. Children who have difficulty sleeping at night may become less restless if they nap during the day. Sleeping near older siblings or parents can also be comforting.

At age 4 or 5, children resist daytime sleep. Children who cannot sleep during the day often need a rest period. Parents can promote rest by darkening a room and providing restful or quiet activities. Day-care centers and kindergartens commonly schedule such rest periods. By age 5, children usually sleep restfully through the night but may require occasional daytime naps if activities are overly stimulating. Nightmares may persist but are to be expected.

School-Age Children

A peaceful night's sleep is often not possible for school-age children. Although their sleep requirements are less (9 to 13 hours), they may have nightmares, often associated with fears of death, a concept they are beginning to understand. Parents can expect questions, discussions, and confidences from children of this age.

Growing children increasingly want a say about the time they go to bed. Parental judgment is still required, however. Parents need to set limits on the child's activities and schedule specific bedtimes to ensure sufficient rest. More flexible schedules are possible with older children.

Adolescents

Adolescents usually sleep from 8 to 10 hours a day. Because adolescents are very active, they need rest and sleep. Sometimes adolescents are unaware of their needs, and adults must set limits so teenagers can obtain the necessary rest and sleep. Reading and other restful activities help the adolescent avoid fatigue. Adolescents seldom wake spontaneously in the night.

Young Adults

Young adults' need for sleep is largely determined by such factors as emotional and physical health, amount of activity, pregnancy, and personality. Although most young adults require 7 to 8 hours, it is also normal for adults to sleep less than 6 hours or more than 9.

Sometimes young adults find their sleep disturbed by young children. Sleeping a few hours at a time produces the same effect as sleeping less, even though the total time is the same. Stage IV sleep is most often disturbed, and the sleeper obtains little REM sleep. When such a young adult gets the opportunity to sleep undisturbed, he or she gets more REM sleep than usual. **Insomnia** (inability to get enough sleep) in young adults is an increasing problem. Commonly, the difficulty is getting to sleep rather than waking midsleep.

Middle-Age Adults

Middle-age adults normally sleep on an average of 7 hours a day and get more non-REM (deep and restful) sleep than young adults. The 90-minute REM cycle remains relatively constant; however, there is a marked decrease in the amount of Stage IV sleep.

Elderly Adults

People 60 and older take longer to go to sleep and tend to awaken earlier. Older adults also experience changes in sleep patterns. The amount of Stage IV sleep decreases by about 15% to 30% (Hayter 1980, p. 460). Elderly people awaken more often during the night—six times per night at age 60 compared to once a night in young adulthood (Hayter 1980, p. 460). It is also believed that women's sleep patterns change about 10 years later than men's.

Factors Affecting Sleep

Both the quality and the quantity of sleep are affected by several factors. *Quality of sleep* means the individual's ability to stay asleep and to get appropriate amounts of REM and non-REM sleep. Sleep stages can be differentiated and measured only in a laboratory. *Quantity of sleep* is the total time the individual sleeps.

Some of the most common factors that affect sleep adversely are illness, environment, exercise, fatigue, psychologic stress, medications, alcohol and stimulants, and nutrition. See Table 40–2.

Illness

People who are ill require more sleep than normal, and the normal rhythm of sleep and wakefulness is also disturbed. People deprived of REM sleep subsequently spend more sleep time than normal in this stage. Pain also can

Table 40–2 Factors Influencing Sleep

Factor	Effect
Liver failure	Day–night reversal
Encephalitis	Day–night reversal
Hypothyroidism	Decreases NREM Stage IV sleep
Antidepressant	Decreases REM sleep
Amphetamine	Decreases REM sleep
Alcohol	Speeds onset of sleep, but decreases REM sleep and disrupts other stages
Depression	Decreases or increases REM sleep
Sedative-hypnotic drug	Suppresses REM sleep and decreases NREM Stages III and IV. On withdrawal, causes rebound REM sleep with vivid dreams and increased awakening
Tranquilizer	Interferes with REM sleep
Bedtime snack of protein food	Induces and maintains sleep

affect sleep—either preventing sleep or awakening the sleeper.

Respiratory conditions can disturb an individual's sleep. Shortness of breath often makes sleep difficult, and people frequently need to lie in bed with two or more pillows elevating their heads and chest in order to ease breathing. In addition, people who have nasal congestion or sinus drainage may have trouble breathing and hence a difficult sleep.

People who have gastric or duodenal ulcers may find their sleep disturbed because of pain, often a result of the increased gastric secretions that occur during REM sleep. Certain endocrine disturbances can also affect sleep. Hyperthyroidism lengthens presleep time, often making it difficult for a client to fall asleep. Hypothyroidism, on the other hand, decreases Stage IV sleep.

The need to urinate during the night (enuresis) also disrupts sleep, and people who awaken at night to urinate sometimes have difficulty getting back to sleep.

Environment

Environment can promote or hinder sleep. People usually become accustomed to the sleeping environment in their home, and any change—e.g., in the noise level—can inhibit sleep. People often become accustomed to certain noises, lights, etc., and the absence of these or the presence of unfamiliar stimuli can keep them from sleeping. A nurse may hear a client say, "I can't sleep here; it is too quiet," or "I can't sleep because of the bell that rings every hour."

Exercise and Fatigue

It is generally believed that a person who exercises during the day is more likely to sleep well at night and that a person who exercises just before retiring will have difficulty getting to sleep. Research in this area is limited; however, it is thought that a person who is moderately fatigued usually has a restful sleep. Fatigue can also affect a person's sleep pattern. The more tired the person is, the shorter the first period of paradoxical (REM) sleep. As the person rests, the REM periods become longer.

Psychologic Stress

Anxiety and other emotional problems can disturb sleep. A person preoccupied with personal problems may be unable to relax sufficiently to get to sleep.

Medications

Medications, especially hypnotics and sedatives, affect the sleep pattern. Hypnotics and barbiturates decrease REM sleep, even though they may increase total sleep time. Amphetamines and antidepressants decrease REM sleep abnormally. Long-term use of amphetamines can produce abnormal behavior, attributable to long-term REM sleep deprivation.

A client withdrawing from any of these drugs gets much more REM sleep than usual and as a result may experience upsetting nightmares. Nurses need to be aware of this possibility and give the client support.

Alcohol and Stimulants

People who drink an excessive amount of alcohol often find their sleep disturbed. Excessive alcohol disrupts REM sleep, although it may hasten the onset of sleep. While making up for lost REM sleep after some of the effects of the alcohol have worn off, clients often experience nightmares. Tolerance to alcohol also affects sleep; the alcohol-

Research Note

In this study of sleep behaviors, questionnaires were mailed to 212 healthy, noninstitutionalized subjects ages 65 to 93 years. The self-reported behaviors revealed that with age there was a significant increase in the amount of time spent in bed (total sleep time, with naps included). For those over age 75 there was also an increase in the number of naps and the amount of time spent napping, as well as an increase in the number of times awake and the amount of wake time after onset of sleep. For those over age 85 there was a significant increase in total sleep time and sleep latency, as well as a change to an earlier bedtime. The researcher concluded that changes in sleep behavior are to be expected as age advances. (Hayter 1983)

tolerant person may be unable to sleep well and may become irritable as a result.

Nutrition

Weight loss and weight gain have been found to affect sleep. Crisp and Stonehill (1976, p. 166) found that weight loss is associated with reduced total sleep time as well as broken sleep and earlier awakening. Weight gain, on the other hand, was associated with an increase in total sleep time, less broken sleep, and later waking.

The amino acid L-tryptophan is thought to affect sleep. Dietary L-tryptophan—found, for example, in cottage cheese, milk, beef, and canned tuna—may be sleep-inducing, which might explain why warm milk helps some people get to sleep.

Common Sleep Disorders

The two most common sleep disorders are insomnia in adults and parasomnias in children. Less common sleep disorders are hypersomnia, narcolepsy, and sleep apnea.

Insomnia

Insomnia is the inability to obtain adequate quality or quantity of sleep. It is *not* the lack of sleep; in fact, people with insomnia often obtain more sleep than they realize. There are three types of insomnia: inability to fall asleep (initial insomnia), inability to stay asleep because of frequent waking (intermittent insomnia), and early awakening and subsequent inability to return to sleep (terminal insomnia). Terminal insomnia is characteristic of depressed people. Insomniacs do not feel refreshed on arising.

Insomnia can result from physical discomfort but more often is a result of mental overstimulation due to anxiety. People sometimes become anxious because they think they might not be able to sleep. People who become habituated to drugs or who drink large quantities of alcohol are likely to have insomnia.

Treatment for insomnia frequently requires the client to develop new behavior patterns that induce sleep. The usefulness of sleeping medications is questionable. Such medications do not deal with the cause of the problem, and their prolonged use creates drug dependencies.

Nurses need to encourage insomniacs to develop an effective sleep/rest and exercise routine. Insomniacs should (a) get adequate exercise during the day; (b) avoid excitement during the evening; (c) establish a relaxing pastime before sleep, such as reading or playing solitaire; (d) go to bed only when sleepy, not when the time seems appropriate; and (e) when unable to sleep at night, get up and pursue some relaxing activity until they feel drowsy (or if unable to sleep in the early morning get up and pursue an activity that provides a sense of accomplishment).

Hypersomnia

Hypersomnia, the opposite of insomnia, is excessive sleep of more than 9 hours at night. The afflicted person often sleeps until noon and takes many naps during the day. Hypersomnia is generally related to psychophysiologic problems, such as psychiatric disorders (depression or anxiety), central nervous system damage, and certain kidney, liver, or metabolic disorders.

Parasomnias

Parasomnias refer to a cluster of disorders that interfere with children's sleep, such as **somnambulism** (sleepwalking), **night terrors** (*pavor nocturnus*), and **nocturnal enuresis** (bedwetting). These disorders often appear together in the same child, run in families, and tend to occur during Stages III and IV of NREM sleep.

Somnambulism is not uncommon in children—about 1% to 6% of children between the ages of 5 and 12 years walk in their sleep (Malasanos et al. 1986, p. 128). It is normally outgrown without incident. A sleepwalker may not awaken if she or he walks only 3 or 4 minutes; if the walk lasts any longer, then some awakening is usually shown. The main concern is to protect the somnambulist from injury. Usually the sleepwalker can be awakened and quietly led back to bed.

Night terrors are frightening to both parents and children. Children 6 and younger are most often afflicted. After having slept for a few hours, the child bolts upright in bed, shakes and screams, appears pale and terrified, but is difficult to arouse. In contrast to nightmares, night terrors are not remembered the next morning.

Nocturnal enuresis can occur in preadolescent children. Its cause is unknown, although in preschool children it may be due to bladder training that is too severe or too early, or to overtraining. If the child is 3 or 4 years old, environmental factors such as a dark hall may contribute to the child's reluctance to go to the bathroom. In the school-age child, enuresis may be caused by inadequate bladder capacity or jealousy over a new brother or sister. Parents should rule out physical abnormalities first and provide an environment in which the child feels loved. Restricting fluids before bedtime may reduce the incidence of bedwetting but does not address the cause of the problem.

Narcolepsy

Narcolepsy—from the Greek *narco,* meaning "numbness," and *lepsis,* meaning "seizure"—is a sudden wave of overwhelming sleepiness that occurs during the day; thus it is referred to as a "sleep attack." Its cause is unknown, although it is believed to be a genetic defect of the central nervous system in which the REM period cannot be controlled. In narcoleptic attacks, sleep starts with the REM phase. Even though narcoleptics sleep well at night, they nod off several times a day.

Many narcoleptics have bouts of **cataplexy,** that is, partial or complete muscle paralysis. Sometimes the person's jaw slackens or the head falls to the chest. These cataplectic bouts are often preceded by moments of exertion or strong emotion, such as laughing or crying.

Narcoleptics are often accused of laziness, disinterest in life and work, and even drunkenness. Their handicap, however, is life-threatening in a world fraught with potential hazards. Drug therapy is used with some success to treat narcolepsy. Stimulants such as amphetamines or methylphenidate hydrochloride (Ritalin) prevent attacks; and antidepressants such as imipramine hydrochloride (Tofranil) prevent the muscle weakness and paralysis of cataplexy. Narcoleptics should avoid liquor, which increases drowsiness.

Sleep Apnea

Sleep apnea is the periodic cessation of breathing during sleep. This disorder needs to be assessed by a sleep expert, but it is often suspected when the person has obstructive snoring, excessive daytime sleepiness, and sometimes insomnia. The periods of apnea, which last from 10 seconds to 3 minutes, occur during REM or NREM sleep. Frequency of episodes ranges from 50 to 600 per night. These apneic episodes drain the person of energy and lead to excessive daytime sleepiness.

Obstructive apnea is caused by defects that temporarily obstruct the air passages and deplete the supply of oxygen to the lungs—for instance, an excessively thick palate, enlarged tonsils, or a jaw deformity. *Central apnea* is caused by defects in the respiratory centers of the brain that cause a transient diaphragmatic arrest, and the lungs stop moving. When carbon dioxide in the blood reaches a certain level, the person is jolted to near-wakefulness (e.g., sitting up with a sudden start) but does not regain consciousness.

Sleep apnea profoundly affects a person's work or school performance. In addition, prolonged sleep apnea can cause a sharp rise in blood pressure and may also lead to cardiac arrest. Over time, apneic episodes can cause pulmonary hypertension and subsequent left-sided heart failure.

The treatment of sleep apnea depends on the cause. Central apnea is sometimes treated with powerful tranquilizers. Some obstructive types are treated by a tracheostomy, a permanent, surgical opening of the trachea; the opening is uncapped during sleep but capped during the day to allow normal breathing.

Assessment

Assessment relative to a client's sleep should include a sleep history and any clinical signs of sleep problems.

Sleep History

A sleep history should include questions about a client's usual sleeping habits and any sleep problems. Suggested content for a sleep history is listed on page 1109. Sometimes clients can provide more precise information if they keep a written record of their sleep pattern and the habits associated with it. Such a sleep log can be kept by clients who are sleeping at home and should be maintained for about a week, particularly if the client has sleeping problems.

Clinical Assessment of Sleep Problems

Some of the early signs and symptoms of insufficient sleep are:

1. Expressing a feeling of fatigue
2. Irritability and restlessness
3. Lassitude and apathy
4. Darkened areas around the eyes, puffy eyelids, reddened conjunctivae, and burning eyes
5. Marked periods of inattention
6. Headache
7. Nausea

Sleep deprivation or prolonged loss of sleep triggers certain biochemical changes in the body. Sleeplessness lowers the seizure threshold. Consequently, people with epilepsy should not go without sleep for prolonged periods. Some of the clinical signs of sleep deprivation are:

1. Behavior and personality changes, such as aggressiveness, withdrawal, depression
2. Increased restlessness
3. Distorted perceptions
4. Visual or auditory hallucinations

Research Note

Pediatric nurses frequently are asked to assist parents in coping with the sleep problems of young children, one of the difficulties parents cite most frequently. The authors of this study sought to identify both the sleep behaviors that are experienced as problematic and various intrafamilial factors that may affect infants' sleep or parents' perception of their sleep patterns. The most striking finding was that 70% of the children with sleep problems were first-born. In addition, night waking was found to be the complaint most frequently cited. Mothers were intensely interested in and concerned about sleep problems, though they paradoxically reported that these sleep problems only caused little-to-moderate disruption in family functioning. The authors suggest that further study is needed to determine the effectiveness of anticipatory guidance in preventing sleep problems. (Edgil et al. 1985)

5. Confusion and disorientation as to time and place
6. Impaired coordination
7. Slurred speech or inappropriate speech and tone

Sleep History

- Usual times of retiring, falling asleep, and waking
- Number of naps taken during the day, as well as their time and duration
- Whether the client's sleep time varies—for example, because of shift work
- Typical day's activities, with specific reference to exercise and recreation
- Usual sleep habits and environment
- Use of rituals before sleep and special equipment, e.g., pillows
- Whether the client sleeps alone
- Medications used for sleeping, either over-the-counter or prescription drugs
- Intake of stimulants, e.g., caffeinated coffee
- How well the client feels she or he sleeps
- Any difficulty sleeping
- Any changes in the client's sleep pattern

Nursing Diagnosis

Examples of nursing diagnoses for clients who have sleep problems are listed on page 1110.

Planning

Planning for sleep disturbances involves nursing interventions that:

1. Identify the causative or contributing factors
2. Reduce environmental distractions and sleep interruptions
3. Increase daytime activities
4. Try to induce sleep
5. Reduce potential injury during sleep
6. Provide teaching and referrals as indicated

Intervention

Identifying Causal or Contributing Factors

The causes of sleep disturbance are varied. Sometimes the client will readily identify the cause, e.g., "pain in my leg" or "the man snoring next door." Other times the nurse and client together may be able to identify the causes or contributing factors after reviewing the sleep history.

For hospitalized clients, sleep problems are often related to the hospital environment or their illness. Assisting the client to sleep in such instances can be challenging to a nurse, often involving scheduling activities, administering analgesics, and providing a supportive environment. Explanations and a supportive relationship are essential for the fearful or anxious client.

Examples of Nursing Diagnoses for Clients with Sleep Problems

- Sleep pattern disturbance related to immobility
- Sleep pattern disturbance related to disturbing roommate
- Sleep pattern disturbance related to pain in left leg
- Sleep pattern disturbance related to fear of surgery

Reducing Environmental Distractions and Sleep Interruptions

Environmental distractions are particularly problematic for hospitalized clients. The noises are strange to most clients, and it is usually impossible to eliminate all sounds. Some of the interventions that may help are listed to the right.

To reduce sleep interruptions, nurses can schedule activities so the client has the fewest possible interruptions while resting or sleeping. For example, if a client requires an intramuscular injection during the night, other interventions may be carried out at the same time, such as assessing vital signs or changing a position. Nurses should also avoid waking a sleeping client for unnecessary care, such as to ask if she or he wants a sleeping medication. To help reduce the number of times a client needs to void at night, fluids taken after the dinner meal can be limited. Also, visits just prior to sleeping should be limited and perhaps rescheduled to another time.

Increasing Daytime Activities

Establishing a schedule of daytime actvities can often assist a client. This schedule must consider the client's health status as well as her or his sleep and rest needs. Sometimes clients cannot sleep at night because they sleep too much during the day. If the nurse schedules activities for the daytime, the client remains awake and may be able to sleep better at night. Or the nurse can arrange for other people, during daytime, to communicate with the client or share an activity such as watching television or playing cards. This way a client is often stimulated sufficiently to remain awake.

Helping to Induce Sleep

There are a number of comfort measures that help clients sleep. For the client accustomed to bedtime rituals, such as a soothing bath or a glass of milk, adherence to these rituals is often helpful. Some people read before going to sleep; others like to watch the nighttime news on television. Provided these practices are not contraindicated because of a client's health status, nurses should help clients maintain their habitual practices. Also, sleep is often aided by encouraging or providing hygienic care, such as brushing teeth, partial bath, a clean bed. For example, for the client who has a painful leg, pillows can be provided to support the leg in a comfortable position.

How to Reduce Environmental Distractions

- Close the door of the client's room.
- Pull curtains around the client's bed.
- Unplug the telephone.
- Provide soft music.
- Reduce or eliminate lighting.
- Provide a night light.
- Decrease the amount and type of stimuli, e.g., staff conversations, television.
- Place the client with a compatible roommate.

Reducing the Potential for Injury

Some clients are afraid to go to sleep for fear of rolling off the bed, or they are afraid to walk to the bathroom at night in an unfamiliar environment because of the danger of tripping over furniture. Specific safety measures are listed below.

Health Teaching and Referrals

Health teaching regarding exercise and stress reduction, as appropriate, are important for the client and her or his health status. It is also helpful to enlist support persons in assisting a client to deal with a sleep problem, including interventions that can relieve the symptoms (Carpenito 1983, pp. 444–45). When a client requires further teaching or counseling, the nurse should make the appropriate referral.

Safety Measures

- Use night lights.
- Place the bed in low position.
- Employ side rails if appropriate.
- Place the call bell within easy reach.
- Instruct the client on how to obtain assistance.
- Instruct the client attached to IV tubing or drainage tubing on how to move about.
- Provide long enough tubing to permit the client to move.

Specific Nursing Interventions

Specific nursing interventions should be safe, supportive of healthy sleep patterns and habits, and appropriate to the individual's age.

Age-Appropriate Interventions

Newborns and Infants

1. Provide a firm mattress covered with thick plastic material that cannot be pulled over the face and cause suffocation. A flat surface provides the best alignment for bone development.
2. Avoid pillows. They, too, can cause accidental suffocation.
3. Position the infant appropriately according to age. Newborns should not be placed on their abdomens unless they are observed very closely. They are unable to turn their heads from side to side and may suffocate if their noses press down firmly against the mattress. The side-lying position is safe, but the infant must be shifted from one side to the other every 2 or 3 hours. Alternating the infant's position prevents flattening of the bones of the skull. The back-lying position is also avoided for newborns and young infants, because of the danger that the child may aspirate fluids if he or she vomits. When able to turn the head from side to side, the infant may be positioned on the back, abdomen, or side. It is recommended that various positions be used.
4. Ensure a comfortable room temperature, approximately 18 to 21 C (65 to 70 F) in the daytime and 15.5 to 18 C (60 to 65 F) at night. Place the child away from drafts, and tuck blankets under the mattress to minimize danger of suffocation.
5. Provide soft lighting directed away from the eyes. Sleeping infants dislike both darkness and bright light and like to face a dim light. One way to reposition a sleeping child and still have the child face a stationary light is to place the child's head alternately at the foot and the head of the crib instead of turning the child from left to right.
6. Ensure that the infant is dry and comfortable. Provide dry diapers and warm, soft clothing.
7. Provide quieting activities before putting the infant to bed, such as cuddling or rocking the infant, talking in soothing tones, and establishing consistent routines and a quiet environment.

Toddlers

To promote sleep in toddlers:

1. Provide consistent bedtime or naptime rituals.
2. Adhere firmly to sleeping schedules.
3. Encourage quieting activities before sleep.
4. Support tension-reducing activities, such as head-rolling or talking. Give the child only one toy at bedtime; too many toys are over-stimulating.
5. Never put the toddler to bed as a disciplinary measure.

Preschoolers

Measures to promote sleep and rest in preschoolers are similar to those for toddlers. Preschoolers show increasing independence during the presleep ritual, but must be encouraged to express fears, which also increase at this age. The nurse usually can reassure the child by listening to the child's expressed fears and making it clear that nurses will be nearby.

Sometimes preschoolers have difficulty getting to sleep because they are so highly stimulated. Often they need time to settle down before sleep, for example, a quiet time during which the nurse reads bedtime stories.

If a child fears going to sleep, reassurance that others are nearby will help allay fears. Some children feel less afraid when there is a night light in the room.

School-Age Children

School-age children require considerable rest; however, they often want to stay up longer than is wise. As children grow, they should have a greater say about when to go to bed.

Adolescents

The nurse must sometimes set limits so that hospitalized or ill adolescents get enough rest and sleep. Adolescents often need time before sleep to tend to grooming and personal hygiene, which is frequently important to them.

Adults (Young, Middle-Aged, Elderly)

The following measures frequently help promote the sleep of adults.

1. Help the client relax before sleep by providing diversions, pain relief, a clean, comfortable bed, and an odor-free room.
2. Provide an environment in which clients feel safe and are assured that help is nearby even when they sleep.
3. Provide sufficient covers so the client does not feel cold. Elderly people often need additional covers because normal body temperature drops as people age.

4. Encourage progressive relaxation exercises. These are particularly helpful for persons who have mild or moderate insomnia. See the relaxation techniques described in Chapter 41.
5. Provide a light snack or glass of warm milk before the client sleeps. Milk and most protein foods as well as some vegetables contain an amino acid (L-tryptophan) that is a precursor of the neurotransmitter serotonin. Serotonin is thought to induce and maintain sleep.
6. Provide a hypnotic or sedative if it is ordered by the physician and needed by the client. If the client also requires an analgesic, administer the analgesic before the sedative so she or he feels comfortable when becoming sleepy.
7. Assist the client to his or her normal sleeping position if this is possible.
8. Give the client a backrub to reduce psychologic stress and promote muscular relaxation.

Evaluation

Examples of outcome criteria appropriate for clients who have sleep problems are listed to the right.

Examples of Outcome Criteria for Clients Who Have Sleep Problems

The client will:

- Sleep 8 hours without awakening
- Have restored strength and the energy to walk unaided to the end of the corridor and back
- Describe factors that prevent or inhibit sleep
- Describe techniques that induce sleep
- Demonstrate a balance of rest and activity appropriate to the client's health status

Nursing Care Plan

Assessment Data

Nursing Assessment

Jack Harrison is a 36-year-old police officer assigned to a high-crime police precinct. One week ago he received a surface bullet wound to his arm and has now come to the outpatient clinic to have his wound redressed. While speaking with the nurse, he mentions that he has recently been promoted to the rank of detective and has assumed new responsibilities. He states that since his promotion, he has experienced an increasing amount of difficulty falling asleep and sometimes staying asleep. Mr. Harrison expressed considerable concern over the danger of his occupation and also his desire to do well in his new position. He complains of waking up feeling tired and of becoming quite irritable.

Physical Examination

Height: 185.4 cm (6′1″)
Weight: 85.7 kg (189 lb)
Temperature: 37.0 C (98.6 F)
Pulse rate: 80 BPM
Respirations: 18 per minute at rest
Blood pressure: 144/88 mm Hg
Pale, drawn with dark circles under eyes

Diagnostic Data

CBC within normal range
X-ray film of left arm: Evidence of superficial soft tissue injury

Nursing Diagnosis	Client Goals and Outcome Criteria	Nursing Interventions and Rationales	Evaluation
Sleep pattern disturbance related to anxiety and overstimulation resulting in difficulty falling asleep and remaining asleep, fatigue, irritability, yawning, drawn appearance with dark circles under eyes.	Client Goal: Establish a satisfactory sleep-rest pattern and awaken feeling rested. Outcome Criteria: Describes one or two factors that cause insomnia. Identifies two or three measures that induce sleep. Sleeps 7–8 hours a night by day 14. Demonstrates less irritability and a greater sense of well-being by day 21.	Assist client in identifying factors that cause or contribute to insomnia. *Rationale:* Knowledge of causative factors can enable client to begin to control these factors. Encourage client to establish and maintain a bedtime routine. *Routine:* A routine may assist in inducing sleep. Encourage client to utilize sleep aids such as reading, getting a back rub, or listening to soft music. *Rationale:* This promotes emotional and muscle relaxation. Instruct the client in use of soporifics, e.g., milk and protein foods at bedtime. *Rationale:* Milk and protein foods contain tryptophan, a precursor of serotonin which is thought to induce and maintain sleep. Instruct client in use of relaxation techniques. *Rationale:* Relaxation techniques provide distraction and comfort and induce sleep. Instruct client to avoid caffeine stimulants in the evening before bedtime. *Rationale:* Stimulants inhibit sleep.	Client is able to identify the stress and anxiety of his occupation and promotion as a source of his insomnia. He is practicing relaxation techniques each night at bedtime. Client drinks warm milk at bedtime. He sleeps 7 hours approximately 3–4 days a week and has experienced a greater sense of well-being.
Anxiety (mild) related to promotion and change in socioeconomic status resulting in insomnia, elevated blood pressure, apprehension, and irritability.	Client Goal: Identify source of anxiety and cope effectively with the situation. Outcome Criteria: Recognizes his coping patterns by day 7. Experiences a decrease in insomnia by day 14. Uses effective coping mechanisms.	Assist client in identifying and acknowledging his anxiety/stressors. *Rationale:* Feelings are real, and it is best to bring them out in the open so that they may be worked through. Be available as a listener and provide reassurance and comfort. *Rationale:* Establishes a rapport and allows client to express himself. Assist client with adaptive coping mechanisms, e.g., talking with wife or counselor about problem. *Rationale:* Adaptive coping mechanisms will assist client in dealing effectively with his anxiety/stressors.	Client acknowledges his insomnia is a somatic expression of his anxiety over his new promotion and a fear of failing. Uses coping mechanism of talking with police department counselor when difficulties arise in the department.

Chapter Highlights

- Sleep is a period when a person's level of consciousness is reduced.
- The sleep cycle is controlled by the reticular activating system (RAS) and the bulbar synchronizing region (BSR) in the brain stem.
- During a normal night's sleep a person has four to six sleep cycles, each with five stages—four stages of NREM sleep and a stage of REM sleep.
- NREM (slow-wave) sleep composes most of a sleep cycle.
- The ratio of NREM to REM sleep varies with age.
- Many factors can affect sleep, including psychologic stress, exercise and fatigue, medications, and alcohol.
- Common sleep disorders include insomnia, hypersomnia, parasomnias, narcolepsy, and sleep apnea.
- A sleep history helps the nurse plan interventions to assist clients to sleep.
- People usually develop their own rituals to help prepare them for sleep.
- Pain control and comfort are important for sleeping.
- L-tryptophan, a component of dairy products and meat, may help induce sleep.

Suggested Readings

Fabijan, L., and Gosselin, M. D. April 1982. How to recognize sleep deprivation in your ICU patient and what to do about it. *The Canadian Nurse* 78:20–23.
The authors discuss the key signs of sleep deprivation and make eight related recommendations to incorporate in an intensive care client's nursing care plan.

Hayter, J. March 1980. The rhythm of sleep. *American Journal of Nursing* 80:457–61.
Hayter describes the five stages of sleep, diseases that alter sleep rhythm, and factors related to REM deprivation.

Hoch, C., and Reynolds, 3rd, C. January/February 1986. Sleep disturbances and what to do about them. *Geriatric Nursing* 7:24–27.
Hoch and Reynolds describe the normal sleep cycle and potential altered sleep–wake patterns. Included is how physical illness, psychologic factors, and medications can affect sleep. Sleep assessment is covered, as are nursing interventions that aid sleep. Specific reference is made to elderly clients.

Selected References

Bahr, R. T. October 1983. Sleep–wake patterns in the aged. *Journal of Gerontological Nursing* 9:534–37, 540–41.

Bellack, J. P., and Bamford, P. A. 1984. *Nursing assessment. A multidimensional approach.* Monterey, Calif.: Wadsworth Health Sciences Div.

Block, A. J. November/December 1980. Respiratory disorders during sleep. Part I. *Heart and Lung* 9:1011–24.

Carpenito, L. J. 1983. *Nursing diagnosis. Application to clinical practice.* Philadelphia: J. B. Lippincott Co.

Crisp, A. N., and Stonehill, E. 1976. *Sleep, nutrition and mood.* New York: John Wiley and Sons.

Deters, G. E. July/August 1980. Circadian rhythm phenomenon. *Maternal Child Nursing* 5:249–51.

Edgil, A. E.; Wood, K. R.; and Smith, D. P. March/April 1985. Sleep problems of older infants and preschool children, *Pediatric Nursing* 11:87–89.

Guyton, A. C. 1986. *Textbook of medical physiology.* 7th ed. Philadelpha: W. B. Saunders Co.

Hayter, J. March/April 1985. To nap or not to nap? *Geriatric Nursing* 6:104–6.

———. July/August 1983. Sleep behaviors of older persons. *Nursing Research* 32:242–46.

———. March 1980. The rhythm of sleep. *American Journal of Nursing* 80:457–61.

Malasanos, L.; Barkauskas, V.; Moss, M.; and Stoltenberg-Allen, K. 1986. *Health assessment.* 3d ed. St. Louis: C. V. Mosby Co.

Miles, L. E., and Dement, W. C. 1980. Sleep and aging. *Sleep* 3(2):119–20.

Milne, B. April 1982. Sleep–wake disorders and what we can do about them. *The Canadian Nurse* 78:24–27.

Narrow, B. W. August 1967. Rest is . . . *American Journal of Nursing* 67:1646–49.

Oswald, I. March 13, 1980. Sleep: No place for the worried. *Nursing Mirror* 150:34–35.

Schirmer, M. S. January 1983. When sleep won't come. *Journal of Gerontological Nursing* 9:16–21.

Walsleben, J. June 1982. Sleep disorders. *American Journal of Nursing* 82:936–40.

Weaver, T., and Millman, R. P. February 1986. Broken sleep. *American Journal of Nursing* 86:146–50.

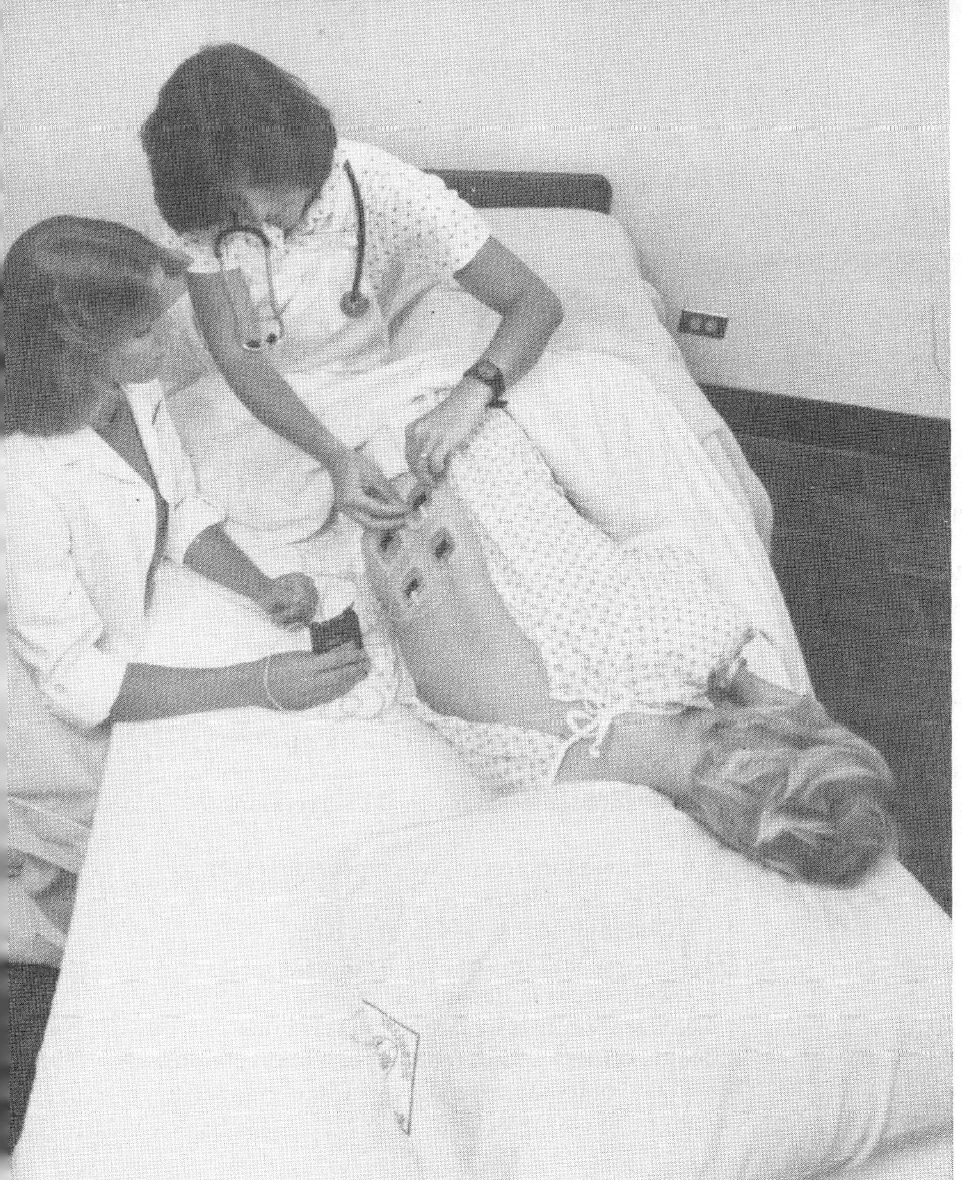

CHUCK SAVADELIS

CHAPTER **41**

Pain

Contents

41 *Pain*

Objectives

1. Know essential facts about pain physiology, perception, and response.
   1.1 Identify various types of pain.
   1.2 Describe pain pathways to the brain.
   1.3 Describe three theories of pain perception.
   1.4 Describe the relationship of endogenous opioids to pain perception.
   1.5 Contrast *pain threshold* and *pain tolerance*.
   1.6 Identify physiologic manifestations of the response to pain.
2. Know information required to assess a client's pain.
   2.1 Identify characteristics by which pain is assessed.
   2.2 Identify essential facts to obtain for a pain history.
   2.3 Identify factors influencing the experience of pain.
3. Understand essential facts about interventions to relieve pain.
   3.1 Explain how to decrease factors that amplify the pain experience.
   3.2 Explain methods used to reduce pain intensity.
   3.3 Explain how distraction relieves pain.
   3.4 Identify situations in which relaxation techniques can relieve pain effectively.
   3.5 Identify essential steps of one relaxation technique.
   3.6 Explain essential aspects of the conscious-suggestion technique.
   3.7 Identify selected skin stimulation techniques used to relieve pain.
   3.8 Identify major types of analgesics.
   3.9 Identify the rationale for using placebos and four ways of maximizing a positive response to them.
   3.10 Identify two drugs commonly used to control intractable cancer pain.
   3.11 Outline essential guidelines for pain management.
   3.12 Identify selected medical interventions to control pain.
4. Apply the nursing process when providing care to selected clients experiencing pain.
   4.1 Obtain necessary assessment data.
   4.2 Analyze and relate assessment data.
   4.3 Write relevant nursing diagnoses.
   4.4 Plan appropriate nursing interventions.
   4.5 Implement appropriate nursing interventions.
   4.6 State outcome criteria by which to evaluate a client's progress.

Terms

acute pain
aching pain
acupuncture
analgesic
biofeedback
burning pain
chronic pain
cordotomy
distraction
dorsal column stimulator
dynorphins
endogenous opioid
endorphins
enkephalins
hyperalgesia
narcotic
narcotic agonist-antagonist
nerve block
neurectomy
nociceptor
pain threshold
pain tolerance
percutaneous electric stimulator
peripheral nerve implant
phantom pain
potentiator
psychogenic (functional) pain
pricking pain
referred pain
rhizotomy
slow pain
somatogenic (organic) pain
substance P
sympathectomy
transcutaneous electric stimulation

Nature of Pain

Pain is a highly unpleasant and very personal sensation that cannot be shared with others. It can occupy all of one's thinking, direct one's activities, and change one's life. Pain often is an important sign that something is physiologically wrong, e.g., tissues are damaged. As such, pain is useful because it prompts the client to seek help for a health problem that might otherwise go unnoticed. Pain is usually accompanied by other bodily sensations, such as pressure, heat, or perhaps cold. Engel (1970, p. 45) defines pain as "a basically unpleasant sensation referred to the body which represents the suffering induced by the psychic perception of real, threatened, or phantasized injury."

McCaffery (1979, p. 11) defines pain as "whatever the experiencing person says it is, existing whenever he says it does." Basic to this definition is the caregiver's willingness to believe the client's pain.

Types of Pain

Pain can be described as either acute or chronic. **Acute pain** is generally of relatively short duration, such as the pain of a fracture or abdominal surgery. A client with acute pain normally exhibits one or two of the following clinical signs: increased perspiration, increased cardiac rate or blood pressure, and pallor. Clients may respond to acute pain by crying, moaning, or rubbing the painful area, although the absence of these behaviors does not mean a client is not experiencing pain. **Chronic pain** develops more slowly and lasts much longer than acute pain, and sufferers may find it difficult to remember when such pain first started. Clients with chronic pain may present few if any clinical signs of pain. Some find a way to handle the pain or are so accustomed to it that their reaction is minimal.

Pain has also been described as either somatogenic or psychogenic. **Somatogenic**, or **organic**, **pain** has a physical origin, whereas **psychogenic**, or **functional**, **pain** has a psychic or mental origin. Most people with localized pain experience a combination of somatogenic and psychogenic pain. Acute pain is frequently associated with anxiety, whereas chronic pain is associated with reactive depression (McCaffery 1979, p. 16). Anxiety and depression generally exacerbate pain.

Intractable pain is resistant to cure or relief. An example is the pain of arthritis, for which narcotic analgesics are contraindicated because of the long duration of the disease and the risk of addiction. Behavior modification is used in some cases of intractable pain. Behavior that is not pain-oriented is rewarded, and pain-oriented behavior is ignored. The aim of this technique is to change behavior so the client can live more comfortably and productively.

Guyton (1986, p. 592) classifies pain into two types: acute pain and slow pain. **Acute pain** occurs within 0.1 second of the application of a pain stimulus. Guyton also describes acute pain by names such as **pricking pain** and sharp pain, which is the type of pain felt when a needle is inserted into the skin or a knife cuts the skin. Acute sharp pain is seldom felt in the deeper tissues of the body (Guyton 1986, p. 592).

Slow pain begins a second or more after a pain stimulus is applied and increases slowly over a period of seconds or even minutes. Slow pain can be described as **burning pain**, **aching pain**, throbbing pain, nauseous pain, or chronic pain. This type of pain is associated with tissue destruction and can occur, according to Guyton (1986, p. 592), in the skin or in deeper tissues of the body.

Sometimes a client feels pain in an area other than the site of the source of the pain. This is called **referred pain**. For example, cardiac pain may be felt radiating to the left shoulder and down the left arm, or the pain from an inflamed appendix may be felt throughout the abdomen. Referred pain is the result of a synapse between nerve fibers that carry the pain impulses in the spinal cord and neurons that carry pain impulses from the skin. Thus the individual perceives the pain as originating in the skin or internal tissues.

Phantom pain is pain felt in a body part that is no longer present, such as an amputated foot. It is thought that stimulation of a severed dendrite rather than stimulation of the usual receptor causes the individual to perceive the pain in the removed part.

Pain Threshold and Pain Tolerance

An individual's **pain threshold** is the amount of pain stimulation a person requires before feeling pain. A person's pain threshold is generally fairly uniform, although it can be dramatically altered by the person's state of consciousness. For instance, an anesthetized client feels no pain; an unconscious client may or may not react to suborbital pressure, that is, pain on the lower aspect of the eye. Reaction to suborbital pressure is, in fact, one way to test a person's level of consciousness. It is also possible for a person's pain threshold to change. For example, the same stimuli that once produced mild pain can produce intense pain. Such excessive sensitivity to pain is called **hyperalgesia.**

Pain tolerance is the maximum amount and duration of pain that an individual is willing to endure. Some clients are unwilling to tolerate even the slightest pain, whereas others are willing to endure severe pain rather than be treated for it.

Initiation of Pain

The skin and other body tissues have pain receptors. The skin, certain internal tissues such as the periosteum, the joint surfaces, and the arterial walls have many receptors, whereas most other deep tissues have few pain receptors. The alveoli of the lungs have no pain receptors.

A pain receptor, called a **nociceptor**, is stimulated either directly by damage to the receptor cell or secondarily by the release of chemicals such as bradykinin, histamine, prostaglandins, acids, and potassium ions from the damaged tissues. Basically, there are three types of

Table 41–1 Types of Pain Stimuli

Stimulus Type	Physiologic Basis
Mechanical	
1. Trauma to body tissues, e.g., surgery	Tissue damage; direct irritation of the pain receptors; inflammation
2. Alterations in body tissues, e.g., edema	Pressure on pain receptors
3. Blockage of a body duct	Distention of the lumen of the duct
4. Tumor	Pressure on pain receptors; irritation of nerve endings
5. Muscle spasm	Stimulation of pain receptors (also see *Chemical*)
Thermal	
Extreme heat or cold, e.g., burns	Tissue destruction; stimulation of thermosensitive pain receptors
Chemical	
1. Tissue ischemia, e.g., blocked coronary artery	Stimulation of pain receptors because of accumulated lactic acid (and possibly other chemicals, such as bradykinin) in tissues
2. Muscle spasm	Secondary to mechanical stimulation (see above), causing tissue ischemia

stimuli that excite corresponding types of nociceptors: mechanical, thermal, and chemical. See Table 41–1.

Pain signals are transmitted along two types of fibers: delta type A fibers and type C fibers. Type A fibers transmit the signal relatively quickly, i.e., between 6 and 30 meters per second. It is thought that type A fibers chiefly transmit sharp pain. Type C fibers transmit signals more slowly, i.e., 0.5 to 2 meters per second, and it is believed they transmit burning and aching pain. Therefore, a sudden pain can give a double sensation: a sharp, fast pain sensation followed by a slow burning sensation. The latter tends to become more painful over time (Guyton 1986, p. 594).

Pain fibers enter the spinal cord through the dorsal roots. From there they ascend or descend one or two cord segments to terminate in neurons in the dorsal horns of the gray matter called the *substantia gelatinosa.* Type A fibers terminate in the gray matter of laminae I and V, type C fibers in that of laminae II and III. Most signals pass through one or more neurons before reaching long-fibered neurons that cross to the opposite side of the cord. The stimulus then passes upward via the anterolateral spinothalamic tract to the brain. See Figure 41–1.

Both the slow and fast fibers are differentiated in the lateral spinothalamic tract. Both types of pain fiber enter the brain stem. About 75% to 90% of all acute, fast pain fibers terminate in the reticular formation of the medulla, pons, and mesencephalon. From there some of the acute fast fibers connect with higher-order neurons, transmitting the pain signals to the thalamus, hypothalamus, and other areas of the diencephalon and cerebrum. See Figure 41–2.

Almost all of the slow chronic fibers terminate in the reticular formation. However, some signals are relayed to the thalamus. Because these fibers activate the reticular system, they arouse the entire nervous system, even when a person is asleep (Guyton 1986, p. 596).

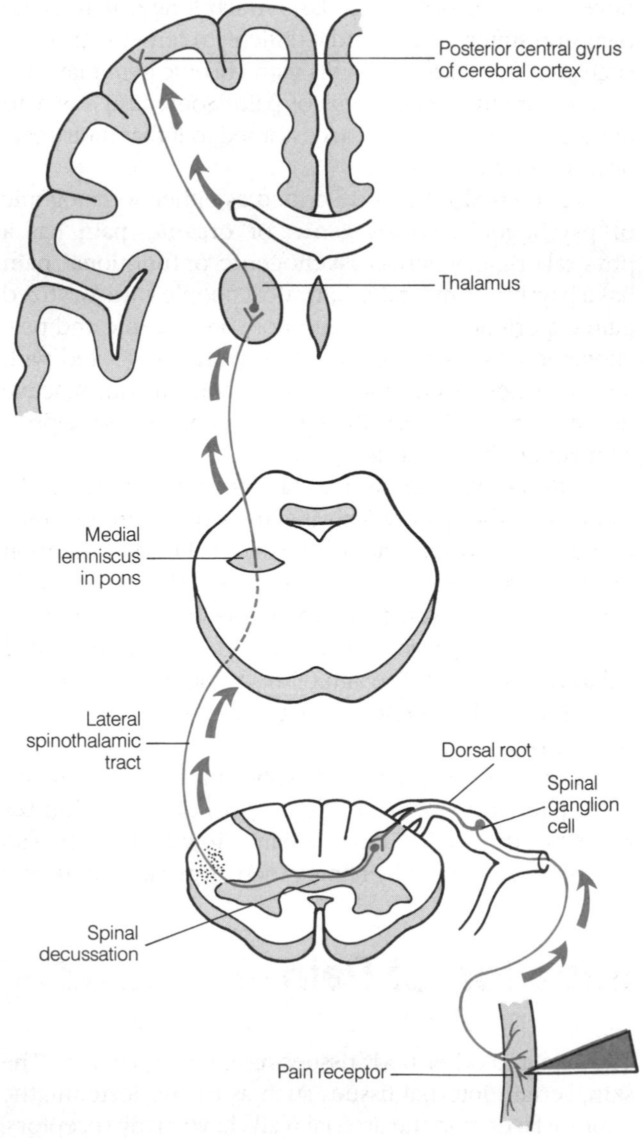

Figure 41–1 Acute pain pathway

There is also a proprioceptive reflex that occurs with the stimulation of pain receptors. Impulses travel along sensory pain fibers to the spinal cord. There they synapse with motor neurons, and the impulses travel back via motor fibers to a muscle near the site of the pain. See Figure 41–3. The muscle then contracts in a protective action. For example, when a person touches a hot stove the hand reflexively draws back from the heat even before the person is aware of the pain.

Pain Perception

Pain perception involves both physiologic and psychosocial factors. Consequently, individuals vary widely in their perception of pain; for instance, some people perceive a cut finger as exceedingly painful, whereas others hardly notice such a cut.

Physiologic Factors

Pain impulses that originate at a nociceptor travel to the spinal cord and up the lateral spinothalamic tract to the reticular formation of the medulla, pons, and mesencephalon. From there some impulses continue to the cerebrum, which makes the individual consciously aware of the pain—its location, severity and type. The stimulation of the reticular formation arouses the person to the pain and motivates the individual to take steps in response. The involvement of the cerebrum permits the individual to know about the pain.

Theories of Pain Perception

There are a number of theories that explain how pain is transmitted and perceived, including the pattern theory, and specificity theory, and the gate-control theory.

Pattern theory The *pattern theory* actually combines several pain concepts. According to this theory the pain impulses generated by the nociceptors form a pattern or code that conveys to the central nervous system information that a particular pain is present. A key concept in this theory is that, following tissue injury, circuits can be established in the spinal interneurons that enable the pain to be perceived even though the stimuli that initiated the pain are no longer present. This *reverberating circuit* might explain phantom pain.

Specificity theory The *specificity theory,* which originated about 200 years ago, assumes that pain travels from a specific nociceptor to a pain center in the brain. Although this theory helps in understanding the transmission of impulses along pathways, in light of current knowledge it appears to have limitations. First of all it assumes that specific fibers carry pain impulses only; however, research has shown that the nerve fibers that carry pain impulses also carry pressure and temperature sensations (Nursing Now 1985, p. 16). Two other assumptions of this theory are in conflict with current research: it assumes a direct relationship between the intensity of the pain stimulus and the perceived intensity of pain; and it assumes that only one structure in the brain is involved in a pain response. In addition, this theory does not explain the psychologic factors involved in pain (see following section).

Gate-control theory In 1965, Melzack and Wall proposed the *gate-control theory* (Melzack and Wall 1982, p. 232). According to this theory, the synapses in the dorsal horns act as gates that close to keep impulses from reaching the brain or open to permit impulses to ascend to the brain. Melzack and Wall further hypothesize that when there are a great number of impulses along the thick nerve fibers, which carry impulses of heat, cold, touch, etc., the gates close to the pain impulses on the thinner fibers, thus blocking the pain. (Pain impulses are thought to travel along these thinner fibers.) Only when the synaptic gates are open, as when impulses on the pain fibers predominate, does the person feel pain.

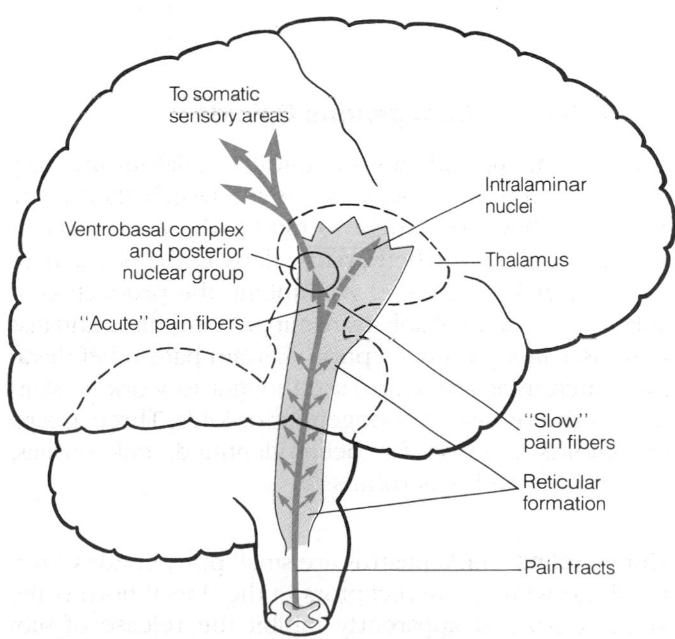

Figure 41–2 Transmission of pain signals to the higher brain centers. Redrawn from *Textbook of Medical Physiology* by A. C. Guyton. © 1986 W. B. Saunders Company, p. 595.

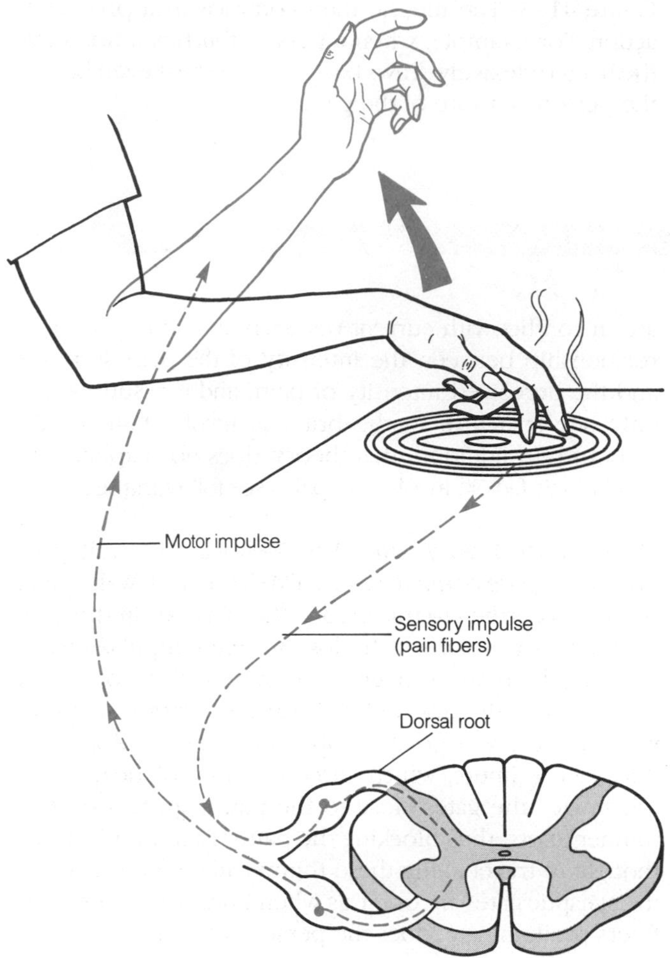

Figure 41–3 Protective reflex to a pain stimulus

The Effects of Endogenous Opioids

Endogenous opioids are chemical regulators that may modify pain. Their exact action is still largely theoretical; however, they are thought to bind with opiate receptor sites throughout the body, particularly in the dorsal horn of the spinal cord, thereby inhibiting the production of substances that probably transmit pain impulses and that may also alter pain perception. Certain pain relief therapies, such as acupuncture, are thought to work by stimulating the release of endogenous opioids. Three groups of opioids have so far been identified: enkephalins, endorphins, and dynorphins.

Enkephalins **Enkephalins** are small polypeptides. They combine with opiate receptors in the dorsal horn of the spinal cord and apparently inhibit the release of substance P. **Substance P** is a neurotransmitter that acts to enhance transmission of pain impulses across synapses. Enkephalins are also found outside the spinal cord—in the brain stem, limbic system, hypothalamus, adrenal glands, and gastrointestinal tract.

Endorphins **Endorphins** are larger polypeptides. They may be synthesized and stored by the pituitary gland. They are also found in the hypothalamus, midbrain, and limbic system of the central nervous system. There are several subgroups of endorphins, including beta-endorphins, which are highly concentrated in the hypothalamus and pituitary gland. The beta-endorphins have been found to be more potent than the enkephalins.

Dynorphins **Dynorphins**, only recently discovered, are compounds found in the pituitary gland, hypothalamus, and spinal cord. They seem to have an analgesic effect, one that is 50 times greater than that of the beta-endorphins.

Psychosocial Factors

Numerous psychosocial factors can affect a person's perception of pain. These include past experience, values regarding pain, family expectations, environment, emotions, and a person's culture.

Past Experience

Past experience can certainly influence a person's present perception of pain. It is known that people who have had previous experience with pain, either their own or that of a significant other, are more threatened by anticipated pain than people who have had no such pain experience (Nursing Now 1985, p. 20). In addition, clients often view interventions in light of past experience. For example, a client who in the past has found certain analgesics to be ineffective is likely to have little faith in their effectiveness in the present. Or, if a client has had prior experience with severe pain, she or he may perceive a present pain as less intense, even though another person with a similar injury might perceive severe pain.

Values

How a client values pain can also affect her or his perceptions and responses. If a person views pain as a weakness or a necessary evil, she or he may withstand the pain well. If benefits are associated with the pain, e.g., absence from a distasteful job or sympathy from a spouse, then the pain will most likely be tolerated well. On the other hand, if a client perceives the pain as unnecessary or as a threat to her or his comfort, well-being, or valued lifestyle, it will likely be tolerated less well.

Family Expectations

Family expectations can affect a person's perceptions of and responses to pain. In many cultures, for example, girls are permitted to express pain more openly than boys. Family role can also affect how a person perceives or responds to pain. For instance, a single mother supporting three children may ignore pain because of her need to stay on the job. The presence of support persons often changes a client's reaction to pain. For example, toddlers tolerate pain more readily when supportive parents or nurses are nearby. Adults, too, handle pain better when supportive, trusted people are present.

Environment

An individual's environment affects pain perception and response. For instance, the woman entertaining her husband's co-workers at home may have decreased perceptions and responses to the pain while the guests are present; but in a hospital she may perceive the pain as more severe and respond more openly.

Emotions

Emotions influence the perception of pain. Think of the client so absorbed in playing basketball that he or she may be unaware of the pain of an injury until after the game is over. On the other hand, a person who is bored or depressed is more likely to think about his or her pain and be more aware of it. Also, a highly anxious client is more likely to have a heightened perception of pain, and a less anxious person will tolerate pain more effectively.

Culture

Response to pain is in part culturally determined; thus, the meaning of pain and the expected interventions vary from culture to culture. A number of research studies in the 1950s and 1960s indicate that culture affects a person's tolerance and reaction to pain. Some groups, such as native American Indians and the Chinese, were found to respond stoically to pain. Other groups, such as Italians and Jews, tended to react more expressively (Blaylock 1968, p. 270).

More recently it has been recognized that although culture has a role to play in a person's perceptions of and reactions to pain, generalizations about an individual client should not be made. A multicultural society influences individuals in many ways, and although a knowledge of cultural orientation to pain can be helpful, each client should be assessed individually.

It is important that nurses recognize the wide variety of learned responses considered appropriate by different cultural groups. For instance, the stoical response to pain is largely accepted in North American society; however, because of the many ethnic groups in North America, nurses will observe a variety of responses to pain, none of which should be judged as good or bad. It is also true that a stoical person probably will not tell the nurse when he or she is in pain, making nonverbal clues important during assessment.

Pain Response

The body's response to pain occurs in three stages: activation, rebound, and adaptation.

Activation

After pain is first perceived, the body assumes a fight-or-flight reaction, initiated by the sympathetic nervous system. See Table 41–2 and Chapter 17 for further information.

Rebound

During the rebound stage, the pain experienced is intense but brief. It is at this stage that the parasympathetic nervous system takes over. Its effects, the opposite of the sympathetic system's, include decreased cardiac rate and decreased blood pressure.

Adaptation

When pain is long-lasting, the physiologic response is adaptation, i.e., a decreased sympathetic response. Adaptation may be due to endorphins counteracting the pain; see the earlier discussion of pain perception. The body experiences a general adaptive reaction when the pain lasts for many hours or days. See the section on the general adaptation syndrome, Chapter 17, page 336, and Figure 17–5, page 338, for current concepts of physiologic reactions to stress.

Changes in body chemistry due to pain influence a person's behavior. The secretion of excessive norepinephrine causes the individual to feel powerful, in control, confident, and excited. However, when norepinephrine is depleted—for example, when the pain is prolonged—the individual may feel helpless, worthless,

Table 41–2 Responses to Pain

Sympatho-Adrenal Responses	Muscular Responses	Emotional Responses
Increased pulse rate	Increased muscle tension or rigidity	Excitement
Increased systolic blood pressure	Writhing	Irritability
Increased respiratory rate	Restlessness	Behavior change
Excessive perspiration	Knees drawn up to abdomen or other unusual postures	Extreme quietness
Nausea and vomiting due to blood flow shift from viscera to muscles of the lungs, heart, and striated body muscles	Rubbing	Groaning
Pallor	Scratching	Crying
Bronchial dilation	Immobility	Increased alertness
Conversion of stored glycogen to glucose		
Release of erythrocytes from the spleen		
Pupil dilation		

and lethargic. Stimulation of the inhibitory system increases the production of serotonin. This reaction is seen in clients after they meditate or take narcotics. The individual feels secure, serene, and safe. Depleted serotonin levels, seen in clients with chronic pain, produce tension, agitation, anxiety, hypersensitivity, and a variety of sleep disorders (Booker 1982, p. 49). Clients with depleted levels of both norepinephrine and serotonin may demonstrate agitated depression. In addition, depression may be aggravated by narcotics, which block the norepinephrine and serotonin receptor sites in the central nervous system (Booker 1982, p. 49).

Assessment

Assessment relative to pain should include a pain history and clinical signs and symptoms of pain.

Pain History

It is important for nurses to obtain from the client a history of pain experience, including pain location, intensity, and duration. The nurse can establish how long the client had experienced the pain; what effects the pain had on normal activity; how the pain occurred, e.g., quickly or slowly; and what events precipitated it. The history should also include a description of measures employed in the past to relieve pain. An outline of a pain history is shown to the right.

While taking the pain history, the nurse must include an opportunity for the client to express in his or her own words how the client views the pain and the situation. This will help the nurse understand what the pain means to the client and how the client is coping with it. Copp (1985, p. 69) sees a relationship between different coper types, their self-image, and the way each type describes their pain.

Pain History

- Location
- Intensity
- Quality, e.g., aching, piercing
- Time of onset and duration
- Precipitating factors
- Associated symptoms
- Effect on activities of daily living
- Measures taken to relieve pain
- Analgesics history

Clinical Signs and Symptoms

Assessment of the clinical signs and symptoms of a client's pain should include: pain location, intensity, time of onset and duration, quality, behavioral response, precipitating factors, associated symptoms, effect of the pain on activities of daily living, measures used to relieve pain, and coping resources.

Location

Superficial pain usually can be located quite accurately by a client; however, pain arising from the viscera is perceived more generally. Nurses need to ascertain where the client experiences pain. The various body landmarks for describing pain location are shown in Chapter 35. In addition, the nurse needs to use such terms as *proximal, distal, medial,* and *lateral* when describing the location of pain. See Chapter 37. The term *diffuse pain* refers to pain perceived over a large area.

When assessing the location of a child's pain, the nurse needs to understand the child's vocabulary. For example, *tummy* might refer to the abdomen or part of the chest. It is wise for a nurse to ask a child to point to the pain rather than to rely on the child's description, which may be highly idiosyncratic. Parents can help nurses interpret the meaning of a child's words. Observing when a smaller child or baby cries in response to movement can help the nurse establish the location of a baby's pain.

Intensity

The intensity or severity of pain is also important. Although this is subjective, it is also true that certain tissues are more sensitive than others. Several factors affect the perception of intensity. One is amount of distraction, or the client's concentration on another event; a second is the client's state of consciousness, and a third is the person's expectations.

Pain may be described as slight, mild, medium, severe, or excruciating. Two simple descriptive scales are shown in Figure 41–4. The client is asked to indicate the scale point that best represents her or his pain intensity. It is very important to note and report any change in intensity described by the client, which may indicate a change in the client's pathologic condition. For example, the abrupt cessation of acute abdominal pain may indicate a ruptured appendix.

A client's reports of pain must be considered in relation to the client's ability and need to report. The elderly or confused may distort the intensity of pain; a child may minimize pain to avoid admission to the hospital or unpleasant tests. The pain ruler shown in Figure 41–5 was designed to assist clients in describing the intensity of their pain.

0 1 2 3 4 5 6 7 8 9

No pain — Moderate pain — Severe pain

No pain	Mild pain	Moderate pain	Severe pain	Unbearable pain

Figure 41–4 Two simple descriptive pain-intensity scales

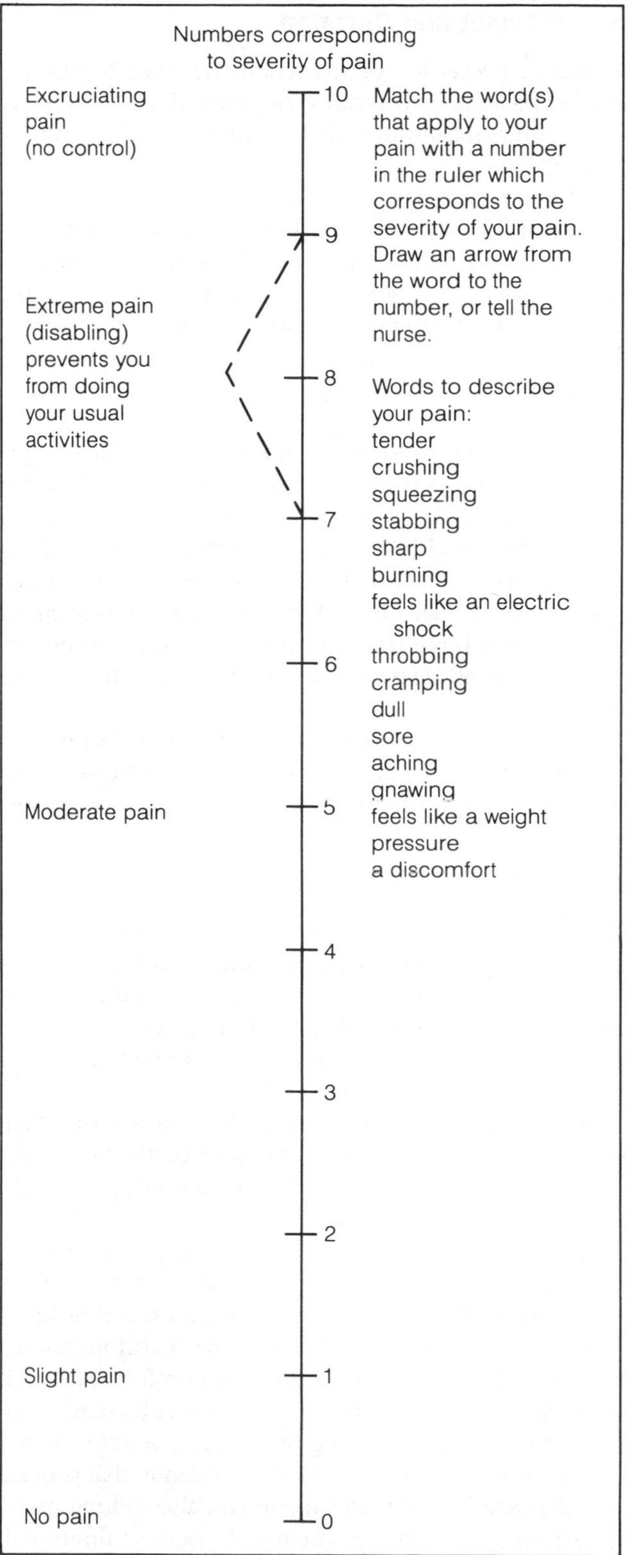

Figure 41–5 The pain ruler. Clients match the words that describe their pain to a number that corresponds to the intensity of their pain.

Source: F. Bourbonnais, "Pain assessment: Development of a tool for the nurse and the patient," *Journal of Advanced Nursing,* 1981, 6:280. Reprinted with permission of Blackwell Scientific Publications Ltd.

Time of Onset and Duration

The nurse needs to record when the pain began; how long the pain lasts; whether it recurs and, if so, the length of the interval without pain; and when the pain last occurred.

The interval between pains can be very important. For example, the intervals between labor contractions help the maternity nurse assess the client's progress in labor. As birth becomes more imminent, labor pains become more frequent and more severe.

Quality

Descriptive adjectives help people communicate the quality of pain. Clients use the terms they know: A headache may be described as "hammerlike" or an abdominal pain as "piercing like a knife." Sometimes clients have difficulty describing pain because they have never experienced any sensation like it. This is particularly true of children, and of adults who have pain originating within the nervous system. Some of the terms used to describe pain are listed on the right.

Nurses need to record the exact words clients use to describe pain. A client's words are more accurate and descriptive than an interpretation in the nurse's words.

Terms That Describe Pain Quality

- Aching
- Burning
- Constant
- Cramping
- Crushing
- Cutting
- Diffuse
- Dull
- Excruciating
- Gnawing
- Hammering
- Heavy
- Intermittent (spasmodic)
- Irritating
- Jabbing
- Knifelike
- Knotting
- Lancing
- Piercing
- Pinching
- Pounding
- Prickly
- Radiating
- Searing
- Sharp
- Shifting
- Squeezing
- Stabbing
- Tearing
- Throbbing
- Tingling
- Viselike

Behavioral Response

Behavioral responses are of particular importance in assessing pain experienced by clients unable to communicate verbally. The very young, the aphasic, and confused or disoriented persons often communicate their experience of pain only nonverbally. There are several types of nonverbal behavior to watch for.

Facial expression is often the first indication of pain and may be the only one. Clenched teeth, tightly shut eyes, open somber eyes, biting of the lower lip, and other facial grimaces are indicative of pain.

Body movement can help the nurse assess pain. Immobilization of the body or a part of the body may indicate pain. The client with chest pain often holds the left arm across the chest. A person with abdominal pain may assume the position of greatest comfort, often with the knees and hips flexed, and move reluctantly. Even babies flex their hips and legs when experiencing abdominal pain, although they tend not to remain in that position.

Purposeless body movements can also indicate pain—for example, tossing and turning in bed or flinging the arms about. Involuntary movements such as a reflexive jerking away from a needle inserted through the skin indicate pain. An adult may be able to control this reflex; however, a child may be unable or unwilling to do so.

Rhythmic body movements or rubbing may indicate pain. The teething baby likes to chew on an object; an adult or child may assume a fetal position and rock back and forth when experiencing abdominal pain. During labor a woman may massage her abdomen rhythmically with her hands.

Speech and vocal pitch can help the nurse assess pain. Rapid speech and elevated pitch reflect anxiety, and slow speech and monotonous tone can signal intense pain. For additional information on nonverbal behavior see Chapter 27.

Precipitating Factors

The nurse needs to report any factors that precipitate pain. Certain activities sometimes precede pain; for example, physical exertion may precede chest pain, or abdominal pain may occur after eating. These observations are helpful not only in preventing the pain but also in determining its cause.

Environmental factors can increase pain in those who are well or ill. Extreme cold or heat and extremes of humidity can affect some types of pain. For example, sudden exercise on a hot day can cause muscle spasm.

Physical and emotional stressors can precipitate pain. Emotional tension frequently brings on a migraine headache. Intense fear or physical exertion can cause angina.

Associated Symptoms

Also included in the clinical appraisal of pain are any other associated symptoms, such as vomiting, dizziness, and constipation. Sometimes clients experience such a symptom immediately prior to the pain.

Effect on Activities of Daily Living

Knowing how activities of daily living are affected by the pain helps the nurse understand the client's perspective on the pain's severity. A number of tools have been developed to assist the nurse with this assessment, including a scale measuring the effects of pain on daily life. See Table 41–3.

Table 41–3 Scale for Assessing the Effects of Pain on Daily Life

On a scale of 0 (no pain) to 5 (maximum pain) the client should indicate the areas of life (listed below) currently affected and the severity of the interference. If the client's current level of pain is less than that usually felt, the client should be asked to rate the most pain ever experienced in these areas.

Sleep	Home activities
Appetite	Driving/walking
Concentration	Leisure activities
Work/school	Emotional status (mood, irritability, depression, anxiety)
Interpersonal relationships	
Marital relations/sex	

Source: From E. Matassarin-Jacobs, unpublished presentation, "Pain Assessment," Chicago, Illinois, May 1981. Used by permission.

Measures for Relieving Pain

Included in this area of assessment are analgesics taken, rest, and applications of heat or cold. The nurse should also explore how long such measures were employed before relief was obtained and whether they had any effect at all or even made the pain worse. The McGill-Melzack Pain Questionnaire (see Figure 41–6) is meant to assess a client's level of pain and the effectiveness of pain interventions.

Coping Resources

Clients sometimes learn highly effective ways of coping with pain. These methods may modify the pain to such a degree that assessment of pain will be incomplete unless the nurse is aware of them. For example, a client may tell a nurse that his abdominal pain lasted only a few minutes and neglect to say that he took an antacid when the pain started.

People in pain often display coping strategies and styles learned in childhood (Copp 1985, p. 69). When a person experiences pain, she or he must acknowledge vulnerability, which threatens some people more than others. The person coping with pain may see himself or herself as victim, combatant, responder, reactor, or interactor (Copp 1985, p. 69).

Nursing Diagnosis

Examples of nursing diagnoses for clients experiencing pain can be found to the right. By identifying the specific kind of pain, the location, and any implications, the nurse becomes better able to plan nursing interventions. For example, for a client diagnosed as having a self-care deficit related to inability to move the arms secondary to shoulder joint pain, the nurse can help arrange the client's bathing, dressing, and eating practices to accommodate the pain.

Examples of Nursing Diagnoses for Clients Experiencing Pain

- Alterations in comfort: acute pain related to fracture of the right hip
- Alterations in comfort: chronic pain related to arthritis
- Impaired mobility related to pain in right foot
- Self-care deficit related to inability to move arms secondary to pain in shoulder joints

Planning

The overall client goals for the client experiencing pain include:

1. Reducing or eliminating factors that augment the pain experience
2. Learning noninvasive techniques to modify the pain experience
3. Learning about measures for optimal pain relief, e.g., prescribed analgesics

Figure 41–6 **A,** McGill Pain Questionnaire. The descriptors fall into four major groups: sensory, 1 to 10; affective, 11 to 15; evaluative, 16; and miscellaneous, 17 to 20. The rank value of each descriptor is based on its position in the word set. The sum of the rank values is the pain rating index (PRI). The present pain intensity (PPI) is based on a scale of 0 to 5. **B,** Spatial display of pain descriptors based on intensity ratings by clients. The intensity scale values range from 1 (mild) to 5 (excruciating).

Source: A and B reprinted with permission from: R. Melzack, *Pain measurement and assessment.* (New York: Raven, 1983).

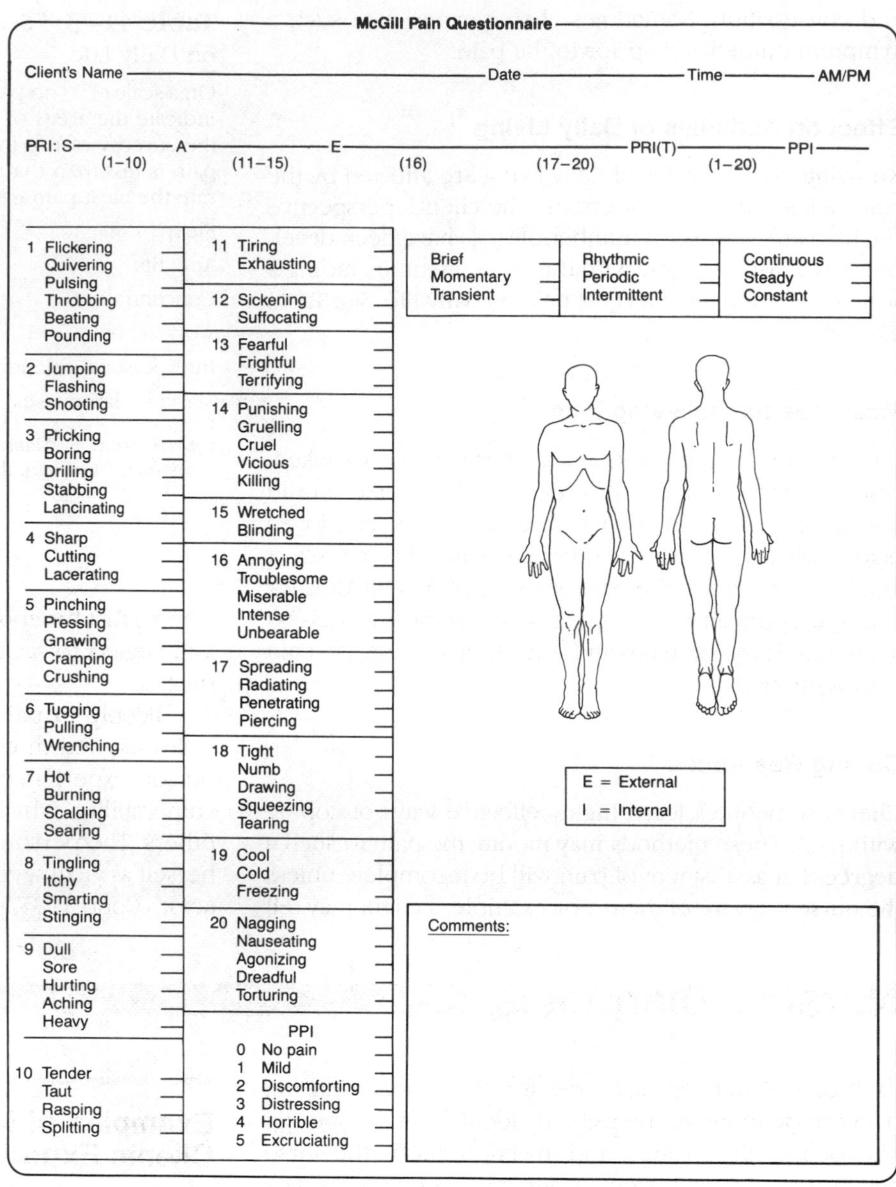
McGill Pain Questionnaire
Client's Name ______ Date ______ Time ______ AM/PM
PRI: S ______ A ______ E ______ ______ PRI(T) ______ PPI ______
(1–10) (11–15) (16) (17–20) (1–20)

1 Flickering, Quivering, Pulsing, Throbbing, Beating, Pounding
2 Jumping, Flashing, Shooting
3 Pricking, Boring, Drilling, Stabbing, Lancinating
4 Sharp, Cutting, Lacerating
5 Pinching, Pressing, Gnawing, Cramping, Crushing
6 Tugging, Pulling, Wrenching
7 Hot, Burning, Scalding, Searing
8 Tingling, Itchy, Smarting, Stinging
9 Dull, Sore, Hurting, Aching, Heavy
10 Tender, Taut, Rasping, Splitting
11 Tiring, Exhausting
12 Sickening, Suffocating
13 Fearful, Frightful, Terrifying
14 Punishing, Gruelling, Cruel, Vicious, Killing
15 Wretched, Blinding
16 Annoying, Troublesome, Miserable, Intense, Unbearable
17 Spreading, Radiating, Penetrating, Piercing
18 Tight, Numb, Drawing, Squeezing, Tearing
19 Cool, Cold, Freezing
20 Nagging, Nauseating, Agonizing, Dreadful, Torturing

PPI
0 No pain
1 Mild
2 Discomforting
3 Distressing
4 Horrible
5 Excruciating

Brief, Momentary, Transient
Rhythmic, Periodic, Intermittent
Continuous, Steady, Constant

E = External
I = Internal

Comments:

A

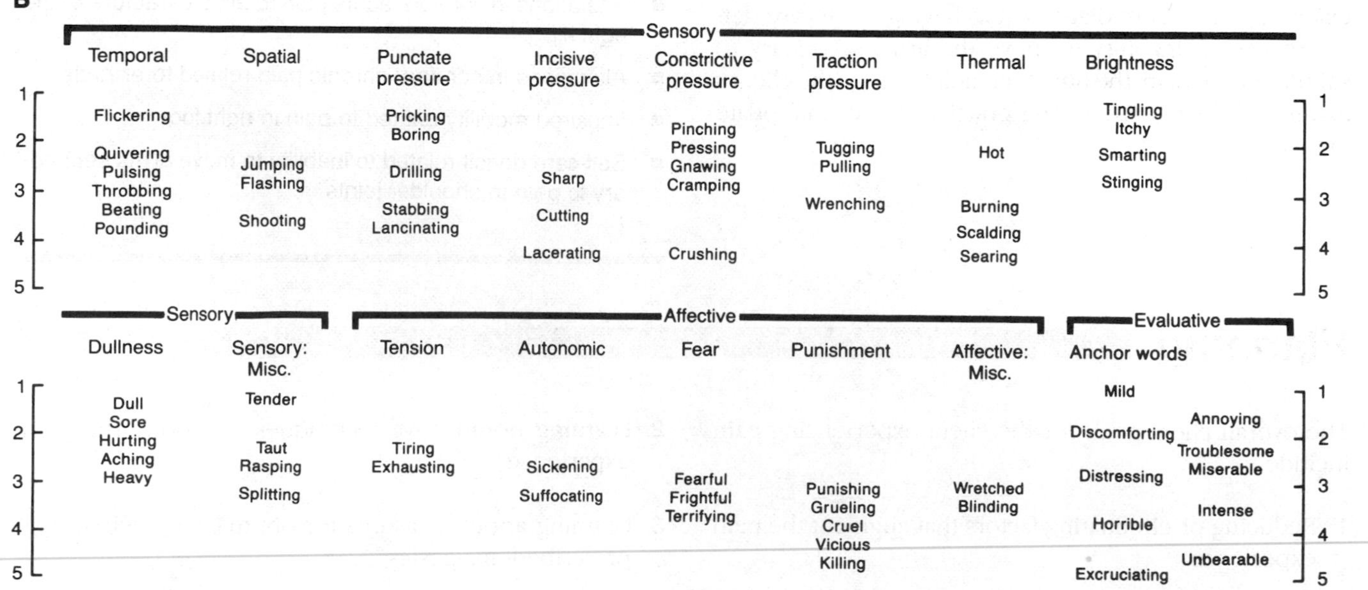

4. Positive response by support persons to the pain experience

Scheduling measures to prevent pain is far more supportive of the client than trying to deal with pain when the client perceives it. Many postoperative clients need regularly administered analgesics as well as other nursing measures. In this way, the client's pain is anticipated and avoided, and recovery is often hastened. When planning, nurses need to choose pain relief measures appropriate for the client. Heat stimulates serotonin production; cold, norepinephrine production. One of these measures may be appropriate (if it is not contraindicated for other health reasons). The nurse may need a physician's order before applying heat or cold.

Intervention

Factors That Augment Pain

Many factors can augment pain, including others' disbelief that the client is in pain, misconceptions about pain, fear, fatigue, and monotony.

Disbelief

Nursing measures that convey to the client belief about the presence of the pain include the following:

1. Verbally acknowledge the presence of the pain. "I understand your leg is very painful, how do you feel about the pain?"
2. Listen attentively to what the client says about the pain.
3. Convey to the client that you are assessing her or his pain to understand it better, *not* to determine if the pain is real. For example: "How does your pain feel now?" or "Tell me how it feels compared to an hour ago."

Clients experiencing pain need to be convinced that the nurse believes them and can be trusted. When clients have no opportunity to talk about their pain and associated fears, their reactions to the pain can be intensified. The client may become angry or complain about the nurse's care when the problem really is that she or he believes the pain is not being attended to. If the nurse is honest and sincere and promptly attends to the client's needs, the client is much more likely to know that the nurse does believe she or he is in pain.

Misconceptions

Reducing a client's misconceptions about his or her pain and its treatment will avoid intensifying the pain. The nurse should explain to the client that pain is a highly individual experience and that it is only the client who really experiences the pain, although others can understand and emphathize. Misconceptions are also dealt with when nurse and client discuss why the pain has increased or decreased at certain times. For example, a client whose pain increases in the evening may mistakenly think this is the result of dinner rather than fatigue.

Fear

By providing accurate information, a nurse also can reduce many of the client's fears, such as a fear of addiction or a fear that she or he will always have pain. It also helps many clients to have privacy when they are experiencing pain. It is always wise to encourage clients to share their fears and concerns about how they are handling the pain.

Fatigue

Because fatigue can intensify pain, nurses should assist clients in developing patterns of activity that provide them sufficient rest, including ordered analgesics at bedtime. Clients may be relieved to know that pain is a stressor and as such can be a cause of fatigue.

Monotony

Monotony can increase pain. Distraction can often be used therapeutically to reduce pain. **Distraction** draws the person's attention away from the pain and lessens the perception of pain. In some instances, distraction can make a client completely unaware of pain. For example, a client recovering from surgery may feel no pain while watching a football game on television, yet feel pain again when the game is over. The way in which distraction decreases pain can be explained by the gate-control theory. In the spinal cord, the receptor cells receiving the peripheral pain stimuli are inhibited by stimuli from other peripheral nerve fibers carrying different stimuli. Because pain messages are slower than diversional messages, the spinal cord gate, which controls the amount of input to the brain, closes and the client feels less pain (Cummings 1981, p. 62). Distraction is most effective when pain is mild or moderate, but intense concentration on other subjects can also relieve acute pain. An example of the latter is an adolescent who feels pain from a fractured foot bone only after she finishes playing a basketball game. A person who is anxious, lonely, or bored feels pain more intensely. In addition, disturbing stimuli such as loud noises, bright lights, unpleasant odors, and an argumentative visitor can increase pain perception. Therefore, the nurse needs to reduce disturbing stimuli.

Some distraction techniques include (McCaffery 1980b, p. 56):

1. *Slow, rhythmic breathing.* The nurse has the client stare at an object; inhale slowly through the nose while the nurse counts 1, 2, 3, 4; and exhale slowly through the mouth while the nurse counts 1, 2, 3, 4. The nurse encourages the client to concentrate on the sensation of breathing and to picture a restful scene. This process is continued until a rhythmic pattern is established. When the client feels comfortable, he or she can count silently and perform this technique independently.
2. *Massage and slow, rhythmic breathing.* The client breathes rhythmically as in step 1 but at the same time massages a painful body part with stroking or circular movements.
3. *Rhythmic singing and tapping.* The client selects a well-liked song and concentrates attention on its words and rhythm. The nurse encourages the client to mouth or sing the words and tap a finger or foot. Loud, fast songs are best for intense pain.
4. *Active listening.* The client listens to music and concentrates on the rhythm by tapping a finger or foot.
5. *Guided imagery.* The nurse asks the client to close his or her eyes and imagine and describe something pleasurable. As the client describes the image, the nurse asks about the sights, sounds, and smells imagined.

Reducing Pain Intensity Through Noninvasive Techniques

The intensity of pain can be reduced through a number of techniques, including relaxation and cutaneous stimulation.

Relaxation

Relaxation techniques are effective primarily for chronic pain, and thus provide many benefits:

1. Reduce anxiety related to pain or stress
2. Ease muscle tension pain
3. Help the person dissociate from pain
4. Promote maximum benefits from rest and sleep periods
5. Enhance the effectiveness of other pain therapies
6. Relieve hopelessness and depression associated with pain

For many years, nurses on maternity units have encouraged women in labor to relax and breathe rhythmically. These techniques, however, can be useful for any client in pain.

Three requisites to relaxation are correct posture, a mind at rest, and a quiet environment. The client must be positioned comfortably, with all body parts supported (e.g., pillow supporting neck), joints slightly flexed, and no strain or pull on muscles (e.g., arms and legs should not be crossed). To rest the mind, the client is asked to gaze slowly around the room, i.e., across the ceiling, down the wall, along a window curtain, around the fabric pattern, back up the wall, etc. This exercise focuses the mind outside of the body (away from the pain) and creates a second center of concentration. To relax the face, the client is encouraged to smile slightly or let the lower jaw sag.

Stewart (1976, p. 959) describes this relaxation technique as follows.

1. The client takes a deep breath and fills the lungs with air.
2. The client slowly hisses out the air while letting the body go limp and concentrating on how good this feels.
3. The client breathes in natural rhythm a few times.
4. The client takes another deep breath and releases it slowly, this time letting only the legs and feet go limp. The nurse asks the client to concentrate on how each leg feels—loose, heavy, and warm.
5. The client repeats step 4, concentrating on the arms, abdomen, back, and other muscle groups.
6. After the client is relaxed, slow, rhythmic breathing is added. Either abdominal or chest breathing may be used. If pain becomes intense, the client can use a more rapid, shallow breathing pattern.

There are several relaxation methods. Some recommend that separate muscle groups (e.g., neck, shoulder, back, arm, leg) be first tensed and then relaxed. After all muscle groups are tensed and relaxed, the whole body is tensed and then relaxed.

Others suggest a stretching form of relaxation. The client lies supine, points the toes toward the knees, presses the back of the knees against the mattress or floor, flattens the hollow of the back and neck as much as possible, holds this position for several minutes, and then relaxes completely for several minutes.

Conscious suggestion by the nurse can help relax an anxious, frightened client in pain. It involves skillful use of the voice, body language, and word choice. A calm, soft, but distinct voice makes the client listen and gives a sense of security. Bending near the client, establishing eye contact, and placing a hand on the client's shoulder communicates the nurse's concern and calmness to the client. Positive, affirmative words help to convey the suggestion of relaxation to the client. During the session, the nurse, after calming and reassuring the client, might make this suggestion: "You will allow yourself to relax as the doctors and nurses treat you." For further information see Holderby (1981).

Cutaneous Stimulation

Stimulation of the skin by cold packs, analgesic ointments, counterirritants, and contralateral stimulation can reduce pain intensity.

1. *Cold packs* slow the conduction of pain impulses to the brain and of motor impulses to muscles in the painful area. They provide quicker and longer-lasting pain relief than hot packs (McCaffery 1980b, p. 57). Cold packs help relieve headaches, muscle strains, joint pain, muscle spasm, and back pain during childbirth.
2. *Analgesic ointments* containing menthol relieve pain, but the analgesic mechanism is unknown. These ointments produce immediate sensations of warmth that last for several hours, and even longer if the body part is wrapped in plastic. They are very commonly used to relieve joint or muscle pain. However, menthol ointment rubbed into the neck, scalp, or forehead sometimes relieves tension headaches, and some cultures (e.g., Filipino) use it on the abdomen to relieve gas pains or on the abdomen or lower back to relieve the pain of labor or delivery (McCaffery 1980b, p. 57).
3. *Counterirritants,* such as mustard plasters, flaxseed poultices, and liniments, relieve the aching joint pain of rheumatoid arthritis and osteoarthritis. Counterirritants are thought to relieve pain by increasing circulation to the painful area. Increased circulation removes trapped tissue metabolites, lessens muscle spasm, and improves joint mobility.
4. *Contralateral stimulation* is stimulation of the skin in an area opposite to the painful area (e.g., stimulating the left knee if the pain is in the right knee). The contralateral area is scratched for itching, massaged for cramps, or treated with cold packs or analgesic ointments. This method is useful when the painful area cannot be touched because it is hypersensitive, because it is made inaccessible by a cast or bandages, or because the pain is felt in a missing part (phantom pain) (McCaffery 1980b, p. 57).

Providing Optimum Relief Through Analgesics

Analgesics alter perception and interpretation of pain by depressing the central nervous system at the thalamus and cerebral cortex. Analgesics are more effective when given before the client feels severe pain than when given after the pain is severe. For this reason, analgesics are given at regular intervals, such as every 4 hours (q4h) after surgery.

Types of Analgesic

There are two major classifications of analgesics: narcotic (strong analgesics) and nonnarcotic (mild analgesics). **Narcotic** *analgesics* include opiate derivatives, such as morphine and codeine. Narcotics relieve pain largely by altering the emotional aspect of the pain experience (i.e., pain perception). Changes in mood and attitude and feelings of well-being make the person feel more comfortable even though the pain persists. *Nonnarcotic analgesics* include derivatives of salicylic acid such as aspirin; para-aminophenols such as phenacetin (Empirin); and pyrazolon derivatives such as phenylbutazone (Butazolidin). In addition, several combinations of analgesic drugs are available, e.g., a combination of a strong analgesic and a mild analgesic. An example is Tylenol #3, which combines acetaminophen, a nonnarcotic, with codeine, 30 mg. The specific way in which nonnarcotic analgesics relieve pain is unknown. It is thought that their primary site of action is the peripheral nervous system (PNS), where sensitization of the pain receptors is prevented.

A newer type of injectable analgesic is the **narcotic agonist-antagonist.** This type has *agonistic* properties in that it acts like a narcotic and relieves severe pain, but it also has *antagonistic* properties in that it also acts against a narcotic. When given to a client who has taken a pure narcotic, these drugs reverse its effects; when given to a narcotic-free client, they have a narcotic effect. Examples are butorphanol (Stadol), nalbuphine (Nubain), and pentazocine (Talwin, Fortal).

Choice of Analgesic

When choosing an analgesic, the health team member considers the quality and intensity of the pain and the specific actions of each analgesic. Narcotics should not be given when nonnarcotics will suffice, but they must be used when potent analgesia is required. Some nurses hesitate administering narcotics even when warranted because they fear causing addiction. See the section on "Guidelines for Pain Management," page 1130. Narcotics are essential in such situations as acute heart attack, renal or biliary colic, vascular occlusion anywhere in the body, fractures, burns, postoperative pain, and terminal malignancies. It is essential that the nurse review the side-effects. For example, narcotic analgesics depress respiration and must be used cautiously in clients with respiratory problems. Nonnarcotics such as aspirin, however, may aggravate gastrointestinal bleeding and therefore are contraindicated in clients with peptic ulcers.

Placebos

A placebo is any form of treatment, e.g., medication or nursing intervention, that produces an effect in the client because of its intent rather than its physical or chemical properties (McCaffery 1982, p. 22). A medication that contains no analgesic properties (e.g., sugar, normal saline, or water) but is intended to relieve pain is a placebo. Years ago, the client who claimed the placebo gave relief was assumed to be malingering or falsely claiming pain. These assumptions have been proved wrong. Placebos do provide pain relief. Thirty-six percent of subjects in a study of 446 clients with severe postoperative pain reported relief after taking a placebo (Goodwin et al. 1982, p. 25). Placebos may help clients return to health and do have a physiologic effect; in some instances they cause the body to release endorphins, which are powerful analgesics (McCaffery 1982, pp. 23–24). It has also been proposed that placebos relieve pain by relieving anxiety or by classical conditioning. In the latter instance the client is conditioned to pain relief and responds positively to the placebo (Nursing Now 1985, p. 95).

Before administering a placebo, nurses must have a physician's order. Just because there are no active chemical ingredients in a placebo does not mean that nurses can administer them independently. It is important that nurses know why a placebo is being given before they give it. Placebos should not be used to punish a "difficult" client. Nor can they be used to prove that a client does not really have pain. Since it is legal to administer placebos, nurses must also examine their own values relative to the ethics of giving placebos. Nurses have at least four choices:

1. They can deceive the client by giving the placebo and saying it is another medicine.
2. They can refuse to give the placebo.
3. They can inform the client about the placebo and obtain his or her consent to use it.
4. They can set up a double-blind situation, explaining the double blind to the client and requesting his or her consent. Neither the nurse nor the client knows whether a placebo or an active drug is being administered, because both have been packaged identically by the pharmacist.

McCaffery (1982) suggests that there is greater probability of a positive response to a placebo if:

1. The treatment makes sense to the client and includes stimuli that convince him or her that the pain will be relieved. For example, intravenous administration is more likely than oral to elicit a positive placebo response.
2. The treatment is administered by an expert whom the client trusts.
3. There is a focus on the client's pain—thorough pain assessment and explanations that the treatment will relieve the pain.
4. The intent of the measure is explained to the client (e.g., "This is another way to relieve your pain").

Assisting Support Persons

Support persons often need assistance to respond positively to the client experiencing pain. Nurses can help support persons by giving them accurate information about the pain and by providing opportunities for them to discuss their emotional reactions, which may include anger, fear, frustration, and feelings of inadequacy. Enlisting the aid of support persons in the provision of pain relief to the client, such as massaging the client's back, may diminish their feelings of helplessness and foster a more positive attitude toward the client's pain experience. Support persons also may need the nurse's verbal recognition of their concern and participation in the client's care.

Guidelines for Pain Management

1. Determine the cause of pain, and try other palliative measures before administering drugs, or use palliative measures as well as administering analgesics. For example, proper positioning, massage, relief of anxiety, or heat can often negate the need for analgesics or can enhance their effects in clients with muscle spasm.
2. Involve the client and support persons in planning, carrying out, and evaluating the pain management program. It is obvious that the participation and cooperation of the client is essential for distraction and relaxation techniques and for evaluation of the selected intervention. They also need information about the effects of certain therapies and need to be involved in planning what best suits them. Support persons may need education in helping the client continue selected therapies at home, e.g., education in guided imagery or distraction techniques.
3. Use nonnarcotic analgesics rather than narcotics if the pain is mild to moderate, since these drugs do not have the adverse side-effects of narcotics—sedation, respiratory depression, constipation, and increased tolerance to the drug (reduced effectiveness over time).
4. Learn to not avoid using narcotics for fear of causing addiction. Studies show that less than 1% to 3% of clients become addicted, and people stop taking nar-

cotics when pain stops (McCaffery 1980a, p. 38). Narcotics are essential for the management of severe pain.

5. Assess the client's response to analgesics, and note the degree and duration of pain relief and side-effects. If pain is not relieved within an hour after administration or if the client is in too much pain to perform activities required for recovery, such as coughing, deep breathing, and ambulation, the dosage is insufficient. If the client complains of pain before the next dose is scheduled, the interval between doses may be too long. If the client experiences significant respiratory depression (e.g., a drop from 18 to 12) or is overly sedated, the dosage is excessive. *Before* administering narcotics, the nurse needs to assess a client's respiratory rate and level of alertness, for baseline data. The nurse also needs to note other side-effects, such as nausea and vomiting.

6. Give analgesics at regular, scheduled intervals rather than as needed (p.r.n.). This is particularly essential for oral analgesics, which may take 1 hour to act. The client on an inadequate schedule could be in pain a substantially long time before feeling relief.

7. Give analgesics *before* the client feels pain or *as soon as* pain starts to return. Higher doses are needed to alleviate severe pain than to prevent it. Clients often need to be encouraged to inform nurses before pain becomes too severe.

8. Individualize the drug and the dosage for each client. This is normally done by the physician. Clients vary considerably in the amount of analgesic they require. No two persons have the same intensity of pain, nor is the absorption, metabolism, or excretion of the drug identical in any two clients.

9. Beware of so-called potentiators of analgesia. Most potentiators sedate the client. Commonly prescribed **potentiators** (drugs that are said to increase the effectiveness of analgesics or the duration of pain relief) are hydroxyzine (Vistaril and Atarax) and promethazine (Phenergan). Neither of these drugs potentiates narcotic analgesia (McCaffery 1980a, p. 39).

10. Keep in mind the client's disease process and allergies when administering analgesics. Clients with certain respiratory diseases are at increased risk from respiratory depression induced by narcotics, and clients with bleeding gastrointestinal ulcers need to avoid aspirin. Those with liver or kidney disease may not metabolize or excrete drugs appropriately. Those with intestinal problems may not absorb oral medications appropriately. Thus, the nurse always needs to bear in mind the side-effects of analgesics in relation to the client's disease.

11. Schedule required activities, such as physical therapy, ambulation, or diagnostic procedures, at times when analgesics are having their fullest effect.

12. When possible, stay with clients who are in pain unless they prefer to be left alone. Some clients with migraine headaches desire minimal stimulation, and others may fear loss of control or be embarrassed about sharing their coping methods of cursing or shouting. Usually, however, the nurse's presence is comforting and may distract them and help them focus attention externally rather than internally.

13. Record the response of the client to the pain. Some nurses use pain medication flowsheets for this purpose. See Figure 41–7.

Management of Intractable Pain

The management of intractable cancer pain presents a challenge to nurses. Drugs commonly used are methadone, Brompton's mixture, and continuous morphine infusion.

Methadone is advantageous because it is effective orally, has a long duration of action, has a cumulative effect that can maintain steady analgesic levels, and does not substantially alter mood (Maxwell 1980, p. 1606).

Brompton's mixture, developed in the 1930s at Brompton's Hospital, London, was originally used as an oral analgesic for postoperative clients. This medication was valued because it relieves pain without clouding the mind. Several different preparations are called Brompton's mixture, since these mixtures are prepared in hospice and hospital pharmacies. The original mixture contained heroin (narcotic analgesic), cocaine (CNS stimulant to counteract the sedation and respiratory depression of the narcotic), alcohol (flavor enhancer), and syrup and chloroform water to improve the taste and texture (Gever 1980, p. 57). In many places in North America, morphine or methadone is substituted for heroin, and amphetamine is used in place of cocaine, since cocaine is poorly absorbed and its importation is curtailed. The alcohol component may be ethanol, gin, or brandy. Fruit-flavored syrups are used to improve the flavor. In some hospitals, an antiemetic is also added for its tranquilizing effect.

Brompton's mixture is prescribed every 3 to 4 hours if it contains morphine or every 6 to 8 hours if it contains methadone, which has a longer action. It is given on schedule rather than as needed (p.r.n.) to prevent, not relieve, pain. Because Brompton's mixture is stable for only 2 weeks, the nurse needs to check the preparation

Date	Time	Medication	Pain level (0 = no pain; 10 = worst pain imaginable) and ct. comments	Respirations
10/1	12:30 p.m.	---------	8 "can't stand the pain"	22 (baseline)
	12:55 p.m.	morphine, 5 mg, I.V. push	8	22
	1:00 p.m.	morphine drip, 5 mg in 25 ml to run over 1 hour	7 "beginning to ease somewhat"	18
	1:30 p.m.	---------	7	18
	2:00 p.m.	morphine drip, 5 mg in 25 ml to run over 1 hour	5 (ct. has slept some)	17
	2:30 p.m.	---------	5	20
	3:00 p.m.	morphine drip, 5 mg in 25 ml to run over 1 hour	5 "feel sore"	17
	3:30 p.m.	---------	6 "more cramping and aching"	22
	4:00 p.m.	morphine drip, 7 mg in 25 ml to run over 1 hour	6	22
	4:30 p.m.	---------	4 "pain is easing"	18
	5:00 p.m.	morphine drip, 28 mg in 100 ml to run over 4 hours	3 "much more comfortable" (ct. sleeping intermittently)	18
	9:00 p.m.	morphine drip, 28 mg in 100 ml to run over 4 hours	3	18

Figure 41–7 Pain medication flowsheet

Source: From L. McGuire and A. Wright, Continuous narcotic infusion. It's not just for cancer patients, *Nursing 84,* December 1984, 14:53. Used by permission.

date before administering the mixture. Because the narcotic depresses respiration, the nurse must monitor the respirations of clients receiving Brompton's mixture.

Continuous morphine infusion is used for clients with end-stage terminal illness who are suffering extreme pain, who have built up a tolerance to other pain medication, who have difficulty taking anything orally, and who cannot tolerate repeated injections. The goals of this method of pain control are (a) to provide continuous pain relief, (b) to allow the client limited functional capacity, (c) to make the client as comfortable as possible as long as he or she survives, and (d) to support the desire to die with dignity (O'Donnell and Papciak 1981, pp. 69–71).

Morphine infusions are administered through an infusion control pump with a microdrip infusion set and usually through a secondary intravenous line, although a primary line may be used. See Chapter 46 for a description of this equipment. A physician's order for dosage and infusion rate is essential. Starting dosages are based on the client's previous pain medication, the client's level of tolerance, and the severity of the pain. Generally, morphine is mixed in solutions of 5% dextrose in water (D5W), but it can be mixed with any intravenous solution. If other medications are being infused, drug incompatibilities must be ascertained. Some incompatible drugs are heparin, aminophylline, and sodium bicarbonate. Dosages may range from 4 to 40 mg of morphine in 100 ml of solution; 8 to 80 mg in 200 ml of solution; and 10 to 100 mg of morphine in 250 ml of solution (O'Donnell and Papciak, p. 72). Nurses need to follow agency policies and guidelines for use of continuous morphine infusions. Policy statements and guidelines should include (O'Donnell and Papciak, p. 72):

1. *Which clients can be selected for the procedure.* For example, a client may be eligible only if he or she has intractable pain and requires injectable narcotics.
2. *The responsibilities of the attending physician.* For example, the physician (a) records the terminal nature of the illness and justifies the intravenous morphine infusion on the client's progress notes, (b) discusses the potential side-effects with the client or support persons, (c) supplies a written signed request specifying the dosage and rate of infusion to the pharmacist, and (d) supplies a daily written order for the infusion.

3. *Who prepares the infusion.* In some agencies, the pharmacist or nurse prepares the infusion solution.
4. *How the infusion is to be administered.* For example, it may be administered by microdrip infusion set and infusion control pump.
5. *The responsibilities of the nurse, with emphasis on measures to prevent an overdose.* For example, the nurse (a) records a baseline blood pressure and respiratory rate prior to the infusion, (b) initiates the infusion, and (c) monitors blood pressure and respiration rates at specified intervals, such as every 30 minutes for the first 2 or 3 hours and then as nursing assessments warrant.
6. *The changes in rates of blood pressure and respiration during infusion that are acceptable and the actions to take when unacceptable changes occur.* For example, if the respiratory rate falls below 14, the infusion rate may be slowed by 50% and the respiration rate monitored every 10 or 15 minutes. The infusion is discontinued with continued decreases in respiratory rate.
7. *How respiratory depression is managed, should it occur.* Naloxone hydrochloride (Narcan), a narcotic antagonist, should be available at the nursing station for administration by the physician, or nurse, if ordered, in the event of respiratory depression.

Medical Management of Pain

Nerve Blocks

A **nerve block** is a chemical interruption of a nerve pathway, effected by injecting a local anesthetic—e.g., lidocaine (Xylocaine) or procaine (Novocain) into the nerve. Nerve blocks are widely used during dental work: The injected drug blocks nerve pathways from the painful tooth, thus stopping the transmission of pain impulses to the brain. Nerve blocks are often used to relieve the pain of whiplash injury, low-back disorders, bursitis, and cancer. Sometimes alcohol blocks are used. These, however, destroy nerve fibers and as a result are usually used for peripheral blocks, since peripheral nerve fibers regenerate.

Electric Stimulation

Electric stimulation is sometimes used to combat certain intractable pain. There are several methods. In **transcutaneous electric stimulation**, electrodes are placed on the surface of the skin over the painful area and over peripheral nerve pathways. In **percutaneous electric stimulation**, needles are inserted near a major peripheral nerve (e.g., the sciatic nerve). In both methods, an electric charge blocks the pain impulse by stimulating the gate-control mechanism. The percutaneous method is used primarily to determine whether a client should consider having a permanent implant inserted.

Two implantable devices are the **peripheral nerve implant** and the **dorsal column stimulator**. The peripheral implant is an electrode attached to a major sensory nerve. The column stimulator is an electrode attached to the dorsal column of the spinal cord. Both devices have a transmitter that the client wears externally. The transmitter sends an impulse that blocks the transmission of the pain impulse (Gaumer 1974, pp. 504–05). The blocking of pain impulses is generally within the scope of a physician's practice only. However, some nurses functioning in expanded roles may have responsibility for such procedures.

Acupuncture

Acupuncture has been practiced for centuries in China and is receiving increasing attention in North America. It is currently being used selectively in North America to treat chronic pain. The acupuncturist inserts long, slender needles into the body at various sites, which are not necessarily near the body parts to be treated. The needles can be heated, attached to a mild electric current, or twirled continuously with the hand.

Traditional acupuncturists believe acupuncture corrects a disharmony between the life forces of yin and yang. See Chapter 18. Western scientists, puzzled by the effectiveness of acupuncture, theorize that it closes the gate mechanism to pain or stimulates sites near pain fibers leading to the brain, thereby blocking the perception of pain. It is also possible that there are neurologic links between body sites; stimulation of one site may affect pain at another. This idea is supported by the fact that organic pain is often referred to a distant body part. Cardiac pain, for example, is often referred to the shoulder, back, or lower jaw.

Hypnosis

Hypnosis has been used to treat psychogenic pain, to achieve anesthesia, and to enhance the effectiveness of medications given for pain aggravated by tension. The susceptible person accepts positive suggestions, which tend to alter perceptions. The success of hypnosis depends to a large degree on the person's openness to suggestion, emotional readiness, and faith in the effectiveness of the hypnosis (American Journal of Nursing 1974a, p. 515).

Surgery

Pain conduction pathways can be interrupted surgically. Because this disruption is permanent, surgery is performed only as a last resort, generally for intractable pain. Several surgical procedures may be performed:

1. In **cordotomy**, the spinothalamic portion of the anterolateral tract is severed. This procedure obliterates pain and temperature sensation below the level severed, and is usually done for pain in the legs and trunk.
2. In **rhizotomy**, the anterior or posterior nerve root between the ganglion and the cord is interrupted. Interruption of anterior *motor* nerve roots stops spasmodic movements that accompany paraplegia. Interruption of posterior *sensory* nerve roots eliminates pain in areas innervated by that specific nerve root. Rhizotomies are generally performed on cervical nerve roots to alleviate pain of the head and neck from cancer or neuralgia.
3. In **neurectomy**, peripheral or cranial nerves are interrupted to alleviate localized pain, such as pain in the lower leg or foot arising from a vascular occlusion.
4. In a **sympathectomy**, pathways of the sympathetic division of the autonomic nervous system are severed. This procedure eliminates vasospasm, improves peripheral blood supply, and thus is effective in treating painful vascular disorders such as angina and Raynaud's disease.

Biofeedback

Biofeedback is a method of controlling certain physiologic functions by providing information normally unavailable to the individual. In the past, most physiologic processes were considered involuntary. However, it has been discovered that many of these processes are partially subject to voluntary control. Studies show that muscle tension, heart rate, blood flow, and pain, for example, can be controlled voluntarily. The feedback is usually provided through auditory or visual means, e.g., the client sees an electromyogram that shows the electric potential created by the contraction of muscles.

Biofeedback allows the client to be fully involved in his or her treatment. The responsibility in biofeedback training lies primarily with the client. The client may require months or even years of training before the optimum level of response is reached. Therefore, clients must usually be highly motivated to participate in biofeedback programs.

Evaluation

Examples of outcome criteria for clients experiencing pain are listed below.

Examples of Outcome Criteria for Clients Experiencing Pain

The client will:

- State that he or she feels no postoperative pain
- Carry out deep-breathing exercises and cough without severe pain
- Walk to the end of the corridor and back without discomfort
- Perform relaxation exercises as scheduled

Nursing Care Plan

Assessment Data

Nursing Assessment

Mr. Harvey Jones is a 57-year-old businessman who was admitted yesterday morning to the surgical unit at the hospital for the treatment of a possible strangulated inguinal hernia. Yesterday afternoon he went to surgery, and a partial bowel resection was performed. This morning, Mr. Jones is NPO. He has an intravenous infusion in the left arm, a nasogastric tube attached to low intermittent suction, and a clear dermal dressing applied to his large abdominal incision. He is in a dorsal recumbent (supine) position and is attempting to draw up his legs. Mr. Jones appears to be somewhat restless and pale. He is grimacing and appears to be generally uncomfortable.

Physical Examination

Height: 188 cm (6′2″)
Weight: 90.9 kg (200 lb)
Temperature: 37 C (98.6 F)
Pulse rate: 90 BPM
Respirations: 24 per minute

Blood pressure: 158/82 mm Hg
Skin pale and moist
Midline abdominal incision—sutures dry and intact
Pupils dilated

Diagnostic Data
Chest x-ray film: Negative
WBC: 12,000
Urine: Negative

Nursing Diagnosis	Client Goals and Outcome Criteria	Nursing Interventions and Rationales	Evaluation
Alteration in comfort: pain due to surgical incision/ stimulation of mechanosensitive receptors resulting in grimacing; pallor; restlessness; elevated pulse, respirations, and systolic blood pressure; dilated pupils; and verbalization of abdominal pain and discomfort.	Client Goal: Experience minimal abdominal pain and discomfort. Outcome Criteria: States that postoperative discomfort is relieved within 20–30 minutes of verbalization of pain. Practices one relaxation technique for relief of pain by end of first day. Practices one distraction technique for relief of pain by day 2. Requests medication for relief of pain before pain becomes severe. Turns, coughs, and deep breathes with a minimum amount of discomfort by day 2.	Assess and record the description, location, duration, and characteristics of client's pain. *Rationale:* Pain is a personal experience, and the nurse will need to rely on the client's description of pain in order to treat it effectively. Maintain frequent contact with client and listen attentively to his complaints of pain. *Rationale:* This will reduce anxiety, and anxiety increases pain. Reduce or eliminate pain-producing factors, e.g., fear, anxiety, lack of knowledge, a wet dressing, improper positioning. *Rationale:* Eliminating precipitating factors decreases incidence of pain. Employ distraction techniques, e.g., slow rhythmic breathing and guided imagery, to provide pain relief. *Rationale:* Distraction draws the client's attention away from the pain and lessens the perception of pain. Provide cutaneous stimulation, e.g., back rub. *Rationale:* Cutaneous stimulation provides pain relief by blocking pain impulses along the thinner nerve fibers in the synapses in the dorsal horn (gate control theory). Administer prescribed analgesics. *Rationale:* Analgesics alter perception and interpretation of pain by depressing the central nervous system at the thalamus and cerebral cortex. Note response to medication. *Rationale:* The medication dose may not be adequate to raise the client's pain threshold, or side-effects, e.g., respiratory depression, may occur. Instruct client to request analgesic before pain becomes severe. *Rationale:* Severe pain is more difficult to control and increases client's anxiety and fatigue. Instruct client in relaxation techniques, e.g., tensing and relaxing muscle groups and rhythmic breathing. *Rationale:* Relaxation techniques enhance the effect of other pain therapies, reduce anxiety, and relieve depression.	Client requests analgesics at onset of pain. States, "Pain is practically gone" 20 minutes after administration of analgesic. Reads, watches TV, and listens to his favorite music frequently throughout the day. Practices rhythmic breathing q3 to 4 hrs during his waking hours by day 2. Requests analgesic 30 minutes before turning in bed and assuming new position. Coughs and deep breathes q1 to 2 hrs after analgesic is administered.

(continued)

Nursing Diagnosis	Client Goals and Outcome Criteria	Nursing Interventions and Rationales	Evaluation
Impairment in skin integrity due to surgical incision resulting in disruption of skin layers.	Client Goal: Healed surgical wound without complications. Outcome Criteria: Edges of surgical wound remain approximated throughout healing phase (21 days). No evidence of reddened skin in immediate area of wound after day 7. Vital signs remain within normal range. Splints abdominal incision with hands and/or pillow when turning, coughing, and deep breathing first post-op day.	Monitor vital signs frequently, especially increased temperature/pulse and respirations. *Rationale:* Increased temperature may indicate wound infection, which will delay healing. Employ surgical asepsis in dressing changes. *Rationale:* Sterile technique will decrease chance of wound infection and subsequent delayed healing. Splint incision with hands and/or pillow during coughing and deep-breathing exercises. *Rationale:* Incisional support decreases stress on healing wound edges. Monitor laboratory data such as WBC. *Rationale:* An elevated leukocyte count may indicate infection and subsequent delayed wound healing. Encourage adequate protein and vitamin C intake. *Rationale:* Protein and vitamin C are essential for tissue repair.	Wound edges remain approximated and intact. There is no evidence of redness or swelling of the wound. Vital signs are within normal range. Mr. Jones splints his abdomen with his pillow before making position changes. He supports his abdominal wall with his hands or a pillow when coughing.

Chapter Highlights

- Pain is a personal experience.
- Pain warns the individual of tissue injury.
- The pain experience has three components: pain stimulation, perception, and response.
- Nociceptors are initially stimulated if pain is to be perceived.
- Three types of pain stimuli are mechanical, thermal, and chemical.
- There are three types of endogenous opioids: enkephalins, endorphins, and dynorphins.
- Many psychosocial factors influence pain perception.
- The pain response has three stages: activation, rebound, and adaptation.
- Assessment of a client who is experiencing pain should include a pain history and the clinical signs and symptoms of pain.
- Nursing diagnoses regarding pain include the pain itself, the effect of the pain on the client, and a component of the pain experience.
- Planning for intervening with a client in pain must include reducing or eliminating factors that intensify pain.
- Specific noninvasive techniques can modify pain experience.
- Distraction lessens the perception of pain.
- Relaxation techniques are helpful in reducing the intensity of chronic pain.
- A regular schedule for analgesic administration can help prevent pain.
- Evaluating the client's pain therapy includes the response of the client, the changes in the pain, and the client's perceptions of the effectiveness of the therapy.

Suggested Readings

Copp, L. A. Summer 1985. Pain coping model and typology. *Image: The Journal of Nursing Scholarship* 17:69–71.
Copp relates the self-image of the person experiencing pain to the nature of that person's perception of the pain. Five types of self-image are described: victim, combatant, responder, reactor, interactor. Copp also presents a coping model that includes a guideline for assessing pain from the client's point of view. Copp also presents coping strategies used by each type.

Dolan, M. B. January 1982. Controlling pain in a personal way. *Nursing 82* 12:68.
Palliative measures such as positioning, massage, and "guided imagery" need to be implemented before analgesics are administered. Thirteen rules for pain management are given.

Doyle, J. E. April 1981. If your patient's legs hurt the reason may be arterial insufficiency. *Nursing 81* 11:74–78.
The author provides a guide for assessing peripheral arterial insufficiency. Physical examination of the feet is discussed, and color photographs of some of the signs of arterial insufficiency are included, such as gangrene, ulcers, and atrophic skin. Pulse evaluation is also discussed.

Fagerhaugh, S. Y., and Strauss, A. February 1980. How to manage your patient's pain . . . and how not to. *Nursing 80* 10:44–47.
These authors, after surveying 20 hospital units, discovered that each nurse follows his or her own pain philosophy. The result is confusion among clients. They recommend clearly defined drug policies and suggest ways in which nurses can build pain management into a surgical unit's client care system.

Holderby, R. A. May 1981. Conscious suggestion: Using talk to manage pain. *Nursing 81* 11:44–46.
This chaplain and crisis counselor discusses essential aspects of the conscious suggestion technique used to manage pain.

McCaffery, M. September 1980. Understanding your patient's pain. *Nursing 80* 10:26–31.
The author defines pain and describes the signs of acute pain. The causes of pain are discussed together with descriptions of psychogenic and somatogenic pain. Duration, severity, and client tolerance are considered.

———. November 1980. How to relieve your patients' pain fast and effectively . . . with oral analgesics. *Nursing 80* 10:58–63.
The author outlines guidelines that help nurses choose and administer oral analgesics effectively. Equianalgesic lists are provided for commonly used oral analgesics.

———. June 1981. When your patient's still in pain don't just do something: Sit there. *Nursing 81* 11:58–61.
This article outlines the advantages of staying with clients in pain, tells when not to be there, and describes problems the nurse may encounter by being there.

Selected References

American Journal of Nursing. March 1974a. Hypnotic suggestion. *American Journal of Nursing* 74:515.

———. March 1974b. Chemical and surgical intervention. *American Journal of Nursing* 74:511.

Barrett-Griesemer, P.; Meisel, S.; and Rate, R. April 1981. A guide to headaches—and how to relieve their pain. *Nursing 81* 11:50–57.

Bellack, J. P., and Bamford, P. A. 1984. *Nursing assessment. A multidimensional approach.* Monterey, Calif.: Wadsworth Health Sciences Div.

Beyerman, K. February 1982. Flawed perceptions about pain. *American Journal of Nursing* 82:302–4.

Blaylock, J. 1968. The psychological and cultural influences on the reaction to pain: A review of literature. *Nursing Forum* 7(3):262–74.

Booker, J. E. March 1982. Pain: It's all in your patient's head (or is it?). *Nursing 82* 12:46–51.

Breeden, S. A., and Kondo, C. November 1975. Using biofeedback to reduce tension. *American Journal of Nursing* 75:2010–12.

Broome, A. April 16–22, 1986. Coping with pain: Strategies for relief. *Nursing Times* 82:43–44.

Carpenito, L. J. 1983. *Nursing diagnosis application to clinical practice.* Philadelphia: J. B. Lippincott.

Copp, L. A. March 1974. The spectrum of suffering. *American Journal of Nursing* 74:491–95.

———. Summer 1985. Pain coping model and typology. *Image: The Journal of Nursing Scholarship.* 17:69–71.

Cummings, D. January 1981. Stopping chronic pain before it starts. *Nursing 81* 11:60–62.

Dernham, P. January/February 1986. Phantom limb pain. *Geriatric Nursing* 7:34–37.

Escobar, P. L. January 1985. Management of chronic pain. *Nurse Practitioner* 10:24–25, 29–30, 32.

Engel, G. L. 1970. Pain. In MacBryde, C. M., and Blacklow, R. S., editors. *Signs and symptoms: Applied physiologic physiology and clinical interpretation.* 5th ed. Philadelphia: J. B. Lippincott Co.

Gaumer, W. R. March 1974. Electrical stimulation in chronic pain. *American Journal of Nursing* 74:504–5.

Gever, L. N. May 1980. Brompton's mixture. How it relieves pain of terminal cancer. *Nursing 80* 10:57.

Goodwin, J. S.; Goodwin, J. M.; and Vogel, A. V. February 1982. Placebo misuse. *Nursing 82* 12:24–25.

Guyton, A. C. 1986. *Textbook of medical physiology.* 7th ed. Philadelphia: W. B. Saunders Co.

Hamm, B. H., and King, V. Spring 1984. A holistic approach to pain control with geriatric clients . . . guided imagery. *Journal of Holistic Nursing* 2:32–37.

Holderby, R. A. May 1981. Conscious suggestion: Using talk to manage pain. Part 9. *Nursing 81* 11:44–46.

Lara, M. J. July/August 1985. Intractable pain: Is more medication the only answer? Emotional distress may be the culprit. *Nursing Life* 5:44–47.

McCaffery, M. 1979. *Nursing management of the patient with pain.* 2d ed. Philadelphia: J. B. Lippincott Co.

———. October 1980a. Patients shouldn't have to suffer. How to relieve pain with injectable narcotics. *Nursing 80* 10:34–39.

———. December 1980b. Relieving pain with noninvasive techniques. *Nursing 80* 10:55–57.

———. February 1982. Would you administer placebos for pain? These facts can help you decide. *Nursing 82* 12:22–27.

McGuire, L. March 1981. A short, simple tool for assessing your patient's pain. *Nursing 81* 11:48–49.

McGuire, L., and Wright, A. December 1984. Continuous narcotic infusion. It's not just for cancer patients. *Nursing 84* 14:50–55.

Maxwell, M. B. September 1980. How to use methadone for the cancer patient's pain. *American Journal of Nursing* 80:1606–9.

Meissner, J. E. January 1980. McGill-Melzack pain questionnaire. *Nursing 80* 10:50–51.

Melzack, R., and Wall, P. D. 1982. *The challenge of pain.* New York: Penguin Books.

———. 19 November 1965. Pain mechanisms: A new theory. *Science* 150:971–79.

———. 1983. *The challenge of pain.* New York: Basic Books.

Nursing Now. 1985. *Pain.* Hicksville, N.Y.: Nursing 85 Books, Spring House Corp.

O'Donnell, L., and Papciak, B. August 1981. When all else fails: Continuous morphine infusion for controlling intractable pain. *Nursing 81* 11:69–72.

Perry, S. W., and Heidrich, G. April 1981. Placebo response: Myth and matter. *American Journal of Nursing* 81:720–25.

Stewart, E. June 1976. To lessen pain: Relaxation and rhythmic breathing. *American Journal of Nursing* 76:958–59.

Warfield, C. A. July 15, 1985. Patient-controlled analgesia. *Hospital Practice* 20:32L, O–P.

West, B. A. February 1981. Understanding endorphins: Our natural pain relief system. *Nursing 81* 11:50–53.

Wilson, R. W., and Elmassian, B. J. April 1981. Endorphins. *American Journal of Nursing* 81:722–25.

CHAPTER **42**

Nutrition

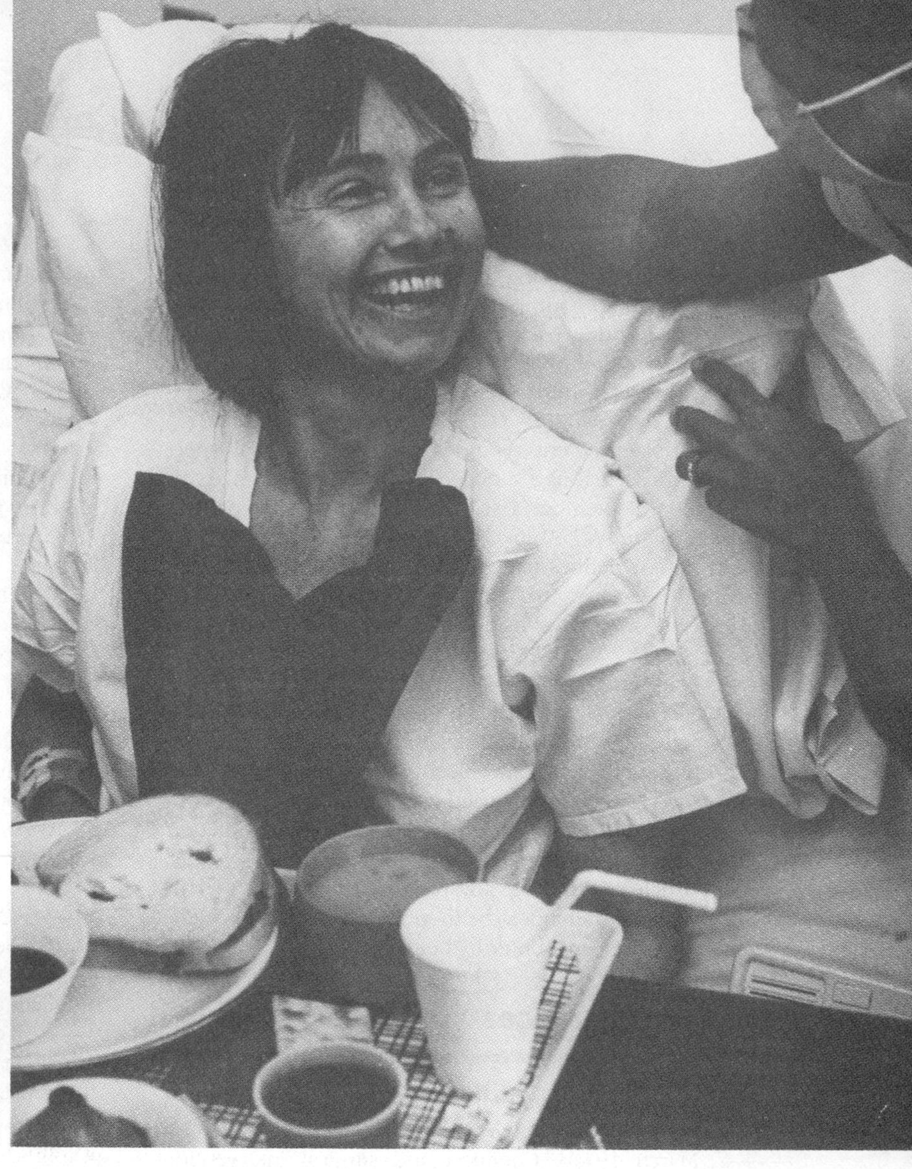
WILLIAM THOMPSON

Contents

(continued)

Contents *(continued)*

Objectives

1. Understand essential facts about nutrition, metabolism, energy balance, and essential nutrients.
   1.1 Define selected terms.
   1.2 Differentiate nutrition from metabolism.
   1.3 Identify factors that influence a person's energy requirements.
   1.4 Identify ways that nutrients are classified.
   1.5 Identify good sources of required nutrients.
   1.6 Identify mechanisms involved in the digestion of nutrients.
   1.7 Describe mechanisms involved in the absorption of nutrients.
   1.8 Describe how nutrients are stored in the body.
   1.9 Identify essential mechanisms involved in the metabolism of nutrients.
   1.10 Identify functions and food sources of various nutrients and some clinical signs of deficiency and excess.
   1.11 Describe the effects of food storage, processing, and cooking methods on nutrients.
2. Understand essential aspects of standards developed to ensure a healthy diet.
   2.1 Describe essential aspects of daily food group guides.
   2.2 Describe the purpose of recommended dietary allowances or recommended nutrient intake guides.
   2.3 Differentiate recommended dietary allowances (RDAs) developed by the Food and Nutrition Board from U.S. RDAs.
   2.4 Describe the dietary recommendations of the U.S. Senate Select Committee on Human Needs.
   2.5 Identify potential nutritional problems of vegetarians and ways to avoid them.
3. Understand essential facts about developmental variables in nutrition.
   3.1 Identify the benefits of mature breast milk for infants.
   3.2 Describe various commercial infant milk feedings.
   3.3 Identify supplement requirements for various milk feedings.
   3.4 Describe a recommended sequence for introducing solid foods to infants.
   3.5 Describe essential aspects of nutrition for children and adolescents.
   3.6 Compare the nutritional needs of young, middle-age, and older adults.
4. Know essential information and methods required to assess nutritional status and establish nursing diagnoses.
   4.1 Describe anthropometric techniques.
   4.2 Describe various biochemical measurements used to detect subclinical malnutrition.
   4.3 Identify clinical signs of inadequate nutritional status.
   4.4 Describe essential aspects of a dietary history.
   4.5 Identify factors that influence a person's eating patterns.
   4.6 Identify nursing diagnoses and contributing factors associated with the client's nutritional status.
5. Understand essential aspects of nursing interventions that maintain, promote, and restore good nutrition.
   5.1 Describe the process of nutritional counseling.
   5.2 Identify the essentials of progressive hospital diets.
   5.3 Identify interventions to stimulate a client's appetite.
   5.4 Describe ways to assist clients with meals.
   5.5 Describe essential aspects of feeding clients.
   5.6 Describe some aids that enable self-feeding.
   5.7 Discuss some special nutritional services available for selected subgroups of the population.
   5.8 Identify essential steps in administering nasogastric or gastrostomy feedings.

Terms

adenosine triphosphate (ATP)
amino acid (essential and nonessential)
anabolism
anthropometric measurement
basal metabolic rate (BMR)
caloric density
caloric value
calorie (small calorie)
carbohydrate
catabolism
cholesterol

(continued)

chyme
citric acid cycle (Krebs cycle)
colostrum
deamination
disaccharide
emulsification
enzyme
ester
fad
fat
fatty acids (saturated, unsaturated, and polyunsaturated)
fiber
gastrostomy feeding
gluconeogenesis
glycogen
glycogenesis
glycogenolysis
glycolysis
hematocrit
hydrolysis
hyperlipidemia
jejunostomy feeding
ketogenesis
ketosis
kilocalorie (Calorie, large calorie)
lipids
macromineral
mastication
mature milk
metabolism
metabolite
micromineral
micronutrient
monosaccharide
nasogastric feeding (gastric gavage)
nitrogen balance (positive and negative)
nutrient
nutrition
nutritive value
obesity
osteoporosis
overweight
peristalsis
phosphorylation
polysaccharide
protein (complete and incomplete)
protein complementing (mutual supplementation)
segmentation contractions
sodium cotransport theory
transitional milk
triglyceride
vitamin (fat-soluble and water-soluble)

The Nurse's Role in Nutrition

Throughout life, people develop their own unique ideas and feelings about food and nutrition—by being consumers; by participating in family, ethnic, religious, and regional traditions; and by being exposed to advertising. Today, North Americans are becoming more aware of the importance of a healthy diet and of the effect of certain nutrients on health and well-being. Unfortunately, however, advice about nutrition is often conflicting, and people end up confused about which food choices are best. Many people worry that certain foods may be unsafe, especially since commonly used additives (e.g., cyclamates and saccharin) have been linked with cancer and birth defects and banned by the Food and Drug Administration (FDA). As a result, growing numbers of individuals, believing that "natural" and "organic" foods are the safest foods to eat, are shopping in health food stores. In addition, the public is being given the message that overconsumption of fats, cholesterol, and sugar is unhealthy and shortens lives. As a result, people are learning to cut down on major sources of cholesterol (e.g., eggs), calories, and fat and to use vegetable oils (polyunsaturated fats) rather than animal fats (saturated fats) to prevent cardiovascular diseases.

Health professionals have a major role in promoting health by helping people make informed food choices. Nutritionists and dietitians provide nutritional and dietary counseling to the public. Effective education emphasizes an understanding not only of essential nutrients but also of methods to change eating habits. To be an effective promoter of health, the nurse has these specific responsibilities to clients: (a) to assess the client's nutritional status; (b) to observe the client's nutritional intake; (c) to reinforce nutritional and dietary instruction; (d) to consider the many factors, e.g., emotions, culture, life-style, and financial resources, that affect the person's food choices; (e) to help the client effect beneficial changes in eating behaviors; and (f) to evaluate the client's response to prescribed therapy or planned changes.

Nutrition, Metabolism, and Energy Balance

Nutrition

Nutrition is the sum of all the interactions between an organism and the food it consumes (Christian and Greger 1985, p. 4). In other words, nutrition is what a person eats and how the body uses it.

People require food or essential nutrients for the growth and maintenance of all body tissues and the normal functioning of all body processes. **Nutrients** are the organic and inorganic chemicals found in foods and required for proper body functioning. An adequate food intake consists of a balance of essential nutrients: water, carbohydrates, proteins, fats, vitamins, and minerals. Foods differ greatly in their **nutritive value** (the nutrient content of a specified amount of food), and no one food provides all essential nutrients.

Nutrients have three major functions (Suitor and Hunter 1980, p. 4):

1. They provide energy for body processes and movement.
2. They provide structural material for body tissues, e.g., bones and muscles.
3. They regulate body processes.

The amount of energy that nutrients or foods supply to the body is their **caloric value.** A **calorie** is a unit of heat energy. A **small calorie** is the amount of heat required to raise the temperature of 1 g of water 1 degree C. A **large calorie** (**Calorie, kilocalorie**, or kcal) is the amount of heat required to raise the temperature of 1 kg of water 1 degree C and is the unit used in nutrition. The energy liberated from each gram of carbohydrate and protein after it is metabolized is about 4 kcal; that liberated from each gram of fat, about 9 kcal. The average North American receives approximately 45% of energy from carbohydrates, 40% from fat, and 15% from protein (Guyton 1986, p. 861). In most other parts of the world, people derive far more energy from carbohydrates than from fats and proteins. People in Mongolia, for example, derive 80% to 85% of energy from carbohydrates (Guyton 1986, p. 861).

Metabolism

Metabolism refers simply to all cellular chemical reactions that make it possible for body cells to continue living (Guyton 1986, p. 844). It consists of anabolic and catabolic reactions. Anabolic reactions build substances and body tissues. Catabolic reactions break down substances.

Many of the chemical reactions in the cells make the energy in foods available to the various physiologic systems of the cell. For instance, energy is required for (a) muscular activity, (b) secretion by the glands, (c) maintenance of membrane potentials by the nerve and muscle fibers, (d) synthesis of substances in the cells, (e) absorption of foods from the gastrointestinal tract, and (f) many other functions (Guyton 1986, p. 844).

The energy in food, expressed as Calories (kcal), maintains the basal metabolic rate of the body and provides energy for activities such as running and walking. Metabolic rate is normally expressed in terms of the rate of heat liberated during chemical reactions. The **basal metabolic rate** (BMR) is the rate at which the body metabolizes food to maintain the energy requirements of a person who is awake and at rest.

A person's energy requirements beyond the BMR are influenced by many factors, e.g., age, body size, activity, body temperature, environmental temperature, growth, sex, and emotional state.

When energy requirements are completely met by calories taken in as food, people maintain their activity level without weight change. When caloric intake exceeds energy needs, the person gains weight. When caloric intake fails to meet energy requirements, the person burns body fat for energy and loses weight. Energy requirements vary from day to day, reflecting changes in the factors that influence them. For example, illness frequently increases energy requirements because of increased body temperature, increased metabolic rate, and stress.

Energy Balance

A person's weight depends on calories taken in and energy expended. To maintain a specific weight, a person needs to balance caloric (energy) intake and energy output. See Table 35–3 on page 809 for recommended weights. There is a higher incidence of diabetes mellitus, gallbladder disease, and cardiovascular disease among overweight people. Obesity decreases life expectancy and may negatively affect the quality of life. As a result, health authorities in recent years have stressed maintaining normal weight as a preventive health measure. The caloric requirements of individuals vary with age and growth, sex, climate, health, sleep, food, and activity.

Age and Growth

During periods of growth, the body uses more energy. Rapid growth during the first 2 years of life, adolescence, and pregnancy increases the need for calories. For example, an active adolescent body may need 3600 kcal, whereas a 70-year-old woman may require only 1800 kcal or less. See Appendix E for caloric intake variables by age.

Sex

Men usually have higher basal metabolic rates than women, a fact largely explained by the greater proportion of muscle in men's bodies. Pregnant women also have higher basal metabolic rates.

Climate

Climate affects heat production. People in cold climates have a higher (about 20%, on average) metabolic rate than people in hot climates. This fact may be due to increased thyroxine levels in people who live in cold climates.

Health

Some illnesses, such as those accompanied by high temperature or infection, increase metabolic rate. In malnourished people, however, the metabolic rate is lowered.

Sleep

People need less energy during sleep, when the muscles are relaxed and physiologic processes are slowed. The metabolic rate drops about 10% to 15% during sleep.

Food

The body's metabolism is stimulated by all foods, but by some more than others. Proteins increase heat production about 30%, carbohydrates and fats about 5%.

Activity

Muscular activity affects metabolic rate more than any other factor; the more strenuous the activity, the greater the stimulation. Mental activity, which requires only about 4 kcal per hour, provides very little stimulation.

Obesity is a major problem in the United States and Canada. See page 1178 later in this chapter.

Essential Nutrients

Essential nutrients include water, carbohydrates, proteins, fats, vitamins, and minerals. The most basic nutrient need is water. Because every cell requires a continuous supply of fuel, the body's most urgent nutritional need, after water, is for nutrients that provide fuel, or energy. The energy-providing nutrients are carbohydrates, fats, and proteins. Hunger impels people to eat enough energy-providing nutrients to satisfy their energy needs.

No clear-cut body signals lead a person to ingest certain vitamins or minerals, both of which are often referred to as **micronutrients**. Lack of such signals, however, does not mean that people do not need these nutrients. Micronutrients are essential for vital structures and regulatory functions of the body.

Water

Water is the most abundant compound in the body and vital to all body processes. Fortunately, people are impelled by thirst to drink water long before the body's water levels are too low. Chapter 46 provides detailed information about this nutrient.

Carbohydrates

Definition and Description

Carbohydrates are composed of the elements carbon, hydrogen, and oxygen and are of two basic kinds: sugars (simple carbohydrates) and starches (complex carbohydrates). The sugars may be **monosaccharides** (single molecules), which include glucose, fructose, and galactose, or **disaccharides** (double molecules), which include sucrose or table sugar (a combination of glucose and fructose), maltose or grain sugar (two glucose molecules), and lactose or milk sugar (a combination of glucose and galactose). Starches are **polysaccharides** because they are composed of branched chains of dozens of molecules of glucose. Nearly all carbohydrates (with the exception of those in milk and milk products, which contain the disaccharide lactose) are derived from plants.

Carbohydrates are also categorized as natural (those found in foods as they come from the earth, e.g., fruits, vegetables, wheat) and refined or processed (those extracted from their natural sources and added to foods, e.g., cookies, candy, cakes, and pies). The natural carbohydrates supply vital nutrients such as protein, vitamins, and minerals and an important nonnutrient, dietary fiber.

Fiber, a carbohydrate derived from plants, cannot be digested by humans and has few or no calories but supplies roughage or bulk to the diet. This bulk not only satisfies appetite but also helps the digestive tract to function effectively and to eliminate wastes. Refined carbohydrates are relatively low in nutrients in relation to the large number of calories they contain and thus are often referred to as empty calories.

Digestion

Ingested food must be altered physically and chemically before the body can absorb it from the gastrointestinal tract.

Physical alterations Physical alterations include mechanical breakdown and mixing of food. Mechanical breakdown results from the **mastication** (chewing) of food, which breaks down cell walls, releases their nutrients, and increases the surface area of food, thus facilitating chemical digestion. Mixing of food with secretions occurs in the mouth, stomach, and intestines. Initial mixing of food with saliva in the mouth begins the chemical digestion of carbohydrates and aids the passage of all swallowed food to the stomach. Mixing waves usually start at the midpoint of the stomach but are very vigorous in the antrum (portion of the stomach between the fundus or body and the pylorus). Food is churned with gastric secretions. In the intestine, mixing of **chyme** (mixture of food and secretions passing from the stomach into the duodenum) is continued by **segmentation** (local) **contractions** and to a lesser degree by **peristalsis.** These contractions mix the chyme with digestive secretions and bring the chyme into contact with the intestinal mucosa, thus facilitating absorption of nutrients.

Chemical alterations Chemical alterations include the digestive processes that convert food nutrients to a form the body can absorb. Energy nutrients (carbohydrates, fats, and proteins) and vitamins are altered chemically by **hydrolysis**, a process that involves the splitting of a molecule in the presence of particular digestive enzymes with the addition of water. (**Enzymes** are biologic catalysts that speed up chemical reactions.) Very large molecules can be hydrolyzed hundreds of times to much smaller molecules suitable for absorption. Digestive enzymes, which break down nutrients chemically into smaller compounds

Table 42–1 Actions of Major Digestive Enzymes

Name	Source	Site of Action	Agents Acted Upon	Resulting Products
Carbohydrate enzymes				
Ptyalin (salivary amylase)	Saliva (secretions from parotid and submaxillary glands)	Mouth; some in body of stomach	Starch, e.g., grains, potatoes, legumes	Dextrins, maltose, glucose
Pancreatic amylase	Pancreatic secretions	Small intestine	Starch	As above
			Dextrins	Maltose, glucose
Disaccharidases	Small intestine	Brush border of small intestine	Disaccharides	Monosaccharides
a. Lactase			Lactose in milk	Glucose and galactose
b. Maltase			Maltose in corn syrup	Glucose
c. Sucrase			Sucrose in table sugar, fruits	Glucose and fructose
Protein enzymes				
Pepsin	Peptic cells of stomach; inactive proenzyme pepsinogen is activated to pepsin by hydrochloric acid	Stomach	Large protein molecules	Proteoses, peptones, and large polypeptides
Rennin (in infants only)	Gastric mucosa	Stomach; calcium is necessary for activity	Casein in milk	Coagulated milk
Trypsin	Pancreatic cells; inactive proenzyme trypsinogen activated to trypsin by enterokinase (hormone produced in duodenal wall)	Lumen of small intestine	Whole and partially digested proteins, e.g., proteoses, peptones	Smaller polypeptides and dipeptides
Chymotrypsin	Pancreatic cells; inactive proenzyme chymotrypsinogen is activated to chymotrypsin by trypsin	Lumen of small intestine	Same as trypsin	Same as trypsin; also coagulates milk
Carboxypeptidase	Pancreatic cells; inactive proenzyme procarboxypeptidase is activated to carboxypeptidase by trypsin	Lumen of small intestine	Same as trypsin	Same as trypsin plus some amino acids
Aminopeptidase	Glands in intestinal wall	Brush border of small intestine	Polypeptides	Short chain peptides and amino acids
Dipeptidase	Glands in intestinal wall	Brush border of small intestine	Dipeptides	Amino acids
Fat enzymes				
Pancreatic lipase	Pancreas	Small intestine	Triglycerides, diglycerides	Diglycerides, monoglycerides, fatty acids

by hydrolysis, are categorized according to the types of nutrients on which they act. See Table 42–1.

The desired end products of carbohydrate digestion are monosaccharides (glucose, fructose, and galactose). Some simple sugars, therefore, require no digestion. Of the three monosaccharides, glucose is by far the most abundant. Major enzymes of carbohydrate metabolism include ptyalin (salivary amylase), pancreatic amylase, and the disaccharidases: maltase, sucrase, and lactase.

Absorption and Transport

The small intestine provides an extremely large mucosal surface area, since it is covered with tiny projections (villi) that in turn have smaller projections (microvilli), referred to as the brush border. These projections increase the surface area of the mucosa enormously, making possible the absorption of large amounts of nutrients.

In healthy persons, essentially all digested carbohydrate is absorbed by the small intestine. The precise mechanism by which monosaccharides are absorbed is not known. It is thought that a carrier for transport of glucose and some other monosaccharides (e.g., galactose) is present in the brush border of the epithelial cells. This carrier, however, will not transport the glucose in the absence of the transport of sodium. (See the section on active transport of sodium, Chapter 46, page 1351.) Thus, it is thought that the carrier has receptor sites for both a glucose molecule and a sodium ion and will not transport glucose to the inside of cells unless the receptor site for sodium is simultaneously filled (Guyton 1982, p. 516). This hypothesized carrier mechanism for glucose transport is the basis of the **sodium cotransport theory.**

Monosaccharides are absorbed into the portal blood and, after passing through the liver, are transported everywhere in the body by the circulatory system. Fructose and galactose undergo chemical changes in the liver, which converts them into glucose. Thus, essentially all of the monosaccharides that circulate in the blood are glucose.

Transport of glucose through the cell membrane into the tissue cells occurs by facilitated diffusion. Because glucose is too large a molecule to diffuse through cell membranes, it first combines with a carrier substance (thought to be a protein of small molecular weight) that makes glucose soluble in the cell membrane and able to diffuse readily to the cell interior. After passage through the cell membrane, glucose is dissociated from the carrier.

The rate of glucose transport through the cell membrane is greatly increased by insulin. In the absence of insulin, the amount of glucose that diffuses to the cell interior is far too little to supply normal requirements for energy (with the exception of the liver and brain cells). Glucose metabolism is therefore controlled by the rate at which insulin is available from the pancreas.

After entry into the cells, glucose combines with phosphate by an irreversible process called **phosphorylation**. This process captures the glucose in the cell; i.e., once in the cell, glucose cannot diffuse back out. Three exceptions to this irreversible process are liver, renal tubular epithelial, and intestinal epithelial cells, where specific enzymes (phosphatases) are available to reverse the reaction. Once in the cell, glucose is either used for immediate release of energy or stored.

Storage

Glucose is stored in cells in the form of **glycogen** (a large polymer of glucose). Although all cells of the body are capable of storing some glycogen, certain cells—liver and muscle—can store large amounts. The process of glycogen formation is called **glycogenesis**, and the breakdown of glycogen to re-form glucose is called **glycogenolysis**. Two hormones activate glycogenolysis: glucagon from the alpha cells of the pancreas, and epinephrine from the adrenal medulla. Glucagon is secreted when blood glucose concentrations fall to low levels; glucagon stimulates glycogenolysis mainly in the liver. The liver delivers large amounts of glucose into the bloodstream, thus elevating the blood glucose. Epinephrine is released whenever the sympathetic nervous system is stimulated. Epinephrine stimulates glycogenolysis in both liver and muscle cells, thereby releasing energy needed by the body for action during sympathetic stimulation. Most of the glucose formed in the liver as a result of glycogenolysis passes directly into the bloodstream; thus liver glycogenolysis always causes an increase in the blood glucose concentration. In most other cells of the body, however, particularly muscle cells, the glucose from glycogenolysis is used inside that cell and does not enter the bloodstream.

When the body's stores of carbohydrates fall below normal, certain quantities of glucose are formed from protein (amino acids) and fat reserves by **gluconeogenesis**, a process that occurs in the liver. Up to 60% of the amino acids in the body's protein can be converted into glucose. Some types of amino acids cannot be converted. During periods of starvation, the body depletes its fat first and later its protein reserves.

Metabolism

Once in the cells, glucose undergoes a series of reactions to produce energy for the body's varied demands. There are two major pathways for breaking down glucose into the end products of carbon dioxide and water, thus producing energy:

1. Glycolysis and the formation of pyruvic acid (Embden-Meyerhof glycolytic pathway)
2. Citric acid cycle (Krebs cycle or tricarboxylic acid cycle)

Glycolysis is the release of energy through the **catabolism** (breaking down) of a glucose molecule into two molecules of pyruvic acid. This is a complex process involving 10 successive steps of chemical reactions, each of which is catalyzed by specific enzymes. During the process, the end-products of glycolysis are oxidized, and energy is released in small packets to form **adenosine triphosphate** (ATP). ATP is a compound with high-energy bonds that stores the energy produced during glucose oxidation. Not all of the energy is stored, however. Some of it is lost in the form of heat. Because of the formation of ATP, the body's energy supply is conserved rather than dissipated all at once. During the cycle, two ATP molecules are formed from one glucose molecule (Guyton 1982, p. 528). The formation of pyruvic acid ends this glycolytic pathway; however, pyruvic acid provides the gateway to the next pathway, the citric acid cycle. The pyruvic acid is first broken down into two molecules of acetyl coenzyme A (acetyl-CoA).

The **citric acid cycle** is a complex series of chemical reactions by which the acetyl portion of acetyl-CoA is broken down to carbon dioxide and hydrogen atoms. The hydrogen atoms are subsequently oxidized, thus releasing more energy to form ATP. In the initial stage of the citric acid cycle, acetyl-CoA combines with oxaloacetic acid to form citric acid, which gives this cycle its name. For each molecule of glucose metabolized in the citric acid cycle, two molecules of ATP are formed (Guyton 1982, p. 530). See also Figure 37–69 on page 999.

Proteins

Definition and Description

Proteins are organic substances that upon hydrolysis or digestion yield their constituent building blocks—amino acids (Williams 1981, p. 51). Like carbohydrates, proteins are composed of carbon, hydrogen, and oxygen, but proteins also contain nitrogen. Every cell in the body contains some protein, and about three-quarters of body solids are proteins. Protein is part of muscle, bone, cartilage, skin, blood, and lymph. Many hormones and all enzymes are proteins. The only body substances normally lacking protein are urine and bile.

Proteins can be categorized by chemical structure as simple or compound.

Simple proteins contain only amino acids or their derivatives. **Amino acids** are nitrogen-containing chemicals, the building blocks of protein. Examples of simple proteins are (Williams 1981, p. 52):

1. Albumin, e.g., lactalbumin in milk and serum albumin in blood
2. Albuminoid, e.g., keratin in hair and skin, and gelatin
3. Globulin, e.g., ovoglobulin in egg and serum globulin in blood
4. Glutelin, e.g., gluten in wheat
5. Prolamin, e.g., zein in corn and gliadin in wheat

Compound proteins are composites of simple protein and another nonprotein group. Examples are (Williams 1981, p. 52):

1. Chromoproteins composed of a protein and a chromorphic or pigmented group, e.g., hemoglobin
2. Glycoproteins and mucoproteins composed of a protein and carbohydrate, e.g., mucin found in mucous membrane secretions
3. Lipoproteins composed of a triglyceride or other lipid, e.g., cholesterol or phospholipid
4. Nucleoproteins composed of one or more proteins and nucleic acid, e.g., purines found in glandular tissue

Amino acids are categorized as essential or nonessential. **Essential amino acids** are those that cannot be manufactured in the body and must be supplied in their final form as part of the protein ingested in the diet. They are essential for tissue growth and maintenance. Ten essential amino acids are threonine, leucine, isoleucine, valine, lysine, methionine, phenylalanine, tryptophan, histidine, and arginine. Histidine and arginine are necessary during growth but not during adulthood (Brody 1981, p. 36; Williams 1981, p. 53).

Nonessential amino acids are those that the body can manufacture. The body takes apart amino acids derived from the diet and reconstructs new ones from their basic elements (carbohydrates and nitrogen). Nonessential amino acids include glycine, alanine, aspartic acid, glutamic acid, proline, hydroxyproline, cystine, tyrosine, and serine (Williams 1981, p. 53).

Proteins are categorized as complete or incomplete. **Complete proteins** contain all of the essential amino acids plus many nonessential ones. Most animal proteins, including meats, poultry, fish, dairy products, and eggs, are complete proteins. Some animal proteins, however, contain less than the required amount of one or more essential amino acids and therefore alone cannot support continued growth. These proteins are sometimes referred to as partially complete proteins. Examples are some fish, which have small amounts of methionine, and the milk protein casein, which has little arginine.

Incomplete proteins are deficient in one or more essential amino acids and include those derived from vegetables. Incomplete proteins are most commonly deficient in lysine, methionine, or tryptophan. If, however, an appropriate mixture of plant proteins is provided in the diet, a balanced ration of essential amino acids can be created. Because protein is not stored, these mixtures must be eaten at the same meal. For example, a combination of corn (low in tryptophan and lysine) and beans (low in methionine) is a complete protein. Such combinations of two or more vegetables are called complementary proteins.

Another way to take full advantage of vegetable proteins is to eat them with a small amount of animal protein. Examples are spaghetti with cheese, rice with pork, noodles with tuna, and cereal with milk.

Digestion

Physical alterations Like carbohydrates, protein foods are altered physically by mechanical breakdown in the mouth and mixing with secretions in the stomach and intestine.

Chemical alterations Chemical digestion of protein begins in the stomach by three agents present in gastric secretions: pepsin, hydrochloric acid, and rennin. Pepsin is the main gastric enzyme specific for proteins. It is formed inside the peptic cells as pepsinogen, which has no digestive action. When, however, pepsinogen comes in contact with hydrochloric acid, it immediately forms active pepsin. This active pepsin then breaks the protein down into proteoses, peptones, and large polypeptides, smaller but still relatively large protein derivatives. Complete digestion of proteins to amino acids (the desired end products of protein digestion) could occur in the stomach if protein were held in the stomach longer. However, because the stomach normally empties in a relatively short time, only the beginning stages of protein breakdown are activated by pepsin. Protein breaks down into successively smaller molecules in this sequence: proteins, proteoses, peptones, polypeptides, dipeptides, and finally amino acids.

Hydrochloric acid, which converts inactive pepsinogen to the active enzyme pepsin, is secreted by the parietal cells and is an essential catalyst for protein digestion.

Rennin is a gastric enzyme necessary for infants to digest milk. Rennin is lacking in the gastric secretions of adults. Rennin and calcium act on the casein in milk, coagulate it, and delay its passage from the stomach.

Chemical digestion of protein continues in the intestine, where proteolytic enzymes from pancreatic and intestinal secretions break down large complex proteins into progressively smaller peptide chains and ultimately into the end products of water-soluble amino acids. Pancreatic enzymes include trypsin, chymotrypsin, and carboxypeptidase. Intestinal enzymes include aminopeptidase and dipeptidase. See Table 42–1.

Absorption and Transport

Amino acids are absorbed from the small intestine directly into the portal blood. It is thought that amino acids are absorbed by the same sodium cotransport system that facilitates carbohydrate diffusion (Guyton 1982, p. 516).

Amino acids are transported into the cells only by active transport or facilitated diffusion through carrier mechanisms. The nature of these carrier mechanisms is still poorly understood.

Storage

Soon after entry into the cells, amino acids are converted by intracellular enzymes into cellular protein. Thus, amino acids are not stored in the cells as amino acids but as actual proteins. Many of these intracellular proteins, however, can be decomposed again into amino acids and transported back out of the cell into the blood when blood levels fall below normal. Some tissues decompose stored protein more than others; for example, the liver, kidney, and intestinal mucosa reverse protein storage more readily than muscle, brain, and skin tissues.

Several hormones regulate the balance of amino acids in the cells (tissues) and the amino acid concentration of plasma. Insulin and growth hormone increase the formation of tissue proteins (anabolism); adrenocortical glucocorticoid hormones and thyroxine increase the concentration of plasma amino acids (catabolism).

The plasma proteins (albumin, globulin, and fibrinogen) are produced primarily in the liver and can be used for the rapid replacement of tissue proteins. Whole plasma proteins can be transferred (under the influence of the reticuloendothelial system) into the tissue cells, where they are split into amino acids, transported back into the blood, and used throughout the body to build cellular proteins. Plasma proteins, therefore, act as a labile protein storage medium.

Metabolism

Metabolic activities of protein can be categorized into three broad divisions of **anabolism** (building tissue), catabolism (breakdown of tissue), and balance (Williams 1981, p. 58).

Anabolism Proteins are synthesized in all cells of the body provided the appropriate amino acids are present. The types of proteins formed depend on the functional characteristics of each cell and are controlled basically by the genes of the cells.

Breakdown of tissue Because there is a limit to the amount of protein that can accumulate in a cell, additional amino acids are degraded and used for energy or stored as fat. This degradation occurs primarily in the liver and begins with the process of **deamination**—the removal of the amino (NH_2) groups by hydrolysis from the amino acids. Ammonia (NH_3) is a toxic byproduct of this process. Ammonia is removed from the blood almost entirely by the liver, which converts ammonia to urea. Urea is then excreted by the kidney.

After deamination, keto-acid products are released. These acids may be oxidized to release energy for metabolism. Because some of the deaminated amino acids are similar to the breakdown products of glucose and fat metabolism, they may also be converted to glucose or fatty acids. For example, deaminated alinine is pyruvic acid, which can be converted into glucose or glycogen (gluconeogenesis) or converted into acetyl-CoA. Acetyl-CoA can then be converted into fatty acids by a process called **ketogenesis**.

An obligatory loss of proteins occurs daily if a person eats no proteins. Certain proportions of body proteins (20 to 30 g) continue to be degraded into amino acids, then deaminated and oxidized. Thus, to prevent a net loss of protein, a person must ingest at least 20 to 30 g of protein each day (Guyton 1982, p. 544).

Balance All body protein is in a dynamic state of breakdown and renewal. Free amino acids present in the liver and plasma comprise an amino acid pool. This pool is a supply of essential and nonessential amino acids that can be used for protein synthesis in any part of the body. The supply of amino acids in the pool is maintained by dietary intake of protein and by catabolism of body proteins.

The state of protein nutrition is usually referred to as the state of **nitrogen balance**, since nitrogen is the element that distinguishes protein from carbohydrate and fat. Almost all nitrogen ingested is in the form of protein. However, most of the nitrogen lost from the body is in the form of nonprotein nitrogen compounds, i.e., the end products of protein catabolism. These end products include urea, creatinine, uric acid, and ammonia salts.

The state of nitrogen balance is the net result of intake and loss of nitrogen. When intake of nitrogen equals output, a state of nitrogen balance exists. Nurses can assume that a person is in nitrogen balance if he or she is (Suitor and Hunter 1980, p. 75):

1. Ambulatory and healthy
2. Not growing or replenishing body tissue
3. Consuming a diet adequate in essential amino acids, calories, and micronutrients

Positive nitrogen balance exists when nitrogen input exceeds output; in other words, when the total anabolism of protein and other nitrogenous substances exceeds catabolism and loss. Nurses can assume that a state of positive nitrogen balance exists (Suitor and Hunter 1980, p. 175):

1. During periods of growth, such as:
   a. During childhood and adolescence, when there are increases of height and lean body mass
   b. During pregnancy, when there are increases in maternal and fetal tissues
   c. During phases of physical exercise, when there are increases in muscle growth
2. During periods of tissue replacement, such as:
   a. During convalescence from an illness that caused protein depletion, when body tissues are regenerated
   b. After fasting or inadequate intake of protein and calories, when body tissues are regenerated

Eating more protein than is necessary to meet body needs does *not* result in an increase in positive nitrogen balance or lean body mass in healthy adults. However, excess protein intake can lead to weight gain (positive caloric balance). Generally, a surplus of nitrogen intake is balanced by increased excretion of nitrogen as urea.

Negative nitrogen balance exists when nitrogen output exceeds intake (when catabolism exceeds anabolism). This state occurs when (Suitor and Hunter 1980, p. 175):

1. The diet is inadequate in essential amino acids and calories.
2. A person is immobilized.
3. A person is exposed to unusual stress as a result of trauma (e.g., surgery or disease).

Fats

Definition and Description

Fats are groups of organic substances (fats, oils, waxes, and related compounds) that are greasy and insoluble in water but soluble in alcohol or ether (Williams 1981, p. 34). These organic substances are **lipids**. Fats have the same elements (carbon, hydrogen, and oxygen) as carbohydrates, but the hydrogen content of fats is higher. Fats are actual or potential esters of fatty acids, which are used in metabolism. **Fatty acids** are the basic structural units of fats. **Esters** are compounds of an alcohol and an acid.

Fats can be classified as simple lipids or compound lipids. Simple lipids or neutral fats are known also as **triglycerides**, since they are esters of fatty acids with glycerol in the ratio of three fatty acids to each glycerol base. Neutral fat is found in food of both animal and plant origin. Compound lipids are various combinations of neutral fat with other components. Three compound lipids important in nutrition are:

1. Phospholipids, which are compounds of neutral fat, phosphoric acid, and a nitrogen base.
2. Glycolipids, which are compounds of fatty acids combined with carbohydrates and nitrogen. Because these are found mainly in brain tissue they are also referred to as cerebrosides.
3. Lipoproteins, which are compounds of various lipids with protein. They contain mixtures of triglycerides, phospholipids, cholesterol, and protein. There are three major classes of lipoproteins:
   a. Very-low-density lipoproteins contain high concentrations of triglycerides and moderate concentrations of phospholipids and cholesterol.
   b. Low-density lipoproteins contain few triglycerides but very high concentrations of cholesterol.
   c. High-density lipoproteins contain small concentrations of lipids but high concentrations of protein (about 50%).

Cholesterol is also classified as a lipid. Although cholesterol does not contain fatty acid, it does have many of the physical and chemical properties of other lipids and is capable of forming esters with fatty acids. Large quantities of cholesterol and phospholipids are present in cell membranes and are essential for the structural elements of cells. Exogenous cholesterol is ingested in the diet and absorbed; endogenous cholesterol is formed in the body's cells, principally in liver cells.

High blood levels of one or more of the lipids, particularly cholesterol or triglycerides, is called **hyperlipi-**

demia. Hyperlipidemia puts people at risk of coronary heart disease. The precise relationship between plasma cholesterol levels and cardiovascular disease, however, has not been established.

Fatty acids are described as saturated or unsaturated. The degree of saturation is determined by the relative number of hydrogen atoms in the fatty acid. **Saturated** fatty acids are saturated with hydrogen. All carbon atoms are filled to capacity with hydrogen. An example of a saturated fatty acid is butyric acid found in butter. **Unsaturated** fatty acids have less hydrogen attached to the available carbon atoms. When several carbon atoms in a fatty acid are not bonded to a hydrogen atom, the fatty acid is **polyunsaturated.** An example of a polyunsaturated fatty acid is linoleic acid found in vegetable oil.

Williams (1981, p. 37) gives a list of food fats, with the most saturated first:

Saturated (animal fat)	*Unsaturated (plant fat)*
beef suet	olives, olive oil
mutton tallow	vegetable oils (peanut, soybean, cottonseed, corn, safflower)
red meats	
poultry	
seafood	
egg yolk	
dairy fat	

Digestion

Physical alterations Like carbohydrates and proteins, fats are altered physically by mechanical breakdown in the mouth and mixing with secretions in the stomach and intestine. In addition, fats are emulsified in the small intestine by bile salts, which are produced in the liver and released in bile. **Emulsification** is the process by which lipids are broken up and evenly dispersed in an aqueous medium. Bile salts promote the breakdown of fat globules into minute particles by lowering the surface tension of the globules. Emulsification greatly increases the surface area of lipids, thus enhancing their digestion and absorption. Bile is released from the gallbladder whenever fats are present in the duodenum. Fats in the duodenum stimulate the secretion of cholecystokinin from glands in the intestine. Cholecystokinin stimulates the gallbladder to contract and secrete bile via the common bile duct into the duodenum.

Chemical alterations Although chemical digestion of fats begins in the stomach, fats are digested mainly in the small intestine. Enzymes that break down fats include lipase, a pancreatic enzyme, and enteric lipase, an intestinal enzyme. Most chemical digestion is facilitated by pancreatic lipase. See Table 42–1. The desired end products of chemical digestion of fats are monoglycerides, fatty acids, and glycerol.

Absorption

Some end products of fat digestion (e.g., glycerol and some free fatty acids) are absorbed into the portal blood system and carried to the liver. Other end products (e.g., monoglycerides and cholesterol) are absorbed into the abdominal lacteals and transported through the lymphatic system to the thoracic duct, where they enter the blood through the left subclavian vein.

Storage

Large quantities of fat are stored in two major tissues: adipose tissue and the liver. Adipose tissue, referred to as the fat depot, stores triglycerides until they are needed for energy. Adipose tissue also has the subsidiary function of providing body insulation.

Metabolism

Large quantities of lipases are present in adipose tissue. Some lipases facilitate the deposition of triglycerides; others cause splitting of the triglycerides to release fatty acids into the blood.

The liver functions in lipid metabolism are (a) to degrade fatty acids into smaller compounds that can be used for energy, (b) to synthesize triglycerides from carbohydrates and to a lesser extent from proteins, and (c) to synthesize other lipids from fatty acids, such as cholesterol and phospholipids (Guyton 1982, p. 536). Triglycerides are used for energy. More than half of all the energy used by the cells is supplied by fatty acids derived from triglycerides or indirectly from carbohydrates. Oxidation of fatty acids produces acetyl-CoA, which enters the citric acid cycle discussed earlier.

Release of fatty acids from fat tissue is facilitated by the stress hormones epinephrine and norepinephrine from the adrenal medulla, corticotropin from the anterior pituitary gland, and glucocorticoids from the adrenal cortex. In addition, growth hormone and thyroid hormone cause rapid mobilization of fat.

Vitamins

Definition and Description

A **vitamin** is an organic compound that cannot be manufactured by the body and is needed in small quantities to catalyze metabolic processes. Thus, when vitamins are lacking in the diet, metabolic deficits result.

Vitamins are generally classified as fat soluble or water soluble. **Fat-soluble** vitamins include A, D, E, and K. **Water-soluble** vitamins include C and the B-complex vitamins: B_1 (thiamine), B_2 (riboflavin), B_3 (niacin or nicotinic acid), B_6 (pyridoxine), B_9 (folic acid), B_{12} (cobalamin), pantothenic acid, and biotin. The body cannot store water-soluble vitamins; thus, people must get a daily supply in the diet. The body can store fat-soluble vitamins, although there is a limit to the amounts of vitamins E and K the body can store. A daily supply of fat-soluble vitamins is therefore not absolutely necessary.

Vitamins are contained in many foods. Water-soluble vitamins, in particular, can be affected by food processing, storage, and preparation. Vitamin content is highest in fresh foods that are consumed as soon as possible after harvest.

Daily Requirements

Table 42–2 indicates the usually recommended daily requirement of vitamins. These requirements, however, vary considerably, as follows (Guyton 1982, p. 563):

1. The greater a person's size, the greater the vitamin requirement.
2. Growing persons require greater quantities.
3. Exercise increases vitamin requirements.
4. Disease and fever increase vitamin requirements.
5. Pregnancy and lactation increase the requirement for vitamin D.
6. Greater than normal metabolism of carbohydrates increases the requirement for B vitamins, e.g., thiamine and other B-complex vitamins.

In addition, some medications interfere with vitamin absorption (e.g., aspirin interferes with vitamin C absorption).

Food Sources and Functions

A balanced diet of carbohydrate, fat, and protein contains the necessary vitamins. See Table 42–2 for food sources, functions, and signs of deficiencies and excesses of major vitamins.

Units of Measurement

In the past, vitamins were quantified by their mass, which meant that milligrams and micrograms were the usual units of measurement. For a few vitamins, the international units (IUs) that pharmacists use were the standard units. Since scientists became aware that different forms of some vitamins have varying potencies, a new unit called equivalents is increasingly being used. The unit of equivalents reflects the vitamin activity that various forms provide in the body. The recommended dietary allowance (RDA) for each vitamin is shown in Table 42–2. RDAs of vitamins A, E, and niacin are measured in the new equivalents. The new unit for vitamin A is the retinol equivalent (RE); for vitamin E, the alpha tocopherol equivalent; and for niacin, the niacin equivalent (NE).

Minerals

Definition and Description

Minerals are found in organic compounds, as inorganic compounds, and as free ions. Upon oxidation, minerals leave an ash, which can be acid or alkaline. Calcium and phosphorus make up 80% of all the mineral elements in the body. There are two categories of minerals: macrominerals and microminerals. **Macrominerals** are those that people require daily in amounts over 100 mg. They include calcium, phosphorus, sodium, potassium, magnesium, chloride, and sulfur. **Microminerals** are those that people require daily in amounts less than 100 mg. They include iron, zinc, manganese, iodine, fluoride, copper, cobalt, chromium, and selenium. Different minerals have different biochemical functions. They can be grouped into four general categories (Christian and Greger 1985, p. 334):

1. They form part of tissue structure.
2. They help maintain water and acid-base balance.
3. They form components of important organic molecules, such as enzymes and hormones, that regulate body processes.
4. They facilitate nerve impulse transmission and muscle contraction.

Common problems associated with the mineral nutrients are iron deficiency resulting in anemia, and osteoporosis resulting from loss of bone calcium, discussed next. Key information about many essential minerals is shown in Table 42–3. Additional information about major minerals associated with the body's fluid and electrolyte balance is given in Chapter 46.

Iron Deficiency

Like many other minerals, iron is a component of many enzymes. It is also a part of hemoglobin, a carrier protein in the blood, and myoglobin, its counterpart in muscle. Iron enables these proteins to perform essential tasks of transporting oxygen and carbon dioxide to and from all body cells. Major clinical signs of iron deficiency are fatigue and a hematocrit or hemoglobin level below normal. Most North Americans, however, usually consume enough iron to prevent deficiency. The RDA of iron for adult men and postmenopausal women is 10 mg per day; for menstruating women, it is 18 mg per day. Women require more dietary iron than men do because of losses of iron during menstruation and childbirth.

The RDA of iron for adolescent males and females is also 18 mg daily. These high iron recommendations reflect physiologic changes that occur during the teenage years. Teenage males use the extra iron primarily to form additional lean body mass; females use it to replace iron lost during menstruation.

Table 42–2 Key Information About Vitamins

Vitamin	RDAs* for Healthy Adults (per day)	Major Food Sources	Major Functions	Signs of Severe Prolonged Deficiency	Signs of Extreme Excess
Water-soluble					
C (ascorbic acid)	35–60 mg	Citrus fruits, cantaloupe, strawberries, tomatoes, potatoes, broccoli, green pepper, spinach	Still under intense study. Thought to aid in metabolism of certain amino acids, aid collagen formation for healing, enhance iron absorption, aid in formation of red blood cells, and maintain integrity of capillary walls.	Scurvy (bleeding gums, loose teeth, skin spots, and bruising); delayed wound healing; impaired immune response	Gastrointestinal upsets, poorer immune response, confounds certain lab tests
B_1 (thiamine)	Females: 1.1 mg; males: 1.5 mg	Pork, liver, whole grains, peas, eggs, milk, peanuts, oatmeal, pasta	Function as coenzymes in metabolism of carbohydrates, fats, amino acids, and alcohol.	Beriberi (nerve changes; sometimes edema, heart failure, muscle weakness)	Unknown
B_2 (riboflavin)	Females: 1–3 mg; males: 1–7 mg	Milk and milk products; eggs; Cheddar cheese; organ meats (liver, heart, kidney); whole grains; green vegetables	As above for thiamine.	Skin lesions, e.g., inflammation and cracking at angles of mouth, dermatitis at angles of nares, keratitis of corneas	Unknown
B_3 (niacin or nicotinic acid)	Females: 14 NE (niacin equivalents; males: 19 NE	Beef, pork, fish, liver, whole grains, peanuts, green vegetables, dairy products	As above for thiamine.	Pellagra (diarrhea, dermatitis, dementia)	Flushing of face, neck, hands; liver damage
B_6 (pyridoxine)	Females: 2 mg; males: 2.2 mg	High-protein foods (e.g., meat, liver, tuna, poultry, nuts); some vegetables (e.g., green beans, potatoes; bananas)	Protein metabolism, acts in transport of some amino acids across cell membranes, converts tryptophan to niacin.	Nervous and muscular problems, e.g., depression, confusion, weakness, convulsions	Unstable gait, numb feet, poor hand coordination, abnormal brain function
B_9 (folacin or folic acid)	400 μg (microgram)	Green leafy vegetables, broccoli, green beans, whole grains, nuts, orange juice, cottage cheese, peanuts	Maturation of red blood cells; acts as coenzyme in metabolism of certain amino acids and DNA and RNA; essential during growth periods.	Megaloblastic anemia (large, immature red blood cells), gastrointestinal disturbances	None known
B_{12} (cobalamin)	3 μg	Animal products (meats, chicken, fish, eggs, liver, milk)	As above for folacin.	Megaloblastic anemia, pernicious anemia when due to inadequate intrinsic factor, nervous system damage	Unknown

Table 42–2 *(continued)*

Vitamin	RDAs* for Healthy Adults (per day)	Major Food Sources	Major Functions	Signs of Severe Prolonged Deficiency	Signs of Extreme Excess
Pantothenic acid	4–7 mg	Widely distributed in foods	Assists in metabolism of carbohydrates and fats.	Fatigue, sleep disturbances, nausea, poor coordination	Unknown
Biotin	100–200 μg	Widely distributed in foods	As above for pantothenic acid.	Fatigue, depression, muscular pain, dermatitis	Unknown
Fat-soluble					
A (retinol, retinoic acid, carotene, palmitate)	Females: 800 RE (retinol equivalents), 4000 IU (international units); males: 1000 RE, 5000 IU	Dark green and deep orange fruits and vegetables: apricots, broccoli, cantaloupe, carrots, pumpkin, winter squash, sweet potatoes, spinach and other dark leafy greens	Still under intense study: known to maintain health and normal functioning of cartilage, bone, and body coverings and linings (e.g., corneas, mucous membrane, skin); is a component of rhodopsin, a colored and light-sensitive substance in retina.	Keratinization of epithelial tissues, opacity of the cornea, night blindness, dry and scaling skin	Damage to liver, kidney, bone, headache, irritability, vomiting, hair loss, blurred vision, yellow skin from carotene
D (cholecalciferol, ergocalciferol)	5 μg or 200 IU	Fortified and full-fat dairy products, egg yolk; synthesized in the skin on exposure to sunlight	Increases calcium absorption from gastrointestinal tract; helps control calcium deposition in bones.	Rickets (bone deformities in children, osteomalacia (bone softening) in adults	Gastrointestinal upset; lethargy; cerebral, cardiovascular, and kidney damage; kidney stones
E (tocopherols: alpha, beta, gamma, and delta)	8–10 mg as alpha tocopherol equivalents	Vegetable oils and their products (e.g., salad dressings, many margarines); peanuts	Antioxidant, i.e., prevents oxygen from combining with other substances (vitamins A and C and polyunsaturated fatty acids) and damaging them; prevents cell membrane damage.	Possible anemia	In anemic children, blood abnormalities may develop
K (menadione, phylloquinone)	70–40 μg	Green leafy vegetables (e.g., lettuce, cabbage, spinach, peas, asparagus); meat	Necessary for formation of prothrombin in liver; prothrombin is essential for blood clotting.	Severe bleeding on injury; internal hemorrhage	Liver damage and anemia from high doses of synthetic forms

*RDAs are recommended daily allowances.

Sources: Adapted from National Research Council, Committee on Dietary Allowances, Food and Nutrition Board, *Recommended dietary allowances,* 9th ed. (Washington, D.C.: National Academy of Sciences, 1980) and J. L. Christian and J. L. Greger, *Nutrition for living* (Menlo Park, Calif.: Benjamin/Cummings Publishing Co., 1985).

Table 42–3 Key Information About Many Essential Minerals

Mineral	RDA for Healthy Adults	Major Dietary Sources	Major Functions	Signs of Severe, Prolonged Deficiency	Signs of Extreme Excess
Major minerals					
Calcium	800 mg	Milk, cheese, dark green vegetables, legumes	Bone and tooth formation; blood clotting; nerve transmission	Stunted growth; maybe bone loss	Depressed absorption of some other minerals
Phosphorus	800 mg	Milk, cheese, meat, poultry, whole grains	Bone and tooth formation; acid-base balance; component of coenzymes	Weakness; demineralization of bone	Some forms depress absorption of some minerals
Magnesium	Females: 300 mg; males: 350 mg	Whole grains, green leafy vegetables	Component of enzymes	Neurologic disturbances	Neurologic disturbances
Sulfur	(Provided by sulfur amino acids)	Sulfur amino acids in dietary proteins	Component of cartilage, tendon, and proteins; acid-base balance	(Related to protein deficiency)	Excess sulfur amino acid intake leads to poor growth; liver damage
Sodium	1100–3300 mg*	Common salt, soy sauce, cured meats, pickles, canned soups, processed cheese	Body water balance; nerve function	Muscle cramps; reduced appetite	High blood pressure in genetically predisposed individuals
Potassium	1875–5625 mg*	Meats, milk, many fruits and vegetables, whole grains	Body water balance; nerve function	Muscular weakness; paralysis	Muscular weakness; cardiac arrest
Chloride	1700–5100 mg*	Common salt, many processed foods (as for sodium)	Plays a role in acid-base balance; formation of gastric juice	Muscle cramps; reduced appetite; poor growth	Vomiting
Trace minerals					
Iron	Females: 18 mg; males: 10 mg	Meats, eggs, legumes, whole grains, green leafy vegetables	Component of hemoglobin and enzymes	Iron-deficiency anemia, weakness, impaired immune function	Acute: shock, death; chronic: liver damage, cardiac failure
Iodine	0.15 mg	Marine fish and shellfish; dairy products; iodized salt; some breads	Component of thyroid hormones	Goiter (enlarged thyroid)	Iodide goiter
Fluoride	1.5–4.0 mg*	Drinking water, tea, seafood	Maintenance of tooth (and maybe bone) structure	Higher frequency of tooth decay	Mottling of teeth; skeletal deformation
Zinc	15 mg	Meats, seafood, whole grains	Component of enzymes	Growth failure; reproductive failure; impaired immune function	Nausea; vomiting; diarrhea; adversely affects copper metabolism
Selenium	0.05–0.2 mg*	Seafood, meat, whole grains	Component of enzyme; functions in close association with vitamin E	Muscle pain; maybe heart muscle deterioration	In animals: liver damage; depressed growth
Copper	2–3 mg*	Seafood, nuts, legumes, organ meats	Component of enzymes	Anemia; bone changes	Liver and neurologic damage
Cobalt	(Required as vitamin B_{12})	Vitamin B_{12} (animal products)	Component of vitamin B_{12}	Not reported except as vitamin B_{12} deficiency	Diseases of red blood cells

Table 42–3 *(continued)*

Mineral	RDA for Healthy Adults	Major Dietary Sources	Major Functions	Signs of Severe, Prolonged Deficiency	Signs of Extreme Excess
Chromium	0.05–0.2 mg*	Brewers' yeast, liver, seafood, meat, some vegetables	Involved in glucose and energy metabolism	Impaired glucose metabolism	Lung, skin, and kidney damage (occupational exposures)
Manganese	2.5–5.0 mg*	Nuts, whole grains, vegetables and fruits	Component of enzymes	Abnormal bone and cartilage	Neuromuscular effects
Molybdenum	0.15–0.5 mg*	Legumes, cereals, some vegetables	Component of enzymes	Disorder in nitrogen excretion	Inhibition of enzymes; adversely affects cobalt metabolism

*Estimated safe and adequate daily dietary intake.

References: (1) Shils, M. E. 1980. Magnesium. In *Modern nutrition in health and disease*, ed. R. S. Goodhart and M. E. Shils. Philadelphia: Lea and Febiger. (2) National Research Council, National Academy of Sciences (NAS), 1980. *Recommended dietary allowances*, 9th ed. Washington, DC: NAS. (3) Scrimshaw, N. J. and V. R. Young. 1976. The requirements of human nutrition. *Scientific American* 235:50–64. (4) Underwood, E. J. 1977. *Trace elements in human and animal nutrition*. New York: Academic Press.

The recommended intakes of iron for pregnant and lactating women are the highest of all due to the demands of growing fetal, placental, and maternal tissues. Because it is almost impossible to meet these needs through diet alone during pregnancy, the 1980 RDA committee recommended 30–60 mg of supplemental iron daily for this group. The iron needs of lactating women are not substantially different from those of nonpregnant women, but continued supplementation for 2–3 months after delivery is advisable to replenish stores depleted during pregnancy. Adult men and postmenopausal women develop iron deficiency only because of apparent or occult bleeding.

Food sources of iron are shown in Table 42–4. Meat, fish, and poultry are superior sources because the iron in meat is absorbed better than the iron in vegetables.

Eating meat or fish with other iron-containing foods increases the amount of iron that is absorbed. Foods rich in vitamin C, e.g., citrus fruits, cabbage, and potatoes, also enhance iron absorption. Fiber, antacids, and tea interfere with iron absorption (Russell and Naccarto 1982, p. 115).

Calcium and Osteoporosis

Most of the calcium in the body (99%) is deposited in the bones and teeth. Calcium also performs other critical functions: With other elements, it plays a part in neural transmission; with vitamin K, in blood clotting.

In healthy persons, the amounts of minerals leached from bone into the bloodstream and entering bone from the bloodstream are equal; a state of dynamic equilibrium exists. When more mineral salts leave the bone than are replaced, the bones "soften" and weaken. **Osteoporosis** is a condition in which the mineral deposits, principally calcium, are lost from bone, thus decreasing the total amount of bone and weakening the skeleton. This condition is four times more prevalent in women than in men and usually begins during the third decade of life. Disability results if the weakened bone fractures. Fractures most often occur in the vertebrae, arms, and hips.

Although it has been theorized that osteoporosis may be a calcium deficiency disease, its actual causes are still under study. It is suggested that women, especially after menopause, have a dietary intake of 1500 mg/day of calcium to achieve calcium balance. This is almost double the current RDA of 800 mg/day (Heaney et al. 1982, p. 987). Exercise has also been found to delay some of the loss in bone mineral associated with aging. Several methods have been implemented to prevent osteoporosis in younger women and to halt the progress of existing disease: exercise regimens; estrogen (female hormone) therapy; and supplements of calcium. Although each of these methods has shown some benefits (Heaney et al. 1982, p. 1111), there is currently no known guaranteed preventive or curative treatment. Still, some physicians advocate exercise regimens and daily intakes of calcium in the 1200–1500 mg range for females over age 35.

Because calcium plays a part in blood clotting and neural transmission, it could be expected that low calcium intake might interfere with these processes. Blood calcium levels, however, are largely unaffected by dietary calcium intake. When dietary intake of calcium is low, several hormones work together to withdraw calcium from the bone as it is needed in the bloodstream. Thus, blood calcium levels are normally maintained.

Major food sources of calcium are shown in Table 42–5. Three important sources are milk, yogurt, and cheese. A person who consumes 2 cups of milk per day ingests almost 600 mg of calcium, just 200 short of the RDA. That amount is relatively easy to obtain from other foods. In an attempt to consume larger amounts of calcium, many women take the antacid Tums to supplement food sources. One tablet of Tums provides about 200 mg of calcium.

Table 42–4 Major Food Sources of Iron

Foods	Household Measure	Iron (mg)	Foods	Household Measure	Iron (mg)
Meat and alternates			*Vegetables*		
Beef	3½ oz	3.2	Spinach		
Beef liver	3½ oz	8.2	raw	½ cup	2
Beef heart	3½ oz	5.9	cooked	½ cup	2.2
Beef kidneys	3½ oz	7.4	Beet greens	⅔ cup	1.9
Chicken			Chick peas	½ cup	3
light meat	3½ oz	1.3	Kidney beans	½ cup	2.2
dark meat	3½ oz	1.7	Soybeans	3½ oz	2.8
Canned beans with pork	½ cup	2.3	*Fruits*		
Ham	3½ oz	2.6	Dates (pitted)	½ cup	3
Pork chops	3½ oz	3.4	Prunes	six	1.8
Turkey	3½ oz	1.8	Prune juice	½ cup	4.1
Veal	3½ oz	3.3	Raisins	⅔ cup	3.5
Sausage			*Wheat products*		
Bologna	3½ oz	1.8	Bread		
Frankfurter	2 medium	1.9	white	1 slice	0.6
Liverwurst	3½ oz	5.4	whole wheat	1 slice	0.8
Pork sausage	3½ oz	2.4	Corn muffins	1	0.6
Fish			Enriched pasta	½ cup	2.0
Clams	3½ oz	4.1	Kellogg's Special K	1 oz	4.5
Oysters	5–8 medium	5.5	Shredded wheat	1 biscuit	0.9
Scallops	3½ oz	3.0	*Other*		
Shrimp	3½ oz	3.1	Tofu (soybean curd)	½ cup	1.9
Tuna			Eggs	2 medium	2.3
in oil	3½ oz	1.9	Peanuts	⅔ cup	2.1
in water	3½ oz	1.6	Corn syrup	⅓ cup	4.1
			Molasses	1 tbsp	0.9

References: J. L. Christian and J. L. Greger, *Nutrition for living* (Menlo Park, Calif.: Benjamin/Cummings Publishing Co., 1985), pp. 348–49; A. B. Natow and J. Heslin, *Nutritional care of the older adult* (New York: Macmillan Publishing Co., 1986), p. 212; and E. N. Whitney and C. B. Cataldo, *Understanding normal and clinical nutrition* (St. Paul: West Publishing Co., 1983), pp. H49–H77.

Effects of Inadequate and Excessive Intakes of Nutrients

The effects of inadequate and excessive intakes of nutrients depend on the type and numbers of nutrients involved, the duration of inadequate or excessive consumption, and the age of the person. If all or some nutrients are totally missing, the person stops growing, fails to thrive, is incapable of reproduction, and eventually dies. If all of the nutrients are present but are generally available in inadequate amounts, the consequences are less severe. In children, limited growth is the likely result. In adults, the effect is likely to be a loss of body weight and a decreased capacity for work.

If intake of just one nutrient is inadequate, a more specific effect is likely to be apparent. For example, an insufficient intake of vitamin C over a period of months may cause a person's gums to bleed when the teeth are brushed. Over a period of years, a deficiency of vitamin A can cause night blindness (loss of visual acuity at night) or eye damage severe enough to cause permanent blindness. Although severe vitamin deficiencies are not usual in developed countries, they are not uncommon in developing countries.

Table 42–5 Major Food Sources of Calcium

Foods	Household Measure	Calcium (mg)
Milk and milk products		
Milk, buttermilk	1 cup	296
Milk, nonfat dry (reconstituted)	1 cup	298
Milk, skim (1% fat)	1 cup	300
Milk, skim plus milk solids (protein fortified)	1 cup	349
Milk, whole	1 cup	291
Cheese, American	1 oz (1 slice)	195
Cheese, Cheddar	1 oz	204
Cheese, cottage, creamed	½ cup	68
Cheese, Swiss	1 oz	259
Custard	½ cup	161
Ice cream	½ cup	99
Yogurt	1 cup	293
Other		
Tofu	3 oz	128
Fish		
Salmon	3 oz	167
Sardines	3 oz	372
Shrimp	3 oz	98
Vegetables		
Collards	1 cup	357
Beet greens	1 cup	144
Okra	10 pods	98
Fruits		
Rhubarb	1 cup	211

References: A. B. Natow and J. Heslin, *Nutritional care of the older adult* (New York: Macmillan Publishing Co., 1986), p. 212; and E. N. Whitney and C. B. Cataldo, *Understanding normal and clinical nutrition* (St. Paul: West Publishing Co., 1983), pp. H49–H77.

Substantial overdoses of nutrients can also produce ill effects. Generally, vitamin supplements are beneficial in certain situations, as in pregnancy, if taken in appropriate amounts. Overdoses of vitamins and minerals are most often caused by indiscriminate use of nutritional supplements. Examples of vitamin overdoses are:

1. Consumption of vitamin A in much higher than recommended amounts for a period of many months may result in nausea, vomiting, and headaches.
2. Consumption of vitamin B_6 in amounts 1000 times the recommended intake can cause nerve problems that make small and large muscle control difficult. For example, a person who takes extreme overdoses may have difficulty walking or typing (Christian and Greger 1985, p. 10). See Table 42–2 for signs of excesses of other vitamins.

The effects of nutrient deficits or excesses may take weeks, months, or even years to manifest themselves. Vitamin deficiencies and excesses generally take weeks or months. Surplus kilocalories or excesses of the energy nutrients, especially carbohydrates and fats, also become apparent as extra body fat in weeks or months.

Some effects may take much longer to become apparent. For example, links between certain nutrients and the development of health problems such as cancer and heart disease may take years or even decades to become apparent. Many factors, however, are involved in the development of such diseases, e.g., inborn or genetic predisposition, stress, level of exercise, and detrimental environmental substances.

Effects of Storage, Processing, and Cooking

Many factors change the vitamin and mineral values of foods, thus affecting the nutrient values shown in food composition tables. Four major factors are storage of foods, processing of foods, preservation methods, and cooking methods.

Storage

When fresh fruits and vegetables are not consumed immediately after harvesting, progressive vitamin degradation occurs. Vitamin C and the fat-soluble vitamins are particularly vulnerable. Generally, the vitamin losses are greater in vegetables than in fruits and meats. Storage and processing factors influencing this vitamin degradation include (Christian and Greger 1985, pp. 373–87):

1. *Temperature.* The higher the temperature, the greater the losses. Various vegetables lose from 30% to 40% of vitamin C when stored for 1 day at room temperature. In contrast, they lose only about 10% in the same time when stored at near-freezing temperatures.
2. *Moisture.* The greater the moisture loss during storage, the greater the vitamin losses.
3. *Light.* Losses of riboflavin can occur from fluid milk, since riboflavin is vulnerable to light. As much as 50%

of the riboflavin in milk can be lost in 2 hours of exposure to sunlight. Such losses were not uncommon in the days when milk was delivered to the doorstep in clear glass bottles. Current use of waxed cardboard or plastic containers conserves much of the riboflavin content.

The implications of these situations are apparent: Vitamin values are best retained by placing vegetables in airtight packages and immediately chilling them after harvest.

Processing

Various processing techniques promote or retard nutrient losses:

1. *Dividing*. The B vitamins are relatively stable in the presence of oxygen, whereas vitamin C is very vulnerable to destruction by oxygen. Vitamins that are vulnerable to oxygen are partially destroyed when the food is chopped or cut. Dividing foods into smaller pieces exposes a larger surface area to oxygen. For example, cantaloupe cut into pieces and refrigerated for 24 hours can lose up to 35% of its vitamin C; tomato pulp can lose up to 40% of its vitamin C content.
2. *Soaking*. Water-soluble vitamins and minerals are lost from foods that are soaked, since these micronutrients diffuse into the water. For example, the loss of water-soluble vitamins from peeled potatoes soaked for about a day at room temperature is about 10%. When peeled potatoes are stored in water and refrigerated for the same length of time, the loss of vitamin C is minimal.
3. *Trimming and peeling*. Nutrient losses occur when parts of foods are trimmed or discarded. Some of the loss occurs because the remaining part is exposed to oxygen. However, the discarded parts often have higher vitamin contents per weight unit than the parts kept for eating. For example, the vitamin C content of potatoes is highest in the layer just beneath the skin. After peeling, a potato loses 12% to 15% of its vitamin C. The sometimes discarded, darker outer leaves of cabbage, spinach, lettuce, and other green leafy vegetables contain more vitamins than the inner leaves. To avoid these losses, people should eat the edible skins and peels of fruits and vegetables and salvage the outer leaves of green leafy vegetables.

Preservation

Food preservation methods also produce changes in micronutrients.

1. *Canning*. Vitamin losses from canning are high. Only about 50% of the vitamins in fresh cooked vegetables or fresh fruits are retained in canned products. Canned products retain more of their vitamins if stored at temperatures of about 50–65 F. Lower temperatures are needed if they are stored longer than 1 year.
2. *Freezing*. Freezing retains the nutrient value of foods relatively well, although some destruction of vitamins C and E occurs. Nutrient retention is better in fruits than in vegetables. Up to 30% of the vitamins in vegetables are lost in the blanching process that precedes freezing. For best vitamin conservation, frozen products should be maintained at 0 F or less.
3. *Blanching*. Blanching is the brief heating of foods to destroy many of the enzymes that adversely affect color, flavor, and texture. Foods are often blanched before freezing, dehydration, or canning. The nutrient loss varies with the blanching method. Vitamin losses are greatest when vegetables are blanched in boiling water; fewer vitamins are lost when vegetables are steamed. Microwave blanching seems to produce the least significant loss.
4. *Drying*. Drying procedures vary. The oldest method involves drying foods in the sun for several days. Commercial techniques involve the faster methods of oven-drying, freeze-drying, and spray-drying. Vitamins A and C and thiamine are the vitamins most affected by drying. The greatest losses occur with sun-drying; the least with freeze-drying. Dried items stored with minimum exposure to oxygen and moisture and at a temperature close to freezing retain more nutrients.

Cooking

Cooking causes the largest loss of vitamins. Nutrient losses during cooking vary according to the type of food, the stability of nutrients, the amount of water used in preparation, the size of food pieces, the cooking time, and the method of cooking used.

1. *Boiling*. Immersion in boiling water can cause significant nutrient losses, especially when the volume of water is large. Up to 25% of the mineral content is leached from vegetables covered with water and boiled. Use of less water reduces the loss. Significant losses of vitamin C (45%) and carotene (20%) can occur when a large volume of water is used. Waterless cooking reduces the loss by 20%; boiling in less water (e.g., ½ cup) reduces the loss by 10%. Cooking time is also a factor in vitamin losses. The shorter the cooking time, the smaller the loss. Vegetables, therefore, should be boiled in just enough water to prevent the pan from scorching, in a pan with a tight-fitting lid, and only until tender but crisp.
2. *Steaming*. Steaming causes much lower nutrient losses than boiling does. Mineral losses are only about 50%

of the losses that occur during boiling. Vitamin C losses are also about 50% less.

3. *Pressure cooking.* Because processing time is short, fewer nutrients are lost during pressure cooking than during either boiling or steaming. Mineral losses are minimal, and vitamin C losses are lower.
4. *Microwave cooking.* More research is required to determine the effects of microwave cooking on nutrients. Because microwave cooking time is short, people generally expect more nutrients to be retained after microwaving than after other cooking methods. To date, some studies support this idea, but others do not (Christian and Greger 1985, p. 387).
5. *Roasting, frying, grilling.* Roasting, frying, and grilling cause approximately a 20% loss of vitamins. However, stewing or boiling the same foods doubles these losses.

Standards for a Healthy Diet

Several guides have been developed to provide standards for an adequate or healthy diet that includes all nutrients needed by the average person. These include: daily food group guides; Recommended Dietary Allowances; Guidelines for Americans by the Senate Select Committee on Nutrition and Human Needs; and vegetarian food guides.

Daily Food Group Guides

Various daily food group guides have been developed over the past four decades to help healthy people meet the daily requirements of essential nutrients and to facilitate meal planning. These food group plans emphasize the general types or groups of foods eaten rather than the specific foods eaten, since related foods are similar in composition and often have similar nutrient values. For example, all grains, whether wheat, oats, or other grains, are significant sources of carbohydrate, iron, and the B vitamin thiamine. Although the nutrients in each grain food are not identical, they are similar.

Daily food group plans that have been in use recently include the Basic Four Food Guide, the Hassle-Free Guide to a Better Diet, and the SANE Guide.

The Basic Four Food Guide

The Basic Four Food Guide was introduced by the USDA in 1956. This plan is based on four basic food groups: milk and milk products; meats and alternates; breads and cereals; and fruits and vegetables. Foods selected from the guide generally supply 1000 to 1400 kcal. Numbers and sizes of servings are listed for each group. See Tables 42–6 and 42–7. Because individual needs vary with age, sex, and activity, additional calories to meet energy requirements can be acquired by increasing the number and size of servings from the various food groups and/or by adding other foods that are not listed in the food groups. Examples are butter, margarine, sugars, flour, or products made from them; unenriched cereals; jelly, carbonated beverages; and bacon. The major ingredients of these foods are fats, sugar, starch, and unenriched refined grains. Most of these foods are high in calories and low in nutrients. Critics of the Basic Four Food Guide point out that it does not provide guidance on judicious choices of these low-nutrient-density foods and beverages. In addition, it does not provide guidelines about convenience foods such as hamburgers, milk shakes, and pizzas, which have become so much a part of the North American diet.

Another criticism is that the Basic Four Food Guide does not address fluid intake. A daily intake of 4 to 6 cups or more from any source is recommended. Users of the Guide also need to pay attention to adequate iodine intake. In areas of the country where the iodine content of food is low, iodized salt should be used. Unless there is an adequate supply in drinking water, fluoride, too, should be supplemented. Also, it is possible to follow the Guide and still eat insufficient fiber, which is found in raw fruits, vegetables, and whole grains.

Use of the Basic Four Food Guide has the advantage that the four groups are easily remembered. Although the plan does not guarantee that a person will consume the recommended levels of essential nutrients, it suggests that people are likely to come close to recommended levels, especially if they eat more than the minimum amounts recommended.

See Appendix C for the 1983 Canada Food Guide, which also uses four food groups.

The Hassle-Free Guide to a Better Diet

In 1979, the USDA replaced the Basic Four Food Guide with the Hassle-Free Guide. This plan adds a fifth group to the basic four. The fifth group includes foods high in fats, sugar, and alcohol. Moderation in consumption of these foods is recommended. Critics of this plan say that people may misinterpret the purpose of the fifth group and believe that the foods in the fifth group are being recommended for regular consumption rather than being restricted.

The SANE Guide

The SANE Guide, developed by Christian and Greger (1985, p. 38), is an attempt to build on the strengths of previous

Table 42–6 The Basic Four Food Guide for Adults

Food Group	Foods	Major Nutrients	Recommended Servings
Milk and milk products	All milk and milk drinks, cheese, yogurt, ice cream	Protein, fat, vitamins A and D, riboflavin, B_{12}, calcium, and phosphorus	2 or more servings. One serving is 1 cup (8 oz) of milk or designated equivalent.*
Meats and alternates	All meats, poultry, fish, and shellfish; eggs; dried peas and beans; soybeans and other meat substitutes; peanut butter	Protein; carbohydrate in plant alternates; fats except in legumes; B_{12} in meat, fish, and poultry; niacin; iron; zinc	2 or more servings. One serving is 2 to 3 oz cooked lean meat, fish, poultry, liver, or designated equivalent.†
Breads and cereals	All whole-grain or enriched bread and cereal products	Carbohydrate, some protein, thiamine, niacin, iron, fiber	4 or more servings daily. One serving is 1 slice bread or ½ to ¾ cup cereal or designated equivalent.‡
Fruits and vegetables	All fruits and fruit juices; all vegetables, including potatoes	Carbohydrate, vitamin C in citrus fruits and tomatoes, vitamin A in dark green or deep yellow vegetables, folacin, iron, calcium, fiber	4 or more servings. One serving is ½ cup fruit or vegetables or juice or designated equivalent.§ Include at least one citrus fruit or juice or tomato or tomato juice. Include one dark green or deep yellow vegetable daily or every other day.

*Milk equivalents: 1½ oz cheese or processed cheese, ¾ cup yogurt, ½ cup dry skim milk, ½ cup evaporated milk, 1⅔ cups ice cream, 1 cup ice milk.

†Meat equivalents: 2 eggs, 1 cup cooked dried peas or beans, 4 Tbsp. (60 ml) peanut butter, ½ cup nuts or seeds, ½ cup cottage cheese, 2 oz Cheddar cheese.

‡Bread and cereal equivalents: ½–¾ cup cooked cereal; 1 cup ready-to-eat cereal; ½–¾ cup cooked rice, macaroni, spaghetti, or noodles; ½ hamburger or wiener bun; 1 roll or muffin; 5 Saltine crackers; 2 squares Graham crackers.

§Fruit and vegetable equivalents: 1 medium apple, orange, peach, or banana; ½ medium grapefruit or melon; 1 medium potato.

Sources: Minister of National Health and Welfare, Department of Health and Welfare, *Canada's food guide* (Ottawa: Department of Health and Welfare, 1983); Chicago Dietetic Association and South Suburban Dietetic Association of Cook and Wills County, *Manual of clinical dietetics* (Philadelphia: W. B. Saunders Co., 1981), pp. 1–2; S. Williams, *Nutrition and diet therapy,* 4th ed. (St. Louis: C. V. Mosby Co., 1984).

guides and add other useful information. SANE is an acronym for Sound Approach to Nutritious Eating. The SANE Guide recommends the same major food groups found in the Basic Four Food and Hassle-Free Guides and the same numbers of daily minimum servings for an adult. The SANE Guide recommends different intakes of milk products by people of different ages. Unique aspects of the SANE Guide are:

1. It includes a fifth group called *limited extras.* The foods in this group are not needed for good nutrition, since they do not contain the essential nutrients in significant amounts. Therefore, they should be used as limited supplements rather than as mainstays of the diet. Many of these foods, e.g., fatty foods, sugary foods, alcoholic beverages, and unenriched baking goods, are high in calories. Examples are salad dressings, cream cheese, bacon, chocolate, sour cream, soy sauce, olives, ketchup, jam, jellies, and cakes. Overweight people should eat fewer of these foods. Other foods in this group are low both in calories and nutrients but contribute water. Examples are tea, coffee, broth, low-calorie soft drinks, and diet gelatin desserts.
2. It recommends that plant sources of protein be substituted for meat sources several times each week. The plant sources are richer in certain nutrients, e.g., magnesium and the B vitamin folacin, than meats are. Plant sources include legumes (e.g., garbanzo, kidney, lima, navy, and pinto beans; soybeans; lentils; and split peas), nuts, seeds, and nut or seed butters.
3. It lists serving sizes for some representative foods within each group.
4. It indicates the relative content of fat, sodium, and added sugar of certain foods in each group, allowing the user to reduce the amounts of fat, sodium, and added sugar in the diet.
5. It shows how people can count common combination foods, e.g., casseroles and sandwiches, when they use this system. Each ingredient must be identified by group. For example:
   a. 1 cup spaghetti with meatballs includes: 1 serving meat (2 oz); 1 serving grain (¾ cup spaghetti); and ½ serving vegetable (¼ cup tomato sauce).
   b. ¼ of a 12-inch cheese pizza includes: 1½ servings

milk (2 oz cheese); 3 servings grain (pizza dough); ½ serving vegetable (¼ cup vegetables).

Recommended Dietary Allowances

The Committee on Dietary Allowances of the Food and Nutrition Board of the National Academy of Sciences in Washington D.C. publishes lists of recommended dietary allowances (RDAs). RDAs are the levels of intake of essential nutrients that, to the best available scientific knowledge, adequately meet the known nutritional needs of most healthy persons (National Research Council 1980, p. 1). About every 5 years, the findings of recent studies are reviewed, and daily nutrient intake recommendations are updated. This process is undertaken by a group of leading nutritional scientists who compose the Recommended Dietary Allowances Committee. A table of the 1980 RDAs is in Appendix D. RDAs are recommended for 10 different age groups and pregnant and lactating women. The nutrients are measured in metric units. The macronutrients are expressed as gram (g) amounts; there are about 30 grams in an ounce. Most micronutrients are quantified in milligrams (mg); a mg is a thousandth of a gram. The recommended intakes for some vitamins and minerals are so small that they are given in micrograms (μg); a μg is a millionth of a gram.

Because a person's actual need for any given nutrient can be influenced by sex, body size, growth, and reproductive status, separate recommendations are made for various subgroups, defined by sex, age, pregnancy, and lactation. Recommended nutrient levels are usually set high enough (a) to include the needs of 97.5% of the people in that group and (b) to allow for some loss of the nutrient as it makes its way through the body. For example, the RDA allows for losses that occur during absorption or conversion from one chemical form to another, when some of the nutrient's activity may be decreased.

Factors not taken into account in the RDAs are:

1. The effect of illness or injury, which increases the body's need for nutrients
2. The variability among individuals within any given group, i.e., variability in energy requirements. The RDAs reflect an average need by each age group to avoid overconsumption.

The U.S. Recommended Daily Allowances

U.S. RDAs differ from the RDAs, although the U.S. RDAs were derived from the RDAs. U.S. RDAs usually reflect the highest recommended level of intake for most nutrients on the RDA table for any person over 4 years old with the exception of pregnant and lactating women. The U.S. RDA is a standard developed for use only on food product labels. U.S. RDAs provide information about nutrient content and allow comparisons between products.

Table 42–7 The Basic Four Food Guide for Children and Adolescents

Food Group	Recommended Servings*
Milk and milk products	Children up to 9 years: 2–3 servings Children 9 to 12 years: 3 or more servings Adolescents: 4 or more cups
Meats and alternates	All ages: 2 or more servings
Breads and cereals	All ages: 4 or more servings
Fruits and vegetables	All ages: 4 or more servings

*Serving sizes and foods are shown in Table 42–6.

References: J. L. Christian and J. L. Greger, *Nutrition for living* (Menlo Park, Calif.: The Benjamin/Cummings Publishing Co., 1985), p. 41; and S. Williams, *Nutrition and diet therapy,* 4th ed. (St. Louis: C. V. Mosby Co., 1984).

Nutrition labeling is required on foods that have added nutrients or whose labeling or advertising makes a nutritional claim. Many food processors voluntarily provide this information for other products as well. Certain nutrients *must* appear on the label: protein, vitamins A and C, thiamine, riboflavin, niacin, calcium, and iron. Nutrients that *may* appear include vitamins D and E; other B vitamins; and such minerals as phosphorus, iodine, magnesium, and zinc.

The U.S. RDA enables the consumer to see at a glance the nutrients a serving of food contains. Amounts of nutrients present are expressed as a percentage of the U.S. RDAs. For example, if a nutrition label states that a serving of skim milk contains 25% of the U.S. RDA for calcium, a person who consumes a serving will get at least 25% of the U.S. RDA for calcium. See Figure 42–1. Nutrition labels must specify the serving size, which may vary from product to product.

Recommended Nutrient Intakes for Canadians

A process similar to the National Research Council's setting of recommended dietary allowances is undertaken by the Canadian Department of National Health and Welfare. They prepare standards called the recommended daily nutrient intakes, which are published by the Committee for Revision of the Canadian Dietary Standard, Bureau of Nutritional Sciences, Health and Welfare. These Canadian standards provide nutrient intakes for 15 different age groups, for each trimester of pregnancy, and for lactating women. See Appendix E.

Dairy Darling
Skim Milk

Nutrition information per serving

Serving size	1 cup
Servings per container	1
Calories	90
Protein	8 g
Carbohydrate	13 g
Fat	0 g

Percentage of U.S. RDA

Protein	18
Vitamin A	10
Vitamin C	4
Thiamin	8
Riboflavin	30
Niacin	*
Calcium	25
Iron	*

*Contains less than 2% of the U.S. RDA for these nutrients.

Figure 42–1 A U.S. RDA nutrition label

Dietary Goals/Guidelines for Americans

In the late 1970s and early 1980s, dietary recommendations were issued by various governmental bodies other than the USDA. In addition to emphasizing self-responsibility for health and reinforcing the importance of getting enough essential nutrients, these recommendations also addressed concerns about the overabundant diet, specifically excessive consumption of fat, sugar, sodium, and alcohol. Increasingly, overabundant diets are being associated with cancer, heart disease, hypertension, diabetes mellitus, dental caries, gastrointestinal disorders, and other health problems. Because these diseases have been associated with the life-styles and diets of people in certain developed countries, they have been called the "diseases of overabundance." Some physicians and nutritionists suggest that certain prudent changes in diet benefit the individual, even though it cannot be said at this point that such a diet prevents disease.

In December 1977, the U.S. Senate Select Committee on Nutrition and Human Needs (1977, p. 4) released the second edition of *Dietary Goals for the United States,* which recommended *specific* reductions in fats, refined and processed sugars, cholesterol, and salt and suggested caloric intakes to achieve or maintain desirable body weight. Critics of these guidelines said that such specific restrictions were unnecessary for the general population. They thought such restrictions should be prescribed only for persons at risk for certain health problems and that the recommendations were difficult for people to incorporate into meal planning.

As a result, in 1980 the USDA and the Department of Health and Human Services jointly produced *Nutrition and Your Health: Dietary Guidelines for Americans.* These recommendations were based on the *Dietary Goals* but were less specific. Key points of the *Dietary Guidelines* are:

1. Eat a variety of foods daily.
2. Maintain ideal weight.
3. Avoid too much fat, saturated fat, and cholesterol.
4. Eat foods with adequate starch and fiber.
5. Avoid too much sugar.
6. Avoid too much sodium.
7. If you drink alcohol, do so in moderation.

Vegetarian Diets

In the United States and Canada, there are increasing numbers of vegetarians. There are two basic vegetarian diets: those that allow only plant foods and those that include milk, eggs, and dairy products. Some people, not strictly vegetarians, eat fish and poultry but not beef, lamb, or pork; others eat only fresh fruit, juices, and nuts; and still others eat plant foods and dairy products but not eggs. See Table 42–8.

People may become vegetarians for economic, health, religious, ethical, and ecologic reasons. Increased meat prices during the last decade have forced some people to become vegetarians or eat meat infrequently. Some people avoid meat because they believe it is healthy to do so. They cite as evidence that vegetarians tend to be less obese than others and that blood cholesterol levels of vegetarians tend to be lower, two factors that reduce the probability of heart disease. Among those who practice vegetarianism for religious reasons are Seventh-Day Adventists and followers of certain Oriental religious philosophies. Some people are vegetarians for ethical reasons: They object to the killing of animals or the way they are raised. People who follow vegetarian diets for ecologic reasons point out the wastefulness of eating animals that consume a large part of the world's supply of grain when this grain could be better used for people.

Vegetarian diets have several advantages:

1. Fiber in the diet is increased.
2. Total caloric intake is usually decreased.
3. Fat and cholesterol intake is decreased.
4. Protein sources are more economical.

Table 42–8 Types of Vegetarian Diets

Kind	Description
Vegans	Strict vegetarians, use no animal or milk products
Lacto-ovo-vegetarians	Drink milk and eat eggs but eat no other products of animals
Lacto-vegetarians	Drink milk but do not eat eggs or other products of animals
Ovo-vegetarians	Eat eggs but do not drink milk or eat other meat products
Pesco-vegetarians	Eat milk, eggs, and fish but no other meat products
Partial vegetarians (semivegetarians)	Eat chicken and fish but do not eat red meat
Fruitarians	Eat only fresh (raw) fruits, juices, and nuts

Vegetarian diets can be nutritionally sound if they include a wide variety of legumes, grains, fruits, vegetables, nuts, milk, and milk products and if proper protein complementation and vitamin-mineral supplementation is provided. Diets such as the fruitarian diet do not provide sufficient amounts of essential nutrients and are not recommended for long-term use.

Nutritional Concerns

Nutritional concerns of vegetarian diets relate to insufficient intake of protein, vitamin B_{12}, iron, and, with vegans, also calcium. Protein intake can be insufficient in the vegan diet if complementary protein relationships are not understood and followed. Although plant foods contain amino acids, many do not contain them in sufficient quantity or variety. When *eaten together,* however, certain foods often contain about the right proportions of amino acids. This phenomenon of one food supplementing low levels of amino acids in another is called **protein complementing** or **mutual supplementation**. Examples of foods that contain complementary amino acids are shown in Table 42–9. Generally, legumes (starchy beans, peas, lentils) have complementary relationships with grains and with nuts and seeds. Protein complementing is of particular importance for growing children and pregnant and lactating women whose protein needs are high.

Because foods of animal origin provide vitamin B_{12}, vegans need to eat other sources of vitamin B_{12}: brewer's yeast, foods fortified with vitamin B_{12}, or a direct vitamin supplement. Iron deficiency is also a possibility if red meat is not eaten because plant sources of iron are not absorbed efficiently. Vegans, therefore, are advised to consume (a) a vitamin-C–rich food with each meal to enhance iron absorption from plant sources, (b) many iron-rich foods, e.g., green leafy vegetables, whole grains, raisins, and molasses, and (c) iron-enriched foods. Calcium deficiency is a concern for strict vegetarians. It can be prevented by including in the diet soybean milk fortified with calcium, leafy green vegetables, and tofu (soybean curd) that has added calcium.

Table 42–9 Complementary Protein Relationships

Food Groups	Complementary Food Combinations
Legumes	Legumes with rice
	Soybeans with:
	Rice and wheat
	Corn and milk
	Wheat and sesame seeds
	Peanuts and sesame seeds
	Beans with corn or wheat
Grains	Rice with:
	Legumes
	Milk and milk products
	Brewer's yeast
	Corn with legumes
	Wheat with:
	Legumes
	Milk and milk products
	Peanuts and milk
	Sesame seeds and soybeans
Vegetables	Lima beans, peas, Brussels sprouts, cauliflower, or broccoli with sesame seeds, Brazil nuts, and mushrooms
Nuts and seeds	Sesame seeds with:
	Beans
	Soybeans and wheat
	Peanuts with:
	Sesame seeds and soybeans
	Milk and milk products
	Sunflower seeds
	Wheat and milk

Source: Adapted from R. B. Howard and N. H. Herbold, ***Nutrition in clinical care,*** 2d ed. (New York: McGraw-Hill Book Co., 1982), p. 352. Used by permission.

Vegetarian Food Guide

A good guide for vegetarians is shown in Table 42–10. It includes four basic food groups: milk group; vegetable protein foods; fruits and vegetables; and breads and cereals. In addition, eggs and fats are advised.

Table 42–10 Vegetarian Food Guide

Food Group	Recommended Serving per Day	Examples of Foods
Milk group	2 or more servings. One serving is 1 cup or designated equivalent.	Whole, skim, or soy milk; yogurt; cheese (1 oz); cottage cheese (¼ cup); powdered soy milk (4 Tbsp); evaporated milk (½ cup)
Vegetable protein foods	2 or more servings.	Beans, lentils, peas, and garbanzos (1 cup); peanut butter (4 Tbsp); nuts or seeds (1½ Tbsp); tofu (4 oz); dry textured vegetable proteins (20–30 g)
Fruits and vegetables	4 or more servings (include 1 serving vitamin-C–rich foods and 1 or 2 servings carotene-rich foods). One serving is ½ cup cooked vegetables or fruits, ½ cup juice, or 1 cup raw vegetables.	Vitamin-C–rich foods: orange, grapefruit, cabbage, tomatoes, melon, green pepper, strawberries Carotene-rich foods: dark yellow vegetables and fruits and leafy green vegetables
Breads and cereals	4 or more servings. One serving is 1 slice of bread or ½ to ¾ cup cereal or pasta.	Whole wheat or enriched bread; hamburger bun (½); Graham crackers (2); Saltines (5); Wheat Thins (8); enriched or whole rice; enriched spaghetti, macaroni, noodles; granola
Other: Eggs and fats	3 or 4 eggs per week, 1 Tbsp oil or soft margarine per day.	

Source: Adapted from I. B. Vhymeister, U. D. Register, and L. M. Sonnenberg, Safe vegetarian diets for children, *Pediatric Clinics of North America,* February 1977, 24(1):207. Used by permission.

Developmental Variables in Nutrition

Infants

Full-term newborns are able to digest and absorb simple carbohydrates, proteins, and moderate amounts of fat. Simple carbohydrates are required since the starch-splitting enzyme amylase is not present at birth. The newborn's diet must be balanced and supply all essential nutrients discussed earlier to meet the energy requirements of rapid growth. Caloric requirements are about 110–120 kcal/kg/day. Water requirements are high (140–160 ml/kg/day) because of the infant's inability to concentrate urine. Fluids must be increased in hot weather or if the infant is ill. Essential amino acids are required for body tissue growth and maintenance. Too much protein can cause dehydration; too little, nutritional inadequacy. Fats provide long-lasting energy and carry essential nutrients. Too much fat can cause a poor appetite; too little, a hungry and unsatisfied baby. Carbohydrates provide quick energy, spare protein for building and repair, and help burn body fat. Too much carbohydrate contributes to a diet that does not satisfy the infant; too little contributes to low energy levels, fails to spare protein, and contributes to **ketosis** (accumulation of waste products from the incomplete metabolism of fat). Adequate vitamins and minerals are also needed to prevent deficiency states. Iron intake is affected by the amount of iron stored during fetal life and by the mother's iron intake during pregnancy and when nursing.

During the first year of life, the infant passes through three distinctive feeding periods (Satter 1983, p. 126):

1. Birth to 6 months: milk feeding
2. Four to 12 months: transition stage (beginning solid foods)
3. Eight months on: beginning to eat adult foods.

The ages for these feeding periods overlap to some extent, since infants spend varying amounts of time in each period.

Because milk is the infant's major or only food during first 6 months, it must be appropriate for his or her needs. Breast milk, commercial formulas (cow's-milk-based and soy-based), and evaporated milk formula all meet the infant's needs. Hypoallergenic and premature infant formulas are also available to meet special needs. Breast milk and all standard infant formulas have an appropriate balance of protein, fat, and carbohydrate. Pasteurized milk (whole, 2%, or skim), however, has too much protein for infants and, with the exception of whole milk, too little fat. Although whole milk contains sufficient fat, the infant has difficulty digesting and absorbing the fat in whole milk. Foods and nutritional supplements for infants during the first 6 months are shown in Table 42–11.

Because breast milk has some characteristics that cannot be duplicated by even the most sophisticated formula, breast-feeding is considered better than infant formula for most babies (Satter 1983, p. 73) and is the recommended method of feeding. Formula feeding, however, is a highly acceptable substitute.

Whether a woman chooses to breast-feed or bottle-feed her baby depends on many factors. Some are (a) the influence of husband, relatives, and friends, (b) social acceptability of breast-feeding, (c) home and work demands, (d) personal preference, (e) nutritional and

Table 42–11 Feeding Recommendations for the First 6 Months

Milk Feeding	Nutritional Supplements
Breast milk	Vitamin D—400 IU
	Fluoride—0.25 mg
Commercial formula	Fluoride if none in water—0.25 mg
	Iron (5–10 mg) at 4 months*
Evaporated milk formula	Fluoride if none in water
	Vitamin C—35 mg or 3 oz orange juice
	Iron (5–10 mg) at 4 months
Avoid pasteurized milk. It is inappropriate for infant feeding.	

*The preterm baby on all feedings needs iron at 2 months.

Source: E. Satter, *Child of mine: Feeding with love and good sense* (Palo Alto, Calif.: Bull Publishing Co., 1983), p. 127. Used by permission.

physiologic considerations for both mother and infant, and (f) economic reasons. Evaporated milk formulas are least expensive, followed by breast-feeding, then commercial formulas. The cost of food needed by a nursing mother is higher than the cost of evaporated milk formula (Satter 1983, p. 86).

Breast-Feeding

Three types of breast milk are produced: (a) colostrum, (b) transitional milk, and (c) mature milk. **Colostrum** is a yellowish or creamy fluid that is thicker than later milk and contains more protein, fat-soluble vitamins, and minerals. It also contains high levels of immunoglobulins, which may be a source of immunity for the newborn. **Transitional milk** is produced from 2 to 4 days after delivery (during which colostrum is produced) until approximately 2 weeks postpartum. This milk contains higher levels of fat, lactose, water-soluble vitamins, and calories than colostrum does. **Mature milk** has a high percentage of water, and although it appears similar to skim milk it has more calories: 20 calories per ounce, whereas skim milk provides only 10 calories per ounce.

Breast-feeding is advantageous to both the mother and the baby because:

1. Sucking stimulates the release of oxytocin in the mother so that uterine involution (retrogression) occurs more quickly after delivery.
2. It is convenient and economical, negating the need to purchase and prepare formula.
3. It fosters psychologic closeness between the mother and the baby.

Unique benefits of mature breast milk for the infant include (Christian and Greger 1985, p. 439; Satter 1983, p. 76):

1. Breast milk is nutritionally very nearly complete for the full-term newborn infant; it needs to be supplemented only with vitamin D and fluoride.
2. *Lactobacillus bifidus,* a beneficial microorganism found in breast milk, prevents the growth of dangerous bacteria in the intestine. Lactoferrin, an iron-containing protein in breast milk, also discourages the growth of potentially harmful bacteria.
3. The proteins in breast milk are mostly lactalbumins. These are easier for the infant to digest than the casein proteins of non-heat-treated cow's milk.
4. Lactose, the main carbohydrate in human and animal milks, is more abundant in human milk than in cow's milk. It promotes the absorption of calcium and some other minerals.
5. Some unique lipids (triglycerides) supply about half of the calories in breast milk. The structure of the triglycerides makes them highly absorbable.
6. The mineral content of breast milk is well suited to the infant's needs. The ratio of calcium to phosphorus, approximately 2:1, facilitates absorption. The iron content of breast milk, although low, is very readily absorbed by the infant.
7. Breast milk contains lipose, an enzyme that helps the infant's immature intestine digest other fats.
8. Provided the mother is well nourished, the vitamin content of breast milk is adequate for the baby's needs. Inadequacies in the mother's diet are reflected in lower quantities of some vitamins in her milk.
9. Proteins in human milk do not cause allergies as often as the proteins in other milks or foods.

One disadvantage of breast milk is that a small but variable percentage of every drug taken by the mother is transmitted through her breast milk. It is extremely important, therefore, for nursing mothers to be cautious about drug selection and consumption. Certain antacids, anticoagulants, hormones, anticonvulsants, laxatives, and other drugs are contraindicated for breast-feeding mothers. Any drug, over-the-counter or otherwise, should be carefully checked before use by the breast-feeding mother. A few foods, such as rhubarb and chocolate, should not be eaten by breast-feeding mothers because they contain an active ingredient that is laxative (Satter 1983, p. 84).

Within a breast-feeding period, the composition of the mother's milk changes somewhat. Initially, the water content of milk is high, and the milk appears thin and bluish. Thus, the infant gets relatively dilute milk at the beginning of the feeding, when he or she is very thirsty. As feeding progresses, the fat content increases and the milk is more concentrated. Most of the fat is produced in the last minute of nursing. The infant then stops nursing and resumes feeding only if the lower fat milk from the other breast is offered. It is thought these changes may signal the infant to stop nursing and may have an effect on food and weight regulation (Hall 1975, p. 780).

Formula (Bottle) Feeding

Several types of infant milk feedings are available: cow's milk formulas, soy formulas, and predigested formulas. These products are designed to resemble human milk as closely as possible but have different types and amounts of protein, fats, and carbohydrates. Many are fortified with vitamins A and D.

Cow's milk formulas Most formulas are made from modified cow's milk. The major protein in cow's milk—casein—produces a tough curd in the stomach and is difficult for the infant to digest; thus, most milk-based formulas are heat-treated to make the casein easier to digest. The butterfat is replaced by more readily absorbed polyunsaturated vegetable oils. Additional lactose or other carbohydrate is included and vitamins and most minerals are added in amounts resembling those in human milk. Because there is some debate about the infant's need for iron, most infant formula producers make two products—one fortified with iron and one not fortified. Some experts believe that the healthy newborn has sufficient iron stores in the liver to last for about 6 months; others believe that infants who receive an iron-supplemented formula will not deplete their own stores. The new mother needs to be advised to seek her pediatrician's advice when deciding which product to choose.

The most commonly used commercial formulas are the standard casein-based formulas, e.g., Enfamil and Similac. Increasingly, the trend is toward whey-based formulas, e.g., SMA and Similac with Whey. The protein in these formulas has been modified to make it more like the protein in human milk. The casein content is decreased and the whey is increased. Another product used for infant formulas is whole evaporated milk formula fortified with vitamins A and D. Evaporated milk is a canned cow's milk product that has been concentrated by removing half of the water. It is *not* the same as condensed milk, which has added sugar and is used in baking. Evaporated milk must be supplemented with 35 mg of vitamin C or 3 oz of orange juice daily. Most formulas are available as a powder, a liquid concentrate, or a ready-to-use product. Before use, powders and liquid concentrates, including evaporated milk, require reconstitution with water.

Soy formulas Soy formulas are made from the protein of soybeans. These formulas may be recommended for infants who are potentially allergic to cow's milk protein. Because infants can also be allergic to soy protein, it is not recommended for infants who have already shown signs of an allergy. Infants may be allergic to both types of protein.

Predigested formulas In predigested formulas the protein, fat, or carbohydrate, or all three, are modified to suit the infant with allergies or digestive problems. They are based on a nonallergic and highly digestible protein. Examples are Pregestimil and Nutramigen.

Introduction of Solid Foods

The introduction of solid foods to an infant's diet is based on (a) the infant's need for nutrients that solid foods provide, and (b) developmental stage or readiness to handle solid foods. Both of these phenomena occur at about the same time—4 to 7 months of age. See below for a summary of the infant's developmental abilities in relation to feeding.

At 4 to 6 months, infants begin to lose their iron stores if they have not received iron supplements. In addition, the rapid growth of the infant demands foods that provide more energy than breast milk or formula. Table 42–12 shows a common sequence for introducing solid

The Infant's Developmental Abilities in Relation to Feeding

- The extrusion reflex is normally present for the first 4 months. This reflex causes young infants to spit out solids rather than swallow them. At 4 months, because infants can reach their mouths with their hands, the hands may get in the way during feeding.
- By 5 to 6 months, infants can sit with support, can grasp objects in a mittenlike fashion, can bring their lips to the rim of a cup and begin drinking, and can begin to chew.
- At 7 months, infants can feed themselves a biscuit, like to play with food and smear it, bang cups and objects on the table, and enjoy finger foods (e.g., pieces of banana).
- At 9 months, infants can hold their bottles, sit erect unsupported in a high chair, and develop finger-to-thumb (pincer) movements to pick up food.
- At 10 months, infants poke at food with their index fingers, reach for food and utensils, and like to hold a spoon and push objects with it.
- Beyond 10 months, infants show an increased desire to feed themselves. They begin to use a spoon and to hold a cup with both hands, but frequently spill food. Between 2 and 3 years of age, self-feeding is completed with only occasional spilling.

Table 42–12 Feeding Schedule: 6 to 12 Months

	4–7 Months*	6–8 Months	7–10 Months	10–12 Months
Milk feeding	Breast milk or formula	Breast milk or formula	Breast milk or formula	Breast milk or formula Evaporated milk diluted 1:1 with water Whole pasteurized milk *or combination*
Cereal and bread	Begin iron-fortified baby cereal mixed with milk feeding.	Continue baby cereal. Begin other breads and cereals.	Continue baby cereal. Other breads and cereals from the table.	Continue baby cereal until 18 months. Total of four servings bread and cereal from table.
Fruit and vegetables (including juice)	None	Begin juice from cup: 3 oz vitamin C source Begin fork-mashed, soft fruits and vegetables	3 oz juice Pieces of soft and cooked fruits and vegetables from table.	Table-food diet to allow four servings/ day, including juice
Meat and other protein sources	None	None	Gradually begin milled or finely-cut meat. Casseroles, ground beef, eggs, fish, peanut butter, legumes, cheese	Two servings daily; 1 oz total, meat or equivalent

*Ages overlap and are given as ranges because of variations in rate of infant development.

Source: E. Satter, *Child of mine: Feeding with love and good sense* (Palo Alto, Calif.: Bull Publishing Co., 1983), p. 227. Used by permission.

foods. Iron-fortified infant rice cereal mixed with breast milk or formula is usually introduced as the first solid food. It provides iron and has a smooth, semiliquid texture that the infant can readily handle. (Between 4 and 6 months of age, the infant learns to transfer soft foods from the front of the tongue to the back.) As the child develops oral skills and is able to eat foods of a thicker consistency, less milk is added to the cereal. The next addition recommended at 6 to 8 months is mashed or chopped cooked or soft fruits and vegetables. These foods provide vitamins A and C and have a lumpier texture that encourages more chewing and tongue movements. At this time, other cereals and "finger" breads, which provide B vitamins and iron, can also be added since the infant's palmar and pincer grasp begins to develop. By 8 months of age, most infants can grab a spoon. When the infant is about 7 to 10 months old, minced or finely cut meat casseroles and table foods can be added. The infant who is able to sit in a high chair at this age should be encouraged to adhere to the family eating schedule. When the infant is 10 months old, he or she begins to handle a cup and manipulate a spoon. Children do not learn to master a spoon until they are 15 to 16 months old. The final transition is a change from breast milk or formula to whole pasteurized milk. This change occurs when the child is about 1 year old, gets a good assortment of foods from the basic four food groups, and eats three meals a day.

New foods are introduced one at a time and in small amounts to permit recognition of allergies. The adult places 2 ml (¼ tsp) of food well back on the infant's tongue without exerting pressure that would cause the infant to gag. New foods are offered when the infant is hungry and before the formula or food to which the baby is accustomed. No sweetener or medications should be added. Initially, the foods need to be soft and smooth (strained or pureed) and at moderate temperatures. When their teeth begin to erupt (at 6 months of age), infants prefer foods that they can chew, e.g., teething biscuits or chopped cooked vegetables. The shift from pureed to chopped foods needs to be gradual.

At about 7 months of age or later, the infant can be introduced to using a cup at meals. Some infants begin self-feeding with a cup at 9 months of age, when they are also beginning to manipulate a spoon.

By the end of the transition period, all of the infant's nutritional requirements can be met by a mixed diet of table foods. See Table 42–7 for recommended numbers of servings of the four basic food groups per day.

Toddlers and Preschoolers

More teeth erupt during the infant's second and third year of life. By age 3, when most of the deciduous teeth have emerged, the child is able to bite and chew adult table foods well. Manipulative skills are sufficiently developed for self-feeding, although the child still needs some adult assistance and small utensils. Children should be taught table manners only after they master manipulative skills. The average toddler or preschooler generally requires:

1. The milk group: two to three servings per day (one serving equals ½ to ¾ cup)
2. The meat group: two or more servings per day (one serving equals 3 to 4 Tbsp)
3. Cereals and breads: four or more servings per day (one serving equals ½ to 1 slice of bread or ½ to ¾ cup of dried or cooked cereal)
4. Vegetables and fruits: four or more servings per day, to include at least one or more servings of citrus fruit and one or more servings of green or yellow vegetables (one serving equals 3 to 4 Tbsp)

It is important that children develop good food habits early. They should be seated comfortably. Appetite will vary from one meal to the next, so it is better to serve less than more of what they will eat. Overly large servings can discourage children from eating. Children need forks and spoons they can handle; fork tines should be blunt to prevent harm.

Children should be served new foods at the beginning of a meal along with well-liked foods. If a child refuses a food, it is best to remove it without discussion. Children quickly learn to attract attention by not eating.

School-Age Children

Children of school age need the same number of servings per day of the four basic food groups as preschoolers do, but in larger amounts to meet growth needs. For example, one serving of milk is 1 cup; one serving of meat is 6 to 8 Tbsp; one serving of vegetable or fruit is ⅓ to ½ cup; and one serving of bread and cereal equals 1 to 2 slices or ½ to 1 cup.

Adolescents

Teenage boys and girls have high energy requirements due to their rapid growth and need a diet plentiful in milk, meats, and green and yellow vegetables. Adults should encourage teenagers to eat nutritious snacks, e.g., fresh fruit and vegetables. Food fads are common among teenagers, some of which may be extreme and a cause for concern.

The pregnant adolescent often requires special counseling about nutrition and related issues. Worthington-Roberts et al. (1981, pp. 135–37) outline these issues as follows: (a) acceptance of pregnancy, (b) body image, (c) living conditions, (d) relationship with the father, (e) peer acceptance, (f) nutritional state, (g) prenatal care, (h) nutrition attitudes and knowledge, (i) food resources, (j) previous reproductive experience/contraceptives, and (k) preparation for child feeding.

Pregnant adolescents may need to learn to eat regular, well-balanced meals. Their energy requirements are usually very high because of their own growth needs as well as those of the fetus. They also need extra protein, iron, and calcium.

Young Adults

Young adults require balanced diets and caloric intakes appropriate to energy output. Of special consideration, however, is the pregnant and lactating woman. In addition to the basic diet for an adult, the pregnant woman needs:

1. Increased protein because of the growth of the fetus and accessory tissues of the woman
2. Double the usual calcium and phosphorus requirements
3. An additional 150 mg of magnesium daily
4. Iron to build sufficient hemoglobin and provide iron for the fetus
5. Iodine (175 mg), found commonly in iodized salt, seafood, and milk
6. Zinc (5 mg above the normal daily requirement) to meet the needs of newly forming maternal and fetal tissue

Some physicians also recommend folic acid supplements; however, the need for general vitamin supplements is questionable unless the woman is at nutritional risk.

Middle-Age Adults

Both men and women in the middle years need to reduce their caloric intakes primarily because metabolic rates decrease, growth is complete, and activity slackens. Therefore, middle-age adults need to eat less or increase activity to prevent obesity.

People in their middle years need to choose their foods from the four food groups and at the same time adhere to a prudent diet (Howard and Herbold 1982, p. 35). The latter includes more low-fat milk products, poultry, fish, and beans and limits eggs to three times per week. Vegetables, fruit, cereals, and whole-grain breads are recommended for their fiber and protein content.

Elderly Adults

Metabolic rate and physical activity decrease with age; therefore, elderly people require fewer calories than previously, but nutrient requirements remain relatively unchanged. Such physical changes as tooth loss and impaired sense of taste and smell may also affect eating habits. Other physical deficiencies that may affect eating habits and nutritional status are (Raab and Raab 1985, p. 24):

1. Decreased bile/gastric juice secretion
2. Decreased peristalsis
3. Impaired circulation
4. Decreased glucose tolerance
5. Loss of bone density
6. Loss of lean body mass

In addition, psychosocial factors contribute to nutritional problems. Some elderly people who live alone do not want to cook for themselves or eat alone. As a result, the elderly person may adopt poor dietary habits and is at risk of malnourishment. Loss of spouse, living alone, anxiety, depression, dependence on others, and lowered income all affect eating habits.

Nutrient intakes of people 50 to 74 years old and people 75 and older are indicated in the Recommended Nutrient Intakes of Canadians (Department of National Health and Welfare Canada, pp. 179–181). See Appendix E. More specific guidelines, however, are still needed (Raab and Raab 1985, p. 25). Guidelines need to reflect the need for high-nutrient foods that are compatible with the diminished chewing and swallowing abilities and other problems of these age groups. Raab and Raab (1985, pp. 25, 58) recommend the following guidelines for older adults:

1. Reduce fat consumption by drinking low-fat milk, eating more poultry and fish rather than red meats, limiting meat portions to 4 to 6 oz per day, and limiting the intake of added fats, e.g., butter, margarine, and oil-based salad dressings.
2. Consume desserts such as fresh or canned fruit and puddings made with low-fat milk rather than pies, cookies, cakes, or ice cream.
3. Make sure that intake of meat, poultry, fish, eggs, and cheese is sufficient, since intakes of these foods are often decreased in the older population.
4. Because of a lowered glucose tolerance, consume more complex carbohydrates, e.g., breads, cereals, rice, pasta, potatoes, and legumes, rather than sugar-rich foods.
5. Ensure an intake of at least 800 mg of calcium to prevent bone loss. Milk and milk products, e.g., cheese, yogurt, cream soups, milk puddings, and frozen milk products, are principal sources of calcium.
6. Make sure that intake of vitamin D is sufficient. Vitamin D is essential to maintain calcium homeostasis. To meet vitamin D requirements, include some milk in the diet, since such dairy products as cheese, cottage cheese, and yogurt are not usually fortified with vitamin D. If milk or milk products cannot be tolerated due to a lactose deficiency, supplements should be provided.
7. Because sodium may be restricted for older adults who have hypertension or other cardiac problems, avoid such foods as canned soups; ketchup; mustard; and salted, smoked, cured, and pickled meats, poultry, and fish. No salt should be added during the cooking of foods.
8. Due to the increased incidence of gastrointestinal disturbances and chronic diarrhea, the regular aspirin use among some elderly women, and the possible reduction in meat intake, the need for iron may be increased. See Table 42–4 for iron-rich foods.
9. Difficulties with chewing raw fruits and vegetables may lead to a deficiency in vitamins A and C, minerals, and fiber. Adaptions in food preparation may be necessary. The elderly may need to chop fruits and vegetables finely, shred green leafy vegetables, and substitute pâtés of meat, poultry, or fish for foods that are more difficult to chew.
10. Consume fiber-rich foods to prevent constipation and minimize use of laxatives. See Table 42–13 for examples of fiber-rich foods. Fiber-rich foods also provide bulk and a feeling of fullness. They are therefore useful in helping people control their appetites and lose weight.

Table 42–13 Fiber-Rich Foods

Food	Portion	Approximate Fiber Content (g)
Bran	50 grams (1½ oz)	22
Prunes	5 medium	8
Peas, fresh	1 cup	8
Apple	1 medium	7
Whole-wheat bread	2 slices	5
Potato	1 medium	5
Broccoli	1 cup	5
Lentils, cooked	½ cup	4
Pear	1 medium	4
String beans	1 cup	3

Source: Adapted from C. Wade, The fiber diet, Alive, *Canadian Journal of Health and Nutrition,* 41:12. Used by permission.

Additional measures for those who provide meals for elderly people include:

1. Serving food attractively, providing color contrast for visual appeal
2. Cooking food well so that it can be easily chewed by denture wearers
3. Serving essential foods first and providing sweet foods (carbohydrates) in moderation afterward
4. Noting foods that cause indigestion and not serving them again
5. Serving the heaviest meal at noon to those who have difficulty sleeping at night after a heavy meal
6. Not serving tea, coffee, or other stimulants in the evening to those who have difficulty sleeping

Assessment

To assess the nutritional status of a person, the nurse follows the "ABCD" approach: she or he takes *anthropometric measurements* (A), looks at *biochemical data* (B), assesses the *clinical signs* of nutritional status (C), and obtains a *dietary history* (D). The dietary history should include factors that influence the client's eating patterns.

Anthropometric Measurements

Anthropometric measurements provide a quick and easy way to assess a person's protein and calorie reserves. Protein-calorie malnutrition (PCM) is a common problem among hospitalized clients; it is estimated to occur in as many as 50% (Bistrian et al. 1974, p. 858; Weinsier et al. 1979, p. 418).

Anthropometric measurements are measurements of the size and composition of the body. They include measurements of height, weight, skin folds (fat folds), and arm circumference. The triceps, subscapular, biceps, and suprailiac skin folds can be measured with special calipers. The site most commonly used is the triceps fold. This section includes only mid-upper-arm circumference and triceps and subscapular skin fold measurements. The arm muscle circumference is calculated from the triceps skin fold and upper-arm circumference.

Assessment of height and weight is discussed in Chapter 35. Normal weight ranges by age, sex, and frame for adults are given in Table 35–3. An inadequately nourished person can be underweight, overweight, or obese: in every case his or her caloric intake is not in balance with expenditure of energy.

Mid-Upper-Arm Circumference

The mid-upper-arm circumference (MUAC) provides information about the individual's muscle mass. To measure the MUAC, make sure the client's upper arm hangs freely in a dependent position and his or her forearm is positioned horizontally. Locate the midpoint of the upper arm, i.e., halfway between the acromial process and the olecranon process. See Figure 42–2. Use a flexible steel tape measure calibrated in millimeters to measure the circumference of the arm at the midpoint. Read the measurement to the nearest millimeter. Maintain the tape in a horizontal plane and avoid distortion of the skin surface.

Triceps Skin Fold

A skin fold measurement indicates the amount of body fat, the main form of stored energy. The fold of skin includes the subcutaneous tissue but not the underlying muscle. This measurement can be considered an index of the body's energy stores. To measure the triceps skin fold the nurse first locates the midpoint of the upper arm, then

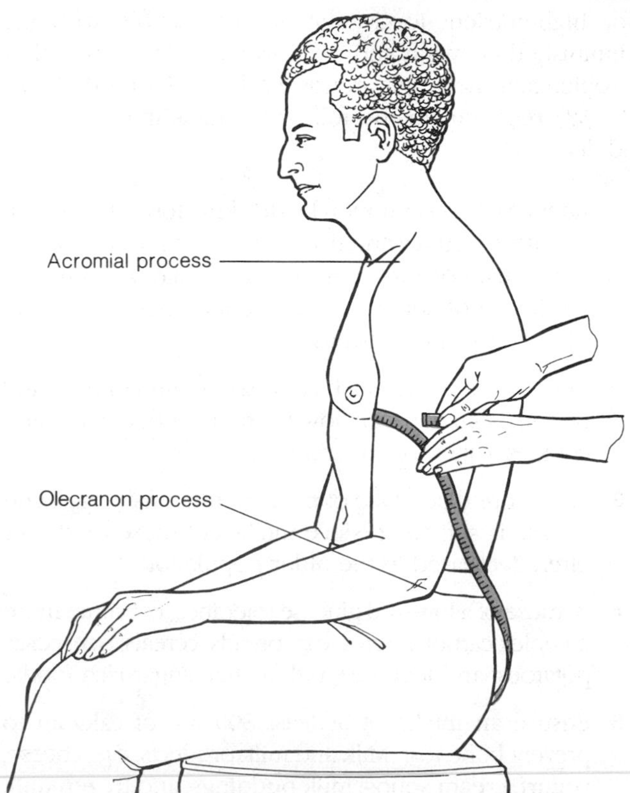

Figure 42–2 Measuring mid-upper-arm circumference

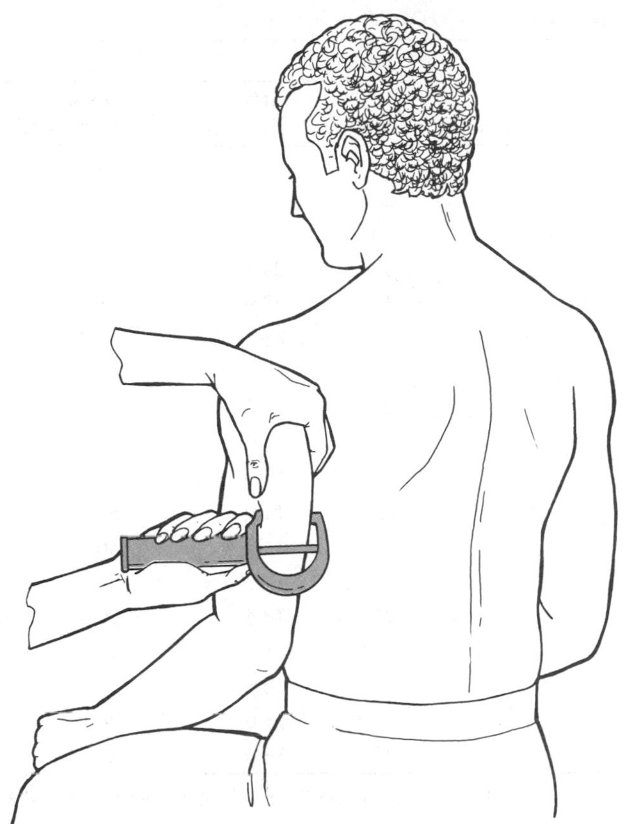

Figure 42–3 Measuring the triceps skin fold

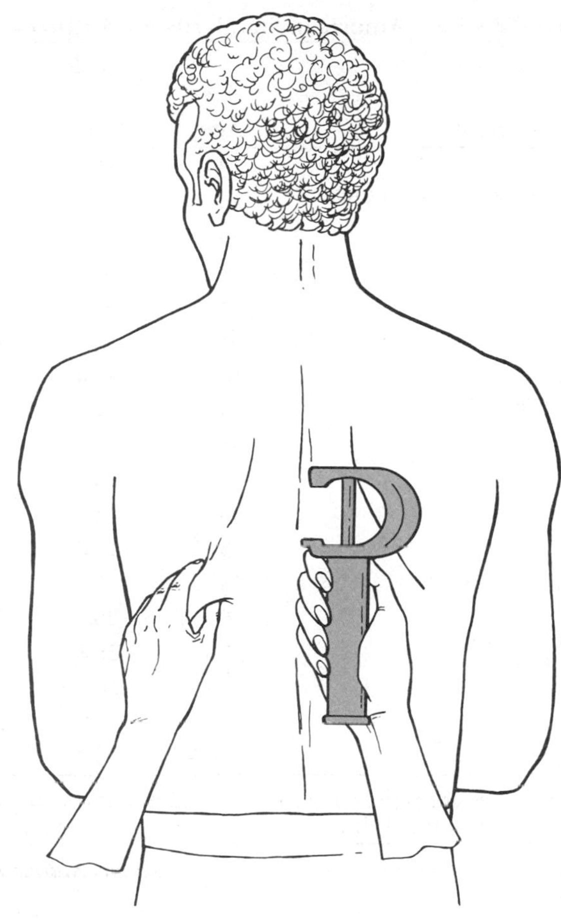

Figure 42–4 Measuring the subscapular skin fold

grasps the skin on the back of the upper arm along the long axis of the humerus. See Figure 42–3. Placing the calipers 1 cm (0.4 in) below her or his fingers, the nurse measures the thickness of the fold to the nearest millimeter.

Subscapular Skin Fold

To measure the subscapular skin fold, the nurse picks up the skin below the scapula. Three fingers should be on top of the fold just below the scapula, the thumb below the fold, and the forefinger at the lower tip of the scapula. The skin fold should be angled about 45° from the horizontal, upward medially and downward laterally. See Figure 42–4. The nurse places the calipers about 1 cm (0.4 in) above or below her or his fingers and measures the skin fold.

Arm Muscle Circumference

Since muscle serves as the major protein reserve of the body, the arm muscle circumference (AMC) can be considered an index of the body's protein reserves. Use the following formula to calculate the AMC in millimeters:

$$AMC = MUAC\ (mm) - [3.14 \times \text{triceps skin fold (mm)}]$$

Tables can be used instead. See Table 42–14 for standards for these measurements.

Biochemical Data

Biochemical measurements can be used to detect subclinical malnutrition. In contrast to anthropometric measures, which let the nurse assess observable changes in the body, laboratory tests help the nurse determine what is happening inside the body. Blood and urine samples are taken to measure a nutrient or a **metabolite** (end product or enzyme) that is affected by that nutrient. Blood tests are often ordered in packages referred to as SMAs (simultaneous multiple analysis) followed by a number, e.g., SMA-12 or SMA-18. Each package includes several biochemical measurements; the number following SMA indicates the number of tests that will be done.

The laboratory studies most commonly used today to assess nutrition include hemoglobin and hematocrit, albumin, transferrin, total lymphocyte count, nitrogen balance, and creatinine excretion tests. Although less commonly used, other laboratory tests can be performed to assess vitamins, minerals, and trace elements. Because many factors can influence these laboratory tests, it is important to realize that no single test can confirm a nutritional problem.

Table 42–14 American Standards for Anthropometric Measures*

		Male			Female		
Measurement	Age	Mean	5th Percentile	95th Percentile	Mean	5th Percentile	95th Percentile
Mid-upper-arm circumference in centimeters	18–24	30.9	25.7	37.4	27.0	22.1	34.3
	25–34	32.3	27.0	37.6	28.6	23.3	37.2
	35–44	32.7	27.8	37.1	30.0	24.1	38.5
	45–54	32.1	26.7	37.6	30.7	24.3	39.3
	55–64	31.5	25.6	36.6	30.7	23.9	38.2
	65–74	30.5	25.3	36.5	30.1	23.8	37.2
Triceps skin fold thickness in millimeters	18–24	11.2	4.0	23.0	19.4	9.4	34.0
	25–34	12.6	4.5	24.0	21.9	10.5	37.0
	35–44	12.4	5.0	23.0	24.0	12.0	39.0
	45–54	12.4	5.0	25.5	25.4	13.0	40.0
	55–64	11.6	5.0	21.5	24.9	11.0	39.0
	65–74	11.8	4.5	22.0	23.3	11.5	36.0
Mid-upper-arm muscle circumference in centimeters	18–24	27.4	23.5	32.3	20.9	17.7	24.9
	25–34	28.3	24.2	32.9	21.7	18.3	26.6
	35–44	28.8	25.0	33.0	22.5	18.5	27.4
	45–54	28.2	24.0	32.6	22.7	18.8	27.8
	55–64	27.8	22.8	31.8	22.8	18.6	28.1
	65–74	26.8	22.5	30.7	22.8	18.6	28.1

*These values are representative of the adult noninstitutionalized civilian population of the United States as of November 1, 1972, and were developed from measurements obtained from the right arm.

Source: National Center for Health Statistics, *Health and Nutrition Examination Survey of 1971 to 1974,* DHEW Pub No. (PHS) 79-1310, n.d. Used by permission.

Hemoglobin and Hematocrit Indices

A low hemoglobin level may be evidence of iron-deficiency anemia. **Hematocrit** (Hct), or packed cell volume, is a measure of the percentage of a given volume of whole blood occupied by red blood cells. Thus, a hematocrit of 45% indicates that 45 ml of each deciliter of peripheral blood is composed of red blood cells. An elevated hematocrit level is evidence of dehydration.

Serum Albumin

Albumin, which accounts for over 50% of the total serum proteins, helps to maintain fluid and electrolyte balance and to transport many nutrients, hormones, and drugs. Albumin synthesis depends on healthy, functioning liver cells and on an appropriate supply of amino acids. Albumin is a useful indicator of prolonged protein depletion. Because there is so much albumin in the body and because it is not broken down very quickly, albumin concentrations change slowly.

Many conditions besides malnutrition can depress albumin concentration, however. These include liver disease, advanced kidney disease, infection, cancer, and malabsorption disorders. Thus serum albumin level is used as only one indicator among several to determine protein status.

Transferrin

Transferrin is a blood protein that binds with iron and transports it throughout the body. Transferrin level is considered a more sensitive indicator of protein malnutrition than albumin level, because transferrin responds more promptly to changes in protein intake and has a smaller body pool (Whitney and Cataldo 1983, p. 691).

Most transferrin is synthesized in the liver. Transferrin levels are high when iron stores are low and low when iron stores are excessive. Certain diseases, e.g., liver disease, advanced kidney disease, and burns also cause decreases in transferrin levels.

Because some laboratories do not have the equipment required to determine transferrin levels directly, an estimate of a client's transferrin level is obtained by measuring his or her total iron-binding capacity (TIBC). The TIBC test is more widely available. The equation for converting the TIBC reading to a transferrin measurement is determined in each laboratory.

Total Lymphocyte Count

Certain nutrient deficiencies and forms of PCM (protein-calorie malnutrition) can depress the immune system. The total number of lymphocytes decreases as protein depletion occurs.

Nitrogen Balance

Nitrogen balance is discussed earlier, on page 1147. Nitrogen balance studies are useful in estimating the degree to which protein is being depleted or replaced in the body. Tests to measure nitrogen balance include the blood urea nitrogen (BUN) and the urine urea nitrogen (UUN), which requires the collection of urine excreted by the client during a 24-hour period. Urea is the chief end product of protein and amino acid metabolism. It is formed from ammonia detoxified by the liver and transported to the kidneys for excretion in urine. Urea concentrations in the blood and urine, therefore, are directly influenced by the intake and breakdown of dietary protein, the rate of urea production in the liver, and the rate of urea removal by the kidneys. Elevated BUN levels may be caused by excessive protein intake, severe dehydration, or general ill health and malnutrition; however, the most common cause is inadequate excretion of urea due to kidney disease or urinary obstruction. Decreased BUN levels may be caused by a low-protein diet. Elevated UUN levels may occur with starvation.

Creatinine Excretion

Creatinine is the chief end product of the creatine produced when energy is released from phosphocreatine, an energy-storing compound, during skeletal muscle metabolism. The rate of creatinine formation is directly proportional to the total muscle mass. Creatinine is removed from the bloodstream by the kidneys and excreted in the urine at a rate that closely parallels its formation. Creatinine excretion, therefore, reflects a person's total muscle mass. As skeletal muscle atrophies during malnutrition, creatinine excretion decreases.

Measurement of urinary creatinine requires collection of urine excreted by the client during a 24-hour period. Standards for creatinine excretion are developed on the basis of sex and height. These standards are used with the creatinine measurement to determine the creatinine height index (CHI) expressed as a percentage. For example, a CHI of 70% means that the client's skeletal muscle mass is approximately 70% of that expected in a person of the same size.

Clinical Signs

Since nutrition affects most body systems, an assessment of these systems can reveal nutritional problems. Table 42–15 lists some of the data that can be collected to assist nursing personnel in determining a client's nutritional status. This list is not exhaustive; for more detailed information, consult nutrition and assessment texts. A thorough assessment is usually done with the initial physical examination when the client is admitted to a health care agency. The data obtained serve as baseline data for comparison with later findings during the client's stay.

Dietary History

A dietary history generally includes data about the client's usual eating patterns and habits, food preferences and restrictions, daily fluid intake, use of vitamin or mineral supplements, any dietary problems (e.g., difficulty chewing or swallowing), physical activity, health history, and concerns related to food buying and preparation. See Figure 42–5 for a sample nutritional history tool for an adult. Although the tool shown is relatively structured and condensed to accommodate space limitations of this text, it indicates major areas included in most dietary history tools. To obtain data about eating patterns and habits, the nurse elicits a typical 24-hour diet history. More detailed records of the client's food intake can be kept over a

Table 42–15 Clinical Signs Indicating Nutritional Status

Body Part or System	Normal Signs	Abnormal Signs
Hair	Shiny, neither dry nor oily	Oily, dry, dull, patchy in growth
Skin	Smooth, slightly moist, good turgor	Dry, oily, broken out in rash, scaly, rough, bruised
Eyes	Bright, clear	Dry, reddened
Tongue	Pink, moist	Reddened in patches, swollen
Mucous membranes	Reddish pink, moist	Reddened, dry, cracked
Cardiovascular	Heart rate and blood pressure within normal ranges, heart rhythm regular	Rapid heart rate, elevated blood pressure, irregular heart rhythm
Muscles	Firm, well developed	Poor in tone, soft, underdeveloped
Gastrointestinal	Appetite good, elimination regular and normal	Manifesting anorexia, indigestion, diarrhea, constipation
Neurologic	Reflexes normal, alert, good attention span, emotionally stable	Reflexes decreased, irritable, inattentive, confused, emotionally labile
Vitality	Vigorous, energetic, able to sleep well	Lacking energy, tired, apathetic, sleeping poorly
Weight	Normal for age, build, and height	Overweight, underweight

NUTRITIONAL HISTORY

Name ______
Age ______ Height ______

WEIGHT
Current weight ______
Weight history (obesity, onset, fluctuations) ______
Percentage of
Overweight ______
Underweight ______

OTHER ANTHROPOMETRIC DATA
Triceps skin fold measurement ______
Arm muscle circumference ______

EATING PATTERNS AND HABITS
1. Typical day's food intake

Time	Item	Portion

2. Food likes ______
3. Food dislikes ______
4. Food allergies ______
5. Foods considered harmful or beneficial to health
   Harmful ______
   Beneficial ______
6. Food restrictions
   Special diet ______
   Religious ______
   Cultural ______
7. Fluid intake
   Number of glasses of water per day ______
   Number of cups of tea or coffee per day ______
   Number of soft drinks per day ______
   Amount of alcohol or wine per day ______
8. Use of vitamins
   Kind ______
   Frequency ______
9. Use of minerals (eg, calcium, iron)
   Kind ______
   Frequency ______
10. Perception of diet
   Nutritionally balanced ______
   Not nutritionally balanced ______

DIETARY PROBLEMS
1. Describe appetite (usual, increased, decreased) ______
2. Foods causing indigestion, diarrhea, or gas ______
3. Difficulty following special diet
   Yes ______ No ______
   If yes, how ______
4. Chewing difficulties
   Number of teeth
   Upper ______ Lower ______
   Dentures
   Partial ______
   Complete ______
   Fit of dentures ______
5. Swallowing difficulties ______
6. Usual bowel movements ______

HEALTH HISTORY
1. Physical activity
   Type ______
   Frequency ______
2. Medication intake
   Name ______
   Time ______
3. History of diseases, surgical procedures, or weight problems

	Yes	No
Diabetes	___	___
Heart problems	___	___
Surgery (specify) ______	___	___
Cancer	___	___
Kidney stones	___	___
Gallstones	___	___
Ulcers	___	___
Intestinal disorder	___	___
Allergies other than food (specify) ______	___	___
Weight problems	___	___

4. Perception of general health
   Good ______
   Satisfactory ______
   Poor ______

FOOD BUYING AND PREPARATION
1. Ingredients used
   Salt ______
   Soy ______
   MSG ______
   Other ______
2. Methods most used
   Boil ______
   Bake ______
   Fry ______
   Broil ______
   Steam ______
   Other ______
3. Shopping/cooking capabilities
   Is able to shop ______
   Relies on others ______
   Is able to cook ______
   Relies on others ______
4. Living situation
   Number of family members ______
   Lives alone ______
5. Do food costs affect diet?
   Yes ______ No ______
   How? ______

Figure 42–5 A sample adult nursing history tool

3-day period, including 1 weekend day. Such a record enables the nurse and the client to compare the data listed with recommended daily allowances or to determine whether the client is receiving a nutritionally balanced diet.

The nurse also acquires the client's perspective of his or her nutritional status. It is important not to judge differences from the nurse's own practices. A question about what foods the client considers harmful or helpful to health is beneficial in eliciting cultural data. For example, people of Asian and Hispanic origins may classify foods as *hot* or *cold* on the basis of inherent characteristics of the food, and not on their actual temperature. According to these cultures, the hot and cold foods need to be balanced for optimum health. If a person has a "cold" illness or condition, such as colic or earache, he or she should eat "hot" foods to balance the condition. Data about the client's medication intake are also important, especially in relation to mealtimes. Many medications are to be taken only before or after meals, so variations from the usual breakfast–lunch–dinner mealtimes need to be documented.

Analyzing the Client's Diet

Several approaches can be used to analyze the client's dietary history. Two commonly used approaches involve (a) use of daily food group guides, and (b) use of food composition tables.

Using Daily Food Groups

Using daily food group guides to analyze the client's diet is a relatively workable approach for the nurse. The nurse simply determines whether the client is receiving the daily recommended servings of the four basic food groups.

Using Food Composition Tables

Dietary analyses using food composition tables provide more specific data about specific nutrient intake. To do a dietary analysis using food composition tables (Christian and Greger 1985, p. 32):

1. Look up the foods the client ate on a food composition table and record the amounts of nutrients in them. For each food, record across the page the amounts of protein, fat, carbohydrate, calcium, iron, vitamins A and C, and thiamine. Adjust the nutrient values for different serving sizes. For example, if the client drank ½ cup of milk but the table gives the values for 1 cup, divide all values by 2 before recording them.
2. After entering each food eaten, calculate the totals for each nutrient.
3. Enter the RDA for the client's sex, age, and reproductive status on the line below the sums.
4. Compare the client's sums to the RDAs. Calculate what percentage of the client's RDA he or she obtained for each nutrient by dividing the sum for a given nutrient by its RDA. Multiply the answer by 100 to get the percentage. If the client's intake is less than the RDA for a nutrient, the percentage will be less than 100; if more, the percentage will be over 100.

This calculation method takes time. Fortunately, computerized nutrient databases and diet analysis software are increasingly being developed and used in nutrition education and health care.

Factors Influencing Dietary Patterns

It is important to determine the factors that affect an individual's eating habits. Some of these are culture, religion, economic status, personal preference, emotions, hunger, appetite, satiety, and health. All factors act in combination, influencing each other.

Culture

Ethnicity often determines food preferences. The diversity of cultures in the United States bears out this fact. Traditionally foods—for example, rice for Orientals, pasta for Italians, curry for Indians—are eaten long after other traditional customs are abandoned. Often clients readily explain their food practices when asked. See page 1174 for some examples of typical foods of various ethnic groups. Although food patterns vary from region to region and person to person, these examples illustrate the diversity of food patterns among people.

Religion

Religion also affects diet. Some Roman Catholics avoid meat on certain days, and some Protestant faiths prohibit tea, coffee, or alcohol. Both Orthodox Judaism and Islam prohibit pork. Orthodox Jews observe kosher customs, eating certain foods only if they are inspected by a rabbi and prepared according to dietary laws. Examples of Jewish Dietary Laws are (Whitney and Cataldo 1983, p. 732):

1. Dairy foods such as milk, cheese, and butter cannot be eaten with meat.
2. Meat is allowed from the forequarters of cattle, deer, goats, and sheep.
3. Animals and poultry are soaked and salted after slaughter to remove as much blood as possible.
4. Only fish with scales and fins are permitted; shellfish are forbidden.
5. Animal fats are prohibited unless specially certified.
6. Separate sets of cooking utensils and dishes must be used for dairy foods and meats.

Examples of Foods Preferred by Selected Ethnic Groups

Chinese	Rice
	Green tea
	Mixtures of fish, pork, or chicken and vegetables (bamboo shoots, broccoli, cabbage, mushrooms, onions, and pea pods)
Italian	Dishes made with pasta
	Bread
	Cheese
	Vegetables such as artichokes, eggplant, greens, tomato, and zucchini
Japanese	Rice
	Green tea
	Raw fish and soy sauce
	Abundance of vegetables
Mexican	Dried beans
	Tortillas made from wheat or corn flour instead of bread
	Tacos, burritos, enchiladas
	Chili peppers, especially in sauces
Polish	Highly salted and seasoned foods
	Sausages; smoked and cured meats
	Noodles, potatoes, dumplings
	Bread
	Coffee with sugar and cream
Puerto Rican	Rice and beans with spicy sauce
	Plantain (vegetable similar in appearance to a large banana)
	Coffee with large amount of milk
Southern black	Pork and chicken
	Dried peas, beans, squash, and greens cooked with fatback or salt pork

(Whitney and Cataldo 1983, pp. 730–31)

The nurse must be sensitive to such religious dietary practices. See Chapter 18 for further information.

Economic Status

What, how much, and how often a person eats are frequently affected by economic status. For example, people with limited income, including some elderly people, may not be able to afford beef and fresh vegetables. Such people may purchase and eat more complex carbohydrates and less protein than recommended. In contrast, people with higher incomes may purchase more proteins and fats and fewer complex carbohydrates. Regardless of economic status, people may not purchase foods containing essential nutrients. Many other factors are involved.

Peer Groups

Peer groups or other subgroups distinguished by age, sex, occupation, or other interests also influence a person's food choices. For example, certain foods may become "in" with teenagers and certain eating places may become teenage hangouts. Members of any group may change their food choices to align themselves more closely with an influential group member. For example, when a financially successful member of a group of business executives shows a strong preference for decaffeinated coffee, some associates are likely to recognize its benefits as well. Sexism may also influence food choices. Some men, for example, may not choose a salad as an entree because such a choice may be perceived as feminine to some people.

Personal Preference and Uniqueness

What an individual likes and dislikes significantly affects eating habits. People often carry childhood preferences into adulthood. Father dislikes curry, thus does his son; mother loves oysters, and so does her daughter. People also develop likes and dislikes based on associations with a typical food. A child who loves to visit his grandparents may love pickled crabapples because they are served in the grandparents' home. Another child who dislikes a very strict aunt grows up to dislike the chicken casserole she often prepares.

Individual likes and dislikes can also be related to familiarity, particularly for children. Children often say they dislike a food before they sample it. Some adults are very adventuresome and eager to try new foods. Others prefer to eat foods they have had many times before.

Preferences in the tastes, smells, flavors (blends of taste and smell), textures, temperatures, colors, shapes, and sizes of food influence a person's food choices uniquely. For example, some people may prefer sweet and sour tastes to bitter or salty tastes. Textures play a great role in food preferences. Some people prefer crisp food to limp food, firm to soft, tender to tough, smooth to lumpy, or dry to soggy. Many people like certain combinations of taste and textures.

Life-Style

Certain life-styles are linked to food-related behaviors. People who are always in a hurry probably buy convenience grocery items or eat restaurant meals. People who spend many leisurely hours at home may take time to prepare more meals "from scratch."

Individual differences also influence life-style patterns. Is the person skilled in cooking? Is the person willing to learn to make new things? Does the person thrive on routine and familiarity? Does the person skip meals and eat whenever it is convenient? Is the person concerned about health foods and adequate exercise that enhances well-being?

Beliefs About Health Effects of Food

Beliefs about effects of foods on health and well-being can affect food choices. For example, a person who feels stomach pain after eating spicy foods or gassiness after eating cabbage or onions may avoid these foods or eat them less often and in smaller amounts. Many beliefs about effects of food on health arise from what a person learns about nutrition through other sources such as radio, television, magazines, newspapers, and books, whether these sources are accurate or not. For example, many people are reducing their intake of animal fats in response to evidence that excessive consumption of animal fats is a major risk factor in cardiovascular disease.

Food fads that involve nontraditional food practices are relatively common. A **fad** is a widespread but short-lived interest or a practice followed with considerable zeal. Often the truth about a food is exaggerated or used out of context to support the rationale behind the fad. A fad may be based either on the belief that certain foods have special curative powers or on the notion that certain foods are harmful.

Food fads appeal, for example, to the individual seeking a miracle cure for a disease or the person who desires superior health and wants to delay aging. Food fads also appeal to people who follow fashion and to people who distrust the medical profession. Persons in the latter group hope that the diet will allow them to avoid medical treatment.

Some fad diets are harmless, but others are potentially dangerous. An example that has received considerable publicity is the liquid protein diet, which has been linked to several deaths. It is important for the nurse to consider what needs the fad diet fills for the client. The nurse can then both support these psychologic needs and suggest a more nutritious diet.

Nurses have these further responsibilities to clients who are considering or following food fads:

1. If a client is thinking about following some advertised practice, it is the nurse's responsibility to suggest that the client discuss it with the physician.
2. Fads that are contrary to accepted nutritional practice need to be investigated further, perhaps with a nutritionist or nurse.
3. Fads that promise improbable results need to be considered in light of the advice of a physician, nutritionist, or nurse.
4. People who believe in fads based on false statements require correct information. People often need information on the possibly toxic effects of taking very large doses of certain vitamins and education on the importance of balanced diet to health.

Examples of food beliefs that are myths rather than fact are:

1. Eating large amounts of yogurt and vitamin E retards aging. (Scientific evidence does not support this belief.)
2. Honey is healthier than sugar, more readily digested, and a cure for the common cold. (There are no significant differences in digestion, and honey does not have curative powers.)
3. Cabbage and onions "turn" breast milk. (Breast milk is not affected by maternal food intake other than by insufficient nutrient intake.)
4. Raw eggs, rare lean beef, and oysters increase sexual potency or fertility. (No single food affects sexual potency or fertility.)
5. Yogurt is more nutritious than milk. (Yogurt has essentially the same nutritional value as milk.)

Advertising

Food producers try to persuade people to change from the product they currently use to the brand of the producer. Often popular actors and actresses are used to influence television viewers' or radio listeners' choices. Although more research is needed to determine whether and to what extent such messages affect people's food choices, advertising is thought to influence people's food choices and eating patterns to a certain extent. Of note is that such products as alcoholic beverages, cake and other dessert mixes, soups, tea, coffee, frozen dinners, and soft drinks are more heavily advertised than such products as milk, canned seafood, bread, cheese, poultry, vegetables, and fruits (Christian and Greger 1985, p. 216).

Psychologic Factors

Anorexia and weight loss can indicate severe stress or depression. Although some people overeat when stressed, depressed, or lonely, others eat very little under the same conditions. Anorexia nervosa and bulimia are severe psychophysiologic conditions seen most frequently in female adolescents. These are discussed in Chapter 24.

Health Status

An individual's health status greatly affects his or her eating habits and nutritional status. The lack of teeth, ill-fitting teeth, or a sore mouth make the mastication of food difficult. Difficulty swallowing (dysphagia) due to a painfully inflamed throat or a stricture of the esophagus can discourage a person from obtaining adequate nourishment.

Many disease processes and surgery of the gastrointestinal tract and related structures can affect digestion, absorption, metabolism, and excretion of essential nutrients. For example, inflammatory disease, tumors, or ulcers often impair digestion and absorption of nutrients. Gastrointestinal and other diseases also create anorexia, nausea, vomiting, and diarrhea, all of which adversely affect a person's eating habits and nutritional status. Gallstones, which can block the flow of bile, are a common cause of impaired digestion of fat.

Many other disease processes affect nutrition. Disease of the liver can impair metabolic processes. Disease of the kidney can impair excretion of the end products of metabolism. Disease of the pancreas can affect glucose metabolism or fat digestion. Malignancies anywhere in the body increase metabolic needs, since malignant cells compete with normal cells for nutrients. Disease of endocrine glands, e.g., thyroid, parathyroid, and adrenal glands, can result in severe hormonal imbalances that affect the client's nutritional status.

Therapies prescribed for certain diseases may also adversely affect eating patterns and nutrition. For example, cancer clients who receive chemotherapy and radiation are at risk of nutritional deficits. Normal tissue cells, e.g., those of the bone marrow and the gastrointestinal mucosa, are naturally very active and particularly susceptible to antineoplastic agents. Oral ulcers, intestinal bleeding, or diarrhea resulting from the toxicity of antineoplastics can diminish a person's nutritional status seriously.

The effects of radiotherapy depend on the area that is treated. For example, radiotherapy of the head and neck may cause decreased salivation, taste distortions, and swallowing difficulties; radiotherapy of the abdomen and pelvis may cause malabsorption, nausea, vomiting, and diarrhea. Many clients feel profound fatigue and anorexia.

Alcohol and Drugs

Excessive consumption of alcohol contributes to nutritional deficiencies if alcohol constitutes a large part of the person's food intake. Chronic consumption of alcohol often leads to protein, thiamine, folacin, niacin, and vitamin B_6 deficiencies as a result of interruptions in the body's normal nutritional processes anywhere from ingestion through excretion.

The effects of drugs on nutrition vary considerably. They may alter appetite, disturb taste perception, or interfere with nutrient absorption or excretion. Nurses need to be aware of the nutritional effects of specific drugs when evaluating a client for nutritional problems. The nursing history interview should include questions about the medications the client is taking. Nutrients can also affect drug utilization. Some nutrients can decrease drug absorption; others enhance absorption. For example, the calcium in milk hinders absorption of the antibiotic tetracycline but enhances the absorption of the antibiotic erythromycin. Selected drug and nutrient interactions are shown in Table 42–16.

Identifying Clients at Risk of Nutritional Problems

To identify clients at risk of nutritional problems, the nurse needs to consider data from the client's dietary history, medication history, and medical history. A summary of risk factors for altered nutrition status is shown below.

Summary of Risk Factors for Nutritional Problems

Diet history

- Chewing or swallowing difficulties (including ill-fitting dentures, dental caries, and missing teeth)
- Inadequate food intake
- Restricted or fad diets
- No intake for 10 or more days
- Intravenous fluids (other than total parenteral nutrition for 10 or more days)
- Inadequate food budget
- Inadequate food preparation facilities
- Inadequate food storage facilities
- Physical disabilities
- Elderly living and eating alone

Medical history

- Overweight
- Underweight
- Recent weight loss or gain
- Recent major illness
- Recent major surgery
- Surgery of the GI tract
- Anorexia
- Nausea
- Vomiting
- Diarrhea
- Alcoholism
- Cancer
- Liver disease
- Kidney disease
- Diabetes
- Thyroid or parathyroid disease
- Adrenal disease
- Mental disability
- Teenage pregnancy
- Multiple pregnancies
- Pancreatic insufficiency
- Radiation therapy

Medication history

- Aspirin
- Antibiotics
- Antacid
- Antidepressants
- Antihypertensives
- Antiinflammatory agents
- Antineoplastic agents
- Digitalis
- Laxatives
- Diuretics (thiazides)
- Potassium chloride
- Vitamin or other nutrient preparations

Table 42–16 Selected Drug-Nutrient Interactions

Drug	Effect on Nutrition
Acetylsalicylic acid (aspirin)	Decreases serum folate and folacin nutrition
	Increases excretion of vitamin C, thiamine, potassium, amino acids, and glucose
	May cause nausea and gastritis
Antacids containing aluminum or magnesium hydroxide (Maalox)	Decrease absorption of phosphate and vitamin A
	Inactivate thiamine
	May cause deficiency of calcium and vitamin D
Thiazide diuretics (Diuril, HydroDIURIL)	Increase excretion of sodium, potassium, chloride, calcium, magnesium, zinc, and riboflavin
	May cause anorexia, nausea, vomiting, diarrhea, or constipation
Potassium chloride (Kaochlor, K-Lor, Slow-K)	Decreases absorption of vitamin B_{12}
	May cause diarrhea, nausea, or vomiting
Digitalis	Increases excretion of potassium, magnesium, and calcium
	May cause anorexia, nausea, or vomiting
	Is incompatible with protein hydrolysates
Laxatives	May cause calcium and potassium depletion
	Mineral oil and phenolphthalein (Ex-lax) decrease absorption of vitamins A, D, E, and K.
Antihypertensives	Hydralazine (Apresoline) may cause anorexia, vomiting, nausea, and constipation
	Methyldopa (Aldomet) increases need for vitamin B_{12} and folate
	May cause dry mouth, nausea, vomiting, diarrhea, constipation
Antiinflammatory agents	Colchicine decreases absorption of vitamin B_{12}, carotene, fat, lactose, sodium, potassium, protein, and cholesterol
	Prednisone decreases absorption of calcium and phosphorus
Antidepressants	Amitriptyline (Elavil) increases food intake (large amounts may suppress intake)

References: A. B. Natow and J. Heslin, *Nutritional care of the older adult* (New York: Macmillan Publishing Co., 1986), pp. 252–255; and D. Raab and N. Raab, Nutrition and the aging: An overview, *Canadian Nurse*, March 1985, 81: 3.

Nursing Diagnosis

Nursing diagnoses for clients with nutritional problems may be broadly stated as alterations in nutrition and further categorized as:

1. Less than body requirements or nutritional deficit (insufficient intake)
2. More than body requirements or obesity (excessive intake)

Either of these problems may be actual or potential.

Nutritional Deficit

Nutritional deficit is insufficient intake of one or more nutrients required to meet metabolic needs (Gordon 1982, p. 68). When possible, the nurse should state the specific deficit, e.g., inadequate protein, iron, or vitamin C intake.

Indications of nutritional deficits of specific vitamins are outlined in Table 42–2. The following signs may indicate other generalized deficits:

1. Weight 20% or more under the ideal for height and frame
2. Loss of weight with adequate food intake
3. Food intake less than that recommended by food guides or evidence of lack of food
4. Eating difficulties
5. Gastrointestinal signs, such as abdominal pain, cramping, diarrhea, and hyperactive bowel sounds
6. Muscle weakness and reduced energy level
7. Excessive loss of hair
8. Pallor of skin, mucous membranes, and conjunctiva

A very severe protein deficit results in kwashiorkor, a disease seen in many Eastern undernourished populations. It is characterized by retarded growth and development; mental apathy; extreme muscular wasting, which may be masked by edema; depigmentation of the hair and skin; and scaly changes in skin texture. Many of the factors previously discussed contribute to nutritional deficits. See the section on factors influencing dietary patterns on page 1173.

Obesity

Obesity is the result of calorie intake that exceeds metabolic need. People become obese by eating too much food or eating too many foods of high caloric density. **Caloric density** describes the number of kilocalories per unit weight of food. Fats and oils have the highest caloric density, whereas vegetables such as celery and lettuce have low densities. Energy expenditure is also a factor in weight control. By increasing activity, the individual increases energy expenditure and often decreases weight. Obesity is evidenced by weight 20% greater than the ideal for height and frame and by triceps skin folds greater than 15 mm in men and 25 mm in women (Kim and Moritz 1982, p. 300). **Overweight** refers to weight 10% greater than the ideal for height and frame (White and Schroeder 1981, p. 550). Obesity is currently one of the most prevalent health problems in North America. It is associated with hypertension, cardiovascular diseases, and diabetes. Factors contributing to obesity include:

1. Sedentary habits (low activity level)
2. Inappropriate eating patterns (e.g., eating large amounts of carbohydrates and saturated fats)
3. Depression or anxiety (often accompanied by stressors such as a death in the family or a change in marital or work status)
4. Eating the largest meal at the end of the day

Factors placing a person at risk for obesity may include sedentary habits, genetic predisposition, obesity in one or both parents, and a pattern of excessive food intake in early infancy and childhood.

Examples of Nursing Diagnoses Related to Nutrition

- Potential alteration in nutrition: less than body requirements related to lack of knowledge about increased requirements during pregnancy
- Potential alteration in nutrition: less than body requirements related to lack of knowledge about necessary requirements for growth
- Potential alteration in nutrition: less than body requirements related to lack of knowledge about ways to get essential proteins on vegetarian diets
- Potential alteration in nutrition: less than body requirements (iron) related to pregnancy
- Alteration in nutrition: less than body requirements related to inability to chew secondary to ill-fitting dentures
- Alteration in nutrition: less than body requirements related to inability to procure food associated with financial and transportation problems
- Alteration in nutrition related to self-imposed starvation secondary to denial of being underweight and desire to remain slender
- Alteration in nutrition: less than body requirements (calcium) related to age and potential osteoporosis
- Alteration in nutrition: more than body requirements related to compulsive overeating
- Alteration in nutrition: more than body requirements related to excessive intake of carbohydrates and sedentary habits

Examples of Nursing Diagnoses

Examples of nursing diagnoses for clients with nutritional problems are shown above.

Planning

The nurse's overall responsibilities in relation to a client's nutrition include:

1. Maintenance or restoration of the client's nutritional status
2. Prevention of nutritional problems
3. Making the client's mealtimes pleasurable

When planning measures to meet the client's nutrition needs, the nurse needs to consider the learning needs of the person and to implement measures to help him or her obtain nourishment. A client may need to learn information about a healthy or newly prescribed therapeutic diet and even new skills for eating. For example, the client with limited ability to move the arms may need to learn to eat with a spoon with a long handle.

Planning also involves establishing outcome criteria. For suggestions, see the section on evaluation later in this chapter.

Intervention

Counseling About Nutrition

People frequently need nutrition counseling. Nurses need to know the special nutritional needs of different age groups and sources of nutrients, especially inexpensive sources.

Nurses may also be asked about common problems, such as feeding problems of babies and children and nutritional needs of pregnant and lactating women. Many clients need information about therapeutic diets and ways to prepare foods that meet the restrictions of these diets. In community health care settings, the nurse shares responsibility for nutritional counseling with nutritionists.

Nutrition counseling involves much more than simply providing information. The nurse must help the client integrate diet changes into the client's life style and provide strategies to motivate the client to change his or her eating habits. Counseling can be likened to the teaching-learning process discussed in Chapter 29. First, a thorough assessment of the client's nutritional status and nutrient intake is necessary. From this assessment, the nurse determines the client's educational requirements. At this point, the nurse must assess her or his own knowledge of the subject to be discussed and if necessary obtain the appropriate information or refer the client to an expert on the subject. Then the client and nurse set goals or objectives, plan strategies to achieve the goals, and establish criteria to evaluate achievement of the goals. Because it is the client's responsibility to make the necessary dietary changes and to change his or her behavior, the nurse's role is to support and encourage the client. Ways the nurse can enhance behavior change are discussed in Chapter 20.

Teaching About Special Diets

Assisting clients and support persons with special or therapeutic diets prescribed by the physician is a function shared by the dietitian and the nurse. The dietitian, for example, informs the client and support persons about the specific foods allowed and not allowed and assists the client with meal planning. The nurse reinforces this instruction, assists the client to make beneficial changes, and evaluates the client's response to the planned changes.

Physicians order special diets for clients who cannot eat the usual foods. A special or therapeutic diet is one in which the amount of food, the kind of food, or the frequency of eating is prescribed. Special diets are used for one or more of the following reasons:

1. To treat a disease process, e.g., a low-salt diet for high blood pressure
2. To prepare for a special examination or surgery
3. To promote health, e.g., a low-calorie diet for an overweight client

Some diets are temporary, observed perhaps for one meal or 1 week, but some clients must follow certain diets (e.g., the diabetic diet) for a lifetime. If the diet is long term, the client must not only understand the diet but also develop a healthy, positive attitude toward it. The client needs to know that failure to follow the diet for even 1 day, perhaps because of anger, could result in acute illness.

Progressive hospital diets are often unique to institutions, and nurses need to be familiar with the diets prescribed in their agencies.

Regular Diet

Clients who do not have special needs eat the regular diet, whose quantity and content are designed to meet the needs of most clients. In some agencies, the regular diet is referred to as the normal, house, standard, or regular diet. Some hospitals offer clients a daily menu from which to select their meals for the next day. Other hospitals provide standard meals to each client on the general diet. Certain foods (e.g., cabbage, which tends to produce flatus, and highly seasoned and fried foods, which are difficult for some people to digest) are usually omitted from the regular diet.

Light Diet

A variation of the regular diet is the light diet, designed for postoperative and other clients who are not ready for the regular diet. Foods in the light diet are plainly cooked. Foods containing large amounts of fat are usually omitted, as are bran and foods containing a great deal of fiber. Not all agencies provide a light diet.

Soft Diet

A soft diet is easily chewed and digested. It is often ordered for clients who have difficulty chewing and swallowing (dysphagia). A soft diet is a lightly seasoned, low-residue (low-fiber) diet. Many nonhospitalized clients often require a soft diet. Suggestions of foods that can be selected for a soft or semisoft diet are shown on the next page.

Full Liquid Diet

A full liquid diet contains only liquids or foods that turn to liquid at room temperature, such as ice cream. Full liquid diets are eaten by clients who have gastrointestinal disturbances or are otherwise unable to tolerate solid or semisolid foods. Full fluid foods are free of cellulose, irritating condiments such as mustard or ketchup, and spices such as black pepper or chili powder. This diet is not recommended for long-term use. Its iron content, protein content, and caloric density are low, and its cho-

Food Suggestions for a Soft Diet

Meats and Alternates
- Any tender meat, fish, poultry (chopped or shredded)
- Chopped meat in cream sauce
- Omelet or scrambled egg
- Spaghetti sauce with chopped meat over small shaped pasta
- Cottage cheese

Vegetables
- Rice in cream or cheese sauce
- Mashed potatoes
- Mashed sweet potatoes
- Mashed squash
- Mashed potatoes with chopped spinach
- Vegetables in cream or cheese sauce
- Vegetables pureed with diced vegetables (e.g., carrot or turnip puree with baby peas)
- Avocado
- Cauliflower
- Asparagus tips
- Spinach

Fruits
- Chunky apple sauce
- Ripe banana
- Cooked, peeled fresh fruits
- Canned fruits

Desserts
- Pudding
- Custard
- Ice Cream
- Yogurt
- Pudding cake
- Junket
- Gelatin
- Sherbet
- Soft cake

Cereals and Breads
- Cooked cereal
- Crustless bread

Liquids
- All allowed (except when restricted by physician)

lesterol content is high because of the amount of milk offered. Clients who must receive only liquids for longer periods are usually given a nutritionally balanced oral supplement, e.g., Sustacal. The full liquid diet is monotonous and difficult for clients to accept. Planning six or more feedings per day may encourage a more adequate intake.

Clear Liquid Diet

The clear liquid diet is often limited to water, tea, coffee, clear broths, ginger ale or other carbonated beverages, apple juice, and plain gelatin. It does not permit milk. This diet provides the client with fluid and carbohydrate (in the form of sugar), but it does not supply adequate protein, fat, vitamins, minerals, or calories. No more than 600 kcal/day are provided. It is usually a short-term diet (24 to 36 hours) provided for clients after certain surgery or clients in the acute stages of infection, particularly of the gastrointestinal tract. The major objective of this diet is to relieve thirst, prevent dehydration, and minimize stimulation of the gastrointestinal tract. Clear fluids are offered throughout the day as tolerated by the client.

Other Special Diets

There are many other special diets, sometimes especially devised for individual clients. Common ones are:

1. A reducing diet provides a limited number of calories so that the client will lose weight.
2. A diabetic diet provides protein, fat, and carbohydrate in accordance with the individual's ability to produce insulin.
3. A low-salt (NaCl) or sodium-restricted diet is designed to limit the client's sodium (Na) intake. Some low-salt diets merely limit the salt added to food during cooking or eating. Others restrict certain foods because they are naturally high in sodium. These diets are usually prescribed for clients with certain cardiovascular diseases.
4. Allergy diets omit the particular foods to which a client is allergic. Some foods that commonly produce allergic reactions are cow's milk, wheat, and eggs.

Details about these diets are provided in nutrition and medical surgical nursing textbooks.

Clients often need assistance adapting their diets to their cultural, religious, ethnic, and economic patterns. Helping the client adapt the diet to food habits is of great importance. Most diets in North America are devised for the Anglo-American taste and omit many otherwise acceptable ethnic foods. Such a diet may be unfamiliar or unpalatable to the ethnic client. Nutritionists and dietitians can often assist nurses to adapt a diet to suit a person's life-style.

Another important aspect is adapting a diet to a person's economic status. Often, less costly foods can be substituted for recommended foods, such as powdered milk for fresh milk.

Motivation is highly important for the success of a dieter. If a client does not accept the need for a diet, she or he will probably not adhere to it, and its therapeutic value is lost. Understanding is also important. A client may understand that sugar in coffee is not allowed on a low-calorie diet, but may not understand that bread also contains sugar and is also restricted. A teenager may understand that a diet applies to what is eaten at meals, but may not understand that it also applies to between-meal snacks. An elderly client may understand that she is not to add salt to foods when cooking but salts her food at the table. This client does not really understand the importance or the reason for salt restriction.

Stimulating Appetite

Many hospitalized clients have poor appetites for a variety of reasons:

1. An accompanying physical illness
2. Unfamiliar food or food the client finds unpalatable
3. Environmental factors, e.g., unpleasant odors or an elevated room temperature
4. Psychologic factors, e.g., anxiety or depression
5. Physical discomfort or pain

Lowered food intake of a few days' duration is not often a problem for adults; however, a prolonged decreased food intake leads to weight loss, decreased strength and stamina, and subsequent nutritional problems. Decreased food intake is often accompanied by decreased fluid intake, which may cause fluid and electrolyte problems. See Chapter 46 for further information.

Increasing a person's appetite requires determining the reason for the lack of appetite and then dealing with the problem. Some nursing interventions that may improve client's appetites are:

1. Relieving illness symptoms that deaden appetite prior to mealtime, e.g., giving an analgesic for pain or an antipyretic for a fever or allowing rest for fatigue.
2. Providing food that the person likes and with which the client is familiar. Often the relatives of clients are pleased to bring food from home but may need some guidance about special diet requirements. It is also important to present the food in sufficiently small quantities so as not to discourage the anorexic client.
3. Making the environment conducive to eating. It needs to be fresh and free of unpleasant odors. Unpleasant or uncomfortable treatments should not be carried out immediately before or after a meal. A tidy, clean environment that is free of unpleasant sights is also important. A soiled dressing, a used bedpan, an uncovered irrigation set, or even used dishes can destroy appetite.
4. Reducing psychologic stress. A lack of understanding of therapy, the anticipation of an operation, and fear of the unknown can cause anorexia. Often, the nurse can help by discussing feelings with the client, giving information and assistance, and allaying fears.

Assisting Clients with Meals

Provision of Meals in Hospital

Arrangements for the provision of food to clients vary considerably. Some hospitals serve meals to ambulatory clients in a special dining area, and the clients are expected to go there to eat. Other agencies, e.g., day-care centers, have a coffee shop for food or machines from which clients can obtain sandwiches and beverages. However, because clients are frequently confined to their beds, particularly in acute care settings, most hospitals must have meals brought to the client. Often the client receives a tray that has been assembled in a central hospital kitchen or a kitchen adjacent to the nursing unit. Nursing personnel may be responsible for giving out and collecting the trays; in some settings this is done by special personnel. In either case, nurses have the following responsibilities associated with the provision of meals for clients:

1. Check on the client's chart or Kardex whether the client is fasting for laboratory tests or surgery or whether the physician has ordered "nothing by mouth" (NPO). For clients who are fasting or on NPO, ensure that the appropriate signs are placed on either the room door or the client's bed, according to agency practice.
2. For clients who are experiencing considerable pain, check the nursing care plan, and arrange for analgesics to be provided about 30 minutes before the meal. Pain usually takes away a client's appetite.
3. Some clients require medications before or with their meals. Check the client's chart, and provide the prescribed medication, or check that this has been done.
4. If there is a change in the type of food the client is to receive, notify the dietary staff. Some hospitals have a form with the client's name that indicates any change in diet. This form is placed in a special location for the dietary staff.
5. Prior to mealtime, determine if the client needs to urinate or defecate. Assist him or her to the bathroom or onto a bedpan or commode, as appropriate.
6. Ensure that the client washes his or her hands prior to a meal. If the client has problems with oral hygiene, brushing the teeth or using a mouthwash can improve the taste in his or her mouth and hence the appetite.
7. Provide good ventilation and good light, and remove any unpleasant room odors. A spray deodorizer can help.
8. Remove any unpleasant sights, such as a full bedpan or a soiled dressing, which could disturb the client's appetite.
9. Assist the client to a comfortable position for eating. Most people sit during a meal; if it is permitted, assist the client to sit in bed (see Figure 42–6) or in a chair, whichever is appropriate. Make sure that a client who must remain in a supine or lateral position is comfortable.
10. Overbed tables are often used for clients sitting in bed or on bedside chairs. Clear the table so that there is space for the tray. If the client must remain in a

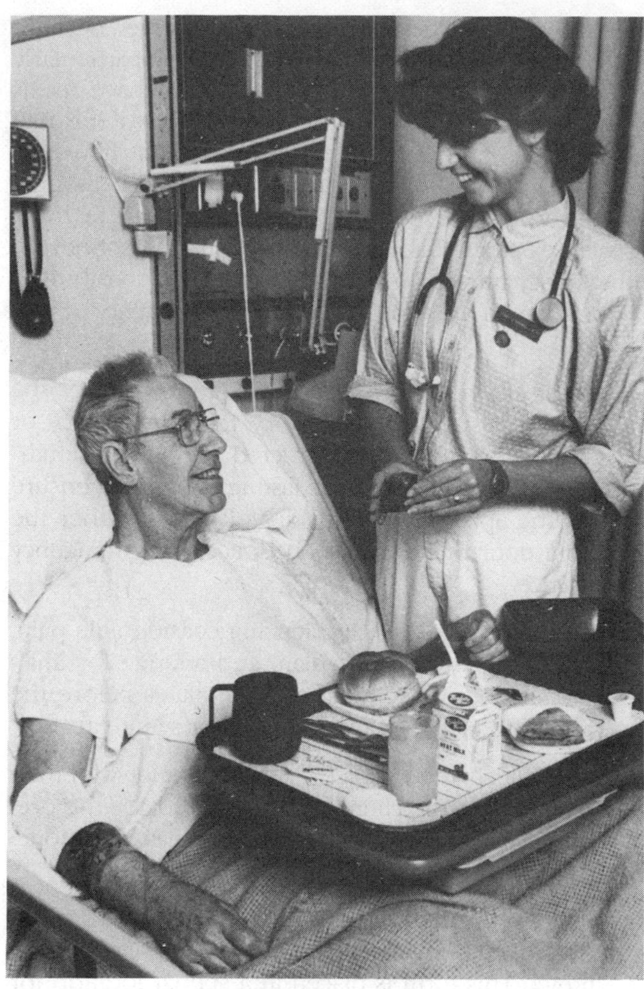

Figure 42–6 A supported sitting position contributes to a client's comfort while eating.

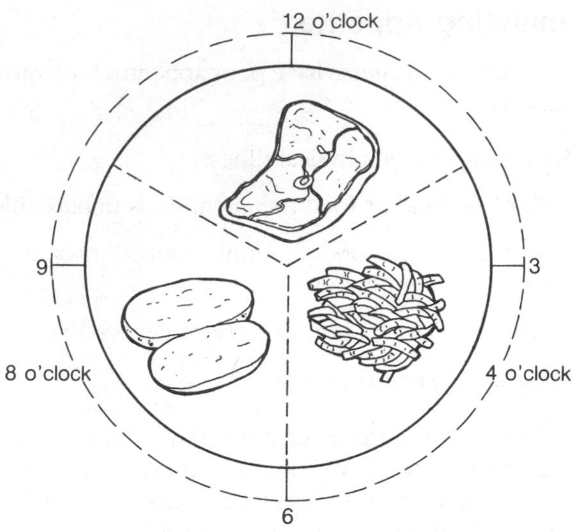

Figure 42–7 If the client is blind, the nurse can use the clock system to describe the location of food on the plate.

lying position in bed, arrange the overbed table close to the bedside, so that the client can see the food.

11. Trays are usually delivered to the nursing unit on a movable trolley or a special lift. If nursing personnel are expected to deliver the trays, the unit will have a method of notifying the nurses that the trays have arrived.

12. Check each tray for the client's name, the type of diet, and completeness. In some agencies, the client's name and bed number are written on a colored card. Different colors are used to represent different diets, e.g., white for the general diet and blue for the soft diet. If the diet does not seem to be correct, check it against the client's chart. Confirm the client's name by checking the wristband before leaving the tray. Do not leave an incorrect diet for a client to eat.

13. Assist the client as required, e.g., to remove the food covers, butter the bread, pour the tea, and cut the meat.

14. For a blind person, identify the placement of the food as you would describe the time on a clock. For instance, the nurse may say, "The potatoes are at eight o'clock; the beef steak at 12 o'clock; and the green beans at 4 o'clock. See Figure 42–7. If the blind client is a child, the nurse may say, "Think of the plate as a face. The potatoes are where the mouth would be."

15. Clients who need to be fed may receive their trays before or after other clients. It is important that the clients be fed as soon as the trays are out and while the food is hot. Some agencies arrange for these trays to come out 30 minutes earlier, and nursing personnel are designated to feed specific clients.

16. After the client has completed the meal, replace the food covers, and note how much and what the client has eaten and the amount of fluid taken. If the client's intake and output of fluid is being recorded, record the fluid ingested. See Chapter 46. If a calorie count has been ordered, record the exact amount of each food eaten. A special form is usually provided by the dietitian.

17. Assist the client to a comfortable position. For some clients eating is a tiring process, and they will need to rest after a meal.

18. If the client is on a special diet or is having problems eating, record on the chart the pertinent data, such as amount of food eaten and any pain, fatigue, or nausea experienced.

19. If the client is not eating, notify the responsible nurse so that the diet can be changed or other nursing measures can be taken, e.g., rescheduling the meals, providing smaller, more frequent meals, or obtaining special self-feeding aids.

Assisting Clients with Feeding

The amount and kind of assistance a client needs with eating depend on the physical and mental limitations of the client. Two groups of people frequently require help: the elderly, who are weakened and quickly fatigued when they are ill; and the handicapped, e.g., blind clients, those who must remain in a back-lying position, or those who do not have use of their hands. The client's nursing care plan will indicate that assistance is required with meals.

Because all clients except infants are usually accustomed to feeding themselves, the nurse must be sensitive to feelings of embarrassment, resentment, and loss of autonomy in clients who cannot feed themselves. Young children who have learned to feed themselves only recently and are proud of their new accomplishment may be especially resentful of the need for help. Whenever possible, the nurse should help incapacitated clients feed themselves rather than feed them. Some clients become depressed because they require help and because they believe they are burdensome to busy nursing personnel. It is very important not to convey, either verbally or nonverbally, impatience or annoyance with clients who require assistance eating. Rather, appear unhurried and convey that you have ample time.

Although normal utensils should be used whenever possible, the nurse may need to use special utensils to assist a client to eat. Straws help many people who have difficulty drinking from a cup or glass. Straws often permit the client to obtain liquids with less effort and with less spillage, which can be embarrassing to many clients. Special drinking cups are also available. One model has a spout; another is specially designed to permit drinking with less tipping of the cup than is normally required. See Figure 42–8.

Before feeding the client, the nurse should ask the client in which order he or she desires to eat the food. The nurse always warns the client if the food is hot or cold. If the client cannot see, tell him or her which food you are giving. Always allow ample time for the client to chew and swallow the food before offering more. Provide the client with fluids as requested, or, if he or she is unable to tell you, offer fluids after every three or four mouthfuls of solid food. Make the time a pleasant one, choosing topics of conversation that are of interest to the client if he or she wants to talk.

Special Self-Feeding Aids

Many adaptive feeding aids are available to help maintain the independence of clients who are having difficulty handling regular utensils. A standard eating utensil with a built-up or widened handle helps clients who cannot grasp objects easily. Utensils with wide handles can be purchased, or a regular eating utensil can be modified by wrapping foam around the handle or slipping a foam rubber hair curler over the handle. The foam increases friction and thus steadies the client's grasp. Handles may be bent or angled to compensate for limited motion. Collars or bands can be attached to the end of the handle. These fit over the client's hand and prevent the utensil from being dropped.

Plates with rims and plastic or metal plate guards enable the client to pick up the food by first pushing it against this raised edge. A suction cup or damp sponge or cloth can also be placed under the dish to keep it from moving while the client is eating.

Cups and glasses can be adapted, or special aids can be purchased. No-spill mugs and two-handled drinking cups are especially useful for persons with impaired hand coordination. Stretch terry cloth or hand-knitted or crocheted glass covers can help the client keep a secure grasp on a glass. To hold a straw steady and in place, attach a pen clip to a glass or cup and thread the straw through where the pen was originally held. Lidded tip-proof glasses are also available. Figures 42–9 and 42–10 show some of these eating aids.

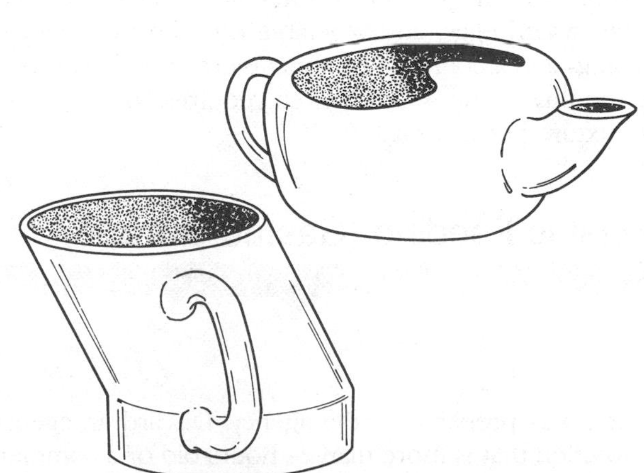

Figure 42–8 Two types of special drinking cups

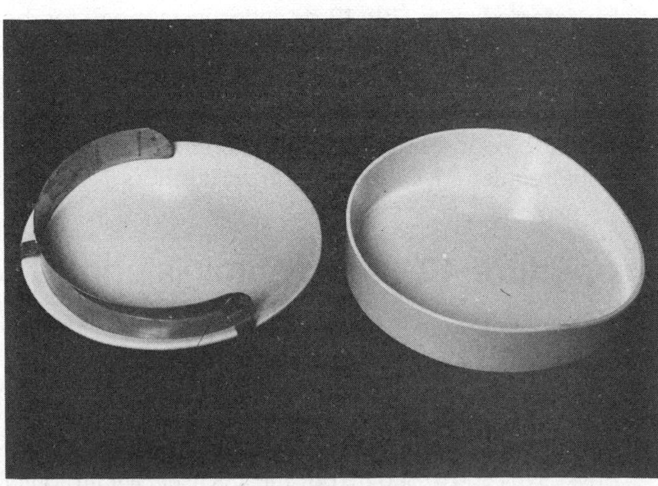

Figure 42–9 A, Dinner plate with plate guard attached; **B,** lipped plate

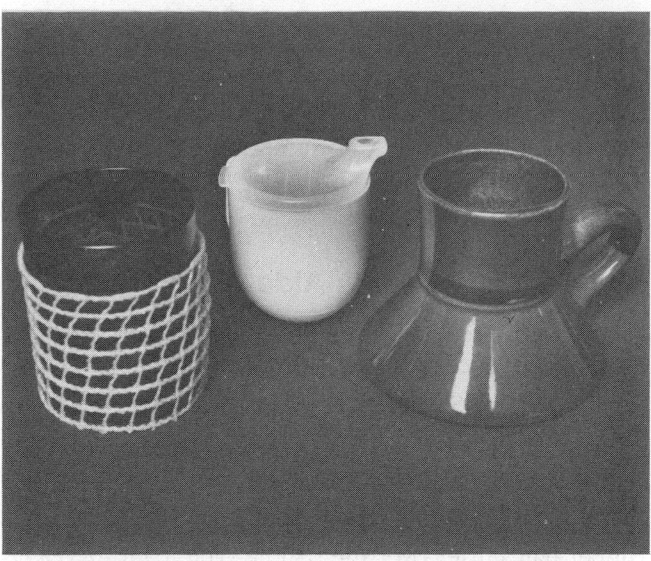

Figure 42–10 Left to right: **A,** Stretch terry cloth or knitted glass cover; **B,** lidded, tip-proof glass; and **C,** no-spill mug

Special Community Nutritional Services

Various programs in the community are designed to help special subgroups of the population meet their nutritional needs. For the elderly who cannot prepare meals or leave their homes, ready-to-eat meals or frozen dinners are delivered to the home by local organizations. Meals-on-wheels is one such well-known organization. For people who can prepare meals but are physically handicapped and unable to shop for groceries, some organizations provide grocery delivery services.

The Nutrition Program for Older Americans, administered by the Department of Health and Human Services, provides community-based noon meals at an optional nominal fee for mobile people over age 60. This program is also referred to as Title III or congregate meals for the elderly. The Title III meals are designed to provide one-third of the RDAs. In addition to providing a nutritious meal, this program offers nutrition education and health and welfare counseling. An added benefit for the participants is regular social interaction with others.

For the impoverished, the U.S. Department of Agriculture funds a food stamp program. People with low incomes can use stamps to purchase food at any approved grocery store. The value of the food stamps provided depends on the size and income of the family.

Many industries have established health maintenance programs for their employees. These programs generally include exercise facilities, stress reduction education, and nutritional counseling. In some companies, the food service departments make a special effort to adhere to the recommendations of the *Dietary Guidelines.* Such programs are thought to be cost effective, since illness is reduced and less time is lost from work and employee satisfaction increases work productivity.

Alternate Feeding Methods

Nasogastric Feeding

A **nasogastric feeding,** or **gastric gavage,** is the instillation of specially prepared nutrients into the stomach through a nasogastric tube. It usually requires a physician's order. A tube is inserted through one of the nostrils, down the nasopharynx and esophagus, into the stomach. In some instances, the tube is passed through the mouth and pharynx into the esophagus and stomach, although this route may be more uncomfortable for the adult client and cause gagging. This approach is often used for infants who are obligatory nose breathers (who must breathe through the nose) and premature infants who have no gag reflex.

Nasogastric feedings are indicated for clients who cannot eat by mouth or swallow a sufficient diet without aspirating food or fluid into the lungs. Feedings may be given continuously over a 24-hour period or at prescribed intervals, e.g., four times per day. Feeding mixtures are available commercially or may be prepared by the dietary department in accordance with the physician's orders. The preparations are liquid and contain a variety of nutrients, depending on the physician's order. The standard solution contains 1 kcal per milliliter of solution with protein, fat, carbohydrate, minerals, and vitamins in specified proportions. The foods commonly included are milk, sugar, water, eggs, and vegetable oil. The frequency of feedings and amounts to be administered are also ordered by the physician. An adult often requires 300 to 500 ml of mixture per feeding.

Procedure 42–1 ▲ Administering a Nasogastric Feeding (Gastric Gavage)

Equipment

1. The correct amount of feeding solution ordered by the physician (300 to 500 ml per meal is usual for an adult). Check the expiration date on a commercially prepared formula or the preparation date and time if the solution was prepared in the agency. Discard an agency solution that is more than 24 hours old or a commercial formula that has passed the expiration date. Feedings are usually administered at room temperature

unless the order specifies otherwise. Warm the specified amount of solution in a basin of warm water or let it stand for a while until it reaches room temperature. Continuous feeding should be kept cold (see item 7 below). Excessive heat coagulates feedings of milk and egg, and hot liquids can irritate the mucous membranes. On the other hand, excessively cold feedings can reduce the flow of digestive juices by causing vasoconstriction and may cause cramps. Commercially prepared feedings are available in cans and bottles ready for administration. Some containers are designed so that ice chips can be placed in an outer section to keep the formula cooled.

2. A 20 to 50 ml syringe with an adapter. The syringe is used to check that the tube is in the stomach.

3. An emesis basin to collect the aspirated stomach contents.

4. If an intermittent feeding is being given, a bulb syringe. The bulb is removed from the syringe, and the barrel is attached to the tube.

   or

   A burette (calibrated plastic bag) and a drip chamber, which can be attached to the tubing.

   or

   A prefilled bottle with a drip chamber, tubing, and a flow regulator clamp.

5. A measuring container from which to pour the feeding if the syringe or burette method is used.

6. Water at room temperature (60 ml unless otherwise specified) to clean the inside of the tube after the feeding.

7. Optional: a feeding pump, which can be used with a prefilled tube-feeding set to regulate the exact amount of feeding for the client. See Figure 42–11. The pump can also be used to administer the feeding in instances when smaller-bore gastric tubes are used or when gravity flow is insufficient to instill the feeding. Because the feeding is administered over a long time, a formula that is warmed can grow microorganisms. It should not hang longer than the manufacturer recommends, e.g., 3 to 4 hours. If it will hang longer, it should be kept cool with ice chips.

Intervention

1. Before administering the feeding assess the client for:
   a. Any feeling of abdominal distention, belching, loose stools, flatus, or pain. The lack of bulk in liquid feedings may cause constipation. The presence of concentrated ingredients may cause diarrhea and flatulence. A distended abdomen could indicate the client's intolerance to a previous feeding.
   b. Bowel sounds, by auscultating the client's abdomen. Bowel sounds reflect intestinal movement.
   c. Hydration status. Dehydration may cause constipation. Note complaints of thirst and make sure the client's fluid intake and output are in balance.
   d. Allergies to any foods, such as eggs. Check the contents of the feeding for these foods. Report any significant problems to the responsible nurse.
   e. Glucose tolerance and response to the feedings, as ordered. Assess glucose tolerance by monitoring the client's blood and urine glucose levels. Assess response to therapy by monitoring serum electrolytes, doing other ordered blood tests, and taking anthropometric measurements.

2. Explain the technique to the client. A feeding should not cause any discomfort, but it may cause a feeling of fullness. For an adult, the usual intermittent feeding takes about 10 minutes; the exact duration depends largely on the volume of the feeding.

3. Provide privacy for this procedure if the client desires it. Nasogastric feedings are embarrassing to some people.

4. Assist the client to a Fowler's position in bed or a sitting position in a chair, the normal position for eating. If a sitting position is contraindicated, a slightly elevated right side-lying position is acceptable.

   Rationale These positions enhance the gravitational flow of the solution and prevent aspiration of fluid into the lungs.

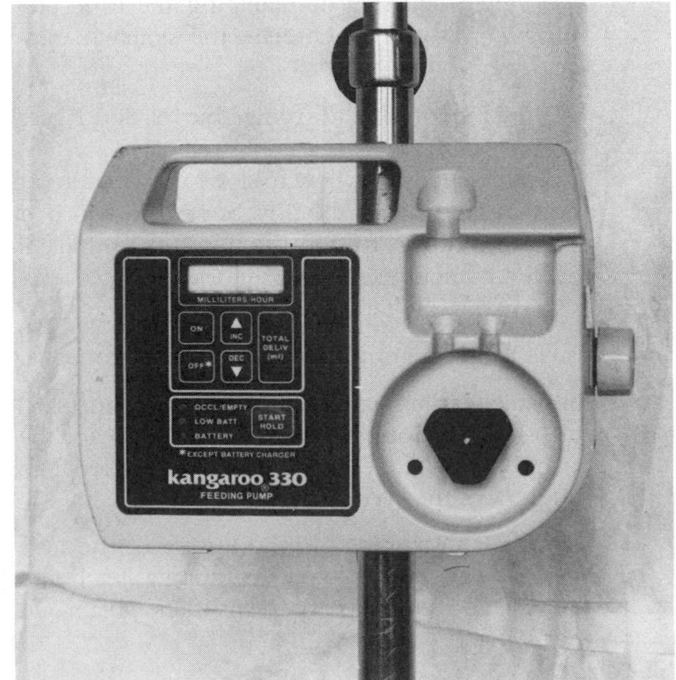

Figure 42–11

5. If the client does not have a nasogastric tube in place, insert one. See Procedure 53–3.
6. Confirm that the nasogastric tube is in the stomach. Attach the syringe to the open end of the nasogastric tube, and aspirate stomach contents. See Table 53–4 for other methods to determine placement of a nasogastric tube.
7. If the nasogastric tube is maintained in the client:
   a. Aspirate all the stomach contents and measure the amount prior to administering the feeding.

      Rationale This is done to evaluate absorption of the last feeding, i.e., whether undigested formula of a previous feeding remains.

   b. If 50 ml or more of undigested formula is withdrawn, check with the responsible nurse before proceeding.

      Rationale In some agencies, a feeding is withheld if 50 ml or more of formula remains in the stomach.

   c. Reinstill the gastric contents into the stomach if this is the agency or physician's practice. Remove the syringe bulb or plunger, and pour the gastric contents via the syringe into the nasogastric tube.

      Rationale Removal of the contents could disturb the client's electrolyte balance.

8. If a bulb syringe is being used:
   a. Remove the bulb from the syringe, and connect the syringe to a pinched or clamped nasogastric tube.

      Rationale Pinching or clamping the tube prevents excess air from entering the stomach, causing distention.

   b. Add the feeding to the syringe barrel. See Figure 42–12.
   c. Permit the feeding to flow in slowly. Raise or lower the syringe to adjust the flow as needed. Pinch or clamp the tubing to stop the flow for a minute if the client experiences discomfort.

      Rationale Quickly administered feedings can cause flatus, crampy pain, and/or reflex vomiting.

   d. After the feeding has been administered, instill 60 ml of water through the tube. Be sure to add the water before the feeding solution has drained from the neck of the syringe.

      Rationale Water cleans the lumen of the tube and prevents future blockage. Adding water before the syringe is empty prevents instillation of air into the stomach.

   e. Clamp the tube before removing the syringe.

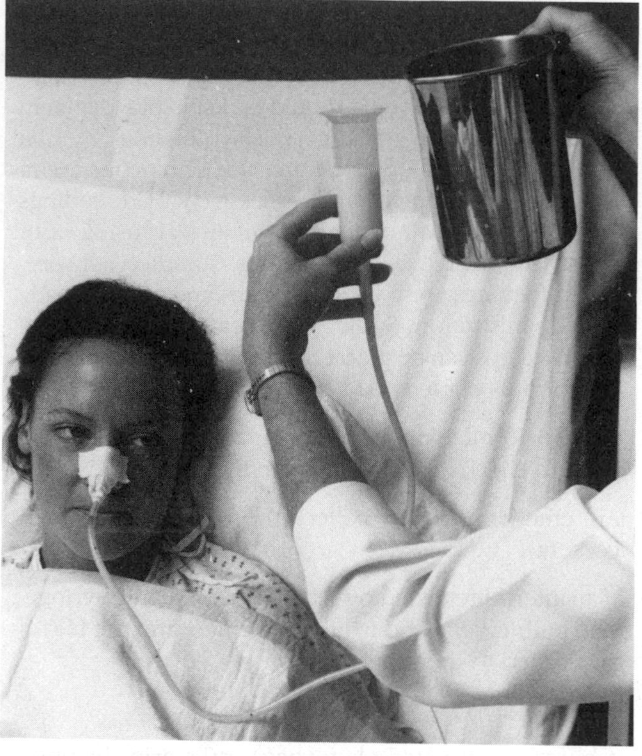

COURTESY SWEARINGEN PHOTO-ATLAS

Figure 42–12

      Rationale Clamping prevents any reflux of the feeding.

9. If a burette is being used:
   a. Hang the burette from an infusion pole about 30 cm (12 in) above the tube's point of insertion into the client.
   b. Clamp the tubing, and pour the formula into the burette.
   c. Open the clamp, run the formula through the burette tubing, and reclamp the tube.

      Rationale The formula will displace the air in the burette and its tubing, thus preventing the instillation of excess air into the client's stomach.

   d. Confirm placement of the nasogastric tube by withdrawing stomach contents (see step 6) or injecting air through the nasogastric tube while listening for a whooshing sound with a stethoscope placed over the client's stomach.
   e. After completing step 6, attach the burette tubing to the nasogastric tube and regulate the drip by adjusting the clamp.
   f. Just before all the formula has run through and the burette is empty, add 60 ml of water to the burette and run it through the nasogastric tube.

      Rationale The water rinses the nasogastric tube and maintains its patency by removing sticky formula that can occlude the tube.

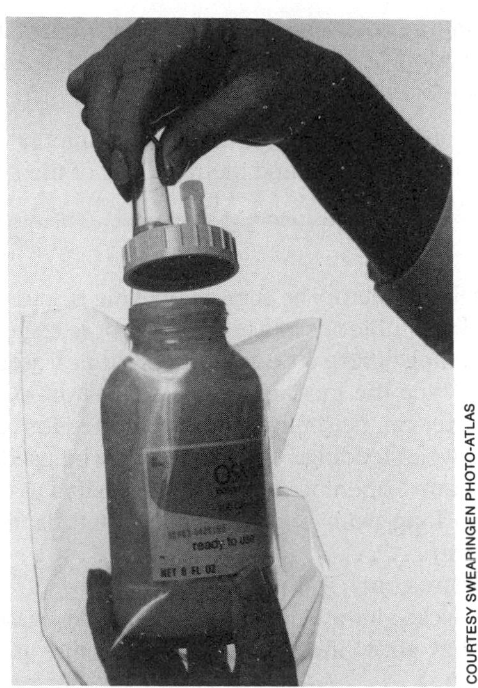

COURTESY SWEARINGEN PHOTO-ATLAS

Figure 42–13

g. Clamp the burette tube before all the water has gone through the tube.

   Rationale Clamping the tube prevents air from entering the stomach.

10. If a prefilled tube-feeding set is being used:
   a. Remove the sealed cap from the container, and replace it with the screw-on cap to which the drip chamber and tubing are attached. See Figure 42–13.
   b. Close the clamp on the tubing.
   c. Hang the container on an intravenous pole about 30 cm (12 in) above the tube's insertion point into the client.

      Rationale At this height the formula should run at a safe rate into the stomach.

   d. Squeeze the drip chamber to fill it to one-third to one-half its capacity.
   e. Open the tubing clamp, run the formula through the tubing, and reclamp the tube.

      Rationale The formula will displace the air in the tubing, thus preventing the instillation of excess air into the client's stomach.

   f. Follow step 7 above. Then attach the feeding set tubing to the nasogastric tube, and regulate the drip rate to deliver the feeding over the desired length of time. Some prefilled tube-feeding sets can be attached to a feeding pump.
   g. Just before all the formula has run through the tubing, clamp the feeding tube and the nasogastric tube and disconnect the two.
   h. Using a 50 ml syringe, instill 30 to 50 ml of water through the nasogastric tube to rinse it.

11. If the feeding is a continuous-drip tube feeding, discontinue the feeding at least every 6 hours, or as indicated by agency policy, and aspirate and measure the gastric contents. Then flush the tubing with 30 to 50 ml of water.

    Rationale This ensures adequate absorption and verifies correct placement of the tube.

12. After the feeding and tube rinsing, clamp the client's tube, if this is agency practice; some tubes are left unclamped.

    Rationale Clamping prevents leakage from the tube.

13. Cover the end of the tube with gauze held by an elastic band, and pin the tubing to the client's gown. See Figure 42–14.

    Rationale Covering the tube end prevents contamination.

14. Have the client remain sitting upright, in Fowler's position, or in a slightly elevated right lateral position for at least 30 minutes.

    Rationale These positions facilitate digestion. A right lateral position facilitates movement of the feeding from the stomach into the small intestine.

15. If the equipment is to be reused, wash it thoroughly with soap and water so that it is ready for reuse.

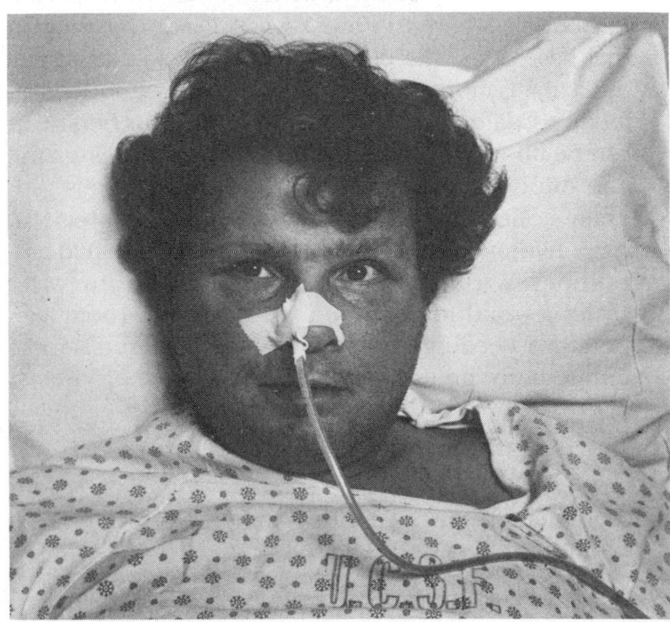

Figure 42–14

Change equipment every 24 hours or according to agency policy.

16. Check the agency's policy on the frequency of changing the nasogastric tube and the use of smaller-lumen tubes.

Rationale These measures prevent irritation and abrasion of the pharyngeal and esophageal mucous membrane.

17. Record the feeding, including the amount and kind of solution taken and the response of the client.

Gastrostomy or Jejunostomy Feeding

A **gastrostomy feeding** is the instillation of liquid nourishment through a tube that enters a surgical opening (called a gastrostomy) through the abdominal wall into the stomach. A **jejunostomy feeding** is the instillation of liquid nourishment through a tube that enters a surgical opening (a jejunostomy) through the abdominal wall into the jejunum. These feedings are usually temporary measures. When there is an obstruction in the esophagus, they may become permanent measures, for example, after removal of the esophagus.

For gastrostomies and jejunostomies, a surgeon inserts a plastic or rubber tube or catheter into either the stomach or the jejunum. The surgical opening is sutured tightly around the tube or catheter to prevent leakage. Care of this opening before it heals requires surgical aseptic technique. When the incision heals (10 to 14 days), the tube or catheter can be removed and reinserted for each feeding. Between feedings, a prosthesis may be used to close the "ostomy" opening. It consists of a shaft 4 to 6 cm (1½ to 2 in) long, with internal and external flanges and a screw cap.

Gastrostomy and jejunostomy feedings are used as alternatives to intravenous infusions and nasogastric feedings. They allow the client greater mobility and enable self-feeding.

Procedure 42–2 ▲ Administering a Gastrostomy or Jejunostomy Feeding

Equipment

1. The correct amount of feeding solution. Amounts are gradually increased from about 200 to 800 ml. Check the expiration date on a commercially prepared formula or the preparation date and time if the solution has been prepared in the agency. Discard a solution that has passed the expiration date or an agency formula that is more than 24 hours old. Gastric and jejunal feedings differ. Jejunal feedings contain nutrients that can be absorbed in the small intestine without gastric and duodenal digestive processes. All feedings generally contain 1 kcal/ml of solution with protein, fat, carbohydrate, minerals, and vitamins in specified proportions. Warm the solution in a basin of warm water or let it stand for a while until it reaches room temperature. Feedings are generally administered at room temperature unless the order specifies otherwise.
2. A large bulb syringe.
3. A graduated container to hold the feeding.
4. A graduated container with 60 ml of water to flush the tubing.
5. For a tube sutured in place:
   a. Some 4 × 4 gauze squares to cover the end of the tube.
   b. An elastic band.
6. For tube insertion:
   a. Water-soluble lubricant to lubricate the tube.
   b. Clean disposable gloves.
   c. A #18 French whistle-tip catheter or other feeding tube.
   d. A tubing clamp.
   e. A moisture-proof bag.
7. For a prosthesis:
   a. Water-soluble lubricant.
   b. A #18 French whistle-tip catheter or other feeding tube.
8. For cleaning the peristomal skin and dressing the stoma:
   a. Mild soap and water.
   b. Petrolatum, zinc oxide ointment, or other skin protectant.
   c. Precut 4 × 4 gauze squares.
   d. Uncut 4 × 4 gauze squares.
   e. Abdominal pads.
   f. An abdominal binder or Montgomery straps.

Intervention

1. Provide privacy for this procedure. Gastrostomy and jejunal feedings involve exposing the abdomen, which is embarrassing to many people, and this method of feeding may in itself be embarrassing.

2. Before administering the feeding, assess the client for:
   a. Allergies to any food in the feeding. Commonly included foods are milk, sugar, water, eggs, and vegetable oil.
   b. Bowel sounds before each feeding to determine intestinal activity.
   c. Abdominal distention at least daily. Measure the client's abdominal girth at the umbilicus.
   d. Regurgitation and feelings of fullness after a feeding.
   e. Hydration status. Measure the client's fluid intake and output, and note complaints of thirst.
   f. Changes in anthropometric measurements, i.e., weight, triceps skin fold, and arm muscle circumference. See page 1168.
   g. Dumping syndrome. Jejunostomy clients may experience nausea, vomiting, diarrhea, cramps, pallor, sweating, heart palpitations, increased pulse rate, and fainting after a feeding. These are signs of dumping syndrome, which results when hypertonic foods and liquids suddenly distend the jejunum. To make the intestinal contents isotonic, body fluids shift rapidly from the client's vascular system. Smaller, more frequent feedings and a longer adjustment period may relieve dumping.

3. Assist the client to a Fowler's position in bed, a sitting position on a chair, or, if sitting is contraindicated, a slightly elevated right lateral position.

   Rationale These positions promote digestion and prevent esophageal reflux of a gastric feeding.

4. If a tube is already in place:
   a. Remove the gauze from the end of the tube.
   b. Remove the clamp from the tube unless agency policy indicates otherwise. Some agencies leave the tube clamped until the syringe is attached.

      Rationale A clamped tube prevents excess air from distending the stomach or duodenum and causing discomfort.

   c. Attach the bulb syringe to the tube.
   d. Pour 15 to 30 ml of water into the syringe, remove the tube clamp, and allow the water to flow into the tube.

      Rationale This determines the patency of the tube. If water flows freely, the tube is patent; if it does not, notify the responsible nurse and/or physician.

5. If a tube is not in place, and one needs to be inserted:
   a. Lubricate the insertion end of the tube.
   b. Wearing gloves, remove the ostomy dressing and discard the dressing and gloves in the moisture-proof bag.
   c. Insert the tube into the ostomy opening about 10 to 15 cm (4 to 6 in).
   d. Attach the bulb syringe to the tube.

6. If a prosthesis is in place:
   a. Remove the screw cap on the prosthesis.
   b. Lubricate and insert the feeding tube into the ostomy opening about 10 to 15 cm (4 to 6 in).
   c. Attach the syringe to the end of the feeding tube.

7. Aspirate and measure the stomach or jejunal contents as follows:
   a. Compress the bulb on the syringe, and withdraw the stomach or jejunal contents.
   b. Measure the amount of aspirated contents in a graduated pitcher.

      Rationale To evaluate absorption of the previous feeding, the aspirated amount is compared with the amount instilled. If the amount is significant (e.g., more than half of the last feeding) the amount or frequency of the feeding may be changed.

   c. If 50 ml or more of undigested formula is withdrawn, check with the responsible nurse before proceeding.

      Rationale At some agencies a feeding is withheld if 50 ml or more of formula remains in the stomach.

   d. Reinstill the gastric or jejunal contents if this is the agency or physician's practice. Remove the bulb and pour the contents via the syringe into the tube.

      Rationale The removed formula is reinstilled to prevent electrolyte imbalance.

8. To administer the feeding solution:
   a. Hold the syringe about 7 to 15 cm (3 to 6 in) above the ostomy opening.
   b. Slowly pour the solution into the syringe, and allow it to flow through the tube by gravity.
   c. Just before all the formula has run through and the syringe is empty, add 30 ml of water.

      Rationale Water rinses the tube and preserves its patency.

   d. If the tube is sutured in place, hold it upright, remove the syringe, and then clamp the tube to prevent leakage. Cover the end of the tube with a 4 × 4 gauze, and secure the gauze with a rubber band.
   e. If the tube was inserted for the feeding, remove it, and either apply the screw cap to a prosthesis or apply a dressing over the ostomy.

9. After the feeding, have the client remain in the sitting position, or a slightly elevated right lateral position, for at least 30 minutes.

   Rationale This prevents leakage and enhances the normal digestive process.

10. Assess the status of the peristomal skin. Gastric or jejunal drainage contains digestive enzymes that can

irritate the skin. Any redness and broken skin areas need to be reported and recorded.

11. Check agency policy about cleaning the peristomal skin, applying a skin protectant, and applying appropriate dressings. Generally, the peristomal skin is washed with mild soap and water at least once daily. Petrolatum, zinc oxide ointment, or other skin protectant may be applied around the stoma, and precut 4 × 4 gauze squares may be placed around the tube. The precut squares are then covered with regular 4 × 4 gauze squares, and the tube is coiled over them. The coiled tube is covered with abdominal pads and secured with either an abdominal binder or Montgomery straps.
12. Record the date, the time, the type and amount of each feeding, the amount of water instilled, and any relevant assessment data.
13. When appropriate, instruct the client in how to care for the stoma and tube and how to administer a feeding.

Hyperalimentation

A more recently developed method of administering nutrients to a client is intravenous hyperalimentation (IVH) or total parenteral nutrition (TPN). See Chapter 46 for a discussion of intravenous hyperalimentation.

Evaluation

Examples of outcome criteria to evaluate the client's goal achievement and effectiveness of nursing interventions are shown to the right.

Examples of Outcome Criteria Related to Nutritional Status and Nutrient Intake

The client will:

- Have a triceps skin fold measurement within predetermined range or at baseline level
- Have an arm muscle circumference (AMC) within predetermined range or at baseline level
- Have a stable daily weight
- Maintain fluid intake at prescribed level or 1500 ml/day
- Demonstrate planned weekly weight loss while on reducing diet
- Demonstrate planned weekly weight gain
- Have normal blood and urine glucose
- Have normal serum electrolytes
- Feed self independently using self-feeding aid
- Tolerate entire meal without feeling nauseated
- Plan a balanced meal using the diet information provided
- Identify foods high in calcium

Nursing Care Plan

Assessment Data

Nursing Assessment

Mrs. Rose Santini, a 59-year-old homemaker, attends a community-hospital–sponsored health fair. She approaches the nutrition information booth, and Miss Pamela Norris, the nurse clinical specialist in nutritional support, gathers a nursing history of Mrs. Santini's nutritional problems. Mrs. Santini is very upset about her 9-kg (20-lb) weight gain. She relates to Miss Norris that since the death of her husband a month ago, she has lost interest in many of her usual physical and social activities. She no longer attends the YMCA exercise and swimming sessions and has all but lost contact with her couples bridge group at her church. She states that she is bored and depressed and very unhappy about her appearance. She has a small frame and has always prided herself on her "girlish figure." Mrs. Santini says her eating habits have changed considerably. She tends to snack a great deal while watching TV, and she rarely prepares a complete meal.

Physical Examination

Height: 162.6 cm (5′4″)
Weight: 63.6 kg (140 lb)
Temperature: 37 C (98.6 F)
Pulse rate: 76 BPM
Respirations: 16 per minute at rest
Blood pressure: 144/84 mm Hg
Triceps skin fold 27 mm
Small frame, weight in excess of 10% over ideal for height and frame

Diagnostic Studies

CBC: Normal
Urine: Negative
Chest x-ray film: Negative
Thyroid profile: Within normal limits

Nursing Diagnosis	Client Goals and Outcome Criteria	Nursing Interventions and Rationales	Evaluation
Alternation in nutrition: More than body requirements, related to excess intake and decreased activity expenditure, resulting in weight gain of 20 lbs, triceps skin fold greater than 25 mm, undesirable eating patterns.	Client Goal: Ideal body weight for height and frame. Outcome Criteria: Loses 2 kg (4 lbs) in 14 days. Plans 3 menus each day that result in a 500-calorie reduction in intake. Engages in physical exercise for 15 to 20 minutes by day 3. Identifies eating habits that lead to weight gain.	Assess for causes of excessive weight gain. *Rationale:* Excessive food intake is a complex problem with physical and psychosocial aspects. Encourage client to keep a 24-hour diet log. *Rationale:* Increases client's awareness of activities and foods that contribute to excessive intake. Encourage client to set realistic goals, e.g., decrease caloric intake by 500 calories each day. *Rationale:* A reduction of 500 calories per day will result in a 1 to 2 lb weight loss per week. Encourage client to knit or sew instead of eating snacks while watching TV. *Rationale:* Activity may distract the client from thinking about and taking snacks. Instruct client in behavior modification techniques, e.g., drink 8 oz of water before each meal, eat slowly and chew thoroughly. *Rationale:* Behavior modification may assist client in losing weight. Encourage client to increase physical exercise and/or to enroll in physical fitness program. *Rationale:* Exercise produces weight loss by increasing caloric requirements of the body.	Client kept a dietary log for 5 days and as a result now plans balanced meals each day, resulting in a daily loss of 400–500 calories. She is aware that she eats excessively because she is bored and depressed, and is now attempting to reestablish some of her former social contacts and activities. She has purchased a stationary bicycle and exercises 15 to 30 minutes each day. This past week she has enrolled in a knitting class as well, and she hopes this will help to keep her hands busy while she is watching TV. She has lost 1½ lbs in the past week.
Alteration in self-concept: disturbance in body image related to excessive weight gain resulting in withdrawal from social contacts and expressions of disgust with bodily appearance.	Client Goal: Achieve realistic concept of body image. Outcome Criteria: Verbalizes a realistic self-concept by day 14. Begins to assume responsibility for weight loss by day 7.	Establish a good nurse/client rapport. *Rationale:* A good nurse/client rapport will allow client to vent her feelings about her self-concept. Encourage client to reestablish social contacts. *Rationale:* Social acceptance can increase self-esteem.	Client states she hopes her old friends will accept her changed appearance. She has joined Weight Watchers and finds the persons in her group to be supportive and very helpful.

(*continued*)

Nursing Diagnosis	Client Goals and Outcome Criteria	Nursing Interventions and Rationales	Evaluation
	Expresses confidence in ability to change body image by losing weight by day 14.	Refer client to a weight-loss support group. *Rationale:* Support groups can provide companionship, increase motivation, and offer practical solutions to common problems. Discuss the client's view of being fat. *Rationale:* A mental image includes the ideal and is not always realistic.	She states that she knows she can lose weight if she "puts her mind to it," but that she may not be a size 8 by the end of 6 months.

Chapter Highlights

- Nutrition is the sum total of all interactions between an organism and the food it consumes.
- Although people are continually bombarded with information about what to eat and what not to eat, each person is responsible for selecting foods that provide essential nutrients.
- Nurses can assist people to evaluate the information they receive about nutrients.
- Essential nutrients are grouped into six categories: water, carbohydrates, fats, proteins, vitamins, and minerals.
- The first four classes are macronutrients; vitamins and minerals are micronutrients.
- Nutrients serve three basic purposes: (a) They form body structures (such as bones and blood); (b) they provide energy, which is measured in kilocalories; and (c) they help to regulate the body's biochemical reactions, collectively called metabolism.
- Both inadequate and excessive intakes of nutrients result in malnutrition.
- The effects of malnutrition can be general or specific, depending on which nutrients and what level of deficiency or excess are involved.
- The effects of deficits or excesses of nutrients become apparent in anywhere from a few weeks or months to years.
- Some of the long-range effects of certain nutrients excesses are among the many factors involved in certain diseases, e.g., coronary artery disease and cancer.
- Methods of food storage, processing, preserving, and cooking can significantly influence the micronutrient content of foods; use of selected methods can substantially decrease losses of micronutrients.
- Many standards of diet adequacy have been developed.
- Nutritional needs vary considerably according to age, growth, and energy requirements.
- Although breast milk has unique benefits for infants, many commercial infant milk preparations resemble human milk closely. Each, including breast milk, must be supplemented.
- Whether a woman chooses to breast-feed or bottle-feed depends on such factors as influence of others, personal preference, home and work demands, social customs, and economics.
- The infant is introduced to solid foods when the infant needs nutrients that solid foods provide and is ready to handle them.
- Iron-fortified rice cereal is the first solid food introduced, followed by mashed or chopped cooked soft fruits and vegetables and then finely cut meat.
- Toddlers, preschoolers, and school-age children require a variety of foods from the four basic food groups.
- Adolescents have high energy requirements due to their rapid growth; a diet plentiful in milk, meats, green and yellow vegetables, and fresh fruits is required.
- Middle-age adults and older adults often need to reduce their caloric intake because of decreases in metabolic rate and activity levels. Fats, sugary foods, and sodium must often be limited.
- Pre- and postmenopausal women, in particular, need to consume extra calcium to prevent bone loss.
- To assess the nutritional status of a person, the nurse follows the ABCD approach: anthropometric measurements are taken, biochemical data are assessed, clinical signs of nutritional status are assessed, and a dietary history is obtained.
- During the assessment stage and when planning nursing interventions to help clients reach nutritional goals, nurses must consider the many factors that influence a person's dietary patterns.

- Nursing diagnoses for clients with nutritional problems are broadly stated as alterations in nutrition and are further categorized as less than body requirements or more than body requirements.
- Obesity is a common nutritional problem of North Americans.
- Nurses can assist obese clients by recommending increased activity and intake of foods that have a low caloric density.
- Counseling about nutrition involves more than simply providing information. It can be likened to the teaching-learning process, which includes assessing specific learning needs, setting goals, planning strategies to meet goals, and establishing outcome criteria to evaluate goal achievement.
- Assisting clients and support persons with therapeutic diets is a function shared by the nurse and the dietitian. The nurse reinforces the dietitian's instructions, assists the client to make beneficial changes, and evaluates the client's response to planned changes.
- Because many hospitalized clients have poor appetites, a major responsibility of the nurse is to provide nursing interventions that stimulate their appetites.
- Whenever possible, the nurse should help incapacitated clients to feed themselves; a number of self-feeding aids help clients who have difficulty handling regular utensils.
- Various community programs help special subgroups of the population meet their nutritional needs. The nurse can be instrumental in referring clients to such services.

Suggested Readings

American Journal of Nursing. March 1981. Overeaters Anonymous: A self-help group. *American Journal of Nursing* 81:560–63.
Hyperphagia (compulsive overeating) is a chronic illness. Overeaters Anonymous provides a plan that includes 12 steps and 6 tools to control the problem for the rest of one's life.

Barclay, V. May/June 1980. How to eat on $1.18 per day. *Geriatric Nursing* 1:50–51.
Finances are a problem for many elderly people on fixed incomes. Barclay offers suggestions about foods that are economic but nutritious.

Christian, J. L., and Greger, J. L. 1985. A synthesized approach: The sound approach to nutritious eating (SANE). In *Nutrition for living*. Menlo Park, Calif.: Benjamin/Cummings Publishing Co., pp. 38–45.
Details of the SANE guide are provided. Charts of each food group are shown, and graphs indicate the fat, salt, and sugar in various foods.

Glaser, S. September/October 1981. How to improve the first stage of digestion. *Geriatric Nursing* 2:350–53.
Glaser describes ways to help ill, elderly people eat. Included is a discussion of how to serve the food and how to assess cough, gag, bite, and suck reflexes as well as neck and jaw control.

Hill, M. May 1979. Helping the hypertensive patient control sodium intake. *American Journal of Nursing* 79:906–9.
Hill discusses the importance of sodium, alternatives to sodium restriction, and teaching guidelines for those on sodium-restricted diets. A table shows the sodium content of selected foods.

Kornguth, M. L. March 1981. When your client has a weight problem: Nursing management. *American Journal of Nursing* 81:553–54.
This article includes realistic weekly weight loss goals, nutrition education information, and general tips for dieters.

White, J. H., and Schroeder, M. A. March 1981. When your client has a weight problem: Nursing assessment. *American Journal of Nursing* 81:550–52.
These authors are consultants who work with overweight clients in the community. Guidelines for an assessment interview are outlined along with a concise assessment tool.

Yen, P. K. May/June 1980. What is an adequate diet for the older adult? *Geriatric Nursing* 1:64, 71, 73.
Yen describes the recommended dietary allowances (RDAs) for elderly people including energy, protein, vitamin, and mineral requirements. These are related to the physiologic changes of the elderly person. The authors give nurses six suggestions for promoting good nutrition in elderly people.

———. July/August 1984. Nutrition, Fat, Cholesterol, and a healthy older heart. *Geriatric Nursing* 5:254–57.
Yen summarizes information about the relationship of a high-fat diet to coronary artery disease and cancer. She discusses which qualities of fat are good, how much fat is too much, which levels of cholesterol are safe, and which people should lower their cholesterol levels.

Selected References

Bechtel, S. November 1981. B_{12} for healthy nerves and blood. *Prevention* 33:63–67.

———. May 1982. Look to nutrition for sharper vision. *Prevention* 34:103–7.

Bishop, C. W.; Bowen, P. E.; and Ritchey, S. J. November 1981. Norms for nutritional assessments of American adults by upper arm anthropometry. *American Journal of Clinical Nutrition* 34(11):2530–39.

Bistrian, B. R., et al. Protein status of general surgical patients. *JAMA* 1974; 230–258.

Bowen, E., and Mondshein, N. November/December 1980. Give your patients a portion of good nutrition education. *Journal of Practical Nursing* 30:23–24, 65.

Brody, J. E. 1981. *Jane Brody's nutrition book*. New York: W. W. Norton and Co.

Byrne, C. J.; Saxton, D. F.; Pelikan, P. K.; and Nugent, P. M. 1986. *Laboratory tests: Implications for nursing care*. 2d ed. Menlo Park, Calif.: Addison-Wesley Publishing Co.

Caly, J. C. October 1977. Helping people eat for health: Assessing adult's nutrition. *American Journal of Nursing* 77:1605–10.

Chicago Dietetic Association and South Suburban Dietetic Association of Cook Will County. 1981. *Manual of Clinical Dietetics.* 2d ed. Philadelphia: W. B. Saunders Co.

Christian, J. L., and Greger, J. L. 1985. *Nutrition for living.* Menlo Park, Calif.: Benjamin/Cummings Publishing Co.

Crim, S. R. September 1969. Nutritional problems of the poor. *Nursing Outlook* 17:65–67.

Endres, J. B., and Rockwell, R. E. 1980. *Food, nutrition, and the young child.* St. Louis: C. V. Mosby Co.

Fennema, O. 1977. Loss of vitamins in fresh and frozen foods. *Food Technology* 31:32–36.

Frisancho, A. R. November 1981. New norms of upper limb fat and muscle areas for assessment of nutritional status. *American Journal of Clinical Nutrition* 34(11):2540–45.

Glaser, S. September/October 1981. How to improve the first stage of digestion. *Geriatric Nursing* 2:350–53.

Gordon, M. 1982. *Manual of nursing diagnosis.* New York: McGraw-Hill Book Co.

Grall, E. September/October 1981. It was easier, but . . . benefits of congregate eating far outweigh the drawbacks. *Geriatric Nursing* 2:353–54.

Gray, E. G., and Gray, L. K. November 1980. Anthropometric measurements and their interpretation: Principles, practices, and problems. *Journal of the American Dietetic Association* 77(5):534–39.

Griggs, B. A., and Hoppe, M. C. March 1979. Update: Nasogastric tube feeding. *American Journal of Nursing* 79:481–85.

Guyton, A. C. 1982. *Human physiology and mechanisms of disease.* 3d ed. Philadelphia: W. B. Saunders Co.

———. 1986. *Textbook of medical physiology.* 7th ed. Philadelphia: W. B. Saunders Co.

Hall, B. April 5, 1975. Changing composition of human milk and early development of appetite control. *Lancet* 779–81.

Halpern, S. L. 1979. *Quick reference to clinical nutrition.* Philadelphia: J. B. Lippincott Co.

Hayter, J. January/February 1981. Diabetes and the older person. *Geriatric Nursing* 2:32–36.

Heaney, R. P.; Gallger, J. C.; Johnson, C. C.; et al. 1982. Calcium nutrition and bone health in the elderly. *American Journal of Clinical Nutrition* 36:986–1013.

Howard, R. B., and Herbold, N. H. 1982. *Nutrition in clinical care.* 2d ed. New York: McGraw-Hill Book Co.

Keithley, J. C. February 1979. Proper nutritional assessment can prevent hospital malnutrition. *Nursing 79* 9:68–72.

Kim, M. J., and Mortiz, D. A., editors. 1982. *Classification of nursing diagnoses: Proceedings of the third and fourth national conferences.* New York: McGraw-Hill Book Co.

Konstantinides, N. N., and Shronts, E. September 1983. Tube feeding: Managing the basics. *American Journal of Nursing* 83:1312–18.

Lambert, M. L. March 1975. Drug and diet interactions. *American Journal of Nursing* 75:402–6.

Langford, R. W. March 1981. Teenagers and obesity. *American Journal of Nursing* 81:556–59.

Mazer, E. March 1982. Vitamin A: Good health insurance. *Prevention* 34:18, 22–24.

Mertz, W. 1981. The essential trace elements. *Science* 213:1332–38.

Metheny, M. M. January 1985. 20 ways to prevent tube-feeding complications. *Nursing 85* 15:47–50.

Montoye, H. J. 1984. Exercise and osteoporosis. In *Proceedings of the American Academy of Physical Education.* Champaign-Urbana, Ill.: Human Kinetics Publications.

National Center for Health Statistics. n.d. *Health and nutrition examination survey of 1971 to 1974.* DHEW Pub No. (PHS) 79-1310.

———. 1979. *Plan and operation of the health and nutrition examination survey (HANES), United States, 1971–1973.* Vital and Health Statistics, Series 1: Programs and Collection Procedure, No. 10a, DHEW Pub No. (PHS) 79-1310.

National Research Council, Committee on Dietary Allowances: Food and Nutrition Board. 1980. *Recommended dietary allowances.* 9th ed. Washington, D.C.: National Academy of Sciences.

Natow, A. B., and Heslin, J. 1986. *Nutritional care of the older adult.* New York: Macmillan Publishing Co.

Pechter, K. March 1982. Riboflavin is ready to help. *Prevention* 34:107–12.

Pipes, P. L. 1981. *Nutrition in infancy and childhood.* 2d ed. St. Louis: C. V. Mosby Co.

Raab, D., and Raab, N. March 1985. Nutrition and the aging: An overview. *Canadian Nurse* 81:24–26.

Rose, J. C. July 1978. Nutritional problems in radiotherapy patients. *American Journal of Nursing* 78:1194–96.

Russell, R. M., and Naccarto, D. V. October 1982. Current perspectives on trace elements. *Drug Therapy* 7:115–18.

Satter, E. 1983. *Child of mine: Feeding with love and good sense.* Palo Alto, Calif.: Bull Publishing Co.

Suitor, C. W., and Hunter, M. F. 1980. *Nutrition: Principles and application in health promotion.* Philadelphia: J. B. Lippincott Co.

Todd, B. September/October 1981. When the patient has a potassium deficiency. *Geriatric Nursing* 2:373.

U.S. Congress. Senate Select Committee on Nutrition and Human Needs. 1977. *Dietary goals for the United States.* 2d ed. Washington, D.C.: Government Printing Office.

U.S. Department of Agriculture. 1979. *The Hassle-free guide to a better diet.* Science and Education Administration Leaflet No. 567: U.S. Government Printing Office.

———. 1981. *Nutritive value of foods.* Home and Garden Bulletin No. 72: U.S. Government Printing Office.

U.S. Department of Agriculture and U.S. Department of Health and Human Services. 1980. *Nutrition and your health: Dietary guidelines for Americans.* Home and Garden Bulletin No. 232: U.S. Government Printing Office.

Vhymeister, I. B.; Register, U. D.; and Sonnenberg, L. M. February 1977. Safe vegetarian diets for children. *Pediatric Clinics of North America* 24(1):207.

Weinsier, R. I., et al. 1979. Hospital malnutrition: A prospective evaluation of general medical patients during the course of hospitalization. *American Journal of Clinical Nutrition* 32:418.

White, J. H. M., and Schroeder, M. A. March 1981. When your client has a weight problem: Nursing assessment. *American Journal of Nursing* 81:550–52.

Whitney, E. N., and Cataldo, C. B. 1983. *Understanding normal and clinical nutrition.* St. Paul: West Publishing Co.

Williams, S. R. 1981. *Nutrition and diet therapy.* 4th ed. St. Louis: C. V. Mosby Co.

Worthington-Roberts, B. S.; Vermeersch, J.; and Williams, S. R. 1981. *Nutrition in pregnancy and lactation.* 2d ed. St. Louis: C. V. Mosby Co.

43 *Fecal Elimination*

Contents *(continued)*

Objectives

1. Know essential facts about the lower intestinal tract and the development of bowel control.
   1.1 Define selected terms.
   1.2 Identify the anatomy of the lower intestinal tract.
   1.3 Describe the functions of the large intestine.
   1.4 Identify the age at which bowel control is achieved.
   1.5 List measures that promote the development of bowel control.
2. Know essential information and methods required to assess a person's fecal elimination status.
   2.1 Identify factors that influence fecal elimination.
   2.2 Identify factors that influence patterns of defecation.
   2.3 Identify normal characteristics and constituents of feces.
   2.4 Identify abnormal characteristics and constituents of feces.
   2.5 Describe methods used to assess the intestinal tract.
3. Understand essential facts about common fecal elimination problems and nursing diagnoses.
   3.1 Differentiate among specific common fecal elimination problems.
   3.2 Identify common causes and effects of selected fecal elimination problems.
   3.3 Identify assessment data indicative of common fecal elimination problems.

Terms

acholic
adsorbent
astringent
atony
bilirubin
borborygmi
bowel diversion ostomy
carminative
cathartic
chyme
constipation
defecation
demulcent
diarrhea

The colon's main functions are the absorption of water and nutrients, the mucal protection of the intestinal wall, and fecal elimination.

The colon absorbs water and significant amounts of sodium and chloride as food passes along it. As much as 1500 ml of chyme passes into the large intestine daily, and all but about 100 ml is absorbed in the proximal half of the colon. The 100 ml of fluid is excreted in the feces (Guyton 1986, p. 796).

The colon also serves a protective function in that it secretes mucus. This mucus contains large amounts of bicarbonate ions. The mucus secretion is stimulated by excitation of parasympathetic nerves. Therefore, during extreme stimulation—e.g., as a result of emotions—large amounts of mucus are secreted, resulting in the passage of stringy mucus as often as every 30 minutes with little or no feces (Guyton 1986, p. 785). Mucus serves to protect the wall of the large intestine from trauma by the acids formed in the feces, and it serves as an adherent for holding the fecal material together. Mucus also protects the intestinal wall from bacterial activity.

The colon acts to transport along its lumen the products of digestion, which are eventually eliminated through the anal canal. These products are flatus and feces. Flatus is largely air and the by-products of the digestion of carbohydrates.

The colon additionally serves to eliminate waste products, that is, feces. Three types of movements propel the chyme along the colon: haustral shuffling, contractions of the haustra, and peristalsis. See Figure 43–3. *Haustral shuffling* involves movement of the chyme back and forth within the haustra. In addition to mixing the contents, this action aids in the the absorption of water and moves the contents forward to the next haustra.

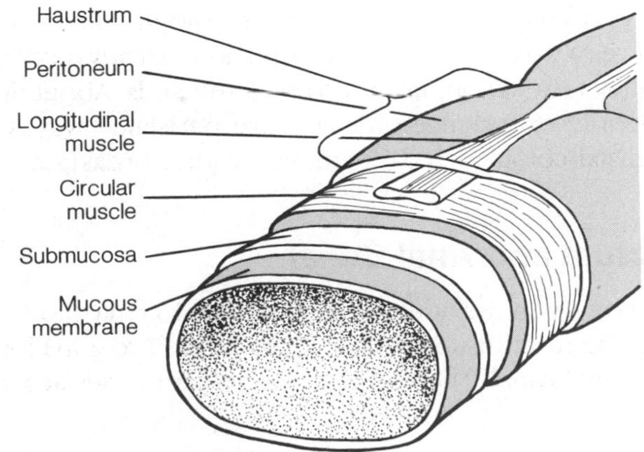

Figure 43–2 The layers of the wall of the large intestine

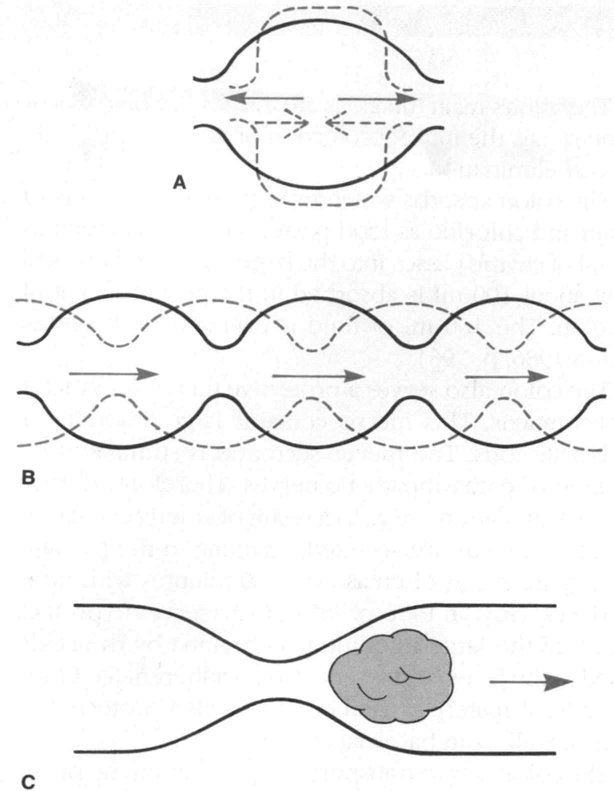

Figure 43–3 Three types of intestinal movements: **A,** haustral shuffling; **B,** contraction of the haustra; **C,** peristalsis

Contractions of the haustra, also called *segmentation,* help propel the liquid and semisolid contents along the colon. This kind of movement is less effective when it involves formed feces (Vick 1984, p. 738). These contraction movements normally occur intermittently, averaging one every 2 hours during fasting and about one every hour after a meal (Vick 1984, p. 739).

Peristalsis, the third type of colonic movement, involves a wave of muscular contraction that advances the length of the colon, usually toward the anus. About 50% of people experience one or more peristaltic waves in the distal colon each day, commonly after breakfast.

Rectum and Anal Canal

The rectum in the adult is usually 10 to 15 cm (4 to 6 in) long; the most distal portion, 2.5 to 5 cm (1 to 2 in) long, is the anal canal. The length of the rectum varies according to age:

1. Infant: 2.5 to 3.8 cm (1 to 1.5 in)
2. Toddler: 4 cm (2 in)
3. Preschooler: 7.6 cm (3 in)
4. School-age: 10 cm (4 in)

In the rectum are three folds of tissue that extend across the rectum and several folds that extend vertically. Each of the vertical folds contains a vein and an artery. It is believed that these folds help retain feces within the rectum. When the veins become distended, as can occur with repeated pressure, a condition known as *hemorrhoids* occurs (see discussion later in the chapter).

The anal canal is bounded by an internal and an external sphincter muscle. See Figure 43–4. The *internal sphincter* is under involuntary control, and the external sphincter normally is voluntarily controlled. The *external sphincter's* action is augmented by the levator ani muscles of the pelvic floor. The internal sphincter muscle is innervated by the autonomic nervous system; the external sphincter is innervated by the somatic nervous system.

Defecation

The frequency of **defecation** is highly individual, varying from several times per day to two or three times per week. The amount defecated also varies from person to person. When peristaltic waves move the feces into the sigmoid colon and the rectum, the sensory nerves in the rectum are stimulated and the individual becomes aware of the need to defecate.

Defecation is normally initiated by two defecation reflexes. When feces enter the rectum, distention of the rectum initiates a signal that spreads through the mesenteric plexus to initiate peristaltic waves in the descending and sigmoid colons and in the rectum. These waves force the feces toward the anus. As the peristaltic waves approach the anus, the internal anal sphincter becomes inhibited from closing and, if the external sphincter is relaxed, defecation occurs. This is called the *intrinsic defecation reflex.*

The second reflex, called the *parasympathetic defecation reflex,* is also actively involved in defecation. When nerve fibers in the rectum are stimulated, signals are transmitted to the spinal cord and then back to the descending and sigmoid colons and the rectum. These parasympathetic signals intensify the peristaltic waves, relax the internal anal sphincter, and intensify the intrinsic defecation reflex.

The *internal* anal sphincter relaxes, and feces move into the anal canal. After the individual is seated on a toilet or bedpan, the *external* anal sphincter is relaxed voluntarily. Expulsion of the feces is assisted by contraction of the abdominal muscles and the diaphragm, which increases abdominal pressure, and by contraction of the levator ani muscles of the pelvic floor, which moves the feces through the anal canal. See Figure 43–5. Normal defecation is facilitated by (a) thigh flexion, which increases the pres-

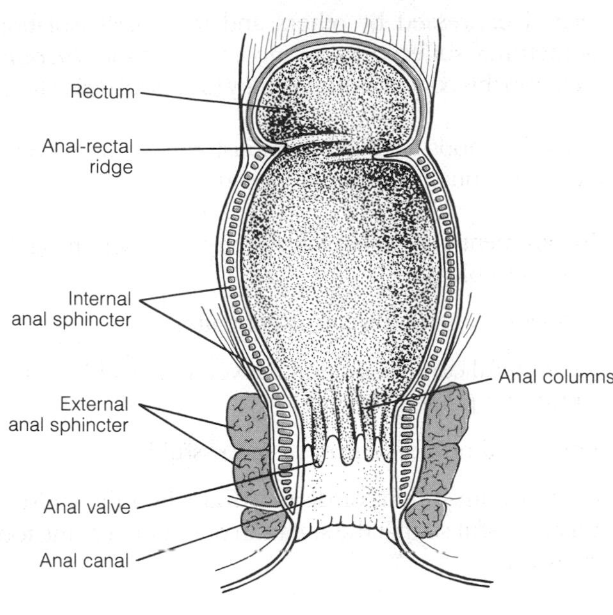

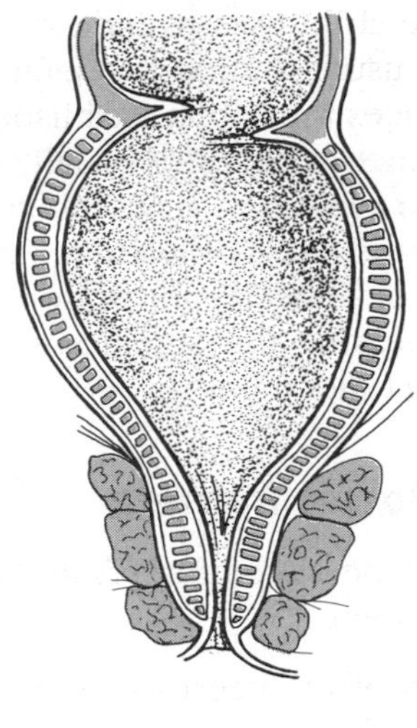

Figure 43–4 The rectum, anal canal, and anal sphincters: **A,** open; **B,** closed

sure within the abdomen, and (b) a sitting position, which increases the downward pressure on the rectum.

If the defecation reflex is ignored, or if defecation is consciously inhibited by contracting the external sphincter muscle, the urge to defecate normally disappears for a few hours before occurring again. Repeated inhibition of the urge to defecate can result in expansion of the rectum to accommodate accumulated feces and eventual loss of sensitivity to the need to defecate. Constipation can be the ultimate result.

Bowel Training

Bowel training usually can begin after a child learns to walk, at about age 1½ to 2. At this age, the child can ask to go to the toilet during the day when the need is felt. At this age, too, the child's nervous and muscular systems are sufficiently well developed to allow some degree of control.

Guidelines for the Bowel Training of Children

When children are being toilet trained, it is important for them to be as independent as possible in this function. The following measures are helpful.

1. Pants they can easily remove themselves.
2. An easily accessible training toilet. This can be a portable toilet or a special seat on the toilet with steps up to it so the toddler can reach it.

When a child is admitted to the hospital, it is important that the nurse learn from the parents the child's stage of toilet training. In particular, it is important to know

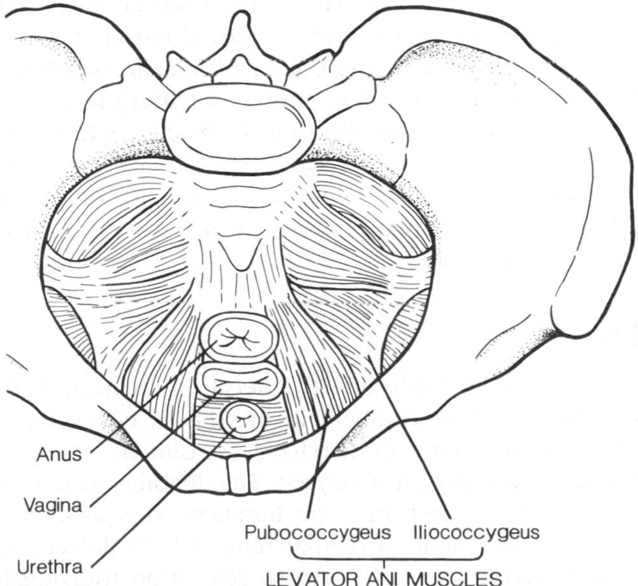

Figure 43–5 The levator ani muscles of the pelvic floor aid in expulsion of feces

what words the child uses to indicate his or her needs and the child's usual routine for defecation. It is best if the child continues the habits established at home. If the child is not trained, training is usually not begun in the hospital, for two reasons: A sick or anxious child will not readily tolerate the stress of learning new habits, and the child's mother or a significant person is not present in the hospital. Pleasing the significant person motivates children during toilet training.

Stages of Bowel Training

1. Awareness of the discomfort created by an incontinent bowel movement
2. Identification of the need to eliminate as the reason for the discomfort
3. Awareness of the body sensation that indicates the need to defecate
4. Desire to avoid the discomfort caused by involuntary defecation. This discomfort can be physical and/or sociologic. The latter is demonstrated by the disapproval expressed by others and the social isolation sometimes suffered by an incontinent child. *Incontinence* in this context is the inability to control defecation.

The methods used to accomplish toilet training vary; usually they must incorporate five aspects:

1. Involvement of a significant person—a person the child wishes to please
2. Sufficient time and a consistent pattern
3. Meaningful communication between the child and the significant person
4. Praise and reinforcement of successful behavior
5. Lack of punishment or disapproval when the child is unsuccessful so that the situation does not become too stressful

If any of these is absent, the child may have difficulty during training. Daytime bowel control is normally attained by the age of 30 months.

Factors that Affect Defecation

Age

Age affects not only the character of fecal elimination but also its control. The very young are unable to control elimination until the neuromuscular system is developed, usually between the ages of 2 and 3 years. The elderly also experience changes that can affect bowel evacuation. Two of these are **atony** (lack of normal muscle tone) of the smooth muscle of the colon, which can result in a slower peristalsis and thus hardened (drier) feces, and decreased tone of the abdominal muscles, which also decreases the pressure that can be exerted during bowel evacuation. Some elderly people also have lessened control of the anal sphincter muscles, which can result in an urgency to defecate.

Diet

Food is a major factor affecting fecal elimination. Sufficient bulk (cellulose, fiber) in the diet is necessary to provide fecal volume. Certain foods are difficult or impossible for some people to digest. This inability results in digestive upsets and, in some instances, the passage of watery stools. Eating at regular times affects defecation; irregular eating can impair regular defecation. Individuals who eat at the same times every day have a regularly timed, physiologic response to the food intake and a regular pattern of peristaltic activity in the colon.

Fluid

Fluid intake also affects fecal elimination. When fluid intake is inadequate or output (urine or vomitus, for example) is excessive for some reason, the body continues to reabsorb fluid from the chyme as it passes along the colon. As a result the chyme becomes drier than normal, resulting in hard feces. In addition, reduced fluid intake slows the chyme's passage along the intestines, further increasing the reabsorption of fluid from the chyme.

Muscle Tone

Well-toned abdominal and pelvic muscles and the diaphragm are important in defecation. Activity also stimulates peristalsis, thus facilitating the movement of chyme along the colon. Weak muscles are often ineffective in increasing the intraabdominal pressure during defecation or in controlling defecation. Weak muscles can result from lack of exercise, immobility, or impaired neurologic functioning.

Psychologic Factors

It appears that psychologic stress can affect defecation. Certain diseases that involve severe diarrhea, such as ulcerative colitis, may have a psychologic component. It is also known that some people who are anxious or angry experience increased peristaltic activity and subsequent diarrhea. In addition, people who are depressed may experience slower intestinal motility, resulting in constipation.

Life-Style

Life-style influences fecal elimination in a number of ways. Early bowel training may establish the habit of defecating at regular times, such as daily after breakfast, or it may lead to an irregular pattern of defecation. The availability of toilet facilities, embarrassment about odors, and the need for privacy also affect fecal elimination patterns. A client who shares a room in a hospital may be unwilling to use a bedpan because of the lack of privacy and embarrassment about odors.

Medications

Some drugs have side effects that can interfere with normal elimination. Some cause diarrhea; others, such as large doses of certain tranquilizers and repeated administration of morphine and codeine, cause constipation.

Some medications directly affect elimination. **Laxatives** are medications that stimulate bowel activity and so assist fecal elimination. There are medications that soften stool, facilitating defecation. Certain medications, such as dicyclomine hydrochloride (Bentyl), suppress peristaltic activity and sometimes are used to treat diarrhea.

Diagnostic Procedures

Certain diagnostic procedures, such as visualization of the sigmoid colon (sigmoidoscopy), require no food or fluid after midnight preceding the examination and often involve a cleansing enema prior to the examination. In these instances the client will not usually defecate normally until she or he has resumed eating.

Barium (used in radiologic exams) presents a further problem. It hardens if allowed to remain in the colon, producing constipation and sometimes an impaction. For additional information see Chapter 54.

Anesthesia and Surgery

General anesthetics cause the normal colonic movements to cease or slow down by blocking parasympathetic stimulation to the muscles of the colon. Clients who have regional or spinal anesthesia are less likely to experience this problem.

Surgery that involves direct handling of the intestines can cause temporary cessation of intestinal movement. This is called *paralytic ileus,* a condition that usually lasts 24 to 48 hours. Listening for bowel sounds that reflect intestinal motility is an important nursing assessment following surgery. See Chapter 35 for assessment of bowel sounds.

Pain

Pain can affect defecation. Clients who experience discomfort when defecating, e.g., following hemorrhoid surgery, will often suppress the urge to defecate to avoid the pain. Such clients can experience constipation as a result.

Irritants

Substances such as spicy foods, bacterial toxins, and poisons can irritate the intestinal tract and produce diarrhea and often large amounts of flatus.

Sensory and Motor Disturbances

Spinal cord injuries and head injuries, for example, can decrease the sensory stimulation for defecation. Impaired mobility may limit the client's ability to respond to the urge to defecate when she or he is unable to reach a toilet or summon assistance. As a result, the client may experience constipation. Or a client may experience fecal incontinence because of poorly functioning anal sphincters (see discussion later in the chapter).

Common Fecal Elimination Problems

There are six common problems of fecal elimination: constipation, fecal impaction, diarrhea, fecal incontinence, flatulence, and hemorrhoids.

Constipation

Constipation refers to the passage of small, dry, hard stool or the passage of no stool for a period of time. It occurs when the movement of feces through the large intestine is slow, thus allowing time for additional reabsorption of fluid from the large intestine. Associated with constipation are difficult evacuation of stool and increased effort or straining of the voluntary muscles of defecation. It is important to define constipation in relation to the person's regular elimination pattern. Some people normally defecate only a few times a week and therefore are not necessarily constipated when they miss a day or two. Other people defecate more than once a day, and to them a movement only once a day can indicate constipation. Careful assessment of the person's habits is necessary before a diagnosis of constipation is made.

There are many causes of constipation:

1. *Irregular defecation habits.* One of the most frequent causes of constipation is irregular defecation habits. When the normal defecation reflexes are inhibited or ignored, these conditioned reflexes tend to be progressively weakened. When habitually ignored, the urge to defecate is ultimately lost. Children at play may ignore these reflexes; adults ignore them because of the pressures of time or work. Hospitalized patients may suppress the urge because of embarrassment about using a bedpan or because defecation is too uncomfortable. Change of routine and diet can also contribute to constipation. The best way to prevent constipation is to establish regular bowel habits throughout life.
2. *Overuse of laxatives.* Laxatives frequently are used to relieve bowel irregularity. Overuse of laxatives has the same effect as ignoring the urge to defecate—natural defecation reflexes are inhibited. The habitual user of laxatives eventually requires larger or stronger doses, since they have a progressively reduced effect with continual use.
3. *Increased psychologic stress.* Strong emotion is thought to cause constipation by inhibiting intestinal peristalsis through the action of epinephrine and the sympathetic nervous system. Stress can also cause a spastic bowel (spastic or hypertonic constipation or an irritable colon). Associated with this type of constipation are abdominal cramps, increased amounts of mucus, and alternating periods of constipation and diarrhea.
4. *Inappropriate diet.* Bland diets and low-roughage diets are lacking in bulk and therefore create insufficient residue of waste products to stimulate the reflex for defecation. Low-residue foods such as rice, eggs, and lean meats move more slowly through the intestinal tract. Increasing fluid intake with such foods increases their rate of movement.
5. *Medications.* Many drugs have side effects that cause constipation. Some of these, such as morphine or codeine as well as adrenergic and anticholinergic drugs, slow the motility of the colon through their action on the central nervous system, thus causing constipation. Others, such as iron tablets, have an astringent effect and act more locally on the bowel mucosa to cause constipation. Iron also has an irritating effect and can cause diarrhea in some people.
6. *Insufficient exercise.* The effects of lack of exercise are discussed in Chapter 37. In clients on prolonged bed rest, generalized muscle weakness extends to the muscles of the abdomen, diaphragm, and pelvic floor, which are used in defecation. Indirectly associated with lack of exercise is lack of appetite and possible subsequent lack of roughage, which is necessary to stimulate defecation reflexes.
7. *Age.* The muscle weakness and poor sphincter tone that occur in elderly people contribute to constipation.
8. *Disease processes.* Several disease conditions of the bowel can produce constipation. Among these are bowel obstruction; painful defecation due to hemorrhoids, which makes the person avoid defecating; paralysis, which inhibits the client's ability to bear down; and pelvic inflammatory conditions, which create paralysis or atony of the bowel.

Constipation can be hazardous to clients. Straining in order to defecate can place stress on abdominal or perineal sutures, rupturing them if the pressure is sufficiently great. In addition, straining often is accompanied by holding the breath. This Valsalva maneuver (explained earlier) can present serious problems to people with heart disease, brain injuries, or respiratory disease. Holding the breath increases the intrathoracic and the intracranial pressures. To some degree this pressure can be reduced if the person exhales through the mouth while straining. However, avoiding any straining is the best precaution.

Fecal Impaction

Fecal impaction can be defined as a mass or collection of hardened, puttylike feces in the folds of the rectum. Impaction results from prolonged retention and accumulation of fecal material. In severe impactions the feces accumulate and extend well up into the sigmoid colon and beyond. Fecal impaction is recognized by the passage of liquid fecal seepage (diarrhea) and no normal stool. The liquid portion of the feces seeps out around the impacted mass. See Figure 43–6. Impaction can also be assessed by digital examination of the rectum, during which the hardened mass can often be palpated.

Along with fecal seepage and constipation, symptoms include frequent but nonproductive desire to defecate and rectal pain. A generalized feeling of illness results; the client becomes anorexic, the abdomen becomes distended, and nausea and vomiting may occur.

The causes of fecal impaction are usually poor defecation habits and constipation. Certain medications (see page 1201) also contribute to impactions. The barium used in radiologic examinations of the upper and lower gastrointestinal tracts can be a causative factor. Therefore, after these examinations, measures are taken to ensure removal of the barium. In the elderly, a combination of factors contribute to impactions: poor fluid intake, insufficient bulk in the diet, lack of activity, and weakened muscle tone. In some people, impactions tend to occur regardless of the measures taken to prevent them.

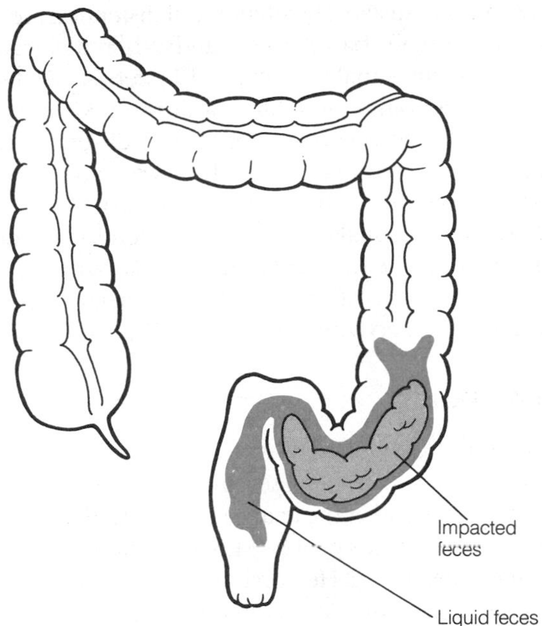

Figure 43–6 A fecal impaction with liquid feces passing around the impaction

When a nurse suspects an impaction, it can sometimes be palpated through the client's abdomen. Also, digital examination of the impaction through the rectum may be indicated. Digital examination should be done gently and carefully because stimulation of the vagus nerve in the rectal wall can slow the client's heart. Some nurses advise against digital rectal examination without a physician's order.

Diarrhea

Diarrhea refers to the passage of liquid feces and an increased frequency of defecation. It is the opposite of constipation and results from rapid movement of fecal contents through the large intestine. Rapid passage of chyme reduces the time available for the large intestine to reabsorb water and electrolytes. Some people pass stool with increased frequency, but diarrhea is not present unless the stool is relatively unformed and excessively liquid. The person with diarrhea finds it difficult or impossible to control for very long the urge to defecate. Diarrhea and the threat of incontinence are a source of concern and embarrassment. Often, spasmodic and piercing abdominal cramps are associated with diarrhea. Sometimes the client passes blood and excessive mucus; nausea and vomiting may also occur. With persistent diarrhea, irritation of the anal region extending to the perineum and buttocks generally results. Fatigue, weakness, malaise, and emaciation are the results of prolonged diarrhea.

When the cause of diarrhea is irritants in the intestinal tract, diarrhea is thought to be a protective flushing mechanism. It can create serious fluid and electrolyte losses in the body, however, that can develop within frighteningly short periods of time, particularly in infants and small children. See Chapter 46 for further information concerning fluid and electrolyte losses in the body. Table 43–1 lists some of the major causes of diarrhea and the physiologic response of the body.

Fecal Incontinence

Incontinence refers to loss of voluntary ability to control fecal and gaseous discharges through the anal sphincter. The incontinence may occur at specific times, such as after meals, or it may occur irregularly.

Fecal incontinence is generally associated with impaired functioning of the anal sphincter or its nerve supply, such as in some neuromuscular diseases, spinal cord trauma, and tumors of the external anal sphincter muscle.

Fecal incontinence is an emotionally distressing problem that can ultimately lead to social isolation. Afflicted persons withdraw into their homes or, if in the hospital, the confines of their room to minimize the embarrassment associated with soiling. Such people may come to prefer easily washable night garments to street clothes. Incontinent feces are acidic and contain digestive enzymes that are highly irritating to skin. Therefore, the area around the anal region should be protected with zinc oxide or some other protective ointment. These areas should also be kept clean and dry.

Table 43–1 Major Causes of Diarrhea

Cause	Physiologic Response
Psychologic stress, e.g., anxiety	Increased intestinal motility and mucus secretion
Medications	
Antibiotics	Inflammation and infection of mucosa due to overgrowth of normal intestinal microorganisms
Iron	Irritation of intestinal mucosa
Cathartics	Irritation of intestinal mucosa
Allergy to food or fluid	Incomplete digestion of food or fluid
Intolerance of food or fluid	Increased intestinal motility and mucus secretion
Diseases of the colon	
Malabsorption syndrome	Reduced absorption of fluids
Crohn's disease	Inflammation of the mucosa often leading to ulcer formation

Flatulence

Air or gas in the gastrointestinal tract is called **flatus.** There are three primary causes of flatus: (a) action of bacteria on the chyme in the large intestine, (b) swallowed air, and (c) gas that diffuses from the bloodstream into the intestine. Normally all but 0.6 liters of this gas is absorbed into the intestinal capillaries (Guyton 1986, p. 805).

Flatulence is the presence of excessive flatus in the intestines and leads to stretching and inflation of the intestines **(intestinal distention).** This condition is also referred to as **tympanites.** Large amounts of air and other gases can accumulate in the stomach, resulting in gastric distention.

An adult usually forms 7 to 10 liters of flatus in the large intestine every 24 hours. The gases include carbon dioxide, methane, hydrogen, oxygen, and nitrogen. Some are swallowed with food and fluids taken by mouth, and others are formed through the action of bacteria on the chyme in the large intestine (Guyton 1986, p. 805).

The gases that are swallowed are most expelled through the mouth, by **eructation** (belching). The gases formed in the large intestine are chiefly absorbed, through the intestinal capillaries, into the circulation. Flatulence can occur in the colon, however, from a variety of causes, such as abdominal surgery, anesthetics, and narcotics. If this gas cannot be expelled through the anus, it may be necessary to insert a rectal tube or provide a return flow enema to remove it.

Common causes of flatulence and distention are constipation; codeine, barbiturates, and other medications that decrease intestinal motility; and anxiety states during which large amounts of air are swallowed. Most people have experienced some flatulence and distention after eating such gas-forming foods as beans or cabbage. Postoperative distention after abdominal surgery is commonly seen in hospitals. This type of distention generally occurs on about the third postoperative day and is caused by the effects of anesthetics, narcotics, dietary changes, and reduction in activity. See Chapter 53.

Hemorrhoids

Hemorrhoids, also called *piles,* are distended veins in the anal area. They can be internal or external. Internal hemorrhoids occur in the anal canal, where they remain. External hemorrhoids prolapse through the anal opening and can be seen there. Hemorrhoids can occur as a result of increased pressure in the anal area, often secondary to chronic constipation, straining during defecation, pregnancy, or obesity.

Some hemorrhoids are asymptomatic; others cause pain, itching, and sometimes bleeding. Hemorrhoids are often treated conservatively with **astringents** (to shrink the tissues) and local anesthetics (to provide relief from the pain). Stool softeners may also be used, to decrease irritation during defecation. In some instances hemorrhoids are removed surgically.

Assessment

Assessment of fecal elimination includes taking a nursing history that determines the pattern of defecation and includes physical examination of the abdomen, with specific reference to the intestinal tract. The feces are also assessed; the presence of flatus is determined. The nurse also should review any data obtained from relevant diagnostic tests.

Nursing History

A nursing history for fecal elimination will help the nurse ascertain the client's normal pattern. Most nursing histories include the following.

1. *Defecation pattern.* The frequency and time of day of the client's defecation. Has this pattern changed recently? Does it ever change? If so, does the client know what factors affect it? See "Pattern of Defecation" later in this chapter.
2. *Behavioral patterns.* The use of laxatives, fluids, and the like to maintain the normal defecation pattern. What routines does the client follow to maintain her or his usual defecation pattern (e.g., a glass of hot lemon juice with breakfast or a long walk before breakfast)?
3. *Description of feces.* How does the client describe her or his feces, including color, texture (hard, soft, watery), shape, odor?
4. *Diet.* What foods does the client believe affect defecation? What foods does the client typically eat? What food does he or she always avoid? Are meals taken at a regular time?
5. *Fluid.* What amount and kind of fluid is taken each day (e.g., 6 glasses of water, 5 cups of coffee)?
6. *Exercise.* What is the client's usual daily exercise pattern? Obtain specifics about exercise rather than asking whether it is sufficient or not, since people have different ideas of what is sufficient.
7. *Medications.* Has the client taken any medications that could affect the gastrointestinal tract (e.g, iron, antibiotics)?

8. *Stress.* Is the client experiencing any long-term or short-term stress? Determine what stresses the client experiences and how she or he perceives them.

9. *Pertinent illness or surgery.* Has the client had any surgery or illness that affects the intestinal tract? The presence of any ostomies must be explored (e.g., a colostomy or ileostomy).

Physical Examination of the Abdomen

Intestines

During assessment of the abdomen, with specific reference to the intestinal tract, the client assumes a supine position and is draped so that only the abdomen is exposed. The nurse should first identify the landmarks that are to be used as reference points for describing the findings. See page 859.

Inspection Nurses observe the abdominal wall for visible waves indicating peristalsis. Except in exceedingly thin people peristalsis is not normally observable. When the waves can be seen, they often start in the upper left quadrant and move inferiorly and medially over the abdomen. Observable peristalsis may indicate an intestinal obstruction.

Observe the abdomen for shape, symmetry, and distention. The abdomen should be evenly shaped without any apparent protuberances or distention. Protuberances such as masses will appear as a bulging of the abdominal shape. Distention will appear as an overall outward protuberance, with the skin appearing tight and tense.

A distended abdomen should be measured at the level of the umbilicus by placing a tape measure around the body. Repeated measurements will indicate whether the distention is increasing or decreasing.

Auscultation Bowel sounds are assessed with a stethoscope. Bowel sounds chiefly reflect small intestine peristalsis; they are described according to intensity, pitch, and frequency or degree of activity. Intensity indicates the force of the sounds or the rate of peristalsis. Pitch is the vibration of the intestinal wall as a result of the peristaltic waves; with intestinal distention there may be an increased pitch. The degree of activity or frequency of the bowel sounds is also assessed. See Chapter 35 for how to assess bowel sounds. Cessation of or decreased peristalsis can occur for several reasons: extensive handling of the intestines during surgery; electrolyte disorders, such as abnormally low serum-potassium levels; and peritonitis. Abnormally intense and frequent bowel sounds (**borborygmi**) occur in enteritis and with obstructions of the small intestine.

Percussion The abdomen is percussed to detect fluid in the abdominal cavity, distention of the intestines due to flatus, and masses such as an enlarged spleen or liver.

The entire abdomen is percussed, first in the upper right quadrant and clockwise from there. Flatus produces resonance (tympany), whereas fluid and masses produce a dull sound.

When abdominal fluid is present, percussion produces dullness below the fluid level. When the client lies on one side, the ascitic fluid flows to that side. Percussion reveals a line of demarcation between dullness and tympany; this line indicates the level of the fluid. A line drawn on the abdomen lets the nurse gauge if fluid amount is increasing or decreasing when the abdomen is next percussed. See Chapter 35 for percussion technique.

Palpation Both light and deep palpations are carried out, usually to detect and explore any tender areas and masses. The four quadrants of the abdomen are palpated. The abdominal muscles should be relaxed for successful palpation. The nurse should first palpate lightly and then deeply. Sensitive areas should be palpated last because of tightening of the muscles (abdominal guarding) that often occurs when painful areas are touched.

Rectum and Anus

For an anorectal examination the client usually needs to assume a left Sims's position or a genupectoral position. A female client can also assume a lithotomy position. See Chapter 35.

Inspection The perianal region is inspected for discolorations, inflammations, scars, lesions, fissures, fistulas, or hemorrhoids. The color, size, location, and consistency of any lesion is noted.

Palpation See Chapter 35 for palpation of the anal canal and rectum. During the rectal examination it is important that palpation be gentle so as not to stimulate the vagus nerve reflex, which could depress the cardiac rate.

Pattern of Defecation

The time of defecation and the amount of feces expelled are as individual as the frequency of defecation. Some people normally defecate once a day; others defecate only three or four times a week. Some defecate after breakfast; others do so in the evening. Often the patterns individuals follow depend largely on early training and on convenience. Most people develop the habit of defecating after breakfast, when the gastrocolic and deudenocolic reflexes cause mass movements in the large intestine. The presence of flatus should also be assessed.

Feces

Special containers may be provided for a fecal sample. It is important that the nurse know why the specimen is being obtained and that the correct container be used. Sometimes containers hold preservatives specific to the tests to be performed. Attached to or written on the container may be special directions, which need to be followed when obtaining the specimen.

Clients often can obtain their own specimen if given adequate information. The feces should not be mixed with urine or water, thus the client defecates in a bedpan or a commode.

A wooden or plastic tongue depressor is used to transfer the specimen, and about 2.5 cm (1 in) is placed into the container. If the stool is liquid, 15 to 30 ml is collected. The container is then closed securely and the appropriate requisitions completed. The fact that the specimen has been obtained is entered on the client's record.

For certain tests, fresh stool samples are needed. If so, the specimen is taken immediately to the laboratory. A stool specimen should not be left at room temperature for long because bacteriologic changes take place. Specimen containers usually have directions for storage; these should be followed if the specimen cannot be delivered immediately to the laboratory. In some instances refrigeration is indicated.

To secure a stool specimen from a baby or young child who is not toilet trained, the specimen is taken from newly passed feces. When the stool is being cultured for microorganisms, it is transferred to the container with a sterile applicator.

Normal feces are brown, due to the bilirubin derivatives stercobilin and urobilin and to the action of the normal bacteria within the intestine. **Bilirubin** is a yellow pigment in the bile.

Feces may have other colors, especially when there are abnormal constituents. For example, black, tarry feces may indicate the presence of blood from the stomach or small intestine; clay-colored (**acholic**) feces usually indicate the absence of bile; and green or orange stools may indicate the presence of an intestinal infection. Food may also affect the color of feces; for example, beets can color stool red or sometimes green. Medications, too, can alter the color of feces; iron, for example, can make stool black. See Table 43–2.

Consistency

Normally feces are formed but soft and contain about 75% water if the person has an adequate fluid intake. The other 25% is solid materials. See Table 43–3.

Watery feces contain more than the normal 75% water. The stool has moved more quickly than normal through the intestine; thus less water and fewer ions were reabsorbed into the body.

Hard stool contains less water than normal and in some instances may be difficult and painful to excrete. Some people, in particular babies and young children, may pass stool containing undigested food.

Shape

Feces are normally the shape of the rectum. Abnormalities in the shape must be noted. A stringlike stool may indicate a pathologic condition of the rectum.

Table 43–2 Characteristics of Normal and Abnormal Feces

Characteristic	Normal	Abnormal	Possible Cause
Color	Adult: brown	Clay or white	Bile obstruction
	Infant: yellow	Black; tarry	Drug, e.g., iron; upper gastrointestinal bleeding
		Red	Lower gastrointestinal bleeding; some foods, e.g., beets
		Pale	Malabsorption of fat
Consistency	Formed; moist	Hard	Constipation
		Watery	Diarrhea, e.g., intestinal irritation
Odor	Aromatic: affected by ingested food	Pungent	Infection, blood
Frequency	Adult: varies from 1–3 movements per day to once every 3 days	More than 3 movements per day; fewer than 1 movement per week	
	Infant: 1–6 movements per day	More than 6 movements per day; fewer than 1 movement every 2 days	
Shape	Cylindrical (contour of rectum)	Narrow	Obstruction
Amount	100–400 g per day (varies with diet)		

Odor

The odor of feces results from the action of bacteria in the intestine, and it normally varies somewhat from person to person. It is important for the nurse to note any changes in odor that the client notices. A putrid (rotten, distasteful) odor may indicate a digestive disorder.

Blood

Blood in feces is abnormal. The blood may be frank and bright red, meaning that the blood colored the feces late in the eliminative process. Black, tarry feces may mean that blood entered the chyme in the stomach or small intestine. Some medications and foods, however, can make feces red or black; therefore, the presence of blood should be confirmed by a test. Blood in the stool need not be visible. Such blood is referred to as *occult* (hidden).

Tests for the presence of blood in feces are routinely performed in clinical areas. There are several tests available commercially. The *Hematest* uses reagent tablets, whereas the *Guaiac* and *Hemoccult* tests use reagent solutions. Every test calls for a stool specimen (see the earlier discussion on obtaining samples). The Guaiac test is commonly used: A thin layer of feces is applied to a filter paper or paper towel. The reagent is then applied and the color noted; blue indicates the presence of blood. The manufacturer's directions should be followed for each test.

Abnormal Constituents

Sometimes feces contain foreign objects that have been ingested accidentally; accidental ingestion of foreign objects is most common in young children. Other abnormal constituents include pus, mucus, parasites, fat in large quantities, and pathogenic bacteria. Tests for the presence of any of these are usually performed in a laboratory.

Table 43–3 Composition of Normal Feces

Constituent	Percentage of Feces	Percentage of Solid Constituents
Water	75	
Solid materials	25	
Dead bacteria		30
Fat		10 to 20
Inorganic matter		10 to 20
Protein		2 to 3
Undigested roughage and dried constituents of digestive juices (e.g., bile pigment and sloughed epithelial cells)		30

Adapted from A. C. Guyton, *Textbook of medical physiology*, 7th ed (Philadelphia: W. B. Saunders Co., 1986), p. 796.

Diagnostic Tests

Direct Viewing

Direct viewing techniques include anoscopy, the viewing of the anal canal; proctoscopy, the viewing of the rectum; and proctosigmoidoscopy, the viewing of the rectum and sigmoid colon. These tests are discussed further in Chapter 54.

Roentgenography

Roentgenography of the large intestine requires the introduction into the colon of barium, a radiopaque substance. Barium permits the viewing of the outline of the colon by either fluoroscopy or roentgenography. For further discussion, see Chapter 54.

Nursing Diagnosis

Nursing diagnoses are determined from the assessment data collected by the nurse. Examples of nursing diagnoses related to fecal elimination are shown to the right.

Examples of Nursing Diagnoses Related to Alterations in Bowel Elimination

- Constipation related to ingestion of barium
- Constipation related to immobility
- Constipation related to spinal cord injury
- Diarrhea related to stress
- Diarrhea related to travel
- Diarrhea related to excessive consumption of coffee

Planning

The primary client goals in planning interventions often include:

- Understanding normal elimination
- Understanding the appropriate food and fluids required
- Maintaining skin integrity
- Establishing regular defecation habits
- Establishing a regular exercise program
- Understanding measures to relieve stress

Intervention

Normal Defecation

Normal defecation can be helped by a number of nursing interventions, including providing privacy, assisting a client to assume a squatting position, and administering cathartics or antidiarrheal medications, as ordered and needed, as well as providing enemas.

Privacy is extremely important to many people while they defecate. If this is true for a client, the nurse should provide as much privacy as possible. After defecating, some clients also prefer to wipe, wash, and dry themselves. A nurse may need to provide water and a washcloth and towel for this purpose.

Clients who are confined to bed may need assistance to sit on a bedpan. Squatting is the best position for defecation.

There are two main types of bedpans, the regular high-back pan (see Figure 43–7, *A*) and the slipper or fracture pan (see Figure 43–7, *B*). The slipper pan has a low back and is used for clients unable to raise their buttocks because of physical problems or therapy that contraindicates such movement. Female clients use a bedpan for both urine and feces; male clients use a bedpan for feces and a urinal for urine (see Chapter 44).

A *commode* is sometimes used instead of a bedpan when the client can get out of bed but is unable to go to a bathroom. A commode is like an armchair with an open, toiletlike seat and a receptacle underneath for receiving the urine and feces. The receptacle may be specially fitted to the commode or simply a bedpan that fits under the toiletlike seat. A commode may or may not be on wheels and freely movable. Some commodes have an additional plain seat, thus doubling as a regular chair.

If a client has difficulty raising off a toilet, an elevated toilet seat can be attached to a regular toilet. The client then does not have to lower herself or himself as far onto the seat and does not have to lift as far off the seat.

A client confined to bed may require assistance getting on and off a bedpan. Nurses should bear in mind that a client using a bedpan should not exert herself or himself unduly and therefore provide support while the client is seated on the bedpan to avoid muscle strain. For the client who can raise her or his buttocks, the nurse can place the bedpan under the client after she or he has flexed the knees and raised the buttocks. A client can be assisted in this movement if the nurse places a hand, palm up, under the client's lower back, resting the elbow on the mattress and using the forearm as a lever. The nurse then can place a regular bedpan under the client's buttocks, with the narrow end toward the foot of the bed and the client's buttocks resting on the smooth, rounded rim. A slipper (fracture) pan should be placed with the flat end under the client's buttocks. For helpless clients who cannot raise their buttocks on and off a bedpan, do the following.

1. Assist the client to a side-lying position, backside toward you.
2. Place the bedpan against the client's buttocks, with the open rim toward the foot of the bed.

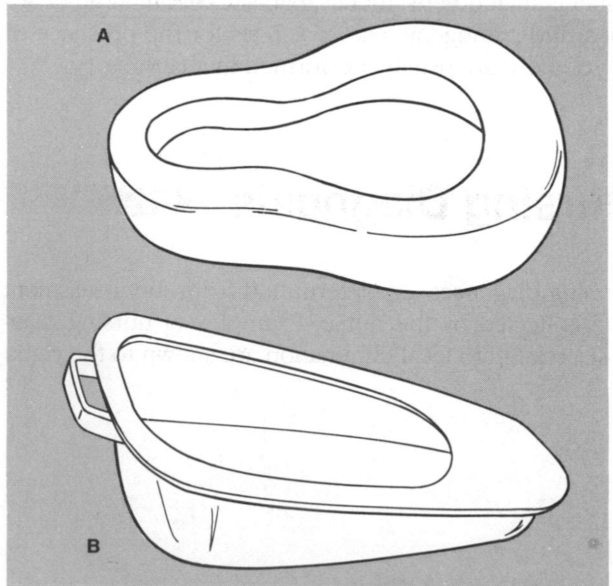

Figure 43–7 Two types of bedpans: **A,** the high-back or regular pan; **B,** the slipper or fracture pan

3. Hold the far hip with one hand and the bedpan with the other. Smoothly roll the client toward you and onto his or her back, with the bedpan in place (see Figure 43–8). Assume a wide stance and shift your weight from the front leg to the back leg when moving the client. The use of appropriate body mechanics prevents undue muscle exertion and strain. A bedpan should never be shoved under a client, because this can injure the client's skin.
4. Elevate the head of the bed to a semi-Fowler's position. This position relieves strain on the client's back and permits a more normal position for elimination.
5. If the client is unable to assume a semi-Fowler's position, place a small pillow under his or her back for support.

After placing tissues and the call light within easy reach, the nurse then leaves the client in privacy. The nurse should return to remove the bedpan when the client signals. If assistance cleaning the perineal area is required, the nurse should wrap toilet tissue several times around his or her hand and wipe the client from the pubic area to the anal area, using one stroke for each piece of tissue. (Cleaning from the less soiled to the more soiled area helps prevent the spread of microorganisms.) The nurse then turns the client on his or her side, spreads the buttocks, and cleans the anal area in the same manner. The anal area should be washed with soap and water, as indicated, and then thoroughly dried. Adequate washing and drying help prevent skin irritation and excessive accumulation of microorganisms.

For helpless clients, do the following:

1. Return the bed to flat position, if health permits.
2. Fold the top bed linen down to the client's thighs.
3. Holding the bedpan securely with one hand, gently roll the client to a side-lying position, either facing you or away from you. If you are alone, it is safer and easier to roll the helpless client toward you rather than away from you. If you are planning to turn the client away from you, raise the side rail or have another nurse present to prevent a fall.

Clean the anal area as described above. If the bed linens have become soiled they should be changed.

Before the pan is emptied (either in the client's toilet or in a receptacle in the utility room) the contents should be observed and perhaps measured. Most hospitals have spray faucets to rinse the bedpan thoroughly.

Cathartics and Antidiarrheal Medications

Cathartics are drugs that induce defecation. They vary in their degree and method of action. Cathartics can have a laxative effect or a purgative effect. A laxative effect is mild in comparison to a purgative effect, which produces frequent movements of the bowel, soft liquid stools, and sometimes abdominal cramps. Different cathartics have different effects, but even the same cathartic may have either a purgative or laxative effect depending on the dosage taken. A large dose of a cathartic may have a purgative effect, whereas a small dose of the same cathartic may have a laxative effect and produce a normal bowel movement.

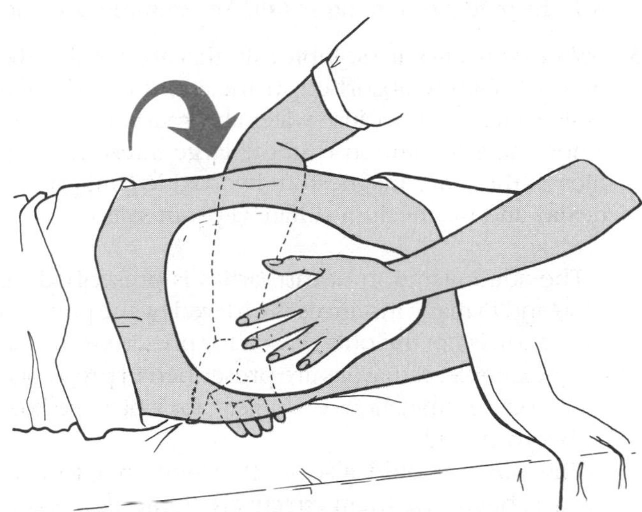

Figure 43–8 Placing a regular bedpan on the buttocks of an immobilized client

Cathartics induce defecation in several ways:

1. *Bulk-forming cathartics* act by increasing the fluid, gaseous, or solid bulk of the intestinal content. The increased bulk stimulates peristalsis, and defecation occurs. Fluids must be taken with this type of cathartic. An example is psyllium hydrophilic mucilloid (Metamucil).
2. *Emollient cathartics,* such as liquid petrolatum, act to soften and delay the drying of the fecal mass. Prolonged use of liquid petrolatum is contraindicated, since it inhibits the absorption of some fat-soluble vitamins.
3. *Chemical irritants* irritate the bowel mucosa and cause rapid propulsion of the contents from the small intestine. Considerable fluid is passed with the stool because of the rapid movement of the feces, which does not allow the normal absorption of fluid from the bowel. Castor oil is an example of a chemically irritating cathartic. It causes complete evacuation of the bowel, and no movements may occur for a day or two after its administration. Another example is cascara, although its irritant effect occurs primarily in the large intestine.
4. *Moistening or wetting agents* act by lowering the surface tension of the fecal matter, thus allowing water to

penetrate and become well mixed with the feces. A soft, formed stool is the result. An example is Colace.

5. *Saline cathartics* are soluble salts that are not absorbed or only slightly absorbed in the intestine. The fluid bulk is increased because water absorption is decreased when the salt solution is in the large intestine. Examples of these are magnesium hydroxide (milk of magnesia) and magnesium sulfate (Epsom salts).

The administration of carthartics is prescribed with caution and in many instances is ordered by the physician. Constipation is not the only reason for prescribing cathartics. For example, cathartics are prescribed in preparation for radiologic examinations or surgery, for which the bowel must be evacuated.

The nurse should also teach clients not to abuse cathartics, but to use them effectively. Some clients come to rely on cathartics and need help to learn how to change this habit. Others may need to take cathartics regularly or periodically. An example is the elderly person who has difficulty increasing bulk in the diet because of being edentulous or whose physical health prohibits appropriate exercise.

Before administering cathartics, the nurse also needs to be aware of any other pathologic condition the client may have. The classic example is the person with an inflamed appendix. Giving this person a cathartic can rupture the appendix as a result of the increased peristaltic action of the bowel. Some other contraindications are ulcerative conditions of the intestine, pathologic obstructions, or severe debilitation from electrolyte imbalances.

Suppositories

Some cathartics are given in the form of suppositories. These act in various ways: by softening the feces, by releasing gases such as carbon dioxide to distend the rectum, or by stimulating the nerve endings in the rectal mucosa. Suppositories need to be inserted beyond the internal anal sphincter. A finger cot or disposable glove is worn by the nurse, and the suppository is well lubricated prior to insertion, to prevent friction and tissue damage. For an adult the suppository is inserted gently 7.5 to 10 cm (3 to 4 in), or the length of the nurse's index finger; less for a child or baby. The client is instructed to breathe through the mouth, because mouth breathing may relax the anal sphincter. To be effective, the suppository needs to be placed along the wall of the rectum rather than lodged in the feces. Immediately after inserting the suppository, the nurse can help dispel any urge the client has to expel the suppository by pressing the client's buttocks together for a few seconds. After the procedure, the nurse removes the glove or finger cot (by turning it inside out) and discards it. Nondisposable gloves are washed in soap and water. See Chapter 54 for rectal insertion.

Generally, suppositories are effective within 30 minutes. The best results can be obtained by inserting the suppository 30 minutes before the client's usual defecation time or when the peristaltic action is greatest, such as after breakfast.

Antidiarrheal Medications

Clients who have diarrhea may require antidiarrhetics. Some of these mechanically coat the irritated bowel and act as protectives (**demulcents**). Others absorb gas or toxic substances from the bowel (**adsorbents**) or shrink swollen and inflamed tissues (**astringents**). In certain situations, sedatives and antispasmodics may also be required.

Enemas

An **enema** is a solution introduced into the rectum and sigmoid colon. Its function is to remove feces and/or flatus.

Types of Enemas

Enemas are classified into four groups, according to their action: cleansing, carminative, retention, or return flow. A *cleansing enema* stimulates peristalsis by irritating the colon and rectum and/or by distending the intestine with the volume of fluid introduced. Two kinds of cleansing enemas are the high enema and the low enema. The *high enema* is given to clean as much of the colon as possible. Often about 1,000 ml (1 liter) of solution is administered to an adult, and the client changes from the left lateral to the dorsal recumbent position and then to the right lateral position during the administration so that the fluid can follow the large intestine. See Figure 43–1. The fluid is administered at a higher pressure than for a low enema; that is, the container of solution is held higher. Cleansing enemas are most effective if held for 5 to 10 minutes. The *low enema* is used to clean the rectum and the sigmoid colon only. About 500 ml (0.5 liters) of solution is administered to an adult, and the client maintains the left side-lying position during its administration.

A **carminative** *enema* is given primarily to expel flatus. The solution instilled into the rectum releases gas, which in turn distends the rectum and the colon, thus stimulating peristalsis. For an adult, 60 to 180 ml of fluid is instilled.

A *retention enema* introduces oil into the rectum and sigmoid colon. The oil is retained for a relatively long period of time (e.g., 1 to 3 hours). It acts to soften the feces and to lubricate the rectum and anal canal, thus facilitating passage of the feces.

A *return flow enema,* sometimes referred to as the *Harris flush* or *colonic irrigation,* is used to expel flatus. This is a repetitive instillation of fluid into and drainage of fluid from the rectum. First a solution (100 to 200 ml for an adult) is instilled into the client's rectum and sigmoid colon. Then the solution container is lowered so that the fluid flows back out through the rectal tube into the container. This alternating flow of fluid into and out of the large intestine stimulates peristalsis and the expulsion of flatus. The inflow–outflow process is repeated five or six times, until gas bubbles cease or abdominal distention and discomfort is relieved. The solution may need to be replaced several times during the procedure if it becomes thick with feces. Because the solution is replaced, a total of about 1000 ml is usually used for an adult.

Various solutions are used for enemas. The specific solution may be ordered by the physician or dictated by agency practice. Table 43–4 lists some of these solutions, giving the quantity and proportions frequently used.

An enema is a relatively safe procedure for the client. The chief dangers are irritation of the rectal mucosa by too much soap or an irritating soap and negative effects of a *hypertonic solution* (possessing a greater tonicity than blood) or *hypotonic solution* (possessing a lesser tonicity than blood) on the body fluid and electrolytes. A hypertonic solution, such as the phosphate solutions of some commercially prepared enemas, is slightly irritating to the mucous membrane, and it causes fluid to be drawn into the colon from the surrounding tissues. The process by which this happens is called *osmosis*. Because only a small amount of fluid is normally administered, the advantages of comfort, retention for only 5 to 7 minutes, and convenience generally outweigh these disadvantages. However, electrolyte and fluid imbalances can occur, particularly in infants under 2 years of age. The solution can cause hypocalcemia (a decreased amount of calcium in the blood serum) and hyperphosphatemia (an excessive amount of phosphate in the blood).

The repeated administration of hypotonic solutions, such as tap water enemas, can result in absorption of the water from the colon into the bloodstream. This increases the blood volume and can produce water intoxication. For this reason, some health agencies limit to three the number of tap water enemas given consecutively. This is of particular concern when the order is "enemas until returns are clear"—for example, prior to a visual examination of the large intestine. Hypotonic solutions can also be unsafe for patients with decreased kidney function or acute heart failure.

Guidelines for Administering Enemas

1. The appropriate-size rectal tube needs to be used. For adults this is usually #22 to #30 Fr. Children use a smaller tube, such as #12 Fr. for an infant and #14 to #18 Fr. for the toddler or school-age child.
2. Rectal tubes must be smooth and flexible, with one or two openings at the end through which the solution flows. They are usually made of rubber or plastic. Any tube with a sharp or ragged edge should not be used because of the possibility of damaging the mucous membrane of the rectum. The rectal tube is lubricated with a water-soluble lubricant to facilitate insertion and decrease irritation of the rectal mucosa.
3. Enemas for adults are usually given at 40.5 to 43 C (105 to 110 F); those for children are given at 37.7 C (100 F), unless otherwise specified. Some oil retention enemas are given at 33 C (91 F). High temperatures can be injurious to the bowel mucosa; cold temperatures are uncomfortable for the client and may trigger a spasm of the sphincter muscles.
4. The amount of solution to be administered depends on the kind of enema, the age and size of the person, and the amount of fluid that can be retained.
   a. Infant, 250 ml or less
   b. Toddler or preschooler, 250 to 350 ml or less
   c. School-age child, 300 to 500 ml
   d. Adolescent, 500 to 750 ml
   e. Adult, 750 to 1000 ml
5. When an enema is administered, the client usually assumes the left lateral position, so that the sigmoid colon is below the rectum, thus facilitating instillation of the fluid. During a high cleansing enema, the client changes position from left lateral to dorsal recumbent and then to right lateral. In this way the entire colon is reached by the fluid.
6. The distance to which the tube is inserted depends on the age and size of the client. In adults, it is normally inserted 7.5 to 10 cm (3 to 4 in). In children it is inserted 5 to 7.5 cm (2 to 3 in) and in infants only 2.5 to 3.75 cm (1 to 1.5 in). If any obstruction is encountered when the tube is inserted, the tube should be withdrawn and the obstruction reported.
7. The force of flow of the solution is governed by:
   a. Height of the solution container
   b. Size of the tubing
   c. Viscosity of the fluid
   d. Resistance of the rectum

   The higher the solution container is held above the rectum, the faster the flow and the greater the force

Table 43–4 Types of Enemas Commonly Used for Adults

Name	Constituents
Commercially prepared enema	90–120 ml of a hypertonic solution, such as sodium phosphate (see directions on the package)
Saline	9 ml of sodium chloride to 1,000 ml of water
Tap water	1,000 ml of tap water
Soap	5 ml of white bland soap to 1,000 ml of water
Oil, e.g., olive oil	90–120 ml of oil (commercially prepared): mineral, olive, or cottonseed

(pressure) in the rectum. During most adult enemas, the solution container should be no higher than 30 cm (12 in) above the rectum. During a high cleansing enema, the solution container is usually held 30 to 45 cm (12 to 18 in) above the rectum, because the fluid is instilled farther to clean the entire bowel. For an infant, the solution container is held no more than 7.5 cm (3 in) above the rectum.

8. The time it takes to administer an enema largely depends on the amount of fluid to be instilled and the client's tolerance. Large volumes, such as 1,000 ml, may take 10 to 15 minutes to instill; small volumes require less time.
9. The length of time that the enema solution is retained depends on the purpose of the enema and the ability of the client to contract the external sphincter to retain the solution. Oil retention enemas are usually retained 2 to 3 hours. Other enemas are normally retained 5 to 10 minutes. To assist an incontinent person to retain the solution, the nurse can press the buttocks together, providing pressure over the anal area.
10. While the enema solution is in the body, the client may have a feeling of fullness and some abdominal discomfort.
11. When it is time for the client to defecate, the nurse may assist her or him to a commode or toilet, depending on the client's preference and physical condition.
12. For self-administration of an enema, an adult can assume a back-lying position (see Figure 43–9).
13. When administering an enema to an infant, the infant's legs can be immobilized with a diaper (see Figure 43–10).

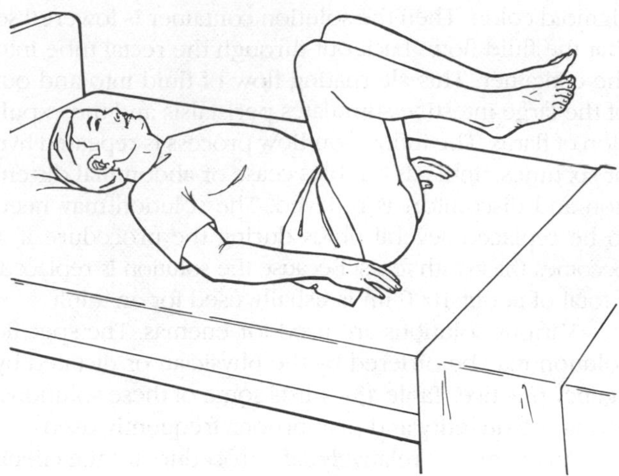

Figure 43–9 A back-lying position for self-administration of an enema

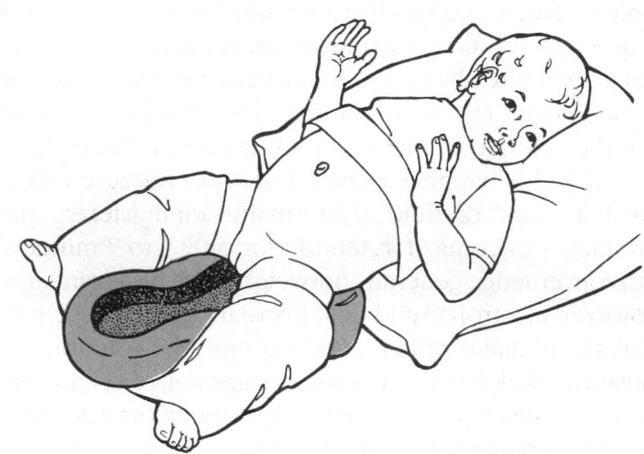

Figure 43–10 An infant's legs are immobilized for an enema by placing a diaper under the bedpan and over the thighs

Procedure 43–1 ▲ Administering an Enema

Before administering an enema, determine if a physician's order is required. At some agencies, a physician must order the kind of enema and sometimes the temperature of the enema and the time to give it, e.g., the evening before surgery or the morning of the examination. When the client has rectal pathology, the physician may also specify the size of the rectal tube to use. At other agencies, enemas are given at the nurses' discretion, i.e., as necessary on a p.r.n. order.

It is important that the nurse be aware that prepackaged enemas have their own instructions, which should be followed unless there are other instructions from the physician or the agency.

Equipment

1. A disposable enema unit (see Figure 43–11)

   or

2. An enema set containing:
   a. A container to hold the solution
   b. Tubing to connect the container to the rectal tube
   c. A clamp to compress the tubing, to control the flow of solution into the client
   d. A rectal tube of the correct size. See Guideline 1 on page 1211.

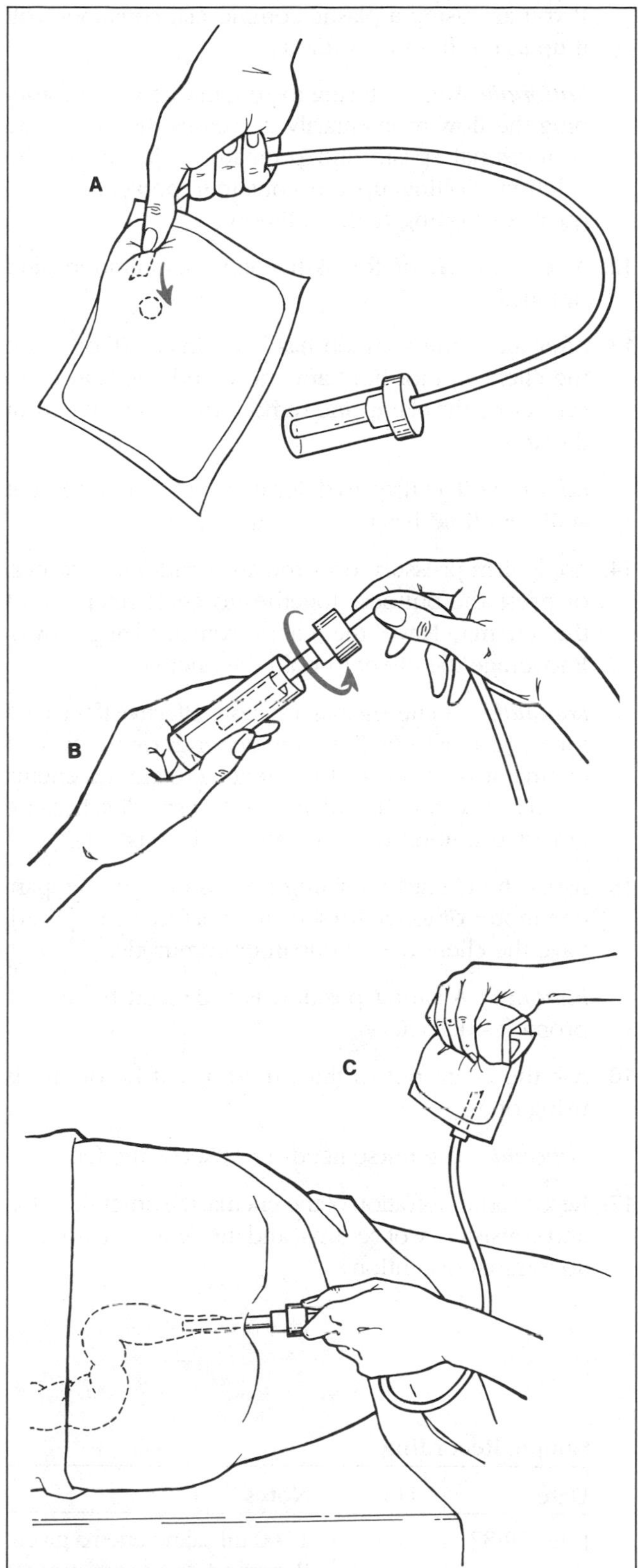

Figure 43–11 One type of commercially prepared disposable enema: **A,** the bead that seals the tube is expelled from the tube into the bag so the solution can flow through the tubing; **B,** the protector cover of the insertion tip is rotated to distribute the lubricant on the tip before the cover is removed; **C,** after the tube has been inserted, the bag is inverted and compressed

e. Lubricant to apply to the rectal tube before it is inserted
f. A bath thermometer to check the temperature of the solution
g. Soap, salt, or other ingredients as required
h. The prescribed amount of solution at the correct temperature. The nurse places the solution in the container, checks that the temperature and amount of solution are correct, and then adds the soap, salt, or other ingredients as needed.

3. A bath blanket to drape the client
4. A waterproof absorbent pad to protect the bed
5. Tissue wipes
6. A bedpan or commode if the client is unable to reach the bathroom

Intervention

1. Explain the procedure to the client. Indicate that he or she may experience a feeling of fullness while the solution is being administered.
2. Assist the adult or school-aged client to a left lateral position, with the right leg acutely flexed, and drape her or him with the bath blanket.

   Rationale This position facilitates the flow of solution by gravity into the sigmoid and descending colon, which are on the left side. Having the right leg acutely flexed provides for adequate exposure of the anus.

   For infants and small children, the dorsal recumbent position is frequently used. Position them on a small padded bedpan with support for the back and head. Secure the legs by placing a diaper under the bedpan and pinning it around the thighs. See Figure 43–10.
3. Place the waterproof pad under the client's buttocks to protect the bed linen.
4. Lubricate 5 cm (2 in) of the rectal tube if the enema is for an adult and 2.5 cm (1 in) if it is for a child. Some commercially prepared enema sets already have lubricated nozzles.

   Rationale Lubrication facilitates insertion through the sphincters and minimizes trauma.
5. Open the clamp, and run some solution through the connecting tubing and the rectal tube; then close the clamp.

   Rationale The tubes are filled with solution to expel any air in them. Air instilled into the rectum causes unnecessary distention.
6. Inspect the anal area for the presence of hemorrhoids.
7. Insert the rectal tube smoothly and slowly into the rectum, directing it toward the umbilicus. See Figure

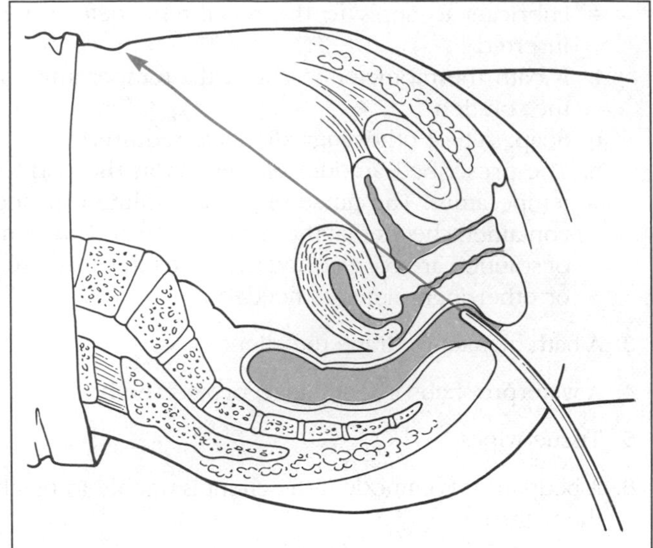

Figure 43–12

43–12. Insert the tube an appropriate distance. See Guideline 6 on page 1211. Note any sign of discomfort on inserting the tube and any obstruction to the passage.

Rationale Inserting the tube toward the umbilicus guides the tube along the length of the rectum. The rectum of the average adult is 10 to 20 cm (4 to 6 in) long, but the size varies with age. The rectal tube is inserted beyond the internal sphincter.

8. If resistance is encountered at the internal sphincter, ask the client to take a deep breath, and run a small amount of solution through the tube. If the resistance persists, withdraw the tube and report the resistance to the responsible nurse.

   Rationale Deep breathing by the client and inserting a small amount of solution may relax the sphincter.

9. If there is no resistance, open the clamp, and raise the solution container to the appropriate height above the rectum: 30 to 45 cm (12 to 18 in) for an adult, 7.5 cm (3 in) for an infant.

   Rationale At this height, the solution does not exert enough pressure to damage the lining of the rectum.

   or

10. Compress a pliable commercial container by hand.

11. Administer the fluid slowly. If the client complains of fullness or pain, use the clamp to stop the flow for 30 seconds and then restart the flow at a slower rate. If you are using a plastic commercial container, roll it up as the fluid is instilled.

    Rationale Administering the enema slowly and stopping the flow momentarily decreases the likelihood of intestinal spasm and premature ejection of the solution. Rolling up the container prevents subsequent suctioning of the solution.

12. Assess the client for skin color, perspiration, and dyspnea.

13. After all of the solution has been instilled, or when the client cannot hold any more and wants to defecate, close the clamp and remove the rectal tube from the anus.

    Rationale The urge to defecate usually indicates that sufficient fluid has been administered.

14. Apply firm pressure over the anus with tissue wipes, or press the buttocks together to assist retention of the enema. Have the client remain lying down. Encourage the client to hold the enema.

    Rationale Some enemas are more effective if retained for 5 to 10 minutes. The time depends on the type of enema. It is easier for the client to retain the enema when lying down than when sitting or standing because gravity promotes drainage and peristalsis.

15. Assist the client to a sitting position on the bedpan, commode, or toilet. If a specimen of feces is required, have the client use a bedpan or commode.

    Rationale A sitting position is preferred because it promotes defecation.

16. Ask the client not to flush the toilet if he or she is using one.

    Rationale The nurse needs to observe the feces.

17. Record administration of the enema; the amount, color, and consistency of returns; and the relief of flatus and abdominal distention.

Sample Recording

Date	Time	Notes
June/29/87	2100	1,000 ml saline enema given. Returned large amount of hard, white stool and large amount of flatus. Abdomen soft and less distended. P 72. —Roxy-Ann B. Stanley, NS

Administering an Enema to an Incontinent Client

Occasionally a nurse needs to administer an enema to a client who is unable to control his or her external sphincter muscle and thus cannot retain the enema solution for even a few minutes. In that case the client assumes a supine position on a bedpan. The head of the bed can be elevated slightly, e.g., to 30° if necessary, and the client's head and back are supported by pillows. The nurse wears a glove over the hand that holds the rectal tube, to prevent direct contact with the solution and feces that are expelled over the hand into the bedpan during administration of the enema.

Siphoning an Enema

In some instances a client may be unable to expel the solution after administration of an enema. The solution must then be siphoned off. In siphoning, the nurse uses the force of gravity to draw the fluid out of the rectum and colon.

The equipment required is a bedpan, a funnel and rectal tube, lubricant, and a container of water at 40 C (105 F). During siphoning, the client assumes a right side-lying position so that the sigmoid colon is uppermost, thus facilitating drainage of the solution from the rectum and the colon. The client lies on the bed with hips close to the side of the bed. The nurse places a bedpan on a chair at the side of the bed near the client's hips. The chair must be lower than the bed. The rectal tube is lubricated and attached to the funnel. The tube and half of the funnel are filled with solution, then the tube is pinched and gently inserted into the rectum as for an enema. The nurse holds the funnel about 10 cm (4 in) above the anus, releases the pinched rectal tube, and quickly lowers the funnel over the bedpan. This action should draw the fluid from the colon and rectum, permitting it to flow through the rectal tube and funnel into the bedpan. The nurse then notes the amount of fluid siphoned off as well as the color, odor, and presence of any feces or abnormal constituents, such as blood or mucus.

Digital Removal of a Fecal Impaction

Digital removal of a fecal impaction is sometimes necessary. The nurse breaks up the fecal mass digitally and then removes portions of it. This procedure is distressing and uncomfortable, and clients may desire the presence of another nurse or family member for support. Care must be taken to avoid injuring the bowel mucosa and thus to prevent bleeding. Also, rectal stimulation is contraindicated for some clients, since it may cause an excessive vagal response, resulting in cardiac arrhythmia. For these reasons, agency policies vary about who may break up impactions digitally. After disimpaction, follow-up measures to encourage normal defecation, such as administering enemas or suppositories, are implemented for a few days.

The procedure for digital removal of a fecal impaction is as follows.

1. Help the client assume a side-lying position, with the knees flexed and the back toward you. Although some clients may prefer to stand by a toilet, the bed position is advised because disimpaction can be exhausting.
2. Place a waterproof bedpad under the client's buttocks and a bedpan nearby to receive stool.
3. Put on a pair of plastic or rubber gloves and liberally lubricate the index finger to be inserted.
4. Gently insert the index finger into the rectum and move the finger toward the client's umbilicus, moving along the length of the rectum.
5. Loosen and dislodge stool by gently massaging around it. Break up stool by working the finger into the hardened mass. Take care to avoid injury to the mucosa of the rectum.
6. Carefully work stool downward to the end of the rectum and remove it in small pieces. Continue to remove as much fecal material as possible. Periodically assess the client for signs of fatigue, such as facial pallor, diaphoresis, or change in pulse rate. Manual stimulation should be minimal, since excessive vagal nerve stimulation could result in cardiac arrhythmia.
7. Following disimpaction, assist the client to clean the anal area and buttocks. Then assist him or her onto a bedpan or commode for a short time, because digital stimulation of the rectum often induces the urge to defecate.

Food and Fluids

The diet a client needs for normal elimination varies, depending on the kind of feces the client currently has, the frequency of defecation, and the types of foods that the client finds assist normal defecation.

For the client who is constipated:

1. Increase daily fluid intake, and have the client take a hot drink upon arising, if health permits.
2. Include bulk in the diet, that is, foods such as prunes, raw fruit, and bran products.

For the client who has diarrhea, encourage oral intake of fluids and food. Because ingestion of foods and fluids stimulates the gastrocolic and duodenocolic reflexes, thus inducing more stool, the client may be reluctant to eat or drink. Eating small amounts of bland foods can be helpful, since they are more easily absorbed. Potassium losses may be great with diarrhea, and the ingestion of food or fluids containing potassium should be encouraged. See the discussion of hypokalemia in Chapter 46. Excessively hot or cold fluids should be avoided, because they stimulate peristalsis.

For the client who has flatulence, limit carbonated beverages, the use of drinking straws, and chewing gum—all of which increase the ingestion of air.

Skin Integrity

A client who has diarrhea or fecal incontinence is predisposed to skin irritation when the fecal material remains on the skin. Liquid stool is acidic and contains digestive enzymes; therefore it is highly irritating to skin. When a client has become soiled, the skin should be washed with a mild soap, rinsed, and dried. Often, protective ointments such as zinc oxide or petrolatum jelly also will protect the skin.

Exercise

Regular exercise for the constipated client will help her or him develop a more normal defecation pattern and feces. Walking and swimming, for example, help stimulate normal motility of the intestines. Postsurgical clients often are encouraged to ambulate, with regaining normal intestinal motility as one of the reasons.

If a client has weak abdominal and pelvic muscles (thereby impeding normal defecation), she or he may be able to strengthen them with the following isometric exercises.

1. In a supine position the client tightens the abdominal muscles as though pulling them inward, holding them for about 10 seconds and then relaxing them. This should be repeated five to ten times, four times a day, depending on the client's health.
2. Again in a supine position, the client can contract the thigh muscles and hold them contracted for about 10 seconds, repeating the exercise five to ten times, four times a day. This helps the client confined to bed gain strength in the thigh muscles, thereby making it easier to use a bedpan.

Flatulence

There are several ways to reduce or prevent flatulence: avoiding gas-producing foods, exercise, and repositioning clients are recommended. Another way involves inserting a rectal tube into the rectum and leaving it there for varying lengths of time—generally no longer than 30 minutes, to prevent undue irritation to the rectal lining. The tube can then be reinserted, as needed, every 2 to 3 hours. Some nurses advocate connecting the open end of the rectal tube, via another tube, to a collecting receptacle containing water. By noting gas bubbles in the water, the passage of flatus can be assessed. The required equipment is listed above.

Equipment for Relieving Flatulence

- A rectal tube (#22 to #30 Fr. for adults; #14 to #18 Fr. for children, according to their age)
- Lubricant for the tip of the rectal tube
- A towel in which to carry the lubricant and rectal tube to the bedside
- Tape to attach the rectal tube to the buttock (optional)
- Either a waterproof absorbent pad (e.g., an abdominal or incontinence pad) to wrap around the open end of the rectal tube, or a connecting tube and a receptacle containing water

Before inserting the rectal tube the nurse should assess the flatulence in the following manner.

1. Palpate the client's abdomen to determine the amount of distention.
2. Auscultate the abdomen for bowel sounds.
3. Determine whether the client is experiencing any abdominal discomfort.
4. Assess the respiratory rate. Flatulence can cause pressure upward on the diaphragm, resulting in difficult respirations.
5. Assess signs associated with flatulence, such as eructations and their frequency and the passage of flatus by rectum.

Assist the client to a left lateral position and expose the anus. Then liberally lubricate the insertion tip of the rectal tube for 5 cm (2 in). Gently insert the rectal tube into the rectum—for an adult, 10 to 15 cm (4 to 6 in); for a child, 5 to 10 cm (2 to 4 in), depending on the child's age. The rectal tube can be inserted farther for this procedure than is recommended for an enema, since fluid will not be administered. Tape the rectal tube to the client's buttock, to prevent dislodging the tube. Place the open end of the rectal tube in a folded absorbent pad to catch any liquid fecal material that seeps through the tube, *or* attach the open end of the rectal tube to a connecting tube and a drainage receptacle filled with water. Place the distal end of the tubing below the level of the water in the collecting receptacle. Gas bubbles can be noted only if the tubing is below water level. Leave the client in a comfortable lateral position. After 30 minutes, remove the rectal tube. Determine whether flatus has been expelled.

Evaluation

Examples of outcome criteria for fecal elimination are listed on the right.

Outcome Criteria for Fecal Elimination

The client will:

- Establish a regular time for defecation
- Participate in a regular exercise program
- Eat the diet explained
- Defecate without discomfort
- Ingest 2000 ml of fluid daily

Bowel Diversion Ostomies

There are many types of ostomies, depending on the organs involved. A *gastrostomy* is an opening through the abdominal wall into the stomach. A *jejunostomy* is an opening through the abdominal wall into the jejunum. An *ileostomy* is an opening into the ileum (small bowel). A *colostomy* is an opening into the colon (large bowel). See Figure 43–13, which shows a colostomy stoma with the surgical incision to the right and retention sutures supporting the incision. A *ureterostomy* is an opening into the ureter. Gastrostomies and jejunostomies are generally performed to provide an alternate feeding route. The purpose of bowel and urinary ostomies is to divert and drain fecal or urinary material. **Bowel diversion ostomies** are often classified according to (a) whether they are permanent or temporary, (b) their anatomic location, and (c) the construction of the **stoma** (artificial opening in the abdominal wall).

Permanence

Colostomies can be either temporary or permanent. Temporary colostomies are generally performed for traumatic injuries or inflammatory conditions of the bowel. They allow the distal diseased portion of the bowel to rest and heal. Permanent colostomies are performed to provide a means of elimination when the rectum or anus is nonfunctional as a result of disease or birth defect. They are commonly performed for diseases such as cancer of the bowel. The diseased portion may or may not be removed.

Anatomic Location

An ileostomy generally empties from the distal end of the small intestine. A cecostomy empties from the cecum (the first part of the ascending colon). An ascending colostomy empties from the ascending colon. A transverse colostomy empties from the transverse colon. A descending colostomy empties from the descending colon. A sigmoidostomy empties from the sigmoid colon. See Figure 43–14.

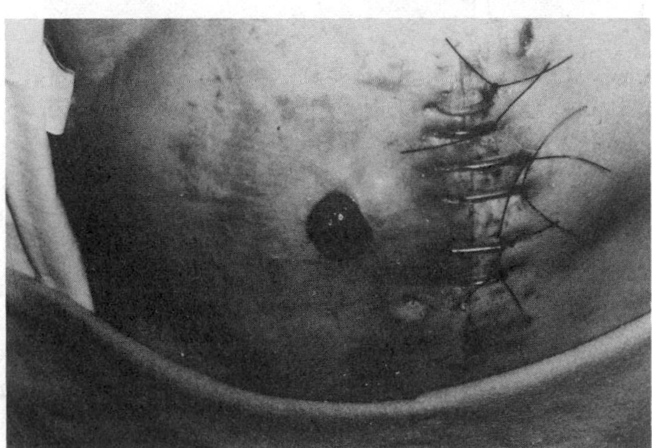

Figure 43–13 A colostomy stoma, with the surgical incision to the right. Note the retention sutures supporting the incision.

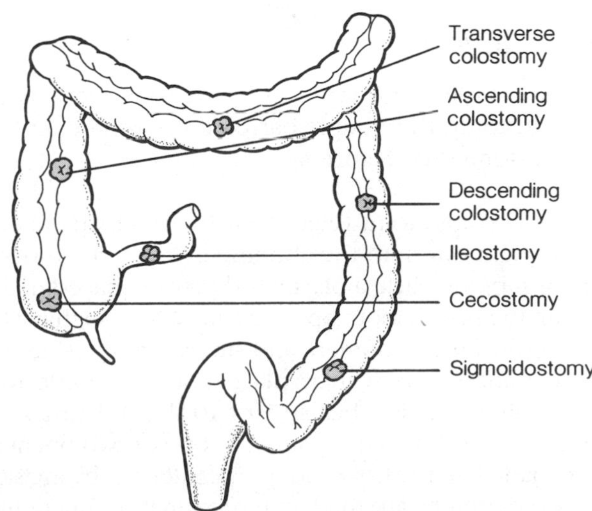

Figure 43–14 The locations of bowel diversion ostomies

The location of the ostomy influences the character and management of the fecal drainage. The farther along the bowel, the more formed the stool, since the large bowel reabsorbs water from the fecal mass. In addition, more control over the frequency of stomal discharge can be established. For example:

1. An ileostomy produces liquid fecal drainage that drains continuously and cannot be regulated. Ileostomy drainage contains some digestive enzymes, which are damaging to the skin. Ileostomy clients must wear an appliance continuously and take special precautions to prevent skin breakdown. Odor is minimal, however, compared to colostomies, because fewer bacteria are present.
2. An ascending colostomy is similar to an ileostomy in that the drainage is liquid and cannot be regulated. However, digestive enzymes are present, and odor is a problem requiring control (e.g., a deodorant inside the appliance).
3. A transverse colostomy produces a malodorous, mushy drainage because some of the liquid has been reabsorbed. There is usually no control.
4. A descending colostomy produces increasingly solid fecal drainage. Stools from a sigmoidostomy are of normal consistency, and the frequency of discharge can be regulated. Clients with sigmoidostomies may not have to wear an appliance at all times, and odors can usually be controlled.

The length of time an ostomy is in place also helps determine the consistency of the stool, particularly with transverse and descending colostomies. Over time, the stool becomes more formed because the remaining functioning portions of the colon tend to increase water reabsorption in compensation.

Construction

There are three major types of stoma constructions: the loop colostomy, the double-barreled colostomy, and the end colostomy. See Figure 43–15.

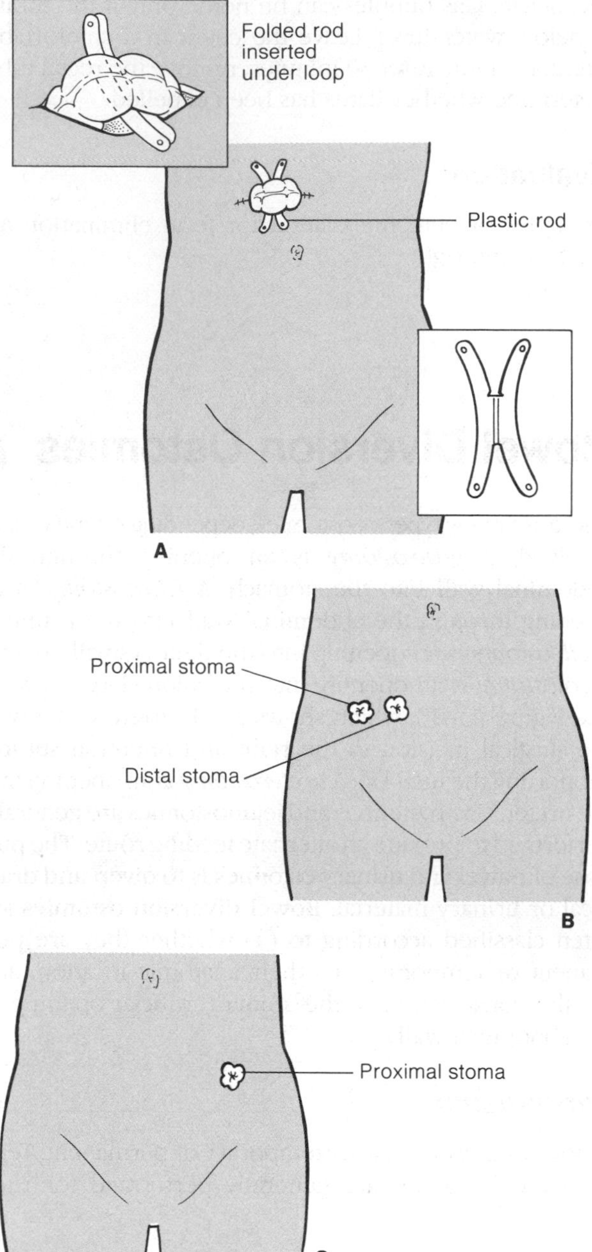

Figure 43–15 Three types of colostomies: **A,** the loop colostomy using a plastic rod; **B,** the double-barreled colostomy; **C,** the end colostomy

1. For a loop colostomy (Figure 43–15, *A*), a loop of bowel is brought out onto the abdomen. To keep the bowel from slipping back, a plastic rod may be placed underneath the bowel loop, opened (unfolded) so that it lies flat against the abdomen, and sutured to the skin. The rod holds the bowel in place until the underlying abdominal incision heals (7 to 10 days). During surgery or 2 or 3 days after surgery, one or two openings are made into the bowel loop by cautery or by incision. If two openings are made the proximal or functioning opening discharges fecal material. The other opening is the distal or nonfunctioning end. It discharges only mucus unless emergency surgery was performed without the usual bowel preparation. In this instance some fecal matter may be discharged. When only one opening is made, it connects to both proximal and distal parts of the bowel. The loop colostomy is relatively large and cumbersome. It is created generally in an emergency, e.g., an acute bowel obstruction or bowel injury. Complete diversion of fecal matter is not achieved with this procedure because the bowel is not separated.
2. In the double-barreled colostomy (Figure 43–15, *B*), two separate stomas are constructed. One is the prox-

imal or functioning stoma, and the other is the distal or resting stoma. The stomas are generally adjacent to one another—one above the other or side by side.

3. An end colostomy has only one stoma (Figure 43–15, *C*), which arises from the end of the proximal portion of the bowel. The distal end of the bowel and rectum is either resected by an abdominoperineal resection (removal through abdominal and perineal incisions) or is closed off by sutures and remains in the abdominal space. The latter is often referred to as an *end colostomy and Hartmann pouch,* the pouch referring to the remaining distal portion of the bowel.

Assessment

Assessment pertaining to a bowel diversion ostomy should include the following.

1. *Stoma color.* The stoma should appear red, similar in color to the mucosal lining of the inner cheek. Very pale or darker-colored stomas with a bluish or purplish hue indicate impaired blood circulation to the area.
2. *Stoma swelling.* Most stomas protrude slightly from the abdomen. New stomas normally appear swollen, but this generally decreases postoperatively over 2 or 3 weeks. Changes may occur for as long as 6 weeks postoperatively. The size of the stoma varies with the kind and location. For example, a loop colostomy of the transverse colon can be expected to be larger than an end colostomy of the sigmoid colon. Lack of decrease in the size of a stoma may indicate a problem, e.g., blockage.
3. *Redness and irritation of peristomal skin.* Peristomal skin is the 5 to 13 cm (2 to 5 in) of skin surrounding the stoma.
4. *Amount and type of feces.* For ileal effluent and feces (colostomy effluent), assess the amount, color, odor, and consistency. Inspect for abnormalities, such as pus or blood.
5. *Tape allergy.* The client may have a documented allergic reaction to the tape used to secure the ostomy appliance to the abdomen. If so, do a 24-hour tape-patch test, experimenting with at least three or four different types of tape (silk, paper, and foam). Cut strips of each type, label them with a marking pen, and place them on the client's abdomen. See Figure 43–16. A 24-hour tape-patch test is best done *before* the client has surgery and on the nonoperative side. The abdomen, rather than the inner arm, is used, since abdominal skin is more sensitive. Abdominal hair may first need to be removed (using scissors or an electric razor or clippers). During the next 24 hours, note complaints of itching or burning, and at the end of the period remove the tape and inspect the abdomen for redness and swelling. Document specific allergies, if present, on the client's chart, and provide the client with an allergic-alert arm band.

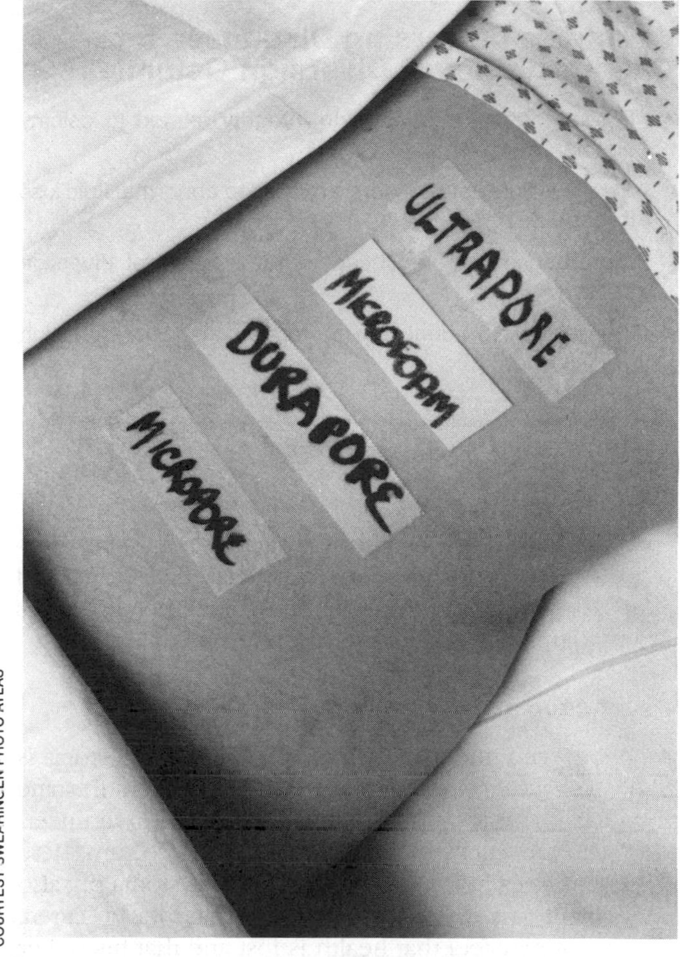

Figure 43–16 A 24-hour tape-patch allergy test

6. *Presence of abdominal discomfort and/or abdominal distention.*

Nursing Diagnosis

Examples of nursing diagnoses appropriate for clients with bowel diversion ostomies are given on page 1220.

Planning

The primary client goals in planning interventions often include the following.

- Understanding how the ostomy functions.
- Changing the ostomy dressing as shown.
- Being able to discuss the ostomy with other.s
- Establishing a regular diet as shown.

Examples of Nursing Diagnoses for Client with Bowel Diversion Ostomies

- Potential impairment of skin integrity related to ostomy discharge
- Potential fluid volume deficit related to abnormal fluid loss through ostomy
- Disturbance in self-concept related to bowel diversion ostomy
- Ineffective individual coping related to bowel diversion ostomy

Intervention

A client who has a stoma usually requires nursing assistance in four major areas: psychosocial, diet, stoma and skin care, and odor control. Enterostomal therapy nurses are recognized specialists for such clients.

Psychosocial Factors

A person who undergoes surgery resulting in a stoma is likely to have strong reactions to the operation. In some instances the ostomy is palliative treatment for an underlying disease, such as a malignancy of the rectum. Here the client faces not only adjustment to the stoma but also adjustment to a disease process that may not be cured. The client may feel that health is lost and that his or her life-style must change. Some clients and family members go through a process of grieving before accepting the ostomy and learning to deal with it.

A stoma means changes in both the method and pattern of defecation, which is a highly personal function. Most clients are very aware of other people's reactions to the stoma and particularly sensitive to any negative behavior that could be interpreted as meaning she or he is offensive. It is important for nurses to communicate acceptance and understanding and to provide the same privacy during care that is normally provided for elimination.

In some instances an ostomy brings relief from pain. For example, for a person who has experienced years of discomfort and difficulty due to ulcerative colitis, the creation of an ileostomy may mean that he or she will be able to lead a more normal life than has been possible in the past.

Diet

The client who has had intestinal surgery will usually be on nothing by mouth until bowel function returns and then a liquid or low-residue diet until the bowel has healed, or as tolerated. After that, the client can ingest most or all pre-illness foods and fluids and should maintain a well-balanced diet. Clients are generally encouraged not to restrict their diets but rather to use discretion. For example, if gas or odor production are of concern before a specific social engagement, gas- and odor-forming foods can be avoided prior to the event. In addition, a gas-filtering pouch can be used. Odor-forming foods do not need to be restricted, because an intact appliance will contain odor. Clients often are concerned about gas formation because they believe the excessive gas that forms postoperatively when bowel function returns will become their usual pattern. They need to be assured that this is temporary.

The following guidelines may be helpful in controlling gas and odor by dietary means.

1. Certain foods, such as cheese, onions, and cucumbers, are known to produce a definite odor in feces.
2. Cabbage, brussels sprouts, garlic, onions, sauerkraut, broccoli, corn, cauliflower, and legumes are known to be gas-forming foods.
3. Sucking carbonated drinks through a straw can result in the ingestion of air, which will cause gas.
4. Certain foods, such as parsley and yogurt, are thought to reduce the odor of feces.

The client with an ileostomy may encounter two problems that can usually be prevented by diet: (a) blockage near the stoma due to the accumulation of cellulose, and (b) fluid and electrolyte imbalance. Cellulose (fiber, roughage) is normally not digested but passes along the gastrointestinal tract for expulsion through the anus. Prior to defecation, cellulose and other waste products accumulate in the sigmoid colon and rectum, which expand to accommodate them. However, with an ileostomy, the accumulated waste products can block the ileum, often at the point where it passes through the abdominal wall. Blockage is best prevented by teaching the client to chew potentially obstructing foods well and introducing them one at a time, so that if a problem results the offending food can be avoided. Examples of potentially obstructing foods are corn, celery, and whole grains.

Fluid and electrolyte imbalance can occur because the client is without a functioning colon. The colon normally functions to allow water and sodium to be reabsorbed through its wall into the blood circulation. Clients who have ileostomies tend to lose excessive amounts of sodium and fluid through the ileal effluent. Therefore, their diet should be high in fluids, sodium, and potassium, especially when diarrhea is present or if losses are significant from other routes, such as a high sodium loss from excessive perspiration. Clients need to be taught to respond to thirst and the signs and symptoms of fluid electrolyte imbalance. Major sources of sodium and are listed in Table 42–3, page 1152. Foods rich in potassium include bananas, chard, avocados, and fish.

Stoma and Skin Care

Care of the stoma and skin is important for all clients who have ostomies. With a colostomy or ileostomy, the fecal material is irritating to the peristomal skin. This is particularly true of ileal effluent, which contains digestive enzymes.

It is important that the peristomal skin be assessed for irritation each time the appliance is changed. Any irritations or skin breakdown need to be treated immediately. The skin is kept clean by washing off any excretion, then drying it thoroughly. A barrier such as karaya is applied over the skin around the stoma, to prevent the skin from coming into direct contact with any excretion. An appliance (bag) is then fitted to the stoma so there is no leakage around it. It is exceedingly important that the skin be dry before the appliance is attached, because the pouch will not adhere to moist skin and will cause effluent to leak onto the skin.

Odor Control

Because fecal odor is generally considered socially unacceptable, odor control is essential. As soon as the client is out of bed, he or she can learn to work with the ostomy in the bathroom so that the odor of feces remains there and not at the bed.

For odor control, it is necessary to use the appropriate kind of appliance. An intact appliance is odor-proof and will contain odor within it. The appliance should be rinsed thoroughly when it is emptied. Deodorizers can be placed in the pouch of the appliance, or pouches with charcoal filter discs are available. Oral intake of charcoal or bismuth subcarbonate are thought by some to help and can be taken with the physician's approval.

Procedure 43–2 ▲ Changing a Bowel Diversion Ostomy Appliance

Disposable ostomy appliances can be applied for up to 7 days. They need to be changed whenever the effluent leaks onto peristomal skin or when it cannot be rinsed completely away. Many people prefer to change them daily or whenever they become soiled, but this practice can be detrimental to the integrity of the peristomal skin and is expensive. Check agency practice in this regard.

Many types of appliances are available commercially. See Figure 43–17. All appliances have three things in common: a pouch to collect the effluent, an outlet at the bottom for easy emptying, and a faceplate. Temporary, disposable pouches are made of transparent plastic and have a peel-off adhesive square into which a hole the size of the stoma is cut. Permanent pouches are made of an opaque rubber or vinyl and have a solid ring faceplate that fits around the stoma.

It is important to select an appliance designed for the particular type of stoma. Some agencies employ an enterostomal therapy nurse who can assist in selecting the appliance. An appliance should have the following characteristics.

1. The appliance needs to be odor-resistant.
2. The opening needs to be just large enough to fit closely around the stoma.
3. If the bag has an adhesive-backed disc, it must be nonallergenic.
4. If the appliance has a belt, it should fit comfortably around the client's waist (this depends on the model used). Many clients do not use belts unless absolutely necessary.

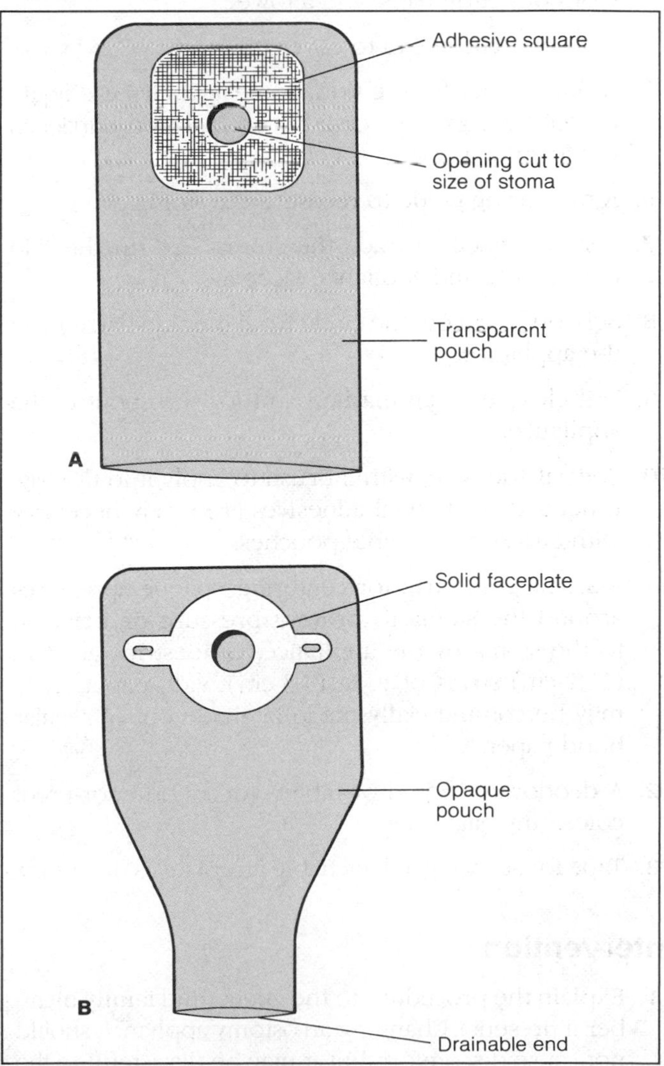

Figure 43–17 Ostomy appliances: **A,** temporary, disposable; **B,** permanent, reusable

Disposable postoperative pouches should be:

1. Transparent, to enable assessment of the stoma

2. Odorproof, to enhance client acceptability
3. Drainable, so the pouch can be emptied without removing it.
4. Adjustable, so the size of the opening can be altered to accommodate changes in stoma shape and size as edema resolves.

Equipment

1. Solvent (presaturated sponges or liquid) for removing the appliance. This is not needed in most cases and should be used only when absolutely necessary.
2. A receptacle for the soiled appliance. To minimize odor, a waterproof bag can be used to wrap the bag prior to disposal. If the agency uses plastic bags to line wastebaskets, this receptacle can be used and then removed after the procedure.
3. Cleaning materials, including tissues (to wipe away the stool), warm water, mild soap (optional), a washcloth or cotton balls, and a towel.
4. Tissue or gauze pad to cover the stoma.
5. A skin barrier for the skin. Some agencies use liquid protective coverings or a peristomal skin barrier in the form of a disc or sheet.
6. A measuring guide to measure the stoma.
7. Pen or pencil to trace the stoma size on the skin barrier disc and appliance faceplate.
8. Scissors to cut out the circle from the skin barrier and the appliance.
9. Tail closure or an elastic band for the spout of the appliance.
10. Special adhesive, with a brush to apply it to the bag, if needed. Additional adhesives are rarely necessary with currently available pouches.
11. A stoma guidestrip for centering opaque appliances around the stoma to prevent pressure or irritation to the stoma by the appliance. Guidestrips are 6-in (15.2-cm) strips of ½-in (1.3-cm) wide paper. They may be commercially made or made out of regular bond paper.
12. A deodorant (liquid or tablet) for a non-odor-proof colostomy bag.
13. Tape for securing a detachable faceplate as necessary.

Intervention

1. Explain the procedure to the client (and family member if present). Changing an ostomy appliance should not cause discomfort, but it may be distasteful to the client.

   Rationale Family members can be supportive and helpful to the client if properly informed.
2. Communicate acceptance and support of the client. Colostomy effluent may have an unpleasant odor, and the client may feel "dirty." It is important to change the appliance competently and quickly and not to convey disgust. Timing is also an important factor. Avoid times close to meal hours whenever possible.
3. Provide privacy, preferably in the bathroom, where the client can learn to deal with the ostomy as he or she would at home.
4. Assist the client to a comfortable sitting or lying position, and expose only the stoma area.
5. Unfasten the belt if one is being worn.
6. Empty the pouch when it is one-third to one-half full. Assess the consistency and amount of effluent.

   Rationale When the fluid level in the bag becomes too high, the weight of it may loosen the faceplate and separate it from the skin, causing the effluent to leak and irritate the peristomal skin.
7. Remove the appliance. Apply solvent with an applicator if needed. Peel the bag off slowly while holding the client's skin taut.

   Rationale Occasionally adhesives require the application of a solvent before removing. Holding the skin taut minimizes client discomfort and prevents skin abrasion.
8. If the appliance is disposable, discard it in a moistureproof bag.
9. Using warm water and mild soap, clean the peristomal skin and the stoma. Check agency practice on the use of soap.

   Rationale Soap is sometimes not advised because it can be irritating to the skin.
10. Dry the area thoroughly by patting with a towel or cotton swabs.

    Rationale Excessive rubbing can abrade the skin.
11. Assess the stoma for color and size.
12. Assess the peristomal skin for any redness, ulceration, or irritation. Transient redness is normal after the removal of adhesive.
13. Place a piece of tissue or gauze pad over the stoma, and change it as needed.

    Rationale The tissue will absorb any seepage from the stoma.

    There are two methods for preparing and applying the skin barrier (peristomal seal) and ostomy appliance. One method is described in steps 14–15; the other is described in step 16.

14. Prepare and apply the skin barrier. There are many types of skin barriers, so read the manufacturer's directions as well as the steps below. If using a sheet or disc type, such as Stomahesive, Reliaseal, Colly-Seel ring, HolliHesive, Crixiline, or Premium Barrier:
    a. Use the stoma measuring guide to measure the size of the stoma. See Figure 43–18.

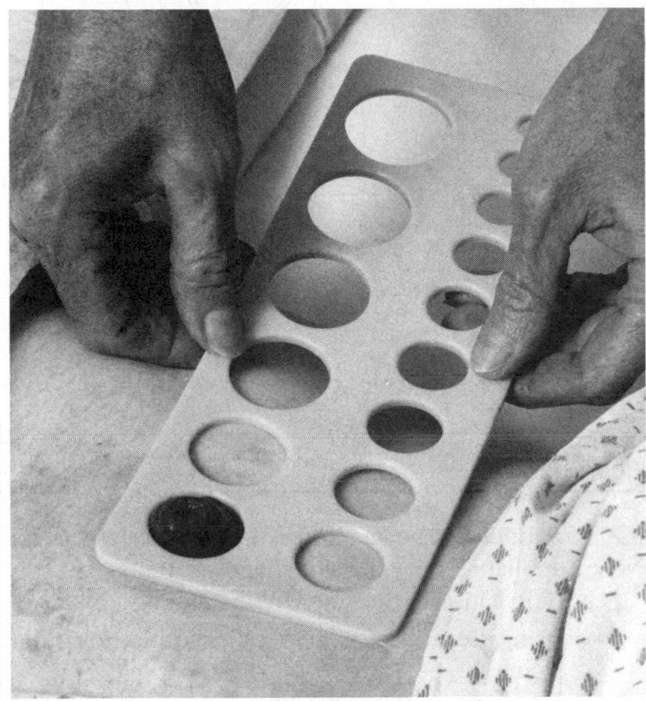
COURTESY SWEARINGEN PHOTO ATLAS

Figure 43–18

b. Trace a circle on the backing of the skin barrier the same size as the stomal opening.
c. Make a template of the stoma pattern.

Rationale A template aids other nurses and the client with future appliance changes but will need to be adjusted as the stoma size decreases.

d. Cut out the traced stoma pattern to make an opening in the skin barrier.
e. Remove the backing to expose the sticky adhesive side on certain products, such as Stomahesive or Reliaseal. Moisten and rub a Colly-Seel ring with tap water until the ring becomes sticky; knead the ring to make it more flexible.
f. Center the skin barrier over the stoma and gently press it onto the client's skin, smoothing out any wrinkles or bubbles. See Figure 43–19.

If using Skin Prep liquid or wipes or a similar product, e.g., Stomahesive:

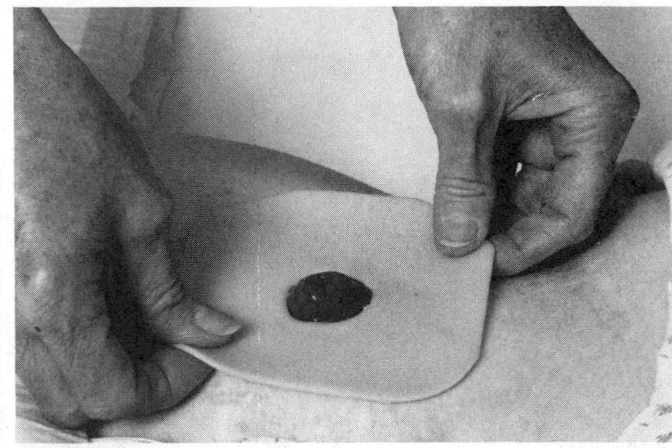
COURTESY SWEARINGEN PHOTO ATLAS

Figure 43–19

g. Cover the stoma with a gauze pad to avoid getting the Skin Prep on the stoma.
h. Either wipe the product evenly around the peristomal skin or use a brush to apply a thin layer of the liquid plastic coating to the same area.
i. Allow the skin barrier to dry until it no longer feels tacky.

If applying a karaya ring seal:

j. Select a seal with an opening the same size as the stoma.
k. Place the ring around the stoma, ensuring that it fits snugly around its base.
l. Gently press the seal to the skin.

15. Prepare and apply the clean appliance. Remove the tissue over the stoma before applying the pouch. To apply a *disposable pouch* with *adhesive square:*
    a. If the appliance does not have a precut opening, trace a circle ⅛ to ⅙ inch larger than the stoma size on the appliance's adhesive square.

    Rationale The opening is made slightly larger than the stoma to prevent rubbing, cutting, or trauma to the stoma.

    b. Cut out a circle in the adhesive. Take care not to cut any portion of the pouch. See Figure 43–20.
    c. Peel off the backing from the adhesive seal.
    d. Center the opening of the pouch over the client's stoma and apply it directly onto the skin barrier. See Figure 43–21.
    e. Gently press the adhesive backing onto the skin and smooth out any wrinkles, working from the stoma outward.

    Rationale Wrinkles allow seepage of effluent, which can irritate the skin or soil clothing.

    f. Remove the air from the pouch.

    Rationale Removing the air helps the pouch lie flat against the abdomen.

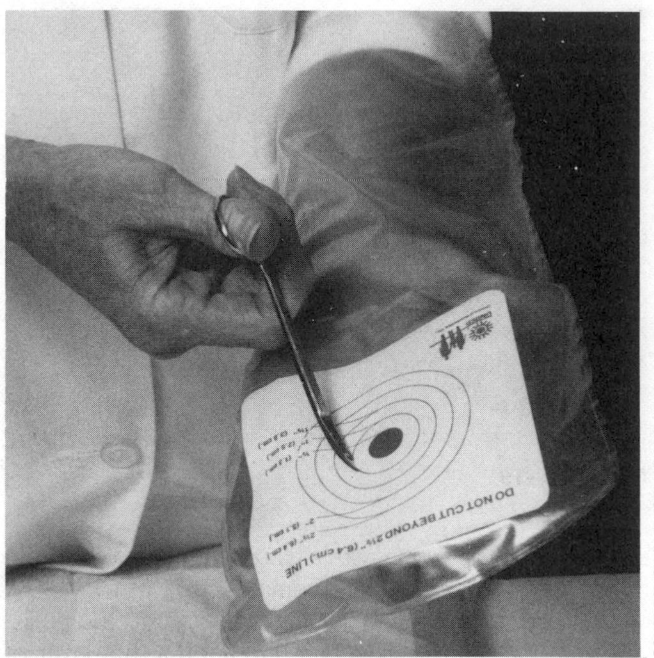

COURTESY SWEARINGEN PHOTO ATLAS

Figure 43–20

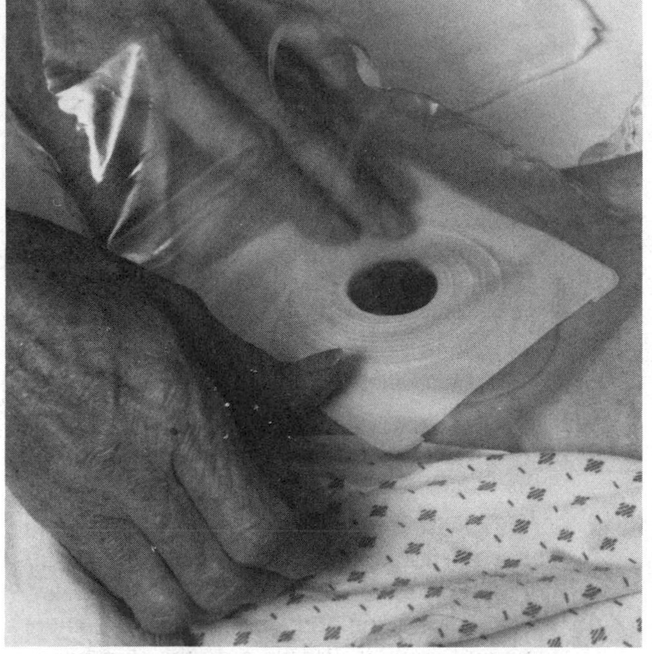

COURTESY SWEARINGEN PHOTO ATLAS

Figure 43–21

g. Place a deodorant in the pouch (optional).
h. Close the pouch by turning up the bottom a few times, fanfolding its end lengthwise, and securing it with a rubber band or tail closure clamp.

To apply a *reusable pouch* with *faceplate attached:*

i. Apply either adhesive cement or a double-faced adhesive disc to the faceplate of the appliance, depending on the type of appliance being used. Follow the manufacturer's directions.
j. Insert a coiled paper guidestrip into the faceplate opening. The strip should protrude slightly from the opening and expand to fit it. See Figure 43–22.

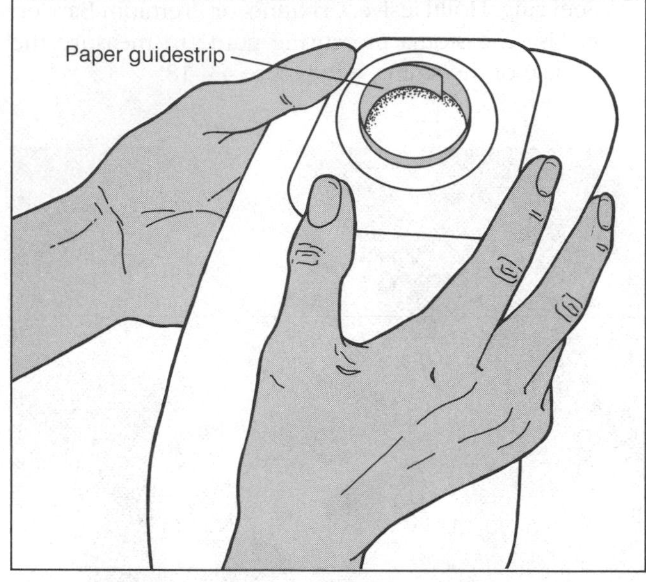

Figure 43–22

Rationale The guidestrip helps you center the appliance over the stoma and prevents pressure or irritation to the stoma by an ill-fitting appliance.

k. Using the guidestrip, center the faceplate over the stoma.
l. Firmly press the adhesive seal to the peristomal skin. The guidestrip will fall into the pouch; commercially prepared guidestrips will dissolve in the pouch.
m. Place a deodorant in the bag if the bag is not odor-proof. Most pouches are odor-proof.
n. Close the end of the pouch with the designated clamp. See Figure 43–23.

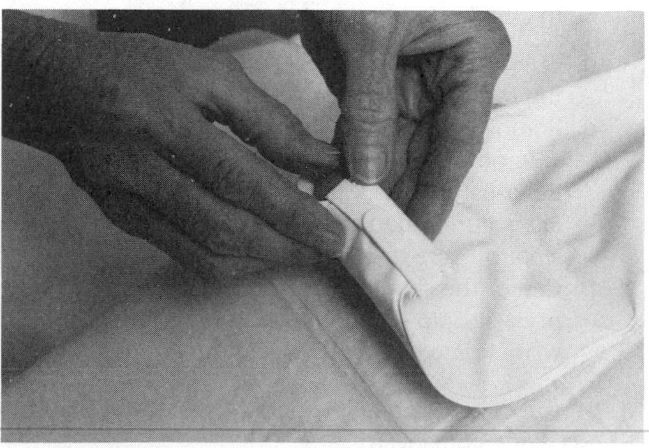

COURTESY SWEARINGEN PHOTO ATLAS

Figure 43–23

o. Attach the pouch belt and fasten it around the client's waist (optional).

To apply a *reusable pouch* with *detachable faceplate:*

p. Apply a skin sealant (e.g., Skin Prep) to the faceplate.

   Rationale This makes it easier to remove the adhesive disc from the faceplate.

q. Remove the protective paper strip from one side of the double-faced adhesive disc.

r. Apply the sticky side to the back of the faceplate.

s. Remove the remaining protective paper strip from the other side of the adhesive disc.

t. Center the faceplate over the stoma and skin barrier, then press and hold the faceplate against the client's skin for a few minutes to secure the seal. See Figure 43–24.

u. Press the adhesive around the circumference of the adhesive disc.

v. Tape the faceplate to the client's abdomen using four or eight 7.5-cm (3-in) strips of tape. Place the strips around the faceplate in a "picture-framing" manner, one strip down each side, one across the top, and one across the bottom. See Figure 43–25. The additional four strips can be placed diagonally over the other tapes to secure the seal.

w. Stretch the opening on the back of the pouch and position it over the base of the faceplate. Ease it over the faceplate flange.

x. Place the lock ring or "bead-o-ring" (see Figure 43–26) between the pouch and the faceplate flange (see Figure 43–27) to seal the pouch against the faceplate.

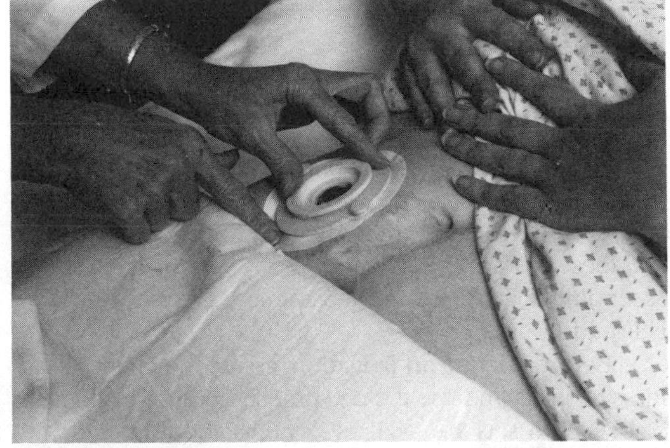

COURTESY SWEARINGEN PHOTO ATLAS

Figure 43–24

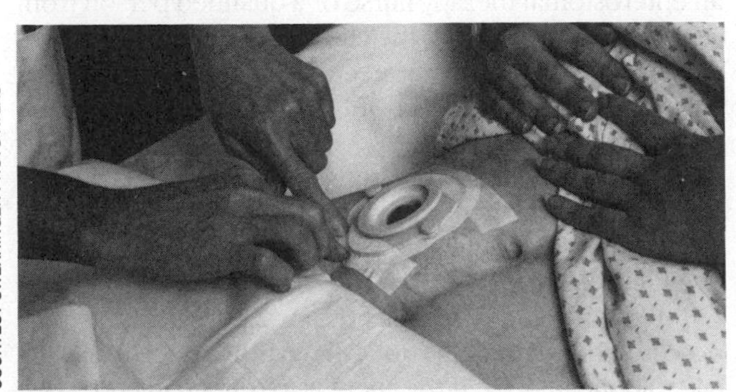

COURTESY SWEARINGEN PHOTO ATLAS

Figure 43–25

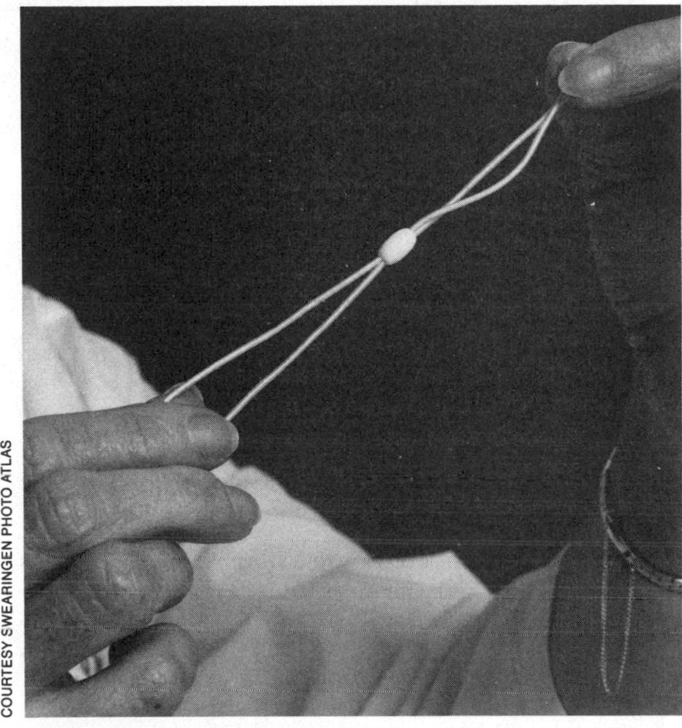

COURTESY SWEARINGEN PHOTO ATLAS

Figure 43–26

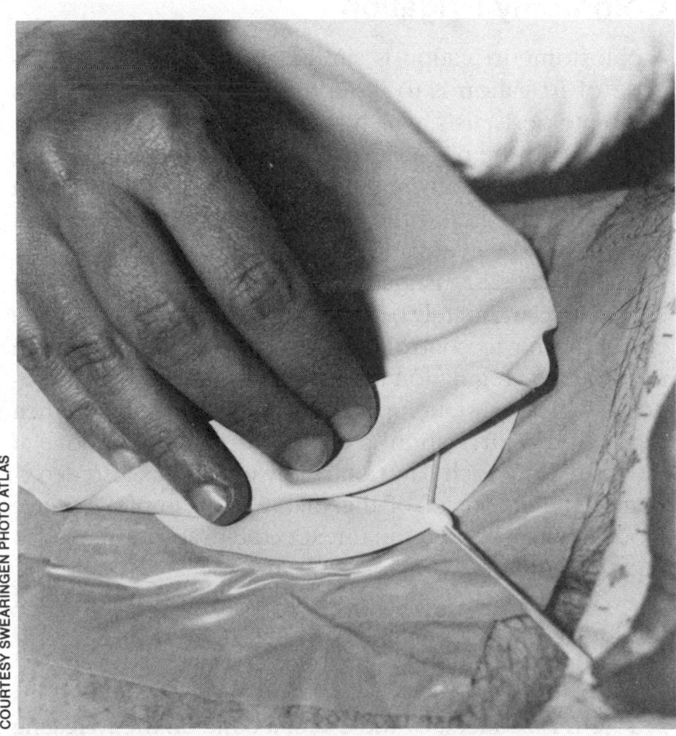

COURTESY SWEARINGEN PHOTO ATLAS

Figure 43–27

y. Close the base of the pouch with the appropriate clamp.

z. Attach the pouch belt and fasten it around the client's waist (optional).

16. If a disc or wafer-type skin barrier is used, an alternate method can be used to replace steps 14 and 15. For this method, the ostomy appliance is put onto the skin barrier and then applied in one assembled unit to the client's skin.

    Rationale Applying the skin barrier and the appliance together is not only quicker but thought by some to reduce the chance of wrinkles. It also is easier for the client to apply without help.

    To apply *skin barrier and appliance as one unit:*

    a. Prepare the skin barrier as in steps 14a–14d.
    b. Prepare the appliance as in steps 15a–15c.
    c. Center the opening of the pouch over the skin barrier.
    d. Remove the backing to expose the sticky adhesive side on the skin barrier.
    e. Center the skin barrier and appliance over the stoma, and press it onto the client's skin.

17. Assess the client's response to the technique in terms of skills learned; the amount, color, and consistency of the drainage; the condition of the skin; and the client's fatigue, discomfort, and behavior about the ostomy.

18. Discard the bag, or clean it if it is to be used again. Measure liquid feces, then empty the feces into a toilet or hopper. If the bag is to be reused, wash it with cool water and mild soap, rinse, and dry.

19. Wash a soiled belt with warm water and mild soap, rinse, and dry.

20. Record on the client's chart any discoloration of the stoma; the appearance of the peristomal skin; the amount and type of drainage; and the client's fatigue, discomfort, and significant behavior about the ostomy.

21. Adjust the client's teaching plan and nursing care plan as needed. Include on the teaching plan the equipment and procedure used.

    Rationale Learning to care for the ostomy is facilitated for the client if procedures implemented by nurses are consistent.

Sample Recording

Date	Time	Notes
Oct/5/87	1400	Colostomy appliance changed. 350 ml dark brown liquid feces. Stoma pink, 8 cm. Peristomal skin intact. No discomfort. Helped to clean the peristomal skin.——— —Ramona L. de Santo, NS

Colostomy Irrigation

A colostomy irrigation is similar to an enema. The purpose of irrigation is to distend the bowel sufficiently to stimulate peristalsis, which stimulates evacuation.

Initially the physician is responsible for determining whether a colostomy should be irrigated, what solution should be used, and the type of irrigation to be given. The last may be preestablished by agency policy, however.

Routine daily irrigations for control of the time of elimination ultimately become the client's decision. Some clients prefer to control the time of elimination through rigid dietary regulation and not be bothered with irrigations, which can take up to an hour to complete. When regulation by irrigation is chosen, it should be done at the same time each day. Control by irrigations also necessitates some control of the diet. For example, laxative foods that might cause an unexpected evacuation need to be avoided.

For most clients, a relatively small amount of fluid (300 to 500 ml) stimulates evacuation. For others, up to 1000 ml may be needed, since a colostomy has no sphincter and the fluid tends to return as it is instilled. This problem is reduced by the use of a cone on the irrigating catheter. The cone helps to hold the fluid within the bowel during the irrigation.

Irrigations are commonly used for end colostomies and descending colostomies; they are not advised for ascending colostomies or ileostomies, where the effluent is liquid in nature.

Before starting an irrigation, assess the client's readiness to select and use the equipment. Because many types of irrigation sets are available, clients should begin with a "starter set" until they are familiar with the colostomy and the problems of irrigating it. Later, with the help of an enterostomal therapy nurse or a qualified person from a surgical supply house, the client can select the set most appropriate for his or her needs. The nurse next auscultates the abdomen for bowel sounds and palpates the abdomen for distention.

The equipment commonly used for a colostomy irrigation is listed on page 1227. Both commercially prepared equipment and standard equipment are available. See Figure 43–28.

First the nurse explains the procedure and its purpose to the client. The total irrigation process usually takes about an hour. If the client is to remain in bed, assist

Equipment for a Colostomy Irrigation

- A moisture-resistant bag
- A clean colostomy appliance or dressings
- Irrigation equipment
    1. A bag to hold the solution. With routine irrigations for regulation, the bag is usually filled with 500 ml of warm (body temperature) tap water, or other solution as ordered. For a bowel preparation, 1000 ml of solution is needed.
    2. Tubing attached to the bag
    3. A tubing clamp or flow regulator
    4. A #28 rubber colon catheter, calibrated in either centimeters or inches, with a stoma cone or seal
    5. A disposable stoma-irrigation drainage sleeve with belt to direct the fecal contents into the toilet or bedpan
- Lubricant
- Clean rubber gloves (optional) to protect the nurse's hands from contamination, and one glove to dilate the stoma if ordered by the physician
- A bath blanket
- An IV pole
- A disposable bedpad, bedpan, and cover, if the client is to remain in bed

him or her to a side-lying position. Place a disposable bedpad on the bed in front of the client, and place the bedpan on top of the disposable pad, beneath the stoma. If the client is ambulatory, assist him or her to sit on the toilet or on a commode in the bathroom. Ensure that the client's gown or pajamas are moved out of the way to prevent soiling, and cover the client appropriately with the bath blanket, to prevent undue exposure. Throughout the technique provide explanations, and encourage the client to participate as much as he or she desires.

Hang the solution bag on an IV pole so the bottom of the container is at the level of the client's shoulder, or 30 to 45 cm (12 to 18 in) above the stoma. This height provides a pressure gradient that allows fluid to flow into the colon. The rate of flow can be regulated with the tubing clamp. Attach the colon catheter securely to the tubing. Open the regulator clamp, and run fluid through the tubing to expel all air from it. Close the clamp until ready for the irrigation. Air should not be introduced into the bowel because it distends the bowel and can cause cramps. Remove the soiled colostomy bag, and place it in the moisture-resistant bag so that microorganisms are contained and odor is reduced. Center the irrigation

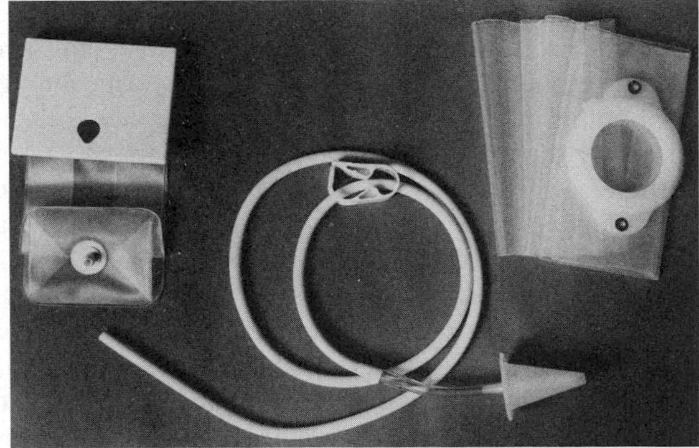

Figure 43–28 A commercially prepared colostomy irrigation set. The irrigation solution bag is on the left and the collecting bag (irrigation drainage sleeve) on the right; the stoma cone is fitted to the catheter.

drainage sleeve over the stoma, and attach it snugly to prevent seepage of the fluid onto the skin. Direct the lower open end of the drainage sleeve into the bedpan or between the client's legs into the toilet. If ordered by the physician, dilate the stoma:

1. Put on a glove.
2. Lubricate the tip of the little finger.
3. Gently insert the finger into the stoma, using a massaging motion. See Figure 43–29. A massaging motion relaxes the intestinal muscles.
4. Repeat steps 2 and 3 above, using progressively larger fingers until maximum dilation is achieved. Stoma dilation helps to stretch and relax the stomal opening and enables the nurse to assess the direction of the proximal colon prior to an irrigation.

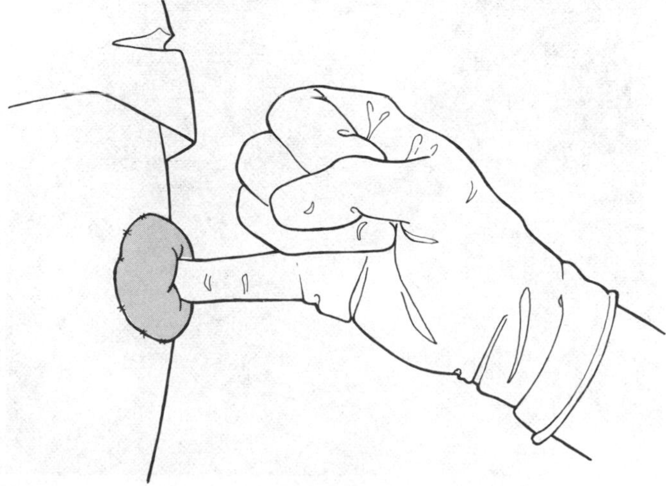

Figure 43–29 Dilating a colostomy stoma

Lubricate the tip of the stoma cone or colon catheter to ease its insertion and prevent injury to the stoma. Using a rotating motion, insert the catheter or stoma cone through the opening in the top of the irrigation drainage sleeve and gently through the stoma. See Figure 43–30. Insert a catheter only 7 cm (3 in); insert a stoma cone just until it fits snugly. Many practitioners prefer using a cone to avoid the risk of perforating the bowel. If you have difficulty inserting the catheter or cone, do not apply force. A rotating motion on insertion helps to open the stoma. Forcing the cone or catheter may traumatize or perforate the bowel. Open the tubing clamp, and allow the fluid to flow into the bowel. If cramping occurs, stop the flow until the cramps subside; then resume the flow. Fluid that is too cold or administered too quickly may cause cramps. If the fluid flows out as fast as you put it in, press the stoma cone or seal more firmly against the stoma to occlude it. If a stoma cone or seal is not available, press around the stoma with your fingers to close the stoma against the catheter. After all the fluid is instilled, remove the catheter or cone and allow the colon to empty. Although not always indicated, you may ask the client to gently massage the abdomen and sit quietly for 10 to 15 minutes until initial emptying has occurred. Massaging the abdomen encourages initial emptying. In some agencies the stoma cone is left in place for 10 to 15 minutes before it is removed.

Clean the base of the irrigation drainage sleeve, and seal the top and bottom with a drainage clamp, following the manufacturer's instructions. Encourage an ambulatory client to move around for about 30 minutes, since complete emptying of the colon takes up to half an hour and moving around facilitates peristalsis. Empty the irrigation drainage sleeve and remove it. Clean the area around the stoma and dry it thoroughly. See Figure 43–31. Put a colostomy appliance on the client as needed.

Promptly report to the responsible nurse any problems, such as no fluid or stool returns, difficulties inserting the tube, peristomal skin redness or irritation, and stomal discoloration. Record the irrigation on the client's chart. Include the time of the irrigation, the type and amount of fluid instilled, the returns, and the client's response.

Sample Recording

Date	Time	Notes
Dec/5/87	0900	Colostomy irrigated with 750 ml warm tap water. Water and large amount soft brown stool expelled. Stoma is pink, and tube inserted without difficulty. Peristomal skin intact. Asked questions about irrigation, looked at stoma for first time. Observed stoma care and pouch application.——————Chung-Hao Jen, NS

Evaluation

Examples of outcome criteria are listed on page 1230.

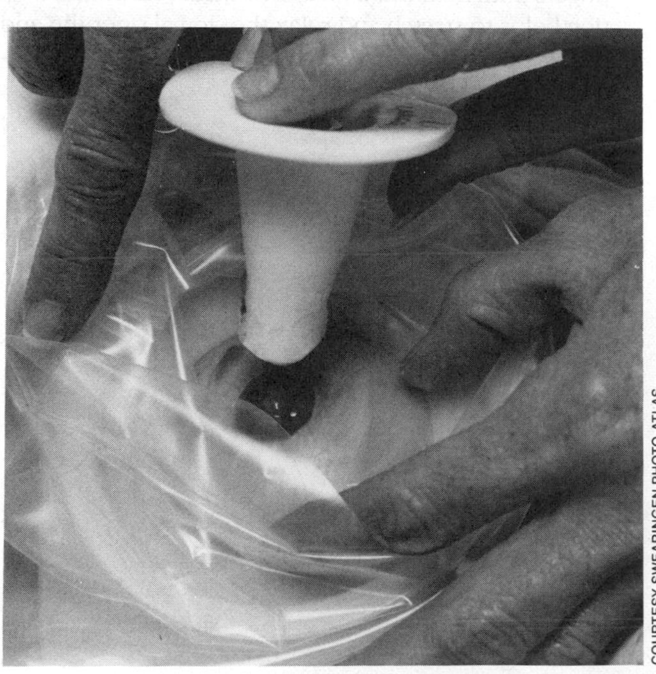

Figure 43–30 Inserting a stoma cone into a colostomy.

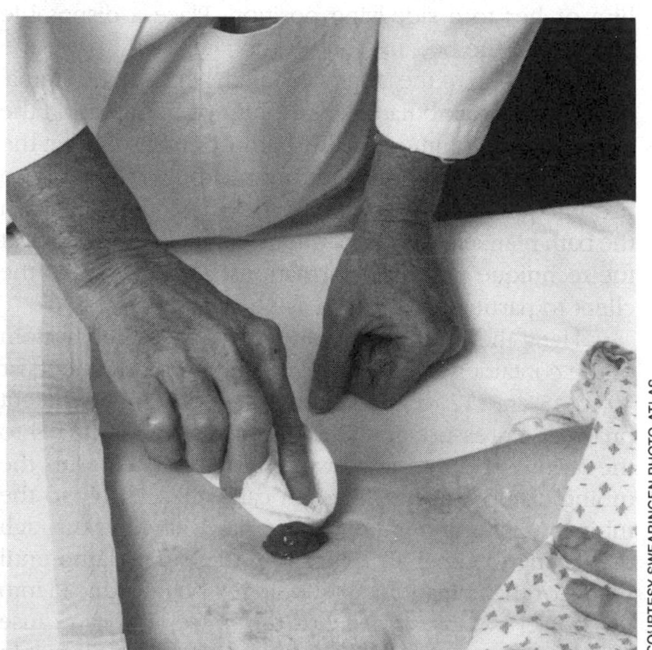

Figure 43–31 Wiping around a stoma to remove any solution or feces.

Nursing Care Plan

Assessment Data

Nursing Assessment

Mrs. Emma Brown is a 78-year-old widow of 9 months. She lives alone in a low-income housing complex for the elderly. Her two children live with their families in a city approximately 150 miles away. She has always enjoyed cooking for her family in the past; however, now that she is alone, she does not enjoy cooking for herself. As a result, she has developed irregular eating patterns and tends to prepare soup-and-toast meals. She does not walk or exercise very much. She has bouts of insomnia since her husband's death. As of late, Mrs. Brown has been having a problem with constipation. She has a bowel movement approximately every 3 or 4 days and her stools are hard and painful to excrete. When the housing complex sponsors a health fair, Mrs. Brown attends and seeks some assistance with her elimination problem from Laura Anderson, the county public health nurse.

Physical Examination

Height: 162 cm (5′4″)
Weight: 65 kg (143 lb)
Temperature: 36.2 C (97.2 F)
Pulse rate: 82 BPM
Respirations: 20 per minute at rest
Blood pressure: 128/74 mm Hg
Active bowel sounds
Abdomen slightly distended

Diagnostic Data

CBC: Hgb 10.8
Urine: Negative

Nursing Diagnosis	Client Goals and Outcome Criteria	Nursing Interventions and Rationales	Evaluation
Alteration in bowel elimination: constipation related to low fiber intake and inactivity resulting in infrequent hard stools, painful defecation, abdominal distention.	Client Goal: Relief of constipation Outcome Criteria: Drinks 2000 to 3000 ml of fluid daily Eats bran flakes for breakfast 3 times per week. Eats 3 complete meals each day.	Encourage warm fluids, e.g., warm lemonade or coffee, early each morning. *Rationale:* Increased fluid intake decreases incidence of constipation and hot fluid stimulates peristalsis. Encourage foods such as bran, fresh fruits, and vegetables in daily diet. *Rationale:* High-fiber foods provide bulk that increases fecal volume. Discuss need to eat 3 or 4 regularly scheduled meals a day. *Rationale:* Eating at regular times promotes regular defecation. Increase physical activity through exercise, e.g., walking. *Rationale:* Exercise increases appetite and peristalsis.	Passes soft and formed stools daily. She drinks warm lemonade each morning before a breakfast that frequently includes bran flakes and prune juice. She now participates in the "Meals on Wheels" program and has joined the Seniors Exercise Club.
Alteration in nutrition: less than body requirements, resulting in weight loss, inadequate intake of fiber, vitamins, and proteins.	Client Goal: Maintain normal body weight. Outcome Criteria: Identifies factors related to inadequate food intake. Gains weight at rate of 1 pound per month. Identifies two food sources high in fiber.	Instruct client to keep a diet log for 1 week. *Rationale:* A diary can identify types of foods eaten. Refer client to nutritionist regarding diet. *Rationale:* Proper food sources of protein and fiber can be identified and recommended. Discuss ways to modify eating behavior pattern. *Rationale:* Behavior modifications may assist in changing eating habits.	Client identifies two food sources high in fiber, protein, and vitamins after consulting with dietitian. She has gained 2 pounds in past month and feels less fatigued.

Examples of Outcome Criteria for Clients with Bowel Diversion Ostomies

The client will:

- Have intact skin around the ostomy
- Change his own ostomy appliance as demonstrated
- Discuss plans for looking after his ostomy at home
- Describe foods that should be avoided

Chapter Highlights

- Patterns of fecal elimination vary greatly among people; regular fecal elimination is usually important.
- The main functions of the colon are absorption, protection, and elimination.
- Bowel training can only occur after a child's muscular and nervous systems are sufficiently developed.
- A variety of factors affect defecation, including age, diet, fluid intake, muscle tone, and psychologic factors.
- Anesthesia and surgical procedures often impair intestinal movements temporarily.
- Sufficient fluid and fiber intake helps keep feces soft.
- Lack of exercise, irregular defecation habits, stress, and bland diets are all thought to contribute to constipation.
- Constipation can cause straining during defecation, which can lead to the Valsalva maneuver and subsequent cardiac problems.
- With a fecal impaction the excreted feces is usually liquid or loose.
- Digital removal of an impaction should be carried out gently because of vagal nerve stimulation and subsequent depressed cardiac rate.
- Diarrhea can be serious because of the resulting fluid and electrolyte imbalance that can occur.
- Flatulence occurs chiefly as a result of gas formed in the intestines.
- Hemorrhoids can occur as a consequence of constipation.
- Assessment relative to fecal elimination includes a nursing history, physical health examination, pattern of defecation, feces, and diagnostic test data.
- Normal defecation is often facilitated by providing privacy and by assisting the client to a normal squatting position.
- An enema involves the instillation of fluid into the rectum and sigmoid colon.
- The position of a bowel diversion ostomy greatly affects the character and management of the fecal drainage.
- Assessment of a bowel diversion ostomy includes the color of the stoma, stoma swelling, peristomal skin, amount and type of feces, tape allergy, and the presence of abdominal discomfort or distention.
- Clients who have a bowel diversion ostomy require considerable instruction in order to manage the ostomy.
- Psychosocial factors must be considered for clients who have ostomies.
- Protecting the peristomal skin is important in the care of ostomies because fecal effluent is irritating to skin.
- A colostomy irrigation is similar to an enema except that the client cannot control the expulsion of fluid and feces.

Suggested Readings

Alterescu, V. November 1985. The ostomy. What do you teach the patient? *American Journal of Nursing* 85:1250–53.
This article includes a discussion of some of the psychosocial implications of a colostomy. Preoperative and postoperative teaching is also included. Eleven do's and don'ts of ostomy-client teaching are provided as well as sample discharge instructions.

Blackwell, A. K., and Blackwell, W. January 1975. Relieving gas pains. *American Journal of Nursing* 75:66–67.
The authors describe five positions clients can assume to relieve their gas pains; these positions facilitate the expulsion of flatus through the rectum.

Corman, M. L., Veidenheimer, M. C., and Coller, J. A. February 1975. Cathartics. *American Journal of Nursing* 75:273–79.
The authors discuss the use of different cathartics and make recommendations for improving bowel function. Over-the-counter laxatives are listed, together with sites of action.

Habeeb, M. C., and Kallstrom, M. D. April 1976. Bowel program for institutionalized adults. *American Journal of Nursing* 76:606–8.
This article describes a program by which incontinent clients can achieve fecal continence. The program includes low-residue diet, medications, rectal examinations, and enemas when needed.

Smith, D. B. November 1985. The ostomy, how is it managed? *American Journal of Nursing* 85:1246–49.
This article describes how to assess a new colostomy and how to irrigate a colostomy. Ileostomy care is also covered. Includes a number of color photographs.

CHAPTER 44

Urinary Elimination

KAREN STAFFORD RANTZMAN

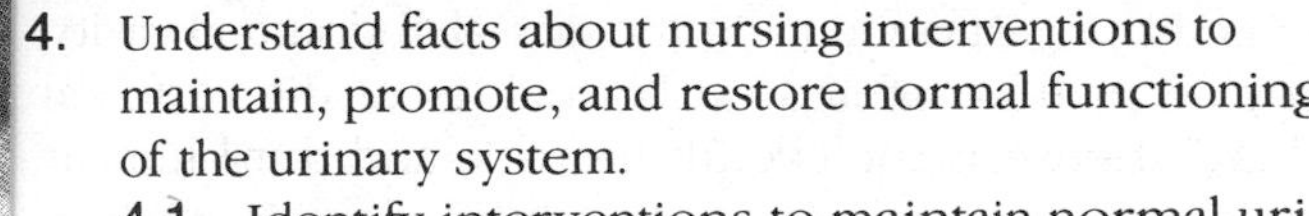

4. Understand facts about nursing interventions to maintain, promote, and restore normal functioning of the urinary system.
   - 4.1 Identify interventions to maintain normal urinary elimination.
   - 4.2 Identify measures that promote the development of bladder control in children.
   - 4.3 Outline common interventions for urinary incontinence and retention.
   - 4.4 Identify ways to prevent urinary infection.
   - 4.5 Describe interventions required for clients with retention catheters.
5. Perform selected urinary procedures safely.
   - 5.1 Assist clients to use bedpans and urinals.
   - 5.2 Perform a urinary catheterization for a male client and a female client.
   - 5.3 Apply a condom device and drainage apparatus.
   - 5.4 Measure residual urine.
   - 5.5 Obtain a sterile specimen from a retention catheter.
   - 5.6 Collect urine specimens.
   - 5.7 Perform urinary catheter and bladder irrigations.

Contents

nephron
nocturia
neurogenic bladder
oliguria
plasma
polydipsia
polyuria
proteinuria
pyuria
reflux
renal pelvis
residual urine
retention
retroperitoneal
specific gravity
sphincter
stasis
stricture
suppression
trigone
urethritis
urgency
ureterostomy
urinalysis

tion

through the ureters to the bladder, where it is held until the urge to urinate is felt, and then eliminated from the body through the urethra.

Kidneys

The kidneys are located in the **retroperitoneal** space (behind the peritoneum) in the dorsal abdominal cavity. They lie in front of and on both sides of the vertebral column, between the twelfth thoracic and third lumbar vertebrae. See Figure 44–1. An adult kidney is approximately 5 to 7 cm wide, 11 to 13 cm long, and 2.5 cm thick; it is shaped like a red kidney bean. Usually, kidneys of women and older persons are smaller than those of men. Each kidney is covered with a thin fibrous capsule, similar to cellophane, and is surrounded by fat. An adrenal gland lies above each kidney. The outer renal surface is convex, except for the medial aspect, the **hilum**, which is concave. The renal vessels, lymphatics, nerves, and ureter enter and exit through the hilum.

The kidneys are protected anteriorly by abdominal muscles, fascia, fat, and intestine. The right kidney is protected superiorly by the liver; the left kidney is protected by the spleen. Because of the large size of the liver above the right kidney, the right kidney is lower than the left. Posteriorly, the kidneys are protected by large back muscles and ribs. Several ribs guard the upper third of the kidneys. The kidneys move with ventilation, since they are in contact with the diaphragm. They also move slightly with changes in body position: When the body is supine, the kidneys are positioned slightly higher and more posterior than when the body is erect.

The kidneys filter from the blood any products for which the body has no use. Each kidney has one *renal artery* that originates from the abdominal aorta and enters the kidney at the hilum. (See Figure 44–1.) The renal vein exits through the hilum and joins the inferior vena cava. It is estimated that, in the average adult, 1200 ml of blood passes through the kidneys every minute. This figure represents about 21% of the cardiac output (5600 ml per minute). The body's total blood supply circulates through the kidneys approximately 12 times per hour (Richard 1986, p. 13).

From this blood, the **nephron** (the functional unit of the kidney—see Figure 44–2) forms a fluid called **glomerular filtrate** (about 180 liters daily, or 25 ml per minute). This volume–time ratio is referred to as the *glomerular filtration rate (GFR).* The **glomerulus** is a tuft or cluster of blood vessels surrounded by Bowman's capsule. Because the glomerular membrane is relatively porous, water and all of the dissolved constituents of **plasma** (the fluid portion of the blood) proteins do not filter through to Bowman's capsule. Thus, the glomerular filtrate is chemically almost the same as plasma, except that it has only minute quantities of protein (0.03%) compared to plasma (7%). **Proteinuria** is a sign of glomerular injury. Glomerular filtrate consists of water, electrolytes, creatinine, glucose, urea, amino acids, uric acid, bicarbonate, and other electrolytes.

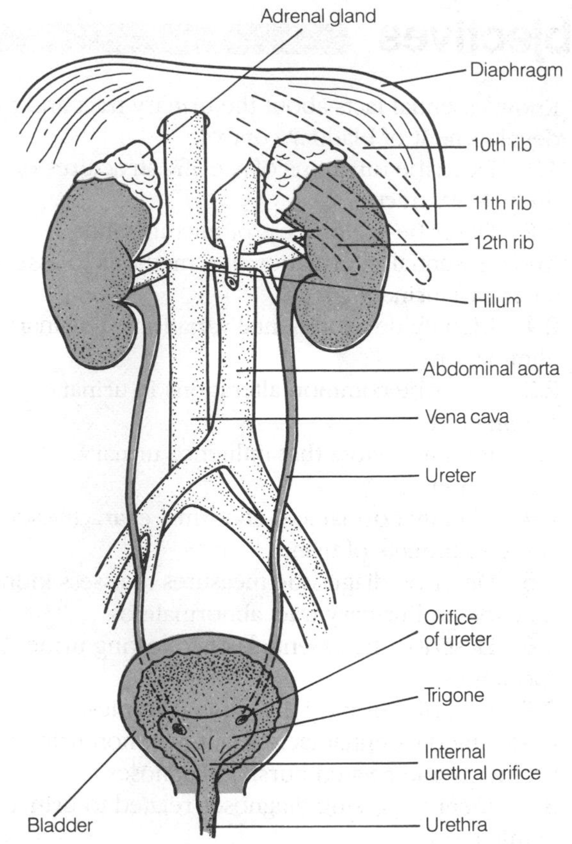

Figure 44–1 Anatomic structures of the urinary tract

After the filtrate enters Bowman's capsule, it passes into the tubular system, where about 99% of it is reabsorbed into the bloodstream. The remaining 1% forms the urine to be excreted from the body (Guyton 1986, p. 398). The function of the nephron, thus, is to return the majority of glomerular filtrate to the circulation. Therefore the kidneys are the most important organs in regulating body fluid balance.

The normal range of urine production for an adult is 0.6 to 1.6 liters a day. Various factors, such as fluid intake and body temperature, may affect urine production. An output of 50 ml of urine per hour is generally normal, and an output of less than 30 ml per hour may indicate kidney failure. Normal and abnormal constituents of urine are shown later in this chapter in Table 44–3.

Ureters

Once the urine is formed in the kidneys, it enters the ureters via collecting ducts and then passes on to the bladder. See Figure 44–1. The ureters are from 25 to 30 cm (10 to 12 in) long in the adult and about 1.25 cm (0.5

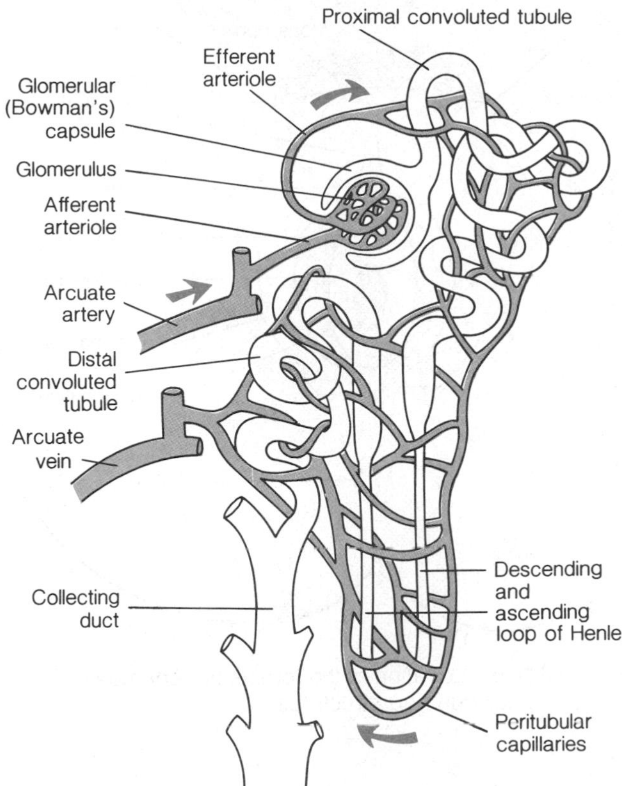

Figure 44–2 The nephrons of the kidney are composed of five parts: Bowman's capsule, proximal convoluted tubule, loop of Henle, distal convoluted tubule, and collecting duct.

in) in diameter. The upper end of each ureter is funnel-shaped as it enters the kidney, forming what is referred to as the **renal pelvis.** The lower ends of the ureters enter the bladder at the posterior corners of the floor of the bladder. At this junction between the ureter and the bladder there is a flaplike fold of mucous membrane that acts as a valve to prevent the backflow (**reflux**) of urine up the ureters to the kidneys.

The walls of the ureters consist of three layers: (a) the lining layer of mucous membrane that is continuous with the lining of the renal tubules and urinary bladder; (b) a middle layer of smooth muscle fibers that helps transport urine through the ureters into the bladder by peristaltic waves occurring at the rate of about 1 to 5 per minute; and (c) an outer layer of fibrous connective tissue that provides support to the ureters.

Stones known as *renal calculi* (singular: **calculus**) sometimes develop within the kidney. Urine may wash them into the ureter, where they may cause extreme pain if they are large enough to distend its walls. Ureteral obstructions from calculi result in strong peristaltic waves that attempt to move the stone into the bladder.

Bladder

The urinary bladder is a hollow, muscular organ that serves as a reservoir for urine and as the organ of excretion. When empty it lies behind the symphysis pubis. In the male it lies in front of the rectum and above the prostate gland (see Figure 44–3); in the female it lies in front of the uterus and vagina (see Figure 44–4). The wall of the bladder is made up of four layers: (a) an inner mucous layer that is continuous with that of the ureters and the urethra; (b) a submucous connective tissue layer; (c) a muscular layer consisting of three layers of smooth muscle fibers, some of which extend lengthwise, some obliquely, and some more or less circularly; and (d) an outer serous layer. The smooth muscle layers are collectively called the **detrusor muscle**. The base of the bladder, called the **trigone**, is a triangular area marked by the ureter openings at the posterior corners forming the base and the opening of the urethra at the anterior inferior corner forming the apex. Urine exits from the bladder through the urethra.

The amount of urine normally stored in the bladder varies to some degree among individuals and with age. For an adult, the desire to void is normally experienced when the bladder contains between 250 and 450 ml of urine. Normal output of urine for an adult is about 1500 ml/day.

The bladder is capable of considerable distention because of *rugae* (folds) in the mucous membrane lining and because of the elasticity of its walls. When full, the dome of the bladder may extend above the symphysis pubis; in extreme situations it may extend as high as the umbilicus.

During pregnancy the growing fetus puts pressure on the bladder, causing increased sensitivity and reduced

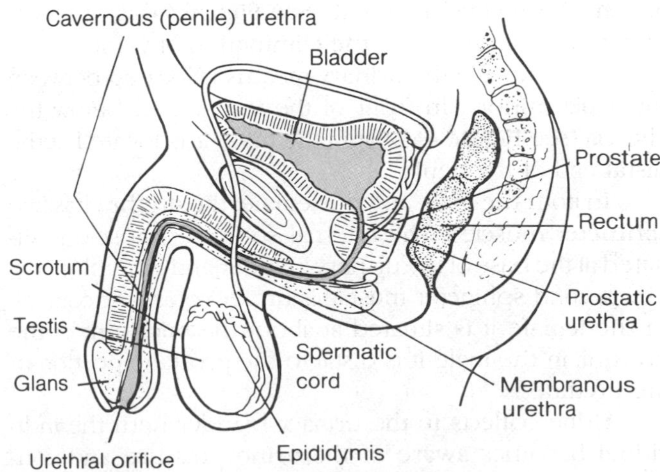

Figure 44–3 The male urogenital system

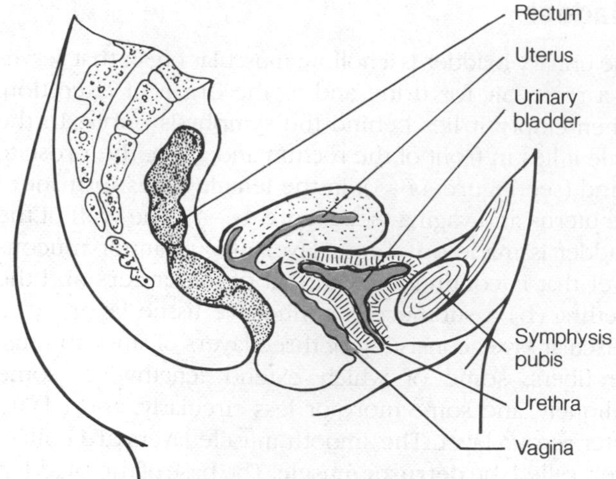

Figure 44–4 The female urogenital system

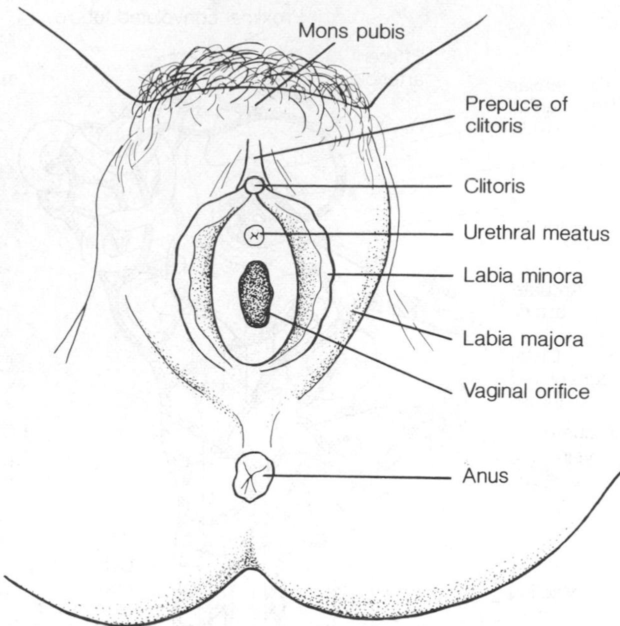

Figure 44–5 Location of the female urinary meatus in relation to surrounding structures

storage capacity. This often causes urgency and frequency (see the discussion of these problems later in this chapter).

Urethra

The urethra extends from the bladder to the urinary **meatus** (opening, or passage) and is the exit passageway for the urine. It is lined with mucous membrane. In the adult male the urethra—which functions as a passageway for reproductive fluid (semen) as well as urine—is about 20 cm (8 in) in length. It is divided into three parts: the prostatic urethra, which starts at the bladder and extends through the prostate gland; the membranous urethra, which extends from the prostatic section to the penis; and the cavernous (penile) urethra, which extends from the base of the penis to the urethral orifice. See Figure 44–3.

In the adult female the urethra lies directly behind the symphysis pubis, anterior to the vagina, and is about 3.7 cm (1.5 inches) in length. See Figure 44–4. It serves only as a passageway for the elimination of urine.

In the female the urinary meatus is located between the labia minora, in front of the vagina and below the clitoris (see Figure 44–5); in the male it is located at the distal end of the penis.

In both the male and the female, the urethra has two **sphincter** muscles. The internal sphincter muscle is situated at the base of the urinary bladder and is involuntary. The second sphincter muscle is under voluntary control. In the female it is situated at about the midpoint of the urethra; in the male it is distal to the prostatic portion of the urethra.

Urine collects in the urinary bladder until the individual becomes aware of the urine pressure and consciously releases it, or voids. Babies have no such conscious control, so their urine is released involuntarily after only a small amount accumulates in the bladder.

In both males and females, the urethra has a mucous membrane lining that is continuous with the bladder and the ureters. Thus, an infection of the urethra can readily extend through the urinary tract to the kidneys. Women are particularly prone to urinary tract infections because of the shortness of their urethras.

Urination

Micturition, **voiding**, and **urination** all refer to the process of emptying the urinary bladder. Urine collects in the bladder until pressure stimulates special sensory nerve endings in the bladder wall called *stretch receptors*. This occurs when the adult bladder contains between 250 and 450 ml of urine. In children, a considerably smaller volume, 50 to 200 ml, stimulates these nerves.

Once excited, the stretch receptors transmit impulses to the spinal cord, specifically to the voiding reflex center located at the level of the second to fourth sacral vertebrae. Some impulses continue up the spinal cord to the voiding control center in the cerebral cortex. If the time is appropriate to void, the brain then sends impulses through the spinal cord to the motor neurons in the sacral area, causing stimulation of the parasympathetic nerves. The parasympathetic nervous system innervates the detrusor muscle and the internal urethral sphincter muscle, producing (a) contraction of the detrusor muscle, and (b) relaxation of the internal sphincter muscle. As a result, urine can be released from the bladder, but it is still impeded by the external urinary sphincter. If the time and place are appropriate for urination, the conscious portion of the brain relaxes the external urethral sphincter muscle, and urination takes place. If the time and place are inappropriate, the micturition reflex usually subsides until the bladder becomes more filled and the reflex is stimulated again.

The sympathetic nervous system also innervates the bladder, causing it to relax. However the nerves do not normally enter into micturition control.

Voluntary control of micturition is possible only if the nerves supplying the bladder and urethra, the projection tracts of the cord and brain, and the motor area of the cerebrum are all intact. Injury to any of these parts of the nervous system—by, for example, a cerebral hemorrhage or spinal cord injury above the level of the sacral region—results in intermittent involuntary emptying of the bladder. Involuntary micturition is called **incontinence.** When there is damage to the spinal cord above the sacral vertebrae, the micturition reflex may remain intact and urination may occur reflexively. This situation is referred to as an *automatic bladder.*

Occasionally a person is unable to void even though the bladder contains an excessive amount of urine. This condition is known as **retention.** Catheterization (introduction of a rubber tube—known as a **catheter**—through the urethra into the bladder to remove urine) relieves the discomfort that accompanies retention. A more serious complication, which is also characterized by the inability to void, is called **suppression.** In this situation the person cannot void because the kidneys are not secreting any urine; the bladder is empty.

Assessment

To assess a client's urinary elimination patterns and function the nurse (a) considers developmental variables, (b) determines patterns of urination, (c) determines any alterations in urinary elimination and influencing or associated factors, (d) performs a physical assessment, (e) assesses volumes and characteristics of the client's urine, (f) reviews data obtained from diagnostic tests and examinations, and (g) determines past illnesses or surgery.

Developmental Variables

Urinary elimination functioning changes throughout the life cycle. These changes are shown in Table 44–1.

Patterns of Urination

The nurse determines the client's pattern and frequency of urination by asking the client the approximate times that voiding occurs each day and about any changes in usual elimination patterns. Although people's patterns of urination are highly individual, most people void about five or more times a day. People usually void when they first awaken in the morning, before they go to bed, and around meal times. Most people void about 70% of their daily urine during the waking hours and do not need to void during the night.

Alterations in Urinary Elimination

To determine recent changes and/or problems in urinary elimination patterns the nurse asks the client whether he or she has experienced any of the following clinical signs.

Polyuria

Polyuria, or **diuresis,** refers to the production of abnormally large amounts of urine by the kidneys, such as 2500 ml/day, without any increase in fluid intake. This can happen as a result of (a) excessive fluid intake, (b) the ingestion of substances containing caffeine and alcohol, (c) diabetes mellitus, (d) hormone imbalances (e.g., deficiency of antidiuretic hormone, or ADH), or (e) chronic kidney disease. Alcohol inhibits the release of antidiuretic hormone (ADH) and thus promotes urine formation. Coffee, tea, and cola drinks, which usually contain caffeine, increase the frequency and volume of micturition. Other signs often associated with diuresis are **polydipsia** (intense thirst), dehydration, and weight loss.

Oliguria and Anuria

Oliguria refers to voiding scant amounts of urine, such as 100 to 500 ml/day. **Anuria** refers to voiding less than 100 ml/day. The terms *complete kidney shutdown, renal failure,* and *urinary suppression* have the same meaning. Oliguria may result from an extremely low fluid intake but may also follow disease. Both anuria and oliguria can result from kidney disease, severe heart failure, burns, and shock. These clinical signs can be fatal if some other means—such as an artificial kidney—is not used to remove body wastes.

Oliguria may also normally accompany fever and heavy perspiration. Because of excessive fluid losses via the skin, urine production is decreased. Urine that is produced during febrile conditions is usually concentrated. The elevated metabolism associated with fever increases the accumulation of body wastes.

Frequency and Nocturia

Frequency is generally considered voiding at frequent intervals, that is, more often than usual. Normally with an increased intake of fluid there is some increase in the frequency with which a person voids. Frequency without

Table 44–1 Changes in Urinary Elimination Through the Life Cycle

Stage	Variations
Fetus	The fetal kidney begins to excrete urine between the 11th and 12th week of development. Fetal urine is hypotonic to plasma. The placenta serves as a pseudo-kidney in regulating fetal fluid and electrolyte balance. The kidney does not function independently until after birth.
Infant	Ability to concentrate urine is minimal; therefore urine appears light yellow. Voluntary urinary control is absent.
Children	Kidney function reaches maturity between the first and second year of life; urine is concentrated effectively and appears a normal amber color. Voluntary control of urine begins at 18 to 24 months of age, when the child starts to recognize bladder fullness, holds urine beyond the urge to void, and warns parents of the urge to void. Full urinary control is not gained until age 4 or 5 years; daytime control is usually achieved by age 2 years. Boys are slower than girls in gaining control. The kidneys grow in proportion to overall body growth.
Adults	The kidneys reach maximum size between 35 and 40 years of age. After age 50 the kidneys begin to diminish in size and function. Most shrinkage occurs in the cortex of the kidney, due primarily to the loss of glomeruli.
Elderly Adults	There is an estimated 30% loss of glomeruli by age 80 (Richard 1986, p. 38). Renal blood flow decreases because of vascular changes and a decrease in cardiac output. Urine concentratability declines. Excessive urination at night and increased frequency of urination occur because of loss of concentratability and diminished bladder muscle tone. Residual urine may increase due to diminished bladder muscle tone and contractability, which increases the risk of bacterial growth and infection. Urinary incontinence may occur due to mobility problems or neurologic impairments.

an increase in fluid intake may be the result of **cystitis** (an acutely inflamed bladder), stress, or pressure on the bladder (because of pregnancy, for example).

With frequency, the total amount of urine voided may be normal, since the amounts voided each time are small, such as 50 to 100 ml.

Nocturia, or *nycturia,* is increased frequency at night that is not a result of an increase in fluid intake. Like frequency, it is usually expressed in terms of the number of times the person gets out of bed to void, for exmaple, "nocturia ×4."

Urgency

Urgency is the feeling that the person *must* void. There may or may not be a great deal of urine in the bladder, but the person feels a need to void immediately. Often the person hurries to the toilet with the fear of being incontinent if he or she does not urinate. Urgency accompanies psychologic stress and irritation of the trigone and urethra. It is also common in young children who have poor external sphincter control.

Dysuria

Dysuria means voiding that is either painful or difficult. It can accompany a **stricture** (decrease in caliber) of the urethra, urinary infections, and injury to the bladder and/or urethra. Often clients will say they have to push to void or that burning accompanies or follows voiding. Burning during micturition is often due to an irritated urethra; burning following urination may be the result of a bladder infection when the irritated rugae (ridges) of the trigone rub together. The burning may be described as severe, like a hot poker, or more subdued, like a sunburn. Often, **hesitancy** (a delay and difficulty in initiating voiding) is associated.

Enuresis

Broadly speaking, **enuresis** is defined as repeated involuntary urination in children beyond the age when voluntary bladder control is normally acquired, usually 4 or 5 years of age (Whaley and Wong 1983, p. 662).

Enuresis can also be described as *primary,* meaning there has never been a long, dry, symptom-free period, or *secondary* (*acquired*), meaning the enuresis occurs after a dry period of at least a year. It is also described as *nocturnal* (nighttime), *diurnal* (daytime), or both. The incidence is approximately 5% to 17% in otherwise normal children between 3 and 15 years of age, with a male predominance (Whaley and Wong 1983, p. 662). Diurnal enuresis without nocturnal enuresis is unusual. There are many reasons for enuresis; several causes or contributing factors may exist in each individual situation. Some of these factors are listed here.

- Heredity. There appears to be a high frequency of bed-wetting among parents, siblings, and other near relatives of the involved child. It is thought that these persons have difficulty inhibiting the mechanisms that regulate bladder emptying.
- Smaller-than-normal bladder capacity.
- Child is a sound sleeper. Signals from the bladder indicating the need to urinate go unnoticed until it is too late for the child to get out of bed and to the bathroom.
- Irritable bladder. Such a bladder is unable to hold large quantities of urine.
- Socioeconomic conditions. There is a higher frequency among children who live in homes where toilet facilities are not readily accessible, the temperature is cold at night, the child sleeps with a bed-wetting sibling, and cleanliness practices are poor.
- Too early and too vigorous bladder training. If training occurs before the child is physiologically ready, enuresis may express an unconscious desire to regress and to receive the attention and care the child had when younger. It may also be an expression of resentment toward the parents.
- Parents who believe the child will outgrow the habit. Such parents do not try to train the child.
- Infections of the urinary tract, or physical or neurologic defects of the urinary system.
- Foods too rich in salts and minerals, or spicy foods. Foods such as pickles and relishes are irritating to the urinary system.
- Child who fears the dark. Walking down a dark corridor to the bathroom at night is fearful for such a child.

In most children, enuresis ceases between ages 6 and 8, although it may continue into adolescence.

Incontinence

Incontinence is involuntary leakage or loss of urine from the bladder. Four specific types of incontinence are differentiated: total incontinence, stress incontinence, urgency incontinence, and overflow incontinence (McConnell and Zimmerman 1983, p. 47). In *total incontinence* there is nearly continuous urine leakage. Common causes are injury to the external urinary sphincter in the male, injury to the perineal musculature or a fistula between the bladder and vagina in the female, and congenital or acquired neurogenic disease. In *stress incontinence,* leakage of urine is a result of a sudden increase in intraabdominal pressure that occurs when the person coughs, sneezes, laughs, or otherwise exerts physical strain. This type of incontinence occurs most frequently in females who suffer pelvic relaxation due to childbirth trauma, loss of tissue tone, or aging.

Urgency incontinence follows a sudden strong desire to urinate. The client is unable to stop urine flow when it starts and often fails to get to the bathroom on time. Urgency incontinence is different from stress incontinence in that loss of urine occurs at any time—not just with straining. It often occurs with **cystitis** (inflammation of the bladder) in women and other bladder diseases, such as calculi and tumors, in both men and women. Psychologic factors may also stimulate voiding. There is a high incidence of urgency incontinence in older adults, although the reasons are not completely understood. Inhibitory impulses that normally calm the bladder may be too weak, or some other imbalance of voiding reflexes may exist due to central nervous system pathology such as cerebral arteriosclerosis.

Overflow incontinence is a dribbling incontinence that results when the client's bladder is greatly distended with urine because of an obstruction at the bladder level or below or because of a flaccid neurogenic bladder. The term **neurogenic bladder** describes any voiding problem relating to neurologic impairment or dysfunction. A flaccid type of neurogenic bladder occurs following spinal injury or other pathology at the sacral level (below T_{12}). With this type of pathology the client is unaware of bladder-filling; the bladder walls become overstretched and atonic. Urine "overflows" or dribbles when the pressure increases in the bladder to a point where it surpasses the urethral sphincter's resistance to urine. A highly distended bladder can be palpated, and urine retained in the bladder may increase up to 3000 ml.

In addition to these types of incontinence, the nurse needs to consider problems the client may have with mobility. Diseases such as rheumatoid arthritis or other degenerative musculoskeletal or neurologic disorders that impair the client's mobility may cause accidental incontinence. Clients who have impaired mobility of the lower extremities may have difficulty in reaching and using toilet facilities. Clients who have impaired hand coordination may have difficulty manipulating clothing fasteners.

Retention

Urinary retention is the accumulation of urine in the bladder with associated inability of the bladder to empty itself. Because urine production continues, retention distends the bladder. An adult urinary bladder normally holds 250 to 450 ml of urine when the micturition reflex is triggered. With urinary retention, some adult bladders may distend to hold 3000 ml of urine. Distention of 1000 ml or more can mean weeks or months until full recovery of bladder tone; in some cases the result is permanent loss of bladder tone (McConnell and Zimmerman 1983, p. 40).

Occasionally a client will have *urinary retention with overflow.* (See "overflow incontinence" described earlier.) The client voids small amounts of urine frequently, or dribbles urine, while the bladder remains distended. Prolonged retention leads to **stasis** (a slowing of the flow of urine) and stagnation of urine, which increase the possibility of urinary tract infection.

Retention can be identified by several clinical signs: discomfort in the pubic area, bladder distention, inability to void or frequent voiding of small volumes (25 to 50 ml), a disproportionately small amount of fluid output in relation to intake, and increasing restlessness and need to void. It is distinguished from oliguria or anuria by the bladder distention. Bladder distention can be assessed by palpation and percussion above the symphysis pubis. See bladder palpation in Chapter 35 and see Figure 35–101. Percussion of the suprapubic area produces a "kettledrum" or dull sound when the bladder is full.

There are several causes of urinary retention: surgical procedures, postpartum perineal trauma, medication side effects, and psychosocial factors.

Postoperative retention The most common type of retention is *postoperative retention*; the exact etiology is unclear. Higher incidences of postoperative retention occur in certain clients (Innes and Bruga 1977, pp. 13–16):

- Those who have had a spinal anesthetic either alone or in combination with general or regional anesthesia.
- Those over age 70.
- Those for whom the time period between administration of preoperative medications and the beginning of anesthesia was short. The shorter the interval the greater the risk for retention. This variable may be related to the time needed to metabolize the medication.
- Those who have had certain types of surgery, e.g., intraabdominal, spinal, total hip replacement, lower extremity surgery, and to a lesser degree hemorrhoidectomy, and hernia repair.
- Those whose activity is minimal between the end of anesthesia and the time of voiding. Clients who remained on bed rest before voiding have an increased incidence of retention; those with some ambulatory activity have a lower incidence.
- Those who do not void spontaneously in 2 to 10 hours postoperatively. Clients who void spontaneously within 2 to 10 hours postoperatively have a lower incidence of retention than those who do not. However, many clients *do* void *after this time period,* which suggests that factors such as the amount of intravenous fluids administered during surgery and the amount of distention detected on bladder palpation need to be considered *before* decisions are made to catheterize clients.
- Those whose postoperative fluid intake is low. Over time, a low fluid intake may result in retention because the detrusor muscle accommodates to a slowly increasing volume in such a way that the stretch receptors are not fully activated. When the detrusor muscle fibers are stretched beyond a certain point, their contractability is hindered and voiding does not occur.

Postpartum retention *Postpartum retention* is most commonly due to swelling of the urinary meatus that results from perineal trauma associated with vaginal delivery. It is also caused by conditions that contribute to spasm of the perineal musculature.

Medication Side-Effects

Many medications interfere with the normal urination process and may cause retention. Examples are:

- Anticholinergic–antispasmodic medications such as atropine, belladonna, Donnatol, papaverine.
- Antidepressant–antipsychotic agents such as phenothyazines and MAO inhibitors.
- Antiparkinsonism drugs such as levodopa, artane, and cogentin.
- Antihistamine preparations such as Actifed and Sudafed.
- Beta-adrenergic blockers such as Inderal.
- Antihypertensives such as Apresoline and Aldomet.

Psychosocial Factors

Certain psychosocial factors may be associated with retention. Many people have developed a set of behaviors that help stimulate the micturition reflex. Examples are privacy, normal position, sufficient time, and, occasionally, running water. North Americans in contrast to many Europeans expect private toilet facilities; many Europeans more readily accept communal toilet facilities. There are also sex differences in privacy needs. Women are used to enclosed cubicles in public facilities; men are used to sharing more open facilities. Circumstances that counter the client's usual set of behaviors may produce anxiety and muscle tension. In persons who are unable to relax abdominal and perineal muscles and the external urethral sphincter, voiding may be incomplete and result in urinary retention. A summary of altered urinary patterns and influencing factors the nurse should assess in relation to them is shown in Table 44–2.

Table 44–2 Assessing Factors Associated with Altered Urinary Elimination Patterns

Altered Pattern	Selected Influencing and Associated Factors to be Determined
Polyuria	Increases in fluid intake and ingestion of fluids containing caffeine or alcohol
	Whether diuretics are prescribed (note type and dosage)
	Presence of thirst, dehydration, and weight loss
	Presence of, or familial history of, diabetes insipidus or kidney disease
Oliguria, anuria	Decreases in fluid intake and signs of dehydration (see Chapter 46)
	Presence of known kidney disease or familial history of kidney disease
	Signs of renal failure, such as the presence of uremic frost (urea crystals) on the skin, an elevated BUN, and an aromatic odor to the skin, and signs of fluid and electrolyte imbalances (see Chapter 46)
	Presence of febrile condition
Frequency or Nocturia	Whether client is pregnant
	Increases in fluid intake
	Presence of known urinary tract inflammation or infection
	Any known contributing or initiating causes, such as stress
Urgency	Presence of psychologic stress
	Presence of known urinary tract inflammation or infection
Dysuria	Presence of known urinary tract inflammation, infection, or injury
	Presence of other signs that may accompany dysuria, such as hesitancy, hematuria, pyuria, and frequency.
Enuresis	Family history of enuresis
	Access to toilet facilities and home cleanliness habits
	Home stresses
	Bladder training methods used
Incontinence	Whether urine leakage is continuous, occurs as a result of increased intraabdominal pressure, follows a strong desire to urinate, or is dribbling associated with a distended bladder
	Medical history and surgery for associated causes
	Presence of known bladder inflammation or other disease
	The client's age and mobility
Retention	Amounts and frequency of voiding
	Presence of distended bladder by palpation and percussion
	Associated signs, such as pubic discomfort, restlessness
	Whether fluid intake is low
	Recent anesthesia and type
	Type of surgery
	Time period between administration of perspective medications and anesthesia
	Amount of activity after recovery from anesthesia
	Presence of perineal swelling
	Types of medications prescribed
	Whether sufficient privacy or other factors that initiate micturition are lacking

Physical Assessment

Physical assessment of the urinary tract is discussed in Chapter 35. The kidneys are percussed to detect areas of tenderness and palpated for contour, size, tenderness and lumps. (See Procedure 35-9, pages 865 and 867.) Palpation and percussion of the bladder is described on page 868. The urethral meatus of both male and female clients are inspected during examination of the genitals (see pages 872 and 876 in Chapter 35). The meatus is inspected for swelling, discharge, and inflammation.

Assessment of Urine

Normal urine consists of 96% water and 4% solutes. Organic solutes include urea, ammonia, creatinine, and uric acid. Urea is the chief organic solute. Inorganic solutes include sodium, chloride, potassium, sulfate, magnesium, and phosphorus. Sodium chloride is the most abundant inorganic salt.

Assessment of urine involves measuring the volume of urine in relation to the client's intake; inspection of urine for color, clarity, and odor; testing of urine for specific gravity, glucose, ketone bodies, blood, and pH; and review of data obtained from diagnostic tests. Characteristics of normal and abnormal urine are summarized in Table 44–3.

Measurement or Inspection of Urine

Volume Urine volume depends on the amount of solutes to be excreted, loss of fluid in perspiration and exhaled air, the cardiac status and renal status of the client, hormonal influences, and the amount of fluid ingested. Normally the kidneys produce urine continuously at the rate of 30 to 60 ml per hour (720 to 1440 ml per day) in the adult, but the rate may be as high as 2000 ml per day if fluid intake is high. Fluid balance and measurement of all fluid intake and output are discussed in Chapter 46. Urine outputs below 30 ml per hour may indicate kidney malfunction and must be reported immediately. Urine excretion of more than 2000 ml per day or 80 ml per hr constitutes polyuria. In children normal values for urine volumes are 300 to 1500 ml per day.

Color Normal urine is straw-colored or amber-colored. The latter is most likely early in the morning, when urine is most concentrated. Increased fluid intake throughout the day normally makes the urine less concentrated, so it becomes paler in color.

Table 44–3 Characteristics of Normal and Abnormal Urine

Characteristic	Normal	Abnormal	Possible causes
Amount in 24 hours (adult)	1,200–1,500 ml	Under 1,200 ml	Decreased fluid intake
			Kidney failure
		Over 1,500 ml	Diabetes
			Diuretics
			Increased fluid intake
Color	Straw, amber	Dark amber	Insufficient fluid intake resulting in concentrated urine
	Transparent	Cloudy	Infectious process
		Dark orange	Drugs, e.g., pyridium
		Red or dark brown	Disease process causing blood in urine
Consistency	Clear liquid	Mucous plugs, viscid, thick	Infectious process
Odor	Faint aromatic	Offensive	Infectious process
Sterility	No microorganisms present	Microorganisms present	Infection of the urinary tract
pH	4.5 to 8	Under 4.5	Uncontrolled diabetes
		Over 8	Urinary tract infections
			Starvation
			Dehydration
Specific gravity	1.010 to 1.025	Under 1.010	Diabetes insipitus
			Kidney disease
			Overhydration
		Over 1.025	Diabetes mellitus
			Underhydration
Glucose	Not present	Present	Diabetes mellitus
Ketone bodies (acetone)	Not present	Present	Diabetic coma
			Starvation
			Prolonged vomiting
Blood	Not present	Occult	Kidney disease
		Bright red	Hemorrhage

Abnormal urine colors can occur for several reasons:

- Although color changes due to foods are rare, certain foods, such as beets, may make the urine appear red.
- Bleeding from the urinary tract makes the urine appear dark or bright red. Usually, bleeding from the kidneys and ureters appears dark red; bleeding from the bladder or urethra appears bright red. Blood in the urine is called **hematuria.**
- High concentrations of bilirubin in the urine make the urine appear yellow-brown or greenish-brown. Bilirubin appears in the urine in obstructive biliary or liver disease that causes jaundice. Urine with bilirubin can be distinguished from dark, concentrated urine by the appearance of yellow foam when a sample is shaken. Normal urine has a white foam.
- Special dyes used in some intravenous diagnostic studies are excreted by the kidneys. Some of these dyes may discolor urine.
- Menstrual contamination of urine produces a red or reddish-brown color.
- Some medications also alter urine color. See Table 44–4.
- Acid urine that contains hemoglobin becomes dark brown or black on standing. Black colors may also be caused by melanin which is associated with melanotic sarcoma. Table 44–4 summarizes some causes of urine discoloration.

Clarity Normal, freshly voided urine is clear or transparent. Urine may become cloudy due to the presence of mucus or pus, or when urine has a high protein concentration as a result of kidney disease. Urine that is left to stand for a while *normally* becomes cloudy.

Odor Normal, freshly voided urine has a characteristically faint aromatic odor but acquires a stronger odor the more concentrated it becomes. The odor may be modified after urine stands for any length of time by bacterial decomposition, which produces the characteristic pungent odor of ammonia. Additional odors may be due to a variety of causes (Byrne et al. 1986, p. 9):

- A sweet or fruity smell occurs from acetone and acetoacetic acid formed in starvation, diabetes mellitus, or dehydration.
- An offensive odor results from bacterial action on pus in heavily infected urine (**pyuria**).
- Certain ingested foods, such as garlic or asparagus, produce characteristic odors.
- Certain medications, such as menthol, antibiotics, paraldehyde, and vitamins, give characteristic odors.

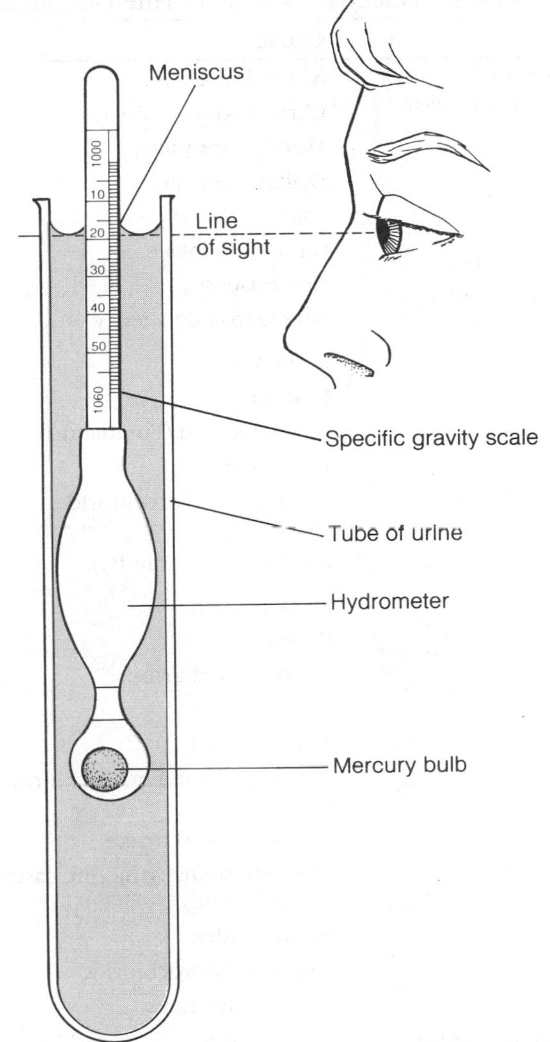

Figure 44–6 A urinometer measurement of specific gravity is taken at the base of the meniscus.

Routine Urine Testing

Several urine tests are simple to perform and are often done by nurses on the nursing units or are taught to clients, who perform them on their own urine. Tests commonly performed on urine include those for specific gravity, pH, presence of glucose and ketone bodies, and presence of occult blood.

Specific gravity **Specific gravity** is the weight or degree of concentration of a substance compared with that of an equal volume of another, such as distilled water, taken as a standard. The specific gravity of distilled water is 1.00 g/ml (in other words, 1 ml of water weighs 1 g). The specific gravity of urine can be measured by a urinometer (**hydrometer**), calibrated in units of 0.001. The instrument is placed in a glass cylinder containing the urine. See Figure 44–6. The scale on the urinometer progresses from 1.000 at the top to 1.060 at the bottom. The specific gravity of urine is normally about 1.010 to 1.025 g/ml. A

Table 44–4 Selected Causes of Urine Discoloration

Color	Cause
Almost colorless (very pale greenish yellow)	Alcohol ingestion
	Chronic kidney disease
	Diabetes insipidus
	Diabetes mellitus
	Diuretic therapy
	Large fluid intake
	Nervousness
	Severe iron deficiency
Yellow	Acriflavine
	Cascara
	Nitrofurantoin (Furadantin)
	Phenacetin
	Quinacrine hydrochloride (Atabrine)
	Riboflavin (vitamin B_2)
Orange	Azo Gantrisin
	Bilirubin
	Concentrated urine
	Multivitamins
	Nitrofurantoin
	Phenazopyridine hydrochloride (Pyridium)
	Restricted fluid intake
	Rhubarb, senna, santonin, cascara (in acid urine)
	Sulfonamides
	Thiamine hydrochloride
	Urobilin in excess
Pink, red, or reddish orange	Azo Gantrisin
	Beets
	Cascara (in alkaline urine)
	Chlorpromazine hydrochloride (Thorazine)
	Dorbantyl
	Doxidan
	Ex-Lax
	Hemoglobin
	Phenothiazine
	Phenytoin (Dilantin)
	Porphyrin
	Rifampin (Rifadin)
Green or blue-green (often blue mixed with yellow urine)	Amitriptyline (Elavil hydrochloride)
	Azuresin (Diagnex Blue)
	Bilirubin-biliverdin
	Methocarbamol (Robaxin)
	Phenylsalicylate
	Vitamin B complex
	Yeast concentrate
Pale blue	Pyrenium
Brown or black	Bilirubin-biliverdin
	Cascara (in acid urine)
	Chloroquine phosphate (Aralen)
	Furazolidone (Furoxone)
	Iron compounds (injectable)
	Levodopa (L-dopa)
	Melanin
	Nitrofurantoin
	Phenol
	Phenylhydrazine
	Porphyrin
	Sinemet
Cloudy	Bacteria
	Calculi "gravel"
	Clumps, pus, tissue
	Fecal contamination
	Leukocytes
	Mucin, mucous threads
	Phosphates, carbonates
	Prostatic fluid
	Red blood cells (smoky)
	X-ray contrast media
Milky	Fat (lipuria, opalescent; chyluria, milky)
	Pyuria

Adapted from C. J. Byrne, D. F. Saxton, P. K. Pelikan, and P. M. Nugent, *Laboratory Tests Implications for Nursing Care* 2d ed. (Menlo Park, Calif.: Addison-Wesley Pub. Co., 1986), pp. 10–12. Used by permission.

low specific gravity is often the result of overhydration or a disease that affects the kidneys' ability to concentrate solutes in the urine. A high specific gravity is often the result of dehydration or a disease that increases water reabsorption by the kidneys, causing concentrated urine. False positive results are caused by drugs such as dextran and radiopaque materials used in x-ray examination of the urinary tract.

To measure specific gravity with a urinometer, the nurse can do the following.

1. Pour at least 20 ml of a fresh urine sample in a glass cylinder, or fill the cylinder three-quarters full.
2. Place the urinometer into the cylinder and give it a gentle spin to prevent it from adhering to the sides of the cylinder.

3. Hold the urinometer at eye level, and read the measurement at the base of the meniscus at the surface of the urine. See Figure 44–6.

The concentration of the urine affects the degree to which the urinometer will float. The depth to which it sinks indicates the specific gravity.

Specific gravity can also be measured with a spectrometer or refractometer. In this instance the nurse places one or two drops of urine on a slide, turns on the instrument light, and looks into the instrument. The specific gravity appears on a scope. Manufacturer's directions are usually available for specific models.

pH (acid–base) pH is a measurement of the concentration of hydrogen ions, which indicates the acidity or alkalinity of a substance. Discrete measurements of pH are made on a scale of 1 to 14, in which the value 7 is neutral, below 7 is acid, and above 7 is alkaline (base). Such quantitative measurements, however, are conducted in the agency laboratory, where specific reactive agents are used.

Urine becomes increasingly acidic when increasing amounts of sodium and excess acid are retained in the body. Ingestion of various foods also affects urinary pH. A diet rich in animal protein and cranberry juice decreases the pH and produces an acid urine. A diet high in citrus fruits, most vegetables, milk, and other dairy products increases the pH and produces an alkaline urine. Urine that is left at room temperature for several hours will gradually become alkaline because of bacterial action.

Control of the urine pH is an important factor in certain medical therapies. For example, the formation of renal stones is partially dependent on the urinary pH; therefore, clients being treated for stones are often given diets or medications to alter the pH and prevent stone formation. Certain medications, such as streptomycin, neomycin, and kanamycin, are more effective for treating urinary tract infections if the urine is alkaline.

Measurement of pH involves dipping a strip of either red or blue litmus paper into the urine specimen, observing the color of the litmus paper, and comparing it to a standardized color chart on the bottle. The blue litmus paper, more commonly used, remains blue if the urine is alkaline and turns red if it is acidic. The red litmus paper remains red in the presence of acid urine and turns blue if the urine is alkaline. Whichever litmus strip is used, red always indicates acid urine and blue alkaline urine.

Presence of glucose Urine is tested for glucose to screen clients for diabetes mellitus or to follow the progress of a known diabetic. Normally the amount of glucose in the urine is negligible, although individuals who have ingested large amounts of sugar may show small amounts of glucose in their urine.

Several commercial products are commonly used to test for the presence of glucose, e.g., Clinitest tablets and Clinistix, Diastix, and Tes-Tape reagent strips. Each uses a color scale to measure the quantity of glucose in the urine, but the scales are not interchangeable from one product to the other. The scales grade the results as negative, trace, one plus (1+ or +), two plus (2+, or ++), three plus (3+ or +++), etc. Each grade reflects a specific percentage of glucose, which varies from one testing product to another. For example, a 2+ result from a Clinitest reaction indicates 75% glucose in the urine, whereas a 2+ result from a Tes-Tape strip indicates 25% glucose.

False readings can arise from medications a client is receiving, depending on the type of chemical product used to test the urine for glucose. For example, tetracycline and large doses of ascorbic acid and chloral hydrate can generate false positive results from Clinitest tablets. For this reason, many agencies stock more than one testing product. Nurses need to compare the medications a client is receiving with the literature about each product, and choose the appropriate product for the test.

To test urine for glucose the nurse carries out the following steps:

1. Obtain a freshly voided specimen. Most agencies require a *second-voided specimen:* Have the client void, and in 30 minutes have the client void again, providing a specimen for the test this time. A second-voided specimen more accurately reflects the present condition of the body. Urine that has accumulated in the bladder, e.g., overnight, reflects the condition of the body at the time the urine was produced, e.g., 0300 hours.
2. Select the appropriate equipment and testing product for the client. If Clinitest tablets are used, obtain a clean test tube and dropper. Follow the directions specified by the manufacturer to carry out the test. If Clinitest tablets are used, be careful not to touch the bottom of the test tube, because this becomes extremely hot when the tablet boils in the presence of urine and water.
3. Compare the results with the appropriate color chart, and record them on the client's chart. Most agencies now record the findings in percentage of glucose in the urine rather than 2+ or 3+.

Presence of ketone bodies Ketone bodies are products of incomplete fat metabolism and appear in the urine in instances of fasting, very low intake of carbohydrates, and uncontrolled diabetes mellitus. Usually the urine is tested for ketone bodies at the same time it is tested for glucose. Tablets or reagent strips are used.

For this test one or two drops of urine are placed on a reagent tablet (e.g., an Acetest tablet), or a reagent test strip (e.g., Ketostix) is dipped into the urine. The results are observed and compared with the appropriate color chart to determine the quantity of ketones present. The results may be graded as negative, small, moderate, or large amounts, or as negative, positive, or strongly positive. Record the results in accordance with the product used and agency practice.

Presence of occult blood Normal urine is free of blood. When blood is present, it may be clearly visible or not visible (occult). Commercial reagent strips are used to test for occult blood in the urine. The nurse dips the reagent strip (e.g., Hemastix) into a sample of urine and compares the color change with a color chart, in the same manner as for other reagent strips.

Diagnostic Tests

A number of diagnostic tests and procedures are carried out to determine urinary tract pathology. These include laboratory analysis of urine (**urinalysis**), urine culture, radiographic examinations (KUB and IVP), cystoscopy, and blood tests. Intravenous pyelogram (IVP) and cystoscopy are discussed in Chapter 54.

Urinalysis

A routine screening urinalysis is usually performed on all clients when they are admitted to a health care agency. Routine urine examination is usually done on the first voided specimen in the morning, because it tends to have a higher, more uniform concentration and a more acid pH than specimens later in the day (Byrne et al., 1986, p. 5). A clean specimen voided into a urinal, bedpan, or clean urine cup is usually adequate for routine examination. Collection of routine urine samples is discussed later in this chapter. In addition to the routine tests discussed previously (i.e., specific gravity, pH, presence of glucose, ketone bodies, and blood), the urinalysis also includes data about the presence of other abnormal constituents, such as protein, bilirubin, urobilinogen, and nitrite determinations.

Protein The presence of protein in the urine, often albumin, can be tested for with a reagent strip or by using other, more sophisticated measurement devices. Normally, large protein molecules such as albumin, fibrinogen, and globulin are not filtered through the kidneys into the urine. However, in cases of damaged kidneys, albumin, the smallest molecule of the three, can filter into the urine from the blood. The presence of protein in the urine is called **proteinuria**; the presence of albumin is referred to as **albuminuria**.

A benign transitory proteinuria that is unrelated to organic disease can occur following nonpathologic activities such as strenuous exercise, severe emotional stress, or prolonged exposure to cold. However, continued proteinuria in an apparently healthy person usually is a sign of at least minimal kidney damage.

Bilirubin *Bilirubin,* the chief bile pigment, is derived from the breakdown of red blood cells by the reticuloendothelial cells of the liver and spleen. This free bilirubin travels to the liver, where it is linked (conjugated) with glucuronic acid and excreted with bile into the gastrointestinal tract. Normally, only very small amounts of conjugated bilirubin are found in the blood, although any obstruction to the flow of the bile causes this concentration to increase.

Conjugated bilirubin is water-soluble and easily passes the glomerular barrier of the kidney to appear in the urine (bilirubinuria). Bilirubin may be present in the urine before jaundice becomes visible; this has the same significance as jaundice in the detection of liver disease. Laboratory screening tests for urine bilirubin frequently are included in routine urinalysis to detect latent or unsuspected liver disease, especially disorders that do not produce recognizable jaundice.

Urobilinogen *Urobilinogen* is a substance produced by the degradation of bilirubin. Its formation in the intestines results from bacterial activity on the conjugated bilirubin excreted in the bile. Intestinal bacteria reduce the bilirubin to a series of colorless compounds known collectively as urobilinogen, which are further oxidized to orange-brown urobilin.

About half of the urobilinogen formed in the intestine is excreted with the feces. The remainder passes into the bloodstream via the portal system. Most of this reabsorbed urobilinogen returns to the liver for reexcretion with the bile, but a minute amount enters the urine as the blood passes through the kidneys.

If obstruction or severe liver disease prevents or interrupts the flow of bile, bilirubin cannot reach the intestine, preventing the formation of urobilinogen and causing urobilinogen levels to decrease. Conversely, urine urobilinogen levels increase when abnormally large amounts accumulate in the intestine or when the liver cannot adequately dispose of the reabsorbed urobilinogen. Laboratory tests for urine urobilinogen help to differentiate obstructive jaundice from the jaundice associated with hemolytic anemia.

Nitrite Nitrite determinations are performed to detect the presence of asymptomatic **bacteriuria** (bacteria in the urine). Because the only way nitrite can appear in the urine is through the bacterial metabolism of nitrates, positive test results always indicate significant bacterial infection. Laboratory tests for urine nitrite are used to determine if urine culture and identification of organisms are needed.

Other abnormal constituents Other abnormal constituents of urine include large amounts of mucus, crystals, pus (**pyuria**), epithelial cells, and red and white blood cells. A few of these in the urine may be normal, but large numbers are generally indicative of a pathologic process such as **calculi** (solidified masses of mineral salts or stones), tumors, or infection.

Tests for these constituents are usually made with a microscope. The urine is centrifuged to separate the sediment from the liquid. The sediment is placed on a slide and examined under a microscope. Although these tests are usually carried out in a laboratory, nurses are frequently responsible for collecting the urine specimen. Many other tests are performed on urine specimens. See "Tests Using Timed Urine Specimens" later in this chapter.

Urine Culture

Urine culture and sensitivity tests are done to identify specific causative microorganisms of urinary tract infections. Culture and sensitivity (C & S) is described in Chapter 32, page 692. The nurse's role in bacteriologic urine culture tests is to obtain a clean-catch specimen, also referred to as a clean voided midstream urine (CVMS). See Procedure 44–1 later in this chapter.

In the past, catheterization was the preferred method for acquiring specimens for culture that were free from contamination, particularly from females. These days, even though the clean-catch specimen may be somewhat contaminated by skin bacteria, it is considered better to have a contaminated specimen than to cause infection to the client's urinary tract. A bacterial count can generally reveal whether the bacteria in CVMS specimens came from the skin or from a urinary infection. Bacterial counts below 10,000 per ml of urine generally mean skin contamination of the specimen and not a true urinary tract infection. Counts above 100,000 per ml generally indicate a true infection of the urinary tract. Analyses showing counts between 10,000 and 100,000 are usually repeated.

It is obvious that a CVMS specimen cannot be obtained from clients with indwelling catheters. If a client has an indwelling catheter, the aspiration method is used. This involves inserting a sterile needle with a syringe into a disinfected port on the catheter, withdrawing urine, and transferring the urine into a sterile specimen container.

X-ray Examinations and Scanning

Radiographic examinations involving the urinary tract include intravenous pyelogram (IVP), x-ray films of the kidneys, ureters, and bladder (KUB), and renal scans. These examinations provide data about the presence of tumors or other obstructions within the organs and distortions in the shapes or densities of the organs. The nurse's role in assisting clients with these examinations and descriptions of these tests are described in Chapter 54.

Blood Tests

Two blood tests commonly conducted to examine renal function are the blood urea nitrogen (BUN) clearance test and the creatinine clearance test. These measure how effectively the kidneys are excreting the respective substances. A normal range of BUN is 8 to 28 mg per 100 ml of blood. The normal range for creatinine is 0.5 to 1.2 mg per 100 ml of blood. A former blood test for kidney function was the nonprotein nitrogen (NPN) test. Nonprotein nitrogen compounds are small-molecule crystaloids of body fluids. They are normally present in the blood at levels of 10 to 40 mg per 100 ml of blood. This test has been largely replaced by more specific tests of the constituent compounds, such as creatinine, urea nitrogen, and uric acid.

Collecting Urine Specimens

The nurse is responsible for collecting urine specimens for a number of types of tests: clean voided specimens for routine urinalysis, clean-catch or midstream urine specimens for urine culture, and timed urine specimens for a variety of tests that depend on the client's specific health problem.

Clean Voided Specimens

Clients need varying degrees of instruction and assistance to provide clean voided specimens. Many clients are able to provide the specimen independently. Male clients generally have little difficulty voiding directly into the specimen container, but female clients usually need to stand over a toilet bowl and hold the container between their legs during the process of voiding. About 120 ml (4 oz) of urine is generally required. Clients who are seriously ill, physically incapacitated, or disoriented may need to use a bedpan or urinal in bed; others may require supervision and/or assistance in the bathroom. Whatever the situation, explicit directions are required.

Explain that all specimens must be free of fecal contamination, so voiding needs to occur at a different time from defecation. Instruct female clients to discard the toilet tissue in the toilet or in a waste bag rather than in the bedpan, since tissue in the specimen makes laboratory analysis more difficult. When the specimen is obtained, put the lid tightly on the container to prevent spillage of the urine and contamination of other objects. If the outside of the container has been contaminated by urine, clean it with a disinfectant. Make sure that the specimen label and the laboratory requisition carry the correct information, and attach them securely to the specimen. Inappropriate identification of the specimen can lead to errors of diagnosis or therapy for the client. Refrigerate the specimen, or take it immediately to the laboratory. Urine left at room temperature deteriorates relatively rapidly because of bacterial contamination.

Clean-Catch Specimens

Clean-catch or mid-stream specimens must be as free as possible from external contamination by microorganisms near the urethral opening. Sterile specimen containers and lids are used for these specimens. Procedure 44–1 describes the steps involved in obtaining these specimens.

Procedure 44–1 ▲ Collecting a Urine Specimen for Culture and Sensitivity by Clean Catch

Equipment

Equipment used varies from agency to agency. Some agencies use commercially prepared disposable clean-catch kits. See Figure 44–7. Others use agency-prepared sterile trays. Both prepared trays and kits generally contain the following items:

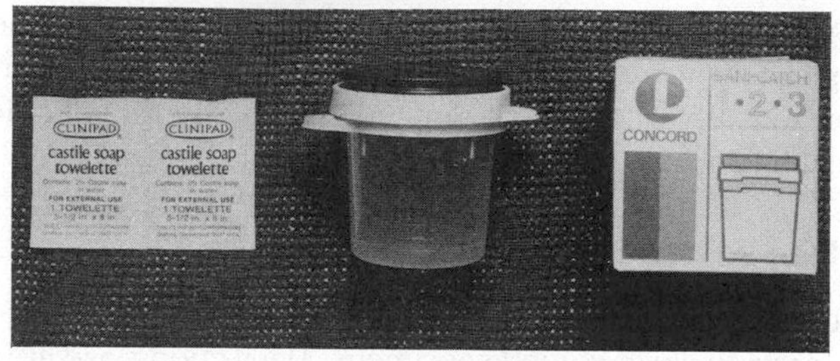

Figure 44–7 A commercially prepared disposable clean-catch kit.

1. Sterile cotton balls in a container, to clean and dry the genitals and perineal area.
2. An antiseptic, such as aqueous Zephiran 1:700. The antiseptic may need to be added to an agency-prepared tray.
3. A container of sterile water to rinse the perineal area after cleaning.
4. Sterile gloves to wear when swabbing and cleaning.
5. A urine receptacle.
6. A sterile specimen container for the urine specimen.
7. A specimen identification label.

Additional supplies:

8. A completed laboratory requisition form.
9. A bath blanket, if the client is not ambulatory.
10. A disinfectant.

Intervention

1. Inform the client that a urine specimen is required; give the reason for it, and explain the method to be used to collect it.
2. Ask the client to wash and dry his or her genitals and perineum thoroughly with soap and water. A clean perineum is essential, to reduce the number of skin bacteria and to minimize contamination of the specimen.
3. Assist the ambulatory client to the bathroom. The preferred method to collect the specimen from ambulatory clients is to have them provide the specimen while standing over the toilet in the bathroom.
4. Assist nonambulatory clients to an upright sitting position on a urine receptacle. Provide appropriate covers for the client: Fold back the top bed linen to the bottom of the bed and drape the client in a bath blanket, exposing only the perineal area.
5. Assist female clients to spread their legs enough to ensure that the urine does not touch the legs.
6. Open the sterile kit or tray, using sterile technique.

   Rationale Sterile technique is essential to maintain the sterility of the specimen container.
7. Put on the sterile gloves.
8. Pour the antiseptic solution over the cotton balls.
9. Clean the client's vulvar area or the tip of the penis with the antiseptic.

   Rationale The antiseptic reduces the number of bacteria near the urethral opening and minimizes contamination of the urine specimens.
10. For female clients:
    a. Swab the labia minora from front to back, using one swab for each wipe.

       Rationale Swabbing from front to back cleans from the area of least contamination to the area of greatest contamination.

    b. Spread the labia minora well apart, using the thumb and another finger, e.g., the third finger, of one hand.
    c. Swab between the labia minor over the urethra from front to back.

       Rationale The urethra is considered less contaminated than the vagina and anus.

    d. Rinse the area with sterile water.

       Rationale Rinsing removes the antiseptic and other external contaminants.

    e. Dry the area with sterile cotton balls.
11. For male clients:
    a. Hold the penis with one hand and clean the urinary meatus using a circular motion. Retract the foreskin of an uncircumcised male.

b. Wash outward from the meatus in a circular motion, using one swab for each wipe.

Rationale This cleans from the area of least contamination to the area of greatest contamination.

c. Rinse the area with sterile water.

d. Dry the area with cotton balls, in the same manner used for cleaning.

12. Ask the client to start voiding.

Rationale Initial voiding clears additional external contaminants at the urethral opening.

13. After the client has begun to void, place the specimen container under the stream of urine to collect 30 to 60 ml of midstream urine. Handle only the outside of the container.

Rationale Handling only the outside protects the sterility of the inside.

14. Put the sterile cap tightly on the specimen container, touching only the outside of the cap.

Rationale Capping the container prevents spillage of urine and contamination of other objects. Touching only the outside of the cap retains the sterility of the inside of the cap.

15. Inspect the urine for normal and abnormal characteristics. See Table 44–3 earlier.

16. Clean the outer surface of the container with a disinfectant.

Rationale Cleaning the outer surface prevents the transfer of microorganisms to others.

17. Remove your gloves and wash hands.

18. Ensure that the specimen label and the laboratory requisition carry the correct information. Attach them securely to the specimen.

Rationale Inaccurate indentification and/or information on the specimen container can lead to errors of diagnosis or therapy.

19. Arrange for the specimen to be sent to the laboratory immediately.

Rationale Bacterial cultures must be started immediately, before any contaminating organisms can grow, multiply, and produce false results.

20. Record collection of the specimen, any pertinent observations of the urine in terms of color, odor, or consistency, and any difficulty in voiding that the client experienced.

Timed Urine Specimens

Several urine tests require timed specimens. Urine specimens are collected at timed intervals, for short periods (1 to 2 hours) or long periods (12 to 24 hours). All timed urine specimens need to be refrigerated, to prevent bacterial growth and decomposition of the urine components, which can affect the findings. For some timed specimens, large collection containers are kept in a refrigerator, often in the laboratory, not at the bedside. Each voiding of urine is collected in a small, clean container and then emptied immediately into the large refrigerated bottle. In most instances the entire amount of urine voided is collected.

For some tests, a chemical urine preservative, e.g., toluene or acetic acid, is added to the large collection container. Other tests require different preservatives, since certain additives invalidate the results for certain tests. It is wise to contact the laboratory prior to the specimen collection to confirm the additive for a test.

Tests using timed urine specimens Some of the tests performed on timed urine specimens include:

1. Quantitative albumin test (24 hours) to determine the daily amount of albumin lost in the urine in such conditions as kidney disease, hypertension, drug toxicity, or severe heart failure involving kidney damage.
2. Amino acid tests (24 hours) to determine acquired or congenital disease of the kidneys.
3. Amylase test (2, 12, or 24 hours). Amylase is a pancreatic enzyme that may be excreted in the urine in certain diseases of the pancreas.
4. Quantitative chlorides test (24 hours) to determine the total excretion of chloride. This test may be performed in the management of cardiac clients who are on low-salt diets.
5. Concentration and dilution tests to determine disorders of the kidney tubules in concentrating and diluting urine. These specimens are collected over varying periods of time. Specimens are commonly collected at hourly intervals for two to four hours after the client has been given a specified amount of clear fluid to drink. Check agency procedures.
6. Creatinine test or creatinine clearance test (24 hours) to reflect the degree of kidney impairment. Creatinine is formed in the muscles from creatine in relatively constant daily amounts and is excreted in the urine. Elevated creatinine content indicates a disturbance in kidney function.
7. Estriol determination test (24 hours) to measure the level of this hormone in the urine of high-risk pregnant women such as those with toxemia or diabetes.

Estriol is the major form in which estrogen is excreted in the urine. Low levels can indicate inadequate function of the placenta and possible fetal distress.

8. Glucose tolerance test (24 hours) to determine disorders of glucose metabolism that may arise from malfunction of the liver or pancreas. Tests are performed on both the blood and the urine after the client is given a large amount of glucose orally or intravenously.
9. 17-hydroxycorticosteroid test (24 hours) to assess the functioning of the adrenal cortex. Corticosteroids are hormones that are produced in the adrenal cortex, altered, and then excreted in the urine.
10. Urobilinogen test (random times or 2 hours) to determine obstruction of the biliary tract, excessive destruction of red blood cells, or liver damage. These specimens are collected in brown bottles because they need to be protected from light.

Specimen Collection Technique

Appropriate specimen containers with or without preservative in accordance with the specific test are generally obtained from the laboratory and placed in the client's bathroom or in the utility room. Alert signs are placed in the client's unit to remind staff of the test in progress. Specimen identification labels need to indicate the date and time of each voiding in addition to the usual identification information. They may also be numbered sequentially, e.g., 1st specimen, 2nd specimen, 3rd specimen.

Clients need to be given explicit instructions about the purpose of the test and how they can assist. Tell the client when the specimen collection will begin and end; for example, a 24-hour urine test commonly begins at 0700 hours and ends at the same hour the next day. Instructions should include the following facts:

1. All urine must be saved and placed in the specimen containers once the test starts.
2. The urine must be free of fecal contamination and toilet tissue.
3. Each specimen must be given to the nursing staff immediately so that it can be placed in the appropriate specimen bottle.

The collection period is started by having the client void in the toilet or bedpan or urinal. This urine is usually discarded, but agency procedure needs to be checked. All subsequent urine specimens are collected, including the one at the end of the period.

The nurse needs to make sure that the client ingests the required amount of liquid for certain tests and instructs the client to void all subsequent urine into the bedpan or urinal and to notify the nursing staff when each specimen is provided. Some tests require that the client void at specified times. Each specimen must be placed into the appropriately labeled container. For some tests each specimen is not kept separately but is poured into a large bottle in the laboratory refrigerator. Each specimen is refrigerated throughout the timed collection period to prevent bacterial decomposition of the urine. Ask the client to provide the last specimen 5 to 10 minutes before the end of the collection period and inform the client that the test is completed. The starting time of the test and completion of the specimen collection are recorded on the client's chart. In addition, if indicated for the specific test, the time each urine specimen was collected is noted, as are the volume of each specimen, the appearance of the urine, and other relevant data such as fluid intake or restrictions.

Past Illnesses or Surgery

The nurse determines the client's past history of elimination problems and urinary tract disease or surgery and other diseases that may affect urinary elimination. Some of these are:

- Hematuria, frequency, or other urinary elimination alterations discussed previously
- Urinary tract infections of the kidney, bladder, or urethra
- Urinary calculi
- Urinary track surgery, such as kidney surgery, bladder surgery, prostate removal, or other surgical procedures that alter urinary routes, e.g., ureterostomy (see "Urinary Diversion Ostomies," discussed next)
- Cardiovascular disease such as hypertension or heart disease
- Chronic diseases that alter urinary characteristics or impair urinary function, such as diabetes mellitus, neurologic disease, e.g., multiple sclerosis, and cancer

For clients who have urinary diversion ostomies the nurse determines the type of ostomy and the client's method of managing it. Essential data include:

1. Type of appliances or pouch used
2. Type of skin barriers or applications and other methods used to reduce or prevent skin irritation
3. Frequency of appliance changes
4. Type of nighttime drainage system
5. Status of peristomal skin
6. History or presence of urinary infection

Urinary Diversion Ostomies

There are four main types of urinary diversion ostomies:

1. Cutaneous ureterostomy
2. Ileal conduit
3. Vesicostomy
4. Ureterosigmoidostomy or ureteroileosigmoidostomy

Permanent urinary diversion stomas are indicated for any condition that requires a total cystectomy, e.g., cancer of the bladder. Temporary urinary diversion stomas are indicated for any condition requiring partial cystectomy, trauma to the lower urinary tract, or severe chronic urinary tract infections.

Ureterostomy

In cutaneous **ureterostomy**, the ureters are diverted to the abdominal wall or flank, and a ureteral stoma is formed. Ureterostomies are small compared to colostomies (about 0.5 mm, or 1/4 in, in diameter) and drain continuously. They may involve the right or left ureter (*unilateral ureterostomy,* Figure 44–8, *A*) or both ureters (*bilateral ureterostomy,* Figure 44–8, *B*), in which case each one is covered by a separate appliance, unless they are placed close to each other.

Variations of the bilateral ureterostomy include:

1. The *double-barreled ureterostomy,* in which both ureters are brought to the skin surface to form side-by-side stomas. See Figure 44–8, *C.*
2. The *loop ureterostomy,* in which the ureters are looped out to the skin surface of each flank to form the stomas. See Figure 44–8, *D.*
3. The *transureteroureterostomy,* in which one ureter is first connected to the other, and then the receiving ureter is brought to the skin surface to form a stoma. See Figure 44–8, *E.*

Ileal Conduit

The ileal (ileo) conduit is also referred to as *ileal (ileo) loop, ileal (ileo) bladder, ureteroileostomy,* or *Bricker's loop*. See Figure 44–9. In this procedure, a segment of the ileum is removed and the intestinal ends are reattached. One end of the portion removed is closed with sutures to create an ileal pouch, and the other end is brought out through the abdominal wall to create a stoma. The ureters are implanted into the ileal pouch, and the bladder is usually removed. The advantages of this procedure over ureterostomies are that the ileal stoma is larger and more readily fitted with an appliance; there is less chance of an ascending kidney infection, since the mucous membrane lining of the ileum acts as a barrier to microorganisms; and the stoma is less likely to stenose, a major problem with ureterostomy stomas. For these reasons, the ileal conduit is one of the most commonly used urinary diversion procedures.

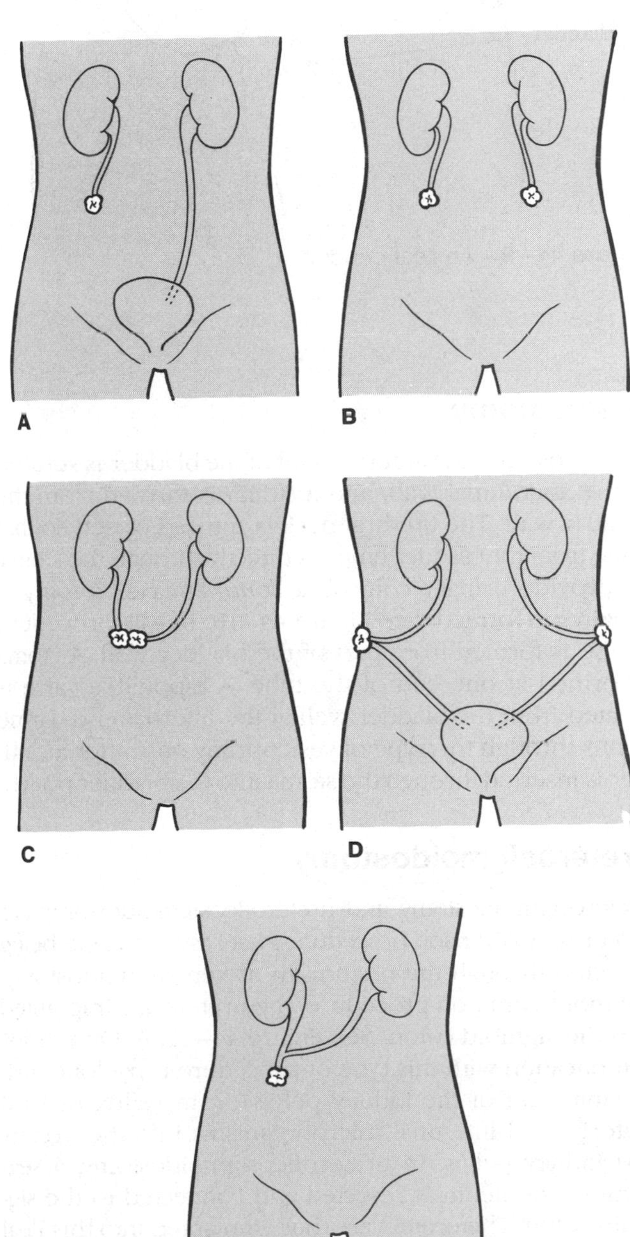

Figure 44–8 Five types of ureterostomies: **A,** right unilateral ureterostomy; **B,** bilateral ureterostomy; **C,** double-barreled ureterostomy; **D,** flank loop ureterostomy; **E,** transureteroureterostomy.

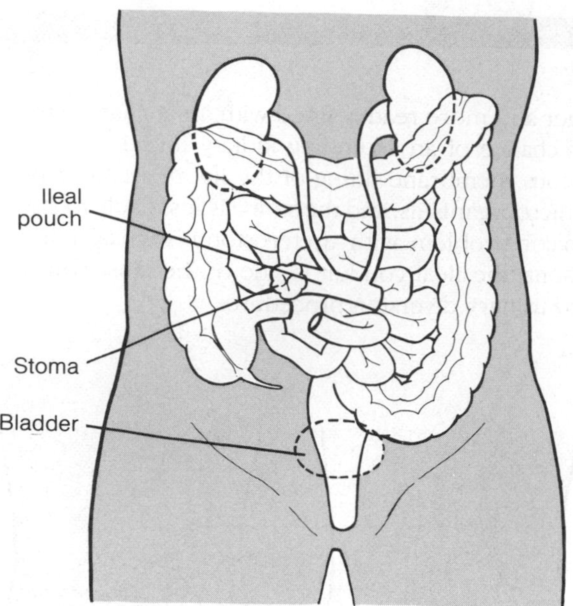

Figure 44–9 An ileal conduit.

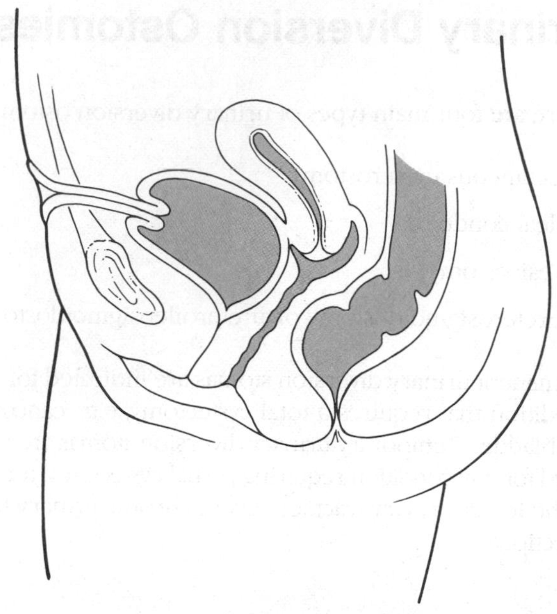

Figure 44–10 A continent vesicostomy.

Vesicostomy

In vesicostomy, the anterior wall of the bladder is sutured to the abdominal wall, and a stoma is formed from the bladder wall. The urethral neck is sutured closed so that urine from the bladder empties directly through the stoma. To provide urinary control, a *continent vesicostomy* is usually performed. See Figure 44–10. In this procedure a tube is formed from part of the bladder wall. A stoma is formed at one end of the tube. A nipplelike valve is created from the bladder wall at the internal end. Urine drains through this type of vesicostomy only after a catheter is inserted through the stoma into the bladder pouch.

Ureterosigmoidostomy

Ureterosigmoidostomy and ureteroileosigmoidostomy are two urinary diversion procedures that result in urine being excreted through the rectum. In ureterosigmoidostomy, the more common procedure, the ureters are implanted into the sigmoid colon. See Figure 44–11, *A*. One major complication with this type of procedure is pyelonephritis (infection of the kidney pelvis) from reflux of fecal material and intestinal microorganisms into the ureters and kidney pelvis. In ureteroileosigmoidostomy, a segment of the ileum is resected and connected to the sigmoid colon. The ureters are then implanted into this ileal pouch. See Figure 44–11, *B*. This procedure is thought to reduce the incidence of pyelonephritis. In both of these procedures, urine mixes with fecal material, resulting in very liquid stools and possible anal leakage of urine.

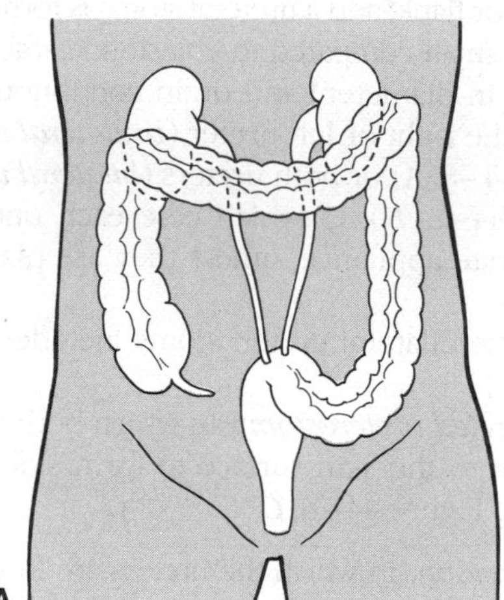

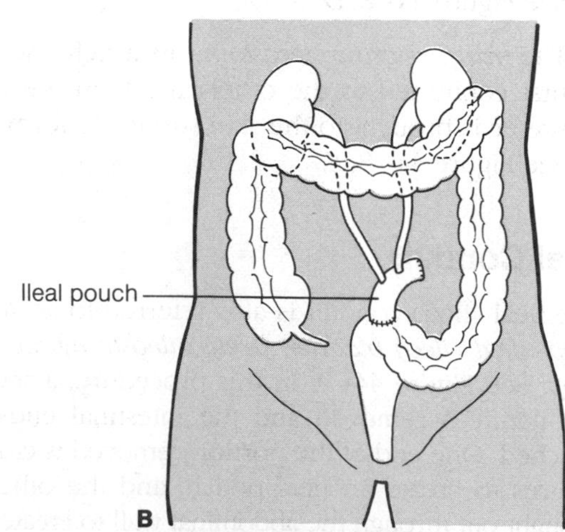

Figure 44–11 **A,** Ureterosigmoidostomy; **B,** ureteroileosigmoidostomy.

Nursing Diagnosis

Nursing diagnoses that relate to urinary tract function and urinary patterns include alteration in urinary elimination pattern, stress incontinence, reflex incontinence, functional incontinence, total incontinence, urge incontinence, urinary retention, potential for infection, altered comfort, potential fluid volume deficit or excess, disturbance in self-concept, and potential impairment of skin integrity.

Common urinary alterations the nurse encounters are urinary incontinence, urinary retention, and lower urinary tract infection. Incontinence can be physically and emotionally distressing to clients because it is considered socially unacceptable. Often the client is embarrassed about dribbling or about having an accident and may restrict normal activities for this reason. Emotional support and understanding need to be provided. With incontinence there is also risk of skin breakdown. Bed linens and clothes saturated with urine irritate and excoriate the skin. Prolonged skin dampness leads to **dermatitis** (inflammation of the skin) and subsequent decubitus ulcer formation.

Clients who have urinary retention not only experience discomfort but are also at risk of urinary tract infection. Distention of the bladder reduces blood flow to the mucosal layers, and tissues become more susceptible to bacterial invasion. Stasis of urine in the bladder provides an ideal media for bacterial growth and reproduction. Depending on the acidity and urea concentration of this urine in the bladder, infection may occur. Bacteria favor an alkaline media and a certain concentraiton of urea.

The most common cause of urinary tract infection is an invasive procedure such as catheterization or cystoscopic examination. In catheterization a urine drainage tube is inserted through the urethra into the bladder; in cystoscopic examination a diagnostic lighted instrument is inserted. These procedures provide a direct route for microorganisms to ascend through the urethra to the bladder and beyond into the ureters and kidneys. A catheter may also irritate urethral and bladder tissues, thus predisposing them to further risk of bacterial invasion.

Females in particular are prone to ascending urinary tract infections because of their short urethras. Microorganisms are normally present in the perineal area surrounding the urinary meatus, in the distal urethra, and in the vagina. Males, who have longer urethras and prostatic secretions containing antibacterial substances, are less prone. Factors contributing to urinary infections in females, e.g., cystitis or **urethritis**, include poor perineal hygiene, failure to wipe from the front to the back after voiding or defecating, inadequate handwashing, and frequent sexual intercourse.

With lower urinary tract infections clients often experience **dysuria** (burning during urination) due to passage of urine over inflamed tissues; frequency and urgency resulting from irritated tissues and disruption of normal micturition mechanisms; and, if the infection is acute, fever, chills, nausea, vomiting, and malaise. Urine appears cloudy due to the presence of pus (**pyuria**). With upper urinary tract infections the client experiences flank pain and tenderness, and chills.

Examples of nursing diagnoses are shown below. The North American Nursing Diagnosis Association uses the definitions of incontinence that follow (NANDA 1986):

Examples of Nursing Diagnoses Related to Urinary Elimination Problems

- Stress incontinence related to weak pelvic muscles and structural supports associated with increased age
- Functional urinary incontinence related to mobility deficit
- Reflex incontinence related to spinal cord lesion
- Total incontinence related to dysfunction causing triggering of micturition at unpredictable times
- Total incontinence related to independent contraction of detrusor reflex associated with surgery
- Total incontinence related to fistula between bladder and vagina
- Total incontinence related to trauma affecting spinal cord nerves
- Urge incontinence related to decreased bladder capacity
- Urge incontinence related to irritation of bladder stretch receptors, causing spasm
- Urge incontinence related to overdistention of bladder
- Urinary retention related to urethral blockage associated with enlarged prostate gland
- Urinary retention related to inhibition of micturition reflex arc
- Potential for urinary tract infection related to indwelling urethral catheter
- Potential for urinary tract infection related to urinary retention and stasis of urine
- Potential for impaired skin integrity related to incontinence
- Disturbance in self-concept related to inability to control urine
- Disturbance in self-concept related to enuresis
- Potential for fluid imbalance related to urinary retention

- *Stress incontinence:* a loss of urine of less than 50 ml occurring with increased abdominal pressure.
- *Reflex incontinence:* an involuntary loss of urine occurring at somewhat predictable intervals when a specific bladder volume is reached.
- *Functional incontinence:* an involuntary, unpredictable passage of urine.
- *Total incontinence:* a continuous and unpredictable loss of urine.
- *Urge incontinence:* an involuntary passage of urine occurring soon after a strong sense of urgency to void.

Planning

The overall goals for clients with potential or actual urinary elimination problems are maintenance or restoration of the client's normal urinary elimination pattern and prevention of potential associated risks such as infection, skin breakdown, fluid and electrolyte imbalance, and lowered self-esteem. For young children, promotion of urinary control and self-esteem may be included. The client's need for education must also be considered. For example, a female may need education about perineal hygiene; a male about self-care in regard to catheter care or insertion; and new parents about appropriate ways to toilet train their child.

Planning also involves the establishment of outcome criteria. For suggestions, see the "Evaluation" section later in this chapter.

Intervention

Maintaining Normal Urinary Elimination

Most interventions to maintain normal urinary elimination are independent nursing functions. These include maintaining an adequate fluid intake and maintaining normal voiding habits.

Fluid Intake

Increasing fluid intake increases urine production, which in turn stimulates the micturition reflex. A normal, average daily intake of 1200 to 1500 ml of measurable fluids is adequate for most clients. Additional amounts are required for clients whose fluid demands are great, e.g., those who have abnormal fluid losses from other routes, such as excessive perspiration, vomiting, or diarrhea. Immobilized clients who are susceptible to calculi formation require daily intakes of 2000 to 3000 ml per day. Dilute urine prevents urinary tract stones and infection. Increased fluid intakes are contraindicated in clients who require fluid restrictions, e.g., those with renal impairment or congestive heart failure. Measurement of a client's fluid intake is discussed in Chapter 46. Fluid intake can also be increased by encouraging the client to eat plenty of raw fruits and vegetables, which have a high water content.

Maintaining Normal Voiding Habits

Hospital routines and prescribed medical therapies can interfere with a client's normal voiding habits. The nurse can help clients maintain their normal voiding habits in a number of ways:

1. *Positioning.* Assist the client to a normal position for voiding: standing for males; for females, squatting or sitting. Use bedside commodes as necessary for females and urinals for males standing at the bedside. Voiding in a lying position is hindered because (a) movement of urine through the tract is not aided by gravity and, (b) intraabdominal pressure cannot be increased. To further enhance voiding in the standing or sitting positions, encourage the client to push over the pubic area with the hands or to lean forward. These measures increase intraabdominal pressure and external pressure on the bladder.
2. *Relaxation.* Relaxation is essential to initiate micturition. The nurse can help to promote relaxation by:
   a. Providing privacy for the client. Even children may be accustomed to privacy and may be unable to void in the presence of another person other than family members.
   b. Allowing the client sufficient time to void. Hurrying the client produces anxiety and tension.
   c. Providing sensory stimuli that may help the client relax. Although these methods do not have well-established rationales, they often succeed through the power of suggestion or other conditioned responses: Pour warm water over the perineum of a female or have the client sit in a warm bath to

promote muscle relaxation. Application of a hot-water bottle to the lower abdomen of both men and women may also foster muscle relaxation. Turn on running water within hearing distance of the client. Running water masks the sound of voiding for persons who find this embarrassing. And by the power of suggestion, flowing water may induce micturition. Stroke the inner thighs with light pressure or apply ice to stimulate sensory nerves that activate the micturition reflex. Place the client's hands in warm water. Offer the client some fluids. Some clients find that a drink of coffee or beer promotes urination. Allow the client to read or to listen to music.

d. Relieving physical and emotional discomfort that creates muscle tension and prevents the mental concentration that may be needed for micturition. Make sure that ordered analgesics and emotional support are provided the client.

3. *Timing.* When clients have the urge to void, nurses need to assist them immediately. Delays only increase the difficulty in starting to void, and the desire to void may pass. Timing is also important in offering toileting assistance to the client at his or her usual times of voiding, e.g., on awakening, before or after meals, and at bedtime.

4. *Bed-confined clients.* For bed-confined females who must use a bedpan, make sure the bedpan is warm. A cold bedpan may prompt contraction of her perineal muscles and inhibit voiding. Elevate the head of the client's bed to Fowler's position, place a small pillow or rolled towel at the small of the back to increase physical support and comfort, and have the client flex her hips and knees. This position simulates the normal voiding position as closely as possible. Assisting clients to use bedpans is discussed in Chapter 43. Some female clients may prefer to use a female urinal. Figure 44–12, *B,* shows a female urinal; Figure 44–12, *A,* shows a male urinal.

Assisting the Hospitalized Child to Urinate

Children who are hospitalized and separated from their parents may regress in their ability to control the bladder and may wet occasionally. On the child's admission to the hospital, the nurse records the child's stage of development and determines the methods of training that were or are being used. For example, the nurse finds out what equipment is being used, what words the child uses about urinating, and the times the child habitually urinates in the toilet each day. The child's customary methods of urinating should be continued in the hospital as much as possible. However, some children will have to use bedpans or urinals for a period of time. This equipment is

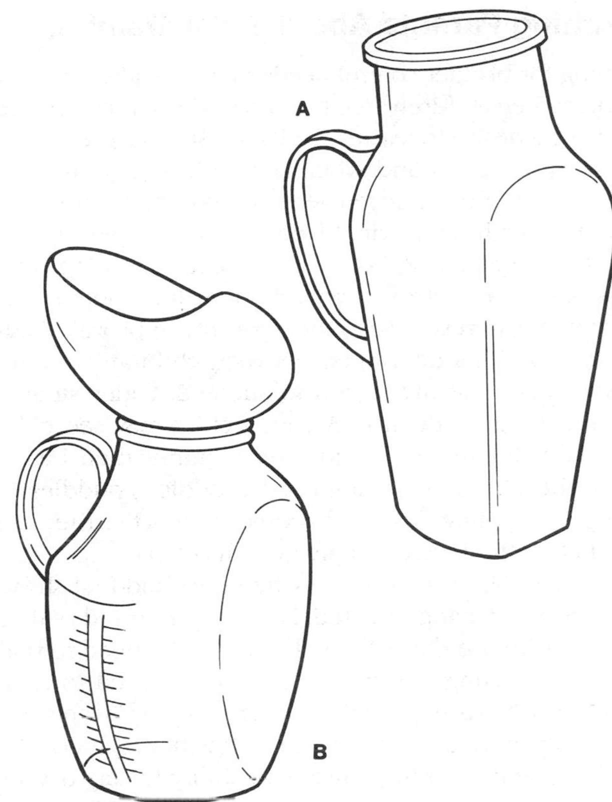

Figure 44–12 Two types of urinals: **A,** male urinal; **B,** female urinal.

best shown to the child in the parents' presence, with the hope that their approval will encourage the child to cooperate in using it.

Even children who are toilet trained have accidents. Children who wet accidentally in the hospital generally are upset and need understanding help and acceptance from the nurse. It is important that nurses examine their own feelings about children who wet or soil their beds or clothing. Feelings of repugnance need to be controlled.

If children are not toilet trained, it is advised that toilet training not be started while they are in the hospital, unless they are to have an extended stay. When young children are hospitalized, they feel abandoned by their parents and suffer enough emotional strain without adding the stress of toilet training. During a prolonged hospitalization, toilet training is planned and carried out by the parents and preferably by a nurse who is liked by the child.

A few children in the hospital use soiling as a means of gaining attention or getting even with their parents for abandoning them. In these instances the nurse needs to avoid censuring the child, accept this behavior in a matter-of-fact fashion, and determine the reason for the behavior. Together the nurse and the child need to work out a way to meet the child's love and attention needs more appropriately.

Teaching Parents About Toilet Training

Training for bladder control needs to be a gradual process, starting when children are physiologically mature enough and have a desire to learn. Usually it is started after bowel control has begun and when the child is able to hold urine for 2 hours. Children generally communicate when they are ready to begin bladder training, perhaps by pointing or gesturing before they begin urinating. Toddlers learn to control their urination, like their bowel movements, in response to their parents' approval. Trusting relationships developed between child and parents thus facilitate the motivation to succeed. Older siblings can also be an influence. A young child may see older children using the toilet and want to mimic their behavior, or the siblings may laugh at the toddler's puddles on the floor. As young children become more active they also find wet clothing increasingly uncomfortable.

Praise should be offered when the child first shows awareness of having urinated. However, a period of time must pass before the child will indicate the need to void prior to urinating. Specific words will be used to communicate what is expected, such as "pee" or "wee-wee." When the child has been dry for a few hours, he or she needs to be put on the toilet. The ability to stay dry for this amount of time generally occurs at about 18 months of age. Parents who say their children are trained before this age have probably trained themselves to catch the child's urination at regular times. The child can be helped to keep dry during the day by observing the usual times of urination and by taking the child to the toilet at these times, for example, before or after meals, before or after naps, before or after going outside, and before bedtime. It is not necessary for the child to remain on the toilet longer than a few minutes. The bladder will empty relatively quickly, since it is just starting to fill up to near capacity.

Training pants during the day and suitable clothing also assist the child. Changing the pants when they are even slightly wet helps the child to become accustomed to being dry, and being out of diapers can make him or her feel more grown up. A sense of independence is achieved with the use of pull-down trousers that the child can manage alone. Steps to enable the child to climb up to the adult toilet and an attachable child's seat may be helpful. Little boys first learn to urinate sitting down and learn to stand up to urinate by watching other males. Thus the age at which boys stand to urinate varies with their contact with older males. Little girls may also want to urinate in the standing position but soon realize the problems this creates.

A casual, patient, matter-of-fact attitude is required by parents for bladder training their children. This skill is learned more slowly than bowel control, and it has periods of success alternating with periods of failure or accidents. Growing children are active and busy, and, although they may have learned the signals of a full bladder, these signs may go unnoticed during play until an accident occurs. They then generally run to their parents to tell them about it, an indication that some responsibility about urinating has been learned. Wetting may also occur when children are excited.

Each time a child urinates in the toilet or training chair, praise and cuddling should be given. When the child fails to do so, it is best not to display disapproval or disappointment, or the child may develop feelings of fear or inferiority.

Nighttime bladder control takes even more time than daytime control. It is recommended that this not be hurried. Some advise that the child's intake of fluids be restricted in the late afternoon and evening; however, the child may then cry of thirst during the night. Getting the child up to urinate between 2200 and 2400 hours may help, but it is not advised if the child is antagonized by being wakened or has long periods of sleeplessness following. Increasing maturity generally brings nighttime control. Even when the child has acquired good control, there normally may be lapses in control when the child is too fatigued or is suffering emotionally.

Nursing Interventions for Urinary Incontinence

Nursing interventions for clients with urinary incontinence include a bladder-training program, meticulous skin care, and for males, application of an external drainage device (**condom**).

Bladder Training

A bladder-training program requires involvement of the nurse, the client, and support persons and includes the following steps:

1. Determine the client's voiding pattern and encourage voiding at those times, or establish a regular voiding schedule and help the client to maintain it, for example, every 1 or 2 hours, whether feeling the urge or not. Often when the client finds that voiding can be controlled this way, the intervals between voiding can be lengthened slightly without loss of continence. The stretching–relaxing sequence of such a schedule tends to increase bladder muscle tone and promote more voluntary control.
2. Regulate fluid intake, particularly before the client retires, to help reduce the need to void during the night. Fluids may be encouraged about half an hour before the voiding time; at other times they are carefully regulated. Usually fluids are encouraged between the hours of 0600 and 1800, or allow two hours between the last fluid and bedtime. Large amounts of fruit juices

and carbonated beverages are avoided, since fruit juice alkalizes the urine and soda pops cause bladder irritation. Due to the diuretic effects of stimulants, tea, coffee, and alcoholic beverages are avoided at bedtime to decrease the possibility of nocturia. A sufficient daily fluid intake (at least 2000 ml) is essential. Some incontinent clients have a tendency to reduce their fluid intake because they believe that the less fluids taken the less urine there is to void. Nurses need to explain to these clients that adequate urine production is needed to stimulate the micturition reflex. Clients who have fluid restrictions due to medical condition may be maintained on 1500 ml per day.

3. As a protective measure, apply protector pads to keep the bed linen dry, and provide specially made waterproof underwear to contain the urine and decrease the client's embarrassment. Avoid using "diapers," which are demeaning and also suggest that incontinence is permissible.
4. Assist the client with an exercise program to increase the tone of abdominal and pelvic muscles, which will aid micturition. Sit-ups with the knees bent can increase abdominal muscles, although these may be too strenuous for many clients. Kegel's exercises strengthen pubococcygeal muscles, thus increasing the ability to start and stop the urinary stream. To perform Kegel's exercises the client alternately contracts or tightens the perineal muscles as if trying to stop urination and then relaxes the muscle as if trying to void. Exercises should be performed three or four times each waking hour. The advantage of Kegel's exercises is that they can be performed anytime, anywhere, sitting or standing—even when voiding. The client is asked to intentionally stop and restart the urine stream. Increasing ability to start and stop the urinary stream is one indicator of voiding control.
5. Provide a system of positive and negative reinforcements to encourage continence. Such systems are commonly referred to as *behavior modification* and require the cooperation of all persons involved in the client's care. A positive reward, for example, might be allowing a client to watch a favorite television program each day he is continent for a specified number of hours.

Skin Care

Skin that is continually moist becomes macerated. Over a period of time urine that accumulates on the skin is converted to ammonia, which is very irritating to the skin. Since both skin irritation and maceration predispose the client to skin breakdown and decubiti, meticulous skin care is required for the incontinent person. To prevent alterations in skin integrity, wash the client's perineal area with soap and water after periods of incontinence, dry it thoroughly, and provide clean, dry clothing or bed linen. If the skin is irritated, apply barrier creams such as zinc oxide ointment to protect it from contact with urine. If it is necessary to pad the client's clothes for protection, use products that absorb wetness and leave a dry surface in contact with the skin.

Research Note

A study to determine the incidence of urinary incontinence and to demonstrate the results of nursing intervention that focused on assessment and retraining strategies was conducted within an acute geriatric assessment unit at a Veteran's Administration Medical Center on clients (primarily males) over 75 years of age. Of all clients admitted over a 7-month period, 19% were identified as incontinent of urine and were placed on a bladder-retraining program. At the time of discharge, 79% of these incontinent clients were continent.

Nurses play a leading role in preventing and treating urinary incontinence. The researcher concluded that nursing research must continue to explore and validate nursing interventions identified as successful for incontinence. Nursing practice based on reliable research findings will play an important part in minimizing urinary incontinence in the elderly. (Long 1985)

Research Note

A study was conducted using a sample of 43 females over the age of 60 who lived in a community setting. It aimed to:

1. Identify urinary incontinence.
2. Identify hidden urinary incontinence.
3. Identify the self-concept of these elderly females.

It was hypothesized that a negative self-esteem would result in hiding the symptoms of being incontinent. This hypothesis was not supported, since there were no statistical differences between the self-esteem scores in the continent and incontinent groups. The concept of hidden incontinence *was* supported in that 11 subjects (50%) identified as being incontinent did not reveal the symptom to a health care provider. The study also revealed that elderly women perceive the problem of urinary incontinence as a common problem that is inevitable with age, implying that elderly women need to be informed that incontinence is not normal. It was found, in addition, that physicians lack interest in the problem. (Simons 1985)

External Urinary Devices

The application of a *condom,* also referred to as a *urinary sheath* or *external catheter,* and attachment of its base to a urinary drainage system are commonly prescribed for males who experience incontinence. Use of a condom appliance is preferable to insertion of a retention catheter, because it avoids entrance into the urethra and bladder and minimizes the risk of urethral or bladder infection.

Methods of applying condoms vary with the length of time the condom is to be worn. Condoms that are to be worn for short periods are generally applied with elastic tape only; condoms that are to be worn for longer periods (e.g., a few days) require additional measures to protect the foreskin and to ensure secure attachment. The manufacturer's instructions need to be followed when applying a condom. Before applying the condom, the nurse assesses when the client experiences incontinence. Some clients may require a condom appliance at night only, others continuously. Procedure 44–2 describes how to apply and remove a drainage condom.

Procedure 44–2 ▲ Applying and Removing a Drainage Condom

Equipment

1. A condom drainage kit containing:
   a. A drainage condom made of plastic or rubber
   b. Elastic tape. Ordinary tape is contraindicated because it is not flexible and can stop blood flow.
   c. Skin paste or tincture of benzoin. A plasticized skin spray may also be used; it is more readily removed and less likely to irritate the skin.
   d. Skin bonding cement, also called *skin prep*
   e. Applicator swabs or tongue depressors
   f. A razor
   g. Extension tubing
   h. A leg drainage bag and straps
2. Soap, a basin of warm water, a washcloth, and a towel

Some commercially prepared appliances (e.g., Texas Catheter Navy drainage) are equipped with an adhesive foam strip. For these, skin spray, skin bonding cement, and elastic tape are not used. Instead, the adhesive foam or plastic strip is attached below the rolled edge of the condom and not against the skin. The following equipment is then required in addition to item 2:

3. The condom
4. A skin protector
5. A leg drainage bag and straps
6. Extension tubing

Intervention

Applying the Condom

1. Position the client in either a supine or a bed-sitting position, and cover the client's body with the bedclothes, exposing only the penis.
2. Inspect the penis for skin irritation (contact dermatitis), excoriation, swelling, or discoloration.
3. Clean the genital area, and dry it thoroughly, to minimize skin irritation and excoriation after the condom is applied.
4. Shave or trim any hair on the base of the penis unless a skin protector is being applied.

   Rationale Hair will adhere to the condom and cause discomfort when the condom is removed.
5. Remove the protective film from the underside of the plastic skin protector and apply the protector to the base of the penis. Then remove the protective film from the anterior surface of the skin protector.

   or

   Apply skin paste, tincture of benzoin, or plasticized skin spray around the base of the penis where the elasticized tape is to be applied. After the paste, tincture, or spray feels dry, apply a thin layer of skin bonding cement.
6. Roll the condom smoothly over the penis, leaving 2.5 cm (1 in) between the end of the penis and the rubber or plastic connecting tube. See Figure 44–13. Make sure that no pubic hair is caught in the condom. On some models the condom is rolled first so that the inner flap is exposed, which is applied around the urinary meatus to prevent the reflux of urine. See Figure 44–14.
7. Optional (depending on the kind of condom): Secure the condom firmly but not too tightly to the penis by wrapping a strip of elastic tape spirally around two-thirds the length of the penis, making sure that the spirals do not overlap.

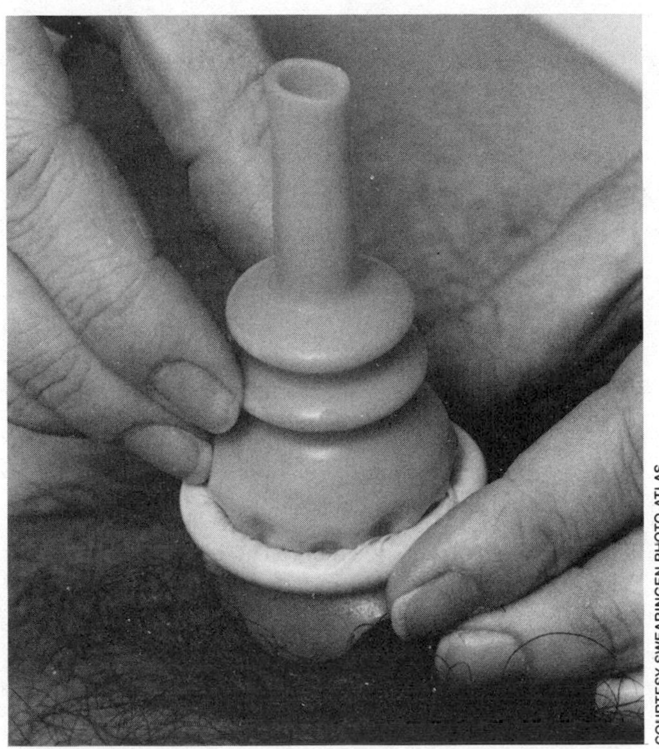

Figure 44–13

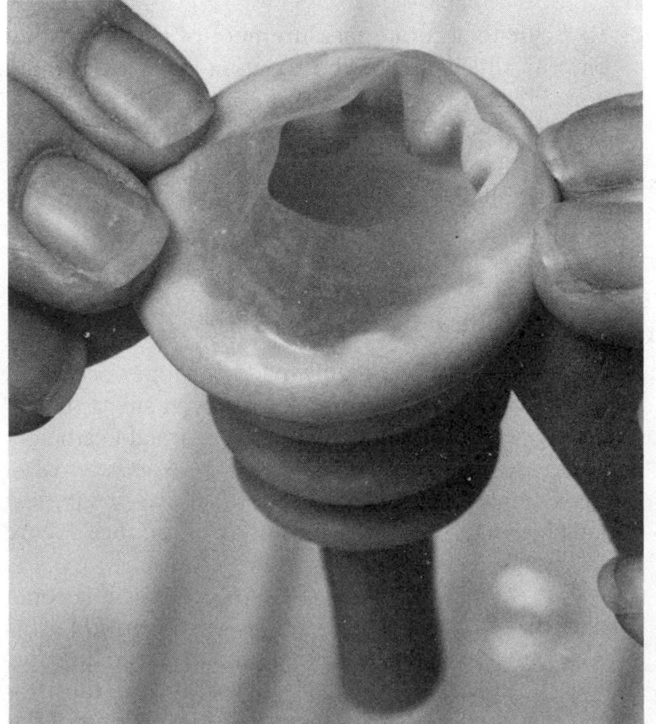

Figure 44–14

Rationale Overlapping spirals prevent the tape from stretching and could impede the blood circulation in the penis.

8. Attach the urinary drainage system securely to the condom. Make sure that the tip of the penis is not touching the condom and that the condom is not twisted.

   Rationale The condom could irritate the tip of the penis, and a twisted condom could obstruct the flow of urine.

9. Attach the urinary drainage bag to the bed frame if the client is to remain in bed, or to the client's leg if he is ambulatory. See Figure 44–15.

   Rationale Attaching the drainage bag to the leg helps control the movement of the tubing and prevents twisting of the thin material of the condom appliance at the tip of the penis.

10. Teach the client about attaching the drainage system to his leg, keeping the drainage bag below the level of the condom, and avoiding loops or kinks in the tubing.

11. Assess the urine for color and characteristics, e.g., clarity, odor.

12. Record the application of the condom, the time, and pertinent observations, such as irritated areas on the penis.

13. Observe the penis for swelling and discoloration 30 minutes following the application of the condom. Also check urine flow.

    Rationale Swelling and discoloration could indicate that the condom is too tight. Normally some urine will be present in the tube if the flow is not obstructed.

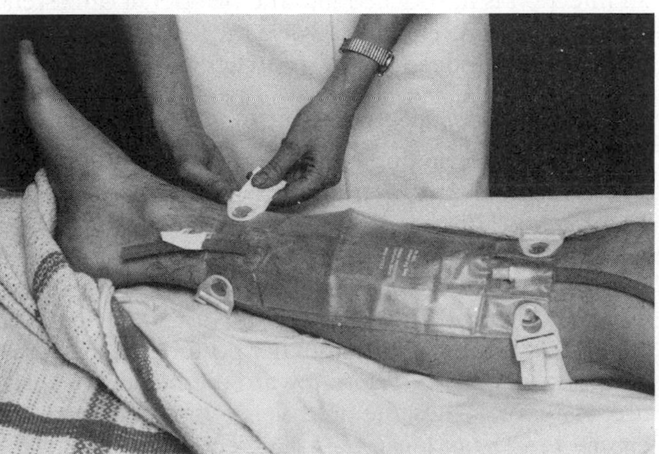

Figure 44–15

Removing the Condom

14. Remove the tape, if it was applied, and roll off the condom. Remove the plasticized skin spray (it peels off readily) or the skin protector every one or two days to provide skin care to the penis. Wash the penis with soapy water, rinse, and dry it thoroughly.
15. Change the condom daily, and assess the foreskin for signs of irritation, swelling, and discoloration.

Nursing Interventions for Urinary Retention

Interventions that assist the client to maintain a normal voiding pattern, discussed on page 1254, are applicable when dealing with urinary retention. If these actions are unsuccessful, the physician may order a cholinergic drug such as bethanecol chloride (Urecholine) to stimulate bladder contraction and facilitate voiding. For clients who have bladder **flaccidity** (weak, soft, and lax bladder muscles), manual exertion of pressure on the bladder may be necessary to force urine out. This is known as **Credé's maneuver** or *method*. It is not advised without the order of a physician and is used only for clients who have lost and are not expected to regain voluntary bladder control. For clients who are expected to regain control, this maneuver does not promote increased bladder muscle tone and may cause damage to the urethral sphincters. When all measures fail to initiate voiding, urinary catheterization may be necessary. See the next section.

Urinary Catheterization

Urinary catheterization involves the introduction of a catheter through the urethra into the urinary bladder. This is usually performed only when absolutely necessary, since certain hazards are incurred. Because the urinary structures are normally sterile except at the end of the urethra, the danger exists of introducing microorganisms into the bladder. This hazard is greatest for clients who have lowered resistance due to disease processes. Once an infection is introduced into the bladder, it can ascend the ureters and eventually involve the kidneys. Even after the catheter has been inserted and left in place for a time, the hazard of infection remains, since pathogens can be introduced through the catheter lumen. Thus, strict surgical asceptic technique is used for catheterizations.

Another hazard is trauma, particularly in the male client, whose urethra is longer and more tortuous. It is important to insert a catheter along the normal contour of the urethra. Damage to the urethra can occur if the catheter is forced through strictures or at an incorrect angle. For females, the urethra lies posteriorly, then takes a slightly anterior direction toward the bladder. See Figure 44–4. For males, the urethra is normally curved (see Figure 44–3), but it can be straightened by elevating the penis to a position perpendicular to the body.

Procedures to catheterize males and females are described later in this chapter.

Purposes of Catheterization

Clients are catheterized for a variety of reasons:

1. To relieve discomfort due to bladder distention and to provide gradual decompression of a distended bladder
2. To assess the amount of residual urine if the bladder is emptied incompletely
3. To obtain a urine specimen to assess the presence of abnormal constituents and the characteristics of the urine
4. To empty the bladder completely prior to surgery, to prevent inadvertent injury to adjacent organs such as the rectum or vagina
5. To manage incontinence when all other measures have failed
6. To provide for intermittent or continuous bladder drainage and irrigation
7. To prevent urine from contacting an incision after perineal surgery
8. To facilitate accurate measurement of urinary output for critically ill clients whose output needs to be monitored hourly

A straight or single-lumen catheter is usually used, except for purposes 4–8 above or as ordered by the physician.

Types of Urethral Catheters

Catheters are tubes commonly made of rubber or plastic, although certain types are made of woven silk or metal. Two categories of urinary catheters are straight catheters and retention catheters. The *straight* or *Robinson catheter* is a single-lumen tube with a small eye or opening about 1¼ cm (½ in) from the insertion tip. See Figure 44–16, *A*.

The *retention* or *Foley catheter* contains a second, smaller tube throughout its length on the inside. This tube is connected to a balloon near the insertion tip. After catheter insertion, the balloon is inflated to hold the catheter in place within the bladder. The outside end of the retention catheter is bifurcated, that is, it has two openings, one to drain the urine, the other to inflate the balloon. See Figure 44–16, *B*.

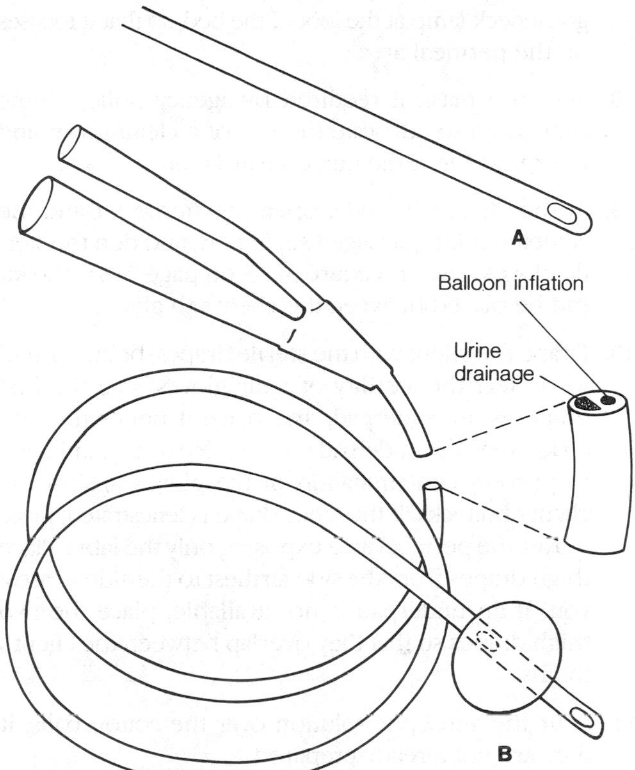

Figure 44–16 Two types of commonly used catheters: A, a straight (Robinson) catheter; B, a retention (Foley) catheter with the balloon inflated.

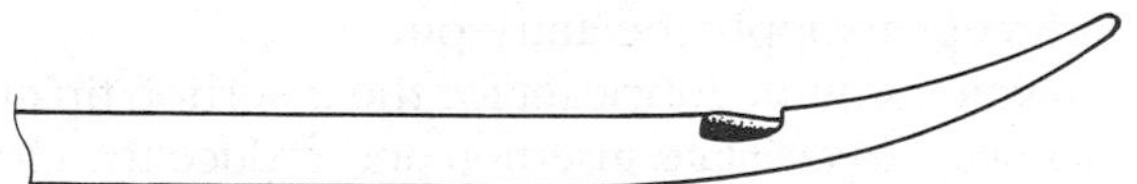

Figure 44–17 The catheter coudé, a urethral catheter with a curved tip.

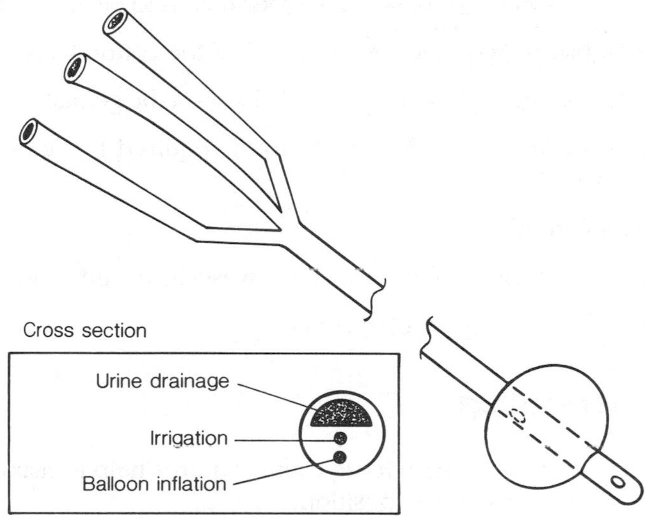

Figure 44–18 A three-way Foley catheter.

Another type of straight catheter is the *catheter coudé* (elbowed catheter), which has a curved tip. See Figure 44–17. This is sometimes used for elderly men who have a hypertrophied prostate, because its passage is often less traumatic to the gland than other types of straight catheters. It is somewhat stiff and is more readily controlled.

There are several other types of retention catheters. One that is frequently used for a client requiring continual or periodic bladder irrigations is the *three-way Foley catheter.* It is similar to the two-way Foley catheter described earlier, except that it has a third channel through which sterile fluid can flow into the urinary bladder. From the bladder, the fluid then flows through a second channel into a receptacle. See Figure 44–18.

Catheters are sized by the diameter of the lumen and are graded on a French scale of numbers; the larger the number, the larger the lumen. Small sizes, such as #8 or #10, are used for children; #14, #16, and #18 are commonly used for adults. Men frequently require a larger size than women. Only even numbers are available.

The balloons of retention catheters are sized by the volume of fluid or air used to inflate them. The two commonly used sizes are 5 ml and 30 ml balloons. The size of the balloon is indicated on the catheter along with the diameter, e.g., "#18 Fr.—5 ml."

Catheterization of males and females, using straight catheters, is described in Procedures 44–3 and 44–4, respectively.

Procedure 44–3 ▲ Female Urinary Catheterization Using a Straight Catheter

Equipment

1. A sterile catheterization kit containing:
   a. Gloves
   b. Drapes to protect the bed and to provide a sterile field
   c. A fenestrated drape (optional) to place over the perineum
   d. An antiseptic solution recommended by agency policy, e.g., aqueous benzalkonium chloride (Zephiran Chloride) 1:750, to clean the labia and urinary meatus
   e. Cotton balls or gauze squares to apply the antiseptic

f. Forceps to apply the antiseptic
g. A water-soluble lubricant for the insertion tip of the catheter to facilitate insertion and reduce the chance of trauma to the mucous membrane lining the urethra
h. A catheter of appropriate size (#14 or #16)
i. A receptacle for the urine. Often the base of the kit serves this purpose.
j. A specimen container if a specimen is to be acquired

2. A bag or receptacle for disposal of the cotton balls
3. A flashlight or lamp to provide light on the genital area
4. A mask, clean gown, and cap, if required by agency policy
5. A bath blanket
6. Soap, a basin of warm water, a washcloth, and a towel
7. Disposable gloves (optional)

Intervention

1. Obtain assistance if the client requires help to maintain the required position.
2. Explain the technique to the client, and provide support as needed. Some clients fear pain and need to learn that they will experience no pain, only a slight sensation of pressure.
3. Provide privacy. Exposure of the genitals is embarrassing to most clients.

   Rationale Relieving the client's tension can facilitate insertion of the catheter, because the urinary sphincters are more likely to be relaxed.
4. Assist the client to a supine position with knees flexed and thighs externally rotated. Pillows can be used to support the knees and elevate the buttocks.

   Rationale Raising the client's pelvis gives the nurse a better view of the urinary meatus.
5. Drape the client. Use a bath blanket to cover the client's chest and abdomen. Pull the client's gown up over her hips. Cover her legs and feet with the bed sheet or another blanket. Place it diagonally on the client with a corner around each foot. See Figure 35–3 on page 803.
6. Wash the perineal–genital area with warm water and soap; rinse and dry. Disposable gloves may be used.

   Rationale Cleanliness reduces the possibility of introducing microorganisms with the catheter. Appropriate rinsing removes soap that could inhibit the action of the antiseptic used later.
7. Adjust the light for vision of the urinary meatus. It may be necessary to use a flashlight or to place a gooseneck lamp at the foot of the bed, so that it focuses on the perineal area.
8. Put on a mask if required by agency policy. Some agencies also advocate the use of a clean gown and a surgical cap if the nurse's hair is long.
9. At the client's bedside, open the sterile kit and the catheter, if it is packaged separately, and don the sterile gloves (see Procedure 32–3 on page 718). The kit can be placed between the client's thighs.
10. Drape the client with the sterile drapes, being careful to protect the sterility of your gloves. Use the first drape as an underpad, and place it under the buttocks. Keep the underpad edges cuffed over your gloves to prevent contamination of the gloves against the client's buttocks. If the other drape is fenestrated, place it over the perineal area exposing only the labia. Place thigh drapes from the side farthest to the side nearest you. If an underpad is not available, place the two thigh drapes so that they overlap between the client's thighs.
11. Pour the antiseptic solution over the cotton balls, if they are not already prepared.
12. Lubricate the insertion tip of the catheter liberally. Place it aside in the sterile container ready for use.

    Rationale Water-soluble lubricant facilitates insertion of the catheter by reducing friction. It is important to lubricate at this point, because the nurse will subsequently have only one sterile hand available.
13. Separate the labia majora with the thumb and index or other finger of one hand, and clean the labia minora on each side using forceps and cotton balls soaked in antiseptic. Use a new swab for each stroke, and move downward from the pubic area to the anus. See Figure 44–19. Then separate the labia minora with two other fingers, still using the same hand. See Figure 44–20.

    Rationale The hand that touches the client becomes contaminated. It remains in position exposing the urinary meatus, while the other hand remains sterile holding the sterile forceps. Cleaning from anterior to posterior cleans from the area of least contamination to the area of greatest contamination.
14. Expose the urinary meatus adequately by retracting the tissue of the labia minora in an upward (anterior) direction. See Figure 44–20. Clean first from the meatus downward and then on either side, using a new swab for each stroke. Once the meatus is cleaned, do not allow the labia to close over it.

    Rationale Keeping the labia apart prevents the risk of contaminating the urinary meatus.
15. Assess any signs, such as excoriation of the tissues surrounding the urinary meatus, swelling of the uri-

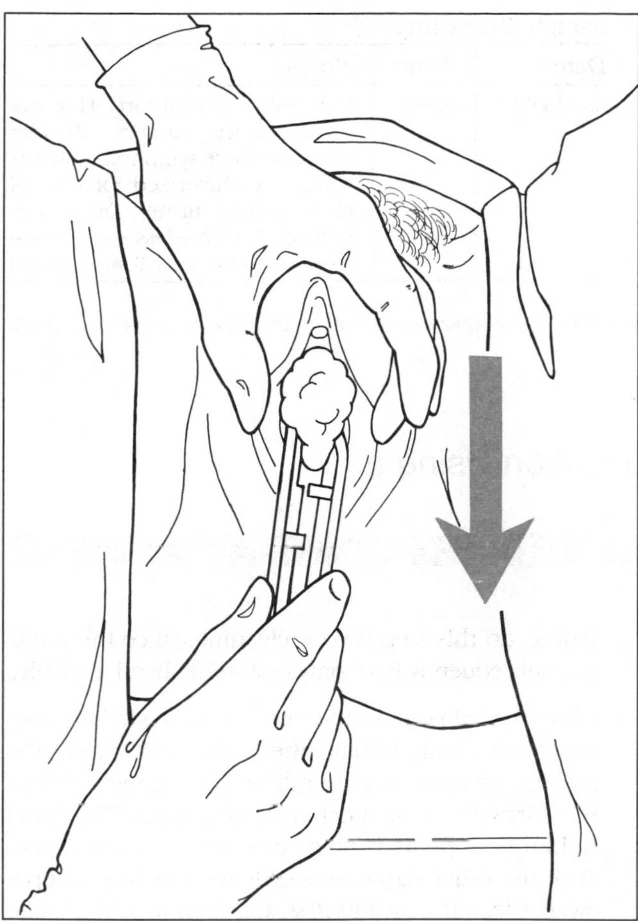

Figure 44–19

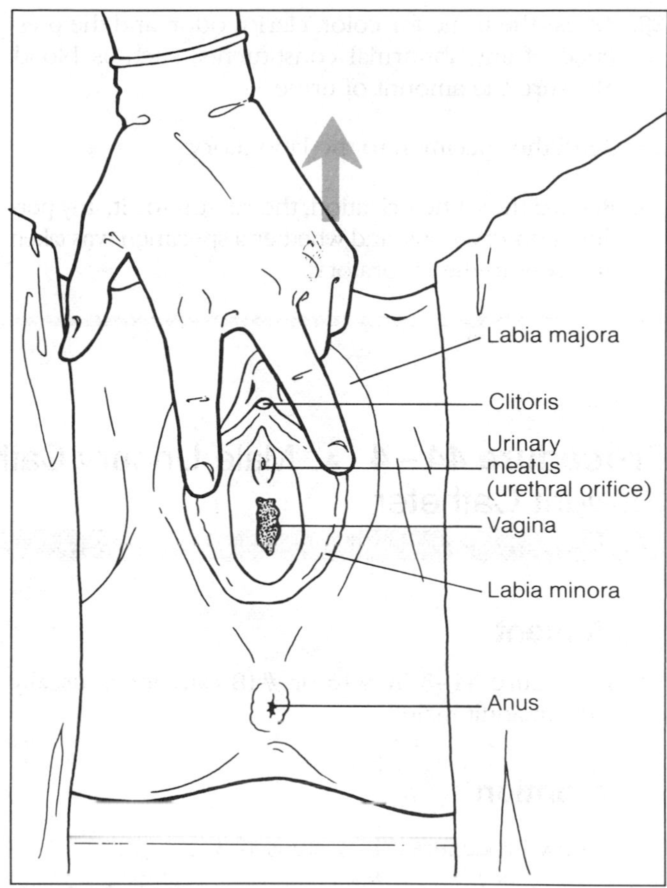

Figure 44–20

nary meatus, or the presence of discharge around the urinary meatus.

16. Place the drainage end of the catheter in the urine receptacle. Then pick up the insertion end of the catheter with your uncontaminated, sterile, gloved hand, holding it 5 to 8 cm (2 to 3 in) from the insertion tip for an adult and 2 to 3 cm (1 in) for an infant or small child. If agency policy requires, use sterile forceps to pick up the catheter.

    Rationale The adult female urethra is approximately 4 cm (1.5 in) long. The nurse holds the catheter far enough from the end to allow full insertion into the bladder and to maintain control of the tip of the catheter so it will not accidentally become contaminated.

17. Gently insert the catheter into the urinary meatus about 5 cm (2 in) for an adult, 2.5 cm (1 in) for a small child, or until urine flows. Insert the catheter in the direction of the urethra. If the catheter meets resistance during insertion, do not force it. Ask the client to take deep breaths. If this does not relieve the resistance, discontinue the procedure, and report the problem to the responsible nurse. Exercise caution to prevent the catheter tip from becoming contaminated. If it becomes contaminated, discard it.

    Rationale Forceful pressure exerted against the urethra can produce trauma. Deep breaths by the client may relax the external sphincter.

18. When the urine flows, transfer your hand from the labia to the catheter to hold it in place at the meatus.
19. Collect a urine specimen. Pinch the catheter, and transfer the drainage end of it into the sterile specimen bottle. Usually 30 ml of urine is sufficient for a specimen.
20. Empty the bladder or drain the amount of urine specified in the order. For adult clients experiencing urinary retention, it is recommended that no more than 750 ml be removed at one time. Remove the catheter slowly.

    Rationale Removing large amounts of urine too quickly can induce engorgement of the pelvic blood vessels and hypovolemic shock. Usually the physician prescribes the amount to be removed and times at which the remaining urine is to be withdrawn.

21. Dry the client's perineum with a towel or drape.

22. Assess the urine for color, clarity, odor, and the presence of any abnormal constituents, such as blood. Measure the amount of urine.

23. Send the specimen to the laboratory.

24. Record the catheterization, the reason for it, any pertinent observations, and whether a specimen was taken and sent to the laboratory.

Sample Recording

Date	Time	Notes
Jan/26/87	1900	C/o pubic discomfort. Has not voided since surgery. Bladder palpable above symphysis pubis. Is restless. Catheterized for 650 ml clear amber urine. Discomfort relieved. Less restless.——— ———Sylvia F. Tompkins, RN

Procedure 44–4 ▲ Male Urinary Catheterization Using a Straight Catheter

Equipment

See Procedure 44–3. A #16 or #18 catheter is usually used for an adult male.

Intervention

1. Follow Procedure 44–3, steps 1–3.
2. Assist the client to a supine position with the knees slightly flexed and the thighs slightly apart.

   Rationale This allows greater relaxation of the abdominal and perineal muscles and permits easier insertion of the catheter.
3. Drape the client by folding the top bedclothes down so that the penis is exposed and the thighs are covered. Use a bath blanket to cover the client's chest and abdomen.
4. Follow Procedure 44–3, steps 6–8.
5. Open the sterile tray, and don the sterile gloves (see Procedure 33–3). Place the tray directly on the client's thighs, if he is not restless.
6. Place a drape under the penis and a second drape above the penis over the pubic area. If a fenestrated drape is available, place it over the penis and pubic area, exposing only the penis.
7. Pour the antiseptic solution over the cotton balls, if they are not already prepared.
8. Lubricate the insertion tip of the catheter liberally for about 5 to 7 cm (2 to 3 in). Place it aside on the sterile tray ready for insertion.

   Rationale Water-soluble lubricant facilitates insertion of the catheter by reducing friction. It is important to do this step before cleaning, since the nurse will subsequently have only one sterile hand available.
9. Clean the urinary meatus with antiseptic swabs. Grasp the penis firmly behind the glans, and spread the meatus between the thumb and forefinger. Retract the foreskin of an uncircumcised male. The hand holding the penis is now considered contaminated. With the other hand use sterile forceps to pick up a swab. Clean the meatus first, and then wipe the tissue surrounding the meatus in a circular fashion. Discard each swab after only one wipe.

   Rationale To avoid stimulating an erection, firm pressure rather than light pressure is used to grasp the penis. Using forceps maintains the sterility of the nurse's glove.
10. Place the drainage end of the catheter in the urine receptacle. Then pick up the insertion end of the catheter with your uncontaminated, sterile, gloved hand, holding it about 8 to 10 cm (3 to 4 in) from the insertion tip for an adult or about 2.5 cm (1 in) for a baby or small boy. In some agencies the catheter is picked up with forceps.

    Rationale The male urethra is approximately 20 cm (8 in) long. The nurse holds the catheter far enough from the end to maintain control of the tip of the catheter so it will not accidentally become contaminated.
11. To insert the catheter, lift the penis to a position perpendicular to the body (90° angle) and exert slight traction (pulling or tension upward). Insert the catheter steadily about 20 cm (8 in) or until urine begins to flow. To bypass slight resistance at the sphincters, twist the catheter or wait until the sphincter relaxes. Have the client take deep breaths or try to void. If

difficult resistance is met, discontinue the procedure, and report the problem to the responsible nurse.

Rationale Lifting the penis perpendicular to the body straightens the downward curvature of the urethra. Slight resistance is normally encountered at the external and internal urethral sphincters. Deep breaths by the client can help to relax the external sphincter. Forceful pressure exerted against a major resistance can traumatize the urethra.

12. While the urine flows, lower the penis and transfer your hand to hold the catheter in place at the meatus.
13. Collect a urine specimen (if required) after the urine has flowed for a few seconds. Pinch the catheter, and transfer the drainage end of the catheter into the sterile specimen bottle. Usually 30 ml of urine is sufficient for a specimen.
14. Empty the bladder or drain the amount of urine specified in the order. For adult clients experiencing urinary retention, it is recommmended that no more than 750 ml be removed at one time. Remove the catheter slowly.

    Rationale Removing large amounts of urine too quickly can induce engorgement of the pelvic blood vessels and hypovolemic shock. Usually the physician prescribes the amount to be removed and times at which the remaining urine is to be withdrawn.
15. Dry the client's penis with a towel or drape.
16. Follow Procedure 44–3, steps 22–24.

Measuring Residual Urine

Residual urine is normally nil or only a few milliliters. However, whenever there is a bladder outlet obstruction (e.g., enlargement of the prostate gland) or loss of bladder muscle tone, there can be large amounts of residual urine. Loss of bladder tone may be the result of spinal or cranial neurologic disorders affecting the nerve and muscle regulation of the bladder, following pelvic surgery, or prolonged indwelling catheterization of the bladder. The consequence of incomplete emptying of the bladder is urinary stasis and, ultimately, infection.

Measurement of residual urine may be prescribed by the physician or responsible nurse in accordance with agency policy. Incomplete emptying of the bladder may be suspected when the client experiences frequency and when only small amounts of urine are voided at a time (e.g., 100 ml in an adult). The purposes of measuring the residual urine are: (a) to determine the degree to which the bladder is emptying, and (b) to assess the need to establish therapy that will empty the bladder (e.g., insertion of a retention catheter).

To measure the residual urine, the nurse asks the client to void and then immediately catheterizes the client. Both the amount of urine voided and the amount of residual urine are measured and recorded. Generally, if the amount of residual urine exceeds 50 ml, an in-dwelling catheter is inserted.

Procedure 44–5 ▲ Inserting a Retention Catheter

The procedure for inserting a urinary retention catheter is similar to the basic catheterization procedure, with differences occurring primarily after the catheter is inserted. Prior to insertion of the catheter, the nurse needs to test the balloon of the retention catheter to see that it is intact, and following the insertion, the nurse inflates the balloon and attaches a urinary drainage system.

Equipment

In addition to the equipment used for a straight catheterization, the following equipment is needed:

1. A retention catheter, #14 or #16 for adults, #8 or #10 for children. The catheter may be supplied separately from the sterile set in some agencies. The catheter may be attached to sterile tubing and a receptacle for the urine (closed drainage system). See Figure 44–21. If these are not in the set, acquire a drainage bag and tubing.
2. A prefilled syringe to inflate the balloon of the catheter. Sterile water is often used.
3. Nonallergenic tape to secure the catheter to the client.
4. A safety pin or clip to attach the catheter tubing to the bedding.

Intervention

1. Explain to the client the reason for inserting the retention catheter, how long it will be in place, and the ways in which the urinary drainage equipment

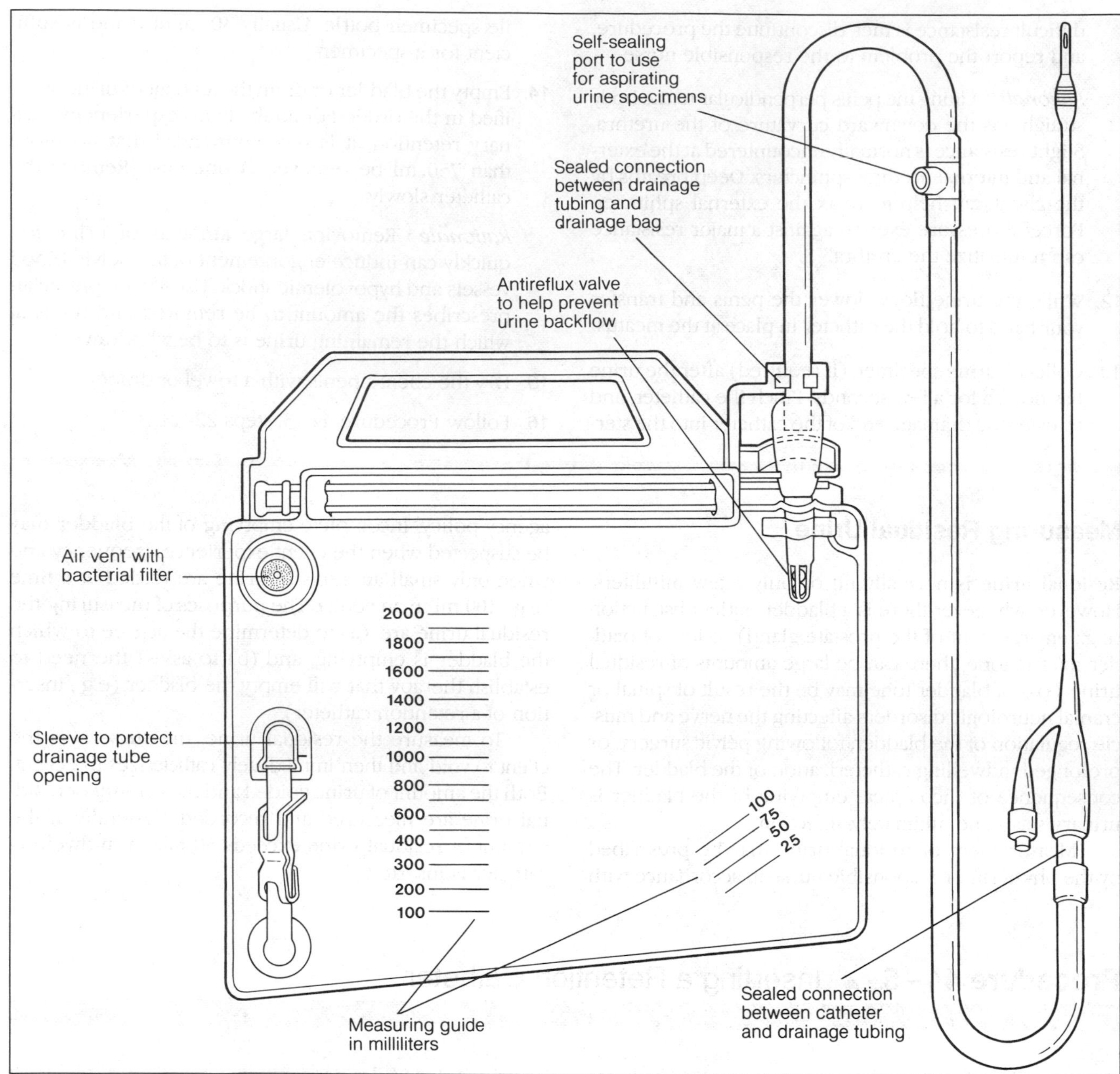

Figure 44–21 A closed urinary drainage system.

needs to be handled to maintain and facilitate the drainage of urine. Reassure the client that the procedure is painless. Some clients fear spillage of urine when they experience the urge to void during insertion of the catheter and for a short period of time after the catheter is in place. Reassure these clients that the catheter drains the urine and that the urge to void will disappear.

2. Follow procedure as for straight catheterization up to and including draping the client.

3. Test the catheter balloon by attaching the prefilled syringe to the balloon valve and injecting the fluid. The balloon should inflate appropriately and should not leak. Withdraw the fluid, and set aside the catheter with the syringe attached for later use. If the balloon leaks or does not inflate adequately, replace the catheter. In such a case, withdraw the fluid, and detach the syringe for later use. Ask another nurse to obtain a second catheter and open the package for you, then test the new balloon.

or

Remove the equipment and obtain another catheter. Then start the Intervention over with the new sterile equipment.

4. Follow steps as for straight catheterization to:
   a. Lubricate the injection tip of the catheter.
   b. Remove the sterile cap from the specimen container.
   c. Separate and clean the urinary meatus and surrounding tissues.
   d. Insert the catheter.
   e. Collect a urine specimen as required.

5. Insert the catheter an additional 2.5 to 5 cm (1 to 2 in) beyond the point at which urine began to flow.

   Rationale The balloon of the catheter is located behind the opening at the insertion tip, and sufficient space needs to be provided to inflate the balloon. This ensures that the balloon is inflated inside the bladder and not in the urethra, where it could produce trauma.

6. Inflate the balloon by injecting the contents of the prefilled syringe into the valve of the catheter. See Figure 44–22, *A*. Placement of the catheter and balloon in a male client is shown in Figure 44–22, *B*. If the client complains of discomfort or pain during the balloon inflation, withdraw the fluid, insert the catheter a little farther, and inflate the balloon again. Insert no more fluid than the balloon size indicates (e.g., 5 ml or 30 ml), and remove the syringe. A special valve prevents backflow of the fluid out of the catheter. When 30-ml balloons are used, some agency policies state that only 15 ml of fluid is injected for inflation.

7. When the balloon is safely inflated, apply slight tension on the catheter until you feel resistance. Then move the catheter slightly back into the bladder.

   Rationale Resistance indicates that the catheter balloon is inflated appropriately, and the catheter is well anchored in the bladder. Moving the catheter slightly back into the bladder keeps the balloon from exerting undue pressure on the neck of the bladder.

8. If the drainage bag and tubing are not already attached to the end of the catheter, remove the protective cap or plug from the tubing, and attach the catheter. Handle the ends of both the catheter and the drainage tube at least 2.5 cm (1 in) away from their tips.

   Rationale The sterility of the tips of both the catheter and the drainage tube must be maintained so that microorganisms do not enter the system and move to the bladder.

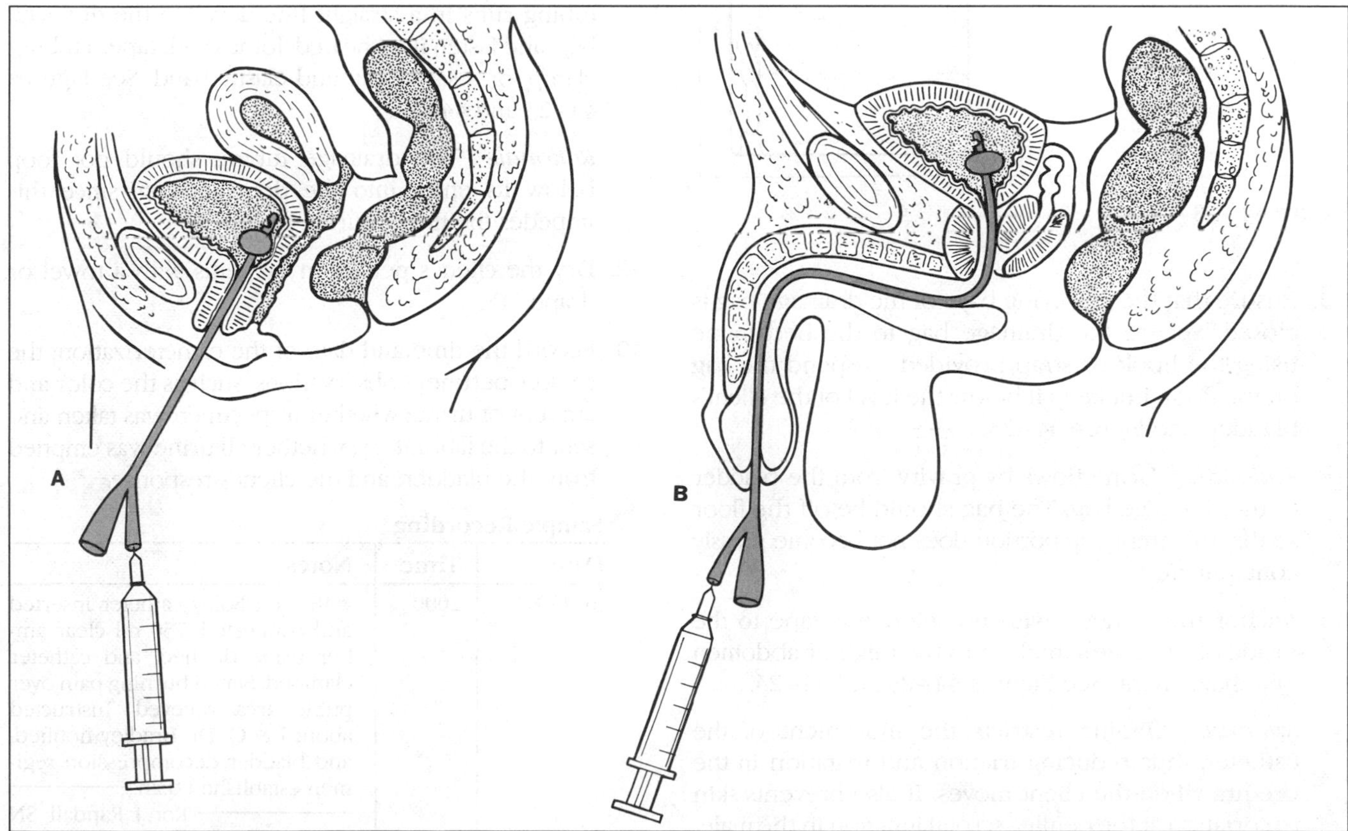

Figure 44–22

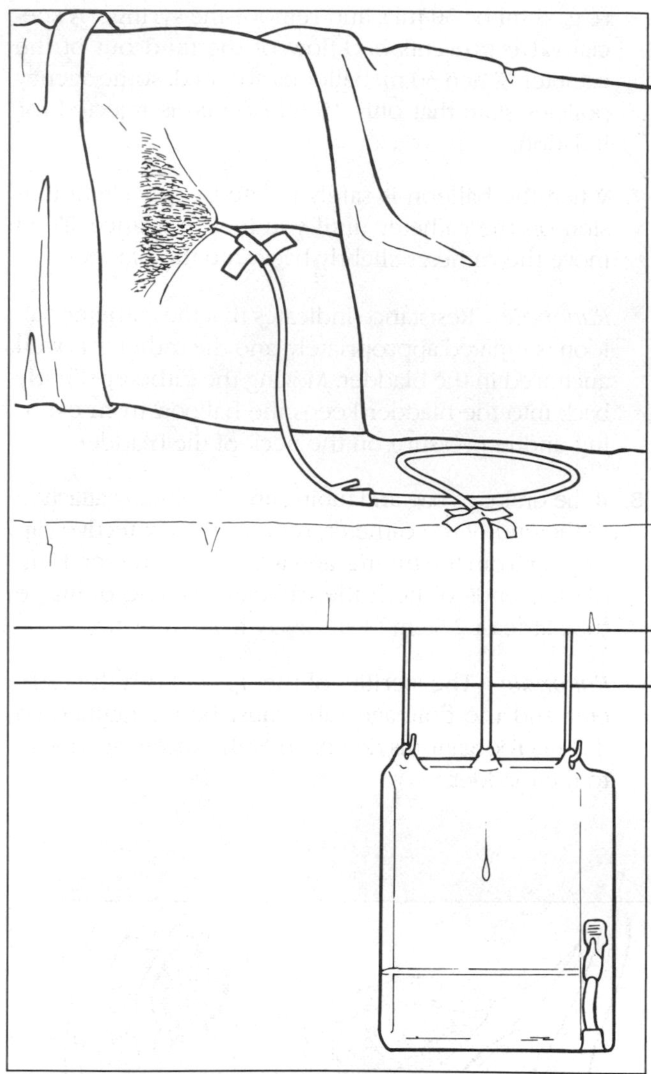

Figure 44–23

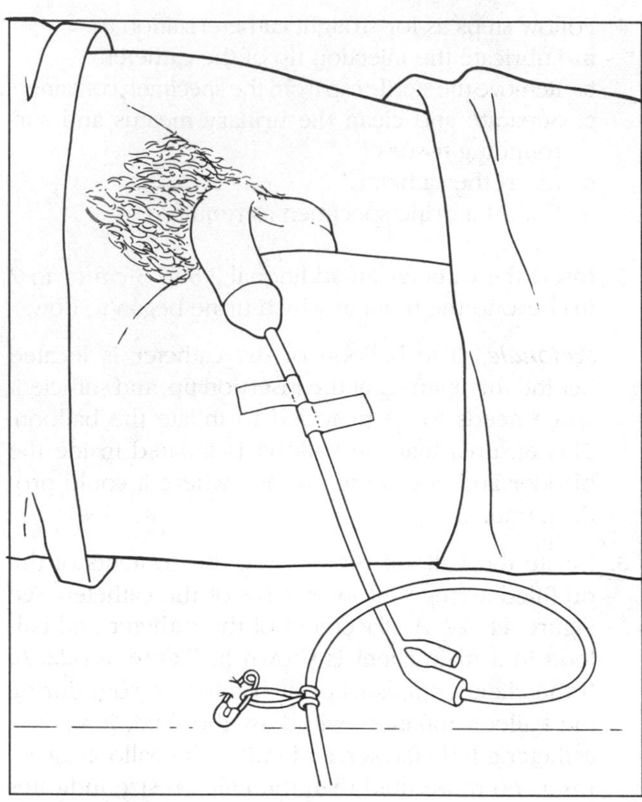

Figure 44–24

9. Ensure that the emptying base of the drainage bag is closed. Secure the drainage bag to the bed frame using the hook or strap provided. Suspend the bag off the floor, but keep it below the level of the client's bladder. See Figure 44–23.

   Rationale Urine flows by gravity from the bladder to the drainage bag. The bag should be off the floor so that the emptying portion does not become grossly contaminated.

10. Anchor the catheter with nonallergenic tape to the inside of a female's thigh or to the thigh or abdomen of a male client. See Figures 44–23 and 44–24.

    Rationale Taping restricts the movement of the catheter, thus reducing friction and irritation in the urethra when the client moves. It also prevents skin excoriation at the penile–scrotal junction in the male.

11. Coil the drainage tubing beside the client so that the tubing runs in a straight line down to the drainage bag, and fasten it to the bedclothes with tape, a tubing clamp, or a safety pin and elastic band. See Figures 44–23 and 44–24.

    Rationale The drainage tubing should not loop below its entry into the drainage bag, since this impedes the flow of urine by gravity.

12. Dry the client's perineum or penis with a towel or drape.

13. Record the time and date of the catheterization; the reason; pertinent observations, such as the color and amount of urine; whether a specimen was taken and sent to the laboratory; whether all urine was emptied from the bladder; and the client's response.

Sample Recording

Date	Time	Notes
Jul/12/87	2000	#18 5-ml Foley catheter inserted and connected. 750 ml clear amber urine drained, and catheter clamped. Stated burning pain over pubic area relieved. Instructed about I & O. Dr. Bradley notified, and bladder decompression regimen established q.2h.——————Ron J. Randall, SN

Nursing Intervention for Clients with Retention Catheters

Nursing care of the client with an indwelling catheter and continuous drainage is largely directed toward preventing infection of the urinary tract and encouraging urinary flow through the drainage system. It includes encouraging large amounts of fluid intake, accurate recording of the fluid intake and output, providing perineal–genital care, providing catheter care, changing the retention catheter and tubing, maintaining the patency of the drainage system, preventing contamination of the drainage system, and teaching these measures to the client.

Fluids and Fluid Balance

An appropriate fluid balance is essential for the client with a retention catheter to minimize the risk of infection. Encourage the client to drink up to 3000 ml per day if permitted. Large amounts of fluid ensure a large urine output, which keeps the bladder flushed out and decreases the likelihood of urinary stasis and subsequent infection. Large volumes of urine also minimize the risk of sediment or other particles obstructing the drainage tubing. Accurate recording of fluid intake and output is discussed in Chapter 46.

Dietary Measures

Many agencies implement prophylactic measures to acidify the client's urine to prevent urinary infection. By changing the composition of the diet, the urine can be made either acid or alkaline. Most vegetables and fruits yield an alkaline urine, whereas meat, fish, fowl, eggs, and cereals yield an acid urine. Alkalinization of the urine may be warranted to soothe an irritated bladder.

Perineal–Genital Care

Perineal–genital care is recommended at least twice daily or as needed for the client with an indwelling catheter. It is considered one of the most significant measures for reducing the incidence of infection. Any secretions or encrustations that accumulate at the urethral orifice provide an excellent medium for pathogens, which can ascend the tract. Most agencies recommend specific cleaning methods. Some advocate routine perineal–genital care with warm water and soap. For the uncircumcised male client, the foreskin is retracted to clean well under it.

Catheter Care

Clients with retention catheters require special catheter care once or twice a day in addition to the perineal–genital care described in Chapter 36. This is because microorganisms on the catheter and at the urinary meatus can ascend into the urethra and bladder and cause an infection. Catheter care is usually given directly after perineal–genital care. Because catheter care varies considerably from agency to agency, check agency practice. Agencies provide different types of equipment and solutions for cleaning clients who have catheters. See Procedure 44–6 for steps in providing catheter care.

Procedure 44–6 ▲ Providing Catheter Care

Equipment

1. A sterile catheter care kit containing:
   a. A drape to cover the legs and perineal area around the catheter and the urinary meatus
   b. Gloves to wear during the procedure
   c. An antiseptic solution, such as a water-soluble iodine solution
   d. Cotton balls or applicator swabs
   e. An antibiotic ointment, such as neomycin, or hydrocortisone
   f. Sterile forceps
   g. A small receptacle for the discarded balls or swabs
2. A bath blanket (optional)

Intervention

1. Discuss the possibility that the client may provide his or her own care. Because of exposure of the genital area, some clients find this procedure embarrassing and often prefer to learn to do it themselves.
2. Arrange the bedclothes or bath blanket so that only the perineal area is exposed.
3. Open the sterile catheter care kit using surgical asceptic technique.
4. Don the sterile gloves.
5. Drape the client.

6. Pour antiseptic on the cotton balls or swabs.
7. Put some sterile ointment on one cotton ball or swab.
8. Assess the area around the urinary meatus for inflammation, swelling, and discharge. Determine the color, amount, and consistency of any discharge. Note any odor from the area.
9. Clean the perineal–genital area, using forceps and cotton balls or swabs. Use each swab only once.
   a. For a female client, clean the labia majora, moving downward. Then separate the labia majora with your thumb and fourth finger, and clean the labia minora. Then separate them with the index and middle fingers of the same hand. Expose the urinary meatus adequately by retracting the tissue of the labia minora in an upward (anterior) direction. Clean first from the meatus and catheter downward and then on either side.
   b. For a male client, clean the meatus by grasping the penis behind the glans and spreading the urinary meatus between your thumb and forefinger. Retract the foreskin of an uncircumcised male. Clean the meatus around the catheter first, and then wipe the tissue surrounding the meatus in a circular fashion.
10. Assess the area around the urinary meatus for:
    a. Discomfort experienced by the client.
    b. Inflammation or swelling.
    c. Discharge (note the color, amount, and consistency).
    d. Odor.
11. Using a new swab, clean along the catheter for about 10 cm (4 in). Use a circular motion to ensure that all sides of the catheter are cleaned.
12. Apply antiseptic ointment around the base and along about 2.5 cm (1 in) of the catheter.

    Rationale This protects the urethra from infection.
13. Inspect the patency of the drainage system.
14. Record on the client's chart the procedure, the time, and pertinent assessment data. Report any problems to the responsible nurse.

Sample Recording

Date	Time	Notes
Apr/30/87	0900	Catheter care given. No apparent urethral redness or swelling. Small amount of thick white discharge around base of catheter. No complaints of discomfort.——Yvonne A. Able, NS

15. Check and adjust the nursing care plan, if necessary, to include regular catheter care.

Changing the Catheter and Tubing

Agency policies may specify the frequency of catheter and tubing changes. Some agencies advocate that both be changed weekly or every other week; others change the catheter only when sediment accumulates at the distal end. Sediment is present if you feel sandy particles when rolling the end of the catheter between your thumb and fingers. The drainage bag and tubing are generally changed along with the catheter but need to be changed more frequently if sediment accumulates, if leakage occurs, or if a strong odor is evident. Recommendations for changes are made on the basis of reducing the incidence of infection and preventing unpleasant odors. Some authorities recommend that catheters be changed as infrequently as possible.

During tubing changes, strict sterile technique is essential to prevent contamination of the distal lumen of the catheter. The nurse acquires a new sterile drainage bag and tubing, a sterile towel or sterile gauzes, clamp, and antiseptic solution. The steps involved are:

1. Wash hands using surgical aseptic technique.
2. Open the sterile towel or sterile gauze.
3. Open the new drainage and tubing package.
4. Remove the protective cap from the drainage tube, and place the open end of the tubing on the sterile towel or gauze.
5. Clamp the catheter above the tubing connector, clean the catheter–tubing junction with an antiseptic solution, and disconnect the catheter from the old tubing, being careful to not contaminate the end of the catheter.
6. Connect the catheter to the new tubing.
7. Unclamp the catheter, and establish drainage by securing the tubing and drainage receptacle to the bed at an appropriate level.
8. Apply waterproof tape around the connection site of the catheter and the tubing, if recommended, to ensure a closed drainage system.

Maintaining Patency of the Drainage System

To ensure continual patency of the system, nurses need to:

1. Ensure that there are no obstructions in the drainage. For example, check that there are no kinks in the tubing, the client is not lying on the tubing, and the tubing is not clogged with mucus or blood.

2. Check that there is no tension on the catheter or tubing, that the catheter is securely taped to the thigh or abdomen, and that the tubing is fastened appropriately to the bedclothes.
3. Ensure that gravity drainage is maintained. For example, check that there are no loops in the tubing below its entry to the drainage receptacle and that the drainage receptacle is below the level of the client's bladder.
4. Ensure that the drainage system is well sealed or closed. For example, check that there are no leaks at the connection sites in open systems. You may apply waterproof tape around the connection site of the catheter and tubing to ensure closure.
5. Observe the flow of urine every 2 or 3 hours, and note color, odor, and any abnormal constituents. If blood clots are present, check the catheter more frequently to ascertain whether it is plugged.

Preventing Contamination of the Drainage System

Some agencies recommend instillation of hydrogen peroxide in the drainage bag of open systems to prevent the growth of microorganisms in the bag and to reduce odor. Agency policies vary, however.

When emptying the drainage bag, the nurse must maintain surgical aseptic technique. The bag is emptied usually at the end of each shift of duty, and the tube at the bottom of the bag is used to drain the bag. The amount of drainage is noted in accordance with calibrations on the bag, or a graduated pitcher is brought to the bedside to assess the output. It is important for the nurse not to contaminate the end of the tubing and to reattach it appropriately when the bag is emptied.

Guidelines to prevent catheter-associated urinary tract infections are given to the right.

Client Education

Usually nurses need to teach the client some principles about the gravity drainage system and the importance of maintaining a closed system. The client has to understand that the drainage tubing and drainage bag need to be kept lower than the bladder at all times. The client also needs to know how to prevent tension on the catheter tubing, to prevent loops or kinks in the drainage tubing, and to avoid lying on the tubing. Understanding how to manipulate the system when ambulating can give the client a sense of independence. Some clients will also benefit from instruction about fluid intake measurement and self perineal–genital care. Clients who wish to be involved in recording fluid intake measurements will need information about how to compute these values and which foods are considered fluids.

Guidelines to Prevent Catheter-Associated Urinary Tract Infections

- Have an established infection control program.
- Catheterize clients only when necessary, by using aseptic technique, sterile equipment, and trained personnel.
- Maintain a sterile closed-drainage system.
- Do not disconnect the catheter and drainage tubing unless absolutely necessary.
- Remove the catheter as soon as possible.
- Follow and reinforce good handwashing technique.
- Changing indwelling catheters at arbitrary, fixed intervals and regular bacteriologic monitoring of catheterized clients are not cost-effective practices and should not be performed.
- Avoid other measures until further data are available. New products that appear to be questionable or gimmicky probably should be avoided.
- Although instillation of H_2O_2 into the outlet tube of the drainage set or into the drainage bags has been associated with a reduction in bag contamination, studies indicate no difference in the rate of bag-source infection in clients with the suggested instillation of H_2O_2 into the drainage bag when compared with clients who had conventional closed-drainage systems. (Epstein 1985)

Catheter Removal

Retention catheters are removed after their purpose has been achieved, usually on the order of the physician. A few days prior to removal the catheter may be clamped for specified periods of time (e.g., 2 to 4 hours) and then released. This causes some distention of the bladder and stimulation of the bladder musculature. See Procedure 44–7 for steps to remove a retention catheter.

Procedure 44–7 ▲ Removing a Retention Catheter

Equipment

1. A receptacle for the catheter after its removal, e.g., a kidney basin
2. A syringe to deflate the balloon. A needle may also be required to deflate some types of balloons.

3. Cotton balls to dry the genital area
4. Disposable gloves, if desired, to protect the nurse

Intervention

1. Clamp the catheter.

   Rationale This prevents spillage of urine that might remain in the catheter.

2. Insert the syringe into the balloon inflation tube of the catheter and draw out all the fluid.

   Rationale The balloon needs to be completely deflated to prevent trauma to the urethra when the catheter is withdrawn.

3. Gently withdraw the catheter from the urethra.
4. Place the catheter in the kidney basin or other receptacle.
5. Dry the genital area with cotton balls.
6. Measure the urine in the drainage bag.
7. Record the time the catheter was removed and the amount, color, and consistency of the urine in the drainage bag.
8. Adjust the nursing care plan to:
   a. Encourage the client to drink up to 3,000 ml of fluid daily if not contraindicated.

      Rationale If the urethra has been irritated by the catheter, the client may experience some burning when voiding. This problem is minimized by diluting the urine with an increased fluid intake.

   b. Monitor the client's fluid intake and output.
9. Assess the frequency of voiding, or any unusual symptoms related to voiding following the procedure. Prolonged, continuous drainage of urine through an indwelling catheter causes loss of bladder tone. The bladder remains relatively empty and thus is never stretched to its capacity. When a muscle fails to be stretched regularly, atrophy develops. When a catheter is removed, the client may have difficulty regaining urinary control.
10. Assess fluid intake and output following the technique.

Obtaining a Urine Specimen from a Retention Catheter

Sterile urine specimens can be acquired from closed drainage systems by inserting a sterile 1-in needle (#21 to #25 gauge), attached to a 3-ml syringe, into the end of the catheter or through a drainage port in the tubing. See Figure 44–25. Note that aspiration of urine from catheters can be done only with self-sealing rubber catheters, not plastic, silicone, or silastic catheters.

First the nurse cleans the entry point of the needle with a disinfectant swab. The needle is then inserted at an angle, to facilitate self-sealing of the rubber, and at a place where it will not puncture the tube leading to the balloon. If the urine is not readily available, the drainage tubing is elevated slightly to return urine to the area or the catheter is pinched or clamped about 5 to 7 cm (3 in) from its tip for a short period until urine appears.

After the urine is drawn into the syringe, the nurse transfers it to a *sterile* specimen container, caps the container, labels it, and sends it to the laboratory immediately for analysis or refrigeration.

Urinary Irrigations and Instillations

An *irrigation* is a flushing or washing-out using a specified solution. A *bladder irrigation* is carried out on a physician's order, usually to wash out the bladder and/or apply an antiseptic solution to the bladder lining to treat a bladder infection. Sterile technique is used. *Catheter irrigations* are usually carried out to maintain or restore the patency of a catheter, e.g., to remove pus or blood clots that have formed in the bladder and are blocking the catheter. A physician's order may or may not be required, depending on agency policy.

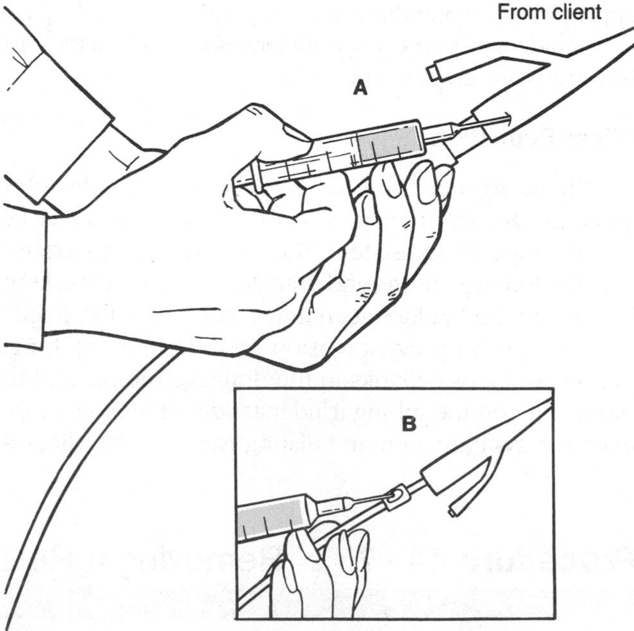

Figure 44–25 Obtaining a urine specimen from a retention catheter: **A,** from a specific area, sometimes designated by a patch, near the end of the catheter; **B,** from a drainage port in the tubing.

In a bladder *instillation,* a small amount of liquid is placed in the bladder and allowed to remain there for a specific period of time. For example, an antiseptic solution may be instilled through a catheter, which is then clamped for 30 minutes so that the antiseptic will remain in contact with the walls of the bladder. Bladder instillations and irrigations are rarely performed because of the danger of transmitting microorganisms into the urinary bladder.

In the usual bladder irrigation or instillation, either a two-way Foley catheter is already in place or a straight catheter is inserted.

For a bladder irrigation, the frequency, and the type, amount, and strength of solution to be used are ordered by the physician. If the physician has not specified these on the client's chart, check agency policies. Some agencies recommend the use of sterile normal saline at room temperature for both catheter and bladder irrigations. To irrigate an adult bladder, 1,000 ml is commonly used; for a catheter irrigation, 200 ml is normally required. The strength, amount, and kind of medication for a bladder instillation are specified by the physician.

Irrigations performed via straight gravity drainage are referred to as *plain irrigations.* A variation of the plain irrigation is the intermittent irrigation, in which one lumen of a three-way catheter is connected by tubing to a drip chamber and then to a container of sterile solution. The second lumen is attached to tubing and then to a urine receptacle. See Figure 44–26. There are clamps on both tubes. The clamp from the solution container (*A*) is released while the clamp to the urine bag (*B*) is closed. The fluid enters and remains in the bladder. The container tubing is then reclamped, and the urine receptacle tubing is unclamped, permitting the solution to flow out of the bladder. This process is carried out regularly. The same system can be used for continuous irrigations by carefully regulating the flow of fluid leaving the solution container and permitting it to flow freely out of the bladder into the urine bag.

There are several variations of this irrigation system. One requires a specific fluid pressure to build up in the urinary bladder before the irrigation system "trips," allowing the solution to flow out of the bladder into a receptacle. These systems are usually set up by a physician and monitored by nurses.

Before irrigating a bladder or catheter, the nurse can do the following. Assess whether the catheter and tubing are indeed blocked. Compare the amount of urine in the bag with the drainage on the previous shift or with the client's fluid intake. If urine does not appear to be running freely, "milk" the catheter and tubing, working from the client toward the drainage bag. This can dislodge an obstruction, avoiding the necessity of an irrigation to remove it. It is important to milk away from the client so that the obstruction, e.g., a blood clot, is forced into the drainage bag and not into the urinary bladder.

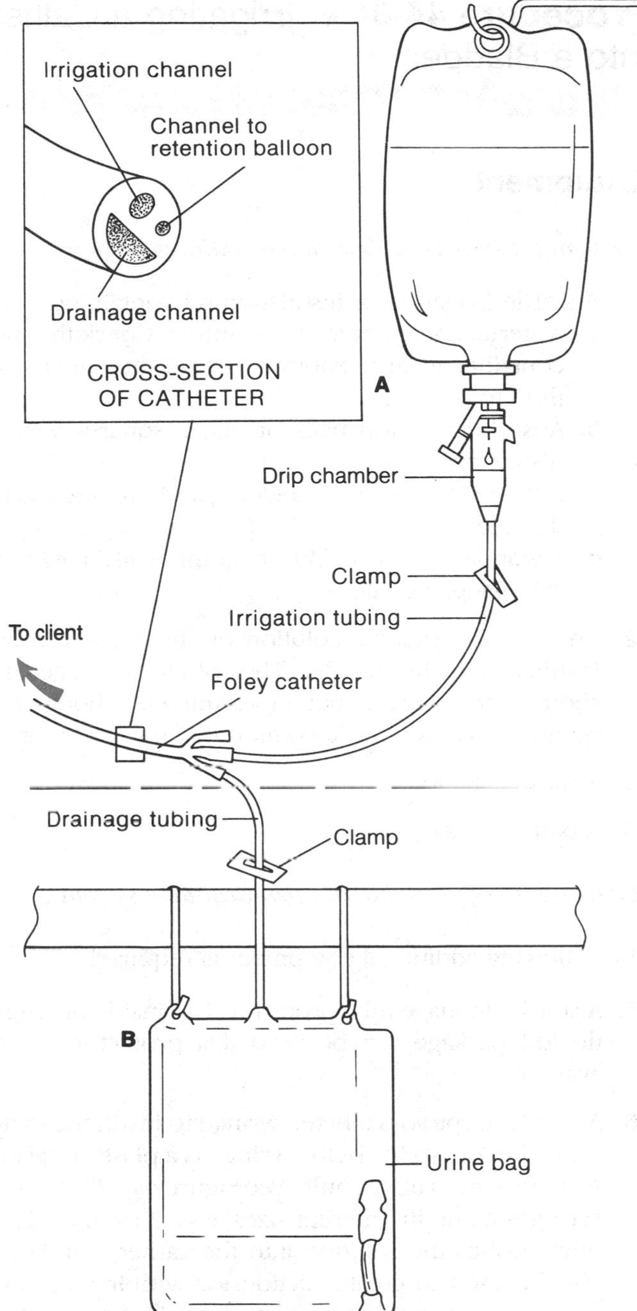

Figure 44–26 An intermittent bladder irrigation.

Equipment required for plain catheter or bladder irrigation varies, depending on whether the urinary drainage system is closed or open. For closed drainage systems a sterile syringe and needle are used to insert the fluid through tubing injection ports. For open drainage systems the drainage tubing is separated from the catheter and fluid is inserted using an Apseto or catheter syringe. Procedure 44–8 describes the steps involved in irrigating a catheter or bladder and instilling a medication into a bladder.

Procedure 44-8 ▲ Irrigating a Catheter or Bladder and Instilling Medication into a Bladder

Equipment

For using a syringe with a closed drainage system

1. A sterile irrigation or instillation set containing:
   a. A sterile container for the solution. Check that the container is large enough to hold the amount of fluid to be used.
   b. Absorbent cotton balls or gauze squares with a disinfectant
   c. A drape to protect the bedding and provide a sterile field
   d. A standard syringe (30 or 50 ml) with a #18 or #19 gauge needle
2. The sterile irrigating solution or medication to be instilled into the bladder. The solution is generally room temperature, although warming it to body temperature makes it more comfortable for the client.
3. A tubing clamp
4. A bath blanket

For using a syringe with an open drainage system

The following additional equipment is required:

5. A sterile drainage tube protector. The inside of a sterile foil package can be used if a protector is not available.
6. A sterile Asepto or catheter syringe to instill the solution. The Asepto (or bulb) syringe is a plastic or glass syringe with a rubber bulb. See Figure 44–27, *A.* Bulb syringes come in different sizes, e.g., 2 oz, 4 oz. The bulb pushes the solution into the catheter and can also be used to create suction for withdrawing the solution. A second type of syringe is the catheter syringe with an adapter tip. See Figure 44–27, *B.*
7. A sterile drainage receptacle, if an irrigation is being performed

For intermittent irrigations using a Y-connector and a two-way Foley catheter

8. A container of sterile irrigating solution
9. A sterile Y-connector, with sterile tubing to connect to the solution container, a drip chamber, and a clamp
10. An IV pole
11. A two-way Foley catheter inserted into the client's bladder
12. Sterile drainage tubing, a clamp, and a drainage receptacle. The tubing connects the catheter to the receptacle.
13. A bath blanket

For continuous irrigations using a three-way Foley catheter

14. A container of sterile irrigating solution
15. Sterile irrigation tubing, a drip chamber, and a clamp
16. An IV pole
17. A three-way Foley catheter inserted into the client's bladder
18. Sterile drainage tubing and a drainage bag. The tubing connects the catheter to the bag.
19. A bath blanket

Intervention

1. Determine the amount of urine in the urine bag.

   Rationale This amount has to be deducted from subsequent measurements of the irrigating fluid returns.

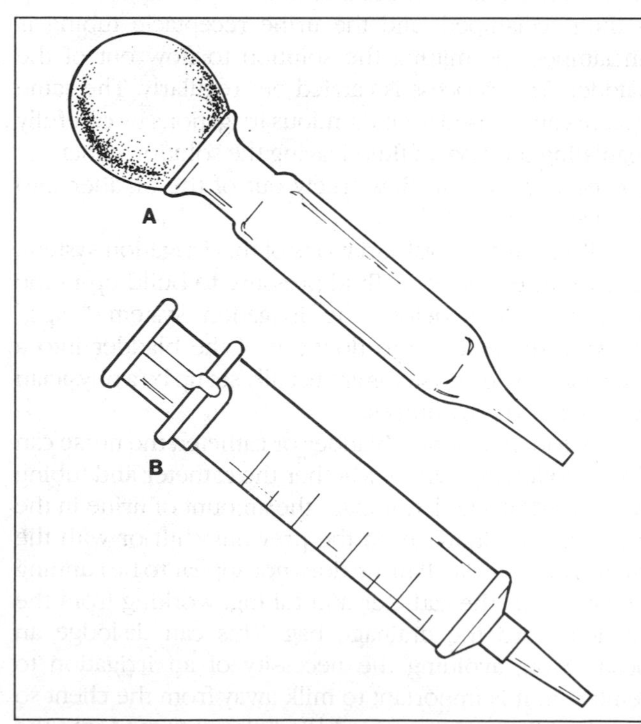

Figure 44–27 Two types of irrigating syringes: **A,** an Asepto syringe; **B,** a catheter syringe with an adaptor tip.

2. Assist the client to a dorsal recumbent position, to facilitate the flow of the irrigating fluid into the bladder.

3. Fold back the top bedclothes to expose the retention catheter. Place a bath blanket across the client's chest and abdomen to prevent undue exposure.

For a Closed Drainage System

4. Open the sterile set beside or between the client's thighs, using sterile technique.

5. Place the drape under the end of the catheter.

6. Clamp the drainage tubing for a bladder irrigation or bladder instillation. Leave it unclamped for a catheter irrigation.

   Rationale Clamping prevents the urine and solu tion from draining through the tubing.

7. Draw the irrigation solution into the syringe, maintaining the sterility of the syringe and the solution.

8. Attach the needle to the syringe, maintaining the sterility of the needle.

9. Using the disinfectant swab, wipe the place on the catheter lumen or the port on the drainage tubing through which the solution is to be instilled. The correct place on the catheter lumen is usually marked.

10. Insert the needle into the port. See Figure 44–25, earlier.

11. Infuse the solution gently into the catheter. For a catheter irrigation, instill about 30 to 40 ml of fluid for an adult; for a bladder irrigation, instill about 100 to 200 ml. Use smaller amounts for children. For a bladder instillation, instill the amount of medication specified in the order.

    Rationale Gentle instillation avoids injury to the lining of the bladder and bladder spasms.

12. Remove the needle from the port.

13. For a *catheter irrigation,* immediately lower the catheter so that the fluid will run toward the distal end of the catheter into the drainage tubing.

    or

    For a *bladder instillation,* leave the catheter clamped so the fluid will remain in the bladder.

    or

    For a *bladder irrigation,* unclamp the drainage tubing so the solution will run out of the bladder through the catheter and tubing.

14. For an irrigation, repeat steps 6–13 until all of the solution has been used or until the purpose of the irrigation has been accomplished.

15. Empty the urine bag. Record on the appropriate records (e.g., the bedside output record) the amount of urine drained by subtracting the amount of solution used from the volume of fluid in the bag.

16. Assess the response of the client to the irrigation or instillation in terms of discomfort and the color and clarity of the irrigating fluid and the urine flow.

17. Record on the client's chart the procedure, the time, the color and clarity of the irrigation returns, the presence of any abnormal constituents, and any discomfort experienced by the client. Add the amount of fluid instilled to the intake and output record.

For an Open Drainage System

18. Follow steps 4–5.

19. After disinfecting the ends, separate the catheter from the drainage tubing, and place the tubing protector over the end of the tubing. Hold the catheter and the tubing at least 2.5 cm (1 in) from their ends.

    Rationale This distance avoids contaminating the ends of the catheter and tubing.

20. Draw the fluid into the syringe, then gently inject it into the catheter, maintaining the sterility of the end of the catheter, the syringe, and the solution.

21. For a *bladder or catheter irrigation:*
    a. Remove the syringe, and allow the fluid to return through the catheter into the drainage receptacle.
    b. Repeat steps 20–21a until the catheter is running freely or until the purpose of the irrigation has been accomplished.

22. For a *bladder instillation,* clamp the catheter after instilling the solution. Leave the clamp in place for the time ordered.

    Rationale The solution will remain in the bladder for the designated time.

23. Reattach the catheter to the tubing, maintaining the sterility of the ends of the tubing and the catheter. For a bladder instillation, open the catheter clamp at the designated time, and drain the bladder contents into the receptacle.

24. Coil the drainage tubing carefully on the bed so that the urine can flow through it freely.

25. Empty the irrigation drainage receptacle.

26. Follow steps 16–17.

For an Intermittent Irrigation Using a Y-Connector

This system uses a two-way catheter with a Y-connector attached to the catheter end. See Figure 44–28.

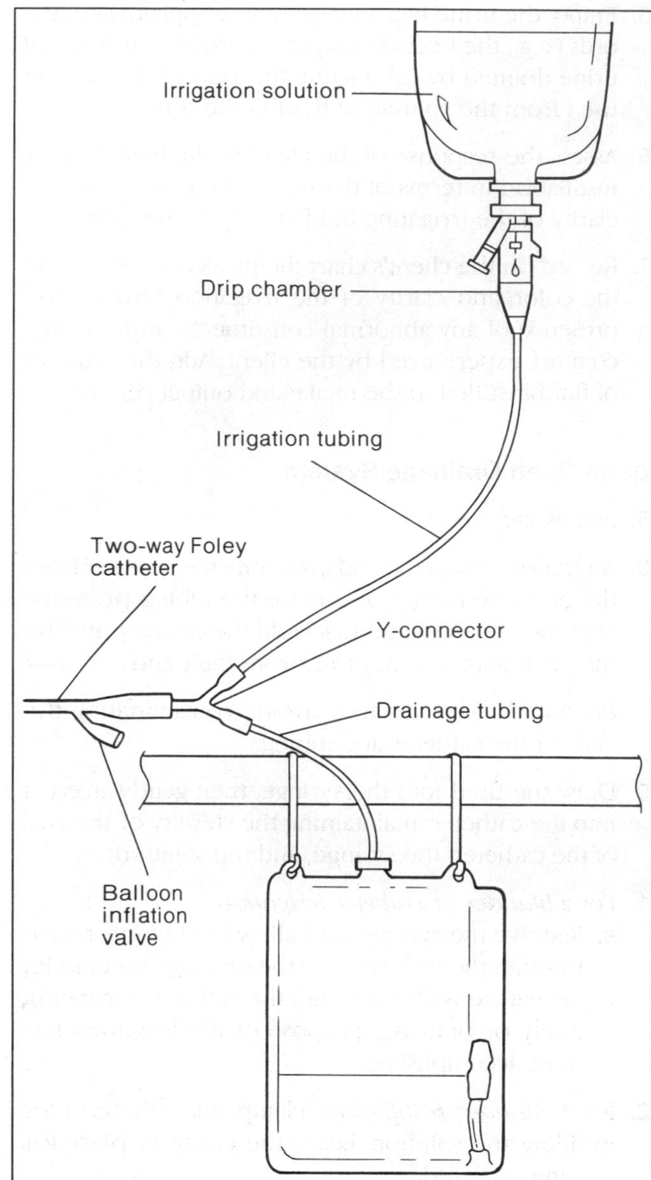

Figure 44–28

27. Insert the sterile irrigation tubing into the sterile solution bag.

28. Close the clamp on the irrigation solution, and hang the container on the IV pole.

29. Attach the stem of the sterile Y-connector to the catheter, maintaining the sterility of the inside of the catheter.

30. Open the clamp, permit some solution to run through the tubing, then close the clamp.

Rationale The solution expels the air from the tubing.

31. Attach one arm of the Y-connector to the irrigation tubing.

32. Attach the other arm of the Y-connector to the sterile drainage tubing.

33. Clamp the drainage tubing.

Rationale Urine and irrigating solution then cannot flow out of the bladder.

34. Open the clamp on the tubing from the solution container, and let the prescribed amount of fluid run into the bladder at the prescribed rate. If the amount is not specified by the physician, instill about 100 ml for an adult.

35. Close the irrigation clamp.

36. Open the drainage clamp, and permit the fluid and urine to flow into the receptacle.

37. Repeat steps 33–36 until the returning fluid is clear or as ordered by the physician.

38. Assess the response of the client in terms of any discomfort and the color and clarity of the return flow.

39. Record the procedure on the client's chart, including your assessments.

For a Continuous Irrigation Using a Three-Way Foley Catheter

40. Using sterile technique, assemble the equipment as for an intermittent irrigation, except that one port of the three-way catheter is connected to the irrigation tubing and the other is connected to the drainage tubing. See Figure 44–26. In some closed systems, the tubings are already connected to the catheter.

41. Open the flow clamp on the drainage tubing.

42. Adjust the flow rate, using the clamp on the irrigation tubing, as specified by the physician. If the order does not specify, the rate should be 40 to 60 drops per minute.

43. Inspect the fluid returns for amount, color, and clarity. The amount of returning fluid should correspond to the amount of fluid entering the bladder.

44. Record the procedure and your assessments on the client's chart.

Sample Recording

Date	Time	Notes
April/24/87	1400	Catheter irrigated with 200 ml normal saline at room temperature. Returns slightly blood-tinged with some small blood clots. Catheter running freely. No discomfort.—Sandi R. Bailey, NS

Suprapubic Catheter Care

A suprapubic catheter is inserted through the abdominal wall above the symphysis pubis into the urinary bladder. See Figure 44–29. The physician inserts the catheter using local anesthesia, in the client's bed unit, or using general anesthesia in conjunction with bladder or vaginal surgery, in the operating room. The catheter may be secured in place either with sutures or with a commercial retention body seal, or with both sutures and a body seal. It is then attached to a closed drainage system. When the catheter is removed, the muscle layers of the bladder contract over the insertion site to seal off the opening. Suprapubic catheters are advantageous over urethral catheters because:

1. They are associated with a lower rate of urinary tract infections.
2. They are more comfortable for the client.
3. They allow the opportunity to evaluate the client's ability to void normally; the client is asked to void normally when the suprapubic catheter is clamped. To assess the client's ability to void normally with a urethral catheter, you must first remove the catheter.
4. They facilitate evaluation of the client's residual urine.

Two commonly used suprapubic catheters are the *Cystocath* and the *Bonanno catheter.* See Figure 44–30. These are narrow-lumen catheters with a curl at the distal end that prevents the catheter from being expelled by the bladder through the urethra. The Cystocath has a disc that holds the catheter in place on the abdominal wall; the Bonanno catheter has wings for that purpose. Attachments of the catheter to the drainage system tubing also vary: The Cystocath is joined with a stopcock; the Bonanno with a Luer-Lok adapter.

The most common problem with the suprapubic catheter is blockage of drainage due to sediment, clots, or the bladder wall itself obstructing the catheter or catheter tip. Dislodgement of the catheter and hematuria following the use of a large-bore catheter are less common problems. Care of clients with suprapubic catheters includes regular assessments of the client's urine, fluid intake, and comfort; maintenance of a patent drainage system; skin care around the insertion site; periodic clamping of the catheter preparatory to removing it; and measurement of residual urine. The physician's order about management of the catheter is followed. Orders generally include: leaving the catheter open to drainage for 48 to 72 hours, then clamping the catheter for 3- to 4-hour periods during the day until the client can void satisfactory amounts. Satisfactory voiding is determined by measuring the client's residual urine after voiding.

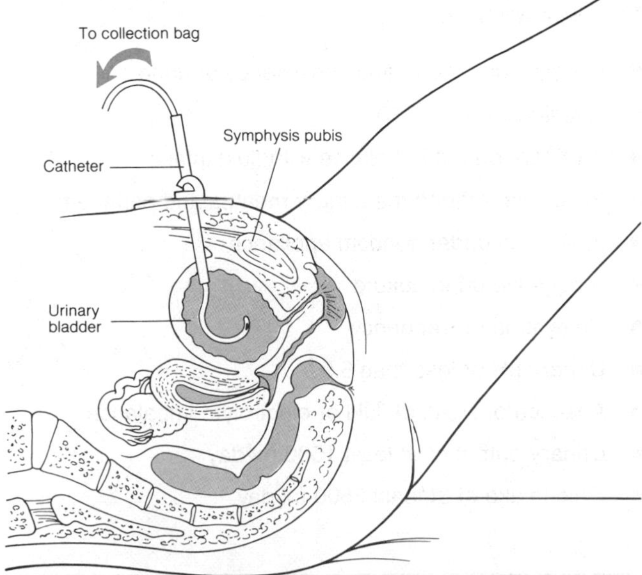

Figure 44–29 A suprapubic catheter in place.

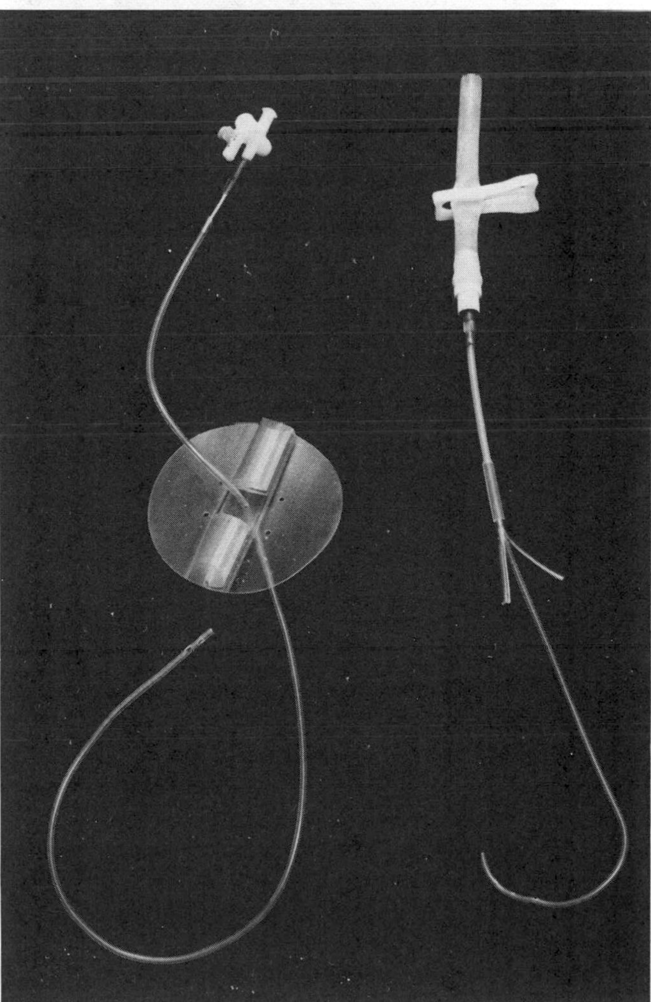

Figure 44–30 Two types of suprapubic catheters: a Cystocath (left) and a Bonanno (right).

The client's urine needs to be assessed for color, consistency, clarity, and amount of urine drained, hourly for the first 24 hours and then at least three times daily. Fluid intake is carefully monitored to ensure it is adequate to maintain a satisfactory urine output. Bladder discomfort may occur because of bladder spasms. Bladder spasms may occur during the first 24 to 48 hours. Spasms are identified by the presence of intermittent pain that does not affect the amount of urinary output.

Patency of the drainage system is maintained in the same manner as an indwelling catheter urinary drainage system. For example, the nurse makes sure that the catheter and drainage tubes are securely connected and taped, to avoid separation of the tubes, and ensures that the tubing is not kinked, that it runs straight up from the collection bag, and that excess tubing is coiled appropriately and taped to the client's abdomen or leg. Obstruction in the drainage system is identified by distention and tenderness of the bladder (assessed by palpation), feelings of fullness, pubic pain, and a reduction in urinary output.

Dressings around the suprapubic catheter are changed whenever they are soiled with drainage to prevent bacterial growth around the insertion site and reduce the potential for infection. A small amount of povidone-iodine ointment is applied around the insertion site and the site covered with gauze dressings. Procedures for cleaning wounds and changing dressings are discussed in Chapter 52. Any redness and discharge at the skin around the insertion site must be reported.

To ascertain the residual urine the suprapubic catheter is first closed with a clamp for 2 to 4 hours. The client then voids by the normal route, emptying the bladder as completely as possible. After this the residual urine is obtained by releasing the suprapubic catheter and allowing any remaining urine to drain into the drainage bag. Both the amount of urine voided and the amount of residual urine are measured. If the client can void a satisfactory amount (e.g., 150 to 350 ml) and the residual urine is less than 50 to 100 ml or volume specified by the physician, the catheter is removed.

To remove a suprapubic catheter the nurse first removes the dressing and any sutures holding the catheter in place. Suture removal is described in Chapter 52. The nurse then removes the catheter with a steady, continuous pull, applies pressure over the insertion site with gauze squares, cleans the site with antiseptic solution or swabs, and applies povidone-iodine ointment and an Elastoplast bandage.

Evaluation

Examples of outcome criteria to evaluate the client's goal achievement and the effectiveness of nursing interventions are shown to the right.

Examples of Outcome Criteria to Evaluate the Client's Urinary Elimination and Associated Problems

The client will have:

- Normal color, odor, and consistency of urine
- A residual urine of 30 ml
- A urinary output in balance with fluid intake
- Intact skin around the urinary meatus and perineum
- Intact skin under condom appliance
- A negative urine culture
- No dysuria or frequency
- Urinary pH of less than 5.5
- Absence of signs of fluid or electrolyte imbalance
- Urinary output of at least 1500 ml/day
- Fluid intake of at least 2500 ml/day

Nursing Care Plan

Assessment Data

Nursing Assessment

Mr. John Baker is a 68-year-old shopkeeper who was admitted to the hospital early this morning because he has been unable to void since 7 o'clock last evening. Mrs. Fran Wittmer, the nurse, gathers the following information when taking a nursing history. He states he has noticed that for the past few weeks he has had to go to the bathroom more frequently during the day and that he doesn't always feel he has emptied his bladder after voiding. He has also noticed that he must get up a few times during the night to urinate. As of the past few days, he has noted some problems in starting urination and then dribbling urine afterward. He states that this is very embarrassing to him since he must deal with his customers during the day. Mr. Baker wonders what is causing his urinary problems.

Physical Examination

Height: 185.4 cm (6′1″)
Weight: 85.7 kg (189 lb)
Temperature: 37 C (98.6 F)
Pulse rate: 78 BPM
Respirations: 20 per minute
Blood pressure: 146/86 mm Hg
Retention catheter to closed drainage bag draining 800 ml amber urine

Diagnostic Data

CBC: Within normal range
Urine: Amber, clear, pH 7.5, specific gravity 1.025, negative for glucose, protein, ketone, RBC and bacteria
IVP: evidence of enlarged prostate gland

Nursing Diagnosis	Client Goals and Outcome Criteria	Nursing Interventions and Rationales	Evaluation
Alteration in urinary elimination patterns: retention and incontinence related to bladder neck obstruction/enlarged prostate gland resulting in urgency, dysuria, frequency, nocturia, dribbling, hesitancy, and bladder distention.	Client Goal: Establish normal urination pattern. Outcome Criteria: Experiences relief of urinary retention within 24 hrs. Output will balance intake by day 2. Experiences absence of dysuria by day 5. Verbalize increased self-esteem by day 5. Maintain negative urine culture by day 3.	Observe amount, color, and character of urinary output. *Rationale:* Determines adequacy of urinary tract function. Encourage fluid intake of approximately 3000 ml per day. *Rationale:* Increased fluids will increase urinary output and discourage bacterial growth. Encourage fluids, e.g., cranberry juice, that acidify urine. *Rationale.* Acidification of urine inhibits growth of bacteria. Maintain accurate I&O. *Rationale:* Serves as indicator of urinary tract and renal function and fluid balance. Maintain patency of retention catheter. *Rationale:* Prevents urinary stasis and bladder spasms. Provide perineal-genital care. *Rationale:* Cleanliness of area will decrease chance of urinary infection. Tape retention catheter to lower abdomen. *Rationale:* Prevents erosion and pressure on penile-scrotal junction. Maintain drainage receptacle below level of client's bladder. *Rationale:* Prevents reflux flow to bladder.	Mr. Baker's retention catheter remained patent and his urinary output for the first 24 hrs was 2050 ml. For the past 48 hrs his fluid intake has been 2000 to 3000 ml, and his urinary output has been 2500 ml. The results of his repeat urinalysis were negative. Mr. Baker's retention catheter was removed on day 4 and he is voiding in the amounts of 200 to 300 ml q4–5 hrs. At times, he experiences some difficulty initiating a urinary stream, as well as some dribbling after voiding.

(continued)

Nursing Diagnosis	Client Goals and Outcome Criteria	Nursing Interventions and Rationales	Evaluation
Knowledge deficit related to health problem (enlarged prostate gland and urinary retention) and its treatment resulting in anxious behavior, increased verbalization, inability to concentrate.	Client Goal: Understand prostatic hypertrophy and its treatment. Outcome Criteria: Describes function and anatomical location of gland by day 3. Describes 1 or 2 aspects of treatment for his condition by day 3. Experiences less anxiety as evidenced by use of coping mechanism by day 3.	Establish a good rapport with client by being supportive and empathetic. *Rationale:* Encourages client to ask questions and seek assistance. Encourage verbalization of concerns. *Rationale:* Assists client in working through his feelings and fears. Assess client's learning needs. *Rationale:* Will permit building upon client's present understanding of his condition. Adapt teaching to client's abilities. *Rationale:* Learning will be more meaningful to client. Reduce client's anxiety by explaining health problem. *Rationale:* Knowledge may decrease anxiety. Instruct client regarding dietary and activity restrictions. *Rationale:* Knowing what foods or activities to avoid will decrease symptoms of disease.	Mr. Baker was able to relate his urinary problems to his enlarged prostate gland by day 3. He states he now knows to avoid spicy foods, alcohol, and coffee. He was able to verbalize his fears regarding his difficulty in voiding and the possibility of future surgery "to stop this dribbling."

Chapter Highlights

- Urinary elimination depends on normal functioning of the urinary, cardiovascular, and nervous systems.
- Urinary control is a learned response that occurs after bowel control is established. Daytime control is generally achieved by the age of 2 years, but nighttime control may not be achieved until age 4.
- The normal process of micturition includes sufficient accumulation of urine in the bladder to stimulate the sensory stretch nerves in the bladder wall. Impulses from these stretch receptors then travel to the spinal cord to the voiding reflex center and to the voiding control center in the cerebral cortex, where conscious control of micturition is regulated.
- In the adult, micturition generally occurs after 250 to 450 ml of urine has collected in the bladder.
- Many factors influence a person's urinary elimination. Increased amounts of urine may be excreted when large amounts of fluid are ingested, during stress, when activity is increased, or when diuretics are prescribed. Various disease processes may increase or decrease the amount of urine eliminated.
- When assessing a person's urinary function, the nurse considers (a) pattern and frequency of urination, (b) problems with urinary elimination and influencing factors, (c) physical assessment data, (d) characteristics of the urine, such as color and odor, (e) past illnesses or surgery, and (f) data obtained from diagnostic tests and examinations.
- From the assessment data obtained, the nurse establishes the nursing diagnoses, sets nursing goals, and plans nursing interventions.
- Nursing diagnoses that relate to urinary tract function and urinary patterns include alteration in urinary elimination pattern, stress incontinence, reflex incontinence, functional incontinence, total incontinence, urge incontinence, urinary retention, potential for infection, altered comfort, potential fluid volume deficit or excess, disturbance in self-concept, and potential impairment of skin integrity.
- Common urinary alterations the nurse encounters are urinary incontinence, urinary retention, and lower urinary tract infection.
- Incontinence can be physically and emotionally distressing to clients because it is considered socially unacceptable.
- Clients who have urinary retention not only experience discomfort but are also at risk of urinary tract infection.

- The most common cause of urinary tract infection are invasive procedures such as catheterization and cystoscopic examination.
- Females in particular are prone to ascending urinary tract infections because of their short urethras.
- Nursing interventions related to urinary elimination are generally directed toward facilitating the normal functioning of the urinary system or toward assisting the client with particular problems.
- Interventions include (a) assisting the client to maintain an appropriate fluid intake, (b) assisting the client to maintain normal voiding patterns, (c) monitoring the client's daily fluid intake and output, and (d) maintaining cleanliness of the genital area.
- Bladder-training programs can effectively reduce incontinence.
- Urinary catheterization is frequently required for clients with urinary retention but is only performed when all other measures to facilitate voiding fail. Sterile technique is essential to prevent ascending urinary infections.
- Care of clients with in-dwelling catheters is directed toward preventing infection of the urinary tract and encouraging urinary flow through the drainage system.

Suggested Readings

Birdsall, C. November 1985. How do you teach female self-catheterization? *American Journal of Nursing* 85:1226–27.
Birdsall discusses positions for self-catheterization, ways to locate the urinary meatus, aseptic techniques to use, tips for inserting the catheter, and other information the client should know.

Greengold, B. A., and Ouslander, J. G. June 1986. Bladder retraining: Program for elderly patients with post-indwelling catheterization. *Journal of Gerontological Nursing* 12:31–35.
Greengold and Ouslander describe differences among three bladder training programs and provide a seven-step bladder retraining program to use after the removal of an indwelling catheter. An incontinence monitoring record is included.

Kneip-Hardy, M. J.; Votava, K.; and Stubbings, M. J. September/October 1985. Managing indwelling catheters in the home. *Geriatric Nursing* 6:280–85.
These authors provide a comprehensive guide to managing the everyday decisions and problems in the long-term care of clients requiring a Foley catheter. Instructions to the family and client are provided about catheter care, changing the catheter, catheter irrigation, and how to manage leaks around the catheter.

Selected References

Autry, D.; Lauzon, F.; and Holiday, P. January/February 1984. *Geriatric Nursing* 5:22–25.

Baum, M. E. February 1978. "I want to be dry": The (almost) carefree way to conquer urinary incontinence. *Nursing 78* 8:75–76, 78.

Beber, R. March 1980. Freedom for the incontinent. *American Journal of Nursing* 80:482–484.

Brogna, L., and Lakaszawski, M. L. February 1986. The continent urostomy . . . the Kock pouch. *American Journal of Nursing* 86:160–63.

Byrne, C. J.; Saxton, D. F.; Pelikan, P. K.; and Nugent, P. M. 1986. *Laboratory tests implications for nursing care.* 2d ed. Menlo Park, Calif. Addison-Wesley Pub. Co.

Caring for a patient with a urinary diversion stoma. July 1984. *Nursing 84* 14:20–22.

Clark, R., Creamer, L.; Lawson, E.; and Tracey, P. December 1978. Infection control: A team approach that really works. *Canadian Nurse* 74:16–19.

DeGroot, J. August 1976. Catheter-induced urinary tract infections: Can we prevent them? *Nursing 76* 6:34–37.

DeGroot, J. December 1976. Urethral catheterization: Observing "niceties" prevents infections. *Nursing 76* 6:51–55.

DeGroot, J., and Kunin, C. M. March 1975. Indwelling catheters. *American Journal of Nursing* 75:448–49.

Demmerle, B., and Bartol, M. A. November/December 1980. Nursing care for the incontinent person. *Geriatric Nursing* 1:246–50.

Epstein, S. E. December 1985. Cost-effective application of the Centers for Disease Control Guideline for prevention of catheter-associated urinary tract infections. *American Journal of Infection Control* 13:272–75.

Frye, S., and Melman, A. January 15, 1985. Urinary tract infection: Aspects of asymptomatic UTI in elderly patients. *Consultant* 25:51–2, 62–3.

Garner, J., February 1974. Urinary catheter care: Doing it better. *Nursing 74* 4:54–56.

Graber, R. F. March 1985. Passing a urinary catheter. *Patient Care* 19:162–63, 167, 171.

Grant, R. July/August 1982. Washable pads or disposable diapers? *Geriatric Nursing* 3:248–51.

Gurevich, I. July 1985. Selection of closed urinary drainage systems—an update. *Infection Control* 6:289–90.

Guyton, A. C. 1986. *Textbook of Medical Physiology,* 7th ed. Philadelphia: W. B. Saunders Co.

Hart, J. A. 1985. The urethral catheter: A review of its implication in urinary tract infection. *International Journal of Nursing Studies* 22(1):57–59.

Hart, M., and Adamek, C. July/August 1984. Do increased fluids decrease urinary stone formation? *Geriatric Nursing* 5:245–48.

Home Teaching Aid. July/August 1985. Testing your urine for glucose and ketones. *Nursing Life* 5:32.

Home Teaching Aid. July/August 1985. Urine Self-testing: What your patient needs to know. *Nursing Life* 5:31.

Innes, B., and Bruga, M. 1977. Postoperative voiding patterns and related contributing factors. *Washington State Journal of Nursing 49,* 3:13–16.

Killon, A. May 1982. Reducing the risk of infection from indwelling urethral catheters. *Nursing 82* 12:84–88.

Kinney, A. B.; Blount, M.; and Dowell, M. November/December 1980. Urethral catheterization: Pros and cons of an invasive but sometimes essential procedure. *Geriatric Nursing* 1:258–63.

Kniep-Hardy, M. J.; Votava, K.; and Stubbings, M. J. September/October 1985. Managing indwelling catheters in the home. *Geriatric Nursing* 6:280–85.

Long, M. L. January 1985. Incontinence: Defining the nursing role. *Journal of Gerontological Nursing* 11:30–35, 41.

McConnell, J. November/December 1984. Preventing urinary tract infections. *Geriatric Nursing* 5:361–62.

McConnell, E. A., and Zimmerman, M. I. 1983. *Care of patients with urologic problems.* Philadelphia: J. B. Lippincott.

McGuckin, M. B. January 1981. Getting better urine specimens with the clean-catch midstream technique. *Nursing 81* 1:24–25.

Peterson, H. January 1985. When the patient is incontinent. *Patient Care* 19:49–52, 54, 57.

Peterson, H. March 1985. Tips on using a urinary catheter. *Patient Care* 19:155–56, 158–60.

Richard, C. J. 1986. *Comprehensive nephrology nursing.* Boston: Little, Brown & Co.

Simons, J. June 1985. Does incontinence affect your client's self-concept? *Journal of Gerontological Nursing* 11:37–40, 42.

Swearingen, P. L. 1984. *The Addison-Wesley Photo-Atlas of Nursing Procedures.* Menlo Park, Calif.: Addison-Wesley Pub. Co.

Voith, A. M., and Smith, D. A. December 1985. Validation of the nursing diagnosis of urinary retention. *Nursing Clinics of North America* 20:723–29.

Whaley, L. F., and Wong, D. L. 1983. *Nursing care of infants and children,* 2d ed. St. Louis: C. V. Mosby Co.

Whyte, J. F., and Thistle, N. A. September 1976. Male incontinence: The inside story on external collection. *Nursing 76* 6:66–67.

Woodrow, M. October 1976. Suprapubic catheters, part 1: A direct line to better drainage. *Nursing 76* 6:40–45.

Woodrow, M. November 1976. Suprapubic catheters, part 2: A direct line to better drainage. *Nursing 76* 6:40–42.

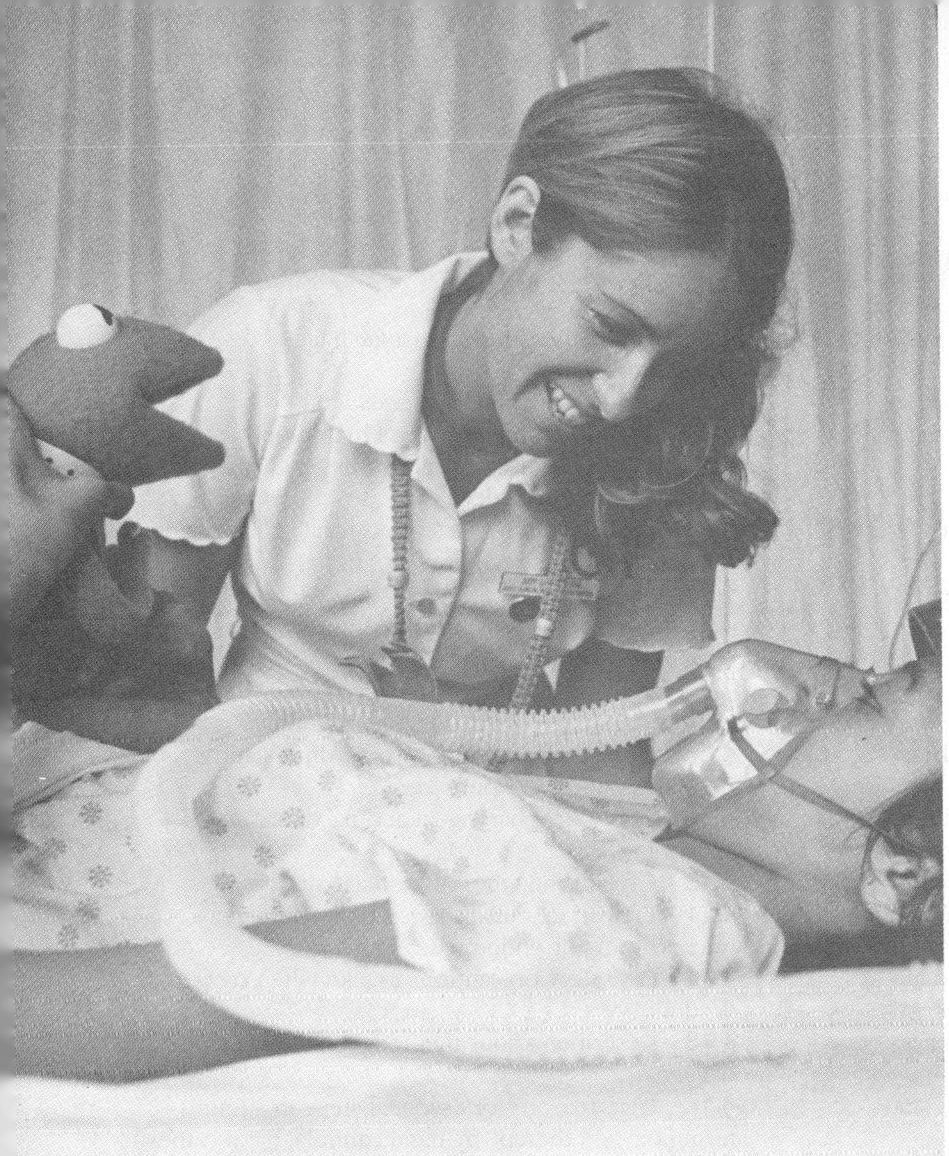

CHAPTER 45

Oxygenation

Contents

45 *Oxygenation*

Objectives

1. Know essential terms and facts about oxygenation.
   1.1 Define selected terms.
   1.2 Explain the three phases of respiration.
   1.3 Describe the basic mechanics of breathing.
   1.4 Identify major pulmonary volumes.
   1.5 Identify major pulmonary capacities.
   1.6 Relate changes in pulmonary pressures to the act of the breathing.
   1.7 Identify the requirements of adequate ventilation.
   1.8 Explain mechanisms regulating the respiratory process.
   1.9 Identify factors that influence the rate of diffusion of gases through the respiratory membrane and give examples of each.
   1.10 Describe how oxygen is transported to the tissues and how carbon dioxide is transported from the tissues.
   1.11 Explain major factors influencing oxygen transport.
2. Know information and methods required to assess a person's oxygenation status.
   2.1 Identify terms used to describe respiratory and circulatory status.
   2.2 Identify factors influencing respiratory and circulatory function.
   2.3 Explain clinical signs of hypoxia.
   2.4 Explain selected altered breathing patterns.
   2.5 Explain the signs of an obstructed airway.
3. Know essential facts about nursing diagnoses related to oxygenation.
   3.1 Identify responses to alterations in respiratory and circulatory status.
   3.2 Identify manifestations of and factors contributing to ineffective airway clearance.
   3.3 Identify manifestations of and factors contributing to ineffective breathing patterns.
   3.4 Identify manifestations of and factors contributing to decreased cardiac output.
4. Understand facts about nursing intervention required to maintain, promote, and restore oxygenation.
   4.1 Explain the position that facilitates oxygenation.
   4.2 Explain breathing exercises.
   4.3 Explain the importance of hydration.
   4.4 Explain the use of blow bottles and sustained maximal inspiration devices.
   4.5 Explain the purposes of postural drainage and the accompanying techniques of percussion and vibration.
   4.6 Identify positions used to drain specific lung segments by gravity.
   4.7 Identify areas to percuss (or vibrate) during postural drainage of various lung segments.
   4.8 Identify various types of humidifiers and nebulizers and their purposes.
   4.9 Explain oropharyngeal and nasopharyngeal suctioning.
   4.10 Explain the types of artificial airways.
   4.11 Explain essential aspects of suctioning a tracheostomy or endotracheal tube.
   4.12 List safety precautions to take when oxygen is administered.
   4.13 Describe various methods to administer oxygen.
   4.14 Give reasons for essential steps in administering oxygen therapy by nasal cannula, nasal catheter, and face mask.
   4.15 Describe essential steps in cardiopulmonary resuscitation.
   4.16 Describe steps in clearing foreign-body airway obstructions.
5. Apply the nursing process for clients with oxygenation problems.
   5.1 Obtain necessary assessment data.
   5.2 Analyze and relate assessment data.
   5.3 Write relevant nursing diagnoses.
   5.4 Plan appropriate nursing strategies.
   5.5 Implement appropriate nursing interventions.
   5.6 State outcome criteria against which to evaluate client progress.

Terms

airway
anemia
anoxia
apnea
artificial respiration
atelectasis
adventitious sounds
basic life support (BLS)
bradypnea
carbaminohemoglobin
carbonic acid
cardiac arrest
cardiac output
cardiopulmonary resuscitation (CPR)
carina

chemoreceptors
Cheyne-Stokes breathing
cilia
cough
cyanosis
cytology
deep breathing
diffusion
diffusion coefficient
dyspnea
emphysema
erythrocytes
erythropoiesis
eupnea
expectorate
expiration (exhalation)
expiratory reserve volume
external cardiac massage
flail chest
functional residual capacity
Heimlich maneuver
hematocrit
hemoglobin
hemoptysis
hemothorax
hypercarbia (hypercapnia)
hyperventilation
hypocarbia (hypocapnia)
hypoventilation
hypoxemia
hypoxia
inhalation (aerosol) therapy
inspiration (inhalation)
inspiratory capacity
inspiratory reserve volume
intercostal retraction
intermittent positive pressure breathing (IPPB)
intrapleural pressure
intrapulmonic pressure
Kussmaul breathing
lingula
lung compliance
lung recoil
morphology
nebulizer
nonproductive cough
orthopnea
oxyhemoglobin
$Paco_2$
Pao_2
paradoxical breathing
partial pressure
percussion
Pco_2
pneumothorax
Po_2
postural drainage
productive cough
pulmonary capacities
reduced hemoglobin
residual volume
respiration
respiratory arrest
respiratory membrane
resuscitation
substernal retraction
suctioning
surfactant
tachypnea
tidal volume
total lung capacity
ventilation
vibration
vital capacity

Physiology of Respiration

Respiration is the transport of oxygen from the atmosphere to the body cells and the transport of carbon dioxide from the cells back to the atmosphere. The process has three parts:

1. Pulmonary ventilation, or the inflow and outflow of air between the atmosphere and the alveoli of the lungs
2. Diffusion of gases (oxygen and carbon dioxide) between the alveoli and pulmonary capillaries
3. Transport of oxygen and carbon dioxide via the blood to and from the tissue cells

Pulmonary Ventilation

Ventilation of the lungs includes the basic mechanics or act of breathing (inspiration and expiration). The degree of chest expansion during ventilation is minimal with normal breathing but can reach maximum capacities during strenuous activity. These normal pulmonary volumes and capacities are described and considered in this section. The relationship of the pulmonary pressures to inspiration and expiration is also included. Many factors are essential for adequate ventilation: adequate atmospheric oxygen, clear air passageways, adequate pulmonary compliance, and regulation of respiration.

Mechanisms of Breathing

The act of breathing is like the working of a bellows. Breathing consists of **inspiration (inhalation)**, the inflow of air from the atmosphere to the lungs, and **expiration (exhalation)**, the outflow of air from the lungs to the atmosphere. Inspiration normally lasts 1 to 1.5 seconds, and expiration 2 to 3 seconds, including a short resting phase. **Eupnea** (normal breathing) is silent and effortless. It is accomplished largely by movement of the diaphragm. The diaphragm contracts or flattens on inspiration, thus lengthening and pulling the lower chest cavity downward. On expiration, the diaphragm simply relaxes, moving upward. This upward movement of the diaphragm is enhanced by contraction of the abdominal muscles, which push the abdominal organs up against the bottom of the diaphragm. See Figure 45–1.

Breathing during strenuous exercise or illness requires greater chest expansion and effort. The greater chest expansion of heavy breathing is accomplished by intercostal and other muscles that elevate or depress the rib cage. During inspiration, the rib cage is pulled upward by the action of the anterior neck muscles and contraction of the external intercostals. During expiration, the rib cage is pulled downward by the anterior abdominal muscles. Active use of these muscles and noticeable effort in breathing are seen in clients with obstructive respiratory disease. See the section on inspecting the shape and sym-

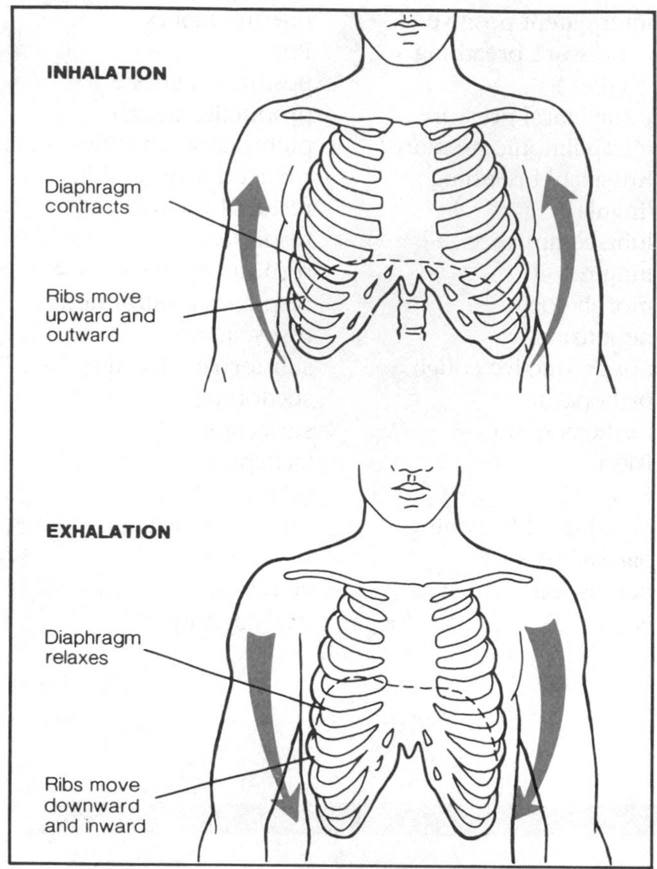

Figure 45–1 Inhalation and exhalation

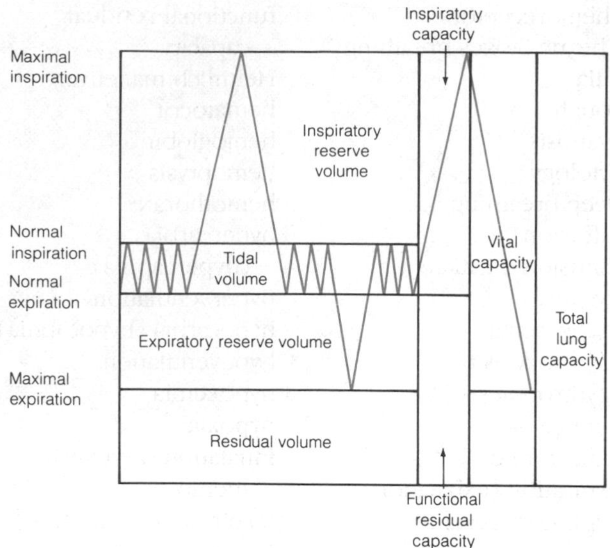

Figure 45–2 Pulmonary volumes and capacities

metry of the chest, Chapter 35, p. 841. The changes in thoracic diameters during ventilation are associated with changes in pulmonary volumes and pulmonary pressures.

Pulmonary volumes The volume to which the lungs expand during ventilation depends on whether breathing is normal and whether maximum inspiration and expiration occur. The normal volume of air inspired and expired is referred to as the **tidal volume**. See Figure 45–2. In the young male adult, the tidal volume is about 500 ml. *Note:* This volume is about 20% to 25% smaller in the female. Volumes may be smaller in small persons or greater in large or athletic persons. There are three other volumes: the **inspiratory reserve volume, the expiratory reserve volume**, and the **residual volume**. These three volumes added to the tidal volume yield the **total lung capacity**, which is the maximum volume to which the lungs can expand. See Table 45–1.

Pulmonary capacities Pulmonary volumes are often grouped in combinations of two or more. These combined volumes are referred to as the **pulmonary capacities** and include total lung capacity plus the **inspiratory capacity**, the **functional residual capacity**, and the **vital capacity**. See Table 45–2. The residual volume is normally about 20% of the total lung capacity.

Individual vital capacity varies with (a) anatomical build, (b) position, (c) strength of the respiratory muscles, (d) distensibility of the lungs and thorax, and (e) age. An adult's vital capacity is normally about 4500 to 5000 ml. A tall, thin person has a higher capacity than an obese person. Athletes may develop vital capacities up to 7000 ml. Standing increases vital capacity, whereas lying down reduces it. When a person is lying down, the abdominal organs tend to push against the diaphragm and the volume of pulmonary blood increases, both of which effects reduce pulmonary space and air. Weakness or paralysis of respiratory muscles, such as occurs in quadriplegics, can decrease the vital capacity to a point that is just adequate to sustain life or lower (500 to 1000 ml). Diseases that impair lung distensibility, such as pulmonary edema and lung cancer, seriously reduce vital capacity.

Measurement of the pulmonary volumes and capacities is frequently done by *spirometry*. The client breathes a mixture of air and oxygen, through a mouthpiece, from a drum suspended over a chamber of water. As the client breathes in and out, the gas drum rises and falls in the water, and a recording is made on another drum (spirogram). All lung volumes and capacities can be measured by spirometry except for the residual volume and, consequently, the functional residual capacity and total vital capacity, which include the residual volume. See Figure 45–2.

Pulmonary pressure Breathing produces changes in **intrapulmonic pressure** (pressure within the lungs) and in **intrapleural pressure** (pressure outside or around the lungs). These pressure changes are related to the changes in the lung volumes in accordance with Boyle's Law, which states that the volume of a gas at constant temperature varies inversely with its pressure. In other words, at a constant temperature, as the volume increases the pressure decreases, and vice versa.

Table 45–1 Terms Related to Lung Volume

Term	Definition	Normal Value, Average Adult Male[1]
Inspiratory reserve volume (IRV)	The maximum amount of air inhaled after a normal inspiration	3000 ml
Expiratory reserve volume (ERV)	The maximum amount of air exhaled after a normal exhalation	1200 ml
Residual volume (RV)	The amount of air remaining in the lungs after maximal exhalation, i.e., after exhaling the ERV and TV	1200 ml
Tidal volume (TV)	The normal volume of air inhaled or exhaled	600 ml

[1]Female lung volumes are 20% to 25% smaller.

Source: Adapted from R. L. Vick, *Contemporary medical physiology* (Menlo Park, Calif.: Addison-Wesley Publishing Co., 1984).

Table 45–2 Terms Related to Lung Capacity

Term	Definition	Normal Value, Average Adult Male[1]
Total lung capacity (TLC)	Amount of air in the lungs after a maximal inhalation	6000 ml
Inspiratory capacity (IC)	Maximum amount of air that can be inhaled after a normal exhalation	3600 ml
Functional residual capacity (FRC)	Volume of air remaining in the lungs after a normal expiration	2500 ml
Vital capacity (VC)	Maximum amount of air that can be exhaled following a maximal inhalation	4800 ml
Timed vital capacity (TVC)	Percentage of vital capacity that can be exhaled in 1, 2, and 3 seconds	—

[1]Female lung volumes are 20% to 25% smaller.

Source: Adapted from R. L. Vick, *Contemporary medical physiology* (Menlo Park, Calif.: Addison-Wesley Publishing Co., 1984).

Boyle's Law applies to respiration in this way: On inspiration the volume of the lungs increases, and thus the intrapulmonic pressure decreases. This decreased pressure allows atmospheric air to enter, since its pressure is greater. Conversely, on expiration the volume of the lungs decreases, and the intrapulmonic pressure increases. This allows the air to escape to the atmosphere, whose pressure is low relative to the lungs'. At sea level, atmospheric pressure is about 760 mm Hg. Only very small pressure changes are required to move air in and out of the lungs. On inspiration, the intraalveolar pressure drops to less than 1 mm Hg below atmospheric pressure, whereas on expiration it rises to 1 mm Hg above atmospheric pressure. Although very little pressure is required to move air in and out of the lungs, pressures can increase substantially, as, for example, in certain lung diseases. In a healthy man, a maximum expiratory effort can raise the intraalveolar pressure to as high as 140 mm Hg; a maximum inspiratory effort can depress the intraalveolar pressure to as low as − 100 mm Hg (Guyton 1986, p. 46).

Unless the chest cavity is damaged or opened, the intrapleural pressure is always negative. This negative pressure is essential because it creates the suction that holds the visceral pleura and the parietal pleura together as the chest cage expands and contracts. The recoil tendency of the lungs is a major factor responsible for this negative pressure. The fluid in the intrapleural space, however, provides even more negative pressure. Intrapleural fluid causes the pleura to adhere together, much as a film of water can cause two glass slides to adhere together.

Essential Requirements for Ventilation

Ventilation of the lungs depends on (a) adequate atmospheric oxygen, (b) clear air passages, (c) adequate pulmonary compliance and recoil, and (d) regulation of respiration.

Adequate atmospheric oxygen The presence of atmospheric oxygen in adequate concentration is basic to adequate respirations. Concentrations of oxygen are lower at high altitudes than at sea level. In some instances people at very high altitudes need supplementary oxygen.

Clear air passages During inspiration, air passes through the nose, pharynx, larynx, trachea, bronchi, and bronchioles to the alveoli, and expiration reverses that course. The nose performs three important functions. It warms, moistens, and filters the air. These functions are appreciated by people required to breathe directly through a tube into the trachea (tracheostomy); dry, unfiltered air can lead to infections of the lung. Large particles in the air are filtered by the hairs at the entrance of the nares, and smaller particles are filtered by nasal turbulence. Each time air contacts the nasal turbinates or nasal septum it must change direction, and in the process small particles are trapped.

Air passages are cleared by the mucous membrane lining, which contains **cilia** (hairlike projections of the respiratory mucous membrane). Mucus entraps organisms or other small foreign material while the cilia move the material from the trachea, for example, toward the pharynx. The cilia beat continually at a rate of 10 to 20 times per second, directed toward the pharynx. Thus the cilia in the lower respiratory passageways (e.g., the bronchi) beat upward, and the cilia in the nose beat downward. Material can be moved as much as 1 cm per minute along the trachea (Guyton 1986, p. 475). The cough reflex and the sneeze reflex are also essential cleaning mechanisms. The **cough** reflex is triggered by irritants that send nerve impulses through the vagus nerve to the medulla. Any foreign matter in the larynx, trachea, or bronchi initiates the cough reflex. A particularly sensitive area is the **carina**, the ridge or junction where the main bronchi meet at the trachea. The cough reflex process is described below. The sneeze reflex is to the nasal passages as the cough is to lower respiratory passages. Sneezing is initiated when irritating impulses pass by way of the fifth cranial nerve to the medulla. Sneezing involves a series of reactions similar to the cough reflex; however, the uvula is depressed so that a large volume of air passes rapidly through the nose as well as the mouth, thus helping to clear the nasal passages (Guyton 1986, p. 475).

Adequate pulmonary compliance and recoil **Lung compliance** is expansibility or stretchability. It generally includes expansibility of both the lungs and the thorax but sometimes denotes compliance of the lungs alone. Compliance can be measured by noting the increase in lung volume produced by units of increased intraalveolar pressure. Expansibility is obviously essential to adequate inspiration.

The Cough Reflex Process

1. 2.5 liters of air is inspired.
2. The epiglottis closes.
3. The vocal cords shut tightly to entrap air in the lungs.
4. The abdominal muscles contract forcefully, pushing against the diaphragm.
5. Simultaneously, the thoracic expiratory muscles—e.g., internal intercostal muscles—contract forcefully.
6. As a result the pressure in the lungs rises to as high as 100 mm Hg or more.
7. The vocal cords and epiglottis open suddenly.
8. The pressure in the lungs explodes outward, sometimes at a velocity as high as 75 to 100 mph.
9. The compression of the lungs collapses the bronchi and trachea, causing their noncartilaginous parts to invaginate inward, and the exploding air therefore passes through bronchial and tracheal slits. (Guyton 1986, p. 475)

Inadequate compliance can result from any condition that destroys lung tissue, such as edema or tumors, or any condition that inhibits thoracic expansion, such as paralysis or kyphosis.

In contrast to lung compliance is **lung recoil**. The lungs have a continual tendency to collapse away from the chest wall. Two factors are responsible for this recoil tendency: (a) elastic fibers present in lung tissue and (b) surface tension of the fluid lining the alveoli. The latter accounts for two-thirds of the recoil phenomenon. Counterbalancing this surface tension in the alveoli is a lipoprotein mixture called **surfactant**. When surfactant is absent, lung expansion is exceedingly difficult and the lungs collapse. Normally, the secretion of surfactant by the alveoli is stimulated several times each hour by yawning, sighing, or deep breaths. Surfactant stimulation is important for clients on automatic ventilation. The alveoli must be stretched several times every hour by a sigh mechanism on the respirator.

Diffusion of Gases

After the alveoli are ventilated, the second phase of the respiratory process—the diffusion of oxygen from the alveoli and into the pulmonary blood vessels—begins. **Diffusion** is the movement of gases or other particles from an area of greater pressure or concentration to an area of lower pressure or concentration. Carbon dioxide diffuses in the opposite direction, from the pulmonary blood vessels and into the alveoli. Because the alveolar walls are very thin and are surrounded by a closely intertwined network of blood capillaries, these membranes together are often referred to as the **respiratory membrane**.

Four factors influence the rate of diffusion of gases through the respiratory membrane: (a) thickness of the membrane, (b) surface area of the membrane, (c) diffusion coefficient of the gas, and (d) pressure difference on each side of the membrane (Guyton 1986, p. 488).

The thickness of the respiratory membrane increases in clients with pulmonary edema or certain other pulmonary diseases. Any increase in the thickness of this membrane can seriously decrease gaseous diffusion. The surface area of the membrane can also be altered. Conditions such as **emphysema**, in which alveoli coalesce, or lobectomy, the surgical removal of a portion of the lung, impede gaseous exchange. In clients at rest, the loss of some surface area is not a serious deficit. However, a loss of more than 25% is serious. Also, when for some reason (e.g., exercise or certain diseases) there is increased pulmonary demand, a loss of less than 25% can be a serious deficit.

The diffusion coefficients of oxygen and carbon dioxide are also a significant factor. The **diffusion coefficient** depends on the gas's molecular weight and solubility in the membrane. Carbon dioxide diffuses about 20 times more rapidly than oxygen. Thus, in some situations an oxygen lack is seen without a carbon dioxide build-up. Oxygen diffuses about twice as rapidly as nitrogen.

Pressure differences in the gases on each side of the respiratory membrane obviously affect diffusion. When the pressure of oxygen is greater in the alveoli than in the blood, oxygen diffuses into the blood. The reverse happens with carbon dioxide. Normally the oxygen pressure gradient between the alveoli and the blood entering the pulmonary capillaries is about 40 mm Hg. The **partial pressure** (the pressure exerted by each individual gas in a mixture according to its concentration in the mixture) of oxygen (PO_2) in the alveoli is about 100 mm Hg, whereas the PO_2 in the entering venous blood of the pulmonary arteries is about 60 mm Hg. These pressures equalize very rapidly, however, so that the arterial pressure (PaO_2) also reaches about 100 mm Hg. By contrast, carbon dioxide in the venous blood entering the pulmonary capillaries has a partial pressure of about 45 mm Hg, whereas that in the alveoli has a partial pressure of about 40 mm Hg. These partial pressures frequently are used diagnostically to assess deficiencies or excesses of oxygen and carbon dioxide in persons with pulmonary disease.

The partial pressure of oxygen in arterial blood is abbreviated **PaO_2**. The partial pressure of oxygen in the air or in venous blood is written as **PO_2**. **PCO_2** and **$PaCO_2$** denote pressures of carbon dioxide in venous and arterial blood, respectively.

Transport of Oxygen and Carbon Dioxide

The third part of the respiratory process involves the transport of respiratory gases. Oxygen needs to be transported from the lungs to the tissues, and carbon dioxide must be transported from the tissues back to the lungs.

Oxygen Transport

Normally, most of the oxygen (97%) combines loosely with the **hemoglobin** (oxygen-carrying red pigment) in the red blood cells and is carried to the tissues as **oxyhemoglobin** (the compound of oxygen and hemoglobin). The remaining oxygen is dissolved and transported in the fluid of plasma and cells. The amount of oxygen that the blood will absorb before reaching saturation is about 20 ml per 100 ml of blood. This ratio is expressed as 20 vol%. Hemoglobin after it has released oxygen to the tissues is referred to as **reduced hemoglobin.** Normally, only about 25%—or 5 ml (¼ of 20 ml)—of oxygen per 100 ml of blood is diffused to the tissues (utilization coefficient). However, this rate of release can increase to 75% during periods of stress or increased exercise, since more oxygen is utilized by the cells. In situations of extreme oxygen lack in the tissues caused by a sluggish blood flow or a very high metabolic rate, the tissues can remove 100% of the oxygen from the blood (Guyton 1986, pp. 496–97).

Influencing Factors

Several factors affect the rate of oxygen transport from the lungs to the tissues. The major factors are (a) cardiac output, (b) number of erythrocytes, (c) exercise, and (d) blood hematocrit.

Normal **cardiac output** (amount of blood pumped by the heart) is approximately 5 liters per minute. In the person at rest, 250 ml of oxygen is transported per minute. Any pathologic condition that decreases cardiac output diminishes the amount of oxygen delivered to the tissues. Disease such as myocardial infarction (heart attack) weakens the pumping motion of the heart and thus inhibits the transport of oxygen. Hemorrhage or dehydration can significantly reduce the blood volume and subsequently the cardiac output. A backlog of blood in the venous system—for any reason—prevents adequate return of blood to the heart. These all reduce cardiac output and thus diminish oxygen transport. Generally, the heart compensates for inadequate output by increasing its pumping rate. Normally, compensatory cardiac output can increase the oxygen transport fivefold; but when disease conditions exist, this is not possible.

The second factor influencing oxygen transport is the number of **erythrocytes** (red blood cells, or RBC). In men the number of circulating erythrocytes is normally about 5 million per cubic milliliter of blood, and in women, about 4½ million per cubic milliliter. Reductions in these normal values can be brought about by anemia of any cause.

Exercise also has a direct influence on oxygen transport. In well-trained athletes, oxygen transport can be increased up to 20 times normal, due in part to an increased cardiac output and to increased utilization of oxygen by the cells (utilization coefficient).

The **hematocrit** is the percent of the blood that is erythrocytes. It is also referred to as the packed cell volume per 100 ml. Normally this ratio is about 40% to 50% in men and 35% to 45% in women. Excessive increases in the blood hematocrit increase the blood viscosity, reduce the cardiac output, and therefore reduce oxygen transport. Excessive reductions in the blood hematocrit, such as occur in anemia, also reduce oxygen transport. It is interesting to note that persons who develop elevated hematocrits when acclimatizing to high altitudes seldom have oxygen transport problems, probably because of an associated increase in the numbers and sizes of peripheral blood vessels, thus preventing a fall in cardiac output.

Carbon Dioxide Transport

On the return trip to the lungs, the hemoglobin, having released its oxygen, carries carbon dioxide. (Hemoglobin has the ability to combine with carbon dioxide as **carbaminohemoglobin.**) However, only a moderate amount of carbon dioxide (30%) is transported this way. The largest amount (about 65%) is carried in the form of bicarbonate (HCO_3^-) inside the red blood cells. Smaller amounts (5%) are transported in solution in the plasma and as **carbonic acid** (the compound formed when CO_2 combines with water). In the normal resting person, about 4 ml of CO_2 in each 100 ml of blood is transported from the tissues to the lungs. Carbon dioxide is an important factor in the acid-base balance of the body. This function is discussed in Chapter 46.

Respiratory Regulation

Respiratory regulation includes both neural and chemical controls.

Neural Controls

The nervous system of the body adjusts the rate of alveolar ventilations to meet the needs of the body so that Po_2 and Pco_2 remain relatively constant.

The "respiratory center" is actually a number of groups of neurons located in the medulla oblongata and pons of the brain. There are three main groups: a dorsal respiratory group, a ventral respiratory group, and the pneumotaxic center.

The *dorsal respiratory group* is located in the medulla. Stimulation of this group causes inspiration. Expiration, on the other hand, is produced passively, by elastic recoil of the distended lungs and chest. A second function of the dorsal group is the control of respiratory rhythm.

The *ventral respiratory group* is also located in the medulla of the brain. These neurons become active when there is a need for increased respiratory ventilation, and they then contribute to increased respiratory inspiration and expiration. This group of neurons remains inactive during normal, quiet respiration.

The *pneumotaxic center* is located in the upper part of the pons. Impulses from this area function primarily to control the duration of inspiration. Therefore the main function of the pneumotaxic center is to limit inspiration.

Chemical Controls

Respiratory control basically functions to maintain the correct concentrations of oxygen, carbon dioxide, and hydrogen ions in the body fluid. Respiratory activity is highly responsive to changes in the concentration of any one of these. There is believed to be a chemosensitive center in the medulla oblongata that is highly responsive to changes in blood CO_2 or hydrogen ion concentration. By influencing other respiratory centers, this center can increase the activity of the inspiratory center, the rate of respirations, and the rate and depth of inspirations.

In addition to direct chemical stimulation of the respiratory center in the brain, there are special receptors located outside the central nervous system, in the carotid and aortic bodies. Impulses from these **chemoreceptors** travel along Hering's nerves to the glossopharyngeal nerves and on to the dorsal respiratory area in the medulla. Changes in arterial oxygen concentrations have no direct effect on the respiratory center. Instead, such changes stimulate the chemoreceptors in the aortic and carotid bodies. For instance, when oxygen levels fall, these chemoreceptors are stimulated, and they in turn stimulate the respiratory center to increase ventilation. Of the three blood gases that can trigger chemoreceptors (carbon dioxide, hydrogen ions, and oxygen), it is an increase in carbon dioxide concentration that stimulates respiration most strongly. However, in clients with certain lung ailments, such as pneumonia and emphysema, oxygen concentrations—*not* carbon dioxide concentrations—play the major role in regulating respiration.

Voluntary Control

Respirations can also be controlled voluntarily. It is generally believed that impulses from the cerebral cortex pass directly along the corticospinal tract to the neurons that stimulate the respiratory muscles, making it possible for a person to increase her or his respiratory rate if she or he so desires.

Factors Affecting Oxygenation

Factors that influence oxygenation include altitude, environment, emotions, exercise, health, and life-style.

Altitude

The higher the altitude, the lower is the partial pressure of the oxygen (Po_2) an individual breathes. Consequently, the arterial blood has a lower Pao_2. As a result, the person at high altitudes has increased respiratory and cardiac rates and increased respiratory depth, which usually become most apparent to the individual upon exercising.

Environment

The need for oxygen is affected by the environment. In response to heat, the peripheral blood vessels dilate; consequently, blood flows to the skin, increasing the amount of heat lost from the body surface. Also, because of vasodilation, the lumens of blood vessels enlarge, thus decreasing the resistance to the blood flow. In response, the heart increases output to maintain blood pressure. The increased cardiac output requires additional oxygen; thus the rate and depth of breathing increase.

By contrast, in a cold environment the peripheral blood vessels constrict, raising the blood pressure, which decreases cardiac action, thereby reducing the need for oxygen.

Emotions

An accelerated heart rate is one body response to emotions such as fear, anxiety, and anger. It is thought that cardiac action is influenced by impulses from the higher centers in the cerebrum by way of the hypothalamus, which stimulates the cardiac centers (cardioinhibitory and cardioaccelerator) in the medulla of the brain. Motor fibers from those centers carry the impulses to parasympathetic and sympathetic neurons, which then transmit the impulses to the heart. For further information on stress reactions, see Chapter 17, page 336.

Exercise

Physical exercise or activity increases respirations and hence the supply of oxygen in the body. The mechanism underlying this effect is not completely known; however, it is thought that a number of factors are involved, including chemical, neural, and temperature changes.

Health

In the healthy person, the cardiovascular and respiratory systems can normally provide the oxygen the body needs. However, diseases of the cardiovascular system often affect the delivery of oxygen to the cells of the body. In addition, diseases of the respiratory system can adversely affect the oxygenation of the blood. In both instances, hypoxemia can result.

One cardiovascular condition that affects oxygenation is **anemia**, which is a deficiency in erythrocytes. When an individual's erythrocyte count is low—e.g., below 4.2 million per ml in men—the amount of hemoglobin normally present in the erythrocytes is often low. There are many reasons for anemia, including malnutrition, loss of blood, and the effect of chemicals. Because hemoglobin carries oxygen and carbon dioxide, as explained earlier, anemia can affect the delivery of these gases to and from the body cells. Terms associated with anemia are given in Table 45–3.

Table 45–3 Terms Related to Anemia

Term	Definition
Aplastic	Lack of functioning bone marrow
Hemolytic	Fragile erythrocytes that rupture easily
Hypochromic	Abnormal decrease in the amount of hemoglobin in the erythrocytes
Macrocytic	Abnormally large erythrocytes
Microcytic	Abnormally small erythrocytes
Normocyte	An erythrocyte of normal size, shape, and color
Pernicious	A type of anemia resulting from a deficiency in vitamin B_{12} or folic acid, which are necessary for normal erythrocyte development
Sickle cell	An anemia in which the erythrocytes contain abnormal hemoglobin

Life-Style

It is important to assess the life-style of the person with special oxygen needs. Data about smoking and the inhalation of polluted air can provide some indication of the condition of the client's lungs. Certain occupations predispose to lung disease. For example, silicosis is seen more often in sandstone blasters and potters than in the rest of the population; asbestosis in asbestos workers; anthracosis in coal miners; and organic dust disease in farmers and agricultural employees who work with moldy hay.

Alterations in Respiratory Function

Respiratory function can be altered by conditions that affect three areas of function: the movement of air into or out of the lungs, the diffusion of oxygen and carbon dioxide between the alveoli and the pulmonary capillaries, and the transport of oxygen and carbon dioxide via the blood to and from the tissue cells. Three major alterations in respiration are hypoxia, altered breathing pattern, and obstructed or partially obstructed airway.

Hypoxia

Hypoxia is a condition of insufficient oxygen anywhere in the body, from the inspired gas to the tissues. **Hypoxemia** is a condition of low partial pressure of oxygen or low saturation of oxyhemoglobin in the arterial blood (Vick 1984, p. 526). Hypoxia can be related to any of the three parts of respiration: ventilation, diffusion of gases, or transport of gases by the blood.

Ventilation. At high altitudes the partial pressure of oxygen is low; therefore, the alveolar Po_2 and the arterial Pao_2 are low. This form of hypoxia is called *hypoxic hypoxia.* Another cause of hypoxia is **hypoventilation,** that is, a decreased tidal volume. Whatever the reason for a decreased tidal volume (diseases of the respiratory muscles, drugs, or anesthetics, for example), carbon dioxide will often also accumulate in the blood. This condition is

Terms Related to Hypoxia

- *Respiratory insufficiency*—inability of the lungs to maintain normal arterial blood gas levels when the individual is breathing 21% oxygen (at sea level).
- *Hyperpnea*—excessively high rate of alveolar ventilation
- *Hypopnea*—low rate of alveolar ventilation, i.e., under-respiration
- *Hypocarbia (hypocapnia)*—depressed blood carbon dioxide level
- *Acapnia*—absence of carbon dioxide in the blood (this state is incompatible with life)

called **hypercarbia** (**hypercapnia**). Additional terms relating to hypoxia are given above.

Diffusion. Hypoxia can develop when the lungs' ability to diffuse oxygen into the arterial blood decreases, as with pulmonary edema.

Transport. Hypoxia can also result from problems in the delivery of oxygen to the tissues—for example, anemia, cardiac failure, and embolism.

Hypoxia may be acute or chronic. Early clinical signs of hypoxia are increased pulse rate, increased rate and depth of respirations, and slight increase in systolic blood pressure. Later signs include a slower pulse rate and lower systolic blood pressure, dyspnea, cough, and hemoptysis. **Cyanosis** (bluish discoloration of the skin, nail beds, and mucous membranes, due to reduced blood oxygen levels) may be present; however, a client can be hypoxic without exhibiting cyanosis. Cyanosis of the skin and mucous membranes requires these two conditions: (a) the blood must contain about 5 g or more of unoxygenated hemoglobin per 100 ml of blood, and (b) the surface blood capillaries must be dilated. Any factors that interfere with either of these conditions, e.g., severe anemia or the administration of adrenaline, will eliminate cyanosis as a sign even if the client is experiencing hypoxia.

Other clinical signs of acute hypoxia are nausea, vomiting, oliguria, and possibly anuria. Hypoxia can affect the central nervous system, resulting in headache, apathy, dizziness, irritability, and memory loss. The cerebral cortex can tolerate hypoxia for only 3 to 5 minutes before permanent damage occurs.

The face of the acutely hypoxic person usually appears anxious, tired, and drawn. Such a person usually assumes a sitting position, often leaning forward slightly to permit greater expansion of the thoracic cavity. The hypoxic client may or may not experience pain on breathing. Although lung tissue lacks pain receptors, pain can arise from the pleura, chest wall, or upper respiratory tract.

In long-term hypoxia, the client often appears fatigued. He or she is lethargic. The body often adapts to the lack of oxygen in the following manner: (a) pulmonary ventilation increases, (b) the red blood cell count increases, and (c) the hemoglobin concentration increases. The client's fingers are often clubbed as a result of long-term lack of oxygen in the arterial blood supply to the fingers. With clubbing, the base of the nail becomes swollen and the ends of the fingers and toes increase in size. The angle between the nail and the base of the nail increases to more than 160°. See Figure 35–16, page 812.

Altered Breathing Patterns

Breathing patterns refer to the rate, volume, rhythm, and relative ease or effort of respiration.

Alterations in Rate

Normal respiration (eupnea) is quiet, rhythmic, and effortless. Variations in rate include tachypnea and bradypnea. **Tachypnea** (rapid rate) is seen with fevers, metabolic acidosis (see Chapter 46), and pain and with hypercapnia (elevated blood CO_2) or anoxemia (decreased oxygen in the blood). **Bradypnea** is an abnormally slow respiratory rate, which may be seen in clients who have taken drugs such as morphine sulphate (which is a respiratory depressant), who have metabolic acidosis (see Chapter 46), or who have increased intracranial pressure, e.g., from brain injuries.

Alterations in Volume

There are two types of abnormal breathing volume: hyperventilation and hypoventilation. **Hyperventilation** is an excessive amount of air in the lungs. It is often called *alveolar hyperventilation* because the amount of air in the alveoli exceeds the body's metabolic requirements; that is, more CO_2 is eliminated than is produced, resulting in hypocapnia. Hyperventilation usually results from an increase in the rate and depth of respirations. One particular type of hyperventilation that accompanies metabolic acidosis is **Kussmaul breathing**, by which the body attempts to give off excess body acids by blowing off the carbon dioxide through deep and rapid breathing. Hyperventilation can occur after the administration of amphetamines because of the increased metabolic rate such drugs induce.

Hypoventilation is inadequate alveolar ventilation, i.e., ventilation that does not meet the body's requirements. As a result, carbon dioxide is retained in the bloodstream (hypercapnia) and hypoxemia results. Hypoventilation can occur, for example, as a result of collapse of the alveoli, leaving too few functioning alveoli to meet the body's ventilation needs; or from airway obstruction or the side-effects of some drugs. Hypoventilation is indicated when the arterial $Paco_2$ is above 35 to 45 mm Hg (Byrne et al. 1986, p. 285). Elevated $Paco_2$ levels may occur with pneumonia, asthma, and emphysema, for example.

Alterations in Rhythm

Abnormal respiratory rhythms create an irregular breathing pattern. There are a number of abnormal rhythms. See Chapter 34, page 787.

Alterations in Ease

Normal breathing is effortless. When breathing is difficult or labored, the condition is called **dyspnea.** The dyspneic person often appears anxious and may say, "I can't catch my breath." Often the nostrils will appear flared because of the increased effort of inspiration. The skin may appear dusky; heart rate is increased. **Orthopnea** is being able to breathe only in an upright sitting or standing position.

Obstructed Airway

A complete or partially obstructed **airway** can occur anywhere along the upper or lower respiratory passageways. An upper airway obstruction—i.e., in the nose, pharynx, larynx, or trachea—can rise because of a foreign object, such as food; because the tongue falls back into the oropharynx when a person is unconscious; or when secretions collect in the passageways. In the latter instance, the respirations will sound gurgly or bubbly as the air attempts to pass through the secretions. Lower airway obstruction involves partial or complete occlusion of the passageways in the lungs, i.e., the bronchi.

Maintaining an open (patent) airway is a frequent nursing intervention, and one that often requires immediate action. See "Opening the Airway" later in this chapter. Partial obstruction of the upper airway passages is indicated by a low-pitched snoring sound during inhalation. Complete obstruction is indicated by extreme inspiratory effort that produces no chest movement. Such a client, in an effort to obtain air, may also exhibit marked sternal and intercostal contractions. Lower airway obstruction is not always as easy to observe. The client may have altered arterial blood gas levels, restlessness, dyspnea, and **adventitious** (abnormal) breath **sounds**. See Table 35–12, page 847.

Assessment

Assessment regarding oxygenation includes taking a nursing history, performing a physical health examination, and collecting relevant data from records and reports.

Nursing History

A nursing history relevant to oxygenation should include the following areas. Terms describing oxygenation are given on page 1294.

1. *Respiratory problems.* Has the client experienced a problem such as wheezing or shortness of breath? Which of the client's activities might cause these symptoms to occur?
2. *History of respiratory diseases.* Has the client had colds, asthma, croup, bronchitis, or pneumonia? How frequently have these occurred? How long did they last? And how were they treated?
3. *The presence of a cough.* Is it productive or nonproductive? A **productive cough** is accompanied by expectorated secretions. To **expectorate** is to cough and spit out secretions from the lungs, bronchi, and trachea. When a client has a productive cough, a sputum specimen is usually obtained and sent to the laboratory for examination. See "Diagnostic Records and Reports" later in this chapter. When a cough is productive, the nurse should question the client about the sputum: When is sputum produced? What is the amount, color, thickness, and odor?
4. *Life-style.* Does the client smoke? If so, how much? Does any member of the client's family smoke?
5. *Cardiovascular problems.* Does the client have a history of cardiac or blood circulation problems?
6. *Pain.* Does the client experience any pain associated with breathing or activity? Pain that is a result of activity may reflect a cardiovascular problem. Pain associated with breathing can indicate any number of problems, including infections of the lungs or pleura, injured ribs, and trauma to the chest muscles. Where is the pain located? What words does the client use to describe the pain? How long does it last? What activities precede the pain? And what is the effect of the pain on respiration? See Chapter 41, page 1122, for additional information on assessing pain.
7. *Risk factors.* Are there present any risk factors that can impair oxygenation? Some of these are listed on page 1295. Also see Chapter 20, page 430.
8. *Medication history.* Has the client taken or does the client take any over-the-counter or prescription medications for heart, blood pressure, or breathing? Which ones? And what are the dosages, times taken, and effects on the client, including side-effects?
9. *Stressors.* What stressors exist in the client's life? For example, the alcohol problems of a partner may affect respiratory and cardiac problems.
10. *Health status.* What are the client's perceptions of her or his health status? Even though a client may present numerous problems, she or he may consider herself or himself to be well or even healthier than in previous years.

Terms Describing Oxygenation

Breathing Patterns

Rate

- *Eupnea*—normal respiration that is quiet, rhythmic, and effortless
- *Tachypnea*—rapid respiration marked by quick, shallow breaths
- *Bradypnea*—abnormally slow breathing
- *Apnea*—cessation of breathing

Volume

- *Hyperventilation*—an increase in the amount of air in the lungs characterized by prolonged and deep breaths; may be associated with anxiety
- *Hypoventilation*—a reduction in the amount of air in the lungs; characterized by shallow respirations

Rhythm

- *Cheyne-Stokes breathing*—rhythmic waxing and waning of respirations, from very deep to very shallow breathing and temporary apnea; often associated with cardiac failure, increased intracranial pressure, or brain damage

Ease or effort

- *Dyspnea*—difficult and labored breathing during which the individual has a persistent, unsatisfied need for air and feels distressed
- *Orthopnea*—ability to breathe only in upright sitting or standing positions

Breath Sounds

Audible without amplification

- *Stridor*—a shrill, harsh sound heard during inspiration with laryngeal obstruction
- *Stertor*—snoring or sonorous respiration, usually due to a partial obstruction of the upper airway
- *Wheeze*—a whistling respiratory sound on expiration that usually indicates a narrowing of the bronchial tree
- *Bubbling*—gurgling sounds heard as air passes through moist secretions in the respiratory tract

Audible by stethoscope

- *Rales*—rattling or bubbling sounds generally heard on inspiration as air moves through accumulated moist secretions
- *Rhonchi*—coarse, dry, wheezy, or whistling sound more audible during expiration as the air moves through tenacious mucus or narrowed bronchi
- *Creps* (crepitation)—a dry, crackling sound (like crumpled cellophane) produced by air in the subcutaneous tissue or by air moving through fluid in the alveoli
- *Pleural rub*—coarse, leathery, or grating sound produced by the rubbing together of the pleura; also called *friction rub*

Chest Movements

- *Intercostal retraction*—indrawing between the ribs
- *Substernal retraction*—indrawing beneath the breast bone
- *Suprasternal retraction*—indrawing above the breast bone
- *Supraclavicular retraction*—indrawing above the clavicles
- *Tracheal tug*—indrawing and downward pull of the trachea during inspiration
- *Flail chest*—the ballooning out of the chest wall through injured rib spaces; results in *paradoxical breathing,* during which the chest wall balloons on expiration but is depressed or sucked inward on inspiration

Secretions and Coughing

- *Hemoptysis*—the presence of blood in the sputum
- *Productive cough*—a cough accompanied by expectorated secretions
- *Nonproductive cough*—a dry, harsh cough without secretions

11. *Strengths.* What are the client's strengths at this time? For instance, does the client have any insight into her or his health problems? Does she or he comply with therapeutic regimens?

Clinical Examinations

Clinically examining a client with reference to oxygenation should include four examination techniques: inspection, palpation, percussion, and auscultation.

Respirations. Respirations are assessed for rate, depth, rhythm, and quality. See Chapter 34, page 786.

Posture. The position the client assumes for breathing is also important. Some clients with chronic respiratory problems prefer to bend forward at the waist to ease breathing. Often a client prefers to sit leaning over a table, which position permits maximal lung expansion as compared to lying on the back or on either side, which restricts expansion of part of the thorax (the underlying portion). Although the decreased expansion is small to a dyspneic

Risk Factors Relative to Oxygenation

- Family history of hypertension, heart disease, or cerebrovascular accident
- Smoking
- Middle age or older
- Overweight or obesity
- Sedentary life-style
- Diet high in saturated fats
- Elevated serum cholesterol or triglycerides (Bellack and Bamford 1984, p. 362)

Terms Describing Circulatory Status

Heart rate

- *Tachycardia*—excessively rapid heart rate; over 100 beats per minute in the adult
- *Bradycardia*—abnormally slow heart rate; below 60 beats per minute in the adult
- *Pulse deficit*—difference between the apical and radial pulses

Blood pressure

- *Hypertension*—elevated arterial blood pressure
- *Hypotension*—abnormally low arterial blood pressure

Oxygenation

- *Anoxia*—systematic absence or reduction of oxygen below physiologic levels in body tissues; frequently accompanied by increased pulse rate, rapid or deep respirations, cyanosis, restlessness, anxiety, dizziness (vertigo), or faintness (synscope)
- *Hypoxemia*—deficient oxygenation of the blood, as measured by laboratory tests
- *Hypoxia*—diminished availability of oxygen for body tissues due to internal or external causes
- *Cyanosis*—bluish color of mucous membrane, nail beds, or skin due to excessive deoxygenation of hemoglobin

client, it may be important. See "Positioning," page 1299.

Thorax shape. The shape of the thorax should be inspected. See Chapter 35, page 840.

Lungs. The lungs should be palpated for breath sounds and voice sounds; auscultated; and assessed for diaphragmatic excursion. See Chapter 35, page 843.

Heart. The heart should be palpated and auscultated for indications of problems that might impede blood flow and the delivery of oxygen to the tissues. See Chapter 35, page 853, for heart assessment. Terms significant to circulatory assessment are given to the right.

Diagnostic Records and Reports

A number of diagnostic tests are frequently performed relative to oxygenation. Often it is a nurse who collects the specimens that are sent to the laboratory for analysis.

Sputum

Sputum is the mucous secretion from the lungs, bronchi, and trachea. It is important to differentiate it from *saliva,* the clear liquid secreted by the salivary glands in the mouth, sometimes referred to as "spit." Healthy individuals do not produce sputum. Clients need to cough to bring sputum up from the lungs, bronchi, and trachea into the mouth in order to expectorate it into a collecting container.

Sputum specimens are usually collected for one or more of the following reasons:

1. For "culture and sensitivity," that is, to identify a specific microorganism and its drug sensitivities.
2. For "cytology." **Cytology** is the study of the origin, structure, function, and pathology of cells. Specimens for cytology often require serial collection of three early morning specimens and are tested to identify cancer in the lung and its specific cell type. Specimens for "acid-fast bacillus (AFB)," which also require serial collection, often for three consecutive days, are obtained to identify the presence of this particular organism, also known as the tubercle bacillus (TB). Some agencies use a special glass container when the presence of AFB is suspected.
3. To assess the effectiveness of therapy. Sputum specimens are often collected in the morning, for upon awakening, the client can cough up the secretions that have accumulated during the night. The client rinses his or her mouth with water but does not eat or drink until the sputum has been expectorated. Sometimes specimens are collected during postural drainage, when the client can usually produce sputum. When a client cannot cough, the nurse must sometimes use pharyngeal suctioning to obtain a specimen.

In order to collect a sputum specimen, the nurse should have the client breathe deeply and cough up 1 to 2 tablespoons of sputum (15 to 30 ml, or 4 to 8 fluid drams). The client then expectorates into the specimen container, taking care that the sputum does not contact the outside of the container (see Figure 45–3). If the outside of the container should become contaminated,

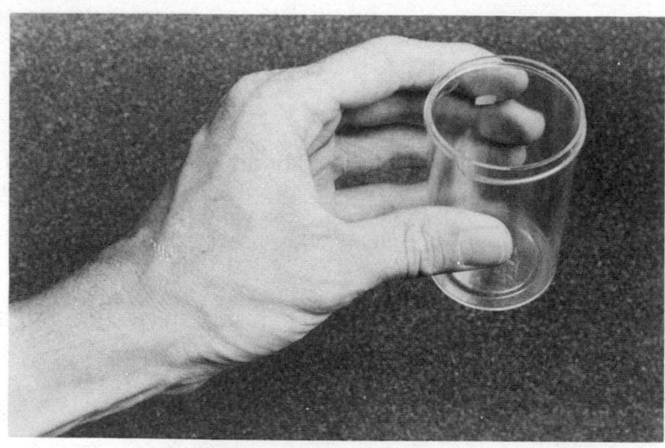

Figure 45–3 Sputum specimen container

the nurse washes it with a disinfectant. The client might wish a mouth wash after producing the specimen, to remove any unpleasant taste. When recording the collection of the sputum specimen the nurse should include the amount, color, odor, consistency (thick, tenacious, watery, etc.), and the presence of any blood (hemoptysis). Normal sputum often contains the same kinds of microorganisms found in the upper respiratory passages. The normal flora found in sputum are listed to the right.

Normal Flora of Sputum

Bacteria

- *Bacteroides* species
- *Borrelia* species
- *Corynebacterium diphtheriae*
- *Fusobacterium* species
- *Haemophilus influenzae*
- *Neisseria catarrhalis*
- *Staphylococcus aureus*
- *Staphylococcus epidermidis*
- *Streptococcus* species (groups A, B, D)
- *Streptococcus pneumoniae*
- *Streptococcus viridans*

Fungi

- *Candida albicans* (Byrne et al. 1986, p. 513)

Nose and Throat Specimens

Nose and throat specimens are collected from the mucosa of the nose and throat and then cultured and examined for the presence of disease-producing microorganisms.

To obtain a specimen a nurse will need the following equipment:

1. Four sterile swabs or applicators. Swabs are sterilized and then stored in a manner that keeps them from contact with the air and any unsterilized materials.
2. A tongue blade, to depress the client's tongue and expose the pharynx.
3. Four containers of growing medium or four sterile containers to hold the specimens. Frequently, glass tubes with securely attachable caps are used. Some agencies use special tubes containing about 2 ml of broth, which keeps the air in the tube moist so the specimen will not dry out. The swab is suspended without touching the broth.
4. A source of light, to illuminate the inside of the mouth and throat.
5. An otoscope with a nasal speculum, to light the inside of the nose and provide access to the area to be swabbed.
6. A moisture-resistant waste container in which to discard the tongue blade.
7. A container for the nasal speculum, e.g., a kidney basin.
8. Completed labels for each specimen container, including client identification information and the exact source of the specimen, e.g., right nostril or left tonsil.
9. A completed requisition to accompany the specimens to the laboratory.

Taking a throat specimen Assist the client to a sitting position if health permits. This is the most comfortable position for many clients and one in which the pharynx is clearly visible. Ask the client to open her or his mouth and say "ah." Assess the pharynx and tonsils for redness, swelling, and discharge. Extending the tongue exposes the pharynx. Saying "ah" relaxes the throat muscles and helps minimize contraction of the constriction muscle of the pharynx (the gag reflex). If the posterior pharynx cannot be seen, use a light and depress the tongue with a tongue blade. Depress the tongue firmly without touching the throat, to avoid stimulating the gag reflex. See Figure 45–4. Insert a swab into the mouth, taking care not to touch any part of the mouth or tongue. Quickly run the swab along the tonsils, making sure to contact any areas on the pharynx that are particularly erythematous (reddened) or that contain exudate. Erythematous areas and areas with exudate will likely have the most microorganisms. The swab should not pick up microorganisms in the mouth. The swab is moved quickly to avoid initiating the gag reflex or causing discomfort.

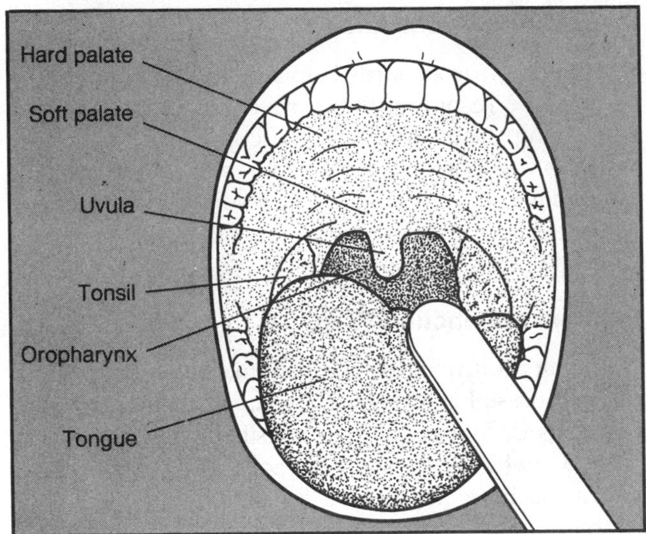

Figure 45–4

Remove the swab without touching the mouth or lips, to avoid transmitting microorganisms to the mouth.

Insert the swab into the sterile tube or container of growing medium without allowing it to touch the outside of the container. Make sure the swab is placed in the correctly labeled tube. Touching the outside of the tube could transmit microorganisms to it and then to others. Place the top securely on the tube, taking care not to touch the inside of the cap so as to avoid transmitting additional microorganisms into the tube. Repeat with the second swab. Discard the tongue blade in the waste container.

Taking a nasal specimen Gently insert the lighted nasal speculum up one nostril. Observe the inside of the nostril for redness, discharge, and swelling. Insert the sterile swab carefully through the speculum without touching the edges. Wipe along the reddened areas or areas with the most exudate. Remove the swab without touching the speculum, and place it in a sterile tube. Repeat for the other nostril.

Venous Blood Samples

Specimens of venous blood are taken for a complete blood count (CBC), which includes hemoglobin and hematocrit measurements, erythrocyte (RBC) count, leukocyte (WBC) count, and a differential red cell and white cell count. For the venipuncture technique, see Chapter 46, page 1346. See Table 45–4 for normal values.

The hematocrit is the packed cell volume. It denotes the percent of a given volume of whole blood occupied by erythrocytes (RBCs). Therefore, a hematocrit level of 25% indicates that erythrocytes make up 25% of the total volume of whole blood. Hematocrit levels are usually related to hemoglobin values.

Erythrocyte counts show the number of red blood cells in 1 ml or 1 ml^3 of whole blood. The level of red blood cells is regulated by their rate of formation in the bone marrow. The rate of red blood cell formation normally remains relatively constant; however, in clients with hypoxia, **erythropoiesis** (the formation of red blood cells) is stimulated.

A white blood cell count determines the number of circulating leukocytes (white blood cells) in 1 ml or 1 ml^3 of whole blood. Above-normal WBC counts indicate increased production of leukocytes by the bone marrow, often in response to the presence of bacterial pathogens in the body. Decreased WBC levels, by contrast, are due to decreased production of leukocytes, often because of the presence of viruses or toxic chemicals in the body.

Differential leukocyte and erythrocyte counts enumerate the different kinds of white and red blood cells in the blood specimen. A number of white blood cells are identified and classified according to their **morphology** (their form and structure). The percentage distribution of the different kinds of white blood cells can assist in diagnosis because characteristic patterns of distribution

Table 45–4 Normal Values of a Complete Blood Count

Age	Hemoglobin (g/dl*)	Hematocrit (%)	RBC (million/μl†)	WBC (/μl‡)
Newborn	18–27	42–68	4.8–7.0	9000–30,000
1 year	9.0–14.6	29–41	3.6–5.5	6000–17,500
3 years	9.4–15.5	29–44	3.8–5.4	4500–13,500
10 years	10.7–15.5	34–45	3.9–5.2	4500–13,500
Adult man	14–18	40–54	4.5–6.2	4500–11,000
Adult woman	12–16	37–47	4.0–5.5	4500–11,000

*g/dl = grams per deciliter (1/10 of a liter, metric equivalent)
†million/μl = million per microliter (10^{-3} ml, metric equivalent)
‡/μl = per microliter (10^{-3} ml, metric equivalent)

Source: Adapted from C. J. Byrne, D. F. Saxton, P. K. Pelikan, and P. M. Nugent, *Laboratory tests: Implications for nurses and allied health professionals*, 2d ed. (Menlo Park, Calif.: Addison-Wesley Publishing Co., 1986), pp. 67–74.

are consistent with certain disorders. Red blood cells are examined for their size, shape, color, maturation, and content.

Arterial Blood Samples

Specimens of arterial blood are normally taken by specialty nurses or medical technicians. Tests performed on arterial blood can indicate a client's respiratory status: Arterial blood is often tested for partial pressure of oxygen (PaO_2), partial pressure of carbon dioxide ($PaCO_2$), oxygen saturation (SO_2 or O_2Sat), hydrogen ion concentration (pH), and the amount of bicarbonate (HCO_3^-) and base excess (BE). For further information about these tests, see Chapter 46.

Blood for these tests is taken from the radial, brachial, or femoral arteries. Because of the relatively great pressure of the blood in these arteries, it is important to prevent hemorrhaging by applying pressure to the puncture site for about 5 minutes after removing the needle.

Visualization Procedures

A number of procedures help medical personnel view parts of the respiratory tract: roentgenography, fluoroscopy, lung scan, and bronchoscopy. For further information about these procedures and the nursing assessment and interventions involved, see Chapter 54.

Pulmonary Function Tests

Pulmonary function tests measure many of the lung functions discussed earlier in this chapter. Pulmonary function tests do not require an anesthetic and are usually carried out by a respiratory therapist. The client breathes into a machine. The tests are painless, but the client's cooperation is essential. Nurses need to explain the tests to people beforehand and help them get rest afterward, because the tests are often tiring.

Nursing Diagnosis

There are four main categories of nursing diagnoses relative to oxygenation: (a) alterations in respiratory function, (b) ineffective airway clearance, (c) ineffective breathing patterns, and (c) alterations in cardiac output. Examples of nursing diagnoses related to oxygenation are given to the right.

Examples of Nursing Diagnoses Related to Oxygenation

- Alterations in respiratory function related to pain secondary to abdominal incision
- Alterations in respiratory function related to smoking 2 to 3 packs of cigarettes for 15 years
- Alterations in respiratory function related to allergy to unknown pollens
- Ineffective airway clearance related to ineffective coughing
- Ineffective airway clearance related to fear of pain
- Ineffective breathing pattern related to activity
- Alterations in cardiac output related to anemia
- Alterations in cardiac output related to medications

Planning

Planning for a client's actual or potential oxygenation problems relates to one or more of the following:

1. Facilitating pulmonary ventilation
2. Facilitating the diffusion of gases
3. Facilitating the transport of oxygen and carbon dioxide

Facilitating pulmonary ventilation may include ensuring a patent airway, positioning, deep breathing and coughing, and ensuring adequate hydration. Other nursing interventions helpful to ventilation are suctioning, lung inflation techniques, postural drainage, and percussion and vibration.

Nursing strategies that can facilitate the diffusion of gases through the alveolar membrane include coughing and deep breathing, and suitable activity. To promote the transport of oxygen and carbon dioxide, cardiac output can be optimized by reducing stress, planning appropriate activities, and positioning the client so as to promote vascular blood flow.

A client's nursing care plan should also include dependent nursing interventions such as oxygen therapy, tracheostomy care, and maintenance of a chest tube.

Nursing Interventions

Positioning

Normally, adequate ventilation is maintained by frequent changes of position, ambulation, and exercise. When persons become ill, however, their respiratory functions may be inhibited, for a variety of reasons. One common reason is immobility induced by surgery or medical therapy. Lying too long in one position compresses the thorax, limits chest expansion, and thus inhibits the movement of air through the lungs. Sitting in a slumped position also inhibits chest expansion, since the abdominal contents are pushed up against the diaphragm. Another frequent cause of limited chest expansion is abdominal pain or chest pain. The client often voluntarily limits chest movements to relieve the pain. Shallow respirations inhibit both diaphragmatic excursion and lung distensibility. The result of inadequate chest expansion is stasis and pooling of respiratory secretions, which ultimately harbor microorganisms and promote infection. This situation is often compounded in the hospitalized client who receives narcotics for pain, because narcotics further depress the rate and depth of respiration.

Interventions by the nurse to maintain the normal respirations of clients include (a) positioning the client to allow for maximum chest expansion, (b) encouraging or providing frequent changes in position, (c) encouraging ambulation, and (d) implementing measures that promote comfort, such as giving pain medications. The semi-Fowler's or high-Fowler's position encourages maximum chest expansion in bedfast clients, particularly dyspneic clients. The nurse needs to encourage clients unable to assume this position to turn from side to side frequently, so that alternate sides of the chest are permitted maximum expansion.

In-hospital dyspneic clients often sit in bed and lean over their overbed tables (which are raised to a suitable height), usually with a pillow for support. This position, referred to as an *orthopneic position,* is an adaptation of the high-Fowler's position. It has a further advantage in that, as with high-Fowler's, the abdominal organs are not pressing on the diaphragm. Also, in the orthopneic position a client can press the lower part of the chest against the table to help in exhaling.

Deep Breathing and Coughing

In addition to positioning clients, the nurse can facilitate respiratory functioning by encouraging **deep-breathing** exercises and coughing to remove secretions. Breathing exercises are frequently indicated for clients with restricted chest expansion, i.e., people with chronic obstructive pulmonary disease (COPD) or recovering from thoracic surgery. Commonly employed breathing exercises are abdominal (diaphragmatic) and pursed-lip breathing, apical expansion, and basal expansion exercises. Deep-breathing and coughing exercises for the postoperative client are discussed in Chapter 53. Procedure 45–1 details how to teach such exercises.

Research Note

Nurses bathe clients or assist them with bathing during all phases of illness. Nurses, therefore, can profit greatly from increased knowledge of the physiologic changes and "costs" during this activity. Winslow, Love, and Gaffney compared 22 normal subjects with 18 stable, acute postmyocardial infarction (MI) clients while they bathed themselves in a tub, in a shower, or from a basin. Oxygen consumption, EKG tracings via a Holter monitor, and subjective symptoms all were measured. The investigators found that, in clients taking all three types of baths, oxygen consumption increased less than threefold and there were no ischemic changes noted in the heart. There were some rhythm disturbances, which were as expected in postinfarction clients. Both control subjects and postinfarction clients decidedly preferred tub baths or showers. In fact, a self-administered basin bath created more exertion for many subjects. In general, this study supports the idea that many stable, acute MI clients who can tolerate the upright position and are able to get in and out of a tub can safely take either a tub bath or a shower if the water is about body temperature. (Winslow, Lane, and Gaffney 1985)

Procedure 45–1 ▲ Teaching Deep-Breathing Exercises

Intervention

Abdominal (Diaphragmatic) and Pursed-Lip Breathing

1. Explain to the client that diaphragmatic breathing can help her or him to breathe more deeply and with less effort.

2. Have the client assume a comfortable semi-Fowler's position with knees flexed, back supported, and one head pillow, or a supine position with one head pillow and knees flexed. After learning the exercise, the client can practice, first in either supine or semi-Fowler's position and then when sitting upright, standing, and walking.

   Rationale The supine and semi-Fowler's positions with knees flexed help relax the abdominal muscles.

3. Have the client place one or both hands on the abdomen, just below the ribs. See Figure 45–5.

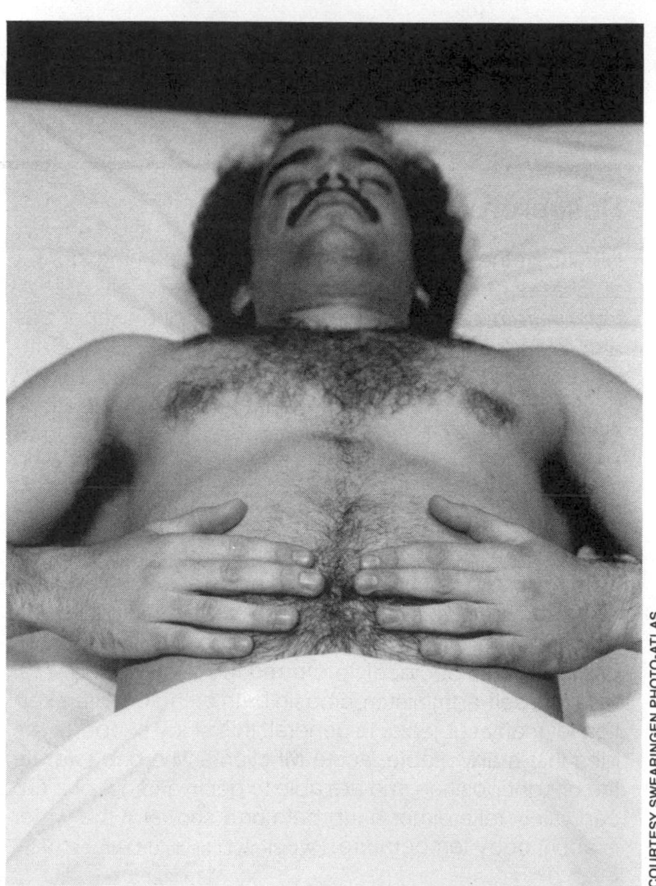

Figure 45–5

4. Instruct the client to breathe in deeply through the nose, with the mouth closed, to stay relaxed, not to arch the back, and to concentrate on feeling the abdomen rise as far as possible.

   Rationale When the client breathes in, the diaphragm contracts (drops), the lungs fill with air, and the abdomen rises or protrudes. See Figure 45–1 on page 1286.

5. If the client has difficulty raising the abdomen, have him or her take a quick, forceful inhalation through the nose.

   Rationale With a quick sniff, the client will feel the abdomen rise.

6. Instruct the client to purse the lips as if about to whistle, to breathe out slowly and gently, making a slow "whooshing" sound, not to puff out the cheeks, to concentrate on feeling the abdomen fall or sink, and to tighten (contract) the abdominal muscles while breathing out.

   Rationale Pursing the lips creates a resistance to air flowing out of the lungs, increases pressure within the bronchi, and minimizes the collapse of smaller bronchioles, a common problem for clients with COPD. While the client breathes out, the diaphragm relaxes (rises) and the abdomen sinks. See Figure 45–1 on page 1286. Tightening the abdominal muscles helps the client exhale more effectively.

7. If the client has COPD, teach her or him the "double cough" technique. Have the client:
   a. Breathe in through the nose and inflate the lungs to the midinspiration point rather than to the full, deep inspiration point
   b. Simultaneously exhale and cough two or more abrupt, sharp coughs in rapid succession

   Rationale A very forceful cough by a client with COPD can cause small-airway collapse. With two or more abrupt coughs, the first one loosens secretions, and subsequent coughs facilitate movement of secretions toward the upper airways.

8. Instruct the client to use this exercise whenever feeling short of breath and to increase it gradually to 5 to 10 minutes four times a day.

   Rationale Regular practice enables the client to eventually do this type of breathing without conscious effort.

Apical Expansion Exercises

Apical expansion exercises are often required for clients who restrict their upper chest movement because of pain from a severe respiratory disease or surgery, e.g., lobectomy (removal of a lung lobe) or mastectomy (removal of a breast).

9. Place your fingers below the client's clavicles and exert moderate pressure, or have the client place her or his hands over the same area. See Figure 45–6.

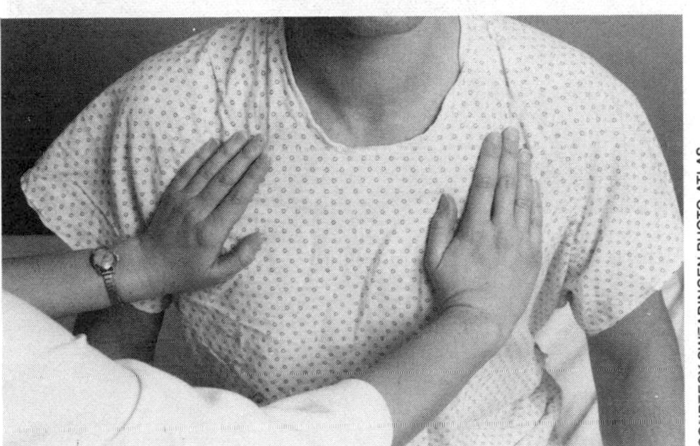

Figure 45–6

Rationale This hand position enables evaluation of the depth of apical inhalation.

10. Instruct the client to inhale through the nose and to concentrate on pushing the upper chest upward and forward against the fingers.

    Rationale This helps to aerate the apical areas of the upper lung lobes.

11. Have the client hold the inhalation for a few seconds.

    Rationale This promotes aeration of the alveoli.

12. Have the client exhale through the mouth or nose slowly, quietly, and passively while concentrating on moving the upper chest inward and downward.

13. Instruct the client to perform the exercise for at least five respirations four times a day.

    Rationale Repeating the exercise helps to reexpand lung tissue, eliminate secretions, and minimize flattening of the upper chest wall.

Basal Expansion Exercises

Basal expansion exercises are often required for clients who have restricted bilateral chest movements because of pain from a respiratory disorder or chest surgery.

14. Place the palms of your hands in the area of the client's lower ribs, along the midaxillary lines, and exert moderate pressure, or have the client place her or his hands over the same area. See Figure 45–7.

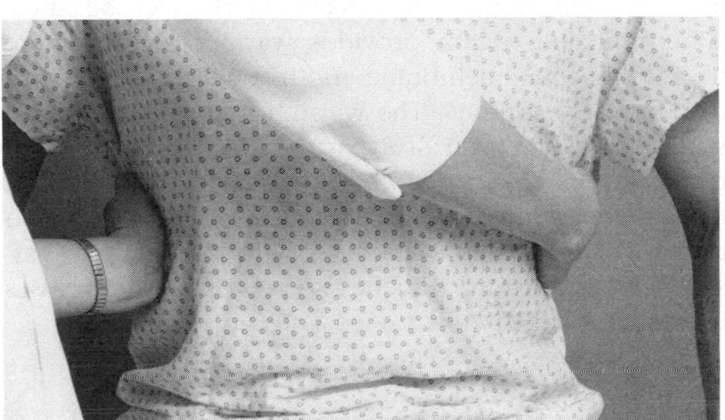

Figure 45–7

Rationale This hand position enables evaluation and comparison of the depth of bilateral basal inspiration.

15. Instruct the client to inhale through the nose and to concentrate on moving the lower chest outward against the hands.
16. Have the client hold the inhalation for a few seconds.
17. Have the client exhale through the nose or mouth slowly, quietly, and passively. If the client has COPD, observe the rate and character of the exhalation. Normal exhalation is slow, and the upper chest appears relaxed. If the exhalation appears difficult or there is indrawing of the upper chest, encourage pursed-lip exhalation. See step 6 above.
18. Instruct the client to perform this exercise for at least five respirations four times a day.

    Rationale Repetition helps to reexpand lung tissue and eliminate secretions.

Hydration

Adequate hydration maintains the moisture of the respiratory mucous membranes. Normally, respiratory tract secretions are thin and therefore moved readily by ciliary action. However, when the client is dehydrated or when the environment has a low humidity, the respiratory secretions can become thick and tenacious. The mucous membranes then become irritated and prone to infection. Nursing measures to increase and monitor fluid intake are discussed in Chapter 46. If the air lacks humidity, humidifiers may be necessary.

There are also several types of steam inhalators available. In the home, an electric kettle can be used. When inhaled, steam provides warmth and moisture to the mucous membrane. Both facilitate the expectoration of secretions. The warmth increases the blood supply and hydration of the respiratory membranes by transudation. *Transudation* is the passage of body fluid through a membrane or tissue surface. Warmth also relaxes the smooth muscles of the respiratory passages. The moisture liquefies secretions and decreases irritation.

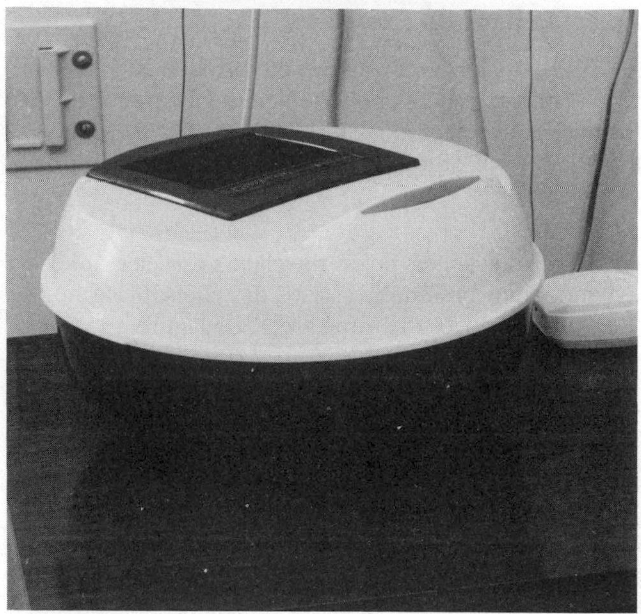

Figure 45–8 A room humidifier

Humidifiers and Nebulizers

Humidifiers are devices that add water vapor to inspired air. Their purposes are to prevent mucous membranes from drying and becoming irritated and to loosen secretions for easier expectoration. All humidifiers employ the simple method of passing the gas through sterile water so that water vapor is picked up before the gas reaches the client. The more bubbles are created during this process, the more water vapor is produced. Some humidifiers heat the water vapor, which increases the humidity provided. There are several kinds of humidifiers; three main types are the room humidifier (for home use most often), the cascade humidifier, and the cold bubble diffuser (humidifier).

A *room humidifier* (see Figure 45–8) can provide either cool mist or steam. Some types can be used with gas lines, e.g., oxygen, to provide moistened air directly to the client.

A *cascade humidifier* can deliver 100% humidity at body temperature. The temperature of the vapor can be controlled, and the machine can be used to provide humidified oxygen to clients on ventilators.

A *cold bubble diffuser* or *humidifier* (see Figure 45–9) is used with all oxygen equipment to moisten the oxygen before it is inhaled. This device provides 20% to 40% humidity. The oxygen passes through sterile distilled water and then along a line to the device through which the moistened oxygen is inhaled (e.g., a cannula, nasal catheter, or oxygen mask). See "Oxygen Therapy" later in this chapter.

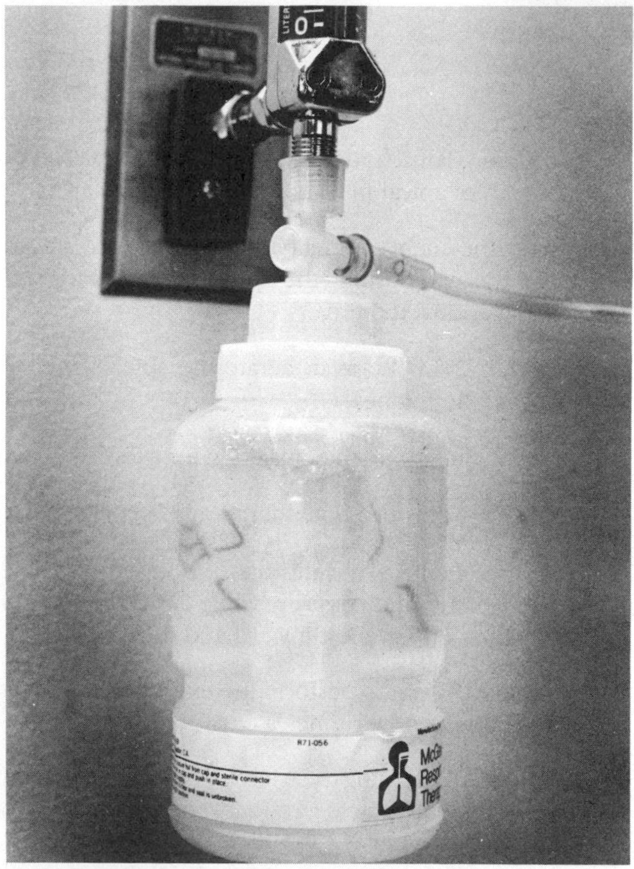

Figure 45–9 A cold bubble humidifier

A *nebulizer* is used to deliver a fine spray of medication or moisture to a client. *Nebulization* is the production of a fog or mist. There are two kinds: atomization and aerosolization. In *atomization,* a device called an *atomizer* produces rather large droplets for inhalation. When the droplets are suspended in a gas, such as oxygen, the process is **inhalation (aerosol) therapy**. The smaller the droplets, the further they can be inhaled into the respiratory tract. When a medication is intended for the nasal mucosa, it is inhaled through the nose; when it is intended for the trachea, bronchi, and/or lungs, it is inhaled through the mouth.

Nebulization can be provided by a large-volume nebulizer, ultrasonic nebulizer, hand nebulizer, mini-nebulizer (Maxi-mist), or side-stream nebulizer. A *large-volume nebulizer* can provide a heated or cool mist. It is used for long-term therapy, such as that following a tracheostomy. These nebulizers have a 250-ml capacity and deliver oxygen or room air.

The *ultrasonic nebulizer* (see Figure 45–10) provides 100% humidity and can provide particles small enough to be inhaled deeply into the respiratory tract. There are two types: One has a cup that is filled with sterile distilled water; the other requires a continuous supply of sterile distilled water from a bag connected by tubing to the nebulizer bottle.

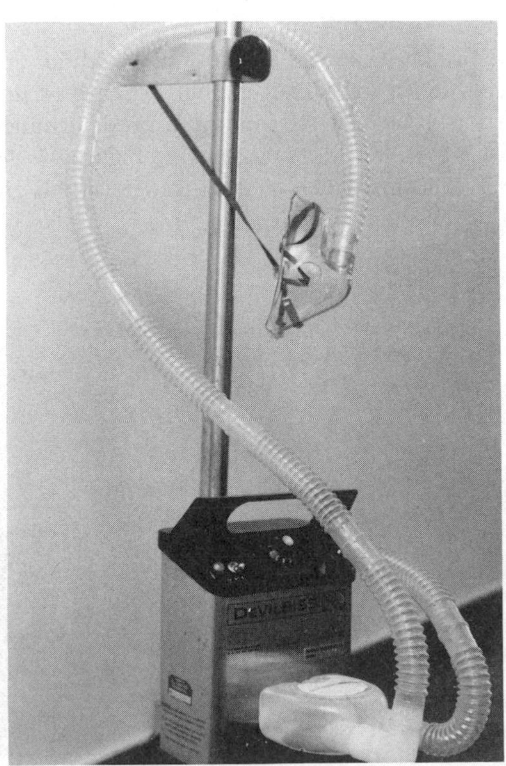

Figure 45–10 An ultrasonic nebulizer

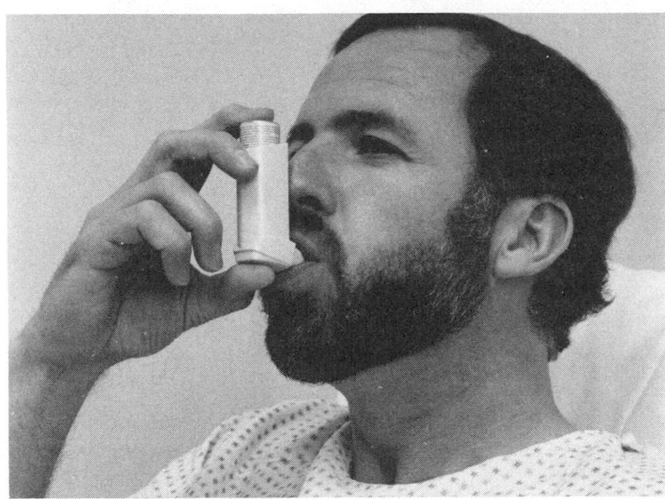

Figure 45–11 A hand nebulizer

The *hand nebulizer* (see Figure 45–11) is a container of medication that can be compressed by hand to release the medication through a nosepiece or mouthpiece. The force with which the air moves through the nebulizer causes the large particles of medicated solution to break up into finer particles, forming a mist or fine spray.

The *mini-nebulizer* is used with oxygen or a pressurized gas source, e.g., air. With this device, the client inhales and exhales independently. Medication is administered during inhalation. These units are available commercially and are disposable.

A *side-stream nebulizer* provides a medication to a client on a ventilator or receiving IPPB therapy. The gas, e.g., oxygen, passes through a device containing the medicated solution and then into the ventilator and to the client.

Lung Inflation Techniques

Lung inflation techniques are meant to assist the client increase her or his lung inflation. Three types are: blow bottles, sustained maximal inspiration (SMI) devices, and volume-oriented SMIs.

Blow Bottles and Sustained Maximal Inspiration Devices

Blow bottles are two bottles half filled with water and connected by tubing. They provide feedback about a client's respiratory *exhalation.* The client moves the water from one bottle to the other by blowing into a short tube connected to the first bottle. See Figure 45–12. Lung inflation

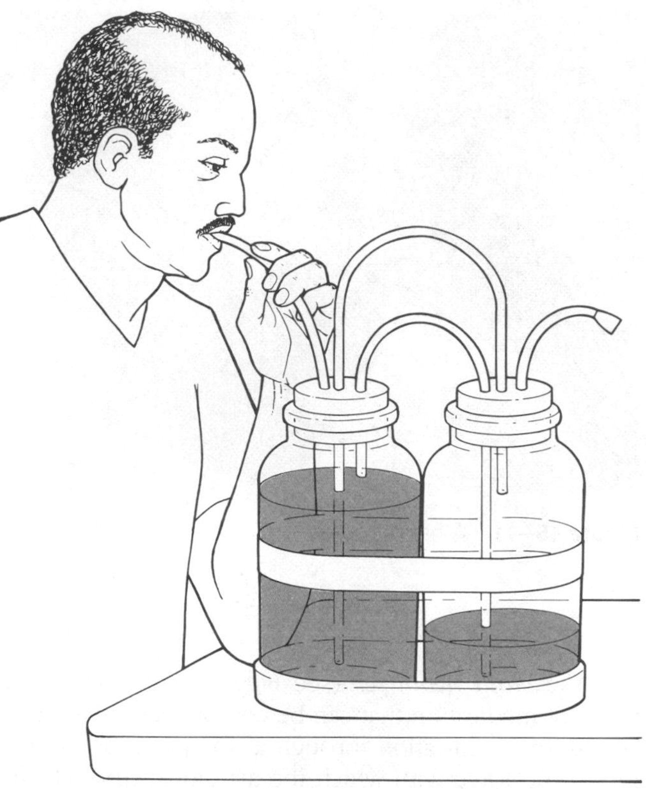

Figure 45–12 Blow bottles

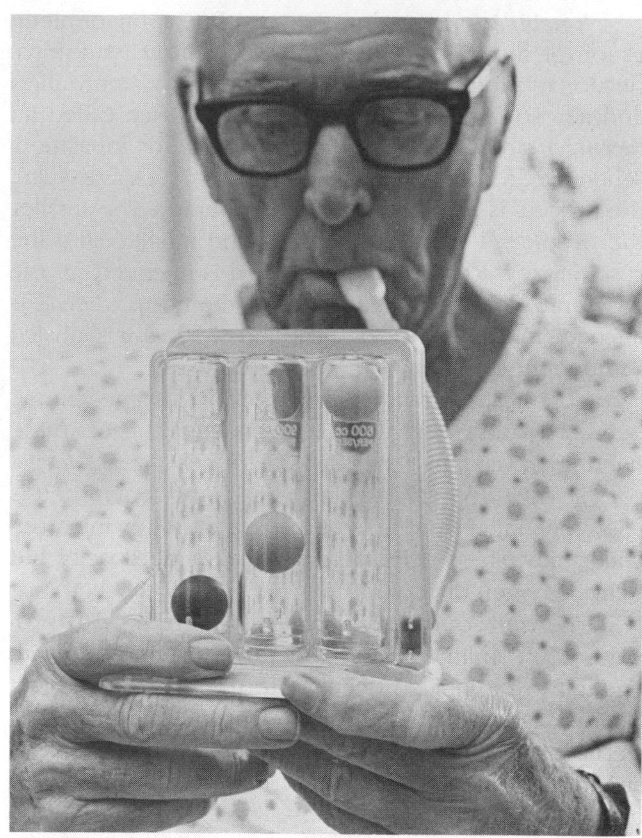

Figure 45–13 Sustained maximal inspiration device (SMI)

is encouraged by the deep breath the client needs before blowing into the bottle. After the client transfers the fluid from the first bottle, the set is reversed, and the procedure is repeated. A single blow bottle may also be used; it is a gallon bottle half filled with water. In this case the client is asked to "blow bubbles," e.g., for 5 minutes every hour.

Sustained maximal inspiration devices (SMIs) measure the flow of air inhaled through the mouthpiece. They therefore offer an incentive to improve *inhalation*. Two general types are the flow-oriented spirometer and the volume-oriented spirometer. The *flow-oriented SMI* consists of one or more clear plastic chambers that contain freely movable, colored balls or discs. The balls or discs are elevated as the client inhales. The client is asked to keep them elevated as long as possible with a maximal sustained inhalation. Figure 45–13 shows a Triflo II SMI. Flow-oriented SMIs are low-cost devices, are often disposable, and can be used independently by clients. They do not measure the specific volume of air inhaled, however.

The more expensive *volume-oriented SMIs* precisely measure the inhalation volume maintained by the client. These devices contain pistons or bellows that are raised by the client's inhalation to a predetermined volume. Some volume-oriented devices are designed with an achievement counter or light. The light will not turn on until the inspiration is held at the minimum predetermined volume for a specified time period. See Figure 45–14. The details of assisting clients to use these devices is given in Procedure 45–2.

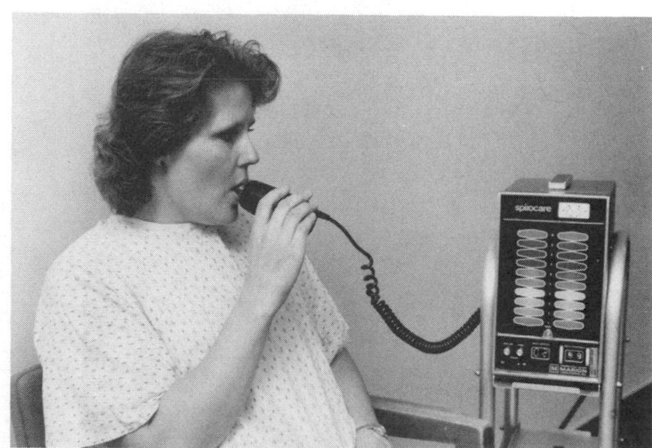

Figure 45–14 Volume-oriented SMI

Procedure 45–2 ▲ Assisting Clients to Use Blow Bottles or a Sustained Maximal Inspiration Device

Equipment

1. Blow bottles

   or

   A flow-oriented SMI

   or

   A volume-oriented SMI
2. A mouthpiece or breathing tube
3. A nose clip (optional)

Intervention

1. Assist the client to an upright sitting position in bed or in a chair. If the client is unable to assume a sitting position for a flow spirometer, have him or her assume any position.

   Rationale A sitting position facilitates maximum ventilation.

For Blow Bottles

2. Instruct the client to:
   a. Take in a slow, deep breath.

      Rationale A deep breath ensures maximum inflation of the alveoli, which facilitates gaseous exchange.

   b. Seal the lips tightly around the mouthpiece, exhale slowly and steadily as long as possible into the bottle, and concentrate on moving the fluid from one bottle to the other.

      Rationale A tight lip seal prevents leakage of exhaled air outside the mouthpiece and ensures adequate movement and measurement of the fluid. As the client exhales, pressure in the bottle is increased and displaces the water with air. A prolonged exhalation against resistance creates an increase in alveolar pressure, reexpanding collapsed alveoli, preventing atelectasis (collapse of the lung), and strengthening the muscles of expiration.

   c. Establish a goal of moving a certain portion of water into the second bottle with each exhalation (e.g., ¼, ⅓, ½, ¾). Provide practice periods about five times every hour, and set progressive increases in the volume of fluid to be moved.

      Rationale Initially the client may be unable to move the entire contents of one bottle to the other with one breath. The nurse and the client need to establish realistic goals. Practice helps to increase the expiratory volume.

For a Flow-oriented SMI

3. If the spirometer has an inspiratory volume level pointer, set the pointer at the prescribed level. Check the physician's or respiratory therapist's order.
4. Instruct the client to:
   a. Hold the spirometer in the upright position.

      Rationale A tilted spirometer requires less effort to raise the balls or discs.

   b. Exhale normally.
   c. Seal the lips tightly around the mouthpiece, take in a slow, deep breath to elevate the balls, and then hold the breath for 2 seconds initially, increasing to 6 seconds (optimum), to keep the balls elevated if possible. Instruct the client to avoid brisk, low-volume breaths that snap the balls to the top of the chamber. The client may use a noseclip if he or she has difficulty breathing only through the mouth.

      Rationale A slow, deep breath ensures maximal ventilation. Greater lung expansion is achieved with a very slow inspiration than with a brisk, shallow breath, even though it may not elevate the balls or keep them elevated while the client holds his or her breath (Luce, Tyler, and Pierson 1984). Sustained elevation of the balls ensures adequate alveolar ventilation.

   d. Remove the mouthpiece, and exhale normally.
   e. Cough after the incentive effort.

      Rationale Deep ventilation may loosen secretions, and coughing can facilitate their removal.

   f. Relax, and take several normal breaths before using the spirometer again.
   g. Repeat the procedure several times and then four or five times hourly.

Rationale Practice increases inspiratory volume, maintains alveolar ventilation, and prevents atelectasis.

For a Volume-oriented SMI

5. Set the spirometer to the predetermined volume. Volume ranges vary from 0 to 5000 ml depending on the type of spirometer. Check the physician's or respiratory therapist's order.
6. Since some SMIs are battery-operated, ensure that the spirometer is functioning. Place the device on the client's bedside table.
7. Instruct the client to:
   a. Exhale normally.
   b. Seal the lips tightly around the mouthpiece, and take in a slow, deep breath, until the piston is elevated to the preset level. The piston level may be visible to the client, or lights or the word "Hold" may be illuminated to identify the volume obtained.
   c. Hold the breath for 6 seconds to ensure maximal alveolar ventilation.
   d. Remove the mouthpiece, and exhale normally.
   e. Follow steps 4e–g above.

For All Devices

8. Clean the mouthpiece with sterile water and shake it dry. Label the mouthpiece and a disposable SMI with the client's name, and store them in the client's bedside unit. Only the mouthpiece of a volume SMI is stored with the client, since volume SMIs are used by many clients. Disposable mouthpieces are changed every 24 hours.
9. Auscultate the client's lungs to compare with the baseline data.
10. Record the technique, including type of spirometer, number of breaths taken, volume or flow levels achieved, and results of auscultation. For a flow SMI, calculate the volume achieved by multiplying the setting by the length of time the client kept the balls elevated. For example, if the setting was 500 ml and the balls were kept suspended for 2 seconds, the volume is 500 × 2 = 1000 ml. For a volume SMI, take the volume directly from the spirometer, e.g., 1500 ml.

Sample Recording

Date	Time	Notes
July/6/87	1100	Instructed in use of Triflo II spirometer. 5 breaths taken at volume of 1000 ml (500 ml × 2 sec). Bilateral breath sounds normal on auscultation before and after spirometry.————Nicholas Coscos, SN

Intermittent Positive Pressure Breathing

Intermittent positive pressure breathing (IBBP) is the delivery of air or oxygen into the lungs at positive (above atmospheric) pressure during inspiration and automatic release of the pressure when the predetermined positive pressure level is reached in the air passages, so that expiration occurs passively. Some IPPB machines can exert pressure during expiration, and the abbreviations IPPB/I (inspiratory) and IPPB/E (expiratory) are sometimes used to differentiate the two methods. Generally, however, IPPB refers to positive pressure therapy administered during inspiration, a safer and more common practice.

Use of IPPB therapy has decreased since the advent of incentive spirometers. Advocates of IPPB therapy, however, believe that IPPB devices are more effective in expanding the lungs, moving secretions, promoting coughs, and delivering aerosol medications into the deeper, smaller air passages, and they require less effort by the client.

Various IPPB machines are marketed. Two commonly used types are the Bird respirator and the Bennett respirator. Assembly and maintenance of respirators is usually handled by respiratory therapists. The machine is connected to an oxygen supply and is equipped with an in-line humidifier, which must be filled with distilled water. The client breathes through a mouthpiece or a mask attached to the end of the respirator tubing.

Usually, IPPB treatments are given by respiratory therapists or by nurses who have had special education. However, the general nurse needs to understand the reason for IPPB therapy and its principles, to assist clients, as needed, in the absence of special therapists. The nurse must also observe the client's progress and response to such therapy. Therapy can be client-activated and given on an intermittent basis. Controlled or time-cycled continuous therapy is used for clients unable to initiate inspiration. The breathing of such clients is maintained entirely by machine.

Percussion, Vibration, and Postural Drainage (PVD)

Percussion, sometimes called *clapping,* is forcefully striking the skin with cupped hands. To percuss a client's chest, hold your fingers and thumb together, and flex them slightly to form a cup, as you would to scoop up water. With both hands in this position, alternately flex and extend the wrists rapidly to slap the chest. See Figure 45–15. The

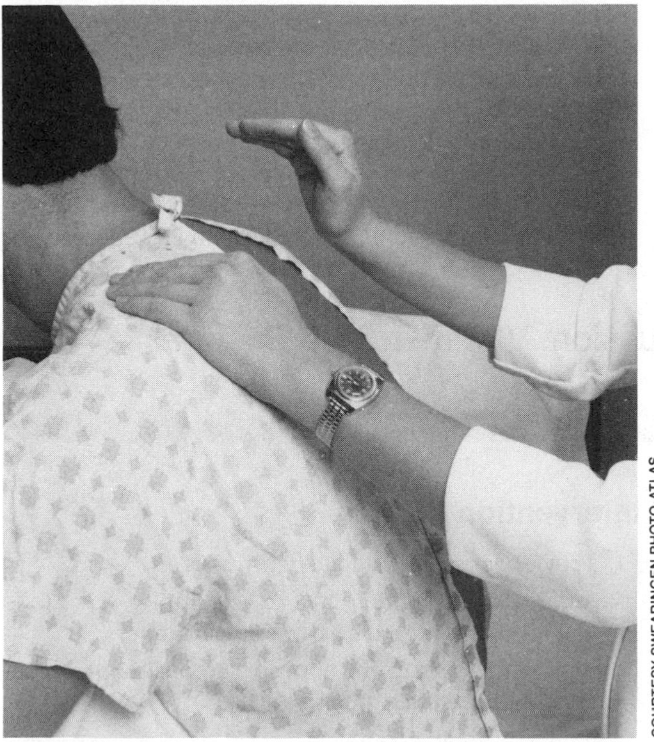

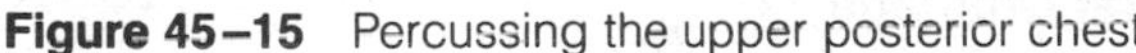
Figure 45–15 Percussing the upper posterior chest

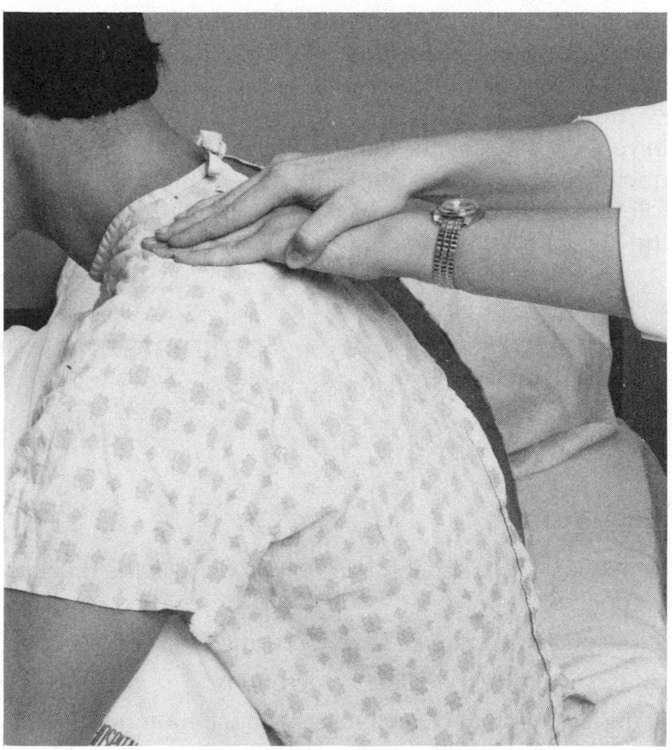

Figure 45–16 Vibrating the upper posterior chest

hands must remain cupped so the air cushions the impact, to avoid injuring the client.

Percussion is usually carried out for only 1 or 2 minutes, or up to 5 minutes over each area, according to the order. It is done over specific congested lung areas, to mechanically dislodge tenacious secretions from the bronchial walls. Percussion is avoided over certain areas, such as the breasts, sternum, spinal column, and kidneys, to prevent injury.

Vibration is a series of vigorous quiverings. It is used after percussion to increase the turbulence of the exhaled air and thus loosen thick secretions. It is often done alternately with percussion. It can replace percussion if the client is experiencing chest pain. The orders will specify.

To vibrate, place your hands palms down, one hand over the other, with fingers together and extended, on the chest area to be drained. See Figure 45–16. Alternatively, the hands may be placed side by side. Ask the client to inhale deeply and exhale slowly. During the exhalation, tense all your hand and arm muscles, and, using mostly the heel of the hand, vibrate (shake) your hands, moving them downward. Stop the vibrating when the client inhales. Vibration is often done four or five times during postural drainage.

Postural drainage is the drainage, by gravity, of secretions from various lung segments. Secretions that remain in the lungs or respiratory airways facilitate bacterial growth and subsequent infection. They also can obstruct the smaller airways and can cause atelectasis. Secretions in the major airways, such as the trachea and the right and left main bronchi, are usually coughed into the pharynx, where they can be expectorated, swallowed, or effectively removed by suctioning.

A wide variety of positions is necessary to drain all segments of the lungs, but not all positions are required for every client. Only those positions that drain specific affected areas are used. The lower lobes require drainage most frequently, since the upper lobes drain during normal daily activities. The exception occurs in immobilized clients. The sequence for PVD is usually: positioning, percussion, vibration, and removal of secretions by coughing or suction. Each position is usually assumed for 10 to 15 minutes, although beginning treatments may start with shorter times and gradually increase. Prior to postural drainage, the client may be given a bronchodilator medication or nebulization therapy to loosen secretions.

Scheduling Postural Drainage

Frequently, postural drainage treatments are scheduled two or three times daily, depending on the degree of lung congestion. The best times include before breakfast, before lunch, in the late afternoon, and before bedtime. It is best to avoid hours shortly after meals because postural drainage at these times can be tiring and can induce vomiting.

The length of treatments must also be considered. Usually, the entire treatment, including preparatory nebulization and deep breathing as well as all postures, takes 30 minutes. Some clients can tolerate long, relatively infrequent treatments. Others require shorter, more frequent treatments. The nurse needs to evaluate the client's tolerance of these treatments by assessing the stability of the client's vital signs, particularly the pulse and respiratory rates, and by noting signs of intolerance, such as pallor, diaphoresis, dyspnea, and fatigue.

Some clients do not react well to certain drainage positions, and the nurse must make appropriate adjustments. For example, some become dyspneic in Trendelenburg's position and require only a moderate tilt or a shorter time in those positions.

How to administer PVD is detailed in Procedure 45–3.

Procedure 45–3 ▲ Administering Percussion, Vibration, and Postural Drainage (PVD) to Adults

Equipment

1. Pillows to comfortably support the client in the required positions
2. A sputum container for expectorated secretions
3. Tissues for expectorated secretions
4. Mouth wash to clean and freshen the mouth following the treatment
5. A specimen label and requisition, if a specimen is required
6. A hospital bed that can be placed in Trendelenburg's position
7. A hospital gown or pajamas to prevent undue exposure and to protect the skin during percussion and vibration
8. A towel to place over the area to be percussed, if needed, to prevent discomfort

Intervention

1. Provide visual and auditory privacy.

   Rationale Coughing and expectorating secretions can embarrass the client and disturb others.
2. Assist the client to the appropriate position for postural drainage. See steps 3–11.

Postural Drainage

Drainage of the *upper lobes:* The upper lobes consist of three segments—the apical or uppermost segments and the anterior and posterior segments, below.

3. To drain the *apical segments* of the upper lobes, have the client lie back at a 30° angle. See Figure 45–17. Percuss and vibrate between the clavicles and above the scapulae.

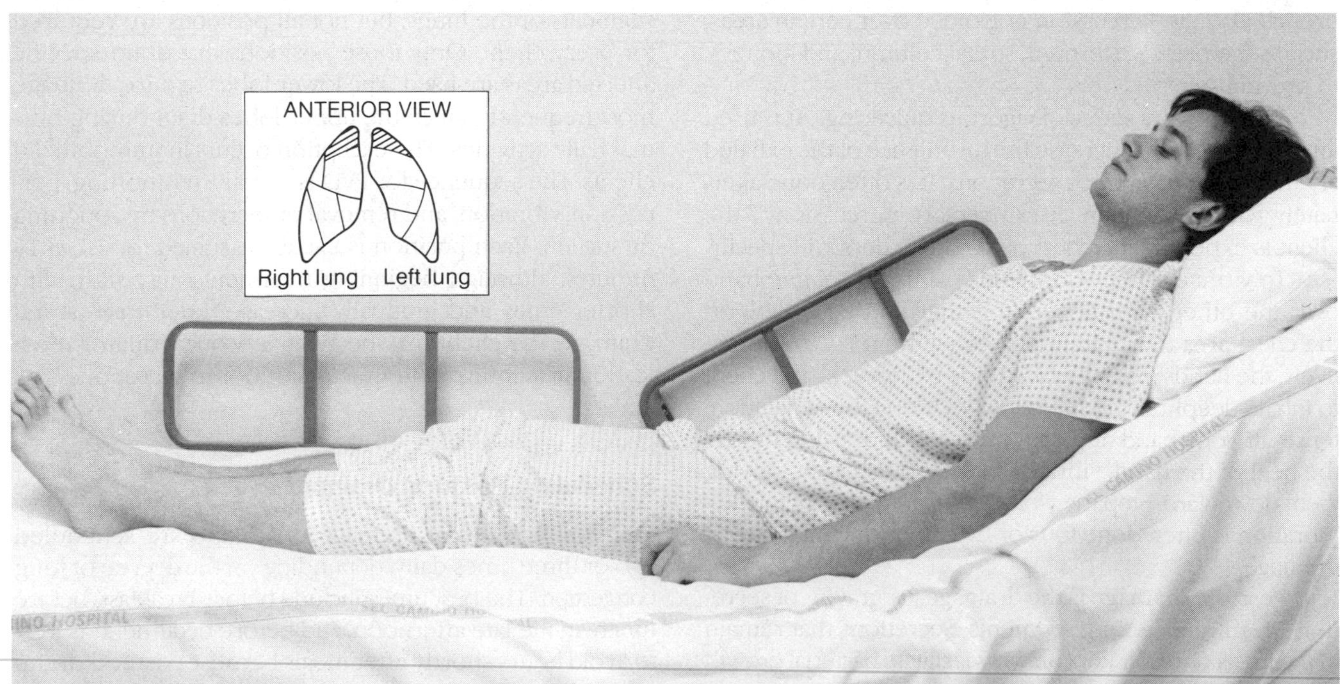

Figure 45–17

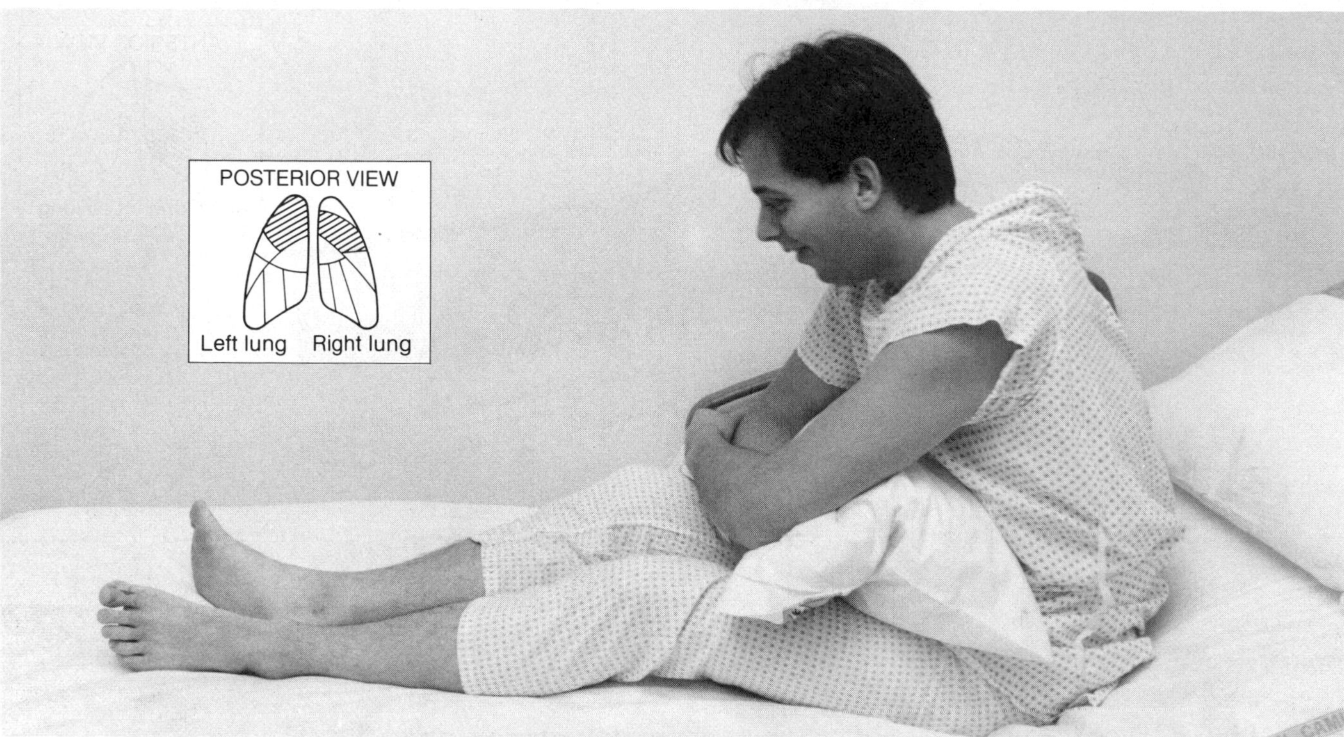

Figure 45–18

4. To drain the *posterior segments* of the upper lobes, have the client sit upright in a chair or in bed with the head bent slightly forward. See Figure 45–18. Percuss and vibrate the area between the clavicles (collarbones) and the scapulae (shoulder blades). For percussion, see steps 12–16; for vibration, see steps 17–20.
5. To drain the *anterior segments* of the upper lobes, have the client lie on a flat bed with pillows under the knees to flex them. See Figure 45–19. Percuss and vibrate the upper chest below the clavicles down to the nipple line, except for women. The breasts of women are not percussed, because percussion may cause pain.

Drainage of the *right middle lobe and lower division of the left upper lobe:* The right middle lobe has two segments—lateral and medial. The lower division of the left

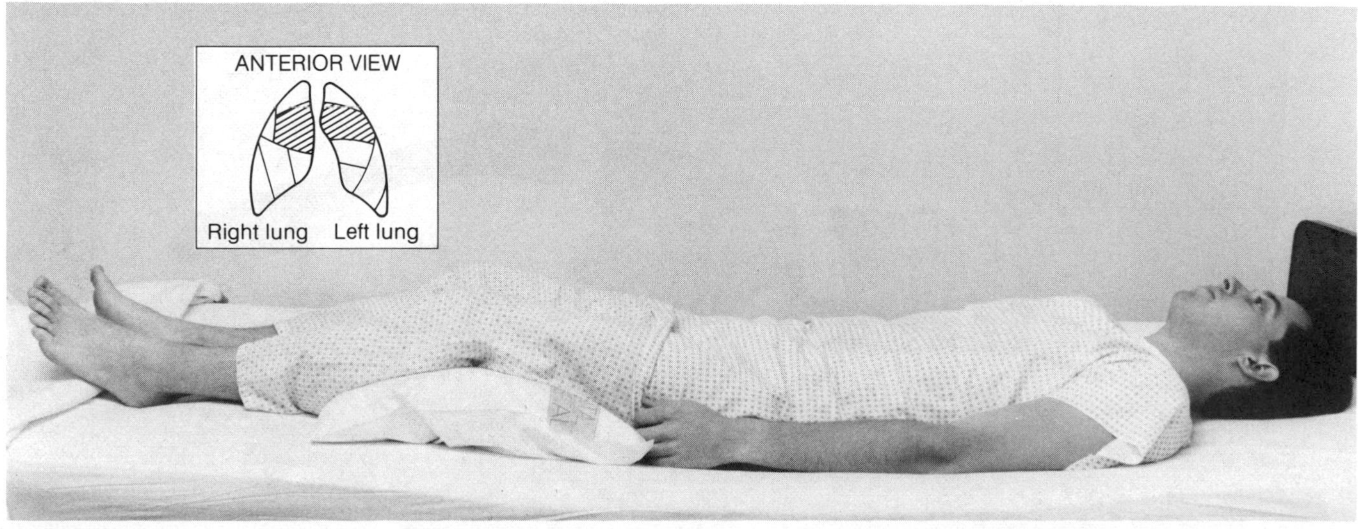

Figure 45–19

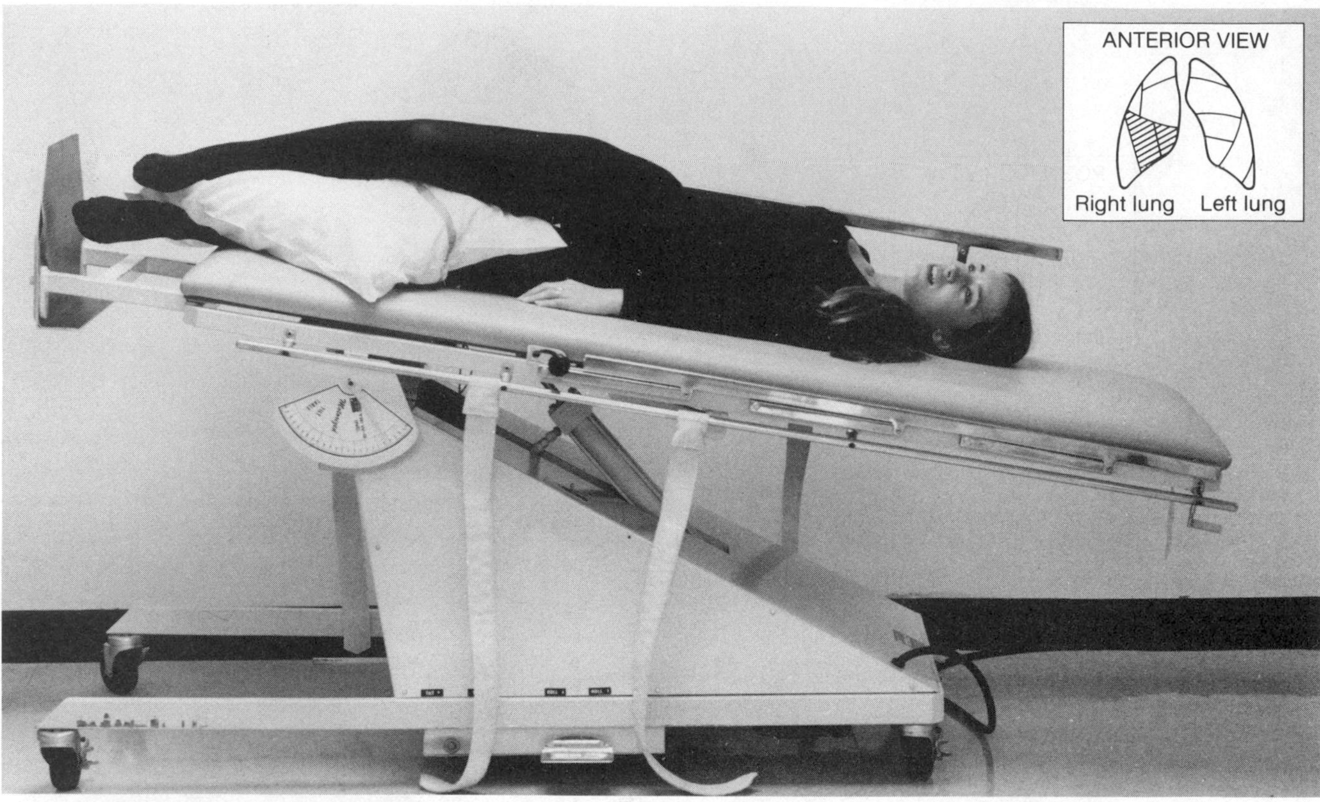

Figure 45–20

upper lobe, called the **lingula** of that lobe, has two segments—superior and inferior.

6. To drain the *right lateral and medial segments,* elevate the foot of the bed about 15° or 40 cm (15 in), and have the client lie on the left side. Help the client to lean back slightly (about a quarter turn) against pillows extending at the back from the shoulder to the hip. See Figure 45–20. If the client is male, percuss and vibrate over the right side of the chest at the level of the nipple between the fourth and sixth ribs. If the client is female, position the heel of your hand toward her axilla, with your cupped fingers extending forward beneath her breast to percuss and vibrate beneath the breast.
7. To drain the *left lingular segments,* elevate the foot of the bed as in step 6, and have the client lie as in step 6, but on the right side. See Figure 45–21.

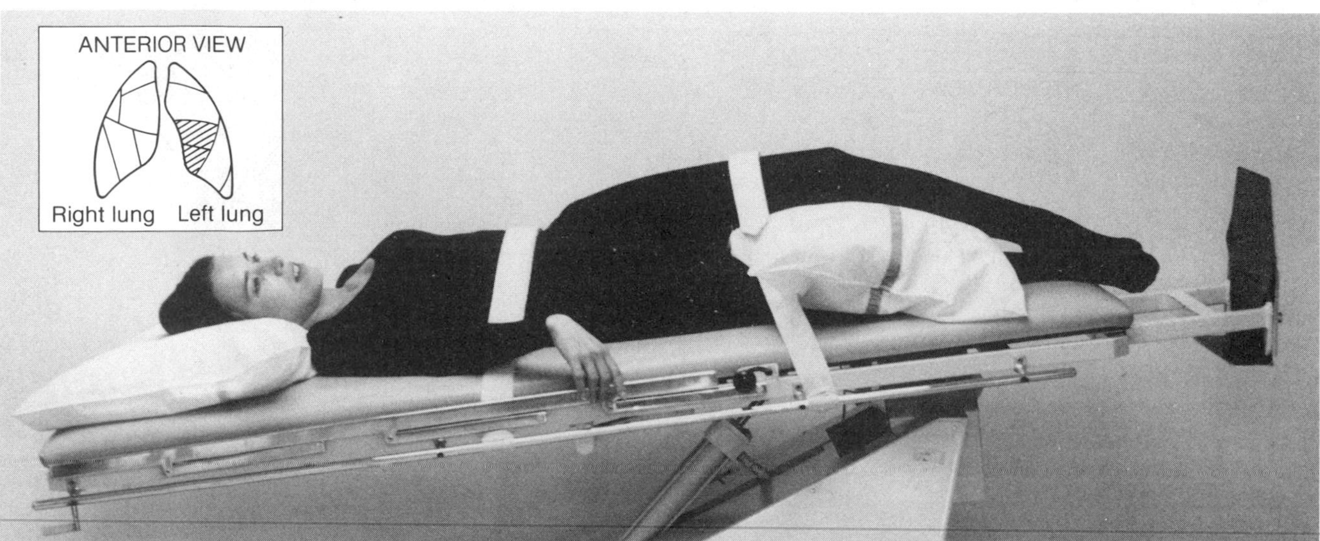

Figure 45–21

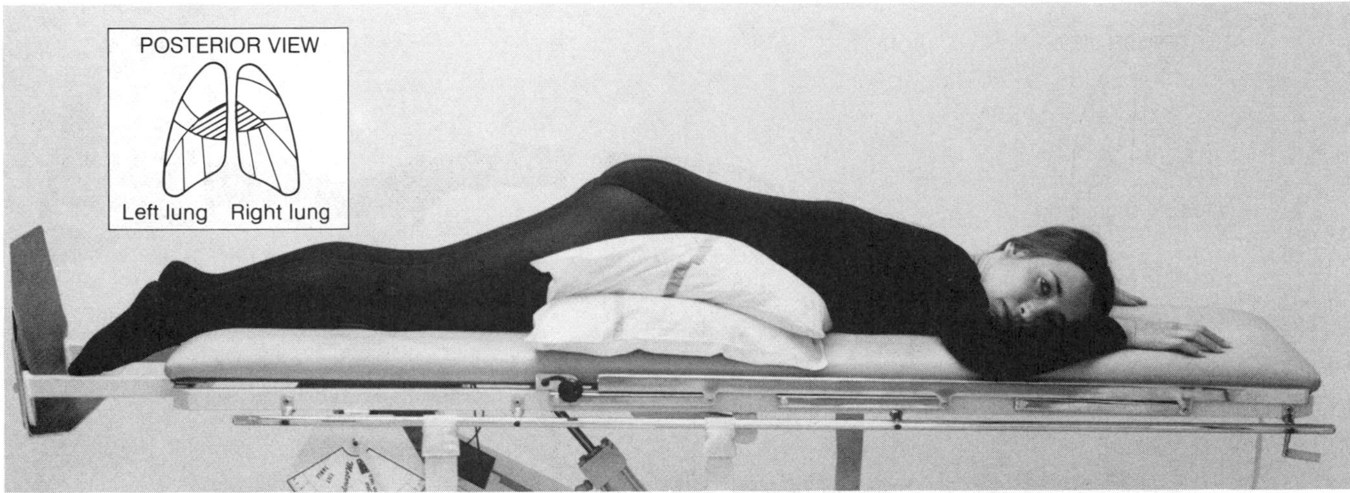

Figure 45–22

Percuss and vibrate the right side of the chest as in step 6.

Drainage of the *lower lobes:* The lower lobes have four segments—superior, anterior basal, lateral basal, and posterior basal.

8. To drain the *superior segments,* have the client lie on the abdomen on a flat bed, and place two pillows under the hips. See Figure 45–22. Percuss and vibrate the middle area of the back (below the scapulae) on both sides of the spine.
9. To drain the *anterior basal segments,* have the client lie on the unaffected side, with the upper arm over the head. Elevate the foot of the bed about 30° or 45 cm (18 in), or to the height tolerated by the client. Place one pillow between the client's knees. Another under the head is optional. See Figure 45–23. Percuss and vibrate the affected side of the chest over the lower ribs, inferior to the axilla.
10. To drain the *lateral basal segments,* have the client lie partly on the unaffected side and partly on the abdomen. Elevate the foot of the bed about 30° or 45 cm (18 in), or elevate the client's hips with pillows. See Figure 45–24. Percuss and vibrate the uppermost side of the lower ribs.
11. To drain the *posterior basal segments,* have the client lie prone. Elevate the foot of the bed about 45 cm (18 in), and elevate the client's hips on two or three pillows to produce a jackknife position from the knees to the shoulders. See Figure 45–25. Percuss and vibrate over the lower ribs on both sides close to the spine, but not directly over the spine or kidneys.

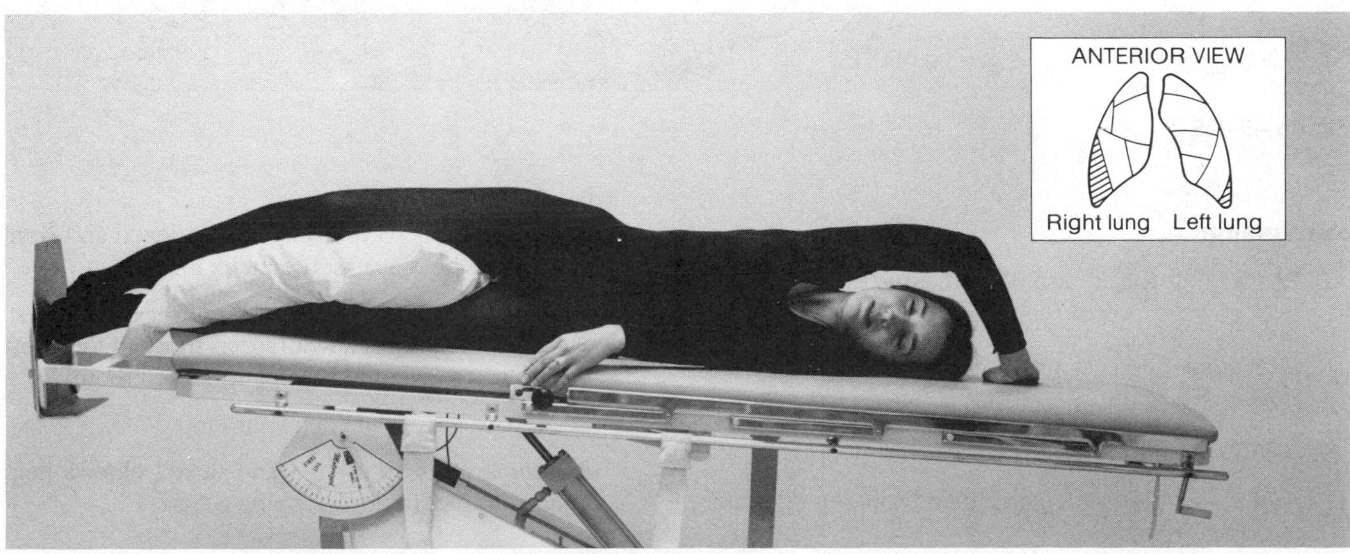

Figure 45–23

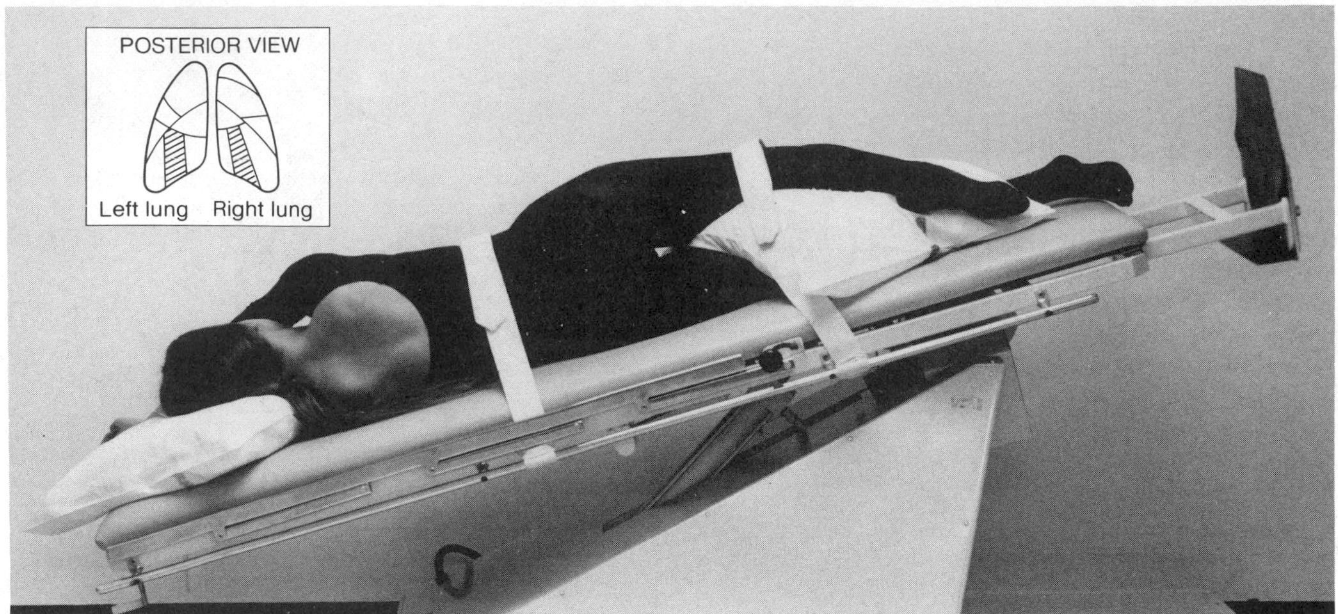

Figure 45–24

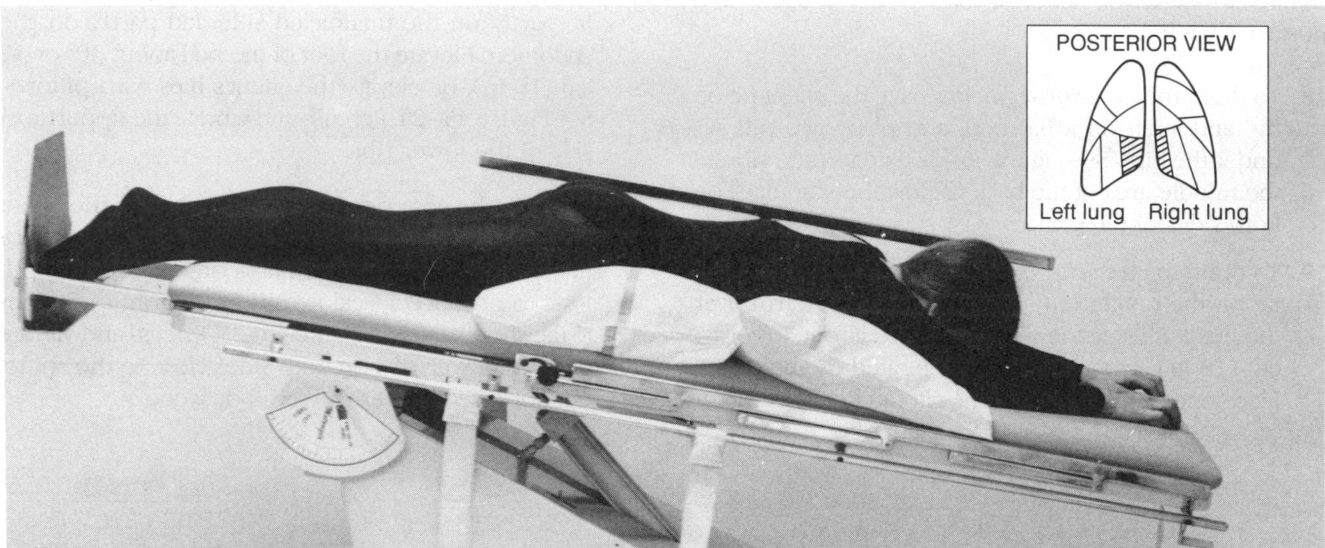

Figure 45–25

Percussion

12. Ensure that the area to be percussed is covered, e.g., by a gown or towel.

    Rationale Percussing the skin directly can cause discomfort.

13. Ask the client to breathe slowly and deeply.

    Rationale Slow, deep breathing promotes relaxation.

14. Cup your hands so your fingers are flexed and your thumbs are held against the index fingers.

    Rationale Cupped hands trap the air against the chest. The trapped air sets up vibrations through the chest wall to the secretions, helping to loosen them.

15. Relax your wrists, and flex your elbows.

    Rationale Relaxed wrists and flexed elbows help obtain a rapid, hollow, popping action.

16. Alternating hands rapidly, percuss each affected lung segment for 1 to 2 minutes. The percussing action should produce a hollow, popping sound when done correctly. See Figure 45–15, earlier.

Vibration

17. Ask the client to inhale deeply through the mouth and exhale slowly through pursed lips or the nose.

18. During exhalation, press your hands flatly one over the other (or side by side) against the affected chest area. See Figure 45–16, earlier.

19. Straighten your elbows, and lean slightly against the client's chest while tensing your arm and shoulder muscles in isometric contractions.

    Rationale Isometric contractions will transmit fine vibrations through the client's chest wall.

20. Vibrate during five exhalations over one affected lung segment.

21. Encourage the client to cough and expectorate secretions into the sputum container. Offer the client mouth wash.

22. Auscultate the client's lungs, and compare the findings to the baseline data.

23. Observe the amount, color, and character of expectorated secretions.

Oropharyngeal and Nasopharyngeal Suctioning

The nurse must sometimes apply suction to the oropharynx and nasal passages of clients who have difficulty swallowing or expectorating secretions. **Suctioning** is the aspiration of secretions, often through a rubber or polyethylene catheter connected to a suction machine or wall outlet. There are several types of catheters used for suctioning. They vary in size from #14 to #18 Fr. for adults and from #8 to #18 Fr. for children. The tip of a suction catheter has several openings along the sides. These openings distribute the negative pressure of the suction over a wide area, thus preventing excessive irritation to any one area of the respiratory mucous membrane. The suction apparatus includes a collection bottle, a tubing system connected to the suction catheter, and a gauge that registers the degree of suction. These gauges are either portable or wall mounted. See Figure 45–26.

Oropharyngeal or nasopharyngeal suctioning removes secretions from the upper respiratory tract. Deeper suctioning, called *endotracheal suctioning,* removes secretions from the trachea and the bronchi. Deep suctioning requires considerably more skill and is usually carried out by a critical-care nursing specialist or an experienced nurse.

It is recommended that sterile technique be used for all suctioning, so that microorganisms are not introduced into the pharynx, where they can multiply and move into the trachea and bronchi. This is particularly important for debilitated clients, who are more susceptible to infection.

Suctioning of the upper respiratory airways is indicated when the client (a) is unable to cough, (b) is unable to swallow, and (c) makes light bubbling or rattling breath sounds that signal the accumulation of secretions.

How to perform oropharyngeal and nasopharyngeal suctioning is described in Procedure 45–4.

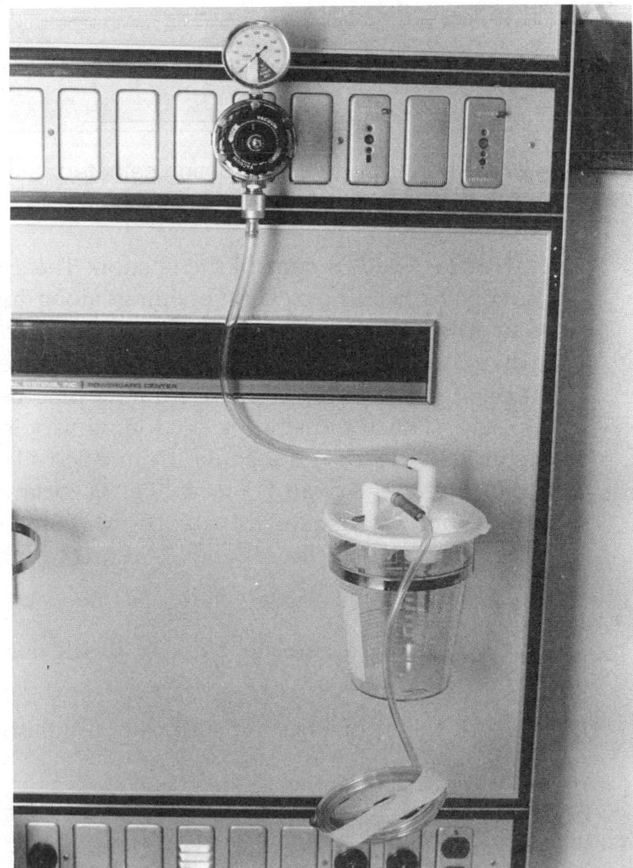

Figure 45–26 A wall suction unit

Procedure 45–4 ▲ Oropharyngeal and Nasopharyngeal Suctioning

Equipment

1. A suction machine or a gauge to attach to wall suction equipment with tubing and a collection receptacle. See Figure 45–26, earlier.
2. A sterile suction package that includes:
   a. A suction catheter. Several types of catheters are available. The open-tipped catheter has an opening at the end and several openings along the sides. See Figure 45–27, *A*. It is effective for thick mucous plugs, but it can irritate tissue. The whistle-tipped catheter has a slanted opening at the tip. See Figure 45–27, *B*. Some catheters have a thumb port on the side, which is used to control the suction. The tip of a suction catheter has several openings along the sides to distribute the negative pressure of the suction over a wide area, thus preventing excessive irritation of any one area of the respiratory mucous membrane. Catheters used for suctioning vary in size from #12 to #18 Fr. for adults, from #8 to #10 Fr. for children, and from #5 to #8 Fr. for infants. If both the oropharynx and the nasopharynx are to be suctioned, one sterile catheter is required for each.
   b. A glove.
   c. A cup or container for sterile water or sterile normal saline.

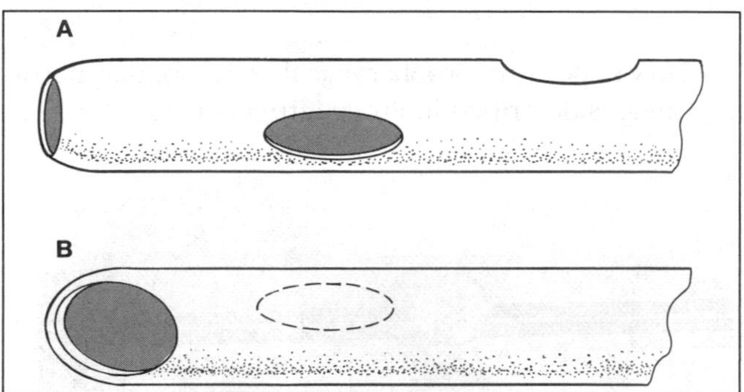

Figure 45–27 Types of pharyngeal suction catheters: **A,** open-tipped; **B,** whistle-tipped

3. Sterile normal saline or water to lubricate and flush the catheter.
4. A Y-connector to regulate the suction system if the catheter does not have a thumb port.
5. Sterile gauzes to wipe the catheter and the client's mouth or nose (optional).
6. A moisture-resistant bag for disposable catheters and gloves.
7. A towel to protect the client's gown and pillows.
8. A sputum trap, if a specimen is to be collected during suctioning.

Intervention

1. Explain to the client that suctioning will relieve his or her breathing difficulty and that the procedure is painless but may stimulate the cough, gag, or sneeze reflex.

   Rationale Knowing that the procedure will relieve breathing problems often reassures the client and enlists cooperation.

2. Position a conscious client who has a functional gag reflex in the semi-Fowler's position, with the client's head turned to one side for oral suctioning or with the neck hyperextended for nasal suctioning.

   Rationale These positions facilitate the insertion of the catheter and help prevent aspiration of secretions.

3. Position an unconscious client in the lateral position, facing you.

   Rationale This position allows the client's tongue to fall forward so that it will not obstruct the catheter on insertion. Lateral position also facilitates drainage of secretions from the pharynx and prevents the possibility of aspiration.

4. Place the towel over the pillow or under the client's chin.
5. Set the pressure on the suction gauge, and turn on the suction. Some suction devices are calibrated to three pressure ranges: high (120 to 150 mm Hg), medium (80 to 120 mm Hg), and low (0 to 80 mm Hg). Generally a pressure of 100 to 120 mm Hg is used for adults and 50 to 75 mm Hg for infants and children.
6. Open the sterile suction package.
   a. Set up the cup or container, touching only its outside.
   b. Pour sterile water or saline into the container.
   c. Don the sterile glove.
7. With your sterile gloved hand, pick up the catheter and attach it to the suction unit. See Figure 45–28.
8. Make an approximate measure of the depth for the insertion. Mark the position on the tube with the fingers of your gloved hand. An appropriate measure is the distance between the tip of the client's nose and the earlobe, or about 13 cm (5 in) for an adult.

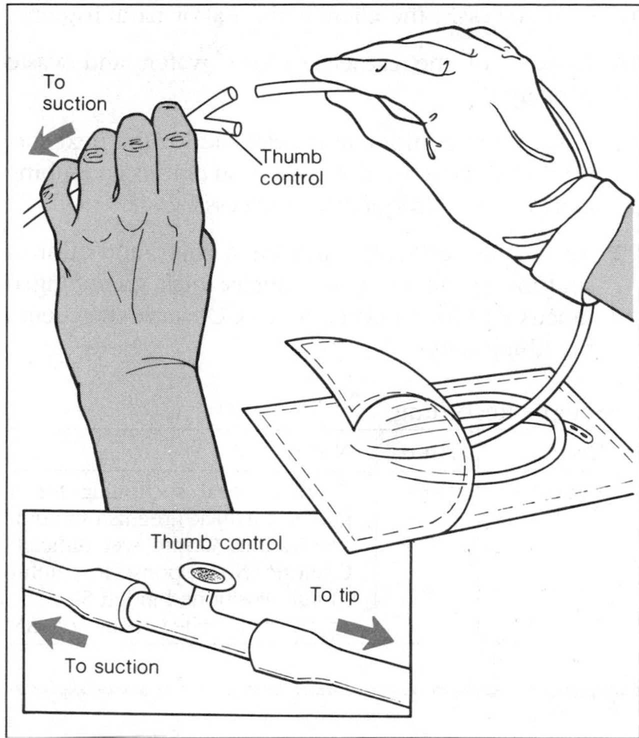

Figure 45–28

9. Moisten the catheter tip by dipping it in the container of sterile water or saline.

   Rationale Moistening reduces friction and eases insertion.

10. Test the suction and the patency of the catheter by applying your finger to the thumb port or open branch of the Y-connector (the suction control) to create suction.

11. For a nasopharyngeal suction, insert the catheter gently through one nostril with your thumb away from the suction control (i.e., not applying suction). Direct the catheter along the floor of the nasal cavity. If one nostril is not patent, try the other. Never force the catheter against an obstruction.

    or

    For an oropharyngeal suction, insert the catheter through the mouth, along one side, into the oropharynx, without applying suction.

    Rationale Gentle insertion and not applying suction during insertion prevent trauma to the mucous membrane. Directing the catheter along the floor of the nasal cavity avoids the nasal turbinates. Directing the catheter along one side of the mouth prevents gagging.

12. Apply your finger to the suction control port, and gently rotate the catheter. Apply suction for 5 to 10 seconds, then remove your finger from the control and remove the catheter. It may be necessary during oropharyngeal suctioning to apply suction to secretions that collect in the vestibule of the mouth and beneath the tongue. A suction attempt should last only 15 seconds. During this time the catheter is inserted, the suction applied and discontinued, and the catheter removed.

    Rationale Placing the finger over the suction control port starts the suction. Gentle rotation of the catheter ensures that all surfaces are reached and prevents trauma to any one area of the respiratory mucosa due to prolonged suction.

13. Wipe off the catheter with sterile gauze if it is thickly coated with secretions, flush it with sterile water or saline, and repeat steps 9, 11–12, until the air passage is clear, but do not apply suction for more than 5 minutes total.

    Rationale Applying suction for too long can decrease the client's oxygen supply.

14. Encourage the client to breathe deeply and cough between suctions.

    Rationale Coughing and deep breathing help carry secretions from the trachea and bronchi into the pharynx, where they can be reached with the suction catheter.

15. If a specimen is required, use a sputum trap (see Figure 45–29):

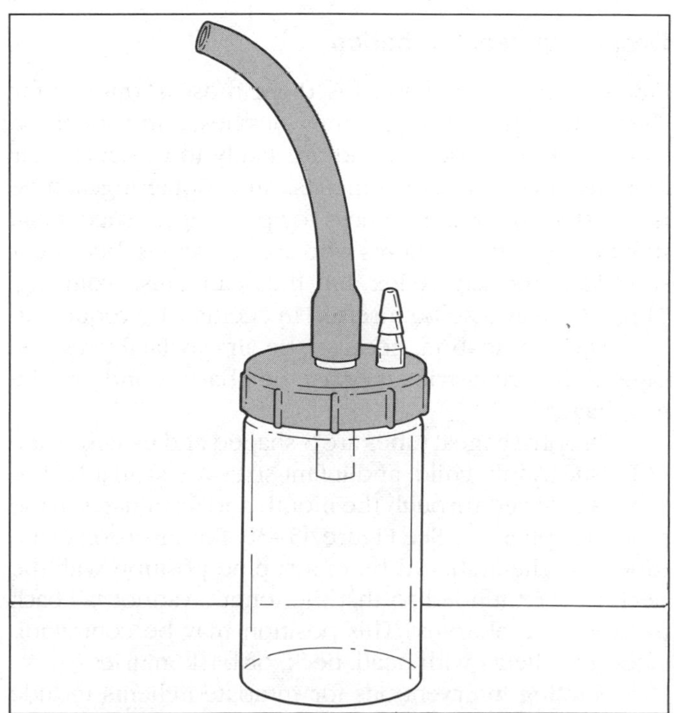

Figure 45–29

a. Attach the suction catheter to the rubber tubing of the sputum trap.
b. Attach the suction tubing to the sputum trap air vent.
c. Suction the client's nasopharynx or oropharynx. The sputum trap will collect the mucus during suctioning.
d. Remove the catheter from the client. Disconnect the sputum trap rubber tubing from the suction catheter. Remove the trap air vent from the suction tubing.
e. Connect the rubber tubing of the sputum trap to its air vent.

Rationale This prevents the spread of microorganisms from the sputum.

16. When the catheter has been removed, rinse the catheter by flushing it with water.

Rationale Rinsing the catheter removes secretions from the tubing.

17. Offer, or assist the client with, oral or nasal hygiene.

18. Dispose of the catheter, glove, water, and waste container.

19. Ensure that equipment is available for the next suctioning. Change suction collection bottles and tubing daily or more frequently as necessary.

20. Record the amount, consistency, color, and odor of sputum, e.g., foamy, white mucus; thick, green-tinged mucus; or blood-flecked mucus. Observe the client's breathing status.

Sample Recording

Date	Time	Notes
May/12/87	0200	Oropharyngeal suctioning for 5 min. 35 ml thick, greenish sputum. Respirations 30/min, wet, difficult. Cyanotic. No response to painful stimuli. Positioned in left Sims'.——————Rozelle L. Schwartz, RN

Artificial Airways

Artificial airways are inserted to maintain a patent air passage for clients whose airway has become or may become obstructed. A patent airway is necessary so that air can flow to and from the lungs. Airways are usually inserted by physicians. Four of the more common types of intubation are oropharyngeal, nasopharyngeal, endotracheal, and tracheostomy.

Oropharyngeal Intubation

Oropharyngeal intubation is done most frequently for clients who have had general anesthesia and for those who are semiconscious and are likely to obstruct their own airways with their tongues. An oropharyngeal tube is inserted in some instances for pharyngeal suctioning. It is not inserted in clients who are conscious, because it stimulates the gag reflex and thus can cause vomiting. This tube may also be inserted in clients who require an orogastric intubation, because the airway facilitates passage of the orogastric tube past the pharynx and into the esophagus.

Oropharyngeal tubes are S-shaped and usually made of plastic. Adult, child, and infant sizes are available. The tube is inserted through the mouth and terminates in the posterior pharynx. See Figure 45–30. For insertion of the tube, the client should be in a supine position with the neck hyperextended so that the tongue cannot fall back to block the pharynx. This position may be contraindicated for clients with head, neck, or back injuries.

Nursing interventions for intubated clients include the following.

1. Remove the tube every 4 hours, or more often if necessary, and provide oral hygiene to maintain the health of oral mucosa.

2. Make sure a bite block is in place if the client is likely to bite the tube and thus obstruct the airway.

3. Maintain the client in a lateral or semiprone position so that blood, vomitus, and mucus will drain out of the mouth and not be aspirated.

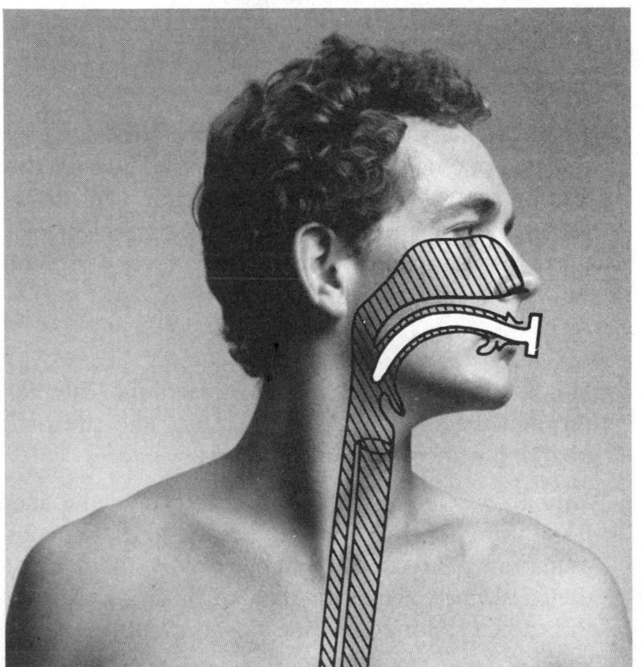

COURTESY SWEARINGEN PHOTO-ATLAS

Figure 45–30 An oropharyngeal tube in place

4. Remove the airway once the client has regained consciousness and has the swallow, gag, and cough reflexes.

Nasopharyngeal Intubation

Nasopharyngeal intubation is carried out if the oropharyngeal route is contraindicated, e.g., following oral surgery. A nasopharyngeal tube may also be inserted to protect the nasal and pharyngeal mucosa during nasopharyngeal or nasotracheal suctioning. The tube is inserted through a nostril and terminates in the pharynx, below the upper edge of the epiglottis. See Figure 45–31. Tubes vary in size for adults, children, and infants. They are usually made of latex rubber.

Nursing interventions include the following.

1. Lubricate the tube with a water-soluble lubricant and/or a topical anesthetic prior to insertion, to prevent irritation of the nasopharyngeal mucosa and undue discomfort. The local anesthetic will be specified in the order.
2. Remove the tube, and insert it in the other nostril at least every 8 hours, or as ordered by the physician, or more often to prevent irritation of the mucosa.
3. Provide nasal hygiene every 4 hours, or more often if needed.
4. Monitor the client closely for stimulation of the vagus nerve if nasotracheal suctioning is carried out. Vagal stimulation can lead to cardiac arrest.

Endotracheal Intubation

Endotracheal tubes are most commonly inserted for clients who have had general anesthetics, or in emergency situations where mechanical ventilation is required. An endotracheal tube is a curved polyvinyl chloride tube that is inserted through either the mouth or the nose and into the trachea. See Figure 45–32. It terminates just superior to the bifurcation of the trachea into the bronchi. Tubes come in various lengths and diameters. The lengths are measured in centimeters and the inner and outer diameters in millimeters.

Nursing interventions include the following.

1. Maintain the client in a lateral or semiprone position so that blood, vomitus, or secretions can drain from the mouth and are not aspirated.
2. Provide oral or nasal hygiene every 3 hours or as needed.
3. For an oral insertion, provide a bite block so the client cannot bite the tube and occlude the airway.
4. Change the tube's position to the opposite side of the mouth or to the other nostril every 8 hours, or as ordered by the physician, or as needed to prevent irritation of the mucosa.
5. Closely monitor the air pressure in the endotracheal cuff. If it is greater than 20 mm Hg, necrosis of the tracheal tissues can result.
6. Tape the airway in place to prevent accidental slippage or extubation.

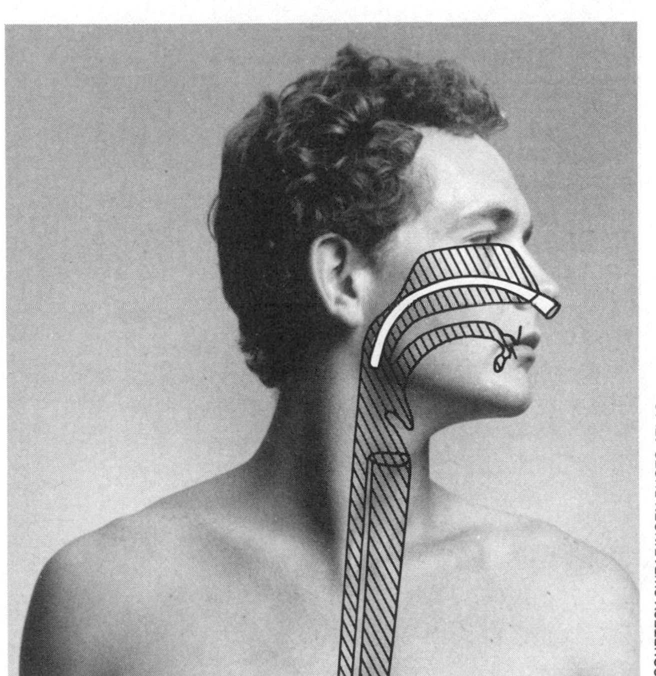

COURTESY SWEARINGEN PHOTO-ATLAS

Figure 45–31 A nasopharyngeal tube in place

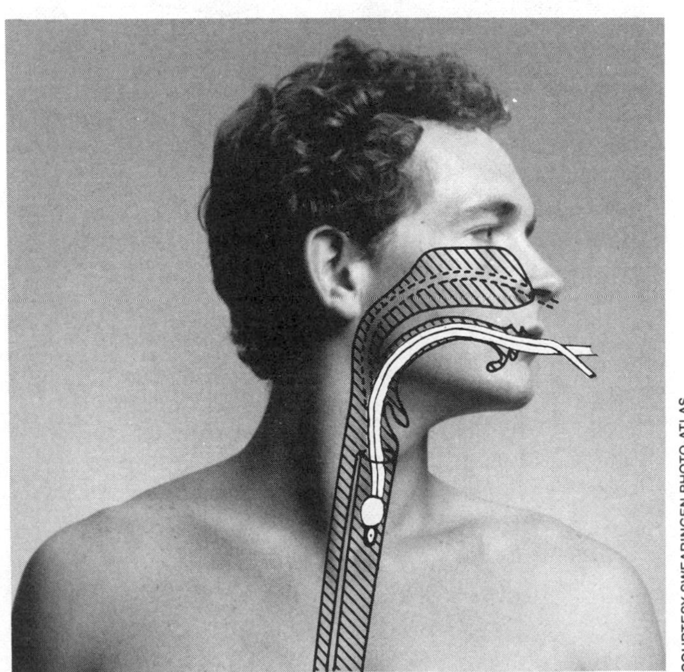

COURTESY SWEARINGEN PHOTO-ATLAS

Figure 45–32 An endotracheal tube in place

7. Provide continuous humidification or aerosol therapy to prevent undue drying and irritation of the mucous membranes, if the tube is left in for more than a short time, e.g., for days or weeks.

Tracheostomy Intubation

Tracheostomy tubes are inserted to provide and maintain a patent airway, to remove tracheobronchial secretions from clients unable to cough, to replace endotracheal tubes, to permit the use of positive pressure ventilation, and to prevent unconscious clients from aspirating secretions. A tracheostomy tube is a curved tube that is inserted into a tracheostomy (a surgical incision in the trachea just below the first or second tracheal cartilage). See Figure 45–33. The tube may be metal, plastic, or foam. Plastic tubes are increasingly popular, because they are lightweight, their parts are interchangeable, and crusting from the tissues rarely forms on plastic materials. The tracheostomy tube extends through the tracheostomy stoma into the trachea. See Figure 45–34. Tubes come in different sizes.

The main parts of a tracheostomy set are the outer tube, the inner tube or inner cannula, and the obturator. See Figure 45–35. The obturator is used only to insert the outer tube. It is removed once the outer tube is in place. The outer tube usually has ties to secure it around the client's neck, although many plastic tubes are cuffed with a soft balloon that can be inflated to hold the tube in place. Fitted inside the outer tube is an inner cannula. (Some plastic sets do not have this, because it is unnecessary to change the tube. They are called *single-cannula tubes.*) In double-cannula sets, the inner cannula is inserted and locked in place after the obturator is removed; it acts as a removable liner for the more permanent, outer cannula. The inner tube is withdrawn for brief periods to be cleaned.

An adaptation of the tracheostomy tube is the *tracheostomy button.* This is a very short tube that extends from the tracheostomy stoma to just inside the tracheal wall. The button enables a client to breathe and cough more easily than a tracheostomy tube. It has a closure plug, which can be removed for suctioning and/or ventilating. When the plug is inserted, the client can speak.

Nursing interventions for a client who has a tracheostomy button include the following.

1. Clean the cannula regularly by washing it in hydrogen peroxide solution and rinsing it with sterile water.
2. Clean the stoma regularly to prevent skin irritation and the formation of crusts. Cleaning is usually done with a solution of hydrogen peroxide. The stoma is then rinsed with sterile water and dried with sterile gauze. It is important that no solution enter the tracheostomy, where it could irritate the mucosal lining and/or be aspirated into the respiratory tract.

How to suction a tracheostomy or endotracheal tube is detailed in Procedure 45–5.

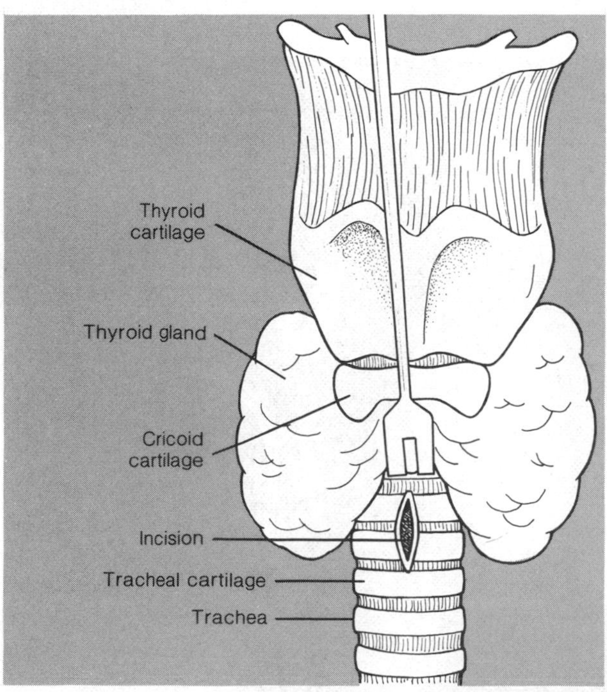

Figure 45–33 A site of a tracheostomy incision

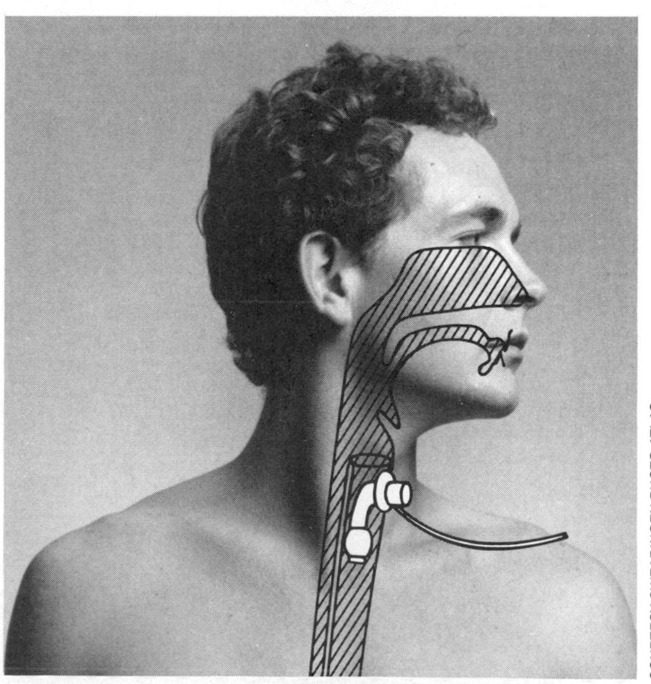

COURTESY SWEARINGEN PHOTO-ATLAS

Figure 45–34 A tracheostomy tube in place

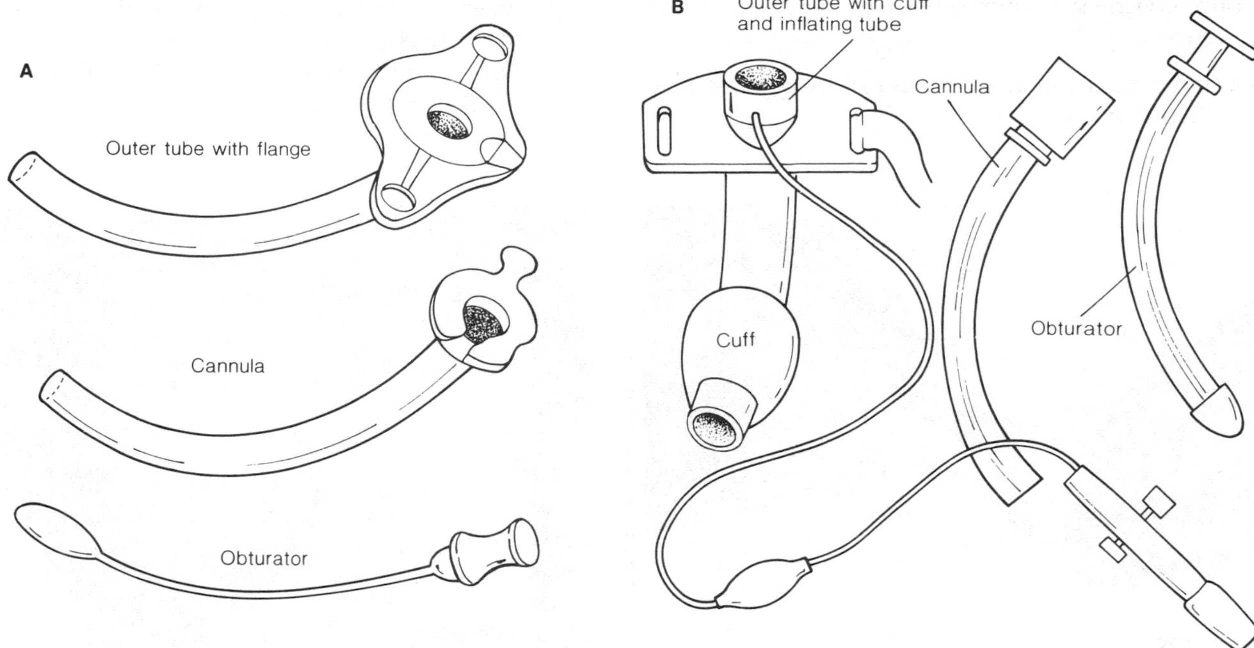

Figure 45–35 Two types of tracheostomy sets: **A,** noncuffed; **B,** cuffed

Procedure 45–5 ▲ Suctioning a Tracheostomy or Endotracheal Tube

Equipment

1. Suction equipment, including a collection receptable.
2. A sterile suction catheter. The diameter should be about half the inside diameter of the tracheostomy tube, to prevent hypoxia. Adults often require a #12 or #14 Fr. and children a #8 or #10 Fr. Some catheters have a thumb port on the side to control the suction.
3. A Y-connector to join the catheter to the suction tubing if the catheter does not have a thumb port. One arm of the Y is then used to control the suction. A straight connector is used if the catheter has a thumb port.
4. A container with sterile normal saline to lubricate and flush the catheter.
5. A sterile 2- to 10-ml syringe and sterile normal saline without a bacteriostatic preservative for a tracheal lavage, if this is agency practice and/or is ordered. Lavage can liquefy tenacious secretions so that they are more easily suctioned out. The amount used is generally 0.5 to 1 ml for infants, 2 ml for children, and 2 to 5 ml for adults.
6. Sterile gloves.
7. A moisture-resistant bag in which to discard the disposable catheter and gloves.
8. A sterile towel to provide an additional sterile area (optional).
9. An oxygen source flowmeter with a ventilator, or a manual resuscitator, e.g., an Ambu or Laerdal bag.

Intervention

1. Inform the client that suctioning usually causes intermittent coughing and that this assists in removing the secretions.
2. If not contraindicated because of health, place the client in semi-Fowler's position to promote deep breathing, maximum lung expansion, and productive coughing. Place an unconscious client in the supine position.

   Rationale Deep breathing oxygenates the lungs, counteracts the hypoxic effects of suctioning, and may induce coughing. Coughing helps to loosen and move secretions.

3. Attach the resuscitation apparatus to the oxygen source. See Figure 45–36.

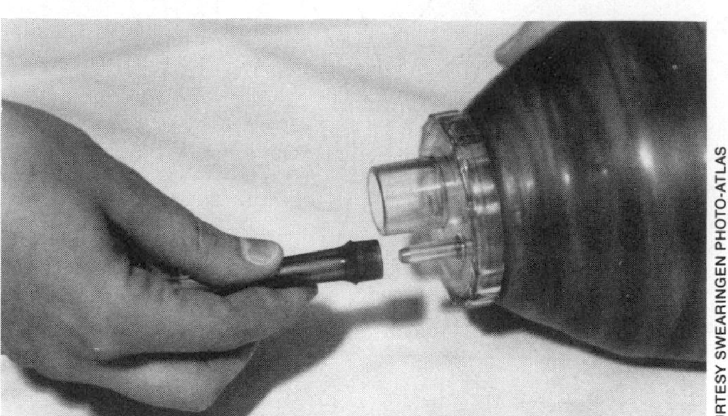

Figure 45–36

4. Open the sterile supplies in readiness for use.
5. Place the sterile towel, if used, across the client's chest, below the tracheostomy.
6. Turn on the suction, and set the pressure in accordance with agency policy. Usually 100 to 120 mm Hg pressure is used for adults, 50 to 75 mm Hg for infants and children.
7. Put a sterile glove on your dominant hand. Some agencies recommend putting a sterile glove on the nondominant hand also, to protect you and the client.
8. Holding the catheter in the dominant hand and the connector in the ungloved hand, attach the catheter to the Y-connector or straight connector. See Figure 45–28, earlier.
9. Using the gloved hand, place the catheter tip in the sterile saline solution; using the thumb of the ungloved hand, occlude the thumb control, and suction a small amount of sterile solution through the catheter.

   Rationale This ensures that the suction equipment is working properly and lubricates the outside and the lumen of the catheter. Lubrication eases insertion and reduces tissue trauma during insertion. Lubricating the lumen helps prevent secretions from sticking to the inside of the catheter.

10. If the client does *not* have copious secretions, hyperventilate the lungs with a resuscitation bag before suctioning:
    a. Using your nondominant hand, turn on the oxygen to 12 to 15 liters per minute.
    b. Attach the tracheostomy adapter of the resuscitator to the tracheostomy or endotracheal tube.
    c. Compress the Ambu or Laerdal bag (see Figure 45–37) as the client inhales, or every 5 seconds for an adult and every 3 seconds for an infant. This is best done by a second person who can use both hands to compress the bag, providing a greater inflation volume.
    d. Observe the rise and fall of the client's chest to assess the adequacy of the ventilation.

    or

    If the client has copious secretions, do not hyperventilate with a resuscitator because the secretions can be forced deeper into the respiratory tract. Instead, keep the client on the regular wall-outlet oxygen delivery device, and increase the liter flow for a few minutes before suctioning.

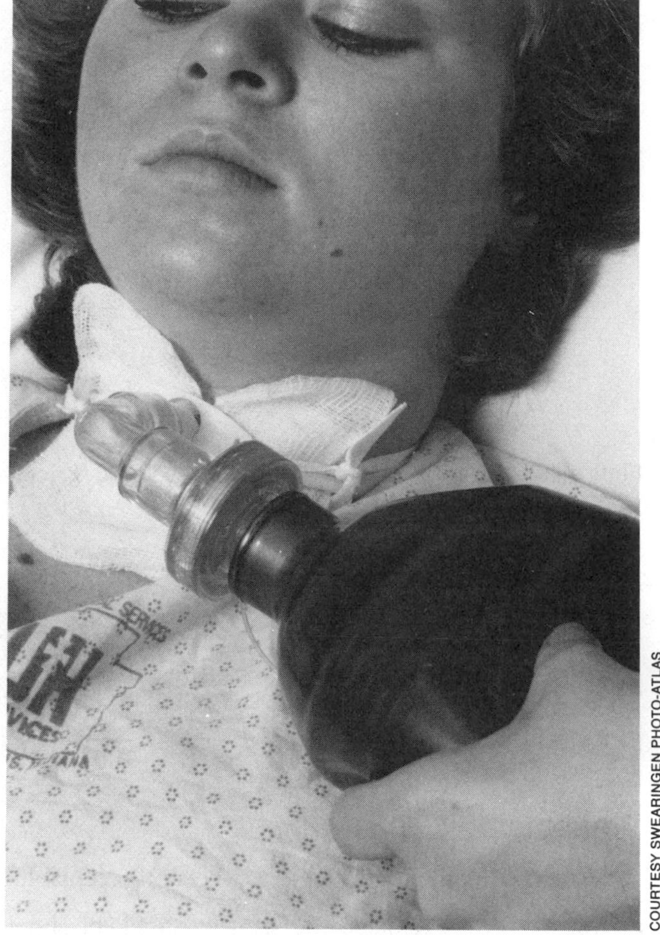

Figure 45–37

11. Remove the oxygen device.

12. With your nondominant thumb off the suction port, quickly but gently insert the catheter into the trachea through the tracheostomy or endotracheal tube. See Figure 45–38. Insert the catheter about 10 to 12.5 cm (4 to 5 in) or until the client coughs.

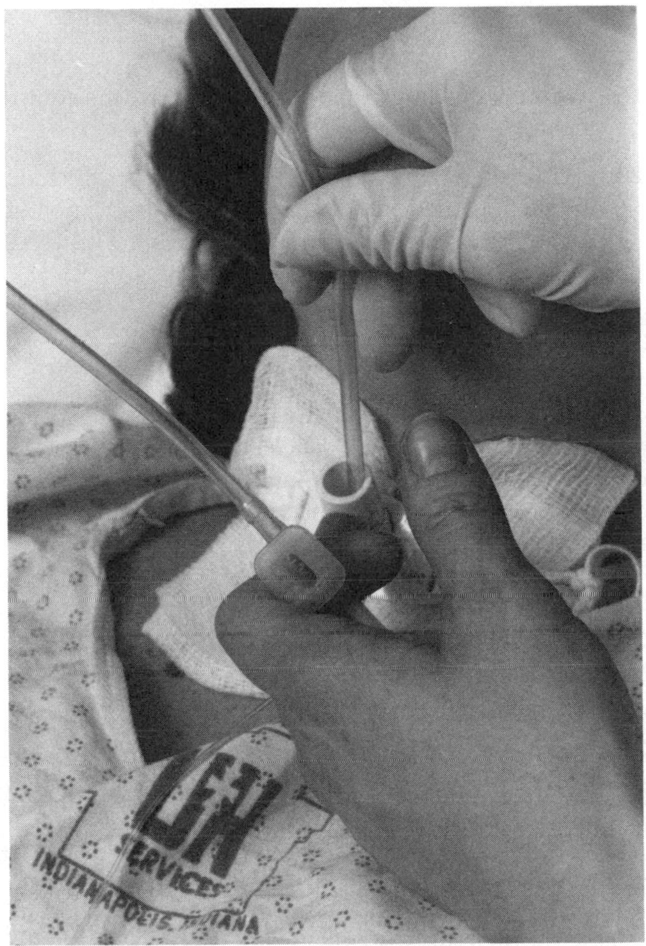

COURTESY SWEARINGEN PHOTO-ATLAS

Figure 45–38

Rationale To prevent tissue trauma and oxygen loss, suction is not applied during insertion of the catheter.

13. Apply suction for 5 to 10 seconds by placing the nondominant thumb over the thumb port. Rotate the catheter by rolling it between your thumb and forefinger while slowly withdrawing it.

    Rationale Suction time is restricted to 10 seconds or less to minimize oxygen loss. Rotating the catheter as it is withdrawn prevents tissue trauma by minimizing the suction time against any part of the trachea.

14. Withdraw the catheter completely, and release the suction.

15. If secretions are thick, flush the catheter in the sterile solution and insert 3 to 5 ml of sterile saline solution into the trachea. See Figure 45–39. Then suction.

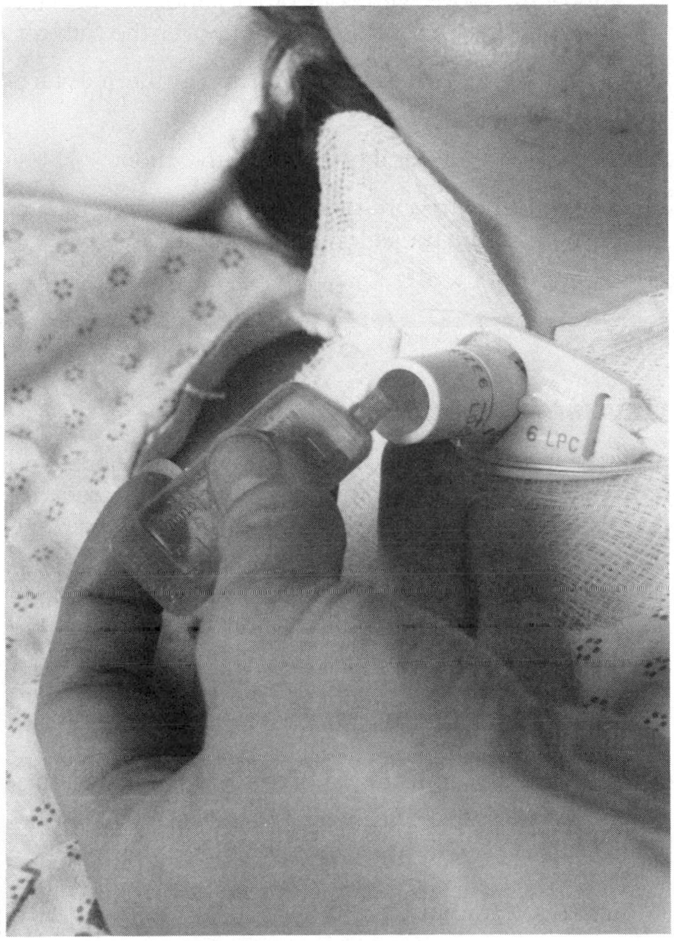

COURTESY SWEARINGEN PHOTO-ATLAS

Figure 45–39

16. Reapply the client's source of supplementary oxygen if appropriate. Observe the client's respirations and skin color, and allow him or her to rest for a few minutes.

17. Encourage the client to breathe deeply and cough. Repeat steps 10–14 until the air passage is clear and the client's breathing is relatively effortless and quiet. Do not suction for more than 3 to 5 minutes total.

    Rationale Suctioning too long can decrease the client's oxygen supply.

18. If agency policy indicates, and if the client's condition warrants it, hyperoxygenate the client's lungs for a few minutes after each suction attempt and on completion of the suctioning procedure.

Rationale This relieves hypoxia that may be created by suctioning.

19. Turn off the suction, and disconnect the catheter from the suction tubing.
20. Holding the catheter in your gloved hand, grasp the cuff of the glove with your other hand, and peel the glove off so that it turns inside out over the catheter.
21. Discard the glove and the catheter in the moisture-resistant bag.
22. Provide oral or nasal hygiene for the client.
23. Observe the amount of secretions obtained by suction, including the color, odor, and thickness.
24. Assist the client to a comfortable, safe position that aids breathing. If the client is conscious, a semi-Fowler's position is frequently indicated. If the client is unconscious, Sims' position can assist the drainage of secretions from the mouth.
25. Replenish the sterile fluid and supplies so that the suction is ready to be used again.

    Rationale Clients who require suctioning often require it quickly, so it is essential to leave the equipment at the bedside ready for use.
26. Record the technique on the client's chart. Include the suction, the route, the amount and description of suction returns, the amount of sterile saline instilled, and the client's breathing, breath sounds, etc.

Oxygen Therapy

Additional oxygen is indicated for numerous clients who have *hypoxemia,* for example, people who have reduced lung diffusion of oxygen through the respiratory membrane, heart failure leading to inadequate transport of oxygen, or substantial loss of lung tissue due to tumors or surgery. In most situations, oxygen therapy is prescribed by the physician, who specifies the specific concentration, method, and liter flow per minute. The concentration is of more importance than the liter flow per minute.

When the administration of oxygen is an emergency measure, the nurse may initiate the therapy. The signs of hypoxemia generally include, in order of occurrence:

1. Increased rapid pulse
2. Rapid, shallow respirations and dyspnea
3. Increased restlessness or lightheadedness
4. Flaring of the nares
5. Substernal or intercostal retractions
6. Cyanosis

Difficult breathing creates apprehension and panic. The nurse, therefore, needs to be competent in providing support and appropriate therapy.

Safety Precautions During Oxygen Therapy

Oxygen by itself will not burn or explode, but it does facilitate combustion. For example, a bed sheet ordinarily burns slowly when ignited in the atmosphere; however, if saturated with free-flowing oxygen and ignited by a spark, it will burn rapidly and explosively. The greater the concentration of the oxygen, the more rapidly fires start and burn, and such fires are difficult to extinguish. Because oxygen is colorless, odorless, and tasteless, people are often unaware of its presence. Safety measures must therefore be taken by the staff, the client, and visitors. These include the following.

1. Place cautionary signs reading "No Smoking: Oxygen in Use" on the client's door, at the foot or head of the bed, and on the oxygen equipment.
2. Remove matches and cigarette lighters from the bedside.
3. Request other clients in the room and visitors to smoke in areas provided elsewhere in the hospital.
4. Remove or store electric equipment, such as razors, hearing aids, radios, televisions, and heating pads, in case short-circuit sparks occur.
5. Avoid materials that generate static electricity, such as woolen blankets and synthetic fabrics. Cotton blankets are used, and nurses are advised to wear cotton fabrics.
6. Avoid the use of volatile, flammable materials, such as oils, greases, alcohol, and ether, near clients receiving oxygen. Lip ointments, if required, should have a water-soluble base such as K-Y jelly or glycerin. Alcohol back rubs are avoided, and nail polish removers or the like are taken away from the immediate vicinity.
7. Ground electric monitoring equipment, suction machines, and portable diagnostic machines. Oxygen therapy should be discontinued temporarily if portable radiographic equipment is required. Monitoring and suction equipment is placed on the bedside opposite the oxygen source.
8. Make known the location of fire extinguishers, and make sure personnel are trained in their use.

Oxygen Supply

Oxygen is supplied in hospitals in two ways: by liquid portable systems (cylinders) and from wall outlets. Oxygen cylinders are made of steel. Large ones contain 244 cubic feet of oxygen stored at a pressure of 2200 pounds per square inch (psi). Smaller cylinders that are readily portable on stretchers are often used. Piped-in oxygen is stored at much lower pressure, usually 50 to 60 psi.

Oxygen administered from a cylinder or wall-outlet system is dry. When dry gases are given to clients, dehydration of the respiratory mucous membranes occurs. Humidifying devices are thus an essential adjunct of oxygen therapy. See page 1302.

Oxygen cylinders Oxygen cylinders are generally encased in metal carriers equipped with wheels for transport and a broad flat base on which the cylinder stands at the bedside to prevent it from falling. A cap on the top protects the valves and outlets. Oxygen cylinders should be placed near the head of the bed and away from traffic areas and heaters. A regulator and a humidifier must be attached before the cylinder is used. The purpose of the regulator is to reduce the pressure in the oxygen cylinder to a safe level. The regulator consists of two parts: a flowmeter and a pressure-reducing valve. The flowmeter regulates the gas flow in liters per minute. Two types of regulators are shown in Figure 45–40.

To assemble the oxygen cylinder for use:

1. Remove the protector cap.
2. Remove any dust in the outlets by slightly opening the handwheel at the top of the cylinder. See Figure 45–41. Turn the handwheel clockwise slowly, and then close it quickly. This is called "cracking the cylinder." People can be frightened if not forewarned of the loud hissing sound it makes.
3. Connect the flow-regulator gauge to the cylinder outlet, and tighten the inlet nut with a wrench. This will ensure that the regulator is held firmly.
4. Stand at the side of the cylinder and open the cylinder valve very slowly until it is fully open. Then turn it back one quarter turn.
5. Regulate the flowmeter to the desired rate of flow in liters per minute. For the Thorpe tube, turn the flow-adjusting valve. For the Bourdon tube, slowly turn the flow-adjusting handle clockwise.
6. Fill the humidifier bottle with distilled water to the mark indicated, and attach it below the flowmeter. For humidifying devices, see page 1302.
7. Attach the specific oxygen tubing and equipment prescribed for the client, e.g., nasal catheter, nasal cannula, or face mask.

Using wall outlet oxygen For oxygen piped in to a wall outlet, only a flowmeter and a humidifier are required.

1. Attach the flowmeter to the wall outlet, exerting firm pressure. The flowmeter should be in the off position. See Figure 45–42.

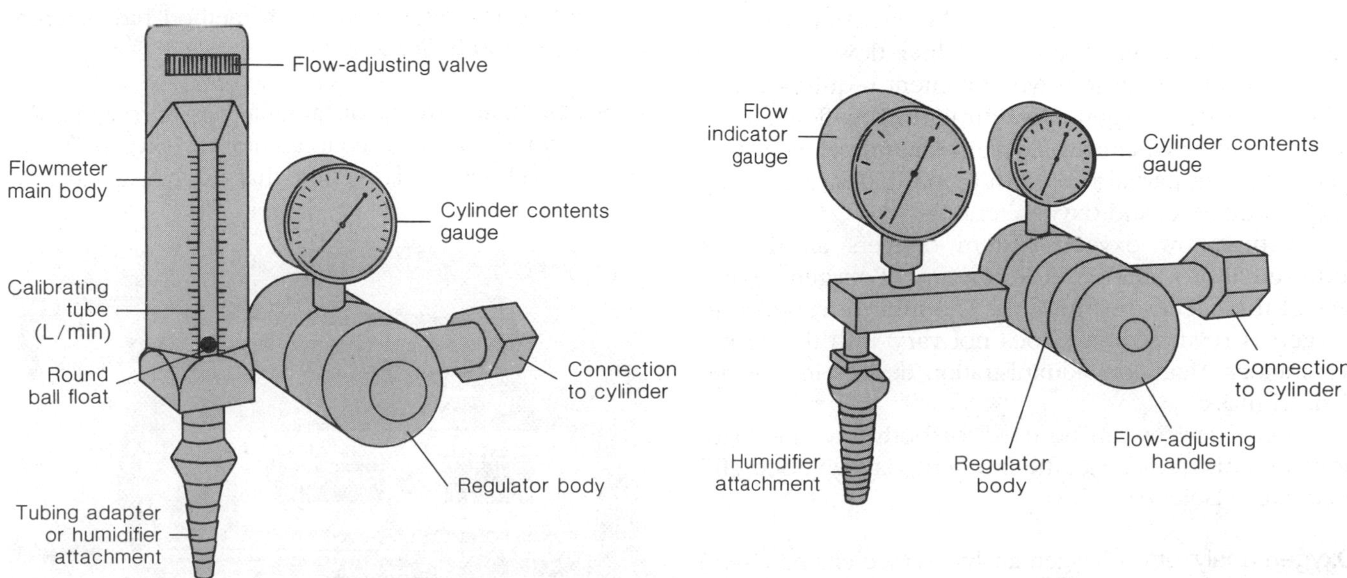

Figure 45–40 Two types of oxygen regulators: **A,** Thorpe tube; **B,** Bourbon tube

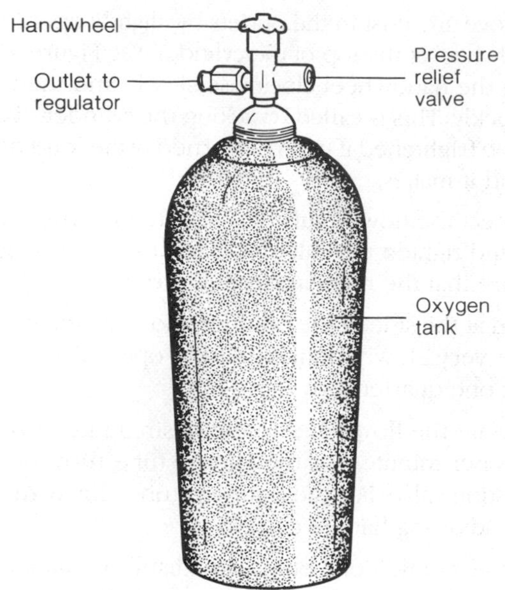

Figure 45–41 The basic parts of an oxygen tank

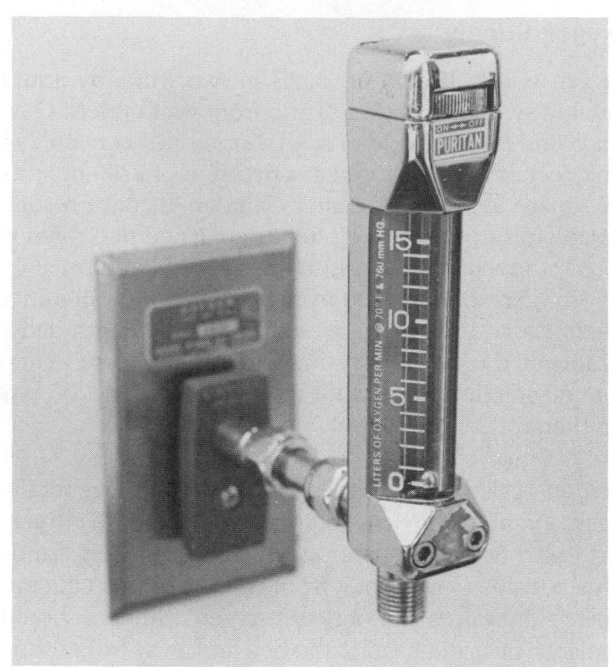

Figure 45–42 An oxygen flowmeter attached to a wall outlet

2. Fill the humidifier bottle with distilled water. (This can be done before coming to the bedside.)
3. Attach the humidifier bottle to the base of the flow meter. See Figure 45–9, on page 1302.
4. Attach the prescribed oxygen tubing and delivery device to the humidifier.
5. Regulate the flowmeter to the prescribed level.

Delivery devices Oxygen is administered by either low-flow or high-flow systems. Both systems can deliver oxygen as well as room air. The fraction of inspired oxygen (FiO_2) is variable, depending on the client's respiratory rate and volume and the oxygen liter flow. A low-flow system is contraindicated when a client requires a carefully monitored oxygen concentration. Low-flow administration devices include nasal cannula, simple face mask, nasal catheter, partial rebreathing mask, nonrebreathing mask, Croupette, and oxygen tent.

A high-flow oxygen system delivers all the gas required. It provides a precise amount of oxygen, regardless of the client's respirations. The ratio of room air to oxygen is regulated and does not vary with the client's respirations. High-flow administration devices include the Venturi mask.

Some devices can be used for both low- and high-flow administration, e.g., the face tent, oxygen hood, and incubator (Isolette).

Oxygen analyzers Oxygen analyzers (see Figure 45–43) measure the concentration of oxygen being received by the client. The analyzer is first used to measure the concentration of oxygen in the room. It should register 0.21 (21%). If it does not, the nurse adjusts the dial to this calibration. Then the sampling tube is placed next to the client's nose, and the reading on the analyzer is monitored. The nurse adjusts the oxygen flow rate to obtain the desired fraction of inspired oxygen (FiO_2).

Oxygen Administration

Oxygen can be administered by nasal cannulae, nasal catheters, oxygen masks, Croupette and other oxygen tents, incubators, and respirators. Each method has different advantages and indications.

Nasal cannula The nasal cannula (nasal prongs) is the most common device used to administer oxygen. It consists of a rubber or plastic tube that extends around the

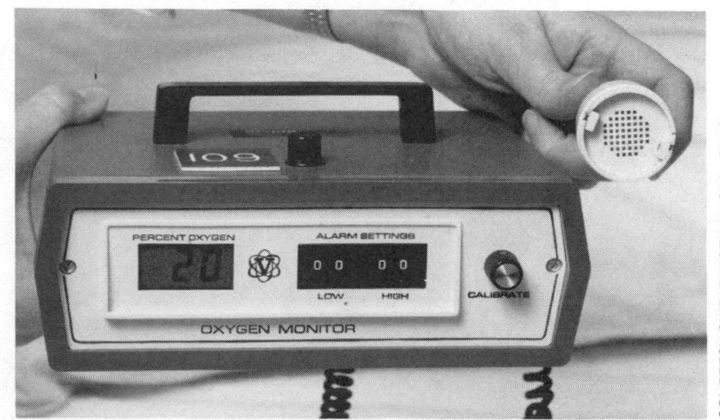

COURTESY SWEARINGEN PHOTO-ATLAS

Figure 45–43 An oxygen analyzer

face, with 0.6- to 1.3-cm (¼- to ½-in) curved prongs that fit into the nostrils. One side of the tube connects to the oxygen tubing and oxygen supply. The cannula is often held in place by an elastic band that fits around the client's head or under the chin. For clients who are confused or particularly active, it may be helpful to secure the cannula in place with small pieces of tape on each side of the face.

The nasal cannula is easy to apply and does not interfere with the client's ability to eat or talk. It also is relatively comfortable and permits some freedom of movement. It delivers a relatively low concentration of oxygen (23% to 44%) at flow rates of 2 to 6 liters per minute. Higher concentrations and flow rates can be administered; however, above 6 liters per minute there is a tendency for the client to swallow air and for the nasal and pharyngeal mucosa to become irritated.

Administering oxygen by cannula is detailed in Procedure 45–6.

Procedure 45–6 ▲ Administering Oxygen by Cannula

Equipment

1. An oxygen supply with a flowmeter
2. A humidifier with sterile distilled water
3. A nasal cannula and tubing
4. Tape, if needed, to secure the cannula in place
5. Gauzes to pad the tubing over the cheekbones

Intervention

1. Assist the client to a semi-Fowler's position if possible.

   Rationale This position permits easier chest expansion and hence easier breathing.

2. Explain that oxygen is not dangerous when safety precautions are observed and that it will ease the discomfort of dyspnea. Inform the client and support persons about the safety precautions connected with oxygen use.

3. Set up the oxygen equipment and the humidifier. See page 1323.

4. Turn on the oxygen at the flow rate ordered, e.g., 2 to 6 liters per minute for clients who have a regular respiratory pattern, a respiratory rate less than 25 breaths per minute, and a tidal volume of 300 to 700 ml. Higher concentrations and flow rates can be administered, but above 6 liters per minute there is a tendency for the client to swallow air and experience irritation of the nasal and pharyngeal mucosa.

5. Check that the oxygen is flowing freely through the tubing. There should be no kinks in the tubing, and the connections should be airtight. There should be bubbles in the humidifier as the oxygen flows through the water. You should feel the oxygen at the outlets of the cannula.

6. Put the cannula over the client's face, with the outlet prongs fitting into the nares and the elastic band around the head. Some models have a strap to adjust under the chin. Make sure the prongs are turned upward so the oxygen is directed into the nasal passages and not into the tissues at the base of the nares. See Figure 45–44.

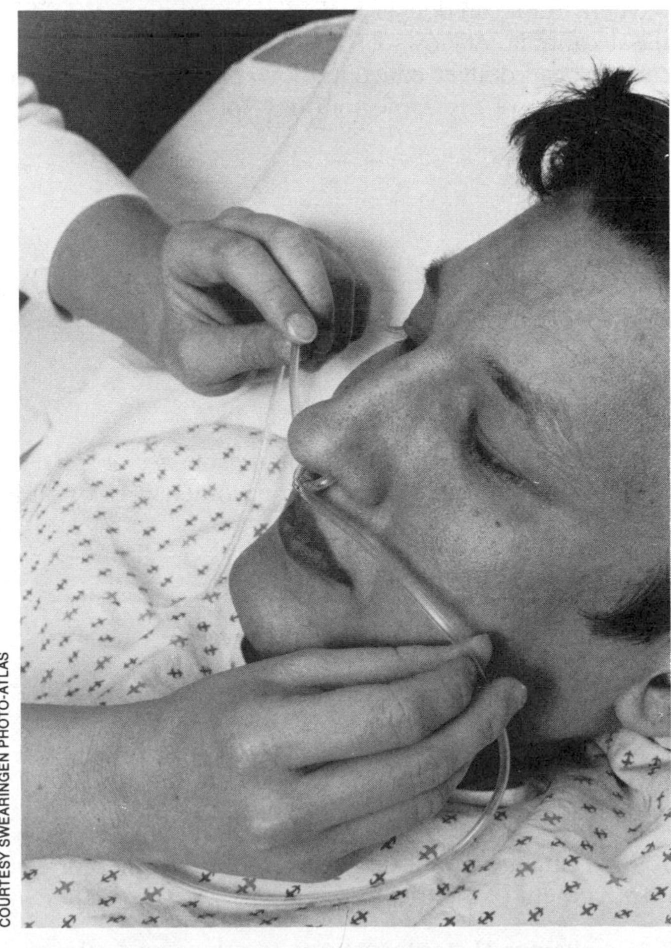

COURTESY SWEARINGEN PHOTO-ATLAS

Figure 45–44

7. If the cannula will not stay in place, tape it at the sides of the face. Slip gauze pads under the tubing over the cheekbones to prevent skin irritation.

8. Assess the client's immediate response to the oxygen, in terms of color, respirations, discomfort, etc., and provide support while adjusting to the cannula.

9. Assess the client's response to the therapy in 15 to 30 minutes, depending on the client's condition, and regularly thereafter. Assess vital signs, color, breathing patterns, and chest movements.

10. Make sure that safety precautions are being followed.

11. Check the liter flow and the level of water in the humidifier in 30 minutes and whenever providing care to the client.

12. Assess the client regularly for clinical signs of hypoxia: tachycardia, confusion, dyspnea, restlessness, and cyanosis.

13. Assess the client's nares for encrustations and irritation. Apply a water-soluble lubricant as required to soothe the mucous membranes.

14. Record initiation of the therapy and the assessment data.

Sample Recording

Date	Time	Notes
Dec/5/87	0730	O_2 by cannula at 3 L/min. P 96, R 24. Slightly cyanotic, dyspneic on exertion, and restless. ——— Susan de Camillis, SN
	0800	Cyanosis improved. P 84, R 16. Dyspnea and restlessness reduced. ——— Susan de Camillis, SN

Nasal catheter The nasal catheter (low-flow device) is a rubber or plastic tube about 39 cm (16 in) long, with six or eight holes at the tip to disperse the oxygen. It is used to administer low to moderate concentrations of oxygen, but it can deliver higher concentrations than the nasal cannula. At flows of 1 to 5 liters per minute, the catheter can deliver concentrations of oxygen of 30% to 35%. It allows the same mobility for the client as the cannula.

Major problems associated with nasal catheters are laryngeal ulceration, from the constant flow of oxygen into the larynx, and gastric distention, caused by air and oxygen entering the stomach. Gastric distention can be relieved by inserting a nasogastric tube. Laryngeal ulceration may be prevented by moving the catheter from one nostril to the other every 8 hours (Fuchs 1980, p. 39).

The details of administering oxygen by catheter are given in Procedure 45–7.

Procedure 45–7 ▲ Administering Oxygen by Catheter

Equipment

1. A nasal catheter of the appropriate size: #8 or #10 Fr. for children; #10 or #12 Fr. for women; #12 or #14 Fr. for men

2. An oxygen supply with a flowmeter

3. A humidifier with sterile distilled water

4. Water-soluble lubricating jelly, to facilitate catheter insertion, and a gauze square to apply it

5. Adhesive tape (nonallergenic is preferred) to secure the catheter to the client's face

6. A flashlight and a tongue blade for assessing correct placement of the catheter

7. A container of sterile water to test the oxygen flow

Intervention

1. Follow Procedure 45–6, steps 1–3. Test the oxygen flow by turning on the flowmeter to 3 liters per minute and inserting the tip of the catheter into a container of sterile water. Bubbling indicates that oxygen is flowing.

2. Determine how deep to insert the catheter by placing the end of the catheter in a straight line between the tip of the client's nose and the earlobe. See Figure 45–45. This distance can be marked with tape.

   Rationale This external distance approximates the distance from the nares to the oropharynx.

3. Lubricate the tip of the catheter with water-soluble jelly. Squeeze the lubricant onto a gauze square, and rotate the catheter tip through it. Do *not* use mineral oil or petroleum jelly.

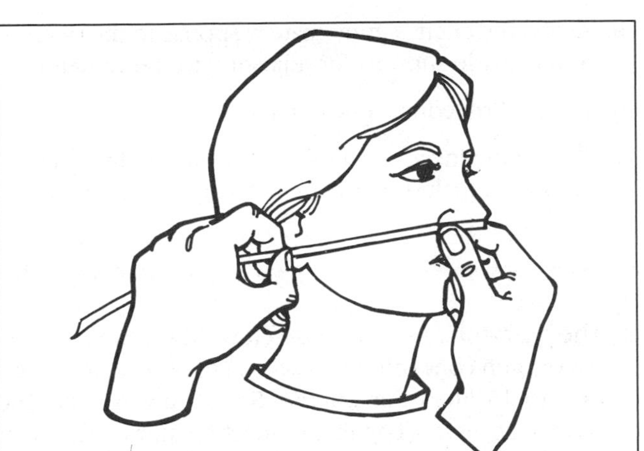

Figure 45–45

Rationale Lubrication facilitates insertion and prevents injury to the nasal mucosa. If aspirated, mineral oil or petroleum jelly can cause severe lung irritations or lipoid pneumonia.

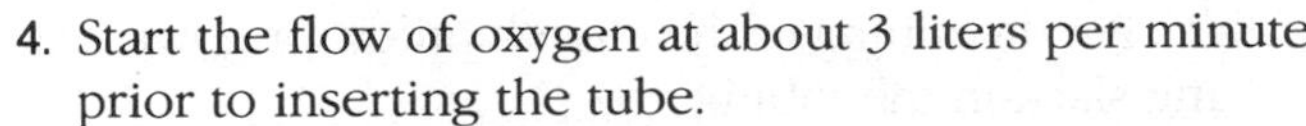

4. Start the flow of oxygen at about 3 liters per minute prior to inserting the tube.

   Rationale The flow of oxygen prevents the catheter from becoming plugged with secretions during insertion.

5. Introduce the catheter slowly through one nostril until the tip is at the entrance to the oropharynx (the marked distance). See Figure 45–46, *A*. Look into the client's mouth, using the flashlight and tongue blade, to check placement. The tip of the catheter will be visible beside the uvula. See Figure 45–46, *B*.

6. Withdraw the tip slightly so that it can no longer be seen.

   Rationale When the catheter is in this position, the client is less likely to swallow oxygen.

7. Tape the catheter to the client's face at the side of the nose and the cheek (see Figure 45–47, *A*) or at the tip of the nose and the forehead (see Figure 45–47,

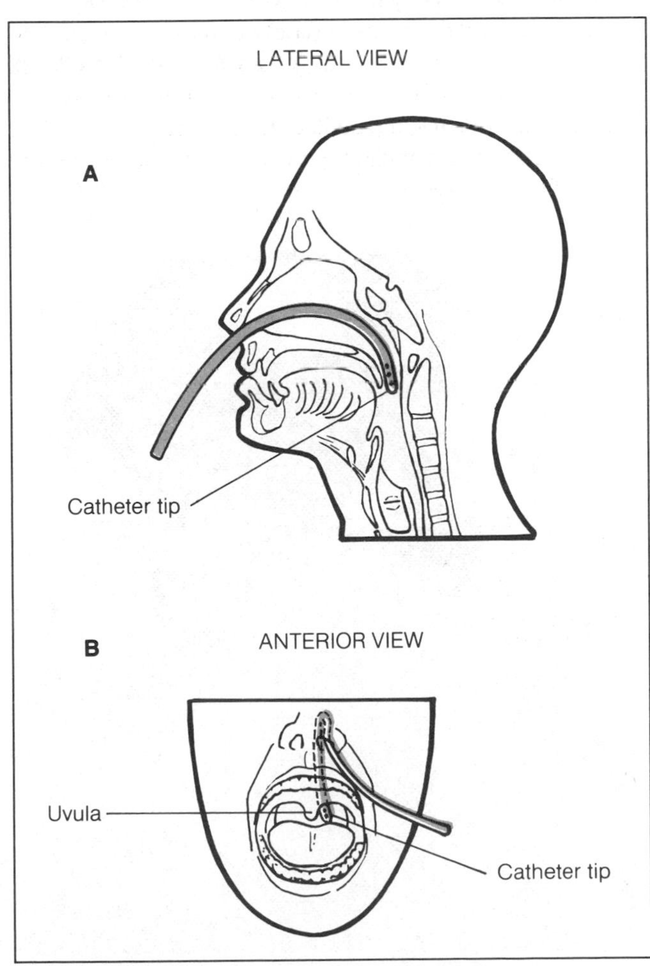

Figure 45–46

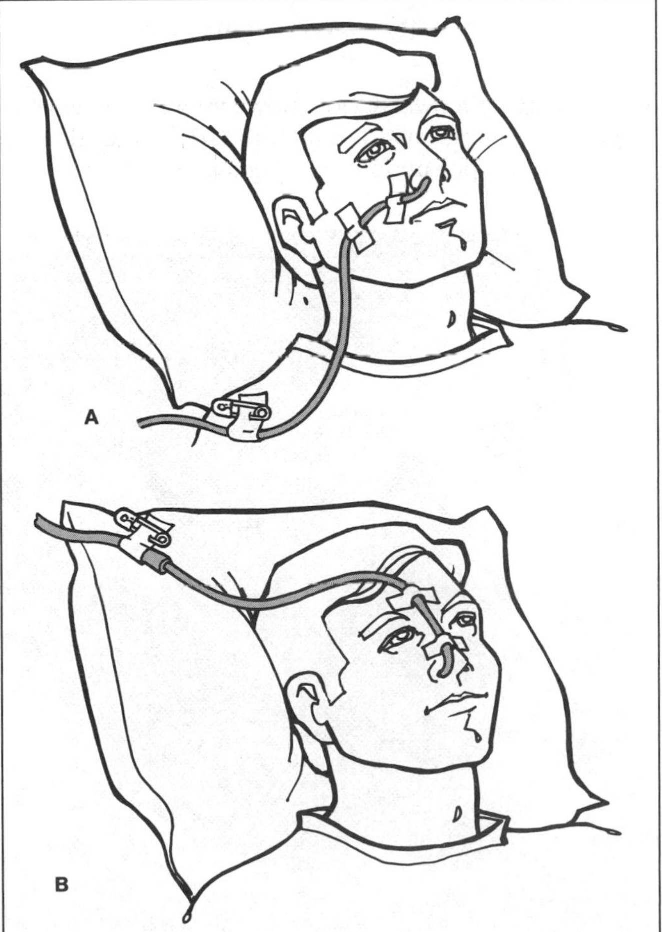

Figure 45–47

B). Pin the tubing to the client's pillow or gown, leaving slack in the tubing.

Rationale If taped and pinned, the catheter will not be displaced when the client moves. Slack allows the client to move without pulling on the tubing.

8. Adjust the flow to the prescribed rate.
9. Assess the client's immediate response to the oxygen, and provide support for adjusting to the catheter.
10. Follow Procedure 45–6, steps 9–12.
11. Record the initiation of oxygen therapy and the client's response, including the method and the flow rate.

Face mask Face masks that cover the client's nose and mouth may be used for oxygen inhalation. Most masks are made of clear, pliable plastic or rubber that can be molded to fit the face. They are held to the client's head with elastic bands. Some have a metal clip that can be bent over the bridge of the nose for a snug fit. There are several holes in the sides of the mask (exhalation ports) to allow the escape of exhaled carbon dioxide.

Some masks have reservoir bags, which provide higher oxygen concentrations to the client. A portion of the client's expired air is directed into the bag. Because this air comes from the upper respiratory passages (e.g., the trachea and bronchi), where it does not take part in gaseous exchange, its oxygen concentration remains the same as that of inspired air.

A variety of oxygen masks are marketed:

1. The *simple face mask* (low-flow system) delivers oxygen concentrations from 40% to 60% at liter flows of 5 to 8 liters per minute. See Figure 45–48.
2. The *partial rebreather mask* (low-flow system) delivers oxygen concentrations of 35% to 60% at liter flows of 6 to 15 liters per minute. See Figure 45–49. The oxygen reservoir bag that is attached allows the client to rebreathe about the first third of the exhaled air. The partial rebreather bag must not totally deflate during inspiration. If this problem occurs, increase the liter flow of oxygen.
3. The *nonrebreather mask* (low-flow system) delivers the highest oxygen concentration possible by means other than intubation or mechanical ventilation, i.e., 60% to 90% at liter flows of 6 to 15 liters per minute. See Figure 45–50. Using a nonrebreather mask, the client breathes only the source gas from the bag. One-way valves on the mask and between the reservoir bag and the mask prevent the room air and the client's exhaled air from entering the bag. The nonrebreather bag must not totally deflate during inspiration. If it does, this problem can be corrected by increasing the liter flow of oxygen.

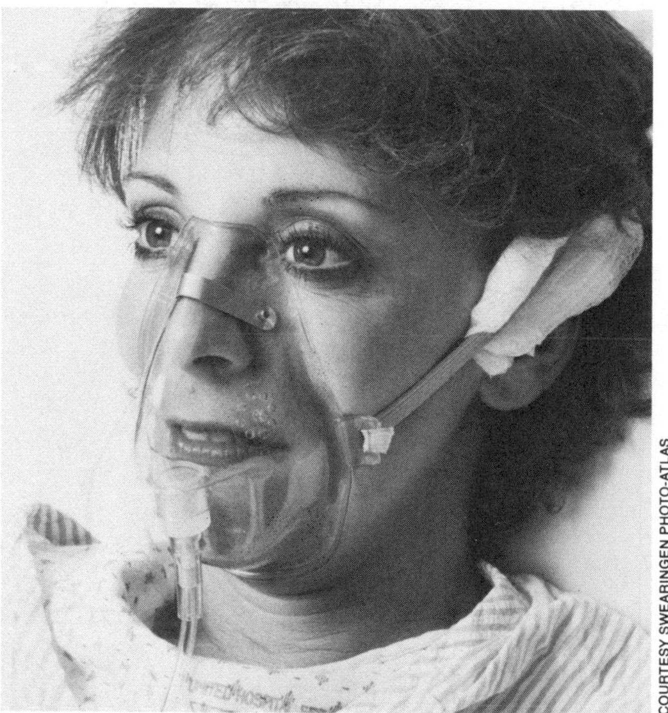

COURTESY SWEARINGEN PHOTO-ATLAS

Figure 45–48 A simple face mask for a low-flow oxygen system

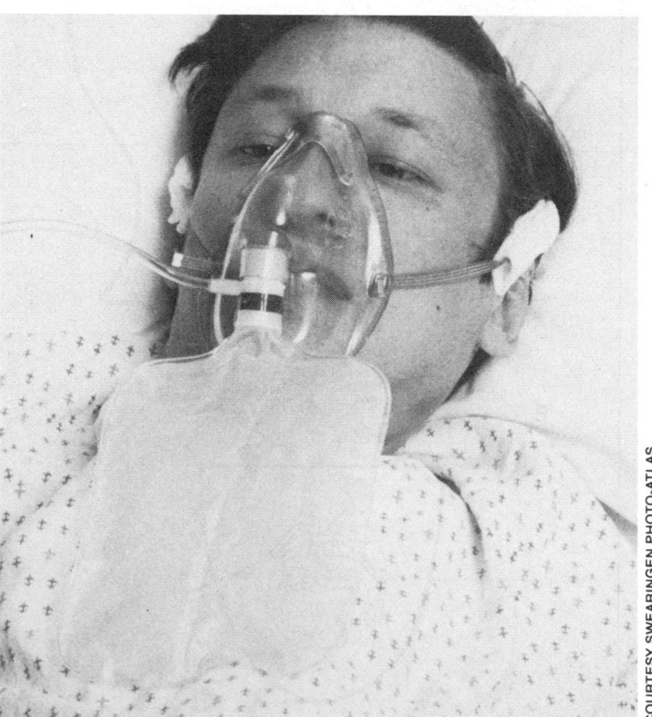

COURTESY SWEARINGEN PHOTO-ATLAS

Figure 45–49 A partial rebreathing mask for a low-flow oxygen system

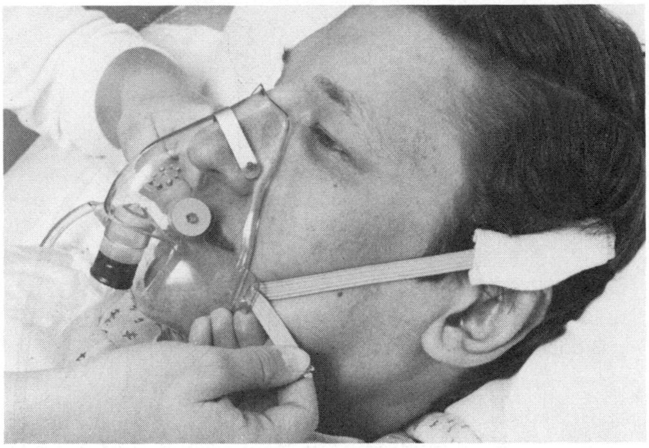

COURTESY SWEARINGEN PHOTO-ATLAS

Figure 45–50 A nonrebreathing mask for a low-flow or a high-flow oxygen system

4. The *Venturi mask* (high-flow system) delivers oxygen concentrations precise to within 1% and is often used for clients with COPD. See Figure 45–51. Oxygen concentrations vary from 24% to 40% or 50%, depending on the brand, at liter flows of 4 to 8 liters per minute. The Venturi mask is designed with wide-bore tubing and various color-coded jet adapters. Each color code corresponds to a precise oxygen concentration and a specific liter flow. For example, a blue adapter delivers a 24% concentration of oxygen at 4 liters per minute, and a green adapter delivers a 35% concentration of oxygen at 8 liters per minute. Optional humidification adapters are also available for clients who require them, e.g., those receiving oxygen concentrations in excess of 30%.

The Venturi system operates as follows.

1. Oxygen enters the tubing at a prescribed flow rate.
2. When the gas reaches the jet adapter of the Venturi device, which is essentially a restricted orifice, the velocity of the oxygen increases to maintain the same (prescribed) flow rate.
3. As the velocity of the gas increases, less pressure is exerted at the jet outlet.
4. With less pressure, the higher-pressure room air is drawn in through the air entrainment ports.
5. This room air dilutes the oxygen to a certain concentration (the percentage specified for the particular jet adapter).

The amount of air drawn in is determined by the size of the orifice (jet adapter). The smaller the orifice, the greater the increase in velocity of oxygen, the greater the decrease in tubing pressure, and the larger the amount of room

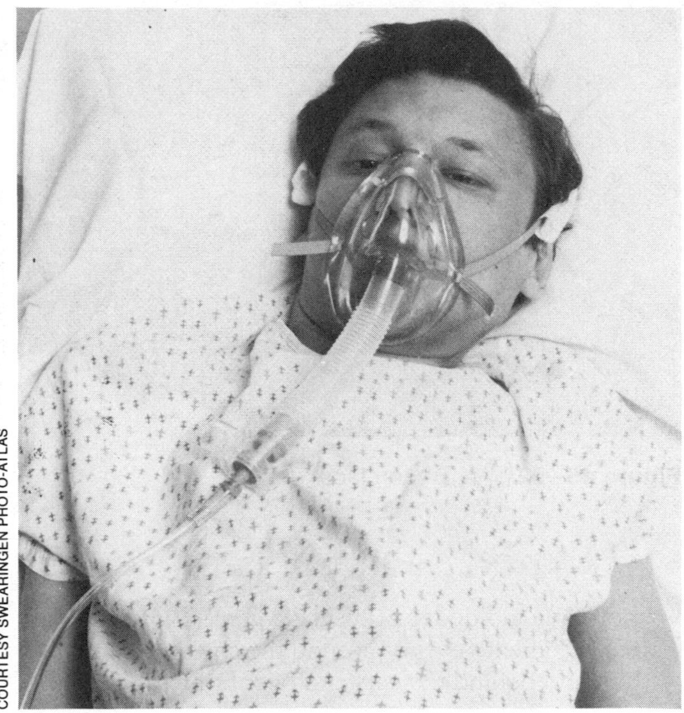

COURTESY SWEARINGEN PHOTO-ATLAS

Figure 45–51 A Venturi mask for a high-flow oxygen system

air drawn in through the entrainment ports. Thus, the narrower the jet adapter, the greater the air dilution, and the lower the concentration of oxygen.

When using a Venturi mask it is important to prevent occlusion of the air entrainment ports by bed linen, clothing, or other objects. Blood gas measurements are taken frequently to monitor the effectiveness of therapy. Changes in the blood gas measurements may necessitate changing the jet adapter and the oxygen concentration.

Initiating oxygen by mask is much the same as initiating oxygen by cannula or catheter, except that the nurse must find a mask of appropriate size. Smaller sizes are available for children. When fitting a client with a face mask, the nurse needs to:

1. Familiarize the client with the mask when possible. Allow the client to hold the mask, guide it toward the face, and get used to the sensation of the mask covering the nose and mouth. Instruct the client to put on the mask from the nose downward during expiration.
2. Turn on the oxygen to the prescribed rate of flow. When the mask has a reservoir bag, the nurse should first flush the mask with oxygen until it is partially inflated.
3. Gradually fit the mask to the contours of the face, and encourage the client to breathe normally. The mask

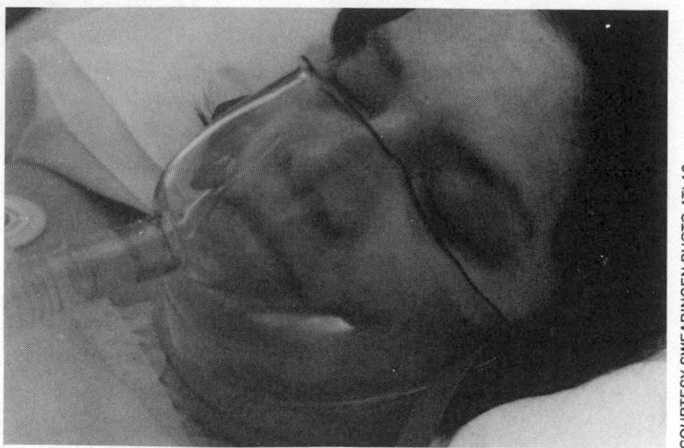

Figure 45–52 An oxygen face tent

should be molded to prevent oxygen escaping upward into the client's eyes or around the cheeks or chin. Pad the band behind the ears and over bony prominences to prevent skin irritation.

Face tent Face tents can replace oxygen masks when masks are poorly tolerated by clients (e.g., children). When a face tent alone is used to supply oxygen, the concentration of oxygen varies; therefore, it is often used in conjunction with a Venturi system. Face tents can provide 30% to 55% concentration of oxygen at 4 to 8 liters per minute. When using a face tent, frequently inspect the client's facial skin for dampness or chafing, and dry and treat as needed. See Figure 45–52.

Chest Tubes

Chest tubes are made of pliable plastic or rubber. They are usually inserted through an intercostal space into the pleural cavity. See Figure 45–53. A **pneumothorax** is the collection of air in the pleural cavity. A **hemothorax** is an accumulation of blood in the pleural cavity. Chest tubes that are used to remove air are usually inserted superiorly, i.e., through the second intercostal space, and anteriorly, because air tends to rise in the pleural cavity. Tubes used to drain fluid are inserted more inferiorly, often in the eighth or ninth intercostal space, and more posteriorly. Sometimes a tube used to drain air is inserted inferiorly and threaded superiorly in the pleural space. When a client requires drainage of both fluid and air, two chest tubes may be inserted. These are sometimes joined externally by a Y-connector.

Chest tubes are inserted during surgery and in nonsurgical situations, e.g., in emergency treatment of injuries. When a chest tube is inserted during surgery, it may extrude through the incision or through a stab wound (a small, deep wound made with a scalpel for insertion of the tube).

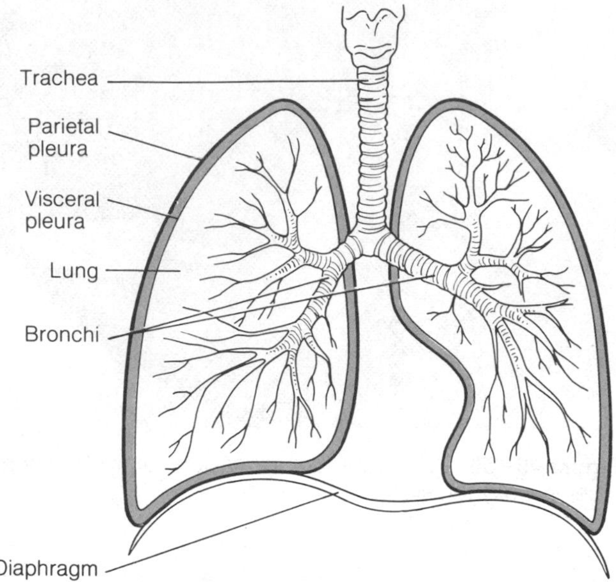

Figure 45–53 The pleural cavity is a potential space that lies between the visceral pleura and the parietal pleura. Chest tubes are inserted into this space.

Drainage Systems

Because the pleural cavity normally has negative pressure, any drainage system connected to it must be sealed so that air or liquid cannot enter. Such a drainage system is called a *water-sealed (underwater) drainage* or a *disposable pleural drainage system.* In water-sealed drainage, fluid in the bottom of the container prevents air from entering the chest tube and thus entering the pleural cavity. The system must be kept below the level of the client's chest so that the fluid in the container is not drawn into the pleural cavity by gravity. It is also very important to maintain the patency of the tubing.

Drainage systems use three mechanisms to drain fluid and air from the pleural cavity: positive expiratory pressure, gravity, and suction. When the pleural cavity contains some air or fluid, a positive pressure develops during expiration. This positive pressure is abnormal, but it does help expel the air and to some extent fluid from the space. Gravity acts as an evacuation force when the tubing is placed so that it descends from the insertion site to the drainage receptacle. Suction is used in conjunction with the other two forces in some drainage systems.

There are several kinds of water-sealed drainage systems: one- and two-bottle gravity systems, two- and three-bottle suction systems, and disposable unit systems.

Evaluation

Examples of outcome criteria related to oxygenation are listed to the right.

Examples of Outcome Criteria Related to Oxygenation

The client will:

- Have full lung expansion during deep breathing exercises
- Expectorate secretions when coughing
- Exhibit no adventitious breath sounds
- Have no chest retractions
- Have a blood pressure within normal range
- Have a normal Pao_2 and $Paco_2$

Resuscitation

Basic life support (BLS) is a phase of emergency cardiac care that is intended to prevent circulatory or respiratory arrest or, through cardiopulmonary resuscitation, to externally support circulation and ventilation of a person who has had a cardiac or respiratory arrest. When a victim's heart and lungs stop functioning, **cardiopulmonary resuscitation (CPR)** needs to be performed quickly and efficiently. It is a life-saving measure that may be needed in a hospital or any place where there are people. A delay of 4 minutes or more can result in permanent brain damage due to cerebral anoxia. Recognizing the need for CPR and skill in performing it quickly and competently are essential functions of nurses. More and more laypersons are also being encouraged to learn CPR. Courses are available at national Red Cross and Heart Associations throughout the country. Learning to perform these procedures correctly requires instruction from a certified instructor at these associations and supervised practice.

Cardiac and Respiratory Arrests

A **cardiac arrest** is the cessation of cardiac function; the heart stops beating. Often a cardiac arrest is unexpected and sudden. When it occurs, the heart no longer pumps blood to any of the organs of the body. Breathing then stops, and the person becomes unconscious and limp. Within 20 to 40 seconds of a cardiac arrest, the victim is clinically dead. After 4 to 6 minutes, the lack of oxygen supply to the brain causes permanent and extensive damage.

Causes of cardiac arrest are many and include electrocution, myocardial infarction (heart attack), respiratory failure, extensive hemorrhage, and brain injury. The three cardinal signs of a cardiac arrest are apnea, absence of a carotid or femoral pulse, and dilated pupils. The person's skin appears pale or grayish and feels cool. Cyanosis is evident when respiratory function fails prior to heart failure.

A **respiratory** (pulmonary) **arrest** is the cessation of breathing. It often occurs as a result of a blocked airway, but it can occur following a cardiac arrest and for other reasons. A respiratory arrest is preceded by short, shallow breathing. The breathing becomes increasingly labored. Then the person becomes flushed and disoriented and experiences feelings of suffocation. If the respiratory problem persists, the person becomes cyanotic, becomes comatose, and goes into cardiac arrest. Respiratory arrest leads to cardiac arrest because of the lack of oxygen to vital organs, especially the heart and the brain.

Life Support

Resuscitation is restoration to consciousness or life; it includes all measures to revive individuals who have stopped breathing due to either respiratory or cardiac failure. **Artificial respiration** (e.g., oral resuscitation) is used when the victim's breathing has stopped while the heart continues to beat. **External cardiac massage** (or compression) is used when both the heartbeat and breathing have stopped; then both artificial respiration and external cardiac massage are applied at the same time. These combined measures are often called **cardiopulmonary resuscitation (CPR)** or **basic life support (BLS)**. Basic life support must be complemented by a rapid delivery of advanced cardiac life support (ACLS). ACLS includes:

1. Establishing an effective airway: endotracheal intubation is preferable
2. Establishing an IV line
3. Administering epinephrine intravenously
4. Administering sodium bicarbonate
5. Defibrillation
6. Administering other intravenous bolus drug therapy as indicated, e.g., atropine, calcium chloride, lidocaine, isoproterenol (Isuprel), norepinephrine (Levophed), or digoxin

The survival rate from cardiac arrest due to ventricular fibrillation clearly depends on the promptness of the initiation of CPR and ACLS. Studies show that there is a 43% survival rate if CPR is initiated within 4 minutes and ACLS within 8 minutes. Only 10% survive if ACLS is not initiated until 16 minutes have elapsed (McIntyre and Lewis 1983, p. 9).

ABCs of Cardiopulmonary Resuscitation

The ABCs of cardiopulmonary resuscitation (CPR) are:

A. Clear the *airways*.

B. Initiate artificial *breathing* (oral resuscitation).

C. Initiate *cardiac* compression (artificial *circulation*).

This sequence is recommended because spontaneous breathing can occur after any one action, such as after the airway is opened or after a few artificial respirations are provided. **External cardiac compression** is meant to provide artificial circulation. Compression reproduces the normal intermittent heart contractions that pump blood through the body. External cardiac compression is manual, intermittent, rhythmic compression applied to the victim's sternum with the heel of your hand. The heart is squeezed between the sternum and the vertebrae lying posteriorly. Cardiac compression is ineffective unless there is simultaneous artificial respiration to oxygenate the bloodstream.

External cardiac compression should never be practiced on a person with a functioning heart, because it could interfere with normal cardiac contractions.

Assessment

The assessment phases of BLS are of extreme importance. Each of the ABCs of CPR begins with an assessment phase:

A. *Airway*. Determine the person's responsiveness.

B. *Breathing*. Determine the person's breathlessness.

C. *Circulation*. Determine the person's pulselessness.

Performing each assessment step ensures that the victim will not be subjected to any intrusive procedure (e.g., positioning, opening the airway, rescue breathing, external cardiac compression) until the need for it is determined. Table 45–5 provides a summary of the recent changes in the CPR standards of the American Heart Association.

Initial Steps

Initial steps when a rescuer arrives at the scene of the emergency include the following.

1. Assess any injury, and determine whether the victim is responsive or not. To ascertain whether the victim has lost consciousness, tap or gently shake the victim and shout, "Are you all right?" If there is no response, the victim is unconscious. If injury to the head or neck is evident or suspected, avoid moving the victim inappropriately, to prevent further injury and potential paralysis.
2. If the victim does not respond, call for help. When another rescuer arrives, have him or her call an ambulance or that particular community's emergency medical services (EMS).
3. Position the victim supine on a flat firm surface, with the arms alongside his or her body. If the victim is lying face downward, roll him or her as a unit (head, shoulders, and trunk simultaneously), to prevent twisting and injury of the spine.
4. Kneel beside the victim's shoulders so you can perform rescue breathing and chest compression without moving your knees. If the victim is in bed, you may have to kneel on the bed.

Opening the Airway

The tongue and epiglottis are the most common airway obstructions in the unconscious victim. Without sufficient muscle tone the tongue will obstruct the pharynx and the epiglottis may obstruct the larynx. Moving the lower jaw forward lifts the tongue away from the back of the throat. See Figure 45–54. This can be accomplished by using the head-tilt/chin-lift or jaw-thrust maneuver.

Digital removal of foreign material If foreign material is visible in the mouth it must first be expediently removed. To digitally remove foreign material from the mouth the rescuer should do the following.

1. Open the person's mouth by grasping the tongue and lower jaw between your thumb and fingers and lifting

Table 45–5 Summary of New and Old CPR Standards

New Standards	Old Standards
OPENING THE AIRWAY	
1. Lay rescuers are to be taught only the *head-tilt/chin-lift* method, since: (a) it is simple, easily learned, and safe; (b) it is more effective than the head-tilt/neck-lift; and (c) the jaw thrust, though very effective, is technically difficult and fatiguing. 2. Professional rescuers (nurses, physicians, emergency medical technicians) are to learn both the head-tilt/chin-lift and the jaw-thrust method; the latter is the safest method for victims with suspected neck injury.	Lay and professional rescuers were taught (a) the head-tilt/neck-lift, (b) the head-tilt/chin-lift, and (c) the jaw-thrust method.
WHEN BREATHLESSNESS IS DETERMINED	
For persons over 1 year of age	
Deliver two full breaths lasting 1 to 1½ seconds each, pausing to inhale before delivering the second breath. This allows adequate time for good chest expansion and decreases the possibility of gastric distention. A duration of 1 to 1½ seconds for each breath more closely matches the victim's inspiratory time.	Deliver four quick, full or "staircase" breaths, with no pause between breaths.
For infants under 1 year of age*	
Deliver two *slow* breaths lasting 1 to 1½ seconds, with a pause between breaths.	Deliver four quick, full puffs of air, with no pause between puffs.
In two-person CPR for an adult	
Deliver one breath, lasting 1 to 1½ seconds, *during a pause* after every fifth chest compression. The pause may be shorter than each breath. Slower breaths reduce the risk of gastric distention, regurgitation, and aspiration.	Deliver one breath on the upstroke of every fifth chest compression, with no pause in the chest compressions.
WHEN AIRWAY OBSTRUCTION IS DETERMINED	
In persons over 1 year of age	
Perform *only* the Heimlich maneuver (subdiaphragmatic abdominal thrusts).	Deliver four back blows and perform the Heimlich maneuver (subdiaphragmatic abdominal thrusts).
For women in late pregnancy or markedly obese individuals	
Deliver chest thrusts, since there is no room between the enlarged uterus or adipose tissue and the rib cage.	Same as new standard
For infants under 1 year of age*	
Provide a combination of chest thrusts and back blows. In this age group there is potential for intraabdominal injury from the Heimlich maneuver.	Same as new standard
WHEN PULSELESSNESS IS DETERMINED	
For an infant*	
Using two or three fingers, compress the sternum *one finger width below* the nipple line. Evidence has shown that the infant's heart is lower in relation to the external chest landmarks than previously thought.	Using two or three fingers, compress the sternum *at* the nipple line.
In one-person CPR for an adult	
Perform external cardiac compressions at the rate of 80 to 100 per minute. This increased compression rate increases blood flow from the heart.	Perform cardiac compressions at the rate of 60 to 80 per minute.

(continued)

Table 45–5 *(continued)*

New Standards	Old Standards
In two-person CPR for an adult	
Deliver one breath, lasting 1 to 1½ seconds, *during a pause* after every fifth chest compression. Slower breaths reduce the risk of gastric distention, regurgitation, and aspiration.	Deliver one breath on the upstroke of every fifth chest compression, with no pause in the chest compressions.
RESCUER INSTRUCTION	
1. Only one-person CPR will be taught to laypersons, because (a) two-person CPR has not been used that often, and (b) knowledge of only one technique makes for both better retention and improved performance. When one rescuer becomes tired, the second rescuer should relieve him or her.	All rescuers were taught both one-person and two-person CPR.
2. Both one-person and two-person CPR will be taught to professional rescuers, since two-person CPR is less fatiguing and can be performed for longer periods.	

*Cardiopulmonary resuscitation and removal of foreign-body obstructions in the upper airways of infants and children are included in the Procedures Supplement for *Fundamentals of Nursing*.

Source: Adapted from American Heart Association, Standards and guidelines for cardiopulmonary resuscitation (CPR) and emergency cardiac care (ECC), *Journal of the American Medical Association*, June 6, 1986, 255:2841–3044.

the jaw upward. See Figure 45–55. This pulls the tongue away from the back of the throat.

2. Remove solid material by inserting the index finger of your free hand along the inside of the person's cheek and deep into the throat. With your finger hooked, use a sweeping motion to try to dislodge and lift out the foreign material.
3. Clear out liquid material, such as mucus, blood, and emesis, with a scooping motion, using two fingers wrapped with a tissue or piece of cloth.

Head-tilt/chin-lift maneuver The head-tilt/chin-lift maneuver is the method recommended for establishing an open pharynx (American Heart Association 1986, p. 2916). Tilt the victim's head backward by placing one hand on the victim's forehead and applying firm pressure backward with the palm. Lift the chin forward by placing the fingers of your other hand under the bony part of the lower jaw near the chin. The teeth should then be almost closed. See Figure 45–56. Moving the jaw forward will

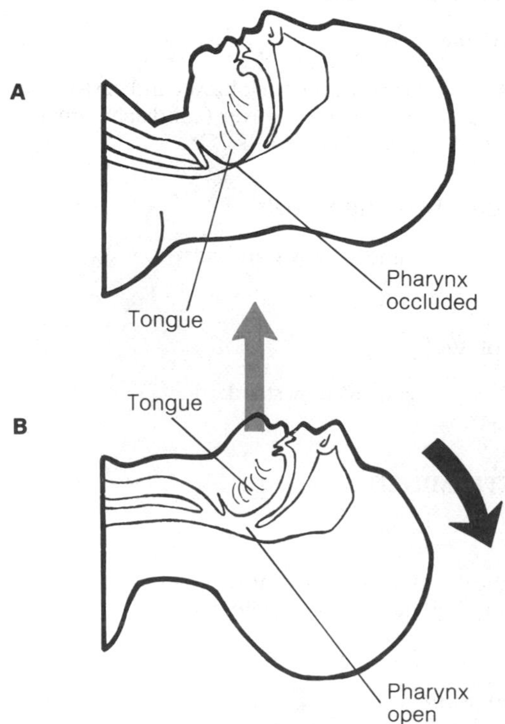

Figure 45–54 The position of an unconscious person's tongue: **A,** pharynx occluded; **B,** pharynx open

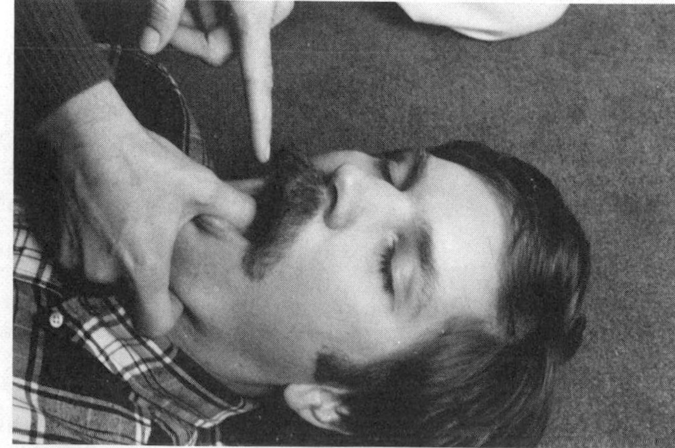

Figure 45–55 Finger sweep to remove an obstruction from the mouth or throat

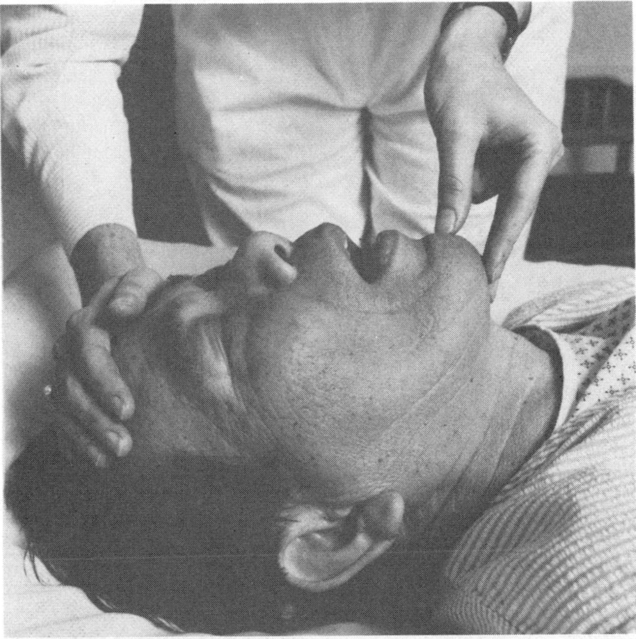

Figure 45–56 The head-tilt/chin-lift maneuver

lift the tongue away from the back of the throat and open the airway. The mouth should *not* be closed completely. Avoid pressing the fingers deeply into the soft tissues under the chin, for too much pressure can obstruct the airway. Remove dentures if they cannot be maintained in place. However, dentures that can be managed in place make a mouth-to-mouth seal easier should rescue breathing be required.

Jaw-thrust maneuver The jaw-thrust, an alternate method of opening the airway, is more difficult to perform but is the safest method when a neck injury is suspected. Grasp the angles of the victim's lower jaw and lift the jaw with both hands (see Figure 45–57). The rescuer's elbows should be resting on the firm surface on which the victim is lying. If the jaw-thrust is not successful, the head may be tilted back slightly.

Breathing

Assess the victim's breathing in 3 to 5 seconds by doing the following.

1. *Observe* the rise and fall of the chest.
2. Listen for air escaping from the nose or mouth during exhalation.
3. Feel for the flow of air against your cheek.

When the victim is trying to breathe but there is no air moving, then the airway may still be obstructed. Ensure that the airway is open. See "Opening the Airway," above. If the victim resumes breathing, continue to help maintain an open airway. If the victim is breathless, mouth-to-mouth rescue breathing must be initiated.

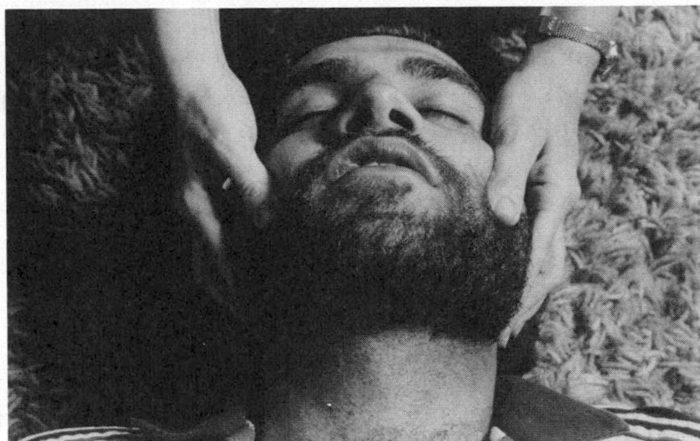

Figure 45–57 The jaw-thrust maneuver

Mouth-to-mouth rescue breathing To perform mouth-to-mouth rescue breathing:

1. Maintain the airway open by using the head-tilt/chin-lift maneuver.
2. Pinch the victim's nose closed by using the thumb and index finger of the hand on the forehead. This prevents air from escaping through the victim's nose during ventilation.
3. Take a deep breath and seal your lips around the outside of the victim's mouth, creating an air-tight seal. See Figure 45–58.

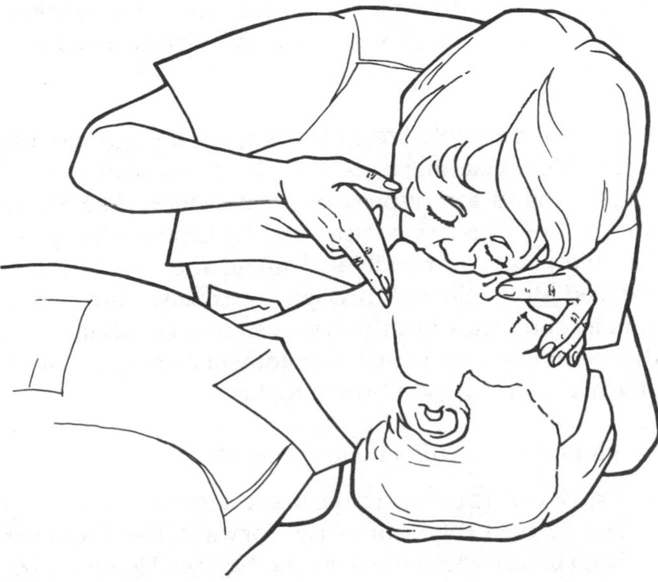

Figure 45–58 Mouth-to-mouth rescue breathing

4. Exhale two full breaths (1 to 1½ seconds per breath). Pause and take a breath after the first ventilation. Breaths lasting 1 to 1½ seconds closely match the victim's inspiratory time, give adequate time for good chest expansion, and decrease the possibility of gastric distention. Excessive air volumes and rapid inspiratory flow rates can cause pharyngeal pressures great enough to open the esophagus, thus allowing air to enter the stomach.

Each ventilation (about 800 ml air) should make the chest rise. Adequate ventilation has been obtained when the chest rises and falls and air can be heard and felt during exhalation.

If the initial ventilation attempt is unsuccessful, reposition the victim's head and repeat the rescue breathing as above. If the victim still cannot be ventilated, proceed to clear the airway of any foreign bodies. See "Foreign-Body Airway Obstruction," later in this chapter.

Mouth-to-nose rescue breathing Mouth-to-nose rescue breathing is performed when it is impossible to ventilate through the victim's mouth, e.g., when the mouth cannot be opened or when the mouth is injured. To perform mouth-to-nose ventilation:

1. Maintain the head-tilt/chin-lift.
2. Close the victim's mouth by pressing the palm of your hand against the victim's chin. The thumb of the same hand may be used to hold the bottom lip closed.
3. Take a deep breath and seal your lips around the victim's nose.
4. Blow into the victim's nose.
5. Remove your mouth from the nose and allow the victim to exhale passively. It may be necessary to separate the victim's lips or to open the mouth for exhaling, since the nasal passages may be obstructed during exhalation.

Hand-compressible breathing bag Many agencies use rubberized breathing bags (e.g., the Ambu bag) attached to face masks for respiratory resuscitation. See Figure 45–59. The bags are compressed by hand to deliver air into the mask and rapidly self-inflate after compression. Exhaled air is released through an exhaust valve to prevent its entry back into the bag. A significant advantage of the breathing bag is that supplemental oxygen can be attached to it. To use a breathing bag:

1. Stand at the victim's head and nose.
2. Use one hand to secure the mask at the top and bottom and to hold the victim's jaw forward. Use the other hand to squeeze and release the bag. See Figure 45–60.
3. Compress the bag until sufficient elevation of the victim's chest is observed. Then release the bag.

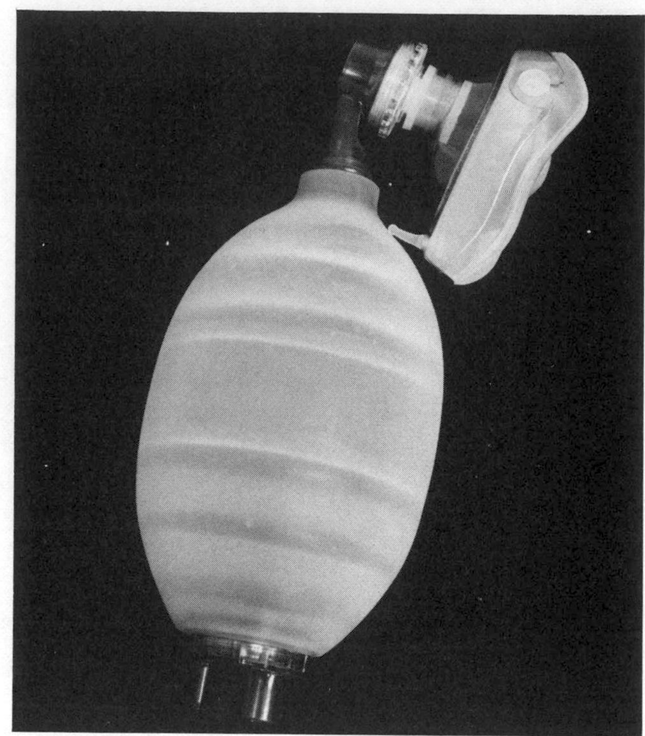

Figure 45–59 An Ambu bag with a face mask

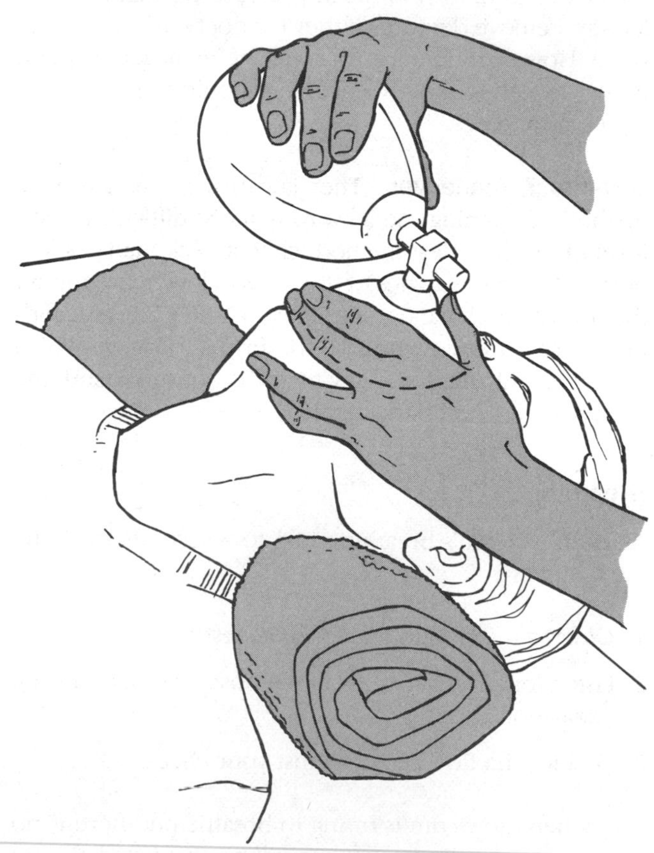

Figure 45–60 An Ambu bag in position

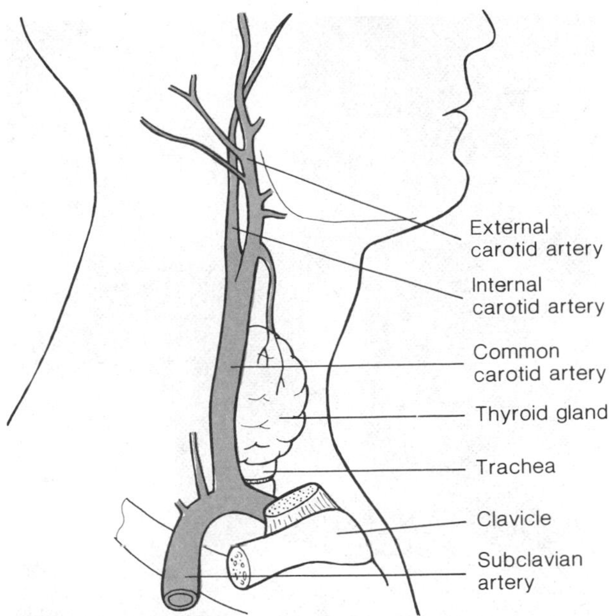

Figure 45–61 Location of the carotid artery

Circulation

To determine pulselessness, which is indicative of cardiac arrest, assess the carotid artery pulse. See Figure 45–61.

1. Maintain the head-tilt by holding one hand on the victim's forehead.
2. Locate the victim's larynx with two or three fingers of the other hand.
3. Slide these fingers into the groove between the trachea and the muscles at the side of the neck. The carotid pulse can be felt at this spot when the area is gently pressed. Gentle pressure avoids compressing the artery. Adequate time is needed for this pulse check (about 5 to 10 seconds), since the victim's pulse may be very weak and rapid, irregular, or slow. The carotid pulse is assessed because it can be palpated when more peripheral pulses cannot.

In hospitals, health care practitioners can use the femoral pulse instead of the carotid pulse. This pulse is difficult to locate on a fully clothed person. See Chapter 34, page 779.

It is essential to accurately assess the victim's pulse, since performing external chest compressions on victims who have a pulse can lead to serious medical complications. If the pulse is present but breathing is absent, rescue breathing should be initiated at a rate of 12 times per minute (every 5 seconds) after the initial two breaths.

If palpation reveals no pulse, then a cardiac arrest is confirmed. The nurse should then have another person call for emergency medical service (EMS). In many communities the emergency telephone number is 911. The person who calls the local EMS should be able to impart all of the following information (American Heart Association 1986, p. 2918):

- Location of the emergency
- Telephone number from which the call is being made
- What happened
- Number of people needing assistance
- Condition of the victim(s)
- What aid is being given
- Any other information that is requested

If no help comes and the rescuer is alone, CPR should be performed for 1 minute and then help summoned again.

External chest compression The external chest compression procedure consists of sequential, rhythmic applications of pressure over the lower half of the sternum. These compressions provide circulation to the lungs, heart, brain, and other organs through increased intrathoracic pressure and/or direct compression of the heart. For effectiveness the victim must be placed supine on a firm surface. Blood flow to the brain will be inadequate during CPR if the victim's head is positioned higher than the thorax. A hard surface facilitates compression of the heart between the sternum and the hard surface. If the victim is in bed in a health care facility, place a cardiac board—preferably the full width of the bed—under his or her back. If necessary, place the victim on the floor. Elevating the lower extremities may promote venous return and augment circulation during external cardiac compressions (American Heart Association 1986, p. 2919).

Hand placement Proper hand placement is essential for effective cardiac compression. Position the hands as follows.

1. With the hand nearest the victim's legs locate the lower margin of the rib cage using the middle and index fingers.
2. Move the fingers up the rib cage to the notch where the ribs meet the sternum. See Figure 45–62.
3. Place the heel of the other hand (nearest the victim's head) along the lower half of the victim's sternum, close to the index finger that is next to the middle finger in the costal-sternal notch.
4. Then place the first hand on top of the second hand so that both hands are parallel. The fingers may be extended or interlaced.

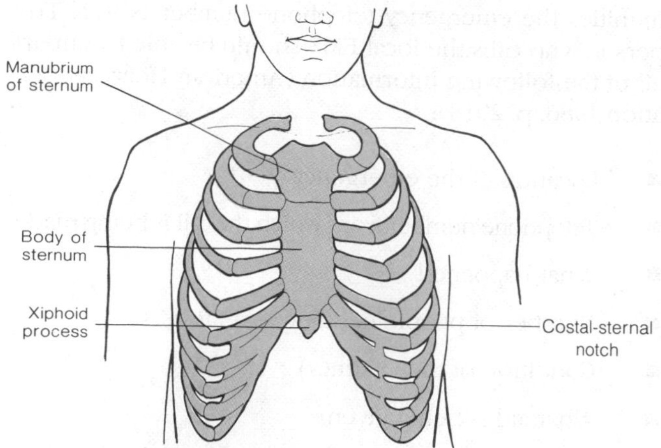

Figure 45–62 The sternum and ribs

Compression technique Effective cardiac compression is achieved as follows (American Heart Association 1986, p. 2921):

1. Lock your elbows into position, straighten your arms, and position your shoulders directly over your hands.
2. For each compression, thrust *straight down* on the sternum (see Figure 45–63) until the sterum is depressed 3.8 to 5.0 cm (1.5 to 2 in) (in the normal-size adult).
3. Completely release the compression pressure, to permit blood to flow into the heart. However, do *not* lift your hands from the chest or change their position, to avoid losing correct hand placement.
4. Provide external cardiac compressions at the rate of 80 to 100 per minute.

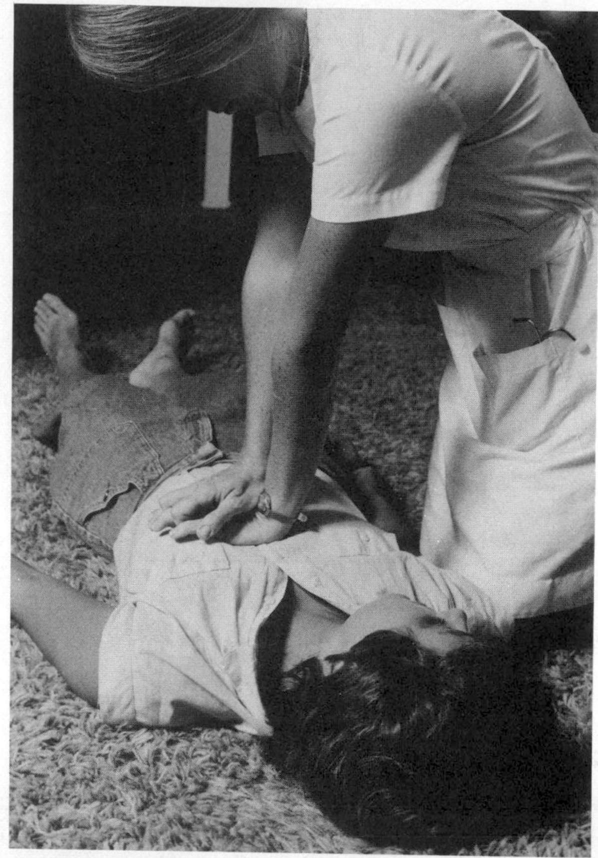

Figure 45–63 Arm and hand position for external cardiac massage

CPR Performed by One Rescuer

Airway

1. Assess responsiveness.
2. Call for help.
3. Position the victim.
4. Open the airway with the head-tilt/chin-lift maneuver.

Breathing If the victim is breathing, then monitor the breathing, maintain an open airway, and call for EMS. If the victim is *not* breathing, then:

5. Perform rescue breathing by giving two initial breaths.
6. If unable to give two breaths, then reposition the head and attempt to ventilate again.
7. If still unsuccessful, remove foreign bodies from the victim's airway. See "Foreign-Body Airway Obstruction," later in this chapter.

Circulation Determine pulselessness as described earlier, using the carotid pulse or, in a health care facility, the femoral pulse.

8. If pulse is present:
   a. Continue rescue breathing at 12 times per minute.
   b. Call for EMS.
9. If pulse is absent:
   a. Call for EMS.
   b. Begin external chest compression.
   c. Perform chest compression: 15 external chest compressions at the rate of 80 to 100 per minute. Count, "One and, two and, three and . . ." up to 15.
   d. Open the airway and give two rescue breaths.
   e. Repeat 15 chest compressions.
   f. Perform four complete cycles of 15 compressions and two ventilations.

Reevaluate the victim

10. Check for the return of the carotid pulse. If it is absent, resume CPR with two ventilations followed by compressions. If the carotid pulse is present, monitor breathing and pulse. If breathing is absent, resume rescue breathing at 12 times per minute, and monitor pulse.
11. If CPR is continued, check for the carotid pulse every few minutes, but do *not* interrupt CPR for more than 7 seconds.

CPR Performed by Two Rescuers

The AHA recommends that all health care practitioners learn one-rescuer and two-rescuer techniques. One rescuer is positioned at the victim's side and performs external chest compression. The second rescuer remains at the victim's head to maintain an open airway, monitor the carotid pulse, and provide rescue breathing.

The compression rate for two-rescuer CPR is 80 to 100 per minute. The compression:ventilation ratio is 5:1, with a pause for ventilation (1 to 1½ seconds). When the person compressing the chest becomes fatigued, positions should be exchanged.

Terminating CPR

A rescuer terminates CPR only when one of the following events occurs:

1. Another person takes over.
2. The victim's heartbeat and breathing are reestablished.
3. Adjunctive life-support measures are initiated.
4. A physician states that the individual is dead and that CPR is to be discontinued.
5. The rescuer becomes exhausted and there is no one to take over.

CPR in a Hospital

Most acute care health agencies have established practices and policies governing cardiopulmonary resuscitation. Nurses need to learn immediately the following information:

1. The agency procedure for external cardiac massage
2. Where the emergency equipment is kept
3. The agency's method of notification of a cardiac arrest
4. The advised compression rates for adults, children, and infants

Practices commonly include the following.

1. The person who discovers a client who has had a cardiac arrest is responsible for obtaining assistance. The nurse may simply call out to others or may telephone the hospital switchboard. The person then starts CPR immediately.
2. Many hospitals have a special team that answers the call (the crash team). The team usually consists of physicians and nurses who have had special training in CPR. The team will have a crash cart stocked with the special supplies and equipment required for CPR.
3. Hospitals with a loudspeaker system to summon the special team ordinarily use a code to notify the staff without alarming visitors and clients. Some agencies use a number, such as "99"; others use a color, such as "blue." The announcement may be "Code blue, West 8" or "Doctor 99, West 8" to tell the members of the team that the cardiac arrest is on the eighth floor of the west wing.
4. When the special team arrives, it takes over the care of the client. The nursing staff may stay to assist or continue with other nursing responsibilities, depend ing on the agency's policies.
5. If external cardiac compression does not produce a heartbeat, the physician may decide to defibrillate the client. There are many types of defibrillators; most function by passing an electric current through the client's heart to establish normal cardiac rhythm. The two paddles of the defibrillator are lubricated and then placed on the client's chest: one to the right of the sternum, the other near the apex of the heart along the left axillary line. The axillary line extends inferiorly from the anterior axillary fold. Before the current is activated, all persons stand away from the client so as not to receive the electric current from the client. The effectiveness of the defibrillation can be determined by checking the carotid pulse, the movement of the pupils of the eyes, and the return of respirations.

Foreign-Body Airway Obstruction

There are several possible causes of upper airway obstruction and, as a result, different ways of clearing an obstructed airway. Causes include:

1. Aspirated food, mucus plug, or foreign bodies, such as partial dentures or small toys. Food is the most common cause.
2. Unconsciousness or seizures, which cause the tongue to fall back and block the airway.

3. Severe trauma to the nose, mouth, or neck that produce blood clots that obstruct the airway, especially in unconscious victims.
4. Acute edema of the trachea, from smoke inhalation, facial and neck burns, or anaphylaxis. In these instances, a tracheostomy is often indicated.

Food is the most common cause of choking, particularly meat that has been poorly chewed.

Foreign bodies may cause either partial or complete airway obstruction. When an airway is partially obstructed, the victim may have either good or poor air exchange. If she or he is able to obtain sufficient air, even if wheezing frequently between coughs, do *not* interfere with his or her attempts to expel the foreign object. If the partial obstruction remains, then call for EMS. Partial obstructions with poor air exchange are dealt with as if they were complete obstructions.

The victim with complete airway obstruction is unable to speak, breathe, or cough and may clutch at her or his neck. The **Heimlich maneuver** (subdiaphragmatic abdominal thrusts) is recommended to relieve the obstruction. By elevating the diaphragm, this maneuver forces air from the lungs, creating an artificial cough to expel the obstruction. To clear the airway, it may be necessary to perform the Heimlich maneuver six to ten times. It can be performed when the victim is conscious and standing or sitting or when the victim is unconscious and lying flat.

Heimlich Maneuver (Victim Standing or Sitting)

To perform the Heimlich maneuver on a conscious person who is standing or sitting:

1. Stand behind the person and wrap your arms around his or her waist.
2. Make a fist with one hand, tuck the thumb inside the fist, and place the flexed thumb against the person's epigastrium, i.e., below the xiphoid process. A protruding thumb could inflict injury.
3. With your other hand, grasp the fist (see Figure 45–64) and press it into the person's abdomen with a firm, quick upward thrust (see Figure 45–65). Avoid tightening your arms around the rib cage, and thrust in the direction of your chin. Deliver one quick thrust.
4. Deliver successive thrusts as separate and complete movements.

Heimlich Maneuver (Victim Lying Flat)

To perform the Heimlich maneuver on an unconscious person who is lying on the ground:

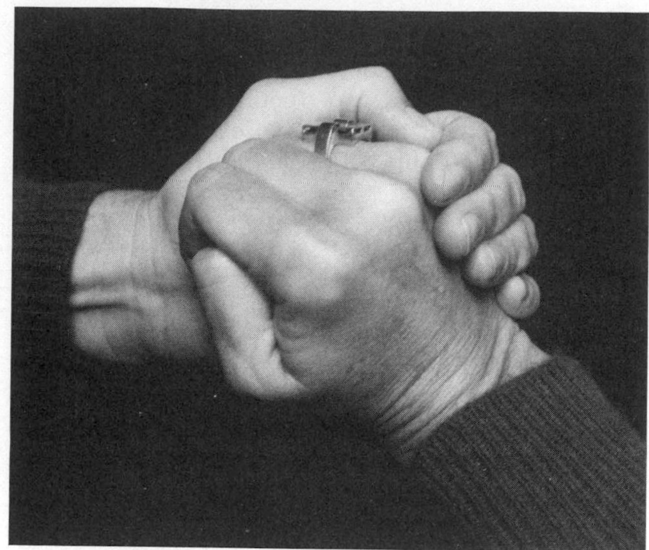

Figure 45–64 Making a fist for the Heimlich maneuver

1. Place the person supine, and kneel, preferably astride or to the side of the person's thighs.
2. Place the heel of one hand slightly above the person's navel and well below the tip of the xiphoid process, i.e., in the epigastric area.
3. Place your other hand directly on top of the first. Make sure your shoulders are over the person's abdomen and your elbows are straight.

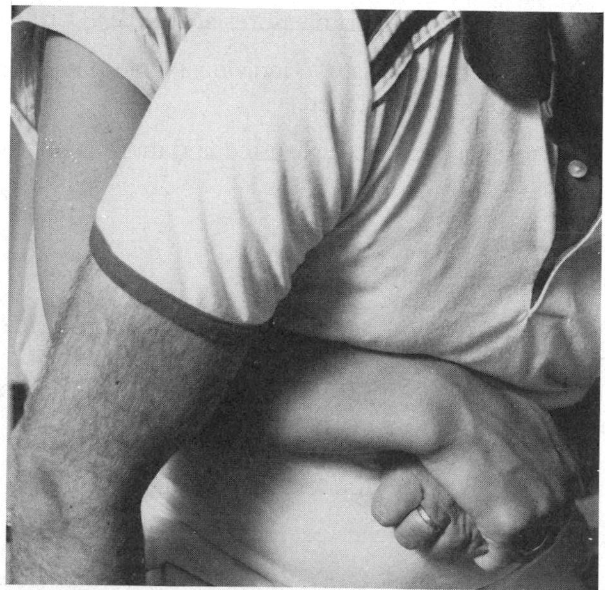

Figure 45–65 Arm position for the Heimlich maneuver

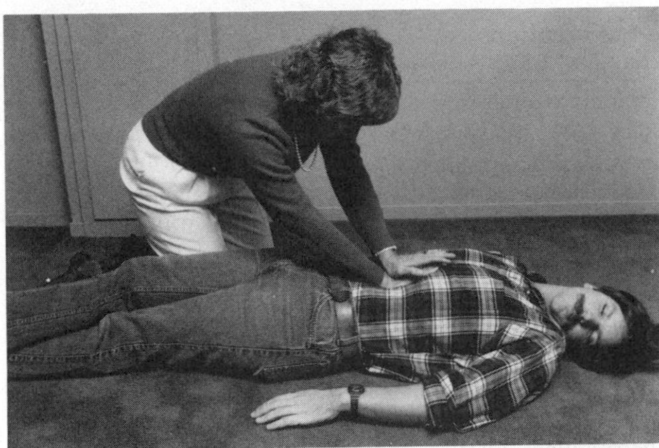

Figure 45–66 Position for the Heimlich maneuver when the victim is lying down

4. Press the heel of the first hand into the abdomen with a quick upward thrust. See Figure 45–66. Be sure to direct the thrust in the midline of the abdomen, not to the left or right. The weight of your shoulders and trunk supplies power for the thrust.

Chest Thrusts (Victim Standing or Sitting)

Chest thrusts are administered only to women in advanced stages of pregnancy or markedly obese persons who cannot receive the Heimlich maneuver. To administer chest thrusts:

1. Stand behind the person, with your arms under the person's armpits and encircling the person's chest.
2. Place the thumb side of your fist on the *middle* of the breast bone, *not* on the xiphoid process.
3. Grab your other fist and deliver a quick backward thrust.
4. Repeat thrusts until the obstruction is relieved.

Chest Thrusts (Victim Lying Flat)

Chest thrusts to an unconscious person lying on the ground are administered only to women in advanced stages of pregnancy or markedly obese persons. To administer this maneuver:

1. Position the person supine, and kneel close beside the person's trunk.
2. Position your hands as for cardiac compression, with the heel of the hand on the lower half of the sternum.
3. Administer downward thrusts, each one slowly and distinctly.

Finger Sweep

The finger sweep should be used only on unconscious persons. See "Digital Removal of Foreign Material," earlier in this chapter, p. 1332.

Nursing Care Plan

Assessment Data

Nursing Assessment

Miss Mary Ellen Martin is a 19-year-old secretary who was admitted to the hospital yesterday with an elevated temperature, a productive cough, and rapid, labored respirations. In taking a nursing history, Miss Helen Hayes finds that Miss Martin had a "bad cold" for several weeks that just wouldn't go away. She has been dieting for several months and skipping meals in order to decrease her caloric intake. Miss Martin mentions that in addition to her full-time job as a secretary, she is attending college classes 2 evenings a week and a dance class on Saturdays. Miss Martin, who is a smoker, states she has been unable to smoke for several days because of her cough and cold.

Physical Examination

Height: 167.6 cm (5′6″)
Weight: 54.4 kg (120 lb)
Temperature: 39.4 C (103 F)
Pulse rate: 28 BPM
Blood pressure: 118/70 mm Hg
Skin pale, cheeks flushed, chills
Nasal flaring
Use of accessory muscles
Inspiratory rales with diminished breath sounds right base

Diagnostic Data

Chest x-ray film: R lobar infiltration
WBC: 14,000

Nursing Diagnosis	Client Goals and Outcome Criteria	Nursing Interventions and Rationales	Evaluation
Ineffective airway clearance related to thick sputum/pneumonia resulting in frequent productive cough, rapid respirations, nasal flaring, adventitious breath sounds, stabbing chest pain.	Client Goal: Normal breath sounds in right lung. Outcome Criteria: Coughs and deep breathes q1 hr within first 24 hrs. Ineffective coughing is eliminated by day 2. Expectorates secretions from airway whenever necessary. Increases fluid intake to 3000 ml to liquefy secretions by day 2.	Assess respirations and respiratory movements. *Rationale:* Aids in determining whether ventilation is adequate. Encourage coughing and deep breathing q1h. *Rationale:* Coughing in conjunction with deep breathing facilitates the movements and expectoration of respiratory tract secretions. Demonstrate effective coughing while splinting client's chest. *Rationale:* Ineffective coughing is tiring and will exhaust the client. Encourage fluid intake of 3000 ml/day. *Rationale:* Hydration will aid in liquefying thick, tenacious secretions and make them easier to expectorate as well as to replace fluid loss due to fever. Position client in semi-Fowler's or high Fowler's position. *Rationale:* Encourages maximum chest expansion. Assist with postural drainage 3 times daily. *Rationale:* Postural drainage will drain secretions from lung segments into tracheobronchial tree, from where they can be removed. Assist with IPPB and/or nebulizer treatments. *Rationale:* Facilitates the clearing of bronchial secretions by thinning secretions.	Miss Martin coughs and deep breathes purposefully q1–2 hrs during the day. While coughing, she splints her chest with her hands or a pillow. She coughs forcefully after taking a deep breath, using her abdominal and accessory respiratory muscles. Her fluid intake is approximately 3000 ml each day. Cough continues to be productive of moderately thick, rusty sputum. Inspiratory rales still present in right lung. Adventitious breath sounds still audible at base of right lung.
Impaired gas exchange related to accumulation of secretions in airways resulting in dyspnea, tachypnea, pallor, tachycardia, decreased activity tolerance, decreased PaO_2.	Client Goal: Increase O_2 and CO_2 exchange. Increase activity tolerance without experiencing dyspnea and chest pain. Outcome Criteria: Relief of symptoms of chest pain, tachypnea, dyspnea by day 5. Improved activity tolerance by day 5. Improved Pao_2 by day 2.	Assess respiratory status and vital signs. *Rationale:* Vital signs and respiratory status will indicate adequacy of ventilation. Maintain oxygen 30% per nasal cannula at 5 liters. *Rationale:* Additional oxygen will reduce hypoxemia. Maintain bedrest and assist with ADLs. *Rationale:* Rest decreases metabolic rate and oxygen demand by tissues, thereby decreasing dyspnea. Monitor arterial blood gases. *Rationale:* Indicates adequacy of ventilation and perfusion.	On day 5, Miss Martin is able to sit at the beside 4 × daily without chest pain and dyspnea. Her respirations are 22 per minute. She is assisting with her bedbath. Her Pao_2 is 85 mm Hg.

Chapter Highlights

- The cells of the body tissues require oxygen.
- The alveolar membrane of the lungs serves as site for the exchange of oxygen and carbon dioxide between the alveoli and the bloodstream.
- Compliance is the ability of the lungs to expand.
- Elastic recoil is the tendency of the lungs to collapse away from the chest wall.
- Most oxygen is transported to the body tissues as oxyhemoglobin.
- Inspiration (inhalation) is an active process, and expiration (exhalation) is a passive process.
- Three relatively common problems of oxygenation are hypoxia, abnormal respiratory patterns, and obstructed airway.
- Planning for a client with oxygenation problems includes dependent and independent nursing strategies.
- Positioning and hydration are important in maintaining oxygenation.
- Cardiac or respiratory arrest is an emergency requiring immediate action.

Suggested Readings

Foley, M.; Tomashefski, J.; and Underwood, E., Jr. September 1977. Pulmonary function screening tests in industry. *American Journal of Nursing* 77:1480–84.
Screening tests help detect early signs of pulmonary disease. However, individual variations need to be considered in calculating the test results. The tests are reviewed, and the steps are given for interpreting results.

Sandham, G., and Reid, B. October 1977. Some Q's and A's about suctioning, with an illustrated guide to better techniques. *Nursing 77* 7:60–65.
A series of questions and answers about suctioning equipment, preparation for suctioning, and suctioning. Photographs illustrate the steps.

Waterson, M. March 1978. Teaching your patients postural drainage. *Nursing 78* 8:51–53.
This article includes a client teaching aid showing six commonly prescribed positions. Client reminders are outlined in a Do-and-Don't format.

Wimsatt, R. November 1985. Unlocking the mysteries behind the chest wall. *Nursing 83* 15:58–63.
Wimsatt describes the importance of oxygenation and what to observe about a client. The techniques of chest palpation, percussion and auscultation are explained. Adventitious breath sounds are described, as well as a respiratory distress syndrome that requires an immediate nursing response.

Selected References

Acee, S. July/August 1984. Helping patients breathe more easily. *Geriatric Nursing* 5:230–33.

Administering oxygen safely. October 1980. When, why, how. *Nursing 80* 10:54–56.

D'Agostino, J. S. July 1983. Set your mind at ease on oxygen toxicity. *Nursing 83* 13:54–56.

Albanese, A. J., et al. April 1982. A hassle-free guide to suctioning a tracheostomy. *RN* 45:24–29.

American Heart Association. 1986. Standards and guidelines for cardiopulmonary resuscitation (CPR) and emergency cardiac care (ECC). *Journal of the American Medical Association* 255:2841–3044.

Bellack, J. P., and Bamford, P. A. 1984. Nursing assessment: A multidimensional approach. Monterey, Calif.: Wadsworth Health Sciences Div.

Brown, I. May 1982. Trach care? Take care—infection's on the prowl. *Nursing 82* 12:44–49.

Byrne, C. J.; Saxton, D. F.; Pelikan, P. K.; and Nugent, P. M. 1986. *Laboratory tests: Implications for nursing care.* 2d ed. Menlo Park, Calif.: Addison-Wesley Publishing Co.

Carroll, P. F. January 1985. Action stat dislodged trach tube. *Nursing 85* 15:46.

Dalrymple, D. June 1984. Setting up for thoracic drainage. *Nursing 84* 14:12–14.

Ellmyer, P., and Thomas, N. J. January 1982. A guide to your patient's safe home use of oxygen. *Nursing 82* 12:56–57.

Flatter, P. A. January 1968. Hazards of oxygen therapy. *American Journal of Nursing* 68:80–84.

Foss, G. April 1973. Postural drainage. *American Journal of Nursing* 73:666–69.

Fuchs, P. I. July 1984. Streamlining your suctioning techniques, part 3: Tracheostomy suctioning. *Nursing 84* 14:39–43.

———. May 1984. Streamlining your suctioning techniques, part I: Nasotracheal suctioning. *Nursing 84* 14:55–61.

Fuchs, P. L. Nebulizers. 1983a. *The nurse's reference library: Procedures.* Nursing 83 Books, Intermed Communications. pp. 462–66.

———. Humidifiers. 1983b. *The nurse's reference library: Procedures.* Nursing 83 Books, Intermed Communications, pp. 458–62.

———. December 1980. Getting the best out of oxygen delivery systems. *Nursing 80* 10:34–43.

———. December 1979. Understanding continuous mechanical ventilation. *Nursing 79* 9:26–33.

Guyton, A. C. 1986. *Textbook of medical physiology.* 7th ed. Philadelphia: W. B. Saunders Co.

LeFort, S. February 1978. Cardiopulmonary resuscitation (CPR): Step-by-step. *Canadian Nurse* 74:38–47.

Luce, J. M.; Tyler, M. L.; and Pierson, D. J. 1984. *Intensive respiratory care.* Philadelphia: W. B. Saunders Co.

McIntyre, K. M., and Lewis, A. J. (editors). 1983. *Textbook of advanced cardiac life support.* American Heart Association.

Manzi, C. C. March 1978. Cardiac emergency! How to use drugs and C.P.R. to save lives. *Nursing 78* 8:30–39.

Mason, T. N. November/December 1982. A hand ventilation technique for neonates. *American Journal of Maternal Child Nursing* 7(6):366–69.

Nielsen, L. December 1980. Mechanical ventilation: Patient assessment and nursing care. *American Journal of Nursing* 80:2191–217.

Nursing 80 Photobook Series. 1980. *Dealing with emergencies.* Intermed Communications.

Nursing 80 Photobook Series. 1979. *Providing respiratory care.* Intermed Communications.

Nussbaum, G. B., and Fisher, J. C. January 1978. A crash cart that works. *American Journal of Nursing* 78:45–48.

O'Donnell, B. March 1978. How to change tracheostomy ties—easily and safely. *Nursing 78* 8:66–69.

Promisloff, R. A. October 1980. Administering oxygen safely: When, why, how. *Nursing 80* 10:54–56.

Rifas, E. M. June 1980. How you—and your patient—can manage dyspnea. *Nursing 80* 10:34–41.

Ryan, M. A. August 1974. Helping the family cope with cardiac arrest. *Nursing 74* 4:80–81.

Sandham, G., and Reid, B. October 1977. Some Q's and A's about suctioning, with an illustrated guide to better techniques. *Nursing 77* 7:60–65.

Sumner, S. M., and Gran, P. E. July 1982. Emergency! First aid for choking. *Nursing 82* 12:40–49.

Teaching your patient to live with C.O.P.D. May/June 1985. *Nursing Life* 5:31–32.

Techniques of cardiopulmonary resuscitation in infants. February 1978. *American Journal of Nursing* 78:265.

VanMeter, M. March 1981. Keeping cool in a code. *RN* 44:29–35.

Ventilators and how they work. December 1980. *American Journal of Nursing* 80:2202–5.

Vick, R. L. 1984. *Contemporary medical physiology.* Menlo Park, Calif.: Addison-Wesley Publishing Co.

Wade, J. F. 1981. *Respiratory nursing care physiology and technique.* 3d ed. St. Louis: C. V. Mosby Co.

Waldron, M. W. February 1979. Oxygen transport. *American Journal of Nursing* 79:272–75.

Waterson, M. (consultant). March 1978. Teaching your patients postural drainage. *Nursing 78* 8:51–53.

Weaver, T. May 1985. Chronic ineffective gas exchange when your patient goes from bad to worse. *Nursing 85* 15:7.

Weaver, T. E. February 1981. New life for lungs through incentive spirometers. *Nursing 81* 11:54–58.

Winslow, E. H.; Lane, L. D.; and Gaffney, F. A. May/June 1985. Oxygen uptake and cardiovascular responses in control adults and acute myocardial infarction patients during bathing. *Nursing Research* 34(3):164–69.

Worthington, L. May 1980. Hypoxemia. *RN* 43:48–53.

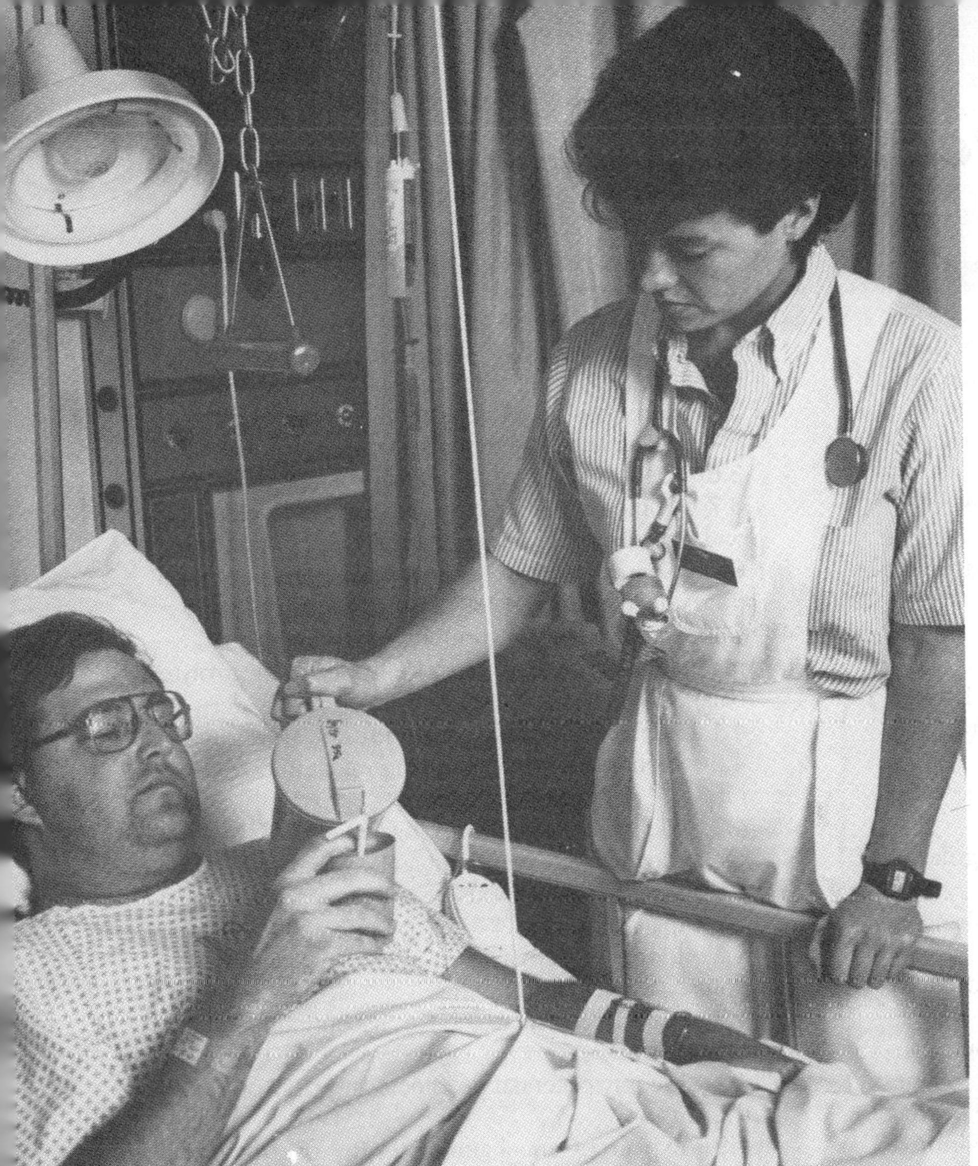
KAREN STAFFORD RANTZMAN

CHAPTER **46**

Fluid and Electrolytes

Contents

46 *Fluid and Electrolytes*

Objectives

1. Know essential terms and facts about body fluid and fluid, electrolyte, and acid-base balance.
   1.1 Define selected terms.
   1.2 Describe factors affecting the proportion of body weight that is fluid.
   1.3 Name the body's fluid compartments.
   1.4 Identify major constituents (electrolytes) of intracellular and extracellular fluid compartments and body secretions.
   1.5 Describe ways in which fluids and electrolytes move through the body.
   1.6 Identify ways in which osmotic and hydrostatic pressures influence movement of fluid through membranes.
   1.7 Identify mechanisms that regulate the body's fluid and electrolyte volume.
   1.8 Describe how these mechanisms regulate fluid and electrolyte balance.
   1.9 Identify the role of the kidneys and lungs in regulating acid-base balance.
   1.10 Identify three major sources of body fluid.
   1.11 Identify sources of fluid output.
   1.12 Identify normal fluid intakes and outputs.
2. Know information and methods required to assess a person's fluid, electroltye, and acid-base balance.
   2.1 Identify essential information to obtain in a health history.
   2.2 Identify ways in which selected factors influence fluid and electrolyte balance.
   2.3 Describe clinical signs of the well-hydrated person.
   2.4 Identify essential steps in measuring a person's fluid intake and output.
   2.5 Identify essential diagnostic tests and their significance.
3. Understand essential facts about fluid, electrolyte, and acid-base imbalances.
   3.1 Identify the types of fluid imbalances.
   3.2 Identify causes of extracellular deficits and excesses.
   3.3 Contrast clinical signs and laboratory findings of all types of fluid imbalances.
   3.4 Identify causes of specific electrolyte deficits and excesses.
   3.5 Identify clinical signs and laboratory findings of specific electrolyte imbalances.
   3.6 Identify four acid-base disturbances.
   3.7 Compare respiratory acidosis and alkalosis with metabolic acidosis and alkalosis.
   3.8 Give examples of nursing diagnoses related to fluid, electrolyte, and acid-base imbalances.
4. Understand facts about nursing interventions to maintain, promote, and restore fluid and electrolyte balance.
   4.1 Explain how to calculate infusion flow rates.
   4.2 Identify factors influencing infusion flow rates.
   4.3 Identify common sites for venipuncture.
   4.4 Identify four main human blood groups.
   4.5 Explain why various blood groups are incompatible.
   4.6 Identify essential steps in changing intravenous containers and tubing.
   4.7 Identify essential steps in discontinuing an IV infusion.
   4.8 Identify potential problems and risks of blood transfusions.
   4.9 Explain essential guidelines for assisting with blood transfusions.
   4.10 Explain essential nursing responsibilities associated with monitoring TPN.
5. Apply the nursing process when providing care to selected clients with actual or potential fluid and electrolyte problems.
   5.1 Obtain necessary assessment data.
   5.2 Analyze and relate assessment data.
   5.3 Write relevant nursing diagnoses.
   5.4 Plan appropriate nursing strategies.
   5.5 Implement appropriate nursing interventions.
   5.6 State outcome criteria essential for evaluating the client's progress.

Terms

acidosis (acidemia)
active transport
agglutination
agglutinins
agglutinogen
alkalosis (alkalemia)
anasarca
anion
anuria
blood transfusion
cation
circulatory overload
colloids
crystalloids
dehydration
dialyzing membrane
diaphoresis
diffusion
drop (drip) factor
edema

electrolyte
excretion
extracellular fluid (ECF)
exudate
hemolysis
hydrostatic pressure (filtration force)
hyperalimentation
hypercalcemia
hyperchloremia
hyperkalemia
hypermagnesemia
hypernatremia
hypertonic
hypervolemia
hypocalcemia
hypochloremia
hypodermoclysis
hypokalemia
hypomagnesemia
hyponatremia
hypotonic
hypovolemia
insensible fluid loss
interstitial fluid
intracellular (cellular) fluid (ICF)
intravascular fluid (plasma)
ion
isotonic
Kussmaul breathing
milliequivalent
obligatory loss
oliguria
osmolarity (osmolality)
osmosis
osmotic pressure
overhydration
parenteral
pH
phlebitis
pitting edema
Rh factor
secretion
sodium-potassium pump
solute
solvent
tetany
thrombophlebitis
total parenteral nutrition (TPN)
universal donor
universal recipient

Distribution of Body Fluid

Fluids and electrolytes are necessary to maintain good health, and their relative amounts in the body must be maintained within a narrow range. The balance of fluids and electrolytes in the body is a part of physiologic homeostasis. See Chapter 17.

A great deal has been learned about the roles of fluids and electrolytes in both health and disease. This delicate balance is maintained in health by the body's physiologic processes. Almost every illness, however, threatens the balance. Even in normal daily living, excessive temperatures or excessive activity can disturb the balance if adequate water or salt intake is not maintained. Some therapeutic measures for clients, such as the use of diuretics, can also disturb the body's homeostasis unless water and electrolytes are replaced.

The body's fluid is divided into two major reservoirs, intracellular and extracellular. The **intracellular fluid (ICF)**, also referred to as the **cellular fluid**, is found within the cells of the body. It comprises two-thirds to three-quarters of the total body fluid. The **extracellular fluid (ECF)** is found outside the cells; it is subdivided into two compartments, **intravascular** (plasma) and **interstitial. Plasma** is fluid found within the vascular system; **interstitial fluid** is fluid that surrounds the cells, and it includes lymph. Extracellular fluids comprise one-third to one-fourth of the total body fluid.

Extracellular fluid is in constant motion throughout the body. Although it is the smaller of the two compartments, it is the transport system that carries nutrients to and waste products from the cells. Plasma carries oxygen from the lungs and glucose from the gastrointestinal tract, for example, to the capillaries of the vascular system. From there, the oxygen and glucose move across the capillary membranes into the interstitial spaces and then across the cellular membranes into the cells. The opposite route is taken for waste products, such as carbon dioxide going from the cells to the lungs and metabolic acid wastes going eventually to the kidneys. Interstitial fluid transports wastes from the cells by way of the lymph system as well as directly into the blood plasma through capillaries. Lymph circulation ultimately enters the vascular circulation through the thoracic duct into the venous system.

Interstitial fluid comprises three-quarters of extracellular fluid. Normal body functioning requires that the volume of each fluid compartment remain relatively constant. Regulating mechanisms are discussed later in this chapter.

Secretions and excretions are also part of the body's total fluid volume and serve essential functions. They are part of the extracellular fluid. A **secretion** is the product of a gland, for example, the salivary glands. Examples are cerebrospinal fluid, synovial fluid, pericardial fluid, and alimentary secretions. An **excretion** is waste produced by the cells of the body. Just as balances exist between cellular and extracellular compartments, special balances exist between plasma and secretions and excretions. Alimentary secretions for an adult, for example, are estimated to be about 6700 ml per day. See Table 46–1.

Table 46–1 Secretions of the Adult Alimentary Tract

Secretion	Volume (ml/day)
Saliva	1000
Gastric secretion	1500
Pancreatic secretion	1000
Bile	1000
Small-intestine secretion	1800
Brunner's gland secretion	200
Large-intestine secretion	200
Total	6700

Source: Adapted from A. C. Guyton, *Textbook of medical physiology,* 7th ed. (Philadelphia: W. B. Saunders Co., 1986), p. 772.

Proportions of Body Fluid

The proportion of the human body composed of fluid is surprisingly large, considering that the external appearance suggests mostly solid tissue such as muscle and bone. Fluid comprises about 57% of the average healthy adult man's weight. In health, this volume (about 40 liters) of body fluid remains relatively constant. In fact, a healthy person's weight varies less than 0.2 kg (0.5 lb) in 24 hours, regardless of the amount of fluid ingested. Some diseases cause serious excesses or deficiencies of body fluid. For example, a client with heart failure can retain fluid in the tissues and may suffer a fluid excess. A person with kidney disease may not be able to excrete the required amount of urine and also suffer a fluid excess. Another person with a mouth injury may not be able to drink and may suffer a fluid loss.

The percentage of total body fluid varies according to the individual's age, body fat, and sex. See Table 46–2. Infants have the highest proportion of fluid; as people grow older, the proportion decreases. Body fat is essentially free of fluid; therefore, the amount of fat a person has alters the proportion of body fluid to body weight. In other words, the less body fat present, the greater the proportion of body fluid. For example, a thin man's body may be 70% fluid, whereas an obese man's may be only 55%. This variable, body fat, also accounts for the difference in total body fluid between the sexes. After adolescence, women have proportionately more fat than men. Thus, they have a smaller percentage of fluid in relation to total body weight than do men.

Large volumes of fluid also carry dissolved waste materials through the kidneys and through the gastrointestinal tract. However, in both instances, most of this fluid is reabsorbed into the vascular spaces and reused by the body. For example, of 6700 ml produced in the alimentary tract, only 100 ml is usually excreted in the feces, just enough to keep the feces lubricated. Of 180 liters of glomerular filtrate that filters through the kidneys per day, only 1.4 liters are excreted from the body under normal conditions. See Table 46–3.

Nurses need to be aware of abnormal amounts of secretions and excretions. Excessive losses can seriously deplete first the extracellular fluid volume and then the intracellular fluid volume. Excessive or inadequate secretions interfere with a number of body processes, e.g., digestion and elimination.

Table 46–2 Fluid Percentage of Body Weight, by Age

Developmental Stage	Percentage of Water
Newborn infant	75
Adult male	57
Adult female	55
Elderly adult	45 (approx.)

Note: As age increases, proportion of body water decreases.

Table 46–3 Average Daily Fluid Output for an Adult

Route	Amount at Normal Temperature (ml)
Urine	1400
Insensible losses:	
Lungs	350
Skin	350
Sweat	100
Feces	100
Total	2300

Source: Adapted from A. C. Guyton, *Textbook of medical physiology,* 7th ed. (Philadelphia: W. B. Saunders Co., 1986), p. 383.

Body Electrolytes

Extracellular and intracellular fluids are similar in their content of electrolytes and other substances. These fluids contain oxygen from the lungs; dissolved nutrients, from the gastrointestinal tract; excretory products of metabolism, of which carbon dioxide is the most abundant; and particles called **ions**.

Many salts dissociate in water, i.e., break up into electrically charged ions. The salt sodium chloride breaks up into one ion of sodium (Na^+) and one ion of chloride (Cl^-). These charged particles are called **electrolytes** because they are capable of conducting electricity. Ions that carry a positive charge are called **cations**, and ions carrying a negative charge are called **anions**. Examples of cations are sodium (Na^+), potassium (K^+), calcium (Ca^{2+}), and magnesium (Mg^{2+}). Anions include chloride (Cl^-), bicarbonate (HCO_3^-), monohydrogen phosphate (HPO_4^{2-}), and sulfate (SO_4^{2-}).

Electrolyte Composition of Body Fluids

The electrolyte composition of fluids varies from one compartment to another. Principal ions of extracellular fluid are sodium and chloride; principal ions of cellular fluid are potassium and phosphate. See Figure 46–1. The ion composition of the two extracellular fluid reservoirs (intravascular and interstitial) is similar; the main difference is that intravascular fluid (plasma) has a greater quantity of protein than interstitial fluid does. This is because large particles of protein have difficulty passing through the vascular (capillary) membranes into the interstitial fluid. All other electrolytes move readily between these two extracellular compartments.

The higher quantity of protein in plasma plays a significant role in maintaining the intravascular fluid volume and blood pressure. When quantities of plasma protein are low in the body, the blood volume diminishes noticeably and results in a state of hypotension (low blood pressure). This is particularly manifest in people with diseases of the liver (the source of body plasma proteins), who are unable to produce sufficient quantities of plasma proteins.

Just as fluid volumes must be maintained within compartments, so must the electrolyte composition of the various compartments. Balances of electrolytes are maintained in proportion to the quantities of fluid in the compartments. Although the specific numbers of cations and anions may differ in the fluid compartments, in a state of homeostasis the total number of cations equals the number of anions within each compartment.

Body secretions and excretions also contain electrolytes. This is of particular concern when excretions are abnormally increased or decreased or when a secretion is lost from the body (for example, when gastric suction removes the gastric secretions). Fluid and electrolyte imbalance can result from prolonged loss through these routes. See Table 46–4 for the electrolyte composition of body secretions and excretions.

Measurement of Electrolytes

Electrolytes are measured in milliequivalents per liter of water (mEq/liter) or milligrams per 100 milliliters (mg/100 ml). The term **milliequivalent** means one thousandth of an equivalent; equivalent refers to the *chemical combining power* of a substance, or the power of cations to unite with anions to form molecules. This chemical combining activity is measured in relation to the chemical combining activity of the hydrogen ion (H^+). Sodium and chloride ions are equivalent, since they combine equally: 1 mEq of Na^+ equals 1 mEq of Cl^-. However, these cations and anions are not equal in weight: 1 mg of Na^+ does not equal 1 mg of Cl^-; rather, 3 mg of Na^+ equals 2 mg of Cl^-.

Clinically, the milliequivalent system is commonly used. However, nurses need to be aware of the different systems of measurement when interpreting laboratory results. It is also important to realize that a laboratory examination usually indicates the findings of blood plasma, since intracellular fluid is not easily accessible for examination. Examination of extracellular fluid (plasma) can frequently reflect the state of the intracellular fluid, though not always precisely.

Movement of Body Fluid and Electrolytes

Movement of fluid and transport of substances occur in three phases. First, blood plasma moves around the body within the circulatory system, and nutrients and fluids are picked up from the lungs and the gastrointestinal tract. Second, interstitial fluid and its components move between the blood capillaries and the cells. Third, fluid and substances then move from the interstitial fluid into the cells. In the reverse direction, fluid and its components move back from the cells to the interstitial spaces and then to the intravascular compartment. The intravascular fluid then flows to the kidneys, where the metabolic by-products of the cells are excreted.

Table 46–4 Electrolyte Composition of Secretions and Excretions Compared to Plasma

	Electrolyte (mEq/L)			
Substance	**Sodium (Na^+)**	**Potassium (K^+)**	**Chloride (Cl^-)**	**Bicarbonate (HCO_3^-)**
Plasma	135–145	3.6–5.0	95–108	21–28
Gastric secretions	70	5+	140	5
Pancreatic juice	140+	5	35	115+
Hepatic duct bile	140+	5	100+	40
Jejunal secretions	140	5	135	30
Perspiration	80	5	85	—

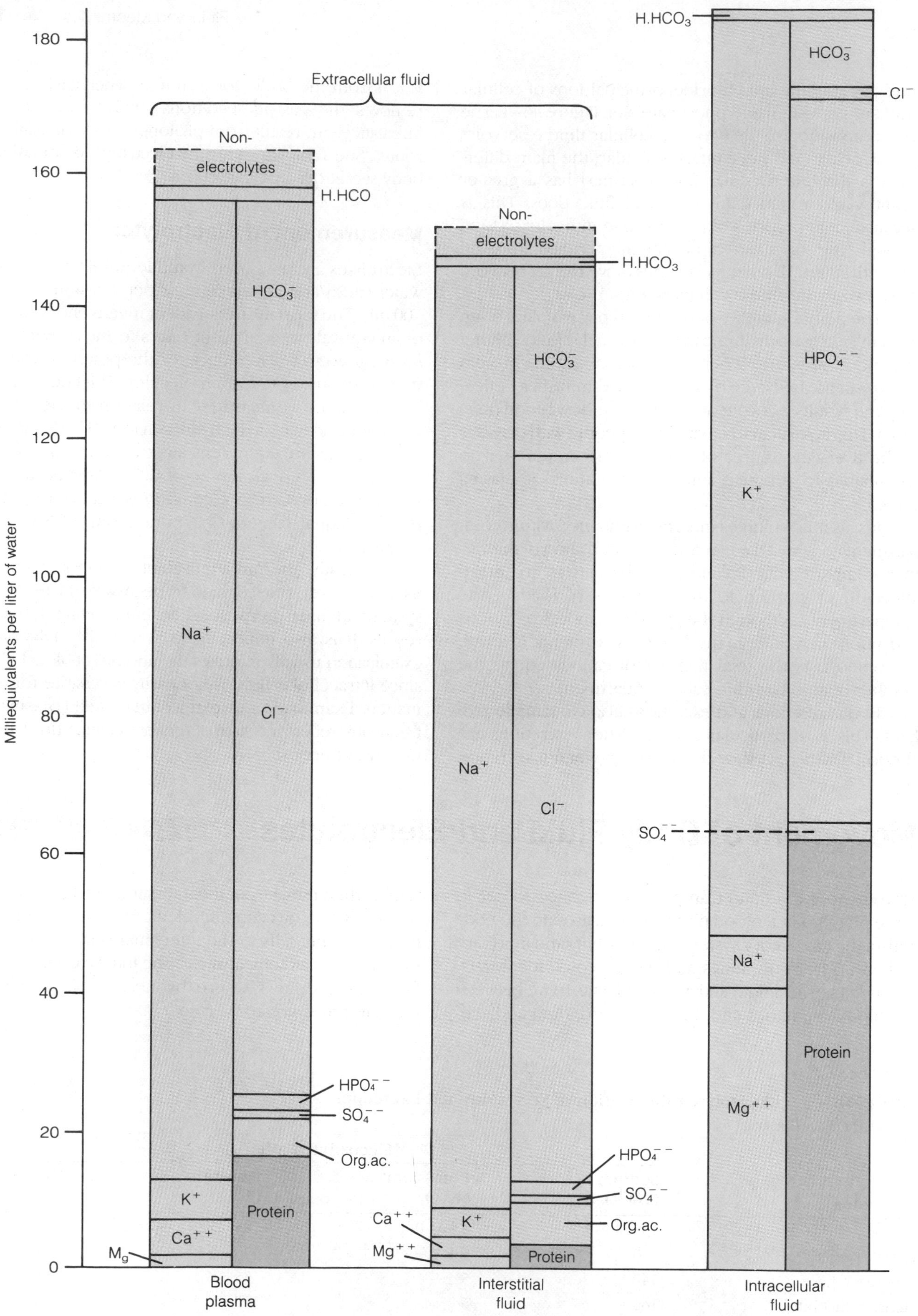

Figure 46–1 The composition of plasma, interstitial fluid, and intracellular fluid

Source: Adapted from A. C. Guyton, *Textbook of medical physiology,* 7th ed. (Philadelphia: W. B. Saunders Co., 1986), p. 386. Used by permission.

Methods of Movement

The methods by which body fluids and electrolytes move are: diffusion, osmosis, and active transport.

Diffusion

Diffusion is the continual intermingling of molecules in liquids, gases, or solids brought about by the random movement of the molecules. For example, two gases become mixed by the incessant motion of their molecules. The process of diffusion occurs even when two substances are separated by a thin membrane. In the body, diffusion of water, electrolytes, and other substances occurs through the "slit pores" of capillary membranes.

The rate of diffusion of substances varies according to (a) size of the molecules, (b) concentration of the solution, and (c) temperature of the solution. Larger molecules move less quickly than smaller ones, since they require more energy to move about. Molecules move more rapidly from a solution of higher concentration to a solution of lower concentration. Increases in temperature increase the rate of motion of molecules and therefore the rate of diffusion.

Osmosis

Osmosis is the movement of water across cell membranes, from the less concentrated solution to the more concentrated solution. In other words, water moves toward the higher concentration of solute. A **solute** is a substance dissolved in a solution. A **solvent** is the component of a solution that can dissolve a solute. In a salt solution, water is the solvent, and sodium chloride (NaCl) is the solute. Osmosis is important in maintaining proper balance in the volumes of extracellular and intracellular fluid.

Osmolarity is a measure of the concentration of a solution, expressed in a unit called the osmol: 1 osmol is the number of particles in 1 gram molecular weight of dissociated solute. Osmolarity is expressed in osmols per liter of solution.

Active Transport

Substances can move across cell membranes from a less concentrated solution to a more concentrated one by **active transport**. This process differs from diffusion and osmosis in that metabolic energy is expended. In active transport, the substance combines with a carrier on the outside surface of the cell membrane. The combined carrier and substance then move to the inside surface. Once inside, they separate, and the substance is released to the inside of the cell. A specific carrier is required for each substance, and enzymes are required for active transport.

This process is of particular importance in maintaining the differences in sodium and potassium ion concentrations of extracellular and intracellular fluid. Under normal conditions, sodium concentrations are higher in the extracellular fluid, while potassium concentrations are higher inside the cells. To maintain this balance, the active transport mechanism (the **sodium-potassium pump**) is activated, moving sodium from the cells and potassium into the cells.

Fluid Pressures

A number of pressures are exerted as part of the movement of fluid and electrolytes from one compartment to another. Two of these are osmotic pressure and hydrostatic pressure, each of which can cause a flow of fluid through the capillary membranes.

Osmotic Pressure

Osmotic pressure is the pressure exerted by a solution to stop osmosis. The osmotic pressure exerted by particles, e.g., ions or molecules, that cannot penetrate the membrane depends on the number of particles per unit of volume, not the total mass of the particles. The reason is that each particle in a solution exerts the same amount of pressure on the membrane regardless of its mass.

Osmotic pressure is the force exerted by solute particles drawing water across membranes. The solute particles may be **crystalloids** (salts that dissolve readily into true solutions) or **colloids** (substances such as large protein molecules that do not readily dissolve into true solutions). Normally, the net movement of fluid across cell membranes is nil; i.e., the distribution of electrolytes on both sides of membranes is even. If the concentration of solute on one side of a membrane becomes greater, the osmotic pressure and attraction for water increase on that side, and water flows toward the solution of greater concentration until the concentration gradient disappears.

The principle of osmosis can be applied clinically in the administration of intravenous solutions. Usually, the solutions given are **isotonic**, having the same concentration (osmolarity) as blood plasma. This prevents sudden shifts of fluids and electrolytes. In some cases, however, hypertonic or hypotonic solutions are infused. **Hypertonic** solutions have a greater concentration of solutes than plasma does; **hypotonic** solutions have a lesser concentration of solutes. An example of a hypertonic solution is 50% glucose, which may be given to reduce cerebral edema. The high concentration of glucose temporarily draws fluid from interstitial spaces in the brain into the blood compartment. Use of hypotonic solutions is rare.

The osmotic pressure of plasma is greater than the osmotic pressure of interstitial fluid because (a) the protein concentration (solute) in plasma is greater than that in interstitial fluid and (b) protein molecules are large, resemble colloids, and do not readily pass through capillary membranes. This greater colloid osmotic pressure of plasma is extremely important in maintaining the intravascular fluid volume.

Hydrostatic Pressure

Counterbalancing the osmotic pressure of plasma, which attracts fluid, is the hydrostatic pressure of the blood flowing through the capillaries, which pushes fluid out of the vascular space. **Hydrostatic pressure** is the pressure exerted by a fluid within a closed system. Thus, the hydrostatic pressure of blood is the force exerted by blood against the vascular walls, e.g., the artery walls. It is also referred to as **filtration force.** The principle involved in hydrostatic pressure is that fluids move from the area of greater pressure to the area of less pressure. For this reason, fluid moves out of blood vessels.

The net movement of water from plasma to tissue spaces thus depends on which force is greater: hydrostatic pressure, which forces fluid out of the blood vessels, or osmotic pressure, which draws fluid into the blood vessels. Normally, fluid moves out of capillaries at the arterial end, where the intravascular hydrostatic pressure exceeds the colloid osmotic pressure. At the venous end of the capillaries, where the colloid osmotic pressure is greater, fluid is drawn from the interstitial compartment into the intravascular compartment.

Selective Permeability of Membranes

Capillary and cellular membranes in the body are described as selectively permeable, because not all substances move with the same ease across the membranes. Compounds such as proteins and glycogen do not readily cross capillary and cellular membranes. Organic compounds such as glucose and amino acids move freely across capillary walls, although they often require active transport. Certain membranes, called **dialyzing membranes**, allow water molecules and particles in true solution (crystalloids), but not particles in colloid dispersion, to pass through. Most of the membranes that surround cells are dialyzing membranes.

Cellular (not capillary) membranes are particularly selective in regard to sodium and potassium ions. Movement of potassium across cell membranes depends on metabolic cellular activities. Administration of glucose or insulin accelerates the movement of potassium into the cells. Sodium enters in greater quantities when the cells lose potassium. Any factor that alters the properties of the cell membranes brings about changes in the distribution of sodium and potassium. Some of these factors are excitation of nerve and muscle cells, changes in pH, and anoxia.

Regulating Fluid Volume

Health is usually maintained as long as the fluid volume and chemical composition of the fluid compartments stay within narrow safe limits. Normally, a person's fluid intake is counterbalanced by fluid loss. Illness can upset this balance so that the body has too little or too much fluid.

Fluid Intake

During periods of moderate activity at moderate temperature, the average adult drinks about 1500 ml per day but needs 2500 ml per day, an additional 1000 ml. This added volume is acquired from foods (referred to as preformed water) and from the oxidation of these foods during metabolic processes. Interestingly, the water content of food is relatively large, contributing about 750 ml per day. The water content of fresh vegetables is approximately 90%, of fresh fruits about 85%, and of lean meats around 60%.

Oxidative water, which is formed as a by-product of the body's oxidation of food, accounts for most of the remaining fluid volume required. This quantity ranges from 150 to 250 ml per day for the average adult (Guyton 1986, p. 382).

The primary regulator of fluid intake is the body's thirst mechanism. The thirst center is situated in the supraoptic nuclei in the lateral preoptic area of the hypothalamus. A number of stimuli trigger this center: intracellular dehydration, excess angiotensin II (a hormone released into the blood in response to very low blood pressure) in the body fluids, hemorrhage, and low cardiac output resulting in lowered blood volume. Angiotensin II is a potent vasoconstrictor. It forms largely in the small blood vessels in the lungs, in response to release of renin to the bloodstream from the kidneys.

Dryness of the mouth is often associated with thirst but can occur independently (for example, when a person's salivary glands do not secrete saliva). Thirst is normally relieved immediately after drinking a small amount of fluid, even before it is absorbed from the gastrointestinal tract. However, this relief is only temporary, and the thirst returns in about 15 minutes. The thirst is again temporarily relieved after the ingested fluid distends the upper gastrointestinal tract. These mechanisms protect the individual from drinking too much, because it takes from 30 minutes to 1 hour for the fluid to be absorbed and distributed throughout the body. If a person continued to drink during that time, the fluid ingested would overdilute the body fluids. See Table 46–5 for average daily water requirements.

Fluid Output

Fluid losses counterbalance the adult's 2300-ml daily intake of water. The main channel of excretion is the kidneys, which are responsible for an output of about 1500 ml per day in the adult. This approximates the amount of fluid an adult drinks per day. Oral intake and kidney output are frequently and easily measured in nursing practice.

Three other routes of fluid output are:

1. Insensible loss through the skin as perspiration and through the lungs as water vapor in the expired air
2. Noticeable loss through the skin as sweat
3. Loss through the intestines in feces

See Table 46–3 for the average daily fluid output for an adult. The normal loss from skin and lungs accounts for about two-thirds of the urinary loss, whereas loss in the feces is minimal. It is important to remember that daily intake equals daily output.

Obligatory loss is the essential fluid loss required to maintain body functioning. Water lost as vapor in expired air and as vapor from the skin, a minimum volume of about 500 ml from the kidneys, and the fluid required to excrete the solid metabolic wastes produced daily are the obligatory losses, totaling about 1300 ml per day.

Since the vaporized losses are not readily measured, the measured obligatory kidney loss becomes of prime importance in critical illness. An adult hourly urine volume of less than 30 ml or daily volume under 500 ml is serious. Clients with inadequate output require immediate attention, and such a finding by the nurse must therefore be reported promptly. Although losses from the skin, lungs, and intestines in health account for approximately half of the daily loss, they can account for a much larger percentage of loss from a client who has a fever or accelerated respiration. Increases in respiratory rate, fever, **diaphoresis** (sweating), and diarrhea can magnify fluid loss from the normal routes immensely. Other routes of loss, such as from the stomach through emesis or suction or from abnormal body openings such as fistulas or surgically implanted drainage tubes, often account for significant losses, all of which require intake replacements.

In health, the output volumes shown in Table 46–3 may vary noticeably from day to day and throughout the day. For example, sweat gland activity can increase when the environmental temperature increases. Urinary volume automatically increases as the amount of fluids ingested increases, e.g., on a hot summer day. If fluid loss from the skin is large, however, the urinary volume may decrease to maintain the fluid volumes in the body. Balance is maintained between the intake and output by the homeostatic mechanisms already discussed in this chapter.

Table 46–5 Average Daily Water Requirements, by Age and Weight

Age	Water Requirement	
	ml	ml/kg Body Weight
3 days	250–300	80–100
1 year	1150–300	120–135
2 years	1350–1500	115–125
4 years	1600–1800	100–110
10 years	2000–2500	70–85
14 years	2200–2700	50–60
18 years	2200–2700	40–50
Adult	2400–2600	20–30

Sources: R. E. Behrman and V. C. Vaughan, *Nelson textbook of pediatrics,* 12th ed. (Philadelphia: W. B. Saunders Co., 1983), p. 138; and R. B. Howard and N. H. Herbold, *Nutrition in clinical care,* 2d ed. (New York: McGraw-Hill, 1982), p. 153.

Urine

The formation of urine by the kidneys and its subsequent excretion from the urinary bladder is the major avenue of fluid output. The two kidneys each contain about 2,400,000 nephrons (Guyton 1986, p. 393). The nephron was described in Chapter 44. The glomerulus filters glomerular fluid into a long tubule, where most of the fluid is reabsorbed into the bloodstream. The remainder of the fluid that is not absorbed becomes urine. The formation of urine and the control of that process are highly complex. One of the major controls of urine formation is blood volume. When the volume of circulating blood becomes excessive, the stretch receptors in the walls of the left and right atria are triggered to transmit impulses to the brain. The brain reacts by inhibiting sympathetic nervous impulses to the kidneys, reducing the secretion of antidiuretic hormone (ADH), and dilating the body's peripheral capillaries. As a result of these mechanisms, the rate of urine output is increased and excess blood volume filters temporarily into the tissue spaces.

Another control mechanism is the osmoreceptor of sodium and antidiuretic hormone system. This feedback system controls the concentration of sodium in the extracellular fluid, the fluid's osmolarity, and thus urine formation. An increase in the osmolarity (sodium concentration) of the extracellular fluid stimulates osmoreceptors, which are located in the supraoptic nuclei of the hypothalamus. These stimulate the production of antidiuretic hormone (ADH) by the hypothalamus and release of ADH by the posterior pituitary gland. ADH acts on the cells of the distal and collecting tubules of the glomeruli to make them more permeable to water. As a result, more fluid is reabsorbed into the bloodstream to dilute the sodium and other substances in the extracellular fluid, and less urine is formed. When the extracellular fluid becomes sufficiently diluted, the osmoreceptors respond to the decreased sodium concentration by reducing the production of ADH. Consequently, the antidiuretic effect ceases, and additional urine is produced.

Insensible Losses

Insensible fluid loss occurs through the skin and lungs. It is called *insensible* because it is usually not noticeable. The insensible loss through the skin is by diffusion. It is normally controlled by the outer layer of the epidermis, the stratum corneum. However, when the skin layers are destroyed by burns and abrasions, fluid loss can increase considerably.

Another type of insensible loss is the water in exhaled air. In an adult, this is normally 300 to 400 ml per day. When respiratory rate accelerates, e.g., due to exercise or an elevated body temperature, this loss can increase.

Sweat

Sweating occurs when the body becomes overheated. The sweat glands secrete large quantities of sweat onto the surface of the body to provide cooling by evaporation. Sweating occurs in response to stimulation of the preoptic area in the anterior hypothalamus. Impulses are transmitted to the spinal cord and via the sympathetic nervous system to the skin.

The rate of flow of sweat can vary from none in a cold environment to 1.5 to 2 liters per hour in an adult acclimatized to a hot environment (Guyton 1986, p. 853).

Large amounts of sweat contain large amounts of sodium chloride, whereas small amounts of sweat contain lower concentrations of sodium chloride. Sweat also contains urea, lactic acid, and potassium ions. The concentrations of these substances can be very high when the rate of sweat secretion is low and are lower when the rate of sweat secretion is high (Guyton 1986, p. 852).

Feces

The chyme that passes from the small intestine into the large intestine is composed of water and electrolytes. The volume of chyme that passes through the ileocecal valve in an adult is normally about 1500 ml per day (Guyton 1986, p. 796). Of this amount, all but about 100 ml is reabsorbed in the proximal half of the large intestine. Sodium and chloride ions are also actively absorbed, and bicarbonate ions are secreted by the mucosa of the large intestine. The bicarbonate helps to neutralize the acidic end products of bacterial action in the colon. For further information about the composition of feces, see Chapter 43.

Regulating Electrolytes

The major electrolytes of the body are the cations sodium, potassium, and calcium and the anion chloride.

Sodium (Na^+)

The sources of sodium for the body are largely table salt (NaCl) and foods high in sodium, e.g., cheese, pork products, salted meats, bread, potato chips, and cereals.

Normal sodium concentrations in the extracellular fluid are regulated by ADH and aldosterone. Aldosterone, a hormone produced by the adrenal cortex, acts to maintain sodium concentrations, although its action can be overridden by ADH and the thirst mechanism described earlier. ADH regulates the amount of water absorbed into the blood from the renal tubules. Aldosterone regulates the amount of sodium reabsorbed into the blood. When aldosterone is secreted and the reabsorption of sodium is increased, the sodium concentration of the extracellular fluid rises. In a feedback mechanism, the increased extracellular sodium causes the adrenal cortex to decrease the secretion of aldosterone. If the body must conserve sodium for any reason, it can excrete sodium-free urine.

Sodium not only moves into and out of the body but also moves in careful balance among the three fluid compartments. It is found in most body secretions, e.g., saliva, gastric and intestinal secretions, bile, and pancreatic fluid. Therefore, continuous excretion of any of these fluids, e.g., via intestinal suction, can result in a sodium deficit.

Sodium functions largely in the control and regulation of the body fluids. When sodium is reabsorbed into the blood from the tubules of the glomeruli, chloride is reabsorbed with it. The combined reabsorption increases the fluid held in the body. Sodium also helps maintain blood volume and interstitial fluid volume through this mechanism. With potassium, sodium helps maintain the electrolyte balance of intracellular and extracellular fluids by means of the active transport mechanism, the sodium-potassium pump. For additional information about sodium see Table 42–3, page 1152.

Hyponatremia

Hyponatremia is a sodium deficit in the blood plasma. This condition occurs with overhydration. (**Overhydration** is an excess of fluid in the body.) Two situations can precede hyponatremia:

1. Sodium loss that exceeds corresponding water loss, e.g., due to prolonged, excessive sweating or to the prolonged use of strong diuretics
2. Intake of water that exceeds corresponding intake of sodium, e.g., due to drinking excessive quantities of water

Excessive sodium loss can be the result of profuse sweating. Also, clients can lose abnormally large amounts of sodium through the gastrointestinal tract. The sodium content of pancreatic secretions and gastric mucus is especially high. Severe, prolonged diarrhea or a draining pancreatic fistula can result in abnormally high sodium loss. Gastric suction, which withdraws gastric mucus along with other gastric fluids, can be the cause as well. The clinical signs of hyponatremia are listed below.

Hypernatremia

Hypernatremia is sodium excess in the blood plasma. Hypernatremia occurs with dehydration. (**Dehydration** is insufficient fluid in the body.) Hypernatremia can occur when:

1. Sodium intake greatly exceeds water intake, e.g., when a person mistakenly ingests a large number of sodium chloride tablets.
2. Water loss exceeds sodium loss. For example, a client may lose more water than sodium through a draining intestinal wound and as a result become hypernatremic. A client who is not treated for watery diarrhea may experience hypernatremia on about the fifth or sixth day after onset.

The clinical signs of hypernatremia are listed to the right.

Potassium (K^+)

Potassium is the major cation of intracellular fluid (see Figure 46–1, earlier). Major sources of potassium are bananas, broccoli, canteloupe, citrus fruits, and potatoes.

Potassium balance is regulated in the kidneys by two mechanisms: exchange with sodium ions in the kidney tubules and secretion of aldosterone. Aldosterone is extremely important in controlling potassium concentrations in extracellular fluids. The aldosterone-potassium feedback system works in three steps:

1. Increased potassium concentration in extracellular fluid causes an increase in the production of aldosterone.
2. The elevated aldosterone level increases the amount of potassium excreted by the kidneys.
3. As potassium excretion increases, the concentration of potassium in the extracellular fluid decreases. In turn, aldosterone production decreases.

Potassium affects the functions of most body systems, including the cardiovascular system, the gastrointestinal system, the neuromuscular system, and the respiratory system. Of particular importance is potassium's role in transmitting electrical impulses to the heart and other muscles, to lung tissues, and to intestinal tissues. Most of the body's potassium is found inside the cells. A small amount is found in the plasma and interstitial fluids. See Table 42–3, page 1152, for additional information about potassium.

Potassium is usually excreted by the kidneys. However, the kidneys do not regulate potassium excretion as effectively as sodium excretion. Therefore, an acute potassium deficiency can develop rapidly. Of the body's secretions, the gastrointestinal secretions are high in potassium.

Like other electrolytes, potassium moves continually in and out of the cells. This movement from the interstitial fluid, which has less potassium, to the intracellular fluid, which has a greater concentration, is influenced by the adrenal steroids, testosterone, pH changes, glycogen formation, and hyponatremia. If tissues are damaged, the body can lose potassium quickly.

Hypokalemia

Hypokalemia is a potassium deficit in the blood plasma. Hypokalemia can develop quickly in people who are

---

Clinical Signs of Hyponatremia

Observations

- Feelings of apprehension
- Fatigue
- Abdominal cramps and diarrhea
- Weakness
- Postural hypotension
- Personality change
- Cold, clammy skin

Laboratory data

- Plasma sodium level below 135 mEq/L

Clinical Signs of Hypernatremia

Observations

- Extreme thirst
- Dry, sticky mucous membrane
- Tongue red and dry
- Flushed skin
- Elevated body temperature
- Agitated behavior

Laboratory data

- Plasma sodium level about 145 mEq/L

Clinical Signs of Hypokalemia

Observations

- Muscle weakness
- Chronic fatigue
- Anorexia and abdominal distention
- Cardiac arrhythmia
- Decreased bowel sounds

Laboratory data

- Plasma potassium level below 3.5 mEq/L
- Electrocardiogram may show flattening of the T waves and depression of the S-T segment

starving. The combined effects of inadequate potassium intake and potassium loss because of prolonged diarrhea can deplete potassium stores acutely. The leading cause of potassium deficit is thought to be the use of powerful diuretics (Metheny and Snively 1983, p. 48). Surgical procedures, particularly those involving the digestive tract, often result in a potassium deficit unless supplemental potassium is supplied. See above for the clinical signs of hypokalemia.

Hyperkalemia

Hyperkalemia is a potassium excess in the blood plasma. Hyperkalemia is most often caused by a leakage of potassium from the body's cells, e.g., after severe burns. It can also occur as a result of excessive ingestion of potassium or the intravenous administration of excessive amounts of potassium when kidney function is impaired. The clinical signs of hyperkalemia are shown below.

Clinical Signs of Hyperkalemia

Observations

- Gastrointestinal hyperactivity
- Cardiac arrhythmia
- Weakness
- Anxiety and irritability

Laboratory data

- Plasma potassium level greater than 5 mEq/L

Calcium (Ca^{2+})

The richest sources of calcium are milk and milk products. Smaller amounts are found in grains, fruits, nuts, shellfish, and eggs. Drinking water in some parts of the country also contains an absorbable calcium. See Table 42–3 on page 1152.

Calcium functions in bone formation and in the transmission of nerve impulses, muscle contraction, blood coagulation, and activation of certain enzymes, e.g., pancreatic lipase and phospholipase.

Calcium is excreted in urine, feces, bile, digestive secretions, and sweat. The concentration of body calcium is controlled indirectly by the effect of parathyroid hormone on bone reabsorption. When calcium levels in extracellular fluid fall too low, the parathyroid glands are stimulated to increase parathyroid hormone (parathormone) secretion. This hormone acts directly on the bones to increase the release of calcium into the blood. When the bones run out of calcium, parathyroid hormone acts on both the kidney tubules and the intestinal mucosa to increase the reabsorption of calcium from the kidneys and the intestine.

Another hormone, calcitonin, has an effect nearly opposite that of the parathyroid hormone. Calcitonin reduces the concentration of calcium ions in the blood. Calcitonin, which is secreted by the thyroid gland, stimulates the deposition of calcium in bone and depresses the formation of osteoclasts in the bone. However, the effect of calcitonin on plasma concentration levels of adults is minimal (Guyton 1986, p. 947) because the parathyroid hormone counteracts the effect of calcitonin within hours. In adults, the daily absorption and deposition of calcium are minimal. See below.

An adult excretes about five-sixths of the daily intake of calcium in feces and the remaining one-sixth in urine. Calcium is poorly absorbed from the intestine. However, vitamin D greatly potentiates the absorption of calcium from the intestine.

Absorption and Excretion of Calcium

Intake	800 mg
Intestinal secretion	190 mg
Intestinal absorption	350 mg
Net absorption	170 mg
Loss in feces	630 mg
Loss in urine	170 mg
Total	800 mg

Hypocalcemia

Hypocalcemia is a calcium deficit in the blood plasma. Two common causes of hypocalcemia are removal of the parathyroid glands and excessive loss of intestinal secretions, which contain a great deal of calcium. Mild hypocalcemia may be reflected as a tingling sensation in the fingers and around the mouth, and as abdominal and skeletal muscle cramps. Severe depletion can cause **tetany** (muscle spasms, sharp flexion of the wrists and ankles, cramps), which can lead to convulsions. Adults experience hypocalcemia when the serum calcium level falls below 4.3 mEq/liter.

Hypercalcemia

Hypercalcemia is an excess of calcium in the blood plasma. It can be due to, for example, drinking too much milk or a tumor of the parathyroid glands. The clinical signs of hypercalcemia are given below.

Chloride (Cl^-)

Chloride is the major anion of extracellular fluid (see Figure 46–1, earlier). Chloride is found in blood, interstitial fluid, and lymph. A very small amount is found in intracellular fluid. It functions as sodium does to maintain the osmotic pressure of the blood. Its reabsorption in the kidney is secondary to that of sodium; i.e., each sodium ion reabsorbed is accompanied by a chloride or bicarbonate ion. Because aldosterone controls the reabsorption of sodium, it controls the reabsorption of chloride indirectly.

The chief dietary sources of chloride are dairy products and meat. Chloride is also found with sodium as salt (NaCl) in food. See Table 42–3, page 1152.

Hypochloremia (a deficit in serum chloride) and **hyperchloremia** (an excess serum chloride) usually develop along with sodium disturbances. The normal serum chloride of an adult is 95 to 108 mEq/liter.

Clinical Signs of Hypercalcemia

Observations

- Deep bone pain
- Relaxed muscles
- Flank pain caused by kidney stones
- Hypercalcemic crisis preceded by nausea, vomiting, dehydration, and coma

Laboratory data

- Serum calcium level more than 4.3 mEq/L

Magnesium (Mg^{2+})

Magnesium is the fourth most abundant cation in the body. The average adult body contains about 20 g (Metheny and Snively 1983, p. 59). Like calcium, magnesium is regulated by the parathyroid glands. It is absorbed from the intestinal tract. The magnesium content of the body is affected by the potassium concentration. If magnesium is deficient, the kidneys tend to excrete more potassium. It is known that increased extracellular magnesium depresses nervous system activity and skeletal muscle contractions. Low magnesium concentrations, by contrast, cause increased irritability of the nervous system, peripheral vasodilation, and cardiac arrhythmias (Guyton 1986, p. 872). For clinical signs of **hypomagnesemia** (magnesium deficit) and **hypermagnesemia** (magnesium excess), see below.

Bicarbonate (HCO_3^-)

The anion bicarbonate is one of the major base buffers of the body, i.e., a main component of the carbonic acid-bicarbonate ion buffering system. For additional information, see the section on acid-base balance later in this chapter.

Phosphate (PO_4^-)

The phosphate anion is found both in intracellular and extracellular fluid. See Figure 46–1, earlier. Together with calcium, phosphate is involved in bone and tooth for-

Clinical Signs of Magnesium Disturbances

Hypomagnesemia

Observations

- Neuromuscular irritability with tremors
- Leg and foot cramps
- Tachycardia
- Hypertension
- Disorientation and confusion

Laboratory data

- Serum magnesium below 1.5 mEq/L

Hypermagnesemia

Observations

- Lethargy
- Coma
- Impaired respirations

Laboratory data

- Serum magnesium above 2.5 mEq/L

mation. It is also involved in many chemical actions of the cells. Many of the B vitamins are effective only when combined with phosphate (Metheny and Snively 1983, p. 58). Phosphate is absorbed exceedingly well from the intestine, and it is excreted in the urine. Phosphate is a threshold substance because none is lost in urine when blood plasma concentrations fall below a critical level. When the concentration is above the critical level, however, it is excreted in proportion to the increase. Therefore, the kidneys regulate the concentration of phosphate in the extracellular fluid. In addition, phosphate excretion is regulated by the parathyroid hormone.

Fluid Volume Disturbances

The two major fluid volume disturbances are deficits and excesses. A fluid volume disturbance can be the result of excesses or deficits in *both* water and electrolytes.

Extracellular Fluid (ECF) Deficit

An extracellular fluid deficit is also called a fluid deficit, **hypovolemia**, or dehydration. In the strict sense, dehydration is not an ECF deficit but a water deficit only.

ECF deficit can occur because of an abrupt decrease in fluid intake or a marked increase in fluid output, i.e., an acute loss of secretions or excretions. The body's initial response to a fluid deficit is depletion of the intravascular compartment. Then fluid is drawn into the intravascular compartment, depleting the interstitial compartment. To compensate for the decreased interstitial volume, the body then draws intracellular fluid out of the cells. This depletion of fluid volume can occur with diarrhea and vomiting.

Three types of extracellular volume deficits or dehydration are recognized: isotonic, hypertonic, and hypotonic. *Isotonic dehydration* occurs when proportionate amounts of fluid and electrolytes are lost. *Hypertonic dehydration* occurs when there is a greater loss of water than of electrolytes. *Hypotonic dehydration,* the least common type, is a greater loss of electrolytes than of water.

Changes brought about by extracellular fluid losses are (a) reduced ECF volume (hypovolemia) and (b) elevated hematocrit. Because of the isotonic loss of both water and sodium, serum sodium concentration and serum osmolality remain normal, i.e., isotonic. However, the hematocrit is elevated because the volume of ECF is reduced. In early stages, there is no shift of fluid from the intracellular fluid (ICF) spaces because the body osmolality remains the same. When the condition persists longer than several days, urea nitrogen and creatinine are also elevated, and the body draws water from intracellular fluids to restore the blood volume. Long-term extracellular fluid loss, then, results in depletion of intracellular fluid as well.

Fluid deficits can develop slowly or quickly and are not always readily detected. The clinical signs of a fluid volume deficit in an adult are listed to the right.

Causes

Isolated water deficits may occur because of insufficient water intake, excessive solute intake, profuse and prolonged sweating, and certain disorders creating large renal fluid losses (Harvey et al. 1980, pp. 53–54).

Insufficient intake Dehydration due to insufficient intake of water is usually confined to the very young, the very old, and persons too debilitated to satisfy their own water needs. Insufficient intake is especially likely during hot weather, when there is increased loss through the skin. When the greatest fluid loss is through perspiration, the sweating person may also lose significant amounts of sodium, resulting in a coexisting sodium deficit.

Excess solute intake Excess solute intake is most commonly seen in ill, elderly clients who receive nasogastric tube feedings, which have high protein and sodium chloride contents (e.g., 120 g of protein and 10 g of salt). Such solute intakes result in obligatory excretion of urine in volumes between 1200 and 1500 ml per day (Harvey et

Clinical Signs of ECF Deficit

Observations

- Postural hypotension
- Weight loss
- Decreased tearing and salivation
- Dryness in the axillae and groin
- Inelastic skin
- Oliguria
- Increased pulse and respiratory rates

Laboratory data

- Increased specific gravity of urine

al. 1980, p. 54). Urine volumes may exceed 2000 to 2500 ml per day in elderly people, who often have significant impairments in renal concentrating ability. Thus, a greatly increased water intake (e.g., up to 3 or 4 liters per day) may be required to meet the demand created by a high solute intake.

Prolonged sweating Profuse, prolonged sweating can rapidly lead to fluid deficits (and moderate sodium deficits) if the sweating person does not drink sufficient fluids. Work in extremely hot environments, vigorous sports in hot weather, and prolonged exposure to sunlight may all produce profuse sweating and large water losses (e.g., up to 8 liters per day).

Disorders creating renal loss Normally, water deficits by renal loss are rare, since antidiuretic hormone (ADH) acts promptly to decrease the rate of loss when any significant water deficit elevates the osmolarity of plasma. However, certain disorders of the hypothalamus, posterior pituitary gland, and kidney can lead to excessive fluid loss through the kidneys. These include diabetes insipidus and impairments in the ability of the kidneys to concentrate urine.

Many illnesses are characterized by excessive losses of gastrointestinal fluids. Fluid loss accompanies vomiting, diarrhea, fistulas, tube drainages, and bowel obstructions (in which fluids are not reabsorbed). With such losses, varying amounts of solutes (electrolytes) are also lost. Urine and sweat losses also create deficits in electrolytes. For practical purposes, it is wise to assume that in other than mild dehydration, the body also loses sodium, chloride, and potassium.

Effects

The effects of dehydration depend on the rate and volume of loss. Dehydration can be categorized as mild, moderate, severe, or very severe. See Table 46–6.

Changes brought about by dehydration of the extracellular fluid compartment are: (a) reduced extracellular fluid (ECF) volume and (b) hypertonicity or a hyperosmolar fluid imbalance. These changes occur because with dehydration there is more solute in proportion to fluid. When the body is deprived of water, the extracellular fluid compartment, including interstitial fluid, is reduced. However, water passes into plasma immediately. The water gained passes by osmosis from the intracellular compartments through interstitial fluid to the plasma. This transfer of water tends to preserve the circulating blood plasma volume. If the kidneys are functioning normally, they will attempt to retain water and salt by reducing the excretion of sodium chloride and water to minimal amounts. As dehydration progresses, the concentrations of the sodium ion (Na^+) and the chloride ion (Cl^-) in plasma rise, thus increasing blood concentration (increased serum osmolarity).

Clients go into shock when intravascular fluid compartments become greatly depleted. Shock indicates that the deficits are so great that the regulatory mechanisms of the body can no longer maintain the plasma volume. This blood volume reduction, called hypovolemia, is responsible for such manifestations as a rapid weak pulse, fall in blood pressure, and increased concentration of blood solutes. Since the kidneys rely on sufficient arterial blood pressure to produce urine, hypovolemia results in **oliguria** (decreased urine output). Oliguria progresses to **anuria** (absence of urine). As a consequence, metabolic

Table 46–6 Severity of Fluid Deficit and Excess

Severity	Magnitude of Deficit or Excess (liters)	% of Body Water Deficit or Excess	Serum Na* (mEq/L)	Serum Osmolality* (mOsm/kg)
Fluid deficit				
Mild	1.5–2	3–4.5	149–151	294–298
Moderate	2–4	4.5–10	152–158	299–313
Severe	4–6	10–15	159–166	314–329
Very severe	>6	>15	>166	>330
Fluid excess				
Mild	1.5–4	3–8	139–132	275–261
Moderate	4–6	8–13	131–127	262–251
Severe	6–10	13–22	126–118	250–233
Very severe	>10	>22	<118	<233

*Normal serum Na is 144 mEq/liter and normal serum osmolality is 285 mOsm/kg.

Source: From A. M. Harvey, R. J. Johns, V. A. McKusick, A. H. Owens, and R. S. Ross, ***The principles and practice of medicine,*** 20th ed. (New York: Appleton-Century-Crofts, 1980), pp. 53, 57.

wastes accumulate, the client quickly becomes disoriented and comatose, and death ensues due to the effects of the acid waste products on the cells.

Extracellular Fluid (ECF) Excess

A fluid volume excess, also called overhydration, is characterized by an excessive amount of extracellular fluid. Excesses of extracellular fluid lead to (a) **hypervolemia** (increased blood volume) and (b) **edema** (excess fluid in the interstitial compartment). Normally, the interstitial fluid compartment is not bogged with water but compact, elastic, and expandable, with just enough fluid to fill the crevices between tissues. This compact state facilitates diffusion of nutrients from the plasma to the intracellular fluid (ICF) and diffusion of the metabolic wastes from the cells to the plasma. Edema increases the distance between the blood capillaries and the cells and thus hinders cell nutrition.

Pitting edema is edema that leaves a small depression or pit after finger pressure is applied to the swollen area. The pit is caused by movement of fluid to adjacent tissue, away from the point of pressure. Within 10 to 30 seconds, the pit normally disappears. Pitting edema is never seen in clients with a pure water excess (Harvey et al. 1980, p. 56). (In nonpitting edema, the fluid in edematous tissues cannot be moved to adjacent spaces by finger pressure. Nonpitting edema is not a sign of ECF excess but often accompanies infections and traumas that cause fluid to collect and coagulate in tissue spaces. The coagulation prevents displacement of fluid to other areas by pressure.)

Overloading of the vascular fluid compartment increases blood hydrostatic pressure, which forces fluid into the interstitial spaces. **Anasarca** (edema that is generalized throughout the body) is the result. Greatly increased hydrostatic pressure forces large amounts of fluid through the alveolar-capillary membrane into the alveoli of the lungs, causing pulmonary edema, a serious problem that can result in death by suffocation. Manifestations of pulmonary edema are frothy sputum, dyspnea, cough, and gurgling sounds on respiration. The most common cause of pulmonary edema is left-sided heart failure, with resulting increases in the pressure of the pulmonary blood capillaries and the interstitial spaces of the lung tissue.

Clinical Signs of ECF Excess

Observations

- Peripheral edema (pitting)
- Puffy eyelids
- Ascites
- Moist rales in the lungs
- Full, bounding pulse
- Sudden weight gain

Laboratory data

- Not significant

Nurses need to exercise caution when administering intravenous fluids to clients with cardiac problems because of the danger of overload of the lung capillaries. Caution is also necessary with infants and elderly persons. Infants, because of their small lungs and small extravascular reserves, cannot handle large amounts of fluid. Elderly people have inelastic blood vessels and tolerate only small increases in blood volume before the hydrostatic pressure is substantially increased.

Because there is no change in the tonicity of body fluids in ECF volume excess, fluid does not move into the ICF compartment. Thus, clients with ECF excess do not develop cerebral signs as do clients with isolated water excess. The serum sodium level and serum osmolarity also remain normal. The hematocrit may be normal or decreased. In persistent ECF excesses associated with heart failure or cirrhosis, the client's hematocrit is usually normal. In acute ECF excesses, however, the hematocrit decreases in proportion to the severity of the problem.

When fluid moves from the vascular compartment into the interstitial spaces, the blood volume drops. In response, the body releases antidiuretic hormone (ADH) and aldosterone, which stimulate the kidneys to retain fluid and sodium. This response adds to the existing problem because the retained fluid can also move into the interstitial spaces, thus augmenting the edema. Therefore, generalized edema is a self-perpetuating condition. See above for the clinical signs of ECF excess.

Acid-Base Balance

The body's cellular activity requires an alkaline medium. Alkalinity and its opposite, acidity, are measured in terms of hydrogen ion concentration, expressed on a scale called **pH**. Body fluids are normally maintained at a pH of about 7.4. Alterations of pH of even a few tenths can be incompatible with cellular activity.

Opposing the body's alkalinity are cellular chemical processes that are constantly producing large amounts of acid as by-products of metabolism. Fortunately, precise control mechanisms maintain the pH of body fluids within a very narrow range. The pH is controlled by buffer systems in all body fluids and by respiratory and kidney regulatory systems.

Three major buffer systems of the body fluids are the bicarbonate buffer, the phosphate buffer, and the protein buffer. Discussion here is limited to the bicarbonate buffer system, since the phosphate and protein buffer systems operate in almost the same manner.

Bicarbonate Buffer System

The bicarbonate buffer system consists of sodium bicarbonate ($NaHCO_3$) or potassium bicarbonate ($KHCO_3$) and carbonic acid (H_2CO_3) in the same solution. Buffers do not neutralize; acid-base buffers decrease the effect of strong acids and strong bases, so that the pH of a body fluid falls or rises only slightly. For example, if a strong acid such as hydrochloric acid (HCl) is introduced into a glass of water, the pH of the fluid drops significantly to 1 or 2. However, if a bicarbonate buffer system is already present in the water, the HCl quickly combines with the buffer, producing a weaker acid (carbonic acid), and the pH drops only slightly. The reaction is:

$$\underset{\text{(hydrochloric acid)}}{HCl} + \underset{\text{(sodium bicarbonate)}}{NaHCO_3} \rightarrow \underset{\text{(carbonic acid)}}{H_2CO_3} + \underset{\text{(sodium chloride)}}{NaCl}$$

A strong acid is a compound that completely dissociates its hydrogen ions; for example, HCl yields H^+ and Cl^-. A weak acid frees only some of its hydrogen ions; for example, H_2CO_3 yields H^+ and HCO_3^-. One hydrogen ion is free, the other is not.

Alkalis undergo a similar change. When a strong base such as sodium hydroxide is added to body fluids, it combines with carbonic acid to form a weaker base, sodium bicarbonate:

$$\underset{\text{(sodium hydroxide)}}{NaOH} + \underset{\text{(carbonic acid)}}{H_2CO_3} \rightarrow \underset{\text{(sodium bicarbonate)}}{NaHCO_3} + \underset{\text{(water)}}{H_2O}$$

Although the bicarbonate buffer system is not the strongest buffer system in the body (the most powerful and plentiful one consists of the proteins of plasma and cells), it is important, because the concentration of sodium bicarbonate is regulated by the kidneys and the concentration of carbonic acid by the respiratory system.

Respiratory Regulation

Elimination of carbon dioxide by the lungs also regulates acid-base balance. The carbon dioxide that a person exhales comes from carbonic acid as follows:

$$H_2CO_3 \rightarrow CO_2 + H_2O$$

The more CO_2 exhaled, the more H_2CO_3 is removed from the blood, thus elevating the blood pH to a more alkaline level. Hyperventilation is an example of this shift. Increasing the ventilation rate raises the pH. By contrast, holding one's breath, or hypoventilating, causes the body to retain CO_2, which is then available to form carbonic acid, reducing the pH and acidifying body fluids. Respiratory alterations, therefore, change the pH of body fluids significantly.

Renal Regulation

The kidney's role in maintaining acid-base balance is complex. A simplified account of the process follows. The kidneys excrete hydrogen ions and form bicarbonate ions in specific amounts as indicated by the pH of the blood. When the plasma pH drops (becomes more acidic), hydrogen ions (acid) are excreted, and bicarbonate ions (base) are formed and retained. Conversely, when the plasma pH rises (becomes more alkaline), hydrogen ions are retained in the body, and bicarbonate ions are excreted.

Imbalances

The normal pH range of extracellular fluid is 7.35 to 7.45. See Figure 46–2. This precise balance is maintained as long as the ratio of 1 carbonic acid molecule to 20 bicarbonate ions is maintained in the extracellular fluid. The ratio, rather than the specific amount of each, is important.

Imbalances in pH can result in either acidosis or alkalosis. *Acidosis* occurs with increases in blood carbonic acid or with decreases in blood bicarbonate. *Alkalosis* occurs with increases in blood bicarbonate or decreases in blood carbonic acid. A client will not become acidotic or alkalotic, however, unless the normal ratio of 1 carbonic acid molecule to 20 bicarbonate ions is altered. Compensatory (adaptive) mechanisms operate to maintain this balance.

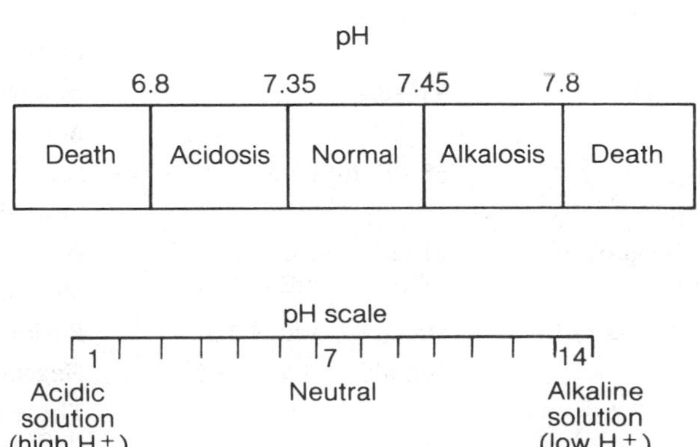

Figure 46–2 Body fluids are normally slightly alkaline, between a pH of 7.35 and 7.45.

Two adjectives describe the general cause or origin of a pH imbalance: metabolic and respiratory. Metabolic acidosis and metabolic alkalosis are imbalances brought about by changes in bicarbonate levels as a result of metabolic alterations. Respiratory acidosis and respiratory alkalosis are imbalances brought about by changes in carbonic acid levels as a result of respiratory alterations. See Table 46–7 for laboratory indications of acid-base imbalances.

Acidosis

Acidosis, also referred to as **acidemia,** is a blood pH below 7.35.

Respiratory acidosis (carbonic acid excess) Respiratory acidosis occurs when exhalation of carbonic dioxide is inhibited, creating a carbonic acid excess in the body. Hypoventilation is its general cause. Two major conditions that cause hypoventilation are central nervous system depression and obstructive lung disease. Morphine poisoning and anesthesia are examples of central nervous system depression, whereas asthma and emphysema are obstructive lung diseases. Hypoventilation, whatever its cause, makes the body retain carbon dioxide and therefore carbonic acid. Thus, acidosis ensues.

Clinical signs

1. Hypoventilation evidenced by shallow respirations, poor exhalation, or respiratory embarrassment
2. Loss of mental alertness and disorientation progressing to stupor, indicating central nervous system depression

Laboratory findings

1. Low plasma pH (below 7.35) or a normal pH if compensated (compensation discussed subsequently)
2. Low urine pH (below 6)
3. High $Paco_2$ (above 45 mm Hg) (carbonic acid concentration measured as partial arterial pressure exerted by carbon dioxide)
4. Normal or high plasma bicarbonate (HCO_3^-)
   a. Above 28 mEq/L in adults
   b. Above 25 mEq/L in children
5. Base excess (BE) is 0 or positive (for example, +6) with chronic conditions that are compensated

Metabolic acidosis (base bicarbonate deficit) Metabolic acidosis occurs when levels of base bicarbonate are low in relation to carbonic acid blood levels. The kidneys normally retain bicarbonate (HCO_3^-) or excrete hydrogen ions (H^+) in response to altered blood pH. Starvation, renal impairment, and diabetes mellitus are among the conditions that deluge the plasma with acid metabolites. Prolonged diarrhea can decrease bicarbonate.

Clinical signs

1. **Kussmaul breathing** (deep rapid breathing), a compensatory mechanism, though absent in infants
2. Weakness
3. Disorientation
4. Coma

Table 46–7 Laboratory Indications of Acid-Base Imbalance

Sign	Normal	Interpretation
Plasma pH	7.35–7.45	Less than 7.35 → acidosis More than 7.45 → alkalosis
Urine pH	4.6–8.0	Below 6 → acidosis Above 7 → alkalosis
$Paco_2$	35–45 mm Hg	Less than 35 → respiratory alkalosis More than 45 → respiratory acidosis
Bicarbonate (HCO_3^-)	21–28 mEq/L (about 25 mEq/L)	Less than 21 → metabolic acidosis More than 28 → metabolic alkalosis
Base excess (BE)	Male: −3.3 to +1.2 Female: −2.4 to +2.3	Positive results → alkaline excess Negative results → alkaline deficit These values do not always indicate a state of acidosis or alkalosis but show deficits or excesses of base.
Pao_2	80 to 100 mm Hg	May be greater than 100 mm Hg if client is on oxygen and less than 75 if there is a pulmonary problem.

Laboratory findings

1. Low plasma pH (below 7.35) or a normal pH if compensated
2. Low urine pH (below 6)
3. Normal Pa_{CO_2} or low if compensated (an attempt by the lungs to blow off more acid)
4. Low plasma bicarbonate
   a. Below 21 mEq/L in adults
   b. Below 20 mEq/L in children
5. Base excess with negative results (for example, −6)
6. Hyperkalemia usually associated with metabolic acidosis

Alkalosis

Alkalosis, also referred to as **alkalemia,** is a blood pH above 7.45.

Respiratory alkalosis (carbonic acid deficit) Respiratory alkalosis occurs when exhalation of carbonic dioxide is excessive, resulting in a carbonic acid deficit. Its root cause is hyperventilation, which can be due to fever, anxiety, or pulmonary infections. Hyperventilation blows off abundant carbon dioxide, resulting in lowered carbonic acid blood levels.

Clinical signs

1. Hyperventilation (deep and/or rapid breathing)
2. Unconsciousness

Laboratory findings

1. High plasma pH (above 7.45)
2. High urine pH (above 7)
3. Low plasma bicarbonate as a compensatory measure (body compensation depends on the kidneys and is often slow)
   a. Below 21 mEq/L in adults
   b. Below 20 mEq/L in children
4. Low Pa_{CO_2} (below 35 mm Hg)
5. Base excess: 0

Metabolic alkalosis (bicarbonate excess) Metabolic alkalosis occurs when the level of base bicarbonate is high. Metabolic alkalosis may be due to excess intake of baking soda and other alkalis, prolonged vomiting, and other conditions that flood plasma with the bicarbonate anion. Prolonged vomiting causes the body to lose chloride (Cl^-) and hydrogen (H^+) ions. Loss of chloride ions causes an increase of bicarbonate in the blood.

Clinical signs

1. Depressed respiration (compensatory)
2. Hypertonic muscles
3. Tetany
4. Mental dullness

Laboratory findings

1. High plasma pH (above 7.45)
2. High urine pH (above 7)
3. High plasma bicarbonate
   a. Above 28 mEq/L in adults
   b. Above 25 mEq/L in children
4. Normal or high Pa_{CO_2} (above 45 mm Hg)—compensatory elevation
5. Base excess—positive results indicating an excess (for example, +8)
6. Low K^+

Compensation

In all acid-base imbalances, there is a corrective body response by both the kidneys and the lungs. Any given acid-base imbalance can be described as compensated until body reserves are used up. Then the condition is described as uncompensated.

In compensated acidosis or alkalosis, the kidneys and lungs are able to restore the altered ratio of 1 carbonic acid molecule to 20 bicarbonate ions, thereby maintaining a normal pH. In respiratory acidosis, the plasma pH is maintained at normal even though there is an increase in the Pa_{CO_2} (carbonic acid) because the kidneys retain bicarbonate.

When the plasma pH is not maintained, the condition is uncompensated. In uncompensated respiratory acidosis, there is an increase in the Pa_{CO_2} (carbonic acid), the pH is lower (more acid) than normal, and the kidneys can no longer retain enough bicarbonate. See Table 46–8 for an overview of fluid and electrolyte data.

Clinical Situations

When interpreting laboratory results, the nurse can find a systematic method helpful. To determine whether the client has acidosis or alkalosis, the nurse looks first at the plasma pH. If it is high or low, the interpretation is straightforward. However, if the pH of the plasma is normal, the client may still have a compensated acid-base imbalance. The nurse then needs to note the Pa_{CO_2}. Pa_{CO_2} values above or below normal indicate, respectively, a respiratory acidosis or alkalosis. If the Pa_{CO_2} is normal,

Table 46–8 Summary Data Regarding Fluid and Electrolytes

Clinical Factor	Body Normal	Predisposing Conditions	Deficit Symptoms	Excess Symptoms	Food Source
Extracellular fluid	Infant: 29% of body weight Adult: 15% of body weight	*Deficit:* Insufficient fluid intake, vomiting, diarrhea *Excess:* Excess administration or intake of fluid with NaCl	Weight loss, dry skin and mucous membrane, thirst, oliguria, low blood pressure, plasma pH above 7.45, urine pH above 7.0	Weight gain, edema, puffy eyelids, high blood pressure	Meats, fruits, vegetables, liquids
Bicarbonate (HCO_3^-)	Plasma bicarbonates 21–29 mEq/L, urine pH 4.6–8.0, plasma pH 7.35–7.45 (arterial blood)	*Deficit:* Uncontrolled diabetes mellitus, starvation, severe infectious disease, renal insufficiency *Excess:* Loss of Cl^- and H^+ through vomiting, gastric suction, hyperadrenalism, prolonged insertion of alkali	Metabolic acidosis, disorientation, weakness, shortness of breath, sweet fruity odor to breath, plasma pH below 7.35, HCO_3^- below 25 mEq/L	Metabolic alkalosis, slow and shallow respirations, tetany, hypertonic muscles, plasma pH above 7.45, HCO_3^- above 30 mEq/L	
Carbonic acid (H_2CO_3)	$Paco_2$ 35–45 mm Hg, plasma pH 7.35–7.45 (arterial blood)	*Deficit:* Oxygen lack, fever, anxiety, pulmonary infections, hyperventilation *Excess:* Hypoventilation, chronic asthma, emphysema, barbiturate poisoning	Respiratory alkalosis, deep and rapid breathing, unconsciousness, plasma pH above 7.45, low $Paco_2$	Respiratory acidosis, disorientation, shallow respirations, plasma pH below 7.35, high $Paco_2$	
Sodium (Na^+)	135–145 mEq/L (plasma)	*Deficit:* Excessive perspiration, gastrointestinal suction, diarrhea *Excess:* Inadequate water intake	Apprehension, abdominal cramps, rapid and weak pulse, oliguria, plasma sodium below 135 mEq/L	Dry and sticky mucous membranes, fever, thirst, firm rubbery tissue turgor, plasma sodium above 145 mEq/L	Table salt (NaCl), cheese, butter and margarine, processed meat (ham, bacon, pork), canned vegetables, vegetable juice
Potassium (K^+)	3.6–5.0 mEq/L (plasma)	*Deficit:* Diarrhea, vomiting, some kidney disease, diuretic therapy, increased stress *Excess:* Renal failure, burns, excessive administration	Muscle weakness, abnormal heart rhythm, anorexia, abdominal distention	Oliguria, intestinal colic, irritability, irregular pulse, diarrhea	Nuts, fruits, vegetables, poultry, fish
Calcium (Ca^{2+})	4.3–5.3 mEq/L (plasma)	*Deficit:* Removal of parathyroid glands, excessive loss of intestinal fluids, massive infections *Excess:* Overactive parathyroid gland, excessive ingestion of milk	Muscle cramps, tingling in the fingers, tetany, convulsions	Relaxed muscles, flank pain, kidney stones, deep bone pain	Dairy products, meat, fish, poultry, whole grain cereals, greens, beans

Table 46–8 *(continued)*

Clinical Factor	Body Normal	Predisposing Conditions	Deficit Symptoms	Excess Symptoms	Food Source
Chloride (Cl^-)	98–108 mEq/L	*Deficit:* Increased HCO_3^-, loss through vomiting, excessive ECF loss through intestinal fistula *Excess:* Increased Na^+, excessive fluid loss through kidneys, severe dehydration	*See* sodium	*See* sodium	Table salt, dairy products, meat

the nurse needs to look at the plasma bicarbonate level. An elevation of this value indicates a metabolic alkalosis, whereas a deficit indicates a metabolic acidosis. The nurse also needs to be aware that chronic disease conditions are usually compensated. Therefore the $PaCO_2$ and bicarbonate values may be altered accordingly. Examples follow:

Problem 1. Respiratory acidosis

Acute

pH = 7.25	(low)
$PaCO_2$ = 60 mm Hg	(high)
HCO_3^-) = 25 mEq/L	(normal)
Base excess (BE) = 0	(normal)
PaO_2 = 60 mm Hg	(low)

Chronic (compensated)

pH = 7.36	(normal)
$PaCO_2$ = 70 mm Hg	(high)
HCO_3^-) = 32 mEq/L	(high)
BE = +7	(excess)
PaO_2 = 80 mm Hg	(normal)

Problem 2. Metabolic acidosis

Acute

pH = 7.30	(low)
$PaCO_2$ = 40 mm Hg	(normal)
HCO_3^-) = 19 mEq/L	(low)
BE = −6	(deficit)
PaO_2 = 75 mm Hg	(low)

Chronic (compensated)

pH = 7.38	(normal)
$PaCO_2$ = 31 mm Hg	(low)
HCO_3^-) = 18 mEq/L	(low)
BE = −6	(deficit)
PaO_2 = 80 mm Hg	(normal)

Problem 3. Respiratory alkalosis

Acute

pH = 7.52	(high)
$PaCO_2$ = 31 mm Hg	(low)
HCO_3^-) = 25 mEq/L	(normal)
BE = 0	(normal)

Problem 4. Metabolic alkalosis

Acute

pH = 7.50	(high)
$PaCO_2$ = 40 mm Hg	(normal)
HCO_3^-) = 31 mEq/L	(high)
BE = +8	(excess)

Factors Affecting Fluid and Electrolyte Balance

Age

Fluid intake requirements vary with age. Intake requirements have been determined for various ages in relation to body surface area, metabolic requirements, and body weight.

Infants and growing children have much greater fluid turnover than adults, i.e., greater water needs and greater water losses. This is due to their greater metabolic rate, which increases fluid loss through the kidneys. Because immature kidneys are less efficient than adult kidneys, infants lose more fluid through the kidneys. Infant losses from both the lungs and the skin are also greater in proportion to body weight, essentially because respirations are more rapid and the body surface area is proportionately greater. The more rapid turnover of fluid plus the losses produced by disease can create critical fluid imbalances in children much more rapidly than in adults. See Table 46–5, earlier, for approximate fluid requirements at different ages according to body weight.

In elderly people, fluid and electrolyte imbalances are often associated with kidney or cardiac problems. Because the kidneys are less able to concentrate urine, the elderly person may need to take in additional fluid to meet his or her fluid needs. Whereas water comprises 60% of the body weight of young males, it comprises only 52% of the body weight of elderly males and 46% of the body weight of elderly females (Metheny and Snively 1983, p. 371).

Environmental Temperature

Excessive heat stimulates the sympathetic nervous system and causes the person to sweat. When the person is not acclimatized to the heat, the sweat glands are strongly stimulated, and he or she can lose as much as 700 ml to 2 liters per hour by sweating. The sodium chloride (NaCl) in the sweat is also lost. An unacclimatized person can lose as much as 15 to 30 g of salt each day (Guyton 1986, p. 853).

Diet

A person's diet obviously affects the intake of fluids and electrolytes. When nutritional intake is inadequate or unbalanced, the body tries to preserve stored protein by breaking down glycogen and fat. Once these resources are gone, the body draws on protein stores, and the serum albumin level decreases. Serum albumin plays an important role in drawing fluid from the interstitial body compartment into the blood through osmosis. When fluid is not drawn normally into the bloodstream, it remains in the interstitial space, causing edema.

Stress

Stress affects a person's fluid and electrolyte balance. Stress can increase cellular metabolism, blood glucose concentration, and muscle glycolysis. These mechanisms can lead to sodium and water retention. In addition, stress can increase production of the antidiuretic hormone, which in turn decreases urine production. The overall response of the body to stress is to increase the blood volume. See Chapter 17, page 339, for additional information.

Illness

Extensive surgical procedures can change a person's fluid and electrolyte balance through a number of mechanisms. The stress response mentioned above is one of these. In addition, tissue trauma can cause the loss of fluid and electrolytes from within the damaged cells. An example of such trauma is severe burns. The burned person loses plasma and interstitial fluid as exudate. (An **exudate** is material that has escaped from the blood vessels and is deposited in the tissues or on the tissue surfaces.) Also, water vapor is lost from the burn site, blood leaks from damaged capillaries, and water and sodium move into the tissue cells (Metheny and Snively 1983, pp. 204–5).

Cardiac and renal disorders also affect the body's fluid and electrolyte balance. For example, impaired heart function can decrease blood flow to the kidneys and thus hinder the elimination of the waste products of metabolism. When urine output decreases, the body retains sodium, and circulatory overload (hypervolemia) can result. Fluid retention can also lead to pulmonary edema (fluid in the lungs).

Assessment

To assess a client's fluid and electrolyte balance, the nurse takes a nursing history, performs a physical examination, and refers to data in laboratory reports.

Nursing History

A client's nursing history should include data about elimination patterns (see Chapters 43 and 44), oxygenation (see Chapter 45), and food and fluid intake (see Chapter 42).

In addition, data specifically relative to fluid and electrolyte balance should be gathered. See list to the right.

Nursing History Data About Fluid and Electrolyte Balance

- Amount, type, and frequency of fluid intake
- Recent changes in health, e.g., draining wound
- Medications
- Dietary restrictions
- Health problems that affect fluid or electrolyte balance, e.g., vomiting

Physical Examination

The client is examined for clinical signs of fluid, electrolyte, and acid-base imbalances. The nurse needs a knowledge of significant signs as well as the normal clinical picture presented by the client. Specific assessments should include body weight and assessment of each body system where potential or actual problems exist. Tables 46–7 and 46–8, earlier, describe some common clinical signs of fluid, electrolyte, and acid-base imbalances. For information on the assessment of urine, see Chapter 44, page 1242.

The well-hydrated person shows the following signs:

1. Stable weight from day to day
2. Moist mucous membranes
3. An appropriate food intake
4. Straw-colored urine with a specific gravity of 1.010 to 1.030
5. Good tissue turgor
6. Mental orientation
7. No complaint of thirst
8. An appropriate amount of excreted urine in relation to fluid intake
9. No evidence of edema
10. No evidence of dehydration, such as depressed periorbital spaces

Laboratory Reports

Electrolyte Levels

Serum electrolyte levels are frequently tested to determine the acid-base and electrolyte balance of the body fluids. The most commonly ordered serum tests are for sodium, potassium, carbon dioxide (bicarbonate), and chloride. Serum sodium and potassium tests are done to determine changes in fluid and sodium balances in clients who have fluid imbalances, have endocrine disorders, or are receiving intravenous infusions with electrolytes. Variations in the serum chloride level usually occur with changes in sodium level. Elevated serum chloride is found in such disorders as prostatic obstruction and renal failure. Decreased chloride levels may be found in clients with congestive heart failure or burns.

The carbon dioxide content of plasma reflects the body's ability to control acid-base balance. The total carbon dioxide content of the blood consists of: dissolved carbon dioxide gas (CO_2), carbonic acid (HCO_3) and bicarbonate ions (HCO_3^-). In the past, carbon dioxide content was determined in terms of carbon dioxide combining power—that is, the amount of CO_2 gas that could

Research Note

Nurses must often make critical assessments as to the fluid status of their clients, particularly after surgery, or in cases of trauma or sepsis. A group of investigators studied 50 clients who had become hypovolemic, either with or without shock. By infusing 100 ml of colloid solution every 10 minutes up to at least 500 ml total, the researchers could carefully observe the cardiac and fluid status of each client and avoid overloading the heart or lungs.

The group of clients whose hearts were functioning poorly did not benefit from the fluid infusion and in many cases became worse. The group with adequate heart performance improved on such indices as urine output, mental alertness, warmth of extremities, and O_2 saturation of the blood. Volume loading with colloid solution is somewhat controversial but, according to these authors, is highly desirable with certain clients if this particular protocol is utilized. (Howard et al. 1984)

be absorbed by a specimen of plasma. However, it is now thought that this measure is not accurate because the CO_2 is combined at a constant pressure of 40 mm Hg rather than at the varying pressures that exist in the client (Byrne et al. 1986, p. 260). Therefore, this test is being replaced by tests such as the bicarbonate ion concentration test. A normal plasma bicarbonate level is 21 to 28 mEq/liter.

Acid-Base Balance

Tests normally carried out to determine acid-base balance are called blood-gas determinations and routinely include: blood pH, $Paco_2$ (carbonic acid concentration), total CO_2 (bicarbonate ion plus carbonic acid), Pao_2, and O_2 saturation. Specimens of arterial blood are taken for these tests.

The pH is a measure of the concentration of hydrogen ions, indicating the blood's acidity or alkalinity. Normally, arterial blood has a pH of 7.35 to 7.45. Any variation from normal can reflect a problem in the bicarbonate and carbonic acid buffer system.

The $Paco_2$ is a measure of the pressure exerted by carbon dioxide gas dissolved in the blood. The Pa stands for partial arterial pressure—here, the pressure exerted by CO_2 in the arterial blood. This pressure is regulated by the lungs and reflects the amount of carbonic acid available to the bicarbonate and carbonic acid buffer system. A normal $Paco_2$ is 35 to 45 mm Hg.

Total CO_2 content is the measure of both the bicarbonate ion and carbonic acid in the blood. The total CO_2 measure provides an accurate guide to the functioning of the bicarbonate and carbonic acid buffer system. The combined measurement in arterial blood is normally 21 to 30 mEq/liter.

Partial pressure of oxygen (PaO_2) is the pressure exerted by the small amount of oxygen that is dissolved in the plasma. This oxygen is separate from the oxygen carried by the hemoglobin of the erythrocytes. Normal values of PaO_2 are 80 to 100 mm Hg in arterial blood.

Oxygen saturation (O_2 Sat) is the ratio of the oxygen in the blood to the maximum amount of oxygen the blood can carry. Normal values are 95% to 98% in arterial blood and 60% and 85% in venous blood. Oxygen saturation provides some indication of the functioning of the client's lung ventilation.

Nursing Diagnosis

Examples of nursing diagnoses for clients who have fluid and electrolyte disturbances are given to the right.

Examples of Nursing Diagnoses Related to Fluid and Electrolyte Problems

- Fluid volume deficit related to inability to swallow
- Fluid volume deficit related to diarrhea
- Fluid volume deficit related to depression
- Fluid volume excess: edema related to decreased cardiac output
- Fluid volume excess related to excessive intake of fluid intravenously

Planning

When planning interventions for a client who has fluid and electrolyte imbalances, nurses should consider the following:

1. Monitoring fluid intake and output
2. Correcting fluid and/or electrolyte imbalance
3. Maintaining fluid and/or electrolyte balance
4. Preventing problems as a result of imbalances or therapy

For outcome criteria, see the section on evaluation later in this chapter.

Intervention

Fluid Intake and Output

Clients who have actual or potential fluid and/or electrolyte imbalances need to have their fluid intake and output monitored. The following clients are commonly monitored in this way:

1. Postoperative clients
2. Clients who are permitted nothing by mouth (NPO) and have intravenous infusions
3. Clients who have retention catheters and urinary drainage systems
4. Clients who have special drainages or suctions, such as a nasogastric suction
5. Clients receiving diuretics
6. Clients who have excessive fluid losses and require increased intake
7. Clients who retain fluids and whose intake may need to be restricted
8. Clients who may not be taking in the fluids they need, e.g., the elderly

Units of Measurement

The unit used to measure intake and output (I & O) is the milliliter (ml) or cubic centimeter (cc); these are equivalent metric units of measurement. In household measures, 30 ml is roughly equivalent to 1 fluid ounce, 500 ml is about 1 pint, and 1000 ml is about 1 quart. To measure fluid intake, nurses must convert household measures such as a glass, cup, or soup bowl to metric units. Most agencies provide conversion tables, since the sizes of dishes vary from agency to agency. A table is often provided on or with the bedside I & O record. Examples of equivalents are given to the right.

Intake and Output Forms

Most agencies have a form for recording I & O, usually a bedside record on which the nurse lists all items measured and their quantities per shift (see Figure 30–7 on page 643). Some agencies have another form for recording the specifics of intravenous fluids, such as the type of solution, additives, time started, amounts absorbed, and amounts remaining per shift.

Commonly Used Fluid Containers and Their Volumes

Water glass	200 ml
Juice glass	120 ml
Cup	180 ml
Soup bowl	
Adult	180 ml
Child	100 ml
Teapot	240 ml
Creamer	
Large	90 ml
Small	30 ml
Water pitcher	1000 ml
Jello, custard dish	100 ml
Ice cream dish	120 ml
Paper cup	
Large	200 ml
Small	120 ml

Procedure 46–1 ▲ Measuring Fluid Intake and Output

Equipment

1. A bedside I & O form and a pencil
2. A bedside bedpan, commode, or urinal
3. A calibrated container in which to measure the urine

Intervention

1. Explain to the client that an accurate measurement of his or her fluid intake and output is required. Explain the reason for it, and the need to use a bedpan or urinal (unless a urinary drainage system is in place). Many clients wish to be involved in recording these measurements and need to be given further information about how to compute the values and what foods are considered fluids.
2. Establish with the client a plan for ingesting the required amount of fluid. Generally, half the total volume is ingested during the day shift, and the other half is divided between the evening and night shifts, with the majority on the evening shift.

To Measure Fluid Intake

3. Following meals, record on the I & O form the amount of each fluid item taken, if the client has not already done so. Specify the kind of fluid and the time. Measure all obvious fluids, such as water, milk, juice, soft drinks, coffee, tea, cream, soup, sherry, and wine. Also include such foods as ice cream, sherbet, custard, and gelatin (Jello). Do *not* measure foods that are pureed.

   Rationale Purees are simply solid foods prepared in a different form.
4. Ascertain if the client ingested any other fluids between meals, and add the amounts to the form. Include water that is taken with medications. To assess the amount of water used from a water pitcher, measure what remains and subtract this amount from the volume of the full pitcher. Then refill the pitcher.
5. Total the measurements at the end of the shift (every 8 or 12 hours), and place these totals on the client's record. Include the total volumes of intravenous fluids, including blood transfusions. In some critical care settings, you may need to record intake hourly.

To Measure Fluid Output

6. Following each voiding, pour the urine into the measuring container, observe the amount, and record it and the time of voiding on the bedside I & O form. Clean the bedpan and measuring container, and return the bedpan to the client.

7. For clients with retention catheters, note and record the amount of urine at the end of the shift, and then empty the drainage bag. Drainage bags are usually calibrated to indicate the amount of urine. If there is any doubt about the amount in the drainage bag, empty it into an accurate measuring container.

8. Record any other output, such as emesis, liquid feces, and other drainage. Specify the type of fluid and the time.

9. If the client is incontinent of urine or is extremely diaphoretic, estimate and record these outputs. For example, of an incontinent client you might record "Incontinent × 3," or "Drawsheet soaked in 12-in diameter." Of a diaphoretic client you might record "Perspiring profusely [or + + +]. Gown and drawsheet changed × 2." Follow agency practices in this regard.

10. At the end of the shift (every 8 to 12 hours), total the measurements, and transfer the totals to the correct column on the permanent record. In some critical care units, you may need to total the fluid measurements hourly.

11. Compare the total fluid output measurement with the total fluid intake measurement to previous measurements.

    Rationale Determine whether the fluid output is proportional to fluid intake. Note any changes in fluid balance.

12. Observe the client for signs of dehydration or overhydration. Weigh the client daily, if indicated. See Chapter 35, page 807.

13. Report to the responsible nurse inadequate intakes and outputs. In an adult, urine output of less than 500 ml in 24 hours is considered inadequate.

14. Adjust the nursing care plan as needed to ensure appropriate fluid intake for the client and appropriate measurement of I & O.

Providing Fluids and Electrolytes Orally

When the client's health permits, fluid and electrolytes may be replaced orally. Some clients may need to drink a large volume of fluid, e.g., over 3000 ml daily. For others, oral intake may be restricted. Fluid restrictions vary from "nothing by mouth" to a precise amount ordered by a physician. In addition, a client may be limited to only fluids or only clear fluids. See Chapter 42, page 1179. It is important that the client and support persons understand the fluid requirements and the reasons for them so that the client does not mistakenly take fluids that are not permitted.

Electrolytes can often be provided orally through food and fluids. Potassium commonly needs to be supplemented. See Table 46–9 for foods high in specific electrolytes. Nurses can often help clients by giving them a list of foods and fluids high in the electrolyte they require. See Chapter 42 on page 1155 for foods high in calcium.

Intravenous Therapy

Fluid therapy can also be administered by nasogastric tube or by the **parenteral** routes (not through the alimentary canal) of intravenous infusion or subcutaneous infusion (**hypodermoclysis**). Nasogastric feedings are discussed in Chapter 42.

Intravenous (IV) fluid therapy is a common practice today. It is an efficient and effective method of supplying fluids directly into the extracellular fluid compartment, specifically the venous system. Hypodermoclysis is not as commonly used, but it is useful in the very young or elderly person whose veins are too small or difficult to enter. Parenteral fluid therapy is ordered by the physician. The nurse is responsible for administering and maintaining the therapy.

Purposes of Intravenous Therapy

1. To supply fluid when clients are unable to take in an adequate volume of fluids by mouth
2. To provide salts needed to maintain electrolyte balance
3. To provide glucose (dextrose), the main fuel for metabolism

Table 46–9 Major Food Sources of Selected Electrolytes

Electrolyte	Sources
Sodium (Na)	Table salt, cheese, ham, processed meats, canned foods, fish
Potassium (K)	Dark leafy greens, bananas, oranges, nuts, meat, fish, liver
Calcium (Ca)	Milk, cheese, yogurt
Magnesium (Mg)	Nuts, peanut butter, whole grains
Phosphorus (P)	Milk, poultry, fish, cereals

4. To provide water-soluble vitamins and medications
5. To promote a lifeline for rapidly needed medications

Common Types of IV Solutions

Common IV solutions include nutrient solutions, electrolyte solutions, alkalizing and acidifying solutions, and blood volume expanders.

Nutrient solutions Nutrient solutions contain some form of carbohydrate (e.g., dextrose, glucose, or levulose) and water. Water is supplied for fluid requirements and carbohydrate for calories and energy. For example, 1 liter of 5% dextrose provides 170 calories. Common nutrient solutions are:

1. 5% dextrose in water (D5W)
2. 3.3% glucose in 0.3% sodium chloride (NaCl) (glucose in saline)
3. 5% dextrose in 0.45% sodium chloride (dextrose in half-strength saline)

Nutrient solutions are useful in preventing dehydration and ketosis but do not provide sufficient calories to promote wound healing, weight gain, or normal growth in children.

Electrolyte solutions Electrolyte solutions are either saline (NaCl) or multiple electrolyte solutions containing varying amounts of cations and anions. Commonly used solutions are:

1. Normal saline (0.9% sodium chloride solution).
2. Ringer's solution, which contains sodium (Na^+), chloride (Cl^-), potassium (K^+), and calcium (Ca^{2+}).
3. Lactated Ringer's solution, which contains sodium, chloride, potassium, calcium, and lactate. Lactate is a salt of lactic acid that is metabolized in the liver to form bicarbonate (HCO_3^-).

Normal saline solutions are frequently used as initial hydrating solutions. Multiple electroltye solutions approximate the ionic profile of plasma and are used to prevent dehydration or to restore or correct fluid and electrolyte imbalances.

Alkalizing and acidifying solutions Alkalizing solutions are administered to counteract metabolic acidosis. One commonly used solution is lactated Ringer's solution. Acidifying solutions, in contrast, are administered to counteract metabolic alkalosis. Examples of acidifying solutions are 5% dextrose in 0.45% sodium chloride, and 0.9% sodium chloride solution.

The body fluids are normally maintained within a precise pH range of 7.35 to 7.45. This state is slightly alkaline. However, conditions such as prolonged diarrhea, starvation, or renal impairment can cause metabolic acidosis. Metabolic alkalosis can occur with prolonged vomiting and other conditions that result in an excessive amount of bicarbonate ions in the bloodstream.

Blood volume expanders Blood volume expanders are used to increase the volume of blood following severe loss of blood (e.g., from hemorrhage) or plasma (e.g., from severe burns, which draw large amounts of plasma from the bloodstream to the burn site). Common blood volume expanders are:

1. Dextran
2. Plasma
3. Human serum albumin

Venipuncture Sites

The site chosen for venipuncture varies with the client's age, the infusion time, the type of solution used, and the condition of the veins. For adults, veins in the arm are commonly used; for infants, veins in the scalp are used. The larger veins of the forearm are preferred to the meta carpal veins of the hand for infusions that need to be given rapidly and for solutions that are hypertonic, are highly acidic or alkaline, or contain irritating medications.

Adults The most convenient veins for venipuncture in the adult are the basilic and median cubital veins in the crease of the elbow (antecubital space). See Figure 46–3. Laboratory technicians often withdraw blood for examination from these large superficial veins. Unfortunately, use of these veins for prolonged infusions limits arm mobility, because a splint is needed to stabilize the elbow joint. For prolonged therapy, veins on the back of the hand and on the forearm are preferred. The metacarpal, basilic, and cephalic veins are commonly used. The ulna and radius act as natural splints at these sites, and the client has greater freedom of arm movement for activities such as eating.

Ideally, for long-term therapy, sites at the distal end of the arm should be used first. If these veins have been used for prolonged periods or have developed thrombi, other more proximal sites may be used. If arm veins are inaccessible, veins in the feet and legs may be used, although they are more prone to thrombus formation and subsequent emboli.

Infants Because infants do not have large veins in the antecubital fossa, blood specimens for examination are usually taken from the external jugular vein and femoral veins. If an infusion is to be maintained for a long period, veins in the temporal region of the scalp, or sometimes the back of the hand or the dorsum of the foot, are used.

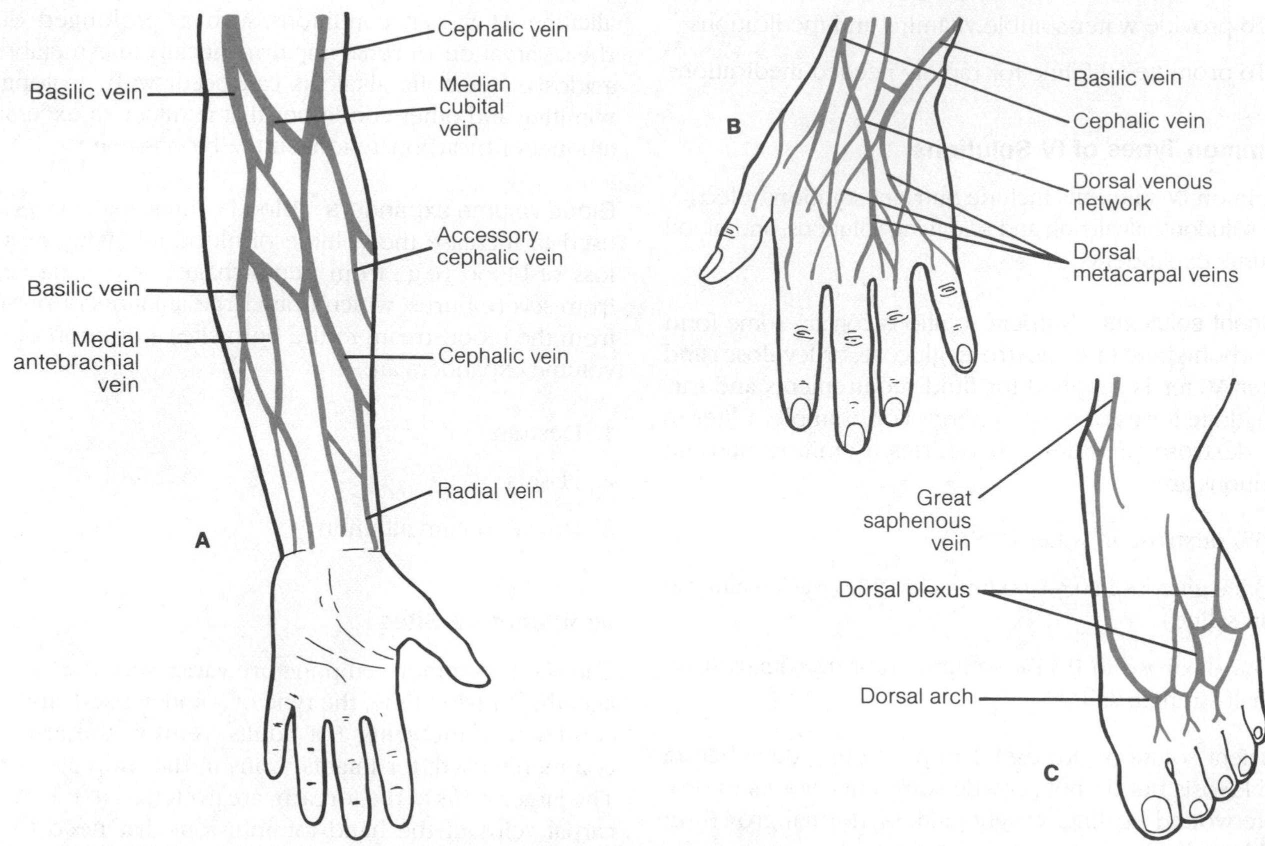

Figure 46–3 Commonly used venipuncture sites of the **A,** arm; **B,** hand; **C,** foot

Procedure 46–2 ▲ Setting Up an Intravenous Infusion

Equipment

1. The container(s) of sterile intravenous solution. See Figure 46–4.
   a. Select the size ordered. Do not select containers with greater volumes than ordered. For example, if 750 ml 5% D/NS (750 ml of 5% dextrose in normal saline) has been ordered, obtain one 500-ml container and one 250-ml container, which total 750 ml. Do not obtain a 1000-ml container with the intention of stopping the solution after 750 ml has been administered. Too often the incorrect amount can be instilled. If a 1000-ml solution container *must* be used, remove 250 ml before starting the IV.
   b. Some solution bottles have a tube inside the bottle that serves as an air vent so that, as the solution runs out of the bottle, it is replaced with air. See Figure 46–5. Containers without air vents require a vent on the administration set. See Figure 46–6. Air vents usually have filters to remove any contamination from the air that enters the container.
2. An administration set, consisting of an insertion spike, a drip chamber, a roller valve or screw clamp, tubing, and a protective cap over the needle adapter. See Figure 46–7. The insertion spike is kept sterile and inserted into the solution container when the IV is set up and ready to start. The drip chamber permits a predictable amount of fluid to be delivered. A commonly used drip chamber is the macrodrip, which provides 10 to 20 drops per ml of solution. This information will be on the package. There are also microdrip sets, which provide 60 drops per ml of solution. The roller valve or screw clamp is used to control the rate of flow of the solution by compressing the lumen of the tubing. The protective cap over the needle adapter maintains the sterility of the end of the tubing so that it can be attached to a sterile needle inserted in the client's vein.
3. IV poles (rods) for hanging the solution container. Some poles are attached to hospital beds. Others stand on the floor or hang from the ceiling. There are floor models with casters that can be pushed along when

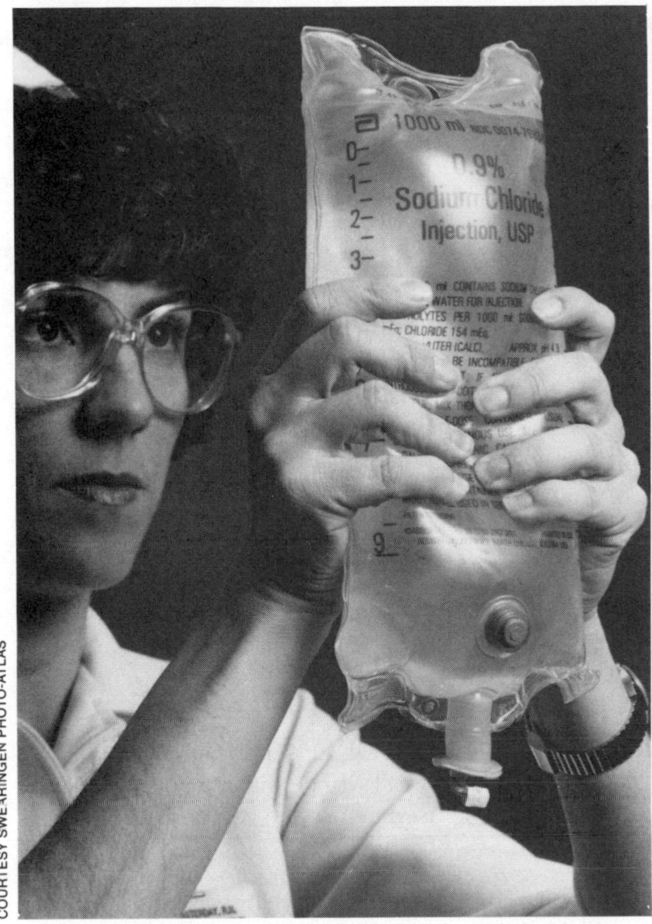

COURTESY SWEARINGEN PHOTO-ATLAS

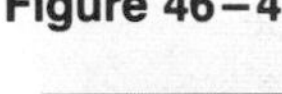

Figure 46–4

Figure 46–6

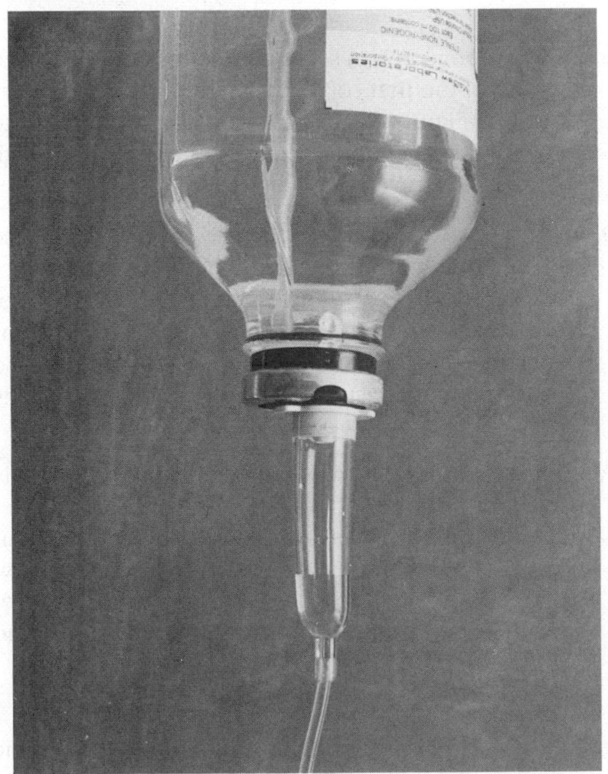

Figure 46–5

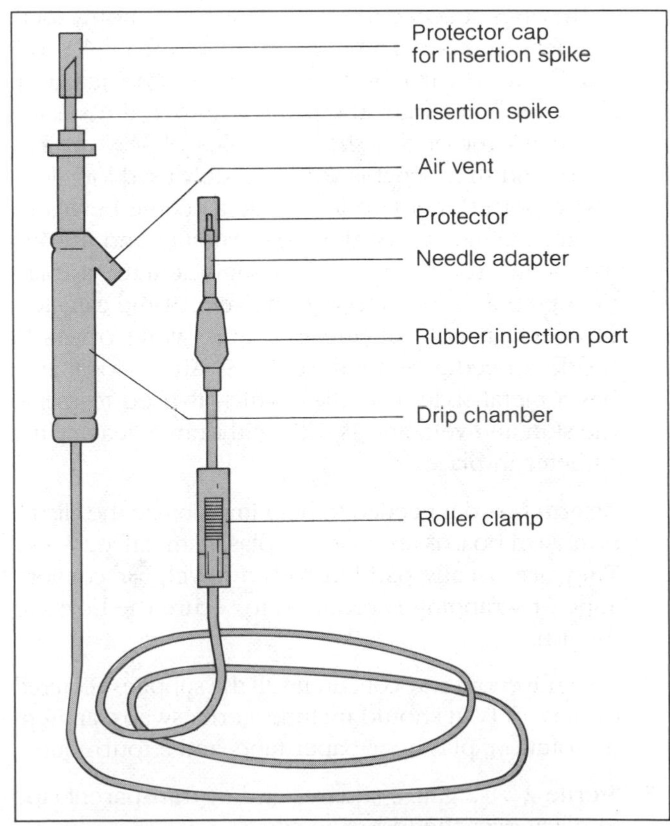

Figure 46–7

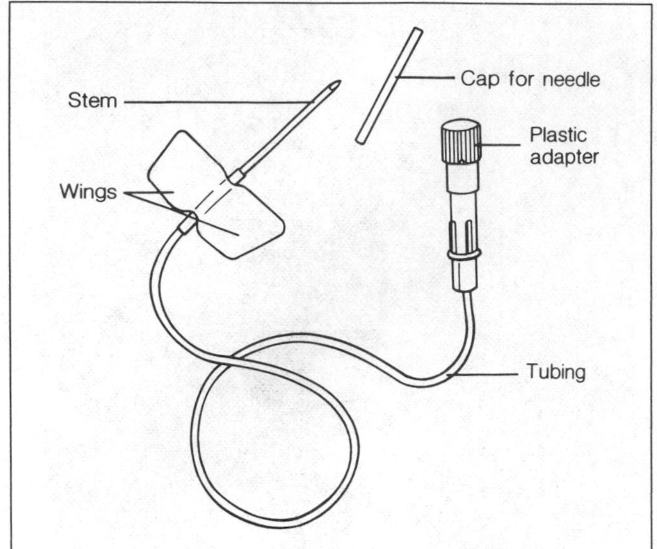

Figure 46–8

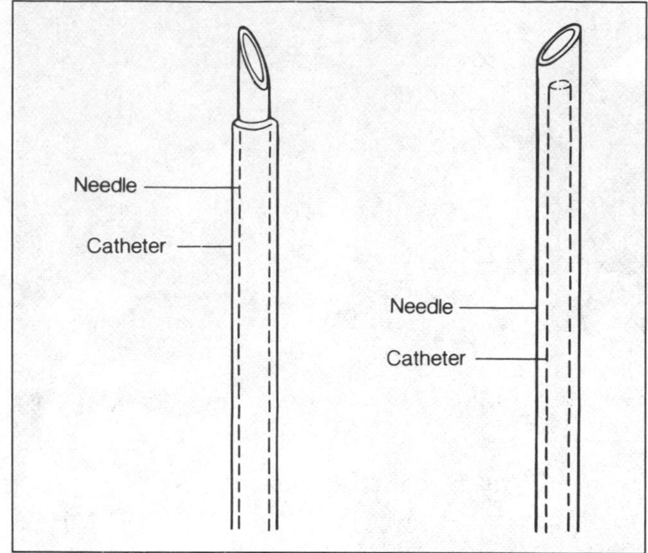

Figure 46–9

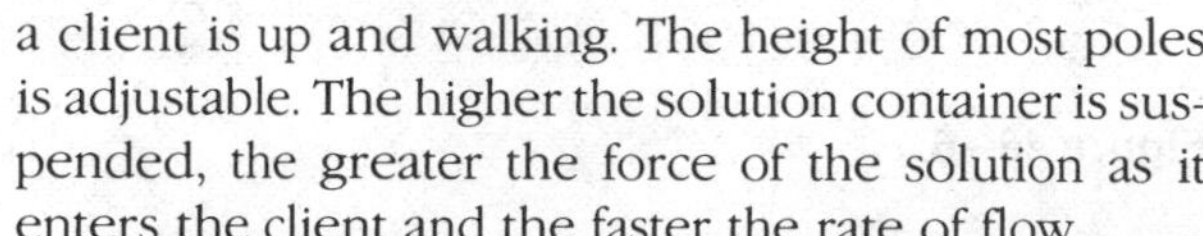

a client is up and walking. The height of most poles is adjustable. The higher the solution container is suspended, the greater the force of the solution as it enters the client and the faster the rate of flow.

4. An intravenous needle or catheter. These are usually packaged separately. Butterfly or wing-tipped needles, with wings attached to the shaft, are commonly used. See Figure 46–8. They vary in length from 1.5 to 3 cm (½ to 1¼ in), and from #25 to #17 gauge in diameter. The larger the gauge number, the smaller the diameter of the shaft. Needles of #20 to #22 gauge and short lengths are commonly used for adults. Some practitioners prefer to use a needle bevel that is short, to minimize injury to the tissues and discomfort on insertion. A catheter or angiocatheter is a plastic tube that is inserted into the vein. Some catheters fit over a needle during insertion, while others fit inside a needle. See Figure 46–9. An angiocatheter has a metal stylet (needle), which is used to pierce the skin and vein and is then withdrawn, leaving the catheter in place.
5. An arm board if needed to help immobilize the client's arm. Arm boards are made of plastic, metal, or wood. They are usually padded with a towel, for comfort. Tape or wrapping is required to secure the board to the arm.
6. An intravenous tray containing all the supplies required to start an IV. It should include sterile swabs, antiseptic solution, plastic or paper tape, and a tourniquet.
7. Sterile 2 × 2 gauze squares and/or transparent tape to place over the insertion site.
8. A local anesthetic, e.g., 1% lidocaine without epinephrine, and a small syringe with a #27 gauge needle, if this is to be used before the venipuncture.

Additional equipment is required for variations from the standard infusion. Secondary sets are required when more than one solution is running at the same time.

9. In a tandem setup, a second container is attached to the line of the first container at the lower, secondary port. See Figure 46–10, *A*. It permits medications to be administered intermittently or simultaneously with the first solution.
10. In the piggyback alignment, a second set connects the second container to the tubing of the first at the upper port. This setup is used solely for intermittent drug administration. See Figure 46–10, *B*. Various manufacturers describe these sets differently, so check the manufacturer's labeling and directions carefully.
11. Another variation is a volume-control set, which is used if the volume of fluid administered is to be carefully controlled. The set is attached below the solution container, and the drip chamber is placed below it. See Figure 46–11. Volume control sets are frequently used in pediatric settings, where the volume administered is critical.

Agencies have different policies about when to take the equipment to the bedside prior to starting an intravenous

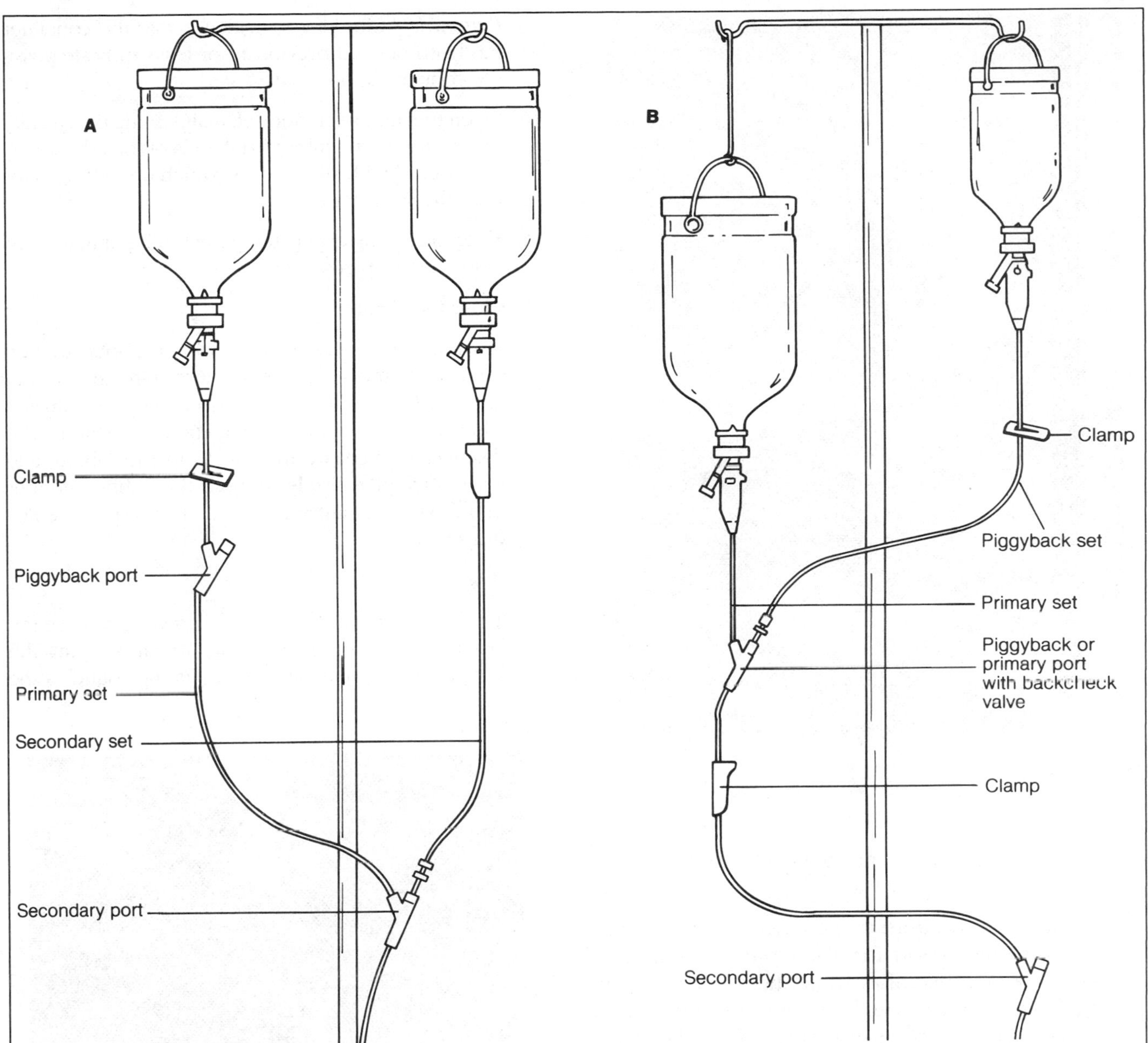

Figure 46–10 Secondary intravenous lines: **A**, a tandem intravenous alignment; and **B**, a piggyback intravenous alignment.

infusion. Normally it is not taken to the bedside in advance if it will produce anxiety in the client.

Intervention

1. Check the client's record for the physician's order indicating the type of solution, the amount to be administered, and the rate of flow of the infusion.
2. Determine the types of solutions used by the agency and the container sizes that are available. Intravenous solutions are supplied in 150-ml, 250-ml, 500-ml, and 1000-ml sizes. Some agencies use abbreviations to describe commonly used solutions, e.g., DW (distilled water), NS (normal saline), D5W (5% dextrose in water), D5NS (5% dextrose in normal saline). Check the abbreviations used by the agency.
3. Check the order for any special equipment required, e.g., a microdrip set is usually required if the fluid is to be administered at a rate of 50 to 75 ml/hr or less, for accurate regulation.
4. Determine the agency practice or the physician's order about the type of needle or catheter to be used for intravenous infusions.
5. Determine what equipment is contained in an intravenous set. Some agencies have special trays for use by personnel who start infusions. These are normally

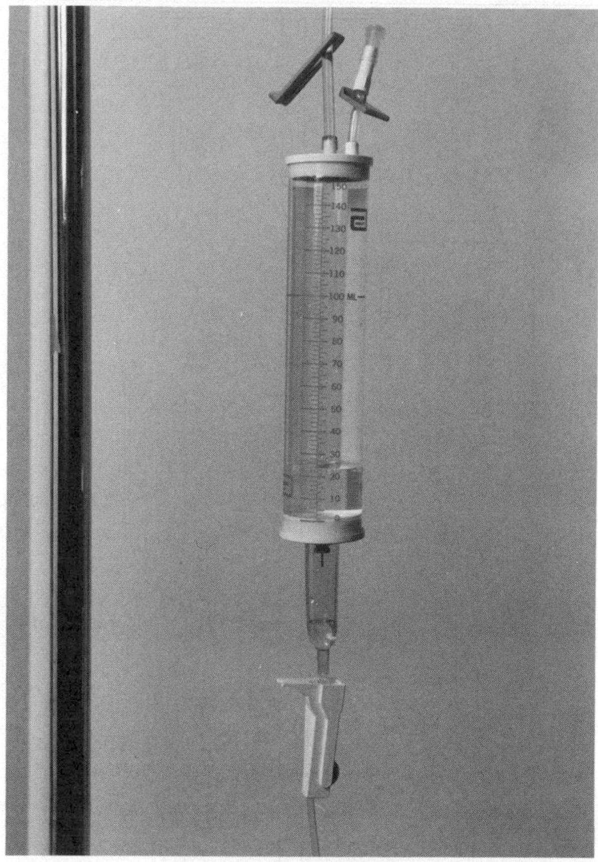

Figure 46–11

kept in a central place and taken to the bedside when the infusion is to be started.

6. Explain the procedure to the client. A venipuncture can cause discomfort for a few seconds, but there should be no discomfort while the solution is flowing. Clients often want to know how long the process will last. The physician's order may specify the length of time of the infusion, e.g., 3000 ml over 24 hours.
7. Provide any scheduled care before establishing the IV, to minimize movement of the affected limb during the procedure, since moving the limb after the IV is established could dislodge the needle.
8. Make sure that the client's gown can be removed over the IV apparatus if necessary. Some agencies provide special gowns that open over the shoulder and down the sleeve for easy removal.
9. Determine that the solution is sterile and in good condition, i.e., clear. Check the expiration date on the label. Examine the other packages to confirm their sterility. Squeeze a plastic solution bag and inspect it for leaks or hairline cracks. Return any unsatisfactory container to the central supply or distributing department, indicating the reason for the return.

   Rationale Cloudiness, evidence that the container has been opened previously, or leaks indicate possible contamination.
10. Open the administration set, maintaining the sterility of the ends of the tubing. The ends of the tubing may be covered with plastic caps, which are left in place until the IV is started.
11. Slide the tubing clamp along the tubing until it is just below the drip chamber.
12. Close the clamp.
13. If using an intravenous bottle with a rubber stopper, remove the metal disc while maintaining the sterility of the stopper. If the stopper becomes contaminated while you are removing the metal disc, swab it with disinfectant. Remove the cap from the tubing, and insert the spike firmly through the rubber stopper into the port, maintaining sterile technique. See Figure 46–12.

    or

    If using a bottle with an indwelling vent, remove the metal disc and the rubber diaphragm, keeping the stopper sterile, and listen for a hissing sound as the

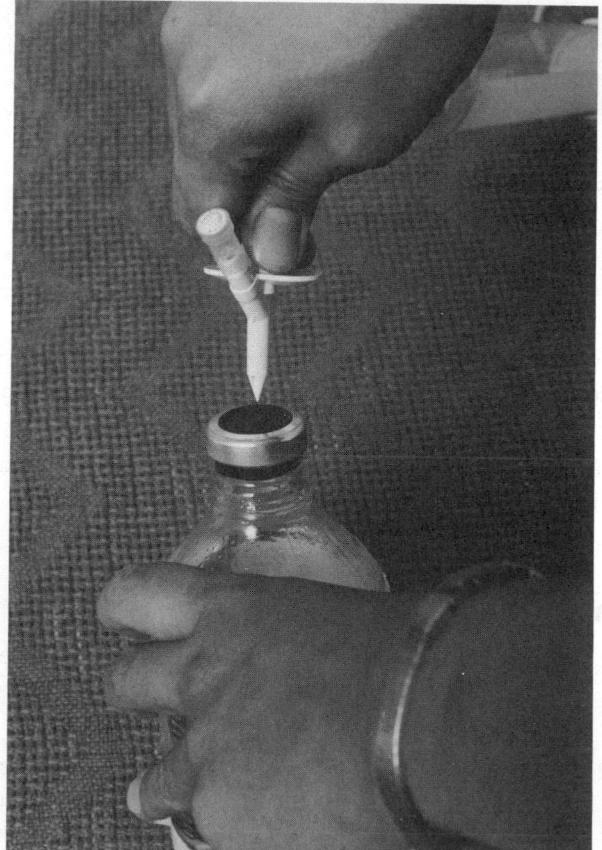

Figure 46–12

air rushes into the bottle. If there is no hissing sound, discard the container because it was probably not sealed. Insert the spike into the larger hole (the one without the vent.)

or

For spiking a plastic bag, read the manufacturer's directions. Some bags are hung on the pole before spiking.

14. Hang the solution container on the pole, usually about 1 m (3 ft) above the client's head.

    Rationale This height is needed to enable gravity to overcome venous pressure and facilitate flow of the solution into the vein.

15. If using a flexible drip chamber, squeeze it gently until it is half full of solution. See Figure 46–13.

    or

    If the drip chamber is firm, it will usually fill automatically.

    Rationale The drip chamber is partly filled with solution to prevent air from moving down the tubing.

16. To prime the tubing, remove the protective cap, and hold the tubing over a cup or basin. Maintain the sterility of the end of the tubing and the cap. Release the clamp and let the fluid run through the tubing until all bubbles are removed. Tap the tubing with your fingers to help the bubbles move.

    Rationale The tubing is primed to prevent the introduction of air into the client, because air bubbles can act as emboli in the bloodstream.

17. Reclamp the tubing.

18. Replace the tubing cap, maintaining sterile technique.

19. Label the solution container, applying the label upside down on the container. Include the following information: the client's name, identification number, room, and/or bed number; any medication and dosage; the drip rate; the date and the time the container is started; the container number; and the name of the person starting it. See Figure 46–14. Labeling may be done when the IV is started.

    Rationale The label is applied upside down so it can be read easily when the container is hanging up. The IV bottles are numbered consecutively.

20. Apply a timing label on the solution container. The timing label may be applied at the time the IV is started. Follow agency practice.

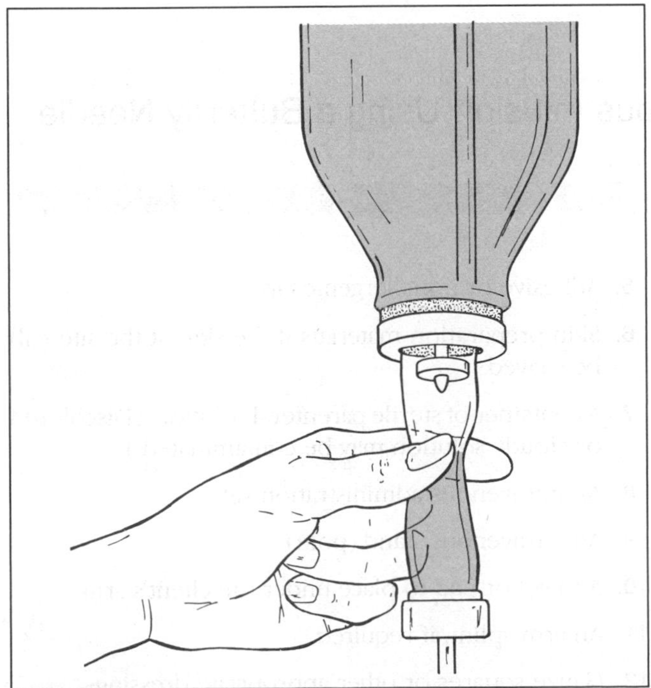

Figure 46–13

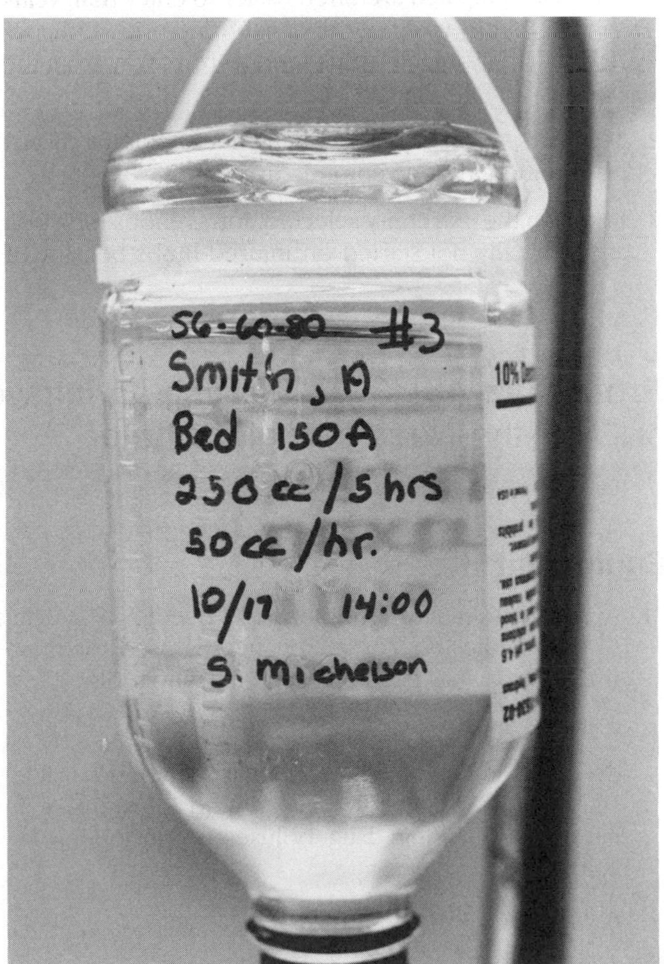

Figure 46–14

21. Label the IV tubing with the date and time of attachment. This labeling may also be done at the time the IV is started.

    Rationale The tubing is labeled to ensure that it is changed every 48 hours or sooner (Centers for Disease Control 1982, p. 62).

22. Assess the client's reaction to the setting up of the IV. If he or she expresses anxiety and fear, assist the client to deal with these emotions, and record the reaction on the chart.

23. Notify the responsible nurse when the intravenous infusion has been set up.

Initiating an Intravenous Infusion

Agency practices vary about which nurses perform venipunctures and start intravenous infusions. In many settings, nurses must be supervised and approved before they are permitted to start infusions on their own. Some agencies have teams of specially prepared nurses who initiate all intravenous infusions. Before starting an infusion, the nurse should assess the client for:

1. Veins that would be satisfactory venipuncture sites. Veins that are continually distended with blood, have been damaged by previous venipunctures, or have become knotted and tortuous are normally not used. Veins that are easily palpated are often easier to enter than veins that are highly visible or deeply buried under adipose tissue. Highly visible veins tend to roll away from the needle.
2. Tendency to bleed easily. Such clients require special observation after a venipuncture.
3. Injury to the extremity selected. Intravenous infusions are normally not started on injured limbs because of possible impaired circulation, discomfort for the client, and obstruction of the site by dressings.
4. Any abrasions in the skin area chosen for the venipuncture. If an abraded area must be used, record the abrasions.
5. Hydration and electrolyte status for baseline data. See the section on assessment, earlier in this chapter.

The nurse also determines:

1. Whether the client has any allergies, e.g., to tape or povidone-iodine.
2. Which solution is to be used, how much is to be infused, and how long the infusion is to run.
3. What agency policy is about shaving the area before a venipuncture. Some agencies advise against shaving because of the possibility of nicking the skin and subsequent infection.

Procedure 46–3 ▲ Starting an Intravenous Infusion Using a Butterfly Needle or Over-the-Needle Angiocatheter

Equipment

1. A sterile butterfly (wing-tipped) needle. A 2.5-cm (1-in) needle, #21 or #23 gauge, is used for most infusions; a #19 needle is used for whole blood.

   or

   An over-the-needle angiocatheter (ONC) of suitable size, e.g., #22 gauge for clear liquid infusions, #20 gauge for infusing drug boluses or peripheral fat solutions.
2. Antiseptic swabs.
3. A tourniquet.
4. A receptacle for discarded fluid.
5. Adhesive or nonallergenic tape.
6. Skin preparation materials if the skin at the site will be shaved.
7. A container of sterile parenteral solution. (Discolored or cloudy solution may be contaminated.)
8. An intravenous administration set.
9. An intravenous stand (pole).
10. A towel or pad to place under the client's arm.
11. An arm splint, if required.
12. Gauze squares or other appropriate dressings.
13. Antiseptic ointment, e.g., povidone-iodine (Betadine).

Intervention

Preparing the Infusion Equipment

1. Follow Procedures 46–2, steps 1–21, on pages 1375 to 1378, if the equipment has not already been prepared.

Selecting and Preparing the Venipuncture Site

2. Prepare strips of adhesive tape to stabilize the IV needle once it is inserted.
3. Select a site, starting at the distal end of the vein.

   Rationale Veins can become sclerotic from irritation by the infusion or the needle. Sclerosis may then interfere with venous flow. If so, more proximal parts of the veins can be used.
4. If necessary, shave the skin where adhesive tape will be applied. Check agency policy.

Dilating the Vein

5. Place the extremity in a dependent position (lower than the client's heart).

   Rationale Gravity slows venous return and distends the veins. Distending the veins makes it easier to insert the needle properly.
6. Apply a tourniquet firmly 15 to 20 cm (6 to 8 in) above the venipuncture site. The tourniquet must be tight enough to obstruct venous flow but not so tight that it occludes arterial flow. If a radial pulse can be palpated, the arterial flow is not obstructed.

   Rationale Obstructing arterial flow inhibits venous filling.
7. If the vein is not sufficiently dilated:
   a. Massage or stroke the vein distal to the site and in the direction of venous flow toward the heart.

      Rationale This action helps fill the vein.

   b. Encourage the client to rapidly clench and unclench the fist.

      Rationale Contracting the muscles compresses the distal veins, forcing blood along the veins and distending them.

   c. Lightly tap the vein with your fingertips.

      Rationale Tapping may distend the vein.
8. If steps 5–7 fail to distend the vein, remove the tourniquet and apply heat to the entire extremity for 10 to 15 minutes. Then repeat steps 5–7.

   Rationale Heat dilates superficial blood vessels, causing them to fill.
9. Clean the skin at the site of entry with a topical antiseptic swab, e.g., alcohol, and then an anti-infective, e.g., povidone-iodine (Betadine) solution.
10. Use one thumb to pull the skin taut below the entry site.

    Rationale This action stabilizes the vein and makes the skin taut for needle entry. It can also make initial tissue penetration less painful.

Inserting a Needle

11. Hold the needle, pointed in the direction of the blood flow, at a 30° angle, with the bevel up, and pierce the skin beside the vein about 1 cm (½ in) below the site planned for piercing the vein. See Figure 46–15.

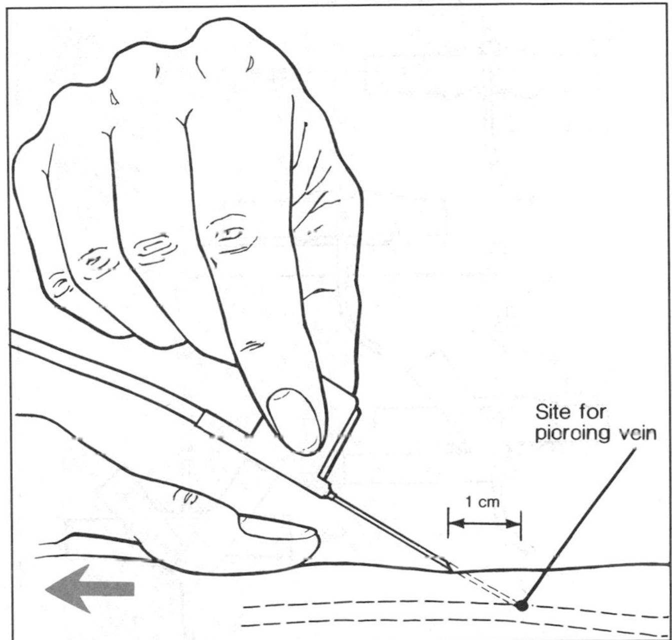

Figure 46–15

12. Once the needle is through the skin, lower the needle so it is almost parallel with the skin. Follow the course of the vein and pierce one side of the vein.

    Rationale Lowering the needle reduces the chances of puncturing both sides of the vein.
13. When blood flows back into the needle tubing, insert the needle farther up the vein 2 to 2.5 cm (¾ to 1 in) or to the hub of the butterfly needle. Sudden lack of resistance can be felt as blood enters the needle.
14. Release the tourniquet, attach the infusion, and initiate flow as quickly as possible.

    Rationale Attaching the tubing quickly prevents blood from clotting and obstructing the needle.

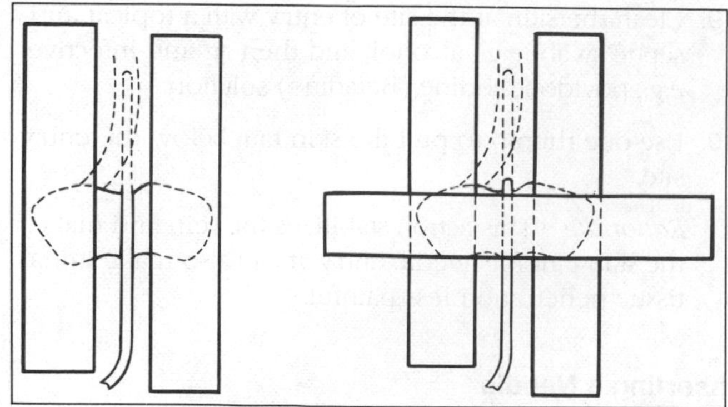

Figure 46–16

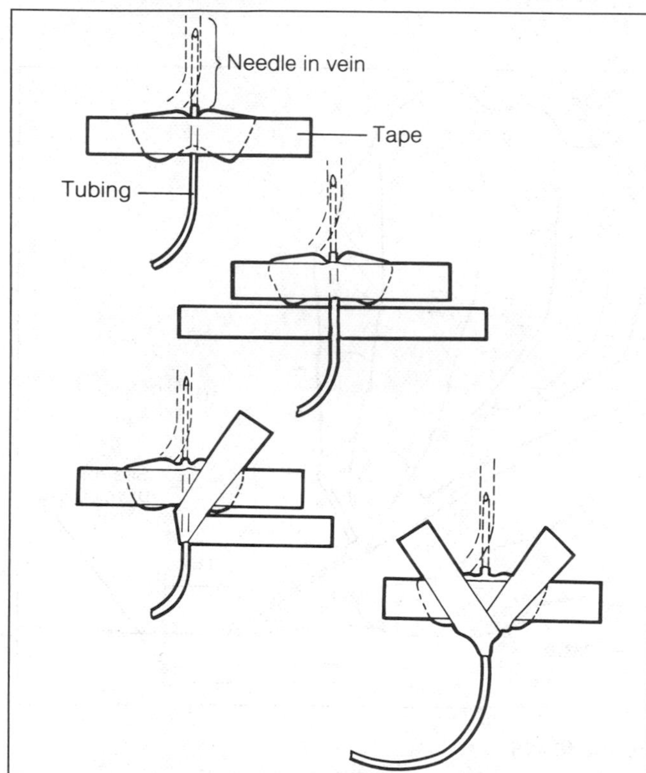

Figure 46–17

15. Tape the needle securely by the H method (see Figure 46–16) or crisscross (chevron) method (see Figure 46–17). You may need to place a cotton ball or small gauze square under the needle to keep it in position in the vein. Go to step 27.

Inserting an Over-the-Needle Angiocatheter

16. Insert the catheter by the direct or indirect method. For the direct method, hold the catheter bevel up, at a 15° to 20° angle, and thrust the catheter through the skin and into the vein in one thrust. For the indirect method, first pierce the skin, then reduce the angle, and advance the catheter into the vein. Sudden lack of resistance is felt as the catheter enters the vein.

    Rationale The direct method is preferred for large veins and the indirect method for smaller veins (Peck 1985, p. 40).

17. Once blood appears in the catheter or you feel the lack of resistance, advance the catheter another 0.6 cm (¼ in).

    Rationale The catheter is advanced to ensure that it, and not just the metal needle, is in the vein.

18. Release the tourniquet.
19. Remove the protective cap from the distal end of the tubing, and hold it ready to attach to the catheter, maintaining the sterility of the end.
20. Grasp the hub of the catheter with your thumb and index finger, and withdraw the needle. See Figure 46–18.

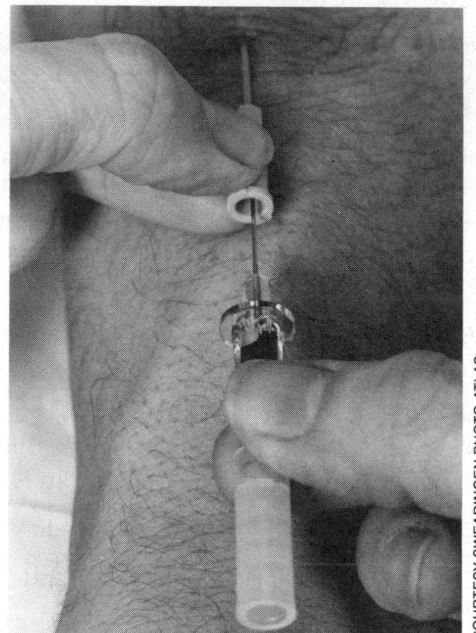

Figure 46–18

21. Advance the catheter up to the hub or until you feel resistance.
22. Attach the end of the infusion tubing to the catheter hub.
23. Initiate the infusion.
24. Inspect the insertion site for signs of infiltration, e.g., swelling.

25. Tape the catheter in place.
    a. Place the first tape, sticky side up, under the catheter hub, and fold the sides as shown in Figure 46–19.

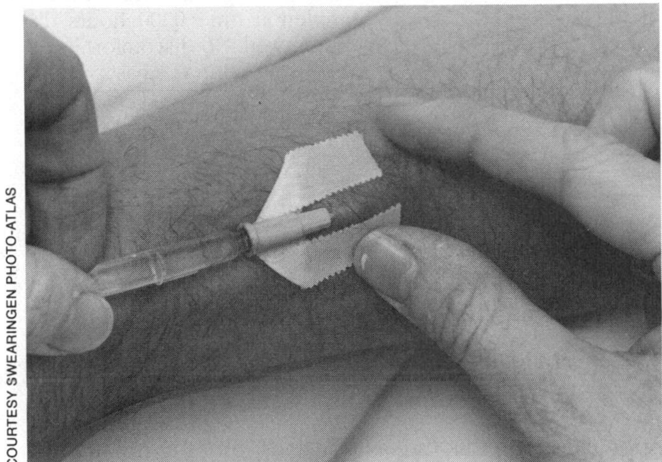
COURTESY SWEARINGEN PHOTO-ATLAS

Figure 46–19

    b. Place the second strip, sticky side down, across the catheter hub. See Figure 46–20.

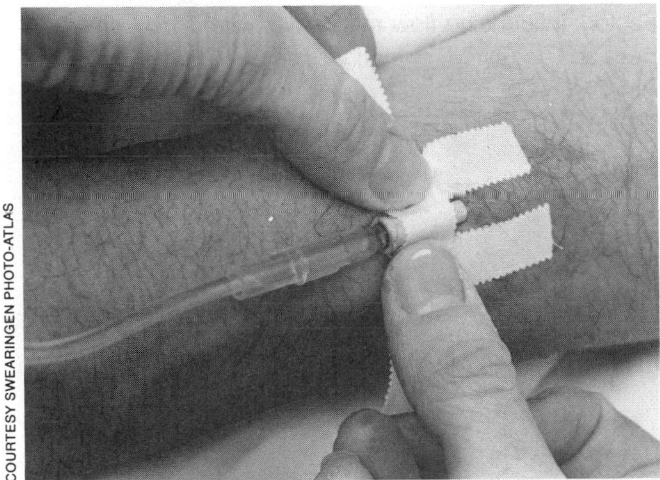
COURTESY SWEARINGEN PHOTO-ATLAS

Figure 46–20

    c. Place the third strip, sticky side up, under the catheter hub distal to the second strip, and fold each side diagonally across the catheter. See Figure 46–21.

26. Dress the venipuncture site according to agency policy. In some agencies, the nurse puts a small amount of antiseptic ointment, e.g., povidone-iodine, over the venipuncture site, then a gauze square. In other agencies, a sterile transparent occlusive dressing is applied. This permits assessment of the site without disturbing the dressing. This type of dressing can be left on for 72 hours unless there are complications (Peck 1985, p. 32).

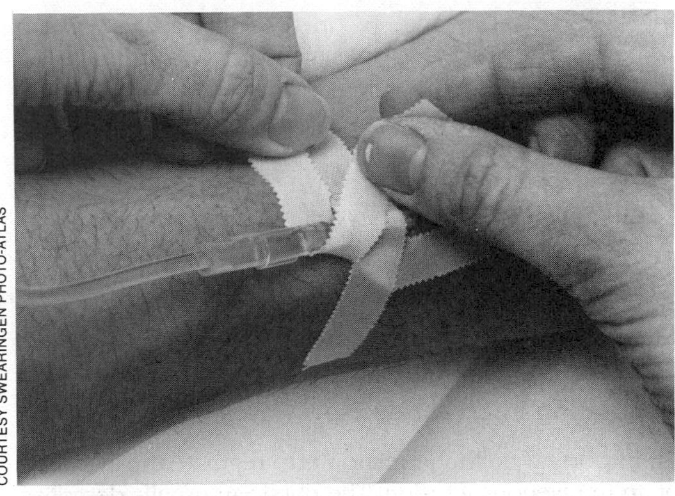
COURTESY SWEARINGEN PHOTO-ATLAS

Figure 46–21

For a Butterfly Needle or Angiocatheter

27. Loop the tubing, and secure it to the dressing with tape.

    Rationale Looping and securing the tubing prevents the weight of the tubing or any movement from pulling on the needle or catheter.

28. Apply a padded armboard to splint the elbow or wrist joint if needed.

29. Adjust the infusion rate of flow according to the order.

30. Label a piece of tape with the date and time of insertion, type and gauge of needle or catheter used, and your initials. Apply the tape label over the venipuncture dressing. See Figure 46–22.

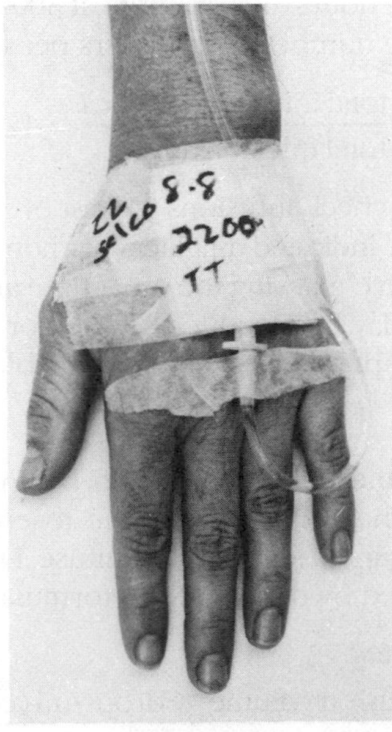

Figure 46–22

31. Record starting the IV on the client's chart. Some agencies provide a special form for this purpose. Include the date and time of the venipuncture, amount and type of solution used, including any additives (e.g., kind and amount of medications), absorption time, container number, drip rate, type and gauge of the needle or catheter, venipuncture site, and client's general response.

Sample Recording

Date	Time	Notes
Jun/8/87	1800	IV #1–1000 ml D5W started in the right basilic vein. BF needle #21G inserted. Drip rate 125 ml/hr. Completion time 0200 hours. IV running well. No discomfort.——— ———Dino C. Anastasio, NS

Regulating Intravenous Flow Rates

An important nursing function is to regulate the flow rate of an intravenous infusion. The physician usually describes in the IV order how long an infusion should last, e.g., 3000 ml over 24 hours. It is then a nursing responsibility to calculate the correct flow rate and regulate the infusion. Problems that can result from incorrectly regulated infusions are discussed next in this chapter.

There are a number of commercially prepared infusion sets, and each has its own type of drip chamber, so it is important to know the number of drops per ml of solution for a particular drip chamber before calculating a drip rate. This rate is called the **drop** or **drip factor** and is printed on most commercially prepared packages. Common drop factors are 10, 15, and 20 for macrodrips and 60 for microdrips.

There are two methods of calculating flow rates: the number of milliliters per hour and the number of drops per minute.

Milliliters per hour Hourly rates of infusion can be calculated by dividing the total infusion volume by the total infusion time in hours. For example, if 3000 ml is infused in 24 hours, the number of milliliters per hour is

$$\frac{3000\text{ ml (total infusion volume)}}{24\text{ hr (total infusion time)}} = 125\text{ ml/hr}$$

Nurses need to check infusions at least every 30 minutes to assure that the indicated milliliters per hour have infused. A strip of adhesive marking the exact time and/or amount to be infused may be taped to the solution bottle. Some agencies make premarked labels available. See Figure 46–23.

Drops per minute The nurse who begins an infusion must regulate the drops per minute to ensure that the prescribed amount of solution will infuse. Drops per minute are calculated by the following formula:

Drops per minute

$$= \frac{\text{Total infusion volume} \times \text{drops/ml (or drop factor)}}{\text{Total time of infusion in } \textit{minutes}}$$

If the requirements are 1000 ml in 8 hours (480 minutes) and the drip factor is 20 drops/ml, the drops per minute should be:

$$\frac{1000\text{ ml} \times 20\text{ drops/ml}}{480\text{ min}} = 41\text{ drops/min}$$

Approximating this rate as 40 drops/min, the nurse must then regulate the drops per minute by tightening or releasing the intravenous tubing clamp and counting the drops the same way a pulse is counted. Devices such as battery-operated rate meters and infusion pumps with alarm systems facilitate a regulated flow.

Factors influencing flow rates No matter how often flow rates are regulated, several factors can change the rate of

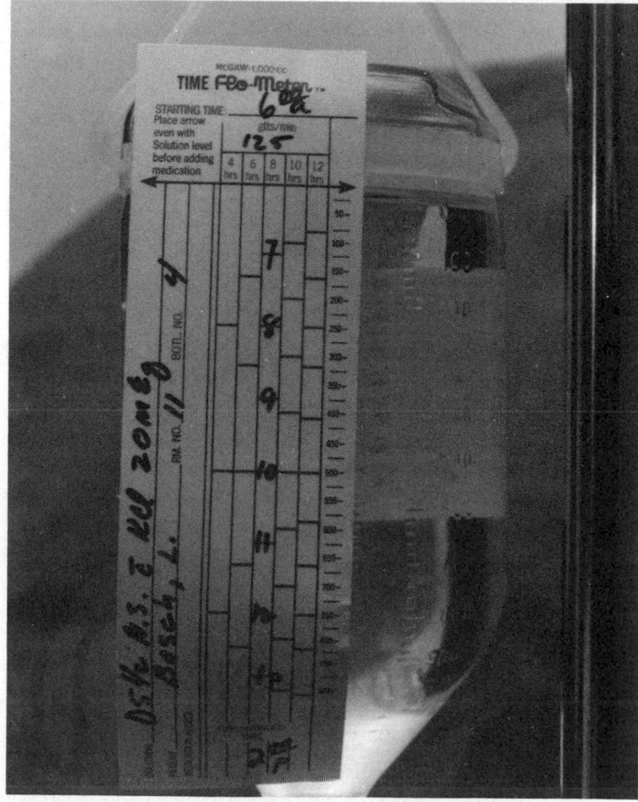

Figure 46–23 Timing label on an intravenous container

flow of an IV infusion. If an infusion is too fast or too slow, the nurse needs to consider several factors:

1. *The position of the forearm.* Sometimes a change in the position of the client's arm increases flow. Slight pronation, supination, extension, or elevation of the forearm on a pillow can increase flow.

2. *The position and patency of the tubing.* Not infrequently, the tubing is obstructed by the client's weight, a kink, or a clamp closed too tightly. The flow rate also diminishes when part of the tubing dangles below the puncture site.

3. *The height of the infusion bottle.* Elevating the height of the infusion bottle a few inches can speed the flow by creating more pressure.

4. *Possible infiltration or fluid leakage.* Swelling, a feeling of coldness, and tenderness at the venipuncture site may indicate infiltration.

Monitoring and Maintaining an Intravenous Infusion

Check the physician's order on the client's chart to determine the type and sequence of solutions to be infused. Then determine from the nursing care plan the rate of flow, infusion schedule, and any relevant problems. See Table 46–10 for an intravenous infusion checklist.

Inspect the client's infusion site for fluid infiltration, i.e., the escape of intravenous fluid into the interstitial tissues, usually near the insertion site, in case the needle has become dislodged from the client's vein, allowing the intravenous fluid to flow into the subcutaneous tissue. The clinical signs are swelling, coolness, pain, pallor at the site, and discomfort. To ascertain the presence of infiltration:

1. Palpate the surrounding tissue for edema.

2. Feel the surrounding skin for changes in temperature.

If infiltration is not evident, the following measures can determine whether the needle is dislodged from the vein:

1. If the tubing does not have a backcheck valve, lower the infusion bottle below the level of the venipuncture site to see if blood returns. Blood may indicate that the intravenous needle is still in the vein. This method is not foolproof, however, because the needle may be penetrating the vein wall partially.

2. Use a sterile syringe of saline to withdraw fluid from the rubber at the end of the tubing near the venipuncture site. If blood does not return, discontinue the intravenous infusion.

Table 46–10 Checklist for an Intravenous Infusion

Component	Data
Solution container	
Name of solution	______
Amount of solution	______
Number of container	______
Date and time	______
Time of completion	______
Next solution	
Name of solution	______
Amount of solution	______
Number of container	______
Date and time	______
Time of completion	______
Tubing	
Intact	______
Coiled smoothly	______
Unobstructed	______
Drip chamber	
Appropriately filled	______
Dripping at correct rate	______
Client	
Venipuncture site	______
Dry or wet	______
Bleeding	______
Swelling	______
Skin color	______
Skin temperature	______
Pain	______
Respirations	______
Pulse	______
Urine output	______
Edema	______
Sputum and cough	______
Psychologic concerns	______

3. Try to stop the flow by applying a tourniquet 10 to 15 cm (4 to 6 in) above the insertion site and opening the roller clamp wide. If the infusion continues to flow slowly, the needle is in subcutaneous tissue (it has infiltrated).

4. If the client is elderly or hypovolemic, it may be necessary to combine steps 2 and 3 to check for blood return before discontinuing the infusion.

Inspect for the presence of **phlebitis** (inflammation of a vein), which can occur with or without a blood clot. If a blood clot exists, the condition is called **thrombophlebitis.** Phlebitis can occur as a result of injury to a vein, e.g., because of mechanical trauma or chemical irritation. Chemical injury to a vein can occur from intravenous electrolytes and medications. The clinical signs are redness, warmth, and swelling at the intravenous site and burning pain along the course of a vein. A new venipuncture site is usually selected, and the injured vein is not used for further infusions.

Be alert to signs of circulatory overload. **Circulatory overload** means that the circulatory system contains more fluid than normal. An adult normally has about 6 liters of blood in circulation. A significant increase in this volume, e.g., when an IV is administered too quickly, can cause circulatory overload, which may result in pulmonary edema and cardiac failure. The clinical signs of cardiac failure are dyspnea, reduced urine output, edema, weak and rapid pulse, and shallow, rapid respirations. The clinical signs of pulmonary edema are dyspnea, coughing, and frothy sputum.

Inspect for bleeding at the intravenous site. This can occur during an IV but is more likely to occur after the needle has been removed from the vein. The site of the needle or catheter insertion should always be inspected for evidence of blood, particularly in clients who bleed readily, e.g., clients receiving heparin.

Ensure that the correct solution is being infused. If the solution is incorrect, slow the rate of flow to a minimum to maintain the patency of the needle or catheter. If the IV is terminated, the client will have to have another venipuncture before the new solution is administered. Report the matter to the responsible nurse. Change the solution to the correct one. Agencies have different policies about how and to whom to report an incident.

Inspect the system to make sure that it is intact. If there is leakage, locate the source. If the leak is at the needle connection, tighten the tubing into the needle. If the leak cannot be stopped, slow the IV as much as possible without stopping it, and replace the tubing with a new sterile set. Report any leaks to the responsible nurse. Estimate how much solution was lost if the amount was substantial.

Compare the rate of flow regularly, e.g., every hour, against the schedule. If the rate is too fast, slow it so that the infusion will be completed at the planned time. If it is too slow, check agency practice. Some agencies permit nursing personnel to adjust a rate of flow 3 ml/min or less. Adjustments above 3 ml/min require a physician's order. If the rate of flow is 150 ml/hr or more, the rate of flow must be checked more frequently, e.g., every 15 to 30 minutes. IV infusions that are off schedule can be harmful to a client. Solution that is administered too slowly can supply insufficient fluid, electrolytes, or medication for a client's needs. Solution administered too quickly may cause circulatory overload and possibly pulmonary edema or cardiac failure.

Inspect the system for blockages. The flow of solution can be blocked or impeded for several reasons.

1. Inspect the tubing for any kinks. Arrange the tubing so that it is lightly coiled and under no pressure. Sometimes the tubing becomes caught under the client's arm, and the weight of the arm blocks the flow.
2. Determine whether the bevel of the needle or catheter is blocked against the wall of the vein. If it is blocked, pull back gently on the needle or catheter, and turn it slightly. Do not turn a butterfly needle; instead, raise or lower the angle of the needle slightly, using a sterile gauze pad under the wings. Turning a butterfly needle can injure the vein. The sterile gauze pad protects the skin and changes the position of the bevel of the needle.
3. Examine the tubing clamp. If it is closed, adjust it to the open position.
4. Observe the position of the solution container. If it is less than 1 m (3 ft) above the IV site, readjust it to the correct height on the pole. If the container is too low, the solution may not flow into the vein because there is insufficient gravitational pressure to overcome the pressure of the blood within the vein.
5. Observe the position of the tubing. If it is dangling below the venipuncture, coil it carefully on the surface of the bed. The solution cannot flow upward into the vein against the force of gravity.

Observe the drip chamber. If it is less than half full, squeeze the chamber to allow the correct amount of fluid to flow in. Implement corrective measures for problems, as outlined or recommended by the agency.

If the client is able, teach him or her when to call for assistance, e.g., if the solution stops dripping or the venipuncture site becomes swollen. In addition, to help the client maintain an intravenous infusion, instruct her or him to:

1. Avoid sudden twisting or turning movements of the arm with the needle or catheter.
2. Avoid stretching or placing tension on the tubing.
3. Try to keep the tubing from dangling below the level of the needle.
4. Notify a nurse if:
   a. There is a sudden change in the flow rate.
   b. The solution container is nearly empty.
   c. There is blood in the IV tubing.
   d. He or she feels discomfort at the IV site.

Changing Intravenous Containers

Intravenous solution containers are changed when only a small amount of fluid remains in the neck of the container and fluid still remains in the drip chamber. The Centers for Disease Control (CDC) (1982) recommend that tubing be changed every 48 hours to decrease the incidence of phlebitis. Usually the tubing is changed at a time when the container is being changed.

It is important to know agency practices regarding the frequency of changing infusion tubing and cleaning venipuncture sites.

1. Compare the number of the new container against the number of the used container. Read the label of the new container.
2. Remove the cover of the new container so that it is ready for spiking. Maintain the sterility of the container top. Follow the manufacturer's directions in setting up the container. Sometimes it is hung on the IV pole before the spike is inserted, and sometimes it is placed on a table.
3. Close the clamp on the tubing to stop the flow of solution.
4. Take the used solution container off the pole, and invert it.
5. Remove the spike from the container, maintaining its sterility.
6. Hold the new container with one hand so it will not slip, and insert the spike into the container with the other. Do not twist the tubing; twisting can sever the connections.
7. Hang the container on the pole if it is not already hung.
8. Adjust the clamp, and regulate the rate of flow of the solution according to the order on the chart.
9. Label the solution container if this was not done prior to changing the container.
10. Record the change of solution container in the client's record. Record the number of the container if the containers are numbered.

Procedure 46–4 ▲ Changing an Intravenous Container and Tubing

The CDC (1982) recommends that tubing be changed every 48 hours to decrease the incidence of infection. However, nurses should follow agency policy regarding this. Tubing is changed most easily when a new container is added.

Equipment

To Change the Container

1. A container with the correct kind and amount of sterile solution.

To Change the Tubing

2. An administration set with sterile tubing, drip chamber, etc.
3. Tape for taping the needle and new tubing.
4. A sterile gauze square for positioning the needle.
5. Antiseptic solution and/or ointment for cleaning the site. Check agency practice.
6. Sterile swabs.
7. A receptacle (e.g., a kidney basin) for discarded fluid.

Intervention

Before starting, compare the number on the new container against the number on the used container. Read the label of the new container.

1. Open the administration set, and attach it to the container, using sterile technique.
2. Tighten the clamp and hang the container on the pole if it is not already hung.
3. Remove the protective cap from the end of the tubing, and prime the tubing. See Procedure 46–2, step 16. Clamp the tubing, and replace the protective cap.

   Rationale Replacing the cap maintains the sterility of the end of the tubing.
4. Remove the tape and the dressing carefully from around the needle. Take care not to dislodge the needle from the vein.
5. Place a sterile swab under the hub of the catheter to absorb any leakage that might occur when the tubing is disconnected. Clamp the old tubing.
6. Holding the hub of the needle with the fingers of one hand, remove the tubing with the other hand, using a twisting, pulling motion. Place the end of the tubing in the kidney basin or other receptacle.

Rationale Holding the needle firmly but gently maintains its position in the vein.

7. Continue to hold the needle, and grasp the new tubing with the other hand. Remove the protective cap, and, maintaining sterility, insert the tubing end tightly into the needle hub.
8. Open the clamp to start the solution flowing.
9. Clean the venipuncture site, working from the insertion point outward in a circular manner. Iodine or ethyl alcohol is frequently used. Some agencies also place water-soluble iodine ointment, e.g., Betadine, at the site.
10. Apply a sterile dressing over the site and tape the needle in place. See Procedure 46–3, step 15. Apply a labeled tape over the dressing. The label should include: the date and time the dressing is applied; the original date and time of the venipuncture; the size of the catheter or needle; and your initials, as the nurse who changed the dressing.
11. Tape a label on the new tubing with the date and time of the change and your initials. See Figure 46–24.
12. Regulate the rate of flow of the solution according to the order on the chart.
13. Record the change of the solution container and/or tubing in the appropriate place on the client's chart. Also record the fluid intake according to agency practice. Some agencies have special flow sheets or intake and output records for recording IVs. Record the number of the container if the containers are numbered at the agency. Also record your assessments.

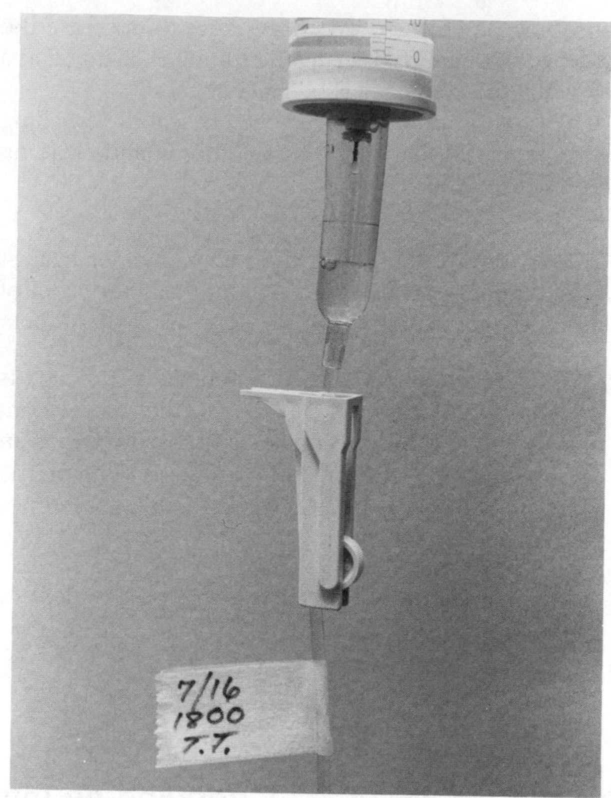

Figure 46–24

Discontinuing an Intravenous Infusion

Discontinuing an infusion is not an uncomfortable procedure; in fact, it is usually a relief for the client and takes only a couple of minutes. IVs are usually discontinued for one of two reasons:

1. The client's oral fluid intake and hydration status are satisfactory, so that no further intravenous solutions are ordered.
2. There is a problem with the infusion that cannot be fixed. Consult with the responsible nurse before discontinuing an IV because of such a difficulty.

Procedure 46–5 ▲ Discontinuing an Intravenous Infusion

Equipment

1. A small sterile dressing and tape to cover the site temporarily
2. Dry or antiseptic-soaked swabs, according to agency practice

Intervention

1. Clamp the infusion tubing.

Rationale Clamping the tubing will prevent the fluid from flowing out of the needle onto the client or bed.

2. Loosen the tape at the venipuncture site while holding the needle firmly and applying countertraction to the skin.

   Rationale Movement of the needle can injure the vein and cause discomfort to the client. Countertraction prevents pulling the skin and causing discomfort.

3. Hold a swab above the venipuncture site.

4. Withdraw the needle or catheter by pulling it out along the line of the vein.

   Rationale Pulling out in line with the vein avoids injury to the vein.

5. Apply firm pressure immediately to the site, using the swab, for 2 to 3 minutes.

   Rationale Pressure helps stop the bleeding and prevents hematoma formation.

6. Hold the client's arm or leg above his or her body if any bleeding persists.

   Rationale Raising the limb decreases blood flow to the area.

7. Inspect the needle or catheter to make sure it is intact. Report a broken needle or catheter to the responsible nurse immediately.

   Rationale A piece of needle or tubing that remains in the client's vein could move centrally (toward the heart or lungs) and cause serious problems.

8. Apply the sterile dressing.

   Rationale The dressing continues the pressure and covers the open area in the skin, preventing infection.

9. Assess the client's response to the IV in terms of the appearance of the venipuncture site; the client's pulse, respirations, color, edema, sputum, cough, and urine output; and the client's perception of his or her physical and psychologic status.

10. Discard the IV solution container, if infusions are being discontinued, and discard the used supplies appropriately.

11. Record the amount of fluid infused on the intake and output record and on the client's chart, according to agency practice. Include the container number, type of solution used, time of discontinuing the infusion, and client's response.

Pumps and Controllers

Several kinds of pumps and controllers are used with IV infusions. Each should be set up according to the manufacturer's directions. A pump delivers a measured amount of IV solution or medication at a constant high pressure. A controller, by contrast, operates by gravitational force (see Figure 46–25). The IV container must be at least 76 cm (30 in) above the venipuncture site for a controller to work. Because controllers do not provide the same pressure as pumps, they cannot be used to keep an arterial line open or to administer highly viscid fluids.

Pumps measure the flow rate in milliliters per hour. Some pumps are volumetric and are very precise. Controllers regulate the gravitational flow by counting the drops and compressing the IV tubing to obtain the desired infusion rate. Because drops vary in size, controllers are not as accurate as pumps.

Some pumps and controllers are equipped with alarm systems, which are triggered when there is a change in the flow rate, when there are air bubbles in either the drip chamber or the intravenous tubing, when battery power is low, or when an occlusion is present. If the equipment has an alarm system, explain the alarm to the client, and let the client hear it so that he or she will know what to expect if the alarm comes on later.

Blood Transfusions

A **blood transfusion** is the introduction of whole blood or components of the blood, e.g., plasma serum, erythrocytes, or platelets, into the venous circulation. See Table 46–11 for types of blood and blood products, and indications for their use.

Blood transfusions are given for the following reasons:

1. To restore blood volume after severe hemorrhage
2. To restore the red blood cell level after severe and chronic anemias and to maintain blood hemoglobin levels
3. To provide plasma factors, e.g., antihemophilic factor (AHF) or factor VIII, which controls bleeding

Blood Matching

Blood groups Human blood is classified into four main groups (A, B, AB, and O) on the basis of polysaccharide antigens on the erythrocyte surface. These antigens, type A and type B, commonly cause antibody reactions and are called **agglutinogens**. In other words, group A blood contains type A agglutinogen, group B blood contains type B agglutinogen, group AB blood contains both A and

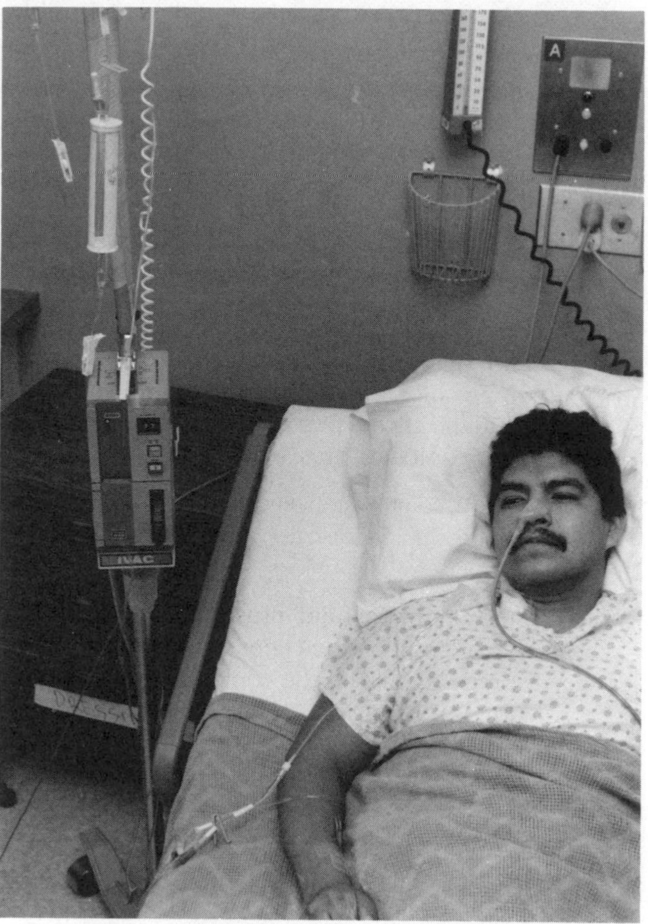

Figure 46–25 An intravenous infusion controller

B agglutinogens, and group O blood contains neither agglutinogen.

In addition to agglutinogens on the erythrocytes, **agglutinins** (antibodies) are present in the blood plasma. The agglutinins are referred to as alpha (anti-A) agglutinins, which agglutinate type A cells, and beta (anti-B) agglutinins, which agglutinate type B cells. No individual can have agglutinins and agglutinogens of the same type; that person's system would attack its own cells. Thus group A blood does not contain agglutinin A but does contain agglutinin B. Group B blood does not contain agglutinin B but does contain agglutinin A. Group AB blood contains neither agglutinin, and Group O contains both anti-A and anti-B agglutinins. Blood transfusions must be matched to the recipient's blood type in terms of compatible agglutinogens. Mismatched blood will cause a hemolytic reaction. The most common blood types are A and O. Type B blood is found in 20% of the black population and only 9% of the white population. Almost 50% of both populations have type O blood. See Table 46–12.

Rhesus (Rh) groups Rh antigens, also on the surface of erythrocytes, are present in about 85% of the population and can be a major cause of hemolytic reactions. Persons who possess the **Rh factor** are referred to as *Rh positive;* those who do not are referred to as *Rh negative.* Some other blood factors are the Hr, Kell, Lewis M, N, and P factors. These rarely cause major reactions because their antigenic properties are poor.

The Rh factor differs from the A and B agglutinogens in that it cannot cause a hemolytic reaction on the first

Table 46–11 Blood Products and Indications for Use

Type of Blood Product	Indications
Whole blood (Type A, B, AB, O, and/or Rh positive or negative)	To treat blood volume deficiencies, e.g., in acute hemorrhage; not indicated for correction of chronic anemia
Plasma	To expand blood volume; to restore circulation and renal blood flow when plasma volume is decreased but red cell mass is adequate, as in acute dehydration or burns; to replace deficient coagulation factors in bleeding disorders
Packed red cells (high hematocrit, since approximately 80% of plasma is removed)	Used when blood volume is adequate but red cell mass is inadequate, as in chronic anemia
Platelets	For clients with severe thrombocytopenia (reduced platelets); platelets plug small vascular leaks prior to clotting
Albumin	To expand blood volume when volume is reduced in clients in shock or with burns; to increase level of albumin in clients with hypoalbuminemia
Prothrombin complex (Konyne, Proplex)—contains factors VII, IX, and XI and prothrombin	For bleeding associated with deficiencies of those factors
Factor VIII fractions	For hemophiliacs
Fibrinogen preparations	For bleeding associated particularly with congenital hypofibrinogenemia (deficiency of fibrinogen, necessary for blood coagulation)

exposure to mismatched blood. This is because the Rh antibody is *not* normally present in the plasma of persons who are Rh negative.

Transfusion Reactions

Transfusion reactions can be categorized as hemolytic, febrile, and allergic. The signs, symptoms, and nursing actions for each type of reaction are outlined in Table 46–13. The hemolytic reaction, a fatal response, occurs when agglutinins and agglutinogens of the same type come in contact; e.g., A agglutinogen and anti-A agglutinin, or type B agglutinogen and anti-B agglutinin. **Agglutination** (clumping) and **hemolysis** (rupture) of the red cells result from such contact. It is essential, therefore, to match the donor's blood type to the recipient's. Otherwise, the

Table 46–12 Survey of Information on Blood Groups

Blood Type (Red Blood Cell Agglutinogens)	Agglutinins in Plasma	Possible Donors	Percentage of Human Population
A	Anti-B (beta)	Types A and O	41
B	Anti-A (alpha)	Types B and O	9
AB	None	Types AB, A, B, and O	3
O (no agglutinogen)	Anti-A and anti-B	Type O	47

Source: Adapted from A. C. Guyton. *Textbook of Medical Physiology,* 7th ed. (Philadelphia: W. B. Saunders Co., 1986) p. 70.

Table 46–13 Transfusion Reactions: Clinical Signs and Nursing Interventions

Reaction	Clinical Signs	Nursing Interventions
Hemolytic reaction	Chills, fever, headache, back pain, hemoglobinemia, hemoglobinuria, oliguria, jaundice, dyspnea, cyanosis, chest pain, vascular collapse, hypotension	1. Observe client closely for first 10 minutes of transfusion, since these reactions occur rapidly 2. Discontinue blood immediately when reaction is assessed 3. Notify physician of client's symptoms and vital signs 4. Notify laboratory to type and cross-match blood and confirm diagnosis; send donor blood back to laboratory and have specimen of recipient's blood retested 5. Maintain intravenous infusion with D5W or saline 6. Monitor vital signs every 15 minutes to assess shock and temperature 7. Record fluid intake and output to assess degree of kidney functioning 8. Save first voided specimen for laboratory analysis 9. Implement treatment as prescribed by physician
Febrile reaction	Fever, shaking, chills, warm flushed skin, headache, backache, nausea, hematemesis, diarrhea, red shock, confusion or delirium	*For mild reaction:* 1. Observe client closely for first 30 minutes of transfusion *For severe reaction:* 1. Stop transfusion 2. Maintain intravenous infusion with saline or D5W 3. Monitor client's vital signs every 30 minutes 4. Notify physician 5. Notify laboratory to take culture of client's and donor's blood 6. Implement therapy as prescribed by physician 7. Apply alcohol sponges for fever if necessary
Allergic reaction	Urticaria, occasional wheezing, arthralgia, generalized itching, nasal congestion, bronchospasm, severe dyspnea, circulatory collapse	*For mild reaction:* 1. Slow transfusion 2. Implement therapy as prescribed by physician *For severe reaction:* 1. Stop transfusion 2. Notify physician immediately 3. Maintain intravenous infusion with saline or D5W 4. Monitor vital signs frequently

agglutinins present in the recipient's plasma will agglutinate the red cells donated. Because type O blood has neither A nor B agglutinogens, it can be donated to recipients with any of the four types of blood; a person with this type is called a **universal donor.** A person with type AB blood, because it has neither anti-A nor anti-B agglutinins in plasma, is referred to as a **universal recipient**, able to receive any of the four blood types. Table 46–12 summarizes compatibility among blood groups.

Febrile reactions (bacterial reactions) are rare. They occur as a result of contaminated blood or sensitivity to the donor's white blood cells. Allergic reactions are relatively common and are thought to be due to allergenic substances or antibodies in the donor's plasma.

Procedure 46–6 ▲ Initiating, Maintaining, and Terminating a Blood Transfusion

Equipment

1. A unit of whole blood. Blood is usually provided in plastic bags by the blood bank. One unit of whole blood is 500 ml of blood in a container.
2. A blood administration set. There are two types: a straight line and a Y-set. The Y-set is preferred because the infusion can be maintained with saline if any adverse effects arise from the transfusion. The infusion tubing has a filter inside the drip chamber. The tubing clamp should be just under the drip chamber. A Y-set can also be used when a saline solution needs to be infused with the blood (e.g., when giving packed cells) or to flush the line before the blood enters the tubing (e.g., when a running IV infusion is not saline).
3. A venipuncture set containing a #18 needle or catheter, if one is not already in place, alcohol swabs, and tape. When blood is to be administered quickly, a #15 needle or a larger catheter, e.g., #14, is often used.
4. A container of 250 ml of saline solution. Some agencies recommend that saline be run through the tubing before and after a blood transfusion.
5. An IV pole.

Intervention

1. Check that there is a signed consent form from the client, if required by the agency. If the client is a Jehovah's Witness, written permission is required.
2. If the client has an IV running, check whether the needle and solution are appropriate to administer blood. The needle should be #18 gauge or larger, and the solution must be saline. If the infusion is not compatible, remove it, and cap the bottle to maintain sterility. Dextrose, Ringer's solution, medications and other additives, and hyperalimentation solutions are incompatible.
3. When obtaining the blood, check the requisition form and the blood bag label with a laboratory technician or according to agency policy. Specifically check the client's name, identification number, blood type (e.g., A, B, AB, or O) and Rh group, the blood donor number, and the expiration date of the blood.
4. With another nurse (the agency may require an RN) compare the laboratory blood type record with:
   a. The client's name and identification number.
   b. The number on the blood bag label.
   c. The ABO group and Rh type on the blood bag label.
5. Sign the appropriate form with the other nurse according to agency policy.
6. Make sure that the blood is not left at room temperature for more than 30 minutes before starting the transfusion because red blood cells deteriorate after 2 hours at room temperature. Agencies may designate different times at which the blood must be returned to the blood bank if the transfusion has not been started.

Initiating a Transfusion

If the client does not have an IV running, you need to perform a venipuncture on a suitable vein and start an IV infusion of normal saline. In some agencies, an IV must be running before the blood is obtained from the blood bank.

7. Obtain a Y-set for blood administration. See Figure 46–26.
8. Ensure that the attached blood filter is suitable for whole blood or the blood components to be transfused.
9. Close all the clamps on the Y-set.

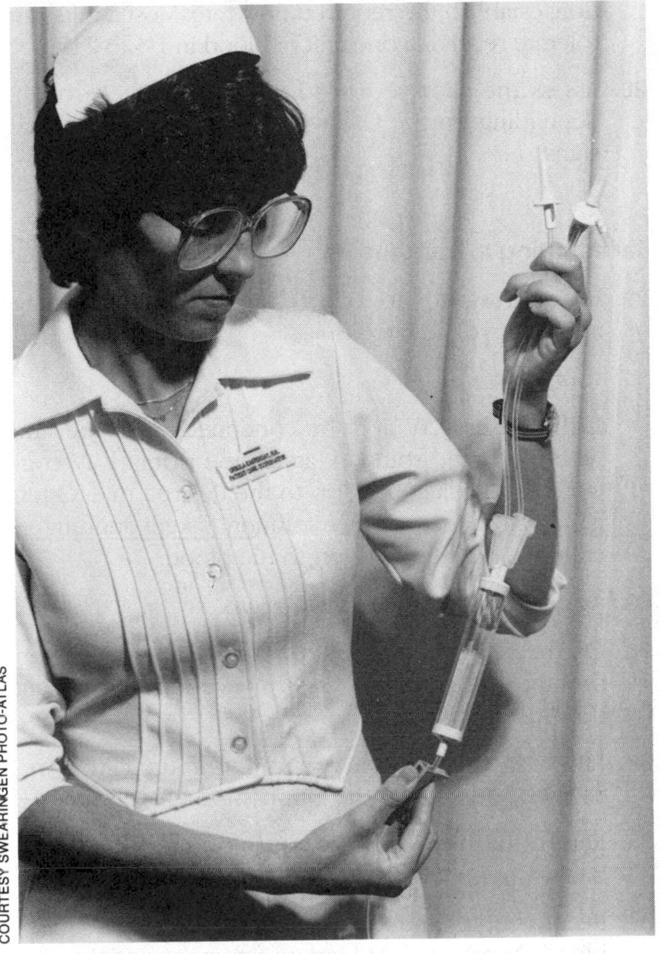

COURTESY SWEARINGEN PHOTO-ATLAS

Figure 46–26

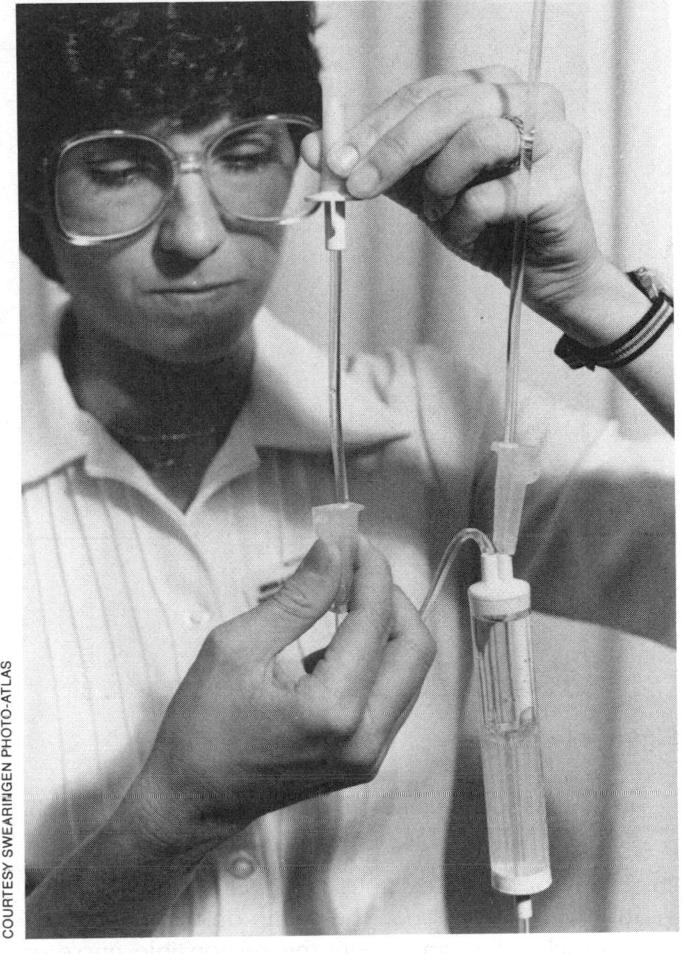

COURTESY SWEARINGEN PHOTO-ATLAS

Figure 46–27

10. Spike a container of 0.9% saline solution with one of the Y-set spikes, and hang the container about 1 m (36 in) above the planned venipuncture site.

11. Open the clamp on the normal saline tubing, and squeeze the drip chamber. Tap the drip chamber as needed to remove any residual air.

    Rationale This primes the upper saline line and blood filter.

12. Open the clamp on the empty Y-set line that is to receive blood. See Figure 46–27.

    Rationale This primes the empty part of the line, because normal saline then flows up the blood line.

13. When the blood line is primed, close the clamp on it.

14. Leave the clamp on the normal saline line open.

15. Open the main roller clamp below the filter, and prime the lower tubing.

16. Close the main roller clamp.

17. Invert the blood bag gently several times to mix the cells with the plasma.

    Rationale Rough handling can damage the cells.

18. Perform a venipuncture. See Procedure 46–3.

19. Expose the port on the blood bag by pulling back the tabs. See Figure 46–28.

20. Insert the remaining Y-set spike into the blood bag.

21. Hang the blood bag at the same level as the saline container.

22. Attach the primed infusion tubing to the needle, and tape it securely.

23. Close the upper roller clamp on the normal saline line, open the upper roller clamp on the blood line, and open the main roller clamp below the filter to infuse the blood.

24. Run the blood for the first 15 minutes at 20 drops per minute. Observe the client closely for signs of adverse

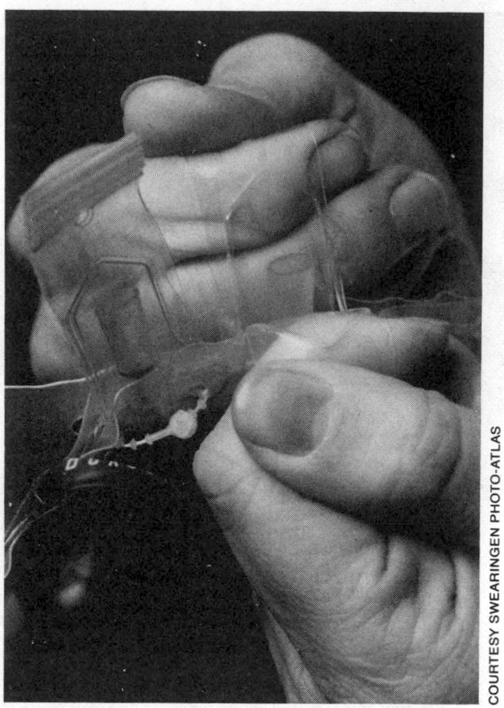
COURTESY SWEARINGEN PHOTO-ATLAS

Figure 46–28

reactions such as chilling, nausea, vomiting, skin rash, or tachycardia.

25. If any of these reactions occur, close the clamp on the transfusion, open the clamp on the tubing with normal saline, and notify the responsible nurse or physician immediately. Follow agency procedure about obtaining urine specimens, etc.

26. Record starting the blood, including vital signs, type of blood, blood unit number, sequence number (e.g., #1 of three ordered units), site of the venipuncture, size of the needle, and drip rate.

Maintaining a Transfusion

27. Fifteen minutes after initiating the transfusion, check the client's vital signs. If there are no signs of a reaction, establish the required flow rate. Most adults can tolerate receiving one unit of blood in 1½ to 2 hours.

28. Assess the client every 30 minutes, or more often, depending on the client's condition, including vital signs.

Terminating a Transfusion

29. If no infusion is to follow, clamp the blood tubing and remove the needle.

    or

    If the primary IV is to be continued, flush the line with the saline solution, attach the primary IV container, and adjust the drip to the desired rate. Often a normal saline or other solution is kept running in case of a delayed reaction to the blood.

30. Again assess the client's vital signs.

31. On the requisition attached to the blood unit, fill in the time the transfusion was completed and the amount transfused.

32. Attach one copy of the requisition to the client's record and another to the empty blood bag.

33. Return the blood bag and requisition to the blood bank.

34. Record completion of the transfusion, the amount of blood absorbed, the blood unit number, and the vital signs. If the primary IV infusion was continued, record connecting it.

Sample Recording

Date	Time	Notes
Dec/12/87	1100	1 unit whole blood administered. No adverse reactions. BP stable at 120/70, TPR 37, 88, 14. 500 ml saline started at 10 gtt/min.——————— ——————Selina L. Ward, SN

Total Parenteral Nutrition

Total parenteral nutrition (TPN), also referred to as **intravenous hyperalimentation** (IVH), is the parenteral administration of solutions of dextrose, water, fat, proteins, electrolytes, vitamins, and trace elements. TPN is the provision of all needed calories. PN is the provision of nutritional solutions, with additional calories coming from other sources, e.g., tube feeding. TPN is a means of achieving an anabolic state in clients who are unable to maintain a normal nitrogen balance. Such clients may include those with severe malnutrition, severe burns, bowel disease disorders (e.g., ulcerative colitis or enteric fistula), acute renal failure, hepatic failure, metastatic cancer, or major surgeries where nothing may be taken by mouth for more than 5 days.

Many of the sepsis problems associated with conventional IV therapy are also associated with TPN. Moreover, the problems are magnified because: (a) clients receiving TPN therapy are often critically ill, may be malnourished, and are sometimes immunosuppressed, (b) TPN catheters are left in place for long periods of time, (c) the intralipids used in TPN therapy support the growth of a wide variety of microorganisms, and (d) the therapy uses the central venous system because of the osmolarity of the fluid. Infection control is therefore of utmost importance during TPN therapy. The nurse must always observe surgical aseptic technique when changing solutions, tubing, dressings, and filters.

TPN (IVH) Sites

Because TPN solutions are **hypertonic** (highly concentrated in comparison to the solute concentration of blood), they are injected only into high-flow central veins, where they are diluted by the client's blood. This prevents injury to the intimal layer of these blood vessels. Clients receiving TPN are thought to be predisposed to thrombophlebitis and possibly bacteremia.

Typically, TPN solutions are administered through a central IV line that rests in the client's superior vena cava. This may be a standard line or a Hickman, Broviac, or other catheter (see "Types of Central Venous Lines," later). After the catheter is inserted, it is attached to IV tubing previously primed with a solution of 5% dextrose in water or normal saline, which is infused until catheter placement is confirmed. The catheter is secured in place by suture, appropriate taping, or both. An antimicrobial ointment and a temporary dressing are then applied over the insertion site until placement of the catheter is confirmed by x-ray examination. Because an improperly placed catheter may cause a pneumothorax, the nurse must assess the client for signs of chest pain and labored breathing and auscultate the lungs for abnormal breath sounds. If the catheter is misplaced, the physician will either manipulate it or remove it and insert another catheter. When correct catheter placement is confirmed, the nurse places a secure occlusive dressing over the insertion site and then commences infusion of the TPN solution.

Administering TPN (IVH) Solutions

TPN is a mixture of 10% to 50% dextrose in water, amino acids, and special additives such as vitamins (e.g., B complex, C, D, K), minerals (e.g., potassium, sodium, chloride, calcium, phosphate, magnesium), and trace elements (e.g., cobalt, zinc, manganese). Additives are adapted to each client's nutritional needs. Fat emulsions may be given to provide essential fatty acids to correct and/or prevent essential fatty acid deficiency or to supplement the calories for clients who, for example, have high calorie needs or cannot tolerate glucose as the only calorie source.

Because TPN solutions are high in glucose, infusions are started gradually to prevent hyperglycemia. The client needs to adapt to TPN therapy by increasing his or her insulin output from the pancreas. For example, an adult client may be given 1 liter (40 ml/hr) of TPN solution the first day, if the infusion is tolerated; the amount may be increased to 2 liters (80 ml/hr) for 24 to 48 hours, and then to 3 liters (120 ml/hr) within 3 to 5 days. When TPN therapy is to be discontinued, the TPN infusion rates are decreased slowly to prevent hyperinsulinemia and hypoglycemia. Weaning a client from TPN may take up to 48 hours but can occur in 6 hours as long as the client receives adequate carbohydrates either orally or intravenously.

Nursing Assessment and Interventions

Meticulous client assessment is necessary during TPN therapy. The assessment should focus on the client and on the TPN system. Observe the client for signs of thrombosis or thrombophlebitis at the catheter insertion site (e.g., edema or redness) and along the course of the vein (e.g., pain or swelling of the arm, neck, or face). Purulent thrombophlebitis may result in a purulent discharge, which appears at the insertion site with slight pressure. If such signs are observed, notify the physician, who may order removal of the catheter and initiation of a heparin infusion at a peripheral vein site. Also observe the client for signs of air embolism (apprehension, dyspnea, tachycardia, chest pain, hypotension, cyanosis, and loss of consciousness). If air embolism is suspected, administer oxygen and place the client on his or her left side with the head lowered. Lowering the head increases intrathoracic pressure, decreasing the flow of air into the vein during inhalation. A left side lying position helps prevent the air from moving to the pulmonary artery.

Monitor vital signs every 4 hours or more often, depending on the client's health. An elevated temperature is one of the earliest indications of catheter-related sepsis. Change the TPN tubing every 48 hours or according to agency practice.

Never use the TPN infusion line to (a) take central venous pressure (CVP) measurements, (b) take blood samples, (c) piggyback other solutions, (d) infuse blood or blood products, or (e) inject medications. Before administering any TPN solution, check its expiration date. Most solutions must be used within 24 hours of preparation, unless they are refrigerated. Carefully monitor the infusion flow rate and the laboratory test results to detect such complications as hyperglycemia or electrolyte imbalance. Use of an infusion pump keeps the infusion rate regular. Collect double-voided urine specimens at least every 6 hours or in accordance with agency policy, and test the urine for specific gravity and glucose and acetone levels. If the specific gravity is abnormal, notify the physician, who may alter the constituents of the TPN solution. Also notify the physician if the glucose level is elevated to ¼% (+ +). Supplementary insulin may be ordered and given subcutaneously or added directly to the TPN solution by pharmacy personnel. Glucosuria is often the first sign of catheter-related sepsis.

Record the client's daily fluid intake and output and calorie intake as baseline data. Precise replacement for fluid and electrolyte deficits can then be more readily determined. Weigh the client daily, at the same time and in the same garments. A gain of more than 0.5 kg (1.1 lb) per day indicates fluid excess and should be reported. Measure arm circumference and triceps skin fold thickness to assess the client's physical changes. Monitor the results of laboratory tests (e.g., serum electrolytes, blood glucose, and blood urea nitrogen) and report abnormal findings to the physician.

Change the TPN dressing at least every 48 hours or more often if it is moist or loose, in accordance with agency policy. Changing TPN dressing requires strict sterile technique and special practices to ensure that microorganisms do not enter the incision.

Central Venous Lines

A central venous line is a catheter inserted into a large vein located centrally in the body. The tip of the catheter may terminate in the vein, e.g., the superior vena cava, or in the right atrium of the heart. Insertion of the line may be a nonsurgical or a surgical procedure. Central venous lines are usually inserted by physicians, although some nurses who are specially prepared insert central venous lines that exit peripherally in the antecubital fossa of the arm.

Central venous lines are inserted primarily for the following reasons:

1. To administer nutritional solutions that are highly irritating to smaller veins
2. To administer irritating medications
3. To monitor central venous pressure (CVP)
4. To withdraw central venous blood

Types of Central Venous Lines

Standard central venous lines are catheters of variable length that are inserted in a nonsurgical procedure. They are usually made of polyethylene or silicone rubber and vary in size. A 20-cm-long #16 gauge catheter is frequently used. The catheters are radiopaque so that they will show up on fluoroscopy or x-ray films. Short lines are used when the tip is inserted to the superior vena cava or subclavian vein; longer lines are used when the tip is inserted to the right atrium of the heart. A peripherally inserted line is a long venous catheter; two kinds are the Intrasil catheter and the Drum catheter.

Catheters are also inserted surgically. Examples are the Hickman catheter and the Broviac catheter. The Hickman is a single- or double-lumen catheter, with a 1.6-mm internal diameter of the lumen. It is therefore large enough for the passage of nutritional substances, blood, and antibiotics. The drawbacks of the single-lumen Hickman catheter are that the administration of nutritional substances must be interrupted if the catheter needs to be used for measuring central venous pressure or to administer blood, and the risk of infection is increased. A double Hickman catheter is used for this reason. It is the fusion of two Hickman catheters or a Hickman and a Broviac catheter. The Broviac line has an internal diameter of 1.0 mm, narrower than the Hickman but still large enough to administer nutritional substances. With the double-lumen catheter, the administration of TPN can be continued through the smaller lumen while antibiotics, for example, can be administered through the larger lumen. The Broviac catheter used alone is like a single Hickman catheter. However, because its lumen is narrower, blood cannot be withdrawn through it. These surgically inserted lines are intended for use over an extended period.

Nonsurgical Insertion

The insertion of a standard central venous line is normally considered a nonsurgical procedure. Commonly, the line is inserted below the clavicle (the infraclavicular approach) into the right or left subclavian vein, and the tip of the catheter remains in the subclavian vein or the superior vena cava (see Figure 46–29, *A*), i.e., a short line is used.

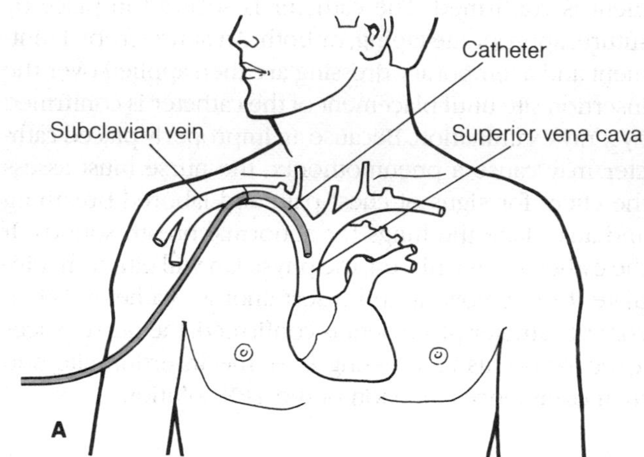

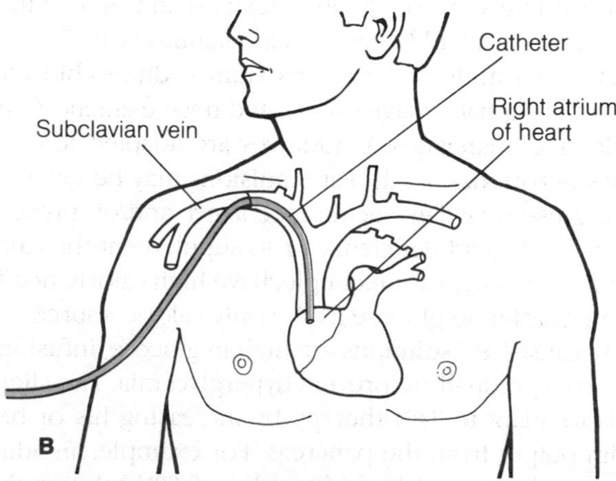

Figure 46–29 A central venous line with the exit site on the chest below the clavicle: **A,** the tip of the catheter is in the superior vena cava; **B,** the tip of the catheter is in the right atrium of the heart.

It can also be extended into the atrium of the heart (see Figure 46–29, *B*), i.e., a long line can be used. This site permits freedom of movement for ambulation, but a pneumothorax can occur during insertion. Another approach for a standard central venous line is through the right or left jugular vein (the supraclavicular approach). This site hinders head and neck movement somewhat but provides a straight line to the subclavian vein (and superior vena cava). See Figure 46–30. This is an especially useful approach for children.

When the infra- and supraclavicular approaches are used, a local anesthetic is usually applied to the site prior to the catheter insertion. While the physician is inserting the catheter, the nurse monitors the client's pulse rate. The onset of arrhythmia may indicate that the catheter tip is irritating the heart and placement requires adjustment.

Another type of central venous line, i.e., the Intrasil catheter, is inserted more peripherally, e.g., into a vein in the antecubital fossa of the arm, and threaded up the vein in the arm into the right atrium of the heart. The position of the catheter is verified by fluoroscopy. See Figure 46–31. This type of line can be used to administer nutritional solutions, to obtain blood specimens, and to measure pressure in the right atrium of the heart.

The exit of this catheter (at the antecubital fossa) looks like that of an intravenous line. It is important for nurses to know that the catheter extends farther into the vein and that its purpose and care differ.

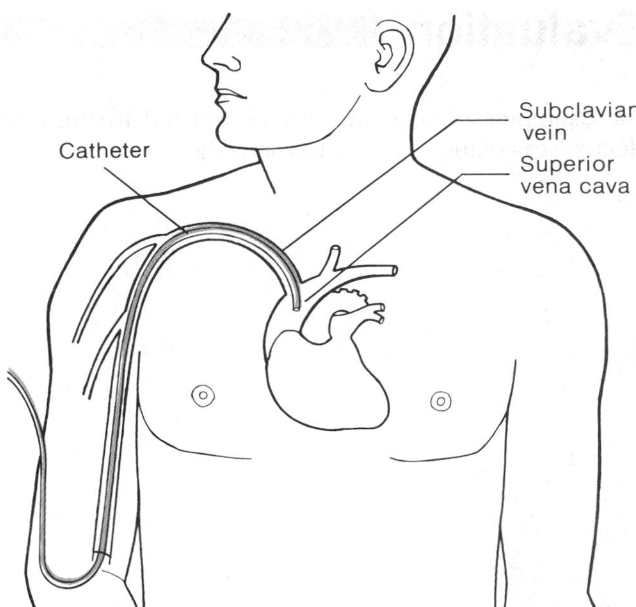

Figure 46–31 A central venous line inserted peripherally at a point in the antecubital fossa of the right arm, with the tip of the catheter in the superior vena cava

Surgical Insertion

The surgical insertion of a central venous catheter (e.g., a Hickman, Quinton, or Corcath catheter) involves an incision into the tissue of the chest. The catheter is inserted under the subcutaneous tissue to a centrally located vein, e.g., the subclavian vein. It is then inserted into the vein and extended into the atrium of the heart. See Figure 46–32. These catheters usually have Dacron cuffs that promote growth of the subcutaneous tissue around the catheter, thus helping to prevent infection. With this type of insertion, the exit site of the catheter is on the chest some distance from its insertion site into the venous system.

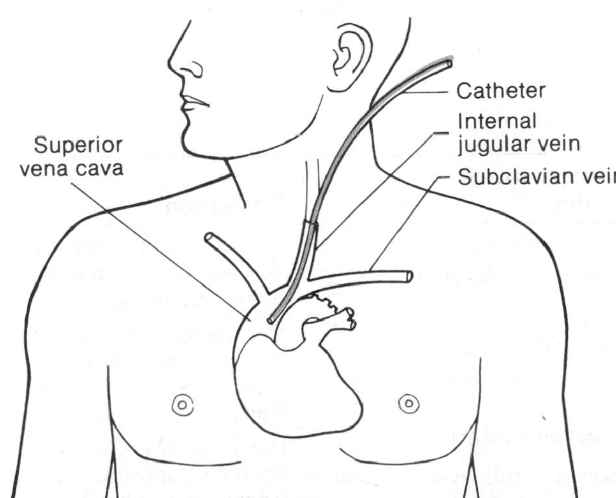

Figure 46–30 A central venous line inserted into the left jugular vein, with the tip of the catheter in the superior vena cava

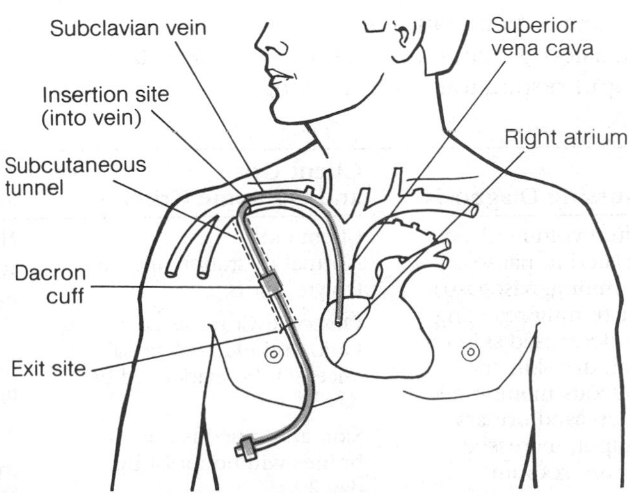

Figure 46–32 A Hickman catheter inserted surgically into the chest wall, entering the subclavian vein, and extending into the right atrium

Evaluation

For examples of outcome criteria related to fluid and electrolyte balance, see list to the right.

Examples of Outcome Criteria for Clients with Fluid and Electrolyte Imbalances

The client will:

- Drink 3000 ml of fluid daily
- Have good tissue turgor
- Have a normal serum potassium
- Lose 3 pounds in 2 days
- Have a normal urine specific gravity
- Have a normal $Paco_2$

Nursing Care Plan

Assessment Data

Nursing Assessment

Mrs. Joan O'Brien is a 46-year-old waitress who underwent a cholecystectomy yesterday for treatment of acute cholecystitis/cholelithiasis. She has had an intolerance of fatty foods and indigestion for several months. For 2 days prior to surgery, she had experienced acute pain and tenderness in the upper right abdomen and severe nausea and vomiting. In addition, she has been anorexic for several days. Mrs. O'Brien returned from surgery with a nasogastric tube connected to low intermittent suction and a T-tube to gravity drainage. She is NPO and is receiving intravenous infusions at an 8-hour rate. Her skin and mucous membranes are dry. Her subcostal abdominal incision is painful, and as a result she is taking shallow, rapid respirations with splinting.

Physical Examination

Height: 160 cm (5′3″)
Weight: 66.2 kg (146 lb)
Temperature: 38.1 C (100.6 F)
Pulse rate: 96 BPM
Respirations: 28 per minute
Blood pressure: 110/70 mm Hg
Skin turgor poor
Skin dry and mucous membranes dry and sticky
Dark amber urine

Diagnostic Data

Chest x-ray film: Negative
Serum Na: 155 mEq/liter
Serum Osmolarity: 298 mOsm/kg
Serum Potassium: 3.2 mEq/liter
Serum Bicarbonate: 33 mEq/liter
Plasma pH 7.48

Nursing Diagnosis	Client Goals and Outcome Criteria	Nursing Interventions and Rationales	Evaluation
Fluid volume deficit related to nausea, vomiting, nasogastric suctioning resulting in decreased skin turgor, dry skin and mucous membranes, decreased urinary output, increased serum sodium.	Client Goal: Normal hydration and electrolyte status. Outcome Criteria: Fluid and electrolyte balance will be evidenced by day 3. Skin and mucous membranes will be moist by day 2. Urinary output will be approximately 2000 ml per day.	Maintain accurate I&O. *Rationale:* Provides data about fluid balance. Assess client for dry skin, dry mucous membranes, and poor skin turgor. *Rationale:* Denotes dehydration. Irrigate nasogastric tube with normal saline. *Rationale:* Keeps tube patent and decreases chance of further electrolyte imbalance.	On day 3, Mrs. O'Brien's skin and mucous membranes are moist. Her nasogastric tube has been removed, and she is taking sips of water and ice chips. Her 24-hr IV intake has been 2000 ml, and her urinary output has been 1500 ml.

(continued)

Nursing Diagnosis	Client Goals and Outcome Criteria	Nursing Interventions and Rationales	Evaluation
		Administer IV fluids and electrolytes as ordered. *Rationale:* Replaces fluids and electrolytes and maintains hydration and nutrition. Assess wound and T-tube drainage. *Rationale:* Excessive drainage may increase fluid imbalance and need for increase in fluid replacement.	Her lab values are Potassium: 3.8 mEq/liter Sodium: 137 mEq/liter Serum osmolarity: 287 mOsm/kg
Ineffective breathing pattern due to subcostal abdominal incision resulting in shallow respiration, ineffective coughing, splinted/guarded respirations.	Client Goal: Maintain effective breathing pattern and have no respiratory complications. Outcome Criteria: Coughs and deep breathes q1 hr within first 48 hrs. Absence of adventitious breath sounds by day 2. Splints abdomen when coughing or deep breathing by day 2.	Assess for shallow breathing and adventitious breath sounds. *Rationale:* Ineffective breathing may result in atelectasis or pneumonia. Encourage coughing, turning, and deep breathing q1–2 hrs. *Rationale:* Assists in mobilizing secretions and decreasing development of atelectasis and other complications. Instruct client to splint incision while coughing and deep breathing. *Rationale:* Splinting incision provides support and decreases pain. Assist client with use of incentive spirometer. *Rationale:* Use of incentive spirometer will improve the volume of inspiration.	On day 2, Mrs. O'Brien splints her abdominal incision while coughing and deep breathing a minimum of every 2 hrs. Her breath sounds are clear; no adventitious breath sounds are noted.

Chapter Highlights

- A balance of both fluids and electrolytes in the body is necessary for health and life.
- The younger the person, the higher the proportion of water in the body.
- Extracellular fluid (ECF) is subdivided into two compartments: intravascular (plasma) and interstitial.
- ECF comprises about one-quarter to one-third of total body fluid.
- Intracellular fluid (ICF) is the fluid inside the cells.
- There are two types of body electrolytes (ions): positively charged ions (cations) and negatively charged ions (anions).
- The principal ions of ECF are sodium and chloride.
- The principal ions of ICF are potassium and phosphate.
- Fluids move among the body compartments by diffusion, osmosis, and active transport.
- The major fluid pressures are osmotic pressure and hydrostatic pressure.
- The three sources of body fluid are fluids taken orally, food ingested, and the oxidation of food.
- Fluid intake is regulated by the thirst mechanism.
- Fluid output is chiefly through the excretion of urine, although body fluid is also lost through sweat, feces, and insensible vapor loss.
- The acid-base balance of the body is controlled by three buffer systems: bicarbonate, phosphate, and protein.
- Fluid and electrolyte imbalance is most accurately determined through laboratory examination of blood plasma.
- The most common electrolyte imbalances are deficits or excesses in sodium, potassium, and calcium.
- Acid-base imbalance occurs when the body fluids are higher or lower than the normal pH range: 7.35 to 7.45.

- There are two types of acid-base disturbance, respiratory and metabolic, which can result in acidosis or alkalosis.
- Parenteral therapy includes the administration of fluids and electrolytes intravenously (IV).
- Preventing complications is an important aspect of IV therapy and blood transfusions.
- Assessment of a client's hydration and electrolyte status is an important nursing responsibility.

Suggested Readings

Feldstein, A. January 1986. Detect phlebitis and infiltration before they harm your patient. *Nursing 86* 16:44–47.
More than 70% of hospitalized clients receive IV therapy. Preventing phlebitis and infiltration necessitates selecting the right cannula and right vein. Feldstein explains these two problems, indicates the clinical signs, and explains what nurses should do in the event they identify any of the clinical signs.

Folk-Lighty, M. February 1984. Solving the puzzles of patients' fluid imbalances. *Nursing 84* 14:34–41.
Folk-Lighty identifies clients at greatest risk of developing fluid and electrolyte imbalances, explains the physiology underlying imbalances, and details the nursing assessment of clients.

Nelson, R., and Miller, H. March 1986. Keeping air out of IV lines. *Nursing 86* 16:57–59.
Nelson and Miller describe ways to prevent air emboli in IV lines. Suggested techniques included using a roller clamp, priming the drip chamber, priming the IV tubing, removing air from the line, circumventing a back check valve, and removing air from a secondary line.

Scarlato, M. February 1978. Blood transfusions today: What you should know and do. *Nursing 78* 8:68–70, 72.
Scarlato outlines the nurse's responsibilities and nursing guidelines for transfusions. Checklists are provided to help the nurse minimize the risks of transfusing whole blood, packed red blood cells, platelets, and plasma fractions.

Twombly, M. June 1978. The shift into third space. *Nursing 78* 8:38–41.
Twombly describes fluid shifts into the interstitial fluid compartment (a process called *third spacing*), the physiologic changes that occur during two phases, and the interventions the nurse can take.

Selected References

Anderson, M. A.; Aker, S. N.; and Hickman, R. O. February 1982. The double-lumen Hickman catheter. *American Journal of Nursing* 82:272–73.

Beaumont, E. July 1977. The new IV infusion pumps. *Nursing 77* 7:31–35.

Behrman, R. E., and Vaughan, V. C. 1983. *Nelson textbook of pediatrics.* 12th ed. Philadelphia: W. B. Saunders Co.

Bellack, J. P., and Bamford, P. A. 1984. *Nursing assessment: A multidimensional approach.* Monterey, Calif.: Wadsworth Health Sciences Division.

Burke, S. R. 1980. *The composition and function of body fluids.* 3d ed. St. Louis: C. V. Mosby Co.

Burrows, C. W. December 1984. Take a step toward better IV needle selections. *Nursing 84* 14:32–33.

Byrne, C. J.; Saxton, D. F.; Pelikan, P. K.; and Nugent, P. M. 1986. *Laboratory tests: Implications for nursing care.* 2d ed. Menlo Park, Calif.: Addison-Wesley Publishing Co.

Centers for Disease Control. 1982. Guidelines for prevention of intravascular infections. *Infection Control* 3:61–72.

Christian, J. L., and Greger, J. L. 1985. *Nutrition for living.* Menlo Park, Calif.: Benjamin/Cummings Publishing Co.

Feldstein, A. G. March 1985. Action stat catheter embolus. *Nursing 85* 15:59.

Frawley, L. W. December 1985. Cost-effective application of the Centers for Disease Control guideline for prevention of intravascular infections. *American Journal of Infection Control* 13:275–77.

Goldberg, P. B. September/October 1980. Medications that contain sodium. *Geriatric Nursing* 1:204–5.

Grant, M. M., and Kubo, W. M. August 1975. Assessing a patient's hydration status. *American Journal of Nursing* 75:1306–11.

Guyton, A. C. 1986. *Textbook of medical physiology.* 7th ed. Philadelphia: W. B. Saunders Co.

Harvey, A. M.; Johns, R. J.; McKusick, V. A.; Owens, A. H.; and Ross, R. S. 1980. *The principles and practice of medicine.* 20th ed. New York: Appleton-Century-Crofts.

Howard, M.; Puri, V.; and Paidipaty, B. November 1984. The effects of fluid resuscitation in the critically ill patient. *Heart and Lung* 13(6):649–54.

Howard, R. B., and Herbold, N. H. 1982. *Nutrition in clinical care.* 2d ed. New York: McGraw-Hill.

Huey, F. L. 1983. Setting up and troubleshooting. *American Journal of Nursing* 83:1026–28.

Intermed Communications. 1980. *Managing IV therapy.* Nursing 80 Photobook Series. Horsham, Pa.: Intermed Communications.

———. 1981. *Monitoring fluid and electrolytes precisely.* Nursing Skillbook Series. Horsham, Pa.: Intermed Communications.

Karrei, I. December 1982. Hickman catheters: Your guide to troublefree use. *Canadian Nurse* 78:25–27.

Keithley, J. K., and Fraulini, K. E. March 1982. What's behind that IV line? *Nursing 82* 12:32–42.

Lee, C. A.; Stroot, V. R.; and Schaper, C. A. August 1975. What to do when acid-base problems hang in the balance. *Nursing 75* 5:32–37.

Metheny, N. M., and Snively, W. D. 1983. *Nurses' handbook of fluid balance.* 4th ed. Philadelphia: J. B. Lippincott Co.

Munro-Black, J. February 1984. The ABC's of total parenteral nutrition. *Nursing 84* 14:50–56.

Peck, N. 1985. Perfecting your IV therapy techniques. (3 parts.) *Nursing 85* (May) 15:38–43, (June) 15:48–51, and (July) 15:32–35.

Reed, G. M. March 1974. Confused about potassium? Here's a clear concise guide. *Nursing 74* 4:21.

Sharer, J. E. June 1975. Reviewing acid-base balance. *American Journal of Nursing* 75:980–83.

Speciale, J. L. October 1985. Infuse-a-port new path for IV therapy. *Nursing 85* 15:40–43.

Taylor, D. L. October 1984. Respiratory acidosis: Physiology, signs, and symptoms. *Nursing 84* 14:44–45.

———. November 1984. Respiratory alkalosis: Physiology, signs, and symptoms. *Nursing 84* 14:44–45.

Tripp, A. July 1976. Hyper- and hypocalcemia. *American Journal of Nursing* 76:1142–45.

Ungvarski, P. J. December 1976. Parenteral therapy. *American Journal of Nursing* 76:1974–77.

Vick, R. E. 1984. *Contemporary medical physiology.* Menlo Park, Calif.: Addison-Wesley Publishing Co.

Whitney, E. N., and Cataldo, C. B. 1983. *Understanding normal and clinical nutrition.* West.

Wiseman, M. April 1985. Setting standards for home IV therapy. *American Journal of Nursing* 85:421–23.

Wittig, P., and Semmler-Bertanzi, D. J. July 1983. Pumps and controllers: A nurse's assessment guide. *American Journal of Nursing* 83:1022–25.

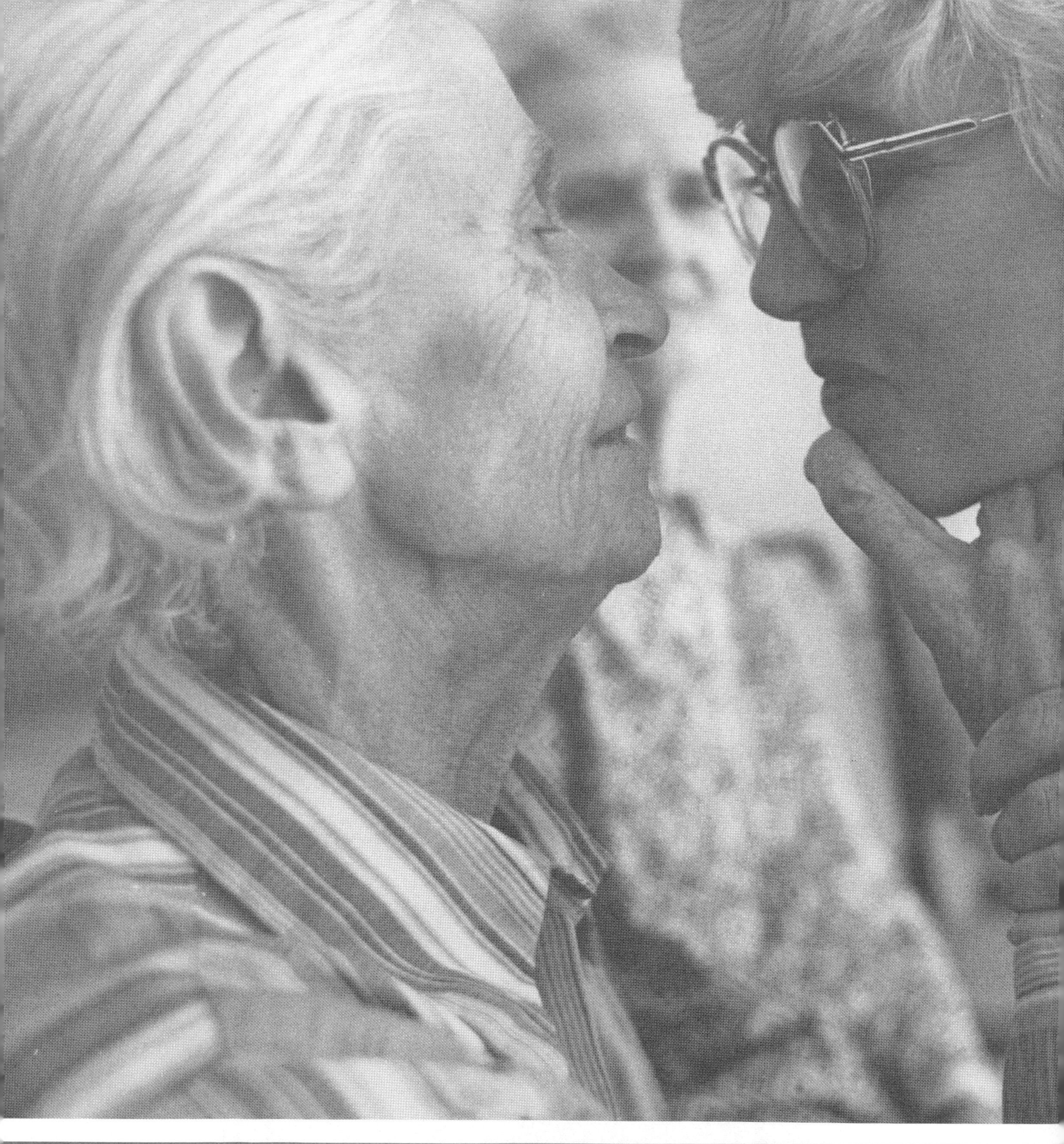

Nursing puts us in touch with being human. Nurses are invited into the inner spaces of other people's existence without even asking, for where there is suffering, loneliness, the tolerable pain of cure or the solitary pain of permanent change, there is the need for the kind of human service we call nursing. (Donna Diers)

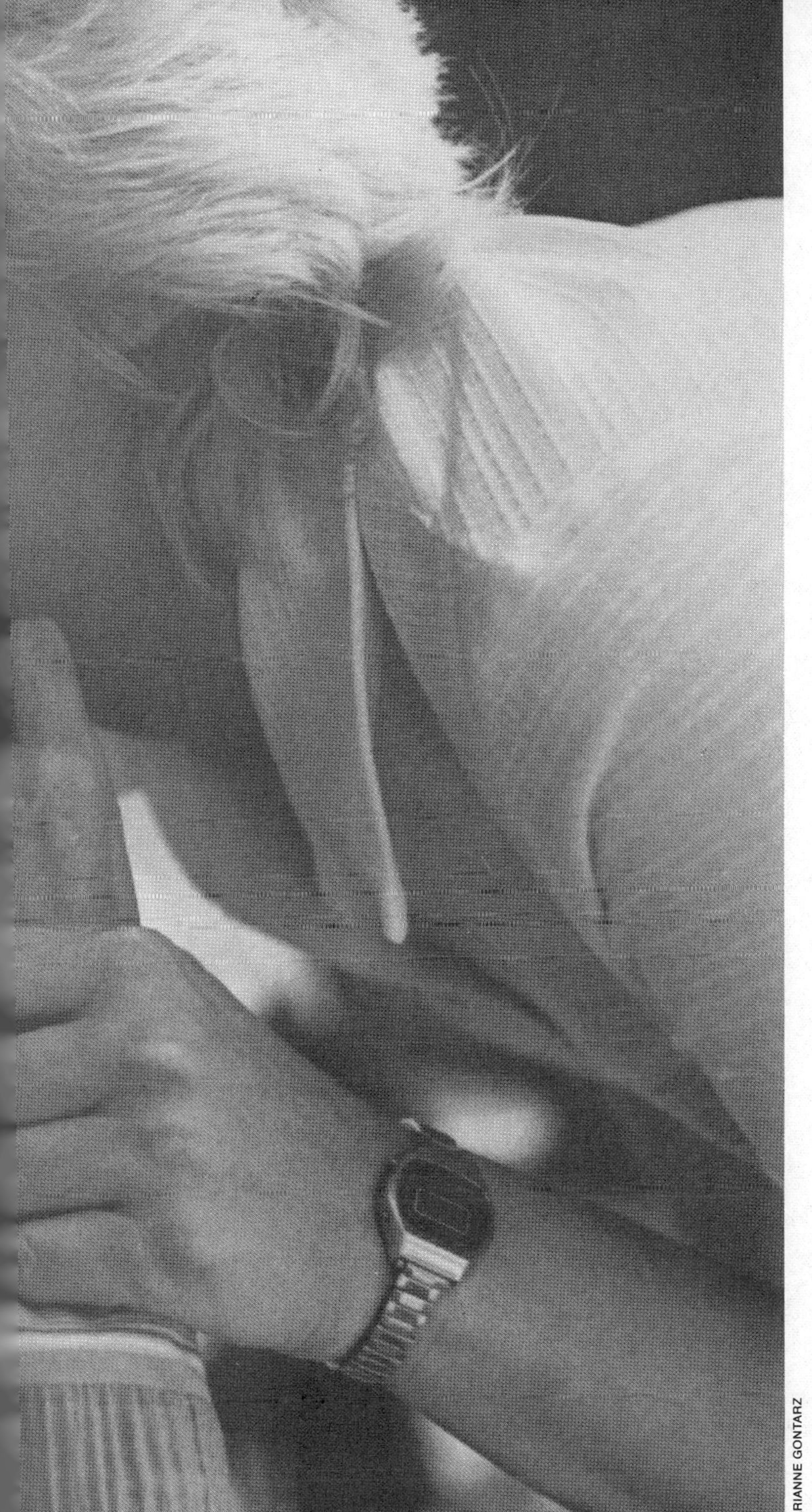

UNIT **10**

Psychosocial Concepts

Contents

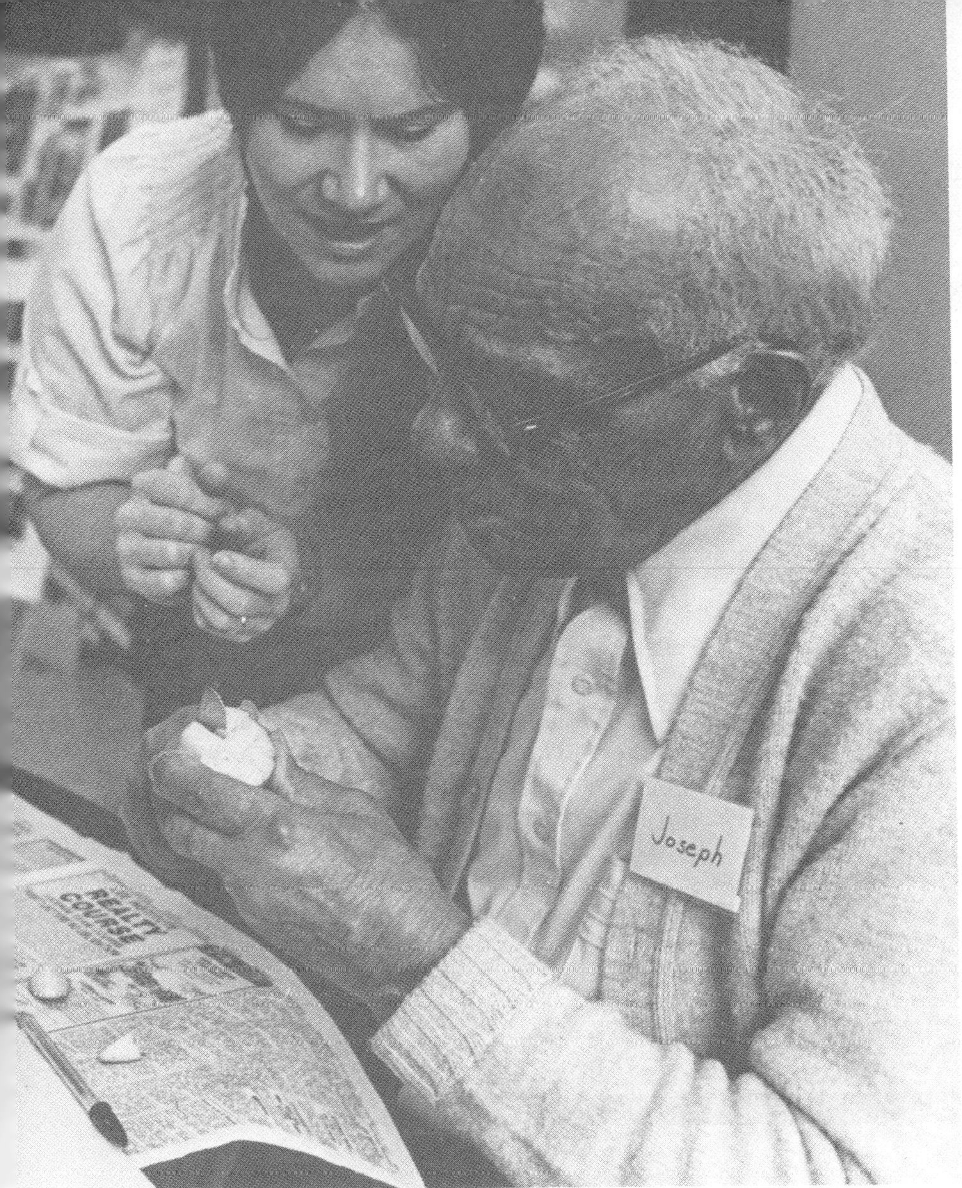

MARIANNE GONTARZ

CHAPTER 47

Stimulation

Contents

47 *Stimulation*

Objectives

1. Know essential facts about sensory stimulation and the sensory-perceptual process.
   1.1 Define selected terms.
   1.2 Identify stages of awareness and consciousness.
   1.3 Identify structural and physiologic elements of the sensory-perceptual process.
   1.4 Identify various types of sensation.
   1.5 Identify causes and signs of three kinds of sensory disturbance.
2. Know information and methods required to assess and diagnose sensory-perceptual status.
   2.1 Identify clients most at risk of sensory disturbances.
   2.2 Identify data to obtain in the health history.
   2.3 Identify factors influencing sensory function.
   2.4 Identify physical examinations that assess sensory function.
   2.5 Identify clinical signs of sensory dysfunction.
   2.6 Identify nursing diagnoses of sensory disturbances.
3. Know facts about nursing interventions to maintain and promote optimal sensory stimulation.
   3.1 Explain nursing interventions to adjust environmental stimuli.
   3.2 Explain interventions that promote functioning of existing senses.
   3.3 Explain interventions that help the client adapt to altered sensory function.
   3.4 Identify interventions that decrease further sensory loss.
   3.5 Explain ways of providing a safe environment.
4. Apply the nursing process when providing care to selected clients with sensory disturbances.
   4.1 Obtain necessary assessment data.
   4.2 Analyze and relate assessment data.
   4.3 Write relevant nursing diagnoses.
   4.4 Plan appropriate nursing strategies.
   4.5 Implement appropriate nursing interventions.
   4.6 State outcome criteria against which to evaluate the client's progress.

Terms

aphasia
auditory stimulus
awareness
consciousness
decussate
disengagement
engagement
gustatory stimulus
hallucination
illusion
kinesthesia
kinesthetic stimulus
olfactory stimulus
self-engagement
sensoristasis
sensorium
sensory adaptation
sensory deficit
sensory deprivation (input deficit)
sensory overload
stereognosis
tactile stimulus
visceral stimulus
visual stimulus

Sensory Perception

Sensory perception starts with a stimulus that triggers a receptor. The stimulus travels along a neuron (sensory neuron I) to the central nervous system. From the spinal cord or brain stem, the impulses travel along sensory neuron II to the thalamus. These neurons synapse with sensory neurons III, which conduct the impulses from the thalamus to the somatosensory area of the postcentral gyrus of the parietal lobe of the brain, also called the primary sensory area. See Figure 47–1. In most instances, sensory pathways **decussate** (cross over) and register sensations from the opposite side of the body. Usually, decussation takes place at the level of sensory neuron II.

Sensory pathways carry information about heat, cold, touch, and pressure. **Stereognosis** (awareness of an object's size, shape, and texture), **kinesthesia** (ability to perceive muscle movement), vibratory sense, and two-point and weight discrimination are also sensory abilities that terminate in the primary sensory area. See Figure 47–2. Other special sensory areas are: visual, auditory, and olfactory association areas. The gustatory area is located in the parietal lobe deep in the lateral fissure.

Consciousness requires continuous stimulation of cortical neurons by impulses conducted through a relay of neurons called the reticular activating system. This system consists of centers in the brain stem that receive impulses from the spinal cord and relay them to the thalamus and from there to all parts of the cerebral cortex. For additional information about perception, see Chapter 10, pages 224 to 225.

The need for sensory stimulation is called **sensoristasis.** Humans need constant and varied sensory stimuli. Insufficient stimuli cause sensory deprivation. Overstimulation at any one site causes **sensory adaptation,** a result of the ability of sensory receptors to adapt partially or completely to a repeated stimulus. At first, receptors respond at a very high impulse rate; with continued stimulation, the receptors respond less rapidly and finally many do not respond at all. For this reason, the brain ceases to perceive the repeated stimulus. Extreme concentration produces a similar effect: The brain does not perceive extraneous stimuli.

Sensory stimuli are either external or internal. External stimuli arise from outside of the person. They are **visual** (sight), **auditory** (hearing), **olfactory** (smell), **tactile** (touch), and **gustatory** (taste). Gustatory stimuli can be internal as well. Internal stimuli are kinesthetic or visceral. **Kinesthetic** refers to awareness of the position and movement of body parts. **Visceral** refers to any large organ in the body's interior.

Certain problems create sensations that do not arise from normal external or internal stimuli. For example, a client who has a disease of the auditory nerve may hear sounds that correspond to no external stimulus. **Hallucinations** (perceptions of external stimuli in the absence of such stimuli) can result, for example, from a disease process or hallucinogenic drugs. **Illusions** are misinterpretations of external stimuli. For example, a person may interpret a shadow cast by a lamp as a person.

States of Awareness

Awareness is the ability to perceive environmental stimuli and body reactions and to respond appropriately through thought and action. The normal, alert person can assimilate many kinds of information at one time. The restaurant patron who dines with friends appreciates odors, tastes, conversation, and company at the same time. The normal person perceives reality accurately and acts on those perceptions. Part of this process is separating necessary stimuli from extraneous ones and reaching logical conclusions by correlating information. Most people do this with little or no awareness of the mental processes involved. Occasionally, normal persons exhibit abnormalities of thought; they become absent minded, lose their sense of direction, and so on. Often these episodes are due to intense concentration on one subject to the exclusion of others.

Consciousness is awareness of environment, self, and others. Illness and age can affect consciousness, as can hospitalization. Mildly confused hospitalized clients may momentarily forget they are not at home, wander from their rooms, misplace personal belongings, and so forth. Severely confused (disoriented) persons may not know family members or may think the nurse is a relative. Such persons may act atypically: Confused, normally docile people may become combative with nurses and others. Severely confused people do not know where they are or what time of day or day of the week it is.

Level of consciousness also affects awareness. See Table 35–29, page 897, for levels of consciousness.

Sensory Alterations

Sensory Deprivation

Sensory deprivation is a level of sensory input too low to permit normal functioning. Sensory deprivation, also called emotional-touch deprivation, is situational; i.e., it occurs when clients are confined in a stressful environment and interpersonal interactions are reduced (Gioiella and Bevil 1985, p. 537). Ebersole and Hess (1985, p. 321) describe three sources of sensory deprivation: (a) restricting the environment, (b) reducing sensory input, and (c) eliminating order and meaning from input.

When a person experiences sensory deprivation, the balance of the reticular activating system (RAS) is disturbed. The RAS is unable to maintain normal stimulation of the cerebral cortex. Because of this reduced stimulation, the person becomes more acutely aware of the remaining stimuli and perceives these in a distorted manner.

Maintaining some contact with the environment is considered to be essential for self-esteem (Ravish 1985, p. 10). Through **engagement,** a process that occurs from childhood through middle age, relationships are formed.

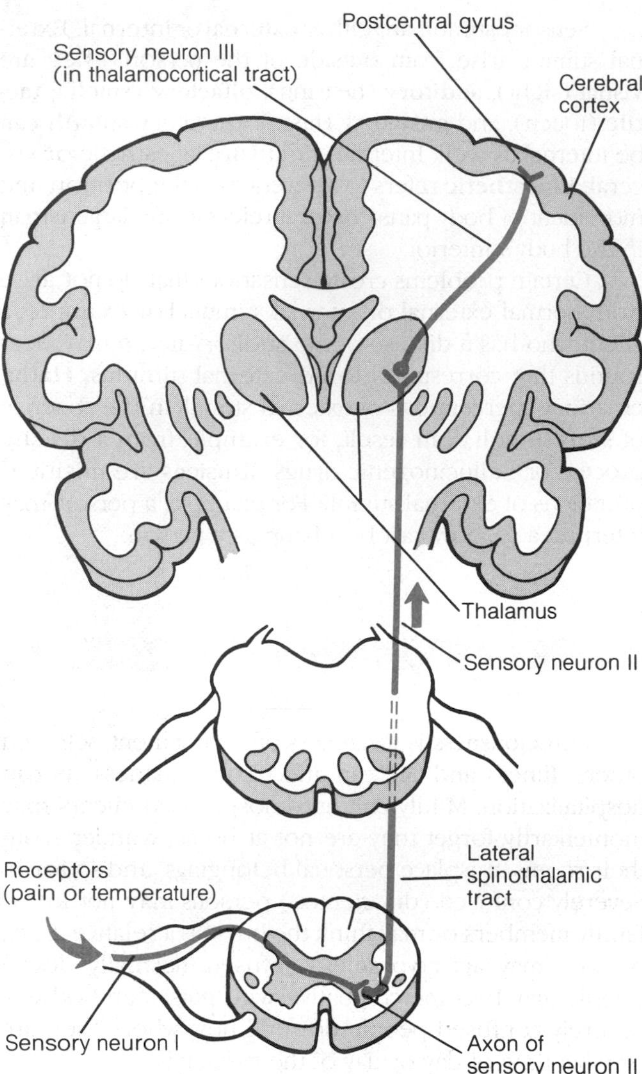

Figure 47–1 The lateral spinothalamic tract transmits impulses of crude touch, pain, and temperature up the spinal cord to the thalamus. The thalamocortical tract transmits impulses from the thalamus to the somatic sensory area of the cortex (postcentral gyrus).

Disengagement begins as the person enters old age. **Disengagement** is the process of narrowing social contacts and reducing the number of roles a person assumes. Disengagement, however, does not mean severing all contacts. Normally, disengagement is intentional and voluntary. **Self-engagement** is the final aspect of disengagement. At this time, the elderly individual becomes more self-directed and participates in solitary, though creative and enjoyable, activities (Ravish 1985, p. 11). The elderly person at this time normally maintains contact with the environment through family and friends.

Elderly people are particularly susceptible to social isolation and a restricted environment. The elderly person can become socially isolated for a number of reasons, e.g., limited physical mobility, death of a spouse and/or friends, and changed living arrangements.

Sensory Overload

Sensory overload is more sensory stimulation in a given period than one can tolerate. Hospitalized clients, exposed to bright lights, noise, unfamiliar machinery, and too many visits from friends and health personnel, may suffer sensory overload. A continuous barrage of stimuli can produce in clients many of the symptoms of sensory deprivation. The person may appear fatigued, agitated, and confused and may have hallucinations.

Sensory Deficit

A **sensory deficit** is impaired functioning of a sensory or perceptual process. Blindness and deafness are sensory deficits. A sensory deficit may also be considered a type of sensory deprivation. When only one sense is affected, other senses may become more acute to compensate for the loss. However, sudden loss of eyesight can result in total disorientation.

When there is gradual loss of sensory function, individuals often develop behavioral alterations to compensate for the loss; sometimes the behaviors are unconscious. For example, a person with gradual hearing loss in the right ear may unconsciously turn the left ear toward a speaker. When the loss is sudden, compensatory behaviors take days or weeks to develop.

Some neurologic diseases cause changes in kinesthetic sense and tactile perceptions. Disease of the inner ear, for example, can cause loss of kinesthetic sense. Spinal cord injuries and cerebrovascular accidents cause paralysis and loss of tactile perception.

Factors Affecting Sensory-Perceptual Function

Age

Perception of sensation is critical to the intellectual, social, and physical development of infants and children. As children grow, they learn that certain sensations provide cues for behavior already learned, e.g., stopping and looking both ways before crossing a street. Adults have many learned responses to sensory cues. Loss or impairment of any sense, therefore, has profound effects on both the child and young adult. The gradual diminishing of sensory perception that comes with age does not have as profound an effect.

Vision, hearing, and touch decline with age. Sight usually declines after age 45. Vision accuracy (both near and far perception), adaptation to light and dark, color discrimination, adaptation to glare, and visual acuity all diminish (Crandall 1980, p. 142). Hearing begins to decline at about 25 years. Generally, elderly people experience loss of volume perception and loss of pitch perception. At about 55 years, people become less sensitive to changes in touch, temperature, and pain. Loss of sensitivity usually

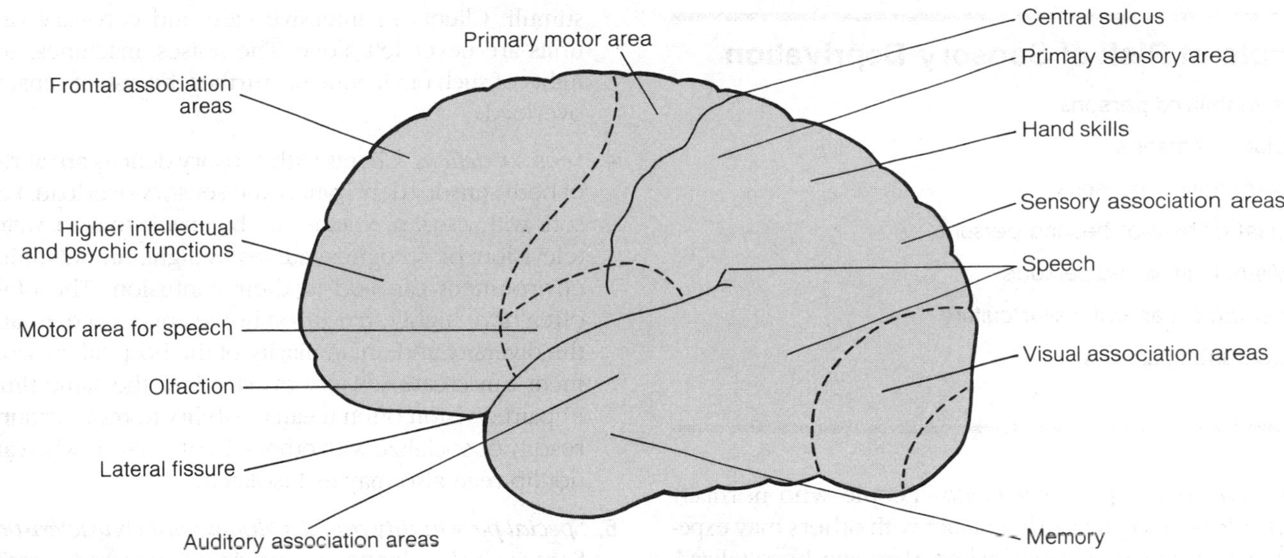

Figure 47–2 The lateral aspect of the functional areas of the left cerebral cortex.

begins on the lower half of the body and spreads upward (Crandall 1980, p. 145). Taste and smell do not seem to change with age. It is thought that changes are more probably due to disease or to chronic smoking.

Illness

Certain illnesses affect sensory function. Atherosclerosis, arteriosclerosis, and similar disorders restrict blood flow to the receptor organ or the brain, decreasing awareness and slowing responses. Uncontrolled diabetes mellitus can impair vision. Central nervous system disease causes varying degrees of paralysis and sensory loss.

Cognitive and Emotional Resources

Individuals' cognitive and emotional resources also affect their capacity to deal with sensory deprivation and sensory overload. Mitchell and Loustau (1981, p. 317) found that intelligent and creative people can cope with sensory deprivation better than others.

Medications

Certain medications can affect a person's sensory perceptions, e.g., streptomycin can cause injury to the auditory nerve. Narcotics and sedatives can alter a person's perceptions of sensory stimuli, making people lethargic and less aware of their environments.

Environment

Because sensory stimuli come from the environment, the environment is a major factor in sensory deprivation and sensory overload. Suedfeld (1985, p. 84) describes environmental stimulation as including all environmental inputs that are sensed or received at some level. Environmental stimuli can be social or nonsocial. There are three actions that people may or may not be able to take in response to stressful stimuli. The first is to change environments, e.g., move away from a noisy machine. This solution may not be practical, e.g., when a client needs a "noisy" respirator in order to breathe. The second is to modify the environment, i.e., increase or decrease the level of stimulation. This solution is workable only if the person has control over the environment. The client on a respirator, for example, cannot adjust the noise of the machine. The third is to change one's perception or reaction to the stimuli, e.g., by reinterpreting the stimuli, changing one's attentional focus, or raising or lowering one's threshold to the stimuli. For example, the client on a respirator might interpret the noise of the machine as soothing rhythm (reinterpreting the stimuli), turn his or her attention to a television program (changing attentional focus), or cognitively raise his or her internal threshold so that he or she does not hear the machine, much as a man who works in a noisy factory trains himself not to notice the noise.

Clients at Risk

Some people are particularly at risk of sensory deprivation (see page 1408). Others are at risk of sensory overload.

Nurses need to be aware of those people who are particularly susceptible to sensory disturbances. By anticipating possible problems, the nurse can often implement measures to prevent them. The following circumstances may predispose to sensory disturbances.

People at Risk of Sensory Deprivation

- Immobilized persons
- Elderly persons
- Terminally ill persons
- Deaf or hard-of-hearing persons
- Visually impaired persons
- Persons in an unfamiliar culture
- Confused persons

1. *Nonstimulating environments.* People who normally live alone and have little contact with others may experience sensory overload when they are hospitalized. This is particularly true of the elderly and of people who work at home alone. In their homes, these persons are at risk of sensory deprivation. People who live in institutions with unchanging social and perceptual stimuli are also at risk of sensory deprivations.
2. *Therapeutic isolation.* Therapeutic isolation, either in the hospital or at home, can predispose to sensory disturbance. Clients on protective asepsis are often confined to a room, and their primary social contacts are with gowned, masked personnel. Clients confined to bed, even though in rooms with other clients and allowed visitors, are also prone to sensory deprivation.
3. *Medically intensive environments.* Clients in constantly staffed environments are often overloaded with stimuli. Clients in intensive care and coronary care units are never left alone. The noises, machines, and lights of such environments further the risk of sensory overload.
4. *Sensory deficits.* Clients with sensory deficits are at risk of both sensory deprivation and sensory overload. Persons with visual problems may be unable to read, watch television, or recognize nurses by sight. An unfamiliar environment can add to their confusion. The blind often have highly structured home environments, and the diversity and unfamiliarity of the hospital environment can create sensory overload. At the same time, impaired vision often means inability to move around readily or socialize with others. Deaf persons who cannot lip-read also may feel isolated.
5. *Special personality and developmental characteristics.* Some people tolerate sensory deprivation and sensory overload better than others. People whose developmental levels are characterized by short attention spans, need for physical activity, and dependence on others for amusement are more susceptible to sensory deprivation than people who are more self-reliant and contemplative (Mitchell and Loustau 1981, p. 326). Likewise, persons who are stressed and anxious have more difficulty coping with sensory deprivation. Certain drugs, e.g., narcotics, decrease awareness of the environment, and people taking such drugs may be susceptible to sensory deprivation. People tolerate sensory overload differently. For example, a mother accustomed to six active, noisy children may hardly notice the noise of her environment, whereas another person would find the noise bothersome.

Assessment

When assessing for sensory disturbances, nurses should take a health history, examine the client for signs of sensory disturbance, and refer to laboratory reports.

Nursing History

The nursing history includes not only the client's present sensory perceptions but also his or her usual functioning. What is normal for one person may be abnormal for another. In some instances, significant others can provide data the woman cannot. For example, a woman may observe her partner's hearing loss long before the partner is aware of it.

The nursing history should include the **sensorium** (consciousness or mental clarity), the sensory realm, and the affective realm. See Table 47–1. The nurse must also consider the sensory-perceptual environment. Obviously,

Table 47–1 Perceptual-Sensory History Outline

Sensorium
Consciousness (awareness of internal and external stimuli)
Orientation (person, place, time)
Attention span
Memory (recent and remote)
Cognitive skills (e.g., ability to learn, abstract, and compute)
Sensory
Visual changes
Auditory changes
Gustatory changes
Tactile changes
Olfactory changes
Kinesthetic changes
Affective
Reaction to change
Decision making
Illusions or delusions

changes in environment affect sensory input. The elderly woman who moves from her daughter's busy home to a room in a boarding house experiences a change in level of sensory input. This change may affect cerebral functioning. See detailed nursing history outlines for the various senses in Chapter 35.

Physical Examination

Vision, hearing, as well as olfactory, gustatory, tactile, and kinesthetic status are examined. Some examiners also test vocal status (voice quality). See Chapter 35 for additional information about these examinations and Table 47–2 for a summary.

To assess sensory deprivation or overload, the nurse needs to know the level of sensory input the person is accustomed to and tolerates best. This level is highly individual. The child who has five brothers and sisters may be accustomed to a different level of sensory input than the only child.

Sensory Deprivation

A person experiencing sensory deprivation may manifest boredom, inactivity, slowness of thought, daydreaming, increased sleeping, thought disorganization, anxiety, panic, or hallucinations (Cameron et al. 1972, p. 33).

Both activity and inactivity can signal boredom. If active, the bored person occupies time with unimportant matters. The bored person may ask for assistance unnecessarily. An inactive person may appear apathetic and withdrawn. This person may also be irritable and exhibit childish emotional responses (Heron 1971, p. 358).

Slowness of thought is demonstrated by difficulty grasping ideas and slowness in communicating. Reaction time is slow, and the person may appear clumsy.

Persons who are daydreaming appear absorbed in their own thoughts and may talk and laugh to themselves. It may be difficult to engage such a person in conversation. These persons may confuse a daydream with reality and imagine a conversation that did not take place. Increased sleeping is another manifestation of sensory deprivation. The person who lacks external stimulation may have difficulty staying awake and may sleep to pass time.

Difficulty remembering what one was saying may be evidence of thought disorganization. The person may start a sentence on one subject and end it with an unrelated subject. Thought disorganization may also be reflected in confusion about the time of day or the day of the week. The person may react inappropriately, e.g., by laughing at bad news, or experience sensory distortions, e.g., mistaking the smell of food for the smell of smoke.

Anxiety and panic are similar. Panic is severe anxiety. See the signs of increased stress listed in Chapter 17. Hallucinations can also be a result of sensory deprivation. The person may hear nonexistent voices or see nonexistent sights. The client may misinterpret stimuli and, for example, see a shadow as a man with a knife. These misinterpreted stimuli are called illusions.

Table 47–2 Clinical Signs of Sensory Deficits

Auditory
Is the person able to locate the direction of sounds? (Persons with hearing aids often have difficulties locating the direction.)
Can the person distinguish and differentiate voices?
Does the person report a humming, ringing, or buzzing in the ears?
Does the person speak loudly or shout?
Visual
Is the person able to see objects or persons nearby and at a distance?
Does the person hold reading material close or far away?
Does the person report unusual distortions in vision?
Does the person have a full field of vision? Does the person see objects only directly in his or her line of vision?
Does the person report seeing spots, colored areas, or halos around objects?
Gustatory
Does the person report persistent, unusual tastes, e.g., bitterness or metallic tastes?
Can the person differentiate between sweet, sour, salty, and bitter tastes?
Olfactory
Can the person distinguish foods by their odors?
Does the person report nonexistent odors, e.g., smoke when nothing is burning?
Tactile
Does the person discriminate between dull and sharp?
Does the person perceive heat, cold, and pain?
Does the person perceive unusual sensations such as pins and needles?
Kinesthetic
Is the person aware of the position of the parts of his or her body?
Visceral
Does the person report unusual internal sensations, e.g., pain or pressure?

Sensory Overload

Sensory overload may have the same symptoms as sensory deprivation. In addition, the client may appear agitated and restless. If symptoms worsen when the client's social contacts increase, sensory overload is probable.

Sensory Deficits

Sensory deficits are generally assessed during initial health assessment. In addition, nurses need to observe and note behaviors that may reflect impairment of any of the senses. See Table 47–2.

Nursing Diagnosis

Examples of nursing diagnoses related to sensory alterations appear to the right.

Examples of Nursing Diagnoses Related to Sensory Disturbances

- Social isolation related to inability to walk
- Social isolation related to death of husband
- Sensory-perceptual alteration: visual deficit related to surgery
- Sensory-perceptual alteration: auditory deficit related to aging
- Sensory-perceptual alteration: taste deficit related to radiation therapy
- Sensory-perceptual alteration: sensory overload related to hospitalization

Planning

Nursing strategies are planned around all or some of the following:

1. Adjusting environmental stimuli
2. Promoting the function of existing senses
3. Helping the client to adapt to altered sensory function
4. Decreasing further sensory alterations
5. Providing a safe environment

Intervention

Stimulation During Growth

Children require tactile, auditory, and visual stimulation. Nurses need to teach parents the importance of these stimuli. When infants and children are hospitalized, these needs are met largely by nurses, although in some settings volunteers play with children. Some agencies have playrooms where a play therapist helps meet children's play and stimulation needs.

The following provide stimulation:

1. Holding, talking to, and playing with infants who are not asleep, rather than leaving them alone in cribs
2. Placing bright objects of varied design near infants' cribs and giving children stimulating toys of different textures, sizes, and colors
3. Changing infants' environments by taking them for walks or scheduling play in a variety of settings
4. Providing music and auditory stimuli at suitable intervals
5. Providing foods with a variety of tastes, textures, and colors

Constant sensory stimulation without adequate sleep and rest periods can result in sensory overload. A child needs to rest in a quiet, dark, odor-free room. Sensory stimulation needs continue when the infant or child is hospitalized or confined to bed at home.

Adjusting Environmental Stimuli

When a client is at risk of overstimulation or understimulation, nurses should adjust the environmental stimuli. A client who is understimulated should be provided with meaningful stimuli for all the senses. Clients who are overstimulated need a reduction in the number and type of stimuli. When a client is overstimulated, the nurse can counteract sensory overload by blocking stimuli, helping the client organize the stimuli, and helping him or her alter responses to the stimuli.

Blocking Stimuli

There are many ways of blocking stimuli. Dark glasses can partially block light rays, and a sun screen or a drape over a window can reduce visual stimulation. Ear plugs reduce auditory stimuli, as do soft background music and earphones. Odors, too, can contribute to sensory overload. Odors from a draining wound can be an unpleasant, constant stimulus. The odor can often be minimized by keeping the dressing dry and clean and applying a liquid deodorant on a gauze near the wound.

Another method of reducing sensory overload is to establish daily routines that reduce novelty and surprise. These routines should provide long rest intervals free of interruptions. Sometimes the number of visitors and the length of visits must be restricted. A nurse can organize care so that the client has long periods of little stimulation. If the nurse carries out several nursing measures together, the client can have a scheduled quiet period before the next activity.

Organizing Stimuli

If the nurse explains the sounds in the environment, the client can organize them mentally: A bell signals a change of shift; a buzzer, a change of IV. When clients understand their meaning, stimuli are frequently less confusing and more easily ignored.

Altering Responses

People can learn to alter their responses to stimuli. Clients can employ relaxation techniques to reduce anxiety and stress despite continual sensory stimulation.

Promoting the Function of Existing Senses

Providing significant and meaningful stimuli can help the client use existing senses. Nurses should provide a variety of stimuli that appeal to different senses, e.g., newspapers, varied foods, and music. Clocks that differentiate night from day by color can help orient a client. Nurses can help by providing objects that are pleasant to touch. For example, many people obtain great joy from holding and stroking a pet.

When a client is understimulated, nurses need to determine the reasons before planning nursing intervention. Deprivation is usually due to inadequate stimuli, inability to receive stimuli, or inability to process stimuli.

Inadequate stimuli can mean insufficient stimuli. Stimuli are also inadequate when they are monotonous, infrequent, or too weak. A client confined to bed in a private room without television or radio and receiving visitors only once a week is inadequately stimulated. After a month, this client may experience sensory deprivation. The nurse can anticipate and prevent deprivation by arranging for visits from other clients or personnel, a radio or television, a variety of foods, and books and magazines.

Acute sensory deprivation indicates a need for more interaction with nursing staff and health personnel as well as other stimuli. When the client is hallucinating, the nurse must first acknowledge the emotional component of the client's experience: "I recognize that you are afraid." The nurse might then explain that there is nothing present to cause the fear: "There is only a clothes hamper in the corner, not an animal."

The understimulated client usually benefits from being touched by nurses and others. The elderly client, in particular, might suffer from touch deprivation. Most clients are reassured by this gesture of warmth, but some people dislike being touched. The nurse needs to observe each client's desire for touching.

Many hospitals for adults, particularly long-term care facilities, have libraries and occupational or recreational facilities that provide stimulation for the inactive or underactive person.

Adapting to Altered Sensory Function

Nursing intervention for clients with sensory deficits includes helping clients develop compensatory skills and preventing sensory deprivation.

Impaired Vision

The following nursing interventions may help clients with impaired vision:

1. Arrange for suitable lighting, including night lights.
2. Encourage the client to have his or her eyes examined.
3. Obtain books with large printing and "reading tapes"—recorded books—for the client.
4. Provide written instructions in print large enough for the client to read.
5. Support the client in any decision that gives mobility and independence, e.g., using a white cane or acquiring a seeing-eye dog.

Impaired Hearing

People may or may not tell others when their hearing begins to fail. The loss may not always be evident, but the person begins to feel isolated as he or she has difficulty conversing, using the telephone, and listening to television. As a result, the person with impaired hearing can withdraw and become depressed. Significant others should be involved in planning for her or him.

The following interventions are appropriate:

1. Obtain the person's attention before speaking.
2. Speak distinctly while facing the person.
3. Assume a position that allows the person to see your face clearly, e.g., do not stand against the light or far away.
4. Rephrase your message if the individual does not understand it the first time.
5. Encourage the client to have hearing tests and to obtain a hearing aid if one will be helpful.
6. Keep conversational groups small; the hearing-impaired find it difficult to follow conversation in large groups.

Decreased Gustatory or Olfactory Senses

The following measures may assist clients with gustatory or olfactory impairment:

1. Serve hot food hot and cold food cold.
2. Serve well-seasoned, not bland, foods.
3. Serve meals that offer a variety of smells, tastes, and textures.

Decreasing Further Sensory Loss

An individual's life-style can worsen existing sensory loss. One example is hazards, e.g., noise, in the workplace. In this instance, wearing protective ear covers may prevent further hearing loss. Often, people with sensory deficits, e.g., impaired hearing or eyesight, can feel isolated. Nurses can plan time to communicate in a meaningful way with such a client.

A client with aphasia (impaired speech) may find it frustrating to be unable to express her or his thoughts coherently. Such a person can frequently think clearly even though his or her speech is impaired. Nurses can help aphasic clients communicate their needs and thoughts in writing or with a communication board. Some communication boards have pictures to which the person can point to express her or his needs. An important aspect of the aphasic client's care is teaching support persons how to enhance the client's independence. Sometimes people think it is kind to speak for the asphasic client, not realizing that he or she should be encouraged to communicate by whatever means are available.

Providing a Safe Environment

Clients with sensory deficits are particularly susceptible to injury. As a result, they may require assistance from nurses in taking precautions to prevent accidents.

A client with loss of vision may require assistance walking. A nurse should stand on the client's nondominant side about one step ahead of the client. A blind person should grasp the nurse's arm with his nondominant arm. In addition, nurses can make the environment safe by:

1. Arranging furniture and other objects so the client will not trip over them and explaining the location of furniture
2. Leaving bedside articles as the client arranges them and within easy reach.

For further information, see Chapter 33, pages 735 and 748.

For Altered Level of Consciousness

Nursing intervention for the client with altered level of consciousness has three main objectives:

1. To provide emotional support to the client and support persons
2. To provide a safe environment and otherwise ensure the client's safety
3. To provide assistance with daily activities the client cannot accomplish alone

Emotional Support

Altered levels of consciousness can be frightening to both clients and their support persons. Often people know that something is wrong and that they need help. The following interventions may help clients and support persons:

1. Reorient the confused client to self, time, and place.
2. Listen carefully to the client's and support person's concerns. Often they simply want to express them.
3. Maintain the same schedule each day. Routine gives the client a sense of security and sometimes decreases confusion.
4. Touch and stroke the unconscious client.
5. Explain what is happening to the support persons and encourage them to talk to and touch the unconscious client as if he or she were conscious. This auditory and tactile stimulation supports the client and may restore some degree of consciousness.

Safety

The client whose level of consciousness is altered needs protection. Side rails to prevent falls, appropriate positioning in bed, appropriate lighting, and reduced noise level are all common safety measures.

Activities of Daily Living

The client whose level of consciousness is altered may need assistance with activities of daily living. If the client is unconscious, necessary nursing interventions include bathing, giving skin care, feeding, and meeting elimination needs. If the client is disoriented but conscious, the nurse may need to give instructions on how to perform these activities. Unless the person is totally incapacitated, it is preferable to foster independence and feelings of self-worth by helping the individual care for himself or herself than to give complete care to a passive client.

Evaluation

Examples of outcome criteria for clients who have sensory alterations are given to the right.

Examples of Outcome Criteria for Sensory Disturbances

Sensory-perceptual overload

The client will:

- Sleep for 6 hours without awakening
- Verbalize feelings of well-being

Sensory-perceptual deprivation

The client:

- Knows the day of the week and place when questioned
- Expresses interest in watching television

Sensory deficit

The client will:

- Read for 1 hour using new glasses
- Walk safely to the bathroom and back
- Talk while using hearing aid

Nursing Care Plan

Assessment Data

Nursing Assessment

Mrs. Julia Hagstrom is an 80-year-old widow who has recently become a resident of an extended care facility. Just prior to her admission to the extended care facility, she had undergone surgery for the removal of cataracts. She had also experienced increased difficulty in hearing. Her children were concerned about her physical safety and also her lack of socialization and consequently urged her to enter a nursing home. Up until the time Mrs. Hagstrom entered the extended care facility, she had lived alone in her home for 15 years and cared for herself independently. Three days after she was admitted to Valley View Home, her nurse, Marie Carter, finds Mrs. Hagstrom to be somewhat confused and disoriented to person, place, and time. She appears restless and withdrawn and her syntax is sometimes confused. She states, "I'm afraid of all these strange creatures in this orphanage."

Physical Examination

Height: 160 cm (5′3″)
Weight: 55.3 kg (122 lb)
Temperature: 37 C (98.6 F)
Pulse rate: 72 BPM
Respirations: 18 per minute
Blood pressure: 128/74 mm Hg
Rinne test: Negative

Diagnostic Data:

Chest x-ray film: Negative
CBC: Negative
Urine: Negative

(continued)

Nursing Diagnosis	Client Goals and Outcome Criteria	Nursing Interventions and Rationales	Evaluation
Sensory-perceptual alterations (sensory overload) related to change in environment/hearing loss resulting in disorientation to time, place, and person; restlessness; fear; and altered behavior.	Client Goal: Demonstrate decreased symptoms and increased level of orientation to reality. Outcome Criteria: Is oriented to place, month, and year when questioned by day 3. Participates in self-care activities by day 3. Identifies 1 or 2 caregivers by name by day 4.	Assess for factors contributing to confusion. *Rationale:* Identification of contributing factors will assist in eliminating such factors. Establish daily routine. *Rationale:* Decreases novelty, surprise, and overstimulation. Provide for adequate rest periods. *Rationale:* Reduces overstimulation and fatigue. Attempt to assign same caregiver as often as possible. *Rationale:* Familiarity reduces confusion. Encourage caregivers to speak slowly and as one adult to another. *Rationale:* Enhances communication and client's dignity and self-esteem. Provide for meaningful sensory input. *Rationale:* Increases client's orientation to person, place, and time. Encourage client's participation in ADLs. *Rationale:* Increases client's self-esteem and sense of control.	Mrs. Hagstrom identifies Miss Carter by sight and name. On December 3rd, during the course of the morning's conversation, she questions whether any shopping trips are planned for next week "since Christmas is only three weeks from now." She bathes herself each morning and makes her own bed.
Impaired verbal communication related to auditory impairment resulting in decreased comprehension, inattention to voices/noises, and confusion.	Client Goal: Demonstrate improved ability to communicate. Outcome Criteria: Wears hearing aid during waking hours by day 2. Communicates effectively with care provider by day 5. Indicates feeling of well-being by day 5.	Assess ability to hear and speak. *Rationale:* Identifies client's specific problems of communication. Obtain client's attention before speaking. *Rationale:* Aids in establishing first step in communication. Speak slowly and distinctly while facing client. *Rationale:* Client will be better able to lip-read and comprehend speech. Assume a position for good eye contact. *Rationale:* Conveys interest and promotes better contact between client and caregiver. Establish therapeutic relationship. *Rationale:* Therapeutic relationship is necessary when dealing with communication problems.	Mrs. Hagstrom's daughter has brought new batteries for her hearing aid, and she now wears her hearing aid during the day. She recognizes Miss Carter by name and talks to her about her family and her former home. She states, "I guess at my age, it's best to have someone nearby at all times."

Chapter Highlights

- Awareness includes the ability to perceive environmental stimuli and respond appropriately.
- Sensoristasis is the need for sensory stimulation.
- Sensory stimuli can be visual, auditory, olfactory, tactile, gustatory, kinesthetic, and visceral.
- Sensory deprivation is a level of stimulation that is too low to permit normal functioning.
- Sensory overload is more sensory stimulation than a person can tolerate.

- Sensory deficit is an impairment in the sensory or perceptual processes.
- A sensory deficit can contribute to sensory deprivation.
- The nurse needs to identify clients at most risk of developing sensory disturbances.
- A person who appears bored and sleeps excessively may be experiencing sensory deprivation.
- Sensory overload may be manifested as agitation and restlessness but can produce some of the same clinical signs that sensory deprivation produces.

Suggested Readings

Bolin, R. H. 1974. Sensory deprivation: An overview. *Nursing Forum* 13(3):240–58.
Bolin provides a theoretical framework for concepts of sensory deprivation. Also included are an overview of clinical records of deprivation and the nursing implications.

Brozian, M. W., and Clark, H. M. March 1980. Counteracting sensory changes in the aging. *American Journal of Nursing* 80:473–76.
Aging causes changes in hearing; vision and depth perception; position sense; and response to temperature, smell, taste, light touch, vibration, and deep pressure. Nursing measures can help clients adjust to these changes.

Lindenmuth, J. E.; Breu, C. S.; and Malooley, J. A. August 1980. Sensory overload. *American Journal of Nursing* 80:1456–58.
In this study of sensory overload in a coronary care unit, the researchers found that the three major client problems were potential for disorientation, potential for physical discomfort, and loss of privacy. Nursing interventions for each of these problems are given.

Selected References

Amacher, N. J. May 1973. Touch is a way of caring and a way of communicating with an aphasic patient. *American Journal of Nursing* 73:852–54.

Brown, I. A. October 1985. The widespread influence of olfaction. *Journal of Neurological Nursing* 17:273–79.

Brown, J., and Hepler, R. April 1976. Stimulation: A corollary to physical care. *American Journal of Nursing* 76:578–81.

Burnside, I. M. December 1973. Touching is talking. *American Journal of Nursing* 73:2060–63.

Cameron, C. F., et al. November 1972. When sensory deprivation occurs. *Canadian Nurse* 68:32–34.

Carpenito, L. J. November 1985. Altered thoughts or altered perceptions? *American Journal of Nursing* 85:1283.

Chodil, J., and Williams, B. 1970. The concept of sensory deprivation. *Nursing Clinics of North America* 5(3):544–48.

Cohen, S. October 1981. Programmed instruction: Sensory changes in the elderly. *American Journal of Nursing* 81:1851–80.

Crandall, R. C. 1980. *Gerontology: A behavioral science approach.* Reading, Mass.: Addison-Wesley Publishing Co.

DeForest, J., and Porter, A. July/August 1981. Cuddlers: A volunteer infant stimulation program. *Canadian Nurse* 77:38–40.

Downs, F. S. March 1974. Bed rest and sensory disturbances. *American Journal of Nursing* 74:434–38.

Ebersole, P., and Hess, P. 1985. *Toward healthy aging: Human needs and nursing response.* 2d ed. St. Louis: C. V. Mosby Co.

Gioiella, E. C., and Bevil, C. W. 1985. *Nursing care of the aging client: Promoting healthy adaptation.* Norwalk, Conn.: Appleton-Century-Crofts.

Heron, W. 1971. The pathology of boredom. In *Readings from Scientific American: Physiological psychology.* San Francisco: W. H. Freeman and Co.

Kopac, C. A. June 1983. Sensory loss in the aged: The role of the nurse and the family. *Nursing Clinics of North America* 18:373–84.

MacKinnon-Kesler, S. May 1983. Maximizing your ICU patient's sensory and perceptual environment. *Canadian Nurse* 79: 37–39.

McCorkie, R. March/April 1974. Effects of touch on seriously ill patients. *Nursing Research* 23:125–32.

Mitchell, P. H., and Loustau, A. 1981. *Concepts basic to nursing.* 3d ed. New York: McGraw-Hill.

Perron, D. M. June 1974. Deprived of sound. *American Journal of Nursing* 74:1057–59.

Ravish, T. October 1985. Prevent social isolation before it starts. *Journal of Gerontological Nursing* 11:10–13.

Smith, M. J. March/April 1975. Changes in judgment of duration with different patterns of auditory information for individuals confined to bed. *Nursing Research* 24:93–98.

Suedfeld, P. 1985. Stressful levels of environmental stimuli. *Issues in Mental Health Nursing* 7:83–104.

Sullivan, N. April 1983. Vision in the elderly. Declining visual function in old age. Parts 1 and 2. *Journal of Gerontological Nursing* 9:228–35.

Thomson, L. R. February 1973. Sensory deprivation: A personal experience. *American Journal of Nursing* 73:266–68.

Watson, C. A., and Wyatt, N. N. 1981. Altered levels of awareness. In Hart, L. K.; Reese, J. L.; and Fearing, M. O., editors. *Concepts common to acute illness: Identification and management.* St. Louis: C. V. Mosby Co.

Wolanin, M. O., and Phillips, L. R. F. 1981. *Confusion: Prevention and care.* St. Louis: C. V. Mosby Co.

Wyness, M. A. April 1985. Perceptual dysfunction: Nursing assessment and management. *Journal of Neurological Nursing* 17:105–10.

CHAPTER **48**

Self-Concept

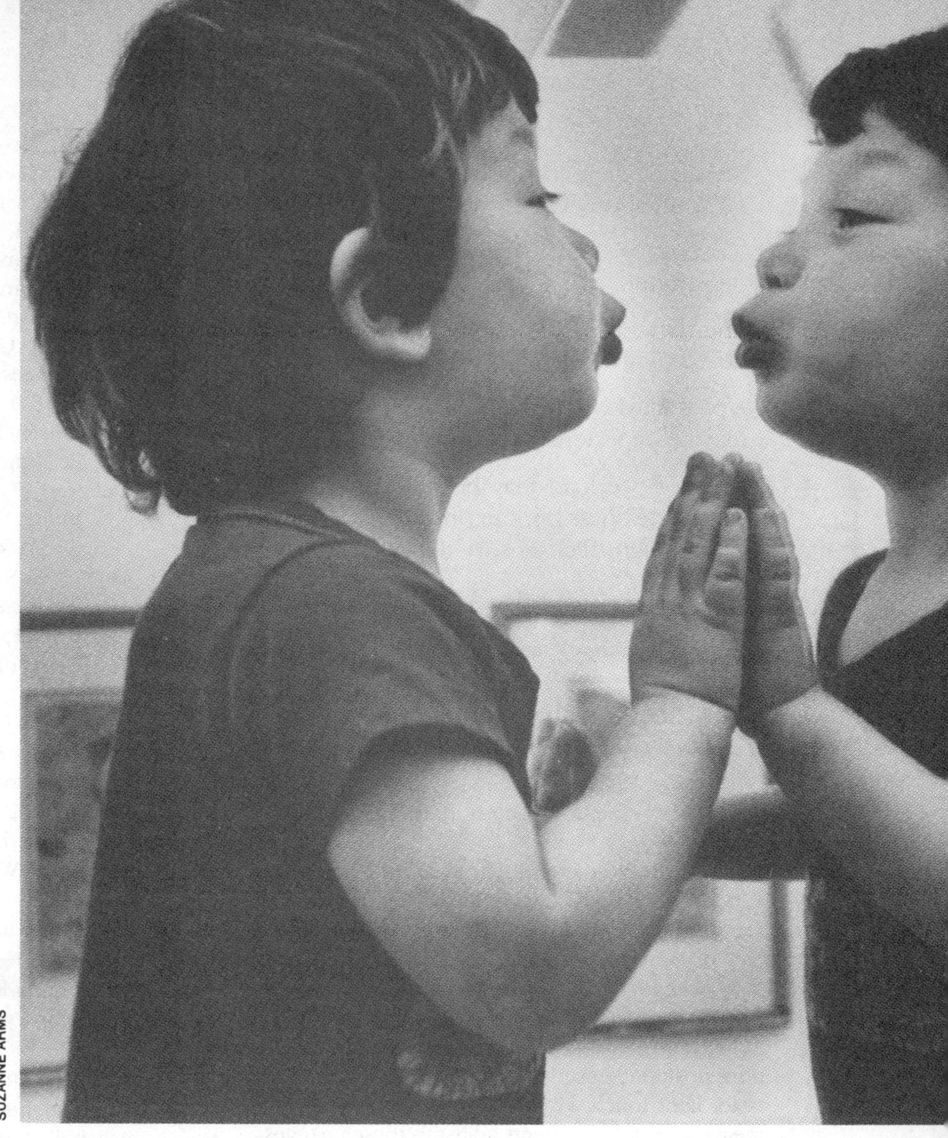

SUZANNE ARMS

Contents

Objectives

1. Understand essential aspects of self-concept.
   1.1 Define selected terms.
   1.2 Describe the importance of self-concept.
   1.3 Differentiate between *self-concept* and *self-esteem.*
   1.4 Identify areas of performance on which people base their self-concept.
   1.5 Identify three positions of self-concept.
   1.6 Describe the components of self-concept.
   1.7 Differentiate between *basic self-esteem* and *functional self-esteem.*
   1.8 Describe how self-esteem is maintained and evaluated.
   1.9 Identify four elements of experience that are pertinent to the development of self-esteem.
   1.10 Describe the effects of Erikson's psychosocial crises on self-concept and self-esteem.
   1.11 Describe the effects of communication/coping styles on self-esteem.
2. Understand the essentials of assessment and nursing diagnoses related to altered self-concept.
   2.1 Identify four areas involved in the nursing assessment of self-concept.
   2.2 Describe essential aspects of assessment of self-perception.
   2.3 Describe the essentials of assessing roles and relationships.
   2.4 Describe aspects essential to assessing stressors and coping strategies.
   2.5 Identify common stressors affecting self-concept and self-esteem.
   2.6 Identify behaviors suggestive of altered self-concept.
   2.7 Identify nursing diagnoses related to altered self-concept.
3. Understand the essentials involved in planning and implementing nursing interventions to maintain, promote, and restore a person's self-concept and self-esteem.
   3.1 Identify types of client goals.
   3.2 Describe the advantages of identifying a client's strengths.
   3.3 Identify the essential components of a framework for identifying personality strengths.
   3.4 Describe strategies for developing behavior specificity.
   3.5 Describe how to change a client's language patterns from passive to active phrases.
   3.6 Describe ways to encourage a client's positive self-evaluation.
   3.7 Describe ways to enhance a child's and adolescent's self-esteem.
   3.8 Describe ways to enhance the self-esteem of older adults.

Terms

aggressiveness
assertiveness
body image
core self-concept
ego integrity
generativity
global self
global self-esteem
ideal self
perceived self
role
role ambiguity
role conflict
role mastery
role performance
role strain
self-concept
self-esteem
self-identity
significant other
specific self-esteem

Importance of a Healthy Self-Concept

A healthy self-concept—that is, positive self-esteem—is essential to psychologic well-being; it is something everyone wants and everyone needs. The following outlines the influences of a person's self-concept or self-esteem (Sanford and Donovan 1984, p. 3):

1. It affects everything one thinks, says, or does.
2. It affects how others in the world see and treat one.
3. It affects the choices one makes, such as who one will be involved with and what to do with one's life.
4. It affects one's ability to give and receive love.
5. It affects one's ability to take action to change things that need to be changed.

A healthy self-concept enables a person to find happiness in life and to cope with life's disappointments and changes. People who do not have a healthy self-concept are less able to live as fully or be as happy as they might be. People with an unhealthy self-concept generally express feelings of worthlessness, self-dislike or self-hatred, and, on some occasions, hatred for others. They often feel sad or hopeless and are drained of energy.

The ideas of *self-concept, self-esteem,* and *self-image* are important for the nurse to understand. They are essential to a person's mental and physical health. Individuals with a positive self-concept or high self-esteem are better able to develop and maintain warm interpersonal relationships and resist psychologic and physical illness. Failure to achieve a positive self-image presents major obstacles in the treatment of common disorders such as depression, eating disorders, postvictimization syndrome (abuse or rape), and crisis reactions. One of the nurse's major responsibilities is to identify persons with a negative self-concept or low self-esteem and to assist them in developing a more positive view of themselves.

Self-concept is also of personal relevance to the nurse. Nurses who have difficulty meeting their own needs have difficulty meeting the needs of clients. Nurses who feel positive about themselves are better equipped to meet the needs of others. Such nurses feel good, look good, are effective and productive, and respond to people (including themselves) in healthy and positive ways.

Research Note

Although a number of studies have shown the importance of self-esteem and social support to health status, few have related them to specific positive health practices. Muhlenkamp and Sayles studied how social support and self-esteem are interrelated and how their interrelation influences positive health practices. They found that respondents with high self-esteem perceived their social support as highly adequate. More important, respondents with high self-esteem were found to maintain more positive health practices than those with lower levels of self-esteem and social support. (Muhlenkamp and Sayles 1986)

Concept of Self and Self-Esteem

The terms *self-concept, self-image, self-esteem, self-worth, sense of self-worth, self-respect,* and *self-love* are often used interchangeably. *Self-concept* has been referred to as the *cognitive* component of the self system, and self-esteem as the *affective* component (Hamachek 1978). In other words, **self-concept** is "how I *see* myself," and **self-esteem** is "how I *feel about* myself." Stanwyck (1983, p. 11), however, says these two constructs are inseparable, since self-esteem is based on self-concept. To Stanwyck, self-esteem is "how I feel about how I see myself," even though most researchers use the terms interchangeably. Others view self-concept as a broad generic term that encompasses many smaller constructs, e.g., body-image, self-esteem, self-identity, and role performance and relationships. See "Components of Self-Concept" on the facing page.

Global and Specific Self-Concept/ Self-Esteem

The term **global self** refers to the aggregate beliefs and images one holds about oneself. It is the most complete description that an individual can give of himself or herself at any one time. It is also a person's frame of reference for experiencing and viewing the world. Some of these beliefs and images represent statements of fact, for example: "I am a woman"; "I am a mother"; "I am black"; "I am short"; "I am a student"; "I am poor." Others refer to less tangible aspects of self, for instance: "I am stupid"; "I am competent"; "I am clumsy"; "I am lovable"; "I am no good"; "I am shy"; "I am strong"; "I am outgoing."

Each separate image and belief a person holds about himself or herself has a bearing on self-esteem. However, self-concept is not simply a sum of its parts, for the various images and beliefs a person holds about himself or herself are not given equal weight and prominence (Sanford and Donovan 1984, p. 9). Each person's self-concept is like a collage. At the center of the collage are the beliefs and images that are most vital to the person's identity and self-esteem. They constitute **core self-concept.** For example: "I am competent/incompetent"; "I am pretty/ugly"; "I am rich/poor"; "I am male/female." Images and beliefs that are less important to the person are on the periphery. For example: "I am left-/right-handed"; "I am athletic/unathletic"; "I am a good/poor cook"; "I have brown/blue eyes."

The way a person perceives and structures his or her self-concept can result in either positive or negative self-esteem. There are two types of self-esteem, global and specific (Sanford and Donovan 1984, p. 9). **Global self-esteem** is how much the person likes his or her perceived self as a whole. **Specific self-esteem** is how much a person approves of a certain part of himself or herself (Sanford and Donovan 1984, p. 9). Global self-esteem is influenced by specific self-esteem. For example, if a man values his looks, then how he looks will strongly affect his global self-esteem. On the other hand, if the man places little value on his cooking skills, then how well or badly he cooks will have little influence on his global self-esteem.

According to Goldin (1985, p. 33), people base their self-concept on how they perceive and evaluate themselves in the areas of:

1. Vocational performance
2. Intellectual functioning

3. Personal appearance and physical attractiveness
4. Sexual attractiveness and performance
5. Being liked by others
6. Ability to cope with and resolve problems
7. Independence
8. Particular talents

Self-esteem categories for children include (Stanwyck 1983, p. 12):

1. School performance
2. Peer relationships
3. Family relationships
4. Emotional well-being
5. Physical self-perception

A person's perception of himself or herself in any of these areas becomes a self-fulfilling prophecy: The person actually behaves as he or she perceives himself or herself (Goldin 1985, p. 34).

Positions of Self-Concept

Three positions of self-concept have been delineated (Burns 1979, p. 50):

1. *Cognized self,* or self as known to the individual: "How I am," or, "How I perceive me."
2. *Other self,* or social self: "How I perceive others perceiving me."
3. *Ideal self:* "How I would like to be."

People who value most "how I perceive me" can be termed "me-centered." They try hard to live up to their own expectations and compete only with themselves, not others. In contrast, "other-centered" people have a high need for approval from others and try hard to live up to the expectations of others, constantly comparing, competing, and evaluating themselves in relation to others. They tend to avoid personal shortcomings, are unable to assert themselves, and continually fear disapproval. The healthy self-concept, therefore, is me-centered and is formed without reference to other persons.

Components of Self-Concept

The North American Nursing Diagnosis Association suggests four components of self-concept: body image, role performance, self-identity, and self-esteem (Kim et al. 1984, p. 47). Self-esteem has already been discussed.

Body Image

The image of physical self, or **body image**, is how a person perceives the size, appearance, and functioning of his or her body and its parts. It includes clothing, makeup, hairstyle, jewelry, and other things intimately connected to the person, e.g., artificial limb or wheelchair. A person's body image develops partly from others' attitudes and responses to his or her body. Cultural and societal values also influence a person's body image. For instance, Western societies value beauty, youth, and wholeness. Generally, a person has developed a stable body image over a long time; thus, actual or potential threats to alterations in body image can create considerable anxiety.

Role Performance

Throughout life people undergo numerous role changes. A **role** is a set of expectations about how the person occupying one position behaves toward a person occupying another position (Roy 1984, p. 285). Expectations, or standards of behavior, are set by society or the smaller group to which the person belongs. Each person usually has several roles, e.g., husband, parent, brother, son, employee, friend, golf club member. Some roles are assumed for only limited periods, e.g., client/nurse, student/instructor, and the sick role.

To act appropriately, people need to know who they are in relation to others and what society expects for the positions they hold. When there is **role ambiguity**, expectations are unclear, and the person does not know what to do or how to do it and is unable to predict the reactions of others to his or her behavior. This creates confusion and stress. In addition, to relate or interact appropriately with others, people need to know the role positions that others occupy.

Role performance relates what a person does in a particular role to the behaviors expected of that role. **Role mastery** means that the person's behaviors meet social expectations. Failure to master a role creates frustration and feelings of inadequacy, often with consequent lowered self-esteem.

Self-concept is also affected by role strain and role conflicts. **Role strain** means a person is frustrated because he or she feels or is made to feel inadequate or unsuited to a role. Role strain often is associated with sex role stereotypes. For example, women in occupations traditionally held by men may be thought less knowledgeable and less competent than men in the same roles. As a result, these women feel the need to surpass the level expected for role mastery by male counterparts.

Role conflicts arise from opposing or incompatible expectations. In an *interpersonal conflict,* different people have different expectations about a particular role. For example, a mother's parents may have different expectations about how the mother should care for her children. In an *interrole conflict,* one person's or group's role expectations differ from the expectations of another person or group. For example, a woman who works in an office 8 hours a day may have a role conflict if her husband expects her to be home with the children. In a *person-role conflict,* role expectations violate the beliefs or values of the role occupant. For example, a woman who values her right to choose abortion will have a conflict if this right is denied.

Self-Identity

A person's **self-identity** is the conscious sense of individuality and uniqueness that is continually evolving throughout life. People often view their identity in terms of name, sex, age, race, ethnicity or culture, occupation or roles, talents, and other situational characteristics, such as marital status and education. People usually first identify themselves by name and occupation or roles. When interactions progress beyond the superficial, other characteristics may be revealed, e.g., special talents or interests. However, self-identity also includes a person's beliefs and values, personality, and character. For instance, is the person outgoing, friendly, reserved, generous, kind, honest, ruthless, selfish? Self-identity, thus, encompasses both the tangible and factual, such as name and sex, and the intangible, such as values and beliefs. In brief: Identity is what distinguishes self from others.

Maintenance and Evaluation of Self-Esteem

By the time people reach adulthood, their *basic* self-concept and *basic* level of self-esteem are relatively well established, and they already have some idea about their **perceived self**, i.e., how they see themselves and how they are seen by others. In addition, they have an idea about their **ideal self**, i.e., how they should be or would prefer to be. Sometimes this ideal self is realistic; sometimes it is not. When perceived self is close to ideal self, people do not wish to be much different from what they believe they already are. When there is a discrepancy between ideal self and perceived self, this can be an incentive to self-improvement. However, when the discrepancy is large, low self-esteem can result.

Basic self-esteem refers to the foundation for self-esteem that is established during early life experiences, usually within the family. However, an adult's functional level of overall self-esteem may change markedly from day to day and moment to moment. *Functional self-esteem* is a result of the person's ongoing evaluation of interactions with people and objects. Functional self-esteem can exceed basic self-esteem, or it can regress to a level below that of basic self-esteem. Severe stress—for example, prolonged illness or unemployment—can substantially lower a person's basic self-esteem.

Perceptions of self (both as is and as desired) generally arise from self-evaluation in accordance with certain criteria. Four basic criteria by which people judge themselves are:

1. *Power*—the ability to influence significant others and control events that are personally important
2. *Significance*—the acceptance, attention, and affection of others who communicate to the person a clear sense of being valued and cared about as a worthwhile human being
3. *Competence*—successfully meeting demands for achievement, particularly personally important goals
4. *Virtue*—adherence to moral and ethical standards

Self-evaluation is usually a covert mental process. Frequently, people label themselves negatively or project failures into the future. Positive self-credit is usually less frequent.

Development of Self-Esteem

Four elements of experience that are pertinent to the development of self-esteem are: (a) significant others, (b) social role expectations, (c) crises of psychosocial development, and (d) communication/coping style (Stanwyck 1983, p. 13).

Significant Others

The crucial role of social interaction in the development of self-esteem is recognized by most social psychologists. Because some people exert more influence than others on the development of an individual's self-esteem, Sullivan's term *significant other* has been generally accepted (Sullivan 1950). A **significant other** is an individual or group that takes on special importance for the development of self-esteem during a particular life stage. Significant others may include parents, siblings, peers, teachers, and the like. During various stages of development one or several significant others may be identified. Through social interaction with significant others and the resultant interpreted feedback on how others perceive and label him or her, a person develops attitudes toward himself or herself. Put more simply, "as a person is judged by others, so he comes to judge himself" (Burns 1979, p. 184). Many components of a person's self-evaluation are established early in life under the influence of significant others. These values often get so strongly reinforced that they are difficult to change later, even though it may benefit the person to do so.

Social Role Expectations

At the various stages of life, people are strongly influenced by general societal expectations regarding role-specific behavior. The larger society and smaller societal groups have expectations that differ in clarity and are communicated with varying degrees of force. Expectations differ by age, sex, socioeconomic status, ethnicity, and career identification. Smaller societal groups such as the family, school, armed forces, work groups, and recreational groups also expect certain behaviors and performance levels of people. Success in meeting such expectations has profound implications for self-esteem.

Because North American society is highly achievement oriented, everything a person does is evaluated, e.g., earning capacity, social skills, performance at school, athletic performance, and sexual performance. A high level of performance is rewarded; poor performance is belittled. As a result people tend to focus on their failures and shortcomings rather than on their strengths. In many instances a person's actual performance is superior to his or her *perception* of that performance. Compliance with the social expectations for role-specific behavior therefore leads to judgments of personal worth; noncompliance often leads to judgments of personal worthlessness.

Crises of Psychosocial Development

Throughout life people face certain developmental tasks that, if not successfully achieved, may lead to problems with self, self-concept, and self-esteem. Several developmental theories are discussed in Chapter 22. The eight psychosocial stages described by Erikson (1963) provide a convenient and familiar theoretic framework with obvious implications for self-esteem. The success with which a person copes with these developmental crises largely determines the development of self-concept. Inability to cope results in self-concept problems, at the time and often later in life. See Table 48–1 for behaviors indicating successful and unsuccessful resolution of these developmental crises.

Infancy

Erikson labels the psychosocial crisis of the first year of life the crisis of *trust versus mistrust*. Through experience the infant comes to a "decision" about the extent to which the environment, including people, can be trusted to provide for his or her basic needs—nourishment, dryness, warmth, safety, and love. From experiences with having needs met, the infant develops trust in the external environment—confidence in the sameness, continuity, and predictability of the environment. Although some frustration for the infant is inevitable, since needs cannot always be met promptly, these first interactions shape the infant's behavioral patterns, and they may come to characterize the infant's later interpersonal style. From trust in the external environment the infant learns to trust himself or herself. Infants who do not develop trust in the environment and the self may be unable to trust or rely on themselves or others in later years.

The primary caretaker, usually the mother, provides the most important input by which the infant determines whether the environment is positive, reliable, consistent, and therefore trustworthy. What is expected of the infant is also a major influence during this stage. Each parent has an image of what the infant should be and how he or she should behave. Demands on the infant and sanctions imposed for nonperformance may be more stringent than for adults (Stanwyck 1983, p. 15). For example, if the parents expect a quiet baby and get a noisy one, or vice versa, or if they expect a healthy baby and get a sick one, they may respond by withholding the type of physical and psychologic supports that are essential to the infant's developing a sense of trust in the world as "an okay place."

Infants take their place in a family system and learn to behave in ways that not only provide temporary self-satisfaction but serve the family's needs as well. If the family functions in an open and esteem-enhancing fashion, the infant will come to trust rather than mistrust his or her world.

Toddlerhood

An infant who has developed a sense of trust is ready to develop autonomy, or a sense of "I." At this stage, the child will use the words *no* and *I* a great deal. The major barrier to a person's autonomy is the rejection of his or her right to exist in whatever form he or she presents. It can cause a child who in infancy developed an attitude of mistrust to believe that "It is not only the world that is not okay; it is me as well" (Stanwyck 1983, p. 16). During early childhood, children have many opportunities to increase their competence in mastering the world, e.g., learning to walk, speak, control their elimination. If the family or significant others respond with encouragement and patience, the child learns to trust his or her own capability and to take pride in it. If, on the other hand, the family responds with impatience and punishment, the child experiences shame and comes to mistrust his or her own capabilities.

Positive self-esteem is a result of genuine autonomy. A family that prizes each person's individuality and appreciates and encourages each person's autonomy and independence assists the growing child toward positive self-esteem.

Erikson labels the toddler's developmental crisis as *autonomy versus shame and doubt*. Children need enough

Table 48–1 Examples of Behaviors Associated with Erikson's Stages of Psychosocial Development

Stage: Developmental Crisis	Behaviors Indicating Positive Resolution	Behaviors Indicating Negative Resolution
Infancy: Trust vs mistrust	Requesting assistance and expecting to receive it Expressing belief of another person Sharing time, opinions, and experiences	Restricting conversation to superficialities Refusing to provide a person with information Being unable to accept assistance
Toddlerhood: Autonomy vs shame and doubt	Accepting the rules of a group but also expressing disagreement when it is felt Expressing one's own opinion Easily accepting deferment of a wish fulfillment	Failing to express needs Not expressing one's own opinion when opposed Overconcern about being clean
Early childhood: Initiative vs guilt	Starting projects eagerly Expressing curiosity about many things Demonstrating original thought	Imitating others rather than developing independent ideas Apologizing and being very embarrassed over small mistakes Verbalizing fear about starting a new project
Early school years: Industry vs inferiority	Completing a task once it has been started Working well with others Using time effectively	Not completing tasks started Not assisting with the work of others Not organizing work
Adolescence: Identity vs role confusion	Asserting independence Planning realistically for future roles Establishing close interpersonal relationships	Failing to assume responsibility for directing one's own behavior Accepting the values of others without question Failing to set goals in life
Early adulthood: Intimacy vs isolation	Establishing a close, intense relationship with another person Accepting sexual behavior as desirable Making a commitment to that relationship, even in times of stress and sacrifice	Remaining alone Avoiding close interpersonal relationships
Middle-age adults: Generativity vs stagnation	Being willing to share with another person Guiding others Establishing a priority of needs, recognizing both self and others	Talking about oneself instead of listening to others Showing concern for oneself in spite of the needs of others Being unable to accept interdependence
Elderly adults: Integrity vs despair	Using past experience to assist others Maintaining productivity in some areas Accepting limitations	Crying and being apathetic Not accepting changes Demanding unnecessary assistance and attention from others

freedom to develop autonomy without experiencing serious harm (e.g., to skin his or her knees but not break a leg). Too little freedom stifles the child.

Early Childhood

From about 3 to 5 years of age children need to be allowed the initiative to develop plans and ideas and put them into action, explore the world, and live out various roles through play. Failure to achieve a sense of initiative can result in feelings of guilt. Hence Erikson calls the developmental crisis of this stage *initiative versus guilt*. Although some guilt feelings are normal, they must be balanced by a sense of initiative. Also, at this stage children start to develop a conscience. They attempt to sort out actions labeled "good" or "bad." Discipline that uses shame creates feelings of guilt and decreases feelings of self-worth.

Early School Years

School offers children a set of new rules and expectations and as a result many more opportunities for success or failure. The teacher now becomes important. Although teachers may redefine familiar aspects of the child's experience, they may also introduce rules about new role behaviors that can conflict with the rules and customs learned at home. Parents often are faced with a child who says, "But my *teacher* says . . ."

School-age children are faced with substantial challenges to their sense of autonomy. Prior to the school years, children's activities are loosely structured, and they generally make their own decisions about what to do, when to do it, and when to stop. In school, however, it is the teacher who controls the selection, duration, and sequence of activities. Because a sense of autonomy contributes to self-esteem, this change in the locus of decision making has important implications for the child's self-esteem.

Almost every behavior of the child in school is subject to evaluation. A pattern of success or failure set in the early school years is likely to persist throughout the child's school career. In children who have a high *external* locus of control (LOC), teacher evaluations may either confirm the existing level of self-esteem or require the child to adjust self-esteem toward the majority evaluation. A child with a high *internal* locus of control is likely to reject evaluations that are inconsistent with his or her self-esteem and to accept only those that do not challenge it (Stanwyck 1983, p. 18).

Erikson labels the developmental crisis of this period *industry versus inferiority.* Taking things apart to see how they work, putting them back together again, and physically manipulating things helps the child achieve a sense of competence and mastery. Projects that test intellectual as well as physical competence need to be offered. Such projects provide the child the opportunity to not only explore the world but to change it as well. Completing projects is important. Lack of opportunity to do so is frustrating and reduces the child's sense of competence and autonomy. If the child's experiences during this period lead to feelings of inferiority, later years are likely to be characterized by lack of initiative and low levels of achievement.

About the age of 8 to 10 the peer group becomes an important factor in the child's life. Special same-sex chumships develop. Chums offer important and often frank feedback that contributes to the development and maintenance of more stable self-esteem.

Adolescence

Erikson's term *identity crisis,* now commonly used by laypersons, describes the developmental crisis of adolescence. According to Erikson the best way to resolve the problems of the teen years is to develop a general "sense of psychosocial well-being" (Erikson 1968, p. 165). For Erikson, identity includes a physical self-acceptance, sense of vocational commitment, and clarification and acceptance of long-term social goals and roles. Individuals who fail to achieve this sense of identity will experience role confusion and difficulty meeting the later challenges of adulthood.

Opposite-sex and same-sex relationships are important in adolescence. The adolescent's overall self-esteem is likely to be maintained at its previous level if his or her choice of partners complements and reinforces esteem-confirming behavior patterns. Sexual identity and orientation is discussed in detail in Chapter 19.

Achieving autonomy is another major source of adolescent self-esteem. Like many other struggles, the struggle for autonomy begins in the home. If parents encourage dependence on the family, then full autonomy by the adolescent is impeded. The result is a low self-esteem that can be carried into adulthood.

Early Adulthood

Self-esteem in early adulthood is supported largely by growth in social relationship and career. A major task of adulthood affecting self-esteem is developing a close interpersonal relationship. Erikson calls this developmental crisis *intimacy versus isolation.* Achieving intimacy with another person involves a deeper level of trust than did previous relationships. It includes committing the self to another person and abandonment of self in intimate relationship. Failure to achieve intimacy can lead to a sense of isolation and self-absorption, with concomitant difficulty perceiving feedback from others and impeding the subsequent development of a fuller sense of self.

Societal pressures—for instance, to get married and have children—can also affect a person's self-esteem. For some people, establishing a household and beginning a family can enhance self-esteem by increasing the person's sense of autonomy, satisfying social role expectations, and leading to a greater sense of personal security. Others, however, may not adapt well to the responsibilities and challenges of marriage and childrearing. Increased dissatisfaction and frustration coupled with inability to break out of ineffective behavior patterns may contribute to lowered self-esteem. If divorce occurs, then the ensuing sense of failure, frustration of personal and social expectations, and loss of a significant other can severely threaten self-esteem.

Satisfaction of career goals can enhance self-esteem because employment introduces another set of significant others, i.e., employers, superiors, colleagues. The individual's self-esteem in the work setting becomes somewhat dependent on the evaluation of superiors, on promotions, and on pay raises. Failure to achieve promotion and prolonged unemployment can each have serious consequences on a person's self-esteem. Intense, all-pervasive depression can result.

Middle-Age Adults

Erikson labels the crisis of middle age as *generativity versus stagnation.* **Generativity** means concern with establishing and guiding the next generation. It includes both productivity and creativity. Generativity is not restricted to producing children, for it can also include producing something to be passed on to another generation, such as writing, health, or ideas. When a person creates nothing to pass along, stagnation results; the person becomes concerned chiefly with self rather than others. If the middle-age person experiences no major stresses (e.g., divorce, unemployment), this can be a time of relatively stable self-esteem. Many middle-age adults see themselves as having made progress toward achieving long-range goals. Some, however, may recognize that they are not going to realize their adolescent dreams and refuse to accept this conclusion or set more realistic goals. Such persons are likely to become frustrated and depressed and to have low self-esteem.

Elderly Adults

Older adults tend to look more toward past accomplishments than future goals. The last of Erikson's psychosocial crises is *integrity versus despair.* **Ego integrity** means feeling satisfied with one's life-style and accepting the inevitability of the life cycle. The person who does not achieve integrity experiences despair and feels too little time is left to start anew.

Old age, however, is a time of loss. Deteriorating health, coupled with increasing sensory impairment, reduces autonomy and independence. Retirement separates many from their most important productive activity. Deaths of friends and relatives, including spouse, can seriously alter support systems. Perhaps the most damaging thing to an elderly person's self-esteem is the assumption by some people that old people have little to contribute. This is expressed in many ways: impatience with performance deficits, treating them as children, failure to involve them in decision making. Feelings of uselessness and rejection are the result. Self-esteem cannot survive without being nourished by the esteem of others.

Communication/Coping Styles

A person's choice of strategies to cope with a stress-producing situation is important in determining how successfully a person adapts to that situation and whether self-esteem is maintained, enhanced, or decreased. Reactions to stressful situations that threaten self-esteem include problem-solving reactions, assertive reactions, and defensive reactions.

Problem-Solving Reactions

Problem solving is a conscious, action-oriented response in which the person uses his or her cognitive skills to deal with a stressor. First the person cognitively appraises the threatening situation by asking questions such as:

> "What is the exact nature of the threatening situation?"
>
> "What unfavorable consequences can I expect from the situation should it occur?"
>
> "What courses of action can I use to cope with the threat?"
>
> "What courses of action are most likely to succeed, i.e., cause the least personal loss or problem?"

After a realistic appraisal, the person chooses the most effective course of action, e.g., talking to a friend, calling a crisis center, doing nothing, or seeking out professional help.

Assertive Responses

Everyday interpersonal interactions can produce stress. In such situations, assertive behavior is useful. **Assertiveness** involves expressing oneself openly and directly without hurting others. It provides feelings of control and self-confidence for the communicator and is based on the belief that each person is important. Assertive people are able to present their feelings and values, stand up for themselves, and claim their rights. Assertiveness is prerequisite to building self-esteem. Because it enables the person to actively cope with a stressful event, it enhances self-esteem.

Assertiveness with individuals and groups facilitates:

1. Prompt coping with problems
2. Achievement of group goals
3. Communication of power within oneself
4. Communication of competence and self-confidence
5. Reduction of anxiety or tenseness in key situations

Assertiveness, nonassertiveness, and aggressiveness compared Assertive behavior can be described as falling between nonassertiveness and aggressive behavior on a continuum. Nonassertive, or passive, persons appear hesitant and unsure of themselves. Their feelings are hidden, for fear of hurting others or being hurt. Because nonassertive persons do not ask or know how to ask, they often do not obtain what they want and thus become frustrated. After a time, this frustration often results in explosively aggressive behavior, which helps the person feel better, but only briefly. Through **aggressiveness**, at the other extreme, people can make their feelings known, but often at others' expense. Although this behavior can result in change, it can be harmful to the individual eventually, as others respond negatively to the aggressive behavior.

Nurses, too, can benefit from using assertive responses. The example that follows illustrates the different types of responses in a typical nursing situation.

> *Situation*
> Charge nurse: Miss Eammons, why can't you ever take your blood pressures on time? This is the fourth day this week that they have not been taken.
>
> *Aggressive response*
> Nurse: It's not my fault they are late. You're always interrupting my work with extra duties.
>
> *Nonassertive response*
> Nurse: Yes, I'm sorry. We've been short staffed, and I have a very heavy load.

Assertive response
Nurse: I didn't know that all the blood pressures were late. I'd like to check that further. Could we discuss this in your office before you leave today?

Assertive techniques The following assertive techniques can help the nurse.

1. Include positive and negative information in a statement: "I like your plan but . . . ."
2. Start the statement with "I," and avoid generalizations such as "we all believe" or "it seems like a good idea."
3. Express your own beliefs and rights: "I believe that . . . ."
4. Express your thoughts and feelings directly, to reinforce your identity: "I feel you are . . ." or "I want you to . . . ."
5. When replying negatively, state, "I won't . . ." not "I can't . . . ." The latter implies lack of power, whereas the former communicates assumption of responsibility.
6. Make assertive statements (Bakdash 1978, p. 1712):
   a. Simple assertive: "I think . . . ."
   b. Empathic assertive: "I realize you are very tired, but . . . ."
   c. Confrontive assertive: "You said you could bathe Mr. Greene, but you didn't . . . ."
   d. Soft assertive: "I am very grateful you did that for me, and I think . . . ."
   e. Persuasive assertive: "I agree with most of what you said, but I also think . . . ."

When an individual says something that the nurse perceives as negative or a "put-down," the following assertive responses can be given to provide time:

1. "I need to think about this for a few minutes."
2. "It seems to me that . . ." and a clear statement of personal feelings.
3. Silence as an answer, giving no verbal response.

Three assertive methods of coping with criticism are fogging, negative assertion, and negative inquiry (Smith 1975, pp. 104–32). *Fogging* is agreeing in principle to a statement made by another. In this technique, the nurse listens carefully to the criticism and accepts it without becoming defensive or anxious:

Client: You can't do anything right.

Nurse: You're not satisfied with my work, Mr. Milos.

Negative assertion is the assertive expression of those attributes that are negative about oneself:

Client: You didn't give that injection well.

Nurse: I didn't give it very smoothly.

Negative inquiry asks for additional information about the critical statements:

Charge nurse: You look messy today.

Nurse: What do you mean?

Charge nurse: You look untidy.

Nurse: Do you mean my uniform is wrinkled?

To learn assertiveness, nurses can take workshops or study articles on the subject.

Defensive Responses

Defensive responses are generally used when other responses have been unsuccessful in adapting to the stressful event and anxiety or other feelings remain high. Specific defensive coping behaviors are called ego-defense mechanisms. These are discussed in Chapter 17, page 346.

Assessment

Assessment of problems related to self-concept is normally indicated if (a) the client or support persons present cues that could reflect problems, or (b) the client's illness is one often associated with self-concept problems. Problems with self-concept and self-esteem are frequently manifested by expressions of anxiety, fear, anger, hostility, guilt, and/or powerlessness. Behaviors reflecting excessive role conflict may also indicate the need for meaningful intervention by nurses.

The nursing assessment involves four areas: (a) self-perception or self-awareness, (b) role performance and relationships, (c) major stressors and coping strategies, (d) behaviors suggestive of altered self-concept.

A trusting client–nurse relationship is essential for an effective assessment of self-concept. Clients tend not to share personal feelings unless the nurse has established an empathetic, nonjudgmental relationship. Potential disclosure of personal data can be threatening. Some people, particularly those with low self-esteem, may fear that the nurse will not accept or like them if they reveal their true performance capabilities, thoughts, and feelings.

Self-Perception

Assessment of self-perception involves (a) determining the client's perception of physical self, personal self, and worth, and (b) observing for nonverbal cues that reflect the client's self-perception.

Physical Self

To determine the client's perception of physical self, or body image, the nurse either listens to comments made by the client about his or her physical self or asks the client questions. For example:

> "How do you feel about your personal appearance (or physical features)?"
>
> "What do others say about your personal appearance (or physical features)?"
>
> "How would you describe your physical movements?"
>
> "What changes in your body do you expect as a result of this illness (or surgery, or treatment)?"
>
> "What changes have you noticed in how your body looks (or functions)?"
>
> "How have important persons in your life (e.g., spouse, parent, partner) reacted to changes in your body?"
>
> "How do you think the important people in your life will react to the anticipated change in your body?"

Responses such as "I feel ugly," "I'm awkward and clumsy," "I can't do anything now," "No one will like me now," and "I'm afraid my husband won't love me any more" indicate that the client's self-esteem is threatened or low. The client is focusing on particular disabilities or shortcomings and blocking out accurate perception of the total self.

Personal Self

Some people may volunteer clearly self-deprecating or over-critical comments about self indicating low self-esteem—e.g., "People don't like me," or "I'm no good." For other clients, the nurse may consider asking some of the following questions:

> "How would you describe your personal characteristics?" or, "How do you see yourself as a person?"
>
> "What do you like about yourself?"
>
> "How do others describe you as a person?"
>
> "What do you do well?"
>
> "What are your personal strengths, talents, and abilities?"
>
> "What would you change about yourself if you could?"
>
> "Does it bother you a great deal if you think someone doesn't like you?"
>
> "Is it difficult for you to say no when you want to say no?"
>
> "How do you feel about your educational achievements?"
>
> "Do you ever feel inadequate with certain people? Who?"
>
> "How easily can you express your opinion when it differs from that of others?"
>
> "Do you make friends easily?"
>
> "Generally, do you feel liked by your peers and co-workers?"
>
> "How do you feel about your occupation?"
>
> "Do you feel appreciated by your employer?"

Nonverbal Cues

Nonverbal behaviors—such as body posture, movements, gestures, tone of voice, speech pattern, and general appearance—tend to be more spontaneous than verbal messages and can provide important clues to the person's self-concept. Nonverbal cues that can indicate low self-esteem include stooped shoulders, lack of attention to hygiene or grooming, avoiding eye contact, hesitant speech, and withdrawing from social interaction. Nonverbal cues can help the nurse confirm the reliability of the client's verbal messages.

Roles and Relationships

The nurse assesses the client's satisfactions and dissatisfactions associated with role responsibilities and relationships: family roles, work roles, student roles, social roles. Family roles are especially important to clients, since family relationships are particularly close. Relationships can be supportive and growth-producing or, at the opposite extreme, highly stressful if violence and abuse permeate relationships. Assessment of family roles and relationships may begin with structural aspects such as number in the family group, ages, and residence location. There are a number of frameworks for studying the family. See Chapter 21. To obtain data related to the client's self-esteem in the family setting the nurse might ask some of the following questions. Keep in mind, however, that questions need to be tailored to the individual and his or her age and situation.

> "Tell me about your family."
>
> "What is home like?"

"Who are you closest to in the family?"

"Who are you most distant from in the family?"

"What are your relationships like with your other relatives?"

"What are your responsibilities in the family?"

"How well do you feel you accomplish what is expected of you?"

"What about your role or responsibilities would you like changed?"

"Do you see yourself as frequently getting the short end of things and coming out second best?"

"Are you proud of your family members?"

"Do you feel your family members are proud of you?"

"Tell me how you spend your time each day."

In determining the client's satisfaction or dissatisfaction with work roles and social roles, the nurse might ask questions such as:

"Do you like your work?"

"How do you get along at work?"

"What about your work would you like to change if you could?"

"How do you spend your free time?"

"Are you involved in any community groups?"

"Are you most comfortable alone, with one other person, or in a group?"

"Who is most important to you?"

"Whom do you seek out for help?"

Major Stressors and Coping Strategies

It is important for the nurse to identify stressors that challenge the client's self-worth. Common stressors that influence a client's self-concept and self-esteem are shown on the right. Most people face numerous stress-producing events simultaneously. Illness and hospitalization can compound the effects.

When stressors are identified, the nurse needs to determine how the client perceives the stressor. A positive, growth-oriented perception of stressful events reinforces self-worth; a negative, hopeless, defeatist perception leads to decreased self-esteem.

The nurse also determines the client's usual pattern of coping or choice of coping strategies. See "Communication/Coping Styles," earlier in this chapter, and ["Manifestations of the Stress Experience"] in Chapter 17. To determine the client's coping style, the nurse needs to ask the client two questions: (a) "When you have a problem or face a stressful situation, how do you usually deal with it?" (b) "Do these methods work?"

Stressors Affecting Self-Concept and Self-Esteem

Body-Image Stressors

- Loss of body parts, e.g., amputation, mastectomy, hysterectomy
- Loss of body functions, e.g., from heart disease, renal disease, spinal cord injury, cerebrovascular accident, neuromuscular disease, arthritis, declining mental or sensory abilities
- Disfigurement, e.g., through pregnancy, severe burns, facial blemishes, colostomy, ileostomy, tracheostomy, laryngectomy

Role Stressors

- Loss of parent, spouse, child, or close friend
- Change or loss of job
- Retirement
- Divorce or separation
- Illness
- Hospitalization
- Ambiguous role expectations
- Conflicting role expectations
- Inability to meet role expectations

Identity Stressors

- Change in physical appearance
- Declining physical, mental, or sensory abilities
- Inability to achieve goals
- Relationship concerns
- Sexuality concerns
- Unrealistic ideal self
- Membership in a minority group

Behaviors Suggestive of Altered Self-Concept

Some of the verbal and nonverbal behaviors that can indicate altered self-concept or low self-esteem were discussed earlier in this section. Other behaviors associated with low self-esteem are listed on the next page.

Behaviors Associated with Low Self-Esteem

The client:

- Avoids eye contact
- Stoops in posture and moves slowly
- Is poorly groomed and has an unkempt appearance
- Is hesitant or halting in speech
- Is overly critical of self, e.g., "I'm no good," "I'm ugly," or "People don't like me."
- May be overly critical of others
- Is unable to accept positive remarks about self
- Encourages reprimands from others, to punish self
- Apologizes frequently
- Verbalizes feelings of hopelessness, helplessness, and powerlessness, such as "I really don't care what happens," "I'll do whatever anyone wants," "Whatever is destined will happen."
- Verbalizes feelings of worthlessness, such as "Nobody cares about me," "I'm just a burden to everyone," "I'm not worth all that trouble."
- Verbalizes feelings of guilt, such as "It's all my fault," "I am to blame."
- Withdraws from or changes social involvements or relationships
- Fails to complete or follow through with activities
- Avoids initiating conversation or interaction with others
- Exhibits self-destructive behavior, such as excessive use of alcohol, drugs, smoking
- Has negative feelings about own body, e.g., avoids looking at or touching body part, or hides body part; emphasizes previous appearance or function; talks excessively about loss or change
- Is indecisive, e.g., "I can't make up my mind what to do," "I don't understand what's happening."
- Cannot solve problems effectively and does not ask for help
- Displays overdependence, e.g., asks for assistance unnecessarily, seeks attention by speaking loudly, asks irrelevant questions, seeks approval and praise
- Displays lack of energy, e.g., "I feel tired all the time."
- Verbalizes inability to cope
- Expresses or manifests anxiety, fear, anger
- Does not meet role expectations.

(North American Nursing Diagnosis Association 1986, pp. 534, 537–40; Carpenito 1983, pp. 389–94)

Distorted Thinking

People with low self-esteem generally exhibit illogical and distorted thinking. Some cognitive therapists (Ellis and Harper 1975, p. 100; Beck 1979, p. 54) assert that illogical and distorted thinking causes or perpetuates low self-esteem. Common types of irrational, illogical, or muddled thinking include the following (Crouch and Straub 1983, p. 72).

Catastrophizing This is the tendency to think the worst. For example, the person says, "If something bad can happen it will," or, "Things are bad now, but they will get worse."

Minimizing and maximizing This is the tendency to minimize the positive, to overlook partial successes, to magnify the significance or meaning of the negative, and to emphasize mistakes.

Black-and-white thinking This is the tendency to attribute things to one of two extremes. Things are either perfect or no good. Activities must be performed without mistake or the performance is a failure.

Overgeneralization This is the tendency to believe that something that applied in one situation or that happened once will apply in all situations.

Self-reference This is the tendency to believe that what others are thinking, saying, or doing relates to self. The person believes that others are highly concerned with his or her thoughts and actions and are particularly aware of his or her shortcomings and mistakes.

Filtering This is the tendency to support beliefs or conclusions by selectively pulling certain details out of context and neglecting other facts. Usually, it is the negative details that are selected while positive facts are neglected.

Nursing Diagnosis

Nursing diagnoses for clients with problems related to self-concept include disturbance in body image, disturbance in self-esteem, disturbance in role performance, and disturbance in personal identity (Kim et al. 1984, pp. 47–50). Other diagnoses that relate to self-concept include ineffective individual coping, social isolation, powerlessness, sexual dysfunction, anticipatory grieving, and dysfunctional grieving. Sexual dysfunction is discussed in Chapter 19, and grieving in Chapter 50. Further examples of nursing diagnoses related to self-concept are shown below.

Examples of Nursing Diagnoses Related to Altered Self-Concept

- Disturbance in body image related to mastectomy
- Disturbance in body image related to colostomy
- Disturbance in body image related to amputation
- Disturbance in body image related to massive facial scarring
- Disturbance in body image related to pregnancy
- Disturbance in self-esteem related to loss of job
- Disturbance in self-esteem related to unrealistic self-expectations
- Disturbance in self-esteem related to unrealistic parental expectations
- Disturbance in self-esteem related to divorce
- Disturbance in role performance related to change in physical capacity to assume role
- Disturbance in role performance related to newly assumed work and family roles
- Disturbance in personal identity related to loss of job
- Ineffective individual coping related to divorce and change in financial status
- Ineffective individual coping related to death of mother
- Ineffective individual coping related to inadequate personal resources and social support
- Ineffective coping related to need for mutilating surgery
- Social isolation related to alteration in body image
- Powerlessness related to inability to perform activities of daily living secondary to arthritis
- Powerlessness related to inability to perform role responsibilities secondary to progressive debilitating disease

Planning

The nurse's focus in the planning phase is on assisting the client to set goals that reflect a positive resolution of the problem or stressors identified in the nursing diagnosis. Goals should emphasize strengths rather than weaknesses or impairments. Broadly speaking, goals may be stated as follows. The client will:

1. Have increased awareness of strengths and weaknesses
2. Have improved feelings of self-worth
3. Perceive and respond to stressors in a constructive manner
4. Improve interpersonal relationships

Two types of self-image goals can be considered: tangible and personality (Goldin 1985, p. 35). Tangible goals are those that can be measured by objective means, for example, improve personal appearance, improve educational level, improve fund of information. Personality goals are more subjective in nature, for example, increase assertiveness, enhance ability to reach out for new friendships, become more independent and self-sufficient, develop self-pride. Once goals for changing self-image are set, the process of modifying self-image begins.

Planning also involves establishing outcome criteria by which to measure goals achievement. For examples of outcome criteria, see the Evaluation section later in this chapter.

Intervention

Assisting people with self-concept disturbances requires skills in communicating and in developing helping relationships (see Chapter 27). Helping clients with self-concept disturbances is akin to promoting health, as discussed in Chapter 20. The client assumes responsibility for implementing the plans. The nurse provides information, education, and on-going support; suggests strategies to encourage behavioral change; and implements techniques that help the client gain a realistic and acceptable view of self. Selected interventions to help clients with self-concept disturbances follow. Numerous community self-improvement programs are also available, many of them emphasizing the need for individuals to take charge of their lives, to take responsibility for their actions, to think positively rather than negatively, and to become more assertive.

It is important for both the nurse and the client to realize that changes in self-concept require an extended period of time. Although varying from person to person, this may take several months or years. It is essential for the client to learn that self-concept or self-image is not etched in stone; it can change and improve in progressive small steps, particularly if the client desires such change.

Identifying Areas of Strength

Healthy or "normal" people of any age often perceive their problems and weaknesses more clearly than their assets and strengths. The average well-functioning person with some college education, when asked to write down his or her strengths, is able to list only five or six; however, the same person can list three to four times as many problems or areas of weakness (Otto 1965, p. 34).

Research Note

An increase in violent, self-destructive, and risk-taking behaviors among adolescents has caused concern for the health of American youth. A cross-sectional survey of 138 white, secondary-school adolescents ages 14 to 18 was conducted to ascertain the prevalence of psychologic symptoms among adolescents in the general population and to identify any predictive relationships among sets of personality, demographic, and symptom variables. Findings indicated that subjects' reported symptoms were highly correlated with personality variables associated with Erikson's notions of identity confusion. Based on these findings the authors propose for adolescents a nursing diagnosis of identity confusion. For future study they propose four nursing diagnoses related to developmental difficulties among adolescents: identity confusion related to problems of intimacy; identity confusion related to problems of negative identity; identity confusion related to problems of time perspective; and identity confusion related to diffusion of industry. (Oldaker 1985)

Because people with low self-esteem tend to focus on their limitations, one of the nurse's major responsibilities is to help the client identify his or her personality resources and assets. Personality strengths are present in latent or unused form in all people; they exist as *potentialities* (Otto 1965, p. 32). An inventory of one's strengths is in itself strengthening. Such an inventory has the following advantages.

1. It can result in a more well-rounded self-concept and more positive self-esteem.
2. It can help mobilize health and regenerative processes.
3. It can help the person to become more aware of the strengths of others and thus facilitate relationships. The person begins to see others' previously unrecognized strengths or "good side."

Because the client may be unclear about personality strengths and assets, the nurse must provide the client with a framework to follow. Interests, abilities, and past accomplishments and experiences need to be included. An abbreviated framework for identifying personality strengths has been developed at the University of Utah. It is shown on the facing page.

Developing Behavior Specificity

Many people overgeneralize and think in unspecific ways. The nurse can assist clients to think more clearly and to become more behavior specific in language and thought. Crouch and Straub (1983, p. 71) offer the following strategies for developing behavior specificity.

Defining Goals Clearly

The first step is to help clients clearly define goals. For example, in response to the question "How would you like to feel differently about yourself?" the client may give an unspecific, subjective, and unmeasurable answer such as "better," "happier," or "not so uptight." To help the client become more behavior specific the nurse needs to bring unspecific answers into focus. This can be done by inquiring, for example, "How will you know you are better?" or "What do you mean by 'uptight'?" or "If I were to observe you now in your usual activities and then after you had made these changes, how could I tell you had achieved them?" Open-ended questions that probe into the who, what, how much, when, where, and how of thought and behavior help the client and the nurse develop a clearer understanding of the individual, the problem, and the goals.

When formulating goals, and strategies for achieving them, the nurse needs to assess the client's ideal self and perceived self, along with the amount of discrepancy between them. Teaching the client about perceived self

Framework for Identifying Personality Strengths

Spectator sports and similar activities The rationale here is that the client's current interest or participation in spectator sports, as well as past interests which he recalls with pleasure, constitutes a vital spark, is evidence of his creative engagement with life, and, in most instances, presages a movement in the direction of health.

Sports and activities Taking part in a program of bodybuilding, conditioning, or rehabilitative exercises or similar physical regimens, including an interest (and anticipated future participation) in sports and outdoor activities.

Hobbies and crafts Participating, or having participated in, some hobby or craft activity, and having the desire to start or resume a hobby, craft, or similar pursuit.

Expressive arts Past or current interest in writing, painting, sketching, or music appreciation with a desire to participate in one of the expressive arts.

Health status Desire to maintain or regain his health, as well as having an interest or ability to carry through with regimens and treatments designed to foster and facilitate health.

Education, training, and related areas Any education is seen as a personality asset—vocational trade or technical training, scholastic honors, self-education or a desire to obtain further education or training.

Work, vocation, job, or position Successful on-the-job performance or enjoyment in his work, a sense of pride in work or duties, earned seniority or recognition for work performed.

Special aptitudes or resources Included here are such diverse factors as sales ability, aptitude for mathematics or some other subject, ability to fix mechanical things, a "green thumb," ability to construct or teach, knowing how to make a good impression on people.

Strengths through family and others Such sources of strengths as a spouse or children, relationships with parents, in-laws, or relatives who give love and understanding.

Intellectual strengths Ability to apply reason to problem solving, do original, creative, and critical thinking, accept new ideas, work on broadening his mind through reading, conversation, and sharing ideas; the capacity to learn and enjoy learning.

Aesthetic strengths Recognizing and enjoying beauty, and being able to use the sense of beauty to enhance the physical environment.

Organizational strengths Capacity for systematic planning, developing sound short- and long-range goals, and organizing resources, energy, and time to achieve such goals; the ability to assign and carry out priorities and to coordinate or lead the efforts and labor of others in relation to specific tasks.

Imaginative and creative strengths Such characteristics as creativity, imagination, and inventiveness for the development of new and different ideas in connection with his home, family, work, or social relationships.

Relationship strengths Ability to make people feel comfortable and the capacity to enjoy being with people, being aware of people's needs and feelings, being able to listen, and being patient with children as well as with adults.

Spiritual strengths Religious faith or love of God, membership and participation in church and related activities, and the capacity to express moral and religious values in living, that is, "living what one believes."

Emotional strengths Capacity to give and receive warmth, affection, and love; ability to "take" anger, and to feel and express a wide range of emotions; capacity for empathy.

Other strengths Included here are the ability to use humor, to "laugh" at oneself and take "kidding"; having a liking for adventure or pioneering; having sticktoitiveness, perseverance, and the drive or will needed to get things done.

(Otto 1965, reprinted with permission)

and ideal self can assist the client in exploring areas in which he or she may be unduly biased. It is also of value for subsequent exploration and assessment. For example, if a client expresses discouragement about the way he or she behaved in a situation, the nurse could say, "Ideally, how do you think you should have acted or reacted?" and then "How do you perceive you actually acted?" Some situations involve complications that are beyond the person's control; such questioning will help clarify that for the client.

Thinking Clearly

The second step in developing behavior specificity is to help the client think clearly. Clients with low self-esteem tend to think negatively and irrationally. (Behaviors indicating low self-esteem are discussed earlier in this chapter.) For example, a client with low self-esteem who has followed through on homework for three out of seven days might say, "There was no excuse; I failed," or "I didn't follow through; I can't do anything right." When responding, the nurse should avoid contradicting the client but need not accept the client's evaluation as accurate. The nurse might ask, "Specifically, how did you fail?" or "What exactly did you not follow through with?" or "How does not doing the homework perfectly mean you can't do anything right?"

Changing Language Patterns

Helping a client to change language patterns from passive phrases to more active phrases can help the client assume greater responsibility for his or her power. Examples of passive phrases and alternate active phrases are:

It makes me . . . (passive)
I choose to . . . *or* I do. (active)

I have to . . . (passive)
I want to . . . (active)

I can't . . . (passive)
I won't . . . *or* I choose not to . . . (active)

It scared me. (passive)
I scared myself. (active)

Changing language patterns does not alter a person's beliefs, but the process of recognizing and modifying language helps the person consider habitual as well as alternate ways of thinking and believing. When a client uses passive language, the nurse can ask for more specificity. For example, if the client says, "It really made me angry when . . ." the nurse might respond by asking, "How was it that you made yourself angry when . . . ?" or "What did you say to yourself to make yourself angry when . . . ?"

To encourage the use of more active language, the nurse may have the client initially listen for passive language without modifying it and then deliberately notice passive language and modify it. It is also important for the client to gain awareness of his or her overall feeling states when using passive or active language.

Encouraging Positive Self-Evaluation

Persons with high self-esteem express positive self-evaluation more frequently than negative self-evaluation. Persons with low self-esteem, on the other hand, frequently make negative self-evaluations and rarely give themselves positive feedback. Therefore, clients with low self-esteem need help in developing more positive thoughts and images about themselves. Several strategies are available for this, including modeling, praise or recognition, positive self-feedback, and visualization.

Modeling The nurse can model positive self-statements for the client by saying such things as "I did a good job painting my recreation room last weekend," or "I am improving my cooking," or "I am proud of the produce I'm getting from my vegetable garden."

Praise To help the client make the transition to self-recognition, the nurse provides honest, positive feedback. For example, the nurse might say, "I think you did a really fine job," or "It sounds like you worked very hard and have done well."

Positive self-feedback To help clients begin making positive self-statements the nurse may implement some of the following strategies.

1. Ask the client: "Tell me some things you have done recently that you feel good about," or "Tell me some things you like about yourself."
2. Have the client develop a list of accomplishments he or she feels good about and a list of characteristics he or she likes about himself or herself. Accomplishments, behaviors, and characteristics that hold high significance for the person are preferred, since they incorporate a sense of competence, virtue, and power. Frequent reference to this list or to one attribute on the list is encouraged.
3. Reduce negative self-feedback through thought-stopping techniques. For example, every time the client begins to think negatively about self, ask him or her to say mentally, "Stop," or "No," or "Think about now," and then attend to the details of the present experience.

Visualization Because strong positive images or expectations often become self-fulfilling, visualization, or imagery procedures, can be used to enhance self-esteem. In visualization, positive images of desired changes are consciously imagined. This can be a powerful tool for achieving goals and gaining a positive self-concept. To strengthen goals with visualization, the client:

1. Sets a positive goal or image, such as "I am talking with someone at a party" or "I am saying to my family that I need some help from them to be able to manage work and home responsibilities"
2. Relaxes and slowly repeats the goal-phrase several times
3. Closes his or her eyes and visualizes the goal-phrase on a written page
4. Envisions self as having accomplished the goal

Because a person's receptivity to positive suggestions is greater when that person is deeply relaxed, deep-breathing exercises, progressive relaxation techniques, meditation, and self-hypnosis are often introduced before imagery techniques are used in individual and group self-involvement programs. The nurse may refer clients to specific community programs.

Enhancing Self-Esteem in Children and Adolescents

The roles of parents and teachers are of great significance in determining children's self-concept. Children are able to grow in self-confidence, personal competence, and independence if they can develop five basic attitudes, involving (a) security and trust, (b) identity, (c) belonging, (d) purpose, and (e) personal competence (Reasoner 1983, p. 55). Parents and teachers have specific roles and responsibilities in helping children develop these five basic attitudes. The nurse can be instrumental in helping parents learn their supportive role.

Security and Trust

This first step in the development of self-esteem can be achieved by providing the child with well-defined limits, i.e., what is expected in terms of behavior and what has to be done to get approval. Limits need to be consistently enforced by all involved adults. Inconsistency tends to create anxiety and weakens feelings of security. Rules or standards need to be reasonable and broad enough to serve as general guidelines in new situations, such as in a neighbor's house, a friend's yard, or school classroom. Standards needs to be established for the treatment of others, respect for the property of others, the value of honesty, and routines such as getting ready for school in the morning, doing homework, completing chores, and going to bed at night.

Systems such as checklists, charts, and calendars can serve as reminders of what is expected and also enable the child to monitor his or her own performance. Conformance to expectations builds positive self-esteem. Self-monitoring builds a sense of pride and provides opportunities for positive recognition as opposed to only negative feedback for uncompleted chores.

Preparing the child for what to expect if standards are *not* met is also effective in encouraging desired behavior and discouraging misbehavior. Restricting privileges tends to be more effective than scolding or lecturing, and it helps the child learn the consequences of his or her behavior.

To feel secure, children also need to believe that the adults responsible for them are dependable and can be counted on. Adults, therefore, must serve as role models for appropriate behavior.

Identity

The second step in developing self-esteem is a strong sense of identity. Children need to feel they are unique. A child's identity is strengthened when the child is given positive feedback, recognition of his or her strengths, demonstrated love and acceptance, and help in assessing his or her strengths and shortcomings.

Children need positive feedback from the people of greatest significance to them: parents, grandparents, older siblings, teachers, and close friends. The kind of feedback given can be more significant than the child's actual level of performance. Positive feedback enhances a child's sense of identity and self-concept. No feedback is likely to make a child hesitant and unsure in new situations. Predominantly negative feedback can give a child a negative self-image.

Adults foster a strong self-concept by recognizing a child's strengths. Parents and teachers who focus on the child's shortcomings and devote extra time to only those areas considered weak contribute to the child's negative feelings. Adults need to point out the child's special talents and qualities, such as an attractive smile, skill at playing games, desire to help others, and a strong sense of right and wrong.

Before they can accept themselves, children need to feel loved and accepted. Adults can demonstrate this by taking time to be with the child, to listen, to read, to play, or to just be there. Physical contact—a hand on the shoulder, or a hug—usually conveys warmth and caring more tellingly than words.

Children need to learn to assess their own level of performance and to build confidence in their own judgment. Even though positive feedback from others is always important, children also need to learn to rely on their own judgment. They can be encouraged to evaluate their performance through test results, grades, or other objective measures.

Belonging

Feeling socially accepted is important to children. Just as children need to feel unique, so do they need to feel just like everyone else. They need to dress the same, talk the same, and be in the same club. A sense of belonging can be developed through a family that is united. The family unit enables children to learn how to function as group members, to learn that they cannot always be first or have their way, and to learn that they need to handle their own share of responsibilities. In the family unit and in groups children learn sensitivity and concern for others. Parents and group leaders can foster this concern by encouraging children to express empathy for others and to find ways to help others. Learning how to be of service to others and how to be a friend builds a sense of belonging and reduces feelings of alienation.

Purpose

Children need a sense of purpose, to give direction to their lives and as a basis for success, fulfillment, and, therefore, a positive self-concept. Adults can help a child develop a sense of purpose by setting reasonable expectations and by helping the child set realistic goals, by conveying faith and confidence in the child's ability to achieve the goals, and by helping the child expand his or her interests, talents, and abilities.

Children tend to work toward expectations that are set for them by parents or teachers, especially if the goals are within their capabilities and the adults are confident they can achieve them. If expectations are too high or too low, motivation is reduced. Expectations that are long-term and relatively general put less pressure on the child and tend to enhance motivation (Reasoner 1983, p. 60). For example, expecting a child to improve his general math skills is more motivating and less stressful than expecting an A on the next math test. To encourage children to try new challenges and reach new levels of performance, adults can expose children to new experiences. For instance, watching a demonstration on how to cook Chinese food, observing a highly skilled gymnast's performance, or talking with a fireman can help children identify their own goals. The more opportunities a child has, the more likely that he or she will be motivated to learn and to acquire new skills.

Children need help to be specific in defining what they want to learn or how to solve a problem. Parents can help by assisting children to identify the sequence of steps needed to achieve a goal or solve a problem. When a child sets a goal for himself or herself, involved adults should convey faith in the child's ability to achieve the goal. Children who sense a parent's or teacher's confidence in them tend to increase their efforts toward, and their chances for, success.

Personal Competence

A sense of personal competence grows out of a sequence of successes. This gives the child a feeling of being able to cope with problems or meet goals. Children with a sense of personal competence have a positive approach to solving problems, tend to achieve success, and feel responsible for their own actions. Children who lack a sense of personal competence are overwhelmed by problems and may attribute lack of success to fate or being victimized. Parents can foster a feeling of competence by helping the child achieve the goals he or she has set. To do this the parent needs to do the following.

1. Develop a plan of action by having the child list the steps to be taken or review alternatives for achieving the goals. Parents should avoid prescribing what to do. Directing tends to foster dependency rather than independence. The child needs the freedom to make final decisions on how a plan should proceed.
2. Provide encouragement and support while monitoring the child's progress. From time to time the parent needs to check on the child's progress, helping assess what might still need to be done, fostering consideration of other resources, or—most important—praising the child's efforts and achievement.
3. Provide feedback that will help the child determine whether the goal has been achieved. This should include more sharing of the joy of accomplishment and factual comparative information than judgment or praise, although some children value an extrinsic reward more highly. However, children need to learn to become less dependent on extrinsic or tangible rewards. Excessive praise also can make some children more rather than less dependent (Reasoner 1983, p. 62).

Enhancing Self-Esteem in Older Adults

There is a wide variation in the way older adults perceive themselves; most, however, benefit from having their independence fostered. Low self-esteem is often associated with the dependence that accompanies the declining physical and mental capacities related to aging. The nurse can foster the older adult's independence and a more positive self-concept by doing the following (Hirst and Metcalf 1984, p. 76):

1. Encourage the person to participate in planning his or her care, and involve him or her in decision making. For example, allow the person to choose what to wear or what activities to participate in, and consult him or her about food preferences.
2. Allow the person to collect numerous objects around him or her. These establish the person's territory or physical space as his or her own.
3. Ask permission before putting the person's clothing (e.g., dressing gown, nightclothes) or other objects into his or her locker or closet. To do so without permission would deny the existence of the person's personal space and can be perceived as disrespectful.
4. Listen to what the person is saying. Elderly people need to know their comments are valued.
5. Allow the person sufficient time to complete an interaction or activity. Older adults are often slow to respond. Attempts to hurry their responses can create anxiety and embarrassment and can lower self-esteem.
6. Receive contributions of thanks or appreciation (e.g., candy or fruit) graciously and sincerely. Having something to contribute helps older adults maintain or enhance their self-esteem.

Evaluation

Examples of outcome criteria for clients with self-concept disturbance are shown to the right.

Examples of Outcome Criteria Related to Disturbance in Self-Concept

The client will:

- Discuss limitations in physical mobility
- Express feelings and thoughts about body changes
- Look at and touch a body deformity
- Make decisions regarding a job change and financial arrangements
- Participate in self-care
- Accept offers of help
- Continue preexisting socialization pattern
- Begin to assume role-related responsibilities
- Discuss own strengths and talents with another person
-  Share feelings about self with significant others
- Discuss options and alternatives when trying to solve problems

Nursing Care Plan

Assessment Data

Nursing Assessment

Mr. David Ginsberg is a 30-year-old married lawyer who has been treated for ulcerative colitis for the past few years. Recently, his symptoms have become exacerbated, and it was determined that surgery (an ileostomy) needed to be performed. Since his surgery, Mr. Ginsberg has been embarrassed and angry about his ostomy and refuses to see any of his friends and colleagues. He has refused to look at his stoma and has not permitted his wife to see it either. He has not actively participated in self-care activities. On his fourth post-operative day, his newly assigned nurse, Judy Wright, enters his room and introduces herself. Mr. Ginsberg replies, "If you're here to give me my morning care, I don't prefer any. What's the use of all this? The pouch will get filled up in a short time anyway. I don't particularly feel up to looking at it this morning, and I don't want you or anyone else to see it either. It's disgusting. Please leave me alone."

Physical Examination

Height: 190.5 cm (6′3″)
Weight: 76 kg (165 lb)
Temperature: 37 C (98.6 F)
Pulse rate: 76 BPM
Respirations: 20 per minute
Blood pressure: 126/80 mm Hg
Skin warm, dry, and pale
Ileostomy stoma 2.5 cm midline; skin of lower abdomen pink and intact

Diagnostic Data

RBC: 3.4 ml/μL
Hgb: 10.2 grams/L
Hematocrit: 34%
Urine: Negative
Colon x-ray film: Diffuse lesions left colon

Nursing Diagnosis	Client Goals and Outcome Criteria	Nursing Interventions and Rationales	Evaluation
Alteration in self-concept: disturbance in body image related to ileostomy (fecal diversion) resulting in refusal to touch or look at body part, refusal to participate in self-care, withdrawal from social contacts and signs of grieving.	Client Goal: Accept altered body image. Outcome Criteria: Client will view stoma by day 3. Client will begin to participate in stoma care by day 5. Participates in self-care activities like bathing and shaving by day 4. Verbalizes feelings about body changes by day 2.	Establish a trusting relationship with client. *Rationale:* Trust in the caregiver will encourage the client to express the way he feels, thinks, or views himself. Encourage client and significant others to verbalize their feelings about an ostomy. *Rationale:* Feelings must be recognized before they can be dealt with effectively. Provide client and significant others with a listening ear, interest, and concern rather than advice. *Rationale:* People generally clarify problems and solutions if they are permitted to express their thoughts and feelings. Allow the client to respond to loss of body function and changed body image with denial, shock, anger, and depression. *Rationale:* These are normal reactions in the grieving process. Support client's strengths and assist him to look at himself in totality. *Rationale:* Focuses attention away from limitations and increases awareness of strengths. Encourage and provide opportunities for self-care of ostomy. *Rationale:* Independence in self-care increases self-esteem. Provide for opportunity for client to meet with other ostomates. *Rationale:* Provides a good support system and reinforcement.	He voiced his concern regarding his wife's reaction to his stoma and fecal diversion. He feared she may find him unattractive and perhaps repulsive. He also felt he would not be socially acceptable to his friends, colleagues and his profession with his ileostomy bag, possible odors, etc. He started looking at his stoma when Miss Wright changed his pouch on day 3. On day 5 he empties his pouch whenever necessary and he is beginning to participate in his stoma care. He showers and shaves each morning.
Ineffective coping related to depression in response to body image change resulting in verbalization of inability to cope; inability to ask for help; insomnia, lack of grooming, lack of social contact, and anger.	Client Goal: Identify problem and become involved in problem solving. Outcome Criteria: Verbalizes feelings of anger and sadness by day 2. Focuses attention on things that must be done, e.g., stoma care, by day 3. Expresses feelings about body changes by day 2. Shares feelings with wife by day 5.	Assess for causes of depression. *Rationale:* Identification of causes allows for more effective interventions. Assess client's coping status. *Rationale:* Will aid in determining whether coping behaviors are effective or ineffective in client's problem-solving process. Use active listening. *Rationale:* Aids in identifying client's needs and problems. Provide a nonthreatening environment. *Rationale:* Client will be less fearful of verbalizing concerns.	Mr. Ginsberg has begun to verbalize his feelings about his altered physical state with his wife, the nurses, and the social worker. He now participates in the care of his ostomy. He has accepted social visits from a few close friends. He states, "I think this condition is manageable. I'll just have to work at it."

(continued)

Nursing Diagnosis	Client Goals and Outcome Criteria	Nursing Interventions and Rationales	Evaluation
		Determine support persons and resources available to client and the responses of support persons. *Rationale:* These responses influence the client's acceptance of his altered appearance and behavior. Allow for client's input regarding sequence of care. *Rationale:* Gives client sense of control and decreases sense of helplessness. Be supportive of client's effective coping behaviors. *Rationale:* Will assist client with maintaining self-concept and his relationship with others. Initiate referrals as necessary. *Rationale:* Will provide support system and aid client in coping.	

Chapter Highlights

- A healthy self-concept, or positive self-esteem, is essential to a person's physical and psychologic well-being.
- Self-concept is sometimes referred to as the cognitive component of the self system and self-esteem as the affective component.
- Self-concept and self-esteem are closely related, since self-esteem is "how I feel about how I see myself."
- Components of self-concept include body image, role performance, self-identity, and self-esteem.
- A person's self-perception can differ from the person's perception of how others see him or her and from how the person would like to be.
- From the hour of birth, interactions with significant others create the conditions that influence self-esteem throughout life.
- When individuals are able to conceptualize the self, they begin a lifelong process of deciding whether and to what extent they are valuable and worthy.
- Individuals who grow up in families whose members value each other are likely to feel good about themselves.
- Most individuals feel good about themselves in some ways and bad about themselves in other ways.
- The development of self-esteem can be seen as a process of establishing a sense of security, a sense of identity, and a sense of belonging.
- When children feel secure and accepted they can be encouraged to set goals for themselves.
- If adults help children to accomplish goals that are important to them, children begin to develop a sense of personal competence and independence.
- Four elements of experience that affect the development of self-esteem are: significant others, social role expectations, psychosocial development crises, and communication/coping style.
- Adults base their self-concept on how they perceive and evaluate their performance in the areas of work, intellect, appearance, sexual attractiveness, particular talents, ability to cope and to resolve problems, independence, and interpersonal interactions.
- An individual's functional level of overall self-esteem may change markedly from day to day and moment to moment.
- Because a healthy self-concept is basic to health, one of the nurse's major responsibilities is to assist clients whose self-concept is disturbed to develop a more positive and realistic image of themselves.
- A trusting client–nurse relationship is essential for the effective assessment of a client's self-concept, for providing help and support, and for motivating client behavior change.

Suggested Readings

Bond, M. October 13, 1982. Dare you say no? *Nursing Mirror* 155:40–43.

Describes methods for making and refusing requests, to help the nurse become more assertive and avoid stress. A table includes the characteristics of aggressive, submissive, manipulative, and assertive behaviors in terms of speech content, eye contact, posture, gestures, facial expression, timing, and voice tone.

Bush, M. A., and Kjervik, D. K. April 26, 1979. The nurse's self-image: By being assertive, nurses will no longer grossly underrate their abilities. *Nursing Times* 75:697–701.

This is a discussion of ways that nurses can increase their self-esteem.

Hein, E., and Leavitt, M. May 1977. Providing emotional support. *Nursing 77* 7:38–41.

According to these authors, nurses can learn to be supportive just as they learn any other nursing technique. Concrete ways in which the nurse can provide support as a planned process are described.

Meissner, J. E. February 1980. Semantic differential scales for assessing patients' feelings. *Nursing 80* 10:70–71.

This article presents a semantic differential scale on which the client is asked to check the boxes that most closely describe his or her feelings, e.g., "lonely," "nervous," "indifferent," "calm," and "dejected."

———. May 1980. Uncovering your patient's hidden psychological problems. *Nursing 80* 10:78–79.

The author provides a concise assessment tool for clients to answer so that nurses can plan helpful nursing interventions related to the client's psychosocial needs.

Singleton, E. K. October 1984. Role clarification. A prerequisite to autonomy. *Journal of Nursing Administration* 14:17–22.

Because autonomy in nursing practice can become a reality, nurses must clearly identify their roles. A plan to help concretize role clarification is discussed.

Selected References

Antonucci, T. C., and Jackson, J. S. August 1983. Physical health and self-esteem. *Family and Community Health* 6:29–49.

Beck, A. T. 1979. *Cognitive theory of depression.* New York: The Guilford Press.

Burns, R. B. 1979. *The self concept in theory, measurement, development, and behavior.* London: Longman Group Ltd.

Carpenito, L. J. 1983. *Nursing diagnosis. Application to clinical practice.* Philadelphia: J. B. Lippincott Co.

Clarke, J. I. 1978. Self-esteem: A family affair. Minneapolis: Winston Press.

Crosby, R. September 1982. Self-concept development. *The Journal of School Health* 52:432–36.

Crouch, M. A., and Straub, V. August 1983. Enhancement of self-esteem in adults. *Family and Community Health* 6:65–78.

Ellis, A., and Harper, R. A. 1975. *A new guide to rational living.* North Hollywood, Calif.: Wilshire Book Co.

Erikson, E. H. 1963. *Childhood and society.* 2d ed. New York: W. W. Norton and Co.

———.1968. *Identity, youth, and crisis.* New York: W. W. Norton and Co.

Gilbert, R. August 1983. The evaluation of self-esteem. *Family and Community Health* 6:29–49.

Gillies, D. A. September/October 1984. Body image changes following illness and injury. *Journal of Enterostomal Therapy* 11:186–89.

Goldin, J. November/December 1985. The influence of self-image upon the performance of nursing home staff. *Nursing Homes* 34:33–38.

Hamachek, D. E. 1978. *Encounters with self.* 2d ed. New York: Holt, Rinehart and Winston.

Hirst, S. P., and Metcalf, B. J. February 1984. Promoting self-esteem. *Journal of Gerontological Nursing* 2:72–77.

Kim, M. J.; McFarland, G. K.; and McLane, A. M. 1984. *Pocket guide to nursing diagnoses.* St. Louis: C. V. Mosby Co.

Muhlenkamp, A. F., and Sayles, J. A. November/December 1986. Self-esteem, social support, and positive health practices. *Nursing Research* 35:334–38.

Norris, J., and Kunes-Connell, M. December 1985. Self-esteem disturbance. *Nursing Clinics of North America* 20:745–61.

North American Nursing Diagnosis Association. 1986. Classification of nursing diagnoses. Proceedings of the sixth national conference. Mary E. Hurley, editor. St. Louis: C. V. Mosby Co.

Oldaker, S. M. December 1985. Identity confusion. Nursing diagnoses for adolescents. *Nursing Clinics of North America* 20:763–73.

Otto, H. A. August 1965. The human potentialities of nurses and patients. *Nursing Outlook* 13:32–35.

Reasoner, R. W. August 1983. Enhancing self-esteem in children and adolescents. *Family and Community Health* 6:51–64.

Roy, S. C. 1984. *Introduction to nursing. An adaptation model.* 2d ed. Englewood Cliffs, N.J.: Prentice-Hall, Inc.

Sanford, L. T., and Donovan, M. E. 1984. *Women and self-esteem.* New York: Penguin Books.

Smith, M. J. 1975. *When I say no, I feel guilty.* New York: Bantam Books.

Stanwyck, D. J. August 1983. Self-esteem through the life span. *Family and Community Health* 6:11–28.

Sullivan, H. S. 1950. *The interpersonal theory of psychiatry.* New York: W. W. Norton and Co.

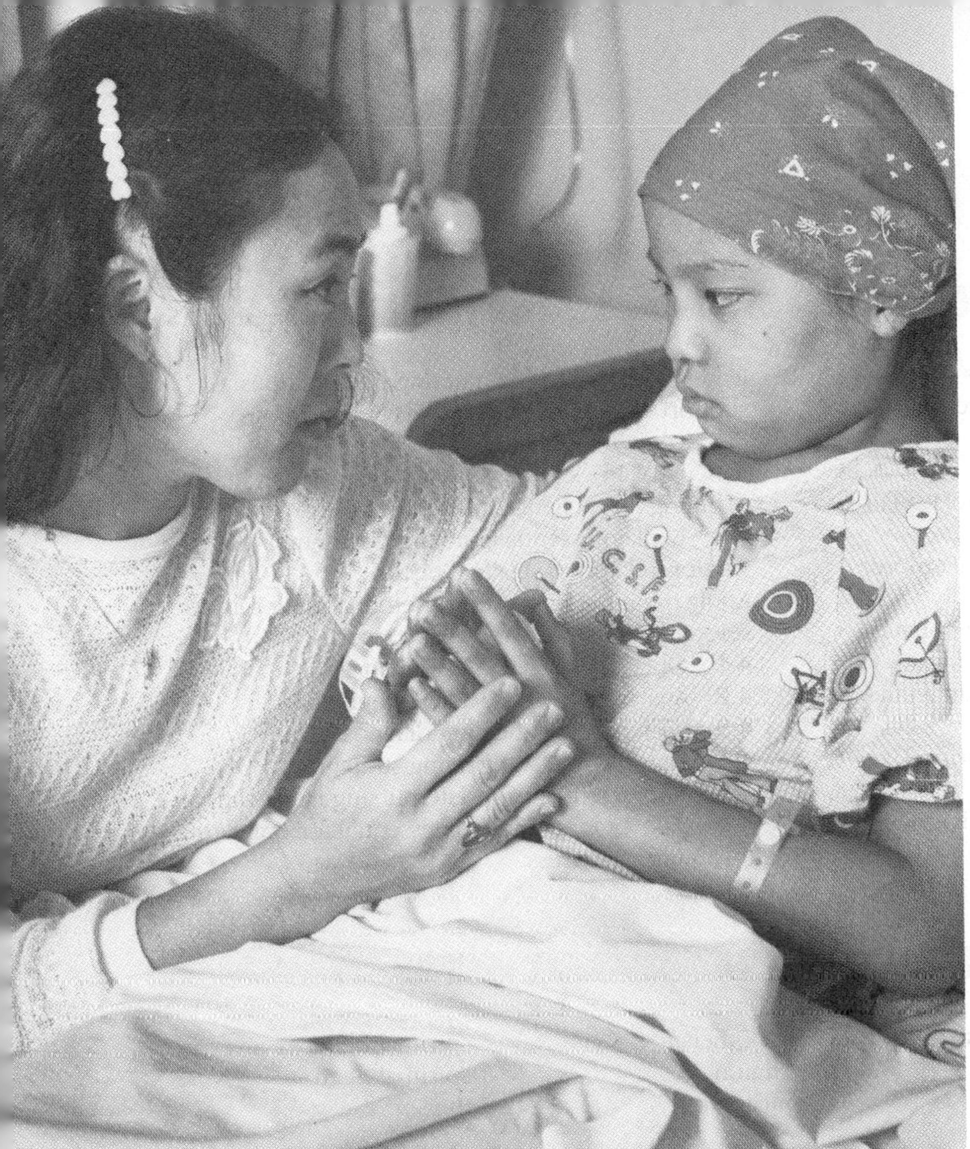

KAREN STAFFORD RANTZMAN

CHAPTER 49

Spirituality

Contents

49 *Spirituality*

Objectives

1. Know essential facts about spiritual beliefs and religious practices and doctrines as they relate to health care.
   1.1 Define selected terms.
   1.2 Identify significant religious beliefs related to health care.
2. Know information requires to assess and diagnose a client's spiritual needs and problems.
   2.1 Identify clients who can benefit from spiritual assistance.
   2.2 Identify essential information to obtain in the nursing history.
   2.3 Identify clinical signs indicating a spiritual need.
   2.4 Identify essential aspects of nursing diagnoses related to spiritual distress.
3. Understand facts about nursing interventions to support client's spiritual beliefs and religious practices.
   3.1 Explain essential aspects to consider when planning for a client's spiritual support.
   3.2 Explain essential guidelines for nursing intervention related to spiritual needs.
4. Apply the nursing process when providing care to selected clients with spiritual concerns.
   4.1 Obtain necessary assessment data.
   4.2 Analyze and relate assessment data.
   4.3 Write relevant nursing diagnoses.
   4.4 Plan appropriate nursing strategies.
   4.5 Implement appropriate nursing interventions.
   4.6 State outcome criteria essential for evaluating the client's progress.

Terms

agnostic
atheist
clergy
extreme unction (last rites)
faith
Holy Communion
monotheism
religion
spirituality
spiritual belief
spiritual need
theism

Spirituality and Religion

Spirituality and religion are separate entities, yet some people use the words interchangeably. **Spirituality** is a belief in some higher power, creative force, divine being, or infinite source of energy. For example, a person may believe in "God," in "Allah," or in a "higher power." "The spiritual dimension tries to be in harmony with the universe, strives for answers about the infinite" (Murray and Zentner 1985, p. 475). A **religion** is an organized system of worship. Religions have central beliefs, rituals, and practices usually related to birth, death, marriage, and salvation. **Faith**, according to Fowler and Keen (1985, p. 18), is a universal—a feature of living, acting, and self-understanding. To have faith is to believe in or be committed to something or someone. In a general sense, religion or spiritual beliefs are an individual's attempt to understand his or her place in the universe, i.e., how that person sees himself or herself in relation to the total environment.

Religion and Illness

Spiritual and religious beliefs are important in many people's lives. They can influence life-style, attitudes, and feelings about illness and death. Some organized religions specify practices about diet, birth control, and appropriate medical therapy. Some religious groups condemn modern science because of "false teachings," such as evolution. Other groups support medical therapy in general but object to specific practices, e.g., the Seventh Day Adventist Church urges its members to avoid all drugs unless they are exceedingly ill.

Spiritual beliefs may assume greater importance at a time of illness than at any other time in a person's life. **Spiritual beliefs** may help some people accept illness, and beliefs may explain illness for others. Some clients may look upon illness as a test of faith, i.e., "If I have enough faith I will get well." Viewed from this perspective, illness is usually accepted by the client and his or her support persons and does not present a threat to their religious beliefs.

Other people may look upon illness as punishment and think, "What have I done to deserve this?" These people associate disease with immoral behavior and believe their illness is punishment for past sins. They may believe that through prayer, promises, and perhaps penance, the cause of the disease will disappear. Such people believe that health professionals treat only the symptoms of disease and that they will become well if they are forgiven. If such an individual does not get well, then the support persons either accept the "punishment" or view the "punishment" as unfair.

Usually, spiritual beliefs help people to accept illness and to plan for the future. Religion can help people prepare for death and strengthen them during life.

Religion can provide any of the following:

1. A meaning to life and to death
2. A haven of strength, serenity, and faith at a time of crisis
3. A sense of security
4. A tangible network of social support.

Certain spiritual beliefs are in conflict with accepted medical practice. When a person's faith leads him or her to reject certain medical treatment, life may be threatened. For example, many practicing Jehovah's Witnesses will not accept blood transfusions because of religious doctrine.

Summary of Spiritual Development

Infants and Toddlers

Infants do not have a sense of right or wrong, spiritual beliefs, or convictions that guide their activities. Toddlers may follow certain rituals, such as saying their prayers at night, but they are only imitating to conform to the expectations of their parents. They may attend a church nursery school, but the emphasis of the teaching is typically on play and enhancing their positive self-image by having them accomplish simple tasks and telling them what they have accomplished.

Preschoolers

The greatest influence on preschoolers is their parents. Parental attitudes toward moral codes and religion convey to children what is considered good and bad. At this age, children are imitators and tend to copy what they see rather than what they are told. If what they see and what they are told are contradictory, problems arise.

Preschoolers often ask questions about morality and religion, e.g., "Why is (some action or word) wrong?" and "What is heaven?" They think that their parents are like God: omnipotent. Two methods of spiritual education are used with preschool children: indoctrinating them and letting them choose their own way. Children will follow a religion at this age not because they understand it but because it is part of their daily life. Three-year-olds like prayers at night and before meals. Five-year-olds often make up prayers themselves.

Children 3 to 5 years old believe that God or actual human beings are responsible for such natural events as rain and wind. They may reason, "The rain is God crying; the wind is God blowing air out of His mouth." At this age, children are old enough to go to church school and to participate in religious holidays. They ask many questions about the meaning of the holidays and need explanations about them. However, they are more occupied with such rituals as Santa Claus coming at Christmas than with the reason behind the holiday. When children begin to question such myths as the Easter Bunny, they are ready for a more sophisticated explanation about Easter.

School-Age Children

During the school years, children learn more about religion. Six-year-olds expect that their prayers will be answered, good rewarded, and bad punished. They have reverence for many thoughts and matters.

During the prepuberty stage, children become aware of spiritual disappointments. They realize that their prayers are not always answered on their own terms, and they begin to reason rather than accept a faith blindly. At this age, some children drop or modify certain religious practices (e.g., praying for tangible benefits); others continue to follow religious practices because of dependence on their parents.

During adolescence, children compare the standards of their parents with others and determine which ones they want to incorporate into their own behavior. At this age, children may keep parental standards. Adolescents also compare the scientific viewpoint with the religious viewpoint and try to bring the two together. By 16 years, many adolescents have decided whether to accept the family religion. They may experience personal religious awakenings, such as being saved or converted, either suddenly or gradually. Adolescents with parents of different faiths may choose one faith over the other or no faith. For some, a firm faith provides strength during these turbulent years.

Adults

Young adults who need to answer the religious questions of their own children may find that the teachings of their own early childhood are more acceptable to them now than during adolescence. During the middle years, adults often find that they have more time for religious activities because their children are older. Older adults who have developed religious values often endeavor to broaden them and to understand the newer values of younger people. They are comfortable with their own values but appreciate those of others. Elderly adults who do not have mature religious beliefs may experience a feeling of deprivation as they become less active, e.g., because of retirement. During these years, people face death—both their own and that of a spouse. This recognition may make them despondent. The development of a mature religious philosophy can often help older people face reality, participate in life, have feelings of self-worth, and accept death as inevitable. For additional information, see the sections on spiritual development in Chapters 22 to 26.

Religious Beliefs Related to Health Care

Meeting the spiritual needs of clients and their support persons is part of the function of nurses as well as designated chaplains and other clergy. The term **clergy** refers to priests, rabbis, ministers, church elders, deacons, and other spiritual advisers. Some religious groups, such as the Church of Latter-Day Saints and the Christian Scientists, do not have ordained clergy; they usually do have people whose role it is to minister to the ill, and these people must be recognized by nurses as having appropriate functions. In Christian Science, the role of ministering to the sick is carried out by a practitioner (reader).

Although nurses cannot expect to be well versed about the practices of all the religious groups in the United States or Canada, it is important to be familiar with the major religious groups of the community. Representatives of a religion are usually pleased to give nurses information required in the care of clients. Some of the larger religious groups are discussed briefly here. Other reference texts can supply greater detail and information not included in this summary.

The major religions of the United States and Canada are Protestantism, Catholicism, and Judaism. There are many Protestant denominations, e.g., Episcopalians, Methodists, and Baptists. The denominations share some doctrines, but each denomination has its own interpretation of scripture and its own religious practices. Catholicism also encompasses several groups, e.g., the Roman Catholic Church, the Greek Orthodox Church, and the Russian Orthodox Church.

Major religions, denominations, and some spiritual groups are listed alphabetically below. Selected facts about each group are included, but no attempt has been made to discuss broad philosophical beliefs or issues.

Agnosticism and Atheism

An **agnostic** is a person who doubts the existence of God or a supreme being or believes the existence of God has not been proven. An **atheist** denies the existence of God. **Theism** is the belief in the existence of a god or gods. **Monotheism** is the belief in the existence of one God. The moral and ethical codes of agnostics and atheists are not derived from theistic beliefs.

Baha'i

People following the Baha'i faith use prayer at times of illness. Their beliefs permit use of alcohol and drugs only on a physician's order. It is written in the scriptures that ill persons are to seek competent medical assistance.

Baptist

Baptists believe in the possibility of cure of illness by the "laying on of hands." Although some believe in faith healing to the exclusion of medical therapy, most seek competent medical help. Generally no restrictions are placed on the use of drugs, blood, or vaccines; biopsies or amputation of limbs; transplants; autopsies; or burial or cremation. Birth control, sterilization, and abortion (therapeutic or demand) are left to individual choice. When clients are clearly terminally ill, artificial prolongation of life is discouraged. Full-term stillborn babies are buried; less than full-term fetuses are not. Infant baptism is not practiced.

Some Baptists do not drink coffee or tea, and many Baptists do not take alcohol. The clergy ministers to individuals and support persons at times of illness.

Black Muslim (Nation of Islam)

The Black Muslim religion is not the same as Islam, although their beliefs are similar. Members emphasize black independence and are encouraged to obtain health care provided by the black community.

Black Muslims have a special procedure for washing and shrouding the dead and special funeral rites. Dietary considerations include prohibitions against alcoholic beverages and pork. Personal cleanliness is of great importance.

Buddhism

The doctrine of avoidance of extremes is practiced by Buddhists and applied to the use of drugs, blood, or vaccines. Buddhism does not condone the taking of lives in any form, but, if a client is beyond recovery and can no longer strive toward "enlightenment," euthanasia *may* be permitted. Likewise, certain circumstances may warrant abortion. Buddhists approve either burial or cremation. Last rite chanting is frequently practiced at the bedside of the deceased. Cleanliness is very important.

Buddhists generally do not practice any dietary restrictions, although members of some sects are strict vegetarians. Many Buddhists do not use tobacco, alcohol, or drugs. Buddhists have special holy days: January 1, February 15, March 21, April 8, May 21, July 15, September 1 and 23, and December 8 and 31. Clients may need to be asked how they feel about tests and treatments on those days.

Church of Christ, Scientist

Members of the Church of Christ, Scientist, oppose human intervention to cure illness, seeing it as God's will. Sickness and sin are errors of the human mind and can be changed by altering thoughts rather than by medicine. People who strictly follow this religion will not accept a physician's consultation or medical treatment and rarely, if ever, enter a hospital. Christian Scientists do not permit psychotherapy, because in this process the mind is altered by others. A Christian Science "practitioner" can be called to minister to the sick, and spiritual healing is practiced. Physicians and midwives may be used during childbirth, however.

Drugs and blood transfusions are not used, and biopsies and physical examinations are not sought. Tobacco, alcohol, and coffee are considered drugs and not used. Vaccines are accepted only as required by law. Christian Scientists do not have strictly defined policies about birth control, sterilization, or abortion. Autopsy is discouraged but accepted in sudden deaths, and Christian Scientists are unlikely to seek or donate organs for transplant. Whether a person wishes to rely completely upon Christian Science is up to the individual. In some areas, the church operates nursing homes in which there is complete reliance on church doctrine.

Eastern Orthodox

There are a number of Eastern Orthodox denominations, including Greek Orthodox, Russian Orthodox, and Armenian. Most believe in infant baptism by immersion 8 to 40 days after birth. The last rites may be obligatory if death is impending. Dietary restrictions depend on the particular sect. Eastern Orthodox beliefs and practices generally do not restrict medical science; however, the Russian Orthodox church discourages autopsy as well as donation of body parts.

The Greek Orthodox church opposes abortion. The church advocates confession at least yearly. The last rites include administration of **Holy Communion** (also referred to as the *Eucharist* or the *Lord's Supper*), a memorial sacrament in which the worshipper receives consecrated bread (or a thin wafer) representing the body of Jesus Christ, and wine or grape juice representing the blood of Jesus. The church advocates fasting, usually on Wednesdays, Fridays, and during Lent; the church encourages prolonging life, even for terminally ill clients. Abortion is prohibited.

Episcopalian (Anglican)

The Episcopal or Anglican religion places no restrictions on the use of drugs, blood, or vaccines; biopsies; or amputations or transplants for saving life. It permits birth control and sterilization, autopsy, therapeutic abortion as a life-saving measure, burial or cremation, and genetic counseling. Abortion on demand, however, is regarded as unacceptable. Anglicans celebrate Holy Communion. Some members of this church fast before receiving Communion and abstain from meat on Fridays. The church advocates confession. The rite for anointing of the sick may be performed but is not mandatory. For information about anointing see page 1445.

Hinduism

Hindus have many dietary variations. Veal and beef and their derivatives are not eaten by some Hindus. Some are strict vegetarians. Alcohol may be consumed at western social functions. Most Hindus accept modern medical practices; artificial insemination is rejected, however, because sterility reflects divine will. When giving a Hindu medications, the nurse avoids touching the client's lips, if possible.

Hindus practice special rites at death. Death is considered rebirth. The priest pours water into the mouth of the corpse and ties a thread around the wrist or neck to indicate blessing. This thread must not be removed. The body undergoes cremation, and the ashes are disposed of in holy rivers. Some injuries, such as loss of a limb, are considered signs of wrongdoing in a previous life, although the afflicted person is not an outcast from society. Hindus do believe there is a natural division among people, so that little mixing occurs among classes.

Jehovah's Witness

Jehovah's Witnesses are opposed to blood transfusions and organ transplants, although some individuals do agree to them in a crisis. When parents refuse to have an infant transfused, a court order may be sought transferring custody to the courts or to an official of the hospital.

Members of the church eat meat that has been drained of blood. Some oppose modern medicine. Infant baptism is not practiced.

Jehovah's Witnesses generally have a neutral attitude toward birth control, believing it is a matter of individual conscience, but sterilization is condemned and prohibited. Both therapeutic and demand abortions are forbidden. Practices such as masturbation and homosexuality are condemned. Both burial and cremation are approved. Autopsy is approved only as required by law, and no parts of the body are to be removed. This restriction has implications for donor transplants.

Judaism

There are three main Jewish groups: the Orthodox is the most strict; the Conservative and Reform groups are less strict. Jewish law demands that Jews seek competent medical care. Jews allow the use of drugs, blood, and vaccines; biopsies and amputations are also permitted. Some Orthodox Jews believe that the entire God-given body must be returned to the earth, and they require any body tissue to be buried. Donor transplants may therefore not be acceptable to Orthodox Jews. The nurse must ensure that amputated limbs or organs are made available to such Orthodox families for burial. Cremation is discouraged. Autopsy may be permitted in less strict groups as long as parts of the body are not removed. Bodies, even those of fetuses, are washed by the ritual burial society and buried as soon as possible after death.

Therapeutic abortion is permissible if the mother's physical or psychologic health is threatened. Demand abortion is prohibited. Vasectomy is not permitted.

Orthodox and Conservative Jews observe kosher dietary laws, which prohibit pork, shellfish, and other foods and the eating of milk products and meat products in the same meal. Reform Jews usually do not observe kosher dietary regulations.

Circumcision is performed by Orthodox and Conservative Jews on the eighth day of a male baby's life, although it may be delayed if medically contraindicated. The rabbi and male synagogue members may be present, and a Jewish physician or mohel (ritual circumciser acquainted with Jewish law and hygienic medical technique) performs the circumcision. Special arrangements generally need to be made for the ceremony and the physician's approval obtained.

Orthodox and some Conservative Jews observe the Sabbath from sundown Friday to sundown Saturday and may resist hospital admission or medical procedures during that period or during major Jewish festivals, unless the treatment is necessary to preserve life. Rosh Hashanah is the first day of the Jewish new year, which occurs in September. Ten days later, Yom Kippur marks the end of the time devoted to reflecting upon life.

Lutheran

The Lutheran church imposes no restrictions on medical procedures, including autopsies and therapeutic abortions, and no dietary restrictions. Abortion on demand is not approved, however. Marriage and procreation are discouraged when offspring are likely to inherit severe physical or mental deficits. Birth control and sterilization are left to the individual's conscience. Members are baptized 6 to 8 weeks after birth, and those who wish may be anointed and blessed before death. Burial rites are generally performed on infants who die after 6 to 7 months' gestation.

Mennonite

Members of the Mennonite church are baptized in their middle teens. The church advocates no special dietary restrictions, although some congregations require abstinence from alcohol. No restrictions are placed on medical procedures, although demand abortion is not approved in some sects of the church; in others, it is left to individual conscience. Mennonites oppose the laying on of hands.

Mormon (Church of Jesus Christ of Latter-Day Saints)

Some Mormons believe in cure by the "laying on of hands"; however, there is no prohibition on medical therapy—in fact, the church operates health facilities. Alcohol, tobacco, tea, and coffee are prohibited, and meat is eaten sparingly. Some members of the church wear a special undergarment at all times unless seriously ill. Mormon clients in the hospital may request the Sacrament of the Lord's Supper by a church priesthood holder.

Muslim/Moslem (Islam)

Islam is a major religion of North Africa and the Near East. There are over 70 sects of the Islamic faith. It emphasizes strict rituals and prayers.

All pork products are prohibited, and some oppose alcoholic beverages. There is a fasting period in the ninth month of the Mohammedan year (Ramadan), but people who are ill are exempt from it. Circumcision is practiced, and cleanliness is very important.

If a fetus is aborted 130 days or more after conception, it is treated as a fully developed human being. Before that time, it is looked upon as discarded tissue.

The dying person must confess sins and beg forgiveness. Only relatives and family can touch the body after death. They wash and prepare it and turn it toward Mecca. Islam encourages prolonging life, even for the terminally ill.

Native American

There are several hundred Native American tribes in the United States and Canada, each with its own religious culture. Most have medicine men or shamans, who perform various actions against illness. Believers look to superhuman powers for protection from disease. Many Native Americans today follow modern Christian religions; however, some follow traditional beliefs, and some hold a combination of Christian and traditional beliefs. See Chapter 18, page 371, for additional information.

Pentecostalist (Assembly of God, Foursquare Church)

The Pentecostal church has no doctrine against modern medical science, including blood transfusions. Members are encouraged to abstain from use of alcohol and tobacco and from eating strangled animals. Some members do not eat pork. Members may pray for divine healing, and in some congregations anointing with oil is practiced.

Roman Catholic

It is a Catholic belief that an infant has a soul from the moment of conception; therefore, a fetus must be baptized unless it is obviously dead, and so must all babies whose health or life is endangered. Baptism may be performed by any person (e.g., a physician or nurse in the absence of a priest) who does what the church requires. A valid baptism requires pouring water on the baby's head while repeating the prescribed Trinitarian invocation: "I baptize thee in the name of the Father, of the Son, and of the Holy Spirit." When performed by a nurse or physician, the baptism should be recorded on the infant's chart and the family and priest informed.

The Roman Catholic church encourages anointing of the sick. The sacrament of anointing is now considered both a source of strength or healing and a preparation for death. The priest anoints several areas of the body with oil. Before changes were instituted by the Second Vatican Council in 1963, this Catholic sacrament was administered to persons only when death was imminent and was referred to as **extreme unction** or the **last rites**, since it was one of the last rites of the church. Today, possibility of death may still be a reason for this sacrament, but death need not be the immediate concern. Catholics can now be anointed more than once. Many older Catholics, however, may respond to this sacrament with fear or dread, considering it a sign of imminent death. Thus, before a reluctant client is anointed, the nurse or priest should interpret its current meaning to the client, to minimize apprehension. Anointing of the sick may be preceded by confession and Holy Communion. These sacraments are also performed by a priest or other commissioned person. Receiving viaticum (Holy Communion) as a last rite before death is considered an obligation, but anointing is not.

The Roman Catholic belief in the "principle of totality" underlies a general acceptance of medical procedures. A donor transplant is accepted as long as loss of the organ does not deprive the donor of life or functional integrity of the body. Biopsies and amputations are accepted in the same light, but some dioceses require burial of the amputated limb. Autopsy is also accepted; again, all major parts of the body (those retaining human quality) must be given an appropriate burial or cremation.

Strict laws govern birth control, sterilization, and abortion. The only approved method of birth control is abstinence; artificial means are illicit. Sterilization is forbidden unless there is a sound medical indication for it. Both demand and therapeutic abortions are prohibited, even to save the mother's life.

Some Catholics observe certain dietary and fasting practices but are excused from otherwise obligatory fasting or abstaining from meat on Ash Wednesday and Good Friday when in the hospital. Sunday is the day of worship, although church services are held in some churches other days of the week as well.

Salvation Army

The Salvation Army places no restrictions on medical procedures, including transplants and autopsies. Birth control and sterilization are acceptable within marriage. Demand abortions are opposed, but therapeutic ones are approved.

Seventh-Day Adventist (Church of God, Advent Christian Church)

The Adventist church is opposed to infant baptism but conducts baptism of adults by immersion. In dietary matters, it prohibits alcohol, tobacco, narcotics, and stimulants, and some members advocate ovolactovegetarian diets. Some sects practice divine healing and anointing with oil. Saturday is considered the Sabbath by some.

Adventists are encouraged to avoid drugs, but they recognize that blood transfusions, vaccines, and drugs are sometimes necessary. Birth control and sterilization are left to individual conscience. Abortion is approved if the mother's life is endangered or if pregnancy is due to rape or incest. The use of hypnotism is opposed.

Shinto

Some members believe in healing through prayer, and the family is important in providing care and providing emotional support. Shintoists believe in tradition, and they worship ancestors and nature. Physical health may be valued.

Sikh

The Sikhs are a relatively new sect that opposes the caste system in India. Sikhs hold weekly religious services at their temple, from Friday morning through Sunday, in which each member in turn reads the holy scripture (the Granth Sahib) for 2-hour periods until the entire scripture is read.

Baptized male Sikhs wear unshorn hair and turbans, which symbolize dedication and group consciousness. A steel bracelet on the right wrist symbolizes restraint, a reminder not to do wrong. No significant dietary restrictions are imposed by the Sikh faith, but many Sikhs are vegetarians. Use of tobacco and alcohol is discouraged.

Taoism

Taoists view illness as part of the health/illness duality. They may accept illness and view medical treatment as interference. Death is seen as a natural part of life, and the body is kept in-house for 49 days. Taoists believe in an esthetically pleasing environment for meditation.

Unitarian/Universalist

Unitarian/Universalists emphasize reason, knowledge, individual responsibility, and personally established values. There are no dietary restrictions or official sacraments in the church, and no medical practices are prohibited. The Unitarian/Universalist church encourages its members to donate parts of their bodies to research and to medical banks.

United Church of Canada

The United Church of Canada is the largest Protestant denomination in Canada. It was formed in 1925 by the amalgamation of the Methodist, Presbyterian, and Congregationalist Churches. It operates some hospitals in under-serviced areas of Canada.

Zen

Adherents of Zen practice meditation, with the goal of discovering simplicity. When a client is ill, he or she may wish to see a Zen master.

Clients Most Likely to Desire Spiritual Assistance

Any client or support person may desire spiritual assistance. The following people are often desirous of it, but nurses should not limit their attention to these clients. At times of illness, support persons may be stressed and may wish spiritual assistance. The client facing death may have accepted it, but not necessarily the family and support persons. Often relatives are grateful for spiritual support by a nurse or pastor. Assisting them may indirectly assist the client. People often desirous of spiritual help include:

1. Clients who appear lonely and have few visitors
2. Clients who express fear and anxiety
3. Clients whose illness is related to the emotions or to religious attitudes
4. Clients who face surgery
5. Clients who must change their life-style as a result of illness or injury
6. Clients who are preoccupied about the relationship of their religion and health
7. Clients who are unable to have their pastor visit or who would not normally receive pastoral care
8. Clients whose illness has social implications
9. Clients who are dying

Assessment

A **spiritual need** is a person's need to maintain, increase, or restore his or her beliefs and faith, and to fulfill religious obligations. It is often the nurse who identifies a need for spiritual assistance and obtains the desired help. Sometimes clients ask directly for a visit from the hospital chaplain or their own clergyman. Others want to discuss their concerns with the nurse and ask about the nurse's beliefs as a way of seeking an empathic listener. Some people are embarrassed to ask for spiritual counsel but may hint at their concern in such statements as, "I've been wondering what really will happen to me when I die," or "Do you got to a church?" The nurse may also obtain clues about a client's concerns through observation. Does the client read a prayer book or the Bible each day? Does he or she wear or use religious medals, medallions, or symbols?

In a hospital, the admission record and the nursing history usually record the client's religion. The nurse also can ask if the client follows any religious practices and if he or should would like a visit from the appropriate clergy. It is important to ask the individual before obtaining assistance. Some people profess to have no religious beliefs and may be angered if the nurse makes arrangements for a chaplain to visit. The nurse needs to respect the client's wishes and not make a judgment of right or wrong, good or bad.

Nursing History

Nurses may elicit data about a client's spiritual beliefs as part of the general history. Often the information elicited is limited to the client's religious affiliation. Nurses should never assume, however, that a client follows all the practices of his or her stated religion.

Stoll (1979, p. 1574) suggests a spiritual history guide to elicit information in four areas: (a) the person's concept of God or deity, (b) the person's source of hope and strength, (c) the significance of religious practices and rituals to the person, and (d) the relationship the person perceives between his or her spiritual beliefs and his or her state of health. Stoll further cautions that each person has a right to his or her own values and beliefs and that people have a right not to discuss or reveal these beliefs to others.

When a nurse has developed a relationship with the client and/or support persons and feels that it is appropriate to discuss spiritual matters, the following questions may be suitable:

1. Are any particular religious practices important to you? If so, could you please tell me about them?
2. Will being here interfere with your religious practices?
3. Do you feel your faith is helpful to you? In what ways is it important to you right now?
4. In what ways can I help you to carry out your faith? For example, would you like me to read your prayer book to you?
5. Would you like a visit from your spiritual counselor or the hospital chaplain?
6. What are your hopes and your sources of strength right now?

Clinical Assessment

Spiritual distress may be revealed by one or more of the following:

1. *Affect and attitude.* Does the client appear lonely, depressed, angry, anxious, agitated, apathetic, or preoccupied?
2. *Behavior.* Does the client appear to pray before meals or at other times? Does the client read religious literature? Does the client complain frequently, need unusually high doses of sedation, pace the halls at night, joke inappropriately, have nightmares and sleep disturbances, or express anger at religious representatives or a diety?
3. *Verbalization.* Does the client mention God, prayer, faith, the church, or religious topics (even briefly)? Does the client ask about a visit from the clergy? Does the client express fear of death, concern with the meaning of life, inner conflict about religious beliefs, concern about a relationship with the deity, questions about the meaning of existence, the meaning of suffering, or the moral/ethical implications of therapy?
4. *Interpersonal relationships.* Who visits? How does the client respond to visitors? Does a minister come? How does the client relate to other clients and nursing personnel?
5. *Environment.* Does the client have a Bible, prayer book, devotional literature, religious medals, a rosary, or religious get-well cards in the room? Does a church send altar flowers or Sunday bulletins? (Fish and Shelley 1978, p. 61).

Nursing Diagnosis

Examples of nursing diagnoses for clients experiencing spiritual distress are given to the right.

Examples of Nursing Diagnoses for Clients Experiencing Spiritual Distress

- Spiritual distress related to inability to attend religious services
- Spiritual distress related to conflict between religious doctrine and recommended therapy
- Spiritual distress related to death of husband

Planning

Planning in relation to spiritual distress should be designed to meet one or more of the following needs:

1. To provide spiritual resources otherwise unavailable
2. To help the client fulfill religious obligations
3. To help the client draw on and use inner resources more effectively to meet the present situation
4. To help the client maintain or establish a dynamic, personal relationship with the deity in the face of unpleasant circumstances
5. To help the client find meaning in existence and the present situation

Planning also involves establishing outcome criteria. For suggestions, see the section on evaluation, later in this chapter.

Intervention Guidelines

1. Examine and clarify the personal spiritual or religious convictions and beliefs that may influence your interactions with clients and support persons. Ask yourself:
   a. Are all religions and beliefs equally valid for the persons holding them, or is there only one true religion?
   b. What do I believe about life after death, euthanasia, birth control, sterilization, therapeutic and demand abortion, prolonging life, autopsy, burial or cremation, nonmedical modes of healing, donation of body parts, care of excised body tissue, and amputated limbs?
   c. Do I see any relationship among sin, punishment, suffering, and illness?
   d. How often have I read a Bible to or prayed with a person, and how comfortable would I be doing so with a client? Would I feel frightened, uneasy, ambivalent, sure, or comfortable?
   e. If there is conflict between medical practice and religious doctrine, which should take precedence?
   f. How will I respond if a client tries to convert me to his or her beliefs and practices?
   g. How will I respond if a client's beliefs and practices conflict with my own or are unacceptable to me? To help a client who is experiencing spiritual distress, a nurse must be aware of her or his own beliefs and values. It is also important that a nurse recognize and accept that her or his own beliefs may not be right for others and be able to place these aside when assisting clients with their own perceived spiritual needs.
2. Focus attention on the client's perception of his or her spiritual needs rather than the practices or beliefs of the religious affiliation stated on the client's record. The spiritual beliefs of a given religion may vary greatly among members. People join religious groups for many reasons, e.g., to have a place of worship, to find an avenue for social action such as helping the poor or homeless, to gain friends for recreational purposes, or to have a place for important life events such as weddings and funerals. Often, different sects within a religious denomination have varying practices.
3. Do not assume that a client has no spiritual needs because the record states no religious affiliation or specifies atheist or agnostic.
4. Acknowledge and respond to the client's nonverbal cues about spiritual need, such as visible devotional materials, religious articles, or visits from the clergy. Your interest in and questions about religious objects show that you care about the clients' spiritual concerns.
5. Respond to the client's verbal cues with brief, specific, factual answers. Responding involves:
   a. Active listening: attempting to enter into the other person's frame of reference so as to understand more fully his or her feelings and experiences.
   b. Support: accepting the person, even though his or her beliefs may not agree with yours, by being there, showing genuine concern, asking questions, providing information, reflecting feelings, and acknowledging strengths.
   c. Awareness: being sensitive to what the client is saying and not saying and to the client's emotional tone.
   d. Empathy: understanding and experiencing the client's feelings.
   e. Nonjudgmental understanding: accepting and understanding the person without approving or disapproving.
6. Determine the meaning the client attributes to the situation. Such meanings can influence the client's response to an illness or condition and may either hinder nursing intervention or provide hope, cour-

age, and strength. For example, a person who believes that illness is God's punishment may feel powerless and demonstrate little interest in therapy designed to prevent illness.

7. Help the client meet religious obligations:
   a. Prepare the client and the environment for visits by the clergy.
   b. Ensure privacy for prayer and meditation.
   c. Greet the clergy when they enter the nursing unit and assist them as required.
   d. Protect the client's religious objects from loss or damage.
   e. Help the client meet religious dietary obligations.
   f. Allow helpless clients to say grace, if desired, before feeding them.
   g. Arrange for appropriate care of the body after death.
8. Inform clients about the services provided by the hospital to meet spiritual needs, and arrange for clients to participate in these as they are able. Many large hospitals have full-time chaplains who assist clients, support persons, and staff with spiritual needs. Chaplains of several faiths usually participate, including a rabbi, a Roman Catholic priest, and Protestant ministers, from denominations such as Episcopalian, Methodist, Lutheran, Baptist, and Presbyterian. For smaller hospitals that do not have chaplains, clergy in the community usually provide this service. Many nursing units have a list of clergy who are on call when needed.

   The chaplain functions in a variety of ways. Usually a newly admitted client is visited, and spiritual needs are assessed. The chaplain then may read spiritual literature aloud, conduct special sacraments, or simply visit—whatever is appropriate for the person.

   Some agencies have a chapel where regular religious services are held for clients, support persons, and staff. Most hospitals also have quiet rooms that can be used for meditation, counsel, and even worship services. Sometimes a client prefers to meet the chaplain in a quiet room where there is privacy. This is particularly true when a client is sharing a room.

   A hospital may hold nondenominational religious services or several services for different denominations. If a client expresses a desire to attend services, the nurse needs to help organize the client's care so that attendance is possible if health permits.
9. Determine whether the client wishes to receive Holy Communion. Communion is celebrated by most Christian churches (Protestant and Catholic), but practices and underlying theologic concepts vary considerably from denomination to denomination. When a hospitalized client is to receive Holy Communion, determine what preparations are necessary. Some clients fast for several hours prior to this sacrament, but fasting is not required during periods of ill health. Medications are allowed if needed. Some agencies supply communion sets containing a white tablecloth, a candle, a spoon, and a small glass. Many clergy carry small communion sets with them.
10. Determine whether the client wants a visit from religious groups that visit hospitals. If the client does not want such a visit, respect this wish and communicate it tactfully to visitors.
11. In some instances, members of religious groups will chant or wail at the client's bedside during times of grief. If this is disturbing to others, intervene tactfully. It may be possible to move roommates temporarily to another room or provide a private place for the client and visitors.
12. If you feel uncomfortable assisting the client spiritually (e.g., reading devotional material or praying with the client on request), verbalize this discomfort, and offer to obtain assistance for him or her. It is important to respect the client's beliefs and maintain a supportive relationship. It is equally important not to feel guilty about your discomfort.
13. If a client attempts to convert you to his or her beliefs and practices, tell him or her honestly that you have other beliefs and feel uncomfortable with this request. At the same time, acknowledge respect for the client's beliefs.
14. If a client appears to be misinformed or lack information about health and spiritual matters, discuss the possibility of contacting a spiritual leader who could provide such information.
15. If you determine that there is a true conflict between spiritual beliefs and medical therapy, encourage the client and physician to discuss the conflict and consider alternative methods of therapy. Support the client's right to make an informed decision. If the client's beliefs conflict with your own values, discuss this conflict with the responsible nurse and your own spiritual leader. It may be preferable for the client to receive nursing from a nurse with compatible views. It may also be desirable to discuss your feelings with other health professionals, e.g., other nurses on the team.
16. If, during an emergency, a client chooses or is given medical therapy contrary to his or her spiritual practices (e.g., if a Jehovah's Witness is given a blood transfusion following injury from an automobile accident), anticipate a reaction from the client and/or support persons and prepare to deal with:
    a. Anger, depression, or fear
    b. Slower recovery and impaired recovery
    c. Refusal to accept care

Evaluation

Examples of outcome criteria for clients who have spiritual distress are listed to the right.

Examples of Outcome Criteria for Clients in Spiritual Distress

The client will

- Express comfort with spiritual beliefs
- Continue spiritual practices appropriate to health status
- Express decreased feelings of guilt
- State acceptance of moral decision
- Display positive affect
- Express finding positive meaning in the present situation and in his or her own existence

Nursing Care Plan

Assessment Data

Nursing Assessment

Mrs. Sally Horton is a 60-year-old hospitalized homemaker who is recovering from a right radical mastectomy. Yesterday, she was told by her physician that due to widespread metastases of the cancer, her prognosis is poor. This morning Marilyn Fleener, her primary nurse, finds her to be tearful and obviously upset and depressed. She asks Miss Fleener, "Why has God done this to me? Perhaps it's because I have sinned in my life. I've not gone to church or spoken to a minister in a number of years. Is there a chapel in the hospital where I could go and maybe pray? I'm terribly afraid of dying and what awaits me."

Physical Examination

Height: 165.1 cm (5′5″)
Weight: 54.0 kg (119 lb)
Temperature: 36.6 C (98 F)
Pulse rate: 88 BPM
Respirations: 22 per minute
Blood pressure: 146/86 mm Hg
Large surgical dressing to right chest wall and axillary region dry and intact
Slight edema of right hand and arm

Diagnostic Data

RBC: 3.5 ml/uL
Hgb: 10.5 grams/L
Hematocrit: 35%
Mammography reveals large right breast mass in upper outer quadrant

Nursing Diagnosis	Client Goals and Outcome Criteria	Nursing Interventions and Rationales	Evaluation
Spiritual distress related to separation from religious rituals resulting in questioning credibility of beliefs, depression, expressions of fear of death and relationship to deity.	Client Goal: Express sense of spiritual satisfaction. Outcome Criteria: Expresses comfort with relationship with deity by day 4. Visits with clergyman by day 2. Displays absence of feelings of guilt by day 5.	Assess for factors contributing to spiritual distress. *Rationale:* Enables the nurse to deal more effectively with problem when client's needs are known. Acknowledge and respond to client's verbal and nonverbal cues about spiritual needs. *Rationale:* Demonstrates interest in the client's religious concerns. Determine the meaning the client attributes to his physical/spiritual situation.	Mrs. Horton has been visited on several occasions by her clergyman. She reads scripture each day and has found consolation, especially in reading the Book of Psalms. She states, "God is merciful and will help me bear my suffering."

(continued)

Nursing Diagnosis	Client Goals and Outcome Criteria	Nursing Interventions and Rationales	Evaluation
		Rationale: Spiritual care may directly influence a client's recovery. Provide for the client's meeting of her spiritual obligations. *Rationale:* This will aid in reducing her spiritual distress. Inform client of spiritual services provided by the institution to assist her to meet her spiritual needs. *Rationale:* Permits client to choose to avail herself of these spiritual services. Encourage and provide for client's preferred spiritual rituals. *Rationale:* All people have basic spiritual dimensions, and spiritual practices assist in meeting their spiritual needs.	
Fear related to terminal illness and dying resulting in feeling of loss of control; increased pulse, respirations, and blood pressure; and increased questioning.	Client Goal: Experience greater psychologic and physiologic comfort. Outcome Criteria: Clearly identifies actual source of fear by day 2. Distinguishes between ineffective and effective coping behaviors by day 5. Identifies individual coping response by day 5.	Acknowledge client's fear. *Rationale:* Feelings are real, and discussing them may assist in resolving them. Reduce or eliminate factors contributing to fear. *Rationale:* Will reduce intensity and/or incidence of fear. Encourage normal coping mechanisms. *Rationale:* Enhances control and diffuses fear. Be available and provide a nonthreatening atmosphere. *Rationale:* Establishes rapport and permits client to voice her feelings.	Mrs. Horton talked about her fear of dying and her concern for her husband, who is disabled with Parkinson's disease and cannot care for himself. She feels her coping response is her spiritual renewal and her visits with her clergyman. Reverend MacLeod has arranged for Mr. Horton to be admitted to the Presbyterian Nursing Home.

Chapter Highlights

- The spiritual needs of clients and support persons often come into focus at a time of illness.
- Nurses must respect the rights of people to hold their own spiritual beliefs and to communicate or not communicate these to others.
- Spiritual beliefs and practices are highly personal.
- Spiritual and religious beliefs can influence life-style, attitudes, and feelings about illness and death.
- Spiritual beliefs often help people accept illness and plan for the future.
- When taking a nursing history, a nurse can often obtain information about a client's concept of God or deity, the client's source of hope and strength, the significance of religious practices and rituals, and the relationship the client perceives between his or her health and his or her spiritual beliefs.
- Spiritual distress may be reflected in a number of behaviors, including depression, anxiety, and verbalizations of fear of death.
- Nurses should be aware of their own spiritual beliefs in order to be comfortable assisting others.
- Nurses may intervene directly to help clients, support persons, and clergy to meet spiritual needs.

Suggested Readings

Carson, V. January-February 1980. Meeting the spiritual needs of hospitalized psychiatric patients. *Perspectives in Psychiatric Care* 18:17–20.

Carson describes how a prayer group for psychiatric clients promoted such benefits as increased support among members for each other.

Morris, K. L., and Foerster, J. D. December 1972. Team work: Nurse and chaplain. *American Journal of Nursing* 72:2197–99.

The authors describe a program in which nurses and clergy worked together and the benefits to both clients and personnel.

Piepgras, R. December 1968. The other dimension: Spiritual help. *American Journal of Nursing* 68:2610–13.

Piepgras suggests that little emphasis is placed on spiritual needs of clients, yet some clients need this help more than any other. Five manifestations of the need for spiritual help are outlined, and client examples are included.

Ruffing-Rahal, M. A. March/April 1984. The spiritual dimension of well-being: Implications for the elderly. *Home Healthcare Nurse* 2:12–13, 16.

Ruffing-Rahal introduces the concept of holistic health care and the spiritual dimension. The losses of the elderly are briefly outlined together with an explanation of holistic well-being. Religion and spirituality are defined as separate entities. Ruffing-Rahal then describes the nurse's role in hospital and home care. The author discusses how to assess and assist clients.

Selected References

Baasher, T. October 1982. The healing power of faith . . . across a wide range of cultures. *World Health* ( ): 5–7.

Berkowitz, P., and Berkowitz, N. S. November 1967. The Jewish patient in hospital. *American Journal of Nursing* 67:2335–37.

Carpenito, L. J. 1983. *Nursing diagnosis: Application to clinical practice.* Philadelphia: J. B. Lippincott Co.

Dickinson, C. October 1975. The search for spiritual meaning. *American Journal of Nursing* 75:1789–93.

Drakulic, L., and Tanaka, W. March 1981. The East Indian family in Canada. *Canadian Nurse* 77:24–26.

Ellis, D. September 1980. What happened to the spiritual dimension? *Canadian Nurse* 76:42–43.

Fish, S., and Shelley, J. A. 1978. *Spiritual care: The nurse's role.* Downers Grove, Ill.: InterVarsity Press.

Fowler, J. W., and Keen, S. 1985. *Life maps: Conversations on the journey of faith.* Waco, Texas: Word.

Hogan, R. M. September 1982. Influences of culture on sexuality. *Nursing Clinics of North America* 17:365–76.

Kelsey, M. T. 1973. *Healing and Christianity.* Toronto: Fitzhenry and Whiteside.

Maslow, A. H. 1970. *Religious values and peak experiences.* Markham, Ont.: Penguin Books.

Murray, R. B., and Zentuen, J. P. 1985. *Nursing Concepts for Health Promotion.* 3d ed. Englewood Cliffs, N.J.: Prentice-Hall, Inc.

Naiman, H. L. November 1970. Nursing in Jewish law. *American Journal of Nursing* 70:2378–79.

Perk, D. 1975. *Man's quest for meaning, faith, identity.* Johannesburg: Aegis Press.

Pumphrey, J. B. December 1977. Recognizing your patient's spiritual needs. *Nursing 77* 7:64–69.

Stoll, R. T. September 1979. Guidelines for spiritual assessment. *American Journal of Nursing* 79:1574–77.

VanKaam, A. 1976a. *Dynamics of spiritual direction.* Denville, N.J.: Dimension Books.

———. 1976b. *In search of spiritual identity.* Denville, N.J.: Dimension Books.

———. 1976c. *Spirituality and the gentle life.* Denville, N.J.: Dimension Books.

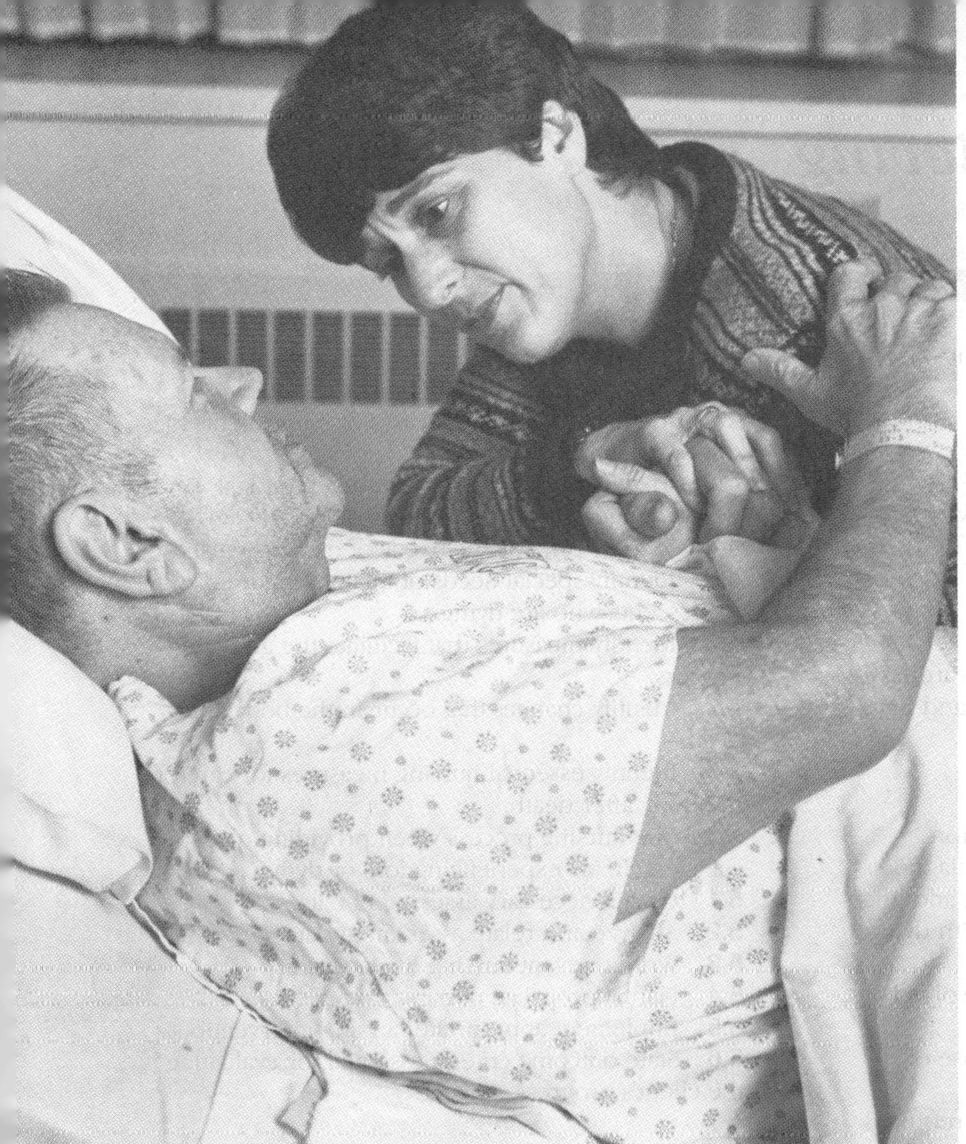

CHAPTER 50

Loss and Grieving

Ross A. Stewart
Thomas Eoyang

Contents

50 *Loss and Grieving*

Objectives

1. Know essential facts about loss, grief, dying, and death.
   1.1 Define selected terms.
   1.2 Identify types of loss.
   1.3 Identify characteristics of grieving.
   1.4 Identify Kübler-Ross's, Engel's, and Martocchio's stages of grieving.
   1.5 Identify legal implications of death.
2. Know information and methods required to assess dying and grieving clients.
   2.1 Identify the dying client's level of awareness.
   2.2 Identify clinical signs of impending and imminent death.
   2.3 Identify clinical signs of death.
   2.4 Identify clinical symptoms of grief.
   2.5 Identify factors affecting a loss reaction.
3. Understand essential facts about nursing diagnoses for clients with problems related to dying and grief.
   3.1 Identify common fears associated with dying.
   3.2 Identify types of grief.
   3.3 Identify factors contributing to unresolved grief.
   3.4 Identify factors contributing to a sense of hopelessness.
4. Understand facts about nursing measures required to assist people with dying, grief, and care of the body after death.
   4.1 Identify the significance of developing self-awareness about death and dying.
   4.2 Identify essential aspects of helping clients to die with dignity.
   4.3 Identify measures to meet the emotional needs of clients in various stages of dying.
   4.4 Identify physiologic needs of dying clients.
   4.5 Identify special needs of infants, children, and adolescents who are dying.
   4.6 Identify measures that facilitate the grieving process.
   4.7 Identify changes that occur in the body after death.
   4.8 Identify essential nursing measures for care of the body after death.
5. Apply the nursing process when providing care to selected clients experiencing loss or dying.
   5.1 Obtain necessary assessment data.
   5.2 Analyze and relate assessment data.
   5.3 Write relevant nursing diagnoses.
   5.4 Plan appropriate nursing strategies.
   5.5 Implement appropriate nursing interventions.
   5.6 State outcome criteria essential for evaluating the client's progress.

Terms

actual loss
algor mortis
anticipatory loss
autopsy (postmortem examination)
bereavement
cerebral death
grief
hospice
livor mortis
loss
mortician (undertaker)
mourning
palliative care
perceived loss
rigor mortis
shroud

Loss

Loss is an actual or potential situation in which a valued object, person, or the like is inaccessible or changed so it is no longer perceived as valuable. People can experience the loss of body image, a significant other, a sense of well-being, a job, personal possessions, beliefs, a sense of self, and so on. Illness and hospitalization often produce losses. The sources of loss arc discussed further in the next section.

Death is a fundamental loss, both for the dying person and for those who survive. Although death is inevitable for everyone, it is a lonely experience that each person ultimately faces alone. Yet even death, like loss, can stimulate people to grow in perception of both themselves and others. Death can be viewed not simply as loss of life, but as the dying person's final opportunity to experience life in ways that bring meaning and fulfillment.

Types of Loss

There are two general types of loss, actual and perceived. Both actual losses and perceived losses can be anticipatory. An **actual loss** can be identified by others and can arise either in response to or in anticipation of a situation. For example, a woman whose husband is dying may experience actual loss in anticipation of his death. A **perceived loss** is experienced by one person but cannot be verified by others. Psychologic losses are often perceived losses, in that they are not directly verifiable. For example, a woman who leaves her employment to care for her children at home may perceive a loss of independence and freedom. An **anticipatory loss** is experienced before the loss really occurs.

Sources of Loss

There are many sources of loss:

1. Loss of an aspect of oneself—a body part, a physiologic function, or a psychologic attribute
2. Loss of an object external to oneself
3. Separation from an accustomed environment
4. Loss of a loved or valued person

Aspect of self The loss of an aspect of self changes a person's body image even though the loss may not be obvious to others. A face scarred from a burn is generally obvious to people; loss of part of the stomach or loss of ability to feel emotion may not be as obvious. The degree to which these losses affect a person largely depends on the integrity of the person's body image (part of self-concept). Sometimes changes in self-image affect a person's social roles, such as employee, father, and husband. Any change that is perceived by the person as negative in the way he or she relates to the environment can be considered a loss of self.

Another aspect of loss of self occurs as a result of growth and development. See the discussion of development of the self-concept in Chapter 48. Failure to develop a normal self-concept can occur for many reasons. At each stage of growth, lack of the conditions essential for development can impair the self-concept. An infant learns to distinguish self from the environment through experience with tactile and auditory stimuli. Parents provide touch by holding, feeding, and bathing the infant; auditory stimuli come from talk and other environmental sounds. The toddler needs to learn about body parts through feeling them and requires an accepting attitude rather than a judgmental one. Schoolchildren need peer contact and feedback that they are normal. Without such reassurance, they can develop a negative or uncertain self-image.

In adulthood, losses such as divorce can have considerable impact. A divorce may mean loss of financial security, a home, daily routines, etc. Therefore, even when the divorce was desired, the sense of loss can last for some time afterward.

Old age is another time when dramatic changes occur in physical and mental capabilities. Again the self-image is vulnerable, and support and reassurance are important. Old age is when people usually experience many losses: of employment, of usual activities, of independence, of health, of friends, of family, etc.

External objects Loss of external objects includes (a) loss of inanimate objects that have importance to the person, such as the loss of money for a person without financial means, or the burning down of a family's house, and (b) loss of animate objects such as pets that provide love and companionship.

Accustomed environment Separation from an environment and people who provide security can result in a sense of loss. The 6-year-old who has had the protection of home and family is likely to feel loss when first attending school and relating to more people. The university student who moves away from home for the first time also experiences a sense of loss.

Loved ones The loss of a loved one or valued person through illness, separation, or death can be very disturbing. In illness such as brain damage from viral infection or stroke, a person may undergo personality changes that make friends and family feel they have lost that person.

The death of a loved one is a permanent and complete loss. In primitive societies, death was considered a normal, natural event, and life was seldom long. The death of a young man brought greater grief than the deaths of women, children, or elderly people. In contemporary North American society, death is considered unacceptable and usually occurs in private, unless there is an accident. Death often happens in a hospital or in a home in the presence of immediate family. There is a tendency to prolong and preserve life. The culture reveres youthfulness; although people expect to live to old age, this is not considered as attractive as youth.

Loss as Crisis

Loss, especially loss of life or a loved one, can be viewed as a crisis event, either situational or developmental. The loss of a job or the loss of a young child, for example, is usually an unexpected situational crisis. On the other hand, losses incurred in the process of normal development—such as the departure of grown children from the home, retirement from a career, and the death of aged parents—are developmental crises that can be anticipated and, to some extent, prepared for.

How individuals deal with loss is closely related to their stage of development, personal resources, and social support systems. In dealing with loss of life, the nurse needs to consider the influence of these factors on the dying person and the surviving loved ones. As with all people in crisis, the experience of a dying person cannot be properly understood apart from the social context (Hoff 1984). In crisis situations, including the crisis of death, it is important for the nurse to consider the entire family as the client of care.

Bereavement and Grief

Bereavement is the subjective response to a loss through the death of a person with whom there has been a significant relationship. **Grief** is the total response to the emotional experience of the loss and is manifested in thoughts, feelings, and behaviors (Martocchio 1985, p. 327). **Mourning** is a behavioral process through which grief is eventually resolved or altered; it is often influenced by culture and custom.

Although loss and death can be seen in the context of crisis theory, some feel that bereavement and grief cannot be viewed as a single crisis but rather are a series of crises that constitute a "life transition period" (Demi and Miles 1986). To view death as a single crisis can mislead caregivers into believing that short-term crisis intervention will bring positive resolution of the grief experience. In fact, normal bereavement can last as long as a year or more. Dealing with death loss is complex and intensely emotional and should not be oversimplified.

Age and the Impact of Loss

Age affects a person's understanding of and reaction to loss. With experience, people usually increase their understanding and acceptance of life, loss, and death. As in other aspects of human development, children show more rapid and dramatic variation and changes in their understanding of death. Their understanding is susceptible to influence by outside events, such as life-threatening illness, which usually deepens the child's understanding of death and makes it more like that of an adult (Fetsch 1984). Table 50–1 outlines the development of the concept of death through the life span.

People do not usually experience the loss of life or loved ones at regular intervals. As a result, preparation for these experiences is difficult. Coping with other of life's losses, such as the loss of a pet, the loss of a friend, and the loss of youth or a job, can help people anticipate the more severe loss of death by teaching them successful coping strategies.

Childhood

Children differ from adults not only in their understanding of loss and death, but also in how they are affected by the loss of others. The child's patterns progress rapidly; adult patterns of growth and development are generally stable. The loss of a parent or other significant person can threaten the child's ability to develop, and regression sometimes results. Assisting the child with the grief experience includes helping the child regain the normal continuity and pace of emotional development.

Table 50–1 Development of the Concept of Death

Age	Beliefs/Attitudes
Infancy to 5 years	Does not understand concept of death
	Infant's sense of separation forms basis for later understanding of loss and death
	Believes death is reversible, a temporary departure, or sleep
	Emphasizes immobility and inactivity as attributes of death
5 to 9 years	Understands that death is final
	Believes own death can be avoided
	Associates death with aggression or violence
	Believes wishes or unrelated actions can be responsible for death
9 to 12 years	Understands death as the inevitable end of life
	Begins to understand own mortality, expressed as interest in afterlife or as fear of death
	Expresses ideas about death gathered from parents and other adults
12 to 18 years	Fears a lingering death
	May fantasize that death can be defied, acting out defiance through reckless behaviors, e.g., dangerous driving, substance abuse
	Seldom thinks about death, but views it in religious and philosophic terms
	May seem to reach "adult" perception of death but be emotionally unable to accept it
	May still hold concepts from previous developmental stages
18 to 45 years	Has attitude toward death influenced by religious and cultural beliefs
45 to 65 years	Accepts own mortality
	Encounters death of parents and some peers
	Experiences peaks of death anxiety
	Death anxiety diminishes with emotional well-being
65 years +	Fears prolonged illness
	Encounters death of family members and peers
	Sees death as having multiple meanings, e.g., freedom from pain, reunion with already deceased family members

Adults often assume that children do not have the same need as an adult to grieve the loss of others. In situations of crisis and loss, children are sometimes pushed aside or protected form the pain. They can feel afraid, abandoned, and lonely. Careful work with bereaved children is especially necessary, because experiencing a loss in childhood can have serious effects later in life. Research suggests a connection between early loss of a parent through death or divorce and increased risk of depression or suicide in adulthood (Taylor 1983–84).

Early and Middle Adulthood

As people grow, loss comes to be experienced as part of normal development. By middle age, for example, the loss of a parent through death seems a normal occurrence compared to the death of a younger person. Coping with the death of an aged parent has even been viewed as a necessary developmental task of the middle-age adult. Society does not support intense or prolonged mourning for such a normal event (Moss and Moss 1983–84).

For the middle-age adult the loss of a parent can signal the disintegration of the family of origin. It is also a forceful reminder that the adult child is part of the older generation and therefore closer to death. The challenge of this developmental crisis for adult children is to assess the psychologic legacy of the parent, integrating what is valuable into their own identity. If the relationship with the parent was full of conflict, the parent's death can help release the child's energy for more productive use.

Late Adulthood

For older adults, the loss through death of a long-time mate is profound. Though individuals differ in their ability to deal with such a loss, research suggests an increase in health problems for widows and widowers during the first year following (Richter 1984). Because the majority of deaths occur among the elderly, and because the number of elderly is increasing in North America, nurses will need to be especially alert to the potential problems of older grieving adults.

Educating the Nurse About Loss

People in North America are socialized to think of death as the worst occurrence in life. They therefore do their best to avoid thinking or talking about death—especially their own. Death is thought about rarely, and almost exclusively in negative terms. Nurses are not immune to such attitudes. They need to take time to analyze their own feelings about death before they can effectively help others with a terminal illness. Nurses who are unconsciously uncomfortable with dying clients tend to impede the clients' attempts to discuss dying and death by:

1. Changing the subject, e.g., "Let's think of something more cheerful," or "You shouldn't say things like that."
2. Offering reassurance, e.g., "You are doing very well."
3. Denying what is happening, e.g., "You don't really mean that," or "You're going to live until you are a hundred."
4. Being fatalistic, e.g., "Everyone dies sooner or later," or "God will take you when He wants you."
5. Blocking discussion, e.g., "I don't think things are really that bad," conveying an attitude that stops further discussion of the subject
6. Being aloof and distant or avoiding the client
7. "Managing" the client's care and making the client feel increasingly dependent and powerless

The curricula of many nursing schools include education about death. Agencies and associations sponsor continuing education programs aimed at reducing death anxiety among nursing staff. Other programs help nurses explore the specific problems of direct contact with terminally ill clients and around-the-clock responsibility for their care. In all such programs nurses learn not only their own attitudes and concerns but also ways to support and comfort each other when they experience anger and frustration in the grief that follows the death of clients whom they not only cared for but cared about.

Caring for the dying and the bereaved is one of the nurse's most complex and challenging responsibilities, bringing into play all the skills needed for holistic physiologic and psychosocial care. To be effective, nurses must come to grips with their own attitudes toward loss, death, and dying, because these attitudes will directly affect their ability to provide care. No single textbook chapter can give nursing students all the information and guidance needed to prepare them to care for dying clients and their families. Each nurse is personally responsible for actively engaging in a career-long process of education through reading, listening, and self-examination.

Grief

Grieving, the normal subjective emotional response to loss, is essential for good mental and physical health. It permits the individual to cope with the loss gradually and to accept it as part of reality. Grief is a social process, in that it is best shared and carried out with the assistance of others.

Grief work is important, because bereavement has been shown to have potentially devastating effects on health.

Among the symptoms that can accompany grief are anxiety, depression, weight loss, difficulties in swallowing, vomiting, fatigue, headaches, dizziness, fainting, blurred vision, skin rashes, excessive sweating, menstrual disturbances, palpitations, chest pain, dyspnea, and infection (Gonda and Ruark 1984). The bereaved may also experience alterations in libido, concentration, and patterns of eating, sleeping, activity, and communication.

Although bereavement can threaten health, a positive resolution of the grieving process can enrich the individual with new insights, values, challenges, openness, and sensitivity. This applies to both the dying person and surviving loved ones, for the dying person is also living. If the quality of life permits, the dying person also should have the opportunity to grow emotionally and spiritually in the time that remains

Stages of Grieving

Many authors have described stages or phases of grieving, perhaps the most famous of them being Kübler-Ross, who has described five stages: denial, anger, bargaining, depression, and acceptance. (Kübler-Ross 1969, pp. 38–137). See Table 50–2. Engel (1964, pp. 94–96) has identified six stages of grieving: shock and disbelief, developing awareness, restitution, resolving the loss, idealization, and outcome. See Table 50–3.

Recently, nurses have begun to write about the components of grief. Clark (1984) describes a three-phase course through which the bereaved progresses, lasting 6 months to 2 years. Martocchio (1985) discusses five clusters of grief and maintains that there is no single correct way, nor a correct timetable, by which a person progresses through the grief process. Whether a person can succeed in integrating the loss, and how this is accomplished, is related to that person's individual development and personal makeup. And individuals responding to the very same loss cannot be expected to follow the same pattern or schedule in resolving their grief, even while they support each other. Martocchio's five clusters of grief follow (Martocchio 1985).

Shock and Disbelief

A feeling of numbness is a common response immediately following the death of a loved one. The bereaved may feel depressed, angry, guilty, and sad. Disbelief or denial may persist even though the loss has been accepted intellectually.

Table 50–2 Kübler-Ross's Stages of Grieving

Stage	Behavioral Responses	Nursing Implications
Denial	Refuses to believe that loss is happening Is unready to deal with practical problems, such as prosthesis after loss of leg May assume artificial cheerfulness to prolong denial	Verbally support client's denial for its protective function Examine your own behavior to ensure that you do not share in client's denial
Anger	Client or family may direct anger at nurse or hospital staff, about matters that normally would not bother them	Help client understand that anger is a normal response to feelings of loss and powerlessness Avoid withdrawal or retaliation with anger; do not take anger personally Deal with needs underlying any angry reaction Provide structure and continuity to promote feelings of security Allow client as much control as possible over his or her life
Bargaining	Seeks to bargain to avoid loss May express feelings of guilt or fear of punishment for past sins, real or imagined	Listen attentively and encourage client to talk to relieve guilt and irrational fears If appropriate, offer spiritual support
Depression	Grieves over what has happened and what cannot be May talk freely (e.g., reviewing past losses such as money or job), or may withdraw	Allow client to express sadness Communicate nonverbally by sitting quietly without expecting conversation Convey caring by touch Help support persons understand importance of being with the client in silence
Acceptance	Comes to terms with loss May have decreased interest in surroundings and support persons May wish to begin making plans, e.g., will, prosthesis, altered living arrangements	Help family and friends understand client's decreased need to socialize and need for short, quiet visits Encourage client to participate as much as possible in the treatment program

Table 50–3 Engel's Stages of Grieving

Stage	Behavioral Responses
Shock and disbelief	Refusal to accept loss
	Stunned feelings
	Intellectual acceptance but emotional denial
Developing awareness	Reality of loss begins to penetrate consciousness
	Anger may be directed at hospital, nurses, etc.
	Crying and self-blame
Restitution	Rituals of mourning, e.g., funeral
Resolving the loss	Attempts to deal with painful void
	Still unable to accept new love object to replace lost person
	May accept more dependent relationship with support person
	Thinks over and talks about memories of the dead person
Idealization	Produces image of dead person that is almost devoid of undesirable features
	Represses all negative and hostile feelings toward deceased
	May feel guilty and remorseful about past inconsiderate or unkind acts to deceased
	Unconsciously internalizes admired qualities of deceased
	Reminders of deceased evoke fewer feelings of sadness
	Reinvests feelings in others
Outcome	Behavior influenced by several factors, such as: importance of lost object as source of support, degree of dependence on relationship, degree of ambivalence toward deceased, number and nature of other relationships, and number and nature of previous grief experiences (which tend to be cumulative)

Source: From G. L. Engel, Grief and grieving, *American Journal of Nursing,* September 1964, 64:93–98. Used by permission.

Yearning and Protest

The anger that the bereaved feel may be directed at the deceased for having died, at God, at others whose loved ones are still alive, or at the caregivers. The bereaved may begin to fear their own mental deterioration, and withdraw from sharing their thoughts and feelings with others.

Anguish, Disorganization, and Despair

When the reality of the loss is genuinely admitted, depression can set in. Weeping is common at this time. The bereaved lose interest and motivation in pursuing the future, are unable to make decisions, and lack confidence and purpose. Activities that were once enjoyed with the deceased are now without attraction. Coping strategies such as excessive drinking may compromise health.

Identification in Bereavement

The bereaved may take on the behavior, personal traits, habits, and ambitions of the deceased. Sometimes they may also experience the same symptoms of physical illness.

Reorganization and Restitution

Achieving stability and a sense of reintegration can take a period of time that ranges widely, from less than a year to several years. Although the bereaved are able to experience a sense of well-being and can resume most normal patterns of functioning, the feelings of grief do not simply cease. For many the pain of loss, though diminished, recurs for the rest of their lives.

Research Note

Bereaved people are at much higher risk for physical and mental problems and as such are likely to come into contact with nurses, who must understand the bereavement process in order to help them. Cowan and Murphy studied 69 bereaved subjects and a matched control group of 50 nonbereaved. The authors conceptualized bereavement as a complex, multivariate phenomenon, an approach they feel provides more accurate predictors of which persons among the bereaved are most at risk for physical illness, depression, or somaticization. The authors hypothesized that the variables of age, gender, concurrent life stresses, social support, closeness of relationship to the deceased, and belief in the preventability of the loss would to varying degrees account for the outcomes of bereavement. They found stress to be the most important risk factor. In addition, their findings supported the overall hypothesis. Cowan and Murphy present persuasive evidence that the long-accepted but largely untested "stage" model of the grieving process (Kübler-Ross 1969) is simply inadequate.
(Cowan and Murphy 1985)

Assessment

States of Awareness

In cases of terminal illness, the state of awareness shared by the dying person and the family is a major influence on the nurse's role. The state of awareness affects the nurse's ability to communicate freely with clients and other health care team members and to assist in the grieving process. Three types of awareness that have been described are (a) closed awareness, (b) mutual pretense, and (c) open awareness (Strauss et al. 1970, p. 300). One study indicates that nurses prefer the state of open awareness and prefer to become emotionally involved with their clients, since it "allows them to fully implement their ideal of nursing care" (Field 1984, p. 67).

Closed awareness In closed awareness the client and family are unaware of impending death. They may not completely understand why the client is ill, and they believe he or she will recover. The physician may believe it is best not to communicate a diagnosis or prognosis to the client or family. Nursing personnel are confronted with an ethical problem in this situation, and they have several choices. One course is to answer questions evasively or falsely. But ultimately the client and family will know the truth, and when they do they may recognize that information given them earlier was false. See Chapter 8 for further information on ethical dilemmas.

Mutual pretense With mutual pretense, the client, family, and health personnel know that the prognosis is terminal but do not talk about it and make an effort not to raise the subject. Sometimes the client refrains from discussing death to protect the family from distress. The client may also sense discomfort on the part of health personnel and therefore not bring up the subject. Mutual pretense permits the client a degree of privacy and dignity, but it places a heavy burden on the dying person, who then has no one to whom to confide fears.

Open awareness With open awareness, the client and people around know about the impending death and feel comfortable about discussing it, even though it is difficult. This awareness provides the client an opportunity to finalize affairs and even participate in planning funeral arrangements.

Not all people can handle open awareness. For example, a 45-year-old man who knows he is dying may be unable to discuss his forthcoming death without becoming angry at people around him.

Whether to inform dying clients of their terminality is a difficult issue for physicians. Some authorities believe that terminal clients acquire knowledge of their condition even if they are not directly informed. Others believe that many clients remain unaware of their condition until the end. It is difficult, however, to distinguish what a client knows from what he or she is willing to accept. A study by Cappon (1970) asked groups of healthy persons, physically ill clients, psychiatric clients, and dying clients whether they would like to know if a serious illness were terminal. The majority responded yes; however, of the four groups, the dying least desired this information (33% did not want to be told). Cappon concluded that physicians should be cautious and not give more information than the client wants.

Reaction to the Loss

The nurse assesses the grieving client and/or family members following a loss to determine the phase or stage of grieving. The following clinical symptoms of grief are described by Schulz (1978, pp. 142–43).

1. Repeated somatic distress
2. Tightness in the chest
3. Choking or shortness of breath
4. Sighing
5. Empty feeling in the abdomen
6. Loss of muscular power
7. Intense subjective distress

Physiologically, the body responds to a current or anticipated loss with a stress reaction. The nurse can assess the clinical signs of this response. See Chapter 17.

Factors Influencing a Loss Reaction

The influence of age and developmental level on how a person reacts to loss has already been discussed. Other factors include the personal significance of the loss, culture, spiritual beliefs, sex role, and socioeconomic status.

Significance of the loss The significance of a loss depends on the perceptions of the individual experiencing the loss. One person may experience a great sense of loss over a divorce; another may find it only mildly disrupting. A number of factors affect the significance of the loss: the age of the person; the value placed on the lost person, body part, etc.; the degree of change required because of the loss; and the person's beliefs and values.

Expectations can also greatly affect significance. For elderly people who have already encountered many losses (e.g., family, health, independence), an anticipated loss such as their own death may not be important; they may be apathetic about it instead of reactive. More than fearing death, some may fear loss of control or becoming a burden (Charmaz 1980, p. 77).

Culture Culture influences an individual's reaction to loss. How grief is expressed is often determined by the customs of the culture. It has been suggested that the Protestant ethic—individualism, self-reliance, independence, and hard work—leads to the practice of handling grief only with significant others, not a larger community (Charmaz 1980, p. 284). In the United States and Canada, unless an extended family structure exists, grief is handled by the nuclear family, which, because of its small size, emphasizes self-reliance and independence.

Many Americans appear to have internalized the belief that grief is a private matter to be endured internally.

Therefore, feelings tend to be repressed and may remain unidentified. People who have been socialized to "be strong" and "make the best of the situation" may not express deep feelings or personal concerns when they experience a serious loss.

Some cultural groups value social support and the expression of loss. In certain black churches the expression of emotion plays a prominent part. In Hispanic American groups where strong kinship ties are maintained, support and assistance are provided by family members, and the free expression of grief is encouraged.

Spiritual beliefs Spiritual beliefs and practices greatly influence both a person's reaction to loss and subsequent behavior. Most religious groups have practices related to dying, and these are often important to the client and support persons. For additional information, see Chapter 49. For nurses to provide support at a time of death it is important that they understand the client's particular beliefs and practices.

Sex role The sex roles into which many people are socialized in the United States and Canada affect their reactions at times of loss. Men are frequently expected to "be strong" and show very little emotion during grief, whereas it is acceptable for women to show grief by crying, etc. Often when a wife dies, the husband, who is the chief mourner, is expected to repress his own emotions and to comfort sons and daughters in their grieving.

Sex roles also affect the significance of body image changes to clients. A man might consider a facial scar to be "macho," but a woman might consider it ugly. Thus, the woman, but not the man, would see it as a loss.

Socioeconomic status The socioeconomic status of an individual often affects the support system available at the time of a loss. A pension plan or insurance, for example, can offer a widowed or disabled person choices of ways to deal with a loss: A woman who loses a hand and can no longer do her previous work may be able to pursue vocational reeducation; a man whose wife has died can afford to take a cruise or visit relatives in Europe. Conversely, a person who is confronted with both severe loss and economic hardship may not be able to cope with either.

Nursing Diagnosis

Many of the accepted nursing diagnoses are applicable to grieving clients, depending on the information obtained from individual assessment. Three diagnoses that may be particularly appropriate are "dysfunctional grieving," "impaired adjustment," and "social isolation."

Dysfunctional Grieving

A normal grief reaction may be abbreviated or anticipatory. Unhealthy grief—that is, *pathologic grief*—may be unresolved or inhibited. Both normal and unhealthy grief may be delayed. Many factors can contribute to pathologic grief, including a prior traumatic loss in childhood and the circumstances of the present loss. For instance, the sudden, untimely death of an adolescent or young adult can complicate the expression and resolution of grief. Other influences include family or cultural barriers to the emotional expression of grief.

Abbreviated grief is brief but genuinely felt. The lost object may not have been sufficiently important to the grieving person or may have been replaced immediately by another, equally esteemed object.

Anticipatory grief is experienced in advance of the event. The wife who grieves before her ailing husband dies is anticipating the loss. A beauty queen may grieve in advance of an operation that will leave a scar on her body. Because many of the normal symptoms of grief will have already been expressed in anticipation, the reaction when the loss actually occurs may be quite abbreviated.

Unresolved grief is extended in length and severity. The same signs are expressed as with normal grief, but the bereaved may also have difficulty expressing the grief, may deny the loss, or may grieve beyond the expected time.

With *inhibited grief* many of the normal symptoms of grief are suppressed, and other effects, including somatic, are experienced instead.

Burgess and Lazare (1976a, p. 100) state that the diagnosis of pathologic grief may be inferred from the following data or observations:

1. The client fails to grieve following the death of a loved one; e.g., a husband does not cry at, or absents himself from, his wife's funeral.
2. The client becomes recurrently symptomatic on the anniversary of a loss or during holidays (especially Thanksgiving and Christmas).
3. The client avoids visiting the grave and refuses to participate in religious memorial services of a loved one, even though these practices are a part of the client's culture.
4. The client develops persistent guilt and lowered self-esteem.
5. Even after a prolonged period, the client continues to search for the lost person. Some make the search while in fugue states. Others may wander from town to town or act as if they were expecting the deceased to return. Some may consider suicide to effect reunion.
6. A relatively minor event triggers symptoms of grief.
7. Even after a period of time, the client is unable to discuss the deceased with equanimity, e.g., the client's voice cracks and quivers, eyes become moist.
8. An interview of the client is characterized by themes of loss.

9. After the normal period of grief, the client experiences physical symptoms similar to those of the person who died.
10. The client's relationships with friends and relatives worsen following the death.

Many factors contribute to unresolved grief. Some of these are (Burgess and Lazare 1976a, pp. 97–100):

1. Ambivalence (intense feelings of both love and hate) toward the lost person. The bereaved is often afraid to grieve for fear of discovering unacceptable negative feelings.
2. A perceived need to be brave and in control; fear of losing control in front of others.
3. Endurance of multiple losses, such as the loss of an entire family, which the bereaved finds too overwhelming to contemplate.
4. Extremely high emotional value (overcathexis) invested in the dead person. Failure to grieve in this instance helps the bereaved avoid the reality of the loss.
5. Uncertainty about the loss—for example, when a loved one is "missing in action."
6. Lack of support persons.
7. Subjection to socially unacceptable loss that cannot be spoken about, e.g., suicide, abortion, or giving a child up for adoption.

Impaired Adjustment

When changed health status demands modifications in life-style and behavior that the person cannot make, the appropriate nursing diagnosis may be "impaired adjustment." This diagnosis can be applied to either the person suffering the loss or a significant other. For instance, the husband of a woman hospitalized with a life-threatening illness may feel unable to assume unaccustomed domestic duties such as childcare. And he may be resentful that the disease has removed the person who maintained the stability of family life. The athlete who suffers a sudden heart attack might also be diagnosed with impaired adjustment. The reduced capacity for physical exertion that the condition imposes may threaten self-image and self-esteem.

Social Isolation

The painful nature of grief can cause those experiencing it to withdraw from their normal social support systems, which is the opposite of what they should be doing. Some people feel the need to display mastery of the situation or wish not to burden friends. They may be afraid to test the strength of friendships. A new widow, for example, might feel awkward maintaining social relationships in the circle of married couples she had participated in with her husband.

Social support is a major positive influence on the successful resolution of grief (Richter 1984). Social isolation, as a nursing diagnosis, can therefore be useful in directing nursing interventions that help the client to build the necessary support network.

Planning and Intervention

Helping the Bereaved

The goals of grieving are to be able to remember the lost object or person without intense pain and to be able to redirect emotional energy into one's own life and regain the capacity to love. More specifically, the client needs to feel (a) free from emotional bondage to the deceased person, (b) adjusted to the changed environment, (c) capable of developing new relationships and renewing old ones, and (d) comfortable with both positive and negative memories of the deceased (Martocchio 1985).

The following nursing guidelines can help the client achieve these goals (Benoliel 1985, p. 445).

1. Provide opportunity for the persons involved to "tell their story."
2. Recognize and accept the varied emotions that people express in relation to a significant loss.
3. Provide support for the expression of difficult feelings, such as anger and sadness, recognizing that people must do this in their own way and at their own pace.
4. Include children in the grieving process.
5. Encourage the bereaved to maintain established relationships.
6. Acknowledge the usefulness of mutual-help groups.
7. Encourage self-care by family members—in particular, the primary caregiver.
8. Acknowledge the usefulness of counseling for especially difficult problems.

Communication

Effective communication skills are an essential part of nursing care of the dying client and his or her family. See Chapter 27. The skills most relevant to situations of loss and grief are attentive listening, silence, open and closed questioning, paraphrasing, clarifying and reflecting feelings, and summarization. Less helpful to clients are responses that give advice and evaluation, those that interpret and analyze, and those that give unwarranted reassurance (Martocchio 1985). To ensure effective communication, the nurse needs to accurately assess what is appropriate for the client.

Poor communication can have seriously harmful consequences. Mistrust may result when clients receive conflicting messages about vital matters. Clients may also feel powerless, isolated, or abandoned if they believe important information is being withheld. Anger and resentment can be the consequences of mistrust and powerlessness. Finally, poor communication can prevent clients from taking care of important final business, whether it be financial, emotional, or spiritual (Gonda and Ruark 1984).

Dying clients sometimes have an urgent need to be listened to; yet because they are dying they are often avoided by caregivers and family members. One student nurse who overcame her fear and self-doubt to spend time listening to a dying woman summarized her experience this way: "She needed someone to listen as she reviewed her life and verbally expressed her fears through her questions. She needed to be accepted for her humanness. She wanted to feel a sense of dignity and meaning in her life" (Wagg and Yurick 1983, p. 502).

Communication with grieving clients needs to be tuned to their stage of grief. Whether the client is angry or depressed will affect how he or she hears messages and how the nurse interprets the client's statements. Implications for nurse–client communication are related to Kübler-Ross's five stages in Table 50–2, page 1458.

Evaluation

Evaluating the effectiveness of nursing care of the grieving client is difficult because of the long-term nature of the life transition. Criteria for evaluation must be based on goals set by the client and family, and not on an arbitrary standard of success (Benoliel 1985). A follow-up visit to the surviving family members may be an appropriate nursing measure not only to obtain information for evaluation, but to assist nurses in working through their own grief by expressing their continuing concern for the family.

Examples of outcome criteria for grieving clients are:

1. Verbalizes feelings of sorrow (or anger or loss)
2. Verbalizes understanding of feelings experienced
3. Has resumed usual activities
4. Has established new relationships

Care of the Dying Client

Assessment

Nursing care and support for the dying client and his or her family include making an accurate assessment of the physiologic signs of approaching death.

Clinical Signs of Impending Death

In addition to signs related to the client's specific pathology, certain other physical signs are indicative of impending death.

1. *Loss of muscle tone,* which results in:
   a. Relaxation of the facial muscles (e.g., the jaw may sag)
   b. Difficulty speaking
   c. Difficulty swallowing and gradual loss of the gag reflex
   d. Decreased activity of the gastrointestinal tract, with subsequent nausea, accumulation of flatus, abdominal distention, and retention of feces, especially if narcotics or tranquilizers are being administered
   e. Possible urinary and rectal incontinence due to decreased sphincter control
   f. Diminished body movement
2. *Slowing of the circulation,* which results in:
   a. Diminished sensation
   b. Mottling and cyanosis of the extremities
   c. Cold skin, first in the feet and later in the hands, ears, and nose (the client, however, may feel warm due to elevated temperature)
3. *Changes in vital signs:*
   a. Decelerated and weaker pulse
   b. Decreased blood pressure
   c. Rapid, shallow, irregular, or abnormally slow respirations; mouth breathing, which leads to dry oral mucous membranes
4. *Sensory impairment:*
   a. Blurred vision
   b. Impaired senses of taste and smell

Various levels of consciousness are seen just before death. Some clients are alert, whereas others are drowsy, stuporous, or comatose. Hearing is thought to be the last sense lost.

Clinical Signs of Imminent Death

1. Dilated, fixed pupils
2. Inability to move
3. Loss of reflexes
4. Faster, weaker pulse
5. Cheyne-Stokes respirations

6. Noisy breathing, referred to as the *death rattle,* due to collection of mucus in the throat
7. Lowered blood pressure

Eyes may be either partly open or closed.

Clinical Signs of Death

The traditional clinical signs of death were cessation of the apical pulse, respirations, and blood pressure. However, since the advent of artificial means to maintain respirations and blood circulation, identifying death is more difficult. In 1968 the World Medical Assembly adopted the following guidelines for physicians as indications of death (Benton 1978, p. 18):

1. Total lack of response to external stimuli
2. No muscular movement, especially breathing
3. No reflexes
4. Flat encephalogram

In 1968 a committee of the Harvard Medical School also published criteria indicating death (Benton 1978, p. 18):

1. Unreceptivity and unresponsivity
2. No movement or breathing
3. No reflexes
4. Flat encephalogram

In instances of artificial support, the Harvard committee stated, absence of electric currents from the brain (measured by an electroencephalogram) for at least 24 hours is an indication of death. Only a physician can pronounce death, and only after this pronouncement can life support systems be shut off.

Another definition of death is **cerebral death,** which occurs when the higher brain center, the cerebral cortex, is irreversibly destroyed. The client may still be able to breathe but is irreversibly unconscious. People who support this definition of death believe the cerebral cortex, which holds the capacity for thought, voluntary action, and movement, *is* the individual (Schulz 1978, p. 92).

Nursing Diagnosis

The full range of nursing diagnoses, addressing both physiologic and psychosocial needs, can be applied to the dying client, depending on the assessment data. Two diagnoses that may be particularly appropriate are "fear," and "hopelessness."

Fear

Many fears are associated with death, and the nurse needs to determine a client's specific fears. Gonda and Ruark (1984, pp. 31–32) discuss three objects of the dying person's fear: the process of dying, nonexistence, and what comes after death. The nurse is usually better able to assist a client with the complex process of dying than with the spiritual fears of nonexistence and the hereafter.

Schulz (1978, p. 27) outlines the following fears related to a person's own death: pain, body misfunction, humiliation, rejection or abandonment, nonbeing, punishment, interruption of goals, and negative impact on survivors (e.g., psychologic suffering, economic hardship).

Sheehy (1981, pp. 27–62), in his discussion about common fears of dying, includes fear of pain, loneliness, dependence, the moment of death, and annihilation. Although there is no pain at the moment of death and the transition from life to death seems easy, many people fear this moment. Sheehy believes that fear of the moment of death is the result of the emotional sting and pain experienced during the death of a parent. People remember this previous pain and, therefore, believe that dying is painful. Fear of annihilation, or being reduced to nothingness after death, and questions about immortality need to be faced. Does immortality rest in what the individual achieved in this life or does the soul survive after death? Whatever a person believes about life after death, both body and mind may be viewed as reentering the universe and becoming part of it as some form of energy.

Hopelessness

The very nature of a terminal illness or any other dying process can lead to a client's loss of hope. The nurse can identify this subjective state by noting some of the following behaviors (North American Nursing Diagnosis Association 1986, p. 1).

1. Passivity
2. Decreased verbalization
3. Decreased affect
4. Verbal cues (sighing, "I can't," or "Why bother?")
5. Lack of initiative
6. Decreased response to stimuli

Feelings of hopelessness often follow an awareness of the reality of the loss and may be expressed in the despair phase of mourning (Gonda and Ruark 1984, p. 38). Real or perceived abandonment can also mean a diagnosis of hopelessness. A loss of belief in religious and spiritual values or powers may be related to the development of hopelessness. The return of realistic hope can be facili-

Research Note

Rothlis suggests that persons with reactive depression share a common experience, namely, external loss accompanied by feelings of hopelessness and helplessness. This experience, she believes, is amenable to treatment through a self-help group. She hypothesized that persons with reactive depression who have experienced a loss and who participate in a self-help group will show a greater decrease in feelings of hopelessness and helplessness. The sample consisted of 28 clients, 21 who lost a significant person, and 7 who lost a job. The hypothesis was supported by the research results. (Rothlis 1984)

tated by the nurse through assisting the client and/or family to focus on the outcomes of specific, short-term goals (Gonda and Ruark 1984, pp. 89–90).

Planning and Intervention

The major nursing responsibility for clients who are dying is to assist the client to a peaceful death. More specific responsibilities are:

1. To provide relief from from loneliness, fear, and depression
2. To maintain the client's sense of security, self-confidence, dignity, and self-worth
3. To maintain hope
4. To help the client accept his or her losses
5. To provide physical comfort

People facing death need help facing the fact that they will have to depend on others. Some dying clients require only minimal care and can be cared for at home; others need continuous attention and the services of a hospital and its staff. People need help, well in advance of death, in planning for the period of dependence. They need to consider what will happen and how and where they would like to die.

Planning also involves establishing outcome criteria based on the client's nursing diagnosis. For examples of outcome criteria, see the "Evaluation" section later in this chapter.

Helping Clients Die with Dignity

Dignity may be defined as the ability to function as a significant and integrated person (Sheehy 1981, p. 56). True dignity comes from within. Generally, dependence on others and loss of control over oneself and interactions with the environment are associated with loss of dignity. Dying clients often feel they have lost control over their lives and over life itself. By introducing options available to the client and significant others, nurses can restore and support feelings of control. Some choices that clients can make are: the location of care, e.g., hospital, home, or hospice; times of appointments with health professionals; activity schedule; use of health resources; and times of visits from relatives and friends.

Most clients interviewed about dying indicate that they want to be able to manage the events preceding death so they can die peacefully. Nurses can help clients to find meaning and completeness and to determine their own physical, psychologic, and social priorities. Dying people often strive for self-fulfillment more than self-preservation, and they need to find meaning in continuing to live while suffering. Part of the nurse's challenge, then, is to help maintain, day to day, the client's will and hope.

Salter (1982, p. 21) believes it is important for nurses and clients to focus not on the end, but on three stages of living fully until death:

1. *Developing and growing.* In this stage the client can be assisted to paint, sculpt, go to a library, visit an art gallery, etc. An occupational therapist can help clients do what they still can do and what is pleasurable.
2. *Lying fallow.* In this stage, physiotherapy measures, such as breathing exercises and passive exercises, help the client to relax and enhance self-esteem.
3. *Letting go and becoming dependent.* In this stage, nursing intervention is usually required to meet both physical and psychologic needs.

Hospice and Home Care

Hospice care, palliative care, and home care focus on support and care of the dying person and his or her family, with the goal of facilitating a peaceful and dignified death. The following list of characteristics of **hospice** caregiving highlights the holistic nature of the concept and the contrast to cure-oriented hospital care (Hadlock 1983, pp. 108–10).

1. Total care
2. Symptom control
3. Pain management
4. Emotional support
5. Support for families
6. Support for staff and staff stress

The principles of hospice care can be carried out in a variety of settings, the most common being the autonomous hospice and the hospital-based **palliative-care** unit. Services range from fully comprehensive to a focus on selected areas, such as symptom control and pain management, in some palliative care units. Home care services for the dying client maintain the client in the natural home environment until that is no longer possible or until death. See Chapter 4 for further information on Home Health Care. Hospice care is always provided by a team of both health professionals and nonprofessionals, to ensure a full range of care services. In the United States these services have been delivered primarily through autonomous, community-based hospices, such as the Connecticut Hospice. In Canada one finds hospital-based palliative care programs, such as the Palliative Care Services of the Royal Victoria Hospital in Montreal. This difference may be a function of different methods for funding health care (Corless 1983, pp. 336–39). Both countries have established standards and guidelines for the development and operation of hospice programs (Health and Welfare Canada 1981; National Hospice Organization 1981).

Meeting Physiologic Needs of the Dying Client

The physiologic needs of the dying are related to a slowing of body processes and to homeostatic imbalances. Interventions include personal hygiene measures, pain control, relief of respiratory difficulties, assistance with movement, nutrition, hydration, and elimination, and measures related to sensory changes. See also Table 50–4.

Personal hygiene measures Cleanliness of the skin, hair, and mouth is essential. Excessive diaphoresis may necessitate frequent baths and linen changes. Some clients wish to wear daytime clothes and should be encouraged to do so if comfortable. Secretions may gather in the eyes, which may necessitate cleaning the eyelids with absorbent cotton and saline. Due to elevated body temperature, the client's mouth may become dry, requiring mouth care.

Pain control Many drugs have been used to control the pain associated with terminal illness: morphine, heroin, methadone, alcohol, marijuana, and LSD. In hospitals the most frequently used agents are morphine, methadone, and alcohol. See Chapter 41. Usually the physician deter-

Table 50–4 Physiologic Needs of Dying Persons

Problem	Nursing Interventions
Ineffective airway clearance	Fowler's position: conscious clients
	Throat suctioning: conscious clients
	Low-Fowler's position: unconscious clients
	Oxygen therapy as needed
Impaired physical mobility	Assist client out of bed periodically, if client able
	Regularly change bedridden clients' position
	Support client's position with rolls of blankets or towels as needed
	Lateral position in bed, to decrease aspiration of saliva
	Elevate client's legs when sitting up, to prevent pooling of blood
Alteration in nutrition, less than body requirements	Antiemetics or alcoholic beverages, to stimulate appetite
	High-calorie, high-vitamin diet
Fluid volume deficit, actual or potential	Semisolid, soft, or liquid foods because of decreased gag reflex
	Continuing assessment of gag reflex
Alteration in bowel elimination	Laxatives as needed to prevent constipation
Alteration in urinary elimination	Skin care because of incontinence of urine or feces
	Bedpan, urinal, or commode chair within easy reach
	Call light within reach for assistance onto bedpan or commode
	Absorbent pads placed under incontinent client; linen changed as often as needed
	Catheterization in some cases
	Keep room as clean and odor-free as possible
Sensory-perceptual alteration (visual, tactile)	Clients prefer a light room
	Hearing is *not* diminished; speak clearly and do not whisper
	Touch is diminished, but client will feel pressure of touch

Source: C. R. Kneisl and S. W. Ames, ***Adult health nursing. A biopsychosocial approach*** (Menlo Park, Calif.: Addison-Wesley Publishing Co., 1986), p. 492. Used by permission.

mines the dosage, but the client's opinion should be considered; the client is the one ultimately aware of personal pain tolerance and fluctuations of internal states. Because of decreased blood circulation, analgesics may be administered by intravenous infusion rather than subcutaneously or intramuscularly.

Relief of respiratory difficulty Respiratory difficulties are likely to alarm support persons as well as the client. For conscious clients, Fowler's position and throat suctioning are indicated. For the unconscious, a semiprone position facilitates drainage of mucus from the mouth and throat. Oxygen therapy by cannula or mask may be necessary in some instances.

Movement When possible, dying clients should be assisted out of bed periodically. Bedridden clients need regular changes of position to prevent decubitus ulcers. With progressive loss of muscle tone, the client requires increasing support to maintain a comfortable position. Lateral positions are preferable to supine positions so that saliva, which cannot be swallowed, will drain from the mouth.

When clients are positioned in a chair, it is important to elevate the lower extremities to prevent pooling of blood due to reduced circulation.

Nutrition and hydration Dying clients are often anorexic and nauseated, because of reduced peristalsis and accumulation of flatus. Antiemetics or alcoholic beverages may be given to control nausea and to stimulate appetite. High-calorie, high-vitamin diets are indicated. Because of loss of muscle tone, the client may be dysphagic and require semisolid or liquid foods or even intravenous infusions. To swallow effectively, the gag reflex must be present; the nurse, therefore, assesses the client's gag reflex as required.

Elimination Due to loss of muscle tone, the client may develop constipation, incontinence (fecal and urinary), or urinary retention. Laxatives may be necessary to prevent constipation. For skin irritation due to incontinence, a soothing ointment can be applied around the anus and perineum. A bedpan, urinal, or commode should be readily available for incontinent clients, or the nurse should assist or position the client onto the bedpan or urinal at scheduled intervals. Bed linens should be changed as often as necessary. If the client is incontinent, absorbent pads are used and changed frequently. For urinary retention, catheterization may be necessary; in some cases, an indwelling catheter may be inserted. The environment needs to be kept free of unpleasant odors, using deodorants and adequate ventilation.

Measures related to sensory changes As death approaches and the client's vision becomes blurred, many prefer a light to a darkened room. The dying client usually turns his or her head to the light. Although the sense of touch will be diminished, the client will sense pressure. A dying client may hear what people are saying after he or she can no longer see or respond. When talking to a dying client, nurses and visitors need to speak clearly and avoid whispering, since clients tend to become disturbed when unable to hear.

Spiritual Support

Spiritual support is of great importance in dealing with death. Although not all clients identify with a specific religious faith or belief, the majority have a need for meaning in their lives, particularly as they experience a terminal illness. Conrad (1985, pp. 417–19) has categorized the spiritual needs of the dying as follows:

1. Search for meaning
2. Sense of forgiveness
3. Need for love
4. Need for hope

The nurse has a responsibility to ensure that the client's spiritual needs are attended to, either through direct intervention or by arranging access to individuals who can provide spiritual care. The nurse needs to be aware of her own comfort with spiritual issues and be clear about her own ability to interact supportively with the client. Nurses have a responsibility to not impose their own religious/spiritual beliefs on a client, but to respond to the client in relation to his or her own background and needs. The categories of spiritual need noted above should be addressed by the nurse in the context of a careful assessment of the client's religious or spiritual belief system. Communication skills are most important in helping the client articulate his or her needs and in developing a sense of caring and trust.

Specific interventions may include facilitating expressions of feeling, prayer, meditation, reading, and discussion with appropriate clergy/spiritual advisor. It is important for nurses to establish an effective interdisciplinary relationship with spiritual support specialists.

For a further discussion of spiritual issues, see Chapter 49. Death-related beliefs and practices of selected religious groups are shown in Table 50–5.

Special Needs of the Dying Child

Infants A dying infant requires comforting and care, as do the parents. Parents' grief about their infant's death goes beyond comprehension. Parents often internalize their feelings of helplessness and act them out in their marriage and social life (Kavanaugh 1976, p. 44).

Parents can become obsessed with questions about genetic and family heritage and parental inadequacy, such as "Did I really want the baby?" or "Did he die because I smoked during pregnancy?" Both parents require

Table 50–5 Death-Related Beliefs and Practices of Selected Religious Groups

Group	Afterlife	Rituals/ Funerals	Autopsy	Organ Donation	Cremation	Prolonging Life
American Indian	Beliefs vary	Practices vary; most want family present	Prohibited		Practices vary	
Black Muslim		Special procedures for washing and shrouding the dead; special funeral rites				
Buddhist in America	Reincarnation; after reaching state of enlightenment, may attain nirvana	Last rite; chanting at bedside	No restriction		No restriction	Permit euthanasia in hopeless illness
Church of Christ Scientist	Yes	No last rites	Only in sudden death	No	Individual decision	
Church of Jesus Christ of Latter Day Saints (Mormon)	Yes	Baptism essential; preaching gospel to dead also practiced	No restriction	No restriction	Discouraged	
Eastern Orthodox (Greek and Russian Orthodox)	Yes	Last rites (administration of Holy Communion obligatory)	Discouraged		Discouraged	Encouraged
Episcopal (Anglican)	Yes	Last rites not mandatory	No restriction	No restriction	No restriction	
Hindu	Reincarnation; after leading a perfect life, may join Brahma	Priest pours water into mouth of corpse and ties string around wrist or neck as sign of blessing; string must not be removed; family washes body	No restriction	No restriction	Preferred; ashes cast in holy river	
Islam (Moslem, Muslim)	May join Allah by being a good Moslem and observing rituals daily	Dying person must confess sins and ask forgiveness in presence of family; family washes and prepares body (female body cannot be washed by male) and turns body toward Mecca	Prohibited unless required by law	Prohibited	Prohibited	Encouraged

Table 50–5 *(continued)*

Group	Afterlife	Rituals/ Funerals	Autopsy	Organ Donation	Cremation	Prolonging Life
Jehovah's Witness			Prohibited unless required by law. No body parts may be removed	Prohibited	No restriction	
Judaism	Dead will be resurrected with coming of Messiah; man lives on through survival of memory	Body ritually washed by members of Ritual Burial Society; burial as soon as possible after death; dead not left unattended; five stages of mourning extending over a year; no embalming; no flowers at funeral because flowers are a symbol of life	Orthodox prohibit; some liberals permit; no body parts removed	Beliefs vary	Largely prohibited; beliefs vary	
Lutheran	Yes	Last rites optional	No restriction	No restriction	No restriction	
Roman Catholicism	Yes; resurrection with second coming of Christ	Rites for anointing the sick not mandatory; receiving Holy Communion mandatory	Permitted, but all body parts must be given appropriate burial	No restriction	No restriction	Discouraged
Seventh Day Adventist	Dead are asleep until return of Christ, when final rewards and punishments will be given					
Unitarian	Beliefs vary		No	No	Encouraged	Preferred

Sources: H. M. Ross, Societal/cultural views regarding death and dying, *Topics in Clinical Nursing*, 1981, 3(3):1–16 by permission of Aspen Publishers, Inc.; *Nursing 77,* Dec. 1977, 7:64–70. Used by permission of Springhouse Corporation.

encouragement to verbalize these feelings and to find their own answers. Parents often vent their anger at nurses and the care the infant is receiving. It is important for nurses to accept this anger openly and then assist the parents to see beyond it.

The birth of a handicapped child, an infant who requires intensive care after birth, or a stillborn infant produces a grief reaction. Frequently parents ask themselves, "What have I done that this should happen?" Working through the grief is very important, and nurses can support the parents while they do so. See the description of stages of grieving, earlier in this chapter.

Children Nursing intervention for the dying child needs to include the parents and siblings. Parents are generally exceedingly emotionally involved in the death of a child, more so than in the death of an older person.

It is important to listen carefully to a child's questions and to answer them truthfully. To a question such as "Will I be home for Christmas?" nurses can truthfully answer, "I really don't know, but I hope so." Children may ask questions about death; simple answers often suffice, such as "It means not living anymore."

Parents of a dying child may have guilt feelings and may need to talk out their feelings to help each other and the child (Northrup 1974, p. 1068). Parents often fear that the child will suffer more as death nears. Honest reassurance that the child will not suffer unduly is important.

Part of a young child's fear of death is aloneness, being away from the parents. Parents should be encouraged to interact with nurses in the child's presence so that the nurses can be identified as trustworthy substitute caretakers (Betz and Poster, 1984).

Adolescents Dying adolescents need to deal not only with the reality of dying but also with developmental tasks of their age. Because hospitalization imposes many restrictions on normal activity, adolescents are apt to feel frustrated and resentful. They need supportive understanding for their behavior. Like children, adolescents require honest answers to their questions, support in their thinking, and encouragement to accept the reality of death.

Evaluation

Examples of outcome criteria for clients who are dying are:

1. Is free of pain
2. Participates in self-care activities
3. Verbalizes feelings of anger, sorrow, or loss
4. Participates in plans for therapy
5. Maintains open relationships with support persons and staff

Care of the Body after Death

Body Changes

Rigor Mortis

Rigor mortis is the stiffening of the body that occurs about 2 to 4 hours after death. It results from a lack of adenosine triphosphate (ATP), which is not synthesized because of a lack of glycogen in the body. ATP is necessary for muscle fiber relaxation. Its lack causes the muscles to contract, which in turn immobilizes the joints. Rigor mortis starts in the involuntary muscles (heart, bladder, etc.), then progresses to the head, neck, and trunk, and finally reaches the extremities.

Because the deceased's family often wants to view the body, and because it is important that the deceased appear natural and comfortable, nurses need to position the body, place dentures in the mouth, and close the eyes and mouth *before* rigor mortis sets in. Rigor mortis usually leaves the body about 96 hours after death.

Algor Mortis

Algor mortis is the gradual decrease of the body's temperature after death. When blood circulation terminates and the hypothalamus ceases to function, body temperature falls about 1 C (1.8 F) per hour until it reaches room temperature. Simultaneously, the skin loses its elasticity and can easily be broken when removing dressings and adhesive tape.

Postmortem Decomposition

After blood circulation has ceased, the skin becomes discolored. The red blood cells break down, releasing hemoglobin, which discolors the surrounding tissues. This discoloration, referred to as **livor mortis**, appears in the lowermost or dependent areas of the body, such as the buttocks in a sitting position.

Tissues after death become soft and eventually liquefied by bacterial fermentation. The hotter the temperature, the more rapid the change. Therefore, bodies are often stored in cool places to delay this process. Embalming reverses the process through injection of chemicals into the body to destroy the bacteria (Pennington 1978, p. 847).

Legal Aspects of Death

Of the many legal ramifications of human death, the most basic for the nurse is that death must be certified by a physician. In circumstances of unusual death, an **autopsy** (postmortem examination) may be required. Nurses have a responsibility to be aware of the legal ramifications of death in the jurisdiction in which they practice. Chapter 7 provides legal information about death certificates, labeling the deceased, autopsy, organ donation, and inquest. Wills, euthanasia, and the right to die (living wills) are also discussed in Chapter 7.

Nursing Intervention

Nursing personnel may be responsible for care of a body after death. If the deceased's family or friends wish to view the body, it is important to make the environment as clean and pleasant as possible and to make the body appear natural and comfortable. All equipment and supplies should be removed from the bedside. Some agencies require that all tubes in the body be clamped and remain in place; in other agencies, tubes may be cut to within 2.5 cm (1 in) of the skin and taped in place. Soiled linen is removed so that the room is free from odors.

The body is normally placed in a supine position with the arms either at the sides, palms down, or across the abdomen. The wristband is left on unless it is too tight. One pillow is placed under the head and shoulders to prevent blood from discoloring the face by settling in it. The eyelids are closed and held in place for a few seconds so they remain closed. If they will not stay closed, a moistened cotton fluff will hold them in place. Dentures are usually inserted to help give the face a natural appearance. The mouth is then closed; a rolled towel under the chin will hold it closed.

Soiled areas of the body are washed; however, a complete bath is not necessary, since the body will be washed by the **mortician** (also referred to as an **undertaker**), a person trained in care of the dead. Absorbent pads are placed under the buttocks to take up any feces and urine released because of relaxation of the sphincter muscles. A clean gown is placed on the client and the hair is brushed and combed. All jewelry is removed, except a wedding band in some instances, which is taped to the finger. The top bed linens are adjusted neatly to cover the client to the shoulders. Soft lighting and chairs are provided for the family. All the client's valuables, including clothing, are listed and placed in a safe storage area for the family to take away.

After the body has been viewed by the family, additional identification tags are applied, one to the ankle and one to the wrist if the client's wrist identification band was not left in place. The body is wrapped in a **shroud**, a large rectangular or square piece of plastic or cotton material used to enclose a body after death. Another identification band is then applied to the outside of the shroud. The body is taken to the morgue for cooling, if arrangements have not been made to have a mortician pick it up from the client's room. Agencies vary in their policies about transporting bodies. Some close all room doors before transporting a deceased client through corridors, and service elevators are often used.

Nursing Care Plan

Assessment Data

Nursing Assessment

Stephanie Smith is a 58-year-old widow whose husband died of a heart attack 6 months ago. Her children are grown and are either pursuing careers in other cities or are away at school. Mrs. Smith's husband was a prominent physician who served on the faculties of a number of medical schools. As his wife, she was largely responsible for the rearing of the children. She was always perceived as a strong person who made the best of most situations. Mrs. Smith's interests were focused primarily on her husband's work and career and her family. Immediately after his death she continued to be a source of strength to her children and close friends. Now, 6 months later, her daughter comes home to find her mother depressed, withdrawn, and tearful. She complains of being ill and on occasion having headaches, backaches, chest pains, and gastrointestinal disturbances. She states that she has not been able to socialize with her friends because of her poor health and constant fatigue. She spends her days alone, reading her husband's papers or looking through photo albums. Her daughter insists that Mrs. Smith seek medical attention.

Physical Examination

Height: 167.6 cm (5′6″)
Weight: 50.3 kg (111 lb)
Temperature: 37 C (98.6 F)
Pulse rate: 78 BPM
Blood pressure: 112/72 mm Hg
Skin warm, dry, and pale

Diagnostic Data

Urine: Negative
Chest x-ray film: Negative
Electrocardiogram: Normal
Gastrointestinal series: Essentially negative

Nursing Diagnosis	Client Goals and Outcome Criteria	Nursing Interventions and Rationales	Evaluation
Grieving related to actual loss of spouse resulting in crying, depression, withdrawn behavior, and somatic complaints.	Client Goal: Experience a resolution of grief. Outcome Criteria: Expresses her grief by day 2. Verbalizes understanding of feelings experienced by day 3. Resumes usual activities by day 14.	Assess for factors that prolong grieving. *Rationale:* Identification of such factors will assist in determining appropriate intervention. Provide a safe, secure environment. *Rationale:* Less threatening to client and allows client to ventilate feelings. Establish a trusting relationship with client. *Rationale:* Client will feel more secure in discussing her grief. Encourage client to express her sorrow, sense of loss, and feelings of guilt. *Rationale:* Promotes the work of grieving. Ensure that the bereaved client has support persons.	Mrs. Smith has cried and expressed her sorrow and pain over the death of her husband to her children and her caregivers. Her children have provided loving support and have requested that she spend time visiting each of them for extended periods. She is considering the possibility of rejoining her bridge club.

(*continued*)

Nursing Diagnosis	Client Goals and Outcome Criteria	Nursing Interventions and Rationales	Evaluation
		Rationale: Support persons are essential in assisting the bereaved client with the work of grieving. Encourage client to seek spiritual assistance from clergy. *Rationale:* During the grieving process, spiritual assistance aids the client in dealing with her sorrow. Encourage the client to continue in familiar roles and to accept new ones. *Rationale:* Will increase client's self-esteem and decrease incidence of unresolved grief.	
Social isolation related to death of spouse resulting in increased signs of illness, underactivity, failing to interact with others.	Client Goal: Reestablish old contacts and partake in usual activities. Outcome Criteria: Identifies causes of feelings of isolation by day 3. Identifies means of increasing social contacts by day 3. Identifies 1 or 2 diversional activities of interest by day 5.	Identify factors that contribute to social isolation. *Rationale:* Appropriate interventions can be taken when causative factors are identified. Enlist aid of family members and significant others. *Rationale:* Promotes social interaction and decreases sense of isolation. Encourage participation in outside activities of interest to client, e.g., golf and bridge club. *Rationale:* Activity increases sense of well-being and self-esteem. Initiate referrals as needed. *Rationale:* Socially isolated clients are not always able to initiate or undertake social activities on their own.	Mrs. Smith states that she has been depressed since her husband's death, and she didn't want to burden her friends or family with her sorrow and pain. She now acknowledges this has only increased her grief and grieving. She has accepted visits from several good friends, who have urged her to rejoin their bridge club. She hopes to get a new puppy for companionship while the children are away at school.

Chapter Highlights

- Nurses help clients deal with all kinds of losses, including loss of body image, loss of a loved one, loss of a sense of well-being, and loss of a job.
- Loss, especially loss of a loved one or a valued body part, can be viewed as a crisis event, either situational or developmental, and either actual or perceived (both of which can be anticipatory).
- How an individual deals with loss is closely related to the individual's stage of development, personal resources, and social support systems.
- Caring for the dying and the bereaved is one of the nurse's most complex and challenging responsibilities.
- Nurses' attitudes about death and dying directly affect their ability to provide care.
- Nurses must consider the entire family as the client of care in situations involving loss, especially the crisis of death.
- Grieving is a normal, subjective emotional response to loss; it is essential for mental and physical health. Grieving allows the bereaved person to cope with loss gradually and to accept it as part of reality.
- Knowledge of different stages or phases of grieving and factors that influence the loss reaction can help the nurse understand the responses and needs of clients.
- Effective communication skills are essential to the nursing of clients who are suffering loss or dying.
- Dying clients require physical help and emotional support to ensure a peaceful and dignified death.

Suggested Readings

Benoliel, J. Q. June 1985. Loss and terminal illness. *Nursing Clinics of North America* 20(2):439–48.

The leading nurse-scholar writing on loss and grief presents a succinct overview of loss and the implications for the individual, the family, and nursing care.

Mina, C. F. March/April 1985. A program for helping grieving parents. *Maternal Child Nursing* 10:118–21.

A program to improve care given to parents after the loss of an infant is described. Emphasis is placed on education and support. A checklist for nurses to ensure that parents are offered all available options to assist grief is presented.

Wagg, B., and Yurick, A. G. September 1983. Care enough to hear. *Journal of Gerontological Nursing* 9(9):498–503.
Written by a nursing student and her instructor, this article describes the student's successful experience in supporting a person during the final stages of living. The implications for the student's personal growth and for the death-education needs of all nurses are mentioned.

Whelan, E. January/February 1985. Support for the survivor. *Geriatric Nursing* 6(1):21–23.
The author examines the grief process as experienced by bereaved spouses. Reactions of the spouses to the attention given by nurses are used to indicate useful nursing strategies in helping survivors deal with their loss.

Selected References

Alexander, J., and Kiely, J. March/April 1986. Working with the bereaved. *Geriatric Nursing* 7(2):85–86.

Benoliel, J. Q. June 1985. Loss and terminal illness. *Nursing Clinics of North America* 20(2):439–48.

Benton, R. E. 1978. *Death and dying: Principles and practices in patient care.* New York: D. Van Nostrand Co.

Betz, C. L., and Poster, E. C. June 1984. Children's concepts of death: Implications for pediatric practice. *Nursing Clinics of North America* 19(2):341–49.

Burgess, A. W., and Lazare, A. 1976a. *Community mental health: Target populations.* Englewood Cliffs, N.J.: Prentice-Hall.

Cantor, R. C. 1978. *And a time to live.* New York: Harper and Row.

Cappon, D. February 1970. Attitudes towards death. *Coast Graduate Medicine* 47:257.

Charmaz, K. 1980 *The social reality of death.* Reading, Mass.: Addison-Wesley Publishing Co.

Clark, M. D. December 1984. Healthy and unhealthy grief behaviors. *Occupational Health Nursing* 32(12):633–35.

Conrad, N. L. June 1985. Spiritual support for the dying. *Nursing Clinics of North America* 20(2):415–26.

Corless, I. B. 1983. The hospice movement in North America. In Corr, C. A., and Corr, D. M. (editors). *Hospice care: Principles and practice.* New York: Springer Publishing Co.

Cowan, M. E.; Murphy, S. A.; et al. March/April 1985. Identification of postdisaster bereavement risk predictors. *Nursing Research* 34(2):71–75.

Demi, A. S., and Miles, M. S. 1986. Bereavement. *Annual Review of Nursing Research* 4:105–23.

Engel, G. L. September 1964. Grief and grieving. *American Journal of Nursing* 64:93–98.

Enlow, P. M. July 1986. Coping with anticipatory grief. *Journal of Gerontological Nursing* 12(7):36–37.

Fetsch, S. H. November/December 1984. The 7- to 10-year-old child's conceptualization of death. *Oncology Nurses' Forum* 11(6):52–56.

Field, D. January 1984. "We didn't want him to die on his own"—Nurses' accounts of nursing dying patients. *Journal of Advanced Nursing* 1:59–70.

Gonda, T. A., and Ruark, J.E. 1984. *Dying dignified: The health professional's guide to care.* Menlo Park, Calif.: Addison-Wesley.

Hadlock, D. C. 1983. Physician rules in hospice care. In Corr, C. A., and Corr, D. M. (editors). *Hospice care: Principles and practice.* New York: Springer Publishing Co.

Health and Welfare Canada. 1981. Palliative care services in hospitals: Guidelines. Ottowa: Ministry of National Health and Welfare.

Hoff, L. A. 1984. *People in crisis.* Menlo Park, Calif.: Addison-Wesley.

Kavanaugh, R. E. 1976. Children's special needs. In *Dealing with death and dying,* pp. 33–46. Nursing 77 Skillbook Series. Horsham, Pa.: Intermed Communications.

Kennedy, S. R. January/February 1985. Sharing, caring, living, dying. *Geriatric Nursing* 6(1):12–17.

Kübler-Ross, E. 1969. *On death and dying.* New York: Macmillan Publishing Co.

———. 1974. *Questions and answers on death and dying.* New York: Macmillan Publishing Co.

———. 1975. *Death: The final stage of growth.* Englewood Cliffs, N.J.: Prentice-Hall.

———. 1978. *To live until we say good-bye.* Englewood Cliffs, N.J.: Prentice-Hall.

Martocchio, B. C. June 1985. Grief and bereavement: Healing through hurt. *Nursing Clinics of North America* 20(2):327–41.

Moss, M. S., and Moss, S. Z. 1983–84. The impact of parental death on middle-aged children. *Omega* 14(1):65–75.

National Hospice Organization. 1981. Standards of a hospice program of care. Arlington, Va.: National Hospice Organization.

North American Nursing Diagnosis Association. Summer 1986. New diagnoses accepted. *Nursing Diagnosis Newsletter* 13(1):1.

Northrup, F. C. June 1974. The dying child. *American Journal of Nursing* 74:1066–68.

Pennington, E. A. May 1978. Postmortem care: More than ritual. *American Journal of Nursing* 78:846–47.

Peterson, E. A. October 1985. The physical . . . The spiritual . . . Can you meet all of your patients' needs? *Journal of Gerontological Nursing* 11(10):23–27.

Richter, J. M. July 1984. Crisis of mate loss in the elderly. *American Nursing Society* 6(4):45–54.

Rothlis, J. Spring 1984. The effect of a self-help group on feelings of hopelessness and helplessness. *Western Journal of Nursing* 6:157–69.

Salter, R. March 1982. The art of dying. *Canadian Nurse* 78:20–21.

Schulz, R. 1978. *The psychology of death, dying and bereavement.* Reading, Mass.: Addison-Wesley Publishing Co.

Sheehy, P. F. 1981. *On dying with dignity.* New York: Pinnacle Books.

Strauss, A. L., et al. 1970. Awareness of dying. In Schoenberg, B., et al., editors. *Loss and grief.* New York: Columbia University Press.

Taylor, D. A. 1983–84. View of death from sufferers of early loss. *Omega* 14(1):77–82.

Wagg, B., and Yurick, A. G. September 1983. Care enough to hear. *Journal of Gerontological Nursing* 9(9):498–503.

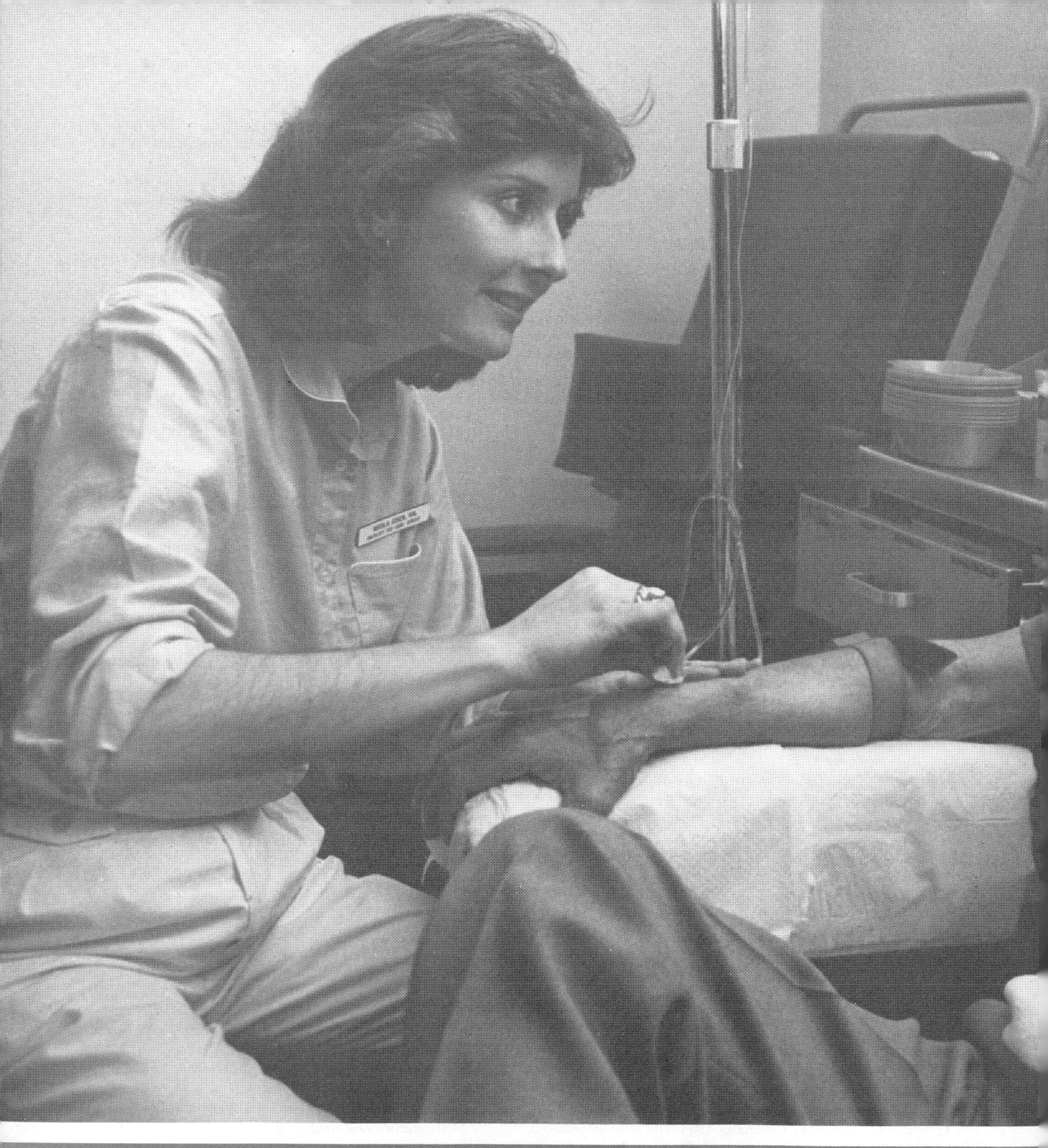

The horizon for nursing expands exhilaratingly. The depth has not been sounded. So we explore depths and distances. The nugget of truth lies in the nurse-patient relationship. The distant star is the health of all people. (Lucille Petry Leone)

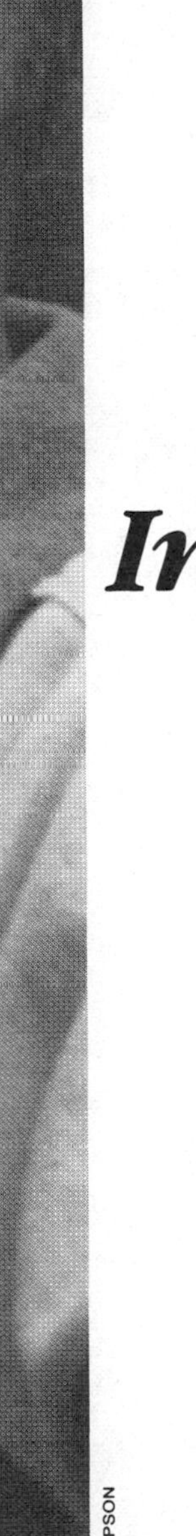

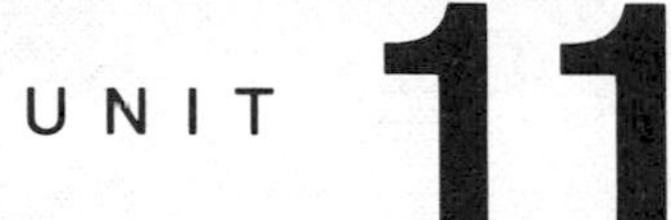

UNIT 11

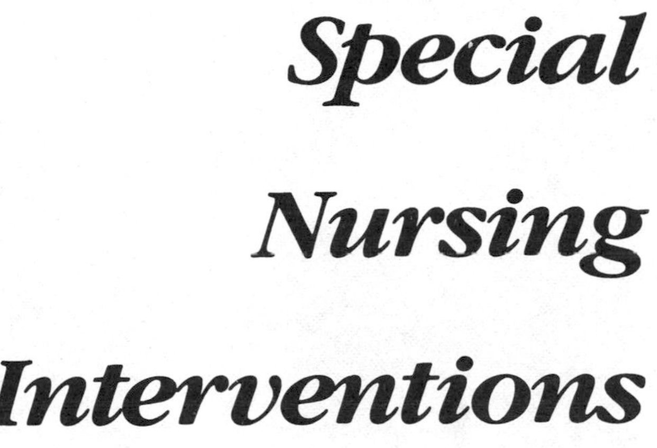

Special Nursing Interventions

Contents

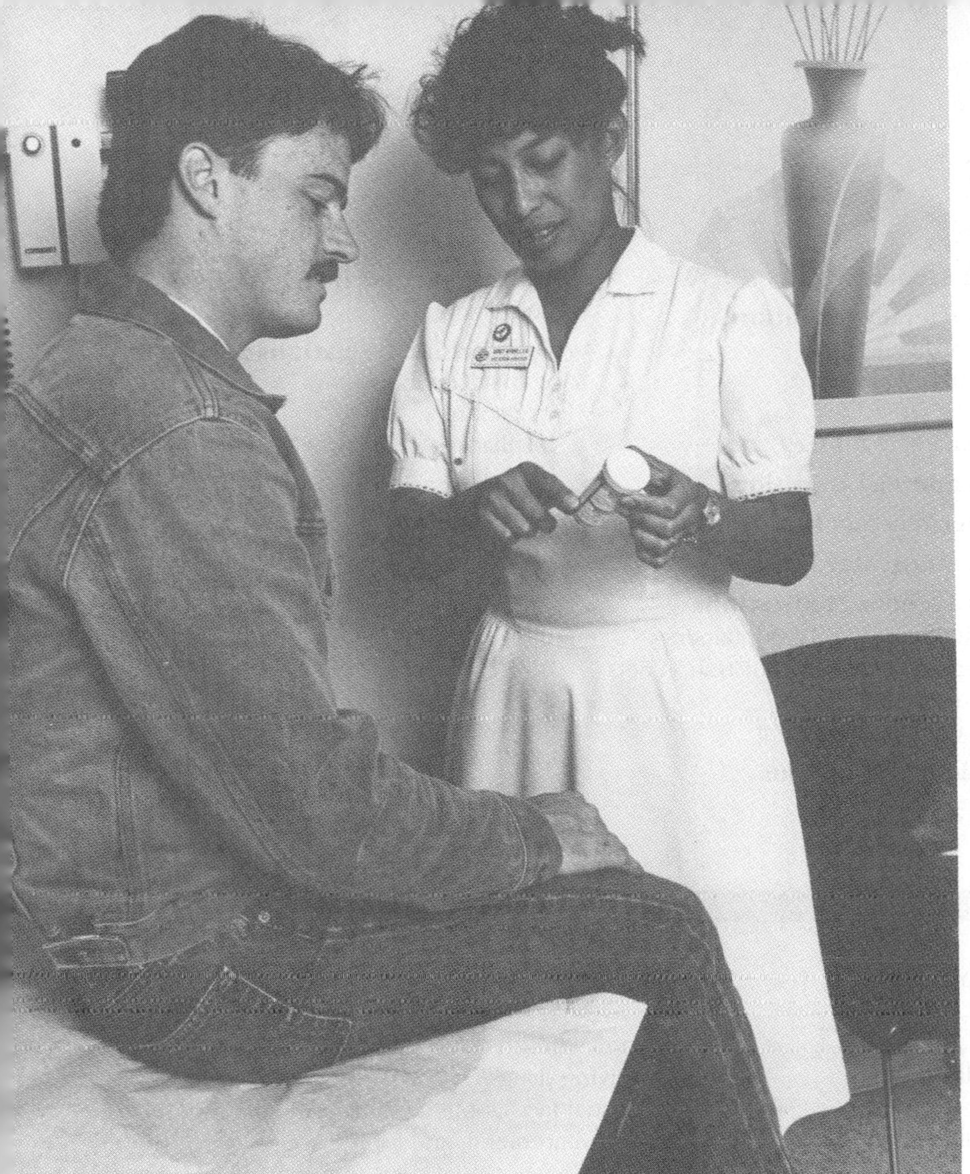

KAREN STAFFORD RANTZMAN

CHAPTER **51**

Medications

Contents

(continued)

51 *Medications*

Contents *(continued)*

Objectives

1. Know essential terms and facts about drugs.
   1.1 Define selected terms.
   1.2 Identify official drug listings.
   1.3 Describe major federal acts controlling drugs in the United States and Canada.
   1.4 Identify legal aspects of administering drugs.
   1.5 Identify drug preparations by type.
   1.6 Identify physiologic factors affecting drug action.
   1.7 Identify individual variables influencing drug action.
   1.8 Identify various effects of drugs.
   1.9 Differentiate between noncompliance, drug misuse, and drug abuse.
   1.10 Describe three types of drug supply systems.
2. Understand essential facts about the administration of medications.
   2.1 Identify various routes of drug administration.
   2.2 Identify various types of medication orders.
   2.3 Identify essential parts of a drug order.
   2.4 Identify abbreviations commonly used in medication orders.
   2.5 Identify basic units of weight and volume of the metric, apothecaries', and household systems.
   2.6 Identify approximate equivalents within each system of measurement and among systems.
   2.7 Calculate fractional dosages of drugs.
   2.8 Use body surface area and body weight to calculate fractional dosages of medications for infants and children.
3. Know essential assessment information pertinent to medications and their administration.
   3.1 Identify essential data to obtain in the nursing history.
   3.2 Identify clinical data required to assess the client receiving drugs.
4. Know essential facts about administering medications by oral, parenteral, and topical routes.
   4.1 Identify five essential steps to follow when administering drugs.
   4.2 Identify essential guidelines for administering medications, including the five "rights."
   4.3 Identify variations in methods of administering drugs to infants, children, and elderly persons.
   4.4 Identify physiologic changes in elderly persons that alter the effects of drugs.
   4.5 Outline steps required to administer oral medications safely.
   4.6 Identify equipment required for parenteral medications.
   4.7 Identify essential steps in mixing selected drugs from vials and ampules, and in preparing powdered drugs.
   4.8 Identify sites used for subcutaneous, intramuscular, and intradermal injections.
   4.9 Identify essential steps in safely administering a subcutaneous injection, an intramuscular injection, and an intradermal injection.
   4.10 Give reasons for steps in administering medications.
   4.11 Describe the Z-track technique.
   4.12 Identify essential steps in safely administering topical medications: dermatologic, ophthalmic, otic, nasal, vaginal, and rectal.

Terms

agonist
ampule
anaphylactic reaction
bioavailability
bioequivalent
biotransformation
buccal
clinical pharmacist
compliance
cumulative effect (of drug)
dermatologic preparations
drug (medication)
drug abuse
drug allergy
drug dependence
drug habituation
drug interaction
drug misuse
drug tolerance
drug toxicity
formulary
iatrogenic disease
idiosyncratic effect (of drug)
illicit drug
immunologic reaction
individual-client supply system
inhalation
irrigation (lavage)
instillation
intraarterial
intracardiac
intradermal
intramuscular
intraosseous
intrathecal (intraspinal)
intravenous
inunction
meniscus
metabolite
minim
noncompliance
parenteral
peak plasma level
pharmacist
pharmacology
pharmacokinetics
pharmacopoeia
pharmacy
pharmacy assistant
physiologic dependence
prescription
psychologic dependence
reconstitution
side-effect
stock supply
subcutaneous
sublingual
therapeutic effect
topical
unit-dose system
vial

Names and Types of Medications

Medications have been known and used since antiquity. Crude drugs such as opium, castor oil, and vinegar were used in ancient times. Knowledge about these drugs was relatively limited and pragmatic. Over the centuries the number of drugs available has increased greatly, and knowledge about these drugs has become correspondingly more accurate and detailed. It is estimated that some 25,000 drugs and drug products are available in North America today, and new ones are being added daily.

A **drug (medication)** is a substance administered to people or animals for the diagnosis, cure, treatment, mitigation (relief), or prevention of disease. In the health care context, the words *drug* and *medication* are generally used interchangeably. Lay people often use the term *drug* for illicitly obtained substances such as heroin, cocaine, or amphetamines. Lay people often refer to medications as medicines.

Pharmacology is the study of the effect of drugs on living organisms. Drugs are prepared by a **pharmacist**, a person licensed to prepare and dispense drugs and to make up prescriptions. A **clinical pharmacist** is a specialist who often guides the physician in prescribing drugs. A **pharmacy assistant** is a member of the health team who in some states administers drugs to clients. **Pharmacy** is the art of preparing, compounding, and dispensing drugs. The word also refers to the place where drugs are prepared and dispensed.

In the United States and Canada, drugs are usually dispensed on the order of physicians and dentists. In some states in the United States, nurse practitioners under a physician's license also prescribe drugs. The written direction for the preparation and administration of a drug is a **prescription**.

1. *Names.* One drug can have as many as four kinds of names: its generic name, official name, chemical name, and trademark or brand name. The *generic name* is given before a drug becomes official. The *official name* is the name under which it is listed in one of the official publications. The *chemical name* is the name by which a chemist knows it; this name describes the constituents of the drug precisely. The *trademark*, or *brand name*, is the name given by the drug manufacturer. Because one drug may be manufactured by several companies, it can have several trade names; for example, the drug hydrochlorothiazide (official name) is known by the trade names Esidrix, Diuril, Lexor, and Thiuretic.
2. *Classifications.* Drugs are classified according to their effect, their composition, and their purposes. Most classifications according to effect lack exactness because some drugs act on several systems of the body and may be used for different purposes for different people.
3. *Types of preparations.* Medications are differently prepared. The kind of preparation may determine the method of administration; an elixir, for example, is taken by mouth. It is important to administer the type of preparation specified in the medication order. See Table 51–1.

Table 51–1 Types of Drug Preparations

Type	Description	Type	Description
Aqueous solution	One or more drugs dissolved in water	Paste	A preparation like an ointment, but thicker and stiffer, that penetrates the skin less than an ointment
Aerosol spray or foam	A liquid, powder, or foam deposited in a thin layer on the skin by air pressure	Pill	One or more drugs mixed with a cohesive material, in oval, round, or flattened shapes
Aqueous suspension	One or more drugs finely divided in a liquid such as water	Powder	A finely ground drug or drugs; some are used internally, others externally
Capsule	A gelatinous container to hold a drug in powder, liquid, or oil form	Spirit	A concentrated alcoholic solution of a volatile substance
Cream	A nongreasy, semisolid preparation used on the skin	Suppository	One or several drugs mixed with a firm base such as gelatin and shaped for insertion into the body; the base dissolves gradually at body temperature, releasing the drug
Elixir	A sweetened and aromatic solution of alcohol used as a vehicle for medicinal agents	Syrup	An aqueous solution of sugar often used to disguise unpleasant-tasting drugs
Extract	A concentrated form of a drug made from vegetables or animals	Tablet	A powdered drug compressed into a hard small disc; some are readily broken along a scored line; others are enteric-coated to prevent them from dissolving in the stomach
Fluid extract	An alcoholic solution of a drug from a vegetable source; the most concentrated of all fluid preparations	Tincture	An alcoholic or water-and-alcohol solution prepared from drugs derived from plants
Gel or jelly	A clear or translucent semisolid that liquefies when applied to the skin		
Liniment	An oily liquid used on the skin		
Lotion	An emollient liquid that may be a clear solution, suspension, or emulsion used on the skin		
Lozenge (troche)	A flat, round, or oval preparation that dissolves and releases a drug when held in the mouth		
Ointment	A semisolid preparation of one or more drugs used for application to the skin and mucous membrane		

Drug Standards

Drugs may have plant, mineral, and animal (all natural) sources or they may be synthesized in the laboratory. For example, digitalis and opium are plant derived, iron and sodium chloride are minerals, insulin and vaccines have animal or human sources, and the sulfonamides and propoxyphene hydrochloride (the analgesic Darvon) are the products of laboratory synthesis. Early drugs were derived from the three natural sources. During the past 45 years, however, more and more drugs have been produced synthetically.

Drugs vary in strength and activity. Drugs derived from plants, for example, vary in strength according to the age of the plant, the variety, the place in which it is grown, and the method by which it is preserved. Drugs must be pure and of uniform strength if drug dosages are to be predictable in their effect. Drug standards have therefore been developed to ensure uniform quality.

In the United States, official drugs are those so designated by the Federal Food, Drug, and Cosmetic Act. These drugs are officially listed in the *United States Pharmacopeia (USP)* and described according to their source, physical and chemical properties, tests for purity and identity, method of storage, assay, category, and normal dosages. A **pharmacopoeia** is a book containing a list of products used in medicine, with descriptions of the product, chemical tests for determining identity and purity, and formulas for certain mixtures. Two other publications, the *National Formulary* and the *Homeopathic Pharmacopoeia of the United States,* also list official drugs. In Canada the *British Pharmacopoeia* is used for the same purpose, although some drugs used in Canada conform to the *USP* because they are obtained from the United States.

Under the auspices of the World Health Organization, the *Pharmacopoeia Internationalis (Ph. I.)* is published in Spanish, French, and English. It has improved drug standards throughout the world.

A **formulary** is a collection of formulas and prescriptions. The United States *National Formulary* and the *Canadian Formulary* are published in North America. The *National Formulary* lists drugs and their therapeutic value and can include drugs that may still be used but not listed in the *USP*. The *Canadian Formulary* lists drugs used extensively in Canada but not necessarily listed in the *British Pharmacopoeia*.

Pharmacopoeias and formularies are invaluable reference sources for nurses and nursing students. Nurses not only administer thousands of medications but also are responsible for assessing their effectiveness and recognizing unfavorable reactions to drugs. Since it is impossible to commit to memory all pertinent information about a very large number of drugs, nurses must have a reliable reference readily available.

Legal Aspects of Drug Administration

The administration of drugs in both the United States and Canada is controlled by law. In the United States the major federal acts controlling drugs are the Food, Drug, and Cosmetic Act (1938) and its amendments and the Comprehensive Drug Abuse Prevention and Control Act (1970) (Controlled Substances Act). The Food, Drug, and Cosmetic Act and its amendments require proof of both safety and efficacy before a drug can be sold. The first federal narcotic act was the Harrison Narcotic Act of 1914; it was replaced by the Controlled Substances Act, which was enacted to prevent drug abuse and drug dependence, to provide treatment and rehabilitation for drug users and drug-dependent people, and to strengthen drug abuse laws. This act makes it illegal to possess a controlled substance without a valid prescription. Controlled substances such as narcotics, amphetamines, barbiturates, and tranquilizers are covered by this act. See Table 51–2 for additional information.

In Canada three federal acts control drugs: the Food and Drugs Act (1953), the Proprietary or Patent Medicine Act (1908), and the Narcotic Control Act (1961). The Food and Drugs Act controls the sale of food, drugs, and cosmetics. It also provides for appropriate labeling, including expiration date and recommended single and daily adult dose, and directions for use. The Proprietary or Patent Medicine Act protects the public against unsafe or ineffective home remedies (over-the-counter medications). The dosage, efficiency, compatibility, directions for use, and claims of patent medicines such as cough syrups are controlled. The Canadian Narcotic Control Act governs the possession, sale, manufacture, production, and distribution of narcotics. This law applies to all narcotics, including cocaine, morphine, opium, and marijuana. The Canadian Mounted Police enforce these laws. See Table 51–3 for additional information.

Nursing legislation also controls the administration of medications by nurses. Nurse-practice acts describe legitimate nursing activity. The nurse-practice acts of Alaska, Maine, New Mexico, Idaho, New Hampshire, North Carolina, Oregon, Tennessee, Vermont, and Washington

Table 51–2 United States Drug Legislation

Legislation	Content
Food, Drug, and Cosmetic Act (1938)	Implemented by Food and Drug Administration (FDA); requires that labels be accurate and that all drugs be tested for harmful effects
Durkham-Humphrey Amendment (1952)	Differentiates clearly between drugs that can be sold with and without a prescription
Kefauver-Harris Amendment (1962)	Requires proof of safety and efficacy of a drug for approval
Comprehensive Drug Abuse Prevention and Control Act (1970) (Controlled Substances Act)	Categorizes controlled substances and limits how often a prescription can be filled

Table 51–3 Canadian Drug Legislation

Legislation	Content
Proprietary or Patent Medicine Act (1908)	Protects the public against unsafe and ineffective over-the-counter drugs
Canada Food and Drugs Act (1953)	Prohibits advertising any food, drug, cosmetic, or device as a cure for certain specified diseases. Prohibits the sale of certain drugs unless approved by the federal government
Canadian Narcotic Control Act (1961)	Allows only authorized people to possess narcotics. Specifies records about narcotics that must be kept

include prescription writing as a nursing function for nurse-practitioners, although in some states there must be a supervising physician. In other jurisdictions, prescription writing is the responsibility of the physician. Another change in some jurisdictions is the administration by nurses with the appropriate order of small volumes of intravenous medications by IV "push" or into IV tubing, a task previously carried out by physicians.

It is important for nurses to know how nursing acts in their areas define and limit their functions; it is equally important for them to recognize the limits of their own knowledge and skill. To function beyond the limits of nursing acts or one's ability is to endanger clients' lives and leave oneself open to malpractice suits.

Under the law, nurses are responsible for their own actions regardless of whether there is a written order. If a physician writes an incorrect order—for example, Demerol 500 mg instead of Demerol 50 mg—a nurse who administers the written incorrect dosage is responsible for the error. Therefore, nurses should question an order that appears unreasonable or refuse to give the medication until the order is clarified.

Another aspect of nursing practice governed by law is the use of narcotics and barbiturates. In hospitals, narcotics are kept under double lock in a drawer or cupboard. Other medications, including barbiturates, are kept under single lock, although in some places barbiturates are kept with narcotics. Agencies have special forms for recording narcotics. The information required usually includes the name of the client, date and time of administration, name of the drug, dosage, and signature of the person who prepared and gave the narcotic. The name of the physician who ordered the narcotic may also be part of the record.

Included on the record are narcotics wasted during preparation. In most agencies, narcotic and barbiturate counts are taken at the end of each shift. The count total should tally with the total at the end of the last shift minus the number used. If the totals do not tally, the discrepancy must be reported immediately.

The keys for drug and narcotic cupboards are carried by a nurse on duty. They should never be left in the lock, even if a nurse leaves the cupboard for only a minute.

Narcotics and barbiturates are closely controlled because they are highly addictive. The illegal sale of the opiate heroin receives much publicity. It is more potent than either morphine or codeine. Heroin, however, has not been used in health agencies because of the danger that a client may become dependent on the drug. Related drugs such as morphine, meperidine hydrochloride (Demerol), hydromorphinone hydrochloride (Dilaudid), and codeine are more frequently used in hospitals and prescribed by physicians.

In the United States, drugs used in clinical areas should be officially listed in the *United States Pharmacopeia (USP)* or the *National Formulary*. Drugs used in Canadian agencies should be listed in the *British Pharmacopoeia*, the *USP*, or the *Canadian Formulary*. In the United States, a new drug must have investigational new-drug exemption (IND) before it can be tested on people.

Systems of Delivery

Systems to deliver medications to clients vary among health care agencies and with their facilities and equipment, supply systems, and procedural policies and practices. All systems are designed to ensure the safe storage and administration of medications.

Facilities and Equipment

Nursing units have at least one area designated for stocking drugs ready to dispense to clients. Many agencies have specially designed central medications rooms with locked cupboards containing the medications for all clients on the unit. Other agencies have locked wall cupboards near clients' rooms or mobile carts with locked drawers. In all facilities, narcotics are kept in a double-locked drawer, box, or cupboard.

Supply Systems

Procedures for delivering medications are based on three supply systems: the stock supply, the individual-client supply, and the unit dose systems.

In the **stock-supply** system, medications are kept on the unit in relatively large quantities, and individual doses are taken from it and administered by nursing personnel. For example, individual doses of a certain laxative or antibiotic are taken from a large stock-supply bottle. Sedatives and narcotics are commonly provided as stock-supply medications on each nursing unit.

In the **individual-client supply** system, the medications for each client are supplied separately in specified doses and quantities for a specified period of time. For example, 20 250-mg tetracycline capsules are supplied in a separate container or envelope only for Mr. John Brown. This supply is not used for other clients.

The **unit-dose** system is increasingly used, since pharmacy personnel have begun to participate in administering medications to clients and in evaluating their effects. In this system, pharmacy personnel prepackage and label an individual dose, called the unit dose, for each client. The unit dose is the ordered amount of medication the client is to receive at a prescribed hour. Depending on agency practice, the medications are administered by pharmacy personnel or nursing personnel from the pharmacy or on the nursing unit. Many believe that the unit-dose system makes error less likely and saves time for nursing personnel.

Policies and Practices

Dispensing medications, i.e., preparing and packaging medications, is the responsibility of pharmacists. The pharmacist may dispense directly to the client or to a person who will administer the drug. In some agencies, a senior nurse may be delegated the responsibility of dispensing drugs in the absence of a pharmacist, e.g., on the night shift or on a holiday.

In most agencies, graduate nurses administer all types of medications (oral, topical, and parenteral), unless pharmacy personnel are delegated this function. Agency practice determines who is permitted to administer intravenous medications; agency practices vary. Licensed vocational nurses are often permitted to administer oral medications only, and registered nurse students who have demonstrated competence are generally allowed to administer all types of medications. It is essential that the nursing student check agency policies and practices governing medications before administering them.

Kinds of Drug Actions

Drugs can have a number of actions or effects on a client; some of them may be desirable and others undesirable.

Therapeutic Effect vs. Side-Effect

The **therapeutic effect** of a drug, also referred to as the *desired effect,* is the primary effect intended, that is, the reason the drug is prescribed. For example, the therapeutic effect of morphine sulphate is analgesia, and the therapeutic effect of diazepam is relief of anxiety. See Table 51–4 for different types of therapeutic drugs.

A **side-effect**, or secondary effect, of a drug is one that is unintended. Side-effects are usually predictable and may be either harmless or potentially harmful. For example, digitalis increases the strength of myocardial contractions, but it can have the side-effect of inducing nausea and vomiting. Some side-effects are tolerated for the drug's therapeutic effect; hazardous side-effects justify the discontinuation of a drug. The side-effects of some drugs have led to a therapeutic value of the drug for another condition. Some major side-effects are discussed next.

Toxic Effect

Drug toxicity (deleterious effects of a drug on an organism or tissue) results from overdosage, ingestion of a drug intended for external use, and buildup of the drug in the blood because of impaired metabolism or excretion (cumulative effect). Almost every drug can have toxic effects. Some toxic effects are apparent immediately; some are not apparent for weeks or months. Fortunately most drug toxicity is avoidable if careful attention is paid to dosage and monitoring for toxicity. An example of a toxic effect is respiratory depression due to the cumulative effect of morphine sulphate in the body.

Drug Allergy

A **drug allergy** is the immunologic reaction to a drug to which a person has already been sensitized. When a client is first exposed to a foreign substance (antigen), the body may react by producing antibodies. This is called an **immunologic reaction**. See Chapter 32. A client can react

Table 51–4 Types of Therapeutic Drugs

Drug Type	Description	Examples
Palliative	Relieves the symptoms of a disease but does not affect the disease itself	Morphine sulphate, aspirin for pain
Curative	Cures a disease or condition	Penicillin for infection
Supportive	Supports body functions until other treatment or the body's response can take over	Levophed for low blood pressure; aspirin for high body temperature
Substitutive	Replaces body fluids or substances	Thyroxin for hypothyroidism; insulin for diabetes mellitus
Chemotherapeutic	Destroys malignant cells	Busulfan for leukemia
Restorative	Returns the body to health	Vitamin, mineral supplements

to a drug as to an antigen and thus develop symptoms of an allergic reaction.

Allergic reactions can be either mild or severe. A mild reaction has a variety of symptoms, from skin rashes to diarrhea. See Table 51–5. It can occur anytime from a few hours to 2 weeks after the administration of the drug.

A severe allergic reaction usually occurs immediately after the administration of the drug; it is called an **anaphylactic reaction**. This response can be fatal if the symptoms are not noticed immediately and treatment is not obtained promptly. The earliest symptoms are acute shortness of breath, acute hypotension, and tachycardia.

Table 51–5 Common Mild Allergic Responses

Symptom	Description/rationale
Skin rash	Either an intraepidermal vesicle rash or a rash typified by an urticarial wheal or macular eruption; rash is usually generalized over the body
Pruritus	Itching of the skin with or without a rash
Angioedema	Edema due to increased permeability of the blood capillaries
Rhinitis	Excessive watery discharge from the nose
Lacrimal tearing	Excessive tearing
Nausea, vomiting	Stimulation of these centers in the brain
Wheezing and dyspnea	Shortness of breath and wheezing upon inhalation and exhalation due to accumulated fluids and swelling of the respiratory tissues
Diarrhea	Irritation of the mucosa of the large intestine

Drug Tolerance

Drug tolerance exists in a person who has unusually low physiologic activity in response to a drug and who requires increases in the dosage to maintain a given therapeutic effect. Drugs that commonly produce tolerance are opiates, barbiturates, ethyl alcohol, and tobacco.

Cumulative Effect

A **cumulative effect** occurs when a person is unable to metabolize (break down) one dose of a drug before another dose is given. As a result, the amount of the drug builds up in the client's body unless the dosage is adjusted. This can be to the client's benefit unless it produces toxic effects.

Idiosyncratic Effect

An **idiosyncratic effect** is unexpected and individual. Underresponse and overresponse to a drug may be idiosyncratic. Also, the drug may have a completely different effect from the normal one or cause unpredictable and unexplainable symptoms in a particular client.

Drug Interaction

A **drug interaction** occurs when administration of one drug before, at the same time as, or after another drug alters the effect of one or both drugs. The effect of one or both drugs may be either increased (*potentiating effect*) or decreased (*inhibiting effect*). Drug interactions may be beneficial or harmful. Combination drug therapy exploits beneficial drug interactions. For example, Probenecid, which blocks the excretion of penicillin, is often given with penicillin to increase blood levels of the penicillin for longer periods (potentiating effect). Two analgesics, such as aspirin and codeine, are often given together because together they provide greater pain relief (additive effect). Other drugs are used in combination to prevent or minimize certain side-effects. For example, two diuretics may be administered together because one depletes the body's potassium levels while the other spares potassium.

Some drugs when given together, however, are antagonistic because the combination either exerts an inhibiting effect or increases toxicity. Changes in dosage or timing of one or both drugs can avoid the problem. One incompatible combination is tetracycline and certain antacids (in fact, any substance that is high in calcium, such as milk). Calcium reduces the absorption of tetracycline, inhibiting its efficacy; thus, tetracycline should be given 1 hour before or 2 hours after products containing calcium. There are many incompatible combinations. The nurse needs to check incompatability charts or ask a clinical pharmacologist about such combinations when any new drug is added to the client's regimen. Some drugs are incompatible with foods. For example, ampicillin and erythromycin should not be taken with fruit juices, and antihistamines should not be taken with alcohol.

Iatrogenic Disease

Iatrogenic disease (disease caused unintentionally by medical therapy) can be due to drug therapy. Five major syndromes can be induced by drug therapy (Hahn et al. 1982, p. 55).

1. Blood dyscrasias from bone marrow depression, resulting in anemia and thrombocytopenia
2. Hepatic toxicity resulting in biliary obstruction or hepatic necrosis
3. Renal damage, especially of the glomerulus
4. Dermatologic effects such a eczema, acne, and psoriasis
5. Malformations of the fetus as a result of drugs taken during pregnancy

Drug Use

Two terms describe how an individual follows the directions of drug therapy. **Compliance** is careful adherence to the prescribed drug therapy. The individual takes the correct drug and dosage at the times prescribed and follows other suggested measures, such as taking milk with the medication. **Noncompliance** is failure to follow the prescribed therapy. There are many reasons for noncompliance, although no reason should be assumed unless explicitly stated by the client. Some reasons are:

1. Insufficient money to purchase the medications
2. Not understanding the medication order
3. Belief that the medication will not help
4. Perception of wellness, i.e., lack of symptoms

For additional information about compliance, see Chapter 2, page 67.

Drug Misuse

Drug misuse is the improper use of common medications in ways that lead to acute and chronic toxicity. Drug misuse leads to such problems as gastrointestinal bleeding, kidney damage, and liver damage. Both over-the-counter drugs and prescription drugs may be misused. Some people who are stressed or ill take unprescribed medications in the hope of saving time and money or perhaps because they do not want to bother the physician. Self-medication poses the danger of masking symptoms but not treating the cause. As a result, problems can go undetected for prolonged periods.

Laxatives, antacids, vitamins, headache remedies, and cough and cold medications are often self-prescribed and overused. Most people suffer no harmful effects from these drugs, but some people do. A persistent cough may go undiagnosed until the underlying problem is serious and advanced. Persistent use of some over-the-counter or prescribed drugs can also damage body parts that were initially healthy. For example, prolonged use of headache remedies containing phenacetin can cause kidney damage and even death.

Drug Abuse

Drug abuse is inappropriate intake of a substance, either continually or periodically. By definition, drug use is abusive when society considers it abusive. For example, the intake of alcohol at work may be considered alcohol abuse, but intake at a social gathering may not. Frequently abused drugs are alcohol, amphetamines, caffeine, tobacco, sedatives, and tranquilizers.

Drug abuse in North America is growing. It has two main facets, drug dependence and habituation. **Drug dependence** is a person's reliance on or need to take a drug or substance. There are two types of dependence: physiologic and psychologic. They may occur separately or together. **Physiologic dependence** is due to biochemical changes in body tissues, especially of the nervous system. These tissues come to require the substance for normal functioning. When the person no longer takes the drug, he or she experiences withdrawal symptoms. Withdrawal symptoms vary with the drug used, the amount used, and the duration of use. The client taking opiates may manifest elevated mood, relief of anxiety, and pinpoint pupils. On withdrawal, the client may be restless, feel chilly, yawn, sneeze, and have increased nasal and lacrimal secretions, for example. Sometimes withdrawal is sufficiently severe to cause cardiovascular collapse.

Psychologic dependence is emotional reliance on a drug to maintain a sense of well-being, accompanied by feelings of need or cravings for that drug. There are varying degrees of psychologic dependence, ranging from mild desire to craving and compulsive use of the drug. In severe cases, the dependent person gives up other goals and satisfactions to satisfy his or her dependence. For example, a man highly dependent on tobacco may give up his job and increase a health problem rather than stop smoking.

Drug habituation denotes a mild form of psychologic dependence. The individual develops the habit of taking the substance and feels better after taking it. The habituated individual tends to continue the habit even though it may be injurious to his or her health. However, the average, emotionally stable person can deal with its discontinuance and does not seek out the substance compulsively or manifest other behaviors typical of the psychologically dependent person.

In regard to problems of dependence and substance habituation, nurses have these broad responsibilities:

1. To identify when a client is becoming dependent and to report this
2. To observe for symptoms of habituation to or dependence on substances and to identify withdrawal symptoms
3. To make available information on drug habituation and to help clients develop healthy habits

Another source of drug misuse is the unnecessary use of prescription drugs, for example, sedatives and tranquilizers. Clients dependent on drugs are often people with low self-esteem who have distorted views of their environments and are manipulative in human relationships. Nurses can assist these clients in overcoming their dependence by doing the following.

1. Convey a nonjudgmental and positive attitude that the dependence can be overcome.
2. Engage in mutual setting of goals and limits.

3. Share responsibility with the client (Reiss and Melick 1984, p. 132).

Illicit Drugs

Illicit drugs, also called *street drugs*, are those sold illegally. Illicit drugs are of two types: (a) drugs unavailable for purchase under any circumstances, e.g., heroin (in the United States), and (b) drugs normally available with a prescription that are being obtained through illegal channels. Illicit drugs often are taken because of their mood altering effect; i.e., they make the person feel happy or relaxed.

Illicit drugs are the basis for considerable crime in some parts of the United States and Canada. People dependent on heroin, for example, may have to pay $500 a day to support their habit with money they may obtain through illegal activities such as theft. Regular use of illicit drugs can cause both psychologic and physiologic damage to the body. In addition, illicit drugs can be diluted with dangerous substances without the purchaser's knowing.

Nurses who have clients dependent on illicit drugs often see symptoms of withdrawal when a client is admitted to a hospital for another reason. The clinical signs of heroin withdrawal appear within 8 hours of the last dose. They include restlessness, chills, sneezing, hot flashes, abdominal cramps, nausea, and an elevated pulse rate and blood pressure. Any of these signs must be reported immediately so that supportive therapy can be commenced for the client.

Variables Influencing Drug Action

Age and Weight

Very young people and elderly people often are highly responsive to drugs and thus require lower doses. Immature liver and kidney function as well as diminished renal functioning due to aging can affect the action of a drug. See the section on "Developmental Considerations," page 1501, later in this chapter. Body weight also directly affects drug action—the greater the body weight, the greater the dosage required.

Sex

Differences in the way men and women respond to drugs are chiefly due to two factors: differences in distribution of fat and water and hormonal differences. Because women usually weigh less than men, equal drug dosages are likely to affect women more than men. Women usually have more fatty pads than men, and men have more body fluid than women. Some drugs may be more soluble in fat, whereas others are more soluble in water. Thus, men absorb some drugs more readily than women, and vice versa.

Genetic Factors

Individuals may react differently to drugs as a result of genetic factors. A client may be abnormally sensitive to a drug or may metabolize a drug differently than most people because of genetic influences. Sometimes these reactions are mistaken for allergic reactions.

Psychologic Factors

How one feels about a drug and what one believes it can do influence its effect. A traditional example is the reaction of some people to a placebo, a substance (such as normal saline) often given to relieve pain. For some clients, the placebo has the same effect as an analgesic. See Chapter 41, page 1129, for further information.

Illness and Disease

Illness and disease can affect the action of drugs. For example, a person with chronic severe pain may require large quantities of morphine before feeling relief, yet there is little likelihood the client will become psychologically dependent on it. The same amount of morphine given to a person who does not have this pain may produce **psychologic dependence**, emotional reliance on a drug to maintain well-being. See the earlier section on "Kinds of Drug Actions." Another example is aspirin. Aspirin can reduce the body temperature of a feverish client but has no effect on the body temperature of a client without fever. Drug action is altered in clients with circulatory, liver, or kidney dysfunction. Diabetics need larger doses of insulin than usual if the condition is complicated by fever or infection.

Time of Administration

The time of administration of oral medications affects the relative speed with which they act. Orally administered medications are absorbed more quickly if the stomach is empty. Thus, oral medications taken 2 hours before meals act faster than those taken after meals. However, some medications irritate the gastrointestinal tract and need to be given after a meal, when they will be better tolerated. An example is iron (ferrous sulphate).

A client's sleep–wake rhythm may affect the action of a drug. Circadian variations in urine output and blood circulation, for example, may affect a client's response to a drug.

Environment

The client's environment can affect the action of drugs, particularly those used to alter behavior and mood. Therefore, nurses assessing the effects of a drug need to consider the drug itself as well as the client's personality and milieu. An example of a drug that needs to be considered in this context is amitriptyline hydrochloride (Elavil).

Environmental temperature may also affect drug activity. When environmental temperature is high, the peripheral blood vessels dilate, thus intensifying the action of vasodilators. On the other hand, a cold environment and the consequent vasoconstriction inhibit the action of vasodilators but enhance the action of vasoconstrictors.

Pharmacokinetics of Drug Action

Pharmacokinetics is the study of the absorption, distribution, biotransformation, and excretion of drugs.

Absorption

Absorption is the process by which a drug passes into the bloodstream. Unless the drug is administered directly into the bloodstream, absorption is the first step in the movement of the drug through the body.

For absorption to occur, the correct form of the drug must be given by the route intended (see "Routes of Administration," later in this chapter). When a drug in solid form, such as a tablet, is taken orally it must dissolve in the fluid of the stomach or intestines before it can be absorbed into the bloodstream. Giving fluids with a solid-form drug generally will increase its rate of absorption. The rate at which drugs are absorbed varies considerably. **Bioavailability** is the term used to describe the efficiency with which a particular drug preparation is absorbed. Two different preparations of the same drug, e.g., a liquid and a tablet, will in all likelihood have a different bioavailability. When two different versions of the same drug have the same bioavailability, they are said to be **bioequivalent**.

Many factors affect the absorption of a drug in the stomach. Food, for example, can delay the dissolution and absorption of some drugs as well as their passage into the small intestine, where most drug absorption occurs. Food can also combine with molecules of certain drugs, thereby changing their molecular structure and subsequently inhibiting or preventing their absorption. Another factor that affects the absorption of some drugs is the acid medium in the stomach. Acidity can vary according to the time of day, the food ingested, and the age of the client. In addition some drugs are unable or have limited ability to dissolve in the gastrointestinal fluids. This also affects absorption into the bloodstream. Some administered drugs are absorbed by tissues before they reach the stomach. For example, nitroglycerine is administered sublingually (under the tongue), where it is absorbed into the blood vessels that carry it directly to the heart, the intended site of action. If swallowed, this drug will be absorbed into the bloodstream and carried to the liver, where it will be destroyed.

Drugs injected into tissues, i.e., into subcutaneous or muscle tissue, are then absorbed into the bloodstream. Because subcutaneous tissue has a poorer blood supply than muscle tissue, absorption from subcutaneous tissue is slower. The rate of absorption of a drug can be accelerated by the application of heat, which increases blood flow to the area; conversely, absorption can be slowed by the application of cold. In addition, the injection of a vasoconstrictor drug such as epinephrine into the tissue can slow absorption. Some drugs intended to be absorbed slowly are suspended in a low-solubility medium such as oil, to be absorbed slowly over a long period of time.

The absorption of drugs from the rectum into the bloodstream tends to be unpredictable. Therefore, this route is used when other routes are unavailable or when the intended action is localized to the rectum or sigmoid colon (Reiss and Melick 1984, p. 16). In contrast, a drug administered directly into the bloodstream, i.e., intravenously, is immediately in the vascular system without having to be absorbed. This then is the route of choice for rapid action.

Distribution

Distribution is the second step in the pharmacokinetic process. It is the step during which a drug is transported from its site of absorption to its site of action. When a drug enters the bloodstream it is carried most rapidly to the most vascular organs, i.e., liver, kidneys, and brain. Body areas with lower blood supply, i.e., skin and muscles, receive the drug later. The chemical and physical properties of a drug largely determine the area of the body to which the drug will be attracted. For example, drugs that are fat soluble will accumulate in fatty tissue, whereas other drugs may bind with plasma proteins. In situations where two drugs given at the same time both bind to the plasma protein, one bound drug can be displaced by the other. As a result there will be more of one drug unbound in an active state in the blood plasma, causing a greater drug response in the client. Therefore, careful assessment of the client is essential (Reiss and Melick 1984, p. 17).

Biotransformation

Biotransformation, also called *detoxification*, is a process by which a drug is converted to a less active form. Most biotransformation takes place in the liver. There are many drug-metabolizing enzymes in the liver cells that detoxify the drugs. The products of this process are called **metabolites**. There are two types of metabolites: active and inactive. An *active metabolite* has a pharmacologic action itself, whereas an *inactive metabolite* does not.

Drugs are delivered to the liver via the hepatic portal vein, which also carries nutrients from the digestive system. At the same time, the hepatic artery delivers blood rich in oxygen to the liver. The oxygen and nutrients are used by the liver to metabolize and detoxify substances, including drugs. Once the drugs have been detoxified, the metabolites leave the liver via the hepatic veins, which empty into the vena cava.

The biotransformation capability of a client's liver may be impaired. For example, an elderly client, just like a client with hepatic damage, may have a decreased ability to metabolize drugs. In these situations, nurses must be alert to the accumulation of the active drug in the client and to subsequent toxicity.

Excretion

Excretion is the process by which metabolites and drugs are eliminated from the body. Most metabolites are eliminated by the kidneys in the urine; however, some are excreted in the feces, the breath, perspiration and saliva and in breast milk. Certain drugs, e.g., general anesthetics, are excreted in an unchanged form via the respiratory tract. In addition to metabolites, alcohol is eliminated, unchanged, through the lungs.

The efficiency with which the kidneys excrete drugs and metabolites diminishes with age. Elderly people may require smaller doses of a drug because the drug and its metabolites may accumulate in the body. Also, kidney disease can impair excretion of drugs and metabolites.

Drug Action

The action of a drug in the body can be described in terms of its *half-life* or *elimination half-time,* i.e., the time interval required for the body's elimination processes to reduce the concentration of the drug in the body by one half. For example, if a drug's half-life is 8 hours, then the amount of drug in the body:

Initially = 100%
After 8 hours = 50%
After 16 hours = 25%
After 24 hours = 12.5%
After 32 hours = 6.25%

Since the purpose of most drug therapy is to maintain a constant drug level in the body repeated doses are required to maintain that level. When an orally administered drug is absorbed from the gastrointestinal tract into the blood plasma, its concentration in the plasma increases, from zero, and rises until the elimination rate equals the rate of absorption. This point is known as the **peak plasma level**. See Figure 51–1. Unless the same dosage of the drug is continued, its concentration steadily decreases.

It is usual for a number of doses of a drug to be given before a steady concentration is reached in the plasma. The intent in prescribing most drugs is to choose the dose and the interval between doses that will achieve a concentration in the blood plasma that is above the *minimum effective concentration (MEC);* at the same time it should be below the *minimum toxic concentration (MTC).* Often, a drug must be administered a number of times before the concentration in the blood plasma reaches a plateau.

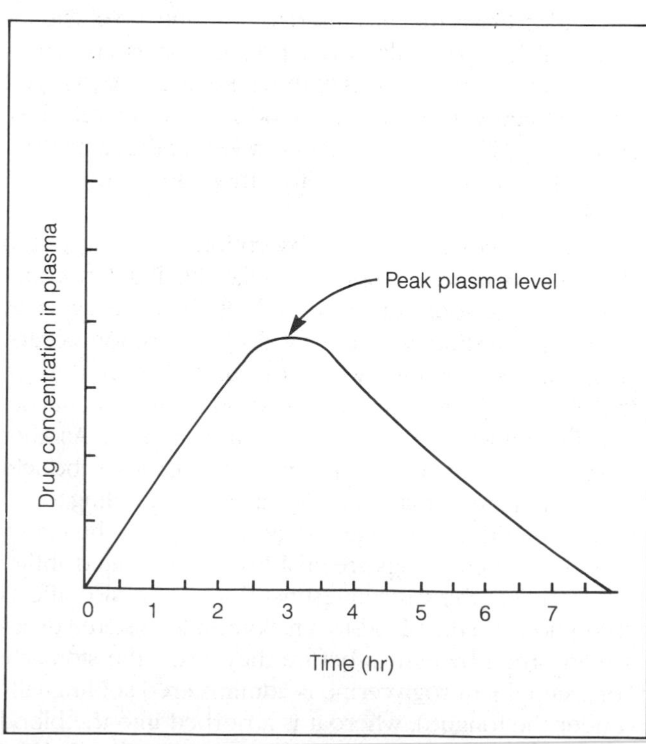

Figure 51–1 A graphic plot of the concentration of a drug in the blood plasma following a single dose.

It has been observed that about four elimination half-times must be allowed before this concentration is reached (Reiss and Melick 1984, p. 19). It is therefore extremely important that nurses administer the exact prescribed dosage of a drug on the prescribed schedule for it to have maximum effectiveness. Key terms related to drug action are listed and described to the right.

Principles of Drug Action

The actions of drugs on the body can be described in terms of four general principles (Reiss and Melick 1984, pp. 14–15).

1. Drugs act on existing cellular functions; they do not create new cellular function. For example, an antibiotic can slow microbial growth; laxatives can increase peristalsis.
2. Drugs act on the body in a number of ways. Some drugs alter the chemical composition of a body fluid; e.g., an antacid decreases the acidity of the gastric contents. Other drugs accumulate in certain body tissues because of their attraction to that tissue; e.g., propylthiouracil (PTU) is an antithyroid drug with an affinity for the thyroid gland, which thereby prevents the formation of thyroid hormones in the gland. Still other drugs act by forming a chemical bond with a receptor in the body. This binding occurs only when the drug and the receptor are compatible.
3. Drugs that reach the same receptor can be expected to produce a similar drug response in a client. For example, most penicillins, such as amoxicillin and cyclacillin, have a similar action.
4. A drug that interacts with a receptor to produce a response is known as an **agonist**. Drugs that have no special pharmacologic action of their own but that inhibit or prevent the action of an agonist are called *specific antagonists*. There are also *partial agonists*, that is, drugs that interact with a receptor to elicit some response but that at the same time have an antagonistic action. For example, morphine—an agonist in depressing the central nervous system—will have its action blocked if a client is also given an antagonist, such as naloxone. However, if the client is given a partial antagonist, such as levallorphan tartrate, the depressant action of the morphine is decreased.

Key Terms Related to Drug Action

■ Onset of action	The time after administration when the body initially responds to the drug
■ Peak plasma level	The highest plasma level achieved by a single dose when the elimination rate of a drug equals the absorption rate
■ Drug half-life (elimination half-life)	The time required for the elimination process to reduce the concentration of the drug to one half what it was at initial administration
■ Plateau	When a drug's concentration in the plasma is maintained during a series of scheduled doses

Routes of Adminstration

Pharmaceutical preparations are generally designed for one or two specific routes of administration. Normally, the route of administration is ordered when the drug is ordered. If a nurse is administering the drug, it is essential that the pharmaceutical preparation be appropriate to the route ordered. For example, phenobarbital is taken orally; phenobarbital sodium may be taken parenterally. See Table 51–6.

Oral

Most commonly, drugs are administered orally. Oral administration is usually least expensive and most convenient for most clients. It is also a safe method of administration in that the skin is not broken as it is for an injection.

The major disadvantages of oral administration are that the drugs may have an unpleasant taste, irritate the gastric mucosa, be absorbed irregularly from the gastrointestinal tract, be absorbed slowly, and, in some cases, harm the client's teeth. For example, hydrochloric acid can damage the enamel of teeth.

Sublingual

A drug may be placed under the tongue (**sublingual**), where it dissolves. See Figure 51–2. In a relatively short time the drug is largely absorbed into the blood vessels on the underside of the tongue. The medication should not be swallowed. Drugs such as nitroglycerine are commonly given in this manner.

Table 51–6 Routes of Administration

Route	Advantages	Disadvantages
Oral	Most convenient Usually least expensive Safe, does not break skin barrier Administration usually does not cause stress	Inappropriate for clients nauseated or vomiting Drug may have unpleasant taste or odor Inappropriate when gastrointestinal tract has reduced mobility Inappropriate when client cannot swallow or is unconscious Cannot be used before certain diagnostic tests or surgical procedures Drug may discolor teeth, harm tooth enamel Drug may irritate gastric mucosa Drug can be aspirated by seriously ill clients
Sublingual	Same as for oral, *plus*: Drug can be administered for local effect Drug is rapidly absorbed into the bloodstream Ensures greater potency because drug directly enters the blood and bypasses the liver	If swallowed, drug may be inactivated by gastric juice Drug must remain under tongue until dissolved and absorbed
Buccal	Same as for sublingual	Same as for sublingual
Rectal	Can be used when drug has objectionable taste or odor Drug released at slow, steady rate	Dose absorbed is unpredictable
Skin	Provides a local effect Few side-effects	May be messy and may soil clothes Drug can rapidly enter body through abrasions and cause systemic effects
Subcutaneous	Onset of drug action faster than oral	Must involve sterile technique because breaks skin barrier More expensive than oral Can administer only small volume Slower than intramuscular administration Some drugs can irritate tissues and cause pain Can be anxiety-producing
Intramuscular	Pain from irritating drugs is minimized Can administer larger volume than subcutaneous Drug is rapidly absorbed	Breaks skin barrier Can be anxiety-producing
Intradermal	Absorption is slow (this is an advantage when testing for allergies)	Amount of drug administered must be small Breaks skin barrier
Intravenous	Rapid effect	Limited to highly soluble drugs Drug distribution may be inhibited by poor circulation
Inhalation	Introduces drug throughout the respiratory tract Rapid localized relief Drug can be administered when client is unconscious	Drug intended for localized effect can have systemic effect Only of use for the respiratory system

Buccal

Buccal means "pertaining to the cheek." In buccal administration, a medication (e.g., a tablet) is held in the mouth against the mucous membranes of the cheek until the drug dissolves. See Figure 51–3. The drug may act locally on the mucous membranes of the mouth or systemically when it is swallowed in the saliva.

Parenteral

Parenteral administration is administration other than through the alimentary tract, i.e., by needle. Some of the more common routes for parenteral administration are:

- **Subcutaneous** (hypodermic): into the subcutaneous tissue, just below the skin
- **Intramuscular**: into a muscle
- **Intradermal**: under the epidermis (into the dermis)
- **Intravenous**: into a vein

Some of the less commonly used routes for parenteral administration are **intraarterial** (into an artery), **intracardiac** (into the heart muscle), **intraosseous** (into a bone), and **intrathecal** or **intraspinal** (into the spinal canal). These less common injections are normally carried out by physicians. All parenteral therapy utilizes ster-

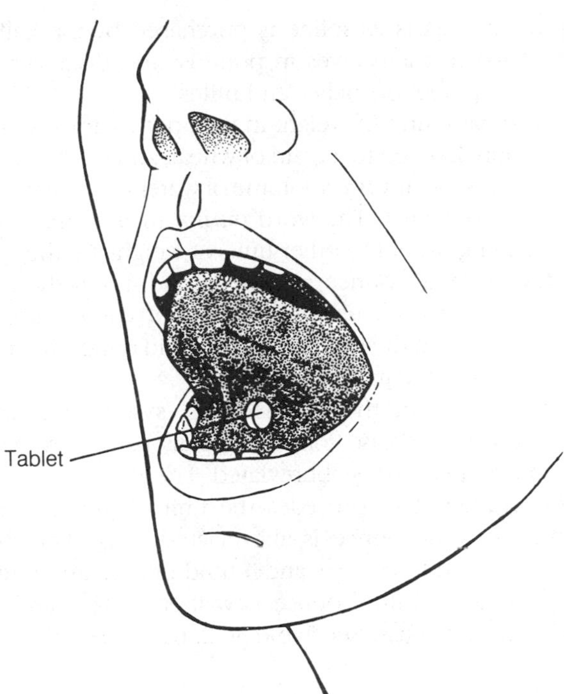

Figure 51–2 Sublingual administration of a tablet.

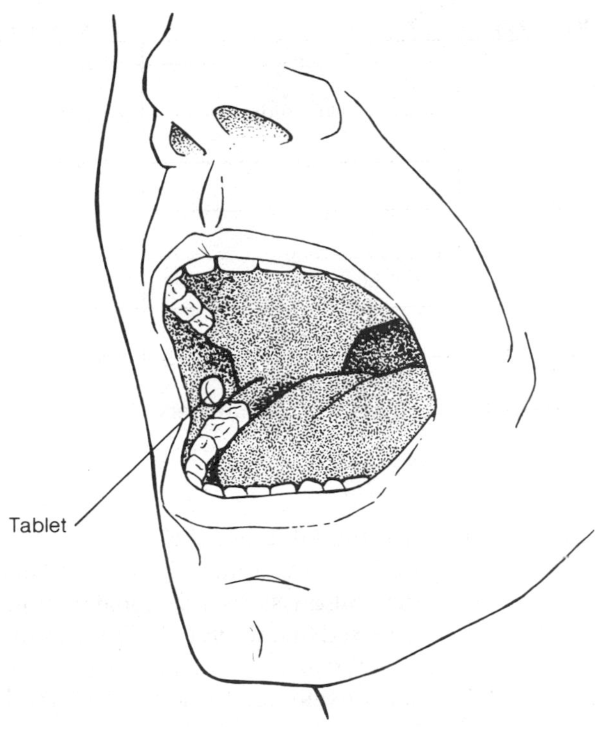

Figure 51–3 Buccal administration of a tablet.

ile equipment and sterile drug solutions. Parenteral therapy has the primary advantage of fast absorption of a measured amount of drug.

Topical

Topical applications are those applied to a circumscribed surface area of the body. They affect only the area to which they are applied. Topical applications include:

- **Dermatologic preparations**, medications applied to the skin.
- **Instillations**, medications applied into body cavities or orifices such as the urinary bladder, eyes, ears, nose, rectum, or vagina.
- **Inhalations**, medications administered into the respiratory tract by nebulizers or positive pressure breathing apparatuses. Air, oxygen, and vapor are generally used to carry the drug into the lungs. See Chapter 45.

Systems of Measurement

Three systems of measurement are used in North America: the metric system, the apothecaries' system, and the household system, which is similar to the apothecaries' system. It would be much simpler for everyone if one system were universally accepted; however, because all systems are in current use, it is necessary for nurses to become familiar with the three systems and to be able to convert from one to the other as necessary. In recent years Canada has officially adopted the metric system, which is being used increasingly in the United States.

Metric System

The metric system, devised by the French in the latter part of the 18th century, is the system prescribed by law in most European countries. The metric system is very logically organized into units of ten; it is a decimal system. Basic units can be multiplied or divided by ten to form secondary units. Multiples are calculated by moving the decimal point to the right, and divisions by moving the decimal point to the left.

Basic units of measurement are the meter, the liter, and the gram. Prefixes derived from Latin designate subdivisions of the basic unit: deci (1/10 or 0.1), centi (1/100 or 0.01), and milli (1/1000 or 0.001). Multiples of the basic unit are designated by prefixes derived from Greek: deka (10), hecto (100), and kilo (1000). Only the measurements of volume (the liter) and of weight (the gram) are discussed in this chapter. These are the measures used in medication administration. See Figure 51–4. In medical

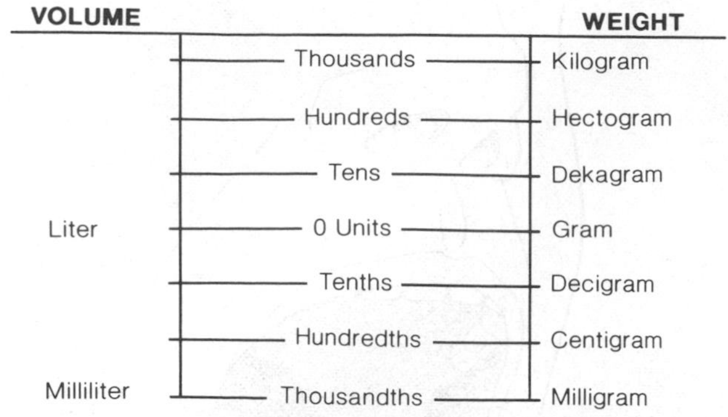

Figure 51–4 Basic metric measurements of volume and weight.

and nursing practice the kilogram (kg) is the only multiple of the gram used, and the milligram (mg) and microgram (mcg or μg) are subdivisions. Fractional parts of the liter are usually expressed in milliliters (ml), for example, 600 ml; multiples of the liter are usually expressed as liters or milliliters, for example, 2.5 liters or 2500 ml.

Apothecaries' System

The apothecaries' system, older than the metric system, was brought to the United States from England during the colonial period. North Americans are familiar with most units of measure in the apothecaries' system, since they are used in everyday life. For example, milk is bought in pints or quarts, gasoline is purchased by the gallon, people weigh themselves in pounds, and distances are measured in feet or inches and miles.

The basic unit of weight in the apothecaries' system is the grain, likened to a grain of wheat, and the basic unit of volume is the **minim**, a volume of water equal in weight to a grain of wheat. The word *minim* means "the least." In ascending order the other units of weight are the scruple, the dram, the ounce, and the pound. Today the scruple (scr) is seldom used. The units of volume are, in ascending order, the fluid dram, the fluid ounce, the pint, the quart, and the gallon.

Quantities in the apothecaries' system are often expressed by lowercase Roman numerals, particularly when the unit of measure is abbreviated. The Roman numeral follows rather than precedes the unit of measure. For example, a fluid ounce is abbreviated as f℥. Two fluid ounces are written as f℥ii, and 4 fluid ounces are written as f℥iv. One half fluid ounce is written as f℥ss, and 1½ fluid ounces as f℥iss. See Table 30-2, page 641.

Household System

Household measures may be used when more accurate systems of measure are not required. Included in household measures are drops, teaspoons, tablespoons, cups, and glasses. Although pints and quarts are often found in the home, they are defined as apothecaries' measures. Equivalent units of the household system are in Appendix F.

Converting Units of Weight and Measure

Sometimes drugs are dispensed from the pharmacy in grams when the order specifies milligrams, or they are dispensed in milligrams though ordered in grains. The nurse preparing a medicated irrigation may find that the order calls for quarts and that the solution is dispensed in liter containers. In all situations it is the nurse's responsibility to convert units of measure or weight, and thus nurses must be aware of approximate equivalents within each system of measurement and among systems.

Converting Weights Within the Metric System

It is relatively simple to arrive at equivalent units of weight within the metric system, since the system is based on units of ten. Only three metric units of weight are used for drug dosages, the gram (g), milligram (mg), and microgram (mcg or μg): 1000 mg or 1,000,000 mcg equals 1 g. Equivalents are computed by dividing or multiplying; e.g., to change milligrams to grams, milligrams are divided by 1000. The simplest way to divide by 1000 is to move the decimal point three places to the left:

1000 mg = 1 g

500 mg = 0.5 g

Conversely, to convert grams to milligrams, the grams are multiplied by 1000, or the decimal point is moved three places to the right:

0.006 g = 6 mg

Converting Weights and Measures Among Systems

When preparing client medications, a nurse may find it necessary to convert weights or volumes from one system to another. As an example, the pharmacy may dispense milligrams or grams of chloral hydrate, yet the nurse must administer an order that reads chloral hydrate grains viiss. To prepare the correct dose, the nurse must convert from the apothecaries' to the metric system. The nurse may have to convert from the apothecaries' or metric system to the household system to give clients a useful, realistic measure to use at home. All conversions are approximate, that is, not totally precise.

Converting Units of Volume

It is advisable for a nurse to learn some commonly used approximate equivalents, such as those in Table 51–7.

By learning the equivalents in Table 51–7, the nurse can make many conversions readily. For example, 15 minims = approximately 15 drops; therefore 1 minim is approximately 1 drop. Similarly, 1 quart approximates 1000 ml, and 1 gallon approximates 4000 ml; therefore 4 quarts is approximately 1 gallon.

The following are some situations in which nurses need to apply a knowledge of volume conversion.

1. Milliliter dosages may need to be fractionalized. The nurse can fractionalize milliliter dosages by remembering that 1 ml contains 15 drops or minims.
2. Fluid drams and ounces are commonly used in prescribing liquid medications, such as cough syrups, laxatives, antacids, and antibiotics for children. The fluid ounce is frequently converted to milliliters when measuring a client's fluid intake or output.
3. Liters and milliliters are the volumes commonly used in preparing solutions for enemas, irrigating solutions for douches, bladder irrigations, and solutions for cleaning open wounds. In some situations, the nurse needs to convert the volumes of such solutions.

Converting Units of Weight

The units of weight most commonly used in nursing practice are the gram, milligram, and kilogram and the grain and the pound. Household units of weight are generally not applicable.

Table 51–8 shows metric and apothecaries' approximate equivalents. Learning these equivalents helps the nurse make weight conversions readily.

Nurses need to convert units of weight in the following situations:

1. Converting a person's body weight from kilograms to pounds and vice versa
2. Converting grams and milligrams to grains and vice versa, for example, when preparing medications

When converting units of weight from the metric system to the apothecaries' system, the nurse should keep in mind that a milligram is smaller than a grain (1 mg = 1/60 grain and 1 grain = 60 mg). The result of converting a smaller unit (milligram) to a larger unit (grain) is a smaller number. Thus, the nurse must divide (by 60 if converting from milligrams to grains). Conversely, when converting from a larger unit to a smaller unit, the nurse multiplies (by 60 if converting from grains to milligrams), and the product is a larger number. In other words:

Small units (mg) to large units (grains) = a smaller number

Large units (grains) to small units (mg) = a larger number

$$\frac{3000 \text{ mg}}{60} = 50 \text{ grains}$$

$$50 \text{ grains} \times 60 = 3000 \text{ mg}$$

When converting pounds to kilograms, the nurse applies the same rule. The pound is a smaller unit than the kilogram, and the nurse converts by dividing or multiplying by 2.2:

$$\frac{110 \text{ lb}}{2.2} = 50 \text{ kg}$$

$$50 \text{ kg} \times 2.2 = 110 \text{ lb}$$

The conversion of milligrams to grams was previously discussed. The decimal point is moved three spaces to the left:

$$3000 \text{ mg} = 3 \text{ g}$$

Table 51–7 **Equivalent Measures: Metric, Apothecaries', and Household**

Metric		Apothecaries'		Household
1 ml	=	15 minims (min or m)	=	15 drops (gtt)
15 ml	=	4 fluid drams (fʒ)	=	1 tablespoon (Tbsp)
30 ml	=	1 fluid ounce (f℥)	=	same
500 ml	=	1 pint (pt)	=	same
1000 ml	=	1 quart (qt)	=	same
4000 ml	=	1 gallon (gal)	=	same

Table 51–8 **Approximate Weight Equivalents: Metric and Apothecaries' Systems**

Metric		Apothecaries'
1 mg	=	1/60 grain
60 mg	=	1 grain
1 g	=	15 grains
4 g	=	1 dram
30 g	=	1 ounce
500 g	=	1.1 pound (lb)
1000 g (1 kg)	=	2.2 lb

Calculating Fractional Dosages

The need to calculate fractional dosages arises chiefly when small dosages must be administered to infants and children. Such calculation may also be necessary in preparing preoperative medications, injectable analgesics, and intravenous medications for adult clients.

Dosages for Children

Although dosage is stated in the medication order, nurses must understand something about the safe dosages for children. Unlike adult dosages, children's dosages are not always standard. There are several formulas to determine pediatric dosages using body surface area and weight.

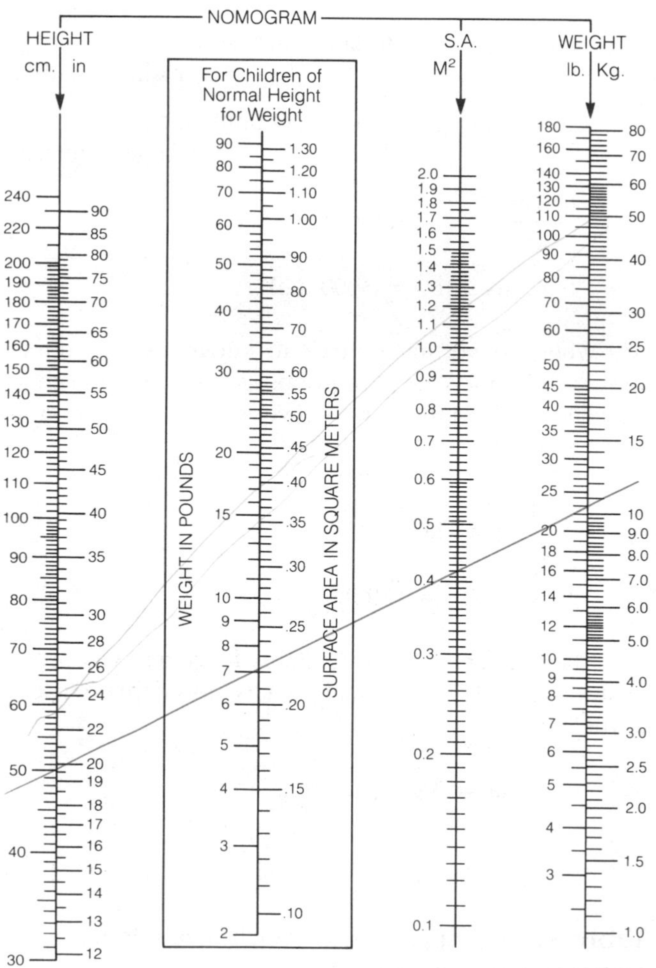

Figure 51–5 Nomogram with estimated body surface area. A straight line is drawn between the child's height (on the left) and the child's weight (on the right). The point at which the line intersects the surface area column is the estimated body surface area.

Source: Courtesy of the Commonwealth Fund and Harvard University.

Body Surface Area

Body surface area is determined by using a nomogram and the child's height and weight. This is considered to be the most accurate method of calculating a child's dose. Standard nomograms give a child's body surface area according to weight and age. See Figure 51–5. The formula is the ratio of the child's body surface area to the surface area of an average adult (1.7 square meters, or 1.7 m^2), multiplied by the normal adult dose of the drug:

$$\text{Child's dose} = \frac{\text{Surface area of child } (m^2)}{1.7\ m^2} \times \text{normal adult dose}$$

For example, if a child weighs 10 kg and his height is 50 cm, then he has a body surface area of 0.4 m^2. Therefore, the child's dose of tetracycline corresponding to an adult dose of 250 mg would be:

$$\text{Child's dose} = \frac{0.4\ m^2}{1.7\ m^2} \times 250\ \text{mg}$$

$$= 0.23 \times 250 = 58.82\ \text{mg}$$

Clark's Rule

Clark's rule, which applies to children of all ages, is less accurate than the above method for calculating pediatric dosages. It compares the child's body weight to the weight of a 150-pound (68-kilogram) adult and multiplies this ratio by the adult dose:

$$\text{Child's dose} = \frac{\text{Child's weight (lb)}}{150\ \text{lb}} \times \text{adult dose}$$

For example, for a child weighing 30 pounds and requiring Demerol, for which the adult dose is 100 mg:

$$\text{Child's dose} = \frac{30\ \text{lb}}{150\ \text{lb}} \times 100\ \text{mg}$$

$$= 0.2 \times 100 = 20\ \text{mg}$$

Fractional Dosages from Vials or Ampules

Many medications are already in liquid form and ready for use. For example, meperidine hydrochloride (Demerol) is often distributed in large vials and prepared in dilutions of 50 mg per ml. Thus if the order calls for 100 mg, the nurse injects 2 ml, and if it calls for 75 mg, the nurse injects 1½ ml. To calculate the volume of solution that contains a certain milligram dosage, the nurse uses this formula:

$$\frac{\text{D (amount desired)}}{\text{H (amount on hand)}} = \text{Amount (volume) wanted}$$

$$\frac{40\text{ mg}}{50\text{ mg}} = \frac{4}{5}\text{ml}$$

Example problem Prepare 4 mg of a drug from a vial containing 20 mg in a 5-ml solution. Formula:

$$\frac{\text{Drug available}}{\text{Amount of solution}} = \frac{\text{Dose wanted}}{x\text{ ml}}$$

$$\frac{20\text{ mg}}{5\text{ ml}} = \frac{4\text{ mg}}{x\text{ ml}}$$

Therefore

$$\frac{20}{5} = \frac{4}{x}$$

Cross multiply:

$$20x = 20$$

$$x = \frac{20}{20} = 1\text{ ml}$$

Medication Orders

A physician is the person who usually determines the clients' medications needs and orders medications, although in some settings nurse-practitioners now order some drugs. Usually, the order is written, although telephone and verbal orders are acceptable in a number of agencies. Nursing students need to know the agency policies about medication orders. In some hospitals, for example, only graduate nurses are permitted to accept telephone and verbal orders.

Types of Medication Orders

Four common medication orders are the stat order, the single order, the standing order, and the p.r.n. order.

1. A *stat* order indicates that the medication is to be given immediately and only once, e.g., Demerol 100 mg IM stat.
2. The *single* order is for a medication to be given once at a specified time, e.g., Seconal 100 mg h.s. before surgery.
3. The *standing* order may or may not have a termination date. A standing order may be carried out indefinitely (e.g., multiple vitamins daily) until an order is written to cancel it, or it may be carried out for a specified number of days (e.g., Demerol 100 mg IM q.4h. × 5 days). In some agencies, standing orders are automatically canceled after a specified number of days and must be reordered.
4. A *p.r.n.* order permits the nurse to give a medication when in her or his judgment the client requires it, e.g., Amphojel 15 ml p.r.n. The nurse must use good judgment as to when the medication is needed and when it can be safely administered.

Policies about physicians' orders vary considerably from agency to agency. Generally, there is an order as to which medicines are to be given to a client by nurses and which medications a client can keep at the hospital bedside to self-administer. Hospitals also have varying policies regarding orders. It is not unusual for a client's orders to be automatically canceled after surgery or an examination involving an anesthetic. New orders must then be written. This policy is a safety measure to ensure that physicians are aware of their clients' conditions, particularly at critical times. Most agencies also have lists of abbreviations officially accepted for use in the agency. Both nurses and physicians may need to refer to these lists if they have been working in a different agency. These abbreviations can be used on legal documents, such as clients' charts. See Table 51–9.

Drug Order: Essential Parts

The drug order has six essential parts: (a) full name of the client, (b) date the order is written, (c) name of the drug to be administered, (d) dosage of the drug, (e) method of administration, and (f) signature of the physician or nurse-practitioner. In addition, unless it is a standing order, it should state the number of doses or the number of days the drug is to be administered.

Full Name of the Client

A client's full name, that is, the first and last names and middle initials or names, should always be used to avoid

Table 51–9 Common Abbreviations Used in Medication Orders

Abbreviation	Explanation	Example of Administration Time
a.c.	before meals	0700, 1100, and 1700 hours
ad lib	freely, as desired	
agit	shake, stir	
aq	water	
aq dest	distilled water	
b.i.d.	twice a day	0900 and 2100 hours
c̄	with	
cap	capsule	
comp	compound	
dil	dissolve, dilute	
elix	elixir	
h.	an hour	
h.s.	at bedtime	
I.M.	intramuscular	
I.V.	intravenous	
M. or m.	mix	
no.	number	
non rep	do not repeat	
OD	right eye	
OS or o.l.	left eye	
OU	both eyes	
p.c.	after meals	0900, 1300, and 1900 hours
p.o.	by mouth	
p.r.n.	when needed	
q.	every	
q.d.	every day	
q.AM (o.m.)	every morning	1000 hours
q.h. (q.1h.)	every hour	
q.2h.	every 2 hours	0800, 1000, 1200 hours, etc
q.3h.	every 3 hours	0900, 1200, 1500 hours, etc
q.4h.	every 4 hours	1000, 1400, 1800 hours, etc
q.6h.	every 6 hours	0600, 1200, 1800, 2400 hours
q.h.s.	every night at bedtime	
q.i.d.	four times a day	1000, 1400, 1800, 2200 hours
q.o.d.	every other day	0900 hours on odd dates
q.s.	sufficient quantity	
rept	may be repeated	
Rx	take	
s̄	without	
s.c.	subcutaneous	
Sig. or S.	label	
s.o.s.	if it is needed	
ss or s̄s̄	one half	
stat	at once	
sup or supp	suppository	
susp	suspension	
t.i.d.	three times a day	1000, 1400, and 1800 hours
Tr. or tinct	tincture	

confusion between two clients who have the same last names. In some agencies the client's admission number is put on the order as further identification.

Some hospitals imprint the client's name and hospital number on all forms. This imprinter is on the nursing unit; it is much like the credit card imprinters used in shops.

Date

Shown on an order are the day, the month, and the year the order was written; some agencies also require that the time of day be written. Writing the time of day on the order can eliminate errors when nursing shifts change. Putting the time of day on the order also makes it clear when certain orders automatically terminate. For example, in some settings, narcotics can be ordered only for 48 hours after surgery. Therefore a drug that is ordered at 1600 hours February 1, 1988 is automatically canceled at 1600 hours February 3, 1988.

Many agencies use the 24-hour clock, which eliminates confusion between morning and afternoon times. Time with the 24-hour clock starts at midnight, which is 0000 hours. See Figure 30–5, page 639.

Name of the Drug

The name of the drug ordered must be clearly written. In some settings only generic names are permitted; however, trade names are widely used in hospitals and health agencies. In most settings where drug orders are written, nurses and physicians can refer to the *Physician's Desk Reference*, the *Compendium of Pharmaceuticals and Specialties*, and similar sources. A nurse who is unsure about a drug that is ordered needs to look it up in a suitable reference before preparing or administering the drug. Some hospitals provide their own formulary listing all drugs stocked in the hospital.

In some situations, hospital clients may continue to take medications prescribed before they were admitted.

To know what drug the client is taking, the nurse needs to check the drug label or check with the physician or the pharmacy if the bottle is unlabeled.

Dosage

The dosage of the drug includes the amount, the times or frequency of administration, and in many instances the strength; for example, tetracycline *250 mg* (amount) *four times a day* (frequency); hydrochloric acid *10%* (strength) *5 ml* (amount) *three times a day with meals* (time and frequency).

Dosages can be written in apothecaries' or metric systems, but the metric system is being used increasingly in North America.

Method of Administration

Also included in the order is the method of administering the drug. This part of the order, like other parts, is frequently abbreviated. See Table 51-9 for abbreviations of routes of administration. It is not unusual for a drug to have several possible routes of administration; therefore, it is important that the route be included in the order. If the nurse believes the client's condition makes the ordered route of administration inappropriate, the nurse must notify the physician to change the order. Changes in clients' conditions sometimes make it impossible to carry out a standing order. For example, if a client becomes unconscious, a standing order for an oral medication must be changed.

Signature

The signature of the ordering physician or nurse makes the drug order a legal request. An unsigned order has no validity, and the ordering physician or nurse needs to be notified if his or her order is unsigned.

In agencies where telephone orders are taken, the nurse usually indicates the name of the person who phoned in the order. The nurse signs the order, but usually the person who ordered the drug must also sign at a later date. Some hospitals have policies that those who give orders by telephone must sign those orders within a certain time, for example, 48 hours after they have communicated the order.

When a physician writes a prescription for a client, the prescription also includes information for the pharmacist. Therefore, a prescription's content differs from that of a medication order in a hospital. Compare the parts of a prescription listed above on the right with Figure 51-6.

Parts of a Prescription

- Descriptive information about the client: name, address and, sometimes, age
- Date on which the prescription was written
- The R symbol meaning "take thou"
- Medication name, dosage, and strength
- Route of administration
- Dispensing instructions for the pharmacist, e.g., "Dispense 30 capsules"
- Directions for administration to be given to the client, e.g., "Sig. Tab ī tid with meals"
- Refill and/or special labeling, e.g., "Refill × 1" or "Do not label"
- Prescriber's signature

Communicating a Medication Order

A drug order is written by a physician, usually on the client's chart or in a special book. From there it is copied by a nurse or clerk to a Kardex and to a medication card. Increasingly nurses are being provided with computer printouts of a client's medications instead of copying the physician's order. This method avoids errors of copying and saves nursing time.

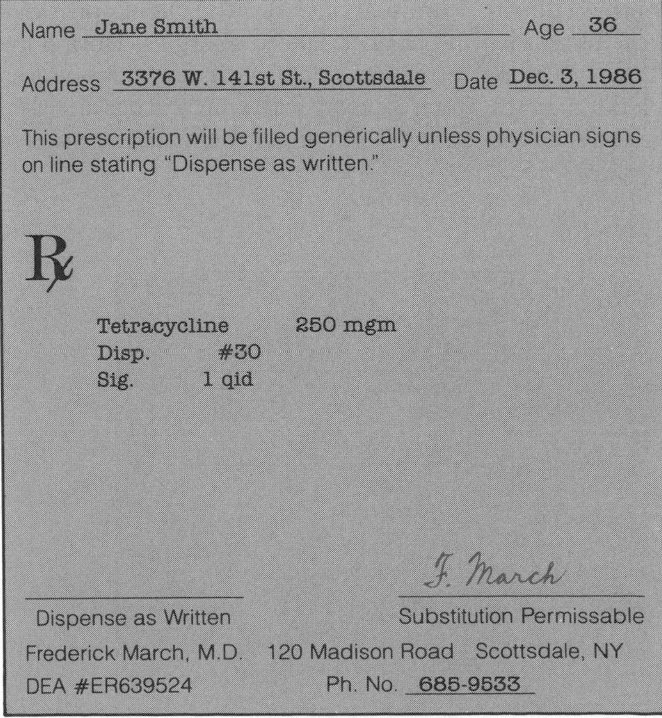
Name Jane Smith Age 36
Address 3376 W. 141st St., Scottsdale Date Dec. 3, 1986
This prescription will be filled generically unless physician signs on line stating "Dispense as written."
℞
Tetracycline 250 mgm
Disp. #30
Sig. 1 qid
F. March
Dispense as Written Substitution Permissable
Frederick March, M.D. 120 Madison Road Scottsdale, NY
DEA #ER639524 Ph. No. 685-9533

Figure 51–6 A prescription filled out for a client by a physician.

Medication cards (see Figure 51–7) vary in form but include the client's name, room, and bed number; drug name and dose; and times and method of administration. In some agencies the date the order was prescribed and the date the order expires are also included, along with the signature of the person writing the order.

Assessment

Assessment relative to medications includes:

1. A medication history
2. Assessing the client's condition
3. Assessing the client's learning needs regarding the medication

Medication History

The medication history includes information about the drugs the client is taking currently or has taken recently. This includes prescription drugs, over-the-counter drugs such as antacids, alcohol and tobacco, and nonsanctioned drugs such as marijuana. Sometimes one or more of these drugs may affect the choice of another, different medication, since they may be incompatible.

An important part of the history is the client's knowledge of his or her drug allergies. Some clients can tell a nurse, "I am allergic to penicillin, adhesive tape, and curry." Other clients may not be sure about allergic reactions. An illness occurring after a drug was taken may not be identified as an allergy, but the client may associate the drug with an illness or unusual reaction. The client's physician can often give information about allergies. During the history, the nurse tries to elicit information about drug dependencies. The frequency with which drugs are taken and the client's perceived need for them are measures of dependence.

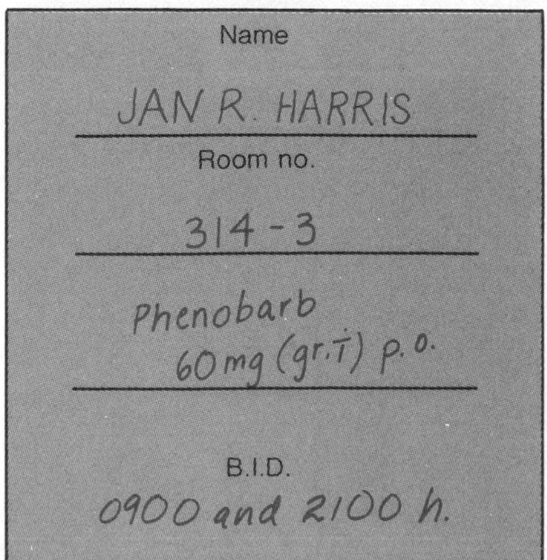

Figure 51–7 A sample medication card containing essential information.

Also included in the history is the client's normal eating habits. Sometimes the medication schedule needs to be coordinated with mealtimes or the ingestion of foods. Where a medication must be taken with food on a specified schedule, clients can often adjust their mealtime or have a snack, e.g., with a bedtime medication. In addition, certain foods are incompatible with certain medications, e.g., milk is incompatible with tetracycline.

Any problems the client may have in self-administering a medication must also be identified. If a client has poor eyesight, for example, special labels may be required for the medication container; an elderly client with unsteady hands may not be able to hold a syringe or to inject herself or himself or another.

Client Assessment

The nurse should always assess a client's physical status prior to giving any medication. The exact nature of this assignment depends on the client's illness, his or her condition, and the intended drug and route of administration. Clients who are dyspneic, for example, need to have their respirations assessed before being given any medication that could affect their respirations. Or, a client who says that she or he is nauseated may not be able to swallow a capsule and retain it.

In general the nurse assesses the client's condition before giving *any* medication that could affect her or his condition. Not only may the findings contraindicate providing the medication, they can also serve as baseline data against which to compare the effects of the medication. For example, a nurse should assess a client's respirations (see Chapter 34, page 786) as well as auscultate for chest sounds before administering a bronchodilator or an expectorant.

In addition, a nurse must sometimes assess the client's need for a drug. This is particularly true of analgesics and p.r.n. medications.

Learning Needs

A client's learning needs relate to what she or he desires to learn and what she or he needs to know. For example, one client may not want to know about the medications, whereas another may want to know everything available about his or her drugs. Clients who need to follow a medication regimen may need to have specific knowledge and skills, e.g., assessing their own pulse rate as part of this regimen. See Chapter 2, page 65, for additional information about compliance and Chapter 29, "Teaching and Learning."

Some clients are given prescriptions while they are in hospital for medications they are to take after discharge. This is also an important area of client teaching. This type of prescription usually contains more information than the usual medication order because the client will need to know when to take the medicine and any other directions, such as after meals. See "Parts of a Prescription," page 1497.

Medications may be prescribed by trade name or generic name. In 45 states of the U.S. the law permits the pharmacist to select which of these to dispense unless the prescriber specifies brand name by signing above the drug name the words "Dispense as written." When a drug is marketed by more than one company, significant amounts can often be saved, particularly if a generic product can be purchased.

Administering Medications Safely

Process of Administering Medications

When administering any drug, regardless of the route of administration, the nurse must do the following.

1. Identify the client.
2. Administer the drug.
3. Provide adjunctive interventions as indicated.
4. Record.
5. Evaluate the client's response to the drug.

The five "rights" listed below on the right are guides to accurate drug administration.

Identifying the Client

Identifying a client sounds simple—and usually is. But errors can and do occur, usually because one client gets a drug intended for another. In hospitals, most clients wear some sort of identification, such as a wristband with name and hospital identification number. To prevent mistakes, nurses also ask the client's name, or they state the name clearly and then listen to the client's response, before administering any medication.

Administering the Drug

Equally important is giving the correct drug. Medication orders and cards or lists need to be read carefully and checked against the name on the medication envelope or on the drawer in which the client's medications are kept if a medication cart is used. The medication is then administered in the dosage and by the route ordered.

Adjunctive Nursing Intervention

Clients may need help when receiving medications. They may require physical assistance, for instance, in assuming positions for intramuscular injections, or they may need explanations about the medications and guidance about measures to enhance drug effectiveness and prevent complications, e.g., drinking fluids. Some clients convey fear about their medications. The nurse can allay fears by listening carefully to clients' concerns and giving correct information. Clients may give the nurse information regarding their drugs. One client may say that an analgesic is effective for only 10 or 15 minutes, another may feel nauseated about 20 minutes after ingesting a drug, a third may feel dizzy each afternoon at about the same time, and a fourth may have pain in the right leg. This type of information needs to be recorded and, when appropriate, relayed to the physician. In some cases, simple nursing interventions can relieve the problem; for instance, the nurse can provide milk with a medication to a client with nausea. In other instances, it may be necessary for the physician to reassess the needs of the client.

Recording

Once complete, the intervention is recorded on the client's record. The facts recorded are name of the drug, dosage, method of administration, specific relevant data such as pulse rate (taken in most settings prior to the administration of digitalis), and any other pertinent information. The record should include the exact time of administration and in most agencies the signature of the nurse providing

---

Five "Rights" of Drug Administration

- Right drug
- Right dose
- Right time
- Right route
- Right client

---

the medication. Often medications that are given regularly are recorded on a special flow record, whereas p.r.n. or stat medications are recorded separately on the nurse's notes.

Evaluating Client Response

The client's response to a medication can often be detected directly after intravenous administration, 10 to 20 minutes after an intramuscular or subcutaneous injection, and anywhere from immediately to several days after oral administration. For example, the ingestion of aluminum hydroxide gel (Amphojel) often provides almost immediate relief to a client with epigastric pain; on the other hand, the effects of an antibiotic may not be noticeable for 3 or 4 days.

The kinds of behavior that reflect the action or lack of action of a drug are as variable as the purposes of the drugs themselves. The anxious client may show the effects of a tranquilizer by behavior that reflects a lowered stress level—for example, slower speech or fewer random movements. The effectiveness of a sedative can often be measured by how well a client slept; the effectiveness of an antispasmodic, by how much pain the client feels. In all nursing activities, nurses need to be aware of the medications that a client is taking and record their effectiveness as assessed by the client and the nurse on the client's chart. If appropriate, the nurse may also report the client's response directly to the senior nurse and physician.

Guidelines for Administering Medications

1. Although medications are prescribed chiefly by physicians, the nurses who administer them are responsible for their own actions. Therefore you should question any order you consider incorrect. The physician's order should include the client's full name, the order date, the name of the medication, the dosage, the method and frequency of administration, and the physician's signature. The order may include additional directions, e.g., "Withhold dosage if pulse is below 60."
2. Before administering a medication, make sure you are knowledgeable about the drug. Most nursing units have drug reference books.
3. Federal laws govern the use of narcotics and barbiturates. Narcotics and barbiturates are kept in a drawer or cupboard with a double lock. Special forms are used for recording them. The data usually required are the client's name, drug, and physician; date; time of administration; dosage; and signature of the person who prepared and administered the drug.
4. Medication cards are used in some agencies as guides for preparing medications. A card normally includes the client's name, room and bed number; name of the drug; dosage; and times and method of administration. In some agencies, the date on which the order was prescribed and the date on which it expires are also included.
5. To avoid errors while preparing and giving medications, concentrate on the task. Use the five "rights" as a guide: right drug, right dose, right route, right client, right time.
6. To prevent an error when preparing medications, read the label on the container three times: before taking it off the shelf, while pouring the medication, and after placing it back on the shelf.
7. Ensure that the drug preparation is appropriate to the route prescribed.
8. If you prepare medications, you must also administer and chart them. You are the only person who can confirm the medication.
9. When preparing medications, do *not* use the following:
   a. Medications from unmarked containers or containers with illegible labels—even though you think you can identify the drug.
   b. Medications that are cloudy or have changed color.
   c. Medications that have a sediment at the bottom, unless the medication normally requires shaking before use.

   Return such medications to the pharmacy. Write the reason for their return on the label.
10. Never return a medication to a container or transfer a medication from one container to another. This practice avoids mixing drugs or placing a drug in the wrong container.
11. Identify the client correctly and carefully, using the appropriate means of identification, e.g., the identification bracelet.
12. With rare exceptions, clients have the right to know the name and the action of the drug they are taking, and they have the right to refuse a medication. Medications that are refused must be discarded and the reason for refusal recorded.
13. Provide the correct adjunctive nursing interventions with the medication; e.g., measure a pulse rate before giving a digitalis preparation, or notify the physician before giving the drug if the apical pulse is below 60.
14. Medications should not be left at the bedside, with the exception of antacids, nonnarcotic cough syrups, nitroglycerine, lotions or ointments, certain eye medications, and inhalants. Check agency policies about each of these. When medications are left at the bedside, determine from the client when she or he takes or applies them.

15. Give medications within 30 minutes of the time ordered, except for preoperative medications, which must be given at the exact time ordered, or medications that are ordered to be given hourly or every 2 hours (e.g., eye medications prior to surgery).
16. If a client vomits after taking an oral medication, report the fact to the responsible nurse, and state the names of all medications given. Withhold the medication(s). Often the physician will reorder the same drug by a different route, e.g., subcutaneously or intramuscularly.
17. Special precautions must be observed for certain drugs. Most agencies require that two qualified nurses double-check the dosages of anticoagulants, insulin, digitalis preparations, and certain IV medications. Check agency policies.
18. After a medication has been administered, record it on the client's chart. The recording should include the time, the name of the drug, the dosage, the route of administration, and any related data.
19. Most agencies have an official list of abbreviations used in medication orders and in recording. See Table 51–9 and *Learning Guide* for commonly used abbreviations.
20. Evaluate the effectiveness of a medication a suitable time after its administration. For example, the initial effectiveness of an intramuscularly injected analgesic can be evaluated at the time it reaches its peak plasma level—for example, 20 minutes after administration. The duration of its effectiveness must also be evaluated.
21. Medications are usually discontinued before surgery, and the physician writes new orders after the surgery. New orders are generally given for drugs a newly admitted client takes at home or when a client is transferred to another service within an agency or outside the agency. Check agency policies.
22. When medications are intentionally omitted, e.g., before surgery or a diagnostic test, record the omission and the reason on the client's chart. It may also be necessary to notify the prescriber.
23. Medication errors sometimes occur. When an error is made, report it immediately to the responsible nurse so that corrective measures can be implemented promptly. Errors are usually documented on an unusual incident form that becomes a part of the agency's file. Check the policies and practices of the agency.
24. Be aware of your clients' rights regarding medications. These are listed above on the right.

Client's Rights According to the Patient's Bill of Rights

1. To be informed of the drug's name, purpose, action and any possible adverse side effects.
2. To refuse any medication.
3. To have a qualified person, ie, nurse or physician assess your medication history including allergies.
4. To have complete information about the experimental use of any drug and to refuse or consent to its use.
5. To receive labelled medications safely.
6. To receive appropriate therapy adjunctive to the drug therapy.
7. Not to be given unnecessary medications.

(American Hospital Association 1973, p. 82)

Developmental Considerations

Knowledge of growth and development is essential for the nurse administering medications to children. The nurse needs to know how to approach a child and what explanations and methods are required. Adolescents, pregnant women, and elderly clients also have special needs.

Infants and Children

Oral medications Oral medications for children are usually prepared in sweetened liquid form to make them more palatable. Some drugs are unpalatable, and the nurse can mask the taste with honey, jam, juice, or any suitable sweetener. The parents may provide suggestions about what method is best for their child. Necessary foods such as milk or orange juice should not be used to mask the taste of medications because the child may develop unpleasant associations and refuse that food in the future. Artificial sweeteners may be used for diabetic children. Not all children reject unsweetened medicine. Some may be content with a sip of juice or a mint before and after taking a medication. Nurses are encouraged to be aware of the tastes of the medications they are giving, which allows them to answer questions honestly. For example, in response to "Will it taste bad?" the nurse may reply, "It tastes like strawberry to me" or ". . . like sour lemon. Tell me what you think it tastes like." Most children accept this challenge to experiment and learn.

Toddlers who are in the independent "no" stage challenge the nurse's ability to gain the child's cooperation. It is common for toddlers to push medications away or to close their mouths in refusal. This behavior may reflect dislike of medicines, a need to control the situation, or a desire to take the medicine independently. A nurse can offer encouragement by holding the child, acknowledging the child's distaste for the medicine, offering a simple explanation about why it is needed, and expressing faith in the child's ability to manage this situation independently. A spoon, a glass, or a straw may help toddlers take medications. A few words of praise go a long way. The nurse should encourage the child to participate as much as possible—for example, by holding the glass or by choosing between a straw or a spoon. Forcing medications is futile; it communicates hostility and engenders distrust. If the child does not spit out the medication in response to force, the child will no doubt intentionally vomit the medication soon after. It is important, too, that nurses not convey to the child, either verbally or nonverbally, negative attitudes they may have about the medication.

By the age of 4 to 6 years, children are generally able to take pills. Some children of 2 years have already learned to swallow pills. To teach children to swallow pills, the nurse tells them to put the pill near the back of the tongue and then to wash it down with water, milk, or juice. Recognition and praise elicit the cooperation of most young children, and seeing other children taking medications may help.

When older children refuse to take medications, the nurse encourages them to discuss their feelings about the drugs and to share suggestions they have. Coaxing and bribing will not get the child to cooperate. It is better to convey an attitude of expectancy and helpful cooperation. For example, it is better to say, "I have your green pill for you, Johnny" than "Johnny, will you please take your green pill?" If given a few choices, such as whether to take a pill or a liquid, most children cooperate more readily. On rare occasions children resist all strategies to get them to take a medication. In that case, the situation needs to be analyzed individually. If all attempts fail, the physician needs to be consulted.

Injectable medications Children tend to fear any procedure in which a needle is used because they anticipate pain or because the procedure is unfamiliar and threatening. The nurse needs to acknowledge that the child will feel some pain. Denying this fact only deepens the child's distrust. Very young infants may not experience painful stimuli with the same sensitivity as children because infants have delayed reactions to stimuli. They also have limited experiences and thus feel less anticipatory fear or anxiety. By the age of approximately 6 months, infants have memory of past pain and therefore begin to anticipate pain and cry when they see a needle and syringe. By the age of 10 months or a year, the infant may make active attempts to wriggle away or to push the equipment aside. Thus when administering injections to young children, the nurse restrains them to protect them from injury. After the injection, it is important for the nurse (or the parent) to cuddle and speak softly to the infant and give the child a toy to dispel the child's association of the nurse only with pain.

The reasoning ability of toddlers and preschoolers is immature. They often view an injection as punishment for some "bad" behavior, real or imagined, particularly if they are hospitalized. They may believe their parents abandoned them and therefore do not want them or want them punished. Although it is difficult for children of this age to understand why the procedure is necessary, even when they receive simple explanations, children who are prepared can and usually do muster coping mechanisms. For example, one child who was to receive an immunization found the situation easier to deal with when he was encouraged to tell the nurse, "You better be quick!" All injections should be given as rapidly as possible, and children must be adequately restrained. Even though a child says, "I'll hold still," another nurse needs to be present for safety. Two nurses may be required to restrain some 4-year-olds. See Figure 51–8 for one method of holding a child during an intramuscular injection.

Children should be told about an injection shortly before it is given. Even if this knowledge increases anxiety, the child should be told the truth. It is also important to find out how the child copes with pain and to support those coping methods. By recognizing the child's developmental level, the nurse can formulate an approach that provides meaningful support. For example, a preschooler (5 years old) who is developing a conscience could view an injection as punishment. By telling the child that injections are never used as punishment and giving the child a simple, honest explanation of the injection, the nurse allays guilt and fear.

Children and adolescents should be encouraged to vent their feelings before and after the treatment. Young children may do this in play; adolescents may require support for open discussion.

Participation of parents often can be elicited, although many parents choose not to be involved in restraining their children. If they do participate, they can often con-

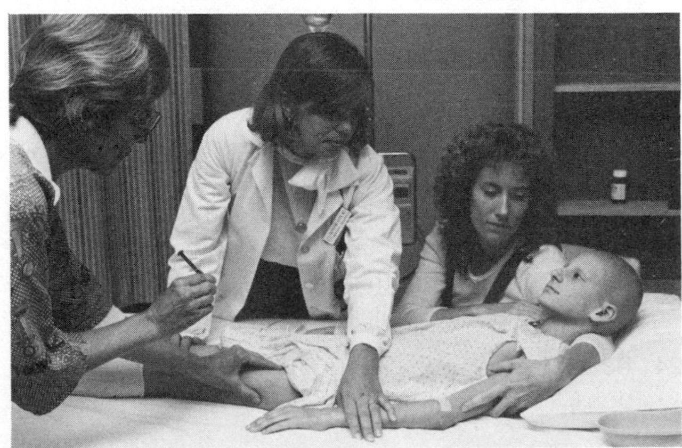

Figure 51–8 Holding a child during an intramuscular injection.

sole or divert their children during the injection. The nurse may gain children's cooperation by involving them in the procedure—for instance, by asking them on which side they want the injection, or by allowing them to swab the site.

Elderly People

Older people can present special problems in relation to medications. Most of their problems are related to physiologic changes, to past experiences, and to established attitudes toward medications.

Physiologic changes in elderly persons may involve:

1. Altered memory
2. Less acute vision
3. Decrease in kidney function resulting in slower elimination of drugs and higher drug concentrations in the bloodstream for longer periods
4. Less complete and slower absorption from the gastrointestinal tract
5. Increased proportion of fat to lean body mass, which facilitates retention of fat-soluble drugs and increases potential for toxicity
6. Decreased liver function, which hinders biotransformation of drugs
7. Decreased organ sensitivity, which means that the response to the same drug concentration in the vicinity of the target organ is less in older people than in the young
8. Altered quality of organ responsiveness, resulting in adverse effects becoming pronounced before therapeutic effects are achieved; for example, in older people, digitalis often produces arrhythmia, nausea, or vomiting, before slower and stronger cardiac contractions are achieved.

Many of these changes enhance the possibility of cumulative effects and toxicity. For example, impaired circulation delays the action of medications given intramuscularly or subcutaneously. Digitalis, which is frequently taken by elderly people, can accumulate to toxic levels and be lethal.

It is not uncommon for elderly clients to take several different medications daily. The possibility of error increases with the number of medications taken, whether self-administered at home or administered by nurses in a hospital. The greater number of medications also compounds the problem of drug interactions, because much is yet to be learned about the effects of drugs given in combinations. A general rule to follow is that elderly clients should take as few medications as possible.

Like the very young, elderly persons usually require smaller dosages of drugs, especially sedatives and other central nervous system depressants, because their effects are greater on older clients. Reactions of the elderly to medications, particularly sedatives, are unpredictable and often bizarre. It is not uncommon to see irritability, confusion, disorientation, restlessness, and incontinence as a result of sedatives. Nurses therefore need to observe clients carefully for untoward reactions. Chloral hydrate is an effective sedative for elderly people. The use of alcohol (e.g., brandy) as a bedtime relaxant and as an appetizer before meals is becoming more common. The moderate use of alcohol by people who are accustomed to it can contribute to a sense of well-being.

Attitudes of elderly people toward medical care and medications vary. Elderly people tend to believe in the wisdom of the physician more readily than younger people. Some older people are bewildered by the prescription of several medications and may passively accept their medications from nurses but not take them. Others may be suspicious of medications and actively refuse them. For this reason, the nurse is advised to stay with clients until they have taken the medications.

Elderly people are mature adults capable of reasoning. Therefore, the nurse needs to explain the reasons for and effects of medications, particularly to ambulatory geriatric clients. This education can prevent the common occurrence of clients taking medications long after there is a need for them, or it can prevent clients from discontinuing a drug too quickly. For example, clients should know that diuretics will cause them to urinate more frequently and may reduce ankle edema. Instructions about medications need to be given to all clients prior to discharge from a hospital. These instructions should include when to take the drugs, what effects to expect, and when to consult a physician.

Because some clients are required to take several medications daily and because visual acuity and memory may be impaired, it is important for the nurse, in consultation with the physician if necessary, to develop simple, realistic plans for clients to follow at home. For example, most people, including elderly people, can have difficulties remembering to take drugs. If they are scheduled to be taken with meals or at bedtime, clients are not as likely to forget. Some clients may take their medications and then an hour later not remember whether they took them. One solution to forgetfulness is to use a special container or glass strictly for medications. If the container or glass is empty, the person knows that he or she took the pills. Loss of visual acuity presents problems that can be overcome by writing out the plan in a print large enough to be read. In some situations the help of a spouse, son, or daughter can be enlisted.

Oral Medications

The oral route is the most common route by which medications are given. As long as a client can swallow and retain the drug in her or his stomach, this is the route of choice. See Procedure 51–1.

Oral medications are contraindicated when a client is vomiting, has gastric or intestinal suction, or is unconscious and unable to swallow. Such clients in a hospital usually are on orders "nothing by mouth" (NPO, nothing per ora, nil per os).

Procedure 51–1 ▲ Administering Oral Medications

Equipment

1. A medication tray or cart
2. Medication cards or computer printout. To save time and avoid retracing steps, arrange the cards in the order in which you will give the medications. Plan to give medications first to clients who do not require assistance and last to those who do.
3. Disposable medication cups. Small paper or plastic cups are needed for tablets and capsules; for liquids, waxed or plastic calibrated medication cups are needed.

Intervention

1. Check the date on the medication order, and verify the order for accuracy. It should contain the following:
   a. Client's name
   b. Name and dosage of the drug
   c. Time for administration
   d. Route of administration, e.g., oral (p.o.), subcutaneous or hypodermic (s.c. or H), intramuscular (IM), or intravenous (IV)

   Records of medication orders include the physician's order, which is usually on the client's chart, the Kardex record, and the medication card. The surest check is to compare the medication card against the physician's order. In some settings a medication Kardex or computer printout is used instead of medication cards. This Kardex or printout is usually kept in the medications room or in the medication cart. Any discrepancies in the order should be brought to the notice of the responsible nurse or the physician, whichever is appropriate in the agency.
2. Read the medication card or printout, and take the appropriate medication from the shelf, drawer, or refrigerator. The medication may be dispensed in a bottle, box, or envelope.
3. Compare the label of the medication container against the order on the medication card. If these are not identical, recheck the client's chart. If there is still a discrepancy, check with the responsible nurse.
4. Prepare the correct amount of medication for the required dose, without contaminating the medication.
   a. If administering tablets or capsules from a bottle, pour the required number into the bottle cap, and then transfer the medication to the disposable cup. Do not touch the tablets. See Figure 51–9. Usually all tablets or capsules to be given to the client are placed in the same cup. Medications that require specific assessments, e.g., pulse measurements, respiratory rate or depth, or blood pressure, must be kept separate from the others.

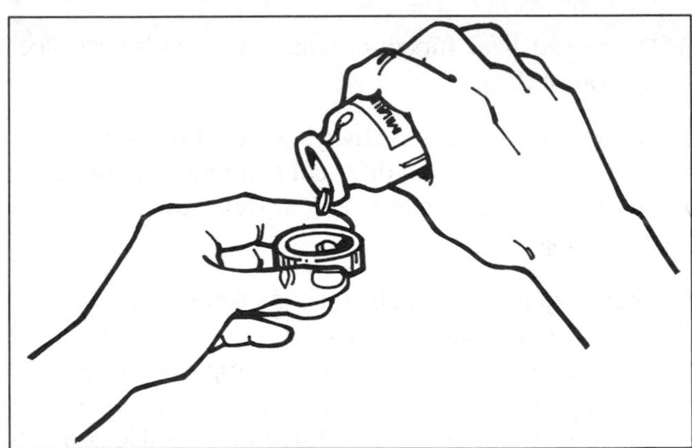

Figure 51–9

   b. If administering a liquid medication, remove the cap, and place it upside down on the countertop to avoid contaminating it. Hold the bottle with the label next to your palm so that if any spills, the label will not become soiled and illegible. See Figure 51–10. Hold the medication cup at eye level and fill it to the desired level, using the bottom of

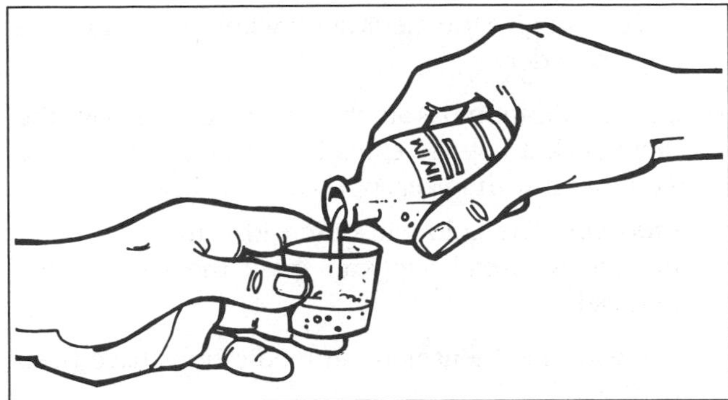

Figure 51–10

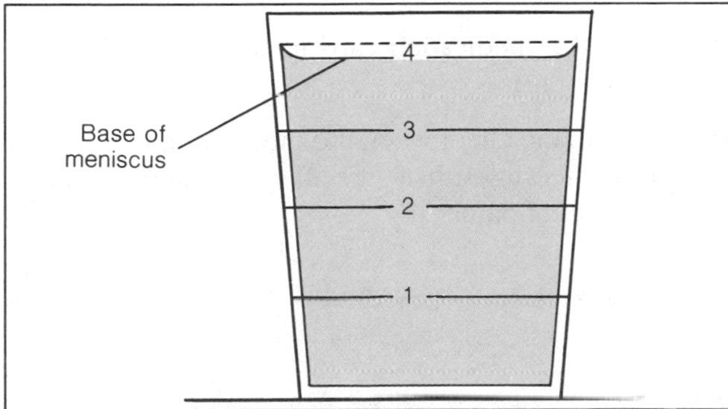

Figure 51–11

the **meniscus** (crescent-shaped upper surface of a column of liquid) as the measurement guide. See Figure 51–11.

c. If administering an oral narcotic from a narcotic dispenser, expose the tablet by turning the dial or sliding out the numbered dose, and drop it into the cup. These containers are sectioned and numbered. See Figure 51–12. After removing a tablet, you must record the fact on the appropriate narcotic control record and sign it.

d. Open unit-dose medications at the client's side.

5. Place the prepared medication and medication card together on the tray or cart.

6. Check the label on the container again, and return the bottle, box, or envelope to its storage place.

7. Identify the client by comparing the name on the medication card, printout, or medication package with the name on the client's identification bracelet or by asking the client to tell you his or her name.

8. Explain to the client the purpose of the medication and how it will help, using language that she or he can understand. Include relevant information about effects, e.g., tell the client receiving a diuretic that she or he can expect an increase in urine.

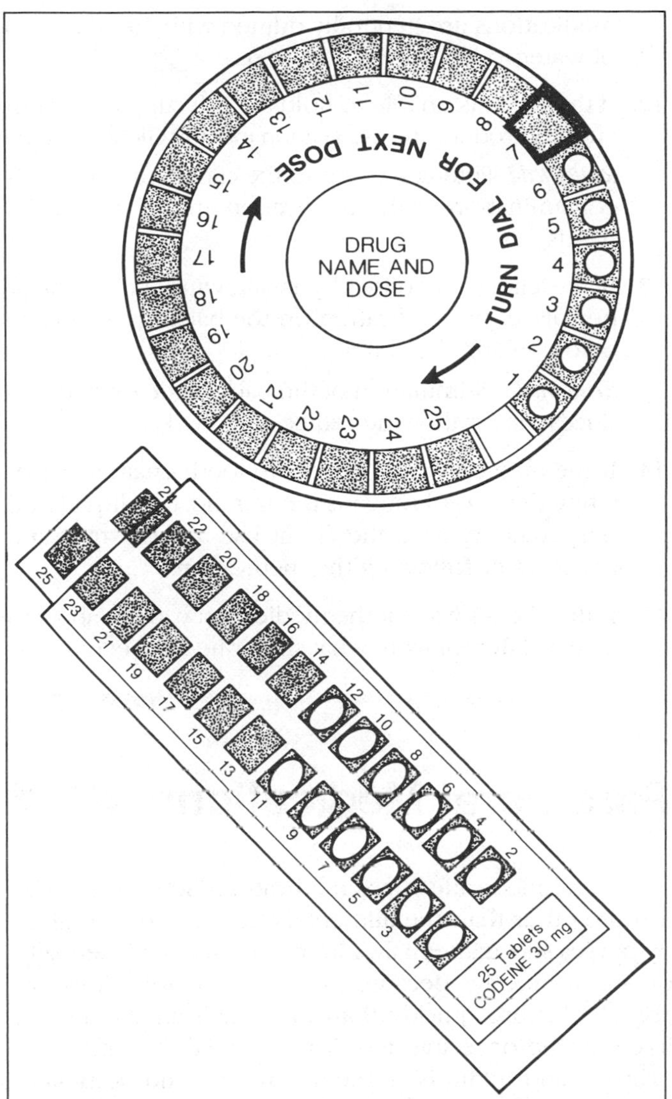

Figure 51–12

9. Assist the client to a sitting position or, if not possible, to a lateral position.

   Rationale These positions facilitate swallowing and prevent aspiration.

10. Take the required assessment measures, e.g., pulse and respiratory rates or blood pressure. The pulse rate is taken before administering digitalis preparations. Blood pressure is taken before giving hypotensive drugs. The respiratory rate is taken prior to administering narcotics, since narcotics depress the respiratory center. If the rate is below 12, the responsible nurse should be consulted before giving the medication.

11. Give the client sufficient water or juice to swallow the medication if appropriate.

    Rationale Fluids ease swallowing and facilitate absorption from the gastrointestinal tract. Liquid medications are generally diluted with 15 ml (½ oz) of water to facilitate absorption.

12. If the client is unable to hold the pill cup, use the pill cup to introduce the medication into the client's mouth.

    Rationale Putting the cup to the client's mouth avoids contamination of the medication and of the nurse's hands.

13. If the client has difficulty swallowing, have him or her place the medication on the back of the tongue before taking the water.

    Rationale Stimulation of the back of the tongue produces the swallowing reflex.

14. If the medication is harmful to tooth enamel or irritating to the oral mucous membrane, e.g., liquid iron preparations, have the client use a glass straw and drink water following the medication.

15. If the client says that the medication you are about to give is different from what she or he has been receiving, do not give the medication without checking the original order.

16. If the medication has an objectionable taste, have the client suck a few ice chips beforehand, or give the medication with juice, applesauce, or bread.

    Rationale The cold will desensitize the taste buds, and juices, bread, etc. can mask the taste of the medication.

17. Stay with the client until all medications have been swallowed.

18. Record the medication given, dosage, time, any complaints or assessments of the client, and your signature.

19. Return the medication card to the slot of the next time it is due.

20. Return to the client when the medication is expected to take effect to evaluate the effects of the medication, e.g., relief of pain.

Parenteral Medications

Parenteral medications are medications administered by a route other than the alimentary canal. They are given by nurses subcutaneously, intramuscularly, intradermally, or intravenously. Because parenteral medications are absorbed more quickly than oral medications and are irretrievable once injected, it is essential that the nurse prepare and administer them carefully and accurately. Administering parenteral drugs requires the same nursing knowledge as for oral and topical drugs, plus considerable manual dexterity and the use of sterile technique.

Equipment

Syringes

All syringes have three parts: the tip, which connects with the needle; the barrel, or outside part, on which the scales are printed; and the plunger, which fits inside the barrel. See Figure 51–13. Most syringes used today are made of plastic and are individually packaged for sterility in a paper wrapper or a rigid plastic container. They may be prefitted with needles. These syringes and needles may be disposable or nondisposable.

Types of Syringes

There are several kinds of syringes, differing in size, shape, and material. The three most commonly used types are the standard hypodermic syringe, the insulin syringe, and the tuberculin syringe. See Figure 51–14.

Hypodermic syringes come in 2, 2.5, and 3 ml sizes. They usually have two scales marked on them: the minim and the milliliter. The milliliter scale is the one normally used; the minim scale is used for very small dosages, such as "epinephrine minims iii H."

Insulin syringes are similar to hypodermic syringes, except that they have a scale specially designed for insulin: a 100-unit calibrated scale intended for use with U-100 insulin. This scale is replacing the U-40 and U-80 scale used for 40-unit and 80-unit insulins.

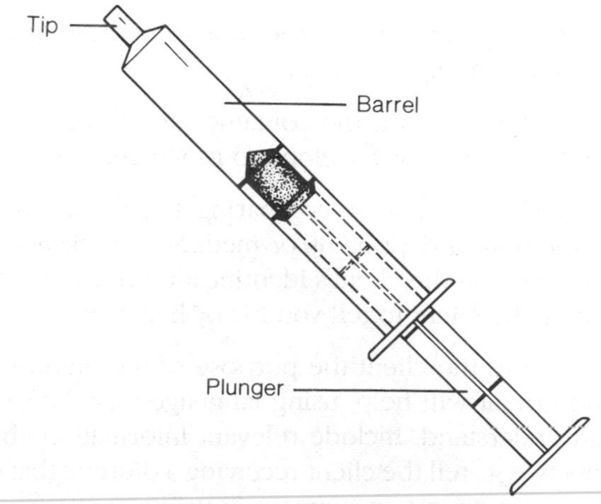

Figure 51–13 The three parts of a syringe.

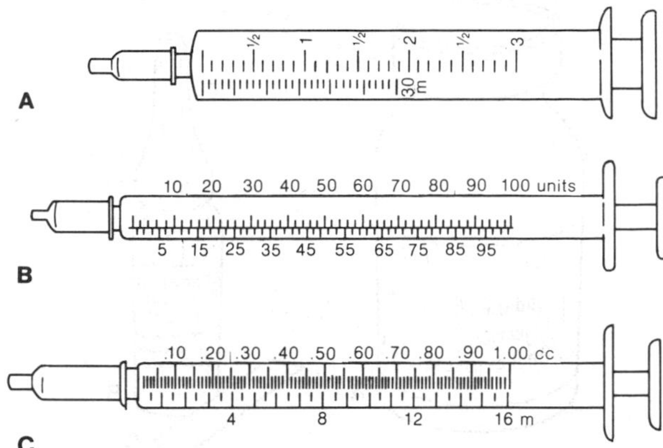

Figure 51–14 Three kinds of syringes: **A**, hypodermic; **B**, insulin; **C**, tuberculin.

The *tuberculin syringe* was designed to administer tuberculin. It is a narrow syringe, calibrated in tenths and hundredths of a milliliter (up to 1 ml) on one scale and in sixteenths of a minim (up to 1 min) on the other scale. This type of syringe can also be useful in administering other drugs, particularly when small or precise measurement is indicated—for example, pediatric dosages.

Syringes are made in other sizes as well, for example, 5, 10, 20, and 50 milliliters. These are not generally used to administer drugs directly but can be useful for adding sterile solutions to intravenous flasks or for irrigating wounds.

Glass Syringes

Nondisposable glass syringes are less widely used. However, because glass syringes can be sterilized, they are often placed in sterile treatment sets for special procedures, e.g., administering a local anesthetic. Glass syringes, like disposable syringes, can be fitted with special Luer-Lok tips. These have threaded seals, so the needle connects more securely to the syringe than on a standard type of syringe. See Figure 51–15. The Luer-Lok tips can be attached to devices other than needles, e.g., irrigators.

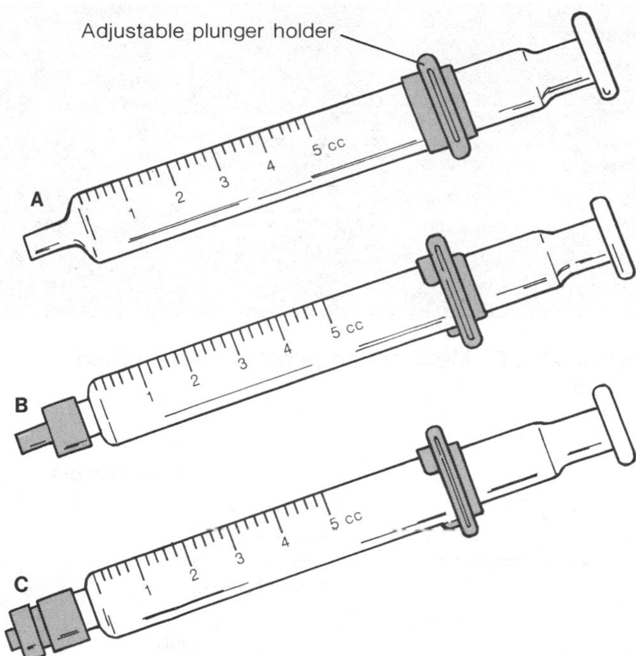

Figure 51–15 Glass syringes: **A**, with a glass tip; **B**, with a metal tip; **C**, with a Luer-Lok.

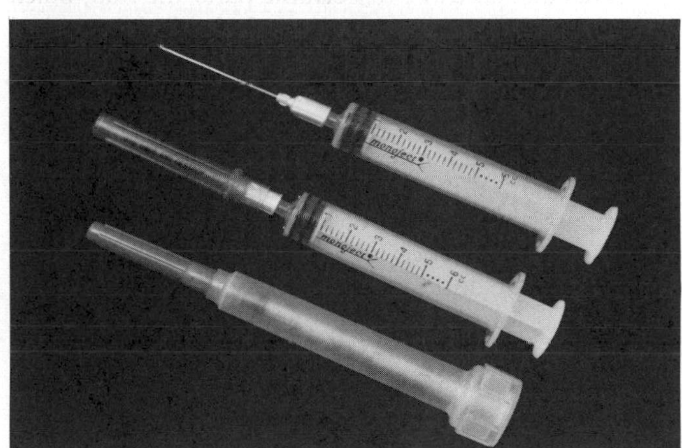

Figure 51–16 Disposable plastic syringes and needles: **top**, with syringe and needle exposed; **middle**, with plastic cup over the needle; **bottom**, with plastic case over the needle and syringe.

Disposable Plastic Syringes

Most frequently used today is the disposable plastic syringe. The syringe is supplied with a needle, which may have a plastic cap over it. The syringe and needle may be packaged together or separately in a paper wrapper or in a rigid plastic container. See Figure 51–16.

Disposable Prefilled Syringes and Cartridges

Injectable medications are frequently supplied in prefilled unit-dose syringes with needles or cartridge-needle units. These prefilled syringes and cartridge-needle units are disposable. The cartridge-needle units, however, require special metal or plastic cartridge holders or syringes for administration. These syringes and cartridges come with manufacturer's directions for use. See Figure 51–17.

Needles

Needles are made of stainless steel and may or may not be disposable. Reusable needles need to be sharpened periodically before resterilization, because the points become dull with use and are occasionally damaged or acquire burrs on the tips. A dull or damaged needle should *never* be used.

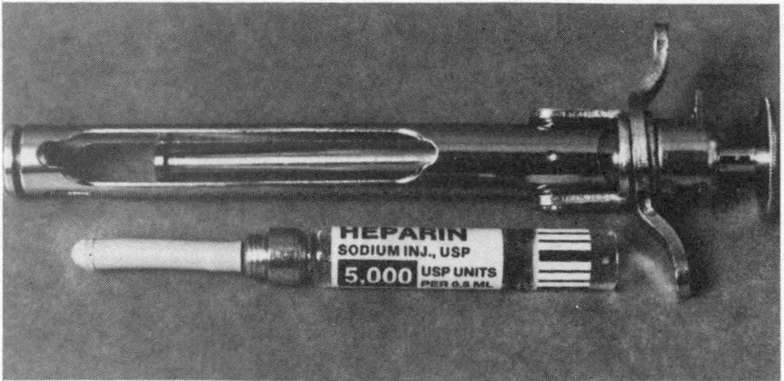

Figure 51–17 Metal cartridge holder and prefilled cartridge.

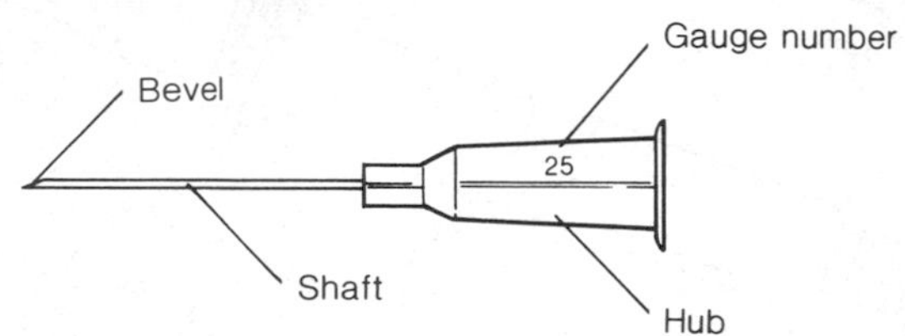

Figure 51–18 The parts of a needle.

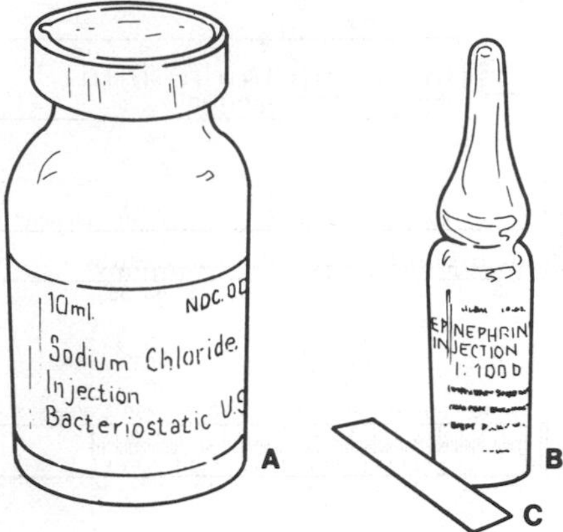

Figure 51–19 **A**, vial; **B**, ampule; **C**, ampule file.

A needle has three discernible parts: the hub, which fits onto the syringe; the cannula, or shaft, which is attached to the hub; and the bevel, which is the slanted part at the tip of the needle. See Figure 51–18. A disposable needle has a plastic hub.

Needles used for injections have three variables: the slant or length of the bevel, the length of the shaft, and the gauge (or diameter) of the shaft. The bevel of the needle may be short or long. Longer bevels provide the sharpest needle and cause less discomfort and are commonly used for subcutaneous and intramuscular injections. Short bevels are used for intradermal and intravenous injections, because a long bevel can become occluded if it rests against the side of a blood vessel.

The shaft length of commonly used needles varies from ¼ to 5 in, and the gauge varies from 14 to 27. The larger the gauge number, the smaller the diameter of the shaft. Smaller gauges produce less tissue trauma, but larger gauges are necessary for viscous medications, such as penicillin. For subcutaneous injections, it is usual to use a needle of 24 to 26 gauge and ⅜ to ⅝ in long. Obese clients may require a 1-in needle. For intramuscular injections, a longer needle, e.g., 1 to 1½ in, with a larger gauge, e.g., gauge 20 to 22, is used.

Ampules and Vials

Ampules and vials are frequently used to package sterile parenteral medications. See Figure 51–19. An **ampule** is a glass container usually designed to hold a single dose of a drug. It is made of clear glass and has a particular shape with a constricted neck. Some ampule necks have colored marks around them, and some are prescored for easy opening. If the neck is not scored, it is filed with a small file, then broken off at the neck.

A **vial** is a small glass bottle with a sealed rubber cap. Vials come in different sizes, from single to multidose vials. They usually have a metal cap that protects the rubber seal; it is easily removed.

Procedure 51–2 describes how to prepare medications from ampules and vials.

Procedure 51–2 ▲ Preparing Medications from Ampules and Vials

Equipment

1. The vial or ampule of sterile medication
2. Sterile gauze
3. A needle and syringe
4. Special filter needle (optional) for withdrawing premixed liquid medications from multidose vials
5. Antiseptic solution
6. Sterile water, if necessary. Some vials contain only a powder, and it is necessary to instill a liquid such as sterile water to prepare the medication. The manufacturer specifies preparation directions.
7. File if required to open the ampule
8. Medication card or computer printout

Intervention

1. Check the label on the ampule or vial carefully against the medication card or the client's chart to make sure the correct medication is being prepared.
2. Follow the three checks for administering medications. Read the label on the medication before it is taken off the shelf, before pouring the medication, and after placing it back on the shelf.

Ampules

3. Flick the upper stem of the ampule several times with a fingernail, or, holding the upper stem of the ampule, make a large circle with the arm extended.

   Rationale This will bring all the medication down to the main portion of the ampule.
4. Partially file the neck of the ampule, if it is not prescored, to start a clean break.
5. Place a piece of sterile gauze on the far side of the ampule neck, and break off the top by bending it toward the gauze. See Figure 51–20.

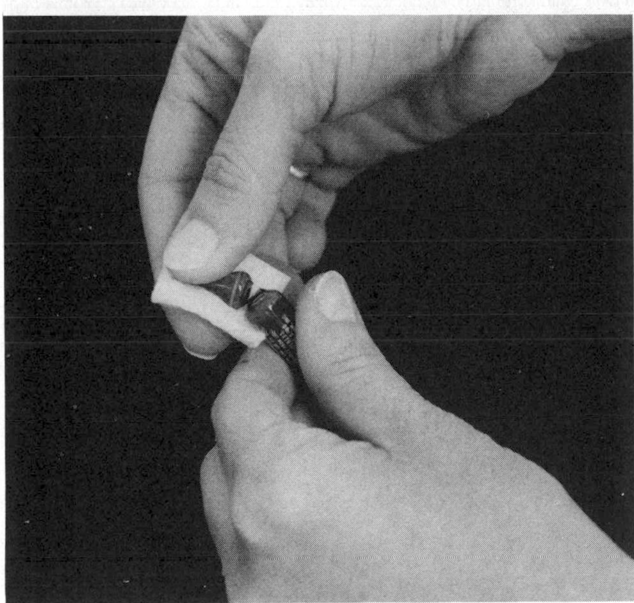

Figure 51–20

   Rationale The sterile gauze protects the nurse's fingers from the broken glass.
6. Assemble the syringe and needle, if not preassembled. Hold the barrel of the syringe in the middle and insert the plunger, maintaining the sterility of the plunger except at its uppermost end (which you are holding). Attach the needle to the barrel by holding the hub of the needle and maintaining the sterility of the remainder of the needle and the tip of the syringe. Many needles have protective caps to help maintain their sterility.
7. Remove the cap from the needle, insert the needle in the ampule, and withdraw the amount of drug required for the dosage. See Figure 51–21. With a single-dose ampule, hold the ampule slightly on its side, if necessary, to obtain all the medication.

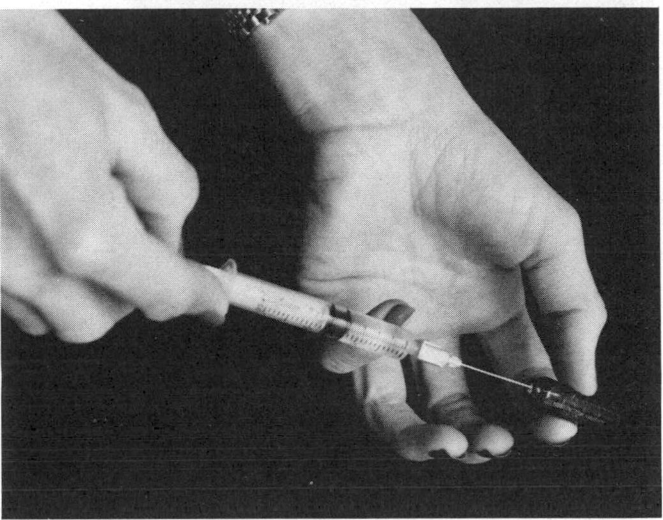

Figure 51–21

Vials

8. Mix the solution, if necessary, by rotating the vial between the palms of the hands, *not* by shaking.

   Rationale Some vials contain aqueous suspensions, which settle when they stand. In some instances shaking is contraindicated, because it may cause the mixture to foam.
9. Remove the protective metal cap, and clean the rubber cap with an antiseptic, such as 70% alcohol, on a sterile gauze, rubbing in a rotary motion.

   Rationale The antiseptic cleans the cap so the needle will not be contaminated when inserted.
10. Remove the cap from the needle; then draw up into the syringe an amount of air equal to the volume of the medication to be withdrawn. In some agencies, a special filter needle is used to draw up premixed liquid medications from multidose vials. The filter needle is then replaced by a regular needle to inject the medication into the client. The filter prevents any solid material from being drawn up through the needle.
11. Carefully insert the needle into the vial through the center of the rubber cap, maintaining the sterility of the needle.

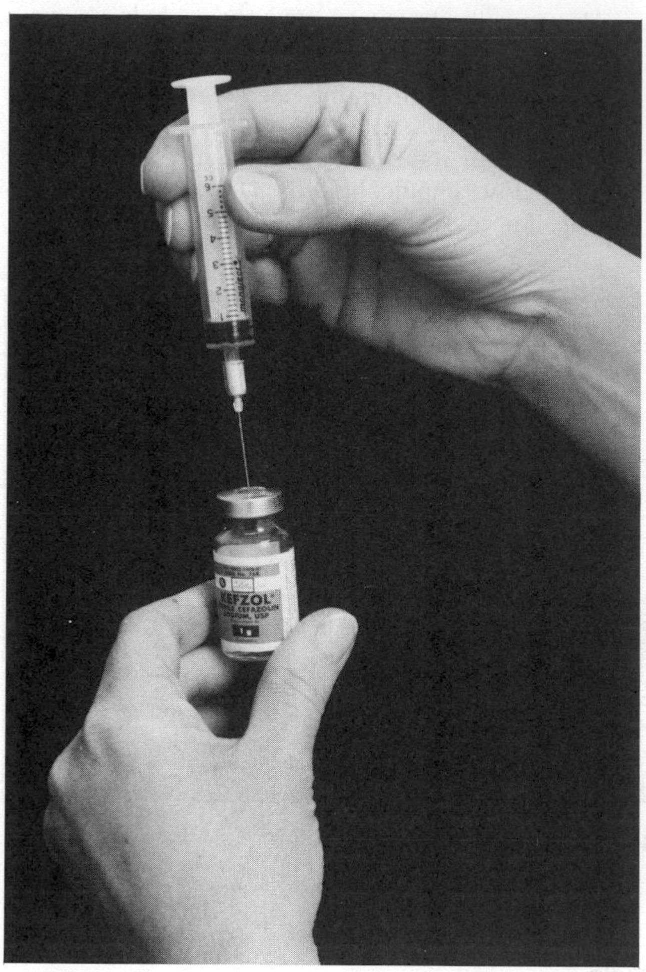

Figure 51–22

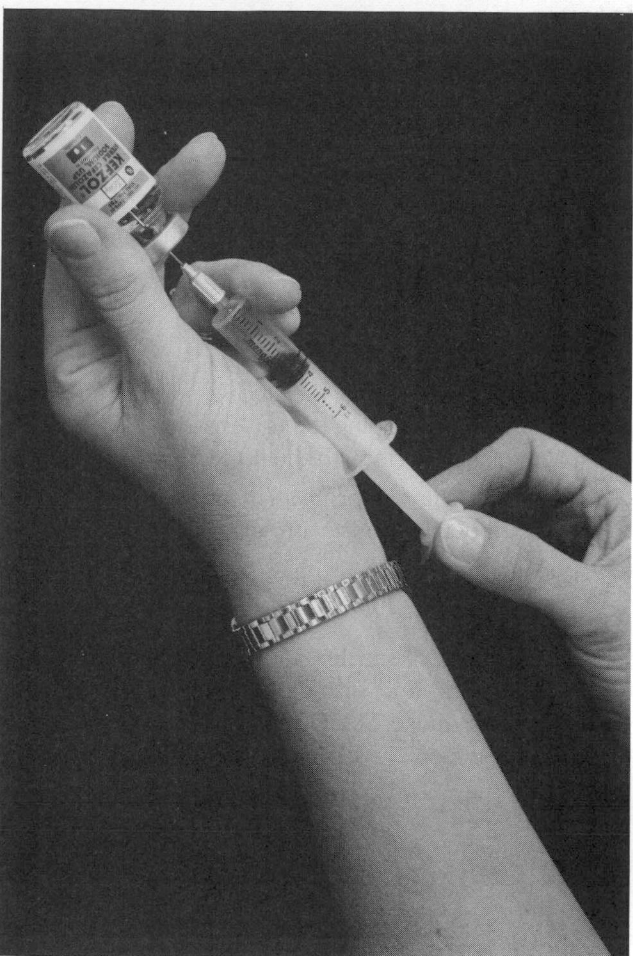

Figure 51–23

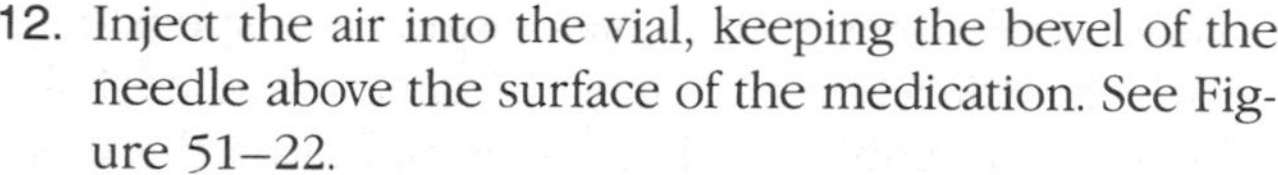

12. Inject the air into the vial, keeping the bevel of the needle above the surface of the medication. See Figure 51–22.

    Rationale The air will allow the medication to be drawn out easily, since negative pressure is not created inside the vial. The bevel is kept above the medication to avoid creating bubbles in the medication.

13. Invert the vial and hold it at eye level while withdrawing the correct dosage of the drug into the syringe. See Figure 51–23.

14. Withdraw the needle from the vial, and replace the cap over the needle, thus maintaining its sterility. If a filter needle was used to withdraw the medication, replace it with a regular needle before injecting the client.

Preparing Powdered Drugs

Several drugs (e.g., penicillin) are dispensed as powders in vials. A liquid (solvent, or diluent) must be added to a powdered medication before it can be injected. The technique of adding a solvent to a powdered drug to prepare it for administration is called **reconstitution**. Powdered drugs usually have printed instructions (enclosed with each packaged vial) that describe the amount and kind of solvent to be added. Commonly used solvents are sterile water or sterile normal saline. Some preparations are supplied in individual-dose vials; others come in multidose vials.

15. Read the manufacturer's directions. The following are two examples of the preparation of powdered drugs:
    a. *Single-dose vial:* Instructions for preparing a single-dose vial direct that 1.5 ml of sterile water be added to the sterile dry powder, thus providing a single dose of 2 ml. The volume of the drug powder was 0.5 ml.
    b. *Multidose vial:* A dose of 750 mg of a certain drug is ordered. On hand is a 10-g multidose vial. The directions for preparation read: "Add 8.5 ml of sterile water, and each milliliter will contain 1.0 g or 1,000 mg." Thus, after adding the solvent, the

nurse will give 750/1,000, or ¾, ml (0.75 ml) of the medication.

16. Withdraw an equivalent amount of air from the vial before adding the solvent, unless otherwise indicated by the directions.
17. Add the amount of sterile water or saline indicated in the directions.
18. If a multidose vial is reconstituted, label the vial with the date it was prepared, the amount of drug contained in each milliliter of solution, and your initials. Time is an important factor to consider in the expiration of these medications.
19. Once reconstituted, store the medication in the vial in a refrigerator, if indicated.

Mixing Drugs

Frequently clients need more than one drug injected at the same time. To spare the client the experience of being injected twice, two drugs (if compatible) are often mixed together in one syringe and given as one injection. It is common, for instance, to combine two types of insulin in this manner or to combine injectable preoperative medications such as morphine or meperidine (Demerol) with atropine or scopolamine. Drugs can also be mixed in intravenous solutions. When uncertain about drug compatibilities, the nurse should consult a pharmacist before mixing the drugs.

Mixing Drugs from Two Vials

When withdrawing and mixing medications from two different vials, the nurse takes care not to contaminate the medication remaining in one vial with the other medication. To do this safely, the nurse inserts into vial A a needle attached to a syringe containing the needed volume of air and injects a volume of air equal to the volume of medication to be withdrawn. The tip of the needle must not touch the solution. The nurse withdraws the needle and repeats the procedure with vial B; the nurse again injects a volume of air equal to the volume of medication to be withdrawn. The nurse then withdraws the required amount of medication from vial B. In this way vial B is not contaminated by medication from vial A. The nurse then attaches a new, sterile needle to the syringe, inserts it into vial A, and withdraws the required amount of medication into the syringe. The syringe now contains a mixture of medications from vials A and B, and neither vial is contaminated by microorganisms or by medication from the other vial. For information on mixing two types of insulin, see the section on "Preparing Insulin."

Mixing Drugs from One Vial and One Ampule

Because ampules do not require the addition of air prior to withdrawal of the drug, it is recommended that the nurse prepare the medication from the vial first, and then withdraw the medication from the ampule.

Mixing Drugs from a Vial or Ampule and a Cartridge

Ensure that the correct dose of the medication is in the cartridge. Any excess medication should be withdrawn and discarded as if in a vial. Then the nurse should draw up in a syringe the required medication from a vial or ampule and add this into the cartridge.

Preparing Insulin

Insulin is prepared in units rather than milligrams or grains. It is available in 40, 80, and 100 units per milliliter of solution. Insulin syringes are described earlier in this chapter. It is essential when preparing insulin that the appropriate calibrations on the syringe be used; for example, the 40-unit scale on the syringe is used only when administering 40-unit insulin and the 80-unit scale only for 80-unit insulin.

Because insulin is watery, the needle gauge used can be as small as possible (26 gauge). Insulin preparations are stored in the refrigerator to prevent deterioration. Preparations that have changed in appearance should never be used, and the solution should be well mixed prior to administration to ensure an accurate concentration and dose. Because shaking the vial can make the medication frothy, a vial of insulin is usually rotated between the palms of the hands and inverted end to end to mix it thoroughly.

Mixing Insulin from Two Vials

Although there are several types of insulin available, all have the same basic action. However, they vary in their time of action; some act within 2 hours and last for 8 to 10 hours, whereas others act within 6 hours and last for 24 to 36 hours. Often clients are given two types of insulin, short- and long-acting; these two types vary in content. Chemically, insulin is a protein, which, when hydrolyzed in the body, yields a number of amino acids. Some insulin preparations contain an additional modifying protein, such as globulin or protamine, that slows absorption. This fact is relevant to the mixing of two insulin preparations for

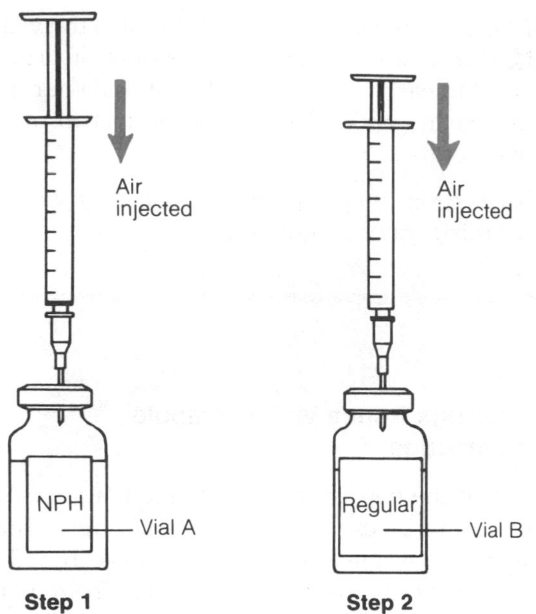

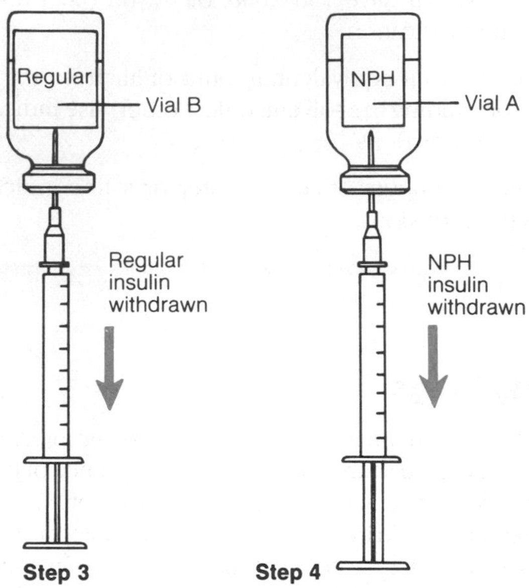

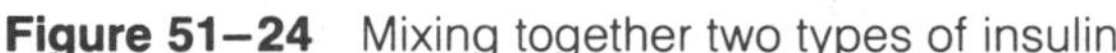
Figure 51–24 Mixing together two types of insulin.

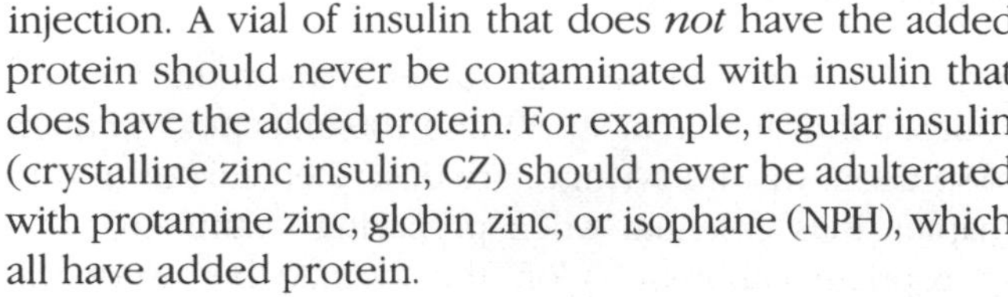
injection. A vial of insulin that does *not* have the added protein should never be contaminated with insulin that does have the added protein. For example, regular insulin (crystalline zinc insulin, CZ) should never be adulterated with protamine zinc, globin zinc, or isophane (NPH), which all have added protein.

Example At 0730 hours the nurse is to administer to a client 10 units of CZ and 30 units of NPH insulin, which contains protamine.

1. Inject 30 units of air into the NPH vial and withdraw the needle. (There should be no insulin in the needle.) The needle should not touch the insulin.
2. Inject 10 units of air into the CZ vial and immediately withdraw 10 units of CZ insulin.
3. Reinsert the needle into the NPH insulin vial and withdraw 30 units of NPH insulin. (The air was previously injected into the vial.) See Figure 51–24.

By using this method, the nurse does not add NPH insulin to the CZ insulin.

Intradermal Injections

An **intradermal** (intracutaneous) injection is the administration of a drug into the dermal layer of the skin just beneath the epidermis. Usually only a small amount of liquid is used, for example, 0.1 ml. This method of administration is frequently indicated for allergy and tuberculin tests and for vaccinations.

Common sites for intradermal injections are the inner lower arm, the upper chest, and the back beneath the scapulae. See Figure 51–25.

The equipment normally used is a 1-ml syringe calibrated into hundredths of a milliliter. The needle is short and fine, frequently a #25, #26, or #27 gauge, ¼ inch to ⅝ inch long. The preparation is similar to that for a subcutaneous injection.

After the site is cleaned, the skin is held tautly, and the syringe is held at about a 15° angle to the skin, with the bevel of the needle upward. The bevel is thrust through the epidermis into the dermis, and then the fluid is injected. The drug produces a small bleb just under the skin. See Figure 51–26. The needle is then withdrawn quickly, and the site is very lightly wiped with an antiseptic swab. The area is not massaged because the medication may disperse into the tissue or out through the needle insertion site. Intradermal injections are absorbed slowly through blood capillaries in the area.

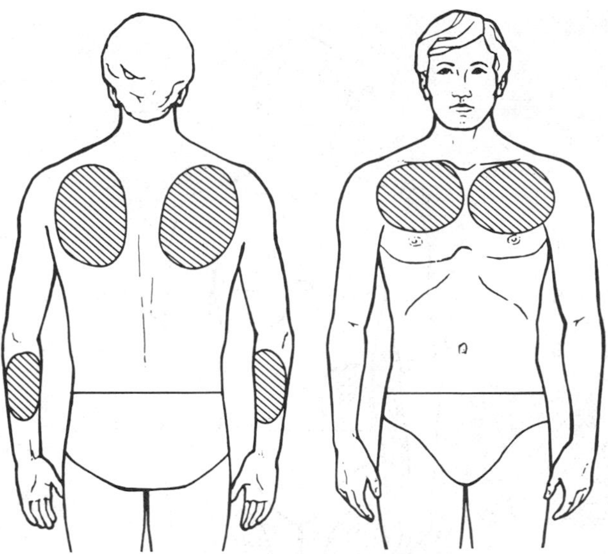

Figure 51–25 Body sites commonly used for intradermal injections.

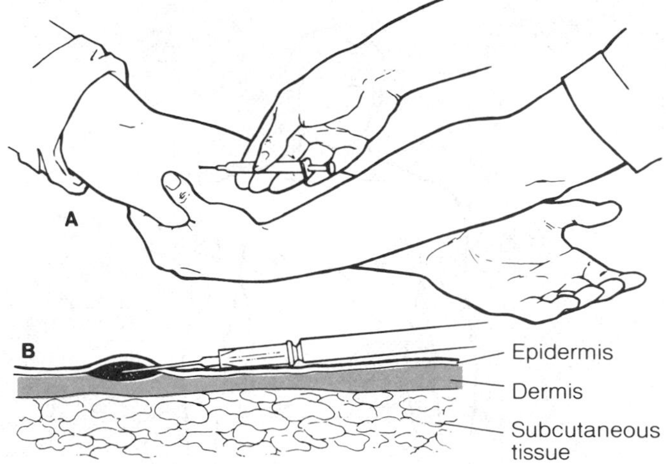

Figure 51–26 For an intradermal injection: **A**, the needle enters the skin at a 15° angle; and **B**, the medication forms a bleb under the epidermis.

Subcutaneous Injections

A **subcutaneous** injection is the introduction of a medication into the subcutaneous tissues. It is also referred to as a *hypodermic* injection. Among the many kinds of drugs administered subcutaneously are vaccines, preoperative medications, narcotics, insulin, and heparin.

Common sites for subcutaneous injections are the outer aspect of the upper arms and the anterior aspects of the thighs. These areas are convenient and normally have good blood circulation. Other areas that can be used are the abdomen, the scapular areas of the upper back, and the upper ventro/dorsal gluteal areas. See Figure 51–27. Clients who administer their own injections, such as diabetics requiring insulin, usually use the abdomen and anterior thigh sites.

Subcutaneous sites need to be rotated in an orderly fashion to minimize tissue damage, aid absorption, and avoid discomfort. This is especially important for clients who must receive repeated injections, e.g., diabetics. To accomplish this, the nurse or client can prepare a diagram indicating the sites to be used and after each injection mark its location on the diagram. See Figure 51–28. The steps for administering a subcutaneous injection are described in Procedure 51–3.

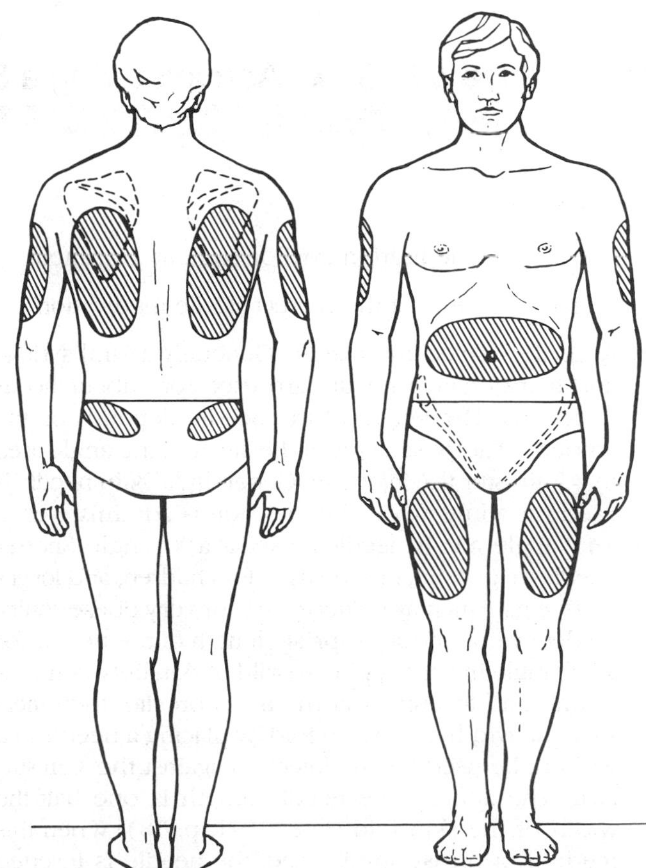

Figure 51–27 Body sites commonly used for subcutaneous injections.

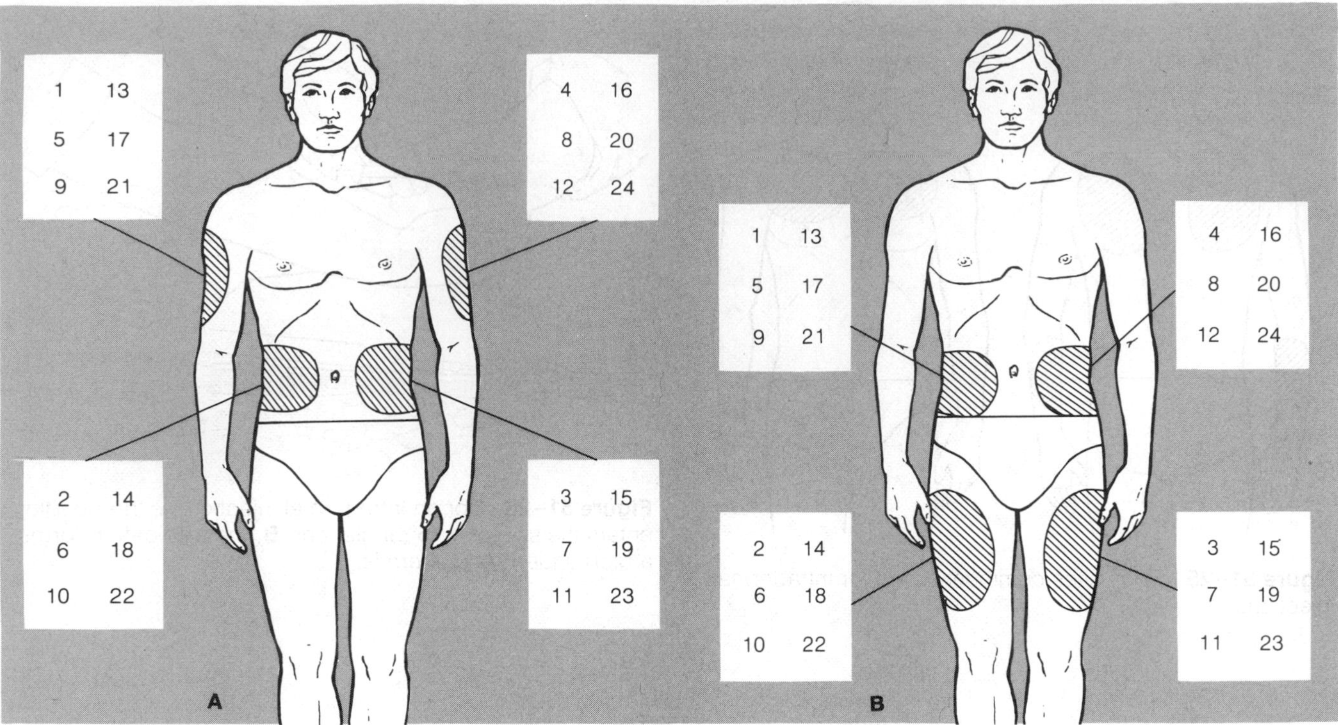

Figure 51–28 A commonly used system of rotating body injection sites for injecting insulin: **A**, sites used by the nurse; **B**, sites used by the client.

Procedure 51–3 ▲ Administering a Subcutaneous Injection

Equipment

1. The client's medication card or computer printout
2. A vial or ampule of the correct sterile medication
3. A sterile syringe and needle. Generally a 2-ml syringe and a #25 gauge needle are used for subcutaneous injections. The length of the needle depends on the amount of adipose tissue at the site and the angle used to administer the injection. Generally, a ⅝-in needle is used for adults when the injection is administered at a 45° angle; a ½-in needle is used at a 90° angle. Shorter needles, e.g., ⅜-in, may be used for children, and longer ones, e.g., 1 in, may be necessary for very obese adults. To determine the appropriate length of the needle for a 90° angle injection, pinch a fold of skin between your thumb and forefinger at the injection site, then measure the width of the skin fold by placing a needle that will not be used for the injection against the skin surface. The appropriate needle length is one half the width of the skin fold (Pitel 1971, p. 78). When this method of measuring is used, the needle is inserted without pinching the skin.
4. Sterile antiseptic-soaked swabs to clean the top of a medication vial and the injection site
5. Dry sterile gauze for opening an ampule

Intervention

1. Check the medication order. See Procedure 51–1, "Administering Oral Medications," steps 1 and 2, on page 1504.
2. Prepare the drug dosage from a vial or ampule. See earlier discussion in Procedure 51–2.
3. Select a site free of tenderness, hardness, swelling, scarring, itching, burning, or localized inflammation. Select a site that has not been used frequently.

   Rationale These conditions could hinder the absorption of the medication and also increase the likelihood of an infection at the injection site.
4. As agency policy indicates, clean the site with an antiseptic swab. Start at the center of the site and clean in a widening circle. Allow the area to dry thoroughly.

Place the swab between the third and fourth fingers of the nondominant hand for later use.

Rationale Recommendations differ about the necessity of cleaning the skin prior to injections. Some believe that the antiseptic lessens the number of microorganisms on the skin; others (Dann 1966, p. 1121; Lacey 1968, p. 212) think that cleaning destroys the normal antibacterial properties of the skin. The swab's mechanical action does remove skin secretions, which contain microorganisms.

5. Remove the needle cap while waiting for the antiseptic to dry. Pull the cap straight off to avoid contaminating the needle by the outside edge of the cap.

   Rationale The needle will become contaminated if it touches anything but the inside of the cap, which is sterile.

6. Expel any air bubbles from the syringe by inverting the syringe and gently pushing on the plunger until a drop of solution can be seen in the needle bevel. If air bubbles still remain, flick the side of the syringe barrel.

   or

7. When it is important that the entire amount of medication be administered, Wong (1982 p. 1237) recommends leaving 0.2 ml of air in the syringe. This is referred to as the ***air-bubble technique***. Others (Chaplin, Shull, and Welk 1985, p. 59) do not recommend this technique.

   Rationale Users of the air bubble technique believe this small amount of air ensures that only air remains in the needle bore and that all the medication is injected into the client. Nonusers believe that the risk of medication error is increased when the "dead-space volume" (residual amount of drug in the syringe hub and needle) is expelled during injection, since it is *not* part of the syringe barrel calibration.

8. Grasp the syringe in your dominant hand by holding it between your thumb and fingers with palm facing upward for a 45° angle insertion or with the palm downward for a 90° angle insertion. See Figure 51–29.

9. Using the nondominant hand, pinch or spread the skin at the site, and insert the needle, using a firm steady push. See Figure 51–30.

   Rationale Recommendations vary about whether to pinch or spread the skin. Pinching the skin is thought to desensitize the area somewhat and thus lessen the sensation of needle insertion. Spreading the skin can make it firmer and facilitate needle insertion. Some recommend neither pinching nor spreading the skin (Pitel 1971, p. 79). The nurse needs to judge which method to use depending on the client's tissue firmness.

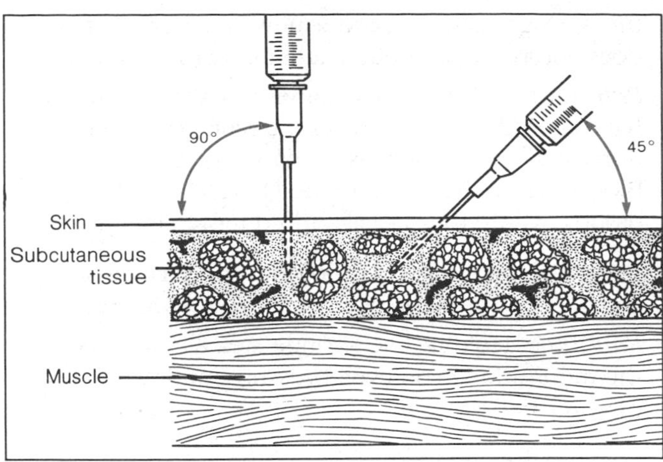

Figure 51–29

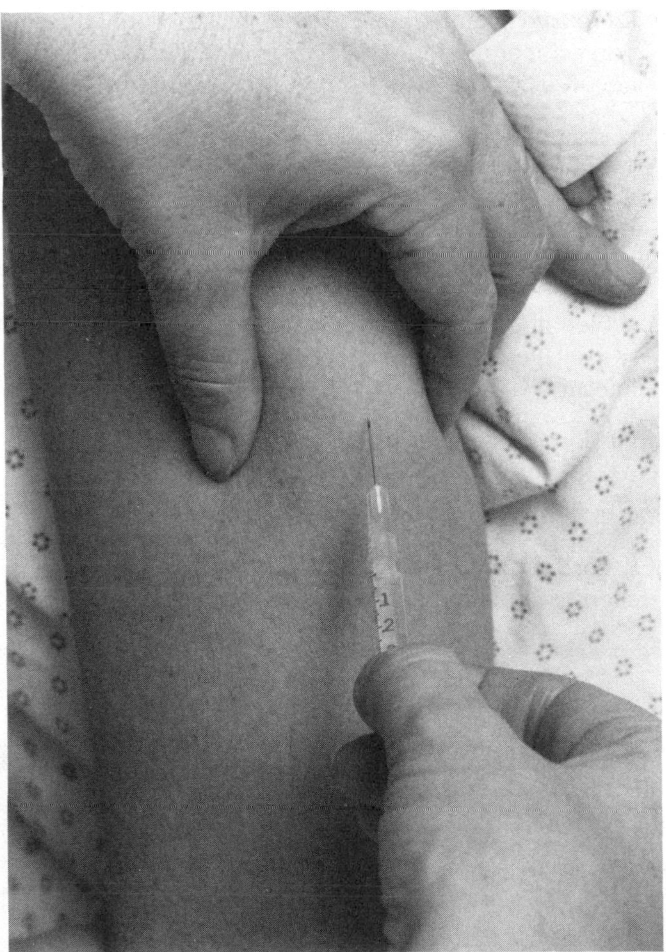

Figure 51–30

10. When the needle is inserted, move your nondominant hand to the barrel of the syringe and your dominant hand to the end of the plunger.

11. Aspirate by pulling back on the plunger. If blood appears in the syringe, withdraw the needle, discard

the syringe, and prepare a new injection. If blood does not appear, continue to administer the medication.

Rationale This step determines whether the needle has entered a blood vessel. Subcutaneous medications may be dangerous if placed directly into the bloodstream; they are intended for the subcutaneous tissues, where they are absorbed more slowly.

12. Inject the medication by holding the syringe steady and depressing the plunger with a slow, even pressure.

    Rationale Holding the syringe steady and injecting the medication at an even pressure minimizes client discomfort.

13. Remove the needle quickly, pulling along the line of insertion while depressing the skin with your nondominant hand.

    Rationale Depressing the skin places countertraction on it and minimizes client discomfort when the needle is withdrawn.

14. Massage the site lightly with a sterile antiseptic-soaked swab, or apply slight pressure.

    Rationale Massage is thought to disperse the medication in the tissues and facilitate its absorption. Massaging is omitted with heparin injections.

15. If bleeding occurs, apply pressure to the site until it stops. Bleeding rarely occurs after subcutaneous injection.

16. Dispose of supplies according to agency procedure.

    Rationale Proper disposal protects the nurse and others from injury and contamination.

17. Record the medication given, dosage, time, route, any client complaints, and your signature.

18. Assess the effectiveness of the medication as appropriate for the medication.

Variations for a Heparin Injection

The subcutaneous administration of heparin requires special precautions because of the drug's anticoagulant properties.

19. Select a site on the abdomen above the level of the iliac crests.

    Rationale These areas are away from major muscles and are not involved in muscular activity, as the arms and legs are; thus, the possibility of hematoma is reduced.

20. Use a ½-in, #25 or #26 gauge needle, and insert it at a 90° angle. Draw 0.1 ml of air into the syringe when preparing the heparin, and inject it after the heparin.

    Rationale This step fills the needle with air and prevents any leakage of heparin into the intradermal layers when the needle is inserted and when the needle is withdrawn, thus minimizing the possibility of a hematoma.

21. Check agency practices regarding aspiration.

    Rationale Some nurses recommend against aspirating to determine needle placement because this can cause the needle to move, possibly damaging tissue and rupturing small blood vessels, causing bleeding and severe bruising.

22. Do not massage the site after the injection.

    Rationale Massaging could cause bleeding and ecchymoses.

23. Alternate sites of subsequent injections.

Intramuscular Injections

The intramuscular (IM) injection route is ordered for the following reasons:

1. Medications that irritate subcutaneous tissue, for example, penicillin and paraldehyde, may safely be given by intramuscular injection.
2. The speed of absorption is faster than by the subcutaneous route because of the greater blood supply to the body muscles.
3. Muscles can usually take a larger volume of fluid without discomfort than subcutaneous tissues, although the amount varies among people, chiefly with muscle size and condition.

Sites

A number of body sites are used for intramuscular injections. Frequently used sites are the dorsogluteal, ventrogluteal, vastus lateralis, rectus femoris, deltoid, and triceps muscles. Only healthy muscles should be used for injections.

Dorsogluteal Site

The dorsogluteal site is composed of the thick gluteal muscles of the buttocks. See Figure 51–31. The injection site must be chosen carefully to avoid striking the sciatic nerve, major blood vessels, or bone. There are two methods of establishing the exact site, which is the upper outer

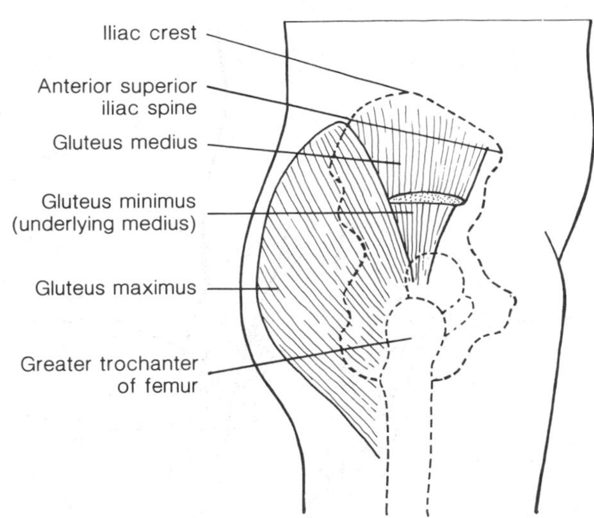

Figure 51–31 Lateral view of the right buttock showing the three gluteal muscles used for intramuscular injections.

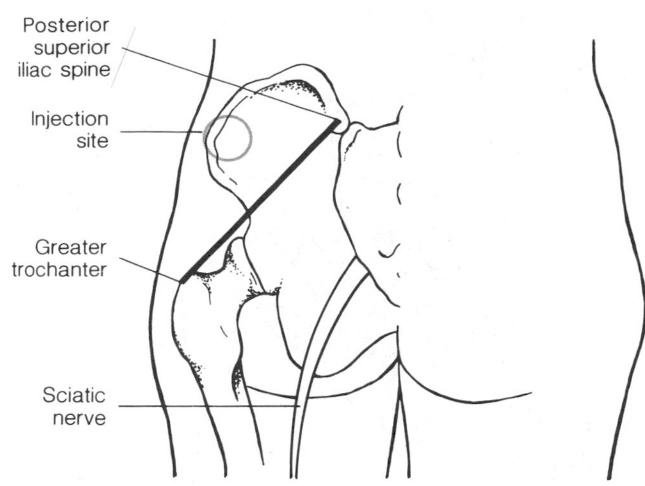

Figure 51–33 A second method for establishing the dorsogluteal site for an intramuscular injection.

aspect of the upper outer quadrant of the buttock, about 5 to 8 cm (2 to 3 in) below the crest of the ilium:

1. Divide the buttock by imaginary lines as in Figure 51–32. The vertical line extends from the crest of the ilium to the gluteal fold. The horizontal line extends from the medial fold to the lateral aspect of the buttock. From these landmarks, the upper outer aspect of the upper outer quadrant is established. See Figure 51–32. It is important to palpate the crest of the ilium so the chosen site is high enough. Visual calculations alone can result in an injection that is placed too low and injures other structures.
2. Palpate the posterior superior iliac spine, then draw an imaginary line to the greater trochanter of the femur. This line will be lateral to and parallel to the sciatic nerve. The injection site is then lateral and superior to this line. See Figure 51–33.

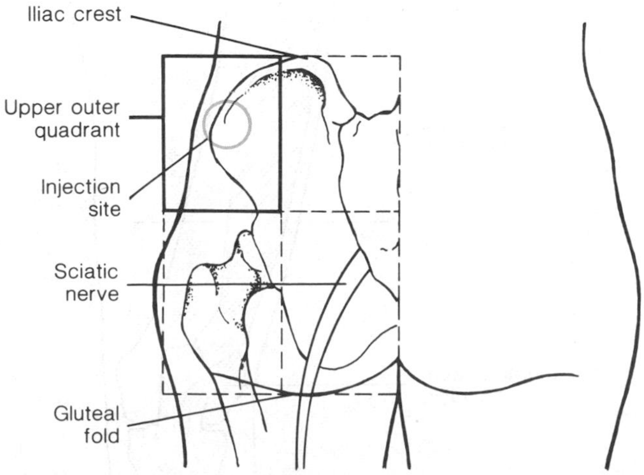

Figure 51–32 One method to establish the dorsogluteal site for an intramuscular injection.

In the past, the dorsogluteal site was most commonly used for intramuscular injections. However, because of the problems caused by inaccurately locating the site, it is losing favor as the best intramuscular site.

The dorsogluteal site can be used for adults and for children with well-developed gluteal muscles. Because these muscles are developed by walking, it is generally not used for infants under 3 years.

To administer an injection into this site, have the client assume a prone position with the toes pointing medially. A side-lying position can also be used, with the upper leg flexed at the thigh and the knee and placed in front of the lower leg. Both positions promote relaxation of the gluteal muscles.

Ventrogluteal Site

The ventrogluteal site, also known as von Hochstetter's site, uses the gluteas medius muscle, which lies over the gluteus minimus. See Figure 51–31. Use of this site is gaining favor because there are no large nerves or blood vessels in the area and less fat than in the buttock area. It is also farther from the rectal area and tends to be less contaminated, which is a consideration when giving injections to infants and incontinent adults.

To establish the exact site, the heel of the nurse's hand is placed on the greater trochanter, with the fingers pointing toward the client's head. The right hand is used for the left hip, and the left hand for the right hip. With the index finger on the anterior superior iliac spine, the middle finger is stretched dorsally, palpating the crest of the ilium and then pressing below it. The triangle formed

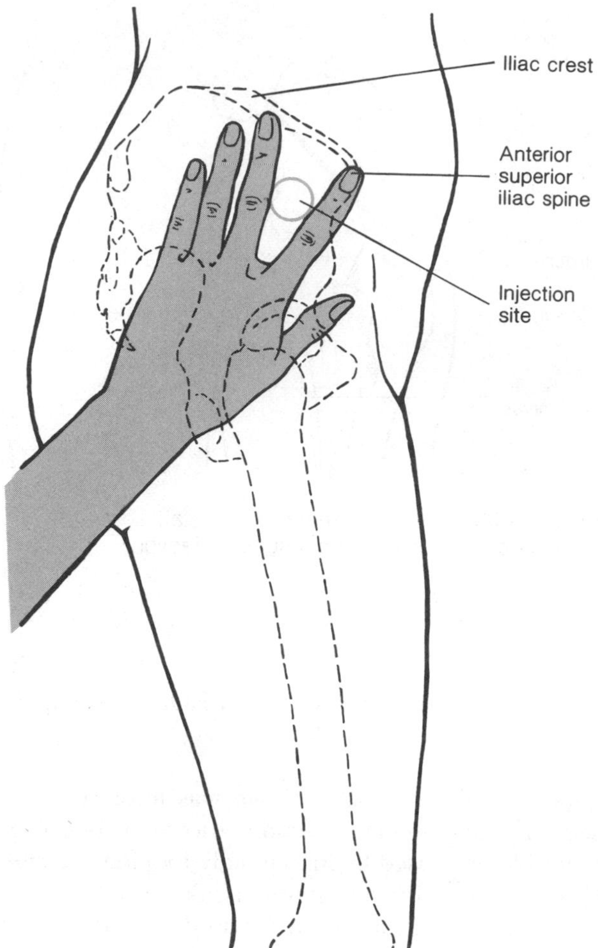

Figure 51–34 The ventrogluteal site for an intramuscular injection.

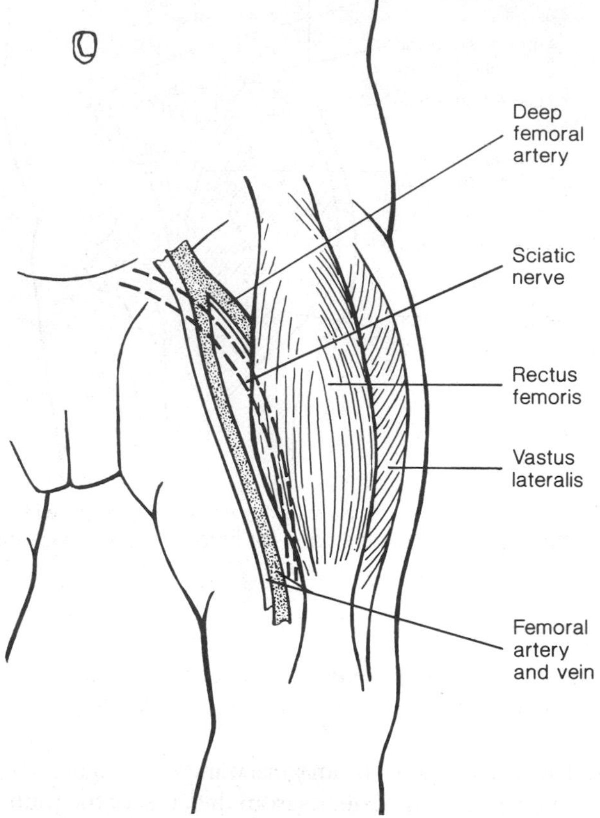

Figure 51–35 The vastus lateralis muscle of the upper thigh, used for intramuscular injections.

by the index finger, the third finger, and the crest of the ilium is the injection site. See Figure 51–34.

This site is suitable for infants, children, and adults. The client position for the injection can be a back- or side-lying position with the knee and hip flexed to relax the gluteal muscles.

Vastus Lateralis Site

The vastus lateralis muscle is usually thick and well-developed in both adults and children. It is increasingly recommended as the site of choice for intramuscular injections because there are no major blood vessels or nerves in the area. It is situated on the anterior lateral aspect of the thigh. See Figure 51–35. The middle third of the muscle is suggested as the site. It is established by dividing the area between the greater trochanter of the femur and the lateral femoral condyle into thirds and selecting the middle third. See Figure 51–36. The client can assume a back-lying or a sitting position for an injection into this site.

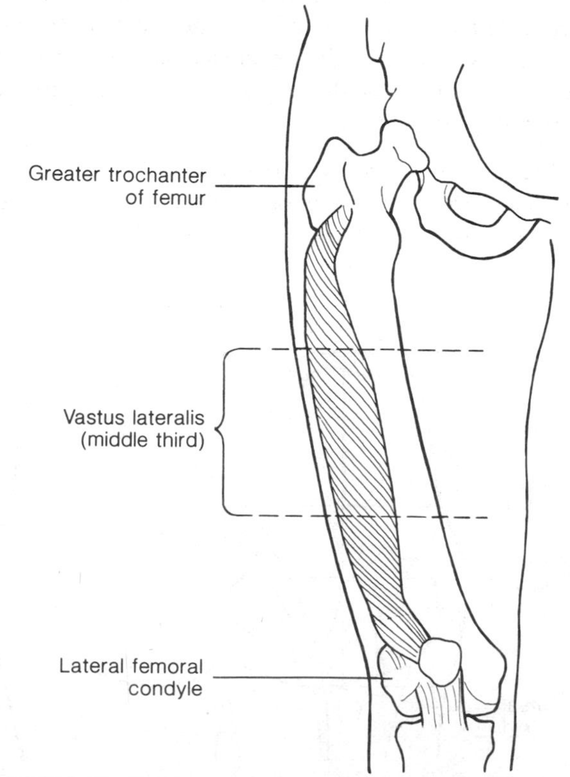

Figure 51–36 The vastus lateralis site for an intramuscular injection.

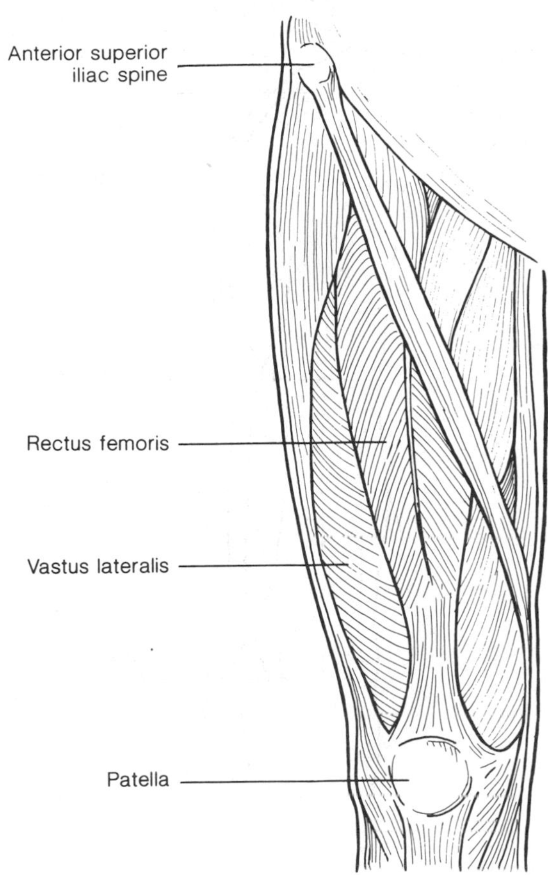

Figure 51–37 The rectus femoris muscle of the upper right thigh, used for intramuscular injections.

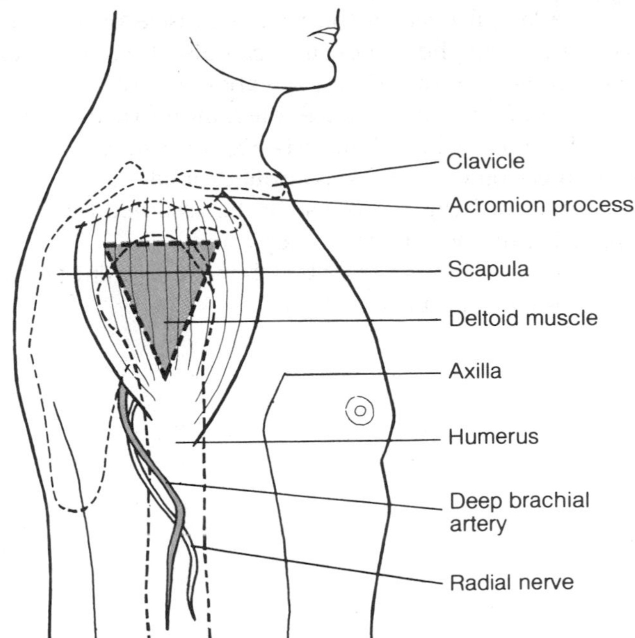

Figure 51–38 The deltoid muscle of the upper arm, used for intramuscular injections.

Rectus Femoris Site

The rectus femoris muscle, which belongs to the quadriceps muscle group, can also be used for intramuscular injections. It is situated on the anterior aspect of the thigh. See Figure 51–37. This site can be used for infants and children generally and for adults when other sites are contraindicated. Its chief advantage is that the client who administers his or her own injections can reach this site easily. Its main disadvantage is that an injection here may cause considerable discomfort for some people. The client assumes a sitting or back-lying position for an injection at this site.

Deltoid and Triceps Sites

The deltoid muscle is found on the lateral aspect of the upper arm. It is not used often for intramuscular injections because it is a relatively small muscle and is very close to the radial nerve and radial artery. To locate the densest part of the muscle, the nurse palpates the lower edge of the acromion process and the midpoint on the lateral aspect of the arm that is in line with the axilla. A triangle within these boundaries indicates the deltoid muscle about 5 cm (2 in) below the acromion process. See Figure 51–38. Another method of establishing the deltoid site is to place four fingers across the deltoid muscle, with the first finger on the acromion process; i.e., the site is three finger breadths below the acromion process. See Figure 51–39.

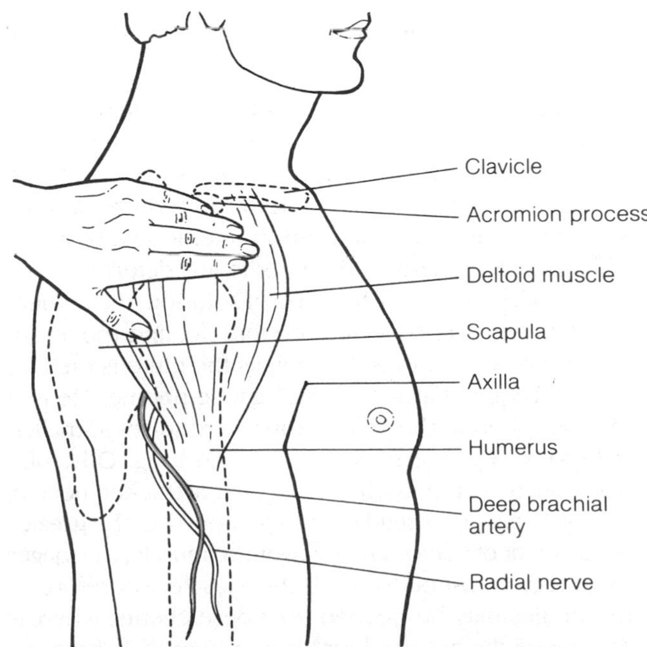

Figure 51–39 A method for establishing the deltoid muscle site for an intramuscular injection.

The lateral head of the triceps muscle on the posterior aspect of the upper arm can also be used as an injection site. The site of choice is about midway between the acromion process and the olecranon process of the ulna (the elbow). See Figure 51–40. This site is not often used unless other sites are contraindicated.

Sitting or lying positions can be assumed for injections using the deltoid and triceps sites.

Procedure 51–4 describes how to administer an intramuscular injection.

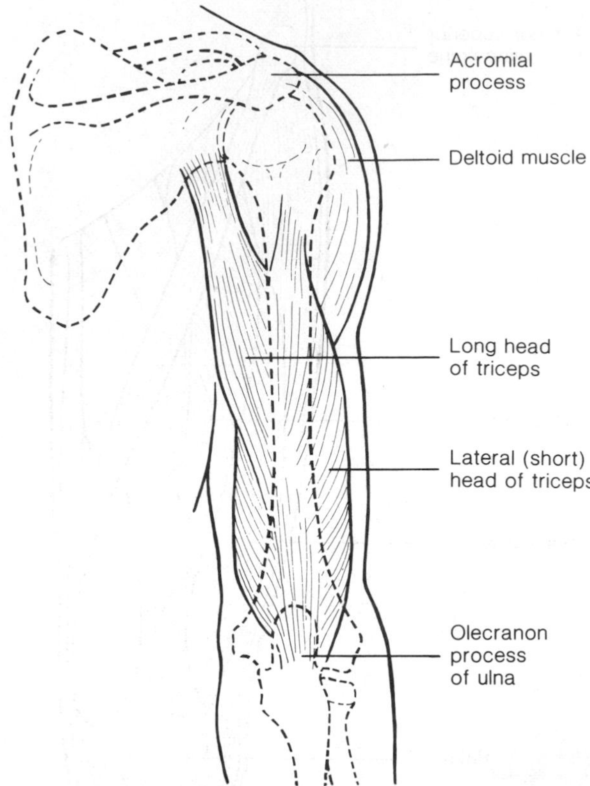

Figure 51–40 Posterior view of the upper right arm showing the triceps muscle, used for intramuscular injections.

Procedure 51–4 ▲ Administering an Intramuscular Injection

Equipment

1. The medication card or computer printout
2. The sterile medication. This is usually provided in an ampule or vial.
3. A sterile syringe and needle. Choose the size of syringe appropriate for the amount of solution to be administered. Usually a 2- to 5-ml syringe is needed. Some medications, such as paraldehyde, require a glass syringe, because the medication interacts with plastic. The size and length of the needle are determined by the muscle to be used, the type of solution, the amount of adipose tissue covering the muscle, and the age of the client. A large muscle, such as the gluteus medius, usually requires a #20 to #23 gauge needle, 1½ to 3 in long, whereas the deltoid muscle requires a smaller, #23 to #25 gauge needle, ⅝ to 1 in long. Oily solutions such as paraldehyde require a thicker needle, e.g., #21 gauge instead of #23 gauge. Also, the greater the amount of adipose tissue over the muscle, the longer the needle must be to reach the muscle. Therefore, 3-in needles may be needed for obese clients, whereas 1½-in needles are used for thinner people. Infants and young children usually require smaller, shorter needles, such as #22 to #25 gauge, ⅝ to 1 in long.
4. A swab saturated in an antiseptic solution for cleaning the site
5. Dry sterile gauze, if an ampule must be opened

Intervention

1. Check the medication order. See Procedure 51–1, "Administering Oral Medications," page 1504.
2. Prepare the correct dosage of the drug from a vial or ampule. See earlier discussion.
3. If the medication is particularly irritating to subcutaneous tissue, change the needle on the syringe before inserting it.

   Rationale Because the outside of the new needle is free of medication, it does not irritate subcutaneoous tissues as it passes into the muscle.
4. Select the intramuscular site for adequate muscle mass. The skin surface over the site should be free of bruises, abrasions, and infection. Determine if the size of the muscle is appropriate to the amount of medication to be injected. An average adult's deltoid muscle can usually absorb 0.5 ml of medication, although some authorities believe 2 ml can be absorbed by a well-developed deltoid muscle, and the gluteus medius

muscle can absorb 1 to 5 ml (Newton and Newton 1979, p. 19), although 5 ml may be very painful. The site should not have been used frequently. If injections are to be frequent, sites should be alternated. If necessary, discuss an alternate method of providing the medication with the person prescribing it.

5. Establish the exact site for the injection and assist the client to an appropriate position. See discussion of "Sites," page 1516.

6. Clean the site with an antiseptic swab. Using a circular motion, start at the center and move outward about 5 cm (2 in).

7. Remove the needle cover.

8. Invert the syringe and expel any excess air that may have accidentally entered the syringe, leaving only 0.2 ml of air if the air-bubble technique is being used. See Figure 51–41, *A*. It may be necessary to flick the syringe to move the bubbles out. The remaining air will rise to the plunger end when the needle is pointed downward. See Figure 51–41, *B*.

   Rationale Users of the air-bubble technique for IM injections believe that, in addition to clearing the medication from the bore of the needle, this technique prevents medication from leaking into subcutaneous tissue and onto the skin surface, where it can cause pain and tissue damage (Wong 1982, p. 1237). Nonusers believe that the best way to prevent leakage is to use the Z-track method described below. However, if the nurse is administering (a) Wyeth's vaccines of diphtheria and tetanus toxoids prepared with aluminum adjuvant, or (b) diphtheria and tetanus toxoids and pertussis vaccine, or (c) tetanus toxoid, it is recommended that the air-bubble technique be used to prevent abscess formation (Chaplin, Shull, and Welk 1985, p. 59).

9. Use the nondominant hand to spread the skin at the site.

   Rationale Spreading the skin makes it firmer and facilitates needle insertion. Under some circumstances, e.g., when the client is emaciated or an infant, the muscle may be bunched.

10. Holding the syringe between the thumb and forefinger, pierce the skin quickly at a 90° angle (see Figure 51–42), and insert the needle into the muscle (see Figure 51–43).

    Rationale Using a quick motion lessens the client's discomfort.

11. Aspirate by holding the barrel of the syringe steady with your nondominant hand and by pulling back on the plunger with your dominant hand. If blood appears in the syringe, withdraw the needle, discard the syringe, and prepare a new injection.

    Rationale This step determines whether the needle is in a blood vessel.

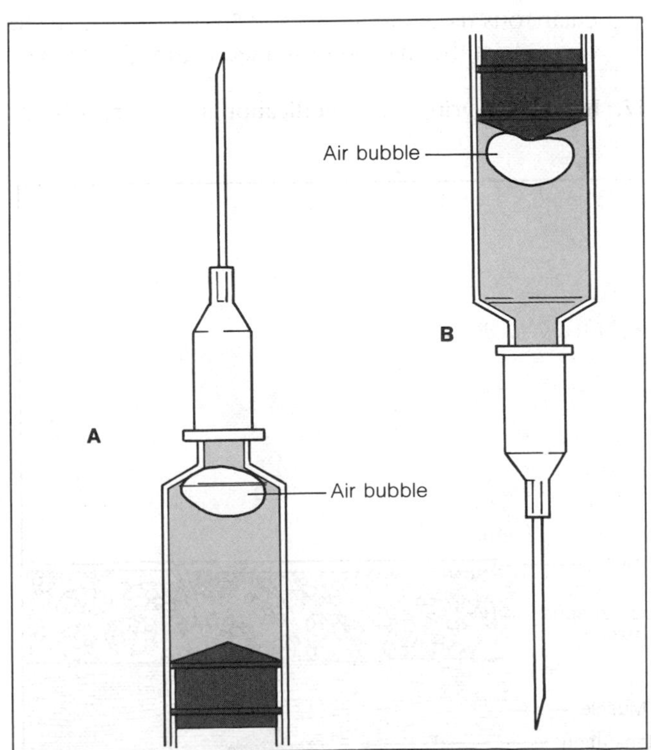

Figure 51–41

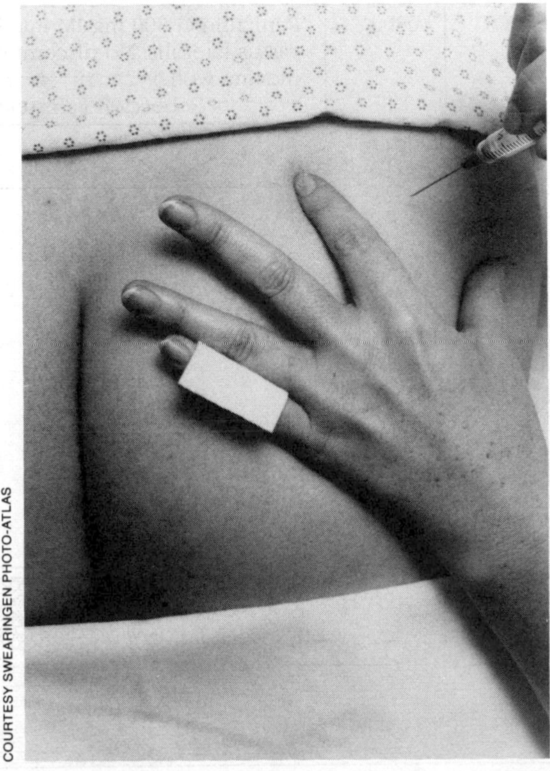

Figure 51–42

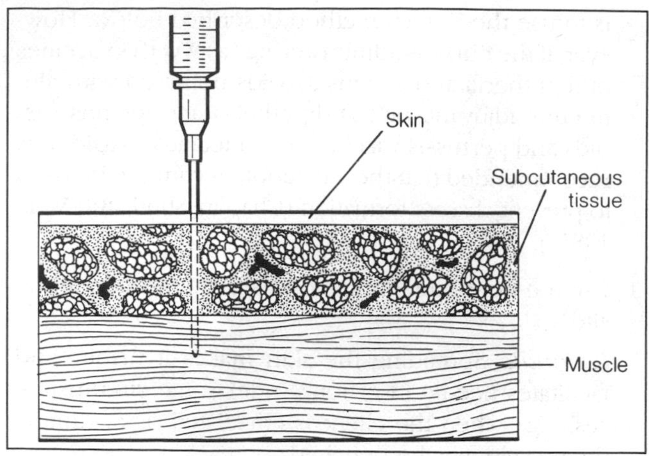

Figure 51–43

Research Note

This study compared the Z-track intramuscular injection technique and the stardard injection technique as to severity of discomfort and lesions at the injection sites. Each of 50 subjects received both types of injection every 3 to 4 hours, for a total of two to eight injections per subject. The substance injected was either meperidine hydrochloride alone or meperidine hydrochloride in combination with promethazine hydrochloride. The Z-track technique was found to significantly decrease the incidence of stated discomfort and the severity of lesions. (Keen 1986)

12. If blood does not appear, inject the medication steadily and slowly, holding the syringe steady.

    Rationale Injecting medication slowly permits it to disperse into the muscle tissue, thus decreasing client discomfort. Holding the syringe steady minimizes discomfort.

13. See Procedure 51–3, "Administering a Subcutaneous Injection," steps 12–18, page 1516, for withdrawing the needle, massaging the site, disposing of supplies, recording, and conducting follow-up assessment.

Sample Recording

Date	Time	Notes
Dec 5/87	0800	Penicillin G 500 mg IM into left vastus lateralis. No discomfort, moving well.——— ———Rebecca I. Feinstein, NS

Variation for a Z-track Injection

This variation of the standard intramuscular technique is used to administer intramuscular medications that are highly irritating to subcutaneous and skin tissues.

14. Follow steps 1–8.

15. Attach a clean sterile needle to the syringe.

    Rationale A new needle will not have any medication adhering to the outside that could be irritating to tissues.

16. With the nondominant hand, pull the skin and subcutaneous tissue about 2.5 to 3.5 cm (1 to 1½ in) to one side at the injection site (see Figure 51–44, *A*).

17. Insert the syringe and medication as in steps 10–12.

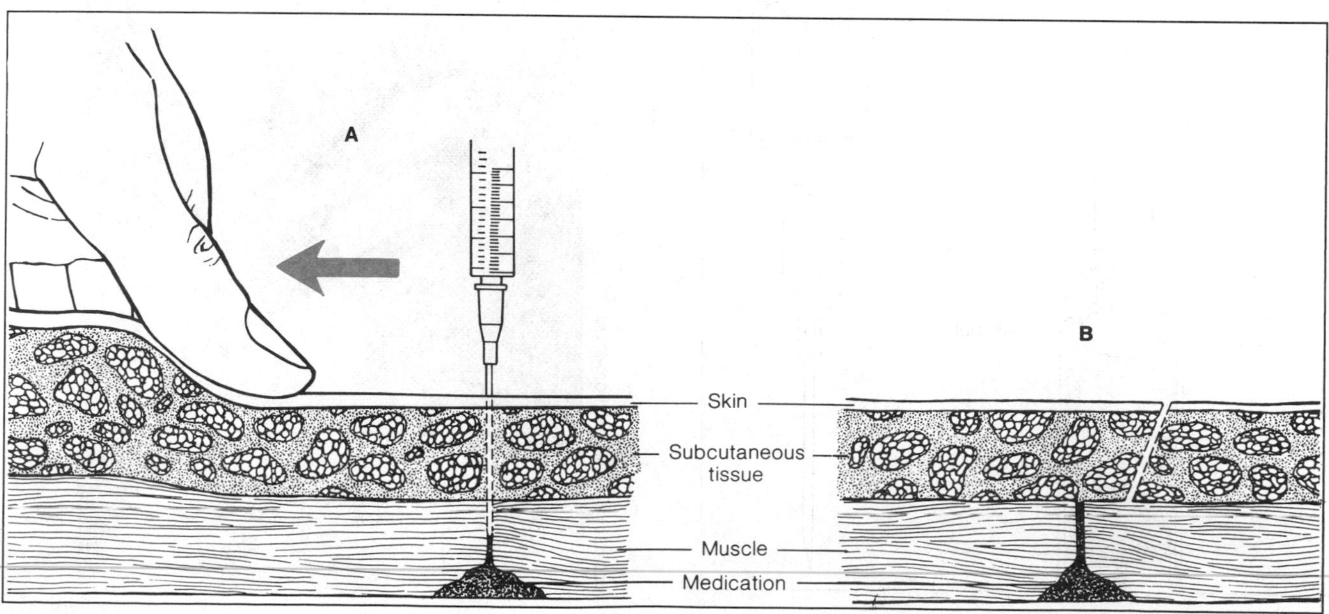

Figure 51–44

18. Maintain the traction for 10 seconds; then remove the needle and permit the skin to return to its normal position.

    Rationale During this time, muscle tissues relax and begin to absorb the medication. When the skin returns to its normal position, the needle track is interrupted, and the medication does not seep into the needle track or subcutaneous tissue. See Figure 51–44, *B*.

19. Do not massage.

    Rationale Massage might cause seepage into delicate tissue.

Intravenous Medications

Medications are administered intravenously via:

1. Intravenous bottle or bag
2. Additional intravenous container
3. Volume-control administration set
4. Intravenous push (bolus)

Because intravenous (IV) medications enter the client's bloodstream directly, they are appropriate when a rapid effect is required (e.g., in a life-threatening situation such as cardiac arrest). The IV route is also appropriate when medications are too irritating to tissues to be given by other routes, e.g., levarterenol bitartrate (Levophed) for acute hypotension. When an IV line is already established, this route is desirable because it avoids the discomfort of other parenteral routes.

There are, however, potential hazards in giving IV medications: infection and rapid, severe reactions to the medication. To prevent infection, sterile technique is used during all aspects of IV medication techniques. To safeguard the client against severe reactions, the nurse must administer the drug slowly, following the manufacturer's recommendations. The client is assessed closely during the administration, and the medication is discontinued immediately if an untoward reaction occurs.

IV medications can be added to a new fluid container prior to hanging it or to a fluid container that is already attached and running. Electrolytes (e.g., potassium chloride) and vitamins (e.g., Solu-B) are commonly administered by this method.

Before administering the medication, inspect and palpate the intravenous insertion site for signs of infection, infiltration, or a dislocated needle. Also, inspect the surrounding skin for redness, pallor, or swelling. Palpate the surrounding tissues for coldness and presence of edema, which could indicate leakage of the IV fluid into the tissues. Then take the vital signs for baseline data. It is also important to make sure that the drug and solutions are compatible. A nurse may need to consult a physician for this information. An *incompatibility* is an undesired chemical or physical reaction between a drug and an infusion solution, between two or more drugs, or between a drug and the container or tubing.

See Procedure 51–5.

Procedure 51–5 ▲ Adding an IV Medication to an IV Bottle or Bag

Equipment

1. The correct solution container, if a new one is to be attached. Confirm its sterility by ensuring that there are no container cracks or leaks, fluid discoloration, or seal damage.
2. The physician's order or medication card
3. The correct sterile medication. If the medication is in a powdered form, a diluent (e.g., sterile saline solution or water) will also be necessary.
4. Antiseptic swabs
5. A sterile syringe of appropriate size (e.g., 5 or 10 ml) and a 1- to 1½-in, #20 or #21 gauge sterile needle.
6. A medication label to attach to the IV solution container.

Intervention

1. Prepare the medication from a vial or ampule as described earlier. Check the agency's practice about whether a special filter needle is to be used when withdrawing the medication. A filter needle may be used to draw up premixed liquid medications from multidose vials. The filter prevents any solid material from being drawn up. If a filter needle is used, replace it with a regular needle to inject the medication into the solution container.
2. Compare the name on the medication card with the client's identification band.
3. For a glass IV container, remove the metal cap and the rubber disc, if the bottle is vented. Locate the injection port.

or

4. For a plastic container, locate the separate, self-sealing, soft rubber injection port. An injection port may be designated in several ways, e.g., by a triangular indentation or by the word *add*. It is important not to inject medication through the port for the administration spike or through an air vent port if there is an injection port. (See Chapter 46 for further information about infusion equipment.)
5. Clean the injection port with an antiseptic swab.
6. Remove the needle cover from the medication syringe, and inject the medication into the port. See Figure 51–45.
7. Remove the needle. For a glass container, cover the top immediately with either:
   a. An antiseptic swab with the metal IV cap taped over it

      or

   b. The special sterile cap provided by the manufacturer
8. Gently rotate the solution container to mix the drug with the solution.
9. Attach the medication label upside down to the fluid container. See Figure 51–46 for the information to be included on the medication label.

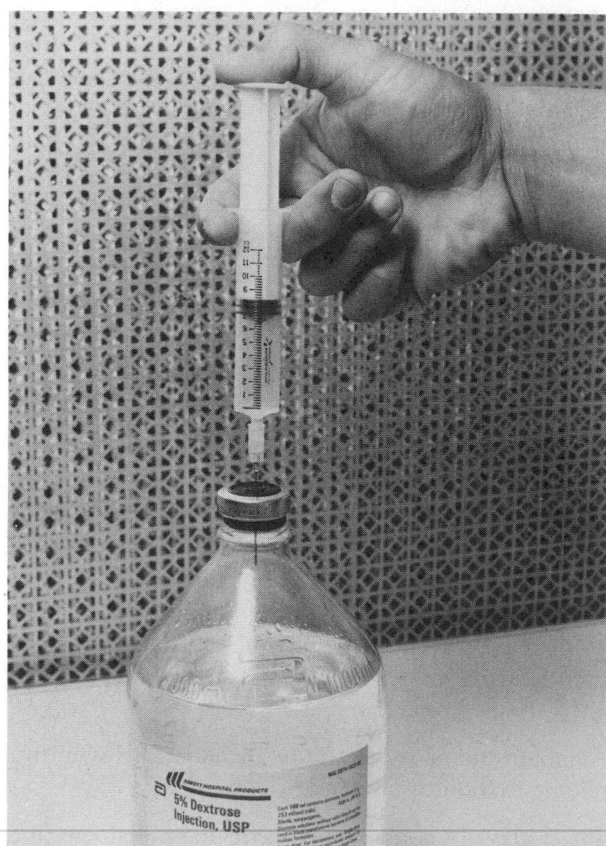

Figure 51–45

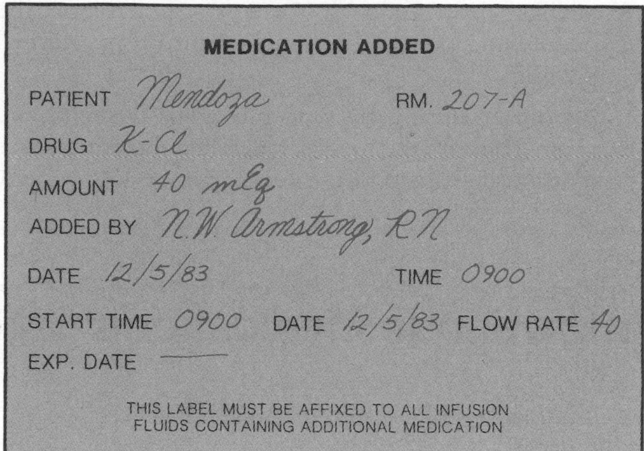

MEDICATION ADDED

PATIENT Mendoza RM. 207-A

DRUG K-Cl

AMOUNT 40 mEq

ADDED BY N.W. Armstrong, RN

DATE 12/5/83 TIME 0900

START TIME 0900 DATE 12/5/83 FLOW RATE 40

EXP. DATE ——

THIS LABEL MUST BE AFFIXED TO ALL INFUSION FLUIDS CONTAINING ADDITIONAL MEDICATION

Figure 51–46

Rationale This makes the label easy to read when the container is hanging.

10. Spike and hang the container, and regulate the flow rate according to the dosage required when the medication is to be administered. See Chapter 46, pages 1376 and 1382.
11. Record the IV infusion and medication.
12. Carefully monitor the IV infusion to maintain delivery of the medication and IV fluid at the specified rate.
13. During the administration, observe the client for signs of an adverse reaction, such as noisy respirations, changes in pulse rate, chills, nausea, or headache. If any adverse sign occurs, notify the physician or responsible nurse. Also monitor the client for signs of the intended action of the medication.

Variations for Adding Medications to an Infusing Container

See chapter 46 for additional information about intravenous infusion equipment.

14. *For an IV bottle with a vented administration set:*
    a. Make sure there is sufficient solution in the bottle to maintain proper dilution of the drug.
    b. Close the IV flow clamp.

       Rationale Closing the clamp is essential to prevent the medication from infusing to the client before it is properly diluted with the solution. Undiluted medication can produce a severe reaction.
    c. Detach the air vent cap, taking care not to contaminate the end. See Figure 51–47.
    d. Insert the tip of the medication syringe *without the needle* into the air vent port. See Figure 51–48.
    e. Instill the medication.
    f. Reattach the air vent.

       or

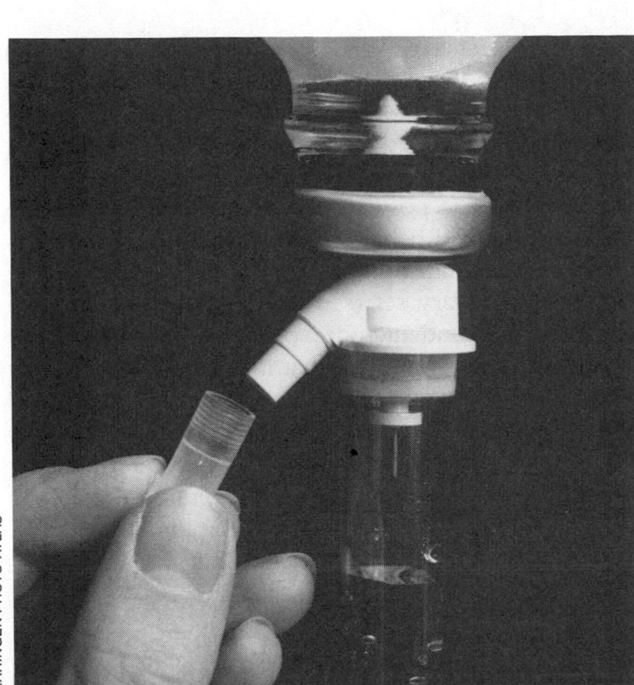

Figure 51–47

For a vented IV bottle:

g. After ensuring that there is sufficient solution in the bottle, close the IV flow clamp.
h. Clean the medication port with an antiseptic swab.
i. Insert the syringe needle through the port and instill the medication. The medication port is usually marked by a triangular imprint.

or

For a plastic IV bag:

j. After ensuring that there is sufficient solution in the bag, close the IV flow clamp.
k. Clean the medication port with an antiseptic swab.
l. While supporting and stabilizing the bag with your thumb and forefinger, carefully insert the syringe needle through the port and inject the medication. See Figure 51–49.

Rationale The bag is supported while injecting the medication to avoid puncturing the bag.

15. Gently lift and rotate the container.
Rationale This mixes the solution and medication.
16. Open the IV flow clamp and regulate the rate as ordered.
17. Attach a medication label to the IV container.
18. Follow steps 11–13 above.

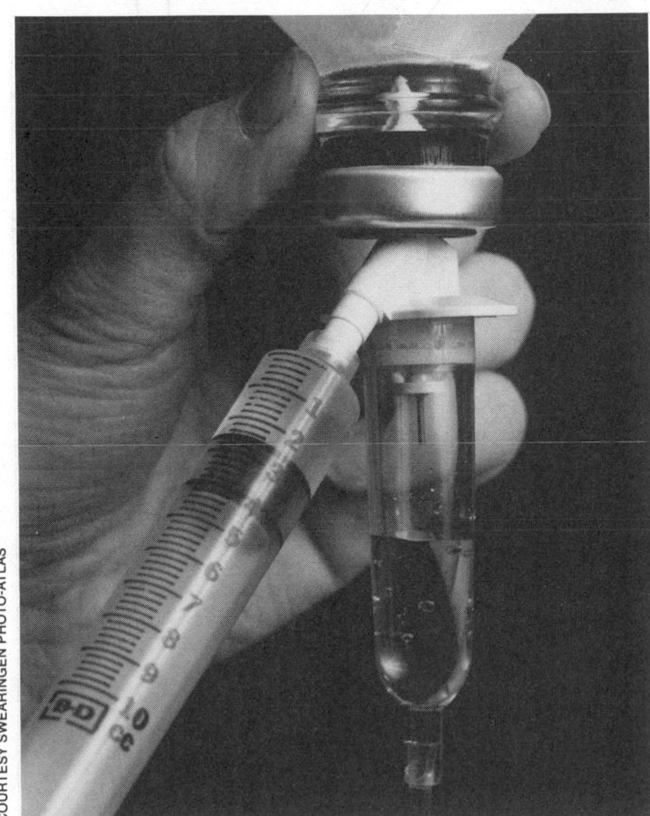

Figure 51–48

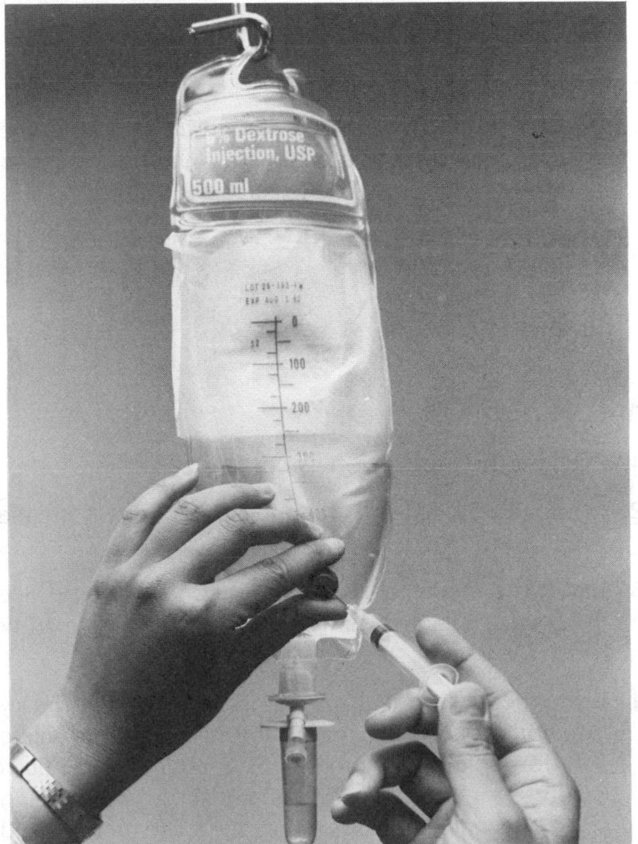

Figure 51–49

Using Additional IV Containers

Additional fluid containers and sets are sometimes attached to a primary infusion set to administer IV medications. They may be used to administer IV drugs intermittently that cannot be mixed with the primary solution for reason of incompatibility, or to maintain peak levels of a medication in the client's bloodstream and at the same time maintain a constant total infusion rate by simultaneous infusion of the primary line. Examples of two medications commonly administered in this manner are the bronchodilator aminophylline and antibiotic cephalothin sodium (Keflin).

There are two methods of attaching additional containers: the piggyback set and the secondary set. The piggyback set (see Figure 46–10, *B*, on page 1375) consists of a small IV bottle (minibottle) and a short tubing line that is connected to the upper Y-port (the piggyback port) of the primary line. Either a macrodrip or a microdrip system may be used. The term *piggyback* refers to the positioning of the additive bottle, which is higher than the primary infusion bottle. Manufacturers provide an extension hook to position the primary bottle below the piggyback bottle. The piggyback set is used for intermittent IV drug administration.

The secondary set (see Figure 46–10, *A*, on page 1375) uses a second microdrip or macrodrip bottle of any size and a long tubing line that it attached to the lower Y-port (secondary port) of the primary line. The primary and secondary bottles are positioned at the same height. This system is used to administer IV drugs intermittently or continuously with the primary IV solution.

Procedure 51–6 gives the steps for administering an IV medication using additional containers.

Procedure 51–6 ▲ Administering an IV Medication Using Additional Containers

Equipment

1. The appropriate additive set
2. The physician's order or the medication card
3. The correct sterile medication
4. A sterile syringe and needle. Generally a #20 gauge, 1-in needle is used, because longer needles can puncture the tubing and cause leakage of IV fluid.
5. A medication label
6. An antiseptic swab
7. Adhesive tape

Intervention

1. Prepare the medication as described earlier.
2. Compare the client's identification band with the medication card.
3. Insert the medication into the secondary bottle. See Procedure 51–5, "Adding an IV Medication to an IV Bottle or Bag."
4. If the medication is not compatible with the primary infusion, flush the primary line with a sterile saline solution before attaching the secondary set. To flush the line, wipe the port with an antiseptic swab, clamp the primary line, and, using a sterile needle and syringe, instill a few milliliters of sterile saline through the port to wash any primary infusion fluid out of the infusion tubing.

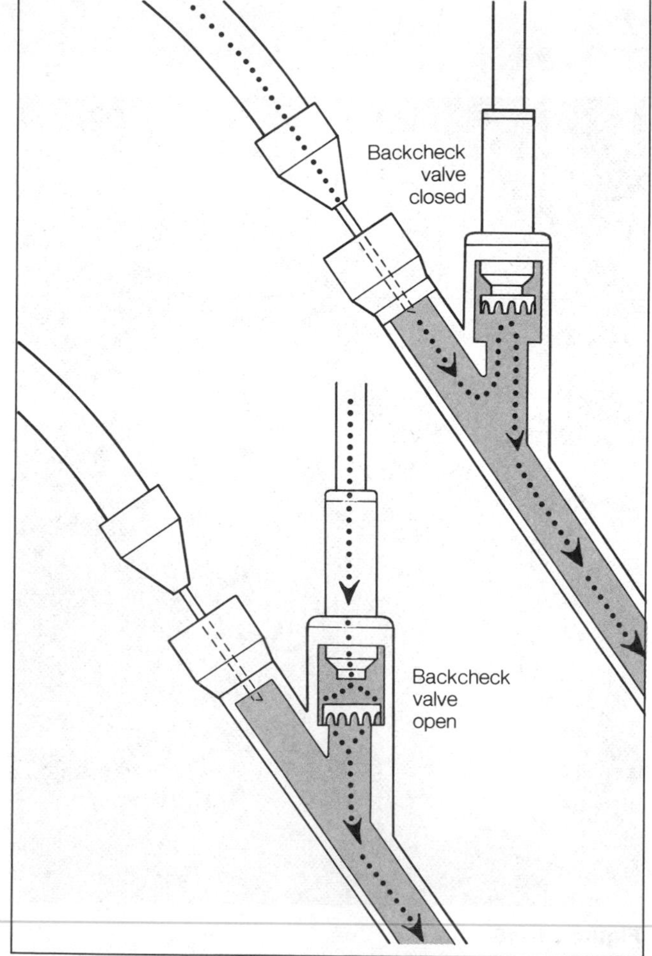

Figure 51–50

5. Wipe the port with an antiseptic swab.
6. Insert the needle of the secondary set into the port on the primary line, and secure it with adhesive tape. Some agencies recommend that a needle guard be taped alongside the needle to support the needle placement and keep the needle guard handy for use when discontinuing the secondary attachment.
7. Open the clamp on the secondary line, and regulate it in accordance with the recommended rate for that medication.
8. If a secondary set is used, clamp off the primary infusion, if necessary. When a piggyback set is used, a backcheck valve in the port automatically stops the flow of the primary infusion so that only the additive set infuses. See Figure 51–50. After the piggyback solution has infused and the level of the solution is below the level of the primary infusion drip chamber, the backcheck valve is released and the primary infusion automatically starts running.
9. Record the IV infusion and medication.
10. Carefully monitor the IV infusion to maintain delivery of the medication and the IV fluid at the specified rate.
11. Assess the client's response to the medication in terms of the intended action of the medication, adverse reactions to it, discomfort, etc.
12. When the medication has infused, readjust the flow of the primary line at the correct rate.
13. Either retain the secondary line for subsequent use or detach it and dispose of the equipment.

Volume-Control Administration Sets

Controlled volume administration sets have different names, depending on the manufacturer, e.g., Buretrol, Soluset, Volutrol, Pediatrol. They are small fluid containers (100 to 150 ml in size) attached below the primary infusion container. Volume-control sets are equipped with either a stationary membrane filter or a floating valve filter at the base of the container and are designed to finely control the amount of infusing fluid. See Figure 51–51.

Volume-control administration sets serve the following purposes.

1. To administer IV medications (such as some antibiotics) that do not remain stable for the length of time it takes an entire solution container to infuse
2. To administer medications intermittently
3. To avoid mixing medications that are incompatible
4. To dilute a drug so that it is less irritating to the veins than if given by direct intravenous push
5. To deliver medications diluted in precise amounts of fluid

See Procedure 51–7 for a description of the steps involved in adding an IV medication to a volume-control set.

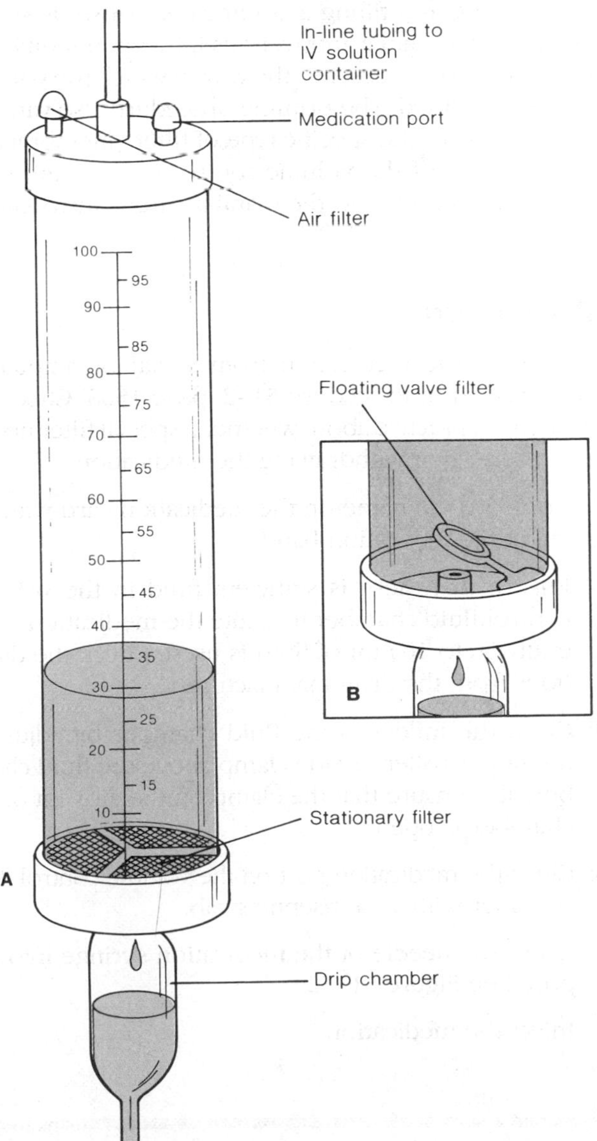

Figure 51–51 A volume-control intravenous infusion set: **A**, with a stationary filter; **B**, with a floating valve filter.

Procedure 51–7 ▲ Adding an IV Medication to a Volume-Control Administration Set

Equipment

1. The correct solution container
2. A volume-control administration set
3. The physician's order or the medication card
4. The correct sterile medication
5. Antiseptic swabs
6. A sterile syringe of appropriate size (e.g., 5 or 10 ml); a 1- to 1½-in, #20 or #21 gauge, sterile needle; and a sterile filter needle if needed to withdraw the medication
7. A medication label for the volume-control set

Attaching and filling a volume-control set is similar to setting up a regular intravenous infusion but differs in the priming procedure, i.e., the way in which the volume-control set is filled. The priming procedure also varies in accordance with the specific type of filter (membrane or floating valve) of the volume-control set. Assemble the equipment according to the manufacturer's instructions.

Intervention

1. Prepare the medication from a vial or ampule as described in Procedure 51–2, page 1508. Check the agency's practice about whether a special filter needle is used when withdrawing the medication.
2. Compare the name on the medication card with the client's identification band.
3. Ensure that there is sufficient fluid in the volume-control fluid chamber to dilute the medication. Generally 50 to 100 ml of fluid is used. Check the directions from the drug manufacturer.
4. Close the inflow to the fluid chamber by adjusting the upper roller or side clamp above the fluid chamber; also ensure that the clamp on the air vent of the chamber is open.
5. Clean the medication port on the volume-control fluid chamber with an antiseptic swab.
6. Insert the needle of the medication syringe into the port. See Figure 51–52.
7. Inject the medication.

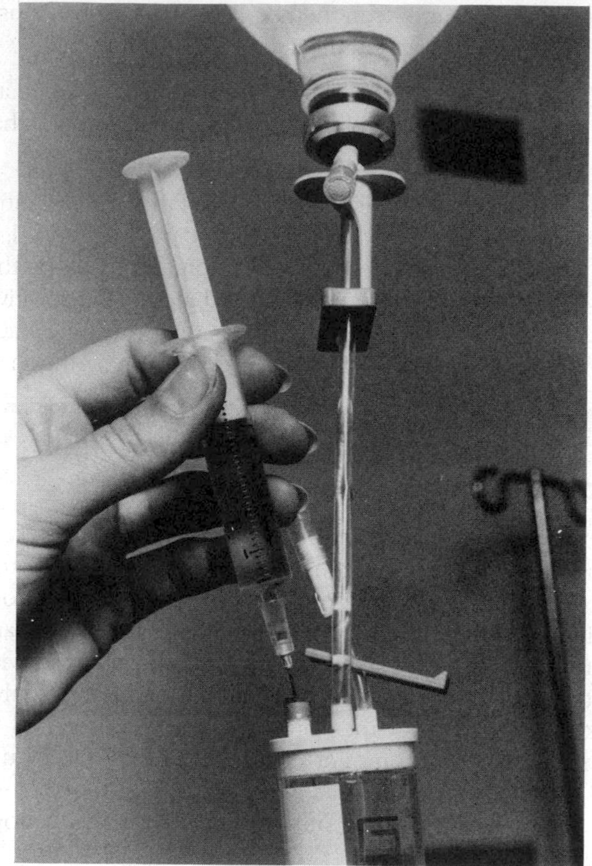

Figure 51–52

8. Gently rotate the fluid chamber until the fluid is well mixed.
9. Regulate the flow by adjusting the lower roller or side clamp below the fluid chamber.
10. Attach a medication label to the volume control fluid chamber.
11. Record the IV infusion and medication.
12. Carefully monitor the IV infusion to maintain delivery of the medication and IV fluid at the specified rate.
13. Assess the client's response to the medication in terms of the intended action of the medication, adverse reactions to it, discomfort, etc.

IV Push (Bolus)

An IV push is the intravenous administration of a medication that cannot be diluted or that is needed in an emergency. Also, certain drugs are administered this way to achieve maximum effect. It is important to remember that the medication is administered rapidly with an IV push, which could be dangerous for the client. Some agencies allow only physicians or specially trained nurses to administer IV push medications. Check agency policy.

An IV push can be administered directly into a vein through venipuncture, into an existing intravenous apparatus through an injection port (see Figure 51–53 below), or through an intermittent infusion set (heparin lock) when the client does not have an IV running but does have a heparin lock in place. The heparin lock, also referred to as a male adapter plug (MAP), is used primarily for clients who require regular intermittent IV medications but not the fluid volume of an intravenous infusion. The set usually consists of an indwelling needle or catheter attached to a plastic tube with a sealed injection tip. See Figure 51–55 later in this chapter. It is called a *heparin lock* because small amounts of heparin are injected into it to maintain its patency. The infusion set is generally inserted into the client's arm or hand.

Administration via IV push is described in Procedure 51–8.

Procedure 51–8 ▲ Administering an IV Medication by Intravenous Push (Bolus)

Equipment

1. The physician's order or the medication card
2. The correct sterile medication
3. A sterile syringe of the appropriate size for the volume of medication and a sterile 2.5-cm (1-in) #25 gauge needle to prevent large puncture holes in the injection port
4. Alcohol swabs

In addition, for a heparin lock,

5. A sterile syringe and needle with a heparin flush solution. Check agency practice. Many hospitals advocate the use of 100 units per milliliter of solution, and 0.5 ml is generally used. Prepackaged heparin syringes and needles are available.
6. A sterile syringe and needle with 4 ml (or amount prescribed by the agency) of normal saline

Intervention

1. Prepare the medication as described earlier in this chapter. Label the syringe with the name of the medication and the dosage.
2. In a separate syringe, prepare the heparin solution according to agency policy, if needed. Label this syringe.
3. In another syringe, prepare the saline solution. Label this syringe.
4. Compare the name on the client's identification band with the name on the medication card.

IV Push into an Existing IV

5. Identify an injection port nearest the client. Some ports have a circle indicating the site for the needle insertion.

   Rationale An injection port must be used because it is self-sealing. Any puncture to the plastic tubing will leak.
6. Clean the port with an antiseptic swab.
7. Stop the IV flow by closing the clamp or pinching the tubing above the injection port (see Figure 51–53).
8. While holding the port steady, insert the needle into the port.
9. Draw back on the plunger to withdraw some blood into the IV tubing (not into the syringe).

   Rationale This shows that the needle is in the vein.

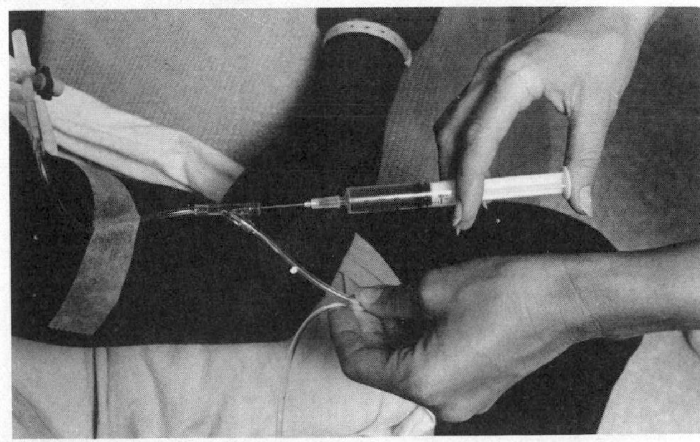

Figure 51–53

10. Inject the medication at the correct rate, withdraw the needle, reopen the clamp, and reestablish the intravenous infusion at the correct rate. If the medication is particularly irritating to the veins, run the IV rapidly for about a minute to dilute the medication, and then adjust the rate.

IV Push into an Intermittent Infusion Set

11. Swab the injection port with an antiseptic swab.
12. Insert the needle with the normal saline into the port and aspirate for blood return. See Figure 51–54.

    Rationale This ensures that the heparin lock catheter is in the vein. In some situations blood will not return even though the heparin lock is patent.
13. Inject 2 ml of the normal saline solution. This step is optional. Check agency practice.

    Rationale This is done to flush the heparin from the catheter.

    If the client experiences burning or stinging sensations, it may be that the needle or catheter is not in the vein and the fluid is infiltrating the tissue. In this case withhold the medication until the heparin lock is replaced.
14. Remove the saline-filled syringe, and cap the needle to maintain its sterility.

    Rationale This syringe is used again, so it must be kept sterile.
15. Insert the needle attached to the medication syringe.
16. Inject the medication slowly at the recommended rate of infusion. Observe the client closely for adverse reactions. Remove the needle and syringe when all medication is administered.
17. Reattach the saline syringe, and inject the recommended amount of saline.

    Rationale The saline injection flushes the medication through the catheter and prepares the lock for the heparin.
18. Insert the heparin syringe, and inject the heparin slowly into the set. See Figure 51–55 for a prepackaged heparin syringe.
19. Check the patency of the heparin lock at least every 8 hours or according to agency practice.
    a. Aspirate for return blood flow.
    b. Flush the catheter with 2 to 3 ml of normal saline.
    c. Refill the heparin lock with heparin solution.

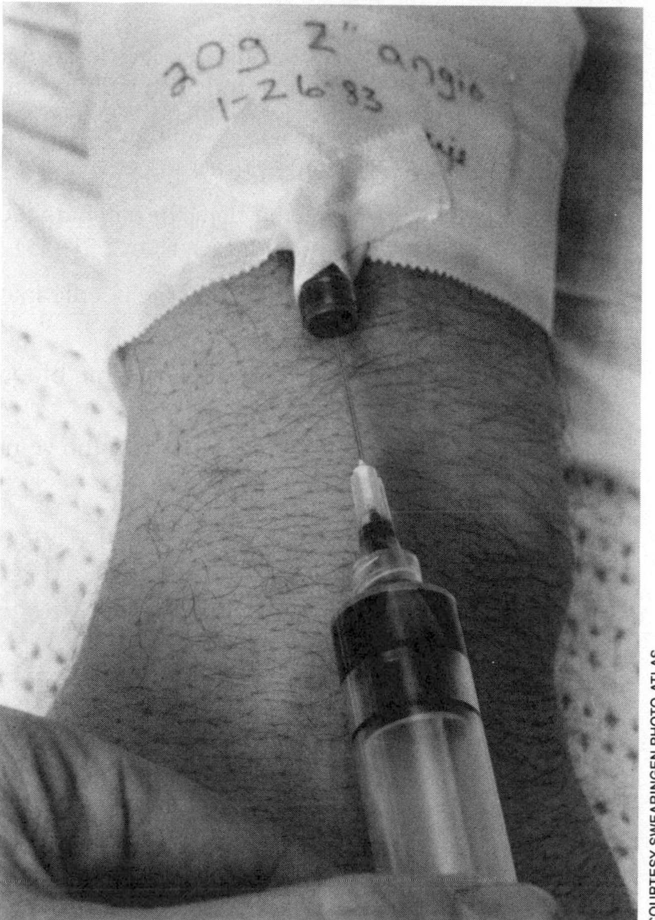

COURTESY SWEARINGEN PHOTO-ATLAS

Figure 51–54

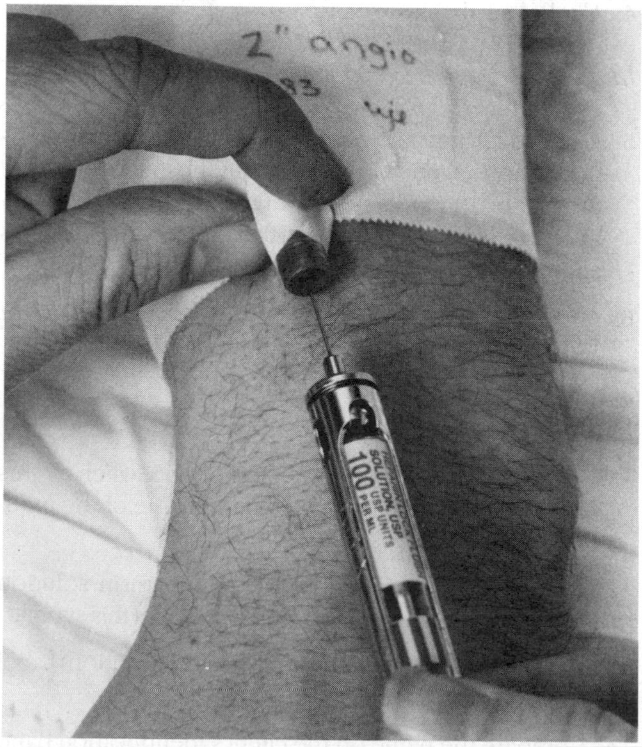

COURTESY SWEARINGEN PHOTO-ATLAS

Figure 51–55

20. Check agency practice about recommended times for changing the heparin lock. Some agencies advocate a change every 48 to 72 hours.

IV Push Directly into a Vein

21. Perform a venipuncture. See Chapter 46, page 1378.
22. Slowly inject the medication into the vein. The rate of the injection will vary according to the medication, the physician's order, and/or the manufacturer's directions. Many medications are injected slowly over a period of several minutes. Check drug reference information.
23. Withdraw the needle, and apply pressure to the site to prevent bleeding.

For All Types of Intravenous Medications

24. Record the medication given, dosage, time, route, any complaints of the client, and your signature.
25. Carefully assess the client's response to the medication in terms of the intended action of the medication, adverse reactions to it, discomfort, etc. Because the medication is administered relatively quickly and directly into the bloodstream, it can produce sudden and severe reactions.

Disposal of Equipment

Needles that have been inserted into a client may be contaminated with microorganisms, such as the hepatitis virus, that can be passed along to other people if the contaminated needle pricks their skin. In addition, needles and syringes have value in the illicit drug market.

Nurses should carefully break off a needle at the hub and discard needles and syringes in designed containers. There are needle breakers available commercially to break needles after use.

Topical Medications

Dermatologic medications are commonly applied for one of the following reasons:

1. To decrease itching (pruritus)
2. To lubricate and soften the skin
3. To cause local vasoconstriction or vasodilation
4. To increase or decrease secretions from the skin
5. To provide a protective coating to the skin
6. To apply an antibiotic or antiseptic to treat or prevent infection

Inunction is the application of topical drugs meant to be absorbed through the epidermis. Such drugs must be rubbed in. Drugs are not readily absorbed through the epidermis; however, they can be absorbed into the lining of the sebaceous glands and sweat pores. Absorption is facilitated by washing the area well before the application, using a pharmaceutical preparation with a base that mixes with fat, such as alcohol, and using a drug that is fat soluble.

Dermatologic preparations include lotions, emollients, liniments, ointments, pastes, and powders. See Table 51–1, earlier in the chapter.

Unless contraindicated by an order, always wash and carefully dry the area, using a patting motion, before applying a dermatologic preparation. Skin encrustations and discharges harbor microorganisms and cause local infections. They can also prevent the medication from coming in contact with the area to be treated.

Nurses should always use sterile technique when an open wound is present. If a client has lesions, the preparation must be applied using gloves or tongue depressors. In this way the nurse's hand will not come in direct contact with microorganisms in and around the lesions. See Table 51–10.

Table 51–10 Topical Applications

Medication	Application
Lotion	Shake before use to distribute suspended particles. Pour onto sterile gauze and pat onto affected area. Do not rub, to avoid aggravating affected area.
Liniment	Pour onto hands and rub into client's skin with long, smooth strokes.
Ointment and paste	Usually applied with a tongue blade or with gloves. Some must be applied thinly over the area, e.g., cortisone. Sterile dressing may be applied over ointment.
Powder	Sprinkle over the surface and cover with a dressing.

Irrigations and Instillations

Irrigation (lavage) is the washing out of a body cavity by a stream of water or other fluid. **Instillation** is the insertion of a medication into a body cavity.

Irrigation is performed for one or more of the following reasons:

1. To clean the area, i.e., to remove a foreign object or discharge
2. To apply heat or cold
3. To apply a medication, such as an antiseptic
4. To prepare an area for surgery, e.g., the eye

Irrigations necessitate the use of sterile technique whenever there is a break in the skin, for example, in a wound irrigation, or whenever a sterile body cavity, such as the bladder, is entered. However, some irrigations, e.g., an eye irrigation to remove foreign material, or a vaginal, rectal, or gastric irrigation, are safely conducted using clean technique. Instillations are performed to apply medication to an area.

Equipment

A number of different kinds of syringes are used for irrigations. The most common are the Asepto, the rubber bulb, the Toomey, and the Pomeroy. The syringes are often calibrated.

The *Asepto syringe* is a plastic (or glass) syringe with a rubber bulb. See Figure 51–56, *A*. Squeezing the air out of the bulb produces negative pressure, and fluid can be sucked into the syringe. When the bulb is squeezed again, the fluid is ejected from the syringe. Asepto syringes come in several sizes, e.g., 30 ml (1 oz), 60 ml (2 oz), and 120 ml (4 oz).

The *rubber bulb syringe*, also called the *ear syringe*, is often used for irrigating the ears. See Figure 51–56, *B*. Like the Asepto syringe, it comes in a range of sizes.

The *Toomey syringe*, which is made of plastic or glass, is also calibrated. See Figure 51–56, *C*. This syringe has a removable tip of metal or plastic that can fit into the end of tubing such as a catheter. Toomey syringes are used for deep-wound irrigations that require a catheter and for some types of bladder irrigations.

The *Pomeroy syringe* is a metal syringe commonly used for ear irrigations. A shield near the tip prevents the solution from spraying outward (see Figure 51–56, *D*). In the home an eye cup is frequently used for eye irrigation. See Chapter 52, page 1564, for wound irrigation.

For an instillation, a syringe or a dropper is usually used. Liquid eye, ear, and nose medications are commonly instilled using the plastic container in which the drug is packaged or a small eye dropper. Ointments are applied directly from their small tube.

Ophthalmic Irrigations and Instillations

The client is assisted to either a sitting or lying position with her or his head tilted toward the affected eye so that any solution will not run into the other eye but to the basin at the side of the client's head. Clean the eyelid and lashes with sterile cotton balls moistened with sterile irrigating solution or sterile normal saline. Wipe from the inner to the outer canthus to prevent contamination of the other eye and the lacrimal duct. While wiping the eye,

1. Assess the eye for redness, the location and nature of any discharge, lacrimation, and swelling of the eyelids or of the lacrimal gland.
2. Assess any client complaints, e.g., itching, burning, pain, blurring of vision, or photophobia.
3. Assess the client's behavior, e.g., squinting, blinking excessively, frowning, or rubbing the eyes.

The equipment required is described on page 1533.

Irrigation

For an irrigation, expose the lower conjunctival sac by separating the lids with the thumb and forefinger (see Figure 51–57). Or, to irrigate in stages, first hold the lower lid down, then hold the upper lid up. Exert pressure on the bony prominences of the cheekbone and beneath the eyebrow when holding the eyelids. Separating the lids prevents reflex blinking. Exerting pressure on the bony prominences minimizes the possibility of pressing the eyeball and causing discomfort.

Hold the irrigator about 2.5 cm (1 in) above the eye so the pressure of the solution will not damage the eye and so the irrigator cannot touch the eye. Irrigate the eye, directing the solution onto the lower conjunctival sac, from the inner canthus to the outer canthus. Directing the solution in this way prevents possible injury to the cornea and prevents fluid and contaminants from flowing down the nasolacrimal duct. Irrigate until the solution leaving the eye is clear (no discharge is present) or until

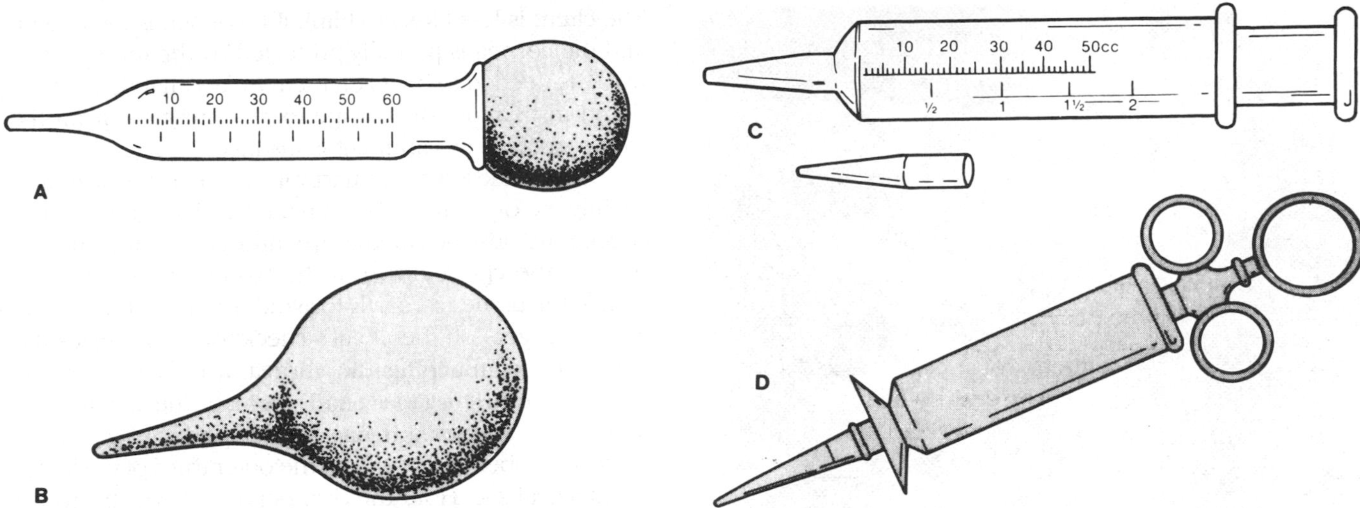

Figure 51–56 Four types of syringes commonly used for irrigations: **A**, Asepto; **B**, rubber bulb; **C**, Toomey with adaptor tip to fit into tubing; **D**, Pomeroy.

all the solution has been used. Instruct the client to close and move the eye periodically so that secretions move from the upper to the lower conjunctival sac. Dry around the eye with cotton balls.

Instillation

Check the ophthalmic preparation as to name, strength, and number of drops if a liquid is used. Then draw the correct number of drops into the dropper if a dropper is used. If ointment is used, discard the first bead, because it is considered to be contaminated. Ask the client to look up to the ceiling and give him or her a piece of tissue.

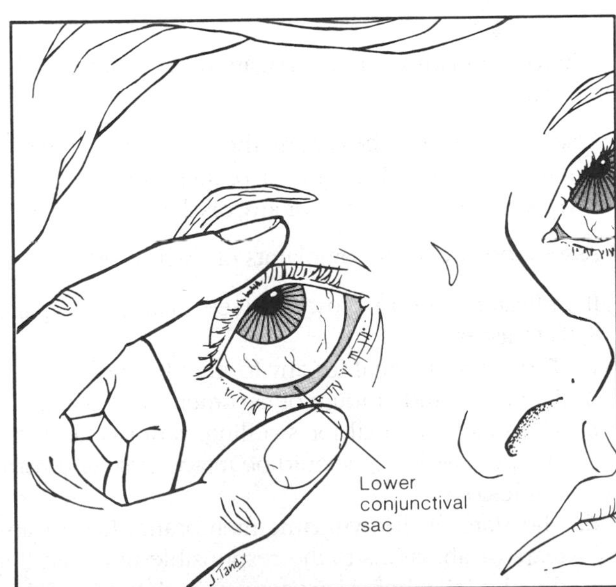

Figure 51–57 Exposing the lower conjunctival sac.

Ophthalmic Equipment

For an irrigation

- A sterile container for the irrigating solution
- Irrigating solution. Usually 60 to 235 ml (2 to 8 oz) of solution at 37 C (98.6 F) is appropriate.
- A sterile eye syringe or eye irrigator. An eyedropper can be used if only small amounts of solution are required.
- A sterile kidney basin
- Sterile cotton balls
- Sterile normal saline (optional)
- A moisture-proof drape
- Sterile gloves (optional)

For an instillation

- The medication. Some eye medications are packaged in plastic containers that are also used to administer the preparation. Ointments are usually supplied in small tubes.
- A sterile eyedropper, if needed
- Sterile absorbent sponges. Soak some sponges in sterile normal saline for cleaning the eyelid and eyelashes.
- A sterile eye dressing (pad), as needed, and paper eye tape to secure it

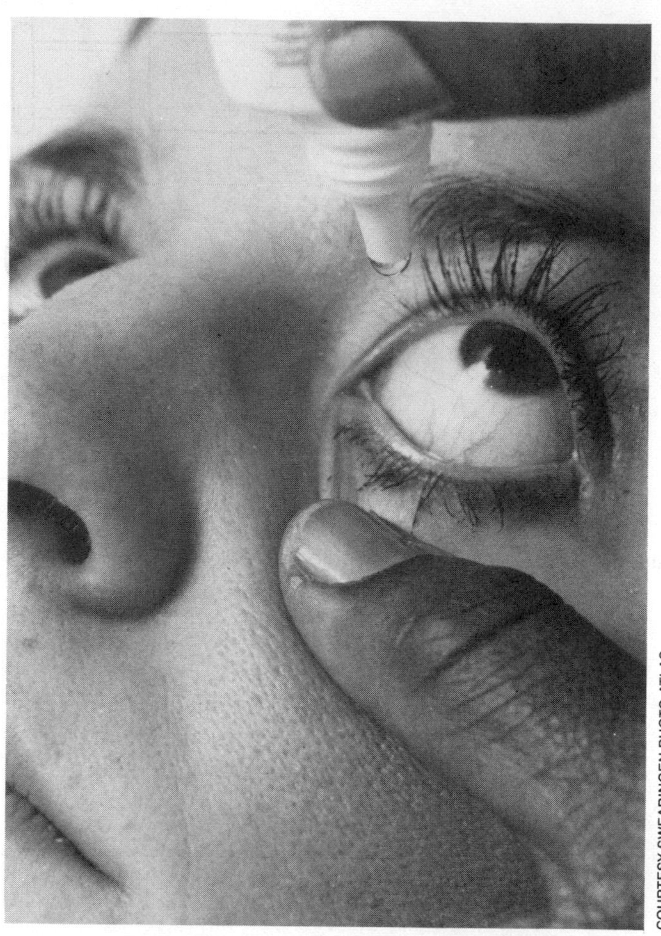

Figure 51–58 Instilling an eye drop into the lower conjunctival sac.

The client is less likely to blink if he or she is looking up and the cornea is partially protected by the top eyelid. A tissue is needed to press on the nasolacrimal duct after a liquid instillation, or to wipe excess ointment from the eyelashes after an ointment is instilled.

Expose the lower conjunctival sac by placing the thumb or fingers of your nondominant hand on the client's cheekbone, just below the eye, and gently drawing the skin on the cheek down. If the tissues are edematous, handle the tissues carefully to avoid damaging them. Placing the fingers on the client's cheekbone minimizes the possibility of touching the cornea, avoids putting any pressure on the eyeball, and prevents the client from blinking or squinting. Using a side approach, instill the correct number of drops onto the outer third of the lower conjunctival sac. Hold the dropper 1 to 2 cm (0.4 to 0.8 in) above the sac. See Figure 51–58. The client is less likely to blink if a side approach is used. When instilled into the conjunctival sac, drops will not harm the cornea as they might if dropped directly on it. The dropper must not touch the sac or the cornea.

When instilling an ointment, hold the tube above the lower conjunctival sac, squeeze 3 cm (0.8 in) of ointment from the tube into the lower conjunctival sac, from the inner canthus outward. The client should then close her or his eyes but not squeeze them, because squeezing can injure the eye and push out the medication. For liquid medications, press firmly or have the client press firmly on the nasolacrimal duct for at least 30 seconds so that the medication is held in the eye and does not run down the nasolacrimal duct.

Otic Irrigations and Instillations

Irrigation

Irrigations of the external auditory canal are generally carried out for cleaning purposes, although applications of heat and of antiseptic solutions are sometimes prescribed. Irrigations usually are performed in a hospital, with sterile supplies and equipment so that microorganisms will not be introduced into the ear. If done at home, sterile supplies usually are not necessary because the client is accustomed to the microorganisms in the home environment. Medical aseptic technique is used to instill medications to the ear unless the tympanic membrane is damaged, in which case sterile technique is used.

The position of the external auditory canal varies with age. In the child under 3 years of age, it is directed upward on the inside. In the adult, the external auditory canal is an S-shaped structure about 2.5 cm (1 in) long. Hairs grow along the outer third of the canal.

Before initiating an otic irrigation or instillation the nurse must:

1. Assess the pinna of the ear and the meatus of the external auditory canal for signs of redness and abrasions and the type and amount of any discharge.
2. Assess the client for complaints of discomfort.
3. If indicated, use an otoscope (see Chapter 35, page 830) to assess:
   a. The external canal for any foreign bodies
   b. The color and amount of cerumen in the canal
   c. The external canal for swelling, redness, and discharge. The lining should be intact, pink, and without lesions.
   d. The state of the tympanic membrane. Report any tears or abrasions to the responsible nurse and/or the physician before proceeding with the irrigation or instillation.

The equipment required is listed to the right.

Explain to the client that she or he may experience a feeling of fullness, warmth, and occasionally dizziness and discomfort when the fluid comes in contact with the tympanic membrane. Assist the client to a sitting or lying position, with head turned toward the affected ear. The solution can then flow from the ear canal to a basin. Place the moisture-resistant towel around the client's shoulder, and position the basin under the ear to be irrigated.

Clean the pinna of the ear and the meatus of the ear canal with applicator swabs and solution. Remove any discharge so it will not be washed into the ear canal. Fill the syringe with solution.

Alternatively, the nurse can do the following. Hang up the irrigating container, and run solution through the tubing and the nozzle to remove any air. Straighten the client's auditory canal so the fluid can flow the entire length of the canal. See Chapter 35, page 830. Insert the tip of the syringe or nozzle into the auditory meatus, and direct the solution gently upward against the top of the canal. The solution will flow around the entire canal and out at the bottom. The solution is instilled gently because strong pressure from the fluid can cause discomfort and damage the tympanic membrane. Continue instilling the fluid until all the solution is used or until the canal is cleaned, depending on the purpose of the irrigation. Take care not to block the outward flow of the solution with the syringe or nozzle. Dry the outside of the ear with absorbent cotton balls. Place a cotton fluff in the auditory meatus for about 15 minutes to absorb the excess fluid. Assist the client to a side-lying position on the affected side so that excess fluid will drain by gravity.

Assess the client's response to the irrigation in terms of discomfort, dizziness, and the appearance and odor of the fluid returns. Record the irrigation; the type, concentration, amount, and temperature of the solution used; the appearance of the returns; and the client's response in terms of discomfort and dizziness.

Equipment for an Otic Irrigation and Otic Instillation

For an irrigation

- A container for the irrigating solution
- Irrigating solution. About 500 ml (16 oz) of solution is required. Normal saline is frequently used. Solution temperature should be body temperature: for an adult, 37.0 C (98.6 F).
- A syringe. A rubber bulb or Asepto syringe is frequently used.
- A basin to receive the irrigating solution
- A moisture-resistant towel
- Applicator swabs for cleaning the external ear
- Absorbent cotton balls to dry the pinna of the ear after the irrigation

For an instillation

- The correct medication bottle, with a dropper. To make the instillation more comfortable for the client, warm the container in your hand or place it in warm water for a short time.
- A cotton-tipped applicator to wipe the auditory meatus
- A flexible rubber tip (optional) for the end of the dropper, which prevents injury from sudden motion, e.g., by a child or disoriented client
- A cotton fluff to cover the auditory meatus following the instillation

Instillation

The client assumes a side-lying position, with the ear to be treated uppermost. Wipe the external auditory meatus with a cotton-tipped applicator and then straighten the ear canal as for an irrigation. Instill the required number of drops of medication, which should be at room temperature unless otherwise ordered. Insert a small cotton fluff in the auditory meatus for 15–20 minutes to help retain the medication.

Nasal Instillations

Nose drops usually are instilled for their astringent effect (to shrink swollen mucous membranes) or to treat infections of the nasal cavity or sinuses. Equipment required: the medication solution, which usually comes in a bottle with an attached dropper; disposable tissues; and a tray for the equipment. Prior to the instillation, the client blows his or her nose to clear the nasal passages.

The client assumes a back-lying position. For treating the opening of the eustachian (auditory) tube, the client can assume a dorsal recumbent position. The drops flow into the pharynx, where the eustachian tube opens. To treat the ethmoid and sphenoid sinuses, the client assumes a back-lying position, with the head over the edge of the bed or a pillow under the shoulders so the head is tipped backward. To treat the maxillary and frontal sinuses, the client assumes the same back-lying position, with the head turned toward the side to be treated. This is the Parkinson position. The nurse makes sure the client is positioned so the correct side is accessible if only one side is to be treated. If the client's head is over the edge of the bed, it must be supported by the nurse's hands so the neck muscles are not strained.

Once the client has assumed one of the above positions, the nurse administers the drops. The dropper is held just above the nostril, and the drops are directed toward the midline of the superior concha of the ethmoid bone as the client breathes through his or her mouth. If the drops are directed toward the base of the nasal cavity, they will run down the eustachian tube. The mucous membranes of the nostrils should not be touched, to avoid injury to tissue and contamination of the dropper. The nurse has the client remain in this position for 5 to 10 minutes so the solution will flow into the desired area. The nurse discards any medication remaining in the dropper before returning the dropper to the bottle.

To administer nose drops to an infant, the nurse places a pillow under the infant's shoulders and allows the child's head to fall back slightly over the edge of the pillow onto the nurse's arm. This arm can also be used to restrain the infant's arms. The other hand can be used to administer the nose drops.

Vaginal Instillations and Irrigations

Vaginal medications are inserted as creams, jellies, foams, suppositories, or irrigations (douches). Medical aseptic technique should be used. Vaginal creams, jellies, and foams are applied with a tubular applicator and plunger. Suppositories are inserted with the index finger of a gloved hand. Vaginal medications are inserted to treat a vaginal infection topically or to relieve vaginal discomfort, e.g., itching or pain.

Prior to the instillation, the nurse asks the client to urinate, since a full bladder can make treatment uncomfortable. Privacy is essential for this procedure. The nurse assists the client to a back-lying position, with the knees flexed and the hips rotated laterally. The client is draped as for catheterization. Adequate lighting on the vaginal orifice is necessary.

Instillation of a Vaginal Suppository

Suppositories are designed to melt at body temperature, so they are generally stored in the refrigerator to keep them firm for insertion. The nurse unwraps the suppository, puts it on the opened wrapper, and dons gloves to prevent contamination. Next, the nurse lubricates the smooth or rounded end of the suppository to facilitate its insertion. The rounded end is inserted first.

To insert the suppository, the nurse lubricates the gloved index finger and exposes the vaginal orifice by separating the labia with the nondominant hand. The suppository is placed about 8 to 10 cm (3 to 4 in) along the posterior wall of the vagina, or as far as it will go. See Figure 51–59. (The posterior wall of the vagina is about 2.5 cm [1 in] longer than the anterior wall because the cervix protrudes into the uppermost portion of the anterior wall. The anterior wall is usually about 6 to 7.5 cm [2½ to 3 in] long.) The nurse withdraws the finger, removes the gloves by turning them inside out, and places them on a paper towel. Turning the gloves inside out prevents the spread of microorganisms. The client remains in the supine position for 5 to 10 minutes after the insertion. Her hips may also be elevated on a pillow. The client remains lying down to allow the melted medication to flow into the posterior fornix.

Instillation of a Vaginal Cream

The nurse fills the applicator with the prescribed cream, jelly, or foam. Directions are provided with the manufacturer's applicator. With the gloved nondominant hand, the nurse exposes the vaginal orifice. A second glove may also be worn to protect the nurse's hands from micro-

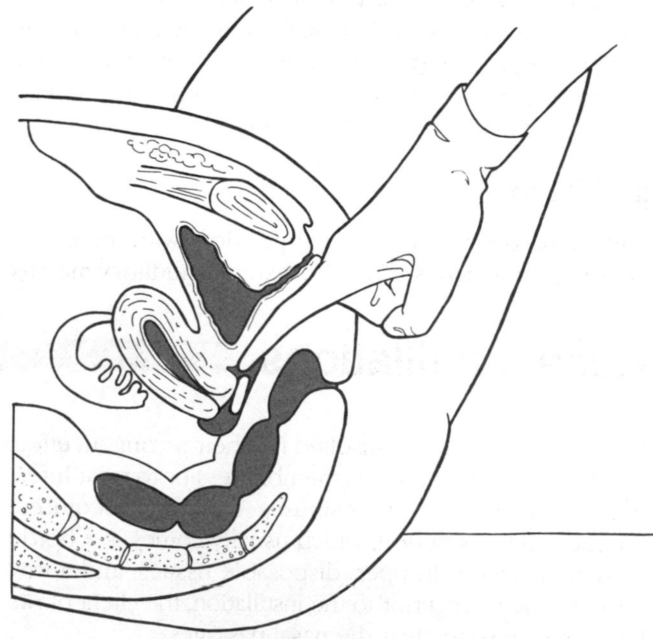

Figure 51–59 Instilling a vaginal suppository.

organisms. The nurse gently inserts the applicator about 5 cm (2 in) and pushes the plunger until the applicator is empty. See Figure 51–60. The applicator is removed and placed on a paper towel to contain microorganisms and prevent their spread. Next, the nurse removes the glove, turns it inside out, and places it on the paper towel. The client needs to remain supine for 5 to 10 minutes following the instillation. Finally, the nurse applies a clean perineal pad and a T-binder if there is excessive drainage.

Procedure 51–9 describes how to perform a vaginal irrigation.

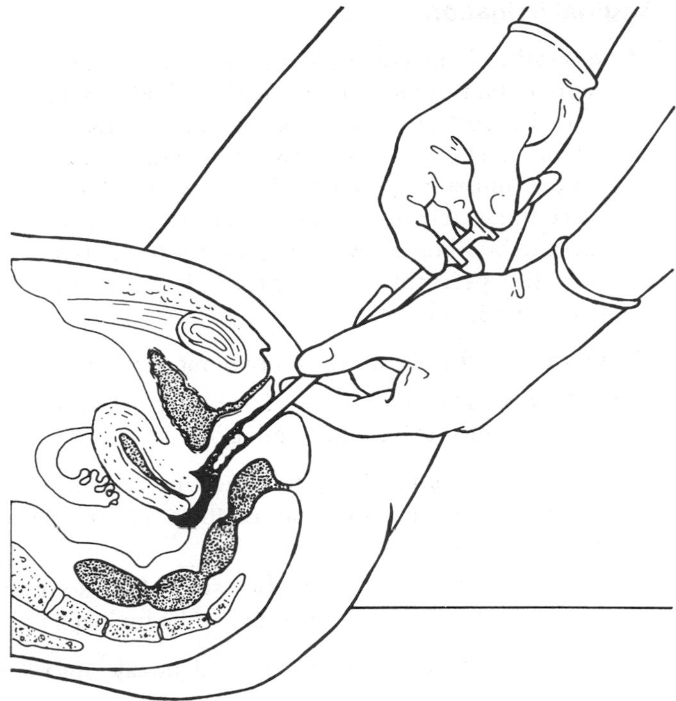

Figure 51–60 Instilling a vaginal cream using an applicator.

Procedure 51–9 ▲ Administering a Vaginal Irrigation

Equipment

In hospitals, sterile supplies and equipment are used; in a home, sterility is not usually necessary because clients are accustomed to the microorganisms in their environments. Sterile technique is indicated if there is an open wound.

1. A vaginal irrigation set (these are often disposable) containing:
   a. A nozzle
   b. Tubing and a clamp
   c. A container for the solution
   d. A moisture-resistant drape
2. Irrigating solution. Usually 1000 to 2000 ml at 40.5 C (105 F) is required. Check agency practice. Normal saline, tap water, sodium bicarbonate solution (8 ml of sodium bicarbonate to 1000 ml of water), and vinegar solution (8 ml of vinegar to 1000 ml of water) are commonly used.
3. A thermometer to check the temperature of the solution. This is usually measured before the equipment is taken to the client.
4. A moisture-proof pad to protect the bedding and a drape to cover the client's legs
5. A bedpan to receive the irrigation returns
6. Tissues to dry the perineum
7. Gloves (optional). They may be required to protect the nurse from infection.
8. An IV pole on which to hang the solution container

Intervention

1. Explain the technique to the client. A vaginal irrigation is normally a painless procedure and in fact may bring relief from itching and burning if an infection is present. It usually takes about 10 minutes. Many clients feel embarrassed about this procedure, and some may prefer to perform the procedure themselves if instruction is provided.
2. Carefully check the physician's order for the specific medication or solution ordered, its dosage, and the time of administration.
3. Provide privacy, and ask the client to void.

   Rationale The client will have less discomfort during the treatment, and the possibility of injuring the vaginal lining is decreased, if the bladder is empty.

Vaginal Irrigation

4. Assist the client to a back-lying position, with the hips higher than the shoulders so the solution will flow into the posterior fornix of the vagina. Position the client on a bedpan, and provide comfortable support for the lumbar region of the back with a roll or pillow. Place the waterproof drape under the bedpan to protect the bedding. Provide a drape for the legs so that only the perineal area is exposed. See "Draping," Chapter 35, page 802.

5. Provide perineal care to remove microorganisms.

   Rationale This decreases the chance of flushing microorganisms into the vagina.

6. Clamp the tubing. Hang the irrigating container on the IV pole so the base is about 30 cm (12 in) above the vagina.

   Rationale At this height the pressure of the solution should not be great enough to injure the vaginal lining.

7. Run fluid through the tubing and nozzle into the bedpan.

   Rationale Fluid is run through the tubing to remove air and to moisten the nozzle.

8. Run some fluid over the perineal area, then insert the nozzle carefully into the vagina. See Figure 51–61. Direct the nozzle toward the sacrum, following the direction of the vagina.

9. Insert the nozzle about 7 to 10 cm (3 to 4 in), and rotate it several times.

   Rationale Rotating the nozzle irrigates all parts of the vagina.

10. Use all of the irrigating solution, permitting it to flow out freely into the bedpan.

    Rationale Obstructing the flow of the returns could result in pressure injury to the tissues.

11. Remove the nozzle from the vagina.

12. Assist the client to a sitting position on the bedpan. tion; any discomfort, etc.; and the client's response to the irrigation.

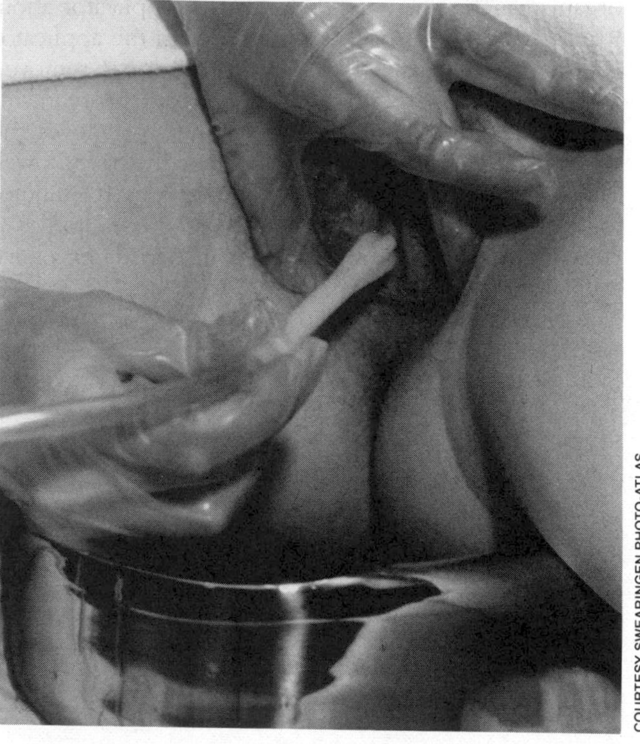

COURTESY SWEARINGEN PHOTO-ATLAS

Figure 51–61

Rationale Sitting on the bedpan helps drain the remaining fluid by gravity.

13. Dry the perineum with tissues.

14. Remove the bedpan.

15. Assess the client's response in terms of the color of the fluid returns and the presence of any flecks, discomfort, redness of the vagina, and odor from the vagina.

16. Remove the moisture-resistant pad and the drape.

17. Apply a dressing if indicated.

18. On the client's chart, record the irrigation; the amount, type, strength, and temperature of the irrigating solution; and all nursing assessments.

Rectal Instillations

Rectal suppositories are a convenient and safe method of giving certain medications. The advantages of rectal instillation include:

1. It avoids irritation of the upper gastrointestinal tract.
2. Some medications are well-absorbed across the mucosal surface of the rectum.
3. Rectal suppositories are thought to provide higher bloodstream levels (titers) of medication, since the venous blood from the rectum is not transported through the liver (Hahn et al. 1982, p. 99).

Rectal medications may have a local effect (e.g., a laxative suppository will soften feces and stimulate defecation) or a systemic effect (e.g., an aminophylline suppository will dilate the client's bronchi and ease breathing).

Prior to the insertion, the nurse helps the client to a lateral position, with the upper leg acutely flexed. Next, the nurse unwraps the suppository, puts it on the opened wrapper, and dons a glove or fingercot on the hand that will insert the suppository. The glove or fingercot prevents contamination of the nurse's hand by rectal microorganisms and feces. The nurse lubricates the smooth, rounded end of the suppository to prevent anal friction and tissue damage during insertion and lubricates the gloved index finger as well. To relax the client's anal sphincter, the nurse asks the client to breathe through the mouth. The suppository is inserted gently into the anus and along the wall of the rectum with the gloved index finger. In adults, suppositories are inserted to a depth of 10 cm (4 in); in children or infants, 5 cm (2 in) or less. See Figure 51–62. To be effective, the suppository needs to be placed along the wall of the rectum rather than embedded in feces. The nurse withdraws the finger, removes the fingercot or glove by turning it inside out, and places it on a paper towel. Turning it inside out contains the rectal microorganisms and prevents their spread. To dispel the client's urge to expel the suppository, the nurse presses the client's buttocks together for a few seconds. If a laxative suppository has been given, the nurse asks the client to retain it for as long as possible (e.g., 15 to 20 minutes). The call signal should be within easy reach so the client can summon assistance to use the bedpan or toilet.

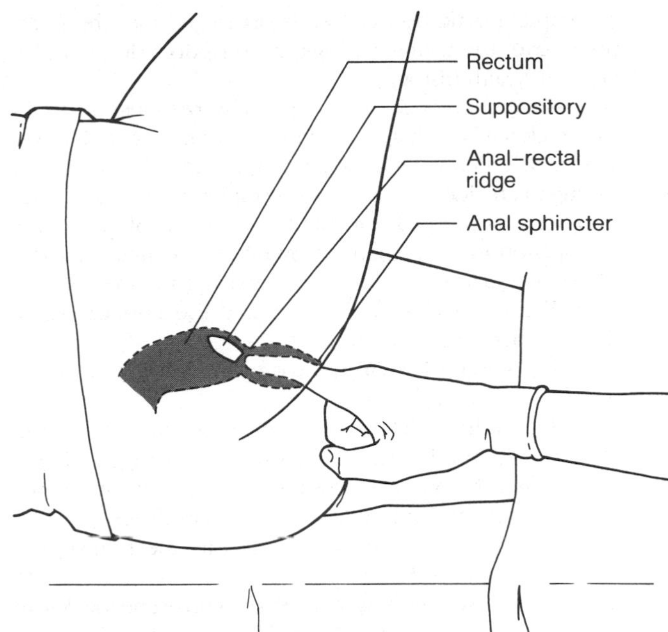

Figure 51–62 A rectal suppository is inserted along the rectal wall beyond the internal anal sphincter.

Chapter Highlights

- Nurse-practice acts set out limits on the nurse's responsibilities regarding medications.
- Federal drug legislation in the United States and Canada regulates the production, prescription, distribution, and administration of drugs.
- Drugs are classified according to their overall action in the body.
- Primary actions of drugs in the body are stimulation and inhibition of tissue or organ functions.
- Many factors influence a client's response to a drug.
- The effects of a drug are characterized as therapeutic, side-effects, allergic, tolerance, cumulative, and idiosyncratic.
- A drug may be incompatible with another drug or a particular food or an intravenous solution.
- Repeated doses of a drug will achieve a sustained level in the bloodstream.
- Obese clients require a larger dose of a drug than thin clients.
- Drugs given parenterally act more quickly than drugs given orally.
- The metric system is the standard system of measurement used by most countries in the world.
- The five "rights" help ensure accurate administration of a drug.
- A nurse should administer only the drugs that she or he has prepared.
- Clients have a right to refuse a drug.
- Administered drugs must be recorded immediately after they have been given.
- Medications should be given at the time they are ordered.
- Drug errors must be reported immediately upon occurrence.
- Parenteral administration of medications employs sterile technique.
- Clients receiving a series of injections should have the injection sites rotated.
- The Z-track method of intramuscular injections protects subcutaneous tissues from medications that are irritating.

Suggested Readings

Bell, S. K. March 1980. Guidelines for taking a complete drug history. *Nursing 80.* 10:10–11.

A complete drug history tool is organized into three sections: over-the-counter drugs, prescription drugs, and a general health history.

Hayter, J. November/December 1981. Why response to medication changes with age. *Geriatric Nursing* 2:411–16, 441.
This article describes how absorption and distribution of a drug in an elderly person's body differs from that of other people. It is pointed out that the duration of action of a medication may be changed by decreased liver function. Also covered are the toxic effects of drugs in older persons as well as their changing senses and the implications of these changes on drug dosages.

Lambert, M. L. March 1975. Drug and diet interactions. *American Journal of Nursing* 75:402–6.
Included in this article are food malabsorption, drug malabsorption, and the interactions between drugs and food and fluids. A helpful list gives the nurse a guide at a glance as to how and when to administer certain drugs.

Lenz, C. L. February 1983. Make your needle selection right to the point. *Nursing 83* 13:50–51.
The author describes how to select the correct needle length so an intramuscular injection will be introduced into the center of the muscle. The article describes the pinch test, which can be used to calculate muscle size. It also considers the effect of the client's overall size and points out that correct needle length prevents some of the complications of intramuscular injections.

Selected References

Allen, M. D. August 1980. Drug therapy in the elderly. *American Journal of Nursing* 80:1474–75.

American Hospital Association. February 1973. A patient's bill of rights. *Nursing Outlook* 21:82.

Budd, R. February 1971. We changed to unit-dose system. *Nursing Outlook* 19:116–17.

Chaplin, G.; Shull, H.; and Welk, P. C. September 1985. How safe is the air-bubble technique for I.M. injections? *Nursing 85* 15:59.

Clark, J. B.; Queener, S. F.; and Karb, V. B. 1982. *Pharmacological basis of nursing practice.* St. Louis: C. V. Mosby Co.

Cohen, M. R. April 1981. Medication errors. *Nursing 81* 11:9.

Dann, T. C. August 1966. Routine skin preparation before injection—is it necessary? *Nursing Times* 62:1121–22.

Davis, N. M., and Cohen, M. R. March 1982. Learning from mistakes: 20 tips for avoiding medication errors. *Nursing 82* 12:65–72. Canadian ed. 12:23–30.

Evans, M. L., and Hansen, B. D. May/June 1981. Administering injections to different-aged children. *Maternal Child Nursing* 6:194–99.

Gaerlan, M. November 1980. Living and working with drugs. *The Canadian Nurse* 76:35–42.

Galton, L. August 1976. Drugs and the elderly: What you should know about them. *Nursing 76* 6:39–43.

Geolot, D. H., and McKinney, N. P. May 1975. Administering parenteral drugs. *American Journal of Nursing* 75:788–93.

Gilman, A. G.; Goodman, L. S.; and Gilman, A. 1980. *The pharmacological basis of therapeutics,* 6th ed. New York: Macmillan Pub. Co.

Hahn, A. B.; Barkin, R. L.; and Oestreich, S. J. K. 1982. *Pharmacology in nursing,* 15th ed. St. Louis: C. V. Mosby Co.

Hays, D. June 1974. Do it yourself the Z-track way. *American Journal of Nursing* 74:1070–71.

Hayter, J. November/December 1981. Why response to medication changes with age. *Geriatric Nursing* 2:411–16.

Keen, M. F. July/August 1986. Comparison of intramuscular injection techniques to reduce site discomfort and lesions. *Nursing Research* 35:207–10.

Kennedy, B. March 1981. Self-medication. *Canadian Nurse* 77:36–37.

Kolesar, G. November 1980. It could happen to you—nurses, physicians and pharmacists. Part 1. *The Canadian Nurse* 76:20–22.

Lacey, R. W. April 1968. Antibacterial action of human skin. *British Journal of Experimental Pathology* 49:209–15.

Lambert, M. L. March 1975. Drug and diet interactions. *American Journal of Nursing* 75:402–6.

Matus, N. R. (consultant). November 1977. Topical therapy: Choosing and using the proper vehicle. *Nursing 77* 7:8–10.

Mayers, M. H. November/December 1981. Legal guidelines. *Geriatric Nursing* 2:417–21, 441.

Monahan, F. D. March/April 1984. When swallowing pills is difficult. *Geriatric Nursing* 5:88–89.

Motz-Harding, E., and Good, F. February 1985. The right solution: Mixing I.V. drugs thoroughly. *Nursing 85* 15:62–64.

Newton, D. W., and Newton, M. July 1979. Route, site, and, technique: Three key decisions in giving parenteral medication. *Nursing 79* 9:18–21, 23, 25.

Paech, G. November 1980. Drug abuse: A health-oriented approach . . . use? or abuse? *The Canadian Nurse* 76:18–19.

Pavkov, J., and Stephens, B. December 1981. Special considerations for the community-based elderly. *Geriatric Nursing* 2:422–28.

Pitel, M. January 1971. The subcutaneous injection. *American Journal of Nursing* 71:76–79.

Reiss, B. S., and Melick, M. E. 1984. *Pharmacological aspects of nursing care.* Albany, New York: Delmar.

Skeist, R., and Carlson, G. November/December 1981. Storing medications safely. *Geriatric Nursing* 2:429–32, 441.

Sklar, C. L. December 1981. You and the law: Accidents, imponderables, what is foreseeable and what is not: What constitutes nursing negligence in the administration of medications? *The Canadian Nurse* 77:48, 50.

Stewart, D. Y; Kelly, J.; and Dinel, B. A. August 1976. Unit-dose medication: A nursing perspective. *American Journal of Nursing* 76:1308–10.

Todd, B. January/February 1983. Drugs and the elderly: Using eye drops and ointments safely. *Geriatric Nursing* 4(1):53–56.

———. May/June 1983. Drugs and the elderly: Topical analgesics. *Geriatric Nursing* 4(3):152, 192, 196.

———. July/August 1985. Drugs and the elderly: Identifying drug toxicity. *Geriatric Nursing* 6:231, 234.

Winfrey, A. July 1985. Single-dose I. M. injections: How much is too much? *Nursing 85* 15:38–39.

Wong, D. L. August 1982. Significance of dead space in syringes. *American Journal of Nursing* 82:1237.

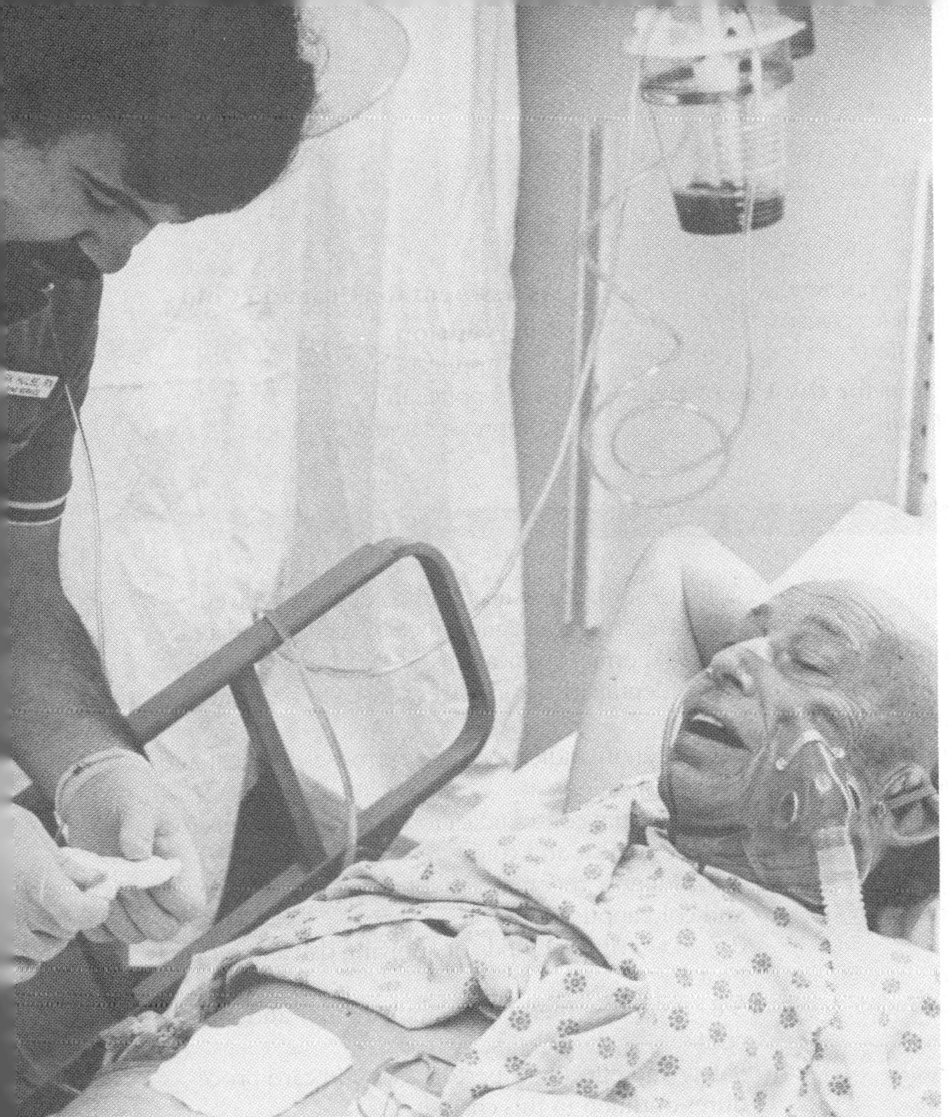

CHAPTER **52**

Wound Care

Contents

(continued)

52 *Wound Care*

Contents *(continued)*

Objectives

1. Know essential facts about wounds and wound healing.
   1.1 Define terms commonly used to describe wounds.
   1.2 Identify two basic ways in which wounds heal.
   1.3 Identify factors that affect wound healing.
   1.4 Identify the main complications of wound healing.
   1.5 Identify assessment criteria of a clean, healing wound.
2. Understand essential facts about interventions for wound care.
   2.1 Identify seven purposes of wound care.
   2.2 Compare open and closed methods of wound care.
   2.3 Identify commonly used dressing materials.
   2.4 Identify commonly used types of binders.
   2.5 Identify basic turns used in bandaging.
   2.6 Identify reasons for implementing selected wound care procedures.
   2.7 Identify essential aspects of wound care procedures outlined in this chapter.
   2.8 Give reasons for selected steps of wound care procedures outlined in this chapter.
   2.9 Identify appropriate assessment and recording data for selected procedures.
3. Know essential terms and facts about hot and cold applications.
   3.1 Describe how heat and cold are perceived.
   3.2 Describe the significance of receptor adaptation to thermal applications.
   3.3 Identify physiologic responses to heat and cold.
   3.4 Identify indications and purposes for heat and cold applications.
   3.5 Identify contraindications and precautions for the use of heat and cold.
   3.6 Identify recommended temperatures for hot and cold applications.
   3.7 Describe methods of applying dry and moist heat.
   3.8 Describe methods of applying dry and moist cold.
4. Safely and effectively perform wound care procedures outlined in this chapter.
   4.1 Change a dry surgical dressing.
   4.2 Change a wet-to-dry dressing.
   4.3 Clean a Penrose drain site.
   4.4 Shorten a Penrose drain.
   4.5 Remove skin sutures.
   4.6 Irrigate a wound.
   4.7 Apply wound suction.
   4.8 Apply common types of binders.
   4.9 Apply bandages.

Terms

abrasion
approximation
bandage
binder
cicatrix
collagen
compress
consensual response
contusion
debridement
dehiscence
ecchymotic
eschar
evisceration
exudate
granulation tissue
hemorrhage
hemostasis
hyperemia
incision
irrigation (lavage)
ischemia
laceration
Montgomery straps (tie tapes)
paresthesia
Penrose drain
primary intention healing
purulent
rebound phenomenon
regeneration
retention (stay) suture
sanguineous
secondary intention healing
sitz bath
suppuration
suture
vasoconstriction
vasodilation
viscosity

The Integument

The skin, subcutaneous and adipose tissues, and immune system superbly protect the body from trauma (injury). The skin, or integument, encloses the body structures—i.e., organs and bones—and the body fluids, thereby protecting them from external assault. See Figure 52–1. The skin's composition is described in Chapter 36, page 907.

The immune system further protects the body from invasion by undesirable foreign material such as microorganisms and metal. The inflammatory process of the immune response eliminates the foreign material, if it can, and prepares the body area for healing. See Chapter 32, page 677, for additional information.

Types of Wounds

The body can receive wounds that are either intentional or unintentional. *Intentional* traumas occur during therapy such as an operation, venipuncture, or radiation. Although it is therapeutic to remove a tumor, the surgeon must cut into body tissues, thus traumatizing them. *Unintentional* wounds are acquired by accident; for example, an arm may be fractured in an automobile accident. If the tissues are traumatized without a break in the skin, the result is a *closed wound.* A blow from a hard instrument causes bruising, called a **contusion**, which is considered a closed wound. An *open wound* occurs when the skin or mucous membrane surface is broken.

Wounds can be further described according to the likelihood and degree of wound contamination (Garner 1986, p. 73).

Clean wounds. These are uninfected wounds in which no inflammation is encountered and the respiratory, alimentary, genital, and urinary tracts are not entered. Clean wounds are primarily closed wounds; or, if necessary, they are drained with closed drainage (see "Wound Drains," later in this chapter).

Clean-contaminated wounds. These are surgical wounds in which the respiratory, alimentary, genital

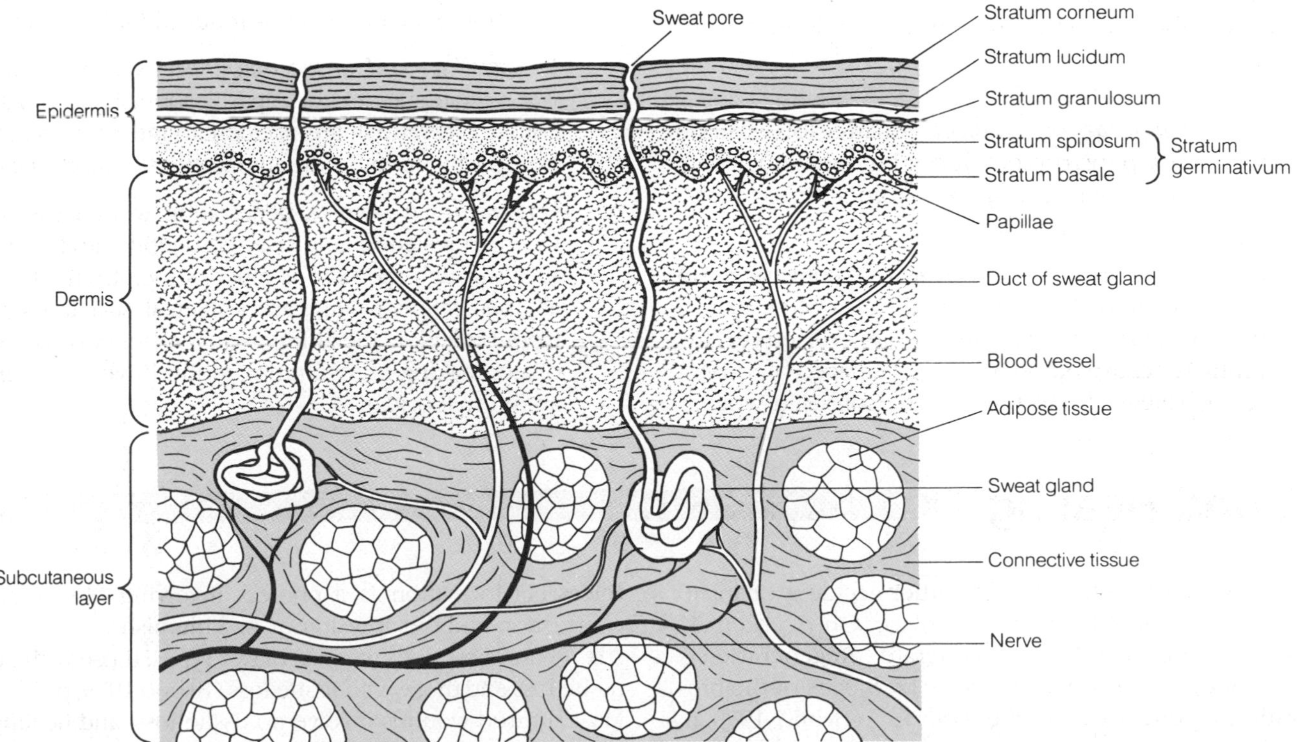

Figure 52–1 Structure of the epidermis, dermis, and subcutaneous layers of the skin

or urinary tract has been entered. Such wounds show no evidence of infection.

Contaminated wounds. These include open, fresh, accidental wounds and surgical wounds involving a major break in sterile technique or a large amount of spillage from the gastrointestinal tract. Contaminated wounds show evidence of inflammation.

Dirty or infected wounds. These include old, accidental wounds containing dead tissue and wounds with evidence of a clinical infection, e.g., purulent drainage.

Table 52–1 Probability of Infection for Different Types of Wounds

Type of Wound	Probability of Infection
Clean	1% to 5%
Clean-contaminated	3% to 11%
Contaminated	10% to 17%
Dirty	over 27%

Source: J. S. Garner, CDC guidelines for the prevention and control of nosocomial infections: Guideline for prevention of surgical wound infections, 1985, *American Journal of Infection Control,* April 1986, 14:73.

"Surgical wound infections are the second most frequent nosocomial infection in most hospitals and are an important cause of morbidity, mortality, and excess hospital costs" (Garner 1986, p. 72). It is estimated by the Centers for Disease Control (CDC) that 60% to 70% of infections are incisional. In general, a wound is considered infected, according to the CDC, if purulent material is draining from it. This definition has the advantage over a definition based on the presence of microorganisms from a wound culture, in that (1) a positive culture does not necessarily indicate an infection, and (2) infected wounds may not reveal pathogens by culture because either the pathogen is fastidious, the culture technique is inadequate, or the client has received antimicrobial therapy (Garner 1986, p. 73). See Table 52–1 for the predicted probability of a wound's becoming infected.

Wounds are frequently described according to the manner in which they are acquired: (a) incised, (b) contused, (c) abraded, (d) punctured, (e) lacerated, or (f) penetrating.

Incised wound, or incision. An **incision** is made with a sharp instrument. It can be intentional, such as a cut made with a surgeon's scalpel, or accidental, such as a cut from a sharp knife.

Contused wound, or contusion. A **contusion** is a closed wound that is the result of a blow from a blunt instrument. The skin appears bruised (**ecchymotic**) because blood from the damaged blood vessels is released into the tissues. Contused wounds are usually unintentional, although they may result from surgical manipulation.

Abraded wound, or abrasion. An **abrasion** is an open wound that results from friction, such as a scraped knee from a fall on a road surface. It involves the skin only. Abraded wounds can also be intentional; for example, in a dermal abrasion, the superficial layers of the skin are removed, either by sandpapering or by an abrasive machine, to obliterate scars and pockmarks.

Punctured wound, stab wound, or puncture. This is an open wound made by a sharp instrument that penetrates the skin and underlying tissues. Puncture wounds can be accidental, such as a wound made by stepping on a nail, or intentional, such as a wound made by a surgeon for insertion of a drain. Venipuncture and intramuscular injections are other common puncture wounds induced intentionally.

Lacerated wound, or laceration. A **laceration** results when the tissues are torn apart, producing irregular edges. Lacerations are accidental and often result from accidents involving automobiles or machinery.

Penetrating wound. A penetrating wound results when an instrument is inserted deeply into the tissues through the skin or mucous membrane. Usually, penetrating wounds are accidental, such as those from bullets or metal fragments. A bullet or other object making a penetrating wound may lodge in an internal organ.

Wound Healing

Following injury to the skin by either accident or intention, the process of healing takes place. Only certain tissues of the body are able to regenerate. "**Regeneration** is the restoration of normal structure by means of the proliferation of undamaged 'like' cells . . ." (Bruno 1979, p. 667). Tissues incapable of regeneration form scars. *Scar* (**cicatrix**) formation is a process involving fibroplasia contraction and the appearance of a blemish.

Bruno describes wounds of two types: those with no tissue loss and those with tissue loss (Bruno 1979, p. 667). Most sutured wounds involve no tissue loss, and healing is by primary (first) intention. **Primary intention healing** occurs in a wound in which the tissue surfaces are or have been approximated and there is minimal or no tissue loss; it is characterized by the formation of minimal granulation tissue and scarring. It is also called *primary union* or *first intention healing*. Wounds with tissue loss—e.g., decubitus ulcers and burns—heal by secondary intention. **Secondary intention healing** occurs in a wound in which the tissue surfaces are not approximated and there is extensive tissue loss; it is characterized by the formation of excessive granulation tissue and scarring. It is also called *secondary union*. Secondary intention healing takes longer than primary intention healing; therefore, the chance of infection is greater.

Healing by Primary Intention

Bruno (1979) describes three stages of primary intention healing: defensive, reconstructive, and maturative.

Defensive Stage

The defensive stage begins at the time of injury and lasts 4 to 6 days. It has three major mechanisms: hemostasis, inflammation, and cell migration.

Hemostasis **Hemostasis** (the cessation of bleeding) results from vasoconstriction of the blood vessels in the affected area, retraction (drawing back) of injured blood vessels, as well as the deposition of fibrin and the formation of blood clots in the area. The blood clots provide a matrix of fibrin that becomes the framework for cell repair. A scab also forms on the surface of the wound. Consisting of clots and dead and dying tissue, this scab serves to aid hemostasis and inhibit contamination of the wound by microorganisms. Below the scab, epithelial cells migrate into the wound from the edges. This process of epithelization is slowed if the tissue becomes excessively dry (Pollack 1981, p. 16). The epithelial cells, which move from both sides of the wound and meet within 48 hours (Pollack 1981, p. 17), serve as a barrier between the body and the environment, preventing the entry of microorganisms.

Inflammation Inflammation involves vascular and cellular responses intended to remove any foreign substances and dead and dying tissues. The blood supply to the wound is increased, bringing with it substances and nutrients needed in the healing process. The area appears reddened and edematous as a result.

Cell migration Leukocytes move into the interstitial space (emigration), and erythrocytes pass through the blood vessel walls by a process known as diapedesis. Leukocytes (neutrophils) appear first and are replaced by monocytes. Leukocytes engulf bacteria and cellular debris by a process known as phagocytosis. Fibroblasts also migrate into the wound beginning about the second or third day as the inflammatory process subsides. New blood capillaries then form in the wound.

Reconstructive Stage

The reconstructive stage commences before the defensive processes are completed. The fibroblasts in the wound synthesize mucopolysaccharides, glycoproteins, and collagen. This process, called fibroplasia, requires 2 to 4 weeks, depending on the size and site of the wound. **Collagen** is a whitish protein substance that adds tensile strength to the wound. As the amount of collagen increases, so does the strength of the wound; thus, there is progressively less chance that the wound will open. During this time the wound appears as a purplish, irregular, raised scar.

Maturative Stage

During the maturative stage, the scar changes in shape and size. This can take months or even years. The collagen fibers change to preinjury configuration. Although the wound gets progressively stronger, a healed wound usually does not attain the strength of preinjured tissue (Bruno 1979, p. 677). However, visceral wounds, e.g., to the stomach, regain strength sooner than skin wounds.

Healing by Secondary Intention

A wound heals by secondary intention when it is extensive and there is considerable tissue loss. Secondary intention healing differs from primary intention healing in three ways:

1. The repair time is longer.
2. The scarring is greater.
3. The susceptibility to infection is greater.

The healing process takes longer because dead tissue in the wound must be removed and because the wound must become filled with connective scar tissue to replace the previous tissue framework, which has been lost. As a result of this scarring, contracture and loss of function can occur. In addition, inflammation tends to develop during secondary healing. With inflammation, it is macrophages and lymphocytes (not neutrophils) that usually predominate. Fibroblasts and capillary buds move slowly toward the center of the wound. As the capillary network develops, the tissue becomes a translucent red color. This tissue, called **granulation tissue**, is fragile, bleeds easily, may protrude above the wound margins, and may have a mucin covering. When the granulation tissue matures, marginal epithelial cells migrate to it, proliferating over this connective tissue base to fill the wound. If the wound does not close by epithelization, the area becomes covered with dried plasma proteins and dead cells. This is called **eschar**. Initially, wounds healing by secondary intention seep serosanguineous drainage. Later, if they are not covered by epithelial cells, they become covered with thick, gray, fibrinous tissue that is eventually converted into dense scar tissue.

Kinds of Wound Drainage

There are three major types of **exudate** (material, such as fluid and cells, that during the inflammatory process has escaped from blood vessels to be deposited in tissue or on tissue surfaces): serous, purulent, and sanguineous.

A *serous exudate* is comprised chiefly of serum (the clear portion of the blood) derived from the blood and serous membranes of the body, such as the peritoneum, pleura, pericardium, and meninges. It is watery in appearance and has few cells. An example is the fluid in a blister from a burn.

A **purulent** *exudate* is thicker than a serous exudate due to the presence of pus. It consists of leukocytes, liquefied dead tissue debris, and dead and living bacteria. The process of pus formation is referred to as **suppuration**, and the bacteria that produce pus are called *pyogenic bacteria*. Not all microorganisms are pyogenic. Purulent exudates vary in color, some acquiring tinges of blue, green, or yellow. The color may depend on the causative organism.

A **sanguineous**, or *hemorrhagic, exudate* consists of large amounts of red blood cells, indicating damage to capillaries that is severe enough to allow the escape of red blood cells from plasma. This type of exudate is frequently seen in open wounds. Nurses often need to ascertain whether the sanguineous exudate is dark or bright. A bright sanguineous exudate indicates fresh bleeding, whereas dark sanguineous exudate denotes older bleeding.

Mixed types of exudates are often observed. A serosanguineous exudate is commonly seen in surgical incisions; it consists of serous and sanguineous drainage.

Factors That Affect Wound Healing

Many factors can affect wound healing, either positively or negatively, and they can be divided into internal and external factors. Internal factors include vasculature, anemia, age, compromised host, nutrition, obesity, drugs, smoking, and stress. External factors include preoperative stay, preoperative preparation and intraoperative elements (Flynn and Rovee 1982, pp. 1550–52).

Internal Factors

Vasculature Without an adequate blood supply to a wound, healing is delayed or does not occur at all. The blood brings with it white blood cells and fibrinogen, whose roles have already been explained. In addition, the blood brings nutrients required for the building of new tissues. Interference in the blood supply due to vascular changes can interfere with the inflammatory response.

Anemia Whether anemia affects wound healing is somewhat controversial. It is known, however, that if the anemia is caused by hypovolemia (reduced blood volume) in which the erythrocyte count falls below 15%, collagen synthesis is slowed (Flynn and Rovee 1982, p. 1550). Also, anemia accompanied by diabetes mellitus or atherosclerosis may affect healing because of the reduced blood supply to the area.

Age According to Flynn and Rovee (1982), recent research indicates that healing is slower in the elderly. However, Bruno and Craven (1982, p. 687) write that this has not been verified. Poor nutrition may accompany aging, possibly resulting in low blood cell counts.

Compromised host A *compromised host* is a person at risk for some other reason. Clients who have diabetes mellitus or acid–base imbalances, for example, may be more likely to get an infection. Some cancer therapies may also delay healing and increase susceptibility to infection.

Nutrition A poorly nourished person often has weakened T-lymphocytic protection. See Chapter 32, page 682, for additional information about the immune system. In addition, insufficient glucose can reduce cellular energy. This energy is required by leukocytes and fibroblasts (Pollack 1982b, p. 28). Vitamins are also thought to play a role in healing; specifics are detailed on page 1547. Trace elements and minerals also are required for wound healing. Iron is necessary for collagen synthesis (Pollack 1982b, p. 32). Zinc has been found to be associated with RNA and DNA biosynthesis, i.e., protein synthesis. Copper also is necessary for collagen synthesis, and manganese is required for the activation of enzymes such as phosphatases, kinases, and decarboxylases. Some of these enzymes are necessary for the synthesis of protein.

Obesity Obesity predisposes the individual to a number of problems. Adipose tissue has a limited blood supply; thus, an obese client is more likely to acquire an infection. In addition, adipose tissue is difficult to suture, increasing the likelihood of wound **dehiscence** (separating of the wound edges).

Drugs Some medications may retard healing, e.g., immunosuppressive agents can affect collagen synthesis, and antiinflammatory drugs such as the corticosteroids can suppress the inflammatory reaction. In addition, the prolonged use of antibiotics can increase the likelihood of infection because of their effect on glucose metabolism and electrolyte balance, for example.

Smoking People who smoke have a reduced amount of functional hemoglobin, with a resultant reduced level of oxygen in the circulating blood. Also, smoking is possibly related to increased aggregation of platelets, resulting in hypercoagulability (Schumann 1979, p. 685).

Stress Stress associated with accidental or intentional wounds can have a negative affect on healing. See Chapter 17 for additional information.

External Factors

Preoperative stay Cruse and Foord (1980) recommend that preoperative hospital stay be short in order to reduce the likelihood of postoperative wound infection.

Preoperative preparation The Centers for Disease Control recommend the following (Garner 1986, p. 77):

1. Bacterial infections should be treated before surgery.
2. The preoperative hospital stay should be as short as possible.
3. Malnourished clients should receive enteral or parenteral nutrition preoperatively if the surgery is not urgent.

Vitamins and Wound Healing

- *Vitamin A:* Needed for epithelization, wound closure, and collagen synthesis
- *Vitamin B complex:* Act as cofactors in enzyme systems. Their absence disturbs protein, carbohydrate, and fat metabolism
- *Vitamin C:* Needed for fibroblast function, resistance to infection, and capillary formation
- *Vitamin K:* Required for the synthesis of prothrombin and clotting factors II, VII, IX, and X.

(Pollack 1982b)

4. Clients having elective surgery should bathe with an antimicrobial soap the night before surgery.
5. Hair near the operative site should not be removed unless absolutely necessary.
6. If hair must be removed, it should be clipped or should be removed with a depilatory, rather than being shaved.

In addition, the preoperative use of antibiotics is recommended where there is a high risk of infection (Nichols 1982). The timing and dosage of the antibiotics is important to the prevention of postoperative infections in clients who are at high risk. Nichols recommends administering parenteral antibiotics within 1 hour of surgery and continuing for 24 to 72 hours. This allows time for drugs to reach therapeutic levels in the tissues but does not permit bacterial resistance to develop (Nichols 1982, p. 34).

Intraoperative elements Many factors during the intraoperative period can affect a client's postoperative healing, including operating room ventilation, operating room cleaning, and the sterilization of surgical instruments. Also, considerations regarding wound care can affect healing. These are discussed later in this chapter.

Complications of Wound Healing

There are four main complications of wound healing: hemorrhage, infection, dehiscence, and evisceration.

Hemorrhage

Some bleeding from a wound is normal intraoperatively and postoperatively. **Hemorrhage**, however, is abnormal. It may be caused by a dislodged clot, infection, a slipped ligature, or erosion of a blood vessel, for example. The latter can result from the irritation of a drain or from the action of escaping enzymic fluids (Flynn and Rovee 1982, p. 1550). Hemorrhage can occur outside the body (external hemorrhage) or inside the body (internal hemorrhage).

Because of the danger of hemorrhage, client wounds should be observed closely. The clinical signs of hemorrhage are given on page 1548. Excessive bleeding should be reported immediately.

Infection

Infection of a surgical wound may become obvious 2 to 11 days postoperatively (Wright 1983, p. 143). The clinical

Clinical Signs of Hemorrhage

- Increased pulse rate
- Increased respiratory rate
- Lowered blood pressure
- Restlessness
- Thirst
- Cold, clammy skin

signs of wound infection include redness, swelling, pain, induration (hardening of the tissues), fever, and an increased leukocyte count. Wounds should always be observed regularly for signs of infection, and these must be reported so that therapy can be commenced. When a wound that is suspected of being infected has any drainage, it should be cultured and smeared for Gram stain (Garner 1986, p. 79).

Dehiscence and Evisceration

Dehiscence is the partial or total rupturing of a wound. Dehiscence often refers specifically to the opening of an abdominal wound in which the layers below the skin also separate. **Evisceration** is the protrusion of the internal viscera through an incision. Both of these are serious and frightening wound complications.

A number of factors put a client at risk of wound dehiscence, including obesity, poor nutrition, multiple trauma, failure of suturing, excessive coughing, vomiting, and dehydration (American Journal of Nursing 1982, p. 1555). Wound dehiscence is more likely to occur when no healing ridge has appeared within 4 to 5 days postoperatively. This ridge normally develops the entire length of an incision and is a sign that fibroplasia has occurred (LeMaitre and Finnegan 1980, p. 76).

The early clinical signs of dehiscence are: unexplained fever, unexplained tachycardia, unusual wound pain, prolonged and paralytic ileus. Wound dehiscence may become obvious when a client describes a sudden gush of serosanguineous fluid or a sudden release of abdominal pressure (LeMaitre and Finnegan 1980, pp. 78–79).

If dehiscence occurs, the area should immediately be covered with sterile towels soaked in sterile saline in order to maintain tissue moistness, and the physician should be notified immediately. Wound dehiscence is an emergency situation requiring surgical resuturing. A nurse should remain with the client and support the wound, often with the hands, to prevent evisceration.

Wound Assessment

Untreated versus Treated Wounds

Untreated wounds usually are seen shortly after an injury, e.g., at the scene of an accident or in an emergency center. The kind of wound largely determines how extensive the assessment should be. For example, since a puncture wound that has penetrated further than 2.5 cm (1 inch) can cause serious internal bleeding, whereas a skin abrasion is superficial, the client with a puncture wound should be assessed for signs of internal bleeding, such as pallor and tachycardia. All untreated wounds should be assessed for bleeding and the presence of foreign material such as glass. The following guidelines apply to untreated wounds.

1. Control bleeding if it is severe. Apply a sterile dressing over the wound. If sterile supplies are unavailable, then use material that is clean. Wrap the wound tightly enough to apply pressure. When the first layer of dressing becomes saturated with blood, apply a second layer, and do so without removing the first layer of dressing, because blood clots might be disturbed, resulting in more bleeding.
2. Permit wounds that are bleeding minimally to continue bleeding. This will help remove dirt.

Treated wounds, that is, sutured wounds, are usually assessed at the time a dressing is changed. If a physician has not ordered dressing changes, the wound itself is not directly inspected; however, the dressing is inspected and other data regarding the wound, e.g., the presence of pain, are determined. Some surgical wounds are covered with a transparent occlusive dressing that permits observation of the wound without exposing it to the air.

Clinical Assessment

Wounds are assessed by visual inspection, palpation, and the sense of smell. They are assessed as to appearance, drainage, swelling, odor, dehiscence, and pain. The client is assessed for any of the clinical signs of complications, as described earlier in the chapter.

Appearance Inspect the wound itself for signs of healing and approximation of the wound edges. **Approxi-**

mation means being close together. Taylor (1983, p. 44) and Bruno (1979, p. 670) outline the following *sequential* signs of primary wound healing:

1. *Absence of bleeding and a clot binding the wound edges together.* After tissue is damaged, blood fills the area. A clot is formed from blood platelets, and the wound edges are well approximated and bound together by fibrin in the clot within the first few hours after surgical closure.
2. *Inflammation (redness and swelling) at the wound edges* for 1 to 3 days. An inflammatory reaction begins after the clot sets, bringing white blood cells to ingest bacteria and cellular debris, and to demolish the clot.
3. *Reduction in inflammation when the clot diminishes,* as granulation tissue starts to bridge the area. Healthy tissue at the wound edges secretes nutrients, fibroblasts, and other building materials, e.g., epithelial cells, to bridge and close the wound within 7 to 10 days. Increased inflammation associated with fever and drainage is indicative of wound infection; the wound edges then appear brightly inflamed and swollen.
4. *Scar formation.* Fibroblasts in the granulation tissue secrete collagen, which forms scar tissue. Collagen synthesis starts 4 days after injury and continues for 6 months or longer.
5. *Diminished scar size* over a period of months or years. Collagen fibers shorten, and wound strength increases. An increase in scar size indicates keloid formation.

Drainage Assess the location and type (color, consistency) of wound drainage, and the number of gauzes saturated or the diameter of drainage collected on the dressings. Also assess the wound drainage for odor. Old blood typically has a pungent odor. A strong, offensive odor can indicate infection. See "Kinds of Wound Drainage," earlier in the chapter.

Swelling The area around a wound should be assessed for swelling. It is not unusual for a surgical incision area to be swollen the first few days postoperatively. Wear sterile gloves when palpating a wound for swelling. Palpate just to the side of the wound's edge, feeling for tenseness of the tissues.

Odor Wounds normally have no odor, except perhaps for the pungent, musty smell of old blood. A wound with an offensive, strong odor may indicate infection.

Dehiscence Assess for the presence of dehiscence, or wound gaping. Determine the exact location and size of any dehiscence.

Pain The client may complain of discomfort; if so, determine the location of the discomfort. Generally, incisional pain is severe for up to 3 days postoperatively and is relieved with narcotic analgesics. After that, milder analgesics provide relief. When clients complain of persistent severe pain, an infection or other problem may be the cause.

Laboratory Data

Laboratory data can often tell nurses whether or not healing is taking place. A deficient leukocyte count can delay healing and increase the possibility of infection. Blood coagulation studies can also impart information about healing. Prolonged coagulation times can result in excessive blood loss and prolonged clot absorption. Hypercoagulability can lead to intravascular clotting. Intraarterial clotting can result in ischemia to the wound area.

Nursing Diagnosis

Nursing diagnoses for wound care are largely concerned with preventing complications. Examples of nursing diagnoses are provided to the right.

Examples of Nursing Diagnoses for Wound Care

- Potential impairment of skin integrity related to wound drainage
- Potential for injury related to an open wound
- Potential for injury related to the presence of a Penrose drain
- Alterations in comfort related to abdominal incision
- Impaired physical mobility related to trauma

Planning

Just as there are many types of wounds, there are many ways of caring for wounds. In general, the care varies with the type of wound, its size, the amount of exudate present, whether it is an open or closed wound, the location, the personal preference of the physician, and the presence of complicating factors.

Planning includes both independent and dependent nursing strategies. Dependent strategies are those that stem largely from the wound care orders written by the surgeon. Both independent and dependent strategies are intended chiefly to promote healing and prevent infection.

Preventing infection Infection from microorganisms entering a wound through the broken protective barriers of the skin and mucous membranes can be prevented by using sterile technique when caring for the wound, using antiseptic on the skin, and, on occasion, administering antibiotics as prescribed by the physician.

Preventing further tissue damage Fragile healing wounds can be damaged by friction or injury. This is prevented by protecting the wound with dressings and by immobilizing the part with slings or binders.

Promoting healing This is accomplished by approximating wound edges with sutures (a physician's function), ensuring a good blood supply, supplying essential nutrients, and keeping the area free from body excretions.

Cleaning wounds of foreign debris Debris such as pieces of glass can act as irritants; excessive exudate can harbor microorganisms. **Debridement** is the cleaning of an injured area to remove debris, and it is usually performed by the physician. Wounds may be irrigated with water or cleaning solution such as hydrogen peroxide to clear away organic material prior to cleaning with antiseptics.

Promoting drainage Rubber or plastic tubes or drains are frequently put into wounds or ducts by the physician during surgery to promote drainage. Some of these drains, commonly referred to as **Penrose drains**, are shortened progressively throughout the healing process. They ensure removal of inflammatory exudates and blood prior to closure of the overlying skin. Other drains are placed in ducts, such as the ureter or common bile duct, to ensure patency of the duct and to prevent adhesion or closure of the duct during healing. Drains or tubes may be attached to suction apparatus to facilitate drainage. A portable vacuum suction (Hemovac) is sometimes used to drain blood and serous exudate from deep surgical wounds, such as those from orthopedic surgery. With this kind of suction, a vacuum is created in an evacuator bag, which gently draws the drainage out of the wound.

Preventing hemorrhage Occlusive pressure dressings may be applied to surgical incisions for the first few days, until a dressing change is ordered by the physician. In certain body areas, such as the rectum or vagina, long strips of gauze in varying widths are packed into the orifice to apply pressure on blood capillaries and prevent bleeding. This *packing* is usually removed 2 to 3 days after surgery.

Preventing skin excoriation around draining wounds This is accomplished by changing saturated dressings as required and by cleaning and drying wounds and surrounding skin areas. When drainage is excessive, as in some bowel (colostomy) or urinary surgery, protective ointments or pastes may be applied to surrounding skin to prevent irritation and excoriation. The frequent removal of tape can also be irritating to the skin; thus, Montgomery straps, or tie tapes, or newer tape products that have minimal adhesive and are porous are frequently used. These cause the least skin disruption.

For examples of outcome criteria, see the "Evaluation" section later in this chapter.

Intervention

Care of Open versus Closed Wounds

The *open method* of wound care uses no dressings. The *closed method* involves applying a dressing.

Dressings have the following advantages:

1. They promote wound healing by absorbing drainage and debriding a wound.
2. They protect the wound from external microbial contamination.
3. They can aid in hemostasis if applied with elastic bandages.
4. They can assist in approximating wound edges.
5. They support and splint the wound site, thus reducing its mobility and trauma.
6. They cover unpleasant disfigurements.

In some situations, the physician applies a protective covering such as collodion spray instead of a gauze dressing.

This spray hardens like nail polish and can be either peeled from the skin when the wound is healed or removed with a special solution. A spray covering is often preferred to a dressing, since friction is eliminated and the wound is always observable through the translucent covering. The wound is protected from external contamination because the spray is moisture-proof. For children, who are active and who heal quickly, spray is frequently used. It is not advised for wounds that have drainage.

The open method avoids certain disadvantages of dressings. For example: (a) dressings produce dark, warm, moist environments in which resident and nonresident microorganisms can multiply; and (b) dressings can irritate wounds by friction. Exposing wounds to the air produces drying. This discourages the growth of microorganisms, which need moisture. The open method is frequently employed for burns.

Dressing Materials

Materials to Clean Wounds

Some nurses prefer cotton balls to clean wounds because of their absorbent qualities; others prefer gauze squares, claiming that threads of cotton balls can stick to sutures. Cleaning agents vary considerably. Some of the common ones are:

Alcohol 70%

Aqueous and tincture of chlorhexidine gluconate (Hibitane)

Hydrogen peroxide

Materials to Cover Wounds

Several sizes of gauze are available to cover wounds. See Figure 52–2. The standard sizes are 10 × 10 cm (4 × 4 in) and 10 × 20 cm (4 × 8 in). The size and the number of pads used depend on the nature of the wound, the amount of exudate, and the location of the wound. These decisions are left to the nurse's judgment. Sometimes the gauze is precut halfway through one side to make it fit around a drain, or it is folded in a special way. See Procedure 52–3, step 10.

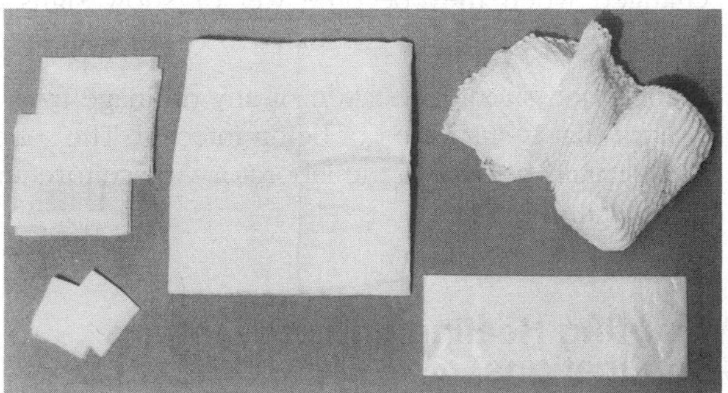

Figure 52–2 Some frequently used dressing materials (clockwise from bottom left): 2 × 2 gauze, 4 × 4 gauze, surgipad or abdominal pad, roller gauze, and nonadherent absorbent dressing

Telfa gauze is a special type. It has a shiny, nonadherent surface on one or both sides and is applied with the shiny surface on the wound. Exudate seeps through this surface and collects on absorbent material on the other side or sandwiched between the two nonadherent surfaces. Since the dressing does not adhere, it does not cause injury to the wound when removed. Petrolatum gauze, another nonadherent type, is impregnated with petroleum jelly. It is placed against the wound and usually covered with 4 × 4 gauze.

Larger and thicker gauze dressings, called *surgipads* or *abdominal pads,* are used to cover small gauzes. They not only hold the other gauzes in place but also absorb and collect excess drainage. Surgipads are more absorbent on one side, and this side is placed toward the wound; the less absorbent, more protective side is placed outward to protect the wound from external contamination. The outer side is often indicated with a blue stripe.

Materials to Secure Dressings

Tapes After abdominal or other types of surgery, an elastic adhesive tape may be applied over wounds because of its ability to compress, thereby controlling hemorrhage. The original tape is removed during the initial dressing change, and a lighter dressing is applied. Various tapes are available in strips to apply across a dressing, e.g., nonallergenic tape and paper tape. It is important to secure the dressing at both ends and across the middle and to use tape of a sufficient width for the dressing and the wound. See "Taping Dressings," below.

Montgomery straps **Montgomery straps (tie tapes)** are commonly used for wounds requiring frequent dressing changes. See Figure 52–3. These straps prevent skin irritation and discomfort caused by removing the adhesive each time the dressing is changed. Nonallergenic tie tapes are available for people who have sensitive skin. If these are not available, tincture of benzoin applied to the skin where the adhesive is to be placed protects the skin.

Bandages and binders There are numerous types of roller bandages and binders that may be used to secure dressings, as well as to support or immobilize a wound. See later in this chapter.

Taping Dressings

It is important to tape a dressing over a wound so (a) the dressing is maintained over the entire wound, and (b) the tape does not become dislodged. The correct type of

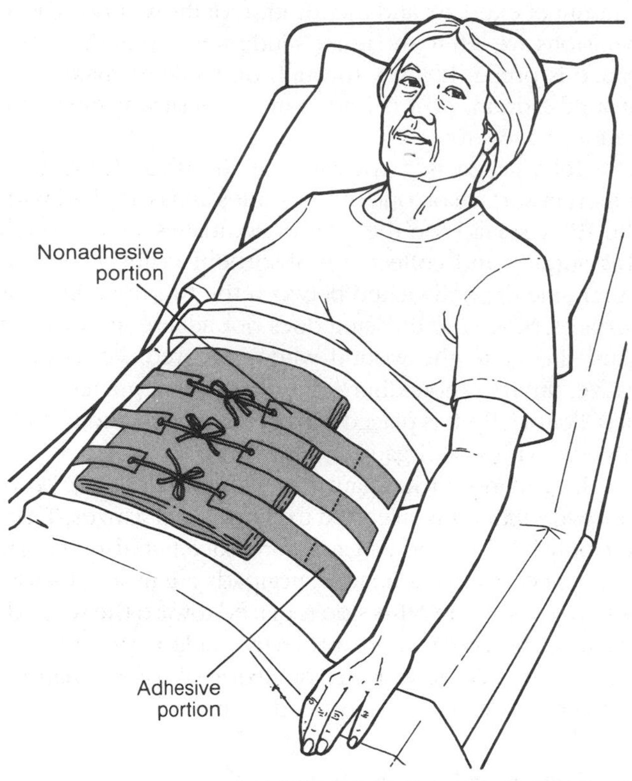

Figure 52–3 Montgomery straps, or tie tapes, are used to secure large dressings that require frequent changing.

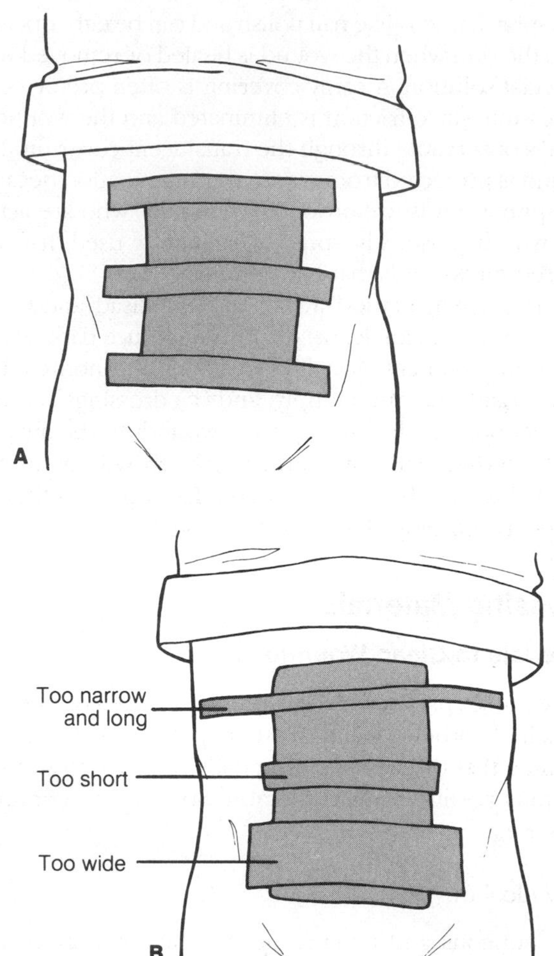

Figure 52–4 The strips of tape should be placed at the ends of the dressing and must be sufficiently long and wide to secure the dressing. **A,** Correct taping; **B,** incorrect taping.

tape must be selected for the purpose. Elastic tape can provide pressure; nonallergenic tape can be used if a client is allergic to other tape.

1. Place the tape so the dressing cannot fold back to expose the wound. Place strips at the ends of the dressing, and space tapes evenly in the middle. See Figure 52–4.
2. Ensure that the tape is long and wide enough to adhere to the skin but not so long or wide that it loosens with activity. See Figure 52–4.
3. Place the tape in the opposite direction from the body action, e.g., across a body joint or crease, not lengthwise. See Figure 52–5.

Preventing Infection

The Centers for Disease Control recommend the following wound care practices for preventing wound infection (Garner 1986, pp. 78–79).

1. Wash hands before and after caring for surgical wounds.
2. Touch an open or fresh surgical wound only when wearing sterile gloves or using sterile forceps. After the wound is sealed, sterile gloves are no longer required.
3. Dressings over closed wounds should be removed or changed when they become wet or show signs of infection.
4. A specimen should be taken of any drainage from a wound that is suspected of being infected. The specimen should be sent to the laboratory for culture and Gram stain.

Promoting Healing and Preventing Complications

Adequate nutrition is essential to wound healing. Proteins, vitamins, and trace metals are recognized to play a major role in the healing process. In addition, adequate

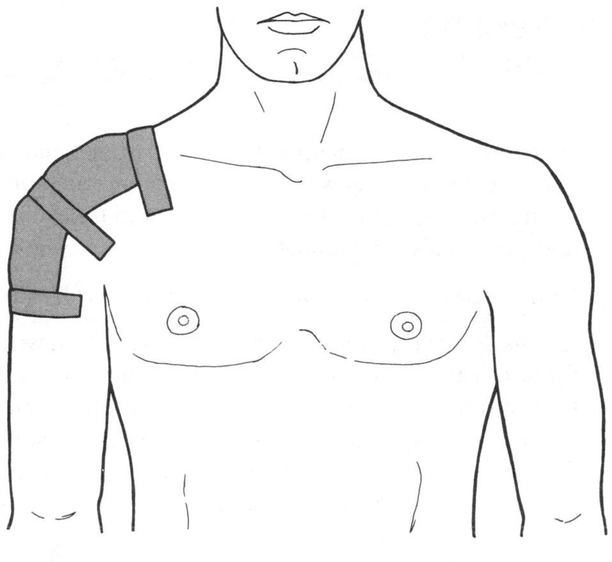

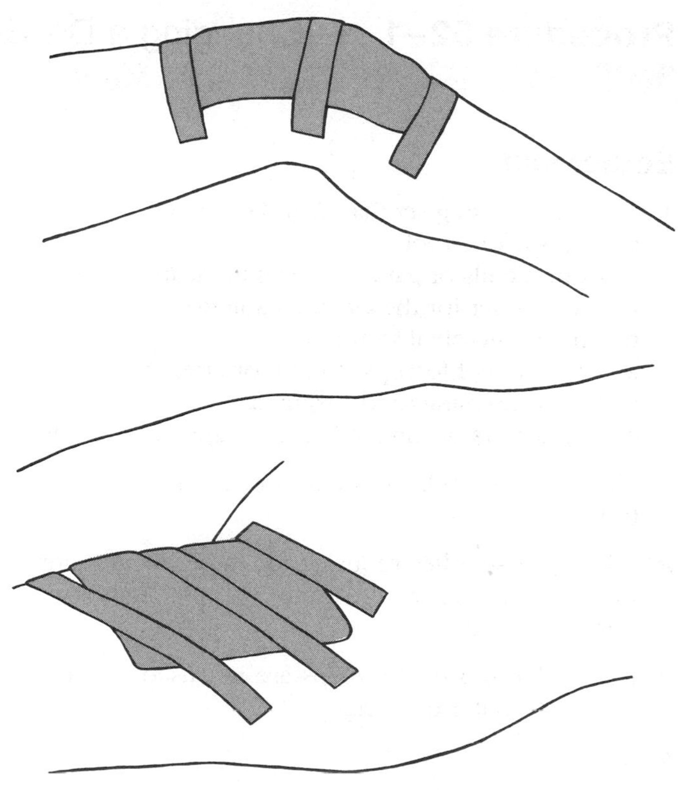

Figure 52–5 Dressings over moving parts must remain secure in spite of the movement.

nutrition, especially protein intake, promotes a positive nitrogen balance. See "Wound Healing," earlier in the chapter.

During the healing process, it is important to prevent stress on a wound, e.g., vomiting, abdominal distention, or strenuous coughing. Vomiting is often prevented by withholding food and oral fluids until there is no nausea; or a nasogastric tube may be inserted.

Abdominal distention often can be prevented by frequent changing of the client's position and by frequent early ambulation. Electrolyte imbalance also can contribute to abdominal distention and delayed wound healing (Cooper and Schumann 1979, p. 716). Specifically, imbalances due to hydrogen ion loss through gastric suctioning and excessive loss of potassium through the kidneys contribute to smooth muscle inactivity and abdominal distention. Ambulation helps improve blood circulation and respirations, which aid the delivery of nutrients and oxygen to the wound area. In addition, a distended urinary bladder can impair wound healing by displacing affected tissue and stretching an incision. Therefore, careful monitoring of fluid intake and output is important. See Chapter 53, Perioperative Care, for additional information.

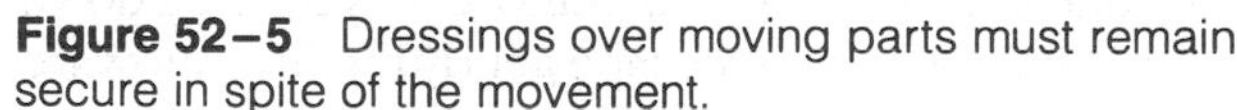

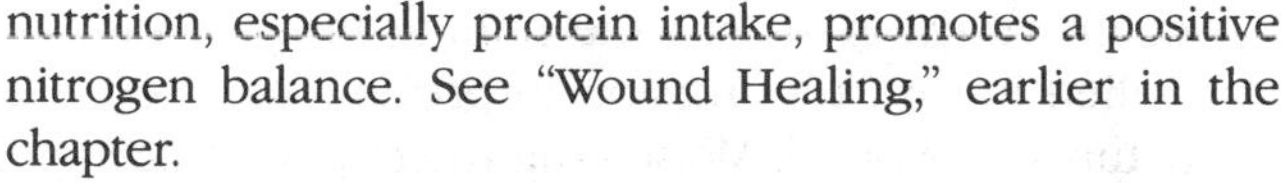

Dry Surgical Dressings

Sterile dry dressings are used for wounds such as surgical incisions that have minimal drainage and no tissue loss and that heal by *primary intention*. Most dressings have three layers:

1. A contact dressing that covers the incision and part of the surrounding skin and that collects fibrin, blood products, and debris from the wound
2. A gauze absorbent dressing that acts as a reservoir for excess secretions
3. A thicker outer dressing that protects the wound from external contamination

Not all surgical dressings require changing. Sometimes the surgeon applies a dressing in the operating room that remains in place until the sutures are removed, and no further dressings are required. In many situations, however, surgical dressings are changed regularly. Changing the dressing helps to prevent the growth of microorganisms that flourish in a damp, dark environment.

In some instances, a client may have a Penrose drain inserted. The main surgical incision is considered to be cleaner than a subsidiary surgical stab wound, which usually has considerable drainage. Therefore the main incision is cleaned first, and under no circumstances are materials moved from the stab wound *to* the main incision. The main incision is kept free of the microorganisms that are around the stab wound.

How to change a dry sterile dressing is detailed in Procedure 52–1.

Procedure 52–1 ▲ Changing a Dry Sterile Dressing

Equipment

1. A sterile dressing set that includes:
   a. A drape or towel
   b. Cotton balls or gauze squares to clean the wound
   c. A container for the cleaning solution
   d. An antimicrobial solution
   e. Two pairs of forceps (thumb or artery)
   f. Gauze dressings and surgipads
   g. Applicators or tongue blades to apply ointments

   If a set is not available, gather these items from a central supply cart.
2. Additional supplies required for the particular dressing, e.g., extra gauze dressings and ointment or powder, if ordered
3. Disposable gloves if forceps are not used to remove the soiled outer dressings
4. A mask
5. A moisture-proof bag for disposal of the old dressings and the used cleaning gauzes
6. Tape or tie tapes to secure the dressing
7. A bath blanket, if necessary, to cover the client and prevent undue exposure
8. Acetone or another solution to loosen adhesive, if necessary

Intervention

Preparing the Client

1. Acquire assistance for changing a dressing on an infant or young child.

   Rationale The child might move and contaminate the sterile field or the wound.
2. Assist the client to a comfortable position, one in which the wound can be readily exposed. Expose only the wound area, using a bath blanket to drape the client, if necessary.

   Rationale Undue exposure is physically and psychologically distressing to most clients.
3. Make a cuff on the moisture-proof bag for disposal of the soiled dressings, and place the bag within reach. It can be taped to the bedclothes or bedside table.

   Rationale A cuff keeps the outside of the bag free from contamination by the soiled dressings and prevents subsequent contamination of the nurse's hands. Placement of the bag within reach prevents the nurse from reaching across the sterile field and the wound and potentially contaminating these areas.
4. Don a face mask, if required, and wash your hands.

   Rationale Many agencies require that a mask be worn for surgical dressing changes to prevent contamination of the wound by droplet spray from the nurse's respiratory tract. The mask is donned *before* washing the hands because the hands will become contaminated when they touch the hair.

Removing the Soiled Dressing

5. Remove binders, if used, and place them aside. Untie Montgomery straps, if used.
6. If adhesive tape was used, remove it by holding down the skin and pulling the tape gently but firmly toward the wound. Use a solvent to loosen the tape, if required.

   Rationale Pressing down on the skin provides countertraction against the pulling motion. Tape is pulled toward the incision to prevent strain on the sutures or wound. Moistening the tape with acetone or a similar solvent lessens the discomfort of removal, particularly from hairy surfaces.
7. Remove the outer abdominal dressing or surgipad by hand if the dressing is dry, or by using a disposable glove if the dressing is moist. Lift the dressing so the underside is away from the client's face.

   Rationale The outer surgipad is considered contaminated by the client's clothing and linen. The appearance and odor of the drainage may be upsetting to the client.
8. Place the soiled dressing in the waterproof bag without touching the outside of the bag.

   Rationale Contamination of the outside of the bag is avoided to prevent the spread of microorganisms to the nurse and subsequently to others.
9. Open the sterile dressing set using the technique for opening sterile packages described in Chapter 32.
10. Place the sterile drape beside the wound.
11. Remove the under-dressings with tissue forceps or gloves, taking care not to dislodge any drains. If the gauze sticks to the drain, use two pairs of forceps, one to remove the gauze and one to hold the drain, or secure the drain with one sterile gloved hand.

Rationale Forceps or gloves are used to prevent contamination of the wound by the nurse's hands and contamination of the nurse's hands by wound drainage.

12. Assess the location, type (color, consistency), and odor of wound drainage, and the number of gauzes saturated or the diameter of drainage collected on the dressings. See "Kinds of Wound Drainage," earlier in this chapter.
13. Discard the soiled dressings in the bag. To avoid contaminating the forceps tips on the edge of the bag, hold the dressings 10 to 15 cm (4 to 6 in) above the bag, and drop the dressings into it. After the dressings are removed, discard the forceps, or set them aside from the sterile field.

Cleaning and Dressing the Wound

14. Clean the wound, using the second pair of artery or tissue forceps and gauze swabs moistened with antimicrobial solution. Keep the forceps tips lower than the handles at all times. Use a separate swab for each stroke, cleaning from the top of the incision downward. Discard each swab after use.

    Rationale The wound is cleaned from the least to the most contaminated area, i.e., from the top of the incision, which is drier, to the bottom, where any drainage will collect and which is considered more contaminated. Forceps tips are always held lower than the handle to prevent their contamination by fluid traveling up to the handle, which is contaminated by the nurse's bare hand, and back.

    a. Clean with strokes from top to bottom, starting at the center and continuing to the outside. See Figure 52–6.

       or

       Clean with strokes outward from the incision on one side and then outward on the other side. See Figure 52–7.

    b. If a drain is present, clean it *after* cleaning the incision. See Procedure 52–3.

    c. For irregular wounds, such as a decubitus ulcer, clean from the center of the wound outward, using circular strokes.

15. Repeat the cleaning process until all drainage is removed.
16. Dry the wound with dry gauze swabs, using the strokes described in step 14.
17. Assess the overall appearance of the wound.
18. Assess the presence of dehiscence.
19. Apply powder or ointment if required. Shake powder directly onto the wound; use sterile applicators or tongue blades to apply ointment.

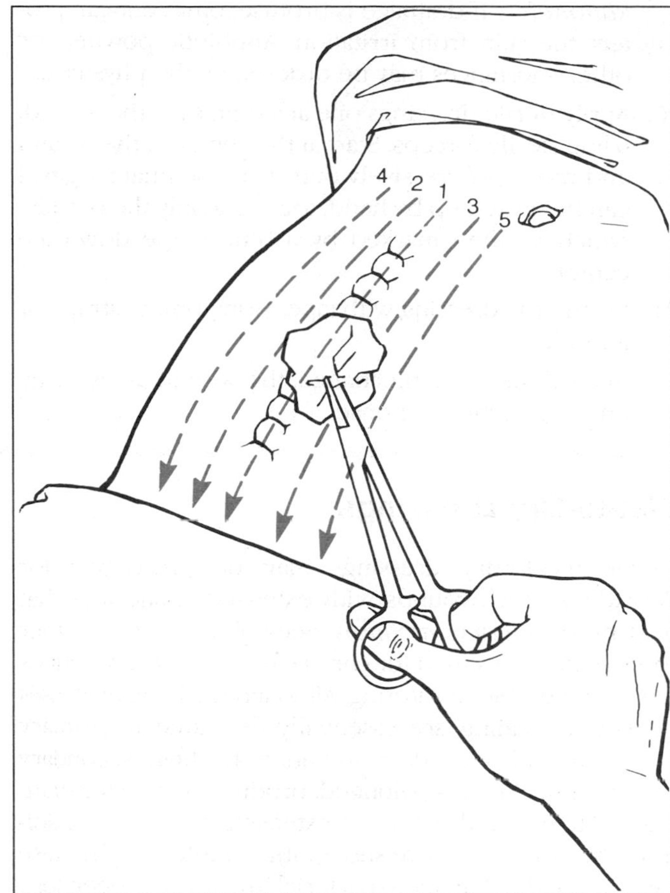

Figure 52–6

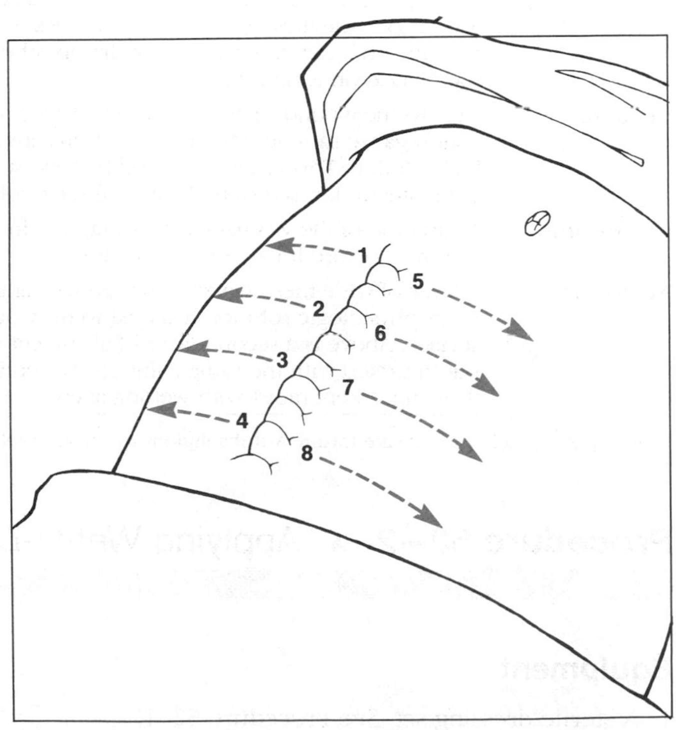

Figure 52–7

Rationale If drainage is profuse, ointment can protect the skin from irritation. Antibiotic powders or other substances may be ordered by the physician.

20. Apply sterile dressings one at a time over the wound, using sterile forceps. Start at the center of the wound and move progressively outward. The final surgipad can be picked up by hand, touching only the outside, which is often marked by a blue stripe down the center.
21. Secure the dressing with tape, Montgomery straps, or a binder.
22. Record the dressing change, the wound assessment, and the client's response.

Sample Recording

Date	Time	Notes
Dec/5/87	1500	Perineal dressing changed. Incision cleaned with Tr. Hibitane. Two 4 × 4 gauzes saturated with serous drainage at base of incision. Wound clean, edges closely approximated. No redness on incision line or surrounding tissue. 4 × 4 gauze and surgipads secured with T-binder. No discomfort.——— ———Evangeline R. Puritos, RN

Wet-to-Dry Dressings

Sterile wet-to-dry dressings may be prescribed for debridement of wounds with extensive tissue loss that heal by *secondary intention*. See Table 52–2 for other types of dressings used for chronic wounds. These wounds are not amenable to suturing. Although the basic processes of wound healing are essentially the same in primary intention and secondary intention healing, secondary intention healing is prolonged, produces extensive granulation tissue, and results in extensive scarring. In addition, the wound is more susceptible to infection because the normal skin barrier to bacterial invasion has been lost.

Wet-to-dry dressings consist of a moistened contact dressing layer that touches the wound surface. This layer is allowed to dry between dressing changes every 4 to 6 hours. Wet-to-dry dressings are the treatment of choice for wounds requiring debridement, i.e., cleaning of infected and necrotic material from the wound. The wet gauze traps necrotic material in its spaces as it dries. Dry dressings do not trap the debris as effectively. Wet dressings that do not dry out enough to trap debris promote bacterial growth in the damp environment and can cause tissue breakdown.

Procedure 52–3 describes how to apply wet-to-dry dressings.

Table 52–2 Dressings for Chronic Wounds

Dressing	Description	Purpose
Dry-to-dry	A layer of wide-mesh cotton gauze lies next to the wound surface. A second layer of dry absorbent cotton or Dacron is on top.	Necrotic debris and exudate are trapped in the interstices of the contact (gauze) layer. These are removed when the dressing is removed.
Wet-to-dry	Next to the wound surface is a layer of wide-mesh cotton gauze saturated with saline or an antimicrobial solution. This layer is covered by a moist absorbent material, i.e., moistened with the same solution.	Necrotic debris is softened by the solution and then adheres to the mesh gauze as it dries. It is removed when the dressing is removed. Also, moisture helps dilute viscous exudate.
Wet-to-damp	A variation of the wet-to-dry dressing, this dressing is removed before it has completely dried.	The wound is debrided when the gauze is removed.
Wet-to-wet	A layer of wide-mesh gauze saturated with antibacterial or physiologic solution lies next to the wound surface. Above is a second layer of absorbent material saturated with the same solution. The entire dressing is kept moist with wetting agent.	The wound surface is continually bathed. Moisture dilutes viscous exudate.

Source: J. Z. Cuzzell, Wound care forum: Artful solutions to chronic problems, *American Journal of Nursing,* February 1985, 85:162–66.

Procedure 52–2 ▲ Applying Wet-to-Dry Dressings

Equipment

1. A sterile dressing set. See Procedure 52–1.
2. Sterile thin, fine-mesh gauze. Generally 4 × 4 non-cotton-filled gauze dressings are used. Cotton fibers are contraindicated because they can pull loose and remain in the wound, encouraging bacterial growth and contamination.
3. A sterile round or kidney-shaped container for the solution.

4. The ordered solution. The type used depends on the condition of the wound and the purpose of the dressings. Normal saline often is used to moisten necrotic tissue and help loosen and remove it. Betadine (10% solution) frequently is used for draining wounds infected with *Staphylococcus* or aerobic bacteria; it can cause burning and stinging, and some clients may be allergic to it. Acetic acid (0.25% solution) often is used for wounds infected with *Pseudomonas* or gram-positive and gram-negative organisms; it can be irritating to the skin surrounding the wound. Hydrogen peroxide (3% solution), not used as frequently today as in the past, is a debriding agent that facilitates removal of necrotic tissue. Sodium hypochlorite (Dakin's solution) is an antiseptic that dissolves necrotic tissue and retards *Pseudomonas* growth. Dakin's solution can cause skin breakdown, so it is used only on necrotic tissue.
5. Clean disposable gloves to remove soiled dressings.
6. Sterile gloves for cleaning the wound and applying dressings.
7. A mask.
8. A moisture-proof bag for soiled dressings.
9. Tape or tie tapes.

Intervention

1. Assemble all equipment, prepare the client, and remove the soiled dressings as in Procedure 52–1, steps 1–13.
2. If the dressing adheres to underlying tissue, do not moisten it but gradually free the dressing as gently as possible.

   Rationale Wet-to-dry dressings are intended to clean wounds by debridement of the exudate or necrotic tissue.
3. Assess the character and amount of drainage on the dressings and the appearance of the wound, i.e., the progress of healing by secondary intention. Observe the development and amount of granulation tissue. In wounds with extensive tissue loss, fibroblasts and capillary buds move slowly toward the center of the wound. As the capillary network develops, the tissue becomes a translucent red color. See "Healing by Secondary Intention," earlier in this chapter.
4. Remove the disposable gloves and discard them in the bag.
5. Wash your hands.
6. Open the packages of the sterile dressing set, fine-mesh gauze, and sterile solution container.
7. Pour the ordered solution into the solution container.
8. Don the sterile gloves.
9. Place the fine-mesh gauze dressings into the solution container and thoroughly saturate them with solution.

   Rationale The entire gauze must be moistened to enhance its absorptive abilities.
10. If agency policy indicates, clean the wound gently using a circular motion. Work outward from the center of the wound to its edge and beyond. Use a separate gauze swab for each cleaning stroke.
11. Wring out excess moisture from the saturated fine-mesh gauze dressings.

    Rationale Dressings that are too wet will not dry in 4 to 6 hours.
12. Pack the moistened dressings into all depressions and grooves of the wound, ensuring that all exposed surfaces are covered. If necessary, use forceps to feed the gauze gradually into deep depressed areas.

    Rationale Necrotic tissue is usually more prevalent in depressed wound areas and needs to be covered with the wet-to-dry gauze.
13. Apply a dry 4 × 4 gauze over the wet dressings.

    Rationale The dry gauze absorbs excess drainage.
14. Cover the dressings with a surgipad or abdominal pad.

    Rationale The pad protects the wound from external contaminants.
15. Remove your gloves.
16. Secure the dressing at the edges only, with tape, Montgomery ties, bandage, or binder. Do not apply an airtight occlusive covering.

    Rationale Occlusive dressings prevent air circulation and hinder drying of the fine-mesh gauze.
17. Record the dressing change, the wound assessment, and the client's response.

Wound Drains

Frequently, flexible rubber drains, called *Penrose drains,* are inserted during abdominal surgery to provide drainage of excessive serosanguineous fluid and purulent material and promote healing of underlying tissues by obliterating dead space. These drains may be inserted and sutured through the incision line, but they are most commonly inserted through stab wounds a few centimeters away from the incision line so the incision is kept dry.

Without a drain, some wounds would heal over on the surface and trap the discharge inside. Then the tissues under the skin could not heal because of the discharge, and an abscess might form.

Drains vary in length and width. The length inserted can be 25 to 35 cm (10 to 14 in), and the width 2.5 to 4 cm (0.5 to 1.5 in). To facilitate drainage and healing of tissues from the inside to the outside, or from the bottom to the top, the physician commonly orders that the drain be pulled out or shortened 2 to 5 cm (1 to 2 in) each day. When a drain is completely removed, the remaining stab wound usually heals within a day or two. In some agencies this shortening procedure is performed only by physicians; in others, it is ordered by the physician and performed by nurses. Shortening of a drain is done in conjunction with a dressing change. See Procedure 52–3.

Procedure 52–3 ▲ Cleaning a Drain Site and Shortening a Penrose Drain

Equipment

1. A sterile dressing set, including:
   a. Gauzes for cleaning the wound.
   b. A container for the cleaning solution.
   c. A towel or drape.
   d. Surgipads and/or gauze dressings.
   e. Antimicrobial solution.
   f. Two pairs of forceps, including at least one hemostat.
   g. Cotton-tipped applicators.
2. Sterile dressing materials sufficient to cover the surgical incision and the drain site. At least two 4 × 4 gauzes are usually needed to dress the drain site; more are required if drainage is copious. A sterile precut gauze is needed to apply first around the drain site.
3. Sterile scissors to cut the drain.
4. A sterile safety pin. Add this to the sterile dressing set.
5. Sterile gloves (optional) for removing a moist outer dressing or shortening the drain if you prefer gloves to forceps.
6. A moisture-proof bag to receive the old dressings.
7. Tape, tie tapes, or other binding supplies.
8. A mask for the nurse and one for the client, if necessary.

Intervention

1. Inform the client that the drain is to be shortened and that this procedure should not be painful. Explain that she or he may feel a pulling sensation for a few seconds when the drain is being drawn out before it is shortened.
2. Ask the client not to speak unnecessarily or touch the wound during the dressing change, so as not to contaminate the wound. If the client will likely want to talk, provide him or her with a mask.
3. Follow Procedure 52–1, steps 1–18.

   Rationale The incision is cleaned first, since it is considered cleaner than the drain site. Moist drainage facilitates the growth of resident skin bacteria around the drain.

Cleaning the Drain

4. Clean the skin around the drain site by swabbing in half or full circles from around the drain site outward, using separate swabs for each wipe. See Figure 52–8. Forceps may be used in the nondominant hand to hold the drain erect while cleaning around it. Clean as many times as necessary to remove the drainage.
5. Assess the amount and character of drainage, including odor, thickness, and color.

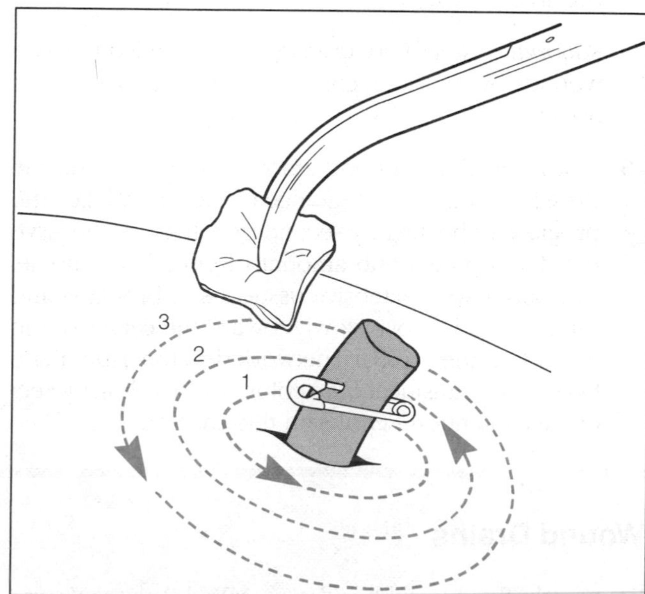

Figure 52–8

Shortening a Drain

6. If the drain has not been shortened before, cut and remove the suture. See Procedure 52–4. The drain is sutured to the skin during surgery to keep it from slipping into the body cavity.
7. With a hemostat, firmly grasp the drain by its full width at the level of the skin, and pull the drain out the required length.

   Rationale Grasping the full width of the drain ensures even traction.
8. Put on sterile gloves, and insert the sterile safety pin through the base of the drain as close to the skin as possible, holding the drain tightly against the skin edge and inserting the pin above your fingers. See Figure 52–9.

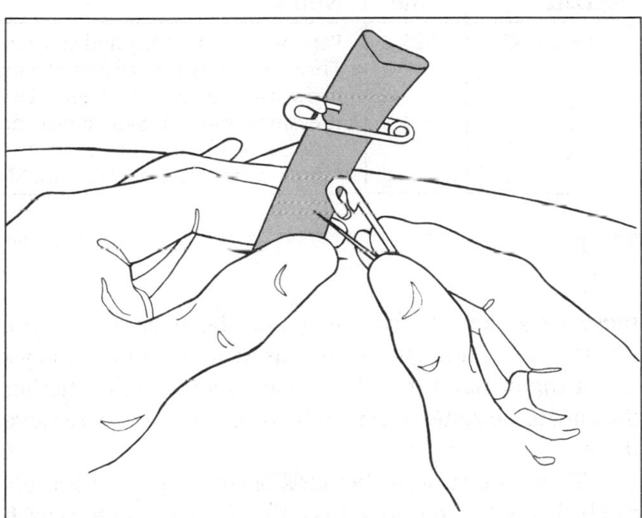

Figure 52–9

   Rationale The pin keeps the drain from falling back into the incision. Holding the drain securely in place at the skin level and inserting the pin above the fingers prevents the nurse from pulling the drain farther out or pricking the client during this step.

   or

   Use two pairs of sterile forceps instead of wearing sterile gloves to shorten the drain. This procedure requires manipulative skill.
   a. After pulling out the drain, pick up the sterile safety pin at the clasp end using one pair of forceps held in the nondominant hand.
   b. Securely grasp the base of the pin with the hemostat held in the dominant hand. See Figure 52–10.

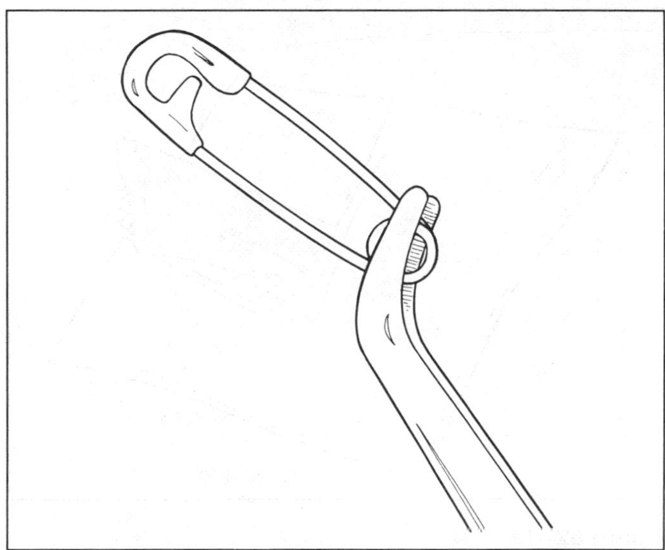

Figure 52–10

   c. Holding the pin securely with the hemostat, open the pin using the other forceps.
   d. Use those forceps to hold the drain at the skin level while inserting the pin through the drain over the forceps.
   e. Close the pin using the forceps.
9. Cut off the excess drain so that about 2.5 cm (1 in) remains above the skin. See Figure 52–11. Discard the excess in the waste bag.
10. Place a precut 4 × 4 gauze snugly around the drain (see Figure 52–12); or open a 4 × 4 gauze to 4 × 8, fold it lengthwise to 2 × 8, and place the 2 × 8 around the drain so the ends overlap.

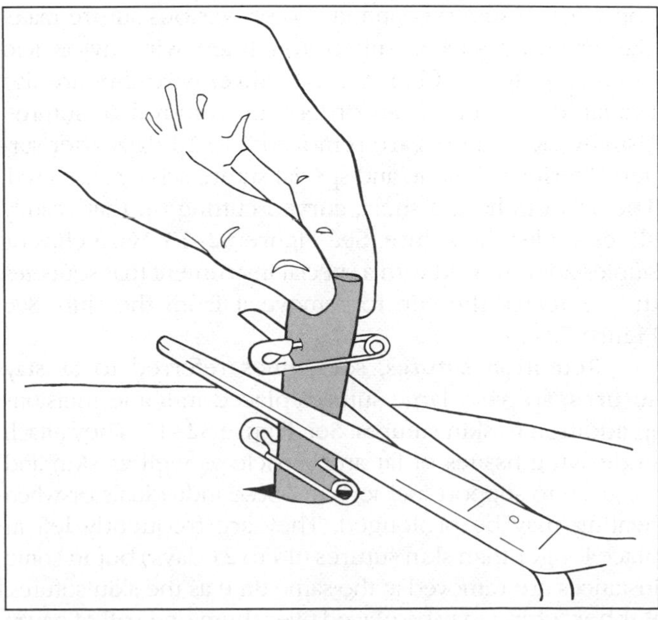

Figure 52–11

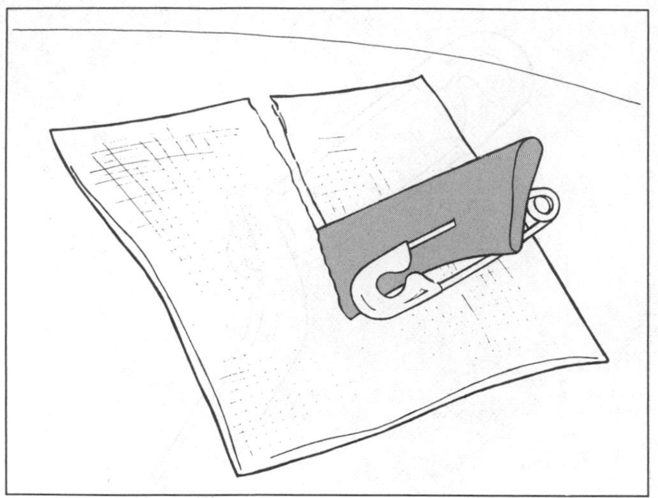

Figure 52–12

Rationale This dressing absorbs the drainage and helps prevent it from excoriating the skin. Using pre-cut gauze or folding it as described instead of cutting the gauze prevents any threads from coming loose and getting into the wound, where they could cause inflammation and provide a site for infection.

11. Apply the sterile dressings one at a time using sterile gloved hands or sterile forceps. Take care that the dressings do not slide off and become contaminated. Place the bulk of the dressings over the drain area and below the drain, depending on the client's usual position.

    Rationale Layers of dressings are placed for best absorption of drainage, which flows by gravity.

12. Apply the final surgipad by hand, touching only the outside unless using sterile gloves, and secure the dressing with tape or ties.

13. Record the technique on the client's record, including the amount the drain was shortened and the type and amount of drainage present. Also see the Sample Recording at the end of Procedure 52–1.

Sample Recording

Date	Time	Notes
Dec/5/87	1025	Penrose drain shortened 2.5 cm. Three 4 × 4 gauzes saturated with brownish yellow drainage. Dry dressings applied. Skin intact; no redness or irritation.——— ———Maria L. Antonio, RN

Sutures

Sutures are stitches used to sew body tissues together. *Suture* can also refer to the material used to sew the stitch. Policies vary about the personnel who may remove skin sutures. In some agencies, only physicians remove sutures; in others, registered nurses and student nurses with appropriate supervision may do so. Various suture materials are used, such as silk, cotton, linen, wire, nylon, and Dacron (polyester fiber) threads. Silver wire clips are also available. The physician orders the removal of sutures. Usually, skin sutures are removed 7 to 10 days after surgery. Sterile technique and special suture scissors are used. The scissors have a short, curved cutting tip that readily slides under the suture. See Figure 52–13. Wire clips or staples are removed with a special instrument that squeezes the center of the clip to remove it from the skin. See Figure 52–14.

Retention sutures, sometimes referred to as **stay sutures**, are very large sutures placed in some incisions in addition to skin sutures. See Figure 52–15. They attach underlying tissues of fat and muscle as well as skin and are used to support incisions in obese individuals or when healing may be prolonged. They are frequently left in place longer than skin sutures (14 to 21 days) but in some instances are removed at the same time as the skin sutures. Rubber tubing may be placed over them or a roll of gauze under them extending down the incision line, to prevent these large sutures from irritating the incision. Several forms of retention sutures are used, and agency policies about them may vary. The nurse should verify whether they are to be removed and which personnel may remove them.

There are various methods of suturing. Skin sutures can be broadly categorized as either (a) interrupted (each stitch is tied and knotted separately), or (b) continuous (one thread runs in a series of stitches and is tied only at the beginning and at the end of the run). Common sutures

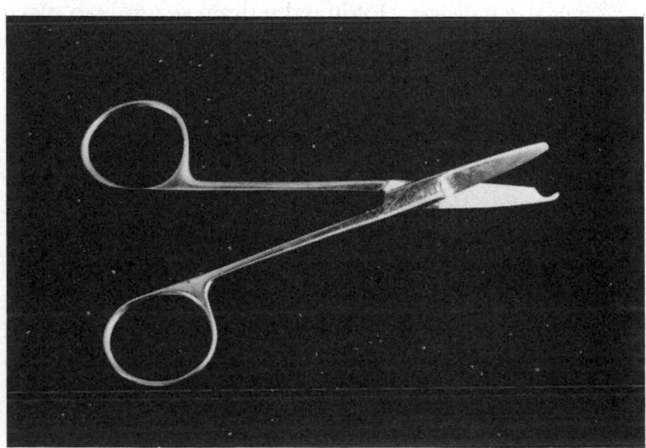

Figure 52–13 Suture scissors

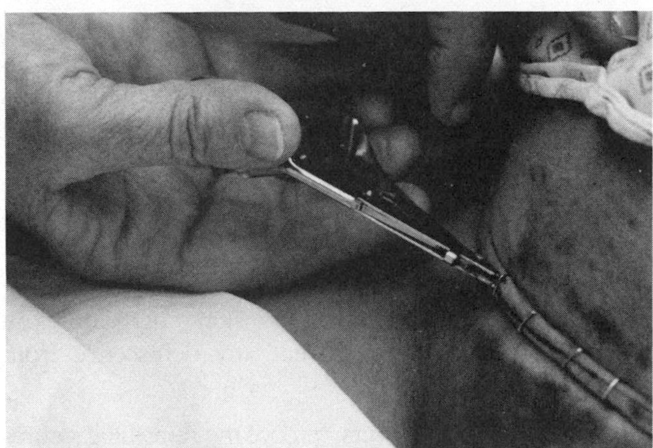

Figure 52–14 Removing metal clips (staples) with a clip remover

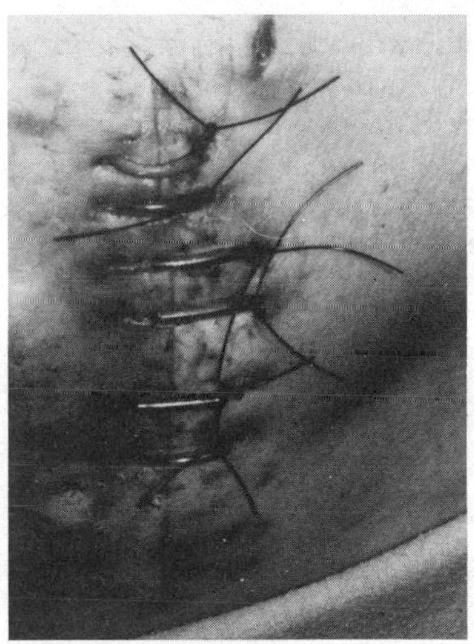

Figure 52–15 A surgical incision with retention sutures

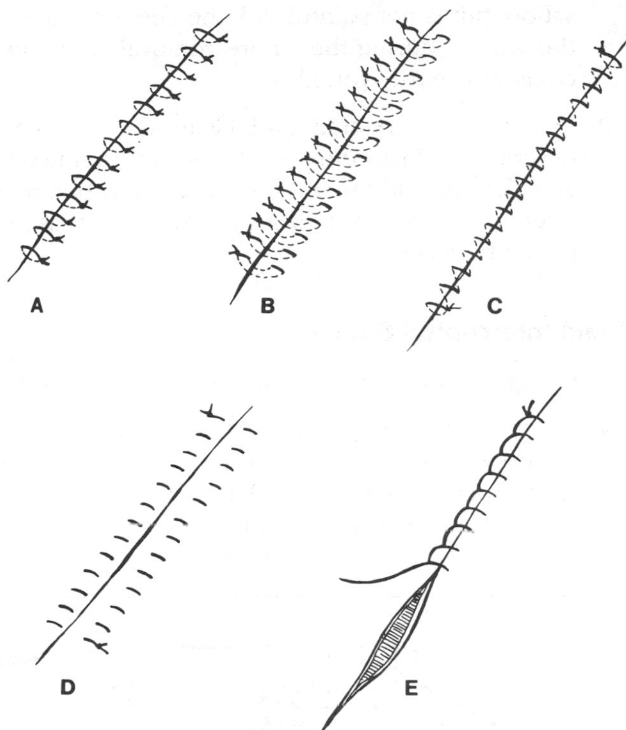

Figure 52–16 Common methods of suturing: **A,** plain interrupted; **B,** mattress interrupted; **C,** plain continuous; **D,** mattress continuous; **E,** blanket continuous

include plain interrupted (see Figure 52–16, *A*), mattress interrupted (see Figure 52–16, *B*), plain continuous (see Figure 52–16, *C*), mattress continuous (see Figure 52–16, *D*), and blanket continuous (see Figure 52–16, *E*).

The technique for removing skin sutures is described in Procedure 52–4.

Procedure 52–4 ▲ Removing Skin Sutures

Equipment

1. A sterile dressing set. See Procedure 52–1, page 1554.
2. Sterile suture scissors.
3. Sterile butterfly tape (optional) to hold the wound edges together if wound dehiscence occurs.
4. A moisture-proof bag to receive used dressings and supplies.
5. A light, sterile gauze pad and tape if a dressing is to be applied.

Intervention

Refer to the client's record for the physician's orders for suture removal. Many times only *alternate* interrupted sutures are removed one day, and the remaining sutures are removed a day or two later. The record should also say whether a dressing is to be applied following the suture removal. Some physicians order no dressing; others prefer a small, light gauze dressing to prevent friction from clothing.

1. Inform the client that suture removal may produce slight discomfort, such as a pulling or stinging sen-

sation, but is not painful. Ask the client not to touch the wound during the suture removal, so as not to contaminate the wound.

2. Remove the dressing and clean the incision, as described in Procedure 52–1. The suture line is usually cleaned with antimicrobial solution before and after suture removal as a prophylactic measure to prevent infection.

Plain Interrupted Sutures

3. Grasp the suture at the knot with a pair of forceps.
4. Place the curved tip of the suture scissors under the suture as close to the skin as possible, either on the side opposite the knot (see Figure 52–17) or directly under the knot. Cut the suture.

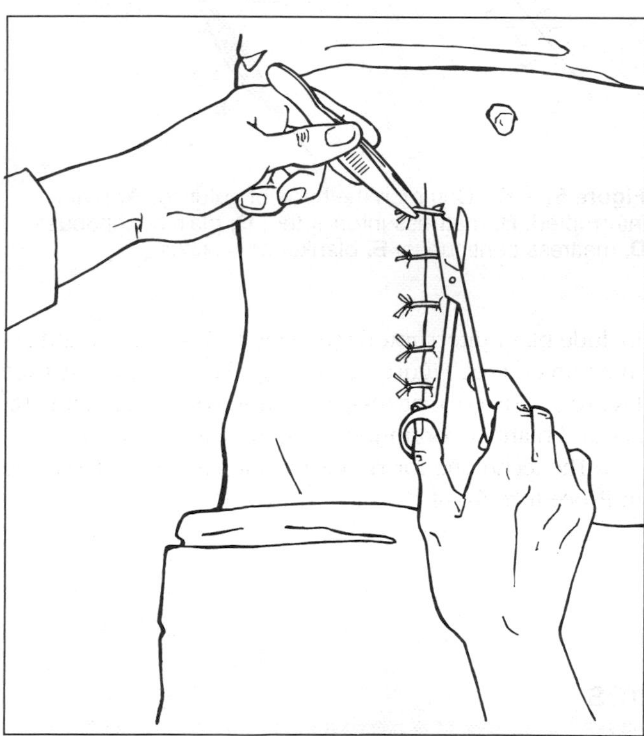

Figure 52–17

Rationale Suture are cut as close to the skin as possible on one side of the visible part because the suture material visible to the eye is in contact with resident bacteria of the skin and must not be pulled beneath the skin during removal. Suture material that is beneath the skin is considered free from bacteria.

5. With the forceps, pull the suture out in one piece. Be sure that all suture material is removed.

   Rationale Suture material left beneath the skin acts as a foreign body and causes inflammation.

6. Discard the suture onto a piece of sterile gauze or into the moisture-proof bag, being careful not to contaminate the forceps tips. Sometimes the suture sticks to the forceps and needs to be removed by wiping the tips on a sterile gauze.
7. Continue to remove *alternate* sutures, i.e., the third, fifth, seventh, etc.

   Rationale Alternate sutures are removed first so that remaining sutures keep the skin edges in close approximation and prevent any dehiscence from becoming large.

8. If no dehiscence occurs, remove the remaining sutures if ordered. If dehiscence does occur, do *not* remove the remaining sutures; and report the dehiscence to the responsible nurse.
9. a. If a little wound dehiscence occurs, apply a sterile butterfly tape over the gap:
   - Attach the tape to one side of the incision.
   - Press the wound edges together.
   - Attach the tape to the other side of the incision. See Figure 52–18.

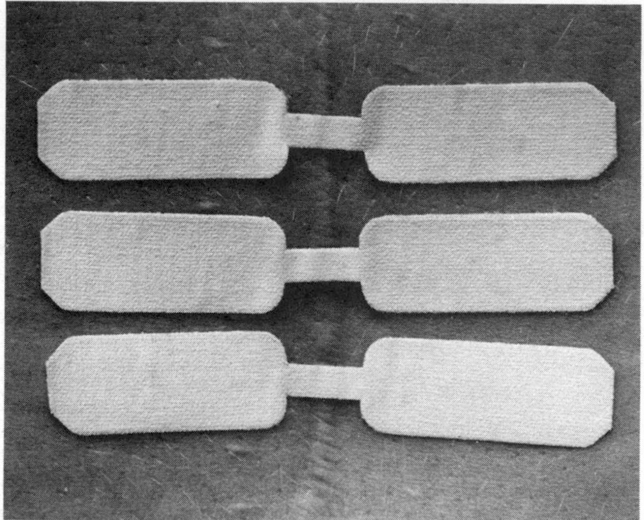

Figure 52–18

Rationale The butterfly tape holds the wound edges as close together as possible and promotes healing.

   b. If a large dehiscence occurs, cover the wound with sterile gauze; and report the problem immediately to the responsible nurse or physician.

10. Clean the incision again with skin antimicrobial solution.
11. Apply a small, light, sterile gauze dressing if any small dehiscence has occurred or if this is agency practice.

12. Instruct the client about follow-up wound care. Generally, if a wound is dry and healing well, the client can shower in a day or two. Instruct the client to contact the physician if wound discharge appears.

13. Record the suture removal and relevant assessment data on the appropriate records.

Sample Recording

Date	Time	Notes
Dec/5/87	1105	Abdominal sutures were removed. Wound dry, edges approximated closely. No signs of inflammation. Gauze dressing applied.———— ————Gwen E. Owens, NS

Mattress Interrupted Sutures

See Figure 52–19. Mattress interrupted sutures do not cross the incision line outside the skin and have two threads underlying the skin.

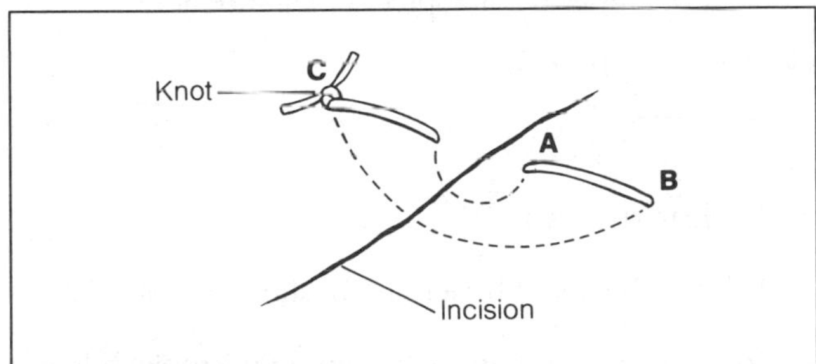

Figure 52–19

14. When possible, cut the visible part of the suture close to the skin at *A* and *B* in Figure 52–19, opposite the knot, and remove this small visible piece. Discard it as in step 6. In some sutures, the visible part opposite the knot may be so small that it can be cut only once.

15. Grasp the knot (*C*) with forceps. Remove the remainder of the suture beneath the skin by pulling out in the direction of the knot.

16. Follow steps 7–13.

Plain Continuous Sutures

See Figure 52–20.

17. Cut the thread of the first suture opposite the knot at *A* in Figure 52–20. Then cut the thread of the second suture on that same side at *B*.

18. Grasp the knot (*C*) with the forceps, and pull. This removes the first stitch and the piece of thread beneath

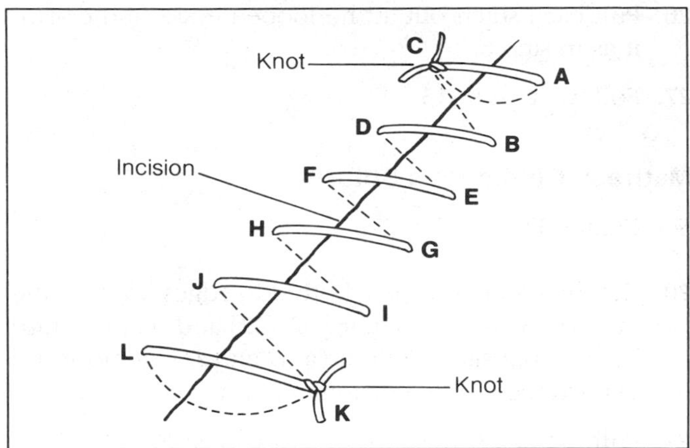

Figure 52–20

the skin, which is attached to the second stitch. Discard the sutures as in step 6.

19. Cut off the visible part of the second suture at *D*, and discard it.

20. Grasp the suture at *E*, and pull out the underlying loop between *D* and *E*.

21. Cut the visible part at *F*, and remove it.

22. Repeat steps 19–21 at *G–J*, until the last knot is reached. Note: after the first stitch is removed, each thread is cut down the same side, below the original knot.

23. Cut the last suture at *L*, and pull out the last suture at *K*.

24. Follow steps 9–13.

Blanket Continuous Sutures

See Figure 52–21.

25. Cut the threads that are opposite the looped blanket edge; i.e., cut at *A–F* in Figure 52–21.

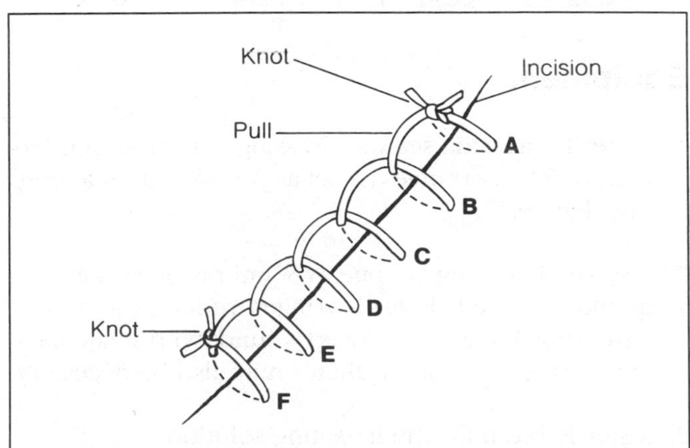

Figure 52–21

26. Pull each stitch out at the looped edge, and discard it as in step 6.
27. Follow steps 9–13.

Mattress Continuous Sutures

See Figure 52–22.

28. Cut the visible suture at both skin edges opposite the knot (at *A* and *B* in Figure 52–22) and on the suture below opposite the knot (at *C* and *D*). Remove and discard the visible portions as in step 6.
29. Pull the first suture out by the knot at *E*.
30. Lift the second suture between *F* and *G* to pull out the underlying suture between *G* and *C*. Cut off the visible part at *F* as close to the skin edge as possible.
31. Go to the opposite side between *H* and *I*. Lift out the suture between *F* and *I*, and cut off all the visible part close to the skin at *H*.
32. Lift the suture between *J* and *K* to pull out the suture between *H* and *K*, and cut the suture close to the skin at *J*.

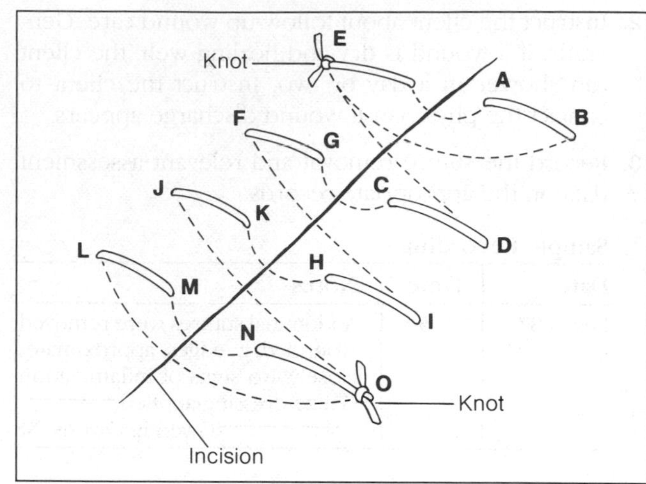

Figure 52–22

33. Repeat steps 31–32, working from side to side of the incision, until the last suture is reached.
34. Cut the visible suture opposite the knot at *L* and *M*. Pull out all remaining pieces of suture at *O*.
35. Follow steps 9–13.

Wound Irrigation

An **irrigation (lavage)** is the washing or flushing out of an area. Sterile technique is required for a wound irrigation, because there is a break in the skin integrity. Wounds are usually irrigated for one or more of the following reasons:

1. To clean the area
2. To apply heat and hasten the healing process
3. To apply a medication, such as an antimicrobial solution

See Procedure 52–5.

Procedure 52–5 ▲ Irrigating a Wound

Equipment

1. A sterile dressing set and dressing materials. See Procedure 52–1. Arrange the set as you would for a dressing change.
2. A sterile irrigating syringe. A 50-ml piston syringe frequently is used. Piston syringes reduce the risk of aspirating drainage. For deep wounds with small openings, a sterile straight catheter may also be necessary.
3. A sterile basin for the irrigating solution.
4. A sterile basin to receive the irrigation returns.
5. Irrigating solution, usually 200 ml (6.5 oz) of solution at 32 to 35 C (90 to 95 F), according to the agency's or physician's practice. Sterile normal saline, Dakin's solution, hydrogen peroxide, or antimicrobial solutions frequently are used.
6. Sterile gloves to wear if you will touch the wound.
7. A moisture-proof sterile drape to protect the client and the bed.
8. Sterile petroleum jelly to protect the surrounding skin from irritation by certain solutions (e.g., Dakin's solution).
9. A sterile tongue blade to apply the petroleum jelly.

Intervention

1. Remove the old dressing, and clean the wound. See Procedure 52–1, steps 1–18.

2. Assist the client to a position in which the irrigating solution will flow by gravity from the upper end of the wound to the lower end and then into the basin.

3. Place the waterproof drape over the client and the bed, and position the sterile basin on it below the wound, to catch the irrigating solution.

4. If an irrigating solution, such as Dakin's solution, is being used, apply sterile petroleum jelly to the skin around the wound, using the sterile tongue blade.

5. Using the syringe, gently instill a steady stream of irrigating solution into the wound. Make sure all areas of the wound are irrigated. If you are using a catheter, insert the catheter into the wound until you feel resistance. Do not force the catheter, since this can damage tissue.

6. Continue irrigating until the solution becomes clear (no exudate is present) or until all the solution has been used.

   Rationale The irrigation washes away tissue debris and drainage so that later returns are clearer.

7. Using dressing forceps and sterile gauze, dry the area around the wound.

   Rationale Moisture left on the skin promotes the growth of microorganisms and can cause skin irritation.

8. Assess the appearance of the wound, noting in particular the type and amount of exudate, and the presence and extent of granulation tissue.

9. Apply a sterile dressing to the wound. See Procedure 52–1, steps 20–21.

10. Record the irrigation, the solution used, the appearance of the wound, and the appearance of any exudate and sloughing tissue.

Wound Suction

The plastic bellows wound suction (Hemovac) is used to suction excessive drainage from surgical wounds. Suction is created by manually compressing and releasing the sides of the apparatus.

The Hemovac is increasingly being used by surgeons after various operations, e.g., spinal surgery, hip surgery, radical mastectomy, head or neck surgery, and perineal surgery. This type of suction is advantageous in that it exerts a *gentle,* even pressure on tissues, is quiet and lightweight, and moves easily with the client. The unit consists of an evacuator bag, evacuator tubing with a Y-connector, and wound tubing with a needle. See Figure 52–23.

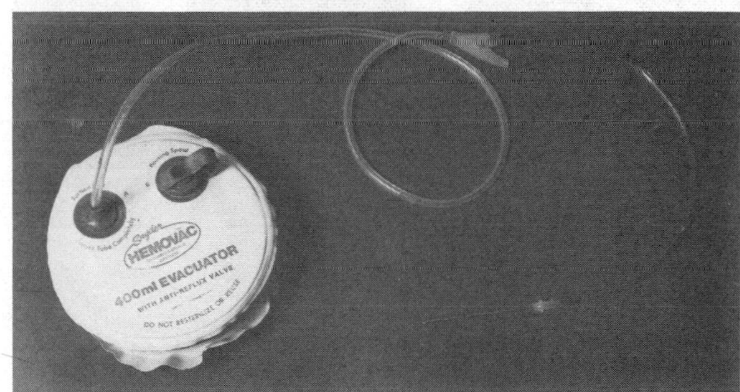

Figure 52–23 A wound suction (Hemovac)

The surgeon inserts the wound drainage tube during surgery. Generally the suction is removed from 3 to 7 days postoperatively or when the wound is free from drainage. Nurses are responsible for maintaining the patency of the wound suction, which hastens the healing process by draining excess exudate that might otherwise interfere with the formation of granulation tissue in a wound. See Procedure 52–6.

Procedure 52–6 ▲ Establishing and Maintaining a Plastic Bellows Wound Suction (Hemovac, Portable Wound Suction)

Equipment

To empty the evacuator bag

1. A drainage receptacle, e.g., a solution basin.

2. A calibrated pitcher to measure the drainage.

To irrigate the tubing

3. A sterile 50-ml syringe.

4. A sterile #18 or #20 needle with a blunt bevel. The needle needs to fit snugly into the drainage tubing.

5. Sterile irrigating solution as ordered, e.g., normal saline.
6. A sterile set with a sterile receptacle, e.g., a kidney basin or solution basin and a sterile towel.

Intervention

Establishing Suction

Establish suction if it was not initiated by the physician.

1. Place the evacuator bag on a solid, flat surface.
2. Open the drainage plug (marked *B*) on top of the bag, without contaminating it.
3. Compress the bag; while it is compressed, close the drainage plug to retain the vacuum. See Figure 52–24.

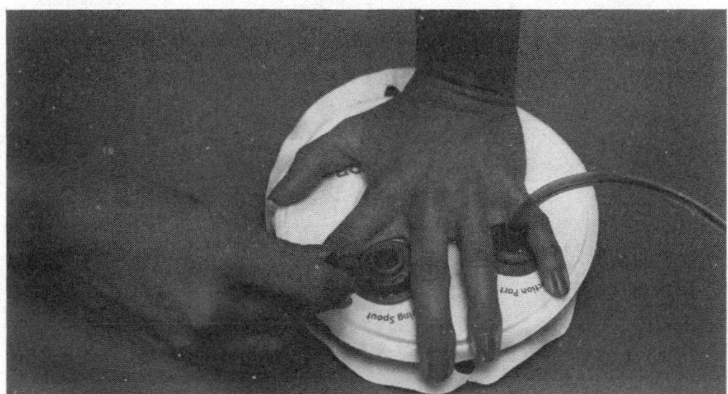

Figure 52–24

Emptying the Evacuator Bag

4. When the drainage fluid reaches the line marked *Full,* open the drainage plug marked *B*.
5. Invert the bag, and empty it into the collecting receptacle. See Figure 52–25.

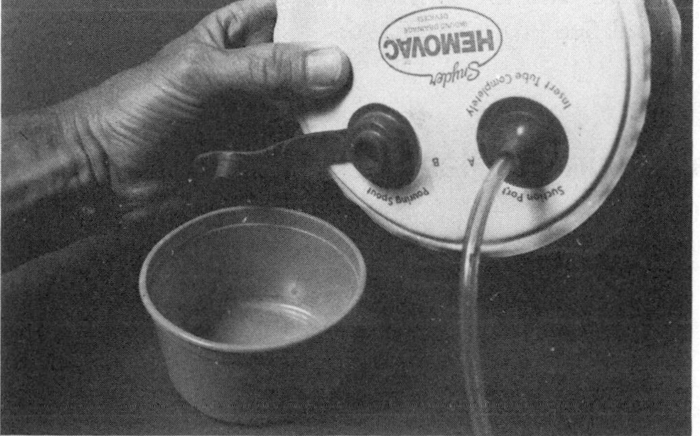

Figure 52–25

6. Reestablish suction as in steps 1–3.
7. Measure the amount of drainage, and note its characteristics.

Irrigating the Evacuator and Wound Tubing

Because the wound tubing of a portable wound suction is siliconized and perforated with many holes, occlusions of the tubing are rare. However, when the evacuator bag is compressed and no drainage appears, either the wound is free of exudate or the tubing is clogged. In the latter instance, notify the responsible nurse and/or the physician; an irrigation *may* be ordered.

8. Open the sterile set, and prepare a sterile field.
9. Fill the irrigating syringe with irrigating fluid, keeping the needle and plunger sterile.
10. Disconnect the wound tubing from the tubing connector, keeping the ends sterile to prevent contamination of the wound.
11. Insert the needle into the wound tubing, taking care not to perforate the tubing with the needle.
12. Instill the prescribed amount of irrigating fluid slowly and gently.

    Rationale Too much force could injure the tissues.
13. Detach the syringe from the tubing and place the end of the wound tubing in a sterile container.
14. Refill the syringe, if necessary, and insert the needle into the Y-connector opening. See Figure 53–26.
15. Irrigate the evacuator tubing until the fluid that runs into the evacuator bag is clear.
16. Reconnect the tubes securely, and empty the bag. Calculate the amount of drainage by subtracting the amount of irrigating fluid used.

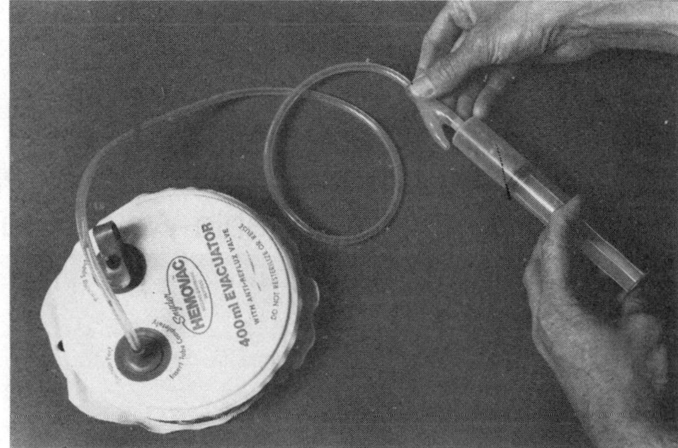

Figure 52–26

17. Reestablish the suction as in steps 1–3.
18. Assess the client's response to the technique in terms of discomfort, relief from discomfort, etc.
19. Record the emptying of the evacuator bag, irrigation of the tubing, etc., on the client's record.
20. Record on the appropriate records the response of the client and the amount, appearance, etc., of the drainage. For example, the amount and type of drainage should be included on the client's intake and output record and on the nursing notes.

Wound Drainage Specimens

Specimens of wound drainage are obtained when it is suspected that a client's wound is infected. The specimen usually is obtained when the dressing is changed, and it is then sent to the laboratory for culture and sensitivity.

After removing the old dressing as in changing a surgical dressing, the nurse removes her or his gloves and then opens a package of sterile swabs or applicators. The nurse then dons sterile gloves and opens the sterile specimen tube. Using a sterile swab, the nurse wipes the drainage at a designated point or where it is heaviest and nearest the wound. As much drainage as possible is absorbed onto the swab. The nurse then carefully inserts the swab into the sterile container, taking care not to touch the top or outside of the tube so they remain free of pathogenic microorganisms.

If a specimen is required from another site, a second swab is used. Only one wipe is taken with each swab, to prevent contamination of the wound. Each specimen is correctly labeled, including the exact site from which it was taken. The specimens are then sent to the laboratory.

Evaluation

Examples of outcome criteria for wound care are listed to the right.

Examples of Outcome Criteria for Wound Care

The client will:

- Exhibit less inflammation and drainage from the wound
- Have no discomfort in the wound area
- Have a normal body temperature
- Exhibit no signs of wound infection

Supporting and Immobilizing Wounds

A **bandage** is a strip of cloth used to wrap some part of the body. Bandages are available in various widths, most commonly 1.5 to 7.5 cm (0.5 to 3 in). They are usually supplied in rolls for easy application to a body part. A **binder**, a type of bandage, is designed for a specific body part; for example, the triangular binder (sling) fits the arm. Binders are used to support large areas of the body, such as the abdomen, arm, or chest.

Bandages and binders serve a variety of purposes:

1. To support a wound, e.g., a fractured bone
2. To immobilize a wound, e.g., a strained shoulder
3. To apply pressure; e.g., elastic bandages apply pressure to the lower extremities to improve venous blood flow
4. To secure a dressing, e.g., for an extensive abdominal surgical wound
5. To retain splints (this applies chiefly to bandages)
6. To retain warmth, e.g., a flannel bandage on a rheumatoid joint

Support and immobilization are the most common purposes.

Materials

For Bandages

The materials used in bandaging vary widely, according to the purpose of the bandage. *Gauze* is one of the materials used most commonly because it is light and porous and readily molds to the body. It is also relatively inexpensive, so it is generally discarded once it becomes soiled. Gauze frequently is used to retain dressings on wounds and to bandage the fingers, hands, toes, and feet. It supports dressings well and at the same time permits air to circulate, and it can be impregnated with petroleum jelly or other medications for application to wounds.

Flannel is a soft, pliable material that provides warmth to a body part. It is strong and fairly heavy and can be washed and reused.

Muslin (a plain woven cotton) is lighter than flannel but is also strong and supplies good support. Like flannel, muslin can be washed and reused.

Crinoline and *Kling* are types of woven gauze. Kling is woven in such a manner that it will stretch and mold to the body. Crinoline is loosely woven yet strong. It is impregnated with plaster of paris for use as the base for casts.

There are many kinds of *elasticized* bandages that are applied to provide pressure to an area. They are commonly used as tensor bandages or as partial stockings to provide support to the legs and improve the venous circulation (see Chapter 53). Some elasticized bandages have an adhesive backing and can be secured to the skin. These are most frequently used to retain dressings and at the same time provide some support to a wound.

Plastic adhesive bandages also are used to retain dressings. They are waterproof and thus retain wound drainage or keep an area dry. They have some elastic properties and therefore provide some pressure.

For Binders

Most binders are made of muslin, flannel, or a synthetic that may or may not be elasticized. Some abdominal binders are made of an elasticized, netlike material that fits the body contours and permits air to circulate around the body part.

Bandaging

Assessment for Bandaging

Before applying a bandage it is important to know its purpose and the area of the body to which it needs to be applied. The client should be assessed for:

1. Abrasions or wounds. Open areas will require dressing before a bandage is applied.
2. The color and temperature of the skin and any numbness, tingling, or pain in the area. Pale or cyanotic skin, cool temperature, tingling, or pain can indicate impaired circulation in the area. Data from the client's record or comparison of the skin temperature of, for example, one extremity with that of the other can provide baseline information against which to judge the assessment data.

Guidelines for Bandaging

1. Whenever possible, bandage the part in its normal position, with the joint slightly flexed, to avoid putting strain on the ligaments and the muscles of the joint.
2. Pad between skin surfaces and over bony prominences to prevent friction from the bandage and consequent abrasion of the skin.
3. Always bandage body parts by working from the distal end to the proximal end, to aid the return flow of the venous blood.
4. Bandage with even pressure so as not to interfere with blood circulation.
5. Whenever possible, leave the end of the body part (e.g., the finger) exposed so you will be able to determine the adequacy of blood circulation to the extremity.
6. Cover dressings with bandages at least 5 cm (2 in) beyond the edges of the dressing to prevent the dressing and wound from becoming contaminated.
7. Face the client when applying a bandage, to maintain uniform tension and the appropriate direction of the bandage.

Basic Bandaging

Applying bandages to various parts of the body involves one or more of five basic bandaging turns: circular, spiral, spiral reverse, recurrent, and figure-eight.

Circular turns Circular turns are used to anchor bandages and to terminate them. They are also used to bandage certain areas, such as the proximal aspect of a finger or a wrist. Circular turns usually are not applied directly over a wound because of the discomfort the bandage would cause.

Spiral turns Spiral turns are used to bandage parts of the body that are fairly uniform in circumference, e.g., the upper arm or upper leg.

Spiral reverse turns Spiral reverse turns are used to bandage cylindrical parts of the body that are not uniform in circumference, e.g., the lower leg or forearm.

Recurrent turns Recurrent turns are used to cover distal parts of the body, e.g., the end of a finger, the skull, or the stump of an amputation.

Figure-eight turns Figure-eight turns are used to bandage an elbow, knee, or ankle, because they permit some movement after they are applied. The *spica* bandage is a variation of the figure-eight turn.

Procedure 52–7 details how to apply a basic bandage.

Procedure 52–7 ▲ Applying Basic Bandages

Equipment

1. A clean bandage of the appropriate material and width. The width of the bandage depends on the size of the body part to be bandaged. For example, a 2.5-cm (1-in) bandage is used for a finger, a 5-cm (2-in) bandage for an arm, and a 7.5 cm or 10-cm (3-in or 4-in) bandage for a leg. The larger the circumference of the part, the wider the bandage.
2. Padding for bony prominences and for between skin surfaces. Abdominal dressings (ABD pads) and gauze squares frequently are used to cover bony prominences, such as the elbow, or to separate skin surfaces, such as the fingers.
3. Tape, special metal clips, or a safety pin to secure the end of the bandage.

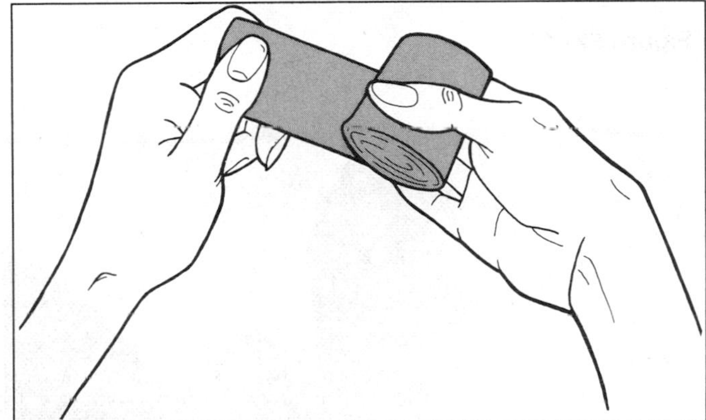

Figure 52–27

Intervention

1. Provide the client with a chair or bed, and arrange support for the area to be bandaged. For example, if a hand needs to be bandaged, have the client place his or her elbow on a table so the hand does not have to be held up unsupported.

   Rationale Because bandaging takes time, holding up a body part without support can be very tiring.

2. Make sure the area to be bandaged is clean and dry. Wash and dry the area if necessary.

   Rationale Washing and drying remove microorganisms, which flourish in warm, moist areas.

3. Align the part to be bandaged with slight flexion of the joints, unless this is contraindicated.

   Rationale Slight flexion places less strain on the ligaments and muscles of the joint.

Circular Turns

4. Hold the bandage in your dominant hand, with the roll uppermost (see Figure 52–27), and unroll the bandage about 8 cm (3 in).

   Rationale This length of unrolled bandage allows good control for placement and tension.

5. Apply the end of the bandage to the body part to be bandaged. Hold the end down with the thumb of the other hand. See Figure 52–28.
6. Encircle the body part as often as needed, each turn directly covering the previous turn. See Figure 52–29.

   Rationale This provides even support to the area.

7. Secure the end of the bandage with tape, metal clips, or a safety pin over an *uninjured* area.

   Rationale Clips and pins can be uncomfortable when situated over an injured area.

Spiral Turns

8. See steps 1–5.
9. Make two circular turns.

   Rationale Two circular turns anchor the bandage.

10. Continue spiral turns at about a 30° angle, each turn overlapping the preceding one by two-thirds the width of the bandage. See Figure 52–30.

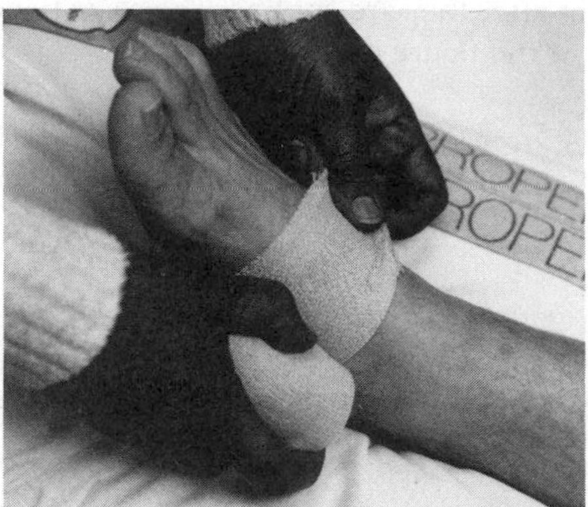

Figure 52–28

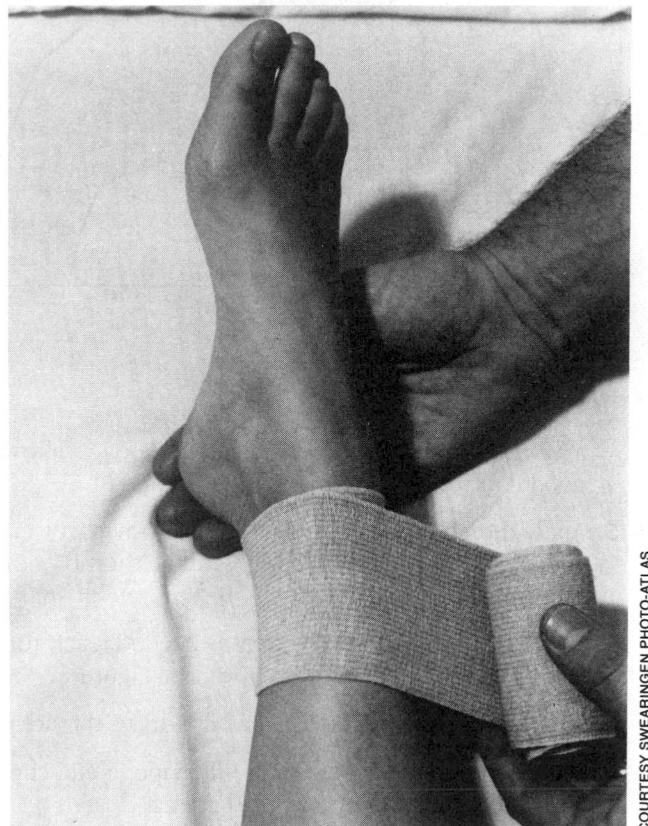

COURTESY SWEARINGEN PHOTO-ATLAS

Figure 52–29

11. Terminate the bandage with two circular turns, and secure the end with tape, metal clips, or a safety pin over an uninjured area.

Spiral Reverse Turns

12. See steps 1–5.
13. Anchor the bandage with two circular turns, and bring the bandage upward at about a 30° angle.

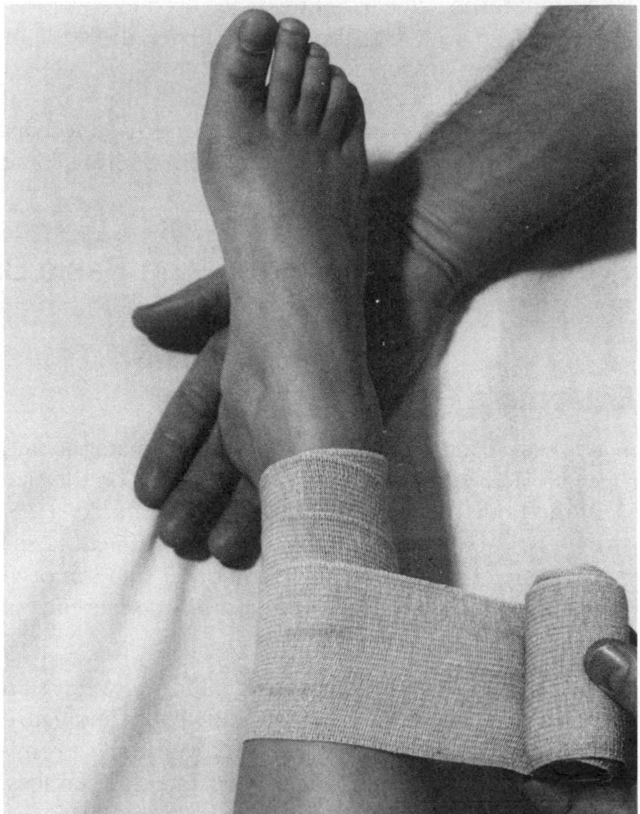

COURTESY SWEARINGEN PHOTO-ATLAS

Figure 52–30

14. Place the thumb of your free hand on the upper edge of the bandage. See Figure 52–31, *A*.

    Rationale The thumb will hold the bandage while it is folded upon itself.

15. Unroll the bandage about 15 cm (6 in), then turn your hand so the bandage falls over itself. See Figure 52–31, *B*.
16. Continue the bandage around the limb, overlapping each previous turn by two-thirds the width of the bandage. Make each bandage turn at the same position on the limb so the turns of the bandage are aligned. See Figure 52–31, *C*.
17. Terminate the bandage with two circular turns, and secure the end with tape, metal clips, or a safety pin over an uninjured area.

Recurrent Turns

18. See steps 1–5.
19. Anchor the bandage with two circular turns.
20. Fold it back on itself and bring it centrally over the distal end to be bandaged. See Figure 52–32.

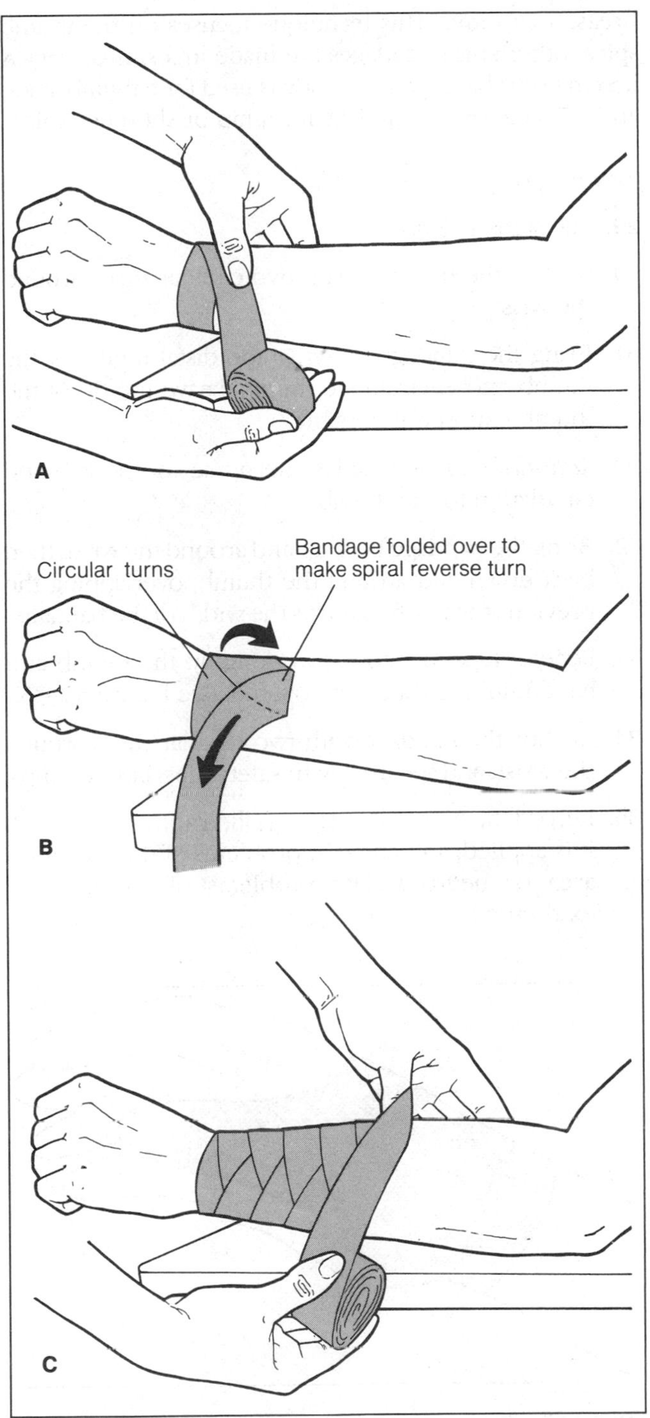

Figure 52–31

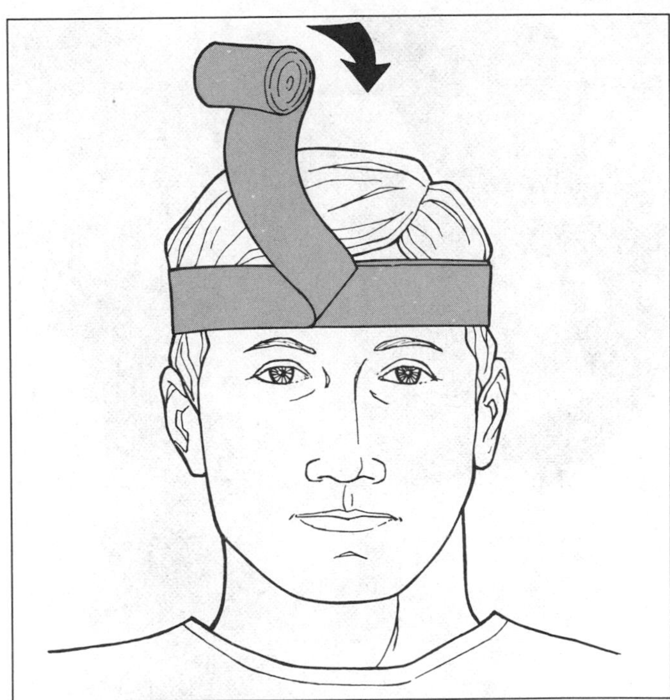

Figure 52–32

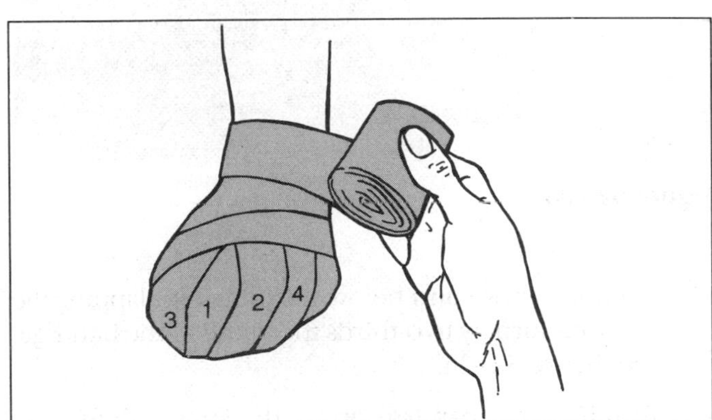

Figure 52–33

21. Holding it with the other hand, bring it back over the end to the right of the center bandage but overlapping it by two-thirds the width of the bandage.
22. Bring the bandage back on the left side, also overlapping the first turn by two-thirds the width of the bandage.
23. Continue this pattern of alternating right and left until the area is covered. Overlap the preceding turn by two-thirds the bandage width each time.
24. Terminate the bandage with two circular turns. See Figure 52–33. Secure the end with tape, metal clips, or a safety pin over an uninjured area.

Figure-Eight Turns

25. See steps 1–5 and then anchor the bandage with two circular turns.
26. Carry the bandage above the joint, around it, and then below it, making a figure eight.

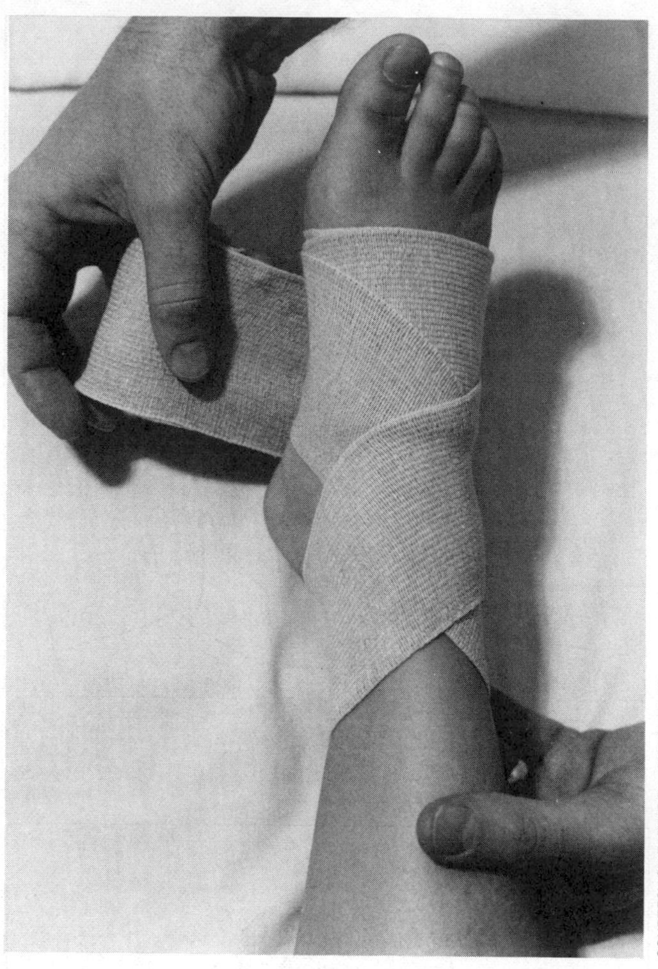

Figure 52–34

27. Continue above and below the joint, overlapping the previous turn by two-thirds the width of the bandage. See Figure 52–34.
28. Terminate the bandage above the joint with two circular turns, and secure it with tape, metal clips, or a safety pin over an uninjured area.

Spica Bandage

A spica bandage is a variation of the figure-eight bandage. It is commonly used to bandage the hip, groin, shoulder, breast, or thumb. This technique focuses on the thumb spica; other spica bandages are made in a similar way. A 2.5-cm (1-in) bandage frequently is used for a thumb spica, and a 7.5-cm (3-in) bandage for a hip or shoulder spica.

Thumb spica

29. See steps 1–5 above.
30. Anchor the bandage with two circular turns around the wrist.
31. Bring the bandage down to the distal aspect of the thumb and encircle the thumb. Leave the tip of the thumb exposed if possible.

    Rationale This enables the nurse to check blood circulation to the thumb.
32. Bring the bandage back up and around the wrist, then back down and around the thumb, overlapping the previous turn by two-thirds the width of the bandage.
33. Repeat steps 31 and 32, working up the thumb and hand until the thumb is covered. See Figure 52–35.
34. Anchor the bandage with two circular turns around the wrist, and secure it with safety pins, tape, or clips.
35. Record the type of bandage applied, the area to which it is applied, and any skin problems of the bandaged area or neurovascular problems of the involved extremity.

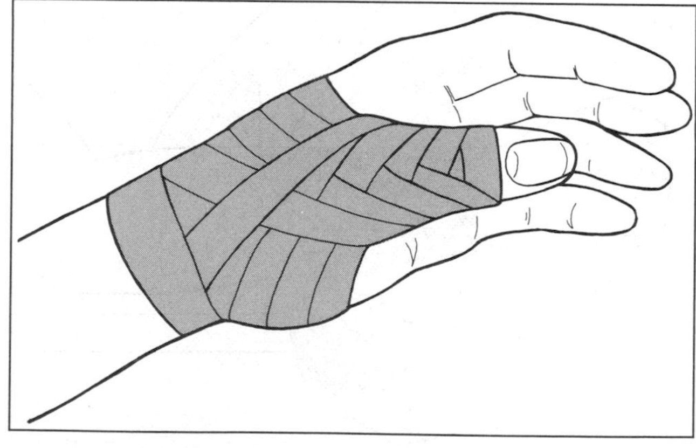

Figure 52–35

Binders

Binders are used to provide support, to apply pressure, to prevent or reduce swelling, or to retain dressings.

Triangular arm binder (sling) This is usually applied as a full triangle to support the arm, elbow, and forearm or to reduce or prevent swelling of a hand. See Figure 52–36.

Breast binder This type of binder provides pressure on the breasts, for example, when drying up the milk flow after childbirth, or to support the breasts, for example, after surgery. Breast binders are pinned in the front and usually have shoulder straps to prevent the binder from slipping down. See Figure 52–37.

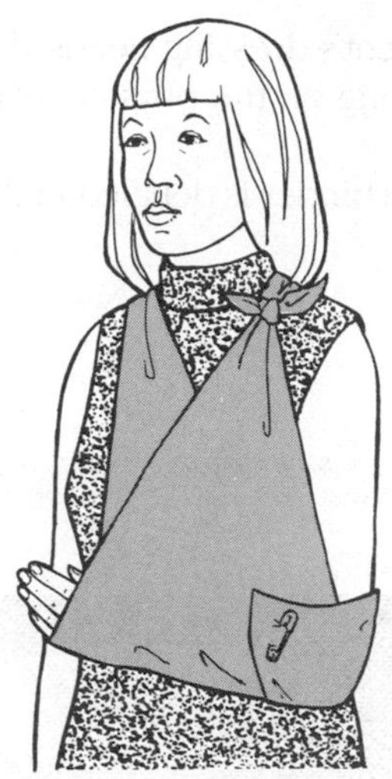

Figure 52–36 A large arm sling

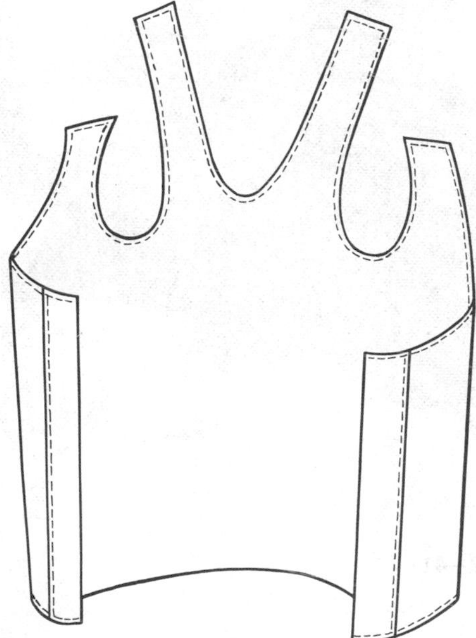

Figure 52–37 A breast binder

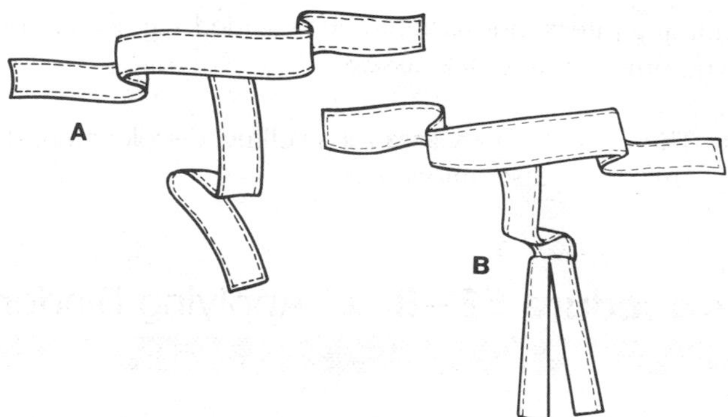

Figure 52–38 T-binders: A, single T; B, double T

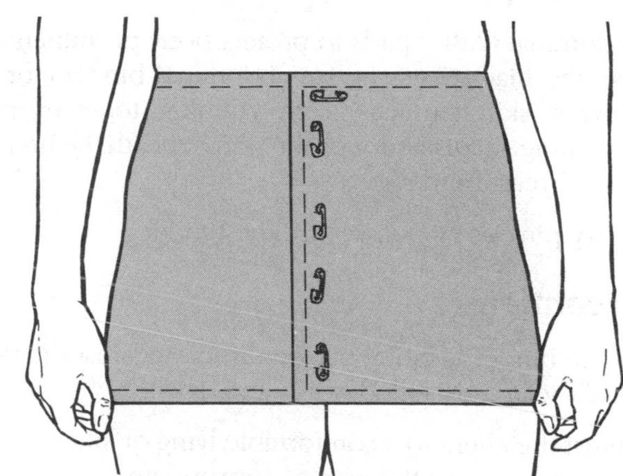

Figure 52–39 A straight abdominal binder

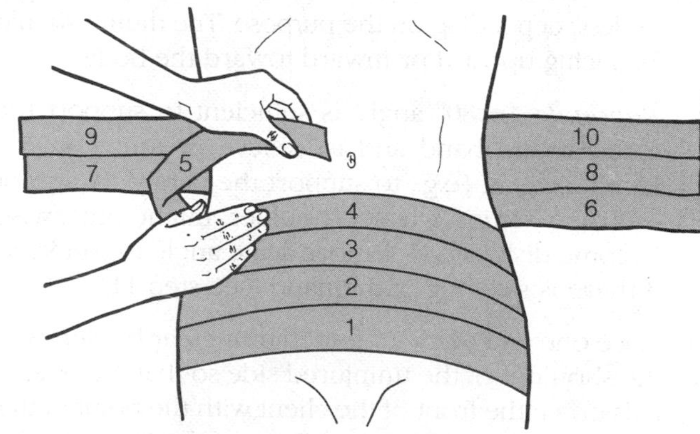

Figure 52–40 A scultetus (many-tailed) binder

T-binder (single or double T) This binder is used to retain pads, dressings, or packs in the perineal area. Single T-binders are often used for females, and double T-binders for males to prevent undue pressure on the penis. See Figure 52–38. The double T-binder can also provide greater support for large dressings on both males and females.

Straight abdominal binder This binder, which is used to provide support to the abdomen, is a rectangular piece of material long enough to encircle the abdomen with some overlap. See Figure 52–39. It can be made from any material, e.g., a bath blanket or towel.

Scultetus (many-tailed) binder A scultetus binder is used to provide support to the abdomen and, in some instances, to retain dressings. See Figure 52–40.

Assessment for Binders

Before applying a binder, the nurse should refer to the client's nursing care plan for the binder type needed, when it should be applied, and whether other adjunctive nursing interventions are to be provided, e.g., a cold pack. The nurse should also assess:

1. The involved body area for swelling, discoloration, skin abrasions, discomfort, etc.
2. Whether the client's dressing needs changing or reinforcing, depending on the physician's orders

How to apply a binder is detailed in Procedure 52–8.

Procedure 52–8 ▲ Applying Binders

Equipment

1. The appropriate binder
2. Abdominal (ABD) pads to protect bony prominences, e.g., the iliac crests (for an abdominal binder), or to prevent skin surfaces from rubbing together and becoming excoriated, e.g., the skin beneath the breasts (for a breast binder)
3. Safety pins or tape to secure the binder

Intervention

1. If the binder is being placed directly against the skin and the area is soiled, wash and dry it.
2. Assist the client to a comfortable lying or sitting position, supporting the area as appropriate.

Triangular Arm Sling

3. Have the client flex his or her elbow to an 80° angle or less, depending on the purpose. The thumb should be facing upward or inward toward the body.

   Rationale An 80° angle is sufficient to support the forearm and hand and to relieve pressure on the shoulder joint (e.g., to support the paralyzed arm of a stroke victim whose shoulder might otherwise become dislocated). A more acute angle is preferred if there is swelling of the hand (see step 11).

4. Place one end of the unfolded triangular binder over the shoulder of the uninjured side so that the binder falls down the front of the client with the point of the triangle (apex) under the elbow of the injured side. See Figure 52–41.
5. Take the upper corner and carry it around the neck until it hangs over the shoulder on the injured side.
6. Bring the lower corner of the binder up over the arm to the shoulder of the injured side. Using a reef knot, secure this corner to the upper corner at the side of the neck on the involved side. See Figure 52–42.

   Rationale A reef knot will not slip. Tying the knot at the side of the neck prevents pressure on the bony prominences of the vertebral column at the back of the neck.

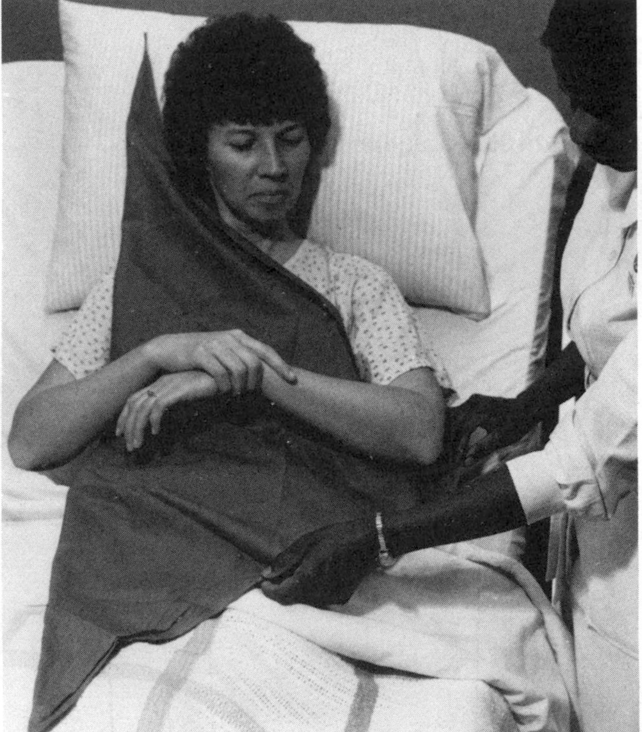
COURTESY SWEARINGEN PHOTO-ATLAS

Figure 52–41

7. Make sure the wrist is well supported, to maintain alignment.
8. Fold the sling neatly at the elbow, and secure it with safety pins or tape. It may be folded and fastened at the front. See Figure 52–36, on page 1573.
9. Remove the sling periodically to inspect the skin for indications of irritation, especially around the site of the knot.

Other Uses of the Triangular Binder

10. *Small arm sling (cravat binder)*
    a. Make a cravat binder by folding the triangular binder in on itself, starting at the apex. See Figure 52–43, *A*.
    b. Apply the sling as in Figure 52–43, *B*, with the knot on the affected side.

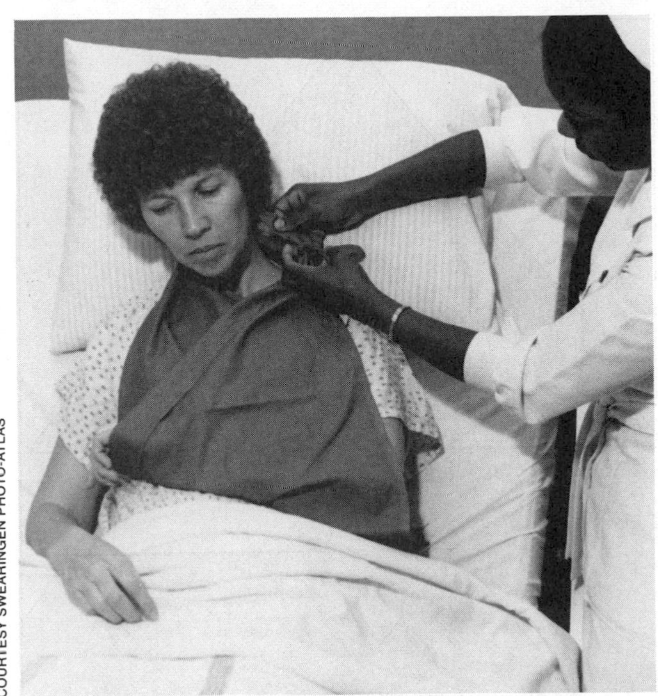

Figure 52–42

11. *Triangular arm sling for maximum hand elevation*
    a. Flex the client's arm so his or her hand rests on the clavicle of the uninjured side.

       Rationale This position provides maximum elevation of the hand.

    b. Place the binder over the shoulder of the uninjured side and *over the arm* (i.e., in front of the arm) so the apex of the binder extends beyond the elbow of the injured side. See Figure 52–44, *A*.

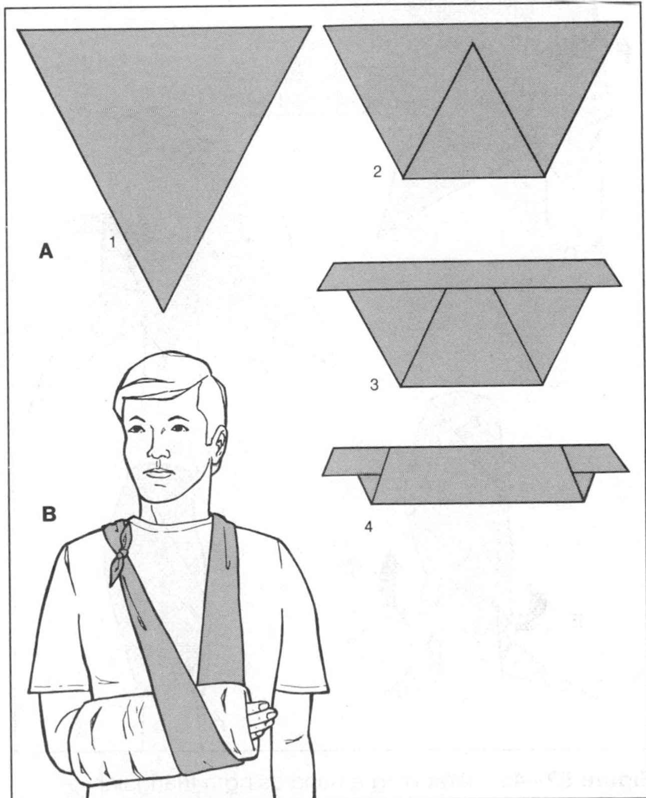

Figure 52–43 **A,** Making a cravat: (1) lay the triangular bandage on a flat surface; (2) fold the point up toward the base of the bandage; (3) fold the base over on itself to make a smooth edge; (4) fold the cravat from the other side to the desired width. **B,** The cravat applied as a small arm sling

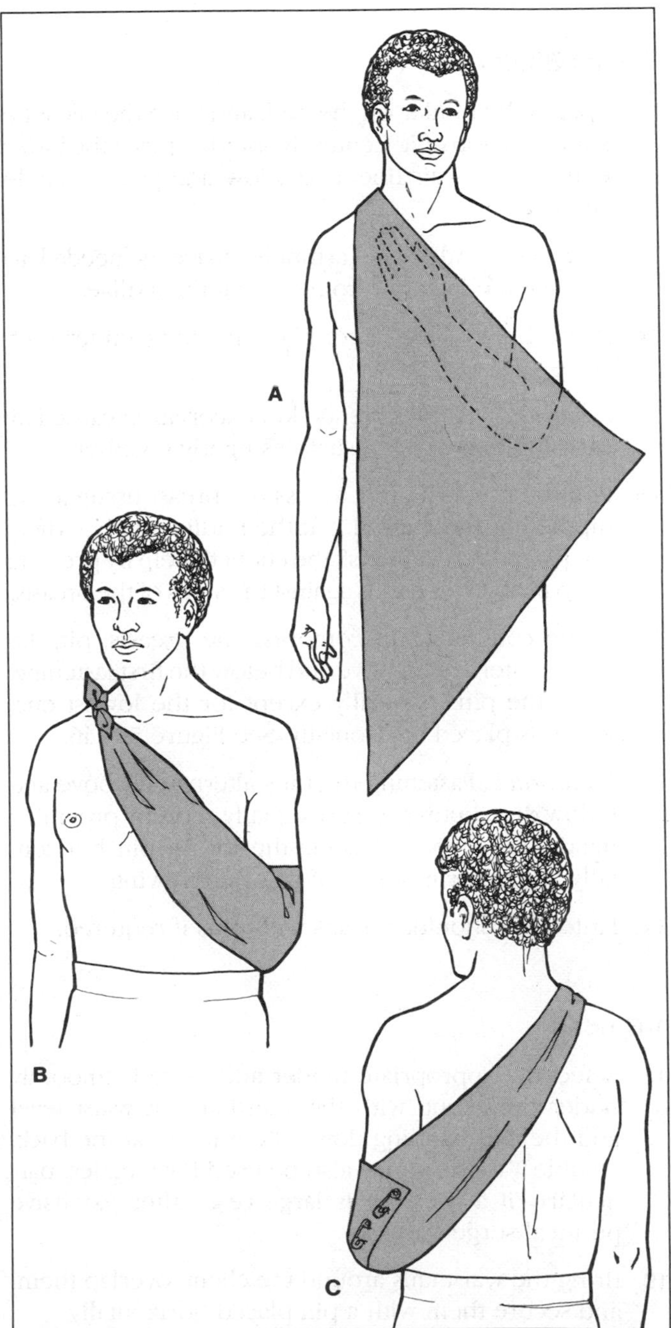

Figure 52–44

c. Tuck the base of the binder under the client's arm, bring the free end across the client's back, and, using a reef knot, tie it to the other free end at the shoulder *on the uninjured side*. The knot should rest in the hollow of the clavicle to prevent pressure on the clavicle. See Figure 52–44, *B*.

d. Bring the apex of the sling toward the client's back, tuck it in, and secure it with a safety pin or pins. See Figure 52–44, *C*.

12. *Hand or foot mitt*
Apply the triangular bandage as a mitt to cover hand or foot dressings. See Figure 52–45.

Breast Binder

13. Spread the binder on the bed, and have the client lie supine on top of it. Center the binder, place the lower edge at the waistline, and allow adequate armhole space.

    Rationale Adequate armhole space is needed to prevent the material from chafing the axillae.

14. If the breasts are large, place padding under each breast.

    Rationale This prevents skin excoriation caused by pressing the two skin surfaces tightly together.

15. Pull the binder tightly across the breast tissue at the nipple line, and fasten it at the midline with a safety pin placed vertically. Ask the client to help by pressing the palms of her hands against the sides of the breasts.

16. While continuing to compress the breasts, pin the binder alternately above and below the first fastening. Place the pins vertically except for the lowest one, which is placed horizontally. See Figure 52–46.

    Rationale Fastening the pins alternately above and below distributes pressure equally, thereby providing maximum support. Placing the lowest pin horizontally allows for more comfort when moving.

17. Fasten the shoulder straps with pins if required.

T-Binder

18. Select the appropriate binder and place it smoothly under the client, with the waistband at waist level and the tails running down the midline at the back. Double T-binders may also be used for females, particularly if a dressing is large (e.g., after extensive perineal surgery).

19. Bring the waist tails around the client, overlap them, and secure them with a pin placed horizontally.

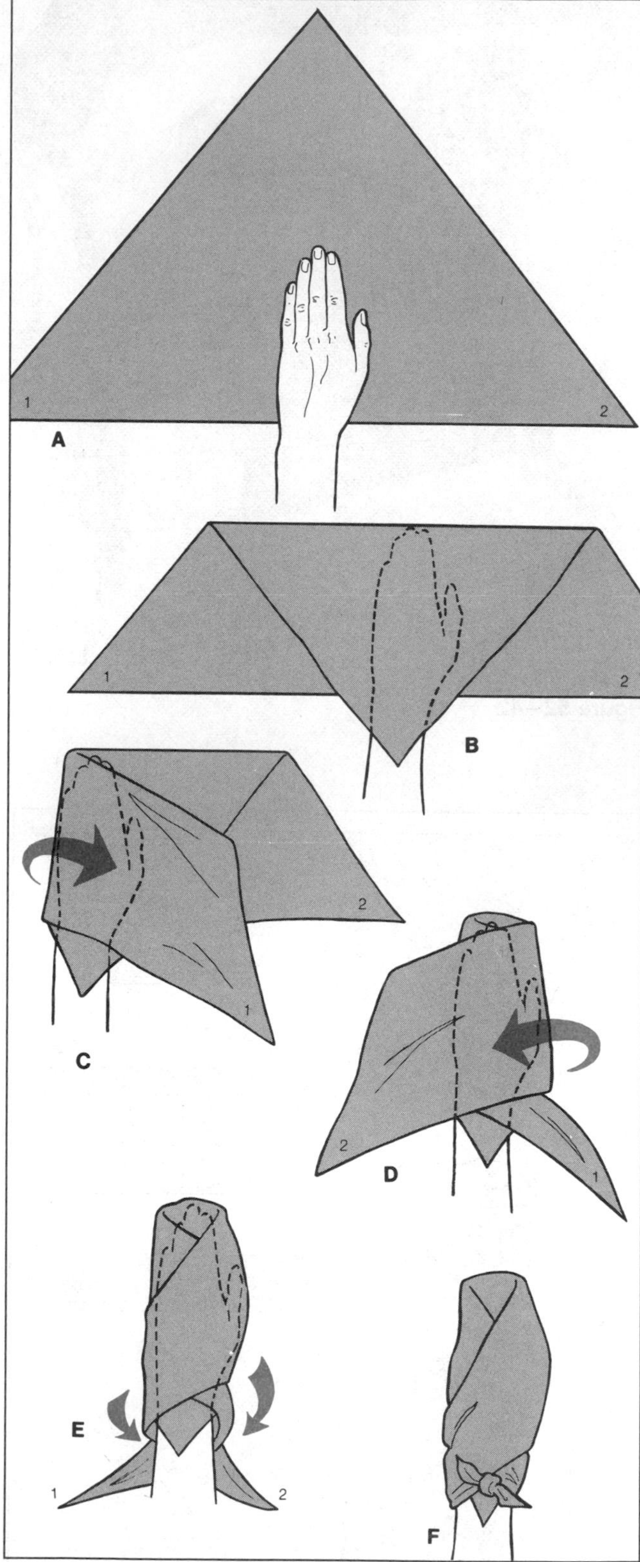

Figure 52–45 Wrapping a hand using a triangular bandage: **A,** lay the hand in the center of the triangular bandage; **B,** fold the apex over the wrist; **C, D,** wrap the corners (1 and 2) around the hand; **E,** bring the corners around the wrist; **F,** tie a reef knot on the dorsum of the wrist.

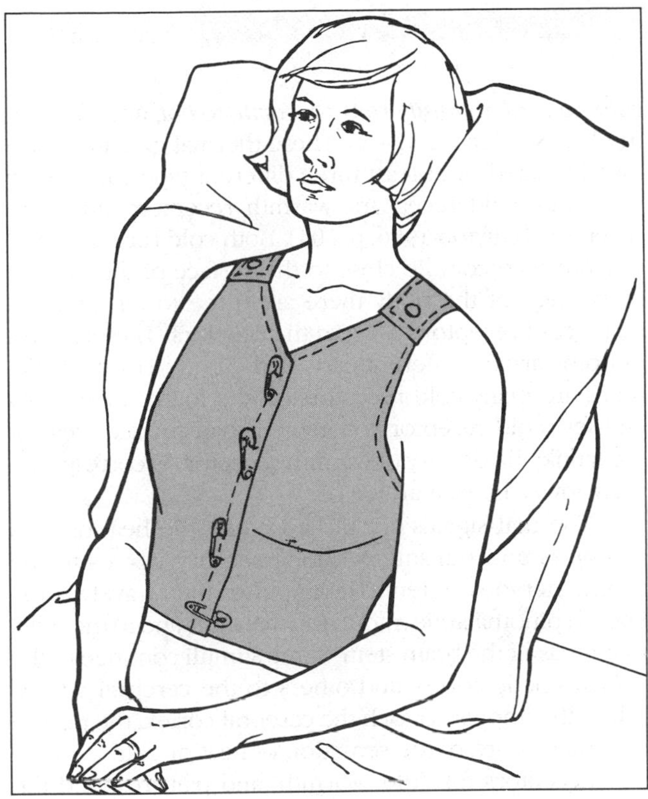

Figure 52–46

Rationale Horizontally placed pins allow comfort when bending at the waist and moving.

20. Bring the center tail up between the client's legs. See Figure 52–47, *A*. The two tails of the double T-binder are brought up on either side of the penis. See Figure 52–47, *B*. When dressings are in place, take care to touch only the outside of the dressings to prevent contamination of the wound or yourself.

21. Fasten the ties at the waist with a safety pin placed horizontally.

Straight Abdominal or Scultetus Binder

22. With the client in a supine position, place the binder smoothly under the client, with the upper border of the binder at the waist and the lower border at the level of the gluteal fold.

    Rationale A binder placed above the waist interferes with respiration; one placed too low interferes with elimination and walking.

23. Apply padding over the iliac crests if the client is thin.

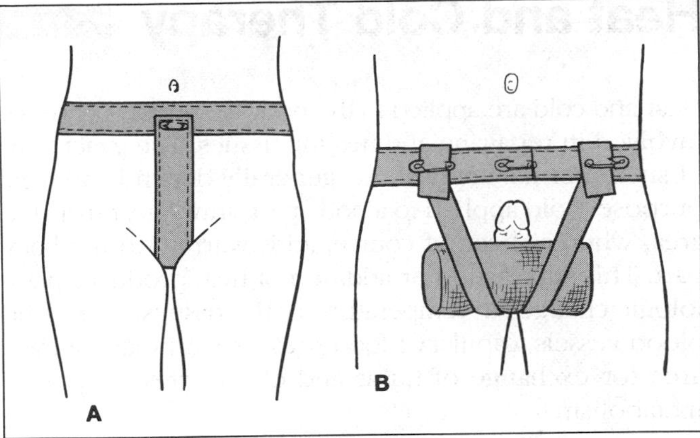

Figure 52–47

24. For a straight abdominal binder, bring the ends around the client, overlap them, and secure them with pins. See Figure 52–39, on page 1573.

25. Place the top pin horizontally at the waist to allow for comfort when moving.

26. For a scultetus binder, bring the tails over to the center from alternate sides. See Figure 52–40, on page 1573. The last tail is secured with a safety pin. Each tail should overlap the preceding one by about half the width of the tail for maximum support. In thin people, the tails may extend beyond the other side and require folding back.
    a. For clients who have had abdominal surgery, lace the tails from the bottom up.

       Rationale This provides maximum upward support.

    b. For the postpartum client, lace the tails from the top down.

       Rationale This provides downward pressure on the uterus.

For All Binders

27. Ensure that there are no wrinkles or creases in the binders.

    Rationale Wrinkles and creases put pressure on the skin, producing subsequent excoriation.

28. Check the agency's policies on recording the application of a binder. It generally goes unrecorded when the binder is applied to hold a dressing in place. However, application of an arm sling, a breast binder, or an abdominal binder may be recorded together with assessment and evaluation data.

Heat and Cold Therapy

Heat and cold are applied to the body to support processes involved in repairing and healing tissues. The exact form of such thermal applications generally depends on their purpose. Cold applied to a body part draws heat from the area, whereas heat, of course, adds warmth to the body part. This subtraction or addition of heat produces physiologic changes in temperature of the tissues, size of the blood vessels, capillary blood pressure, capillary surface area for exchange of fluids and electrolytes, and tissue metabolism.

Mechanisms of Heat Transfer

Heat is transferred from one source to another by conduction, convection, conversion, and evaporation. These processes are described in Chapter 34, page 766. Heat is lost from the body via the same four processes. When heat is applied, all of these processes except evaporation are involved.

Conductive heat is provided by the direct application of heat, e.g., a hot water bag or immersion in heated bath water. Heat is transferred directly to the skin and then to underlying tissues. Conductive heat is relatively superficial; it penetrates 1 to 2 mm and requires about 20 to 30 minutes to produce the desired effect.

Conversive or radiant heat is provided by a heat lamp, e.g., a standard lamp with a 40-watt bulb or an ultraviolet lamp. Infrared rays penetrate from 1 to 3 mm, depending on whether the wavelengths are near or far. Near wavelengths are 7700–14,000 angstroms (Å); far wavelengths are 14,000–120,000 Å. (The angstrom is a unit of wavelength of electromagnetic radiation.) Near infrared radiation penetrates about 3 mm, and far infrared about 1 mm. Luminous bulbs produce more near infrared radiation and thus have greater penetration than nonluminous filaments, which produce far infrared radiation.

Convective heat is easily applied by heating the surrounding air. Within the body, *forced convection* is brought about by the circulatory system, with heat being transferred or distributed by the bloodstream. This is the method by which heat from external applications reaches other body parts.

Perception of Heat and Cold

The skin is well supplied with nerves, blood vessels, and lymph vessels. The temperature receptors in the skin are sensitive to temperatures that are either higher or lower than that of the skin surface itself, which is 33.9 C (93.0 F). Humans can perceive different gradations of temperature, progressing from *very* or *freezing cold,* to *cold,* to *cool,* to *indifferent,* to *warm,* to *hot,* and to *burning hot.* See Figure 52–48. These thermal gradations are discriminated by at least three different types of sensory receptors: cold receptors, warmth receptors, and pain receptors (Guyton 1986, p. 603). Both cold receptors and warmth receptors lie close to the surface of the skin. In most areas of the body there are three to ten times as many cold receptors as warmth receptors. The densities of both vary on different parts of the body. For example, there are many cold receptors on the forehead and lips and few cold receptors on some broad surface areas of the trunk; the density of warmth receptors is correspondingly lower in each area.

Thermal signals are picked up by the heat or cold receptors and transmitted along sensory nerves to the central nervous system. The impulses then travel via the lateral spinothalamic tract to the thalamus and to the reticular areas of the brain stem. Some stimuli continue to the somatesthetic cortex and others to the cerebral cortex. When the impulses reach the cerebral cortex, the person becomes aware of the sensation of heat or cold.

Receptors for cold, warmth, and pain respond differently at different temperatures. For example, the pain receptors are stimulated only in the *very* cold regions. As the temperature rises to 10 to 15 C (50 to 59 F), pain impulses cease and cold receptors are stimulated. Above approximately 30 C (85 F), the warmth receptors are stimulated; the cold impulses decline and cease at about 43 C (109 F). Around 45 C (112 F), pain fibers are again stimulated by heat. Temperatures of approximately the temperature of the skin—between 30 and 35 C (85 and 95 F)—are normally undifferentiated. In elderly persons there is decreased sensitivity to localized temperature changes, such as those from hot or cold applications.

Adaptation of Thermal Receptors

When a cold receptor is subjected to an abrupt fall in temperature, or a warmth receptor is subjected to an abrupt rise in temperature, the receptor is initially strongly stimulated. This strong stimulation declines rapidly during the first few seconds and then more slowly during the next half hour or more as the receptor adapts to the new temperature (Guyton 1986, p. 604). This adaptive mechanism explains why people feel much colder when they go outdoors from a heated room on a cold day or feel very warm when they go from a cold environment to a heated room or from a warm room to a hot tub.

It is essential that nurses understand this adaptive response when applying heat and cold. Clients may be tempted to change the temperature of a thermal application to colder or hotter because of the change in ther-

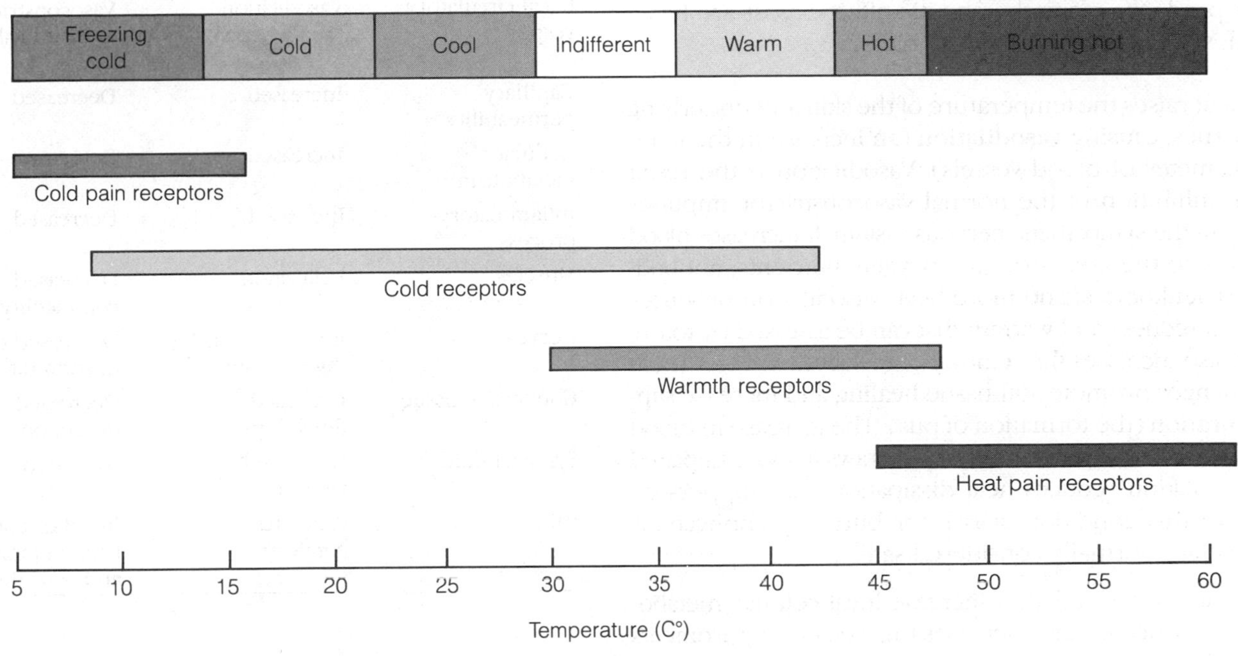

Figure 52–48 Approximate temperatures at which receptors for cold, warmth, and pain respond.
Source: Adapted from A. C. Guyton, *Textbook of medical physiology,* 7th ed. (Philadelphia: W. B. Saunders Co., 1986), p. 604.

mal sensation following adaptation. Increasing the temperature of a hot application after adaptation has occurred can result in serious burns. Decreasing the temperature of a cold application can result in pain and serious impairment of circulation to the body part.

Tolerance to Heat and Cold

The physiologic tolerance of the body to heat and cold varies according to the following factors:

Body part. The back of the hand and foot are not very temperature-sensitive. In contrast, the inner aspect of the wrist and forearm, the neck, and the perineal area are temperature-sensitive.

Size of the exposed body part. The larger the area exposed to heat or cold, the lower the tolerance.

Individual tolerance. Tolerance to heat and cold is to some degree affected by age and the condition of the skin, nervous system, and circulatory system. The very young and the very old generally have the lowest tolerance. Persons who have neurosensory impairments may have a high tolerance, but the risk of injury is great.

Length of exposure. People feel hot and cold applications most while the skin temperature is changing. After a period of time, tolerance is increased.

Intactness of skin. Damaged skin areas are more sensitive to temperature variations.

Physiologic Responses to Heat and Cold

The physiologic responses of body tissues to heat and cold form the basis for the therapeutic effects of hot and cold applications. Local, consensual, and systemic responses occur. In addition, the duration of the application affects the response (see "Rebound Phenomenon," later in this section).

Local Effects of Heat

Heat is an old remedy for aches and pains; people often equate heat with comfort and relief. The application of heat produces many therapeutic effects: most are beneficial; some are adverse. See Table 52–3.

1. Heat raises the temperature of the skin and underlying tissues, causing **vasodilation** (an increase in the inner diameter of blood vessels). Vasodilation is the result of inhibition of the normal vasoconstrictor impulses from the sympathetic nervous system. It increases blood flow to the area, bringing oxygen, nutrients, antibodies, leukocytes, and more heat. Vasodilation produces skin redness and warmth that can be assessed by touch. It also increases the removal of metabolic wastes. These changes promote soft-tissue healing and increase **suppuration** (the formation of pus). The increase in blood flow also dissipates the heat, or draws it away. Impaired circulation reduces heat dissipation, making persons with this condition at risk for burns by applications that are normally considered safe.
2. Heat and vasodilation increase local cellular metabolism, which in turn increases the oxygen requirements of the tissues.
3. Heat increases capillary permeability, which allows extracellular fluid and substances such as plasma proteins to pass through the capillary walls. Increased permeability can produce edema (excessive amounts of fluid in the tissues) or an increase in preexisting edema. This is one of the adverse effects of heat.
4. Heat accelerates the inflammatory process by increasing both the action of phagocytic cells that ingest microorganisms and other foreign material and the removal of the waste products of infection.
5. Heat promotes muscle relaxation, relieves muscle spasm, and decreases joint stiffness. Muscle relaxation is the result of an increase in sensory nerve conduction and vasodilation (Lehmann and DeLateur, 1982b). Heat stimulates the thermal receptors and increases the conduction speed of sensory nerve impulses and the speed of cutaneous circulation. Heat also makes connective tissue more flexible and decreases the **viscosity** (thickness) of synovial fluid, i.e., the fluid found in joint cavities.
6. Heat to the abdomen decreases peristalsis, decreases blood flow to the gastrointestinal tract and mucous membrane, and decreases the secretion of hydrochloric acid in the stomach (Kottke et al. 1982).
7. Heat relieves pain. The exact mechanisms for the analgesic effects of heat are unknown. Heat may raise the pain threshold or may equalize temperatures from superficial to deep tissues. The relaxation effect of heat obviously promotes comfort. The vasodilation effect is particularly useful in relieving pain from muscle spasm caused by **ischemia** (lack of blood supply to a body part).

Table 52–3 Physiologic Effects of Heat and Cold

Body Part or Process	Effect of Heat	Effect of Cold
Local circulatory response	Vasodilation (reddened skin)	Vasoconstriction (pale, bluish skin)
Capillary permeability	Increased	Decreased
Cellular metabolism	Increased	Decreased
Inflammatory process	Increased	Decreased
Muscles	Relaxation	Decreased contractility
Nerves	Increased conduction rate	Decreased conduction rate
Connective tissue	Increased flexibility	Decreased distention
Synovial fluid	Decreased viscosity	Increased viscosity
Pain	Promotes comfort	Initial discomfort; later, numbness and paresthesia

Local Effects of Cold

Cold therapy is more recent than heat therapy. Generally, its physiologic effects are opposite to the effects of heat. See Table 52–3.

1. Cold lowers the temperature of the skin and underlying tissues and causes **vasoconstriction** (a decrease in the inner diameter of blood vessels). Vasoconstriction reduces blood flow to the area and thus reduces the supply of oxygen and metabolites, decreases the removal of wastes, and produces skin pallor, or a bluish discoloration, and coolness. Vasoconstriction and its consequent lowered blood flow to an area help control bleeding after injury.
2. Cold and vasoconstriction decrease local cellular metabolism, thus reducing the oxygen needs of the tissues.
3. Cold decreases capillary permeability, thereby preventing the extravasation of fluid into the tissues. Cold therefore prevents swelling associated with the inflammatory process.
4. Cold, like heat, can reduce muscle spasm. It is thought to reduce the activity of nerve endings supplying the muscles.

5. Cold alters tissue sensitivity, leading to numbness of the arm or **paresthesia** (abnormal skin sensations such as burning, prickling, and decreased sensation). This effect is evident when handling ice cubes or snow with the bare hands.
6. Cold relieves pain, particularly that associated with muscle spasm, since it decreases muscle contractility. It may also be used as a counterirritant to relieve pain (see the "gate theory" of pain in Chapter 41).
7. Prolonged exposure to cold results in impaired circulation, cell deprivation, and subsequent damage to the tissues from lack of oxygen and nourishment. The signs of tissues damaged by cold are a bluish-purple mottled appearance of the skin, numbness, stiffness, pallor, and sometimes blisters and pain.

Rebound Phenomenon

The **rebound phenomenon** occurs at the time the maximum therapeutic effect of the hot or cold application is achieved and the opposite effect begins. For example, heat produces maximum vasodilation in about 20 to 30 minutes; continuation of the application beyond 30 or 45 minutes brings tissue congestion, and the blood vessels then *constrict* for reasons unknown. If the heat application is continued further, the client is at risk for burns, since the constricted blood vessels are unable to adequately dissipate the heat via the blood circulation.

With cold applications, maximum vasoconstriction occurs when the involved skin reaches a temperature of 15 C (60 F). Below 15 C, vasodilation begins. This rebound phenomenon is thought to be the result of paralysis of the mechanism that contracts the vessel wall, or blockage of the nerve impulses to the vessels, or inactivation of the vasoconstrictor chemicals (Lehmann and DeLateur 1982a). This mechanism is protective because it helps to prevent freezing of body tissues normally exposed to cold, such as the nose and ears. It also explains the ruddiness of the skin of a person who has been walking in cold weather.

An understanding of the rebound phenomenon is essential for the nurse. Thermal applications must be halted *before* the rebound phenomenon begins.

Consensual Response

Heating (or cooling) one part of the body produces vasodilation (or vasoconstriction) not only in the involved body part but also in other body parts. For example, if heat is applied to the right arm, vasodilation occurs in the left arm as well as the right. This phenomenon is called the **consensual response** or *consensual reaction* (Lehmann and DeLateur 1982a). The speed with which this occurs indicates that it is a reflex and not the result of a change in the body's core temperature. The consensual response occurs less quickly than the direct response at the area of application, and it neither lasts as long nor is as strong. Whether it occurs depends on the intensity of the applied temperature and the involved surface area.

Systemic Effects

Heat applied to a localized body area, particularly a large body area, may increase cardiac output and pulmonary ventilation. These increases are a result of excessive peripheral vasodilation, which diverts large supplies of blood from the internal organs and produces a drop in blood pressure. A significant drop in blood pressure can cause fainting. Clients who have heart or pulmonary disease and who have circulatory disturbances such as arteriosclerosis are more prone to this effect than healthy persons.

With extensive cold applications and vasoconstriction, a client's blood pressure can increase, because blood is shunted from the cutaneous circulation to the internal blood vessels. This shunting of blood, a normal protective response to prolonged cold, is the body's attempt to maintain its core temperature. Shivering, another generalized effect of prolonged cold, is a normal response as the body attempts to warm itself.

Indications for the Use of Heat and Cold

Heat and cold applications are appropriate in a number of situations. See Tables 52–4 and 52–5. Heat is often used for clients with musculoskeletal problems such as joint stiffness from arthritis, contractures, and low back pain; and for those with open wounds needing debridement. Heat is used to relieve pain, relieve muscle spasm, decrease joint stiffness, increase blood flow, resolve inflammation, hasten healing, and increase the distensibility of connective tissue.

Cold is most often used for active young people with sports injuries (e.g., sprains, strains, fractures) to limit postinjury swelling and bleeding. It is increasingly being used for clients with rheumatoid arthritis, since it is thought to inhibit the activity of certain destructive enzymes that accelerate joint problems (Lehmann and DeLateur 1982b). Cold can produce the same outcomes for muscle spasm and pain as heat does. Cold is also used to reduce tissue trauma from burns.

Table 52–4 Selected Indications for Heat

Indication	Effect of Heat
Muscle spasm	Relaxes muscles and increases their contractility
Inflammation	Increases blood flow, bringing more phagocytes (to facilitate exudate formation) and essential nutrients for healing; also enhances removal of wastes and debris formed in the inflammatory process. Moist heat softens exudates
Contracture	Reduces contractures and increases joint range of motion by allowing greater distention of muscles and connective tissue
Joint stiffness	Reduces joint stiffness by decreasing the viscosity of synovial fluid and increasing tissue distensibility
Pain	Relieves pain, possibly by promoting muscle relaxation, increasing circulation to ischemic areas, promoting psychologic relaxation and a feeling of comfort, and acting as a counterirritant

Source: P. S. Tepperman and M. Devlin, Therapeutic heat and cold. A practitioner's guide. *Postgraduate Medicine,* January 1983, 73:69.

Table 52–5 Selected Indications for Cold

Indication	Effect of Cold
Traumatic injury	Decreases bleeding by constricting blood vessels; decreases edema by reducing capillary permeability
Inflammation	Decreases inflammation by causing vasoconstriction, decreasing capillary permeability, decreasing blood flow, decreasing cellular metabolism, and slowing phagocytosis
Muscle spasm	Increases muscle relaxation by decreasing muscle contractility
Pain	Decreases pain by slowing nerve conduction rate and blocking nerve impulses, by producing numbness, by acting as a counterirritant, and by increasing the pain threshold

Source: P. S. Tepperman and M. Devlin, Therapeutic heat and cold. A practitioner's guide. *Postgraduate Medicine,* January 1983, 73:69.

Assessment for Heat and Cold

Before applying heat or cold, the nurse assesses the area to be treated and the client's history and current health status to (a) determine the client's ability to tolerate the therapy, and (b) identify conditions that contraindicate the therapy.

The nurse inspects the area to be treated for color and alterations in skin integrity, such as the presence of edema, bruises, open lesions, discharge, and bleeding. Alterations in skin integrity increase the client's risk for injury. Although some forms of heat and cold may be prescribed by the physician for traumatized areas, the nurse's observations serve as baseline data to evaluate changes after the application. For example, if drainage is present, the nurse determines its amount, color, and character. Before applications to large body areas the nurse should also take the client's pulse, respirations, and blood pressure to provide baseline data against which to compare later assessments.

To determine the circulatory status of the area, the nurse inspects and palpates the involved skin, comparing its temperature with that of the corresponding body part on the opposite side of the body. Tissues that feel cold, have a pale or bluish hue, and lack sensation or feel numb indicate circulatory impairment. Assessment of sensory function is described in Chapter 35, page 888. Contraindications and precautions for the application of heat and cold are shown on the next page.

Intervention: Heat and Cold

Heat Applications

Heat is applied to the body in both dry and moist forms. Dry heat is applied locally, for heat conduction, by means of a hot water bottle, electric pad, aquathermia pad, or disposable heat pack. The heat lamp and bed cradle provide dry heat by radiation. Moist heat can be provided, through conduction, by compress, hot pack, soak, or sitz bath.

Because heat is often supplied by electrically operated equipment, it is important for nurses to understand some of the properties and dangers of electricity. For information about electricity, see Chapter 33, page 743. Before electrically operated equipment is used, it should be checked to see that it is in proper working order.

Recommended temperatures for hot and cold applications are shown in Table 52–6.

Contraindications and Precautions for the Use of Heat

Contraindications

- *During the first 24 hours after traumatic injury.* Heat increases bleeding and swelling.
- *Active hemorrhage.* Heat causes vasodilation and increases bleeding.
- *Noninflammatory edema.* Heat increases capillary permeability and edema. Because heat enhances the inflammatory process, heat is *not* contraindicated for inflammatory edema but may not be the therapy of choice.
- *Acutely inflamed areas.* Heat on such areas can increase edema; for example, it can rupture an appendix.
- *Localized malignant tumor.* Because heat accelerates cell metabolism and cell growth and increases circulation, it may accelerate metastases (secondary tumors).
- *Testes.* Heat can inhibit the development of and destroy sperm.
- *Developing fetus.* Heat to the abdomen of a pregnant woman can cause mutation in the fetal germinal cells and affect fetal growth.
- *Skin disorder causing redness or blisters.* Heat can burn or cause further damage to the skin.
- *Metallic implants* (such as pacemakers, knee or hip replacements). Because metal is a good conductor of heat, medical diathermy—which uses electric current to heat deep tissues—can burn deep tissues.

Precautions

- *Sensory impairment.* Persons with sensory impairments are unable to perceive that heat is damaging the tissues and are at risk for burns.
- *Impaired mental status.* Confused persons and persons with an altered level of consciousness lack full awareness and are unable to cooperate during the application, making such therapy unsafe for them.
- *Impaired circulation.* Persons with peripheral vascular disease, diabetes, or congestive heart failure lack the normal ability to dissipate heat via the blood circulation, which puts them at risk for tissue damage.
- *Low heat tolerance.* Infants, children, and older clients tolerate temperature changes poorly. Precautions are needed to prevent burning.
- *Open wounds.* Because tissues around an open wound are more sensitive to heat and cold, only low temperatures should be used.

Contraindications and Precautions for the Use of Cold

Contraindications

- *Open wounds.* Cold can increase tissue damage by decreasing blood flow to an open wound.
- *Impaired circulation.* Cold can further impair nourishment of the tissues and cause tissue damage. In clients with Raynaud's disease, cold increases arterial spasm.
- *Allergy or hypersensitivity to cold.* Some clients have an allergy to cold that may be manifested by an inflammatory response, i.e., erythema, hives, swelling, joint pain, and occasional muscle spasm. Some react with a sudden increase in blood pressure, which can be hazardous if the person is hypertensive.

Precautions

- *Sensory impairment.* Persons with sensory impairments are unable to perceive discomfort from cold and are unable to prevent tissue injury.
- *Impaired mental status.* Persons who are confused or have an altered level of consciousness need monitoring and supervision during cold applications to ensure safe therapy.
- *Low cold tolerance.* Infants, children, and older clients tolerate temperature changes poorly. Precautions are needed to prevent adverse effects.

Hot Water Bottles/Bags

A hot water bottle or bag is a common source of dry heat for localized effect. It is convenient and relatively inexpensive. However, because of a danger of burning from improper use, agencies may require the client to sign a release absolving the agency and its employees from responsibility for injury incurred with the use of hot water bottles.

The following temperatures of the water in the bag are considered safe in most situations and provide the desired effect:

Normal adult, 52 C (125 F)

Debilitated or unconscious adult, 40.5 to 46 C (105 to 115 F)

Child under 2 years, 40.5 to 46 C (105 to 115 F)

Hot water bags usually are filled about two-thirds full. The remaining air is expelled and the top secured. The hot water bag can then be readily molded to a body part. Before application, the bag is dried and held upside down

Table 52–6 Recommended Temperatures for Hot and Cold Applications

Description	Centigrade	Fahrenheit	Application
Very cold	Below 15	Below 59	Ice bags
Cold	15–18	59–65	Cold pack
Cool	18–27	65–80	Cold compress
Tepid	27–37	80–98	Alcohol and tepid sponges
Warm	37–40	98–105	Warm bath
Hot	40–46	105–115	Aquathermia, soaks, sitz baths, irrigations, moist sterile compresses, hot water bags for debilitated or young clients
Very hot	Above 46	Above 115	Hot water bags for adults, heat cradles

to test for leakage. If it is secure, it is then wrapped in a towel or cover and placed on the body site. A hot water bottle will usually stay hot for 45 minutes before needing to be replaced.

Electric Pads

Electric pads have become less popular in recent years. The pad provides a constant, even heat, is lightweight, and can be molded to a body part. Electric pads, however, can burn if the setting is too high. In some agencies the controls on the pads are set to a specific temperature to prevent burning.

When using electric pads, caution needs to be taken to ensure that the body area is dry, since electricity in the presence of moisture can conduct a shock. Some models have waterproof covers for use when the pad is placed over a moist dressing. The nurse should also caution the client not to insert any sharp, pointed object, e.g., a pin, in the pad. A pin might strike a wire, damaging the pad and giving an electric shock to the client.

Aquathermia (Water-Flow) Pad

The aquathermia or aquamatic pad is a device in which warm distilled water circulates, providing heat to a body part. The pad is attached by tubing to an electrically powered control unit that has an opening for water and a temperature gauge. See Figure 52–49. Some aquathermia pads have an absorbent surface through which moist heat can be applied. The other surface of the pad is waterproof. These pads are disposable.

The reservoir of an aquathermia unit is filled two-thirds full. The desired temperature is set, the pad is covered, placed on the body part, and maintained in place with roller gauze if needed. The nurse may need to regulate the temperature with a key if it has not been preset. Check the manufacturer's instructions. Normal temperature is 40.5 C (105 F), and treatment is usually continued for 10 to 15 minutes. If unusual redness or pain occurs, treatment is discontinued and the client's reaction reported and recorded.

Commercial Hot Pack

Dry heat can be supplied by commercially prepared disposable hot packs. See Figure 52–50. Directions on the package tell how to initiate the heating process, e.g., strike, squeeze, or knead the pack. Hot packs provide a specified amount of heat for a specified time.

Heat Lamp

A heat lamp is often a gooseneck lamp with either a special or an ordinary 40-watt or 60-watt bulb. Also used is the infrared lamp, which has an infrared element rather than a bulb. Both lamps provide dry heat to a localized area. See Figure 52–51. Before a heat lamp is used, the area to be heated should be cleaned and dried, to lessen the likelihood of burning. A heat lamp with a 40- or 60-watt bulb or a small infrared lamp is usually placed 45 to 60 cm (18 to 24 in) from the client. A large infrared lamp

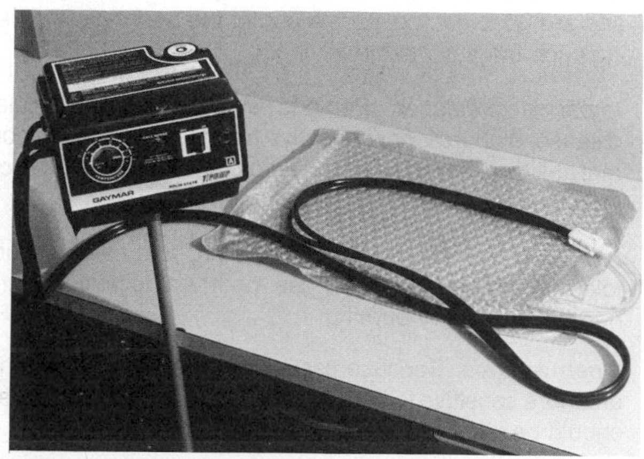

Figure 52–49 An aquathermia heating unit

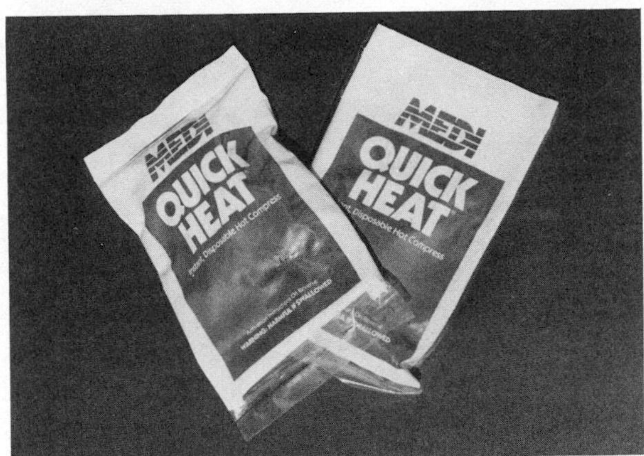

Figure 52–50 Commercially prepared disposable hot packs

is placed 60 to 75 cm (24 to 30 in) away. The treatment usually lasts 15 to 20 minutes, provided the client is tolerating the heat. The client should be checked every 5 minutes for discomfort, burning, or any untoward reaction. It is important to caution the client not to touch the infrared lamp, and the lamp should not be draped or placed under any bedclothes because of the risk of fire. At the first sign of skin redness or discomfort, the treatment should be terminated and the reaction reported and recorded.

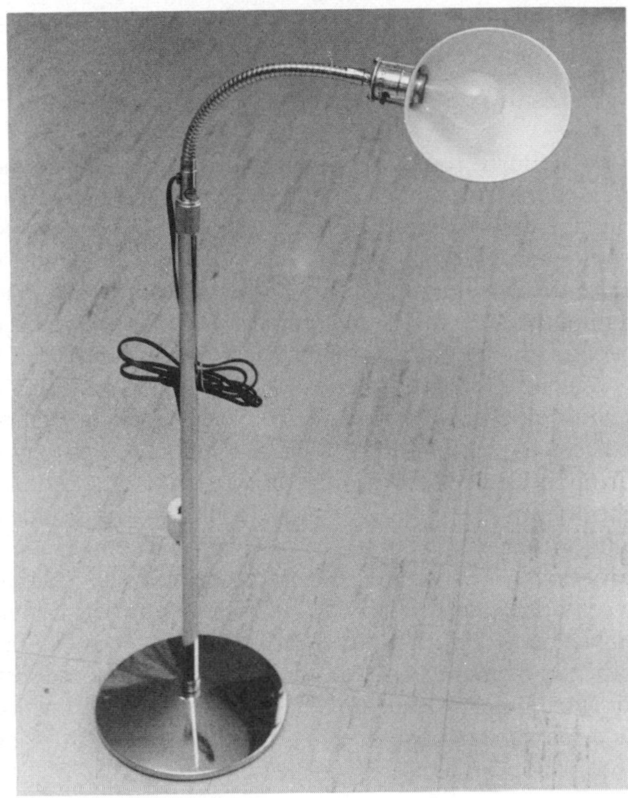

Figure 52–51 A heat lamp used to provide dry heat

Heat Cradle

A heat cradle is a metal frame with a row of 25-watt light bulbs used to provide less localized dry heat than a heat lamp. The cradle is placed over the client and usually covered with a bath blanket or sheet. The temperature inside the cradle normally should not exceed 51.6 C (125 F), and the treatment normally lasts 10 to 15 minutes. The heat source inside the cradle should be 45 to 60 cm (18 to 24 in) away from the client. The client should be checked every 10 minutes for discomfort or any untoward reaction.

Hot Soaks

A *soak* refers either to immersing a body part, e.g., an arm, in a solution or to wrapping a part in gauze dressings and then saturating the dressing with a solution. Soaks may employ clean technique or sterile technique. Sterile technique is generally indicated for open wounds, e.g., a burn or an area that has had surgery. Dry dressings are usually applied between the soaks.

Soaks are usually indicated for the following reasons:

1. To apply heat, thus hastening suppuration and softening exudates
2. To apply medications
3. To clean a wound in which there is sloughing tissue or an exudate.

The physician's order usually specifies the site for the soak, the type of solution, the temperature of the solution, the length of time for the soak, the frequency, and the purpose. Whether to use sterile technique is usually a nursing judgment; if there is a break in the skin, sterile technique is indicated.

The equipment required for a soak is:

1. A container such as a small basin to soak a finger or hand, a special arm or foot bath, or a sitz tub or chair.
2. The specified solution at the correct temperature. If a temperature is not ordered, check agency policy; 40 to 43 C (105 to 110 F) is usually indicated, as tolerated by the client. Fill the container at least one-half full.
3. A thermometer to test the temperature of the solution.
4. Towels to support the limb against the sharp edge of a basin and to dry the body part following the soak.

5. The required dressing materials, e.g., gauze squares and roller gauze.
6. A moisture-resistant bag for discarded dressings.

The nurse removes any dressings from the area and assesses the amount, color, odor, and consistency of the drainage before discarding them. The client is assisted to a well-aligned, comfortable position to prevent muscle strain; the position adopted will be maintained for 15 to 20 minutes. After the temperature of the solution has been checked, the part is slowly immersed in the solution. If it is a sterile soak, the open container is covered with a sterile drape or the container wrapper. Assess the client and test the temperature of the solution at least once during the soak. Assess for discomfort, need for additional support, and the client's response to the soak. Additional solution may be required to maintain the temperature. Immediately report any unexpected responses, such as increased discomfort, to the responsible nurse, and terminate the soak. At completion of the soak remove the body part from the basin and dry it thoroughly. If the soak was sterile, use a sterile towel for drying. Carefully assess the appearance of the body part, and reapply a dressing if required.

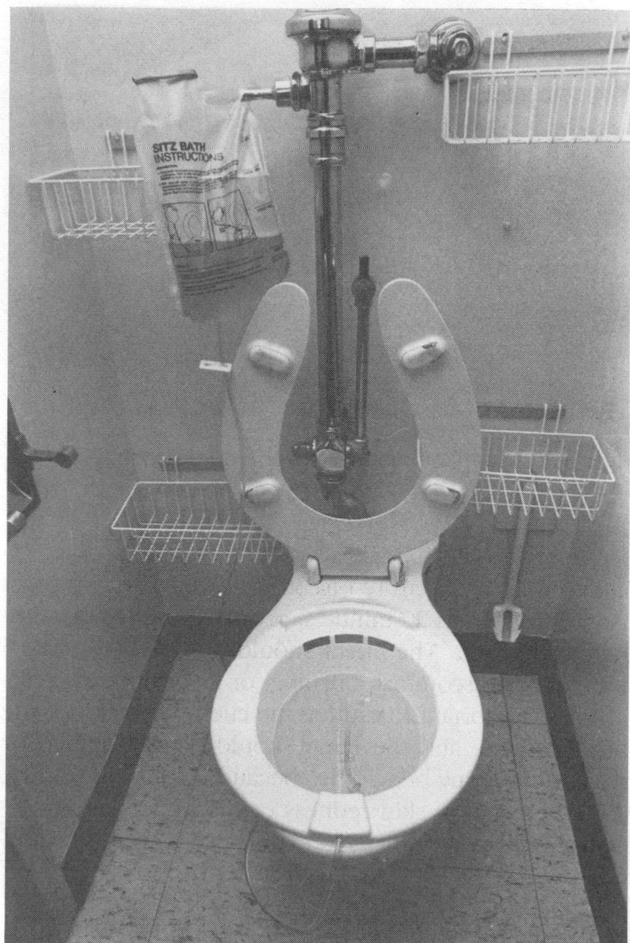

Figure 52–53 A disposable sitz bath commonly used in the home

Sitz Bath

A **sitz bath**, or hip bath, is used to soak a client's pelvic area. The client sits in a special tub or chair, usually immersed from the midthighs to the iliac crests or umbilicus. Special tubs or chairs are preferred to the regular bathtub, which immerses the legs and results in less effective blood circulation to the perineum or pelvic area. See Figure 52–52. Disposable sitz baths are also available; they are commonly used in homes but may be used in hospitals as well. See Figure 52–53.

The temperature of the water should be from 40 to 43 C (105 to 110 F), unless otherwise ordered by the physician, or unless the client is unable to tolerate the heat. Some sitz tubs have temperature indicators attached to the water taps. The duration of the bath is generally 15 to 20 minutes, depending on the client's condition.

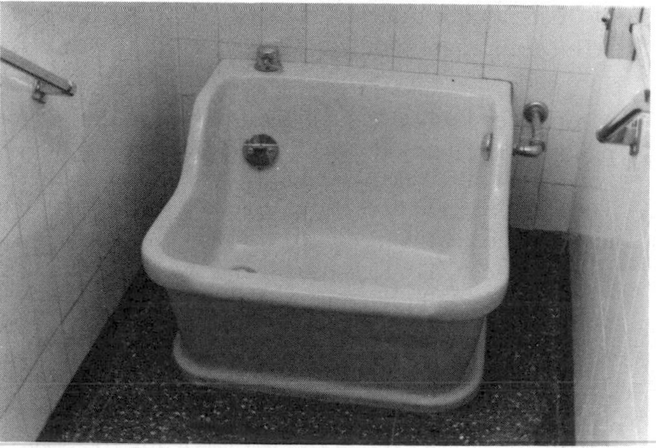

Figure 52–52 A hospital sitz bath

To prevent undue pressure on the sacrum or posterior aspects of the thighs, towels can be placed in or on the edges of a sitz tub. When a disposable sitz bath is used, a footstool can prevent pressure on the back of the thighs. Precautions also need to be taken to prevent chilling, burning, or fainting. Often a bath blanket over the client's shoulders and measures to eliminate drafts during the bath will prevent chilling. Maintaining the temperature of the bath is important. The water temperature should be tested at least once during the bath, adjusting it as necessary.

Some clients feel faint and dizzy during a sitz bath, particularly those who have just had surgery. Therefore, close observation of the client is necessary during the sitz bath. An accelerated pulse or extreme pallor may precede fainting. If the feeling of faintness or untoward signs persist, the bath should be terminated. Clients need to be instructed beforehand to signal for the nurse if they feel weak.

Following the sitz bath, the nurse assists the client to dry the area and reapply dressings (e.g., a perineal pad and T-binder) and garments. The perineal area is reassessed before dressings are reapplied.

Cold Applications

Cold may be applied dry or moist. Dry cold is administered for localized effect with ice bags, ice collars, ice gloves, or disposable cold packs. Moist cold is applied for either localized or systemic effects. Cold moist compresses are administered to body parts for a localized effect; a tepid sponge bath is given for a systemic cooling effect.

Ice Bag, Collar, or Glove

The *ice bag,* a common device in many homes and hospitals, is a moderate-sized rubber or plastic bag, with removable cap, into which pieces of ice can be inserted. Commercially prepared ice bags are available in some agencies. Such bags are filled with an alcohol-base solution and sealed; they are kept in freezing units in a central supply area.

An *ice collar* is similar to an ice bag but is long and narrow. It is designed for use around the neck, though it can be used for other areas of the body.

The *ice glove* is simply a rubber or plastic glove filled with ice chips and tied at the open end. Gloves are generally used for small body parts, e.g., an eye.

To prepare an ice bag, ice collar, or ice glove, the nurse places crushed ice inside the container until it is one-half to two-thirds full, expels excess air, and secures the top to prevent leakage. The container is then covered with a soft cloth, if it is not already equipped with such a cover, and placed on the client so it molds to the body part. The covering, which absorbs moisture from condensation, needs to be changed when it becomes wet. The device can be held in place with roller gauze, a binder, or a towel secured by safety pins as necessary. The bag or other pack should be removed 30 to 60 minutes after application and reapplied an hour later for maximum effectiveness.

The nurse assesses the client's reaction in terms of comfort, the purpose of the cold application, and skin reaction (e.g., pallor, mottled appearance). Assess the client's response as frequently as necessary for the client's safety. Factors such as previous responses to applications and the client's ability to report any problems need to be considered.

Commercial Cold Pack

Disposable cold packs are similar to disposable hot packs. They come in a variety of sizes and shapes and provide a specific degree of coldness for a specified period of time, as indicated on the package. By striking, squeezing, or kneading the package, chemical reactions are activated that release the cold. The manufacturer's instructions must be followed. Most commercially prepared cold packs have soft outer coverings so they can be applied directly to the body part. See Figure 52–54.

Cooling Sponge Bath

A cooling sponge bath is given to reduce a client's fever. It promotes body heat loss through conduction and vaporization. The cooling sponge bath uses water or a combination of alcohol and water that is below body temperature. Alcohol evaporates at a low temperature and therefore removes body heat rapidly. However, alcohol-and-water sponge baths are used less frequently than in the past, because alcohol has a drying effect on the skin. The temperatures for cooling sponge baths range from 18 to 32 C (65 to 90 F). A *tepid* sponge bath generally refers to one in which the water temperature is 32 C (90 F) throughout the bath. For a *cool* sponge bath, the water temperature is 32 C (90 F) at the beginning of the bath and is gradually lowered to 18 C (65 F) by adding ice chips.

Before the bath, the nurse assesses the client's body temperature, pulse, and respirations, if they are not already recorded, to provide comparative baseline data. The decision to give a tepid sponge bath is generally made only after a marked fever is noted or after a temperature increase of 1 to 2 C (2 or 3 F). Other signs of fever, e.g., skin warmth, flushing, complaints of heat or chilling, diaphoresis, irritability, restlessness, general malaise, or delirium, are also noted.

Procedure 52–9 describes how to administer a cooling sponge bath.

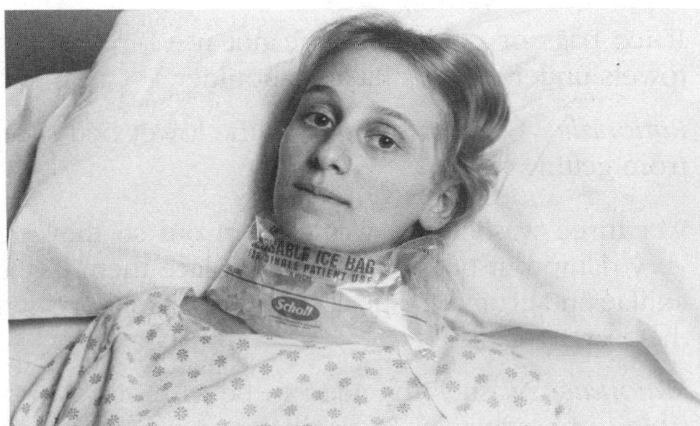

Figure 52–54 A disposable ice collar provides dry cold to the neck area—for example, to control bleeding after a tonsillectomy.

Procedure 52–9 ▲ Administering a Cooling Sponge Bath

Equipment

1. A basin for the solution.
2. A bath thermometer to check the temperature of the solution.
3. A solution at the correct temperature. Water or equal portions of 70% alcohol and water are used.
4. Ice chips for a cool sponge bath.
5. Several washcloths and bath towels. Fewer are needed if ice bags or cold packs are used.
6. A bath blanket.
7. A thermometer to measure the client's temperature.

A fan is sometimes used to increase air movement around the client, which lowers the body temperature through convection. In this case, drafts are not usually eliminated during the sponge bath.

Intervention

1. Explain to the client that the face, arms, legs, back, and buttocks will be sponged, but not the chest and abdomen. The procedure takes about 30 minutes.
2. Minimize drafts by closing the room door and windows as indicated.
3. Remove the client's gown and assist him or her to a comfortable supine position. Place a bath blanket over the client.
4. First sponge the client's face with plain water only, and dry it. An ice bag or cold pack may be applied to the client's head for comfort.
5. If ice bags or cold packs are not used, place bath towels under each axilla and shoulder.

   Rationale Bath towels protect the lower bed sheet from getting wet.

6. Wet three washcloths, wring them out so they are very damp but not dripping, and place them in the axillae and groins. Or place ice bags or cold packs in these areas.

   Rationale Washcloths need to be as moist as possible to be effective. The axillae and groins contain large superficial blood vessels, which aid the transfer of heat.

7. Leave the washcloths in place for about 5 minutes, or until they feel warm. Rewet and replace them as required during the bath.

   Rationale Washcloths warm up relatively quickly in such vascular areas.

8. Place a bath towel under one arm. Sponge the arm slowly and gently for about 5 minutes or as tolerated by the client. Or place a saturated towel over the extremity, and rewet it as necessary. Give the client enough time to adjust to the initial reaction of chilliness and for the body to cool.

   Rationale Slow, gentle motions are indicated because firm rubbing motions increase tissue metabolism and heat production. Cool sponges given rapidly or for a short period of time tend to increase the body's heat production by causing shivering.

9. Dry the arm, using a patting motion rather than a rubbing motion.
10. Repeat steps 8 and 9 for the other arm and the legs.
11. When sponging the extremities, hold the washcloth briefly over the wrists and ankles.

    Rationale The blood circulation is close to the skin surface in the wrists and ankles.

12. After 15 minutes check the client's vital signs. Compare with data taken before the bath.

    Rationale The vital signs are checked to evaluate the effectiveness of the sponge bath.

13. Ask the client to turn on his or her side, and sponge the back and buttocks for 3 to 5 minutes. Pat these areas dry.
14. Remove the washcloths from the axillae and groins, and dry these areas.
15. Recheck the client's vital signs.
16. Record the vital signs, type of sponge bath given, and responses of the client.

Sample Recording

Date	Time	Notes
Dec/5/87	1600	C/o headache, appears restless, is flushed and diaphoretic. T 104, P 110, R 24. Tepid sponge given.—
	1615	T 102, P 105, R 22.—
	1630	T 100, P 100, R 20. Sponge bath discontinued.—
		—Marya A. Shapiro, NS

Compresses and Moist Packs

Compresses and moist packs can be either hot or cold. A **compress** is a moist gauze dressing applied frequently to an open wound. When hot compresses are ordered, the solution is heated to the temperature indicated by the physician, e.g., 40.5 (105 F). When there is a break in the skin or when the body part is vulnerable to microbrial invasion (e.g., an eye), compresses are applied using sterile technique; therefore sterile gloves or sterile forceps are needed for their application. A hot or cold pack is a hot or cold moist cloth applied to an area of the body. Hot packs are also referred to as foments. Frequently, wool flannel is used because it holds heat or cold well. Packs are usually unsterile; after application, they are covered with a water-resistant material (e.g., plastic wrap) to contain the moisture and prevent the transfer of airborne microorganisms to the area.

Hot compresses usually are applied to hasten the suppurative process and healing. Cold compresses are applied to either decrease or prevent bleeding or to reduce inflammation. Hot packs are applied to relieve muscle spasm or pain, to reduce the pressure of accumulated fluid in a tissue or joint, and to reduce congestion in an underlying organ. Cold packs are used to prevent swelling due to tissue trauma and inflammation, and to anesthetize tissues and temporarily reduce pain.

After a compress or a pack has been applied, it is advisable to apply external heat or cold, such as a hot water bottle, heating pad, or ice bag, to help maintain the temperature of the application.

Application of compresses and moist packs is described in Procedure 52–10.

Procedure 52–10 ▲ Applying Compresses and Moist Packs

Equipment

Compress

1. A container for the solution
2. The solution at the strength and temperature specified by the physician or the agency
3. A thermometer to test the temperature of the solution
4. Gauze squares to soak with the solution and apply to the client
5. Plastic to insulate the compresses, to retain the temperature and moisture
6. An insulating towel to help maintain the temperature of the compress
7. A hot water bottle (optional) to provide additional heat and maintain the heat of a hot compress

   or

8. An ice bag (optional) to maintain the cold of a cold compress
9. Ties, e.g., roller gauze, to fasten the compress in place

For a sterile compress, the solution, container, thermometer, towels, and gauze squares must be sterile. In addition, sterile forceps or sterile gloves are required to maintain the sterility of the gauze when it is wrung out and applied. If a sterile thermometer is not available, pour a small amount of the solution into a clean basin, measure the temperature with a bath thermometer, and then discard the solution, since it is no longer sterile. Adjust the temperature of the solution according to your findings.

Moist pack

10. Flannel pieces or towel packs
11. A hot-pack machine for heating the packs

    or

12. A basin of water with some ice chips to cool the water
13. Plastic for insulation
14. Insulating material, e.g., flannel or towels
15. A hot water bottle (optional) to provide additional heat and maintain the heat of the pack

    or

16. An ice bag (optional) to maintain the cold of the pack
17. A thermometer if a specific temperature is ordered for the pack (e.g., a cold pack of 24 C [75 F] may be ordered)
18. Petroleum jelly to apply to surrounding skin areas if the pack tends to irritate them
19. Ties, e.g., roller gauze, to fasten the pack

For a sterile moist pack, the container, solution, thermometer, and all materials must be sterile. In addition, sterile gloves or forceps are required to maintain the sterility of the pack when it is wrung out and applied.

Intervention

1. Assist the client to a comfortable position, expose the area for the compress or pack, and provide support for the body part requiring the compress or pack.

Compress

2. Place the gauze in the solution.
3. Remove the wound dressing, if present. A dry, sterile dressing is often placed over open wounds between applications of moist heat or cold. To remove a sterile dressing, see Procedure 52–1, page 1554.
4. Assess:
   a. The area to which the compress or pack is to be applied for any signs of redness, abraded skin, or discharge. If the wound is open, assess its size, appearance, and type and amount of discharge.
   b. Any discomfort, swelling, or bleeding, to provide baseline data for comparison.
   c. Whether the blood circulation to the area is impaired. Clinical signs of impairment are numbness or tingling, cyanosis, and coolness to the touch. Areas with poor blood circulation are less tolerant of heat and cold, so therapy may be contraindicated. Report any impairment to the responsible nurse before starting the treatment.
5. Wring out the gauze so the solution does not drip from it. For a sterile compress, use sterile forceps or sterile gloves.
6. Apply the gauze to the designated area, molding the compress close to the body.

   Rationale Air is a poor conductor of cold or heat, and molding excludes air.
7. Optional: Apply a hot water bottle or ice bag over the gauze, if the compress is not sterile. If a hot water bottle is used, the temperature of the water should be lower than usual, e.g., 40 to 43 C (105 to 110 F), because a moist compress can burn the client if it is too hot.
8. Quickly cover the gauze (and hot water bottle or ice bag, if used) with the plastic and the insulating material, e.g., a towel.

   Rationale The compress is insulated quickly to maintain its temperature.
9. Secure the compress in place with ties.

Moist Pack

10. Assess the client's pulse, respirations, and blood pressure for baseline data if moist packs are to be applied over a large area of the body, e.g., the posterior trunk.
11. Heat the flannel or towel.
12. Apply petroleum jelly to the surrounding skin if it appears reddened.
13. Wring out the flannel. For a sterile pack, use sterile gloves.
14. Apply the flannel to the body area, molding it closely to the body part.
15. Optional: Apply a hot water bottle or ice bag over the pack, if it is an unsterile pack.
16. Quickly cover the flannel (and ice bag or hot water bottle, if used) with the plastic insulating material, e.g., a towel.
17. Secure the pack in place with ties.
18. Record on the client's chart the technique, the time, the type and strength of the solution if appropriate, and the appearance of the wound and surrounding skin area.
19. Frequently assess the client's level of comfort. If the client feels any discomfort, assess the area for erythema, numbness, etc. For applications to large areas of the body, note any change in the client's pulse, respirations, or blood pressure. In the event of unexpected outcomes, terminate the treatment and report to the responsible nurse.
20. Remove the compress or pack at the specified time. Compresses and packs with external heat or cold usually retain their temperature anywhere from 15 to 30 minutes. Without external heat or cold, they need to be changed every 5 minutes.
21. Apply a sterile dressing if one is required.
22. When the compress or pack is removed, record the appearance of the area and any other responses of the client.

Sample Recording

Date	Time	Notes
Dec/12/87	0910	Sterile normal saline compress with K-Matic 37.7 C applied to sacral ulcer. Pink tissue surrounding ulcer. Small amount of serosanguineous discharge. No discomfort.——— Olga R. Resnicoff, NS
Dec/12/87	0940	Compress removed. No further discharge. Dry dressing applied.— Olga R. Resnicoff, NS

Chapter Highlights

- Nurses commonly care for wounds. This may involve changing dressings, shortening and maintaining drains, applying heat and cold, and applying bandages and binders.
- Wounds may be intentional or unintentional. There are six types of wounds: incisions, contusions, abrasions, lacerations, punctures, and penetrating wounds.
- Wounds may also be categorized according to the likelihood and degree of wound contamination: clean, clean-contaminated, contaminated, and dirty or infected.
- Wounds heal by either primary intention or secondary intention, depending on the extent of tissue loss.
- Many internal and external factors affect wound healing, either positively or negatively. Internal factors include vasculature, presence of anemia, age, whether the person is compromised, nutrition, obesity, smoking, stress, and medications. External factors include preoperative stay, preoperative preparation, and intraoperative factors.
- Four main complications of wound healing are hemorrhage, infection, dehiscence, and evisceration.
- The nurse assesses wounds by visual inspection, palpation, and the sense of smell. Wound assessment is an ongoing process to evaluate healing.
- Nursing diagnoses related to wound care include potential impairment of skin integrity, potential for injury, alterations in comfort, and impaired physical mobility.
- Major responsibilities of the nurse related to wound care include preventing infection, preventing further tissue damage, preventing hemorrhage, promoting healing, and cleaning wounds of foreign debris. Skin excoriation around draining wounds must also be prevented.
- The care of wounds varies considerably in accordance with the type of wound, size and location, amount of exudate, presence of complicating factors, and sometimes the personal preference of the physician. Open and closed methods of wound care have advantages and disadvantages that make them appropriate for different circumstances.
- Various dressing materials are indicated for cleaning, covering, and supporting wounds.
- Before changing dressings the nurse needs to ascertain the physician's orders, the presence of drains, the amount of wound drainage, and the cleaning solutions to be used.
- In some agencies, registered nurses may be responsible for shortening a Penrose drain; proper technique is essential to prevent client discomfort and to keep the drain from falling back into the incision.
- In some agencies, registered nurses may be responsible for removing skin sutures. There are five common types of sutures: plain interrupted, mattress interrupted, plain continuous, mattress continuous, and blanket continuous. Each is removed by a specific procedure.
- Bandages and binders serve several purposes in the care of wounds, but support and immobilization are the two most common ones. Materials used vary widely and relate to the purpose of the bandage. Examples are flannel, muslin, gauze, and elastic adhesive.
- There are five basic turns required for bandaging specific body parts: spiral, circular, spiral reverse, recurrent, and figure-eight.
- There are five commonly used types of binders: the triangular binder, the breast binder, the scultetus (many-tailed) binder, the T-binder, and the abdominal binder.
- Heat and cold can be applied in either dry or moist forms.
- Because of the adaptive nature of the body's thermal receptors, the nurse must use caution when applying heat and cold.
- Heat and cold produce specific local physiologic responses that form the basis for their therapeutic effects.
- An understanding of the rebound phenomenon is essential for the nurse; thermal applications must be halted before this phenomenon begins.
- Before applying heat or cold, the nurse must determine the client's ability to tolerate the therapy and identify conditions that contraindicate the therapy.
- Clients who have sensory impairments, impaired mental status, or low heat or cold tolerance must be closely supervised and assessed during hot and cold therapies.

Suggested Readings

Cuzzell, J. Z. February 1985. Wound care forum: Artful solutions to chronic problems. *American Journal of Nursing* 85:162–66.

According to Cuzzell, there are two general purposes to the care of chronic wounds: (1) cleaning a dirty, infected wound to prepare for surgical closure, and (2) protecting a clean wound until it can heal by the processes of contracture and epithelization. Different types of dressings are described: dry-to-dry, wet-to-dry, wet-to-damp, and wet-to-wet, as well as synthetic dressings, topical enzyme preparations, and products that absorb exudates and cleanse a wound surface.

———. May 1986. Wound care forum: Tell it like it is. A realistic approach to wound documentation. *American Journal of Nursing* 86:600–601.
Cuzzell presents a "wound assessment flowsheet." The article includes two assessment guides, one for a wound without tissue loss and one for a wound with tissue loss.

Neuberger, G. B., and Reckling, J. B. February 1985. A new look at wound care. *Nursing 85* 15:34–41.
The article explains the chain of infection. Preoperative care is described, including skin disinfection, hair removal, antibiotic prophylaxis, and parenteral hyperalimentation. Laminar airflow devices and wound stapling are described as aspects of intraoperative care. Postoperative suture-line care and suture (staple) removal are discussed. A separate section on wound and skin cleaners is included.

Selected References

Alterescue, V. May/June 1983. Toward a physiologic approach to the topical treatment of opened wounds. *Journal of Enterostomal Therapy* 10:101–7.

Bauman, B. January 1982. Update your technique for changing dressings: Dry to dry. *Nursing 82* 12:64–67.

———. February 1982. Update your technique for changing dressings: Wet to dry. *Nursing 82* 12:68–71.

Brozenec, S. April 1985. Caring for the postoperative patient with an abdominal drain. *Nursing 85* 15:55–57.

Brubacher, L. L. March 1982. To heal a draining wound. *RN* 45:30–35.

Bruno, P. December 1979. The nature of wound healing: Implications for nursing practice. *Nursing Clinics of North America* 14(4):667–82.

Bruno, P., and Craven, R. F. December 1982. Age challenges to wound healing. *Journal of Gerontological Nursing* 8:686–91.

Cooper, D. M., and Schumann, D. December 1979. Postsurgical nursing intervention as an adjunct to wound healing. *Nursing Clinics of North America* 14:713–26.

Cruse, P. J. E., and Foord, R. February 1980. The epidemiology of wound infections. A ten-year prospective study of 62,939 wounds. *Surgical Clinics of North America* 60:27–40.

Flynn, M. E., and Rovee, D. T. October 1982. Wound healing mechanisms. *American Journal of Nursing* 82:1544–50.

Garner, J. S. April 1986. CDC guidelines for the prevention and control of nosocomial infections: Guideline for prevention of surgical wound infections, 1985. *American Journal of Infection Control* 14:71–80.

Guyton, A. C. 1986. *Textbook of medical physiology.* 7th ed. Philadelphia: W. B. Saunders Co.

Influencing repair and recovery. October 1982. *American Journal of Nursing* 82:1550–57.

Kottke, F. J.; Stillwell, G. K.; and Lehmann, J. F. 1982. *Krusen's handbook of physical medicine and rehabilitation.* 3d ed. Philadelphia: W. B. Saunders Co.

Lehmann, J. F., and DeLateur, B. J. 1982a. *Therapeutic heat and cold.* 3d ed. Baltimore: Williams and Wilkins Co.

———. 1982b. Diathermy and superficial heat and cold therapy. In Kottke, F. J.; Stillwell, G. K.; and Lehmann, J. F. *Krusen's handbook of physical medicine and rehabilitation.* 3d ed. Philadelphia: W. B. Saunders Co.

LeMaitre, G. D., and Finnegan, J. A. 1980. *The patient in surgery: A guide for nurses.* 4th ed. Philadelphia: W. B. Saunders Co.

Montgomery, B. A. November/December 1981. Techniques for use of a new dressing: A moisture vapor permeable film. *Journal of Enterostomal Therapy* 8:26–29.

Reckling, J. B., and Neuberger, G. B. February 1985. A new look at wound care. *Nursing 85* 15:1 (Canadian ed., pp. 34–41).

Nichols, R. L. January/February 1982. Techniques known to prevent post-operative wound infection. *Infection Control* 3:34–37.

Pollack, S. V. November/December 1981. Wound healing: A review: I. The biology of wound healing. *Journal of Enterostomal Therapy* 8:16–18, 19, 21, 39.

———. January/February 1982a. Wound healing: A review: II. Environmental factors affecting wound healing. *Journal of Enterostomal Therapy* 9:14–16, 35.

———. March/April 1982b. Wound healing: A review. III. Nutritional factors affecting wound healing. *Journal of Enterostomal Therapy* 9:28–29, 32–33.

Schumann, D. December 1979. Preoperative measures to promote wound healing. *Nursing Clinics of North America* 14:683–99.

Slahetka, F. May/June 1984. Dakin's solution for deep ulcers. *Geriatric Nursing* 5:168–69.

Taylor, D. L. May 1983. Wound healing: Physiology, signs and symptoms. *Nursing 83* 13(5):44–45.

Tepperman, P. S., and Devlin, M. January 1983. Therapeutic heat and cold. A practitioner's guide. *Postgraduate Medicine* 73:69.

Wright, N. E. July/August 1983. Abdominal wounds: Breakdown and dehiscence. *Journal of Enterostomal Therapy* 10:143–44.

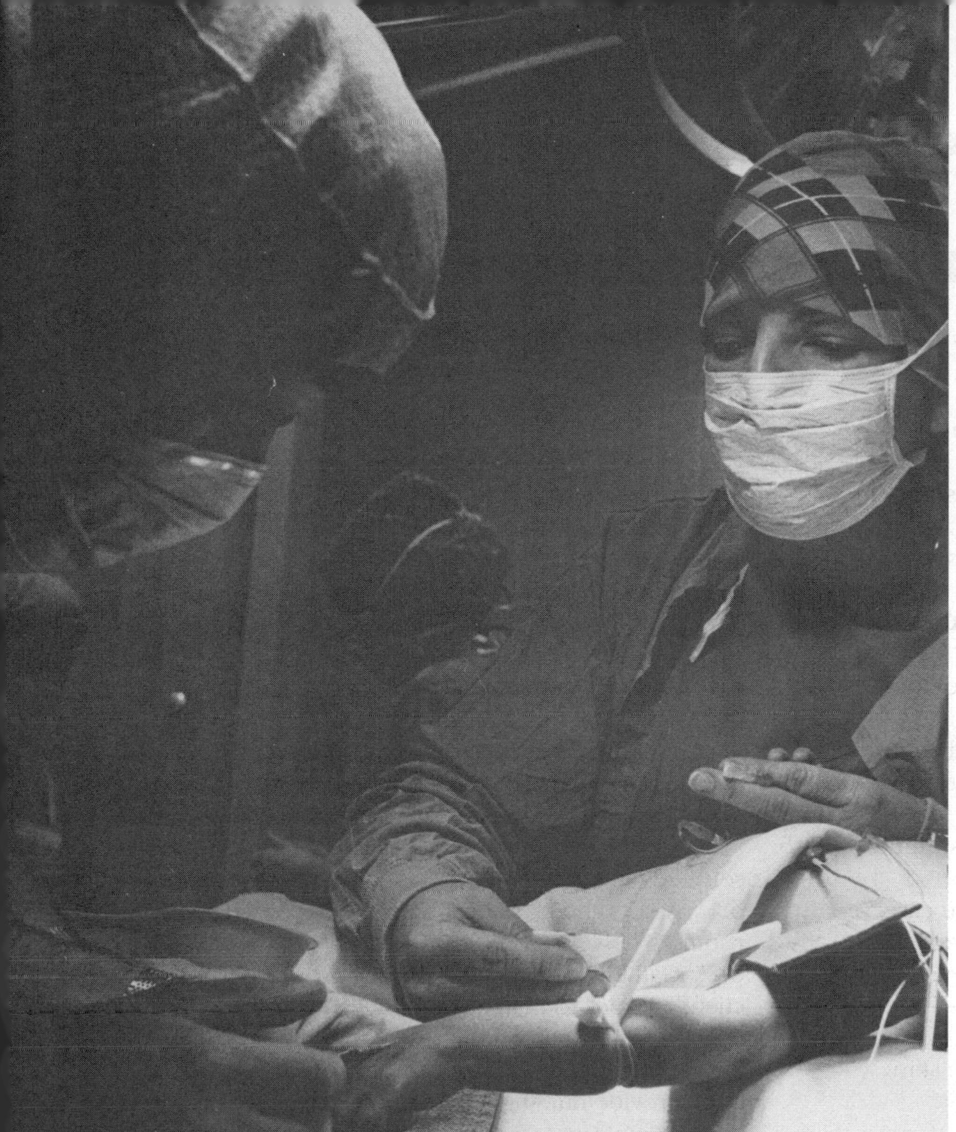

CHAPTER 53

Perioperative Care

Contents

53 *Perioperative Care*

Objectives

1. Know essential terms and facts about surgery, anesthesia, and perioperative nursing care.
   1.1 Define selected terms.
   1.2 Describe the phases of the perioperative period.
   1.3 Differentiate among the various types of surgery.
   1.4 Describe the different types of anesthesia.
   1.5 Discuss the legal aspects of surgery.
   1.6 Describe the elements involved in surgical risk.
   1.7 Outline the various aspects of preoperative assessment.
   1.8 Give examples of pertinent nursing diagnoses.
2. Understand essential information about preoperative planning and intervention.
   2.1 Identify the essential nursing responsibilities included in planning.
   2.2 Explain the essentials of perioperative care.
   2.3 Describe how to teach clients to move, perform leg exercises, and perform coughing and deep breathing exercises.
   2.4 Describe preoperative preparation.
   2.5 Identify the essentials of preoperative skin preparation.
   2.6 Explain gastric intubation.
   2.7 Give the essentials of preparing for the postoperative client.
3. Understand essential facts about the intraoperative phase.
   3.1 Describe some of the ways to protect a client from injury.
   3.2 Identify circumstances in which the nurse monitors a client.
   3.3 Describe intraoperative documentation.
   3.4 Identify the various nursing roles during the intraoperative period.
4. Understand essential facts about the postoperative phase.
   4.1 Describe nursing interventions required during the postoperative phase.
   4.2 Identify potential postoperative complications and nursing interventions to prevent them.
   4.3 Identify possible nursing diagnoses.
5. Provide effective postoperative nursing care to selected clients.
   5.1 Assess clients returning from the recovery room.
   5.2 Gather necessary information from the client's record to plan postoperative care.
   5.3 With assistance, establish a nursing care plan for the client.
   5.4 Provide nursing interventions to relieve discomfort and prevent complications.
   5.5 Evaluate the effectiveness of nursing interventions.

Terms

ablative surgery
bronchopneumonia
Cantor tube
caudal anesthesia
constructive surgery
dehiscence
diagnostic surgery
elective surgery
embolus
evisceration
exploratory surgery
general anesthesia
Harris tube
hypostatic pneumonia
hypovolemic shock
intraoperative phase
Levin tube
lobar pneumonia
local anesthesia
lumbar epidural anesthesia
major surgery
Miller-Abbott tube
minor surgery
nasogastric tube
nerve block
optional surgery
orogastric tube
palliative surgery
perioperative
postoperative phase
preoperative phase
reconstructive surgery
regional anesthesia
Salem sump tube
singultus
spinal anesthesia
thrombophlebitis
thrombus
tissue perfusion
tympanites
urgent surgery

The Perioperative Period

Operations are traumatic for both clients and their support persons. Today most operations take place in hospitals, which many people associate with pain and death. Many clients equate operations with disfigurement and pain, so the nurse must be sensitive to the psychologic needs of clients having operations.

The **perioperative** period is the time before, during, and after an operation; it encompasses three phases: preoperative, intraoperative,and postoperative. The **preoperative phase** begins when the decision for surgical intervention is made, and it ends when the client is transferred to the operating room bed. The preoperative client is prepared psychologically and physically for surgery. An important aspect of preoperative nursing is teaching the client what he or she needs to know. The preoperative period can vary from hours to months. The **intraoperative phase** is the time of surgery. It begins when the client is transferred to the operating room bed, and it terminates when she or he is admitted to the postanesthetic area. The main intraoperative nursing function is to maintain the client's safety. The **postoperative** (postsurgical) **phase** is the time following surgery. It begins with admission to the postanesthesia area and ends when the client has completely recovered from her or his surgery. Major postoperative nursing functions are to help the client recover from the anesthetic, maintain the client's body systems, prevent postoperative complications, and prevent undue discomfort. The postoperative period is sometimes divided into the initial postoperative period, during which the client recovers from the anesthetic, and the continuing postoperative period, after the client returns to a clinical nursing unit.

The nurse is an essential member of the health team caring for the surgical client. The nurse prepares clients before operations; often the nurse is responsible for explaining to client and support persons what the operation will entail. After surgery, the nurse helps the client return to health. Before they leave the hospital, some postoperative clients need to learn skills such as walking with crutches. Clients also need to learn how to prevent postoperative complications such as pneumonia. Teaching is an important aspect of nursing intervention. For a summary of nursing practice during each phase of the perioperative period see Table 53–1.

Types of Surgery

Surgical procedures are commonly grouped into three general categories according to (a) urgency, (b) risk, and (c) purpose.

Degree of Urgency

In terms of urgency, surgery can be classified into three types: urgent, elective, and optional. **Urgent surgery** is surgery performed for reasons of health, such as the removal of an inflamed appendix. Urgent surgery is always essential but not always an emergency. An emergency operation to control internal hemorrhaging is one kind of urgent surgery; another type is breast surgery for a malignancy. **Elective surgery** is surgery performed for the client's well-being though not absolutely necessary for life, such as straightening a bent finger. It may be planned weeks or months ahead. **Optional surgery** is that requested by the client, though not necessary for physical health. Usually an operation such as facial plastic surgery is optional, being performed for psychologic reasons.

Degree of Risk

Surgery is classified as major or minor according to the degree of risk to the client. **Major surgery** involves a high degree of risk, and for a variety of reasons: it may be complicated or prolonged; large losses of blood may occur; vital organs may be involved; or postoperative complications may be likely. Examples of major surgery are organ transplant, open heart surgery, and removal of a kidney. In contrast, **minor surgery** involves little risk, produces few complications, and may be performed in a "day surgery." Examples are breast biopsy, removal of tonsils, and removal of polyps from the nose. See also "Assessing Surgical Risk" on page 1597.

Purpose

Surgical procedures are also categorized according to their purpose:

1. **Diagnostic surgery** enables the surgeon to confirm a diagnosis. Sometimes a surgeon awaits laboratory

Table 53–1 Major Areas of Nursing Practice During the Perioperative Period

Preoperative Phase	Intraoperative Phase	Postoperative Phase
Preoperative assessment	Maintain client safety	Communicate intraoperative information
Preoperative preparation	Monitor client's vital signs	Assess client's physical condition
Preoperative teaching	Provide support to client prior to anesthetic	Provide nursing interventions
Support for client and support persons		Support client and support persons

Adapted from Association of Operating Room Nurses, *AORN standards and recommended practices for perioperative nursing* (Denver: Association of Operating Room Nurses, Inc., 1986), p. 1:1-4.

analysis of tissue removed during the operation before proceeding with further surgery. A common example is a breast biopsy, in which a specimen of tissue is excised and sent to the laboratory during or after the surgery for analysis. The diagnosis determines how the surgeon will proceed.

2. **Exploratory surgery** is frequently performed to determine the extent of a pathologic process and sometimes to confirm a diagnosis. For example, an exploratory laparotomy (opening into the abdomen) may be done to assess the extent of a cancerous growth.

3. **Palliative surgery** is performed to relieve symptoms of a disease process without correcting the disease causing the symptoms. For example, if a client has an inoperable, obstructive malignant tumor of the bowel, an intestinal bypass operation (colostomy) may be done to relieve the discomfort caused by the obstruction.

4. **Reconstructive surgery** refers to the repair of tissues or organs whose appearance or function has been damaged. Two examples are a vaginal repair and plastic surgery to repair a body part following extensive scarring from a burn.

5. **Constructive surgery** is performed to a congenitally malformed organ or tissue, such as a harelip.

6. **Ablative surgery** refers to the removal of a diseased organ such as the gallbladder or appendix. The term *ablate,* of Latin derivation, means "take away or cut off."

Types of Anesthesia

General Anesthesia

General anesthesia is the loss of all sensation and consciousness. A general anesthetic acts by blocking awareness centers in the brain so that amnesia (loss of memory), analgesia (insensibility to pain), hypnosis (artificial sleep), and relaxation (rendering a part of the body less tense) occur. General anesthetics are administered by intravenous infusion, or by inhalation of gases or vapors delivered through a mask or through an endotracheal tube inserted into the trachea. Often an intravenous drug such as thiopental sodium (Pentothal) is used to render the client unconscious and is then supplemented with other agents to produce surgical anesthesia.

General anesthesia has certain advantages. Because the client is unconscious rather than awake and anxious, respiration and cardiac function are readily regulated. Also, the anesthesia can be adjusted to the length of the operation and the client's age and physical status. Its chief disadvantage is that it depresses the respiratory and circulatory systems. Some clients become more anxious about a general anesthetic than about the surgery itself. Often this is because they fear losing the capacity to control their own bodies.

Regional Anesthesia

Regional anesthesia is the loss of sensation in one area of the body due to the blockage of sensory impulses to the brain. The client remains conscious. A number of methods are employed, such as spinal anesthesia, nerve block, and epidural block. **Spinal anesthesia** requires a lumbar puncture. See Figure 53–1 and the section on lumbar puncture in Chapter 54. The physician injects the anesthetic into the spinal canal (subarachnoid space). One type of spinal anesthesia is the saddle anesthesia, a "low spinal," which affects the lower lumbar nerves (L1–5) and sacral nerves (S1–4). Commonly used anesthetic agents are lidocaine hydrochloride (Xylocaine) and tetracaine hydrochloride (Pontocaine).

A **nerve block** involves the injection of an anesthetic agent into a nerve plexus to anesthetize part of the body.

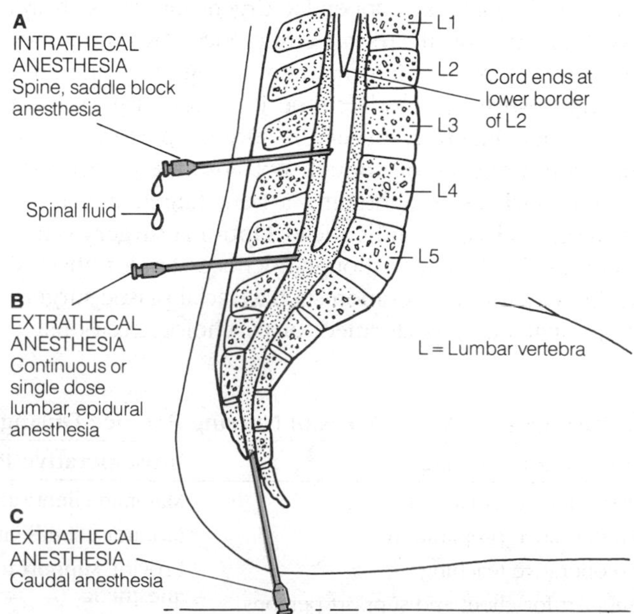

Figure 53–1 Anatomic sites for local anesthetics

For instance, injecting tetracaine into the brachial plexus interrupts the nerve impulses and anesthetizes the arm.

For **lumbar epidural anesthesia**, the agent is injected through the lumbar interspace into the epidural space, i.e., outside the spinal canal. See Figure 53–1. The agent infiltrates the tissues and affects a band around the client's body at the level of the injection. In **caudal anesthesia** the needle is inserted through the sacral hiatus into the caudal canal. See Figure 53–1. The client may assume a lateral or knee–chest position for the administration of a caudal anesthetic.

Local Anesthesia

Local anesthesia is the loss of sensation in a small area of tissue. An anesthetic agent may be sprayed onto the skin or mucous membrane or injected into the tissue. For instance, proparacaine hydrochloride (Alcaine) commonly is used in a 0.5% solution to anesthetize the eye. Tetracaine, lidocaine (Xylocaine), and bupivacaine hydrochloride (Marcaine) are commonly used as injectable anesthetic agents. The chief advantage of this method is that the anesthetic acts quickly and has few side-effects.

Legal Aspects of Surgery

Prior to any surgical procedure clients must sign a surgical consent form. See Figure 53–2. This requirement protects clients from having any surgical procedure they do not want or do not know about. It also protects the hospital and the health personnel from a claim by client or family that permission was not granted. The consent form becomes a part of the client's record and goes to the operating room with the client.

Obtaining legal, informed consent to perform surgery is the responsibility of the surgeon. Informed consent is possible only when the client is told in advance of the character and importance of the surgery, its probable consequences, the chances for success, and alternative measures. Often a nurse is responsible for witnessing a consent. The nurse must be aware of his or her responsibilities regarding consents and be aware of the particular hospital's policies.

Adults sign their own forms unless they are mentally incompetent or unconscious, in which case a spouse or next of kin signs for them. Children 19 or younger (18 or younger in some jurisdictions) cannot sign consent forms. A parent or guardian must sign instead. However, some jurisdictions allow teenagers to give consent. In Ontario, a 16-year-old can give consent for surgery. In Quebec, a minor of 14 years can give consent (and be operated on without parents' knowledge), provided the minor is not hospitalized longer than 12 hours and treatment is not prolonged (Creighton 1981, p. 274). If a minor's parents cannot be found, a court order can be obtained to permit surgery. See Chapter 7, page 163, for information about informed consent.

Preoperative Assessment

Assessing Surgical Risk

The degree of risk involved in a surgical procedure is affected by the client's age, nutritional status, fluid and electrolyte balance, general health, use of medications, and mental health and attitude.

Age

Very young and elderly clients are greater surgical risks than children and adults. A neonate's physiologic response to surgery is substantially different from an adult's. Factors that affect the risk are the neonate's circulation, which is largely central, and renal function, which is not fully developed until about 6 months of age. The neonate can respond to an additional need for oxygen only with an increased respiratory rate, and limited blood volume results in a limited fluid reserve.

Elderly persons are at additional risk from surgery because of their often impaired circulation due to arteriosclerosis and limited cardiac function. Energy reserves are frequently limited, and hydration and nutritional status may be poor. In addition, elderly people can be highly sensitive to medications such as morphine sulfate and barbiturates, frequently used preoperatively and postoperatively. Special hazards to which the elderly surgical client is subject are listed on page 1599.

Nutritional Status

Two nutritional problems that can increase surgical risk are obesity and malnutrition due to protein, iron, and vitamin deficiencies. Surgery for obese clients is often deferred, except in emergencies. The obese often have overtaxed hearts and elevated blood pressures. In addi-

EL CAMINO HOSPITAL DISTRICT

Pt. Name
Hosp. No.
Rm. No.

AUTHORIZATION AND CONSENT TO SURGERY, ANESTHESIA, DIAGNOSTIC OR THERAPEUTIC PROCEDURES

YOUR DOCTOR IS ______________________________

THE OPERATION(S) OR PROCEDURE(S) TO BE PERFORMED IS/ARE:

____
(MEDICAL TERMINOLOGY)

____
(LAY TERMINOLOGY)

1. The hospital maintains personnel and facilities to assist your doctor in his performance of various surgical operations and other special diagnostic and therapeutic procedures. These operations and procedures may all involve risks of unsuccessful results, complications, injury, or even death, from both known and unforeseen causes, and no warranty or guarantee is made as to result or cure. You have the right to be informed of such risks as well as the nature and purpose of the operation(s) or procedure(s) and the available alternative methods of treatment and this form is not a substitute for such explanations which are provided by the above named physician. Except in cases of emergency, the operation(s) or procedure(s) is/are not performed until the patient has had the opportunity to receive such explanations. You may refuse any proposed operation or procedure anytime prior to its performance.

2. Your doctor has recommended the operation(s) or procedure(s) set forth above. Upon your authorization and consent, such operation(s) or procedure(s), together with any different or further procedure(s) which in the opinion of your doctor may be indicated due to any emergency, will be performed on you. The operation(s) or procedure(s) will be performed by the doctor named above together with associates and assistants, including anesthesiologists and radiologists from the medical staff of El Camino Hospital. Your attending physician, surgeon, assistant surgeon, anesthesiologist, and other physicians are not agents, servants or employees of the hospital or your doctor but are independent contractors, and therefore your agents.

3. Your signature below authorizes the hospital pathologist to use his or her discretion in disposition of any member, organ or other tissue removed from your person during the above-named procedure(s).

4. Your signature below constitutes your acknowledgement (1) that you have read and agree to the foregoing; (2) that the operation(s) or procedure(s) set forth above has/have been adequately explained to you by your doctor and that you have received all of the information you desire concerning such operation(s) or procedure(s); (3) that you authorize and consent to the performance of the operation(s) or procedure(s); (4) and that you acknowledge receipt of a copy of this authorization.

SIGNATURE: ______________________________ PATIENT/PARENT/LEGAL GUARDIAN

______________________________ DATE AND TIME

______________________________ RELATIONSHIP

______________________________ WITNESS (NOT PATIENT'S DOCTOR)

______________________________ REASON PATIENT UNABLE TO SIGN

Figure 53–2 A sample surgical consent form

Source: Courtesy of El Camino Hospital, Mountain View, California.

tion, incisions in overly fatty tissue are difficult to suture and prone to infection. Nutritional deficiencies are particularly common among elderly clients and chronically ill clients. Protein and vitamins are needed for wound healing; vitamin K is essential for blood clotting.

Fluid and Electrolyte Balance

Dehydration and hypovolemia predispose a client to problems during surgery. Electrolyte imbalances often accompany fluid imbalances. Imbalances in calcium, magnesium, potassium, and hydrogen ions are of particular concern during surgery. See Chapter 46.

General Health

Surgery is least risky when the client's general health is good. Any infection or pathophysiology increases the risk. Of particular concern are upper respiratory tract infections, which together with a general anesthetic can adversely affect respiratory function.

A recent myocardial infarction or any cardiovascular disease also can make surgery more dangerous than usual. Renal function is essential for the excretion of body wastes. In addition, the kidneys help regulate the body's fluids and electrolytes. Any renal impairment can affect blood pressure and the ability of the body to respond to the additional stress of surgery. Metabolic and liver function affect healing and the detoxification and elimination of medications. When liver function is impaired, the liver cannot detoxify drugs and metabolize carbohydrates, proteins, and fats efficiently. Untreated diabetes mellitus predisposes to infection and impaired healing. A person whose blood does not coagulate normally may bleed more than normal or even hemorrhage and go into shock.

Medications

The regular use of certain medications can increase surgical risk. These include:

1. *Anticoagulants,* which increase blood coagulation time
2. *Tranquilizers,* which can cause hypotension and thus contribute to shock
3. *Heroin and other depressants,* which decrease central nervous system responses
4. *Antibiotics incompatible with anesthetic agents,* which result in untoward reactions
5. *Diuretics,* which can create electrolyte (especially potassium) imbalances

In addition, some medications interact adversely with other medications and with anesthetic agents.

Special Hazards for the Elderly Surgical Client

- Contractures
- Osteoporosis
- Urinary calculi
- Dehydration
- Decubitus ulcers
- Venous thrombosis

Mental Health and Attitude

Extreme anxiety can increase surgical risk. The level of anxiety does not always correspond to the seriousness of the surgical procedure. The surgeon needs to know if a person fears that he or she will die during surgery. In some instances, professional counseling and a delay in the surgery are indicated.

Clients who have shown poor psychologic adjustment for some time may not be able to cope with the additional stress of surgery. People who cope only minimally in a stable, familiar environment can develop emotional problems postoperatively.

See Table 53–2 for at-risk factors for the elderly surgical client.

Nursing History

The nursing history obtained before surgery provides client data that help the nurse to plan preoperative and postoperative care. Although forms vary considerably among agencies, essential preoperative information includes the following.

Physical condition. The client's general appearance is noted—color, weight, hydration status, and energy level. Problems such as obesity, malnutrition, dehydration, and marked fatigue may indicate the need for therapy prior to surgery. For instance, the dehydrated client may need fluids administered intravenously.

Mental attitude. Anxiety is a normal response to surgery. However, extreme anxiety can increase surgical risk and needs to be reported to the physician.

Understanding the surgery. Determining the client's knowledge about the surgery helps the nurse plan appropriate instruction. A well-informed client knows what to expect and in general accepts and copes more effectively with surgery and convalescence.

Table 53–2 Risk Factors for the Elderly Surgical Client

Physiologic Change	Preoperative Nursing Interventions
Integumentary System	
Vulnerable skin due to venous stasis and poor venous return	Teach passive and active exercises. Measure the client for antiemboli stockings.
Cardiovascular System	
Reduced cardiac reserve due to changes in the myocardium	Determine usual pattern of ADLs and how quickly the client tires.
Tachycardia from anxiety, which is tolerated poorly in the elderly heart	Teach about and support anxiety reduction.
Decreased compliance of blood vessels due to atherosclerosis	Teach leg exercises and turning. Obtain baseline data re vital signs. Monitor blood pressure closely for hypertension.
Respiratory System	
Reduced vital capacity due to lowered expansibility of the rib cage	Teach deep breathing and coughing. Obtain baseline data re respirations.
Urinary System	
Reduced blood flow to the kidneys	Obtain baseline urine output for 24 hours.
Reduced ability to excrete toxins due to reduced glomerular filtration	Initiate fluid intake and output recordings.
Fluids and Electrolytes	
Dehydration from repeated enemas	Assess hydration status for baseline data.
Hypokalemia due to diarrhea	Monitor fluid intake and output.
Neurologic System	
Reduced sensory acuity	Orient client to surroundings.
Decreased reaction time	Allow time for client to proceed at own pace.

Experience with previous surgeries. Some previous experiences may influence the client's physical and psychologic responses to the planned surgery. For example, a client who has developed a wound infection that has caused a gape in a previous incision may demonstrate acute anxiety when sutures are removed and may be unwilling to move, believing that movement will cause the wound to gape.

Expected outcomes of surgery. Surgery alters a client's body image and life-style to varying degrees. A middle-age woman about to have a hysterectomy may feel she will no longer be valued or adequate as a wife and mother; a young man having a hernia repair may worry that he will miss his chance to play in a championship football game. To provide the necessary support for adjustment, nurses need to determine each client's concerns.

Use of medications. Because some medications react with anesthetics or other drugs, the nurse needs to list all medications that the client takes (birth control pills, diuretics, vitamins, anticonvulsants, insulin, etc.). Certain medications, such as anticonvulsants and insulin, must be continued throughout the operative period to prevent adverse effects. A physician's order to this effect is required, however.

Smoking habits. The lung tissue of a person who smokes is chronically irritated, and a general anesthetic irritates it further. When possible, nurses should discourage clients from smoking on the day of surgery and be alert for respiratory complications following surgery.

Use of alcohol. Moderate use of alcohol does not usually present a surgical hazard; but heavy, consistent use can lead to problems during anesthesia, surgery, and recovery.

Coping resources. Because surgery is a stressful experience it is important that nurses assess a client's individual coping resources. A client who has had previous surgery may be able to describe how she or he coped with that surgery. Diversional activities such as reading and relaxation exercises may be helpful. See Chapter 17 for more information about stress and coping methods. Family members and friends often provide considerable support to the surgical client. They need to be recognized and often included in explanations and in health instruction or follow-up care.

Self-concept. A client with a healthy, positive self-concept is most likely to approach a surgical experience with confidence that she or he can handle it successfully. A client with a negative self-concept may view surgery as a tremendous hurdle and may doubt her or his ability to handle it.

Body image. A client's image of her or his body can be of concern prior to surgery. A scar can be devastating to the person who prizes physical appearance; to another person a scar may be of no consequence. Some clients believe surgical intervention will affect their sexuality. For example, a client whose breast is to be removed may believe she will no longer be sexually attractive to her partner; or a man about to undergo a prostatectomy may believe that sexual intercourse will be impossible after surgery. It is important that such concerns be expressed. Providing accurate information, e.g., about a prostectomy, will often allay fears based on misconceptions. In addition, talking about their concerns often helps a client put them in perspective and enables the nurse to provide support during the perioperative period.

Physical Health Examination

If surgery is elective or optional, a physical examination is usually done in the physician's office prior to admission to the agency; however, it is done on admission before emergency surgery. In some settings, nurses perform a physical health examination. For information about physical health examinations, see Chapter 35. Knowledge of the client's overall health is essential in preventing complications and reducing surgical risk.

Common health problems that increase surgical risk and may lead to the decision to postpone or cancel surgery include the following.

1. Conditions such as angina pectoris, recent myocardial infarction, severe hypertension, and severe congestive heart failure. Well-controlled cardiac problems generally pose minimal operative risk.
2. Blood coagulation problems that may lead to severe bleeding, hemorrhage, and subsequent shock.
3. Upper respiratory tract infections or chronic obstructive lung diseases, such as emphysema. These conditions, especially when exacerbated by the effects of a general anesthetic, adversely affect pulmonary function. They also predispose the client to postoperative lung infections.
4. Renal disease that impairs the regulation of the body's fluids and electrolytes, e.g., renal insufficiency.
5. Diabetes mellitus, which predisposes the client to wound infection and delayed healing.
6. Liver disease, such as cirrhosis, which impairs the liver's abilities to: detoxify medications used during surgery; produce the prothrombin necessary for blood clotting; and metabolize nutrients essential for healing.
7. Uncontrolled neurologic disease, such as epilepsy.

Screening Tests

The physician is responsible for ordering all the radiologic and laboratory tests and examinations the client needs. The nurse's responsibility is to check the orders carefully, to see that they are carried out, and to ensure that the results are obtained prior to surgery. Screening tests conducted prior to surgery include the following.

1. *Chest roentgenography,* to determine the condition of the client's lungs and in some situations heart size and location. The results may influence the physician's choice of both the preoperative sedation and the anesthetic.
2. *Blood analysis,* on the day before surgery when possible. Analysis may include: red blood cell count (RBC), hemoglobin (Hb or Hgb), and hematocrit (Hct). If substantial blood loss is anticipated during surgery, the physician may order a blood typing and cross-match and sufficient units of blood for a replacement transfusion. When the physician anticipates bleeding problems, an analysis of bleeding time, clotting time, or prothrombin time may also be ordered. The results of blood tests are important in ruling out many problems that could increase the surgical risk. For example, a high white blood cell count (WBC) may signal an infection; a low RBC or low hemoglobin may indicate anemia. Both conditions can delay healing. Other blood tests usually routinely included are fasting blood sugar, blood urea nitrogen, and creatinine.
3. *Urine analysis* for all clients before surgery. The results may indicate urinary infection, diabetes, or other abnormalities that warrant treatment prior to surgery.
4. *Electrocardiogram* for all middle-age and elderly clients and for clients suspected of having cardiac disease (LeMaitre and Finnegan 1980, p. 54). See Table 53–3 for routine preoperative screening tests.

In addition to these routine tests, diagnostic tests directly related to the client's pathology are usually appropriate (e.g., stomach roentgenography to clarify the pathology before gastric surgery). See Chapter 54.

Records and Reports

The surgeon has usually indicated the type of surgery in the preoperative orders on the client's chart. From this information, the nurse determines the kind and extent of skin preparation required (if not already specified on the order) and the teaching needed. Agencies often have protocols to follow regarding skin preparation areas and some aspects of perioperative care. Special surgeon's orders, such as an enema or the insertion of a catheter or Levin tube, are given before certain surgeries, e.g., "Saline enema the night before surgery."

Nursing Diagnosis

Examples of nursing diagnoses for the surgical client are given to the right. Because surgery can both directly and indirectly involve many body systems and is a complex experience for a client, the nursing diagnoses focus on a wide variety of problems the client may encounter postoperatively.

Examples of Nursing Diagnoses for the Surgical Client

- Knowledge deficit about need for leg exercises
- Anxiety related to perceived inability to deal with possible pain
- Alterations in respiratory functions related to smoking
- Alterations in thought process related to fear of the unknown
- Potential skin impairment related to immobility secondary to surgery
- Sleep pattern disturbance related to hospitalization
- Disturbance in self-concept related to surgery
- Potential ineffective breathing patterns related to pain secondary to surgery
- Potential fluid volume deficit related to decreased fluid intake secondary to surgery

Planning

Planning for the perioperative period should involve the client, support persons, and the nurse. The following are essential nursing responsibilities.

1. Identify and meet the client's and support persons' learning needs.
2. Promote the client's peace of mind.
3. Meet fluid and nutritional needs, or correct nutritional deficiencies.
4. Promote rest.
5. Reduce the number of skin microorganisms and potential for postoperative infection.
6. Prevent bowel or bladder incontinence during anesthesia.
7. Prevent aspiration of vomitus and respiratory obstruction by oral prostheses during anesthesia.
8. Prevent physical trauma to the client during anesthesia.
9. Protect the client's personal property during the intraoperative period.
10. Ensure that the client's physical status (e.g., circulation) can be assessed appropriately during the intraoperative period.

Planning also involves the establishment of outcome criteria. For suggested examples, see the later section on "Evaluation," page 1631.

The duration of the preoperative period often affects preoperative care and planning. When the preoperative period lasts several days, nurses can draw up a nursing care plan and a teaching plan. See Chapter 29. When the preoperative period is just an hour, only the essentials can be carried out. In this case the learning needs of the client must be met during the postoperative period.

The Association of Operating Room Nurses' outcome standards for perioperative nursing are given on page 1603.

Preoperative Intervention

Explanation of Perioperative Care

An explanation of perioperative care includes informing the client and her or his support persons about the perioperative period. Usually people are anxious at this time, and many have misconceptions about surgery and surgical care. The surgeon has the responsibility of obtaining an informed consent from the client. See Chapter 7, page 163, and "Legal Aspects of Surgery" earlier in this chapter.

Informed Consent: The surgeon is responsible for determining the surgical procedure and obtaining the client's written permission for it. The nurse is responsible for witnessing the informed consent, including the exchange between the client and the surgeon and the client's affixing of signature. The nurse is also responsible for establishing that the client was truly informed. (Northrop 1984, p. 223)

Clients often ask nurses about the operation after the surgeon has gained informed consent and left the client's room. If the client is anxious about the procedure or has questions about the surgery that are unrelated to the nurse, the surgeon should be notified.

The client also may have specific learning needs regarding postoperative care. For example, learning to attend to a colostomy or the like requires preparation *before* surgery.

Pain is common postoperatively, and clients are reassured to learn *beforehand* how to minimize it (e.g., by holding a pillow against the abdomen when moving after abdominal surgery). It also is important that clients know they will receive analgesics postoperatively to minimize discomfort. Most surgical clients need to learn how to move, breathe deeply, cough, and do leg exercises after surgery. These are discussed later in the chapter.

Clients and their support persons need to know the time and type of surgery. The surgeon usually arranges the date and may specify it in the orders. The exact time may not be known until the surgical schedule for the hospital is distributed. When a nurse does not know the exact time of surgery this lack of information should be explained to the client, and when the time becomes known the client and support persons should be told.

It is important to listen attentively and carefully to the client to help him or her identify specific concerns or fears and talk them through. Typical questions are: What will happen during surgery? How will I feel after the operation? What will the surgeon find? How long will the hospital stay be? Some clients may worry about finances. Those whose surgery involves disfigurement of some kind may have problems with their self-image.

This is also the time to clarify any misconceptions the client may have. Providing accurate information and acting supportively will help the client deal with identified concerns. Do not dismiss the client's concerns by saying, "Everything will be all right." Unknowns or misconceptions can produce unrealistic fears and anxiety.

Outcome Standards for Perioperative Nursing

- The client demonstrates knowledge of the physiologic and psychologic responses to surgery.
- The client is free from infection.
- The client's skin integrity is maintained.
- The client is free from injury related to positioning, extraneous objects, or chemical, physical, and electrical hazards.
- The client's fluid and electrolyte balance is maintained.
- The client participates in the rehabilitation process.

(AORN 1986)

Table 53–3 Routine Preoperative Screening Tests

Test	Rationale
Urinalysis	To detect urinary tract infections and glucose in the urine
Chest roentgenography	To identify lung pathology and heart size and location
Electrocardiography (usual for clients who have cardiac pathology)	To determine cardiac pathology
Complete blood count (CBC)	To determine Hgb, Hct, RBC (i.e., the blood's ability to carry oxygen), and WBC, which signals infection when elevated
Blood grouping and cross-matching	To establish blood type for possible blood transfusion
Serum electrolytes (Na^+, K^+, Mg^{2+}, Ca^{2+}, H^+)	To determine electrolyte imbalances
Fasting blood sugar	To detect the presence of glucose in the blood, which may indicate metabolic disorders, e.g., diabetes mellitus
Blood urea nitrogen (BUN) or creatinine	To assess urinary excretion

When children are involved, the nurse should provide explanations in a language they can understand and at a rate that keeps their attention and does not overwhelm them. It will also help to show the child the anesthetic equipment and the postanesthesia room ("wake-up room") before surgery, explaining all postoperative care and discomfort clearly and simply, for example, "You will have a sore tummy." Confirm when the parents will visit, because this is the most essential piece of information the nurse can give the child (Luciano 1974, p. 65).

Preoperative Teaching

Preoperative teaching includes moving, leg exercises, and coughing and deep-breathing exercises. See Procedure 53–1.

Procedure 53–1 ▲ Teaching Moving, Leg Exercises, and Coughing and Deep-Breathing Exercises

Intervention

Moving

After surgery, turning in bed and early ambulation are encouraged to help clients maintain blood circulation, stimulate respiratory functions, and decrease the stasis of gas in the intestines (and its resulting discomfort). Clients who practice turning before surgery usually find it easier to do postoperatively.

1. Show the client ways to turn in bed and ways to get out of bed. Have the client start from the supine position.
   a. Instruct a client who will have a right abdominal incision or a right-sided chest incision to turn to the left side of the bed and sit up as follows:
      - Flex the knees.
      - Hold the left arm and hand or a small pillow against the incision to splint the wound.
      - Turn to the left while pushing with the right foot and grasping the side rail on the left side of the bed with the right hand.
      - Raise himself or herself to a sitting position on the side of the bed by using the right arm and hand to push down against the mattress.
   b. For a client with a left abdominal or left-sided chest incision, reverse the procedure.
   c. For clients with orthopedic surgery (e.g., hip surgery), use special aids, such as a trapeze to assist with movement.

Leg Exercises

2. Teach the client the following three exercises, which contract and relax the quadriceps muscles (vastus intermediatius, vastus lateralis, rectus femoris, and vastus medialis) and the gastrocnemius muscles (see Figure 53–3).
   a. Alternate dorsiflexion and plantar flexion of the feet. This exercise is sometimes referred to as *calf pumping,* since it alternately contracts and relaxes the calf muscles, including the gastrocnemius muscles.
   b. Flex and extend the knees, and press the backs of the knees into the bed. See Figure 53–4. Clients

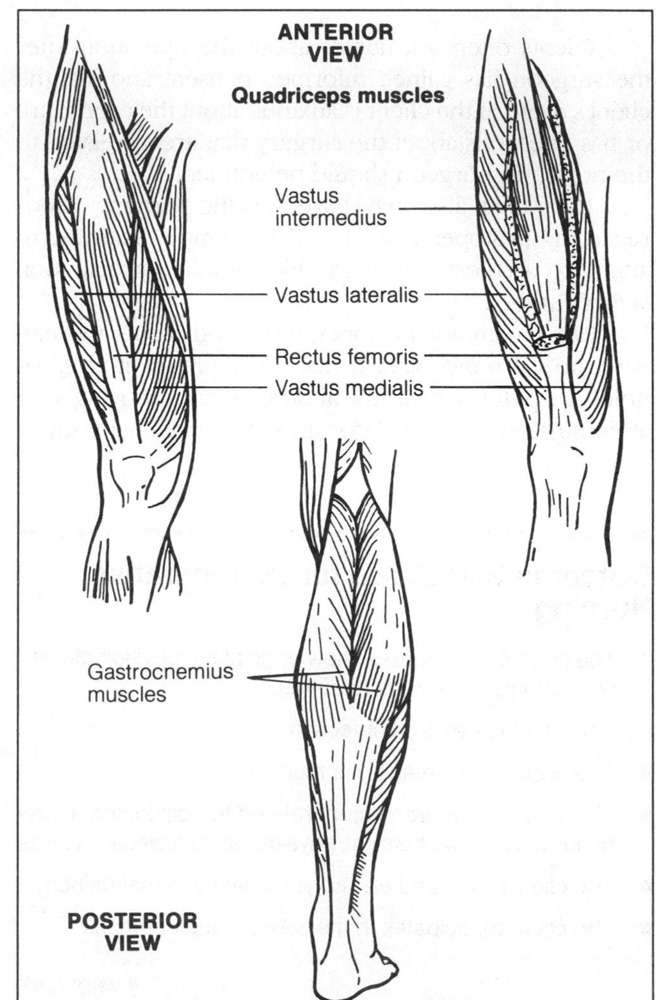

Figure 53–3

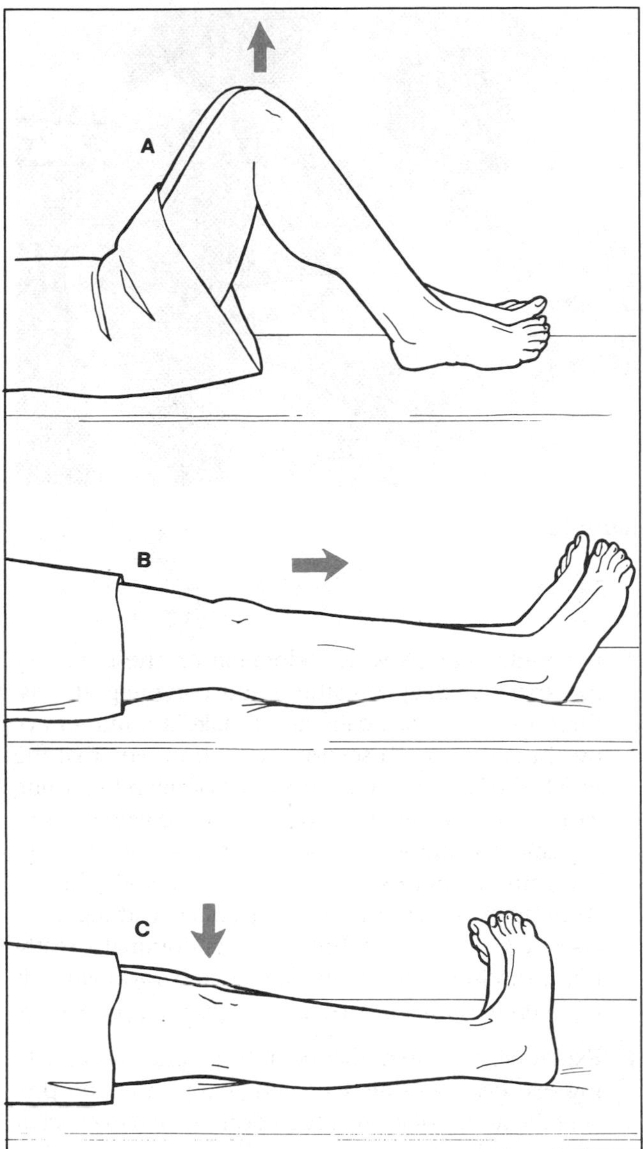

Figure 53–4

who cannot raise their legs can do isometric exercises that contract and relax the muscles (see Chapter 37, page 1000).

c. Raise and lower the legs alternately from the surface of the bed. Extend the knee of the moving leg. See Figure 53–5. This exercise contracts and relaxes the quadriceps muscles.

Rationale Leg exercises help prevent thrombophlebitis due to slowed venous circulation (venous stasis). The major danger of thrombophlebitis is that thrombi can become emboli and lodge in the arteries of the heart, brain, or lungs, causing serious injury or death.

3. Instruct the client to start exercising as soon after surgery as she or he is able.

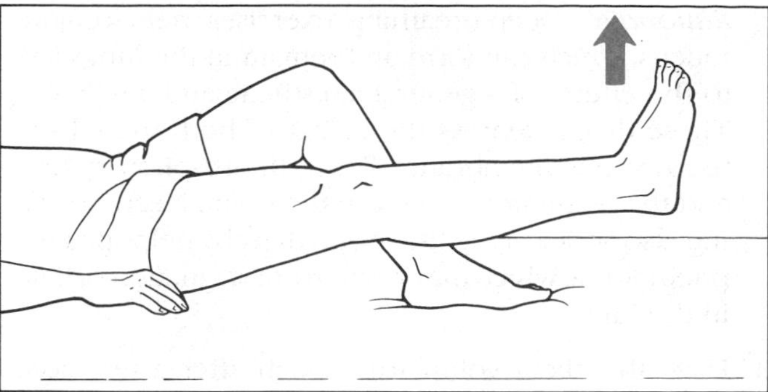

Figure 53–5

4. Encourage the client to do exercises at least once every waking hour. Note, however, that the frequency of exercising depends on the client's condition and the agency's practices.
5. Explain to the client that these muscle contractions will compress the veins and promote venous circulation.

Coughing and Deep-Breathing Exercises

6. Demonstrate deep (diaphragmatic) breathing exercises as follows:
   a. Place your hands palm down on the border of your rib cage, and inhale slowly and evenly through the nose until the greatest chest expansion is achieved. See Figure 53–6.
   b. Hold your breath for 2 to 3 seconds.
   c. Exhale slowly through the mouth.
   d. Continue exhalation until maximum chest contraction is achieved.
7. Have the client assume a sitting position and perform deep-breathing exercises while placing the palms of your hands on the border of the client's rib cage.

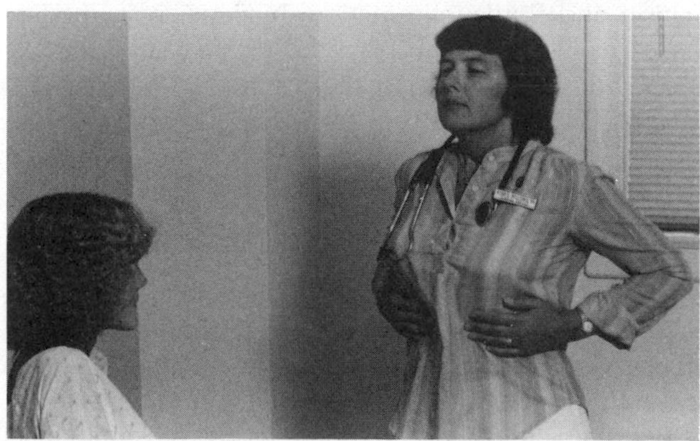

Figure 53–6

Rationale Deep-breathing exercises help remove mucus, which can form and remain in the lungs due to the effects of a general anesthetic and analgesics. These drugs depress the action of both the cilia of the mucous membranes lining the respiratory tract and the respiratory center in the brain. Deep breathing also aerates lung tissue and thereby helps prevent pneumonia, which may result from stagnation of fluid in the lungs.

8. Have the client voluntarily cough after a few deep inhalations. Have the client inhale deeply, hold the breath for a few seconds, and then cough one or two times. Make sure the client coughs deeply and does not just clear the throat. Splinting the abdomen with clasped hands and a pillow held against the abdomen helps coughing be effective.

   Rationale Deep breathing frequently initiates the coughing reflex. Voluntary coughing in conjunction with deep breathing facilitates the movement and expectoration of respiratory tract secretions.

9. If the client will have an incision that will be painful when coughing, demonstrate how the nurse or client can support (splint) it as the client coughs. Place the palms of your hands on either side of the incision or directly over the incision, holding the palm of one hand over the other. Also instruct the client with an abdominal incision how to splint the incision independently with a firmly rolled pillow. See Figure 53–7.

   Rationale Coughing uses the abdominal and other accessory respiratory muscles. Splinting the incision may reduce pain while coughing if the incision is near any of these muscles.

10. Instruct the client to start the exercises as soon after surgery as he or she is able.

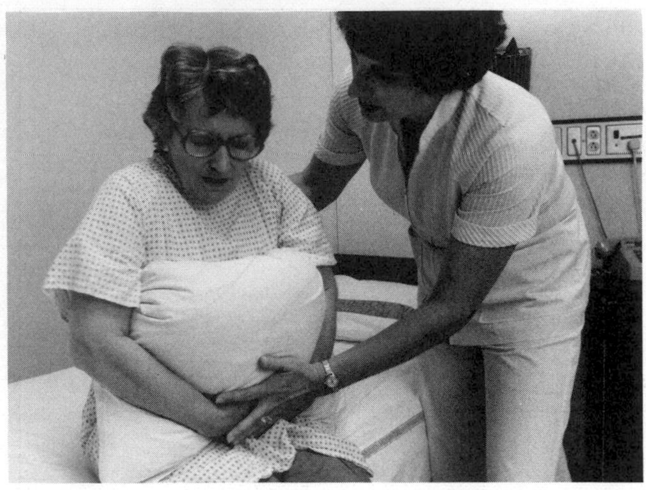

Figure 53–7

11. Encourage clients with abdominal or chest surgery to carry out deep breathing and coughing at least three or four times daily and to take a minimum of five breaths at each session. Note, however, that the number of breaths and frequency of deep breathing varies with the client's condition. Those who are susceptible to pulmonary problems may need deep-breathing exercises every hour. Those with chronic respiratory disease may need special breathing exercises, e.g., pursed-lip breathing, abdominal breathing, exercises using blow bottles and various kinds of incentive spirometers. See Chapter 45, page 1303.

12. Explain to the client that deep-breathing and coughing exercises will increase lung expansion and prevent the accumulation of secretions, which may occur after anesthesia.

Preoperative Preparation

Preoperative preparation includes the following areas: nutrition and fluids, elimination, hygiene, rest, medications, care of valuables and prostheses, surgical skin preparation, vital signs, and special orders.

Nutrition and Fluids

Adequate hydration and nutrition promote healing. Nurses need to record any sign of malnutrition. A perioperative record of the client's weight is one way to determine one aspect of nutritional status. If the client is on intravenous fluids or on measured fluid intake, nurses must ensure that the fluids are carefully measured. See Chapter 46.

Because anesthetics depress gastrointestinal functioning and because there is a danger the client may vomit and aspirate vomitus during administration of a general anesthetic, the client usually fasts at least 6 to 8 hours before surgery. The surgical client and support persons need to understand the necessity of fasting. Usually, the nurse removes food and fluids from the bedside and places a fasting sign at the bed the evening before surgery. The client can use a mouthwash if her or his mouth feels dry but must not swallow any. If the client ingests food or fluids during the fasting period, the nurse must notify the surgeon.

Elimination

The nurse should ascertain whether the client has emptied her or his bowels and bladder the day of surgery. If an enema is ordered, the order will specify whether it should be given the evening prior to or the day of surgery. If it is ordered for the day of surgery, it should be administered soon enough on that day so the client has time to expel it. A series of enemas may be needed if surgery on the bowel is planned. Sometimes a rectal suppository is ordered instead of an enema. An enema or suppository is given because anesthesia and abdominal surgery decrease bowel activity for a few days postoperatively.

If a retention catheter is ordered, this is usually inserted the day of surgery. The purpose of the catheter is to ensure that the bladder remains empty, to prevent inadvertent injury to the bladder, particularly during pelvic surgery.

Hygiene

Nurses may assist the client with a complete or partial bath. In some settings clients are asked to have a bath or shower using an antimicrobial agent the evening or morning of surgery (or both). The bath includes a shampoo whenever possible. The client's nails should be trimmed and free of polish, and all cosmetics should be removed, so the nail beds, skin, and lips are visible when assessing circulation during and following surgery.

Antiemboli stockings and surgical caps are donned the day of surgery by clients in some hospitals. Antiemboli stockings compress the peripheral veins and increase venous return during the inactive period, thereby preventing the formation of thrombi or emboli. See later in this chapter, page 1625. The surgical caps are to contain the client's hair and any microorganisms on the hair and scalp.

On the day of surgery it is important to remove, or ask the client to remove, all hair pins and clips. Long hair can be braided and fastened with elastic bands to keep it in place. Hair pins and clips may cause pressure or accidental damage to the scalp when the client is unconscious.

Rest

Nurses should do everything to help the client sleep the night before surgery. See Chapter 40. Adequate rest helps the client manage the stress of surgery.

Medications

The nurse should check the preoperative medications the evening prior to surgery. Often a sedative is ordered to help the client get a good sleep. Preoperative medications also may be ordered for the day of surgery. Usually a narcotic (e.g., morphine) and a medication to dry the secretions of the mouth and respiratory tract (e.g., atropine) are given by injection. Sometimes the surgeon orders oral sedatives (e.g., secobarbital) or tranquilizers to be administered before the injectable medications are given. A newer trend is to give *no* preoperative medications. It is essential to administer preoperative medications, if ordered, exactly at the time specified.

A narcotic, sedative, or tranquilizer calms the client before general anesthesia and enhances a smooth anesthesia induction. Atropine or a similar drying drug minimizes the danger of aspirating secretions into the lungs. Giving preoperative medications on time is essential because of their desired effect in combination with the anesthetic.

After giving the preoperative medications, inform the client that the medication will cause drowsiness and instruct him or her to remain quietly in bed. Raise the side rails and lower the bed for safety. Place the call light within reach. Also, explain that scopalomine or atropine may cause thirst and that although a mouth wash may be used, he or she must not have anything to drink.

Valuables and Prostheses

Valuables such as jewelry and money should be labeled and placed in safekeeping if support persons cannot take them home. In most hospitals valuables can be kept in special envelopes and locked in a storage area on the unit. If a client wishes not to remove a wedding band, the nurse can tape it in place. Wedding bands must be removed, however, if there is danger of the fingers swelling after surgery. Situations warranting removal of a wedding band include surgery of or cast application to an arm and a mastectomy that involves removal of the lymph nodes. Mastectomies may cause edema of the arm and hand.

All prostheses (artificial body parts, such as partial or complete dentures, contact lenses, artificial eyes, and artificial limbs), as well as eyeglasses, wigs, false eyelashes, and hearing aids, must be removed before surgery. Also, check for the presence of chewing gum or loose teeth, a common problem with 5- or 6-year-olds having tonsils removed. In some hospitals dentures are placed in a locked storage area; in others they are kept at the client's bedside. Partial dentures can become dislodged and obstruct an unconscious client's breathing. Loose teeth can become dislodged and be aspirated during anesthesia. Other prostheses may become damaged.

Surgical Skin Preparation

The purpose of preparing the skin before surgery (preoperative skin preparation) is to destroy microorganisms and thus reduce the chance of infection.

It is recommended that the hair near the operative site not be removed unless absolutely necessary. In some agencies the client's skin is "prepped" in a special room just before surgery. The Centers for Disease Control recommend, if hair must be removed, that it be clipped or a depilatory used and the area cleansed with antimicrobials just before surgery (Garner 1986, p. 77).

The area prepared is generally larger than the incision area. This practice minimizes the number of microorganisms in the areas adjacent to the incision. Hospital policy describes how the skin is prepared before various operations.

The Association of Operating Room Nurses recommends that hair removal only be done as necessary. Studies have shown that the method of hair removal affects skin infection rates. One study showed an infection rate of 2.5% in clients shaved with an electric razor, whereas clients neither clipped nor shaved had an infection rate of 0.9% (Cruse and Foord 1980, pp. 27–40).

Studies also have shown that the amount of time between the preoperative shave and the operation has a direct effect on the infection rate (Association of Operating Room Nurses 1986, p. 111:9-1). One study found a postsurgical infection rate of 3.1% when the shave was done immediately prior to surgery, whereas it was 7.4% when done within 24 hours of surgery and 20% when it was done more than 24 hours in advance of surgery (Seropian and Reynolds 1971, pp. 251–54).

Prior to any skin preparation it is important to carefully inspect the prospective surgical area for growths, moles, rashes, pustules, irritations, exudate, abrasions, bruises or any broken or ischemic areas. These should be recorded and reported to the surgeon. In addition, the nurse must determine whether the client is allergic to any of the solutions used in the skin preparation, e.g., iodine in the antiseptic.

The details of preparing a client's skin for surgery are given in Procedure 53–2.

Procedure 53–2 ▲ Surgical Skin Preparation

Equipment

1. Adequate lighting for clear visibility of the hair on the skin
2. A bath blanket to drape the client

Clipping

3. Electric clippers with sharp heads and unbroken teeth
4. Scissors for long hair, if needed
5. Antimicrobial solution and applicators, if needed

Wet Shave (not recommended by CDC, 1986)

6. Skin preparation set, which contains a disposable razor, compartmentalized basin for solutions, moisture-proof drape to protect the bedding, soap solution, sponges for applying the soap solution, and cotton-tipped applicators for cleaning areas such as the umbilicus
7. Warm water to make the soap solution

Intervention

Before Clipping

1. Drape the client. Expose only the area to be clipped at one time. You will clip about 15 cm (6 in) at a time.

Clipping

2. Make sure the area is dry.
3. Remove hair with clippers; do not apply pressure.

   Rationale Pressure can cause abrasions, particularly over bony prominences.
4. Move the drape, and repeat steps 2 and 3 until the entire area to be prepared is clipped. If applying antimicrobial solution, follow the steps in the section below on "Cleaning and Disinfecting."

Wet Shaving

5. Place the moisture-proof towel under the area to be prepared.
6. Lather the skin well with the soap solution.

   Rationale One research study showed that soaking the skin hair in lather for 4 minutes allows the keratin to absorb water and thereby makes the hair easier and softer to remove (Tkach et al. 1979).
7. Stretch the skin taut and hold the razor at about a 45° angle to the skin. Shave in the direction in which the hair grows. Use short strokes and rinse the razor frequently.

   Rationale Rinsing removes hairs and lather that can obstruct the blade.
8. Wipe excess hair off the skin with the sponges.
9. Move the drape and repeat steps 6–8 until the entire area to be prepared is shaved.

Cleaning and Disinfecting

10. Clean any body crevices, such as the umbilicus, nails, and ear canals, with applicators and solutions. Dry with swabs.
11. If an antimicrobial solution is used, apply to the area immediately after it is clipped. Leave it for the designated time, then dry the area with clean swabs. Agency policy will guide you on whether to use an antimicrobial solution and, if so, which to use and how long to leave it on.

After Clipping

12. After clipping, the skin preparation may need to be checked by the responsible nurse. Report to the responsible nurse any abrasions, including those made by the clippers or razor.
13. Remove the waterproof towel and bath blanket carefully so as not to spill the clipped hairs onto the bed.
14. Record the skin preparation on the client's chart.

Sample Recording

Date	Time	Notes
Dec/5/87	0830	Hair clipped on left lower extremity. Skin intact. Appeared tense. Stated: "I hope the scar won't show much."———Eunice L. Lentz, NS

Vital Signs

Take vital signs to obtain comparative baseline data against which to assess the client's responses during and following surgery. Because any abnormality can cause postponement of surgery, report promptly abnormalities in any of these signs—e.g., an elevated temperature—to the responsible nurse and to the surgeon.

Special Orders

Check the surgeon's orders for special requirements, such as the insertion of a nasogastric tube prior to surgery or the administration of medications, such as insulin. For the technique of inserting and removing a nasogastric tube see Procedure 53–3.

Recording

In most agencies, personnel use a preoperative checklist to record interventions. See Figure 53–8. Check the agency's forms, and follow appropriate recording procedures. It is essential that all pertinent records (laboratory records, x-ray films, consents, etc.) be assembled and completed so that operating and recovery room personnel can refer to them.

Transferring the Client to Surgery

When the operating room transport person arrives for the client, carefully check the client's identification bracelet against his or her chart. Generally, one staff member reads the identifying data from the bracelet while another checks it against the client's record. Do not rely on a drowsy client to identify himself or herself.

Gastric Intubation

Gastric intubation is the insertion of a tube into the stomach, through either the nose, the mouth, or a gastrostomy opening. A **nasogastric tube** can be passed through either the mouth or the nose; however, the nose is preferred because there is less discomfort from the gag reflex. A tube passed through the mouth is often called an **orogastric tube**.

Several types of nasogastric tubes are used for irrigation and gastric decompression. *Gastric decompression* is the reduction of the pressure within the stomach, e.g., by removal of the gastric contents. The **Levin tube** is commonly used for nasogastric intubation. It is a flexible, rubber or plastic, single-lumen tube with holes near the tip. See Figure 53–9, *A*. Inserting a Levin tube is often the nurse's responsibility. The **Salem sump tube**, also frequently used, is a nasogastric tube with a double lumen.

Some tubes pass through the client's mouth or nose, through the stomach and into the intestines. Physicians and nurse-specialists usually insert such tubes. The **Miller-Abbott tube** is a double-lumen tube; one lumen leads to a balloon near the tip, and the other lumen leads to the end of the tube opening into the intestine. See Figure 53–9, *B*. This tube is inserted into the small intestine, usually (a) to obtain secretions for diagnostic study or (b) for irrigation. The external end of the tube has a metal adapter with two openings. One inflates or deflates the balloon; the other drains intestinal secretions. The **Cantor tube** is a single-lumen tube with an inflatable bag at the tip and several holes along the distal end. See Figure 53–9, *C*. The bag is filled with mercury before the tube is inserted. The weight of the mercury causes the tube to move into the intestines. The **Harris tube**, a single-lumen tube with a metal tip, is used for irrigations and suctions of the small intestines. See Figure 53–9, *D*.

The main reasons for inserting a gastric tube are:

1. To prevent nausea, vomiting, and gastric distention following surgery
2. To provide a route for feeding the client
3. To remove stomach contents for laboratory analysis
4. To lavage the stomach in cases of poisoning or overdose of medications

Procedure 53–3 gives detailed steps for gastric intubation.

Form NS-68

ST. PAUL'S HOSPITAL
Vancouver, B.C.

PRE-OPERATIVE PREPARATION

EVENING PRIOR TO SURGERY—CHECK	Yes	Not Applicable
1. History—completed with signature		
2. Consultation (when necessary) on chart		
3. Treatment and operative consents—signed and witnessed		
4. Telephone no. of next of kin or friend:		
5. Identaband on wrist		
6. Allergy sign on chart and wristband		
7. Operative area prepared		
8. Pre-op bath or shower		
9. Pre-op teaching: a. Attended "Operation Tomorrow"		
b. Demonstrated deep breathing, coughing, and leg exercises		
c. Stated approximate time to OR and return to ward		
d. Stated expectations: • surgery planned		
• incision and dressing area		
• activity progression		
• pain and effect of analgesic		
• NPO, intravenous, diet progression		
• pre-op urine specimen		
e. Verbalized probable discharge plans		
10. H.S. sedation administered or refused—charted on anesthetic record		
11. Fasting sign posted		

DATE ________ SIGNATURE ________________

IMMEDIATELY PRIOR TO SURGERY	Yes	Not Applicable
1. Pre-operative urine specimen sent		
2. Reports attached to chart—Lab, X-ray, ECG		
3. Old chart		
4. Addressograph plate attached		
5. Contact lens, wig, jewelry, make-up removed, prosthesis off		
6. Dentures and partial plates removed		
7. Voided ______ Catheterized—time ______ amount ______		
8. Patient in hospital gown		
9. Blood pressure, pulse and respirations taken at least an hour prior to pre-op medication—charted on clinical record		
10. Pre-medication administered and charted on the anesthetic record		
11. Notation made in nurses notes of time to surgery		

DATE ________ SIGNATURE ________________

OPERATING ROOM	Yes	Not Applicable
1. Patient identified by circulating nurse		
2. Site of surgery checked by circulating nurse a. Left side ______ Right side ______		
b. Slate ______ Surgeon ______ History ______ Consent ______		

SIGNATURE ________________

Figure 53–8 A sample preoperative checklist
Source: Courtesy of St. Paul's Hospital, Nursing Department, Vancouver, British Columbia.

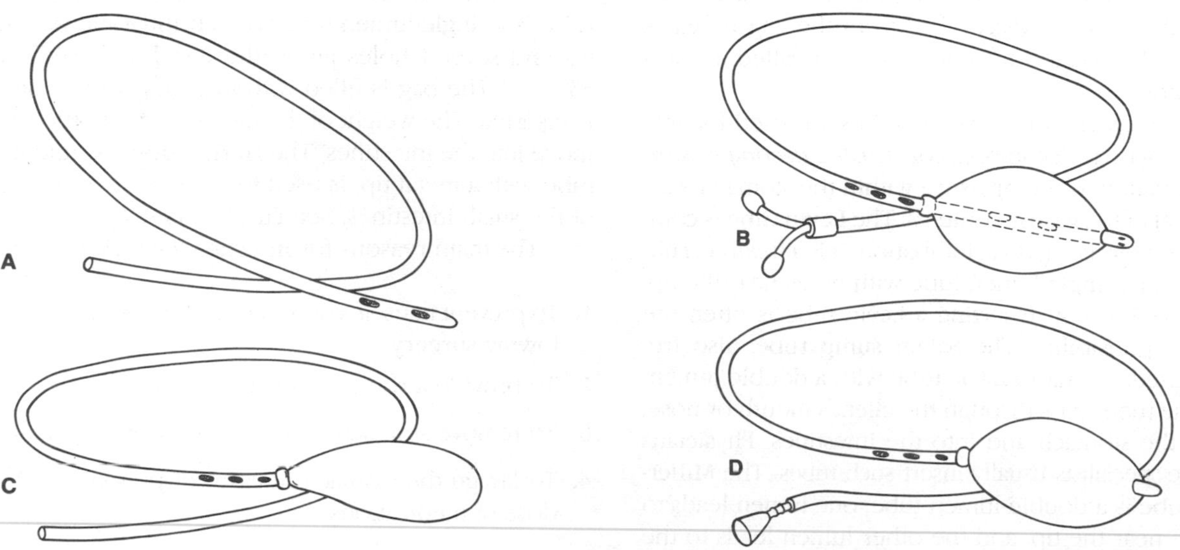

Figure 53–9 Four types of tubes used for gastric and intestinal suction and irrigations: **A,** Levin; **B,** Miller-Abbott; **C,** Cantor; **D,** Harris

Procedure 53–3 ▲ Inserting and Removing a Nasogastric Tube

Some clients, for instance, those having gastric or duodenal surgery, require the insertion of a Levin (gastric) tube preoperatively. The tube removes fluid and flatus from the stomach, thereby preventing nausea, vomiting, and distention due to reduced peristaltic action after surgery. In many agencies, insertion of a nasogastric tube is done by a registered nurse or a student with supervision. However, for the following clients the passing of the tube is the responsibility of the physician.

1. All unconscious clients
2. Confused or delirious clients
3. Clients who have abnormalities of or who have undergone surgery of the mouth or esophagus
4. Clients with gastric hemorrhage
5. Pre- or postoperative gastric surgery clients

Assessment

Assess the client for:

1. Any obstruction or deformities of the nostrils. Ask the client to hyperextend the head, and observe the nares, either with a flashlight or by asking the client to breathe through one nostril while occluding the other. Select the nostril that has the greatest air flow.
2. Intactness of the tissues of the nostrils, including any irritations or abrasions
3. Abdominal distention. Palpate the abdomen for hardness and swelling.

Other data include:

1. Whether the tube is to be attached to suction
2. The size of tube to be inserted

Equipment

1. A gastric tube (plastic or rubber)
2. A solution basin filled with warm water or ice. Rubber tubes are placed on ice to stiffen them for easier insertion. Plastic tubes are placed in warm water to make them more flexible for insertion.
3. A water-soluble lubricant
4. A 20- to 50-ml syringe with an adapter to attach to the tube, to withdraw stomach contents
5. A basin in which to collect gastric contents
6. Nonallergenic adhesive tape, 2.5 cm (1 in) wide, to secure the tube to the face
7. A clamp (optional) to close the tube after insertion
8. Suction apparatus, if ordered
9. A gauze square or a plastic specimen bag and an elastic band to cover the end of the tube
10. A safety pin and an elastic band to secure the nasogastric tube to the client's gown
11. A bib or towel to protect the client's gown
12. A glass of water and drinking straw to help the client swallow the tube
13. Facial tissues in case the client's eyes water during the procedure
14. A stethoscope to help assess placement of the tube

Intervention

Inserting a Nasogastric Tube

1. Explain to the client what you plan to do.

   Rationale The passage of a gastric tube is not painful, but it is unpleasant because the gag reflex is activated during insertion.

2. Assist the client to a high-Fowler's position, if health permits, and support the client's head on a pillow.

   Rationale It is often easier for the client to swallow in this position, and gravity helps the passage of the tube.

3. Hyperextend the client's head to examine the nostrils. Have the client breathe through each nostril while compressing the other nostril, to select the more patent one.

   Rationale The tube is inserted through the nostril that is more patent.

4. Determine how far to insert the tube in the following manner: Use the tube to mark off the distance from the tip of the client's nose to the tip of the earlobe and then from the tip of the earlobe to the tip of the sternum. See Figure 53–10. Mark this length with adhesive tape if the tube does not have markings.

   Rationale This length approximates the distance from the nares to the stomach. The distance varies among individuals.

5. Lubricate the tip of the tube well with water-soluble lubricant to ease insertion.

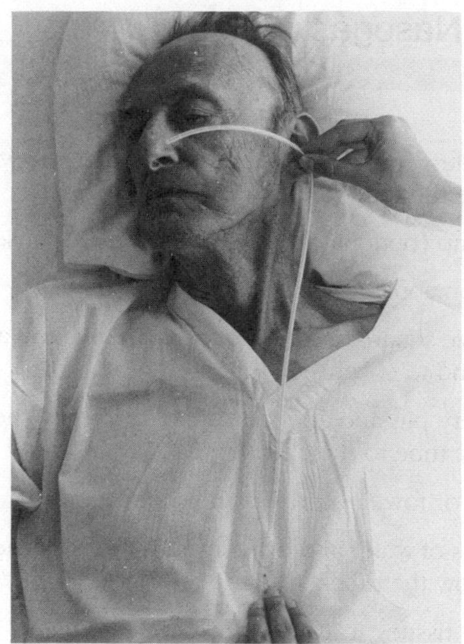

Figure 53–10

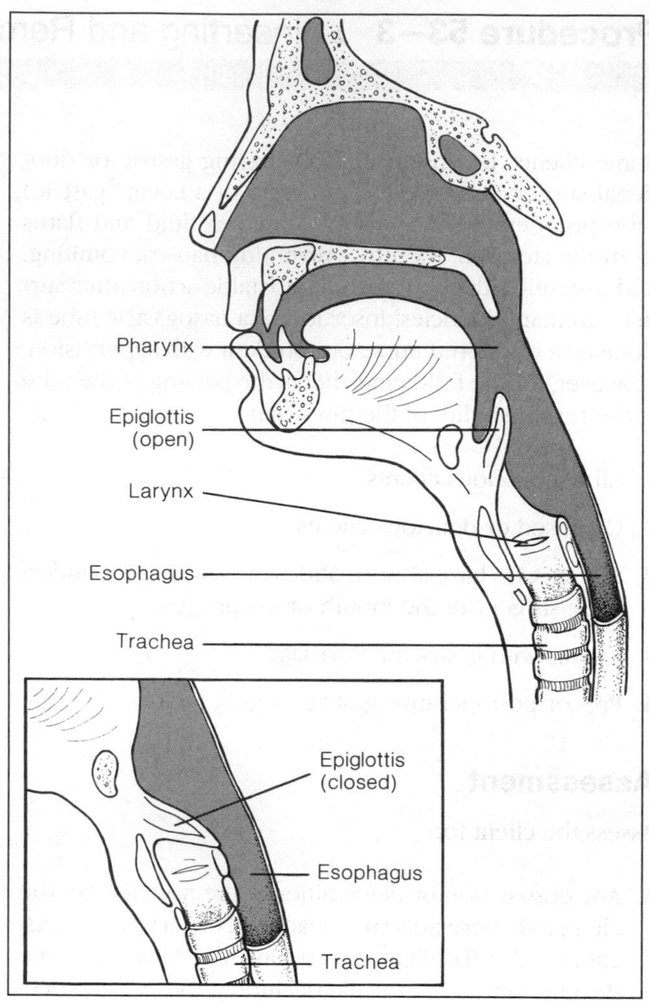

Figure 53–11

Rationale A water-soluble lubricant dissolves if the tube accidentally enters the lungs. An oil-based lubricant, such as petroleum jelly, will not dissolve and could cause respiratory complications if it enters the lungs.

6. Insert the tube, with its natural curve toward the client, into the selected nostril.

7. Have the client hyperextend his or her neck, and gently advance the tube toward the nasopharynx. Direct the tube along the floor of the nostril and toward the ear on that side. Provide tissues if the client's eyes water. If the tube meets resistance, withdraw it, relubricate it, and insert it in the other nostril.

   Rationale Hyperextension reduces the curvature of the nasopharyngeal junction. Directing the tube along the floor avoids the projections (turbinates) along the lateral wall. Slight pressure is sometimes required to pass the tube into the nasopharynx, and some clients' eyes may water at this point. Tears are a natural body response. The tube should never be forced against resistance because of the danger of injury.

8. Once the tube reaches the oropharynx (throat), have the client tilt the head forward and encourage him or her to drink and swallow. If the client gags, stop passing the tube momentarily. Have the client rest, take a few breaths, and take sips of water to calm the gag reflex.

   Rationale The client will feel the tube in his or her throat and may gag and retch. Tilting the head forward facilitates passage of the tube into the posterior pharynx and esophagus rather than into the larynx; swallowing moves the epiglottis over the opening to the larynx. See Figure 53–11.

9. In cooperation with the client, pass the tube 5 to 10 cm (2 to 4 in) with each swallow, until the indicated length is inserted. If the client continues to gag and the tube does not advance with each swallow, withdraw it slightly and inspect the client's throat by looking through the mouth.

   Rationale The tube may be coiled. If so, it is withdrawn until it is straight, and the nurse tries again to insert it.

10. Aspirate the stomach contents with a syringe to determine placement of the tube. See Table 53–4 for other methods.

    Rationale If fluid is removed, it is assumed that the tube is in the stomach. (Stomach contents are usually clear or yellow with mucus.)

11. If the signs do not indicate placement in the stomach, advance the tube 5 cm (2 in) and repeat the tests.

Table 53–4 Placement of a Nasogastric Tube

Nurse's Action	If Tube Is in the Stomach	If Tube Is in the Lungs
To Assess Placement		
Attach distal end of tube to syringe, and withdraw plunger.	Some gastric contents will fill tube.	No fluid will be in tube.
Other Indications of Placement		
Using a stethoscope, listen over the epigastric area of the abdomen while injecting 10 ml of air into tube.	Air will make a rushing sound.	There will be no sound.
Listen to distal end of tube.	There will be no sound.	There will be a crackling sound.
Ask conscious client to talk and hum.	Client will be able to talk and hum.	Client will be unable to talk or hum and will cough and/or choke.
Note unconscious client's skin color.	Color will be normal.	Client will be cyanotic.
Place end of tube in a glass of water while client exhales.	Few, if any, bubbles will appear in water.	Steady stream of bubbles will appear.

12. Secure the tube by taping it to the bridge of the client's nose.
    a. Cut 7.5 cm (3 in) of tape and split it at one end, leaving a 2.5-cm (1-in) tab at the end.
    b. Place the tape over the bridge of the client's nose, and bring the split ends under the tubing and back up over the nose.

    Rationale Taping in this manner prevents the tube from pressing against and irritating the edge of the nostril.

13. Attach the end of the tubing securely to suction, if ordered. See "Suction" later in this chapter.

    or

14. Clamp the end of the tubing and cover it with a gauze square or plastic specimen bag and an elastic band. If inserted preoperatively, the tube is usually clamped.
15. Attach the end of the tube to the client's gown by one of these two methods:
    a. Loop an elastic band around the end of the tubing and attach the elastic band to the gown with a safety pin.

    or

    b. Attach a piece of adhesive tape to the tube, and pin the tape to the gown. See Figure 53–12.

    Rationale The tube is attached to prevent it from dangling and pulling.

16. Record the insertion of the tube and the client's response (discomfort, etc.).
17. Establish a plan for providing daily nasogastric tube care, including:
    a. Inspecting the nostril for discharge and irritation
    b. Cleaning the nostril and tube with moistened, cotton-tipped applicators
    c. Apply water-soluble lubricant to the nostril if it appears dry or encrusted
    d. Changing the adhesive tape as required
    e. Giving frequent mouth care, since the client may breathe through the mouth and cannot drink
18. If suction is applied, ensure that the patency of both the nasogastric and suction tubes is maintained. Irrigations of the tube with 30 ml of normal saline may

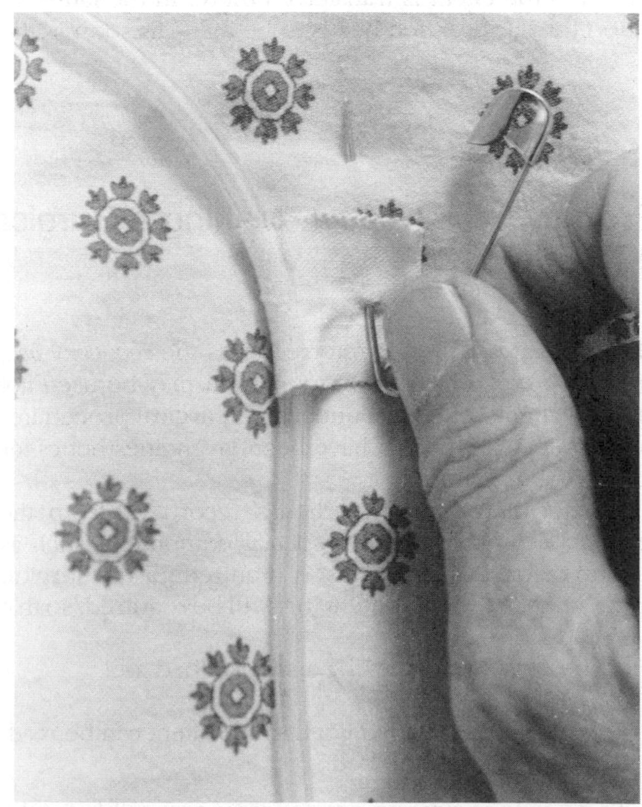

Figure 53–12

be required at regular intervals. In some agencies, irrigations must be ordered by the physician.

19. Keep accurate records of the client's liquid intake and output, and record the amount and characteristics of the drainage.

Removing a Nasogastric Tube

The removal of a nasogastric tube is ordered by a physician.

20. Turn off the suction, and disconnect the tube from suction apparatus.
21. Remove the adhesive tape securing the tube to the client's nose. Unpin the tube from the client's gown.
22. Have the client take a deep breath and hold it.
23. Steadily and quickly remove the tube while the client is holding breath.
24. Dispose of the tube in a bag.
25. Provide tissues for the client to blow his or her nose, and offer mouth wash if desired.
26. Remove the suction apparatus from the bedside. Measure the amount of fluid drained. Then empty and clean the drainage bottle.
27. Record the removal of the tube, the client's response, and the amount of fluid drained.

Preparing for the Postoperative Client

While the client is in the operating room the client's bed and room are prepared for the postoperative phase; that is, the surgical bed is made. See Procedure 53–4. In some agencies, the client is brought back to the unit on a stretcher and transferred to the bed in her or his room. At other agencies, the surgical bed is brought to the recovery room (RR), and the client is transferred there. In the latter situation the surgical bed needs to be made as soon as the client goes to the operating room so that it can be taken to the RR at any time. In addition, the nurse must obtain and set up special equipment as needed, such as an intravenous pole, suction, oxygen equipment, and orthopedic appliances (traction, etc.). If these are not requested on the client's record, the nurse should consult with the responsible nurse.

Procedure 53–4 ▲ Making a Surgical Bed

The surgical bed is also referred to as the *recovery bed, anesthetic bed,* or *postoperative bed.* It may be used not only for clients who have undergone surgical procedures but also for clients who have been given anesthetics for certain examinations.

Determine from the client's record or from the responsible nurse whether special equipment, such as suction or oxygen apparatus, is required for the surgical unit. Connect any equipment that will be required, so that it is ready for use.

The reasons for making a surgical bed are:

1. To arrange the top bed linen so the client can be readily transferred to the bed
2. To provide as clean an environment as possible for the client
3. To provide a bed foundation that can be changed quickly and easily if it becomes soiled
4. In some instances, to provide extra warmth through the use of flannelette sheets

Equipment

Though supplies vary from one agency to another, the following are generally needed:

1. Two clean sheets
2. A clean cotton drawsheet
3. A clean flannelette sheet for the foundation of the bed, if this is agency practice

4. A clean bedspread
5. A disposable incontinence or drainage pad (optional)

At some agencies these supplies are arranged in a surgical bundle.

Intervention

1. Place the supplies within easy reach and in the order in which they will be used.
2. Place and leave the pillows on the bedside chair.

   Rationale Pillows are not put onto the bed to facilitate transferring the client into the bed.
3. Arrange the furniture and equipment so there is room near the bed for a stretcher or room to move the bed out of the room if the bed is to be transported to the operating room.
4. Strip the bed according to Procedure 36–9 on page 955.
5. Make the foundation of the bed as shown in Procedure 36–9.
6. Place the flannelette sheet on the foundation of the bed, if this is needed.

   Rationale A flannelette sheet provides additional warmth.
7. Place a disposable pad for the client's head (optional).
8. Spread the top covers on the bed. Do *not* tuck them in, miter the corners, or make a toe pleat.
9. Fold the hanging edges of the top covers up over the top of the bed so the folds are at the mattress edge (fold the sides first, then the top and bottom). Then fanfold the covers in either of the following ways:
   a. Fanfold them lengthwise at one side of the bed. See Figure 53–13.

      or

   b. Fanfold them crosswise at the bottom of the bed. See Figure 53–14.

   Rationale The covers are fanfolded for ease in transferring the client into bed.
10. Lock the wheels of the bed if the bed is not to be moved, and leave the bed in the high position to meet the level of the stretcher.

    Rationale Locking the wheels keeps the bed from rolling. The high position facilitates the transfer of the client.
11. Notify appropriate people that the surgical bed is ready. In some hospitals, a porter service or the like takes the bed to the recovery room.
12. Place any additional equipment, e.g., suction, in readiness for use when the client returns from surgery.

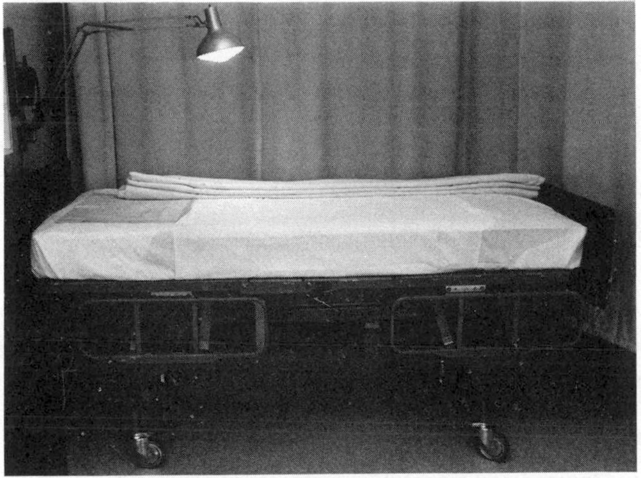

Figure 53–13

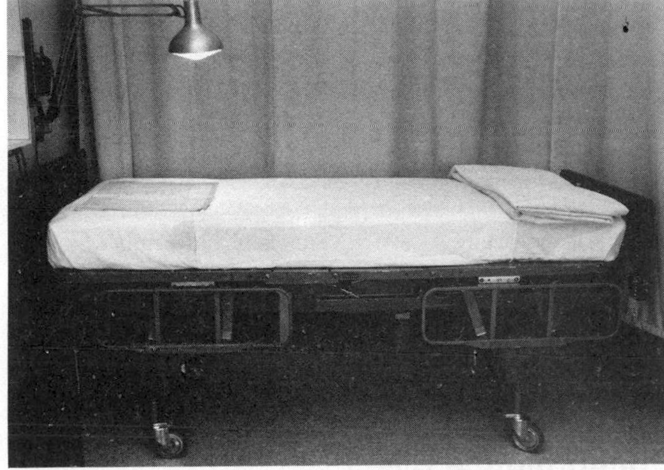

Figure 53–14

Some surgeons have postoperative routines requiring certain equipment. In some instances, nursing personnel in the RR will notify the nursing unit before the client's arrival if special equipment is required. A sphygmomanometer and cuff and a stethoscope must also be available. In some agencies, sphygmomanometers are attached to the wall at the head of the bed. The nurse should make sure that an intake and output record are nearby. When the client is returned to the unit, he or she is carefully assisted or lifted into the bed, if not already in it.

Intraoperative Phase

There are thousands of surgical procedures performed in hospitals. Some clients have *day surgery;* arriving at the hospital on the day of the operation and leaving that same day, after the operation. Other surgical procedures necessitate a longer hospital stay, from a few days to several weeks. The prefixes and suffixes of the names of surgical procedures help the student understand the nature of the operation. See Appendix B.

During the intraoperative phase, nurses in the operating room should protect the client from injury and infection, monitor the client, and maintain appropriate documentation.

Protecting the Client from Injury

The client who has had an anesthetic is vulnerable to injury because she or he is unaware of the surroundings and cannot protect herself or himself. For example, a client may be placed in any of a variety of positions to afford access to the operative area. However, the position should not impair the neuromuscular system or injure the skin. Because the client's operating position often is maintained for hours, some clients feel stiff and sore postoperatively. If a client's joint—e.g., hip—is extended further than normal range for that joint, the muscles surrounding it will be painful later and could be injured. The following should be considered when nurses are positioning clients in preparation for surgery.

1. Protect the client's skin from injury while moving and positioning him or her.

2. Maintain the client's position within the limits of any involved joint's range of motion.

3. Use appropriate safety devices, e.g., side rails of a gurney and safety straps.

4. Ensure that equipment that should be sterile is kept sterile. See basic aseptic technique to the right.

Monitoring the Client

Monitoring the client's physiologic responses is the responsibility of an anesthetist or anesthesiologist when one is present. However, when a client receives a local anesthetic from the surgeon and no anesthesiologist or anesthesist is present, a nurse is usually responsible for monitoring the client. "Each client should be monitored for reaction to drugs and for behavioral and physiological changes" (Association of Operating Room Nurses 1986, p. 111:16-1).

Maintaining Documentation

Documentation during the intraoperative phase includes the intraoperative record, which focuses on nursing interventions, often including notes about: sponges; instrument and needle counts; grounding location for the electrosurgical unit; monitors used; tourniquet location, times, and pressure set; implant and lot numbers; dressings; drains; specimens and cultures; medications; client position on the operating room table; and types of safety devices, e.g., hand restraints (Kneedler and Dodge 1983, p. 463).

Nursing Roles

During surgery there are usually two types of nurses, the scrub nurse and the circulating nurse. The scrub nurse is attired in a sterile gown, cap, mask, and gloves. The scrub nurse's responsibilities include:

1. Handing the surgeon sterile instruments and supplies from the sterile tray. Because many instruments are required during certain operations, a scrub nurse must have an extensive knowledge of all instruments and how they are used.

2. Counting sponges, needles, and instruments. Counting is done before the surgeon closes the incision so that none are left inside the client.

3. Disposing of used instruments.

The circulating nurse's responsibilities include:

1. Helping position the client on the operating room table

2. Helping drape the client, and assisting the surgeon and scrub nurse to don sterile gowns and gloves

Basic Aseptic Technique

- **All items used within a sterile field should be sterile.**
- **Gowns used by scrub persons should be sterile.**
- **Draped tables should be considered sterile only at table level.**
- **All personnel moving within or around a sterile field should do so in a manner consistent with maintaining the sterility of the field.**

(Association of Operating Room Nurses 1986, pp. 111:2-1–111:2-3)

3. Opening supply packages so the scrub nurse can remove the sterile supplies
4. Arranging for transfer of biopsy specimens to the laboratory
5. Adjusting operating room lights
6. Obtaining additional supplies and equipment

Postoperative Phase

Nursing during the postoperative phase is especially important for the client's recovery. An anesthetic impairs the ability of clients to respond to environmental stimuli and to help themselves, although the degree of consciousness of clients will vary. Moreover, surgery itself traumatizes the body by decreasing the body's energy and resistance. Nursing interventions include monitoring the client's cardiovascular status, fluid balance, and neurologic status; providing comfort and safety; encouraging mobility; and preventing complications. The postoperative phase can be divided into two stages: immediate postanesthetic stage and continuing postoperative stage.

Immediate Postanesthetic Stage

Immediate postanesthetic care is usually provided in a postanesthetic room (PAR), also referred to as the recovery room (RR). Recovery room nurses have specialized skills to care for clients recovering from anesthetics and surgery. Once a client's health status has stabilized, he or she is returned to the nursing unit, or in the case of a day-surgery client, to the day-surgery area before discharge.

Assessment

Recovery room care includes regular, systematic assessment of:

1. Dressings, tubes, and drains
2. Respiratory function
3. Cardiovascular function (circulation)
4. Fluid and electrolyte balance
5. Neurologic status
6. Pain
7. Safety

Dressings, tubes, and drains An unconscious client is positioned on his or her side, with the face slightly down. A pillow is not placed under the head. In this position, gravity keeps the tongue forward, preventing occlusion of the pharynx and allowing drainage of mucus or vomitus out of the mouth rather than down the respiratory tree. Maximum chest expansion is ensured by elevating the client's upper arm on a pillow. The upper arm is supported because the pressure of an arm against the chest reduces chest expansion potential. Once the client's reflexes return, she or he can usually assume a back-lying position. An artificial airway is maintained in place, and suction is supplied until reflexes for controlling coughing and swallowing return. Generally, the client spits out an oropharyngeal airway when coughing returns. Endotracheal tubes are not removed until the client is awake and able to maintain his or her own airway. Before removing any artificial airway, suction is applied to the airway and the pharynx. The client is then helped to turn, cough, and take deep breaths, provided vital signs are stable. See Chapter 45 for information about artificial airways.

Respiratory function A nurse must assess the rate, depth, and quality of respirations as well as the client's chest movements. See Chapter 34, page 786. The nurse then compares the findings with the baseline data on the client's record. If respirations appear extremely shallow, the nurse should hold her or his hand in front of the client's mouth to feel for exhaled air. If exhalations are not detected, the lungs should be auscultated and any bilateral air movement noted. Oxygen should be supplied to hypoventilating clients as necessary.

The nurse should assess the client for signs of respiratory obstruction, the most common recovery room emergency. It may be due to occlusion of the pharynx by the tongue, spasm or edema of the airway, accumulation of secretions in the airway, or aspiration of regurgitated vomitus. Signs of respiratory obstruction include:

1. Restlessness (early sign)
2. Rapid, thready pulse (early sign)
3. Noisy, irregular respirations
4. Use of accessory muscles for breathing (e.g., the muscles in abdomen or neck) and intercostal retractions (indrawing between the ribs)
5. Apprehension or anxiety
6. Attempts to sit upright
7. Pallor or cyanosis (late signs)

Cardiovascular function The client's pulse must be assessed for rate, rhythm, and quality every 15 minutes until signs stabilize and then every 30 minutes. Generally, the pulse is slightly faster after surgery, but a pulse above 110 beats per minute or below 60 beats per minute should be reported. Also, a pulse rate markedly above or below the client's preoperative rate is abnormal; it may indicate internal hemorrhage or some other physiologic problem. If the radial pulse is thready, the nurse should take the apical pulse. And the client's blood pressure should be assessed every 15 minutes until stable and then every 30 minutes. The surgeon must be informed if the client's blood pressure falls more than 20 mm Hg after surgery or falls 5 or 10 mm Hg at each reading. This is because certain anesthetic agents and muscle relaxants may cause postoperative hypotension; it may also be a sign of hemorrhage and shock. The patient's skin color and condition, particularly that of the lips and nail beds, should be assessed, because the color of the lips and nail beds are indicators of **tissue perfusion** (passage of blood through the vessels). Pale, cyanotic, cool, and moist skin may be a sign of circulatory problems. In addition, the client should be assessed for signs of common circulatory problems: hemorrhage and shock, cardiac arrest, and postoperative hypotension. Cardiac arrest is discussed in Chapter 45. Disruption of sutures and insecure ligation of blood vessels can cause hemorrhage. Shock occurs as a result of massive hemorrhage or cardiac insufficiency. Signs of hemorrhage and shock include:

1. Increased pulse and respiratory rates
2. Restlessness
3. Lowered blood pressure
4. Cold, clammy skin
5. Thirst
6. Pallor

The nurse must inspect the client's dressings and the bedclothes underneath the client. Excessive bloody drainage on dressings or on bedclothes, often appearing underneath the client, can indicate hemorrhage. The amount of drainage on dressings is recorded by describing the diameter of stains. It is extremely important for the nurse to ensure that there is adequate replacement of fluids lost during surgery, to maintain blood pressure. Elastic (antiemboli) stockings should be applied, if ordered, to prevent pooling of blood in peripheral blood vessels. See page 1625.

Fluid and electrolyte balance The client's fluid intake and output are monitored. The client should also be assessed for signs of circulatory overload. See Chapter 46, page 1360. During surgery, aldosterone production increases, and as a result the body conserves sodium and fluid. Therefore, care must be taken not to overload the body with fluid. In addition, the client is assessed for signs of fluid or electrolyte imbalance. If the client is receiving blood, the assessment must include signs of adverse reactions. See Chapter 46, page 1389. Nurses in the RR also must determine the color, consistency, and amount of drainage from all tubes and suction apparatuses. All tubes should be patent, and tubes and suction equipment should be functioning properly.

Neurologic status After general anesthesia, clients awaken in the following sequence: respond to stimuli, i.e., to loud noises or to their names spoken loudly; become drowsy; are awake but not oriented; are alert and oriented (McConnell 1977a, p. 34). The return of the client's reflexes, such as swallowing and gagging, indicates that anesthesia is ending. Time of recovery from anesthesia varies with the kind of anesthetic used, its dosage, and the individual's response to it. Nurses should arouse the client by calling her or him by name, and in a normal tone of voice repeatedly tell the client that the surgery is over and that she or he is in the recovery room.

Pain As the client emerges from anesthesia, it is important to assess any need for analgesics and to administer them as ordered. Analgesic dosages given in the RR are often reduced from normal levels by one quarter to one third, but their effects are closely evaluated. Smaller dosages of analgesics are given because respiratory and cardiovascular function are depressed by anesthesia and can be impaired further by analgesic dosages that are too high. Nurses should use judgment in withholding pain medications from hypotensive clients, for pain may be the cause of hypotension (McConnell 1977a, p. 36).

Safety A client in the RR should have the side rails of her or his bed elevated, if the client is unconscious. Drainage tubings should be frequently monitored to make sure the client has not changed position in a way that occludes the tubing.

Continuing Postoperative Stage

As soon as the client returns to the nursing unit from the RR, the nurse conducts an initial assessment. See Figure 53–15 for a postoperative checklist. The sequence of these activities varies with the situation. For example, the nurse may need to check the physician's stat orders before conducting the initial assessment; in such a case, nursing interventions to implement the orders can be carried out at the same time as assessment. Initial assessment activities include the following.

Postoperative Assessment

1. Determine the time of arrival at the nursing unit.
2. Measure vital signs—pulse, respirations, and blood pressure—and compare them with RR data.

POSTOPERATIVE INITIAL ASSESSMENT CHECKLIST

1. **Time of arrival** ______
2. **Vital signs**
   Pulse ____ Respirations ____ Blood pressure ____
3. **Skin**
   Color ______
   Condition ______
4. **Level of consciousness**
   Conscious ____ Semiconscious ____ Unconscious ____
5. **Dressing**
   Dry ____ Drainage present ______
   Blood ______ Intact ______
6. **Intravenous**
   Type of solution ______
   Amount in bottle ______ Drip rate ______
   Venipuncture site ______
7. **Drainage tubes**
   Type ______
   Attached to suction or drainage container ______
   Appearance and amount of drainage ______
8. **Patient position** ______
9. **Side rails** ______
10. **Pain**
    Type of analgesic ______
    Time last given ______
11. **Other discomforts** ______

Figure 53–15 A sample postoperative checklist

3. Observe the color and condition of the client's skin (e.g., diaphoresis, coldness).
4. Assess the client's level of consciousness. At this point, most postoperative clients are conscious but drowsy. A fully conscious person responds verbally, is alert, and is aware of time, place, and person. A semiconscious person has fluctuating states of awareness. An unconsciousness person does not respond verbally, has variable responses to stimuli such as noise or pain, and may be incontinent of urine or feces.
5. Inspect dressings for moisture or bleeding. Feel under the client for pooled blood. Report blood immediately to the responsible nurse.
6. Observe any intravenous infusions. Record the type of solution, the amount in the bottle, the drip rate, and the venipuncture site. Obtain additional solutions as ordered. See Chapter 46.
7. Inspect drainage tubes, such as urinary catheters, and connect them appropriately, e.g., to drainage containers or suction. Verify that fluids are draining and that tubes are not obstructed. Observe the amount, color, etc., of the drainage.
8. Determine what position is ordered for the client. This information is in the client's record, in the surgeon's orders, or in RR records. Clients who have had spinal anesthetics usually lie flat for 8 to 12 hours. Follow established nursing practice in the agency about how long the client lies flat. If the client is unconscious or semiconscious, place the client on his or her side, if possible, or in a position that allows fluids to drain from the mouth. Otherwise, follow the client's preference. Most people prefer a back-lying position.
9. For the client's safety, raise the side rails on the bed.
10. Assess the client's pain or discomfort, and note when the client last had an analgesic.
11. Record the client's condition, including your assessment, on the chart. Many hospitals have postoperative routines for regular assessment of clients. In some agencies, assessments are made every 15 minutes until vital signs stabilize, every hour thereafter the same day, and every 4 hours for the next 2 days. It is very important that the assessments be made as often as the client's condition requires.
12. Notify the client's support persons that she or he has returned from surgery. It may be necessary to caution them about the client's drowsiness and about not staying too long.

Postoperative Nursing Diagnoses

Nursing diagnoses for postoperative clients depend on the health status and needs of the particular client. Many nursing diagnoses are stated in terms of potential problems. Most people recover from surgery without incident. Complications or problems are relatively rare, yet nurses must be aware of such possibilities and their clinical signs. See Table 53–5. Many postoperative nursing interventions are intended to prevent complications. Examples of postoperative nursing diagnoses are listed below.

Examples of Postoperative Nursing Diagnoses

- Alteration in comfort related to surgical incision
- Potential fluid volume deficit related to excessive wound drainage
- Impaired mobility related to incisional pain
- Potential disturbance in self-concept related to loss of right breast
- Knowledge deficit about need for breathing exercises
- Alterations in oral mucous membrane related to taking no oral fluids
- Potential for infection related to surgery
- Potential altered skin integrity related to immobility secondary to surgery

Table 53–5 Potential Postoperative Problems

Problem	Description	Cause	Clinical Signs	Preventive Interventions
Respiratory				
Pneumonia	Inflammation of the alveoli	Commonly *Diplococcus pneumoniae*, a resident bacteria in the respiratory tract	Elevated temperature, cough, expectoration of blood-tinged or purulent sputum, dyspnea, chest pain	Deep-breathing and coughing exercises, moving in bed, early ambulation
Lobar pneumonia	Involves one or more lobes			
Bronchopneumonia	Originates in bronchi and involves patches of lung tissue	Poor lung expansion and circulation, resulting in stagnation of secretions		
Hypostatic pneumonia	Poor or stagnant circulation causing inflammation of lung tissue			
Atelectasis	Collapse of the alveoli, with retained secretions	Mucous plugs blocking bronchial passageways, inadequate lung expansion, analgesics, immobility	Marked dyspnea, cyanosis, pleural pain, prostration, tachycardia, increased respiratory rate, fever, productive cough, auscultatory crackling sounds	Deep-breathing and coughing exercises, turning, early ambulation, adequate fluid intake
Pulmonary embolism	Blood clot that has moved to the lungs and obstructs a pulmonary artery, thus inhibiting blood flow to one or more lung lobes	Stasis of venous blood from immobility, venous injury from fractures or during surgery, use of oral contraceptives high in estrogen, preexisting coagulation or circulatory disorder	Sudden chest pain, shortness of breath, cyanosis, shock (tachycardia, low blood pressure)	Deep-breathing and coughing exercises, turning, ambulation, anti-emboli stockings
Circulatory				
Hemorrhage	Bleeding internally or externally	Disruption of sutures, insecure ligation of blood vessels	Rapid weak pulse, increasing respiratory rate, restlessness, lowered blood pressure, cold clammy skin, thirst, pallor, reduced urine output	Early recognition of signs
Hypovolemic shock	Markedly reduced volume of circulating blood resulting in inadequate tissue perfusion	Hemorrhage	Same as for Hemorrhage	Early recognition of signs
Thrombophlebitis	Inflammation of the veins, usually of the legs and associated with a blood clot	Slowed venous blood flow due to immobility or prolonged sitting; trauma to vein, resulting in inflammation and increased blood coagulability	Aching, cramping pain; affected area is swollen, red, and hot to touch; vein feels hard; discomfort in calf when foot is dorsiflexed or when client walks (Homan's sign)	Early ambulation, leg exercises, anti-emboli stockings, adequate fluid intake
Thrombus	Blood clot attached to wall of vein or artery, most commonly the leg veins	Venous stasis; vein injury resulting from surgery of legs, pelvis, abdomen; factors causing increased blood coagulability, e.g., use of estrogen	Same as for Pulmonary Embolism; if lodged in heart or brain, cardiac or neurologic signs	Same as for Thrombophlebitis
Embolus	Clot that has moved from its site of formation to another area of the body, e.g., the lungs, heart, or brain	Same as for Thrombus	Same as for Thrombus	Same as for Thrombophlebitis

Table 53–5 *(continued)*

Problem	Description	Cause	Clinical Signs	Preventive Interventions
Urinary				
Urinary retention	Accumulation of urine in the bladder and inability of the bladder to empty itself	Depressed bladder muscle tone from narcotics and anesthetics; handling of tissues during surgery on adjacent organs (rectum, vagina)	Fluid intake larger than output; inability to void or frequent voiding of small amounts, bladder distention, suprapubic discomfort, restlessness	Monitoring of fluid intake and output, interventions to facilitate voiding
Urinary infection	Inflammation of bladder	Immobilization and limited fluid intake	Burning sensation when voiding, urgency, cloudy urine, lower-abdominal pain	Adequate fluid intake, early ambulation, good perineal hygiene
Gastrointestinal				
Constipation	Infrequent or no stool passage for abnormal length of time, e.g., within 48 hours after solid diet started	Lack of dietary roughage, analgesics (decrease intestinal motility)	Absence of stool elimination, abdominal distention and discomfort	Adequate fluid intake, high-fiber diet, early ambulation
Singultus	Intermittent spasms of the diaphragm	Irritation of the phrenic nerve—for a variety of reasons, e.g., abdominal distention	Hiccups	Prevent the cause
Tympanites	Retention of gases within the intestines	Slowed motility of the intestines due to handling of the bowel during surgery and the effects of anesthesia	Obvious abdominal distention, abdominal discomfort (gas pains), absence of bowel sounds	Early ambulation, IV fluid progressing to clear fluids, full fluids and regular diet when peristalsis returns
Nausea and vomiting		Pain, abdominal distention, ingesting food or fluids before return of peristalsis, certain medications, anxiety	Complaints of feeling sick to the stomach, retching or gagging	IV fluids until peristalsis returns; then clear fluids, full fluids, and regular diet; antiemetic drugs if ordered; analgesics for pain
Wound				
Wound infection	Inflammation and infection of incision or drain site	Poor aseptic technique; laboratory analysis of wound swab identifies causative microorganism	Purulent exudate, redness, tenderness, elevated body temperature, wound odor	Keeping wound clean and dry, surgical aseptic technique when changing dressings
Wound dehiscence	Separation of a suture line before the incision heals	Malnutrition (emaciation, obesity), poor circulation, excessive strain on suture line	Increased incision drainage, tissues underlying skin become visible along parts of the incision	Adequate nutrition, appropriate incisional support and avoidance of strain
Wound evisceration	Extrusion of internal organs and tissues through the incision	Same as for Wound Dehiscence	Opening of incision and visible protrusion of organs	Same as for Wound Dehiscence
Psychologic				
Postoperative depression	See Clinical Signs	News of malignancy, severely altered body image	Anorexia, tearfulness, loss of ambition, withdrawal, rejection of others, feelings of dejection, sleep disturbances (insomnia, excessive sleeping)	Adequate rest, physical activity, opportunity to express anger and other negative feelings

Postoperative Planning

There are many sources of data for planning a client's postoperative nursing—for example, the preoperative nursing history, postoperative orders, the RR report (see significant data from the recovery room record to the right), and the client. From the surgeon's postoperative orders the nurse should be aware of:

1. Food and fluids permitted by mouth
2. Intravenous solutions and intravenous medications
3. Position in bed
4. Medications ordered, e.g., analgesics, antibiotics
5. Laboratory tests
6. Intake and output, which in some agencies are monitored for all postoperative clients
7. Activity permitted, including ambulation

The purposes of planning at this stage are primarily:

1. To prevent complications
2. To provide comfort and rest for the client
3. To maintain the client's safety
4. To facilitate the client's return to the highest possible level of wellness
5. To encourage exercises learned preoperatively
6. To help the client maintain a healthy attitude toward self

For examples of outcome criteria for the postoperative client see the Evaluation section later in this chapter.

Recovery Room Record: Significant Data

- Operation performed
- Presence and location of any drains
- Anesthetic used
- Postoperative diagnosis
- Estimated blood loss
- Medications administered in the recovery room

Postoperative Interventions

Vital Signs

The client's vital signs need to be taken at least every 4 hours, or more frequently if they are abnormal. An elevated temperature along with other signs can indicate infection of the respiratory tract, urinary tract, or incision. A rapid, weak pulse and increased respiratory rate along with other signs can indicate infection, hemorrhage, or shock. A lowered blood pressure along with other signs can indicate hemorrhage, shock, or pulmonary embolism. The nurse should assess the client's respiratory rate, depth, and rhythm every 4 hours, or whenever the vital signs are taken, remaining alert to signs of respiratory problems. See Table 53–5. The client's skin color and temperature must be assessed. Extreme pallor and a cold, clammy skin are signs of shock.

Deep-Breathing and Coughing Exercises

The client should be encouraged to do deep-breathing and coughing exercises hourly, or at least every 2 hours, during waking hours for the first few days. The nurse should assist the client to a sitting position in bed or on the side of the bed. The client should splint the incision with a pillow when coughing, or the nurse should splint the incision for the client. These exercises help prevent respiratory complications such as hypostatic pneumonia and atelectasis. See Table 53–5. To assist clients who have difficulty with deep-breathing and coughing exercises, the nurse should check about the use of blow bottles and incentive spirometers (see Chapter 45, page 1303). For clients unable to cough up secretions, suction may be necessary (see Chapter 45, page 1313).

Leg Exercises

The client should be encouraged to do leg exercises every hour, or at least every 2 hours, during waking hours. Muscle contractions compress the veins, preventing the stasis of blood in the veins, a cause of thrombus formation and subsequent thrombophlebitis and emboli. See Table 53–5. Contractions also promote arterial blood flow.

Moving and Ambulation

The client must be turned from side to side every 2 hours. Turning allows alternating maximum expansion of the uppermost lung. Avoid placing pillows or rolls under the client's knees because pressure on the popliteal blood vessels can slow the blood circulation to and from the lower extremities. The client should ambulate as soon as possible after surgery in accordance with the surgeon's orders. Generally, clients begin ambulation the evening of the day of surgery or the first day after surgery, unless the surgeon orders otherwise. Early ambulation prevents respiratory, circulatory, urinary, and gastrointestinal complications. It also prevents general muscle weakness. See Table 53–5. Ambulation should be scheduled for periods after the client has taken an analgesic or when she or he is comfortable. And it should be gradual; starting with the client sitting on the bed and dangling the feet over the side. The nurse should assess the client's tolerance by noting skin color, respirations, diaphoresis, pulse rate, etc. The pulse should be taken before the client is moved and again after. Next, the client should be helped to stand at the bedside and take a few steps, increasing the distance gradually as the client's tolerance grows.

Supportive measures need to be provided as required—for example, a pillow to support an abdominal incision, or moving a urinary drainage bag or IV pole during ambulation. Verbal encouragement and reassurance, as necessary, can aid this. Clients with cardiovascular problems need tensor bandages up to the knees or antiemboli stockings. See Procedure 53–5, page 1625. These devices support superficial veins and prevent stasis of venous circulation. If the client cannot ambulate, he or she should be periodically assisted to a sitting position in bed, if allowed, and turned frequently. The sitting position permits the greatest lung expansion.

Hydration

The nurse should maintain IV infusions as ordered. IV infusions are given to balance loss of body fluids during surgery (e.g., blood loss, perspiration, vomiting, and fasting). Only small sips of water should be offered to clients who can have fluids by mouth, until they establish tolerance. Large amounts of water can induce vomiting, since anesthetics and narcotic analgesics temporarily inhibit the motility of the stomach. Ice chips, if permitted, may be offered. The client who cannot take fluids by mouth *may* be allowed to suck ice chips. Check the surgeon's orders. Mouth care should be provided, and a mouth wash should be placed at the client's bedside. Postoperative clients often complain of thirst and a dry, sticky mouth. These discomforts are a result of the preoperative fasting period, preoperative medications (such as atropine or scopolamine), and loss of body fluid.

The client's fluid intake and output should be measured for at least 2 days, or until fluid balance is stable without an IV. It is important to ensure adequate fluid balance. Sufficient fluids keep the respiratory mucous membranes and secretions moist, thus facilitating the expectoration of mucus during coughing. Also, an adequate fluid balance will prevent dehydration and the resulting concentration of the blood that, along with venous stasis, is conducive to thrombus formation.

The client should be assessed for signs of dehydration. See Chapter 46, page 1358, for additional information about dehydration.

Nutrition

The surgeon orders the client's postoperative diet. Depending on the extent of surgery and the organs involved, some clients may be given intravenous fluids and nothing by mouth for a few days, whereas others may progress from a diet of clear liquids to full fluids, to a light diet, and then to a regular diet within a few days. See Chapter 42. The nurse should also check the surgeon's orders carefully regarding diet. The return of peristalsis can be assessed by auscultating the abdomen. Gurgling and rumbling sounds indicate peristalsis (see Chapter 35, page 861). Anesthetics, narcotics, handling of the intestines during abdominal surgery, changes in fluid and food intake, and inactivity all inhibit peristalsis. Oral fluids and food are usually started after the return of peristalsis. The nurse may need to assist the client to eat if she or he is very weak. In addition, observe the client's tolerance of the food and fluids ingested.

Urinary Elimination

The nurse may provide measures that promote urinary elimination. For example, help male clients stand at the bedside, ensure that clients are free from pain, ensure that fluid intake is adequate, and help clients walk. Determine if the client has any difficulties voiding, and assess him or her for bladder distention (see Chapter 44). Report promptly to the responsible nurse if a client does not void within 8 hours following surgery. Anesthetics temporarily depress urinary bladder tone, which usually returns within 6 to 8 hours after surgery. Surgery in the pubic area, vagina, or rectum, during which the surgeon may manipulate the bladder, often causes urinary retention. Catheterize a client if all measures to promote voiding fail. See Chapter 44. In some agencies, catheterization requires a physician's or surgeon's order. Measure the liquid intake and output of all clients with urinary catheters or other drainage devices. Keep I & O records for at least 2 days and until the client reestablishes fluid balance without a catheter in place.

Comfort and Rest

Pain is usually greatest 12 to 36 hours after surgery, decreasing on the second or third day. Analgesics are usually administered every 3 or 4 hours the first day; by the third day most clients require only oral analgesics. Some may refuse to take analgesics on a regular schedule because they are not in severe pain. In this situation, assess the need for analgesics (see Chapter 41); if indicated, inform the client that analgesics are most effective if given *before* pain becomes severe. Provide comfort measures to relax the client, e.g., back rubs, position changes, rest periods, and diverting activities, since tension increases pain perception and responses. Administer analgesics as ordered and as required, for analgesics relieve pain and therefore also help the client to do deep-breathing and coughing exercises effectively and to ambulate.

Research Note

Nurses play a role in the prevention, observation, and treatment of postoperative pain. In this study, postoperative distress was compared for cholecystectomy and hysterectomy clients. Only hysterectomy clients who reported lower pain levels were found to benefit from relaxation training. Earlier studies also have supported the idea that relaxing becomes more difficult as pain sensations increase in intensity. Thus, the value of relaxation training appears to be only in relieving the distress caused by painful sensations, not in ameliorating their intensity. The authors were somewhat surprised by their findings. This study emphasizes the demonstrated value of relaxation training and suggests preliminary definition of those clients who will benefit most from such a program. (Mogan et al. 1985)

Observe the client for signs of acute pain, e.g., pallor, perspiration, tension, and reluctance to perform deep-breathing and coughing exercises or to move or ambulate. Move and position the client to minimize discomfort. Plan to give analgesics *before* activities (e.g., ambulation or meals) or rest periods (e.g., at bedtime). Assess the effectiveness of the analgesics. Listen attentively to the client's complaints of pain; note the location and type of pain, and determine the cause. Do not assume that the pain is caused by the incision. Often the cause can be tight dressings, irritation from drainage tubes, or muscle strains resulting from positioning on the operating table.

Fecal Elimination

Note and report the passage of flatus. Abdominal distention due to reduced peristalsis is very common after surgery. Many people who have had abdominal surgery start experiencing this discomfort about the third day after surgery. The passage of flatus indicates the return of peristalsis. Auscultate the client's abdomen to confirm the return of peristalsis. See Chapter 35, page 861. Administer a rectal tube, enema, or suppository as required and if ordered. See Chapter 43.

Wound Protection

Inspect dressings regularly to ensure that they are clean and dry. Excessive drainage can indicate hemorrhage, infection, or dehiscence. See Table 53–5. Ensure that the dressing is fastened securely, because an intact, secure dressing prevents infection of the wound. Apply abdominal binders for support as ordered. Change dressings, using sterile technique as required, when they are soiled with drainage or in accordance with the surgeon's or nursing orders. See Chapter 52. Note that the first dressing change postoperatively may be done by the physician. Inspect the wound for signs of local infection if the wound is exposed. Also, assess the client for signs of generalized infection, e.g., elevated temperature and increased pulse and respiratory rates. Report wound separations promptly. If a large dehiscence or evisceration occurs, cover the wound with sterile, moist saline towels or dressings and apply an abdominal binder for support of the internal organs. Notify the physician immediately. See Chapter 52.

Recording

All aspects of the nursing process should be recorded on the appropriate client record.

Sample Recording: Initial Assessment on Return to Unit

Date	Time	Notes
Dec/22/87	1100	Transferred from PAR. Appears pale, tense, and drowsy. Is responding verbally and aware of time and surroundings. Complaining of severe abdominal pain. BP 140/70, P 88, R 18. Dressing dry and intact. IV of D5W infusing. IV site intact and dry. Foley catheter attached to closed drainage bag. Urine clear amber color.———
	1115	Demerol 75 mg IM administered. Family notified.——— ———Terrence G. Fox, SN

Sample Recording: Ongoing Postoperative Intervention

Date	Time	Notes
Jan/26/87	1500	Vital signs stable at 125/72, T 37, P 76, R 16. Performing deep-breathing and coughing exercises well q.2h. Performing leg exercises q.1h. Ambulated first time to bathroom. Tolerated well. Voided 250 ml clear amber urine.———
	1600	IV 1,000 ml D5W infused: 1,000 ml Ringer's lactate started. Tolerating sips of water and ice chips. No bowel sounds evident.
	1630	Demerol 75 mg IM given for abdominal pain. Dressing dry and intact.———Trudy Jones, SN

Antiemboli Stockings

Antiemboli (elastic) stockings are indicted for clients who have problems with circulation to their feet and legs. The elastic material compresses the veins of the legs and thereby facilitates the return of venous blood to the heart. These stockings are frequently applied preoperatively and/or postoperatively.

There are several types of stockings. One type extends from foot to knee and another from foot to midthigh. Women sometimes prefer to wear garters with the longer type, although garters are not necessary to hold elastic stockings in place. Another type of stocking extends to the waist and fastens with an adjustable belt and its own garters. Stockings have a partial foot that exposes either the heel or toes so that extremity circulation can be assessed. See Figure 53–16. Elastic stockings usually come in small, medium, and large sizes.

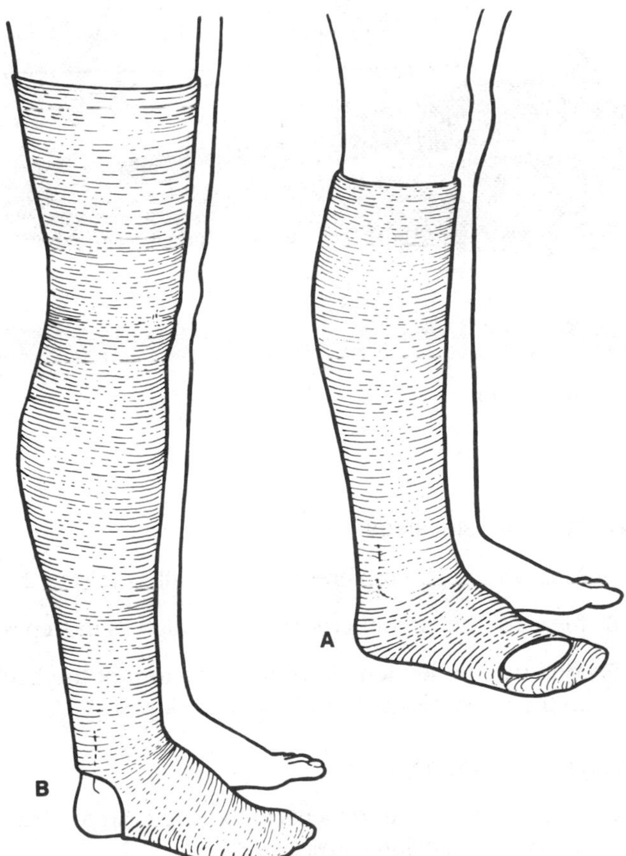

Figure 53–16 Two types of antiemboli stockings: **A,** extending to the knee, with an opening above the toes; **B,** extending to midthigh, with the heel exposed.

Before applying antiemboli stockings, assess the client's legs for:

1. Inadequate arterial blood circulation:
   a. Cool skin temperature in a warm environment
   b. Pallor
   c. Shiny taut skin
   d. Mild edema
2. Insufficient venous blood return:
   a. Thickening of the skin
   b. Increased pigmentation around the ankles
   c. Pitting edema (edema in which firm finger pressure on the skin produces an indentation, or pit, that remains for several seconds)
   d. Peripheral cyanosis
3. Posterior tibial and dorsalis pedis pulse rates, volumes, and rhythms. See Chapter 34, page 779.
4. Pain in the calf of the leg. Dorsiflex the foot abruptly and firmly while the knee is straight or slightly flexed (see Figure 53–17) to assess pain in the calf (Homan's sign). The presence of pain is a positive Homan's sign.
5. The appearance or presence of distended superficial veins in the legs. Normally veins may appear distended in a dependent position but collapse when the limb is elevated.

Procedure 53–5 describes how to measure and apply antiemboli stockings.

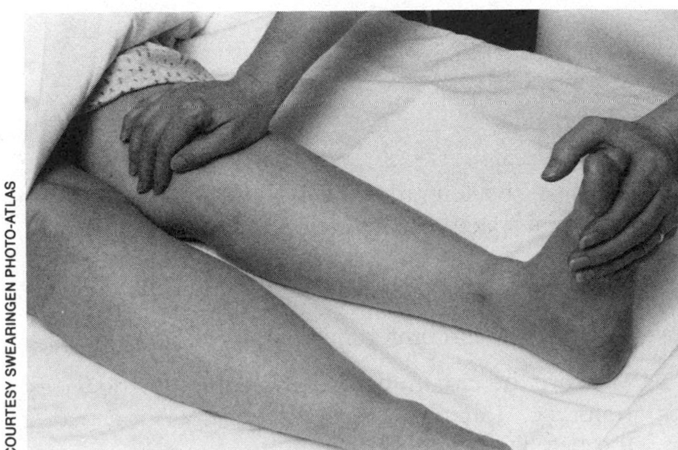

COURTESY SWEARINGEN PHOTO-ATLAS

Figure 53–17 Assessing Homan's sign

Procedure 53–5 ▲ Measuring and Applying Antiemboli Stockings

Equipment

1. Measuring tape
2. Size chart
3. Correct size of elastic stockings

Intervention

1. Assist the client to a lying position in bed. Stockings should be applied before the client arises.

   Rationale The stockings should be donned before the veins become distended and edema occurs.

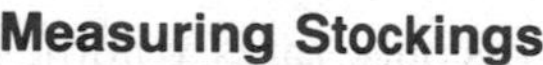

Measuring Stockings

Knee-length stockings

2. Measure the circumference of the calf at the widest point, i.e., 15 cm (6 in) below the inferior aspect of the patella. See Figure 53–18.

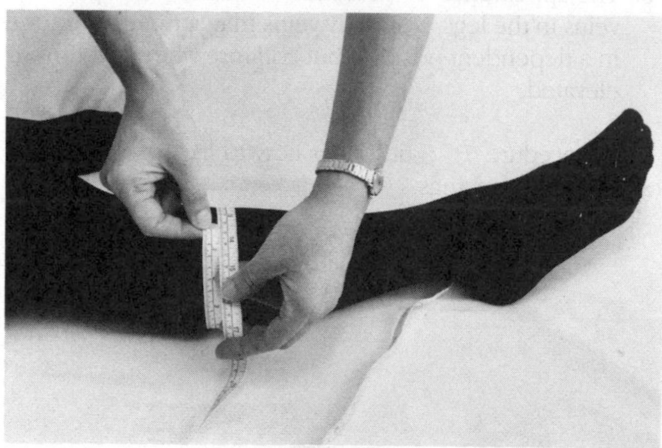

Figure 53–18

3. Measure the length of the leg from the heel to the popliteal space. See Figure 53–19.

Thigh-length stockings

4. Measure the circumference of the calf as in step 2.
5. Measure the circumference of the thigh at the widest point, i.e., 15 cm (6 in) above the superior aspect of the patella.
6. Measure the length of the leg from the heel to the gluteal fold. See Figure 53–20.

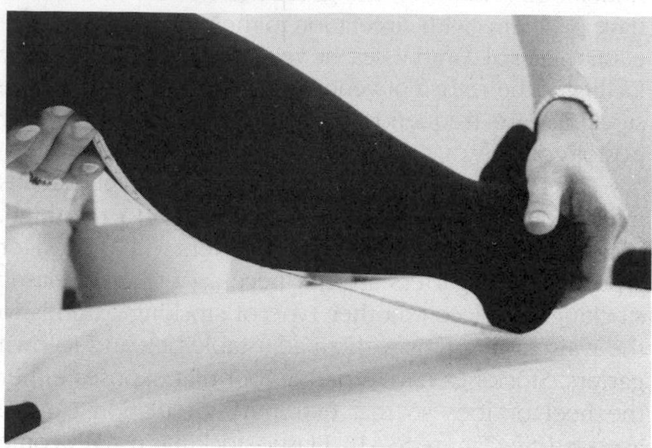

Figure 53–19

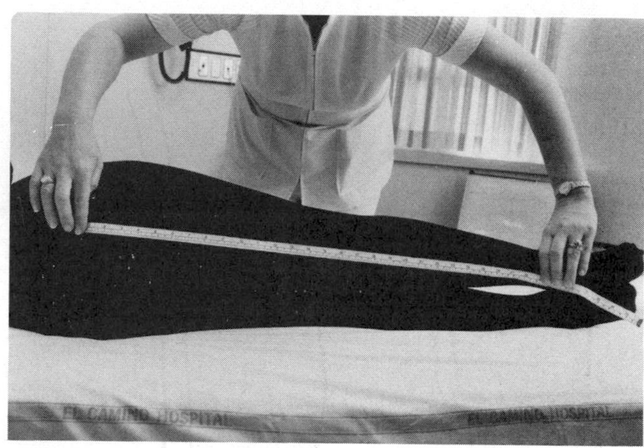

Figure 53–20

Waist-length stockings

7. Measure the circumference of the calf as in step 2.
8. Measure the circumference of the thigh as in step 5.
9. Measure the leg length from the bottom of the heel to the waist, along the side of the body.

All types of stockings

10. Compare the measurements to the size chart to obtain the correct stocking size.

Applying Elastic Stockings

11. Make sure the stocking is inside out; then grasp the foot and heel of the stocking, and invert the stocking

over your hand, so as to turn the leg and foot portions inside out to the heel portion.

12. Remove your hand, and slip the foot portion of the stocking over the toes, foot, and heel. See Figure 53–21. Make sure the foot fits into the toe and heel portions of the stocking.
13. Pull the leg portion of the stocking over the foot and up the leg.
14. Pull the stocking up the leg evenly to its full length. Make sure there are no wrinkles or creases. Observe the lines in the material to make sure the stocking is not twisted.

    Rationale Wrinkles and creases can irritate the skin and impede blood circulation.
15. Repeat for the other leg.
16. Inspect the stocking periodically to see that the top has not rolled and that the leg above the stocking is not swollen.

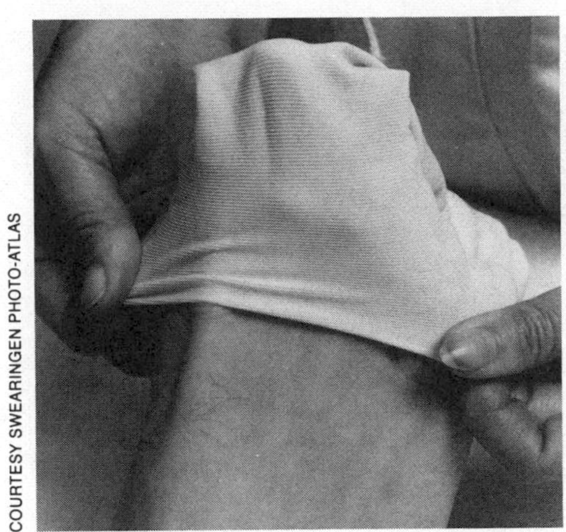

Figure 53–21

Removing a Stocking

17. Hold the top of the stocking with both hands and pull it down to thc foot.
18. Supporting the foot at the ankle with one hand, pull the stocking over the foot and off.
19. Repeat for the other leg.
20. Record assessments and the time and application of the elastic stockings.

Suction

The manner in which suction is applied to drainage tubes depends on the type of equipment available in the agency and the amount of suction required. The following are the most commonly used.

Wall suction. In some agencies, wall suction units with piped-in negative pressure are available. See Figure 45–26, page 1313. These units consist of a suction pressure regulator and a drainage receptacle, which needs to be checked regularly to prevent overflow.

Portable electric motor suction. Portable electric units are plugged into electric wall outlets. The units have an on–off switch, a motor that generates the negative pressure, and a drainage bottle. The bottle needs to be monitored regularly to prevent overflow of drainage into the motor, which can cause irreparable damage to the apparatus.

Gomco thermotic pump. The Gomco pump is electrically operated but consists of a pump rather than a motor. See Figure 53–22. It provides intermittent suction by alternating the air pressure, i.e., expanding and contracting the air. As the pressure alternates, red and green lights flash on and off. The amount of suction is regulated by a "high" or "low" pressure button. The pump is commonly used to suction gastrointestinal tubes.

Plastic bellows wound suction. Plastic bellows suction equipment is commonly referred to as the *Hemovac,* or portable wound suction, since it is used to suction drainage from surgical wounds. See Procedure 52–6, page 1565. Suction is created by manually compressing and releasing the sides of the apparatus.

Before gastric suction is initiated, the nurse should assess the client for:

1. Abdominal distention. Palpate the abdomen (see Chapter 35).
2. Bowel sounds. Auscultate the abdomen (see Chapter 35).
3. Nostril irritation, produced by the tube

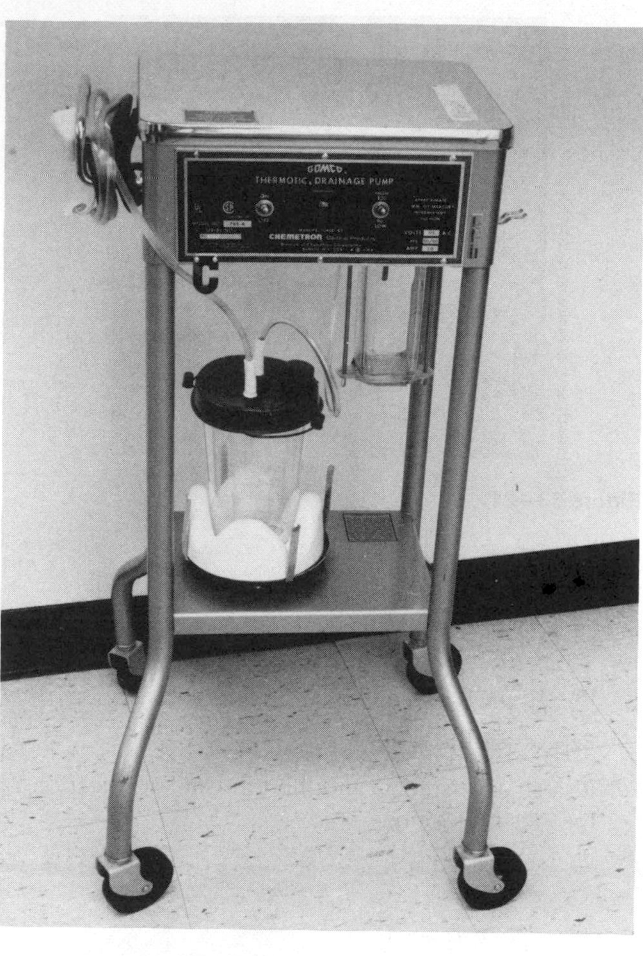

Figure 53–22 A Gomco thermotic pump

4. Abdominal discomfort
5. Vital signs, for baseline data

In addition the nurse needs to know the following.

1. Whether the suction is continuous or intermittent
2. The ordered suction pressure. A low suction pressure is between 80 and 100 mm Hg; high pressure is between 100 and 120 mm Hg for an adult.
3. Whether there is an order to irrigate the gastrointestinal tube; and if so, the type of solution to use

Procedure 53–6 details how to manage gastrointestinal suction.

Procedure 53–6 ▲ Managing Gastrointestinal Suction

Some clients return from surgery with a gastric or intestinal tube in place and orders to connect the tube to suction. The suction ordered can be continuous or intermittent. Intermittent suctioning is less likely to harm the mucous membrane lining near the tip of the suction tube.

Equipment

Initiating and Maintaining Suction

1. A gastrointestinal tube in place in the client. This may have been inserted prior to or following surgery (or prior to establishing the suction on a nonsurgical client).
2. A suction device for either continuous or intermittent suction
3. A 50-ml syringe with an adapter to aspirate the stomach and the tube
4. A basin to collect the aspirated fluid
5. A connector to connect the gastrointestinal tube to the suction tubing
6. Connecting tubing
7. Cotton-tipped applicators
8. Ointment or lubricant to decrease irritation of the nostrils
9. A moisture-resistant pad

Irrigating a Gastrointestinal Tube

10. A disposable irrigating set:
    a. A 50-ml syringe
    b. A moisture-resistant pad
    c. A basin to collect the irrigating solution
    d. A graduated container

11. Sterile normal saline (500 ml) or the ordered solution
12. A stethoscope

Intervention

Initiating Suction

1. Assist the client to the required position or to semi-Fowler's position if it is not contraindicated.

   Rationale In semi-Fowler's position the tube is not as likely to lie against the wall of the stomach and will therefore suction most efficiently. Semi-Fowler's position also prevents reflux of gastric contents, which could lead to aspiration.

2. Confirm that the tube is in the stomach by aspirating the stomach contents with the syringe and adapter. See Table 53–4.

   Rationale The most accurate way to confirm the placement of the tube in the stomach is by withdrawing stomach contents using a syringe. Other methods listed in Table 53–4 are supplemental.

3. Connect the gastrointestinal tube to the tubing from the suction, using the connector.
4. Set the suction at the recommended pressure and turn the suction on.
   a. Adjust the suction machine for the recommended suction pressure, in accordance with agency policy or the surgeon's order. Some suctions are preset and cannot be adjusted. If using a Gomco thermotic pump, the suction is usually set on intermittent "low" suction for a single-lumen nasogastric tube or on "high" suction for a double-lumen nasogastric tube (e.g., Salem sump tube).
   b. Turn on the suction machine, and check that the suction is working. The Gomco thermotic drainage pump has a red indicator light in the middle of the front panel; it blinks continuously when the machine is functioning. When using other suction machines, test for proper suctioning by holding the open end of the suction tube to your ear. Proper suctioning is confirmed by a sucking noise.
5. Watch the tubing for a few minutes until the gastric contents appear to be running through the tubing into the receptacle.
6. If the suction is not working properly, check that the rubber stopper in the collection bottle and all tubing connections are tightly sealed and that the tubing is not kinked.
7. Coil and pin the tubing on the bed so that it does not loop below the suction bottle.

   Rationale If the tubing falls below the suction bottle, the suction may be obstructed because of the pressure required to push the fluid against gravity.

8. If the gastrointestinal tube has an air vent, place it beside or above the client's head. If the vent becomes blocked with gastric contents, inject 10 cc of air with a syringe to clear the vent.

   Rationale If the vent is below the client's head, i.e., in a dependent position, the gastric contents can flow into the vent and block it.

9. Assess the amount, color, odor, and consistency of the drainage. Normal gastric drainage has a mucoid consistency and is either colorless or yellow-green due to the presence of bile. A coffee-grounds color and consistency may indicate bleeding. Test the gastric drainage for pH and blood (Hematest) when indicated. A client who has had gastrointestinal surgery can be expected to have some blood in the drainage.
10. Record initiating the suction and the time. Also record the pressure established, the color and consistency of the drainage, and assessments of the client.

Sample Recording

Date	Time	Notes
Sept/18/87	1400	Suction initiated 100 mm Hg. Returns bright red. Abdomen firm and slightly distended. Bowel sounds irregular and high pitched. ——————Molly Jones, RN

Maintaining Suction

11. Assess the client regularly (every 30 minutes until the system is running well and then every 2 hours) to ensure that the suction is functioning properly. If the client complains of fullness, nausea, or epigastric pain, or if the flow of gastric secretions is not evident in the tubing or the collection bottle, ineffective suctioning or blockage of the nasogastric tube is likely.
12. Inspect the suction system for patency of the system, e.g., kinks or blockages in the tubing, and tightness of the connections.

    Rationale Loose connections can permit air to enter and thus decrease the effectiveness of the suction by decreasing the negative pressure.

13. To relieve blockages:
    a. Milk the suction tubing.
    b. Check the suction equipment. To do this, disconnect the nasogastric tube from the suction over a collecting basin (to collect gastric drainage), and

then, with the suction on, place the end of the suction tubing in a basin of water. If water is drawn into the drainage bottle, the suction equipment is functioning properly, but the nasogastric tube is either blocked or positioned incorrectly.

c. Reposition the client, e.g., to her or his other side if permitted. This may facilitate drainage.
d. Rotate the nasogastric tube and reposition it. This step is contraindicated for clients with gastric surgery because moving the tube may interfere with gastric sutures.
e. Irrigate the nasogastric tube as agency policy advocates or on the order of the physician. See steps 20–30 later in this procedure.

14. Clean the client's nostrils every 3 hours or as needed, using the cotton-tipped applicators and water. Apply a water-soluble lubricant or ointment.
15. Provide mouth care every 3 hours or as needed. See Chapter 36, page 932. Some postoperative clients are permitted to suck ice chips or a moist cloth to maintain the moisture of the oral mucosa.
16. Check the drainage bottle regularly to ensure that it does not overflow.
17. Empty the drainage receptacle every 8 hours or whenever it becomes three quarters full. To empty:
    a. Clamp the nasogastric tube and turn off the suction.
    b. If the receptacle is graduated, determine the amount of drainage.
    c. Disconnect the receptacle.
    d. If not already measured, empty the contents into a graduated container and measure.
    e. Inspect the drainage carefully for color, consistency, and presence of substances, e.g., blood clots.
    f. Rinse the receptacle with warm water.
    g. Reattach the receptacle to the suction.
    h. Turn on the suction and unclamp the nasogastric tube.
    i. Observe the system for several minutes to make sure it is functioning well.
18. Encourage the client to turn from side to side and ambulate when permitted. To ambulate:
    a. Turn off the suction.
    b. Disconnect the gastrointestinal tube from the connector.
    c. Clamp the gastrointestinal tube, and attach it to the client's gown. See Procedure 53–3, steps 14–15, on page 1613. Some agencies use a catheter plug, which is inserted into the lumen of the tube.
    d. Ambulate the client.
    e. Reestablish the suction after the client returns to bed.
19. Record assessments of the client, supportive care, and any problems with the suction system.

Sample Recording

Date	Time	Notes
Mar/7/87	800	250 ml light brown drainage. No complaints of pain. Bowel sounds hyperactive, increased pitch. Abdomen soft upon palpation. No irritation in nostrils. Nostrils cleaned with water and lubricant applied. Vital signs q.2h. BP 140/80, P 90, R 18 and stable—R. Woo, SN

Irrigating a Gastrointestinal Tube

Nasogastric tubes are generally irrigated (a) before and after the instillation of medications, (b) before and after tube feedings, and (c) as ordered to prevent clogging. Check agency policies and practices. Nasogastric irrigation may require a physician's order. Excessive irrigation can lead to metabolic alkalosis.

20. Place the moisture-resistant pad under the end of the gastrointestinal tube.
21. Turn off the suction.
22. Disconnect the gastrointestinal tube from the connector.
23. Determine that the tube is in the stomach by aspirating gastric contents using a syringe. If no contents can be aspirated, inject 10 ml of air while listening over the epigastric region using a stethoscope. See Table 53–4.

    Rationale This ensures that the irrigating solution enters the stomach.
24. Draw up the ordered volume of irrigating solution in the syringe; 30 ml of solution per instillation is usual, but up to 60 ml may be given per instillation if ordered.
25. Attach the syringe to the nasogastric tube and *slowly* inject the solution.
26. Gently aspirate the solution.

    Rationale Forceful withdrawal could damage the gastric mucosa.
27. If you encounter difficulty in withdrawing the solution, inject 20 ml of air and aspirate again, and/or reposition the client or the nasogastric tube.

    Rationale Air and repositioning may move the end of the tube away from the stomach wall.

    If aspirating difficulty continues, reattach the tube to intermittent low suction and notify the responsible nurse or physician.

28. Repeat steps 23–25 until the ordered amount of solution is instilled.
29. Reconnect the nasogastric tube to suction. If a Salem sump tube is used, inject the air vent lumen with air after reconnecting the tube to suction.
30. Observe the system for several minutes to make sure it is functioning well.
31. Record verification of tube placement; the time of the irrigation; the amount and type of irrigating solution used; the amount, color, and consistency of the returns; the patency of the system following the irrigation; and assessments of the client.

Sample Recording

Date	Time	Notes
Sept/19/87	1600	Tube placement confirmed by injecting 10 ml air. Tube irrigated with 30 ml normal saline × 2. 30 ml × 2 returns cloudy, pink with small clots. Suction running well. Abdomen soft, no discomfort, vital signs stable.——R. Woo, SN

Evaluation

Examples of outcome criteria for a postoperative client are given on the right.

The client will:

- Carry out leg exercises every 4 hours as instructed
- Turn from side to side in bed independently
- Cough and deep breathe every 2 hours as instructed
- Walk to the end of the corridor each morning, with assistance
- Have normal vital signs
- Have no abdominal distention

Chapter Highlights

- The perioperative period includes three phases: preoperative, intraoperative, and postoperative.
- Surgery is classified according to degree of urgency, degree of risk, and purpose.
- There are three broad types of anesthesia: general, regional, and local.
- Nurses should determine the risk factors prior to a client's surgery whenever possible.
- Nursing history data are an important source for planning preoperative and postoperative care.
- The surgical excision of a part of the body may affect a client's self-image.
- Preoperative teaching should include moving, leg exercises, and coughing and deep-breathing exercises.
- Many aspects of preoperative teaching are intended to prevent postoperative complications.
- A surgical skin preparation should be carried out as close to the time of surgery as possible.
- Antiemboli stockings are intended to facilitate venous blood return.
- A preoperative checklist provides a guide and documentation of a client's preparation before surgery.
- A postoperative initial assessment checklist provides the nurse with a concise guide.
- Nurses may need to set up a gastric suction postoperatively.

Suggested Readings

Blackwood, S. January 1986. Back to basics: The preop exam. *American Journal of Nursing* 86:39–44.
Blackwood describes the preoperative examination, including essential methods, e.g., palpation, percussion, and auscultation. Included are illustrations of late clubbing, the location of the jugular veins, and measuring the legs for edema. A table summarizes the assessment techniques and normal and abnormal data.

Montanari, J. August 1985. Documenting your postop assessment findings. *Nursing 85* 15:31–35.
Montanari describes the transfer of a postoperative client from the RR to the nursing unit. The article includes a detailed description of postoperative assessment, including a two-page postoperative assessment form.

Smith, B. J. October 1978. Safeguarding your patient after anesthesia. *Nursing 78* 8:53–56.
This author outlines guidelines to help nurses deal with the effects of various types of anesthetic agents, drug abuse, and general situations.

Steele, B. G. March 1980. Test your knowledge of postoperative pain management. *Nursing 80* 10:70–72.
A self-test about postoperative pain management includes 26 multiple-choice questions and answers.

Selected References

Association of Operating Room Nurses. 1986. *AORN standards and recommended practices for perioperative nursing.* Denver: Association of Operating Room Nurses, Inc.

Creighton, H. 1981. *Law every nurse should know.* 4th ed. Philadelphia: W. B. Saunders Co.

Croushore, J. M. April 1979. Postoperative assessment: The key to avoiding the most common nursing mistakes. *Nursing 79* 9:46–50.

Cruse, P. J., and Foord, R. February 1980. The epidemiology of wound infection: A 10-year prospective study of 62,939 wounds. *Surgical Clinics of North America* 60:27–40.

Dossey, B., and Passons, J. M. March 1981. Pulmonary embolism: Preventing it, treating it. *Nursing 81* 11:26–33.

Drain, C. B. August 1984. Managing postoperative pain . . . It's a matter of sighs. *Nursing 84* 14:52–55.

Dziurbejko, M. M., and Larkin, J. C. November 1978. Including the family in preoperative teaching. *American Journal of Nursing* 78:1892–94.

Erickson, R. July 1982. Tube talk principles of fluid flow in tubes. *Nursing 82* 12:54–61.

Garner, J. S. April 1986. CDC guidelines for the prevention and control of nosocomial infections: Guideline for prevention of surgical wound infections, 1985. *American Journal of Infection Control* 14:71–80.

Healy, K. M. January 1968. Does preoperative instruction make a difference? *American Journal of Nursing* 68:62–67.

Keithley, J. K., and Tasic, P. W. April 1982. A united approach to assessment of the surgical patient. *American Journal of Nursing* 82:612–14.

Kneedler, J. A., and Dodge, G. H. 1983. *Perioperative patient care.* Boston: Blackwell Scientific Publications, Inc.

Laird, M. August 1975. Techniques for teaching pre- and postoperative patients. *American Journal of Nursing* 75:1338–40.

LeMaitre, G. D., and Finnegan, J. A. 1980. *The patient in surgery: A guide for nurses.* 4th ed. Philadelphia: W. B. Saunders.

Luciano, K. November 1974. The who, when, where, what and how of preparing children for surgery. *Nursing 74* 4:64–65.

McConnell, E. A. September 1975. All about gastrointestinal intubation. *Nursing 75* 5:30–37.

———. March 1977a. After surgery. *Nursing 77* 7:32–39.

———. September 1977b. Ensuring safer stomach suctioning with a Salem sump tube. *Nursing 77* 7:54–57.

———. April 1979. Ten problems with nasogastric tubes . . . and how to solve them. *Nursing 79* 9:78–81.

Mogan, J.; Wells, N.; Robertson, E. 1985. Effects of preoperative teaching on postoperative pain: A replication and expansion. *International Journal of Nursing Studies* 22(3):267–80.

Northrop, C. 1984. Legal aspects of nursing. In McCann Flynn, J. B., and Heffron, P. B. *Nursing: From concept to practice.* Bowie, Md.: Robert J. Brady Co.

Parsons, M. C., and Stephens, G. J. February 1974. Postoperative complications: Assessment and intervention. *American Journal of Nursing* 74:240–44.

Rau, J., and Rau, M. April 1977. To breathe, or be breathed: Understanding IPPB. *American Journal of Nursing* 77:613–17.

Ryan, R. October 1976. Thrombophlebitis: Assessment and prevention. *American Journal of Nursing* 76:1634–36.

Seropian, R., and Reynolds, B. March 1971. Wound infections after preoperative depilatory versus razor preparation. *American Journal of Surgery* 121:251–54.

Tkach, J. R.; Shannon, A. M.; and Beasfrom, R. November 1979. Pseudofolliculitis due to preoperative shaving. *AORN Journal* 30:881–84.

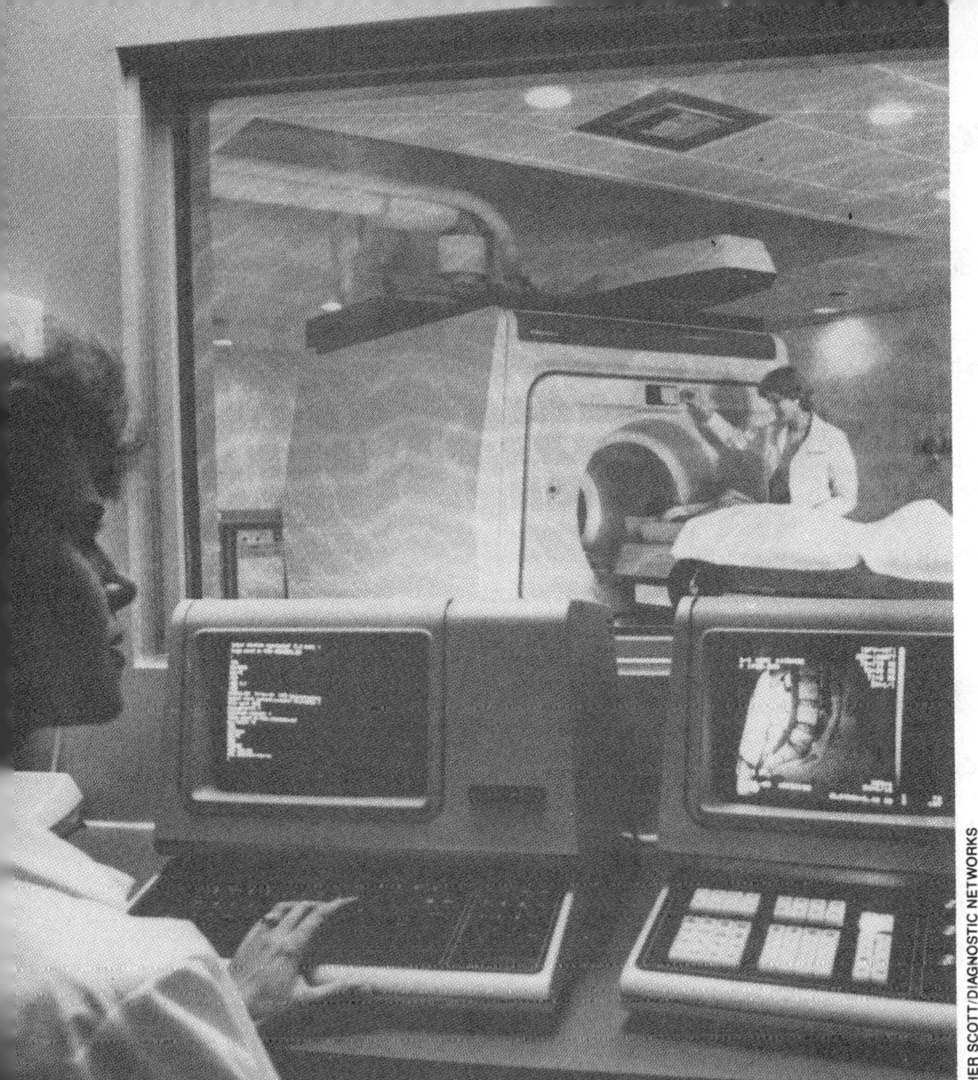

CHAPTER 54

Special Procedures

Contents

54 *Special Procedures*

Objectives

1. Understand essential terms and facts related to assisting clients undergoing special procedures.
   1.1 Define selected terms.
   1.2 Describe various procedures.
   1.3 Identify purposes of specific procedures.
   1.4 Identify assessment data required for specific procedures.
   1.5 Identify education needs of clients about to have certain tests and treatments.
   1.6 Outline measures to prepare the client physically for specific procedures.
   1.7 Give reasons for essential aspects of specific procedures.
   1.8 Outline essential follow-up measures for specific procedures.

Terms

abdominal paracentesis
angiography
anoscopy
ascites
atrioventricular (AV) node
barium enema
barium swallow
bronchogram
bronchoscopy
cannula
cardiac monitor
cholangiography
cholecystography
cisternal puncture
colonoscopy
computed tomography (CT scan)
contrast (ductal injection) mammography
cystoscopy
depolarization (cardiac)
duodenoscopy
electrocardiogram (ECG, EKG)
electrocardiograph
electroencephalogram
electroencephalograph
electromyogram
electromyograph
endoscope
esophagoscopy
fasciculation
fluoroscopy
gastroscopy
intravenous pyelography (IVP) or urography (IVU)
laryngoscopy
lumbar puncture (LP)
mammography
myelography
nerve conduction study
pneumoventriculogram
polarization (cardiac)
proctoscopy
Purkinje's fibers
radioisotopes
repolarization (cardiac)
retrograde pyelography
scan
scintillation camera
scintillation counter
sigmoidoscopy
sinoatrial (SA) node
soft-tissue mammography
thermography
thoracocentesis (thoracentesis)
tomogram
trocar
ultrasonography
ventriculogram
xerography (xeromammography)

General Nursing Guidelines

Psychologic Preparation

Tests and treatments are frightening to many people. People may fear pain, the results of tests, or their reactions to either the pain or the findings of a test. Fear of the unknown increases these misgivings. It is important for nurses to be aware of the needs of clients and their support persons and to help them meet these needs.

The client and possibly the support persons need explanations of why a test or treatment is necessary and what it will entail. This explanation needs to be adjusted to the client's needs. A small child requires a different explanation than a curious adult. Some persons want to know every detail, but others need only a general explanation. It is important that the nurse be honest with the client; if the client will feel sharp pain during the test, it is better to say so than to not mention it.

Often clients want to know where the test will take place, who will do it, how long it will last, and when the results will be available. The last question is often associated with fear. The nurse can base answers on knowledge of the test and on experience.

Informed Consent

It is important that the client sign a consent form before any procedure. Obtaining the client's informed consent is the responsibility of a physician. To give truly informed consent, the client must understand what the procedure

Research Note

Schuster and Jones explored possible differences in nurse versus client opinions about what client education is appropriate before the barium enema procedure. Twenty-eight nurses and 30 clients participated in the study. Findings showed that nurses believed clients need more information than clients believed they needed, and that clients wanted only minimal detailed information about events that will happen *during* the procedure. Rather, clients were interested in knowing the benefits and purpose of the procedure, while nurses believed that such information should be provided by the physician, not the nurse. Finally, nurses were dissatisfied, in general, about the education given to clients in the past before a barium enema procedure. (Schuster and Jones 1982)

entails, what the risks are, and what the alternatives are. Before procedures that are invasive, e.g., lumbar puncture, the client must often sign a special consent form in addition to the general consent signed upon admission to a health agency. See Chapter 7 for more information about informed consent.

Physical Preparation

Some tests require special preparation, e.g., a cleaning enema before a barium enema or sedation before a bronchoscopy. In some instances, special lighting and drapes are required at the client's unit. Just before paracentesis and several other treatments, the patient needs to assume a special position. When a physician orders sedatives or tranquilizers as needed (p.r.n.) before a test, the nurse often decides when or whether to administer them.

Many clients undergo these procedures at a hospital clinic or a physician's office. They prepare themselves at home before they come to the clinic for the procedure. It is important for the nurse to verify that the client has followed preparation instructions correctly before the procedure begins. Most clients are given written directions about their preparation; however, confirming the preparation is essential.

Assembling Equipment

It is usually the nurse's responsibility to assemble the equipment for tests and treatments carried out at a hospitalized client's bedside or in an adjacent clinical treatment room. It is also a nursing responsibility to maintain the sterility of sterile equipment. When a client goes to another unit, such as the radiology department, that department assumes responsibility for assembling the equipment.

Many agencies use prepackaged disposable sets, which require a minimum of setting up. The nurse should check that the set contains all the required equipment. If the nurse is unsure about what equipment is needed, it is important to ask the physician before the procedure and make any necessary adjustments to the set.

Assessing before the Procedure

Before any procedure, nurses should obtain information that can be used as baseline data for assessment during and following the procedure. Before a lumbar puncture, for example, it is important to record the client's vital signs (temperature, pulse, blood pressure) as well as any client complaints of headache or neurologic signs, e.g., tingling in the feet or legs. These clinical signs will be assessed after the lumbar puncture.

In addition, signs that the client's life is threatened—e.g., falling blood pressure; irregular, weak pulse; or dyspnea—must be reported to the physician before the procedure.

If a client appears unduly anxious about the procedure, the nurse should report the anxiety to the physician. The physician may reduce excessive anxiety by giving additional information and reassurance and in some instances ordering a tranquilizer or other medication.

Intervening during the Procedure

During the treatment or test, the nurse needs to assess the client and provide emotional support. The nurse should be sensitive to signs of distress, such as pallor, profuse sweating, accelerated pulse, or signs of nausea or acute

Research Note

Hartfield, Cason, and Cason conducted a study to examine how receiving information about an impending threatening event (barium enema) affected subjects' expectations and the intensity of their emotional response to the event. The group of subjects who received sensation information, i.e., information about the feelings they would experience, reported significantly less anxiety than the group of subjects who received only procedural information. In addition, the expectations of subjects who received sensation information were more congruent with their actual experiences. Sensation information may reduce emotional responses by decreasing the incongruence between reports of what individuals expect to feel and reports of what they actually feel. Procedural information does not appear to affect the individual's expectations about feelings or anxiety level during the procedure. (Hartfield et al. 1982)

pain. Any distress needs to be reported immediately to the physician conducting the procedure. The nurse can support the client by providing information, for instance: "It will be only 2 minutes more," "The needle is all the way in now," or "You won't feel any additional discomfort." Sometimes the nurse can distract the client by asking questions; however, some clients do not respond well to this tactic, and the nurse must be sensitive to the client's wishes.

Assisting with the Procedure

In some instances, the nurse hands equipment to the person carrying out the procedure or makes notes on findings made during the procedure, such as the spinal fluid pressure of a client having a lumbar puncture. Nurses need to know what the physician will expect of them.

Intervening After the Procedure

The nurse assesses the client after any test or treatment. The interval between assessments depends on the client's condition. Even if there are no adverse reactions, in many instances clients should be assessed immediately after the procedure and 30 minutes thereafter. Data obtained during the assessments are compared with the baseline data to determine any changes in the client's health status. Sometimes clients feel nauseated after some procedures, such as a barium swallow.

After a procedure, the nurse must assist the client to a prescribed or comfortable position. For example, after a lumbar puncture, the client must assume a dorsal recumbent position. Support persons need to be told when a procedure is completed and when they can see the client or take the ambulatory client home. It is best to remove equipment before support persons enter the treatment room because many people find long needles and similar equipment disquieting.

The ambulatory client who is returning home after the procedure should receive written directions for any follow-up measures. People are often anxious and preoccupied at these times and find it difficult to remember verbal directions.

Caring for Equipment and Specimens

After the test or treatment, the nurse returns the equipment to the appropriate area or discards disposable equipment. Reusable equipment is washed and rinsed and sent for disinfection or sterilization.

Specimens must be appropriately labeled. Hospital specimens usually are marked with the client's name, identification number, and date. Some specimens require special care if not sent directly to the laboratory. Some urine specimens are refrigerated, and some fecal specimens are kept warm to keep microorganisms alive.

Recording

Preprocedure assessments and nursing interventions are recorded before the procedure starts. After the procedure, the nurse records what treatment or test was performed, when it was done, who carried it out, and whether a specimen was taken. The nurse also records specific information, such as spinal fluid pressures, and any assessments and nursing interventions carried out during and after the procedure.

Examinations Involving Electric Impulses

A number of machines measure and record electric impulses. The **electrocardiograph** receives impulses from the heart, the **electroencephalograph** from the brain, and the **electromyograph** from muscles. All these machines have electrodes that attach to body parts. The electrodes are sensitive to electric activity, which is recorded graphically. The graphic reading can also be shown on an oscilloscope screen.

Electrocardiography

An **electrocardiogram** (ECG or EKG) is a graph of electric impulses from the heart. The heart muscle is said to be **polarized** or charged when it is at rest. When the muscle cells of the ventricles and the atria contract, they **depolarize** or lose their charge. During a resting stage, they regain their electric charge or **repolarize**. Cardiac depolarization and repolarization are recorded on an electrocardiogram.

The heartbeat is normally initiated at the **sinoatrial (SA) node,** which is located in the upper aspect of the right atrium. The SA node is often referred to as the pacemaker of the heart. The impulse it initiates radiates over the atria, causing them to contract. It is then picked up by the **atrioventricular (AV) node,** situated at the base of the atrial septum. The impulse travels from the AV node down two bundle branches throughout the ventricles of the heart. The SA and AV nodes and the bundle branches have dense nctworks of **Purkinjc's fibers,** modified cardiac tissue that helps conduct the impulse. As the impulse travels throughout this system, the ventricles contract or depolarize. Figure 54–1 shows a normal electrocardi-

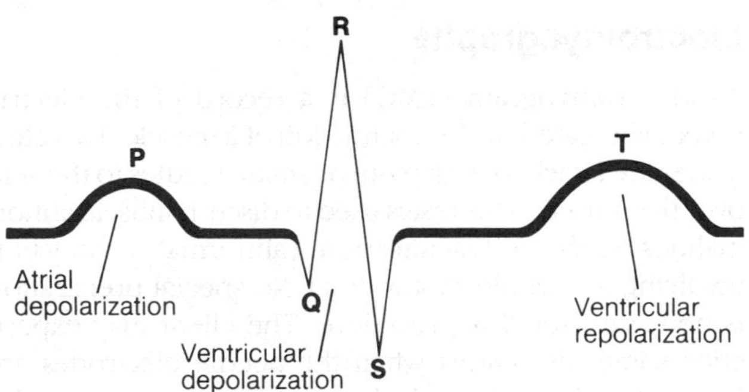

Figure 54–1 Schematic of a normal electrocardiogram

ogram and indicates the intervals of depolarization and repolarization. The P wave arises when the impulse from the SA node causes the atria to contract or depolarize. The QRS wave occurs with contraction and depolarization of the ventricles. The T wave represents the resting or repolarization of the ventricles. Repolarization of the atria occurs during the QRS segment of the graph; it is normally not seen on an ECG. The ECG is produced on finely lined paper. The horizontal lines represent the voltage of the electric impulse, and the vertical lines represent time. See Figure 54–2. The graph waves can be abnormal in size, position, and form when cardiac pathology exists.

Clients who require ECGs may go to a special department of a hospital or laboratory. If the client is very ill, a portable ECG machine can be brought to the bedside in a home or hospital. If the client is critically ill, the heart may be monitored continually. For such clients, a **cardiac monitor** is used. This machine shows cardiac waves on an oscilloscope.

Electrocardiography is painless and usually takes about 10 minutes. Some physicians order an electrocardiogram as part of routine physical examinations of clients over age 40. No special preparation is required before the test unless the physician so specifies, e.g., "exercise strenuously for 5 minutes just prior to ECG."

An electrocardiogram is usually taken by a specially trained technician or by a physician. Electrodes are attached by leads to the electrocardiograph. The electrodes are attached to the client's body with paste, suction cups, or tape. One electrode is attached to the lower part of each limb, and a fifth electrode is moved to six different positions on the chest. The first position is on the right sternal border; subsequent positions follow the general outline of the heart around to the left sternal border and laterally as far as the midaxillary line. See Figure 54–3. The heart's electric impulses register on a graph that the machine produces during the procedure. A physician interprets the graph after the test.

Before the test, the nurse assesses the client's vital signs (body temperature, pulse, respirations, and blood pressure) for baseline data, if not already available. The nurse also determines whether the client has had an electrocardiogram before and explains the procedure, as the client requires. The client may be anxious, not about the test, which is painless, but about the results, which might indicate a problem with the heart. Generally, nursing assistance is not required during the procedure. Following the test, the nurse assesses the client's response to the test, including reported discomfort, pulse, respirations, and blood pressure. The nurse then records on the client's chart the time the ECG was carried out, the person who performed it, and the client's response.

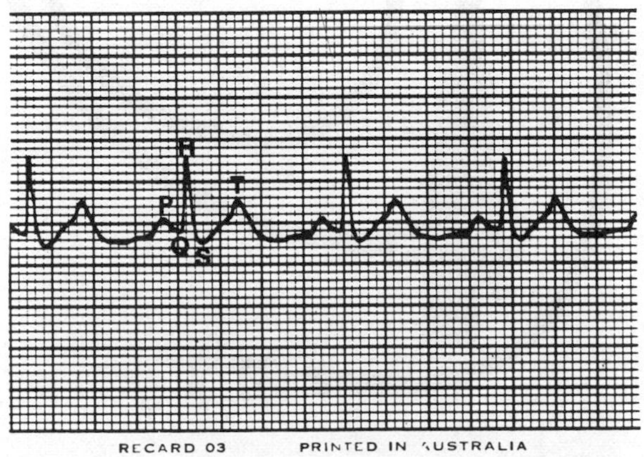

Figure 54–2 A normal electrocardiogram

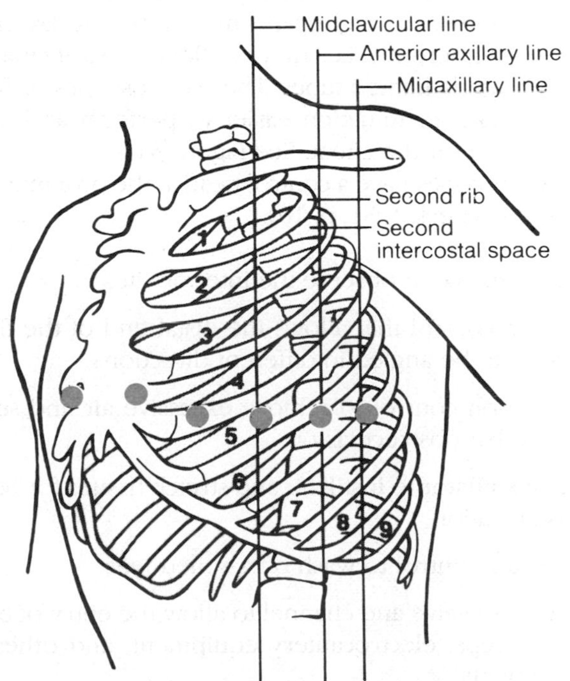

Figure 54–3 The placement of electrodes on the chest of an adult for electrocardiography

If the client is particularly anxious about the test, the nurse notifies the physician so that the results can be explained as soon as possible.

Electroencephalography

Electroencephalograms (EEGs) are recordings of electric activity in the brain. Electroencephalographs have leads to electrodes that attach to the client's scalp with paste or small needles. The client lies in a dorsal recumbent position in a darkened room. The client may be asked to hyperventilate, and readings may also be taken while the client sleeps. If performed on a sleeping client, the test may take 2 hours; otherwise it lasts no more than 1 hour. Figure 40–1 shows brain wave patterns that occur during sleep. The test is normally painless, although the client may feel occasional pinpricks if needle electrodes are used in the scalp.

Preparation for an EEG varies. Some agencies advise that, on the day of the test, the client may not take stimulants such as coffee or depressants such as alcohol. Usually the client takes no medications prior to the test, and the nurse shampoos the client's hair, which should be free of hair spray, hair creams, and the like.

Electromyography

An **electromyogram** (EMG) is a record of the electric potential created by the contraction of a muscle. Two electrodes are attached with paste or small needles to the skin over the muscle. This test is used to discern muscle abnormalities such as **fasciculation** (abnormal contraction involving the whole motor unit). No special preparation is necessary for this procedure. The client may experience some discomfort when the needle electrodes are inserted and some residual discomfort if many muscles are tested.

Often a **nerve conduction study** is done in conjunction with the EMG. This procedure determines the excitability and conduction velocities of motor and sensory nerves and the presence of disease of the peripheral nerves. A stimulating electrode and a recording electrode are placed over specific sites to test a specific nerve. The distance between the electrodes and the time required for a nerve impulse to pass from the point of stimulation to the point of recording are precisely measured. Conduction velocity is then calculated. The client will experience the discomfort of mild electric shock during this procedure, but there should be no residual discomfort.

Examinations Involving Visual Inspection

Visual inspection or direct visualization techniques involve the use of special instruments called **endoscopes**, through which interior parts of the body can be seen. Originally, endoscopes were straight, rigid, metal tubes. Today, endoscopes are fiberoptic, i.e., they are flexible, easily maneuvered, brightly lighted tubes. These endoscopes or fiberscopes make examination easier to perform and more comfortable for the client. See Figure 54–4.

Endoscopes have a control head at the proximal end containing (Beck 1981, p. 10):

1. An eyepiece to observe the interior sites
2. A lens control that allows the distal end of the fiberscope to be angled in different directions
3. A suction control to remove excessive air and secretions that obstruct vision
4. An insufflator to instill air and stretch tissues for better visualization
5. A water control to wash off a soiled lens
6. A biopsy valve and channel to allow the entry of biopsy forceps, electrocautery equipment, and other instruments

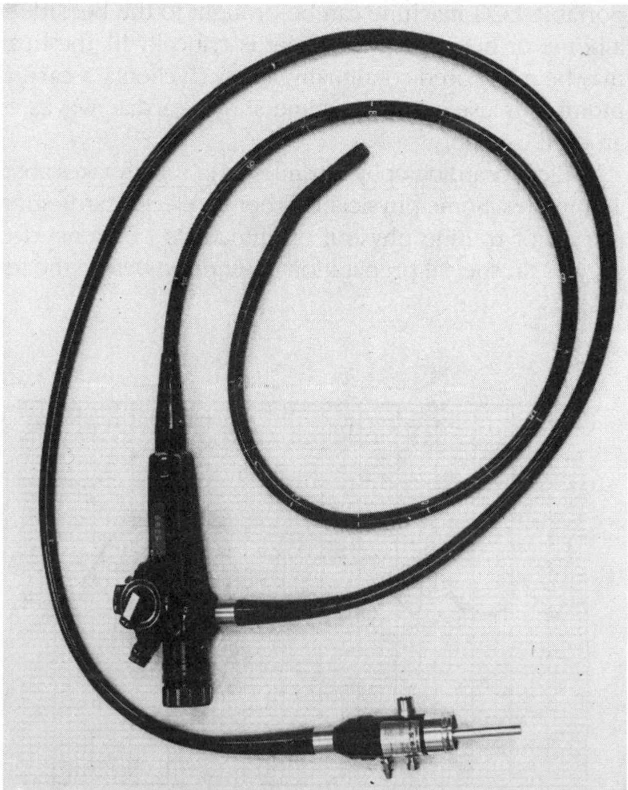

Some endoscopes are equipped with a camera that takes color photographs, which can be studied following the

Figure 54–4 A proctoscope

examination; others allow the attachment of a second eyepiece so that another diagnostician can observe the procedure simultaneously.

Endoscopes and the examinations performed with them assume their names from the body part to be examined. For example, a bronchoscope is used to visualize the bronchi of the lungs, and the examination is called a bronchoscopy. "Scope" denotes the instrument used for visual examination and "scopy" denotes the examination. Endoscopic examinations are usually performed in surgery or special treatment rooms. They generally take about 30 to 60 minutes to complete.

Laryngoscopy and Bronchoscopy

Laryngoscopy and **bronchoscopy** are sterile procedures using a laryngoscope and bronchoscope, respectively. A general or local anesthetic may be given before the examination. If a general anesthetic is given, routine preoperative care is given. See Chapter 53. If a general anesthetic is not given, a local anesthetic is sprayed on the client's pharynx to prevent gagging; alternatively, the client gargles with an anesthetic to anesthetize the throat. The bronchoscope is then inserted to visualize the larynx or bronchi. In some cases, a section of tissue is taken for biopsy. For this procedure, the client usually lies supine on the examining table. See Table 54–1 for nursing interventions before, during, and after the examination.

Esophagoscopy, Gastroscopy, and Duodenoscopy

Esophagoscopy (visual examination of the esophagus), **gastroscopy** (visual examination of the stomach), and **duodenoscopy** (visual examination of the duodenum) are performed with a gastroscope. This is a clean rather than a sterile procedure. See Figure 54–5. If the duodenum is examined, the procedure may last 1 hour. The preparation and care of the client are the same as for laryngoscopy and bronchoscopy. During these procedures, a tissue sample may be taken for biopsy, and samples of secretions may be taken for study of digestive enzymes. See Table 54–1 for nursing interventions.

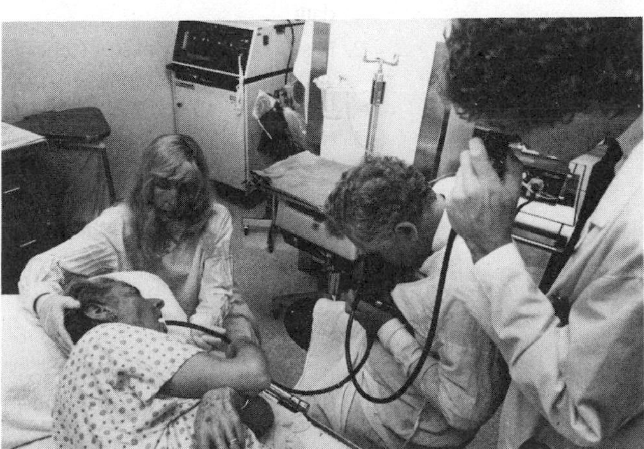

Figure 54–5 An endoscopic procedure in progress

Cystoscopy

Cystoscopy is the visualization of the interior of the urinary bladder; this examination requires insertion of a cystoscope into the bladder via the urethra. It is a sterile procedure. A general or local anesthetic is given, and the preparation is similar to that for bronchoscopy. During cystoscopy, catheters may be inserted up the ureters into each kidney. Contrast medium is then injected into the kidneys, and x-ray photographs are taken. This procedure is known as **retrograde pyelography**. The x-ray film shows the kidney calyces, the kidney pelvis, the ureters, and the urinary bladder. When a pyelogram is to be taken, the client is given laxatives and enemas to free the intestines of feces and gas. **Intravenous pyelography** (IVP) or **urography** (IVU) is roentgenography of the kidneys after the injection of dye into the arterial system. An intravenous pyelogram shows the same structures as a retrograde pyelogram. This examination does not require an anesthetic and normally lasts about 1 hour.

Cystoscopy is a sterile procedure. It may be performed both for diagnostic and for therapeutic purposes. Diagnostic purposes include:

1. Direct inspection for tumors, calculi, ulcers, or other defects
2. Biopsy of the bladder and urethra
3. Measurement of bladder capacity
4. Collection of urine directly from each kidney separately
5. X-ray visualization as described above

Therapeutic purposes include:

1. Removal of stones
2. Emptying of the renal pelvis
3. Removal of tumors
4. Dilation of urethra, bladder, or uretus
5. Cautery of bleeding areas

See Table 54–1 for nursing interventions.

Anoscopy, Proctoscopy, Sigmoidoscopy, and Colonoscopy

Anoscopy, **proctoscopy**, **sigmoidoscopy**, and **colonoscopy** are endoscopic procedures of the mucosa of the anus, rectum, sigmoid colon, and colon, respectively. A

Table 54–1 Nursing Interventions for Endoscopic Examinations

Examination	Preprocedure	During Procedure	Postprocedure
Laryngoscopy or bronchoscopy	Explain the procedure and clarify concerns of the client. Explain that a local spray or gargle will be given or that some medications will be injected through a needle in the vein, that the client will rest the teeth against a small plastic mouthpiece, that the procedure is painless but some pressure may be felt. Explain that the test will take about 30–60 minutes. Assess vital signs, sputum, and character of respirations for baseline data. Remove dentures, necklaces, earrings, hairpins, and combs. Ensure good oral hygiene. Ensure nothing by mouth 6 to 8 hours beforehand. Confirm that the client is not allergic to any medications that will be given. Administer analgesic, sedative, antianxiety agent, and medication to dry secretions, if ordered.	Assist the physician as required, e.g., to hold the head piece or to move the client's head. Monitor the client's pulse and respirations. Support the client using touch and verbal communication.	1. Monitor vital signs every 30 minutes during the recovery period and compare results to baseline data. 2. Withhold fluids until the gag reflex is restored and the client is conscious. 3. Position the client as ordered or indicated. Place the unconscious client in the lateral position so that secretions are not aspirated. 4. Inspect the client's sputum for blood caused by tissue damage. 5. Observe the client for signs of dyspnea, stridor, and shortness of breath, which may result from laryngeal edema or laryngospasm. 6. Provide ice chips and warm saline gargles or throat lozenges and administer ordered analgesics as required for throat discomfort. 7. Advise the client to contact the physician if client has persistent difficulty with breathing, blood in sputum, fever, or pain.
Esophagoscopy, gastroscopy, and duodenoscopy	As above for bronchoscopy, with the exception of assessing sputum. Explain that the client may feel pressure in the stomach as the tube is moved about and fullness or bloating, like that after eating a large meal.	As above for bronchoscopy. Administer oral simethicone (Mylicon) before test if ordered; it decreases air bubbles in the stomach. If atropine is given intravenously to reduce gastrointestinal spasm, carefully monitor the client's pulse rate. Atropine increases the heart rate.	1. Follow steps 1 to 3 and 6, as for bronchoscopy. 2. Inspect emesis for blood and test it for occult blood if agency practice indicates. 3. Advise the client to contact the physician if client has persistent difficulty swallowing, pain, fever, blood in vomitus, or black stools.
Cystoscopy	Assess vital signs, frequency of urination, dysuria, amount and consistency of urine for baseline data. Administer enema if ordered. A clear bowel is necessary if x-ray films are planned. Ensure nothing by mouth for 6 to 8 hours or only IV fluids if general anesthetic is being given. Ensure appropriate fluid intake, if ordered, for the client having a local anesthetic to ensure an adequate flow of urine for the collection of specimens. Administer sedative and medication to dry secretions, if ordered.	Support the client emotionally. Monitor vital signs. Label specimens, if taken, appropriately. Assist the physician as requested.	1. Monitor vital signs, urination, and urine and compare with baseline data. 2. Position the unconscious client appropriately (as above for bronchoscopy). 3. Inspect the client's urine for blood and report bright red bleeding. 4. Report inability to urinate by 8 hours. 5. Encourage increased fluid intake to decrease irritation of urinary tissue. 6. If dyes were used in the procedure, warn the client that the urine may be an unusual color.

Table 54–1 *(continued)*

Examination	Preprocedure	During Procedure	Postprocedure
			7. Administer analgesics, as ordered, for pain. 8. If the client is discharged, advise him or her to report persistent difficulty passing urine, bright blood in urine, pain, or fever.
Anoscopy, proctoscopy, sigmoidoscopy, and colonoscopy	Assess vital signs and consistency of feces for baseline data. Ensure appropriate preexamination diet and fluid intake. Some agencies provide a light evening meal the day before and only fluid the day of the examination. Administer laxative, if ordered, the evening before. Administer enemas until returns are clear or suppository as ordered the morning of the examination. Ensure that the client voids before the examination. The pressure of the procedure may injure a full bladder. Administer sedative beforehand, if ordered. Just before the endoscope is inserted explain (a) that the client will experience the sensation of having to move the bowels due to the pressure of the instrument, and (b) that the client may experience some abdominal cramping when air is introduced to distend the bowel.	Support the client physically in the knee-chest position, as needed. Monitor pulse and respiratory rates. Label specimens, if taken, appropriately. Support the client emotionally. Acknowledge feelings the client experiences, e.g., cramps, and assure him or her that they are expected.	1. Monitor vital signs and compare with baseline data. 2. Inspect the next few stools for blood. 3. Allow the client to rest. This procedure is physically and emotionally tiring. 4. Provide fluids and food.

proctoscope or sigmoidoscope is used to examine the anus, rectum, and sigmoid colon. A colonoscope is used to examine the large bowel.

Preparation generally includes the administration of laxatives or enemas begun the evening before to clear the bowel of feces. General anesthesia is usually not necessary, although the client may experience some discomfort. The client assumes a knee-chest position on a special examining table during the examination.

Examinations Involving Removal of Body Fluids and Tissues

Certain body fluids and tissues can help physicians diagnose disease. Table 54–2 lists some common procedures for removing body fluids and tissues. The procedures are normally performed by a physician at the bedside, in an examining room, or sometimes in the emergency department of a hospital. All the procedures described here involve inserting an instrument, often a needle, through the skin and withdrawing some fluid or tissue. The fluid or tissue is usually placed in a special container and sent to the laboratory for examination.

Lumbar Puncture

A **lumbar puncture** (LP, spinal tap) is the insertion of a needle into the subarachnoid space of the spinal canal to withdraw cerebrospinal fluid (CSF). An adult normally has about 150 ml of CSF (Guyton 1986, p. 374). The major function of the spinal fluid is to cushion the brain within the skull. The site of a lumbar puncture is usually between the third and fourth or the fourth and fifth lumbar vertebrae. Inserted at this level, the needle does not damage

Table 54–2 Common Aspiration Studies

Name	Type of Specimen	Source	Key Postprocedure Assessments
Lumbar puncture	Spinal fluid	Subarachnoid space of the spinal canal	Vital signs, neurologic signs, headache
Cisternal puncture	Spinal fluid	Subarachnoid space of the cisterna magna	As for lumbar puncture
Abdominal paracentesis	Ascitic fluid	Peritoneal cavity	Blood pressure, pulse, skin color, weight, abdominal girth
Thoracocentesis	Pleural fluid	Pleural cavity	Pulse, respirations, skin color
Pericardial aspiration	Pericardial fluid	Pericardial sac	As for thoracocentesis
Bone marrow biopsy	Bone marrow	Iliac crest, posterior superior iliac spine, or sternum	Leakage at site, pain
Liver biopsy	Liver tissue	Liver	Blood pressure, pulse, respirations, bleeding at site

the spinal cord and major nerve roots. See Figure 54–6. The fourth lumbar interspace is the most common lumbar puncture site for adults, but the site is usually lower for infants and small children, whose spinal cord extends almost into the sacral region.

About 500 ml of cerebrospinal fluid (about three times the total volume of fluid in the CSF cavity) is formed daily. About two-thirds of this is formed by the choroid plexus in each of the four ventricles of the brain. The remainder comes from the ependymal surfaces of the ventricles and from the brain directly (Guyton 1986, p. 375). The fluid normally circulates freely through the ventricles, through the subarachnoid space around the brain and spinal cord, and through the central canal of the cord. It is continually reabsorbed into the venous circulation through villi from the arachnoid layer, which extend into the superior sagittal sinus.

Lumbar punctures are carried out for the following diagnostic and therapeutic reasons:

1. To analyze the constituents of the CSF
2. To test the pressure of CSF
3. To relieve pressure by removing CSF
4. To inject a spinal anesthetic, dye, or air into the spinal canal

Equipment

A lumbar puncture requires sterile technique. Many hospitals have disposable lumbar puncture kits. The equipment required includes:

1. Sterile sponges
2. Antiseptic solution
3. Local anesthetic and 21- and 24-gauge needles and syringes for its injection
4. Lumbar puncture needle 5 to 12.5 cm (2 to 5 in) long, depending on the age and size of the client (infants require a 5 cm needle)
5. Specimen containers
6. Manometer to measure spinal fluid pressure
7. Three-way stopcock
8. Small dressing to put over the puncture site
9. Sterile gloves
10. Masks (optional)

Medical Technique

The physician applies an antiseptic to the area, injects local anesthetic, and inserts the needle into the intravertebral space. When the flow of CSF is established, the stopcock and manometer are attached to obtain an initial CSF pressure reading. Normal opening pressures are 60 to 180 mm of water. Pressures above 200 mm are considered abnormal.

A Queckenstedt-Stookey test may also be done while the manometer is attached. Someone (often the nurse) exerts digital pressure on one or both of the client's internal jugular veins. If the client is normal, digital pressure temporarily increases the manometer reading. If there is a blockage in the spinal canal, digital pressure on the veins affects CSF pressure very little or not at all.

The physician usually takes specimens of CSF and hands the specimen tubes to the nurse, who numbers them in the sequence taken. The physician collects a total of 10 ml of fluid and places 2 to 3 ml of fluid in each specimen tube. Specimens of CSF are often tested in the laboratory for sugar, bacteria, cell count, etc. Normal CSF is a clear, colorless fluid. Blood may give the fluid a reddish cast, and infection may make the fluid cloudy.

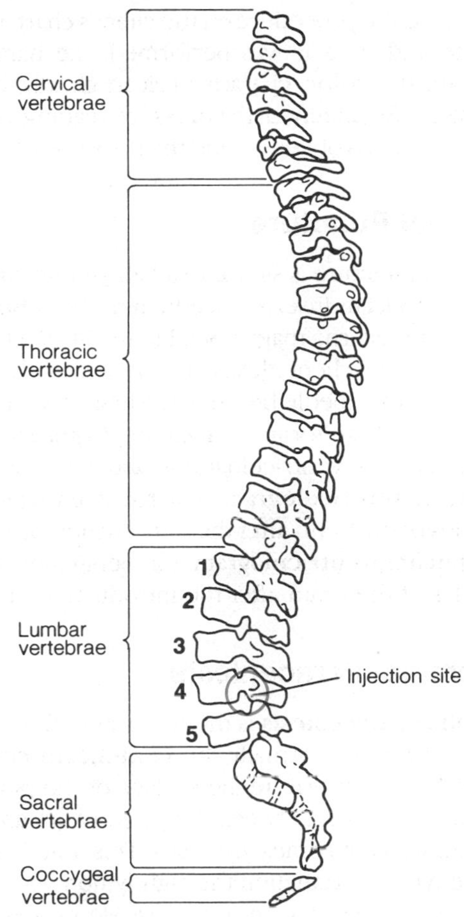

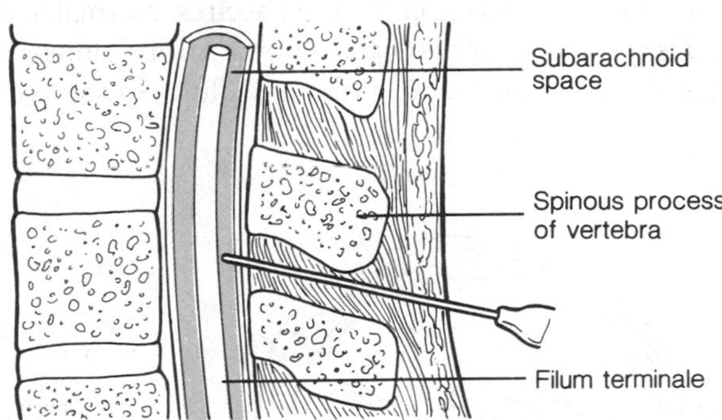

Figure 54–6 A diagram of the vertebral column, indicating the site for a lumbar puncture

After collecting the specimens, the physician may take a final (closing) CSF pressure reading before removing the spinal needle.

Nursing Intervention

Preprocedure Assess the client's vital signs, pertinent health status, e.g., level of consciousness and neurologic status, to obtain baseline data. Determine drug allergies, particularly to local anesthetics and skin antiseptics.

Explain the following to the client, even if he or she appears stuporous or confused:

1. That the physician will be taking a small sample of spinal fluid from the lower spine
2. That a local anesthetic will be given so that the client will feel no pain
3. When and where the procedure will occur, e.g., at the bedside or in the treatment room
4. Who will be present, i.e., the physician and the nurse
5. The time involved, e.g., about 15 minutes

In addition, tell the client what to expect during the procedure. The client may feel slight discomfort (like a pinprick) when the local anesthetic is injected and a sensation of pressure when the spinal needle is being inserted. Remind the client that it is important to remain still and in one position throughout the procedure. A restless client or a child will need to be held to prevent movement.

Have the client empty his or her bladder and bowels prior to the procedure to prevent unnecessary discomfort.

Position the client laterally with the head bent toward the chest, the knees flexed onto the abdomen and the back at the edge of the bed or examining table. See Figure 54–7. Place a very small pillow under the client's head to maintain the horizontal alignment of the spine. In this position, the back is arched, increasing the spaces between the vertebrae so that the spinal needle can be inserted readily. Drape the client to expose only the lumbar spine.

Open the lumbar puncture set, and supply the physician with the sterile gloves and antiseptic, in a container or poured onto sterile gauze squares, if necessary.

During the procedure Stand in front of the client, and support the back of the client's neck and knees if the client

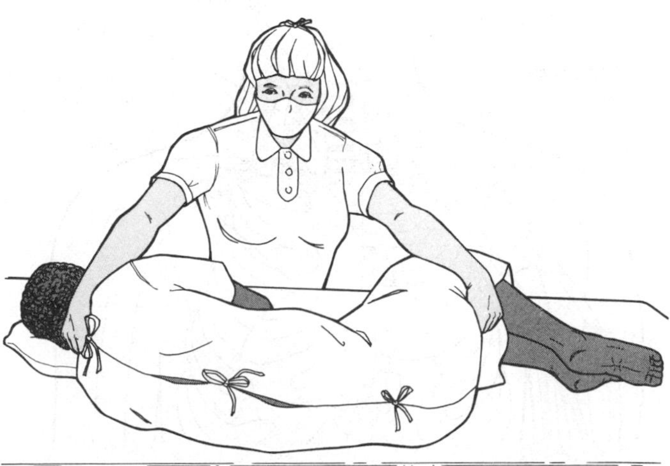

Figure 54–7 Positioning the client for a lumbar puncture

needs help remaining in this position without moving. See Figure 54–7. Reassure the client throughout the procedure by explaining what is happening. Encourage him or her to breathe normally and relax as much as possible because excessive muscle tension, coughing, or changes in breathing can increase CSF pressure, resulting in a false reading.

If the Queckenstedt-Stookey test is being done, place digital pressure on the client's jugular veins. See Figure 54–8. Label the specimen tubes in sequence if they are not already labeled. While handling the tubes, take care to prevent contamination of the physician's sterile gloves, the sterile field, and yourself, since the CSF may contain virulent microorganisms, e.g., those that cause meningitis. Place a small sterile dressing over the site of the puncture to help prevent infection after the needle is removed.

Postprocedure Assist the client to a dorsal recumbent position with only one pillow under the head. The client should not sit up for 8 to 24 hours, until the CSF is replenished. Determine the recommended time this position should be maintained. Some clients experience a headache after a lumbar puncture, and the dorsal recumbent position tends to prevent or alleviate it. Often analgesics are ordered and can be given for headaches.

Assess the client's pallor, changes in pulse rate and other vital signs, changes in neurologic status, swelling or bleeding at the puncture site, and complaints of faintness or headache. Be alert for complaints of numbness, tingling, or pain radiating down the legs, which may be due to nerve irritation. Observe the puncture site for leakage of CSF.

Ensure that the CSF specimens are correctly labeled and send them immediately to the laboratory, with the completed requisition.

Record the procedure on the client's chart, including the date and time it was performed; the name of the physician; the color, character (clear, cloudy, etc.), and amount of CSF obtained; the pressure readings; the number of specimens obtained; and the response of the client.

Cisternal Puncture

A **cisternal puncture** is similar to a lumbar puncture except that the physician inserts a needle into the subarachnoid space of the cisterna magna. See Figure 54–9. During this procedure, the client flexes the neck acutely to allow insertion of the needle between the first cervical vertebra and the rim of the foramen magnum. Cisternal puncture is necessary for ventriculograms and pneumoventriculograms. A **ventriculogram** is a roentgenogram of the ventricles of the brain after the introduction of an opaque dye. A **pneumoventriculogram** is a roentgenogram of the ventricles of the brain after the introduction of air.

Abdominal Paracentesis

Abdominal paracentesis is the removal of fluid from the peritoneal cavity. Normally the peritoneum creates just enough fluid to lubricate the surface of the peritoneum and reduce friction between the peritoneum and the tissues with which it comes in contact. This fluid is absorbed into the lymph circulation through lymph vessels in the peritoneum. However, in some disease processes, such as cirrhosis of the liver, large amounts of fluid collect in the cavity; this condition is called **ascites**. Normal ascitic fluid is serous (clear and light yellow). An abdominal paracentesis is carried out to obtain a fluid specimen for

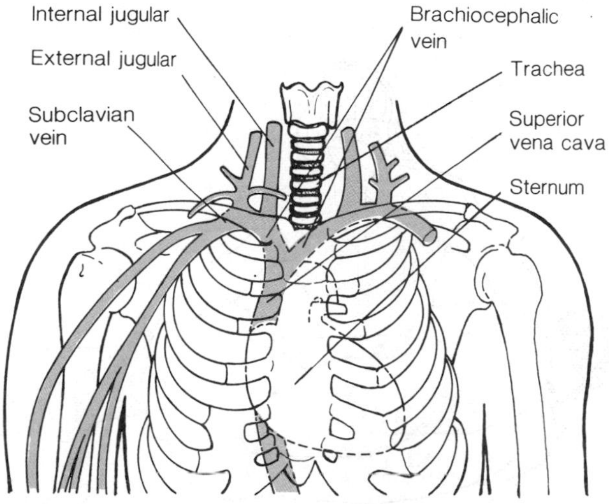

Figure 54–8 Location of the internal jugular vein, where digital pressure is applied during the Queckenstedt-Stookey test

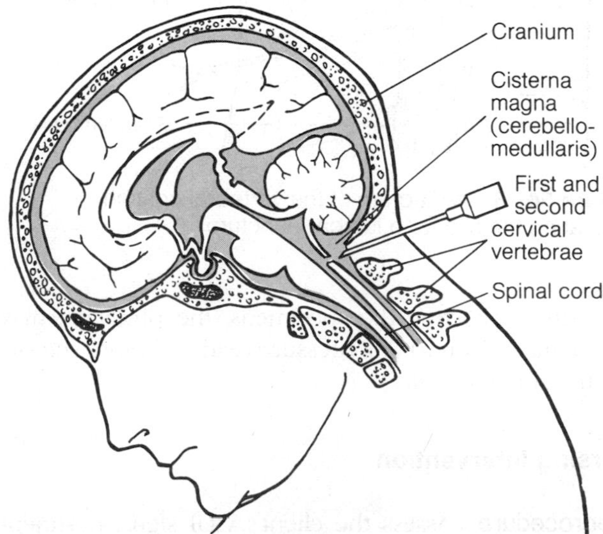

Figure 54–9 During a cisternal puncture, a needle is inserted into the subarachnoid space of the cisterna magna.

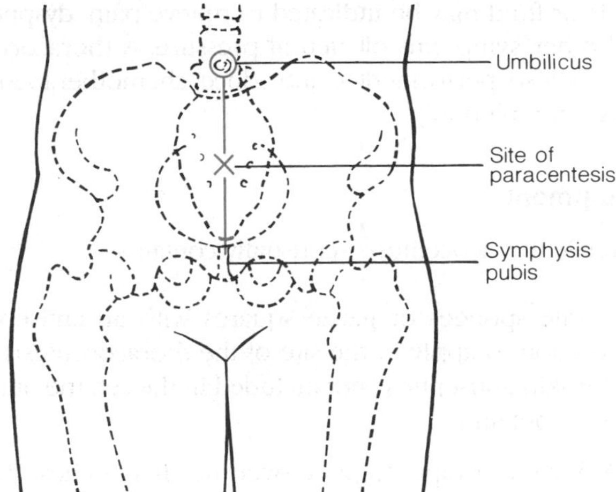

Figure 54–10 A common site for an abdominal paracentesis

laboratory study and to relieve pressure on the abdominal organs due to excess fluid. A common site for an abdominal paracentesis is midway between the umbilicus and the symphysis pubis in the midline. See Figure 54–10.

Equipment

Abdominal paracentesis requires sterile technique. Paracentesis sets are usually available. These contain:

1. Antiseptic
2. Sponges
3. Local anesthetic
4. Syringe and 24- and 22-gauge needles to administer the anesthetic
5. Fenestrated drape
6. Small scalpel to make an incision in the abdomen
7. A needle holder and sutures to sew the incision
8. Specimen containers
9. Dressings
10. Aspirating set

The aspirating set generally includes a receptacle for the fluid, tubing, and a trocar and cannula. A **trocar** is a sharp, pointed instrument that fits inside the cannula and pierces, in this case, the peritoneal cavity. A **cannula** is a tube through which plastic tubing can be threaded to drain fluid. The trocar and cannula (and the scalpel, sutures, and needle holder) are needed only if the purpose of paracentesis is to drain fluid. If the purpose is to obtain a specimen, an incision is not made. A long aspirating needle attached to a syringe is used in place of a trocar and cannula. Masks are optional. Also needed are sterile gloves for the physician.

Medical Technique

The physician applies an antiseptic to the site of the incision, drapes the area with sterile drapes, and administers a local anesthetic. After the area is numbed, the physician makes a small incision with a scalpel, inserts the trocar and cannula (the trocar inside the cannula), and then withdraws the trocar. Tubing is attached to the cannula, and the fluid flows through the tubing into a receptacle. Normally about 1500 ml is the maximum amount of fluid drained at one time, to avoid hypovolemic shock. The fluid is drained very slowly for the same reason. Some fluid is placed in the specimen container before the cannula is withdrawn. The small incision may or may not be sutured; in either case, it is covered with a small sterile bandage.

Nursing Intervention

Preprocedure Assess the client's vital signs to obtain baseline data. Weigh the client and measure the client's abdominal girth at the level of the umbilicus to obtain an indication of the amount of ascites. (See Figure 54–11.) Determine any allergies, in particular to local anesthetics and antiseptics. Record your findings.

Explain the procedure to the client. Normally an abdominal paracentesis is not painful, and, when a client

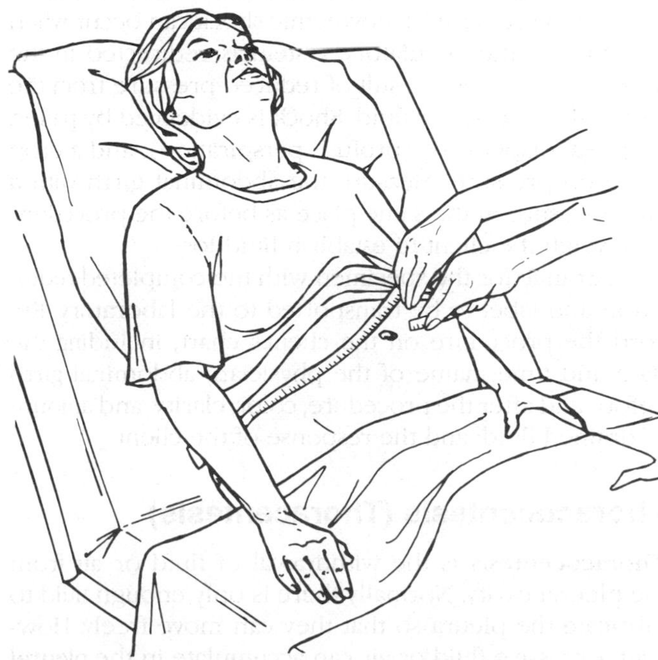

Figure 54–11 Measuring the abdominal girth at the level of the umbilicus

has considerable ascites, the procedure can relieve discomfort caused by the fluid. The procedure to remove ascitic fluid usually takes 30 to 60 minutes. Obtaining a specimen usually takes about 15 minutes. Emphasize the importance of remaining still during the procedure. Explain when and where the procedure will occur and who will be present.

Have the client void just before the paracentesis to lessen the possibility of puncturing the urinary bladder. Notify the physician if the client cannot void prior to the procedure.

Help the client assume a sitting position in bed so that the fluid will accumulate in the lower abdominal cavity and so that gravity and the pressure of the abdominal organs will help the flow of the fluid from the cavity. Some clients may be able to sit on the edge of the bed with pillows to support the back. Cover the client to expose only the necessary area.

During the procedure Open the paracentesis set, and supply the physician with the sterile gloves and antiseptic in a container or poured onto sterile gauze squares. Open and hold the ampule or vial of local anesthetic, if it is not part of the sterile set.

Support the client verbally, and describe the steps of the procedure, if the physician does not do so. Observe the client closely for signs of distress. A major concern is hypovolemic shock induced by the loss of fluid. See postprocedure interventions.

Place a small sterile dressing over the site of the incision after the cannula is withdrawn.

Postprocedure Assess the client's pulse rate, skin color, and blood pressure. Hypovolemic shock can occur when the fluid in the circulatory system is redirected to the abdominal area as a result of reduced pressure from the removal of the ascitic fluid. Shock is evidenced by pallor, dyspnea, diaphoresis (profuse perspiration), and a drop in blood pressure. Measure the abdominal girth with a tape measure in the same place as before the procedure and weigh the client to establish fluid loss.

Arrange for the specimen with the completed requisition and label to be transported to the laboratory. Record the procedure on the client's chart, including the date and time; name of the physician; abdominal girth before and after the procedure; color, clarity, and amount of drained fluid; and the response of the client.

Thoracocentesis (Thoracentesis)

Thoracocentesis is the withdrawal of fluid or air from the pleural cavity. Normally there is only enough fluid to lubricate the pleura so that they can move freely. However, excessive fluid or air can accumulate in the pleural cavity as a result of injury or disease. Pleural fluid is removed for both diagnostic and therapeutic purposes. Aspiration of air or fluid may be indicated to relieve pain, dyspnea, and other symptoms of pleural pressure. A thoracocentesis is also performed to introduce chemotherapeutic drugs intrapleurally.

Equipment

A sterile thoracocentesis set usually contains:

1. Sterile sponges or gauze squares with an antiseptic solution to apply to the site of the thoracocentesis. If the skin antiseptic is not included in the set, the nurse must obtain it.
2. A drape or drapes to place over the client's chest. The drape is often fenestrated, and the opening is placed at the site of the thoracocentesis.
3. A 2 ml syringe and 24- and 22-gauge needles to administer the anesthetic. If these are not in the set, the nurse needs to obtain them.
4. A receptacle for the fluid. This may be a syringe (50 ml) and 16-gauge needle or an airtight container with negative pressure created by a pump or a suction machine. The negative pressure in the container must be greater than that of the pleural space. Negative pressure also prevents air from entering the pleural space and causing a pneumothorax (air in the pleural cavity).
5. A three-way stopcock to prevent air from entering the pleural space.
6. A two-way stopcock with connecting tubing to maintain the negative pressure in the receptacle and to direct the flow of pleural fluid into the container.
7. A thoracocentesis needle, usually a 15-gauge needle about 5 to 7.5 cm (2 to 3 in) long.
8. A specimen container.
9. A local anesthetic. The anesthetic is usually packaged in an ampule.

Sterile gloves for the physician are required. Masks for the nurse and the physician are optional. A completed laboratory requisition and label for the specimen are needed.

Medical Technique

The physician dons sterile gloves, cleans the site with an antiseptic solution, and administers a local anesthetic. The physician attaches a syringe and/or stopcock to the aspirating needle. The stopcock must be in the closed position so that no air will enter the pleural space. The physician inserts the needle through the intercostal space into the pleural cavity. In some instances, a small plastic tube is threaded through the needle and the needle is then withdrawn. (The tubing is less likely to puncture the pleura.) If a syringe is used, the plunger is pulled out to draw out the pleural fluid as the stopcock is opened. If a large container is used to receive the fluid, the tubing is attached from the stopcock to the adapter on the receiving bottle. When the adapter and stopcock are opened, negative pressure in the container draws the fluid from the pleural cavity. After the fluid has been withdrawn, the physician removes the needle or plastic tubing.

Nursing Intervention

Preprocedure Assess (a) vital signs (body temperature, pulse, respirations, and blood pressure) to obtain baseline data, if these are not already available; (b) respiratory depth and the movement of both sides of the chest during inspiration, to note differences between the two sides; (c) complaints of chest pain; (d) breath sounds; (e) dyspnea; (f) type and frequency of cough, if present; and (g) character and amount of sputum.

Also determine if the client has drug allergies, particularly allergies to the medications contained in local anesthetics and skin antiseptics. Administer any ordered cough medicine 30 minutes before the thoracocentesis to suppress coughing during the procedure.

Explain the procedure to the client. Normally a thoracocentesis is not painful, although the client may experience a feeling of pressure when the needle is inserted. The client may experience considerable relief if breathing has been difficult. The procedure takes only a few minutes, depending primarily on the time it takes the fluid to drain from the pleural cavity. It is important for the client not to cough while the needle is inserted, to avoid puncturing the lungs. Explain when and where the procedure will occur and who will be present.

Help the client assume a comfortable position. This is usually a sitting position with the arms above the head, which spreads the ribs and enlarges the intercostal space. Two positions commonly used are: arm elevated and stretched forward (see Figure 54–12*A*), and leaning forward over pillows (see Figure 54–12*B*). To make sure that the needle is inserted below the fluid level when fluid is to be removed (or above any fluid if air is to be removed), the physician palpates the chest and selects the exact site for insertion of the needle. A site on the lower posterior chest is often used to remove fluid, and a site on the upper anterior chest is used to remove air.

During the procedure Open the thoracocentesis set, and supply the sterile gloves to the physician. Pour antiseptic solution into a container or onto sterile gauze squares if necessary. Open and hold the ampule or vial of local anesthetic if it is not part of the sterile set.

Support the client verbally, and describe the steps of the procedure if the physician does not do so. Observe

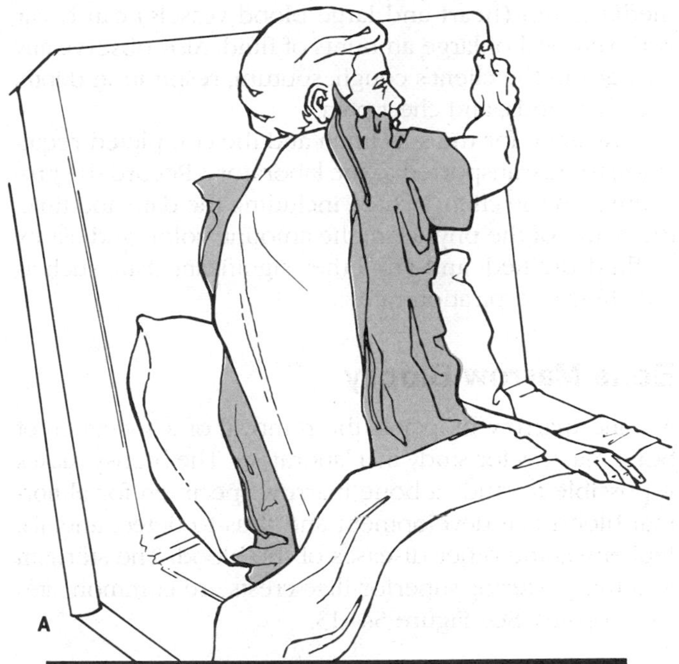

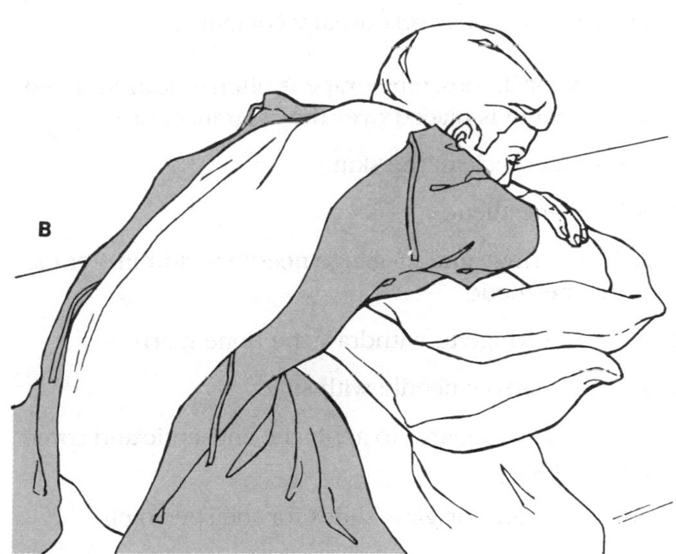

Figure 54–12 Two positions commonly used for a thoracocentesis: **A,** arm held in front and up; **B,** sitting and leaning forward over pillows

the client closely for signs of distress, such as dyspnea, pallor, and coughing. If the client becomes distressed or has to cough, the procedure is halted briefly. The physician may withdraw the needle slightly to avoid puncturing the pleura.

Following the removal of the needle, place a small sterile dressing over the puncture site.

Postprocedure Assess the client's blood pressure, pulse, respiration rate, and skin color, because a shift in the mediastinum (heart and large blood vessels) can occur with removal of large amounts of fluid. Also observe any changes in the client's cough, sputum, respiration depth, breath sounds, and chest pain.

Arrange for the specimen and the completed requisition to be transported to the laboratory. Record the procedure on the client's chart, including the date and time; the name of the physician; the amount, color, and clarity of fluid drained; and any other significant data, such as the client's respiration rate.

Bone Marrow Biopsy

A bone marrow biopsy is the removal of a specimen of bone marrow for study in a laboratory. The biopsy makes it possible to study a bone marrow specimen for abnormal blood cell development and thus to detect anemia, leukemia, and other diseases of the blood. The sternum and the posterior superior iliac crests are common sites for biopsies. See Figure 54–13.

Equipment

Bone marrow biopsy sets usually contain:

1. A drape or drapes. One drape is often fenestrated, and the opening is placed over the aspiration site.
2. Antiseptic to clean the skin.
3. A local anesthetic.
4. A 2 ml syringe and 25-gauge needle to administer the local anesthetic.
5. A 10 ml syringe to withdraw the bone marrow.
6. A bone marrow needle with stylet.
7. Sterile gauze squares to apply the antiseptic and cover the wound.
8. Test tubes and/or glass slides for the specimen.

Also needed are masks for the nurse and physician (optional), sterile gloves for the physician, and a completed laboratory requisition and labels for the specimen.

Medical Technique

The physician dons sterile gloves, applies a drape, and cleans the skin with antiseptic. The physician administers a local anesthetic into the skin and the periosteum of the bone. Then the physician introduces a bone marrow needle with stylet through the skin and bone into the red marrow of the spongy bone. Once the needle is in the marrow space, the physician removes the stylet, attaches a 10 ml syringe to the needle, and draws the plunger back until 1 or 2 ml of marrow has been withdrawn. The physician replaces the stylet in the needle, withdraws the needle, and places the specimen in test tubes and/or on glass slides.

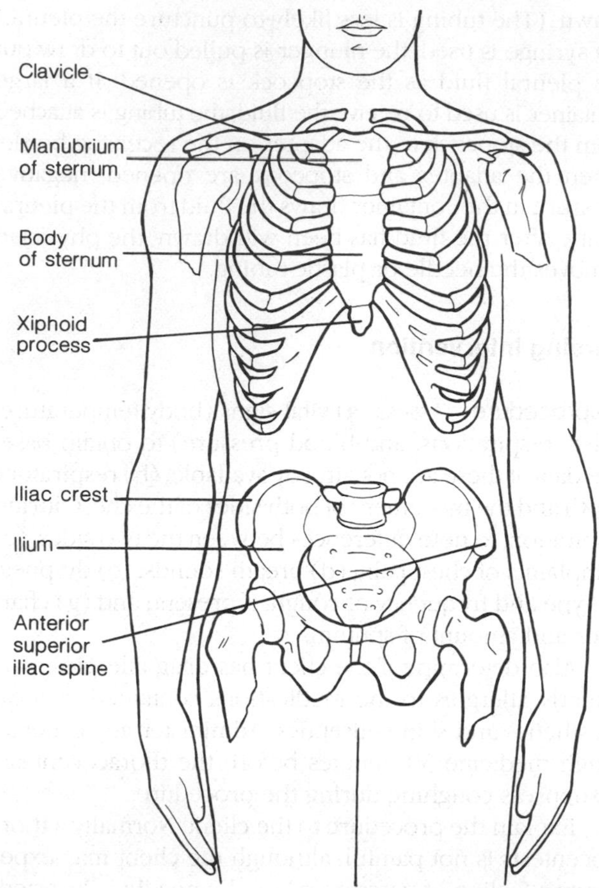

Figure 54–13 The sternum and iliac crests are common sites for bone marrow biopsies.

Nursing Intervention

Preprocedure Assess the client's vital signs for baseline data. Determine any client allergies, in particular to local anesthetics and skin antiseptics.

Explain the procedure to the client. The client may experience pain when the marrow is aspirated. There may be a crunching sound when the needle is pushed through the cortex of the bone. The entire procedure usually takes 15 to 30 minutes. Explain when and where the procedure will occur and who will be present.

Help the client assume a supine position (with one pillow if desired) for a biopsy of the sternum (sternal puncture) or a prone position for a biopsy of either iliac crest. Fold the bedclothes back to expose the area.

During the procedure Open the bone marrow set, and supply the sterile gloves to the physician. Pour the antiseptic into a container in the set or over sterile gauze squares. Open and hold the ampule or vial of local anesthetic, if it is not in the set.

Describe the steps of the procedure to the client, and provide verbal support. Observe the client for pallor, diaphoresis, and faintness. Place a small dressing over the site of the puncture after the needle is withdrawn.

Postprocedure Assess the client's discomfort and any bleeding from the site. The client may experience some tenderness in the area. Bleeding and hematoma formation need to be assessed for several days. Provide an analgesic if required by the client and ordered by the physician.

Arrange for the specimen with the completed requisition and label to be transported to the laboratory. Record the procedure on the client's chart, including the date and time of the procedure, the name of the physician, and the response of the client.

Liver Biopsy

A liver biopsy is a short procedure, generally performed at the client's bedside. It requires sterile technique. The physician inserts a needle into the liver to aspirate a sample of liver tissue. The site of insertion is either between two of the right lower ribs (see Figure 54–14) or through the abdomen below the right rib cage (subcostally). Liver biopsies are usually conducted to facilitate diagnosis of liver disease and to gain information about changes in liver tissue.

Equipment

A sterile liver biopsy set containing:

1. Sterile sponges or gauze squares with an antiseptic solution to apply to the skin site

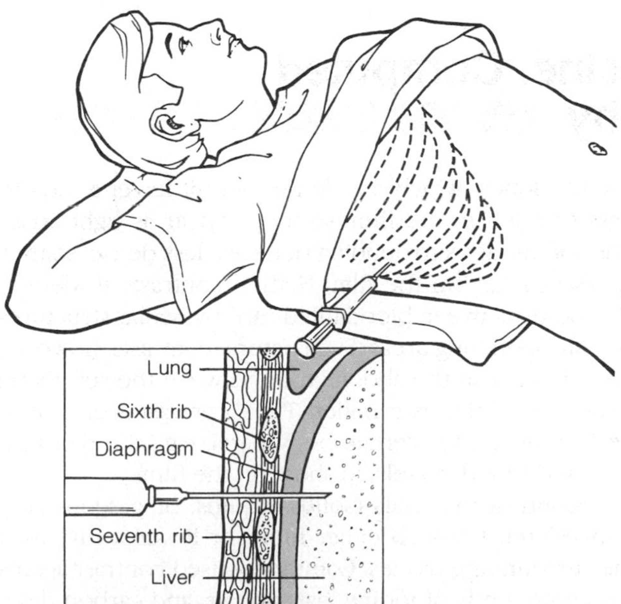

Figure 54–14 The site for a liver biopsy

2. A 2 ml syringe and 22- and 25-gauge needles (¾ in) to inject the local anesthetic
3. A large biopsy syringe and needle
4. Drapes
5. A local anesthetic
6. Sterile normal saline to clean the biopsy needle after insertion
7. A specimen container with formalin to preserve the liver tissue

Also needed are face masks for the physician and the nurse (optional), sterile gloves for the physician, and a laboratory requisition and a specimen label.

Medical Technique

The physician puts on sterile gloves, applies an antiseptic to the biopsy site, drapes the area with sterile drapes, and injects the local anesthetic. When the area feels numb, the client holds his or her breath, and the physician inserts the biopsy needle, injects a small amount of sterile normal saline to clear the needle of blood or particles of tissue picked up during insertion, and aspirates liver tissue by drawing back on the plunger of the syringe. After the needle is withdrawn, the nurse applies pressure to the site to prevent bleeding.

Nursing Intervention

Preprocedure Assess the client's vital signs (body temperature, pulse, respirations, and blood pressure) for baseline data. Determine any drug allergies, particularly allergies to medications contained in the local anesthetics and skin antiseptics. Also assess the client's ability to hold his or her breath for up to 10 seconds. It is vitally important that the client do so and remain still while the biopsy needle is inserted.

Also determine the prothrombin time and platelet count from the client's record. Ensure that these are normal. Because many clients with liver disease have blood clotting defects and are prone to bleeding, prothrombin time and platelet count are normally determined well in advance of the test. If the test results are abnormal, the biopsy may be contraindicated. Also determine if any preprocedural medications are required. Ensure that ordered medications have been given. Several days before the test, vitamin K may be administered intramuscularly to reduce the risk of hemorrhage. Vitamin K may be lacking in some clients with liver disease. It is essential for the production of prothrombin, which is a requisite for blood clotting.

Explain the procedure to the client, including what the physician will do, i.e., take a small sample of liver tissue by putting a needle into the client's side or abdomen; what will be done to prevent pain, i.e., a sedative and local anesthetic will be given; when and where the procedure will occur; who will be present; how long the procedure will last; and what to expect as the procedure is performed, i.e., the client may experience mild discomfort when the local anesthetic is injected and slight pressure when the biopsy needle is inserted.

Ensure that the client fasts for at least two hours before the procedure. Administer the appropriate sedative about 30 minutes beforehand or at the specified time. Help the client assume a supine position, with the upper right quadrant of the abdomen exposed. Cover the client with the bedclothes so that only the abdominal area is exposed.

During the procedure Open the sterile set and provide the sterile gloves for the physician. Pour antiseptic solution over the sterile sponges or gauze, or into a container, as required.

Support the client in a supine position. Instruct the client to take a few deep inhalations and exhalations and to hold his or her breath after the final exhalation for up to 10 seconds as the needle is inserted, the biopsy obtained, and the needle withdrawn. Holding the breath after exhalation immobilizes the chest wall and liver and keeps the diaphragm in its highest position, avoiding injury to the diaphragm and laceration of the liver. Instruct the client to resume breathing when the needle is withdrawn. Apply pressure to the site of the puncture. Pressure will help stop any bleeding. Apply a small dressing to the site of the puncture site.

Postprocedure Assist the client to a right side-lying position with a small pillow or folded towel under the biopsy site. See Figure 54–15. Instruct him or her to remain in this position for several hours. The right lateral position compresses the biopsy site of the liver against the chest wall and minimizes the escape of blood or bile through the puncture site. Send the labeled specimen immediately to the laboratory along with the completed requisition.

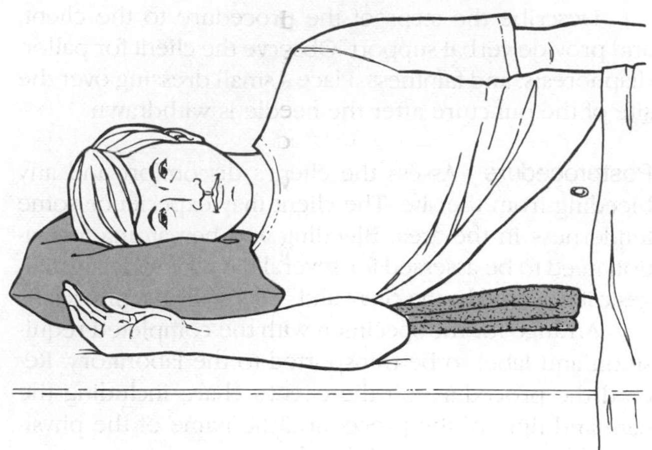

Figure 54–15 A position to provide pressure on the site after liver biopsy

Assess the client's pulse, respirations, and blood pressure every 15 minutes for the first hour following the test or until they are stable. Complications of a liver biopsy are rare, but hemorrhage from a perforated blood vessel can occur. Determine whether the client is experiencing abdominal pain. Severe abdominal pain may indicate bile peritonitis (an inflammation of the peritoneal lining of the abdomen caused by bile leaking from a bile duct). Observe the biopsy site for localized bleeding. Pressure dressings may be required if bleeding occurs. Record the procedure, including the date and time it was performed, the name of the physician, and the client's responses.

Roentgenography, Nuclear Medicine, Computed Tomography, and Ultrasonography

Roentgenography

Roentgen rays (x rays) are part of the spectrum of electromagnetic radiation. They travel at the speed of light and have considerably shorter wavelengths than light or radio waves. This distinctive property enables radiation to penetrate organs and tissues according to their thickness and density. High-voltage x rays have shorter wavelengths and produce a more penetrating (harder) radiation; low-voltage x rays have logner wavelengths and produce a more easily absorbable (softer) radiation. X rays that are not absorbed pass through the tissue to form an image on the photographic film (a plain, or static, radiograph) or on a fluorescent screen (fluoroscopy).

It is the differential absorption of x rays by the various tissues that makes roentgenography diagnostically useful. Bones, which are dense, permit fewer x rays to pass through to the film, so they appear as light areas. The soft tissues surrounding bone are less dense, so they appear darker on the film. Natural contrasts in density also occur between blood-filled cardiovascular structures and air-filled lung areas. Such natural contrasts, however, do not occur in the abdomen or between the soft tissue structures of the extremities. Thus, contrast agents must be introduced for certain body parts, e.g., the digestive tract and blood vessels, to show on the film.

Contrast materials (solids, liquids, or gaseous substances) must absorb either more or fewer x rays than the surrounding tissues. Commonly used contrast agents are compounds of iodine, barium, air, and carbon dioxide. Iodine and barium absorb more x rays than soft tissues; air and carbon dioxide absorb fewer.

Contrast materials are introduced into the body in four ways to view specific organs:

1. Orally or rectally for the digestive tract (esophagus, stomach, intestines) and gallbladder. See Figure 54–16.
2. Intravenously for the blood vessels, bile ducts, and kidneys.
3. Into the subarachnoid space for the spine and the ventricles of the brain.
4. Through a nasotracheal tube or bronchoscope for the bronchial tree. This method is used infrequently now, since the advent of fiberoptic bronchoscopy, which has increased the area available to direct visual examination.

Radiographic studies can be carried out on many body systems. Nonhospitalized people undergo these studies in the radiographic department of a hospital or at a physician's office. In these instances, the individual usually prepares for the examination at home, sometimes with the help of support persons or a home health care nurse. For example, an 84-year-old man may be unable to give himself an enema. When the client is responsible for his or her own preparation, it is important for the nurse to provide written instructions, explain the instructions, and verify that they have been carried out before the study begins. A simple question—for instance, "How did you prepare for this test?"—usually elicits the required information. It is also important to give the client a written statement and explanation of followup care after the study.

Radiography of the gastrointestinal tract often involves fluoroscopy as well as a radiographic examination. **Fluoroscopy** is an examination during which x rays are used to visualize body structures on a screen. A fluoroscope is a machine for examining internal structures by viewing the shadows they cast on the fluorescent screen after x rays travel through the structures. For example, a physician uses fluoroscopy to view the esophagus on a screen as barium passes through it.

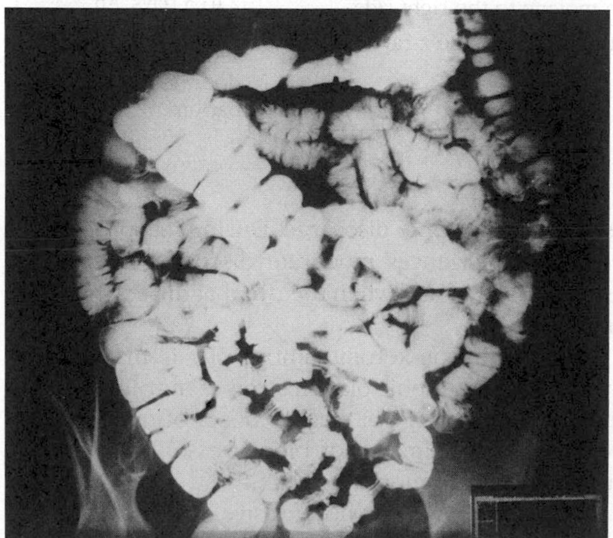

Figure 54–16 An x-ray film of the small and large intestines filled with a contrast medium

Radiographic studies are frequently carried out on:

1. Gastrointestinal tract—pharynx and esophagus (**barium swallow**), upper gastrointestinal tract, and lower gastrointestinal tract (**barium enema**). See Table 54–3.
2. Gallbladder (**cholecystography**) and bile ducts (**cholangiography**). See Table 54–4.
3. Urinary tract (IVP or IVU). See Table 54–5.
4. Central nervous system (**mylelography**). See Table 54–5.
5. Musculoskeletal system.
6. Vascular system (**angiography**). See Table 54–5.

Mammography

Mammography is radiologic examination of breast tissue. See Figure 54–17. It may be done with or without injec-

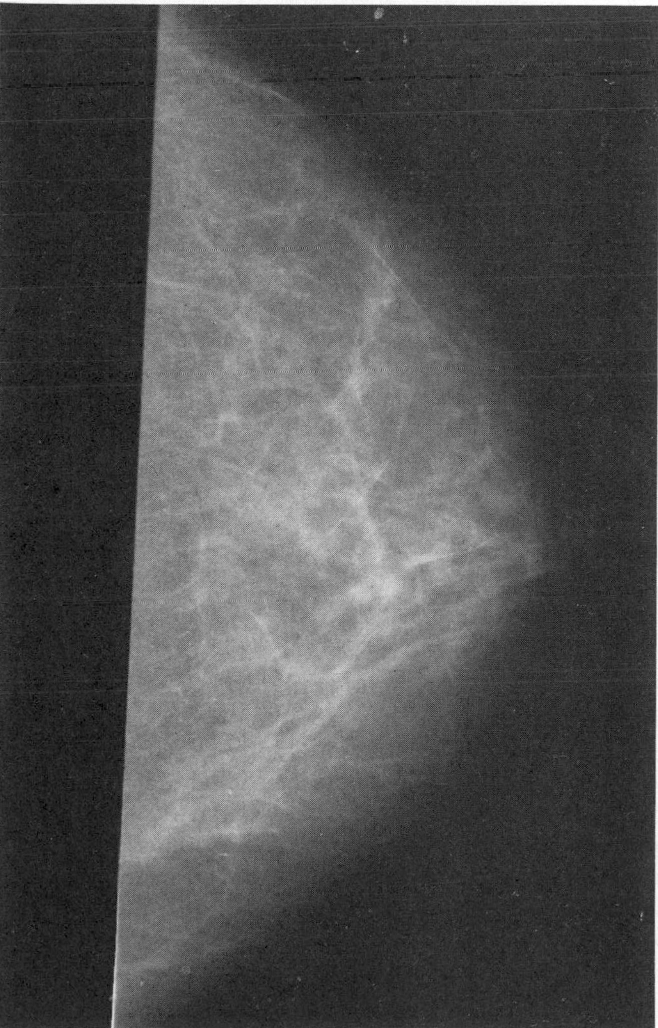

Figure 54–17 A normal mammogram of the breast

Table 54–3 Studies of the Gastrointestinal Tract

Name	Description	Nursing Intervention *Preprocedure Teaching*	*Postprocedure*
Barium swallow (usually part of an upper GI series)	The client swallows barium, and the pharynx and esophagus are outlined.	Procedure lasts 30 minutes. Client will be given a chalky substance (liquid barium) to drink.	Encourage fluids and activity to prevent constipation. Observe stool for whitish color, indicating client has passed barium in stool. Notify physician if barium not passed in 2 to 3 days (a laxative may be required).
Upper gastrointestinal (GI) series	The client swallows barium, and x-ray films are taken of its course through the esophagus, stomach, and duodenum.	Client must fast 4 to 6 hours before the examination. The client will be given a chalky substance (liquid barium) to drink. Procedure lasts from 30 minutes to 1 hour. Client may experience a feeling of fullness. Client may need to assume several positions on the x-ray table.	Encourage fluids and activity to prevent constipation. Observe stool for whitish color, indicating client has passed barium in stool. Client may require a laxative or enema if client is constipated or does not pass barium in 2 to 3 days
Lower gastrointestinal series (barium enema)	A barium enema is given, and x-ray films are taken of the large intestine.	A laxative may be given the night before the test. Liquids are restricted after midnight before the test. Enemas or suppositories are given on the morning of the test to clean the bowel. The barium enema creates a feeling of fullness, and the client will feel the urge to defecate. Test usually lasts 30 to 45 minutes. There may be some cramping. Special tubes with balloons are often used to help the client retain the barium. The client will be asked to assume various positions, e.g., lying on the left side, then moving to the right side. Client will probably pass the barium at the x-ray department.	Provide a rest period afterward because procedure is fatiguing. Encourage fluids to prevent constipation. Observe stool for passage of barium and assess regularity of movements. Notify physician if barium not passed in 2 to 3 days. An enema may be required if client does not pass all the barium.

tion of a contrast agent and is performed as a screening test or to study suspicious areas before a mass is distinguishable. **Soft-tissue mammography** is done without a contrast medium; the procedure is the same as a standard x-ray examination. Side and top-to-bottom views are taken of each breast. In **contrast** (or **ductal injection**) **mammography**, a small-gauge needle is inserted successively into each mammary duct to be examined and a radiopaque dye is injected before the x-ray films are taken. This test is usually performed to detect an intraductal mass if there is nipple discharge. During this procedure, the client experiences moderate discomfort when the needle is inserted and when the dye that dilates the ducts is injected.

Xerography or xeromammography is mammography using a xerographic plate instead of film. The advantage of xerography is that smaller doses of radiation are used and that the images of blood vessel patterns and tissue densities are more distinct.

Thermography is a noninvasive screening proce-

Table 54–4 Studies of the Gallbladder and Bile Ducts

Name	Description	Nursing Interventions *Preprocedure*	 *Postprocedure*
Cholecystography (oral cholecystography)	X-ray films are taken of the gallbladder after a contrast dye has been given orally.	A fat-free supper is given the evening before. Check for allergy to the contrast dye, which contains iodine. A laxative may be given the evening before, or an enema the morning of the test. Six or more contrast pills (e.g., Telepaque) are given at 5-minute intervals the evening before the test, each with 4 to 6 oz water. The client fasts from midnight the evening before but may drink water. Explain that: • A fatty drink may be given during the test. • No discomfort is usually felt. • The procedure lasts about 30 to 45 minutes.	Provide a rest period. The client resumes a regular diet. A snack can be provided if the client is hungry. Assess allergy to the contrast dye.
Intravenous cholangiography	X-ray films are taken of the bile ducts after dye has been administered intravenously.	The client fasts from midnight the evening before the test but may drink water. The bowel is cleaned with a laxative the evening before or with an enema the morning of the test. Check for allergy to iodine contained in the dye. Explain that: • Iodine dye is given intravenously in the x-ray department. A test for allergy is given in the arm before the test. • Study lasts 3 to 4 hours.	Assess for allergy to the dye. Observe I.V. site for bleeding, tenderness.
Percutaneous transhepatic cholangiography	A needle is inserted through the abdominal wall into the biliary radicle, and a contrast agent is injected. Test distinguishes between obstructive and nonobstructive jaundice.	See *Intravenous cholangiography* for preparation. Explain that procedure lasts about 30 minutes.	Monitor vital signs q15 minutes for 1 hour, q30 minutes for 4 hours, and then q4 hours until client is stable. Encourage bed rest. Position client on right side to place pressure on the puncture site to prevent bleeding. Monitor puncture site for bleeding.
Postoperative cholangiography	Dye is injected through the T-tube, and x-ray films are taken and fluoroscopy is done to determine if common bile duct is unobstructed.	See *Intravenous cholangiography.*	If T-tube is in place, clamp or attach to drainage as ordered. If T-tube is removed, apply sterile dressing.

Table 54–5 Radiographic Studies: Intravenous Pyelography, Angiography, Myelography

Name	Description	Nursing Interventions: *Preprocedure*	Nursing Interventions: *Postprocedure*
Intravenous pyelography or urography (IVP, IVU)	An intravenous injection of radiopaque material is given to examine the kidneys and ureters.	A strong laxative (e.g., castor oil) is given the afternoon before the test to clear the bowel of fecal material, which can obstruct the view of the urinary structures. The client fasts from midnight prior to the test. Check for allergy to iodine. Explain that: • An intravenous injection will be administered in the x-ray department. • The procedure lasts about 1 hour.	Encourage fluid intake. The client resumes a regular diet. Provide for rest, since the laxative and fasting can cause weakness. Observe for reactions to the radiopaque dye.
Angiography, e.g., cerebral angiography (vascular system of the brain), coronary arteriography (coronary arteries of the heart), renal angiography (vascular system of the kidneys), pulmonary angiography (vascular system of the lungs).	A radiopaque material is injected into an artery or vein to examine portions of the vascular system.	For some of these procedures, a catheter may be inserted into an artery or vein prior to the injection of radiopaque material. Before some procedures, the client is given a sedative. The client fasts from midnight prior to the test. A strong laxative may be given the evening before certain tests (e.g., renal arteriography). Client will be tested for allergy to iodine. The time needed for these procedures varies. Some may take up to 3 hours.	Bed rest is generally maintained for up to 12 hours. Monitor the client's radial pulse, respirations, and blood pressure every 15 to 30 minutes until they stabilize. Monitor peripheral pulses distal to the injection site. Observe the injection site for bleeding and swelling. Cold pack may prevent swelling. Determine any discomfort experienced by the client.
Myelography	A contrast material is injected into the subarachnoid space, and x-ray films are taken of the spinal cord, nerve roots, and vertebrae.	Fasting may be required from midnight prior to the test. The client may be given a sedative prior to the procedure. Explain that: • A radiopaque oil dye is injected via a lumbar puncture or a cisternal puncture in the x-ray department. • The client will assume various positions, e.g., on the side for a lumbar puncture, then prone, and then tilted on x-ray table equipped with shoulder and foot supports. • Some pain may be felt when the oil is removed, due to irritation of the nerve roots. • The procedure may last about 2 hours.	The client is generally positioned flat in bed for 24 hours to minimize headache and/or nausea, but may be positioned with the head elevated above the level of the spine if the dye has not been completely removed. This prevents the dye from moving to the head and causing an inflammation of the meninges (meningitis). Monitor vital signs and neurologic status, e.g., complaints of numbness, pain, or tingling in the extremities; muscle weakness. Monitor urinary output.

dure usually done before mammography. It measures and records the temperature distribution, especially areas of heat, of breast tissue. For this examination, the temperature of the breast skin must be as close as possible to room temperature. The woman usually must sit with her breasts exposed 5 to 10 minutes before the test. There are various types of thermography (Wilcox 1981, p. 1647):

1. Color or black-and-white thermography, in which infrared photos are taken. "Hot spots" in breast tissue

are indicated by either red or black in color photos and either white or black in black-and-white photos. Because a rapidly processed film is used, results of this thermogram are readily available.

2. Mammometry, in which electrodelike skin thermometers are applied to the breast. Results are recorded on an ECG-like printout. Skin temperature elevations of more than 2.5 F are considered abnormal. The results of this test are usually not available for at least 1 week.
3. Thermal scan, in which the thermoscope is passed over the breast skin, set at the median temperature of the breast, and then passed over breast tissue again to identify the temperature variables. Results of this test are available immediately after interpretation

Mammography is the chief method of detecting breast lesions. Extremely small, nonpalpable breast lesions that would otherwise not be detected can show up in this examination. An initial mammograph to yield baseline data is recommended for all women between 35 and 40 years. Asymptomatic women are then advised to have a mammographic examination every 2 years between ages 40 and 49 and annually after age 50 (Mammography Guidelines 1983, p. 255).

Procedure 54–1 ▲ Assisting with Roentgenography

The nurse's role in assisting with an x-ray procedure is largely one of preparing the client (or teaching the client how to prepare) for the examination and providing follow-up care (or teaching the client to provide follow-up care). The reasons for roentgenography are:

1. To determine abnormalities in the structure or appearance of body organs, e.g., ulcerations in the stomach, tumors, bone fractures, or consolidated infectious material in the lungs
2. To determine disruptions in the function of body organs, e.g., decreased function of the gallbladder or thyroid gland
3. To determine the presence of obstructions to body ducts or vessels, e.g., stones in the bile ducts or urinary system, or blood clots in the arteries
4. To determine the extent or spread of malignant tumors

Intervention: Preprocedure

1. Check the physician's order sheet to determine the specific examination ordered. For example, cholecystography and cholangiography may appear similar, but they involve different preparations: Before cholecystography, contrast material is taken orally; before cholangiography, the contrast material is given intravenously. See Table 54–4.
2. Explain the specific preparatory measures required for the x-ray procedure or scan. For example, before certain x-ray films are taken, a strong laxative needs to be administered to clear the bowel of fecal material, which could prevent proper visualization of a body organ, e.g., the kidney or the gallbladder. For other x-ray films, the client needs to fast for a specific time and/or take tablets containing contrast material at prescribed times. Some clients are given a sedative beforehand.
3. Explain where the examination is to be carried out. Most x-ray examinations are performed in a radiology department. However, some scanning procedures that use radioactive materials are carried out in the nuclear medicine department of a hospital.
4. Explain when the examination is scheduled and approximately how long it will last. The anxiety of the client and support persons can be reduced if they are informed about time schedules.
5. Explain whether medications the client is receiving are to be given or are canceled prior to the test. For example, a diabetic client whose diet is altered before a barium enema may have his or her insulin canceled the morning of the test. For a diabetic client, the roentgenography may be scheduled early in the day to prevent undue disruption of routine insulin administration and diet.
6. Determine that all preparation was carried out.

Intervention: Postprocedure

1. Suggest adequate rest periods for the client following the procedure. Many diagnostic procedures are tiring, and in some instances several procedures are carried out on consecutive days. For example, a sigmoidoscopy may be done one day, a barium enema the next day, and a barium swallow the third day.
2. Monitor the client closely for discomfort and potential complications related to the procedure. These are outlined in Tables 54–3, 54–4, and 54–5.

3. Provide the follow-up care that is recommended for the procedure.
4. Record the procedure in accordance with agency practices, including:
   a. Preparatory measures carried out
   b. The procedure itself
   c. The time the client is transported to the radiology or nuclear medicine department
   d. The time the client returns to the unit
   e. Follow-up measures provided
   f. The assessment of the client

Sample Recording

Date	Time	Notes
Dec/15/86	0700	Clear liquid breakfast given. ——— ——— Adrian L. Stewart, NS
	0800	3 saline enemas given until returns were clear. Large amount of soft, dark brown stool obtained. — ——— Adrian L. Stewart, NS
	0930	Transported to radiology for barium enema. ——— Adrian L. Stewart, NS
	1030	Returned to unit. States is tired. No complaints of discomfort. ——— ——— Adrian L. Stewart, NS

Nuclear Medicine (Radioisotopes)

The instruments and **radioisotopes** (radioactive tracers) used in nuclear medicine are constantly changing, but the fundamental principles remain the same. A basic principle is that body constituents are dynamic, not static. Isotopes enter into the same chemical reactions and metabolic processes as stable elements.

In nuclear medicine techniques, radioactive substances that have an affinity for specific body tissues are introduced orally or intravenously. For example, radioactive iodine may be given to measure the function of the thyroid gland. The thyroid gland normally picks up and uses iodine to produce the hormone thyroxine. When radioactive iodine is introduced, how much iodine the thyroid picks up and how it is distributed can be detected by a scanning device, allowing the examiner to detect any deficiencies in thyroid function. The scanning device may be a **scintillation counter** or a **scintillation camera.** The scintillation scanner has a probe that is passed back and forth over the body area being studied; the scintillation camera produces many images in rapid sequence, showing the transit of the isotope through blood vessels.

Radioisotopes are administered in extremely small doses, e.g., one billionth of a gram. For this reason, the body absorbs minimal amounts of radiation, and normal body cells are not damaged. The procedure is painless and has three steps:

1. Oral or intravenous intake of the radioisotope
2. A waiting period from 1 to 48 hours, during which the isotope is assimilated by the organ being studied
3. The scanning procedure, during which the client must remain still

Scintillation scanning (scintiscans) can be used to assess the function of an organ or detect a tumor. Organs commonly studied by nuclear medicine procedures include the thyroid, heart, brain, lungs, liver, spleen, bone marrow, bones, and kidneys. Radioisotopes are also used to measure blood volume, blood circulation rate, red blood cell turnover, cardiac output, and lung blood flow.

Computed Tomography (CT Scan)

Computed tomography is a painless, noninvasive x-ray procedure with the unique capability of distinguishing minor differences in the radiodensity of soft tissues. See Figure 54–18. For example, CT scans can be used to distinguish between liver tissue and tumor or brain tissue and hematoma. Dense substances appear white; low-density substances appear dark. The organ to be studied gives the scan its name, e.g., brain scan, liver scan, lung scan.

In this technique, a planar slice of the body is subjected to sequential sweeps or **scans** of a narrow x-ray beam. The unabsorbed beam emerging through the tissues is measured by a radiation detector. Data obtained are stored in a computer, which produces an image, called a **tomogram,** on a viewing apparatus or printout machine. Photographs of the image can be reproduced.

The CT scan provides a three-dimensional view of the area under study. The scanner rotates 1° at a time through a 180° arc in about 5 minutes. At least five consecutive scans or "cuts" are taken of sequential parts of the organ. Following this initial scan, the client is usually given an intravenous injection of an iodine-containing contrast material, and the entire scan is repeated. This second scan is referred to as a "contrast enhancement" scan. The entire scanning procedure takes about 1 hour. The client must remain still throughout the scan to prevent false computer results.

The only risk involved with a CT scan is the possibility of allergic reaction to iodine; thus the client must always be asked about any known allergy to iodine before the test. Usually no special preparation is required. In some agencies, no food or fluids may be given 4 to 6 hours beforehand because the iodine-containing contrast medium may cause nausea.

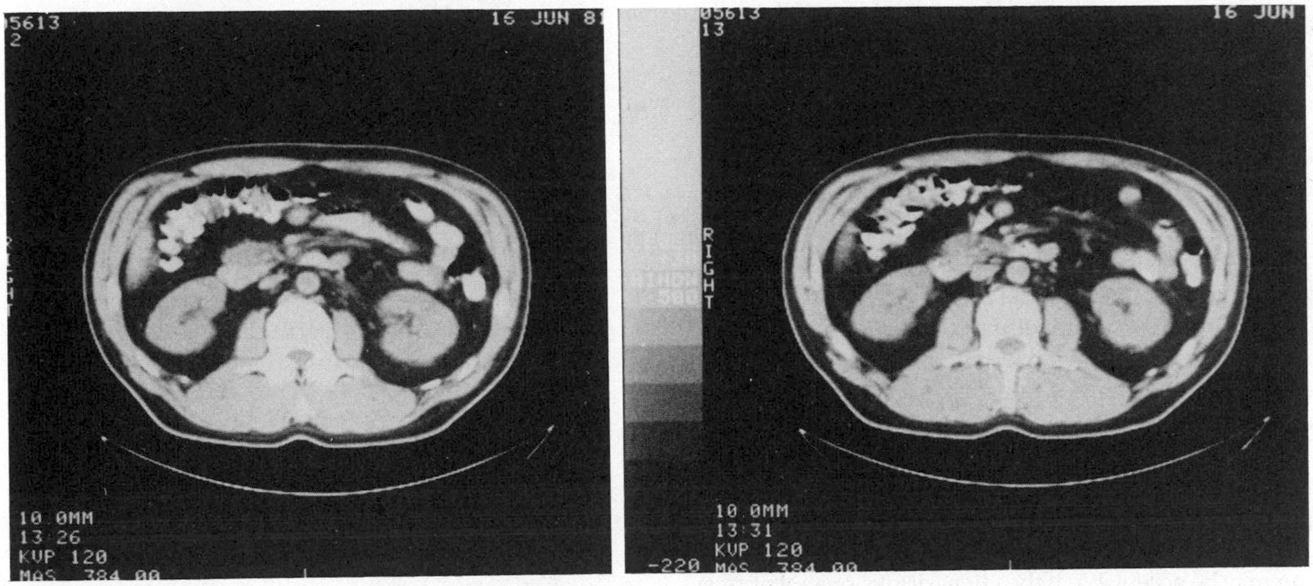

Figure 54–18 A CT scan showing a midabdomen cross section of a client. The spine is at the base; the kidneys are to the left and right of the spine.

Other preprocedure nursing considerations include:

1. Restless clients, e.g., children, may be given a sedative prior to the procedure so that they will lie still during the procedure.
2. The nurse assures the client that there is no need to fear exposure to radiation; a CT scan exposes the client to less radiation than the usual x-ray procedure. A radioactive substance is given orally or intravenously.
3. Depending on the substance used, a blocking agent may also be given to prevent uptake of the radioactive substance by organs other than the one being studied, and to ensure that the substance goes into the organ being studied, e.g.:
   a. Lugol's solution (iodine) may be given to block uptake by the thyroid (given orally with juice, since its taste is unpleasant), or a potassium compound may be given to clients allergic to iodine.
   b. Mercaptomerin sodium is given intramuscularly to block uptake by the kidneys.

   Check for allergies to the blocking agents used.
4. The nurse explains that:
   a. The scan is performed in the nuclear medicine department.
   b. There will be a waiting period while the radioactive substance is taken up by the body.
   c. There is no discomfort.
   d. The client will be asked to assume various positions and must remain still while the scans are taken.

After the procedure, there are usually no side-effects or limitations on client activity. Additional scans may be performed at subsequent intervals, e.g., 2 hours, 24 hours, 48 hours, and 72 hours. Observe for allergic reactions to the blocking agent.

Ultrasonography (Ultrasound)

Ultrasonography, another noninvasive technique, uses high-frequency sound waves well above the upper limit of human hearing. During this procedure, which has no known harmful effects, acoustic densities of tissues are measured. In contrast to usual radiography, ultrasound reveals the depth of a structure below the skin and the anteroposterior dimension of masses. Sound waves travel at different speeds, depending on the density of the structures through which they pass. Because sound is poorly conducted by gases and is well reflected by bone, structures containing air (such as the lung) or surrounded by bone (such as the pelvis) are difficult to examine with ultrasound.

In this technique, a transducer or probe is used as both an emitter and a receiver. The probe is moved over the structure being examined, and an ultrasound beam is directed into the body. Echoes (sounds reflected back to the probe) are translated into a display unit for observation and photographic recording. The test usually takes 20 to 45 minutes.

Ultrasound can:

1. Reveal the size, shape, and consistency of internal structures

2. Show masses, fluid inflammation, and stones
3. Differentiate between cystic and solid masses
4. Outline the boundaries of lesions and displacement of surrounding tissues
5. Depict motion

Many ultrasound examinations require no physical preparation of the client. Food and fluids are withheld 8 to 10 hours before examination of the abdominal organs, and some physicians may order an enema or other agent to decrease the amount of intestinal gas, which impedes the sound reflection. For examinations of the pelvic organs, the client must have some urine in the bladder to enable better visualization. Inform the client to void 4 hours before the procedure and then not to void until after the procedure. If this is difficult for the client, 2 hours without voiding may be acceptable if the client drinks several glasses of fluid before the examination.

The client also needs to know that:

1. Mineral oil or water-soluble jelly will be spread over the skin. The oil prevents air from becoming trapped between the probe and the skin and facilitates acoustic contact.
2. The procedure is painless. The client will merely feel the probe moving over the skin.
3. He or she will be asked to change positions on the table to allow visualization of the organ from different angles.
4. During a scan of upper abdominal organs, the client may be asked periodically to inhale deeply and hold the breath for a few seconds. Inspiration displaces upper abdominal organs downward.

Chapter Highlights

- Tests and treatments are frightening for many people; they may fear pain, the findings of the tests, or their reactions to either the pain or the findings.
- The nurse must identify the concerns of the client and provide information and support to alleviate concern.
- To give informed consent before a procedure, the client must understand what the procedure entails, what the risks are, and what the alternatives are.
- The nurse ensures that the client has been informed prior to any special procedure.
- Appropriate physical preparation before the test ensures its effectiveness. The nurse is largely responsible for ensuring that appropriate physical preparation is carried out.
- Baseline assessment data are collected before the test and compared with the client's responses during and after the test.
- During the procedure, the nurse, if present, is usually the client's primary support person.
- The nurse is responsible for ensuring that specimens taken during the procedure are appropriately labeled, handled, and transported to the laboratory for study.
- Knowledge of the procedure and complications that may arise helps the nurse provide necessary interventions following the procedure to ensure the recovery and safety of the client.

Suggested Readings

Beck, M. L. January 1981. Preparing your patient psychologically for an esophagogastroduodenoscopy. Part 1. *Nursing 81* 11:28–29. (Canadian edition, pp. 10–11).
Beck discusses the esophagogastroduodenoscopy (EGD) procedure, indications for it, client education, and ways to provide emotional support to the client. Five photographs are included.

Beck, M. L. February 1981. Preparing your patient physically for an esophagogastroduodenoscopy. Part 2. *Nursing 81* 11:88–89. (Canadian edition, pp. 15–16).
In Part 2, Beck discusses the physical preparation of a client before this procedure and lists the precautions to take following it. Beck also discusses the endoscopic retrograde cholangiopancreatography (ERCP) that may be conducted during the procedure.

Berger, M. E., and Hubner, K. F. August 1983. Hospital hazards: Diagnostic radiation. *American Journal of Nursing* 83:1155–59.
The authors discuss what the nurse can do to foster radiation safety in the hospital and detail radiation hazards, including unnecessary procedures and poor technique.

Blackwell, C. A. February 1975. PEG and angiography: A patient's sensations. *American Journal of Nursing* 75:264–66.
Knowing what a client feels during a carotid arteriogram and a pneumoencephalogram can help the nurse prepare clients for such procedures.

Hansen, B. D., and Evans, M. L. November/December 1981. Preparing a child for procedures. *The American Journal of Maternal Child Nursing* 6:392–97.
The authors suggest general principles for preparing children before medical procedures. In addition, specific guidelines that outline the child's developmental stage and the nurse's role are provided.

Haughey, C. April 1981. Understanding ultrasonography. *Nursing 81* 11:36–40.
Haughey describes ultrasonography, lists the body structures that can be examined by it, discusses the client prep-

aration necessary before the procedure, and outlines the steps taken during the examination. Thirteen photographs are included.

Luciano, K., and Shumsky, C. J. January 1975. Pediatric procedures: :The explanation should always come first. *Nursing 75* 5:49–52.
Explanations are important and must be suited to the age of the client. Infants, toddlers, and their parents need reassurance before pediatric procedures. Ways to communicate with each age group are shown with examples.

Markus, S. April 1981. Taking the fear out of bone marrow examinations. *Nursing 81* 11:64–67.
At most hospitals, bone marrow biopsies are done only by physicians. However, an increasing number of hospitals are authorizing qualified nurses to do the procedure. Markus describes the technique for obtaining a bone marrow specimen and provides helpful hints for nurses preparing the client psychologically for this procedure.

Shearer, D.; Collins, B.; and Creel, D. January 1975. Preparing a patient for EEG. *American Journal of Nursing* 75:63–64.
Physical and psychologic preparation of the client improve the quality of EEG recordings.

Van Meter, M., and Lavine, P. G. April 1975. What every nurse should know about EKGs. Part 1. *Nursing 75* 5:19–27.
Included are the interpretation of EKG readings, the 12-lead system, and types of rhythms. The electric impulses of the heart's conduction system are explained on pages 26 and 27.

Selected References

Beck, M. L. January 1981a. Preparing your patient psychologically for an esophagogastroduodenoscopy. Part 1. *Nursing 81* 11:28–29. (Canadian edition, pp. 10–11).

———. February 1981b. Preparing your patient physically for an esophagogastroduodenoscopy. Part 2. *Nursing 81* 11:88–89. (Canadian edition, pp. 15–16).

Byrne, C. J.; Saxton, D. F.; Pelikan, P. K.; and Nugent, P. M. 1986. *Laboratory tests: Implications for nursing care.* 2d ed. Menlo Park, Calif.: Addison-Wesley Publishing Co.

Contrast radiography fact sheet: Update your knowledge of these contrast radiography studies. August 1984. *Nursing 84* 14:22–23.

Diagnostic scanning procedures and ultrasonography: Test yourself. November 1980. *American Journal of Nursing* 80:2005.

Donaldson, R. February 19, 1981. Echocardiography: Sounding out the heart. *Nursing Mirror* 152:40–41.

Guyton, A. C. 1986. *Textbook of medical physiology.* 7th ed. Philadelphia: W. B. Saunders Co.

Hartfield, M. T.; Cason, C. L.; and Cason, G. J. July/August 1982. Effects of information about a threatening procedure on patient's expectations and emotional distress. *Nursing Research* 31:202–5.

Harvey, A. M.; Johns, R. J.; McKusick, V. A.; Owens, A. H.; and Ross, R. S. 1980. *The principles and practice of medicine.* 20th ed. New York: Appleton-Century-Crofts.

Haughey, C. April 1981. Understanding ultrasonography. *Nursing 81* 11:36–40.

Mammography Guidelines. 1983. Background statement and update of cancer related check-up guidelines for breast cancer detection in asymptomatic women age 40 to 49. *Cancer* 33:255.

Marici, F. N. October 1973. The flexible fiberoptic bronchoscope. *American Journal of Nursing* 73:1776–78.

Markus, S. April 1981. Taking the fear out of bone marrow examinations. *Nursing 81* 11:64–67.

The Nurses' Reference Library. 1981. *Diagnostics.* Springhouse, Pa.: Intermed Communications.

Questions and answers about the CT scan exam: Patient education aid. April 15, 1985. *Patient Care* 19:185.

Schuster, P., and Jones, S. November 1982. Preparing the patient for a barium enema: A comparison of nurse and patient opinions. *Journal of Advanced Nursing* 7:523–27.

Shearer, D.; Collins, B.; and Creel, D. January 1975. Preparing a patient for EEG. *American Journal of Nursing* 75:63–64.

Shetler, M. G., and Bartos, H. January 1981. Spinal and peritoneal taps: When quick action counts. *RN* 44:50–53.

———. December 1980. Thoracentesis . . . and pericardiocentesis, too. *RN* 43:50–53.

Stiklorius, C. April 1982. When patient preparation is the key to success: In barium enemas and small bowel studies, timely prep is the decisive factor. *RN* 45:64–65.

———. May 1982. Large bowel diagnostics challenge your stress-reduction skills. *RN* 45:56–57.

———. June 1982. 'Fair warnings' for patients facing esophagoscopy and gastroscopy. *RN* 45:64–65.

Weir, J., and Abrahams, P. September 25, 1980. X-ray anatomy. Part 5. *Nursing Times* 76:center pages.

———. November 27, 1980. X-ray anatomy: Computerized axial tomograms of head . . . body . . . xeromammogram. Part 6. *Nursing Times* 76:center pages.

Wilcox, P. M. September 1981. Benign breast disorders. *American Journal of Nursing* 81:1644–51.

Appendices

Contents

Appendix A Rights of Special Groups

Appendix A–1 Declaration on the Rights of Disabled Persons

1. The term "disabled person" means any person unable to ensure by himself or herself wholly or partly the necessities of a normal individual and/or social life, as a result of a deficiency, either congenital or not, in his or her physical or mental capabilities.
2. Disabled persons shall enjoy all the rights set forth in this Declaration. These rights shall be granted to all disabled persons without any exception whatsoever and without distinction or discrimination on the basis of race, colour, sex, language, religion, political or other opinions, national or social origin, state of wealth, birth or any other situation applying either to the disabled person himself or herself or to his or her family.
3. Disabled persons have the inherent right to respect for their human dignity. Disabled persons, whatever the origin, nature and seriousness of their handicaps and disabilities, have the same fundamental rights as their fellow-citizens of the same age, which implies first and foremost the right to enjoy a decent life, as normal and full as possible.
4. Disabled persons have the same civil and political rights as other human beings; article 7 of the Declaration of the Rights of Mentally Retarded Persons applies to any possible limitation or suppression of those rights for mentally disabled persons.
5. Disabled persons are entitled to the measures designed to enable them to become as self-reliant as possible.
6. Disabled persons have the right to medical, psychological and functional treatment, including prosthetic and orthetic appliances, to medical and social rehabilitation, education, vocational education, training and rehabilitation, aid, counselling, placement services and other services which will enable them to develop their capabilities and skills to the maximum and will hasten the process of their social integration or reintegration.
7. Disabled persons have the right to economic and social security and to a decent level of living. They have the right, according to their capabilities, to secure and retain employment or to engage in a useful, productive and remunerative occupation and to join trade unions.
8. Disabled persons are entitled to have their special needs taken into consideration at all stages of economic and social planning.
9. Disabled persons have the right to live with their families or with foster parents and to participate in all social, creative or recreational activities. No disabled person shall be subjected, as far as his or her residence is concerned, to differential treatment other than that required by his or her condition or by the improvement which he or she may derive therefrom. If the stay of a disabled person in a specialized establishment is indispensable, the environment and living conditions therein shall be as close as possible to those of the normal life of a person of his or her age.
10. Disabled persons shall be protected against all exploitation, all regulations and all treatment of a discriminatory, abusive and degrading nature.
11. Disabled persons shall be able to avail themselves of qualified legal aid when such aid proves indispensable for the protection of their persons or property. If judicial proceedings are instituted against them, the legal procedures applied shall take their physical and mental condition fully into account.
12. Organizations of disabled persons may be usefully consulted in all matters regarding the rights of disabled persons.
13. Disabled persons, their families and communities shall be fully informed, by all appropriate means, of the rights contained in this Declaration.

Adopted by the General Assembly of the United Nations, December 1975.

Appendix A–2 The Dying Person's Bill of Rights

- I have the right to be treated as a living human being until I die.
- I have the right to maintain a sense of hopefulness however changing its focus may be.
- I have the right to be cared for by those who can maintain a sense of hopefulness, however changing this might be.
- I have the right to express my feelings and emotions about my approaching death in my own way.
- I have the right to participate in decisions concerning my care.
- I have the right to expect continuing medical and nursing attention even though "cure" goals must be changed to "comfort" goals.
- I have the right not to die alone.
- I have the right to be free from pain.
- I have the right to have my questions answered honestly.
- I have the right not to be deceived.
- I have the right to have help from and for my family in accepting my death.
- I have the right to die in peace and dignity.
- I have the right to retain my individuality and not be judged for my decisions which may be contrary to beliefs of others.
- I have the right to discuss and enlarge my religious and/or spiritual experiences, whatever these may mean to others.
- I have the right to expect that the sanctity of the human body will be respected after death.
- I have the right to be cared for by caring, sensitive, knowledgeable people who will attempt to understand my needs and will be able to gain some satisfaction in helping me face my death.

From Amelia J. Barbus, The dying person's bill of rights, *American Journal of Nursing,* January 1975, 75:99.

Appendix A–3 Declaration on the Rights of Mentally Retarded Persons

1. The mentally retarded person has, to the maximum degree of feasibility, the same rights as other human beings.
2. The mentally retarded person has a right to proper medical care and physical therapy and to such education, training, rehabilitation and guidance as will enable him to develop his ability and maximum potential.
3. The mentally retarded person has a right to economic security and to a decent standard of living. He has a right to perform productive work or to engage in any meaningful occupation to the fullest possible extent of his capabilities.
4. Whenever possible, the mentally retarded person should live with his own family or with foster parents and participate in different forms of community life. The family with which he lives should receive assistance. If care in an institution becomes necessary, it should be provided in surroundings and other circumstances as close as possible to those of normal life.
5. The mentally retarded person has a right to a qualified guardian when this is required to protect his personal well-being and interests.
6. The mentally retarded person has a right to protection from exploitation, abuse and degrading treatment. If prosecuted for any offence, he shall have a right to due process of law with full recognition being given to his degree of mental responsibility.
7. Whenever mentally retarded persons are unable, because of the severity of their handicap, to exercise all their rights in a meaningful way or it should become necessary to restrict or deny some or all of these rights, the procedure used for that restriction or denial of rights must contain proper legal safeguards against every form of abuse. This procedure must be based on an evaluation of the social capability of the mentally retarded person by qualified experts and must be subject to periodic review and to the right of appeal to higher authorities.

Adopted by the General Assembly of the United Nations, December 1971.

Appendix A–4 United Nations Declaration of the Rights of the Child

Preamble

Whereas the peoples of the United Nations have, in the Charter, reaffirmed their faith in fundamental human rights, and in the dignity and worth of the human person, and have determined to promote social progress and better standards of life in larger freedom,

Whereas the United Nations has, in the Universal Declaration of Human Rights, proclaimed that everyone is entitled to all the rights and freedoms set forth therein, without distinction of any kind, such as race, colour, sex, language, religion, political or other opinion, national or social origin, property, birth or other status,

Whereas the child, by reason of his physical and mental immaturity, needs special safeguards and care, including appropriate legal protection, before as well as after birth,

Whereas the need for such special safeguards has been stated in the Geneva Declaration of the Rights of the Child of 1924, and recognized in the Universal Declaration of Human Rights and in the statues of specialized agencies and international organizations concerned with the welfare of children,

Whereas mankind owes to the child the best it has to give,

Now therefore,

The General Assembly

Proclaims this Declaration of the Rights of the Child to the end that he may have a happy childhood and enjoy for his own good and for the good of society the rights and freedoms herein set forth, and calls upon parents, upon men and women as individuals, and upon voluntary organizations, local authorities and national Governments to recognize these rights and strive for their observance by legislative and other measures progressively taken in accordance with the following principles:

Principle 1

The child shall enjoy all the rights set forth in this Declaration. Every child, without any exception whatsoever, shall be entitled to these rights, without distinction or discrimination on account of race, colour, sex, language, religion, political or other opinion, national or social origin, property, birth or other status, whether of himself or of his family.

Principle 2

The child shall enjoy special protection, and shall be given opportunities and facilities, by law and by other means, to enable him to develop physically, mentally, morally, spiritually and socially in a healthy and normal manner and in conditions of freedom and dignity. In the enactment of laws for this purpose, the best interests of the child shall be the paramount consideration.

Principle 3

The child shall be entitled from his birth to a name and a nationality.

Principle 4

The child shall enjoy the benefits of social security. He shall be entitled to grow and develop in health; to this end, special care and protection shall be provided both to him and to his mother, including adequate pre-natal and post-natal care. The child shall have the right to adequate nutrition, housing, recreation and medical services.

Principle 5

The child who is physically, mentally or socially handicapped shall be given the special treatment, education and care required by his particular condition.

Principle 6

The child, for the full and harmonious development of his personality, needs love and understanding. He shall, whenever possible, grow up in the care and under the responsibility of his parents, and, in any case, in an atmosphere of affection and of moral and material security; a child of tender years shall not, save in exceptional circumstances, be separated from his mother. Society and the public authorities shall have the duty to extend particular care to children without a family and to those without adequate means of support. Payment of State and other assistance towards the maintenance of children of large families is desirable.

Principle 7

The child is entitled to receive education, which shall be free and compulsory, at least in the elementary stages. He shall be given an education which will promote his general culture, and enable him, on a basis of equal opportunity, to develop his abilities, his individual judgement, and his sense of moral and social responsibility, and to become a useful member of society.

The best interests of the child shall be the guiding principle of those responsible for his education and guidance; that responsibility lies in the first place with his parents.

The child shall have full opportunity for play and recreation, which should be directed to the same purposes as education; society and the public authorities shall endeavour to promote the enjoyment of this right.

Principle 8

The child shall in all circumstances be among the first to receive protection and relief.

Principle 9

The child shall be protected against all forms of neglect, cruelty and exploitation. He shall not be the subject of traffic, in any form.

The child shall not be admitted to employment before an appropriate minimum age; he shall in no case be caused or permitted to engage in any occupation or employment which would prejudice his health or education, or interfere with his physical, mental or moral development.

Principle 10

The child shall be protected from practices which may foster racial, religious and any other form of discrimination. He shall be brought up in a spirit of understanding, tolerance, friendship among peoples, peace and universal brotherhood and in full consciousness that his energy and talents should be devoted to the service of his fellow men.

Adopted by the General Assembly of the United Nations, November 20, 1959.

Appendix A–5 The Pregnant Patient's Bill of Rights

1. The Pregnant Patient has the right, prior to the administration of any drug or procedure, to be informed by the health professional caring for her of any potential direct or indirect effects, risks or hazards to herself or her unborn or newborn infant which may result from the use of a drug or procedure prescribed for or administered to her during pregnancy, labor, birth or lactation.
2. The Pregnant Patient has the right, prior to the proposed therapy, to be informed, not only of the benefits, risks and hazards of the proposed therapy but also of known alternative therapy, such as available childbirth education classes which could help to prepare the Pregnant Patient physically and mentally to cope with the discomfort or stress of pregnancy and the experience of childbirth, thereby reducing or eliminating her need for drugs and obstetric intervention. She should be offered such information early in her pregnancy in order that she may make a reasoned decision.
3. The Pregnant Patient has the right, prior to the administration of any drug, to be informed by the health professional who is prescribing or administering the drug to her that any drug which she receives during pregnancy, labor and birth, no matter how or when the drug is taken or administered may adversely affect her unborn baby, directly or indirectly, and that there is no drug or chemical which has been proven safe for the unborn child.
4. The Pregnant Patient has the right if cesarean section is anticipated, to be informed prior to the administration of any drug, and preferably prior to her hospitalization, that minimizing her and in turn, her baby's intake of nonessential preoperative medicine will benefit her baby.
5. The Pregnant Patient has the right, prior to the administration of a drug or procedure, to be informed of the areas of uncertainty if there is no properly controlled follow-up research which has established the safety of the drug or procedure with regard to its direct and/or indirect effects on the physiological, mental and neurological development of the child exposed, via the mother, to the drug or procedure during pregnancy, labor, birth or lactation (this would apply to virtually all drugs and the vast majority of obstetric procedures).
6. The Pregnant Patient has the right, prior to the administration of any drug, to be informed of the brand name and generic name of the drug in order that she may advise the health professional of any past adverse reaction to the drug.
7. The Pregnant Patient has the right to determine for herself, without pressure from her attendant, whether she will accept the risks inherent in the proposed therapy or refuse a drug or procedure.
8. The Pregnant Patient has the right to know the name and qualifications of the individual administering a medication or procedure to her during labor or birth.
9. The Pregnant Patient has the right to be informed, prior to the administration of any procedure, whether that procedure is being administered to her for her

or her baby's benefit (medically indicated) or as an elective procedure (for convenience, teaching purposes or research).

10. The Pregnant Patient has the right to be accompanied during the stress of labor and birth by someone she cares for, and to whom she looks for emotional comfort and encouragement.

11. The Pregnant Patient has the right after appropriate medical consultation to choose a position for labor and for birth which is least stressful to her baby and to herself.

12. The Obstetric Patient has the right to have her baby cared for at her bedside if her baby is normal, and to feed her baby according to her baby's needs rather than according to the hospital regimen.

13. The Obstetric Patient has the right to be informed in writing of the name of the person who actually delivered her baby and the professional qualifications of that person. This information should also be on the birth certificate.

14. The Obstetric Patient has the right to be informed if there is any known or indicated aspect of her or her baby's care or condition which may cause her or her baby later difficulty or problems.

15. The Obstetric Patient has the right to have her and her baby's hospital medical records complete, accurate and legible and to have their records, including Nurses' Notes, retained by the hospital until the child reaches at least the age of majority, or alternatively, to have the records offered to her before they are destroyed.

16. The Obstetric Patient, both during and after her hospital stay, has the right to have access to her complete hospital medical records, including Nurses' Notes, and to receive a copy upon payment of a reasonable fee and without incurring the expense of retaining an attorney.

It is the obstetric patient and her baby, not the health professional, who must sustain any trauma or injury resulting from the use of a drug or obstetric procedure. The observation of the rights listed above will not only permit the obstetric patient to participate in the decisions involving her and her baby's health care, but will help to protect the health professional and the hospital against litigation arising from resentment or misunderstanding on the part of the mother.

Written by Doris B. Haire, published by the International Childbirth Education Association.

Appendix B Root Words, Prefixes, and Suffixes

Word element	Meaning
ROOT WORDS	
Circulatory system	
cardio	heart
angio, vaso	vessel
hem, hema, hemato	blood
vena, phlebo	vein
arteria	artery
lympho	lymph
thrombo	clot (of blood)
embolus	moving clot
Digestive system	
bucca	cheek
os, stomato	mouth
gingiva	gum
glossa	tongue
pharyngo	pharynx
esophago	esophagus
gastro	stomach
hepato	liver
cholecyst	gallbladder
pancreas	pancreas
entero	intestines
duodeno	duodenum
jejuno	jejunum
ileo	ileum
caeco	cecum
appendeco	appendix
colo	colon
recto	rectum
ano, procto	anus
Skeletal system	
skeleto	skeleton
Respiratory system	
naso, rhino	nose
tonsillo	tonsil
laryngo	larynx
tracheo	trachea
bronchus, broncho	bronchus (pl. bronchi)
pulmo, pneuma, pneum	lung (sac with air)
Nervous system	
neuro	nerve
cerebrum	brain
oculo, ophthalmo	eye
oto	ear
psych, psycho	mind
Urinary system	
urethro	urethra
cysto	bladder
uretero	ureter
reni, reno, nephro	kidney
pyelo	pelvis of kidney
uro	urine
Female reproductive system	
vulvo	vulva
perineo	perineum
labio	labium (pl. labia)
vagino, colpo	vagina
cervico	cervix
utero	womb; uterus
tubo, salpingo	fallopian tube
ovario, oophoro	ovary
Male reproductive system	
orchido	testes
Regions of the body	
crani, cephalo	head
cervico, tracheo	neck
thoraco	chest
abdomino	abdomen
dorsum	back
Tissues	
cutis, dermato	skin
lipo	fat
musculo, myo	muscle
osteo	bone
myelo	marrow
chondro	cartilage
Miscellaneous	
cyto	cell
genetic	formation, origin
gram	tracing or mark
graph	writing, description
kinesis	motion
meter	measure
oligo	small, few
phobia	fear
photo	light
pyo	pus
scope	instrument for visual examination
roentgen	x-ray
lapar	flank; through the abdominal wall
PREFIXES	
a, an, ar	without or not
ab	away from
acro	extremities
ad	toward, to
adeno	glandular

Word element	Meaning
aero	air
ambi	around, on both sides
amyl	starch
ante	before, forward
anti	against, counteracting
bi	double
bili	bile
bio	life
bis	two
brachio	arm
brady	slow
broncho	bronchus (pl. bronchi)
cardio	heart
cervico	neck
chole	gall or bile
cholecysto	gallbladder
circum	around
co	together
contra	against, opposite
costo	ribs
cyto	cell
cysto	bladder
demi	half
derma	skin
dis	from
dorso	back
dys	abnormal, difficult
electro	electric
en	into, in, within
encephal	brain
entero	intestine
equi	equal
eryth	red
ex	out, out of, away from
extra	outside of, in addition to
ferro	iron
fibro	fiber
fore	before, in front of
gastro	stomach
glosso	tongue
glyco	sugar
hemi	half
hemo	blood
hepa, hepato	liver
histo	tissue
homo	same
hydro	water
hygro	moisture
hyper	too much, high
hypo	under, decreased
hyster	uterus
ileo	ileum
in	in, within, into
inter	between
intra	within
intro	in, within, into
juxta	near, close to
laryngo	larynx
latero	side
lapar	abdomen
leuk	white
macro	large, big
mal	bad, poor
mast	breast

Word element	Meaning
medio	middle
mega, megalo	large, great
meno	menses
mono	single
multi	many
myelo	bone marrow, spinal cord
myo	muscle
neo	new
nephro	kidney
neuro	nerve
nitro	nitrogen
noct	night
non	not
ob	against, in front of
oculo	eye
odonto	tooth
ophthalmo	eye
ortho	straight, normal
os	mouth, bone
osteo	bone
oto	ear
pan	all
para	beside, accessory to
path	disease
ped	child, foot
per	by, through
peri	around
pharyngo	pharynx
phlebo	vein
photo	light
phren	diaphragm, mind
pneumo	air, lungs
pod	foot
poly	many, much
post	after
pre	before
proct	rectum
pseudo	false
psych	mind
pyel	pelvis of the kidney
pyo	pus
pyro	fever, heat
quadri	four
radio	radiation
re	back, again
reno	kidney
retro	backward
rhin	nose
sacro	sacrum
salpingo	fallopian tube
sarco	flesh
sclero	hard, hardening
semi	half
sex	six
skeleto	skeleton
steno	narrowing, constriction
sub	under
super	above, excess
supra	above
syn	together
tachy	fast
thyro	thyroid, gland
trache	trachea
trans	across, over

Word element	Meaning
tri	three
ultra	beyond
un	not, back, reversal
uni	one
uretero	ureter
urethro	urethra
uro	urine, urinary organs
vaso	vessel
SUFFIXES	
able	able to
algia	pain
cele	tumor, swelling
centesis	surgical puncture to remove fluid
cide	killing, destructive
cule	little
cyte	cell
ectasia	dilating, stretching
ectomy	excision, surgical removal of
emia	blood
esis	action
form	shaped like
genesis, genetic	formation, origin
gram	tracing, mark
graph	writing
ism	condition
itis	inflammation
ize	to treat
lith	stone, calculus
lithiasis	presence of stones
lysis	disintegration
megaly	enlargement
meter	instrument that measures
oid	likeness, resemblance
oma	tumor
opathy	disease of
orrhaphy	surgical repair
osis	disease, condition of
ostomy	to form an opening or outlet
otomy	to incise
pexy	fixation
phage	ingesting
phobia	fear
plasty	plastic surgery
plegia	paralysis
rhage	to burst forth
rhea	excessive discharge
rhexis	rupture
scope	lighted instrument for visual examination
scopy	to examine visually
stomy	to form an opening
tomy	incision into
uria	urine

Sources: Courtesy of Margaret Ling, Director of Vocational Nursing, Santa Rosa Junior College, Santa Rosa, Calif.; B Kozier, G Erb: *Fundamentals of Nursing: Concepts and Procedures,* 2nd ed., Addison-Wesley, 1983. Used by permission.

Appendix C Canada's Food Guide (1983)

Variety. Choose different kinds of foods from within each group in appropriate numbers of servings and portion sizes.

Energy balance. Needs vary with age, sex, and activity. Balance energy intake from foods with energy output from physical activity to control weight. Foods selected according to the Guide can supply 1000–1400 kilo-calories. For additional energy, increase the number and size of servings from the various foods groups and/or add other foods.

Moderation. Select and prepare foods with limited amounts of fat, sugar and salt. If alcohol is consumed, use limited amounts.

Food group	Recommended number of servings (adults)	Some examples of one serving
Milk and milk products	2[a]	1 cup milk; ¾ cup yogurt; 1½ oz cheddar or process cheese
Meat, fish, poultry, and alternates	2	2–3 oz cooked lean meat, fish, poultry, or liver; 4 T peanut butter; 1 cup cooked dried peas, beans, or lentils; ½ cup nuts or seeds; 2 oz cheddar cheese; ½ cup cottage cheese; 2 eggs
Breads and cereals[b]	3–5	1 slice bread; ½ cup cooked cereal; ¾ cup ready-to-eat cereal; 1 roll or muffin; ½–¾ cup cooked rice, macaroni, spaghetti or noodles; ½ hamburger or wiener bun
Fruits and vegetables	4–5[c]	½ cup vegetables or fruits—fresh, frozen, or canned; ½ cup juice–fresh, frozen, or canned; 1 medium-sized potato, carrot, tomato, peach, apple, orange, or banana

[a]For children up to 11 years, 2–3 servings; adolescents, 3–4 servings; pregnant and nursing women, 3–4 servings.

[b]Whole grain or enriched. Whole grain products are recommended.

[c]Include at least two vegetables. Choose a variety of both vegetables and fruits—cooked, raw, or their juices. Include yellow, green, or green leafy vegetables.

Source: Minister of National Health and Welfare, Ottawa. Reproduced by permission of the Minister of Supply and Services Canada.

Appendix D Recommended Daily Dietary Allowances (revised 1980)

Food and Nutrition Board, National Academy of Sciences—National Research Council Recommended Daily Dietary Allowances,[a] (revised 1980)*

	Age (years)	Weight (kg)	Weight (lb)	Height (cm)	Height (in)	Protein (g)	Fat-Soluble Vitamins: Vitamin A (μg RE)[b]	Vitamin D (μg)[c]	Vitamin E (mg α-TE)[d]
Infants	0.0–0.5	6	13	60	24	kg × 2.2	420	10	3
	0.5—1.0	9	20	71	28	kg × 2.0	400	10	4
Children	1–3	13	29	90	35	23	400	10	5
	4–6	20	44	112	44	30	500	10	6
	7–10	28	62	132	52	34	700	10	7
Males	11–14	45	99	157	62	45	1000	10	8
	15–18	66	145	176	69	56	1000	10	10
	19–22	70	154	177	70	56	1000	7.5	10
	23–50	70	154	178	70	56	1000	5	10
	51 +	70	154	178	70	56	1000	5	10
Females	11–14	46	101	157	62	46	800	10	8
	15–18	55	120	163	64	46	800	10	8
	19–22	55	120	163	64	44	800	7.5	8
	23–50	55	120	163	64	44	800	5	8
	51 +	55	120	163	64	44	800	5	8
Pregnant						+30	+200	+5	+2
Lactating						+20	+400	+5	+3

*Designed for the maintenance of good nutrition of practically all healthy people in the U.S.A.

[a]The allowances are intended to provide for individual variations among most normal persons as they live in the United States under usual environmental stresses. Diets should be based on a variety of common foods in order to provide other nutrients for which human requirements have been less well defined.

[b]Retinol equivalents. 1 retinol equivalent = 1 μg retinol or 6 μg β carotene.

[c]As cholecalciferol. μg cholecalciferol = 400 IU of vitamin D.

[d]α-tocopherol equivalents. 1 mg *d*-α tocopherol = 1 α-TE.

[e]1 NE (niacin equivalent) is equal to 1 mg of niacin or 60 mg of dietary tryptophan.

Water-Soluble Vitamins							Minerals					
Vitamin C (mg)	Thiamin (mg)	Riboflavin (mg)	Niacin (mg NE)[e]	Vitamin B-6 (mg)	Folacin[f] (μg)	Vitamin B-12 (μg)	Calcium (mg)	Phosphorus (mg)	Magnesium (mg)	Iron (mg)	Zinc (mg)	Iodine (μg)
35	0.3	0.4	6	0.3	30	0.5[g]	360	240	50	10	3	40
35	0.5	0.6	8	0.6	45	1.5	540	360	70	15	5	50
45	0.7	0.8	9	0.9	100	2.0	800	800	150	15	10	70
45	0.9	1.0	11	1.3	200	2.5	800	800	200	10	10	90
45	1.2	1.4	16	1.6	300	3.0	800	800	250	10	10	120
50	1.4	1.6	18	1.8	400	3.0	1200	1200	350	18	15	150
60	1.4	1.7	18	2.0	400	3.0	1200	1200	400	18	15	150
60	1.5	1.7	19	2.2	400	3.0	800	800	350	10	15	150
60	1.4	1.6	18	2.2	400	3.0	800	800	350	10	15	150
60	1.2	1.4	16	2.2	400	3.0	800	800	350	10	15	150
50	1.1	1.3	15	1.8	400	3.0	1200	1200	300	18	15	150
60	1.1	1.3	14	2.0	400	3.0	1200	1200	300	18	15	150
60	1.1	1.3	14	2.0	400	3.0	800	800	300	18	15	150
60	1.0	1.2	13	2.0	400	3.0	800	800	300	18	15	150
60	1.0	1.2	13	2.0	400	3.0	800	800	300	10	15	150
+20	+0.4	+0.3	+2	+0.6	+400	+1.0	+400	+400	+150	*h*	+5	+25
+40	+0.5	+0.5	+5	+0.5	+100	+1.0	+400	+400	+150	*h*	+10	+50

[f]The folacin allowances refer to dietary sources as determined by *Lactobacillus casei* assay after treatment with enzymes (conjugases) to make polyglutamyl forms of the vitamin available to the test organism.

[g]The recommended dietary allowance for vitamin B-12 in infants is based on average concentration of the vitamin in human milk. The allowances after weaning are based on energy intake (as recommended by the American Academy of Pediatrics) and consideration of other factors, such as intestinal absorption.

[h]The increased requirement during pregnancy cannot be met by the iron content of habitual American diets nor by the existing iron stores of many women; therefore the use of 30–60 mg of supplemental iron is recommended. Iron needs during lactation are not substantially different from those of nonpregnant women, but continued supplementation of the mother for 2–3 months after parturition is advisable in order to replenish stores depleted by pregnancy.

Source: Committee on Dietary Allowances Food and Nutrition Board, National Research Council, National Academy of Sciences. Washington, D.C.: 1980.

Appendix E Summary Examples of Recommended Nutrient Intakes for Canadians[a,b] (1982)

Age	Sex	Average weight (kg)	Average energy needs (kcal/day)[c]	Protein (g/day)[d]	Fat-soluble vitamins: Vitamin A (RE/day)[e]	Vitamin D (µg/day)[f]	Vitamin E (mg/day)[g]	Water-soluble vitamins: Vitamin C (mg/day)	Folacin (µg/day)[h]	Vitamin B-12 (µg/day)	Minerals: Calcium (mg/day)	Magnesium (mg/day)	Iron (mg/day)	Iodine (µg/day)	Zinc (mg/day)
Months															
0–2	Both	4.5	500	11[i]	400	10	3	20	50	0.3	350	30	0.4[j]	25	2[k]
3–5	Both	7.0	700	14[i]	400	10	3	20	50	0.3	350	40	5	35	3
6–8	Both	8.5	800	16[i]	400	10	3	20	50	0.3	400	45	7	40	3
9–11	Both	9.5	950	18	400	10	3	20	55	0.3	400	50	7	45	3
Years															
1	Both	11	1100	18	400	10	3	20	65	0.3	500	55	6	55	4
2–3	Both	14	1300	20	400	5	4	20	80	0.4	500	65	6	65	4
4–6	Both	18	1800	25	500	5	5	25	90	0.5	600	90	6	85	5
7–9	M	25	2200	31	700	2.5	7	35	125	0.8	700	110	7	110	6
	F	25	1900	29	700	2.5	6	30	125	0.8	700	110	7	95	6
10–12	M	34	2500	38	800	2.5	8	40	170	1.0	900	150	10	125	7
	F	36	2200	39	800	2.5	7	40	170	1.0	1000	160	10	110	7
13–15	M	50	2800	49	900	2.5	9	50	160	1.5	1100	220	12	160	9
	F	48	2200	43	800	2.5	7	45	160	1.5	800	190	13	160	8
16–18	M	62	3200	54	1000	2.5	10	55	190	1.9	900	240	10	160	9
	F	53	2100	47	800	2.5	7	45	160	1.9	700	220	14	160	8
19–24	M	71	3000	57	1000	2.5	10	60	210	2.0	800	240	8	160	9
	F	58	2100	41	800	2.5	7	45	165	2.0	700	190	14	160	8
25–49	M	74	2700	57	1000	2.5	9	60	210	2.0	800	240	8	160	9
	F	59	1900	41	800	2.5	6	45	165	2.0	700	190	14[l]	160	8
50–74	M	73	2300	57	1000	2.5	7	60	210	2.0	800	240	8	160	9
	F	63	1800	41	800	2.5	6	45	165	2.0	800	190	7	160	8
75+	M	69	2000	57	1000	2.5	6	60	210	2.0	800	240	8	160	9
	F	64	1500	41	800	2.5	5	45	165	2.0	800	190	7	160	8
Pregnancy (additional															
1st Trimester				15	100	2.5	2	0	305	1.0	500	15	6	25	0
2nd Trimester				20	100	2.5	2	20	305	1.0	500	20	6	25	1
3rd Trimester				25	100	2.5	2	20	305	1.0	500	25	6	25	2
Lactation (additional)				20	400	2.5	3	30	120	0.5	500	80	0	50	6

[a]Recommended intakes of energy and of certain nutrients are not listed in this table because of the nature of the variables upon which they are based. The figures for energy are estimates of average requirements for expected patterns of activity. For nutrients not shown, the following amounts are recommended: thiamin, 0.4 mg/1000 kcal (0.48 mg/5000 kJ); riboflavin, 0.5 mg/1000 kcal (0.6 mg/5000 kJ); niacin, 7.2 NE/1000 kcal (8.6 NE/5000 kJ); vitamin B_6, 15µg, as pyridoxine, per gram of protein; phosphorus, same as calcium.

[b]Recommended intakes during periods of growth are taken as appropriate for individuals representative of the mid-point in each age group. All recommended intakes are designed to cover individual variations in essentially all of a healthy population subsisting upon a variety of common foods available in Canada.

[c]Requirements can be expected to vary with a range of ±30%.

[d]The primary units are grams per kilogram of body weight. The figures shown here are only examples.

[e]One retinol equivalent (RE) corresponds to the biological activity of 1 µg of retinol, 6 µg of β-carotene or 12 µg of other carotenes.

[f]Expressed as cholecalciferol or ergocalciferol.

[g]Expressed as *d*-α-tocopherol equivalents, relative to which β- and γ-tocopherol and α-tocotrienol have activities of 0.5, 0.1 and 0.3 respectively.

[h]Expressed as total folate.

[i]Assumption that the protein is from breast milk or is of the same biological value as that of breast milk and that between 3 and 9 months adjustment for the quality of the protein is made.

[j]It is assumed that breast milk is the source of iron up to 2 months of age.

[k]Based on the assumption that breast milk is the source of zinc for the first 2 months.

[l]After the menopause the recommended intake is 7 mg/day.

Source: Bureau of Nutritional Sciences, Food Directorate, Health Protection Branch, Ottawa. Reproduced by permission of the Minister of Supply and Services Canada.

Appendix F Equivalents

Metric Equivalents

Weights

1 picogram	=	10^{-12} gram
1 nanogram	=	10^{-9} gram
1 microgram	=	10^{-3} milligram = 10^{-6} gram
1 milligram	=	1000 micrograms = 10^{-6} gram
1 centigram	=	10 milligrams = 10^{-1} decigram = 10^{-2} gram
1 decigram	=	100 milligrams = 10 centigrams = 10^{-1} gram
1 gram	=	1000 milligrams = 100 centigrams = 10 decigrams
1 kilogram	=	1000 grams

Volume

1 milliliter	=	1 gram
1 liter	=	1 kilogram = 1000 grams (milliliters)

Approximate Weight Equivalents: Metric and Apothecaries' Systems

Metric	Apothecaries'	Metric	Apothecaries'
0.1 mg	1/600 grain	30 mg	1/2 grain
1.12 mg	1/500 grain	40 mg	2/3 grain
0.15 mg	1/400 grain	50 mg	3/4 grain
0.2 mg	1/300 grain	60 mg	1 grain
0.25 mg	1/250 grain	100 mg (0.1 gm)	1-1/2 grains
0.3 mg	1/200 grain	150 mg (0.15 gm)	2-1/2 grains
0.4 mg	1/150 grain	200 mg (0.2 gm)	3 grains
0.5 mg	1/120 grain	300 mg (0.3 gm)	5 grains
0.6 mg	1/100 grain	400 mg (0.4 gm)	6 grains
0.8 mg	1/80 grain	500 mg (0.5 gm)	7-1/2 grains
1 mg	1/60 grain	600 mg (0.6 gm)	10 grains
1.2 mg	1/50 grain	1 gram	15 grains
1.5 mg	1/40 grain	1.5 gm	22 grains
2 mg	1/30 grain	2 gm	30 grains
3 mg	1/20 grain	3 gm	45 grains
4 mg	1/15 grain	4 gm	60 grains (1 dram)
5 mg	1/12 grain	5 gm	75 grains
6 mg	1/10 grain	6 gm	90 grains
8 mg	1/8 grain	7.5 gm	120 grains (2 drams)
10 mg	1/6 grain	10 gm	2-1/2 drams
12 mg	1/5 grain	30 gm	1 ounce (8 drams)
15 mg	1/4 grain	500 gm	1.1 pounds
20 mg	1/3 grain	1000 gm	2.2 pounds 1 kilogram)
25 mg	3/8 grain		

Approximate Volume Equivalents: Metric, Apothecaries', and Household Systems

Metric	Apothecaries'	Household
0.06 ml	1 minim (m)	1 drop (gt)
0.3 ml	5 minims	
0.6 ml	10 minims	
1 ml	15 minims	15 drops (gtt)
2 ml	30 minims	
3 ml	45 minims	
4 ml	60 minims (1 fluid dram [fʒ])	60 drops (1 teaspoon [tsp])
8 ml	2 fluid drams	2 teaspoons
15 ml	4 fluid drams	4 teaspoons (1 tablespoon [Tbsp])
30 ml	8 fluid drams (1 fluid ounce [f℥])	2 tablespoons
60 ml	2 fluid ounces	
90 ml	3 fluid ounces	
200 ml	6 fluid ounces	1 teacup
250 ml	8 fluid ounces	1 large glass
500 ml	16 fluid ounces (1 pint)	1 pint
750 ml	1½ pints	
1000 ml (1 liter)	2 pints (1 quart)	1 quart
4000 ml	4 quarts	1 gallon

Glossary

abdominal paracentesis removal of fluid from the peritoneal cavity
abduction movement of a bone away from the midline of the body
abductor muscle a muscle that moves a bone away from the midline of the body
ablative surgery surgery to remove a diseased organ
abrasion wearing away of a structure, such as the skin or teeth
abscess a localized collection of pus and disintegrating body tissues
abstracting forming a summary; isolating or considering separately a particular aspect of an object
acapnia a decreased level of carbon dioxide in the blood
acatalasia a disease characterized by absence of the enzyme catalase, occurring mostly in Japanese people
accommodation (Piaget) the process of change in which a person's cognitive processes are sufficiently matured so that he or she can solve problems that could not be solved previously
accountability being responsible for one's actions involving clients and/or colleagues and accepting the consequences for one's behavior
accreditation a process by which a nongovernmental agency appraises institutions or programs to determine whether they meet established standards for service or training
acetone a flammable, colorless liquid with an ethereal odor, used to remove nail polish
acetylcholine an acetic acid ester of choline, which has an important function in the transmission of nerve impulses at the myoneural junction
aching pain a deep pain of varying degrees of intensity
acholic clay colored and free from bile
acidosis (acidemia) a condition that occurs with increases in blood carbonic acid or with decreases in blood bicarbonate; blood pH below 7.35
acne an inflammatory condition of the sebaceous glands
acromion (acromial process) the lateral projection of the scapula extending over the shoulder joint
active assistive exercise exercise carried out by the client with some assistance by the nurse
active euthanasia acts performed to shorten a person's life
active exercise exercise carried out by the client, who supplies the energy to move the body parts
active transport movement of substances across cell membranes against the concentration gradient
activity energetic action or being in a state of movement
actual health problem a health problem that currently exists
actual loss a loss identifiable by others
acupuncture a Chinese practice of piercing specific superficial nerves with needles, often to treat pain
acute sharp or severe; describing a severe condition with a sudden onset and short course (as opposed to *chronic*)
adaptation the process of modifying to meet new, changing, or different conditions
adaptation (Piaget) the coping behavior of a person who has the ability to handle the demands of the environment
adaptive mechanisms learned behaviors that assist an individual to adjust to the environment
addiction a term used previously to describe dependence on a drug or habit
adduction movement of a bone toward the midline of the body
adductor muscle a muscle that moves a bone toward the midline of the body
adenohypophysis the anterior part of the pituitary gland
adenosine triphosphate (ATP) a compound that stores energy from glucose oxidation
adherent sticking together, clinging
adhesion a fibrous band or structure by which parts are abnormally held together
adipose fat; of a fatty nature
adolescence a period of life beginning with the appearance of secondary sex characteristics and terminating with somatic growth, usually between ages 11 and 19
adolescent parents teenagers who assume the responsibilities of parenthood
adrenal gland an endocrine gland that is located on the superior aspect of the kidney
Adrenalin a trademark name for preparations of epinephrine
adrenocortical arising from the cortex of the adrenal gland
adrenocorticotrophic hormone (ACTH) a hormone produced by the pituitary gland that stimulates the adrenal cortex to produce hormones
adsorbent an agent that attracts other materials or particles to its surface, e.g., charcoal in the stomach and intestines
adventitious breath sounds abnormal breath sounds
advocate one who pleads the cause of another or argues or pleads for a cause or proposal
advocate (nurse) one who supports the rights of clients by making sure that they know their rights and that they have the necessary knowledge to make informed decisions about their care
aeration the process by which the blood exchanges carbon dioxide for oxygen in the lungs
aerobe an organism that requires oxygen to live
aerobic requiring oxygen
affect feelings, emotions
agglutination the process of clumping together
agglutinin a specific antibody formed in blood
agglutinogen a substance that acts as an antigen and stimulates the production of agglutinin
aggression an unprovoked attack or hostile, injurious, or destructive behavior or outlook
agnostic one who believes that the existence of God is unknown
air hunger dyspnea occurring in paroxysms
airway a passageway through which air normally circulates; a device that is inserted through the client's mouth to maintain the patency of air passages such as the trachea
alarm reaction (Selye) the initial reaction of the body to a stressor
albuminuria the presence of albumin in the urine
aldosterone a hormone produced by the adrenal cortex that regulates the level of sodium in the body
alerting as an element of anger, the act of engaging another's attention
algor mortis the gradual decrease in body temperature after death
alignment (posture) the position of body parts that facilitates body function
alkalosis (alkalemia) a condition that occurs with increases in blood bicarbonate or decreases in blood carbonic acid; blood pH above 7.45
allergy a hypersensitive state
alopecia abnormal loss of hair
altruism selfless concern for others
alveolus saclike dilation or cavity in the body (plural: alveoli)
ambulation the act of walking
amino acid one of a group of organic acids containing nitrogen that are considered the components of protein
ammonia dermatitis diaper rash
amphetamine a drug used to stimulate the central nervous system
ampule a small, sealed glass flask, usually designed to hold a single dose of a medication

anabolism a process in which simple substances are converted by the body cells into more complex substances, e.g., building tissue; positive nitrogen balance

anaerobe an organism that does not require oxygen to live

anal canal the terminal aspect of the rectum

analgesic a medication used to alter the perception and interpretation of pain

anal stage (Freud) a stage of human development usually occurring during the 2nd and 3rd years when the child is learning toilet training

analyzing (or analysis) breaking down a whole into component parts

anaphylaxis (anaphylactic shock, anaphylactic reaction) a severe allergic reaction

anasarca generalized edema throughout the body

anastomose to join or connect

anatomic position the position of normal body alignment

androgen any substance producing male characteristics

andropause (climacteric) the period of change in men when sexual activity decreases

androsperm sperm bearing a Y chromosome

anemia a condition in which the blood is deficient in red blood cells or hemoglobin

aneroid containing no liquid

anesthesia loss of sensation or feeling; induced loss of the sense of pain

anesthesiologist a physician specializing in the administration of anesthetics

anesthetic bed *see* surgical bed

anesthetist a person such as a nurse who specializes in administering anesthetics

aneurysm dilation of the wall of an artery, a vein, or the heart

anger an emotional state or a subjective feeling of animosity or strong displeasure

angiogram a diagnostic procedure enabling x-ray visualization of the vascular system after injection of a radiopaque dye

angstrom (Å) a unit of wavelength of the electromagnetic spectrum

anilingus anal stimulation provided orally

anion an ion carrying a negative charge

ankylosis permanent fixation of a joint; stiffening of a joint

anodyne a medication that relieves pain

anogenital referring to the area around the anus and the genitals

anonymity the right of a client participating in research to not be linked to the information gathered

anorexia lack of appetite

anorexia nervosa a psychologic condition in which the person eats little or nothing, leading to emaciation

anoscopy visual examination of the anal canal using a lighted instrument called an anoscope

anoxemia a condition in which the level of oxygen in the blood is below normal

anoxia systemic absence or reduction of oxygen in the body tissues below physiologic levels

answer (legal) a written response to a complaint

antagonist muscle a muscle that acts in the opposite manner to another muscle

antecubital space the area in front of the elbow

anterior of, toward, or at the front

anthelmintic destructive to worms

anthropometric measurement measurement of the size and composition of the body, e.g., height, weight, and skin folds

antibiosis an antagonistic association between organisms

antibiotic a substance produced by microorganisms that has the capacity to inhibit the growth of or kill other microorganisms

antibody a protective substance produced in the body to counteract antigens

anticipatory loss a loss experienced before it actually occurs

antidiuretic hormone (ADH) a hormone that is stored and released by the posterior pituitary gland and that controls water reabsorption from the kidney tubules; also referred to as *vasopressin*

antigen a substance capable of inducing the formation of antibodies

antipyretic a substance that is effective in relieving fever

antiseptic an agent that inhibits the growth of some microorganisms

antiserum (immune serum) a serum that contains antibodies

antrum the portion of the stomach between the fundus and the pylorus

anuria the failure of the kidneys to produce urine, resulting in total lack of urination or output of less than 100 ml per day in an adult

anus the opening of the rectum, the posterior opening of the gastrointestinal tract

anxiety a state of mental uneasiness, apprehension, or dread producing an increased level of arousal due to an impending or anticipated threat to self or significant relationships

apathy lack of interest or feeling

Apgar score a system of numerically rating the condition of a newborn infant

aphasia the inability to communicate by speech, signs, or writing, resulting from an injury or disease

apical beat the heartbeat as heard over the apex of the heart

apical-radial pulse measurement of the apical beat and the radial pulse

apnea cessation of breathing

apocrine gland a large sweat gland whose duct usually opens into a hair follicle

appetite a pleasant sensation in which one desires and anticipates food

appliance (ostomy) a device or bag that is secured to the abdomen to collect either urine or feces

approximate to bring close together (referring to wound or incision edges)

areola the circular area of different color around a central point, such as the circular pigmented area surrounding the nipple of the breast

aromatic having a spicy odor

arrector pili muscle the erector muscle attached to the hair follicle

arrhythmia an irregular pulse rhythm

arteriography x-ray filming of an arterial system after injection of a radiopaque material

arteriosclerosis a condition in which the walls of the arteries become hardened and thickened

artery forceps *see* hemostat

artificial intelligence area of computer science focusing on how computers can be used for tasks requiring human characteristics of intelligence

artificial respiration forceful movement of air into and out of the lungs by means external to the person

ascites the accumulation of fluid in the abdominal cavity

asepsis the absence of disease-producing microorganisms

asphyxia a condition resulting from a lack of oxygen in the inspired air

asphyxiation (suffocation) lack of oxygen due to interrupted breathing

aspirate to remove gases or fluids from a cavity by using suction

assault an attempt or threat to touch another person unjustifiably

assertiveness expression of oneself openly and directly without hurting others

assessing collecting, verifying, and organizing data about a client's health status

assessment in general, an organized collection of data about a client; in relation to the problem-oriented medical record, the third step of SOAP—that is, analysis and interpretation of the data or diagnosis of a specific problem

assimilation (of a group) the blending of attitudes and beliefs of the members

assimilation (Piaget) the process whereby humans are able to encounter and react to new situations by using the mechanisms they already possess

associative thinking a type of thinking that has little direction and often involves random thoughts (e.g., daydreaming)

asthma a disease characterized by spasmodic dyspnea, coughing, and a sense of constriction of the bronchi

astigmatism a refractive error of the eye due to an uneven curvature of the cornea
astringent an agent that causes contraction or shrinkage of tissue; usually applied topically
asymmetric lacking symmetry; showing dissimilarity of corresponding organs on opposite sides of the body
atelectasis collapse of lung tissue
atheist one who denies the existence of God
athetosis involuntary twisting and writhing movements
athlete's foot (tinea pedis) a fungal injection of the foot; ringworm
atony lack of normal muscle tone
atresia absence, closure, or degeneration of a passageway or cavity such as the primordial follicles of the ovaries
atrioventricular (AV) node the neuromuscular tissue of the heart at the base of the atrial septum that conveys impulses to the ventricles
atrioventricular valves cardiac valves between the atria and the ventricles; also referred to as the *tricuspid* and *mitral* valves
at-risk aggregate subgroup of a population who are at greater risk of illness or poor recovery
atrophy a wasting away or decrease in size of a cell, tissue, body organ, or muscle
attenuate to make thin or to weaken
attitude a feeling tone; a concomitant of behavior
audit an examination or review of records
auditory related to or experienced through hearing
auricle a chamber of the ear or the heart
auscultation the practice of examining the body by listening to body sounds
authority the right to act and command
autoantigen an antigen that originates in the person's own body
autoclave an apparatus that sterilizes, using steam under pressure
autogenous (infection) originating from the patient's own microbial flora
autonomic self-controlling; capable of independent function
autonomy the state of being independent and self-directed without outside control
autopsy (postmortem examination) the examination of a body after death; performed by a physician
axilla the armpit (plural: axillae)
axillary line an imaginary line extending vertically from the anterior fold of the axilla

babbling prelinguistic repetitive sounds produced by infants
Babinski (plantar) reflex in infants up to 1 year, the normal fanning out of toes and dorsiflexion of the big toe elicited by stroking the sole of the foot (positive Babinski); after 1 year the normal curling of the toes at this stroking (negative Babinski)
bacteriocide an agent capable of destroying some microorganisms
bacteriostatic agent an agent that prevents the growth and reproduction of some microorganisms
balance stability; steadiness; a state of equipoise in which opposing forces counteract each other
Balkan frame a metal frame extending lengthwise over a bed and supported at either end for attaching traction or providing a means of mobility to bedridden clients
bandage a material used to wrap a body part
barbiturate a drug commonly used as a hypnotic and sedative
barium a metallic element commonly used in solution as a contrast medium for x-ray filming of the gastrointestinal tract
barium enema x-ray filming of the large intestine using a contrast medium; also called a *lower gastrointestinal series*
barium swallow x-ray filming of the esophagus, stomach, and duodenum; also referred to as an *upper gastrointestinal series*
barrel chest a chest shape in which the ratio of the anteroposterior diameter to the lateral diameter is 1 to 1
barrier technique *see* reverse protective asepsis
basalis the layer of endometrium of the uterus closest to the myometrium
basal metabolic rate (BMR) the rate at which the body metabolizes food to produce the energy required to maintain body functions at rest
base of support the area on which an object rests
basic human need those things humans require to maintain physiologic and psychologic homeostasis
basic services a level of home care in which clients require supportive services, maintenance care, or personal care as an alternative to long-term institutionalization
basilic vein a superficial vein that arises on the ulnar side of the dorsum of the hand, goes up the forearm, and joins the brachial vein to form the axillary vein
battery willful or negligent touching of a person or a person's clothes, which may or may not cause harm
Beau's line a deep line visible across a nail after its growth has been halted and then renewed
bedpan a receptacle used to collect urine and feces from a person confined in bed
behavioral contact a written commitment by a client to follow through with selected actions
behavior modification eliciting and rewarding externally desired behavioral responses to reduce, modify, or eliminate ineffective adaptive coping responses
belief something accepted as true by a judgment of probability rather than actuality
bereavement the state of a person who has experienced the loss of a significant other through death
beriberi a condition due to deficiency of thiamine (vitamin B_1)
bevel a slanting edge
bilateral affecting two sides
bilirubin orange pigment in the bile
bill of rights a summary of fundamental rights and privileges guaranteed to people
binder a type of bandage applied to large body areas, e.g., the abdomen or chest
biofeedback conscious control of physiologic responses under the control of the autonomic nervous system, such as heart rate and blood pressure
biologic sex sexual gender genetically determined at conception from the XX or XY chromosomal combination
biopsy the removal and examination of tissue from the living body
biorhythm an inner rhythm that appears to control a variety of biologic processes
biorhythmology study of the biologic rhythms of the body
bisexual experiencing sexual attraction to people of both genders
bleb (wheal) a small, smooth, slightly raised area on the skin, usually filled with fluid
blended family family composed of two previously existing family units; also called *reconstituted family*
blister a collection of fluid between the epidermis and the dermis
blood pressure the pressure of the blood as it pulsates through the arteries
body image an individual's perception of his or her own physical attributes, body functioning, sexuality, appearance, and state of wellness
body image disturbance negative feelings or perceptions about characteristics, functions, or limits of one's own body or body part
body mechanics the efficient and coordinated use of the body during resting activities and movement
body temperature the internal temperature of the human body
bolus a mass of food or pharmaceutical preparation ready to be swallowed; a mass passing along the gastrointestinal tract; a concentrated mass of pharmaceutical preparation given intravenously
borborygmi abnormally intense and frequent bowel sounds
boundary (of a system) a real or imaginary line that differentiates one system from another system or a system from its environment

brachial pulse a pulse located on the inner side of the biceps muscle just below the axilla; usually palpated medially in the antecubital space
bradycardia an abnormally slow heart rate, below 60 beats per minute in an adult
bradypnea abnormally slow respirations; usually fewer than 10 respirations per minute
brainstorming technique to generate ideas in which one person's idea elicits an idea from another person and so on
Braxton Hicks contractions painless, intermittent contractions of the uterus during pregnancy
bronchial sounds normal loud, harsh, hollow blowing sounds heard by auscultation over the trachea and major bronchi
bronchodilator an agent that dilates the bronchi of the lungs
bronchogram an x-ray film of the bronchial tree taken after injection of an iodized oil dye, used as a contrast medium
bronchophony an increase in vocal resonance; an abnormal voice sound heard on auscultation of the chest wall
bronchopneumonia an infection that originates in the bronchi and involves patches of lung tissue
bronchoscope a lighted instrument used to visualize the bronchi of the lungs
bronchoscopy visual examination of the bronchi using a bronchoscope
bronchovesicular sounds combination of bronchial and vesicular sounds heard by auscultation over parts of the chest where a bronchus is near lung tissue
bronchus a large air passageway of the lungs (plural: bronchi)
bruit abnormal blowing, swishing, or rippling sounds heard during auscultation
bubbling gurgling sounds produced as air passes through moist secretions in the respiratory tract
buccal pertaining to the cheek
buffer an agent or system that tends to maintain constancy or that prevents changes in the chemical concentration of a substance
bulimia an uncontrollable compulsion to consume enormous amounts of food and then expel the food by self-induced vomiting
burden of proof (legal) evidence of the defendant's wrongdoing presented by the plaintiff
burning pain pain like the pain of burning skin

cachexia a state of weakness, emaciation, and malnutrition often seen in wasting diseases and terminal malignancies
calcitonin a hormone secreted by the thyroid gland that regulates blood calcium levels
calculus a stone composed of minerals that is formed in the body, e.g., a renal calculus formed in the kidney
calipers an instrument used to measure the thickness of folds of skin
callus hyperplasia or thickening of the horny layer of the epidermis, usually due to pressure
caloric density the number of kilocalories per unit weight of food
caloric value the amount of energy that nutrients or foods supply to the body
Calorie (large calorie, kilocarie, C.) the amount of heat required to raise the temperature of 1 kilogram of water 1 degree centigrade
calorie (small calorie) the unit of heat required to raise the temperature of 1 gram of water 1 degree centigrade
calyx (calix) a cup-shaped organ or cavity
cancellous bone bone of spongy or latticelike structure
cannula a tube with a lumen (channel), which is inserted into a cavity or duct and is often fitted with a trocar during insertion
canthus the angle formed by the upper and lower eyelids; each eye has an inner and an outer canthus
Cantor tube a single-lumen tube inserted through the mouth into the intestines
capillary action the movement of fluid in a tube, caused by the adhesion of the fluid to the wall of the tube
capsule a soft, soluble container for a medication; an anatomic structure enclosing an organ or part of the body; (of a cell) a well-defined, gelatinous layer surrounding a bacterial cell
caput succedaneum edematous swelling of the soft tissues of the part of a newborn's scalp that was encircled by the cervix before it dilated
carbaminohemoglobin the chemical combination of carbon dioxide and hemoglobin
carbohydrate a nutrient composed of carbon, hydrogen, and oxygen, e.g., starches and sugars
carbonic acid the compound formed when carbon dioxide combines with water
cardiac arrest the cessation of heart function
cardiac board a flat board placed under a person's chest when that person requires cardiac massage and is lying on a soft surface
cardiac monitor a machine that measures and records the heart function
cardiac output the amount of blood ejected from the heart per minute by ventricular contraction
cardiopulmonary resuscitation (CPR) artificial stimulation of the heart and lungs
caries decay of a tooth or bone
carina the ridge or junction where the main bronchi meet the trachea
carminative an agent that promotes the passage of flatus from the colon
carotid arteries major arteries lying on either side of the trachea and larynx
carotid receptors nerve endings that are found in the carotid bodies and carotid sinuses and that are sensitive to blood pH, changes in blood pressure, and excessive blood CO_2
carrier a person who harbors pathogens but is not ill
cartilage a firm connective tissue found throughout the body
caster a small wheel, often made of rubber or plastic, that permits furniture such as a bed to be moved easily
catabolism a destructive process in which complex substances are broken down into simpler substances, e.g., breakdown of tissue
cataplexy partial or complete muscle paralysis that can occur during narcolepsy
cataract opacity of the lens of the eye or its capsule
catarrh inflammation of the mucous membrane accompanied by a discharge
cathartic a drug that induces evacuation of feces from the large intestine
catheter a tube of plastic, rubber, metal, or other material used to remove or inject fluids into a cavity such as the bladder
cation a positively charged ion
cauda a tail or taillike appendage
caudal anesthetic an anesthetic injected into the caudal canal, below the spinal cord
cavity a hollow space within the body or one of its organs
CD ROM compact disks with read-only memory for storage of computer-generated data
cecum a dilated pouch that constitutes the first part of the large intestine adjoining the small intestine
cellular fluid *see* intracellular fluid
cellulitis inflammation of cellular tissue
Celsius *see* centigrade
cementum a bonelike connective tissue surrounding the root of a tooth
center of gravity the point at which the mass (weight) of the body is centered
centigrade (Celsius) a thermometer scale used to measure heat; the freezing point of water is 0 C and the boiling point is 100 C
central venous pressure (CVP) a measurement of the pressure of the blood, in millimeters of water, within the vena cava or the right atrium of the heart
cephalhematoma swelling of the scalp due to an effusion of blood between the periosteum and the bone
cephalocaudal proceeding in the direction from head to toe
cerebral death death that occurs when the cerebral cortex is irreversibly destroyed
cerebrospinal fluid fluid contained within the four ventricles of the brain, the subarachnoid space, and the central canal of the spinal cord

certification the practice of determining minimum standards of competence in specialty areas
cerumen waxlike material that protects the auditory canal
cervix the lower end or neck of the uterus; projects into the vagina
Chadwick's sign a change of the mucous membrane of the vagina to a bluish or violet color during pregnancy
chancre a papular lesion (sore) occurring at the entry of infection in some diseases; the primary sore of syphilis
change process that leads to modifications in behavior
change agent an individual, such as a nurse, or group who operates to change the status quo in another individual or in a system
chart (medical record) a written account of a client's health history, current health status, treatment, and progress
charting (recording) the process of making written entries about a client on the medical record
cheilosis cracks or scaling at the corners of the lips
chemical thermogenesis the production of heat by chemical means, e.g., production and circulation of ephinephrine
chemoreceptor a receptor that is sensitive to chemical substances
chemosensitive pain receptors pain receptors stimulated by chemicals
chemotaxis the movement of a cell or an organism in response to a chemical gradient
Cheyne-Stokes respirations rhythmic waxing and waning of respirations from very deep breathing to very shallow breathing with periods of temporary apnea, often associated with cardiac failure, increased intracranial pressure, or brain damage
childbearing family stage of family development during which the husband and wife assume the roles of parents
childrearing family stage of family development during which the primary focus is the nurturing, education, and socialization of children
chill shivering and shaking of body with involuntary contractions of the voluntary muscles
cholangiogram an x-ray film of the biliary tract taken after the injection of a dye
cholecystogram an x-ray film of the gallbladder after the ingestion of a contrast dye; also called *oral cholecystography*
cholesterol a lipid that does not contain fatty acid but possesses many of the chemical and physical properties of other lipids
chordotomy *see* cordotomy
chorionic gonadotropin (HCG) a hormone produced by the placenta
chorionic somatomammotropin (human placental lactogen) a hormone secreted by the placenta that influences fetal growth
choroid plexus projections of the pia mater into the ventricles of the brain that secrete cerebrospinal fluid
chromosome a structure in the nucleus of a cell that contains DNA and transmits genetic information
chronic persisting over a long time
chyme semifluid material produced by gastric digestion of food in the stomach; it is found in the small and large intestines
cicatrical tissue *see* scar tissue
cicatrix scar
cicatrization formation of a scar
cilia hairlike projections from cells, e.g., of the mucous membrane of the respiratory tract
circadian rhythm rhythmic repetition of certain phenomena each 24 hours
circa dies about a day
circulatory overload a state in which the intravascular fluid compartment contains more fluid than normal
circumcision surgical removal of part or all of the foreskin of the penis; usually performed during infancy
circumduction movement of the distal part of a bone in a circle, with the proximal end remaining fixed
circumference the outer measurement or perimeter, e.g., the distance around the chest
cisterna an enclosed space that serves as a reservoir for body fluid
cisternal puncture insertion of a needle into the subarachnoid space of the cisterna magna
citric acid cycle (Krebs cycle) a complex series of chemical reactions by which the acetyl portion of acetyl coenzyme A is broken down into carbon dioxide and hydrogen
civil action a legal action between two or more individuals
civil (private) law rules that regulate or control relationships between people rather that between persons and governments
clavicle the bone commonly known as the collarbone; it articulates with the scapula and the sternum
clean free of pathogenic organisms
clean technique a technique that maintains an area or articles free from pathogens
clergy priests, rabbis, ministers, church elders, deacons, and any other spiritual advisers
client (patient) a person seeking, waiting for, or undergoing health care
client contract a written agreement between a client and a nurse regarding a behavior change
client goal statement about the expected or desired change in a client's status after he or she receives nursing interventions
climacteric the point in development when reproduction capacity in the female terminates (menopause) and the sexual activity of the male decreases (andropause)
clinical pharmacist a person who specializes in drugs that are used for treatment, prevention, and diagnosis of disease
clitoris a small round mass of erectile tissue, blood vessels, and nerves located behind the junction of the labia minora; homologous to the penis
closed questions restrictive questions requiring only short answer
closed system a system that does not exchange energy or matter with its environment
closed wound a wound in which there is no break in the skin
clubbing (of nails) an elevation of the proximal aspect of the nail and softening of the nail bed
coagulate to clot
coccidioidomycosis a fungus disease with an acute, benign respiratory infection in the primary stage and a virulent, progressive secondary stage
cochlea a tubular structure in the inner ear that contains the organ for hearing
code of ethics formal guidelines for professional action
coercive power power derived from the perception of one's ability to threaten, harm, or punish others
cognition the process of knowing, including judgment and awareness
cognitive referring to intellectual processes such as remembering, thinking, perceiving, abstracting, and generalizing
cognitive appraisal an evaluative process that determines why and to what extent a particular transaction or series of transactions between a person and the environment are stressful
cohabiting (communal) family family unit formed by unrelated individuals or families cohabiting or living under one roof
cohesive sticking together
cohesiveness (of group) the degree of group unity or oneness
coitus sexual intercourse; from Latin, meaning "a coming together"
coitus interruptus a method of contraception during which the penis is withdrawn prior to ejaculation
colic paroxysmal intestinal cramplike pain
collaborative nursing action activity performed jointly with another member of the health care team or as a result of a joint decision by the nurse and another member of the health care team
collagen a protein found in connective tissue
colloid substances, such as large plasma protein molecules, that do not readily dissolve in true solutions
colonoscope a lighted instrument used to visualize the interior of the colon
colonoscopy visual examination of the interior of the colon with a colonoscope

colostomy an artificial abdominal opening into the colon (large bowel)
colostrum a yellow, milky fluid secreted by the mother's mammary glands a few days before or after childbirth
comatose a state of unconsciousness in which the person shows no response to maximum painful stimuli, absence of reflexes, and absence of muscle tone in the extremities
combustible able to burn; flammable
comedo a mass on the skin consisting of keratin, lipids, fatty acids, and bacteria
commitment (of group) an agreement, pledge, or obligation to do something or follow a course of action
commode a portable, chairlike structure used as a toilet
common law unwritten laws that are binding and upheld by precedent in legal cases rather than statutes
communicable disease (infectious disease) a disease that can spread from one person to another
communication exchange of thoughts, ideas, or feelings between two or more people
compensation defense mechanism in which a person substitutes an activity for one that he or she would prefer doing or cannot do
complaint (legal) a document filed by the plaintiff claiming that his or her legal rights have been infringed
compliance in learning, an individual's agreement to learn; in drug therapy, the act of carefully following the prescription
complier a person who follows a therapeutic regimen
compress a moist gauze dressing that is applied frequently to an open wound; it sometimes is medicated
concave hollowed or rounded inward
concept an abstract idea or mental image of phenomena or reality generalized from particular instances
conceptual framework set of concepts and statements that integrate the concepts into a meaningful configuration
conceptual model a basic structure in which a complex of ideas is united to portray a large general idea
concurrent audit an audit to review present practices
concurrent disinfection measures taken while a client is infectious to control the spread of the microorganisms
conditioning learning in which a response previously associated with one stimulus becomes associated with another stimulus
condom a sheath or cover, usually made of rubber or plastic, worn over the penis during coitus to prevent conception or infection; it may also be used to catch urine
conduction the transfer of heat from one molecule or object to another by contact
confer to consult another person or persons for advice, information, ideas, or instructions
confidentiality the right of a client or research subject that any information revealed by that individual will not be made public or available to others
conformity actions in accordance with specified standards
confounding variable *see* uncontrolled variable
confusion a mental state in which a person appears bewildered and may make inappropriate statements and answers to questions
congenital existing at, and often before, birth
congestion excessive accumulation of blood in a part of the body
congruence (communication) a state in which one's verbal and nonverbal communications convey the same message
conjunctiva the delicate membrane that covers the eyeball and lines the eyelids
conjunctivitis inflammation of the conjunctiva
connection power power derived from the perception that one has important contracts or relationships with others
consciousness a person's normal state of awareness of the environment, self, and others
consensual reaction (eyes) a reaction in which one pupil constricts quickly in response to a bright light and the other pupil constricts also, but more slowly
sent permission given voluntarily by a person in his or her right mind; *informed consent* implies that the individual is knowledgeable about the consent and understands it
constant data information that is unchanging
constipation passage of small, dry, hard stool or passage of no stool for an abnormally long time
constitutional law law stated in federal, state, or provincial constitutions
construct abstract concept derived from existing theories or observations
constructive surgery surgery to repair a congenitally malformed organ or tissue.
construct validity the degree to which an instrument measures the abstract concept it was designed to measure
consultation deliberation by two or more people
consumer an individual, group, or community that uses a service or a product
contact a person who has been near an infected person and thus exposed to pathogenic microorganisms
contact lens a small, plastic corrective lens that fits on the cornea of the eye directly over the pupil
contaminated possessing pathogenic organisms
continuum a grid or graduated scale
contour position (of a bed) a position with the head and foot of the bed elevated, creating an angle of about 15°
contraception the prevention of fertilization of the ovum by any method
contract a written or verbal agreement between two or more people to do or not do some lawful act
contracting family stage of family development during which the children leave the family unit, and the adult family members stabilize their roles, age, and prepare for retirement
contraction the normal active shortening or tensing of a muscle
contractual obligation a duty to render service established by a formal or informal contract
contracture permanent shortening of a muscle and subsequent shortening of tendons and ligaments
contusion a closed wound that occurs as a result of a blow from a blunt instrument; a bruise
convection transfer of heat by movement of a liquid or gas, e.g., air currents
conversion a defense mechanism in which a mental conflict is converted into a physical symptom
conversive heat heat that results from the conversion of a primary source of energy
convex curved or rounded like the external surface of a sphere
coping the process through which the individual manages the demands of the person-environment relationship that are stressful
coping behavior behavior learned in response to stress
coping mechanisms physical or emotional adaptive or defensive abilities
coping strategy an innate or acquired way of responding to a changing environment or specific problem or situation
copulation the act of coitus; from Latin, meaning "coupling or joining"
coraje a Hispanic term meaning rage in response to a particular situation
cordotomy (chordotomy) surgical severing of the spinothalamic portion of the anterolateral tract of the spinal cord, usually for the purpose of relieving pain
core-gender identity *see* sexual identity
corium *see* dermis
corn a hardening and thickening of the skin forming a conical mass pointing downward into the corium
cornea the transparent covering of the anterior eye that connects with the sclera
corneal reflex irritation of the cornea resulting in a reflex closing of the eyelids
cornification hardening
coronal plane any line or plane dividing the body into anterior (ventral) and posterior (dorsal) portions at right angles to the sagittal plane
coroner a public official who is responsible for investigating any deaths that appear to be unnatural

corpus albicans a mass of white, scarred tissue that replaces the corpus luteum in the ovary when fertilization does not occur
corpus luteum a yellow body formed in the Graafian follicle after the ovum is discharged
cortical bone compact bone
corticoid a term applied to hormones of the adrenal cortex or substances with similar activity
cortisol the most abundant glucocorticoid; also called hydrocortisone
cortisone a hormone produced by the adrenal cortex that has antiinflammatory properties and is involved in the metabolism of glycogen to glucose
costovertebral angle the angle formed by a rib and the spine
cough a sudden expulsion of air from the lungs
counseling the process of helping a client to recognize and cope with stressful psychologic or coping problems, to develop improved interpersonal relationships, and to promote personal growth
counterirritant an agent that produces an irritation with the intent of relieving some other problem
countershock phase part of the initial stage of the general adaptation syndrome during which the body changes produced in response to a stressor are reversed
CPR *see* cardiopulmonary resuscitation
CPU (central processing unit) the electronic equipment built into a computer that executes program instructions to manipulate data
cradle cap a yellowish, oily crusting of the scalp of infants
creatinine a nitrogenous waste that is excreted in the urine
creative thinking a pattern of thinking involving establishing new relationships and new concepts and solving problems innovatively
credentialing (nursing) the process of determining and maintaining competence in nursing practice
Credé's maneuver manual exertion of pressure on the bladder to force urine out
cremaster the inner layer of striated muscle and connective tissue in the scrotum
crepitus a grating sound caused by bone fragments rubbing together
creps (crepitation) a dry, crackling sound like that of crumpled cellophane, produced by air in the subcutaneous tissue or by air moving through fluid in the alveoli of the lungs
crime an act committed in violation of societal law
criminal action a legal action dealing with disputes between an individual and society as a whole
criminal law law that deals with actions against the safety and welfare of the public
crisis in psychosocial terms, a rapid change or event that disturbs a person's psychologic homeostasis; in fever, the sudden reduction of an elevated body temperature
criteria (of nursing care) indicators of the quality of nursing care or measures by which the nursing care is judged
criterion a standard or model that can be used in judging
critical thinking cognitive processes during which data are reviewed and explanations considered before an opinion is formed
crown (of a tooth) the exposed part of the tooth outside the gum, covered by enamel
crutch a device with hand and arm supports used to facilitate walking
crutch palsy weakness of the hand, wrist, and forearm induced by prolonged pressure of a crutch on the axillary nerves
cryptorchidism failure of the testes to descend from the abdominal cavity to the scrotal sacs
crystalline amino acids refined protein used in hyperalimentation
crystalloid salts that dissolve readily in true solutions
cue fact the nurse acquires by using the five senses
cultural heritage values and beliefs unique to a particular culture that influence the family's structure, methods of interaction, health care practices, and coping mechanisms
culture in microbiology, the cultivation of microorganisms or cells in a special growth medium; in sociology, the beliefs and practices that are shared by people and passed down from generation to generation
culture shock the shock that can occur when an individual changes quickly from one social setting to another where former patterns of behavior are often ineffective
cumulative effect the effect of a drug when the level builds up in the blood
cunnilingus oral stimulation of the clitoris and labia by a partner
cupula a gelatinous dome-shaped structure of the inner ear that contains sensory hair cells
curandero (female: **curandera**) a healer within the Hispanic community
curet a spoon-shaped instrument used for removing material from a body cavity
curettage removal of material from the wall of a cavity, e.g., the uterus, with a curet
cuticle the flat, thin rim of skin surrounding the nail
CVP *see* central venous pressure
cyanosis bluish discoloration of the skin, nail beds, and mucous membranes, due to reduced oxygen in the blood
cybernetics the science that deals with the process of communication and automatic control systems
cyst an enclosed cavity or sac lined by epithelium and containing liquid or semisolid material
cystic fibrosis a hereditary condition marked by the accumulation of thick and tenacious mucus in the lungs and the abnormal secretion of saliva and sweat
cystitis inflammation of the urinary bladder
cystocele protrusion of the urinary bladder through the vaginal wall
cystoscope a lighted instrument used to visualize the interior of the urinary bladder
cytoscopy visual examination of the urinary bladder with a cystoscope
cytology the study of the origin, structure, function, and pathology of cells

Dakin's solution a buffered aqueous solution of sodium hypochlorite used as a bactericide
dandruff a dry or greasy, scaly material shed from the scalp
data information
database (baseline data) all information known about a client; it includes the physician's history and physical examination, the nurse's assessment and history, and material contributed by other members of the health team
database (computer) collections of information on a particular topic
data collection the process of gathering information about a patient or client
deamination the removal of the amino (NH_2) groups by hydrolysis from amino acids
debilitated having lost strength
debride to remove foreign and dying tissue from a wound so that healthy tissue is exposed
deceased dead; a person who is dead
decerebrate posturing a posture indicative of midbrain damage, consisting of extension, adduction, and internal rotation of the arms; extension of the legs with the feet in plantar flexion; and arching of the back
decibel a unit used to measure or describe sound
deciduous teeth temporary teeth that are shed
decision (legal) the outcome of a trial, rendered by a judge
decisional law laws determined by the courts in ruling on cases, rather than by statutes
decoding the process of receiving a communication and converting the message into understandable terms
decortical posturing a posture indicative of damage to the internal capsule and corticospinal tracts above the brain stem; it consists of flexion and adduction of the fingers, wrists, and shoulders; extension and internal rotation of the legs and feet; and rigidity of all extremities
decubitus ulcer an ulcer of the skin and underlying tissues produced by prolonged pressure
decussate to cross over
deductive reasoning making specific observations from a generalization
deductive theory a theory formulated by a process in which the idea

is developed first, followed by observation of relevant supportive phenomena
deep breathing inhaling the maximum amount of air possible, then exhaling
defamation a communication that is injurious to a person
defecation expulsion of feces from the rectum and anus
defendant (legal) person who is alleged to have infringed on the rights of another
defense mechanism unconscious psychologic processes that protect the person from anxiety
dehiscence a splitting open or rupture
dehydration insufficient fluid in the body
delegate to authorize another as one's representative or to entrust authority to another
delegation assigning to another aspect of client care; sharing of responsibility and authority with others and holding them accountable for performance
delirious experiencing mental confusion, restlessness, and incoherence
demineralization excessive loss of minerals or inorganic salts
demography the study of population statistics
demulcent a drug that coats the intestine, thus protecting the lining
denial a defense mechanism in which painful or anxiety-producing aspects of reality are blocked out of consciousness
dental caries tooth decay
dental crown the exposed part of the tooth outside the gum, covered by enamel
dental floss waxed or unwaxed thread used for cleaning between the teeth and the gums
dental plaque deposits on the teeth that serve as a medium for bacterial growth
dental pulp cavity a space in the center of the tooth containing blood vessels and nerves
dental root the part of the tooth that is imbedded in the jaw
dentifrice a paste or powder used to clean or polish the teeth
dentin the internal part of the tooth crown below the enamel
dentures a natural or artificial set of teeth; usually the term designates artificial replacements for natural teeth
deoxyribonucleic acid (DNA) a nucleic acid found in all living cells; it is the carrier of genetic information
dependence reliance
dependent edema edema that collects in the lower parts of the body, where hydrostatic pressure is greatest
dependent nursing action, intervention, or **function** activity by a nurse that is a result of a physician's order
dependent variable (DV) the condition, element, or process that a researcher is attempting to affect by manipulating other variables; also called the *outcome* or *criterion variable*
depolarize to reduce toward a nonpolarized state; to cause loss of charge
depression feelings of sadness and dejection, often accompanied by physiologic change; a decrease of functional activity, as in depression of sensorium
dermatologic preparation a medication applied to the skin
dermis (corium) true skin, containing blood vessels, nerves, hair follicles, and glands
describing as an element of anger, the process of delineating the source of the angry feelings
detrusor muscle the three layers of smooth muscle that make up the urinary bladder
detumescence the process of returning to a flaccid state, e.g., referring to the penis following ejaculation
development an individual's increasing capacity and skill in functioning, related to growth
developmental crisis a crisis that occurs as a result of stressors impeding development
developmental tasks skills and behavior patterns learned during development
developmental theory framework for studying the family unit that views [illegible]ies as having stages of development
dextrose a sugar; also called *glucose*
diagnosis a statement or conclusion concerning the nature of some phenomenon
diagnostic related group (DRG) a predetermined category of illnesses, injuries, surgical procedures, and/or other conditions requiring hospitalization for which the cost of care is established prior to a client's hospitalization
diagnostic surgery surgery performed to confirm a diagnosis
dialyzing membrane a membrane that permits water molecules and crystalloids in true solution to move through it but not particles in a colloid dispersion
diapedesis the movement of blood corpuscles through a blood vessel wall
diaphoresis profuse sweating
diaphragm a musculomembranous partition that separates the abdominal and thoracic (chest) cavities
diarrhea defecation of liquid feces and increased frequency of defecation
diastole the period when the ventricles of the heart are relaxed
diastolic pressure the pressure of the blood against the arterial walls when the ventricles of the heart are at rest
diathermy the production of heat in body tissues by high-frequency electric currents
diet the food and fluid regularly consumed by an individual each day
dietitian a person who is skilled in the use of diets in health and disease
diffusion movement of gases or other particles from an area of greater pressure to an area of lower pressure or concentration; the continual intermingling of molecules in liquids, gases, or solids brought about by the random movement of the molecules
diffusion coefficient the rate of solubility of gases in the respiratory membrane
digital performed with the finger
dildo an artificial penis
diploid number the original number of chromosomes in all cells of the body (23 pairs in humans)
diplopia double vision
direct interview highly structured questioning that elicits specific information
direct nursing activities activities by a nurse that are carried out in the presence of the client
direct services home care activities that involve direct contact between a caregiver and a client for the purpose of administering care measures, teaching, or planning care
directed thinking a pattern of thinking that is purposeful and is used for forming judgments, problem-solving, and decision-making
disaccharide a sugar consisting of double molecules
discharge planners nurses employed by hospitals whose primary responsibility is to assess client's anticipated needs after discharge
discharge planning the process of anticipating and planning for client's needs after discharge from a hospital or other facility
discovery (legal) pretrial activities designed to gain all the facts of a situation
disease a morbid (unhealthful) process having definite symptoms
disequilibrium a disturbed state of equilibrium, either mental or physical; an unbalanced condition
disinfectant an agent that destroys pathogens other than spores
disinfection the process by which an article is rendered free of pathogens
disk (diskette) recordlike device to store computer-generated data
disk drive device that records data onto or reads data from a computer disk
disorientation a state of mental confusion; loss of bearings, time, and place
displacement a defense mechanism in which an emotional reaction is transferred from one object to another less threatening object
distal farthest from the point of reference
distention (abdominal) *see* tympanites
distraction a mechanism for relieving pain in which the person's attention is drawn away from the pain
diuresis *see* polyuria

diuretic an agent that increases the production of urine
dorsal of, toward, or at the back
dorsal column stimulator an electrode attached to the dorsal column of the spinal cord for the purpose of relieving pain
dorsal flexion movement of the ankle so that the toes are pointing up
dorsalis pedis pulse a pulse located on the instep of the foot
dorsal recumbent position a back-lying position with the head and shoulders slightly elevated
dot-matrix printer output device that forms images (e.g., letters) by generating patterns of small dots
drain a substance or appliance (usually made of rubber or gauze) to assist in the discharge of drainage from a wound
drainage a discharge from a wound or cavity
dressing a material used to cover and protect a wound
drug (medication) a chemical compound taken for disease prevention, diagnosis, cure, or relief or to affect the structure or function of the body
drug abuse excessive intake of a substance either continually or periodically
drug allergy a hypersensitivity to a drug; the immunologic reaction to a drug
drug dependence inability to keep the intake of a drug or substance under control
drug habituation a mild form of psychologic dependence on a drug
drug interaction the beneficial or harmful interaction of one drug with another drug
drug misuse improper use of common medications in ways that can lead to acute and chronic toxicity
drug tolerance a condition in which successive increases in the dosage of a drug are required to maintain a given therapeutic effect
drug toxicity the quality of a drug that exerts a deleterious effect on an organism or tissue
DT diphtheria and tetanus toxoid
DTP diphtheria toxoid, tetanus toxoid, and pertussis vaccine
dullness (in percussion) decreased resonance or percussion sound that occurs when large amounts of fluid or pus collect in the alveoli
duodenocolic reflex a mass peristaltic movement of the colon stimulated by the presence of chyme in the duodenum
dura (dura mater) the outermost, fibrous membrane covering the brain and spinal cord
duration (of sound) the length of the sound (long or short)
dyad a two-person group
dynamic electricity moving electric charges
dynamic equilibrium tendency of the body to maintain a state of balance or equilibrium while continually changing
dysfunction impaired functioning
dyspareunia pain experienced by a woman during intercourse
dyspepsia indigestion
dysphagia difficulty or inability to swallow
dysphasia difficulty speaking
dyspnea difficult and labored breathing in which the client has a persistent unsatisfied need for air and feels distressed
dysuria painful or difficult urination

ecchymosis a blotchy area or discoloration of the skin; a bruise
ecchymotic appearing like a bruise
eccrine gland a sweat gland that secretes outward via a duct
echolalia the repetition by a person of words addressed to him or her
eclampsia convulsions and coma associated with hypertension and proteinuria in pregnant women
ecology the study of the relationship of humans and the environment
ectoderm the outermost of the three primary germ layers of the embryo
ectopic pregnancy the implantation of the fertilized ovum outside the uterus
ectropion a rolling out of the eyelid
edema excess interstitial fluid
edentulous without teeth
effector organ a muscle or gland that responds to nerve impulses
efferent conveying away from the center
effluent urine or feces discharged through a stoma
ego (Freud) the part of the psyche that maintains its identity; the conscious sense of self
egocentricity concern about oneself
egocentric speech self-centered, noncommunicative speech
ego integrity feeling satisfied with one's life-style and accepting the inevitability of one's life cycle
egophony a type of bronchophony in which the voice has a nasal, bleating quality
ejaculation expulsion of semen from the penis
ejaculatory ducts short tubes that pass through the prostate gland and terminate in the urethra
elective surgery surgery performed for a person's well-being but not absolutely necessary for life
Electra complex (Freud) the female child's attraction to her father; compare with *Oedipus complex*
electrocardiogram (ECG, EKG) a graph of the electric activity of the heart
electrocardiograph a machine that measures and records impulses from the heart on an electrocardiogram
electroencephalogram (EEG) a graph of the electric activity of the brain
electroencephalograph a machine that measures and records impulses from the brain on an electroencephalogram
electrolyte a chemical substance that develops an electric charge and is able to conduct an electric current when placed in water; an ion
electromyogram (EMG) a record of the electric potential created by the contract of a muscle
electromyograph a machine that measures and records impulses from the muscles on an electromyogram
electron a negatively charged electric particle
emaciation excessive thinness
embalming a process of preserving a body chemically
embolus a blood clot (or a substance, such as air) that has moved from its place of origin and is obstructing the circulation in a blood vessel (plural: emboli)
embryo the derivative of a fertilized ovum that develops into the offspring
embryonic phase the period during which the fertilized ovum develops into an organism; it extends for the first 8–12 weeks after conception
emesis vomit
emmetropia the normal refraction of the eye, which focuses objects on the retina
emollient an agent that soothes and softens skin or mucous membrane; often an oily substance
empacho a Hispanic term for a disease seen primarily in children that includes a swollen abdomen as a result of intestinal blockage
empathy seeing or feeling a situation the way another person sees or feels it
emphysema a chronic obstructive lung disorder in which the terminal bronchioles become distended and plugged with mucus
empirical by observation or experience
empirical data information collected from the observable world
emulsification a process by which lipids are broken up and evenly dispersed in an aqueous medium
emulsion a preparation in which one liquid is distributed throughout another
enamel (of a tooth) the hard, inorganic substance that covers the crown of a tooth
encoding the selection of specific signs and symbols to transmit a message
endemic present in a community all the time
endoderm (entoderm) the innermost of the three primary germ layers of the embryo
endogenous developing from within
endometrium the inner mucous membrane lining of the uterus
endorphin a polypeptide found throughout the body that is thought to relieve pain
endosteum the membrane lining a hollow bone

endothelium the layer of endothelial cells lining the blood vessels, cavities of the heart, and serous cavities
enema a solution injected into the rectum and the sigmoid colon
engorgement excessive fullness of an organ or passage
enkephalin a pentapeptide naturally occurring in the brain that has opiatelike effects
enteric referring to the intestines
enteric-coated surrounded with a special coating used for tablets and capsules that prevents release of the drug until it is in the intestines
enteric feeding a feeding administered directly into the small intestine through a tube
enteritis inflammation of the small intestine
enteroclysis the injection of a nutrient or drug into the colon
enterostomal therapist a person who specializes in ostomy care
enterostomy an opening through the abdominal wall into the intestines
entropion an inturned eyelid
enuresis bedwetting
environmental stimulus anything in the environment that arouses or incites action of a receptor (the terminus of a sensory nerve)
enzyme a biologic catalyst that speeds up chemical reactions
epidemic the occurrence of a disease in many people at the same time or in rapid succession in an area
epidemiology study of the occurrence and distribution of disease
epidermis the outermost, nonvascular layer of skin
epididymis a highly coiled duct between the seminiferous tubules of the testes and the vas deferens
epidural outside the dura mater
epidural block injection of an anesthetic between a lumbar interspace into the spinal canal (external to the dura mater)
epinephrine a hormone produced by the medulla of the adrenal glands; it is also manufactured artificially
epistaxis nosebleed
equilibrium a state of balance
equipoise a state of equilibrium
erection (penile) lengthening, widening, and hardening of the penis as it becomes congested with blood during sexual arousal
erogenous sexually sensitive
erotic stimuli sensations that cause sexual arousal
eructation ejection of gas from the stomach (belching)
erythema redness that is associated with a variety of rashes
erythematous of the nature of erythema
erythroblastosis fetalis a condition produced in second and subsequent infants borne by Rh negative mothers when the father is Rh positive
erythrocyte red blood cell
erythropoiesis the formation of red blood cells
esophagoscopy visual examination of the interior of the esophagus with a lighted instrument
esophagus the muscular tube that extends from the pharynx to the stomach
espanto a Hispanic term for a disease in which the individual is frightened by seeing supernatural spirits or events
ester a compound of alcohol and acid
estrogen a female sex hormone formed by the ovaries, the adrenal cortex, the testes, and the fetoplacental organ
ethics the rules or principles that govern right conduct
ethnic relating to races or to large groups of people with common traits and customs
ethnic group a set of individuals who share a unique cultural and social heritage passed on from one generation to another
ethnicity the condition of belonging to a specific ethnic group
ethnoscience systematic study of the way of life of a designated cultural group to obtain accurate data regarding behavior, perceptions, and interpretations of the universe
etiology cause
Eucharist *see* Holy Communion
eupnea normal respiration that is quiet, rhythmic, and effortless
eustachian (auditory) tube the tube that connects the middle ear with nasopharynx
euthanasia the act or practice of killing for reasons of mercy
evacuator an instrument for removing fluid or small particles from a body cavity
evaluate to judge or appraise; to identify whether or to what degree a client's goals of care have been met
evaluating assessing the client's response to nursing intervention and then comparing the response to predetermined standards
evaluation the process of identifying the client's progress toward achievement of established goals, using well-defined outcome criteria; judgment or appraisal
evaporation conversion of liquid into a vapor
eversion turning outward
evisceration extrusion of the internal organs
examine to inspect or investigate
excise to cut off or out
excoriation loss of the superficial layers of the skin
excretion elimination of a waste product produced by the body cells from the body
exhalation (expiration) the act of breathing out; the outflow of air from the lungs to the atmosphere
exophthalmos protruding eyeballs
exotoxin a toxic substance formed by bacteria and found outside the bacterial cell
expanded role increased responsibility assumed by a nurse by virtue of education and experience
expanding family the stage of family development that includes the childbearing and childrearing phases
expected date of confinement (EDC) the projected date of birth of a baby
expectorate to cough and spit up mucus or other materials
expert power power derived from one's expertise, talents, and skills
expert systems computer-based model that attempts to simulate the way human experts in a particular field gather data and make decisions
expert witness one who by education or experience possesses knowledge that the ordinary layperson does not have
expiration (exhalation) the outflow of air from the lungs to the atmosphere
expiratory reserve volume the maximum amount of air exhaled after a normal exhalation
expired dead
exploratory surgery surgery performed to confirm the extent of a pathologic process and sometimes to confirm a diagnosis
extended family the nuclear family plus other relatives such as uncles, aunts, and grandparents
extension increasing the angle of a joint (between two bones); the act of straightening
extensor (muscle) a muscle that acts to straighten a joint thus increasing the angle between two bones
external cardiac massage rhythmic massage of the heart muscle over the sternum
extracellular outside the cells
extracellular fluid (ECF) fluid found outside the body cells
extraneous variable *see* uncontrolled variable
extrapolating inferring facts or data from known facts or data
extrathecal outside the sheath, e.g., outside the spinal canal
extravasation the escape of blood from a vessel into the body tissues
extreme unction the sacrament of anointing the sick
exudate material, e.g., fluid and cells, that has escaped from blood vessels and is deposited in tissues or on tissue surfaces during the inflammatory process

fad a practice followed for a time with exaggerated zeal
Fahrenheit a thermometer scale used to measure heat; the freezing point of water is 32 F, and the boiling point is 212 F
family-centered nursing nursing that considers the health of the family as a unit in addition to the health of the individual family members
fantasy an adaptive mechanism in which wishes and desires are imagined as fulfilled

fasciculation abnormal contraction of a muscle involving the whole motor unit of the muscle
fastigium the highest point
fasting abstinence from eating
fat an organic substance that is greasy and insoluble in water; adipose tissue, a whitish-yellow tissue that forms soft pads between various body organs and serves as an energy reserve; an ester of glycerol with fatty acids
fatty acid the basic structural unit of fat
fear an emotional response to an actual, present danger
febrile pertaining to a fever; feverish
fecal impaction a mass of hardened feces in the folds of the rectum
fecal incontinence inability to control the passage of feces through the anus
feces body wastes and undigested food eliminated from the rectum
feedback a process that enables a system to regulate itself; the response to some of a system's output, which acts as input for the purpose of exerting influence over a process; in communication, it is the response; in learning, it is the process of relating a person's performance to the desired goal
fellatio the oral stimulation of the male genitals by licking, blowing, or sucking
felony a crime of a serious nature punishable by imprisonment
femoral anteversion the forward tipping or tilting of the femur
femoral pulse the pulse found in the groin at the midpoint of the inguinal ligament
fenestrated perforated to provide a window or opening
fetal heartbeat the heart beat of the fetus, generally heard through the maternal abdominal wall
fetal phase the stage of development from 8 or 12 weeks after conception until birth
fetus the unborn offspring in the postembryonic stage of development
fever elevated body temperature
fiber an indigestible carbohydrate derived from plants
fibrillation involuntary contractions of a muscle; cardiac arrhythmia characterized by extremely rapid, irregular, and ineffective twitchings of the atria or ventricles
fibrin an insoluble protein formed from fibrinogen during the clotting of blood
fibrinous exudate exudate containing large amounts of fibrin
fibroplasia the formation of fibrous tissue
fibrous tissue common connective tissue composed of elastic and collagen fibers
field single data item within a record
figure-eight bandage a bandage turn usually used for flexed joints in which the bandage makes a figure-eight around and over the joint
file collection of data about one area within a database
first intention healing primary healing of a wound, which occurs when the tissue surfaces have been approximated
fissure a groove or deep fold such as that which separates the lobes of the lung
fistula an abnormal communication or passage usually between two organs or between an organ and the body surface
flaccid weak or lax
flaccid paralysis impaired muscle function with loss of muscle tone
flail chest the ballooning out of the chest wall through injured rib spaces during exhalation
flatness (in percussion) absence of resonance; extreme dullness
flatulence the presence of excessive amounts of gas in the stomach or intestines
flatus gas or air normally present in the stomach or intestines
flexion decreasing the angle of a joint (between two bones); the act of bending
flexor muscle a muscle that acts to bend a joint, decreasing the angle between two bones
flowsheet a record used to chart the progress of specific or specialized data, such as vital signs, fluid balance, or routine medications
flushing transient redness of the skin, often of the face and neck; it may be generalized or restricted to a particular area
follicle (hair) a pouchlike depression in the skin in which a hair is enclosed
follicle stimulating hormone (FSH) a hormone produced by the anterior pituitary gland (adenohypophysis) that stimulates the development of the ovarian follicle
follicular stage *see* preovulatory stage
foment *see* hot pack
fomite an inanimate object other than food that can harbor pathogenic microorganisms and transmit an infection
fontanelle an unossified membranous gap in the bone structure of the skull
footboard a board placed at the foot of a bed against which a client can brace the feet
foot drop plantar flexion of the foot with permanent contracture of the gastrocnemius (calf) muscle and tendon
forceps an instrument with two blades and a handle used to grasp sterile supplies and to compress or grasp tissues
forensic medicine the application of medical knowledge to the law
foreplay physical stimulation to increase sexual arousal prior to intercourse; also called *precoital stimulation*
foreskin a covering fold of skin over the glans of the penis; also called the *prepuce*
formal operations stage (Piaget) the fourth cognitive developmental stage during ages 11 to 15 or 16 years
formulary a collection of prescriptions and formulas
Fowler's position a bed sitting position with the head of the bed raised to 45°
fracture a break in the continuity of bone
fracture board a support placed under the mattress of a bed to add rigidity
framework a basic structure supporting anything
fraud false presentation of some fact or facts with the intention that the information will be acted on by another person
frenulum a fold of mucous membrane that attaches the tongue to the floor of the mouth; a fold on the lower surface of the glans penis that connects it with the prepuce
frequency (of urination) voiding at more frequent intervals than usual
friction rubbing; the force that opposes motion
friction rub *see* pleural rub
frigidity a low or nondetectable sex drive, usually applied to females
frontal plane the plane that divides the body into ventral and dorsal sections
frustration increased emotional tension due to inability to meet goals
fulcrum the fixed point of a lever
full disclosure provision of complete and truthful information to a client participating in a research study
functionalis a layer of endometrium that is shed during menstruation
functional residual capacity volume of air remaining in the lungs after a normal expiration
funnel chest (pectus excavatum) a congenital defect in which the sternum is depressed and the anteroposterior diameter of the chest is narrowed

gait the way a person walks
gastric pertaining to the stomach
gastrocolic reflex increased peristalsis of the colon after food has entered the stomach
gastroenteritis inflammation of the stomach and the intestines
gastroscope a lighted instrument used to visualize the interior of the stomach
gastroscopy visual examination of the stomach with a gastroscope
gastrostomy a surgical opening that leads through the abdomen directly into the stomach
gauge (of a needle) the diameter of the shaft of a needle
gavage administration of nourishment to the stomach through a nasogastric or orogastric tube; tube feeding

gay and lesbian families families in which the adult couple are homosexual partners
gelatinous like jelly
gender behavior behavior with masculine or feminine connotations
gender identity a person's sense of being masculine or feminine as distinct from being male or female
gender role (sexual role) all that a person says or does to indicate whether the person is male or female
gene the biologic unit of heredity, located on a chromosome
general adaptation syndrome (GAS) a general arousal response of the body to a stressor that is characterized by certain physiologic events and that is dominated by the sympathetic nervous system
general inhibition syndrome (possum response) a response to a stressor that is characterized by inhibition of physiologic functioning and that is dominated by the parasympathetic nervous system
generativity (Erikson) concern for establishing and guiding the next generation
genitals the reproductive organs, usually the external ones
genital stage (Freud) the final stage of maturity of an adult
genupectoral position a position in which the weight is borne by the knees and chest and the body is at a 90° angle to the hips
genu valgum a condition in which the medial aspects of the knees touch in the standing position while the feet remain apart; knock-knees
genu varum a condition in which, when the feet are held together, the knees remain apart; bowlegs
geographic poverty the existence of poverty in certain geographic areas of the country
geriatrics the branch of medicine pertaining to elderly people
germicidal possessing the ability to kill microorganisms
germicide an agent that kills some pathogens
gerontology the study of all aspects of aging
gingiva the gum tissue
gingivitis inflammation of the gums
glans clitoris the exposed part of the clitoris
glans penis the cap-shaped, expansive structure at the end of the penis
glaucoma an eye disease characterized by an increase in intraocular pressure that produces changes in the optic disc and the field of vision
glomerular filtrate fluid formed in the nephron of the kidney that is similar to plasma in composition; the precursor of urine
glossitis inflammation of the tongue
glottis the vocal apparatus of the larynx
glucagon a hormone produced by the alpha cells of the islands of Langerhans in the pancreas; it stimulates the breakdown of liver glycogen
glucocorticoid a hormone produced by the adrenal glands that influences the metabolism of glucose, protein, and fat
gluconeogenesis the process by which the liver converts proteins and fats into glucose
glucose a monosaccharide occurring in food
glycerol the alcohol components of fats
glycogen the chief carbohydrate stored in the body, particularly in the liver and muscles
glycogenesis formation of glycogen
glycogenolysis the breakdown of glycogen to reform glucose
glycolysis the release of energy through the breakdown of glucose
glycosuria the presence of glucose in the urine; glucosuria
goal the desired outcome of nursing interventions
gonad an ovary or testis
gonorrhea a sexually transmitted (venereal) infection due to *Neisseria gonorrhoeae*
Goodell's sign the softening of the cervix during pregnancy
Good Samaritan act a law that protects physicians and sometimes nurses when rendering aid to a person in an emergency
gout a condition characterized by excessive uric acid in the blood
governance the establishment and maintenance of social, political, and economic arrangements by which practitioners control their practice, self-discipline, working conditions, and professional affairs
Graafian follicle a small sac, embedded in the ovary, that encloses an ovum
granulation tissue young connective tissue with new capillaries formed in the wound healing process
granulosa cells a single layer of cells that surrounds the ovum
graphics a computer application in which data are depicted in graph or illustration form
gravity the force that pulls objects toward the center of the earth
grief emotional suffering often caused by bereavement
grounded theory a highly evolved and explicitly codified method for developing categories of theories and propositions about their relationships from qualitative data
grounding process of making an electrical connection between a conductor and the earth or a large body of zero potential
group two or more persons who have shared needs or goals
group dynamics (process) forces that determine the behavior of the group and its members
growth an increase in weight and height; an increase in physical size; the proliferation of cells
guilt the painful emotion associated with transgression of moral-ethical beliefs
gustatory referring to the sense of taste
gynecology the branch of medicine that deals with processes of the female reproductive tract
gynosperm sperm bearing an X chromosome

habitus physique; body build or body type
hair follicle a pouchlike depression in the skin enclosing the root of a hair
hair shaft the visible part of the hair
halitosis bad breath
hallucinate to perceive through the senses something unreal; such as hearing voices or seeing things that do not exist
hallucinogens drugs that cause distortion of the sensory perception
hangnail a shred of epidermal tissue at either side of the nail
haploid number the number of chromosomes (23 single) found in human sperm and egg cells
hapten a substance free of protein that can interact with other substances on antibodies but does not itself cause the formation of antibodies
hardware the equipment that makes up a computer system
Harris tube a single-lumen tube with a metal tip that is inserted through the mouth into the intestines
haustrum a saclike formation of a part of the colon, produced by contraction of both the longitudinal and the circular muscles (plural: haustra)
head mirror a mirror worn on the examiner's head that directs light onto an area being examined
health a state of being physically fit, mentally stable, and socially comfortable; it encompasses more than the state of being free of disease
health appraisal (family) assessment of the physical and psychosocial health of the family unit and its members
health behavior the action a person takes to understand his or her health state, maintain an optimal state of health, prevent illness and injury, and reach his or her maximum physical and mental potential
health beliefs concepts about health that an individual believes are true
health-illness continuum a continuum (continuous process) with high-level wellness at one end and death at the other
health maintenance organization (HMO) an organization that provides a wide range of health services on a fixed contract basis, usually geared to preventive medicine
health practice an activity that a person carries out as a result of his or her health beliefs and definition of health
health practitioner a person who provides a health care service
health problem any condition or situation in which a person requires help to maintain or regain a state of health or to achieve a peaceful death

health promotion health care aimed at enhancing the wellness of individuals through education and encouragement of behavior changes or changes in the environment
health risk appraisal (HRA) tool that indicates a client's risk of diseases or injury over time by comparing the client with a large national sample with similar demographic data
health status the health of a person at a given time
health team a group of individuals with varying skills whose cooperative efforts are designed to assist people with their health
hectic fever *see* septic fever
Hegar's sign the softening of the lower portion of the uterus during pregnancy
height a vertical measurement extending from the highest point on the head to the surface on which the individual is standing, normally measured in centimeters or inches
hemangioma a large, persistent, bright red or dark purple vascular area of the skin
hematemesis the vomiting of blood
hematocrit the percentage of red blood cell mass in proportion to whole blood
hematoma a collection of blood in a tissue, organ, or body space due to a break in the wall of a blood vessel
hematuria the presence of blood in the urine
hemiplegia the loss of movement on one side of the body
hemoglobin the red pigment in red blood cells that carries oxygen
hemoglobinuria the presence of hemoglobin in the urine
hemolysis rupture of red blood cells
hemopneumothorax a collection of blood and air or gas in the pleural cavity
hemoptysis the presence of blood in the sputum
hemorrhage bleeding; the escape of blood from the blood vessels
hemorrhoids distended veins in the rectum
hemosiderosis deposition of iron in the skin, liver, spleen, and other organs
hemostat (artery forceps) a small pair of forceps used to constrict blood vessels
hemothorax a collection of blood in the pleural cavity
heparin a substance that prevents coagulation of blood
herb a leafy plant that does not have a wood stem and is valued for its medicinal, savory, or aromatic qualities
herbalist an herb doctor; one who prescribes herbs for treating people
hereditary factors risk factors related to genetically transmitted conditions or genetic predispositions to various conditions
Hering-Breuer reflex a reflex that inhibits inspiration
hesitancy (of urination) delay and difficulty initiating voiding
hex a jinx; a spell imposed in witchcraft
high Fowler's position a bed sitting position in which the head of the bed is elevated 90°
hirsutism abnormal hairiness, particularly in women
histology the study of the structure and function of tissues
holism the view that a person is more than the sum of many parts
holistic health a model of health based on the belief that the whole is more than the sum of its parts
holophrastic speech a type of speech in which one word expresses a whole sentence
Holy Communion a memorial sacrament practiced by Christians based on the mandate of Jesus Christ at the Last Supper; it is also called the *Eucharist* or the *Lord's Supper*
home care health services provided to individuals and families in their homes
homeodynamics the continual exchange of energy between humans and the external environment
homeostasis tendency of the body to maintain a state of balance or equilibrium while continually changing
homogamy mating like with like; inbreeding; reproduction resulting from the union of two identical cells
homogeneity a high degree of likeness of attitudes and beliefs among members of a group
homosexual a person whose primary sexual orientation is to a member of the same sex
hormone a chemical substance that is produced by the body and secreted into the bloodstream and that regulates the activity of certain body organs
hospice a health care facility for the dying
hostility overt antagonism; behavior in which the individual tends to be harmful or destructive
hot pack (foment) hot moist cloth applied to an area of the body
human chorionic gonadotropin (HCG) a hormone produced by the placenta in the first trimester of pregnancy
humanism concern for human attributes
human placental lactogen *see* chorionic somatomammotropin
humidity the amount of moisture in the air, expressed as a percentage
hunger an unpleasant sensation caused by deprivation of something, especially food
hyaluronidase an enzyme found in tissues; it catalyzes hydrolysis of hyaluronic acid, the cement substance of tissues
hydration the act of combining or being combined with water
hydraulics the branch of physics that deals with the physical actions of liquids
hydrocephalus a disease process resulting in excessive cerebrospinal fluid within the skull
hydrocortisone an adrenocortical steroid produced by the adrenal glands or produced synthetically; also called *cortisol*
hydrolysates hydrolyzed proteins or amino acids
hydrolysis the process of splitting a molecule in the presence of digestive enzymes with the addition of water
hydrometer an instrument used to determine the specific gravity of a fluid
hydrostatic pressure the pressure a liquid exerts on the sides of the container that holds it; also called *filtration force*
hygiene the science of health and its maintenance
hymen a thin fold of mucous membrane separating the vagina from the vestibule
hyperalgesia extreme sensitivity to pain
hyperalimentation *see* total parenteral nutrition
hypercalcemia excessive calcium in the blood plasma
hypercalciuria excessive calcium in the urine
hypercarbia (hypercapnia) accumulation of carbon dioxide in the blood
hyperemia increased blood flow to an area
hyperextension further extension between two bones or stretching out of a joint
hyperextension position a bed position with the head and foot of the bed lowered to form a 15° angle in the bed foundation
hyperglycemia an increased concentration of glucose in the blood
hyperkalemia excessive potassium in the blood
hypernatremia an elevated level of sodium in the blood plasma
hyperopia farsightedness
hyperphosphatemia increased phosphorus levels in the blood plasma
hyperplasia an abnormal increase in the number of cells in a tissue or an organ
hyperpnea an abnormal increase in the rate and depth of respirations
hyperpyrexia an extremely elevated body temperature
hyperreflexia an exaggeration of the reflexes
hyperresonance a lower-pitched sound than resonance
hypersensitivity an exaggerated response of the body to a foreign substance
hypersommnia excessive sleep
hypertension an abnormally high blood pressure
hyperthermia an abnormally high body temperature, sometimes induced as a therapeutic measure
hypertonicity excessive muscle tone or activity

hypertonic solution a fluid possessing a greater concentration of solutes than plasma has
hypertrophy an increase in size of a cell, tissue, or body organ such as a muscle
hyperventilation an increase in the amount of air entering the lungs, characterized by prolonged and deep breaths
hypervolemia an abnormal increase in the body's blood volume
hypnosis an abnormally induced passive state in which an individual responds to suggestions that do not conflict with the person's conscious or unconscious desires
hypnotic (drug) a drug that induces sleep
hypoalbuminemia reduction in the level of albumin in the blood
hypocalcemia decreased calcium in the blood plasma
hypocarbia (hypocapnia) depressed level of carbon dioxide in the blood
hypochloremia a reduced concentration of chlorides in the blood plasma
hypodermic *see* subcutaneous
hypodermis (subcutaneous tissue) connective tissues beneath the skin
hypodermoclysis the introduction of fluid in the subcutaneous tissues
hypofibrinogenemia an abnormally low level of fibrinogen in the blood
hypoglycemia a reduced amount of glucose in the blood
hypokalemia potassium deficit in the blood plasma
hyponatremia an abnormally low amount of sodium in the blood plasma
hypophosphatemia phosphorus deficiency in the blood
hypophysis *see* pituitary gland
hypostatic pneumonia an infection of lung tissue resulting from poor circulation or stagnation of secretions
hypotension an abnormally low blood pressure
hypothalamus the part of the brain beneath the thalamus that forms the floor and part of the wall of the third ventricle
hypothermia an abnormally low body temperature
hypothesis a statement of the relationship between two or more concepts or variables; an assumption made to test its logical or empirical consequences
hypothesizing technique of predicting which actions will solve a problem or meet a goal
hypotonicity decreased muscle tone
hypotonic solution a fluid possessing a lesser concentration of solutes than plasma has
hypoventilation a reduction in the amount of air entering the lungs, characterized by shallow respirations
hypovolemia reduction in blood volume
hypovolemic shock a state of shock due to a reduction in the volume of circulating blood
hypoxemia low partial pressure of oxygen or low saturation of oxyhemoglobin in the arterial blood
hypoxia insufficient oxygen anywhere in the body

iatrogenic caused by the physician or medical therapy
id (Freud) the unconscious part of the personality that contains primitive desires and urges and is ruled by the pleasure principle
ideational forming images or objects in the mind
identification an adaptative or defense mechanism in which one assumes the attitudes, ideas, and behavior patterns of another person or persons
identifying as an element of anger, the act of seeking a response and support from others
idiosyncratic effect a different, unexpected, or individual effect from the normal one usually expected from a medication; the occurrence of unpredictable and unexplainable symptoms
ileal conduit most commonly used urinary diversion procedure
ileocecal valve membranous folds between the distal ileum and the entrance to the large intestine (cecum)
ileostomy an artificial abdominal opening into the ileum (small bowel)
ileum the distal portion of the small intestine
illness sickness or deviation from a healthy state or the normal functioning of the total person
illness behavior the course of action a person takes to define the state of his or her health and pursue a remedy
illusion a false interpretation of some stimulus
imagination creation by the mind; forming a mental image of something not present to stimulate the senses
imitation copying the behaviors and attitudes of another person
immobility prescribed or unavoidable restriction of movement in any area of a person's life
immunity a specific resistance of the body to infection; it may be natural, endowed resistance or resistance developed after exposure to a disease agent
immunization the process of becoming immune or rendering someone immune
immunoglobulin a part of the body's plasma proteins; also called *immune bodies* or *antibodies*
immunologic reaction production of antibodies in response to an antigen; an allergic reaction
impaction a condition of being firmly wedged or lodged; in reference to feces, a collection of hardened puttylike feces in the folds of the rectum
imperforate abnormally closed; used to describe an opening, such as the anus or the hymen, that is not open
implementing putting the nursing strategies listed in the nursing care plan into action; intervening
impotence inability to achieve or to maintain an erection sufficiently to perform intercourse
impregnation fertilization of the ovum
incision a cut or wound that is intentionally made, e.g., during surgery
incoherent engaging in actions or speech that lacks cohesion, orderly continuity, relevance, or consistency
incontinence inability to control the elimination of urine (enuresis) or feces (fecal incontinence)
incorporation a process by which people or objects are internalized and become a part of one's understanding
incubation period the time between entrance of a pathogen into the body and the onset of symptoms of the infection
incurvated (ingrown) nail a nail that has grown so that it impinges into surrounding soft tissues
independence self-reliance and self-assertiveness
independent nurse practitioner a nurse who practices independently in the health care system
independent nursing action (intervention or function) an activity initiated by a nurse as a result of her or his own knowledge and skills and without the physician's direct order
independent variable (IV) existing conditions or causes or those variables that a researcher manipulates to affect the dependent variable
indirect interview interview in which the nurse allows the client to control the purpose, subject matter, and pacing; also called *nondirect interview*
indirect services measures taken to provide or facilitate direct home care services
individual-client supply system (of drugs) medications supplied separately for each client in specified doses and quantities for a specified period of time
inductive reasoning making generalizations from specific data
inductive theory a theory formulated by a process in which certain phenomena are observed followed by the development of the idea relating the phenomena
induration hardening
infarct a localized area of necrosis (dead cells) usually owing to obstructed arterial blood flow to the part
infection the disease process produced by microorganisms
inference the interpretation of data from knowledge and past experience
inferential reasoning solving problems by means of inference
inferential statistics statistics that are inferred by generalization from other statistics
inferior situated below

infestation invasion of the body by insects, mites, and/or ticks
infiltration the diffusion or deposition into tissue of substances that are not normal to it
inflammation the tissue response to injury or destruction of cells
influence (in a group) the result of the proper use of power
information power power derived from the perception that one controls key information
informed consent *see* consent
infradian rhythm a biorhythm that cycles monthly, such as the human menstrual cycle
infrared heat a radiant type of heat capable of penetrating body tissues to a depth of 10 mm; sources of infrared rays include heat lamps and incandescent light bulbs
infusion the introduction of fluid into a vein or part of the body
ingestion the act of taking in food or medication
ingrown toenail penetration of the edges of the toenail plate into the surrounding tissues
inhalation (inspiration) the act of breathing in; the intake of air or other substances into the lungs
inhalation therapist a respiratory technologist skilled in therapies for individuals with respiratory problems
inhalation (aerosol) therapy deliverance of droplets of medication or moisture suspended in a gas, such as oxygen, by inhalation through the nose or mouth
inner canthus the corner of the upper and lower eyelids near the nose
inorganic having no organs; not of organic origin; in chemistry, acids or compounds that do not contain carbon
input information, material, or energy that enters a system
inquest a legal inquiry into the cause or manner of a death
insensible perspiration unnoticeable sweating that evaporates immediately once it reaches the surface of the skin
insertion (of a muscle) the more movable point of attachment of a muscle
insomnia inability to obtain a sufficient quality or quantity of sleep
inspection visual examination to detect features perceptible to the eye
inspiration (inhalation) the act of drawing air into the lungs
inspiratory capacity the maximum amount of air that can be inhaled after a normal exhalation
inspiratory reserve volume the maximum amount of air inhaled after a normal inspiration
instillation application of a medication into a body cavity or orifice
insufflator an instrument used to blow air into a part of the body, e.g., the rectum
insulator a substance or material that inhibits conduction, e.g., of heat or electricity
insulin a hormone secreted by the beta cells of the islands of Langerhans in the pancreas; also a preparation for administration
integument the skin or covering of the body
integumentary system the skin, hair, and nails
intelligence ability to learn
intensity (in percussion) the loudness or softness of a sound
intensive services level of home care services in which clients require medical and professional nursing care as an alternative to hospitalization of skilled nursing home care
intercostal between the ribs
intercostal retractions indrawing between the ribs
interdependence a balance between dependence and independence
interdigital between the digits (toes and fingers)
intermediate services level of home care services in which clients require professional nursing supervision, direct care, physical or speech therapy, regular and periodic medical supervision, or some combination of these
intermittent (quotidian) fever a fever that recurs daily
intermittent positive pressure breathing (IPPB) delivery of oxygen into the lungs at positive pressure and release of the pressure passively during expiration
intern a graduate of a basic health program who is taking planned practice experience, such as nursing or medicine, usually to obtain a license to practice
internal feedback positive or negative responses from oneself about a communication one has given either in writing or verbally
internal rotation a turning toward the midline, e.g., rotation of the hip joint
interpersonal skills verbal and nonverbal activities that people use when communicating directly with one another
interstitial between the cells of the body's tissues
interstitial cells of Leydig clusters of cells, located between the seminiferous tubules, that secrete male hormones
interstitial fluid fluid surrounding the body cells
intervention activities performed by the nurse and the client to change the effect of a problem
intervertebral between the vertebrae
interview a structured consultation used to obtain information or to evaluate the progress of a person
intestinal distention (tympanites) stretching and inflation of the intestines due to the presence of air or gas
intraarterial within or inside an artery
intracardiac within or into the heart muscle
intracellular within a cell or cells
intracellular fluid (cellular fluid, ICF) fluid found within the body cells
intractable pain pain that is resistant to cure or relief
intradermal (intracutaneous) within the skin
intrafamily communication the pattern of verbal and nonverbally transmitted messages among family members
Intralipid trademark for an intravenous fat solution that provides concentrated calories during total parenteral nutrition
intramuscular within or inside muscle tissue
intraosseous within or into the bone
intrapleural within the pleural cavity
intrapleural pressure pressure within the pleural cavity
intrapulmonic pressure pressure within the lungs
intraspinal *see* intravertebral
intrathecal within or into the spinal canal
intrauterine inside the uterus
intrauterine device (IUD) a device inserted into the uterus for contraception
intravascular within a blood vessel
intravascular fluid plasma
intravenous within a vein
intravenous cholangiogram an x-ray film of the bile ducts after a contrast dye has been administered intravenously
intravenous pyelogram an x-ray film of the kidneys taken after intravenous injection of a radiopaque dye
intravenous pyelography (IVP) x-ray filming of the kidney and ureters after injection of a radiopaque material intravenously; also called *intravenous urography*
intravenous urography (IVU) *see* intravenous pyelography
intravertebral (intraspinal) within the vertebrae
introjection unconscious acceptance and incorporation of the patterns, attitudes, and ideals of another person as one's own
introversion direction of one's energy and interest toward oneself
intubation insertion of a tube
inunction application of a topical drug to the skin or mucous membrane for absorption
inversion a turning inward
invisible poverty social and cultural deprivation
involution a rolling or turning inward of a particular organ or the entire body, e.g., the uterus after the fetus is expelled
ion an atom or group of atoms that carry a positive or negative electric charge; an electrolyte
iris the colored, circular membrane of the eye, situated behind the cornea, in the center of which is the pupil

irradiation exposure to penetrating rays, such as x-rays, gamma rays, infrared rays, or ultraviolet rays
irrational confused as to time, place, and/or person
irrigation (lavage) the washing of a body cavity or a wound
irritant a substance that stimulates unpleasant responses, that is, irritates
ischemia lack of blood supply to a body part
islands of Langerhans clusters of endocrine-secreting cells located in the pancreas
isolation *see* protective asepsis
isometric having the same measure or length
isometric muscle contraction tensing of a muscle against an immovable outer resistance, which does not change muscle length or produce joint motion
isometric static exercise exercise in which a person consciously increases the tension of the muscle without moving the joint
isotonic having the same tonicity as the body fluids; the term is used to compare solutions of the same strength or concentration
isotonic exercise active exercise involving muscle contractions in which there is a marked shortening of muscle length
isotonic muscle contraction shortening of a muscle in the process of doing work that produces joint motion (e.g., range-of-motion exercises or weight lifting)
isthmus a narrow passage connecting two larger parts of an organ

jargon the technical or idiomatic terminology characteristic of a particular group
jaundice a yellowish tinge to the skin and mucous membrane
jejunum the portion of the small intestine that extends from the duodenum to the ileum

Kardex a portable card index file that organizes data about clients in a concise way and often contains nursing care plans
Kelly forceps a type of hemostat
keratin the protein found in epidermis, hair, and nails
keratinized cells dead cells that have been converted to protein
keratotic spots horny growths, such as warts or calluses
ketogenesis the process in which deaminated amino acids are converted into fatty acids, producing ketone bodies (acetone)
ketone any compound containing the carbonyl group, CO, and having hydrocarbon groups attached to the carbonyl group
ketosis a condition in which excessive ketones are formed in the body
kilocalorie (Calorie) the amount of heat required to raise the temperature of 1 kilogram of water 1 degree centigrade
kilogram a unit of weight equal to 1000 grams or approximately 2.2 pounds
kinesiology the study of the motion of the human body
kinesthesia the sense of the position and the movement of the body parts
kinesthetic referring to awareness of body position and movement
knee-chest position *see* genupectoral position
Korotkoff's sounds sounds of blood produced within the artery with each ventricular contraction
kosher sanctioned by Jewish law
Kussmaul breathing (Kussmaul-Kien respiration) deep rapid breathing; a dyspnea occurring in paroxysms often preceding diabetic coma: air hunger
kwashiorkor a condition occurring in children after weaning as a result of protein and calorie malnutrition; evidenced by growth failure, potbelly, edema, and mental apathy
kyphosis an exaggerated convexity in the thoracic region of the vertebral column, resulting in a stooped posture

labia the fleshy edges of a structure, usually the female genitals
labia majora the two longitudinal folds or lips of skin extending downward and backward from the mons pubis that protect the vaginal and urethral orifices
labia minor small folds of skin lying between the labia majora and the vaginal opening
labored breathing difficult or dyspneic breathing
labyrinth a system of interconnecting canals or cavities
lacerate to tear, rather than cut, a body tissue
lacrimal fluid tears produced by the lacrimal glands that lubricate the eye
lacrimal glands organs that are situated in a depression in the frontal bone at the upper, outer angle of the eye orbit, and that secrete tears
lacrimal sac the opening connecting the tear ducts in the inner canthus of the eye to the nasolacrimal duct, which empties into the nasal cavity
lacrimation the secretion and discharge of tears
lactase an enzyme that acts as a catalyst to convert lactose into glucose and galactose
lactate salt of lactic acid that is metabolized in the liver to form bicarbonate
lactation the secretion of milk; the period of milk secretion
lactiferous conveying or producing milk
lactose a carbohydrate found in milk
lalling repetitive sounds infants make based on what they hear
lanugo fine, wooly hair or down on the shoulders, back, sacrum, and earlobes of the unborn child; it may remain for a few weeks after birth
laryngeal mirror an instrument like a dental mirror used to view the pharynx, larynx, or structures of the mouth
laryngeal stridor a harsh, crowing sound heard during expiration when there is a laryngeal obstruction
laryngoscope a lighted instrument used to visualize the larynx
laryngoscopy visual examination of the larynx with a laryngoscope
laryngospasm spasmodic closure of the larynx
larynx a structure composed of nine cartilages guarding the entrance of the trachea and containing the vocal cords
laser printer output device using laser technology that produces high-quality graphics and characters
latch-key children Working parents' school-age children who must care for themselves after school
latency period (Freud) the school-age years (6 to 12 years)
lateral to the side, away from the midline
lateral position a side-lying position
lavage an irrigation or washing of a body organ, such as the stomach
laxative a medication that stimulates bowel activity
leading question question that directs the client's answer
learning a permanent change in behavior
learning need a need to change behavior
learning principle an assumption thought to facilitate and maximize learning
legitimate power power derived from one's formal position or title in an organization
legume the fruit or pod of a leguminous plant, such as a pea or bean
lens a transparent, convex body that is the focusing device of the eye
lesion the traumatic or pathologic interruption of a tissue or the loss of function of a body part
lethargy drowsiness; sleeping much of the time when not stimulated
letter-quality printer output device that produces high-quality, fully formed characters
leukocyte a white blood cell
leukocytosis an increase in the number of white blood cells
lever a rigid bar that moves on a fixed axis called a fulcrum
leverage force applied with the use of a lever
Levin tube a single-lumen nasogastric tube
liability the quality or state of being liable
liable legally responsible for one's obligations and actions and obliged to make financial restitution for wrongful acts
libel defamation by means of print, writing, or pictures
libido (Freud) the urge or desire for sexual activity; the energy form or life instinct; also called *sex drive* and *sexual motivation*
license a legal document authorizing an individual to offer knowledge and skills to the public
life expectancy the age to which a person is expected to live
life-style the values and behaviors adopted by a person in daily life
life-style assessment involves the appraisal of the personal life-style and habits of the client as they affect health

ligament a broad, fibrous band that holds two or more bones together
light pen penlike device that allows inputting of data into a computer by touching the computer display screen
lightening the descent of the uterus into the pelvic cavity, which usually occurs 2 to 3 weeks before labor begins
line of gravity an imaginary vertical line running through the center of gravity
lingula (of the lung) the superior and inferior segments at the lower half of the long upper lobe of the left lung
liniment a topical liquid applied to the skin frequently to stimulate circulation or to relieve pain
lipid *see* fat
lithotomy position a back-lying position in which the feet are supported in stirrups
living will a statement of a person's wish not to be kept alive by artificial means or "heroic measures"
livor mortis discoloration of the tissues of the body after death
lobar pneumonia an infectious disease of one or more lobes of the lung
lobe a well-defined portion of an organ, e.g., of the lung or brain
local adaptation syndrome (LAS) the reaction of one organ or body part to stress
lochia the vaginal discharge that occurs during the 1st week or 2 after the birth of a baby
locus of control a measurable concept that can be used to predict which people are most likely to change their behavior
lordosis an exaggerated concavity in the lumbar region of the vertebral column
loss an actual or potential situation in which a valued ability, object, person, etc., is inaccessible or changed so that it is perceived as no longer valuable
lotion a liquid that often carries an insoluble powder
louse a parasitic insect that infests mammals (plural: lice)
lumbar puncture (LP, spinal tap) the insertion of a needle into the subarachnoid space at the lumbar region
lumen a channel within a tube, such as the channel of an artery in which blood flows
lung compliance expansibility of the lung
lung recoil the tendency of lungs to collapse away from the chest wall
luteal stage *see* postovulatory stage
lymph a transparent, slightly yellow fluid found within the lymphatic vessels
lymphadenitis inflammation of the lymph nodes
lymphangitis the inflammation of a lymphatic vessel or vessels
lymphatic referring to lymph or lymph vessels
lysis (of a fever) the gradual reduction of an elevated body temperature to normal
lysosome a minute body found in many types of cells; it is involved in intracellular digestion
lysozyme an enzyme in saliva and tears that functions as an antibacterial agent

maceration the wasting away or softening of a solid as if by the action of soaking; often used to describe degenerative changes and eventual disintegration
macrocephaly an abnormally large size of the head
macrophage a large phagocytic cell that destroys microorganisms or harmful cells
mainframe the largest, fastest, and most expensive computer system
malaise a general feeling of being unwell or indisposed
mal de ojo among Hispanics, the belief that disease can result from admiring a part of another person's body, e.g., the hair
malignancy abnormal tissue with a tendency to grow and invade other tissues
malingering the willful feigning of the symptoms of illness to avoid facing something unpleasant
malleolus a rounded prominence on the distal end of the tibia or fibula
malnutrition a disorder of nutrition; insufficient nourishment of the body cells
malpractice professional misconduct or unreasonable lack of professional skill
mammary glands breast tissues that secrete nourishment for the young
mandatory licensure laws that require all persons practicing in a field, such as nursing, to be licensed
manometer an instrument used to measure the pressure of fluids or gases
manslaughter an unlawful killing without previous intent; it is a felony
marasmus a condition of children under 1 year as a result of protein and calorie malnutrition; it is evidenced by wasting, wrinkled skin, thinness, eyes appearing large
margination the aggregating or lining up of substances along a surface or edge, e.g., the lining up of white blood cells against the wall of a blood vessel during the inflammatory process
marijuana an intoxicating agent from the leaves and flowers of the plant *Cannabis sativa;* commonly used in cigarettes
marital family the beginning stage of family development when the couple establishes a marital relationship and assumes the roles of husband and wife
mastectomy surgical removal of the breast
masticate to chew, e.g., food
mastication chewing
masturbation self-stimulation of the genitals or other body parts to derive erotic pleasure
material culture objects, such as eating utensils, and the ways these are used by a society
matriarchy a system of social organization in which the mother is the head of the house or family
matrilineal relating to descent through the female line
maturation the process of becoming mature or fully developed; development of inherited traits
meatus an opening, passage, or channel
mechanosensitive pain receptors pain receptors stimulated by mechanical stimuli
meconium a dark green, mucilaginous material found in the intestines of the newborn
medial toward the middle or midline
medical asepsis practices that limit the number, growth, and spread of microorganisms; clean technique
medical examiner a physician who investigates deaths that appear unnatural and who has advanced education in pathology and forensic medicine
medical record (chart) an account of the client's health history, current health status, treatment, and progress
medication (medicine, drug) a chemical or biologic compound administered to humans or animals for disease prevention, cure, or relief, or to affect the structure or function of the body
meditation mental exercise that directs the mind to think inwardly by closing the sense organs to external stimulation
meiosis a specialized type of cell division that occurs in sperm and egg cells
melanin the dark pigment of the skin
menarche the first menstrual period, occurring sometime between the ages of 9 and 17
meniscus the crescent-shaped structure of the surface of a column of liquid; the crescent-shaped cartilage in the knee joint
menopause cessation of menstruation in the human female, usually occurring between ages 45 and 50
menses menstrual flow
mental (defense) mechanism *see* defense mechanism
mental well-being a state of contentment, peace of mind, and satisfaction with living and life
mesoderm the middle layer of the three primary developmental germ layers in the embryo; it lies between the endoderm and the ectoderm
metabolism the sum of all the physical and chemical processes by which

living substance is formed and maintained and by which energy is made available for use by the organism
metacarpal referring to the part of the hand between the wrist and the fingers
metaparadigm of nursing the concepts that influence nursing most significantly and determine its practice: the person, environment, health, and nursing actions
metatarsus adductus adduction of the anterior part of the foot with no deformity of the posterior part of the foot
microcephaly an abnormally small size of the head
microcomputer smallest computer system
microglia a type of nerve tissue with migratory cells that act as phagocytes to the waste products of nerve tissues
micronutrient nutrients, such as vitamins and minerals, required in small quantities by the body
microorganism minute living body visible under a microscope
micturate (urinate, void) to pass urine from the body
micturition (urination, voiding) the voluntary expulsion of urine
midclavicular line an imaginary line that runs inferiorly and vertically from the center of the clavicle
midsternal line an imaginary line that runs vertically through the middle of the sternum
milia (whiteheads) small, white nodules usually found over the nose and face of newborns
miliaria rubra a prickly heat rash of the face, neck, trunk, or perineal area of infants
Miller-Abbott tube a double-lumen tube inserted through the nose or mouth into the intestine
milliequivalent (mEq) one-thousandth of an equivalent, which is the chemical combining power of a substance
milliliter (ml) a unit of volume in the metric system approximating 1 cubic centimeter
millimol one-thousandth of a mol
mineralocorticoid a steroid hormone of the adrenal cortex that acts to retain sodium in the body and to excrete potassium
minicomputer medium-sized computer system
minim the least; the basic unit of volume in the apothecaries' system, equal to 0.0616 ml
minimal services *see* basic services
misdemeanor a crime less serious than a felony and punishable by a fine or short-term imprisonment or both
mitering a method of folding the bedclothes at the bed corners to maintain them securely
mitosis the process of cell division; the process by which the body replaces cells and grows
MMR combined measles, mumps, and rubella vaccine
mobility ability to move about freely
model (paradigm) an abstract outline or a theoretical depiction of a complex phenomenon
modeling observing the behavior of people who have successfully achieved a goal that one has set for oneself and, through observing, acquiring ideas for behavior and coping strategies
modem device that translates the digital signals produced by a computer into modulated signals that the telephone accepts, making it possible to transmit data over the telephone
mol a molar solution of a substance
mongolian spots blue or black spots of varying size found largely in the sacral area of Oriental and black infants
monologue a long speech that occurs when there is no listener or responder
monosaccharide a sugar consisting of single molecules
mons pubis a pillow of adipose tissue situated over the symphysis pubis and covered by coarse hair; also called the *mons veneris*
Montgomery's glands sebaceous glands in the areola of the nipple that become enlarged and prominent during pregnancy
Montgomery straps tie tapes used to hold dressings in place
morbidity incidence of disease
mores values of members in a group
morgue a place where dead bodies are temporarily kept before release to a mortician
morning sickness the nausea and vomiting that occur frequently in the mornings during the first trimester of pregnancy
Moro's reflex the startle reflex of infants, in which the arms and legs are extended outward and retracted in response to a sudden stimulus such as a loud noise
morphology form and structure
mortality death; the death rate
mortician a person trained in the care of the dead; also called an *undertaker*
motivation desire
mourning the process through which grief is eventually resolved or altered
mouse device that allows inputting of data into a computer by rolling the device on a flat surface, which causes corresponding movement of elements on the computer display screen, and by pushing a button to select data
mucin the chief constituent of mucus
mucolytic destroying or dissolving mucus
mucous membrane epithelial tissue that forms mucus, concentrates bile, and secretes or excretes enzymes
mucus the lubricating, free slime of the mucous membranes
murmur (cardiac) harsh, rumbling sounds resulting from turbulent blood flow
mydriatic a medication that dilates the pupils of the eyes
myelogram an x-ray film of the spinal cord, nerve roots, and vertebrae after injection of a contrast media into the subarachnoid space
myocardial infarction cardiac tissue necrosis resulting from obstruction of the blood flow to the heart
myocardium the heart muscle; the middle layer of the heart tissue
myometrium the middle, thick, smooth muscle layer of the uterus
myopia nearsightedness

narcolepsy a condition in which an individual experiences an uncontrollable desire for sleep or attacks of sleep at certain intervals
narcotic a strong analgesic
narcotic agonist-antagonist a drug with properties that simulate a narcotic and with properties that act against the effects of a narcotic
narrative charting a description (narration) of information
narrative notes records of a client's day-to-day progress which may be keyed to the SOAP format in the POMR or keyed chronologically in traditional client-records
nasogastric tube a plastic or rubber tube inserted through the nose into the stomach
nasopharynx the upper part of the pharynx adjoining the nasal passage
naturopath a nonmedical practitioner who uses such things as light, heat, and water in therapy, but not drugs
nausea the urge to vomit
nebulizer an atomizer or sprayer
necessary cause the one factor that must be present for a specific disease to occur
necrosis nonliving cells or tissue in contact with living cells
necrotic dying
need the lack of something requisite, desirable, or useful
negative feedback (homeostasis) a mechanism in which deviations from normal are sensed and counteracted
negative nitrogen balance a nitrogen output that exceeds nitrogen intake
negligence the omission of something a reasonable person would do or the doing of something a reasonable person would not do; an unintentional tort
neonatal mortality infant death within 28 days of birth
neoplasm any growth that is new and abnormal
nephritis inflammation of a kidney
nephron the functional unit of the kidney
nephrosis a disease of the kidney in which there is malfunctioning kidney tissue without inflammation; also called *nephrotic syndrome*

nerve block chemical interruption of a nerve pathway effected by injecting a local anesthetic
neurectomy interruption of the peripheral or cranial nerves, often to relieve localized pain
neurogenous arising in the nervous system
neurohypophysis the posterior part of the pituitary gland
neurologic pertaining to the nervous system
neuron a nerve cell and its processes; the functional unit of the nervous system
neutral question question seeking information without direction or pressure from the interviewer
night terrors (pavor nocturnus) nightmares that the person is unable to recall the next morning
nitrogen balance the state of protein nutrition
nocturia (nycturia) increased frequency of urination at night not as the result of increased fluid intake
nocturnal enuresis involuntary urination at night
noncompliance (drug use) failure to follow a prescription
noncomplier a person who does not follow a therapeutic regimen
nondirect interview *see* direct interview
nonmaterial culture the beliefs, customs, languages, and social institutions of a society
nonpathogen a microorganism that does not produce disease under normal conditions
nonproductive cough a dry, harsh cough without secretions
non-rapid-eye-movement sleep *see* NREM sleep
nonverbal communication (body language) communication other than words, including gestures, posture and facial expressions
norm an ideal or fixed standard; an expected standard of behavior of group members
normal saline an isotonic concentration of salt (NaCl) solution
normocephaly normal head circumference
nosocomial referring to or originating in a hospital or similar institution, e.g., a nosocomial disease
NREM sleep (non-rapid-eye-movement sleep) a deep restful sleep state; also called *slow wave sleep*
nuclear family the family unit composed of parents and children
null hypothesis statement that no relationship other than chance exists between a study's variables
nurse clinician a nurse with advanced skills in a particular area of nursing practice
nurse theorist a person who seeks to define the basis and principles of nursing practice systematically
nursing assessment (nursing history) data collected during an interview between the nurse and client
nursing audit the review of clients' charts to evaluate nursing competence or performance
nursing care conference a meeting of a group of nurses to discuss possible solutions to certain problems of a client
nursing care plan written guide that organizes information about a client's health, focusing on the actions nurses must take to address identified nursing diagnoses and to meet the stated goals
nursing care rounds procedure in which a group of nurses visits all or selected clients at each client's bedside
nursing diagnosis a statement describing a combination of signs or symptoms indicative of an actual or potential health problem that nurses are able, licensed, and accountable to treat
nursing goals goals stated in terms that guide the actions of the nurse
nursing history *see* nursing assessment
nursing order specific action that a nurse takes to help a client meet established health care goals
nursing process a five-step systematic process used in nursing
nursing research research into human responses, clinical problems, and processes of care encountered in the practice of nursing
nursing standards optimum levels of nursing care against which actual performance of a nurse is compared
nursing strategy nursing action designed to achieve established client goals
nutrient an organic or inorganic substance found in food; nutrients are digested and absorbed in the gastrointestinal tract and then used in the body's metabolic processes
nutrition what a person eats and how the body uses it
nutritionist a specialist in food and nutrition
nutritive value the nutrient content of a specified amount of food

obesity weight that is 20% greater than the ideal for height and frame
objective the aim of a maneuver or operation
objective data client information that can be determined by observation or measurement by laboratory or other means
objective symptom a sign; evidence of a disease or body dysfunction that can be observed and described by others
obligatory heat the heat produced by the body as a result of the metabolism of food
obligatory loss the essential fluid loss required to maintain body functioning
observation the act or power of observing; gathering of information by noting facts or occurrences
observe to gather data using the five senses
obstetrics the branch of medicine dealing with the birth process and related events that precede and follow it
obtunded difficult to arouse from sleep; requiring shaking or a painful stimulus to awaken
obturator a disc or instrument that closes an opening; the obturator of a tracheostomy set fits inside and closes off the end of the outer tube
occult hidden
occupation an activity in which one engages
occupational therapist an individual who helps a client develop skills necessary for the activities of daily living
Oedipus complex (Freud) the male child's attraction for his mother and accompanying hostile attitudes toward his father; compare with *Electra complex*
ointment a semisolid preparation applied externally to the body
olfactory referring to the sense of smell
oliguria production of abnormally small amounts of urine by the kidneys
opaque not admitting the passage of light
open-ended question broad question inviting a long answer
open system a system that exchanges matter, energy, and information with the environment
open wound a wound in which the continuity of the skin or mucous membrane has been interrupted
operative (intraoperative) period the time during surgery
ophthalmoscope an instrument used to examine the interior of the eye
optional surgery surgery requested by the client but not necessary for health
oral referring to the mouth
oral stage (Freud) the stage of development during the 1st year of life, when the mouth is the principal area of activity
organic referring to an organ or organs; in chemistry, referring to compounds containing carbon; arising from an organism
orgasm the climax of sexual excitement, during which physiologic and psychologic release occurs; orgasm is characterized by rhythmic spasmodic contractions of the genitals
orgasmic dysfunction the inability of females to achieve orgasm
orgasmic platform an increase in size of the outer one-third of the vagina and the labia minora during precoital stimulation
orientation awareness of time, place, and person
orifice an external opening of a body cavity; e.g., the anus is the orifice of the large intestine
origin (of a muscle) the fixed or least movable point of attachment to a bone
orogastric tube a tube inserted through the mouth into the stomach
oropharynx the part of the pharynx that lies between the upper aspect of the epiglottis and the soft palate
orthopnea the ability to breathe only in the upright position, i.e., sitting or standing
orthostatic hypotension low blood pressure in a standing position

orthostatism the erect standing posture of the body
osmol the number of particles in 1 gram molecular weight of a disassociated solute
osmolarity (osmolality) the concentration of solutes in solution; the osmolar concentration of a solution expressed in osmols per liter of solution
osmosis passage of a solvent through a semipermeable membrane from an area of lesser solute concentration to one of greater solute concentration
osmotic pressure pressure exerted by the number of nondiffusable particles in a solution; the amount of pressure needed to stop the flow of water across a membrane
osseous pertaining to bone
ossification the formation of bone or a bony substance
osteoblast a bone-building cell
osteoclast a cell associated with bone resorption and breakdown
osteomalacia the softening of the bones; decalcification of bones in adults
osteomyelitis inflammation of the bone caused by infection and resulting in bone destruction
osteoporosis decrease in bone density; demineralization of bone
-ostomy a suffix denoting the formation of an opening or outlet
otoscope an instrument used to inspect the eardrum and external ear canal
outcome (evaluative) criteria statements that describe specific, measurable, and observable responses of a client to nursing interventions; expected alterations in the health status of a client
outer canthus the corner of the upper and lower eyelids away from the nose
output the energy, matter, or information released by a system as a result of its processes
outward rotation a turning away from the midline
oval window an opening between the middle and the inner ear
ovary the female gonad (sexual gland); ova are formed in the two ovaries
overbed cradle a frame placed over a client in bed to protect the body from contact with the upper bedclothes
overhydration *see* edema
overnutrition the oversupply of calories
overweight weight that is 10% greater than the ideal for height and frame
ovulation the discharge of a mature ovum from the Graafian follicle of the ovary
ovum (egg) the female reproductive cell, which becomes the embryo after fertilization
oxyhemoglobin the compound of oxygen and hemoglobin
oxytocin a hormone secreted by the posterior pituitary gland; oxytocin helps the uterus to contract before, during, and after delivery

pace the distance covered in a step when one walks or the number of steps taken per minute
packing filling an open wound or cavity with a material such as gauze
$Paco_2$ partial pressure of carbon dioxide (arterial blood)
pain a basically unpleasant sensation, localized or general, mild or intense, that represents the suffering induced by stimulation of specialized nerve endings; pain may be threatened or fantasied and may be induced by disease, injury, or mental derangement caused by disease or injury
pain threshold the amount of stimulation required by a person to feel pain
pain tolerance the maximum amount and duration of pain that an individual is willing to endure
palate the roof of the mouth
palliative affording relief but not cure
palliative surgery surgery to relieve the symptoms of a disease process
pallor absence of normal skin color; a whitish-grayish tinge
palmar grasp reflex a reflex, normally present in newborns, that causes the fingers to curl around a small object placed in the palm of the hand
palpation the act of feeling with the hands, usually the fingers
pandemic an epidemic disease that is widespread
panic severe anxiety
Pao_2 partial pressure of oxygen (arterial blood)
Papanicolaou (Pap) smear a method of taking sample cervical cells for microscopic examination to detect malignancy
papule a small, superficial, round elevation of the skin
paracentesis the insertion of a needle into a cavity (usually the abdominal cavity) to remove fluid
paradigm *see* model
paradoxical breathing the ballooning out of the chest wall during expiration and depression or sucking inward of the chest wall during inspiration
paralysis the impairment or loss of motor function of a body part
paramedical having some connection with the practice of medicine
paraphrasing restating a person's message (thoughts and/or feelings) using similar words
paraplegia paralysis of the lower part of the body (including the legs) affecting both motor function and sensation
parasites plants or animals that live on or within another living organism
parasomnia a disorder that interferes with sleep, e.g., somnambulism
parasympathetic (craniosacral) nervous system a branch of the autonomic nervous system
parathyroid hormone (PTH, parathormone) the hormone produced by the parathyroid glands that regulates the calcium and phosphorus levels in the body
parenchyma the functional or essential elements of an organ
parenteral accomplished by a needle; occurring outside the alimentary tract; injected into the body through some route other than the alimentary canal, e.g., intravenously
paresthesia an abnormal sensation of burning or prickling
paronychia inflammation of the tissue surrounding the nail
parotid glands the large salivary glands located below and in front of the ears
parotitis (parotiditis) inflammation of the parotid salivary gland
paroxysm a sudden attack or sharp recurrence; a spasm
partial pressure the pressure exerted by each individual gas in a mixture according to its percentage concentration in the mixture
passive euthanasia allowing a person to die by withholding or withdrawing measures to maintain life
passive exercise exercise during which the muscles do not contract and the nurse, therapist, or client supplies the energy to move the client's body part
passivity lethargy; receptivity to outside influence; lack of energy or will
paste a semisolid dermatologic preparation that tends to penetrate the skin less than an ointment
pasteurization application of heat to milk to destroy disease-producing microorganisms
pastoral care an interpersonal relationship that focuses on the spiritual component of another person's life during distress
patent open, unobstructed, not closed
pathogen a microorganism capable of producing disease
pathogenic capable of producing disease
pathology a branch of medicine concerned with the nature of disease
patient (client) a person who is waiting for or undergoing medical treatment or care
patient (client) advocate a person who speaks on behalf of a client and can intercede on the client's behalf
patient (client) care standards *see* nursing standards
patient (client) goals goals stated as anticipated client outcomes, not as nursing activities
patriarchy a social system in which the father is the head of the household or family
patrilineal relating to descent through the male line
pavor nocturnus *see* night terrors
Pco_2 partial pressure of carbon dioxide (venous blood)

pectoriloquy exaggerated bronchophony
pediculosis infestation with lice
pediculosis capitis infestation with head lice
peer review an encounter between two persons equal in education, abilities, and qualifications, during which one person critically reviews the practices that the other has documented in a client's record
penetrating wound a wound created by an instrument that penetrated the skin or mucous membranes deeply into the tissues
penis the male organ of copulation and urinary excretion
Penrose drain a flexible rubber drain
perceived loss loss experienced by a person that cannot be verified by others
perception the process of understanding something new and then making it part of one's previous experience or knowledge; a person's awareness and identification of a person, thing, or situation
perception checking (consensual validation) verifying the accuracy of listening skills by giving and receiving feedback about what was communicated
percussion an assessment method in which the body surface is tapped or struck to elicit sound or vibrations from body structures below the struck area
percussion hammer an instrument shaped like a hammer with a head often made of plastic
percutaneous electric stimulation stimulation of major peripheral nerves by electricity
pericardial aspiration the removal of fluid from the pericardial sac via an inserted needle
pericardial sac (pericardium) a fibrous sac that surrounds the heart
perimetrium the thin, outer, serous layer of the uterus
perineum the area between the anus and the posterior aspect of the genitals
periodontal disease inflammation of the tissues that surround and support the teeth
perioperative period the time before, during, and after an operation
periorbital around the eye socket
periosteum the connective tissue covering all bones
periostitis inflammation of the periosteum
peripheral at the edge or outward boundary
peripheral nerve implant an electrode implanted in a major sensory nerve for the purpose of relieving pain
peristalsis wavelike movements produced by circular and longitudinal muscle fibers of the intestinal walls; it propels the intestinal contents onward
peristomal referring to the skin area that surrounds a stoma
peritoneal cavity the area between the layers of peritoneum in the abdomen; a potential space
peritoneum the membrane lining the abdominal walls
peritonitis inflammation of the peritoneum
permissive licensure the policy by which practitioners do not have to be licensed to practice but are not protected by the licensing body
personal space the physical distance people prefer to maintain in their interactions with others
perspiration the fluid secreted by the sweat glands for excreting waste products and cooling the body
petechiae pinpoint red spots on the skin
pH a measure of the relative alkalinity or acidity of a solution; a measure of the concentration of hydrogen ions
phagocyte a cell, e.g., a white blood cell, that ingests microorganisms, other cells, and foreign particles
phagocytosis the process by which cells engulf microorganisms, other cells, or foreign particles
phalanx any bone of the fingers or toes (plural: phalanges)
phallic stage (Freud) the stage of development during the 4th and 5th years when sexual and aggressive feelings come into focus associated with the genital organs
phantom pain pain that remains after the perceived location has been removed, such as pain perceived in a foot after the leg has been amputated
pharmacist an individual licensed to prepare and dispense drugs and to make up prescriptions
pharmacology the scientific study of the actions of drugs on living animals and humans
pharmacopoeia a book containing a list of drug products used in medicine, including their descriptions and formulas
pharmacy the skill of preparing, compounding, and dispensing medicines; the place where medicines are prepared and dispensed
pharmacy assistant a member of the health team who in some situations administers drugs to clients
pharynx a musculomembranous sac behind the nose and mouth that connects with the esophagus and bronchi
phenomenal field the individual's frame of reference
phimosis an extremely narrowed opening of the foreskin of the penis
phlebitis inflammation of a vein
phlebothrombosis intravascular clotting with marked inflammation of a vein
phlebotomy opening a vein to remove blood
phosphorylation the combining of glucose with phosphate inside a cell
photophobia intolerance to light
photosensitive sensitive to light
phrenic referring to the diaphragm
physiatrist a physician who specializes in rehabilitation medicine; physiatrists use physical aids such as light, heat, and apparatuses
physical pertaining to the body or to physics
physical well-being a state of having one's physical needs met appropriately for homeostasis
physiologic pertaining to body function
physiologic dependence biochemical changes occurring in the body as a result of excessive use of a drug
physiology the science concerned with the functioning of living organisms and their parts
physiotherapist (physical therapist) a member of the health team who provides assistance to clients with musculoskeletal problems
pica a craving for unnatural foods, often during pregnancy, some psychologic conditions, or extreme malnutrition
pigeon chest (pectus carinatum) a chest deformity in which there is a narrow transverse diameter, an increased anteroposterior diameter, and a protruding sternum
pilosebaceous follicle the hair follicle and sebaceous gland complex of the skin
pinna the external part of the ear
pitch (in percussion) the number of vibrations per second or the frequency of vibrations
pitting edema edema in which firm finger pressure on the skin produces an indentation (pit) that remains for several seconds
pituitary gland (hypophysis) an endocrine gland (situated in the brain) that secretes a number of hormones, including adrenocorticotropic hormone and thyrotropic hormone
placebo any form of treatment, e.g., medication, that produces an effect in the client because of its intent rather than its chemical or physical properties
placenta the tissue attached to the wall of the uterus; the fetus receives nourishment through the placenta, which is expelled as the "afterbirth" after the child is born
placing reflex a reflex of infants demonstrated when the infant is placed vertically with one foot touching the edge of a table; the infant flexes the knee and hip of the same leg and tries to place the foot on the surface of the table
plaintiff the person who files a legal complaint claiming his or her rights have been infringed
planning establishing a series of steps or designing or arranging the parts of something to achieve an end or goal; process of designing nursing strategies or interventions directed toward resolving health problems
plantar flexion movement of the ankle so that the toes point downward
plantar reflex *see* Babinski reflex

plantar wart a wart on the sole of the foot that is sensitive to pressure and caused by the virus *Papovavirus hominis*
plaque a film of mucus and bacteria that forms on the teeth
plasma the fluid portion of the blood in which the blood cells are suspended
pleura the membrane around the lungs; it consists of an outer layer, the parietal pleura, and an inner layer, the visceral pleura
pleural cavity a potential space between the two layers of pleura
pleural rub (friction rub) a coarse, leathery, or grating sound produced by the rubbing together of the pleura
pleximeter the nondominant hand used in percussion
plexor the dominant hand used in percussion
plexus a network, e.g., of nerves or veins
pneumoencephalogram an x-ray film of the cerebrospinal spaces after the introduction of air
pneumonia inflammation of the lung tissue
pneumothorax accumulation of air or gas in the pleural cavity
pneumoventriculogram an x-ray film of the ventricles of the brain after the introduction of air
Po_2 partial pressure of oxygen (venous blood)
polarity the presence of two opposite poles
polarization (of a group) movement by members of a group toward a goal
polarized (cardiac) electrically charged
poliomyelitis an acute viral disease that may cause paralysis
political action activities aimed toward influencing policies of the government, organizations, community, and in the workplace
politics the process of influencing the allocation of scarce resources in the spheres of government, workplace, organizations, and community
polydipsia excessive thirst
polyneuritis inflammation of many nerves
polypnea an abnormal increase in the respiratory rate
polysaccharide a carbohydrate consisting of dozens of molecules of glucose
polyunsaturated fatty acid a fatty acid that contains two or more double bonds, such as linoleic or arachidonic acid
polyuria (diuresis) the production of abnormally large amounts of urine by the kidneys
POMR (POR) *see* problem-oriented medical record
popliteal referring to the posterior aspect of the knee
population total possible membership of a specified group
population density the number of people per square mile of a given area
port an opening or entrance
portal an entrance
position (in a group) the status or rank one has in a group
positive feedback (homeostasis) a control or regulating mechanism of the body that causes the production of additional hormone
positive nitrogen balance nitrogen input exceeding nitrogen output
positivism the state of being positive; a theory that positive knowledge is based on natural phenomena as verified by empirical sciences
posterior of, toward, or at the back
posterior fornix a vaultlike space at the posterior aspect of the vagina
postmortem examination *see* autopsy
postoperative bed *see* surgical bed
postoperative (postsurgical) period the time following surgery
postovulatory after ovulation
postovulatory stage the part of the female sexual cycle starting immediately after ovulation and lasting about 13 days; also called the *secretory* or *luteal stage*
postpartum occurring after childbirth
possible nursing diagnosis used when evidence about response is unclear or when related factors are unknown
postural drainage drainage of secretions from various lung segments by the use of specific positions and gravity
posture the bearing and position of the body; the relative arrangements of the various parts of the body
potency power; the ability of the male to engage in sexual intercourse
potential health problem the presence of risk factors that predispose persons and families to health problems
potential nursing diagnosis used when a client's responses can be predicted or when health promotion can contribute to well-being
poverty lack of sufficient economic resources to meet basic needs
power capacity to influence another person in some way or to produce change
powerlessness perceived lack of control over events
precedent a prior judicial decision used to justify or confirm a court ruling
precoital stimulation *see* foreplay
precordial thump a sharp blow of the fist to the sternum to restore heart function
precordium the area of the chest over the heart or stomach
preeclampsia an abnormal condition of late pregnancy or the early puerperium characterized by hypertension, albumin in the urine, and generalized edema
prelinguistic pertaining to sounds made by an infant that are not related to language
premature ejaculation the inability to control ejaculation prior to satisfaction of the partner or before 30 to 60 seconds after penetration
preoperational stage (Piaget) the phase of cognitive development that occurs during ages 3 to 7
preoperative period the time before an operation
preoptic center the nerve center anterior to the optic center
preovulatory before ovulation
preovulatory stage the first stage (about 14 days) of the female sexual cycle; also called the *proliferative* or *follicular stage*
prepuberty the period preceding puberty
prepubic urethra the part of the male urethra that is inferior to the pubis
prepuce *see* foreskin
presbycusis loss of hearing due to aging
presbyopia inability of the lens of the eye to accommodate initially to near objects and then to far objects as a result of the aging process
prescription the written direction for the preparation and administration of a remedy
pressoreceptor (baroreceptor) a receptor that is sensitive to changes in pressure, e.g., in the carotid sinus and the arch of the aorta
previable fetus a fetus incapable of extrauterine life
pricking pain pain like the pain of a knife piercing the skin
primary care a type of practice in which the first person to meet the client, e.g., the nurse, assumes responsibility for care
primary group a small, intimate group in which relations among the members are personal
primary nursing a system of nursing in which the client is assigned on admission to one nurse, who has primary responsibility for nursing care 24 hours a day
primary prevention activities directed toward the protection from or avoidance of potential health risks
primary questions questions that introduce topics or new areas in an interview
primary union (wound healing) healing that involves the production of minimal scar tissue
primigravida a woman who is pregnant for the first time
primordial follicle the primitive sac or cavity of the ovary that contains the ovum and the granulosa cells
principle a fundamental law or doctrine; assumption
priority setting process of establishing a preferential order for nursing strategies
privacy a deserved degree of social retreat that provides a comfortable feeling; the right of an individual participating in a research study to behave and think without the possibility of the behavior or thoughts being used to embarass that person later
privileged communication information given to a professional such as a physician, who is not required to disclose it in a court of law

probate proceedings civil actions relating to wills and estates of deceased persons
probing asking for information chiefly out of curiosity
problem *see* health problem
problem-oriented medical record (POMR, POR) a client's chart organized according to the client's problems and recording the reports of several health workers on each problem
process a series of actions directed toward a particular result; in anatomy, a prominence or projection, e.g., of a bone
processing the manipulation of data (e.g., by a computer) to achieve a specific objective
process recording a word-for-word account of a conversation, including all verbal and nonverbal interactions
proctoclysis a slow instillation of fluid into the rectum
proctoscope a lighted instrument used to visualize the interior of the rectum
proctoscopy visualization of the interior of the rectum with a proctoscope
proctosigmoidoscope a lighted instrument used to visualize the rectum and sigmoid colon
proctosigmoidoscopy visual examination of the rectum and sigmoid colon with a proctosigmoidoscope
prodromal period the stage of an illness during which there are early manifestations of the disease
productive cough a cough in which secretions are expectorated
profession work that requires special knowledge, skill, and preparation
professional a person who practices a learned profession
progesterone a hormone produced by the ovaries, placenta, and adrenal cortex
prognosis the medical opinion about the outcome of a disease
program set of instructions that direct a computer to perform certain tasks
projection a defense mechanism by which a person attributes his or her own undesired characteristics to another
prolactin a hormone produced in the anterior pituitary that stimulates lactation
proliferation rapid reproduction of parts or cells
proliferative (follicular) stage *see* preovulatory stage
pronation turning the palm downward; moving the bones of the forearm so that the palm of the hand turns from anterior to posterior in the anatomic position; also, flat feet
prone (prone position) lying on the abdomen with the face turned to one side
prophylaxis preventive treatment; prevention of disease
proposition statement that expresses the relationship between concepts
proprioceptor a sensory receptor that is sensitive to movement and the position of the body
prospective payment system (PPS) federal plan that establishes Medicare reimbursement rates in advance of hospitalization and according to diagnostic related groups
prostate a gland around the base of the urethra of the male
prostatectomy the removal of the prostate gland
prosthesis an artificial part, e.g., a glass eye, an artificial leg, or dentures
prostration extreme exhaustion
protective asepsis (isolation) setting someone or something apart from others; practices that prevent the spread of infections and communicable diseases
protein an organic substance that is composed of carbon, hydrogen, oxygen, and nitrogen and that yields amino acids upon hydrolysis
proteinuria the presence of protein in the urine
protocol written plan specifying the procedures to be followed in a particular situation
protraction moving a part of the body forward in a plane parallel to the ground
proxemics the study of physical distance between people in their interactions
proximal closest to the point of attachment
proximal fragment the part of a fractured bone nearest the individual's head
prudent diet a diet that is likely to benefit the individual even though it may not prevent disease
pruritus intense itching
psychiatry the branch of medicine that treats behavioral, emotional, or mental disorders
psychogenic (functional) pain pain caused by psychologic factors
psychologic dependence (on a drug) a state of emotional reliance on a drug to maintain one's well-being; a feeling of need or craving for a drug
psychologic homeostasis emotional or psychologic balance or a state of mental well-being
psychology the study of mental processes and behavior
psychomotor referring to motor actions related to cerebral or psychic activity
psychosomatic concerning the mind and the body; emotional disturbances manifested by physiologic symptoms
ptyalin an enzyme in saliva
ptyalism excessive secretion of saliva
puberty the age during which the reproductive organs become active and secondary sex characteristics develop
public law rules regulating relationships between individuals and government
pudendum *see* vulva
puerperium the period from delivery to about 6 weeks after delivery
pulmonary referring to the lungs
pulmonary capacities the combinations of two or more pulmonary volumes
pulmonary embolus a blood clot that has moved to the lungs
pulmonary resuscitation *see* respiratory ventilation
pulse the wave of blood within an artery that is created by contraction of the left ventricle of the heart
pulse deficit a difference between the apical and the radial pulses
pulse pressure the difference between the systolic and the diastolic pressures
pulse rate the number of pulse beats per minute
pulse rhythm the pattern of pulse beats and of intervals between beats
pulse tension the elasticity of the arteries
pulse volume the force of the blood with each beat produced by contraction of the left ventricle
pulsus regularis equal lapses of time between beats of a normal pulse
puncture (stab) wound a wound made by a sharp instrument penetrating the skin and underlying tissues
pupil the opening at the center of the iris of the eye
Purkinje fibers a network of fibers in the ventricles of the heart that conduct stimuli from the atria to the ventricles
purulent containing pus
purulent exudate an exudate consisting of leukocytes, liquefied dead tissue debris, and dead and living bacteria
pus a thick liquid associated with inflammation and composed of cells, liquid, microorganisms, and tissue debris
pustule a small elevation of the skin or mucous membrane or a clogged pore or follicle containing pus
putrid rotten
pyelogram an x-ray film of the kidney and ureter, showing the pelvis of the kidney
pyemia a generalized, persistent blood poisoning
pyogenic pus-producing
pyorrhea purulent periodontal disease
pyrexia elevated body temperature; fever
pyrogen a substance that produces a fever
pyuria the presence of pus in the urine

quadriplegia the paralysis of all four limbs
quality (of sound) subjective description of a sound (e.g., whistling, gurgling, or snapping)

quality assessment examination of nursing services
quality assurance the evaluation of nursing services provided and the results achieved against an established standard and the efforts aimed at ensuring quality nursing care
quality assurance criteria *see* criteria (of nursing care)

rabbi a Jew ordained for professional religious leadership
race classification of humans into subgroups according to specific physical and structural characteristics
radial pulse the pulse point located where the radial artery passes over the radius of the arm
radiation the transfer of heat from a warm object to a cooler object by means of electromagnetic waves, without contact between the two objects; electromagnetic waves used in diagnostic tests and some kinds of therapy
radiation therapy therapy involving x-rays, radium, or other radioactive substances
radiology technologist a member of the health team who takes roentgenograms and assists with other related tests
radiopaque able to block the passage of radiant energy, such as x-rays
rales bubbling or rattling sounds audible on inhalation as air moves through accumulated moist secretions in the lungs
random sample a study sample in which all members of a population have an equal chance of being included
range of motion the degree of movement possible for each joint
rationale the scientific reason for selecting a specific nursing action
rationalization a defense mechanism in which good reasons, acceptable to the conscious mind, are given for behavior or circumstances instead of the real reason
reaction formation a defense mechanism in which one behaves exactly opposite to the way one is feeling
readiness the state of being ready; it is used to describe the developmental maturation and growth necessary before one can perform some activities, e.g., walking
receptor (sensor) the terminal of a sensory nerve that is sensitive to specific stimuli
reconstituted family *see* blended family
reconstitution the technique of adding a solvent to a powdered drug to prepare it for injection
reconstructive surgery surgery to repair tissues whose function or appearance is damaged
record a collection of related data items about one file member
recording (charting) the process of making entries on clients' records
recovery bed *see* surgical bed
recovery index the sum of three 30-second pulse rates taken after increasing intervals of activity
recreational therapist a member of the health team who assists clients with activities for recreation
rectocele (proctocele) a protrusion of part of the rectum into the vagina
rectum the distal portion of the large intestine
recumbent length the distance from the soles of the feet to the vertex of the head of a person lying on the back
reduced hemoglobin hemoglobin that has released its oxygen
reduction realignment of fractured bone fragments to their normal position
reexamining (reevaluating) the process of reassessing and replanning
referred pain pain perceived to be in one area but whose source is another area
referrent power power derived from an individual's own vision and sense of self, and his or her ability to communicate these so that others are motivated to follow
referring the transfer of a client's care to another person
reflex an involuntary activity in response to a stimulus
reflexive vocalization nondescriptive sounds infants make in response to various stimuli and environmental conditions
reflexogenic erection an erection of the penis that occurs without apparent sexual stimuli
refractory period the period immediately following orgasm when males cannot respond to sexual stimuli
regeneration the replacement of destroyed tissue cells by cells that are identical or similar in structure and function
regimen a regulated pattern of activity
registration the recording or entering of certain information about individuals
regression a defense mechanism in which one adapts behavior that was comforting earlier in life to overcome the discomfort and insecurity of the present situation
rehabilitation the restoration of a person who is ill or injured to the highest possible capacity
rehabilitative services *see* intermediate services
relapsing fever a fever characterized by periods of normal temperature, lasting 1 or more days, between periods of fever
reliable criterion a criterion that produces consistent results when used by the same person over time or by a different person
reliability the degree to which an instrument produces consistent results on repeated use
religion an organized system of worship
remittent fever a fever characterized by a wide range of temperatures, all above normal, over a 24-hour period
REM sleep sleep during which the person experiences rapid eye movement; also called *paradoxical sleep*
renal relating to the kidney
renal dialysis a process in which blood flows from an artery through an artificial membrane that removes impurities; the blood then returns to the client through a vein
renal pelvis the funnel-shaped upper end of each ureter
renin a substance secreted by the kidneys when blood sodium levels are low; it controls aldosterone secretion
repolarized (cardiac) requiring an electric charge
repression a defense mechanism in which painful events are excluded from consciousness
researchable problem a question that can be investigated using the research process
research ethics one's moral obligations to human subjects and to the development of knowledge
research in nursing study of the nursing profession, including historic, ethical, and political areas
research-practice gap the separation between research and the clinical practice arena
research process a series or steps of phases, which are dynamic, flexible, and expandable, aimed toward generating useful knowledge
reservoir a source of pathogens
residual urine the amount of urine remaining in the bladder after a person voids
residual volume (air) the amount of air remaining in the lungs after a person exhales both tidal and expiratory reserve volumes
resistive behaviors behaviors that inhibit involvement, cooperation, or change
resistive exercise exercise in which the client contracts a muscle against an opposing force, e.g., a weight
resonance a low-pitched, rich sound produced over normal lung tissue when the chest is percussed
respiration the act of breathing; transport of oxygen from the atmosphere to the body cells and transport of carbon dioxide from the cells to the atmosphere
respiratory acidosis (hypercapnia) a state of excess carbon dioxide in the body
respiratory alkalosis a state of excessive loss of carbon dioxide from the body
respiratory arrest the sudden cessation of breathing
respiratory membrane the alveolar walls and the surrounding blood capillaries
respiratory technologist a person who provides diagnostic and therapeutic measures for clients with respiratory problems

respiratory ventilation (pulmonary resuscitation) the inhalation of air into the lungs by artificial means
responsibility reliability and trustworthiness
rest calmness or relaxation without emotional stress
restitution an adaptive mechanism in which one performs restorative acts to relieve guilt
resuscitate to restore life; to revive
resuscitation the application of measures to reestablish breathing
retching the involuntary attempt to vomit without producing emesis
retention (urinary) the accumulation of urine in the bladder and the inability of the bladder to empty itself
retention (stay) suture a large plain suture that attaches to underlying tissues of fat and muscle in addition to the skin; retention sutures are used to support incisions
retina the membrane that lines the back of the eye, receives the image, and is connected to the brain by the optic nerve
retraction moving a part of the body backward in a plane parallel to the ground; the act of drawing back
retrograde pyelogram an x-ray film taken after a contrast medium is injected through ureteral catheters into the kidneys
retroperitoneal behind the peritoneum
retrospective audit an audit of past events
reverse protective asepsis (barrier technique) measures used to prevent certain clients, e.g., those with severe burns, from coming in contact with microorganisms
reverse Trendelenburg's position a position with the head of the bed raised and the foot lowered, while the bed foundation remains unbroken
reward power power derived from the perception of one's ability to bestow rewards or favors on others
Rh factor antigens present on the surface of some people's erythrocytes; persons who possess this factor are referred to as *Rh positive,* while those who do not are referred to as *Rh negative*
rhinitis inflammation of the mucous membrane of the nose
rhizotomy interruption of the anterior or posterior nerve root between the ganglion and the spinal cord, often for the purpose of relieving pain
rhonchi coarse, dry, wheezy, or whistling sounds, more audible during exhalation, as the air moves through tenacious mucus or a constricted bronchus
rickets a bone disorder resulting from a deficiency of vitamin D and calcium; decalcification of bone
right a just claim
rights of human subjects the just claims of individuals who participate in research studies for full disclosure, self-determination, privacy, and confidentiality and to not be harmed
rigidity stiffness or inflexibility of a muscle
rigor mortis the stiffening of the muscles after death
risk assessment *see* health risk appraisal
risk factor a phenomenon that increases a person's chance of acquiring a specific disease
risk of harm exposure to the possibility of injury going beyond everyday situations
risk reduction planning and implementing nursing interventions to reduce health risks when possible or to optimize an individual's current health status when risks cannot be reduced
ritualistic behavior (ritualism) a series of repetitive acts performed compulsively, often to relieve anxiety
roentgen the unit of measurement of gamma rays (γ) or x-radiation
roentgenogram a film produced by photography with x-rays
role the pattern of behavior expected of an individual in a situation or particular group
role conflict a clash between the beliefs, behaviors, etc., imposed by two or more roles fulfilled by one person
rooting reflex a reflex that causes newborns to turn their heads toward the side of a stimulated cheek or lip
rotation turning a bone around its central axis either toward the midline of the body (*internal rotation*) or away from midline of the body (*external rotation*)
round window an opening from the middle ear to the inner ear
rubefacient reddening the skin; a substance that reddens the skin
ruga a ridge or fold in the lining of an organ such as the vagina or the stomach (plural: rugae)

sacrum a triangular bone at the base of the vertebral column
sagittal plane a vertical line or plane dividing the body or its parts into right and left portions
Salem sump tube a double-lumen nasogastric tube
sample a subset of the population selected for study
sanction punishment or a measure used to enforce normative behavior of group members
sanguineous bloody
sanguineous exudate an exudate containing large amounts of red blood cells
saphenous vein either of two superficial veins of the leg; the greater one extends from the foot to the inguinal region, while the lesser one extends from the foot up the back of the leg to the knee joint
sarcoidosis a disease in which affected tissues develop epithelioid cell tubercles; commonly affected organs are the lymph nodes, liver, spleen, lungs, skin, eyes, and small bones in the feet and hands
satiety a feeling of fullness as a result of satisfying the desire for food
saturated fat a fat whose molecular structure is saturated with hydrogen, such as fats in meat, butter, and eggs
scab the crust over a superficial wound
scan a specialized type of x-ray procedure involving the use of a scanning device (probe), a computer, a printout machine, and a viewing apparatus
scapula the shoulder blade, a flat, triangular bone at the back of the shoulder
scar (cicatrical) tissue dense fibrous tissue derived from granulation tissue
scientific inquiry process in which observable, verifiable data are systematically collected to describe, explain, and/or predict events and phenomena
scientific method a logical, systematic approach to solving problems
sclera the white covering of the eye that joins with the cornea
sclerosis a process of hardening that occurs from inflammation and disease of the interstitial substance; the term is used to describe hardening of nervous tissues and arterioles
scoliosis a lateral curvature of a part of the vertebral column
scored marked with a line or groove
scrotum the sac suspended down and behind the penis that contains and protects the testes
scultetus binder an abdominal binder applied in strips that overlap each other
scurvy a condition resulting from vitamin C deficiency
sebaceous gland a gland of the dermis that secretes sebum
seborrheic dermatitis a chronic disease of the skin, characterized by scaling and crusted patches on various body areas, e.g., the scalp
sebum the oily, lubricating secretion of sebaceous glands in the skin
secondary group a group that is generally larger and more impersonal than a primary group
secondary questions probing-type questions
secondary union (second intention) healing that requires the formation of considerable granulation tissue
secretion the product of a gland, e.g., saliva is the secretion of the salivary glands
secretory (luteal) stage *see* postovulatory stage
sedative an agent that tends to calm or tranquilize
segmentation contractions contractions of segments of the intestine in contrast to contractions of large areas of the intestine
self-actualization (Maslow) the highest level of personality development
self-care activities performed by individuals in their own behalf to maintain health and well-being
self-concept the combination of beliefs and feelings one holds about oneself at a given time

self-consistency the aspect of self that strives to maintain a stable self-image
self-determination the right of clients to feel free from undue influence to participate in a study
self-esteem self-acceptance; self-worth
self-expectancy what a person wants to become; the power a person perceives he or she has to meet self-expectations
self-ideal *see* self-expectancy
self-image a person's perception of self at a specific time or over a period of time
self-terminating order on a client's record, an order whose termination time is implicit
semantics the study of the meaning of words
semen seminal plasma combined with sperm
semicircular canals passages shaped like half circles in the inner ear that control the sense of balance by the effect of fluid moving against hairlike nerves
semicomatose pertaining to a state of unconsciousness characterized by reflex movement only when painful stimuli are applied and, in some instances, by decortical or decerebrate posturing
semi-Fowler's position a bed sitting position in which the head of the bed is elevated at least 30°, with or without knee flexion
semilunar valves crescent-shaped valves that guard the entrances from the cardiac ventricles into the aorta and pulmonary trunk
seminal plasma substances that are produced by the seminal vesicles, prostate, and Cowper's glands and that energize the sperm and enhance their transport
seminiferous tubules highly coiled tubes that manufacture sperm within each testis
senescence the process of growing old
senility feebleness or loss of mental, emotional, or physical control that occurs in old age
sensitivity quick response, often referring to the response of microorganisms to an antibiotic
sensorimotor stage (Piaget) the initial phase of cognitive development between birth and 2 years
sensoristasis the need for sensory stimulation
sensorium a sensory nerve center
sensory deficit partial or complete impairment of any sensory organ
sensory deprivation (input deficit) insufficient sensory stimulation for a person to function
sensory overload an overabundance of sensory stimulation
septic produced by putrefaction or decomposition
septic (hectic) fever intermittent fever characterized by wide fluctuations and daily periods when body temperature falls to normal or below normal
serosanguineous composed of serum and blood
serous of or like serum
serous exudate a watery exudate composed mainly of serum
serum (blood) blood plasma from which the fibrinogen has been separated during clotting
sex maleness or femaleness; sexual intercourse
sex behavior the behavior associated with sexual intercourse, including physiologic responses and sexual dysfunctions
sex chromosome pair the pair of chromosomes, one from the sperm and one from the ovum, that determine whether gonads develop into testes or ovaries; the sex chromosome pair is designated XX (female) or XY (male)
sex drive *see* libido
sex-typed behavior the action that typically elicits different rewards for one sex or the other
sexual differentiation biologic sex determination of the fetus, during which male genitals or female genitals develop
sexual dimorphism the average differences between males and females in any given species
sexual dysfunction a perceived problem in achieving desired satisfaction of sexuality
sexual identity (core-gender identity) a person's inner feeling or sense of being male or female
sexuality what constitutes male and female; the constitution of an individual in relation to sexual attitudes or activities
sexually transmitted (venereal) disease a disease that can be passed on through intercourse with an infected person
sexual motivation *see* libido
sexual role behavior sexual behavior and gender behavior
shiatsu form of massage in which firm, gentle pressure is applied to the acupuncture points of the body; also referred to as *acupressure*
shock acute circulatory failure
shock phase initial stage of the general adaptation syndrome during which the stressor may be perceived consciously or unconsciously and large amounts of epinephrine and cortisone are released in the body
show expulsion of the mucous plug during labor
shroud a large rectangular or square piece of plastic or cloth used to enclose a body after death
sick role behavior actions directed at getting well taken by the person who considers himself or herself ill
sickle cell anemia a genetic defect of hemoglobin synthesis that accounts for abnormally crescent-shaped erythrocytes; common to Afro-Americans
side effect (of a drug) an outcome that is not intended, such as an unintended action or complication of a drug
sigmoid colon the lower portion of the descending colon of the large intestine; it is shaped like the letter S
sigmoidoscope a lighted instrument used to examine the sigmoid colon
sigmoidoscopy examination of the interior of the sigmoid colon with a sigmoidoscope
Sims' position semiprone position
single-parent family a family unit in which only one parent is present
sings healing ceremonies or rituals carried out by some Native Americans
singultus hiccups
sinoatrial (SA) node the pacemaker of the heart; the collection of Purkinje's fibers in the right atrium of the heart where the rhythm of contraction is initiated
Skene's glands paraurethral glands that open into the urethra just within the external urinary meatus
slander defamation by spoken words
sleep a state of unconsciousness from which a person can be aroused by appropriate sensory or other stimuli
sleep apnea periodic cessation of breathing during sleep
slipper pan a bedpan with a flattened end to ease placement under the client; also called a *fracture pan*
smear material spread across a glass slide in preparation for microscopic study
smegma a thick, white, cheeselike secretion that collects between the labia and under the foreskin
SOAP the format used in the POR to record the client's progress; it has four components: Subjective data, Objective data, Assessment, and Planning
socialization the process by which individuals learn the knowledge, skills, and dispositions of their social group or society
socialized speech the exchange of thoughts between individuals, including questions, answers, commands, and criticisms of others
social support network others outside the immediate family unit who provide strength, encouragement, and assistance to the family, especially during a crisis
social worker an individual who assists persons and families with social problems
sociogram a diagram of the flow of verbal communication within a group during a specified period
sociology the study of social relationships and social institutions, such as marriage or education
sociopath a person who is unable to follow society's moral and ethical standards; one who has an antisocial personality
sodium cotransport theory a hypothesis about the mechanism for glucose transport in the presence of sodium

software *see* program
soixante-neuf (69) simultaneous oral-genital stimulation between two persons
solute a substance dissolved in a solution
solvent the component of a solution that can dissolve a solute
somatic referring to the physical body
somatogenic (organic) pain pain of physical origin
somnambulism sleepwalking
sordes the accumulation of foul matter (food, microorganisms, and epithelial elements) on the teeth and gums
souffle a blowing sound heard by auscultation
source-oriented medical record a traditional client's chart, organized according to the source of records (i.e., the person or department reporting); it includes separate records for the doctor, the nurse, the social worker, etc.
spasm involuntary contraction of a muscle or muscle group
spastic describing the sudden, prolonged involuntary muscle contractions of clients with damage to the central nervous system
special (therapeutic) diet a diet in which the amount of food, kind of food, or frequency of eating is prescribed
specific gravity the weight or degree of concentration of a substance compared with the weight of an equal amount of another substance used as a standard (e.g., water used as a standard has a specific gravity of 1, while urine in comparison has a specific gravity of 1.010 to 1.025)
speculum a funnel-shaped instrument used to widen and examine canals of the body, e.g., the vagina or nasal canal
sperm the male germ cell (reproductive cell)
spermatogenesis production of sperm
spermicide foam, jelly, or cream inserted in the vagina before intercourse to destroy the sperm chemically
sphincter a ringlike muscle that opens or closes a natural orifice, such as the urethra, when it relaxes or contracts
sphygmomanometer an instrument used to measure the pressure of the blood in the arteries
spinothalamic tract the nerve pathway of the spinal cord in which impulses ascend to the brain
spiral bandage a bandage applied to parts of the body extremities that are of uniform circumference
spiral reverse bandage a bandage applied to extremities of the body that are not of uniform circumference
spiritual belief a belief in a higher power, creative force, divine being, or infinite source of energy; the belief may or may not be associated with an organized religion
spiritual need what a client needs to maintain, increase, or restore his or her beliefs and faith and to fulfill religious obligations
spirometry the measurement of pulmonary volumes and capacities using a spirometer
splint a rigid bar or appliance used to stabilize a body part
spore a round or oval structure highly resistant to destruction that is formed in some bacterial cells
sprain injury of the ligaments and associated structure of a joint by wrenching or twisting; associated structures include tendons, muscles, nerves, and blood vessels
spreader block (bar) a block of wood or metal that spreads traction tape away from the medial and lateral aspects of the foot in a traction such as a Buck's extension
spreadsheet a computer application that permits the manipulation of numbers to produce budgets and similar types of numerical analyses
sputum the mucous secretion from the lungs, bronchi, and trachea that is ejected through the mouth
stability (of a group) the degree of permanence of a group
stab wound *see* puncture wound
stamina staying power or endurance
stammer involuntary repetitions and stops in vocal utterances
standard (norm) a measure of quantity, quality, weight, extent, or value that is set up as a rule
standards in nursing, optimum levels of care against which actual performance is compared
standing order written document about policies, rules, regulations, or orders regarding client care that gives the nurse authority to carry out specific actions under certain circumstances, often when a physician is not available
stasis stagnation or stoppage of flow of body fluids, such as intestinal fluids, urine, or blood
static electricity stationary electric charges
station stance; the way a person stands
stature the height of a standing person
statutory law a law passed by a legislature (state, provincial, or federal)
stenosis constriction or narrowing of a body canal or opening
stepping reflex (walking, dancing reflex) a reflex of infants characterized by an up-and-down walking motion of the legs when the infant is held upright with the feet touching a flat surface
stereognosis ability to recognize objects by touching them
stereotype something that conforms to a fixed pattern; an oversimplified judgment or attitude about a person or group
sterile free from microorganisms, including pathogens
sterile field a specified area that is considered free from microorganisms
sterile technique *see* surgical asepsis
sterilization a process that destroys all microorganisms, including spores
sternum the breastbone, a flat elongated bone lying between the ribs and over the heart
stertor snoring or sonorous respiration, usually due to a partial obstruction of the upper airway
stethoscope an instrument used to listen to various sounds inside the body, such as the heartbeats
stimulus anything that arouses or incites action from a receptor
stock supply (of drugs) medications stocked in relatively large quantities in a nursing unit; individual doses are taken from the large supply
stoma an artificial opening in the abdominal wall; it may be permanent or temporary
stomatitis inflammation of the entire mouth
stool (feces) waste products excreted from the large intestine
stopcock a valve that controls the flow of fluid or air through a tube
storage device equipment used to retain data after processing by a computer
strabismus squinting or crossing of the eyes; uncoordinated eye movements
strain (of a muscle) overexertion or overstretching of a muscle or part of a muscle
stress an event or set of circumstances causing a disrupted response; the disruption caused by a noxious stimulus or stressor
stressor any factor that produces stress or alters the body's equilibrium
stress syndrome *see* general adaptation syndrome (GAS)
stretch receptors nerve receptors sensitive to changes in pressure, i.e., in the aorta and carotid sinus; also called *pressoreceptors* or *baroreceptors*
striae gravidarum colorless streaks or lines on the abdomen, breasts, or thighs caused by pregnancy; stretch marks
stricture a narrowing of a passageway or canal
stridor a shrill, harsh, crowing sound made on inhalation due to constriction of the upper airway or laryngeal obstruction
stroke volume the amount of blood ejected from the heart with each ventricular contraction
stroma tissue that forms the framework or structure of an organ
structural-functional theory a framework for studying the family unit that focuses on family membership and relationships among family members as well as the functions of the family
stupor a condition of partial or nearly complete unconsciousness; stuporous clients are never fully awakened even when painfully stimulated
stuttering a speech problem evidenced by the repetition of letters or words and prolonged pauses
stylet a metal or plastic probe inserted into a needle or cannula to render it stiff and to prevent occlusion of the lumen by particles of tissue

subarachnoid space the area between the arachnoid membrane and the pia mater
subcostal below the ribs
subcutaneous (hypodermic) beneath the layers of the skin
subcutaneous tissue *see* hypodermis
subjective data client information that only the patient personally can give, such as thoughts or feelings
sublimation the channeling of sexual and aggressive desires into socially acceptable forms of behavior
sublingual under the tongue
suborbital beneath the cavity or orbit
subscapular below the scapula
substantia gelatinosa gray matter in the dorsal horns of the spinal cord where pain fibers terminate
substernal retractions indrawing beneath the breastbone
substitution replacing one thing with another; an adaptive mechanism in which unattainable or unacceptable goals are replaced with ones that are attainable or acceptable
subsystem the low-level components of a system
sucking reflex a reflex sucking action in newborns, initiated by touching their lips
suctioning aspiration of secretions by a catheter connected to a suction machine or outlet
sudden infant death syndrome (SIDS) a condition of some children during the first year, resulting in death during sleep
sudoriferous gland a gland of the dermis that secretes sweat
suicide the taking of one's own life
sulcular technique a dental hygiene technique for removing plaque and cleaning under the gingival margins
superego (Freud) an unconscious part of the psyche that monitors the id and the ego; concerned primarily with ethics, conscience, and social standards
supination turning the palm upward; moving the bones of the forearm so that the palm of the hand turns from posterior to anterior in the anatomic position
supine (supine position) lying on the back with the face upward without support for the head and shoulders; also called *dorsal position*
support system the people and activities that can assist a person at a time of stress
suppository a solid, cone-shaped, medicated substance inserted into the rectum, vagina, or urethra
suppression the willful exclusion of a thought or feeling from consciousness; the sudden stoppage of a secretion or an excretion, e.g., urine
suppuration the formation of pus
supraclavicular retractions indrawing above the clavicles
supraoptic above the eye
supraorbital above the orbit of the eye
suprapubic above the pubic arch
suprasternal retractions indrawing above the breastbone
suprasystem the highest level of interrelated subsystems
surfactant a lipoprotein mixture secreted in the alveoli that reduces surface tension of the fluid lining the alveoli
surgical asepsis measures that render and maintain objects free from microorganisms (sterile)
surgical bed (anesthetic, recovery, or postoperative bed) a bed with the top covers fanfolded to one side or to the end of the bed
susto among Hispanics, a disease of emotional origin; fright caused by natural phenomena such as lightning or loud noises
suture in surgery, a surgical stitch used to close accidental or surgical wounds; in anatomy, a junction line of the skull bones
swallowing reflex a reflex that accompanies the infant's sucking reflex and causes the infant to swallow
symbolization an adaptive mechanism by which objects are used to represent ideas or emotions too painful for a person to express; the creation of a mental image to stand for something
sympathectomy the severing of pathways of the sympathetic nervous system, often to relieve pain of a vascular origin
symphysis pubis the fibrocartilagenous line of union of the bodies of the pubic bones in the median plane
symptom (covert data) *see* subjective data
synapse the junction between two neurons, where nerve impulses are transmitted from one neuron to another
syncope fainting or temporary loss of consciousness
syndrome a group of signs and symptoms resulting from a single cause and constituting a typical clinical picture, such as the shock syndrome
synergist an agent that enhances the action of another so that their combined effect is greater than the effect of either
synovial joint a freely movable joint surrounded by a capsule enclosing a cavity that contains a transparent, viscid fluid
synthesis the process of putting together; assembling the parts of a whole
syphilis a sexually transmitted (venereal) disease caused by the microorganism *Treponema pallidum*
syringe an instrument used to inject or withdraw liquids
system a set of identifiable parts or components
systemic pertaining to the body (or other system) as a whole
systems theory a framework applied to studying the family unit that views the family as a system whose members are interdependent, meaning that a change in one member influences the family unit as a whole
systole the period when the ventricles of the heart are contracted
systolic pressure the pressure of the blood against the arterial walls when the ventricles of the heart contract

tablet a medication in solid form that is often compressed and molded
tachycardia an excessively rapid pulse or heart rate, over 100 beats per minute in the adult
tachypnea abnormally fast respirations, usually more than 24 per minute, marked by quick, shallow breaths
tactile pertaining to the sense of touch
tactile (vocal) fremitus vibrations, palpable with the palms of the hands, originating in the larynx and transmitted to the chest wall during speech
talipes equinovarus clubfoot; a foot is malpositioned in plantar flexion at the ankle, with inversion and adduction of the heel and forefoot
Talmud the authoritative written body of Jewish tradition
Taoism Chinese mystical philosophy
tartar the film on teeth, often formed from plaque; dental calculus
taxonomy a classification system or set of categories, such as nursing diagnoses
T-binder a cloth in the shape of a T often used to retain dressings in the genital region
Td combined tetanus and diphtheria toxoid used for people over 6 years of age; it has less diphtheria toxoid than DT
teaching an interactive process between a teacher and one or more learners in which specific learning objectives or desired behavior changes are achieved
team nursing the delivery of individualized nursing care to clients by a nursing team led by a professional nurse
technical assault and battery assault and battery without the intent to injure, e.g., when giving a hypodermic injection
telecommunications process by which computers can exchange information with each other
temporal pulse a pulse point where the temporal artery passes over the temporal bone of the skull
tenacious sticky, adhesive
tendon a fibrous cord that attaches a muscle to a bone
tenesmus straining; painful, ineffective straining during defecation or urination
terminal a combination input-output device that is connected to a computer
terminal hair long, coarse, pigmented body hair
territoriality the pattern of behavior arising from an individual's feeling that certain spaces and objects belong to him or her

testes the male gonads
testosterone a testicular hormone that stimulates the growth of the genitals and the development of male secondary sexual characteristics
tetany a syndrome manifested by muscle twitching, cramps, convulsions, and sharp flexion of the wrist and ankle joints
thalamus the larger and middle portion of the diencephalon of the brain
theory a scientifically acceptable general principle that governs practice or is proposed to explain observed facts
therapeutic healing; supportive of health
therapeutic effect (of a drug) the primary effect desired, or the reason the drug is prescribed
therapy remedial treatment
thermal trauma injury caused by excessive heat or cold
thermosensitive pain receptors pain receptors sensitive to heat and cold
thoracocentesis insertion of a needle into the pleural cavity for diagnostic or therapeutic purposes
thorax the chest cavity
thought disorganization a mental condition evidenced by difficulty remembering what one is saying, confusion about time, inappropriate verbal responses, and sensory distortions
thrombocytopenia an abnormal reduction in the number of platelets in the blood
thrombophlebitis inflammation of a vein followed by formation of a blood clot
thrombosis the development of a blood clot
thrombus a solid mass of blood constituents in the circulatory system; a clot (plural: thrombi)
throughput the process of transforming input so that it is useful to the system
thyroid hormone a hormone produced by the thyroid gland consisting of thyroxine and triiodothyronine
thyroid stimulating hormone (TSH, thyrotropic hormone) a hormone produced by the anterior pituitary gland that stimulates the thyroid gland to produce thyroxine
thyroxine a hormone produced by the thyroid gland
tic a repetitive twitching of the muscles, often of the face or upper trunk
tick a small parasite that bites into tissue and sucks blood
tidal volume the volume of air that is normally inhaled and exhaled
tinea pedis *see* athlete's foot
tinnitus a ringing or buzzing sensation in the ears that is purely subjective
tissue perfusion passage of fluid, e.g., blood, through a specific organ or body part
tolerance the ability to endure without ill effects; the term is often used with reference to taking medications
tomography a scanning procedure during which several x-ray beams pass through the body part from different angles
tone (of a group) the pleasant or unpleasant atmosphere sensed in a group
tonicity the normal condition of tension or tone, e.g., of a muscle
tonic neck reflex a reflex of the newborn, also called the *fencing reflex,* in which, when the head is forcibly turned to one side, the arm and leg on that side are extended while the opposite limbs are flexed
tonometer an instrument used to assess the pressure inside the eye
tonsillectomy the surgical removal of a tonsil or tonsils
tonus the slight, continual contraction of muscles
topical applied externally, e.g., to the skin or mucous membranes
TOPV trivalent oral polio vaccine
torsion twisting
tort a wrong committed by a person against another person or the other person's property
torticollis limited range of motion of the neck, with lateral inclination and rotation of the head away from the midline of the body
tortuous twisted
total lung capacity the maximum volume to which the lungs can be expanded
total parenteral nutrition (TPN) or intravenous hyperalimentation (IVH) administration of a hypertonic solution of carbohydrates, amino acids, and lipds by an indwelling intravenous catheter placed into the superior vena cava via the jugular or subclavian vein
touch screen a device that permits the inputting of data into a computer by touching a certain point on the computer display screen
tourniquet a device, e.g., a rubber strip, that is wrapped around a body area to compress the blood vessels
toxemia a generalized intoxication due to the absorption of toxins in the body
toxemia of pregnancy a metabolic disturbance during pregnancy; *see* eclampsia, preeclampsia
toxin a poison produced by some microorganisms, animals, and plants
toxoid a modified exotoxin that is no longer toxic but still has the ability to stimulate the production of antibodies
trachea a membranous tube, composed of cartilage, descending from the larynx and branching into the right and left bronchi
tracheal tug an indrawing and downward pulling of the trachea during inhalation
tracheostomy a procedure by which an opening is made in the anterior portion of the trachea and a cannula is introduced into the opening
traction the exertion of a pulling force
traditional family family unit in which both parents reside in the home with their children—the mother playing the nurturing role and the father providing necessary economic support
traditional health care mode of health care in which activities are aimed toward identifying and correcting a health problem that already exists
transcutaneous electrical stimulation the placement of electrodes on the surface of the skin over a peripheral nerve pathway for the purpose of relieving pain
transfusion (blood) the introduction of whole blood or its components, e.g., serum, erythrocytes, or platelets, into the venous circulation
transudation the passage of serum or other body fluids through a membrane or tissue
transverse plane a horizontal line or plane dividing the body or its parts into superior and inferior portions
trapeze bar a triangular handgrip suspended from an overbed frame
trauma injury
tremor an involuntary muscle contraction, e.g., quivering, twitching, or convulsions
trend prevailing tendency or approach
Trendelenburg's position a bed position with the head of the bed lowered and the foot raised, while the bed foundation remains unbroken; in some agencies, the position involves elevation of the knees, with the feet lowered and the head lowered
triage picking, choosing, sorting, and selecting
trial legal proceedings during which all relevant facts are presented to a jury or judge
triglyceride a simple lipid or neutral fat consisting of three fatty acids for each glycerol base
trigone the triangular area at the base of the urinary bladder
trimester a period of 3 months
trocar a sharp, pointed instrument that fits inside a cannula and is used to pierce body cavities
trochanter either of two processes below the neck of the femur
trochanter roll a rolled towel support placed against the hips to prevent external rotation of the legs
troche a lozenge
tubal ligation a surgical tying of the fallopian tubes, rendering the female sterile
tubercle a rounded eminence of bone
tumor an uncontrolled and progressive growth of cells
tunica albuginea a dense, white, fibrous capsule encasing each testis

tunica dartos the middle layer of smooth muscle and tough connective tissue in the scrotum
tuning fork an instrument shaped like a two-pronged fork and made of metal; the prongs vibrate when struck
turgor normal fullness and elasticity
two-career family family in which both the husband and wife are employed
tympanic membrane a membrane separating the external and the middle ear
tympanites (distention) swelling of the abdomen due to the presence of excessive flatus in the intestines or peritoneal cavity
tympany a musical drumming sound produced on percussion over organs that contain gas or air

ulcer a localized sloughing of skin tissue or mucous membrane commonly associated with varicosities or hyperactivity of the gastrointestinal tract
ultradian rhythm a biologic cycle completed in minutes or hours
ultrasound high-frequency, mechanical, radiant energy
ultraviolet referring to radiation having wavelengths shorter than violet rays and longer than x-rays; ultraviolet radiation has powerful chemical properties
umbilicus the navel; the site where the umbilical cord was attached to the fetus
unconscious incapable of responding to sensory stimuli; insensible
unconscious mind (Freud) the mental life of which a person is unaware
uncontrolled variable variable other than the independent variable that might affect the outcome of a study
undernutrition inadequate caloric intake or nourishment
unilateral affecting one side
unit dose system (of drugs) prepackaged and labeled individual doses of medication for each client; the amount of medication the client is to receive at a prescribed hour
universal donor a person with type O blood
universal recipient a person with type AB blood
unpalatable distasteful, unpleasant to the taste
unsterile containing microorganisms; unsterile material may be clean or contaminated
untoward adverse
urban relating to or constituting a city
urea a substance found in urine, blood, and lymph; the main nitrogenous substance in blood
urea frost the appearance of the skin when the salt crystals remain after the evaporation of the sweat in urhidrosis
uremia the retention in the blood of excessive amounts of the byproducts of protein metabolism
ureter the fibrous, muscular tube extending from the kidneys to the urinary bladder
ureteroileosigmoidostomy an artificial opening into the ureters in which a segment of the ileum is resected and connected to the sigmoid colon and the ureters are implanted into this ileal pouch
ureterosigmoidostomy an artificial opening into the ureters in which the ureters are implanted into the sigmoid colon
ureterostomy an artificial opening into the ureter
urethra the canal extending from the urinary bladder to the outside of the body
urethritis inflammation of the urethra
urgency a feeling that one must urinate
urgent surgery surgery necessary for the client's health
urhidrosis a condition in which urinous materials, e.g., uric acid and urea, are present in the sweat
urinal a receptacle used to collect urine
urinalysis laboratory analysis of the urine
urinary diversion *see* urostomy
urine the fluid of water and waste products excreted by the kidneys
urobilin the oxidized form of urobilinogen, a compound formed from bilirubin, that is found in feces and occasionally in urine
urostomy (ureterostomy, urinary diversion) an opening through the abdominal wall into the urinary tract that permits the drainage of urine
urticaria an allergic reaction marked by smooth, reddened, slightly elevated patches of skin and intense itching
uterus the womb; the hollow, muscular organ in the female in which the fertilized ovum develops
uvula a small fleshy mass projecting from the soft palate above the base of the tongue

vaccine a suspension of killed, attenuated, or living microorganisms administered to prevent or treat an infectious disease
vagina the canal of the female reproductive tract
vaginal diaphragm a round rubber cup inserted over the cervix of the uterus for contraception
vaginal orifice the external opening of the vagina
vaginal smear vaginal cells placed on a glass slide for laboratory analysis
vaginismus painful, irregular, and involuntary contraction of the muscles around the outer third of the vagina during coitus
valid criterion a criterion that measures what it is intended to measure
validity the degree to which an instrument measures what it is intended to measure
Valsalva maneuver forceful exhalation against a closed glottis, which increases intrathoracic pressure and thus interferes with venous return to the heart
value something of worth; a belief held dearly by a person
values clarification a process by which individuals define their own values
vaporization evaporation; conversion of a solid or liquid into a gas (vapor)
variable data information that is changeable or apt to be changeable
varicosity the state of having swollen, distended, and knotted veins, especially in the legs
vas deferens a long tube that extends from the scrotum, curves around the urinary bladder, and empties into the ejaculatory ducts
vasectomy ligation and cutting of the vas deferens, rendering the male sterile
vasoconstriction a decrease in the caliber (lumen) of blood vessels
vasodilation an increase in the caliber (lumen) of blood vessels
vasopressor an agent that causes the blood pressure to rise
vasospasm spasm or constriction of the blood vessels
vector an insect or other animal that transfers pathogens from one host to another
vehicle a transporting agent or medium
vellus fine, nonpigmented body hair
venereal disease *see* sexually transmitted disease
ventilation the movement of air; the act of breathing
ventral of, toward, or at the front; anterior
ventricle a small cavity, such as those located in the brain or the heart
ventriculogram an x-ray film of the ventricles of the brain taken after the introduction of an opaque medium
ventriculography radiologic examination of the ventricles of the brain following the insertion of air or a radiopaque medium
verbal communication communication by the spoken or written word
verdict (legal) the outcome of a trial rendered by a jury
vermin external animal parasites, e.g., ticks, lice, and fleas
vernix caseosa the white, cheesy, greasy, protective material found on the skin of newborns
vertex the top of the head
vertigo dizziness
vesicostomy an artificial opening into the bladder in which the anterior wall of the bladder is sutured to the abdominal wall and a stoma is formed from the bladder wall
vesicular sounds normal, quiet, rustling or swishing respiratory sounds heard over the terminal bronchioles and alveoli during auscultation
vestibule a space or cavity at the entrance to a canal; the cleft between the labia containing the vaginal and urethral orifices, hymen, and openings of several ducts

viable fetus a fetus capable of extrauterine life
vial a glass medication container with a sealed rubber cap, for single or multiple doses
vibration a technique of rapid agitation of the hands while pressing on a body area
violence exertion of physical force to injure or abuse
virulence ability to produce disease
virus minute infectious agents smaller than bacteria
viscera large interior organs in body cavities, e.g., the liver and stomach (singular: viscus)
visceral referring to viscera
visceral pain pain originating in the viscera
viscosity the quality of being viscous
viscous thick, sticky
visible poverty lack of money or material resources
visual relating to the sense of sight
vital capacity maximum amount of air that can be exhaled following a maximum inhalation
vital (cardinal) signs measurements of physiologic functioning, specifically temperature, pulse, respirations, and blood pressure
vitamins organic chemical substances found in food and essential for normal metabolism and life
vocal resonance vibrations of the larynx transmitted during speech through the respiratory system to the chest wall
vocation the work that a person regularly performs and that especially suits a person
void urinate, micturate
volatile evaporating readily
vomitus material vomited; emesis
voodoo the practice of witchcraft or magic
vulnerable subjects individuals who because of diminished physical or mental capacity may be unable to give free and informed consent
vulva the external female genitals that surround the vaginal orifice and the urethra; also called the *pudendum*

walker a metal, rectangular frame used as an aid to ambulation
weight the heaviness of a body or object, normally measured in kilograms or pounds
well-being active state of an individual in which he or she becomes aware of and makes choices that lead to a more successful existence
wellness the ongoing process of behaving in ways that lead to improved health; subjective perception of balance, harmony, and vitality
wheal *see* bleb
wheeze a whistling sound on exhalation that usually indicates narrowing of the bronchial air passages
will a declaration of how a person wishes to distribute his or her property after death
word processing a computer application that permits the manipulation of words to prepare papers and reports

xiphoid process the lower portion of the sternum
x-rays electromagnetic radiations with extremely short wavelengths

yang in Chinese folk medicine, a positive force that regulates health; it represents the male, warmth, light, and fullness
yin in Chinese folk medicine, a negative force that regulates health; it represents the female, coldness, darkness, and emptiness
yoga an Indian science that involves various physical postures and stationary exercises as well as psychologic measures to improve one's mental, social, and spiritual states

zygote the fertilized ovum

Index

Note: Boldfaced page numbers indicate definitions; italicized page numbers indicate tables and illustrations.

Significant Events in Nursing History

Compiled by Edith P. Lewis, MN, FAAN

1–500 (circa) Care (mostly hygienic and comfort measures) for the destitute, homeless, and sick provided mainly by early Christians, working as committed individuals or in association with an organized church.

500–1500 (circa) Male and female religious, military, and secular orders with the primary purpose of caring for the sick came into being. Conspicuous among them were the Knights Hospitalers of St. John; the Alexian Brotherhood, organized in 1431; and the Augustinian sisters, the first purely nursing order.

1633 Sisters of Charity founded by St. Vincent de Paul in France. It was the first of many such orders with the same name (sometimes Daughters of Charity) organized under various Roman Catholic church auspices and largely devoted to caring for the sick.

1639 Augustinian sisters came to Canada, eventually establishing the Hotel Dieu in Quebec City.

1644 Jeanne Mance, known as the Florence Nightingale of Canada, founded the Hotel Dieu in Montreal.

——Mother Elizabeth Seton established the first American order of Sisters of Charity of St. Joseph, in Maryland.

1738 Mother d'Youville organized a noncloistered group of women to care for the sick in both hospitals and homes. These women became the Soeurs Grises or Grey Nuns.

1836 Theodor Fliedner reinstituted the Order of Deaconesses from earlier days, opening a small hospital and training school in Kaiserswerth, Germany. This was where Florence Nightingale received her "training" in nursing. The deaconess movement spread to four continents, the first motherhouse being established in Pittsburgh, Pennsylvania, in 1849.

1854–56 Florence Nightingale, long concerned with care of the sick, was named Superintendent of the Female Nursing Establishment of the English General Hospitals in Turkey, in charge of the nursing care of the soldiers during the Crimean War.

1859 Publication of *Notes on nursing: What it is and what it is not*, by Nightingale, in London. It was intended for the ordinary woman, not as a text for nurses.

1860 With a fund of 45,000 pounds (over $220,000 at that time) contributed by the grateful British public and soldiers, Nightingale established the first "modern" school of nursing at St. Thomas's Hospital in London. This date is considered the beginning of nursing as an organized profession. Nightingale believed not only in nursing the sick but also in promoting health.

1861–65 Dorothea Lynde Dix, better known for her earlier work in improving conditions of care for the mentally ill, was appointed superintendent of the first nurse corps of the United States Army during the Civil War.

1864 Jean Henri Dunant of Switzerland established the international conference that founded the Red Cross, for the relief of the suffering in war, in the Geneva Convention signed by 14 nations (the United States not among them).

1872 Woman's Hospital, Philadelphia, opened a training school for nurses.

——New England Hospital for Women and Children, Boston, opened a training school for nurses. Linda Richards, who graduated from the school in 1873, became known as America's first trained nurse.

——American Public Health Association established. Its primary concern at that time was with sanitary and environmental conditions. Later nurses became a significant part of its membership.

1873 First three schools of nursing patterned after (but not strictly according to) Nightingale principles were established at Bellevue Hospital, New York; Massachusetts General Hospital, Boston; and New Haven Hospital, Connecticut.

1874 First hospital training school (Mack Training School) for nurses formed in Canada at St. Catharines, Ontario.

1879 Mary Eliza Mahoney, first trained black nurse, graduated from the nursing school of New England Hospital for Women and Children.

1882 American National Red Cross organized by Clara Barton and linked with the international organization when the United States Congress ratified the Geneva Convention.

1885 Publication of *Textbook of nursing for the use of training schools, families and private students*, the first textbook written by an American nurse (Clara Weeks Shaw) for nurses.

1893 Henry Street Settlement, New York, established by Lilian D. Wald and Mary Brewster to care for the sick and poor in their homes.

——American Society of Superintendents of Training Schools for Nurses (renamed the National League of Nursing Education [NLNE] in 1912) became the first organized nursing group in the United States and Canada.

1897 Nurses' Associated Alumnae of United States and Canada organized. Renamed the American Nurses' Association (ANA) in 1911.

——Victorian Order of Nurses established in Canada by Lady Aberdeen. It conducted practically all public health nursing.

1899 International Council of Nurses (ICN) established by Mrs. Bedford Fenwick of Great Britain, United States and Canadian nurses were among its founders, and their national associations were among the first admitted to membership.

1900 *American Journal of Nursing*, first nursing journal in the United States to be owned, operated, and published by nurses, launched. Its publisher, incorporated in 1902, now also publishes *Nursing Research*, established in 1952; *Nursing Outlook*, 1953; *International Nursing Index*, 1966; *MCN: American Journal of Maternal–Child Nursing*, 1976; and *Geriatric Nursing: American Journal of Care for the Aging*, 1980.

1901 United States Army Nurse Corps formally established by act of Congress.

1903 First nurse practice acts passed in North Carolina, New Jersey, Virginia, and New York.

1905 *Canadian Nurse* journal inaugurated. By 1959 it was published in both English and French.

1908 Canadian National Association of Trained Nurses (CNATN) established. It later became the Canadian Nurses' Association (CNA).

——National Association of Colored Graduate Nurses (NACGN) established.

——United States Navy Nurse Corps formed.

1912 National Organization for Public Health Nursing (NOPHN) established.

——United States Children's Bureau created by Congress as part of the Department of Commerce and Labor.

1916 Criteria for a profession, set forth by Abraham Flexner in "Is social work a profession?" (published in *School and society*, volume 1), became yardsticks for nursing and continue to serve this function.

1917 NLNE published its first *Standard curriculum for schools of nursing*; revised editions, under slightly different titles, appeared in 1927 and 1937.

1919 Ethyl Johns established the first baccalaureate degree program in nursing in the British Empire at the University of British Columbia, Vancouver.

1922 Sigma Theta Tau, national honor society of nursing in the United States, founded by six nursing students at Indiana Training School for Nurses.

1923 Publication of *Nursing and nursing education in the United States*, better known as the Goldmark (or Winslow-Goldmark) Report. Originally intended to study education for public health nursing, the study committee extended its work to include all of nursing education, criticizing the low standards, inadequate financing, and lack of separation of education from service.

——Yale University (New Haven, Connecticut) and Western Reserve University (Cleveland, Ohio), each with the aid of endowments, established independent schools of nursing. In 1934, both started requiring a baccalaureate degree for admission to the schools and granted masters of nursing degrees.

1928 Publication of *Nurses, patients, and pocketbooks*, first report of the Committee on Grading of Nursing Schools appointed two years earlier. The report indicated that there was an oversupply of nurses in general but an undersupply of adequately prepared ones.

1929 American Association of Nurse-Midwives formed, It merged in 1969 with the American College of Nurse-Midwifery to become the American College of Nurse-Midwives.

1931 Weir Report in Canada recommended integration of nursing education into the provincial education system.

1932 Association of Collegiate Schools of Nursing (ACSN) established to promote nursing education on a professional and collegiate level and to encourage research.

1933 ANA launched campaign for hospitals to employ graduate nurses instead of relying heavily on nursing students for patient care.

1934 Publication of *Nursing schools today and tomorrow*, final report of the Grading Committee (which never did grade schools publicly). It confirmed the weaknesses in nursing education pointed out in the Goldmark Report, recommended graduate instead of student nursing staffs, and called for public support of nursing education.

1939 Graduate School of Midwifery created by the Frontier Nursing Service, Hyden, Kentucky.

1940 Formation of the Nursing Council on National Defense (retitled the National Nursing Council for War Service [NNCWS] in 1941), with representation from major nursing organizations and nursing service agencies, to unify all nursing activities directly or indirectly related to war.